Current Therapy in Internal Medicine

Medical Titles in the Current Therapy Series

Bardin:
Current Therapy in Endocrinology and Metabolism
Bayless:
Current Management of Inflammatory Bowel Disease
Bayless:
Current Therapy in Gastroenterology and Liver Disease
Brain, Carbone:
Current Therapy in Hematology-Oncology
Callaham:
Current Practice of Emergency Medicine
Charles, Glover:
Current Therapy in Obstetrics
Cherniack:
Current Therapy of Respiratory Disease
Dubovsky, Shore:
Current Therapy in Psychiatry
Eichenwald, Ströder:
Current Therapy in Pediatrics
Foley, Payne:
Current Therapy of Pain
Frohlich, Cooke:
Current Management of Hypertension and Vascular Disease
Garcia, Mastroianni, Amelar, Dubin:
Current Therapy of Infertility
Glassock:
Current Therapy in Nephrology and Hypertension
Horowitz:
Current Management of Arrhythmias
Hurst:
Current Therapy in Cardiovascular Disease
Jeejeebhoy:
Current Therapy in Nutrition
Johnson:
Current Therapy in Neurologic Disease
Kacmarek, Stoller:
Current Respiratory Care
Kass, Platt:
Current Therapy in Infectious Disease
Kassirer:
Current Therapy in Internal Medicine
Lichtenstein, Fauci:
Current Therapy in Allergy, Immunology, and Rheumatology
Nelson:
Current Therapy in Neonatal-Perinatal Medicine
Nelson:
Current Therapy in Pediatric Infectious Disease
Parrillo:
Current Therapy in Critical Care Medicine
Provost, Farmer:
Current Therapy in Dermatology
Rogers:
Current Practice in Anesthesiology
Torg, Welsh, Shephard:
Current Therapy in Sports Medicine

CURRENT THERAPY IN INTERNAL MEDICINE

THIRD EDITION

JEROME P. KASSIRER, M.D.
Professor and Vice Chairman
Department of Medicine
Tufts University School of Medicine

Associate Physician-in-Chief
New England Medical Center
Boston, Massachusetts

B.C. Decker, Inc. • Philadelphia

Publisher

B.C. Decker Inc
320 Walnut Street
Suite 400
Philadelphia, Pennsylvania 19106

Sales and Distribution

United States and Puerto Rico
Mosby–Year Book Inc.
11830 Westline Industrial Drive
Saint Louis, Missouri 63146

Canada
Mosby–Year Book Limited
5240 Finch Ave. E., Unit 1
Scarborough, Ontario M1S 5A2

Australia
McGraw-Hill Book Company Australia Pty. Ltd.
4 Barcoo Street
Roseville East 2069
New South Wales, Australia

Brazil
Editora McGraw-Hill do Brasil, Ltda.
rua Tabapua 1.105, Itaim-Bibi
Sao Paulo, S.P. Brasil

Colombia
Interamericana/McGraw-Hill de Colombia, S.A.
Carrera 17, No. 33-71
(Apartado Postal, A.A., 6131)
Bogota, D.E., Colombia

Europe, United Kingdom, Middle East and Africa
Wolfe Publishing Limited
Brook House
2-16 Torrington Place
London WC1E 7LT England

Hong Kong and China
McGraw-Hill Book Company
Suite 618, Ocean Centre
5 Canton Road
Tsimshatsui, Kowloon
Hong Kong

India
Tata McGraw-Hill Publishing Company, Ltd.
12/4 Asaf Ali Road, 3rd Floor
New Delhi 110002, India

Indonesia
Mr. Wong Fin Fah
P.O. Box 122/JAT
Jakarta, 1300 Indonesia

Japan
Igaku-Shoin Ltd.
Tokyo International P.O. Box 5063
1-28-36 Hongo, Bunkyo-ku,
Tokyo 113, Japan

Korea
Mr. Don Gap-Choi
C.P.O. Box 10583
Seoul, Korea

Malaysia
Mr. Lim Tao Slong
No. 8 Jalan SS 7/6B
Kelana Jaya
47301 Petaling, Jaya
Selangor, Malaysia

Mexico
Interamericana/McGraw-Hill de Mexico, S.A. de C.V.
Cedro 512, Colonia Atlampa
(Apartado Postal 26370)
06450 Mexico, D.F., Mexico

New Zealand
McGraw-Hill Book Co. New Zealand Ltd.
5 Joval Place, Wiri
Manukau City, New Zealand

Portugal
Editora McGraw-Hill de Portugal, Ltda.
Rua Rosa Damasceno 11A–B
1900 Lisboa, Portugal

Singapore and Southeast Asia
McGraw-Hill Book Co.
21 Neythal Road
Jurong, Singapore 2262

South Africa
Libriger Book Distributors
Warehouse Number 8
"Die Ou Looiery"
Tannery Road
Hamilton, Bloemfontein 9300

Spain
McGraw-Hill/Interamericana de Espana, S.A.
Manuel Ferrero, 13
28020 Madrid, Spain

Taiwan
Mr. George Lim
P.O. Box 87–601
Taipei, Taiwan

Thailand
Mr. Vitit Lim
632/5 Phaholyothin Road
Sapan Kwai
Bangkok 10400
Thailand

Venezuela
Editorial Interamericana de Venezuela, C.A.
2da. calle Bello Monte
Local G-2
Caracas, Venezuela

NOTICE

The authors and publisher have made every effort to ensure that the patient care recommended herein, including choice of drugs and drug dosages, is in accord with the accepted standards and practice at the time of publication. However, since research and regulation constantly change clinical standards, the reader is urged to check the product information sheet included in the package of each drug, which includes recommended doses, warnings, and contraindications. This is particularly important with new or infrequently used drugs.

Current Therapy in Internal Medicine, Third Edition

ISBN 1-55664-247-4
ISSN 0899-6865

Library of Congress catalog card number: 87-658603

10 9 8 7 6 5 4 3 2 1

ASSOCIATE EDITORS

To Sheridan L. Kassirer,
who encourages, supports, sustains, and enriches

CONTRIBUTORS

MARTIN D. ABELOFF, M.D.

Professor of Oncology, The Johns Hopkins University School of Medicine; Chief of Medical Oncology, The Johns Hopkins Oncology Center, Baltimore, Maryland

Chemotherapy for Breast Cancer

HAROLD P. ADAMS Jr., M.D.

Professor of Neurology, and Director, Division of Cerebrovascular Diseases, University of Iowa College of Medicine; Attending Neurologist, University of Iowa Hospitals and Clinics, and Consultant Neurologist, Iowa City Veterans Administration Hospital, Iowa City, Iowa

Transient Ischemic Attack

GAIL K. ADLER, M.D., Ph.D.

Assistant Professor, Harvard Medical School; Associate Physician, Brigham and Women's Hospital, Boston, Massachusetts

Primary Aldosteronism

SHARON G. ADLER, M.D.

Adjunct Associate Professor of Medicine, Division of Nephrology, University of California UCLA School of Medicine, Los Angeles; Staff Nephrologist, Harbor-UCLA Medical Center, Torrance, California

Mesangial Proliferative Glomerulonephritis

LLOYD M. AIELLO, M.D.

Associate Clinical Professor of Ophthalmology, Harvard Medical School; Director, William P. Beetham Eye Research and Treatment Unit, The Joslin Diabetes Center, Boston, Massachusetts

Diabetic Retinopathy

GREGORY W. ALBERS, M.D.

Assistant Professor of Neurology and Neurological Sciences, Stanford University School of Medicine, Stanford, California

Principles of Pain Management

ELAINE L. ALEXANDER, M.D., Ph.D.

Assistant Professor of Medicine, The Johns Hopkins University School of Medicine, Baltimore, Maryland

Sjögren's Syndrome

MELODY O'CONNOR ALLEN, M.D., F.A.C.S.

Assistant Professor of Surgery, University of Minnesota Medical School–Minneapolis; Staff Physician, Department of Surgery, Minneapolis Veterans Administration Medical Center, Minneapolis, Minnesota

Acute Cholecystitis

JOHN A. ANDERSON, M.D.

Clinical Professor, Department of Pediatrics, University of Michigan Medical School, Ann Arbor; Head, Division of Allergy and Clinical Immunology, Department of Medicine, Henry Ford Hospital, Detroit, Michigan

Penicillin Allergy

ROBERT J. ANDERSON, M.D.

Professor of Medicine, University of Colorado School of Medicine; Chief, Medical Service, Denver Veterans Administration Medical Center, Denver, Colorado

Hyponatremia

MAUREEN ANDREW, M.D.

Associate Professor of Pediatrics and Pathology, McMaster University Faculty of Medicine; Director, Coagulation Laboratory, McMaster University Medical Center, Hamilton, Ontario, Canada

Vitamin K-Dependent Coagulation Factor Deficiency

GRANT J. ANHALT, M.D.

Associate Professor, Department of Dermatology, The Johns Hopkins University School of Medicine, Baltimore, Maryland

Pemphigus

JOSEPH D. ANSLEY, M.D.

Associate Professor of Surgery, Emory University School of Medicine, Atlanta, Georgia

Acute Thrombophlebitis

ELLIOTT M. ANTMAN, M.D.

Associate Professor of Medicine, Harvard Medical School; Director, Levine Cardiac Unit, Cardiovascular Division, Brigham and Women's Hospital, Boston, Massachusetts

Digitalis Toxicity

DONALD ARMSTRONG, M.D.

Professor of Medicine, Cornell University Medical College; Chief, Infectious Disease Service, and Director, Microbiology Laboratory, Memorial Sloan-Kettering Cancer Center, New York, New York
Antifungal Chemotherapy

VICENTE ARROYO, M.D.

Professor of Medicine, University of Barcelona School of Medicine, Barcelona, Spain
Hepatorenal Syndrome and Ascites

RICHARD H. ASTER, M.D.

Clinical Professor of Medicine and Pathology, Medical College of Wisconsin; President, Blood Center of Southeastern Wisconsin, Milwaukee, Wisconsin
Immune Thrombocytopenia

JOSEPH N. ATTIE, M.D., F.A.C.S.

Clinical Associate Professor of Surgery, New York University School of Medicine, New York, and State University of New York School of Medicine at Stony Brook, Stony Brook; Attending Surgeon and Director, Head and Neck Surgery, Long Island Jewish Medical Center, New Hyde Park, and North Shore University Hospital, Manhasset, New York
Primary Hyperparathyroidism

HOWARD A. AUSTIN III, M.D.

Chief, Clinical Nephrology Service, Kidney Disease Section, National Institute of Diabetes and Digestive and Kidney Diseases, National Institutes of Health, Bethesda, Maryland
Lupus Nephritis

LUIS BAEZ-DIAZ, M.D.

Assistant Professor, University of Puerto Rico School of Medicine; Chief, Hematology-Oncology Section, Veterans Administration Medical Center, San Juan, Puerto Rico
Renal Complications of Carcinoma, Leukemia, Malignant Lymphoma, and Waldenström's Macroglobulinemia

DAIVA R. BAJORUNAS, M.D.

Associate Professor of Clinical Medicine, Cornell University Medical College; Associate Attending Physician, Memorial Hospital, and Associate Member, Memorial Sloan-Kettering Cancer Center, New York, New York
Endocrine Syndromes Associated with Neoplasms

GEORGE L. BAKRIS, M.D., F.A.C.P.

Assistant Professor of Medicine and Physiology, Tulane University School of Medicine; Director of Renal Research, Ochsner Medical Foundation, and Staff Nephrologist, Ochsner Clinic, New Orleans, Louisiana
Hypertension in the Elderly

JAMES E. BALOW, M.D.

Clinical Director and Chief, Kidney Disease Section, National Institute of Diabetes and Digestive and Kidney Diseases, National Institutes of Health, Bethesda, Maryland
Lupus Nephritis

JAMIE S. BARKIN, M.D., F.A.C.P., F.A.C.G.

Professor, University of Miami School of Medicine; Chief, Division of Gastroenterology, Mount Sinai Medical Center, Miami, Florida
Acute Pancreatitis

JOHN B. BARLOW, M.D.

Professor of Cardiology, University of the Witwatersrand Medical School, Parktown; Chief Physician, Johannesburg Hospital, Johannesburg, South Africa
Mitral Valve Billowing and Prolapse

JAMES A. BARROWMAN, Ph.D., M.B., Ch.B., F.R.C.P., FRCPC, F.A.C.P.

Professor of Medicine, Division of Gastroenterology, Memorial University of Newfoundland, St. John's, Newfoundland, Canada
Mesenteric Ischemia

JOHN G. BARTLETT, M.D.

Professor of Medicine, The Johns Hopkins University School of Medicine; Chief, Division of Infectious Diseases, The Johns Hopkins Hospital, Baltimore, Maryland
Gastrointestinal Infection in Patients with the Acquired Immunodeficiency Syndrome

THOMAS G. BAUMGARTNER, M.Ed., Pharm.D., F.A.S.H.P.

Clinical Associate Professor, University of Florida Colleges of Pharmacy and Medicine; Clinical Pharmacy Specialist, Nutritional Support Consult Service, Shands Teaching Hospital, Gainesville, Florida
Total Parenteral Nutrition

THEODORE M. BAYLESS, M.D.

Professor of Medicine, The Johns Hopkins University School of Medicine; Clinical Director, Meyerhoff Digestive Disease–Inflammatory Bowel Disease Center, Baltimore, Maryland
Crohn's Disease of the Colon

ARTHUR C. BEALL Jr., M.D.

Professor of Surgery, Baylor College of Medicine, Houston, Texas
Aortic Aneurysm: Abdominal

THOMAS R. BEAM Jr., M.D.
Associate Professor of Medicine and Microbiology, State University of New York at Buffalo School of Medicine and Biomedical Sciences; Associate Chief of Staff for Education, Buffalo Veterans Administration Medical Center, Buffalo, New York
Bacterial Meningitis

ANN M. BENGER, M.D., FRCPC
Associate Professor of Medicine, Department of Medicine, McMaster University School of Medicine; Hematologist, Hamilton Civic Hospitals, Henderson General Division, Hamilton, Ontario, Canada
Multiple Myeloma and Related Monoclonal Gammopathies

EDWARD H. BERGOFSKY, M.D.
Professor of Medicine, State University of New York Health Sciences Center School of Medicine; Head, Pulmonary-Critical Care Division, University Hospital, Stony Brook, New York
Pulmonary Embolism

PAUL D. BERK, M.D.
Lilian and Henry M. Stratton Professor of Molecular Medicine, Professor of Medicine and Biochemistry, Chief, Liver Diseases, and Director, Hepatic Research Group, Mount Sinai School of Medicine of the City University of New York, New York, New York
Polycythemia Rubra Vera

MICHAEL BESSER, D.Sc., M.D., F.R.C.P.
Professor of Endocrinology, Medical College of St. Bartholomew's Hospital; Consultant Physician, St. Bartholomew's Hospital, London, England
Prolactinoma

JOSÉ BILLER, M.D.
Associate Professor, Division of Cerebrovascular Diseases, Department of Neurology, University of Iowa College of Medicine; Attending Neurologist, University of Iowa Hospitals and Clinics, and Consultant Neurologist, Iowa City Veterans Administration Hospital, Iowa City, Iowa
Transient Ischemic Attack

A. JAY BLOCK, M.D.
Professor of Medicine and Anesthesiology, and Chief, Pulmonary Division, University of Florida College of Medicine; Chief, Pulmonary Division, Shands Hospital, and Staff Physician, Veterans Administration Medical Center, Gainesville, Florida
Drowning and Near Drowning

FRANK G. BOINEAU, M.D.
Associate Professor of Pediatrics, Tulane University School of Medicine; Head, Section of Pediatric Nephrology, Tulane University Medical Center, New Orleans, Louisiana
Poststreptococcal Glomerulonephritis

W. KLINE BOLTON, M.D.
Professor of Internal Medicine, University of Virginia School of Medicine; Chief, Division of Nephrology, University of Virginia Health Science Center, Charlottesville, Virginia
Idiopathic Rapidly Progressive Glomerulonephritis

GIANNI BONADONNA, M.D.
Professor of Hematology, University of Milan School of Medicine; Director, Division of Medical Oncology, National Tumor Institute, Milan, Italy
Hodgkin's Disease

SUSAN E. BORUCHOFF, M.D.
Assistant Professor of Medicine, University of Massachusetts Medical School, Worcester, Massachusetts
Antiviral Chemotherapy

HOMER A. BOUSHEY Jr., M.D.
Professor of Medicine and Vice Chairman, Department of Medicine, University of California School of Medicine, San Francisco, California
Status Asthmaticus

SUZANNE L. BOWYER, M.D.
Assistant Professor of Clinical Pediatrics, University of Southern California School of Medicine; Acting Head, Division of Rheumatology, Children's Hospital, Los Angeles, California
Juvenile Rheumatoid Arthritis

MICHAEL C. BRAIN, D.M., F.R.C.P., FRCPC
Professor of Medicine, McMaster University School of Medicine, Hamilton, Ontario, Canada
Secondary Anemia in Renal Failure and Chronic Disease

NACHMAN BRAUTBAR, M.D.
Clinical Professor of Medicine, Pharmacology and Nutrition, University of Southern California School of Medicine, Los Angeles, California
Hypomagnesemia and Hypermagnesemia

PAUL F. BRENNER, M.D.
Professor of Obstetrics and Gynecology, University of Southern California School of Medicine, Los Angeles, California
Oral Combination Contraceptives

LEONA BRENNER-GATI, M.D.
Assistant Professor of Medicine, Cornell University Medical College; Assistant Attending Physician, New York Hospital, New York, New York
Primary Hypothyroidism

DAVID J. BRILLON, M.D.
Assistant Professor of Medicine, Cornell University Medical College; Associate Program Director, General Clinical Research Center, New York Hospital-Cornell Medical Center, New York, New York
Diabetes Mellitus

ELIOT A. BRINTON, M.D.
Assistant Professor, Laboratory of Biochemical Genetics and Metabolism, The Rockefeller University; Associate Physician, Rockefeller University Hospital, New York, New York
Hyperlipoproteinemia

DAN W. BROCK, Ph.D.
Professor of Philosophy and Professor of Human Values in Medicine, Brown University, Providence, Rhode Island
Respecting Patients' Treatment Preferences

STEVEN L. BRODY, M.D.
Senior Staff Fellow, Pulmonary Branch, National Institutes of Health, Bethesda, Maryland
Cardiac Arrest and Resuscitation from Sudden Death

MARK J. BROWN, M.D.
Professor of Neurology, University of Pennsylvania School of Medicine, Philadelphia, Pennsylvania
Subacute Combined Degeneration and Other Vitamin B_{12} Deficiency-Induced Disorders

ALASTAIR BUCHAN, M.D., FRCPC
Assistant Professor of Neurology, University of Western Ontario Faculty of Medicine; Staff Neurologist, University Hospital, London, Ontario, Canada
Atherothrombotic Cerebrovascular Disease

ROBERT BURAKOFF, M.D.
Associate Professor of Medicine, State University of New York at Stony Brook Health Sciences Center School of Medicine, Stony Brook; Chief, Division of Gastroenterology, Winthrop University Hospital, Mineola, New York
Ulcerative Colitis

JOHN P. BURKE, M.D.
Professor of Medicine, University of Utah School of Medicine; Chief, Infectious Disease Division, LDS Hospital, Salt Lake City, Utah
Urinary Catheter-Associated Infection

KENNETH D. BURMAN, M.D., Col. M.C.
Professor of Medicine, Uniformed Services University of the Health Sciences F. Edward Hébert School of Medicine, Bethesda, Maryland; Assistant Chief, Endocrine Service, Kyle Metabolic Unit, Walter Reed Army Medical Center, Washington, D.C.
Hashimoto's Thyroiditis

THOMAS H. BURNSTINE, M.D.
Fellow in Epilepsy and Clinical Neurophysiology, Department of Neurology and the Epilepsy Center, The Johns Hopkins Hospital, Baltimore, Maryland
Focal Seizure Disorders

JAMES B. BUSSEL, M.D.
Assistant Professor of Pediatrics, Cornell University Medical Center; Assistant Attending Pediatrician, New York Hospital, New York, New York
Immune Neutropenia and Hypersplenism

ALFRED E. BUXTON, M.D.
Associate Professor of Medicine, University of Pennsylvania School of Medicine; Director, Clinical Electrophysiology Laboratory, Hospital of the University of Pennsylvania, Philadelphia, Pennsylvania
Ventricular Premature Depolarizations and Ventricular Tachycardia

RICHARD B. BYRD, M.D.
Clinical Associate Professor of Medicine, University of Washington School of Medicine, Seattle; Consultant in Pulmonary Medicine, Rockwood Clinic, Spokane, Washington
Lung Abscess

JOHN J. BYRNES, M.D.
Chief, Division of Hematology, University of Miami School of Medicine; Chief, Hematology Service, Miami Veterans Administration Medical Center, and Director, The William J. Harrington Center for Blood Diseases, Miami, Florida
Thrombotic Thrombocytopenic Purpura

J. STEWART CAMERON, M.D.
Professor of Renal Medicine and Director, Clinical Science Laboratories, Guy's Campus, United Medical and Dental Schools of Guy's and St. Thomas's Hospitals; Honorary Consultant and Renal Physician, Guy's Hospital, London, England
Schönlein-Henoch Purpura

ROBERT G. CAMPBELL, M.D.

Professor, Department of Medicine, Cornell University Medical College; Program Director, General Clinical Research Center, New York Hospital-Cornell Medical Center, New York, New York

Diabetes Mellitus

ROBERT E. CANFIELD, M.D.

Irving Professor of Medicine and Director, Irving Center for Clinical Research, Columbia University College of Physicians and Surgeons; Attending Physician, Presbyterian Hospital, New York, New York

Paget's Disease of Bone

PETER L. CARLEN, M.D., FRCPC

Professor of Medicine, Division of Neurology, University of Toronto Faculty of Medicine; Head, Neurology Program, Addiction Research Foundation, and Director, Playfair Neuroscience Unit, The Toronto Hospital, Toronto, Ontario, Canada

Wernicke's Encephalopathy and Alcohol-Related Nutritional Disease

EUAN J. F. CARLISLE, M.B., M.D.

Research Associate, Division of Nephrology, St. Michael's Hospital, Toronto, Ontario, Canada

Hypokalemia

HUGH J. CARROLL, M.D.

Professor of Medicine and Director, Electrolyte-Hypertension Division, State University of New York Health Science Center at Brooklyn College of Medicine, Brooklyn, New York

Metabolic Acidosis

RICHARD CASABURI, Ph.D., M.D.

Associate Professor of Medicine, University of California UCLA School of Medicine, Los Angeles; Director, Clinical Physiology Laboratories, Division of Respiratory Physiology and Medicine, Harbor-UCLA Medical Center, Torrance, California

Respiratory Acidosis

DANIEL C. CATTRAN, M.D., F.A.C.P.

Professor of Medicine, University of Toronto Faculty of Medicine; Deputy Director, Division of Nephrology, The Toronto Hospital, Toronto, Ontario, Canada

Membranoproliferative Glomerulonephritis

JERRY CAVALLERANO, O.D., Ph.D., F.A.A.O.

Assistant Professor of Optometry, The New England College of Optometry; Staff Optometrist, William P. Beetham Eye Research and Treatment Unit, The Joslin Diabetes Center, Boston, Massachusetts

Diabetic Retinopathy

JAMES J. CERDA, M.D.

Professor and Associate Chairman, Division of Gastroenterology, Department of Medicine, University of Florida College of Medicine; Chief, Nutrition and Hematology, Shands Teaching Hospital, Gainesville, Florida

Total Parenteral Nutrition

CRAIG E. CHAMBERLAIN, M.D., Maj. M.C.

Faculty of Medicine, Uniformed Services University of the Health Sciences F. Edward Hébert School of Medicine, Bethesda, Maryland; Fellow in Gastroenterology, Walter Reed Army Medical Center, Washington, D.C.

Stress Ulcer and Acute Erosive Gastritis

ALEX Y. C. CHANG, M.D., F.A.C.P.

Associate Professor of Medicine in Oncology, University of Rochester Cancer Center; Director of Cancer Research, Oncology/Hematology Division, The Genesee Hospital, Associate Attending, Strong Memorial Hospital, and Attending, St. Mary's Hospital, Rochester, New York

Prostatic Cancer

R. JEFFREY CHANG, M.D.

Professor and Chairman, Department of Obstetrics and Gynecology, University of California School of Medicine, Davis, California

Polycystic Ovarian Disease

KANU CHATTERJEE, M.B., F.R.C.P.

Professor of Medicine, Lucie Stern Professor of Cardiology, Director, Coronary Care Unit, and Associate Chief, Division of Cardiology, University of California School of Medicine, San Francisco, California

Chronic Congestive Heart Failure

SARAH H. CHEESEMAN, M.D.

Associate Professor of Medicine, Pediatrics, Molecular Genetics, and Microbiology, University of Massachusetts Medical School, Worcester, Massachusetts

Antiviral Chemotherapy

CLARE L. CHERNEY, M.D.

Formerly Instructor in Medicine, The Medical College of Pennsylvania, Philadelphia, Pennsylvania

Bacteriuria and Pyelonephritis

NEIL S. CHERNIACK, M.D.

Professor of Medicine and Physiology, Vice President for Medical Affairs, and Dean, Case Western Reserve University School of Medicine, Cleveland, Ohio

Sleep Disordered Breathing

VICTOR CHERNICK, M.D., FRCPC

Professor of Pediatrics, University of Manitoba Faculty of Medicine; Head, Section of Pediatric Respirology, Children's Hospital of Winnipeg, Winnipeg, Manitoba, Canada

Acute Upper Airway Infection

P. JOAN CHESNEY, M.D., C.M.

Professor of Pediatrics, Division of Pediatric Infectious Diseases, University of Tennessee, Memphis, College of Medicine; Attending Physician, LeBonheur Children's Medical Center, Memphis, Tennessee

Aseptic Meningitis Syndrome

GERALD W. CHODAK, M.D.

Associate Professor, The University of Chicago, Division of the Biological Sciences, Pritzker School of Medicine, Chicago, Illinois

Prostatitis, Epididymitis, and Balanoposthitis

ANTHONY W. CHOW, M.D., FRCPC, F.A.C.P.

Professor and Head, Division of Infectious Disease, Department of Medicine, University of British Columbia School of Medicine, Vancouver, British Columbia, Canada

Vulvovaginitis, Cervicitis, and Pelvic Inflammatory Disease

NICHOLAS P. CHRISTY, M.D.

Writer in Residence and Senior Lecturer in Medicine, Columbia University College of Physicians and Surgeons, New York; Professor Emeritus, State University of New York Health Science Center at Brooklyn, Brooklyn, New York

Corticosteroid Withdrawal

ANDRÉ L. CHURCHWELL, M.D.

Assistant Professor of Medicine (Cardiology), Emory University School of Medicine, Atlanta, Georgia

Ventricular Aneurysm Due to Myocardial Infarction

MICHAEL J. CICALE, M.D.

Associate Professor, Division of Pulmonary Medicine, Department of Medicine, University of Florida College of Medicine; Medical Director, Pulmonary Function Laboratory, Shands Teaching Hospital, and Medical Director, Intensive Care Unit, Gainesville Veterans Administration Hospital, Gainesville, Florida

Drowning and Near Drowning

DAVID C. CLASSEN, M.D.

Assistant Professor of Medicine, University of Utah School of Medicine, Salt Lake City, Utah

Urinary Catheter-Associated Infection

LORA L. CLAWSON, R.N., B.S.N.

ALS Research Coordinator, The Johns Hopkins University School of Medicine, Baltimore, Maryland

Amyotrophic Lateral Sclerosis

THOMAS J. COATES, Ph.D.

Associate Professor of Medicine, and Director, Behavioral Medicine Unit, University of California School of Medicine, San Francisco, California

Behavior Modification

CECIL H. COGGINS, M.D.

Associate Professor of Medicine, Harvard Medical School; Clinical Director, Renal Unit, Massachusetts General Hospital, Boston, Massachusetts

Membranous Nephropathy

ALAN S. COHEN, M.D.

Conrad Wesselhoeft Professor of Medicine, Boston University School of Medicine; Chief of Medicine, Boston City Hospital, and Director, Thorndike Memorial Laboratory, Boston, Massachusetts

Amyloidosis

ARTHUR H. COHEN, M.D.

Professor of Pathology and Medicine, University of California UCLA School of Medicine, Los Angeles; Staff, Department of Pathology and Medicine, Harbor-UCLA Medical Center, Torrance, California

Mesangial Proliferative Glomerulonephritis

MARC S. COHEN, M.D.

Associate Professor, Division of Surgery/Urology, University of Florida College of Medicine, Gainesville, Florida

Organic Impotence

MONROE COLE, M.D.

Associate Professor of Neurology, Case Western Reserve University School of Medicine, Cleveland, Ohio

Intracerebral Hemorrhage

PHILIP C. COMP, M.D., Ph.D.

Associate Professor of Medicine, University of Oklahoma College of Medicine; Director, Thrombosis and Coagulation Laboratory, Oklahoma Memorial Hospital, Oklahoma City, Oklahoma

Deficiency of Naturally Occurring Anticoagulants: Antithrombin III, Protein C, and Protein S

JAMES D. COOK, M.D., F.A.C.P.

Professor of Medicine, University of Kansas Medical Center School of Medicine, Kansas City, Kansas

Iron Deficiency Anemia

BERNARD A. COOPER, M.D.

Professor, Departments of Medicine and Physiology, McGill University Faculty of Medicine; Director, Hematology/Medical Oncology, Royal Victoria Hospital, Montreal, Quebec, Canada

Megaloblastic Anemia

KEVIN D. COOPER, M.D.

Director, Immunodermatology, and Associate Professor, Department of Dermatology, University of Michigan Medical School and Ann Arbor Veterans Administration Hospital, Ann Arbor, Michigan

Atopic Dermatitis

DAVID R. CORNBLATH, M.D.

Associate Professor of Neurology, The Johns Hopkins University School of Medicine, Baltimore, Maryland

Acute Inflammatory Polyneuropathy

HOWARD L. CORWIN, M.D.

Associate Professor of Medicine, Dartmouth Medical School; Associate Director, Critical Care Service, Dartmouth Hitchcock Medical Center, Hanover, New Hampshire

Blood Purification and Exchange

JOSEPH S. COSELLI, M.D.

Assistant Professor of Surgery, Baylor College of Medicine; Surgeon, The Methodist Hospital, Houston, Texas

Aortic Aneurysm: Nondissecting Thoracic

ERNEST K. COTTON, M.D.

Professor Emeritus of Pediatrics (Pulmonary), University of Colorado School of Medicine, Denver, Colorado

Cystic Fibrosis

JEFFREY R. CRAGUN, M.D.

Assistant Professor, Department of Obstetrics and Gynecology, University of California School of Medicine, Davis, California

Polycystic Ovarian Disease

DONALD E. CRAVEN, M.D.

Professor of Medicine and Microbiology, Boston University School of Medicine; Director of AIDS Program, Infectious Disease Section, Boston City Hospital, Boston, Massachusetts

Gram-Negative Rod Bacteremia

E. STANLEY CRAWFORD, M.D.

Professor of Surgery, Baylor College of Medicine; Senior Attending Surgeon, The Methodist Hospital, Houston, Texas

Aortic Aneurysm: Nondissecting Thoracic

EDWARD T. CREAGAN, M.D., F.A.C.P.

Associate Professor of Medical Oncology, Mayo Medical School; Consultant, Division of Medical Oncology, Mayo Clinic, Rochester, Minnesota

Malignant Melanoma

ENRIQUE CRIADO, M.D.

Fellow, Vascular Surgery Department, University of North Carolina at Chapel Hill School of Medicine, Chapel Hill, North Carolina

Chronic Venous Insufficiency

STEVEN R. CUMMINGS, M.D.

Associate Professor of Medicine, and Acting Chief, Division of General Internal Medicine, University of California School of Medicine, San Francisco, California

Behavior Modification

THOMAS R. CUPPS, M.D.

Assistant Professor of Medicine, Division of Rheumatology, Immunology, and Allergy, Georgetown University School of Medicine, Washington, D.C.

Dermatomyositis and Polymyositis
Temporal Arteritis

HARRY E. DASCOMB, M.D.

Professor of Medicine, University of North Carolina at Chapel Hill School of Medicine, Chapel Hill; Professor, Medicine Teaching Service, Wake County Memorial Hospital Area Health Education Centers Program, Raleigh, North Carolina

Biliary Tract Infection

GERALD S. DAVIS, M.D.

Professor of Medicine and Director, Pulmonary Unit, University of Vermont College of Medicine; Attending Physician, Medical Center Hospital of Vermont, Burlington, Vermont

Idiopathic Pulmonary Fibrosis

GERARD M. DEBRUN, M.D.

Professor of Radiology, The Johns Hopkins University School of Medicine; Director of Interventional Neuroradiology, Department of Radiology, The Johns Hopkins Hospital, Baltimore, Maryland

Brain Arteriovenous Malformation

MAHLON R. DELONG, M.D.

Professor of Neurology and Neurosciences, The Johns Hopkins University School of Medicine, Baltimore, Maryland
Parkinson's Disease

ROBERT J. DELORENZO, M.D., Ph.D., M.P.H.

Professor and Chairman of Neurology, and Professor of Pharmacology and Biochemistry and Molecular Biophysics, Medical College of Virginia; Neurologist-in-Chief, Medical College of Virginia Hospitals, Richmond, Virginia
Status Epilepticus

KIERTISIN DHARMSATHAPHORN, M.D.

Associate Professor of Medicine, University of California, San Diego, School of Medicine; Attending Physician, UCSD Medical Center, San Diego, California
Secretory Diarrhea

GERMANO DISCIASCIO, M.D.

Associate Professor of Medicine, Medical College of Virginia, Richmond, Virginia
Myocardial Infarction: Uncomplicated

THOMAS F. DODSON, M.D.

Assistant Professor of Surgery, Emory University School of Medicine; Staff Surgeon, Section of Vascular Surgery, The Emory Clinic, Atlanta, Georgia
Carotid Artery Occlusive Disease

SANDRA M. DONNELLY, M.D.C.M., B.Sc., M.Sc.

Assistant Professor, University of Toronto Faculty of Medicine; Staff Physician, Renal Division, Mount Sinai Hospital, Toronto, Ontario, Canada
Hypokalemia

JEREMIAH P. DONOVAN, M.D.

Assistant Professor of Medicine, University of Nebraska Medical Center, Omaha, Nebraska
Fulminant Hepatic Failure

JOHN S. DOUGLAS Jr., M.D., F.A.C.C.

Associate Professor of Medicine, Emory University School of Medicine; Co-Director, Cardiovascular Laboratory, Emory University Hospital, Atlanta, Georgia
Coronary Angioplasty

HAROLD O. DOUGLASS Jr., M.D., F.A.C.S.

Associate Professor of Research Surgery, State University of New York at Buffalo School of Medicine and Biomedical Sciences; Chief, Gastrointestinal Oncology Service, and Associate Chief, Department of Surgical Oncology, Roswell Park Memorial Institute, Buffalo, New York
Pancreatic Cancer

MARK S. DRAPKIN, M.D.

Associate Professor of Medicine, Tufts University School of Medicine, Boston; Chief of Infectious Disease Service, Newton-Wellesley Hospital, Newton, Massachusetts
Aerobic Gram-Negative Pneumonia

LEONARD S. DREIFUS, M.D.

Professor of Medicine, and Director, Heart Station, Hahnemann University School of Medicine, Philadelphia, Pennsylvania
Sinoatrial Block: Bradycardia-Tachycardia Syndrome

DOUGLAS A. DROSSMAN, M.D.

Associate Professor of Medicine and Psychiatry, University of North Carolina at Chapel Hill School of Medicine; Associate Attending, North Carolina Memorial Hospital, Chapel Hill, North Carolina
Irritable Bowel Syndrome

ASIM K. DUTT, M.D.

Professor of Medicine, Meharry School of Medicine, Nashville; Chief, Medical Service, Alvin C. York Veterans Hospital, Murfreesboro, Tennessee
Tuberculosis

SUDHIR K. DUTTA, M.D.

Associate Professor of Medicine, University of Maryland School of Medicine, Baltimore, Maryland
Chronic Pancreatitis: Exocrine and Endocrine Insufficiency

JOE H. DWEK, M.B., F.A.C.P., F.R.C.P.(E)

Associate Professor of Medicine, Albert Einstein College of Medicine, The Bronx, New York
Drug-Induced Lung Disease

WALTER P. DYCK, M.D.

Professor of Medicine, and Director, Division of Gastroenterology, Texas A & M University College of Medicine, College Station; Senior Staff, Scott and White Clinic, Temple, Texas
Gastric Ulcer

STANLEY W. DZIEDZIC, Ph.D., M.D.

Assistant Clinical Professor of Medicine, Mount Sinai School of Medicine of the City University of New York; Assistant Attending Physician, Mount Sinai Medical Center, New York, New York
Pheochromocytoma

JOHN D. EARLE, M.D.

William H. Donner Professor, Mayo Medical School; Consultant, Division of Radiation Oncology, Mayo Clinic and Mayo Foundation, Rochester, Minnesota
Brain Tumors

JACK ECK, M.D.

Specialist in Internal Medicine, Vail, Colorado
High Altitude Disease

MARK H. ECKMAN, M.D.

Assistant Professor of Medicine, Tufts University School of Medicine; Assistant Physician, New England Medical Center, Boston, Massachusetts
Principles of Therapeutic Decision Making

NORMAN H. EDELMAN, M.D.

Dean, University of Medicine and Dentistry of New Jersey–Robert Wood Johnson Medical School, Piscataway, New Jersey
Cardiopulmonary Syndrome of Obesity

RICHARD M. EFFROS, M.D.

Professor of Medicine, and Chief, Division of Pulmonary and Critical Care Medicine, Medical College of Wisconsin, Milwaukee, Wisconsin
Respiratory Alkalosis

THEODORE C. EICKHOFF, M.D.

Professor of Medicine, University of Colorado School of Medicine; Director of Internal Medicine, Presbyterian-St. Luke's Medical Center, Denver, Colorado
Adult Immunization
Mycoplasmal Pulmonary Infections

LARRY EMPTING-KOSCHORKE, M.D.

Instructor, Department of Neurology, The Johns Hopkins University School of Medicine; Director, Blaustein Pain Treatment Center, The Johns Hopkins Hospital, Baltimore, Maryland
Chronic Low Back Pain and Failed Back Syndrome

RICHARD J. FALK, M.D.

Clinical Professor of Reproductive Endocrinology, Georgetown University School of Medicine and Columbia Hospital for Women, Washington, D.C.
Medical Management of Endometriosis

EVAN R. FARMER, M.D.

Associate Professor of Dermatology and Pathology, The Johns Hopkins Medical Institutions, Baltimore, Maryland
Dermatophyte Infections

GEOFFREY C. FARRELL, M.D., F.R.A.C.P.

Associate Professor of Medicine, University of Sydney; Head, Gastroenterology Unit, Westmead Hospital, Sydney, Australia
Drug-Induced Liver Disease

ANTHONY S. FAUCI, M.D.

Director, National Institute of Allergy and Infectious Disease, National Institutes of Health, Bethesda, Maryland
Systemic Vasculitis

EBEN I. FEINSTEIN, M.D.

Formerly Associate Professor of Clinical Medicine, University of Southern California School of Medicine; Staff Physician, Division of Nephrology, Department of Medicine, Los Angeles County-USC Medical Center, Los Angeles, California
Acute Drug Intoxication

MARK FELDMAN, M.D.

Professor and Vice Chairman, Department of Internal Medicine, University of Texas Southwestern Medical Center at Dallas, Southwestern Medical School; Chief, Medical Service, Dallas Veterans Administration Medical Center, Dallas, Texas
Functional Disorders of the Upper Gastrointestinal Tract

DAVID W. FERGUSON, M.D.

Associate Professor of Medicine/Cardiology, University of Iowa College of Medicine; Director, Cardiovascular Intensive Care Unit and Clinical Cardiovascular Physiology Laboratory, University of Iowa Hospitals and Clinics, Iowa City, Iowa
Cardiogenic Shock

JAMES J. FERGUSON III, M.D.

Assistant Professor, Baylor College of Medicine and University of Texas Medical School at Houston; Associate Director, Cardiology Research, Texas Heart Institute, and Director, Research Catheterization Laboratories, St. Luke's Episcopal Hospital, Houston, Texas
Constrictive Pericarditis

GREGORY A. FILICE, M.D.

Associate Professor of Medicine, University of Minnesota; Staff Physician, Veterans Administration Medical Center, Minneapolis, Minnesota
Toxoplasmosis

LEON G. FINE, M.B., Ch.B., M.D.

Professor of Medicine and Chief, Division of Nephrology, University of California UCLA School of Medicine; Attending Physician, UCLA Medical Center, Los Angeles, California
Hyperkalemia

CHARLES FISCH, M.D.

Distinguished Professor of Medicine, Indiana University School of Medicine; Cardiologist, Indiana University Medical Center, Indianapolis, Indiana
Atrioventricular Block

RICHARD I. FISHER, M.D.

Professor of Medicine and Chief, Section of Hematology/Oncology, Loyola University of Chicago Stritch School of Medicine, Maywood, Illinois

Unfavorable NonHodgkin's Lymphoma

ROBERT S. FONTANA, M.D.

Professor of Medicine, Mayo Medical School; Consultant in Thoracic Diseases and Internal Medicine, Mayo Clinic and Mayo Foundation, Rochester, Minnesota

Lung Cancer

ALPHA A. FOWLER III, M.D.

Associate Professor of Medicine, Medical College of Virginia, Virginia Commonwealth University, Richmond, Virginia

Aspiration of Gastric Contents

NOBLE O. FOWLER, M.D., F.A.C.C.

Professor Emeritus of Medicine and Professor Emeritus of Pharmacology and Cell Biophysics, University of Cincinnati College of Medicine; Chief, Cardiac Clinic, University of Cincinnati Hospital, Cincinnati, Ohio

Acute and Recurrent Pericarditis

STANLEY S. FRANKLIN, M.D.

Clinical Professor of Medicine, Division of Nephrology, University of California UCLA School of Medicine, Los Angeles, California

Hypertensive Emergencies and Urgencies

EDWARD D. FROHLICH, M.D., F.A.C.C.

Professor of Medicine and Physiology, Louisiana State University School of Medicine in New Orleans, Adjunct Professor of Pharmacology and Clinical Professor of Medicine, Tulane University School of Medicine, and Adjunct Clinical Professor of Clinical Laboratory Science, Louisiana Tech; Staff Physician, Ochsner Clinic, New Orleans, Louisiana

Hypertension in the Elderly

STEVEN M. FRUCHTMAN, M.D.

Assistant Professor of Medicine, Polly Annenberg Levee Hematology Center, Mount Sinai School of Medicine of the City University of New York; Assistant Attending Physician, The Mount Sinai Hospital, New York, New York

Polycythemia Rubra Vera

ASHOK M. FULAMBARKER, M.D.

Assistant Professor of Medicine, Division of Pulmonary Medicine, University of Health Sciences/Chicago Medical School; Acting Chief, Pulmonary Disease Section, Veterans Affairs Medical Center, North Chicago, Illinois

Acute Respiratory Failure in Chronic Obstructive Pulmonary Disease

J. TIMOTHY FULENWIDER, M.D.

Clinical Assistant Professor of Surgery, Emory University School of Medicine, Atlanta, Georgia

Raynaud's Syndrome

JACK D. FULMER, M.D.

Professor of Medicine, Division of Pulmonary and Critical Care Medicine, University of Alabama School of Medicine, Birmingham, Alabama

Collagen Vascular Lung Disorders

ROBERT P. GALE, M.D., Ph.D.

Associate Professor of Medicine, University of California UCLA School of Medicine, Los Angeles, California

Acute Lymphoblastic Leukemia

JOHN H. GALLA, M.D.

Professor of Medicine and of Physiology and Biophysics, and Director, Division of Nephrology and Hypertension, University of Cincinnati College of Medicine, Cincinnati, Ohio

Metabolic Alkalosis

DONALD M. GALLANT, M.D.

Professor of Psychiatry and Adjunct Professor of Pharmacology, Tulane University School of Medicine; Veterans Administration Medical Center, New Orleans, Louisiana

Alcoholism

GARY E. GARBER, M.D., FRCPC

Assistant Professor of Medicine, Department of Medicine, University of Ottawa School of Medicine; Head, Division of Infectious Disease, Department of Medicine, Ottawa General Hospital, Ottawa, Ontario, Canada

Vulvovaginitis, Cervicitis, and Pelvic Inflammatory Disease

RENEE E. GARRICK, M.D.

Assistant Professor, Department of Medicine, New York Medical College; Attending Physician, Nephrology and Medicine, Westchester County Medical Center, Valhalla, New York

Hypercalcemia and Hypocalcemia

ELLEN R. GAYNOR, M.D.

Assistant Professor of Medicine, Section of Hematology/Oncology, Loyola University of Chicago Stritch School of Medicine, Maywood, Illinois

Unfavorable NonHodgkin's Lymphoma

JOHN E. GERICH, M.D.

Professor of Medicine and Physiology, University of Pittsburgh School of Medicine; Director, Clinical Research Center and Pittsburgh Diabetes Center, University of Pittsburgh, Pittsburgh, Pennsylvania

Hyperosmolar Nonketotic Coma

MARVIN C. GERSHENGORN, M.D.

Abby Rockefeller Mauzé Distinguished Professor of Endocrinology in Medicine, Cornell University Medical College; Chief, Division of Endocrinology and Metabolism, The New York Hospital, New York, New York
Single Thyroid Nodule

MARK R. GILBERT, M.D.

Instructor, Department of Neurology, The Johns Hopkins University School of Medicine, Baltimore, Maryland
Epidural Spinal Cord Compression and Carcinomatous Meningitis

ALAN R. GILES, M.D., FRCPC

Professor, Departments of Pathology and Medicine, Queen's University Faculty of Medicine; Director, Kingston Regional Hemophilia Program, Director of Hemostasis Laboratory, and Staff Physician, Kingston General Hospital, Kingston, Ontario, Canada
Hemophilia

PERE GINÈS, M.D.

Staff Member, Liver Unit, Hospital Clinic 1 Provincial, Barcelona, Spain
Hepatorenal Syndrome and Ascites

STANLEY E. GITLOW, M.D.

Clinical Professor of Medicine, Mount Sinai School of Medicine of the City University of New York; Attending Physician, Mount Sinai Medical Center, New York, New York
Pheochromocytoma

RICHARD J. GLASSOCK, M.D.

Professor of Medicine, University of California UCLA School of Medicine, Los Angeles; Chairman, Department of Medicine, Harbor-UCLA Medical Center, Torrance, California
Use of Drugs in Renal Failure

STANLEY GOLDFARB, M.D.

Professor of Medicine, University of Pennsylvania School of Medicine; Attending Physician in Medicine and Nephrology, and Co-Chief, Renal Section, Hospital of the University of Pennsylvania, Philadelphia, Pennsylvania
Hypercalcemia and Hypocalcemia

ERNESTO GONZALEZ, M.D.

Assistant Professor of Dermatology, Harvard Medical School; Dermatologist, Massachusetts General Hospital, Boston, Massachusetts
Photoallergic Contact Dermatitis

NORMAN D. GRACE, M.D.

Professor of Medicine, Tufts University School of Medicine; Chief of Gastroenterology, Faulkner and Lemuel Shattuck Hospitals, Boston, Massachusetts
Portal Hypertension

RICHARD D. GRANSTEIN, M.D.

Associate Professor of Dermatology, Harvard Medical School; Assistant Dermatologist, Massachusetts General Hospital, Boston, Massachusetts
Photoallergic Contact Dermatitis

MONTE A. GREER, M.D.

Professor of Medicine and Head, Section of Endocrinology, Oregon Health Sciences University School of Medicine, Portland, Oregon
Diffuse and Multinodular Nontoxic Goiter

GEORGE T. GRIFFING, M.D.

Associate Professor of Medicine, Boston University School of Medicine; Member, Section of Endocrinology and Metabolism, University Hospital, Boston, Massachusetts
Hypoaldosteronism

NICHOLAS J. GROSS, M.D., Ph.D., F.A.C.P., F.R.C.P.(Lond)

Professor, Loyola University of Chicago Stritch School of Medicine, Maywood; Acting Program Director, Pulmonary Medicine, Hines Veterans Administration Hospital, Hines, Illinois
Chronic Bronchitis and Emphysema

ASHLEY GROSSMAN, B.A., B.Sc., M.D., M.R.C.P.

Senior Lecturer in Endocrinology, Medical College of St. Bartholomew's Hospital; Consultant Physician, St. Bartholomew's Hospital, London, England
Prolactinoma

THOMAS GUARNIERI, M.D.

Associate Professor of Medicine, The Johns Hopkins University School of Medicine; Director, Cardiac Arrhythmia Service, The Johns Hopkins Hospital, Baltimore, Maryland
Automatic Implantable Cardioverter Defibrillator

ALAN D. GUERCI, M.D.

Associate Professor of Medicine, The Johns Hopkins University School of Medicine; Director, Coronary Care Unit, The Johns Hopkins Hospital, Baltimore, Maryland
Early Myocardial Infarction: Thrombolytic Therapy

VLADIMIR HACHINSKI, M.D., D.Sc. FRCPC

Professor of Neurology, University of Western Ontario; Staff Neurologist, University Hospital, London, Ontario, Canada
Atherothrombotic Cerebrovascular Disease

THAD C. HAGEN, M.D.

Professor of Medicine and Pharmacology and Associate Dean for Froedtert Memorial Lutheran Hospital, Medical College of Wisconsin, Milwaukee, Wisconsin
Acromegaly

JOSEPH HAIMI, M.D.

Formerly Senior Fellow in Pediatric Hematology/Oncology, The New York Hospital and Memorial Sloan-Kettering Cancer Center, New York, New York
Immune Neutropenia and Hypersplenism

TIMOTHY C. HAIN, M.D.

Assistant Professor of Neurology and Otolaryngology, The Johns Hopkins University School of Medicine, Baltimore, Maryland
Vertigo

RUSSELL P. HALL III, M.D.

Assistant Professor, Department of Medicine, Duke University School of Medicine, Durham, North Carolina
Dermatitis Herpetiformis

MITCHELL L. HALPERIN, M.D.

Professor of Medicine, University of Toronto Faculty of Medicine; Staff Physician, Renal Division, St. Michael's Hospital, Toronto, Ontario, Canada
Hypokalemia

SCOTT M. HAMMER, M.D.

Assistant Professor of Medicine, Harvard Medical School; Director, Research Virology Laboratory, and Member, Infectious Disease Section, New England Deaconess Hospital, Boston, Massachusetts
Herpes Simplex Virus Infections

STEPHEN B. HANAUER, M.D.

Associate Professor of Medicine, University of Chicago, Division of Biological Sciences, Pritzker School of Medicine, Chicago, Illinois
Ulcerative Proctitis and Left-Sided Colitis

E. WILLIAM HANCOCK, M.D.

Professor of Medicine, Cardiology Division, Stanford University School of Medicine, Stanford, California
Cardiac Tamponade

DANIEL F. HANLEY, M.D.

Assistant Professor, The Johns Hopkins University School of Medicine; Director, Neurosciences Critical Care Unit, The Johns Hopkins Hospital, Baltimore, Maryland
Acute Inflammatory Polyneuropathy

MARY ALICE HARBISON, M.D.

Research Fellow in Infectious Diseases, Harvard Medical School; Research Fellow in Infectious Diseases, New England Deaconess Hospital, Boston, Massachusetts
Herpes Simplex Virus Infections

WILLIAM V. HARFORD Jr., M.D.

Assistant Professor of Medicine, University of Texas Southwestern Medical Center at Dallas, Southwestern Medical School; Director, Clinical Gastroenterology Laboratory, Dallas Veterans Administration Medical Center, Dallas, Texas
Functional Disorders of the Upper Gastrointestinal Tract

MARY L. HARRIS, M.D.

Instructor in Medicine, The Johns Hopkins University School of Medicine; Physician, The Johns Hopkins Hospital, Baltimore, Maryland
Crohn's Disease of the Colon

IAN D. HAY, B.Sc.(Hons), M.B., Ch.B., Ph.D., F.A.C.P., F.R.C.P.(Edin, Glasg, & Lond)

Professor of Medicine, Mayo Medical School; Consultant in Endocrinology and Internal Medicine, Mayo Clinic and Medical Center, Rochester, Minnesota
Thyroid Cancer

GEORGE B. HAYCOCK, M.B., B.Chir.

Consultant Pediatric Nephrologist, Guy's Hospital, London, England
Schönlein-Henoch Purpura

PETER S. HEEGER, M.D.

Fellow, Renal-Electrolyte Section, University of Pennsylvania School of Medicine, Philadelphia, Pennsylvania
Acute Interstitial Nephritis

WYLIE C. HEMBREE, M.D.

Associate Professor of Clinical Medicine and Clinical Obstetrics and Gynecology, Columbia University College of Physicians and Surgeons; Associate Attending, Presbyterian Hospital, New York, New York
Hypogonadotropic Hypogonadism: Gonadotropin Therapy

ROBERT M. HERNDON, M.D.

Professor of Neurology, Oregon Health Sciences University; Chief of Neurology, Good Samaritan Hospital and Medical Center, Portland, Oregon

Multiple Sclerosis

SCOTT E. HESSEN, M.D.

Assistant Professor of Medicine, Hahnemann University School of Medicine, Philadelphia, Pennsylvania

Sinoatrial Block: Bradycardia-Tachycardia Syndrome

JOSEPH HOLL, M.D.

Senior Resident, Medical Department II, Klinikum Grosshadern, University of Munich, Munich, Federal Republic of Germany

Biliary Lithotripsy

ROBERT B. HOLTZMAN, M.D.

Clinical Assistant Professor of Surgery, University of Miami School of Medicine, Miami, Florida

Aortic Aneurysm: Abdominal

ANTOINETTE F. HOOD, M.D.

Associate Professor, Department of Dermatology, The Johns Hopkins Medical Institutions, Baltimore, Maryland

Dermatologic Manifestations of the Acquired Immunodeficiency Syndrome

Cutaneous Drug Reactions

HERBERT C. HOOVER Jr., M.D.

Associate Professor of Surgery, Harvard Medical School; Chief, Surgical Oncology Research, Massachusetts General Hospital, Boston, Massachusetts

Colorectal Cancer

CYRUS C. HOPKINS, M.D.

Assistant Professor of Medicine, Harvard Medical School; Hospital Epidemiologist and Physician, Massachusetts General Hospital, Boston, Massachusetts

Intravascular Catheter-Associated Infection

DAVID W. HUDGEL, M.D.

Associate Professor of Medicine, Case Western Reserve University School of Medicine; Director, Pulmonary Division, Metro Health Medical Center, Cleveland, Ohio

Sleep Disordered Breathing

ADAM N. HUREWITZ, M.D.

Associate Professor of Clinical Medicine, State University of New York Health Sciences Center School of Medicine; Staff, Pulmonary-Critical Care Division, University Hospital, Stony Brook, New York

Pulmonary Embolism

JEFFREY S. HYAMS, M.D.

Associate Professor of Pediatrics, University of Connecticut Health Center, Farmington; Director, Division of Pediatric Gastroenterology and Nutrition, Hartford Hospital, Hartford, Connecticut

Carbohydrate Malabsorption

SHAKIR A. HYDER, M.D.

Fellow in Gastroenterology, University of Miami School of Medicine, Miami, and Mount Sinai Medical School, Miami Beach, Florida

Acute Pancreatitis

SIDNEY H. INGBAR, M.D. (Deceased)

Formerly William Bosworth Castle Professor of Medicine, Harvard Medical School; Chief, Thyroid Unit, Beth Israel Hospital, Boston, Massachusetts

Hyperthyroidism in Graves' Disease

GEORGE G. JACKSON, M.D.

Professor, Department of Virology, The London Hospital Medical College, London, England

Viral Respiratory Infections

ANDREW D. JACOBS, M.B., B.S.M.D., M.R.C.P.

Clinical Assistant Professor in Medicine, University of California UCLA School of Medicine, Los Angeles, California

Acute Lymphoblastic Leukemia in Adults

SUSAN J. JACOBSON, M.D.

Infectious Disease Fellow, Tufts University School of Medicine; Geographic Medicine and Infectious Disease, New England Medical Center, Boston, Massachusetts

Malaria

VALERIE J. JAGIELLA, M.D.

Assistant Professor of Medicine, Medical College of Georgia; Assistant Chief, Gastroenterology Section, Veterans Administration Medical Center, Augusta, Georgia

Lower Gastrointestinal Bleeding

JOHN K. JENKINS, M.D.

Instructor, Pulmonary/Critical Care, Medical College of Virginia, Virginia Commonwealth University, Richmond, Virginia

Aspiration of Gastric Contents

PETER G. JESSAMINE, M.D., Hons. B.Sc., FRCPC

Fellow, Section of Infectious Diseases and Medical Microbiology, University of Manitoba Faculty of Medicine, Winnipeg, Manitoba, Canada

Chancroid, Lymphogranuloma Venereum, Granuloma Inguinale, and Condyloma Acuminata

JAMES R. JETT, M.D.

Associate Professor of Medicine, Mayo Medical School; Consultant in Thoracic Diseases and Internal Medicine, Mayo Clinic and Mayo Medical Foundation, Rochester, Minnesota

Lung Cancer

WALDEMAR G. JOHANSON Jr., M.D.

Professor of Medicine, Department of Internal Medicine, University of Texas Medical School, Galveston, Texas

Nosocomial Respiratory Infections

GEORGE JOHNSON, M.D.

Roscoe B. G. Cowper Distinguished Professor of Surgery, and Coordinator, General Surgery Services, University of North Carolina at Chapel Hill School of Medicine, Chapel Hill, North Carolina

Chronic Venous Insufficiency

RICHARD T. JOHNSON, M.D.

Professor and Director of Neurology, and Professor of Microbiology and Neuroscience, The Johns Hopkins University School of Medicine; Neurologist-in-Chief, The Johns Hopkins Hospital, Baltimore, Maryland

Herpes Zoster

RICHARD M. JORDAN, M.D.

Professor, Department of Medicine, East Tennessee State University Quillen College of Medicine; Chief of Medicine, Veterans Administration Medical Center, Johnson City, Tennessee

Hypopituitarism

WILLIAM P. JORDAN Jr., M.D.

Professor of Dermatology, Virginia Commonwealth University, Medical College of Virginia, Richmond, Virginia

Allergic Contact Dermatitis

LOIS JOVANOVIC-PETERSON, M.D.

Senior Scientist, Sansum Medical Research Foundation, Santa Barbara; Clinical Associate Professor of Medicine, University of Southern California, Los Angeles, and Associate Adjunct Professor of Medicine, University of California College of Medicine, Irvine; Director, Diabetes Center, Santa Barbara Cottage Hospital, Santa Barbara, California

Diabetes and Pregnancy

BRUCE A. JULIAN, M.D.

Associate Professor of Medicine, University of Alabama School of Medicine, Birmingham, Alabama

IgA Nephropathy (Berger's Disease)

ANTHONY N. KALLOO, M.D.

Assistant Professor of Medicine, The Johns Hopkins University School of Medicine, Baltimore, Maryland

Sclerotherapy of Esophageal Varices

KAMEL S. KAMEL, M.D., M.B., B.Ch., FRCPC

Assistant Professor, University of Toronto Faculty of Medicine; Staff Physician, Renal Division, St. Michaels Hospital, Toronto, Ontario, Canada

Hypokalemia

MERRILL C. KANTER, M.D.

Assistant Professor, Division of Neurology, University of Texas Health Science Center, San Antonio, Texas

Embolic Stroke of Cardiac Origin

ALLEN P. KAPLAN, M.D.

Professor and Chairman, Department of Medicine, State University of New York at Stony Brook Health Sciences Center School of Medicine, Stony Brook, New York

Hereditary Angioedema

BARRY H. KAPLAN, M.D., Ph.D.

Clinical Assistant Professor of Medicine, Albert Einstein College of Medicine of Yeshiva University; Physician-in-Charge, Medical Oncology, Booth Memorial Medical Center, New York, New York

Head and Neck Cancer

PETER W. KAPLAN, B.Sc.(Hons), M.D., M.B., B.S., M.R.C.P.

Assistant Professor, The Johns Hopkins University School of Medicine; Director of EEG Laboratory and Attending Physician, Francis Scott Key Medical Center, Baltimore, Maryland

Generalized Seizure Disorders

JEROME P. KASSIRER, M.D.

Professor and Chairman, Department of Medicine, Tufts University School of Medicine; Associate Physician-in-Chief, New England Medical Center, Boston, Massachusetts

Principles of Therapeutic Decision Making

TAKAKAZU KATOH, M.D.

Visiting Assistant Professor of Medicine, Fujita Health University School of Medicine, Aichi, Japan

Atrial Premature Depolarization, Atrial Tachycardia, Atrial Flutter, and Atrial Fibrillation

ADRIAN I. KATZ, M.D.

Professor of Medicine, The University of Chicago, Division of the Biological Sciences, Pritzker School of Medicine; Attending Physician, University of Chicago Medical Center, Chicago, Illinois
Hypertension in Pregnancy

PAUL KATZ, M.D.

Associate Professor and Vice Chairman, Department of Medicine, and Chief, Division of Rheumatology, Immunology, and Allergy, Georgetown University School of Medicine, Washington, D.C.
Reiter's Syndrome

DAVID T. KAWANISHI, M.D.

Associate Professor of Medicine, University of Southern California School of Medicine; Director, Griffith Laboratory, Cardiac Catheterization Laboratory, and Pacemaker Center, University of Southern California School of Medicine, Los Angeles, California
Acute Pulmonary Edema

DONALD KAYE, M.D.

Professor and Chairman, Department of Medicine, The Medical College of Pennsylvania, Philadelphia, Pennsylvania
Bacteriuria and Pyelonephritis

JOHN A. KAZMIEROWSKI, M.D.

Clinical Associate Professor of Dermatology, Oregon Health Sciences University School of Medicine, Portland, Oregon
Erythema Multiforme

B. J. KENNEDY, M.D.

Regents' Professor of Medicine and Masonic Professor of Oncology, and Director, Division of Oncology, University of Minnesota Medical School; Staff, Masonic Cancer Center, University of Minnesota Hospital, Minneapolis, Minnesota
Endocrine Therapy for Breast Cancer

JOHN I. KENNEDY Jr., M.D.

Assistant Professor of Medicine, Division of Pulmonary and Critical Care Medicine, University of Alabama School of Medicine and Birmingham Veterans Administration Medical Center, Birmingham, Alabama
Collagen Vascular Lung Disorders

TIMOTHY C. KENNEDY, M.D., F.C.C.P.

Associate Professor of Medicine, Pulmonary Division, University of Colorado Health Sciences Center School of Medicine, Denver, Colorado
High Altitude Disease

THOMAS M. KERKERING, M.D.

Associate Professor of Medicine, Division of Infectious Diseases, Virginia Commonwealth University, Medical College of Virginia, Richmond, Virginia
Localized Infection of the Central Nervous System

KENNETH M. KESSLER, M.D.

Professor of Medicine, University of Miami School of Medicine; Chief, Cardiology Section, Veterans Administration Medical Center, Miami, Florida
Cardiac Arrhythmias Following Myocardial Infarction

BRETT V. KETTELHUT, M.D.

Clinical Assistant Professor of Pediatrics and Internal Medicine, University of Cincinnati School of Medicine, Cincinnati, Ohio
Food Allergy

JOHN G. KIRBY, M.B., M.R.C.P.I., FRCPC

Clinical Fellow, Division of Respirology, Department of Medicine, University of Toronto Faculty of Medicine; Clinical Associate, Wellesley Hospital, Toronto, Ontario, Canada
Bronchiectasis

SAULO KLAHR, M.D.

Joseph Friedman Professor of Renal Diseases, and Director, Renal Division, Washington University School of Medicine; Physician, Barnes Hospital, and Consultant in Nephrology, Jewish Hospital, St. Louis, Missouri
Obstructive Uropathy

IRA W. KLIMBERG, M.D.

Associate Physician in Urology (Private Practice), Ocala, Florida
Organic Impotence

JOHN H. KLIPPEL, M.D.

Clinical Director, National Institutes of Arthritis and Musculoskeletal and Skin Diseases, National Institutes of Health, Bethesda, Maryland
Systemic Lupus Erythematosus

RONICA M. KLUGE, M.D.

Professor and Vice Chair for Educational Affairs, and Director, General Internal Medicine and Geriatrics, Department of Internal Medicine, University of Texas Medical School, Galveston, Texas
Infectious Diarrheas

ADRIENNE N. KNOPF, M.D.

Assistant Professor of Medicine, Tufts University School of Medicine; Director, Emergency Services, New England Medical Center, Boston, Massachusetts
Illicit Drug Intoxication

PETER O. KOHLER, M.D.

President, Oregon Health Sciences University, Portland, Oregon
Hypopituitarism

WILLIAM C. KOLLER, M.D., Ph.D.

Professor and Chairman, Department of Neurology, University of Kansas Medical Center, Kansas City, Kansas
Essential Tremor

RICHARD I. KOPELMAN, M.D.

Associate Professor of Medicine, Tufts University School of Medicine; Director, Medical House Staff Training Program, New England Medical Center, Boston, Massachusetts
Patient Compliance

JOEL D. KOPPLE, M.D.

Professor of Medicine and Public Health, University of California UCLA School of Medicine, Los Angeles; Chief, Division of Nephrology and Hypertension, Harbor-UCLA Medical Center, Torrance, California
Conservative, Nondialytic Management of Acute Renal Failure
Nutritional and Nondialytic Management of Chronic Renal Failure

JOSEPH H. KORN, M.D.

Professor of Medicine, Division of Rheumatic Diseases, University of Connecticut School of Medicine, Farmington; Associate Chief of Staff for Research, Veterans Administration Medical Center, Newington, Connecticut
Ankylosing Spondylitis
Systemic Sclerosis

AMY B. KUHLIK, M.D.

Assistant Professor of Medicine, Tufts University School of Medicine; Chief Medical Resident, New England Medical Center, Boston, Massachusetts
Percutaneous Drainage Procedures

PARVEEN J. KUMAR, B.Sc., M.D., F.R.C.P.

Senior Lecturer, The Medical College of St. Bartholomew's Hospital; Honorary Consulting Physician, St. Bartholomew's Hospital and Homerton Hospital, London, England
Celiac Sprue and Related Problems

RALPH W. KUNCL, M.D., Ph.D.

Associate Professor of Neurology, The Johns Hopkins University School of Medicine; Co-Director, Neuromuscular Clinical Laboratory, The Johns Hopkins Hospital, Baltimore, Maryland
Amyotrophic Lateral Sclerosis

CALVIN M. KUNIN, M.D.

Pomerene Professor of Medicine, Department of Internal Medicine, The Ohio State University College of Medicine, Columbus, Ohio
Urinary Tract Infection

IRA KURTZ, M.D., FRCPC

Associate Professor of Medicine, Division of Nephrology, University of California UCLA School of Medicine; Attending Physician, UCLA Medical Center, Los Angeles, California
Hyperkalemia

NEIL A. KURTZMAN, M.D.

Arnett Professor of Medicine, Professor of Physiology, and Chairman, Department of Internal Medicine, Texas Tech University Health Sciences Center School of Medicine; Chief of Staff, University Medical Center, Lubbock, Texas
Mixed Acid-Base Disturbances

MICHAEL A. KUTCHER, M.D., F.A.C.C.

Associate Professor of Internal Medicine, Bowman Gray School of Medicine of Wake Forest University; Director, Interventional Cardiology, North Carolina Baptist Hospital, Winston-Salem, North Carolina
Angina Pectoris: Stable
Coronary Bypass Surgery

F. MARC LaFORCE, M.D.

Professor of Medicine, University of Rochester School of Medicine and Dentistry; Physician-in-Chief, The Genesee Hospital, Rochester, New York
Health Promotion and Disease Prevention

J. THOMAS LaMONT, M.D.

Professor of Medicine, Boston University School of Medicine; Chief, Section of Gastroenterology, University Hospital, Boston, Massachusetts
Clostridium difficile and Antibiotic-Associated Colitis

GUSTAVE A. LAURENZI, M.D.
Professor of Clinical Medicine, Tufts University School of Medicine, Boston; Chief of Pulmonary Medicine, Newton-Wellesley Hospital, Newton, Massachusetts
Aerobic Gram-Negative Pneumonia

GIORGIO LAVILLA, M.D.
Established Investigator, Clinica Medica II, University of Florence School of Medicine, Florence, Italy
Hepatorenal Syndrome and Ascites

RANDI Y. LEAVITT, M.D., Ph.D.
Senior Investigator, Laboratory of Immunoregulation, National Institute of Allergy and Infectious Diseases, National Institutes of Health, Bethesda, Maryland
Systemic Vasculitis

DESMOND J. LEDDIN, M.B., B.Ch., FRCPC, M.R.C.P.(I.)
Assistant Professor of Medicine, Division of Gastroenterology, Dalhousie University Faculty of Medicine, Halifax, Nova Scotia, Canada
Mesenteric Ischemia

DAVID B. N. LEE, M.D.
Professor of Medicine, University of California UCLA School of Medicine, Los Angeles; Chief, Division of Nephrology, Sepulveda Veterans Administration Medical Center, Sepulveda, California
Hypophosphatemia and Phosphate Depletion

PIERRE J. LEFEBVRE, M.D., Ph.D.
Professor of Internal Medicine and Head, Division of Diabetes, Nutrition and Metabolic Disorders, University of Liege School of Medicine, Liege, Belgium
Hypoglycemia: Postprandial or Reactive

JACK L. LEFROCK, M.D.
Scientific Director, Therapeutic Research Institute, Sarasota, Florida
Bacterial Osteomyelitis

PHILIP I. LERNER, M.D.
Professor of Medicine, Case Western Reserve University School of Medicine; Chief, Infectious Disease Division, Mount Sinai Medical Center, Cleveland, Ohio
Prosthetic Valve Endocarditis

RONALD P. LESSER, M.D.
Associate Professor of Neurology and Neurosurgery, The Johns Hopkins University School of Medicine; Director, The Johns Hopkins Epilepsy Center and The Johns Hopkins EEG Laboratories, The Johns Hopkins Hospital, Baltimore, Maryland
Focal Seizure Disorders

ROLAND A. LEVANDOWSKI, M.D.
Laboratory of Respiratory Viruses, Division of Virology, Center for Biologic Evaluation and Research, Bethesda, Maryland
Viral Respiratory Infections

GAIL LEVEE, M.D.
Formerly Attending Physician, Little Company of Mary Hospital and Torrance Memorial Hospital Medical Center, Torrance, and Ami South Bay Hospital, Redondo Beach, California
Wegener's Granulomatosis

MYRON M. LEVINE, M.D., D.T.P.H.
Professor and Head, Division of Geographic Medicine; Professor and Head, Division of Infectious Diseases and Tropical Pediatrics; and Professor and Director, Center for Vaccine Development, University of Maryland School of Medicine, Baltimore, Maryland
Typhoid Fever and Enteric Fever

JOHN E. LEWY, M.D.
Reily Professor and Chairman, Department of Pediatrics, Tulane University School of Medicine; Chief, Department of Pediatrics, Tulane University Hospital, New Orleans, Louisiana
Poststreptococcal Glomerulonephritis

LOUIS S. LIBBY, M.D., F.C.C.P.
Assistant Clinical Professor of Medicine, Pulmonary Division, Oregon Health Sciences University School of Medicine; Pulmonologist, Thoracic Clinic, Portland, Oregon
Legionellosis

LAWRENCE M. LICHTENSTEIN, M.D., Ph.D.
Professor of Medicine, and Co-Director, Clinical Immunology Division, The Johns Hopkins University School of Medicine, Baltimore, Maryland
Insect Sting Allergy

JACK LIEBERMAN, M.D.
Professor of Medicine, University of California UCLA School of Medicine, Los Angeles; Chief of Pulmonary Ambulatory Care, Veterans Administration Medical Center, Sepulveda, California
Sarcoidosis

MARSHALL D. LINDHEIMER, M.D.

Professor of Medicine and Obstetrics and Gynecology, University of Chicago, Division of the Biological Sciences, Pritzker School of Medicine; Attending Physician, University of Chicago Hospitals and Clinics, and Director, Medical High Risk Clinic, Chicago Lying-In Hospital, Chicago, Illinois

Hypertension in Pregnancy

JOSEPH LINDSAY Jr., M.D.

Professor of Medicine, The George Washington University School of Medicine; Director, Section of Cardiology, Washington Hospital Center, Washington, D.C.

Aortic Dissection

THERA P. LINKS, M.D.

Fellow in Internal Medicine, University Hospital of Gronigen, Gronigen, The Netherlands

Periodic Paralysis

RICHARD K. LO, M.D.

Assistant Professor of Surgery (Urology), Stanford University School of Medicine, Stanford; Chief, Urology Section, Palo Alto Veterans Administration Medical Center, Palo Alto, California

Bladder Cancer

PETER I. LOBO, M.D.

Associate Professor of Internal Medicine, University of Virginia School of Medicine; Physician, Department of Internal Medicine, University of Virginia Health Science Center, Charlottesville, Virginia

Idiopathic Rapidly Progressive Glomerulonephritis

DAN L. LONGO, M.D.

Director, Biological Response Modifiers Program, Division of Cancer Treatment, National Cancer Institute–Frederick Cancer Research Facility, Frederick, Maryland

T-Cell Lymphoma

DAVID L. LONGWORTH, M.D.

Staff Physician, Department of Infectious Diseases, The Cleveland Clinic Foundation, Cleveland, Ohio

Anaerobic Bacterial Pleuropulmonary Infections

DONALD P. LOOKINGBILL, M.D.

Professor of Medicine and Chief, Division of Dermatology, Pennsylvania State University College of Medicine, Hershey, Pennsylvania

Leg Ulcers

BRUCE A. LOWE, M.D.

Assistant Professor of Surgery, and Chief, Urologic Oncology, Division of Urology, Oregon Health Sciences University School of Medicine, Portland, Oregon

Renal and Uroepithelial Cancer

BERTRAM H. LUBIN, M.D.

Adjunct Clinical Professor, Department of Pediatrics, University of California School of Medicine, San Francisco; Director of Medical Research, Children's Hospital Medical Center, Oakland, California

Sickle Cell Anemia

ROBERT G. LUKE, M.B., Ch.B.

Taylor Professor of Medicine, University of Cincinnati College of Medicine; Physician-in-Chief, and Director, Department of Internal Medicine, University of Cincinnati Medical Center, Cincinnati, Ohio

Metabolic Alkalosis

JOHN S. MACDONALD, M.D.

Professor of Medicine, Chief, Division of Medical Oncology, and Director, Temple University Comprehensive Cancer Center, Temple University School of Medicine, Philadelphia, Pennsylvania

Gastric Cancer

ADEL A. F. MAHMOUD, M.D., Ph.D.

The John H. Hord Professor of Medicine and Chairman, Department of Medicine, Case Western Reserve University School of Medicine; Physician-in-Chief, University Hospitals, Cleveland, Ohio

Protozoan and Helminthic Pulmonary Infections

GEORGE D. MALKASIAN Jr., M.D.

Senior Consultant and Professor of Obstetrics and Gynecology, Mayo Graduate School of Medicine; Attending Staff, Mayo Clinic, Rochester, Minnesota

Uterine and Endometrial Carcinoma

RICHARD D. MAMELOK, M.D.

Director of Clinical Pharmacology and Medical Research Operations, Syntex Research, Palo Alto, California

Clinical Pharmacology

ELLIOTT L. MANCALL, M.D.

Professor and Chairman, Department of Neurology, Hahnemann University School of Medicine, Philadelphia, Pennsylvania

Cervical Spondylosis

MICHAEL MANDEL, M.D.
Director, Pulmonary and Critical Care Medicine, Geisinger Medical Group, Wilkes-Barre, Pennsylvania
Cardiopulmonary Syndrome of Obesity

KENNETH MAREK, M.D.
Assistant Professor of Neurology, Yale University School of Medicine, New Haven, Connecticut
Idiopathic Autonomic Insufficiency

JOHN J. MARINI, M.D.
Professor of Medicine, University of Minnesota Medical School, Minneapolis; Director of Pulmonary/Critical Care, St. Paul Ramsey Medical Center, St. Paul, Minnesota
Adult Respiratory Distress Syndrome

BARBARA J. MARTIN, M.D.
Clinical Instructor, Department of Neurology, University of Pennsylvania School of Medicine, Philadelphia, Pennsylvania
Subacute Combined Degeneration and Other Vitamin B_{12} Deficiency-Induced Disorders

MANUEL MARTINEZ-MALDONADO, M.D.
Professor of Medicine and Physiology, Department of Medicine and Physiology, University of Puerto Rico School of Medicine; Chief, Medical Service and Renal Metabolic Laboratory, Veterans Administration Hospital, San Juan, Puerto Rico
Renal Complications of Carcinoma, Leukemia, Malignant Lymphoma, and Waldenström's Macroglobulinemia

LUIGI MASTROIANNI Jr., M.D.
William Goodell Professor, Obstetrics and Gynecology; Director, Division of Human Reproduction, Hospital of the University of Pennsylvania, Philadelphia, Pennsylvania
Menopause

MORTON H. MAXWELL, M.D.
Clinical Professor of Medicine, University of California UCLA School of Medicine, Los Angeles, California
Renovascular Hypertension

KENNETH H. MAYER, M.D.
Associate Professor of Medicine and Community Health, Brown University, Providence; Chief, Infectious Disease Division, Memorial Hospital of Rhode Island, Pawtucket, Rhode Island
Antibacterial Chemotherapy

JOHN H. McANULTY, M.D.
Professor of Medicine, Division of Cardiology, Oregon Health Sciences University School of Medicine, Portland, Oregon
Heart Disease and Pregnancy

JUSTIN C. McARTHUR, M.B., B.S., M.P.H.
Assistant Professor of Neurology, The Johns Hopkins University School of Medicine, Baltimore, Maryland
Neurologic Diseases Associated with HIV-1 Infection

J. A. McBRIDE, M.B., F.R.C.P.(Edin), FRCPC, F.R.C.P.
Professor, Department of Pathology, McMaster University Faculty of Medicine; Head, Hematology Laboratory, Henderson General Hospital, Hamilton, Ontario, Canada
Immediate and Delayed Adverse Reactions to Transfusions

WILLIAM R. McCABE, M.D.
Professor of Medicine and Microbiology, and Director of Infectious Diseases, Boston University School of Medicine; Director, Maxwell Finland Laboratory for Infectious Diseases, Boston City Hospital, Boston, Massachusetts
Gram-Negative Rod Bacteremia

MARTIN C. McHENRY, M.D., M.S.
Staff Physician, Department of Infectious Diseases, The Cleveland Clinic Foundation, Cleveland, Ohio
Anaerobic Bacterial Pleuropulmonary Infections

GUY M. McKHANN, M.D.
Kennedy Professor of Neurology, The Johns Hopkins University School of Medicine, Baltimore, Maryland
Hepatic Encephalopathy

CANDACE MIKLOZEK McNULTY, M.D.
Assistant Professor of Medicine, and Program Director, Combined Program in Cardiology Fellowship, Brown University Program in Medicine, Providence; Director, Doppler-Echocardiography Laboratory at Memorial Hospital of Rhode Island, Pawtucket, Rhode Island
Myocarditis

JAMES C. MELBY, M.D.
Professor of Medicine and Physiology, Boston University School of Medicine; Head, Section of Endocrinology and Metabolism, University Hospital, Boston, Massachusetts
Hypoaldosteronism

WILLIAM W. MERRILL, M.D.

Associate Professor, Yale University School of Medicine; Chief, Pulmonary Section, West Haven Veterans Administration Medical Center, New Haven, Connecticut

Aerobic Gram-Positive Pneumonia

HANS A. MESSNER, M.D., Ph.D., FRCPC

Associate Professor, Department of Medicine, University of Toronto Faculty of Medicine; Staff Physician, and Director, Bone Marrow Transplant Team, Princess Margaret Hospital, Toronto, Ontario, Canada

Allogeneic Bone Marrow Transplantation

DEAN D. METCALFE, M.D.

Head, Mast Cell Physiology Section, Laboratory of Clinical Investigation, National Institute of Allergy and Infectious Diseases, National Institutes of Health, Bethesda, Maryland

Food Allergy

ALAIN MEYRIER, M.D.

Professor of Nephrology, Bobigny Medical School, Paris North University; Chief of Nephrology and Hemodialysis, Hôpital Avicenne, Bobigny, France

Focal Segmental Glomerulosclerosis

P. DAVID MILLER, M.D.

Instructor in Medicine, Boston University School of Medicine; Junior Attending Physician, Section of Gastroenterology, University Hospital, Boston, Massachusetts

Clostridium difficile *and Antibiotic-Associated Colitis*

PHILIP B. MINER Jr., M.D.

Associate Professor of Medicine and Director, Division of Gastroenterology, Department of Medicine, University of Kansas Medical Center, Kansas City, Kansas

Fecal Incontinence

MICHEL MIROWSKI, M.D. (Deceased)

Formerly Professor of Medicine, The Johns Hopkins University School of Medicine, Baltimore, Maryland

Automatic Implantable Cardioverter Defibrillator

MACK C. MITCHELL, M.D.

Associate Professor of Medicine, The Johns Hopkins University School of Medicine; Active Staff, The Johns Hopkins Hospital, Baltimore, Maryland

Alcoholic Liver Disease

HERMAN S. MOGAVERO Jr., M.D.

Assistant Clinical Professor of Medicine and Dermatology, State University of New York School of Medicine; Dermatologist, Buffalo Medical Group, Buffalo, New York

Exfoliative Dermatitis
Granuloma Inguinale

ABDOLGHADER MOLAVI, M.D.

Associate Professor of Medicine, and Chief, Division of Infectious Disease, Hahnemann University School of Medicine, Philadelphia, Pennsylvania

Bacterial Osteomyelitis

WARWICK L. MORISON, M.B., B.S., M.D.

Associate Professor, Department of Dermatology, The Johns Hopkins Medical Institutions, Baltimore, Maryland

Psoriasis

MAURICE A. MUFSON, M.D.

Professor and Chairman, Department of Medicine, Marshall University School of Medicine, Huntington, West Virginia

Pleural Effusion and Empyema

SCOTT MURPHY, M.D.

Professor of Medicine, and Associate Director for Clinical Programs, Cardeza Foundation for Hematologic Research, Jefferson Medical College of Thomas Jefferson University; Attending Physician, Thomas Jefferson University Hospital, Philadelphia, Pennsylvania

Idiopathic Myelofibrosis and Myelophthisic Anemia

FREDERICK T. MURRAY, M.D.

Associate Professor of Medicine, Division of Endocrinology and Metabolism, University of Florida College of Medicine; Staff Physician, Shands Hospital, Gainesville, Florida

Organic Impotence

JAMES A. NEIDHART, M.D.

Professor of Medicine, University of New Mexico School of Medicine; Director, Department of Medicine, University of New Mexico Cancer Center, and Chief, Division of Hematology/Oncology, Department of Medicine, University of New Mexico Hospital, Albuquerque, New Mexico

Renal and Uroepithelial Cancer

ERIC G. NEILSON, M.D.

Associate Professor of Medicine, and Chief, Renal-Electrolyte Section, University of Pennsylvania School of Medicine, Philadelphia, Pennsylvania

Acute Interstitial Nephritis

JACK NEIMAN, M.D., Ph.D.

Assistant Professor and Acting Head, Neuropsychiatry Division, Karolinska Institute, Stockholm, Sweden
Wernicke's Encephalopathy and Alcohol-Related Nutritional Disease

BILL NELEMS, B.A.Sc., M.D., FRCSC

Associate Professor of Surgery, University of British Columbia Faculty of Medicine; Staff, Division of Thoracic Surgery, Vancouver General Hospital, Vancouver, British Columbia, Canada
Pneumothorax

HAROLD S. NELSON, M.D.

Professor of Medicine, University of Colorado Health Sciences Center School of Medicine; Senior Staff Physician, Department of Medicine, National Jewish Center for Immunology and Respiratory Care, Denver, Colorado
Allergic and Nonallergic Rhinitis

MICHAEL T. NEWHOUSE, M.D., M.Sc., FRCPC, F.A.C.P.

Clinical Professor of Medicine, McMaster University Faculty of Health Sciences; Head, Firestone Regional Chest and Allergy Unit, St. Joseph's Hospital, Hamilton, Ontario, Canada
Bronchiectasis

JAMES T. NOBLE, M.D.

Assistant Professor, Tufts University School of Medicine; Director, Clinical AIDS Program, and Assistant Physician, New England Medical Center Hospital, Boston, Massachusetts
Introduction to Acquired Immunodeficiency Syndrome Section
Antiviral Therapy of Human Immunodeficiency Virus Infection
Therapy of AIDS-Related Opportunistic Infections

RICHARD B. NORTH, M.D.

Assistant Professor, Department of Neurosurgery, The Johns Hopkins University School of Medicine, Baltimore, Maryland
Acute Back Pain and Disc Herniation

HARRY C. NOTTEBART Jr., M.D., F.A.C.P.

Clinical Associate Professor of Medicine, University of Virginia School of Medicine, Charlottesville; Associate Clinical Professor of Pathology, Medical College of Virginia, Richmond, Virginia
Syphilis

DENNIS H. NOVACK, M.D.

Associate Professor of Community Health, Brown University Program in Medicine; Associate Physician, Division of General Internal Medicine, Rhode Island Hospital, Providence, Rhode Island
Therapeutic Benefits of the Physician-Patient Interaction

CELIA M. OAKLEY, M.D., F.R.C.P., F.A.C.C., F.E.S.C.

Consultant Cardiologist, and Head, Clinical Cardiology, Department of Medicine, Royal Postgraduate Medical School, London, England
Cardiomyopathy: Dilated

JOHN O'BRIEN, M.D.

Fellow in Gastroenterology, The Johns Hopkins University Medical School, Baltimore, Maryland
Crohn's Disease of the Colon

PAMELA O'HOSKI, A.R.T.

Chief Technologist, Blood Bank, Henderson General Hospital, Hamilton, Ontario, Canada
Immediate and Delayed Adverse Reactions to Transfusions

MARTIN M. OKEN, M.D.

Professor of Medicine, University of Minnesota Medical School; Director, Cancer Day Treatment Center, Veterans Administration Medical Center, Minneapolis, Minnesota
Favorable NonHodgkin's Lymphoma

DALE W. OLLER, M.D.

Associate Professor of Surgery, University of North Carolina at Chapel Hill School of Medicine, Chapel Hill; Director of Trauma and Surgery, Wake County Memorial Hospital Area Health Education Centers Program, Raleigh, North Carolina
Biliary Tract Infection

HANS J. G. H. OOSTERHUIS, M.D., Ph.D.

Professor of Clinical Neurology, University Hospital of Gronigen, Gronigen, The Netherlands
Periodic Paralysis

ROY C. ORLANDO, M.D.

Professor of Medicine, University of North Carolina at Chapel Hill School of Medicine, Chapel Hill, North Carolina
Gastroesophageal Reflux: Medical Treatment

DAVID N. ORTH, M.D., F.A.C.P.

Professor of Medicine and Associate Professor of Molecular Physiology and Biophysics, Vanderbilt University School of Medicine; Director, Division of Endocrinology, Vanderbilt University Medical Center, Nashville, Tennessee
Adrenal Insufficiency

JURAJ OSTERMAN, M.D., Ph.D.

Professor of Medicine, University of South Carolina School of Medicine; Staff Physician, Dorn Veterans Hospital, Columbia, South Carolina
Hypogonadism: Androgen Therapy

DAVID N. OSTROW, B.Sc.(Med), M.D., M.A., FRCPC, F.C.C.P., F.A.C.P.

Associate Professor of Medicine, University of British Columbia Faculty of Medicine; Physician, Vancouver General Hospital, Vancouver, British Columbia, Canada
Pneumothorax

CHARLES Y. C. PAK, M.D.

Professor, Department of Internal Medicine, and Chief, Mineral Metabolism Section, University of Texas Southwestern Medical Center, Southwestern Medical School, Dallas, Texas
Nephrolithiasis

PAUL M. PALEVSKY, M.D.

Assistant Professor of Medicine, University of Pittsburgh School of Medicine; Chief, Hemodialysis, Veterans Administration Medical Center, Pittsburgh, Pennsylvania
Hypernatremia

TALLEY PARKER, M.D.

Instructor, Division of Hepatology, University of Miami School of Medicine, Miami, Florida
Acute Hepatitis: Management and Prevention

JEFFREY PARSONNET, M.D.

Assistant Professor of Medicine, Harvard Medical School; Associate Physician, Department of Medicine, Channing Laboratory, Brigham and Women's Hospital, Boston, Massachusetts
Toxic Shock Syndrome

HANS PASTERKAMP, M.D., FRCPC

Associate Professor of Pediatrics, University of Manitoba Faculty of Medicine; Staff Physician, Section of Pediatric Respirology, Children's Hospital of Winnipeg, Winnipeg, Manitoba, Canada
Acute Upper Airway Infection

HARISH P. PATEL, M.D.

Formerly Assistant Professor, Department of Dermatology, The Johns Hopkins Medical Institutions, Baltimore, Maryland
Bullous Pemphigoid

GUSTAV PAUMGARTNER, M.D.

Professor of Internal Medicine, Medical Department II, Klinikum Grosshadern, University of Munich, Federal Republic of Munich, Germany
Biliary Lithotripsy

J. JASON PAYNE-JAMES, M.B., F.R.C.S.

Research Fellow in Surgery, Department of Gastroenterology and Nutrition, Central Middlesex Hospital, London, England
Enteral Nutrition: Liquid Formula Diets

JOHN R. PERFECT, M.D.

Assistant Professor of Medicine, Duke University School of Medicine, Durham, North Carolina
Cryptococcal Pulmonary Infections

GEORGE DAVID PERKIN, B.A., F.R.C.P.

Consultant Neurologist, Charing Cross and Hillingdon Hospital, London, England
Syncope

STEPHEN J. PEROUTKA, M.D., Ph.D.

Assistant Professor of Neurology and Neurological Sciences, Stanford University Medical Center, Stanford, California
Principles of Pain Management

ROBERT E. PERRILLO, M.D.

Associate Professor of Medicine, Washington University School of Medicine; Director, Gastroenterology, St. Louis Veterans Administration Medical Center, St. Louis, Missouri
Chronic Hepatitis

DEMETRIUS PERTSEMLIDIS, M.D.

Clinical Professor of Surgery, Mount Sinai School of Medicine of the City University of New York; Attending Surgeon, Mount Sinai Medical Center, New York, New York
Pheochromocytoma

CHARLES M. PETERSON, M.D.

Director of Research, Sansum Medical Research Foundation, Santa Barbara; Clinical Professor of Medicine, University of Southern California, Los Angeles; Physician, Santa Barbara Cottage Hospital, Santa Barbara, California
Diabetes and Pregnancy

LAWRENCE D. PETZ, M.D.

Professor, Department of Pathology, University of California School of Medicine, Los Angeles, California
Autoimmune Hemolytic Anemia

DAVID A. PEURA, M.D., F.A.C.P., Col. MC

Associate Professor of Medicine, Uniformed Services University of the Health Sciences F. Edward Hébert School of Medicine, Bethesda, Maryland; Chief, Gastroenterology Service, Walter Reed Army Medical Center, Washington, D.C.
Stress Ulcer and Acute Erosive Gastritis

F. XAVIER PI-SUNYER, M.D.

Professor of Clinical Medicine, Columbia University College of Physicians and Surgeons; Director, Division of Endocrinology, Diabetes and Nutrition, and Obesity Research Center, St. Luke's-Roosevelt Hospital Center, New York, New York

Obesity

PETER E. POCHI, M.D.

Herbert Mescon Professor of Dermatology, Boston University School of Medicine; Visiting Dermatologist, University Hospital, Boston, Massachusetts

Acne

WENDY A. POCOCK, M.B.

Consultant in Cardiology, University of the Witwatersrand Medical School, Parktown; Senior Physician, Johannesburg Hospital, Johannesburg, South Africa

Mitral Valve Billowing and Prolapse

CRAIG M. PRATT, M.D.

Associate Professor of Medicine, Baylor College of Medicine; Director, Coronary Care Unit and Noninvasive Laboratories, The Methodist Hospital, Houston, Texas

Angina Pectoris: Unstable

DANIEL H. PRESENT, M.D.

Clinical Professor of Medicine, The Mount Sinai School of Medicine of the City University of New York; Attending, Mount Sinai Hospital, New York, New York

Crohn's Disease of the Small Bowel

THOMAS T. PROVOST, M.D.

Noxell Professor and Chairman, Department of Dermatology, The Johns Hopkins University School of Medicine, Baltimore, Maryland

Dermatologic Manifestations of the Acquired Immunodeficiency Syndrome

THOMAS C. QUINN, M.D.

Associate Professor of Medicine, The Johns Hopkins University School of Medicine, Baltimore; Senior Investigator, National Institute of Allergy and Infectious Disease, Bethesda, Maryland

Gastrointestinal Infections in Patients with the Acquired Immunodeficiency Syndrome

PETER V. RABINS, M.D., Ph.D.

Associate Professor of Psychiatry, The Johns Hopkins University School of Medicine, Baltimore, Maryland

Dementia

ERIC C. RACKOW, M.D.

Chairman, Department of Medicine, St. Vincent's Hospital and Medical Center of New York, New York, New York

Acute Respiratory Failure in Chronic Obstructive Pulmonary Disease

SHAHBUDIN H. RAHIMTOOLA, M.B., F.R.C.P.

George C. Griffith Professor of Medicine, and Chief, Division of Cardiology, University of Southern California School of Medicine, Los Angeles, California

Acute Pulmonary Edema

KANTI R. RAI, M.D., F.A.C.P.

Professor of Medicine, Albert Einstein College of Medicine of Yeshiva University, The Bronx; Chief, Division of Hematology-Oncology, Long Island Jewish Medical Center, New Hyde Park, New York

Chronic Lymphocytic Leukemia

LAWRENCE G. RAISZ, M.D.

Head, Division of Endocrinology and Metabolism, University of Connecticut Health Center, Farmington, Connecticut

Osteoporosis

ALBERT E. RAIZNER, M.D.

Associate Professor of Medicine, Baylor College of Medicine; Director, Cardiac Catheterization Laboratories, The Methodist Hospital, Houston, Texas

Mitral Regurgitation

DAVID F. RANSOHOFF, M.D.

Associate Professor of Medicine, The Johns Hopkins University School of Medicine; Director of Gastrointestinal Endoscopy, The Johns Hopkins Hospital; Clinical Director, The Johns Hopkins Swallowing Center, Baltimore, Maryland

Cholelithiasis: Medical and Surgical Aspects

T. K. SREEPADA RAO, M.D., F.A.C.P.

Associate Professor of Medicine, State University of New York Health Science Center at Brooklyn School of Medicine; Associate Director, Renal Diseases Division, and Director of Hemodialysis, State University of New York Health Science Center at Brooklyn, Brooklyn, New York

Human Immunodeficiency Virus–Associated Nephropathy

BASIL RAPOPORT, M.B., Ch.B.

Professor of Medicine, University of California School of Medicine; Staff Physician, Veterans Administration Medical Center, San Francisco, California

Myxedema Coma

DAVID P. RARDON, M.D.

Assistant Professor of Medicine, Indiana University School of Medicine; Cardiologist, Indiana University Medical Center, Indianapolis, Indiana
Atrioventricular Block

JONATHAN I. RAVDIN, M.D.

Associate Professor of Medicine and Pharmacology, Division of Clinical Pharmacology, Department of Internal Medicine, University of Virginia School of Medicine, Charlottesville, Virginia
Amebiasis and Giardiasis

NICHOLAS W. READ, M.D., F.R.C.P.

Professor, University of Sheffield; Consultant Physician, Royal Halcamshire Hospital, Sheffield, England
Constipation

ANDREW J. REES, M.D., M.Sc.

Senior Lecturer, Royal Postgraduate Medical School; Consultant Physician, Hammersmith Hospital, London, England
Goodpasture's Syndrome

FREDRIC G. REGENSTEIN, M.D.

Clinical Assistant Professor of Medicine, Tulane University School of Medicine; Physician, Ochsner Medical Institutions, New Orleans, Louisiana
Chronic Hepatitis

STEPHEN G. REICH, M.D.

Instructor in Neurology, The Johns Hopkins University School of Medicine, Baltimore, Maryland
Parkinson's Disease

STUART RICH, M.D.

Associate Professor of Medicine, and Chief, Section of Cardiology, Department of Medicine, The University of Illinois College of Medicine, Chicago, Illinois
Cor Pulmonale

CHARLES T. RICHARDSON, M.D.

Clinical Professor of Internal Medicine, Baylor College of Medicine; Attending Physician, University of Texas Southwestern Medical Center at Dallas, Dallas, Texas
Duodenal Ulcer

STEPHEN P. RICHMAN, M.D.

Professor of Oncology, University of Miami School of Medicine; Chief, Division of Medical Oncology, Sylvester Comprehensive Cancer Institute, Miami, Florida
Kaposi's Sarcoma

JOEL E. RICHTER, M.D.

Professor of Medicine and Director of Clinical Research, Division of Gastroenterology, The University of Alabama at Birmingham School of Medicine, Birmingham, Alabama
Esophageal Motor Disorders and Chest Pain

CAROLINE A. RIELY, M.D.

Professor of Medicine and Pediatrics, College of Medicine, The University of Tennessee; Attending Physician, The William F. Bowld Hospital, Memphis, Tennessee
Liver Disease in Pregnancy

SAFA M. RIFKA, M.D.

Clinical Associate Professor of Reproductive Endocrinology, Georgetown University School of Medicine and Columbia Hospital for Women, Washington, D.C.
Medical Management of Endometriosis

JACOB M. ROBBINS, M.D.

Chief, Clinical Endocrinology Branch, National Institute of Diabetes and Digestive and Kidney Diseases, National Institutes of Health, Bethesda, Maryland
Thyroid Storm

PATRICIA L. ROBERTS, M.D.

Staff Surgeon, Department of Colon and Rectal Surgery, Lahey Clinic Medical Center, Burlington, Massachusetts
Diverticular Disease of the Colon

ROBERT ROBERTS, M.D.

Professor of Medicine and Cell Biology, and Chief of Cardiology, Baylor College of Medicine, Houston, Texas
Angina Pectoris: Unstable

W. NEAL ROBERTS, M.D.

Assistant Professor of Medicine, Division of Rheumatology, Allergy and Immunology, Medical College of Virginia, Richmond, Virginia
Rheumatoid Arthritis

ALAN G. ROBINSON, M.D.

Professor of Medicine and Chief, Division of Endocrinology and Metabolism, University of Pittsburgh School of Medicine, Pittsburgh, Pennsylvania
Diabetes Insipidus

RICHARD J. ROHRER, M.D.

Assistant Professor, Tufts University School of Medicine; Chief, Division of Transplant Surgery, New England Medical Center, Boston, Massachusetts
Organ Transplantation

ALLAN R. RONALD, B.Sc., FRCPC, F.A.C.P.

Professor and Chairman, Department of Internal Medicine, University of Manitoba Faculty of Medicine; Physician-in-Chief, Department of Medicine, Health Sciences Centre, Winnipeg, Manitoba, Canada
Chancroid, Lymphogranuloma Venereum, Granuloma Inguinale, and Condyloma Acuminata

JAMES A. RONAN Jr., M.D.

Clinical Professor of Medicine, Georgetown University School of Medicine, Washington, D.C.; Co-Director, Department of Cardiology, Washington Adventist Hospital, Takoma Park, Maryland
Aortic Stenosis

JESSE ROTH, M.D.

Clinical Professor of Medicine, Uniformed Services University of the Health Sciences F. Edward Hébert School of Medicine, Bethesda, and Associate Clinical Professor, Howard University College of Medicine, Washington, D.C.; Director of Intramural Research and Acting Chief of Diabetes Branch, National Institute of Diabetes and Digestive and Kidney Diseases, National Institutes of Health, Bethesda, Maryland
Insulin Allergy and Insulin Resistance

JEFFREY D. ROTHSTEIN, M.D., Ph.D.

Instructor, Department of Neurology, The Johns Hopkins University School of Medicine, Baltimore, Maryland
Hepatic Encephalopathy

WALTER ROYAL III, M.D.

Instructor, Department of Neurology, The Johns Hopkins University School of Medicine, Baltimore, Maryland
Drug Overdose and Withdrawal

MARY RUBENIS, B.S. (Deceased)

Formerly Senior Research Associate, University of Illinois College of Medicine, Chicago, Illinois
Viral Respiratory Infections

SHAUN RUDDY, M.D.

Professor of Medicine, Microbiology and Immunology, and Chairman, Division of Immunology and Connective Tissue Diseases, Virginia Commonwealth University, Medical College of Virginia, Richmond, Virginia
Rheumatoid Arthritis

ROBERT K. RUDE, M.D.

Associate Professor of Medicine, University of Southern California School of Medicine, Los Angeles, California
Hypocalcemia and Hypoparathyroidism

ZAVERIO M. RUGGERI, M.D.

Associate Member, Scripps Clinic and Research Foundation, La Jolla, California
von Willebrand's Disease

SANDRA SABATINI, M.D., Ph.D.

Professor of Internal Medicine and Physiology, Texas Tech University Health Sciences Center School of Medicine; Attending in Nephrology, University Medical Center, Lubbock, Texas
Mixed Acid-Base Disturbances

R. BRADLEY SACK, M.D., Sc.D.

Professor of International Health and Medicine, and Director, Division of Geographic Medicine, The Johns Hopkins University School of Hygiene and Public Health, Baltimore, Maryland
Traveler's Diarrhea

MICHAEL SACKMANN, M.D.

Senior Resident, Medical Department II, Klinikum Grosshadern, University of Munich, Munich, Federal Republic of Germany
Biliary Lithotripsy

ROBERT A. SALATA, M.D.

Assistant Professor of Medicine, Case Western Reserve University School of Medicine; Attending Physician and Consultant, University Hospitals of Cleveland, Cleveland, Ohio
Protozoan and Helminthic Pulmonary Infections

ALAN SALLIMAN, M.D.

Specialist in Internal Medicine, Glenwood Springs, Colorado
High Altitude Disease

MARTIN A. SAMUELS, M.D.

Associate Professor of Neurology, Harvard Medical School; Chief of Neurology, Brigham and Women's Hospital, Boston, Massachusetts
Disorders of Consciousness

GEORGE W. SANTOS, M.D.

Professor of Oncology and Medicine, The Johns Hopkins University School of Medicine, Baltimore, Maryland
Autologous Bone Marrow Transplantation

TILMAN SAUERBRUCH, M.D.

Associate Professor of Internal Medicine, Medical Department II, Klinikum Grosshadern, University of Munich, Munich, Federal Republic of Germany
Biliary Lithotripsy

DAVID S. SCHADE, M.D.

Professor of Medicine, University of New Mexico School of Medicine, Albuquerque, New Mexico
Diabetic Ketoacidosis

DANIEL F. SCHAFER, M.D.

Associate Professor of Medicine, University of Nebraska Medical Center; Chief, Gastroenterology, Omaha Veterans Administration Medical Center, Omaha, Nebraska
Fulminant Hepatic Failure

EUGENE R. SCHIFF, M.D.

Professor of Medicine, and Chief, Division of Hematology, Center for Liver Diseases, University of Miami School of Medicine; Chief, Hematology Section, Miami Veterans Administration Medical Center, Miami, Florida
Acute Hepatitis: Management and Prevention

ROBERT C. SCHLANT, M.D.

Professor of Medicine (Cardiology), Emory University School of Medicine; Chief of Cardiology, Grady Memorial Hospital, Atlanta, Georgia
Mitral Stenosis

DAVID SCHLOSSBERG, M.D., F.A.C.P.

Professor of Medicine, Temple University School of Medicine; Director, Department of Medicine, Episcopal Hospital, Philadelphia, Pennsylvania
Cellulitis and Soft Tissue Infection

HEINZ-JOSEF SCHMITT, M.D.

Instructor in Medicine, Cornell University Medical College; Fellow in Training, Infectious Disease Service, Memorial Sloan-Kettering Cancer Center, New York, New York
Antifungal Chemotherapy

H. GUNTER SEYDEL, M.D., M.S., F.A.C.R.

Former Clinical Professor of Radiation Oncology, Wayne State University School of Medicine, Detroit, Michigan
Esophageal Carcinoma

PEDER M. SHEA, M.D., F.A.C.C., F.A.C.P.

Assistant Clinical Professor of Medicine, University of California School of Medicine, San Diego, California
Chronic Anticoagulation

DAVID G. SHERMAN, M.D.

Professor, Division of Neurology, University of Texas Health Science Center, San Antonio, Texas
Embolic Stroke of Cardiac Origin

ALAN R. SHULDINER, M.D.

Senior Staff Fellow, Diabetes Branch, National Institute of Diabetes and Digestive and Kidney Diseases, National Institutes of Health, Bethesda, Maryland
Insulin Allergy and Insulin Resistance

LEONARD SICILIAN, M.D.

Assistant Professor of Medicine, Tufts University School of Medicine; Director, Medical Intensive Care Unit, New England Medical Center Hospitals, Boston, Massachusetts
Respirator Care

CRAIG O. SIEGEL, M.D.

Fellow in Cardiology, Baylor College of Medicine and The Methodist Hospital, Houston, Texas
Mitral Regurgitation

MARK SIEGLER, M.D.

Professor of Medicine, and Director, Center for Clinical Medical Ethics, The University of Chicago, Division of the Biological Sciences, Pritzker School of Medicine, Chicago, Illinois
Decisions to Forgo Life-Sustaining Treatment

DAVID B. A. SILK, M.D., F.R.C.P.

Co-Director, Department of Gastroenterology and Nutrition, Central Middlesex Hospital, London, England
Enteral Nutrition: Liquid Formula Diets

DANIEL H. SIMMONS, M.D., Ph.D.

Professor of Medicine Emeritus, Division of Pulmonary and Critical Care Medicine, University of California UCLA School of Medicine; Attending Physician, UCLA Medical Center, Los Angeles, California
Wegener's Granulomatosis

IRWIN SINGER, M.D.

Professor of Medicine, Northwestern University School of Medicine; Chief of Staff, Veterans Administration Lakeside Medical Center, Chicago, Illinois
Hypernatremia

PETER A. SINGER, M.D., M.P.H., FRCPC

Assistant Professor of Medicine, and Associate Director, Centre for Bioethics, University of Toronto Faculty of Medicine, Toronto, Ontario, Canada
Decisions to Forgo Life-Sustaining Treatment

ETHEL S. SIRIS, M.D.

Associate Professor of Clinical Medicine, Columbia University College of Physicians and Surgeons; Associate Attending Physician, Presbyterian Hospital, New York, New York
Paget's Disease of Bone

MICHAEL V. SIVAK Jr., M.D., F.A.C.P., F.A.C.G.

Chairman, Department of Gastroenterology, The Cleveland Clinic Foundation, Cleveland, Ohio
Upper Gastrointestinal Bleeding

ROLAND T. SKEEL, M.D.

Professor of Medicine and Chief, Division of Hematology/Oncology, Medical College of Ohio, Toledo, Ohio
Head and Neck Cancer

MARTHA SKINNER, M.D.

Professor of Medicine, Boston University School of Medicine; Visiting Physician, Boston City Hospital, Boston, Massachusetts
Amyloidosis

PAUL R. SKOLNIK, M.D.

Assistant Professor of Medicine, Tufts University School of Medicine; Director, AIDS Laboratory, and Assistant Physician, New England Medical Center Hospital, Boston, Massachusetts
Antiviral Therapy of Human Immunodeficiency Virus Infection

RAYMOND G. SLAVIN, M.D.

Professor of Internal Medicine and Microbiology, and Director, Division of Allergy and Immunology, St. Louis University School of Medicine, St. Louis, Missouri
Hypersensitivity Pneumonitis

COREY M. SLOVIS, M.D., F.A.C.P., F.A.C.E.P.

Associate Professor, Emergency Medicine, University of Rochester School of Medicine; Chief, Department of Emergency Medicine, Strong Memorial Hospital, Rochester, New York
Cardiac Arrest and Resuscitation from Sudden Death

RICHARD V. SMALLEY, M.D.

Professor of Human Oncology, University of Wisconsin Medical School, Madison, Wisconsin
Ovarian Cancer

BRUCE R. SMITH, Pharm.D.

Associate Director, Therapeutic Research Institute, Sarasota, Florida
Bacterial Osteomyelitis

ROBERT B. SMITH III, M.D.

Professor of Surgery, Emory University School of Medicine; Acting Chairman, Department of Surgery, and Chief, Section of Vascular Surgery, The Emory Clinic, Atlanta, Georgia
Carotid Artery Occlusive Disease

THOMAS W. SMITH, M.D.

Professor of Medicine, Harvard Medical School; Chief, Cardiovascular Division, Brigham and Women's Hospital, Boston, Massachusetts
Digitalis Toxicity

DOROTHY D. SOGN, M.D.

Medical Officer, General Clinical Research Centers Program, National Center for Research Resources, and Staff Physician, The Clinical Center, National Institutes of Health, Bethesda, Maryland
Drug Reactions

RICHARD F. SPARK, M.D.

Associate Clinical Professor of Medicine, Harvard Medical School; Director, Steroid Research Laboratory, Beth Israel Hospital, Boston, Massachusetts
Cushing's Syndrome

ALEXANDER S. D. SPIERS, M.D., Ph.D., F.R.C.P.(E), F.R.A.C.P., F.R.C.Path.A., F.A.C.P.

Professor of Medicine, Division of Medical Oncology, University of South Florida College of Medicine; Director, Leukemia and Lymphoma Center, H. Lee Moffitt Cancer Center and Research Institute, Tampa, Florida
Chronic Granulocytic Leukemia

MARK STACY, M.D.

Clinical Instructor, Department of Neurology, Hahnemann University, Philadelphia, Pennsylvania
Cervical Spondylosis

WILLIAM W. STEAD, M.D.

Professor of Medicine, University of Arkansas School of Medicine; Director, Tuberculosis Program, Arkansas Department of Health, Little Rock, Arkansas
Tuberculosis

BRIAN T. STEELE, M.D., FRCPC

Assistant Professor, McMaster University Faculty of Medicine; Pediatric Nephrologist, McMaster University Medical Center, Hamilton, Ontario, Canada
Hemolytic-Uremic Syndrome

RICHARD A. STEEVES, M.D., Ph.D.

Associate Professor, Department of Human Oncology, University of Wisconsin School of Medicine, Madison, Wisconsin
Radiation Therapy for Breast Cancer

EMIL STEINBERGER, M.D.

President, Texas Institute for Reproductive Medicine and Endocrinology; Professor of Endocrinology, University of Texas Medical School, Houston, Texas
Male Infertility of Undetermined Etiology

WILLIAM M. STRAIN, M.D.

Fellow in Gastroenterology, College of Medicine, University of Tennessee, Memphis, Tennessee
Liver Disease in Pregnancy

DARRYL Y. SUE, M.D.

Associate Professor of Medicine, University of California UCLA School of Medicine, Los Angeles; Director, Medical Intensive Care Unit, and Staff, Division of Respiratory and Critical Care Physiology and Medicine, Harbor-UCLA Medical Center, Torrance, California
Respiratory Acidosis

TIMOTHY J. SULLIVAN III, M.D.

Associate Professor of Internal Medicine and Microbiology, Department of Internal Medicine, University of Texas Southwestern Medical Center, Southwestern Medical School; Head, Allergy and Immunology, Parkland Memorial Hospital, Dallas, Texas
Systemic Anaphylaxis

MARTIN I. SURKS, M.D.

Professor of Medicine and Laboratory Medicine, Albert Einstein College of Medicine of Yeshiva University; Head, Division of Endocrinology and Metabolism, Montefiore Medical Center, The Bronx, New York
Thyroiditis

PATRICK J. SWEENEY, M.D., F.A.C.P.

Associate Clinical Professor of Neurology, Case Western Reserve University School of Medicine; Clinical Neurologist, Department of Neurology, The Cleveland Clinic Foundation, Cleveland, Ohio
Entrapment Neuropathy

IRA B. TAGER, M.D., M.P.H.

Associate Professor of Medicine and Epidemiology and International Health, University of California, San Francisco, School of Medicine; Veterans Administration Medical Center, San Francisco, California
Chronic Bronchitis

ALAIN TAÏEB, M.D.

Assistant des Universités, Université de Bordeaux II; Assistant des Hôpitaux, Service de Dermatologie, Hôpital des Enfants, Centre Hospitalier Universitaire de Bordeaux, Bordeaux, France
Atopic Dermatitis

FRANCIS J. TEDESCO, M.D., F.A.C.P., F.A.C.G.

President and Professor of Medicine, Medical College of Georgia, Augusta, Georgia
Lower Gastrointestinal Bleeding

AMIR TEJANI, M.D.

Professor of Pediatrics, and Director, Renal Division, State University of New York Health Science Center at Brooklyn College of Medicine, Brooklyn, New York
Minimal-Change Disease in Idiopathic Nephrotic Syndrome

RALPH TOMPSETT, M.D.

Professor Emeritus, University of Texas Southwestern Medical Center at Dallas, Southwestern Medical School; Chief, Infectious Diseases, Baylor University Medical Center, Dallas, Texas
Bacterial Arthritis

JOHN H. TOOGOOD, M.D., FRCPC, F.C.C.P.

Professor of Medicine, University of Western Ontario Faculty of Medicine; Director, Allergy Clinic, Victoria Hospital, London, Ontario, Canada
Asthma

VICENTE E. TORRES, M.D.

Associate Professor of Medicine, Mayo Medical School; Consultant, Internal Medicine and Nephrology, The Mayo Clinic, Rochester, Minnesota
Cystic Disease of the Kidney

FRANK M. TORTI, M.D., M.P.H.

Associate Professor of Medicine, Stanford University School of Medicine, Stanford; Chief, Oncology Section, Palo Alto Veterans Affairs Medical Center, Palo Alto, California
Bladder Cancer

KLAUS V. TOYKA, M.D.

Professor and Chairman, Department of Neurology, University of Wurzburg, Wurzburg, Federal Republic of Germany
Myasthenia Gravis

CHARLES B. TREASURE, M.D.

Assistant Professor of Medicine, Emory University School of Medicine; Director, Cardiac Catheterization Laboratory, Grady Memorial Hospital, Atlanta, Georgia
Aortic Regurgitation

DONALD L. TRUMP, M.D., F.A.C.P.

Professor of Medicine, Duke University School of Medicine; Director, Experimental Therapeutics, Duke University Comprehensive Cancer Center, Durham, North Carolina

Testicular Cancer

KENNETH L. TYLER, M.D.

Assistant Professor of Neurology and Neuroscience, Departments of Neurology and Microbiology and Molecular Genetics, Harvard Medical School; Assistant Neurologist, Massachusetts General Hospital, Boston, Massachusetts

Localized Infection of the Nervous System

MARK E. UNIS, M.D.

Dermatologist in Private Practice, Fort Lauderdale, Florida

Erythema Nodosum

WALTER J. URBA, M.D., Ph.D.

Director, Clinical Services, National Cancer Institute-Frederick Cancer Research Facility, Frederick, Maryland

T-Cell Lymphoma

JAIME URIBARRI, M.D.

Assistant Professor of Medicine, State University of New York Health Science Center at Brooklyn College of Medicine; Attending Physician, State University of New York Health Science Center at Brooklyn, Brooklyn, New York

Metabolic Acidosis

JOHN P. UTZ, M.D., F.A.C.P.

Professor of Medicine, Georgetown University School of Medicine; Attending Physician, Georgetown University Hospital, Washington, D.C.

Candidosis

MARTIN D. VALENTINE, M.D.

Professor of Medicine, The Johns Hopkins University School of Medicine; Physician, The Johns Hopkins Hospital and The Johns Hopkins Asthma and Allergy Center at The Francis Scott Key Medical Center, Baltimore, Maryland

Chronic Urticaria

PAUL P. VanARSDEL Jr., M.D.

Professor of Medicine and Head, Section of Allergy, University of Washington School of Medicine; Attending Physician, University Hospital, Seattle, Washington

Drug Reactions

OSWALD van CUTSEM, M.D.

Chest Physician, Clinique Saint Luc, Bouge, Belgium

Aerobic Gram-Positive Pneumonia

A. WARMOLD L. VAN DEN WALL BAKE, M.D., Ph.D.

Associate Professor, Department of Nephrology, University Hospital, Leiden, The Netherlands

IgA Nephropathy (Berger's Disease)

JON A. VANDERHOOF, M.D.

Professor and Chairman, Department of Pediatrics, Creighton University School of Medicine, Omaha, Nebraska

Short Bowel Syndrome

MALCOLM C. VEIDENHEIMER, M.D., C.M., FRCSC, F.A.C.S.

Department of Colon and Rectal Surgery, Lahey Clinic Medical Center, Burlington, Massachusetts

Diverticular Disease of the Colon

JOSEPH G. VERBALIS, M.D.

Associate Professor of Medicine, University of Pittsburgh School of Medicine, Pittsburgh, Pennsylvania

Diabetes Insipidus

UMBERTO VERONESI, M.D.

Professor of Pathological Anatomy, Professor of Surgery, and Director General, National Cancer Institute, Milan, Italy

Surgery for Breast Cancer

GEORGE W. VETROVEC, M.D.

Professor of Medicine, and Associate Chairman of Medicine for Clinical Affairs, Virginia Commonwealth University, Medical College of Virginia; Director, Adult Cardiac Catheterization Laboratory, Medical College of Virginia Hospitals, Richmond, Virginia

Myocardial Infarction: Uncomplicated

ELLIOTT VICHINSKY, M.D.

Associate Director, Hematology/Oncology, and Director, Sickle Cell Program, Children's Hospital Medical Center, Oakland, California

Sickle Cell Anemia

ROBERT A. VIGERSKY, M.D., F.A.C.P.

Clinical Associate Professor of Medicine, Georgetown University; Director, Diabetes Treatment Center, Washington Hospital Center, Washington, D.C.

Anorexia Nervosa and Bulimia

AARON VINIK, M.D.

Professor of Internal Medicine and Surgery, University of Michigan Medical School, Ann Arbor, Michigan

Diabetic Neuropathy

CHARLES L. VOGEL, M.D., F.A.C.P.

Director, South Florida Comprehensive Cancer Centers, Miami, Florida
Kaposi's Sarcoma

C. FORDHAM von REYN, M.D.

Associate Clinical Professor of Medicine, Dartmouth Medical School; Chief, Infectious Disease Section, Hitchcock Medical Center, Hanover, New Hampshire
Infective Endocarditis and Mycotic Aneurysm

JOHN F. WADE III, M.D.

Instructor in Medicine, University of Colorado School of Medicine, Denver, Colorado
Hyponatremia

ABRAHAM U. WAKS, M.D.

Clinical Assistant Professor of Medicine, University of California UCLA School of Medicine, Los Angeles, California
Renovascular Hypertension

STEVEN A. WARTMAN, M.D., Ph.D.

Professor of Medicine and Community Health, Brown University Program in Medicine; Division Director, General Internal Medicine, Rhode Island Hospital, Providence, Rhode Island
Respecting Patients' Treatment Preferences

KARLMAN WASSERMAN, M.D., Ph.D.

Professor of Medicine, University of California UCLA School of Medicine, Los Angeles; Chief, Division of Respiratory and Critical Care Physiology and Medicine, Harbor-UCLA Medical Center, Torrance, California
Respiratory Acidosis

LOUIS R. WASSERMAN, M.D.

Albert A. and Vera G. List Distinguished Professor of Medicine (Hematology) Emeritus, Mount Sinai School of Medicine of the City University of New York, New York, New York
Polycythemia Rubra Vera

YOSHIO WATANABE, M.D.

Professor of Medicine and Director, Cardiovascular Institute, Fujita Health University School of Medicine, Aichi, Japan
Atrial Premature Depolarization, Atrial Tachycardia, Atrial Flutter, and Atrial Fibrillation

DANNY F. WATSON, M.D., Ph.D.

Associate Professor of Neurology, Wayne State University School of Medicine, Detroit, Michigan
Chronic Neuropathy

MAX HARRY WEIL, M.D., Ph.D.

Distinguished Professor of Medicine, Physiology, and Biophysics, and Chairman, Department of Medicine, University of Health Sciences/Chicago Medical School, North Chicago, Illinois
Acute Respiratory Failure in Chronic Obstructive Pulmonary Disease

ETHAN WEINER, M.D.

Assistant Clinical Professor of Medicine, University of Connecticut School of Medicine; Associate Director, Department of Clinical Research, Pfizer Central Research, Farmington, Connecticut
Systemic Sclerosis

JEFFREY I. WEITZ, M.D., FRCPC, F.A.C.P.

Associate Professor, Department of Medicine, McMaster University Faculty of Medicine; Attending Staff, Department of Medicine, Henderson General Hospital, Hamilton, Ontario, Canada
Disseminated Intravascular Coagulation

ALEXANDER WHITE, M.B., M.R.C.P.I.

Clinical Fellow, Tufts University School of Medicine; Research Fellow in Pulmonary Disease, New England Medical Center Hospitals, Boston, Massachusetts
Respirator Care

DAVID O. WIEBERS, M.D.

Associate Professor of Neurology, Mayo Medical School; Head, Section of Neurology, Mayo Clinic and Mayo Foundation, Rochester, Minnesota
Intracranial Aneurysm

PETER H. WIERNIK, M.D.

Gutman Professor and Chairman, Department of Oncology, Montefiore Medical Center; Director, Division of Medical Oncology, Albert Einstein College of Medicine, and Associate Director for Clinical Research, Albert Einstein Cancer Center, The Bronx, New York
Acute Nonlymphocytic Leukemia

ASA J. WILBOURN, M.D.

Assistant Clinical Professor of Neurology, Case Western Reserve University School of Medicine; Director, EMG Laboratory, Department of Neurology, The Cleveland Clinic Foundation, Cleveland, Ohio
Entrapment Neuropathy

JAMES T. WILLERSON, M.D.

Professor and Chairman, Department of Internal Medicine, University of Texas Medical School at Houston; Director, Cardiology Research, and Co-Director, Cullen Cardiovascular Research Laboratories, Texas Heart Institute, Houston, Texas
Constrictive Pericarditis

GORDON H. WILLIAMS, M.D.

Professor of Medicine, Harvard Medical School; Director, Endocrine/Hypertension Unit, Brigham and Women's Hospital, Boston, Massachusetts

Primary Aldosteronism

WILLIAM E. C. WILSON, M.D., C.M., FRCPC, F.A.C.P.

Clinical Professor, Department of Medicine, McMaster University Faculty of Medicine; Service of Clinical Hematology, Department of Medicine, Hamilton Civic Hospitals, Hamilton, Ontario, Canada

Multiple Myeloma and Related Monoclonal Gammopathies

JAMES F. WINCHESTER, M.D., F.R.C.P.(Glas)

Professor of Medicine, and Acting Director, Division of Nephrology, Georgetown University Medical Center, Washington, D.C.

Hypertension in Chronic Renal Failure, Dialysis, and/or Transplantation

GARY P. WORMSER, M.D.

Professor of Medicine and Pharmacology, and Chief, Division of Infectious Diseases, New York Medical College; Chief, Section of Infectious Diseases, Westchester County Medical Center, Valhalla, New York

Lyme Disease

KIRK D. WUEPPER, M.D.

Professor of Dermatology, The Oregon Health Sciences University School of Medicine, Portland, Oregon

Erythema Multiforme

DAVID J. WYLER, M.D.

Professor of Medicine, Tufts University School of Medicine; Physician, New England Medical Center, Boston, Massachusetts

Malaria

ANDREW M. YEAGER, M.D.

Associate Professor of Oncology, Pediatrics, and Neurology, The Johns Hopkins Medical Institutions, Baltimore, Maryland

Autologous Bone Marrow Transplantation

LOWELL S. YOUNG, M.D.

Clinical Professor of Medicine, University of California, San Francisco, School of Medicine; Director, Kuzell Institute for Arthritis and Infectious Diseases; Chief, Division of Infectious Diseases, Pacific Presbyterian Medical Center, San Francisco, California

Infection Complicating Immunosuppression

NEAL S. YOUNG, M.D.

Chief, Cell Biology Section, Clinical Hematology Branch, National Heart, Lung and Blood Institute, National Institutes of Health, Bethesda, Maryland

Aplastic Anemia

GEORGE C. YU, M.D.

Pneumonologist, Ventura County Pulmonary Medical Group, Ventura County, California

Hypophosphatemia and Phosphate Depletion

TS'AI-FAN YU, M.D.

Professor of Medicine Emeritus, Mount Sinai School of Medicine of The City University of New York, New York, New York

Gout

DORI F. ZALEZNIK, M.D.

Assistant Professor of Medicine, Harvard Medical School; Hospital Epidemiologist, Beth Israel Hospital, Boston, Massachusetts

Intra-Abdominal Abscess

JONATHAN M. ZENILMAN, M.D.

Assistant Professor, Division of Infectious Diseases, Department of Medicine; The Johns Hopkins University School of Medicine; Attending Physician, The Johns Hopkins Hospital, Baltimore, Maryland

Disseminated Gonococcal Infection

DEWEY K. ZIEGLER, M.D.

Professor of Neurology, University of Kansas School of Medicine, Kansas City, Kansas

Migraine and Cluster Headache

THEODORE S. ZIMMERMAN, M.D. (Deceased)

Formerly Professor, Department of Basic and Clinical Research, and Director, Coagulation Laboratory, and Staff, Division of Hematology/Oncology, Scripps Clinic and Research Foundation, La Jolla, California

von Willebrand's Disease

STEPHEN H. ZINNER, M.D.

Professor of Medicine, Brown University; Head, Division of Infectious Diseases, Roger Williams General Hospital and Rhode Island Hospital, Providence, Rhode Island

Antibacterial Chemotherapy

PREFACE

Therapeutic decision making is both a science and an art. We base our choices of medical or surgical regimens on complex factors, many of which can be formulated in explicit and precise terms. These factors include the likelihood that a patient has one or more diseases, the efficacy of various treatments for the diseases under consideration, the toxicity of the treatments, and the acceptability of the treatment to the patient. Diets, behavioral modifications, drugs, vaccines, blood products, invasive nonsurgical approaches, and traditional operative procedures constitute many of our current therapeutic modalities. The science of medicine has provided many clear answers about which treatment to use in a given clinical situation, and from fundamental research and clinical trials we have derived specific therapeutic guidelines, often in the form of "treatments of choice." Even when our scientific evidence about a given treatment for a given disorder is "hard," however, experts do not necessarily agree on the optimal approach. And when the evidence is equivocal, or when two or more divergent approaches appear to have similar value, disagreement is often greater. Despite the ambiguity that frequently is embodied in the "optimal" approach for a certain clinical situation, the physician confronted with a patient must make a decision about what to do. This decision may have to be based at once on published data and on an individual's experience, expertise, and judgment. The chapters in this book are based on all of these factors: facts where possible, opinions and judgments where facts fall short. Here we present 361 chapters on therapy of most important problems faced by the practicing internist. We have garnered the expertise of 512 distinguished clinicians who describe their mode of therapy for a specific disease or management problem, as if they were providing that care themselves. Chapter authors were selected not only for their clinical expertise, but also for their contributions to teaching and research and for the clarity of their writing style.

As in the two previous editions of *Current Therapy in Internal Medicine,* the chapters describing treatments for specific disease entities were selected from previously published subspecialty current therapy books (for example, *Current Therapy in Cardiovascular Disease; Current Therapy in Nephrology and Hypertension*). Every chapter in the third edition has been either completely or partially rewritten from the second edition. Even chapters from recent subspecialty books have been updated as necessary.

But this new edition also has a new focus. Two new sections have been added to enhance its usefulness. Recognizing that there is more to therapeutics than the individual prescriptions for each disease entity, we have added an entire section devoted to the principles of therapeutics. Included in this section are chapters devoted to therapeutic decision making, clinical pharmacology, patient compliance, patients' preferences, health promotion and disease prevention, nutritional support, pain management, drug reactions and overdoses, various nonpharmacologic therapeutic modalities, and ethical therapeutic issues. A similar collation of key therapeutic principles is not found elsewhere.

The new structure and content of the book also reflect the increasing importance of the acquired immunodeficiency syndrome in current medical practice. Given the protean manifestations of this increasingly common disease, we have given it special prominence in its own section consisting of eight chapters. Even as we go to press, of course, the management of this disease and its multiple organ manifestations is undergoing evolution.

This book is for the practitioner who identifies a disease or disorder and wishes an authoritative summary of current therapeutic approaches. Its focus should make it valuable to anyone who wishes to understand the principles and pragmatic aspects of medical therapeutics.

Jerome P. Kassirer, M.D.

CONTENTS

INFECTIOUS DISEASES

Cardiovascular Diseases

Gastrointestinal Diseases

Respiratory Diseases

Hematologic Diseases

Neoplastic Disorders

HYPERTENSION AND RENAL DISEASE

THERAPEUTIC PRINCIPLES

PRINCIPLES OF THERAPEUTIC DECISION MAKING

MARK H. ECKMAN, M.D.
JEROME P. KASSIRER, M.D.

Selecting the right treatment at the right time is a prime function of the physician, and a dazzling array of therapeutic approaches is available. Choices lie along a spectrum of dissimilar options: avoidance or cessation of all modalities on the one hand, and the use of accepted drugs and operative approaches or radical new, incompletely effective, and highly risky medical and surgical treatments on the other. The penalties for unwise and inappropriate selection of therapy are formidable, including disappointments, disability, and death.

Needless to say, accurate diagnosis is the critical first step in deciding which treatment to choose; however, many therapeutic decisions must be made before all diagnostic information is available and before we are confident of a diagnosis. In many instances selection of therapy is simple and straightforward because long experience has confirmed the value and safety of a given approach. In such instances we develop comfortable and familiar rules that guide our everyday decisions. For many disease entities we have "treatments of choice" that vary little from year to year.

But not all therapeutic decisions can be based on simple rules or guidelines. In many instances we must return to first principles to make such choices —instances in which we are not guaranteed that a given disease is present or not, instances in which one approach seems only marginally better than another, and instances of newly discovered drugs or novel diseases.

By tradition, we try to select a treatment according to the highest scientific principles: anecdotal reports of therapeutic efficacy and risk are not sufficient because factors such as placebo effect, spontaneous remissions, and regression toward the mean seriously cloud the interpretation of individual responses. To avert these confounding variables, we rely heavily on randomized controlled trials of therapeutic approaches. We insist that for a study to qualify as appropriate, patients must be assigned to treatment randomly, neither the patient nor the physician must know which treatment is being administered, outcomes must be measured and defined with precision, and analysis of data must be done using accepted statistical methods. Such trials are laborious, expensive, and subject to flaws, both in design and implementation, but many such studies have been done well and have provided invaluable therapeutic insights. Even the best of the randomized controlled studies, however, provide only an anchor point or a benchmark when it comes to selecting therapy for an individual patient. To the extent that a patient differs notably from the subjects studied in a randomized trial, that patient's response to the treatment also might well differ. Patients may differ in many ways, including their age, sex, race, genetic makeup, and the stage at which their disease is encountered.

Of course, many instances exist in which no randomized controlled trial has been carried out or is likely ever to be carried out. When the patient fails to match a cohort in a controlled study or when no study is available, the physician's good judgment is the fallback position. The elements of therapeutic judgment become critical in such circumstances, forming the basis for our ability to return to first principles in making decisions in the face of uncertainty.

In the past two decades, the principles of therapeutic decision making have been organized a
codified into a prescriptive method called de-se-
analysis. Although decision analysis is a -bility
ful quantitative approach that app making
and utility theory to therapeuti ciples un-
under conditions of uncertai sis to thera-
derlying the application of applied even
peutic choices can be calculations. To
without reverting describe many of
explicate these monstrate how these
them quali

principles translate into therapeutic decision making, we provide a formal decision analysis for a therapeutic dilemma.

SOME THERAPEUTIC PRINCIPLES

Not surprisingly, the principles of therapy are intertwined inextricably with the principles of diagnosis. Because a diagnosis is only an inference about a patient's illness, we can never be absolutely certain that the disease label we assign to a patient's illness is correct. Even if we have a treatment for a disease that is regularly effective and devoid of risk or cost, we will inevitably give the treatment to some patients who do not have the disease and we will inevitably not give the treatment to some who do have the disease. Both circumstances deprive patients of appropriate therapy. To the extent that the treatment is effective but also harmful to some, patients who have the disease for which the treatment is designated will derive the benefit of therapy, offset to some extent by the risks of therapy. Patients who do not have the disease, however, derive no therapeutic benefit but nonetheless are subjected to the risks.

The interrelations between a diagnosis and the benefits and risks of treatment can be specified in the concept of a therapeutic threshold, a probability of disease above which administering the treatment is optimal and below which withholding the treatment is optimal. The efficacy and risks of a treatment for a given disease determine how confident a physician must be of a given diagnosis before administering therapy as the optimal choice. For treatments with a high ratio of benefits to risks, the treatment can be given even when the probability of disease is relatively low (penicillin for suspected streptococcal pneumonia infections, for example). For these treatments, the therapeutic threshold is quite low. For treatments with a low ratio of benefits to risks, on the other hand, the physician must be quite certain that the patient has the disease before administering therapy (amphotericin B for suspected cryptococcal meningitis, for example). For these treatments, the therapeutic threshold is quite high. Of course, low efficacy of treatment, or high risk, or both can contribute to such a low ratio of benefits to risks.

Independent of diagnosis, decision analysis
kes explicit the tradeoffs between disparate thera-
h choices. Physicians often are compelled to
ter ents choose between short-term and long-
stone in a patient with asymptomatic gall-
be weigh of immediate cholecystectomy must
cholecys the future risk of biliary colic and
artery dis tient with significant coronary
from bypas of early surgical mortality
future risk of st be compared with the
rction. In addition, the

greater efficacy of one therapeutic approach over another must sometimes be measured against its adverse effect on the quality of a patient's life: in a patient with laryngeal carcinoma, the choice between less aggressive, speech-preserving surgery has to be weighed against a more aggressive procedure that results in loss of speech but yields a cure or at least a longer cancer-free interval.

When comparing treatments, both randomized controlled trials and decision analysis disclose the marginal benefits of one therapy over another. In many instances, this benefit is large and the decision is clear. In some instances, however, no clear therapeutic approach emerges. Such decisional "toss-ups" are well known in lay decision making, but physicians have been reluctant to acknowledge their existence in clinical decision making. The principal problem in dealing with therapeutic toss-ups lies in judging the clinical relevance of a small benefit. A difference of several years of life expectancy between treatments seems like quite a lot, whereas when the difference is only several weeks, the physician could easily recommend either treatment. However, even a few weeks' difference could be important to a particular patient. Given these features of therapeutic decision making, patients' preferences must always be taken into consideration. Doing so is especially important when marginal differences in the outcomes of two therapeutic approaches are quite small.

Comparing therapeutic choices quantitatively discloses the benefits of these choices clearly. In some instances the principal benefit of one choice over another lies in a small improvement in the quality of an individual's life. In other instances, it is apparent that no matter which therapeutic choice is made (extensive chemotherapy, for example, versus radical surgery in a patient with metastatic cancer), the outcome will be poor. If nothing more, such an assessment may have important prognostic implications.

As noted before, physicians often conduct their therapeutic reasoning based on experience-proven rules. Given the repetitiveness of our day-to-day patient experiences, this practice generally stands us in good stead. Nonetheless, situations often arise in which the patient or clinical setting is in some way atypical—the operative mortality may be higher than usual because of a patient's other risk factors and illnesses, the diagnosis may be uncertain, or the efficacies of competing therapies may be in doubt. Sometimes we are confronted with innovative techniques for testing or novel therapies, developments in health technology for which we do not yet have adequate information. In these settings, a more formal and quantitative approach to therapeutic decision making is most useful. We illustrate here how decision analysis can be used to deal with a current therapeutic quandary.

FORMAL DECISION-MAKING METHODS

Decision analysis prescribes how decisions should be made rather than describing how they are made. A model of the decision in the form of a decision tree provides a uniform framework around which all of the involved medical caretakers can gather. It makes explicit the questions that are being asked. It provides a common tongue, so that when either a patient or physician asks, for instance, "how will the high risk of this proposed therapy effect our decision?", we can specify clearly the parameter to be discussed and the range of risk to be considered.

Decision analysis quantifies the language of uncertainty. Where one physician's use of the qualifier "likely" may indicate a probability of 90 to 100 percent, another physician's use of the same term in the same clinical setting could well mean 50 to 80 percent. Although no one can rightfully say what "likely" actually means in probabilistic terms, the use of a common model and numerical probabilities as focal points of discussion ensures that all parties are speaking the same language.

The steps in performing a decision analysis include (1) framing the question; (2) structuring the problem; (3) determining the probabilities of each outcome; (4) assigning utilities or values to each outcome; (5) calculating the expected (average) utility for each strategy, thus determining which strategy is best; (6) performing sensitivity analyses to examine the important numerical assumptions used; and (7) interpreting the results.

Here is the problem we illustrate: Should zidovudine or ZDV (formerly known as azidothymidine or AZT) be given to asymptomatic patients who have antibodies to the human immunodeficiency virus (HIV), particularly those with altered T-cell subsets (e.g., T4/T8 ratio less than 1.5)? Let us assume that we are trying to make this decision for an asymptomatic, HIV-positive, 30-year-old white homosexual male.

Structuring the Problem

We first structure the problem, making all of the assumptions, events, and outcomes explicit. This structure usually is provided in the form of a decision tree in which all possible outcomes of each of the choices are laid out and the end branches represent final outcomes. The symbolic notation of a decision tree consists of three basic elements: (1) [square] decision notes, describing the choices to be made by the clinician(s) and patients; (2) [round] chance nodes, representing probabilistic events not under our control; and (3) [rectangular] terminal nodes, representing outcomes (i.e., summaries of events beyond the time horizon of the decision tree). In Figure 1, the initial decision node at the left delineates the two choices—treatment with ZDV ("ZDV") or withholding treatment with ZDV ("No ZDV"). Prognosis is determined by whether the patient ultimately develops the acquired immunodeficiency syndrome (AIDS), whether an opportunistic infection ensues, and whether death occurs as a consequence of such an infection. If ZDV is given, severe bone marrow suppression may occur, in which case the drug is discontinued. In addition, there is morbidity associated with ZDV therapy, generally consisting of nausea, abdominal pains, myalgia, and insomnia.

Probabilities

After the decision tree is structured, the likelihood of each event modeled must next be determined. These probabilities should come from the literature, when available, but if not, they may represent the subjective best estimates of experts. Table 1 describes the probabilities used in this analysis. Severe bone marrow suppression consisting of neutropenia (neutrophil counts less than 1,000 per mm^3) and anemia (hemoglobin less than 7.5 g per deciliter) occur in roughly 20 percent of patients with AIDS and AIDS-related complex treated with ZDV. It is difficult to ferret out which of the patients who die with bone marrow suppression do so solely as a result of the drug toxicity and not from their underlying illness. In this example, we have assumed a value of 0.01 for the probability of death due to bone marrow suppression. In addition, significant morbidity results from treatment with ZDV in about half of the patients.

In a recent study of the efficacy of ZDV in patients with AIDS, opportunistic infections developed in one-third of patients not treated with the drug and in roughly one-sixth of those who received treatment, yielding a 50 percent efficacy in the prevention of opportunistic infections. A significant decrease in mortality also was noted, with death occurring in approximately 40 percent of patients not receiving ZDV and in only 4 percent of those receiving the drug, resulting in an efficacy of 90 percent in the prevention of death due to opportunistic infection. A figure of great dispute as we track the moving target of the AIDS epidemic is the ultimate likelihood of developing AIDS in patients who have antibodies to the HIV. Our uncertainty relates in part to the limited time period over which we have had the opportunity to observe such patients. Early in the course of the epidemic, observations suggested that only 10 percent of antibody-positive patients developed the disease over a 2-year follow-up period. With longer periods of follow-up, some studies have observed that as many as 80 percent of patients develop some symptoms of AIDS or AIDS-related complex over a period of approximately 7 years. There also is evidence that HIV-infected patients with abnormal T-cell subsets are more likely

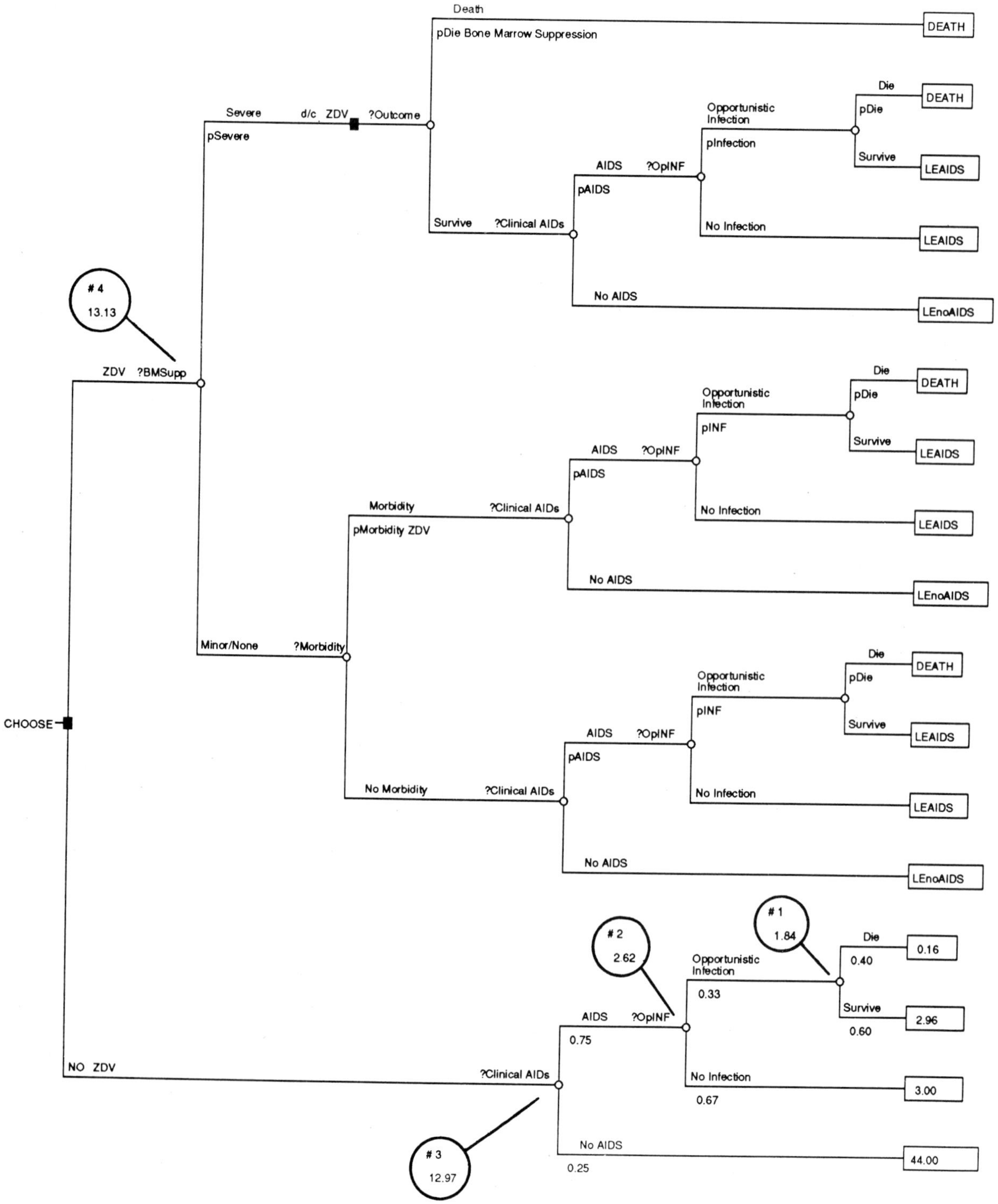

Figure 1 Decision tree examining therapy with zidovudine (ZDV) for an asymptomatic, HIV-positive, 30-year-old white homosexual male. ?BM Supp refers to the chance of bone marrow suppression; ?OpINF refers to the chance of opportunistic infection.

to have their disease progress to AIDS-related complex compared with infected patients with normal T-cell values. For this analysis, we used a probability of 0.75 for the likelihood that a patient with an HIV infection eventually will develop AIDS.

Utilities

The fourth step in performing a decision analysis is to assign values to all of the outcomes in the tree using a single consistent scale. These values are

TABLE 1 Probabilities Used in Decision Tree for Asymptomatic, 30-Year-Old, HIV-Positive Patient

Outcome	*Probability*
Development of AIDS	0.75
Toxicities of ZDV therapy	
Severe bone marrow suppression	0.20
Death from marrow suppression	0.01
Morbidity from drug	0.50
Efficacy of ZDV therapy in prevention of	
Opportunistic infections	0.50
Death	0.90
Untreated patients	
Opportunistic infections	0.33
Death	0.40
Treated patients	
Opportunistic infections	0.17
Death	0.04

TABLE 2 Utilities Used in Decision Tree for 30-Year-Old Male

Outcome	*Average Life Expectancy (yr)*
No Morbidity from ZDV and	
Death	0.2
AIDS	3
No AIDS	44
Long-Term Quality Adjustments:*	
For morbidity from ZDV	0.98
Short-Term Quality Adjustments:†	
For episode of severe bone marrow suppression	0.5 mo
For opportunistic infection	0.5 mo

*Long-term quality adjustments are multiplied by the underlying life expectancy.

†Short-term quality adjustments are subtracted from the underlying life expectancy.

called utilities. There are many possible measures of utility, from simple rank ordering schemes using arbitrary scales (i.e., 0 being the worst outcome to 1 being the best) to more sophisticated utilities that capture multiple attributes of patients' outcomes. A particularly useful utility measure is "quality-adjusted life expectancy," a measure that takes into account not only the quantity of life but also the quality of life. This procedure depreciates the average life expectancy for outcomes that consist of health states with less than ideal quality of life. In this way, patient preferences for the various outcomes in a model can be taken into account. In this example, we depreciated the life expectancy of patients suffering morbidity from treatment with ZDV by 2 percent for that period of time during which they receive the drug. In a similar manner, we debited an amount for patients who suffered an episode of severe bone marrow suppression for the short-term disutility of restriction to a reverse isolation room and all that is entailed by this. Patients who develop opportunistic infections also are debited a small amount for the short-term disutility of that event. For severe bone marrow suppression and opportunistic infection, complications that frequently engender hospitalizations of as long as 1 month, patients' quality of life was depreciated by 50 percent. For this month, therefore, the utility was reduced by one-half month.

We used a declining exponential approximation to calculate average life expectancy for each of the outcomes from survival data (Table 2). In otherwise healthy 30-year-old white males, the average life expectancy is approximately 44 years. The average yearly mortality rate of such an individual is 1/44, or approximately 2 percent. For median survival in patients who ultimately develop AIDS, we used a figure of 2 years. We used these survival data to estimate the average life expectancy in currently asymptomatic patients with HIV infection who ultimately develop symptoms of AIDS. The average mortality rate can be calculated by the equation: $-1/t \times \ln$ (% survival), where t is the length of survival (time). Because 2 years is the median survival, 50 percent of patients are alive at that time. Solving this equation yields $[-(1/2) \times \ln(0.50)]$ or 0.34 deaths per year as the average mortality rate. This mortality rate translates to an average life expectancy for patients with AIDS of (1/0.34), or roughly 3 years. Finally, we made the assumption that patients who die either from ZDV-induced bone marrow suppression or from opportunistic infections live only 3 months (0.2 years).

We also must account for the decreased quality of life experienced by patients who suffer morbidity from therapy with ZDV. There are no established guidelines at present for the duration of ZDV therapy in such patients. Because most patients who ultimately develop AIDS die before 3 years have passed, we selected 3 years as the duration for ZDV therapy. According to this guideline, patients who do not develop AIDS will not continue to be subjected to the toxicities of ZDV. In effect, those who develop AIDS then have a 2 percent depreciation for their entire average life expectancy, as do patients who die from ZDV-related complications. Patients who have been treated with ZDV and do not develop AIDS only suffer this decrement in quality of life for 3 of their 44 years.

Some might argue that if we had long enough periods of observation, all HIV-infected patients would eventually develop clinical manifestations. Models proposed by Roach and his colleagues suggest a constant rate for the development of symptoms in patients who are infected. The simple model described here lacks the fidelity to model such time-dependent events, but examination of the same problem with a Markov recursive model showed nearly identical results.

Evaluation

In evaluating a decision tree, the analyst starts at the distal end of the tree and applies two simple rules. The first rule is that the average or expected value at any chance node is calculated simply as the utility of the events at that chance node weighted by the probability distribution over those events (i.e., branches). This process is demonstrated in Figure 1 for the "No ZDV" strategy. At chance node #1, the utility of the outcome DIE is multiplied by the probability of that event. This quantity is then added to the product of the utility of the outcome SURVIVE and the probability of surviving the opportunistic infection. This calculation results in an expected utility of 1.84 quality-adjusted life years (QALYs) for chance node #1. This same process is carried out for each node in the decision tree, resulting in an expected (average) utility of 12.97 QALYs for the "No ZDV" strategy (see Fig. 1, #3) and 13.13 QALYs for the "ZDV" strategy (see Fig. 1, #4).

The second rule is that whenever a choice must be made (i.e., a decision node), a rational decision maker would select the option with the greatest expected utility. Invoking this rule, we select the "ZDV" strategy as "the best," having a slightly greater expected utility (0.16 year or roughly 2 months) than the "No ZDV" strategy. The small difference is not unexpected because of the overwhelming mortality associated with AIDS.

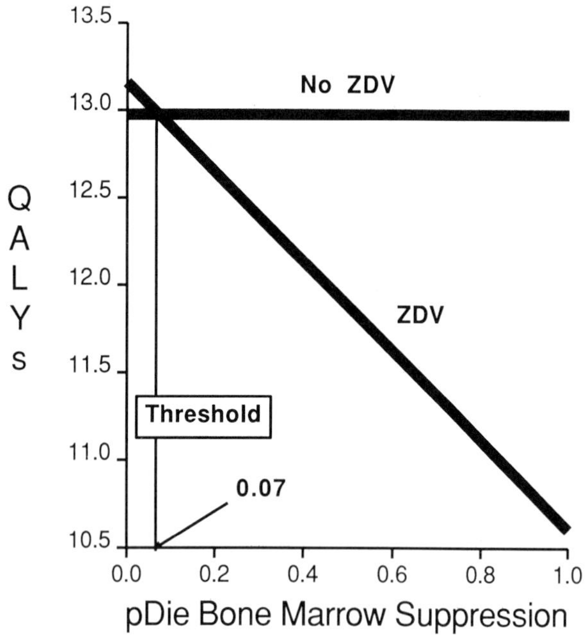

Figure 2 Sensitivity analysis examining the effect of changes in the probability of death from bone marrow suppression (shown on the horizontal axis) on quality-adjusted life years (shown on the vertical axis). The baseline probability of death from marrow suppression is 1 percent. Below a threshold probability of 7 percent it is best to treat with ZDV, whereas above this threshold it is best to withhold therapy.

Sensitivity Analysis

How convincing is this result? If the mortality from bone marrow suppression were greater, would empirical ZDV therapy in asymptomatic patients still be warranted? What if the mortality associated with marrow suppression were as high as 10 percent? Better yet, we can ask, "Above what probability of death from drug-induced marrow suppression would ZDV no longer be the optimal choice?" Attempting to answer such questions allows us to exploit one of the most powerful aspects of decision analysis, namely, sensitivity analysis.

We could perform sensitivity analyses on any or all of the probabilities and utilities in the model, and we could even vary multiple parameters simultaneously. We typically examine the "softest" data first in what are termed one-way sensitivity analyses. Figure 2, for example, demonstrates the effect on the decision of changes in the probability of death from bone marrow suppression. This probability is shown on the horizontal axis in the entire range from zero to one. The vertical axis displays the expected utility of both strategies in units of QALYs. In the strategy "No ZDV," expected utility remains unchanged as the mortality associated with bone marrow suppression increases. This result is to be expected, because patients are not subject to this risk if they are not receiving the drug. However, the strategy in which patients receive "ZDV" is markedly affected by changes in this parameter, with expected utility declining as this mortality increases. At a point where each strategy has the same expected utility, these lines intersect. This point of indifference is termed the threshold. In Figure 2, this threshold occurs at a probability of dying from bone marrow suppression of 7 percent. Therefore, for all values greater than 7 percent, withholding ZDV is preferred, whereas administering ZDV would be favored if the mortality associated with marrow suppression were less than 7 percent. Recall that the baseline value used was 1 percent, a value that lies in the region where administering ZDV is favored.

Any understanding of the problem prompts the observation that the risk of dying from marrow suppression is limited by the probability of developing severe bone marrow suppression. By performing a two-way sensitivity analysis, we can examine the effect of changes in these two parameters simultaneously. Figure 3 demonstrates this analysis. The mortality associated with marrow suppression is shown on the horizontal axis, and the likelihood of severe bone marrow suppression is shown on the vertical axis. In a two-way analysis, the threshold curve divides the space into regions in which the

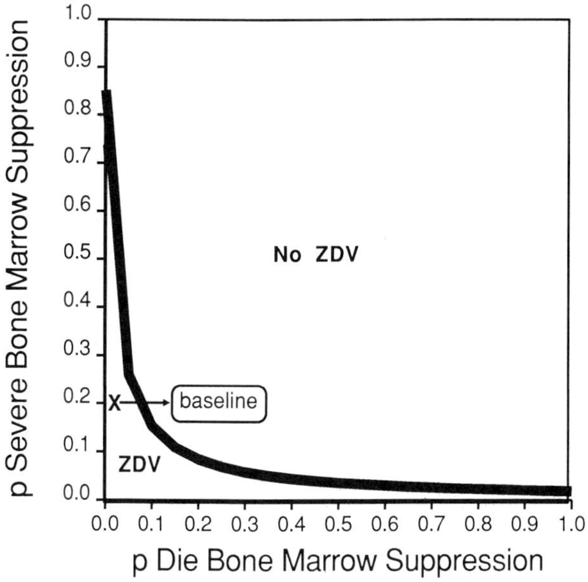

Figure 3 Two-way sensitivity analysis examining both the probability of death from bone marrow suppression (shown on the horizontal axis) and the probability of severe bone marrow suppression (shown on the vertical axis). At the upper right, where both the probability of severe bone marrow suppression and the probability of death given marrow suppression are high, it is best to withhold therapy with ZDV, whereas in the region at the lower left, where both probabilities are low, it is best to treat. The baseline values for these two probabilities are marked by the bold **X**.

different strategies are preferred. In the upper right corner, the mortality associated with marrow suppression is great and the likelihood of marrow suppression is high. In this region, withholding therapy with ZDV is the preferred strategy. In the lower left corner, the mortality and the likelihood of marrow suppression are both low, and in this region administering ZDV is preferable. The bold **X** marking the baseline values for these two parameters falls within the region where therapy is favored.

One final way we can examine the toxicity of ZDV is to assess the effect of changes in the quality adjustment factor describing the severity of the drug's side effects. Figure 4 demonstrates a three-way sensitivity analysis examining, as in Figure 3, the mortality associated with marrow suppression on the horizontal axis and the likelihood of severe bone marrow suppression on the vertical axis. Where in the previous figure there was only a single curve, there is now a family of curves, each representing a different value for the quality adjustment factor describing morbidity from drug toxicity. As in the two-way analysis, the curves separate the graph into regions where one or another strategy is favored. The four curves describe quality adjustment factors of 0.85 through 1.00. (The baseline value for this factor was 0.98.) As this factor gets larger (i.e., less depreciation for ZDV-related morbidity), the area to the lower left in which ZDV is the preferred strategy grows larger.

Figure 4 Three-way sensitivity analysis examining both the probability of death from bone marrow suppression (shown on the horizontal axis) and the probability of severe bone marrow suppression (shown on the vertical axis). Each of the four curves represents the decision threshold given a different quality adjustment for morbidity from ZDV (0.85, 0.90, 0.95, and 1.00). Lower quality adjustments for these side effects diminish the size of the region in which ZDV treatment is best. Even if the quality of life, given the side effects of ZDV, is only 0.85 times that of an otherwise asymptomatic patient, the baseline value still falls within the treatment region.

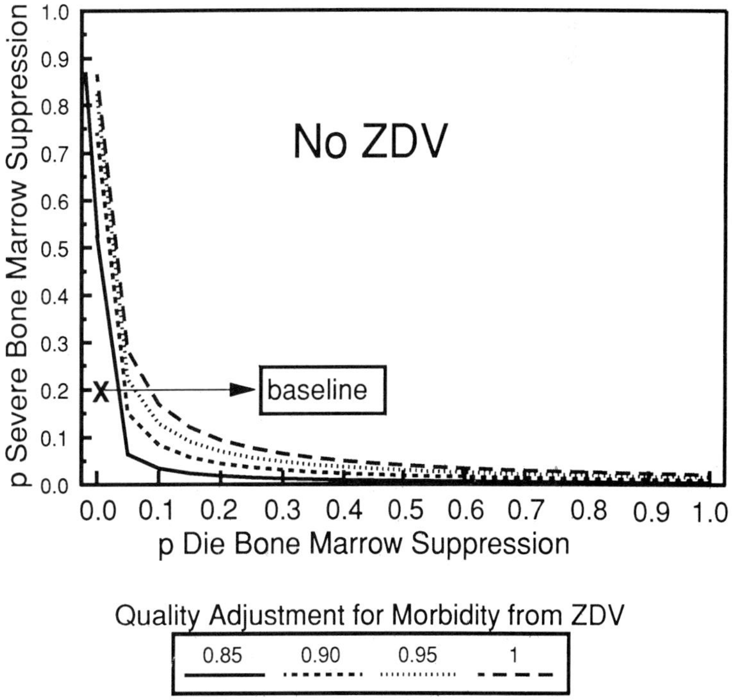

Interpretation of the Results

Although ZDV is favored in this analysis, only a small amount of quality-adjusted life expectancy is gained by this therapy (i.e., ~2 months), primarily because of the overwhelmingly high mortality associated with AIDS. In sensitivity analyses we assessed the effect of different assumptions about the toxicity associated with the drug. As noted earlier, it is difficult to separate out deaths primarily caused by drug-induced marrow suppression as opposed to marrow suppression as a consequence of the immunodeficiency state. This distinction may become known when the results of new clinical trials performed on asymptomatic patients without overt immunodeficiency are available. If the results show that the mortality associated with such marrow suppression is higher than 7 percent, this analysis suggests that ZDV therapy in such a patient would not be warranted.

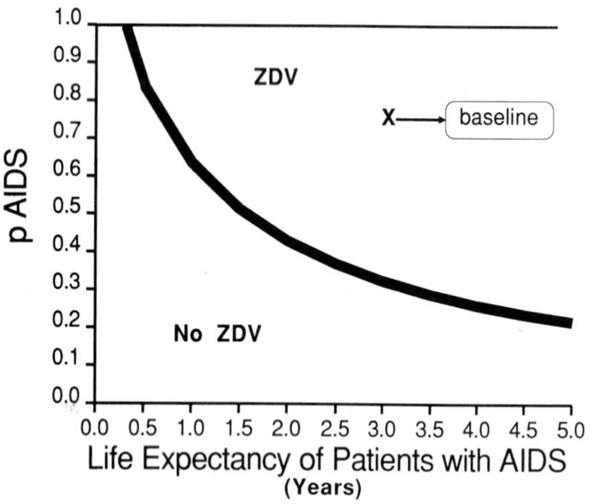

Figure 5 Two-way sensitivity analysis examining the life expectancy of patients with AIDS (shown on the horizontal axis) and the probability of an asymptomatic, HIV-positive patient's developing AIDS (shown on the vertical axis). In the region at the upper right, where the life expectancy of patients with AIDS is greater and the likelihood of developing AIDS is high, treatment with ZDV is best, whereas in the lower left, where the life expectancy of patients with AIDS is poor and the likelihood of developing AIDS is low, withholding therapy is best. Baseline values are marked by a bold **X**, which falls within the treatment region.

A final two-way sensitivity analysis examines uncertainty in two assumptions: (1) the likelihood that these asymptomatic patients will develop AIDS, and (2) the life expectancy of patients who develop AIDS. In Figure 5, the region to the upper right, where both the likelihood of developing AIDS and the life expectancy of patients with AIDS are high, treatment with ZDV is favored. If longer periods of follow-up disclose that higher percentages of HIV-positive patients develop AIDS, empirical treatment of asymptomatic patients with ZDV yields even greater benefits than our analysis concedes. Of course, the life expectancy of these patients will have to be long enough to make the risks of treatment worthwhile.

WHEN TO TURN TO DECISION ANALYSIS

Decision analysis provides a formal quantitative method for considering the tradeoffs between the benefits of therapy and its risks. It is most useful when the patient fails to conform to predetermined rules. Such circumstances include greater than usual uncertainty, poorly established efficacies of treatment, enhanced risks of treatment, unusually expensive treatment, confusion about the optimal timing of a necessary procedure, ambiguity about the optimal sequence of multiple procedures, situations in which patient preferences are critical, or instances in which rare, new, or unique problems are encountered. Analysis can be done, as described here, for individual patients or for complex and controversial choices in classes of patients

SUGGESTED READING

Beck JR, Kassirer JP, Pauker SG. A convenient approximation of life expectancy (The "DEALE"): I. Validation of the method. Am J Med 1982; 73:883–888.

Beck JR, Pauker SG, Gottlieb JE, et al. A convenient approximation of life expectancy (The "DEALE"): II. Use in medical decision making. Am J Med 1982; 73:889–897.

Kassirer JP, Moskowitz AJ, Lau J. Decision analysis: A progress report. Ann Intern Med 1987; 106:275–291.

Pauker SG, Kassirer JP. The threshold approach to clinical decision making. N Engl J Med 1980; 302:1109–1117.

Plante DA, Kassirer JP, Zarin DA, Pauker SG. Clinical decision consultation service. Am J Med 1986; 80:1169–1176.

THERAPEUTIC BENEFITS OF THE PHYSICIAN-PATIENT INTERACTION

DENNIS H. NOVACK, M.D.

Before powerful therapies became available, physicians mainly relied upon the healing power of the physician-patient relationship. Hippocrates observed that "The patient, though conscious that his condition is perilous, may recover his health simply through his contentment with the goodness of the physician." More recently, Balint reaffirmed the importance of doctor-patient interaction, asserting that by far the most frequently used "drug" in medical practice is the physician.

Although physicians use their relationships with patients to enhance therapy, few pause to identify the therapeutic elements of their patient encounters, explaining their effectiveness by their use of the "art of medicine." Yet, if using the healing power of the physician-patient relationship is an art, physicians could become more skillful artists; by identifying the therapeutic elements of their clinical encounters, they might use them more consistently and effectively. Much research has elucidated the therapeutic aspects of clinical encounters. In this chapter, this research is summarized and therapeutic strategies relevant to practicing physicians are discussed.

UNDERSTANDING THE THERAPEUTIC EFFICACY OF THE PHYSICIAN-PATIENT RELATIONSHIP

Two concepts are central to understanding the therapeutic efficacy of the physician-patient relationship: the essential unity of mind and body, and the definitions of and relationships between disease and illness.

Although for historical and scientific reasons it has been useful to separate the concepts of mind and body, the many advances of psychosomatic research have demonstrated their essential unity. One way of understanding this unity is by reflecting that thought, feelings, and abstract reasoning are also neurobiologic processes. While you are reading this chapter, neurochemical processes are being stimulated in your brain. Changes in messenger RNA and neurotransmitter metabolism are occurring as new information is being processed. If your feelings are aroused, neuroendocrine mechanisms are affecting other bodily processes, all of which can, in turn, affect your behavior.

Another central concept is the notion of the differences and relationships between disease and illness. Disease and illness are, respectively, objective and subjective phenomena. Disease can be identified by a laboratory test or a microscopic examination. Illness is a sense of disease, a sense of distress, related to a patient's perceptions and feelings. There can be disease without illness (e.g., hypertension), and illness without disease (e.g., hypochondria). Many patients have a dis-ease and a sense of illness determined not only by the severity of disease but also by a host of psychological and social factors. For the most part, patients come to physicians seeking relief from illness. In contrast to curing disease, which may be accomplished with a scalpel or a drug, to heal illness the physician must often attend to psychosocial issues.

A key therapeutic process by which physicians' communication can affect healing of illness is the reduction of patient anxiety and depression. Significant anxiety and depression are found in up to 35 percent of patients visiting clinicians for physical complaints. Anxiety and depression have a number of deleterious effects. At a biologic level, the neural and neuroendocrine factors associated with anxiety can increase blood glucose levels in the diabetic, increase gastric acid in the patient with an ulcer, or increase cardiac work and tip the compromised heart into congestive failure or induce a fatal arrhythmia. Grief and depression are associated with depressed immune function, which could predispose to infection or neoplasia. At a psychological level, the somatic symptoms of anxiety and depression (e.g., tremor, palpitations, loss of appetite, impotence) may prolong illness and confuse assessment of recovery. Depression is associated with self-defeating thoughts and negative self-images (e.g., "I'm no good, I'll never get better"), which may diminish patients' compliance. At a social level, these effects may undermine relationships with physicians, family, and friends and increase patients' isolation and sense of illness. Thus, to the extent that their interventions relieve anxiety and depression, physicians reduce the negative influences of these effects. With less anxiety and depression, patients begin to feel less ill and are more amenable to the physician's efforts to promote positive attitudes and compliance.

FACTORS CONDUCIVE TO EFFECTIVE THERAPY

Certain factors are conducive to effective therapy, including the clinical setting and physician attitudes, knowledge, and skills.

Clinical Setting

Before patients enter a physician's examining room, they have already had much contact with the physician's setting. The parking facilities, waiting room, administrative procedures, and waiting times affect patients' initial impressions of the physician. The attitudes and practices of receptionists, nurses, and ancillary personnel can either put patients at ease or heighten their anxieties (e.g., a patient did not want to discuss her personal life because she had seen the receptionist reading another patient's chart). A busy practice setting with multiple interruptions can restrain communication. A setting that is comfortable, unhurried, and puts the patient at ease is conducive to effective communication and therapy.

Physician Attitudes and Personal Qualities

Certain attitudes facilitate effective therapy. Accepting the importance of psychosocial factors in illness enhances the evaluation of the patient because more relevant psychological and social data are included. As another benefit of this approach, the physician's active concern for psychological and social issues may convince patients of his or her caring.

Peabody advised, ". . . the secret of the care of the patient is in caring for the patient." Patients want their physicians to be warm and caring. Patients' perceptions of these qualities are related to their evaluations of their physicians' general competence and their satisfaction and compliance with medical visits. Rogers identified an attitude of unconditional positive regard toward patients as the most important of the necessary and sufficient conditions for therapeutic personal change. This attitude implies a nonjudgmental approach, respect for a patient's individuality, and the ability to offer warmth and genuineness. Conversely, if a physician dislikes a patient or feels that a patient is untruthful, these attitudes are likely to be communicated and have a detrimental effect on therapy.

Several authors have commented on the necessity for physicians to be tolerant of ambiguity, uncertainty, and stress in the clinical setting. With all the uncertainty in clinical medicine, this tolerance prevents injudicious use of procedures and laboratory tests and physician anxiety that could undermine patient confidence.

Basic Knowledge and Skills

In addition to biotechnical knowledge and skills, the physician needs to master certain psychosocial knowledge and skills. Examples of key knowledge areas are the somatoform disorders, such as psychogenic pain disorder and conversion disorders, the phenomenology and treatment of depression and anxiety, and the importance of stress and life change in the development of illness. Examples of key skills are the ability to perform an effective patient-centered interview, the ability to interpret and use nonverbal behavior, the ability to recognize and use emotional reactions to patients as data, and skills in patient education and behavior modification techniques.

THERAPEUTIC STRATEGIES

The therapeutic process begins with the patient's decision to seek help. The physician's personal contributions to this process begin with the first interview: attentive listening in itself imparts great therapeutic value. A comprehensive diagnosis guides selection of appropriate therapeutic strategies. This diagnosis involves understanding the contributions of biologic, psychosocial, and personality factors to the onset and maintenance of the illness.

For people to change, they must change the way they think, feel, or behave in their social contexts. Major changes in any of these spheres change the whole person. Interventions, then are presented in four categories: cognitive, affective, behavioral, and social. Although these are categorized for explanatory purposes, there is great overlap in these interventions and in their effects (e.g., giving an explanation often changes the way a person thinks, feels, and behaves). Many of these strategies and interventions have proved useful, as evidenced by their common presence in diverse healing disciplines.

Cognitive Therapeutic Strategies

A patient's thoughts, perceptions, and attitudes are involved in the illness process and can be addressed directly.

Negotiation of Priorities and Expectations

There is value in a negotiated approach to patient care. This approach recognizes the critical importance of eliciting and attending to the patient's perspective, which begins by asking: "How do you hope that I can help?" Physician and patient then negotiate some agreements about the nature of the patient's problems, the patient's requests and expectations, and the goals, methods, and conditions of treatment. Although it may seem obvious that the physician and patient must agree on the problems to be addressed, studies show that physician-patient concordance is often low. In a study of more than 400 patient visits to a medical clinic, physician and patient were fully concordant in the identification of the principal problem only about half the time. Patients often have hidden reasons for visiting doctors, and by focusing too early on chief complaints, physicians often do not elicit patients' real major concerns. Patients report better outcomes when there is physician-patient agreement about problems. In addition to improving physician-patient concordance on a variety of therapeutic issues, the negotiated approach helps both physician and patient to share the responsibility for therapy and prevents unrealistic patient expectations of the relationship.

Giving an Explanation

All healing disciplines give explanations to patients about causes of illness. Patients have intense needs for information and explanations about the causes of illness and are dissatisfied when these are not given. Confusion and uncertainty about diagnosis are noxious emotions for patients. Giving a symptom complex a name and an explanation thus has a salutary effect; patients feel comforted that the physician knows what is wrong and can thus begin appropriate therapy. For instance, one of my patients at first was relieved to learn that he had multiple sclerosis because for years he felt that his doctors were implying that his evanescent neurologic symptoms were not real.

When psychosocial factors are a major part of illness, an effective form of explanation is to tell the patient's story back to him or her in a way that makes the development of illness almost a logical progression. This demonstrates to the patient that the physician has listened and has understood and may help the patient to make sense out of confusing feelings and impressions. In sharing an understanding of the diagnosis, the physician can briefly teach the patient how mind and body work together in the promotion of illness and health. The physician uses his or her authority as an expert to legitimize psychosocial explanations when these are appropriate.

It is often difficult to discuss the etiologic role of psychosocial factors with patients whose long-standing symptoms are related to emotional conflicts and whose "secondary gains" have perpetuated symptoms in their lives. These individuals are often called "problem patients," and many are given psychiatric diagnoses. Although they reject a psychiatric explanation, many such patients are willing to accept that stress plays some role in how they feel, and most would agree that their anxiety and depression about their symptoms make them feel worse. These admissions may be the opening the physician can use to begin to help these patients change their psychosocial situations.

Bringing the Patient to a Crossroad

In some patients, denial contributes to their illness. The business executive who denies that he or she has had a heart attack or the alcoholic who denies his or her drinking habit are examples. Sometimes symptoms of illness serve a purpose in a patient's life. In certain dysfunctional families, illness may help maintain family equilibrium. Symptoms may serve to prevent the recognition of an intrapsychic conflict (which is fantasied to be more painful than the symptoms). Patients frequently hint at or relate interpersonal or intrapsychic conflicts to physicians without recognizing the relation to their symptoms. In these instances, it is often effective for physicians to confront their patients.

For example, when symptoms seem to represent an intrapsychic conflict, sometimes it is effective to discuss conflicts with patients, relate the conflicts to symptoms, and then let patients know that they are at a crossroad; they can begin to work on resolving the conflicts or choose to continue to have symptoms. These confrontations can initiate new relationships between the conflicts, the patients, and the illnesses. In essence, illness has been "reframed" from a biologic problem to a biopsychosocial one.

Suggestion

Suggestion is a powerful therapeutic tool that works in part by influencing patients' expectations of therapy. Suggestion via the placebo response can induce a wide variety of physiologic effects in patients, including release of endorphins. Physicians can use suggestion to enhance the effectiveness of any therapy. If a physician honestly communicates optimism in a therapy, it will often be more effective than if prescribed casually. Prescriptions given with hesitation or uncertainty may have diminished effectiveness. One hypnotic technique that may be useful is to make self-reinforcing positive suggestions. That is, patients may respond to positive suggestions such as, "As you recover from this heart attack and begin to be more active, you will feel less anxious and more optimistic." Suggestions such as this can set up a positive feedback loop: patients may respond to positive suggestions with hope and increased well-being. As their physical conditions improve, these positive emotions not only confirm their sense of recovery but also tend to improve confidence in the physician whose predictions have been accurate. Positive suggestions have limited value for patients with somatoform disorders. Although there may be initial benefits, the predictable recurrence of symptoms may then undermine patient confidence.

Patient Education

Patient education has proven benefits in increasing patient satisfaction and compliance and an overall positive effect on patients' coping. Information can reduce patient anxiety, enhance feelings of personal control, improve a patient's attitude toward a painful procedure, and help patients cope with pain. Presurgical educational interventions increase cooperation with treatment and speed of recovery and decrease postoperative pain and post-hospital complications. In general, physicians spend little time giving information to their patients, overestimate the time they have spent, and underestimate the amount of information the patient wants to receive. Explanations about illness or about tests and procedures should be given in clear language without jargon, using concrete familiar examples and frequently testing for understanding. Careful attention to patient education is important because patients forget or misunderstand so much of what physicians tell them.

Patient education includes correcting misconceptions and incorrect illness attributions. A common example is the belief that hypertension is hyper-tension, that is, feeling too nervous, and that antihypertensive medications can be discontinued when the patient is not feeling stressed. Clinical reality may be viewed quite differently by patient and physician; explanatory models of illness, which are often culturally derived, may give rise to misconceptions that can interfere with therapy. Physicians who elicit these explanatory models can then address points of misunderstanding or disagreement.

Giving a Prognosis

Prognoses should be realistic so that patients do not feel deceived if they become more ill than predicted, and they should be optimistic so as to engender hope. For example, in conveying the diagnosis of a malignancy, many physicians emphasize promising new therapies and describe other patients with the same disease who did well. As in learning a diagnosis, knowledge about prognosis can help patients cope with illness by reducing the dysphoria of uncertainty. Patients told what to expect can prepare and adapt. If the physician can correctly predict certain feelings or physical sensations, patients may avoid misinterpreting these sensations. For example, the patient who returns from the hospital after a heart attack may experience marked tiredness. If the physician explains that this is a natural and common occurrence, the patient will not misinterpret this tiredness as symptomatic of a failing heart.

Affective Therapeutic Strategies

Anger, depression, and anxiety are not only common reactions to illness but also can amplify illness. Physicians can diminish these negative emotions and arouse positive emotional states through a variety of interventions.

Empathy

Expression of empathy is one of the most potent therapeutic interventions. Empathy is sharing in another's emotions or feelings as if they are one's own. All people have a need to be understood, a need made more pressing by illness. Empathy involves accurately identifying a patient's feelings and then communicating this to the patient: "I understand how difficult it is for you to be going through this illness," or "It sounds like your mom's illness has been a real burden to you." Empathy also involves eliciting and responding to the meaning of illness for the patient (e.g., "I can understand your worries about this angina, especially since your brother died of a heart attack"). In addition to strengthening the bond between physician and patient, expression of empathy can aid the diagnostic process. After experiencing physicians' empathy, patients are often encouraged to reveal their most difficult problems. Communication of empathy is a skill that can be effectively learned.

Encouraging Emotional Expression

Many physicians, especially physicians in training, feel uncomfortable when patients cry or grow angry in their offices. However, there are good reasons for encouraging emotional expression, without feeling the need to "resolve" negative feelings. "Ventilation" of strong emotions provides immediate relief for some patients. Conversely, being unable to express emotion makes patients feel alone and creates barriers between patients and physicians. Many forms of psychotherapies and healing disciplines arouse the patient's emotions, recognizing these as the motive power for attitude change. Emotional "catharsis" is considered crucial in some psychotherapies and in many religious and magic healing rituals. In some instances, when a patient realizes that a physician is not threatened or appalled by his or her admissions, a "corrective emotional experience" may take place. The physician can encourage emotional expression by making empathic comments, by inquiring about feelings, or by commenting on nonverbal expressions of affect such as, "You looked sad when you mentioned your son."

Praise

Praise is supportive of patients, conveys respect, and helps give them confidence and hope. Physicians may praise patients' personality strengths, attitudes, or actions (e.g., "You are a bright and conscientious man, and I think you will do fine in dealing with this complicated regimen," or "I think your sensitivity to your wife's feelings is laudable and will help her a lot during these difficult times"). Praise as a reinforcer of desired behaviors is discussed further on. When there is a dearth of personality strengths, the physician may need to resort to paradox and redefine weakness as strength. For example, the physician can redefine a patient's masochism into ability to cope with suffering and thus can encourage and praise a patient's coping abilities.

Offering Hope

Hope is a central coping mechanism; it defends against despair, diminishes anxiety, is energizing, and can stimulate patients to undertake health-promoting activities. On the other hand, hopelessness, the most noxious of emotions both psychologically and physiologically, has been linked to disease onset and sudden death. Patients' hopelessness can engender pessimism in their caregivers, which impedes therapy. Mobilizing hope and instilling "expectant faith" that the physician will help the patient recover is a device used by all healing disciplines. Offering hope is appropriate for patients with diverse illnesses, although the manner in which it is offered varies. Most dying patients maintain some hope until the end, feeling nourished by it in difficult times, and appreciate it when hope is offered despite bad news. Physicians can maintain hope in their dying patients without deception by accepting their hopes and sharing with them the hope that they may have a remission or that they will live longer than expected. For patients with long-standing psychosomatic illness in whom symptoms serve an adaptive function, it is best not to raise hopes for recovery; instead one should assert that these patients deserve and have a good chance for some improvement. In these patients, it is helpful to emphasize coping as the goal rather than cure.

Touch

Placing a hand on his or her shoulder when talking to a hospitalized patient or holding a patient's hand during a moment of reassurance is an important therapeutic intervention. Lewis Thomas calls touching "the oldest and most effective act of doctors." From infancy on, touch is associated with comfort and the relief of anxiety. "Laying on hands" is common to most healing disciplines. It is significant that some patients begin to talk about emotional issues only while the physician is examining them. There is probably an optimal "dose" of touching, however. Too much touching or touching too early in the relationship may be associated with untoward consequences.

Facilitation of Self-Forgiveness

Some symptoms are related to feelings of guilt. Guilt has been linked to the symptoms of conversion disorders, pathologic grief, depression, and psychogenic pain disorders. The associated somatic symptoms are conceptualized as forms of self-punishment to expiate guilty feelings. Guilt may be related to the death of someone close toward whom the patient had harbored angry feelings. Much can be accomplished by exploring these feelings in the context of the past relationship and giving support to the patient about the appropriateness of past behavior and feelings. Often by exploring a patient's feelings of guilt and occasionally by merely listening to a patient's confessions, the physician can help patients forgive themselves. Listening to a patient's confession is a part of many psychotherapies, religious practices, and diverse healing ceremonies in primitive cultures in which sickness is often viewed as punishment for sins.

Reassurance

Most physicians have observed the beneficial effects of reassurance in allaying patient anxiety and diminishing the patient's sense of illness. However, reassurance is a complex phenomenon. It is most ineffective when given prematurely, casually, or without conviction. Reassurance is most effective when it accurately addresses the patient's concerns and personal meanings of illness. It usually cannot be given effectively until the patient senses that the physician has listened to and understood his or her problems and has performed the necessary evaluation. There are several categories of reassurance. The physician can reassure patients that their illnesses are not as severe or threatening as they had imagined. Physicians can help remove the sense of isolation that illness imposes by reassuring patients that they have successfully treated other patients with similar illnesses. Physicians can allay specific fears. It is also reassuring to patients to be told that the physician will continue to work with them whatever the course of the illness.

Behavioral Therapeutic Strategies

One of the major contributions of behavioral therapy research has been the demonstration that accomplishing behavioral changes through successful performance leads to lasting cognitive and affective changes. The emphasis of most behavioral therapies is on changing current determinants of behavior. The therapist focuses on changing environmental cues, thoughts and feelings, and consequences of behavior that make the behavior more likely. Physicians can use specific behavioral approaches in treating obesity, smoking, and noncompliance. Relaxation techniques can be useful in the management of anxiety. In addition, some behavioral therapy principles are applicable in general medical practice.

Emphasis of the Patient's Active Role

Many patients take a passive attitude toward their illnesses, often feeling that their illnesses are controlling them. This contributes to demoralization and depression. On the other hand, a sense of control or mastery has been linked to improved health status. Physicians accomplish much by emphasizing that patients have some control in overcoming illness and by encouraging an "active patient orientation." In this approach, patients are viewed as collaborators in their care; they are given information that will help them discuss diagnostic and management decisions with their physicians, and skill training and technical aids are made available to assist self-care activities (e.g., home blood pressure or glucose monitoring). This approach improves satisfaction, compliance, and functional abilities.

Assigning to the patient self-monitoring of behavior also encourages an active patient role. In asking patients to keep diaries in which they record events relevant to their problems, physicians and patients are provided not only with a useful way to monitor progress but also with valuable information on the determinants of behavior. Other strategies that encourage a patient's role include prescribing physical activity, giving assignments such as books to read or courses to take, and working with patients to delineate conflicts that they must actively resolve.

Praising Desired Behaviors

In behavior modification techniques, praise is recognized as a reinforcer of desired behaviors. When patients successfully perform suggested behaviors, praise encourages them to continue their efforts. Praise can be used in this way to shape a patient's behavior; even when patients have made only small improvements in their behavior, the physician praises these improvements and praises successive approximations of the desired behavior until it is achieved. When treating hypertension or promoting dietary compliance for management of diabetes or hypercholesterolemia, for example, physicians' praise of improving parameters reinforces a patient's progress.

Suggesting Alternative Behaviors

Patients may react to intolerable social situations with an exacerbation of symptoms. Sometimes illness may be in large part a reaction to or solution to an intolerable social situation. Because they are enmeshed in the situations, patients may be unable to perceive alternative strategies for coping. There are several types of responses to intolerable situations: changing the situation, changing one's reaction to the situation, or leaving it. It is often helpful to explore these options with patients and to suggest alternatives the patient is unable to see.

In suggesting alternative behaviors, physicians often engage in covert modeling. They suggest behaviors they feel would be appropriate if they were in a similar situation. Overt modeling in the form of a mini role play is often effective (e.g., "I'll be you for a minute and you be your angry son, and I'll demonstrate one technique that might just work").

Occasionally a patient hesitates to carry out a decision he or she has made that is a viable solution to an intolerable situation. The physician's agreement with and support of a difficult decision may enable the patient to begin to do what is adaptive. A key concept is that only by carrying out feared behaviors can patients compare their dire predictions with the actual events and correct their misapprehensions.

Attending to Compliance

Healing is promoted when patients follow an effective therapeutic plan and take their medications as prescribed. Unfortunately, noncompliance has been found to be as high as 20 to 60 percent, depending on the type of regimen. Physicians typically overestimate rates of compliance among their patients and are often inaccurate in identifying noncompliant individuals. At a most basic level, simply checking with patients about their compliance tends to increase it. When physicians ask about compliance, patients are more likely to express complaints or to admit having problems conforming to a regimen. Other strategies for improving patient compliance have proved effective, such as improving patients' levels of information concerning the specifics of their regimens; reinforcing essential points with review, discussion, and written instruction; emphasizing the importance of the therapeutic plan; simplifying and reducing the cost of the regimen; suggesting behavior prompts (e.g., notes on the refrigerator); and creating physician-patient contracts that include a written outline of behavioral expectations and specified rewards or reinforcements.

Social Therapeutic Strategies

Use of Family and Social Supports

A noxious social environment and a lack of social and community ties have been associated with an overall increase in morbidity and mortality. Conversely, positive family and social supports ameliorate illness and improve compliance. An essential ingredient of many healing rituals is the active participation of family and friends, which begins the reintegration of the ill person into family and community. This reintegration helps to dispel the social isolation frequently imposed by illness. Many rituals also stress mutual service, which counteracts the patient's morbid self-preoccupation and strengthens self-esteem by demonstrating that he or she can do something for others.

Families should be evaluated to see if they are potential resources. Sometimes disengagement from a dysfunctional family is effective therapy. Often, though, families and friends are helpful. As well as providing support and encouragement for patients, they provide valuable perspectives that can help in designing therapy. Family members often have specific informational needs that must be met in order to participate effectively in therapy.

Use of Community Agencies and Other Health Care Providers

Involvement in community agencies, self-help groups such as Alcoholics Anonymous, and religious, cultural, and social groups can play a major role in a patient's recovery. It is helpful for physicians to have a first-hand knowledge of the make-up or workings of the important community agencies to which they can refer patients (particularly programs such as Alcoholics Anonymous, Al-Anon, Overeaters Anonymous, and cardiac rehabilitation programs). Involvement of other members of the health care team, including office staff and pharmacists, increases the patient's social interaction and helps the therapeutic process. Nurses often play essential roles in monitoring compliance, implementing and clarifying health education and attitude change strategies, enlisting family support, and helping with behavior modification strategies.

COMMENT

Although the therapeutic process can be analyzed and studied, medical therapy is also an art. Each physician uniquely synthesizes biopsychosocial knowledge, skills, and attitudes and combines this synthesis with his or her own intuition, natural empathy, and caring for patients. With an organized approach to the therapeutic aspects of the physician-patient relationship, the result is medical care that is both more scientific and more humanistic.

Portions of this chapter appeared originally in Novack DH. Therapeutic aspects of the clinical encounter. J Gen Intern Med 1987; 2:346–355.

SUGGESTED READING

DiMatteo MR, DiNicola DD. Achieving patient compliance. New York: Pergamon Press, 1982.

Engel GL. The need for a new medical model: A challenge for biomedicine. Science 1977; 196:129–135.

Frank JD. Persuasion and healing. New York: Schocken Books, 1977:75.

Novack DH. Psychosocial aspects of illness. South Med J 1981; 74:1376–1381.

Novack DH. Therapeutic aspects of the clinical encounter. J Gen Intern Med 1987; 2:346–355.

CLINICAL PHARMACOLOGY

RICHARD D. MAMELOK, M.D.

This chapter describes some central principles of clinical pharmacology that, if borne in mind by any practitioner of medical therapeutics, should help to support therapeutic discussions on a logical foundation. Although a basic knowledge of pathophysiology, pathogenesis, and therapeutic pharmacology is necessary in order to choose among therapeutic alternatives, these principles of clinical pharmacology can help to determine specific dosing regimens: how much drug to give, how often to give it, and, in some cases, what combination of drugs is likely to succeed in helping a patient. A need to apply these principles arises from the recognition that patients are individuals, that each individual has his or her own dose-response curve, and that individuals vary in their rates of eliminating active drug from the body. The instructions on how to use a drug that appear in a drug's package insert (published in the *Physicians' Desk Reference*) are based on averaged data gathered from hundreds of patients. These instructions should be used as a starting point for planning a therapeutic program but should not be applied without thinking of the characteristics of a particular patient that distinguish that patient from the "average" individual. A poorly tailored therapeutic regimen has the potential to cause serious harm.

ELIMINATION OF A DRUG FROM THE BODY

Drugs are removed from the body by two major processes. The first is by a variety of metabolic pathways in which a drug undergoes a series of chemical reactions resulting in pharmacologically inert compounds. In general, these pharmacologically inactive compounds are also more amenable to excretion in either urine or bile. The second route by which a drug is removed does not involve any chemical modification. Simply, the drug is eliminated from the body in its intact state, usually in the urine. In a particular patient, the sum of the rates by which a drug is metabolized and excreted in an unchanged state determines how frequently that drug needs to be given to that patient.

Metabolism

Most metabolism, the chemical modification of drugs, occurs in the liver. In general, the more lipid-soluble and the less water-soluble a drug is, the larger the role metabolic processes play in eliminating the drug from the body. The two major routes for finally eliminating a drug or its metabolic products from the body are the urine and the bile. Nonpolar, lipid-soluble compounds do not dissolve well in urine and bile. By transforming relatively insoluble compounds into soluble ones, hepatic metabolic pathways increase the efficacy of the body's ability to eliminate a drug. Drugs can be metabolized by oxidation (for example, hydroxylation, N-demethylation, sulfoxidation), reduction, or hydrolysis. These reactions are often called phase I reactions. A second class of reactions, phase II reactions, are biosynthetic in that they involve coupling a drug or a metabolite to an endogenous chemical moiety such as glucuronic acid or acetic acid. Rates of metabolic reaction vary greatly from individual to individual.

Many of the enzymes responsible for catalyzing these metabolic reactions are located on the smooth endoplasmic reticulum. These enzymes are often referred to as microsomal enzymes, because when hepatic cells are mechanically disrupted and centrifuged, pieces of enzyme-rich endoplasmic reticulum settle in a sediment denoted as microsomes. Some drugs have the ability to either enhance or inhibit the activity of these enzymes. Such alteration in enzymatic function is responsible for therapeutically important drug-drug interactions described below.

Although metabolism is important for inactivating drugs, some metabolites also have pharmacologic activity. Accumulation of active metabolites can occur and may contribute to the therapeutic benefit of a drug. In fact, some drugs known as "prodrugs" are administered in an inactive form and are activated by the liver. An example of such a prodrug is the angiotensin-converting enzyme inhibitor, enalapril; the active form is its metabolite, enalaprilat. Metabolites can also have toxicologic activity. The severe hepatotoxicity seen in overdoses of acetaminophen is caused by a metabolite. Finally, some metabolites may contribute to the carcinogenic potential of certain drugs.

Renal Excretion

A number of drugs are eliminated by the kidney in the absence of any preceding metabolic reactions. The kidney has two major mechanisms to achieve such excretion—glomerular filtration and tubular secretion. Most drugs are small enough to pass easily through the glomerular membranes. However, in order for a drug to be filtered, it must be in solution in the plasma. Molecules of a drug that are bound to albumin or other proteins in blood are not filtered. Thus, binding of drugs to proteins in plasma limits the extent to which glomerular filtration accounts for elimination. Whether a drug filtered at the glomerulus ends up in urine is dependent on whether the drug is reabsorbed by the renal tubules. The more polar a drug, the less likely that it will be reabsorbed. Many drugs are weak acids or weak bases and exist in a partly charged and a partly uncharged form at physiologic pH. Since the pH of tubular fluid and urine varies, depending on diet and acid-base status of a patient, changes in urine pH can greatly affect the renal excretion of these drugs. For a weak acid, the higher the pH of tubular fluid, the more ionized a weak acid is. Thus the lower the reabsorption of a weak acid is, the greater the excretion. At a lower pH, a weak acid is less ionized, and thus excretion will diminish because reabsorption is enhanced. The opposite effects occur for a weak base; the lower the pH of tubular fluid, the greater the excretion. An example of a weak acid so affected is salycilate. Amphetamine is an example of a weak base whose renal excretion changes owing to changes in the pH of tubular fluid.

Drugs can also be excreted by secretion from blood, across the epithelium of the proximal tubule and into the tubular fluid. Several transport systems for organic acids and bases have been discovered in the proximal tubule. Examples of some drugs that are excreted unchanged, in part by renal secretion, are penicillin, furosemide, hydrochlorothiazide, ethacrynic acid, methotrexate, procainamide, and cimetidine. Unlike glomerular filtration, secretion is not limited by binding of a drug to protein.

Pharmacokinetics

Pharmacokinetics seeks to describe, in a mathematical way, how the body disposes of a drug. When administered, a drug is distributed to the various tissues of the body. It is also eliminated by the biologic processes described above. The rate at which the drug gets to its site of action, the amount of drug bound to its receptors, the rate at which a drug dissociates from its receptor, and the rate at which the drug is eliminated from the body determine the magnitude and time course of the pharmacologic effect. The equations used for some pharmacokinetic analyses are cumbersome for daily clinical practice, but a few simple principles can be applied to designing a dosing regimen. In order to use these principles, a few terms must be defined.

1. *Steady state* occurs when the rate of administration of a drug is equal to the rate of elimination. When a drug is administered by constant intravenous infusion, the plasma concentration of the drug remains constant. When a drug is administered at regular intervals (e.g., every 8 hours), the highest and lowest concentrations of the drug achieved remain the same from one dosing interval to the next.
2. *Clearance* relates the concentration of a drug

in plasma (or serum) to the rate of elimination of the drug so that

plasma concentration of drug × clearance = rate of elimination = rate of administration (at steady state).

If the clearance of a drug is known, a desired target plasma concentration can be reached by using this equation.

3. *Volume of distribution* relates the total amount of drug in the body to the plasma concentration so that

$$\frac{\text{total amount of drug in body}}{\text{volume of distribution}} = \text{concentration of drug in plasma}$$

When rapid achievement of a target plasma concentration is desired, a loading dose can be calculated by the equation loading dose (equivalent to the total amount of drug in the body) = volume of distribution × concentration of drug. The $\frac{\text{plasma volume}}{\text{volume of distribution}}$ is the fraction of the total amount of drug in the body that actually is in plasma.

4. *Half-life* is the time it takes for the concentration of a drug in plasma to diminish by half. Because the amount of drug in the body is directly proportional to the concentration of the drug in plasma, half-life is also the time it takes for the total amount of drug in the body to diminish by half.

Half-life is directly proportional to the volume of distribution and is inversely proportional to clearance. Although it is intuitive why half-life is inversely related to clearance, which reflects the body's capacity to metabolize and excrete the drug, it may not be obvious why volume of distribution also affects the half-life. As noted above, the volume of distribution determines the fraction of total drug that resides in the plasma. Plasma is the vehicle that delivers drug to the liver and kidneys. If a small fraction of total drug resides in the plasma (a large volume of distribution), only a small fraction of drug can be eliminated in a given period of time and thus the half-life will be long. In contrast, if the volume of distribution is small, a larger fraction of total drug resides in the plasma, and thus there is the potential that a large fraction of total drug could be eliminated in a given period, leading to a short half-life. The half-life of a drug determines how long it takes to reach steady state on any dosing regimen. It takes about four half-lives to reach steady state.

Half-life is often measured, and it is worthwhile clearing up some misconceptions about it. Because it is dependent on both clearance and volume of distribution, a change in half-life could reflect changes in either clearance or volume of distribution. For example, a prolongation of half-life could result from a decreased clearance (slowed elimination) or an increased volume of distribution. Only the former situation would require a change in the maintenance dose of a drug. Thus knowing how the half-life changes in a given disease state does not provide sufficient information to make adjustments to dosing. Similarly, if clearance and volume of distribution change in proportion, no change in half-life would occur; however, changes in dosing regimen would be appropriate because of the changes in clearance. Specific examples of such situations are described in the sections on dosing in disease states.

Another misuse of the measurement of half-life is to use it to determine the dosing interval. One often hears statements such as, "drug X has a half-life of 8 hours; therefore, administer the drug every 8 hours," or "drug Y has a 2-hour half life; therefore, an every-8-hour dosing interval is inappropriate." Neither statement is necessarily correct. In addition to half-life, the amount of drug administered at each dose and the relationship between the amount of drug in the body and the pharmacologic response also contribute to the duration of action of the drug, which in turn dictates an appropriate dosing interval.

DOSING IN DISEASE STATES AND IN THE ELDERLY

Anyone responsible for administering drugs to patients has to choose an initial dosage regimen. A modification in the regimen originally chosen may be required if a toxic effect becomes manifest or if the therapeutic response is not adequate. Recommended dosing regimens as they appear in a drug's package insert are determined from data that are collected from several hundred to a few thousand patients who participated in experimental therapeutic trials required by governmental regulatory agencies such as the Food and Drug Administration in the United States. The best dosing regimen for an individual patient may be different from the recommended dosing regimen for the "average patient." Different patients have different pharmacologic responses to the same dose and even to the same concentration of the drug in plasma. Careful observation of the clinical state of a patient is essential to monitor a response to pharmacologic treatment. However, in general, there is much wider variability among patients with respect to metabolic and excretory function than there is with respect to response to a given concentration of the drug in the body. Thus, it is very useful to account for differences in metabolic and excretory effects when choosing an initial dosing regimen. The most important of these adjustments are made in patients with liver disease, renal disease, or at the extremes of life—the very young and the elderly.

It is beyond the scope of this chapter to give a detailed analysis of how disease states alter the disposition or response to particular drugs. The suggested reading list cites extensive discussions of individual drugs. However, Tables 1 through 4 provide a list of many drugs that require dose adjustments based on easily recognized physiologic and pathophysiologic processes. Fortunately, over the last decade, the Food and Drug Administration and pharmaceutical companies have provided information in a drug's label that gives the physician some guidelines as to dosing adjustments that may be required in particular clinical situations.

Changes in Dose Related to Hepatic Disease

Hepatic disease, both acute and chronic, often decreases the capacity of the liver to metabolize drugs. Also, patients with hepatic disease may have decreased concentrations of serum albumin. Drugs that are bound to albumin may require dosing adjustments because less drug will be trapped in plasma, bound to protein, leading to greater distribution of a drug to other parts of the body. Unfortunately, none of the routinely measured liver function tests predict, in any reliable fashion, the severity of derangements in hepatic metabolic function. Thus any initial adjustment in dose must be refined based on clinical observation of the patient's condition. Measuring the concentration of some drugs can serve as a useful guide, but any change in dose must be done in the context of the actual therapeutic or toxic response. Table 1 lists some drugs that require a change in dosing in patients with liver disease.

TABLE 1 Commonly Used Drugs Requiring a Decreased Dose in Patients with Hepatic Disease

Acetaminophen (avoid; directly hepatotoxic)	Lidocaine
Chloramphenicol	Lincomycin
Chlordiazepoxide	Meperidine (pethidine)
Clindamycin	Methadone
Codeine	Minocycline
Diazepam	Minoxidil
Digitoxin	Morphine
Doxycycline	Pentazocine
Erythromycin	Pentobarbital
Ethacrynic acid	Prazosin
Flurazepam	Propoxyphene
Furosemide	Propranolol
Griseofulvin	Rifampicin
Hydralazine	Sulfasalazine
Isoniazid	Theophylline
Labetalol (oral)	Triamterene
	Verapamil

TABLE 2 Commonly Used Drugs Requiring Dosing Adjustments in Patients with Renal Disease

Acetohexamide	Digoxin
Allopurinol	Disopyramide
Aminoglycoside antibiotics	Encainide
Amoxicillin	Ethambutol
Ampicillin	Hydralazine
Bretylium	Insulin
Carbenicillin	Lincomycin
Cefaclor	Lithium
Cefamandole	Methadone
Cefoxitin	Methicillin
Cefadroxil	Metronidazole
Cephalexin	Penicillin G
Cephaloridine (avoid; nephrotoxic)	Polymixin B
Cephalothin (when glomerular filtration rate <10 ml/min)	Polymixin E
Cephapirin (when gomerular filtration rate <10 ml/min)	Procainamide
Cephradine	Sulfamethoxazole
Cimetidine	Sulfisoxazole
Chlorpropamide	Tetracycline (avoid; may promote negative nitrogen balance)
Clofibrate	Ticarcillin
Clonidine	Tocainide
	Tolazamide
	Trimethoprim
	Vancomycin

Changes in Dosing Related to Renal Disease

Renal disease often necessitates an adjustment in the dose of drugs. In contrast to indices of hepatic function, the serum creatinine level is a good indicator of the ability of the kidney to eliminate drugs from the body. It is important to remember that the normal range of serum creatinine is usually about 0.5 mg per deciliter to 1.5 mg per deciliter. For any individual, a change in serum creatinine from 0.5 mg per deciliter to 1.5 mg per deciliter would indicate a 67 percent reduction in glomerular filtration rate. Thus, whereas a serum creatinine of 1.5 mg per deciliter may be normal for a large, muscular person, it would be distinctly abnormal in a small, nonmuscular person. In theory, a creatinine clearance test would be a more accurate indication of renal function then serum creatinine level, but creatinine clearance as performed in most general hospitals is very inaccurate and often misleading. Use of one of several nomograms or equations that predict creatinine clearance based on a patient's age, weight, and serum creatinine concentration are preferable to actually measuring creatinine clearances. One easily used equation is that of Cockroft and Gault:

$$\text{Creatinine clearance} = \frac{(140 - \text{age}) \times (\text{body weight in kg})}{72 \times (\text{serum creatinine in mg/dl})}$$

The equation would be multiplied by 0.85 for women. In addition to causing a decrease in the elimination of drugs that are normally excreted by

TABLE 3 Commonly Used Drugs Having Active Metabolites That Accumulate in Renal Failure

Acetohexamide	Meperidine (pethidine)
Allopurinol	Nitrofurantoin
Chlorpropamide	Primidone
Clofibrate	Procainamide
Diazepam	Sodium nitroprusside
Digoxin	Verapamil
Hydralazine	

the kidney, renal disease can also cause an accumulation of active metabolites, metabolites of a drug that have pharmacologic activity. The pharmacologic and toxicologic significance of these metabolites can increase when they accumulate. Table 2 lists commonly used drugs requiring a decrease in dose in patients with renal disease, and Table 3 lists some drugs which have active metabolites that accumulate in patients with renal failure.

Changes in Dosing Related to Heart Failure

Heart failure often causes abnormalities in drug elimination and distribution that require adjustments in dose. These changes are produced by a combination of changes in renal and hepatic perfusion, abnormal autonomic activity, altered distribution and binding of drugs to tissues, and hypoxia in tissues. Some drugs affected in heart failure are listed in Table 4.

Effects of Binding of Drugs to Proteins in Plasma

A variety of drugs are bound to plasma protein. There is an equilibrium between the drug bound to proteins and drug in free solution. However, only the drug in free solution (unbound drug) can be distributed to tissues of the body. Thus, the concentration of drug in solution determines the accessibility of drug to its site of action. Because of technical complexities, most clinical laboratories measure the total concentration of drugs in plasma (protein-bound concentration + unbound concentration).

TABLE 4 Dosing of Commonly Used Drugs Affected by Heart Failure

Drug	*Adjustment*
Digoxin	Decrease maintenance dose because of impairment of renal function
Lidocaine	Decrease loading dose (initial bolus) and decrease maintenance infusion rate
Procainamide	Decrease loading and maintenance doses
Theophylline	Decrease maintenance dose

Although this is adequate for many situations, misleading concentrations can be reported in situations in which disease states alter the normal relationship between bound and free drug. Both renal failure and hepatic failure can lead to altered protein binding such that the fraction of the total concentration of the drug in plasma that is unbound increases. The increase in the unbound fraction results from both a decrease in the concentration of albumin and from an accumulation of substances that can displace drug from albumin. A classic and probably the most important example of a drug so affected is phenytoin. The usual therapeutic range of concentrations for phenytoin is decreased when the total concentration is measured. In the absence of renal or hepatic failure, about 90 percent of the total concentration of phenytoin is bound to protein. Thus, at a total concentration of 10 mg per liter (low end of therapeutic range) only 1 mg per liter is in free solution. At a total concentration of 20 mg per liter (high end of therapeutic range), 2 mg per liter is unbound. In severe renal failure, the percent bound can decrease to 75 percent. In this setting, at a total concentration of 10 mg per liter, the free concentration is 2.5 mg per liter. Thus, in severe renal failure the free concentration, which determines the pharmacologic effect, is in a range that is likely to cause toxicity, even though the total concentration could be mistakenly interpreted as being in the lower therapeutic range. In the setting of renal or hepatic failure, it is good practice to consult either a clinical pharmacologist or a clinical pathologist who is knowledgeable about drug assays in order to be sure of the correct interpretation of a reported concentration.

An opposite effect can occur for certain other drugs in the setting of acute inflammation. For example, the protein binding of lidocaine and quinidine may increase in the setting of acute myocardial infarction. Thus, some patients may require a higher than usual total concentration of drug to achieve a therapeutic effect.

The elimination of a drug from the body can be affected by changes of binding. The rates of both renal and hepatic excretion of some drugs can be altered by changes in protein binding. The elimination of other drugs, even some which are bound to a great extent, is not affected by changes in protein binding. In the absence of data from a proper study, it is difficult to predict how the elimination of a drug will be affected by changes in protein binding. It is important to remember that such changes are possible and to consult either an authority on the subject or a good reference.

Changes in Dosing Related to Age

Metabolism and renal function change as people age. These changes become great enough in elderly patients to warrant making modifications in dosing regimens. Renal function declines with age, so that by age 60 the glomerular filtration rate has declined by about 30 percent from the filtration rate of a 20 year old. Tubular function declines at approximately the same rate. As a general precautionary guideline, drugs that require lowering the dose because of renal failure also require lowering the dose in the elderly. However, attention to an individual patient's renal function is the best guide to any adjustment in dosing.

Although there are changes in metabolic activity associated with age, it is difficult to make quantitative generalizations, and thus it is difficult to predict which drugs will have altered metabolism. Changes in body composition, distribution of blood flow, and environmental and genetic factors all affect how the aging process will alter the disposition of drugs. In addition, the actual pharmacologic response to some drugs may change with age, entirely independent of elimination of drug from the body. Thus, an empirical approach is required whereby individual drugs must be studied in an appropriately aged population. Whether general guidelines exist for a particular drug or not, nothing can substitute for careful observation of a patient.

Table 5 lists commonly used drugs that should, in general, be used in the elderly at lower doses than would generally be prescribed in younger patients. However, it cannot be overemphasized that titrating the dose to the desired effect is the best method for dosing.

TABLE 5 Commonly Used Drugs Requiring Decreased Doses in the Elderly*

Drug	*Comments*
Antihypertensive drugs	Possibly increased postural hypotension due to impaired response of baroreceptors
Barbiturates (should be avoided in elderly)	Paradoxical pharmacologic response often leading to restlessness, agitation, or psychosis; decreased rate of elimination
Benzodiazepines	Increased sensitivity to pharmacologic effect; some benzodiazepines may be metabolized more slowly
Cimetidine	Decreased renal function
Digoxin	Decreased renal function
Diuretics	Possible increase in electrolyte disturbances and postural hypotension
Heparin	Increased sensitivity to anticoagulant effects
Narcotic analgesics	Increased sensitivity to analgesic effects; possibly impaired clearance
Tricyclic antidepressants	Increased incidence of cardiac and hemodynamic adverse effects; urinary retention and other anticholinergic effects; decreased drug clearance
Warfarin	Increased sensitivity to anticoagulant effects

*Note: Because of a decline in renal function in the elderly, drugs listed in Table 2 should be used with caution.

DRUG INTERACTIONS

Many patients take more than one drug, and interactions between these drugs often occur. Interactions can lead to enhanced pharmacologic or toxicologic effects, altered binding of drugs to plasma proteins, and either increased or decreased rates of elimination. Any patient taking two or more drugs is subject to a drug-drug interaction. These should be anticipated as much as possible. However, it is impossible to remember all clinically important drug interactions. A good source of information on such interactions should be consulted whenever a new drug is added to a therapeutic regimen. Drug interactions are most important when they involve drugs with low therapeutic ratios (the ratio of toxic dose to therapeutic dose) or when the plasma concentration of a drug is crucial to successful treatment. Such drugs that are commonly used and that are often involved in drug interactions are listed in Table 6. A drug-drug interaction should be included in the differential diagnosis of any unusual or unexpected medical event.

Many drug interactions are caused on purpose and form the basis of rational combination therapy of many diseases and syndromes, including hyper-

TABLE 6 Drugs Frequently Involved in Clinically Significant Drug-Drug Interactions

Aminoglycoside antibiotics	Monoamine oxidase inhibitors
Aminophylline	Oral contraceptives
Antacids	Oral hypoglycemics
Aspirin (and other salicylates)	Penicillin and congeners of penicillin
Barbiturates	Penicillamine
Benzodiazepines	Phenothiazines
Beta-adrenergic blockers	Phenytoin
Carbamazepine	Primidone
Cimetidine	Probenecid
Corticosteroids	Quinidine
Digoxin	Tetracyclines
Erythromycin	Theophylline
Ethanol	Thiazide diuretics
Iron salts	Tricyclic antidepressants
Methotrexate	Warfarin

tension, arrhythmias, cancer, asthma, and heart failure. A good working knowledge of a drug's pharmacology and its mechanism of action is essential to design the most effective combination of drugs.

PHARMACOEPIDEMIOLOGY

Specific information about an individual drug comes from a variety of sources. The controlled clinical trial is the most important for testing whether a drug is efficacious in a particular setting. A second type of information comes under the rubric of pharmacoepidemiology. In the most general sense, pharmacoepidemiology consists of collecting, evaluating, and interpreting data produced by physicians who are using drugs in clinical practice. These data can be collected in a variety of ways. Voluntary reporting of adverse events to the Food and Drug Administration by practicing physicians is an important although sporadic source. Large databases on patients and their diagnoses and treatments are available from government-sponsored medical programs and from large clinics and health maintenance organizations. These databases have also been systematically examined in order to gain more information on a drug's beneficial or harmful effects.

Information from epidemiologic studies can be used to generate hypotheses about a drug's effect. These hypotheses can be tested prospectively in clinical trials. More important, epidemiologic information can complement already existing data on drug efficacy and safety.

When a drug is approved for general use by the Food and Drug Administration, it has usually been studied in 500 to 3,500 people. Some of these studies are double-blind, randomized trials that demonstrated the efficacy of the drug for a particular indication. Other trials examine the drug's pharmacokinetics in patients and in so-called "special populations," such as patients with renal or hepatic disease or in the elderly. Other trials are "safety trials" that attempt to mimic standard clinical practice more closely. However, in all these trials, patients are carefully selected; many patients are excluded because they have too many concurrent conditions that would make it more difficult to draw definite conclusions from the clinical trials. Also, patients in clinical trials are monitored more frequently and in more detail than is done in standard clinical practice. Because of the stringent criteria applied to patients, allowing them to enter clinical trials, a drug is often not tested in patients typical of a general practice population. Because of the small number of patients studied, only the most common adverse reactions caused by the drug are detected. Finally, when the Food and Drug Administration approves a drug for a particular indication, only data specifically pertaining to that indication are evaluated. However, once a drug is approved and available for use, physicians may use the drug for whatever indication they choose. This use of a drug by clinicians for nonapproved indications is often medically appropriate, but the information readily available to physicians in the package insert pertains almost exclusively to patients who had the approved indication. Thus, epidemiologic studies can provide information from many thousand times the number of patients who were studied originally to prove the drug's efficacy and safety. Epidemiologic studies make data available that pertain to a more "typical" clinic population. Also epidemiologic studies can, in theory, provide information on efficacy in indications that are being treated but that are not approved by the Food and Drug Administration. Finally, epidemiologic studies have the potential for discovering beneficial and harmful effects that were not expected or predicted from previous knowledge of the drug.

The proper utility of pharmacoepidemiology, sometimes referred to as postmarketing surveillance, in making both medical and regulatory decisions regarding the proper use of a drug is a subject of active debate. There is little question that such studies provide provocative and exciting information. What is not universally agreed on is how to apply this information in the most judicious fashion. On one side are empiricists who believe that only prospective clinical trials should form the basis of decision making regarding a drug's use. Others are willing to accept fully conclusions from some types of epidemiologic studies, in the absence of prospective trials. It is likely that a combination of the two approaches will yield the most knowledge.

SUGGESTED READING

Anderson RJ, Schrier RW, eds. Clinical use of drugs in patients with kidney and liver disease. Philadelphia: WB Saunders, 1981.

Benet LZ, Sheiner LB. Design and optimization of dosage regimens; pharmacokinetic data. In: Gilman AG, et al, eds. The pharmacological basis of therapeutics. 7th ed. New York: Macmillan, 1985:1663.

Hansten PD. Drug interactions. 6th ed. Philadelphia: Lea & Febiger, 1988.

Shammas FV, Dickstein K. Clinical pharmacokinetics in heart failure. Clin Pharmacokinet 1988; 15:94–113.

Tsujimoto G, Hashimoto K, Hoffman BB. Pharmacokinetic and pharmacodynamic principles of drug therapy in old age. Clin Pharmacol Ther Toxicol 1989; 27:13–26.

PERCUTANEOUS DRAINAGE PROCEDURES

AMY B. KUHLIK, M.D.

Over the past decade, impressive technical advances in radiologic imaging have fostered the development of nonsurgical invasive therapeutic procedures, and in many instances such procedures have replaced surgery as preferred therapeutic modalities. Although many of these procedures are performed by radiologists, they do not fall under the domain of any single specialty. The cardiologist, pulmonologist, gastroenterologist, and surgeon have each become technically involved in invasive therapy.

This explosion in technology has caught the medical profession off guard. Indications have evolved for surgical procedures based on risk-benefit analyses and many years of experience. We now have a variety of therapeutic modalities that offer results comparable to those of surgery but with less risk to the patient. Thus, indications need to be defined on the basis of the benefits and risks of each new procedure.

In this chapter the use of percutaneous catheters for extravascular procedures is examined, focusing on drainage of abdominal and pleural fluid collections, the pericardial cavity, the biliary tree, and the renal collecting system.

DRAINAGE OF ABDOMINAL ABSCESSES

If left untreated, most patients with an intraabdominal abscess die of sepsis or organ failure. Until the middle 1970s, surgical drainage was the only viable therapeutic option. In 1974, percutaneous drainage of intraabdominal abscesses with ultrasonic guidance was first employed. Shortly thereafter, computed tomography (CT) was used to guide abscess evacuation. Although an accurate comparison of surgical and percutaneous drainage procedures has never been reported, successful percutaneous drainage of many types of intraabdominal abscesses is well documented. Percutaneous drainage clearly causes less morbidity than surgery because general anesthesia is avoided, and the patient is able to ambulate soon after the procedure.

Patient Selection

Once a collection of fluid is identified in the abdominal cavity, the route of evacuation needs to be determined expeditiously because an infected fluid collection requires immediate drainage. Consultation among the primary physician, the radiologist, and the surgeon is essential. A series of relative contraindications to percutaneous drainage has evolved in the literature. However, practices vary widely depending on the experience of the invasive radiologist and the available imaging modalities. At our institution, the traditional guidelines are considered too restrictive. We consider the only absolute contraindication to percutaneous abscess drainage to be the absence of a safe route of passage to the abscess. Certain locations and features of an abscess make complete percutaneous drainage technically difficult and less likely to succeed. Table 1 lists these features, each of which is discussed separately. Of note is the fact that the etiology of the intraabdominal abscess is usually not an important determinant of initial therapy (Table 2). A notable exception is an amebic liver abscess, which does not require drainage and should be treated solely with antibiotics.

Multiple Abscess Cavities or Internal Loculations

Although percutaneous drainage of such abscesses has been traditionally contraindicated because of technical difficulty, the following approach is often successful. Contrast material is injected into the dominant cavity to visualize connections between cavities. A guidewire is placed within the cavity and manipulated to remove septations. A catheter is then inserted into the dominant cavity. Multiple catheters and multiple punctures may be required if loculations persist.

Abscesses with Enteric Communication

Abscesses that communicate with the intestine frequently complicate Crohn's disease and diverticulitis. Although it is difficult, percutaneous drainage can be achieved. The underlying bowel is usually severely diseased, and surgical resection is inevitable. However, in the case of a diverticular abscess, percutaneous drainage is particularly desirable because resolution of the infection allows for a single-stage bowel resection with a primary reanastomosis. If percutaneous drainage fails, the patient must undergo surgical drainage and resection with the creation of a temporary enterostomy.

TABLE 1 Intraabdominal Abscesses That Are Difficult to Drain Percutaneously

Abscess with multiple cavities or loculations
Abscess with enteric communication
Interloop abscess
Pancreatic abscess
Infected hematoma

TABLE 2 Abscesses Ideally Suited for Percutaneous Drainage

Unilocular abscess
Location easily accessible without traversing unaffected bowel
Subdiaphragmatic abscess
Perirenal or renal abscess
Pericolic gutter abscess
Hepatic abscess

Interloop Abscesses

It is difficult to gain access to an abscess that is located between loops of bowel without traversing unaffected portions of intestine. However, with proper positioning and CT guidance, safe access often can be attained. Hence, if CT is available, percutaneous drainage of an interloop abscess is preferred over surgery.

Pancreatic Abscesses

A pancreatic abscess is the most lethal type of intraabdominal fluid collection. In addition to pus, it contains thick necrotic tissue debris. The character of the abscess fluid makes complete percutaneous (and even surgical) evacuation difficult. Experience with pancreatic abscesses is limited. Some centers report failure rates of almost 90 percent, and others report high rates of success with percutaneous drainage. Percutaneous drainage of a pancreatic abscess should be attempted because a safe route of entry can usually be achieved. However, the physician should be aware that definitive therapy often requires surgical intervention, and surgical exploration should be done without delay if the patient shows evidence of sepsis.

Infected Hematomas

An infected hematoma is difficult to drain percutaneously because of its high viscosity. Some authors consider its presence to be a contraindication to percutaneous drainage; yet a liquefied hematoma may be amenable to percutaneous drainage. Because one cannot determine radiographically whether or not a hematoma is liquefied, a diagnostic aspiration procedure should be performed before proceeding.

Fluid Collections That Should Not Be Drained Percutaneously

As noted before, intrahepatic abscesses caused by amebae do not require drainage of any sort. Treatment consists solely of antibiotics. Echinococcal cysts should not be aspirated or drained percutaneously because spillage of cyst contents into the peritoneum may cause anaphylaxis.

Procedural Aspects

The abnormal fluid collection may be identified by ultrasonography or CT. CT is the most accurate mode of diagnosis and demonstrates an intraabdominal abscess with 95 percent sensitivity. Once identified, the abscess may be drained using ultrasonic, fluoroscopic, or CT guidance. For abscesses that do not appear to abut vital structures such as bowel or blood vessels, ultrasonic guidance is adequate and less expensive than CT. Retroperitoneal and superficially located intraperitoneal abscesses are usually well suited for drainage under ultrasonography. CT is preferred because it demonstrates the relationship of the abscess to bowel and other vital structures.

Broad-spectrum antibiotics should be administered prior to the drainage procedure. More specific antibiotic therapy is subsequently chosen based on culture results.

Once the route of access has been planned, local anesthesia is applied to the skin and subcutaneous tissue. Needle aspiration of the fluid collection is performed to confirm the presence of pus. A sheathed needle is inserted into the abscess and a guidewire is placed through the needle. A small drainage catheter is then advanced into the abscess over the guidewire. The abscess should be evacuated as completely as possible at the time of the initial aspiration. Saline irrigation may aid in liquefying viscous material. A small catheter is left in the abscess cavity and is placed to dependent drainage. Once the catheter is in place, vigorous irrigation should be avoided because it may result in bacteremia or dislodgement of the catheter. Gentle irrigation with sterile saline may be required on a daily basis to maintain catheter patency.

Repeat radiologic imaging to visualize the abscess should be done at 7 days or earlier if the patient fails to improve. Removal of the drain is based on clinical evidence of improvement, radiologic evidence of abscess resolution, and cessation of drainage from the catheter. On average, this cycle takes from 14 to 21 days; nutritional support and antibiotics represent important adjunctive therapies during this interval. Surgical exploration is warranted if the patient's condition deteriorates or if the patient fails to improve after a trial of percutaneous drainage.

Complications

Death resulting from a complication of percutaneous drainage is exceedingly rare (Table 3). The most common complication of percutaneous drainage is bacteremia (20 percent). Other complications that occur infrequently include puncture of the bowel, creation of a fistulous tract, hemorrhage, and peritoneal contamination.

Percutaneous drainage offers many advantages over surgery. General anesthesia and its associated

TABLE 3 Complications of Percutaneous Abscess Drainage

Bacteremia
Enteric puncture
Fistula formation
Peritoneal contamination
Hemorrhage

complications are avoided. Hospitalization is shorter and thus costs are reduced. The patient is generally able to ambulate within hours after the procedure, and therefore fewer complications are associated with the bedridden state. If modern imaging modalities are available, an effort should be made to drain an intraabdominal abscess percutaneously, with surgical back-up reserved for technical failures.

DRAINAGE OF THE PLEURAL CAVITY

An empyema, hemothorax, or symptomatic pleural effusion is an indication for therapeutic evacuation of the pleural space. In these instances, the mode of drainage depends on the etiology of the fluid collection (Table 4).

Empyema

Once an empyema is discovered, it must be evacuated immediately. Therapeutic options include standard thoracostomy tube drainage, percutaneous drainage under fluoroscopic or ultrasonic guidance, rib excision with open drainage of the pleural space, or surgical thoracotomy with drainage and decortication. The choice of therapy depends on the presence of multiple pockets of infection or loculations within the empyema. If the fluid appears to flow freely according to decubitus-position x-ray film, insertion of a standard chest tube at the bedside should be the initial therapy. Complications of blind chest tube insertion are rare but include bleeding, subcutaneous emphysema, laceration of lung tissue, and injury to the spleen or liver.

Empyemas are commonly multiple or loculated. If multiple pockets are identified, radiographically guided catheter insertion is indicated. Guided drainage is also indicated when a patient remains febrile or has radiographic evidence of undrained fluid despite standard chest tube therapy.

TABLE 4 Indications for Drainage of Pleural Fluid

Empyema
Hemothorax
Large symptomatic effusion

Fluoroscopy, ultrasonography, and CT are all suitable for guiding catheter insertion into the pleural cavity. In this instance, however, contrary to the procedure for drainage of an intraabdominal abscess, fluoroscopy and ultrasonography are often superior to CT because some free-flowing portions of an empyema cannot be drained in the dependent position required for CT imaging.

Radiographic guidance provides distinct advantages over standard chest tube drainage. A multiloculated empyema may be drained by internal manipulation with a guidewire or by the insertion of multiple catheters. The catheter is placed more precisely, lessening the risk of intraabdominal injury from subdiaphragmatic insertion. Also, patients have far less discomfort during guided catheter insertion than with the blind placement of a large-bore chest tube.

The technique of catheter insertion is similar to that described for the drainage of an intraabdominal abscess. Once in place, catheter management is identical to that of a standard chest tube. Repeat fluoroscopy or ultrasonic examination of the chest should be performed within 72 hours to assess the size of the remaining cavity. Definitive surgical therapy is indicated if the patient fails to improve after 5 to 7 days of therapy or if percutaneous access to all infected cavities cannot be achieved.

Hemothorax

Blood in the pleural space is often the consequence of trauma but may develop after a large pulmonary infarct or during anticoagulation therapy. Treatment usually consists of standard chest tube drainage, but if the fluid is infected or loculated, percutaneous catheter drainage is warranted.

Malignant Pleural Effusion

A malignant pleural effusion is most often secondary to metastatic cancer of the lung, breast, or lymphoreticular system. Less commonly, a tumor arising in the pleura is the culprit. If the patient is asymptomatic, fluid removal usually is not indicated. However, if the patient complains of dyspnea, cough, or chest discomfort, palliative therapy to relieve the effusion is warranted. Therapeutic options for symptomatic pleural effusions are listed in Table 5.

TABLE 5 Therapeutic Options for Malignant Pleural Effusions

Repeated thoracentesis
Chest tube drainage
Chemical pleurodesis
Surgical pleurodesis
Pleuroperitoneal shunt

The choice of therapy is determined by taking into account the cause of the effusion, the natural history of the underlying tumor, and the patient's overall state of health. If the patient's prognosis is very unfavorable, with early death inevitable, or the patient is bedridden, therapy should be limited to bedside procedures such as repeated thoracenteses or chest tube drainage. However, if the patient is otherwise ambulatory and the symptoms caused by the effusion impede functional ability, palliative therapy should be aggressively pursued.

Thoracentesis

Thoracentesis should be employed first for malignant effusions because it is safe and can be done in the outpatient setting. If the fluid reaccumulates slowly, repeated thoracenteses on a weekly basis may suffice. Unfortunately, only 20 percent of patients have their symptoms controlled by thoracentesis; therefore other modes of therapy are usually necessary.

Chemical Pleurodesis

Chemical pleurodesis induces an inflammatory response that causes tight adherence of the visceral and parietal pleural surfaces, thus preventing fluid from accumulating in the pleural space. Tetracycline is the preferred chemical agent because it is inexpensive but as efficacious as and less toxic than other agents. The procedure is carried out at the bedside following complete evacuation of the pleural space via chest tube drainage. Tetracycline is instilled into the pleural space through the tube, which is then clamped for 24 hours. Important side effects include fever and pain. Pleurodesis is successful in only 65 percent of attempts. If pleural fluid reaccumulates, the procedure can be repeated. Patients are excluded from therapy if they have infected pleural fluid or if their effusion accumulates so rapidly that the pleural space does not remain empty for 24 hours prior to the procedure.

Surgical Pleurodesis

Surgical pleurodesis or pleurectomy should be reserved for patients who fail to respond to less invasive therapy or those with a significant life expectancy (more than 6 months). The procedure is usually successful, but the thoracotomy and general anesthesia may produce substantial morbidity.

Pleuroperitoneal Shunt

Pleuroperitoneal shunts aid in draining rapidly accumulating effusions or chylous effusions that are often resistant to other types of therapy. The shunt is placed subcutaneously under local anesthesia. Infection in the pleural or peritoneal cavities and renal failure preclude its use.

DRAINAGE OF THE PERICARDIUM

Pericardial effusions result from many disease entities. The most common causes are listed in Table 6. An effusion may be chronic and asymptomatic, in which case no specific therapy is required. Whether or not symptoms of hemodynamic instability develop depends on several factors, including the rate at which the effusion develops, the ability of the pericardium to stretch and accommodate the fluid, and the total volume of the effusion. Patients should be selected for therapy only if they have signs or symptoms of elevated intrapericardial pressure, a potentially life-threatening situation that requires immediate therapy. The procedure of choice is a pericardiocentesis, which can be performed quickly with little morbidity if fluoroscopic or ultrasonic guidance is used. The procedure usually is carried out in the cardiac catheterization laboratory with local anesthesia and sedation. After the fluid is evacuated, a percutaneously placed pigtail catheter is inserted into the pericardial space. The catheter should remain in place until drainage ceases (usually 2 to 3 days). In most cases, catheter drainage proves to be definitive therapy. At other times, it serves as an important temporizing measure while therapy aimed at the underlying cause of the effusion is given an opportunity to work. In a small percentage of cases, the effusion reaccumulates and pericardiectomy is required. There are no absolute contraindications to pericardiocentesis. Even patients with significant coagulation disturbances can safely undergo the procedure, although supportive blood products should be administered. Patients who develop pericardial tamponade within a few days of open heart surgery should be reoperated on immediately, since bleeding that requires surgical control is likely.

DRAINAGE OF THE BILIARY TRACT

Relief of Malignant Biliary Obstruction

The most common malignant causes of biliary obstruction are pancreatic cancer and cholangiocarcinoma, but any tumor that metastasizes to the porta

TABLE 6 Etiologies of Pericardial Effusions

Idiopathic
Neoplastic (lung, breast, lymphoma)
Tuberculosis
Connective tissue diseases
Uremia
Misplaced central venous catheter

TABLE 7 Indications for Percutaneous Biliary Drainage in Malignant Disease

Palliation for patients at high risk for surgery
Palliation for patients with life expectancy less than 6 months
Prior to chemotherapy if drugs are excreted by biliary tract

hepatis can result in obstruction. Biliary obstruction causes significant morbidity and discomfort, and therefore palliative therapy is essential (Table 7).

Therapeutic options include surgical drainage via a biliary-enteric bypass, drainage of the biliary tract via surgically placed stents and decompression by means of endoscopically or percutaneously placed biliary stents. The choice of therapy depends on several factors. If a patient is not at high risk for surgery and has a life expectancy that exceeds 6 months, biliary-enteric bypass provides the best palliation with the least long-term morbidity.

Percutaneous stent insertion is an attractive alternative in patients whose life expectancy is short or in those who are poor surgical candidates. It is not the procedure of choice in good surgical candidates because it carries a high morbidity—the incidence of cholangitis alone is 35 percent.

Percutaneous drainage is also useful in patients who require chemotherapeutic agents that are excreted by the biliary tree. Relief of biliary obstruction in such patients allows for the administration of full-dose chemotherapy.

Technical success usually can be achieved when a catheter is placed transhepatically into the biliary tree under fluoroscopic guidance. Contraindications include severe coagulopathy, massive ascites, and multiple sites of intrahepatic obstruction (which further increases the risk of cholangitis). Cholangitis occurs despite the routine use of prophylactic antibiotics. Other complications include infection at the insertion site and hemorrhage, which is rare.

Percutaneous Biliary Drainage

Previously, percutaneous biliary drainage was performed prior to surgery in patients with obstruction from benign strictures because of the widely held belief that preoperative lowering of the serum bilirubin level lowered the surgical risk. Several prospective trials have not supported this concept; therefore percutaneous drainage is no longer recommended in this circumstance.

Obstruction of the common bile duct by gallstones is addressed elsewhere in this text. Although endoscopic therapy may be preferred to surgery in this instance, percutaneous therapy is not routinely employed.

Percutaneous drainage of the gallbladder can be performed safely in patients with acute cholecystitis as a temporizing measure in circumstances in which the risk of surgery is prohibitively high.

DRAINAGE OF THE URINARY TRACT

Obstruction of the urinary tract threatens both renal function and life. Prior to cystoscopic and percutaneous drainage procedures, surgical nephrostomy and nephrectomy were the only therapeutic options. Percutaneous nephrostomy was first described in 1955. At that time, its use was limited to emergency situations in which retrograde drainage was difficult and surgery was not feasible. It is now the procedure of choice for urinary tract obstruction in many circumstances.

Common causes of urinary tract obstruction include kidney stones, malignancy, and postoperative strictures. The choice of therapy depends on the underlying cause of the obstruction and on whether or not the urinary tract is infected.

Pyonephrosis

In a patient with a dilated collecting system with evidence of an active urinary infection, percutaneous nephrostomy is the procedure of choice because it is technically the fastest, easiest, and safest procedure to perform. Drainage should be achieved urgently to prevent sepsis.

The nephrostomy tube may be of further therapeutic value if a kidney stone is discovered to be the cause of obstruction. Chemical dissolution of the stone may be performed subsequently through the nephrostomy tube. Stents may be inserted in an antegrade fashion through the nephrostomy tract if long-term drainage is required.

There are no absolute contraindications to percutaneous nephrostomy. Because hemorrhage is the most serious complication, patients with severe coagulation disturbances should receive supportive blood products prior to the procedure. Prophylactic antibiotics should be administered because puncture of the infected renal pelvis may result in bacteremia. Pneumothorax and urinoma (a persistent urine leak from the collecting system) are rare complications of percutaneous nephrostomy. Once drainage has been achieved, definitive therapy should be aimed at relieving the underlying cause of obstruction.

Drainage of the Uninfected Urinary Tract

Obstruction of the urinary collecting system in the absence of infection is not immediately life-threatening; however, drainage must be achieved in order to prevent loss of renal function. In this instance, ureteral stents can be inserted under cystoscopic guidance. This procedure is technically more difficult than percutaneous nephrostomy, but it provides a better long-term solution. If retrograde insertion of stents fails to alleviate obstruction, stents may be inserted antegrade using a percutaneous approach. Complications of antegrade stent insertion are the same as those of percutaneous nephrostomy. In addition, patients often complain of urinary frequency from the irritating effect of the pigtail catheter on the trigone of the bladder. The stents should be replaced every 3 months, and the patient should be followed carefully for recurrent urinary tract obstruction.

SUGGESTED READING

Gerzof SG. Percutaneous catheter drainage of abdominal abscesses: A five year experience. N Engl J Med 1981; 305:653–657.

Molner W. Relief of obstructive jaundice through percutaneous transhepatic catheter—a new therapeutic method. Am J Radiol 1974; 122:356–367.

Mueller PR, vanSonnenberg E. Percutaneous drainage of 250 abdominal abscesses and fluid collections. Radiology 1984; 151:343–347.

Reznek RH. Percutaneous nephrostomy. Radiol Clin North Am 1984; Volume 22, Number 2.

Westcott JL. Percutaneous catheter drainage of pleural effusion and empyema. Am J Radiol 1985; 144:1189–1193.

ORGAN TRANSPLANTATION

RICHARD J. ROHRER, M.D.

The ultimate therapy for organ failure is organ replacement. Improvements in donor management, surgical techniques, and immunosuppression over the past decade have led to an improved outcome for the transplant recipient, an enhanced impression of transplantation on the part of clinicians and the public, and rapid growth of transplant programs. This chapter focuses on aspects of kidney, liver, and heart transplantation, as they have by now attained the status of conventional therapy for most patients with the appropriate indications. Transplantation of the single lung, pancreas, and small bowel, although advancing steadily, as yet remain largely experimental.

Although the specifics of kidney, liver, and heart failure differ greatly, several generalizations may be made about organ failure from the transplantation perspective. First, with maturation of each of the transplant fields, the specific diagnosis leading to native organ failure has begun to matter less, whereas the functional status of the potential recipient has begun to matter more. One hardly need make lists of appropriate diagnoses that may lead to organ replacement, since nearly any pathologic process that destroys native kidney, liver, or heart function can, in an appropriate situation, be an indication for transplantation. Second, there has been a natural tendency for yesterday's absolute contraindication to become today's relative contraindication, and for today's relative contraindication to become tomorrow's routine transplant. Barriers such as diabetes in the renal failure patient, a history of alcohol abuse in the liver failure patient, and age over 50 years in the heart failure patient have all been eroded or eliminated. Third, while appropriate initial therapy for all forms of organ failure remains medical, early attention to the transplantation limb of the therapeutic algorithm is imperative. If transplantation with a high degree of success is likely to be the ultimate end anyway, one's threshold for dispensing with bothersome (and occasionally dangerous) medical or surgical temporizing measures should be correspondingly lowered.

KIDNEY TRANSPLANTATION

Pretransplant

Since the first successful kidney transplant in 1954, progressive improvement in this form of renal replacement has made it the therapy of choice for most patients with irreversible renal failure. An enhanced quality of life is the chief benefit of kidney transplantation, although many patients enjoy greater longevity and occupational and economic potential as well. Chronic glomerulonephritis remains the single most common cause of renal failure leading to transplantation, although diabetic nephropathy is the fastest-growing cause. Some forms of renal disease are known for their propensity to recur in a transplanted kidney, but in most cases this propensity is neither so swift nor so sure as to preclude transplantation (Table 1). From a practical point of view, the simple presence of end-stage renal disease in a patient with an adequate social setting and absence of the *relative* contraindications listed in Table 2 constitutes sufficient indication for kidney transplantation. In the United States, advanced age is by far the most common contraindication to transplantation.

Consideration of transplant options should begin simultaneously with consideration of dialysis options, that is, as soon as a chronic, progressive

TABLE 1 Diseases Leading to Transplantation

Glomerulonephritis	24%
Pyelonephritis/interstitial nephritis	17%
Diabetes mellitus	13%
Polycystic kidney disease	9%
Renal vascular disease	8%
Nondiabetic multisystem disease (e.g., lupus erythematosus, nephritis)	5%
Miscellaneous	11%
Unknown	13%

renal condition is diagnosed. This advanced planning allows maximal opportunity for the patient to consider the risks and benefits of transplantation and for any potential living-related donors to be evaluated. No elective dialysis access procedures should be performed without first having explored in at least a preliminary fashion the potential for transplantation. In a significant percentage of patients, access strategy is altered if the potential for a living-related kidney transplant exists. Although virtually all patients should have a distal radiocephalic arteriovenous fistula constructed prior to initiating dialysis if feasible, many patients have poor-quality vessels and a fistula may not be successful. In such instances, if there is a willing family donor, rather than embark on more elaborate permanent access procedures, the patient should be advised to have temporary hemodialysis or peritoneal dialysis as a bridge to transplantation. The success rate with living-related transplantation in 1990 is easily good enough to warrant such a position.

The evaluation of a potential kidney transplant candidate is outlined in Table 3. As post-transplant complications have diminished, so has the requisite list of pretransplant studies. Advances in pharmacologic control of hypertension have been highly effective and have virtually eliminated the need for bilateral nephrectomy. Patients with cardiac disease should have, as a minimum, stable angina and an ejection fraction higher than 40 percent. Cardiac catheterization and invasive coronary artery procedures are pursued only if independent indications for them exist and not as part of a pretransplant routine. In contrast to years gone by, at present it is unusual for a candidate to require some form of surgery to prepare him or her for transplantation; perhaps the only common holdover is sigmoid colectomy for the patient with a history of documented diverticulitis. Peptic ulcer disease is controlled medically prior to transplantation. Cholelithiasis, urolithiasis, polycystic kidneys, and refluxing ureters are all conditions that, although adding to the infectious risks of transplantation, can nonetheless generally be followed expectantly after transplant.

Serologic studies to assess the risk of viral infections are essential. Hepatitis B antigen–positive patients should be counseled that with transplantation they may face a risk as high as 30 percent of progression to chronic liver disease and even death due to liver failure; many would do better with dialysis. Historically, cytomegalovirus (CMV) seronegative recipients of CMV seropositive kidneys have faced a 60 percent risk of morbidity due to CMV syndromes after transplant, and one of several prophylactic measures should be taken to lessen this risk: restricting donors to the CMV seronegative pool or administering prophylactic CMV immune globulin, acyclovir, or ganciclovir. Herpes simplex virus (HSV) seropositivity connotes a risk of reactivation disease which, although rarely a serious illness, can largely be prevented by administration of oral acyclovir after transplant.

Human immunodeficiency virus (HIV) seropos-

TABLE 2 Absolute and Relative Contraindications to Kidney Transplantation

Absolute

Untreated primary malignancy or presence of metastatic disease
AIDS

Relative

Age less than 1 year or more than 70 years
Ongoing alcohol or substance abuse
Unstable cardiac disease
Active serious infection, including HIV seropositivity

TABLE 3 Evaluation of Renal Transplant Candidate

1. Complete history and physical examination (including cervical Papanicolaou smear)
2. Complete blood count with differential, chemistry profile, prothrombin time/partial thromboplastin time, platelet count
3. Titers for hepatitis B surface antigen, cytomegalovirus, herpes simplex virus, HIV antibody
4. ABO grouping
5. Human leukocyte antigen typing and screening for panel-reactive antibodies
6. Urinalysis, urine culture and sensitivity test
7. Electrocardiogram, chest x-ray film
8. Purified protein derivative test
9. Consultation with nephrology, transplant surgery, and social services departments
10. In addition, as indicated:
    - For history of upper abdominal pain or guaiac-positive stools, upper gastrointestinal series, gallbladder ultrasonogram, and upper gastrointestinal endoscopy
    - For history of diverticulitis or unexplained guaiac-positive stools, barium enema, lower gastrointestinal endoscopy
    - For history of symptomatic pyelonephritis or bladder outlet obstruction, a voiding cystourethrogram
    - For history of recent travel or residence in Third World countries or unexplained diarrhea, stool test for ova and parasites
11. Possible consultations with cardiology, psychiatry, hematology, pulmonary, and gynecology departments

itivity is more problematic. Data are scant, but at this time active acquired immunodeficiency syndrome (AIDS) or AIDS-related complex (ARC) patients should be encouraged to stay with dialysis in order to minimize opportunistic infection risks. HIV seropositivity in the absence of ARC or AIDS is more controversial, but at present any such patients interested in transplantation should at least be counseled as to potentially increased infection risk; if transplantation is performed, the patient should be reported to the newly formed registry for HIV-seropositive transplant recipients.

Tuberculin skin testing should be done as a baseline study, but unless independent indications for prophylactic or therapeutic intervention exist, no special pretransplant regimen is needed for reactors.

Management before transplant consists of optimization of the dialysis prescription and control of hypertension. The role of deliberate pretransplant transfusions for immunologic benefit has become controversial, but most centers still recommend that 2 to 6 units be given to cadaver kidney candidates. The evolving use of recombinant erythropoietin and the increasing effectiveness of post-transplant immunosuppression are likely to continue to lessen the incremental benefit seen in prior years with pretransplant transfusions.

Living-related kidney donation is safe for the donor and affords the recipient advantages in scheduling the transplant procedure, early graft function, and long-term immunologic compatibility. Two-thirds of candidates have no suitable parental, sibling, or offspring donors, however, and for them a cadaveric donor is sought. Waiting times vary but generally average from 9 to 12 months. Living-*un*related donation, usually from spouses, is growing in acceptance and confers the same advantages as living-related donation with regard to scheduling and early graft function. Long-term immunologic compatibility is expected to be similar to that attained with cadaveric grafting, however, and for this reason living-unrelated kidney donation is generally pursued after some period of waiting on a cadaver kidney list. In all but the experimental setting, donors and recipients must be blood-group compatible and demonstrate a negative lymphocytotoxic cross-match. Matching of human leukocyte antigens (HLA), particularly at the B and Dr loci, is desirable but not necessary.

Transplant and After Transplant

Whatever their source, kidney allografts are placed retroperitoneally in the right or left iliac fossa with circulation derived from the iliac vessels, and ureteral continuity with native urinary bladder is established by one of several techniques. The most common complication is acute tubular necrosis (ATN) in cadaveric kidney transplantation, which occurs in some 20 percent of cases. This complication is usually manifested by persistent oliguric renal failure in the face of ultrasonography demonstrating a satisfactory technical result, and usually resolves in 7 to 10 days. Dialysis is performed as usual during this time. Other surgical complications, such as wound infection, urinary leakage, and vascular thrombosis, are uncommon. Hospitalization is generally from 1 to 2 weeks.

Prophylactic immunosuppression is begun prior to revascularization of the graft and is continued for the life of the transplant. We prefer "triple" immunosuppression with cyclosporine, azathioprine, and prednisone. Prophylactic anti–T-cell monoclonal antibody, OKT3, is used selectively for the ATN kidney to obviate the need for early post-transplant cyclosporine and its confounding nephrotoxic side effects. In addition, this agent may be used for enhanced prophylaxis in the highly sensitized retransplant patient. Acute rejection most commonly occurs within the first 3 months following transplant and can generally be diagnosed by a rising serum creatinine level in an appropriate clinical setting; percutaneous biopsy is performed in questionable situations. Initial therapy for acute rejection is a high-dose steroid "pulse" over several days; resistant or recurrent rejections are confirmed by biopsy and treated with OKT3. Long-term prophylactic triple immunosuppression is expected in most cases, with variable tapering of the doses of each to minimal levels. Recipients of HLA identical grafts are unique in that cyclosporine is gradually withdrawn over the first 12 months after transplant, leaving them on azathioprine and prednisone alone. Immunosuppressive protocols vary widely from program to program. Follow-up visits are generally on a weekly basis for the first 6 to 12 weeks and then monthly over the remainder of the first year after transplant. Surveillance decreases to once or twice yearly with time.

Overall patient and graft survival 1 year following transplant are 98 percent and 90 percent, respectively. The graft survival data may be stratified by type, with 1-year survival of living-related grafts at 96 percent, first cadaveric transplants at 89 percent, and retransplants at 72 percent. Beyond the first year, chronic rejection exacts a slow but steady toll. Long term, the half-life of living-related kidney transplants is expected to be 15 to 20 years and of cadaveric transplants 10 years, although continuing advances in immunosuppression make prognostication difficult. Upon loss of a transplanted kidney, the patient returns to dialysis; the vast majority seek retransplantation. Those who were able to retain their initial graft longer than 1 year tend to fare better with retransplantation than those who lost their graft sooner, but this factor per se does not greatly affect their candidacy for retransplantation.

LIVER TRANSPLANTATION

Pretransplant

Since a National Institutes of Health Consensus Development Conference concluded in 1983 that liver transplantation had passed from an experimental to a therapeutic modality, there has been rapid growth in the numbers of patients with end-stage liver disease who have received transplants. Because there are no alternative replacement therapies and few effective supports, liver transplantation is lifesaving to those who require it. Native liver diseases leading to end-stage liver disease (Table 4) have been classified as parenchymal, cholestatic, and metabolic, but, as with kidney transplantation, the precise etiology of liver failure is less important than the functional aspects of the patient's condition. From a practical point of view, the simple presence of end-stage liver disease and the absence of the contraindications noted in Table 5 constitute indications for transplantation. Some patients with primary hepatic malignancies (and frequently normal liver function) may be transplant candidates; agreement on this indication for transplantation is not universal.

Alcoholic patients deserve special mention. Most programs have evolved a policy that patients with alcoholic cirrhosis can be considered as candidates for transplantation if they meet strict criteria for abstinence and reform. Criteria to be taken into account in evaluating individual patients include documented abstinence for approximately 6 months or longer, an established record of compliance with medical therapy, absence of a history of abusive, antisocial, or criminal behavior, strong social supports, absence of alcoholic dementia or cardiomyopathy, and documented regular participation in a group or individual counseling program. All such patients should be evaluated by a transplant team psychiatrist as well as by personnel from a substance abuse program. As a practical matter, few of these patients have had the insight to stop drinking before becoming physically ill, and many deteriorate precipitously and require urgent intervention.

TABLE 4 Hepatic Diseases Leading to Transplantation

Non-A, non-B chronic active hepatitis	17%
Biliary atresia	13%
Primary biliary cirrhosis	10%
Sclerosing cholangitis	10%
Cryptogenic cirrhosis	9%
Alpha-1-antitrypsin deficiency	8%
Chronic active hepatitis B	8%
Primary hepatic neoplasm	6%
Alcoholic cirrhosis	4%
Miscellaneous	15%

TABLE 5 Absolute and Relative Contraindications to Liver Transplantation

Absolute
Myocardial infarction within previous 6 months
Advanced cardiac disease
Multiple, uncorrectable, life-threatening congenital abnormalities
Uncontrolled extrahepatic bacterial or fungal infection
Severe chronic obstructive pulmonary disease
Extrahepatic malignancy
Patients with alcoholic liver injury who are still drinking
Active substance abuse
Coexisting severe, life-threatening extrahepatic disease unless it is a direct complication of the underlying liver disease
AIDS
Relative
Age over 60 years
Delta hepatitis, hepatitis B e antigen positivity in patients with hepatitis B
Portal vein thrombosis
Acute or chronic renal failure not associated with liver disease
Intrahepatic or biliary sepsis
Severe hypoxemia resulting from right-to-left shunts
Previous extensive hepatobiliary surgery
Uncontrolled serious psychiatric disorder that would impair the patient's ability to undergo transplantation or to cooperate in immunosuppressive therapy
Anti-HIV seropositivity without AIDS

From the Boston Center for Liver Transplantation, with permission.

The evaluation of a potential liver transplant recipient is outlined in Table 6. It is not always necessary or even desirable to perform all tests on all patients, and clinical judgment is required. A well-known patient with documented primary biliary cirrhosis does not have to be assayed for alpha-1-antitrypsin deficiency, for example, and a previously healthy patient with fulminant hepatic failure may be listed for an emergency transplant after only an ABO grouping and a portal vein sonogram have been done (although further evaluation usually proceeds as conditions permit). The status of the portal vein is the most important anatomic factor to document; for this evaluation, magnetic resonance imaging flow studies may soon surpass Doppler ultrasonography in accuracy and definition but not in convenience. Occult malignancy should also be ruled out, although the occasional incidental hepatoma discovered by pathologists after hepatectomy is usually of no consequence clinically. Viral serologies are important but currently are of less functional significance than in kidney transplantation. Hepatitis B antigenicity and the presence of its related delta virus are bothersome findings because, particularly in the chronic hepatitis patient, they almost always can be detected again after transplant. A substantial percentage of these patients attain long-term survival in spite of antigen-positive status, however. Colonization with CMV and HSV is common, but there is as yet no proven prophylactic regimen to prevent disease. The implications of HIV seropositivity are

TABLE 6 Evaluation of Liver Transplant Candidates

1. Complete history and physical examination (including cervical Papanicolaou smear)
2. Complete blood count with differential
3. Prothrombin time/partial thromboplastin time, platelet count, fibrinogen
4. Electrolytes and blood urea nitrogen, glucose, creatinine, calcium, phosphorus, amylase levels
5. Total and direct bilirubin, aspartate aminotransferase, alanine aminotransferase, gamma-glutamyl transpeptidase, alkaline phosphatase
6. Serum protein electrophoresis, iron, transferrin, ceruloplasmin, hepatitis B surface antigen, hepatitis B core antibody, hepatitis B e antigen, HIV enzyme-linked immunosorbent assay, herpes simplex virus titer, cytomegalovirus titer
7. ABO grouping
8. Human leukocytic antigen typing and screening for panel-reactive antibody
9. Electrocardiogram, chest x-ray film
10. Portal vein Doppler sonogram
11. Computed tomographic scan of abdomen
12. Consultation with hepatology, transplant surgery, anesthesiology, blood bank, psychiatry, and social services departments
13. In addition, as indicated:
    - If patient age over 60 or any question as to cardiopulmonary reserve, pulmonary function tests with arterial blood gases, multigated angiogram
    - If upper abdominal pain or guaiac-positive stool, upper gastrointestinal endoscopy
    - If history of diverticulitis or undiagnosed guaiac-positive stool, barium enema, colonoscopy
    - If abnormal neurologic status, head computed tomographic scan, electroencephalogram
14. Possible consultations with cardiology, infectious diseases, neurology, hematology, and gynecology departments

controversial; patients with antibody alone should be considered on a case-by-case basis, although in the presence of ARC or AIDS, transplantation would be unwise.

The majority of liver transplant candidates have sustained a chronic hepatic insult over a period of months or years and have variable degrees of hepatocellular synthetic dysfunction, cholestasis, and/or cirrhosis with its attendant portal hypertension. Consideration for liver transplantation should begin whenever a patient has been diagnosed with a chronic hepatic condition from which he or she is symptomatic or displays evidence of compromised synthetic function (particularly in the prothrombin time and serum albumin level) or portal hypertension (manifested by varices or hypersplenism). A liver biopsy is of great importance in many cases, as is, to a lesser extent, endoscopic retrograde cholangiopancreatography. The rare patient with a medically treatable form of liver disease, such as autoimmune hepatitis, may be identified in this way. For the patient in whom hepatocellular function is relatively preserved but a biliary or portal venous obstructive process predominates, long-term survival may sometimes be obtained with an alternative surgical procedure such as choledochojejunostomy or splenorenal shunt. Frequently there is uncertainty as to hepatic reserve; in such cases, it is well to complete the pretransplant evaluation before commencing alternative therapy, so that if the patient's condition deteriorates suddenly during (or as a result of) that therapy, minimal time is lost moving on to transplantation. In all cases, it must be remembered that liver transplantation for a stable recipient is successful in the large majority of cases and that many temporizing therapies (surgical and medical alike) risk precipitating an emergency condition from a stable one, in addition to worsening the patient's intrinsic anatomic or immunologic status. As patient survival with transplantation continues to improve, the threshold for dispensing with temporizing therapies should be lowered accordingly.

The decision as to when to proceed with transplantation in the stable patient can be agonizing for patient and physician alike; a patient may be fairly well one day and seriously ill with encephalopathy, spontaneous bacterial peritonitis, or variceal hemorrhage the next. As a general rule, once an appropriate patient with chronic liver disease must curtail full-time employment, requires increasing doses of diuretics to control ascites, or has even one significant episode of bleeding from varices or gastritis, it is time to move ahead no matter how he or she may feel otherwise. Optimization of supportive measures during this time—diet, diuretics, vitamin K, and lactulose—should be supplemented with an oral antifungal agent (clotrimazole or nystatin) to minimize infectious risks after transplant.

Acute hepatic failure takes place over days or weeks and has a character distinct from the chronic liver disorders. Most cases are either viral or idiopathic, although a few result from toxic exposure. A critical point arises early on when one attempts to distinguish acute hepatitis, which may resolve spontaneously, from early fulminant hepatic failure. The pattern of rise and fall in the serum aminotransferase values is of little help and often is completely misleading; much more important is the course of the prothrombin time. Persistent or increasing prolongation of the prothrombin time several days into an otherwise ordinary bout of hepatitis should prompt contact with a transplant center. An orderly series of aggressive, expectant measures is indicated, including intravenous hydration, Foley catheter drainage, lactulose given orally or per nasogastric tube, carafate, fresh frozen plasma to keep the prothrombin time within 7 to 8 seconds of control, central venous pressure monitoring, endotracheal intubation, intravenous antibiotics, and hemodialysis. The advent of encephalopathy and renal dysfunction is an ominous sign, and at this point the patient should be appropriately listed for emergency transplantation if this has not already been done. Intravascular volume must be carefully monitored in the oliguric patient, and generally a continuous infusion of fresh frozen plasma with concentrated dextrose as needed provides the safest regimen. A certain amount of brinksmanship is inevitable, since up to 20 percent of these patients recover without transplantation; nonetheless, the odds strongly favor transplantation if a donor can be found before cerebral edema develops. Therefore, when in doubt, it is best to proceed with transplantation.

Matching in liver transplantation consists of blood group and size compatibility only. Unlike in kidney and heart transplantation, HLA matching and a negative lymphocytotoxic cross-match appear to be of minor (if any) importance in liver transplantation. Until recently, all donors were cadaveric; the technical ability to perform segmental liver grafts has allowed early efforts at living-related transplants to proceed in children.

Transplant and After Transplant

At surgery, the entire diseased liver is removed and the donor organ is placed in an orthotopic position. Depending on anatomy, it is frequently necessary to reconstruct the recipient's biliary drainage system, arterial inflow vessels, or portal vein to attain a satisfactory technical result. In most adults, only 10 to 12 units of banked blood are required: blood loss can be much higher in the face of severe portal hypertension, coagulopathy, and prior right upper quadrant surgery.

The postoperative course in liver transplantation is highly variable, but typically entails 3 to 5 days in an intensive care unit and 3 to 5 subsequent weeks on a transplant floor. Rejection episodes, infections, and technical complications are relatively common compared with other forms of solid organ transplantation. Outpatient visits are at weekly intervals for the first 4 to 8 weeks. Three months after transplant a cholangiogram is obtained and, if it is satisfactory, the indwelling T-tube is removed. Follow-up visits are then at monthly intervals for up to 1 year after transplant and decrease in frequency to twice yearly in the long run.

Triple prophylactic immunosuppression with cyclosporine, azathioprine, and a steroid has become standard at most institutions. For the patient with significant renal dysfunction postoperatively, prophylactic OKT3 or antilymphocyte globulin may be used and cyclosporine withheld temporarily. Acute rejection episodes are treated with high-dose steroids or OKT3. A new drug, FK506, has received promising initial reviews as a potent prophylactic agent, although average follow-up time to date is short.

One-year patient survival is 76 percent at institutions servicing a broad mix of population with an aggressive approach to transplantation. By contrast, 1-year survival without transplantation in this group of patients is less than 10 percent. Early graft loss may be caused by primary graft failure, vascular thrombosis, or rejection. Retransplantation is the only treatment. The most common cause of death is infection, most frequently in the setting of severe pretransplant debility or refractory rejection. Late graft loss months or years after transplantation is predominantly attributable to chronic rejection, often with a progressive histologic picture of "vanishing bile ducts." Cirrhosis of a rejecting liver graft is rare, and the prothrombin time is usually preserved; retransplantation is recommended when constitutional factors such as diminished energy reserves, muscle wasting, and pruritus become debilitating. Five-year patient survival, including those who require retransplantation, is 65 percent.

HEART TRANSPLANTATION

Pretransplant

Improvements in immunosuppression and patient survival in the early 1980s led to explosive growth in the number of institutions performing heart transplants and the number of patients receiving transplants. As with kidney and liver transplantation, almost any pathologic process that causes heart failure can be a reason for transplantation. In fact, the list of cardiac diseases leading to transplantation (Table 7) is substantially shorter than that for renal or hepatic failure, and the "menu" of supportive pharmacologic approaches is substantially longer. Nonetheless, the high prevalence of ischemic cardiomyopathy and the lack of preventive or therapeutic modalities for viral and idiopathic cardiomyopathy make for an estimated need of 15,000 cardiac transplants yearly in the United States alone. That the volume of transplants actually performed yearly is only one-tenth of this number testifies largely to a serious donor shortage.

Candidates for heart transplantation should be classified as New York Heart Association cardiac class IV on maximal medical therapy, or should face an especially poor 6- to 12-month prognosis for survival for other reasons (such as recurrent malignant arrhythmias). Contraindications to heart transplantation are listed in Table 8. Age is the most common exclusionary criterion. Young patients with pulmonary hypertension prohibiting heart transplantation should be considered for a heart-lung transplant.

TABLE 7 Cardiac Diseases Leading to Transplantation

Cardiomyopathy	52%
Coronary artery disease	30%
Congenital heart disease	2%
Miscellaneous	16%

TABLE 8 Absolute and Relative Contraindications to Heart Transplantation

Absolute
Pulmonary vascular resistance in excess of 6 Wood units
Preexisting malignancy
Active drug or alcohol abuse
Relative
Age over 55 years
Serious systemic disease such as severe peripheral vascular disease, insulin-dependent diabetes, systemic lupus erythematosus, or amyloidosis
Active infection or unresolved pulmonary infarction
Other serious irreversible organ diseases such as emphysema or cirrhosis
Marked obesity

The evaluation process is outlined in Table 9. Invasive assessment of cardiac reserve is usual, although the patient with very poor ejection fraction (less than 20 percent), elevated wedge pressure (greater than 25 mm Hg), and normal cardiac valves assessed by echocardiography may not need cardiac catheterization to document the need and timing of transplantation adequately. Medical management of the cardiac transplant candidate is the same as for any other patient with similar cardiac pathophysiology, a progression from simple oral inotropes and diuretics to intra-aortic balloon counterpulsation. In those patients for whom there may be a high-risk surgical option, such as the patient with coronary artery disease and ventricular aneurysm, a difficult decision is faced balancing the likelihood of success with conservative surgery against concerns over local donor availability and post-transplant risks. The role of the prosthetic heart and other ventricular assist or oxygenation devices as "bridges" to transplantation in the acutely deteriorating patient is currently under study.

In the recipient with preformed alloantibody, a pretransplant lymphocyte cross-match is required to prevent antibody-mediated rejection. Otherwise matching is by blood group and size, similar to that for liver transplantation.

TABLE 9 Evaluation of the Heart Transplant Candidate

1. Complete history and physical examination (including cervical Papanicolaou smear)
2. Complete blood count with differential
3. Prothrombin time/partial thromboplastin time, platelet count, bleeding time
4. Chemistry profile
5. Urinalysis, urine culture and sensitivity
6. Hepatitis B surface antigen, HIV enzyme-linked immunosorbent assay, herpes simplex virus titer, cytomegalovirus titer
7. ABO typing
8. Human leukocyte antigen typing and screening for panel-reactive antibodies
9. Electrocardiogram, chest x-ray film
10. Pulmonary function tests with arterial blood gases, multigated angiogram
11. Echocardiogram
12. Cardiac catheterization, pulmonary vascular resistance
13. Routine consultation with cardiology, cardiac surgery, psychiatry, and social services; possible consultation with infectious diseases, pulmonary, nephrology, gastroenterology, and gynecology departments

Transplant and After Transplant

At surgery, the recipient is placed on standard cardiopulmonary bypass and the diseased heart is removed by incising through the right and left atria and through the origins of the aorta and pulmonary artery. The graft is then placed in an orthotopic position, and all air is evacuated from the cardiac chambers and vessels. Contraction of the graft usually begins spontaneously as the recipient is warmed. Implantation must be accomplished within 6 hours of organ procurement.

The postoperative course is variable but generally entails 5 to 10 days in the intensive care unit. Isoproterenol is commonly employed initially for support of heart rate during full recovery from preservation. Renal dysfunction is an almost universal concern given multiple prerenal factors preoperatively and acute tubular necrosis related to surgery; however, dialysis is rarely needed. Three weeks on a standard cardiac hospital floor typically follow. Because there is no reliable biochemical or electrophysiologic assay for rejection, fluoroscopically guided endomyocardial biopsies are performed weekly to monitor for rejection. The preoperative condition of the recipient and the immunologic compatibility of the donor and the recipient are again the major determinants of the length of hospitalization. Outpatient follow-up is weekly for 6 to 12 weeks and tapers down to monthly visits by 1 year after transplant.

Immunosuppression with cyclosporine, azathioprine, and prednisone is now standard procedure. The prophylactic use of antilymphocyte agents soon after transplant, coupled with avoidance of nephrotoxic intravenous cyclosporine, is becoming more common. Rejection episodes are treated with steroid, or, if severe or resistant, with rabbit antilymphocyte globulin or OKT3.

One-year patient survival is 80 percent, with most deaths occurring within the first 3 months following transplant. Heart transplant recipients enjoy the highest rehabilitation rate—over 90 percent—of all solid organ recipients. Early death is usually caused by cardiac failure, infection, or rejection, and late death is the result of coronary artery disease. Graft atherosclerosis is an important cause of long-term graft loss not seen in other solid organ transplants; chronic rejection is a likely component of this phenomenon. Retransplantation is the only treatment. Five-year survival rate, including patients undergoing retransplants, is 75 percent.

LONG-TERM COMPLICATIONS OF IMMUNOSUPPRESSION

Although only kidney transplant recipients have been followed in large numbers for more than a decade, it seems clear that liver and heart transplant patients will experience similar long-term risks of immunosuppression. The tremor associated with cyclosporine and the myelotoxic and hepatotoxic effects of azathioprine are all managed by reduction of the dose. Prolonged corticosteroid use is associated with cushingoid side effects of variable severity, and historically with a 15 percent risk of cataract formation or aseptic necrosis of the hip. In addition, osteoporosis may be exacerbated. These problems can be minimized by use of low-dose steroid protocols, and a slow transition to an alternate-day regimen has proved helpful in those who appear particularly sensitive to corticosteroids.

Infectious risks have already been mentioned, and although they seem to peak at 6 to 12 weeks after transplant, a small long-term risk of opportunistic infection continues. Tumor risk progresses over time, however, and seems to reach approximately 6 percent for development of carcinoma of the skin (basal cell and squamous cell) and 3 percent for lymphomas. There appears to be a negligible increase in risk for other cancers. Skin cancers are simply excised, with no change in the patient's immunosuppression status. Lymphomas are usually of the B-cell line, and if polyclonal may respond to simple reduction in immunosuppression. More often they are monoclonal, however, and require cessation of immunosuppression and chemotherapy or radiotherapy. Stage for stage, the prognosis with transplant-related lymphomas appears to be similar to that for the nontransplant population.

SUGGESTED READING

Keown PA, Stiller CR. Kidney transplantation. Surg Clin North Am 1986; 66:517.

Levey AS, Milford EL. Donor and recipient selection. In: Milford EL, Borchner BM, Stein JH, eds. Contemporary issues in nephrology. Vol. 17, Renal transplantation. New York: Churchill Livingstone, 1989.

Schroeder JS, Hunt S. Cardiac transplantation. JAMA 1987; 258:3142.

Shumway SJ, Kaye MP. The International Society for Heart Transplantation Registry. In: Terasaki P, ed. Clinical transplants 1988. Los Angeles: Regents of the University of California, 1989.

Starzl TE, Demetris AJ, Van Thiel D. Liver transplantation. N Engl J Med 1989; 321:1014 and 1092.

RESPIRATOR CARE

ALEXANDER WHITE, M.B., M.R.C.P.I.
LEONARD SICILIAN, M.D.

Intubation and positive pressure mechanical ventilation are required in critically ill patients when oxygenation and carbon dioxide elimination are severely impaired. Inadequate gas exchange usually results from the rapid onset of respiratory failure in patients with decompensated chronic lung disease (e.g., asthma, emphysema, chronic bronchitis), overwhelming pneumonias, cardiogenic pulmonary edema, and the adult respiratory distress syndrome. Ventilatory support also may be necessary in patients with acute chest trauma, drug overdose, and progressive neuromuscular disease when adequate gas exchange cannot be maintained spontaneously.

In this chapter we discuss the routine management of the ventilated patient and review the possible medical complications of ventilatory support. Complications can arise in ventilated patients from the moment of intubation right through to the time of extubation. The airway, the ventilator, or the interaction between patient and machine can generate problems that must be anticipated, prevented, and treated promptly when present.

MONITORING THE PATIENT

Monitoring the respiratory and cardiac status of mechanically ventilated patients is essential to the successful management of patients with respiratory failure. The physician must ensure adequate gas exchange while minimizing the risks of positive pressure. Even though a vast array of sophisticated equipment can be employed to aid in achieving this goal, direct patient observation by the nurse or physician and the interpretation of the arterial blood gas (ABG) levels remain the mainstays. Thus, any new monitoring device must improve our ability to measure pulmonary and cardiac function accurately, thereby leading to improved gas exchange and ventilation of our patients.

Table 1 lists the four different levels of monitoring. Physical examination (level I) and intermittent monitoring (level II) are most widely used. Although this approach clearly is "low tech" given today's electronics, auscultation of the chest is still the quickest way to detect a pneumothorax, and respiratory rates greater than 30 to 40 breaths per minute (counted at the bedside) actually correlate very well with more invasive measurements of respiratory muscle fatigue. The drawback to monitoring by physical examination is that signs of end-organ damage occur in the later stages of injury. For example, hypoxia is far advanced by the time it results in a

TABLE 1 Monitoring of the Intubated and Ventilated Patient

Level of Monitoring	*Advantages*	*Disadvantages*
Level I—Physical examination	Always available	Physical changes of end-organ damage occur late in critical illness
Level II—Intermittent Arterial blood gas levels Chest x-ray film Spirometry and mechanics (FVC, MIF, $\dot{V}_E$, V_D, C_{dyn}, C_{st}, R_{aw})	Widely available May be automated Equipment simple	Changes occur between measurements Some tests require patient cooperation Measurement "crude" compared to controlled laboratory setting
Level III—Continuous Pneumotachography Capnography ($P_{ET}CO_2$) Oximetry (SaO_2) Skin/transcutaneous (Po_2, Pco_2, pH) Breath sound analysis Diaphragmatic EMG Esophageal balloon	Automated Reduces some invasive measurements Detects trends early	Not always available Frequent calibration and equipment check Clinical usefulness still not proved
Level IV—Computer	Rapid processing and display of data Plot trends	Limited availability Costly Clinical usefulness still not proved

*FVC, forced vital capacity; MIF, maximum inspiratory force; $\dot{V}_E$, minute ventilation; V_D, dead space ventilation; C_{dyn}, dynamic compliance; C_{st}, static compliance; R_{aw}, airways resistance; $P_{ET}CO_2$, partial pressure of end tidal CO_2; SaO_2, arterial oxygen saturation; EMG, electromyography.

change in heart rate or rhythm, blood pressure, or level of consciousness.

The ABG measurement is the most useful and widely used form of intermittent monitoring of ventilated patients. This monitoring level also includes serial chest x-ray films and serial measures of pulmonary mechanics used to determine the state of the patient's lungs and the ability of the patient to breathe spontaneously. Clearly, the major disadvantage of intermittent monitoring is that changes can occur between measurements, thereby going undetected.

Continuous monitoring (level III), now becoming increasingly available, may be less invasive than intermittent monitoring in some instances. The accuracy of continuous monitoring devices (e.g., oximetry) is dependent on frequent quality checks and calibrations, and their efficacy (defined as improvement in patient outcome) has not been proved. Finally, computer monitoring (level IV) is becoming increasingly popular. At present, the role of computerized equipment is to gather, process, and display instantaneously data derived from all levels of monitoring devices. In the future, direct feedback control may be available. In these instances the computer may directly activate changes (e.g., changes in ventilation rate or inspired oxygen concentration) based on computation from the monitored data (e.g., Pco_2 and Po_2). In patients monitored by these high tech approaches, the physician and nurse must resist the tendency to "care for" the equipment rather than the patient. High tech monitoring is truly beneficial to the intubated and ventilated patient only when it facilitates optimal decision making and frees the caretakers for more patient contact. Data collection obviously should not be an end point in itself. A more detailed discussion of monitoring patients (and correcting abnormalities discovered) is found in the section on Ventilator Management.

THE AIRWAY: INTUBATION AND ENDOTRACHEAL TUBE MANAGEMENT

Intubation is indicated for (1) relief of upper airway obstruction; (2) protection from aspiration of oropharyngeal contents in patients with impaired sensorium or neuromuscular disease; (3) clearance of pulmonary secretions in individuals who do not have an effective cough; (4) provision of a closed system for mechanical ventilation; and (5) delivery of inspired oxygen (FiO_2) of greater than 60 percent ($FiO_2 > 0.6$). When any of these indications arise, intubation should be carried out rapidly by an individual skilled in this procedure. The majority of complications associated with endotracheal tubes occur at the time of intubation. Thus, if the patient is not cooperative, sedation must be used. Intubation attempts should last no longer than 1 minute, since prolonged attempts may result in severe hypoxemia, causing grand mal seizures, and intense vagal stimulation, causing bradycardia and a reduction in cerebral perfusion. If the endotracheal tube is not passed in less than 1 minute, the patient should be ventilated with a bag and mask for 2 to 3 minutes before another attempt is made. Rarely, it is necessary to pass the endotracheal tube into the trachea under direct vision; this is accomplished by placing the endotracheal tube over a flexible fiberoptic bronchoscope, then passing the bronchoscope through the vocal cords into the trachea. Once the bronchoscope is in position, the endotracheal tube can be advanced over the bronchoscope directly into the trachea. The bronchoscope is then removed, and the airway is established.

We recommend avoiding paralysis of the patient (with succinylcholine or pancuronium bromide) to achieve intubation in all but extreme circumstances. Once these medications are given, intubation *must* be accomplished in 1 to 3 minutes because the patient will be left with no respiratory muscle activity and will be subject to hypoxemic injury if he or she cannot be connected to a mechanical ventilator.

Once the endotracheal tube is placed, the chest should immediately be auscultated. Absent breath sounds bilaterally with abdominal distention suggest esophageal intubation. The tube should be withdrawn and reinserted after a period of ventilation using an Ambu bag. Even if the tube is successfully placed in the trachea, the potential problem of intubation of only the right main stem bronchus must be considered.

Intubation of the right main stem bronchus can be suspected from markedly reduced breath sounds on the left compared with the right side. Intubation of the right main stem bronchus, if left undiagnosed, may cause a number of problems. Hypoxemia may occur as a result of either inadequate overall ventilation or shunting of blood through the underventilated left lung causing ventilation-perfusion (V-Q) mismatch. Other complications include pneumothorax (because all the ventilator volume will be delivered to only one lung), respiratory alkalosis with subsequent predisposition to cardiac arrhythmias, and an inability to suction secretions from the left lung, predisposing the patient to pneumonia. Right main stem bronchus intubation increases the risk of atelectasis of the left lung. The problem is easily corrected by pulling back the tube a few centimeters and listening to the chest again. A chest x-ray film should be taken to confirm correct tube placement; the distal end of the endotracheal tube should be 2 to 3 cm above the carina. The proximal endotracheal tube should be marked at this optimal position at the gum, lip, or anterior nares so that any movement can be easily observed and corrected.

Which type of tube (orotracheal, nasotracheal, or tracheostomy) should be used when a patient requires intubation? As is often the case in medicine, this answer must be individualized. When rapid establishment of an airway is the major goal, orotracheal intubation is the procedure of choice. The exception to this rule is the patient with actual or suspected cervical spine injury; here, manipulation of the neck during tube placement might cause cervical spinal cord damage. In this situation, nasotracheal intubation without neck manipulation or emergency tracheostomy is indicated. Another benefit of an orotracheal tube is that a larger tube can be utilized. The larger tube allows for better suctioning and reduces airways resistance. Both factors are advantageous, especially for patients with preexisting chronic bronchitis or emphysema, the former because secretions are usually a major problem and the latter because the added airway resistance resulting from a small tube may cause respiratory muscle fatigue during weaning. We recommend the placement of at least an 8-mm internal diameter tube in all patients. Tubes less than 7-mm internal diameter markedly increase airways resistance and limit ability to suction secretions from the lower respiratory tract.

Nasotracheal tubes usually have the advantage of making the tube more stable with less chance of accidental extubation or right main stem bronchus intubation. However, because of the size of the nasal passage, a tube of greater than 7- to 7.5-mm internal diameter rarely can be used. Nasotracheal intubation commonly results in epistaxis, which is usually self-limiting unless the patient has a coagulopathy. Maxillary and sphenoid sinusitis and otitis media are other potential complications seen with nasotracheal intubation. They should be considered in all patients who are intubated and subsequently develop fever or facial and ear pain. Skull x-ray films should be done in such patients, in order to determine the presence of sphenoid sinusitis. Sphenoid sinusitis may be fatal if not promptly diagnosed.

In the successfully intubated patient, a sudden loss of expired volume associated with reduced airway pressure may be due to tube dislodgement or cuff leak. When this occurs with an orotracheal or nasotracheal tube, the tube should be repositioned correctly or, if the cuff is at fault, a new endotracheal tube inserted. In the case of a tracheostomy tube, it may not be possible to replace the tube if the tract is not mature (i.e., less than 72 hours old), and in this case, temporary orotracheal intubation should be performed.

Kinking or blockage of the tube with secretions causes elevation of the peak inspiratory pressure delivered by the ventilator and can usually be corrected by manipulating or repositioning the tube and by suctioning, respectively. Aseptic technique must be followed whenever suction catheters are being utilized to clear secretions from the lower respiratory tract.

Tracheomalacia and tracheal stenosis caused by excessive cuff pressure on the tracheal wall are much less common since the advent of high-volume, low-pressure cuffs. However, it is important to adhere to the correct inflation pressures for endotracheal tubes, i.e., cuff pressure must be below the capillary filling pressure of the trachea, which is less than 25 mm Hg. This goal can be accomplished by attaching an aneroid manometer to the external cuff port and reading the cuff pressure directly to determine if the cuff inflation is in the safe range.

Finally, tracheostomy tubes are usually reserved for elective placement in those patients who require permanent or prolonged intubation. At one time tracheostomy was performed on any patient who was intubated for more than 72 hours. Now, because of new tube material and cuff constructions, oro- or nasotracheal tubes may remain in position for 3 to 4 weeks without the need for tracheostomy. Practically, we recommend early tracheostomy to those patients with acute or chronic neuromuscular disease who will have prolonged or lifelong time on ventilatory support. For other patients whose long-term outlook is unclear, we assess them at the end of 2 weeks. If it appears that extubation will not be accomplished in the next 7 to 10 days, we schedule the patient for an elective tracheostomy.

Table 2 lists the advantages and disadvantages of the three routes of intubation. One can see that, for short periods of intubation, other than tracheostomy, there is little difference among the options. For long-term patients, these differences may become important. Endotracheal and tracheostomy tubes bypass the normal pulmonary defense mechanisms and predispose the ventilated patient to aspiration of material from the nasopharynx. When an intubated patient develops dyspnea, hypoxemia, and radiographic changes in the dependent part of the lung, aspiration pneumonia must be suspected. Care of the oral cavity and oropharynx and good aseptic technique when suctioning help prevent aspiration. Once aspiration occurs, the treatment is mainly supportive, although antibiotics may be required if secondary bacterial infection occurs.

VENTILATOR MANAGEMENT

The ventilator itself is a frequent source of complications. Once successfully intubated and ventilated and sometimes sedated and paralyzed, the patient is dependent on the machine for respiration, literally for life itself. Failure of the machine itself or of the alarms, tubing, valves, or circuitry can seriously impair the patient's respiratory status and may lead to death rapidly. The best way to avoid and treat ventilator problems is to have alert and knowledgeable bedside personnel present at all times. Each patient should be assigned a nurse. In addition, the ventilator (including tubing and equipment) should be checked by a respiratory therapist at least once per nursing shift. The nurse and therapist should check the ventilator more frequently if necessary. A basic hourly checklist for nurses should include FiO_2, tidal volume (V_T), intermittent mandatory ventilation/synchronized intermittent mandatory ventilation rate, peak inspiratory pressure (PIP), positive end-expiratory pressure (PEEP), and alarms. Ventilator malfunctions include mechanical failure, alarm failure, overheating of inspired air, and ventilator alarm left in the "off" position. Repeated sounding of the alarm unfortunately remains the commonest reason for the alarm's being switched off. This must not be allowed to happen! Any alarm warrants immediate evaluation of the patient and the ventilator rather than the alarm's being considered a nuisance and simply switched off. Of the items being serially monitored, changes in PIP, V_T, PEEP, and ABG levels are most important.

TABLE 2 Comparison of the Routes of Intubation

	Endotracheal	*Nasotracheal*	*Tracheostomy*
Ease of tube placement	Good with experience	Good with experience	Poor—need controlled surgery
Tube stability	Fair	Good	Good
Access to lower respiratory tract	Good	Good	Good
Resistance to breathing	Varies—depends on tube size	Most—usually smaller tube	Least
Patient acceptance and communication	Poor	Fair	Good

A sudden rise in airway pressure (PIP) may be due to increased airway resistance or reduced pulmonary compliance. Increased resistance may be a result of malposition or blockage of the tube, as previously discussed, or of bronchospasm. Reduced compliance may result from pneumothorax, pneumomediastinum, or pulmonary edema. Pneumothorax is thought to be due to excessive alveolar pressure resulting in overdistention and rupture of alveoli. Pneumothorax occurs in 3 to 5 percent of patients being given positive pressure ventilation and is more common in those with gram-negative bacterial or *Pneumocystis carinii* pneumonia and those requiring PEEP. Physical examination alone is usually insufficient to detect small pneumothoraces; chest x-ray films therefore are mandatory, both on a daily basis and when there is a change in the patient's cardiopulmonary status. If a pneumothorax is seen, intercostal chest tube drainage is usually mandatory.

Sudden loss of V_T can be noted when a discrepancy is detected between the tidal volume setting on the ventilator and the delivered tidal volume. This results in impaired alveolar ventilation and rises in Pco_2. Loss of V_T is usually due to tube malposition or cuff leak, as previously discussed.

PEEP increases transpulmonary pressure at end-expiration and thereby increases functional residual capacity (FRC) of the lung. Reduced FRC is often the most significant factor in pulmonary disease, resulting in V-Q mismatch and systemic hypoxemia. By increasing FRC, PEEP reduces this mismatch and improves oxygenation. By improving FRC, PEEP also improves lung compliance (although excessive PEEP can paradoxically reduce compliance). PEEP improves gas exchange in pulmonary edema and adult respiratory distress syndrome by increasing alveolar volume, not by moving fluid across the alveolocapillary membrane. At levels of PEEP above 10 cm H_2O, cardiac output can be reduced. Cardiac output falls because of reduced venous return secondary to increased intrapleural pressure and by a direct mechanism of unknown cause. In patients with high PEEP levels, pulmonary capillary wedge pressure readings by Swan-Ganz catheterization become unreliable because the catheter is exposed to high alveolar pressure, resulting in a divergence of wedge and left atrial pressures (i.e., wedge pressure may be read as higher than it actually is). Other effects of PEEP include sodium retention, perhaps from preferential perfusion of juxtamedullary nephrons in the kidney, and changes in atrial natriuretic peptide. Water retention with resultant hyponatremia can occur consequent to increased antidiuretic hormone production. Hypotension may occur following institution of positive pressure ventilation, with or without PEEP, and usually responds to volume expansion with normal saline. If this is unsuccessful, other causes of hypotension should be suspected.

Most clinical problems occur at levels of PEEP greater than 10 cm H_2O, and all patients being treated at these levels of PEEP should have Swan-Ganz catheters placed to monitor cardiac output and fluid status. PEEP should be used to reduce the inspired oxygen concentration and thus to avoid oxygen toxicity. The lowest level of PEEP that keeps the PO_2 in the 60 to 70 mm Hg range (while the FIO_2 is less than 0.5) and maintains adequate cardiac output should be chosen. This approach helps to prevent the superimposition of lung injury owing to oxygen toxicity.

Hyperoxia, a well-known cause of lung damage, acts in two ways: a direct cytotoxic effect mediated by so-called free radicals, and an indirect effect mediated by chemotaxis of polymorphonuclear leukocytes recruited to the site of damage. Development of pulmonary oxygen toxicity is directly related to the partial pressure of inspired oxygen and the duration of exposure. Oxygen toxicity must be suspected in any patient receiving an FIO_2 of greater than 0.5 for more than 48 hours. Early symptoms include cough and chest tightness due to tracheobronchitis. As the process progresses, the PaO_2 falls, bilateral parenchymal infiltrates are seen on chest x-ray film, and pulmonary mechanics show a progressive restrictive pattern with loss of compliance. It is reassuring that short-term high FIO_2, i.e., for 24 to 48 hours, seems to be associated with little risk of oxygen toxicity.

Respiratory acidosis occurring in a mechanically ventilated patient indicates inadequate ventilation; the patient, endotracheal tube, and ventilator system should be quickly evaluated. Once blockage of the endotracheal tube has been ruled out and excessive secretions, pneumothorax, and new parenchymal lung disease are not found, the ventilator system must be inspected. A leak resulting in loss of inspired V_T should first be sought and corrected. The ventilator setting also should be checked to ensure that the V_T or rate has not been accidentally lowered. A common cause of respiratory acidosis in the ventilated patient is poor coordination between patient and machine. Poor coordination results in the machine's being unable to deliver the desired V_T. Occasionally sedation or even paralysis of the patient is necessary to restore ventilatory control. In all cases of respiratory acidosis resulting from a problem with the mechanical ventilator, the patient should be manually ventilated with an Ambu bag until the problem is resolved.

By definition, respiratory alkalosis is a complication of overventilation. It can cause cardiac arrhythmias, reduced cardiac output, seizures, reduced lung compliance, increased airways resistance, and V-Q mismatch; hence it should be corrected rapidly by reducing the V_T or the rate delivered by the ventilator. Agitation caused by the endotracheal tube or the patient's disease can result in increased spontaneous breathing during mechanical ventilation. In this instance, the patient may require sedation or paralysis to control ventilation until the underlying problem can be corrected.

THE VENTILATOR-PATIENT UNIT

In addition to care of the endotracheal tube and care of the ventilator per se, the routine care of the ventilated patient must include the interaction between ventilator and patient. From the physician's point of view, any ventilated patient should be fully examined at least once daily. Patient data must be recorded on a flow sheet hourly (at a minimum), and all recorded information should be assessed at least twice daily by the physician. Limited symptoms may be elicited from the patient by asking questions that can be answered by nodding or shaking the head, or a letter board may be used. Full examination must include extremities, especially if an arterial line is inserted, all intravenous sites, pressure areas, calves, and eyes for ulceration. Daily weight measurements are mandatory and are a useful guide to fluid retention because edema may collect in areas not easily seen; input and output charts also should be carefully assessed for evidence of fluid accumulation. All central lines should be changed every 3 days or sooner if the site appears infected. Swan-Ganz catheters should be removed after 48 hours. ABG levels should be checked 30 minutes after the patient has been intubated and a similar time after any readjustments are made in the ventilator. An ABG determination also should be obtained any time a significant clinical deterioration is observed that might be caused by a change in pulmonary status.

A chest x-ray study must be performed daily and when there is any significant change in the patient's cardiopulmonary status. In particular, the position of the endotracheal tube, Swan-Ganz catheter, and central lines should be noted. The lung pathology should be followed and a pneumothorax and/or pneumomediastinum looked for in all ventilated patients, especially those requiring PEEP. Pleural effusion and lobar collapse are sometimes difficult to spot on films in the supine position that are usually obtained in the intensive care unit. Thus, chest x-ray films should be reviewed daily by the physician with a radiologist. A complete blood count, electrolyte levels, ABG levels, drug levels, urinalysis, and an electrocardiogram usually are ordered on a routine basis.

Other measures that should be performed routinely include moving the endotracheal tube from one side of the mouth to the other and retaping it every 12 hours. Endotracheal tube cuff pressure should be checked every 12 hours to ensure it is less than 25 mm Hg. Suctioning is performed as required to maintain patent airways and should be done with strict aseptic technique. Chest physical therapy performed every 4 hours also helps to mobilize secretions. FIO_2, peak inspiratory pressures, tubing, spirometer alarms, humidifier heat and water levels, and temperature of inspired gas should all be checked every hour by nursing staff and every nursing shift by the respiratory therapists.

The essence of care of the intubated and ventilated patient is regular and routine checking of the patient, the endotracheal tube, and the ventilator. If the physician has the knowledge of all potential problems and the expertise to correct them quickly, the result will be a successful patient outcome.

SUGGESTED READING

Barlett J, Gorbach S. The triple threat of aspiration pneumonia. Chest 1975; 68:560–566.

Bone RC. Monitoring respiratory function in the patient with adult respiratory distress syndrome. Semin Respir Med 1981; 2:140–150.

Deneke SM, Fanburg BL. Oxygen toxicity of the lung: An update. Br J Anaesth 1982; 54:737–749.

Fallat RJ. Respiratory monitoring. Clin Chest Med 1982; 3:181–194.

Jackson RM. Pulmonary oxygen toxicity. Chest 1985; 88:900–905.

Messeter KH, Pettersson KL. Endotracheal intubation with the fiberoptic bronchoscope. Anesthesia 1980; 35:294–297.

Prakash O, Meij S, Zeelenberg C, van der Borden B. Computer based patient monitoring. Crit Care Med 1982; 10:811–822.

Tintinalli JE, Claffey J. Complications of nasotracheal intubation. Ann Emerg Med 1981; 10:142–144.

Tyler DC. Positive end-expiratory pressure: a review. Crit Care Med 1983; 11:300–308.

Weissman IM, Rinaldo JE, Rogers RM. Positive end-expiratory pressure in adult respiratory failure. N Engl J Med 1982: 307:1381–1384.

Zwillich CW, Pierson DJ, Creach GE, et al. Complications of assisted ventilation. A prospective study of 354 consecutive episodes. Am J Med 1974; 57:161–170.

BLOOD PURIFICATION AND EXCHANGE

HOWARD L. CORWIN, M.D.

In many clinical conditions, circulating factors either may be involved in the pathogenesis of the disorder or may be directly responsible for organ damage. Over the last several decades, a variety of methods have been introduced to purify blood of these pathogenic factors. The techniques differ greatly in their ability to remove particular classes of toxins as well as in the side effects associated with toxin removal. The procedure used, therefore, depends on the characteristics of the toxin or toxins to be removed as well as the patient's disease.

This chapter reviews the major techniques utilized for blood purification: hemodialysis, hemofiltration, peritoneal dialysis, hemoperfusion, and plasma exchange/pheresis. The focus of the discussion is on the application of these techniques to acute clinical disorders.

HEMODIALYSIS

Hemodialysis was the first widely employed method of blood purification and is still the most common technique used. In conventional hemodialysis, removal of solute (toxins) occurs by diffusion across a semipermeable membrane. Fluid removal is facilitated by the application of hydrostatic pressure across the membrane. The hydrostatic pressure also results in increased solute removal via convectional forces (solvent drag). However, under most circumstances, diffusion accounts for most of the clearance of toxins. Because of the importance of diffusion for clearance, molecular size is an important determinant in the removal of toxins by hemodialysis. Removal by hemodialysis is best for substances of low molecular weight (less than 500 daltons) as well as those that are not highly protein-bound or lipid-soluble. Other important factors determining clearance include the dialysate and blood flow rate, the surface area and permeability of dialysis membrane, and the concentration gradient between dialysate and blood.

The major advantage of hemodialysis is that clearance is rapid. This characteristic makes it an ideal choice for treatment of drug overdose (if the drug is dialyzable), for life-threatening metabolic abnormalities such as hyperkalemia, or for volume overload. Unfortunately, the rapidity of correction contributes to some of the important complications seen with hemodialysis.

The most common complication associated with hemodialysis is hypotension, occurring in 20 to 50 percent of patients undergoing acute hemodialysis. The etiology of the hypotension is multifactorial. Patients who are hemodynamically unstable, such as those who have sepsis or underlying cardiac disease, are particularly susceptible. Rapid volume removal can clearly lead to hypotension; however, sequential ultrafiltration followed by conventional hemodialysis is often tolerated better than simultaneous ultrafiltration and dialysis, suggesting that factors other than volume are involved. Changes in osmolality induced by dialysis may be an important variable. Raising dialysate sodium concentration has been found by some investigators to be associated with fewer episodes of hypotension. Finally, acetate-containing dialysis fluid may also contribute to hemodynamic instability during dialysis. Although it is still controversial, the use of bicarbonate rather than acetate dialysis fluid is probably best for the hemodynamically unstable patient.

The rapid shifts in fluid and electrolytes that occur during hemodialysis can be associated with the dialysis disequilibrium syndrome. Symptoms of this disorder range from headache, nausea, and restlessness in mild cases to seizure, coma, and death in severe cases. The dialysis disequilibrium syndrome is usually seen after vigorous dialysis of severely uremic patients with acute renal failure. The precise etiology of this syndrome is still not established, but it appears to be related to cerebral edema resulting from idiogenic osmoles in the brain, urea shifts, and/or alterations of cerebrospinal fluid pH. Disequilibrium can be avoided by using shorter, more frequent dialysis treatments when initiating hemodialysis in severely uremic patients. The addition of osmotically active agents such as urea, dextrose, glycerol, or mannitol to the dialysate has also been employed with variable success.

Hypoxemia is often observed during acute hemodialysis, with the PaO_2 falling as much as 10 to 20 mm Hg. This phenomenon is multifactorial and may result from complement-mediated pulmonary leukostasis, the consequences of acetate metabolism, and decreased respiratory drive caused by carbon dioxide loss during dialysis. In most clinical situations, the fall in PaO_2 is not clinically significant; however, in the critically ill patient with borderline pulmonary function, the fall in PaO_2 may produce symptomatic hypoxemia.

To prevent clotting of the dialyzer during dialysis, systemic anticoagulation with heparin is generally used. Of course, anticoagulation presents a significant risk to patients who are actively bleeding or who are at high risk of bleeding. Several approaches to this problem have been employed. In some patients as much as a 50 percent reduction in the total heparin dose can be achieved by low-dose continuous infusion of heparin. Regional heparinization using a protamine infusion on the venous side of the dialyzer to reverse the heparin given on the arterial limb has also been used, but this procedure carries the risk of allergic reactions to protamine as well as rebound anticoagulation attributable to heparin-protamine complexes. More recently, heparin-free dialysis has been utilized effectively, and this procedure represents the best alternative for the patient at risk of bleeding.

The use of hemodialysis requires obtaining vascular access. In patients who require dialysis acutely, access to the circulation is simplest with single-needle dialysis. The catheter can be inserted in either the femoral or the subclavian vein. Femoral catheterization is both easy to perform and generally without serious complication. Nonetheless, these catheters usually must be removed after 24 to 48 hours, and they require that the patient remain in the supine position in bed. Subclavian catheters can be used for longer periods of time, but they are associated with more insertion-related complications (e.g., pneumothorax, hemothorax, and air embolism). Therefore, a femoral catheter is preferable if only one or two dialysis treatments are contemplated (e.g., as in a drug overdose). A subclavian catheter is a better choice if prolonged dialysis is necessary (e.g., in patients with oliguric acute renal failure). If temporary access is required for several months, subclavian catheters with Dacron cuffs can be tunneled through the skin, which minimizes the risk of infection. Scribner shunts are rarely used today.

Hemodialysis is used primarily for removal of uremic toxins and correction of fluid and electrolyte abnormalities associated with renal failure. The ability of hemodialysis to correct fluid and metabolic abnormalities rapidly makes it the ideal treatment for acute renal failure, particularly if life-threatening complications are present. Unfortunately, the rapidity of correction may also lead to the central nervous system problems described above. Absolute indications for initiating dialysis in acute renal failure are severe acidosis, volume overload, hyperkalemia, and uremic encephalopathy. However, dialysis should be initiated, if possible, before the patient develops these metabolic complications. At what point in the course of acute renal failure dialysis should be initiated depends on clinical judgment. Although definitive clinical studies are lacking, my bias is that patients benefit from early and frequent dialysis. When volume overload is a major problem, ultrafiltration alone or sequential ultrafiltration and hemodialysis can be employed for better hemodynamic tolerance.

Hemodialysis has been used for many years for the treatment of intoxications. It is most effective with low molecular weight substances that are not highly protein-bound or lipid-soluble. Hemoperfusion (see further on) has now replaced hemodialysis as the treatment of choice for many intoxications. Hemodialysis still remains the preferred treatment for intoxication with methanol or ethylene glycol or severe salicylate or lithium toxicity.

Because of the high molecular weight of immune complexes, immunoglobulins, and paraproteins, hemodialysis is not effective in removing them.

HEMOFILTRATION

Hemofiltration, an alternative technique to hemodialysis, depends upon convective rather than diffusive forces for the removal of solutes. An ultrafiltrate of plasma is created by exerting a hydrostatic force across a semipermeable membrane, and solutes are carried across the membrane by bulk flow (solvent drag). A substitution fluid is used to replace the lost plasma ultrafiltrate. Clearance of all solutes that cross the membrane is equal to the ultrafiltration rate. This method allows for the removal of larger molecules (up to 15,000 to 30,000 daltons) than can be removed by hemodialysis; however, small solutes are better removed by hemodialysis.

Hemofiltration is better tolerated than hemodialysis in that associated hypotensive episodes are fewer and less severe. In addition, to the extent that large molecules may be involved in causing the uremic syndrome, hemofiltration would be the preferred method of dialysis. The large volume of substitution fluid necessary during hemofiltration makes its use less practical than conventional hemodialysis.

Hemofiltration is still not widely used, and its role in the treatment of the patient with renal failure is still unclear. A derivative technique, however, combining diffusive and convective solute removal termed hemodiafiltration has evoked recent interest. Because of its increased efficiency over conventional dialysis, application of hemodiafiltration has allowed shorter dialysis treatment times for the patient receiving chronic dialysis.

A second technique deriving from hemofiltration, termed continuous arteriovenous hemofiltration (CAVH), has become of major importance in the treatment of acute renal failure. In CAVH, the pressure gradient between artery and vein drives the formation of an ultrafiltrate of plasma across a membrane. Simultaneous with the formation of the ultrafiltrate, the blood volume is reconstituted by the infusion of an electrolyte solution identical to normal plasma. The goal of CAVH is to form at least 500 to 1,000 ml per hour of ultrafiltrate (12 to 24 L per day). If all or most of the ultrafiltrate is replaced, adequate clearance can be provided for most patients. On the other hand, the amount of net volume removal is determined by the difference between the replacement fluid given and the ultrafiltrate formed. Because replacement and ultrafiltration are continuous, CAVH provides a method of removing large fluid volumes gradually over the course of a day or days. For example, if the ultrafiltrate exceeds replacement by as little as 100 ml per hour, 2.4 L of fluid will be removed over a 24-hour period.

CAVH is a particularly effective method for removing large volumes of fluid without causing hemodynamic compromise. It is most useful in the patient who is volume overloaded but too hemodynamically unstable to tolerate hemodialysis. Patients who have undergone major surgical procedures frequently are in this group. Because a patient's obligate daily fluid intake (e.g., antibiotics, hyperalimentation) can be used as part of the replacement fluid, CAVH is particularly valuable in the oliguric patient who requires large amounts of hyperalimentation. It also prevents the large interdialytic volume gains often seen in patients maintained on hemodialysis.

Although CAVH predictably controls volume, it may not provide adequate solute clearance. This difference results in part from the unpredictability in the amount of ultrafiltrate that is formed when blood flow rates are low and blood pressure is low. To improve solute clearance, some investigators have incorporated a continuous flow of dialysate around the CAVH filter, an alternative that adds a component of diffusive clearance (continuous arteriovenous hemofiltration with dialysis, CAVHD). Other modifications that have been attempted to improve the ultrafiltration rate and therefore increase clearance are pre-post dilution and/or the attachment of a vacuum pump for suction on the filtration port. CAVHD is probably the modification of choice if increased clearance is needed. In highly catabolic patients, intermittent hemodialysis treatments are necessary to control uremia. The slow continuous clearance that CAVH provides is not appropriate for the treatment of acute metabolic emergencies, e.g., hyperkalemia. In clinical situations in which immediate treatment is indicated, hemodialysis is the appropriate choice. Once metabolic control is achieved, it can often be maintained using CAVH.

CAVH requires the insertion of both an arterial and a venous catheter. Usually catheterizing the femoral artery and vein works best, although the radial artery is also occasionally used. Because continuous heparinization is required, CAVH must be used with caution in the patient at risk for bleeding.

PERITONEAL DIALYSIS

Peritoneal dialysis (PD) clears solutes from blood predominantly via diffusion across the peritoneal membrane. However, solute clearance also occurs via convection (solute drag) accompanying ultrafiltration. As compared with hemodialysis, PD is better at removing "middle molecules" (500 to 3,000 daltons) but is relatively less effective at removing small solutes (less than 500 daltons). Solute clearance depends upon multiple factors, including dialysate flow rate (number and volume of dialysis exchanges) and characteristics of the peritoneal membrane, such as surface area, thickness, and blood supply. Ultrafiltration similarly depends upon the characteristics of the peritoneal membrane but is predominantly influenced by the osmotic gradient generated by the high concentration of glucose in the dialysate.

To improve clearance in a patient undergoing acute PD, the only variables that can be manipulated easily are the volume of fluid instilled into the peritoneal cavity and the number of exchanges. The maximal dialysate volume instilled is 2 L; however, in the 24 to 48 hours after insertion of a PD catheter, smaller volumes are usually employed. The number of exchanges that can be done is inversely related to dialysate dwell time. A point is reached, however, when a proportionally greater amount of time is spent infusing and draining as opposed to dwelling. At this exchange rate, further increasing the number of exchanges is not helpful. From a practical standpoint, hourly exchange (10-minute infusion, 30-minute dwell, 20-minute drain) is the maximal rate.

As noted before, ultrafiltration is greatly affected by the concentration of glucose in the dialysate. High glucose concentrations lead to a larger osmotic gradient across the peritoneal membrane and thus favor fluid removal. To the extent that ultrafiltration is increased, there may also be increased clearance of solutes via convective forces (solvent drag). Standard glucose concentrations are 1.5 percent, 2.5 percent, or 4.25 percent. Volume removal (ultrafiltration) also can be increased by increasing the rate of exchange; thus to alter the amount of volume removed in a patient undergoing PD, the concentration of glucose, or the number of exchanges, or both, may be varied. Changes in dwell volume have little effect on ultrafiltration.

Because PD allows continuous and gradual correction of metabolic and volume abnormalities, it does not subject the patient to the same risk of hypotension or disequilibrium as acute hemodialysis. A further advantage, in contrast to hemodialysis and CAVH, is that anticoagulation is not required. As with CAVH, however, the slow correction of abnormalities unfortunately also proves to be the major disadvantage of PD. Peritoneal dialysis is not suitable for the acute treatment of intoxications, life-threatening electrolyte abnormalities, or acute volume overload. If technically possible, however, PD is the optimal treatment for the patient with acute renal failure. If initiated early in the course of acute renal failure, PD often prevents uremic complications. If necessary, PD can be initiated simultaneously with either hemodialysis or CAVH. Once the acute problem is stabilized, PD is effective in maintaining metabolic and fluid balance, and then hemodialysis or CAVH can be discontinued.

Insertion of a temporary stylet PD catheter can be done at the bedside under local anesthetic, but even in the most experienced hands this "blind" procedure can be complicated by bowel perforation or major bleeding. Catheter placement is more safely performed under direct visualization through a small abdominal incision under local anesthetic in the operating room or at the bedside. Prior abdominal surgery makes placement under direct visualization mandatory.

Peritoneal dialysis is rarely absolutely contraindicated. Abdominal conditions that limit the surface area of peritoneum available for dialysis or severe adhesions are likely to result in ineffective dialysis. In addition, communication between the pleural space and peritoneal cavity makes it necessary to discontinue PD because the accumulation of dialysate in the pleural space can interfere with respiratory function. Patients with severe pulmonary disease are at risk for further compromise of their pulmonary function by dialysate in the abdomen. This complication usually occurs only if large volumes (2 L) are used. Finally, although it is not absolutely contraindicated, PD should be avoided if possible in the immediate postoperative period following abdominal surgery. Leakage of dialysate through the incision can lead to peritonitis and interfere with wound healing.

The major acute complications of PD are related to catheter insertion (as noted above) and infections of the catheter tract, exit site, or peritoneum. Treatment is initiated for peritonitis if more than 100 white blood cells are seen in the PD fluid, with more than 50 percent polymorphonuclear cells on differential count. Other acute complications include hyperglycemia, dialysate leaks, pancreatitis, hydrothorax, and wound dehiscence. It should be noted that free air may be seen under the diaphragm in patients undergoing PD and does not necessarily indicate bowel perforation.

HEMOPERFUSION

In hemoperfusion, anticoagulated blood is passed over a sorbent system that clears the blood of a toxin by adsorption. These systems have thin, highly porous membranes and a large surface area. Hemoperfusion is most commonly used in the emergency treatment of severe drug intoxications. It has also been used on occasion to clear the blood of "middle molecules" in patients with uremia. Large molecules (up to 40,000 daltons) can be removed, as can lipid-soluble substances. Therefore compared with hemodialysis or peritoneal dialysis, it is more efficient in treating intoxications.

Sorbents that are used include activated charcoal, ion exchange resins, and macroporous resins. The "activation" of charcoal (carbon) induces pores and increases surface area greatly. Toxins will adsorb to the charcoal. Ion exchange resins exchange one ion for another of similar charge, maintaining electrical neutrality. Macroporous resins are non-ionic, gel resins formed into beads. They adsorb organic solutes well and are effective in removing lipid-soluble solutes.

Charcoal hemoperfusion is the most widely utilized and removes most intoxicants. In some situations hemoperfusion may not have as dramatic a clinical effect as would be expected based on high drug extraction ratios. This discrepancy is a result of a variety of factors such as drug distribution in the body and drug movement between body compartments.

Hemoperfusion requires vascular access and anticoagulation and shares many of the complications of hemodialysis. In addition, hemoperfusion results in loss of clotting factors, thrombocytopenia, and occasionally mild hypothermia. Microembolization was a problem in the past but has been eliminated.

Recently, hemoperfusion columns containing particles coated with either antibody or antigen have been used to remove immune proteins from the blood. These immunoadsorbent techniques are of great interest for future treatment of immune-mediated diseases.

PLASMA EXCHANGE AND PLASMAPHERESIS

Plasma exchange or plasmapheresis is a method that clears pathogenic macromolecules from the circulation. Plasma is separated from the cellular elements of whole blood and replaced by either crystalloid (plasmapheresis) or a protein-containing solution (plasma exchange). Initially plasma was separated and removed relatively unselectively, but recently attempts have been made to remove pathogenic components selectively.

Centrifugation methods are available that nonselectively separate plasma from blood. The plasma obtained is then discarded, whereas the cellular elements and replacement fluid are reinfused. Cascade membrane filtration involves the separation of plasma by a membrane into low and high molecular weight fractions. The low molecular weight fraction containing albumin is returned to the patient, whereas the high molecular weight fraction containing the supposed pathogenic macromolecule as well as nonpathogenic macromolecules is discarded. Cryopheresis utilizes cooling to cause cryoprecipitates to form, and these cryoprecipitates are then separated from the plasma. Fractionation based on molecular charge and mobility as well as physiochemical properties has also been employed.

Regardless of the method employed for separation, following plasma exchange the plasma concentration of removed protein quickly begins to rise. This increase is initially the result of redistribution, but the subsequent rise is caused by resynthesis of protein. In immune-mediated diseases, cytotoxic drugs usually are required to blunt the resynthesis.

The clinical value of plasma exchange or pheresis is not well substantiated, largely because evidence of effectiveness has been adduced from case reports and uncontrolled trials. For example, contrary to numerous case reports of dramatic results of plasmapheresis in lupus nephritis, a multicenter controlled trial failed to demonstrate any benefit of plasmapheresis over conventional therapy. Although convincing data are not available in many instances, consensus on the use of plasma exchange has developed for some diseases. In the case of renal diseases, plasma exchange or pheresis appears to be of benefit in anti–glomerular basement membrane disease, cryoglobulinemia, rapidly progressive glomerulonephritis, thrombotic thrombocytopenic purpura, acute renal failure due to myeloma or light-chain disease, and hyperviscosity syndromes. A beneficial effect is less apparent in vasculitis, including Wegener's and polyarteritis, systemic lupus erythematosus, IgA nephritis, and membranoproliferative glomerulonephritis. Plasma exchange or pheresis may also be of benefit in management of myasthenia gravis, multiple sclerosis, Eaton-Lambert syndrome, Guillain-Barré syndrome, chronic inflammatory demyelinating polyneuropathy, and paraprotein-associated neuropathy. More controlled studies are needed to define the role of plasma exchange and plasmapheresis more clearly. Methods to remove proteins from plasma are likely to become increasingly important as more pathogenic proteins are identified.

SUGGESTED READING

Garella S. Extracorporeal techniques in the treatment of exogenous intoxications. Kidney Int 1988; 33:735–754.

Friedman EA. The role of plasmapheresis in nephritic syndromes: Critical assessment of purported benefits. In: Nairins RG, ed.

Controversies in nephrology and hypertension. New York: Churchill Livingstone, 1984:487–493.
Kincaid-Smith P. The role of plasmapheresis in nephritic syndromes: The case for plasmapheresis. In: Nairins RG, ed. Controversies in nephrology and hypertension. New York: Churchill Livingstone, 1984:463–485.
Nissenson AR, Fine RN, Gentile DE. Clinical dialysis. Norwalk, CT: Appleton & Lange, 1990.

DRUG REACTIONS

DOROTHY D. SOGN, M.D.
PAUL P. VanARSDEL Jr., M.D.

The frequency of drug reactions is unknown. By estimate, in excess of 1 million American outpatients have drug reactions, necessitating 50,000 hospitalizations per annum. Additionally some believe that as many as 30 percent of all hospitalized patients (each receiving a mean of nine drugs) develop drug reactions. Most of these clinical events (approximately 75 percent) are nonimmunologic and are outlined in Table 1. According to the Coombs and Gell classification, there are four major types of immune mediated reactions.

CLASSIFICATION OF IMMUNE MEDIATED DRUG REACTIONS

The type I or immediate type of hypersensitivity reaction is responsible for common allergic reactions, including hay fever, some types of asthma, and hives as well as drug reactions leading to urticaria, angioedema, bronchospasm, hypotension, and anaphylactic shock. This type of reaction is mediated by immunoglobulin E (IgE). Drug reactions with clinical manifestations identical to type I reactions but not involving IgE are known as anaphylactoid reactions.

Type II reactions are dependent on complement and involve antibody directed against a cell membrane or cell membrane associated antigen, exemplified by certain drug induced anemias or thrombocytopenias.

Type III reactions are mediated by antigen-antibody complexes and are best illustrated by serum sickness reactions.

In the type IV reactions, sensitized thymus dependent lymphocytes are the mediators. Classic examples are contact dermatitides such as poison ivy, but can include contact type reactions to drugs such as neomycin and drug additives such as parabens and ethylenediamine.

An approach to drug allergy must comprise an understanding of the prevention, diagnosis, and treatment of these reactions. The focus in this article is the management of anaphylactic and anaphylactoid drug reactions.

PREVENTION AND DIAGNOSIS

As with other types of allergies, avoidance of the offending allergen is the best approach to management. Since avoiding a needed drug is not always an option, it is useful to screen patients at high risk for an allergic reaction to a given drug. For these reasons discussions of diagnosis and prevention are virtually inseparable when considering drug allergy.

In diagnosing drug allergy, as a first step a careful history of prior drug reactions must be obtained. Attention must be given to such factors as the nature and timing of the reaction, whether concurrent medications were being taken, and the nature of the underlying illness.

In the many cases when the history is ambiguous or multiple drugs are suspected, a confirmatory immunoassay would be of great help. Unfortunately such assays

TABLE 1 Examples of Nonallergic Drug Reactions*

Overdosage
May result from impaired handling of normal doses or excess intake
Example: theophylline induced vomiting and headaches
Idiosyncratic reactions
May result from unusual resistance to large doses or unexpected responses to ordinary or even low doses
Example: Isoniazid induced polyneuritis
Side effects or unavoidable nontherapeutic effects
Example: Tremulousness induced by metaproterenol (Alupent, Metaprel)
Paradoxical effects or effects opposite those expected
Example: Sedative induced hyperactivity
Drug interactions
Example: Deep sleep induced by simultaneous ingestion of tranquilizers and alcohol

*From Sogn D. How to avoid allergic reactions. Drug Therapy Clinical Therapeutics in the Hospital 1983; 73–81.

are few. The diagnostic value of skin testing with penicillin major and minor determinants has been discussed elsewhere, and as of this writing, a minor determinant mix is not commercially available. Prick and intradermal skin testing also should be employed prior to administration of protein or polypeptide agents such as heterologous antisera, including antithymocyte globulin and the increasingly used therapeutic monoclonal antibodies. Prick and, if negative, intradermal skin testing, read at 20 minutes, with dilutions 1/10 and 1/100, respectively, of these agents will reveal the presence or absence of reaginic antibody to these substances. Such testing is helpful only in predicting the risk of the immediate type of hypersensitivity.

When a convincing history of drug allergy with or without confirmatory immunoassay is obtained, reassessment of the need for the drug should be undertaken. This reassessment may include culture documentation of bacterial or viral infections or the ordering and review of other laboratory data. If the need for the drug is affirmed, consideration of an alternative drug should be pursued. Factors such as efficacy, side effects, and possible cross reactivity with the drug to which the patient is allergic must be weighed in making a decision.

Occasionally a drug can be administered even in the face of a convincing history of reaction to it. Such is the case with known anaphylactoid reactors to injection with radiographic contrast dye who are in need of a repeat procedure. The risk of a repeat reaction in such a patient ranges from 17 to 35 percent. A prophylactic regimen consisting of prednisone, 50 mg orally every 6 hours for three administrations and ending 1 hour prior to the procedure, and diphenhydramine, 50 mg intramuscularly 1 hour before the procedure, has been shown to reduce the risk of repeat reactions to 10.8 percent (usually minor skin reactions). The addition of ephedrine sulfate (25 mg) to this regimen was associated with a lessening of the reaction incidence to 5 percent. The addition of cimetidine hydrochloride was not useful; 14 reactions occurred during 100 procedures (14.0 percent).

A not infrequent clinical situation is that of the egg sensitive individual in need of immunization. Mumps, measles, influenza, typhus, and yellow fever vaccines are grown on materials originating from chickens, such that trace amounts of ovalbumin (0.5 to 1.0 ng) can be detected in these products. Reports of anaphylaxis in children with known egg allergy have occasioned a closer look at this population in which IgE directed against the ovalbumin in the vaccine could be detected. Results of these studies indicate that only patients with histories of anaphylactic reactions to egg are at high risk. These patients should undergo skin testing by the prick or scratch method with a 1/10 dilution of the vaccine, followed by intradermal testing with a 1/100 dilution if the result is negative. Negative responders have safely received the vaccine, but positive responders (with positive histories) should receive the vaccine only by slow incremental dosing.

A variation in the treatment of herniated lumbar disks came with the commercial availability of a papaya tree derived enzyme called chymopapain, which is capable of solubilizing the mucopolysaccharide of the human nucleus pulposus. Some 200,000 Americans are thought to be candidates for this procedure annually. A major drawback to this therapy is the development of anaphylaxis in an estimated 1 percent of the recipients. As a result of this observation, it has been appreciated that a large number of people outside the papain industry are exposed to and become sensitized to this substance through numerous exposures, including debriding ointments, digestive aids, some contact lens solutions, meat tenderizers, and beer. Thus, a careful history for papain hypersensitivity must be obtained. Since the procedure is performed with the aid of radiographic contrast dye, this hypersensitivity must also be ruled out. Premedication of the patient with antihistamines and steroids cannot be relied upon in the prevention of chymopapain induced anaphylaxis. Patterson et al recommend the skin testing of candidates for these injections with chymopapain dilutions in saline with 0.1 percent human serum albumin as a stabilizer, proceeding with the medication only in skin test negative patients. Clinical trials to further study the efficacy of such screening techniques are about to commence.

Anaphylactoid reactions to aspirin affect about 1 million Americans. Reactions usually manifest as either wheezing or urticaria. About 4 percent of all asthmatics demonstrate aspirin sensitivity by exacerbations of wheezing. Another small group of asthmatics suffer from a triad of symptoms consisting of chronic sinusitis, nasal polyposis, and severe (usually late onset) asthma in addition to aspirin sensitivity. Because this reaction is not IgE mediated, patients can tolerate chemically similar compounds, including naturally occurring salicylates, but not certain nonsteroidal anti-inflammatory compounds such as mefenamic acid (Ponstel), ibuprofen (Motrin, Rufen), phenylbutazone, fenoprofen (Nalfon), naproxen (Anaprox, Naprosyn), and flufenamic acid. The diagnosis is usually made through the history; only occasionally is provocation testing needed. Acetaminophen is a useful aspirin substitute in these patients. The possible usefulness of aspirin desensitization for the treatment of asthma in certain aspirin sensitive asthmatics remains an intriguing therapeutic possibility.

DRUG ADDITIVES

Drug reactions may be induced by additives used to color or preserve drug preparations. Of particular concern are additives in medications used to treat allergic conditions, because they not only cause reactions but may confuse the diagnosis.

Certain stabilizing and bacteriostatic additives, such as ethylenediamine, thimerosol, and parabens, which are in some skin preparations, are associated with the induction of contact dermatitis (Coombs and Gell type IV). On re-exposure to these substances, even by another route, the patient may have a reaction.

Fisher described ethylenediamine allergic patients who experienced a hematogenous contact type of dermatitis upon receipt of theophylline ethylenediamine (aminophylline), or certain antihistamines. Patients receiving paraben containing medications can experience similar reactions. Thimerosal is a common contact sensitizer with widespread use, including some contact lens solutions and many vaccines. Very few data exist relating to challenging patients with clinical histories of thimerosal sensitivity or positive skin test results with this chemical.

Metabisulfites, antibrowning agents used in many foods and medications, are increasingly appreciated as inducing asthmatic attacks. Steroid dependent asthmatics are considered at high risk for these reactions.

Desensitization, the administration of a drug by cautious incremental dosing, also can be undertaken when use of an allergy provoking drug is unavoidable. Although termed "desensitization," the exact mechanism(s) explaining this phenomenon is unknown; hypotheses include consumption of IgE in immune complexes, hapten inhibition, mast cell desensitization, and mediator depletion. This procedure is risky and should be undertaken in a controlled setting such as an intensive care unit where full capability for resuscitation is available. Guidelines for the treatment of anaphylaxis are shown in Table 2.

A general scheme for such drug administration consists of the subcutaneous administration of 0.1 ml of the concentration of the material giving the smallest positive skin reaction. The dose is progressively doubled every 15 to 30 minutes if tolerated until 1 ml of the undiluted medication has been administered. At this point the route is switched to intramuscular and then the full dose is given.

Allergic symptoms are treated as they occur and the timing of drug administration is adjusted accordingly, no further dosing being given until symptoms have resolved. Some allergists prefer to premedicate patients undergoing desensitization, hoping to mitigate reactions; others do not premedicate, reasoning that early warning of major allergic reactions may be masked by such therapy.

Desensitization regimens have been tailored for insulin and penicillin allergy and are discussed elsewhere. Of particular interest because of its safety is the successful oral desensitization to penicillin associated with antigen specific desensitization of tissue mast cells.

Because performing a densensitization regimen is likely to be associated with provocation of symptoms, this is a logical point in the discussion to mention treatment modalities.

TABLE 2 Summary Outline of Anaphylaxis Treatment

General
- Epinephrine
- Tourniquet (when physically possible)
- Intravenous line, dextrose, in 0.5 normal saline
- Oxygen and emergency equipment on hand

Hypotension
- Epinephrine, slow intravenous; large volumes of dextrose in 0.5 normal saline
- ECG monitor
- Monitor central venous pressure
- Vasopressor drug (?)

Upper airway obstruction
- Epinephrine
- Diphenhydramine
- Oxygen
- Endotrachial intubation or tracheostomy

Lower airway obstruction
- Epinephrine, isoproterenol
- Oxygen
- Aminophylline, intravenous
- Prepare for treatment of respiratory failure

Cardiac problems
- ECG monitor for dysrhythmias
- Monitor pulmonary artery wedge pressure
- Isoproterenol for cardiogenic shock

Late reactions
- Observe and monitor as necessary for 12 hours
- Glucocorticoid therapy

TREATMENT

Reactions that are thought to be allergic are listed in Table 3. Their clinical features are not discussed here except as they determine the type of treatment needed. In general, if a reaction develops, treatment with the suspected drug or drugs should be stopped unless, in the physician's judgment, the need for treatment is greater than the risk of the reaction and its symptoms can be controlled. Stopping treatment is a necessary step only for nonpruritic skin rashes, drug fever, and most reactions involving the major organ systems.

Pruritus

Urticaria and other pruritic skin rashes are treated with hydroxyzine, 25 to 100 mg by mouth (Atarax) or intramuscularly (Vistaril). Treatment can be repeated every 6 to 8 hours as needed until the eruption subsides. Alternative drugs are diphenhydramine (Benadryl), 25 to 100 mg and cyproheptadine (Periactin), 4 to 8 mg. The main side effect of treatment is drowsiness, not usually a problem with the hospitalized patient, but any ambulatory patient should be warned about the risk of operating a motor vehicle or other machinery while taking one of these drugs. Skin testing for IgE mediated sensitivity cannot be performed for at least 72 hours after the last dose of hydroxyzine and 48 hours after the last dose of the others. If the foregoing treatment is

TABLE 3 Classification of Drug Reactions

Mast cell mediated reactions
Systemic anaphylaxis
Urticaria and angioedema
Some pruritic maculopapular eruptions
Serum sickness (in part)
Anaphylactoid (nonimmunologic)
T-lymphocyte mediated reactions
Allergic eczematous contact dermatitis
Photodermatitis
Other cutaneous reactions (mechanism uncertain)
Maculopapular or exanthematous reactions
Fixed eruptions
Toxic epidermal necrolysis
Drug fever
Systemic lupus erythematosus and other autoimmune reactions
Organ systems reactions
Blood: eosinophilia, hemolytic anemia, thrombocytopenia, granulocytopenia
Lung
Liver
Kidney
Reactions with inconsistent drug associations
Erythema multiforme
Exfoliative dermatitis
Vasculitis

inadequate, one might consider adding an H_2 antihistamine, such as cimetidine or ranantidine, or substituting the tricyclic antihistamine doxepin, but the reaction is more likely to resolve if oral prednisone therapy, 40 mg daily, is given and rapidly tapered to zero when the reaction subsides.

Pain

Pain may be a prominent symptom with some reactions. The arthralgias of serum sickness and systemic lupus erythematosus and the cutaneous pain in vasculitis and some cases of urticaria can be treated with a nonsteroidal anti-inflammatory drug such as indomethacin (Indocin), 25 to 50 mg every 8 hours. If this is inadequate, prednisone treatment should be initiated (to be discussed).

Anaphylaxis

The treatment is summarized in Table 3 according to the usual sequence of events. Since shock and upper airway obstruction are the most likely causes of death, vital signs and the adequacy of respiration should be carefully followed from the onset of the reaction. As indicated in Table 3, epinephrine is effective in alleviating most of the features of anaphylaxis; 0.3 to 0.5 mg in a 1:1000 concentration should be given subcutaneously immediately. If the offending drug (an allergenic extract is a good example) was injected into an extremity, the injection site should be infiltrated with another 0.2 mg and a tourniquet placed above it. This usually is sufficient to prevent progression of the reaction.

Hypotension

If the patient is hypotensive (systolic pressure less than 60 mm), an intravenous line must be placed and a crystalloid solution such as 5 percent dextrose in 0.5 normal saline infused rapidly. Three to 4 liters of fluid may need to be infused to restore the plasma volume. Epinephrine is then infused through a side line at a dilution high enough (e.g., 1:100,000) to allow delivery of the drug at a rate of about 5 to 10 μg per minute, with continuous electrocardiographic monitoring for arrhythmias. Anaphylaxis may occur in a patient who has been taking a beta-adrenergic blocking drug. In such a patient epinephrine resistance may be overcome by increasing the dose, but this maneuver demands careful monitoring for side effects. Ancillary intravenous treatment with both the H_1 antihistamine diphenhydramine (Benadryl), 100 mg and the H_2 antihistamine cimetidine (Tagamet), 300 mg or ranitidine (Zantac), 50 mg, may be advisable. If the blood pressure remains low in the face of a rising central venous pressure, cardiogenic shock may have developed (to be discussed).

Upper Airway Obstruction

Hoarseness, stridor, or the use of accessory respiratory muscles should alert the observer to the possibility of obstructing angioedema. If this happens, diphenhydramine (Benadryl), 100 mg, should be given intravenously in addition to epinephrine, which can be given subcutaneously every 20 minutes. If a number 6 or 7 endotracheal tube cannot be inserted, one must be prepared to perform a tracheostomy or cricothyroid membrane puncture. Oxygen must be provided.

Lower Airway Obstruction

A few patients develop symptoms and signs of asthma as part of the anaphylactic reaction. Their treatment should be supplemented with the intravenous administration of aminophylline, 6 mg per kg over 20 minutes, followed by another 3 mg per kg if necessary. If the symptoms have not subsided, the drug should be continued in a constant infusion of 0.5 mg per kg per hour, adjusted to maintain the blood level at 10 to 20 g per ml. If toxic symptoms or signs appear (nausea, cardiac dysrhythmia), the infusion should be stopped until they subside. If the patient also is hypotensive, the aminophylline dose should be reduced by 50 percent.

Cardiac Problems

Dysrhymias may develop from a combination of factors such as drugs, anaphylactogenic mediators, and hypoxia. If a dysrhythmia develops, it is treated by conventional methods that need not be described here. If hypotension persists despite epinephrine infusion and fluid replacement, the patient is usually maximally vasoconstricted and adding treatment with an alpha-adrenergic vasopressor drug serves no useful purpose. Usually pressure monitoring reveals a reduced cardiac output, which should be treated with isoproterenol (Isuprel), 1 to 5 μg per minute intravenously, with continuous electrocardiographic monitoring. Serving also as a bronchodilator, this drug has a modest advantage over the alternative drugs dopamine and dobutamine.

Prevention of Late Reactions

The acute and potentially life threatening reactions usually resolve within 1 hour. A resurgence of the reaction, less serious but still uncomfortable, may appear 4 to 10 hours later. This may be prevented by giving methylprednisolone (Solu-Medrol), 40 mg intravenously, after all other treatment has been started; this, or 40 mg of prednisone by mouth, can be given again 6 hours later. If no new symptoms develop within 12 hours after the onset, it is unlikely that any will appear later.

Glucocorticoid Treatment

Severe reactions should be treated with oral doses of prednisone or intravenous doses of methylprednisolone, 40 to 60 mg daily, from the start. In addition to the treatment of severe urticaria and serum sickness, and of the late phase of anaphylaxis already discussed, a glucocorticoid may be useful in the treatment of allergic contact dermatitis, erythema multiforme, and exfoliative dermatitis. Glucocorticoid treatment may also hasten recovery from pulmonary, hepatic, and hematologic reactions. Toxic epidermal necrolysis, vasculitis, and interstitial nephritis do not usually respond to glucocorticoids.

SUGGESTED READING

Drug allergy. NIH Publication 82–703, 1982, p. 1. Cited in: Sogn D. How to avoid allergic drug reactions. Drug Therapy Clinical Therapeutics in the Hospital 1983; 73–81.

Fisher AA. Allergic dermatitis medicamentosa: the systemic contact-type variety. Cutis 1976; 18: 637–641.

Greenberger PA, Patterson R, Tapio CM. Prophylaxis against repeated radiocontrast media reactions in 857 cases. Arch Intern Med 1985; 145:2197–2200.

Herman J, Radin R, et al. Allergic reactions to measles (rubeola) vaccine in patients hypersensitive to egg protein. J Pediatr 1983; 102:196–199.

Miller JR, Orgel HA, Meltzer EO. The safety of egg-containing vaccine for egg-allergic patients. J Allergy Clin Immunol 1983; 71:568–573.

Patterson R, Anderson J. Allergic reactions to drugs and biologic agents. In: Salvaggio JE, ed. Primer on allergic and immunologic diseases. JAMA 1982; 248:2643–2644.

Patterson R, DeSwarte RD, Greenberger PA, Grammer LC. Drug allergy and protocols for management of drug allergies. New England and Regional Allergy Proceedings 1986; 325–342.

Stark BJ, Earl HS, Gross GN, et al. Acute and chronic desensitization of penicillin-allergic patients. J Allergy Clin Immunol 1987; 79:523–532.

Sullivan T. Antigen-specific desensitization of patients allergic to penicillin. J Allergy Clin Immunol 1982; 69:500–508.

VanArsdel PP Jr. Diagnosing drug allergy. JAMA 1982; 247:2576–2581.

ACUTE DRUG INTOXICATION

EBEN I. FEINSTEIN, M.D.

Drug overdosage, either suicidal or accidental, is a major health problem in the United States with an estimated incidence of 7.5 million cases per year and more than 10,000 deaths. However, the number of patients who may require extracorporeal methods (hemodialysis or hemoperfusion) for the removal of the toxic agent is considerably smaller. One estimate is that 10 to 15 percent of patients hospitalized for treatment of an overdose have intoxications severe enough to be considered for either hemodialysis or hemoperfusion. The number that receive such therapy is smaller still, based on the estimated 1,000 hemoperfusion devices used each year in this country. The efficacy of extracorporeal removal is well documented for a number of important drugs and poisons. The use of hemodialysis or hemoperfusion in cases of severe poisoning requires no special technical skill, other than that required for the treatment of acute or chronic renal failure. These techniques in most cases entail no significant morbidity. Nonetheless, there is still a difference of opinion as to the role of these techniques in the treatment of poisoning. The arguments pro and con will be considered after a discussion of the therapeutic alternatives, the usual indications for extracorporeal devices, and their side effects.

CLINICAL APPROACH TO THE PATIENT WITH ACUTE DRUG INTOXICATION

The initial evaluation of the patient with suspected or witnessed drug overdosage is outlined in Table 1. A wit-

TABLE 1 Initial Evaluation of the Patient

History
- Witnessed ingestion
- Empty drug bottles

Physical Examination
- Vital signs
- Level of consciousness
- Signs of trauma, especially to the head
- Other neurologic signs, e.g.:
  - Constricted pupils (narcotic overdose)
  - Dilated pupils (anticholinergic drugs)
- Skin
  - Barbiturate-induced skin blisters

Laboratory Tests
- Nonspecific analyses
  - Complete blood count
  - Urinalysis
  - Serum electrolytes
  - Serum urea nitrogen and creatinine
  - Serum glucose
  - Serum bilirubin and transaminases
  - Serum osmolality
- Specific toxicology analyses
  - Qualitative toxicology screening tests of blood or urine
  - Quantitative assays
    - Barbiturates and other sedatives
    - Antidepressants
    - Lithium
    - Cardiac glycosides and other cardiac active drugs, e.g. quinidine, theophylline

ness to the drug ingestion or an empty drug container is helpful in estimating the type and amount of drug ingested. A history of prior ingestion of drugs may be important.

Physical examination reveals crucial information. Vital signs and the level of consciousness should be immediately assessed. If stupor or coma is present, signs of head trauma should be looked for. The size of the pupils is often an important clue: constricted pupils suggest an opiate intoxication, dilated pupils may be due to an anticholinergic agent. The integument should be inspected for needle tracks (from intravenous drug injection) or bullae (secondary to chronic barbiturate use).

Routine laboratory analyses can at times point to a specific intoxicant in addition to supplying important data regarding the general clinical condition of the patient. The clinician should strongly suspect ethylene glycol poisoning in the patient with an acute brain syndrome and acute renal failure who has calcium oxalate crystals in the urine. An elevation of the anion gap may suggest several types of intoxicating substances in the patient with metabolic acidosis. Once uremia and diabetic ketoacidosis are ruled out, salicylate, methanol, and ethylene glycol ingestion should be considered. An osmolal gap (measured plasma osmolality minus calculated osmolality) of greater than 15 mOsm per kilogram is another clue to an alcohol or ethylene glycol intoxication. Finally, analysis of urine and blood can provide qualitative and quantitative information about specific intoxicating agents. These data are usually available several hours after the initial assessment and treatment has been instituted.

The early treatment of acute drug intoxications depends upon the vital signs and level of consciousness of the patient. The comatose patient (Table 2) should be carefully observed for the rate of respiration and the patency of the airway. All patients with coma of unknown cause should receive intravenous glucose and naloxone. Intravenous thiamine is also recommended to treat possible Wernicke's encephalopathy. Supplemental oxygen is helpful in patients with depressed respirations. In many instances these therapies are given by paramedical personnel on the scene where the patient is discovered. Treatment of a suspected intoxication can also begin before arrival at the hospital.

Techniques of Active Drug Removal

The oral administration of activated charcoal is the most commonly used method of enhancing the removal from the body of ingested toxins. Prepared as a slurry of charcoal powder and water (1.0 g of charcoal per kilogram of body weight), the charcoal is either swallowed or given via a gastric tube lavage. If the patient is stuporous, protection of the airway with prior endotracheal intubation is required. Charcoal absorbs many drugs before they can leave the gastrointestinal tract and may later enhance elimination from the body of substances that diffuse back into the gastrointestinal tract from the circulation. However, charcoal may also interfere with the action of orally administered antidotes (e.g., acetylcysteine). A laxative is frequently administered with the sorbent to avoid obstipation; 70 percent sorbitol is effective and avoids possible hypermagnesemia from other laxatives in patients with renal failure.

Enhanced excretion of certain substances by the kidneys can be produced by forced diuresis and alteration in the urinary pH. To be effectively removed in this manner, the substance must be filtered by the glomerulus, must not be highly lipid-soluble or highly protein-bound, and must undergo significant elimination via glomerular filtration and/or tubular secretion. Changing the urinary pH increases drug elimination of those drugs that are weak acids or bases. Their transport across the renal tubular cell depends on the pH of the tubular luminal fluid, which

TABLE 2 Initial Management of the Comatose Patient with a Suspected Drug Overdose

Ensure patent airway

Administer:
- Intravenous glucose
- Intravenous naloxone
- Thiamine hydrochloride
- Oxygen

Prevent gastrointestinal absorption with activated charcoal and a cathartic

Treat hypotension with infusion of normal saline

in turn determines the fraction of the drug existing in a nonionized form. As luminal pH rises, the fraction of a weakly acidic substance that is ionized will increase, thus reducing its tubular reabsorbtion. The ionized fraction of weakly basic drugs similarly is greater at an acidic luminal pH. Forced alkaline diuresis has been advocated for the treatment of *phenobarbital* and *salicylate* overdosage. Acid diuresis is used less frequently; it has been shown to promote renal excretion of amphetamines, fenfluramine, phencyclidine, and quinine. Both methods require administration of large amounts of intravenous fluids and close monitoring of urine flow and systemic and urinary pH. Even with careful monitoring, serious side effects may occur, such as hyponatremia, pulmonary edema, alkalemia, or acidemia. In summary, although a theoretically attractive mode of therapy requiring no invasive techniques, forced diuresis has a minor role in current therapy of most severe intoxications.

Extracorporeal Methods of Drug Removal

Of the extracorporeal methods available for treating intoxication, the two most commonly used are hemodialysis and hemoperfusion. Peritoneal dialysis offers little advantage over forced diuresis. Hemodialysis has been employed for treating intoxications for 30 years. Since its first reported use, data have been gathered concerning the removal of most of the common intoxicating substances. Effective removal by hemodialysis depends upon the nature of the toxin and the properties of the dialysis system. For optimal removal by dialysis, a substance should be of low molecular weight (less than 300 daltons), not highly protein-bound or highly lipid-soluble, and found in adequate concentration in the extracellular fluid. Factors governing removal of poisons by hemodialysis are similar to those affecting removal of uremic toxins; i.e., removal varies with the surface area of the membrane, its permeability, the flow rates of dialysate and blood, and the concentration gradient between blood and dialysate. The removal of molecular weight solutes is usually greatest at blood flow rates of 200 to 300 ml per minute.

Hemoperfusion entered routine clinical use later than hemodialysis and its major use is now for treatment of poisoning. Activated charcoal is the sorbent in common use, but hemoperfusion using the XAD-4 polystyrene resin is also effective, although not in clinical use currently. Charcoal that is "activated" has a large number of pores with multiple ramifications that greatly increase the surface area available for adsorption. Compared to hemodialysis, charcoal hemoperfusion has the capacity to remove both larger molecular weight substances (up to 40,000 daltons) and highly lipid soluble drugs.

Complications of Extracorporeal Therapy

Hemodialysis, whether used in the treatment of renal failure or exogenous intoxication, entails certain risks. Hypotension is one of the most common complications. In most patients, the fall in blood pressure responds to the administration of normal saline. However, there are other causes for dialysis-induced hypotension. The acetate buffer used in dialysate has been implicated as a vasodepressant factor. Therefore, many nephrologists prefer to use a bicarbonate-buffered dialysate in the critically ill patient. It should also be remembered that the poisoning agent may cause hypotension. In such cases it may be necessary to use vasoactive agents such as dopamine to maintain a blood pressure adequate for the patient and for sufficient blood flow through the dialyzer. Another complication of hemodialysis is hypoxemia which is usually not profound. The fall in arterial Po_2 seen with acetate dialysate is reduced when bicarbonate dialysate is used. Dialysis with cellulose-based membranes leads to an early, transient fall in the peripheral leukocyte count. This is usually not clinically significant and can be avoided by using noncellulosic membranes. Bleeding during or after the treatment is another potential problem because heparin is required for anticoagulation during hemodialysis. Finally, in addition to removing the toxic agent, hemodialysis also removes electrolytes, such as potassium, phosphate, and other small, non-protein-bound substances in the circulation. However, hypokalemia and hypophosphatemia are usually not clinically significant problems in the treatment of drug intoxications.

Hemoperfusion shares many of the complications of hemodialysis. Bleeding is a more important concern with hemoperfusion because platelets and clotting factors are absorbed to the cartridge. Although coating of the charcoal with albumin or polymer solutions has reduced the degree of thrombocytopenia, a fall of about 30 percent in the platelet count during the treatment can still be expected. Hemoperfusion is also similar to hemodialysis in removing substances other than those desired for therapeutic effect. Serum glucose, phosphate, and calcium may decline. Hypoglycemia is avoided by infusing dextrose and/or water during the treatment. Clinically important hypocalcemia and hypophosphatemia usually do not occur. Hypotension is less often a problem with hemoperfusion, but it should be kept in mind that vasopressor substances can be taken up by the sorbent. If the blood pressure is being maintained with dopamine or other vasopressor infusions, they should be given into the tubing returning blood to the patient.

There are certain problems with hemoperfusion that are not seen with hemodialysis. Because the blood tubing and sorbent cartridge are usually not heated, body temperature may drop. The alert patient may complain of feeling cold. In the comatose patient, body temperature should be monitored frequently. Another potential problem with charcoal is embolization of the sorbent. With sorbent cartridges now in use, the charcoal is either coated or fixed to a mesh. This method of preparation, along with filters in the blood circuit, have eliminated the danger of significant microembolization.

Access to the circulation is required for both hemoperfusion and hemodialysis. For rapid institution of therapy, insertion of a large catheter(s) into either the femoral or subclavian vein is the commonly used approach. In experienced hands, catheter placement is quick, safe, and relatively painless (many patients will not experience pain in their comatose state). Because of the risks of bleeding during hemoperfusion, particular attention must be paid to adequate hemostasis if the catheters are removed soon after the end of treatment. Large hematomas have developed when adequate local pressure was not applied to the insertion site after catheter removal.

Indications for Extracorporeal Drug Removal

Once the nature of the intoxicant is known and the blood level is determined (where possible), appropriate further therapy can be started. The clinical guidelines for further therapy are given in Table 3. The decision to use an extracorporeal method for drug elimination is based on the clinical condition of the patient and the nature of the drug. Most patients in otherwise good health with blood levels of barbiturates or other hypnotics exceeding those given in Table 4 will survive if treated in an intensive care unit where respiratory and blood pressure support are given. Many physicians, however, prefer to use hemodialysis or hemoperfusion in the deeply comatose patient with profound depression of respiration and blood pressure with the aim of reducing the duration of coma. Certainly, when a patient who is being managed conservatively shows further deterioration or develops other complications such as pneumonia or pneumothorax, then extracorporeal methods are indicated.

Knowledge of the intoxicating substance is also essential for appropriate management. Where specific antidotes or antagonists exist, they should be employed as soon as possible. Examples of such drugs are acetaminophen, methanol, digoxin, and cyanide.

It is generally accepted that intoxications with agents that can cause delayed and often permanent tissue damage should be treated with hemodialysis or hemoperfusion. Ethylene glycol is such a substance; it is metabolized to oxalic acid which can cause irreversible renal failure and central nervous system damage. Methyl alcohol intoxication causes blindness as a result of the toxic effects of its metabolites formaldehyde and formic acid. Other examples of substances with delayed toxic effects include paraquat (pulmonary fibrosis), lithium carbonate, and theophylline (central nervous system damage).

TABLE 3 Indications for the Use of Hemodialysis or Hemoperfusion in Patients with Drug Intoxications

- Clinical condition of the patient
  - Stage III or IV coma
  - Respiratory failure
  - Hypotension
  - Progressive deterioration of vital signs during conservative therapy
  - Development of potentially life-threatening complications
  - Presence of preexisting conditions that may predispose to complications
  - Impaired normal routes of drug excretion
- Nature of the drug
  - The substance can be eliminated by extracorporeal methods at a rate exceeding that of the hepatic or renal routes
  - The drug produces late toxic effects either directly or via a metabolic product
  - Ingestion of more than one intoxicating substance which have similar effects

Treatment of Specific Intoxications

Table 4 lists the common intoxications, the preferred method of removal, and the blood levels above which hemodialysis or hemoperfusion should be considered. The treatment of several commonly encountered intoxications are discussed in this section.

Barbiturates

These drugs are commonly used in attempted suicide. They are prescribed as hypnotic and anticonvulsant agents. Patients who are chronically using barbiturates may develop a tolerance to them and at high blood concentrations may not demonstrate all of the toxic effects that may be seen in a patient who does not have drug tolerance.

Barbiturate overdosage impairs central nervous system function, leading to coma and depression of respiration, blood pressure, and temperature. Treatment of the patient should include prompt gastric lavage and administration of activated charcoal for intestinal adsorption. The patient with coma, respiratory depression, or hypotension needs supportive care in an intensive care unit. Although the overall mortality in barbiturate poisoning is low, patients with profound coma have a mortality rate as high as 34 percent. Therefore these patients should be treated

TABLE 4 Extracorporeal Drug Removal in Common Drug Intoxications

	Potentially Lethal Serum Level (mg/dl)	*Preferred Treatment*
Sedatives and tranquilizers		
Barbiturates		
Long-acting	10	HP
Short-acting	5	HP
Glutethimide	3	HP
Ethchlorvynol	10	HP
Methaqualone	3	HP
Methyprylon	5	HP
Meprobamate	10	HP
Analgesics		
Salicylates	100	HD
Acetaminophen	150 (μg/ml)	HP
Theophylline	50 (μg/ml)	HP
Paraquat	0.2 (μg/ml)	HD
Lithium	3.0 (mEq/L)	HD
Alcohols		
Ethanol	500	HD
Methanol	50	HD
Ethylene glycol		HD

HD= hemodialysis, HP = hemoperfusion

with forced alkaline diuresis, and preferably charcoal hemoperfusion. Forced diuresis will be effective only with phenobarbital-like drugs and not with short-acting barbiturates such as secobarbital.

Other Hypnotics and Sedatives

Glutethimide and ethchlorvynol are nonbarbiturate hypnotic drugs that have significant lipid solubility. Both drugs can cause deep coma, respiratory depression, and hypotension. The treatment of choice for patients with these findings is hemoperfusion. It is important to bear in mind that rebound of blood levels following hemoperfusion can occur. Therefore repetitive treatment with hemoperfusion may be needed as the drug is released from tissue stores.

The benzodiazepine group of drugs includes several commonly prescribed sedatives. Fortunately, severe toxicity following overdosage is rare. When respiratory failure or hypotension occurs, it is likely to be in the setting of a multiple drug overdose. The use of gastric lavage and gastrointestinal absorbtion usually suffices for the treatment of benzodiazepine overdose. Neither hemoperfusion nor hemodialysis has been well studied in this situation.

Lithium

Lithium carbonate is a mainstay of the treatment of bipolar affective disorders. The drug has significant toxic effects on the kidney and central nervous system. Lithium antagonizes the action of antidiuretic hormone, leading to impaired urinary concentrating ability. Some patients may develop chronic interstitial renal disease, but significant renal toxicity is seen only in a small percentage of patients treated with lithium. Central nervous system toxicity includes muscular hyperirritability, parkinsonian movement disorders, delirium, seizures, and coma. Treatment of severe intoxication should include restoration of extracellular fluid volume by saline infusion in the volume-depleted patient. However, enhanced elimination by saline diuresis is not an effective treatment in potentially life-threatening cases. Lithium is highly dialyzable and hemodialysis is indicated in patients with potentially lethal blood levels of the drug. In patients with renal insufficiency, urinary elimination may be impaired; such patients should also be considered for treatment with hemodialysis.

Tricyclic Antidepressants

The tricyclic antidepressants are in common clinical use and are a frequent cause of drug overdosage. The major toxicity of these drugs involves the heart and includes arrhythmias and depressed myocardial contractility. Coma may develop with severe intoxication. Electrocardiographic signs of toxicity include prolongation of the QRS interval, intraventricular conduction defects, and ventricular tachycardia. Patients with serious tricyclic overdosage should have continuous cardiac monitoring. Repeated doses of activated charcoal help to eliminate the drug from the gastrointestinal tract. Alkalinization therapy with intravenous sodium bicarbonate is indicated to control cardiac arrhythmias. Physostigmine is also advocated (2 mg IV given slowly and repeated up to 4 times at 15- to 30-minute intervals), but serious side effects include bradycardia and cardiac arrest. It should not be used when conduction defects are present. Diphenylhydantoin and propranolol may also be used in treatment of ventricular arrhythmias. Extracorporeal therapy to remove these drugs is ineffective owing to their protein binding.

Acetaminophen

Acetaminophen is a widely used analgesic and is a component of numerous over-the-counter medications. The drug itself is nontoxic; however, it is converted to a metabolite which, in high concentrations, causes liver cell necrosis. Since the drug is rapidly absorbed from the gastrointestinal tract, it is imperative that treatment for acute intoxication be instituted within 24 hours (preferably within 16 hours) of ingestion. The plasma level declines sharply in the first 24 hours, so a decision as to the severity of the overdosage must take into account the time interval after the drug was taken. The antidote for acetaminophen poisoning is N-acetylcysteine. This is given orally at an initial dose of 140 mg per kilogram, and 70 mg per kilogram for repeated doses. Signs of liver damage (elevated serum transaminases and bilirubin) should be monitored frequently.

Salicylates

Salicylates can be fairly described as ubiquitous, being found in a myriad of over-the-counter oral analgesics and other preparations. The common symptoms of salicylate poisoning include tinnitus, diaphoresis, and hyperventilation. Agitation is frequently observed, and coma is uncommon. There are several associated disorders of acid-base balance. Respiratory alkalosis occurs as a result of hyperventilation. There may be a concomitant metabolic acidosis producing a mixed acid-base disorder. Salicylate intoxication should be considered (along with ethylene glycol and methanol) in the intoxicated patient with an elevated anion gap acidosis. Salicylates are rapidly absorbed, highly protein-bound, and excreted in a conjugated form in the urine. Treatment of drug overdose includes the standard methods for preventing intestinal absorption. Salicylate excretion in the urine can be effectively enhanced by forced alkaline diuresis. Many patients may require large quantities of sodium bicarbonate to achieve an alkaline urine. For this reason, careful monitoring of the patient is mandatory to prevent circulatory volume overload. In patients with renal insufficiency or pulmonary edema, treatment with hemodialysis should be considered. Hemodialysis not only removes the drug efficiently, but can correct an associated metabolic acidosis.

Theophylline

Theophylline is used mainly in the treatment of acute and chronic obstructive airways disease. Symptoms of toxicity include nausea, seizures, and tachycardia. The liver is the site of theophylline metabolism and the metabolites are excreted in the urine. The treatment of theophylline toxicity should be guided by the serum concentration and the clinical state of the patient. However, in patients who have serum concentrations greater than 50 μg per milliliter, without signs of severe toxicity, hemoperfusion is indicated because of the danger of permanent central nervous system damage. Hemoperfusion is also indicated in elderly patients, and in the presence of heart failure or hepatic insufficiency.

Digoxin

Digoxin toxicity is a common clinical problem. The drug acts as an inhibitor of Na − K − ATPase. Its major toxicity is cardiac: conduction defects, suppression of the sinus node, and stimulation of ectopic pacemaker activity. In severe overdoses, hyperkalemia develops as the Na − K ATPase-dependent cellular transport systems are blocked, preventing cellular uptake of potassium. Treatment for digoxin poisoning includes correction of any precipitating factors, especially hypokalemia. Specific therapy for cardiac arrhythmias may require antiarrhythmic drugs or cardioversion. Hemodialysis and hemoperfusion are not effective owing to the significant tissue binding of the drug. In fact, hemodialysis may be dangerous because it can produce a drop in serum potassium while raising the serum calcium concentration. A specific antidote, digoxin antibody (Fab fragments), reverses digoxin toxicity and enhances drug elimination.

The treatment of acute drug intoxications requires a systematic approach that couples a careful assessment of the individual patient with knowledge of the nature of the intoxicating agent and its metabolism. Extracorporeal methods for drug elimination should be reserved for those situations in which such methods will prevent serious organ damage. In many cases of hypnotic and sedative overdosage, intensive support of the patient during the period of coma and respiratory failure may suffice. In support of this approach, some investigators argue that most of these patients have developed side effects such as aspiration pneumonia before they come to the hospital and their stay in the intensive care unit is usually short. Therefore, extracorporeal drug elimination is largely unnecessary. However, there are no suitable guidelines for predicting which patients will require a lengthy period of intensive care (more than 3 days). With the level of technical expertise that is currently available for the use of extracorporeal methods of drug removal, it is likely that in most cases the risks of the procedure are far smaller than the benefits of accelerated drug removal.

ILLICIT DRUG INTOXICATION

ADRIENNE N. KNOPF, M.D.

The use of illicit drugs has increased greatly over the last several decades. In 1988, approximately 25 percent of all toxic deaths reported to the American Association of Poison Control Centers were related to the use of cocaine, heroin, amphetamines, and other street drugs.

The medical management of these patients is similar to the management of all poisoned patients. Immediate treatment of all life-threatening complications is followed by efforts at decontamination and enhancement of elimination of the poison, use of specific antidotes in the rare poisoning that has a specific pharmacologic antagonist, general supportive care, and appropriate use of laboratory services to corroborate clinical findings.

This chapter describes the treatment of the more common illicit drug intoxications as well as acute alcohol intoxication. The common drugs of abuse are outlined in Table 1.

AMPHETAMINES (CENTRAL NERVOUS SYSTEM STIMULANTS)

Amphetamines are approved for use in the treatment of narcolepsy, hyperkinetic behavior in children, and short-term weight reduction. These agents have strong, long-lasting central nervous system stimulatory effects. “Ice,” a form of methamphetamine, or “speed,” which comes in crystal form and is smoked, creates an 8- to 24-hour “high” and is widely abused.

Amphetamines are taken orally, inhaled, and administered intravenously, subcutaneously, and intravaginally. An acute overdose of an amphetamine or one of its analogues manifests as an enhancement of its usual sympathomimetic and hallucinogenic effects. The major systems affected are the central nervous and cardiovascular systems. The patient may demonstrate hyperactivity, mydriasis, diaphoresis, confusion, hypertension, hyperpyrexia, and rhabdomyolysis. More severe reactions include seizures, acute vascular spasm, arrhythmias, myocardial infarction, hypotension, cardiomyopathy, or coma. Intracranial hemorrhage and transient Gilles de la Tourette-type syndromes have been precipitated by amphetamine use.

TABLE 1 Common Drugs of Abuse

Type	*Street Name*
Hashish	
Marijuana	Sensimilla, pot, Acapulco gold, Mary Jane, MJ, weed, grass
Depressants	
Barbiturates	Barbs
Benzodiazepines	
Chloral hydrate	With alcohol = Mickey Finn
Glutethimide (Doriden)	With codeine = packs, loads
Methaqualone	Quaalude
Hallucinogens	
Lysergic acid diethylamide (LSD)	Acid, blue dots, D
Mescaline-amphetamine hybrids	
MDA	Zen
MDEA	Eve
MDMA	Love pill, ecstasy, Adam
PMA	
Phencyclidine	PCP, angel dust, hog, star search = cocaine and PCP
Narcotics	
Codeine	
Fentanyl (analogues)	China white
Fentanyl (Sublimaze)	"Sub"
Heroin (diacetylmorphine)	H, scag, horse, smack, junk Speedball = heroin and cocaine or heroin and amphetamines
Hydrocodone	
Hydromorphone (Dilaudid)	Little d
Meperidine (Demerol)	Big D
Methadone	Meth, fizzies
Morphine	Dreamer, Miss Emma
MPTP (meperidine analogue)	
MPPP (meperidine analogue)	
Opium	Dover's powder, big O, blackstuff
Oxycodone (Percodan, Percocet	Perks
Pentazocine (Talwin)	t's and blues = Talwin and tripelennamine
Propoxyphene (Darvon)	Dummies
Stimulants	
Amphetamines	Ice
Cocaine (benzoylecgonine)	Coke, flake, snow, speedball = heroin and cocaine Crack = free-base form of cocaine

As is the case with other abused drugs, the amount of the drug ingested and the route of use do not correlate well with the toxic reactions. Blood urine samples can confirm the presence of amphetamines but should not be used to guide patient management.

Treatment consists primarily of stabilization and supportive care aimed at specific manifestations. Stomach emptying and charcoal administration are recommended for those who ingested the drug orally. Amphetamines are weak bases and acidification of the urine increases the excretion of unmetabolized drug, but the major metabolism occurs in the liver. Acid diuresis can worsen seizures, arrhythmias, or rhabdomyolysis and is not recommended.

Supportive treatment is similar to that discussed for cocaine intoxication. The agitation and psychosis seen with amphetamines may be more severe than with cocaine intoxication and may require aggressive treatment. Droperidol (0.1 mg per kilogram given at 2.5 mg per minute) is an intravenous butyrophenone that has been used for amphetamine-associated psychosis. Dystonia, hypotension, and respiratory depression can occur with droperidol.

Inadvertent intra-arterial administration of an amphetamine can cause acute vascular spasm and threaten tissue viability. An axillary nerve block, intra-arterial tolazoline, and intravenous nitroprusside have been used in these instances.

COCAINE (BENZOYLECGONINE)

Cocaine is a local anesthetic as well as a sympathomimetic agent that blocks the presynaptic uptake of norepinephrine and dopamine. It is currently the most abused major stimulant in the United States, with an estimated 22 million users. The major clinical use for cocaine is as a topical anesthetic and vasoconstrictor in rhinolaryngologic procedures. Illicit cocaine may be sold on the streets adulterated with other white powders, such as mannitol, lidocaine, sugars, phencyclidine, or amphetamines. The purity of "street cocaine" ranges from 20 to 70 percent. It is most commonly used intranasally or intravenously. A purer, more potent form of cocaine, crack (the free-base form) is now readily available and has been implicated in many deaths. Crack is not water-soluble and is generally smoked. Complications of cocaine and crack use include angina, myocardial infarction, chest pain syndromes, ventricular arrhythmias, seizures, intracranial hemorrhage, hypertensive emergencies, acute aortic dissection, and rhabdomyolysis.

Cocaine and crack have rapid onsets of action and cause immediate central nervous stimulation with a sense of euphoria and excitement associated with pupillary dilation, tachycardia, and an elevated blood pressure and respiratory rate. There is usually a typical biphasic response, the "caine reaction," characterized by initial excitation followed by depression with coma and circulatory failure.

The major life-threatening risks of cocaine intoxication are intractable seizures, respiratory arrest, hyperthermia, and dysrhythmias. Even at pharmacologic doses used in rhinolaryngologic procedures, cocaine can cause coronary vasoconstriction and a decrease in coronary blood flow despite an increase in myocardial oxygen demand via alpha-adrenergic–mediated stimulation.

Cocaine-induced seizures can be controlled with diazepam, 2 to 10 mg intravenously. Phenobarbital and phenytoin are second-line agents. Pancuronium bromide in combination with a short-acting barbiturate such as thiopental may be required for status epilepticus. Because succinylcholine administration can cause muscle fasciculation and thus worsen hyperthermia, it should be avoided.

Cocaine-induced hypertension probably is the consequence of beta-adrenergic–mediated tachycardia and alpha-adrenergic–mediated vasoconstriction. Mild hypertension does not require treatment. Labetalol is an adrenergic receptor blocking agent that has both alpha-1 and nonselective beta-blocking activity and can be given as an intravenous bolus or infusion, beginning with 20 mg intravenously. Propranolol, 1 mg intravenously every 5 minutes, also can be used. Esmolol is a new, short-acting parenteral beta-blocker agent. Its effects wear off quickly after discontinuance if adverse reactions, such as bradycardia, develop. The usual dose of esmolol is 500 μg per kilogram over 1 minute as a loading dose, followed by 50 to 100 μg per kilogram per minute. The pure alpha-adrenergic blocker, phentolamine, at a dose of 5 mg intravenously or intramuscularly, may be used alone or in conjunction with a beta blocker. Sodium nitroprusside at a dose of 0.5 to 10 μg per kilogram per minute is the best treatment for hypertensive emergencies because its antihypertensive effects can be titrated immediately.

Cocaine-associated tachyarrhythmias can be treated with standard agents, remembering the usefulness of beta-adrenergic blockade to decrease the adrenergic cardiac stimulation. One should recall that lidocaine is not an uncommon adulterant of cocaine, and thus there is the potential for producing lidocaine toxicity when administering this drug. Some evidence suggests that alkalinization protects the myocardium against cocaine-induced arrhythmias.

Hypotension is treated with fluids while other coexisting conditions or toxins are considered. Naloxone should be administered to rule out a coexisting narcotic overdose. If hypotension exists despite aggressive fluid administration (i.e., rapid infusion of 2 L), a vasopressor, such as norepinephrine or dopamine, should be given.

Hyperthermia can be treated with passive cooling with a cooling blanket to keep body temperature lower than 39° C.

Unstable angina related to cocaine use can be treated with nitrates or calcium channel blockers. The use of aspirin, anticoagulant, or thrombolytic therapy must be individualized.

For mild toxic psychosis, sedative doses of diazepam at 2.5 to 5.0 mg intravenously may be used. Providing a quiet environment and reassurance also can be helpful. For schizophreniform psychosis, haloperidol, 2 to 5 mg intramuscularly, can be used. It is generally safe but can lower the seizure threshold.

Treatment of cocaine-associated rhabdomyolysis is with hydration, alkalinization, and metabolic monitoring.

There is no effective means of decreasing absorption or enhancing elimination of cocaine, and there is no specific antidote. Cocaine is rapidly absorbed from all routes and is rapidly metabolized by serum and liver cholinesterases. The serum half-life is approximately 1 hour. Laboratory detection generally depends on detecting a cocaine metabolite in the urine. Blood levels do not correlate well with the severity of the reaction or with the occurrence of death.

DESIGNER DRUGS

Designer drugs are the products of pharmacologic manipulations of legal drugs by black market chemists and are specifically created to mimic the effects of illicit drugs, including narcotics, stimulants, and hallucinogens. As with other illicit drugs, there are no controls over purity or potency.

Fentanyl and Its Derivatives

Fentanyl and its legal derivatives are synthetic opioids that are used as anesthetics and analgesics preoperatively. As a group, they are about 200 times more potent than morphine. Many illicit analogues are available on the streets. "China white," "synthetic heroin," and "Mexican brown" are common street names for fentanyl derivatives.

These drugs are rapidly distributed, metabolized, and excreted by the body. They can cause rapid respiratory depression, bradycardia, hypotension, hypothermia, and seizures. Many deaths have been associated with the most potent of the fentanyl derivatives, 3-methyl-fentanyl, which is 7,000 times more potent than morphine.

The treatment for a fentanyl overdose is identical to that for a heroin overdose, except that very high doses of the narcotic antagonist naloxone hydrochloride (more than 10 mg) may be needed. Laboratory tests are usually not helpful because these drugs are rapidly cleared in the serum.

Meperidine Analogues

Methylphenyltetrahydropyridine (MPTP) and methylphenylpropenylpiperidinol (MPPP) are also synthetic opiate derivatives. Symptoms associated with this group of narcotics are burning along the course of the injection site, blurred vision, a metallic taste in the mouth, myoclonus, athetoid movement, and muscle rigidity. The treatment for the overdose is identical to that for the narcotic overdose.

These drugs resulted in rapid development of a severe, irreversible parkinsonian syndrome in drug abusers in the 1980s.

Mescaline-Amphetamine Hybrids

These hybrids of hallucinogens and stimulants include MDA, 3,4-methylene dioxyamphetamine ("zen"); MDMA, 3,4-methylene dioxymethamphetamine ("ecstasy," "Adam"); MDEA, 3,4-methylene dioxy-ethamphetamine ("Eve"); and PMA, p-methoxyamphetamine.

Many of these drugs were introduced in the 1970s as "disinhibitors," popularized by some therapists as adjuncts to facilitate psychotherapy. MDMA is less hallucinogenic and has less sympathomimetic effects at lower "therapeutic" doses, but in high doses it can cause all the effects of a typical amphetamine overdose, with hypertension, seizures, tachycardia, and dysphoria.

Treatment consists primarily of supportive care. Acidification has been suggested to enhance clearance but can worsen the potential complications of rhabdomyolysis and seizures and should be avoided.

ETHANOL

The most common of all intoxications requiring treatment is the acute ethanol intoxication. Ethanol is a central nervous system depressant. Enhanced toxicity occurs with the coingestion of other central nervous system depressants, such as barbiturates or benzodiazepines. A blood alcohol level of 100 mg per deciliter correlates with the legal level of intoxication in most states, and at this level, most patients have lack of coordination. Higher levels produce stupor. Levels higher than 500 to 700 mg per deciliter can produce coma and death, although chronic alcoholics can tolerate these higher levels.

These patients must be evaluated for associated trauma, coingestions, and other causes of stupor or coma. Airway or circulatory compromise can occur and requires immediate therapy. Treatment then involves thiamine, 100 mg intravenously, to avoid the Wernicke-Korsakoff syndrome, glucose for the comatose patient or the patient with a serum glucose level less than 60 mg per deciliter, hydration, positioning of the patient to help avoid aspiration, administration of benzodiazepines for seizures, and serial neurologic examinations to detect focal abnormalities suggesting a comorbid event that requires additional studies.

A patient may be considered safe for discharge if he or she is fully oriented and ambulatory without ataxia. Ideally, patients should be offered treatment for alcoholism.

MARIJUANA

Marijuana is the most commonly used recreational drug. The active agent is tetrahydrocannabinol. The average marijuana cigarette has 500 mg of marijuana, 1 percent of which is tetrahydrocannabinol. Hashish is a more potent form of marijuana. Marijuana has been used to diminish the nausea and enhance the appetite of patients undergoing chemotherapy and to decrease intraocular pressure in glaucoma patients.

Marijuana produces euphoria, passivity, and an enhanced appetite. Higher doses can produce disturbed thought processes, hallucinations, headache, tachycardia, tremor, and ataxia. The effects begin minutes after inhalation and last for several hours. Urine testing for cannabinoid confirms its presence.

Marijuana users seldom seek medical attention, since their symptoms resolve spontaneously. Treatment of the patient who does seek medical attention involves ruling out other more serious mind-altering toxins, such as phencyclidine (PCP). Benzodiazepines or haloperidol can be used to control agitation. Primary psychiatric illness may need to be excluded.

The toxicity of acute and chronic marijuana use is a subject of great controversy.

NARCOTICS

The clinical effects of a narcotic overdose are pinpoint pupils, depressed respirations, and coma. Seizures may occur, especially with meperidine (Demerol) and propoxyphene (Darvon). Routes of overdose may be intravenous ("mainlining"), subcutaneous ("skin popping"), oral, sniffing, or smoking.

The treatment of the patient with a narcotic overdose and coma begins with establishing an airway, assuring ventilation with initiation of assisted ventilation if necessary and administering 100 mg of thiamine and 50 ml of 50 percent glucose, followed by the specific antidote, naloxone hydrochloride. Gastrointestinal decontamination is useful if the drug was taken orally.

Naloxone (Narcan) is a synthetic congener of oxymorphone and is a specific narcotic antagonist at all three opioid receptors—mu, kappa, and sigma. Ampules containing 0.4, 0.8, and 2.0 mg of naloxone are available. Although naloxone usually is administered intravenously, it can be given subcutaneously, intramuscularly, sublingually, and by endotracheal instillation, an important fact to remember in a comatose intravenous drug user with poor venous access. An initial bolus of 0.4 to 0.8 mg is given, with expected lightening of coma and increased respiratory rate within 15 to 30 seconds. If there is no response, repeated doses should be given every 1 to 2 minutes, up to 10 mg, allowing for assessment of response between doses to avoid using too much naloxone and precipitating acute withdrawal. If acute withdrawal does occur, it can be reversed with cautious administration of 2 mg of morphine sulfate every 2 to 3 minutes until the withdrawal symptoms become tolerable.

If there is no response after 10 mg of naloxone, alternative causes of the coma, such as other toxins or head trauma, must be considered. These higher doses of naloxone (6 to 10 mg) are needed to antagonize the very potent fentanyl derivatives as well as overdoses with meperidine, codeine, propoxyphene, and methadone.

Naloxone has a duration of action of 1 to 3 hours. Repeated doses of naloxone may be required after an initial favorable response. A continuous intravenous infusion may be needed and can easily be formulated by adding 4.0 to 8.0 mg of naloxone to 1,000 ml of 5 percent dextrose in water and administering at 100 ml per hour. Longer-acting narcotics, such as methadone, may require a naloxone infusion for several days. When the infusion is discontinued, the patient should be observed for 2 hours in the intensive care unit for relapse of coma.

A common clinical question arises regarding the appropriate medical disposition of the narcotics user with an accidental overdose who awakens after naloxone and refuses further therapy. Given that the duration of action of naloxone is 2 to 3 hours, it should be safe to allow such a patient to leave the emergency room if he or she has been observed for 4 to 6 hours after the last dose of naloxone and has no other problems necessitating hospitalization.

Naloxone is a well-tolerated and safe drug. The only common adverse reaction is acute withdrawal.

NITRITES

Methemoglobinemia, vasodilation, and hypoxemia complicate nitrite poisoning. Many nitrites are abused as aphrodisiacs ("rush") and stimulants. Stupor, respiratory depression, seizures, and arrhythmias can occur. Venous blood may appear "chocolate brown."

Oxygen should be administered. Levels of methemoglobin higher than 30 percent, as measured by arterial blood gas sample, should be treated with methylene blue, 1 to 2 mg per kilogram of 1 percent solution intravenously. Methylene blue should not be used in glucose-6-phosphate dehydrogenase-deficient patients because it can induce a severe hemolytic anemia in these patients.

PHENCYCLIDINE [1-(1-PHENYLCYCLOHEXYL)PIPERIDINE]

Phencyclidine (PCP) is a synthetic hallucinogen with no medical use. It is the most commonly abused major hallucinogen. A powdered or liquefied form of the drug usually is mixed with tobacco or marijuana and smoked. It is rapidly absorbed, conjugated in the liver, and excreted in its free and conjugated form in the urine. Its half-life varies from 7 to 46 hours.

Nystagmus, hypertension, altered mental status, and psychotic behavior are common manifestations, but other effects occur, including cholinergic, anticholinergic, adrenergic, and dopaminergic reactions. Major intoxication often progresses rapidly to coma.

Treatment must be individualized because of the wide spectrum of manifestations. Gastric lavage and repeated charcoal administration are useful (even when PCP is smoked) because PCP does undergo enterohepatic clearance. Although PCP is a weak base, acidification is generally not indicated because 90 percent is cleared in the liver. Acidification can worsen preexisting metabolic acidosis and is contraindicated if rhabdomyolysis is present.

Behavior modification is an important part of the treatment. Many patients are acutely agitated and require quiet rooms and haloperidol, 5 to 10 mg intramuscularly every hour. Restraints on the extremities can increase the probability of the patient's developing rhabdomyolysis. Phenothiazines should be avoided because they can lower the seizure threshold, accentuate anticholinergic effects, and precipitate hypotension. These patients may be violent and may be potentially harmful to themselves and others.

The laboratory can usually detect urinary PCP, but the clinical severity of intoxication does not correlate well with the drug level.

SEDATIVE-HYPNOTICS

The most serious complications of intoxication with a sedative-hypnotic include respiratory and cardiovascular compromise and hypothermia. Treatment includes airway protection, assisted ventilation, monitoring for sudden apnea, vasopressors and fluids for hypotension, and warming measures for hypothermia. This class of drugs is associated with myocardial depression. Fluid status should be closely monitored to avoid pulmonary edema.

The illicit drugs in this class include methaqualone and glutethimide-codeine combinations.

Methaqualone (Quaalude) is regarded as the street aphrodisiac and creates a sense of indestructibility in the user. In addition to the complications of sedative-hypnotics, methaqualone may induce bleeding diathesis from platelet dysfunction and prolonged prothrombin time and partial thromboplastin time and may require blood product support. Severe muscle rigidity can also occur and can be treated with muscle relaxants.

Glutethimide (Doriden)-codeine combinations are known on the street as "packs" or "loads." Effects such as cerebral edema, seizures, and prominent anticholinergic properties of these agents may require treatment.

SUGGESTED READING

Augenstein L, Kulig K. Management of the poisoned patient. In: Schwartz GR, Bircher N, Hanke BK, et al, eds. Emergency medicine: The essential update. Philadelphia: WB Saunders, 1989:191–209.

Ellenhorn MJ, Barceloux DG. Medical toxicity: Diagnosis and treatment of human poisoning. New York: Elsevier, 1988.

Gross PL. Toxicologic emergencies. In: Wilkins EW, ed. Emergency medicine: Scientific foundations and current practice. 3rd ed. Baltimore: Williams & Wilkins, 1989:395–422.

Litovitz TL, Schmitz BF, Holm KC. 1988 Annual report of the American Association of Poison Control Centers National Data Collection System. Am J Emerg Med 1989; 7:495–545.

Sidford C. Designer drugs. Massachusetts Poison Control System. Clin Toxicol Rev 1989; 11:11

Ungar JR. Current drugs of abuse. In: Schwartz GR, Bircher N, Hanke BK, et al, eds. Emergency medicine: The essential update. Philadelphia: WB Saunders, 1989:210–224.

U.S. Department of Justice, Drug Enforcement Administration. Drugs of abuse. 1988. Available through Superintendent of Documents, U.S. Government Printing Office, Washington, D.C.

ENTERAL NUTRITION: LIQUID FORMULA DIETS

J. JASON PAYNE-JAMES, M.B., F.R.C.S.
DAVID B.A. SILK, M.D., F.R.C.P.

Nutritional support has been provided via the enteral route by tube for many hundreds of years. Formal clinical assessment and scientific evaluation of the enteral route, however, has been undertaken only in the last decade and a half. This almost certainly relates to the emergence of total parenteral nutrition (TPN) as an effective method of nutritional support in the latter half of the 1960s. Much research was based on TPN, and enteral nutrition techniques were to some extent ignored or forgotten. However, enteral nutritional support is considerably cheaper, is more physiologic, and has fewer complications than TPN. Undoubtedly there are situations in which TPN alone is indicated, but our feeling is that overuse does occur, and that TPN is inappropriately prescribed for some patients when they would be better served by the enteral route. Enteral nutritional support has now developed into a technique well supported by basic physiologic experimentation and controlled clinical studies. Our recommendations are based on 10 years of research and clinical experience.

INDICATIONS AND RATIONALE

In our unit, patients who are considered for interventional nutritional support make up three main groups. The first consists of all patients with severe clinical malnutrition as manifested by a weight loss of more than 10 percent in the preceding month, a serum albumin level of less than 30 g per liter, and muscle wasting, with or without peripheral hypoproteinemic edema. The second group includes those who are moderately malnourished and who have had a reduced dietary intake for the previous 2 to 4 weeks. The third group are those who may on initial examination be normally or near-normally nourished, but who may be expected to develop protein energy malnutrition because of their underlying pathologic condition in the absence of nutritional support. Our indications for instituting enteral feeding (in this context taken to mean all feeding administered by tube into some part of the alimentary tract) are based on the belief that *enteral nutrition should be considered for all patients in the above groups with a functioning, accessible gastrointestinal (GI) tract.*

There are three main contraindications to enteral nutrition, which relate to patients with true paralytic ileus, intestinal obstruction, or major intra-abdominal sepsis.

Table 1 lists the widely differing conditions in which enteral nutrition may be used. Enteral nutrition may be considered to be primary treatment in some cases (e.g., malabsorption, fistulae) or supportive (secondary) treatment when it merely supplies adequate nutrient intake. These distinctions are not always absolute. In Crohn's disease, for example, there is evidence that administration of an elemental diet may induce a remission of the disease. However, many Crohn's patients are malnourished, and clearly administration of an enteral feed also improves their nutritional status, which may in itself aid remission. Unfortunately, many studies examining the effects of nutri-

TABLE 1 Pathologic and Other Conditions for Which Enteral Nutrition by the Enteral Route May Be Considered

Anorexia nervosa	Malabsorption syndromes
Burns	Motor neuron disease
Cardiac disease	Neoplastic disease
Cerebrovascular disease	Preoperative
Cystic fibrosis*	Postoperative
Fistulae*	Renal failure
Hepatic failure	Respiratory failure
Inflammatory bowel disease (Crohn's,* ulcerative colitis)	Sepsis
Intensive care	Short bowel syndrome*
	Trauma

* Pathologic conditions for which enteral nutrition may be considered primary treatment.

tional support on inflammatory bowel disease are difficult to interpret because of the concurrent standard medical therapy. At present, we consider that if patients with inflammatory bowel disease are malnourished, or at risk of becoming so during a relapse, they require nutritional support, initially via the enteral route. The evidence now available suggests that patients with Crohn's disease may benefit preferentially with an elemental rather than a polymeric diet, a benefit that is not apparent in ulcerative colitis. These aspects are also discussed in the chapter *Crohn's Disease of the Small Bowel*.

Clearly the list in Table 1 includes patients from most medical specialties and emphasizes the wide potential application of enteral nutritional support.

MANAGEMENT

Administration Techniques

A variety of factors have been identified that are likely to result in inadequate nutritional intake for enterally fed patients. These include poor performance of enteral feeding tubes, the wrong choice of enteral diet, the wrong route of administration, the use of low-volume reservoirs, and the use of starter regimens. All these factors must be considered if optimal enteral nutritional support for individual patients is to be given. The four main areas that need to be taken into account are listed in Table 2.

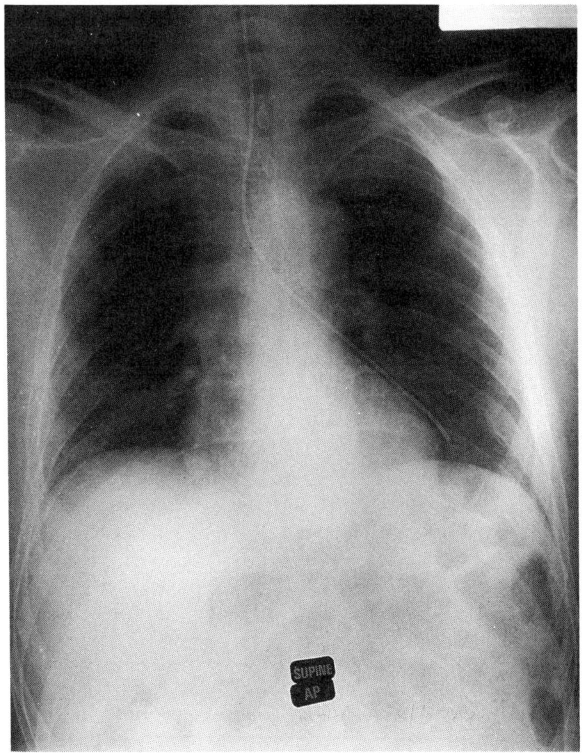

Figure 1 Chest x-ray film showing a fine-bore tube in the left main bronchus.

Route of Administration

Most patients require nutritional support for 4 weeks or less. For these patients the best route of enteral delivery is by means of a fine-bore nasogastric feeding tube. These tubes are virtually free of the complications associated with the Ryle's type of wide-bore nasogastric tube. Therefore, rhinitis, pharyngitis, esophagitis, esophageal erosions and stricture, and upper GI hemorrhage, previously noted in association with nasogastric intubation, are now rarely if ever seen.

Fine-bore tubes with wire stylets should be inserted pernasally by persons trained in the technique. The most important rule with all such tubes is never to use the wire stylet to attempt to resite the tube while the tube is still in the patient, because it is in this situation that the very rare stylet penetration of the esophagus or other viscus is most likely to occur.

The most frequent complication, occurring in approximately 2.5 percent of patients, is tube malposition at initial insertion, most commonly into the trachea and bronchi (Fig. 1). The presence of a fine-bore tube within the bronchus is not in itself a cause of morbidity. If, however, the presence within the bronchus has not been established, accidental intrapulmonary aspiration of feed may occur (Fig. 2), which may be fatal if unrecognized at an early stage. The patients most at risk from this complication are those with altered swallowing or a diminished gag reflex.

TABLE 2 Factors to Consider When Starting Enteral Nutrition

Route (access to GI tract)
Reservoirs and giving sets
Infusion versus bolus administration
Starter regimens

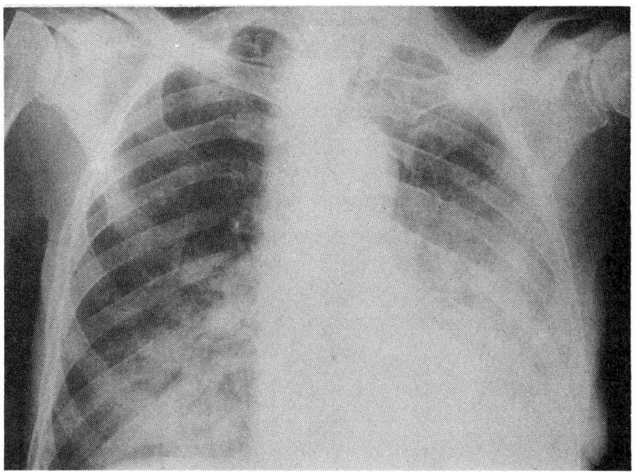

Figure 2 Chest x-ray film demonstrating the typical appearance after pulmonary aspiration of enteral diet.

In patients who are alert and orientated, we confirm correct positioning of the tube by aspiration of gastric contents (pH less than 3) and auscultation of the epigastrium. Aspiration of gastric contents through the tube is not always possible, but controlled trials have demonstrated a significant improvement both in the ability to aspirate via the tube, and in the length of time the tube remains in situ when comparing a polyurethane tube incorporating a modified outflow port (Corpak, Wheeling, IL) and a standard polyvinyl chloride tube. If aspiration or auscultation is unsuccessful, *x-ray confirmation of the position of the tube is essential and must be undertaken routinely in all patients with altered consciousness, with altered cough or gag reflex, or who are mechanically ventilated.* In common with other physicians, we still find that unplanned or nonelective extubations of the fine-bore tubes occur in up to 60 percent of patients and result in interruption of the feeding program. As yet there is no simple and effective method of fixing the fine-bore tube in place. Regular checks and observation of patients is probably the best way of keeping unplanned extubations to a minimum. Suggestions that the addition of a weight to the distal end of the tube may help to keep the tubes in place have not been confirmed in controlled clinical trials.

In some patients nasogastric delivery of nutrients may not be appropriate because of an increased risk of regurgitation or pulmonary aspiration of feed (Table 3). All such patients, as well as those who have gastric atony of paresis for any reason, should be considered for postpyloric nasoduodenal or nasojejunal feeding to reduce the risk of regurgitation or aspiration. Placement of fine-bore tubes beyond the pylorus remains a problem. Tubes with differing distal ends, with and without weights, and with and without bolus tips have all been studied in attempts to find a particular tube that may spontaneously pass (on most occasions) into the duodenum after pernasal passage. As yet no consistently reliable tube has been produced. Other techniques of placing pernasal tubes intraduodenally or intrajejunally have been described. The administration of metoclopramide, manipulation of the tube at the bedside, or manipulation under fluoroscopic control have all been tried with varying success. Our own policy is to introduce a fine-bore tube of appropriate length pernasally, and if spontaneous passage has not occurred after 12 to 24 hours, endoscopic positioning is undertaken. Clearly, confirmatory x-ray studies should be taken at regular intervals, since the tube may migrate proximally into the stomach.

TABLE 3 Patient Groups and Diseases With an Increased Risk of Regurgitation and Aspiration

Diabetes with neuropathy
Hypothyroidism
Intensive Care Unit patients on ventilators
Neuromotor deglutition disorders
Neurosurgical patients
Post-abdominal surgery patients
Stroke

For some patients other routes of administration may be preferable to the nasoenteral route. Pharyngostomy has been described for patients requiring long-term nutritional support, and a technique has been described for insertion under local anesthesia. Esophagostomy may be used in some patients with oropharyngeal neoplasms or after massive facial surgery. Surgically placed gastrostomies are still used for long-term administration of feed in patients with incurable deglutition disorders (e.g., motor neuron disease, multiple sclerosis), but the percutaneous endoscopic gastrostomy (PEG) is probably the technique of choice for planned administration of enteral nutrition for periods of longer than 4 to 6 weeks. Although not yet widely used in the United Kingdom, this technique is now well established in the United States and enables a gastrostomy tube to be inserted under endoscopic control, using local anesthesia. Specially designed PEG sets are now available, which simplify insertion considerably. This technique has proved to be straightforward, with satisfactorily low morbidity and mortality rates compared with the conventional surgical placement of gastrostomy tubes using the Stamm or Depage-Janeway method.

Two specific complications of this technique are reported: (1) necrotizing fasciitis of the anterior abdominal wall, which may be prevented by the use of prophylactic antibiotics; and (2) pneumoperitoneum, which may persist for days and even weeks after tube insertion, but eventually resolves.

Delaney's technique of needle catheter jejunostomy (NCJ) has gained wide acceptance, and newer polyurethane catheters may improve flow characteristics. The catheter is inserted either as a separate surgical procedure or concurrently at the time of abdominal surgery. The fine catheter is inserted into the jejunum and is then brought out through the anterior abdominal wall, away from the laparotomy wound to facilitate postoperative enteral feeding. This procedure is also associated with low morbidity, and has a major complication rate of less than 2 percent. It has been suggested that an NCJ could be recommended for patients (1) malnourished at the time of surgery, (2) undergoing major upper GI surgery, (3) who may receive adjuvant radio- or chemotherapy after surgery, and (4) undergoing laparotomy after major trauma. The availability of this route means that TPN with its attendant risks may be avoided. Our own feelings are that a well-designed, pernasal, fine-bore, double-lumen polyurethane tube with gastric aspiration ports and a jejunal feeding port, positioned during surgery, may be even safer for many of these patients.

Reservoirs and Giving Sets

Enteral feeds were originally administered from 500-ml reservoirs after make-up of feed within a hospital diet kitchen. This does not allow production of sterile feeds, and because of the risk of subsequent bacterial growth and concomitant diarrhea, our policy is to use commercially prepared, sterile enteral diets dispensed from 1- or 1.5-liter containers to reduce the handling required. The policy of using larger reservoirs also improves the ratio of volume of administered diet to volume of prescribed diet, which may be as low as 60 percent with smaller containers. At present we advise a change of giving set every 24 hours, since there is a small but definite risk of ascending contamination of the diet container. However, we are undertaking studies of a closed diet administration system using Tetrabrik 1-liter containers (Corpak, Wheeling, IL), which may reduce both handling time and risk of bacterial contamination and thus allowing prolonged use of giving sets (Fig. 3).

Infusion Versus Bolus Administration

Bolus feeding of enteral diets, in which a volume of perhaps 200 to 400 ml of feed was instilled into the stomach via a nasogastric tube over a period ranging from 15 minutes to 1 hour, was the standard method of administration for many years. As enteral nutrition techniques have developed, it has become clear that bolus administration is not the ideal technique of administering enteral diet, although the side effects such as bloating and diarrhea are similar to those with infusion. In addition, a considerable amount of nursing time is required for bolus feeding, and feeds may often be accidentally omitted. Continuous infusion, either by gravity feed or with a peristaltic pump, is therefore the method of choice. A continuous infusion for 8 to 16 hours overnight, depending on the feed volume, followed by disconnection during the day may be the optimal technique.

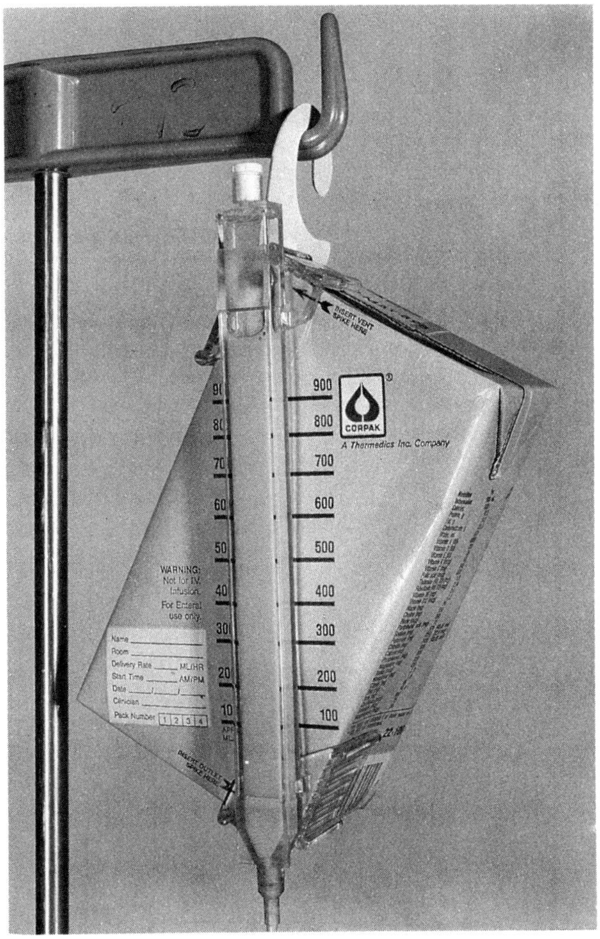

Figure 3 "Closed" diet administration system.

Starter Regimens

It was once thought that in order to minimize GI side effects, the diet should be administered initially in low volumes or in a diluted form, gradually increased to full volume and full strength over a number of days. This concept has now been shown to be incorrect. Controlled clinical trials have demonstrated that the only result of limiting intake of diet in the first few days is to prolong the length of negative nitrogen balance. The incidence of GI side effects is unchanged in patients with normal bowel or those with inflammatory bowel disease when a full-strength, full-volume diet is used at the start of enteral nutrition.

TYPES OF ENTERAL DIETS

Four main groups of diets are produced commercially (Tables 4 and 5).

Polymeric Diets

Polymeric enteral diets are indicated in patients with normal or near-normal GI function. These diets contain whole protein as the nitrogen source and a mixture of carbohydrate and fat as the energy source. The fat component usually makes up 30 to 35 percent of the total energy, and the carbohydrate component consists of a heterogeneous glucose polymer mixture, 49 to 53 percent of total energy content. The polymeric diets are nutritionally complete and thus contain daily electrolyte, vitamin, and trace element requirements. Recent research has questioned whether the recommended daily allowance (RDA) of vitamins and trace elements is sufficient in disease states, and most of the new polymeric diets contain at least 120 percent RDA per 2 liters. At present almost none of the polymeric diets contain omega-3 fatty acids. The potential

TABLE 4 Types of Enteral Diet

Polymeric*
Predigested, chemically defined (elemental)*
Disease specific
Modular

* See Table 5 for suggested composition.

TABLE 5 Suggested Formulation of Polymeric and Predigested Enteral Diets

	Polymeric		
	Standard	*Energy, Nitrogen dense*	*Predigested*
Nitrogen source	Whole protein	Whole protein	Free amino acids or oligopeptide (chain length 2–3 residues)
Concentration (g/L)	6–7	8–10	6–8
Carbohydrate source	Glucose oligomers	Glucose oligomers	Glucose oligomers (purified, chain length <10 residues)
% Energy	49–53	47–51	60–65
Concentration (g/L)	120–140	140–160	145–165
Fat source	LCTs	LCTs	LCTs 12.5%, MCTs 7.5%
% Energy	49–53	49–53	20%
Concentration (g/L)	34–40	40–60	20–25
Na^+ mmol	40–60	40–60	60–80
K^+ mmol	40–60	40–60	40–60
Cl^- mmol	40–60	40–60	40–60
Vitamins (% RDA/2L)	120–130	120–130	120–130
Trace elements (% RDA/2L)	120–130	120–130	120–130
Caloric density (kcal/ml)	1.0	1.0–1.5	1.0
Nonprotein energy Nitrogen ratio (kcal/g nitrogen)	120–150	88–110	130–150
Osmolality	300	350–400	350–550

LCTs=long-chain triglycerides; MCTs=medium-chain triglycerides; RDA=recommended daily allowance.

importance of these is currently under investigation, and future diets may contain a fat source with an omega-6 to omega-3 fatty acid ratio close to 5:1.

Generally, one of two polymeric diets, a "standard" or "energy-nitrogen–dense" diet is prescribed. The standard polymeric diet contains 6 to 7 g nitrogen per liter with an energy density of 1 kcal per milliliter and a nonprotein calorie-to-nitrogen ratio of 120 to 150 kcal per gram of nitrogen. The energy-nitrogen–dense varieties usually contain 8 to 10 g nitrogen per liter and have an energy density of 1 to 1.5 kcal per milliliter, with a nonprotein calorie-to-nitrogen ratio of 88 to 110. A recent study undertaken by our group has stressed the benefits of using an energy-nitrogen–dense diet *routinely* in all patients with normal or near-normal GI function.

Predigested, Chemically Defined Elemental Diets

A small group of patients requiring enteral nutrition have such impaired GI function that luminal hydrolysis becomes rate limiting with respect to nutrient absorption. Examples are patients with nutritionally inadequate short bowel syndrome and those with severe exocrine pancreatic insufficiency. In these, predigested nutrients, presented in the form in which maximal absorption occurs in the absence of luminal or brush border hydrolysis, are indicated. The composition of the predigested, chemically defined elemental diets has been at least partly based on this philosophy. The nitrogen source consists of either free amino acids or oligopeptide mixtures. Our recent research indicates that if an oligopeptide-based nitrogen source is to be used, mixtures of di- and tripeptides rather than longer-chain peptides should be used, since brush border hydrolysis in the absence of luminal hydrolysis becomes rate limiting with respect to absorption if tetra- or higher peptides are used. At present, heterogeneous glucose polymer mixtures with approximately 50 percent of total glucose content as glucose polymers of ten or more molecules constitute the bulk of the energy source. In most clinical situations this is satisfactorily assimilated. In rare instances, however, a purified low-molecular-weight glucose polymer mixture, with glucose present as polymers containing less than ten glucose molecules, is likely to lead to an enhancement of glucose uptake by the gut.

Several of the new predigested diets contain a mixture of long- and medium-chain triglycerides as the fat source. In situations where there are deficient luminal bile salt concentrations (e.g., obstructive jaundice), markedly reduced luminal lipase activity (e.g., severely impaired exocrine pancreatic insufficiency), or very rapid transit through short segments of small intestine with reduced functional absorptive capacity (e.g., the short bowel syndrome), long-chain triglycerides (LCTs) are poorly assimilated. It is doubtful whether the inclusion of more than a small amount of LCTs (10 to 13 percent) is of benefit. Medium-chain triglycerides (MCTs) are assimilated more easily in the presence of reduced luminal bile salt and luminal lipase activity. The ease of assimilation of MCTs under these conditions may have been overestimated, and there seems little point in these diets that contain more than 10 percent total energy content as MCTs.

Many currently available predigested diets contain sodium in concentrations of 30 to 60 mmol per liter. Perfusion studies suggest that water secretion occurs from the gut unless the sodium concentration exceeds 80 mmol per liter. For patients with the short bowel syndrome, therefore, sodium supplements may be required.

Disease-Specific Diets

Specially formulated diets have been developed for patients with specific diseases such as encephalopathy associated with chronic liver disease, and respiratory failure. Malnourished patients with cirrhosis who present with encephalopathy, or who have a previous history of episodes of encephalopathy, pose a difficult problem of nutritional management. From the viewpoint that these individuals have characteristically impaired circulating plasma amino acid profiles, suggestions have been made that an enteral diet based on a modified amino acid nitrogen source (with decreased levels of aromatic amino acids phenylalanine, tyrosine, and tryptophan; decreased methionine; and increased branched-chain amino acids) may be beneficial. At present the results of controlled clinical trials are conflicting, and more research is required before clear clinical recommendations about the use of disease-specific diets in malnourished, encephalopathic cirrhotic patients can be made.

Patients with respiratory failure on ventilators have been shown to be adversely affected by diets containing high carbohydrate loads. The administration of a diet with a higher fat-energy component may be beneficial in allowing earlier weaning off the ventilator. We use this diet particularly in ventilated intensive care patients (Pulmocare, Abbot Laboratories, Ltd.).

Enteral diets are available for use in renal failure. These contain a nitrogen source consisting of all the essential amino acids plus histidine, without the nonessential amino acids. Theoretically these diets promote the reutilization of urea nitrogen for the synthesis of the nonessential amino acids in the liver by transamination. At present there is no firm evidence from controlled clinical trials to support their use.

Other compounds have been advocated for improving nitrogen balance in stressed, postoperative, or septic patients. We are currently undertaking studies on the enteral administration of the ornithine salt of the Krebs-cycle intermediate alpha-ketoglutarate, ornithine alpha-ketoglutarate (Cetornan, Laboratoires Jacques Logeais, Issy-les-Molyneaux, France) to evaluate this substrate further. Intravenous and enteral administration of this compound has demonstrated apparent beneficial effects on nitrogen balance and postoperative skeletal muscle protein synthesis.

Modular Diets

Modular diets are occasionally used (in less than 5 percent of patients) when a particular component of diet requires an increased intake or if a patient requires a special blend of diet.

STARTING ENTERAL FEEDING

Once access is gained to the gut by whatever route and the appropriate diet chosen, enteral nutrition may begin. For patients who are immobile or confined to bed, or who have altered consciousness, our practice is to elevate the head of the bed by 20 or 30 degrees to help reduce the risk of regurgitation and aspiration. In most adult patients with no other metabolic or fluid balance problems, we prescribe 2 to 2.5 liters of diet on a daily basis. This volume is infused from day 1. Only in a small percentage of patients (less than 10 percent) do we need to reduce the rate of administration initially.

We find in our Intensive Therapy Unit (ITU) that approximately 60 percent of patients tolerate enteral feeding. The patients in the ITU in whom we are least likely to prescribe enteral nutrition are those with major abdominal sepsis or who have undergone very major GI surgery. In most cases, if these patients require nutritional support, TPN is appropriate initially. Patients on ventilators often have absent bowel sounds; this alone is not a contraindication to enteral nutrition, although sadly it is often used as a reason not to begin enteral nutrition. However, enteral nutrition is contraindicated in the presence of gross abdominal distention, or more than 400 ml of gastric aspirate in 24 hours. If neither of these are present and the patient is unlikely to feed normally for at least 72 hours, enteral nutrition is indicated. In the first 24 hours of enteral infusion, nasogastric aspiration is undertaken every 2 to 3 hours; if more than 100 ml of feed is aspirated, the infusion should be decreased or stopped temporarily. If after 24 hours there is little residual volume after each aspiration, the regular gastric aspirations can be abandoned.

MONITORING

It is just as important to monitor patients receiving enteral nutritional support as it is to monitor those on TPN, although this need not be done on such a frequent basis, once the feeding regimen is established. Patients who are most likely to develop problems are those with major concurrent illnesses rather than those to whom enteral nutrition is being administered to preserve nutritional status.

Diet charts enable an accurate record to be kept of the *actual* as opposed to *prescribed* intake. As mentioned earlier, there is often a great disparity between these two figures, and the charts will permit correction of intake problems. They are also of importance during the changeover from enteral feeding to per os nutrition.

Weighing is probably the simplest, but most valuable way to ensure that the enteral nutrition regimen prescribed for a particular patient is satisfactory. A steady increase in weight of 1 to 2 kg per week suggests adequate nutrition in those requiring body mass repletion. In those in whom nutritional maintenance is required, over- or underestimates of needs are quickly identified.

Basic hematologic and biochemical parameters should be measured at the start of enteral nutrition. Once nutritional support has been stabilized, weekly measurements are reasonable. Initially, close monitoring of the plasma potassium and phosphate levels is important, along with plasma glucose. One study of tube-fed patients showed an incidence of hyperkalemia in 40 percent, hypophosphatemia in 30 percent, and hyperglycemia in 29 percent. In patients on long-term feeding, checks on vitamin levels or trace element levels may be required if clinically indicated. The plasma proteins albumin, transferrin, and thyroid-binding prealbumin can all be useful markers for indicating a response to nutritional support over a period of time. Urinary urea levels allow an estimate of nitrogen excretion and nitrogen balance to be made, although this is not as accurate as direct determination of urinary nitrogen.

Anthropometric and dynamometric measurements are often considered as research tools, but they offer sensitive and effective demonstrations of the efficacy of nutritional support over a period of time.

COMPLICATIONS

Most potential complications have been discussed above. The potential complications of enteral nutrition are summarised in Table 6.

Tube blockage most commonly occurs after disconnection of the giving set from the feeding tube. As a result, stagnant feeds congeal within the tube. This complication may be prevented by flushing the tube with water after disconnection, and by not allowing crushed tablets to be administered via the tube. Some practitioners recommend flushing enteral tubes up to six times in 24 hours even when continuous infusion is undertaken, although this may be excessive.

Diarrhea is thought to occur in up to 30 percent of patients in some series, although definitions of the term are often unclear. We consider diarrhea to be passage of too loose or too frequent stools, or both, sufficient to have been observed by patient and nursing staff. Because of the difficulty of defining diarrhea in the context of enteral nutrition, its etiology remains unclear. There is, however, a definite association with concomitant antibiotic therapy, and there seems to be increasing evidence that hypoalbuminemia may play a role. For the present, until the cause is clearly established, symptomatic treatment is appropriate, and only rarely does enteral feeding have to be discontinued. Nausea and vomiting may occur in up to 20 percent of enterally fed patients according to some series; our own experience suggests perhaps 5 to 10 percent. The causes are various and may relate to unpalatibility or to the smell of some enteral formula. Other suggested reasons, such as delayed gastric emptying or intolerance because of high osmolality, are difficult to accept in the light of current knowledge of GI physiology. Antiemetics are often helpful. The symptoms of bloating, abdominal distention, and cramps most commonly occur following inadvertent overly rapid administration of feed, and are similar to the symptoms described in association with bolus-type feeding. Finally, mention must be made of the interaction of enteral diets and drugs. Various reports have been published documenting problems with drug therapies in patients being enterally fed. Specifically, problems have been reported with theophylline, warfarin, methyldopa, and digoxin. It is clear that failure of drug therapy in previously stable patients receiving enteral nutritional support must be assumed to be feed related until it is proved otherwise.

We have outlined the methods by which our unit instigates and administers enteral nutritional support and the ways in which we attempt to keep complications to a minimum. Undoubtedly this can be done only with a team approach. A recent report has confirmed the value of an Enteral Nutrition Support team, just as TPN teams have proved invaluable. The continuity provided by such a team (in our case consisting of representatives from clinical medicine, dietetics, nursing, chemical pathology, and pharmacy) enables optimal nutritional support to be given to those patients most in need of it.

TABLE 6 Complications of Enteral Nutrition

Feeding tube related	Malposition
	Unwanted removal
	Blockage
Diet related	Diarrhea
	Bloating
	Nausea
	Cramps
	Regurgitation
	Pulmonary aspiration
	Vitamin, mineral, trace element deficiencies
	Drug interactions
Metabolic-biochemical	
Infective	Diets
	Reservoirs
	Giving sets

SUGGESTED READING

Alpers DH, Clouse RE, Stenson WF. Manual of nutritional therapeutics. Boston: Little, Brown, 1988.

Jeejeebhoy KN, ed. Current therapy in nutrition. Toronto: BC Decker, 1988.

Payne-James JJ, Silk DB. Enteral nutrition: background, management and indications. In: Burns HJ, ed. Nutritional support, Bailliere's clinical gastroenterology. London: Bailliere Tindall, 1988.

Rombeau JL, Caldwell MD, eds. Clinical nutrition. Vol I. Enteral and tube feeding. Philadelphia: WB Saunders, 1984.

Silk DB. Nutritional support in clinical practice. London: Blackwell Scientific Publications, 1983.

TOTAL PARENTERAL NUTRITION

THOMAS G. BAUMGARTNER, M.Ed., Pharm.D., F.A.S.H.P.
JAMES J. CERDA, M.D.

In 1968 the term "hyperalimentation," coined by Dudrick, introduced parenteral feeding using hydrolysates and high-concentration dextrose to the clinical nutritionist. Yet it was not until later, in the 1970s, when the advent of an acceptable fat emulsion (with minimal adverse effects) was added to synthetic amino acid and concentrated dextrose regimens, constituting a truly "total" nutritional regimen.

The literature then pressed onward, and clinicians began to think more and more of parenteral nutrition as a modality to treat disease. The importance of first, parenteral macrosubstrates, and then micronutrients, was appreciated. Today, the important regulatory mechanisms for macronutrient and micronutrient kinetics are receiving aggressive investigation. The spectrum of understanding has turned to substrate interactions and hormonal controls. Furthermore, the role of other factors such as tumor necrosis factor and interleukins on nutritional status is now being actively investigated.

The clinical nutritionist in the twentieth century must have a keen awareness of the ingredients and the monitoring parameters of total parenteral nutrition (TPN) to optimize both institutional and ambulatory nutritional care. The purpose of this chapter is to convey a working knowledge base of both the ingredients (Table 1) and the monitoring of TPN therapy.

PATIENT ASSESSMENT

Initially, anthropometric measurements of midarm muscle circumference to assess muscle mass, and tricep skinfold-scapula determinations of fat stores, were used to grossly assess the anthropometric status of the TPN patient. The assessment of malnutrition by simple methods was studied in 120 patients undergoing elective major abdominal surgery to determine which index was of the most value in predicting postoperative complications. Weight for height and weight loss were of little significant value; serum albumin levels less than 3.5 g per deciliter were more significant ($p < .05$), but were predictive for only one-quarter of patients who developed serious complications. Measurements of muscle stores by anthropometry (arm and forearm muscle circumference) predicted nearly one-half of the patients ($p < .01$). By far the most useful index was hand-grip dynamometry, which predicted 90 percent of those who would develop complications ($p < .001$). The incidence of serious complications was six times greater in patients with a low grip strength. Hand-grip dynamometry appears to be a useful screening test of patients at risk, and a valuable additional test for nutritional assessment.

Anthropometry (the use of body measurements to assess nutritional status) is a practical and immediately applicable technique for assessing developmental patterns for children. However, anthropometric indicators are less accurate than clinical and biochemical techniques when it comes to assessing individual nutritional status. In many field situations in which resources are severely limited, anthropometry can be used as a screening device to identify individuals at risk of undernutrition, followed by a more elaborate investigation using other techniques.

More recently, bioelectric impedance studies have been used to assess lean body mass and lipid body composition through noninvasive conductivity methods. The impedance method has been shown to have a lower predictive error or standard error of the estimates of estimating body fatness than a standard anthropometric technique (2.7 versus 3.9 percent).

Although many other methods (computerized tomography, magnetic resonance imaging, isotopic studies, etc.) have been used to assess the TPN patient, it appears that the monitoring of both anthropometric and biochemical parameters, coupled with clinical nutrition judgment (i.e., global, overt nutritional assessment), may be the preferred eclectic approach for the clinician.

PARENTERAL MACRONUTRIENTS

Protein

Hyperammonemia, hypersensitivity reactions, and the limited animal source of hydrolysates provoked the development of synthetic amino acid solutions in the late 1960s.

The inclusion, and now exclusion, of bisulfite preservatives (in most amino acid products), the recognition that acetate salts–acetic acid buffers were needed to address the acidemia associated with the original chloride salts, and the deletion of several amino acids have been the principal formulation modifications in nonessential and essential amino acid (NEAA/EAA) products.

Special Protein Formulations

Stress/Sepsis Formulations. Stressed adult patients may require as much as 2.5 g AA per kilogram per day. However, most clinicians supply up to 1.5 g AA per kilogram per day and increase to 2.5 AA per kilogram per day with considerable prudence to avoid adverse reactions (e.g., renal solute load and increased respiratory drive to breathlessness).

Burn patients are extremely stressed and may require up to 2.5 g AA per kilogram per day. The systemic metabolic and circulatory alterations following thermal injury are directed to support the healing wound. The open wound is an immediate bodily priority. Structural and functional components of uninjured tissue undergo breakdown to provide energy, substrate, and micronutrients for the healing wound. Glucose is synthesized by the liver and utilized by

Editor's Note: This chapter is more detailed and contains more investigative details than most other chapters in this book because of the thought that an in-depth review of the nutritional literature was warranted. A detailed reference list is available from the authors.

TABLE 1 Total Parenteral Nutrition Formulation Example

Parenteral Macronutrients		
Protein	Empiric: 1.5–2.5 g AA/Kg/day	
Carbohydrate	Empiric	
Lipid	Empiric	
Parenteral Micronutrients		
Electrolytes	Empiric	
	Sodium	80–120 mEq/day
	Potassium	80–120
	Calcium	7–15
	Magnesium	7–24
	Phosphate	7–15
	Acetate	Increase to address acidemia
	Chloride	Increase to address alkalemia
Trace elements	Empiric	
	Chromium	0.020 mg/day
	Copper	0.5–1
	Iodine	0.12
	Manganese	0.5
	Selenium	0.06
	Zinc	3–5
Vitamins	Empiric	
	Multivitamin (12) product* qd	
	Vitamin K	2 mg q wk*

* Available together in pediatric products.

granulation tissue. Wound blood flow is elevated and the injured surface is heated to enhance repair. These changes in systemic metabolism are directed by alterations in neurohumoral control. The exact mechanisms utilized by the wound to initiate these changes are presently unknown.

Combinations of both fat and glucose energy sources with protein supplementation are preferred in burn patients. Early on, infusion of soybean oil emulsion was indistinguishable from low dosage glucose when administered with amino acids. It was shown that a combination of both energy macrosubstrates are preferred in this patient population.

In infected adults, optimal protein intake to produce positive nitrogen balance is 1.5 to 2.0 g of protein per kilogram per day. This appears to reflect the fact that 16 percent of the caloric expenditure comes from protein sources during injury. Since this value is approximately twice that seen during nonstressful situations, the reuse of body protein appears to be decreased. Urinary 3-methylhistidine has been used as a serial measure of relative amount of branched-chain amino acid (BCAA) from muscle that has been metabolized and excreted. Urinary excretion of the post-translationally modified amino acid 3-methylhistidine, derived from the contractile proteins actin and myosin, was measured in patients with conditions associated with nitrogen loss. The ratio of 3-methylhistidine to creatinine excretion, a measure of the fractional catabolic rate of myofibrillar protein, was increased in severe injury, thyrotoxicosis, neoplastic disease, prednisolone administration, and sometimes Duchenne muscular dystrophy. In myxedema, osteomalacia, and hypothermia the ratio was decreased; starvation, elective operations, and rheumatoid arthritis had little effect. Provided that the diet is meat free, measurement of urinary 3-methylhistidine may provide useful information about the cause of protein loss. It was also suggested that increases in urinary 3-methylhistidine above basal levels can be quantitatively accounted for by the 3-methylhistidine content of additional food. In individuals on a constant diet, it should be possible to detect relatively small changes in 3-methylhistidine excretion.

The BCAA have received considerable study in the area of stress and sepsis. Nonetheless, much remains to be learned about their efficacy (safety and effectiveness) in high stress (45 percent BCAA), renal failure (40 percent BCAA), and liver failure (35 percent BCAA).

In addition to the special amino acid formulations, pediatric solutions have been commercialized. In the future, one may envision a special amino acid solution for the aged. As a person ages, there is a progressive diminution of total body protein, due largely to a decline in the size of skeletal muscle mass. These changes are accompanied by a shift in the overall pattern of whole body protein synthesis and breakdown; muscle masses estimated to account for about 30 percent of whole body protein turnover in young adults, compared with 20 percent or less in the elderly. Because skeletal muscle mass plays an important role in the response of body protein and amino acid metabolism to stress, such as infection and trauma, this decline in the contribution of muscle to total body protein metabolism may be responsible for the reduced ability of older people to withstand unfavorable circumstances. Therefore, the protein needs in the elderly are likely to be higher than in the young.

Renal Failure Formulations. The FDA-approved indication for essential amino acids is acute renal failure. EAA are said to be converted to NEAA in vivo as needed, minimizing ureagenesis.

Patients in renal failure require approximately 0.5 to 0.8 g per kilogram per day to avoid excessive renal solute load if creatinine clearance is less than 25 to 30 ml per minute. Usual fluid requirements for TPN patients in general are approximately 1,600 ml per square meter per day for maintenance fluids and up to 70 ml per kilogram per day for replacement fluids. Renal failure patients, who are anuric, require about 500 to 750 ml per day to replace insensible losses. The fluid requirements for hemofiltration, hemodialysis, or peritoneal dialysis are empiric. Protein requirements similarly are empiricly based on nitrogen balances and visceral protein status, but the range is 1.2 to 1.5 g AA per kilogram per day. The higher protein needs are earmarked for the patient on peritoneal dialysis who loses amino acids and intact protein during the filtration procedure.

Nitrogen balance studies were performed by Giordano and colleagues in eight patients undergoing Chronic Ambulatory Peritoneal Dialysis (CAPD). Patients were studied in a metabolic ward for 14 days while eating a diet providing 1.2 g per kilogram per day and supplying 166 to 188 kcal per kilogram. It was concluded that 1.2 g per kilogram per day is a safe intake for patients on CAPD. Nevertheless, it is strongly suggested that patients on CAPD should undergo nitrogen balance studies to verify the correct kilocalorie to nitrogen ratios for repletion and anabolism.

There appear to be insufficient data to support any positive benefits of ketoacids over essential amino acids. On the contrary, evidence on nitrogen balance in children and weight increments in infants clearly indicates that essential amino acids are preferable to ketoacids.

Hepatic Failure Formulations. The hepatic formulations are indicated for grade II encephalopathic patients or patients who have a serum BCAA to aromatic amino acid (AAA) ratio of less than 2. Much has been written about the causes of hepatic encephalopathy, including ammonia, mercaptans, fatty acids, altered levels of plasma amino acid levels, and abnormal neurotransmitter pharmacology. A functional impairment of the amino acid transport systems at the level of the blood-brain barrier seems to play a crucial role in causing deleterious modifications of the synaptic neurotransmission in the central nervous system (CNS) in hepatic encephalopathic syndromes. The reduction of the AAA (said to be a precursor of optopamine, a neurotransmitter that may depress sensorium) transport to the brain usually obtained by parenteral administration of BCAA has been described as of benefit, but the matter is still unresolved. In addition, more concentrated amino acid solutions (15 percent) have been introduced for volume-restricted patients.

Choice of protein requirements for hepatically compromised patients is also empirical, beginning with 0.5 g AA per kilogram per day and increasing to 1 g AA per kilogram per day as tolerated. The synthetic, parenteral amino acids are soy based. It has been suggested that there is less encephalopathy with oral vegetable-based diets. The literature associated with the use of high BCAA and lower concentrations of AAA for hepatic patients has been reviewed recently and the matter is still open to conjecture.

The determination of free amino acids in human tissue is far more complicated than the analysis of plasma amino acids. The concentrations of free amino acids are different in plasma, liver, and muscle. Pathologic conditions such as sepsis, liver failure, and glucagonoma lead to characteristic alterations in the concentrations of free amino acids. However, the relationship between cytosolic amino acid concentrations and protein synthesis is not yet clear. The importance of balanced amino acid solutions is appreciated when one recognizes that reduced levels of even a single amino acid (e.g., glutamine) may lead to a downregulation of protein synthesis.

Dipeptide/Tripeptide Formulations. Parenteral dipeptide and tripeptides have been studied in relation to synthetic amino acids. Ten healthy humans received parenteral nutrition consisting of 80 g of a dipeptide–amino acid mixture and 900 carbohydrate calories infused over 12 hours, and then fasted for another 12 hours. There were no adverse reactions in any of the patients who received the parenteral dipeptide–amino acid mixture. The urinary excretion of the five dipeptides during parenteral nutrition ranged between 1 and 2 percent of the amount infused. The results of this study showed efficient use of glycyl-dipeptides as substrates for parenteral nutrition in man.

Protein-Sparing Therapy

Protein-sparing therapy can be achieved with any one of the three macrosubstrates (amino acid, carbohydrate, and lipid) or any combination thereof. However, the degree of protein sparing is directly associated with the concentration and type of substrate. Since protein is the only macrosubstrate that contains nitrogen, it follows that the best protein-sparing therapy should contain protein and sufficient quantities to prevent endogenous nitrogen losses. Further, since optimal incorporation of nitrogen requires about 100 to 150 kcal of energy for every gram of nitrogen, the higher energy intakes can also be assumed to spare protein more effectively than the lower-energy regimens.

Indeed, it has been shown that albumin synthesis may be related to the higher-calorie regimen. Albumin synthesis rate, nitrogen balance, plasma hormone levels, and selected substrates were measured in 12 patients who underwent colonic operations and who were randomized to receive an intravenous fluid regimen that contained either 3.5 percent amino acids with 20 percent fat and 2.5 percent glucose, or 3.5 percent amino acids with 20 percent fat alone. The albumin synthesis rate was higher in patients who received the first of these intravenous mixtures, but they also had a significantly higher intake of calories.

The mean albumin synthesis rate in the group who received amino acids with glucose and fat was the highest measured. It was thought that the impressive increase in the albumin synthesis rate in those who received supplementary glucose was related to the extra energy infused. In contrast, nitrogen balance was similar in both groups, and thus was not predictive of protein synthesis. Additionally, myofibrillar protein degradation appeared to be equivalent in the two groups, as indicated by 3-methylhistidine output. Plasma albumin synthesis thus may be sensitive, especially to energy intake.

The protein-sparing effects of the peripheral infusion of crystalline amino acids was also studied metabolically in selected surgical patients subjected to various degrees of stress. Twenty-one patients (14 cancer patients receiving chemotherapy or radiotherapy, three with major abdominal traumatic injuries, and four with paralytic ileus) were infused for 21 of 24 hours per day with a solution of 4.2 percent amino acids with only 5 percent glucose as a source of nonprotein calories. One-half of the cancer patients were also allowed ad libitum oral intake of a regular hospital diet or a high-nitrogen elemental diet. The nutritional status was evaluated by measuring changes in body weight, serum albumin levels, and nitrogen balance. Body weight decreased in only the trauma patients. When these solutions were the sole source of nutrients, all patients were in negative nitrogen balance and had significant decreases in serum albumin levels; the latter were preserved only when extra sources of calories were provided. Thus, these studies provided evidence that the infusion of the crystalline amino acids without adequate levels of nonprotein energy does not conserve protein in these stressed patients.

Negative nitrogen balances have also been reported during protein sparing therapy (1 g AA per kilogram per day. Nitrogen balance was significantly less negative (p smaller than 0.01) during amino acid infusion periods (-5.8 ± 1.1 g per day) than during glucose infusion (-9.8 ± 1.8 g per day). No significant differences in nitrogen balance were noted between amino acid infusion periods, despite compositional differences in solutions. Elevated plasma levels of free fatty acids (0.71 ± 0.37 mM) and ketone bodies (1.3 ± 0.3 mM) observed during amino acid infusion periods reflected the availability of body lipids as energy substrate.

In particular, aggressive and early use of adequate (i.e., not solely protein sparing) nutritional support therapies in critically ill patients represents a major advance in critical care medicine. The net protein catabolism and erosion of protein stores that are characteristic of the metabolic response to injury result in significantly higher morbidity and mortality rates in critical care units. Early administration of appropriate protein and energy in support of enhanced demands maintains host defense and preserves organ function, thus allowing time for stabilization of clinical status while life support strategies are implemented. In all circumstances, protein, vitamins, minerals, and nonprotein calories must be provided within fluid and electrolyte restrictions and in conjunction with optimal hemodynamic and pulmonary support.

However, if protein-sparing therapy using only protein is employed in the setting of glucose and fat substrate intolerance, there is a need for greater amounts of protein to provide a positive balance in protein-depleted patients with gastrointestinal (GI) conditions. The data confirm not only that body protein mass can be maintained, but that a net positive nitrogen retention can be achieved in such patients through provision of exogenous amino acids and concurrent mobilization of endogenous energy stores. Of note is that fat mobilization can occur without plasma-free fatty acids or significant blood ketone body elevations. Therefore, an infusion of 2, rather than 3 per kilogram per day for protein sparing seems to be suitable in stressed GI patients.

In sum, parenteral protein supplementation should be approximately 1 to 2.5 g AA per kilogram per day. Monitoring parameters (Table 2) include urea nitrogen production in plasma and urine. Visceral and acute phase reactant proteins provide insight regarding protein status. Adverse effects reported from synthetic soy-based amino acids include azotemia, uremia, abnormal liver function, and anaphylaxis, but azotemia and uremia are the only effects reported with any frequency. There must be a clinical awareness of renal solute load (i.e., 1 g of protein can represent 4 mOsm) and increased ventilatory drive to the point of breathlessness as a consequence of protein excess. Finally, if possible, sufficient calories must accompany protein supplementation to avoid gluconeogenesis of an expensive substrate.

Carbohydrate

The clinical nutritionist must appreciate the profound effect that parenteral nutrition can have on metabolism. One report made an intriguing observation concerning the effect of parenteral nutrition on hepatic phase I oxidative metabolic mechanisms. Patients receiving a postoperative 2,000 kcal TPN regimen, providing all nonprotein calories as dextrose ($n = 16$), showed a 34 percent reduction of mean antipyrine clearance after 7 days of TPN compared with controls ($n = 13$, $p < .05$). This effect was also seen in patients receiving a 1600 kcal dextrose-based regimen ($n = 8$). In patients receiving a 2,000 kcal TPN regimen in which 500 kcal were provided as lipid ($n = 10$), mean antipyrine clearance was not significantly different from that of the control group. This study indicated the sensitivity of hepatic microsomal oxidative function, an important route of drug and nutrition metabolism, to different parenteral nutrition regimens. Further, there is an abundance of reports on the effects of nutrition on other kinetic parameters (absorption, distribution, and excretory function).

The mainstay of carbohydrate energy sources is still dextrose. Although available in various concentrations (5, 10, 20, 50, or 70 percent solutions), dextrose will always be of a low pH (4 to 6) and pyrogen free for parenteral administration. In neonates, fuels in addition to glucose are needed for cerebral metabolism. The chief shortcoming of glucose infusion lies in the possible need for refeeding, which in turn involves (predominantly) hypophosphatemia. Glucose infu-

TABLE 2 Pragmatic Monitoring Parameters for Parenteral Protein*

Plasma
Urea nitrogen
Albumin
Ceruloplasmin
Prealbumin
Retinol-binding protein
Transferrin
Urine
Urea nitrogen
Urinary nitrogen

* Hepatic, pulmonary, renal function testing should be included as needed.

sion drives phosphate (and other important electrolytes) out of the plasma, thereby depleting phosphate availability in the plasma and particularly depleting the erythrocyte content. Low levels of 2,3-diphosphoglycerate in red blood cells leads to increased hemoglobin-oxygen affinity. This action, coupled with decreased body temperature, hypocapnia, or alkalemia, may dramatically shift the oxygen dissociation curve to the left, tightening hemoglobin-oxygen affinity. In fact, fatal hypophosphatemia as a result of end-organ anoxia has been reported. This phenomenon continues to confuse clinicians, since serum phosphates have a circadian rhythm of as much as 2 mg per deciliter (normal levels are 2.5 to 4.6 mg per deciliter in adults), and signs and symptoms associated with low levels are unclear. Infusions in the range of 5 to 7 mg dextrose per kilogram per minute in adults and about 2½ to 3 times that rate in neonates are acceptable rates for glucose oxidation. Rates greater than these have been associated with an inability to metabolize glucose effectively. Hyperglycemia may lead to hyperosmotic dehydration and also has been associated with fatty liver infiltration and decreased liver function. Albumin synthesis regarding positional influences (as much as a 15 percent change), circadian rhythm (as much as 0.75 g per deciliter change in plasma level per day), and assay interferences must be carefully followed since its decreased synthesis may be associated with 75 to 90 percent of liver function compromise. Carbohydrate can be catalyzed to either pyruvate or, with insufficient tissue oxygen, anaerobically, to lactic acid. Ultimately, not unlike amino acid and fat, the end products of carbohydrate metabolism are carbon dioxide, water, and energy. Amino acids can be gluconeogenically converted (40 to 60 percent) to glucose, but the principal amino acid precursors to carbohydrate are alanine and glutamine.

The gut and kidneys (and their glutamine content) may play an important role in the altered glucose dynamics seen in patients with sepsis and other catabolic diseases. One study evaluated the dose-related trophic effects of glutamine, gastrin, and somatostatin on the in vitro growth of human gastric cancer cells and normal human gastric mucosal cells. Glutamine and gastrin stimulated the growth of both normal and malignant gastric mucosal cells. Compared with normal cells, the malignant cells responded to these growth factors at lower concentrations. Somatostatin enhanced growth of gastric cancer cells at all concentrations and inhibited growth of normal cells at high concentrations. Additional studies on the responsiveness of gastric adenocarcinoma to GI tract hormones may elucidate mechanisms of oncogenesis and suggest new therapeutic avenues for patients with gastric cancer.

Studies have also been performed during a postabsorptive basal period and during separate infusions of glutamine, glucose, and beta-hydroxybutyrate. During the basal period there was a significant arterial-portal vein gradient for glucose and glutamine. These substances were taken up by the gut, but there was no significant uptake of beta-hydroxybutyrate as determined in the basal studies. During substrate infusion, gut glucose uptake was unchanged, but consumption of glutamine and beta-hydroxybutyrate increased significantly. During parenteral feedings in patients with GI disorders, circulating levels of beta-hydroxybutyrate and glutamine are often low. It has been suggested that current parenteral formulations (that may contain L-glutamic acid but not glutamine) may not provide appropriate fuels for the GI tract.

Hyperglycemia has long been associated with sepsis, stress, and concentrated solutions of glucose. Many disease states hormonally influence the action of macrosubstrates. It has also been suggested that amino acids may even act as feedback regulators for the protein insulin.

Much work is now being done in the area of polypeptide secretion from the macrophage. These polypeptides, such as tumor necrosis factor or interleukin-I, may be responsible for skeletal proteolysis and lipoprotein lipase inhibition. Tumor necrosis factor may also be related to diarrhea and metabolic acidemia, both often found during the clinical management of the nutrition patient.

Since parenteral amino acids constitute the major expense of parenteral nutrition, the clinician should provide ample monitoring of protein metabolism so that therapy is cost effective. Provision of sufficient glucose and fat to incorporate nitrogen is similarly imperative.

The measurement of gas exchange is valuable in terms of monitoring glucose therapy, since glucose carries with it a respiratory quotient (V_{CO_2} produced ÷ V_{O_2} consumed) of 1 compared with a respiratory quotient for fat of 0.7. It has been suggested that varying the FIO_2 does not significantly affect the accuracy of the calorimeters, but at tidal volumes below 350 ml the difference increases between predicted V_{CO_2} and measured V_{CO_2}

Studies have demonstrated that there is an altered pattern of substrate mobilization and fuel utilization exists in patients who are acutely ill secondary to either injury or infection. These studies have important implications regarding the nutritional support of these patients. They address some of the metabolic sequelae of TPN with hypertonic glucose as the primary source of nonprotein calories, as well as the consequences of administering glucose calories in excess of energy requirements. Administration of glucose in hypercaloric quantities may produce respiratory and a metabolic stress. The former appears to be related to a ventilatory stimulus associated with an increased rate of carbon dioxide production. In acutely ill patients, this response is magnified and there is also a considerable rise in oxygen consumption and free norepinephrine excretion. It is this group of patients that shows the most profound elevation in minute ventilation.

TPN using glucose as nonprotein calories was associated with increases of O_2 consumption (V_{O_2}) and CO_2 production (V_{CO_2}) The magnitude of the changes was a function of the patient's clinical state and glucose load. Depleted patients showed a minimal increase in V_{O_2}, while V_{CO_2} increased 23 percent. Minute ventilation (VE) increased 32 percent. Hypermetabolic patients (major trauma, sepsis) had a 30 percent increase in V_{O_2} and a 57 percent increase in V_{CO_2}, while VE increased 71 percent. Patients with mild to moderate injuries (energy expenditure ± 15 percent of normal) showed a 21 percent increase in V_{O_2} and a 53 percent increase in V_{CO_2}, while VE increased 121 percent.

Large carbohydrate intakes were associated with increases in CO_2 production in all patients, while increases in O_2 consumption were seen primarily in hypermetabolic patients. These changes suggest that the high glucose loads of TPN may be a physiologic stress.

Severely depleted surgical patients were given TPN, providing an average of 34.6 kcal per kilogram and 266 mg nitrogen per kilogram of body weight. Two diets were used, one with glucose as the sole source of nonprotein energy,. the other with a safflower-based fat emulsion substituted isocalorically for one-third of the glucose. The two diets were given alternately, for 1 week at a time, to each patient. Nitrogen (N) balance, at zero energy balance, was estimated to average 50 mg nitrogen per kilogram, indicating that energy intake in excess of expenditure is not required to restore lean body mass in depleted patients. N balance was equally good with either diet. Respiratory quotients and carbohydrate oxidation were lower and fat oxidation was higher with the fat-containing diet. Amino acids and glucose were infused continuously over each 24 hour period, and fat was given for only 6 to 8 hours. Interestingly, during the period of fat infusion, fat oxidation was significantly higher, and carbohydrate oxidation and respiratory quotients were lower than at other times of the day.

One study suggested that intravenous fat emulsions are utilized as an energy substrate in patients with major injury, infection, or nutritional depletion. This observation, along with a relative unresponsiveness to glucose in surgical patients, suggests that fat emulsions may be useful as a calorie source in patients receiving parenteral nutrition.

Other work examined the effect of hypocaloric nutritional regimens on muscle high-energy phosphates in normal individuals and in patients who have received total hip replacement. Results suggested that a series of metabolic changes occur in skeletal muscle after injury such that even small amounts of glucose are important for maintenance of cellular energy levels.

Since high glucose intakes given during administration of TPN have been demonstrated to increase V_{CO_2} production, the alternating use of parenteral fat has been investigated. The workload imposed by the high CO_2 production of glucose may precipitate respiratory distress in patients with compromised pulmonary function. Fat emulsions can serve as a source of nonprotein calories and were associated with lesser degrees of CO_2 production than isocaloric amounts of glucose.

In addition to excess glucose and fat calories, hypertriglyceridemia commonly accompanies sepsis and may be caused by increased hepatic production or decreased clearance of triglyceride from the bloodstream. In contrast, enhanced lipid clearing capacity is usually seen after uncomplicated trauma. It has been found that trauma patients, after several days of 5 percent dextrose in water, have higher lipoprotein lipase (LPL) activity in adipose tissue and higher plasma insulin levels than diet-matched control subjects, but showed no change in skeletal muscle activity. Infected patients with high plasma triglyceride levels had significantly decreased LPL activity in both tissues. A linear relationship was found between insulin concentration and adipose tissue LPL activity in normal individuals. It was concluded that low tissue LPL activity in sepsis may result in diminished lipid clearance and contribute to hypertriglyceridemia; after trauma, changes in tissue LPL activity, as well as other factors such as altered hemodynamics, play a role in determining in vivo lipid clearance, and adipose tissue LPL activity is related to the plasma insulin concentration in normal subjects.

One final comment should be made concerning glucose and its interaction with amino acid solutions: Given the current state of the art with regard to the provision of TPN solution for the home patient, studies have shown that careful attention should be directed to storage conditions for these solutions. Terminal heat sterilization of glucose–amino acid solutions produces Maillard reaction products. Since deleterious effects are associated with these compounds, their presence in parenteral nutrition solutions should be avoided. The addition of electrolytes increased the rate of Maillard product formation at all temperatures. The data indicated that 25 percent glucose plus 4.25 percent amino acid solutions should be stored for only a minimal period, preferably at 4°C, before use.

In summary, glucose is the main energy substrate in most parenteral nutrition formulas. Monitoring parameters (Table 3) include blood sugar, glycosuria, plasma magnesium/phosphate/potassium, pulmonary carbon dioxide production, and liver function. The association of high-amplitude echoes returned from the liver in diffuse fatty infiltration has now become well recognized. Nine out of ten patients with histologically moderate or severe fatty infiltration were shown to have a brightly reflective echo pattern. Computed tomography (CT) and magnetic resonance imaging (MRI) have also played a role in better defining fatty liver infiltration. Since 75 to 90 percent of liver function demise begins to affect albumin synthesis, one may attempt to monitor serial albumin levels to check a fatty liver. However, albumin may be a much better epidemiologic tool than an individual nutritional assessment tool. Positional effects (hemocontraction on sitting or standing can increase plasma values by as much as 15 percent and circadian rhythm (as much as 0.75 g per day) may also limit its usefulness as a monitoring parameter.

Lipids

The fixed oils obtained from the seeds of safflower or soybean have been refined and processed as an oil-in-water emulsion for intravenous administration. These intravenous

TABLE 3 Pragmatic Monitoring Parameters for Parenteral Carbohydrates*

Plasma
Electrolytes (particularly magnesium, phosphate, and potassium)
Glucose
Triglycerides
Urine
Glucose

* Hepatic, pulmonary, and renal function testing should be included as needed.

phospholipids are 0.1 to 0.4-micron molecules designed to mimic chylomicrons, and are used in clinical nutrition to provide a source of energy as well as replete essential fatty acids. They are available as 10 and 20 percent emulsions that are solely soybean, solely safflower, or combinations thereof, for intravenous use. All fat emulsions should be test dosed (0.5 to 1 ml per minute for 15 to 30 minutes) before full rate infusion with patient monitoring for allergic reaction (fever, chills, pain in the chest and back) to the egg emulsifier and avoiding the occurrence of dyspnea or angioedema. Anaphylaxis is, however, very rare. Hypertriglyceridemia and metabolic acidemia have been associated with rapid infusion. The fact that linoleic acid is a precursor of cyclooxygenase (prostaglandin, prostacyclin, thromboxane A) and lipoxygenase (leukotrienes) suggests that there may be advantages to longer infusion time than the longest recommended Center for Disease Control (CDC) infusion hang time (at room temperature) of 12 hours. Several manufacturers have now reversed the 12-hour CDC recommendation for hang time, and have suggested as long as 24 hours. There have also been case reports describing bradycardia, diarrhea, and hyperphosphatemia. The immunologic influences of intravenous fat are still unclear, although the literature is replete with both in vitro and in vivo implications. Carnitine, a vitamin-like protein, has also been said to play an important role in the metabolism of fatty acids and their entry into mitochondria.

Fatty acids or lipids are converted to triglycerides for storage (50 percent of which is in the subcutaneous tissue) or are processed to aceto-acetate as well as β-hydroxybutyrate for energy within the mitochondrion; they then pass to the cell or into the liver as needed. Essential fatty acid deficiency (EFAD) is said to occur (as per package inserts) in 5 days or more without EFA such as linoleic or linolenic acid. Plasma triene/tetraene levels greater than 0.4 have been associated with EFAD. In addition, fat is used to supplement daily calories when there is carbohydrate intolerance. Triglyceride and phosphate levels (fat emulsions contain about 15 mM of phosphate per liter) should be monitored (Table 4), particularly when hypertriglyceridemia (i.e., renal compromise, sepsis) and hypophosphatemia (i.e., trauma, alcohol ingestion/renal compromise, medications) or hyperphosphatemia are of concern. Up to 60 percent of total calories (to include protein in the calorie calculation) can be supplied as fat infusion. In addition to saturated and unsaturated fats, intravenous fats contain cholesterol, glycerol, vitamin E, and selenium. The 2 kcal per milliliter concentration of 20 percent fat emulsions also makes their use attractive in the setting of volume restriction. Of late, medium-chain triglycerides (MCT) are receiving much attention, and replacement of a portion of the long-chain fats (LCTs—linoleic, linolenic, oleic, stearic, and palmitic found in Intralipid, Liposyn, Soyacal, Travamulsion) that are currently commercially available (Table 5) has been suggested by a variety of authors. Lünstedt and colleagues (investigated the effect of a new 20 percent fat emulsion containing 50 percent MCT and 50 percent LCT, in comparison with a 20 percent fat emulsion containing only LCT, in postoperative patients. The possible influence on nitrogen loss, protein synthesis, and fat metabolism was estimated. Twenty patients for elective colon surgery were included in the trial. Parenteral nutrition was provided for 5 days with two isonitrogenic and isocaloric nutritional regimens, including either MCT/LCT or only LCT fat emulsions. Fat emulsions were administered over a period of 12 hours with a total fat supply rate of 0.12 per kilogram per hour. Blood samples for determination of protein synthesis, triglyceride and ketone bodies were sampled during infusion as well as before and after infusion. 24-hour urine samples were taken to measure nitrogen (16 percent protein or amino acid) balance. The results showed no difference in protein levels between the MCT and LCT group. The 5-day nitrogen balance showed a significant increase in the MCT group ($p < 0.5$, Mann-Whitney tank sum test). At the end of the infusion period, triglyceride levels (normal limits 100 to 150 mg per deciliter) in the MCT group (mean value 244 $\pm$ 15 mg per deciliter) differed significantly from those in the LCT group (mean value 190 $\pm$ 24 mg per deciliter) Two-hour triglycerides in both groups fell to basal levels. β- hydroxybutyrate (β-HB) and aceto-acetate (Ac-ac) concentrations showed significant differences between both groups. After 12-hour infusion the MCT group had a mean level of 210 umol per liter β-HB and 180 umol per liter Ac-ac versus 90 umol per liter β-HB and 120 umol per liter Ac-ac in the LCT group. It is important for the clinician to recognize that MCT should not be used to prevent or treat EFAD.

The Harris-Benedict (H-B) equation is used to approximate patient resting metabolic expenditure; it has been said to overestimate energy requirements by 10 to 15 percent. A factor of 1.2 and 1.5 (in some trauma patients as high as 2) is multiplied by these calories to determine maintenance and anabolic needs, respectively. Total calories are approached with the empirical monitoring of ammonemia and ureagenesis (blood and urine) of protein to determine whether anabolism is taking place using the right mix of energy substrates, relative to nitrogen.

Indirect calorimetry metabolic charts and calculations

TABLE 4 Pragmatic Monitoring Parameters for Parenteral Lipid*

Serum
Triglyceride
Glucose
Phosphate

* Cardiovascular, hepatic, pulmonary, and renal function testing should be included as needed.

TABLE 5 Commercially Available Parenteral Fat Emulsions

Safflower
Liposyn
Safflower/Soybean
Liposyn II
Soybean
Intralipid
Soyacal
Travamulsion

involving the oxygen consumption and carbon dioxide production of substrates are used to follow more precisely the energy needs of the dynamically unstable patient. More fat and less carbohydrate are used to reduce carbon dioxide production since the RQ (CO_2 produced/O_2 consumed) for fats is less than carbohydrates or amino acids. Human studies have also shown that lipid infusion may possess a hypoaminoacidemic activity that may be related to a reduced availability of glucose-derived pyruvate or glycerophosphate, as well as enhanced hepatic uptake.

Fatty acids are an important fuel source for neonates. The use of long-chain fatty acids as a fuel source is dependent on adequate concentrations of carnitine. Carnitine also has functions in other physiologic processes critical to the survival of the neonate, such as lipolysis, thermogenesis, ketogenesis, and possibly regulation of certain aspects of nitrogen metabolism. Plasma and tissue carnitine concentrations in neonates are depressed compared with those in older individuals. The capability for carnitine biosynthesis is much less in neonates than in adults. Human milk contains carnitine and appears to be the major source of carnitine to meet neonates' metabolic needs. However, TPN solutions and soy-based infant formulas contain no carnitine. Evidence is accumulating to suggest that all infant diets may need to supply carnitine to meet neonates' metabolic needs. The presence of significant concentrations of carnitine in red blood cells and plasma has been documented.

It has been suggested that neonates, especially premature babies, are born with limited tissue reserves of carnitine and are therefore at an increased risk for developing carnitine deficiency and its adverse effects in the postnatal period, particularly if maintained on carnitine-free intravenous nutrition for prolonged periods. In systemic carnitine deficiency, an early phase of nonketotic hypoglycemia and liver dysfunction may precede a late phase of encephalopathy and myopathy.

When a primary clinical goal is nitrogen conservation, carbohydrate calories should be given in amounts approximating the resting metabolic rate. Additional calories and essential fatty acids then can be safely given as intravenous fat emulsion.

Commercially available intravenous fat emulsions (10 and 20 percent are available in a variety of quantities (50, 100, 200, 250, and 500 ml). All contain egg yolk phospholipid (1.2 percent), glycerin, or glycerol (2.2 to 2.5 percent), and have osmolalities ranging from 260 to 340 mOsm per liter. Parenteral fat monitoring should include plasma triglyceride, phosphates, essential fatty acid deficiencies signs/symptoms (i.e., xerodermia, clinical manifestations of prostaglandin/prostacyclin, thromboxane/leukotriene deficiencies), and major organ function.

PARENTERAL MICRONUTRIENTS

Micronutrients make up approximately 4 percent of total body constituents. Electrolytes, trace elements, and vitamins should be provided daily in the TPN system.

Electrolytes

With the initiation of TPN therapy, both rapid-exchange monovalent (Na, K, HCO_3, Cl) and more metabolic divalent (Mg, PO_4, and Ca) cations should be followed with a daily renal/metabolic battery. Electrolyte kinetics can be found in Table 6.

Ventilator adjustments can change acid-base status abruptly; however, slower modifications are also possible with the use of chloride salts for metabolic alkalemia treatment and acetate, citrate, gluconate, or lactate salts for the treatment of acidemia. Plasma levels of electrolytes may be influenced by acid-base changes (i.e., K, Ca) and may need to be followed several times a day in a rapidly changing setting. Ionized levels may provide more precise information about the actual plasma concentration and minimize the influences of acid-base and protein binding. Plasma levels, however, may not always be a reliable monitoring tool for electrolytes. Although an electrocardiogram (ECG) may be the most sensitive way to monitor plasma levels of electrolytes, tissue stores may be more reliably followed with urine excretion (e.g., more than 80 percent of intake may reflect adequate magnesium tissue stores). The effects of magnesium infusions on urinary and fecal magnesium excretion, serum magnesium, and nitrogen balance were examined in seven well-nourished and three nutritionally depleted adult surgical patients receiving TPN. They were maintained on constant nitrogen and caloric intake for 12 to 16 days. Mag-

TABLE 6 Electrolyte Kinetics

Electrolyte	*Absorption*
Sodium	100%
Potassium	100%
Chloride	100%
Bicarbonate	100% (Na^+)
Calcium	33%; duodenum & proximal jejunum
Magnesium	33% jejunoileal
Phosphate	70–90% jejunum
	Distribution
Potassium	ionic/80% in skeletal muscle
Chloride	ionic
Bicarbonate	20:1 (HCO_3:H_2CO_3)
Calcium	40–50% bound
Magnesium	30% bound to albumin; 50% in bone
Phosphate	buffer; 80% in bone
	Excretion
Potassium	Renal, GI, sweat
Chloride	Renal, GI, sweat
Bicarbonate	Renal, respiratory
Calcium	20% renal, 80% GI
Magnesium	60% renal, 40% GI
Phosphate	60% renal, 40% GI

Abstracted from Baumgartner TG, ed. Clinical guide to parenteral micronutrition. Consultant Pharmacists of America, Inc, 117 W Franklin Building, Suite C-462, Chicago, IL 60605.

nesium doses ranged from 0 to 664 mg per day and were given in varying crossover patterns. In both groups, urinary magnesium excretion increased as the amount of magnesium infused increased, but at comparable magnesium infusions, depleted patients excreted significantly less magnesium. Renal conservation was most pronounced in well-nourished patients on magnesium-free intake and in depleted patients given 70 mg of magnesium daily. Urinary magnesium losses were 40 $\pm$ 5 mg per day and 33 $\pm$ 8 mg per day, respectively, in these two groups. Endogenous fecal magnesium excretion was minimal and ranged from 2 to 38 mg per day. At each level of magnesium intake, serum levels of well-nourished patients were normal. With infusions of less than 200 mg per day, serum magnesium concentrations in depleted patients averaged 1.6 mg per deciliter. In both groups a positive correlation between magnesium and nitrogen balance was noted. An average dosing for parenteral magnesium is approximately 24 mEq per day, but requirements increase in the settings of alcoholism, stress, and excess carbohydrate or protein.

Phosphate must be followed closely, and if plasma levels fall below 2 mg per deciliter, a bolus dose of 0.08 mM phosphate per kilogram must be given (over a period of 4 to 6 hours to minimize abrupt suppression of calcium, unless calcium is simultaneously repleted). There are also circadian rhythms of electrolytes that have been defined; thus, monitoring electrolyte parameters at the same time of day is of importance. Intravenous glucose is a major reason for phosphate shift from the intravascular compartment, thereby depleting the erythrocyte of 2,3-diphosphoglycerate that, in turn, tightens hemoglobin:oxygen affinity.

TABLE 7 Trace Element Monitoring

Chromium

Glucose intolerance, excessive insulin requirement, peripheral neuropathy, metabolic encephalopathy, hyperlipidemia

Plasma chromium, serum chromium, hair, urine

Copper

Avoid use in copper storage disease (i.e., Wilson's), primary biliary cirrhosis; in deficient states: hair depigmentation, skin pallor, ossification changes

Hemogram, WBC/differential, serum copper, serum ceruloplasmin, hair copper, 24-hour urine copper, enzyme assessment, microcytic/hypochromic anemia, neutropenia, possible increase in plasma cholesterol levels

Iron

Avoid with excessive iron accumulation (i.e., hemosiderosis hemochromatosis, thallasemia), multiple transfusions, hypersensitivity, caution in the setting of sepsis

Hypersensitivity (IV test dose, which is 0.1 ml or 5 mg Fe), plasma or serum iron, transferrin, Hgb, Hct, MCV, MCH, MCHC, ferritin, peripheral blood smear

Manganese

Avoid use in cholestatic conditions

Whole blood (neutron activation analysis), potential monitoring tool = manganese-dependent mitochondrial superoxide dismutase

Zinc

Avoid with preexisting zinc toxicity

Plasma zinc, serum zinc, urine-serum alkaline phosphatase, taste acuity, dark adaptation, diarrhea, alopecia, mental depression, impaired wound healing, impaired white cell chemotaxis, impaired T-cell function, growth retardation, hypogonadism, hypospermia

TABLE 8 Biochemical Functions and Manifestations of Deficiency of Essential Trace Elements

Element	*Sites of Action*	*Signs of Deficiency*
Cr	"Glucose tolerance factor"	Impaired glucose clearance (many species) impaired growth, reproduction, and life span (rats and mice)
Co	Coenzyme B_{12}	Pernicious anemia (man), methylmalonic aciduria (humans)
Cu	Metalloenzymes (e.g., cytochrome oxidase, and tryosinase)	Menkes' syndrome (man); anemia, leukopenia, neutropenia (animals and human)
F	Unknown	Anemia (mice); impaired growth and reproduction (rats)
I	Thyroglobulin, thyroxine, triiodothyronine	Thyroid diseases (animals and humans)
Mn	Pyruvate carboxylase; activates many intracellular enzymes	Defective growth, bone anomalies, reproductive dysfunction, and CNS abnormalities in many species
Mo	Flavoenzymes (e.g., xanthine oxidase)	Growth retardation; impaired urate clearance (chicks)
Ni	Ribonucleic acid, serum "nickeloplasmin"	Impaired reproduction (rats), deranged liver lipid and phospholipid metabolism (chicks)
Se	Glutathione peroxidase (erythrocytes); cytochrome" (muscle)	Liver necrosis (rats) "white-muscle disease" (lambs), exudative diathesis (chicks)
Zn	Metalloenzymes (e.g., alcohol dehydrogenase, carboxypeptidase, and DNA polymerase)	Parakeratosis (swine), acrodermatitis enteropathica (humans); ? hypogonadal

Cr, chromium; Co, cobalt; Cu, copper; F, fluorine; I, iodine; Mn, manganese; Mo, molybdenum; Ni, nickel; Se, selenium; Zn, zinc.
Abstracted from Ulmer DD. Trace elements. N Engl J Med 1977; 297:318–321.

TABLE 9 Vitamin Kinetics

Vitamin A
- Absorption: duodenal, upper jejunal areas
- Distribution: various target organs (not heart or skeletal muscle)
- Metabolism: enterohepatic beta-glucuronide, oxidation stored in liver
- Excretion: urine, feces (metabolite and parent vitamin)

Vitamin D
- Absorption: D_2 and D_3 from small intestine, D_3 more completely absorbed; bile necessary for absorption
- Distribution: rapid; chylomicron in lymph; kidneys, adrenals, bones, and intestines
- Metabolism: tl/2 = 19–25 hr for D_2 or D_3, 3–5 days for calcitriol; stores = 6 mo
- Excretion: 40% excreted in 10 days in bile; small amount in urine

Vitamin E
- Absorption: 35% absorbed from small intestine
- Distribution: lymph, all tissues
- Metabolism: urinary tocopheronic acid and gamma lactone glucuronides
- Excretion: 70–80% by liver over 7 days; 20–30% in urine

Vitamin K
- Absorption: small intestine, colon; requires bile
- Distribution: lymph
- Metabolism: glucuronide and sulfate conjugates
- Excretion: bile, urine

Vitamin B_1 (Thiamine)
- Absorption: small intestine (maximal absorption = 8–15 mg/d)
- Distribution: heart, brain, liver, kidneys, skeletal muscles
- Metabolism: degraded by tissues
- Excretion: excess excreted in urine unchanged

Vitamin B_2 (Riboflavin)
- Absorption: small intestine
- Distribution: all tissues, little storage
- Metabolism: phosphorylation to FMN
- Excretion: 9% (inc. with larger doses) unchanged in urine

Vitamin B_3 (Niacin)
- Absorption: throughout GI tract
- Distribution: all tissues, particularly liver
- Metabolism: *N* methyl 2 pyridone 5-carboxamide; *N*-methyl 4-pyridone 3-carboxamide
- Excretion: unchanged in urine

Vitamin B_6 (Pyridoxine)
- Absorption: throughout GI tract (passive transport)
- Distribution: brain, liver, kidneys
- Metabolism: 4-pyridoxic acid in liver
- Excretion: feces, urine

Vitamin B_{12} (Cyanocobalamin)
- Absorption: ileum (distal)
- Distribution: liver, heart, kidney, spleen, brain
- Metabolism: cobalt complex
- Excretion: bile (principally), feces, urine

Pantothenic Acid
- Absorption: throughout GI tract
- Distribution: all tissues
- Metabolism: not metabolized
- Excretion: 70% unchanged in urine

Inositol
- Absorption: throughout the GI tract
- Distribution: all tissues, in particular, brain, heart, and skeletal muscle
- Metabolism: to glucose
- Excretion: small amount in urine

Choline
- Absorption: as lecithin (not fully absorbed)
- Distribution: liver, peripheral tissues liberate into lymphatics
- Metabolism: trimethylamine (metabolized by intestinal bacteria)
- Excretion: feces

Biotin
- Absorption: throughout GI tract
- Distribution: liver and brain
- Metabolism: metabolites in urine
- Excretion: parent compound in feces and urine

Folic Acid
- Absorption: ileum
- Distribution: liver, tissue
- Metabolism: metabolites
- Excretion: urine

Vitamin C (Ascorbic Acid)
- Absorption: intestine
- Distribution: plasma, body cells
- Metabolism: metabolites
- Excretion: urine after 2 mg/dl plasma levels

Abstracted from Baumgartner TG. Total parenteral nutrition therapy. J Pharm Pract 1988; 1:83–91.

Perhaps the most important point to remember is not to replete or curtail electrolytes too abruptly, particularly when reciprocal relationships are apparent.

Trace Elements

Trace element kinetics (Table 7) and deficiencies (Table 8) involve a baseline and periodic assessment of both signs and symptoms. To illustrate, muscle pain and an elevated creatine kinase isoenzyme (secondary to cardiomyopathy) may be associated with selenium deficiency after 1 month on parenteral nutrition without enteral support. Serum tissue or other fluid assessment may not provide enough evidence for deficiency, but enzymes (e.g., glutathione peroxidase) associated with the trace elements may be of monitoring value.

Trace elements must be added to all TPN formulas to ensure supplementation, particularly if patients are only receiving long-term TPN therapy.

Vitamins

Details of deficiencies and their signs and symptoms are plentiful in the literature, but their kinetics are not as easily referenced (Table 9). As is true with other nutrients, an appreciation of any surgical resection or areas of enteral compromise will better define the degree of parenteral supplementation.

In conclusion, the clinical nutritionist must practice in concert with the most current literature. The future surely holds great promise for parenteral feeding and the treatment of malnutrition and disease.

SUGGESTED READING

Alexander WF, Spindel E, Harty RF, Cerda JJ. The usefulness of branched amino acids in patients with acute or chronic hepatic encephalopathy. Am J Gastroenterol 1989; 84:91–96.

Brandl M, Sailer D, Langer K, et al. Parenteral nutrition with an amino acid solution containing a mixture of dipeptides. Evidence for efficient utilization of dipeptides in man. Beitr Infusionsther Klin Ernahr 1987; 17:103–116.

Coran AG, Drongowski RA. Studies on the toxicity and efficacy of a new amino acid solution in pediatric parenteral solution. J Parenter Enteral Nutr 1987; 11:368–377.

Dudrick SJ. Intravenous hyperalimentation. Surgery 1970; 68:726–727.

Foster KJ, Dewbury KC, Griffith AH, Wright R. The accuracy of ultrasound in the detection of fatty infiltration of the liver. Br J Radiol 53:440–442.

Freeman JB, Wittine MF, Stegink LD, Mason ED. Effects of magnesium infusions on magnesium and nitrogen balance during parenteral nutrition. Can J Surg 1982; 25:70–72.

Fukagawa NK, Young VR. Protein and amino acid metabolism and requirements in older persons. Clin Geriatr Med 1987; 3:329–341.

Giordano C, Esposito R, Damiano M. Protein requirement of patients on CAPD: a study on nitrogen balance. Int J Artif Organs 1980; 3:11–14.

Gorstein J, Akre J. The use of anthropometry to assess nutritional status. World Health Stat Q 1988; 41:48–58.

Klidjian AM, Archer TJ, Foster KJ, Karran SJ. Detection of dangerous malnutrition. J. Parenter Enteral Nutr 1982; 6:119–121.

Lünstedt B, Deltz E, Kähler M, Bruhn A. Randomized study comparing long-chain (LCT) and medium-chain (MCT) triglycerides as caloric carriers in postoperative nutritional therapy. Infusionsther Klin Eranhr 1987; 14:61–64.

Muratani H. Kawasaki T, Ueno M, et al. Circadian rhythms of urinary excretions of water and electrolytes in patients receiving total parenteral nutrition (TPN). Life Sci 1985; 37:645–649.

Skillman JJ, Rosenoer VM. Young JB, et al. Energy intake can determine albumin synthesis in man after surgery. Surgery 1985; 97:271–277.

Souba WW, Scott TE, Wilmore DW. Intestinal consumption of intravenously administered fuels. J Parenter Enteral Nutr 1985; 9:18–22.

PRINCIPLES OF PAIN MANAGEMENT

GREGORY W. ALBERS, M.D.
STEPHEN J. PEROUTKA, M.D., Ph.D.

The management of pain is one of the most common and difficult problems facing neurologists. Pain is a nonspecific symptom which may be a manifestation of a diverse array of pathologic conditions. Therefore, identification of the cause of pain is always the first objective of a patient evaluation. Once a tentative diagnosis has been established, a wide variety of treatment options may be considered. In general, the most common and effective mode of treatment for pain is pharmacologic. Surgical options are sometimes available for selected pain syndromes or for conditions refractory to standard treatment approaches. In some patients, therapeutic success may be achieved with alternative modalities such as physical therapy, biofeedback, and/or psychiatric intervention. A summary of the major options available to the physician is provided in Table 1.

DIAGNOSIS

The classification of pain syndromes is difficult, and pain terminology is often confusing. However, some simple generalizations are useful. Pain produced by activation of peripheral pain receptors (somatic or nociceptive pain) usually responds well to standard analgesics. Central pain (pain associated with central nervous system lesions) and neuropathic pain (pain associated with peripheral nerve damage) often respond best to atypical analgesics.

A second important diagnostic consideration concerns the differentiation of chronic pain disorders from acute pain disorders. Chronic pain differs from acute pain both symptomatically and pathophysiologically. For example, patients with chronic pain usually adapt to constant pain and therefore may appear to be quite comfortable. Unfortunately, this lack of apparent distress may lead the physician to question the validity of the patient's complaints.

TABLE 1 Overview of Pain Management Options

Pharmacologic
Prostaglandin inhibitors
Atypical analgesics
Narcotics
Combination analgesics
Surgical
Local anesthesia
Epidural injections
Nerve decompression
Thalamotomy
Alternative options
Psychological/psychiatric intervention
Electrical stimulation (TENS)
Biofeedback
Physical therapy

Generally, pharmacologic therapies aimed at treating patients with chronic pain must avoid the use of addicting substances such as narcotics.

PHARMACOLOGIC OPTIONS

The selection of an appropriate pharmacologic agent for the management of pain can seem quite difficult. Because the number of drugs used for pain may appear overwhelming, it is useful to classify these medications into four major categories: (1) prostaglandin inhibitors, (2) atypical analgesics, (3) narcotics, and (4) combination analgesics. Selection of an appropriate medication for pain relief requires knowledge of the pharmacologic properties and side effect profiles of each of these four drug groups.

Prostaglandin Inhibitors

Prostaglandin inhibitors are the drugs of choice for the management of mild to moderate pain. This group of agents includes aspirin, acetaminophen, and the nonsteroidal anti-inflammatory drugs (NSAIDs). Their mechanism of action involves the inhibition of prostaglandin synthesis primarily through the inhibition of the enzyme cyclooxygenase. These medications have principally analgesic, antipyretic and anti-inflammatory properties. However, it is important to note that the anti-inflammatory potency of acetaminophen is quite weak compared with that of aspirin and the NSAIDs.

Aspirin remains the prototypical prostaglandin inhibitor analgesic. It also remains the drug of choice for mild to moderate pain from headache, neuralgia, or myalgia. Nonetheless, the analgesic potency of aspirin tends to be underrated by most patients and physicians. In blinded studies, for example, 650 mg of aspirin is usually as effective as or more effective than 65 mg of codeine. The extremely low cost and effectiveness of aspirin make it an ideal analgesic for patients who can tolerate its gastrointestinal effects.

Acetaminophen is an excellent alternative for patients who are unable to tolerate aspirin. In general, acetaminophen appears to be equipotent to aspirin in its analgesic effects. However, because of its lack of significant anti-inflammatory actions, it is less effective for pain related to inflammation. Although acetaminophen has minimal gastrointestinal toxicity, it does carry the risk of hepatic necrosis, which may occur with chronic doses as low as 5 to 8 g per day or with an acute overdose of only 10 to 15 g.

NSAIDs offer several potential advantages over aspirin and acetaminophen. First, they have less gastrointestinal toxicity than aspirin. Second, because NSAIDs cause reversible inhibition of cyclooxygenase, their antiplatelet activity is of shorter duration. Third, their analgesic potency is often slightly better than that of aspirin or acetaminophen. Otherwise, NSAIDs have a mechanism of action and side effect profile similar to that of aspirin. Unfortunately, NSAIDs differ from aspirin and acetaminophen also in that they are considerably more expensive.

Although insufficient data are available to differentiate the various NSAIDs in terms of analgesic potency or risk of gastrointestinal hemorrhage, there are many significant differences among agents. For example, piroxicam (Feldene) has the longest half-life (approximately 45 hours), and this allows for once daily dosing. Diflunisal (Dolobid), sulindac (Clinoril), and naproxen (Naprosyn) can be administered in twice daily doses. Indomethacin (Indocin) has superior anti-inflammatory activity but appears to cause more frequent side effects than other NSAIDs. Meclofenamate (Meclomen) is asociated with incidence of diarrhea as high as 30 percent.

All NSAIDs carry a small risk of renal toxicity because of the role of prostaglandins in modulating renal blood flow. This risk is greatly accentuated in patients with pre-existing renal disease, congestive heart failure, or hepatic dysfunction. Several studies have suggested that sulindac (Clinoril) has minimal effects on renal prostaglandin synthesis and therefore appears to carry a relatively reduced risk of renal toxicity.

Since most NSAID side effects are dose-related, a low dose should be chosen initially and increased gradually as required. NSAIDs are highly bound to serum albumin (most are greater than 99 percent bound) and can potentially displace other highly protein-bound drugs such as coumarin anticoagulants, phenytoin, methotrexate, and oral hypoglycemics. Obviously, such interactions could potentially lead to toxicity.

Atypical Analgesics

Several drugs that were originally developed for other conditions such as depression or epilepsy have been found to be useful in pain management. These agents are primarily useful in treating chronic pain syndromes, particularly conditions involving central or neuropathic pain. For example, a substantial amount of data suggest that antidepressants can provide significant pain relief in both depressed and nondepressed patients. Although the exact mechanism remains unclear, effects on descending monoamine pathways involved in the modulation of pain transmission appear to be important.

Before pain therapy with antidepressant drugs is initiated, the rationale for using these agents for pain control, as opposed to depression, should be stressed to the patient. Patients with pain syndromes are often offended by the implication that they are depressed. Therefore, the physician should clearly state the reasons for using these agents for pain. Low doses should be used initially (Table 2). If pain relief is not obtained after 6 to 8 weeks of therapy, the dosage should be increased slowly to full antidepressant doses and continued for at least another 6 to 8 weeks. When a positive response is obtained, drug therapy should be continued for 3 to 6 months, after which a gradual withdrawal of the medication is attempted. If the pain recurs after medication withdrawal, treatment should be reinstituted.

As with the NSAIDs, there are insufficient data to rank the analgesic potency of the antidepressants. Many of the controlled trials have involved the use of agents associated with a high incidence of side effects, such as amitriptyline (Elavil) and imipramine (Tofranil). However, significant analgesic effects also occur with better-tolerated agents such as nortriptyline (Pamelor) and desipramine (Norpramin).

TABLE 2 Commonly Used Analgesics

Drug	*Brand Name**	*Typical Starting Dose*
Prostaglandin inhibitors		
Aspirin		650 mg q4–6h
Acetaminophen	Tylenol	650 mg q4–6h
Ibuprofen	Motrin	400 mg q4–6h
Naproxen	Naprosyn	375 mg q12h
Sulindac	Clinoril	150 mg q12h
Diflunisal	Dolobid	500 mg q12h
Piroxicam	Feldene	20 mg q24h
Atypical analgesics		
Amitriptyline	Elavil	25 mg qhs
Nortriptyline	Pamelor	25 mg qhs
Carbamazepine	Tegretol	100 mg q12h
Narcotics		
Codeine		30 mg q4–6h
Pentazocine	Talwin Nx	1 tab q4–6h
Meperidine	Demerol	100 mg IM q4–6h
Combination analgesics		
Aspirin/ butalbital/ caffeine	Fiorinal	1 tab q4h
Aspirin/ butalbital	Axotal	1 tab q4h
Acetaminophen/ chlorzoxazone	Parafon Forte DSC	2 tabs q6h
Acetaminophen/ codeine	Tylenol #3	1 tab q4h
Acetaminophen/ hydrocodone	Vicodin	1 tab q6h
Aspirin/ oxycodone	Percodan	1 tab q6h

* Several brand names are available for some of these analgesics.

A second major class of atypical analgesics is that of the anticonvulsants. Carbamazepine (Tegretol), phenytoin (Dilantin), valproic acid (Depakene), and clonazepam (Klonopin) are the anticonvulsants most frequently used for pain. These agents may be effective in the treatment of a variety of pain syndromes, including various neuropathies, neuralgias, and pain in multiple sclerosis or Guillain-Barré Syndrome. Carbamazepine (Tegretol) has proven to be the most effective agent for the treatment of trigeminal neuralgia. However, the data are limited on comparisons of the anticonvulsants in treating other painful conditions. Although the exact mechanism of action for pain control is unclear, a reduction of excitatory synaptic transmission within pain-modulating circuits has been postulated.

Several other medications such as anticholinergics, phenothiazines, and baclofen have been advocated for the management of various painful conditions. Unfortunately, very little data from controlled studies are available regarding the use of these drugs. The short-term use of anti-anxiety agents may also be helpful, particularly if pain is accompanied by significant anxiety.

Narcotic Analgesics

Although narcotics are the most effective analgesics available, we strongly believe that narcotic use should be restricted to the short-term relief of moderate to severe pain. We believe that narcotics should rarely be used for chronic pain control in neurologic patients. Quite simply, the problems encountered with long-term narcotic use (e.g., tolerance and addiction) far outweigh their benefits in patients with chronic pain disorders.

For the short-term relief of acute pain, codeine is usually the oral narcotic of choice. Its advantages include a relatively low dependence liability and good oral bioavailability. Unfortunately, like many narcotics, codeine has a short plasma half-life (only about 3.5 hours), necessitating frequent dosing. Codeine, as well as the other orally active narcotics, should generally be administered in combination with a prostaglandin inhibitor, as discussed in the following section of this chapter.

Propoxyphene (Darvon) is one of the least potent narcotics. In many studies it has proven to be less effective than aspirin or acetaminophen. We find that there is little use for this agent in treating neurologic patients. If more potent orally active narcotics are required, hydrocodone (Vicodin) or oxycodone (Percodan) may be considered. These agents are available only in combination with nonopioid analgesics. Of these, oxycodone is the more potent and appears to have higher abuse potential.

For parenteral use, meperidine (Demerol) is a recommended choice because of its relatively low incidence of gastrointestinal side effects. Meperidine hydrochloride (Demerol) can occasionally produce central nervous system side effects, including excitement and seizures, and should not be used for patients on monoamine oxidase inhibitors. Several mixed agonists-antagonists such as pentazocine (Talwin), butorphanol (Stadol), and nalbuphine (Nubain) appear to offer the advantage of less abuse potential than other potent narcotics. Their disadvantages, however, include the risk of precipitation of a withdrawal reaction in patients being treated with other opioids and occasional psychotomimetic effects.

Combination Analgesics

A variety of combination analgesics are available for use in moderate pain disorders. Aspirin or acetaminophen is frequently combined with caffeine and/or a barbiturate for the treatment of headaches (e.g., Excedrin, Fiorinal, Axotal) or with a muscle relaxant for acute musculoskeletal strain (e.g., Norgesic, Soma, Parafon Forte DSC). Certain analgesic combinations appear to offer synergistic effects greater than those obtained by doubling the dose of either individual agent. For example, the most successful combinations involve a prostaglandin inhibitor (usually aspirin or acetaminophen) coupled with an oral narcotic—for example, propoxyphene (Darvon compound), codeine (Tylenol with codeine), hydrocodone bitartrate (Vicodin), and oxycodone (Percodan, Tylox).

SURGICAL OPTIONS

A large variety of surgical or anesthetic procedures are available for specific pain syndromes. Focal neuropathies such as occipital neuralgia, painful neuromas, and carpal tunnel syndrome can be treated with local injections of anesthetic agents and corticosteroids. Occasionally, the pain relief that follows local infiltration is long lasting. Epidural or intrathecal injections may also provide pain relief for selected patients, and standard orthopedic and neurosurgical procedures such as laminectomy and peripheral nerve decompression are available for specific syndromes. For example, reflex sympathetic dystrophy often responds to sympathectomy and/or sympathetic blocking agents. More invasive procedures such as gangliolysis, posterior rhizotomy, cordotomy, or thalamotomy should be performed only in specialized centers.

ALTERNATIVE OPTIONS

A diverse variety of alternative (i.e., nonpharmacologic and nonsurgical) therapies is also available for patients with pain syndromes. In certain chronic pain patients, psychological factors may play a primary role in the pain syndrome and can severely complicate patient management. Fear and depression are also frequently associated with pain and sometimes need to be addressed specifically. For these individuals, psychological and/or psychiatric evaluations may be most appropriate.

Physical therapy and exercise are important options and may be particularly useful in treating pain syndromes related to muscle contraction or spasm. Other therapeutic options such as biofeedback, relaxation training, hypnosis, and transcutaneous nerve stimulation (i.e., TENS) are helpful for selected patients. Depending on the clinical situtation, multimodality therapy may be more successful than any single therapeutic option used alone. For instance, chronic headaches often respond well to a combination of drug therapy, cervical exercises, and psychological or psychiatric intervention.

SUGGESTED READING

Boynton CS, Dick CF, Mayor GH. NSAIDS: an overview. J Clin Pharmacol 1988, 28:512–517.

Beaver WT. Combination analgesics. Am J Med 1984, 77:38–53.

Hackett TP, Bouckoms A. The pain patient: evaluation and treatment. In Hackett TP, Cassem NH, eds. Massachusetts General Hospital handbook of general hospital psychiatry. 2nd ed. Littleton MA: PSG Publishing Co., Inc., 1987:42.

The International Association for the Study of Pain, Subcommittee on Taxonomy. Classification of chronic pain: descriptions of chronic pain syndromes and definitions of pain terms. Pain 1986; 3(suppl):S1–226.

Malone MD, Strube MJ. Meta-analysis of non-medical treatments for chronic pain. Pain 1988, 34:231–244.

PATIENT RESOURCES

International Association for the Study of Pain
909 N.E. 43rd Street, Suite 306
Seattle, Washington 98105
Telephone: (206) 547-6409

American Pain Society
1200 17th Street, N.W. Suite 400
Washington, DC 20036
Telephone: (202) 296-9200

BEHAVIOR MODIFICATION

THOMAS J. COATES, Ph.D.
STEVEN R. CUMMINGS, M.D.

Changing patient behavior is essential to the practice of medicine. The major causes of death and disability in the United States today are chronic diseases (e.g., heart disease, cancer, diabetes) and accidents. Individual behaviors are related strongly to the incidence and course of these causes of death. Tobacco (inhaled, snuffed, or chewed) increases the risk of heart disease, cancers, stroke, accidents (e.g., fires), and influenza. Alcohol is related to heart disease, stroke, some cancers, motor vehicle accidents, cirrhosis, and suicide. Diets high in saturated fats and cholesterol are related to heart disease, cancers, stroke, and arteriosclerosis. High-risk sexual behavior is related to sexually transmitted diseases and pregnancy and increasingly to mortality in diseases such as the acquired immunodeficiency syndrome (AIDS). It is clear that many diseases might be prevented and that the course of disease, once begun, might be altered if individuals were motivated to adopt healthier lifestyles.

In 1974, the Secretary of Health and Human Services of the United States, Joseph Califano, Jr., summarized the challenge as follows:

> We are killing ourselves by our own careless habits. We are killing ourselves by carelessly polluting the environment. We are killing ourselves by permitting harmful social conditions to persist—conditions like poverty, hunger, and ignorance—which destroy health, especially for infants and children. You, the individual, can do more for your own health and well-being than any doctor, any hospital, any drug, any exotic medical device.

Many patients do not feel confident that they can engage in healthful behaviors, and many physicians do not feel confident in their ability to motivate patients to develop and maintain health-promoting behaviors. The task is difficult, the results are not immediate, and formal and systematic training in this aspect of medicine has been lacking. Our objective is to present a guide to the theory and the specific techniques for helping patients to change.

BEHAVIORAL MEDICINE

Behavioral medicine was defined at a National Academy of Sciences meeting as "the *interdisciplinary* field concerned with the development and *integration* of behavioral and biomedical science knowledge and techniques relevant to health and illness and the application of this knowledge and these techniques to prevention, diagnosis, treatment, and rehabilitation." The traditional biomedical sciences and the practice of medicine have been devoted to discovering which biomedical variables affect which other biomedical variables. Thus, identifying the pathogen that causes disease and the chemical or surgical procedure to eradicate disease had yielded considerable growth in treatment of disease in this century. The social and behavioral sciences have been devoted to discovering which social and psychological variables influence behavior and how to modify these variables in order to modify behavior, cognition, or affect of individuals. Education and advertising rely on these sciences to a considerable degree.

Behavioral medicine concerns itself with the interface of the behavioral and biomedical sciences and practices. The objectives are (1) to identify which behaviors are related directly to health and illness; (2) to develop and evaluate methods for modifying these behaviors; and (3) to determine the impact of modifications in these behaviors on the health and illness of various groups of individuals.

Health promotion, disease prevention, and effective use of alternative methods for treating disease require that individuals change their behavior and that medical organizations be reorganized to promote those changes. Effective use of the scientific principles and the strategies derived from them is critical to the success and longevity of these programs.

PRINCIPLES OF BEHAVIORAL CHANGE

The National Academy of Sciences was called upon recently to summarize what is known about how to change behavior to guide work in AIDS prevention. Their study yielded a generic set of principles of behavioral change that apply to virtually any situation in which the desired end is changing behavior to prevent disease. These principles, summarized in Table 1 and explained in the following paragraphs, can provide a guide for the physician in changing patient behavior.

Principle 1: Providing information is the logical starting point in any behavior change effort. Individuals must understand the risks that they incur by engaging in certain behaviors and the benefits they will realize by adopting others. However, the physician should understand that information, although necessary (and sufficient to produce behavior change in some patients), is rarely sufficient by itself to produce significant behavior change in most patients. Significant attention must be paid to how information is presented to patients. Information must be delivered in a manner that is comprehensible and relevant to the patient for whom it is intended. A major impediment to ensuring that information is given appropriately and received by the patient

TABLE 1 Summary of Behavior Change Strategies

Information
- Communication is comprehensible to patient
- Information is relevant to patient
- Patient summarizes information to ensure understanding

Risk Perception and Fear
- Perception of risk is accurate
- Physician relates current symptoms to unhealthful behaviors
- A balance in the level of threat is maintained
- Patient is given specific information on steps to take to protect health

Self-Efficacy: Perceived Ability to Perform Desired Behaviors
- Self-monitoring makes patients aware of behaviors
- Incremental changes
- Substitute new behaviors rather than eliminate old ones
- Provide choices to patient

Skills Training
- Provide opportunities to plan and rehearse new behaviors

Create Environments That Encourage Change
- Help patients to identify environments associated with healthful and unhealthful behaviors
- Plan environments that encourage healthful behaviors

Expect and Plan for Slips
- Advise patients that slips are expected
- Use specific descriptions at slips to plan for future behavioral change

occurs when the physician fails to check whether or not the patient has understood and can act on the information given. This requires more than asking the patient whether or not he or she understands what is to be done. It requires that the physician take the time to ask the patient to summarize the major points that have been discussed and the plans for behavior change developed in the medical encounter.

Principle 2: Individuals are more likely to change if they believe that their behavior will lead to a disease with serious consequences. Most people have optimistic outlooks on life and are likely to deny the possibility of future disease in the absence of personal experience with that disease (e.g., in themselves or in their immediate family). In addition, patients interpret statements about their risk for disease in relation to the value they place on avoiding the health problems in question and on the incentives for engaging in alternative actions. Nonetheless, individuals may be more likely to change if they understand that the risks associated with their lifestyles are serious and likely to lead to important adverse consequences. This can be accomplished in two ways: (1) by relating an individual's family history to his or her current behaviors and risk for disease; and (2) by relating an individual's current disease symptoms to his or her behaviors (e.g., upper respiratory tract infections in a smoker).

Principle 3: Messages to patients that evoke fear about their behavior can be useful in motivating behavioral change. Behavioral change in the context of medical care has the one purpose of helping the patient to avoid the morbid and mortal consequences of his or her lifestyle. A certain level of threat and fear is necessarily involved. However, fear by itself, especially if overwhelming, can hinder rather than help the patient to change. Individuals can deny their risk, point to others who have practiced similar health-threatening behaviors and survived, or avoid medical care altogether. The National Academy of Sciences has proposed three prescriptions for using threatening messages to motivate behavioral change.

1. The messages to the patient should strike a balance in the level of threat that is employed. The level should be sufficiently high to motivate individuals to take action but not so high as to paralyze individuals with fear or cause them to deny their susceptibility. The fear level should be low enough so that it can be effectively managed by the adoption of the desired behavior. For example, telling smokers with upper respiratory tract infections that they may develop emphysema if they continue to smoke may evoke fear. Telling the same smokers that the risk will be lessened if they quit smoking provides an escape within reach.
2. The communication must provide specific information on steps that can be taken to protect the individual from threat to his or her health. Patients must believe that the changes being proposed will do some good. Thus, a reasonable, desirable alternative behavior that protects against the undesired health problem should be offered.
3. Attention should be paid to the short-term adverse consequences of the undesirable behavior and the short-term positive consequences of engaging in the desirable behavior. For example, smokers may know that their tobacco use is related to lung or heart disease but they may deny their risk. Drawing their attention to the respiratory consequences of smoking when they are ill with respiratory tract infections or when they are short of breath may help them to realize the impact that smoking has and will have on their health.
4. Altruism should not be overlooked. Individuals will often do for others what they will not do for themselves. Patients will take steps to avoid adverse consequences to their spouses, children, or parents. Concern for significant others can be a powerful motivator and should not be overlooked. For example, many smokers are motivated to quit because of adverse effects on their children.

Principle 4: If an individual perceives that he or she is capable of performing desired behaviors (self-efficacy), then he or she is likely to engage in those activities. Individuals need to believe that they have a reasonable chance of achieving the changes recommended. People are not likely to engage in activities they feel they will not be able to perform successfully. Expectations of one's abilities can be changed and have been used to increase contraceptive use, help patients stop smoking, or increase sexual activity following myocardial infarctions. A patient's sense of competency and hence his or her willingness to try new behaviors can be increased in the following ways.

Helping patients to become aware of the degree to which they practice unhealthful or healthful behaviors often can motivate behavior change by itself. Self-monitoring is the most effective way to help patients become aware of the degree to which they practice healthful or unhealthful behaviors and the circumstances that are related to the practice of both. Monitoring food intake, exercise, and number of cigarettes smoked per day can help patients to gain control over those behaviors. Monitoring helps patients to set realistic goals for change, to determine the circumstances under which problem behaviors occur, and to measure accurately the degree to which change has occurred. Monitoring is best accomplished when done systematically, that is, when the patient records behaviors on a form using a standardized procedure.

Patients should choose between incremental changes and global lifestyle changes. Modifying rather than eliminating behaviors may be more effective for some patients. Incremental changes provide patients with a way to build new experiences in small steps without too much risk and allow the practitioner to reinforce patient success in accomplishing these early tasks. Incremental changes also allow patients to avoid frustrating failure experiences; they are spared the difficulties involved in aspiring to global changes and then feeling a sense of failure when they are unable to accomplish the impossible. Many patients devalue the importance of small changes such as losing 5 lb in as many weeks, making small changes in dietary intake, or taking small steps in initiating an exercise program. They need to be encouraged that such steps are realistic and important in that they will be more likely to reach long-term goals if the initial steps are successful.

It is often easier to encourage patients to substitute a behavior rather than to eliminate the unhealthful behavior altogether. Individuals engage in unhealthful behaviors because they are reinforcing (i.e., they are satisfying or pleasurable) or because they are popular. To cease engaging in such behaviors is difficult because it means giving up pleasure or behaving contrary to popular norms. Thus, if instead of giving up a behavior altogether individuals can substitute a behavior that is more healthful and at the same time likely to be satisfying or popular, they are more likely to adopt and maintain the practice of that behavior. For example, using condoms may be more acceptable to patients as protection against sexually transmitted diseases than celibacy. Intravenous drug users may be more likely to modify their injection behavior than to give up drug use altogether.

Individuals are more likely to adopt a behavioral change if they are offered choices among alternative behaviors. Patients and physicians together need to negotiate and set goals for behavioral change. Setting goals requires that the physician and patient determine exactly what is to be accomplished and that benchmarks for determining success be established. Vague or unmeasurable goals can lead to the appearance of an agreement without the patient's commitment to take specific actions to change.

Formal contracting can help both patient and physician agree on specific goals and methods for reaching them. Contracting is a process whereby the patient agrees to achieve a specific goal or behavior by a predetermined time in exchange for a reward. An example of contracting is breaking a large goal (e.g., losing 30 lb) into a series of smaller contracts (e.g., losing 5 lb by the next visit) and specifying the reward (e.g., a night out at the movies). All such contracts should be recorded in the medical chart so that follow-up is ensured at the next visit.

Principle 5: Change is more likely if individuals are taught the skills for engaging in the desired behaviors. Behavioral change requires that patients plan and rehearse in advance exactly how they will behave in a specific situation. Rehearsing an activity ahead of time builds confidence and self-efficacy by allowing the person to have the experience of the new behavior before it is actually performed. In one program designed to teach patients how to manage postoperative pain, those who learned what to expect after an operation and rehearsed how to use medication and other techniques required less analgesic medication than unrehearsed patients. Physicians can plan and rehearse difficult situations with patients, such as how to refuse the offer of an alcoholic beverage or caloric food, how to manage the offer of a cigarette, how to fit medication into a busy schedule, or how to manage an asthmatic attack or the symptoms of diabetes mellitus.

Principle 6: The physician should help the patient to create environments that encourage change. Environments influence all of us to behave in healthful and unhealthful ways. For example, it is difficult to refuse alcohol in a bar and to ignore high-calorie foods when they are stocked in the refrigerator. The objective is to avoid settings associated with unhealthful behaviors or to set up the environment so that healthful behaviors are encouraged. For example, when patients are trying to quit smoking, it is often helpful for them to avoid places such as bars or smoking areas where cigarettes are available.

Principle 7: Relapse is expected. It is unreasonable to expect that individuals will change and then maintain new behaviors perfectly. To the contrary, imperfect adherence to desired activities is more likely to be the case. Patients may be reluctant to report relapses to their physician, instead either avoiding medical encounters or seeking other providers. Two attitudes need to be conveyed to the patient by the physician. The first is that one slip does not necessarily lead to complete relapse; patients can slip and then get back on their programs of behavioral change. The second is that talking about relapses does not encourage them to occur. To the contrary, patients can be advised that relapses may occur, and if they do they should not be regarded as "failures" but rather as opportunities to learn how to change behavior more effectively in the future. In the case of smoking, for example, the more times that patients have tried to quit, the more likely they are to be successful at quitting. Advice will be more effective if the relapses are analyzed very specifically, for example, determining where the first cigarettes or drink came from and what circumstances surrounded the "slip," coupled with description and rehearsal of how such slips might be avoided in the future.

THE PHYSICIAN'S PERSPECTIVE

These strategies for behavioral change are based on the optimistic premise that individuals can introduce and maintain changes in their lives. The practicing physician may not always feel such optimism. Change is difficult for anyone, and modifying lifelong habits for the long-term goal of better health may not seem worthwhile for many patients. Two points might help the physician to maintain enthusiasm for this part of medical practice. The first is that the tools available to the physician are limited. Persuasive communication of a limited duration in the confines of the medical office cannot be expected to have an overwhelming influence on patients in comparison with the other influences in their lives. Past histories, personal preferences, the media, the family, and long-standing habits are not overcome easily, even when better health is the motivation. However, the physician can be another voice encouraging the patient to change, and the physician can take advantage of patient vulnerabilities to motivate change. Second, behavioral change should be considered for all patients. Physicians can become discouraged when the patient with extreme chronic obstructive pulmonary disease fails to quit smoking, when the patient with severe diabetes or hypertension fails to lose weight, or when the alcoholic patient cannot stop drinking. Nevertheless, even if success rates are low, these preventive efforts are as worthwhile as any therapy for prevention of chronic disease. Perhaps these patients will never change. Concentrating on patients whose problems are less severe may be more rewarding because their problems are less likely to be out of control and they are more likely to be able to change. In addition, there is the old adage of "trying harder or trying differently." We have attempted to suggest some ways of trying differently and in that way experiencing greater success in an important aspect of medical practice.

SUGGESTED READING

Bandura A. Self-efficacy: Toward a unifying theory of behavioral change. Psychol Rev 1977; 34:191–215.

Becker MH. Patient adherence to prescribed therapies. Med Care 1985; 23:539–555.

Job RFS. Effective and ineffective use of fear in health promotion campaigns. Am J Pub Health 1988; 78:163–167.

Martin AR, Coates TJ. A clinician's guide to helping patients change behavior. West J Med 1987; 146:751–753.

Turner CF, Miller HG, Moses LE. AIDS, sexual behavior and intravenous drug use. Washington, DC: National Academy Press, 1989.

HEALTH PROMOTION AND DISEASE PREVENTION

F. MARC LaFORCE, M.D.

Practicing physicians have become somewhat disenchanted and disappointed with the results of many of the so-called medical miracles. The preponderance of these advances are applied relatively late in the course of a patient's illness, and interventions at that stage, irrespective of their drama and intensity, often yield limited dividends. Some physicians have remarked that we seem to be doing more and more to sicker and sicker patients with gains that are at best marginal. A visit to any intensive care unit attests to at least a partial truth in this assertion. Material in this chapter is aimed at the opposite end of this spectrum and describes primary and secondary preventive measures that are appropriate for the office setting. Primary preventive maneuvers such as immunizations are aimed at asymptomatic persons with no evidence of the condition to be prevented, whereas secondary prevention refers to screening for the early diagnosis of disease in asymptomatic persons. The basic premise is that it is far better, although not necessarily cheaper, to prevent rather than to treat disease.

Most physicians first learned about disease prevention on pediatric services, where the virtues of immunization were emphasized. Training in internal medicine has largely emphasized the diagnosis and treatment of adult diseases with little emphasis on prevention. This attitude is changing with the realization that treatment can be very expensive and may not necessarily result in increased life expectancy or a better quality of life.

The leading causes of death in the United States by age are presented in Table 1, along with modifiable risk factors or interventions that can prevent or delay development of these diseases. Screening and attempts at risk factor modification are appropriate to the office setting but require a change in how medicine is generally practiced. Primary prevention requires that patients assume greater responsibility for their own health. The older paradigm in which the physician assumed total responsibility for the patient's illness has to give way to a model whereby patients become responsible for acts likely to hurt them.

Much of the material presented in this chapter is taken from the 1989 U.S. Preventive Services Task Force report entitled "Guide to Clinical Preventive Services." The Task Force was asked to produce a series of recommendations on health promotion and disease prevention appropriate for the office setting. The Task Force methodology emphasized a rigorous review of the medical literature with the evaluation of specific maneuvers according to strict rules of evidence. More weight was given to results from properly controlled studies, and recommendations from expert groups in the absence of solid experimental data were downgraded. Population benefits were an important consideration when recommending specific maneuvers. For example, because of the small population benefit, a highly effective intervention for a relatively rare disease was deemed less important than a maneuver of moderate or even minor effectiveness that could be applied to a common disease associated with significant morbidity and mortality.

Last, a special effort was made to present recommendations in age-specific packages that recognized the leading causes of morbidity and mortality in specific age groups. A teenager or a young adult is far more likely to die from an automobile accident than

TABLE 1 Leading Causes of Death by Age

Age (yr)	*Condition*	*Risk Factor or Intervention*
19–39	Motor vehicle crashes	Seatbelt noncompliance, alcohol
	Homicide	Gun ownership
	Suicide	Depression
	Injuries (nonvehicular)	Alcohol
40–64	Heart disease	Hypertension, elevated cholesterol level, smoking
	Lung cancer	Smoking
	Cerebrovascular disease	Hypertension, elevated cholesterol level
	Breast cancer	Clinical examination and annual mammogram
	Colorectal cancer	Stool test for occult blood
	Obstructive lung disease	Smoking
65 and over	Heart disease	Hypertension, elevated cholesterol level, smoking
	Cerebrovascular disease	Hypertension, elevated cholesterol level
	Obstructive lung disease	Smoking
	Pneumonia/influenza	Smoking, influenza and pneumococcal vaccines
	Lung cancer	Smoking
	Colorectal cancer	Stool test for occult blood

from any other condition. In 1986, of about 40,000 deaths among persons 15 to 24 years old, half were caused by injuries, and over three-quarters of these injuries occurred in motor vehicle accidents. All forms of cancer accounted for only 6 percent of deaths in this age group. In order to lower mortality rates in teenagers and young adults, it is far more productive for the practitioner to promote seatbelt use and to discourage drinking while driving than to do a comprehensive physical examination.

SCREENING

Most physicians vigorously adhere to the dogma that finding disease early is always good. However, when carefully studied, screening has been shown to have its down side. All procedures, no matter how minor, have side effects, ranging from a direct effect such as sigmoid perforation during a screening sigmoidoscopy to the psychological effects of labeling a person ill after identification by a positive screening test. An example of the negative effect of labeling was a study of asymptomatic steel workers who were screened for hypertension. Some were told they were ill with hypertension, and over the next 2 years they had a significant increase in work absenteeism that was not related to any complications of hypertension but represented a new response to minor illnesses.

Screening for a particular disease or condition, particularly in an asymptomatic person, carries with it a special burden. The person is feeling well, and searching for a particular condition implies an improved outcome as a result of identification of that condition. In an important series of papers, Frame and Carlson set out conditions that had to be met in order that a screening maneuver be recommended: (1) the disease must have a significant effect on quality and quantity of life; (2) acceptable methods of treatment must be available; (3) the disease must have an asymptomatic period during which detection and treatment significantly reduce morbidity and mortality; (4) treatment in the asymptomatic phase must yield a superior therapeutic result; (5) tests must be available at reasonable cost to detect the condition during the asymptomatic period; and (6) the incidence of the condition must be high enough to justify the cost of screening. These conditions are still valid and serve as a convenient standard against which all proposed screening maneuvers should be measured.

In addition, the benefits of screening usually have been overestimated. The phenomenon of lead-time bias is an important confounder, since early diagnosis is invariably associated with improved survival because early diagnosis will always lengthen the time period between diagnosis and death without necessarily having improved survival. Thus early identification of disease may not necessarily improve life expectancy but rather lengthens the time someone is diagnosed as "ill." The effectiveness of screening can also be overestimated because of length-time bias. This refers to the tendency of screening procedures to detect a disproportionately high number of cases of slowly progressive disease. Cases of aggressive disease are less likely to be picked up by a screening maneuver in the population because they are present for a relatively short period of time. Since these cases are underrepresented, results from screening may be associated with a better than average survival rate.

One last problem is the issue of efficacy and effectiveness. A specific screening maneuver may be shown to be effective under study conditions but may lack effectiveness when applied on a population basis. Poor vaccination levels against influenza in the elderly is one such example. Other factors may limit the beneficial impact of screening services. Screening maneuvers are usually furnished free in a study setting, but in the real world they must be billed for, and patients may not be willing to assume this financial burden for a future benefit. Physicians may not be willing to spend the time necessary for counseling because it is considered unreimbursable. Despite all the above limitations, the following screening maneuvers appropriate for the office setting are recommended.

History

Table 2 lists topics that should be reviewed in individuals of all ages. The importance of each of these areas can hardly be overemphasized. General information as to alcohol and drug consumption is easily linked to an inquiry and, if necessary, counseling about the need for seatbelts to be used at all times. Information in any of these areas may help direct the physical examination. Dietary questions that are appropriate for age and sex help direct counseling and educational strategies. The threat of acquired immunodeficiency syndrome (AIDS) and the increasing prevalence of sexually transmitted diseases make it mandatory to inquire into sexual practices. About 30 percent of Americans still smoke, and 390,000 Americans die annually from smoking-related causes. Hence all smokers need to be identified and counseled to stop. Nutrition questions should be age- and gender-specific but should

TABLE 2 Recommended Screening Questions in Patient History (All Ages)

Dietary intake
Physical activity
Use of tobacco, alcohol, or drugs
Sexual practices
Seatbelt use when driving

focus on the need to maintain ideal weight and to limit fat intake in general. These questions logically lead to an inquiry about physical activity. In addition, cancer of the colon, breast, and prostate has been epidemiologically linked with increased fat consumption.

The quality of the information depends on the physician's sensitivity to the patient's concerns. Patients are often uncomfortable about answering questions dealing with sexual practices or drug use for fear of being thought of as deviant, with all that connotation implies. Physicians must be aware of these concerns and in a nonjudgmental manner must attempt to elicit the patient's trust. Several health risk appraisal aids have been developed for the office setting and can serve as instruments to analyze lifestyle in order to provide guidance. Some practitioners have favored use of these instruments because they help to personalize risk and facilitate the prioritization of behavioral changes necessary to reduce risk.

Physical Examination

One of the rituals that has been ingrained into office practice is the annual physical examination. Practitioners expect to do them, and patients have been conditioned to expect them. Nonetheless, a critical review of published studies suggests that the routine physical examination has little screening value in the asymptomatic patient. The Canadian Task Force on the Periodic Examination and the U.S. Preventive Services Task Force have concluded that the annual complete physical examination is unnecessary. Some maneuvers do have screening value and are summarized in Table 3.

Properly conducted randomized or cohort studies have shown that only three maneuvers should be routinely performed: blood pressure determination, clinical breast examination for women over 40 years, and a Papanicolaou test.

TABLE 3 Recommended Screening Maneuvers in the Physical Examination for Individuals at Average Risk

Age in Years		
19–39	*40–64*	*65 and Over*
Height	Height	Height
Weight	Weight	Weight
Blood pressure	Blood pressure	Blood pressure
Papanicolaou smear	Breast examination*	Breast examination*
	Papanicolaou smear	Abdominal examination to detect aneurysm
		Visual acuity
		Hearing

*In association with mammography.

Hypertension is a common disease, and there are excellent supporting data that treating patients with moderate and severe hypertension decreases morbidity and mortality from congestive heart failure, stroke, renal disease, and retinopathy. The Kaiser randomized trial of multiphasic screening showed that there was less mortality in the intervention group, which was screened every 2 years, compared with that of controls, who were screened every 5 years. Therefore blood pressure should be measured at least every 2 years. Blood pressure measurement as an office routine is to be encouraged.

A randomized controlled trial in the United States has shown that breast examination by a physician along with mammography decreases breast cancer mortality in women 50 to 59 years of age. For women over 60 years old, there are case control data supporting annual physical examination and mammography. These data are so persuasive that all practicing physicians should make special efforts to ensure that all women over 40 have an annual breast examination with associated mammography.

Cervical cancer is an ideal disease for screening. The disease can be recognized early and is a relatively slow-growing cancer. Cohort studies have shown that routine screening by Papanicolaou smear tests reduces the incidence and mortality from invasive cervical cancer. The main screening argument has centered on how frequently the test should be done. The U.S. Preventive Services Task Force has suggested that sexually active women should have a Papanicolaou test every 3 years after two initial negative tests obtained 1 year apart.

Because of the frequency of visual and hearing problems with aging, annual examinations are recommended for persons over age 60. There also are excellent data to show that annual dental visits are associated with less dental disease; hence referral for dental care is encouraged. To identify valvular abnormalities requiring antibiotic prophylaxis, cardiac auscultation should be done early in life and again in patients in the middle 60s. Older men should also have an annual abdominal examination to check for the presence of an abdominal aortic aneurysm. Neither the bimanual pelvic examination nor the rectal examination is recommended. Critical review of published data shows that these tests have low sensitivity, specificity, and positive predictive value.

Controversy has surrounded screening recommendations dealing with the physical examination in asymptomatic patients. Thoughtful physicians have argued that the bonding that is essential to the physician-patient relationship is facilitated by the touching that is intrinsic to the physical examination. Nonetheless, an unbiased review of the physical examination suggests that much of it is ritualistic and, in the absence of specific complaints, largely unnecessary. On the positive side is the observation that there are relatively few appropriate screening maneuvers that need to be done when a patient comes to the office with symptoms.

These recommendations should not be overinterpreted. They refer to asymptomatic patients and reflect a paucity of properly conducted clinical trials. In addition, certain maneuvers may be done for other reasons, such as a rectal examination to obtain stool for occult blood testing, and in such circumstances a digital search for rectal masses and prostatic nodules is not being discouraged. The central point that continually needs emphasis is that the time-limited patient-physician encounter requires that the most efficacious activities be carried out. For example, it makes little sense to do a complete physical examination in an asymptomatic 25-year-old patient while not discussing the hazards of AIDS and alcohol and the importance of using seatbelts, counsel that is far more likely to decrease morbidity and increase life expectancy.

Laboratory Procedures

Few laboratory or diagnostic studies are recommended for persons at average risk (Table 4). Periodic measurement of cholesterol levels is recommended, particularly for middle-aged men, because of the large body of epidemiologic, clinical, and animal studies that have linked serum cholesterol levels to coronary atherosclerosis. The ability of cholesterol-lowering drugs to reduce the incidence of coronary atherosclerosis in middle-aged men has been demonstrated in randomized controlled studies. Controversy exists as to whether these results are generalizable to the general population, such as premenopausal women or the elderly. The Framingham data show that coronary artery disease risk augments in a graded fashion, with a sharp increase after cholesterol levels of 220 to 240 mg per deciliter are attained. Asymptomatic adults with cholesterol levels above 240 mg per deciliter should receive dietary counseling and follow-up evaluation.

The need for Papanicolaou testing and mammography in women over age 40 has already been discussed. Early hypothyroidism and hyperthyroidism are difficult diagnoses in the elderly because of the nonspecificity of symptoms. Thyroid screening has been recommended for elderly women on the grounds of clinical prudence, although it has not been proved that adults with thyroid dysfunction who are identified earlier and receive treatment prior to the development of symptoms have a better outcome than those who receive treatment after symptoms have developed. A dipstick urinalysis has been suggested as an appropriate screening measure for older persons because of the higher positive predictive value of renal disease in the elderly. Testing for fecal occult blood in asymptomatic patients is still controversial. Interest in this test is prompted by the well-documented observation that early-stage diagnosis of colorectal cancer is associated with longer survival than in persons with advanced disease. In asymptomatic patients over age 50, the positive predictive value of occult fecal blood is 5 to 10 percent for carcinoma and 30 percent for adenomas. The high proportion of false-positive findings is an important problem because of the complications sometimes associated with follow-up tests, such as barium enema and sigmoidoscopy. However, there are no data showing that screening for colorectal cancer in asymptomatic persons will reduce mortality, although it is hoped that ongoing trials will answer this question.

Persons who fall into high-risk groups for certain diseases are another matter, and in this instance recommendations for screening are far more aggressive (Table 5). For example, breast cancer in a first-order relative significantly increases the risk of breast cancer in the propositus, and for that reason annual breast examinations and mammography have been recommended in women beginning at 35 years. Patients who are sexually active and have multiple partners should be screened for sexually transmitted diseases. Laboratory tests and procedures for high-risk groups are beyond the scope of this review, and readers are referred to the Task Force report for more details.

Some specific screening tests are not recommended because of their poor sensitivity or specificity or, if the condition is identified, the absence of good therapy. Cancer of the lung is the leading cause of cancer deaths in the United States. Screening chest roentgenograms and sputum cytologic examinations have been studied prospectively in smokers and found not to be helpful in early diagnosis. Pancreatic cancer is the fifth most common cancer in the United States, but there are no appropriate screening tests for this disease. Potential screening tests such as computed tomography and endoscopic

TABLE 4 Recommended Screening Laboratory or Diagnostic Studies for Adults of Average Risk

Age in Years		
19–39	*40–64*	*65 and Over*
Blood cholesterol level	Blood cholesterol level	Blood cholesterol level
Papanicolaou smear	Papanicolaou smear	Thyroid function
	Mammogram*	Mammogram*
		Fecal occult blood test
		Dipstick urinalysis

*In association with clinical breast examination.

TABLE 5 Recommended Screening Laboratory or Diagnostic Studies for Adults Deemed to Be at High Risk

Age in Years		
19–39	*40–64*	*65 and Over*
Fasting glucose level	Fasting glucose level	Fasting glucose level
Rubella antibodies	VDRL test	Tuberculin test
VDRL test	Chlamydial testing	Electrocardiogram
Urinalysis (bacteria)	Urinalysis (bacteria)	Sigmoidoscopy
Chlamydial testing	Culture for gonorrhea	Colonoscopy
Culture for gonorrhea	Human immunodeficiency virus testing	Papanicolaou smear
Human immunodeficiency virus testing	Tuberculin test	
Hearing test	Hearing test	
Tuberculin test	Electrocardiogram	
Electrocardiogram	Fecal occult blood/sigmoidoscopy/ colonoscopy	
Mammogram	Bone mineral content scan	
Colonoscopy		

retrograde cholangiopancreatography are expensive, and there is little evidence that early detection lowers morbidity or mortality from the disease. Neither the physical examination nor the Papanicolaou test is accurate enough to be used routinely as a screening test for ovarian carcinoma. Similarly, there are no data to suggest that screening electrocardiograms reduce morbidity or mortality. Neck auscultation and noninvasive testing for carotid artery stenosis have been proposed as screening tests, but neither has been shown to reduce morbidity or mortality in prospective trials.

COUNSELING

As pointed out earlier, patient education and physician-based efforts at influencing cigarette smoking, exercise, nutrition, and alcohol and other drug abuse are more likely to improve life expectancy than more traditional clinically based interventions. However, as any experienced physician will attest, identifying a risk factor is not synonymous with its control. Many physicians do not feel comfortable in their counseling roles. Internists have been trained to diagnose and treat illnesses and have had little formal training in counseling. Studies have compared physician-reported compliance with counseling with medical record reviews and data from consumer surveys. For the most part, physicians either overestimate the amount of counseling they do or do it in such a way that consumers have little realization that they are being counseled. More research in office-based counseling is urgently needed.

The U.S. Preventive Services Task Force proposed ten counseling guidelines.

1. *Develop a therapeutic alliance.* This positions the practitioner as the expert consultant available to patients who remain in control of their own health choices.

2. *Counsel all patients.* Physicians tend to give more information to those who ask questions; middle class whites receive more counseling than working class blacks and Hispanics. Educational efforts must be appropriate to the age, race, sex, and socioeconomic class of the patient.

3. *Ensure that patients understand the relationship between behavior and health.* Physicians should not assume that patients understand the relationship between smoking, poor nutrition, alcohol, and lack of exercise to poor health. Simple terms should be used to explain how these factors affect health singly and together.

4. *Work with patients to assess barriers to behavior change.* Patient beliefs that are not conducive to healthy behavior should be identified and assessed. Obstacles should be identified and patients helped to overcome them.

5. *Gain commitment to change from patients.* This is a key step. If patients do not agree that their behaviors are significantly related to health outcomes, attempts at patient education may be futile.

6. *Involve patients in choosing one risk factor at a time to change.* Let patient need, patient preference, and physician assessment of relative importance to health determine the first risk factor to tackle.

7. *Use a combination of strategies.* Educational efforts that integrate individual counseling, group classes, written materials, and community resources are far more effective than those employing a single technique. However, studies have shown that the practitioner's individual attention and feedback are more important than other communication channels.

8. *Design a behavior modification plan.* Agree on a time-limited goal to be achieved and note it in the medical record. Assist patients in writing action plans and stress your willingness to continue to be involved.

9. *Monitor progress through follow-up contact.* Schedule a follow-up appointment or telephone call within the next few weeks to evaluate progress. Reinforce success and, if unsuccessful, work with patients to identify and overcome obstacles.

10. *Involve office staff.* Use the team approach to patient education. Involve office staff and ensure that patients hear the same message.

IMMUNIZATIONS AND CHEMOPROPHYLAXIS

Recommended immunizations for adults are presented in Table 6. Influenza continues to be an important public health problem in the United States. Ten thousand or more excess deaths were documented in 19 different influenza epidemics from 1957 to 1986. Influenza vaccine contains antigens that are chosen each year on the basis of predictions of which influenza viruses will circulate. In seasons in which the match has been good, vaccine efficacy levels of about 70 percent have been documented. Since 80 to 90 percent of all influenza deaths occur among the elderly, they are a particularly important target. Vaccine should be given annually to all persons above age 65 and to those under 65 who are considered at high risk, predominantly persons with chronic cardiopulmonary disease. To limit disease spread, all health care providers with contact with either the elderly or younger high-risk persons should also receive influenza vaccine annually.

Over 70 percent of reported cases of tetanus in the United States occur in the elderly. Serosurveys in the elderly have shown that about half have tetanus antitoxin levels that are not protective. There is universal need for tetanus immunization in adults, and booster doses should be given every 10 years.

Pneumococcal vaccine should be given once to all persons above age 65 and to all others with medical conditions that put them at special risk of pneumococcal infection. The original 14-valent pneumococcal vaccine was replaced in 1983 by a 23-valent vaccine. The efficacy of pneumococcal vaccine in young populations with high incidence rates of pneumococcal disease is uncontested. However, translation of this efficacy in elderly American populations has yielded conflicting results. The low attack rate of pneumococcal infection and the difficulty in ascribing bacterial etiology in the absence of positive blood cultures have made it difficult to evaluate vaccine efficacy using standard cohort designs. Case-control studies and studies comparing the distribution of pneumococcal serotypes in the blood of vaccinated and unvaccinated persons have shown an efficacy of about 60 percent.

The introduction of measles vaccine more than 20 years ago has been associated with a dramatic decrease in cases in the United States. A major public health effort to eliminate indigenous measles in this country has not succeeded to date. A major problem in this effort has been the occurrence of cases in high school and college students. If given at age 15 months, measles vaccine is 95 percent effective. Over time, the 5 percent vaccine failures have created a pool of susceptible populations in whom epidemics have occurred. In 1989, the Advisory Committee on Immunization Practices adopted a two-dose measles vaccine strategy for all adults born after 1956 who do not have either laboratory evidence of measles immunity or a history of physician-diagnosed measles.

Postexposure prophylaxis has been a useful strategy for preventing certain diseases (Table 7). More information is available in individual disease chapters.

TABLE 6 Immunization by Age Group (Individuals at Average Risk)

Age (yr)	*Antigens*
19–39	Tetanus-diphtheria booster Measles
40–64	Tetanus-diphtheria booster
65 and older	Tetanus-diphtheria booster Influenza vaccine Pneumococcal vaccine

TABLE 7 Recommendations for Chemoprophylaxis or Immunoprophylaxis

Disease	*Chemoprophylactic or Immunoprophylactic Agent*
Meningococcosis	Rifampin
Hepatitis A	Immune globulin
Hepatitis B	Hepatitis B immune globulin*
Rabies	Rabies immune globulin†
Tuberculosis	Isoniazid
Malaria	Chloroquine
Influenza	Amantadine

*With hepatitis B vaccine.
†With rabies vaccine.

SUGGESTED READING

Canadian Task Force on the Periodic Health Examination. The periodic health examination. Can Med Assoc J 1979; 121: 1193–1254.

Frame P, Carlson SJ. A critical review of periodic health screening using specific screening criteria. Parts 1–4. J Fam Pract 1975; 2:29–36, 123–129, 189–194, 283–289.

Morbidity and Mortality Weekly Report. Premature mortality in the United States. MMWR 1986; 35:1S–11S.

Oboler SK, LaForce FM. The periodic physical examination in asymptomatic adults. Ann Intern Med 1989; 110:214–226.

U.S. Preventive Services Task Force. Guide to clinical preventive services. Baltimore: Williams & Wilkins, 1989.

PATIENT COMPLIANCE

RICHARD I. KOPELMAN, M.D.

In the usual physician-patient encounter, one or several medical problems are evaluated and discussed and a plan of action is agreed upon by the physician and patient in an effort to address the problem(s). The plan may be multifactorial, including the prescribing of medications; the pursuit of an alteration in behavior such as losing weight, stopping smoking, or decreasing alcohol consumption; or the scheduling of tests, referrals, or follow-up appointments. Medical compliance is usually defined as the extent to which a patient's behavior is in accord with the advice given by the physician. The term *compliance*, however, has a pejorative flavor because it may imply a subservient role of the patient vis-à-vis an authoritative provider. An alternative term, *adherence*, may better reflect a sense of mutual agreement in the development and implementation of the treatment plan. In this discussion, these terms are used interchangeably.

As physicians we all realize that noncompliance is an everyday problem in our practices. Estimates of its prevalence have ranged from 10 percent to over 90 percent, depending on the clinical setting. For example, among patients who are newly diagnosed as having hypertension, one-half fail to follow up on referral advice and only 50 percent of those who begin therapy are still in treatment at the end of 1 year. Noncompliance can take many forms. It may be intentional in that the patient knowingly does not follow through on the medical advice, even though he or she fully comprehends the rationale behind it. Or noncompliance can be caused by a lack of understanding of the physician's advise owing to a variety of factors to be discussed later. In some studies, poor comprehension has been estimated to be responsible for 20 to 70 percent of noncompliance. In addition, noncompliance can be caused by a variety of errors, most of which occur in the process of taking medications. There can be errors of omission (e.g., a prescribed medication is not taken), errors of commission (the patient may be taking medications of which the physician is not aware), errors in dosing (the wrong dose is taken), and errors in scheduling (the medication is taken at the wrong times of the day). No matter what the defect, compliance should be viewed as the responsibility of both the patient and the provider.

This chapter first discusses some of the factors that have been shown to be associated with noncompliance, then briefly discusses some of the ways in which the physician can better detect noncompliant behavior, and finally provides readers with a list of suggestions to improve adherence to physicians' recommendations.

FACTORS AFFECTING COMPLIANCE

Through the years, numerous studies have attempted to assess the various factors that affect patient compliance. Although there have often been conflicting results, several generalizations still can be made. First, many patient characteristics are worthy of discussion. Numerous investigations have surprisingly shown that demographic variables such as sex, race, education, occupation, income, and marital status usually do not affect compliance. Elderly patients often have problems with compliance because of poor comprehension of advice or even difficulty in opening pill containers. Problems such as alcoholism or drug addiction correlate with noncompliant behavior, as do psychological factors such as feelings of isolation. In addition, obvious barriers such as language difficulties, mental retardation, or major psychological illness increase the risk of noncompliance.

A major factor that affects behavior is the patient's views of his or her illness, especially as they pertain to the perceived susceptibility to the illness, its severity if contracted, and the costs and benefits encountered in pursuing the recommended course of action. These, in turn, are influenced by factors including the patient's family, the cultural background, his or her own value system regarding health, and the presence of any anxiety, hidden fears, or denial. People often have an overly optimistic bias about personal risk ("this won't happen to me"). The patient may be skeptical about the medical profession or be influenced by being told of a previous experience with a similar problem in a friend or relative.

The role of information has been less clearly defined. One would think that better-informed patients would be more likely to follow through with medical advice, but this is not necessarily true. Other factors may have an impact here. Physicians should be aware that patients often receive information from several sources and may be considering advice given by friends or family or information that they have obtained from television or newspapers. Sometimes these other sources are in conflict with the physician's advice.

Patients who have strong support systems including the family network are more likely to be compliant, and those who have been compliant with other regimens are more likely to follow new medical advice.

The effects of specific diseases have been studied extensively. The severity of the illness does not consistently correlate with compliant behavior. Nonetheless, as shown in studies of renal transplant recipients, the more disability that is involved with a medical problem, the more likely the patient is to be compliant. In addition, patients tend to be more compliant with cardiac medications, antihypertensive drugs, and diabetic therapy than they are with drugs used primarily for symptomatic relief such as antihistamines, analgesics, or antacids.

Medical advice involving behavioral changes or alterations in lifestyle such as diet, alcohol intake, or smoking tends to be associated with high rates of noncompliance. Only 15 to 70 percent of such advice is followed. In addition, noncompliant behavior tends to be more common in asymptomatic patients. The importance of preventive care is much more difficult to communicate to patients, many of whom are oriented more to the present than to future risk.

The regimens themselves affect compliance directly. The number of different medications and the number of doses per day are directly associated with nonadherence. As one author stated, "the more drugs the doctor prescribes, the more the patient omits." Another factor relates to the synchrony of dosing. For instance, if the patient has to take one medication three times daily and another four times daily, this regimen is unlikely to be followed appropriately. Not surprisingly, longer courses of treatment are less likely to be followed than shorter courses of therapy: about 75 percent of short-term courses of medication are taken and less than 50 percent of long-term regimens are followed.

Side effects of the medications can be important. Although there has been some debate over the extent of this factor,we are all aware that side effects such as sexual dysfunction from antihypertensive medications are an important part of the compliance problem in the large population of hypertensive patients. Of course, the cost of medications also has become an increasingly difficult problem for many patients.

One of the most important factors affecting compliance is the patient-physician relationship. The ideal relationship is a partnership and not one in which the physician dictates the regimen to the patient. There should be a negotiation between the patient and the physician regarding the medical regimen, with active involvement by the patient. Physicians must be aware that patients often have different value systems and may be anxious and fearful of expressing themselves to the physician. Therefore, open and honest transfer of information must take place, both from the physician to the patient and vice versa. The physician must explain the diagnosis, discuss the rationale for his or her recommendations, encourage questions from the patient, and be willing to discuss openly any differences of opinion. In the long run, a trustful physician-patient relationship is more likely to result in achievement of goals. In chronic conditions, the importance of continuity of care cannot be overemphasized.

Several factors within the medical system affect compliance. If a patient makes an appointment, he or she is more likely to keep it than if a physician initiates the appointment. If a patient spends a long time waiting for a physician at the visit, he or she is much more likely not to return to see that physician. Shorter periods of time between appointments, especially when one is trying to convince a patient of the long-term importance of a problem, are more likely to result in adherence. When a patient is referred to another physician, if that consultation occurs within a short time and if the patient is referred to a specific physician as opposed to a clinic, the patient is more likely to show up.

MEASURING COMPLIANCE

Unfortunately, no gold standard exists with which to measure compliance. Because noncompliant behavior crosses all demographic variables, all patients may be at risk for nonadherence. Several studies have shown that both newly trained and experienced physicians are poor predictors of noncompliant behavior. In one study, physicians accurately predicted only 35 percent of those who were noncompliant, and one-half of the people they thought were nonadherent were in fact compliant. Therefore, the first step to detecting noncompliance is for the physician to have a high index of suspicion for all patients.

The way in which we assess compliance must be careful and diplomatic. The first approach is direct questioning of the patient. If a patient admits to being noncompliant, the report is likely to be accurate, although only about 40 to 80 percent of those shown to be noncompliant admit to it. It is most important that the physician try to be supportive and to deal with the patient in an open-ended way. The physician must come across in a nonthreatening, supportive, and nonjudgmental manner. In general, if a patient admits to noncompliance, that patient is more amenable to modification of such behavior.

Other ways of measuring compliance include counting medications, as is usually done in drug studies. This is far from an optimal way to determine compliance, however. The measurement of drug levels can be helpful, but there are a limited number of medications whose blood levels can be measured, and this approach can be costly. Nonetheless, a nonexistent drug level certainly is strong evidence for noncompliance. A low or subtherapeutic level of medication does not necessarily indicate noncompliance because many factors can affect drug pharmacokinetics in an individual patient.

In a managed health system, monitoring of the frequency of prescription refills can be an additional way to ascertain compliance, but it is not perfect.

One can also attempt to correlate compliance with outcome, but this practice is fraught with error. For instance, just because a patient's blood pressure is normal does not mean that he or she is compliant with recommended medications, because other factors such as weight loss or a decrease in alcohol intake may achieve similar results. Nonetheless, failure to see expected responses to interventions (e.g., a persistent tachycardia in a patient allegedly taking beta-blockers) should arouse suspicion.

Compliance is an ongoing problem, and the issue of adherence to the medical regimen has to be continually reevaluated.

SUGGESTIONS TO IMPROVE COMPLIANCE

1. Much effort should be spent in achieving an optimal physician-patient relationship. The interaction should be one in which both participants feel comfortable with each other and there is free flow of information in both directions. The physician should explain the diagnosis and discuss the rationale behind the treatment, including the benefits to be derived from the therapy. The patient must feel that the physician is willing to listen to his or her point of view and at the same time should be at ease in expressing his or her own anxiety and fears. Medical regimens should be arrived at through mutual negotiation.

2. The physician should be willing to listen to the patient's concerns and allow the patient to make suggestions regarding his or her care. Patients are constantly exposed to and read about many medical controversies (for example, treatments of hypercholesterolemia), and unless these controversial areas are discussed, the patient may follow whatever advice or information is being received from nonmedical sources without a balanced response from the physician.

3. Once a medical regimen is discussed, certain goals should be set by the patient and physician. Often it is not enough to tell a patient to lose weight, but by setting a realistic goal, e.g., losing a certain number of pounds by the next visit, a patient can be given a little more direction. In addition, in the face of multiple goals, partial implementation should be sought. For instance, we often tell our patients to stop smoking, lose weight, and reduce their alcohol intake. To expect a patient to do all three things at once may be unrealistic, and hence patients and physicians should prioritize these goals.

4. Physicians must be explicit in their instructions to patients. When possible, instructions should be both spoken and written. Technical language must be avoided. Studies show that approximately 50 percent of information given to a patient is forgotten in a short time.

5. Planned regimens should be as simple as possible and consistent with the patient's work or lifestyle. It may be impossible for a patient to take a medication while he or she is at work. Pill taking should be integrated with routine daily activities such as toothbrushing or meals whenever possible. To maximize compliance with follow-up appointments, consideration should be given to have appointments available either in the evenings or on weekends in order to avoid forcing patients to take time off from work.

6. At each visit, the medical regimen should be reviewed in detail. It is often helpful to have a patient bring in his or her medications to allow the physician to check compliance with each one. Patients should be asked repeatedly about potential side effects from medications. Although patients may voice many problems, they usually do not bring up certain side effects such as sexual dysfunction. Only if physicians ask about these side effects will important potential causes of noncompliance be discovered. The physician should pay attention to the patient's social system and determine if any changes have occurred. If a patient is under any unusual stress at his or her job or at home, or if there has been a change in economic status, compliance may be affected. The physician should praise the patient for success in achieving goals and at the same time gently explore any problem a patient may have had adhering to a regimen.

7. In certain situations, a physician should encourage the patient to become actively involved in monitoring the course of his or her disease. This practice is successful in patients with diabetes who manage their dosage of insulin and in patients with edema who manage their dosage of diuretics. By having patients keep records of the results, one increases the involvement of the patient in his or her care. In certain patients home blood pressure monitoring can be helpful, although it should be done selectively so as not to make a patient overly fixated on the medical condition.

8. Physicians should be encouraged to use other nonphysician personnel in the treatment of numerous patient problems. By seeing a nurse practitioner or dietitian, the patient can be exposed to complementary views of the disorder. In addition, a patient may be reluctant to raise certain concerns with a physician but may be willing to do so in another setting with another health professional.

9. Care should be taken to prescribe the least number of medications in a practical dosing schedule. If a patient has two disorders, such as hypertension and angina, if possible one should prescribe monotherapy such as a beta-blocker or a calcium channel blocker. In addition, if a patient has to take multiple medications, regimens that permit dosing at the same time each day will be easier to follow.

10. Physicians must pay attention to the costs of medications. An excellent medication does no good

if the prescription is never filled because it is too expensive.

11. The frequency of patient visits should be sufficient to permit the physician to convey the importance of a patient's medical problems. To start a patient on an antihypertensive medication and then follow him or her only every 9 to 12 months does not convey a sense of importance to the patient. Continuity of care should be maximized as much as possible, and long waits should be avoided.

12. Efforts should be made to mobilize support groups, which include both the patient's family and community agencies such as the Visiting Nurses Association. Especially in elderly patients, compliance can be a problem unless these sources of support are in place. Patients may benefit enormously from discussing their problems with people who have the same illnesses through such organizations as Alcoholics Anonymous, smoking cessation groups, or post-myocardial infarction groups.

13. Occasionally, admission to the hospital may be necessary both to monitor compliance and to educate the patient further. We have all had the experience of having had a patient take a growing list of antihypertensive medications, only to find on admission to the hospital that the blood pressure was easily controlled on far fewer medicines.

14. Telephone or written follow-up with a patient after a visit is a helpful means of showing a patient that the physician cares.

15. Follow-up appointments should be made as often as possible at the time of the initial visit. If the physician banks on the patient's making the appointment in the future, the chances are great that it will not be done.

16. Reminders to patients regarding their upcoming appointments result in a small but real increase in attendance.

17. When a patient does not show up for an appointment, a follow-up letter or phone call often ensures that the patient is not lost.

18. When referrals for consultations are made, appointments should be scheduled within a short time with a specific provider.

19. It must be remembered that compliance is an ongoing problem, especially in patients with chronic diseases, and the physician should be constantly on the lookout for potential noncompliant behavior.

SUGGESTED READING

Eraker SA, Kirscht JP, Becker MH. Understanding and improving patient compliance. Ann Intern Med 1984; 100:258-268.

Hatem CJ, Lawrence RS. Improving compliance and health-promoting behavior. In: Branch W, ed. Office practice of medicine. 2nd ed. Philadelphia: WB Saunders, 1987:1075.

Haynes RB, Taylor DW, Sackett DL. Compliance in health care. Baltimore: Johns Hopkins University Press, 1979.

Kern DE, Baile WF. Patient compliance with medical advice. In: Barker LR, Burton JR, Zieve PD, eds. Principles of ambulatory medicine. 2nd ed. Baltimore: Williams & Wilkins, 1986:41.

Matthews D, Hingson R. Improving patient compliance. Med Clin North Am 1977; 61:879-889.

RESPECTING PATIENTS' TREATMENT PREFERENCES

DAN W. BROCK, Ph.D.
STEVEN A. WARTMAN, M.D., Ph.D.

In recent years, physicians and patients have tended to move toward a model of shared treatment decision making. Although this sounds reasonable on the surface, i.e., that patients and physicians collaborate in the process of making decisions regarding medical care, surprisingly little attention has been given to the complex and troubling issues that can arise within this model. In this chapter, we discuss the rationale for the model of shared physician-patient decision making, followed by what that model implies for physicians' responsibilities when an apparently competent patient's preference appears to be irrational. A discussion of this issue requires the development of a taxonomy of the different forms and sources of irrational decision making. These include the bias toward the present and near future; the belief that "it won't happen to me"; fear of pain or the medical experience; patient values or wants that do not make sense; framing effects; and conflicts between individual and social rationality. Our main aim is to develop this taxonomy and thereby to bring out some of the theoretical and practical obstacles in distinguishing irrational patient choices, which physicians might seek to change or override, from merely unusual choices that should be respected.

SHARED DECISION MAKING BETWEEN PHYSICIAN AND PATIENT

Historically, the most common professional ideal of the physician-patient relationship held that the physician directed care and made decisions about treatment, whereas the patient's principal role was to comply with "doctor's orders." Although this paternalistic ideal often did not ignore at least the patient's general preferences and attitudes toward treatment, it nevertheless gave the patient only a minimal role in treatment decision making. This model reflected, on the one hand, the inequality between the medical training, knowledge, and experience of the physician and the average patient, and, on the other, the anxiety, fear, dependency, and regression that can impair or seriously alter sick patients' usual decision-making abilities. When faced with what appeared to be irrational choices or preferences expressed by their patients, this paternalistic model encouraged physicians to overlook or override those choices as not being in the patients' true interests or not what patients would prefer in the absence of their decision-making impairment.

The paternalistic ideal of the physician-patient relation has been challenged by a number of forces from both within and outside of medicine during the last two or three decades and has generally been replaced by an ideal of shared decision making. In this model, health care treatment decisions are a collaborative process in which both physician and patient make active and essential contributions. The physician brings his or her medical training, knowledge, and expertise to the diagnosis and management of the patient's current condition, including available treatment alternatives. The patient brings knowledge of his or her own subjective aims and values through which the risks and benefits of various treatment options can be evaluated. The selection of the best treatment for this particular patient requires the contributions of both parties.

This division of labor oversimplifies, of course, the complexities of the actual roles and contributions of physicians and patients in real instances of treatment decision making, but it does serve to highlight the new, active role of the patient in that process. Some have concluded that in shared decision making, respecting patient autonomy or self-determination requires respecting the patient's treatment preferences no matter how they have been arrived at. However, we believe that such a conclusion is not warranted. It fails to recognize the trade-off between the different, conflicting values involved in the decision to respect or to seek to change or override patients' choices and relies on an inadequate account of the nature and value of self-determination.

Three examples serve to illustrate the kinds of difficulties that can arise when patients are offered the opportunity to participate in the decision-making process and make decisions that appear "irrational" to the physician.

Example No. 1: The Bias Toward the Present or Near Future. A 35-year-old healthy man with a strong family history of heart disease has been found to have hypertension and an elevated cholesterol level. In response to his physician's recommendation of medication to lower blood pressure and a low-cholesterol diet, he responds, "I don't care what happens to me when I'm 65, I know these drugs have side effects, and I want to eat what I like now." This patient seems irrational in caring only about his present situation and disregarding potential future morbidity.

Example No. 2: The Belief That "It Can't Happen to Me." Despite detailed counseling by her physician, an 18-year-old woman with numerous sexual partners continues to practice unsafe sex. When advised again of the risks, she responds by saying that she does not think she will develop any sort of problem. Her seemingly irrational decision appears based on her belief that "It can't happen to me."

Example No. 3: Fear of A Medical Experience. A 44-year-old patient has been admitted to the hospital with a partial bowel obstruction. Despite medical management, his condition steadily worsens. When surgery is repeatedly advised, he refuses because of a fear of "being put to sleep."

How do physicians respect these patients' preferences while trying to offer what they believe is the best medical care? This is especially difficult because, from the physician's point of view, these preferences appear to be "irrational"; that is, they are based on biases, beliefs, or fears that are not necessarily amenable to scientific or medical reasoning. When the physician properly judges the patient's treatment choice to be irrational, attempts to change that choice through persuasion are commonly appropriate. However, it can be difficult to distinguish choices that are truly irrational from those that are merely unusual.

When persuasion fails, the decision to respect or to seek to override a patient's treatment choice is ultimately a question of the patient's competence in making that choice. This is because Anglo-American law holds that a patient's informed and voluntary treatment choice can only be set aside for the patient's own good if that choice is found to be incompetent. Physicians lack both ethical and legal authority unilaterally to override patients' treatment choices. Thus, when we speak of the physician "seeking to override" the patient's choice, we mean initiating the process of determining incompetence and selecting a surrogate, which commonly involves recourse to the courts.

WELL-BEING AND SELF-DETERMINATION

Determining what degree of decision-making impairment on a particular occasion warrants a finding of incompetence involves balancing two principal interests or values of patients. The first value is the patients' own well-being, which can require protecting patients from the harmful consequences of their seriously impaired treatment choices. The second value is respecting patients' self-determination in making significant decisions about their lives for themselves when they are able. When patients appear to be making treatment choices contrary to their own well-being and further discussion is unsuccessful in changing their opinion, these two values will be in conflict.

We use the notion of patient well-being to emphasize that medical care, which relieves pain and suffering, prevents disability, restores function, and prevents loss of life, is ultimately of value to the extent that it serves those aims and purposes that give content and meaning to the patient's overall plan of life. For many conditions, there are alternative treatments that are medically acceptable. These treatment options often have different mixes of risks and benefits, such that the "medical facts" alone will not settle which treatment is best for a particular patient. Moreover, treatment choices usually have an impact on other important values of patients, requiring trade-offs between medical and nonmedical values. The ultimate responsibility of physicians is to use their knowledge, skills, and expertise to serve patients' overall well-being and to facilitate patients' pursuit of their own plans of life. Thus, determining what treatment will best serve a particular patient's well-being has both medical components and patient preference or value components. However, as noted in the examples above, patients can often be mistaken about what best serves their well-being.

Patient self-determination involves patients' making important decisions that shape and affect their lives and having these decisions be respected by others. Self-determination is given great importance throughout American life, and in the field of medicine it has long been the central principle underlying the doctrine of informed consent. Since what serves patients' well-being often depends on their own wishes and values, informed patients are reasonably presumed to be the best judges of how specific treatment choices would contribute to their well-being. In this way, self-determination has instrumental value because respecting patients' self-determination usually serves their well-being. In addition, most persons want to make important decisions about their lives for themselves, even if they believe that others may be able to decide for them better than they themselves can. In this respect, self-determination is valued for its own sake and has noninstrumental value. It is in exercising our capacities to reflect on what kinds of persons we want to be and become and in adopting or affirming our own particular aims and values that we create a unique self and take responsibility for our lives.

It is important to realize that in the physician's decision to respect, attempt to change through persuasion, or seek to override a patient's choice, both the instrumental and noninstrumental values of self-determination vary with different decisions. The more that a patient's decision making is impaired and results in a choice that fails to promote his or her well-being, the less instrumental value self-determination has in promoting well-being; indeed, when the choice is positively harmful, this instrumental value may be thought of as negative. The more far-reaching the effects of the choice for the patient's life and what the patient most cares about, the greater the noninstrumental value of making the choice for oneself. Moreover, the more a choice is based on specific values that have stood some significant test of time in guiding the patient's life, the more weight self-determination deserves in making that choice. The noninstrumental value of self-determination also varies among persons according to how much weight they give to making their own choices, even when those choices are nonoptimal or harmful.

It is common to think that respecting patient self-determination always requires respecting the patient's choice and giving the same weight to all such patient choices. These views, however, are mistaken. First, just because the decision of whether to respect, seek to override, or attempt to change through persuasion a patient's choice sometimes involves weighing patient self-determination against protecting patient well-being, in some cases giving due weight to patient self-determination can be compatible with setting aside patient choices. Second, an assessment is needed in each instance of decision making of how much weight self-determination should properly be given.

Physicians thus have the option of respecting the patient's choice or attempting to override or to change that choice through persuasion, which must reflect both the values of patient well-being and self-determination. It may be the case that these values come into conflict, as in the examples cited above. In these cases, the patients' preferences appear to be irrational, making the physicians' choice to respect, seek to override, or attempt to persuade a difficult one.

THE STANDARD OF RATIONAL DECISION MAKING

Any discussion of irrational decision making must rely on an account of rational decision making. We believe that it is helpful to make that account explicit, even if only in brief outline. Specifically, what is the norm of rational decision making that underlies the ideal of shared decision making between patient and physician? Shared decision making essentially entitles the patient (or surrogate if the patient is incompetent) to weigh the benefits and risks of alternative treatments, including the alternative of no treatment, according to the patient's values and to select the alternative that best promotes those values. In the language of decision theory, the patient's own values determine his or her utility function, and the rational choice is the choice that maximizes expected utility for the patient. Since treatment decisions always involve some degree of uncertainty about both the benefits and harms of alternative treatments, these benefits and harms should be discounted by their probabilities, to the extent that they are known, in calculating the expected utility of different treatment alternatives. When the probabilities are not known, the patient's particular attitude toward risk, including the extent to which the patient is risk-averse or risk-taking, will determine the weight given to uncertain benefits or harms.

Shared decision making requires the physician, in part, to ensure that the patient is well informed. Thus, another aspect of ideal rational decision making is that the patient has and employs correct factual information about relevant alternatives, to the extent that it is available. This sketch of rational decision making ultimately relies on the patient's own aims and values as the ends that guide decision making. Irrational choice then can be conceived instrumentally as a choice that less completely satisfies those aims and values than would some available alternative.

Sometimes physicians employ a second notion of irrational choice that deems a patient's choice irrational if it fails to promote a set of basic aims and values that belong to the physician and/or standard medical practice guidelines. When physicians criticize a patient's choice as irrational in this sense, they express their disagreement with the basic aims and values by which the patient defines his or her own good as opposed to the judgment that the patient's choice will fail to promote best the patient's own aims and values. Since this second notion ignores the patient's own aims and values and thereby fails to respect the patient's self-determination adequately, we rely here on the first account of rational and irrational choice.

FORMS OF IRRATIONAL DECISION MAKING

We turn now to developing a taxonomy of common forms of irrational decision making by patients or their surrogates (but also sometimes physicians) when making treatment choices. In many actual treatment decisions, more than one form of irrationality affects a single choice, but we separate them here for analytic clarity.

Bias Toward the Present and Near Future

The ideal of rational decision making gives equal weight to a benefit or harm whenever it occurs in a person's life, with differences determined only by the size and probability of the benefit or harm. In the case of money, it is rational to apply a discount rate because a dollar received today can then earn interest and so is worth more than a dollar received 10 years from now. Some effects of health care are similar in that it is rational to prefer a restoration of function now rather than in the far future and to prefer that a loss of function occur as far in the future as possible, so as to minimize the period of disability. Similarly, it is rational to prefer that the loss of one's life be postponed as far as possible into the future. For other effects of medical care, however, especially pain and suffering, rational choice would seem to require indifference to when the experience occurs. In particular, it is a paradigm of prudential *ir*rationality to refuse to undergo a bad experience now, when doing so would avoid a much worse experience in the future. The reason such choices are commonly considered irrational is that the choice amounts to preferring that there be more rather than less bad experience or suffering in one's life.

Yet, as clinicians know, medical practice is replete with such irrational choices by patients. Patients who continue heavy smoking or alcohol use or who fail to comply with relatively simple steps to control moderate hypertension are often most plausibly understood as having given inadequate weight in their present decision making to the harms likely to occur to them in the relatively distant future. We call this a bias to the present and near future, because such persons commonly give disproportionate weight to securing benefits or avoiding harms in their present and near future as opposed to their more distant future. The physician's task in such cases is to help the patient fully appreciate the more distant harm or benefit, commensurate with its size or seriousness, so that it can play an appropriate role in the patient's decision making. A variety of methods for doing so may be useful, depending on the particular patient, such as letting the patient see similar effects that have actually occurred in other patients or the use of especially graphic accounts of the nature of the future benefits or harms.

The Belief That "It Won't Happen To Me"

Patients may have differing views as to the nature of the risk or harm to them of not following medical advice. This is especially true for events that have a low probability of occurring. However, what constitutes low probability may vary considerably from patient to patient. Further, since some patients may be greater risk-takers than others, it is often difficult to determine whether a given patient is just more of a risk-taker than most patients or whether this patient has simply failed to give adequate weight to a low-probability, distant event. This situation becomes more complicated by the difficulty of distinguishing among patients who tend to deny the possibility of an untoward event's happening to them, or who have "magical" or illusory beliefs regarding their vulnerability to harm, or who simply have a different way of viewing the medical problem. Adolescents, for example, are commonly subject to feelings of invulnerability to certain harms that are disproportionate to the real risk of those harms.

The physician often needs to gain some understanding of the patient's general attitude toward risk and the extent to which the patient is risk-averse or a risk-taker, perhaps as evidenced by the patient's past behavior. The physician should attempt to distinguish among the possibilities noted above. Sometimes the physician can help the patient more vividly appreciate the risk and relate it to the patient's life. However, in the case of the patient who denies the risk or who uses magical thinking, a more detailed medical and scientific explanation is not likely to be helpful. In these cases, formal counseling or psychiatric evaluation may prove more fruitful.

Fear of Pain or of a Medical Experience

Many patients delay or will not even consider a particular form of treatment for fear of the perceived nature of the experience. In many cases they may even acknowledge that the treatment or procedure is clearly in their best interest. Sometimes their decision is coupled with some form of rationalization— "there's no need to do it yet," or "I'm too busy now with other things." In other cases, when a dreaded experience draws near, a patient may become almost paralyzed by fear. Sometimes the fear may be focused not on pain or suffering but on other dreaded experiences, such as "being cut open" or of "being put to sleep" in surgery. In still other cases, fear of a disease such as cancer or acquired immunodeficiency syndrome can disable a person from making informed decisions about its treatment.

Determining when this form of irrational decision making is present is considerably complicated by the fact that there is no single, correct weight to give to pain or a particular medical experience as measured against the beneficial outcomes for which the experience may be necessary. Patients differ, for example, in the degree to which they are prepared to tolerate painful treatments or conditions for the sake of other ends. Adding to this complexity is the inaccessibility to physicians of other persons' pain. Although we can identify and often quantify the physiologic causes of pain in a particular person as well as the person's associated pain behavior, the person's conscious experience of the pain itself is not accessible to anyone else. As a result, it is often difficult to determine whether a patient gives more or less weight or importance to pain than do most others or is experiencing more or less pain than do others in similar circumstances.

More to the point here, however, is the difficulty of distinguishing persons who give undue weight to certain aspects of treatment because of irrational fear. Physicians may have had prior experience of patients who later were grateful that they were pressured or even forced to undergo such painful or dreaded treatments. The physician's responsibility in these cases is a difficult one—to respect the varying importance different persons give to avoiding pain while helping patients to overcome irrational fears that prevent them from pursuing promising treatment plans. This often involves helping patients to distinguish whether they are experiencing fear of a medical experience which they want to overcome or have instead made a choice with which they are comfortable.

What the Patient Wants Does Not Make Sense

When a competent patient prefers a certain form of treatment or wishes to decline a recommended course of treatment because of an obvious and understandable, although unusual, belief, physicians (and the courts) commonly yield to that belief. Examples include the Jehovah's Witness patient who refuses a blood transfusion, or the Asian patient who requests acupuncture or coining. If the patient's refusal of beneficial treatment is clearly incompetent, such as when a grossly psychotic patient reports that voices told him to refuse therapy, there are institutional and legal mechanisms to transfer medical decision making to another person or to the state. The real difficulties arise when what a competent patient wants does not make sense but is not attributable to something clearly recognizable as a religious belief or cultural preference. It can be extremely difficult in these situations for the physician to determine the basis of a patient's preference. However unusual, the more the preference reflects a deeply held enduring value that is important in the patient's life plan, the stronger the case for respecting it.

In other cases it is what the patient does *not* care about that does not make sense. For example, a patient may state that he or she understands but simply does not care that death or serious disability will result from a refusal of treatment. It may be difficult to determine whether this is an authentic, although unusual, choice or instead a result of a distortion of the patient's values caused by a treatable condition such as depression.

Framing Effects—Avoiding a Harm or Gaining a Benefit

It is well known that the way choices are formulated and presented, or framed, can have major effects on these choices. A simple example is the alternative presentation of a surgical treatment as "substantially extending the lives of 70 percent of patients who select it" or as "killing on the operating table up to 30 percent of the patients who select it." Both characterizations may be true, but which is used, or emphasized, may have a substantial impact on the rate of selection of the surgery.

There are a variety of different and more subtle kinds of framing effects. Some parents in the face of publicity about the diphtheria/pertussis/tetanus (DPT) vaccine refused the vaccine for their children because of the vaccine-related risk of neurologic damage or death. They continued to do so even after being told of the substantially greater risk of the negative outcome from the disease itself without vaccination. If the only relevant outcome of the vaccinate/do not vaccinate choice is the risk of harm to the child, parents' choices not to vaccinate their children are irrational and physicians' responsibilities might then arguably be to seek to persuade those parents to accept vaccination. But attempting to understand such choices of parents is often complex and may not always allow the choices to be so easily and quickly dismissed as irrational. For example, in the case of DPT, one factor affecting some parents' thinking may be a feeling on their part of a greater responsibility for the harm to their child if that harm results from a decision they made as opposed to random bad luck in acquiring the naturally occurring disease.

Work in the psychology of choice shows that losses tend to loom larger than gains in most people's decision making. Of course, whether a particular outcome is viewed as a gain or a loss depends on the status quo or reference point against which the outcome is compared. Many choices in medicine can be framed in either way, as obtaining a gain or avoiding a loss. For example, lowering moderate hypertension can be presented to a patient as adding months to his or her expected life span or as avoiding a shortening of life span from untreated hypertension. Neither framing of the patient's choice is obviously correct or mistaken; instead, each simply relies on different characterizations of the patient's present situation. Tversky and Kahneman have compared the framing effects in decision making to perspective changes in visual judgments; for example, which of two mountains appears higher depends on the position from which one views them. In this case, there is an objective standard by which one mountain could be determined to be higher. But there appears to be no objectively correct framing of many medical decisions, such as that of the patient with moderate hypertension. There are simply the two different but both correct ways of framing the choice, and the one that is used will influence whether some patients choose treatment. Sometimes the best that physicians can do is to present the choice framed in alternative ways in the hope that doing so will at least minimize framing effects.

Individual Versus Social Rationality: Irrational Use of Resources

Sometimes the circumstances that make individual choices rational also make the outcome of those choices irrational when viewed from a different perspective. One factor fueling the intense pressure to control rapidly rising health care costs is the perception that health care resources are often utilized in circumstances in which their expected benefits do not justify their true costs. In the extreme case of a patient's having full insurance coverage with no copayments or deductibles, the patient has no economic incentive to weigh the true costs of medical care under consideration against its expected benefits. Since using that care has no out-of-pocket costs for the patient, it is rational for the patient to choose to use all care with any expected medical benefit, no matter how small the benefit, and without regard for its costs. If the patient's physician employs the commonly accepted professional norm that his or her obligation to patients is to do whatever may be of benefit to them, without regard to cost, then it is rational for the physician also to ignore the cost of care in recommendations and decisions about the patient's treatment. The result will be overutilization of health care as against other goods and services whose benefits are weighed against their true costs. From the perspective of the group paying insurance premiums (for example, employers or the government), the result is an irrational overallocation of resources to health care.

Very different issues are raised by this form of irrational social choice in the use of resources than by the forms of irrational patient choice discussed above. It would be misdirected for physicians to seek to convince insured patients that their choices to employ non-cost-worthy care are irrational. On the contrary, the point is that an insured patient's choice to use non-cost-worthy care *is* rational, although it leads to an irrational social overallocation of resources to health care. Since the irrationality is not at the level of the insured patient's choice of treatment, the response to the irrationality should not be principally at that level. This form of social irrationality in the allocation of resources to health care does not justify a physician's failing to respect the insured patient's individual choice to employ non-cost-worthy care on grounds that the choice is irrational. Instead, this irrationality must be addressed where it exists—in the social and economic health care financing system.

Individual Versus Social Rationality: Public Health Versus Individual Benefit

Often physicians are concerned about the public health benefits of medical interventions, whereas their patients are not. For example, national campaigns to reduce serum cholesterol levels will clearly benefit the nation's health as a whole. However, the beneficial effects for a given individual patient may be minimal or nonexistent. Consequently, some individuals may rationally decide that for them the benefits of the intervention do not outweigh its burdens. This distinction between community-wide and individual benefits has been called the "prevention paradox," whereby a treatment that brings large benefits to the community may offer little to each participating individual. There is no true paradox, however. The society-wide benefit constitutes no reason to view as irrational and to not respect an individual's choice to decline the intervention.

For some infectious diseases, preventing the infection through vaccination (or shortening the period of transmissibility through treatment) of one individual lessens the risk of disease for others. A patient's or parent's refusal of immunization might be rational if the patient or parent is not concerned with the risks for others or believes that because enough of the population is immunized, the threat of the disease is minimal and therefore the risks of immunization outweigh the benefits. In this case, society may adopt mandatory immunization programs or the physician may seek to change the patient's refusal, not because the refusal is irrational but rather because of the social benefit for others.

WHAT SHOULD PHYSICIANS DO?

The model of shared decision making between patient and physician, while respecting the patient's self-determination, does not always require accepting the patient's preferences, particularly when these preferences are irrational. It is appropriate in some cases for the physician to attempt to persuade the patient to change his or her irrational choice or seek to have the patient's choice overridden as incompetent. However, distinguishing when a patient's preferences are truly irrational from when they simply express different attitudes, values, and beliefs can be difficult both in theory and in practice. Physicians need to be sensitive to the complexity of these judgments in helping patients to make sound treatment choices. More research is needed on the frequency and different forms of irrational treatment choices as well as on how physicians and patients can work together to overcome these decision-making irrationalities.

SUGGESTED READING

Forrow L, Wartman SA, Brock DW. Science, ethics and the making of clinical decisions. JAMA 1988; 259:3161–3167.

Gillick MR. Talking with patients about risk. J Gen Intern Med 1988; 3:166–170.

Rose G. Strategy of prevention: Lessons from cardiovascular disease. Br J Med 1981; 282:1847–1851.

Tversky A, Kahneman D. The framing of decisions and the psychology of choice. Science 1981; 211:453–459.

DECISIONS TO FORGO LIFE-SUSTAINING TREATMENT

PETER A. SINGER, M.D., M.P.H., FRCPC
MARK SIEGLER, M.D.

There is a broad consensus in medicine, law, and ethics that mentally competent adult patients may decline all treatments, including life-sustaining treatment (LST). Patients may decide to forgo a treatment that has been proposed (i.e., to have treatment withheld) or one that has already been started (i.e., to have treatment withdrawn). The patient may decide to forgo a wide range of potentially lifesaving treatments, including cardiopulmonary resuscitation, mechanical ventilation, dialysis, antibiotic therapy, and tube feeding. The right of patients to make their own health care decisions regarding LST is founded in the legal right of self-determination and the ethical principle of individual autonomy. It should be noted that the right to forgo LST does not extend to active euthanasia, such as by lethal injection, which remains illegal in all jurisdictions of the United States.

Although in the American legal context the right to forgo LST applies to both competent and incompetent adult patients, the right is effectuated very differently in these two clinical situations. Competent patients can express their wishes regarding life-sustaining treatment directly to their physicians. The situation is much more complex for incompetent patients, who cannot express their wishes regarding LST directly. Ideally, while still competent, the now incompetent patient will have recorded in the form of an advance directive a clearly expressed wish regarding the use of LST. In the absence of an advance directive, the incompetent patient's right to forgo life-sustaining treatment must be exercised by others on the patient's behalf through a process known as "surrogate decision making."

In the 1990s, good clinicians should be prepared to assist patients and families to deal with the following five clinical situations that relate to forgoing

LST: (1) brain death, (2) the use of advance directives, (3) the determination of patient competency, (4) decision making with competent patients, and (5) surrogate decision making for incompetent patients. This chapter aims to describe the principles of management in these five clinical situations.

BRAIN DEATH

If the patient is brain dead, treatment may be discontinued. The family should be informed that the patient has died and that mechanical ventilation and other forms of life support will be stopped. There is no need to ask the family's permission to do so. In three specific circumstances, the physician may choose to continue LST for a limited period even though the patient is brain dead. These circumstances include organ procurement, supporting the patient until the family arrives, and maintaining a brain-dead pregnant woman in an attempt to deliver a viable baby. In all cases of brain death, the physician must remain sensitive to the emotions of the family and should counsel and support them.

Brain death is a clinical diagnosis. The following criteria may be useful in determining brain death in adult patients: (1) absent cortical function as manifested by a patient in a coma who has no spontaneous movement, no response to verbal commands, no response to deep pain, and no seizures; (2) absent brain stem function as manifested by the absence of pupillary, corneal, oculocephalic (doll's eyes), and oculovestibular (ice-water calorics) reflexes and a "negative" apnea test (i.e., absent respiratory effort, hypercarbia, and acidosis in the oxygenated patient who has been taken off the ventilator for 5 to 10 minutes); (3) either the cause of coma is known (e.g., head trauma) and precludes improvement in brain function, or a sufficient period of observation has passed to permit solid prognostication; and (4) other conditions that may be confused with brain death, such as drug intoxications, other metabolic problems, and hypothermia, have been excluded.

The principal clinical justification for using the brain-death standard is futility: no treatment can reverse the pathophysiologic damage in brain-dead patients. Moreover, at least 45 states have laws or judicial opinions recognizing the brain-death standard, and physicians should be familiar with the law in their own state. The specific clinical procedures for determining brain death are generally not prescribed by law. Often, institutional policies outline local guidelines such as those listed above. These policies may also suggest a variety of confirmatory procedures including two or more separate observers, consultation with a neurologist or neurosurgeon, two separate examinations 6 to 12 hours apart, and supplementary tests including an electroencephalogram or cerebral blood flow studies. Most policies suggest that the declaration of death be made by physicians who are not involved in the potential transplantation of the organs of the deceased and who have no other economic or legal conflicts of interest.

ADVANCE DIRECTIVES

Advance directives permit patients to project their wishes regarding LST onto a future situation when they have become incompetent. Therefore, advance directives reduce the vagaries of clinical decision making for incompetent patients who cannot tell the physician at the time what medical care they want. There are two types of advance directives: instruction directives and proxy directives.

Instruction Directives

In an instruction directive, such as a "living will," the now incompetent patient, while still competent, has recorded his or her preferences regarding LST so that these wishes can guide medical care if and when the patient becomes incompetent. The instruction directive focuses on what treatments the patient would want if he or she were unable to participate in decision making in the future. The advantage is that the patient's preferences for withholding and withdrawing care are explicitly stated in the instruction directive. The disadvantage is that these stated preferences may not apply to the patient's actual clinical situation. Written directives have been legally formalized as so-called living wills. Since the first living will law was enacted in California in 1977, 40 states and the District of Columbia have passed legislation, and several other states have had court decisions giving legal force to living wills.

Living wills have been endorsed by many groups, including the President's Commission for the Study of Ethical Problems in Medicine and Biomedical and Behavioral Research. A recent survey showed that almost 80 percent of physicians expressed a positive attitude toward advance directives. Moreover, 67 percent of United States hospitals have institutional policies about advance directives. And, most important, surveys support the concept that the majority of patients welcome advance discussions about elective use of LSTs.

Despite this broad support, living wills have not fulfilled their promise of projecting competent patients' wishes into future clinical circumstances. One survey indicated that only 15 percent of Americans have executed a living will. In our opinion, two main barriers have limited the widespread use of advance directives, including the living will. First, the advance directives themselves are difficult to apply to actual clinical situations that the patient may not have anticipated. Second,most physicians have not been taught how and when to use advance directives.

Advance directives are often too vague to apply to specific clinical situations. They are vague about prognosis; for example, the wording in many living wills requests cessation of treatment when "there is no reasonable expectation of . . . recovery from extreme physical or mental disability." They are also vague about which treatments should be stopped (referring to these as "artificial means" or "life-prolonging procedures"). To address this problem, Emanuel and Emanuel have recently proposed a new advance directive known as the "Medical Directive." A major conceptual advance in medical ethics research, the Medical Directive describes four clinical scenarios, including terminal illness and irreversible coma. For each scenario, the patient is asked whether he or she would want each of 12 specific medical treatments, including cardiopulmonary resuscitation, mechanical ventilation, dialysis, and tube feeding. The patient may request or refuse each treatment, remain undecided, or request a time-limited therapeutic trial. Researchers are currently studying the reliability and validity of the Medical Directive.

In addition to the methodologic problems of designing a more reliable, valid, and clinically sensible advance directive, physicians also face an important public education challenge. Physicians must learn to discuss the elective use of LSTs with patients and to elicit patients' wishes about LST. Physicians should be taught during medical school, postgraduate training, and continuing education how and when to discuss with patients their wishes for end-of-life care. Health care facilities might choose to develop policies of "routine inquiry" regarding elective use of LST, either for all patients or for patients with certain clinical conditions. As a last resort, physician reimbursement incentives might be used to promote greater discussion of advance directives by doctors and patients.

Proxy Directives

In a proxy directive, a now incompetent patient has appointed, while still competent, another person to make health-care decisions on his or her behalf. The focus here is not on the specific details of the decision but rather on having the patient appoint an agent whom he or she trusts to represent his or her values. The advantage of the proxy directive is that decisions about the use of LSTs can be based on the actual clinical circumstances, since a competent decision maker (i.e., the proxy) is at hand. The disadvantage is that although the patient chose the proxy to represent his or her wishes, the proxy's decision on behalf of the patient in a specific clinical situation may not reflect what the patient would choose if he or she were competent. Proxy directives have been legally formalized as "durable powers of attorney for health care." Seventeen states have laws or judicial opinions recognizing the authority of such durable powers of attorney for health care. A formal durable power of attorney has proved particularly valuable in the context of acquired immunodeficiency syndrome in which patients prefer to appoint their friends, rather than their families, as proxy decision makers.

ASSESSMENT OF COMPETENCY

In current clinical practice, advance directives are usually not available. In these situations, when decisions arise about using or forgoing LST, the physician's first task is to determine whether the patient is competent to make decisions for him- or herself. The assessment of competency plays a pivotal role in patient management. Respect for the ethical and legal rights of patients means that physicians accede to the requests of competent patients to forgo treatment, even if it results in the patient's death. On the other hand, physicians may overrule requests to forgo treatment made by incompetent patients because they do not want such patients to suffer serious harm not intended by the patient if he or she were competent. Whether a physician finds a patient competent or incompetent often determines whether or not the doctor accepts the patient's stated wishes about LST or takes steps to override the decision. With so much at stake, it would be desirable to have well-developed clinical standards for the determination of competency. Unfortunately, at present, there are no clearly stipulated criteria for the determination of competency at the bedside.

The President's Commission for the Study of Ethical Problems in Medicine and Biomedical and Behavioral Research has identified three elements of competency: possession of a set of values and goals, the ability to communicate and understand information, and the ability to reason and deliberate about one's choices. The Commission also noted that competency was specific to "the person's actual functioning in situations in which a decision about health care was to be made." In other words, whether the physician acts on a patient's request to stop LST should not depend primarily on whether the patient is oriented to time, place, and person but rather on whether the patient understands that he or she will die without LST. More recently, Appelbaum and Grisso have suggested that the competent patient should be able to communicate choices, understand relevant information, appreciate the situation and its consequences, and manipulate information rationally. An effective clinical index of patient competency to decide about LST, however, would require a listing of specific questions for the physician to ask the patient, clearly stipulated criteria for the appraisal of patient responses, and a mechanism for combining the responses on individual questions into an overall assessment. Until such an index has been developed and evaluated, physicians must continue to rely on ad hoc assessments of competency.

At the extremes, doctors can usually establish whether a patient is competent or incompetent. Moreover, the clinician can sometimes restore patients to a state of competency by treating reversible causes of cognitive dysfunction, including a wide range of metabolic encephalopathies or psychoactive drug use. If uncertainty remains about the patient's competency, we recommend consultation with colleagues. Appropriate consultants include psychiatrists, neurologists, institutional ethics committees, ethics consultation services, or hospital attorneys. At present, it is unclear which of these groups is the preferred consultant, and this may vary in different clinical cases and institutional settings. In controversial cases, judicial review may be indicated. After physicians have determined whether the patient is competent or incompetent, patient management proceeds as described below.

DECISION MAKING WITH COMPETENT PATIENTS

Patients who are competent should be permitted to make their own health care decisions, including the decision to forgo life-sustaining medical treatments. This does not mean that the physician must casually accept the patient's treatment refusal without further discussion. The physician should enter into a dialogue with the patient to ensure that the patient's desire to stop treatment is an authentic reflection of his or her wishes and goals. Further, the physician should try to persuade the patient to pursue a medically reasonable course of treatment. If, after such discussion, the patient remains adamant in refusing treatment, the physician should respect the competent patient's wish and accede to the request to forgo treatment. If conflicts arise, consultation with the institutional ethics committee or even judicial referral may be advisable, but it is preferable to resolve such cases without recourse to a court. If a physician is unable to carry out a competent patient's request to forgo LST on the grounds of the physician's personal conscientious standards, the physician may withdraw from the case after ensuring that another source of care is available to the patient.

SURROGATE DECISION MAKING FOR INCOMPETENT PATIENTS

If the patient is incompetent, the physician should search for reversible causes of cognitive dysfunction. Sometimes, the correction of electrolyte disturbances, acidemia, hypoxemia, uremia, or other metabolic, infectious, or structural causes will restore the patient's competency and allow the patient to speak for him- or herself. Frequently, drugs such as analgesics or sedatives may be the cause of the patient's incompetence.

Incompetent patients whose competency cannot be restored present a troubling ethical problem. This group includes both permanently unconscious patients and patients who are conscious but have severe and irreversible cognitive impairments (such as Alzheimer's disease, congenital mental retardation, or anoxic encephalopathy). Because incompetent patients cannot speak for themselves, courts and legislatures since the 1976 Quinlan decision have developed an approach to end-of-life decisions that allows other parties (surrogates) to make decisions for the incompetent person. The underlying philosophic and legal assumption that permits surrogate decision making is that incompetent patients have the same autonomy claims and right of self-determination (for example, in the refusal of treatment) that competent patients possess. This philosophic and legal fiction views the incompetent person as an autonomous competent decision maker and requires that the surrogate make choices that are in accord with the choices that the now incompetent individual would make if he or she were competent.

In practice, surrogate decision making raises two key questions: who should decide on behalf of the incompetent patient, and on what basis should the decision be made? In addressing these questions, it is important to remember that the goal of surrogate decision making is to project the incompetent patient's wishes onto the current clinical situation.

Who Should Decide?

The best surrogate decision maker is someone identified and trusted by the patient to represent the patient's own wishes. It is the responsibility of the physician to find out whether the patient has appointed such a surrogate. The patient may have done so formally using a durable power of attorney for health care, as discussed previously. In the absence of a formally executed legal document, the physician should still attempt to discover whether the patient had previously designated a surrogate. This may have been done through written or oral statements. Although such surrogates may not have the legal status of a durable power of attorney, they may still have an ethically acceptable standing allowing them to participate in decisions.

In many cases, the patient has not designated a surrogate decision maker. Nonetheless, the physician should attempt to identify a surrogate for the patient, since this can simplify further clinical decision making. The physician may ask the family to identify a surrogate. Alternatively, the physician may try to identify the family member with the closest emotional connection to the patient. Evidence of a close relationship might include frequency of contact, the types of issues the patient discussed with the potential surrogate, and the apparent concern expressed by the potential surrogate about the patients' condition in the hospital. Usually, the surrogate decision maker is the spouse, close relative, or friend of the patient. Several states have enacted laws recognizing the decisional authority of family surrogate decision makers even in the absence of a durable power of attorney.

The patient with no readily identifiable surrogate decision maker presents a particularly difficult clinical management problem. Sometimes an independent physician, such as the department chairman or hospital chief of staff, serves as the surrogate for such patients. Sometimes these cases are referred for judicial review, and the court appoints a surrogate decision maker (known as a guardian ad litem). All too often, no surrogate is appointed and LST is continued, sometimes well beyond the point of benefiting the patient, simply because there is no one to authorize the withholding or withdrawing of LST. There is no consensus on how to manage these difficult cases. Health care facilities should address this situation prospectively through institutional policies. Moreover, it may be desirable to refer such cases to the institutional ethics committee or ethics consultation service.

Another clinically challenging situation occurs when family members disagree about decisions to forgo LST. Some family members may want treatment stopped, whereas others want it continued. In practice, treatment is usually continued in these situations pending the resolution of intrafamily conflicts. When such conflicts arise, ethics committees and consultants may provide an effective, extrajudicial mechanism for mediation. If the "ethical impasse" persists, judicial referral may be necessary.

On What Basis Should the Decision Be Made?

Once a surrogate decision maker has been identified, a second question arises: On what grounds should the surrogate reach a decision? Again, the physician should remember that the goal of surrogate decision making is to project the incompetent patient's wishes onto the current clinical situation. Thus, whenever possible, the surrogate should follow the incompetent patient's general wishes about LST. The practical question becomes: With what level of certainty are the incompetent patient's wishes known? In the absence of explicit written or oral prior wishes, two main standards for surrogate decision making have been developed: substituted judgment and best interests.

Substituted Judgment

With substituted judgment, the surrogate applies the patient's preferences and values to his or her actual clinical situation. The goal of substituted judgment is "to reach the decision that the incapacitated person would make if he or she were able to choose." A fundamental issue in cases that rely on substituted judgment is the quality of information and the surrogate's certainty about the patient's prior wishes.

Two evidentiary standards have evolved. The more stringent one is the "clear and convincing" standard, which requires proof "that the patient held a firm and settled commitment to the termination of life supports under circumstances like those presented." This standard of evidence regarding prior wishes is currently required in New York state to forgo LSTs in incompetent patients. In other states, courts have held incompetent patients and their surrogates to a more lenient standard of evidence about prior wishes, the "trustworthy" standard. Clinicians should consult with legal colleagues about the standards of evidence required in their own state. More important, clinicians should ask the family and close friends of an incompetent patient for specific expressions of the patient's prior wishes. These details represent an important part of the incompetent patient's medical history, and they should be documented in the medical record.

A weakness of the substituted judgment approach is highlighted by recent empirical data that show low rates of agreement between patients and their likely surrogates regarding resuscitation and other end-of-life decisions. Such data raise troubling questions about the adequacy of the substituted judgment approach and should provide impetus for the broader use of advance directives.

Best Interests

When there is no available information about an incompetent patient's prior wishes, physicians and courts have relied on "best interests." This approach is used for patients who have never been competent (such as an adult with severe, congenital mental retardation), for patients who were previously competent but never discussed their wishes regarding end-of-life care, and for patients with no known family or friends. The best interests approach involves a balancing of benefits and burdens: the surrogate chooses as a reasonable person in the patient's circumstance would choose. It requires a set of "objective, societally shared criteria" to rank burdens and benefits.

The problem with the best interests approach is that it requires societal consensus on burdens and benefits. In a pluralistic society, such a consensus is difficult to achieve. The best interests approach requires one person to judge the quality of life of another, opening the door to discrimination against those with disabilities. There is empirical evidence that third parties undervalue the quality of life of chronically ill patients relative to the value these patients place on their own quality of life. The potential for discrimination on the basis of third-party quality-of-life judgments is a serious limitation of the best interests approach.

As a practical matter, the best interests approach may be the only approach available to effectuate the right to refuse treatment of those patients whose prior wishes are unknown. In recent years, a consensus has begun to emerge, based on the best interests standard, that life-sustaining treatment may be withdrawn from patients who are permanently unconscious or in the persistent vegetative state. Health care facilities should develop policies to address the elective use of LSTs in those patients whose prior wishes are unknown. Moreover, clinicians should be encouraged to consult with ethics committees or ethics consultation services about these difficult cases.

THE FUTURE

In the 1990s, several powerful forces will shape policy about decisions to forgo LST. The United States Supreme Court recently issued its opinion in the case of Nancy Cruzan. This landmark case involved a 31-year-old woman in the persistent vegetative state whose family asked the Court to permit the withdrawal of tube feeding. The Court ruled that the state may preserve the life of a comatose patient unless there is "clear and convincing" evidence of the patient's wish to die under such circumstances. As the first "right to die" case involving an adult patient to reach the United States Supreme Court, the Cruzan decision will have important implications for policy.

Attempts to limit the spiraling costs of health care may also influence policies regarding LST. In 1990, the United States will spend about $661 billion on health care, almost 12 percent of its gross national product. An earlier study in the Medicare population showed that almost 30 percent of annual spending flows to the 6 percent of enrollees who die during the year. Physicians can expect cost containment policies aimed to reduce this "high cost of dying." Faced with these policies, the clinical-ethical challenge for physicians will be to maintain their fiduciary commitment to the patient's good.

We believe, however, that enduring solutions to the problems posed by decisions to forgo LST must come from within the profession. Fundamental clinical research challenges remain, for example, the design and evaluation of an index of patient competency or of a clinically sensible advance directive. Despite the immense political, social, and economic importance of clinical policies to guide decisions to forgo LST, this research has not been a high priority for traditional biomedical granting agencies. Moreover, professional education about decisions to forgo LST has been inadequate. We hope that in the 1990s, the medical profession will rise to meet these basic research and educational challenges, before external solutions are imposed by bureaucrats, administrators, and regulators.

SUGGESTED READING

American College of Physicians Ethics Manual. 2nd ed. Part 2: The physician and society; research; life-sustaining treatments; other issues. Ann Intern Med 1989; 111:327–335.

Appelbaum PS, Grisso T. Assessing patients' capacities to consent to treatment. N Engl J Med 1988; 319:1635–1638.

Emanuel LL, Emanuel EJ. The Medical Directive: A new comprehensive advance care document. JAMA 1989; 261:3288–3293.

The Hastings Center. Guidelines on the termination of life-sustaining treatment and the care of the dying. Briarcliff Manor, NY: Hastings Center, 1987.

Jonsen AR, Siegler M, Winslade WJ. Clinical ethics: A practical approach to ethical decisions in clinical medicine. 3rd ed. New York: Macmillan, 1990.

Miles SH, Gomez CF. Protocols for elective use of life-sustaining treatments. New York: Springer, 1989.

Miles SH, Singer PA, Siegler M. Conflicts between patients' wishes to forgo treatment and the policies of health care facilities. N Engl J Med 1989; 321:48–50.

President's Commission for the Study of Ethical Problems in Medicine and Biomedical and Behavioral Research. Deciding to forgo life-sustaining treatment: Ethical, medical, and legal issues in treatment decisions. Washington, DC: US Government Printing Office, 1983.

THE ACQUIRED IMMUNODEFICIENCY SYNDROME

INTRODUCTION

JAMES T. NOBLE, M.D.

Nine years ago, in June of 1981, five cases of *Pneumocystis carinii* pneumonia in ostensibly healthy young men from California were reported to the United States Public Health Service. In the subsequent 2 years, the major clinical and epidemiologic features of the acquired immunodeficiency syndrome (AIDS) were defined through standardized case reporting in a national surveillance system established by the Centers for Disease Control.

The surveillance definition of AIDS, originally elaborated in 1982, included various infections and malignancies, definitively diagnosed, which were characteristically seen in patients with severe cellular immunodeficiency. The discovery of the causative agent of AIDS in 1984 (the human immunodeficiency virus, HIV) led to modifications of the surveillance definition in 1985 and again in 1987 to incorporate other severe morbidity associated with HIV infection. Active surveillance for AIDS in the United States has led to the reporting of approximately 130,000 cases through May, 1990. It is believed that at least several hundred thousand cases of AIDS exist worldwide at the beginning of the decade of the 1990s.

It is now clear, however, that AIDS represents the end stage of a chronic, progressive viral disease that may be present for 10 or more years prior to the development of its terminal stage. Transmitted by sexual intercourse and by exchange of blood or blood products, HIV infection has spread worldwide and affects millions of individuals. In contrast to the clinical manifestations of AIDS, which are reportable in all 50 states and in most countries, HIV infection is not nationally reportable in most countries, including the United States. As a result, the size of the HIV-infected population nationally and worldwide is the subject of much controversy and speculation. In 1986, the United States Public Health Service estimated that 1.0 to 1.5 million HIV infections were present in the United States. Most authorities now believe that this estimate was too high. Consensus values for HIV infections in the United States in 1990 range from 490,000 to 1,500,000, with wide deviations on the high and low sides, depending on the source of the estimate. Predictions about AIDS cases in the 1990s are of course dependent on a proper estimate of the number of existing and new HIV infections for that period.

Regardless of the actual number of cases of AIDS and HIV infection to be diagnosed in the next 10 years, it is clear that the epidemic in the 1990s will far exceed the experience of the 1980s. The demands on physicians and other health care providers to provide timely, effective, and compassionate care will increase accordingly. Results of recent clinical trials clearly indicate that early diagnosis and, in selected cases, early medical intervention can delay and perhaps prevent the development of end-stage HIV disease. Although the science of early anti-HIV intervention is in its infancy, efforts by physicians and requests by patients for early HIV diagnosis by anti-HIV antibody testing should and will increase in the near future.

In view of the foregoing, *Current Therapy in Internal Medicine* has decided to present material on AIDS and HIV disease in a separate section for the first time. Chapters in this year's edition present material on therapy of HIV infection, therapy of AIDS-associated infections, therapy of HIV-related Kaposi's sarcoma, and various organ system manifestations of HIV, including renal, gastrointestinal, neurologic, and cutaneous diseases. It is hoped that this section will serve as a ready reference for physicians who care for HIV-infected individuals at present or who will encounter HIV-infected patients in the future.

ANTIVIRAL THERAPY OF HUMAN IMMUNODEFICIENCY VIRUS INFECTION

PAUL R. SKOLNIK, M.D.
JAMES T. NOBLE, M.D.

Antiviral therapy has become an integral part of infectious disease practice. Acyclovir, ganciclovir, ribavirin, amantadine, and alpha-interferon are useful in the treatment of some herpes simplex viruses, cytomegalovirus, respiratory syncytial virus, influenza A virus, and papillomavirus infections, respectively. Recently, new antiviral agents directed against the human immunodeficiency virus (HIV), the etiologic agent of the acquired immunodeficiency syndrome (AIDS), have been developed (Table 1). One such agent, zidovudine (3′-azido-3′-deoxythymidine or azidothymidine [AZT]), has been licensed by the Food and Drug Administration (FDA) for treatment of patients with certain manifestations of HIV infection. The clinical indications for the use of zidovudine and other antiviral agents with activity against HIV are changing rapidly as new information becomes available. In this chapter, we outline conservative recommendations concerning antiviral therapy of HIV-infected individuals, with the realization that therapeutic recommendations will undoubtedly change as new data become available.

GENERAL CONSIDERATIONS

HIV infection can cause a number of clinical syndromes. It is important to keep these disease categories in mind when planning antiviral therapy. Studies that show effectiveness of a drug during one stage of infection do not necessarily indicate that the drug is useful in another stage of disease. Several systems have been devised to classify the various clinical syndromes associated with HIV infection. These include the Centers for Disease Control classification system (Table 2) and the Walter Reed staging system. The Centers for Disease Control system is a descriptive one, whereas the Walter Reed staging system attempts to include clinical and laboratory parameters that are thought to indicate the relative degree of immunodeficiency.

Clinical staging of disease (and the associated risk of opportunistic infection or disease progression) is a major focus of recent research. Most often used in this connection are absolute CD4 cell number, percentage of CD4 cells in relation to total T-cell count, HIV-1 p24 antigenemia (present in approximately 25 to 45 percent of HIV-infected individuals), and serum beta$_2$-microglobulin and neopterin levels. Recently, quantitative plasma virus cultures have been found to correlate with disease progression and response to therapy with zidovudine. A more detailed understanding of these laboratory correlates of disease progression will help in the design of future drug trials and therapeutic interventions in HIV-infected individuals.

ADVANCED HIV DISEASE

Zidovudine, a nucleoside analogue that inhibits the reverse transcriptase enzyme of HIV, increases survival and decreases the incidence of opportunistic infections in patients with AIDS and a history of *Pneumocystis carinii* pneumonia or AIDS-related complex with fewer than 200 CD4 cells. The dosage used in initial studies was 200 mg by mouth every 4 hours. Beneficial results were obtained at the expense of substantial toxicity; specifically, a macrocytic anemia was common and required ongoing

TABLE 1 Selected Antiviral Agents Under Study for HIV Infection

Proposed Mechanism of Action	*Compound*	*Testing Phase**
Inhibition of binding of HIV to susceptible cells	Soluble CD4	1/2
	CD4-antibody chimeras	Preclinical
	Peptide T	1/2
Inhibition of reverse transcriptase	ddC	Phase 2/3
	ddI	Phase 2/3
	Zidovudine	Phase 2/3/4
	Foscarnet	Phase 1/2
Inhibition of viral protease	Protease inhibitors	Preclinical
Inhibition of viral regulatory proteins	?†	?
Inhibition of viral integrase enzyme	?	?
Inhibition of assembly and/or release	α-Interferon	Phase 1/2
Inhibition of glycosylation	Castanospermine	Phase 1
	Deoxynojirimycin	Phase 1

*As of December 1989.
†? = Active research efforts ongoing.

TABLE 2 Centers for Disease Control Classification System for HIV Infection

Group I	Acute infection
Group II	Asymptomatic infection
Group III	Persistent generalized lymphadenopathy
Group IV	Other disease
Subgroup A	Constitutional disease
Subgroup B	Neurologic diseases
Subgroup C	Secondary infectious diseases
Category C-1	Specified secondary infectious diseases listed in the Centers for Disease Control surveillance definition for AIDS
Category C-2	Other specified secondary infectious diseases
Subgroup D	Secondary cancers
Subgroup E	Other conditions

transfusion in some patients. Adjunctive therapy with human recombinant erythropoietin is being investigated at present to help ameliorate this toxicity. Preliminary data suggest it is most useful in patients with low serum erythropoietin levels. Other growth factors that augment leukocyte production are under active investigation. Granulocyte-macrophage colony stimulating factor may be useful in reducing zidovudine-induced neutropenia. Recently, the FDA has approved a lower dosage of zidovudine for therapy of HIV-infected individuals. These new recommendations are based on as yet unpublished data comparing high (250 mg every 4 hours) and low (100 mg every 4 hours) doses of zidovudine in patients who had recovered from a single episode of *Pneumocystis carinii* pneumonia. Survival rates and frequency of opportunistic infections were similar in the two groups; however, the lower dosage resulted in less hematologic toxicity than the higher dose. Based mostly on theoretical considerations, 1 month of "induction" therapy with zidovudine at 200 mg every 4 hours is recommended, followed by chronic administration of 100 mg every 4 hours. The efficacy of this regimen in most patient groups, especially patients experiencing neurologic dysfunction secondary to HIV infection, is unknown.

Other antiviral agents used to treat HIV-infected individuals with advanced disease must still be considered investigational. Nonetheless, these therapies are often available to physicians and their patients through various mechanisms, including the National Institutes of Health–sponsored AIDS Clinical Trial Groups, pharmaceutical industry–sponsored drug trials, investigational new drug applications, or open label protocols. We therefore briefly review the most promising of these investigational antiviral agents; this list is not inclusive, and additional agents are being developed rapidly.

Nucleoside analogues other than zidovudine have activity against HIV. These include dideoxycytidine (ddC) and dideoxyinosine (ddI). Both of these antiviral agents are currently undergoing clinical testing in large, multicenter trials in the United States. Preliminary results from phase 1 trials to determine appropriate dosing indicate that some surrogate markers of antiretroviral activity are favorably influenced by these agents. Significantly, the toxicities of these two agents do not overlap with those of zidovudine. ddC is associated with rash and peripheral neuropathy (seen especially with higher doses), whereas ddI can induce pancreatitis and peripheral neuropathy. It is important to emphasize that the efficacy of these two agents in any stage of HIV disease remains unproved.

Soluble, recombinant CD4 (srCD4) has been studied in phase 1 trials. The proposed mechanism of action of this agent is competitive blocking of attachment of the HIV gp120 envelope glycoprotein to the cellular CD4 receptor. Again, data about efficacy are not yet available from phase 2 or 3 studies. Toxicities of this agent seem to be minimal and include local pain at the injection site. It is significant that development of anti-CD4 antibodies does not seem to be a common phenomenon. The half-life of this agent is short, and newer recombinant molecules that more faithfully mimic the native CD4 molecule and are combined with other moieties that prolong the serum half-life are being developed.

Inhibitors of glycosylation of the HIV envelope glycoprotein are also in phase 1 studies. The purported mechanism of action of these agents involves alteration of the carbohydrate moieties associated with the HIV envelope glycoprotein. This presumably inhibits binding to the CD4 receptor or the formation of syncytia, which may cause CD4 cell death. Agents in this category include deoxynojirimycin and castanospermine. In vitro data indicate good activity of these agents against HIV-1.

Foscarnet is an antiviral agent with excellent activity against cytomegalovirus and herpes simplex virus; it is also active against HIV-1. This agent may prove useful for the treatment of cytomegalovirus retinitis, acyclovir-resistant strains of herpes simplex virus, and possibly HIV infection. This drug can be nephrotoxic; magnesium and phosphorus electrolyte disorders during therapy have been described. The lack of an oral formulation of foscarnet currently limits its clinical use.

Ribavirin has been in clinical testing for several years. Despite this, no clear evidence of effectiveness in HIV-infected individuals has been garnered. Other agents that have been tested but have not demonstrated effectiveness against HIV or have produced serious toxicity include suramin, HPA-23, ampligen, cyclosporine, and AL-721. Still other compounds show varying degrees of in vitro activity against HIV-1, but await well-designed clinical trials to determine clinical utility (e.g., peptide T and compound Q).

In evaluating all of these drugs, it has become clear that in vitro antiviral activity does not necessarily predict clinical effectiveness. It is also clear that although useful agents have been found that can prolong survival and decrease the incidence of opportunistic infections, no "magic bullet" is available for the treatment of HIV infection.

ASYMPTOMATIC INFECTION AND EARLY AIDS-RELATED COMPLEX

Recent data gathered by the AIDS Clinical Trial Groups indicate that zidovudine may be useful for the treatment of HIV-1-infected individuals who are either asymptomatic or have early symptoms of AIDS-related complex (ARC). These symptoms include one or two mild manifestations of HIV infection such as oral candidiasis, fever, diarrhea, or weight loss. Therapy of the asymptomatic patients utilized a dose of 500 mg each day of zidovudine; the patients with early ARC symptoms were treated with 1,200 mg of zidovudine each day. In the United States, portions of these protocols were stopped when it was found that individuals with less than 500 CD4 cells had a decreased number of opportunistic infections when treated with zidovudine in comparison with those who received placebo. New recommendations therefore include consideration of treatment of asymptomatic and early ARC patients with less than 500 CD4 cells with either 500 or 1,200 mg each day of zidovudine, respectively. It is interesting to note that a joint European and French study and a Veterans Administration study of similar patient populations are continuing after review of the AIDS Clinical Trial Group data. Additional data concerning survival, long-term drug toxicity, and the emergence of drug-resistant mutants of HIV-1 may be available from these studies. In this regard, drug-resistant mutants of HIV-1 have been isolated from individuals treated with zidovudine for prolonged periods of time. This is not surprising in light of our experience with other antiviral agents. Although antiviral therapy may be advisable early in the course of HIV infection, it remains possible that reserving antiviral therapy for later stages of infection, treatment with other antiviral agents, or combination therapy with several antiviral agents may prove superior to zidovudine therapy. At this time, most clinicians in the United States would recommend treating asymptomatic or early ARC patients (those with less than 500 CD4 cells) with zidovudine based on the data supplied so far by the National Institutes of Allergy and Infectious Diseases.

The use of other antiviral agents in these two patient populations has not been rigorously studied. Presumably, trials with the nucleoside analogues ddC and ddI as well as other antiviral agents will eventually be carried out in these two groups.

PROPHYLAXIS OF HIV INFECTION

Interest in prophylactic antiviral therapy of individuals potentially exposed to HIV has received attention, especially in relation to the occurrence of needlestick injuries in health care workers. An attempt to study zidovudine in this situation in a placebo-controlled trial has been stopped. The logistic problems of recruiting a sufficient number of individuals into this trial in light of the low incidence of transmission of HIV infection via needlestick precluded the possibility of finishing the study in a reasonable amount of time. However, based on animal studies showing the effectiveness of zidovudine if administered early after challenge with retrovirus, some clinicians recommend treating individuals with known needlestick injuries from HIV-1-contaminated sources with zidovudine for 6 to 8 weeks. It should be emphasized that the efficacy of prophylactic therapy and the short- and long-term toxicities of this agent have not been defined.

THERAPY OF OTHER HIV-RELATED DISORDERS

When caring for patients with other HIV-related disorders, such as primary (acute) infection, HIV dementia, HIV wasting syndrome, HIV-associated enteropathy, HIV-associated thrombocytopenia, peripheral neuropathy, pediatric infection, HIV-infected pregnant women, or other rarer manifestations of HIV disease, the clinician must make treatment decisions based on very scant data. The Food and Drug Administration has recently approved the use of zidovudine in HIV-infected children over 3 months of age who have HIV-related symptoms or who are asymptomatic with laboratory studies indicating HIV-related immunosuppression. These recommendations were based on two open-label studies of zidovudine therapy in children with symptomatic HIV-related illness. HIV-related thrombocytopenia seems to respond to a number of modalities, including immunoglobulin therapy, splenectomy, and treatment with zidovudine. The decision as to whether treatment is warranted must be based on both the severity of the thrombocytopenia and the toxicities and morbidity associated with these various agents and procedures. It is hoped that further clinical investigation may result in more rational use of antiviral agents in these situations.

TABLE 3 Current Recommendations for Zidovudine Therapy of HIV Infection in Adults (as of January 1990)

*Stage of Infection**	*Therapy*	*Comments*
Acute exposure (e.g., needlestick injury)	100–200 mg q4h × 4–6 wk	Recommendation based entirely on animal data; consider type of exposure and as yet unknown toxicities of therapy
Group I (primary infection)	Investigational therapy†	Self-limited illness; clinical data unavailable
Group II (asymptomatic)		
<500 CD4 cells	100 mg 5 ×/day	AIDS Clinical Trial Groups protocol terminated; other trials continue to determine survival data and long-term toxicities
>500 CD4 cells	Investigational therapy	Clinical trials continue
Group III.	Investigational therapy	Clinical trials continue
Group IV, subgroup A		
<500 CD4 cells	200 mg q4h × 4 wk, then 100 mg q4h	AIDS Clinical Trial Groups protocol terminated; other trials continue to determine survival data and long-term toxicities
>500 CD4 cells	Investigational therapy	Clinical trials continue
Group IV, subgroup B	Investigational therapy	Clinical trials continue
Group IV, subgroup C	200 mg q4h × 4 wk, then 100 mg q4h	Studies to determine optimal dosing regimens ongoing
Group IV, subgroup D	100–200 mg q4h	Can be combined with α-interferon or other chemotherapeutic agents
Group IV, subgroup E	Investigational therapy	Therapy may be valuable for HIV-related thrombocytopenia in selected cases Additional trials in other conditions are ongoing

*Patient selection criteria for the trials on which the recommendations in this table are based frequently do not conform precisely to the Centers for Disease Control classification system; therefore, please see the text (and primary references) for more detailed descriptions of the patient populations that have been studied.

†For all stages of infection (and especially when no proven efficacious therapy exists), consider entry of the patient in a randomized, controlled trial of antiviral theapy.

COMBINATION ANTIVIRAL THERAPY FOR HIV INFECTION

It is likely that combination antiviral therapy for HIV infection will be important in the future care of these patients. This therapy may either alternate antiviral agents or administer them concurrently. Clinical trials are ongoing with zidovudine in combination with acyclovir and ddC. Phase 1 trials with combination zidovudine and ddI are also planned. In addition, antiviral therapy combined with various immunomodulators (e.g., granulocyte-macrophage colony stimulating factor, human recombinant erythropoietin, and interleukin-2) are under way. It is hoped that the results of these studies will allow the rational introduction of combination therapy into clinical practice.

FUTURE TRENDS

Zidovudine therapy may be limited by its known bone marrow toxicity and the recent discovery of drug-resistant variants of HIV-1. Selective use of zidovudine, as outlined above, would therefore appear to be reasonable at this time (Table 3). HIV-infected individuals with other manifestations of disease should be enrolled in well-designed clinical trials. It is hoped that this will allow for the rational development of effective antiviral therapy to benefit all individuals infected with HIV-1. Access to investigational antiviral agents for HIV-infected individuals is being expanded (from that available through the AIDS Clinical Trial Groups and drug company–sponsored protocols) via the so-called parallel track. It is hoped that this greater availability will nonetheless allow for the collection of useful information to assess adequately both the efficacy and the toxicity of the newer antiviral agents. In addition, education to promote behavioral changes and further research on vaccine development and passive immunization may help prevent the transmission of HIV and obviate the need for subsequent antiviral therapy. Current recommendations for antiviral therapy of HIV-infected individuals will undoubtedly change rapidly as new information is accrued. Up-to-date listings of antiviral clinical trials for HIV-infected individuals can be obtained through the National Institutes of Health AIDS Hotline (1-800-TRIALS-A) and the American Foundation for AIDS Research (1515 Broadway, Suite 3601, New York, NY 10036).

SUGGESTED READING

Broder S. Controlled trial methodology and progress in treatment of the acquired immunodeficiency syndrome (AIDS). Ann Intern Med 1989; 110:417–418.

Fischl MA, Richman DD, Causey DM, et al. Prolonged zidovudine therapy in patients with AIDS and advanced AIDS-related complex. JAMA 1989; 262:2405-2410.
Fischl MA, Richman DD, Grieco MH, et al. The efficacy of azidothymidine (AZT) in the treatment of patients with AIDS and AIDS-related complex. N Engl J Med 1987; 371:185-191.
Hirsch MS. Antiviral drug development for the treatment of human immunodeficiency virus infections. Am J Med 1988; 85(Suppl 2A):182-185.
Hirsch MS. The rocky road to effective treatment of human immunodeficiency virus (HIV) infection. Ann Intern Med 1989; 110:1-3.
Hirsch MS, Schooley RT. Resistance to antiviral drugs: The end of innocence. N Engl J Med 1989; 320:313-314.
Yarchoan R, Mitsuya H, Broder S. Clinical and basic advances in the antiretroviral therapy of human immunodeficiency virus infection. Am J Med 1989; 87:191-200.

THERAPY OF AIDS-RELATED OPPORTUNISTIC INFECTIONS

JAMES T. NOBLE, M.D.

Since the initial report of an unusual cluster of cases of *Pneumocystis carinii* pneumonia in 1981, infections associated with cellular immunodeficiency (opportunistic infections) have been the hallmark of the acquired immunodeficiency syndrome (AIDS). Despite revisions to the case definition in 1987 and the increasing recognition of noninfectious complications of human immunodeficiency virus (HIV) infection and pathology caused directly by HIV, opportunistic infections continue to account for the vast majority of diagnosed AIDS cases. In addition, the occurrence of major opportunistic infections continues to represent a strong indicator of poor prognosis in HIV disease.

Somewhat surprisingly, in view of the profound and global nature of severe HIV-induced immune deficiency, five major pathogens account for most AIDS-defining infectious disease. In addition to *Pneumocystis carinii*, they are *Toxoplasma gondii*, *Cryptococcus neoformans*, cytomegalovirus, and *Mycobacterium avium-intracellulare*. These organisms are all pathogens for which an intact T-helper cell network is required for host defense. Therapies for these pathogens are undergoing rapid changes as experience is accumulated and clinical trials are carried out. The current state of diagnosis and therapy of the major opportunistic infections is the subject of this chapter.

PNEUMOCYSTIS CARINII PNEUMONIA

Pneumonia caused by *Pneumocystis carinii* was the first opportunistic infection described in AIDS. It is still the most common and remains responsible for the largest number of AIDS-related deaths. It was the presenting infection in 53 percent of the AIDS cases diagnosed in 1989, and approximately 85 percent of persons with AIDS experience at least one episode.

As of December 31, 1989, approximately 70,000 cases of AIDS-related *Pneumocystis carinii* pneumonia (PCP) had been reported in the United States. The pneumonia typically manifests with fever, hypoxemia, and dyspnea, and the diagnosis is readily confirmed by identification of cysts in induced sputum, bronchoalveolar lavage fluid, or tissue specimen obtained by lung biopsy. In a patient who is known to be infected with HIV or who is a member of a traditional AIDS "risk group," the clinical index of suspicion in the presence of the above symptoms is usually high. However, when a patient whose HIV infection has not been previously diagnosed or who is not a member of a traditional "risk group" presents with symptoms of pneumocystosis, the diagnosis may be delayed. Chest radiographic findings of typical bilateral interstitial infiltrates usually suggest the diagnosis in a symptomatic patient, but the x-ray study findings may be negative in early disease. When the radiologic findings are negative in the presence of compatible symptoms, radionuclide lung scanning with gallium-67 often reveals intense bilateral uptake, leading to confirmation of the diagnosis by examination of appropriate specimens.

Prior to the AIDS epidemic, most clinical experience with pneumocystosis occurred in patients with neoplastic disease. Successful therapy had been described with both trimethoprim-sulfamethoxazole and pentamidine, although the numbers of patients treated with these agents were not large. As a result of treatment of AIDS patients with these two drugs, extensive clinical experience has been accumulated. Both of these "standard" therapies are effective, but both have significant failure rates and significant toxicities. As a result, efforts are under way to develop new therapies for pneumocystosis; these will be reviewed.

Trimethoprim-Sulfamethoxazole

Trimethoprim-sulfamethoxazole (SXT) is considered by most authorities to be the initial treatment of choice for AIDS-associated PCP. A randomized, prospective study of SXT versus pentamidine demonstrated that the drugs were equally effective but that SXT was less toxic. When given intravenously or orally in a dose of 15 to 20 mg per kilogram per day of the trimethoprim component and continued for 14 to 21 days, SXT produces clinical responses in 80 percent of patients. The usefulness of SXT is limited, however, by its toxicity. Common adverse reactions to SXT in AIDS patients include fever, skin rash (which may result in severe, even fatal, exfoliative dermatitis), and neutropenia. Although treatment may be continued in the face of drug-related fever, significant rash and severe neutropenia are usually considered to be indications to interrupt therapy with SXT. The incidence of adverse reactions to SXT is greatly increased in persons with AIDS when compared with patients treated with SXT for other indications. As a result, up to 50 percent of AIDS patients initially treated with SXT for PCP may not be able to complete a full course of therapy.

Some published evidence suggests that lowering the daily dose from 20 mg per kilogram to 15 mg per kilogram reduces toxicity without sacrificing efficacy. Nevertheless, the use of alternative agents is often required for successful therapy of AIDS-associated PCP.

Pentamidine

Pentamidine was recognized as effective therapy for PCP since well before the AIDS epidemic. In fact, an increase in requests for pentamidine to the Parasitic Drug Service of the Centers for Disease Control was one of the first indications of the outbreak of AIDS-associated PCP in the United States. Pentamidine is given intravenously or intramuscularly in a single daily dose of 3 to 4 mg per kilogram and is also given for a total of 14 to 21 days. When pentamidine is given in substitution for SXT because of toxicity of the latter agent, the number of days that SXT has been given is usually included as part of the total course of treatment.

Pentamidine also has significant associated toxicity. The major toxicities of pentamidine are pancreatic islet cell injury (which may be manifest as hyperglycemia, hypoglycemia, or both), renal function abnormalities, and neutropenia. Patients who have experienced toxic reactions to SXT are not thought to be more likely to experience toxicity caused by pentamidine; however, the cumulative risk of toxicity in patients treated with both drugs is very high.

In addition to systemic therapy with pentamidine, investigators have used the drug by aerosol nebulizer to treat PCP. The drug, when delivered by aerosol spray, may achieve very high levels in alveolar lavage fluid when compared with levels achieved with systemic administration. Except in patients on mechanical ventilation, systemic drug levels are negligible when the drug is delivered by aerosol, which should result in decreased toxicity. Dysglycemia has been observed in several patients treated with aerosolized pentamidine, as has pancreatitis, and periodic monitoring is advisable. Pentamidine by aerosol can cure mild to moderate PCP. However, some evidence suggests that it is not as efficacious as systemic therapy for this indication. For this reason, it should be considered an alternative in patients who are refractory to or intolerant of systemic therapy. Clinical studies have been published in a limited number of patients, and further studies are in progress. The optimal dose of pentamidine given by this route for therapy of PCP is not known, but clinical studies have used up to 600 mg per day. Potential limitations of this form of therapy include treatment failure, lack of protection against extrapulmonary pneumocystosis, and pulmonary hemorrhage. The optimal aerosol particle size and type of nebulizer best suited to deliver this therapy are unknown at present. Pentamidine by aerosol is also being widely studied for the prevention of PCP, as discussed further on.

Alternative Therapies

Dapsone-Trimethoprim

Patients with mild PCP have been successfully treated with a regimen of dapsone and trimethoprim. This regimen shares with SXT the potential advantage of an entire course of therapy that can be administered by the oral route. A randomized trial of trimethoprim, 20 mg per kilogram per day in four divided doses, plus dapsone, 100 mg per day in a single dose, has demonstrated comparable efficacy to SXT without a notable increase in toxicity. Although dapsone is a sulfone, patients who are intolerant to SXT can usually tolerate trimethoprim plus dapsone, and patients who have failed to respond to SXT *and* pentamidine have been successfully treated with this combination. The major toxicities of dapsone are methemoglobinemia and anemia.

Trimetrexate

Trimetrexate is an investigational antifolate drug, originally developed for therapy of neoplastic disease. It is related to methotrexate and has been shown to have a much greater ability to inhibit the dihydrofolate reductase present in *Pneumocystis carinii* than does trimethoprim. Because of its potent antifolate activity, it must be given with folinic acid (leucovorin) to prevent hematologic toxicity.

In several studies, trimetrexate plus leucovorin has been shown to be effective for the therapy of PCP. It has produced clinical responses even in patients who have not responded to SXT or pentamidine. It has been noted, however, that patients who have been successfully treated with trimetrexate plus leucovorin tend to relapse earlier than those treated with conventional therapy, which may imply the need for longer courses of therapy than those used in studies to date. It is also noteworthy that studies using very high doses of leucovorin (160 mg per day) have demonstrated inferior results to those using lower doses. This may imply that high concentrations of leucovorin can protect *Pneumocystis carinii* from the inhibitory action of trimetrexate. Further clinical studies to define the proper place of trimetrexate plus leucovorin in the therapy of PCP are currently in progress.

Eflornithine (Difluoromethylornithine, DFMO)

This investigational drug irreversibly inhibits ornithine decarboxylase in several protozoal species, including *Pneumocystis carinii.* It has been successfully used at 400 mg per kilogram per day intravenously for 14 days, followed by 4 to 6 weeks of oral therapy at a reduced dose, for the salvage of patients whose disease is refractory to standard therapy. As would be expected in this patient population, responses to therapy were noted in fewer patients than in those treated with standard therapy, with the poorest prognosis seen in patients dependent on mechanical ventilation. Preliminary data appear to suggest that this drug is not as effective for salvage as trimetrexate, although comparative studies do not exist. The role of DFMO for less severely ill patients is not clear at the present time.

Primaquine/Clindamycin

The combination of primaquine and clindamycin has been found very active in an animal model of PCP. Several humans have been successfully treated with the combination, and further studies are planned.

Corticosteroids

In view of the similarity between fatal cases of PCP and the adult respiratory distress syndrome (ARDS) and the fact that autopsy material from patients dying of PCP often shows an intense pulmonary mononuclear cell infiltrate, many clinicians have attempted to treat severe PCP, in the presence of impending or actual respiratory failure, with short courses of corticosteroids. Two uncontrolled studies and abundant anecdotal experience suggest that steroids may be beneficial in patients with severe PCP and respiratory failure, at least in the first 7 to 10 days of illness. One popular regimen uses a loading dose of 1,000 mg of methylprednisolone, followed by 40 mg every 6 hours for 4 to 7 days. This use remains controversial, however, and concern about the potential for an increased incidence of other opportunistic infections following steroid therapy for PCP as well as nonimmunologic complications of steroid use makes controlled studies on the use of steroids for this indication an urgent necessity. Several small, randomized, prospective studies using steroids or placebo for patients with PCP who develop respiratory failure have not shown convincing evidence of benefit. Preliminary data from a randomized, prospective study that utilized steroids or placebo in combination with anti-PCP therapy from the first day (rather than in the presence of actual or impending respiratory failure) strongly suggested an improved outcome in steroid-treated patients. None of these studies have addressed the issue of long-term toxicity, particularly the potential for worsening of immune dysfunction, after the use of corticosteroids for PCP. The role of corticosteroid therapy in patients with PCP who are not responding to therapy remains controversial at the present time.

Prevention of PCP

It has been known for some time that PCP can be prevented in patients with neoplastic disease who are at high risk (e.g., children with leukemia) by the administration of SXT. Without preventive or antiviral therapy, PCP will recur after an initial episode in persons with AIDS 30 to 70 percent of the time, depending on overall length of survival after diagnosis.

SXT, given as two double-strength tablets daily, is effective in preventing recurrent PCP after a single episode in AIDS. It has also been shown to be effective in preventing initial episodes in patients with AIDS who have Kaposi's sarcoma and fewer than 200 T-helper cells per cubic millimeter. In view of this successful experience and the high morbidity and mortality still associated with AIDS-related PCP, the use of PCP prophylaxis in AIDS and HIV infection has become widespread, despite the lack of placebo-controlled studies demonstrating efficacy for primary prevention. The strong belief on the part of clinicians and patients alike in the efficacy of this therapy has now made it impossible to conduct placebo-controlled studies of this type of therapy.

The high incidence of adverse reactions to SXT, however, makes it suitable prophylaxis for only a minority of patients. Several alternatives are available, and some comparative studies are being performed. Dapsone in a dose of 50 to 100 mg per day probably has comparable efficacy to SXT and is better tolerated. The fixed combination of pyrimethamine/sulfadoxine (Fansidar), given as a single tablet weekly, has produced mixed results in several small series and is associated with a significant risk of life-threatening cutaneous reactions. A higher dose of Fansidar, given more frequently, might ameliorate these difficulties. Pentamidine by intermittent (weekly) intravenous administration is probably effective as well, but most clinical interest now centers on pentamidine by aerosol spray as an alternative to SXT.

Pentamidine has been administered by aerosol nebulizer in several uncontrolled studies for the prevention of PCP. Laboratory studies of nebulized therapy for other indications suggest that particle sizes of 1 to 2 microns are necessary for effective drug delivery to the alveoli. In studies of PCP prevention, multiple different doses and nebulizers producing different particle sizes have been used, making comparisons difficult. Nevertheless, most studies have shown relapse rates of less than 20 percent at 1 year, considerably less than historical controls. The obvious appeal of this type of therapy is the lack of systemic drug absorption and hence reduced toxicity. There is enormous medical and lay enthusiasm for this therapy, and it is not possible to perform placebo-controlled studies. The results of a large study involving over 350 patients and comparing several doses of pentamidine, all delivered by the Respirguard II nebulizer, have led to approval by the United States Food and Drug Administration of aerosolized pentamidine for prevention of PCP at a dose of 300 mg per month. It is currently recommended that patients with HIV infection and less than 200 T4 (helper) lymphocytes be treated with some form of prophylaxis for PCP.

TOXOPLASMIC ENCEPHALITIS

Toxoplasmic encephalitis (TE) is the most common cause of focal central nervous system infection in patients with AIDS. AIDS surveillance data may substantially understate the prevalence of this disease, since the majority of cases are presumptively diagnosed (without brain biopsy) and tend to occur after another AIDS-defining event has led to a case report. TE comes about as a result of reactivation of intracranial cysts, which are present in a widely varying percentage of the population. The likelihood of previous infection with *Toxoplasma gondii* varies by age, sociodemographic status, and geography. In a preliminary study in Boston, 30 percent of a mixed population of HIV-infected individuals were seropositive for toxoplasmosis. Up to 30 percent of *Toxoplasma*-seropositive, HIV-infected individuals develop toxoplasmic encephalitis during the course of their HIV disease.

Definitive diagnosis of TE is possible only by brain biopsy. Serologic methods, although useful for documenting previous exposure, are not sufficiently sensitive in the HIV-infected population to be used for diagnosis. In view of the potential morbidity and inconsistent availability of brain biopsy, however, it is reasonable to begin empirical antitoxoplasmosis therapy in HIV-infected individuals who present with neurologic symptoms and one or more intracerebral mass lesions, reserving biopsy for those who do not improve clinically and radiologically in 10 to 14 days. In the event that a patient is *known* to be *Toxoplasma* antibody negative at presentation, it would be reasonable to proceed directly to biopsy.

Pyrimethamine-Sulfadiazine

The combination of pyrimethamine and sulfadiazine is the only therapy of proven efficacy for TE. There is no agreement among experts on the appropriate dosage or duration of therapy with the combination. Many sources recommend pyrimethamine, 25 mg per day, plus sulfadiazine, 4 g per day, for 4 to 6 weeks. It is our practice to use somewhat higher doses of pyrimethamine (75 to 100 mg per day), as long as they are tolerated, in an attempt to raise intracerebral levels of pyrimethamine. This may be desirable in view of the frequent need to limit or withdraw sulfadiazine therapy before a full course has been administered.

The major toxicities of pyrimethamine are anemia and neutropenia. Folinic acid, 5 to 10 mg per day, is usually coadministered in an attempt to prevent hematologic toxicity. There is considerable interest in the use of hematopoietic growth factors, especially erythropoietin and granulocyte-macrophage colony stimulating factor to prevent these toxicities, but their efficacy and effect on underlying disease have not yet been studied. The major toxicities of sulfadiazine are rash, fever, and renal dysfunction, and cutaneous reactions are especially common.

Clindamycin

Clindamycin has known animal model activity against *Toxoplasma gondii* and has been used as a substitute for sulfadiazine in patients who cannot tolerate the latter agent. It appears that the combination of pyrimethamine and clindamycin has activity comparable to that of the gold standard of pyrimethamine and sulfadiazine. Trials of clindamycin have used doses of 1,200 to 4,800 mg per day, and there is no established dose or course of therapy. The author has limited experience with clindamycin as a single agent in patients with TE and severe pyrimethamine intolerance, and the results have not been encouraging.

Maintenance Therapy

As with other AIDS-related opportunistic infections, relapse is predictable in the absence of ongoing therapy if there is extended patient survival. A French trial suggests that more than 50 percent of TE patients live at least 1 year after diagnosis if the underlying HIV infection is treated with antiretroviral therapy (zidovudine, or AZT). It is common practice to continue one or more antitoxoplasmosis drugs for the life of the patient after an episode of TE, and pyrimethamine, sulfadiazine, and clindamycin have all been used for this purpose. There are insufficient data to prompt preference of one or another maintenance regimen, but the author usually prescribes pyrimethamine alone, 50 to 75 mg per day, if tolerated. Clinical trials comparing various regimens both for acute treatment and maintenance are under way through the National Institute of Allergy and Infectious Diseases AIDS Clinical Trials Group and may provide answers for some of the therapeutic dilemmas in AIDS-associated TE.

CRYPTOCOCCAL MENINGITIS

After PCP and toxoplasmic encephalitis, cryptococcal meningitis (CM) is the third most common opportunistic infection seen in association with AIDS, affecting up to 10 percent of patients. Prior to the outbreak of AIDS, CM was distinctly uncommon and often difficult to diagnose because of the paucity of organisms present in the cerebrospinal fluid. AIDS-associated CM is a subacute or chronic illness associated with fever and subtle alterations in central nervous system functioning. In contrast to the often subtle clinical presentation, examination of cerebrospinal fluid usually reveals a large number of organisms and a very high cryptococcal antigen titer. As is the case with other AIDS-associated opportunistic infections, patients with CM frequently experience relapses, even after prolonged therapy. It is now believed that lifelong therapy is necessary in order to prevent symptomatic disease after initial diagnosis.

Amphotericin B

The gold standard of therapy for CM in the pre-AIDS era was a combination of amphotericin B and 5-flucytosine (5-FC), given until cultures of cerebrospinal fluid were negative and cryptococcal antigen was no longer detectable in cerebrospinal fluid. When these end points were reached, usually no further treatment was required. Many different drug regimens have been used to treat AIDS-associated CM, and none have been carefully evaluated. Several general comments are appropriate, however.

Most AIDS patients are intolerant to 5-FC. As a result, therapy with amphotericin B alone is the mainstay of treatment. Doses higher than the 0.3 mg per kilogram used in combination with 5-FC are required. Typically, patients are treated with 0.5 to 0.8 mg per kilogram per day in order to ameliorate symptoms and lower the cerebrospinal fluid antigen titer. It is very unusual for patients to be "cured" by traditional criteria, but the cerebrospinal fluid antigen titer usually falls to a stable, low titer after approximately 1,000 mg of amphotericin B therapy. At this point, most clinicians prescribe prophylactic therapy to prevent relapse. This therapy is probably more appropriately termed "maintenance," as patients have residual disease that is kept under control by the continued therapy.

Both amphotericin B and ketoconazole, in varying doses, have been used to maintain remission in cryptococcal meningitis. Ketoconazole is now believed to be ineffective for this purpose, and most patients are treated with amphotericin B, 1 mg per kilogram per week in a single dose. Occasionally, patients on this dose of amphotericin B manifest a rising blood or cerebrospinal fluid antigen titer, with or without new symptoms. Clinicians often then increase the frequency of maintenance therapy or resume daily treatment until the status quo is restored.

Adverse reactions to amphotericin B, although not increased in frequency in the AIDS population, remain distressingly common and often present a barrier to continued therapy. Fever, chills, interstitial nephritis, electrolyte abnormalities, and acute renal failure are all seen in patients on this therapy. As a result, there is great interest in possible alternatives.

Fluconazole

Fluconazole is a triazole antifungal agent that has excellent activity against *Cryptococcus neoformans* when tested in animal models. Preliminary clinical studies in Europe and the United States suggested that this agent might be effective in AIDS patients with cryptococcal meningitis, and large studies comparing fluconazole with amphotericin B for both acute therapy and maintenance have been completed and are undergoing analysis. Review of unpublished data from these studies resulted in licensure of fluconazole in the United States in January, 1990. The Food and Drug Administration's approved indications for fluconazole include both therapy of acute CM and maintenance therapy for AIDS-associated CM. A direct report to physicians by the National Institute of Allergy and Infectious Diseases in May, 1990, suggested that, based on preliminary data, fluconazole was at least as effective as and possibly superior to amphotericin B for maintenance therapy of AIDS-associated CM.

As far as is known, the major toxicities of fluconazole are nausea and abnormalities of liver function tests. Symptomatic or icteric hepatitis appears to be rare. The role of fluconazole in AIDS-associated CM is being defined as this chapter is written; it is possible that it will replace amphotericin B for treatment of this disease in the foreseeable future. It is recommended that, when fluconazole is used for therapy of acute CM, a dose of 400 mg per day be administered until the cerebrospinal fluid culture is negative and the patient is asymptomatic. The approved dose for maintenance therapy of AIDS-associated CM is 200 mg per day.

CYTOMEGALOVIRUS DISEASE

Virtually all persons with AIDS and HIV infection have serologic evidence of infection with cytomegalovirus (CMV). CMV disease in AIDS patients ranges from asymptomatic viremia and/or viriuria to fatal multisystem infection. Pneumonitis, hepatitis, and encephalitis are common terminal events when CMV is implicated as the cause of death in AIDS.

CMV also causes retinitis and is the most common opportunistic disease leading to blindness in persons with AIDS. The diagnosis is commonly made on clinical grounds (by ophthalmoscopy), as serologic examination is unreliable and tissue examination is impractical.

Two antiviral agents are undergoing studies for the therapy of serious CMV disease in AIDS patients, especially CMV retinitis. Ganciclovir (9-[1,3 dihydroxy-2-propoxy]methyl)guanine (DHPG) and trisodium phosphonoformic acid (PFA, foscarnet) have both shown activity in preliminary studies. Ganciclovir has received Food and Drug Administration approval for therapy of AIDS-associated CMV retinitis, and both agents are undergoing more extensive evaluation. The unpredictable course of CMV retinitis and the almost uniformly fatal outcome of multisystem CMV infection make objective evaluation of these drugs very difficult.

Many reports exist, however, of substantial improvement in patients treated with DHPG for CMV retinitis. At doses of 7.5 to 15 mg per kilogram per day, arrest of disease and even healing have been reported. After cessation of therapy, however, disease almost uniformly reactivates and progresses, making lifelong therapy a necessity. The safety, efficacy, and patient tolerance of prolonged DHPG are under investigation at present.

The major toxicity of DHPG is leukopenia, particularly neutropenia, which limits the duration of therapy in many patients. Despite the presence of similar toxicity with AZT, the two agents do not appear to exhibit additive toxicity, and therapy with one agent does not alter the pharmacology of the other.

Fewer studies have been performed with PFA, but results similar to those described with DHPG have been reported. PFA will typically arrest or improve active disease, but early relapse after cessation of therapy is common. Asymptomatic elevation of serum creatinine level has been the most commonly described toxicity with PFA, but large clinical studies have not been performed.

Successful therapy for serious CMV disease will probably require the development of agents suitable for chronic oral administration. It is noteworthy that patients enrolled in experimental studies of AZT plus acyclovir for treatment of HIV infection have shown a decreased incidence of new CMV disease, but the significance of this observation is unknown at present.

ATYPICAL MYCOBACTERIAL INFECTIONS

Patients with AIDS are susceptible to an unusual form of disseminated atypical mycobacterial disease. Usually caused by members of the *Mycobacterium avium-intracellulare* complex (MAC), high-grade bacillemia in association with fever, night sweats, and weight loss represents a common presentation. As is the case with CMV, MAC organisms can affect many different organ systems, but infection of the bowel with severe diarrhea and protein-losing enteropathy or infection of the liver and spleen with massive organomegaly appears to be a particularly common clinical pattern.

MAC organisms are resistant to most antituberculous drugs. Even before the advent of AIDS, serious disease caused by MAC was very difficult to treat with drugs, and failure of therapy was common. In a large series of retrospectively analyzed AIDS cases, no benefit from multidrug chemotherapy was found, either in terms of symptoms or survival.

There is much anecdotal evidence, however, of individual responses to therapy, particularly for severe symptoms. The general principles of antituberculous therapy are generally used, e.g., multiple drugs are given over a protracted period of time, and if at all possible, two drugs to which the organism is sensitive in vitro are used. Most MAC isolates from AIDS patients are sensitive in vitro to rifabutin (ansamycin), clofazimine (Lamprene), and ciprofloxacin; in addition, the combination of rifampin and ethambutol shows synergy. In the presence of ethambutol, rifabutin is not notably more active than rifampin. Several studies are in progress to attempt to define a tolerable and effective multidrug regimen for AIDS patients with MAC infection. Before data from such studies are available, however, it seems reasonable to treat severely symptomatic patients with a combination of INH, 300 mg per day, ethambutol, 15 mg per kilogram per day, rifabutin (available from the Centers for Disease Control), 300 mg per day, *or* rifampin, 600 mg per day, and ciprofloxacin, 750 mg per day. If no response is noted after several weeks, clofazimine, 50 to 100 mg per day can be added. If this regimen does not produce clinical improvement or if unacceptable toxicity occurs, therapy can be discontinued after several weeks. The further addition to anti-MAC therapy of amikacin, 7.5 mg per kilogram per day, is advocated by some investigators in the field. A decision to offer therapy for serious MAC disease should be made with a full understanding of the limited potential benefit and the potential for serious drug toxicity.

SUGGESTED READING

Brenner M, Ognibene FP, Lack EE, et al. Prognostic factors and life expectancy of patients with acquired immune deficiency syndrome and *Pneumocystis carinii* pneumonia. Am Rev Respir Dis 1987; 136:1199–1206

Corkery KJ, Luce JM, Montgomery AB. Aerosolized pentamidine for treatment and prophylaxis of *Pneumocystis carinii* pneumonia: An update. Respir Care 1988; 33:676–685

El-Sadr W, Sidhu G, Diamond G, et al. High dose corticosteroids as adjunct therapy in severe *Pneumocystis carinii* pneumonia. AIDS Res 1986; 2:349–355

Hawkins C, Gold JWM, Whimby E, et al. *Mycobacterium avium* complex infections in patients with the acquired immunodeficiency syndrome. Ann Int Med 1986; 105:184–188

Mills J. *Pneumocystis carinii* and *Toxoplasma gondii* infections in patients with AIDS. Rev Infect Dis 1986; 8:1001–1011

Mills J, Jacobson MA, O'Donnell JJ, et al. Treatment of cytomegalovirus retinitis in patients with AIDS. Rev Infect Dis 1988; 10:S522–S531

Sugar AM, Saunders C. Oral fluconazole as suppressive therapy of disseminated cryptococcosis in patients with acquired immunodeficiency syndrome. Am J Med 1988; 85:481–489

Young LS, *Mycobacterium avium* complex infections. J Infect Dis 1988; 157:863–867

DERMATOLOGIC MANIFESTATIONS OF THE ACQUIRED IMMUNODEFICIENCY SYNDROME

ANTOINETTE F. HOOD, M.D.
THOMAS T. PROVOST, M.D.

ETIOLOGY

No treatise on dermatologic treatment in 1990 can be considered complete without a discussion of the cutaneous manifestations of the acquired immunodeficiency syndrome (AIDS). Our knowledge of the spectrum of cutaneous manifestations and etiopathogenesis of AIDS is in a rapid state of evolution. At the time of this writing, three retroviruses (two have yet to be officially designated) of putative simian origin have been found to cause AIDS in man. The virus most commonly associated with the disease has been designated the human immunodeficiency (HIV). Several other closely related retroviruses have been described in addition to the three associated with AIDS. Human T-cell lymphotrophic virus type I (HTLV-I) is a cause of human T-cell leukemia, cutaneous T-cell lymphoma, and adult T-cell leukemia. Human T-cell lymphotrophic virus type II (HTLV-II) causes hairy cell leukemia.

The HIV virus is cytotropic for the T4 (helper-inducer) cell lymphocyte. The virus binds to a specific protein T4 molecule on the T-helper cell, initiating the infection. The HIV virus is also capable of infecting Epstein-Barr virus–infected B lymphocytes, Langerhans' cells, and other macrophage-like cells. Because the virus integrates itself in a latent form into the host DNA, the infection persists for a lifetime.

EPIDEMIOLOGY

In 1979, AIDS, the newest and perhaps the worst epidemic in the history of mankind, was heralded by the recognition of the occurrence of unusual bacterial, protozoan, and fungal infections and Kaposi's sarcoma in homosexual males, Haitians, hemophiliacs, and intravenous drug addicts. Epidemiologic studies have subsequently revealed that the HIV infection is widespread in Africa, affecting an estimated 40 percent of individuals living in the sub-Saharan basin. In Africa HIV was noted to be a heterosexual disease, and the International Congress on the Acquired Immunodeficiency Syndrome held in Washington in June 1987 focused on the heterosexual transmission of this epidemic. Particularly at risk for spreading the disease is the intravenous drug abusing prostitute. In one recent study of a large eastern United States city, 50 percent of randomly screened prostitutes possessed the HIV antibody. Other studies have indicated that 50 to 75 percent of intravenous drug abusers are HIV antibody–positive. Thus, two of the greatest social dilemmas of our era, drug abuse and AIDS, are intimately linked.

It is now known that homosexual men, especially those with many partners and those who practice rectal intercourse, are at greatest risk for infection, as the transmission of the virus sexually is via infected seminal fluid. Male to female infection frequently occurs; the authors of one study estimate that approximately 70 percent of the female sexual partners of HIV-positive males are infected with the virus. However, female to male transmission occurs less frequently. One preliminary report estimates that female transmission to a male sexual partner occurs following intercourse approximately once every 50 times. The infected female also can transfer the virus to her unborn child. An infected child develops poorly and generally dies within the first few years of life.

In the past, contaminated blood supply has been a significant source of infection. This risk has been reduced by vigorous screening of donated blood. It has been estimated that approximately 85 percent of hemophiliacs have contracted the HIV infection from contaminated factor VIII cryoprecipitate.

In contradistinction to the high degree of infectivity associated with sexual contact, blood transfusions, and intravenous drug abuse, the virus has a low degree of infectivity among medical personnel inadvertently injured by needle stick and in individuals who come into close but nonsexual contact with AIDS patients. Apparently the AIDS retrovirus does not survive for long periods of time outside the body.

The clinical features of the AIDS syndrome are many and varied. In general, the development of the opportunistic infections corresponds to the development of a profound lymphopenia. Initially this lymphopenia is indicated by a reversal of the helper T-cell/suppressor T-cell (T4/T8) ratio. As the T helper–inducer lymphocytes disappear from the peripheral circulation, the host becomes more and more susceptible to the development of opportunistic infections. In general, as the T-helper lymphocyte count falls below 100 cells per cubic millimeter of blood, significant opportunistic infections occur.

The cutaneous manifestations of the initial viremia are mild and transient; consequently the exanthem is rarely observed and infrequently diagnosed. It has been demonstrated, however, that following a documented infection several patients have developed a macular and papular (morbilliform) rash accompanied by fever and myalgia. The time lapse between infection and seroconversion ranges from 3 weeks to 6 months after infection. Following the initial infection, most patients develop generalized lymphadenopathy with hypergammaglobulinemia, and some develop thrombocytopenia. This form of disease is known as the AIDS-related complex (ARC). With the development of tumors such as Kaposi's sarcoma or opportunistic infections with organisms such as *Candida albicans* and *Pneumocystis carinii*, the disease is considered to have evolved into AIDS. The length of time between the initial infection and the development of AIDS is unknown, but it appears to be longer than 3 years. Some seropositive patients have not developed AIDS after 7 years of follow-up.

The cutaneous manifestations of AIDS can be divided into the following categories: infections, nonspecific dermatoses, and neoplasia (Tables 1 and 2).

TABLE 1 Mucocutaneous Findings in AIDS

- Infection
  - Viral infections
    - Herpesvirus infection (herpes simplex, herpes zoster varicella)
    - Cytomegalovirus
    - Human papillomavirus
    - Epstein-Barr virus
    - Molluscum contagiosum
    - Oral hairy leukoplakia
  - Fungal infections
    - Oral candidiasis
    - Dermatophytosis
    - Tinea versicolor
    - Cutaneous manifestations of disseminated systemic infection
      - *Cryptococcus neoformans*
      - *Histoplasma capsulatum*
      - *Coccidioides immitis*
      - *Sporothrix schenckii*
  - Bacterial infections
    - Pyoderma, folliculitis, secondary impetiginization
    - Mycobacterium
    - Syphilis
  - Protozoal infections
    - *Acanthamoeba castellani*
- Inflammatory dermatoses
  - Seborrheic dermatitis
  - Papular (pruritic) eruption
  - Drug eruptions
  - Exacerbation of pre-existing skin disease, especially psoriasis
  - Granuloma annulare-like lesions
  - Xerosis, ichthyosis
- Neoplasm
  - Kaposi's sarcoma
  - Lymphoma
  - Other vascular proliferation
    - Angiomas
    - Telangiectasia

INFECTIOUS MANIFESTATIONS

The infectious dermatoses associated with AIDS include manifestations of viral, bacterial, fungal, and protozoan infections. *Herpes simplex infections* are often seen as unusually severe, persistent, or recurrent erosions or ulcerations around the mouth or perineum. They may become secondarily infected with bacteria and if untreated can result in scarring. It is important to note that these lesions frequently do not develop the classic appearance of grouped vesicles on the erythematous base. Identification of these lesions is usually made with either a Tzanck smear preparation or a herpes culture; however, a skin biopsy may be necessary in some cases to establish the diagnosis. Successful treatment requires oral or parenteral administration of acyclovir. A prolonged course of acyclovir may be required for large, deep, or longstanding ulcerations.

Herpes zoster infections may be severe in AIDS patients. In most instances the varicella zoster affliction represents a secondary infection (that is, a recurrence following childhood chickenpox). These pa-

TABLE 2 Cutaneous Manifestations in AIDS

	Common	*Less Common*	*Rare*
Infections	Herpesvirus infection Warts and condylomata acuminata Molluscum contagiosum Oral candidiasis	Dermatophytoses Oral hairy leukoplakia	Cutaneous lesions associated with disseminated systemic fungal infection
Inflammatory dermatoses	Seborrheic dermatitis Drug eruptions	Papular eruption Ichthyosis	Granuloma annulare-like lesions Exacerbation of preexisting dermatoses (psoriasis)
Neoplasms	Kaposi's sarcoma	Lymphoma Basal cell carcinoma Squamous cell carcinoma	Telangiectasias

tients may develop a generalized cutaneous eruption associated with pneumonia. Like their herpes simplex counterparts, the individual lesions of varicella zoster may be clinically atypical in appearance, failing to demonstrate the usual segmental dermatomal eruption or erythema surrounding the vesicles. The Tzanck smear and viral culture are helpful confirmatory diagnostic tests. In general, oral acyclovir treatment is only partially effective in these patients, and intravenous acyclovir therapy is often necessary for individuals with disseminated varicella zoster infection.

Molluscum contagiosum infections are frequently seen in AIDS patients. These lesions can involve any area of the body but most commonly occur on the head, neck, and genitalia. The lesions have a tendency to become very large (i.e., up to 1 cm in diameter). The lesions tend to persist and to recur following therapy. Surgical removal of the viral core with curettage or a shave biopsy technique is recommended, although cryotherapy with liquid nitrogen has also been successfully employed. Although molluscum lesions are fairly distinctive and relatively easy to diagnose in immunocompetent individuals, in AIDS patients other infections such as disseminated histoplasmosis and cryptococcosis may produce similar-looking lesions.

Epstein-Barr virus infection may act synergistically with HIV to produce unusual lymphoproliferations and lymphomas in the AIDS patient. Infectious mononucleosis with a generalized macular dermatitis and a severe hemolytic anemia associated with cold agglutinin antibodies has been described. The diagnosis of this type of dermatosis is difficult; biopsies are of little help. However, serologic studies to examine the patient's serum for antibody responses to early and late Epstein-Barr virus antigens may provide confirmatory data. At this time there is no effective treatment for this Epstein-Barr virus–induced disease.

A distinctive leukoplakia of the tongue, *oral hairy leukoplakia*, has been described in ARC and AIDS patients. The lesions, varying in size from 2 mm to 2 cm, are poorly demarcated, irregular white areas on the lateral surfaces of the tongue, which demonstrate an irregular, corrugated surface or "hairy" appearance. They are generally asymptomatic and clinically may be confused with oral changes seen in cigarette smokers. Histologically the lesions resemble warts, but they are caused by the Epstein-Barr virus. Because of their asymptomatic nature, they usually do not require treatment, but response to oral acyclovir therapy has been reported.

Papillomavirus infections are very frequent in AIDS patients, who may develop warts involving the oral mucosa as well as the genital region. These lesions may be large, recurrent, and very resistant to conventional therapy.

Fungal infection, especially *candidiasis*, is common in patients with AIDS. *Candida albicans* is a saprophyte-commensal organism present in approximately 70 percent of normal individuals. The *Candida* infection in AIDS patients may take the form of plaques on the buccal mucosa and tongue; extension of oral candidiasis to involve the throat and esophagus may produce dysphagia. When *Candida* infections of the mucosa become deep and erosive, they may produce a great deal of discomfort and become difficult to treat. Vaginal candidiasis occurs frequently in women with AIDS and like oral candidiasis may be both extensive and intractable. The diagnosis of candidiasis can be confirmed by microscopic examination of potassium hydroxide preparation of scrapings from lesions or by fungal cultures.

The treatment of AIDS-related oral candidiasis involves the use of nystatin oral suspension, 1 teaspoon three to four times a day. The patient is instructed to swish the material around in the mouth and then to swallow. Amphotericin B, 50 mg suspended in 4 ounces of wild cherry syrup, 1 teaspoon four times a day (swish and swallow), is an effective alternative therapy for the treatment of candidiasis in immunosuppressed patients. (*Note*: It is important to place the amphotericin B in an acid pH to prevent its deactivation; hence, the use of wild cherry syrup.) Vaginal candidiasis is treated with nystatin, miconazole, or clotrimazole suppositories daily. Finally, ketoconazole, 200 mg by mouth daily for 10 to 14 days, may be necessary to control the most severe forms of mucosal candidiasis.

Dermatophyte infections can be extensive, severe, and symptomatic in patients with AIDS. These infections classically involve the genital areas, feet, and toenails but also have been described involving the face and other skin surfaces. The lesions are occasionally very extensive, have a tendency to be hyperkeratotic, and may produce little or no erythema. Potassium hydroxide examination of scrapings from these lesions as well as fungal cultures establish the true nature of the infection. These lesions generally respond poorly to topical treatment with miconazole and clotrimazole. Systemic therapy in the form of griseofulvin or ketoconazole may be necessary, but the infections may be refractory even to this aggressive treatment.

Tinea versicolor has been commonly reported in patients with AIDS. These lesions are usually refractory to topical applications of selenium sulfide, miconazole, or clotrimazole and often require systemic treatment with ketoconazole. Relapses are frequent.

Disseminated deep fungal infections with cutaneous manifestations have been reported in AIDS patients. We have seen several patients with a cutaneous cryptococcal infection that resembled molluscum contagiosum. Histoplasmosis presenting as disseminated papules or necrotic plaques on the trunk and extremities in AIDS patients have also been reported.

Bacterial infections are common in AIDS patients. Cutaneous pyodermas may present as cellulitis, folliculitis, or acneiform lesions. Perirectal ulcerations are frequently infected with *Staphylococcus aureus.* These infections respond well to the appropriate antibiotics

A new and distinctive cutaneous infection has been reported exclusively in AIDS patients that is known as bacillary angiomatosis. The disease is manifested by multiple erythematous to violaceous papules and nodules that may spontaneously resolve. The cat scratch bacillus has recently been discovered as the cause of this disorder.

It should be noted that genital ulcerations in AIDS patients may be a manifestation of *syphilis.* Therefore, in addition to culturing ulcers for viruses and bacteria, a darkfield examination and a serologic test for syphilis should be obtained with all perineal ulcerations. *Secondary syphilis* may present with typical widespread papulosquamous lesions or in atypical forms. Cases of seronegative secondary syphilis have been reported in AIDS patients. In this situation, silver stains demonstrating *Treponema pallidum* in skin biopsy specimens may be necessary to confirm the diagnosis. It should also be noted that secondary syphilis in AIDS patients frequently requires higher doses of penicillin for adequate treatment.

Cutaneous mycobacterial infections have been described in patients with AIDS, including *Mycobacterium scrofulaceum, M. marinum,* and, less commonly, *M. avium-intracellulare.*

Protozoal infections are highly unusual in patients with AIDS. Recently, however, a disseminated protozoal infection caused by *Acanthamoeba castellani* was associated with the development of a papule on the thigh of an AIDS patient.

NONSPECIFIC DERMATOSES

In addition to these viral, fungal, and bacterial infections, AIDS patients may develop nonspecific inflammatory disorders of the skin. For example, seborrheic dermatitis is very common, occurring in approximately 80 percent of AIDS patients. The severity of the seborrheic dermatitis appears to correlate with the severity of the disease. AIDS patients with an explosive onset of erythematous recalcitrant seborrheic dermatitis appear to have the worst prognosis. Xeroderma (dry skin) appears to be frequently associated with the seborrheic dermatitis. Acquired ichthyosis occurs commonly, but usually late in the course of the disease.

A clinically characteristic papular eruption has also been described in both AIDS and the related complex. This condition consists of discrete, skin-colored papules occurring on the head, neck, and upper trunk. These lesions are usually pruritic, and although the condition waxes and wanes, the course of the disease is usually chronic. There appears to be no correlation between the severity of the eruption and systemic signs and symptoms of HIV infection. The histologic appearance of the lesions is nonspecific perivascular mononuclear cell infiltrate with or without eosinophils. A small subpopulation of patients develop widespread, intensely pruritic prurigo nodules; these lesions are notoriously recalcitrant to traditional therapy.

In addition to these cutaneous manifestations of the AIDS syndrome, there is evidence to indicate that AIDS patients may have an increased frequency of cutaneous drug reactions. A high frequency of generalized macular and papular erythematous eruptions has been described in AIDS patients treated with trimethoprim-sulfamethoxazole; dapsone-trimethoprim and pentamidine are also associated with a high incidence of cutaneous eruptions.

Finally, persons with preexisting dermatoses such as psoriasis may experience severe exacerbation of the cutaneous disease as an early manifestation of HIV infection. We have recently seen and cared for two patients with widespread erythrodermic psoriasis. The history of a preceding coronary artery bypass graft requiring blood transfusion alerted the attending physicians to the possibility of HIV-related disease; both patients were antibody-positive, and both have subsequently died of the sequelae of HIV infection.

NEOPLASIA

Immunocompromised patients develop a spectrum of malignant diseases, and it has been estimated that 40 percent of AIDS patients develop neoplasms. The most common tumor is an aggressive form of Kaposi's sarcoma occurring most commonly but not exclusively in homosexuals with HIV infection. In addition to involving the skin (25 percent of the patients with homosexually transmitted AIDS have cutaneous Kaposi's sarcoma), tumors often develop in other organs. In one autopsy series more than 90 percent of AIDS patients had Kaposi's sarcoma involving internal organs.

Typically the cutaneous lesions of AIDS-associated Kaposi's sarcoma occur as small, round, oval papules or plaques on the upper trunk, face, and proximal extremities. The lesions tend to be reddish brown to violaceous and may be extremely subtle in the early stages. Often lesions are oriented along the long axis of skin tension lines on the trunk, in a pityriasis rosea-like pattern. Kaposi's sarcoma has been described as developing a dermatomal distribution following an episode of herpes zoster. Kaposi's sarcoma may be rapid in onset and oral lesions may be prominent. Because early lesions may vary considerably in morphology and because Kaposi's sarcoma is one of the AIDS defining diseases, diagnosis is usually confirmed by biopsy. Treatment is discussed elsewhere in this book.

Lymphomas, usually of B-cell origin, develop in individuals with AIDS. Although skin involvement is not common, when it does occur there is a peculiar disposition in the oral and genital regions.

Other cutaneous tumors described in patients with AIDS include basal cell carcinomas and squamous cell carcinomas (often associated with perianal condyloma).

RECOMMENDATIONS

It is evident that as the AIDS epidemic continues and spreads, recognition of cutaneous abnormalities associated with HIV infection and its subsequent immune deficiencies will play an increasing role in the early diagnosis of this disease. It should be emphasized that many of the characteristic inflammatory features of bacterial, fungal, and viral lesions are muted or nonexistent owing to the underlying immune suppression in these patients. Physicians must be suspicious that any individual lesion may represent an opportunistic infection in an HIV patient. Therefore, viral cultures, Tzanck smears, bacterial cultures (including those for atypical mycobacteria), and biopsies become increasingly important tools in the diagnosis of infections and malignant disease in these patients. If an opportunistic infection is detected, the patient should be referred to an appropriate medical facility for further investigation and treatment. At the present state of development of the medicolegal ramifications in AIDS testing, it is recommended that physicians obtain written permission from the patient prior to obtaining an HIV antibody determination.

Because of the magnitude of the AIDS epidemic, it is currently recommended that physicians wear gloves for all invasive diagnostic or therapeutic procedures, including venipuncture. Careful hand washing with an antiseptic soap before and after each invasive procedure is also advised. If one is inadvertently exposed to a patient's blood, for example, via a needle stick, it is recommended that the following serologic tests be obtained on the patient's blood (with his or her permission): hepatitis antibody and antigen screen, cytomegalovirus antibody screen, and HIV antibody. An infectious disease consultation should also be obtained for up-to-date recommendations regarding follow-up evaluation.

Finally, from a philosophic point of view, it is important to remember that physicians in previous generations have also been placed in potentially dangerous situations. The infectivity and danger to medical personnel posed by an HIV patient are far less than the high infectivity danger to physicians who cared for patients with tuberculosis in previous eras. Good common sense and a healthy respect for the dangers inherent in handling blood and bodily secretions and for performing invasive procedures are of paramount importance for self-protection.

Physicians must realize that they are now and will remain in a "front-line" position in dealing with AIDS and that in this position they are responsible for the recognition and diagnosis of cutaneous diseases that may be early manifestations of the disease. As newer therapies become available for the treatment of HIV infection, early recognition and treatment may be of paramount importance in controlling this epidemic.

GASTROINTESTINAL INFECTIONS IN PATIENTS WITH THE ACQUIRED IMMUNODEFICIENCY SYNDROME

THOMAS C. QUINN, M.D.
JOHN G. BARTLETT, M.D.

Since the recognition of the acquired immunodeficiency syndrome (AIDS) in 1981, over 150,000 cases have been diagnosed in 145 countries of the world. With an estimated 500,000 patients with AIDS-related conditions and 5 to 10 million people infected with the human immunodeficiency virus (HIV), the etiologic agent of AIDS, this disease has become a global pandemic. HIV is a retrovirus with a specific tropism for T-helper (CD4+) lymphocytes, which causes a slow, but progressive cellular immunosuppression secondary to cytolysis of T-helper lymphocytes. With a mean incubation of 8 to 10 years from the time of infection with HIV, disseminated opportunistic infections and malignant conditions characteristic of AIDS usually develop concurrently with further suppression of the cell-mediated immune system. Without an effective vaccine or curative drug, it is evident that the clinical features of HIV infection and AIDS will become even more common in most medical care settings.

HIV is transmitted by three major routes: sexual, parenteral, and perinatal. There is little or no evidence of transmission by casual contact, aerosol, insects, or other indirect means of transmission. The major risk groups for HIV infection include homosexual and bisexual men, intravenous drug abusers, recipients of blood transfusions or factor 8 and factor 9 concentrates before 1985, heterosexual partners of the above risk groups, and children born to HIV-infected mothers. The clinical spectrum of HIV infection is diverse and multiple organ involvement is frequently evident. The gastrointestinal (GI) tract is one of the most common sites of clinical expression, and all levels of the intestine from the oral cavity to the anus are often involved. Epidemiologic and clinical studies indicate that the intestinal tract is a primary site of inoculation with HIV, particularly in homosexual men who engage in anal-rectal intercourse. During acute infection with HIV, GI symptoms are one of the earliest signs of infection, including anorexia, nausea, vomiting, or diarrhea in association with symptoms of fever, sweats, myalgias, adenopathy, and occasionally a diffuse rash. Although most of these symptoms resolve over several months, many HIV-infected individuals develop more severe and prolonged intestinal symptoms, commonly referred to as a "wasting syndrome," or "slim disease." In many of these patients, the appearance of prolonged GI symptoms is highly predictive of the subsequent development of opportunistic infections and the eventual diagnosis of AIDS.

The prevalence of GI symptoms varies among different populations at risk for HIV infection. Among the major risk groups for AIDS in developed countries, homosexual men appear to present most commonly with GI symptoms and signs. Approximately 30 to 50 percent of homosexual men with AIDS have a history of a clinical presentation characterized by progressive loss of more than 10 percent of body weight and chronic diarrhea. This presentation is much less frequent among intravenous drug abusers, transfusion recipients, hemophiliacs, and heterosexual partners of patients at risk for AIDS. It is highly probable that homosexual men appear to be more susceptible to this diarrhea-weight loss syndrome because of their high exposure to GI pathogens as part of the "gay bowel syndrome."

THE GAY BOWEL SYNDROME

Before the AIDS epidemic, it was already evident that in the mid-1970s enteric infections were occurring in epidemic proportions among homosexually active men, and that sexual activities involving fecal contamination and rectal intercourse were the main modes of transmission. Many of these infections included classic sexually transmitted diseases that were known to cause anal-rectal disease such as *Neisseria gonorrhoeae, N. meningitidis, Chlamydia trachomatis, Treponema pallidum,* and herpes simplex virus, while other traditional enteric organisms such as *Shigella, Salmonella, Campylobacter, Giardia lamblia,* and *Entamoeba histolytica* were also found to be endemic among homosexual men. With the subsequent development of AIDS, additional enteric pathogens were identified in homosexual men with GI symptoms. These included *cryptosporidia, Isospora, microsporidia, Mycobacterium avium-intracellulare,* and cytomegalovirus. The list of these pathogens, when added to the other sexually transmitted agents and enteric pathogens, demonstrates the microbial complexity of intestinal infections in homosexual men at risk for HIV infection. The addition of GI malignancies seen in AIDS patients, such as Kaposi's sarcoma, lymphoma, and squamous cell carcinoma of the mouth and rectum, illustrates the diverse presentation of GI disease in this population. Consequently, homosexual men or other individuals at risk for HIV infection who present with GI symptoms must undergo thorough investigation including a full microbiologic evaluation of the GI tract and, in some cases, an assessment of immunocompetence and serologic evidence of HIV infection.

CLINICAL SYNDROMES

It is clinically useful to approach the diagnosis of GI complaints in HIV-infected individuals by dividing the symptoms into five categories: esophagitis, enteritis, proc-

TABLE 1 Clinical Intestinal Syndromes and Associated Infectious Agents Seen in Homosexual Men and AIDS Patients

Syndrome	*Symptoms and Signs*	*Infectious Agents*
Esophagitis	Dysphagia Esophageal ulcers	*Candida albicans* Herpes simplex virus Cytomegalovirus
Enteritis	Diarrhea Abdominal cramps Bloating Normal sigmoidoscopy	*Giardia lamblia* Cryptosporidia *Isospora belli* Microsporidia *Strongyloides stercoralis* *Mycobacterium avium-intracellulare* Cytomegalovirus
Proctocolitis	Diarrhea Low abdominal cramps Abnormal sigmoidoscopy beyond 15 cm	*Campylobacter* spp. *Shigella* spp. *Salmonella* spp. *Entamoeba histolytica* *Clostridium difficile* *Chlamydia trachomatis* (LGV serovar) Cytomegalovirus
Proctitis	Anorectal pain Mucopurulent discharge Abnormal sigmoidoscopy below 15 cm	*Neisseria gonorrhoeae* Herpes simplex virus *Chlamydia trachomatis* (non-LGV serovar) *Treponema pallidum* Cytomegalovirus
Perianal disease	Perianal discomfort Pruritus External lesions	Condyloma acuminatum Herpes simplex virus *Treponema pallidum*

tocolitis, proctitis, and perianal disease. Table 1 lists the wide spectrum of intestinal infections that may be seen in association with each of these clinical syndromes. Esophagitis is frequently associated with odynophagia and retrosternal chest pain. Symptoms of enteritis include diarrhea, abdominal pain, bloating, and cramping. Symptoms of proctitis include anal-rectal pain, mucous bloody discharge, tenesmus, and constipation. Proctocolitis may produce overlapping symptoms of both proctitis and enteritis. Perianal disease due to condyloma acuminatum, herpes simplex virus, or syphilis may result in perianal pain, itching, or discomfort. Clinical presentations characteristic of one of these syndromes may help to narrow the diagnostic evaluation of each patient. However, all high-risk patients should be routinely tested during the initial examination with a rectal Gram stain for evaluation of polymorphonuclear lymphocytes and intracellular gram-negative diplococci, a dark-field examination of any suspicious lesions, and a rapid plasma reagin (RPR) test for syphilis. For high-risk individuals such as homosexual men, other routine tests should include urethral, rectal, and pharyngeal cultures for *N. gonorrhoeae;* rectal cultures for *C. trachomatis;* and a serologic test for HIV. Further diagnostic tests, such as stool examination for ova and parasites and culture for enteric pathogens, should be selected on the basis of the suspected clinical syndrome (Table 1). Frequently, symptomatic patients may have two or more pathogens requiring additional evaluation after the identification and treatment of one pathogen.

In AIDS patients, chronic diarrhea with intermittent symptoms and progressive weight loss are frequently seen. The severity of the diarrhea is highly variable, ranging from intermittent to debilitating diarrhea with large volume losses and the attendant consequences of dehydration, electrolyte imbalance, and emaciation. Extensive studies for microbial agents occasionally yield treatable agents such as *Shigella, Salmonella, Campylobacter,* and *Isospora*, although all of these are likely to recur when treatment is discontinued in HIV-infected patients. Many cases involve untreatable microbial pathogens such as *cryptosporidia, M. avium-intracellulare*, and cytomegalovirus. Overall, specific pathogens may not be identified in 25 to 50 percent of HIV-positive patients with chronic diarrhea. Many of these individuals show histologic evidence of cytomegalovirus infection at autopsy, whereas others have nonspecific inflammation and evidence of chronic malabsorption, such as partial villus atrophy with crypt hyperplasia. Malabsorption is relatively common in all of these patients, and is demonstrated by abnormal D-xylose and ^{14}C-glycerol tripalmitin absorption tests in nearly all of those with GI symptoms. These findings strongly suggest that malabsorption may contribute to the significant weight loss seen in these AIDS patients, and that although individual opportunistic infectious agents may differ from patient to patient, the underlying pathologic process involving the GI tract is similar among most AIDS patients.

After the evaluation of AIDS patients with GI symptoms, specific treatment can be administered if a specific pathogen has been identified. Because of the diversity of infecting agents, treatment should be withheld in patients with mild symptoms until microbiologic results are available. In severe cases of diarrhea, antispasmodic agents such as diphenoxylate hydrochloride and atropine sulfate (Lomotil) or tincture of opium may be required to alleviate symptoms and to avoid further dehydration. Endoscopy with intestinal biopsies is frequently indicated in patients with chronic intestinal symptoms in whom no specific infectious agent has been identified. Contrast studies may also be useful and may reveal multiple lesions. Similarly, abdominal computed tomographic (CT) scans may provide a high diagnostic yield. Patients with AIDS-related conditions commonly show retroperitoneal and mesenteric adenopathy, splenomegaly, and perirectal inflammation. Large intra-abdominal lymph nodes (over 1.5 cm) specifically suggest *M. avium-intracellulare,* Kaposi's sarcoma, or lymphoma. Diagnosis can often be made with a fine-needle percutaneous aspiration or CT-directed biopsy.

Recommendations for specific treatment of infections are summarized in Table 2 and reviewed below.

SPECIFIC INFECTIONS

Oroesophageal Candidiasis

Oral candidiasis, or thrush, is a common complication in debilitated patients and immunosuppressed patients receiving antibiotic therapy. It is one of the most frequent findings in AIDS patients and is a relatively poor prognostic sign. In the absence of other underlining immunosuppressive diseases, the occurrence of thrush in a patient at risk for HIV infection or in association with non-explained chronic diarrhea-wasting syndrome is highly suggestive of HIV infection. The diagnosis is readily established with potassium hydroxide (KOH) stains of exudate from typical oral lesions that show sheets of typi-

TABLE 2 Treatment of Gastrointestinal Infections Associated with AIDS*

Agent	*Initial Treatment*
Candida spp.	Clotrimazole: 1 troche 4–5 times daily *or* nystatin: 500,000 units swish and swallow *or* ketoconazole: 200 mg PO b.i.d. *or* amphotericin B: 0.3 mg /kg/day for total 200–300 mg followed by one of the above regimens indefinitely
Mycobacterium avium-intracellulare	No particular regimen proved effective One regimen includes rifampin, ansamycin, clofazimine, amikacin, ethionamide, ethambutol
Salmonella spp.	Antibiotic chosen on basis of isolate sensitivities Possibilities include: Ampicillin: 6 g/day IV 2–3 wk *or* TMP/SMZ: one double-strength tablet b.i.d. for 2–3 wk *or* ciprofloxacin: 500 mg b.i.d. for 2–3 wk
Shigella spp.	Antibiotic chosen on basis of isolate sensitivities Possibilities include: TMP/SMZ: one double-strength tablet b.i.d. for 7 days *or* ampicillin: 500 mg q.i.d. for 7 days
Campylobacter	Erythromycin: 250 mg q.i.d. for 7 days (gentamycin should be given to patients with bacteremia)
Cryptosporidia	None
Isospora spp.	TMP/SMZ: 2 double-stength tablets b.i.d. for 2 wk
Giardia lamblia	Metronidazole: 250 mg t.i.d. for 10 days
Entamoeba histolytica	Metronidazole: 750 mg t.i.d. for 10 days plus iodoquinol 650 mg t.i.d for 21 days
Microsporidia	None
Herpes simplex virus	Acyclovir: 200 mg PO 5 times daily for 10 days *or* acyclovir: 5 mg/kg IV q8 for 10 days followed by acyclovir: 200 mg PO t.i.d. indefinitely
Cytomegalovirus	DHPG: 5 mg/kg IV b.i.d for 2 wk

* Nearly all infections need chronic suppressive therapy with effective antibiotics to prevent relapses.

cal yeast and pseudomycelial forms. Patients with oral candidiasis usually respond to traditional therapeutic intervention with clotrimazole troches, nystatin, or oral ketoconazole. Despite this response, there is a propensity to relapse as soon as therapy is discontinued. Consequently, chronic administration of one of these drugs is commonly recommended.

Esophageal candidiasis is also relatively common and represents an AIDS-defining diagnosis. Patients with established AIDS and thrush may have esophageal involvement even when the esophageal symptoms are absent. Symptoms, when present, consist of dysphagia with or without retrosternal pain. There usually is oral involvement, but occasionally patients have only esophagitis. Contrast studies of the esophagus show abnormal peristalsis, spasm, and edema with mucosal ulcerations and a cobblestone appearance. The diagnosis is best established by endoscopy that demonstrates dense plaques of white exudate referred to as "cottage-cheese" exudate. Histologic studies of this exudate show yeast and pseudomycelial forms of *Candida*. Biopsies reveal invasion of the mucosa accompanied by an inflammatory response.

The treatment of esophageal candidiasis consists of ketoconazole, 200 mg orally twice daily. Severe or refractory cases should be treated with amphotericin B in a low-dose regimen (0.3 mg per kilogram for 10 to 15 days). Regardless of the initial treatment, patients should subsequently receive an indefinite course of ketoconazole.

Mycobacterium avium-intracellulare

This is an opportunistic organism seen with increasing frequency in the GI tracts of AIDS patients. It often colonizes humans and has been isolated from soil, water, animals, birds, and food. It rarely causes disease except in immunocompromised patients with altered cell-mediated immunity. In patients with AIDS, *M. avium-intracellulare* infection is frequently life-threatening, involving multiple organs including the lung, lymph nodes, spleen, bone marrow, brain, adrenal glands, and gastrointestinal tract, as well as the blood. Disseminated *M. avium-intracellulare* infections are often fatal in patients with AIDS and are somewhat resistant to therapy.

Intestinal involvement with *M. avium-intracellulare* presents as diarrhea, malabsorption, weight loss, and fever. The organism may be detected in the small bowel or colon. Histologic examination shows typical acid-fast organisms, both free and within macrophages of the lamina propria. Pathologic findings of the small bowel are often typical of Whipple's disease, with foamy macrophages that are distended by vesicles containing periodic acid–Schiff (PAS)-positive material in the lamina propria. However, these organisms can be differentiated from Whipple's disease, since they are acid-fast positive. Small bowel radiographic appearances of the two disorders are similar, showing irregular nodularity and distorted villi.

The diagnosis of *M. avium-intracellulare* is based on stool culture identification of the organism with acid-fast stain of the stool, or characteristic histology of small bowel biopsy specimens. Blood cultures using special techniques from mycobacterial organism are frequently positive in AIDS patients who have disseminated *M. avium-intracellulare*. Strains of *M. avium-intracellulare* vary widely in their susceptibility to antibiotics. Most are highly resistant to antituberculous drugs, and current methods of treatment are unsatisfactory. The following drug regimen is sometimes (but not enthusiastically) recommended: rifampin, clofazimine, ethambutol, ethionamide, and amikacin. Other combinations include isoniazid, ethambutol, cycloserine, clofazimine, ethionamide, and ansamycin. These regimens have potential toxicity, and it is not known whether one combination of drugs is more efficacious than others. Reversal of immunosuppression and specific antiviral treatment against HIV may perhaps be more successful therapy for these opportunistic infections than specific treatment of *M. avium-intracellulare*.

Salmonella

Patients with defects in cell-mediated immunity, particularly AIDS, are prone to frequent and more serious infections with *Salmonella*, including gastroenteritis, enteric fever with bacteremia, and extraintestinal sites of infection. It is estimated that the incidence of salmonellosis is increased 20-fold in AIDS patients compared with the general population. The unique features in this patient population include the predominance of *S. typhimurium*, the lack of a clearly identifiable source of infection, the high rates of bacteremia, and the propensity of the infection to persist or recur despite the use of recommended antimicrobial regimens.

Although most authorities do not recommend treatment of nonimmunocompromised *Salmonella* carriers or patients who have only gastroenteritis with this organism, treatment is indicated for *Salmonella* infections in most AIDS patients because of the severe complications associated with these infections. The selection of a specific antimicrobial drug is based on the antibiotic sensitivity of the isolated strain. Some investigators have recommended long-term suppression with amoxicillin after the initial 2- to 3-week course for acute infection.

Shigella

Shigellosis in patients with AIDS appears to be comparable with the experience with salmonellosis, in that there is an unusual propensity for the organism to cause bacteremia and to recur after a therapeutic regimen of antibiotics. Diagnosis is made by selective culture of stool and blood. Treatment includes hydration and trimethoprim-sulfamethoxasole, 160 to 800 mg (double strength) orally twice a day for up to 7 days. Ampicillin can be used if the strain is sensitive.

Campylobacter

Campylobacter jejuni, *C. fetus*, *C. cinaedi*, and *C. fennelliae* have been isolated from homosexual men with and without HIV infection. Studies in symptomatic gay men with diarrhea and proctitis indicate recovery rates of 2 to 6 percent. Similar to *Shigella* and *Salmonella, Campylobacter* bacteremia and recurrent diarrhea following specific therapy has been reported. Selective antibiotic treatment is based on antibiotic sensitivities. Erythromycin, 500 mg orally four times a day for 7 days, is usually successful, except in immunocompromised individuals, who may require more prolonged therapy.

Herpes Simplex Virus

Infection of the oral cavity, esophagus, and anal-rectal area by herpes simplex virus (HSV) is common in homosexual men and some heterosexual women with HIV infection. With increasing immunosuppression, GI infection with HSV, particularly in the anal-rectal area, may become highly progressive and chronic. HSV of the oral region may also be reactivated in immunocompromised patients, resulting in severe oral, pharyngeal, and esophageal herpetic ulcerations. These lesions are usually painful and debilitating, and if left untreated may spread along the entire GI tract. Perianal ulcerations due to HSV may reach up to 10 cm or more in diameter in AIDS patients. Diagnosis is confirmed by viral culture or clinical and histologic criteria.

Treatment of all forms of HSV infection consists of acyclovir, which is available in oral and intravenous preparations. Patients with severe disease should receive the drug intravenously. The usual oral regimen is 200 mg five times daily. After successful treatment, all HIV-infected patients with herpes infection should receive suppressive therapy in the form of oral acyclovir, 200 mg three times daily.

Cytomegalovirus

GI infection with cytomegalovirus (CMV) is an extremely common finding in AIDS patients, being noted in up to 90 percent of autopsy series of AIDS cases. Almost all AIDS patients show serologic evidence of previous CMV infection, and the organism may be isolated from blood, semen, saliva, or intestinal biopsy specimens of most AIDS patients. Histologic or mucosal culture evidence of CMV may be demonstrated in any section of the GI tract. It may be associated with esophagitis, esophageal ulcerations, enteritis, colitis, or proctitis. Patients with CMV infection may present with a diffuse colitis associated with abdominal pain and watery or bloody diarrhea. In some cases, CMV infection may present as a solitary intestinal ulcer, toxic megacolon, or (rarely) intestinal perforation.

Contrast studies of CMV intestinal infection may reveal segmental colitis or pancolitis. A barium enema may show mucosal granularity, thickened folds, spasticity, and superficial erosions. CT studies may demonstrate marked thickening of the intestinal wall with mucosal ulcerations. Endoscopy typically shows focal or diffuse inflammatory changes with superficial ulcerations. Biopsies of lesions show CMV vasculitis with hemorrhagic inflammation in the lamina propria accompanied by typical CMV intranuclear inclusions within endothelial cells.

There currently is no FDA-approved treatment for CMV infection of the GI tract. However, initial studies of treatment with 9-(1,3-dihydroxy-2-propoxymethyl)guanine (DHPG), or Ganciclovir, demonstrate an effective response rate. In one study, 30 of 41 AIDS patients with CMV infection of the GI tract showed clinical improvement following DHPG, 5 mg per kilogram twice daily for 2 weeks; 13 had recurrences at a median time of 9 weeks after initiation of therapy. A similar experience was reported by the collaborative DHPG treatment study group.

Cryptosporidia

Cryptosporidium is a small protozoan parasite that primarily inhabits the microvillus region of intestinal epithelial cells. The parasite has been known to cause diarrhea in various animals, but human infection was not reported until 1976 when it was identified in immunocompromised individuals. Cryptosporidia also appear to be a relatively common cause of infectious diarrhea in immunocompetent patients in whom it causes a self-limited diarrheal illness. It may cause traveler's diarrhea. In immunocompromised patients such as those with AIDS, infection causes a chronic debilitating diarrhea that often results in death. The prevalence of cryptosporidia among AIDS patients is highly variable, depending on symptoms, geographic location, and diagnostic testing. In one study in the U.S., approximately 16 percent of AIDS patients with diarrhea had cryptosporidia, whereas in developing countries the rates of infection range from 8 to 57 percent.

In immunocompetent patients, cryptosporidia cause a diarrhea illness that begins 1 to 2 weeks after contact with an infected source, and lasts 10 to 21 days. Symptoms include nausea, vomiting, low-grade fever, abdominal cramps, pain, anorexia, and watery, frothy bowel movements that may be as frequent as five to ten per day. In immunocompromised individuals the symptoms may be more severe. Bowel movements may occur as often as 25 times a day. The mean duration of diarrhea in such individuals is 4 months, or until their death; weight loss may be as much as 37 percent of total body weight. Complications of cryptosporidial enterocolitis include cholecystitis, pancreatitis, and bronchial infection.

A multicenter trial of Sandostatin, a newly released somatostatin analogue, is now underway for secretory diarrhea in AIDS patients. There are at least two published reports of effectiveness. One of those AIDS patients had cryptosporidia.

Isospora

Isospora belli is another protozoan parasite that invades the microvillus of the small intestine and causes severe protracted diarrhea in patients with AIDS. Although heavily concentrated in the small intestine, *Isospora* can be found throughout the entire GI tract in immunocompromised patients. As with cryptosporidia, major clinical signs and symptoms of *Isospora* include watery diarrhea, abdominal cramps, nausea, vomiting, and weight loss. The diagnosis is made by identification of the oocysts in the stool using the same diagnostic methods described for cyptosporidia. The organism may also be identified on small bowel biopsies.

Unlike cryptosporidia, treatment of *Isospora* infection in immunocompromised individuals may result in marked improvement. In one study 15 patients with isosporiasis were treated with trimethoprim-sulfamethoxazole (IMP/SMZ) for 4 weeks, and in all resolution of diarrhea was noted within 2 days; seven patients relapsed and all responded to retreatment.

Microsporidia

Several AIDS patients presenting with chronic diarrheal illness have been found to have a microsporidial infection of the intestine, as demonstrated by electron microscopy of duodenal-jejunal and ideal biopsy specimens. Microsporidia are ubiquitous spore-forming protozoa that most commonly infect fish, but can also infect other invertebrates and vertebrates, including mammals. The preferred diagnostic method is electron microscopy of small bowel biopsy samples. The role of this organism as an agent of enteric disease is still not clear because of the relatively small number of cases and the lack of any antimicrobial agent to evaluate therapeutic response. The true prevalence of this organism is also unknown owing to the difficulty of diagnosis.

One patient with secretory diarrhea did respond to Sandostatin.

GASTROINTESTINAL NEOPLASMS

Kaposi's Sarcoma

Gastrointestinal involvement with Kaposi's sarcoma has been noted in up to 50 percent of homosexual men with dermatologic lesions of Kaposi's sarcoma. Such lesions can occur anywhere within the GI tract. The oral cavity is frequently involved, and the lesions often are symmetric and resemble submucosal hemorrhages. However, almost any level of the tract may be involved, including the pharynx, esophagus, stomach, small bowel, or colon. Chronic occult blood loss may occasionally occur, but otherwise the intestinal involvement is clinically silent. Sometimes, visceral lesions may predate cutaneous Kaposi's sarcoma, and one report showed that up to 30 percent of AIDS patients with Kaposi's sarcoma lesions in the GI tract have no skin lesions.

Diagnosis is usually confirmed by endoscopy. The characteristic endoscopic appearance is of raised, red nodules measuring several millimeters to 1 or 2 cm in diameter. Larger lesions may show central umbilication. Most of the lesions are clinically silent, although occasional patients have diarrhea, subacute intestinal obstruction, or protein-losing enteropathy. Bleeding is rare and endoscopic biopsies are not often complicated by bleeding, presumably owing to the location in the submucosa.

Treatment for cutaneous and mucosal lesions in the oral cavity is radiation or superficial electron beam irradiation. Chemotherapy with vinca alkaloids, such as vinblastine or vincristine, is also effective in most patients, but there are often complications of nausea, anorexia, vomiting, alopecia, and neutropenia. More recent studies with alpha-interferon in the treatment of cutaneous lesions have been promising, and trials are under way of therapy for GI lesions with this drug. Alternative regimens include combination chemotherapy such as doxorubicin (Adriamycin), bleomycin, and vinblastine; vinblastine and bleomycin; or vinblastine plus methotrexate or alpha-interferon.

Lymphomas

Lymphomas of the GI tract seen in association with AIDs include non-Hodgkin's lymphoma, Burkitt's lymphoma, and occasional cases of small, noncleaved, B-cell, Burkitt's-like lympoma (Table 3). The majority are high-grade B-cell lymphomas that respond poorly to chemotherapy. Patients frequently present with peripheral or abdominal lymphadenopathy and GI symptoms including diarrhea, spasms, constipation, or oral candidiasis. One patient was reported to have small bowel lymphomatous involvement with two spontaneous perforations. Diarrhea is usually secretory without steatorrhea, perhaps reflecting preservation of the villus architecture.

ORAL HAIRY LEUKOPLAKIA

Hairy leukoplakia is a newly recognized disorder that resembles leukoplakia and is seen predominantly in AIDS patients. It has fibrillar projections that extend outward from the surface of the lesion; its gross appearance is of a raised, white thickening on the tongue. Lesions are usually on the lateral border with a corrugated or hairy surface. Initially this may resemble oral candidiasis, and *Candida* or oral thrush is usually associated with these lesions. Histologic changes on biopsy resemble leukoplakia except for the absence of a mononuclear infiltrate. The cause of this lesion is unknown, but various studies have implicated human papillomavirus, herpes, cytomegalovirus, and Epstein-Barr virus (EBV).

Oral hairy leukoplakia is seen exclusively in the presence of HIV infection and represents a relatively poor

TABLE 3 Neoplasms Associated With Intestinal Disorders in Patients With AIDS and Patients at High Risk for AIDS

Kaposi's sarcoma
Diffuse, undifferentiated non-Hodgkin's lymphoma
Small bowel lymphoma
Burkitt's lymphoma
Small, noncleaved, B-cell, Burkitt's-like lymphoma
Squamous cell carcinoma of the tongue
Squamous cell carcinoma of the rectum
Cloacogenic carcinoma of the rectum

prognostic sign for the development of AIDS. There is no known effective treatment, but anecdotal reports have shown dramatic resolution with DHPG or acyclovir therapy.

SUGGESTED READING

Barlett JG, Laughon B, Quinn TC. Gastrointestinal complication of AIDS. In: DeVita VT, Hellman S, Rosenberg SA, eds. AIDS etiology, diagnosis, treatment and prevention. 2nd ed. Philadelphia: JB Lippincott, 1988:227.

Chachous A, Dieterich D, Krasinski K, et al. 9-(1,3-dihydroxy-2-propoxymethyl)guanine (Ganciclovir) in the treatment of cytomegalovirus gastrointestinal disease with the acquired immunodeficiency syndrome. Ann Intern Med 1987; 107:133.

DeHovitz JA, Pape JW, Boncy M, et al. Clinical manifestations and therapy of *Isospora belli* infection in patients with the acquired immunodeficiency syndrome. N Engl J Med 1986; 315:87.

Dobbins WO III, Weinstein WM. Electron microscopy of the intestine and rectum in acquired immunodeficiency syndrome. Gastroenterology 1985; 88:738.

Dworkin B, Wormser GP, Rosenthal WS, et al. Diarrhea and malabsorption associated with the acquired immunodeficiency syndrome (AIDS). Am J Gastroenterol 1985; 80:774.

Gillin JS, Shike M, Alcock N, et al. Malabsorption and mucosal abnormalities of the small intestine in the acquired immunodeficiency syndrome. Ann Intern Med 1985; 102:619.

Gillin JS, Urmacher C, West R, et al. Disseminated *Mycobacterium avium-intracellulare* infection in acquired infection in acquired immunodeficiency syndrome mimicking Whipple's disease. Gastroenterology 1983; 85:1187.

Greenspan D, Greenspan JA, Hearst NG, et al. Relation of oral hairy leukoplakia to infection with the human immunodeficiency virus and the risk of developing AIDS. J Infect Dis 1987; 155:475.

Jacobs JL, Gold JWM, Murray HW, et al. *Salmonella* infections in patients with the acquired immunodeficiency syndrome. Ann Intern Med 1985; 102:186.

Klein RS, Harris CA, Small CB, et al. Oral candidiasis in high risk patients as the initial manifestation of the acquired immunodeficiency syndrome. N Engl J Med 1984; 311:354.

Kotler DP, Gaetz HP, Lange M, et al. Enteropathy associated with the acquired immunodefiency syndrome. Ann Intern Med 1984; 101:421.

Laughon BE, Druckman DA, Vernon A, et al. Prevalence of enteric pathogens in homosexual men with and without AIDs. Gastroenterology 1988; 94:984.

Levinson W, Bennets RW. Cytomegalovirus colitis in acquired immunodeficiency syndrome: a chronic disease with varying manifestations. Am J Gastroenterol 1985; 80:445.

Malebranche R, Arnoux E, Grerin JM, et al. Acquired immunodeficiency syndrome with severe gastrointestinal manifestations in Haiti. Lancet 1985; 2:873.

Navin TR, Hardy AM. Cryptosporidiosis in patients with AIDS. J Infect Dis 1987; 155:150.

Quinn TC. Gastrointestinal manifestations of human immunodeficiency virus. In: Gottlieb MS, Jeffries DJ, Mildran D, et al, eds. Current topics in AIDS. Vol 1. New York: John Wiley, 1987:155.

Quinn TC, Stamm WE, Goodell SE, et al. The polymicrobial origin of intestinal infections in homosexual men. N Engl J Med 1983; 309:576.

Serwadda E, Mugewrwa RD, Sewankambo NK, et al. Slim disease: a new disease in Uganda and its association with HTLV-III infection. Lancet 1985; 2:849.

Totten PA, Fennell CL, Tenover FC, et al. *Campylobacter cinaedi* (sp. nov.) and *Campylobacter fennelliae* (sp. nov.): two new *Campylobacter* species associated with enteric disease in homosexual men. J Infect Dis 1985; 151:131.

HUMAN IMMUNODEFICIENCY VIRUS-ASSOCIATED NEPHROPATHY

T. K. SREEPADA RAO, M.D., F.A.C.P.

First described in the early 1980s, human immunodeficiency virus (HIV)-associated nephropathy—originally called acquired immunodeficiency syndrome-associated nephropathy (AAN)—was met with an initial skepticism by the renal community but is now recognized as a distinct entity with characteristic clinical and pathologic features. It is also becoming clear that patients infected with HIV can develop a variety of kidney diseases, some as a consequence of viral infection, some as a result of the use of therapeutic and diagnostic agents, and some unrelated to the primary disease per se. A classification of renal disorders in patients with HIV is listed in Table 1. Although the clinical experience with HIV-related renal diseases is growing, many issues still remain controversial, and unfortunately little data exist regarding the therapeutic approaches to be used in these patients. Nevertheless, clinicians should be aware of renal problems commonly encountered in HIV disease, especially those forms that are preventable and treatable. This chapter describes briefly the various HIV-associated renal disorders, but focuses mainly on some of the controversies surrounding the subject and on what little is known about the treatment options.

Many forms of acute reversible renal diseases are included in the subcategory of incidental renal disease and HIV infection (Table 2).

The most common form of reversible acute renal failure (ARF) encountered in the clinical management of patients with acquired immunodeficiency syndrome (AIDS) is acute tubular necrosis (ATN). It is not surprising that ATN is frequently seen in hospitalized acutely ill AIDS patients, in view of the natural history and severity of the disorder's multiple infectious complications and the need for the use of nephrotoxic drugs such as pentamidine, aminoglycosides, and radiocontrast agents

TABLE 1 Renal Disorders in Patients with HIV

Incidental renal disease and HIV infection
Various forms of potentially reversible acute renal failure
Fluid-electrolyte and acid-base abnormalities
Infections (bacterial, fungal, viral) of the kidney
Infiltrative diseases of the kidney
Specific renal disease and HIV-associated nephropathy
Focal and segmental glomerulosclerosis
Other forms of glomerulopathy
Unrelated renal disease in HIV-seropositive patients
Heroin-associated nephropathy
Diabetic nephropathy, polycystic kidney disease, and others
Obstructive nephropathy
HIV infection in patients receiving renal replacement therapy
Maintenance dialysis patients acquiring HIV from contaminated blood transfusions, intravenous drug abuse, and sexual contacts
Renal transplant recipients developing HIV infection through renal allograft, contaminated blood transfusions, intravenous drug abuse, and sexual contacts

TABLE 2 Incidental Renal Disorders and HIV

Acute renal failure
Acute tubular necrosis from hypovolemic, anoxic, and toxic injuries
Allergic interstitial nephritis from drugs such as trimethoprim-sulfamethoxazole, phenytoin, and other agents
Acute azotemia from nonsteroidal anti-inflammatory drugs
Renal edema from massive proteinuria and severe hypoalbuminemia
Postinfectious immune complex glomerulonephritis
Crystal-induced renal failure (sulfadiazine and acyclovir)
Plasmacytic interstitial nephritis
ARF from hemolytic-uremic syndrome and thrombotic thrombocytopenic purpura
Fluid, electrolyte, and acid-base derangements
Hyponatremia
Inappropriate secretion of antidiuretic hormone
Hypokalemia and hyperkalemia
Type IV renal tubular acidosis (hyporeninemic hypoaldosteronism)
Metabolic alkalosis
Hypomagnesemia
Infections in the kidney
Renal microabscesses from bacterial infections
Tuberculosis of the kidney (both typical and atypical mycobacterium)
Cytomegalovirus lesions
Cryptococcal, aspergillous, and other fungal diseases
Infiltrative diseases of the kidney
Lymphoma of the kidney
Kaposi's sarcoma
Amyloidosis of the kidney
Calcifications in the kidney

in their management. In many instances, ATN is a terminal event in AIDS patients treated in medical or surgical intensive care units with multiple organ failures and severely compromised hemodynamic status superimposed on sepsis, acidosis, and varying degrees of volume depletion. The majority of such patients die of renal failure from the primary illness, and both conservative and dialytic support fails to alter the prognosis. Nevertheless, when supported with dialysis, some patients recover sufficient renal function to survive the acute event, and a prolonged survival can thus be anticipated. It is therefore important for clinicians to realize that ATN is a potentially reversible and treatable complication in some patients with AIDS, and supportive measures such as meticulous attention to correction of fluid and electrolyte acid-base abnormalities, early dialysis treatment, and nutritional supplements should be employed as indicated. With such an approach, recovery of kidney function is likely, allowing time for the treatment of surviving patients with newer antiviral agents. Physicians caring for AIDS patients should also be cognizant of the fact that ATN may be a complication that can be prevented through the use of prophylactic measures—for example, maintenance of adequate hydration status in patients receiving intravenous contrast agents, being selective in the choice of antibiotics while treating infections, serially monitoring the serum creatinine concentrations and adjusting the dosage of the drug according to blood levels and renal function when aminoglycosides are used.

In renal failure attributable to hypersensitivity nephropathy from various drugs (especially trimethoprim-sulfamethoxazole), renal interstitial edema from massive proteinuria, and intrarenal hemodynamic derangements from nonsteroidal anti-inflammatory drugs the prognosis for recovery of kidney function is good. The clinical features and treatment of these forms of renal failure in AIDS patients are similar to those in the usual nephrologic patient. The problem of crystal-induced renal failure that attends the use of sulfadiazine and intravenous acyclovir is preventable by adequate hydration before their use. One report of an AIDS patient with nephrotic syndrome and renal failure secondary to plasmacytic interstitial nephritis (diagnosed by kidney biopsy) who responded well to corticosteroid therapy underscores the value of identifying treatable disorders and preventing progression to end-stage renal disease (ESRD).

Thrombocytopenia (without renal disease) is a frequently recognized complication of HIV disease. Over the past few years, an increasing number of cases of thrombotic thrombocytopenic purpura (TTP) are being recognized and reported in these patients, raising the question of a specific causal relationship between HIV infection, thrombocytopenia, and kidney failure. Similar speculation surrounds the question of sporadic cases of hemolytic-uremic syndrome (HUS) reported in AIDS patients. In published cases, renal failure from HUS and TTP in AIDS has been associated with a poor patient prognosis. Plasma exchange and infusion, corticosteroids, dialysis, and other supportive measures have been employed with little success in improving survival in HIV patients with TTP.

From the experiences reported over the past decade, it can be concluded that acute renal insufficiency in AIDS patients is incidental to the disease per se and is a consequence of various related and unrelated causes and therapies as might occur in patients with other illnesses complicated by hypotension and requiring nephrotoxic drug regimens. ARF contributes significantly to the morbidity and mortality associated with AIDS. In many patients, it is a terminal morbid event for which aggressive management results in minimal improvement, while in others, it is a reversible complication when appropriately treated. Intervention with early peritoneal dialysis or hemodialysis and other vigorous supportive measures are indicated in AIDS patients with ARF. It is also essential that physicians be aware of this complication and take the steps necessary to prevent the development of ARF in seriously ill AIDS patients by ensuring adequate hydration before administering radiocontrast agents and by either avoiding or minimizing the patients' exposure to nephrotoxic drugs.

One of the most interesting, unusual, and perhaps most controversial aspect of HIV disease in humans is HIV-associated nephropathy. Before the identification of HIV and serologic markers to detect infection, clinicians employed the guidelines adopted by the Centers for Disease Control (CDC) for the diagnosis of AIDS. Consequently, in their original description, Rao et al coined the term AIDS-associated nephropathy to describe a new renal syndrome. Subsequently it became obvious that nephropathy could be found in asymptomatic carriers of the virus (HIV-seropositive individuals), and in those with AIDS-related complex (ARC), and the name was appropriately changed to HIV-associated nephropathy (HIVAN). Although the initial reports of HIVAN were from the New York and Miami areas, several publications have since appeared from many centers in the United States and from other countries including the United Kingdom, Canada, Spain, Brazil, Trinidad, Mexico, and France. The number of cases of HIVAN seen at institutions in both New York and Miami has also increased progressively during recent years.

CLINICAL FEATURES

HIVAN occurs in asymptomatic HIV-seropositive patients and in those with ARC and AIDS. Approximately half of the patients are intravenous drug addicts, and the remainder include homosexual men, recent immigrants from Haiti (mostly in the Brooklyn and Miami areas) who deny intravenous drug use or homosexuality, recipients of contaminated blood products, sexual partners of HIV-infected persons, and children born to infected mothers. The disease is more common in young men (having an incidence of 83 percent), and less than 10 percent of patients are whites. In brief, HIVAN is predominantly a disease of young black men. Approximately 80 cases of renal disease in HIV-afflicted children have been reported. The disease is commonly manifested by heavy proteinuria with the nephrotic syndrome, and at times the onset is sudden. Many of the patients at my institution who have been followed in the HIV clinic with no evidence of renal disease have had explosive presentations with edema and/or severe renal insufficiency during routine follow-up visits.

Massive proteinuria is generally accompanied by either normal creatinine clearance (C_{cr}), or varying degrees of azotemia. Many patients are severely uremic on their initial visit to hospital. Occasionally, the initial features include hematuria, with non-nephrotic range proteinuria, along with normal or impaired C_{cr}. The majority of patients are normotensive and continue to be so despite progression to irreversible uremia. Hypertension, if present at all, is generally mild and not a management problem. Serologic studies reveal HIV seropositivity, with a diminution in the absolute number of circulating CD4 cells and a reversal in the ratio of helper/suppressor T lymphocytes. This finding is observed even in asymptomatic HIV carriers who have the nephropathy. Ultrasonographic examination reveals enlarged and markedly echogenic kidneys during the nephrotic stage of the illness as well as with the onset of ESRD, a finding also substantiated by autopsy studies. Some clinicians have attempted to diagnose HIVAN through ultrasonographic examination of the kidney by grading the echogenecity, but this finding remains to be confirmed by other observers.

The unusual clinical aspect of HIVAN is the fulminant deterioration of renal function to irreversible uremia in the absence of contributing factors such as severe hypertension, volume depletion, or exposure to nephrotoxic agents. Renal histologic examination also fails to explain the malignant nature of renal functional loss. In most reports, the progression to ESRD has been measured in a few weeks to a few months (average of about 4 months), although great variation exists. This observation contrasts strikingly with the clinical course of patients with focal segmental glomerulosclerosis (FSGS) found in association with heroin addiction and idiopathic causes. In patients with HIVAN and ESRD who are only seropositive and who do not meet the CDC criteria for AIDS, maintenance dialysis therapy is tolerated well and prolonged survival and rehabilitation have also been noted. On the other hand, the survival rate and rehabilitation of patients with clinical AIDS and with chronic uremia secondary to HIVAN can only be considered dismal and unsatisfactory at the present time. Despite renal replacement therapy, ESRD in AIDS is generally associated with a patient survival of less than 1 year. During hemodialysis therapy, a major problem is unexplained malnutrition and a wasting phenomenon without evidence for an underlying malignancy and/or an opportunistic infection. AIDS patients manifesting a "failure to thrive" syndrome fail to respond to hyperalimentation, and death results from a combination of cachexia with superimposed opportunistic and or other intercurrent infections. However, this grim prognosis may be changing in recent times because of newer antiviral agents in the therapeutic approaches to HIV patients in the early stages of the disease.

RENAL PATHOLOGIC FEATURES

The typical renal histologic lesion consists of FSGS, with intraglomerular deposition of IgM and C3. Although FSGS is the most common finding, accounting for 82 percent of cases in which renal histology has been included, other infrequently encountered glomerular changes include minimal change disease, mesangial proliferation, and membranous and membranoproliferative glomerulonephritis. In children, mesangial and proliferative glomerular lesions predominate. Nevertheless, if one considers that mesangial changes may represent an early form of and are likely to progress to FSGS, then a sclerosing glomerulopathy accounts for more than 90 percent of patients with HIVAN. The light microscopic features of HIV-associated FSGS are also characterized by hyperplastic visceral epithelial cells with coarse cytoplasmic vacuoles and a greater and widespread collapse of the underlying capillary walls. The most striking pathologic features are seen in the renal tubular alterations and include severe tubular degenerative changes, tubular microectasia commonly referred to as "microcystic dilatation," and lumens filled with pale staining proteinaceous casts. Dilated tubules are present throughout the renal cortex and medulla. There is a notable absence of interstitial infiltrates, interstitial fibrosis, and arteriolar changes of hypertension. The interstitium is mildly and diffusely edematous and contains few lymphocytes, monocytes, and mononuclear cells. Even during late stages of the disease, tubular atrophy and interstitial fibrosis are not prominent.

As demonstrated by immunofluorescence microscopy, there is localization of IgM, C3, and C1q in the sclerosed segments (and sometimes in other mesangial regions), and no other unusual changes have been observed in renal biopsies. However, characteristic ultrastructural lesions considered by some to be distinctive are found in patients with FSGS secondary to HIVAN. These lesions consist of multiple complex inclusions both in the nuclei and cytoplasm in a variety of cells, abundant tubuloreticular inclusions in the vascular (glomerular, peritubular capillary, arterial, and venular) endothelium, and interstitial cell cytoplasm. These inclusions are numerous and readily observable, and their incidental discovery in renal biopsies of otherwise unsuspected patients might suggest a HIV carrier state. Additional changes include the presence of a greater number of complex and heterogenous nuclear bodies, and a peculiar granulofibrillary transformation in the tubular and interstitial cell nuclei. Multiple complex (types III and IV) and budding forms of nuclear bodies are increasingly found in AIDS patients with proteinuria. It should be noted, however, that these peculiar lesions are not limited to renal tissues and resemble those found in lymphocytes, several cell types of different organs from AIDS patients, and in the germinal centers of lymph nodes from patients with ARC. Based on these findings, a viral etiology for HIVAN has been strongly suggested. The recent in situ hybridization studies by Cohen et al demonstrating the proviral HIV DNA in renal tubular and glomerular epithelial cells offer strong support for the viral invasion theory regarding the causation of HIVAN. Whether HIV alone can cause structural and functional changes in the kidney or whether other viral and bacterial agents are also involved remains to be seen. It is also not known whether renal cells contain or manifest receptors for CD4 cells that might facilitate viral entry and subsequent replication.

CONTROVERSIES

Geographic and Racial Differences

The great majority of cases of HIVAN have been reported from urban areas of the United States that treat large numbers of intravenous drug addicts, blacks, and other minorities. For unknown reasons, the nephropathy is extremely rare in San Francisco despite the high prevalence of HIV disease in that city, and at the National Institutes of Health, workers were also unable to discern renal lesions in either clinical or autopsy studies of kidney tissues derived primarily from homosexual men with AIDS. This discrepancy has led not only to questioning of the validity of HIVAN as a distinct entity, but also to several speculations regarding explanations for these divergent observations. The issue of racial and geographic differences is obviously a fundamental question pertinent not only to HIVAN, but also to the complex, poorly understood problem of interaction of the various risk factors that greatly predispose individuals with certain ethnic backgrounds to develop irreversible renal failure. According to the Health Care Finance Administration (HCFA), in 1984, the annual incidence of ESRD for nonwhites (consisting primarily of the American black population) was 217 per million, approximately three times greater than the incidence of 81 per million for whites. Epidemiologic studies have also provided data supporting the fact that hypertensive nephrosclerosis, diabetes mellitus, heroin-associated nephropathy, and certain forms of interstitial nephritis all lead to ESRD in blacks at a higher rate than in whites. Although these findings have been consistently noted over many years of data collection, the factors responsible for this remarkable predisposition to ESRD remains unexplained. Some have suggested a possible genetic factor, while others have speculated that, in blacks, an unknown inherent susceptibility of the kidneys to immunologic, vascular, and other forms of injury accounts for this predisposition. This increased incidence of renal disease in blacks is even more starkly evident in reported cases of HIVAN, especially in the overall context of AIDS in the United States. Of all AIDS cases reported to the CDC, 62 percent occurred in whites, whereas only 24 percent occurred in blacks. By striking contrast, an analysis of the incidence of HIVAN reveals that more than 90 percent of patients are blacks, while less than 10 percent are whites. Both in San Francisco, and in the eastern states, geographic regions with the highest reported incidence of AIDS, HIVAN is rare in white homosexual men and is typically found in black homosexual men. Soni et al found that even though the incidence and severity of proteinuria was equivalent in blacks and hispanics with AIDS, 22.8 percent of blacks as compared with only 6.9 percent of hispanics progressed to renal insufficiency, once again indicating a strong influence of racial factor in ESRD. It seems evident that the black race per se is a major cofactor in the predisposition of patients with HIV infection to acquire a nephropathy and to progress to chronic uremia.

Role of Heroin Addiction

Since approximately half of patients with HIVAN are intravenous drug users and the renal histologic lesions resemble those described previously in narcotic addicts with heroin-associated nephropathy (reported by many workers several years before the AIDS epidemic), it has been argued that the renal disease in HIV patients was related to drug abuse rather than to viral infection. The contribution of intravenous drug abuse to the development of nephropathy in AIDS is clearly evident, as heroin addicts constitute the single largest group of patients with HIVAN; however, they still account for only about half of the reported cases. In a careful survey of published reports, as well as in an analysis by Bourgoignie et al, of the risk factors influencing the occurrence of renal disease in HIV patients in different parts of the country, it has been established that there is a strong correlation between HIVAN and the black race and less of a correlation between HIVAN and intravenous drug use. Critics have misinterpreted the reported studies of patients with HIVAN and ascribed the nephropathy seen in HIV-infected patients almost exclusively to intravenous drug addiction. A closer examination of the data dismisses this notion. The major groups of subjects at high risk for acquiring HIV infection are homosexual men, and intravenous drug addicts who constitute 62 percent and 26 percent, respectively, of all adult AIDS cases in the United States. On the other hand, when one tabulates the numbers of patients with HIVAN, it is found that heroin addicts account for about 55 percent of cases, clearly a majority, emphasizing the foremost although not the only contribution of intravenous drug abuse for the development of renal disease. What is generally not recognized and appreciated is the fact that the remaining 45 percent of patients with HIVAN are comprised of nonaddicts including homosexual men, Haitian immigrants, recipients of contaminated blood products, sexual contacts of HIV-infected persons, and most importantly, children born to infected mothers. The presence of a nephrotic syndrome and FSGS in HIV-infected children in whom intravenous drug abuse can be excluded without a doubt is crucial evidence that there are factors other than heroin abuse in the genesis of nephropathy.

The obvious question that this argument raises is: in an intravenous drug addict with nephrotic syndrome, is it possible to differentiate between HAN and HIVAN, especially in those addicts who are also HIV seropositive and clinically asymptomatic? Although the distinction is not always possible to make, evidence accumulated thus far suggests several criteria for separating the two diseases both on clinical and histopathologic grounds. Features common to both entities as well as their differences are listed in Tàble 3. The natural history of patients with heroin-associated nephropathy (HAN) followed clinically indicates that renal function deterioration is slow and gradual, occurring over a period of years, during which time shrinkage of kidney size occurs that can be demonstrated sonographically. A majority of patients with HAN develop difficult to manage moderate-to-severe hypertension with the onset of renal insufficiency. Drug addicts with ESRD who are treated by either maintenance dialysis or renal transplantation often have a prolonged survival and rehabilitation. Serial renal biopsies in patients with HAN show the evolution of segmental sclerosis to total global glomerulosclerosis, along with severe interstitial fibrosis, marked interstitial infiltration of chronic inflammatory cells, and prominent changes of arteriolosclerosis. These characteristics found in HAN contrast with those seen in HIVAN, including

TABLE 3 Distinguishing HAN from HIVAN

Features	*HAN*	*HIVAN*
Young men	Yes	Yes
90 percent are black	Yes	Yes
Intravenous drug addiction (100% in HAN vs. 55% in HIVAN)	Yes	Yes
Nephrotic syndrome	Yes	Yes
Azotemia of varying degree	Yes	Yes
Focal and segmental glomerulosclerosis	Yes	Yes
Drug addiction	100%	50-60%
Children	No	Yes
Renal sonography	Large	Large
Renal size (ESRD)	Small	Large
Progression to ESRD	2-4 yrs.	3-4 mos.
Hypertension	Yes	No
Renal pathology	FSGS	FSGS with microcystic dilatation of tubules
Electron microscopy		Tubulo-reticular structures
Viral genome	No	Yes
Prognosis of ESRD	Stable course	High mortality

a malignant clinical deterioration in renal function with development of ESRD within weeks of onset of proteinuria, the presence of large kidneys, persistent normotension, and a poor patient prognosis with maintenance dialysis. Many unusual light microscopic and some distinct ultrastructural renal histologic features described above can also distinguish HIVAN from HAN. The localization of HIV p24 antigens in the glomerular capillaries in some cases, and elegant studies by Cohen et al demonstrating HIV genome in the kidney tissues of patients with HIVAN and their absence in HAN are other unique differences between the two diseases. It is also fair to conclude from many studies that in some addicts, drug abuse and HIV infection may exert an additive effect not only in inducing renal disease but also in the fulminant progression to uremia and the subsequent poor survival.

Because a great majority of the AIDS patients studied at San Francisco and at the National Institutes of Health were homosexual white men and only a few were intravenous drug addicts, it is not surprising to find a low incidence of HIVAN at these centers. The regional and racial differences in the attack rate of HIVAN has stimulated speculation that other cofactors strongly influence renal susceptibility, and the conflicting rates of incidence of renal lesions in different parts of the country. These include infection with variant strains of HIV in different high-risk groups, superimposition of other viral infections, the varying nature and type of opportunistic infections present, or (perhaps) the existence of specific immune response genes in the black population. A recent study that found that a higher phenotype frequency of DR4 antigens in those patients with idiopathic forms of FSGS (both whites and blacks) and of BW53 and DR5 in those with HAN (blacks) is consistent with a genetic theory, partially explaining the racial differences without offering insights into the pathogenesis of the disease.

A Spectrum of Renal Pathologic Lesions

FSGS is clearly the most common glomerular pathology in HIVAN, accounting for 82 percent of cases reported in which renal histology was included. However, if one assumes that the mesangial changes represent an early form of the disease and are likely to progress to FSGS with time, the proportion of sclerosing lesion (approximately 90 percent) in HIVAN becomes even more evident. Such a strong association of one type of glomerular alteration is clearly remarkable and is unlikely to be due to chance.

"FSGS" is simply a nonspecific, descriptive term implying a morphologic change, providing no insights into the etiology or pathogenesis of the disease; to this extent, FSGS is like many other glomerular lesions. Our understanding of all forms of FSGS seen in clinical practice, including the most frequently encountered idiopathic variety, has been and continues to be a disorder without an adequate explanation. No evidence proves or disproves a theory of immune pathogenesis in FSGS. Similarly, although an immune-mediated renal response secondary to either HIV or components of the virus (core or the envelope protein) or to other infectious agents has been proposed as a reason for the development of nephropathy in patients with AIDS, data are lacking to support this contention. Compounding this ignorance is a lack of knowledge regarding the role of viruses, including HIV, in the induction of renal disease in general. Cohen et al, who provided objective evidence of a direct viral invasion of the kidneys, suggest that HIVAN is a lesion that involves virtually all renal parenchymal cells and that perhaps a single form of viral injury might directly or indirectly result in diverse morphologic renal lesions. In systemic lupus erythematosus (SLE), considered by some to be a viral-induced disease, it is clear that, when challenged with similar homogeneous antigens (nuclear antigen), the renal response may consist of disparate histologic alterations from minimal change to mesangial hyperplasia, focal, diffuse proliferative, and membranous forms of glomerulonephritis, or it may consist of predominantly interstitial changes. Paradoxically, a wide variety of heterogeneous antigens can induce a glomerular response identical to that seen in patients with membranous glomerulonephritis of such diversified etiologies as idiopathic causes, SLE, syphilis, hepatitis B infection, and drugs such as gold and penicillamine. Obviously in both SLE and membranous glomerulonephritis as well as in experimental forms of glomerulonephritis in animals, the renal lesion evoked is largely determined by the qualitative and quantitative type of host immune response(s) to varying amount(s) and the nature of antigen(s) presented. Patients with HIV disease are prone to infections with a variety of bacterial, viral, fungal, and protozoal agents that can significantly effect the nature of renal response to injury. Therefore it should not be surprising that a wide spectrum of glomerular morphologic changes can also be provoked in patients with HIVAN, while in fact, FSGS is found in 90 percent of patients with HIVAN and massive proteinuria.

Based on the many recently published reviews on HIVAN, it seems appropriate to focus our attention on elucidating the pathogenesis of HIVAN and devising treatment options to prevent what is currently an inexorable renal disease. In this context, the preliminary work of Alpers et al has described FSGS in rhesus monkeys infected with the simian immunodeficiency virus that is similar to that found in humans with HIV. This experimental model offers hope that viral etiology of HIVAN—and possibly the role of other viruses in idiopathic forms of glomerular and nonglomerular renal diseases—may be elucidated.

THERAPEUTIC APPROACHES

Unfortunately, little information exists regarding the treatment of patients with HIVAN. I am aware of anecdotal cases of FSGS secondary to HIVAN (patients without evidence of clinical AIDS or ARC) treated unsuccessfully with short courses of prednisone. Before HIV serologic studies were available, we administered prednisone to two patients with HIVAN, and in both, severe oral candidiasis developed within 2 weeks of therapy and steroids had to be discontinued. Both patients progressed to ESRD rapidly and began receiving maintenance hemodialysis. Thus, because of the possible risks of prednisone therapy in precipitating or aggravating conventional and opportunistic infection in these patients, it seems prudent not to administer prolonged courses of steroids. Because of poor compliance in a majority of our patients with HIVAN, we have generally not employed corticosteroids or other immunosuppressive drugs and have resorted to supportive care only, including nutritional support and salt restriction.

The results of antiviral agents, specifically the effects of zidovudine (AZT) (currently the only agent approved for broad clinical use) on the natural history of HIVAN are unknown. AZT, an analogue of thymidine formed by the substitution of the hydroxyl group with the azide group, is the drug that has been studied the most widely in patients with HIV and is the one with which there is the most clinical experience to date. By undergoing enzymatic phosphorylation inside the host cell, AZT causes the termination of DNA chain synthesis by HIV, thus inhibiting viral replication. The bioavailability of AZT taken orally is 60 percent with an elimination half-life of about 1 hour. AZT is metabolized in the liver to glucuronidated AZT (GAZT), and its half-life parallels that of AZT. Renal clearance of AZT is 350 ml per minute per 70 kg. The drug reaches the spinal fluid rapidly and is not nephrotoxic. After a standard dose of 200 mg in patients with advanced renal insufficiency ($C_{cr} < 20$ ml per minute), and in anuric individuals, neither the plasma AZT levels nor the half-life is significantly altered compared with normals (although in one study, both parameters were increased). GAZT accumulates, however, and the plasma levels are greatly elevated in the presence of renal failure. During hemodialysis, the clearance of AZT ranges from 63 to 102 ml per minute. Since this accounts for about 5 to 8 percent of residual renal clearance, hemodialysis has no appreciable effect on AZT elimination and supplemental doses are not needed in dialysis patients. On the other hand, hemodialyzer clearance of GAZT is 71 to 91 ml per minute, which is much larger than the renal clearance. The biological effects of high levels of GAZT in renal failure patients is unknown. Although studies analyzing the toxicity of AZT in uremic patients are unavailable, limited experience (at our institution and others) indicate that anemia is a major limiting factor in the use of AZT. Anemia secondary to AZT therapy in nonazotemic patients is associated with high levels of serum erythropoietin, and whether or not exogenous erythropoietin therapy can minimize the transfusion requirements in patients with or without renal disease is yet to be determined. Other than mild gastrointestinal intolerances, insomnia, and myalgias, a major side effect of AZT is its effect on the bone marrow. In the original controlled studies, a reduction in the hemoglobin levels, a reduction in the total WBC count, and neutropenia, or a combination of all three were observed in approximately 40 to 45 percent of patients.

A multicenter, double-blind, placebo-controlled trial of AZT in patients with AIDS or advanced ARC clearly demonstrated its efficacy in decreasing the incidence of opportunistic infections, a sixfold reduction in deaths, an increase in CD4 cells, and a return of delayed hypersensitivity reactions. Experimental studies also showed that if AZT is administered immediately after virus exposure, retrovirus infection is prevented and viral replication in previously infected animals is reduced. Human studies have also established the beneficial value of AZT in asymptomatic HIV-seropositive patients.

Until the recent past, there has been a great reluctance on the part of most physicians to prescribe AZT to patients with renal disease, primarily because of a lack of knowledge of pharmacokinetics and the side effect profile of AZT in the presence of renal insufficiency. The Food and Drug Administration's approval of AZT for the treatment of asymptomatic HIV carriers has resulted in its broader usage, including its use in HIV patients with renal failure regardless of whether or not they suffer from clinical AIDS. Although studies dealing with the disposition and half-life of the drug in patients with severe renal impairment and the influence of hemodialysis on the removal of free AZT and metabolites provide us with guidelines for the use of AZT, few data are available regarding its efficacy or adverse consequences on the renal manifestations in HIV disease. It appears that an AZT dose of 200 mg given four times per day with monitoring of GAZT plasma levels may be appropriate in patients with renal failure. The dose may need to be reduced if additional studies reveal GAZT to have toxic effects in uremia. Currently, some studies show that AZT can be effectively used at a dose of 600 mg per day, as compared to the conventional 1.2 g per day in patients with normal renal function. If these findings are confirmed, the dosage may have to be halved in azotemic patients also.

Two issues pertinent to antiviral therapy and HIV disease are (1) whether AZT prevents the development of nephropathy if administered before the onset of renal markers (proteinuria, azotemia, hematuria), and (2) whether the drug alters the course of established HIVAN. In the experience at my institution, many patients with HIV disease (both asymptomatic seropositive carriers and ARC/AIDS patients with no evidence of clinical renal disease), who received AZT subsequently developed typical features of HIVAN and progressed to irreversible uremia. On each occasion, with the onset of renal insufficiency, AZT therapy was discontinued. With regard to the second issue, I am currently treating a patient who has had HIVAN with AZT for more than 2 years with a remission of the nephrotic syndrome (although proteinuria persists) and stable normal C_{cr} for more than 2 years. The use of AZT in two of our pediatric patients with HIV nephropathy was ineffective in inducing a remission and in preventing renal failure. Two reports have appeared indicating the beneficial effects of AZT in HIVAN. In one patient (from the Detroit area) with HIVAN (FSGS, microcystic dilatation of tubules, and tubuloreticular inclusions on biopsy), and a serum creatinine concentration of 8.1 mg per deciliter, AZT in a dose of 200 mg every 4 hours resulted in stabilization of the slope of decline of 1/cr (no additional details given). The second case report from France deals with a patient with HIVAN (massive proteinuria and FSGS on biopsy), who had remission of nephrotic syndrome and normal renal function for 11 months when receiving AZT therapy (800 mg per day). In this patient, AZT was discontinued after 11 months because of severe anemia, resulting in a rapid decline in renal function leading to ESRD within 1 month. These authors also comment on another patient in whom 5 months of AZT therapy led to a temporary discontinuation of chronic hemodialysis therapy. From these anecdotal case reports, we can only suggest that AZT may offer hope for patients with HIVAN. The widespread use of erythropoietin in the successful management of anemia of chronic uremia may circumvent the present limitations and facilitate prolonged administration of AZT treatment to a large number of patients with HIVAN. Since studies suggest that extended AZT treatment is essential in preventing complications of HIV infection, it is hoped that a protracted course of AZT therapy may also alter the natural history of HIVAN, and prevent progression to irreversible renal failure.

UNRELATED RENAL DISEASE AND HIV

Current estimates are that there are more than a million individuals who are carriers of HIV in the United States, and it is logical to expect that these patients can acquire renal diseases secondary to other causes such as diabetes mellitus and polycystic kidneys. We have cared for such patients at our institution, and many centers in the United States have had a similar experience. The increasing availability of serologic screening tests for HIV will undoubtedly uncover more such patients in the future. In addition, ESRD patients undergoing either maintenance hemodialysis or peritoneal dialysis or renal transplantation may contract HIV infection through contaminated blood transfusions, use of intravenous drugs, sexual contacts, and rarely, via renal allograft. The seroprevalence rate in dialysis centers is generally low (0 to 3 percent) except in certain areas where as many as 40 percent of patients may be positive. The exclusion of high-risk individuals as organ and blood donors, refinements in the HIV diagnostic procedures, and the introduction of mandatory screening of transfused blood and organ donors before their use has practically eliminated these modes of transmission of the virus.

Other issues which are also of concern to nephrologists are (1) the effects of maintenance dialysis on the clinical outcome in otherwise asymptomatic HIV-seropositive individuals; (2) the impact that caring for HIV patients has on the renal staff; and (3) renal transplantation in HIV carriers.

The Effects of Maintenance Dialysis on the Clinical Outcome

Many dialysis centers have studied this question, and in summary, it is safe to say that if both hemodialysis and peritoneal dialysis do not adversely affect the progression of the HIV carrier state to ARC or clinical AIDS, prolonged survival can be expected. Uniformly most workers believe that when dialysis patients develop clinical AIDS, the majority are likely to die within less than 1 year. Whether or not AZT therapy will modify these grim statistics in ESRD patients is unknown. In high-risk patients treated by dialysis, screening for HIV is appropriate for the following reasons:

1. Patients should be counseled to prevent further transmission to sexual contacts.
2. To determine the need for antiviral (AZT) therapy, vaccinations against pneumonococcal pneumonia, influenza, and possibly hepatitis B.
3. To provide prophylaxis against *Pneumocystis carinii*, *Candida*, toxoplasmosis, and herpes simplex.
4. To provide early diagnosis and treatment of tuberculosis (both atypical and typical).
5. As surveillance for the onset of lymphomas, Kaposi's sarcoma, and other opportunistic infections, and to provide early intervention.
6. To secure social benefits for patients, obtain epidemiologic data, and diagnose HIV infection.

The Impact That Caring for HIV Patients Has on the Renal Staff

HIV disease has significantly influenced major urban dialysis units in terms of recruiting, and retaining staff members to provide continued care. Although CDC has established precautionary guidelines for providing dialysis care, most centers employ additional modifications to suit their own needs. All published reports to date, which have specifically examined the question of potential risks to staff members, have concluded that the transmissibility of HIV from patients to staff is negligible when appropriate precautions are taken. No cases of nosocomial transmission of HIV has been recorded, even in a high-prevalence dialysis unit.

Renal Transplantation in HIV Carriers

A few cases of transmission of HIV through the renal allograft has been reported in Europe and the United States. In each of these instances, the kidney donor either belonged to a group at high risk for HIV or was the recipient of a large amount of blood before organ harvesting. Some recipients of infected kidney have subsequently developed clinical AIDS, while others have continued to remain asymptomatic with good graft function despite immunosuppressive therapy. The current policy of routine testing of donors before transplantation and exclusion of high-risk individuals as donors should lead to a virtual disappearance of such transmission in the future.

The other question for which data are limited is the feasibility of renal transplantation in asymptomatic HIV seropositive subjects. Few retrospective studies have indicated that the use of immunosuppressive drugs after transplantation in such patients leads to an increased number of infectious complications, resulting in a high patient mortality. Also reported are a few HIV positive transplant recipients who, in spite of receiving corticosteroids and cyclosporine, have survived for longer periods with functioning grafts and no evidence of clinical disease. In view of these uncertainties and lack of adequate information, at present most centers are reluctant to perform renal transplantation in asymptomatic HIV carriers.

SUGGESTED READING

Alpers CE, Baskin GB. Sclerosing glomerulopathy in rhesus monkeys with simian AIDS. Kidney Int 1989; 55:339.

Bourgoignie JJ, Meneses R, Ortiz C, et al. The clinical spectrum of renal disease associated with human immunodeficiency virus. Am J Kidney Dis 1988; 12:131–137.

Carbone L, D'Agati V, Suh JI, et al. Course and prognosis of human immunodeficiency virus associated nephropathy. Am J Med 1989; 87:389–395.

Chander P, Soni A, Suri A, et al. Renal untrastructural markers in AIDS-associated nephropathy. Am J Pathol 1987; 126:513–526.

Cohen AH, Nast CC. HIV-associated nephropathy: a unique combined glomerular, tubular, and interstitial lesion. Modern Pathol 1988; 1:87–97.

Cohen AH, Sun NCJ, Shapshak P, Imagawa DT. Demonstration of human immunodeficiency virus in renal epithelium in HIV-associated nephropathy. Modern Pathol 1989; 2:125–128.

D'Agati V, Suh JI, Carbone L, et al. Pathology of HIV-associated nephropathy: a detailed morphologic and comparative study. Kidney Int 1989; 35:1358–1370.

Rao TKS, Friedman EA. AIDS (HIV)-associated nephropathy: does it exist? An in-depth review. Am J Nephrol 1989; 9:441–453.
Rao TKS, Nicastri AD, Friedman EA. Renal consequences of narcotic abuse. In: Hamburger J, Crosnier J, Grunfeld JP, eds. Nephrology. New York: John Wiley & Sons, 1979:843.
Rao TKS, Nicastri AD, Friedman EA. The nephropathies of drug addiction and acquired immunodeficiency syndrome. In: Tisher CC, Brenner BM, eds. Renal pathology with clinical and functional correlations. Vol. 1. Philadelphia: JB Lippincott Company, 1989:340.
Soni A, Agarwal A, Chander P, et al. Evidence for an HIV-related nephropathy: a clinico-pathologic study. Clin Nephrol 1989; 31:12–17.

NEUROLOGIC DISEASES ASSOCIATED WITH HIV-1 INFECTION

JUSTIN McARTHUR, M.B., B.S., M.P.H.

The nervous system is frequently involved during human immunodeficiency virus type 1 (HIV-1) infection, sometimes before advanced immune deficiency develops. Approximately 40 percent of patients with acquired immunodeficiency syndrome (AIDS) or AIDS-related complex (ARC) will develop one or more neurologic syndromes, and 10 percent of all patients will initially present with nervous system complaints. About half of the neurologic manifestations appear to be related to the direct or indirect effects of HIV-1, and the other half result from secondary complications of the immune deficiency induced by HIV-1. The HIV-1–related neurologic disorders are incompletely understood, and the full spectrum of nervous system involvement with HIV-1 infection remains unclear. However, treatment is available for most of the disorders, particularly if they are recognized at an early stage.

HIV-1–RELATED NEUROLOGIC DISORDERS

Some of these disorders occur early in the incubation period of HIV-1 infection, before any constitutional symptoms have developed. Others typically occur in patients with ARC or AIDS. The timing of these specific disorders, the differences in course, and the pathologic differences clearly suggest that different pathogenetic mechanisms underlie them.

HIV-1–Related Meningitis

One to two percent of recently infected individuals will develop acute aseptic meningitis with headache, meningismus, cranial neuropathies, and occasionally, transient encephalopathy. HIV-1–related meningitis appears to represent the initial response of the central nervous system (CNS) to viral invasion, and there is intrathecal synthesis of antibody to HIV-1. As many as 30 percent of HIV-1 carriers have a more indolent variant of HIV-1–related meningitis with chronic pleocytosis and headaches. Typically the acute symptoms of HIV-1–related meningitis are self-limited, require only symptomatic treatment with analgesics and antipyretics, and resolve within a few weeks. Serologic testing for HIV-1 (and probably human T-cell lymphotrophic virus type 1 [HTLV-1]) should be part of the evaluation of patients with aseptic meningitis or chronic pleocytosis. It is uncertain whether the development of symptomatic meningitis or the detection of silent cerebrospinal fluid (CSF) abnormalities are predictive of subsequent progressive neurologic involvement.

HIV-1 Encephalopathy

Approximately 20 percent of patients with AIDS or ARC will show signs of a progressive subcortical dementia, and this syndrome has now been added to the list of AIDS-defining illnesses (Table 1). Also termed HIV-1–related dementia, AIDS dementia complex, and subacute encephalitis, the mental dulling, intellectual impairment, and memory loss can initially be mistaken for depression or other psychi-

TABLE 1 Major Neurologic Complications of HIV-1 Infection

HIV-1–Related	*Opportunistic Processes*
Acute aseptic meningitis	Cryptococcal meningitis*
Chronic pleocytosis	Toxoplasmosis*
HIV-1 encephalopathy*	CMV retinitis/encephalitis*
Vacuolar myelopathy	Other CNS opportunistic infections*
Predominantly sensory neuropathy	Herpes group radiculitis
Inflammatory demyelinating polyneuropathy	Progressive multifocal leukoencephalopathy*
Mononeuritis multiplex	Primary CNS lymphoma*
Myopathy	Systemic lymphoma*
	Neurosyphilis

* AIDS-defining condition.

atric syndromes. The disorder occurs in all groups at risk for HIV-1 infection, including children. The prevalence in *healthy* HIV-1 carriers is low. Based on current evidence, there is no justification for policies of employment disability based solely on HIV-1 serologic testing. Approximately 20 percent of patients with AIDS will develop a clinically significant dementia; however, during the early stages of dementia, the clinical features are nonspecific and stringent criteria should be used to avoid overdiagnosis of this condition (Table 2). Diagnostic precision is important not only for therapeutic reasons and because this disorder defines a case of AIDS, but also because the diagnosis carries serious prognostic and legal implications. Serial assessments of an individual are important in confirming progressive deterioration and excluding other potentially reversible causes of encephalopathy (see Table 2).

Although the pathogenesis of HIV-1 encephalopathy is unclear, zidovudine should be administered. The full dosage consists of 200 mg every 4 hours, and the drug should be administered in conjunction with the assistance of an internist or an infectious disease specialist because approximately 30 percent of recipients develop bone marrow suppression necessitating blood transfusion and dose reduction. Other side effects include nausea, gastrointestinal upset, and during the first few weeks of treatment, headache. Patients with mild or moderate degrees of HIV-1 encephalopathy will often show improvement within a few weeks, particularly in memory and psychomotor speed. Several studies have demonstrated improvement in neuropsychologic test performance in both adults and children when zidovudine is used; however, the clinical benefits are usually limited to a few months and the disorder then continues to progress. Patients with far-advanced dementia rarely improve with zidovudine therapy. Symptomatic treatment is an important adjunct to antiviral treatment. Patients with mild or moderate dementia and marked apathy may respond to small doses of methylphenidate hydrochloride (Ritalin) starting with 5 mg twice daily. If marked depressive symptoms are present, tricyclic antidepressants may be attempted in a dose 25 to 50 percent of the usual dose. Patients with HIV-1 encephalopathy are extremely susceptible to the adverse effects of psychoactive drugs, and therefore hypnotics and anxiolytics should be avoided. Small doses of neuroleptics, such as haloperidol (Haldol) 0.5 mg administered as necessary, are useful in the agitated patient.

At an early stage before the dementia becomes too severe, one must discuss with patients with progressive dementia medicolegal issues such as arranging for power of attorney, completion of a living will, and arrangement of assets.

TABLE 2 Criteria for Diagnosis of HIV-1-Related Dementia

HIV-1 seropositivity (Western blot confirmation)
History of progressive cognitive/behavioral decline
Neurologic examination: nonfocal or diffuse CNS signs
Neuropsychological assessment: progressive deterioration on serial testing in at least two of the following areas: frontal lobe, motor speed, nonverbal memory
Absence of major affective disorder or active substance abuse
Absence of metabolic derangement (e.g., hypoxia, sepsis)
Absence of CNS opportunistic infections/neoplasms
CT/MRI normal, atrophy, or white matter rarefaction
CSF: negative VDRL and cryptococcal antigen

CT = computed tomography; MRI = magnetic resonance imaging.

HIV-1–Associated Myelopathies

As many as 20 percent of patients with AIDS will be affected by a noninflammatory vacuolar myelopathy manifest by progressive spastic paraparesis and sensory ataxia and often accompanied by progressive dementia. As with HIV-1 encephalopathy, the pathogenetic mechanisms have not been elucidated, and toxic and metabolic factors may be important. The diagnostic approach should consider structural or compressive lesions and correctable nutritional deficiencies such as a vitamin B_{12} deficiency. A sensory level is unusual, so if one is present, particularly with back pain, magnetic resonance imaging of the spine or myelography should be performed to exclude extrinsic cord compression. Nonspecific CSF abnormalities are frequently present, but are not diagnostic. I have not found zidovudine to be useful in reversing the myelopathy, which usually progresses inexorably. Antispasticity agents such as baclofen (Lioresal) may relieve some of the spasticity.

Peripheral Nerve Disorders Associated with HIV-1

Predominantly Sensory Neuropathy

As many as 30 percent of patients with AIDS develop a neuropathy characterized by painful sensory symptoms in the feet. Most individuals develop this neuropathy late in the course of HIV-1 infection, usually in association with systemic opportunistic infections. This disorder can usually be recognized by characteristic complaints of dysesthesias and contact hypersensitivity in the feet with reduced or absent ankle reflexes and elevated sensory thresholds. Although electrophysiologic studies are helpful, they are not essential in the diagnosis and usually reveal a neuropathy affecting both sensory and motor fibers suggestive of a dying back axonopathy. Nerve biopsies are not usually helpful in the clinical setting. Consideration should be given to nutritional and toxic causes of sensory neuropathy, such as alcohol abuse, diabetes, pyridoxine excess, vitamin B_{12} deficiency, and the use of experimental neurotoxic antivirals, such as dideoxycytidine. Patients who develop predominantly sensory neuropathy are often already taking zidovudine because of their advanced immune deficiency. Although occasionally symptoms will stabilize with zidovudine treatment, more often there is no dramatic response, and symptomatic relief with pain-modifying agents such as amitriptyline hydrochloride (Elavil) or phenytoin (Dilantin) is more useful. Because of the potential for delirium, amitriptyline is started at a very small dose, 10 to 25 mg administered at every hour of sleep, and gradually increased to 50 to 100 mg.

Inflammatory Demyelinating Polyneuropathies

Several possibly immune-mediated phenomena have been described in association with HIV-1 infection, including inflammatory demyelinating polyneuropathy (IDP). In contrast to predominantly sensory neuropathy, IDP typically occurs at a relatively early stage of HIV-1 infection, before immunodeficiency develops. Typically there is profound motor weakness, sometimes developing acutely as Guillain-Barré syndrome and associated with CSF pleocytosis. More often, IDP presents as a chronic, sometimes relapsing process. Because of this association between HIV-1 and IDP, a careful search for risk factors for HIV-1 infection and serologic testing should be carried out in any patient presenting with IDP. Plasmapheresis is the treatment of choice because it is less likely to cause additional immunosuppression than corticosteroids. In Guillain-Barré syndrome (GBS), a course of five plasma exchanges is given. With chronic inflammatory demyelinating polyneuropathy (CIDP), an induction course is followed by maintenance exchanges as needed. If plasmapheresis is impractical, short courses of corticosteroids are generally tolerated well without triggering opportunistic infections. For CIDP, I use a 4-day course of methylprednisolone, 15 mg per kilogram intravenously over 4 hours, followed by oral prednisone administered on the basis of an adjustable tapering schedule (60 mg administered over a period of as long as 2 months).

Myopathies

Polymyositis is an uncommon complication of HIV-1 infection that sometimes responds to treatment with immunosuppressive agents. Because of the potential for infectious complications, the use of these agents should be restricted to patients with severe weakness, greatly elevated serum creatine phosphokinase (CPK), and biopsy evidence of fiber necrosis and inflammatory infiltrates. A toxic myopathy can occur with the use of zidovudine, apparently after 6 to 12 months of full-dose treatment. The clinical features of toxic myopathy are not distinguishable from polymyositis. If a "drug holiday" of 2 to 4 weeks is accompanied by clinical improvement and a drop in CPK, I assume that the patient had a toxic myopathy and reduce the dose of zidovudine long-term.

OPPORTUNISTIC PROCESSES

Opportunistic infections and neoplasms of the CNS are common in the setting of HIV-1 infection, reflecting the underlying immune deficiency produced by infection and lysis of CD4 lymphocytes by HIV-1. Patients may have multiple concurrent opportunistic processes, or opportunistic processes may coexist with HIV-1–related neurologic disorders.

Intracranial Focal Lesions

A variety of disorders cause intracranial focal lesions, including toxoplasmosis, primary CNS lymphoma, progressive multifocal leukoencephalopathy, and other bacterial/fungal infections. Multiple concurrent opportunistic processes may coexist. Since specific treatment is available for many of these complications, early detection and accurate diagnosis is critical. A management approach based on empiric toxoplasmosis therapy has evolved (Fig. 1).

Cryptococcal Meningitis

Cryptococcus neoformans, a ubiquitous yeast, produces CNS infection in approximately 10 percent of patients with AIDS, and in some may be the first recognized opportunistic infection. The most common presentation is as meningitis with headache, meningismus, altered mentation, fever, and nausea. This constellation of symptoms mimics cerebral toxoplasmosis, other opportunistic processes, and when more indolent, HIV-1 encephalopathy. The CSF usually has *normal* cellular and protein constituents; however, uniformly cryptococcal antigen is detectable and fungal cultures are positive. A 6-week induction course with amphotericin B (0.6 mg per kilogram per day) is recommended. Flucytosine (Ancobon) is rarely tolerated by patients with AIDS because it causes diarrhea and myelosuppression. During successful treatment, both serum and CSF cryptococcal antigen titers can be expected to fall by at least four dilutions and fungal cultures will become negative. The CSF should be re-examined at the end of induction therapy or with recrudescence of symptoms. An end-of-therapy serum titer or CSF titer $\geq$1:8 implies failure or relapse. Suppressive treatment with amphotericin B administered once or twice weekly via an indwelling Hickman catheter is

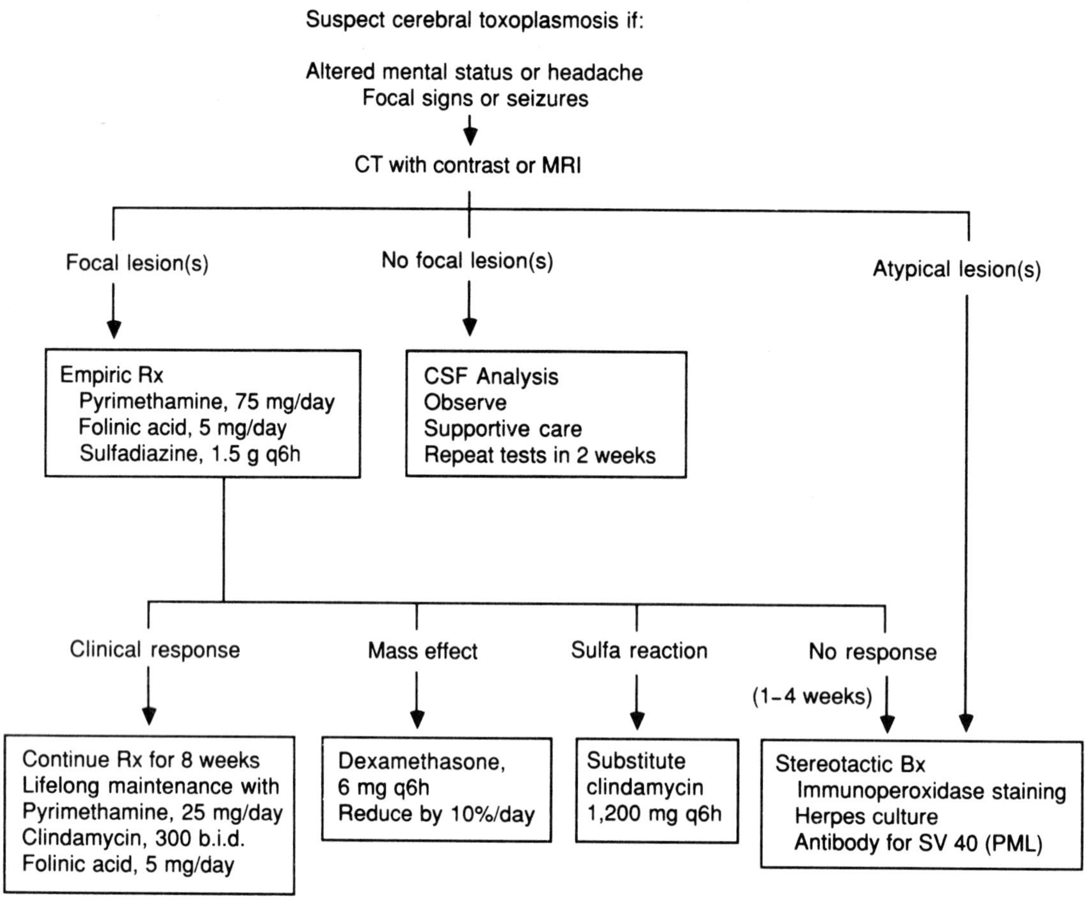

Figure 1 Management of intracranial focal lesions. CT = computed tomography; MRI = magnetic resonance imaging.

necessary for lifelong maintenance. The median survival for patients diagnosed as having cryptococcal meningitis is about 9 months, and relapse occurs in approximately 60 percent. Alternative antifungal agents are being used more widely and include the agents fluconazole and itraconazole, which are still experimental. Fluconazole and itraconazole appear to be far less toxic than amphotericin B, are absorbed orally, and unlike ketoconazole, penetrate the blood brain barrier. They have shown promise both for primary therapy and as maintenance agents.

Cytomegalovirus Encephalitis/Retinitis

Cytomegalovirus (CMV) may cause infection of the retina, producing visual loss in as many as 20 percent of patients with AIDS. Less commonly, CMV produces an encephalitis that is clinically and radiologically indistinguishable from HIV-1 encephalopathy. An acyclovir analog, ganciclovir (Cytovene), is a useful suppressive agent, but frequently causes leukopenia and cannot be given in conjunction with zidovudine.

Cerebral Toxoplasmosis

Infection with *Toxoplasma gondii,* an obligate intracellular protozoan, causes necrotic and inflammatory abscesses that are often multifocal and scattered throughout the cerebral hemispheres with a predilection for the basal ganglia. Toxoplasmosis occurs in 5 to 10 percent of patients with AIDS, typically with fever, altered mentation, seizures, and focal neurologic signs developing over a few days. Imaging studies demonstrate multiple contrast-enhancing mass lesions; however, the radiologic appearances are not specific for toxoplasmosis and can be mimicked by lymphoma or other causes of abscess. Although serologic testing is not diagnostic, most patients with toxoplasmosis have detectable antitoxoplasma immunoglobin G (IgG), and a negative titer (<1:4) suggests an alternate diagnosis. Prompt initiation of antimicrobial therapy leads to clinical and radiologic improvement in approximately 80 percent of patients within 1 to 4 weeks. Corticosteroids should be restricted to patients with large lesions and mass effect. Lifelong

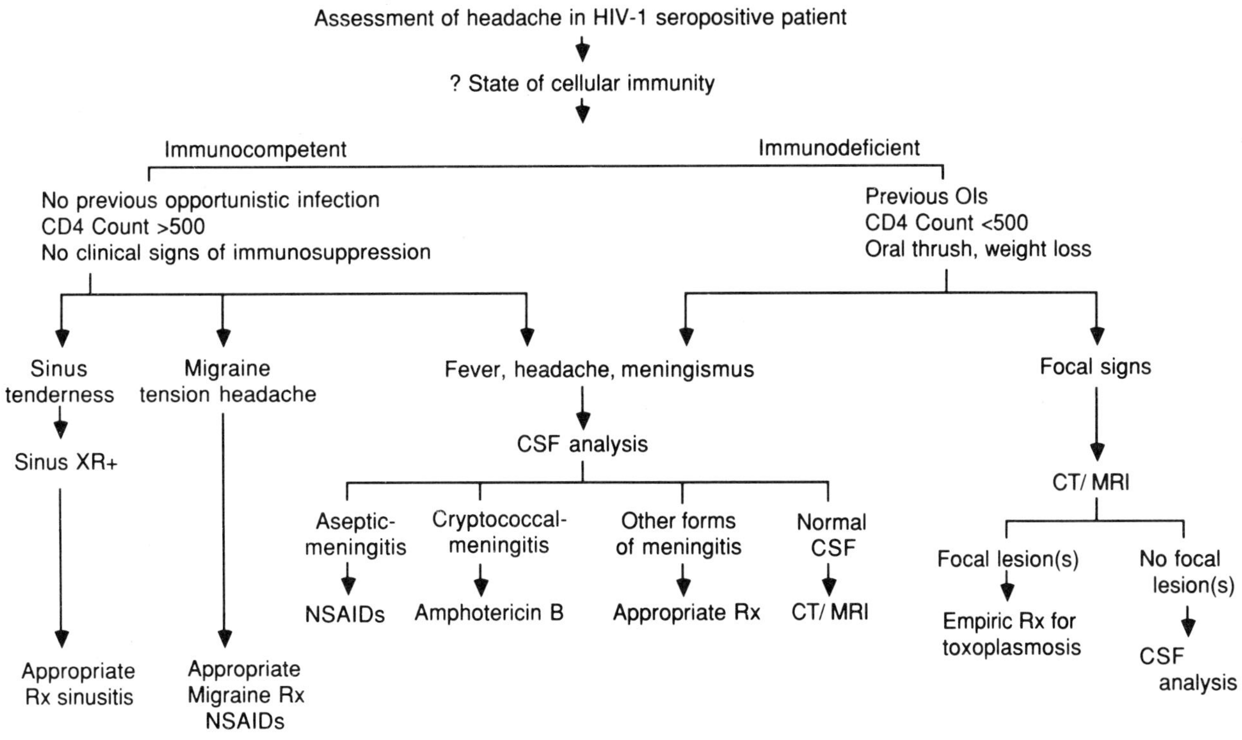

Figure 2 Assessment of headache in the HIV-1 seropositive patient. CT = computed tomography; MRI = magnetic resonance imaging; NSAIDs = nonsteroidal anti-inflammatory drugs; OIs = opportunistic infections.

suppressive therapy with two drugs, is necessary: pyrimethamine, 25 mg daily, and clindamycin (Cleocin), 300 mg twice daily. Relapse occurs in approximately 10 percent of patients.

Primary CNS Lymphoma

About 2 percent of patients with AIDS develop primary CNS lymphoma. The typical presentation is with slowly progressive neurologic deterioration leading to death within 3 months. Because the radiologic appearance cannot be distinguished from that of toxoplasmosis, biopsy is often necessary. CSF cytology is rarely diagnostic, and lumbar puncture may be contraindicated because of mass effect or the risk of herniation. The lymphoma is often multicentric and of B-cell origin, and it behaves aggressively. The response to whole-brain radiation or chemotherapy is poor, with a median survival of 2 months.

Progressive Multifocal Leukoencephalopathy

Progressive multifocal leukoencephalopathy (PML) develops in as many as 2 percent of patients with AIDS and typically presents with a progressive accumulation of focal neurologic deficits. Diagnosis is usually made from the typical clinical course, with imaging studies demonstrating multiple nonenhancing areas within the white matter without mass effect. Biopsy may be necessary to differentiate PML from cerebral toxoplasmosis, other opportunistic infections, or CNS lymphoma (see Fig. 1). Immunostaining with antibody to SV 40 or JC virus is necessary for definitive pathologic diagnosis. There is no effective treatment and the neurologic disorder usually progresses inexorably to death within weeks, or at most, a few months.

Herpes Group Radiculitis

Five to 10 percent of patients with HIV-1 infection develop herpes zoster radiculitis. Dermatomal herpes zoster does not require specific treatment unless cervical or lumbar dermatomes are involved. Here the potential exists for the development of severe myeloradiculitis with permanent motor deficits, and intravenous acyclovir (Zovirax) (30 mg per kilogram per day) should be used. The development of postherpetic neuralgia may necessitate the use of pain-modifying agents such as amitriptyline hydrochloride (Elavil) or carbamazepine (Tegretol). After the vesicles have completely healed, topical capsaicin (Zostrix) can reduce the neuralgic pains, but it must be used for at least 2 weeks. Recently cytomegalovirus has been identified as causing a progressive radiculopathy involving lumbar and sacral roots. Usually there is a polymorphonuclear pleocytosis and cytomegalovirus can often be isolated by culture from the CSF. An acyclovir analog, 9-(1,3-dihydroxy-2-propoxymethyl) guanine (DHPG) (ganciclovir [Cytovene]), has been tried.

Neurosyphilis

While not strictly an opportunistic infection, it has been suggested that the course of syphilis may be accelerated by the disturbance in cellular immunity accompanying HIV-1 infection. The clinical features of neurosyphilis may be modified and the time course from primary to tertiary syphilis shortened. There are reports of false-negative syphilis serology in individuals with biopsy-proven syphilis; however, in general, syphilis serology is reliable. Because of poor CSF penetration, benzathine penicillin should be avoided in patients with neurosyphilis. In a neurologically normal HIV-1 carrier with a history of *treated* syphilis who is sero-fast (rapid plasma reagin [RPR] $\leq$ 1:8 consistently), I do not advocate additional therapy or lumbar puncture. When neurologic symptoms are present, however, even if not typical of neurosyphilis, the CSF should be examined. If CSF Veneral Disease Reference Laboratory (VDRL) is positive or serum RPR is high (>1:16) and clinical features are suggestive of neurosyphilis, I favor treatment with intravenous penicillin, 24 mU for 10 days, or procaine penicillin, 2.4 mU with probenecid for 10 days, followed by re-examination of the CSF.

With an estimated 1.5 million Americans already infected with HIV-1, there is likely to be an increasing burden placed on neurologists for assessment of HIV-1 carriers with symptoms such as headache, memory loss, and neuropsychiatric symptoms. Usually knowledge of the systemic stage of HIV-1 disease and immune status is the most helpful information, and the approach shown in Figure 2 can be followed. One can usually reassure most HIV-1 carriers that serious neurologic complications are unusual at this stage of infection. Neurodiagnostic studies should be limited and lumbar puncture in particular is rarely useful at this stage because of the high frequency of silent HIV-1–related abnormalities.

SUGGESTED READING

AIDS Bibliography. Bethesda, MD: National Library of Medicine.

AIDS Experimental Treatment Directory. New York: American Foundation for AIDS Research (AMFAR).

Aronow HA, Brew BJ, Price RW. The management of the neurologic complications of HIV infection and AIDS. AIDS 2 1988; (suppl 1):S151–S159.

Cornblath DR. Treatment of the neuromuscular complications of human immunodeficiency virus infection. Ann Neurol 1988; 23 (suppl):S88–S91.

Haverkos H. Assessment of therapy for toxoplasma encephalitis. Am J Med 1987; 82:907–914.

McArthur JC. Neurologic manifestations of AIDS. Medicine 1987; 66:407–437.

Zuger A, Louie E, Holzman RS, et al. Cryptococcal disease in patients with the acquired immunodeficiency syndrome: diagnostic features and outcome of treatment. Ann Intern Med 1986; 104:234–240.

PATIENT RESOURCES

American Foundation for AIDS Research (AMFAR)
1515 Broadway 36th floor
New York, New York 10036
Telephone: (212) 333-3118

National Hemophilia Foundation
110 Greene St. Room 406
New York, New York 10012
Telephone: (212) 966-9247

AIDS Clinical Trials Information
Building 10 Room 11B09
Clinical Center NIH
Bethesda, Maryland 20892
Telephone: 1-800-TRIALS-A
Monday–Friday, 9 AM–7 PM EDT

CDC AIDS Hotline
1-800-342-AIDS

Burroughs Wellcome (AZT [zidovudine] manufacturer)
Patient Temporary Assistance Program for Persons with AIDS
Telephone: 1-800-722-9292 (ext. 3633)

National AIDS Information Clearing House
P.O. Box 6003
Rockville, Maryland 20850

National Gay and Lesbian Task Force
Crisis Line
1-800-221-7044

Centers for Disease Control
1-404-639-3311

KAPOSI'S SARCOMA

STEPHEN P. RICHMAN, M.D.
CHARLES L. VOGEL, M.D., F.A.C.P.

Kaposi's sarcoma occurs in four clinical settings: classic Kaposi's sarcoma occurs primarily in elderly men of Mediterranean and Ashkenazic Jewish descent, children and young adults in equatorial Africa, renal transplant patients, and patients with acquired immunodeficiency syndromes (AIDS). Therapy of Kaposi's sarcoma in each of these cases (30,595 in the United States at the end of 1986) and the projected rise to 270,000 by the end of 1991 make AIDS associated Kaposi's sarcoma a major therapeutic concern in contemporary oncology.

APPROACH TO KAPOSI'S SARCOMA ASSOCIATED WITH AIDS (AIDS-KS)

Therapy for AIDS-KS must be administered in the context of the underlying immunologic deficiency and of the opportunistic infections complicating this disease. To permit comparison of patient groups and therapeutic regimens, a staging system has been proposed that is roughly analogous to that used in lymphomas: stage I—cutaneous, locally indolent disease; stage II—cutaneous, locally aggressive disease with or without regional lymphadenopathy; stage III—generalized mucocutaneous and/or lymph node involvement (generalized is defined as more than upper or lower extremity alone and includes minimal gastrointestinal disease); stage IV—visceral disease. Patients are further divided into subtype A consisting of the absence of systemic signs of symptoms and subtype B consisting of the presence of systemic signs involving weight loss greater than 10 percent or fever greater than 100°F orally unrelated to an identifiable source of infection and lasting more than 2 weeks. In practice, stage I is a relatively good prognostic group with 100 percent survival at 18 months, but is relatively rare in epidemic Kaposi's sarcoma. Stage II is encountered even less frequently. Stages IIIA and IVA also have a relatively good prognosis with an 85 percent survival rate at 18 months, but stages IIIB and IVB have a poor prognosis as do patients with opportunistic infections. In addition to extensive disease, systemic signs and symptoms, and opportunistic infection, low T4 levels, low hematocrit, and the presence of acid labile alpha interferon have also had negative prognostic significance.

CHEMOTHERAPY OF AIDS-KS

A number of chemotherapeutic agents are active in AIDS-KS. Vinblastine administered to 22 patients resulted in a 37 percent response rate (one complete and six partial responses in 19 evaluable patients). Therapy was associated with the development of opportunistic infection. Helper-suppressor T-cell ratios showed no significant change. VP-16 administered in a dose of 150 mg per meter squared daily for 3 days to 41 patients resulted in a 30 percent complete response rate, a 46 percent partial response rate, and a mean duration of response of 9 months. Seventeen patients developed opportunistic infections during the course of treatment or within 2 months of terminating therapy. Opportunistic infections occurred in both responders and nonresponders. Vincristine was administered to 23 patients, of whom 22 had received prior therapy. Eighteen were considered evaluable. Eleven patients had a partial response (61 percent) and seven had a minor response. There were no complete responders. Three patients in the treatment group felt to have immune thrombocytopenia experienced tumor regression and increased platelet counts.

Combination chemotherapy has been tested. In particular, a combination regimen consisting of Adriamycin (40 mg per meter squared), bleomycin (15 units times 2), and vinblastine (6 mg per meter squared) was given to 31 patients with advanced AIDS-KS. Twenty-three percent achieved a complete response and 61 percent achieved a partial response. Median survival for complete responders was 20 months and for partial responders was 9 months. Dose reductions of 25 to 50 percent were necessitated by hematologic toxicity in 44 percent of the patients. Sixty-one percent of patients developed opportunistic infections during the treatment or within 2 months of terminating therapy. The authors concluded that therapy was successful from the purely antitumor point of view, but that further treatment was needed to reverse the underlying immune deficiency.

ICRF-159 has recently been tested because of its activity in African Kaposi's sarcoma. However, only one response was seen in 20 evaluable patients. The authors of this study felt that this indicated a difference in the biology of the AIDS-KS compared with that of African-KS. Some chemotherapeutic agents widely used in other malignancies have not been extensively tested in AIDS-KS. Among these are cis-platinum and Adriamycin. Studies with these agents are under way.

In practice, these agents are often administered serially, one at a time in an attempt to achieve palliation with minimal myelosuppression. Vincristine, vinblastine, or VP-16 are generally used as initial therapy with the remaining agents or bleomycin used as secondary and tertiary therapy.

INTERFERONS FOR AIDS-KS

Lymphoblastoid interferon administered intramuscularly daily for 2 months in a dose of 20 MU per meter squared has been reported active in AIDS-KS. Four patients experienced complete remission and four achieved partial remission for a response rate of 67 percent. Minimal tumor burden, the absence of circulating interferon before therapy, and a performance status of greater than 90 percent correlated with an improved response rate. Median duration of response was over 28 weeks. Toxicity consisted of fever, asthenia, weight loss, alopecia, myelosuppresion, and modest abnormalities in liver function tests.

Recombinant alfa-2b interferon has been studied in AIDS-related Kaposi's sarcoma in a series of phase II trials involving a total of 114 patients. Doses of 50 MU, 30 MU, and 1 MU administered subcutaneously all resulted in response rates of 33, 28, and 45 percent in the low, intermediate and high doses, respectively. High dose therapy was associated with a more rapid time to response. Response rates for patients without B symptoms were 38, 44, and 60 percent for the low, intermediate, and high dose groups. Immunologic parameters did not improve during the study. Median survival for nonresponders was 10.5 months and was 33 months for responders. The authors concluded that although the optimum dose of interferon remained to be determined, the high dose was superior to both the intermediate and low dose regimens.

Recombinant alfa-2a interferon has also been studied sequentially in AIDS-related Kaposi's sarcoma. A 38 percent response rate was seen in patients treated with a high dose (36 to 54 MU daily) versus only a 3 percent (3 MU daily) response rate in patients treated with low dose alfa-2a interferon. A 17 percent response rate was seen in those patients in whom the dose was increased after low dose treatment failed. Responders showed a significantly lower rate of opportunistic infection as well as a longer survival rate than did nonresponders.

Although the optimum schedule of interferon and the optimum interferon preparation in AIDS-related Kaposi's may not have been determined, most investigators feel that there is a threshold dose level represented by studies such as those cited above below which response rate falls off. Since treatment goals are primarily palliative, investigators differ regarding the optimum starting time for antitumor therapy in a given patient. The toxicity of the regimen must be weighed against the patient's clinical condition and the fact that the anticipated response rate will fall as the tumor progresses and B symptoms appear. Likewise, the choice between interferons and chemotherapeutic agents varies with the clinical setting, the condition and lifestyle of the patient, cost factors, and the availability of research protocols. Whether tumor response is truly associated with a decreased risk of opportunistic infection is controversial.

Future directions in interferon research with AIDS-KS will involve combined regimens with chemotherapy and antiviral agents. Beta interferon has not yet been extensively tested in this setting. Gamma interferon appears to be inactive. Combined studies with chemotherapy thus far indicate that such regimens are feasible although there has been additive myelosuppressive toxicity. However, it has not yet been demonstrated that response rates are additive or synergistic.

RADIOTHERAPY FOR AIDS-KS

AIDS-associated Kaposi's sarcoma is a radiosensitive tumor. Radiotherapy may be used for the relief of painful, inconvenient, or incapacitating lesions in localized areas. Such lesions might include large nodules on the extremities and oral lesions interfering with dentition. Radiotherapy may also be used for cosmetic purposes, particularly in lesions around the face; although some authors have noted that some residual pigment may interfere with cosmetic goals. Patients who receive chemotherapy soon after receiving radiation to a mucocutaneous area may experience potentiation of toxicity within the radiation field.

CLASSIC KAPOSI'S SARCOMA

This is a disease predominately but not exclusively of elderly males. Frequently, cardiovascular disease and other medical problems prevalent in this age group are major factors in determining therapy. The tumor is viewed as a chronic, multifocal malignancy to be treated primarily with palliative intent. Single or localized lesions may be surgically excised, but multiple or recurrent disease may be successfully palliated with radiotherapy if the disease presentation is not massive. By far the most frequently used palliative agent has been vinblastine as a single agent. Response rates as high as 90 percent have been reported with chronically administered, relatively low dose vinblastine. Newer agents such as doxorubicin, cis-platinum, and the interferons have not been well studied because the medical condition of such patients often precludes the risk of toxicity associated with these agents.

AFRICAN KAPOSI'S SARCOMA

African Kaposi's sarcoma also has a male predominance similar to classic European Kaposi's sarcoma, but in general, the age group is much younger. The disease may present as a nodular, relatively indolent form with primarily dermal involvement; a locally aggressive form which may either be exophytic or infiltrative; or a more disseminated lymphadenopathic form. This last form has the worst prognosis with a 100 percent fatality within 3 years. Regionally localized African Kaposi's sarcoma is sensitive to radiotherapy. African Kaposi's sarcoma has been reported sensitive to a variety of chemotherapeutic regimens including intra-arterial nitrogen mustard, actinomycin D, and combinations of actinomycin D-vincristine and actinomycin D-vincristine-dacarbazine. The actinomycin D regimens have had response rates of 90 percent. Combination chemotherapy appears to be more active than single agent chemotherapy. There has been relatively little reported experience with newer chemotherapeutic and biologic agents in African Kaposi's sarcoma.

KAPOSI'S SARCOMA IN RENAL TRANSPLANT RECIPIENTS

Although disproportionately high amongst renal transplant patients, Kaposi's sarcoma associated with renal transplantation is still relatively rare, and therapy has been individualized. Responses have been seen with reduction in immunosuppressive therapy alone. Localized lesions have been treated with surgery and radiotherapy. The threat of the malignancy to any individual patient (depending upon its extent and aggressiveness) must be balanced against the consequences of losing the transplanted kidney.

SUGGESTED READING

Krigel RL, Friedman-Kien AE. Kaposi's sarcoma in AIDS. In: DeVita VT Jr, et al, eds. AIDS etiology, diagnosis, treatment, and prevention. Philadelphia: JB Lippincott, 1985:185.

Krown SE, Real FX, Vadhan-Raj S, et al. Kaposi's sarcoma and the acquired immunodeficiency syndrome. Cancer 1986; 57:1662–1665.

Odajnyk C, Muggia FM. Treatment of Kaposi's sarcoma: overview and analysis by clinical setting. J Clin Oncol 1985; 3:1277–1286.

Volberding PA, Mitsuyasu RT, Golando JP, et al. Treatment of Kaposi's sarcoma with interferon Alfa-2b (Intron A). Cancer 1987; 59:620–625.

INFECTIOUS DISEASES

ADULT IMMUNIZATION

THEODORE C. EICKHOFF, M.D.

Renewed interest in immunization of adults in the United States began in the early 1980s. Despite the successes of pediatric immunization programs, the utilization of some vaccines recommended primarily for use in adults, such as the vaccines against influenza, pneumococcal infection, and hepatitis B, was poor. The latter two products, introduced in the last decade, were targeted primarily for adult populations and did not receive as much acceptance as was hoped.

Several sources give current information on vaccines for adults. The Advisory Committee on Immunization Practices of the Centers for Disease Control publishes periodic recommendations for the use of vaccines in *Morbidity and Mortality Weekly Report*. Recommendations from MMWR are reprinted regularly in JAMA, and are available as well from other journals. In addition, the American College of Physicians publishes a guide for adult immunization that is available from the American College of Physicians, P.O. Box 7777-R0325, Philadelphia, Pennsylvania 19175. A second edition is planned for release in 1989.

Tables 1 and 2 summarize the vaccines generally recommended for adult use, as well as vaccines recommended in the context of certain occupations or travel. Most of these vaccines are discussed in the chapters in this book that address the specific diseases that may be prevented by the vaccines.

TETANUS AND DIPHTHERIA

Tetanus and diphtheria toxoid (Td) consists of formalinized toxoids, derived from tetanus and diphtheria toxins. It is indicated for use in all adults. Individuals who are primarily immunized as children or earlier in adult life need receive only booster doses at 10-year intervals in order to maintain adequate immunity. Because pediatric immunization schedules generally end with a preschool booster dose of these antigens, the mid-decade birthday (e.g., 15 years, 25, 35) is a convenient recall date to provide the recommended booster dose.

Adults who are not known to have completed a three-dose primary immunization series in childhood should be given three 0.5-ml doses of Td. The second dose should be given 4 weeks after the first, and the third dose given 6 to 12 months after the second.

For wound management, an additional dose of Td is recommended only when there have been major or contaminated wounds and then only if more than 5 years have elapsed since the last dose. Td is preferred to T alone.

MEASLES, MUMPS, RUBELLA

These three vaccines are considered together, inasmuch as the immunizing agents are all attenuated live viruses and are frequently given together. They are available singly as well as in the combination product, MMR vaccine.

All adults should be immune to measles, mumps, and rubella. For measles, a physician-documented diagnosis or laboratory evidence of immunity is acceptable. Individuals vaccinated against measles between 1963 and 1967 may have received inactivated vaccine or vaccine of unknown type and should be reimmunized with live measles vaccine to prevent severe atypical measles, a disease that has occurred among young adults such as college students and military recruits. Adults over the age of 35 years may generally be considered immune to measles and mumps, but younger adults should be investigated more thoroughly.

Since the clinical diagnosis of rubella is too uncertain to be dependable, laboratory evidence of immunity should

TABLE 1 Summary of Vaccines Recommended for Adult Use

	Vaccine					
Age (yr)	*Td*	*MMR*	*Polio*	*Influenza*	*Pneumococcal*	*Hepatitis B*
18–24	+	1	2			3
25–64	+	1	2			3
≥65	+			+	+	

1. Check for documentation of rubella vaccine or serologic test. See text for measles and mumps. MMR vaccine is contraindicated in pregnancy.
2. Inactivated poliovirus vaccine should be used for nonimmune parents of children to be given live oral poliovirus vaccine.
3. Target populations: homosexual or bisexual males, intravenous drug abusers, health care workers at risk of contact with blood or body fluids, and travelers to endemic areas.

TABLE 2 Additional Considerations for Certain Occupations and Travel

Indication	*Vaccine*
Occupation	
Hospital, laboratory, and other health care personnel	Hepatitis B Measles Rubella Influenza Polio
Staff of institutions for the mentally retarded	Hepatitis B
Veterinarians and animal handlers	Rabies
Selected field workers	Plague
International travel, consider:	Polio, yellow fever, hepatitis B, rabies, meningococcal polysaccharide, typhoid, cholera, plague, immune globulin

generally be required unless a record of immunization with rubella vaccine is present. The risks of rubella vaccine during pregnancy are known to be low; nonetheless, women should be counseled not to become pregnant within 3 months after immunization. Transient arthralgias and arthritis after rubella vaccine have been reported in susceptible recipients of rubella vaccine and are believed to be manifestations of the mild vaccine-induced infection.

Most adults are immune to mumps virus; however, a surprising proportion of adults are still susceptible. Since a safe and effective vaccine is available, adults who are not known to be mumps-immune should be immunized.

The combined measles-mumps-rubella (MMR) vaccine is the immunizing agent of choice if the recipient is likely to be susceptible to more than one of the three diseases. There are no adverse effects of giving any of these three components of this vaccine to individuals already immune to one or more of the components.

Since these vaccines are grown in eggs, anaphylactic hypersensitivity to eggs represents a contraindication. Other contraindications include immunoincompetence, pregnancy, and the administration of immune globulin within the preceding 3 months. Commercially available immune globulin provides enough passive antibody directed at measles, mumps, and rubella to inhibit replication of the vaccine virus, thus preventing effective immunization.

POLIOMYELITIS

Two types of poliovirus vaccines are currently available in the United States: live oral poliovirus vaccine (OPV) and inactivated poliovirus vaccine (IPV). An IPV of enhanced potency was introduced in the United States in 1987 and is expected to become the only inactivated poliovaccine available. OPV has been by far the most widely used vaccine in this country. A primary vaccination series with either vaccine produces immunity to all three poliovirus types in over 95 percent of recipients.

Routine polio vaccination of adults living in the United States who have not been primarily immunized is no longer necessary because of the very low risk of poliomyelitis in the United States. When susceptible adults have children, however, they should be immunized against polio at the same time, or preferably before their children are immunized. Since the risk of OPV-associated paralysis is slightly higher in adults than in children, IPV is preferred for susceptible adults who have not received a primary series of polio vaccine in childhood. Similarly, for adults who may be at increased risk of exposure to polioviruses because of international travel or health care occupation, IPV is the preferred product for immunization.

INFLUENZA

Influenza vaccine consists of inactivated influenza virus, either as whole virus or viral subunits. Influenza vaccine differs from other products routinely recommended for use in adults in that its composition is likely to be changed each year, depending on the specific immunologic characteristics of circulating influenza viruses and the fact that the vaccine must be given annually because of the relatively short-lived immunity conferred by the vaccine. The vaccine is recommended for annual use in adults of any age with high-risk conditions such as chronic pulmonary, cardiac, renal, or metabolic diseases, and for all adults over 65 years of age.

Influenza outbreaks in the United States are regularly associated with increased mortality, and the impact of influenza is most severe among elderly persons, who account for 60 to 80 percent of all influenza-associated deaths. Approximately 90 percent of these deaths occur in persons with recognized underlying diseases, but deaths may also occur among apparently healthy elderly adults. For this reason, the annual use of influenza vaccine is strongly recommended to prevent or reduce the excess mortality associated with influenza.

PNEUMOCOCCAL VACCINE

The currently available pneumococcal vaccine consists of 25 μg of each pneumococcal polysaccharide from the 23 pneumococcal capsular types that account for the majority of bacteremic pneumococcal infections in this country. Indications for this vaccine include splenic dysfunction or anatomic asplenia, chronic diseases associated with increased risk of pneumococcal disease, such as chronic cardiopulmonary disease, and all adults over 65 years of age. The indications for pneumococcal vaccine in adults are similar to those for influenza vaccine, but in contrast to influenza vaccine, which is recommended for annual use, pneumococcal vaccine need be given only once. Influenza and pneumococcal vaccines may be given safely and effectively at the same time but in separate sites.

The need for reimmunization of patients at high risk of pneumococcal infection is not clearly defined, but consideration should be given to reimmunizing adults at highest risk who were immunized 6 or more years ago or patients known to have a rapid decline in pneumococcal antibody levels, such as patients with the nephrotic syndrome, renal failure, or organ transplants. It would be prudent to immunize adults at an earlier age, for example, at 55 years, before the age-related increase in frequency of underlying disease occurs, and at a time when a brisk immunologic response might be expected.

HEPATITIS B

The first vaccine directed against hepatitis B consisted of purified, inactivated hepatitis B surface antigen (HBsAg), derived from plasma obtained from chronic HBsAg carriers. A more recently introduced hepatitis B vaccine is derived from yeast cells into which the gene coding for the production of hepatitis B surface antigen has been inserted. This product will eventually fully replace the plasma-derived hepatitis B vaccine.

The vaccine should be administered intramuscularly in the deltoid region in three doses, the second dose 1 month after the first and the third dose 6 months later. The need for booster doses of hepatitis B vaccine after the primary immunizing series is not yet fully clarified. Major target populations for whom the vaccine is recommended include homosexual males, intravenous drug abusers, certain institutionalized populations, household and sexual contacts of chronic carriers of HBsAg, health care personnel who have occupational exposure to blood or blood-contaminated body fluids, and travelers to areas with high endemicity for hepatitis B.

Table 2 should be consulted for additional recommendations relating to certain occupational groups as well as international travel.

SUGGESTED READING

Guide for adult immunization. 2nd ed. Philadelphia: American College of Physicians, 1989.
Morbidity and mortality weekly report. Recommendations of the advisory committee on immunization practices. Atlanta: Centers for Disease Control.
Plotkin, SA, Mortimer EA, eds. Vaccines. Philadelphia: WB Saunders, 1988.

ANTIVIRAL CHEMOTHERAPY

SUSAN E. BORUCHOFF, M.D.
SARAH H. CHEESEMAN, M.D.

The rapid advances being made in antiviral treatment are reflected in the number of chapters in this volume devoted to therapy of specific viral diseases. This chapter provides an overview of the major antiviral agents available or presently under investigation in the United States today, with emphasis on mode of action and pharmacologic properties relevant to clinical use. More detailed discussion of specific therapeutic recommendations are found in other chapters devoted to the individual infections. Zidovudine (AZT) and the many other agents under development for treatment of infections caused by human immunodeficiency virus (HIV) are discussed in the chapter *Antiviral Therapy of Human Immunodeficiency Virus Infection.*

GENERAL PRINCIPLES OF ANTIVIRAL CHEMOTHERAPY

Appropriate and effective use of antiviral agents requires a specific virologic diagnosis, by viral isolation or other laboratory techniques, or at least a strong clinical suspicion based on knowledge of distinctive manifestations of disease. Each available drug has a limited spectrum of activity. The mechanism of action of most antiviral agents involves inhibition of viral replication, either through prevention of uncoating (amantadine/rimantadine) or by interference with nucleic acid replication (acyclovir, ganciclovir, vidarabine, ribavirin, zidovudine). It should be noted that no current therapy can eradicate the latent stage of any viral infection, since the antiviral effects involve interference with active viral multiplication. Another approach to antiviral therapy involves the use of immunomodulatory agents (such as the interferons), which alter the host's immune response to viral infection.

ACYCLOVIR (9-[2-HYDROXYETHOXYMETHYL]GUANINE, ACYCLOGUANOSINE, ZOVIRAX)

Acyclovir is the most important and widely used antiviral agent in clinical practice today. It is a synthetic acyclic analogue of guanosine, with specific activity only against viruses of the herpesvirus family. It has clinical efficacy in the treatment of infections caused by herpes simplex virus (HSV) types 1 and 2 and varicella-zoster virus (VZV). In vitro, the concentrations producing 50 percent inhibition of replication (ID_{50}) of these three viruses are 0.02 to 0.2 μg per milliliter, 0.2 to 0.4 μg per milliliter, and 0.8 to 1.2 μg per milliliter, respectively.

Acyclovir has a unique mechanism of selective action

in virus-infected cells. It is phosphorylated by a virus-encoded thymidine kinase (TK) to acyclovir monophosphate. This, in turn, is phosphorylated to the active form of acyclovir triphosphate by cellular enzymes. Acyclovir triphosphate's antiviral effect is twofold: it inhibits viral DNA polymerase through irreversible binding, and it is incorporated into viral DNA where it acts as a chain terminator. Low levels of acyclovir triphosphate can be found in uninfected cells, indicating that cellular TKs are able to phosphorylate acyclovir to some degree. These levels, although 40- to 100-fold lower than in HSV-infected cells, are enough to produce in vitro inhibition of Epstein-Barr virus, which lacks a viral TK but possesses an especially sensitive DNA polymerase. Viral mutants may become resistant to acyclovir in vitro by alterations in either TK or DNA polymerase. There is as yet little clinical evidence to support the notion that TK deficiency leads to poor outcomes in patients treated with acyclovir; indeed, animal studies suggest that TK-deficient strains of HSV may be less virulent.

Pharmacology and Toxicity

Acyclovir is available in topical, intravenous, and oral forms. Topical administration leads to little percutaneous absorption. Infusions of 5 or 10 mg per kilogram every 8 hours in patients with normal renal function produce average peak concentrations of 9.8 μg per milliliter and 20.7 μg per milliliter, respectively, with corresponding trough levels of 0.9 μg per milliliter and 2.3 μg per milliliter. Only 15 to 30 percent of an oral dose of acyclovir is absorbed. Mean steady-state peak and trough plasma concentrations of 0.7 and 0.4 μg per milliliter, respectively, are achieved in adults taking 200 mg orally five times a day. The bioavailability is further reduced with increasing doses, and 800 mg orally five times a day produces peaks of 1.6 μg per milliliter and troughs of 0.8 μg per milliliter. Cerebrospinal fluid (CSF) concentrations are approximately one-half of plasma levels. Acyclovir and its major metabolite are excreted by the kidneys by glomerular filtration and tubular secretion, with an average plasma half-life of 2.9 hours after intravenous administration in adults with normal renal function. Patients with renal insufficiency require adjustments in dosing (Table 1). Peritoneal dialysis is ineffective in removing acyclovir, but in anuric patients receiving hemodialysis, acyclovir should be given after a dialysis session, as up to 60 percent is removed during each 6-hour dialysis.

Acyclovir is relatively nontoxic. Intravenous acyclovir in doses of at least 5 mg per kilogram every 8 hours has been associated with reversible renal dysfunction caused by tubular crystal deposition in 5 percent of patients. Associated risk factors include dehydration, bolus infusion, and preexisting renal insufficiency. Approximately 1 percent of patients develop encephalopathic changes, including lethargy, tremors, confusion, hallucinations, delirium, seizures, and coma. These changes are more common in the presence of renal insufficiency and resolve when therapy is stopped. Rapid infusion of intravenous acyclovir may cause phlebitis, and extravasation causes blistering and burning at the site. Oral acyclovir is benign and is only infrequently associated with headache and nausea. Topical acyclovir may cause transient burning when applied to genital lesions, especially in females. It is not approved for intravaginal use.

TABLE 1 Dosage Adjustment for Intravenous Acyclovir in Patients With Impaired Renal Function

Creatinine Clearance (ml/min/1.73 m²)	*Percentage of Standard Dose*	*Dosing Interval (hours)*
> 50	100	8
25–50	100	12
10–25	100	24
0–10*	50	24

* Administered after hemodialysis.

Clinical Uses

Acyclovir is most frequently used in treatment of infections caused by herpes simplex viruses, which are the subject of a separate chapter in this volume.

Varicella-Zoster Virus

Acyclovir is the treatment of choice in infections caused by VZV. In immunosuppressed patients with herpes zoster (shingles), treatment with high-dose intravenous acyclovir (500 mg per square meter every 8 hours or 12.4 mg per kilogram every 8 hours) for 7 days significantly reduces the likelihood of cutaneous or visceral dissemination, the duration of viral shedding, the duration of pain, and the time to complete healing of lesions. This is especially true if treatment is begun within 72 hours of onset of lesions. Studies in a similar population of immunosuppressed patients comparing treatment with intravenous acyclovir and intravenous vidarabine found better results in the acyclovir group in all parameters mentioned above. Acyclovir treatment does not seem to decrease the incidence of postherpetic neuralgia. Therefore, although intravenous acyclovir treatment reduces the duration of uncomplicated zoster in adults who are not immunodeficient, its use in this population does not seem worth the cost and inconvenience. Trials of oral acyclovir for herpes zoster are underway, and early results show that oral acyclovir may also reduce the duration of lesions and symptoms in uncomplicated zoster. These require the use of much larger doses (800 mg orally five times daily) than are used for HSV. Intravenous acyclovir is also effective in treatment of immunocompromised children with primary varicella (chickenpox). Administration of 500 mg per square meter every 8 hours for 7 days, beginning within 72 hours of onset of skin lesions, reduces the incidence of pneumonitis and other visceral involvement. We infuse each dose over 1 hour and maintain urine output (in milliliters) equal to the number of milligrams of acyclovir in the total daily dose.

Other Herpesviruses

Despite in vitro sensitivity of Epstein-Barr virus (EBV) to acyclovir at clinically achievable levels, the role of acyclovir in treatment of EBV-associated diseases remains limited. Although a rapid decrease in pharyngeal shedding of EBV occurs in patients with severe infectious mononucleosis given high doses of intravenous acyclovir (10 mg per kilogram every 8 hours), treatment does not significantly shorten the clinical course of the disease. Acyclovir has no proven utility in treatment of infections caused by cytomegalovirus; the related compound, ganciclovir, is much more effective and will be discussed below.

GANCICLOVIR (9-[1,3-DIHYDROXY-2-PROPOXYMETHYL]-GUANINE, DHPG, BW759U)

Ganciclovir, like acyclovir, is an acyclic analogue of guanine, but it is active against all human herpesviruses, especially cytomegalovirus (CMV). Like acyclovir, it is selectively phosphorylated in infected cells to the triphosphate form, which inhibits viral DNA polymerase and acts as a DNA chain terminator. It has had extensive investigational use in treatment of serious CMV infections in immunocompromised hosts and has now been licensed by the U.S. Food and Drug Administration (FDA). The ID_{50} of ganciclovir for CMV is in the range of 1 to 4 μM, a level exceeded several-fold by peak plasma levels in patients treated with the usual dose of 5 mg per kilogram. The drug is excreted unchanged in the urine, and patients with renal insufficiency require adjustments in dosage. The major adverse effect of ganciclovir is neutropenia, which is often dose-related and usually resolves when therapy is stopped. This is a frequent limiting factor in patients with underlying immunosuppressive conditions who are receiving other drugs that suppress the bone marrow.

Studies in immunocompromised patients with serious CMV infections (retinitis, pneumonia, hepatitis, and gastrointestinal tract involvement) have shown that ganciclovir treatment at 5 mg per kilogram every 12 hours rapidly clears viremia and viruria in 70 to 80 percent of patients. Stabilization of retinitis and clearing of gastrointestinal symptoms on therapy are frequent, but CMV pneumonia is more refractory to treatment. Clearing of viral shedding does not always correlate with clinical improvement and, unfortunately, most patients relapse when ganciclovir treatment is stopped. This is especially true of patients with the acquired immunodeficiency syndrome (AIDS), who may respond more poorly than transplant recipients to ganciclovir therapy, in part because reversal of immunosuppression in conjunction with the use of ganciclovir is not possible in AIDS patients. Some studies demonstrate prolongation of clinical improvement with maintenance ganciclovir (5 to 6 mg per kilogram once daily) for an indefinite period following initial therapy, although viremia may recur during maintenance therapy.

VIDARABINE (9-β-D-ARABINOFURANOSYLADENINE, ARA-A, ADENINE ARABINOSIDE, VIRA-A)

Vidarabine was the first drug licensed by the FDA for systemic treatment of life-threatening viral infections. It is active against most herpesviruses, with the exception of CMV, as well as pox viruses and hepatitis B. Multiple clinical studies have documented the efficacy of vidarabine in the treatment of serious infections caused by HSV and VZV. Because of its toxicity, vidarabine has now been replaced by acyclovir as the drug of choice in treatment of infections caused by these viruses.

Vidarabine is an analogue of adenine deoxyriboside, which is phosphorylated in host cells to vidarabine triphosphate. This triphosphate form selectively inhibits viral DNA polymerase and acts as a chain terminator in both viral and cellular DNA. Vidarabine inhibits strains of HSV and VZV that are resistant to acyclovir in vitro.

Pharmacology and Toxicity

Vidarabine is available in intravenous form and as a topical preparation for ophthalmic use. A major problem in the clinical use of intravenous vidarabine is its poor solubility (0.45 mg per milliliter at 25 °C). It is administered in a 12-hour continuous infusion of several liters of fluid daily. This fluid load complicates the management of cerebral edema in herpes simplex encephalitis. Infused vidarabine is rapidly deaminated to hypoxanthine arabinoside (ara-Hx), which is much less active than the parent drug. About 50 percent of a daily infusion is excreted in the urine within 24 hours, most in the form of ara-Hx. Excretion is reduced in the presence of renal insufficiency, and the dose of vidarabine must therefore be reduced. Allopurinol interferes with metabolism of ara-Hx, and its use is contraindicated in patients treated with vidarabine.

At the usual dose range of 10 to 15 mg per kilogram per day, the most common adverse effects involve the gastrointestinal system, including anorexia, nausea, vomiting, diarrhea, and weight loss. These are dose-related and tend to resolve within several days despite continued treatment. Central nervous system toxicity is found in 2 to 10 percent of patients, with manifestations including hallucinations, tremors, ataxia, painful paresthesias, myoclonus, confusion, and coma. These are most common in the presence of renal or hepatic insufficiency and in patients on concurrent interferon therapy. Some of these reactions, especially the pain syndromes, may take several months to resolve. At high doses (20 mg per kilogram per day) vidarabine may cause megaloblastic bone marrow changes and pancytopenia. Rashes, infusion-related thrombophlebitis, and, rarely, syndrome of inappropriate secretion of antidiuretic hormone have also been reported. Vidarabine is teratogenic in some animal systems and is therefore not recommended for use in pregnant women.

Clinical Uses

The use of vidarabine in herpes simplex infections is discussed in a separate chapter. Like acyclovir, vidarabine is effective in limiting the severity of VZV infections in the immunocompromised patient, and it is the only drug that has been shown to reduce the incidence of post-herpetic neuralgia. Vidarabine reduces replication of hepatitis B virus; potential applications of vidarabine in treatment of chronic hepatitis B infection are discussed in the chapter *Chronic Hepatitis.*

RIBAVIRIN (1-β-D-RIBOFURANOSYL-1,2,4-TRIAZOLE-3-CARBOXAMIDE, VIRAZOLE)

Ribavirin is a synthetic guanosine analogue with a broad spectrum of in vitro antiviral activity. It appears to have multiple antiviral mechanisms that are not yet well defined. Ribavirin monophosphate, produced via phosphorylation of ribavirin by host cellular enzymes, competitively inhibits guanine nucleotide synthesis. In addition, ribavirin triphosphate inhibits the capping of viral messenger RNA. Ribavirin is generally ineffective against viruses with single-stranded RNA genomes that act directly as messenger RNA, such as the enteroviruses, but has in vitro activity against a range of other RNA and DNA viruses including influenza A and B viruses, respiratory syncytial virus, HSV, Lassa fever virus, and HIV. Resistance to ribavirin is not known to develop as a result of therapy.

Pharmacology and Toxicity

Ribavirin has been studied in intravenous, oral, and aerosolized forms. The pharmacology of the drug is not well understood. Intravenous and oral treatment have been complicated by a mild, dose-related hemolytic anemia due to accumulation of ribavirin within erythrocytes. This is readily reversible upon cessation of therapy. Aerosolized ribavirin reaches high levels in the lungs, with plasma concentrations only 1 percent of those found in respiratory secretions. No hematologic or other systemic effects are associated with the aerosolized form; with the exception of conjunctival irritation, it is extremely well tolerated. Its use is contraindicated in pregnant women, as it has teratogenic effects in animals.

Clinical Uses

Aerosolized ribavirin is approved by the FDA for treatment of infants with lower respiratory tract disease due to respiratory syncytial virus (RSV). RSV infections are implicated in about 100,000 pediatric admissions yearly in the United States. Ribavirin administered in small-particle aerosolized form (20 mg per milliliter at 12 L per minute for 12 to 20 hours daily over 3 to 7 days) has been shown to decrease the severity of fever and systemic symptoms as well as the duration of viral shedding in both normal infants and those with underlying cardiopulmonary disease, although no study has yet shown that these beneficial effects correlate with shorter hospital stays or with less need for oxygen or ventilatory assistance. Aerosolized ribavirin has generally been used in infants who require hospitalization and who have evidence of severe lower respiratory tract disease and RSV on immunofluorescent staining of nasal wash specimens. Treatment of patients on mechanical ventilators requires the use of prefilters in order to prevent precipitation of drug in the tubing. Measurable quantities of drug in the air around the beds of patients receiving ribavirin aerosol have recently raised concerns about exposure of health care workers to this potentially teratogenic agent. This has led to greatly diminished enthusiasm for the use of this therapy.

Studies in small numbers of young adults with naturally occurring influenza A or B have shown modest decreases in duration of clinical illness when they are treated with oral or aerosolized ribavirin, but the results are not striking. Intravenous or oral ribavirin appears quite effective in the treatment of Lassa fever.

AMANTADINE (1-ADAMANTANAMINE HYDROCHLORIDE, SYMMETREL)

Amantadine is a symmetric tricyclic amine. It is active only against influenza A viruses. The mechanism of action is not entirely clear, but amantadine appears to prevent uncoating of the viral genome following penetration of the virus into the host cell. Most isolates of influenza A are inhibited in vitro at concentrations of 0.2 to 0.6 μg per milliliter. Although strains of influenza A can be made resistant to amantadine by laboratory passage, resistance to amantadine in treated patients is not a clinical problem. There has, however, been a report of isolation of resistant strains from untreated patients during an outbreak in East Germany. Amantadine was the first systemic antiviral drug licensed by the FDA and is indicated for treatment and prophylaxis of influenza A infection.

Pharmacology and Toxicity

Oral amantadine is well absorbed. Steady-state plasma levels in healthy adults taking the usual oral dose of 200 mg daily average 0.7 to 0.8 μg per milliliter, with CSF levels 60 percent of those in plasma. Amantadine also reaches therapeutic concentrations in respiratory secretions. Approximately 90 percent is excreted unchanged in the urine; the mean plasma half-life of 12 to 18 hours in healthy young adults increases to 7.4 days in patients with severely impaired renal function (creatinine clearance less than 10 ml per minute). Hemodialysis removes less than 5 percent of a dose, whereas substantially more is removed by peritoneal dialysis. Dosage adjustment is therefore essential in patients with renal insufficiency.

Oral amantadine is relatively well tolerated. Adverse effects are limited to the gastrointestinal and central nervous systems and appear to correlate with high plasma levels. One to 10 percent of treated patients experience nausea, anorexia, insomnia, difficulty in concentrating, headache, and dizziness, but in several studies the incidence of these complaints was not appreciably different between amantadine and placebo recipients. These minor side effects usually occur within 3 to 4 days of initiation of treatment and may resolve despite continued treatment. Toxic plasma levels (more than 1.0 μg per milliliter) in elderly patients or those with impaired renal function more rarely produce severe central nervous system effects, including delirium, hallucinations, convulsions, and coma. These adverse effects may be related to the dopamine-potentiating effects of amantadine, which are the basis for this drug's other common use, the treatment of Parkinson's disease. Patients with known seizure disorders have an increased risk of seizures with amantadine; this risk may be reduced by decreasing the dose. Oral amantadine is contraindicated in patients with gastric ulceration. High doses of amantadine (50 mg per kilogram daily) are teratogenic in rats; therefore amantadine therapy is not appropriate for pregnant women.

Clinical Uses

Amantadine is useful for treatment and prophylaxis of infections caused by influenza A viruses. When administered prophylactically, amantadine is 50 to 91 percent effective in preventing illness due to influenza A. It is more effective in preventing illness than in preventing infection, as documented by virus isolation or seroconversion. This may in fact be beneficial, as subclinical infection may lead to the development of immune responses that will protect against further exposure to antigenically related strains of influenza A virus. Because flu-like symptoms may be caused by several different infectious agents (only one of which is susceptible to amantadine) and because widespread use of amantadine is quite costly and associated with side effects, amantadine prophylaxis should begin only after there is a documented outbreak of influenza A in the community. The prophylactic efficacies of amantadine and influenza vaccine are roughly equivalent, but amantadine is not a substitute for vaccination as it does not protect against influenza B. In addition, amantadine as sole prophylaxis must be continued for the entire duration of the community outbreak, often 4 to 6 weeks, and the incidence of side effects increases with prolonged use. Thus amantadine prophylaxis should be considered an adjunct to immunization; the combined efficacy of amantadine and vaccine approaches 90 percent.

The target population for prophylaxis includes hospitalized patients; children and adults with chronic cardiovascular, pulmonary, metabolic, or renal disorders; immunodeficient patients; and persons over 65 years of age, especially those in nursing homes. Because of the risk of nosocomial transmission of influenza, vaccination and outbreak-period prophylaxis are recommended for health care workers (both hospital and community based) who have extensive contact with high-risk patients and for the entire staff of chronic care facilities.

High-risk patients who have not been immunized before the beginning of an outbreak of influenza A should begin amantadine as soon as possible and be vaccinated as well. Amantadine should be continued for 2 weeks after vaccination or for the duration of the outbreak if the patient is unable to tolerate vaccination (because of a severe allergy to eggs or a history of severe immediate allergic reaction to a previous dose of vaccine) or is at risk of having a poor antibody response to vaccination (for example, the immunocompromised patient).

Several studies have shown that therapeutic use of amantadine, if begun within 24 to 48 hours of onset of flu-like symptoms, reduces the duration of fever and systemic symptoms by one-third, or 1 to 2 days. It also hastens the resolution of minor small airway abnormalities in patients with uncomplicated influenza A and reduces viral shedding. Its efficacy in the treatment or prevention of primary influenza pneumonia is not clear. Nevertheless, oral amantadine therapy should be considered for high-risk patients with an illness compatible with influenza during a period of known or suspected influenza A activity in the community. Therapy should be initiated within 24 to 48 hours of onset of symptoms and continued for 48 hours after resolution.

The usual dose of oral amantadine for both prophylaxis and therapy in normal adults is 100 mg twice daily. For adults over 65 years of age, the recommended daily dose should not exceed 100 mg. Further dosage reductions are needed for patients with impaired renal function (Table 2) and in patients with known seizure disorders. The approved dosage for children 1 to 9 years of age is 4.4 to 8.8 mg per kilogram per day, up to 150 mg per day. Aerosolized amantadine is also effective in treating uncomplicated influenza A infection, producing therapeutic levels in the lungs with little systemic absorption, but the inconvenience of administration fails to warrant its use, especially in comparison with the equally effective oral form.

RIMANTADINE (α-METHYL-1-ADAMANTANEMETHYLAMINE HYDROCHLORIDE)

Rimantadine is a structural analogue of amantadine. It has the same antiviral spectrum and mechanism of action but is somewhat more effective in vitro than aman-

TABLE 2 Dosage Adjustment for Oral Amantadine in Patients With Impaired Renal Function

Creatinine Clearance ($ml/min/1.73\ m^2$)	*Suggested Oral Maintenance Regimen After 200 mg (100 mg b.i.d.) on the First Day*
≥ 80	100 mg b.i.d.
60–80	100 mg b.i.d. alternating with 100 mg daily
40–60	100 mg daily
30–40	200 mg (100 mg b.i.d.) twice weekly
20–30	100 mg 3 times each week
10–20	200 mg (100 mg b.i.d.) alternating with 100 mg q7d
< 10*	100 mg q7d

* Including patients on hemodialysis.
Modified from Horadan et al. Ann Intern Med 1981; 94:454–458.

tadine. Rimantadine is less well absorbed and more extensively metabolized, with less than 10 percent excreted unchanged in the urine. When given in equal doses, steady-state plasma levels of rimantadine are 61 to 65 percent of amantadine values, and the plasma half-life is twice as long. Central nervous system adverse effects are less frequent with rimantadine, correlating perhaps with lower plasma concentrations. Indeed, comparable plasma concentrations produce comparable symptoms, and the incidence of gastrointestinal complaints is the same with the two drugs. Rimantadine has been used extensively in the Soviet Union. It has been studied in several controlled trials in the United States and found to be as effective as amantadine in prophylaxis and therapy of infections caused by influenza A but is not yet licensed for clinical use.

OTHER AGENTS

Foscarnet (trisodium phosphonoformate) is a DNA polymerase inhibitor that is virustatic for herpesviruses. It has some efficacy in treatment of herpes simplex virus infections and is undergoing trials for therapy of CMV infections in immunosuppressed patients. It may also have activity against HIV. Its use is limited by the need for continuous intravenous infusion, and the major adverse effect appears to be renal dysfunction.

Human interferons (IFNs) have multiple antiviral effects, both in inhibition of viral replication and in modulation of host immune responses. Trials are underway to investigate the efficacy of the various interferons, either alone or in combination with other antiviral agents, in the therapy of several different viral diseases. Intralesional human IFN-α is efficacious in therapy of genital papillomavirus infections (condyloma acuminata).

SUGGESTED READING

Dolin R, Reichman RC, Madore HP, et al. A controlled trial of amantadine and rimantadine in the prophylaxis of influenza A infection. N Engl J Med 1982; 307:580–584.

Dorsky DI, Crumpacker CS. Drugs five years later: acyclovir. Ann Intern Med 1987; 107:859–874.

Hall CB, McBride JT, Walsh EE, et al. Aerosolized ribavirin treatment of infants with respiratory syncytial viral infection. N Engl J Med 1983; 308:1443–1447.

Shepp DH, Dandliker PS, Meyers JD. Treatment of varicella-zoster virus infection in severely immunocompromised patients. N Engl J Med 1986; 314:208–212.

ANTIBACTERIAL CHEMOTHERAPY

STEPHEN H. ZINNER, M.D.
KENNETH H. MAYER, M.D.

The past half century of antibiotic chemotherapy has provided physicians with many choices to treat bacterial infections. Several new antibiotic classes have been introduced in the past decade, and a consideration of the appropriate use of these drugs is important in the current practice of medicine.

While many of the newer, expensive antimicrobial agents are active against a wide range of bacterial pathogens, the physician should use less expensive drugs whenever possible. Often, antibiotics may be given for inappropriate indications (e.g., viral syndromes). Antibiotic resistance continues to cause treatment failures, and any unnecessary use of antibiotics that alters the bacterial ecology and enhances the development of antibiotic resistance should be avoided.

This chapter considers the use of specific classes of antibiotics, their pharmacology, the use of antibiotic susceptibility testing, and studies of antibiotic activity in vitro and in vivo.

GENERAL PRINCIPLES OF ANTIBIOTIC THERAPY

The appropriate use of antibiotics requires an estimation of the likelihood of the presence of bacterial infection. A careful history and physical examination should be performed. Whenever possible, a sample should be obtained from the affected body site or from blood, urine, or other body fluid for stain and culture before the selection of an appropriate antibiotic.

If an empiric antibiotic choice is necessary, this should be based on an evaluation of the most likely pathogen responsible for infection at a given clinical site. The spectrum of activity of the drug, its pharmacology, cost, and the frequency of adverse toxic or side effects all affect the choice of antibiotic. If drugs are administered orally, efforts should be made to ensure patient compliance. In general, it is preferable to use a narrow-spectrum or specific antibiotic whenever the organism is known. The use of broad-spectrum agents can result in the suppression of endogenous, commensal bacterial flora, with resulting diarrhea and overgrowth of resistant pathogens.

The optimal duration of antibiotic therapy has not been clearly established for most infections. In many acute infections, it is appropriate to administer antibiotics for approximately 3 to 5 days after the patient has defervesced. Serious infections such as osteomyelitis, bacterial endocarditis, and septic arthritis require longer therapy, often intravenously, for 4 to 6 weeks. Other infections such as meningitis and gram-negative rod bacteremia are usually treated for 10 to 14 days.

ANTIBIOTIC PHARMACOLOGY

The physician should select a drug that is active against the infecting organism at the site of infection. Antibiotic pharmacology includes consideration of pharmacodynamics, which describe the effects of the drug on the bacteria, and of pharmacokinetics, which consider the absorption, distribution, metabolism, and excretion of these agents.

Pharmacodynamics

Pharmacodynamic considerations include evaluations of the in vitro susceptibility of the bacteria to the antibiotic. Several methods exist to determine antibiotic susceptibility. The Kirby-Bauer-Turck disk test is still commonly used in many hospital microbiology laboratories. This method requires the seeding of an agar plate with the test organism and the application of small disks that have been impregnated with known concentrations of antibiotics. The plates are incubated overnight and the zone of inhibition of bacterial growth around the disk is measured. This method provides an estimate of antibiotic inhibition of bacterial growth and not its bactericidal activity.

The minimal inhibitory concentration (MIC) and minimal bactericidal concentration (MBC) are laboratory tests to determine concentrations of a drug that will inhibit or kill a standard bacterial inoculum (usually 10^4 cfu per milliliter). Several automated methods have been introduced in laboratory microbiology to supply clinicians with specific MICs and MBCs.

In general, bactericidal activity is required in the treatment of bacterial infections that are deep seated or occur in an area of minimal host defense, such as osteomyelitis and endocarditis, as well as infections the treatment of which requires the rapid elimination of the bacterial load, e.g., meningitis or bacteremia in immunocompromised patients. Bactericidal agents include penicillins, cephalosporins, aminoglycosides, quinolones, vancomycin, metronidazole, rifampin, and trimethoprim-sulfamethoxazole. Tetracycline, chloramphenicol, erythromycin, clindamycin, and sulfonamides inhibit bacterial growth and are thus bacteriostatic.

More specialized procedures exist to determine antibiotic pharmacodynamics, such as time-kill curves, in which standard bacterial inocula are exposed to variable concentrations of drugs, usually as multiples of the MIC. The effect of these drug concentrations over time is determined by counting the remaining viable bacteria, usually over an 8- or 12-hour period. Time-kill curves are time- and labor-intensive, usually requiring specially trained technologists, and are not routinely performed for clinical isolates.

The minimum antibiotic concentration (MAC) describes the smallest amount of antibiotic that has any measurable effect on bacteria, such as reduction in bacterial growth rates, bacterial elongation or filamentation, or changes in the adherence of bacteria to various tissues or surfaces. These MACs could result in enhanced phagocytosis at infected tissue sites. Some antibiotics exert an effect on bacteria at concentrations below the MIC. Subinhibitory effects also might enhance local phagocytosis and synergistically abet the activity of other antibiotics when combination chemotherapy is used.

The effect of antibiotics on bacteria can persist after the extracellular drug has been removed. This is known as the postantibiotic effect (PAE) and can be measured in vitro by bacterial exposure to antibiotics, subsequent removal of the drug by washing or enzymatic inactivation, and then comparing the rate of bacterial growth to that of unexposed bacteria. The PAE reflects the difference in time for control and treated bacteria to increase in number by one log. The clinical significance of the PAE is not clearly known, but it may contribute to the clinical activity of aminoglycosides and quinolones.

Local conditions at the site of infection may influence the activity of certain antibiotics. For example, the pH of the surrounding tissues can affect antibiotic activity. Aminoglycosides and erythromycin are more active at an alkaline pH. These drugs are less effective within an abscess or other infected tissues with low pH. Aminoglycosides are not active in an anaerobic environment. Other drugs may be relatively inhibited in the presence of certain urinary components. The activity of aminoglycosides and some of the new quinolone antibiotics may be decreased in the presence of high concentrations of calcium, magnesium, or other cations. All antibiotics may reversibly bind to serum albumin, but tightly bound compounds such as certain cephalosporins may not achieve high concentrations of free or active drug in the central nervous system or in other tissues.

Pharmacokinetics

Some new drugs have been developed in order to take advantage of pharmacokinetic properties. In general, the clinical activity of a drug depends upon the ability to achieve peak serum concentrations of free or unbound drug that are well in excess of the MIC for a given bacterial pathogen. Other important considerations include the time above the MIC, the area under the concentration–time curve above the MIC, as well as the ratio of peak serum concentration to the MIC (Fig. 1). The clinical significance of these variables is especially important with agents such as aminoglycosides, which demonstrate concentration-dependent bactericidal activity.

The route of administration, bioavailability, volume of distribution, and administered dose independently affect the concentration of antibiotic achieved in serum and tissue. The highest serum concentrations usually follow the intravenous administration of an antibiotic. However, some well-absorbed drugs (e.g., chloramphenicol and the fluoroquinolones) achieve similar concentrations by mouth as well as by intravenous administration, although the time to achieve this concentration after oral dosing is delayed by about 1 hour.

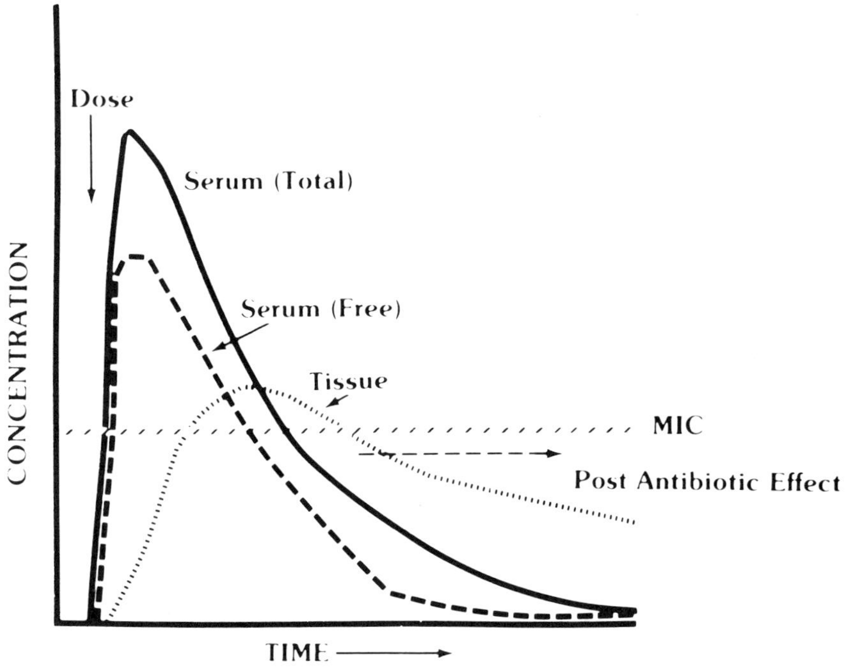

Figure 1 Diagram showing the relation between drug concentrations in serum and those in tissues after a single dose. The postantibiotic effect begins when levels in tissues fall below the MIC. (Reprinted with permission from Kunin CM. Dosage schedules of antimicrobial agents: a historical review. Rev Infect Dis 1981; 3:4–11; by permission of The University of Chicago Press.)

The distribution of antibiotics may also depend on the drug's lipid-partition coefficient. Lipophilic drugs, such as chloramphenicol and rifampin, are more diffusible across cell and tissue membranes. Clinically, this is most important in the treatment of bacterial meningitis where chloramphenicol, rifampin, tetracyclines, sulfonamides, and metronidazole achieve acceptable concentrations even in the absence of inflammation. In the presence of inflamed meninges, adequate therapeutic concentrations are usually achieved with penicillins and most third-generation cephalosporins. Aminoglycosides, clindamycin, erythromycin, and vancomycin cannot reliably achieve therapeutic concentrations in cerebrospinal fluid. Experience with the new quinolones in meningitis is limited.

The absorption of some drugs, notably tetracyclines and the quinolones, may be decreased in the presence of bivalent or trivalent cations. These drugs are less well absorbed following the administration of calcium- or aluminum-containing antacids, respectively.

The volume of distribution of an antimicrobial agent influences the duration of the peak concentration as well as the penetration into tissues. Drugs such as the quinolones, which have a high volume of distribution, have a relatively prompt decrease in their peak concentrations following intravenous administration.

The rate of elimination of an antibiotic is expressed as its elimination half-life (t½). The t½ of antibiotics ranges from less than 1 hour for the penicillins and first-generation cephalosporins to between 3 and 5 hours for some of the new quinolone drugs. In general, the shorter the t½, the more frequently a drug must be administered to achieve an antibacterial effect. Drugs with a very long t½ (e.g., ceftriaxone) may be administered once daily. The dosing of antimicrobial agents that are primarily excreted by the kidney is often reduced in the presence of renal failure. In most cases either each dose is reduced or the interval between doses is prolonged in order to provide appropriate levels and minimize toxicity. Metabolism and excretion of antibiotics are also important factors to consider in determining the ability of active drug to reach the site of infection.

Serum drug concentrations are usually measured for antibiotics having a narrow therapeutic range. Aminoglycosides have variable pharmacokinetics, and their use requires frequent monitoring of serum levels. High trough concentrations of aminoglycosides have been associated with nephrotoxicity.

The serum bactericidal assay utilizes a sample obtained following an antibiotic dose. The ability of successive serum dilutions (e.g., 1:2, 1:4, etc.) to kill a standard inoculum of the patient's infecting organism is determined. The serum bactericidal titer (SBT) is expressed as the highest dilution that kills 99.9 percent of the inoculum. This test describes the relation of achievable drug concentration to the MBC and is useful in the treatment of bacterial endocarditis and osteomyelitis, as well as in bacteremia in the immunocompromised patient. In general, SBTs 1:16 or higher have been associated with good clinical outcome.

ANTIBIOTIC RESISTANCE

Bacteria may become resistant to antibiotics by several mechanisms. Mutations (changes in the bacterial chromosome) may result in antibiotic resistance by alterations in cell wall or membrane components with subsequent drug impermeability. A mutation may result in the alteration of a specific target or binding site of the antibiotic. Mutation in a bacterial regulatory gene may result in overproduction of a substrate or result in the loss of a biochemical intermediate on which the antibiotic acts. Mutations are not readily transferable between species. Although mutated bacteria are resistant to antibiotics, they also have growth disadvantages when compared to their wild-type counterparts. Antibiotic selection pressure clearly may be related to an increase in resistant mutants.

Antibiotic resistance also may be mediated by self-replicating, transferable genetic material called plasmids. These plasmids may contain multiple genes in addition to those mediating antibiotic resistance, and more than one plasmid may exist within a given bacterial cell. In this setting, genetic exchange or recombination can occur, and resistance determinants may move from one plasmid to another or from a plasmid to a chromosome by smaller motile genes called transposons.

Several clinically common mechanisms are responsible for antibiotic resistance in many bacterial species. Enzymes that hydrolyze the β-lactam ring of penicillins and similar compounds render these antibiotics inactive, as they are no longer able to bind specific binding proteins. These β-lactamases may be chromosomally or plasmid-mediated and are common in many species. The ability of bacteria to produce β-lactamases may be constitutive (substrate independent), as in the case of many gram-negative bacilli, or inducible (substrate dependent), as with many gram-positive

TABLE 1 Antibiotics in Clinical Use

Category, Agent	*Available by Oral Route*	*Category, Agent*	*Available by Oral Route*
Penicillins		Other β-lactam drugs	
Penicillin	Yes	Aztreonam	
Ampicillin (±βLI)	Yes	Imipenem-cilastatin	
Amoxicillin (±βLI)	Yes		
Oxacillin	Yes	Aminoglycosides	
Methicillin		Gentamicin	
Nafcillin		Tobramycin	
Cloxacillin	Yes	Amikacin	
Dicloxacillin	Yes	Netilmicin	
Azlocillin			
Mezlocillin		Quinolones	
Piperacillin		Nalidixic acid	Yes
Ticarcillin (±βLI)		Cinoxacin	Yes
Carbenicillin		Norfloxacin	Yes
Amdinocillin		Ciprofloxacin	Yes
		Enoxacin (I)	Yes
Cephalosporins and cefamycins		Ofloxacin (I)	Yes
First-generation*		Lomefloxacin (I)	Yes
Cephalothin		Fleroxacin (I)	Yes
Cefazolin		Pefloxacin (I)	Yes
Cephapirin			
Cephalexin	Yes	Other antibacterial drugs	
Cephradine	Yes	Chloramphenicol	Yes
Cefaclor	Yes	Clindamycin	Yes
Cefadroxil		Erythromycin	Yes
Second-generation†		Metronidazole	Yes
Cefamandole		Nitrofurantoin	Yes
Cefuroxime	Yes	Rifampin	Yes
Cefoxitin		Sulfonamides	Yes
Cefotetan		Trimethoprim	Yes
Cefonicid		Tetracycline (minocycline, doxycycline)	Yes
Ceforanide		Vancomycin	
Third-generation‡		Spectinomycin	
Cefotaxime			
Ceftizoxime			
Ceftriaxone			
Cefoperazone (±βLI)			
Ceftazidime			
Moxalactam			
Cefpiramide			
Cefsulodin			
Cefmenoxime			

Note: (±βLI): may be administered in combination with a β-lactamase inhibitor to enhance antibacterial spectrum; (I): investigational drug.
* First-generation drugs are active against gram-positive cocci and some gram-negative rods.
† Second-generation drugs are also active against *Haemophilus* species and some anaerobic organisms.
‡ Third-generation drugs are more active against gram-negative bacilli and less active against gram-positive cocci, and some have activity against *P. aeruginosa*.

cocci. The β-lactamases may be excreted extracellularly, as in most gram-positive cocci, or may be retained within the periplasmic space between the inner and outer membranes of gram-negative bacilli.

β-Lactam antibiotics also may be inactive against resistant bacteria by means of changes in porins, which are cell wall proteins responsible for the water-filled channels that limit the permeability of the bacterial cells for specific compounds.

Aminoglycosides are most often inactivated because of the production of aminoglycoside-modifying enzymes. These acetylating, adenylating, or phosphorylating enzymes decrease the ability of the aminoglycosides to bind to their ribosomal targets. Some bacteria resist aminoglycosides by mutations in their oxidative phosphorylation mechanisms, which may affect the uptake of aminoglycosides into the bacterial cell. Bacteria also produce enzymes that inactivate chloramphenicol. Resistance to erythromycin is often mediated by ribosomal methylation, which prevents antibiotic binding. Resistance to sulfonamides and trimethoprim may be mediated by plasmid-encoded target enzymes that are not susceptible to these drugs.

ANTIBIOTIC CLASSES

The antibiotics in clinical use are listed in Table 1. Table 2 describes the spectrum of activity of some commonly used antibiotics against prevalent bacterial pathogens.

Penicillins

The penicillins kill bacteria by inhibiting cell wall synthesis. Penicillins bind to specific proteins that prevent peptide cross-linkages, and thus the cell wall becomes osmotically fragile. Some penicillin-binding proteins mediate bacterial lysis, and others, elongation or filament formation. Their spectrum includes the streptococci, clostridia, *Neisseria* species, some anaerobic gram-negative rods, and *Treponema pallidum*. Semisynthetic penicillins, such as nafcillin, oxacillin, methicillin, cloxacillin, and dicloxacillin are bactericidal for *Staphylococcus aureus* and some strains of *Staphylococcus epidermidis*. The extended-spectrum penicillins such as ampicillin and amoxicillin are not active against penicillinase-producing strains of *S. aureus*, but they are active against some gram-negative enteric bacilli such as

TABLE 2 Spectrum of Activity of Some Commonly Used Antibiotics Against Prevalent Bacterial Pathogens

	Organism					
Antibiotic Class	*Nonenterococcal Streptococci*	*Enterococcus**	*S. aureus*†	*Enterobacteriaceae*	*P. aeruginosa*	*Anaerobes*‡
Natural penicillin	++++	+++	+/−	−	−	+++/−
Ampicillin	+++	++++	+/−	+	−	+++/−
Gram-positive semisynthetic penicillin	++	++	++++/−	−	−	+/−
Ureidopenicillin	++	++++	+/−	++++	+++	+++/−
First-generation cephalosporin	++	−	+++/−	++++	−	+/−
Second-generation cephalosporin	++	−	+/−	+++	−	+++
Third-generation cephalosporin§	+	−	+/−	++++	++	+++
Monobactam	−	−	−	+++	++	−
Carbapenem	+++	+++	+++/+	++++	++++	+++
Aminoglycoside#	−	+	++	+++	++	−
Fluoroquinolone	+	−	+++	++++	++++	−
Tetracycline	++	−	+	+	−	+/−
Erythromycin	++	−	++	−	−	+/−
Chloramphenicol	+++	−	++	++	−	+++
Vancomycin	++++	++++	++++	−	−	−
Metronidazole	−	−	−	−	−	++++
Clindamycin	++	−	++	−	−	++++

Specific susceptibilities should be performed on any clinical isolate, since the acquisition of chromosomal- or plasmid-mediated resistance may inactivate a generally efficacious antibiotic. The site of an infection may make an antibiotic with excellent in vitro activity less desirable (e.g., vancomycin for a staphylococcal brain abscess). Allergic reactions and common drug toxicities may limit the use of an agent for a specific infection.

− = no activity
\+ = some activity
++ = moderate activity
+++ = good activity
++++ = first-line agent
* Systemic enterococcal infection requires therapy with a β-lactam or vancomycin (cell wall active compounds) *plus* an aminoglycoside.
† Methicillin susceptible/methicillin resistant.
‡ Anaerobes above the diaphragm/anaerobes below.
§ Specific agents may differ greatly in their activity against gram-negative aerobes.
# Aminoglycosides are rarely used as monotherapy.

Salmonella, *Shigella*, and many urinary tract strains of *Escherichia coli*. In addition, these drugs are active against many strains of *Haemophilus influenzae*. The antipseudomonal penicillins are frequently active against Enterobacteriaceae and include carbenicillin, ticarcillin, piperacillin, azlocillin, and mezlocillin, the latter of which is least active against *Pseudomonas aeruginosa*. These penicillins do not resist the activity of β-lactamases, but amoxicillin, ticarcillin, and ampicillin have been combined with β-lactamase inhibitors such as clavulanic acid and sulbactam, with enhanced activity against many β-lactamase-producing strains of gram-negative rods, including some anaerobic organisms.

Cephalosporins

The cephalosporins have a similar mechanism of action to the penicillins and are active against many gram-negative rods as well as methicillin-sensitive staphylococci and streptococci. The first-generation cephalosporins (cephalothin, cefazolin, cefapirin, and others) are primarily active against staphylococci and urinary isolates of *E. coli*. Newer cephalosporins are also active against β-lactamase-producing *H. influenzae*. Cefotetan and cefoxitin are particularly active against anaerobes. The most recently developed cephalosporins have extended spectra that include most aerobic, multiresistant gram-negative rods. Ceftazidime is also active against *P. aeruginosa*.

Other β-lactam agents include aztreonam, a monobactam agent with activity only against gram-negative bacteria, including *P. aeruginosa*. Imipenem is a carbapenem antibiotic with broad-spectrum activity against most aerobic and anaerobic bacteria. Clinically, it is combined with cilastatin, which inhibits its renal degradation.

Aminoglycosides

The aminoglycoside antibiotics are rapidly bactericidal against gram-negative aerobic bacteria including *P. aeruginosa*. These antibiotics also kill *S. aureus* and, in combination with penicillin or ampicillin, are bactericidal for enterococci. They act on ribosomes and their activity requires metabolic uptake across the bacterial membranes. These drugs are administered intravenously or intramuscularly and are often used in combination with β-lactam agents in the treatment of gram-negative rod bacteremia.

Quinolones

The older quinolones, nalidixic acid and cinoxacin, are primarily limited to the treatment of susceptible urinary tract infections. The new fluoroquinolones, norfloxacin and ciprofloxacin, have enhanced activity against most gram-negative rods, including *P. aeruginosa,* and are active against enteric bacterial pathogens. The new quinolones are also active against staphylococci, *Legionella* species, *Chlamydia trachomatis*, and *Ureaplasma urealyticum*. Some quinolones may be active against some mycobacterial species. These drugs have limited activity against streptococci and no activity against anaerobic gram-negative rods. The quinolones are well absorbed orally, have a large volume of distribution, and act intracellularly. Norfloxacin is clinically limited to urinary and some gastrointestinal infections.

Other Antibacterial Drugs

Chloramphenicol is primarily limited to treatment of bacterial meningitis, brain abscess, and typhoid fever. Clindamycin is a useful antibiotic active against anaerobic gram-negative rods and many gram-positive cocci, including *S. aureus*. Erythromycin is the treatment of choice for Legionnaire's disease and is active against many gram-positive cocci.

Metronidazole's activity is limited to anaerobic organisms, and it is frequently used in the treatment of intra-abdominal infections. Nitrofurantoin is limited to the treatment of urinary tract infections due to susceptible aerobic gram-negative rods. Rifampin is an agent that is usually limited for use in the treatment of tuberculosis but also has activity against gram-positive cocci and many gram-negative rods. It is never used alone because mutational resistance develops rapidly. Its use should be limited to special clinical situations and should be in combination with other antibiotics.

The sulfonamides are primarily used in the treatment of urinary tract infections and in infections caused by *Nocardia asteroides*. They are frequently combined with trimethoprim to enhance activity and bactericidal effects. Tetracyclines are broad-spectrum antimicrobial agents active against a number of intracellular organisms including rickettsiae, mycoplasmas, chlamydiae, and some parasitic infections, as well as some bacteria. Vancomycin is active against most gram-positive organisms, including methicillin-resistant staphylococci. Oral vancomycin may also be used to treat *Clostridium difficile*-related colitis. Spectinomycin is primarily used in the treatment of gonococcal infections.

ANTIBIOTIC COMBINATIONS

Antibiotic synergism occurs with antibiotic combinations in a few clinical circumstances, notably bacteremia in neutropenic patients and enterococcal endocarditis and infections caused by *P. aeruginosa*. Antibiotics may be combined in mixed infections and possibly to limit the emergence of antibiotic-resistant bacteria. Unnecessary antibiotic combinations needlessly contribute to increased costs and could result in drug antagonism.

ANTIBIOTIC PROPHYLAXIS

It is impossible to prevent all infections with antibiotic prophylaxis. However, the preventive use of these agents is clearly valuable in some surgical operations, notably, foreign-body implants, cardiovascular surgery, operations on an infected biliary tract, contaminated intra-abdominal procedures, vaginal and abdominal hysterectomy, and trauma associated with ruptured abdominal viscera or compound fractures. Antibiotic prophylaxis should be started just before surgery and should be stopped within 24 hours after surgery. Two doses of most agents, or one dose of a long-acting agent, are usually sufficient. Longer courses may lead to superinfections and obviously increase costs without benefit to patients.

Prophylactic antibiotics are also used to prevent bacterial endocarditis following instrumentation, surgery, or dental treatment. Prophylaxis is also useful in the prevention of secondary cases of rheumatic fever and following exposure to meningitis caused by *N. meningitidis* and *H. influenzae*. These issues are addressed more fully in other chapters.

CONCLUSIONS

Judicious use of antimicrobial agents requires consideration of the spectrum, pharmacodynamics, and pharmacokinetics, as well as the cost of these frequently expensive drugs. The current trend appears to favor the use of single or twice daily doses of intravenous drugs for serious infections. The use of oral agents with excellent pharmacokinetic properties may minimize hospitalization-associated costs. The utilization of intravenous antibiotics at home is becoming more common, and physicians should closely supervise and monitor the patient's care. Potential adverse effects and pharmacologic interactions of antibiotics should always be considered so that the physician can choose the least expensive and least toxic but most specific and efficacious antibiotic for any given infection.

SUGGESTED READING

Handbook of antimicrobial therapy. New Rochelle, NY: The Medical Letter, 1986.

Kucers A, Bennett N. The use of antibiotics: a comprehensive review with clinical emphasis. Philadelphia: JB Lippincott, 1987.

Neu H. Chemotherapy of infection. In: Braunwald E, ed. Harrison's principles of internal medicine. 12th ed. New York: McGraw-Hill, 1987:485–502.

Sande MA, Mandell GL. Chemotherapy of microbial diseases. In: Goodman and Gilman's the pharmacological basis of therapeutics. 7th ed. New York: Macmillan Publishing, 1980:1066–1198.

Young LS. Antimicrobial therapy. In: Wyngaarden JB, Smith LH, eds. Cecil textbook of medicine 18th ed. Philadelphia: WB Saunders, 1988:112–125.

ANTIFUNGAL CHEMOTHERAPY

HEINZ-JOSEF SCHMITT, M.D.
DONALD ARMSTRONG, M.D.

This chapter reviews antifungal agents that can be used for the treatment of systemic fungal infections. Table 1 shows agents currently available or in various states of clinical evaluation. Ever since its introduction in the 1950s, amphotericin B has been the "gold standard" of treatment of most invasive fungal diseases, despite its considerable toxicity. New agents are on the horizon. The evaluation of their efficacy in human disease, however, as compared with the evaluation of antibacterial agents, is difficult for several reasons:

1. In vitro tests are not standardized, and determination of minimal inhibitory concentrations (MICs) often differs more than 1,000-fold among different laboratories.
2. Animal models more reliably reveal antifungal activity. However, data are sometimes conflicting, and the disease produced may not reflect the counterpart seen in humans (e.g., injection of aspergillus spores intravenously does not produce pulmonary aspergillosis).
3. Clinical trials are difficult to perform because (1) the diagnosis of many systemic fungal infections is difficult to prove without invasive techniques (exception, cryptococcal meningitis); (2) some fungal diseases are rare, and it may take years to complete clinical trials; and (3) in some cases fungal infections heal spontaneously, e.g., when the immune system of a patient recovers or when immunosuppressive therapy is stopped.

These limitations should always be kept in mind when in vitro test results or cases of "successful treatment" of a fungal disease with a new agent are reported. For many diseases the optimal duration of treatment is not known. As a rule of thumb, immunocompromised patients require longer, and sometimes indefinite, treatment.

POLYENES

Polyenes, of which amphotericin B is an example, share a similar structure, mechanism of action, pharmacology, and toxicity. There is practically complete cross-resistance. They are all poorly absorbed from the gastrointestinal tract and remarkably toxic when given parenterally. The common mechanism of action is binding of the lipophilic polyene component to the ergosterol in fungal cytoplasmic membranes, thus causing the membrane to become porous.

Modification of membrane sterols leading to a less efficient binding with amphotericin B and a decrease in membrane ergosterol are mechanisms for resistance. With rare exceptions, however, emergence of resistance is not of major clinical concern. However, a lack of bioavailability of amphotericin B probably contributes to therapeutic failures, especially in immunocompromised patients: Patients dying of invasive aspergillosis and candidiasis had

TABLE 1 Antifungal Agents for Treatment of Systemic Mycoses

Polyenes
Amphotericin B
Nystatin*
5-Fluorocytosine
Azoles
Clotrimazole*
Miconazole
Ketoconazole
Fluconazole†
Itraconazole†
Allylamines
Naftifine*†
Terbinafine†
Lipopeptides
Cilofungin†

* Topical use only.
† Investigational antifungal agents.

amphotericin B concentrations in infected organs that exceeded their MIC by 100-fold, as determined from isolates cultured from the autopsy specimens.

Filipin, trichomycin, candidin, and other compounds of the polyene group have no advantage over amphotericin B, nystatin, and natamycin (pimaricin only as 5 percent ophthalmic suspension), which are the only polyenes marketed in the United States. Nystatin and natamycin are only used topically. None of the others has any proven advantage in terms of clinical efficacy.

Amphotericin B

Amphotericin B is produced by *Streptomyces nodosus*. It is given intravenously in 250 (lower doses) to 1,000 ml of 5 percent dextrose in water (D5W; the recommended final concentration is 0.1 mg per milliliter) over 4 to 6 hours. When it is freshly prepared, protection of amphotericin B from light is not necessary. Addition of electrolytes, sodium, or potassium salts causes aggregation of the amphotericin B suspension and results in decreased effectiveness.

In serum, amphotericin B is separated from the desoxycholate with which it is packaged and binds to β-lipoproteins (probably cholesterol). It leaves the bloodstream rapidly and accumulates in the liver, spleen, and kidneys. The highest amphotericin B concentrations are found in these organs, and lung concentrations are about one-fifth to one-tenth of those found in the liver. Amphotericin B does not penetrate inflamed or normal meninges very well; drug concentrations in inflamed peritoneum, pleura, joints, and vitreous and aqueous humor are about 50 percent of serum concentrations or higher. Serum levels are not helpful in predicting outcome, efficacy, or side effects. Only a small amount of amphotericin B is excreted via the urine. The exact mode of excretion is unknown, although in dogs and rats biliary excretion accounts for some elimination.

No dose-adjustment is necessary in patients with renal failure, except for the purpose of decreasing renal toxicity. Hemodialysis does not change blood levels unless a patient is lipemic and loses amphotericin B because it binds to the dialysis membrane.

Dosage and duration of therapy depend on the type and severity of infection, the underlying disease, the patient's general condition and tolerance, and side effects. Candidal esophagitis usually responds to doses as small as 0.2 to 0.3 mg per kilogram given intravenously for 5 to 7 days. We treat life-threatening fungal infections in immunocompromised patients with 1 mg per kilogram per day, usually for a total dose of 1.0 to 2.5 g. First, a 1-mg test dose is given over 4 hours, and vital signs are monitored at least every 30 minutes. If the dose is tolerated, immediately thereafter 5 mg, followed by 10 mg, 20 mg, and 40 mg, are administered every 4 to 6 hours. Thus, the total dose given on day 1 of amphotericin B treatment is about 1 mg per kilogram, which is the usual dose on the following days.

About 50 percent of all patients receiving amphotericin B experience acute reactions (fevers, chills, malaise), which usually last for a few hours and become less severe with continued therapy. These seem to be due to release of interleukin 1 and tumor necrosis factor and can be ameliorated, if necessary, by premedication with acetaminophen (700 mg orally) and meperidine (50 mg intravenously). Hydrocortisone (50 mg intravenously) can be given if reactions are extreme, but this must be weighed against the possible immunosuppressive effects of glucocorticoids. It is not helpful in patients already receiving steroids for other reasons.

An increase in creatinine level occurs in virtually every patient on amphotericin B. The amount of permanent reduction in the glomerular filtration rate is related to the total dose given. Salt supplementation administered by antibiotic solutions containing large amounts of sodium (e.g., ticarcillin) or by sodium chloride solution (e.g., 1 L of 0.9 percent sodium chloride per day) may minimize amphotericin B–induced nephrotoxicity.

Since only a small amount of amphotericin B is excreted via the kidneys, no dosage adjustment is necessary for patients with a rising creatinine level. For a serum creatinine concentration between 3.0 and 3.5 mg per milliliter, however, a dose reduction may become necessary in order to prevent dehydration and cachexia secondary to nausea and vomiting. In this situation, amphotericin B is often given in a somewhat higher single dose (1.25 mg per kilogram) every other day if the patient is stable and clearly responding. Kidney toxicity is only prevented if the dose given every other day is not doubled.

Electrolytes in serum should be monitored carefully. Hypokalemia and hypomagnesemia occur regularly. Other adverse effects of amphotericin B include anemia, weight loss, headache, phlebitis, renal tubular acidosis, and, in rare cases, thrombocytopenia, leukopenia, burning sensation on the soles of the feet, hypotension, and anaphylaxis. In one report, aggregation of leukocytes by amphotericin B given directly after a white blood cell transfusion was believed to be the cause of acute pulmonary deterioration.

With the first dose, the patient's blood pressure should be checked at least every half hour. Further monitoring should include at least a thrice-weekly determination of the complete blood count, K^+, Na^+, Mg^{++}, and urinalysis. Since amphotericin B is eliminated slowly, its side effects may persist for months after completion of therapy.

Diseases that usually respond to intravenous therapy with amphotericin B include aspergillosis, blastomycosis, candidiasis, coccidioidomycosis, cryptococcosis, histoplasmosis, mucormycosis, paracoccidioidomycosis, and extracutaneous sporotrichosis. In patients with prolonged fever and neutropenia some investigators recommend amphotericin B empirically from day 5 to 7 on, even without documenting a fungal infection. The diagnosis of invasive fungal disease is missed in many of these patients, even when optimal diagnostic approaches are used, and early treatment improves outcome of opportunistic fungal infections.

In order to improve efficacy (bioavailability) or to decrease the amount of adverse effects, local therapy with amphotericin B is used in some instances. Intracisternal or intraventricular amphotericin B is essential for treating meningitis due to *Coccidioides immitis*. In a series from our institution, intraventricular amphotericin B given through an Ommaya reservoir was correlated with improved survival among cancer patients with cryptococcal meningitis. After test doses of 0.05 and 0.1 mg per day on days 1 and 2, a total of 0.2 to 0.5 mg amphotericin B is given once daily to three times a week. More frequent administration is given for more severe disease along with the higher doses. There is no evidence that intrathecal injection in the lumbar area is beneficial. If lumbar injections are used, 10 percent glucose may be preferred for dilution of the stock solution in order to facilitate hyperbaric flow to the brain. Additional intrathecal injection of 5 to 15 mg of hydrocortisone may decrease fever, headache, and nausea. In cystitis due to *Candida*, bladder irrigations with amphotericin B (0.05 mg per milliliter in distilled water) have been suggested. Joint mycosis due to *Sporothrix schenckii* or *C. immitis* may respond favorably to intra-articular injection of amphotericin B (5 to 15 mg). For keratomycoses, corneal baths with amphotericin B (1 mg per milliliter) are used.

New Methods of Delivering Amphotericin B

First reports indicate that amphotericin B encapsulated in liposomes is much better tolerated than amphotericin B desoxycholate. There appears to be virtually no acute toxicity, and adverse reactions occur in only about 3 percent of all patients. The incidence of nephrotoxicity is also decreased. One study group, however, reported somnolence in some patients. The mode of preparation and composition of liposomes may be crucial. The main advantage of liposomal amphotericin B appears to be the increased therapeutic index: much higher doses can be given with fewer adverse effects. Controlled clinical trials will have to show whether there will also be an increased therapeutic efficacy.

Nasal amphotericin B (10 mg per day in three divided doses) given with a sterile atomizer is currently under investigation for prophylaxis of pulmonary aspergillosis in patients with neutropenia and fever. Since the pathogenesis of pulmonary aspergillosis involves direct inhalation of *Aspergillus* spores into distal airways as well as colonization of the upper nasopharynx, we believe that additional measures should be taken. Aerosol amphotericin B has been effective in both preventing and treating pulmonary aspergillosis in our rat model of this disease, and clinical trials are underway.

Amphotericin B in Combination With Other Agents

The rationale in combining amphotericin B with other agents is to increase its efficacy and/or to reduce its toxicity. Many combinations have been shown to act synergistically with amphotericin B in vitro or even in animal models. To date, the only generally accepted indication is cryptococcal meningitis, for which amphotericin B is combined with 5-fluorocytosine (5-FC). Prospective, randomized controlled clinical trials have documented this indication.

Systemic candidiasis due to *Candida tropicalis* we believe to be another indication for the combined use of amphotericin B and 5-FC as suggested from one retrospective study.

In vitro, there is a two- to fourfold reduction in MICs against *Aspergillus, Candida, Cryptococcus, Histoplasma*, and *Mucor* when amphotericin B is combined with rifampin. In our animal model of systemic candidiasis, rifampin acts "synergistically" with amphotericin B, at least in part by increasing about twofold peak serum concentrations of amphotericin B (unpublished data). Clinical studies are needed to further investigate the role of amphotericin B plus rifampin in the treatment of fungal infections.

In various animal models, the combination of ketoconazole and amphotericin B was no better than amphotericin B alone. Some studies even suggested antagonism. Theoretically, antagonism may result when azoles block the synthesis of ergosterol, thus leaving amphotericin B without a target.

Nystatin

Nystatin is available in the United States for topical and oral administration, and it can be used to treat candidal infections of the skin and mucous membranes. Ringworm and subcutaneous fungal infections do not respond. There is no systemic absorption.

Indications for its use are oropharyngeal and esophageal candidiasis (5 ml of the 100,000 U per milliliter suspension four times daily swished in the oral cavity and swallowed thereafter) and vaginal candidiasis (1 tablet with 100,000 U inserted once or twice a day with an applicator high into the vagina for 14 days). For this indication, however, miconazole or clotrimazole cream given for 1 week only might have a lower failure rate. The one-week regimen with clotrimazole or miconazole is more convenient.

Whether nystatin given orally reduces the risk of recurrence of vaginal candidiasis by preventing fecal-vaginal recolonization is less clear. It has been used in doses of up to 30 million U per day in immunocompromised patients in protected environments, and, again, the benefit of this kind of prophylaxis is controversial. We do not use it. The only major side effect, however, is the bad taste of nystatin.

FLUCYTOSINE

5-Fluorocytosine (5-FC) was initially developed to be used as an anticancer agent. Although it was ineffective for this indication, it was found to be effective in experimental fungal infections.

After uptake into a fungal cell by a cytosine permease, 5-FC is deaminated by a cytosine deaminase to 5-fluorouracil (5-FU) and converted to 5-fluorodeoxyuridylic acid monophosphate. The latter is a noncompetitive inhibitor of thymidylate synthetase, interfering with DNA synthesis. Another mechanism of action is replacement of uracil by 5-FU in fungal RNA, leading to a disturbance in protein synthesis.

The two prerequisites for the antifungal activity of 5-FC are enzymatic uptake into the fungal cell and enzymatic conversion to the finally active inhibitor. A decreased permeability (loss of activity of cytosine permease) and a loss of activity of cytosine deaminase as well as other enzymes may lead to resistance to 5-FC. An increase in the amount of de novo synthetized pyrimidines is another mechanism of resistance.

5-FC is marketed in the United States as 250-mg and 500-mg capsules. An intravenous solution is available in other countries, but may only be obtained in the United States for compassionate use from the producer.

5-FC is readily and completely absorbed from the gastrointestinal tract. There is virtually no protein binding, and about 90 percent is excreted unchanged into the urine. In the cerebrospinal fluid (CSF) more than 70 percent of the serum concentration can be achieved. Hemodialysis and peritoneal dialysis remove the medication from the body. In patients with normal renal function, the half-life of 5-FC is about 4 hours, but it is remarkably prolonged in patients with azotemia.

The usual dose is 150 mg per kilogram per day in four divided doses (orally or intravenously). We recommend starting with a daily dose of 100 mg per kilogram per day of 5-FC in order to take into account renal function in older people or those on renally toxic antibiotics, such as aminoglycosides and amphotericin B. Blood levels (see below) should be monitored. It has been suggested to calculate the dose of 5-FC to be given by dividing the usual dose (150 mg per kilogram per day) by the serum creatinine. Patients on hemodialysis should receive a single dose of 37.5 mg per kilogram after each dialysis.

In any case, subsequent doses in all patients should be adjusted according to serum levels obtained before and 2 hours after the administration of 5-FC. A bioassay as well as chemical method give reliable results. Recommended optimal values should range between 50 and 100 μg per milliliter of serum. Levels above 100 μg per milliliter have been associated with severe and even fatal adverse effects. MICs of either *C. neoformans* and *Candida* species are usually in the range of 1 μg per milliliter, so a 5-FC level of 25 to 50 μg per milliliter would be ample.

In patients with normal renal function, adverse effects are rare. Nausea and vomiting (common with the 150 mg per kilogram regimen), rash, diarrhea, and hepatic dysfunction are seen. More severe and even fatal effects may occur in patients with impaired renal function. Thrombocytopenia is often the first sign of bone marrow toxicity, soon followed by neutropenia. Enterocolitis should be suspected in any patient receiving 5-FC and complaining of abdominal pain. If any of these symptoms occur, therapy should be stopped—even if serum levels of 5-FC are within normal limits. These patients usually tolerate lower doses of 5-FC, and it can be restarted after the side effects disappear. Rare cases of permanent marrow aplasia have been reported. It has been assumed that secretion of 5-FC into the gastrointestinal tract, followed by subsequent conversion to 5-FU by intestinal bacteria and reabsorption are the cause of bone marrow and abdominal adverse effects.

Except in treating chromomycosis, 5-FC should never be given as a single agent. It is usually less clinically effective than amphotericin B, and secondary resistance is common. 5-FC in combination with amphotericin B is the treatment of choice for cryptococcal meningitis. Recommended dosages are amphotericin B 0.3 mg per kilogram per day intravenously plus 5-FC 150 mg per kilogram per day by mouth for 4 to 6 weeks. We start out with higher doses of amphotericin B (0.6 to 1 mg per kilogram per day) and lower doses of 5-FC (75 to 100 mg per kilogram per day). We also may treat for longer than 6 weeks if the clinical situation warrants it, which it may in both normal and immunocompromised hosts. Spinal fluid cell counts and sugar and protein levels should be normal, and cryptococcal antigen levels should be absent or should be low (less than 1:16) and stable.

In patients with human immunodeficiency virus infection and cryptococcal meningitis, the antigen levels are much higher and remain higher. Once the patient is stable both clinically and in terms of CSF and serum antigen levels, he is given a maintenance dose of amphotericin B (1 mg per kilogram per week). Relapse rates of 50 percent to 90 percent were evident when this was not done. Many investigators do not use 5-FC in patients with acquired immunodeficiency syndrome (AIDS) because of their poor marrow reserve and because early experience in patients with AIDS suggested that it was not necessary in acute cryptococcosis. Maintenance therapy with ketoconazole and fluconazole have been under study and are discussed below.

Studies in animal models as well as uncontrolled clinical trials suggest that systemic candidiasis may also be an indication for the combination of 5-FC and amphotericin B. We do not use the combination in any other fungal infection except cryptococcosis or candidiasis due to *C. tropicalis*, and especially not in pulmonary aspergillosis, where 5-FC only adds to toxicity without any evidence of benefit for the patient.

AZOLE ANTIFUNGAL AGENTS

The severity and frequency of adverse effects encountered with amphotericin B have stimulated the search for new antifungal agents. Although the antifungal properties of the imidazole benzimidazole have been known since 1944, more extensive research was not done until the 1970s. The common structure of all azole compounds is a five-membered azole ring, which is bound by a carbon nitrogen to other aromatic rings. Triazoles contain a third nitrogen atom in the azole ring as compared with the two nitrogen atoms in imidazoles.

In vitro test results with azoles depend largely upon many factors like culture medium, pH, and inoculum size and may not be helpful in comparing the different compounds. As for other antifungal agents, animal models more reliably allow assessment of the activity of the different agents. The spectrum of activity of azoles is broad, including most clinically relevant species of dermatophytes, yeasts, and dimorphic fungi. Azoles exhibit their antifungal properties by binding to cytochrome P-450, resulting in an inhibition of cytochrome activation and enzyme function. This results in an inhibition of ergosterol synthesis by inhibition of the demethylation of lanosterol. Additional mechanisms of action have been reported. Decreased uptake at the cytoplasmic membrane is a possible mechanism of resistance; however, currently this appears not to be clinically relevant.

Many agents are available or in various stages of laboratory or clinical evaluation. Some are available for topical use only and are not discussed here.

Clotrimazole

Clotrimazole was the first available azole that was shown to be active in fungal infections in experimental animals and in humans. It induces microsomal enzymes in the liver, resulting in increased drug metabolism and decreased antifungal activity. It is used as a 1-percent solution for the treatment of cutaneous fungal infections (candidiasis, ringworm, pityriasis versicolor), as a 1-percent vaginal cream or as 100-mg tablets for vaginal candidiasis, and as 10-mg oral lozenges for oropharyngeal candidiasis.

Miconazole

Miconazole as topical cream or lotion or as a 2-percent vaginal cream can be used interchangeably with clotrimazole for the indications mentioned for clotrimazole. Since ketoconazole has become available, intravenous miconazole is indicated only for severely ill patients with an infection due to *Pseudoallescheria boydii*. There is no rapid metabolism when miconazole is given systemically (an intravenous form is available). However, there are multiple toxic effects such as nausea, vomiting, anaphylactoid reactions, central nervous system reactions (including seizures), pruritus, and cardiorespiratory arrest. The latter may be related to the rate and duration of drug administration, and it is recommended that miconazole be given in at least 200 ml of diluent over a minimum of 2 hours. Some of the adverse effects mentioned have been attributed to the vehicle Cremophor El, which is required for colloidal stabilization.

Ketoconazole

Ketoconazole was the first azole that could be used in a variety of superficial and systemic fungal infections. It is available in 200-mg tablets. Peak serum concentrations of about 2 to 4 μg per milliliter can be observed 2 to 3 hours after oral intake of one tablet. Absorption is markedly decreased in patients with achlorhydria. Only a minimal amount of the drug appears in the CSF. The serum half-life is about 90 minutes (for a 200-mg dose). Ketoconazole is metabolized in the liver and excreted into the bile. Only a small amount appears unchanged in the urine. Serum protein binding is more than 90 percent. Altered liver or kidney function does not result in a change in plasma drug levels. Hemodialysis and peritoneal dialysis do not remove ketoconazole from the body.

Simultaneous therapy with ketoconazole and rifampin leads to decreased plasma levels of both medications; failures of both compounds have been reported. Coadministration of ketoconazole and cyclosporin A prolongs the half-life of the latter, and coadministration with H_2 blockers, such as cimetidine, or with antacids leads to an impaired absorption of ketoconazole.

In contrast to miconazole intravenously administered, oral ketoconazole is well tolerated. Dose-related nausea and vomiting are the most commonly observed side effects. Increases in liver function test values can be seen in up to 2 to 5 percent of patients and usually disappear spontaneously. Progressive hepatotoxicity that is not dose dependent occurs in about 0.01 percent of patients. It may be fatal if the drug is not discontinued. Interference with steroidal hormone production may lead to a dose-related inhibition of testosterone synthesis (resulting in gynecomastia, menstrual irregularity, sexual impotence, oligospermia) and a decreased ACTH-cortisol response.

Ketoconazole, like other azoles, has a broad spectrum of activity. It is not active, however, against molds such as *Aspergillus* species. Response to treatment is usually slow, and therefore ketoconazole should never be used in the initial treatment of systemic fungal infections in critically ill patients, cancer patients, transplant recipients, or patients with AIDS. It should not be used in any form of fungal meningitis because it crosses the blood-brain barrier poorly.

With these limitations in mind, ketoconazole (400 to 800 mg per day for 6 to 12 months) is effective in the treatment of nonmeningeal blastomycosis and pulmonary and disseminated histoplasmosis. If the 400 mg per day dose is not effective, increasing the dose to 600 mg per day or even 800 mg per day may be. Duration of therapy depends on severity of disease and clinical response. Coccidioidomycosis of the skin, soft tissue, bone, and joints and noncavitary lung infection also respond to 400 to 800 mg per day. Patients with paracoccidioidomycosis have responded to daily doses of 200 to 400 mg. Other indications may include griseofulvin-resistant ringworm, onychomycosis, and tinea versicolor. Chronic mucocutaneous candidiasis requires prolonged administration of 3 to 5 mg of ketoconazole per kilogram per day. Oropharyngeal and esophageal candidiasis may not respond better to ketoconazole than to nystatin. We would, however, always try ketoconazole before resorting to amphotericin B. Candidal vaginitis can be treated with 400 mg per day for 5 days, although hepatotoxicity and the possibility for teratogenicity in pregnant women are major concerns.

We do not recommend the use of ketoconazole in patients with prolonged neutropenia and fever, since important fungi like *Aspergillus* species and *Candida glabrata* would not be treated adequately. There is no good evidence that ketoconazole is effective against invasive candidiasis with dissemination. In one animal model, ketoconazole given prophylactically diminished the protective effect of amphotericin B against *Aspergillus fumigatus*.

Azoles Currently Under Clinical Investigation

Itraconazole

Itraconazole is lipophilic, and more than 99 percent is bound to serum proteins. It is well absorbed after oral ingestion, with improved absorption when taken after a meal. It is metabolized, and the (inactive) metabolites are excreted in bile and urine. The area under the curve (AUC) as well as the peak serum concentration increases remarkably with multiple dosages. A steady state is reached after about 2 weeks. Itraconazole is widely distributed throughout the body, with concentrations in lungs, kidneys, and brain being up to five-fold higher than in plasma. Low concentrations are found in saliva and bronchial secretions, and itraconazole does not penetrate into the CSF.

Adverse effects reported so far are rare and not severe. Nausea and vomiting are observed in 1 to 20 percent of patients and elevation of liver enzymes is seen in less than 5 percent. Hypokalemia and pedal edema were noted in some patients. There seems to be no interference with the production of testicular or adrenal steroidal hormones.

First clinical studies suggest that itraconazole may be used for the same indications as ketoconazole. In addition, it may be active in sporotrichosis and aspergillosis. Its activity against aspergilli in vitro is noteworthy, although carefully designed controlled clinical studies will be needed to substantiate the in vitro promise.

Itraconazole is experimental and can only be used in clinical trials or by compassionate-use approval.

Fluconazole

In contrast to other azoles, fluconazole is water soluble and only weakly protein bound. It is well absorbed and undergoes little metabolism, and more than 90 percent of the drug appears unchanged in urine and feces. Two pharmacokinetic properties are of high clinical interest: fluconazole penetrates well into CSF (60 percent and 80 percent of corresponding serum levels are found in uninflamed and inflamed meninges, respectively), and more than 60 percent of the drug can be recovered from urine. The β half-life is 22 hours. There is a slight accumulation with administration over time, and a dosage reduction is necessary in patients with renal impairment.

Fluconazole appears to be well tolerated. Less than 5 percent of patients develop minor side effects such as gastrointestinal symptoms or elevations in liver function tests.

First clinical studies indicate that fluconazole may be used in fungal infections of the skin and in vaginal candidiasis. Its possible use in systemic mycoses is less clear. It appears, however, to be a promising agent for cryptococcal meningitis, and it is currently under evaluation in a randomized trial with once weekly amphotericin B as standard treatment for prevention of relapse of cryptococcal meningitis in patients with AIDS. It is also under prospective, randomized controlled trials in comparison with amphotericin B as initial treatment of cryptococcal meningitis in patients with and without AIDS.

Fluconazole is experimental and can only be used in clinical trials or by compassionate-use approval.

ALLYLAMINES

Naftifine and terbinafine are members of a new group of antifungal agents, the allylamines. They are synthetic naphthalenemethanamines and act as antifungal agents by inhibiting squalene epoxidase, a key enzyme in ergosterol biosynthesis. Their mode of action is highly specific, i.e., they are much more inhibitory to fungal than to mammalian sterol biosynthesis. Lack of bioavailability after systemic administration may be a mechanism of resistance. Naftifine and terbinafine are experimental agents and can only be used in clinical trials or by compassionate-use approval.

Naftifine

The first compound of this group to be discovered was naftifine. It is active in vitro against a wide variety of fungi and can be used for the topical treatment of infections due to dermatophytes and *Candida*. Activity was not seen after oral administration, even with high doses.

Terbinafine

In vitro, terbinafine is even more active than naftifine against a wide variety of fungi. Of high clinical interest is the fact that it showed in vitro activity against *A. fumigatus*, *Aspergillus flavus*, and *Aspergillus niger* that was comparable to or even better than the activity of amphotericin B. In our animal model of pulmonary aspergillosis, however, we could not detect any activity against *A. fumigatus* despite adequate tissue concentrations. Lack of bioavailability may be the explanation for this in vivo resistance. Terbinafine is currently under clinical investigation as topical and oral medication.

CILOFUNGIN (LY121019)

Cilofungin (LY121019), an analogue of echinocandin B, is a novel semisynthetic lipopeptide. Its mode of action is to inhibit the synthesis of the β-(1,3)-glucan cell-wall component of sensitive fungi.

In vitro it is more active than amphotericin B against *C. albicans* and *C. tropicalis* but less active against other *Candida* species. First animal data indicate that intravenous cilofungin is less toxic than intravenous amphotericin B, and it showed efficacy in the treatment of local and systemic infections due to *C. albicans*.

SUGGESTED READING

Heel RC, Brogden RN, Carmine A, et al. Ketoconazole: a review of its therapeutic efficacy in superficial and systemic fungal infections. Drugs 1982; 23:1–36.

Iwatak K, Vanden Bossche H, eds. In vitro and in vivo evaluation of antifungal agents. New York: Elsevier, 1986.

Rev Infect Dis, January/February 1987, Supplement 1. (The whole issue is devoted to itraconazole.)

Rippon JW. Medical mycology. Philadelphia: WB Saunders, 1988.

Schmitt HJ, Bernard EM, Andrade J, et al. MIC and fungicidal activity of terbinafine against clinical isolates of *Aspergillus* spp. Antimicrob Agents Chemother 1988; 32:780–781.

Speller DCE, ed. Antifungal chemotherapy. New York: Wiley, 1980.

Warnock DW, Richardson MD, eds. Fungal infections in the compromised patient. New York: Wiley, 1982.

CHRONIC BRONCHITIS

IRA B. TAGER, M.D., M.P.H.

Chronic bronchitis (CB) refers to the presence of cough and phlegm for 3 months out of the year for more than 2 consecutive years. This definition was developed on the basis of epidemiologic studies performed in the 1950s to provide more precise meaning to a constellation of respiratory symptoms observed in clinical practice and in epidemiologic studies. From its inception, the term CB became synonymous with a disease spectrum that ranged from simple hypersecretion of mucus to airflow obstruction. Although evidence now suggests that the presence and course of mucus hypersecretion are unrelated to long-term deterioration of lung function and mortality, in this chapter, the specific term CB refers to the entire spectrum of illness that includes obstructive lung disease.

EPIDEMIOLOGY

Chronic bronchitis is a common disease that increases in prevalence with age. As a cause of death, CB ranks fifth among all causes and has been rising over the past 25 years. Cigarette smoking is the most important factor that is associated with occurrence of mucus hypersecretion and airflow obstruction. Current estimates indicate that 80 to 90 percent of CB can be attributed to cigarette smoking. Among the number of other factors that have been investigated as causes of CB (Table 1), only the Pi ZZ genotype of α_1-antitrypsin and possibly male sex have been associated with the occurrence of CB. Of note, episodes of acute infection in adult life have not been definitively associated with CB (see below).

PATHOGENESIS

Two epidemiologically derived hypotheses related to the occurrence of CB have dominated the thinking about this disease spectrum. In the "British" hypothesis, mucus hypersecretion results from exposure to a variety of inhaled irritants, which leads to obstructed airways and the occurrence of recurrent infections. These recurrent infections, in turn, were thought to result in further damage to pulmonary airways and parenchyma. A landmark test of this hypothesis has refuted this basic pathophysiologic sequence. The "Dutch" hypothesis proposes that mucus hypersecretion is a manifestation of an allergic hypersensitivity to a variety of environmental insults. Recurrent infections are thought to be a secondary consequence of airways that are already constricted and have a decreased ability to clear microbial insults. Although much indirect evidence has provided support for this hypothesis, a definitive test of its applicability has yet to be completed.

TABLE 1 Risk Factors for Mucus Hypersecretion and/or Chronic Airflow Obstruction in Adults

Clearly established factors
Cigarette smoking (active)
α_1-antitrypsin deficiency
Factors for which some data suggest increased risk
Age
Air pollution
Alcohol
Atopy, allergy or hypersensitivity (bronchial hyperreactivity)
Childhood respiratory illness
Environmental pollution
Familial and/or household
Genetic
Lower social class
Male sex
Occupational exposures
Respiratory illness history in adulthood

In contrast to the above epidemiologic hypotheses, the protease-antiprotease hypothesis derives from the specific pathologic lesion found in patients with CB. In this hypothesis, cigarette smoke is seen as disrupting the normal homeostatic mechanisms that protect the lung from damage by proteolytic enzymes. The role of pulmonary infection is not addressed specifically, but its role can be inferred to be minor relative to the effect of cigarette smoke. Although this hypothesis has a reasonable body of laboratory data to support it, nonetheless, at present it offers incomplete insight into the considerable variability of risk for CB among smokers.

CLINICAL MANIFESTATIONS AND MANAGEMENT

Patients with CB are most likely to present with complaints of shortness of breath with or without complaints of wheeze, cough, and phlegm. Symptoms typically are episodic, especially those related to worsening cough, phlegm, and wheeze (so-called acute exacerbations). In this context, decisions about the management of acute respiratory infections in the context of acute exacerbations of CB require consideration of four issues: (1) the extent to which infections are the cause of acute exacerbations; (2) the susceptibility of patients with CB to respiratory infection and the types of infections involved; (3) the efficacy of antimicrobial therapy; and (4) the relationship of acute infectious exacerbations and their treatment to the long-term course of chronic airflow obstruction.

Although early investigations suggested a unique pathophysiologic role for *Haemophilus influenzae* and *Streptococcus pneumoniae* in the lower respiratory tract secretions of patients with CB, subsequent prospective studies have failed to support such a relationship or have suggested a complex interaction between the occurrence of viral infections and serologic evidence of infection with these bacterial organisms. No consistent associations between other bacteria and acute exacerbations of CB have been identified.

Viruses and *Mycoplasma pneumoniae* also have been implicated as causes of acute exacerbations of CB. Overall, evidence does suggest that patients with CB are somewhat more susceptible to infection with common respiratory viruses and possibly with *M. pneumoniae*. Viral infections are far more common than infections with *M. pneumoniae*, and, together, they account for less than one-half of all exacerbations in patients under the care of physicians. The cause(s) of acute exacerbations in patients without evidence of infection remains unknown, as does the specific role of cigarette smoking in the episodic nature of the clinical manifestations of CB.

Since antiviral agents have been and remain generally unavailable for therapy (with the exception of amantadine/rimantadine for influenza A infection), virtually all of the data that relate to the utility of antimicrobial agents for the treatment of acute exacerbations of CB concern the use of antibacterial agents. These data, and the recommendations that follow, are based on the assumption that radiographically confirmed pneumonia is not present as the cause of the acute exacerbation. During outbreaks of influenza A infection, amantadine/rimantadine can be used in accordance with the usual recommendation for the therapy with these agents.

Until recently, the evidence that antibacterial agents provided a meaningful clinical benefit in the management of acute exacerbations of CB (including those that require hospitalization) was marginal. However, a recent, large placebo-controlled study has suggested that a 10-day course of an antibacterial agent (doxycycline, amoxicillin, or trimethoprim-sulfamethoxazole) in patients with significant airflow obstruction does lead to significantly more rapid resolution of symptoms in exacerbations characterized by increased dyspnea, sputum volume, and sputum purulence. Other types of exacerbations, including those with wheeze in the absence of increased cough and phlegm, were not so benefitted. Peak flows also recovered faster in patients with "responsive" exacerbations, but the effect was observed only for the first 2 weeks of the exacerbation.

Data from well-controlled studies of the prophylactic use of antibacterial agents to suppress the occurrence of acute exacerbations of CB have been uniform in their failure to show any meaningful clinical benefit in terms of the number of such episodes and/or on the rate of deterioration of lung function.

Table 2 provides a suggested approach to the use of antibacterial agents for the management of acute exacerbations of CB. Since only erythromycin and tetracyclines have proven efficacious against *M. pneumoniae* and are also active against *Streptococcus pneumoniae* (both agents) and *H. influenzae* (tetracyclines), no other alternatives are identified in the table. For patients who cannot be given these agents, any antibiotic with activity against the pneumococcus and *H. influenzae* may be given. Since β-lactamase-producing strains are infrequent among the unencapsulated strains of *H. influen-*

TABLE 2 Suggested Approach for the Use of Antibacterial Agents in the Management of Acute Exacerbations of Chronic Bronchitis

General
- Routine Gram stain and culture are not necessary
- Advice on smoking cessation and reduction is essential

Specific
- Exacerbations characterized by new or increased dyspnea with increased cough and purulent sputum: 7–10-d course of a tetracycline or erythromycin (250 mg qid for both: 100 mg bid for doxycycline) (if patient cannot take these agents, choose ampicillin [amoxicillin] (250 mg q4h) or trimethoprim-sulfamethoxazole [80:400 i]
- All other types of exacerbations:
  - Observe patient 3–5 d to determine if improvement occurs without antibacterial therapy
  - If, during observation period, exacerbation meets criteria above or there is clinical deterioration (↓PaO_2 or ↓O_2 saturation, ↑$PaCO_2$, onset or worsening of systemic signs/symptoms), begin 7–10-d course of antibacterial agent as above
- For all exacerbations treated with antibacterial agents, discontinue after 7–10 d and reevaluate if no improvement or continued worsening

Note: This approach assumes that there is no clinical suspicion of pneumonia and/or that pneumonia has been ruled out by radiographic evidence.

zae found in patients with CB, ampicillin (amoxicillin) should be used in preference to more expensive and/or toxic alternatives, including trimethoprim-sulfamethoxazole (sulfonamide toxicity). Recommendations on the role of corticosteroids and bronchodilators in exacerbations of CB are beyond the scope of this chapter.

SUGGESTED READING

Anthonisen NR, Manfreda J, Warren CPW, et al. Antibiotic therapy in exacerbations of chronic obstructive pulmonary disease. Ann Intern Med 1987; 106:196–204.

Gump DW, Philips CA, Forsyth BR, et al. Role of infection in chronic bronchitis. Am Rev Respir Dis 1976; 113:465–474.

Johnston RN, McNeill RS, Smith DH, Legge JS, Fletcher F. Chronic bronchitis-measurements and observations over ten years. Thorax 1976; 31:25–29.

Monto AS, Higgins MW, Ross HW. The Tecumseh Study of respiratory illness. VIII. Acute infection in chronic respiratory disease and comparison group. Am Rev Respir Dis 1975; 111:27–36.

Nicotra MB, Rivera M, Awe JR. Antibiotic therapy of acute exacerbations of chronic bronchitis. Ann Intern Med 1982; 97:18–21.

INFECTIOUS DIARRHEAS

RONICA M. KLUGE, M.D.

Infectious diarrhea is the second most common infection for which medical attention is sought in the United States. It accounts for approximately 20 percent of adult office visits and for nearly one-third of pediatric office visits and admissions to the hospital. From a practical standpoint, it is useful to distinguish noninflammatory from inflammatory diarrhea. The noninflammatory forms are more common, usually arise in the upper small bowel as a result of the effects of enterotoxin or other alterations of absorptive physiology, cause watery diarrhea with or without nausea and vomiting, produce minimal or low-grade fever, and tend to be self-limited, requiring fluid replacement therapy only. The inflammatory forms arise as a consequence of mucosal invasion involving the colon or distal small bowel; cause an inflammatory bloody diarrhea, accompanied by tenesmus, high fever, and abdominal cramps; and generally require specific antimicrobial agents in addition to rehydration.

DECISIONS

Evaluation of the patient should be directed initially toward two critical decisions: first, whether the patient can be managed as an outpatient or will require hospitalization, and second, whether specific antimicrobial treatment will be needed, in addition to supportive measures. The majority of patients with acute diarrhea of infectious origin can be managed satisfactorily as outpatients and require supportive therapy only. Information gained from a detailed history, a thorough physical examination, and examination of a fresh stool for white blood cells will help to differentiate between inflammatory and noninflammatory forms of infectious diarrhea and allow the critical decisions to be reached swiftly.

The age of the patient, season of the year, clinical presentation, and history of specific exposures are helpful clues to the most likely etiologic agent. Exposure history should include facts about foreign travel, antibiotic usage, animals, mountain streams, ingestion of crustaceans, picnics, sexual preferences, and illness in family members or close friends. Such clues can guide early therapy before the causative agent is identified. A summary of the clinical and epidemiologic features of acute infectious diarrheas is provided in Table 1.

A number of factors enter into the decision to hospitalize a patient with acute infectious diarrhea. In general, very young and very old patients with severe diarrhea and patients of any age who manifest significant toxicity, hyperpyrexia, or dehydration require in-hospital management. Some authorities recommend that patients with serious underlying diseases also be hospitalized for management of severe diarrhea. Hospitalized patients with diarrhea thought to be infectious in origin should be placed in enteric isolation.

The presence or absence of stool leukocytes is often of assistance in differentiating the patient who requires antimicrobial therapy from the patient in whom only supportive measures are indicated. The test is easy to perform: Place a small fleck of mucus or a drop of liquid stool on a microscope slide. Add an equal volume of methylene blue to the slide and mix thoroughly with a wooden applicator stick. Place a coverslip over the mixture and examine under high power (not oil) with a simple light microscope. Most bacteria that invade the colonic mucosa are accompanied by stool leukocytes. One toxin-related diarrhea, that due to *Clostridium difficile*, also produces fecal leukocytes. In general, these are the infectious diarrheas that may require specific antimicrobial therapy. Although patients with noninfectious inflammatory bowel disease (Crohn's disease, ulcerative colitis) may have stool leukocytes, their symptoms are more likely to be chronic and/or intermittent rather than acute and isolated. Stool leukocytes are not associated with diarrheal disease due to viruses, most toxigenic bacteria, and parasites. Unless parasites are involved, only supportive therapy is required.

The presence of fecal leukocytes or bloody diarrhea

TABLE 1 Clinical and Epidemiologic Features of Acute Infectious Diarrheas

Agent	Age Group Most Affected	Associated Symptoms			Stool Character			Stool Leukocytes	Epidemiologic Characteristics			Incubation Period	Therapy
		Fever	Vomiting	Cramps	Watery	Mucoid	Bloody		Season	Foreign Travel	Food/Water-Borne		
Noninflammatory													
Rotavirus	6 mo–2 y	+++	++	++	+	±	0	0	Winter	+/0	0	2–4 days	Supportive
Norwalk virus–like agents	School-aged children, adults	+	++++	++	+	0	0	0	Year-round	+/0	0	1–2 days	Supportive
S. aureus, toxin	Any	0	++++	++	+	0	0	0	Summer	0	+	1–6 h	Supportive
B. cereus, diarrheal	Any	0	+	++	+	±	0	0	Year-round	0	+	8–16 h	Supportive
E. coli, toxic	Any	0	+	++	+	+	0	0	Year-round	+/0	+	1–2 days	Supportive
C. perfringens	Any	0	0	+++	+	0	0	0	Year-round	0	+	8–24 h	Supportive
V. cholerae	Any	0	+	+	+	0	0	0	Year-round	+/0	+	2–5 days	Specific*
E. histolytica	Any	++	0	++	+	+	+	0	Year-round	+	+	3 days–3 wk	Specific*
G. lamblia	Any	0	0	++	+	±	0	0	Year-round	+/0	+	3 days–3 wk	Specific*
Cryptosporidia	Any	0	0	+	+	0	0	0	Year-round	0	0	Unknown	Supportive
Inflammatory													
S. aureus, overgrowth	Any	+++	±	+++	+	+	±	Many polys†	Year-round	0	0	1–2 wk	Specific*
Nontyphoid salmonellae	<5 y	++	0	++	+	±	±	Occasional polys, monos‡	Summer	+/0	+	1–2 days	Specific*
Shigellae	<5 y	+++	0	+++	+	+	+	Many polys	Summer	+/0	+	1–3 days	Specific*
Campylobacter	< 5 y, young adults	+++	+	+++	+	+	+	Many polys	Summer	0	+	3–5 days	Specific*
E. coli, invasive	Any	+	+	+++	+	+	+	Many polys	Year-round	+/0	0	8–24 h	Specific*
Y. enterocolitica	5–20 y	++	0	++	+	±	0	Many polys	Winter	+/0	+	1–2 days	Specific*
V. parahaemolyticus	Any	+	+	++	+	±	±	Occasional polys	Summer	0	+	1–4 days	Supportive
C. difficile	Any	++	0	++	+	±	+	Many polys	Year-round	0	0	4–10 days	Specific*

* Specific: may be specific in all or only some instances; see text.
† Polymorphonuclear cells.
‡ Monocytes.

indicates the need for stool cultures and examinations for parasites. The toxic febrile patient should also have blood obtained for culture. Most laboratories prefer a stool specimen to a rectal swab for optimal recovery of pathogens, except in the case of viruses. Special media and/or incubating conditions are required for certain pathogens such as *Campylobacter, Yersinia, Vibrio parahaemolyticus*, and *C. difficile* to grow optimally, so the laboratory must be alerted to your suspicions.

TREATMENT OPTIONS

Fluid and electrolyte replacement therapy is of benefit to most patients with infectious diarrhea, whether administered as the sole means of treatment or in conjunction with specific antimicrobial therapy. The decision to administer oral or parenteral therapy rests on the patient's state of hydration and ability to tolerate oral fluids. Because the oral route offers the most cost-effective method of treating acute infectious diarrhea, its use should be encouraged unless vomiting is a problem or the patient is moderately or severely dehydrated.

In the patient with minimal dehydration, fluid and electrolyte balance can be maintained by intake of fruit juices, caffeine-free soft drinks, and salted crackers. Salty broths should be recommended only for the patient who has had significant vomiting. Milk products, except for breast milk, should be avoided. If the dehydration is more advanced, oral replacement with commercially available Pedialyte is optimal, as it is low in solute and thus avoids the possibility of hypertonicity. Pedialyte contains 25 g of glucose per liter, 45 mEq of sodium per liter, 20 mEq of potassium per liter, 35 mEq of chloride per liter, 30 mEq of citrate per liter, and 100 calories per liter. The World Health Organization's oral fluid replacement has a similar make-up but contains 90 mEq of sodium per liter.

For patients with moderate to severe dehydration, parenteral fluids are indicated. The type of fluid depends on the patient's particular deficits; however, most respond well to an initial solution of 5 percent dextrose with 35 to 40 mEq of potassium per liter and 40 to 50 mEq of sodium per liter. Close monitoring of the patient's electrolytes and fluid status will allow appropriate changes to be made. The total amount of fluid required to replace deficits can be calculated by use of standard formulas.

TABLE 2 Specific Antimicrobial Therapy for Acute Infectious Diarrheas

Agent	*Drug(s) of Choice*	*Alternatives*
Noninflammatory		
V. cholerae	Tetracycline 40 mg/kg/day in 4 divided doses × 2–5 days	Ampicillin, chloramphenicol, or trimethoprim-sulfamethoxazole
E. histolytica	Metronidazole 750 mg t.i.d. × 10 days *followed by* iodoquinol 650 mg t.i.d. × 20 days	Diloxanide furoate (from CDC only) or paromomycin
G. lamblia	Quinacrine 100 mg t.i.d. × 5–7 days	Metronidazole or furazolidone
Inflammatory		
S. aureus, overgrowth	Vancomycin 250 mg q.i.d. × 5–7 days *or* parenteral antistaphylococcal penicillin	Cephalosporin, first-generation
Nontyphoid salmonellae*	Ampicillin 0.5–1.0 g q.i.d. × 10–14 days	Trimethoprim-sulfamethoxazole
Shigellae	Trimethoprim 160 mg *and* sulfamethoxazole 800 mg b.i.d. × 5 days	Tetracycline, ampicillin, or newer quinolone
*Campylobacter**	Erythromycin 250–500 mg q.i.d. × 7 days	Newer quinolone
E. coli, invasive	Trimethoprim 160 mg *and* sulfamethoxazole 800 mg b.i.d. × 5–7 days	Ampicillin
Y. enterocolitica	Gentamicin 3–5 mg/kg/day in 3 divided doses × 7 days	Tetracycline, chloramphenicol, or trimethoprim-sulfamethoxazole
*C. difficile**	Vancomycin 125 mg q.i.d. × 10 days *or* metronidazole 250–500 mg q.i.d. × 10 days	

* See text for additional information.

As indicated in Table 1, the noninflammatory diarrheal diseases require only supportive therapy except in the case of cholera and the protozoal diarrheas. In addition, specific therapy is indicated for each of the inflammatory infectious diarrheas except for that due to *V. parahaemolyticus*. Table 2 outlines the antimicrobial agent(s) of choice and alternatives against those microbes for which specific treatment is required. In general, gastroenteritis caused by the nontyphoidal salmonellae is treated only with supportive measures. However, in a patient with a compromised immune system, foreign bodies such as grafts in place, a known aneurysm, extremes of age, hemolytic anemia, or signs of extreme toxicity, specific antibiotic treatment is recommended. For optimal effect, *Campylobacter* diarrhea must be treated within the first 4 days of symptoms. There is considerable controversy about the effectiveness of antibiotic therapy for diarrheal illness caused by *Yersinia*. In spite of this, specific therapy with an aminoglycoside is suggested in the more toxic-appearing patient. In a patient with *C. difficile* toxin-induced diarrhea without pseudomembrane formation, some success with bismuth subsalicylate has been reported. In every instance of antibiotic-associated diarrhea, it is essential to discontinue the offending antibiotic.

In selected patients, other therapies may be useful. Adsorbents such as Kaopectate act to firm up the stool and may be viewed as important by the individual patient. The patient with a toxin-related diarrhea (except *C. difficile*) may benefit from the administration of bismuth subsalicylate, which has antisecretory properties. Antimotility drugs are used rather indiscriminately for all types of diarrhea. In the presence of an infectious diarrhea, the antimotility drugs are best avoided in children less than 2 years of age and in any patient with high fever or bloody diarrhea.

SUGGESTED READING

Breeling JL. Newly recognized bacterial causes of infectious diarrhea. Infect Dis Pract 1989; 12:1–7.

Cantey JR. Infectious diarrheas. Pathogenesis and risk factors. Am J Med 1985; 78(suppl)6B:65–75.

Consensus conference: Travelers' diarrhea. JAMA 1985; 253:2700–2704.

DuPont HL, Ericsson CD, Johnson PC, et al. Prevention of travelers' diarrhea by the tablet formulation of bismuth subsalicylate. JAMA 1987; 257:1347–1350.

Gorbach SL. Bacterial diarrhoeae and its treatment. Lancet 1987; 2:1378–1382.

Guerrant RL, Wanke CA, Barrett LJ, Schwartzman JD. A cost effective and effective approach to the diagnosis and management of acute infectious diarrhea. Bull NY Acad Med 1987; 63:484–499.

Smith PD, Lane D, Gill VJ, et al. Intestinal infections in patients with acquired immunodeficiency syndrome (AIDS). Etiology and response to therapy. Ann Intern Med 1988; 108:328–333.

TRAVELER'S DIARRHEA

R. BRADLEY SACK, M.D., Sc.D.

Acute diarrheal illnesses are the most common afflictions of travelers from the more developed, sanitized nations who visit the less developed, less sanitized areas of the world. In fact, the diarrheal attack rate of this group is higher than that of any other single population group, with the exception of groups of people involved in common-source outbreaks in which a known, single contaminated food item or beverage has been ingested by all.

Traveler's diarrhea, as we know it today, is a result of the uneven development of sanition in the world over the past century. When all of the world's population was heavily exposed to fecal contaminiation, diarrheal disease was endemic worldwide, occurring frequently regardless of whether or not one traveled widely. As improvements in water supply occurred, certain enteric diseases such as cholera disappeared from Europe and the United States, and cholera thus became a traveler's diarrhea in that it occurred in westerners only when they visited endemic areas. As further improvements in water and sanitation were made, endemic diarrheal diseases, which we now know to be largely bacterial in origin, decreased markedly. Young children in these "developed" areas no longer had frequent diarrheal episodes that would provide immunologic protection from the bacteria in adult life. Furthermore, when these persons traveled to less developed countries, they were highly susceptible to the endemic pathogens of those geographic areas. Thus the clinical and epidemiologic entity, traveler's diarrhea, evolved.

One might describe travelers from a developed country as sentinel markers for the occurrence of endemic diarrheal disease in the children of the country being visited; if the rate of infantile diarrhea is high, the rate of traveler's diarrhea will also be high. The travelers are, in effect, immunologic "infants" in this fecally contaminated environment.

From the first recognition of this clinical entity, approximately 30 to 40 years ago, it was thought to be infectious in origin. But it was not until the late 1960s that enterotoxigenic *Escherichia coli* were described, first as a major cause of severe cholera-like diarrhea in India, and a few years later as the predominant cause of not only traveler's diarrhea, but of endemic infantile diarrhea worldwide.

ETIOLOGY

Enterotoxigenic *E. coli* are responsible for 30 to 70 percent of all episodes of traveler's diarrhea among inhabitants of developed countries who visit less developed parts of the world. The distinction regarding the origin of the travelers is important, for reasons given above. Inhabitants of an underdeveloped country may also develop traveler's diarrhea when visiting another underdeveloped country, but the incidence of the diarrhea will be less, and will usually be caused by enteropathogens other than enterotoxigenic *E. coli*. Other infectious agents that are responsible for traveler's diarrhea include *Shigella, Campylobacter, Salmonella*, and to a lesser entent all the other known etiologic agents of diarrheal disease. Prophylactic and treatment studies using antibiotics, as well as microbiologic studies, strongly indicate that more than 90 percent of episodes of traveler's diarrhea are caused by bacteria.

Some traveler's diarrhea pathogens may be geographically specific, such as *Giardia* in Leningrad, and *Salmonella* in parts of southeast Asia. These unusual associations are undoubtedly due to sanitation problems in water supplies and processed foods. Some diarrheal episodes may also be due to noninfectious causes, such as the ingestion of preformed toxins from fish (e.g., ciguatera toxins).

CLINICAL SYNDROME

Episodes of traveler's diarrhea characteristically begin 2 or 3 days after arrival in the underdeveloped country, and continue at a high rate during the first 3 to 6 weeks, after which the incidence decreases, presumably because of the development of protective immunity to the etiologic agents, most notably enterotoxigenic *E. coli*. The attack rate will be about 25 to 50 percent during the first 3 weeks in the new area, depending on the sanitation of the region. During this period, attack rates of 100 percent have been reported to occur in some areas.

The clinical syndrome is usually characterized by watery diarrhea (three to 10 bowel movements per day), often with abdominal cramping and some nausea, but usually without significant fever. The illness characteristically lasts 2 to 4 days, but it may occasionally last for as long as 10 days. It is usually mild and rarely severe enough to require hospitalization, although there are many anecdotal reports of travelers being hospitalized to receive treatment with intravenous fluids—a situation that the traveler would clearly want to avoid.

Many variations of this clinical syndrome exist, depending on the etiologic agent. Characteristically, *Shigella* infection produces the symptoms of dysentery, and *Giardia* causes a more protracted course.

There are no known long-term sequelae to traveler's diarrhea. It is possible, however, that some episodes may last several weeks or even months after the acute phase. *Giardia* may be one cause of this persistent diarrhea. Tropical sprue and "tropical enteropathy" are other persistent diarrheal syndromes that may respond to either antibiotic therapy or removal from the contaminated environment, respectively. Other noninfectious diarrheas, such as ulcerative colitis, may occur for the first time during travel, and can be confusing because of the temporal relationship to travel.*

Laboratory confirmation of the etiologic agent is usually not possible because of the unavailability of simple diagnostic tests for recognizing enterotoxigenic *E. coli* and the lack of ready access to medical care facilities in underdeveloped countries. However, this is not usually a significant problem. The likely etiologic agents are known from previous studies and appropriate antibiotic therapy, in order to be maximally effective, should not be delayed until culture results become available.

PROPHYLAXIS

Because the etiologic agents of traveler's diarrhea are known to be transmitted by fecally contaminated food and water, the best prevention is avoidance of these vehicles of infection. Carrying one's own water and rations is impossible, and one would not even want to try. Much of the enjoyment of travel comes from the tasteful cuisine of the regions visited. One *can* use practical precautions, when the risks are known. Food that cannot be peeled or cooked is the most likely to be contaminated. This includes fresh vegetable salads. Although these food items can be disinfected by soaking in hypochlorite solution, this is not usually done in restaurants, and these food items should be avoided. Any food that is cooked well and is served hot will be free of any infectious agents. Water, unless it is known to have been boiled or chlorinated, should be avoided. Alternative beverages such as bottled sodas should be drunk instead. Both chlorination tablets and small portable water filters are available for the traveler to purify water, if necessary.

Other more specific preventive measures that have been shown to decrease the attack rate of traveler's diarrhea are shown in Table 1. The only nonantibiotic drug that has been shown to be clinically useful is Pepto-Bismol, the active ingredient of which is bismuth subsalicylate. Regular administration of this agent four times a day will decrease the attack rate by 40 to 60 percent. The exact mechanisms by which the drug acts are not known, although some of the breakdown products of the active ingredient are both antibacterial and antisecretory. Although both bismuth and salicylate toxicity are of concern when one uses this preparation, these are not believed to be significant problems in normal subjects.

Preparations of lactobacilli have been shown not to prevent traveler's diarrhea, although newer formations of lactobacilli are currently being tested. Orally administered immunoglobulin from cow's milk (made by immunizing cows against a wide variety of enterotoxigenic *E. coli* antigens) has been shown to be highly protective against an enterotoxigenic *E. coli* challenge in a volunteer situation; however, this has not yet been tested in travelers.

***Editor's Note:** Some people with preexisting irritable bowel syndrome may be slow to recover over the ensuing weeks or even months. Lactose intolerance may also take weeks or months to improve.

TABLE 1 Prophylaxis of Traveler's Diarrhea

	Dose Frequency	*% Protection Anticipated*
Nonantimicrobials		
Bismuth subsalicylate	2 tablets, four times daily	40–60%
Antimicrobials*		
Doxycycline	100 mg, once daily with breakfast	50–90%
Trimethoprim-sulfamethoxazole (TMP-SMZ)	One double-strength tablet, once daily (160 mg TMP, 800 mg SMZ)	90%
Norfloxacin	One 400-mg tablet, once daily	90%

* Antimicrobials should be started 1 day before one enters the "risk area," (i.e., the underdeveloped country) and discontinued 1 day after leaving. The drugs should not be used for longer than 3 weeks; travelers should be familiar with possible side effects and indications for discontinuing them.

Other antimicrobials that have been shown to be effective, but which are not currently in wide use: trimethoprim alone, erythromycin, amdinocillin, and bicozamycin (investigational).

A number of antimicrobial drugs have been shown to be highly effective in preventing traveler's diarrhea; these are summarized in Table 1. Because all these agents are associated with significant undesirable side effects, although infrequent, we do not recommend that they be used routinely. In certain circumstances, however, in which the traveler clearly understands the potential for adverse reactions and is willing to accept them in return for a high degree of protection (approximately 90 percent) from traveler's diarrhea, they may be prescribed. There is theoretical concern that administering antibiotics prophylactically may make the individual more susceptible to other antibiotic-resistant enteric pathogens, such as *Salmonella,* as has been shown in animal experiments. This has not been observed in practice, however. Another concern is that administering prophylactic antibiotics to large numbers of travelers could conceivably add to the antibiotic pool of the environment, and thus aid in selecting resistant bacterial strains. Yet in practice this does not seem to be significant, because in nearly all the underdeveloped countries, antibiotics are sold over the counter and are used heavily. In this context, the addition of antibiotics from travelers is thought to be insignificant.

Effective vaccines would be an excellent prophylactic measure, but none is available yet. (These are discussed in a later section of the chapter.)

TREATMENT

The treatment of traveler's diarrhea is, in most respects, similar to the treatment of any acute infectious diarrheal disease (Table 2). The main difference is that the etiologic agent is highly likely to be enterotoxigenic *E. coli*, and the therapy has to be self-administered, without medical consultation. It is therefore important that the traveler discuss the indications for treatment and the possibility of any adverse drug reactions before undertaking the travel.

Fluid Replacement

Fluid replacement is the foundation of any diarrheal disease treatment, particularly that of the secretory diarrhea caused by enterotoxigenic *E. coli*. In most cases, diarrheal fluid and electrolyte losses are not great and can be replaced by the usual diet, with perhaps whatever additional liquids are available. If the fluid losses are significant, replacement is best done by using oral rehydration solutions, which have been developed by the World Health Organization and are available as packets containing the appropriate amounts of sodium chloride, sodium citrate, potassium chloride, and glucose to replace diarrheal losses. These are available throughout underdeveloped countries and are inexpensive. However, it is more

TABLE 2 Treatment of Traveler's Diarrhea

Oral rehydration solutions

- WHO packets available in underdeveloped countries, and to a limited extent in the United States*
- Sugar and salt solution (1 tsp of salt and 8 tsp of sugar to 1 qt of drinking water)

Symptomatic therapy

- Antimotility drugs: loperamide hydrochloride or diphenoxylate hydrochloride with atropine sulfate
- Bismuth subsalicylate

Antimicrobial therapy

- Doxycycline, 100 mg tablet b.i.d. for 3 days
- Trimethoprim-sulfamethoxazole (TMP-SMZ), one double-strength trablet (160 mg of TMP and 800 mg SMZ) b.i.d. for 3 days
- Ciprofloxacin, 500 mg b.i.d. for 3 days
- Norfloxacin,* 400 mg b.i.d. for 3 days

* Not specifically studied in traveler's diarrhea therapy, but known to be effective in acute diarrheal diseases of bacterial origin.

Other antimicrobials found to be effective, but not currently used widely: trimethoprim alone, bicozamycin (investigational).

convenient for the traveler to carry several packets along on the trip, to be used as required. The best possible source of uncontaminated water should be used to mix the solution. If the diarrhea is severe, large amounts will need to be taken to prevent significant dehydration. If these solutions are used correctly, the need for hospitalization and intravenous fluids will almost never arise.

Nonantimicrobial Drugs

Antimotility agents, such as diphenoxylate-atropine and loperamide, have proved effective in decreasing the symptoms of traveler's diarrhea. Although these agents have been shown in animal studies to be antisecretory as well, human studies have demonstrated only an antimotility effect. These drugs have a rapid onset of action and will decrease abdominal cramping and frequency of stool. They will not cure the infection, of course, and symptoms will continue until the offending organisms have been eradicated.

These drugs are contraindicated in dysentery syndromes, since the activity of invasive organisms may be enhanced by decrease of the propulsive motility of the bowel. The drugs are also contraindicated in small children because of central nervous system effects and the possibility of developing paralytic ileus.

Pepto-Bismol has also been found useful in reducing symptoms of traveler's diarrhea, but its onset of action is less rapid than that of the antimotility agents.

These nonantimicrobial treatments are most useful in relatively mild diarrhea, and are particularly useful if the traveler is involved in activities in which it may be embarrassing to be interrupted by the need to defecate, such as riding in buses or giving lectures.

Antimicrobial Drugs

Antimicrobial therapy has been shown to be efficacious in a number of studies. The drugs used are directed primarily against enterotoxigenic *E. coli*, but they should also be effective against *Shigella*. The antimicrobials currently recommended are shown in Table 2. Doxycycline is probably less effective now than it was previously because of the continuing development of antibiotic resistance. Nevertheless, outside of areas of Southeast Asia and Central America, its efficacy is still high. At present, trimethoprim-sulfamethoxazole probably is the drug most widely used against *E. coli* and *Shigella*, although the new fluoroquinolones may become more widely used in the future. These latter drugs have the advantage of having a spectrum that includes *Campylobacter*, as well as *Shigella* and enterotoxigenic *E. coli*. All these antibiotics have been shown to shorten the duration of diarrhea to approximately 24 hours, a distinct and significant improvement over the usual 2- to 4-day course of illness.

Antidiarrheal Vaccines

Because there is such a large number of etiologic agents that cause acute diarrhea, no single vaccine will provide protective immunity against all of them. The situation of traveler's diarrhea, however, is unique in that a single group of organisms, enterotoxigenic *E. coli*, cause the majority of episodes. Therefore, a vaccine against these organisms would be useful. Such vaccines are being developed, although none has yet been field-tested. The major difficulty in developing an enterotoxigenic *E. coli* vaccine is the large number of antigens that are produced by these organisms, and therefore the broad-spectrum protection that will be needed.

Parenteral cholera vaccines have been used for almost 100 years, but they are known to provide only short-term protection, and their effects have been studied only in endemic areas. They are not recommended for travelers, unless the nation to be visited requires cholera immunization for entry into the country. Only a few countries still maintain this requirement. The World Health Organization actively discourages cholera vaccine as a "required" vaccine for international travel. A new oral, nonliving cholera vaccine (administered in three doses) has recently been field-tested in Bangladesh, where it was found to give about 60 percent protection for 3 years. This vaccine may be a useful public health tool in the future. Because travelers are at a very low risk for developing cholera, however, even the new cholera vaccine will probably not be useful for them. New oral, living attenuated cholera vaccines that may provide even greater protection are also being developed.

Vaccines against *Shigella* and rotavirus are in the developmental phases. Because rotavirus is an infrequent cause of traveler's diarrhea, this vaccine will not be useful for travelers. *Shigella* vaccine, on the other hand, may be useful for travelers, because these organisms are usually the second most frequent cause of this syndrome.

All of the acute diarrheal vaccines being developed are oral rather than parenteral vaccines. It is now known that the optimal stimulation of protective immunity in the gastrointestinal tract is through the delivery of antigens to the gut mucosa, and particularly to Peyer's patches. Vaccines that can replicate are preferred to nonliving vaccines, because they can be administered in a single dose and, through replication, lead to the delivery of antigens over a prolonged period of time to more effectively induce protective immunity.

SUGGESTED READING

Gorbach SL, Edelman R, eds. Travelers' diarrhea: National Institutes of Health Consensus Development Conference. J Infect Dis 1986; 8:S109–S227.

NIH Consensus Conference. Traveler's diarrhea. JAMA 1985; 253: 2700–2704.

CLOSTRIDIUM DIFFICILE AND ANTIBIOTIC-ASSOCIATED COLITIS

P. DAVID MILLER, M.D.
J. THOMAS LaMONT, M.D.

Administration of antibiotics is frequently associated with diarrhea or colitis. It is now recognized that the most important cause of this disease is the spore-forming, anaerobic bacterium *Clostridium difficile*. Not normally a part of the gastrointestinal (GI) flora in adults, this bacterium is acquired from the environment. It is found in soil and as an environmental contaminant in hospitals reporting outbreaks of *C. difficile*-associated disease. Alteration of the normal colonic microflora by antibiotic therapy is a prerequisite for colonization by *C. difficile* to occur. Colonization of the GI tract by this organism is almost always associated with the administration of antibiotics.

The pathogenesis of *C. difficile* is related to the production of two exotoxins, designated toxins A and B. Toxin A is an enterotoxin that causes intestinal mucosal damage. The pathologic effects of toxin B are less clear: it is a cytotoxin that is detected in stool during the routine cytotoxin assay for *C. difficile*. Invasion of the colonic mucosa by the organism does not occur and blood cultures are negative.

Although almost every currently available antibiotic has been associated in *C. difficile*-associated diarrhea, the most commonly implicated are clindamycin, ampicillin, and the cephalosporins. The highest incidence of diarrhea or colitis is seen when antibiotics are given orally, but parenterally administered antibiotics also are frequently associated with *C. difficile* disease. Curiously, *C. difficile* is sensitive in vitro to most of the antibiotics known to cause antibiotic-associated colitis; indeed, metronidazole, the treatment of choice, may predispose to *C. difficile* colitis. This paradox may be explained by the premise that metronidazole may alter the normal gut flora, allowing *C. difficile* to populate, and is also bactericidal for the same organism.

CLINICAL MANIFESTATIONS

Although the most important manifestation of *C. difficile* infection is pseudomembranous colitis, the physician may encounter a spectrum of disease, ranging from mild diarrhea without colitis to fulminant, fatal colitis. The presenting symptom is invariably diarrhea, which may begin during the course of antibiotic therapy (one-third of patients) or up to 6 weeks after cessation of therapy. Some patients complain only of watery diarrhea without systemic symptoms. These patients have relatively normal-appearing colonic mucosa on sigmoidoscopic examination. Most patients, however, develop colitis with associated fever, leukocytosis, and abdominal tenderness with distention. Stool occult blood is usually positive, but visible rectal bleeding is rare. Sigmoidoscopic examination may reveal changes of acute colitis ranging from mucosal edema to friability and frank ulceration. Pseudomembranes, when present, appear as white to gray plaques, 2 to 8 mm in diameter, that overlie either normal mucosa or mucosa that is reddened and friable. Unlike ulcerative colitis, which involves the colonic mucosa contiguously from the rectum, antibiotic-associated colitis can be associated with patchy involvement of the colon and often spares the rectum.

Electrolyte imbalance, dehydration, and hypoalbuminemia may develop in severe or unrecognized cases of *C. difficile*-associated diarrhea. Although rare, toxic megacolon and perforation have been described.

DIAGNOSIS

The diagnosis of pseudomembranous colitis can be made rapidly at the bedside by sigmoidoscopic examination. The finding of pseudomembranes in a patient recently exposed to antibiotics is highly specific for *C. difficile*-associated colitis. Because pseudomembranes may not be present, or may not involve the rectosigmoid colon, the diagnosis can easily be missed by sigmoidoscopy. For this reason, stool should be sent for *C. difficile* toxin B cytotoxin assay, a widely available, specific, and sensitive test for this pathogen. In some hospital laboratories, assays such as the ELISA and latex agglutination tests are replacing the traditional bioassay for *C. difficile* cytotoxin. We do not believe that these newer assays offer an advantage over the currently available cytotoxin assay.

TREATMENT

All patients with diarrhea and either a positive toxin assay or the finding of pseudomembranes on sigmoidoscopy should be treated for *C. difficile*-associated disease. The major goals of treatment consist of elimination of *C. difficile* from the gut and reestablishment of the normal bowel flora. In every patient the first step is to discontinue all antibiotics. Most patients either will have discontinued antimicrobial therapy before the onset of symptoms or will not have a compelling indication for continued therapy. Patients with serious ongoing systemic infections can be maintained on antibiotics while therapy for *C. difficile* is instituted (Table 1).

C. difficile-infected patients who have moderate to severe diarrhea, with evidence of volume depletion, electrolyte disturbance, or other severe medical conditions, should be hospitalized. Outpatients with mild disease can be treated without hospitalization since all drugs used to treat antibiotic-associated colitis are administered orally. Not all individuals require drug therapy. If the patient is

TABLE 1 Treatment of Antibiotic-Associated Colitis

Discontinue antibiotics, if possible
Correct fluid and electrolyte disturbances
Metronidazole, 250 mg t.i.d. PO for 10 days (use vancomycin, 125 to 500 mg q.i.d. for 10 days for patients with history of adverse reaction to metronidazole, or who will continue drinking alcohol)
Avoid antidiarrheal medications
Contact isolation
Surgical consultation for toxic megacolon or perforation

taking antibiotics when diagnosed with mild *C. difficile*–associated diarrhea or colitis, it is reasonable simply to discontinue the antibiotic and observe. The same approach may be taken with patients whose colitis is symptomatically improving after stopping the offending antibiotic. The rationale for this approach is based on a prospective study that showed complete spontaneous recovery in all patients with *C. difficile*-associated colitis when the antibiotics were promptly discontinued.

Metronidazole

The first-line treatment for symptomatic *C. difficile*–associated diarrhea and colitis is metronidazole, 250 mg three times a day orally for 7 to 10 days. Although intestinal absorption of metronidazole is excellent, fecal concentrations remain bactericidal while colitis is present, and then drop to an undetectable level after recovery. A good initial response is obtained in over 95 percent of patients treated with metronidazole. Fever and abdominal pain resolve within 2 days, and diarrhea generally subsides within 1 week. Stool toxin B assay usually becomes undetectable within 72 hours of instituting therapy. Enteral therapy is not feasible in patients with severe ileus or vomiting. In these patients intravenous metronidazole is used, although response rates are significantly lower than with oral therapy.

Side Effects

Metronidazole is generally well tolerated. The most commonly reported side effects are nausea, vomiting, diarrhea, and abdominal pain. The drug may rarely cause generalized seizures or a sensory peripheral neuropathy. Patients should be warned not to drink alcohol while on metronidazole because of a disulfiram-like effect (nausea, vomiting, and tachycardia). Metronidazole should be avoided in pregnancy because of a possible association with congenital defects.

Vancomycin

Vancomycin, once the mainstay of treatment of *C. difficile* colitis, has been largely replaced by metronidazole as the drug of choice in acute antibiotic-associated colitis. Although response and relapse rates of vancomycin are similar to those of metronidazole, the high cost of vancomycin therapy prohibits its routine use as a first-line agent. At Boston University Medical Center, a 10-day course of vancomycin (250 mg three times a day) costs the patient almost $1,000. Because vancomycin is poorly absorbed from the GI tract, it is virtually without side effects, although nausea, chills, fever, urticaria, and rashes have been reported.

We reserve therapy with vancomycin for patients with previous adverse reactions to metronidazole, those who continue to drink alcohol on therapy, and those who have relapsing diarrhea after metronidazole therapy (see below).

Bacitracin

Bacitracin, a polypeptide antibiotic effective against gram-positive bacteria, has been used in *C. difficile*–associated colitis. At a dose of 25,000 units, four times a day orally for 10 days, the symptomatic response rate equals that of vancomycin. Bacitracin, however, is less effective than vancomycin in eradicating the organism or toxin from stool. Although the high incidence of renal and ototoxicity limits the use of parenteral bacitracin, side effects are not encountered when the drug is administered orally.

Anion-Binding Resins

Cholestyramine and colestipol, anion-binding resins used in the treatment of hypercholesterolemia, have been shown in vitro to neutralize the cytotoxic effects of *C. difficile* toxin. These agents have been used to treat *C. difficile*–associated diarrhea and colitis. In several uncontrolled trials, patients treated with anion-binding resins have had prompt resolution of the diarrhea. A frequent side effect of cholestyramine and colestipol therapy is constipation, which can be severe. It is possible that the symptomatic response is related to this constipating effect and not to a specific effect of the resins on *C. difficile* or its toxins. *C. difficile* is rarely eradicated from the stool after therapy with these drugs, and in some cases may contribute to a carrier state. For this reason, we do not advocate the use of anion-binding resins to treat antibiotic-associated colitis.

Symptomatic Measures

The use of antimotility agents in antibiotic-associated diarrhea or colitis is contraindicated. Diarrhea may actually be beneficial by ridding the colon of *C. difficile* and its toxins. As in salmonellosis and shigellosis, antidiarrheal agents may prolong the carriage of *C. difficile* and predispose to toxic megacolon.

TREATMENT OF RECURRENT DISEASE

Recurrence of *C. difficile*–associated diarrhea or colitis occurs in up to 23 percent of patients treated with either metronidazole or vancomycin. It probably results

TABLE 2 Treatment of Relapsing Antibiotic-Associated Diarrhea or Colitis

Repeat 10-day course of metronidazole or vancomycin
If second relapse occurs: vancomycin 125 mg q.i.d. for 2 weeks, then 125 mg daily for 2 weeks, then 125 mg every third day for 2 weeks; then discontinue.

from failure to clear the spore form of *C. difficile* rather than from reinfection with a new strain. Unlike the vegetative form of the bacterium, *C. difficile* spores are resistant to antibiotics. Most recurrent attacks respond to a second 10-day course of therapy with metronidazole or vancomycin (Table 2). However, a significant number of patients (approximately 20 percent) relapse again after a second course of treatment and may require additional courses of therapy.

Various regimens have been used to eradicate *C. difficile* in patients with recurrent disease. Tapering vancomycin from 125 mg four times a day to 125 mg every third day over 6 weeks has been found to be effective in one uncontrolled trial. One explanation for the efficacy of this regimen is that the antibiotic-resistant spores germinate to the vegetative form during the days that the drug is not given, and these vegetative forms are susceptible to the next dose of vancomycin.

An interesting nondrug therapy for *C. difficile* recurrence is colonization of the bowel with a nontoxogenic strain of the same organism. This presumably prevents colonization by the disease-producing strain, and has been used successfully in two patients. The live organism was administered orally in three doses and both patients appeared to respond without side effects.

SURGICAL THERAPY

The role of surgery in antibiotic-associated colitis is limited. Indications for surgical intervention are fulminant colitis with perforation and toxic megacolon. The procedures most often used are subtotal colectomy or diverting ileostomy.

PREVENTIVE THERAPY

C. difficile can be cultured from environmental surfaces in hospitals and from the hands and stool of health care workers. Most cases of *C. difficile*–associated colitis and diarrhea occur in hospitalized patients, and outbreaks have been reported in several medical centers. It is important, therefore, to take steps to prevent the nosocomial spread of the disease. Care must be taken to avoid contact with feces or soiled bed linen. Hospital personnel should be instructed to wash their hands upon leaving patients' rooms. We routinely place our patients with *C. difficile*–associated disease under this "contact isolation." These measures probably play a major role in decreasing the overall incidence of antibiotic-associated diarrhea and colitis.

TYPHOID FEVER AND ENTERIC FEVER

MYRON M. LEVINE, M.D., D.T.P.H.

Typhoid fever is an acute generalized infection of the reticuloendothelial system, intestinal lymphoid tissues, and gallbladder due to *Salmonella typhi*. A similar disease, paratyphoid fever, follows infection with *S. paratyphi* A and B. These generalized salmonella infections are referred to as enteric fever. Rarely, other serotypes, such as *S. typhimurium*, can cause enteric fever if they infect compromised hosts, young infants, or the elderly.

Humans are both the only natural host and the reservoir of *S. typhi*, and infection is acquired by ingestion of contaminated food or water. Typhoid and paratyphoid bacilli rapidly pass through the intestinal mucosa and reach the systemic circulation by means of lymphatic drainage and the thoracic duct. As a consequence of this primary bacteremia, the fixed phagocytic cells of the reticuloendothelial system become seeded with *S. typhi* as they ingest the bacilli. Following an incubation period of 9 to 14 days, clinical illness appears, accompanied by the characteristic secondary bacteremia of enteric fever. The clinical picture is typified by fever (which increases in stepwise fashion), malaise, headache, and abdominal pain. In adults, constipation is often present, whereas in children diarrhea may occur. Typhoid and paratyphoid infections exhibit a spectrum of clinical illness that includes asymptomatic infection, mild illness with low-grade fever and minimal malaise, or a severe syndrome of very high fever (up to 105 °F to 106 °F), toxemia, and even delirium.

There are many complications that can follow acute enteric fever, but the most important are intestinal perforation and intestinal hemorrhage (which occur in approximately 0.5% of cases) and the chronic biliary carrier state (which occurs in 3% to 5% of cases and is more frequent among females and older patients). In certain areas of the world, such as Indonesia, some patients present with a particularly severe clinical picture of typhoid infection marked by delirium or obtundation.

DIAGNOSIS

Transmission of typhoid or paratyphoid infections within the United States is rare, although occasional outbreaks and sporadic cases still occur. In contrast, enteric fever is a risk for US citizens who travel to less developed areas of the world where these infections are still highly endemic. Microbiology technicians in clinical laboratories comprise another high-risk group because they can acquire the infection while processing cultures. When enteric fever occurs in a very young child in the United States, one should look for a carrier within the household.

If the clinical picture is suspicious, appropriate cultures should be performed. The highest yield of positivity is obtained with a bone marrow culture. This should always be obtained for suspect patients who have had some prior antibiotic therapy; bone marrow cultures in such patients are often positive when blood cultures may be negative. For patients who have not had prior antibiotic therapy, properly performed blood cultures give a high rate of positivity. Three specimens for culture should be obtained, 30 minutes apart, with at least 5 ml of blood per specimen. The blood should be inoculated into a flask containing at least 50 ml of broth to obtain a blood-to-broth ratio of at least 1:10. This dilutes out the factors in blood that may be inhibitory to the salmonellae. Any broth routinely used for blood culture will support the growth of *S. typhi*, but medium containing sodium polyanethol sulfonate is preferred.

Because infection of the gallbladder is usual in acute typhoid fever, culture of bilious duodenal fluid is almost as sensitive as a bone marrow culture. This can easily be accomplished by means of a string-capsule device, the Enterotest (Hedeco; Mountain View, Calif). The string device contained within a gelatin capsule is ingested in the morning by a fasting patient and is removed by gentle traction 3 to 4 hours later. Fluid for culture is expressed from the bile-stained distal 15 cm, using two fingers of a gloved hand. String capsule cultures should be obtained on 2 consecutive days, even if antibiotics have already been started.

Three stool cultures should also be performed as an adjunct to bone marrow, blood, and bile cultures, although they are positive in only about 50 percent of cases (higher if diarrhea is present).

The Widal test, which measures O and H antibodies to *S. typhi*, is not of much practical value. If proper reagents are available and quantitative tube dilutions are performed, elevated titers may be helpful in the nonvaccinated traveler or in children younger than 10 years of age, in endemic areas. However, such Widal serologic techniques are not widely available. Healthy adults in endemic areas often have elevated titers, as do recipients of parenteral typhoid vaccine in the United States; in such patients the Widal titers have no value. Aggressive collection of proper culture specimens should preclude the need for a Widal test.

THERAPY

Historically, the therapy of typhoid fever can be divided into three eras: (*1*) prior to 1948, when effective antibiotic therapy did not exist and the case fatality rate was approximately 10 percent; (*2*) the period from 1948 to 1972, during which oral chloramphenicol was shown to be highly efficacious, practical, and economical, particularly in less developed areas of the world; (*3*) from 1973 to the present, when, as a result of some epidemics due to chloramphenicol-resistant strains of *S. typhi* and the advent of trimethoprim-sulfamethoxazole and amoxicillin, alternative drugs appeared to challenge the preeminent role of chloramphenicol as the mainstay of therapy for typhoid fever.

It is helpful to divide the management of acute typhoid fever into three categories: specific antibiotic therapy, general supportive measures, and treatment of the commoner life-endangering complications.

Antimicrobial Agents

Chloramphenicol has been the mainstay of specific therapy of typhoid fever since its first demonstration of efficacy in 1948. Although many other antibiotics of the 1950s and 1960s (such as tetracycline, streptomycin, kanamycin, and colistin) had impressive in vitro activity against *S. typhi*, only chloramphenicol was clinically effective. Chloramphenicol remains the drug of choice in less developed countries because of its practicality, inexpensiveness, and effectiveness when administered orally. Chloramphenicol had reduced typhoid fever from a 3- to 4-week illness with 10 percent case fatality to an illness of 1 week (or less) with a case fatality well below 1 percent. However, a number of observations make chloramphenicol a less-than-ideal drug: (*1*) relapse occurs in approximately 8 to 15 percent of patients; (*2*) it causes irreversible aplastic anemia in approximately 1 in 40,000 to 100,000 recipients; (*3*) occasional patients treated with this drug develop "toxic crises" (Herxheimer-like reactions); (*4*) in recent years the duration of therapy necessary to achieve an afebrile state has increased; (*5*) the drug is not impressive in preventing development of chronic carriers; and (*6*) epidemics caused by chloramphenicol-resistant strains have occurred (as in Mexico in 1972, in Vietnam in 1973, and in Peru in 1980).

The recommended regimen is 750 mg of chloramphenicol every 6 hours to adults (50 mg per kilogram for children) until the fever subsides (usually 3 to 7 days), followed by 500 mg every 6 hours for adults (50 mg per kilogram for children); the drug is given for a total of 14 days. If the patient is unable to take oral medication, the drug should be given intravenously until the switch to oral medication can be made. Chloramphenicol should not be given intramuscularly because only poor blood levels are achieved. Occasional patients develop a "toxic crisis" following the first doses of drug; it is postulated that this may result from a sudden release of endotoxin secondary to death of the bacteria.

If the *S. typhi* isolate is known to be resistant to chloramphenicol or if epidemiologic data make such infection likely, there are two highly effective alternatives, trimethoprim-sulfamethoxazole and amoxicillin, both of which are administered orally.

Amoxicillin, a congener of ampicillin, shows superior intestinal absorption. Adults are given 1.0 g (children, 100 mg per kilogram) every 6 hours for 14 days. During the 1972 Mexican epidemic caused by chloramphenicol-resistant *S. typhi*, strains began to appear that bore plasmid-mediated resistance to amoxicillin as well. Infections with such strains can be successfully treated with oral trimethoprim-sulfamethoxazole. The dose is 1 tablet of 160 mg trimethoprim and 800 mg sulfamethoxazole twice daily for 14 days. Children should receive 8 mg per kilogram of trimethoprim and 40 mg per kilogram of sulfamethoxazole daily in two divided doses. A large experience with trimethoprim-sulfamethoxazole therapy for typhoid fever caused by chloramphenicol-sensitive strains has shown that it is comparable in efficacy to chloramphenicol in approximately 90 percent of cases. In 8 to 10 percent of infected persons, however, the therapeutic response is retarded, requiring 10 or more days for the body temperature to become normal.

Irrespective of the aforementioned antibiotics selected, the clinical response in typhoid fever is not dramatic. Usually 2 complete days of therapy are required before the fever begins to abate, and a normal temperature is usually not reached for 5 to 7 days.

General Supportive Measures

Because of the high fever, maintenance requirements for water and electrolytes are greatly increased, so the patient should be encouraged to drink fluids liberally. If the patient is too ill to maintain hydration via oral fluids, intravenous fluids must be given; daily maintenance requirements should be increased by 10 percent for each degree of fever above 99 °F (37.2 °C).

Salicylates should not be given to patients with typhoid fever, since they can induce abrupt changes in temperature, hypotension, and even shock. The temperature should be lowered by sponging with tepid water.

Laxatives and enemas should, in general, not be employed because of the danger of precipitating intestinal hemorrhage. If constipation requires relief, oral lactulose should be used; this nonabsorbable disaccharide is a gentle physiologic softener of stool.

COMPLICATIONS

In the preantibiotic era, typhoid fever was a disease marked by a wide array of complications involving virtually every organ system and including intestinal perforation, intestinal hemorrhage, myocarditis, empyema of the gallbladder, encephalopathy, bronchitis, pneumonia, parotitis, osteomyelitis, hepatitis, meningitis, septic arthritis, and orchitis. Since the advent of specific antimicrobial therapy, most of the complications are still encountered with some frequency and are discussed below.

In some areas of the world, such as in Djakarta, Indonesia, an exceptionally virulent form of typhoid fever is seen in a small percentage of patients. These patients with acute typhoid fever present with severe toxemia, delirium, and obtundation and proceed to coma and shock. The case fatality rate in these patients is 55 percent with chloramphenicol alone. However, two days of high-dose dexamethasone drastically reduces the case fatality (to 10%) as the fever and toxemia are reduced. An initial dose of dexamethasone of 3 mg per kilogram should be given intravenously, followed by 1 mg per kilogram every 6 hours for a duration of 48 hours. The use of steroids should be reserved for this rare situation only and otherwise plays no role in the treatment of typhoid fever.

Despite adequate therapy with appropriate antibiotics, 5 to 15 percent of patients manifest relapse. In general, all signs and symptoms are milder in nature than the initial clinical episode, and the treatment is the same as for the initial episode.

Two dreaded complications of typhoid fever are still encountered in approximately 1 percent of cases: intestinal hemorrhage and perforation. When a definitive diagnosis of typhoid fever is made, a unit of blood should be typed and cross-matched as a precaution. Hemorrhage occurs late in the course, often in the second or third week, when the patient is often feeling better. The management of hemorrhage is conservative, utilizing repeated transfusion unless there is evidence of intestinal perforation. In the preantibiotic era, intestinal perforation was almost always fatal. Current consensus favors a combination of medical treatment and surgical intervention. Most surgeons experienced in the treatment of typhoid fever complications favor simple closure of the ulcer. This must be accompanied by additional antibiotics, such as gentamicin, tobramycin, or amikacin (in that order of preference) plus cefoxitin or clindamycin to treat peritoneal contamination by normal enteric flora.

CARRIER STATE

Approximately 3 to 5 percent of persons with acute typhoid fever become chronic biliary carriers. The propensity to carriage increases with age at the time of initial *S. typhi* infection and is greater in females. Most chronic carriers have cholecystitis with stones; occasional carriers lacking gallbladders manifest chronic pathology and infection in the intrahepatic biliary system.

If indicated because of economic or social factors and if the patient is sturdy enough to withstand surgery, cholecystectomy accompanied by 4 weeks of combined intravenous ampicillin and oral amoxicillin therapy can cure the carrier state in approximately 85 percent of instances. When this is not feasible, 3 weeks of high-dose intravenous ampicillin therapy has also shown promising results. Most recently, a moderate success rate has been reported by long-term (at least 4 weeks) oral therapy with ciprofloxacin (750 mg every 12 hours) or norfloxacin (400 mg every 12 hours).

PREVENTION

In multiple controlled field trials in endemic areas, acetone-killed *S. typhi* parenteral vaccine has been shown to confer 75 to 90 percent protective efficacy against typhoid fever. The protection afforded to persons from nonendemic areas appears to be somewhat less. However, the parenteral vaccine causes fever or adverse local reactions (heat, swelling, erythema) in 15 to 25 percent of recipients. Nevertheless, for persons traveling to highly endemic areas, immunization with two 0.5-ml doses 1 month apart is recommended.

A new, live, oral attenuated *S. typhi* vaccine (strain Ty21a) is becoming available in many countries. Three doses of lyophilized vaccine in enteric-coated capsules was recently shown in field trials in Santiago, Chile, to provide approximately 65 percent protection without causing adverse reactions. This vaccine will be licensed in the United States in 1990.

SUGGESTED READING

Avendano A, Herrera P, Horwitz I, et al. Duodenal string cultures: practicality and sensitivity for diagnosing enteric fever in children. J Infect Dis 1986; 153:359–362.

Ferreccio C, Morris JG Jr, Valdivieso C, et al. Efficacy of ciprofloxacin in the treatment of chronic typhoid carriers. J Infect Dis 1988; 157:1235–1239.

Levine MM, Taylor DN, Ferreccio C. Typhoid vaccines come of age. Pediatr Infect Dis 1989; 8:374–381.

Snyder MG, Perroni J, Gonzalez O, et al. Comparative efficacy of chloramphenicol, ampicillin and co-trimoxazole in the treatment of typhoid fever. Lancet 1976; 2:1155–1157.

INTRA-ABDOMINAL ABSCESS

DORI F. ZALEZNIK, M.D.

Intra-abdominal abscesses, either peritoneal or visceral, usually arise as a subacute complication of intra-abdominal sepsis. The most common inciting event for an intra-abdominal abscess is appendicitis with perforation. However, any disruption of the normal integrity of the bowel, for example, surgery, trauma, eroding tumor, diverticulitis, or perforated ulcer, may result in peritonitis and eventual localization into an abscess. Abscesses may arise in an area contiguous to the perforated viscus; may collect in organs such as liver (most common), kidneys, or spleen; or may be located in the subphrenic regions, attached to the peritoneum or within the omentum. Gallbladder perforation may result in peritonitis or liver abscesses via contiguous spread. Abscesses, particularly visceral collections, also may occur following bacteremia.

As will be considered in greater detail below, it is important to consider the origin of peritonitis or bacteremia that has led to abscess development because diagnostic approaches, the need for surgical correction, and the choice of antimicrobial therapy all will be influenced by the initiating events of the infection. Typically, intra-abdominal abscesses represent infections from which many bacterial species are isolated. Anaerobic organisms are found in 96 percent of cases of intra-abdominal sepsis. Knowledge of the normal flora of the human intestine, female genital tract, and gallbladder is helpful in determining likely bacterial species to be involved. Several organisms figure especially prominently in intra-abdominal abscesses, however, and more commonly than one would predict from their numerical representation in the normal flora. The most important of these organisms is *Bacteroides fragilis*, a gram-negative anaerobe which is the most common anaerobic species found in abscess contents and in bacteremia. Among aerobic species, *Escherichia coli* is the most common organism isolated. An exception to the usual polymicrobial content of abscesses may occur when a visceral abscess results from hematogenous spread. A single organism such as *Staphylococcus aureus* or even a viridans streptococcal strain such as *Streptococcus milleri* may cause abscesses under those circumstances. Empiric therapy of suspected intra-abdominal abscess should be directed at both anaerobic and aerobic organisms.

In experimental animal systems mortality in intra-abdominal sepsis is caused by aerobic gram-negative bacilli in the bloodstream. While *B. fragilis* bacteremia is common, mortality from bloodstream infection is rare presumably because the lipopolysaccharide (LPS) component of this anaerobe does not induce the same endotoxin manifestations as gram-negative aerobic LPS. In both animal and human infections, the later manifestation of intra-abdominal sepsis is abscess formation, which usually requires the presence of an anaerobic species. *B. fragilis* given experimentally can cause abscesses, but other anaerobic and aerobic species require a synergistic combination of both anaerobes and aerobes to produce abscesses. For successful antimicrobial prophylaxis against intra-abdominal sepsis in colonic surgery, antibiotics must be active against both aerobic gram-negative bacilli (to prevent gram-negative rod sepsis) and against anaerobes (to guard against later abscess development).

DIAGNOSIS

The presentation of an intra-abdominal abscess may be subtle. Acute peritonitis generally is readily recognized with dramatic abdominal findings of rebound tenderness or guarding. In cases of intra-abdominal abscess, however, physical findings may be absent. Occasionally patients note pleuritic pain from diaphragmatic irritation or shoulder discomfort. Fever and constitutional symptoms, such as malaise or anorexia, suggest a more chronic process and may indicate abscess without any localizing manifestations. Liver abscesses, particularly in elderly patients, may be especially subtle and present only as a fever of unknown origin (FUO). Abdominal findings or antecedent abdominal complaints may be absent. The only abnormal laboratory finding may consist of an elevated alkaline phosphatase. Leukocytosis and other abnormal liver function tests may be absent. An unexplained unilateral pleural effusion can sometimes precipitate an evaluation of the abdomen. Fever is common, and in one-third of patients with a liver abscess, concomitant bacteremia will be found.

In a suspected case of intra-abdominal abscess, several radiologic evaluations are helpful. The most useful specific and sensitive test is computed tomography (CT), which provides a view of the abdomen and pelvis previously obtainable only by exploratory laparotomy. Intravenous or, in the case of examining the bowel, oral contrast enhances the lesions to differentiate from hematomas or tumors. If readily accessible, CT is the single test by which most intra-abdominal abscesses will be diagnosed. Ultrasound studies, if thorough, also can frequently detect abscesses, particularly those in the pelvis. The presence of internal echoes helps to distinguish abscesses from cysts, for example in liver or kidneys. The exact nature of the lesion on ultrasound is more difficult to diagnose than by CT, however. Gallium scans are useful as a broad screen for the evaluation of a patient with an FUO. In the abdomen, however, a gallium scan will never be diagnostic because tumors and other collections take up gallium as well as abscesses, and the bowel concentrates the material, leading to the potential for diagnostic confusion. The test requires a minimum of 48 to 72 hours to perform, limiting its acute diagnostic utility. Gallium can help to pinpoint an area for more specific assessment with CT or ultrasound. On occasion, a single study, even CT, will be negative. If the clinical suspicion for an intra-abdominal abscess is high, a second study should be pursued. The most problematic situation for establishing the diagnosis of intra-abdominal abscess is diverticulitis with abscess. Diverticulitis is a common clinical diagnosis. When perforation occurs, the process will frequently wall off locally rather than causing distant peritonitis. The diagnostic modalities cited above are not ideal for imaging the bowel and a collection contiguous to the bowel may be missed. Diverticula may be seen on CT, but an abscess may not be visualized. In some instances, barium or gastrografin enemas may be necessary to diagnose a diverticular abscess. In rare cases of diverticular abscess, in which the patient experiences recurrent gram-negative bacillary bacteremia without an established focus, exploratory surgery may be required.

TREATMENT

Therapy for intra-abdominal abscess may be divided into two parts. While choice of antimicrobial agents is important, particularly with a number of newer products available, the mainstay of treatment remains drainage of the walled-off pus. In the past, surgical drainage was required. With skilled diagnostic radiologists using CT or ultrasound, however, surgery frequently can be avoided. Percutaneous drainage even of large collections of pus can be performed under CT or ultrasound guidance with insertion of small pigtail catheters that can be left in place to drain and can later be manipulated. There are several clinical situations in which drainage is not required routinely. Diverticulitis with a small, localized abscess can usually be cured medically. The occasional patient with multiple, small liver abscesses not amenable to drainage also may be cured with prolonged antibiotic therapy. Liver abscesses caused by the parasite *Entamoeba histolytica* usually do not require drainage. If an amebic abscess is suspected clinically in a patient, for example, with a travel history, blood serology, which is positive in more than 90 percent of patients with extraintestinal amebiasis, may be diagnostic without aspiration of the lesion. In some patients, mixed amebic and bacterial abscesses occur. In such situations, however, the patients do not respond to therapy for amebiasis alone. Some pelvic collections, such as tubo-ovarian abscesses, may be cured medically without surgical intervention as well.

Some current literature advocates medical therapy of other intra-abdominal abscesses, particularly liver abscesses. While certain patients may be unable to tolerate surgery and have lesions not amenable to the percutaneous approach, the literature is difficult to evaluate. Patients in these studies frequently undergo diagnostic aspiration which may, in some instances, be the equivalent of drainage. While other patients are cured, the length of antibiotic course usually is measured in months rather than weeks. In general, the preferred approach to an intra-abdominal abscess, including liver abscesses, is to establish drainage and use antimicrobial therapy as an important adjunct. Lengthy courses of antibiotics are not without hazard, and patients with prominent constitutional symptoms and fever may take much longer to feel better with a medical approach alone.

As stated above, antimicrobial therapy of intra-abdominal abscesses must be directed at both anaerobic and aerobic species. In general, this dictates combination therapy. It is useful to discuss therapy directed at anaerobes separately as the literature may be confusing and sensitivity testing of anaerobes in most clinical laboratories is not performed routinely. First-line therapy for anaerobes in intra-abdominal sepsis includes three potential choices for which considerable in vitro and clinical data are available. In 1989, the first among these three antibiotics is metronidazole. This agent has a broad anaerobic spectrum, including the more resistant members of the *B. fragilis* group, penetration into abscesses is excellent, and high blood levels can be achieved with oral as well as intravenous administration, raising the possibility of completing therapy with an oral agent. Resistance in clinical isolates has not been reported in the United States. Metronidazole is not active against any aerobic species. If infection with *Clostridium perfringens* is suspected, penicillin is the drug of choice, but that organism is rarely found in intra-abdominal abscesses.

Two other widely used antibiotics are clindamycin and cefoxitin. Both are active against the anaerobic flora below the diaphragm. Clindamycin does not cover aerobic gram-negative bacilli. Cefoxitin can be used as a single agent since it is active against many aerobic gram-negative bacilli as well as against anaerobes such as *B. fragilis*. In some areas of the country, however, there is growing resistance to second-generation cephalosporins among aerobic gram-negative bacilli. In these locales, another agent active against gram-negative organisms should be added to cefoxitin. In recent years reports of growing resistance to clindamycin or cefoxitin by *B. fragilis*, approaching 10 percent, have been published. While these trends are of interest, reports of well-documented clinical failures due to resistant organisms are scarce. Most experts in anaerobic infections still would include both of these antibiotics among first-line therapy. If an individual patient, however, seems to be failing therapy and there is no other focus of infection that needs to be drained, a change of therapy and attempts to perform sensitivity testing on anaerobic isolates are appropriate. There also has been concern that cefoxitin resistance may cross to other β-lactam agents, suggesting that another class of antibiotic should be chosen if cefoxitin resistance is suspected.

Chloramphenicol is another antibiotic that has been used for many years against anaerobes. While *B. fragilis* has not been found to be resistant to this agent in vitro, clinical failures with this drug in experimental and human infections may be as high as 40 percent. Many patients will respond to chloramphenicol, however, and if a patient is improving on the drug, there is no reason to change.

Third-generation cephalosporins, while popular and active against gram-negative aerobic bacilli, are not very effective against *B. fragilis*. Moxalactam displayed the greatest activity of this class of agents but because of bleeding problems is not in widespread use currently. *B. fragilis* has high resistance to cefoperazone and cefotaxime and even to an active metabolite of the latter drug. While there was some initial interest in ceftizoxime, in vitro testing of *B. fragilis* to this antibiotic makes it appear more sensitive than is reflected in clinical results.

The new oral antibiotic class of quinolone agents, such as ciprofloxacin, has a wide antibacterial spectrum but is notable for the absence of anaerobic coverage. Broader-spectrum penicillins, such as ticarcillin or piperacillin, are active against *Bacteroides* species, but the clinical utility of these drugs has not been evaluated widely. Cefotetan, a newer second-generation cephalosporin, is equivalent to cefoxitin in activity against *B. fragilis* but is not as active against other members of the *Bacteroides* group, such as *Bacteroides thetaiotaomicron*. While the half-life of cefotetan allows for less-frequent administration than cefoxitin, thereby decreasing costs, metronidazole is less costly than either of the cephalosporins and is generally preferred.

Several new types of antibiotics appear to be active against anaerobes and bear watching as large clinical trials of intra-abdominal sepsis are completed. These drugs include imipenem, ticarcillin-clavulanic acid, and ampicillin-sulbactam. All are broad-spectrum agents with potential use as monotherapy, although local resistance rates for aerobic gram-negative bacilli need to be assessed in determining the adequacy of single-drug therapy. While clinical trials in known infections involving anaerobic species are not extensive with any of these agents, they are likely to be promising additions in the future.

For treatment of the aerobic components of abscesses, metronidazole or clindamycin usually is used in conjunction with an aminoglycoside. Cefoxitin may be used alone with the proviso that local aerobic gram-negative bacilli are not highly resistant. Chloramphenicol has some aerobic gram-negative spectrum but, as a bacteriostatic antibiotic, generally should be combined with an aminoglycoside. Once the sensitivities of the aerobic species are known, less toxic agents such as cephalosporins can be substituted for the aminoglycoside. Ciprofloxacin also may be considered as oral therapy along with metronidazole, but there are no clinical trials of this regimen in intra-abdominal abscess.

As mentioned above, it is important to consider the site of origin of peritonitis or bacteremia in considering antibiotic coverage. For example, perforation of a duodenal or gastric ulcer or pancreatitis with abscess formation often produces substantial chemical irritation of the peritoneum with less prominent abscess formation.

Much of the consideration for therapy for intra-abdominal infections, usually arising from the colon, takes into account the sensitivities of the *B. fragilis* group. When treating pelvic abscesses arising from the female genital tract, consideration needs to be given to coverage of *Neisseria gonorrhoeae* and *Chlamydia*. When abscesses arise in the pelvic region, as opposed to pelvic inflammatory disease, *B. fragilis* figures prominently as a pathogen as well.

Another location of concern is the gallbladder. Except in cases of multiple episodes of cholecystitis or previous biliary tree surgery, anaerobic organisms do not figure prominently as flora of the gallbladder. Aerobic gram-negative bacilli are the most common organisms found, with enterococci also prominent. Many clinicians will treat to eliminate the enterococcus in intra-abdominal sepsis. Most of the regimens discussed, including metronidazole or clindamycin/gentamicin and cefoxitin, do not include enterococcal coverage. The importance of the enterococcus in mixed intra-abdominal processes has not been established. My practice is not to cover empirically for enterococci except in infections arising in the gallbladder and to consider broadening coverage to include enterococci if the organisms are isolated from blood or repeatedly from abscess contents. Ampicillin usually is added to eliminate the enterococcus (vancomycin in the case of penicillin-allergic patients).

Table 1 summarizes my recommendations about antibiotic regimens for intra-abdominal abscesses. Although an opinion, these recommendations reflect a review of anaerobic susceptibility patterns and the clinical literature at the present time. In general, the technology necessary to perform sensitivity testing on anaerobic species is not available in most clinical laboratories. This should not be viewed as a criticism, since the need for routine susceptibility testing has not been proved. In problematic individual cases, it is helpful to have sensitivity testing accessible. Most of the rele-

TABLE 1 Antibiotics Useful in the Treatment of Intra-Abdominal Abscess

Anaerobic Coverage	*Aerobic Gram-Negative Coverage*
First-line therapy	
Metronidazole 500 mg q8h	Gentamicin 1.5 mg/kg q8h*
Clindamycin 600 mg q8h†	Gentamicin 1.5 mg/kg q8h*
Cefoxitin 2 g q4h	Cefoxitin‡ 2 g q4h
Alternative regimen	
Chloramphenicol 500 mg q6h	Gentamicin 1.5 mg/kg q8h*
Newer antibiotics to be considered	
Imipenem 1 g q6h	Imipenem 1 g q6h
Ampicillin-sulbactam 3 g q6h§	Ampicillin-sulbactam‡ 3 g q6h§
Ticarcillin-clavulanic acid 3.1 g q4h#	Ticarcillin-clavulanic acid‡ 3.1 g q4h#

* Intervals should be adjusted based on creatinine and peak and trough drug levels in renal insufficiency.
† The pharmacokinetics of clindamycin suggest that every 8 hours is a more appropriate dosing interval than every 6 hours.
‡ In areas in which resistance of aerobic gram-negative bacilli to this agent is known to be fairly high, addition of an antibiotic such as gentamicin should be considered.
§ Ampicillin component is 2 g and sulbactam 1 g.
# Ticarcillin component is 3 g and clavulanic acid 100 mg.

vant information can be obtained from studies by experts who have the facilities for susceptibility testing of anaerobes.

SUGGESTED READING

Altemeier WA, Culbertson WR, Fullen WD, Shook CD. Intra-abdominal abscesses. Am J Surg 1973; 125:70–79.

Cuchural GJ, Tally FP, Jacobus NV, et al. Susceptibility of the *Bacteroides fragilis* group in the United States: analysis by site of location. Antimicrob Agents Chemother 1988; 32:712–722.

Gerzof SG, Robbins AH, Johnson WC, Birkett DH, Nabseth DC. Percutaneous catheter drainage of abdominal abscesses. N Engl J Med 1981; 305:653–657.

Tally FP, Gorbach SL. Therapy of mixed anaerobic-aerobic infections. Am J Med 1985; 78:145–153.

Thadepalli H, Gorbach SL, Broido PW, Norsen J, Nyhus L. Abdominal trauma, anaerobes, and antibiotics. Surg Gynecol Obstet 1973; 137:270–276.

BILIARY TRACT INFECTION

HARRY E. DASCOMB, M.D.
DALE W. OLLER, M.D.

The liver, biliary tract, supportive tissue, and serosal membranes receive blood supply from the portal vein and the hepatic artery. Microorganisms that breech the intestinal mucosa from the esophagus to the middle region of the rectum gain access to the portal vein. Since the portal vein contributes two-thirds of the hepatic blood supply, portal vein–borne enteric bacteria or parasites cause the majority of intrahepatic or biliary tract infections. Although portal blood is usually sterile, portal blood cultures of humans and dogs with colitis frequently reveal bacteria. Similarly, patients with acute enteritis, Crohn's disease, ulcerative colitis, diverticulitis, and amebiasis have liver and biliary tract infections as complications. To a lesser extent, the liver, biliary tract, and gallbladder are exposed to systemic bacteremia and viremia conveyed by the hepatic artery or more rarely by the splenic vein (in event of a splenic abscess or septic splenic infarcts). Enteric bacteria also gain access to and colonize the biliary tract via the ampulla of Vater (duodenal papilla), particularly during duodenitis, intestinal obstruction, or common bile duct (CBD) stasis. Intestinal bacteria also gain access to the biliary tract through cholecysto- or choledocho-intestinal fistulae, endoscopic retrograde cholangiopancreatography (ERCP), and transendoscopic surgery. Palliative or diagnostic surgical procedures, such as cholecystotomy or percutaneous transhepatic cholangiography, may contaminate the biliary tract with skin bacteria.

Bile is usually sterile despite these potential sources of hepatic and biliary tract infection. Sterility of the biliary tract is dependent on the phagocytic efficiency of the hepatic Kupffer cells; the daily secretion of 600 to 800 ml of bile, which flushes the biliary system; and the maintenance of a critical balance of bile acids, pigment, cholesterol, and lecithin in the bile, which prevents formation of cholesterol and pigment stones. An imbalance of cholesterol, unconjugated bilirubin, or lecithin and bile acids, together with stasis, causes crystallization of cholesterol micellae or of bilirubinate salts. Bacteria present in the bile may be sequestered in the stones. Indeed, bacteria secreting β-glucuronidase may have a central role in pigmented stone production. Those bacteria capable of producing gas, particularly anaerobes, can cause radiolucent clefts within the stones, which are recognized radiographically as the "Mercedes Benz" sign. The sludge and stones resulting from crystallization usually appear first in the gallbladder and obstruct the cystic duct at the valves of Heister. Stones frequently migrate from the gallbladder (or occasionally from elsewhere) and obstruct the common or hepatic ducts. Biliary obstruction also may occur from primary inflammation and fibrosis as well as malignancy. Stasis due to obstruction permits casual biliary infectious contaminants to flourish, and inflammation results. The inflammatory swelling may cause ischemia, necrosis of adjacent tissue, and complete obstruction of a portion or all of the entire biliary tree; closed space infection can result. In this manner, biliary tract obstruction and infection are expressed in several syndromes: cholecystitis—acute and chronic or acalculous, acute; cholangitis—obstructive (ascending) pyogenic cholangitis, sclerosing cholangitis, and oriental or recurrent cholangitis; pancreatitis—secondary to biliary tract infection; liver abscess—cholangitic or hematogenous; and hepatitis—chronic, granulomatous or acute, nonbacterial. The effective management of biliary tract infections depends on:

1. Identification of the syndrome and specific etiology by clinical examination, clinical laboratory study of blood and urine, and aerobic and anaerobic cultures of venous blood collected from patients with current or recent fever and tissue and bile collected via endoscopy, percutaneous transhepatic aspiration during cholangiography, or cholecystotomy. Serum may be stored (−20°C) for possible subsequent antibody testing of acute phase and convalescent specimens against protozoa, bacteria, and viruses.
2. Investigation of the biliary tract radiographically for confirmation or exclusion of biliary tract obstruction or the presence of intrahepatic or extrahepatic fluid or abscess.
3. Estimation of the etiologic agent(s) based on clinical and initial laboratory findings.
4. Selection of antibiotics based on results of studies 1 through 3—for immediate therapy in acutely ill or septicemic patients or for perioperative prophylaxis against sepsis and wound infection resulting from surgical, endoscopic, or radiologic invasive procedures.
5. Correction or control of metabolic disorders prior to surgery.
6. Performance of surgical, endoscopic, or percutaneous procedures for the prompt removal of biliary tract obstruction, excision, or incision and drainage of localized infection; the collection of tissue, bile, and exudate by surgery or transendoscopic procedure for direct study (wet mount, Gram and special stains), culture for bacteria (identification and antibiotic sensitivity of isolates), culture for viruses when appropriate (e.g., patient with acalculous cholecystitis and sclerosing cholangitis), cytology (special stains for mycobacteria, fungi, protozoa), and histopathology.
7. Revision of the initial antibiotic therapy to attain specificity, optimal dosage, and cost effectiveness, based on the completed microbiologic study results of initial body fluid and surgical specimens, the anatomic diagnosis, and clinical response. Subsequent changes in therapy are determined by the clinical response and the microscopic and culture findings using interval specimens of tissue or exudate.

ACUTE CHOLECYSTITIS

Acute cholecystitis is an emergency that usually presents with symptoms of fever, persistent right upper-quadrant (RUQ) pain extending in a band-like fashion to the infra- or interscapular region, nausea, vomiting, and anxiety. Acute cholecystitis is heralded by fluctuating epigastric cramping pain or colic that persists, with increasing severity, and becomes localized in the right hypochondrium. Occasional episodes of postprandial or nocturnal epigastric pain may occur prior to the acute illness. Physical findings reveal an acutely ill person with elevated vital signs. There is voluntary guarding in the RUQ and tenderness to gentle palpation. Deep inspiration provokes a transient inspiratory arrest and complaint of pain in the subcostal region at the midclavicular line as the tender gallbladder descends against the examiner's hand (Murphy's sign). Gentle pressure with a finger may be required to elicit this sign but fist percussion of the costal margin is unnecessary and elicits excessive patient discomfort. Despite the abdominal muscle guarding, a tender mass or phlegmon may be palpated in the hypochondrium and extend below the paraumbilical line. The skin overlying the inflamed gallbladder radiates heat. Laboratory findings include leukocytosis with moderate left shift and slightly elevated concentrations of serum alkaline phosphatase, bilirubin, and aspartate aminotransferase (AST). Serum amylase elevation may be transient. Persistent serum amylase elevation suggests associated obstruction of pancreatic duct of Wirsung and pancreatitis. Bilirubinuria is frequently present.

Management

Fever or history of rigors, feverishness, and night sweating are indications for the prompt collection of blood and urine for culture. Although the clinical diagnosis of acute cholecystitis is 85 percent accurate, it is helpful to ascertain the gallbladder size and wall thickness and the presence of stones or dilated bile ducts. It is also important to exclude pancreatic, renal, and colonic disease and acute viral hepatitis. Ultrasonography provides excellent definition of the gallbladder, gallstones or bile sludge, and biliary tree dilatation and can exclude extrahepatic disease. Scintigraphy with technetium-99m iminodiacetic acid, such as [^{99m}Tc]Pipida permits visualization of the liver, of segments of the biliary tract, of the duodenum, and of the gallbladder (in the absence of disease). When utilized as an adjunct to ultrasonography, scintigraphy permits accurate diagnosis of gallbladder disease. In cholecystitis the cystic duct is occluded. This prevents or delays the entrance of radioactive bile and a gallbladder image. Radioactivity is apparent, however, in the liver, bile ducts, and duodenum. Scintigraphy may be diagnostic when bowel gas obscures ultrasonographic images. It is helpful also in differentiating acute cholecystitis from acute hepatitis and occasionally from cirrhosis of the liver. Unless ultrasound and scintigraphic findings are incompatible with cholecystitis, no further imaging is necessary. Computed tomography (CT) is considered if an intrahepatic lesion, extra biliary tract compression, renal infection, or pancreatic disease is suspected. Magnetic resonance imaging offers no further advantages over CT at present.

Early surgical correction of biliary tract obstruction is the most effective therapy and at the same time promptly confirms the diagnosis. Surgical removal of the diseased gallbladder and direct examination of the biliary tract usually prevent future problems from stones obstructing extrahepatic bile ducts, the common duct, or the ampulla of Vater. Fortunately, an early inflamed, edematous gallbladder usually presents no major technical difficulties in surgical removal. Surgery is best performed during the first 3 days of acute clinical symptoms. After 3 days of symptoms, inflammatory neovascularity develops, dissection about the gallbladder is more difficult, and the risk of surgical complications increases.

Immediate medical therapy is designed to prepare the patient for surgery. Cardiopulmonary, renal, hematologic, or metabolic diseases are excluded or treated. Nasogastric suction is given to relieve ileus, gastric distention, and vomiting. Meperidine is injected intravenously in doses sufficient to reduce pain and smooth muscle spasm. Intravenous fluids and electrolytes are provided to restore hydration and plasma osmolality.

After blood has been collected for aerobic and anaerobic cultures, antibiotics are initiated immediately if the patient has fever or recent history of fever with or without abdominal pain. A combination of ampicillin 200 mg per kilogram per day (in four divided doses at 6-hour intervals) together with gentamicin 4 mg per kilogram per day (in divided doses at 8-hour intervals) is preferred. These antibiotics give excellent tissue levels that inhibit enterococci as well as most aerobic and anaerobic bacteria associated with acute cholecystitis. If the patient is allergic to penicillin, cefazolin 1 g every 6 hours intravenously or cefoxitin 2 g every 6 hours (or cefotetan 2 g every 12 hours) is effective against *Escherichia coli* and non–hospital-acquired *Klebsiella* species, but these antibiotics are ineffective against enterococci. Adequate perioperative coverage of enterococci and enteric bacilli is accomplished in penicillin-allergic patients by vancomycin 500 mg every 6 hours with cefazolin or cefoxitin, as above. In our experience postoperative infections complicating biliary tract surgery are associated often with enterococci, particularly in patients given a cephalosporin alone perioperatively. For this reason we recommend vancomycin, together with perioperative gram-negative coverage, in patients who are allergic to penicillin. During the surgical procedure, specimens are collected for immediate study. The results of the examination of unstained and stained fresh preparations and the preliminary results of aerobic cultures are often sufficient for tentative identification of infection due to cocci or anaerobes likely to be resistant to the initial choice of antibiotics. For example, immediate identification of gram-negative and -positive pleomorphic rods and coccal bacteria in bile or gallbladder mucosa obtained during surgery suggests anaerobic infection. In this situation, metronidazole should be added to the perioperative antibiotic(s) and the duration of postoperative therapy is extended to prevent appearance later of anaerobic abscesses. When the gallbladder and biliary tract stones have been removed and there is no evidence of obstruction or infection, perioperative antibiotics may be stopped 1 day after surgery. However, if smears and cultures from specimens of bile and tissue collected during surgery contain bacteria, particularly enterococci or highly resistant gram-negative rods, prolonged specific therapy may be needed to eliminate the pathogens and prevent the inflammatory obstruction or extra- or intrahepatic abscess as a late complication. If fever persists or the patient fails to improve, further studies are indicated to exclude biliary obstruction, superimposed biliary tract infection, or a nosocomial infection elsewhere. The bacteria isolated from the T-tube in the common bile duct (CBD), from drainage of the gallbladder bed, or from trans-endoscopic aspirates of CBD may be colonizers only and should not be treated routinely. However, they should be considered in selecting adequate perioperative prophylaxis for any additional postoperative invasive procedure.

Patients with acutely inflamed gallbladders who receive no treatment during the first 10 days of fever may develop pericholecystitis, cholecystoenteritic fistulae, or gallstone ileus. The resulting local and generalized peritonitis and septicemia have a mortality exceeding 30 percent. The complications demand aggressive and often repeated surgical procedures as well as intensive and specific antimicrobial therapy against initial and superimposed pathogens. Piperacillin or imipenem with an aminoglycoside and metronidazole are empirically selected until microbiologic data suggest more effective combinations.

Persons with acute cholecystitis and recent myocardial infarction or other illnesses that increase the risk of immediate cholecystectomy should receive intravenous ampicillin and aminoglycoside or alternate antibiotics for 7 to 10 days or longer, depending on subsidence of symptoms and local signs of gallbladder or liver tenderness. If the operative risks for cholecystectomy or cholecystotomy remain high, surgery may be delayed indefinitely by continuing oral or intramuscular antibiotics. However, surgery should be rescheduled as soon as possible, because cholecystitis will recur until the gallbladder and stones have been removed or cholecystotomy and drainage have been accomplished.

ACUTE ACALCULOUS CHOLECYSTITIS

Acute cholecystitis may occur in the absence of gallstones during a systemic illness. Persons at risk are those with salmonellosis (particularly typhoid fever) and infections due to group A streptococci and disseminated cytomegalovirus (CMV). Acute cholecystitis and gallbladder distention due to insidious development of bile stasis are complications of total parenteral nutrition, acute pancreatitis, trauma, and

Caroli's syndrome. Bile stagnation may result also from inanition, dehydration, fever, CBD obstruction from mesenteric lymphadenopathy due to malignancy or viral infection, or duodenal papillitis. The resulting syndrome of acalculous cholecystitis appears to be due to impaired biliary defenses by atonic smooth muscle, to intrahepatic bile duct dilatation, or to extrinsic or intrinsic CBD obstruction culminating in bile stasis. This permits hematogenous pathogens, indigenous enteric microorganisms, to breach the weakened barriers, to replicate prodigiously within the biliary tract and gallbladder, and to produce acute and chronic inflammation. The clinical and laboratory findings indicate cholecystitis with or without cholangitis.

Management

Successful management of acute acalculous cholecystitis is dependent upon prompt recognition of the etiology of systemic infection and gallbladder pathology, the use of specific antibiotics, and adequate drainage of the gallbladder and biliary tract. Peri- and postoperative antibiotic therapy is selected on the basis of all available clinical and laboratory data. Transendoscopic drainage of the CBD may provide specimens of tissue for parasitic, bacterial, and viral studies as well as relief of pain. Surgery is the most effective procedure to relieve pain and reduce danger of a ruptured gallbladder and peritonitis. When cholecystitis occurs with *Salmonella typhi* or other salmonellae postinfection carrier state often follows as a result of residual biliary tract or splenic foci of infection. This shedding of salmonellae in feces may persist indefinitely despite optimal antibiotic therapy and cholecystectomy. Public health assistance with these patients is required to protect against water and food contamination and community infection. When CMV is identified in symptomatic children or in persons with acquired immunodeficiency syndrome (AIDS), dihydroxypropoxyquanine (ganciclovir) 7.5 to 15 mg per kilogram per day in three divided doses should be considered for its antiviral effect. The appropriate indications for ganciclovir are still being developed.

CHRONIC SYMPTOMATIC CHOLECYSTITIS

Chronic inflammation of the gallbladder is usually associated with cholelithiasis. Complaints of flatulence, anorexia, nausea, hypogeusia, and epigastric abdominal discomfort or pain in the right hypochondrium are common symptoms but are not specific. There may be history of fatty food intolerance with postprandial exacerbation of abdominal colic-like pain and eructations. Usually fever is not present. Physical findings are limited to minimal tenderness in the right upper quadrant of the abdomen. The gallbladder is usually contracted, fibrosed, and not palpable. Occasionally, a palpable fluctuant mass is due to a noninflamed, noncalculous gallbladder that is obstructed and distended with clear to cloudy mucus (hydrops). This, according to Courvoisier's law, suggests carcinoma of the head of the pancreas but occurs in absence of malignancy. Laboratory studies give normal results except for a slight elevation in serum alkaline phosphatase. The differential diagnosis includes functional disorders, systemic diseases (including diabetes mellitus, megaloblastic anemia, myxedema, and malignancies of the biliary tract, pancreas or lymph nodes), or peptic ulcer disease and hiatal hernia.

Gallstones and gallbladder wall thickening are usually readily identified by ultrasonography. These ultrasonographic findings confirm chronic cholecystitis, and at the same time other organs can be visualized to help exclude renal and pancreatic disease. Cholecystography, using a double dose of oral contrast material, is diagnostic if radiolucent stones can be outlined. Cholelithiasis and chronic cholecystitis are confirmed also if the sonogram shows stones and the oral cholecystogram provides no opacification of the gallbladder. ERCP has no role in the diagnosis of confirmed stone-induced chronic cholecystitis, but transendoscopy may have a therapeutic role in removing small gallstones when these have been treated with litholytic chemicals or fragmented by extracorporeal lithotripsy. Stone fragments can be removed from the common duct endoscopically. Endoscopic sphincterotomy after lithotripsy may be a reasonable option in the elderly, poor-risk patient who has gallstones obstructing the duodenal papilla. The major complication of transendoscopic sphincterotomy is hemorrhage into the duodenum, requiring surgical hemostasis. Duodenal or CBD perforations are complications also. Endoscopy-laser fragmentation of stones in the common bile ducts appears to be a promising nonsurgical method of lithotripsy.

Management

Optimal therapy for the majority of patients with chronic symptoms and evidence of cholelithiasis is elective cholecystectomy and thorough exploration of the biliary tract for obscure gallstones. Recent evidence that 40 percent of gallbladders removed for chronic cholecystitis and 80 percent of pigmented stones contain bacteria supports the decision to use perioperative antibiotic prophylaxis for both endoscopic or surgical procedures. Debilitated persons particularly need this protection. Cefazolin is effective against normal skin flora and most aerobic bacteria that may colonize the biliary tract. Cefazolin is ineffective against hospital-acquired *Staphylococcus epidermidis*, all strains of *Enterococcus faecalis*, and most anaerobes. For this reason, ampicillin and gentamicin are preferred initial perioperative therapy and are continued or replaced as determined by the study of the surgical specimen and by the clinical events postoperatively. An alternate perioperative antibiotic is piperacillin in full therapeutic dosage intravenously (Table 1). In the event of penicillin allergy, cefoxitin and vancomycin or vancomycin with an aminoglycoside are options for perioperative prophylaxis against the most common bacterial colonizers of the biliary tract (Table 2).

If the patient is febrile, routine specimens are collected, and ampicillin and gentamicin or alternatives are selected empirically. Both antibiotics are continued postoperatively until the patient is afebrile or the ampicillin and gentamicin are replaced by a more specific single antibiotic or combination of antibiotics. Specificity is determined by in vitro

TABLE 1 Antimicrobial Agents for Specific Problems in Biliary Tract Infections

Antibiotic	Dose (mg/kg/day)	Average Adult Dose: g/h	Route	Total g/day	Indication*
Ceftriaxone	30	2/24	IV IM	2.000	Penicillin allergy Prolonged therapy (3–21 days)
Cefoperazone	60	2/12	IV	4.000	As above; renal failure
Aztreonam	110	2/6	IV	8.000	Gram-negative bacteria, resistant to other antibiotics
Imipenem	50	1/6	IV	4.000	*Pseudomonas* species; *S. aureus*, enteric bacteria resistant to other antibiotics
Metronidazole	15	0.5/6	IV	2.000	Adjunctive therapy for anaerobic bacterial infection
Clindamycin	40	0.9/8	IV	2.700	Penicillin allergy; adjunctive therapy against anaerobes, *S. aureus*
Chloramphenicol	50	1.0/6 1.0/6	IV PO	4.000	Penicillin allergy; liver/renal failure; anaerobic/aerobic; enteric bacteria, enterococcal infection
Sulfamethoxazole-trimethoprim	50 10	1.0/6 0.2/6	IV PO	4.000 0.800	Therapy, penicillin allergy, gram-negative aerobic rods
Ciprofloxacin	21	0.750/12	PO	1.500	Penicillin allergy, prolonged suppressive therapy; *S. aureus*, *Pseudomonas*, *Salmonella*, aerobic enteric gram-negative rods
Ganciclovir (DHPG)	7.5	0.175/8	IV	0.525	Cytomegalovirus†
Amphotericin	0.35–1.00	0.025 to 0.075/24	IV	0.035	Systemic fungal infection
Ansamycin (investigational)	7–9	0.450/24	PO	0.450	*M. avium* complex

* When identity and in vitro sensitivity of pathogen are appropriate for prophlaxis and/or therapy.
† Specific indications for use in this setting are still being developed.

sensitivity tests and by serum bactericidal effect against the isolates from the surgical specimen.

If specimens collected during surgery contain a polymicrobial flora in the stained smear suggesting mixed anaerobic-aerobic infection, and the patient's clinical status worsens, blood is recultured, and piperacillin should replace ampicillin or cefazolin. Aminoglycoside is continued until cultures of intraoperative tissue and bile show no aerobic enterobacteria and those present are sensitive to piperacillin. If *Bacteroides fragilis* or *Bacteroides melaninogenicus* groups are identified, metronidazole is combined with piperacillin.

Chloramphenicol is effective in treating biliary tract infections due to enteric bacteria, including anaerobes and enterococci. It is bacteriostatic and is only curative if drainage has been established. A total daily dose of 4 g is essential in an adult. Polymorphonuclear depression and moderate anemia occur with prolonged therapy but may be monitored by frequent examination of the peripheral blood for polymorphonuclear cells, platelets, and occasional serum iron levels. Chloramphenicol is an excellent choice in patients with renal and liver failure and in β-lactam allergy. It is as effective orally as parenterally. As experienced in treating patients with typhoid fever, chloramphenicol orally has no different depressing effect on the bone marrow than does the intravenous route.

Third-generation cephalosporins should not be used against unidentified bacteria pre- or postoperatively since these may induce resistance in less than bactericidal concentrations. When bacteria in blood or bile are identified and the susceptibilities are known against ceftriaxone or cefoperazone, either is effective. Vitamin K should be given with cefoperazone to prevent prothrombin deficiency. Postoperative therapy with orally administered antibiotics is considered when results of microbiology studies confirm effectiveness of available drugs and as soon as alimentation is tolerated. Ciprofloxacin, ampicillin, clindamycin, metronidazole, and chloramphenicol, alone or combined with one another appropriately, may provide adequate specific therapy. Oral clindamycin has a greater propensity for producing pseudomembranous colitis. Chloramphenicol-treated persons require frequent monitoring of the peripheral blood polymorphonuclear cells and platelets. Chloramphenicol is indicated when biliary tract infection is complicated by renal and/or hepatic disease or in persons allergic to β-lactam antibiotics. Ciprofloxacin is well tolerated orally but has limited effect against anaerobes and enterococci. Specific antibiotic therapy orally or intramuscularly should

TABLE 2 Perioperative Antibiotic Prophylaxis: Dosage and Rationale

		Average Adult Dose	
Antibiotic	*Dose (mg/kg/day)*	*g/h*	*Total g/day*
Ampicillin*	200.0	3.0/6	12.0
Gentamicin	4.3	0.1/8	0.3
Tobramycin	4.3	0.1/8	0.3
Amikacin	15.0	0.5/12	1.0
Piperacillin†	340.0	6.0/6	24.0
Vancomycin‡	30.0	0.5/6	2.0
Cefazolin§	115.0	2.5/8	8.0
Cefoxitin‖	200.0	3.0/6	12.0
Cefotetan#	100.0	3.0/12	6.0

* Ampicillin plus gentamicin, tobramycin, or amikacin: effective against group D enterococci, gram-negative enteric bacteria (not hospital acquired or in a patient previously treated with antibiotics), clostridia and other anaerobes but not for *B. fragilis, B. melaninogenicus*.

† Piperacillin plus gentamicin, tobramycin, or amikacin: effective against the above plus nosocomial gram-negative bacteria and *B. fragilis, B. melaninogenicus*.

‡ Vancomycin, plus gentamicin, tobramycin, or amikacin: effective against enterococci, *S. aureus, S. epidermidis*, gram-negative enteric bacteria, and some anaerobes. Tolerated by persons allergic to β-lactam antibiotics.

§ Cefazolin: effective against *E. coli, Klebsiella* species, *S. aureus, S. epidermidis* (methicillin-sensitive), and some anaerobes. Tolerated by most persons allergic to penicillin.

‖ Cefoxitin plus gentamicin, tobramycin, or amikacin: effective (as are ampicillin and gentamicin) against gram-negative enteric bacteria and anaerobes. Less effective against enterococci. Tolerated by most persons allergic to penicillin. Cefoxitin and vancomycin: effective against enterococci, *S. aureus, S. epidermidis* (methicillin-resistant or -sensitive), gram-negative enteric bacilli, and anaerobes. Tolerated by most persons allergic to penicillin.

\# Cefotetan: alternative for cefoxitin.

be continued in patients with pre- or postoperative infection until signs of local and systemic infection have disappeared. An occasional patient may relapse, with anorexia, fever, weight loss, and anemia even after prolonged postoperative antibiotics. Intra-abdominal infectious complications must be then considered. Aggressive diagnostic studies are initiated. Frequently, exploratory surgery is necessary for both diagnosis and therapy.

CHOLANGITIS

The clinical syndromes of simple obstructive or ascending cholangitis, sclerosing cholangitis, and oriental recurrent cholangitis are the result of biliary tract obstruction. In each of these cholangitides, primary obstruction is due to different combinations of metabolic, infectious, or genetic etiologies.

Obstructive (ascending) pyogenic cholangitis is usually due to gallstones forming in or migrating to the common bile duct (CBD) or to strictures or diverticula of the bile ducts secondary to trauma or infection.

Sclerosing cholangitis is associated with the following conditions:

1. Immunopathy permits opportunistic chronic infection of the biliary tree by viruses, protozoa, bacteria, and fungi that result in biliary tract fibrosis and obstruction, e.g., papillary stenosis associated with cytomegalovirus alone or with protozoa causing CBD obstruction.
2. Viral infection of the ductal mucosa with or without immunodeficiency results in subepithelial fibrosis and obstruction of the CBD and its tributaries, eliminating the secondary and tertiary bile duct branches.
3. Duodenal parasitic infection occludes the distal CBD by periductal fibrosis and lymphadenopathy. The presenting syndrome is intermittent because of acute and chronic pericholangitis resembling chronic active hepatitis.
4. Congenital multifocal dilatation of the segmental bile ducts, CBD and gallbladder, or Caroli's syndrome culminates in polycystic disease of the liver.

Oriental recurrent cholangitis is characterized by intrahepatic bile duct obstruction due to fibrosis. The patients with this impairment have lived in areas in which infection by liver flukes and *Ascaris* species is endemic.

Obstructive (Ascending) Pyogenic Cholangitis

Definition

Calculous biliary obstruction is complicated by a highly concentrated bacteriocholia with enteric, aerobic, and anaerobic bacteria. *E. coli, Klebsiella, Enterobacter, Bacteroides, Clostridium* species, and group D enterococci are most commonly isolated from the bile in pyogenic cholangitis. These pathogens are proteolytic and invasive, causing necrosis, fistulae, abscesses, strictures, and polymicrobial bacteremia.

The cardinal signs of obstructive cholangitis are intermittent pain, fever, and jaundice (Charcot's triad). The attacks are characterized by rigors, fever, moderate RUQ pain, and tenderness. Dark urine and jaundice follow within 3 or 4 days. A cholecystectomy scar is often present in the RUQ, and the liver is enlarged and tender. Clinical evidence of disseminated intravascular coagulation (DIC) may be present, particularly if medical care is delayed. Depending on the severity of the illness, laboratory studies reveal an elevated white blood cell count or leukopenia with granulocytic left shift, consisting of band-formed nucleated cells and metamyelocytes; hyperbilirubinemia; and elevated alkaline phosphatase and transaminases. Often an elevated level of serum amylase is transient. If serum amylase increases and is associated with signs of pancreatitis, obstruction of the duct of Wirsung and/or the CBD at the ampulla of Vater is likely. Increased plasma prothrombin time, partial thromboplastin time, and fibrinogen degradation products, blood urea nitrogen, and creatinine, as well as albuminuria and bacteriuria, confirm endotoxemia and DIC.

Management

Immediate intravenous infusions of fluids and electrolytes are given while blood is collected for hematology, chemistry, and culture. A urine specimen obtained by catheter should be submitted for analysis, Gram stain, and culture. Organisms that cause bacteremia are sometimes also present in the urine. Isolates from cultures of the urine sediment often appear within 18 hours of incubation, permitting antibiotic sensitivity results before positive blood cultures confirm the etiology. Piperacillin, metronidazole, and gentamicin or other aminoglycosides are initiated using one-third of the calculated daily dose of each antibiotic as an initial or loading dose. Piperacillin and metronidazole infusion every 6 hours and gentamicin every 8 hours are continued if results of BUN and creatinine are within normal limits and if there is no clinical or laboratory evidence of hepatocellular dysfunction. At 8 hours of antibiotic therapy, blood samples for trough and 1-hour postinfusion peak aminoglycoside levels are collected. A peak serum level less than 7 to 10 μg per milliliter necessitates a dosage increase. At 24 hours the gentamicin peak and trough levels are again determined, the former to assure continued therapeutic levels, the latter to assure adequate clearance. Piperacillin has been used alone successfully in patients with azotemia since enterococci and most anaerobes are susceptible to it. However, using piperacillin without an aminoglycoside increases the risk of including bacterial resistance, particularly in acute cholangitis. The addition of metronidazole enhances antianaerobe bactericidal activity and prevents persistence and later-appearing abscesses. If biliary obstruction is associated with hepatocellular dysfunction but renal function is normal, metronidazole daily dosage is reduced by 50 percent and divided into two infusions. Piperacillin serum levels are usually not affected during the first 24 hours of therapy in persons with rising BUN and creatinine levels. Dosage reductions of piperacillin recommended by established creatinine clearance nomograms for β-lactam antibiotics should be monitored with peak and trough serum antibacterial levels to assure adequate treatment of patients with severe septicemia. The triple combination of piperacillin, metronidazole, and gentamicin is preferred in severely ill persons to assure optimal bactericidal therapy, resolution of fever, and earliest surgical drainage.

If a patient is allergic to penicillins, cefoxitin or cefotetan may replace piperacillin. If there is allergy to all β-lactam antibiotics and the cephamycins, choramphenicol 1 to 1.5 g every 6 hours for a total daily dose of 4 to 6 g should be used along with metronidazole to prevent inactivation of chloramphenicol by *B. fragilis* or *Clostridium perfringens* that may occur in closed-space infection prior to surgical drainage. Chloramphenicol is also an excellent antimicrobial agent in patients with hepatic and renal impairment. Frequent monitoring of peripheral blood smears and occasionally determining serum levels of chloramphenicol are safeguards against a rapid decrease in leukocytes or platelets observed in occasional patients during therapy.

As the patient improves, further studies are necessary preoperatively to visualize the liver and adjacent organs. Ultrasonography, in the absence of a distended, gas-filled bowel, shows presence or absence of biliary duct dilatation. The site of obstruction is best located by direct visualization using radiopaque substances. If the biliary ducts are dilated, percutaneous transhepatic cholangiography (PTC) is an option. If no biliary tract dilatation is observed in sonograms, ERCP is indicated for diagnosis and occasionally therapy. Common duct stones lodged in the sphincter of Oddi may be removed transendoscopically. Surgery is mandatory if transendoscopic drainage fails. The obstruction may be due to CBD or proximal bile duct pathology such as diverticula, granulomas, extensive fibrosis, or malignancy with or without gallstone impaction. The diagnosis and treatment is best assured by exploration. After the obstruction has been removed or bypassed, a T-tube is emplaced to assure drainage, to provide access for contrast cholangiography and postoperative stone extraction, and to sample bile for bacterial colonization in the event of complications.

Occasionally, emergency measures to drain the biliary tract are necessary prior to definitive surgery when antibiotics fail to control fever and toxemia. This is accomplished by surgical placement of the T-tube in the CBD. Intensive antibiotic therapy is discontinued when the patient improves clinically and is afebrile and laboratory studies reveal no evidence of infection or biliary obstruction. The T-tube is retained for a variable period of time to maintain an access to the biliary tract until convalescence is secured. Occasionally fever persists for 10 or more days postoperatively, associated with anorexia, leukocytosis, and no signs of hospital-acquired infections of the urinary tract, lungs, intravenous access sites, or wounds. This may be due to delayed resolution of the pericholangitis or liver parenchymal infection that will respond to continued antibiotic therapy. Iatrogenic or drug fever must be considered if the persisting fever is unaccompanied by leukocytosis, granulocytic left shift, and toxemia. Effective and less costly antibiotic therapy may be considered for the delayed resolution of cholangitis. Ceftriaxone intramuscularly or ciprofloxacin orally are well tolerated and effective if either inhibits, in vitro, bacteria previously isolated. In most patients with cholangitis and prolonged postoperative fever, further studies are indicated to resolve the cause. These consist of a search for site and cause of intra- or perihepatic infection and biliary tract obstruction. A specimen of bile should be examined for presence of a newly acquired predominant pathogen. T-tube cholangiography is done to determine the existence and location of an obstruction. In the absence of biliary obstruction, CT is necessary to localize abscesses or cysts. Fever and toxemia should improve promptly with surgical or endoscopic relief of obstruction or abscess drainage and effective antibacterial therapy.

Sclerosing Cholangitis

Definition

Sclerosing cholangitis has been an uncommon disease that until recently was not associated with a specific infectious etiology. The biliary tract obstruction is due to subepithelial fibrous thickening of the CBD, gallbladder, and extra- and intrahepatic bile ducts and ductules. Contrast imaging of the biliary tree shows strictures, beading, and fistulae of the bile ducts and decreased arborization and terminal "pruning" of secondary and tertiary radicles. The fibrosis of the common bile duct and gallbladder results in reduced size and thickened walls. The process culminates in biliary obstruction, bacterial infection, and biliary and portal cirrhosis.

Sclerosing cholangitis occurs occasionally in persons with Crohn's disease, ulcerative colitis, Riedel's struma of the thyroid, and lymphoma, suggesting immunopathy as a factor in the pathogenesis. Persons with AIDS develop papillary stenosis and sclerosing cholangitis and present with acalculous cholecystitis. In addition to the immunopathy, CMV has been demonstrated within and isolated from the diseased mucosa cells of the biliary duct in patients with AIDS and sclerosing cholangitis. The localized biliary tract infection with CMV appears in AIDS accompanied by disseminated CMV infection. This complication of AIDS supports a pathogenic role of immunodeficiency in sclerosing cholangitis and suggests that other obligate intracellular pathogens also may initiate damage in the biliary tract that terminates in sclerosing cholangitis. In order to unravel the pathogenicity of sclerosing cholangitis, specimens should be collected at the time of surgery or endoscopy for viral studies particularly in patients with atypical cholangitis and other disease, such as cholangiocarcinoma.

Sclerosing cholangitis also occurs in children following duodenal infection with *Giardia, Ascaris*, and *Strongyloides*. Inadequate antiparasitic therapy or reinfection causes chronic duodenitis, lymphadenitis, and an inflammatory mass adjacent to the duodenum and distal portion of the CBD. The resulting intermittent obstruction causes ascending cholangitis, pericholangitis, and fibrosis. The clinical manifestations are repeated episodes of fever, abdominal pain, hepatosplenomegaly, jaundice, and abnormal serum levels of hepatic enzymes. This syndrome resembles chronic active hepatitis. The diagnosis is usually made during surgery, which offers the most effective means of eliminating the obstruction—a choledochojejunostomy.

Caroli's disease is an autorecessive trait causing multifocal dilatations of the segmental bile ducts and resulting in ectasias and cysts. The biliary ectasia may be diffuse or localized. Spontaneous bacterial cholangitis is the presenting illness as late as 5 to 20 years of age. Prognosis is poor and death ensues 5 to 10 years after the onset of acute cholangitis.

Diagnosis and Management

The clinical and laboratory manifestations of sclerosing cholangitis vary considerably, depending on the underlying disease. In sclerosing cholangitis, Charcot's triad prevails, but gallstones are not the cause of biliary obstruction. Acute bacterial cholangitis frequently is precipitated by endoscopy or surgery, except in Caroli's disease when it may be the presenting illness. Liver enlargement or a palpable gallbladder is often present on examination. Abdominal tenderness in the epigastrium or RUQ of the abdomen is associated with elevated levels of serum bilirubin (direct), alkaline phosphatase, hepatic transaminases, and γ-glutamyl transpeptidase but normal bilirubinemia. Ultrasound study of the upper abdomen is most productive. In absence of signs of stones, grossly dilated bile ducts, or intrahepatic cysts, cholangiography is indicated along with antibiotic prophylaxis. Duodenal endoscopy and retrograde cholangiopancreatography evaluate ampulla of Vater, provide bile and biopsy tissue for study, as well as demonstrate patency or obstruction of the biliary tree. The specimens obtained should be studied for malignancy, bacteria, virus, and parasites.

If the endoscopy and cholangiogram reveal papillary stenosis, dilated CBD, and sclerosed cholangioles in a patient at risk for or proven to be a carrier of human immunodeficiency virus (HIV), a superimposed CMV infection should be considered. The subchondral pain and tenderness may be relieved promptly by biliary tract decompression accomplished by transendoscopic sphincterotomy of the distal CBD. If the gallbladder is distended, cholecystectomy provides permanent relief from pain. Antibiotics specific for bacterial opportunistic infections should be combined with ganciclovir (DHPG) when biopsy reveals cytopathology consistent with CMV or the patient has extensive retinitis. Initial therapy of 2.5 mg per kilogram every 8 hours for 10 to 20 days, followed by prolonged suppressant doses of 5 mg per kilogram per day for 5 to 7 days per week indefinitely are essential in a patient with AIDS. Patients receiving DHPG require monitoring for bone marrow suppression.

Children with symptoms resembling chronic progressive hepatitis, yet equivocal findings in needle biopsy, and previous intestinal parasites should be studied for distal CBD obstruction. Ultrasonography may reveal liver enlargement without dilated bile ducts or gallstones. Endoscopy and ERCP, with periprocedural antibiotic prophylaxis, may confirm obstruction or stenosis of the distal CBD and demonstrate irregular narrowing of its lumen proximally due to chronic inflammation. Choledochojejunostomy is the surgical procedure of choice. These children are acutely and chronically ill and need intensive supportive and antimicrobial therapy pre- and postoperatively. Piperacillin, aminoglycoside, and metronidazole initiated prior to surgery provide a synergistic effect against the most likely bacterial and protozoan pathogens until specific microbes are identified. The prognosis is excellent if biliary tract obstruction is relieved permanently.

Patients with Caroli's disease usually present with acute bacterial cholangitis. Ten to 20 recurrences each year may follow the initial episode. Intensive antibiotic therapy for the infection should be initiated and ultrasound studies of the abdomen should be done. The finding of multiple cysts of varying size and the history are diagnostic of Caroli's disease. Neither antibiotics nor surgical therapy is curative. Antibiotic effect is impaired by polymicrobial infection, multiple intrahepatic biliary tract obstructions, and multiple noncommunicating cysts. Many of the cysts contain stones. Surgery is only palliative and can only drain the larger cysts by converting them to bilioenterostomies. Gallstones in cysts adjacent the liver surface may be removed by transhepatic lithotomy. Although optimal surgical drainage is impossible, suppressant antibiotic using orally administered preparations such as ciprofloxacin, ampicillin, and trimethoprim-sulfamethoxazole reduces the frequency and severity of recurrent cholangitis attacks. These antibiotics are selected empirically due to the multiple sites of infection having no communication with the biliary tree.

When the cystic pathology is localized rather than

diffuse, partial hepatectomy is the procedure of choice. Otherwise, total hepatectomy and liver homotransplantation are the only alternatives for cure.

Oriental Cholangiohepatitis

Definition

Oriental cholangiohepatitis is a form of recurrent pyogenic cholangitis that occurs in 20 to 40 year-old men and women in or from Hong Kong, Taiwan, and Southeast Asia. The etiology is not known. The initial pathology is obstruction by a fibrotic stricture of the intrahepatic bile duct near the junction of its right and left tributaries. This process may have been initiated earlier by infection or trauma. Dilatations of bile ducts, stasis, stones, and cysts are present above and below the stricture. The common bile duct is thickened, dilated, and filled with stones. The ampulla of Vater and the sphincter of Oddi are patulous. This may be the reason for preclinical asymptomatic bacteriocholia and the prodigious bacterial counts during illness.

The clinical presentation is similar to that of recurring, simple, obstructive cholangitis. During an acute attack jaundice usually develops, and severe general abdominal tenderness and guarding prevent localization of the site of infection. Ultrasonography usually demonstrates biliary tree dilatation, stones, and gallbladder distention, but CT provides clearer definition of the hepatic pathology. Gas may be demonstrated in the biliary tract by abdominal x-ray films, particularly if anaerobes or *Proteus* species are present. Percutaneous transhepatic cholangiography should be avoided or delayed until signs of infection have subsided.

Management

Medical and surgical protocols for therapy are as described for ascending pyogenic cholangitis. Complications are more frequent than in simple obstructive cholangitis and include liver abscess, subphrenic abscess, empyema, ruptured gallbladder, bile peritonitis, biliary enteric fistulae, and thrombophlebitis of the hepatic vein.

Surgery should be delayed until toxemia and fever have been controlled, unless the patient continues to deteriorate. The location for emergent biliary drainage (stricture above the bile duct) should be decided from results of ultrasound or CT studies, but surgery may be required to localize obstruction in some cases in spite of the danger of contaminated bile spilling into the peritoneal cavity. The surgical objective is to obtain effective and permanent uninhibited bile flow. Choledochojejunostomy is the most effective surgical procedure. Strictures in bile duct should be dilated, and stones and sludge should be removed. Cholecystectomy is done to prevent further stone formation and perforation of the gallbladder. Transhepatic lithotomy, cyst drainage, and hepaticojejunostomy proximal to the bile duct obstruction are corrections required. Surgical access to the biliary tree via a biliary-enteric bypass should be made to provide endoscopic stone removal, stricture dilatation, or stenting if obstruction reoccurs.

Pancreatitis

Pancreatitis associated with biliary tract infection is usually less severe but as common as that associated with alcohol. In many instances the inflammation is transient, resulting from partial obstruction of the duct of Wirsung during passing of a stone via the ampulla of Vater. Occasionally, it may be chronic, associated with persisting infection about the distal CBD, as in a child with duodenal parasites. In the latter, the biliary tract obstruction, rather than mild pancreatitis, provokes most of the symptoms. Diagnosis is dependent on serum amylase elevations and the ultrasound image. ERCP is preferred by some as the diagnostic procedure since transendoscopic sphincterotomy may relieve the obstruction in the ampulla of Vater and the pancreatic duct. Surgery is the treatment of choice if granuloma or tumor is compressing the pancreatic and common bile ducts.

Hematogenous pancreatitis occurs in disseminated infections that embolize the pancreas and create cellulitis or abscesses. Therapy requires intensive and specific antibiotic therapy. *Staphylococcus aureus, E. coli, Cryptococcus neoformans*, group A streptococci, *Klebsiella*, and *Candida* species require intensive parenteral therapy and appropriate incision and drainage of the primary sites of infection. The patients need monitoring of blood sugars during and after infection for early diagnosis of diabetes mellitus.

Surgical drainage of pancreatic pseudocysts resulting from acute chronic pancreatitis is complicated by peritonitis and intra-abdominal abscess due to released enzymes and secondary infection, usually hospital acquired. Nosocomial strains of *Pseudomonas, Serratia, Acinetobacter*, and *Klebsiella* resist commonly used antibiotics. Piperacillin or imipenem combined with aminoglycoside provides specific therapy. It is essential to recognize recurrent peritoneal abscesses clinically and by CT. Prompt and repeated drainage by needle or laparotomy and smear and culture of exudate are necessary to sustain effective antibiotic therapy. Suppressant therapy using ciprofloxacin orally, ceftriaxone, or other third-generation cephalosporins intramuscularly is continued for several weeks after fever abates to prevent recurrent localized intraperitoneal infections.

Liver Abscess

When acute or chronic febrile illness occurs following cholecystectomy, an extra- or intrahepatic abscess should be suspect, as well as cholangitis. Drainage is necessary if CT or liver-spleen scan confirms the presence of an abscess. An abscess if often accessible to needle aspiration under CT guidance. Percutaneous needle aspiration should be done under antibiotic coverage, such as piperacillin alone or combined with an aminoglycoside, since the bacteria causing the complication are most likely resistant to the previously employed antibiotics. The initial aspirate of the abscess provides excellent material for microbiologic study. Adequate drainage options are by CT-guided pigtail catheter emplacement or open surgery. Surgical drainage is preferred to needle aspiration when multiple macroabscesses are demonstrated within the liver. Ciprofloxacin, ampicillin, and chloramphenicol are effective orally as single antibiotics if the bacteria isolated are sensitive and adequate drainage is assured.

The liver is in jeopardy of infection from bacteremia in addition to that from pyogenic cholangitis or postcholecystectomy infection. Systemic infection with *S. aureus*, β-hemolytic streptococci, yeasts, or fungi may gain access by the hepatic artery and occasionally retrograde from hepatic vein thrombophlebitis. Intra-abdominal infections such as ruptured appendix, diverticulitis, or pericolic abscess may result in multiple abscesses from portal vein thrombophlebitis (pylephlebitis). Amebic liver abscess occurs in persons with asymptomatic colon infections with *Entamoeba histolytica*. Localized bacterial infections in the liver may follow accidents resulting in liver trauma and subsequent cryptogenic bacteremia. The diagnosis of liver abscess is suggested by acute or chronic febrile illness, anorexia, weight loss, and tender, enlarged liver. A chest roentgenogram revealing elevation of the anterior portion of the right diaphragm with or without infiltration in the lower lobe occasionally suggests the diagnosis. Abdominal ultrasonographic liver-spleen scan using technetium-sulfur colloid and gallium scan are diagnostic. CT is more prompt and precise in defining size and location of abscesses.

Management

Therapy of pyogenic abscess within or adjacent to the liver consists of determining etiology of systemic infection and administration of specific antibiotics against bacteria, protozoa, or fungi. Aggressive drainage, surgically or by percutaneous needle aspiration under CT guidance, is necessary to confirm etiology.

E. histolytica liver abscess is suspect in a patient with an illness several weeks in duration and consisting of low-grade fever, night sweats, anorexia, and weight loss. Physical findings include tender, enlarged liver, right anterior subcostal pain on deep breathing, and right-sided inspiratory lag. Leukocytosis with left shift, high level of serum alkaline phosphatase, and moderately increased AST are usually present. If liver-spleen scan and CT suggest a large intrahepatic abscess and CT-guided needle aspiration produces red-brown opaque material having no odor and no microorganisms by wet or stained preparations or culture, the syndrome is characteristic of an amebic abscess. A pig-tailed catheter with side holes should be inserted immediately and the abscess emptied. Further drainage is usually unnecessary. Metronidazole intravenously or orally should be given perioperatively while results of bacterial smear and culture and serologic test results against antigens of *E. histolytica* are awaited. In contrast, if the aspirate is malodorous, has an "anchovy sauce" appearance, and contains coccal and rod-shaped bacteria, the primary etiology may be *E. histolytica* associated with enteric anaerobes. Metronidazole should be given, but in combination with piperacillin, ampicillin, chloramphenicol, or clindamycin. Piperacillin or chloramphenicol with metronidazole is our preferred regimen. *E. histolytica* abscess may be treated also with chloroquine, 1 g orally daily for 2 days then 500 mg for 20 days. Emetine, up to 60 mg per day intramuscularly for 14 days, is effective but is cardiotoxic and the patient should be at bed rest. It is used only if chloroquine is not tolerated. Initial aspiration of nonputrid abscess and continued metronidazole therapy is followed by rapid convalescence. Neither surgical nor indwelling tube drainage is necessary. Metronidazole, 2 g per day orally, is continued for 3 weeks. When anaerobes are present, tube drainage and antibiotics should be continued until odor and bacteria disappear. Metronidazole should be continued for 3 weeks or longer. The patient is followed until the abscess has resolved by CT, usually for 3 to 4 months.

Patients who are immunocompromised may have multiple abscesses, too small and numerous to drain mechanically. These are the result of disseminated disease due to candidiasis, yeast phase of other fungi, *Mycobacteria tuberculosis*, or atypical mycobacteria. Disseminated mycoses and tuberculosis causing miliary granulomata may occur as primary disease in persons without evidence of deficient cellular or humoral immunity. However, miliary abscesses rather than granulomas constitute the pathology in most persons with AIDS. Remittant fever, leukopenia, or rarely leukocytosis, and abnormal levels of liver transaminases are indications for liver biopsy, cytopathology, and staining and culture for fungi, acid-fast bacilli, and other bacteria. The results of liver biopsy studies provide specific diagnoses much earlier than do findings from studies of bronchial washings, spinal fluid, and urine or lung roentgenograms of miliary densities or infiltrates.

Yeast and fungal dissemination demand intensive intravenous therapy using amphotericin B in single daily infusions given over 2 to 3 hours. The dosage is based on the minimal inhibitory concentration as determined in vitro. Daily infusions are necessary until fever abates. Thereafter, alternative-day therapy at no longer than 36- to 40-hour intervals are continued for 6 to 12 weeks, depending on the clinical response. *Candida* species are usually most sensitive (less than 0.8 μg per milliliter) and respond to 20 mg in 250 ml of 5 percent dextrose in water intravenously per day within 3 weeks. Histoplasmosis, blastomycosis, cryptococcosis, and sporotrichosis require 30 to 35 mg in 500 mg dextrose in water 5 percent per day, but 2 to 3 months' therapy is necessary. Coccidioidomycosis and mucormycosis require 50 to 75 mg per day, as tolerated. Most patients tolerate amphotericin B best if the therapeutic dose is attained slowly over 3 to 5 days. Those with severe acute and progressive illness, having received an initial 1-mg dose without hypotension, must receive increased dosage at 6- to 12-hour intervals until the therapeutic dose is attained. When fever, hypotension, and nausea follow a given increment in dose, the drug should be repeated within 6 hours with premedication, using first 25 to 50 mg up to 100 mg hydrocortisone by intravenous bolus. This reduces adverse effects and usually permits progression of amphotericin B to the desired daily dosage. Meperidine, antihistamines, or hydrocortisone should not be mixed with the amphotericin B but given as premedication. (See also *Antifungal Chemotherapy*.)

Combined isoniazid (INH) 300 mg per day, rifampin 600 mg per day orally, and streptomycin 500 mg twice daily intramuscularly are effective against most isolates of *M. tuberculosis* and *M. kansasii*. However atypical mycobacteria, particularly the *M. avium* complex (MAC), resist the first- and most second-line antituberculosis agents. It is impossible to differentiate the resistant atypical strains from sensitive *M. tuberculosis* by morphology alone. For this reason acutely ill persons with acid-fast organisms in liver biopsy should receive INH and rifampin orally plus amikacin intravenously or, if resistance to these drugs is suspected, with ansamycin and INH plus ciprofloxacin until identification has been accomplished. (See discussions of disseminated mycobacterial infections elsewhere in this volume.)

Acute or subacute hepatitis or hepatocellular infection occurs with systemic viral infections in children and adults. Often anorexia, nausea, abdominal pain, and jaundice occur for several days as part of an acute febrile illness with or without an exanthem. Enlarged cervical nodes and hepatosplenomegaly are associated with increased liver enzymes and bilirubin in the liver. Diagnosis is made clinically for the most part, since identifying a virus as the etiologic agent is expensive and is usually not essential. Currently available are acyclovir, gancyclovir, and ribavirin, which are specific against herpesvirus types 1 and 2, cytomegalovirus, and respiratory syncytial virus, respectively (see chapter on viral diseases). The availability of antiviral agents provides a greater incentive to identify the etiologic virus by serologic and/or isolation procedures or the presence of gene protein fragments in tissue. At present only supportive measures are indicated for patients with hepatitis as part of a viral syndrome. However if herpesvirus is identified and disease is progressive, acyclovir intravenously should be initiated (see also *Antiviral Chemotherapy*).

Acknowledgment. The authors wish to thank Walker A. Long, M.D., for editing and Ms. Carolyn T. Sellars for word processing the manuscript.

SUGGESTED READING

Kevin H, Jones RB, Chowdhury L, Kabins S. Acalculous cholecystitis and cytomegalovirus infection in acquired immunodeficiency syndrome. Ann Intern Med 1986; 104:53–54.

Sackmann M, Delius M, Sauerbruch T, et al. Shock-wave lithotripsy of gallbladder stones. N Engl J Med 1988; 318:393–397.

Schiff L, Schiff ER, eds. Diseases of the liver. 6th ed. Particularly sections 42 (Warren K, Williams CI, Tan E); 11 (Zimmon DS); 12 (Pereiras R); and 1 (Rappaport AM). Philadelphia: JB Lippincott, 1987.

Schneiderman D, Cello JP, Laing FC. Papillary stenosis and sclerosing cholangitis in acquired immunodeficiency syndrome. Ann Intern Med 1987; 106:546–549.

Spies JB, Rosen RJ, Lebowitz AS. Antibiotic prophylaxis in vascular and interventional radiology: a rational approach. Radiology 1988; 166:381–387.

Stewart L, Smith AL, Pellegrini C, Matson RW, Way LW. Pigment gallstones form as a composite of bacterial microcolonies and pigment solids. Ann Surg 1987; 206:242–249.

Winkler AP, Gleich S. Acute acalculous cholecystitis caused by *Salmonella typhi* in an 11-year old. Pediatr Infect Dis 1988; 7:125–128.

Young LS, Berlin CG, Inderlied CB. Activity of ciprofloxacin and other fluorinated quinolones against mycobacteria. Am J Med 1987; 82: (Suppl 4A):23.

Young LS, Inderlied CB, Berlin CG, Gottlieb MS. Mycobacterial infections in AIDS patients with an emphasis on the *Mycobacterium avium* complex. Rev Infect Dis 1986; 8:1024.

BACTERIAL MENINGITIS

THOMAS R. BEAM Jr., M.D.

Bacterial meningitis in adults is a disease that remains incompletely described. There is no formal reporting system of meningitis as a disease process other than that caused by meningococci. Thus, the incidence among adults is unknown. Large series of cases have been published, but the etiology often reflects the type of patients seen at a particular medical center and not necessarily the population at large. Meningitis is a reportable disease in New York City, but it is not clear whether the high numbers of cases caused by gram-negative bacilli and *Listeria monocytogenes* reflect the true nature of adult meningitis in other areas of the United States.

The treatment of meningitis in adults is also poorly studied. Rates of meningitis are too low for any single medical center to conduct a controlled clinical trial. Collaborative studies comparing various therapies have never been performed. As a result, data obtained from clinical trials conducted among neonates or children, or from epidemics of disease, are usually extrapolated to adults with sporadic disease. This approach may or may not be able to accurately define optimal chemotherapy.

Given these facts, the clinician should remain wary of bacterial meningitis in adults. Because the disease is almost always fatal when untreated, its presence should always be suspected and a diagnostic spinal tap performed even though many yield negative results. If the clinical circumstances are consistent with a diagnosis of bacterial meningitis, spinal tap should be performed promptly and antimicrobial therapy instituted as soon as possible following the spinal tap. If there is an epidemic of meningitis in the community, the first dose of antibiotic may be given prior to obtaining cerebrospinal fluid for analysis, if any delay in performing the spinal tap is anticipated.

Adults residing in a household that contains a case of meningitis caused by *Neisseria meningitidis* or *Haemophilus influenzae* are at increased risk for acquiring meningitis. Both pathogens spread to vulnerable household contacts with equal efficiency. Rifampin prophylaxis, 600 mg by mouth twice a day for 2 days, should be prescribed. Obtaining nasopharyngeal cultures and/or waiting until culture results become available are inappropriate in this setting. Should the adult develop signs or symptoms of meningitis, treatment with penicillin (meningococci), ampicillin (susceptible *H. influenzae*), or a third-generation cephalosporin such as ceftriaxone (isolate unknown or *H. influenzae*, susceptibility unknown) should be instituted.

Community-acquired adult meningitis is most often identified with a contiguous site of infection or concurrent infection, particularly pneumonia, which seeds the meninges by bacteremic spread. The most common organism isolated from such patients is *Streptococcus pneumoniae*. Penicillin G remains the drug of choice. However, all pneumococci should be tested for penicillin susceptibility, because a small minority of strains will be relatively resistant to penicillin G (minimal inhibitory concentration 0.2 μg per milliliter or more). Susceptibility screening is best done using an oxacillin disc. Chloramphenicol or third-generation cephalosporins may be used as alternative agents if resistance is known to be a problem within the local community, if the patient fails to respond to therapy, or if resistance is documented.

EPIDEMIOLOGIC CONSIDERATIONS AS A GUIDE TO THERAPY

Therapy for adult meningitis should be guided by epidemiologic considerations until a pathogen has been defined (Table 1). Sporadic disease among young adults is distinctly uncommon and most often caused by meningococci. The incidence is 0.6 cases per 100,000 population per year. Type B disease is usually responsible. Armed forces personnel are provided with vaccine against meningococci including types A, C, W135, and Y. These individuals remain vulnerable to type B disease in either sporadic or epidemic form. Pneumococci also occasionally cause meningitis in young adults. Therefore, the drug of choice for treatment is penicillin G.

Recent evidence suggests that the elderly are also susceptible to meningitis. Rough estimates of incidence suggest that the rate may be similar to that seen in young children.

Although pneumococci are the most common cause of meningitis among community-residing elderly individuals, *Escherichia coli*, *Klebsiella pneumoniae*, and *Listeria monocytogenes* are common enough to warrant coverage when empiric therapy is being prescribed. A combination of ampicillin and a third-generation cephalosporin (ceftriaxone, cefotaxime, or ceftizoxime) is preferred.

Certain adults with cutaneous infections caused by *Staphylococcus aureus* may become bacteremic and develop meningitis, particularly if the infection has been present for an extended period. A likely circumstance is the parenteral drug abuser who develops endocarditis and secondarily contaminates the central nervous system by bacteremic spread. Nafcillin is the drug of choice, unless methicillin-resistant staphylococci have been identified or are known to exist in the community at large. Vancomycin should be employed in these latter circumstances.

TABLE 1 Likely Pathogens Responsible for Bacterial Meningitis in Adults

Clinical Parameters	*Pathogens*
No predisposing cause, sporadic	
Young adults	*N. meningitidis, S. pneumoniae*
Elderly (age ≥60 years)	*S. pneumoniae*, Enterobacteriaceae, *L. monocytogenes*
No predisposing cause, epidemic	*N. meningitidis*
Index case in household	*N. meningitidis, H. influenzae*
Predisposing factors:	
Contiguous or comcomitant infection	
Sinusitis, otitis, pneumonia	*S. pneumoniae*
Cutaneous infections	*S. aureus*
Endocarditis	*S. aureus*
Trauma	
Neurosurgery	
Without shunt	Enterobacteriaceae, *S. aureus*
With shunt or intracranial pressure monitor	Staphylococci, Enterobacteriaceae
Frontal fracture with CSF leak	*S. pneumoniae*
CSF leak plus antibiotics	Enterobacteriaceae, *S. aureus*
Skull fracture	*S. aureus*, Enterobacteriaceae
Immune compromise	
Splenic dysfunction, splenectomy	*S. pneumoniae, N. meningitidis*
Alcoholism	*S. pneumoniae, L. monocytogenes*
Hypogammaglobulinemia	*S. pneumoniae*
Immunosuppressive medications	*L. monocytogenes*, Enterobacteriaceae, *S. pneumoniae*
Complement deficiency (late components)	*N. meningitidis*

Adults with trauma to the head should be divided into several different groups. The first is trauma from neurosurgery, which then should be subdivided into procedures involving placement of a shunt or other device versus procedures with no placement of a foreign body. The foreign body strongly enhances the pathogenicity of coagulase-negative staphylococci. *S. aureus* and Enterobacteriaceae also warrant consideration. Vancomycin plus a third-generation cephalosporin, or trimethoprim-sulfamethoxazole as single-agent therapy, should be considered until Gram stain and/or culture information results are available (drugs are listed in order of preference).

Head trauma resulting in a leak of cerebrospinal fluid (CSF) predisposes the individual to pneumococcal meningitis. If the leak persists, recurrent episodes may ensue. If the patient is placed on prophylactic antibiotics to avoid meningitis, which is not advocated, Enterobacteriaceae and *S. aureus* become common pathogens. Treatment should be the same as that advocated for neurosurgical shunt complications.

If there is a skull fracture without rhinorrhea, antibiotic treatment should also be directed against these same pathogens.

The final group of adults vulnerable to bacterial meningitis have various forms of immunologic compromise. Each host-defense–, disease-, or medication-induced defect increases risk of infection caused by certain bacterial pathogens (see Table 1). Presumptive therapy should be directed toward those organisms most likely to be responsible.

DIAGNOSTIC CONSIDERATIONS AS A GUIDE TO THERAPY

In the majority of cases of bacterial meningitis among adults, therapy can be guided by rapidly available diagnostic test results. Following the considerations given to the patient's epidemiologic circumstances, certain clinical features of meningitis should be sought (Fig. 1). Fever, headache, photophobia, nausea and vomiting, and altered level of consciousness are the most important findings. If focal neurologic deficits are elicited on physical examination, a mass lesion must be ruled out before lumbar puncture is performed. In the absence of focal neurologic signs,

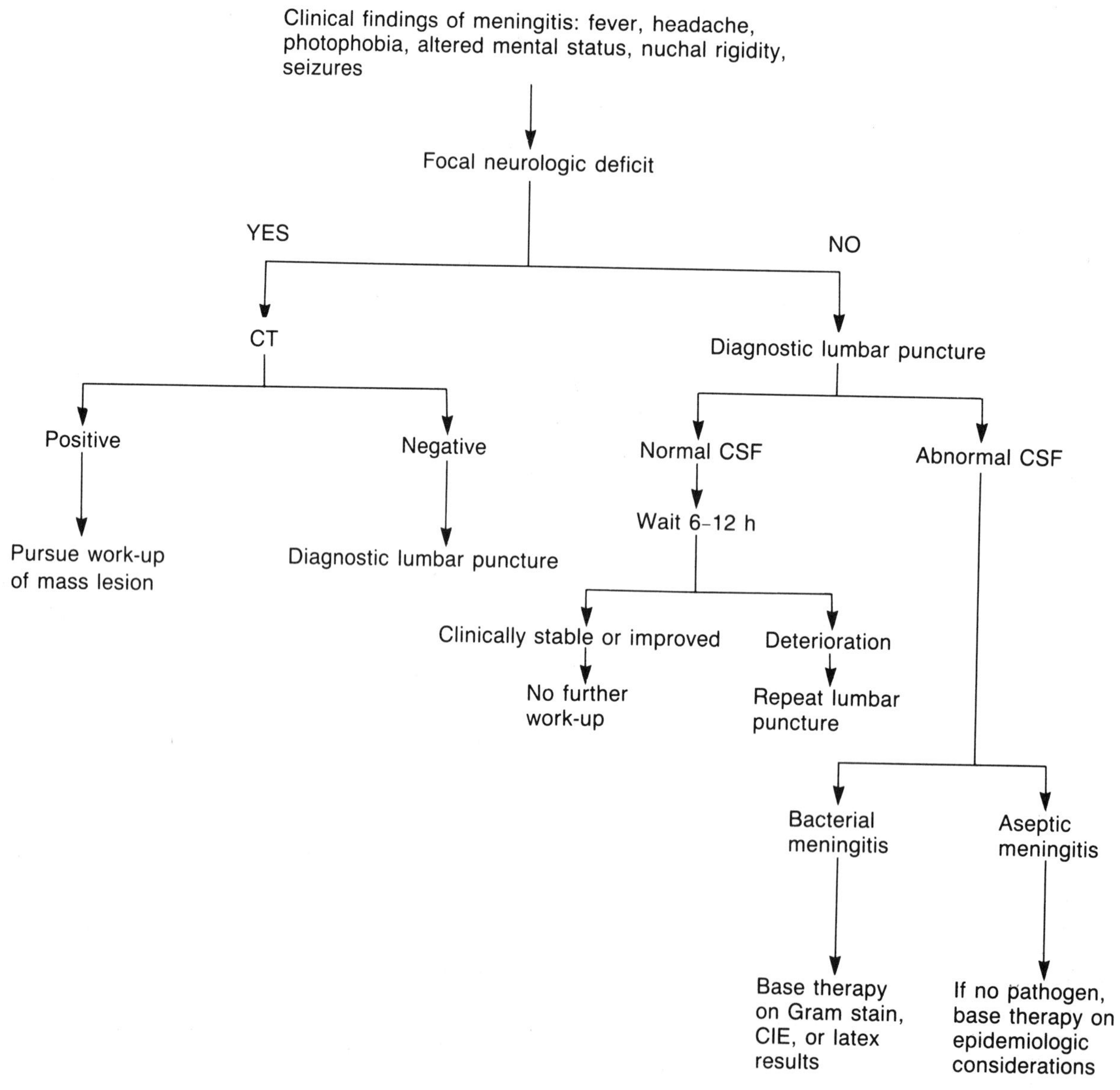

Figure 1 Diagnosing bacterial meningitis in adults.

a diagnostic spinal tap should be done immediately. If lumbar puncture is done without delay, one should await results before starting therapy. If lumbar puncture is delayed because of need for CT scan, time is a critical variable. A 1-hour delay is tolerable; a 6-hour delay is not. In the latter circumstance one dose of ampicillin plus ceftriaxone should be given. Gram stain, culture, glucose and protein levels, and white blood cell and differential counts should be requested. Counterimmunoelectrophoresis (CIE) or latex agglutination studies should be ordered and are particularly useful for diagnosis of bacterial meningitis when the patient has received prior antimicrobial therapy. *S. pneumoniae*, *N. meningitidis*, *H. influenzae*, and *E. coli* can be detected by these techniques. Group B streptococci, pathogens of importance for neonates, rarely cause adult meningitis but can also be detected. Assays take 30 to 45 minutes to perform and report to the clinician. Thus if available, they can be used to confirm or supplement Gram stain information.

If the Gram stain, CIE, and latex agglutination studies do not identify a presumptive pathogen but there is a CSF leukocytosis with polymorphonuclear predominance, hypoglycorrhachia, and elevated protein, empiric therapy should be started based on epidemiologic considerations, as previously described.

ANTIMICROBIAL THERAPY OF BACTERIAL MENINGITIS

As previously noted, therapy should be instituted as rapidly as possible once diagnostic material has been obtained. In addition to CSF, culture of blood, sputum (if available), and urine; complete blood count and differential; and urine for CIE are essential. A summary of recommendations is provided in Table 2.

The choice of antibiotic is based on several factors. It should be bactericidal. It should effectively penetrate into the central nervous system, achieving concentrations that are severalfold in excess of the minimum bactericidal concentration (MBC). Rarely, the nature of the infecting organism and the lack of penetrability of the chemotherapeutic agent may require a route other than parenteral to be chosen. Because of CSF flow dynamics, the optimal site for drug delivery is the cerebral ventricle. Neurosurgical consultation should be called to place a device such as an Ommaya reservoir if interference is anticipated with exchange of CSF from the choroid plexus to other areas.

The issue of bactericidal antibiotics requires clarification. Chloramphenicol is bactericidal for *S. pneumoniae*, *N. meningitidis*, and *H. influenzae* in concentrations achieved in the central nervous system during parenteral therapy. It is bacteriostatic for organisms such as *E. coli* and thus should not be used for meningitis caused by Enterobacteriaceae even when these organisms are reported to be susceptible by in vitro testing.

Combining bactericidal antibiotics can be advantageous. Ampicillin plus chloramphenicol are prescribed because of the potential resistance of *H. influenzae* to either agent alone. One or the other may be discontinued upon determination of the organism's susceptibility pattern. However, combination of a bactericidal and bacteriostatic agent, such as penicillin plus tetracycline, can result in a substantially worse outcome than prescription of penicillin alone for treatment of meningitis caused by *S. pneumoniae*.

The development of third-generation cephalosporins has

TABLE 2 Antibiotic Therapy for Adult Meningitis

Organism	*Preferred Antibiotic*	*Total Daily Dose*	*Dosing Interval*	*Alternative*	*Total Daily Dose*	*Dosing Interval*
S. pneumoniae	Aqueous penicillin G*	24 × 10⁶ U	2 h	Chloramphenicol	4 g	6 h
S. pneumoniae, penicillin-resistant	Chloramphenicol	4 g	6 h	Vancomycin* Cefotaxime	30 mg/kg 12 g	12 h 4–6 h
S. aureus	Nafcillin	12 g	4–6 h	Vancomycin*	30 mg/kg	12 h
S. aureus, methicillin-resistant	Vancomycin*	30 mg/kg	12 h	Trimethoprim-sulfamethoxazole*	12 amps	6 h
N. meningitidis	Aqueous penicillin G*	24 × 10⁶ U	2 h	Chloramphenicol Ceftriaxone Cefotaxime	4 g 4 g 12 g	6 h 12 h 4–6 h
Enterobacteriaceae	Ceftriaxone Cefotaxime	4 g 12 g	12 h 4–6 h	Trimethoprim-sulfamethoxazole*	12 amps	6 h
H. influenzae	Ceftriaxone Cefotaxime	4 g 12 g	12 h 6 h	Ampicillin* ± chloramphenicol	12 g 4 g	4 h 6 h
H. influenzae, ampicillin-resistant	Ceftriaxone Cefotaxime	4 g 12 g	12 h 6 h	Chloramphenicol	4 g	6 h
L. monocytogenes	Ampicillin*	12 g	4 h	Trimethoprim-sulfamethoxazole*	12 amps	6 h
P. aeruginosa	Piperacillin* + tobramycin*	18 g 5.1 mg/kg	4 h 8 h	Ceftazidime* + tobramycin*	6 g 5.1 mg/kg	8 h 8 h

* Requires dose adjustment for elderly or persons with renal dysfunction.

addressed the problem of inadequate therapeutic options available to treat meningitis caused by Enterobacteriaceae. Uncontrolled collections of cases have suggested that morbidity and mortality have been significantly reduced. However, prospective, randomized comparative trials conducted in neonates and children have failed to demonstrate appreciable benefit. This observation was made despite truly remarkable bactericidal activity achieved in CSF.

Although lumbar, cisternal, and direct intraventricular injections of antibiotics have not usually proved helpful (and in certain circumstances they are harmful), there remains a need for local instillation of antibiotics. An organism such as *Pseudomonas aeruginosa* is best treated with a combination of a β-lactam agent (piperacillin or ceftazidime) plus an aminoglycoside (gentamicin, tobramycin, or amikacin) (drugs are listed in order of preference). The β-lactam agent may be delivered parenterally, but the aminoglycoside is rendered more effective by local injection. Preservative-free gentamicin, tobramycin, or amikacin should be delivered through a device such as an Ommaya reservoir. Most experience and FDA approval exist for gentamycin only. The key consideration is to use a preservative-free preparation for local injection. There are, however, no data to recommend one agent in preference to others based on in vitro susceptibility results and correlation to outcome. Gentamicin is administered intrathecally in a dose of 4 mg once per day. A simple alternative to the Ommaya reservoir is to mix gentamicin with CSF in the syringe through which it is administered (barbotage). It should be continued until cultures of CSF are sterile.

Adverse reactions to therapeutic agents employed for treatment of bacterial meningitis are generally those characteristic of the class of drugs to which the specific antibiotic belongs. However, because these agents are used at maximal daily dosing, care must be taken to adjust standard regimens in the presence of impaired renal clearance. The most common problem is β-lactam toxicity attributable to reduced renal function in an elderly patient whose serum creatinine is "normal." The adverse effects that result from accumulation of the drugs include diminished level of consciousness, confusion, and seizure disorder. These drug-related phenomena must be distinguished from the natural history of the disease or failure to respond to therapy.

Although a repeat lumbar puncture is routinely obtained for neonates, infants, and children with bacterial meningitis, this is infrequently done for adults. The only justification is verification that the chosen antibiotic(s) have sterilized the CSF. In neurosurgical cases with direct ventricular access, this evaluation can be performed. Otherwise, it is only required when the patient clinically deteriorates while receiving allegedly effective therapy. Lumbar puncture at the end of treatment yields no useful information for predicting relapse and therefore is unwarranted.

The complications of meningitis are primarily neurologic and include cranial nerve palsies, impaired mental capacity, hearing loss, and a variety of other sequelae. No study has been done to assess the impact of effective antimicrobial therapy on neurologic residua. It is assumed that prompt diagnosis and rapid institution of appropriate therapy play a favorable role in outcome. This appears to be true for postneurosurgical gram-negative bacillary meningitis when contrasted with community-acquired disease caused by the same organisms.

The duration of therapy for effective treatment of bacterial meningitis in adults has not been critically appraised. Thus, arbitrary limits have been established and are both patient- and organism-specific. Defervescence, disappearance of abnormalities in mental status, relief of symptoms such as headache, and normalization of white blood cell count are required. Several additional days of antibiotics are generally prescribed before therapy is stopped. There is no advantage to continued hospitalization to monitor for relapse once antibiotic therapy is complete. In general, adult meningitis is treated for 14 to 21 days.

FUTURE DIRECTIONS: ADJUNCTS TO ANTIBIOTIC THERAPY

Because the development of new antibiotics has not significantly improved morbidity and mortality associated with bacterial meningitis, the role of adjunctive therapy is being explored. It was first noted at the turn of the century that immunoglobulins could treat meningococcal disease. This was verified in the 1930s for *H. influenzae* meningitis. The development of potentially effective antibiotics caused a loss of interest in passive immunotherapy. Interest has regenerated with the development of safer immunoglobulin preparations and the lack of an antibiotic panacea. Under consideration are nonspecific and highly specific (monoclonal) immunoglobulin preparations instilled into cerebrospinal fluid or administered intravenously.

A second area of exploration is reduction of the inflammatory reaction within the central nervous system. Certain neurologic sequelae may be attributed to increased intracranial pressure from impaired CSF flow dynamics due to leukocytes. Also, it has been proposed that leukocyte products may be toxic to nerve cells. Using corticosteroids or nonsteroidal anti-inflammatory agents, it may be possible to reduce the incidence of neurologic sequelae. Since effective antibiotics are available, and since leukocyte function in the central nervous system is impaired by lack of immunoglobulins and complement, an overall reduction in inflammation may be beneficial.

There is insufficient clinical evidence available to consider immunoglobulin therapy, corticosteroid therapy, or nonsteroidal anti-inflammatory drug therapy at this time. Antibiotics may have shortcomings but remain the treatment of choice.

SUGGESTED READING

Beam TR. Cephalosporins in adult meningitis. Bull NY Acad Med 1984; 60:380–393.

McGee ZA, Kaiser AB. Acute meningitis. In: Mandell GL, Douglas RG Jr, Bennett JE, eds. Principles and practice of infectious diseases. 2nd ed. New York: John Wiley and Sons, 1985:560.
Sande MA, Smith AL, Root RK, eds. Bacterial meningitis. Contemporary issues in infectious diseases. Vol 3. New York: Churchill Livingstone, 1985.
Tauber MG, Sande MA. Principles in the treatment of bacterial meningitis. Am J Med 1984; 76(5A):224–230.

ASEPTIC MENINGITIS SYNDROME

P. JOAN CHESNEY, M.D., C.M.

The aseptic meningitis syndrome (AMS) was first defined by Wallgren in 1925. It is a syndrome of multiple etiologies, all of which produce symptoms and signs of meningeal inflammation with no evidence of a pyogenic organism by Gram stain or routine culture of cerebrospinal fluid (CSF). Other characteristics of AMS include an acute or subacute onset, the absence of severe cerebral manifestations, and a self-limited and usually benign outcome, depending on the etiology and the presence of a nonpurulent CSF (Table 1). Although exceptions clearly occur, as a general rule the CSF has a total white blood cell (WBC) count of less than 500 cells per cubic millimeter, a total protein (TP) concentration of less than 100 mg per deciliter, and a glucose concentration that is normal or rarely less than 20 mg per deciliter. The CSF WBC differential depends on the etiology. Although polymorphonuclear cells (PMNs) may predominate in the first 24 hours of a viral infection, Feigin et al found a shift to a lymphocytic predominance in 87 percent of patients within 8 to 12 hours of the first lumbar puncture (LP). Such a rapid shift in cellular morphology does not occur with bacterial meningitis.

The important challenge of AMS is that of identifying, as early as possible, the potentially treatable causes of the syndrome, including unusual presentations of bacterial infections of the central nervous system. Therapeutic strategies, such as the potential use of acyclovir and azidothymidine for the management of some of the viral causes of AMS; the continued availability of amphotericin B, 5-fluorocytosine, and the new imidazoles for fungal causes; antituberculous therapy for acid-fast organisms; and aggressive surgery and therapy for neural neoplasms and parameningeal foci, have created an urgency for establishing a rapid and accurate diagnosis.

In general the term AMS is used to apply to syndromes in which the sole or predominant component is due to meningeal irritation, with other nonneurologic clinical features being less prominent or nonspecific. Thus, once the clinical and diagnostic evaluation establishes the presence of a specific entity such as Kawasaki disease or Rocky Mountain spotted fever, despite the presence of meningeal findings, these entities would no longer be called AMS.

The labels of meningoencephalitis and viral meningitis should be avoided when patients with AMS are initially evaluated. As opposed to the clinical findings of AMS, encephalitis connotes an acute, severe, persistent disturbance of cerebral function. Likewise, early use of the diagnosis of viral meningitis implies a known etiology, which may preclude continued evaluation for the many other, often treatable, causes of this syndrome (Table 2).

Although careful evaluation of body fluids, including the CSF, will provide the answer on occasion (Table 3), most often the diagnosis used to initiate therapy of AMS will be based on the history, a careful review of possible epidemiologic factors, and physical examination.

ETIOLOGY AND EPIDEMIOLOGY

In prospective studies of AMS in which vigorous attempts were made to identify the etiology, a virus was identified in 70 percent of cases. Of those, the enteroviruses accounted for 85 percent of cases, with coxsackievirus B_5 and the echoviruses 4, 6, 9, and 11 as the most common enteroviruses. Arboviruses account for about 5 percent of AMS cases in North America, St Louis encephalitis virus and the California encephalitis virus being the most common. Although mumps used to be a common cause, it has become rare since the advent of the vaccine.

Since 1980, the human immunodeficiency virus (HIV) has become an important cause of virus-associated neuro-

TABLE 1 Clinical and Laboratory Definition of the Aseptic Meningitis Syndrome

Symptoms and signs
Fever and chills
Headache
Vomiting
Nuchal rigidity
Malaise
Fatigue/anorexia
Absence of severe cerebral disturbance
Absence of readily diagnosed systemic syndrome
CSF evaluation
WBC $\leq$500 cells/mm^3 (rarely may be several thousand/mm^3)
WBC differential: either neutrophilic or lymphocytic predominance
Total protein concentration $\leq$100 mg/dl
Glucose concentration $\geq$20 mg/dl and usually normal
Negative Gram stain
Negative routine bacterial cultures

TABLE 2 Differential Diagnosis of the Infectious Etiologies of the Aseptic Meningitis Syndrome

INFECTIOUS ETIOLOGIES

- Viruses
  - Enteroviruses (echo, coxsackie, polio, and others)
  - Human immunodeficiency virus
  - Lymphocytic choriomeningitis virus
  - Varicella-zoster virus
  - Epstein-Barr virus
  - Arboviruses (eastern, western and Venezuelan equine; St. Louis, Powassan, California, and Colorado tick fever in the United States; others in other areas of the world)
  - Mumps virus
  - Herpes simplex type 2 virus
  - Adenovirus
  - Others (encephalomyocarditis virus; cytomegalovirus; measles virus; rubella virus; rhinovirus; coronavirus; parainfluenza virus; influenza A and B virus; rotavirus; variola virus)
- Bacteria
  - Partially treated purulent meningitis
  - Spirochetes
    - *Treponema pallidum* (syphilis)
    - *Borrelia recurrentis* (relapsing fever)
    - *Borrelia burgdorferi* (lyme disease)
    - *Spirillum minor* (rat bite fever)
    - *Leptospira species* (leptospirosis)
  - *Mycobacterium tuberculosis* (tuberculosis)
  - *Nocardia* species (nocardiosis)
  - Suppurative parameningeal focus
    - Brain abscess
    - Sinusitis, mastoiditis, middle ear infection
    - Epidural abscess of cranium or spine
    - Endocarditis or lung abscess with meningeal embolization
    - Cranial osteomyelitis: subdural empyema or suppurative intracranial phlebitis
- Mycoplasmas
  - *Mycoplasma pneumoniae*
  - *Mycoplasma hominis*
- Rickettsia
  - *Rickettsia rickettsii* (Rocky Mountain spotted fever)
  - *Rickettsia prowazeki* (typhus)
- Fungi
  - *Blastomyces dermatitidis* (blastomycosis)
  - *Coccidioides immitis* (coccidioidomycosis
  - *Cryptococcus neoformans* (cryptococcosis)
  - *Histoplasma capsulatum* (histoplasmosis)
  - *Candida* species
  - Other (aspergillosis; mucormycosis)
- Protozoa
  - Amebas
    - *Naegleria fowleri* (primary acute amebic meningoencephalitis)
    - *Entamoeba histolytica* (cerebral amebiasis, secondary)
    - *Acanthamoeba* species (primary subacute or chronic amebic meningoencephalitis)
  - *Trypanosoma* species (sleeping sickness)
  - *Plasmodium* species (malaria)
  - *Toxoplasma gondii* (toxoplasmosis)
- Nematodes
  - *Strongyloides stercoralis* (strongyloidiasis)
  - *Trichinella spiralis* (trichinosis)
  - *Angiostrongylis cantonensis* (eosinophilic meningitis)

NONINFECTIOUS ETIOLOGIES

- Heavy-metal poisoning (lead, arsenic)
- Postvaccination: measles, vaccinia, polio, rabies
- Malignancy: leukemia, meningeal or parameningeal neoplasm
- Unknown etiology:
  - Behçet syndrome; lupus erythematosus; serum sickness; sarcoidosis; Kawasaki syndrome; Mollaret's recurrent meningitis; cat scratch disease; Vogt-Koyanagi-Hanada syndrome
- Miscellaneous:
  - Foreign bodies in the CNS: intrathecal injections (procaine, soaps, or disinfectants)
  - Drug associated (especially nonsteroidal anti-inflammatory drugs): dermoid/epidermoid cysts adjacent to subarachnoid space

logic syndromes. HIV-linked AMS is most often associated with the initial mononucleosis-like acute infection. Clarification of potential host risk factors and of the patient's acute and convalescent enzyme-linked immunosorbent assay (ELISA) and western blot tests and HIV P_{24} antigen status should establish the diagnosis. Ongoing studies will determine whether antiviral therapy of this self-limited stage of the illness will modify the subsequent course.

Epidemiologic factors are important in establishing a tentative etiology for AMS. During the months of July to October, the presence of unexplained fever, rashes, pleurodynia, or pharyngitis in the community suggests the existence of an enteroviral outbreak.

For other agents (see Table 2) the history should include attention to recent travel, recreation, and residence at the time of onset, e.g., southwestern United States (cryptococcosis), southeastern United States (histoplasmosis), or Lacrosse, Wisconsin (California encephalitis virus). Environmental exposures, such as exposure in the woods to animals, insects, or mosquitoes (Lyme disease, relapsing fever, or rickettsial disease); to a beaver pond (blastomycosis); or to a freshwater pond or swimming pool (*Naegleria fowleri*) should be determined. Personal life style should be determined, particularly with respect to drug abuse and sexual activity (syphilis, HIV). Illness in other family members or pets may provide important diagnostic information. Underlying illnesses in the patient, such as those suggesting a recent or current sinusitis or middle ear infection or illness requiring a blood transfusion, dental work, antibiotics, or immunosuppressive agents or placement of intravascular or intracranial foreign bodies, should be determined. Other manifestations of the acute illness, such as a characteristic rash, pharyngitis, cough, adenopathy, conjunctival injection, jaundice, oral or genital ulcers or discharge, or previous episodes of meningeal inflammation, are also important in establishing an etiology.

TABLE 3 Additional Diagnostic Tests That May Assist in Establishing the Diagnosis of Aseptic Meningitis Syndrome

CSF	
Antigen detection*:	for pyogenic bacteria, *Cryptococcus neoformans* and HIV P_{24}
Wet mount or hanging drop†:	amebas
Cytology*:	may demonstrate smudge cells of Mollaret's or malignant cells
Acid-fast stain of sediment* (10 ml CSF):	positive in >80% of cases of tuberculous meningitis
India ink*:	cryptococci and amebas
Limulus lysate‡:	positive result indicates presence of endotoxin
Chloride‡:	<110 mEq/L suggests TB if pyogenic meningitis ruled out
Cultures*	
Bacterial:	*Listeria* may take several days to grow, mycobacteria take several weeks, leptospires grow on special media
Viral:	positive in 70–80% of enteroviral AMS; growth of other viruses from CSF rare
Fungal:	need to culture large volumes of CSF as organisms present at low concentrations and generally take >10 days to grow
Nonspecific tests: lactic acid, C-reactive protein‡:	tend to be higher in bacterial meningitis
CSF antibody†:	Antibody to viruses and *Treponema pallidum* may appear earlier and eventually in higher titer in CSF than in serum
Darkfield examination†:	spirochetes may be seen
Blood	
Antigen detection†:	HIV P_{24}
Acute/convalescent sera*:	obtained ≥3 weeks apart may establish diagnosis in retrospect: ELISA and western blot may be positive with acute HIV infection: viral specific IgM present in 83% of sera by day 3 for Lacrosse strain California encephalitis virus
Culture* (bacterial fungal):	may yield agent when CSF cultures negative
Heavy-metal levels†:	if indicated
Serum/urine electrolytes*:	inappropriate ADH secretion (SIADH) definition
Other body fluids	
Stool viral cultures*:	positive for most enteroviral meningitis: growth in 2–5 days: allows specific serology for coxsackie A viruses
Sputum and bone marrow cultures†:	TB/fungi
Urine culture and antigen detection*:	positive for some viruses (CMV and mumps), TB, and *Candida*: antigen detection for pyogenic bacteria)
Other tests	
Skull and sinus roentgenograms†:	sinusitis or cranial osteomyelitis
CT or brain scan†:	sinus or intracranial abscess or inflammation
EEG†:	diffuse or focal involvement
PPD*:	TB

* Tests routinely performed on every patient with AMS.
† Tests to be performed if a particular agent or diagnosis is strongly suspected.
‡ Tests described in the literature but seldom of diagnostic help.

Initial examination of the CSF will establish the presence of AMS in patients with obvious aberrations, e.g., TP of more than 200 mg per deciliter will immediately indicate further diagnostic tests. Hypoglycorrhachia in AMS suggests either mumps, lymphocytic choriomeningitis, or (in infants) enteroviral infection, the presence of a parameningeal focus, partially treated meningitis, brain tumor, CNS leukemic infiltration, or mycoplasmal, fungal, or acid-fast bacillus infection. Other diagnostic tests that may be utilized for the initial or subsequent CSF examinations are listed in Table 3.

Bacterial cultures of CSF and blood and of any other potentially infected site (urine, skin, catheter) should always be obtained first. If a viral diagnostic laboratory is available, viral cultures of CSF, throat, and stool, particularly during the summer and fall, may prove to be valuable in the management of problematic cases. The enteroviruses that grow in culture will give obvious cytopathogenic changes within 2 to 5 days. The stool culture has the greatest probability of being positive during enteroviral AMS, but CSF culture also has a high yield, with a positive culture 70 percent of the time. Thus, several studies have documented that, based on a positive viral culture result within 5 days of admission, the management of as many as 50 percent of patients with AMS will be changed. Problematic patients with AMS, such as infants or toxic-appearing or partially treated patients initially started on antibiotics, could have the medication stopped or changed on the basis of the positive viral culture.

"Partially treated meningitis" is the most puzzling initial diagnostic and management dilemma posed by patients with AMS, since 25 to 50 percent of patients will already have received antimicrobial therapy at the time of diagnosis. Recent studies have suggested that the only CSF findings altered significantly by prior intramuscular or oral therapy are the Gram stain and culture. Thus, several days of appropriate intravenous therapy are required to decrease the initial high percentage of PMNs and the elevated protein level and to increase the low glucose concentration of the CSF in bacterial meningitis. However, an early or atypical presentation of partially treated bacterial meningitis may initially mimic viral meningitis. In this case, a repeat LP demonstrating a predominance of lymphocytes within 8 to 12 hours, before starting antibiotics, may be justified and useful. Likewise, the CSF TP will not be significantly higher nor the CSF glucose concentration lower. Thus, if the initial physical evaluation and CSF examination strongly suggest either early AMS with a predominance of PMNs or partially treated probable viral AMS, physicians may choose to observe and monitor the patient closely without antimicrobial treatment and to repeat the LP after 8 to 12 hours.

MANAGEMENT

The specific management of the patient with AMS will be determined by the result of the initial evaluation (see Tables 1 to 3). The more general issues of management include the indications for hospitalization, initial cultures and tests to be obtained, isolation procedures, symptomatic therapy, careful fluid management, the need for possible surgical intervention (parameningeal infectious foci or neoplasms), and ongoing diagnostic evaluations including a repeat LP within 8 to 12 hours (Table 4). As with viral culture, the greatest advantage of repeating the LP prior to starting an antibiotic is that of shortening the duration of hospitalization.

Most patients with AMS will be admitted to the hospital with more specific indications for admission, listed in Table 4. Tests to be performed on the initial blood and CSF specimens (see Table 3) will be determined by the epidemiologic factors noted in the history and the possible suspected diagnoses (see Table 2).

Isolation precautions, fluid and electrolyte management, and symptomatic therapy comprise the initial therapy. Careful

TABLE 4 Management of Patients with Aseptic Meningitis Syndrome

Indications for hospitalization
- Toxic-appearing with rapidly progressing symptoms
- High likelihood of treatable cause
- Age <12 mo
- CSF parameters suggesting bacterial etiology despite negative Gram stain
- Positive bacterial antigen test in blood/urine/CSF
- Dehydration or electrolyte imbalance
- Serious underlying disease

Isolation procedures
- Blood, respiratory, and secretion precautions until discharge or etiology clarified; enteroviruses may persist in stool despite clinical improvement

Aggressive and continued diagnostic attempts
- Repeat LPs if indicated
- Repeat bacterial, viral, and fungal cultures and antigen testing if disease progresses
- More complete serologic testing if indicated, i.e., for Epstein-Barr virus, *Mycoplasma* species, Rocky Mountain spotted fever, etc.

Antimicrobial therapy on admission
- Toxic-appearing with progressing symptoms and signs
- No switch to lymphocytic predominance in CSF on repeat 8–12-h LP
- Infant with suspected early or atypical bacterial meningitis or partially treated meningitis
- Immunocompromised individual with possible atypical CSF responses
- Demonstrated parameningeal focus of suspected bacterial etiology
- Selected viral infections

Surgical management
- Parameningeal focus requiring drainage
- CNS shunt manipulation
- Malignancy when indicated

Fluid and electrolyte management
- Intravenous fluid and electrolytes with fluid restriction and ongoing evaluation of serum and urine sodium and specific gravity for evaluation of presence of inappropriate ADH secretion (SIADH)

Symptomatic therapy
- Analgesics for headache, myalgias
- Decreased light, noise, and visitors for photophobia, hyperesthesia
- Antipyretics and antiemetics if indicated

thought should be given to the administration of antimicrobial agents since, once started, they are seldom discontinued before 10 days, thus committing the patient to a potentially unnecessary and expensive hospitalization. Suggested indications for initiating antimicrobial therapy are listed in Table 4. Because of the frequent paucity of clinical manifestations, aberrant CSF findings, and rapid progression of bacterial meningitis in infants and immunocompromised hosts, antimicrobial agents should be started promptly in most of these patients. Likewise, antimicrobial agents should be started in patients who are toxic-appearing, who are strongly suspected of having a parameningeal infection, or who show rapid signs of clinical progression in the hospital. Selected patients with viral causes of AMS may benefit from antiviral drugs. The details of antimicrobial and antiviral therapy are discussed in the chapters devoted to each agent.

The outcome of AMS depends on the etiology. The course of enteroviral meningitis is usually benign and self-limited, with 3 to 5 days of fever and 1 to 2 weeks of neurologic dysfunction. Some patients continue to experience fatigue, irritability and decreased concentration, myalgias, incoordination, and muscle weakness and spasm for several weeks after the acute episode. Infants infected before 3 months of age may experience neurologic sequelae.

The patient with AMS presents a real challenge to the diagnostic and management skills of the physician. Antimicrobial therapy should be initiated soon after admission if the organism is identified or for the indications listed in Table 4. The more difficult and ultimately rewarding path of withholding antimicrobial agents and frequently reevaluating and reassessing the patient, if the etiology is unclear and the patient is stable, may result in a more accurate diagnosis and therapy, shorter hospitalizations, and thus fewer nosocomial infections.

SUGGESTED READING

Cherry JD. Aseptic meningitis and viral meningitis. In: Feigin RD, Cherry JD, eds. Central nervous system infections in pediatric infectious diseases. Philadelphia: WB Saunders, 1987.

Feigin RD, Shackelford PF. Value of repeat lumbar puncture in the differential diagnosis of meningitis. N Engl J Med 1973; 289:571.

Johnson RT, McArthur JC, Narayan O. The neurobiology of human immunodeficiency virus infections. FASEB J 1988; 2:2970–2981.

McGee ZA, Kaiser AB. Acute meningitis. In: Mandell GB, Douglas RG Jr, Bennett JE, eds. Principles and practice of infectious disease. New York: John Wiley, 1985.

Wallgren A. Une nouvelle maladie infectieuse du systeme nerveuse central? Acta Paediatr Scand 1925; 4(Suppl): 158–182.

LOCALIZED INFECTION OF THE CENTRAL NERVOUS SYSTEM

KENNETH L. TYLER, M.D.

Localized infections of the central nervous system (CNS) produce a wide variety of clinical signs and symptoms. Diagnosis of these infections often requires the use and interpretation of specialized diagnostic techniques, including computed tomography (CT scan), cerebral angiography, myelography, and magnetic resonance imaging (MRI). Successful therapy depends on a combination of prompt and aggressive medical management and the use of appropriate neurosurgical intervention. Because of the unique features of each type of infection, they are discussed separately in terms of etiology, pathogenesis, clinical features, laboratory and diagnostic studies, and treatment.

Other CNS infections, including bacterial meningitis, aseptic meningitis, and viral encephalitis, are discussed in separate chapters, as are specific infections such as tuberculosis, syphilis, and certain parasitic diseases.

CEREBRAL SUBDURAL EMPYEMA

Subdural empyema (SDE) can be defined as a collection of pus in the preformed space between the cranial dural and arachnoid membranes. Spinal subdural empyema is a rare form of localized infection of the spinal cord and is discussed separately.

Etiology

Infection of the paranasal sinuses is now the most frequent antecedent to SDE (70 percent of cases). In most cases, the frontal sinuses are involved, but SDE may follow maxillary sinusitis, and sphenoidal sinusitis may precede SDE in the area of the sella turcica (perihypophyseal abscess). SDE usually follows acute rather than chronic sinusitis. In the preantibiotic era, otitic infections were a common antecedent to SDE, but they now account for less than 30 percent of cases; in these cases, SDE often follows an acute exacerbation of chronic otitis. Unusual antecedents of SDE include secondary infection of a subdural hematoma, cranial osteomyelitis, extension through a dural fistula of an epidural abscess, septic thrombophlebitis of the cerebral veins or sinuses, and metastatic spread from a distant primary site of infection. Chronic septic labyrinthitis and petrous apicitis are rare causes of SDE in the posterior fossa. In children, subdural empyema may develop during the course of acute meningitis.

Pathogenesis

Otogenic infections can spread to the subdural space by direct erosion through the adjacent bone of the tegmen tympani and the underlying dura. Infection usually spreads along the tentorium to the falx and may extend into the posterior fossa or laterally over the temporal lobe. Patients with sinusitis may develop septic thrombophlebitis of the mucosal veins, with subsequent spread of infection to the dural veins and venous sinuses, resulting in SDE. SDE may also result from direct extension of infection from the sinuses to the subdural space. In these cases, there is often pathologic evidence of osteomyelitis of the adjacent bone. When associated paranasal sinusitis is present, infection of the subdural space often originates near the frontal pole of the skull and then extends posteriorly.

Clinical Features

The clinical features of SDE are due to (1) signs and symptoms of any antecedent local infection (e.g., sinusitis or otitis), (2) signs and symptoms of increased intracranial pressure, and (3) signs and symptoms of focal neurologic dysfunction. Local pain referred to the region of an infected ear or sinus is quite common. Typically, there is also pain and tenderness over the brow or between the eyes that is exacerbated by percussion of the involved sinus. Orbital swelling and mild proptosis frequently occur and presumably reflect infection involving the orbital veins. Scalp swelling or cellulitis, if present, should suggest the possibility of an associated extradural abscess or of cranial osteomyelitis.

General signs and symptoms include the almost invariable presence of fever, severe headache, and nuchal rigidity. Nausea and vomiting accompany the headache in one-half to two-thirds of cases. Patients generally appear to be severely ill. A change in the level of consciousness occurs with progression of the illness. Early on, patients often seem to be sleepy, confused, or inattentive. With further disease progression, they become somnolent, stuporous, and ultimately comatose. Patients with increased intracranial pressure may develop bradycardia, systolic hypertension, and Cheyne-Stokes breathing. Papilledema is uncommon, and when it appears, there is usually coexisting sinus thrombosis.

Within a few days of the onset of illness, a wide variety of focal signs and symptoms appear. Contralateral hemiparesis or hemiplegia is the commonest focal symptom and eventually develops in almost all patients. Weakness is typically maximal in the face and arm (faciobrachial paresis). The deep tendon reflexes may either be increased or diminished, but the ipsilateral plantar response is usually extensor. Bilaterally upgoing toes should suggest the possibility of transtentorial herniation with compression of the brain stem.

Many patients develop a paresis or palsy of conjugate gaze toward the side opposite the lesion. In more obvious cases, this may result in a resting deviation of the eyes toward the side of the lesion.

Close to 50 percent of patients with SDE develop seizures. Commonly, focal motor or jacksonian seizures antedate more generalized convulsions. Status epilepticus can occur.

Aphasia occurs in many patients with SDE, involving the dominant (typically left) hemisphere. These patients often make naming errors (anomic aphasia), although the full syndrome of either Broca's or, less commonly, Wernicke's aphasia may be seen.

Laboratory and Diagnostic Studies

Computed cranial tomography (CT scanning) has become the cornerstone of diagnosis of SDE. The CT scan is abnormal in virtually all established cases but may be negative in the early stages of infection. Typically, there is a crescent-shaped or lentiform region of decreased attenuation between the inner table of the skull and the cerebral cortex. Midline structures are displaced away from the side of the SDE, and there is typically compression of the ipsilateral lateral ventricle. Contrast injection often produces irregular enhancement of the peripheral margin of the SDE, and in some cases of the adjacent cerebral cortex as well. In cases of intrafalcial empyema, there is a lucent area running sagittally between the cerebral hemispheres. MRI scans may also be useful in identifying the nature and extent of the abscess, although detailed comparisons of the sensitivity and specificity of MRI versus CT in the diagnosis of SDE are not currently available.

In doubtful cases, cerebral angiography may prove valuable. The angiogram typically shows a displacement of vessels away from the inner skull table, suggesting the presence of an extra-axial avascular mass. Particular attention should be paid to the position of the meningeal arteries and the dural sinuses. Displacement of these structures away from the inner skull table suggests extradural, rather than subdural, location of a mass. In the rare cases of intrafalcial empyema, the proximal branches of the anterior cerebral artery are displaced contralaterally and the distal branches ipsilaterally. This results in distinctive S-shaped configuration of the anterior cerebral artery.

Routine radiographic studies are often of value in identifying the presence of sinusitis, mastoiditis, or cranial osteomyelitis. The CT scan may also provide evidence suggesting sinusitis or mastoiditis.

The electroencephalogram is rarely of significant diagnostic value. The electroencephalogram may show decreased voltage and slow waves on the side of the SDE.

Lumbar puncture should be avoided in cases of suspected SDE. The lumbar puncture rarely adds important diagnostic information and can result in cerebral herniation in patients with increased intracranial pressure. When cerebrospinal fluid (CSF) has been obtained in cases of SDE, the findings are quite variable. The CSF pressure is increased in about 70 percent of cases. Pleocytosis is seen in almost all patients, but the cell count varies from 15 to 1,000 cells. In patients with cell counts greater than 1,000, the possibility of rupture of the SDE into the subarachnoid space should be considered. In infants this number of cells suggests that SDE may have resulted as a complication of acute meningitis. The cells may be either predominantly polymorphonuclear leukocytes (PMNs) (60 percent of cases) or predominantly lymphocytes (40 percent). The protein level is typically elevated, but rarely more than 200 mg per deciliter. The glucose level is normal. Organisms are not seen, and CSF cultures are negative unless there is an associated meningitis.

Pathology

A detailed discussion of the pathology of SDE is beyond the scope of this chapter. On gross examination, the subdural exudate usually covers a large part of one cerebral hemisphere. The empyema does not "wall off," and there is no evidence of a limiting membrane surrounding the exudate. Underneath the SDE, the brain is almost always depressed, and there is often evidence of an underlying purulent subarachnoid exudate and thrombosis and/or thrombophlebitis of the subarachnoid veins. Microscopic studies show evidence of infiltration of the dura with inflammatory cells, typically PMNs. The inner surface of the dura is lined with a PMN exudate. The outer layer of the cerebral cortex and subcortical white matter often show evidence of necrosis.

Infecting Agents

The commonest organisms isolated from SDE are aerobic and anaerobic streptococci and *Staphylococcus aureus*. Gram-negative organisms (*Escherichia coli, Proteus* species, *Klebsiella* species; *Pseudomonas* species) may be found in cases that follow otitis or mastoiditis but are rare following paranasal sinusitis. Anaerobic bacteria are often present and may be overlooked unless special culture techniques are utilized.

Therapy

SDE is a fulminating and often life-threatening intracranial infection. Definitive therapy must be initiated without delay. Once the diagnosis is confirmed, operative drainage should be performed urgently. Drainage can be done through burr holes or following craniectomy. In most cases, a surgical approach directed toward the lateral frontal region results in the best drainage of the SDE. Obviously, the surgical approach should be modified according to the best available information on the location of the SDE. Surgical therapy should be combined with high doses of parenteral antibiotics in all cases. The combination (doses are for adults with normal renal function) of nafcillin, 2 g intravenously every 4 hours, or oxacillin, 2 g intravenously every 4 hours (these are therapeutically equivalent), and metronidazole, 15 mg per kilogram intravenously infused over 1 hour, followed by 7.5 mg per kilogram (infused over 1 hour) every 6 hours. Parenteral therapy may be changed to oral therapy with the same dose in the appropriate clinical setting. Antibiotic therapy should be re-evaluated when culture results become available. The semisynthetic broad-spectrum cephalosporin antibiotics are useful in the treatment of certain gram-negative infections. If the patient is allergic to penicillin, vancomycin, 500 mg intravenously every 6 hours, may be used in place of oxacillin or nafcillin.

Anticonvulsants are administered for treatment of seizures, and osmotic agents are used, when necessary, to control increased intracranial pressure.

CEREBRAL EPIDURAL ABSCESS

Etiology and Pathogenesis

Epidural abscess (EA) is the rarest of the localized intracranial suppurative infections. Pus collects between the external layer of the dura and the inner table of the skull. EA is typically associated with an overlying focal cranial osteomyelitis. Infection often spreads across the dura through the emissary veins and produces a subdural empyema as well. EA may follow localized infections of the middle ear or paranasal sinuses. EA may also follow either accidental or surgical penetration of the cranial bones. Implanted foreign bodies (dural grafts, tantalum implants, ventricular shunts, Crutchfield tongs) that penetrate the calvarium may become infected and result in the development of EA. Rare causes of EA include spread of septic dural sinus thrombosis (e.g., infectious cavernous sinus thrombosis), spread of a subdural empyema through a dural fistula, and metastatic spread of infection from a distant site.

Clinical Features

The clinical features of EA do not differ significantly from those described for subdural empyema, and distinction between these two conditions on purely clinical grounds may be difficult. Typically, signs and symptoms of a local infection, such as sinusitis or mastoiditis, are followed by severe generalized headache and high fever. With large abscesses there may be progressive alteration in mental status and focal neurologic signs. In these cases, contralateral hemiparesis is particularly common. Smaller abscesses may produce an isolated contralateral monoparesis. Focal motor convulsions occur with frequency and may generalize. An epidural empyema situated near the petrous pyramid may produce ipsilateral facial pain and sensory loss combined with diplopia due to an ipsilateral lateral rectus palsy (Gradenigo's syndrome).

Laboratory and Diagnostic Studies

The CT scan has become the primary diagnostic study for the diagnosis of EA. The typical picture is one of an extracerebral zone of low density. Evidence of sinusitis or osteomyelitis may be seen. Contrast enhancement of the outer margin of the EA is commonly found. Mass effect—including a contralateral shift of midline structures and compression of the ipsilateral lateral ventricle—is usually seen. It may be impossible to differentiate SDE from EA on CT scan. MRI appears to be of value in the diagnosis of SDE, although its sensitivity and specificity compared with those of the CT scan have not been established.

The typical angiographic features of an epidural mass lesion were discussed in the section on SDE.

Conventional radiographic or polytomographic studies may help suggest the diagnosis of EA by demonstrating the presence of mastoid or paranasal sinus infection or by showing evidence of cranial osteomyelitis.

Lumbar puncture rarely adds valuable diagnostic information and may result in the development of herniation. When the CSF has been examined, it typically shows a mild to moderate pleocytosis in which PMNs or lymphocytes may predominate. The protein is almost invariably elevated. The CSF pressure may be normal or elevated. The CSF glucose levels are normal, and organisms are not seen or cultured.

Pathology

Extradural empyemas are often small and circumscribed, although large lesions are occasionally seen. Pus is found between the outer surface of the dura and the inner table of the skull. The dura itself often shows evidence of inflammation. In autopsy studies, an associated subdural empyema is found in up to 80 percent of cases and an associated brain abscess in 15 to 20 percent.

Infecting Agents

The major infecting agents are similar to those responsible for subdural empyema.

Treatment

Optimal treatment of EA requires the combination of surgical debridement and drainage with parenteral antibiotic therapy. Infected bone should be removed, and the abscess should be drained as completely as possible. Antibiotic therapy is similar to that for SDE and should be modified as indicated by operative cultures.

BRAIN ABSCESS

Etiology

Brain abscesses usually arise from direct extension of infection from contiguous sites (e.g., middle ear, paranasal sinuses), from metastatic spread of distant infections, or from either accidental or surgically induced cranial trauma. Even after careful consideration of each of these possibilities, about 15 to 25 percent of intracranial abscesses are idiopathic in nature.

The two major sources of direct spread of infection are the middle ear/mastoid region and the paranasal sinuses. Otogenic abscesses result when infection in the middle ear erodes through the tegmen tympani or tegmen mastoideum. Spread via the lateral or other sinuses may provide an additional route. Chronic otitis, rather than acute disease, is usually the antecedent infection. Frequently, there is a history of an acute exacerbation of chronic otitis immediately preceding the first symptoms of the brain abscess. In adults otogenic abscesses most commonly occur in the temporal lobe, followed by the cerebellum. In children, a higher percentage of otogenic abscesses are cerebellar. As a corollary to this rule, an otogenic source should always be suspected when an abscess is found in the temporal lobe or cerebellum. The abscesses following infection of the frontal or ethmoid sinuses are commonly located in the frontal lobes. Sphenoidal sinusitis may result in frontal lobe, temporal lobe, or even intrasellar abscesses.

Hematogenous dissemination of infection accounts for about 25 percent of all brain abscesses. In about 20 percent of these cases, multiple abscesses are present. The most frequent site of primary infection is the lung. A wide variety of pulmonary infections, including lung abscesses, pneumonia, empyema, and bronchiectasis, may predispose to brain abscess development. There is also a higher than expected incidence of brain abscesses in patients with cystic fibrosis and pulmonary arteriovenous fistulas (e.g., Osler-Weber-Rendu syndrome). Pulmonary alveolar proteinosis predisposes patients to nocardial brain abscesses. Certain cardiac diseases also predispose to the development of brain abscess. Patients with cyanotic congenital heart disease and a right-to-left shunt are at particular risk. Bacterial endocarditis only rarely results in the production of macroabscesses (more than 1 cm in diameter) in the brain, although microabscesses (less than 1 cm) are quite common. A variety of other primary infections, including peritonsillar abscess, odontogenic abscess, abdominal infections, and infected intrauterine devices, account for occasional cases of metastatic brain abscess. Heroin addicts and other intravenous drug abusers also appear to be at higher risk for developing brain abscesses.

Traumatic brain abscesses may be delayed for years or even decades after the acute trauma. Retained bone or metallic fragments seem to increase the risk.

Clinical Features

The signs and symptoms of brain abscesses are produced by the primary infection, if one is present, by the focal effects of the brain abscess on the CNS, and by increased intracranial pressure.

General symptoms include fever, chills, and malaise. Fever is more commonly present in acute cases and is much less frequent in chronic ones. In most instances the fever appears to be due to the primary infection (e.g., otitis or sinusitis) rather than to the brain abscess. Since fever is present in only about 40 percent of patients and is often low-grade, its absence does not exclude the diagnosis. Signs of increased intracranial pressure can include headache, nausea and vomiting, and alteration in mental status.

Headache may be either generalized or focal and is present in 50 to 70 percent of cases. Its absence does not exclude the diagnosis of brain abscess. Papilledema has been reported in 25 to 50 percent of patients, but it may be a late finding. Paralysis of one or both sixth cranial nerves may result from increased intracranial pressure. Alterations in mental status—ranging from lethargy to stupor or even coma—are found in 50 to 70 percent of patients. Nuchal rigidity occurs in 20 to 50 percent of patients. Seizures may be focal or generalized and occur in about one-third of cases.

A wide variety of focal neurologic signs can occur and may provide a clue to localization. Hemiparesis occurs in about 50 percent of patients, and abnormalities of the visual fields in 5 to 20 percent. Frontal lobe abscesses may produce deterioration in memory function and attention. Temporal lobe abscesses may result in aphasia, hemiparesis, and superior quadrantopsia. Abscesses in the cerebellum often produce suboccipital headache, which radiates to the neck and interscapular area. Signs of cerebellar dysfunction may be subtle and can include incoordination, ataxia, hypotonia, conjugate gaze palsies, and nystagmus.

Laboratory and Diagnostic Studies

The peripheral white blood cell count is about 10,000 per cubic millimeter in about 50 percent of patients but exceeds 20,000 in only 10 percent. The erythrocyte sedimentation rate is increased in about 75 percent of patients and may be a helpful clue in differentiating brain abscess from other mass lesions.

Of the neurodiagnostic tests, the CT scan is unequivocally the most important aid in diagnosis. It permits accurate localization of the abscess, evaluation of its size, and delineation of associated edema and mass effect. The CT scan identifies virtually 100 percent of cases of brain abscesses. The abscess appears as a mass lesion, often with a central lucent zone and a surrounding area of edema. Contrast enhancement is seen as a rim of increased density around the abscess periphery. The development of this pattern of ring enhancement has been attributed to the vascularity of the abscess capsule. Early in its natural history, an abscess appears as a zone of hypodensity without a clear capsule (cerebritis). After 3 to 6 weeks, ring enhancement is seen on CT scan, and after this point, the abscess becomes well demarcated. It is important to remember that ring-enhancing lesions are also produced by primary and metastatic tumors and, occasionally, by hematomas and hemorrhagic infarcts. The visualization on CT scan of septa inside the lesion and of ependymal or meningeal enhancement favors the diagnosis of an abscess. MRI scans appear to be extremely useful in the diagnosis and localization of brain abscess, although their sensitivity and specificity compared to those of CT have not been established.

Angiography is rarely used today to identify or localize brain abscesses. The usual finding is one of an avascular mass, although an area of increased vascularity corresponding to the abscess capsule may be seen. Angiography is reasonably sensitive in localizing abscesses in the temporal lobe, but frontal and parietal abscesses may be missed. The angiogram does not usually allow a precise etiologic diagnosis to be made but simply identifies the presence of a mass lesion.

The electroencephalogram is no longer a primary diagnostic tool in cases of suspected brain abscess. It is abnormal in 75 to 90 percent of cases of supratentorial brain abscesses. The findings may include focal high amplitude slow (delta) waves, epileptiform discharges, or asymmetric fast activity.

Lumbar puncture should be avoided in cases of suspected brain abscess. The lumbar puncture rarely adds useful diagnostic information, and it may result in abrupt neurologic deterioration or death. This type of deterioration occurs in up to one-third of patients within 24 to 48 hours of a lumbar puncture. Reported CSF results generally include increased intracranial pressure, a pleocytosis (more than 10 cells per cubic millimeter) in 70 percent, and an elevated protein level in two-thirds of cases. Cell counts of about 10,000 should raise the possibility that ventricular extension has occurred. Cell counts tend to be higher before the abscess is encapsulated and in abscesses located near the ventricles or subarachnoid space. The glucose levels are normal and cultures are negative unless there is an associated meningitis.

Infecting Agents

The bacteriology of brain abscesses is extremely variable. The most frequently isolated organisms are *S. aureus*, aerobic and anaerobic streptococci, *Streptococcus pneumoniae*, *Bacteroides* species, and gram-negative bacteria. Reports of isolation of a large number of other organisms have appeared. *Listeria monocytogenes* is an important pathogen in immunosuppressed patients. *Clostridium* species and *S. aureus* are often found in post-traumatic abscesses. Multiple pathogens are found in 20 to 30 percent of cases. The reported incidence of anaerobic organisms varies widely and probably depends on the techniques used to culture specimens.

Therapy

The optimal approach to the treatment of brain abscesses is combined medical and neurosurgical therapy. The choice of optimal antibiotic therapy depends on the causative organisms. Every attempt should be made to obtain an aspirate of the abscess material for aerobic, anaerobic, and special cultures. Frequently, a sterotactic aspiration under CT guidance is possible

Prior to identification of the causative organism(s), empirical antibiotic therapy of abscesses associated with paranasal sinusitis should include intravenous penicillin G, 2 million U every 2 hours, plus chloramphenicol, 1.5 g every 6 hours. Nafcillin or oxacillin, 2 g every 4 hours intravenously, should be substituted for penicillin in abscesses of metastatic or traumatic etiology.

Therapy should be continued for a minimum of 4 weeks or until follow-up CT scans demonstrate resolution of the abscess. Several new agents including metronidazole, broad-spectrum semisynthetic cephalosporins, and trimethoprim-sulfamethoxazole may prove to be valuable adjuncts to therapy in specific situations.

The role of medical therapy alone in the treatment of brain abscess remains controversial. We generally reserve this approach for the treatment of surgically inaccessible abscesses, multiple abscesses, or occasional small abscesses. The resolution of medically treated abscesses must be carefully monitored with regular CT or MRI scans.

There remains controversy over the optimal form of surgical therapy for brain abscess. Some neurosurgeons favor repeated aspirations of the abscess, whereas others feel that total excision is the treatment of choice. In general, definitive therapy involves total excision, although careful consideration of both options should be made for each case in consultation with the neurosurgical staff.

In addition to antibiotic therapy, the use of prophylactic anticonvulsants is warranted in most cases because of the high incidence of seizures. Either phenytoin (300 mg per day after an initial loading dose of 1 g in divided doses) or carbamazepine (200 mg twice a day increasing in 200-mg increments every 2 days to 200 mg four times per day) are suitable anticonvulsants. Doses should be adjusted to maintain therapeutic blood levels (phenytoin, 10 to 20 μg per deciliter; carbamazepine, 8 to 12 μg per deciliter). Osmotic agents may be required to control increased intracranial pressure. Steroids should be avoided whenever possible because they may inhibit antibiotic penetration into the abscess cavity.

THROMBOPHLEBITIS OF THE INTRACRANIAL VEINS AND SINUSES

Etiology and Pathogenesis

The etiology of dural sinus or cerebral vein infections varies according to the sinus or vein involved. Infective thrombosis most commonly involves the lateral, cavernous, and petrous sinuses. The superior sagittal sinus and straight sinus are more commonly the sites of noninfective thrombotic processes.

Lateral Sinus Etiology

The lateral sinus includes the transverse and sigmoid sinuses and terminates at the level of the jugular bulb. In many individuals one of the paired lateral sinuses, typically the right, is dominant. The lateral sinus lies in close relation to the middle ear and mastoid bone. Infection that spreads to the sinus commonly begins as mastoiditis or otitis media. A more unusual cause of lateral sinus infection is retrograde spread, via the jugular vein, of infections in the neck or pharynx (e.g., pharyngitis, adenitis, cellulitis, boils).

Clinical Features

Patients with suppurative lateral sinus thrombosis have fever and chills. Septicemia occurs in about 50 percent of cases. Septic emboli to the lungs, joints, or skin can occur. Local signs include retroauricular pain and pain on tilting or rotation of the neck. A firm cord (the jugular vein) may be felt along the anterior border of the sternocleidomastoid muscle. Involvement of the emissary veins results in swelling, erythema, and venous enlargement behind the ear, over the inion, and in the upper neck. If infection involves the dominant sinus, signs of increased intracranial pressure including headache, nausea, and vomiting occur. Papilledema is present in 50 percent of cases. The presence of papilledema or other signs of increased intracranial pressure should suggest the possibility that the contralateral sinus is hypoplastic or that infection has spread to the torcular or superior sagittal sinus. Unilateral papilledema is usually indicative of spread of infection to the ipsilateral cavernous sinus.

Cranial nerve involvement commonly occurs. Involvement of the fifth and sixth nerves (Gradenigo's syndrome) results from petrous apicitis or disease in the inferior petrosal sinus. Sixth cranial nerve involvement can also result from increased intracranial pressure. The clinical findings in Gradenigo's syndrome include facial pain and hypesthesia and diplopia due to lateral rectus muscle palsy. Spread of infection to the jugular bulb can result in paralysis of the ninth, tenth, and eleventh cranial nerves (Vernet's syndrome). Symptoms include hoarseness and dysphagia. There is usually a diminished gag reflex, poor palatal movement on one side, and decreased sensation in the peritonsillar area. Weakness of the ipsilateral sternocleidomastoid muscle and trapezius muscle can occur. Ipsilateral tongue weakness may result from involvement of the twelfth nerve in the hypoglossal canal.

Focal CNS symptoms are uncommon with lateral sinus infection and usually indicate dissemination of infection. Involvement of the inferior anastomotic vein of Labbé can result in contralateral hemiparesis, aphasia, visual field abnormalities, and focal or generalized seizures.

Cavernous Sinus Etiology

Infection of the cavernous sinus (CS) generally occurs via one of three routes. Localized infections in the orbit, paranasal sinuses, or upper half of the face can spread to the CS from the ophthalmic veins. Infections near the teeth, tonsils, or jaw can produce sphenoid sinus infection with subsequent spread to the CS. Finally, ear infections or lateral sinus infections can spread to the CS by way of the petrosal sinuses. Although most cases of CS infection begin unilaterally, they quickly become bilateral because of the interconnection of the two CSs through the circular sinus.

Clinical Features

The onset of CS infection is abrupt, and most patients are acutely ill with high fever. Local signs and symptoms include eye pain, photophobia, proptosis, corneal clouding, orbital swelling and edema, and chemosis of the eyelid and conjunctiva. Cyanosis of the upper face, including the eyelids and the root of the nose, may be seen.

Cranial nerve palsies are invariably found and produce progressive external ophthalmoplegia. The sixth cranial nerve is usually involved initially, with subsequent involvement of the third and fourth nerves. The first division and less commonly the second division of the fifth (trigeminal) nerve can be involved, producing facial pain, paresthesias or hypesthesia, and a diminished corneal reflex. Papilledema results from impaired venous return. Disease of the optic nerve may result in decreased visual acuity and the appearance of scotomas. The pupils may be increased or decreased in size and are commonly sluggish or unreactive.

Superior Sagittal Sinus Etiology

As indicated earlier, septic thrombosis of the superior sagittal sinus is far less common than noninfectious thrombosis. Infection of the superior sagittal sinus may result from nasal infections or infections of the paranasal sinuses. Infection may also spread directly through a contaminated compound skull fracture or from a subdural empyema, epidural abscess, or meningitis. Metastatic infection from a distant primary site and retrograde spread of infection from tributary dural venous sinuses are often causes of superior sagittal sinus infection.

Clinical Features

Patients generally present with headache, fever, and signs of increased intracranial pressure. Edema of the forehead and scalp may result from involvement of emissary veins.

Focal CNS symptoms include paresis of one or both legs, cortical sensory loss, and unilateral seizures. Focal motor seizures or jacksonian seizures are particularly common. When hemiparesis is present, the face is often relatively spared, and the weakness is more pronounced in the legs than in the arms. Many of the focal CNS signs and symptoms reflect thrombosis of cortical veins with subsequent hemorrhagic cortical infarction rather than superior sagittal sinus involvement per se.

Diagnosis of Intracranial Thrombophlebitis

The diagnosis usually depends on a high index of clinical suspicion. The CT scan is often helpful in excluding other causes of intracranial suppuration (e.g., brain abscess). The finding on CT scan of single or multiple hemorrhagic cortical infarctions, especially in the parasagittal area, may suggest cortical vein thrombosis. In some cases a high density serpiginous cord—representing a thrombosed cortical vein—can be seen on nonenhanced scans. This sign is virtually pathognomonic of cerebral vein thrombosis. With superior sagittal sinus occlusion, there may be contrast enhancement of the outer margin of the sinus and a hypodense center ("empty delta" sign).

The most informative test is cerebral angiography. The venous sinuses and cortical veins are well visualized in the late or delayed phases of a cerebral angiogram. Signs of venous sinus occlusion include absent filling, filling defects, dilation or tortuosity of veins, slow venous filling, and reversal of the direction of venous flow. The major venous sinuses are extremely well visualized by digital subtraction angiography. In centers where this test is available, it often replaces conventional angiography as the diagnostic procedure of choice.

Lumbar puncture should be performed only if there are not signs of increased intracranial pressure. The spinal fluid usually shows a mild to moderate lymphocytic pleocytosis and a normal or slightly elevated protein level. The presence of xanthochromia or frank hemorrhage is indicative of cortical vein thrombosis. The glucose is normal and cultures are sterile unless there is an associated meningitis. Manometric studies are not reliable. The Queckenstedt and Toby-Ayer tests of spinal fluid manometrics are only rarely performed but may be valuable in specific situations.

Therapy

Appropriate therapy consists of antibiotics and, in many cases, neurosurgical intervention. Empirical antibiotic therapy is directed toward adequate coverage of aerobic and anaerobic streptococci, *S. aureus*, *S. pneumoniae*, and assorted anaerobes. Gram-negative organisms may be important in certain situations, especially with otogenic infections. Fungal infection (mucormycosis) is a special problem in diabetics. Empirical therapy should consist of nafcillin or oxacillin, 2 g intravenously every 4 hours, plus chloramphenicol, 1.5 g intravenously every 6 hours. Nafcillin and oxacillin are therapeutically equivalent.

Surgery should be performed if there is evidence of localized infection (e.g., osteomyelitis, mastoiditis, sinusitis). The roles of thrombectomy or of ligation of infected sinuses or of the jugular vein have not been established, and these procedures should not be routinely performed. The use of anticoagulants is also controversial. These agents should not be used if there is evidence of cortical vein thrombosis or episodes of septic embolization. Intracranial hypertension may require the use of osmotic agents or ventricular shunting procedures. Anticonvulsants are not used prophylactically but are required in patients who develop focal or generalized seizures, especially in the setting of cortical vein thrombosis.

INTRACEREBRAL MYCOTIC ANEURYSMS

Etiology and Pathogenesis

Mycotic aneurysms are a rare complication of bacterial endocarditis and occur in less than 5 percent of cases. They constitute about 5 percent of all intracranial aneurysms. In acute bacterial endocarditis (e.g., due to *S. aureus*), mycotic aneurysms tend to develop early in the course of infection, whereas in subacute endocarditis (e.g., due to viridans streptococci), they characteristically appear late. Dissemination of infection to a site of arterial damage may produce a mycotic aneurysm even when bacterial endocarditis is not present.

The pathogenesis of these aneurysms remains unclear. In most cases, septic embolization to the vasa vasorum appears to be the inciting factor. In other cases, septic intraluminal aterial emboli appear to produce an endarteritis that subsequently spreads outward through the vessel wall. Spread of infection from contiguous areas to adjacent arteries may be a third mechanism of pathogenesis.

Mycotic aneurysms are solitary in 80 percent of cases and multiple in 20 percent. They tend to involve vessels near their branching points. The distal portion of the middle cerebral artery is probably the most commonly involved site.

Clinical Features

In many cases, mycotic aneurysms, like congenital berry aneurysms, appear to be asymptomatic unless they leak or rupture. Some patients develop severe, unremitting, localized headache. When this symptom develops in a patient with known bacterial endocarditis, aneurysm should be strongly suspected. Many patients have evidence of cerebral embolization of a mycotic aneurysm. Patients with endocarditis who develop focal CNS findings should have a CT scan, followed in most cases by a lumbar puncture. An aseptic CSF pattern (lymphocytic pleocytosis, normal or elevated protein levels, normal glucose level) is usually indicative of embolism, brain abscess, or mycotic aneurysm. The first two possibilities can usually be excluded on the basis of the history and the results of the CT scan. A hemorrhagic spinal fluid (more than 200 red blood cells per cubic millimeter in all tubes after a nontraumatic lumbar puncture) should always suggest mycotic aneurysm.

Diagnostic Studies

Patients who develop severe and persistent focal headache in the setting of endocarditis should undergo cerebral angiography. Patients with endocarditis and hemorrhagic spinal fluid or evidence of intracerebral hemorrhage by CT should also undergo angiography. Angiography remains the definitive diagnostic test for identification of mycotic aneurysms. However, small aneurysms may be missed. Improved techniques for digital subtraction angiography will make this test increasingly valuable in the future. Because of the incidence of multiple aneurysms (about 20 percent), injection of both carotid arteries is advisable. Mycotic aneurysms of the posterior circulation are rare. A vertebral injection is probably not routinely required and should be used only when indicated by the clinical situation or when visualization of the carotid circulation does not reveal an aneurysm. Subtraction and magnification views are essential. Patients with an intracerebral hematoma who have a negative angiogram during the acute stage should have the test repeated after the mass effect of the hematoma has resolved. The small size of aneurysms makes CT of limited value in direct diagnosis. The CT scan may be helpful in excluding other diagnoses (e.g., abscess, infarct) or in indirectly suggesting mycotic aneurysm by demonstrating intracerebral or subarachnoid blood.

The mortality of patients with endocarditis and a ruptured mycotic aneurysm exceeds 80 percent. The goal must be to identify patients with unruptured aneurysms and treat them aggressively. Controversy exists about the appropriate role of antibiotic therapy alone in the treatment of mycotic aneurysms. Antibiotic therapy alone results in resolution of almost 50 percent of recognized peripheral mycotic aneurysms. The mortality rate in patients treated with medical therapy is about 15 percent, although mild to moderate neurologic deficits are seen in 25 to 50 percent of survivors. Patients treated medically should have follow-up angiography on a weekly or biweekly basis. If there is an increase in aneurysm size, any evidence of bleeding, or no decrease in aneurysm size over 4 to 6 weeks, then surgery should be performed. The choice of antibiotics depends on isolation of the etiologic agent from the bloodstream or other sites (e.g., embolic material). Regimens for staphylococci and streptococci are listed blow.

Streptococcal Endocarditis and Mycotic Aneurysm

Administer aqueous penicillin G, 2 million U intravenously every 2 hours, plus streptomycin, 0.5 g intramuscularly every 12 hours. These doses should be modified once organism sensitivities are available. Toxicity may require alteration of the streptomycin dose or dosing interval. Therapy should be continued for a minimum of 4 to 6 weeks. If the aneurysm is decreasing in size but has not resolved, therapy should be continued and a decision about surgical therapy made.

Staphylococcal Endocarditis and Mycotic Aneurysm

Administer nafcillin or oxacillin, 2 g intravenously every 4 hours (for penicillin-allergic patients: vancomycin, 500 mg intravenously every 6 hours). Nafcillin and oxacillin are therapeutically equivalent. Duration of therapy is as noted above.

LOCALIZED INFECTIONS OF THE SPINAL CORD

Localized infections of the spinal cord can be classified according to their anatomic location as epidural, subdural, or intraspinal. Epidural abscesses are considerably more frequent than either subdural or intraspinal infections. Localized infections of the spinal cord are medical and neurosurgical emergencies that require rapid institution of appropriate therapy. Therapeutic delay often results in tragic sequelae for the patient, including permanent paraplegia or quadriplegia and even death.

Pathogenesis

The possible routes of initiation of localized infections of the spinal cord include (1) direct extension from contiguous infection (e.g., vertebral osteomyelitis, perinephric or retroperitoneal abscess); (2) hematogenous spread from a distant site of infection; (3) introduction of infected material (e.g., following knife or gunshot injury, lumbar puncture, operation). In rare cases ("primary"), none of the factors noted above can be identified. Metastatic infection probably accounts for 50 percent of cases of epidural and intraspinal abscess and an even higher percentage of cases of spinal subdural empyema. The primary infection can be in the skin (furunculosis, carbuncles, cellulitis), the lungs (pneumonia, empyema, bronchiectasis), the heart (endocarditis), the genitourinary system (prostatic abscess, purulent cystitis), or the oropharynx (retropharyngeal or tonsillary abscess, dental abscess). Septic abortion may be a site of primary infection in pregnant women.

Clinical Features

Distinction between epidural and subdural infections can rarely be made clinically. These infections appear to occur with increased frequency in immunosuppressed patients, diabetics, and intravenous drug abusers. The initial symptom is usually severe, localized pain, typically in the back. In cases of epidural empyema, pain is increased by percussion or local pressure. Patients with subdural empyema or intraspinal abscess frequently do not have percussion tenderness. With both epi- and subdural infection, patients typically hold the spine rigid and try to avoid any undue motion. At this stage, patients are usually acutely ill. Fever is almost invariably present, and there may be chills or rigors. Headache and meningeal signs are also commonly present. Most patients have radicular pains involving the chest or, less commonly, the arms or legs. Symptoms are followed quickly (in 24 to 48 hours) by signs of an acute transverse spinal cord lesion. Patients develop flaccid paraplegia (or quadriplegia), loss of reflexes, anesthesia with a sensory level, and sphincter disturbances. Babinski's sign is present bilaterally. Flaccidity may subsequently evolve into spasticity with hyperactive reflexes once the period of "spinal shock" is over.

Some patients, especially those whose infections are caused by fungi or mycobacteria (see below), follow a slower ("chronic") course, which can mimic other extradural compressive lesions such as tumors.

Most cases of intraspinal abscesses manifest with a clinical picture similar to that of epidural or subdural lesions. Constitutional symptoms such as fever, malaise, and rigors are followed by back pain with or without meningeal symptoms. Within hours to days, there is paraplegia (flaccid, areflexic), anesthesia with a sensory level, and disorder of bowel and bladder function. Specific signs pointing to an intramedullary lesion (e.g., disassociated sensory loss, sacral sparing) are frequently obscured by the rapid progression of the illness.

Pathology

A complete discussion of pathology is beyond the scope of this chapter. Most epidural and subdural infections are located posterior (dorsal) to the spinal cord. Infections are more common in the thoracic region, although cervical and less commonly lumbar, sacral, or cauda equina lesions occur. In most cases of epidural abscess, the infection extends for several (e.g., three to six) cord segments. Subdural empyema may be present at multiple levels. Intraspinal abscesses are typically located centrally in the cord or in the region of the posterior horns. They are most common in the cervical region and may extend into the brain stem. Abscesses are usually single, but multiple abscesses are not rare. The abscess size is quite variable, from microscopic to the entire length of the cord. Most lesions extend for at least five segments. These abscesses rarely encapsulate.

Infecting Agents

Bacteria are the commonest cause of acute localized spinal infections. Cases of chronic epidural abscess are frequently due to mycobacteria, actinomyces, and fungi (blastomycosis, cryptococcosis, aspergillosis, nocardiosis) and, occasionally, result from other agents (e.g., *Echinococcus*). Of the bacterial agents, *S. aureus* is clearly the most frequently encountered and is responsible for one-half to two-thirds of all cases of localized spinal infection. *Staphylococcus* should be particularly suspected in patients with a history of antecedent trauma or skin infection. Streptococci and pneumococci may be encountered in patients with primary pulmonary infections. In intravenous drug abusers and patients with antecedent genitourinary infections, gram-negative organisms (*Escherichia coli, Pseudomonas aeruginosa, Serratia marcescens, Enterobacter cloacae, Proteus* species) are commonly found.

Laboratory Tests

Patients with acute localized spinal infections almost invariably have a leukocytosis and an elevated erythrocyte sedimentation rate. Radiographs of the spine are often normal but may show evidence of localized osteomyelitis with bone destruction and disk space narrowing. Blood cultures are positive in up to 50 percent of cases. Myelography remains the definitive diagnostic procedure and should be performed immediately in all systemically ill patients who develop severe back pain, radicular symptoms, or signs of spinal cord compression. Ideally, metrizamide myelography should be combined with CT scan of the spine for the best delineation of the lesion. Cervical puncture should be performed for introduction of dye to diminish the risk of entering the abscess if it is located in the lumbar area. In almost all cases of epidural infection or subdural infection, myelography demonstrates either a complete (80 percent) or partial (20 percent) block of the flow of dye. An attempt should be made to define the upper and lower extent of the lesion. CT scan, even without the addition of dye into the subarachnoid space, often demonstrates an epidural abscess. Patients with intraspinal abscess commonly have swelling of the spinal cord seen on myelography or CT. In some cases the swelling is severe enough to result in either partial or complete CSF block. MRI may be a valuable adjunct to diagnosis. Epidural abscesses may manifest as extradural masses with high-intensity signal on spin-echo T_2-weighted images. MRI appears to be superior to routine CT scan but does not appear to be as sensitive as myelography with high-resolution CT.

Lumbar puncture is best deferred until the time of myelography. The CSF in patients with acute epidural or subdural infection usually has a polymorphonuclear pleocytosis (50 to 500 cells), an elevated level of protein, and a normal level of glucose. In patients with epidural abscess, the CSF culture is positive in approximately 20 percent. If the CSF pleocytosis is excessive and the glucose level is depressed, a concomitant spinal meningitis is usually present. Patients with chronic infections may only have an elevated CSF protein level. In cases of suspected epidural abscess, the lumbar puncture needle should be advanced slowly and aspirated frequently. If frank pus is withdrawn, the procedure should be terminated in order to avoid introducing infection into the subdural or subarachnoid space.

Therapy

Once a localized spinal infection has been diagnosed and localized, a bilateral exploratory laminectomy should be performed immediately. In cases of intraspinal abscess, puncture or incision of the cord and aspiration to evacuate pus should be done. In patients with epidural infection, care should be taken to avoid opening the spinal dura. Drains should be placed between the epidural space and the skin surface. Material obtained at operation should be sent for aerobic and anaerobic bacterial cultures and for fungal and mycobacterial cultures in all chronic cases. Pathologic material should be examined microscopically for bacteria, mycobacteria, fungi, and for the presence of granulomas. Gram-stain, Ziehl-Neelsen stain, and other appropriate stains should be performed immediately on some of the available material.

Definitive antibiotic therapy should be based on cultures obtained at operation. Initial antibiotic therapy should be instituted as soon as the diagnosis is suspected. Because of the high frequency of *S. aureus* infections, a semisynthetic penicillin in high does should be used, e.g., nafcillin sodium, 2 g every 4 hours, intravenously, or (therapeutically equivalent) oxacillin sodium, 2 g every 4 hours, intravenously (alternative therapy if patient is penicillin-allergic: vancomycin hydrochloride, 500 mg every 6 hours intravenously).

In drug addicts or patients with preexisting genitourinary disease, a broad-spectrum semisynthetic cephalosporin should be given intravenously in a high dose. Infection caused by tuberculosis should be treated with triple therapy (isoniazid, ethambutol, rifampin, or streptomycin). Amphotericin B or miconazole with or without fluorouracil should be used for fungal infections.

Dr. Tyler is supported by a physician-scientist award from the National Institute of Allergy and Infectious Diseases, by a fellowship grant from the Muscular Dystrophy Association, and by a grant from the William P. Anderson Foundation

SUGGESTED READING

Danner RL, Hartman BJ. Update on spinal epidural abscess: 35 cases and review of the literature. Rev Infect Dis 1987; 9:265–274.

Erntell M, Holtas S, Norlin K, et al. Magnetic resonance imaging in the diagnosis of spinal epidural abscess. Scand J Infect Dis 1988; 20:323–327.

Mapalam TJ, Rosenblum M. Trends in the management of bacterial brain abscesses: A review of 102 cases over 17 years. Neurosurgery 1988; 23:451–458.

Miller ES, Dias PS, Uttley D. Management of subdural empyema: A series of 24 cases. J Neurol Neurosurg Psychiatry 1987; 50:1415–1418.

Morawetz RB, Karp RB. Evolution and resolution of intracranial bacterial (mycotic) aneurysms. Neurosurgery 1984; 15:43–49.

Schliamser SE, Backman K, Norrby SR. Intracranial abscesses in adults: An analysis of 54 consecutive cases. Scand J Infect Dis 1988; 20:1–9.

Silverberg AL, DiNubile. Subdural empyema and cranial epidural abscess. Med Clin North Am 1985; 69:361–374.

Smith BH. Infection of the dura and its venous sinuses. In: Joynt RJ, ed. Neurology. Philadelphia: JB Lippincott, 1988.

BACTERIURIA AND PYELONEPHRITIS

CLARE L. CHERNEY, M.D.
DONALD KAYE, M.D.

Bacteriuria is defined as bacteria in the urine. Bacteriuria is quantitated to ascertain the probability of a truly infected urinary tract. Significant bacteriuria has traditionally been defined as 10^5 or more colony-forming units (cfu) per milliliter of urine, but lesser numbers may have significance in certain situations.

Bacteriuria may be symptomatic or asymptomatic. The clinical syndrome of dysuria, urgency, and frequency—with or without suprapubic tenderness—is defined as cystitis or lower urinary tract infection (UTI). The clinical syndrome of flank pain and/or tenderness and fever, with or without cystitis symptoms, indicates involvement of the kidney in the infectious process (i.e., pyelonephritis). The cystitis syndrome alone in no way excludes upper tract infection and, in fact, kidney involvement is common.

When discussing UTIs, it is important to differentiate reinfection from relapse. A relapse occurs when the same organism persists in the urinary tract so that infection recurs soon after antimicrobial therapy is discontinued. A reinfection is a new infection caused by a different or the same organism.

DIAGNOSIS

Microscopic examination of the urine is a quick, simple office procedure that can yield much useful information. Pyuria is present in many patients with symptomatic and asymptomatic bacteriuria. Pyuria is best defined as more than 10 polymorphonuclear leukocytes per cubic millimeter in a counting chamber. A less accurate definition is more than five to 10 white blood cells (WBCs) per high-power field in a centrifuged (5 minutes at 2,000 rpm) clean-catch urine specimen. It should be emphasized that many patients with pyuria do not have infection and other diagnoses should be entertained.

Methylene blue or Gram staining of the urine can aid in the predictability of significant bacteriuria. One bacterium visualized in each oil-immersion field in an unspun, stained, midstream, clean-catch urine correlates with 10^5 or more cfu per milliliter. If the urine is centrifuged and stained, one visualized bacterium per oil-immersion field correlates with 10^4 or more cfu per milliliter.

Quantitative urine cultures have been used to differentiate true and reproducible bacteriuria from urine contaminated from the urethra or vagina. In the asymptomatic patient, two separate clean-catch specimens, each with 10^5 or more cfu per milliliter of the same organism, are highly predictive of true bacteriuria. Since men and catheterized patients have less chance of contamination, 10^4 or more cfu per milliliter is considered significant in these groups. In women with dysuria and pyuria, 10^2 or more Enterobacteriaceae per milliliter is predictive of infection. Any growth from a suprapubic puncture of the bladder is considered indicative of infection.

MANAGEMENT OF SYMPTOMATIC LOWER URINARY TRACT INFECTION

Since not all patients with dysuria syndromes have UTI, a prerequisite to management is making the correct diagnosis. Herpes, chlamydial, gonococcal, and ureaplasmal infections of the urethra and vaginal infections can all cause dysuria, but routine urine cultures will be negative.

The majority of adults with symptomatic UTIs are young, healthy women. Some of these patients have a predisposition for recurrent UTIs, but few of them have underlying anatomic or surgically correctable abnormalities. Sexual intercourse and use of a diaphragm both increase the frequency of infection in this group. The prognosis is excellent since there is no evidence that recurrent UTIs in nonpregnant women without urinary tract obstruction lead to renal damage.

The majority of UTIs are caused by Enterobacteriaceae, especially *Escherichia coli. Staphylococcus saprophyticus,* a coagulase-negative, novobiocin-resistant staphylococcus, is a common cause of infection in sexually active young women.

Single-dose therapeutic regimens cure 80 to 100 percent of lower tract infections in women. One problem with this approach is the difficulty in identifying patients with asymptomatic upper tract infection, in whom there is a high risk of relapse. Single-dose therapy is applicable only with agents that have a relatively long half-life in serum and therefore provide prolonged urinary levels. Rather than advocate single-dose therapy, we prefer the concept of short-course therapy. This means giving doses of an agent that will provide 1 to 3 days of antimicrobial activity in the urine. This can be achieved, for example, with a single double-strength tablet of trimethoprim-sulfamethoxazole (160 mg of TMP, 800 mg of SMZ) or with 250 mg of amoxicillin or cephalexin every 8 hours for 24 hours. Some authorities prefer to give short-course therapy for 3 days on the assumption that 3 days will cure some patients with asymptomatic upper tract infection. This approach is probably preferable.

Table 1 lists some of the single-dose regimens that have been demonstrated to be effective. Some standard dosing regimens that can be given for short courses (1 to 3 days of therapy) are also listed. Urine cultures are not essential prior to short-course therapy.

Some women with frequently recurring symptomatic UTIs that follow sexual intercourse can be effectively managed with pericoital prophylaxis using a single, low dose of an antimicrobial agent such as one single-strength TMP-

TABLE 1 Some Regimens for Patients Not Seriously Ill

	Therapy	
Condition	*Duration*	*Agent and Dose*
Cystitis	Single-dose therapy for women	TMP 400 mg* TMP-SMZ 320–1,600 mg*† Nitrofurantoin 200 mg Amoxicillin 3 g Tetracycline 2 g‡ Sulfisoxazole 2 g†
	Short-course (1–3 days) therapy for women; 7 days for men; 4–6 wk for relapse	TMP 100 mg q12h* TMP-SMZ 160–800 mg q12h*† Nitrofurantoin 100 mg q6h Amoxicillin 250–500 mg q8h Amoxicillin–clavulanic acid 250–500 mg q8h Sulfisoxazole 500 mg q6h† Cephalexin, Cephradine, Cefaclor } 250 mg q6–8h Norfloxacin 400 mg q12h* Ciprofloxacin 500 mg q12h* Tetracycline 250 mg q6h‡
Prophylaxis for frequently recurring UTIs in female (all in single doses each day)		Nitrofurantoin 50–100 mg/day; children 1–2 mg/kg/day TMP-SMZ 40–200 mg/day or thrice weekly*†; children 2 mg/kg/day of TMP component Trimethoprim 50–100 mg/day*; children 2 mg/kg/day
Children's doses for cystitis	7 days of therapy; 4–6 wk for relapse	TMP 4 mg/kg q12h TMP-SMZ 4–20 mg/kg q12h† Nitrofurantoin 1–2 mg/kg q6h Amoxicillin 20 mg/kg/day up to 20 kg divided q8h Sulfisoxazole 38 mg/kg q6h not to exceed 6 g† Cephalexin 6–12 mg/kg q6h Cephradine 6–12 mg/kg q6h Cefaclor 20 mg/kg/day divided q8h

* Not advocated during pregnancy because of possible teratogenicity.
† Should not be used close to term or in the newborn because of risk of kernicterus.
‡ Not to be used during tooth development, i.e., from the second half of pregnancy through 8 years of age.

SMZ tablet (80 mg, 400 mg) or 100 mg of nitrofurantoin. Women with frequent symptomatic reinfections and children with frequent symptomatic or asymptomatic reinfections with no identifiable precipitating event are candidates for low-dose, long-term prophylaxis, which has been shown to reduce the number of episodes of cystitis by more than 90 percent and is well tolerated in the majority of patients. TMP-SMZ (one-half of one single-strength tablet nightly) or nitrofurantoin (50 mg nightly) have proven to be effective for this purpose. We recommend a trial of 6 months of prophylaxis and then reevaluation.

If patients remain asymptomatic after therapy, follow-up cultures are necessary only in pregnant women and children in whom it is important to treat asymptomatic bacteriuria. For the majority of women, follow-up cultures are not cost effective or warranted. If symptoms persist through therapy, the patient either does not have a UTI or has a UTI with a resistant organism, and a urine culture is indicated for diagnosis and susceptibility patterns.

If a patient responds and then relapses with symptoms after short-course therapy, urine cultures should be obtained and a 14-day course of antimicrobial therapy should be given to treat a possible renal focus. If symptomatic relapse again occurs, evaluation should be obtained to rule out stones and/or obstruction. In the absence of anatomic abnormalities, 4–6 weeks of therapy should be considered. Asymptomatic relapses are probably of little importance except in children and pregnant women.

Any child with a urinary tract infection should have an anatomic evaluation. Vesicoureteral reflux and obstruction are common and important to rule out since progressive renal damage can occur with these abnormalities alone and be accelerated in the presence of bacteriuria. Ultrasonography and radionuclide voiding studies are noninvasive diagnostic techniques that can be used for screening in this situation. Short-course therapy has not been extensively evaluated in children, and we recommend 7-day courses of therapy. Table 1 outlines drugs and dosages for children.

For the child who relapses, 2 weeks of therapy are used, and if relapse occurs again, 4–6 weeks of therapy are indicated. For the child with recurrent reinfections but no surgically correctable abnormality, low-dose, long-term prophylaxis may be indicated. Although new renal scarring in children after the age of 5 years is uncommon, we favor therapy of asymptomatic bacteriuria until young adulthood.

Males with urinary tract infection should be evaluated for structural abnormalities. Urinary tract obstruction is common in males with bacteriuria and, with and without bacteriuria, can lead to progressive renal damage. An ultrasound study with or without a radionuclide bladder-emptying study, may be sufficient. In men, short-course therapy has not been adequately evaluated, and we favor a 7-day course of therapy for lower urinary tract infection. A symptomatic relapse, as with women and children, should be treated for 14 days to cover the possibility of an upper tract focus. A subsequent relapse suggests the possibility of chronic bacterial prostatitis (see the chapter *Prostatitis, Epididymitis, and Balanoposthitis*), obstruction, or calculus. If surgically correctable lesions have been ruled out, longer courses of therapy, such as 4–6 weeks, are indicated at this time. Asymptomatic recurrences in the absence of urinary tract obstruction do not need to be treated in adults.

MANAGEMENT OF SYMPTOMATIC UPPER TRACT INFECTION

Acute pyelonephritis is suspected when a patient presents with fever, flank pain, nausea, and vomiting, with or without abdominal tenderness. Processes such as renal infarct, stones, obstruction, hemorrhage, tumor, spinal or epidural abscesses, intra-abdominal processes, and thoracolumbar herpes zoster can cause similar syndromes. Gram-negative bacteremia complicating pyelonephritis should be suspected when the patient presents with shaking chills, high fever, hypotension, confusion, and/or lethargy.

Patients should be admitted to the hospital when they are seriously ill, elderly, immunocompromised, or unable to take oral medication, or when the diagnosis is not certain. Both blood and urine cultures should be obtained, and the urine should be examined for the presence of pyuria and gram-negative or gram-positive organisms.

Table 2 lists commonly used drugs and dosages, depending on the clinical situation and urine Gram stain. There are many effective options. In the seriously ill patient, when bacteremia is suspected, we favor therapy with a third-generation

TABLE 2 Some Regimens for Seriously Ill Adults

Condition	*Therapy*
Community-acquired gram-negative bacteria in urine	TMP-SMZ 5–25 mg/kg IV q12h or PO*†
	Nonpseudomonal extended-spectrum cephalosporin, e.g., ceftizoxime 2 g IV q8h, cefotaxime 2 g IV q6h, ceftriaxone 2 g IV or IM q24h
	Gentamicin or tobramycin 1.7 mg/kg IV or IM q8h adjusted for renal insufficiency
	Aztreonam 2 g IV q8h†
Nosocomially acquired gram-negative bacteria in urine	Ceftazidime 1–2 g IV q8h
	Gentamicin or tobramycin 1.7 mg/kg IV or IM q8h adjusted for renal insufficiency
	Aztreonam 1–2 g IV q8h†
	Ciprofloxacin 500–750 mg PO q12h†
Community or nosocomially acquired gram-positive bacteria in urine	
Streptococci	Ampicillin 2 g IV q4h plus gentamicin
Staphylococci	Cefazolin 1–2 g IV or IM q8h
	Nafcillin 2 g IV q4h
	or
	Vancomycin 1 g IV q12h adjusted for renal insufficiency if methicillin-resistant†

* Should not be used close to term or in the newborn infant since it can cause kernicterus.
† Not advocated during pregnancy because of possible teratogenicity.

cephalosporin until results of cultures are known. Patients can be switched to oral therapy when they are afebrile and doing well (see dosages in Table 1). Therapy should be given for a total of 14 days.

In the less-severely ill patient with pyelonephritis an oral drug can be administered. Outpatient care is an option when the patient is well enough to take oral medication, the diagnosis is clear, and the patient is reliable enough for adequate follow-up. Oral TMP-SMZ or norfloxacin or ciprofloxacin, or daily intramuscular ceftriaxone or aminoglycoside all are potential outpatient regimens for the moderately ill outpatient. Oral cephalexin, cephradine, and amoxicillin (alone or with clavulanic acid) are other options. Again, therapy should be given for a total of 14 days.

When the patient does not defervesce while being adequately treated for the urine and/or blood isolates, an underlying collection of pus must be suspected. Obstruction with hydropyonephrosis, intraparenchymal renal abscesses, and perinephric abscesses are most important to rule out. Plain films and ultrasonography of the abdomen aid in diagnosis of stones, abnormal gas/fluid patterns, and hydronephrosis, but computed tomography (CT) is the imaging modality of choice to rule out intra-abdominal abscesses.

Intraparenchymal or corticomedullary renal abscesses have been increasingly recognized as more sensitive imaging techniques have been used. In many cases these abscesses represent infected foci that have not yet formed well-encapsulated abscesses. In general, they should be aggressively treated with parenteral antimicrobial agents, and only if no response is noted in 7 days or the patient is doing poorly should percutaneous or surgical drainage be attempted.

Perinephric abscesses probably occur after rupture of a corticomedullary abscess into the space between Gerota's fascia and the kidney. They usually have an insidious onset and are often unsuspected at the time of presentation. As opposed to corticomedullary collections, it is imperative to drain perinephric abscesses.

When upper tract infection is complicated by abscesses, more prolonged therapy is indicated. All patients with pyelonephritis should have at least an ultrasonic study to seek obstruction and/or stones. Follow-up urine cultures are mandatory 2 weeks after therapy is complete in pregnant women and children. In nonpregnant adults without symptoms, follow-up cultures are optional. Symptomatic relapses warrant prolonged antimicrobial therapy (e.g., 4–6 weeks) while anatomic evaluation of the urinary tract is ongoing. In the male, if there are no surgically correctable abnormalities, chronic bacterial prostatitis should be suspected and evaluated and treated as detailed in the chapter on prostatitis. Asymptomatic recurrences need be treated only in pregnant patients, children, and patients with uncorrectable obstructive uropathy.

MANAGEMENT OF ASYMPTOMATIC BACTERIURIA

Asymptomatic bacteriuria is a common finding that increases in frequency with age. Approximately 5 percent of middle-aged women are bacteriuric at any time. In the elderly population, at least 20 percent of women and 10 percent of men have bacteriuria on survey. Excluding pregnant women, patients with obstruction, and young children, the significance of asymptomatic bacteriuria is controversial and unclear. Asymptomatic bacteriuria has been associated with an increased risk of mortality in some community studies but not in others. It is not clear whether the increased mortality (if real) is secondary to bacteriuria itself or secondary to underlying diseases that predispose to bacteriuria. If it were established that bacteriuria definitely increased mortality, it would still be necessary to demonstrate that elimination of bacteriuria lengthened survival before therapy could be advocated in all cases.

With the following exceptions, we favor no therapy for asymptomatic bacteriuria at this time. In the pregnant patient, asymptomatic bacteriuria should be sought and treated (see Management of Bacteriuria During Pregnancy, below). In the presence of obstruction, urinary tract infection probably accelerates destruction of renal tissue and should be treated even if asymptomatic. In children, especially those younger that 5 years, vesicoureteral reflux is common, and in its presence urinary tract infection is likely to lead to renal damage and should be treated. Asymptomatic bacteriuria of lower urinary tract origin can usually be cured with short-course therapy (see Table 1). Asymptomatic bacteriuria of probable upper tract origin, as determined by relapse after short-course therapy, should be treated for 14 days when indicated.

MANAGEMENT OF BACTERIURIA DURING PREGNANCY

Bacteriuria during pregnancy is common (4 to 7 percent) and often asymptomatic. It is well documented that acute pyelonephritis leads to the premature onset of labor and grave risks to the fetus. Since 20 percent of pregnant patients with untreated bacteriuria subsequently develop acute pyelonephritis, asymptomatic bacteriuria during pregnancy should be sought and treated.

Pregnant women are the only group in whom screening for asymptomatic bacteriuria is advocated. Since 75 percent of women who develop bacteriuria during pregnancy are bacteriuric at the first prenatal visit, we recommend a screening urine culture at that time. If positive, a second culture with 10^5 or more cfu per milliliter confirms the diagnosis. In pregnant women, short-course therapy is generally effective (see Table 1). Follow-up cultures about 1 week after therapy are always necessary because of the need to assure eradication of bacteriuria and the consequent risk to the fetus, outlined above.

Table 1 outlines drugs and dosages. Most drugs given to pregnant women carry some risk for the fetus; therefore careful selection of drugs is mandatory. Drugs generally considered safe during pregnancy include ampicillin, amoxicillin, cephalosporins, nitrofurantoin, and sulfonamides. Sulfonamides should not be used near term because of increased risk of kernicterus. Norfloxacin and ciprofloxacin are not approved for use in pregnancy and childhood because of the theoretical risk of teratogenicity and malformations of cartilage.

Patients whose bacteriuria recurs after a short-course of therapy should be treated for 14 days. If a patient relapses after this, more prolonged therapy along with an ultrasound to evaluate for obstruction and/or stones is indicated. Following cure, monthly cultures are indicated for the duration of the pregnancy to detect reinfections.

MANAGEMENT OF CATHETER-RELATED BACTERIURIA

The incidence of bacteriuria in the catheterized patient with a closed, sterile-system indwelling catheter is 5 to 10 percent per day, and virtually everyone with a catheter for more than 30 days becomes bacteriuric. Catheter-induced bacteriuria increases the risk of morbidity and mortality secondary to bacteremia (2 to 4 percent of catheterized patients) (also see the chapter *Urinary Catheter-Associated Infection*). Since bacteriuria in the long-term catheterized patient is unavoidable and treatment of asymptomatic infection only predisposes to colonization with resistant organisms, treatment of asymptomatic bacteriuria in the catheterized patient is not advocated.

The most important preventative maneuvers are to not insert a catheter unless absolutely indicated and to remove the catheter as soon as possible. When this is not feasible, condom catheters for the unobstructed male and intermittent "in and out" catheterization of patients with neurogenic bladders are alternatives that carry definite but lower risks of infection. Prophylactic antibiotics, whether given systemically or placed topically around the catheter, do not decrease the acquisition of bacteriuria in the long-term catheterized patient and should not be used. Closed, sterile, nondisconnectable catheter systems should be used. Indwelling catheters should be changed whenever the flow of urine becomes obstructed.

When the catheterized patient becomes febrile or shows other signs of infection, sources other than the urinary tract should be considered. Obstruction of the catheter should also be ruled out. If the source of infection is likely to be the urinary tract, the infection should be treated with the full realization that relapse and/or reinfection is inevitable.

SUGGESTED READING

Boscia J, Kaye D. Asymptomatic bacteriuria in the elderly. Infect Dis Clin North Am 1987; 1:893–905.

Durbin W, Peter G. Management of urinary tract infections in infants and children. Pediatr Infect Dis 1984; 3:564–574.

Patterson T, Andriole V. Bacteriuria in pregnancy. Infect Dis Clin North Am 1987; 1:807–822.

Sobel J, Kaye D. Urinary tract infections. In:Mandell GL, Douglas RG Jr, Bennett JE, eds. Principles and practice of infectious diseases. New York: John Wiley and Sons, 1985.

Stamey T. Recurrent urinary tract infections in female patients: an overview. Rev Infect Dis 1987; 9(Suppl 2):S195–S210.

Warren J. Catheter-associated urinary tract infections. Infect Dis Clin North Am 1987; 1:823–854.

URINARY CATHETER–ASSOCIATED INFECTION

JOHN P. BURKE, M.D.
DAVID C. CLASSEN, M.D.

The urinary catheter is an ancient device that continues to have an indispensable role in medical care. It is employed in a wide variety of clinical circumstances to permit drainage of the anatomically or functionally obstructed urinary tract, to control drainage in incontinent patients, or to obtain precise measurement of urinary output. The most important clinical distinctions in the use of urinary catheters relate to the duration of use: brief in-and-out catheterization, short periods of indwelling catheterization (1 to 7 days) in postoperative patients, intermediate durations (7 to 30 days) in critically ill medical patients, and long-term (>30 days) catheterization in patients who are incontinent or have incorrectable obstruction of the bladder outlet.

The use of a urinary catheter always entails some risk of both infective and noninfective complications; the former includes the risk of death from gram-negative rod bacteremia and perhaps from other as yet undefined mechanisms. The sequelae of catheter-induced infections include acute and chronic pyelonephritis; perinephric, vesical, and urethral abscesses; bladder and renal stones; renal failure; polyposis and squamous metaplasia; and carcinoma of the bladder, suppurative epididymitis, and urethral strictures. In addition, patients with catheter-associated infections harbor a formidable reservoir of antibiotic-resistant pathogens that may be responsible for cross-infection in health care institutions.

Bacteriuria, i.e., literally the presence of bacteria in urine, is a necessary antecedent of these infectious complications. The normal urinary tract above the distal urethra is free of bacteria and able to clear rapidly small numbers of organisms that may be introduced through urethral trauma or instrumentation. The indwelling urinary catheter breaches this normal mucosal defense mechanism, not only by providing a continuing means of entry for bacteria, but also by serving as a foreign body that promotes infection through a number of additional mechanisms: (1) bacterial adherence to uroepithelial cells may be transiently increased; (2) biofilm production by bacteria adherent to the catheter itself may protect the bacterial colonies from systemic antibiotics as well as from host defenses; and (3) indwelling catheters with retention balloons incompletely empty the bladder, thereby compromising the physical removal of bacteria.

The usual organisms responsible for catheter-associated bacteriuria are gram-negative bacilli and enterococci derived from the fecal flora. Anaerobic bacteria, however, are rarely found. *Candida* and staphylococcal species may account for as many as one-third of the cases. A single infecting species is usual, but serial infections are common; most patients with long-term catheters have polymicrobial bacteriuria with spontaneous turnover of individual species.

There are only two pathways by which microorganisms commonly enter the catheterized urinary tract: through the catheter lumen or through the potential space between the urethral mucosa and the outside surface of the catheter. Candiduria and bacteriuria due to *Staphylococcus aureus* may result from bloodstream infection, but gram-negative rods virtually never infect the urinary tract by the hematogenous route.

Bacteriuria associated with indwelling catheterization may have diverse origins. For example, asymptomatic bacteriuria may precede placement of the catheter, or bacteriuria may arise from organisms pushed into the bladder during transurethral catheter insertion. Bacteriuria may also be acquired through ascent of organisms that are allowed to contaminate the inside of the drainage bag (from improper emptying) or the catheter tubing (from nonsterile disconnection of the catheter drainage tube junction). Finally, bacteria colonizing the perineum and the meatal surface may also migrate to the bladder in the pericatheter space, a pathway that appears to account for 70 percent or more of acquired bacteriurias during short and intermediate durations of catheterization.

Organisms, especially *Pseudomonas* and *Serratia* species, that enter through the intraluminal route are commonly acquired from transient carriage of gram-negative bacilli on the hands of personnel or on collection containers (exogenous infection) and may be transmitted by cross-infection. Organisms that enter through the pericatheter space are generally part of the patient's normal fecal and perineal flora (endogenous infection), although these organisms may become a part of the perineal and meatal flora as a consequence of hospitalization or as a result of cross-infection.

DIAGNOSIS

The diagnosis of catheter-associated bacteriuria in a patient with a standard Foley catheter with a retention balloon depends upon quantitative culture of urine obtained by aseptic needle aspiration from the distal catheter or through a sampling port on the drainage tube. The catheter should not be disconnected from the drainage tube in order to collect a specimen because contamination of the closed system may result.

For occasional sampling, one can avoid the need for clamping the tubing to collect urine by aspirating directly through the catheter itself distal to the channel for inflating the balloon using a 22- or 25-gauge needle. The site should be cleansed with an alcohol wipe before needle puncture, and aseptic precautions should be observed; disposable gloves should be worn and care taken to avoid needle-stick injury.

Despite the concern that continuous drainage through an indwelling catheter may not permit retention of urine in the bladder long enough for bacterial growth to yield high colony counts, especially for organisms with fastidious growth requirements, small numbers of bacteria introduced into the system do generally multiply rapidly and exceed 100,000 or more colonies per milliliter in a day or two in patients not receiving systemic antibiotics. The criterion selected to define bacteriuria depends largely on the purpose to be served. Lower colony counts are commonly selected as a breakpoint in clinical trials of catheter care in order to provide greater sensitivity for detection. Theoretically, any number of bacteria obtained by aspiration should be considered significant. In clinical practice and especially in long-term catheterized patients, the criterion of 100,000 or more colony-forming units (cfu) is quite satisfactory.

Caution in interpreting colony counts is necessary, however, because some rapid tests for bacteriuria are insensitive to low colony counts, and bacteremia does occasionally occur in those with colony counts of less than 100,000 per milliliter. Moreover, colony counts of urine from long-term catheters may not accurately reflect the density of bladder bacteriuria, and some suggest that in these patients the catheter should be changed before a specimen is obtained for culture.

No reliable criteria exist to distinguish bladder colonization from infection. Most patients with catheter-associated bacteriuria also have pyuria and remain asymptomatic. A long-term catheterization patient almost always has pyuria and bacteriuria. Culture of the tip of the Foley catheter has no role in the diagnosis of infection.

PREVENTION OF INFECTION

Although urinary tract infection is an inevitable consequence of long-term catheterization, bacteriuria can be successfully avoided in the majority of patients with short periods of catheterization by the correct use of techniques for closed sterile urinary drainage. In those with intermediate durations, bacteriuria can be successfully postponed. While the benefits of delaying the onset of bacteriuria have not been well defined, complicated infections and urosepsis may be less common and bacteriuria may be better tolerated once the acute stage of the underlying illness has resolved. The prompt removal of catheters that are no longer necessary may result in true prevention. Moreover, cross-infection with antibiotic-resistant organisms can be successfully prevented regardless of the duration of catheterization and is a worthwhile clinical goal.

Nearly all of the commercially available systems for urinary drainage are closed, i.e., the drainage tube is fused to a vented collection bag so that the urine is not exposed to air, and the distal end of the tube is not exposed to the reservoir of urine in the bag. The introduction and widespread use of closed sterile drainage was a major advance and has undoubtedly prevented thousands of deaths from gram-negative bacteremia in the past 25 years. Closed drainage systems represent a passive infection control measure that requires little effort by personnel. However, closed systems must be opened, for example, when urine is emptied from the bag or when the catheter is disconnected from the system for irrigation or by accident.

Unfortunately, the principles of closed drainage are not well understood by all health care workers, and errors in the care of closed systems are commonplace. Improper handling can introduce bacteria that can ascend to the bladder, especially when backflow of urine occurs if the bag is raised above the bladder or placed beside the patient being transported, for example, to the radiology department. Regular and continuing in-service education of personnel, emphasizing the principles of closed drainage, is obviously necessary but appears to hold little promise for major reductions in the rate of catheter-associated bacteriuria, in part because the majority of infections appear to result from the pericatheter pathway. Periodic culture studies as recommended by Kunin (see Suggested Reading) may help individual institutions identify excessive rates of bacteriuria and improper catheter care.

Efforts to block the periurethral pathway of infection by the frequent application of topical antimicrobial agents to the meatal surface have not been cost effective, and the use of povidone-iodine preparations was associated with an increased incidence of bacteriuria in one controlled study.

At present, removal of crusts and debris from the external surface of the catheter, especially around the meatal insertion site, with plain soap and a washcloth during daily bathing is generally recommended and may help to reduce urethral irritation.

Disconnections of the catheter drainage tube can be discouraged by the application of taped seals to the junction, and contamination of the drainage bag can be prevented by the use of disposable gloves for handling the outflow spigot. Other adjuncts to closed drainage have generally been unsuccessful or have had questionable cost benefits.

Modifications of closed drainage have included coating or impregnation of the catheter with proprietary compounds to inhibit bacterial adherence or growth. One such coating using silver oxide has shown promising results in a randomized controlled trial in selected patients; it is currently being evaluated in more broadly representative hospitalized patients. The instillation of antibacterial substances into the drainage bag remains controversial but may have some efficacy in settings where contamination of bags is frequent. This latter approach may become more practical as longer-acting agents are developed so that frequent instillations are not needed. In addition, disinfection of the drainage bag urine could eliminate a reservoir for potential cross-infection.

Urinary drainage equipment is marketed in an aggressively competitive environment in which infection control properties are stressed, usually without supporting clinical evidence of efficacy. Currently the selection of such equipment should be based on factors other than extravagant and unsupported claims for prevention of infection; cost and acceptability to nursing personnel should be the decisive factors.

There seems to be no justification for the use of expensive silicone-coated catheters for patients with brief or intermediate durations of catheterization, although they may be associated with less encrustation, blockage, urethritis, and discomfort with longer-term use. No set interval should be adopted for changing the catheter; in general, patients with long-term catheters will require changing at monthly intervals, but broad individual variation occurs and the "catheter life" of each patient should be determined by examining the removed catheter for encrustations and blocked flow.

The smallest suitable catheter diameter should be selected, and larger catheters are usually needed only for postoperative urologic patients who are passing blood clots. The balloon volume should also be small (5 to 10 ml) since forcible removal of catheters with 30-ml balloons can occur with greater resulting urethral trauma.

In 1983 the Centers for Disease Control (Atlanta) published guidelines for the prevention of catheter-associated infections that represented a consensus of experts and that remain relevant today. Particularly noteworthy is the admonition to catheterize only when necessary and then using correct aseptic technique and closed drainage. Alternatives to indwelling catheterization such as condom catheters, incontinence clothing, or intermittent catheterization should be utilized when possible. At times, the risk of indwelling catheterization may be judged to be more acceptable than the nursing problems associated with incontinence, especially when tissue maceration and decubitus ulcers are present.

The use of suprapubic catheter placement has become prevalent in postoperative gynecologic procedures and appears to be associated with a lower risk of bacteriuria, improved patient comfort, and more rapid restoration of normal voiding mechanisms. Techniques have also been developed for the "nonoperative" placement of small-bore suprapubic catheters without retention balloons. However, further evaluation of the safety, efficacy, and benefits of this approach is needed.

The use of systemic antimicrobial agents to prevent catheter-associated bacteriuria has generally been condemned because of the benign nature of most of these infections and because of the cost, adverse effects, and selection of resistant organisms associated with antibiotic use. A reduced incidence of bacteriuria during the first 4 days of catheterization has been found in patients receiving systemic antibiotics. However, their use for this purpose cannot be recommended except possibly in certain high-risk or immunocompromised patients in whom a short duration of catheterization is anticipated. Suitably controlled studies to define the optimal agents, regimens, and, if present, cost benefits are currently needed. At present, no prophylactic antimicrobial regimen has been found to prevent infection in long-term catheterized patients. Methenamine preparations are not effective in the prevention or treatment of bacteriuria in catheterized patients but may have a role in reducing encrustations and blockage of catheters (by a mechanism unrelated to its antibacterial property), thereby lengthening the interval between required catheter changes in selected patients.

TREATMENT

In the past, investigators have directed less attention to the management than to the prevention of catheter-associated bacteriuria. Consequently, there is a dearth of well-controlled trials to serve as a basis for specific recommendations, in contrast to the many therapeutic trials in other urinary tract infection syndromes. Nonetheless, there is a consensus that catheter-associated bacteriuria should not be treated with systemic antimicrobial agents as long as the patient remains catheterized and asymptomatic.

The basis for this view is that treatment is effective only in making the urine culture-negative while the antibiotic is being given but not in eliminating bacterial colonies adherent to the catheter and protected by the bacterial glycocalyx from exposure to the antibiotic. Relapse of bacteriuria following treatment usually occurs. Replacement of the catheter and drainage bag with a new sterile system within 24 to 48 hours after therapy has begun is a potentially useful strategy that has been incompletely evaluated.

Bacteremia may occur at any time during indwelling catheterization and not only at times of catheter insertion or change. Moreover, fever in a patient with an indwelling catheter should not be attributed to bacteriuria unless other potential causes have been evaluated. Blood and urine specimens should be obtained for culture (a single blood culture should suffice in most instances), and the patient should be empirically treated for bacteremia, usually with either an aminoglycoside or an expanded-spectrum β-lactam antibiotic (see the chapter *Gram-Negative Rod Bacteremia*).

In the nonneutropenic patient who is not in septic shock, there is no adequate justification for the use of combination antimicrobic regimens. However, microscopic examination of a Gram-stained urine specimen can be helpful in selecting empiric therapy, for example, by suggesting the presence of enterococci and the use of ampicillin, either alone or in combination with gentamicin.

A common clinical problem is colonization by yeast, especially in patients receiving systemic antimicrobics. Most often, these patients do not develop invasive disease, and the "infection" clears with removal of the catheter. However, in selected patients, continuous irrigation with amphotericin B (50 mg per liter of sterile water per day) through a triple-lumen catheter for 5 days has been associated with resolution of candiduria and is preferable to systemic antifungal treatment.

Daily monitoring of urine cultures from patients with short or intermediate durations of catheterization has not proved to be a useful strategy to permit the treatment of bacteriuria and, thereby, the prevention of bacteremia. Nonetheless, it seems reasonable to culture the urine at the time of catheter insertion and again immediately before its removal in order to identify asymptomatic infections that require follow-up. In most patients bacteriuria will spontaneously clear after the catheter is removed, but the physician's goal should be to see that the now-noncatheterized urinary tract is left sterile and not to rely on a normal urinalysis or the absence of symptoms for this assurance. A follow-up urine culture 1 to 2 weeks after catheter removal will help to identify persistently bacteriuric patients who are candidates for treatment.

A further indication for urine culture in an asymptomatic catheterized patient occurs when a urologic operation or a surgical procedure involving the placement of prosthetic material or an organ transplant is planned. Systemic antimicrobial treatment selected on the basis of culture and susceptibility data may help to reduce the risk of bacteremia originating from the urinary tract in these patients.

Cultures of urine from asymptomatic long-term catheterized patients may, on the other hand, invite unnecessary antibiotic treatment and lead to antibiotic-resistant infections, adverse effects from the drugs used, and increased costs.

The complications of bacteriuria in long-term catheterized patients are often associated with obstruction and/or stones. Intermittent irrigation, either with normal saline or with antimicrobial solutions, such as 0.25 percent acetic acid, has not proved useful in preventing obstructions or in eradicating established bacteriuria.

Patients with long-term catheters who become febrile ($\geq$ 38.9°C) should be managed as above for possible bacteremia and should also be evaluated for catheter obstruction and local periurethral infection. Patients with recurrent high fevers, bacteremia, or increasing renal dysfunction should be evaluated for urinary tract stones. For such patients, operative intervention may be required.

SUGGESTED READING

Kunin CM. Care of the urinary catheter. In: Detection, prevention and management of urinary tract infections. 4th ed. Philadelphia: Lea & Febiger, 1987:245.

Slade N, Gillespie WA. The urinary tract and the catheter. Infection and other problems. New York: John Wiley & Sons, 1985.

Warren JW. Catheter-associated urinary tract infections. Infect Dis Clin North Am 1987; 1:823–854.

GRAM-NEGATIVE ROD BACTEREMIA

DONALD E. CRAVEN, M.D.
WILLIAM R. McCABE, M.D.

Gram-negative rod bacteremia connotes the isolation of gram-negative bacilli from blood cultures. This term is usually reserved for bacteremia caused by members of the families Enterobacteriaceae and Pseudomonadaceae; *Salmonella* and *Haemophilus* species are not included. By comparison, *gram-negative rod sepsis* is a term often used to described a clinical condition characterized by fever, chills, and impaired tissue perfusion, irrespective of whether bacteremia has been documented.

Gram-negative rod bacteremia was uncommon in the preantibiotic era, but since 1950 it has become one of the commonest infectious disease problems in medical centers throughout the United States. Rates of bacteremia as high as one episode per 100 hospital admissions have been reported in university teaching hospitals, but lower rates have been reported from smaller community hospitals. Common etiologic agents include *Escherichia coli*, species of *Klebsiella, Enterobacter, Serratia, Proteus*, and *Bacteroides*, as well as *Pseudomonas aeruginosa*. Fifteen to 20 percent of gram-negative bacteremias are mixed or polymicrobial. Fatality rates for gram-negative rod bacteremia vary depending on the patient's underlying disease, but overall fatality rates are in the range of 25 percent.

EPIDEMIOLOGY

Gram-negative bacillemia may be categorized as hospital-acquired (nosocomial) or community-acquired. Community-acquired bacteremia usually originates from the genitourinary or gastrointestinal tracts and is frequently caused by *E. coli* sensitive to many antibiotics. Some "community-acquired" bacteremias, acquired during earlier hospitalization or during residence in nursing homes, may be caused by bacteria that are more antibiotic resistant. Hospital-acquired infections that account for approximately 75 percent of cases, may originate from the urinary tract, gastrointestinal tract, respiratory tract, skin, or mucous membranes. Nosocomial bacteremia may be associated with prior surgery or the use of invasive devices and are generally caused by more antibiotic-resistant species of bacteria.

The increasing frequency of gram-negative rod bacteremia over the last three decades can be attributed to several factors. Enteric gram-negative rod bacilli are relatively avirulent and have limited invasive capacity in the normal host, but they comprise the major aerobic flora of the gastrointestinal and female urogenital tract and readily colonize the hospital environment. Nosocomial gram-negative bacilli are known for antibiotic resistance. *P. aeruginosa* is inherently resistant to many antibiotics, whereas other species of gram-negative bacilli acquire antimicrobial resistance from plasmids or R-factors. Plasmids are extrachromosomal fragments of DNA that may rapidly transmit resistance to several antibiotics. Gram-negative bacilli resistant to multiple antimicrobial agents are a continuous problem in hospitals.

The increasing incidence of gram-negative bacteremia over the last 30 years also reflects changes in medical management and the hospital population (Table 1). Patients are older and often have chronic disease. Radical surgery, immunosuppressive therapy, and extensive use of devices that violate natural host barriers have become an integral part of modern medical management.

CLINICAL MANIFESTATIONS

The clinical manifestations of gram-negative rod bacteremia are protean and may vary from fulminant and lethal disease to infections that may go unrecognized for days. Clinical findings suggestive of gram-negative rod bacteremia are shown in Table 2. Many of these symptoms and clinical signs are nonspecific. Therefore, it is imperative to maintain a high index of suspicion and draw blood for cultures whenever bacteremia is suspected.

The classic triad of shaking chills, high fever, and hypotension occurs only in approximately one-third of patients. Fever, although a nonspecific sign, is usually present unless the patient is elderly, uremic, or receiving treatment with corticosteroids. In patients with leukemia or gastrointestinal disease, or those who have had genitourinary tract manipulation, fever may be the only indication of bacteremia.

TABLE 1 Factors That Predispose to Development of Gram-Negative Rod Bacteremia

Underlying host diseases
Diabetes mellitus
Cancer
Congestive heart failure
Hepatic disease
Renal failure
Granulocytopenia
Thermal injury
Multiple organ failure
Devices
Intravascular catheters (peripheral, central, tunneled, and arterial)
Indwelling bladder catheter
Tracheostomy
Endotracheal tube
Nebulization equipment
Prosthetic devices
Treatment factors
Surgery
Steroids
Cytotoxic drugs
Irradiation

TABLE 2 Clinical Manifestations of Gram-Negative Rod Bacteremia

Fever, chills, hypotension
Fever alone (in a patient with a malignancy, hematologic disorder, urinary tract disease, an intravenous or urinary tract catheters)
Hypotension*
Tachypnea, hyperpnea, and respiratory alkalosis*
Change in mental status (confusion, stupor, agitation)*
Oliguria or anuria*
Acidosis*
Hypothermia*
Thrombocytopenia*
Disseminated intravascular coagulation*
Adult respiratory distress syndrome*
Evidence of a urinary tract or pulmonary infection

*Without an alternative cause.

Approximately 40 to 50 percent of patients with bacteremia develop shock—defined as a decrease in blood pressure to 90/60 mm Hg or less. Shock usually occurs 4 to 10 hours after the initial signs of bacteremia caused by gram-negative bacilli. Because of the high frequency of shock associated with gram-negative rod bacteremia, it is essential that the etiology of any episode of shock be clearly elucidated and the possibility of bacteremia considered.

Two types of hemodynamic alterations have been noted in patients with gram-negative rod bacteremia. "Warm shock" is characterized by evidence of a hyperdynamic circulation. Increased cardiac output with decreased peripheral resistance is characteristically associated with a high or normal central venous pressure, hyperventilation, and lactate accumulation in the initial phase of sepsis. Patients in "cold shock" are usually pale, are cyanotic, and have cold and clammy extremities. Cold shock tends to occur late in the course of septic shock. Physiologic alterations in cold shock include decreased cardiac output, increased peripheral vascular resistance associated with decreased central venous pressure, hyperventilation, and lactate accumulation. Respiratory alkalosis usually occurs early and may evolve to a metabolic acidosis, which carries a poorer prognosis.

The combination of hyperpnea, tachypnea, and respiratory alkalosis in the absence of pulmonary abnormalities is an important early clinical sign of bacteremia. In elderly patients, unexplained oliguria, increased confusion, or stupor also may be the only signs of sepsis.

Leukocytosis is common, although some patients may manifest normal or low leukocyte counts. Gram-negative rod bacteremia is a frequent complication of antineoplastic chemotherapy producing granulocytopenia (less than 1,000 neutrophils per cubic millimeter). Neutropenia secondary to bacteremia is an infrequent consequence in patients with normal hematopoietic function.

Mild to moderate thrombocytopenia occurs in about 70 percent of patients. Disseminated intravascular coagulation (DIC), characterized by decreased levels of clotting factors II, V, and VIII, together with hypofibrinogenemia, thrombocytopenia, and circulating fibrin split products is found in approximately 12 percent of patients but only about one-fourth of these patients exhibit clinical manifestations attributable to DIC.

PATHOPHYSIOLOGY

Endotoxin, or lipopolysaccharide (LPS), a major constituent of the gram-negative cell envelope, is generally thought to initiate the changes observed during bacteremia. However, several careful experimental and clinical studies have indicated that factors other than free endotoxin liberated from the bacterial cell wall contribute to the manifestations of such infections. Irrespective of the role of endotoxin, a variety of vasoactive materials have been implicated as potential mediators of the circulatory changes observed in bacteremic shock. These include endogenous pyrogen (interleukin-1), Hageman factor, plasmin, complement components, kinins, serotonin, histamine, prostaglandins, endorphins, catecholamines (epinephrine and norepinephrine), and tumor necrosis factor (cachectin). However, precise delineation of the role and interaction of these mediators in human disease is limited.

Available evidence suggests that the activation of the coagulation, fibrinolysis, kinin, and complement systems may contribute to the hemodynamic and other pathophysiologic alterations seen in gram-negative rod bacteremia. Activation of Hageman factor (Factor XII) by either intact bacilli or endotoxin results in sequential activation of the intrinsic coagulation system and the conversion of plasminogen to plasmin. Circulating gram-negative bacilli, endotoxin, and plasmin are all capable of activating the complement system through the classical or alternate pathways. Anaphylatoxins (C3a and C5a) cause peripheral vasodilation and increased vascular permeability. Plasmin and activated Hageman factor also activate the kinin pathway, resulting in vascular permeability and early peripheral vasodilatation in shock. Bradykinin, in turn, increases the release of prostaglandins PGE_2 and PGF_2.

Endotoxin may also release prostaglandins, prostacycline, or thromboxane. Studies have suggested that prostaglandins and endorphins may contribute to the pathogenesis of septic shock. Inhibitors of prostaglandin synthesis such as ibuprofen and indomethacin have ameliorated endotoxin-induced hypotension in experimental animals and humans.

Endorphins may also contribute to the pathogenesis of shock. The endorphin antagonist noxalone appears to reduce hypotension in animals. One uncontrolled clinical study of patients in shock reported improvement in blood pressure following the intravenous administration of 1.2 mg of the endorphin inhibitor naloxone, but a recent, randomized, placebo-controlled clinical study of patients in septic shock at our institution was unable to confirm any beneficial effect of this dose of naloxone in septic shock.

Cytokines are soluble proteins from stimulated cells that are important mediators of inflammatory response during gram-negative rod bacteremia. Recent interest has been directed at tumor necrosis factor, a 17,000-dalton cytokine released from macrophages that appears to reproduce many of the clinical and metabolic changes observed in gram-negative rod bacteremia and sepsis. Furthermore, antibody to tumor necrosis factor appears to protect animals against shock and death following the administration of endotoxin. Recent data in humans indicate that endotoxin also elicits detectable tumor necrosis factor, which is accompanied by fever, tachycardia, and systemic symptoms, but further studies are needed to define more clearly its role in the pathogenesis of septic shock.

ANTIBIOTIC TREATMENT

Because of the nature of the disease, therapy for gram-negative rod bacteremia is usually initiated before the etiologic agent and antibiotic sensitivities are known. Initial treatment should be based on the type of infection (community-acquired or nosocomial), the probable site of infection, and the bacterial flora residing at that site. Basic principles of management include prompt recognition of the clinical signs and symptoms of bacteremia and identification of the source of infection. Blood cultures, Gram stains, and cultures of infected sites should be performed to identify the etiologic agent and determine antibiotic sensitivity. Fluids, oxygen, and adequate doses of an appropriate antibiotic should be administered promptly. In addition, management of complications such as shock, hypoxia, and hemorrhage is of paramount importance. Any abscess should be drained and infected foreign bodies removed as soon as possible.

Once the source of infection is identified, appropriate antimicrobial therapy designed to cover all the pathogenic flora at that site should be instituted (Table 3). Aminoglycosides such as gentamicin, tobramycin, or amikacin have a broad spectrum of activity against aerobic gram-negative bacilli, including *P. aeruginosa*. The type of aminoglycoside selected (Table 4) will depend on the condition of the patient, the type and location of infection, and the specific antibiotic resistance pattern of the hospital flora. At Boston City Hospital we presently

TABLE 3 Initial Choice of Antibiotics for Suspected Gram-Negative Rod Bacteremia by Site of Infection

Site of Infection	*Likely Etiologic Agent*	*Initial Antibiotic of Choice*
Urinary tract: Community-acquired	*E. coli* *K pneumoniae* *P. mirabilis*	Aminoglycoside* *or* Cephalosporin†‡
Urinary tract: Hospital-acquired	*K. pneumoniae* *Proteus* species *P. aeruginosa*	Aminoglycoside* *or* Aztreonam *or* Third-generation cephalosporin‡
Gastrointestinal tract: Colon	*E. coli* *Bacteroides* species *K. pneumoniae* *Proteus* species *P. aeruginosa*	Aminoglycoside* *or* Aztreonam *plus* Clindamycin *or* Metronidazole *or* Cefoxitin
Biliary tract	*E. coli* *K. pneumoniae* *Proteus species*	Aminoglycoside* *plus* Ampicillin
Female reproductive tract:	*E. coli* *K. pneumoniae* *Bacteroides* species	Aminoglycoside* *plus* Clindamycin *or* Cefoxitin alone
Lower respiratory tract: (patient with tracheostomy or endotracheal tube)	*P. aeruginosa* *Acinetobacter* species *Serratia* species *E. coli* *K. pneumoniae*	Aminoglycoside* *or* Aztreonam *plus* Third-generation cephalosporin‡

Table continues on the following page

TABLE 3 *Continued*

Site of Infection	*Likely Etiologic Agent*	*Initial Antibiotic of Choice*
Aspiration (in hospital)	*E. coli* *Bacteroides* species *Fusobacterium* species *K. pneumoniae* *Acinetobacter* species *Serratia* species	Aminoglycoside* *or* Aztreonam *plus* Penicillin *or* Clindamycin
Decubitus ulcers	*E. coli* *Bacteroides* species *K. pneumoniae* *Proteus* species *P. aeruginosa* *Enterobacter* species	Aminoglycoside* *or* Aztreonam *plus* Clindamycin *or* Cefoxitin *or* Third-generation cephalosporin‡
Burns	*P. aeruginosa* *Enterobacter* species	Aminoglycoside* *or* Aztreonam *or* Aminoglycoside* *plus* Carbenicillin§ *or* Third-generation cephalosporin‡
Intravascular device	*P. aeruginosa* *Acinetobacter* species *Serratia* species	Aminoglycoside* *or* Aztreonam *or* Third-generation cephalosporin‡
Neutropenic patient (< 100 PMN/mm^3)	*E. coli* *Klebsiella* species *P. aeruginosa*	Aminoglycoside* *plus* Carbenicillin§

* Because of their toxicity, aminoglycosides may be replaced by aztreonam or third-generation cephalosporins such as cefotaxime, ceftriaxone, or ceftazidime. An initial loading dose for amikacin = 8 mg/kg, gentamicin = 2 mg/kg, or tobramycin = 2 mg/kg. Modify dosage in patients with renal insufficiency. Reevaluate antibiotic regimen after culture and sensitivity data are available and treat with least toxic drug to which the organism is sensitive.

† Patients having a recent hospitalization or indwelling bladder catheters or residents of nursing homes should initially receive an aminoglycoside.

‡ If the organism is sensitive. Resistant nosocomial gram-negative bacilli or *P. aeruginosa* bacteremia may be treated with an aminoglycoside or aztreonam. Possible third-generation cephalosporins include cefotaxime, cefoperazone, ceftazidime and ceftriaxone.

§ Ticarcillin, mezlocillin, azlocillin, or piperacillin may be used interchangeably with carbenicillin.

recommend gentamicin for initial coverage of gram-negative rods because it is less expensive and the number of gentamicin-resistant gram-negative bacilli is low. Initial therapy with tobramycin or amikacin may be more appropriate in other hospitals, depending on the general patterns of bacterial resistance. Doses of aminoglycosides should be altered for patients with renal failure, and blood levels should be monitored in a person who has impaired renal function or no response to therapy, or in whom long-term therapy is required. Because of their well-known ototoxicity and nephrotoxicity, aminoglycosides may be replaced by less toxic antibiotics if the organism is sensitive.

Infections originating from the gastrointestinal tract or the female reproductive tract may involve aerobic gram-negative bacilli and anaerobic organisms such as *Bacteroides fragilis*. For this reason, combinations of antibiotics such as an aminoglycoside (chosen as indicated above) and clindamycin or metronidazole would be indicated for initial therapy.

A cephalosporin may be used for initial therapy only if the organism is likely to be susceptible. First-generation cephalosporins—such as cephalothin or cefazolin—have activity against community strains of *E. coli*, *Klebsiella pneumoniae*, and *Proteus mirabilis*, but some strains are resistant and activity is lacking against many of the

TABLE 4 Parenteral Antibiotics That May Be Prescribed for the Treatment of Gram-Negative Rod Bacteremia

Antibiotic	*Dose**	*Comments*
Aminoglycosides		
Gentamicin	1.7 mg/kg IM or IV q8h	Aminoglycosides have a good spectrum against aerobic gram-negative bacilli, including *P. aeruginosa*
Tobramycin	1.7 mg/kg IM or IV q8h	
Amikacin	7.5 mg/kg IM or IV q12h	
Cephalosporins		
First-generation		
Cephalothin	2 g IV q4h	Activity limited to *E. coli, K. pneumoniae,* and *P. mirabilus*; should not be used unless sensitivity of organism is known
Cefazolin	2 g IV q8h	
Cephradine	2 g IV q6h	
Cephapirin	2 g IV q4h	
Second-generation		
Cefoxitin	2 g IV q4h	Cefoxitin provides good coverage against *B. fragilis* and most aerobic gram-negative bacilli except *P. aeruginosa*
Cefamandole	2 g IV q4h	
Third-generation		
Cefotaxime	2 g IV q4h	Third-generation cephalosporins have broad-spectrum activity against *P. aeruginosa*; Cefoperazone and ceftazidime have good activity.
Cefoperazone	3 g IV q6h	
Ceftriaxone	1 g IV q12h	
Ceftazidime	2 g IV q8h	
Extended-spectrum penicillins		
Carbenicillin	5 g IV q4h	Useful in combination with an aminoglycoside for treating *P. aeruginosa* bacteremia or for treating patients with neutropenia
Ticarcillin	3 g IV q4h	
Piperacillin	3 g IV q4h	
Mezlocillin	3 g IV q4h	
Azlocillin	3 g IV q4h	
Monobactams		
Aztreonam	2 g IV q8h	Good coverage for gram-negative bacilli, including *P. aeruginosa*
Other beta-lactams		
Imipenem-cilastatin	500 mg of each drug IV q6h	Good coverage for aerobic gram-negative bacilli and *B. fragilis*
Trimethoprim-sulfamethoxazole	2 ampules IV q8h	Effective against many resistant nosocomial gram-negative bacilli

* Doses are the maximum for patients with bacteremia and normal renal flow. Doses should be adjusted after organism and antibiotic activity are known or if patient has impaired renal function.

nosocomial gram-negative bacilli, making this group of agents inappropriate for initial therapy of suspected gram-negative bacteremia. Second-generation cephalosporins, such as cefoxitin, have a greater spectrum of activity against aerobic gram-negative bacilli. Cefoxitin also has activity against *B. fragilis*, but second-generation cephalosporins have no activity against *P. aeruginosa*. Third-generation cephalosporins—such as cefotaxime, ceftriaxone, ceftazidime, and cefoperazone—have activity against a variety of enteric gram-negative bacilli. Cefoperazone and ceftazidime have activity against *P. aeruginosa*. These antibiotics have a high therapeutic-toxicity ratio and serum blood levels do not need to be monitored. Consequently, they are easier to use and are less toxic than aminoglycosides.

Extended-spectrum penicillins—such as ticarcillin, carbenicillin, azlocillin, mezlocillin, and piperacillin—are generally used in combination with an aminoglycoside for treating patients with neutropenia or serious infections caused by *P. aeruginosa*. It should be emphasized that once the sensitivities of the offending organism are known, the least toxic and least expensive antibiotic to which the organism is sensitive should be prescribed. The duration of therapy depends on the source of infection. In general, antibiotics should be continued for a minimum of 5 afebrile days or longer if a local source of infection persists.

Aztreonam is a monobactam that has broad-spectrum activity against all aerobic gram-negative bacilli except *Acinetobacter* species. Aztreonam has activity similar to the aminoglycosides but is less toxic and more expensive.

Imipenem-cilastatin has a wide spectrum of activity against anaerobic and aerobic gram-negative bacilli as well as many gram-positive bacteria. It may be particularly useful for treating some of the more resistant nosocomial pathogens but has a limited spectrum against strains of *P. aeruginosa*.

More recently, the oral quinolone antibiotics have been released, which have excellent activity against most aerobic gram-negative bacilli, and intravenous preparations are being evaluated in clinical trials. Development of resistance may occur and some strains of *P. aeruginosa* may be resistant.

MANAGEMENT OF SHOCK

Shock is the most frequent complication of gram-negative rod bacteremia. Shock in patients with gram-negative rod bacteremia is associated with a sevenfold increase in fatality. Therefore, goals for treating patients with gram-negative rod bacteremia include early diagnosis and therapy to prevent shock and rapid correction of any hemodynamic alterations that occur. Optimal care requires the prompt institution of appropriate antibiotics as well as maintenance of an adequate intravascular volume. A central venous pressure (CVP) catheter or a Swan-Ganz catheter inserted to measure pulmonary artery wedge pressure (PAWP) are valuable aids for monitoring intravascular fluid expansion. Furthermore, an indwelling bladder catheter (using sterile precautions and a closed drainage system) is usually inserted to measure urinary output and renal perfusion.

Initially fluid (5 percent dextrose in normal saline) should be infused at a rate of 10 to 20 ml per minute for 10 to 15 minutes. If the CVP or PAWP does not increase by a level of 5 cm H_2O or 2 mm Hg, respectively, further fluid should be administered. If the need for further fluid volume is established, either colloid or crystalloid may be used at a rate of 10 to 20 ml per minute. Signs of fluid overload and cardiac decompensation include a sudden progressive increase in the CVP of more than 5 cm H_2O, a CVP of more than 12 to 14 cm H_2O, or an increase of PAWP of more than 8 mm Hg or an absolute level of 8 to 12 mm Hg.

If volume expansion does not produce prompt improvement, vasoactive agents should be added to increase cardiac output further. Dopamine is usually given by constant infusion in a dose of 2 to 20 μg per kilogram per minute. If there is no response to dopamine, isoproterenol in a dose of 2 to 8 μg per minute or dobutamine in a dose of 2 to 15 μg per kilogram per minute should be instituted to enhance cardiac output and increase urine output.

In the past, many clinicians have administered corticosteroids to patients in septic shock, but two recent

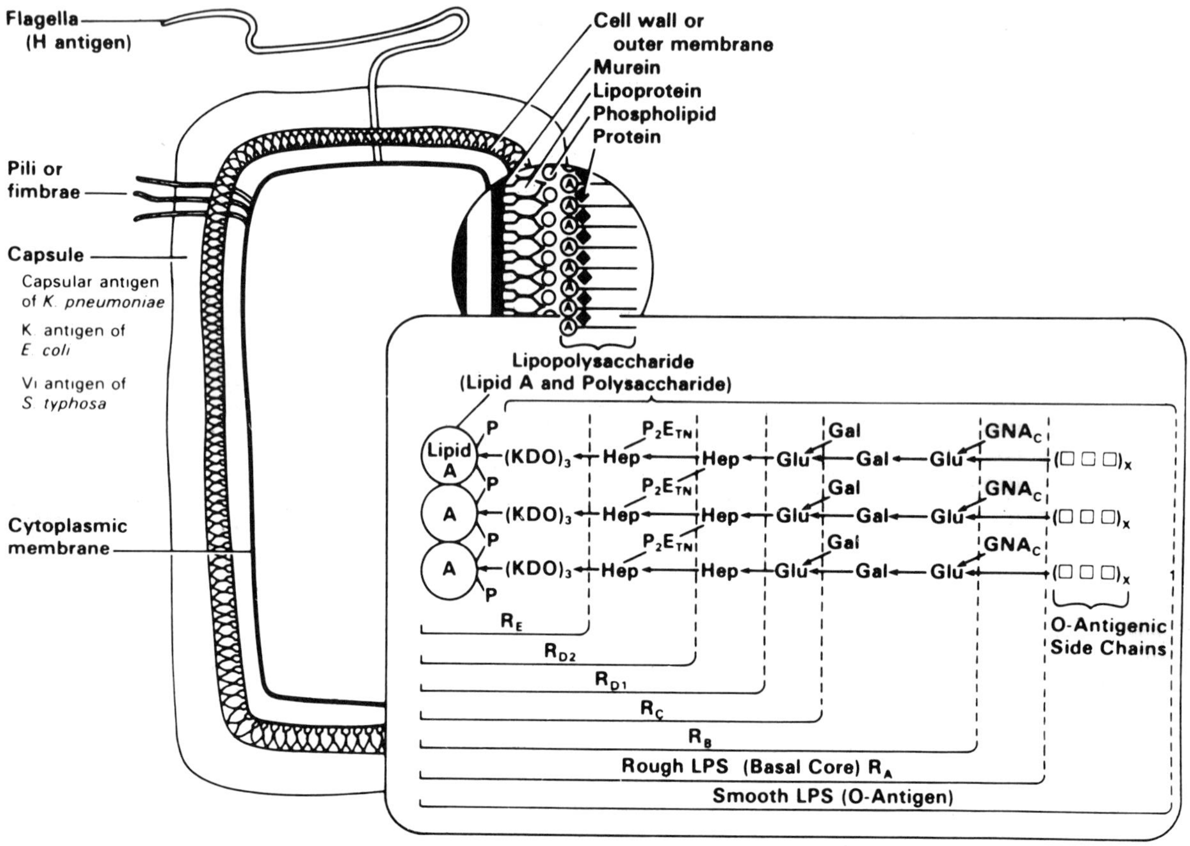

Figure 1 Schematic depiction of structure and antigens of gram-negative bacilli and the chemical structure of the lipopolysaccharide (LPS) of smooth (S) and rough (R) Salmonella. R mutants, Ra, Rb, Rc, Rd_1 Rd_2, and Re are shown in order of increasing roughness produced by progressive deletion of sugars of the core portion of LPS. GNAc = N-acetylglucosamine; Glu = Glucose; Gal = Galactose; Hep = Heptose; KDO = 2-keto 3-deoxyoctulosonate; P = Phosphate. (From McCabe WR. Endotoxin: microbial, chemical, pathophysiological, and clinical correlation. In: Weinstein L, Fields BN, eds. Seminars in infectious disease. New York: Thieme and Stratton, 1980.)

double-blind placebo-controlled studies demonstrated that steroids were no more effective than placebo. Neither study found any beneficial effect in reversing hypotension or increasing survival. Furthermore, there was a suggestion that the patients treated with steroids had more complications with bacterial infections than the patients receiving placebo. Therefore, steroids should only be administered to patients with gram-negative rod bacteremia if there is a suspicion of adrenal insufficiency.

Clinical evidence of disseminated intravascular coagulation (DIC) occurs in less than 5 percent of patients with gram-negative bacteremia, and these patients are invariably in shock. Heparin has been suggested for treatment, but enthusiasm for heparin therapy must be tempered by evidence that such treatment failed to reduce fatalities in either experimental models or humans despite improvement in coagulation factors. For treatment of DIC, we suggest that maximal efforts be directed at replacing blood products and reversing the cause of shock.

Hypoxia occurs frequently in septic shock, and monitoring of arterial blood gases is essential to maintain proper tissue oxygenation. Patients who develop adult respiratory distress syndrome (ARDS) often require mechanical ventilation with a volume-cycled ventilator. Patients who have a progressive decrease in their PaO_2 despite the use of increasing oxygen concentrations, may benefit from positive end-expiratory pressure (PEEP).

Oliguric renal failure is another complication of septic shock. If the urine flow is less than 30 ml per hour, the patient should be treated with an intravenous infusion of 12.5 g of mannitol over 5 minutes. If there is no response, this dose should be repeated in 2 hours. Individuals failing to respond to mannitol can be given furosemide intravenously.

IMMUNIZATION AND PREVENTION

The search for an effective vaccine against gram-negative rod bacteremia has been limited by the large number of distinct organisms causing disease. However, different species of gram-negative bacilli share common antigens present in the core region (Ra-Re) of the lipopolysaccharide in the outer membrane (Fig. 1). There is no program for actively vaccinating humans at risk for gram-negative rod bacteremia. However, hyperimmune serum obtained from persons following immunization with an Rc mutant of *E. coli* has demonstrated increased survival rates of patients in septic shock compared with a controlled group of patients given preimmune serum. Further, multicenter trials of hyperimmune monoclonal antibodies directed against the lipid A portion of the lipopolysaccharide are in progress. Although more research is needed, there may be a role for immunotherapy in addition to antibiotic therapy for the treatment of gram-negative rod sepsis.

Specific efforts should be directed at preventing gram-negative rod bacteremia. Since the majority of gram-negative rod bacteremias are nosocomial in origin, the use of proper handwashing, consideration of barrier precautions in the critical care unit, along with careful evaluation of the need for and care of invasive devices such as the indwelling bladder catheter, endotracheal tube, and central venous and intravenous catheters should reduce the frequency of nosocomial infection and bacteremia. Additional measures should include rational use of antibiotics as well as the appropriate collection and feedback of surveillance data used to monitor nosocomial infection.

SUGGESTED READING

Bone RC, Fisher CJ Jr, Clemmer TP, et al. A controlled clinical trial of high dose methylprednisolone in the treatment of severe sepsis and septic shock. N Engl J Med 1987; 317:653–659.

DeMaria A, Craven DE, Heffernan JJ, et al. Naloxone versus placebo in treatment of septic shock. Lancet 1985; 1:1363–1365.

DuPont HI, Spink WW. Infections due to gram-negative organisms: an analysis of 860 patients with bacteremia at the University of Minnesota Medical Center, 1958–1966. Medicine 1969; 45:307–332.

Klein BS, Perloff WH, Maki DG. Reduction of nosocomial infection during pediatric intensive care by protective isolation. N Engl J Med 1989; 320:1714–1721.

Kreger BE, Craven DE, McCabe WR. Gram-negative bacteremia. III. Re-assessment of etiology, epidemiology, and ecology in 612 patients. Am J Med 1980; 68:332.

Kreger BE, Craven DE, McCabe WR. Gram-negative bacteremia. IV. Re-evaluation of clinical features and treatment in 612 patients. Am J Med 1980; 68:344.

McCabe WR. Endotoxin: microbial, chemical, pathophysiological and clinical correlation. In: Weinstein L, Fields BN, eds. Seminars in infectious disease. Vol III. New York: Thieme and Stratton, 1980:38.

McCabe WR, Jackson CG. Gram-negative bacteremia. II. Clinical, laboratory, and therapeutic observations. Arch Intern Med 1962; 110:856–864.

McCabe WR, Olans RN. Shock in gram-negative bacteremia. In: Remington JS, Swartz MN, eds. Current clinical topics in infectious disease. Vol 2. New York: McGraw-Hill, 1981; 121.

Michie HR, Manogue KR, Spriggs DR, et al. Detection of circulating tumor necrosis factor after endotoxin administration. N Engl J Med 1988; 318:1481–1486.

The Veterans Systemic Sepsis Collaborative Study Group. Effect of high-dose glucocorticoid therapy on mortality in patients with clinical signs of systemic sepsis. N Engl J Med 1987; 317:660–665.

Young LS. Gram-negative sepsis. In: Mandell GL, Douglas RE Jr, Bennett JE, eds. Principles and practices of infectious diseases. New York: John Wiley 1985; 452.

Ziegler EJ. Tumor necrosis factor in humans. N Engl J Med 1988; 318:1533–1535.

Ziegler EJ, McCutchan JA, Fierer J, et al. Treatment of gram-negative bacteremia and shock with human antiserum to a mutant of *Escherichia coli*. N Engl J Med 1982; 307:1225–1230.

VULVOVAGINITIS, CERVICITIS, AND PELVIC INFLAMMATORY DISEASE

GARY E. GARBER, M.D., FRCPC
ANTHONY W. CHOW, M.D., FRCPC, FACP

GENERAL CONSIDERATIONS

Lower genitourinary symptoms are common complaints among adult women in primary care settings as well as in specialty clinics for sexually transmitted diseases. Among such women, vaginal symptoms are more than five times as common as urinary symptoms. Genital and urinary infections may often coexist, and their clinical distinction is not always clearcut. Furthermore, symptoms or signs of an abnormal vaginal discharge may be caused by a diverse variety of conditions or their combination (Table 1). Lack of uniformity in the clinical definition of these conditions, and of a consistent approach to laboratory confirmation also contributes to the diagnostic uncertainties and refractory response to therapy in many instances. Not surprisingly, considerable difficulty is also encountered clinically in differentiating true inflammatory conditions of the female genital tract from physiologic, functional, or psychosomatic causes of symptoms. For these reasons, a systematic approach to the diagnosis and management of urogenital infections is essential. Special emphasis should be given to the following considerations: (1) the history and physical examination should focus primarily on the epidemiology and anatomic localization of the likely sites of infection or inflammation; (2) specific etiologic diagnosis will require additional office or laboratory tests since the clinical diagnosis is imprecise and often misleading; (3) concomitant infection with multiple pathogens at different sites is common; (4) the presence of potentially serious but asymptomatic infection (e.g., cervicitis) should be excluded; (5) an important therapeutic goal should include prevention of upper genital tract infection and its sequelae in addition to eradication of lower genital symptoms and epidemiologic control of major sexually transmitted infections. A critical initial step in the evaluation of all lower genital symptoms, therefore, should be directed to detection and effective treatment of cervicitis or coexisting salpingitis.

An algorithm approach to the management of adult women with lower genital complaints is summarized in Figure 1.

SYSTEMATIC APPROACH TO DIAGNOSIS

History

Historical features are relatively nonspecific, but are useful for defining the epidemiology and natural history of specific infections. Inflammation of the cervix and vagina often produce similar symptoms, such as external dysuria, introital dyspareunia, and increased amount or altered quality of vaginal discharge. Patients with cervicitis often complain of intermenstrual or postcoital spotting. Abdominal pain or systemic complaints are uncommon with vulvovaginitis or uncomplicated cervicitis and should prompt a diligent search for accompanying pelvic inflammatory disease. Presence of fever may suggest acute salpingitis or primary genital herpes. Fever and multisystem involvement beginning during a menstrual period should raise the possibility of toxic shock syndrome.

The color and amount of discharge as perceived by the patient has little value in differential diagnosis. Although trichomoniasis and candidiasis can cause marked vaginal irritation, their clinical presentation can vary greatly from individual to individual. Vaginal odor may be the only symptom in bacterial vaginosis, a condition often associated with little vaginal irritation. The complaint of vaginal discharge does not in itself indicate a pathologic process. Physiologic discharge (mucorrhea) may be heavy enough to stain underwear, but it is not usually associated with external dysuria, vulvar irritation, or odor. The amount of discharge may vary with the phase of the menstrual cycle and may be increased by oral contraceptive use or pregnancy. Because the onset of physiologic discharge often coincides with the onset of sexual activity, women who feel anxious or guilty about their sexual activity may attach inordinate importance to small changes in normal vaginal discharge.

A complete and detailed sexual history is particularly important, since exposure to a new sexual partner increases the likelihood of sexually transmitted disease. The sexual history should include the number of recent new partners, patterns of sexual behavior, previous sexually transmitted diseases, and partner's sexual history. This line of questioning is often disconcerting for both the physician and patient. The patient is far more likely to discuss intimate sexual details freely if the impression projected is that of a routine but necessary and confidential procedure. This skill is acquired only with practice.

TABLE 1 Conditions Associated with Vaginal Discharge

Infectious	*Noninfectious*
Vulvovaginitis Bacterial vaginosis Candidiasis Trichomoniasis	Excessive mucorrhea and physiologic discharge Atrophic vaginitis
Cervicitis Chlamydial infection Gonorrhea Genital herpes	Desquamative inflammatory vaginitis Foreign body, trauma, irradiation, hypersensitivity, or chemical irritation
Salpingitis	
Other sexually transmitted diseases	Endometriosis, neoplasms cysts, or polyps
Toxic shock syndrome	Others
Miscellaneous vulvovaginal pyogenic infections	

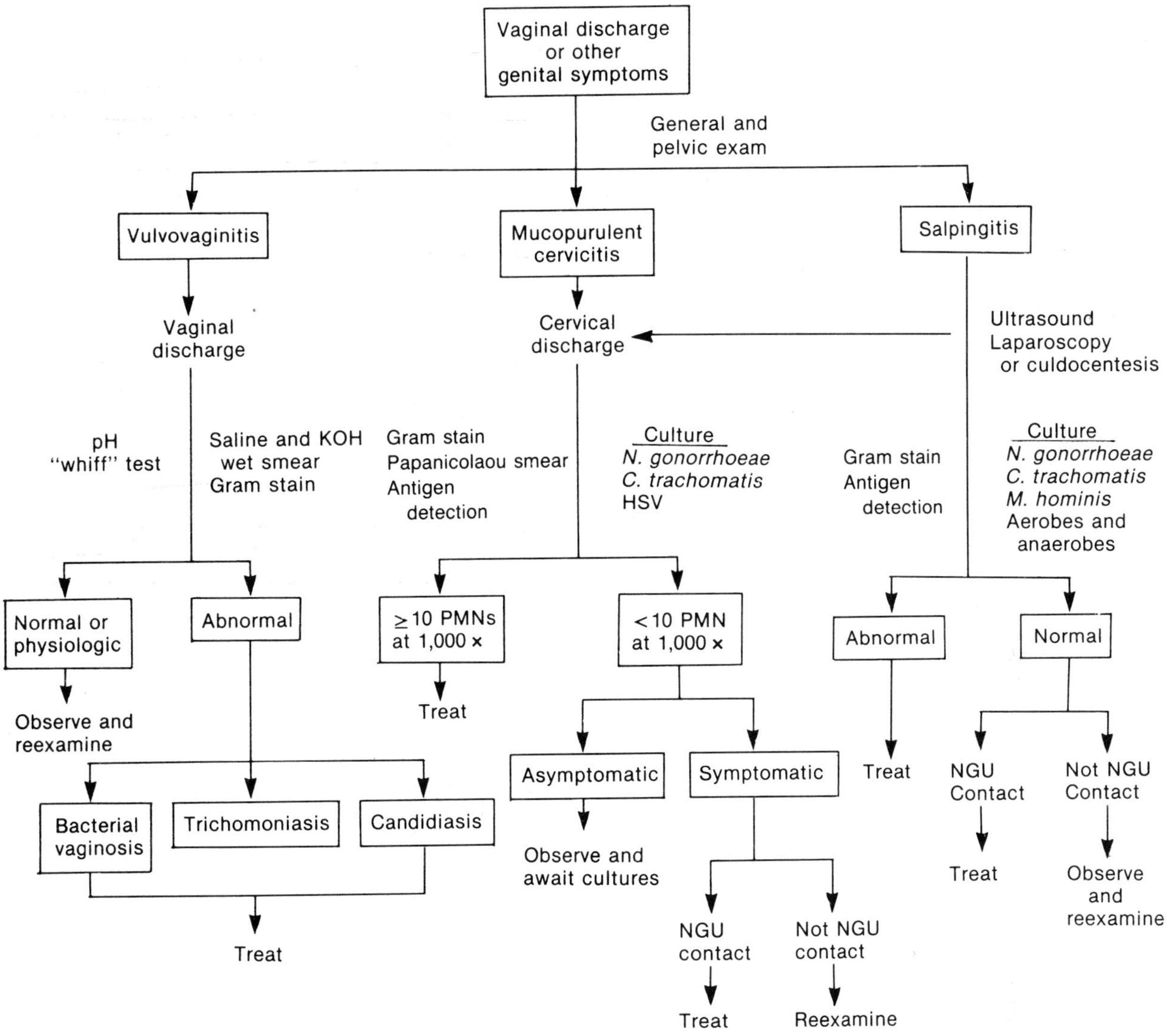

Figure 1 Approach to genital symptoms in premenopausal women.

General Physical Examination

Particular attention should be directed to the skin, palms, soles, eyes, mouth, pharynx, anorectum, pubic hair, lymph nodes, and joints. Examination of the abdomen should include careful listening for diminished bowel sounds and evidence of peritoneal, suprapubic, or perihepatic inflammation. The pubic region should be inspected for lice and other pediculosis. The inguinal and femoral regions should be palpated for adenopathy. An anorectal examination by proctoscopy and digital palpation should be routinely performed.

The Pelvic Examination

The labia and the perineum should be examined for erythema, excoriation, and discrete lesions. Diffuse perineal erythema or edema may accompany trichomoniasis, candidiasis, or early toxic shock syndrome. Examination of extravaginal surfaces may reveal lesions of genital herpes, syphilis, chancroid, condylomata acuminata, molluscum contagiosum, or scabies. Vulvovaginal pyogenic infections such as abscesses involving Bartholin's and Skene's glands, infected labial inclusion cysts, furunculosis, and suppurative hidradenitis are readily apparent.

Next, the urethral meatus is examined and gently stripped with a finger placed inside the introitus. If urethral discharge is expressed, such material should be examined microscopically and cultured. A vaginal speculum, moistened with warm water and without lubricant, is then gently inserted. In the presence of severe genital herpes, or occasionally trichomoniasis, insertion of the speculum may be impossible due to intense discomfort. In such cases, a preliminary etiologic diagnosis is sometimes made from material recovered on a cotton swab gently inserted into the vagina.

After insertion of the speculum, the cervix is first examined, since cervicitis is a serious condition and is often asymptomatic. The cervix should be wiped clean and cotton-tipped swabs of endocervical secretions obtained through the cervical os. Mucoid material is normally observed at the cervical os and is present in increased amounts in women taking oral contraceptives. Normal cervical discharge is usually clear or white and is nonhomogeneous and viscous. Purulent or mucopurulent cervical discharge is associated with infective cervicitis and is readily recognized by the appearance of yellow or green exudate on the white cotton-tipped swab. The cervix should also be observed for erosions, friability, or easy bleeding. Mucopurulent cervicitis is most commonly caused by *Chlamydia trachomatis*, *Neisseria gonorrhoeae*, or both, and must be differentiated from cervicitis caused by herpes simplex virus (HSV), from vaginitis, and from simple cervical ectopy without inflammation. Cervical ectopy represents the presence of columnar endocervical epithelium in an exposed portion of the ectocervix and appears redder than the surrounding stratified vaginal epithelium. Ectopy, when not associated with visible or microscopic endocervical mucopus or with colposcopic epithelial abnormalities, is a normal finding and requires no therapy. Its prevalence is increased at the onset of menarche, by oral contraceptive use, and by pregnancy but gradually declines through later adolescence. Hypertrophic cervicitis manifests as intensely red, congested areas that appear to project from the surface of the cervix. It can be distinguished from ectopy in that it is usually asymmetrical and irregular around the cervical os, is rather friable and bleeds easily, and is usually accompanied by a mucopurulent cervical discharge. Presence of hypertrophic cervicitis is highly suggestive of chlamydial cervicitis, but it is an uncommon clinical finding. Similarly, findings of a "strawberry cervix" in association with increased purulent discharge is highly suggestive of trichomoniasis, but this observation was only 45 percent sensitive by colposcopy, although 99 percent specific. Endocervical scrapings, swabs, or secretions should be collected for Gram stain, for antigen detection, or for culture (or other testing, depending on availability) of *N. gonorrhoeae*, *C. trachomatis*, and HSV. A Papanicolaou smear may identify trichomonads or cytologic findings characteristic of HSV infection.

After establishing the presence or absence of cervicitis, efforts should then be directed to establishing the presence or absence of vaginal infection. Not infrequently, cervicitis coexists with vaginal infection, particularly with bacterial vaginosis or trichomonal vaginitis. The amount, consistency, color, odor, and location of the discharge within the vagina should be noted. The character of vaginal discharge is relatively nonspecific. A yellow or green discharge is suggestive of trichomoniasis, but this occurs in less than one-fifth of infected women. Similarly, a frothy discharge is seen in only one-tenth of women with trichomoniasis, is nonspecific, and is equally suggestive of bacterial vaginosis. The amount of discharge in vulvovaginal candidiasis is highly variable, and one does not always see the classic curdy discharge. The vaginal wall should also be inspected for erythema, edema, and ulceration. Vaginal ulcers tend to occur in the right vaginal fornix, are chronic, and are associated with the use of tampons in some patients. A sample of discharge should be removed with a swab from the vaginal wall, avoiding contamination with cervical mucus. The vaginal pH should be determined directly by rolling the swab containing the specimen onto pH indicator paper. An additional specimen should be removed with a swab and mixed first with a drop of saline, then with a drop of 10 percent potassium hydroxide (KOH) on a microscope slide. The odor released after mixing the specimen with KOH is noted, and separate cover slips are placed on the saline and KOH wet mounts for microscopic examination to detect the presence and quantity of normal epithelial cells, clue cells, polymorphonuclear leukocytes (PMNs), motile trichomonads, or fungal elements.

Finally, the bimanual examination is performed to determine adnexal or cervical motion tenderness, and to exclude the presence of palpable adnexal or cul-de-sac masses. Adnexal tenderness is uncommon with local vaginal infections and suggests salpingitis; palpation of an abnormal adnexal or cul-de-sac mass may indicate tubo-ovarian abscess, ectopic pregnancy, or malignancy that requires prompt gynecologic or surgical consultation.

In most patients, the constellation of symptoms and signs together with the microscopic findings in vaginal secretions will allow a preliminary etiologic diagnosis of vulvovaginitis, and further studies are unnecessary (Table 2). However, it is prudent to request that the patient remain undressed in the examination room in case microscopic examination of the wet smear is unrevealing and further microbiologic studies are indicated. Patients generally do not mind waiting for 2 to 3 minutes for the results of the wet mount before the examination is continued. Depending on the clinical findings, these further studies may include culture for *Candida albicans* and *Trichomonas vaginalis* or Gram stain of vaginal fluid to differentiate between normal flora and the flora characteristic of bacterial vaginosis. In women with prominent vaginal complaints but no abnormal findings, each of these additional microbiologic tests may be indicated to differentiate vaginal infection from functional complaints and other causes of vaginal symptoms.

Routine Office and Laboratory Investigations

A number of bedside and office evaluations of clinical specimens are invaluable in the etiologic diagnosis of vulvovaginitis and cervicitis. These include vaginal pH, KOH "whiff" test, and microscopic examination of wet smears and Gram stains of vaginal and cervical specimens. Cervical and vaginal cultures should be obtained only for specific and selected pathogens and should be interpreted with caution.

Vaginal pH. The pH of vaginal discharge can be estimated at the bedside by use of pH indicators such as nitrazine paper, when the pH is between 4.5 and 7.0. A vaginal pH of 4.5 or less is most consistent with physiologic discharge or with vulvovaginal candidiasis. Vaginal pH greater than 4.5 is seen in patients with trichomoniasis or bacterial vaginosis.

KOH Whiff Test. Vaginal secretions from patients with bacterial vaginosis, when added to several drops of 10 percent KOH on a microscope slide will elicit a pungent fishy, amine-like odor. A positive whiff test can be expected in more than 90 percent of women with bacterial vaginosis and an undefined proportion of patients with trichomoniasis but is absent in women with vulvovaginal candidiasis or physiologic discharge.

Microscopic Examination of Vaginal Specimens. The wet mount of vaginal discharge is the single most useful technique in making an initial etiologic diagnosis of vulvovaginitis (Table 2). The following specific information is sought: (1) the nature of the vaginal epithelial cells and the presence of clue cells; (2) the presence and number of PMNs; (3) the presence of specific and readily identifiable pathogens such as motile trichomonads, budding yeasts, or pseudohyphae. Normal vaginal epithelial cells are flat and clean looking. The edges are sharply defined, and the nuclei, easily visible. Clue cells, which strongly suggest bacterial vaginosis, are squamous epithelial cells covered with coccobacilli, giving them a granular appearance with indistinct cell edges and nucleus. Presence of large numbers of PMNs may be either cervical or vaginal in origin. The number of PMNs is usually normal in bacterial vaginosis (i.e., one would not see an intense inflammatory response) and may be normal or increased in candidal vulvovaginitis or trichomoniasis. The presence of excessive PMNs should prompt further search for an inflammatory genital focus, but the absence of excessive PMNs does not rule out notable infection. The composition and normality of the bacterial vaginal flora is effectively assessed by Gram stain of vaginal fluid. Normal vaginal secretions contain predominantly gram-positive rods resembling lactobacilli, with or without gram-variable coccobacilli resembling *Gardnerella vaginalis*. In bacterial vaginosis, vaginal fluid contains few or no lactobacilli with a predominance of *G. vaginalis* plus other organisms resembling anaerobic gram-negative *Bacteroides* species, gram-positive cocci, or curved rods.

Microscopic Examination of Cervical Specimens. The Gram stain of endocervical secretions examined at 1,000× is the most useful and practical tool for the etiologic diagnosis of symptomatic or asymptomatic cervicitis. Visualization of yellow, mucopurulent endocervical secretions on a white swab or presence of 10 or more PMNs per 1,000× field are positively correlated with cervical *C. trachomatis* infection. Neither *N. gonorrhoeae* nor HSV infection is significantly associated with endocervical PMN leukocyte concentration or presence of macroscopic mucopus. On the other hand, demonstration of intracellular gram-negative diplococci in the Gram stain of endocervical secretions has a sensitivity of 60 percent and specificity close to 100 percent for the diagnosis of gonococcal infection. This compares favorably to isolation of *N. gonorrhoeae* from a single

TABLE 2 Diagnostic Features of Vaginitis in Premenopausal Adults

	Normal or Physiologic Discharge	*Bacterial Vaginosis*	*Candidal Vulvovaginitis*	*Trichomonal Vaginitis*
Etiology	Uninfected; *Lactobacillus* predominant	*G. vaginalis* and various anaerobic bacteria	*C. albicans* and other yeasts	*T. vaginalis*
Predominant symptoms	None	Malodorous discharge	Vulvar itching and/or irritation; increased discharge	Profuse discharge, often malodorous
Vulvitis	None	Rare	Usual	Occasional
Inflammation of vaginal epithelium	None	None	Erythema	Erythema; occasional petechiae
Discharge				
Amount	Variable, but usually scant	Moderate	Scant to moderate	Profuse
Color	Clear or white	White or grey	White	Yellow
Consistency	Nonhomogeneous, flocular	Homogeneous, low viscosity, uniformly coating vaginal walls; occasionally frothy	Clumped, adherent plaques	Homogeneous, low viscosity; often frothy
Usual vaginal pH	<4.5	≥4.5	<4.5	≥5.0
Amine odor with 10% KOH ("whiff test")	None	Positive	None	Often positive
Microscopy (saline or KOH wet smears, Gram stain)	Normal epithelial cells; lactobacilli predominate	Clue cells; few PMNs; lactobacilli outnumbered by profuse mixed flora nearly always including *G. vaginalis* plus anaerobes	PMNs, epithelial cells; yeast or pseudohyphae in up to 80%	PMNs, motile trichomonads in 80–90%

Modified with permission from Holmes KK. Lower genital tract infections in women:cystitis/urethritis, vulvovaginitis, and cervicitis. In: Holmes KK, Mordh P-A, Sparling PF, Wiesner PI, eds. Sexually transmitted diseases. New York: McGraw-Hill, 1984:583.

endocervical culture, which has a sensitivity of 80 to 90 percent. Giemsa-stained smears of endocervical scrapings are of less value for the diagnosis of chlamydial cervicitis since chlamydial inclusions can be identified in only a minority of infected women. Multinucleated giant cells and Cowdry type A intranuclear inclusions suggest HSV cervicitis; but in the presence of extensive tissue necrosis, the cellular architecture is distorted, and the typical cytologic findings are seen in less than one-third of infected patients. Similarly, the typical cytologic findings of HSV infection in Papanicolaou smears are reliable indicators of disease only when observed, but the sensitivity of this technique has been questioned.

Cultures. Prevalence is sufficient to recommend that endocervical, urethral, and anorectal cultures be obtained routinely for confirmation of gonorrhea and for detection of beta-lactamase production by *N. gonorrhoeae* isolates. Although endocervical cultures for *C. trachomatis* and HSV are desirable, they are not readily available in many centers. Routine aerobic and anaerobic vaginal cultures are not recommended, and results should be interpreted with great caution since the vagina is normally colonized by a wide variety of microorganisms. As an example, isolation of *G. vaginalis* from the vagina, even in high concentration, is not specific for the diagnosis of bacterial vaginosis.

Special Diagnostic Procedures

It is important to note that routine office and laboratory investigations are helpful in confirming an etiologic diagnosis of genitourinary infections in only 30 to 60 percent of symptomatic women. Nonroutine and more specialized and comprehensive microbiologic investigations are required to improve the diagnostic yield. Cultural procedures for the isolation of *C. trachomatis* are extremely expensive and labor intensive and may not be readily available. Two immunodiagnostic methods for detection of *C. trachomatis* antigen from cervical specimens, a direct immunofluorescence assay (DFA) and an enzyme immunoassay (EIA), have become widely available. Comparisons of these antigen detection methods in high-prevalence as well as low-prevalence populations have generally supported their usefulness (70 percent as sensitive as culture), although both false-positive and false-negative results can occur. The presence of ectocervical lesions suggestive of HSV infection should warrant laboratory confirmation by viral isolation and differentiation of HSV-1 and HSV-2 serotypes by use of type-specific monoclonal antibodies. Cytologic and immunofluorescent antigen detection techniques for genital herpes are 50 percent and 70 percent, respectively, as sensitive as viral isolation. DNA hybridization has been used to demonstrate human papillomavirus (HPV) in tissue. DNA hybridization is highly specific for demonstrating HPV and has the unique advantage of giving information on the virus serotype. It is much superior to antigen detection for HPV, which has poor sensitivity.

Cultures for *Ureaplasma urealyticum* and *Mycoplasma hominis* from cervical and urethral secretions may be useful for the diagnosis of nongonococcal and nonchlamydial cervicitis, endometritis, or salpingitis. These organisms have been implicated particularly in instances of postpartum fever or recurrent pregnancy loss. A variety of selective media are available for isolation of *T. vaginalis* from vaginal secretions, and culture is the most sensitive method for diagnosis of vaginal trichomoniasis. Vaginal cultures for yeast and *T. vaginalis* are particularly useful when symptoms or signs are suggestive of one or the other, but neither can be demonstrated by direct microscopy of wet smears.

Gas-liquid chromatography of vaginal fluid from women with bacterial vaginosis may show a characteristic pattern of organic acid metabolites: the concentration of lactate, the major metabolite of lactobacilli, is reduced, while succinate, acetate, propionate, butyrate, and other organic acids produced by the abnormal flora are increased. Toxin-producing *Staphylococcus aureus* may be isolated in high concentration from vaginal cultures of women with symptoms and signs suggestive of toxic shock syndrome (TSS). Toxic shock syndrome toxin-1, the major staphylococcal exotoxin implicated in TSS, can be detected in vaginal washings of some patients by solid-phase enzyme-linked immunosorbent assay during the acute illness; serum antitoxin antibodies in such patients are typically low in titer.

Colposcopy is increasingly used to evaluate women with abnormal cytologic smears consistent with cervical intraepithelial neoplasia. Colposcopic examination with magnification of the mucosal surface contour is invaluable for the detection of subclinical HPV infection and for cervicitis. Following application of 3 to 5 percent acetic acid during this procedure, papillomavirus-infected lesions typically appear white and shiny ("acetowhite") with irregular but distinct borders. Asperities (multiple, short, pointed surface projections) and reverse punctation (diffuse pattern of minimally raised white dots against the pink background of the vaginal epithelium) are often seen. If vascular abnormalities are also present, a biopsy should be obtained to exclude the possibility of intraepithelial neoplasia. Laparoscopy is invaluable for the visual diagnosis of salpingitis and is particularly helpful for microbiologic sampling and specific etiologic diagnosis of salpingitis and other pelvic conditions. Ultrasonography, radionuclide scanning, and computed tomography are particularly useful for detection and localization of tubo-ovarian and adnexal inflammatory masses.

MANAGEMENT OF SPECIFIC SYNDROMES

Vulvovaginitis

Vulvovaginitis may be the most frequent cause of genital symptoms in women. The cardinal manifestations are increased yellow or green discharge; vulvar itching, irritation or burning; external dysuria; introital dyspareunia; and malodor that is often increased following sexual intercourse. Treatment should be based on specific etiologic diagnosis that can usually be made at the time of initial clinical evaluation (see Table 2). The commonest cause of all vaginal discharge is bacterial vaginosis, which is also known as nonspecific vaginitis, followed in frequency by vulvovaginal candidiasis and trichomoniasis. Multiple and concomitant vaginal infections are not infrequent, especially trichomoniasis coexisting with *G. vaginalis*-associated bacterial vaginosis. Cervicitis may also present as vaginal discharge and must first be ruled out. Other causes of abnormal vaginal discharge, such as atrophic vaginitis, desquamative inflammatory vaginitis, and vaginal fistula or ulcers, are rare. In a patient with persistent vaginitis for which a specific pathogen cannot be identified, examination of the sexual partner may often provide the answer.

Common pitfalls that lead to misdiagnosis and treatment failure in the management of vulvovaginitis include (1) diagnosis based exclusively on macroscopic appearance of discharge, with failure to perform a wet smear; (2) "telephone" diagnosis and treatment; (3) broad-spectrum, "shotgun" remedies; (4) failure to use appropriate antimicrobial agents; and (5) failure to treat the sexual partner. Recommended therapeutic regimens for the most frequent causes of vulvovaginitis and cervicitis are summarized in Table 3. Adjunctive measures, such as warm tub baths to ease pain and reduce edema, careful attention to personal hygiene, and abstinence from sexual intercourse, are also important. Patients whose symptoms respond promptly to specific therapy should be seen about 1 week after completion of therapy for repeat clinical and microscopic evaluation. Women with physiologic discharge should be given a careful explanation of the con-

TABLE 3 Recommended Regimens for Treatment of Vulvovaginitis, Cervicitis, and Acute Salpingitis

Infection	*Choice*	*Alternative*
Vulvovaginitis		
Bacterial vaginosis	Metronidazole (500 mg PO b.i.d.) for 7 days	Ampicillin (500 mg PO q.i.d.) for 7 days
Candidiasis	Miconazole or clotrimazole vaginal cream (100 mg HS) for 7 days	Nystatin vaginal cream (100,000 units b.i.d.) for 7–14 days *or* Boric acid capsules (600 mg intravaginally HS) for 14 days
Trichomoniasis (sexual partner treated)	Metronidazole or tinadazole (2 g PO) single dose	Clotrimazole vaginal cream (100 mg HS) for 7 days
(sexual partner not treated)	Metronidazole or tinadazole (250 mg PO t.i.d.) for 7-10 days	Clotrimazole vaginal cream (100 mg HS) for 7 days
Cervicitis		
Chlamydial or mucopurulent	Tetracycline (500 mg PO q.i.d.) for 7 days *or* Doxycycline (100 mg PO b.i.d.) for 7 days	Erythromycin (500 mg PO q.i.d.) for 7 days *or* Sulfisoxazole (500 mg PO q.i.d.) for 10 days
Gonococcal		
PPNG not suspected	Ampicillin (3.5 g PO), amoxicillin (3 g PO), or APPG (4.8 mu IM), each with probenecid (1 g PO) and followed by tetracycline (500 mg PO q.i.d.) for 7 days	Tetracycline (500 mg PO q.i.d.) for 5 days
PPNG suspected	Spectinomycin (2 g IM) or ceftriaxone (250 mg IM), each followed by tetracycline (500 mg PO q.i.d.) for 7 days	Trimethoprim-sulfamethoxazole 80-mg/400-mg tablets (9 tablets PO OD) for 3 days
Genital herpes		
Primary or first episode	Acyclovir (5 mg/kg IV q8h or 200 mg PO q4–6h) for 5–7 days	Acyclovir cream topically to external genital lesions, 6 × daily for 7–14 days
Recurrent episodes	Acyclovir (200 mg PO q4–6h) for up to 6 mo for patients with frequent (>6 episodes per yr) and symptomatic recurrences (Routine therapy in immunocompetent hosts not recommended)	
Salpingitis		
Inpatient	Cefoxitin (2 g IV q6h) plus doxycycline (100 mg IV q12h) for 10–14 days	Metronidazole (500 mg IV q6h) plus doxycycline (100 mg IV q12h) for 10–14 days *or* Clindamycin (600 mg IV q6h) plus tobramycin (1.5 mg/kg IV q8h) for 10–14 days
Outpatient	Cefoxitin (2 g IM) plus probenecid (1 g PO), followed by doxycycline (100 mg PO b.i.d.) for 10–14 days	Ampicillin (3.5 g PO), amoxicillin (3 g PO) or APPG (4.8 mu IM), each with probenecid (1 g PO) and followed by doxycycline (100 mg PO b.i.d.) for 10–14 days *or* Trimethoprim-sulfamethoxazole 80-mg/400-mg tablets (2 tablets PO b.i.d.) plus clindamycin (300 mg PO t.i.d.) for 10–14 days

mu = million units.

dition. Persistence of worrisome symptoms in a woman in whom thorough and repeated evaluation has failed to reveal genital pathology may indicate psychosexual problems; such patients may well benefit from counseling provided by a trained therapist.

Bacterial Vaginosis or Nonspecific Vaginitis

Current evidence indicates that *G. vaginalis* (formerly known as *Hemophilus vaginalis* or *Corynebacterium vaginale*) in conjunction with high vaginal concentrations of anaerobic bacteria (particularly *Bacteroides* species, *Peptostreptococcus* species, and motile curved rods known as *Mobiluncus* species) is the primary cause of this condition. It is characterized clinically by symptoms of slightly increased, malodorous, watery vaginal discharge, with little pain or itching. The malodor may increase postcoitally (possibly due to release of amines by semen, which is alkaline). Examination often reveals a nonviscous, homogeneous, gray-white, uniformly adherent vaginal discharge, without gross inflammation of the vaginal mucosa. Bacterial vaginosis should be suspected in the presence of three of four of the following findings: (1) characteristic vaginal discharge; (2) vaginal pH above 4.5; (3) positive whiff test; (4) presence of clue cells. Symptoms alone are not reliable for diagnosis since many patients are asymptomatic. The diagnosis is readily confirmed by the characteristic changes in vaginal flora observed on Gram stain and by demonstration of a high ratio of succinate to lactate (greater than 0.4) or presence of specific amines (putrescine and cadaverine) in vaginal washings of affected patients. The latter two techniques may be useful if confirmation of diagnosis by the four findings above is difficult. The presence or absence of clue cells per se is not helpful since both false-positive (due to adherence by lactobacilli to desquamated vaginal epithelial cells) and false-negative (possibly due to presence of local IgA, which blocks bacterial attachment to vaginal cell surfaces) findings can occur. Culture of vaginal fluid is also not useful since isolation of *G. vaginalis*, even in high concentration, is not specific for bacterial vaginosis.

The recommended therapy of bacterial vaginosis is metronidazole, which appears to eradicate or suppress *G. vaginalis* and obligate anaerobes while promoting recolonization with lactobacilli (Table 3). Single-dose therapy, as used in the treatment of trichomoniasis, is associated with a high failure rate and is not recommended. Treatment with ampicillin is associated with success rates ranging from 33 to 100 percent. Erythromycin and doxycycline are ineffective, as are local measures such as triple-sulfa vaginal cream, or povidone-iodine vaginal tablets. Interestingly, treatment of the male sexual partner with metronidazole does not appear to prevent recurrence of bacterial vaginosis among women who had been treated with metronidazole.

Candidal Vulvovaginitis

This entity accounts for approximately one-third of all cases of vaginitis in office practice. Candidal vulvovaginitis is commoner during menstruation and in pregnancy and is associated with diabetes mellitus, immunosuppression, and use of broad-spectrum antibiotics, corticosteroids, or oral contraceptives. As many as 10 to 27 percent of male sexual partners of infected women may be found to have balanoposthitis. Clinically, candidal vulvovaginitis is characterized by symptoms of vulvar itching, burning, or other irritation, often associated with external dysuria and with scant, nonmalodorous discharge. Examination usually reveals reddened, inflamed vaginal mucosa with a thick, white, "cottage cheese" discharge. The vaginal pH is less than 4.5. Mixed infection with bacterial vaginosis or trichomoniasis is relatively uncommon. The diagnosis is confirmed by the presence of fungal elements either in saline or KOH smears or Gram stain of vaginal secretions. The KOH smear is considered the most sensitive noncultural method of diagnosis. Two drops of 10 percent KOH are mixed with the discharge on a glass slide under a cover slip and heated until boiling. This destroys the PMNs and epithelial cells and leaves intact the candidal budding and pseudohyphal forms. Cultures should be obtained if the clinical presentation is suggestive of vulvovaginal candidiasis but the wet smear is negative. Although *C. albicans* is the commonest isolate, other *Candida* species (e.g., *C. glabrata*) have also been implicated.

The recommended treatment for candidal vulvovaginitis is local application of antifungal imidazoles such as miconazole or clotrimazole nightly for 7 days and is associated with a cure rate of 90 percent over 6 to 8 weeks of follow-up (see Table 3). Three-day therapy with double strength clotrimazole has also been shown to be effective. Intravaginal nystatin cream can also be used, but requires twice-daily applications for 2 weeks and has a slightly lower cure rate of 70 percent. More recently, the use of 600 mg boric acid powder in gelatin capsules, inserted intravaginally each evening for 14 days, has been found to be as effective as nystatin but has the advantage of lower cost. Oral therapy with ketoconazole (200 mg twice daily for 5 days) does not provide added advantage in cure rate or prevention of recurrence and is not recommended except for patients with relapsing vulvovaginal candidiasis or for patients with chronic mucocutaneous candidiasis. The presence of *Candida* species per se in any asymptomatic woman does not require treatment. The need for treatment of the male sexual partner has not been determined.

Trichomonal Vaginitis

Symptoms associated with *T. vaginalis* vaginitis are highly variable and appear to correlate with the severity of the inflammatory response in a given host. *T. vaginalis* may also be associated with asymptomatic infection, which almost invariably leads to symptomatic disease eventually. In patients with minimal or no inflammatory response despite the presence of trichomonads, excessive vaginal discharge may be the only symptom. In more severe cases, the infection is characterized by a profuse, watery, foul-smelling vaginal discharge associated with burning, dysuria, and intermenstrual spotting. Examination shows a foamy, bubbly discharge adherent to an erythematous or often edematous vaginal mucosa with multiple petechiae. The vaginal pH is usually greater than 5.0. Numerous PMNs are seen in the wet smear. Diagnosis is confirmed by the presence of motile trichomonads in the saline preparation of vaginal discharge. In patients with minimal symptoms, the wet smear may not be sufficiently sensitive, and culture for *T. vaginalis* on selective medium (such as Diamond's medium) is highly recommended.

Systemic treatment with oral nitroimidazoles, such as metronidazole or tinidazole, are the only regimens consistently effective for *T. vaginalis* vaginitis (see Table 3). Simultaneous treatment of the male sexual partner is important for prevention of relapse or reinfection and is particularly important if the 2-g single-dose regimen is used. The presence of *T. vaginalis*, even in the absence of vaginal symptoms, should be treated since these women almost invariably develop symptomatic disease eventually. The commonest causes of recurrent *T. vaginalis* infection, or apparent treatment failure, are due to reinfection or patient noncompliance with therapy. Persistent infection despite good compliance and avoidance of reinfection should suggest the possibility of infection due to metronidazole-resistant *T. vaginalis*. Such patients may require 7- to 14-day retreatment regimens consisting of oral metronidazole, 2 to 3 g daily by mouth, together with a vaginal metronidazole tablet, 500 mg, inserted nightly each day until vaginal symptoms have completely subsided. Metronidazole remains the drug of choice for symptomatic trichomonal vaginitis during pregnancy; the dosage is the same as for a nonpregnant woman. Clotrimazole can be administered intravaginally as a topical trichomonicide, but it is clearly less effective than metronidazole.

Cervicitis

Infection of the cervix by sexually transmitted pathogens may lead to several potential complications, including endometritis and salpingitis leading to ectopic pregnancy or infertility; premature rupture of membranes, chorioamnionitis, and puerperal infection during pregnancy; and initiation or promotion of cervical neoplasia. Cervicitis can be difficult to diagnose because many women are asymptomatic, and infection is often discovered only after a sexual partner presents with urethritis. Alternatively, cervical infection may be misdiagnosed as vaginitis if a thorough pelvic examination is not performed. The typical finding of cervicitis is an inflamed cervix, with a mucopurulent exudate emanating from the os. The principal infectious causes are *C. trachomatis*, *N. gonorrhoeae*, and HSV. Although cervical infection with any of these pathogens is more likely to present with a mucopurulent endocervical discharge, only HSV is associated with characteristic ectocervical ulcerations, and only *C. trachomatis* is associated with the presence of mucopus or with 10 or more PMNs per high-power field in cervical mucus. *C. trachomatis* frequently coexists with *N. gonorrhoeae* in cervicitis; treatment for both gonococcal and nongonococcal cervicitis should, therefore, also be effective against *C. trachomatis*.

Mucopurulent or Chlamydial Cervicitis

Chlamydial infection should always be suspected in women with mucopurulent cervicitis whether or not gonorrhea is also found. Similar to the case of gonococcal urethritis in men, women with gonococcal infection treated with 4.8 million units of procaine penicillin G plus probenecid were associated with a significantly higher rate of posttreatment cervicitis and pelvic inflammatory disease as compared with similar women treated with agents effective against both *N. gonorrhoeae* and *C. trachomatis*. Tetracycline or doxycycline at equivalent doses for 7 days is currently the most effective regimen for mucopurulent cervicitis and eradication of *C. trachomatis* from the cervix (see Table 3). If coexisting gonococcal infection is found, additional therapy for gonorrhea should be provided in areas where tetracycline is no longer highly effective against *N. gonorrhoeae*. Erythromycin is recommended for women allergic to tetracycline or during pregnancy. Sulfisoxazole is another alternative for chlamydial cervicitis, but it should be avoided during pregnancy.

Gonococcal Cervicitis

Whenever endocervical gonorrhea is suspected, the urethra as well as paraurethral glands should also be carefully examined. Cultures should be obtained from multiple sites including the anorectum and the oropharynx. A confirmatory test for *C. trachomatis* is also desirable in women with cervicitis, even if gonococcal infection is found, since more than 40 percent of women with gonorrhea have coexisting chlamydial infection. Initial empiric therapy, therefore, should also be effective against *C. trachomatis* (see Table 3). Single-dose ampicillin or amoxicillin plus probenecid followed by 7 days of tetracycline is the regimen of choice for infections in which penicillinase-producing *N. gonorrhoeae* (PPNG) is not suspected. The combined regimen of ampicillin or amoxicillin followed by tetracycline will also eradicate pharyngeal gonococcal infection, for which ampicillin, amoxicillin and spectinomycin are not highly effective. Patients allergic to penicillin or in whom PPNG or pregnancy is suspected may be treated with spectinomycin or ceftriaxone. Trimethoprim-sulfamethoxazole is an alternative to ampicillin-tetracycline combination for dual endocervical infection with *N. gonorrhoeae* and *C. trachomatis*. However, this regimen is poorly tolerated and treatment failure has occurred with both organisms in 10 to 20 percent of cases. The new quinolones show some promise as effective therapy for dual infection with *N. gonorrhoeae* and *C. trachomatis*. Their activity against genital mycoplasmas is quite variable, however.

Herpes Simplex Cervicitis and Genital Infection

The first episode of genital herpes is frequently accompanied by systemic as well as local manifestations. Concomitant cervicitis occurs in the majority of cases (80 to 90 percent), in contrast to recurrent episodes (10 to 20 percent). Several anatomic sites besides the cervix may be involved, including the urethra, vulva, pharynx, and extragenital cutaneous regions. Primary HSV genital infection tends to be more severe in women, and complications occur more frequently than in men. The most prominent local symptoms include pain, dysuria, tender inguinal adenopathy, and neurologic complications such as sacral anesthesia, urinary retention, and constipation. The cervix may show diffuse friability with necrotic and ulcerative lesions of both the exocervix and endocervix. The presence of HSV is confirmed either by culture or direct immunofluorescent staining of scrapings from active lesions. Recurrent genital herpes is less severe and of shorter duration than primary or first episodes of infection. There is, however, considerable variability in the intensity and duration of symptoms and in the frequency of recurrence. Recurrent viral shedding from the cervix can also occur in the absence of symptoms or external genital lesions. This is of clinical importance particularly in late pregnancy because of concern of intrapartum transmission of HSV infection to the neonate. Pregnant women with a history of recurrent genital herpes should be closely monitored virologically or cytologically near term, usually starting between 32 and 36 weeks of gestation. Women with active external genital lesions or cervical viral shedding at the time of labor should be delivered by cesarean section. Women with two sequential negative viral cultures or cytologic studies performed 3 to 4 days apart and absent genital lesions at the time of labor may be delivered vaginally.

Acyclovir is effective in reducing some of the manifestations of primary genital HSV infection and in shortening the duration of viral shedding (see Table 3). Oral acyclovir is also effective in suppressing recurrent episodes among patients receiving continuous therapy and may be indicated in selected patients with severe underlying disease and immunosuppression. Topical acyclovir is useful for the treatment of external genital lesions in women during primary or first episodes of HSV infection. It is not approved for intravaginal use since the polyethylene glycol base is irritating and may cause vaginal erythema. Routine use of topical acyclovir in recurrent genital herpes is not recommended since it has no established role either in prophylaxis of recurrence or in prevention of acquisition of new infection.

Acute Salpingitis

Acute salpingitis, or pelvic inflammatory disease (PID), is believed to result from ascending infection, by contiguous spread of sexually transmitted pathogens and/or indigenous vaginal microflora, from the endocervix and endometrium. Major risk factors for salpingitis include an intrauterine device, previous gonococcal infection, previous episodes of PID, lower socioeconomic status, nulliparity, and number of sexual partners. Use of oral contraceptives appears to have a protective influence. The microbiology of acute PID is complex. Cultures obtained directly from inflamed fallopian tubes either at laparoscopy or laparotomy clearly indicate a polymicrobial etiology, including *N. gonorrhoeae*, *C. trachomatis*, *Mycoplasma hominis*, and mixed aerobes and anaerobes. Clinically, acute PID associated with endocervical gonorrhea tends to occur more frequently during the first 10 days of the menstrual cycle, and affected patients are more severely ill than those with nongonococcal PID. On the other hand, patients with nongonococcal PID are more likely to have a history of previous PID and a less optimal response to conventional antimicrobial therapy, and are more likely to develop late sequelae such as recurrent PID, adnexal abscess, and infertility.

The clinical diagnosis of acute PID by history and physical findings alone is often inaccurate. The classic manifestations include fever, chills, malaise, and bilateral lower abdominal pain that is often aggravated by movement of the iliopsoas muscles. Pelvic examination reveals a mucopurulent cervical discharge, and exquisite tenderness on movement of the cervix. The adnexal regions are tender and thickened, and an adnexal or cul-de-sac mass may be palpable if infection is recurrent or chronic. Visual confirmation of tubal inflammation by colposcopy or laparoscopy can be very helpful and should be undertaken, particularly if the clinical diagnosis of acute PID is in doubt, or when the clinical presentation is atypical. Analyses of specimens obtained by culdocentesis for presence of PMNs and microorganisms by Gram stain and culture are helpful, but not very reliable for the diagnosis of chlamydial salpingitis. Cervical secretions should be routinely examined for PMNs as well as both *N. gonorrhoeae* and *C. trachomatis*. Since appropriate collection and microbiologic testing of specimens from the fallopian tubes are neither practical nor desirable in all cases of PID, treatment is often empiric, based on selection of antimicrobial agents active against the major recognized pathogens (see Table 3). Any IUD should be removed, and all sexual partners within 2 months prior to the patient's illness should be examined and empirically treated with a regimen effective against both *C. trachomatis* and *N. gonorrhoeae* before and irrespective of cultural results. Hospitalization should be considered for acutely ill patients, particularly if pelvic peritonitis is present, if the diagnosis of acute PID is in doubt and other surgical emergencies are possible, if an adnexal or cul-de-sac mass is palpable, or if the patient is pregnant.

It should be noted that none of the currently recommended regimens for acute salpingitis outlined in Table 3 are considered optimal therapy, and their relative efficacy remains to be established by controlled clinical trials. The cefoxitin-doxycycline regimen is theoretically most attractive, since cefoxitin has excellent activity against the anaerobes most frequently isolated in PID, as well as aerobic and microaerophilic streptococci, coliforms, and gonococci, whereas doxycycline is effective against *C. trachomatis* and *M. hominis*. The metronidazole-doxycycline combination is attractive since excellent tissue concentrations can be achieved by oral administration of these agents. However, this regimen may not be reliably effective against Enterobacteriaceae or against *N. gonorrhoeae* in areas where moderate tetracycline resistance is encountered. The clindamycin-aminoglycoside regimen is the least attractive since it does not provide optimal coverage for either *C. trachomatis* or *N. gonorrhoeae*. The combination of trimethoprim-sulfamethoxazole plus clindamycin for outpatient treatment of acute PID appears promising and deserves critical evaluation. Similarly, the combination of a new-generation quinolone plus either clindamycin or metronidazole may prove effective, but results from controlled clinical trials are not yet available. Approximately 5 to 15 percent of women fail to respond to initial antimicrobial therapy, 20 percent have at least one recurrence, and 15 percent are left infertile. It is clear that a comprehensive assessment of any therapeutic regimen for PID must include evaluation for late sequelae such as recurrence, infertility, and ectopic pregnancy, as well as the immediate response to acute symptoms.

Vulvovaginal and Tubo-ovarian Abscess

Pyogenic Vulvovaginal Infections

These include abscess of Bartholin's and Skene's glands, infected labial inclusion cysts, labial abscesses, furunculosis, and hidradenitis. Mixed infection due to both aerobic and anaerobic vaginal bacteria is the general rule, and coliforms, *B. fragilis*, *B. bivius*, and anaerobic cocci are commonly involved. Coexisting *N. gonorrhoeae* should be excluded. Surgical drainage is the primary therapeutic modality, and antimicrobials are of secondary importance. In the absence of specific cultural and antibiotic susceptibility data, initial selection of drugs should include those effective against both aerobic and anaerobic bacteria of vaginal origin (Table 4). Subsequent modification of antimicrobial therapy should be guided by the clinical response and by microbiologic data based on specimens obtained by direct needle aspiration of lesions (avoiding contamination by normal vaginal flora).

Tubo-ovarian Abscess

Tubo-ovarian abscess (TOA) occurring in the absence of obstetric and postoperative infections is generally a consequence of acute or chronic PID. Unilateral presentation of TOA is not uncommon and is not uniquely associated with IUD usage. Tubo-ovarian abscesses are often polymicrobial, caused by mixed aerobes and anaerobes including *Escherichia coli*, *B. fragilis*, *B. bivius*, *Peptostreptococcus* species, and aerobic streptococci. The recommended antimicrobial regimens for initial empiric treatment of TOA are outlined in Table 4. The optimal duration of treatment has not been clearly established. The general recommendation is that antibiotic should be continued by oral administration for 6 to 8 weeks, until the adnexal mass is no longer palpable. Medical therapy with antimicrobial agents alone is successful in 40 to 70 percent of cases. Surgical intervention is indicated if rupture is suspected or imminent or if suboptimal clinical response is observed after 72 hours of initial antimicrobial therapy. Conservative initial management of TOA, particularly in young, nulliparous patients, is indicated in the majority of cases. Serial ultrasonography is particularly useful in assessing the therapeutic response and resolution of mass effect during follow-up.

Genital Warts

Genital warts are caused by specific serotypes of human HPV (types 6, 11, 16, 18, 31, 33, and 35). The association of HPV infection and cervical intraepithelial neoplasia is strong, and unique HPV serotypes are implicated. For example, HPV type 16 or 18, which apparently causes only a small proportion of genital warts, is present in 70 percent of cervical cancers. Conversely, serotype 6, the most common cause of overt genital warts, is rarely found in genital cancer. Serotypes 10, 11, 31, 33, and 35 are also associated with cervical neoplasia but are found in a low percentage of cases.

HPV infection appears to be increasing rapidly in the general population and currently is among the three most

TABLE 4 Recommended Regimens for Treatment of Vulvovaginal and Tubo-ovarian Abscess

Infection	*Choice*	*Alternative*
Vulvovaginal abscess		
Inpatient	Cefoxitin (1.5 g IV q8h) for 5–7 days	Metronidazole (500 mg IV q6h) or clindamycin (600 mg IV q8h) plus gentamicin or tobramycin (1.5 mg/kg IV q8h) for 5–7 days
Outpatient	Ampicillin (500 mg PO q.i.d.) plus metronidazole (500 mg q.i.d.) for 7–10 days	Trimethoprim-sulfamethoxazole 80-mg/400-mg (1 tablet PO b.i.d.) plus clindamycin (300 mg PO t.i.d.) for 7–10 days
Tubo-ovarian abscess		
Inpatient	Clindamycin (600 mg IV q8h) plus tobramycin (1.5 mg/kg IV q8h) for 10–14 days	Metronidazole (500 mg IV q6h) or cefoxitin (1.5 g IV q8h) or ticarcillin (3 g IV q4h), each plus gentamicin or tobramycin (1.5 mg/kg IV q8h) for 10–14 days *or* Cefotaxime (1.5 g IV q6h) ± gentamicin or tobramycin (depending on severity) (1.5 mg/kg IV q8h) for 10–14 days
Outpatient	Ampicillin (500 mg PO q.i.d.) plus metronidazole (500 mg PO q.i.d.) for 6–8 wk	Trimethoprim-sulfamethoxazole 80-mg/400-mg (2 tablets PO b.i.d.) plus clindamycin (300 mg PO t.i.d.) for 6–8 wk

Regimens are applicable after exclusion of endocervical or paraurethral *N. gonorrhoeae* or *C. trachomatis* infection.

common diseases diagnosed in patients attending STD clinics. Most genital warts are subclinical and may be detected only with colposcopy, cytology, biopsy, or DNA hybridization techniques. Infection may be overt, extensive, and symptomatic in immunocompromised individuals, such as in patients with the acquired immunodeficiency syndrome or following bone marrow or solid organ transplantation. Genital warts in women are generally more extensive than might be assumed from overt lesions. The posterior introitus is the most common location for overt warts (73 percent), followed by the vulva (30 percent), the vagina (15 percent), and the cervix (6 percent). However, over 50 percent of women with vulvar warts have colposcopic evidence of cervical HPV infection. As in men, anorectal involvement is not uncommon.

Therapy for HPV infection is primarily directed at symptomatic and overt lesions at present. It remains to be determined whether routine treatment of subclinical infection is warranted and is effective in preventing genital neoplasia. Weekly topical application with podophyllin has been widely used for clearing overt warts and is effective in 75 percent of cases, with an expected relapse rate of 65 to 78 percent within 3 to 12 months. Podophyllin is toxic if absorbed and can cause severe local reactions including ulceration and bleeding. It should be carefully applied under medical supervision, allowed to dry thoroughly, and washed off within 3 to 4 hours after the initial application. This interval may be extended as tolerated during subsequent treatments. Podophyllin should be avoided during pregnancy, and its application to cervical lesions is not recommended. Cryotherapy with liquid nitrogen appears to be an effective alternative and is cost effective for initial therapy of nonextensive warts. Generally, 3 to 6 weekly applications are required. The main adverse effect is pain, but it appears to be better tolerated than electrical cautery. Laser ablation should be reserved for patients with extensive or refractory warts. Topical 5-fluorouracil (1 percent solution) may cause necrosis and sloughing of rapidly proliferating tissue, and its use is more limited. Finally, interferons, either topically, intralesionally, or systemically, have been used experimentally in the treatment of overt genital warts. The type of interferon preparations (leukocyte interferon, α- and β-interferons) and dose and treatment regimens have varied. The early results appear promising, but more careful evaluations are required before their role in the treatment of genital warts is established.

SUGGESTED READING

Berg AO, Heidrich FE, Fihn SD, et al. Establishing the cause of genitourinary symptoms in women in a family practice. JAMA 1984; 251:620–625.

Bruham RC, Paavonen J, Stevens CE, et al. Mucopurulent cervicitis. The ignored counterpart in women of urethritis in men. N Engl J Med 1984; 311:1–6.

Burnakis TG, Hildebrandt NB. Pelvic inflammatory disease. A review with emphasis on antimicrobial therapy. Rev Infect Dis 1986; 8:86–116.

Centers for Disease Control. 1985 STD treatment guidelines. MMWR 1985; 34:75s–108s.

Kirby P, Corey L. Genital human papillomavirus infections. Infect Dis Clin North Am 1987; 1:123–178.

Landers DV, Sweet RL. Current trends in the diagnosis and treatment of tubo-ovarian abscess. Am J Obstet Gynecol 1985; 151:1098–1110.

Noble MA, Kwong A, Barteluk RL, et al. Laboratory diagnosis of *Chlamydia trachomatis* using two immunodiagnostic methods. Am J Clin Pathol 1988; 90:205–210.

Paavonen J, Critchlow CW, DeRouen T, et al. Etiology of cervical inflammation. Am J Obstet Gynecol 1986; 154:556–564.

Paavonen J, Stamm WE. Lower genital tract infections in women. Infect Dis Clin North Am 1987; 1:179–198.

Sobel JD. Recurrent vulvovaginal candidiasis. A prospective study of the efficacy of maintenance ketoconazole therapy. N Engl J Med 1986; 315:1455–1458.

Sweet RL. Pelvic inflammatory disease and infertility in women. Infect Dis Clin North Am 1987; 1:199–215.

Wasserheit JN, Bell TA, Kiviat NB, et al. Microbial causes of proven pelvic inflammatory disease and efficacy of clindamycin and tobramycin. Ann Intern Med 1986; 104:187–193.

TOXIC SHOCK SYNDROME

JEFFREY PARSONNET, M.D.

Despite significant advances in our understanding of the epidemiology, pathogenesis, and treatment of toxic shock syndrome (TSS), this disease continues to strike patients of both sexes, of all ages, and in a variety of clinical settings. TSS remains a clinical diagnosis, defined by the presence of fever, hypotension, rash with late desquamation, and multiple organ system dysfunction. The diagnosis must be made on the basis of clinical criteria alone, without the benefit of diagnostic cultures, antibody titers, or toxicologic studies. The disease is eminently treatable, however, and patients treated early in the course of illness usually recover without sequelae. The burden on the practicing physician is to maintain an awareness of TSS in order to facilitate early recognition, after which options of management are finite and straightforward.

Optimal therapy for TSS is grounded upon an understanding of its epidemiology and pathogenesis, for which reason attention must be directed to these aspects of the disease.

EPIDEMIOLOGY AND PATHOGENESIS

The classic association recognized by most physicians is that between tampon use during menstruation and the development of TSS. This is unfortunate, because it obscures an equally important, and probably more frequent, association between other types of staphylococcal infection and TSS. It is difficult to estimate the relative frequencies with which menstrual and nonmenstrual TSS occur, because of underreporting of the former, underrecognition of the latter, and the absence of a definitive diagnostic test for either. TSS has been reported to occur as a complication of the use of barrier contraceptives, childbirth (by cesarean and vaginal delivery), infections of the upper and lower respiratory tract, infections of prosthetic devices, and a variety of soft tissue and postoperative wound infections. The incidence in men is roughly the same as that in women, if menstrual, postpartum, and contraceptive-associated cases are excluded.

The common denominator in all cases of TSS is infection with a toxin-producing strain of *Staphylococcus aureus* in the absence of protective antibody at the time of infection. In 1981 two groups of investigators independently identified the most common TSS toxin, TSS toxin-1 (TSST-1). Formerly called pyrogenic exotoxin C and staphylococcal enterotoxin F, TSST-1 is now known to cause more than 90 percent of cases of menstrual TSS and about 40 to 60 percent of nonmenstrual cases. Although there is less certainty about what other staphylococcal products cause TSS, it appears that enterotoxins A through E, which heretofore have been recognized only as causing food poisoning, are the most likely candidates to be alternative TSS toxins. This conclusion is based upon the high frequency with which one or several enterotoxins are produced by TSST-1-negative, TSS-associated strains of *S. aureus*, certain biologic properties shared by TSST-1 and the enterotoxins in vitro and in animal models, and serologic data from patients with TSS. Enterotoxin B appears to be the most common TSS toxin among TSST-1-negative strains from cases of nonmenstrual TSS.

Reports of TSS occurring as a consequence of infection with coagulase-negative staphylococci have not been confirmed; only *S. aureus* produces the toxins implicated in TSS, making infection with this organism necessary. The presence of other bacteria, particularly gram-negative bacilli, at sites of infection or mucosal colonization may influence production of toxin or the severity of its effects, but bacteria other than *S. aureus* are not required.

Regardless of the causative toxin, susceptibility to disease correlates with absence of a protective level of antibody to that toxin. The likelihood of an individual having antibody to TSST-1 is a function of age: by age 10 years, about half of all individuals have what is considered to be a protective antibody titer; by age 20, three-quarters of individuals exceed this titer; and by age 30, more than 90 percent of all people are immune. These data suggest that colonization or subclinical infection with TSST-1-producing strains of *S. aureus* is adequate to induce the development of antibody. Antibody to TSST-1 is present at birth (unless the mother is lacking such antibody), making TSS uncommon in infancy. TSS is most common during adolescence, when there is still a relatively large population at risk (by virtue of seronegativity) and health practices come into play that promote infection or enhance production of toxin.

Conditions favoring colonization and infection with toxigenic strains of *S. aureus* have not been identified. At any time, 10 to 20 percent of all individuals are colonized with *S. aureus* at mucosal sites, and about 20 percent of these strains produce TSST-1. On the other hand, factors have been identified that enhance production of TSST-1 at sites of infection; these include an aerobic environment (oxygen being required for production of toxin); a neutral pH; and a low concentration of magnesium ion. The relation of these factors to the development of clinical disease is readily apparent. For example, insertion of a tampon introduces sufficient oxygen to the vagina (which is normally anaerobic) to allow production of TSST-1; vaginal pH, which is acidic in the interval between menses, rises closer to neutrality during menstruation; and certain tampons have been shown to bind magnesium ion, thereby lowering that which is available to the organism to a range that enhances production of TSST-1 in vitro. The relative contribution of each of these factors remains the subject of intense investigation, and the degree to which they apply to nonmenstrual disease and to production of staphylococcal enterotoxins is not known.

Although TSST-1 is potent in its ability to cause disease, it exerts virtually no direct toxicity on human cells. Rather, it appears to act by initiating a cascade of immunologic and nonimmunologic events that centers on binding to and stimulation of mononuclear cells, particularly circulating monocytes and lymphocytes and tissue macrophages. Purified TSST-1 is a potent inducer of interleukin-1 (also known as endogenous pyrogen) production by human monocytes. It also induces production by monocytes of tumor necrosis factor (also known as cachectin), now known to be an important mediator of the lethal effects of endotoxin. Production of these cytokines could account for many of the signs and symptoms of TSS, including fever, shock, and multiple organ system dysfunction, by virtue of direct effects on host cells or by induction of secondary mediators of inflammation. TSST-1 itself is rapidly cleared from the bloodstream when the nidus of infection is removed or drained (which is usually possible) and can be neutralized in vivo by the administration of antibody to the toxin, which may have clinical implications for some patients.

CLINICAL MANIFESTATIONS

The clinical manifestations of TSS are largely encompassed by the case definition, which has remained essentially unchanged over the past decade (Table 1). Fever is invariable. The rash is typically a diffuse, blanching, macular erythroderma, but it may be patchy in distribution. Petechial and papulopustular eruptions have been reported but are distinctly uncommon. The rash is usually present within 48 hours of the onset of illness but may be evanescent and may be mistaken for the flush that may accompany fever. Involvement of the hands and feet is common and is often associated with peripheral edema, which may be severe. Hypotension, defined as a systolic pressure of 90 mm Hg or less or an orthostatic decrease in diastolic pressure of 15 or more mm Hg, is usually present, but a history of orthostatic dizziness or syncope is sufficient to fulfill this criterion. Full-thickness desquamation, especially of the palms, soles, and fingertips, occurs during convalescence, usually 5 to 12 days after onset of illness. (Absence of desquamation at the time of presentation is often mistakenly interpreted as being inconsistent with TSS.) Finally, the diagnosis is contingent on there being "reasonable evidence" for absence of other causes of illness, a criterion satisfied in most cases by a care-

TABLE 1 Case Definition of Toxic Shock Syndrome

Fever: temperature ≥38.9 °C

Rash: typically a diffuse macular erythroderma

Hypotension: systolic blood pressure ≤90 mm Hg for adults or below fifth percentile by age for children <16 yr, orthostatic drop in diastolic blood pressure ≥15 mm Hg, orthostatic syncope, or orthostatic dizziness

Multisystem involvement—three or more of the following:
- Gastrointestinal: vomiting, diarrhea
- Muscular: severe myalgia or CPK ≥ twice the upper limit of normal
- Mucous membrane: vaginal, oropharyngeal, or conjunctival hyperemia
- Renal: BUN or creatinine at least twice the upper limit of normal, or pyuria (≥5 leukocytes per high-power field) in the absence of urinary tract infection
- Hepatic: total bilirubin or serum transaminase at least twice the upper limit of normal
- Hematologic: platelets ≤100,000/mm³
- CNS: disorientation or alterations in consciousness without focal neurologic signs when fever and hypotension are absent

Desquamation: 1–2 weeks after onset of illness

Negative results on the following tests, if obtained; blood, throat, or CSF (blood culture may be positive for *S aureus*); rise in titer to Rocky Mountain spotted fever agent, leptospirosis, or rubeola

From Reingold AL, Hargrett NT, Shands KN, et al. Toxic shock syndrome surveillance in the United States, 1980 to 1981. Ann Intern Med 1982; 96(part 2):875–880.

TABLE 2 Clinical Manifestations and Laboratory Abnormalities in Toxic Shock Syndrome

	Estimated Frequency of Occurrence (%)
Symptoms*	
Myalgia	92
Vomiting	90
Diarrhea	86
Headache	72
Dizziness	70
Sore throat	65
Signs†	
Abdominal tenderness	83
Pharyngitis/strawberry tongue	81
Peripheral edema	73
Conjunctivitis	65
CNS dysfunction	60
Vaginal inflammation	47
Laboratory abnormalities	
Anemia (within first 24 hours)	66
Leukocytosis	70
Thrombocytopenia	52
Increased prothrombin time	70
Increased partial thromboplastin time	43
Increased BUN	68
Increased serum creatinine	69
Increased SGOT	73
Increased total bilirubin	66
Increased CPK	66
Hypocalcemia	80
Hypophosphatemia	60
Hypoalbuminemia	81
Pyuria	77
Hematuria	46

The data are compiled from six reviews of clinical manifestations of TSS.
* Other reported symptoms: chills, cough, dyspnea, arthralgia, abdominal pain, vaginal discharge.
† All patients fulfilled criteria of fever, hypotension, rash, and desquamation. Other reported signs: joint effusion, meningismus, muscle tenderness.

ful epidemiologic history, complete physical examination, and routine cultures, particularly of blood.

Multiple organ-system dysfunction is one of the hallmarks of TSS. Table 2 reflects the frequency with which specific symptoms, signs, and laboratory abnormalities have been noted by various authors. Of note is the nonspecific nature of many features of TSS, including the most frequently reported symptoms of myalgia, vomiting, diarrhea, and headache. In addition to demonstrating signs of illness that are integral to the case definition, physical examination usually reveals a toxic-appearing patient with conjunctival and pharyngeal injection (or a "strawberry tongue"), diffuse abdominal tenderness, muscle tenderness, and peripheral edema. Disorders of the central nervous system, particularly disorientation and a depressed level of consciousness, may be disproportionate to the degree of hypotension. In cases of menstruation-related disease, the pelvic examination is most often normal, with no pelvic tenderness, signs of vaginal inflammation, or purulent discharge, although all have been reported. In nonmenstrual TSS, it is common for the usual signs of pyogenic infection to be lacking; infected surgical wounds, for example, often appear remarkably benign, but nonetheless yield toxigenic *S. aureus* upon culture. Typical manifestations of staphylococcal infection of skin and soft tissues may be evident, but subtle infections are more common. This disparity between the mildness of the local inflammatory response and the severity of systemic toxicity, while not universal, can be an important clue to the diagnosis.

Several aspects of multisystem dysfunction are distinctive enough to serve as diagnostic clues. Myalgias are common and may be severe, for which reason the "influenza-like" features of TSS may predominate. The creatine phosphokinase (CPK) level is often elevated and the degree of elevation may be extreme, with resultant myoglobinuria. The author has treated a young woman with menstrual TSS whose CPK level rose as high as 46,000 units per milliliter, despite rapid correction of what had been relatively mild hypotension. Abnormal clotting parameters and thrombocytopenia are common, which may be useful in distinguishing TSS from Kawasaki disease (in which platelets are either normal or increased) and other disorders. Bleeding is uncommon, however. Hypocalcemia is almost invariable, to the extent that a normal calcium value should prompt reconsideration of the diagnosis. Although the mechanism of hypocalcemia is not known, it appears that both ionized and total calcium are depressed, the latter in part because of hypoalbuminemia. Hypomagnesemia probably occurs more commonly than has been recognized, and hypocalcemia may be refractory to therapy until magnesium stores have been repleted. Despite renal insufficiency, hypophosphatemia is also common, which may be another useful clue to the diagnosis.

The most serious complications encountered in TSS are adult respiratory distress syndrome (ARDS) and progressive renal insufficiency, the pathogeneses of which are multifactorial. The severity and duration of hypotension are probably important determinants of whether these complications ensue, making rapid reversal of hypotension imperative. Cases not associated with a removable focus or with infections amenable to surgical drainage may be associated with an increased rate of complications, presumably because of a longer duration of toxemia. Unfortunately, the ultimate course of the disease is unpredictable in its early stages, making close observation obligatory in all but the mildest cases. Invasive monitoring is useful in guiding early resuscitative measures, particularly when use of a vasopressor is being considered. Consumptive coagulopathy is often present at the time of presentation, the pathogenesis of which is unknown. Rhabdomyolysis, possibly related to massive release of interleukin-1, may be present at the time of presentation or develop subsequent to initiation of therapy. Alopecia and loss of fingernails and toenails 2 to 3 months after the acute illness, a late rash, and persistent neuromuscular and neuropsychiatric abnormalities are commonly seen but ultimately resolve without residual deficits.

Recurrent TSS results from persistent colonization with a toxin-producing staphylococcus in the continued absence of antibody. Before the epidemiology and pathogenesis of menstrual TSS had been elucidated, recurrence rates as high as 66 percent were seen among women who continued to use tampons and were not treated with an antistaphylococcal agent. Some women have a brisk antibody response following an episode of menstrual TSS and are thereby protected from recurrent disease. Unfortunately, some women do not develop protective antibody for several months, and a number have been shown to be antibody-negative a year or more after the first episode (during which time they may have had multiple recurrences). The reasons for this variability are not certain, but failure to develop antibody does not appear to have a hereditary basis nor does it signify a more general immunodeficiency state. As a potent immunomodulator, TSST-1 may actually suppress development of antibody to itself under some circumstances. For reasons that are unclear, recurrent nonmenstrual TSS is uncommon. Regardless of the clinical setting, the risk of recurrence can be determined and influenced by diagnostic and therapeutic measures, as discussed below.

DIAGNOSIS

The diagnosis of TSS is supported by laboratory studies performed at the time of presentation showing evidence of multiple organ–system dysfunction. Routine hematologic and chemistry profiles are usually sufficient for this purpose. For diagnostic purposes, particular attention should be directed to the platelet count; prothrombin time; urinalysis (microscopic and dipstick examinations); tests of renal and hepatic function; serum calcium, magnesium, and phosphate; and CPK—the sum of which often paints the distinctive picture of this syndrome. These data may also have important therapeutic implications for initial management, particularly the coagulation profile, serum electrolytes, and renal parameters. A chest radiograph and electrocardiogram should be performed. Routine cultures of blood and urine, as well as of other appropriate sites (such as the genital tract, throat, respiratory secretions, wounds, or other skin lesions) should be obtained. The isolation of *S aureus* is not an official criterion for diagnosing TSS, but failure to do so should prompt reconsideration of the diagnosis, unless there are mitigating circumstances. There are three reasons why *S. aureus* may not be cultured from a patient with TSS: first, the organism may be overgrown in culture by other organisms, which are often present in abundance; second, TSS-associated strains of *S. aureus* may be misidentified as coagulase-negative staphylococci because they are often not β-hemolytic or pigmented; and third, *S. aureus* may not be sought until after initiation of antimicrobial therapy.

Specialized tests related to detection of TSS toxins and antibody to these toxins are available and can serve three general purposes: first, to support or oppose the diagnosis of TSS in the acute setting, thereby guiding initial management; second, to establish the diagnosis with greater certainty after resolution of the acute process; and third, to provide guidelines for the patient and physician as to the risk of recurrence and the safety of contraceptive and catamenial product use. Such tests are performed by several clinical and research laboratories around the country, including the author's (Channing Laboratory, 180 Longwood Avenue, Boston, MA 02115). Three studies have proved to be of particular utility in the management of patients:

1. Testing for production of toxin by incriminated strains of *S. aureus*. This is especially useful in menstrual TSS, most cases of which are caused by TSST-1, making routine testing advisable. The finding of a TSST-1-positive strain of *S. aureus* in the setting of a compatible clinical illness is moderately supportive of the diagnosis.
2. Testing of acute serum for antibody to TSST-1. This test is also of greater utility in the setting of menstrual illness, in which a low antibody level indicates susceptibility to TSST-1 and a high titer connotes immunity. Some cases of menstrual and many cases of nonmenstrual TSS are caused by other toxins, however, again relegating this analysis to a supportive but nondiagnostic role.
3. Testing of convalescent serum for antibody to TSST-1. When paired with an acute serum sample, this test is of diagnostic utility if seroconversion to TSST-1 (or one of the enterotoxins) is demonstrated. The prognostic and therapeutic implications with regard to the risk of recurrence, and prevention of same, are readily apparent. It is appropriate to obtain a convalescent sample for testing 1 month after the acute illness and thereafter at monthly intervals if necessary.

Some laboratories may also be able to measure TSST-1 in serum and urine samples obtained during the acute illness. These studies (which remain investigational) are of potential diagnostic utility, particularly if arrangements can be made to obtain results quickly. It should be emphasized, however, that the diagnosis of TSS must still be made on clinical grounds and that the greatest utility of specialized testing is to assist the physician in counseling the patient about the risk of recurrence.

The differential diagnosis of TSS includes a large number of disease entities, especially if one considers all illnesses characterized primarily by fever and rash. Many such diagnoses can be effectively ruled out by a careful history, physical examination, and routine laboratory studies. Of prime consideration at the time of initial evaluation are the patient's age, the gynecologic history (including use of tampons and contraceptives), any unusual epidemiologic features, the presence of a possible focus of staphylococcal infection, and, of course, fulfillment of the diagnostic criteria of high fever, rash, hypotension, and multisystem disease. In most instances, these factors will narrow the differential diagnosis to a short list of disease entities (Table 3).

Differentiating between TSS and Kawasaki disease in young children can be difficult, particularly within 24 hours of admission. Like TSS, Kawasaki disease is diagnosed on the basis of clinical criteria, and these criteria are similar in many respects to those of TSS. In the author's experience, the presence of a lesion that could be infected with *S. aureus* (such as a recent burn, wound, or other skin lesion), the pace of the illness, the nature of the rash, the platelet count, and the serum calcium level are useful discriminating parameters in the acute setting. It is not uncommon, however, for patients to be treated for both illnesses while cultures and results of special studies are pending.

Streptococcus pyogenes (group A streptococcus), the etiologic agent of scarlet fever, can cause an illness that is virtually indistinguishable from staphylococcal TSS. This illness, which is mediated principally by streptococcal pyrogenic toxin A, appears to have been increasing in frequency over the past several years. In the author's experience, staphylococcal TSS in children tends to be milder than in adults, thus mimicking scarlet fever, whereas streptococcal infections in adults involving toxigenic strains may be every bit as severe as staphylococcal TSS. It is prudent, therefore, to culture appropriate sites for *S. pyogenes* if staphylococcal infection is not apparent at the time of presentation.

TABLE 3 Differential Diagnosis of Toxic Shock Syndrome at the Time of Presentation

Disease	*Comments*
Kawasaki disease	Can closely resemble TSS in young children. Uncommon in individuals aged >4 yr. More of a subacute illness, with fever ≥5 days required for diagnosis. Swollen, fissured lips, prominent polymorphous rash, adenopathy, cardiac involvement, normal serum calcium level and platelet count, and absence of hypotension may help distinguish from TSS.
Scarlet fever	Exudative pharyngitis (rarely seen in TSS) suggests streptococcal infection. Rash prominent, less evanescent. Severe forms of scarlet fever ("septic scarlet fever," "toxic scarlet fever," "toxic strep syndrome") can be indistinguishable from TSS on clinical grounds.
Staphylococcal scalded skin syndrome	Exudative, bullous lesions with sloughing of skin in acute setting. Leaves extensive denuded areas that are red, raw, and wet. Positive Nikolsky sign (wrinkling of skin in response to gentle friction). Absence of multisystem disease.
Septic shock	Must be considered, for sake of empiric antibiotic coverage, unless clinical setting is classic for TSS or staphylococcal infection is evident (e.g., by Gram stain).
Rocky Mountain spotted fever	Merits consideration because of severe consequences of withholding therapy. Usually distinguishable on epidemiologic grounds or by nature of rash.
Meningococcemia	Merits consideration because of severe consequences of withholding therapy. Petechiae and purpura are uncommon in TSS, but maculopapular eruptions are occasionally seen in meningococcemia.
Viral illness with exanthem	Hypotension uncommon unless patient severely dehydrated.
Drug reactions	Careful history required. May be superimposed on viral or bacterial infection, making distinction from TSS difficult.

TREATMENT

Regardless of the clinical setting, the critical therapeutic measures in TSS are (1) removal of any nidus of infection or surgical drainage of pus; (2) administration of intravenous fluids (the requirements for which may be massive); (3) repletion of serum calcium and magnesium, if necessary; and (4) administration of an antibiotic active against *S. aureus*. When hypotension is severe, vasopressors may be required, but fluids should be considered the mainstay of therapy. In most cases antibiotics should initially be given intravenously, but an oral agent may suffice from the outset in mild cases, particularly if there is a foreign body that can be removed (thereby blocking further absorption of toxin). In such cases, the main rationale for antibiotic use is reduction of the risk of recurrent TSS by eradication of the infecting strain. The response to these measures is usually rapid, unless there has been a prolonged period of hypotension prior to institution of therapy.

The antibiotic used should be the narrowest-spectrum agent having good antimicrobial activity against the infecting strain of *S. aureus*. In most cases oxacillin (or nafcillin) would best meet these criteria at a dose of 6 to 12 g per day, depending on severity of illness (200 mg per kilogram per day for children), given every 4 hours. Penicillin should be used if the organism is shown to be susceptible to it. Cefazolin or vancomycin should be given to patients known to be allergic to penicillin. Vancomycin should be used before sensitivity data are available when there is a higher-than-usual likelihood of infection with a methicillin-resistant strain. Intravenous therapy can be discontinued in favor of an oral antibiotic following resolution of the acute illness, which is usually within 3 days. When TSS complicates a deep-seated focus of infection, intravenous therapy should be continued as long as would otherwise be necessary to treat that infection. Dicloxacillin is the oral drug of choice, assuming the most common susceptibility profile, with a variety of other drugs available for penicillin-allergic patients. A total duration of therapy of 2 weeks is recommended, although this has not been studied systematically.

Two additional forms of therapy, immunoglobulin and corticosteroids, merit consideration under some circumstances. All commercial preparations of immunoglobulin contain high levels of antibody to TSST-1 (and presumably to alternative TSS toxins). The rationale for using immunoglobulin would be to specifically neutralize circulating toxin. In the author's opinion, this treatment is justifiable when there is an undrainable or irremovable focus of infection, such as pneumonia or endometritis, that would result in ongoing toxemia for a considerable period after initiation of therapy. This treatment has not been critically evaluated and should be reserved for the sickest patients. A dose of 400 mg per kilogram, given as a single intravenous infusion over 2 to 3 hours, is reasonable based upon experience with use of immunoglobulin for other diseases (such as Kawasaki disease). A relative contraindication to this mode of therapy is cost; for an average-sized adult, the cost to the patient of immunoglobulin therapy would be more than (U.S.) $2,000.

In a retrospective study, corticosteroids were shown to have a favorable impact on severity of illness and duration of fever if administered within the first few days of illness. In the author's opinion, however, use of steroids on a routine basis cannot be recommended. Unless there is evidence of adrenal insufficiency, steroids should be considered only when a patient's hypotension is not responsive to removal or drainage of the focus of infection and several hours of fluid administration.

The risk of recurrence is low, probably less than 10 percent, among women who are treated with antibiotics for 2 weeks and who refrain from using tampons or barrier contraceptives. Recurrence of nonmenstrual TSS is unusual under any circumstances. The risk of recurrence can be gauged by testing convalescent serum for antibody to TSS toxins, particularly if TSST-1 (about which the most is known) is the causative toxin. If antibody testing is not performed, patients should probably refrain from using tampons or barrier contraceptives for 4 to 6 months, the rationale being that most recurrences take place within several months of the first episode. It may be useful, under some circumstances, to determine whether the patient is still colonized with *S. aureus* and to retreat with antibiotics if it is found, but this course of action is often problematic (and unsuccessful). A sounder approach, in the author's opinion, is to test for the development of antibody and to let these results guide long-term management.

SUGGESTED READING

Chesney PJ, Davis JP, Purdy WK, Wand PJ, Chesney RW. Clinical manifestations of toxic shock syndrome. JAMA 1981; 246:741–748.

Davis JP, Chesney PJ, Wand PJ, et al. Toxic-shock syndrome; epidemiologic features, recurrence, risk factors, and prevention. N Engl J Med 1980; 303:1429–1435.

Parsonnet J. Mediators in the pathogenesis of toxic shock syndrome: overview. Rev Infect Dis 1989; 11:S263–S269.

Reingold AL, Hargrett NT, Dan BB, et al. Nonmenstrual toxic shock syndrome: a review of 130 cases. Ann Intern Med 1982; 96(part 2): 871–874.

Todd J, Fishaut M, Kapral F, Welch T. Toxic-shock syndrome associated with phage-group-I staphylococci. Lancet 1978; 2:1116–1118.

PROSTATITIS, EPIDIDYMITIS, AND BALANOPOSTHITIS

GERALD W. CHODAK, M.D.

PROSTATITIS

Current treatment of inflammatory diseases of the prostate still results in dissatisfied patients and frustrated physicians. Despite significant progress, there is a persistent difficulty in explaining why some patients respond so well to a short course of therapy and others have persistent or recurrent symptoms, even when prolonged therapy is employed. Nevertheless, a systematic approach to evaluation will enable the physician to localize the source of infection and determine whether it is likely to respond to antibiotic therapy.

Diagnostic Evaluation and Culture Techniques

In addition to the routine history and physical examination, information about the prostate can be obtained from microscopy and culture of the prostatic fluid. In order to localize the bacteria to the prostate, samples are taken from different parts of the voided urine as well as from fluid expressed by prostatic massage. At the time of evaluation, the patient should have a relatively full bladder. The urine is divided into the first 10 ml of voided urine (urethral sample) and the midstream urine (bladder sample). A digital examination is then performed, and fluid from the prostate is expressed into the urethra and collected (EPS). Another urine sample is then collected (VB3), which also contains prostatic fluid. The laboratory should be informed of the physician's interest in finding low densities of organisms. Evaluation of this test is difficult, but if pyuria is present, low counts of bacteria can be considered significant if no other diagnostic finding points to a differential diagnosis. The pathogens are usually the same as those causing urinary tract infections and include *Escherichia coli, Klebsiella, Enterobacter, Proteus,* and *Pseudomonas* species.

Microscopic Evaluation of Prostatic Fluid

Two criteria used to diagnose an inflammatory process in the prostate are the presence of leukocytes and lipid-laden macrophages (oval fat bodies) in the expressed prostatic fluid. The fluid must be compared with the first 10 ml of voided urine, which contains urethral contents. Normal prostatic fluid contains fewer than 10 white blood cells (WBC) per high-power field, and more than 15 or 20 WBC per high-power field are considered abnormal. Oval fat bodies are not typically found in the urethra, so that an increase in these cells in the prostatic fluid is also evidence for an inflammatory response.

Interpretation of Cultural Results

A bacterial infection in the prostate may not produce a count of more than 100,000 cfu per milliliter. Therefore, the diagnosis is made by comparing the prostatic cultures with those of the urethra and bladder. A prostatic infection is present when the urine from the bladder (VB2) contains fewer than 10,000 cfu/ml and the prostatic cultures (EPS and VB3) contain 10 times as many bacteria as does the urethral culture (VB1). In order to diagnose bacterial prostatitis when the bladder urine contains significant bacteria, the patient must first be treated for a few days with nitrofurantoin, which sterilizes the urine while not greatly affecting the prostate. Reculture at that time will permit the same comparison between the urethral sample and the VB3 and EPS cultures.

ACUTE BACTERIAL PROSTATITIS

Diagnosis

Patients with acute prostatitis present with fever, chills, and irritative voiding symptoms that include dysuria, frequency, and pain. Examination of the prostate reveals a tender prostate, and prostate massage is not recommended because of the possibility of producing a bacteremia. One underlying cause of this disorder is acute or chronic urinary retention, which is assessed by palpating an enlarged bladder. If significant residual urine is suspected following voiding, then the bladder is catheterized and an indwelling catheter is left in place when more than 100 ml is present.

Treatment

Hospitalization is usually advised for patients with high fever (greater than 101°F) and significant pain. Bed rest, hydration, and analgesics provide symptomatic relief. Antibiotic therapy is instituted with gentamicin (3 mg per kilogram intravenously in three divided doses) and ampicillin (2 g intravenously every 6 hours) until the cultures and sensitivities are available. When the fever has defervesced, the antibiotic can usually be changed to trimethoprim (160 mg) and sulfisoxazole (800 mg) orally twice a day. The usual course of therapy is 2 weeks. More recently, ciprofloxacin (250 to 500 mg twice a day for 7 to 10 days) may also be an excellent choice for treatment.

CHRONIC BACTERIAL PROSTATITIS

Diagnosis

Most men with chronic prostatitis complain of chronic irritative symptoms and pain in the pelvic area or in the penis following ejaculation. Patients may have recurrent urinary infections with the same organism and/or positive EPS or VB3 cultures.

Treatment

Optimal therapy requires obtaining high levels of antibiotic in prostatic secretions rather than in prostatic tissue (Fig. 1). The most effective treatment is trimethoprim (160

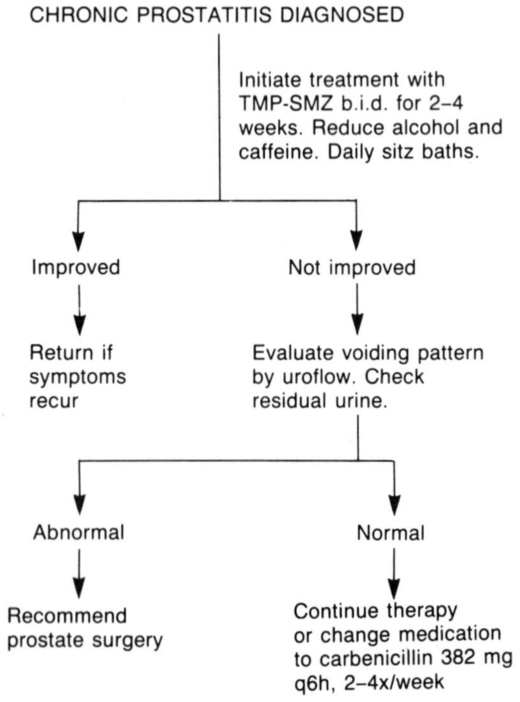

Figure 1 Treatment of chronic prostatitis.

mg) and sulfamethoxazole (800 mg) orally taken in combination twice a day. Patients treated with short courses of therapy are more likely to have recurrences than those taking a longer course. The best approach is to initiate therapy for 2–4 weeks. Patients who develop recurrent symptoms after therapy is discontinued may improve following administration of low-dose daily therapy consisting of 80 mg of trimethoprim and 400 mg of sulfamethoxazole for another 1 to 3 months. An alternative therapy is carbenicillin indanyl sodium (382 mg, two tablets orally four times per day) for 4 weeks, which may be as effective, although it has a substantially higher cost. In some cases, patients fail to obtain prolonged relief of their symptoms, and these may warrant surgical intervention, which involves either transurethral prostatectomy or total prostatovesiculectomy. Although the transurethral procedure has far fewer adverse effects, the patient should be informed that his symptoms may not be totally cured because some residual tissue will still remain. Urologists are generally reluctant to recommend surgery to treat this disorder.

NONBACTERIAL PROSTATITIS

Patients complain of the same symptoms found in bacterial prostatitis, and the prostatic fluid also contains more than 15 to 20 WBC per high-power field; however, the urine, EPS, and VB3 cultures are negative. There is no conclusive evidence that *Chlamydia* is a primary cause of this problem, and, yet, a trial of tetracycline, 500 mg orally every 6 hours for 10 to 14 days, may be warranted. If little or no response occurs, no additional antibiotics are warranted. Patients with negative cultures should not be placed on long-term antibiotic therapy. The optimal treatment is based on symptoms. Patients often feel better by taking hot sitz baths two or three times per day. Prostatic massage has no proven value in the management of this illness. Patients should be encouraged to maintain their normal sexual activity and physical exercise and should be informed that the problem is not serious but the symptoms are likely to persist for a variable period of time. Many patients notice that alcohol and caffeine worsen their symptoms, so that reducing these items from their diet may improve their symptoms.

ACUTE EPIDIDYMITIS

Acute epididymitis is a disorder characterized by an abrupt onset of pain and swelling in the tail of the epididymis and may be followed by diffuse swelling of the entire epididymis, ipsilateral testicle, and hemiscrotum (epididymo-orchitis). The causes may be either sexual or nonsexual; nonsexual causes are more likely to have an anatomic basis. Patients over 40 years of age who develop epididymitis usually have an associated urinary tract infection, which is due to some obstructive process such as a urethral stricture of benign prostatic hypertrophy.

Diagnosis

The initial diagnosis is made based on clinical findings, which include swelling and marked tenderness along the epididymis. As the disease progresses, epididymo-orchitis may develop as the testicle also becomes swollen and tender.

The cause of epididymitis in patients who have a history of sexual exposure may be determined by performing a Gram stain of a urethral smear obtained prior to voiding. If intracellular gram-negative diplococci are identified, then *Neisseria gonorrhoeae* is the cause. If no organisms are identified, then a culture must be performed to rule out gonococcal infection. In the absence of neisseriae, *Chlamydia trachomatis* is usually the responsible organism in this group.

For patients who develop epididymitis secondary to a urinary tract anomaly, a urine culture and sensitivity will identify the causative organism.

An important cause of epididymitis in the older population is urinary obstruction associated with an inability to empty the bladder. When the history or physical examination suggests a significant residual urine, a catheter is passed and left in place if more than 100 ml remains in the bladder following voiding.

Treatment

The optimal treatment of acute epididymitis depends on the underlying cause. Febrile patients with epididymitis secondary to bacteriuria are treated initially with ampicillin, 1 g intravenously every 6 hours, and tobramycin, 3.0 mg per kilogram intravenously in three divided doses, until the results of the urine culture and sensitivity are available. At that time either oral ampicillin, 500 mg orally every 6 hours for 10 days, or a first-generation cephalosporin may be substituted. Patients will usually benefit from symptomatic treatment, which includes hospitalization, bed rest, scrotal elevation, and ice packs to the scrotum to reduce swelling. If significant residual urine is detected, then a prostatectomy should be planned after the acute episode has resolved.

Men who develop acute epididymitis following sexual exposure are treated with ampicillin, 500 mg orally four times per day for 10 days, if *N. gonorrhoeae* has been cultured or found on Gram stain, or with tetracycline, 500 mg orally four times per day for 10 days, if there is no evidence for gonorrhea. In addition, symptomatic relief is provided by bed rest and scrotal elevation. When epididymitis has been caused by sexual transmission, sexual partners must also be treated.

BALANOPOSTHITIS

Infection of the glans penis and foreskin occurs almost exclusively in the uncircumcised male. Usually the foreskin cannot be retracted; this allows smegma and secretions to accumulate and provides a warm, moist culture medium that predisposes to infection. Balanitis and balanoposthitis are commonest in children and may be associated with impaired urination because of a tight phimosis. It also occurs following sexual contact with an infected partner.

Diagnosis

The initial diagnosis is made from physical examination. The foreskin may be difficult to retract over the glans.

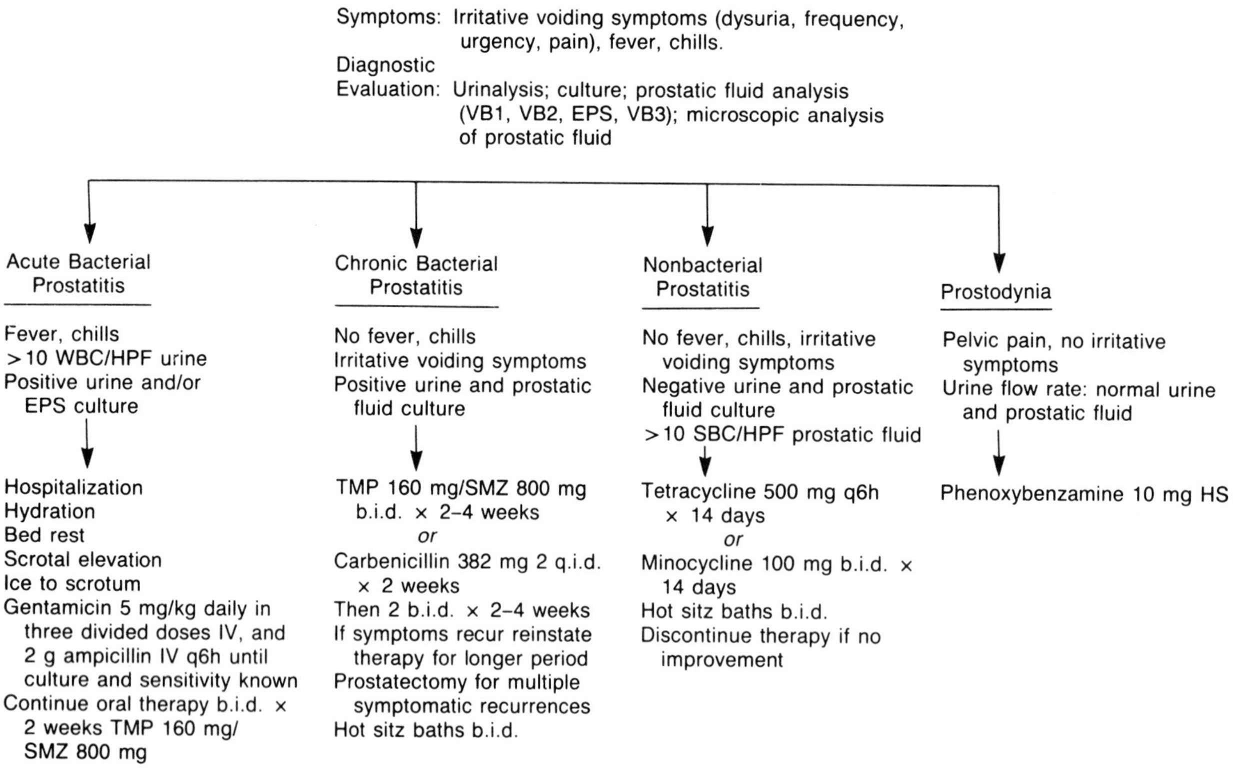

Figure 2 Diagnosis and treatment of prostatitis.

Inflammation and swelling of the glans and/or prepuce are present. A Gram stain of the material under the foreskin will determine the class of organisms present. Sexually active patients who develop balanoposthitis give a history of sexual contact within 6 to 24 hours prior to the onset of symptoms. These patients may have erosive soreness and ulceration of the glans penis. Microscopic examination should reveal the presence of *Candida*.

Treatment

Most cases of balanoposthitis in children can be treated with soap and water cleansing, provided that the foreskin can be retracted over the glans. Acutely, this may not be possible, and a dorsal slit procedure must be performed. This will allow improved hygiene, which helps to rapidly resolve the inflammation and swelling. Once this has resolved, the patient should undergo a circumcision. Antibiotics are usually not required.

Patients who develop balanoposthitis following sexual exposure to women with candidal vaginitis are treated with topical nystatin ointment, 100,000 units per gram, twice a day for 10 days. If phimosis is present and discharge is discovered under the glans, the sexual partner also receives the same treatment. Figure 2 provides a flow chart that summarizes the content of the discussion in this chapter.

DISSEMINATED GONOCOCCAL INFECTION

JONATHAN M. ZENILMAN, M.D.

Disseminated gonococcal infection (DGI) develops in approximately 0.5 to 1.0 percent of patients with gonorrhea, and is the most common cause of septic arthritis in persons under age 45 years. The manifestations of DGI are those of a febrile illness with prominent dermatologic and rheumatologic findings.

DGI has been clinically divided into two major syndromes: the dermatitis-tenosynovitis syndrome and the septic arthritis syndrome. Patients with the dermatitis-tenosynovitis syndrome usually present with chills, fever, polyarthralgias, and tenosynovitis and have three to 20 petechial, papular, pustular, hemorrhagic, or necrotic skin lesions, usually on the extensor surfaces of the distal extremities. The second common syndrome is septic arthritis, usually monoarticular, affecting large joints, most commonly the knee. Cultures of joint fluid are positive in about half the cases with effusion. Overlap between the two syndromes is not uncommon. A small proportion of DGI patients (approximately 1 percent) develop meningitis or endocarditis.

Blood cultures are positive in only half the patients with tenosynovitis dermatitis and in less than 20 percent of patients with septic arthritis. Often, patients with DGI have primary mucosal (either genital or pharyngeal) infection that may be mildly symptomatic or asymptomatic.

DGI should be suspected in sexually active patients with fever and rheumatologic or dermatologic symptoms. The differential diagnosis includes meningococcemia, acute rheumatic fever, Reiter's syndrome and other reactive arthritides, hepatitis B, endocarditis, viral illnesses such as Epstein-Barr or cytomegalovirus disease, and connective tissue diseases such as systemic lupus erythematosis, juvenile rheumatoid arthritis, and gout.

All patients with suspected DGI should have blood cultures performed by use of standard techniques and mucosal cultures at all sites of potential sexual exposure by use of selective medium (such as Thayer-Martin medium). Women should have cultures of the cervix, rectum, and pharynx. Men should have urethral and pharyngeal cultures, and rectal cultures should also be performed in homosexual men. If joint effusion is present, diagnostic arthrocentesis should be performed, with culture on nonselective media, such as chocolate agar. Gram stain and culture should be performed on aspirates of skin lesions; however, the sensitivity of these procedures is low. A confirmed diagnosis of DGI requires a positive culture from blood or synovial fluid; a probable case is defined as one with signs and symptoms of DGI with a positive mucosal site culture. In a small proportion of cases, all cultures may be negative (usually due to prior use of antibiotics). In these cases, the diagnosis is made by evaluating the signs and symptoms presented, ruling out other diseases in the differential diagnosis, and evaluating response to therapy.

CLINICAL AND EPIDEMIOLOGIC CONSIDERATIONS

Since all cases of DGI ultimately result from gonococcal bacteremia (whether or not blood cultures are positive), patients with this disorder must be closely monitored. All patients require daily cardiac evaluation for murmurs and evaluation of affected joints. Joint effusions typically resolve quickly with the institution of antimicrobial therapy. However, in some patients with septic arthritis, periodic arthrocentesis may be indicated, especially early in the course of the disease. Surgical intervention is rarely required.

The basic principle of therapy for DGI (Table 1) is that parenteral therapy is given until the patient defervesces and shows other signs of clinical improvement, including the resolution of joint symptoms and the lack of development of new dermatologic lesions. After the patient is afebrile for 24 hours, most authorities continue oral antibiotics for a total (parenteral plus oral antibiotics) therapy duration of one week.

Most patients with DGI, even those with mild signs and symptoms, should ideally be hospitalized for evaluation and therapy (Table 2). Hospitalization is especially indicated for all patients with joint effusion or those with preexisting cardiac valvular disease or murmurs of uncertain etiology. Occasionally, reliable patients with uncomplicated disease who are not at high risk for complications can be managed with closely supervised daily parenteral outpatient therapy (see below).

Patients who are considered unreliable for compliance with regimens of outpatient therapy or follow-up should be hospitalized. Changes in the epidemiology of gonorrhea over the past 10 years have resulted in a larger proportion of gonorrhea patients from inner-city high-risk groups. Drug abuse, especially intravenous and use of "crack" cocaine, is extremely common in these groups. Clinical differentiation of DGI and bacterial endocarditis in these patients is extremely difficult, and they should be hospitalized.

TABLE 1 Principles of Management

Parenteral antibiotic therapy until defervescence or other measures of clinical improvement
Antimicrobial therapy for 1 week
Frequent (preferably daily) evaluation of cardiac and rheumatologic status
Arthrocentesis if indicated
Hospitalization if indicated (see Table 2)
Initial antibiotic therapy should be effective for treatment of antibiotic-resistant organisms
Clinical isolates should be tested for antimicrobial susceptibility and therapy adjusted accordingly

ANTIMICROBIAL RESISTANCE

Over the past decade, the incidence of *Neisseria gonorrhoeae* isolates resistant to antibiotics has increased geometrically. Multiple types of antimicrobial resistance have emerged (Table 3) and include both plasmid-mediated and chromosomally mediated resistance determinants. As of this writing, most of the major metropolitan areas have had outbreaks of infection due to penicillinase-producing *Neisseria gonorrhoeae* (PPNG) and also have endemic chromosomally mediated resistance. Plasmid and chromosomally mediated tetracycline resistance is especially a problem, leading to recent recommendations that tetracycline not be used as sole therapy for any gonococcal infection. The Centers for Dis-

TABLE 2 Specific Indications for Hospitalization

Uncertain diagnosis
Presence of joint effusion
Unreliable or noncompliant patient
Preexisting cardiac valvular disease or presence of murmur
Altered immune status or complement deficiencies
Meningitis

TABLE 3 Antimicrobial Resistance in *N. gonorrhoeae*

Plasmid-mediated	
Penicillin:	penicillinase-producing *N. gonorrhoeae* (PPNG)
Tetracycline:	High-level tetracycline-resistant *N. gonorrhoeae* (TRNG)
Chromosomally mediated	
Penicillin	
Tetracycline	
Cefoxitin (cefotetan)	
Spectinomycin (rare in the United States; seen primarily in Southeast Asia)	

TABLE 4 Antibiotic Therapy for DGI

Parenteral-Inpatient	*Oral-Outpatient*
Ceftriaxone 1 g/d	Cefuroxime axetil 250 mg–500 mg b.i.d.
Ceftizoxime 1 g q6–8h	Ciprofloxacin 500 mg–750 mg* b.i.d.
Cefotaxime 1 g q6–8h	Amoxicillin 500 mg + clavaulanic acid (Augmentin-500) 1 tab t.i.d.†
Cefoxitin 1 g q6h	
Cefotetan 1 g q12h	Amoxicillin 500 mg t.i.d.
Spectinomycin 2 g q12h	
Ampicillin 1 g q6h‡	

* Contraindicated in pregnancy.

† May be ineffective against organisms with chromosomally mediated resistance.

‡ Should be used only for infections due to organisms with documented sensitivity to penicillin; do not use for initial presumptive therapy except when local incidence of PPNG is less than 1 percent of all *N. gonorrhoeae* isolates.

ease Control (CDC) expects the problem of antimicrobial resistance to get worse in coming years.

A commonly held notion among clinicians and in many textbooks is that the organisms causing DGI are "exquisitely" sensitive to penicillin and other antibiotics. Although true in the 1970s, this is no longer the case. In general, although antibiotic-sensitive isolates among DGI strains are apparently more frequent than those in the general population, antimicrobial resistance is by no means uncommon. PPNG and chromosomally mediated resistant strains causing DGI are occurring with increasing frequency. Additionally, PPNG occurs in DGI patients with approximately the same frequency as in the general population, which has important consequences in areas such as Florida, Detroit, Providence, Southern California, and New York City, where PPNG strains accounted for more than 10 percent of all *N. gonorrhoeae* isolates in 1988. Patients with antibiotic-resistant infection who are not treated appropriately are at risk for treatment failure and secondary complications.

Data on the prevalence of antibiotic-resistant gonorrhea are available from state and local health departments and may help to guide the choice of initial therapy. Unfortunately, in most areas, health department data reflect only the incidence of PPNG, because testing for susceptibility to other antibiotics is rarely performed. Thus, all isolates from patients with DGI should have β-lactamase assays and susceptibility determined to antibiotics that are candidates for therapy.

INITIAL ANTIBIOTIC THERAPY

No large prospective studies on the antibiotic therapy of DGI have been performed since the mid-1970s. Therefore, the following therapy recommendations are based on experience of the author and other experts and the awareness of widespread resistance to antimicrobial agents among *N. gonorrhoeae*. Because of the potentially serious complications of treatment failure, initial therapy should be effective against PPNG and other antimicrobial-resistant strains. Unless isolates are documented to be sensitive to the penicillins, first-generation cephalosporins, or tetracyclines, these drugs should generally not be used as either initial or follow-up therapy in patients with DGI.

Parenteral therapy with third-generation cephalosporins (ceftriaxone, ceftizoxime, cefotaxime) is the cornerstone of initial DGI therapy (Table 4). The author prefers ceftriaxone because its half-life allows once-a-day dosing. In reliable patients with uncomplicated disease, daily supervised in-office intravenous or intramuscular therapy is a practical alternative to hospitalization. Alternatively, cefotaxime or ceftizoxime are equally effective in the appropriate doses. Generally, these drugs can be used in patients with a history of nonanaphylactic penicillin allergy because cross-reactivity is relatively infrequent. Patients with histories of severe allergic reactions to penicillin or anaphylaxis should be treated with spectinomycin.

Third-generation cephalosporins are preferred as initial therapy for several reasons. First, clinically important resistance of *N. gonorrhoeae* to third-generation cephalosporins has not been reported. Second, while second-generation cephalosporins (cefoxitin and cefotetan) are not commonly utilized for treatment of gonorrhea, recent surveillance data from CDC indicate increasing chromosomal resistance to these agents. Last, although spectinomycin resistance is prevalent in Southeast Asia (although still rare in the United States) it is not commonly utilized in inpatients.

Initial therapy with ampicillin or amoxicillin is reasonable in patients with organisms documented to be sensitive to penicillin or in patients residing in geographic areas where resistant infection is rare (less than 1 percent of all gonorrhea, essentially eliminating most U.S. metropolitan areas).

Typically, most patients with DGI respond rapidly to initial therapy, with defervescence and resolution of joint symptoms within 24 to 48 hours. Cases without effusion or other complications can be discharged home to complete their 1-week course of antibiotics with an oral regimen.

In the past, the mainstays of oral therapy have been ampicillin and the tetracyclines. Because of the resistance problem, unless susceptibility data are known, these agents can no longer be recommended as oral therapy options. I recommend that outpatient therapy be completed with either cefuroxime axetil, ciprofloxacin, or amoxicillin–clavulanic acid. Amoxicillin–clavulanate is effective against PPNG. However, theoretically, the drug may be ineffective against chromosomally mediated resistant strains. Ciprofloxacin is contraindicated in pregnant women; ciprofloxacin and other quinolones are also contraindicated in children and adolescents.

SPECIAL PROBLEMS

Pregnant Women

Pregnant women are the group at highest risk for developing DGI. All of the listed inpatient regimens are considered acceptable for use during pregnancy. Spectinomycin should be used only as a last resort because of the higher rates of pharyngeal infection, against which spectinomycin is less effective, in pregnant women. Of the outpatient regimens, only cefuroxime axetil and amoxicillin are considered safe to use in this group.

Public Health Issues

Persons with one sexually transmitted disease (STD) are at high risk for having another. Persons with DGI should also be evaluated for *Chlamydia* with either culture or standardized antigen detection tests, and treated appropriately if positive. Serologic testing for syphilis should be performed. Counseling and testing for human immunodeficiency virus should be strongly considered. Finally, sexual contacts of DGI patients should be treated for gonorrhea and evaluated for other STDs. This process is initiated by reporting of DGI cases to the local health authorities.

SUGGESTED READING

Centers for Disease Control. Disseminated gonorrhea caused by penicillinase-producing *Neisseria gonorrhoeae*—Wisconsin, Pennsylvania. MMWR 1987; 36:161–167.

Centers for Disease Control. 1989 sexually transmitted disease treatment guidelines. MMWR (in press).

Handsfield HH, Wiesner PJ, Holmes KK. Treatment of the gonococcal arthritis-dermatitis syndrome. Ann Intern Med 1976; 84:661–667.

Holmes KK, Counts GW, Beaty HN. Disseminated gonococcal infection. Ann Intern Med 1971; 74:979–993.

Masi AT, Eisenstein BI. Disseminated gonococcal infection and gonococcal arthritis. II. Clinical manifestations, diagnosis, complications, treatment, and prevention. Semin Arthritis Rheum 1981; 10:173–197.

O'Brien JP, Goldenberg DL, Rice PA. Disseminated gonococcal infection: a prospective analysis of 49 patients and a review of pathophysiology and immune mechanisms. Medicine 1983; 62:395–406.

Rompalo AM, Hook EW III, Roberts PL, et al. The acute arthritis-dermatitis syndrome: the changing importance of *Neisseria gonorrhoeae* and *Neisseria meningitidis*. Arch Intern Med 1987; 147:281–283.

SYPHILIS

HARRY C. NOTTEBART Jr., M.D., F.A.C.P.

The Great Pox, the great imitator, the great mimic: syphilis is all of that. There is hardly any medical specialty that does not encounter this disease. It affects and infects people from before birth to old age. Virtually any organ can be involved. The outstanding clinicians of the past said that if one knew syphilis one knew medicine. Today many clinicians think of syphilis in a cookbook fashion: serologic tests and penicillin. The recipes for treatment are even published by the federal government, but, as with most things in the real world, the issues may not be so clear cut.

Syphilis in the past has been described as occurring in stages—primary, secondary, or tertiary. Some of these are so different from one another that they were once thought to be unrelated diseases.

In staging syphilis this way, I think there is the possibility of creating a false mental image of the progression of syphilis. One might think that in the primary stage syphilis is limited to the localized chancre. In secondary syphilis, the disease spreads to the skin and throughout the body. Finally, in tertiary syphilis, the disease is disseminated to deep organs and tissues such as the cardiovascular system or the central nervous system (CNS). This image is not correct.

Studies published 85 or more years ago and those published recently show that *Treponema pallidum* are disseminated by the blood throughout the body, including into the cerebrospinal fluid (CSF) in primary syphilis, and this occurs within minutes of infection. Does that help in understanding the progression and course of the disease?

It certainly could explain why some patients receiving "adequate" therapy have relapses. There are many reports in the literature of patients who have not been cured with "standard" therapy. It is too easy to attribute all of these relapses to reinfection. If the organism were sequestered in the CNS and the low blood levels of penicillin resulted in inadequate CSF levels of penicillin, the organism would not be affected. Afterward, the organism could diffuse back into the bloodstream and disseminate once again.

The fact that there are not more apparent relapses may be due to the functioning of a competent immune system. The severe course of neurosyphilis in human immunodeficiency virus (HIV) infections may then be explained on the basis that the immune system is not functioning appropriately. Perhaps the devastating course of neurosyphilis seen in HIV-infected patients is what would be seen in anyone whose immune system was not functioning properly.

On the same basis, then, the state of "serofast" syphilis may reflect a patient whose infecting organisms are walled off somewhere but still alive and well, much as occurs with the tubercle bacillus in tuberculin-positive individuals. One then might speculate whether high-dose, prolonged intravenous therapy might cure even the so-called serofast state.

It was first described when therapy was arsenicals and

other heavy metals, which may not have been able to diffuse into various sites where the organisms were sequestered.

DIAGNOSIS

The consequences of missing the diagnosis and failing to treat this disease can be devastating not only to the patient and his or her family but also to future children, if the patient is a woman of childbearing age. Because of these dreadful consequences, it is important to diagnose this disease when present.

There are only three ways to diagnose syphilis: dark-field examination for spirochetes, special tissue stains of biopsy material for spirochetes, or serologic testing for antibodies. Routine culturing for the organism that causes syphilis, *T. pallidum*, has not yet been achieved.

The use of dark-field microscopy has been limited because of the lack of dark-field microscopes and of personnel trained to interpret such preparations. Many current clinicians have never seen a positive dark-field preparation. Also, there are treponemes indigenous to various parts of the body, which makes interpretation of the dark-field preparations not as easy as some would indicate.

Biopsy specimens other than those from tertiary gummas or autopsies are rarely obtained, and the special stains for spirochetes are not routinely used.

All of this results in the fact that serologic testing has been the most available and popular diagnostic test for syphilis for many years. Only a small sample of blood is needed, no special preparation of the patient is needed, and no special handling is necessary for the specimen. The physician receives a report that gives the answer in terms of positive or negative. If the result is positive, then most nontreponemal tests such as the VDRL or RPR will be titered so that the result may be reported as "positive, 1:8."

One needs to consider the result of a serologic test in the context of the individual patient's clinical setting since false-positive and false-negative results can occur. The following infectious diseases can give false positives: other spirochetal diseases, such as relapsing fever; parasitic diseases, such as malaria; viral diseases, such as measles and mumps (and their immunizations), and chicken pox; chronic infections, such as leprosy; autoimmune diseases, such as SLE. Even pregnancy is reported to cause false positives. The serologic test may be negative for any of the following reasons: no disease; syphilis acquired and incubating but serology not yet positive; syphilis treated intentionally or inadvertently with reversion of serology; false negative.

The serology may be positive for any of these reasons: current disease; serofast from disease in the past; rising titer reflecting recently acquired disease; falling titer reflecting disease responding to recent therapy—intentional or inadvertent; passively acquired antibody; false positive. It is obvious that the interpretation of positive or negative serologic results depends upon history and physical examination. It is a mistake to rely solely on the serology.

Tests should be used to confirm diagnoses and not to make them.

A positive serologic test in a patient who has a history of contact with a person with syphilis and has one or more physical findings that are compatible with primary or even secondary syphilis confirms the presumptive diagnosis of syphilis. However, a positive serologic test is more likely to be a false positive if the person has no history or physical findings indicative of syphilis. This is true for the nontreponemal tests, such as the VDRL and RPR, and also for the more specific treponemal tests, such as the FTA-ABS and MHA-TP. If there is an unexpected positive test, one needs to repeat the history and physical examination, asking specific questions about sexual contacts and illnesses and looking for chancres and other manifestations that might have been overlooked previously. At the same time serologic testing should be repeated using a treponemal test.

Sexual contacts of the patient should come in for a thorough history, physical, and serologic examination, if this is possible.

A small number of patients have false-positive nontreponemal tests and false-positive treponemal tests. At this point one can temporize by bringing the patient back in several weeks and repeating the history, physical, and serologic testing, or decide on clinical grounds that these test results are false-positives and do nothing more, or decide that the patient has syphilis and treat.

If the patient is pregnant, the nontreponemal test is reactive, and the treponemal test is nonreactive, no therapy is necessary. A repeat test in 4 weeks should show a negative test or constant or falling titers. If titers rise or there is anything in patient's history or physical examination compatible with syphilis, she should be treated. Of course, one should involve the patient so that whether treated or not the patient knows why and what the reasoning was behind such decision. This should be documented in the patient's chart.

From these problems it is obvious that doing serologic testing on unselected patients may result in additional work, more testing, and inconvenience to the patient and his or her sexual contacts for the few cases found.

Special problems arise in attempting to diagnose CNS syphilis. If there are physical signs that the CSF shows increased levels of white blood cells and protein and a VDRL test is positive, the patient should be treated for CNS syphilis. However, there are often no physical signs. One does not do CSF examinations routinely on asymptomatic patients, but sometimes one has CSF results on someone whose blood serology is positive. Then any abnormality in the CSF is a reason for presumptive treatment for CNS syphilis. Patients with completely normal CSF are usually not treated for CNS syphilis, although some studies have obtained organisms even from apparently negative CSF. These patients still need following.

If the patient has positive blood serology and any physical signs compatible with CNS syphilis, a lumbar puncture (LP) should be done for CSF examination. Again, any abnormality provides a reason for treating for CNS syphilis. However, with physical signs, even a completely normal CSF should be treated because 25 percent or more may be negative, even with CNS involvement.

Adequate follow-up for a minimum of 2 years is necessary for all of these patients.

TREATMENT

There is a tendency to believe that the Centers for Disease Control (CDC) recommendations give 100 percent cure rates. However, it has been recognized that not 100 percent of patients would be cured by such a regimen and that follow-up was absolutely necessary to assure that those patients who did not respond to standard therapy were identified and given longer courses with larger doses to effect a cure. In my opinion the importance of follow-up needs to be emphasized.

The dosage schedules publicized by the CDC are to be taken in this context. This is the public health approach in which one tries to cure the greatest number of patients with the shortest course since many patients will not return for multiple doses. In this context, one-dose therapy is ideal as long as it can cure a fairly large proportion of patients. The CDC recommended treatment does this. However, if you are treating patients who are highly motivated and will comply with multiple doses and a longer course, then higher initial cure rates may be obtained. One needs to remember that even healthy people have quite variable antibiotic blood (and CSF) levels after standard doses.

Differences in philosophy can be seen in the different recommendations for the treatment of various stages of syphilis (Table 1). It has long been recognized that the longer *T. pallidum* has had to become established in someone's body, the longer it takes to eradicate and the higher the doses required. This is based on animal experiments decades ago, clinical observations even before the use of penicillin and other potent antibiotics, and more recent observations on the time course of serologic response to therapy. This is reflected also in treatment schedules that recommend higher doses or longer courses or both as the stage of the disease progresses.

For example, in the epidemiologic treatment of possible incubating syphilis, one dose of 2.4 million units of benzathine penicillin intramuscularly (for those not allergic to penicillin) is good therapy. After contact, syphilis may incubate up to 3 months before presenting with a chancre, although on the average the incubation time is about 3 weeks. At this early stage even small doses of penicillin are very effective.

Of course, epidemiologic treatment is offered to contacts of known cases of syphilis, but probably only 50 percent of them would ever present with syphilis, so a fairly large percentage of possible patients will be treated even though they would not develop syphilis. In my opinion, the only appropriate use of benzathine penicillin in syphilis therapy is in incubating syphilis.

In comparing the treatment schedules there are several obvious points. First, there is a surprising amount of unanimity in spite of the fact that there are no long-term comparative studies and the guidelines are based on empirical experience and tradition.

The points of difference are particularly noteworthy. Notice that the Canadian guidelines for the treatment of neurosyphilis recommend only the use of intravenous aqueous crystalline penicillin G. In my opinion this is correct. Since intramuscular benzathine penicillin rarely yields detectable CSF levels, there is no place for the use of such a form of penicillin in the treatment of neurosyphilis. Aqueous procaine penicillin intramuscularly with probenecid four times daily usually yields adequate CSF levels of penicillin but requires a high degree of compliance, and, considering how devastating this disease can be if allowed to progress, this course should be chosen only for highly selected, well-motivated patients in whom there will be adequate follow-up.

The CDC recommendation in neurosyphilis to follow courses of aqueous crystalline penicillin intravenously and aqueous procaine penicillin intramuscularly with a course of benzathine penicillin intramuscularly has no data to justify it.

In congenital syphilis, also note that the Canadian recommendation is for crystalline penicillin intravenously alone. They recommend CSF examination before treatment to provide a baseline but recommend that all neonates be treated as if they had CNS involvement. This is certainly the most conservative approach to management of congenital syphilis.

The World Health Organization (WHO) recommendations are a few years older and rely heavily on aqueous procaine penicillin G in increasingly longer courses of therapy depending on the stage of syphilis. They also specifically recommend against the use of benzathine penicillin G in neurosyphilis.

I would follow the newer recommendations of the Canadian guidelines, although I would use benzathine penicillin intramuscularly only for epidemiologic treatment and use the procaine penicillin regimen for early and late syphilis (but not for neurosyphilis).

ALTERNATE THERAPY

The mainstay of therapy for syphilis is penicillin. No other drug has been studied so well and has such efficacy with so few adverse effects. Many people recommend a course of penicillin desensitization and then treat with penicillin in those patients who are allergic to penicillin. Alternatives to penicillin are oral tetracycline and oral erythromycin. These do not have studies substantiating their doses, course length, or efficacy. Also, tetracycline is not recommended in pregnant patients so one is left with oral erythromycin. Even erythromycin estolate is not recommended in spite of higher achievable blood levels, because there may be liver toxicity associated with its use in pregnancy.

Alternatives to penicillin should be used only when there is documented life-threatening allergy to penicillin and not as a matter of preference for oral or outpatient therapy. Meticulous follow-up is even more important, if that were possible, when drugs other than penicillin are used to treat syphilis.

Some of the newer penicillins and cephalosporins should be effective in treating syphilis; however, there are few studies looking at their efficacy in syphilis.

Cephalothin, 1 g intramuscularly every 12 hours for 20 days, has been effective in primary syphilis, and the same dose for 25 days for secondary syphilis. Cephaloridine intramuscularly seemed to be effective when it was studied 20 years ago; it is no longer available. Cephalexin orally is also effective but does not add anything if the patient can take

TABLE 1 Guidelines for Treatment of Syphilis

Stage of Disease	*CDC Guidelines**	*Canadian Guidelines†*	*WHO Guidelines‡*
Early	Benzathine penicillin G 2.4 x 10^6U IM x 1	Benzathine penicillin G 50,000 U/kg (max 2.4 x 10^6 IM x 1	Aqueous procaine penicillin G 600,000 U IM q.d. x 10 days *or* Benzathine penicillin G 2.4 x 10^6 U IM x 1
If allergic to penicillin	Tetracycline 500 mg PO q.i.d. x 15 days Erythromycin 500 mg PO q.i.d. x 15 days	Tetracycline 500 mg PO q.i.d.; in children under 9 yr desensitization and use of penicillin is preferred *or* erythromycin 40mg/kg/day (max 500 mg) PO q.i.d. x 15 days	Tetracycline 500 mg PO q.i.d. x 15 days Erythromycin (not estolate) 500 mg PO q.i.d. x 15 days
Late§	Benzathine penicillin G 2.4 x 10^6U IM once a week x 3 wk	Benzathine penicillin G 50,000 U/kg (max 2.4 x 10^6) IM weekly for 3 wk	Aqueous procaine penicillin G 600,000 U IM q.d. x 15 days *or* Benzathine penicillin G 2.4 x 10^6U IM weekly x 3 wk
If allergic to penicillin	Tetracycline 500 mg PO q.i.d. x 30 days Erythromycin 500 mg PO q.i.d. x 30 days (if compliance and serologic follow-up can be assured; otherwise manage in consultation with an expert)	Tetracycline 500 mg PO q.i.d. for 30 days; in children under 9 yr desensitization and use of penicillin is preferred *or* erythromycin 40mg/kg/day (max 500 mg) PO q.i.d. x 30 days	Tetracycline 500 mg PO q.i.d. x 30 days Erythromycin (not estolate) 500 mg PO q.i.d. x 30 days
Neurosyphilis	Aqueous crystalline penicillin G 12–24 x 10^6U IV q.d. (2–4 x 10^6U q4h) x 10 days followed by benzathine penicillin G 2.4 x 10^6U IM q.w. x 3 *or* Aqueous procaine penicillin G 2.4 x 10^6U IM q.d. and probenecid 500 mg PO q.i.d. both for 10 days followed by benzathine penicillin G 2.4 x 10^6U IM q.w. x 3 *or* Benzathine penicillin G 2.4 x 10^6U IM q.w. x 3	Crystalline penicillin G 2 to 4 x 10^6U IV q4h (12–24 x 10^6U per day) for at least 10 days	Benzathine penicillin should not be used. Aqueous procaine penicillin G 6 x 10^5U IM q.d. x 20 days
If allergic to penicillin	Confirm allergy and manage in consultation with an expert	(Presumably the same as for late syphilis)	Tetracycline 500 mg. PO q.i.d. x 30 days Erythromycin (not estolate) 500 mg PO q.i.d. x 30 days
Syphilis during pregnancy			
Early	Same as for nonpregnant	Same as for nonpregnant	Same as for nonpregnant
Late	Same as for non-pregnant	Same as for nonpregnant	Same as for nonpregnant
If allergic to penicillin	Erythromycin as for stage of disease; infants then treated with penicillin	Desensitization and then use of penicillin are preferred Early: erythromycin 500 mg PO q.i.d. for 15 days Late: erythromycin 500 mg PO q.i.d. for 30 days Infants treated with penicillin early in neonatal period	Erythromycin (not estolate)
Congenital	Symptomatic or asymptomatic infants with abnormal CSF Aqueous crystalline penicillin G 5 x 10^4U/kg IM or IV q.d. in 2 divided doses for at least 10 days	Crystalline penicillin G 5 x 10^4U/kg/day divided q8–q12h for at least 10 days	Treat infants for congenital syphilis (a) if clinical or x-ray signs of syphilis (b) if serologic titers rise or persist at a high level (c) if mother's treatment was unknown, inadequate, or not penicillin

TABLE 1 *(continued)*

Stage of Disease	*CDC Guidelines**	*Canadian Guidelines*†	*WHO Guidelines*‡
	or Aqueous procaine penicillin G 5 x 10^4U/kg IM q.d. for at least 10 days Asymptomatic infants with normal CSF: no therapy if they can be followed; if no follow-up then many consultants would give benzathine penicillin G 5 x 10^4U/kg IM		Aqueous procaine penicillin G 5 × 10^4U/kg IM q.d. for 10 days If follow-up unlikely, benzathine penicillin G IM, one dose Only penicillin for neonates; no tetracycline under 8 yr
Follow-Up			
Early and congenital	Repeat quantitative nontreponemal tests at least at 3, 6, and 12 mo after treatment	Repeat serologic testing at 1, 3, 6, 12, and 24 mo	Twice in 12 mo after therapy (every 3 mo if not treated with penicillin)
Late	Repeat serologic testing also at 24 mo after treatment	Repeat serologic testing at 1 and 12 mo	At 1, 3, 6, 12, 18, 24 mo, then annually as necessary
Neurosyphilis	Periodic serologic testing, clinical evluation at 6-mo intervals and repeat CSF examinations for at least 3 yr	Repeat serologic testing at 6, 12, and 24 mo and CSF examinations at 6 mo	CSF examinations until 2 yr at least 1 yr apart have normal protein and WBC count; serology may or may not return to normal

* Adapted from Centers for Disease Control 1985 STD Treatment Guidelines, MMWR 34:4S, October 18, 1985.
† Adapted from 1988 Canadian Guidelines for the Treatment of Sexually Transmitted Diseases in Neonates, Children, Adolescents and Adults, Canada Diseases Weekly Report 14S2, April 1988; 7–8 (kindly provided by Dr. G. Jessamine).
‡ Willcox RR. Treatment of syphilis. Bull WHO 1981; 59:655–663.
§ Defined as of greater than 1 year's duration by CDC and Canada; greater than 2 years' duration by WHO.

penicillin. A more recent cephalosporin, ceftriaxone, seems to be effective. Recent studies indicate that 250 mg intramuscularly every day for 10 days or 500 mg intramuscularly every other day for five doses (over 10 days) are effective in early syphilis. In another study, 2 g intramuscularly daily for 2 days or for 5 days were effective and even one dose of 3 g intramuscularly was effective in four of five patients. Future studies may clarify the use of this new agent in the therapy of early syphilis. Ceftriaxone can be used in patients allergic to penicillin who are not allergic to cephalosporins.

Ceftriaxone has even been used successfully in one patient with neurosyphilis who was allergic to penicillin. He was given 1 g intramuscularly daily for 14 days. Since this was done in a carefully controlled situation by a group of experienced venereologists, it cannot yet be recommended for routine use for neurosyphilis, but future studies may point the way to more alternatives in the treatment of syphilis. Another alternative that could be used when cost is not a major consideration is doxycycline.

In those situations in which tetracycline is recommended, there is now a possibility of using doxycycline 200 mg orally twice a day for 21 days. This has the advantage of a shorter course and fewer doses per day, which should yield better compliance and thus higher cure rates. This, however, has been studied in only a small group of patients, and the reported follow-up was not long enough to warrant its routine use.

JARISCH-HERXHEIMER REACTION

The Jarisch-Herxheimer reaction is a systemic response that may occur after the onset of treatment. It often occurs during the first 24 hours following start of therapy. The patient, as well as the physician, needs to be aware of this so that it is not confused with any sort of allergy to the treatment. There may be increases in temperature, pulse, blood pressure, and respiratory rate. This reaction usually begins 2 to 4 hours after the first dose, peaks about 8 hours after the first dose, and resolves by 24 hours after the first dose. No therapy is indicated for this reaction.

FOLLOW-UP

In all stages of syphilis, the mainstay of care for the patient is intensive, adequate follow-up. It is important to ensure that there are clinical improvement and decreasing quantitative serologic titers (or at least stable titers). Patients with early syphilis need to be followed for at least 1 year and patients with late syphilis, a minimum of 2 years. This may seem a great deal for a disease so readily treated, but it is necessary if relapses are to be eliminated and disease progression stopped.

During this follow-up period a quantitative serologic test should show about a fourfold decrease by 3 months after therapy and an eightfold decrease by 6 months. Those patients not falling within these guidelines are probably not responding to therapy, need to be followed carefully for possible relapse, and may need retreatment.

SUGGESTED READING

Nottebart HC Jr. Spirochetes from blood specimens. Spirochetes in CNS specimens. In: Dalton HP, Nottebart HC Jr, eds. Interpretive medical microbiology. New York: Churchill-Livingstone, 1986:132, 227.

Rein MF. General principles of syphilotherapy. In: Holmes KK, Mardh P-A, Sparling PF, Wiesner PJ, eds. Sexually transmitted diseases. New York: McGraw-Hill, 1984:374.

Stokes JH, Beerman H, Ingraham NR Jr. Modern clinical syphilology. 3rd ed. Philadelphia: WB Saunders, 1945.

CHANCROID, LYMPHOGRANULOMA VENEREUM, GRANULOMA INGUINALE, AND CONDYLOMA ACUMINATA

PETER JESSAMINE, HONS. B.Sc., M.D., FRCPC
ALLAN R. RONALD, B.Sc., FRCPC, F.A.C.P.

Chancroid, lymphogranuloma venereum, and granuloma inguinale are infrequent diseases in North America and Europe. They are very common in some developing countries. Condyloma acuminata is prevalent in North America and Europe. Chancroid and possibly condyloma acuminata are important cofactors in the dissemination of human immunodeficiency virus.

CHANCROID

Chancroid is the most important cause of genital ulcer disease in developing countries. In North America and Europe, it occurs in sporadic outbreaks that have become frequent and widespread. The usual incubation period is 2 to 5 days but can be as long as 2 weeks. The initial lesion is a papule that erodes into a painful nonindurated ulcer. Lesions are most frequent on the genitalia. The ulcer has a base of friable granulation tissue that may be covered with a necrotic exudate. Inguinal adenopathy is frequently present, which may suppurate and rupture. Fistulas may drain for prolonged periods and leave sinus tracts.

The causative agent is *Haemophilus ducreyi*. The organism is fastidious, with a requirement for hemin and growing best under humid conditions, at 5 to 10 percent carbon dioxide and 33° C to 35° C. Two media should be used in order to ensure maximal yield. Our laboratory uses gonococcal agar base with bovine hemoglobin and Meuller-Hinton agar base with chocolatized horse blood. These are supplemented with coenzymes, vitamins, amino acids (CVA) enrichment and fetal calf serum, and made selective with vancomycin. Direct gram stain from the ulcer or bubo lacks sufficient sensitivity or specificity to be recommended.

Clinical differentiation of genital ulcers is unreliable, and possible occurrence of mixed infections makes laboratory evaluation essential. The culture of *H. ducreyi* is best done in combination with darkfield microscopy for syphilis. The darkfield should be done first and followed with the swab of the ulcer base of *H. ducreyi*. The media should be inoculated at the bedside as no transport medium exists.

Antimicrobial therapy at the time of presentation may be difficult because there is no rapid diagnostic test for chancroid and syphilis may be difficult to exclude. Specific therapy for chancroid may prevent the diagnosis of syphilis. Figure 1 illustrates treatment strategies. Fluctuant buboes should be aspirated with a large-bore needle, the needle passing through normal skin and then entering the bubo.

At present, the optimal regimen is ceftriaxone, 250 mg intramuscularly as a single dose. It provides the advantage of guaranteed compliance, with greater than 95 percent success. The disadvantages are important: it is ineffective for primary syphilis and may impair the Venereal Diseases Research Laboratory (VDRL) or rapid plasma reagin (RPR) tests.

Sulfamethoxazole-trimethoprim (SMZ-TMP) (800 mg SMZ and 160 mg TMP orally twice a day for 7 days) is more traditional therapy, but its effectiveness is decreasing because of the emergence of resistant strains. It has the advantage of not interfering with the diagnosis of primary syphilis. Single-dose therapy with SMZ-TMP is much less effective than the 7-day regimen and is not recommended.

When an etiologic agent cannot be determined from clinical or epidemiologic data, SMZ-TMP is a reasonable choice. It permits the physician to provide relatively effective therapy for *H. ducreyi* infection and yet not impair the diagnosis of syphilis. If treatment failure occurs, laboratory data will provide the diagnosis, and definitive therapy may be given.

Ciprofloxacin, 500 mg orally twice a day for 3 days, has proved to be effective in treating chancroid with a greater than 95 percent cure rate. This may become the preferred therapy. Effectiveness for syphilis is undetermined.

The patient's sexual partners should be examined, cultured, and treated irrespective of symptoms. An asymptomatic endocervical state has been described.

LYMPHOGRANULOMA VENEREUM

This is a multisystem triphasic disease caused by *Chlamydia trachomatis*, serotypes L1, L2, and L3. It is en-

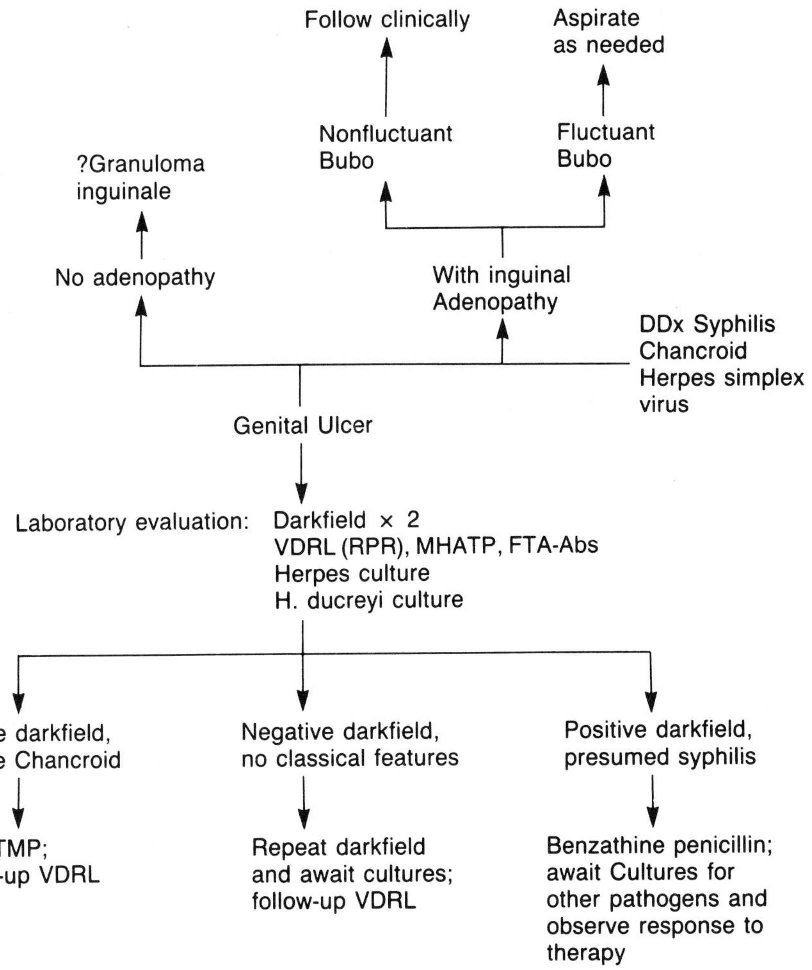

DDx: Differential diagnosis
RPR: Rapid plasma reagin
VDRL: Venereal Disease Research Laboratory
MHATP: Microhemagglutination treponemal antigen
FTA-Abs: Fluorescent treponemal antigen—absorbed

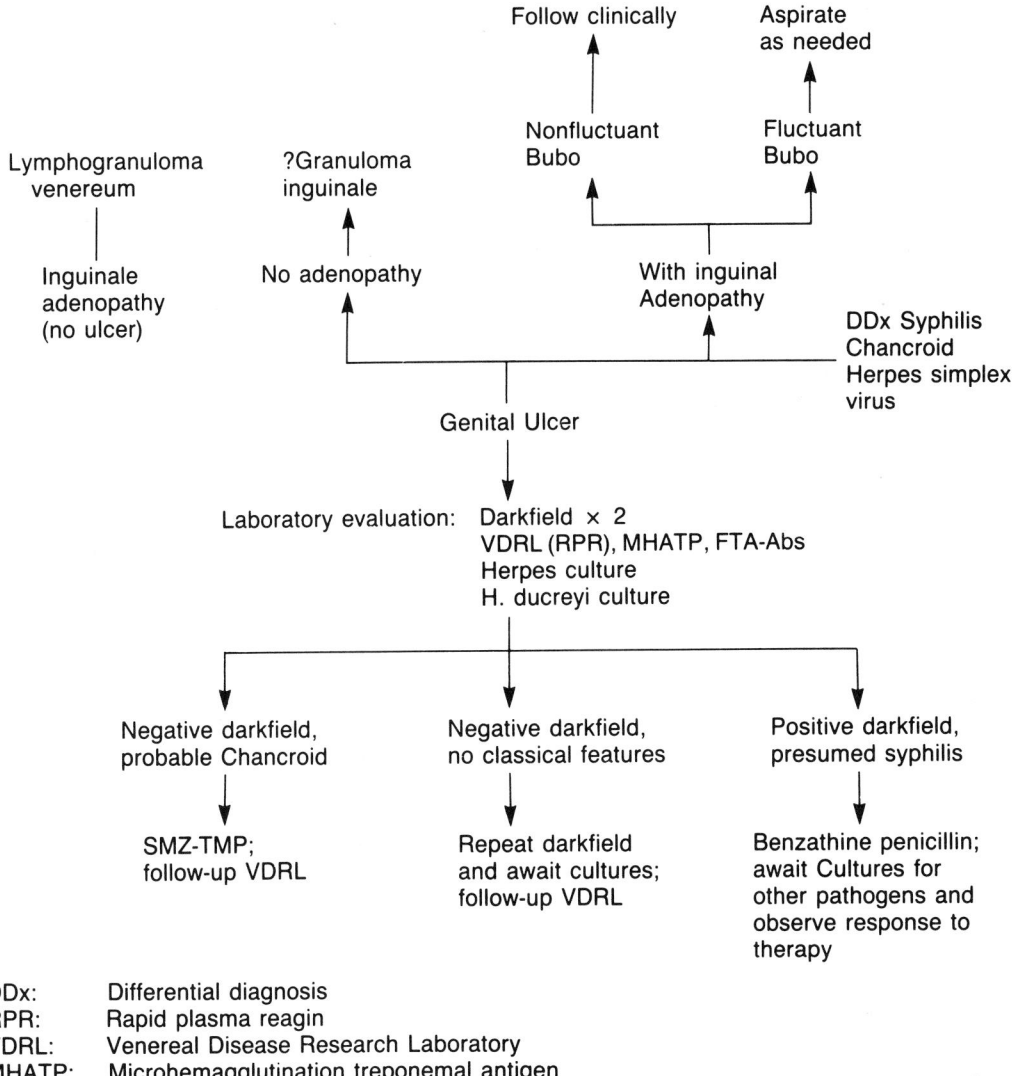

Figure 1 Genital ulcer adenopathy syndromes: management flow chart.

demic in tropical areas and occurs sporadically in North America and Europe. Cases occur in individuals who have had sexual contacts in endemic areas. The primary lesion is a painless papule that resolves without scarring and is often unnoticed. The site of the primary lesion determines the symptoms of subsequent phases.

Men most often develop an inguinal adenitis that may be unilateral or bilateral. Involvement of the corresponding femoral nodes results in the almost pathognomonic "groove sign." The adenitis is suppurative with a propensity to rupture and fistulae formation. In contrast to chancroid and syphilis, the adenitis is not temporally associated with a genital ulcer.

Women and homosexual men who have engaged in anal intercourse can develop a hemorrhagic proctitis. Fistulae may extend through the rectovaginal septum and into the ischiorectal area. Ultimately, fibrosis of the involved areas results in stricture and lymphatic obstruction.

Laboratory diagnosis of lymphogranuloma venereum is difficult. Isolation of the causative organism lacks sensitivity and is not routinely available. The complement fixation test is readily available but lacks specificity as the antigen is genus specific. A high titer (1:64 or greater) usually occurs with active disease. The microimmunofluorescent antibody test is more sensitive and specific, but it is technically demanding.

The unpredictable course of lymphogranuloma venereum makes assessment of uncontrolled clinical trials difficult. Traditional therapy has been with bubo aspiration and tetracycline (500 mg orally four times daily for 14 to 21 days). The former prevents rupture and fistula formation, while the latter treats constitutional symptoms. Buboes may not resolve with antimicrobial agents alone. Alternative antimicrobial regimens include erythromycin (500 mg orally four times daily) or doxycycline (100 mg orally twice daily) for the same duration.

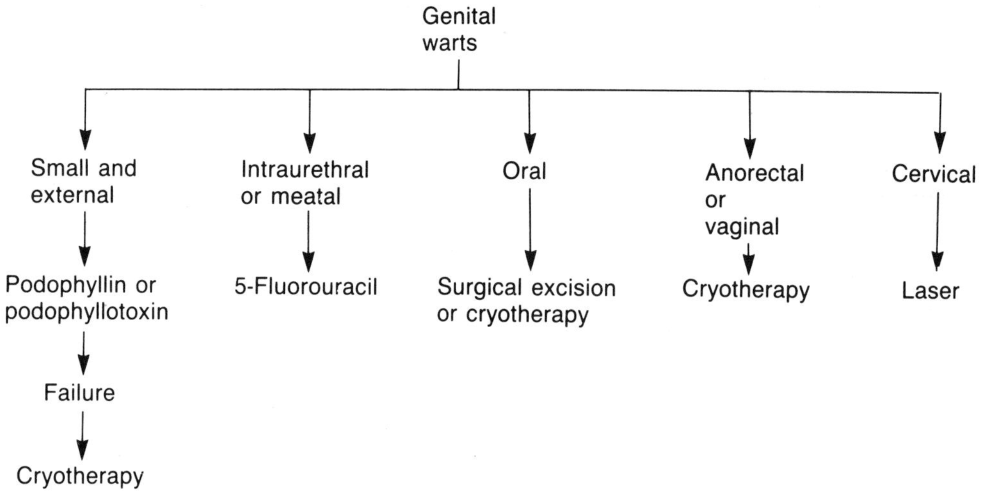

Figure 2 Management of genital warts.

Complications, such as sinus tract or stricture, may require surgery. Sexual partners should be examined and receive prophylactic therapy.

GRANULOMA INGUINALE

This disease is endemic in some tropical countries. It is rarely seen in North America or Europe. It begins as a painless subcutaneous nodule that erodes into a granulomatous ulcer. This is slowly progressive, extending to the fascia and into the groin and perineum. Subcutaneous tissue is primarily limited, and lymph nodes are seldom enlarged. Hematogenous spread to distal sites can occur through poorly understood processes.

The diagnosis is confirmed by examination of crush preparations of granulation tissue for Donovan bodies. The etiologic agent, *Calymmatobacterium granulomatis*, cannot be cultured. Biopsy specimens lack sensitivity. The presence of bipolar-staining bacilli in the cytosol of mononuclear cells establishes the diagnosis.

The traditional therapy has been tetracycline, 500 mg orally four times daily for 3 weeks. Lesions may heal within the treatment period, but this regimen should be completed to prevent recurrences. Alternative regimens include SMZ-TMP (800 mg SMZ and 160 TMP orally twice daily) or chloramphenicol (500 mg orally three times daily) for the same duration.

The disease has limited infectivity. Sexual partners should be examined and treated if lesions are present. In the absence of lesions prophylaxis is not indicated.

CONDYLOMA ACUMINATA

Genital and anal warts are collectively referred to as condyloma acuminata. They are among the commonest sexually transmitted diseases and are caused by specific human papillomaviruses (HPV). These viruses cannot be cultured, and typing is done by DNA hybridization. Twelve of the 45 serotypes are associated with anogenital tract lesions. The viral genome may be incorporated into the infected cell's genome or exist independently within the cell. The most frequent types causing genital infections are 6, 11, 16, 18, 31, 33, and 35.

The HPV lesions are polymorphic, usually multiple, and may coalesce into a larger mass. A subclinical infection was initially described for cervical warts but is now recognized to occur on the vulva, penis, and anus. The association of cervical neoplasia and HPV has been extensively studied. The HPV types most frequently associated with cervical dysplasia and neoplasia are 16 and 18. In several studies, 25 to 30 percent of asymptomatic pregnant women have been found to be infected with HPV, most being subclinical infections. There is increasing association of other genital and anorectal neoplasia with HPV. In addition, laryngeal papillomas occur in the infants of mothers with genital warts.

The diagnosis is usually established clinically but can be confirmed by biopsy. Subclinical infection can be detected by cytology or colposcopy. Cytology has excellent specificity but lacks sensitivity. Colposcopy has significant overlap with dysplasia, therefore necessitating biopsy. DNA hybridization can detect HPV genomes in tissue and cytologic preparations, therefore providing optimal sensitivity. The natural history of HPV infections and role in transformation are not established. The answers to these questions should provide guidelines for diagnosis and patient care.

Spontaneous regression of warts is to be expected, usually within 2 to 6 months. Recurrence is common. As a result, clinical studies must be placebo controlled with an adequate follow-up period. Few studies satisfy these criteria. Therapy should not be overly aggressive or costly.

Traditional therapy has been with podophyllin (10 to 25 percent) in a tincture of benzoin. This preparation is impure and has the potential for serious adverse effects. It should not be used on mucosal surfaces or in large quantities. It should be applied by the physician in small quantities to the lesion and washed off after 3 or 4 hours. Pregnancy contraindicates its use. It is applied at weekly intervals for 3 to 4 weeks and results in approximately a 30 percent cure rate at 3 months.

Podophyllotoxin is the active component of podophyllin. It is more efficacious and less toxic to normal tissue. It can be self-administered and will replace podophyllin when it becomes available.

Intraurethral warts should be treated with 5 percent 5-fluorouracil cream (2 ml) instilled twice per day into the urethra for 7 days. Surgery should be avoided, as stricture may result.

Vaginal, cervical, and anorectal warts should be treated with surgery or cryotherapy rather than podophyllin. Laser therapy has proved effective in cervical lesions and may develop wider applications. Consultation with a specialist should precede treatment of these lesions. Several controlled studies have evaluated the use of interferon either topically or systemically. It is definitely superior to placebo but requires further investigation to determine overall efficacy.

Although not clearly established, it would appear to be prudent to treat visible genital warts in pregnant women prior to delivery. Therapy should be with nontoxic ablative methods (e.g., cryotherapy). This strategy may prevent the development of laryngeal papillomas.

SUGGESTED READING

Eron LJ, Judson F, Tucker S, et al. Interferon therapy for condyloma acuminata. N Engl J Med 1986; 315:1059–1064.

Kirby P, Corey L. Genital papillomavirus infections. Infect Dis Clin North Am 1987; 1:123–143.

Krockta W, Barnes R. Genital ulceration with regional adenopathy. Infect Dis Clin North Am 1987; 1:217–233.

Meanwell CA, Blackledge G, Cox MF, et al. HPV 16 DNA in normal and malignant cervical epithelium: implications for the etiology and behavior of cervical neoplasia. Lancet 1:703–707.

Schmid GP, Sanders LL, Blount JH, Alexander R. Chancroid in the United States. reestablishment of an old disease. JAMA 1987; 258:3265–3268.

Taylor DN, Pitarang SI, Echeverria P, et al. Comparative study of ceftriaxone and trimethoprim-sulfamethoxazole for treatment of chancroid in Thailand. J Infect Dis 1985; 152:1002–1006.

CELLULITIS AND SOFT TISSUE INFECTION

DAVID SCHLOSSBERG, M.D., F.A.C.P.

Localized infection of the skin can be divided conveniently into two categories: localized purulent infection, or pyoderma, and cellulitis. Pyoderma is manifested by folliculitis, furunculitis, carbuncle, and impetigo. Cellulitis comprises various causes of cellulitis and the related entity of erysipelas.

In general, immediate clinical decisions regarding these infections must determine (1) the most appropriate empiric antimicrobial therapy, (2) the need for hospitalization and parenteral therapy, (3) the requirement for surgical intervention for diagnosis or therapy, and (4) the possible presence of a less common infecting organism, requiring therapy different from the usual.

PYODERMA

Folliculitis, furunculitis, and carbuncle are all aspects of the same process, i.e., infection around a hair follicle. Thus, these lesions tend to occur in characteristic areas of the body such as the head, neck, axilla, and groin. Infection of the follicle begins with a small pustule, which may later become crusted. At this stage, local treatment with warm compresses is usually sufficient. Extension of folliculitis results in a deeper nodule called a furuncle (boil). It may become fluctuant and drain spontaneously along the hair shaft.

Further and deeper extension of the furuncle produces a carbuncle. Whereas the furuncle has one site of drainage, a carbuncle usually has multiple drainage sites along many hair follicles and is more likely to be associated with systemic toxicity. As with folliculitis, most furuncles will resolve with application of moist heat. However, when a furuncle is associated with significant inflammation or systemic signs or if it is located on the face, treatment should include a systemic antibiotic and, if the lesion is large and fluctuant, incision and drainage. Similarly, carbuncles should be treated with an antibiotic and incision and drainage when indicated. Since most of these lesions are caused by *Staphylococcus aureus*, appropriate antibiotic therapy is oral dicloxacillin. (Antibiotic dosing regimens are provided in Table 1.) Alternative antibiotics include oral clindamycin and oral erythromycin.

Folliculitis caused by *Pseudomonas aeruginosa* has been described in patients with recreational water exposures such as hot tubs, whirlpools, and waterslides. This entity is self-limited and usually resolves without specific antimicrobial therapy.

Impetigo is characterized by eruption of vesicles, which become purulent and crusted, producing typical honey-colored crusts. They are superficial, grouped, painless lesions that occasionally have an inflammatory halo. Most cases involve the face or extremities. Group A streptococci are the most common cause, but staphylococci may also cause the lesion. Impetigo may be bullous; this form is seen more commonly in the newborn and is characterized by vesicles that become large bullae. These may rupture, the clear fluid producing thin brown crusts. This latter form of impetigo is more frequently caused by staphylococci. Impetigo is contagious and may be spread by direct contact to other patients or by the patient to other areas of the body. Antibiotic therapy should include an antistaphylococcal agent such

TABLE 1 Antibiotic Regimens for Cellulitis and Soft Tissue Infection

Antibiotic	*Children*	*Adults*
Clavulanic acid + amoxacillin (Augmentin)	10 mg/kg q8h PO	0.5 g q8h PO
Cefoxitin	20 mg/kg q6h IV	2 g q6h IV
Cefuroxime	20 mg/kg q8h IV	0.75 g q8h IV
Clindamycin	4 mg/kg q6h, PO 8 mg/kg q8h IV	300 mg q6h PO 600 mg q8h IV
Clotrimazole	Topical 2x/day x 2 wk	Topical 2x/day x 2 wk
Dicloxacillin	25 mg/kg/day PO in 4 equal doses	0.5 g q6h PO
Erythromycin	50 mg/kg/day PO in 4 equal doses	0.5 g q6h PO 1.0 g q6h IV
Gentamicin	2 mg/kg q8h IV	4 mg/kg/day (divided q8h) IV
Nafcillin	30 mg/kg q4h–q6h PO	2 g q6h IV
Penicillin G	25,000 U/kg/day IV in 4 divided doses	2 x 10^6 U q6h IV
Penicillin V	50 mg/kg/day PO in 4 divided doses	500 mg q.i.d. PO
Piperacillin	50 mg/kg q4h IV	3 g q4h IV
Tetracycline	Not recommended	0.5 g q4h IV
Vancomycin	10 mg/kg q6h IV	1 g q12h IV

as oral dicloxacillin, which treats both streptococci and staphylococci. Adjunctive therapeutic measures that may be helpful include gentle removal of crusts by soaking with soap and water. Additionally, patients (or their parents) should be warned about the ability to spread the infection.

ERYSIPELAS AND CELLULITIS

In contrast to the pyodermas discussed above, erysipelas and cellulitis involve large confluent areas of skin with an inflammatory erythema. Erysipelas is a superficial infection involving the dermis, with prominent lymphatic involvement. It most frequently involves the face and is seen particularly in patients with nephrotic syndrome, edema, or lymphatic obstruction. Erysipelas is characterized by an erythematous, indurated, advancing edge. It is usually associated with pain, fever, and toxicity and may be complicated by bacteremia. Recurrences are not unusual. Although usually caused by group A streptococci, other organisms such as group B streptococci, pneumococci, and, rarely, staphylococci may produce this syndrome. If the patient demonstrates significant toxicity or if the erysipelas involves the face, hospitalization is advised and treatment should be initiated with parenteral penicillin G. After clinical improvement, oral penicillin V-K may be employed to complete 10 days of therapy. The oral regimen may suffice for the entire course of therapy if the patient is not toxic, if the erysipelas is not extensive, and if the face is not involved. Alternative antibiotics include erythromycin and clindamycin, both intravenous and oral.

Cellulitis is an acute infection of the skin that extends deeper than erysipelas, to involve the subcutaneous tissue. Erythema (without a discrete advancing edge), pain, and fever are the usual manifestations. Secondary lymphangitis with characteristic red streaks may be seen, and bacteremia may ensue. Patients most prone to develop cellulitis are those with previous trauma or lesions allowing entry of microorganisms into the skin and patients with lymphedema or venous stasis for any reason. Thus, cellulitis may recur in patients who have had a mastectomy, coronary bypass (cellulitis frequently recurs in these patients at the vein-graft donor sites, particularly if tinea pedis is present), and in some women with lower extremity lymphedema (particularly postcoital, the "streptococcal sex syndrome").

The cause of cellulitis is usually *Staphylococcus* or *Streptococcus*, so that initial therapy is safely undertaken with an antistaphylococcal agent such as oral dicloxacillin. As with erysipelas, if the patient is toxic or if the infection is extensive or is in an area of the body where local spread or venous drainage could result in severe complications (e.g., the face or perineum), the patient should be hospitalized. Treatment should then be undertaken with parenteral nafcillin. An oral antistaphylococcal agent like dicloxacillin may be used to complete 10 days of therapy after the patient improves. Alternative antibiotics include erythromycin and clindamycin.

Haemophilus influenzae may cause occasional cases of cellulitis, usually in association with bacteremic respiratory tract infection. The resultant cellulitis is sometimes blue-tinged. Most cases are in children and affect the face and arms. Treatment should include an agent active against staphylococci, streptococci, and *Haemophilus*, such as cefuroxime.

Several warnings must be mentioned regarding cellulitis. First, many clinical entities can mimic or complicate cellulitis (Table 2). Fasciitis and myositis, involving structures deeper than the subcutaneous tissues involved in cellulitis, require immediate surgical debridement as well as antibiotic therapy. This entity is frequently misdiagnosed as cellulitis, with disastrous results. The more invasive process should be suspected when a patient with apparent cellulitis has air in the soft tissues or symptoms out of proportion to the observed inflammation, when blistering develops, or when the cellulitis spreads rapidly in spite of apparently appropriate therapy. An area of apparent cellulitis over the course of a major vessel, particularly in a patient with bacteremia, should raise suspicion of a mycotic aneurysm. Ruptured Baker's cyst and deep vein thrombophlebitis of the calf are often mistaken as cellulitis because of the overlying erythema and the pain and fever. Osteomyelitis involving the long bones may demonstrate an overlying erythema and pain and mislead the clinician to a diagnosis of a simple cellulitis. Herpetic whitlow, infection of the pulp of the finger, may resemble cellulitis with pulp abscess and lead to the unfortunate intervention of incision and attempted drainage. Retro-orbital infection with or without abscess may be misdiagnosed as a simple periorbital cellulitis because of the preseptal inflammation. If there is any question about inflammatory involvement of retro-orbital structures, computed tomography should be performed because drainage might be required.

The other caveat regarding cellulitis is the need for concern for microbial etiologies other than the usual ones. These should be suspected when patients have particular underlying diseases or certain exposures. Although aspiration of cellulitis is not considered productive in most instances, subcutaneous aspiration for Gram stain and culture should always be attempted when an unusual etiology is suspected. An example of an underlying illness that predisposes to less common causes of cellulitis is diabetes mellitus, which may be associated with cellulitis due to *S. aureus*, streptococci, Enterobacteriaceae, and anaerobes.

Frequently, these infections have associated osteomyelitis and/or deep soft tissue extension requiring debridement. Such mixed infections, particularly when the treatment is supplemented by debridement, are usually treated successfully with a drug like cefoxitin, which eradicates the majority of the pathogens present. More extensive coverage in such patients, particularly if they are severely ill, includes a combination of clindamycin and an aminoglycoside.

TABLE 2 Entities That May Mimic Cellulitis

Fasciitis/myositis
Mycotic aneurysm
Ruptured Baker's cyst
Thrombophlebitis
Osteomyelitis
Retro-orbital cellulitis/abscess
Herpetic whitlow

Intravenous drug abusers may develop cellulitis due to unusual organisms or combinations of many organisms, including staphylococci, coagulase-negative staphylococci, streptococci, Enterobacteriaceae, *Pseudomonas*, and fungi, especially *Candida*. Empiric coverage for these patients includes vancomycin and an aminoglycoside until the results of tissue and blood cultures are available. The immunocompromised patient may develop cellulitis due to *Cryptococcus, Pseudomonas,* and *Campylobacter fetus* in addition to the more standard etiologies of cellulitis. Until cultures can be evaluated, initial empiric therapy could include a combination of clindamycin and gentamicin or piperacillin plus gentamicin. Finally, patients with burns may develop cellulitis complicated by infection with *Pseudomonas*, coagulase-negative staphylococci, and fungi in addition to the usual etiologies of cellulitis. Until cultures are available for such patients or if treatment is required prophylactically before manipulation of the wound, therapy would be best undertaken with a combination of vancomycin and gentamicin.

There are certain exposures and crucial points in a patient's history that may also suggest an unusual etiology of cellulitis (Table 3). As with routine etiologies, clinical judgment of severity and extent of infection will determine when hospitalization is necessary, if debridement should be considered, and if parenteral or oral therapy is required. Thus, cellulitis in a patient who has had exposure to fresh water suggests the possibility of infection with *Aeromonas* and is best treated with tetracycline or gentamicin. Exposure to saltwater, on the other hand, may result in severe necrotizing and blistering cellulitis caused by one of several species of vibrios. These patients are also treated with tetracycline or gentamicin. Saltwater fish, shellfish, meat, and hide exposure may result in the syndrome of erysipeloid, caused by *Erysipelothrix*. Penicillin is the treatment of choice for this infection. Aquarium workers and veterinarians who come in contact with seals may develop seal finger; the etiology of this cellulitis is not known but it may respond to treatment with oral tetracycline.

Infections associated with human bites are frequently caused by staphylococci and streptococci, but *Eikenella corrodens* is an important pathogen in this situation and will not be covered adequately by oral cephalosporin or antistaphylococcal antibiotics. Treatment for this form of cellulitis may be undertaken with ampicillin plus clavulanic acid (Augmentin). Similarly, infections from cat and dog bites, though frequently caused by staphylococci and other pathogens, may induce a cellulitis attributable to *Pasteurella multocida* which, like *Eikenella*, is not treated optimally by oral cephalosporins or antistaphylococcal agents. As with human bites, the safest approach to cellulitis resulting from a dog or cat bite is to use ampicillin plus clavulanic acid. Parenteral therapy for both human and dog and cat bites may be achieved with cefoxitin.

Tinea pedis is frequently seen in patients who have recurrent cellulitis of the legs, and the cellulitis stops recurring after the tinea is treated with topical antifungal agents such as clotrimazole. This syndrome is seen frequently in patients who have had coronary bypass and tends to occur at the vein-graft donor site on the legs.

TABLE 3 Less Common Etiologies of Cellulitis

Host Factors	*Organisms(s)*	*Treatment (in order of preference)*
Diabetes mellitus	*S. aureus*, streptococci, Enterobacteriaceae, anaerobes	Until cultures available (a) cefoxitin (b) if patient toxic or infection extensive, clindamycin and gentamicin
Intravenous drug abuse	*S. aureus*, coagulase-negative staphylococci, streptococci, Enterobacteriaceae, *Pseudomonas*, fungi (*Candida*)	Until cultures available: vancomycin and gentamicin
Compromised host	*S. aureus*, streptococci, Enterobacteriaceae, anaerobes, *Pseudomonas*, *Campylobacter fetus*, fungi (*Cryptococcus*)	Until cultures available: clindamycin and gentamicin *or* piperacillin and gentamicin
Burn patients	*S. aureus*, coagulase-negative staphylococci, Enterobacteriaceae, *Pseudomonas*, fungi	Vancomycin and gentamicin
Human bite	*S. aureus*, streptococci, anaerobes, *Eikenella corrodens*	Augmentin (ampicillin + clavulanic acid) Cefoxitin
Dog/cat bite	*S. aureus*, anaerobes, *Pasteurella multocida*, other gram-negative bacilli	Augmentin Cefoxitin
Freshwater exposure	*Aeromonas* *Pseudomonas*	Gentamicin, tetracycline Gentamicin
Saltwater exposure	*Vibrio* species	Gentamicin Tetracycline
Saltwater fish, shellfish, meat, hides	*Erysipelothrix*	Penicillin
Aquarium workers, veterinarians	Seal finger	Tetracycline
Diphtheria (unimmunized patients)	*C. diphtheriae*	Erythromycin
Tinea pedis (frequently seen in patients after vein grafts for coronary bypass)	Streptococci (various types), ? immunologic mechanisms	Penicillin (+ clotrimazole for the tinea)

Finally, one must not forget cutaneous diphtheria, which may produce soft tissue infection, particularly in the unimmunized. This syndrome may resemble cellulitis or impetigo and is documented by methylene blue stain and culture on special media. Both antitoxin and erythromycin constitute appropriate therapy.

Many of the unusual organisms just described show in vitro sensitivity to the quinolone class of antibiotics. At this writing, the role of the quinolones in the treatment of soft tissue infection is undefined, although their wide spectrum may ultimately prove helpful for treatment of both routine and uncommon etiologies of this group of infections.

SUGGESTED READING

Bisno AL. Cutaneous infections: microbiologic and epidemiologic considerations. Am J Med 1984; 76(5A):172–179.
Fitzpatrick TB, Eisen AZ, Wolff K, Freedberg EM, Austin KF. Dermatology in general medicine. New York: McGraw-Hill, 1979.
Hill MK, Sanders CV. Localized and systemic infections due to vibrio species. Infect Dis Clin North Am 1987; 1:687–707.
Mandell GL, Douglas RG Jr, Bennett JE. Principles and practice of infectious diseases. New York: John Wiley and Sons, 1985.

INFECTIVE ENDOCARDITIS AND MYCOTIC ANEURYSM

C. FORDHAM von REYN, M.D.

Optimal management of native valve infective endocarditis (IE) is a multistep process beginning with selection of an appropriate antimicrobial agent and continuing through posttreatment evaluation and counseling (Table 1). Most patients require 4 weeks of intravenous antibiotic therapy, and at least 2 of these weeks of treatment should be under observation in a hospital. Consultation with both an infectious disease specialist and a cardiologist is advisable, and reliable microbiologic support (in-house or reference laboratory) is essential. Patients with congestive heart failure complicating IE should be evaluated by a cardiac surgeon and are generally treated where valve replacement can be performed promptly if necessary. With proper management, overall mortality from infective endocarditis should be 15 percent or less.

SELECTION OF APPROPRIATE ANTIMICROBIAL AGENT(S)

General

The most common organisms causing infective endocarditis are viridans streptococci, enterococci, and *Staphylococcus aureus*. In most cases, antibiotic therapy will ultimately be directed against a specific organism isolated from blood cultures. However, the physician may be required to select an antibiotic before the diagnosis of IE is established, before the infecting organism is identified, or when blood cultures remain negative but IE is suspected. Treatment guidelines will first be offered for specific organisms and then for initial or empiric therapy.

Successful treatment of IE requires sustained serum levels of bactericidal antibiotics, generally 4 weeks of parenteral therapy. Single agents are used against some organisms, but if synergistic combinations are available, two drugs are often used for at least part of the course (Tables 2 to 5).

TABLE 1 Steps in the Management of Infective Endocarditis

Select appropriate antimicrobial agent(s)

Monitor antimicrobial efficacy
- Blood cultures
- Serum antibiotic level
- Serum bactericidal level

Monitor for development of complications
- Cardiac dysfunction requiring valve replacement
- Extracardiac suppurative foci requiring drainage

Monitor for antimicrobial adverse effects

Provide posttreatment evaluation and counseling

Such combinations are recommended for patients with organisms that are difficult to eradicate (e.g., nutritionally deficient viridans streptococci or penicillin-tolerant strains). Congestive heart failure or suppurative foci of infection (e.g., myocardial abscess, extracardiac visceral abscesses, mycotic aneurysms) also are best treated with a combination. More than 4 weeks of treatment may be necessary in patients who have suppurative complications and/or require cardiac surgery.

Except for β-hemolytic streptococci, minimum inhibitory concentrations (MICs) and/or minimum bactericidal concentrations (MBCs) should be determined for all organisms. Since antibiotic adverse effects often necessitate selection of an alternative drug, MICs should be determined for two or more drugs at the outset. The following antibiotics should be tested: (1) viridans streptococci—penicillin, vancomycin, cefazolin, ceftriaxone, and gentamicin; (2) enterococci—gentamicin and vancomycin; (3) *S. aureus*—penicillin, oxacillin, cefazolin and vancomycin; (4) gram-negative bacteria—ampicillin, gentamicin, ceftriaxone, and chloramphenicol.

Several regimens are effective in treating IE caused by penicillin-sensitive streptococci (Table 2). The most potent regimen is intravenous penicillin for 4 weeks plus gentamicin for the first 2 weeks (regimen A). This combination is standard for any patient with complicated IE and for most hospitalized patients. Since gentamicin is given for its synergistic effect, the dosing is lower than in serious gram-negative bacillary infection, and toxicity is less common. Nevertheless, gentamicin can be omitted for uncomplicated

TABLE 2 Antibiotic Treatment of IE Due to Penicillin-Sensitive Streptococci

Standard (4 wk) regimen

Most patients treated in the hospital should receive this regimen. It should always be used in those with complicating factors, including congestive heart failure, prolonged endocarditis ($\geq$3 mo), mycotic aneurysm and other extracardiac foci of infection, nutritionally deficient viridans streptococci, penicillin-tolerant streptococci, or history of long-term penicillin prophylaxis

Penicillin G	4×10^6 U IV q4h $\times$ 4 wk
	and
Gentamicin	1 mg/kg IV q8h (first 2 wk)

Penicillin alone (4 wk) regimen

May be used in patients at special risk for gentamicin toxicity (age 65 yr, underlying renal insufficiency or 8th cranial nerve damage) who do not have complicating factors (see above).

Penicillin	4×10^6 U IV q4h

Penicillin allergic (4 wk) regimen

Convenient and suitable for completing IV treatment in a home setting. Vancomycin should be used if the patient has had an anaphylactic reaction to penicillin.

Ceftriaxone	2 g IV q12h
	or
Vancomycin	1 g IV q12h

Penicillin-sensitive streptococci include viridans streptococci (e.g., *S. sanguis, S. mitior, S. mutans*), β-hemolytic streptococci, *Streptococcus bovis*, and other streptococci with penicillin MIC of ≤ 0.1 μg/ml.

TABLE 3 Antibiotic Treatment of IE Due to Enterococci and Penicillin-Resistant Streptococci

Regimen	Comments
Standard (4 wk)	
Penicillin 4 × 10^6 U IV q4h *plus* Gentamicin 1 mg/kg IV q8h	Both drugs must be given for 4 wk
Penicillin-allergic (4 wk)	
Vancomycin 1 g IV q12h *plus* Gentamicin 1 mg/kg IV q8h	This combination may have an increased risk of nephrotoxicity; renal function should be monitored carefully.

Penicillin MIC of >0.1 μg/ml.

cases in patients considered at significant risk for aminoglycoside toxicity; in this situation, penicillin is given alone (regimen B). Regimen C offers two alternatives for patients who are allergic to penicillin. These regimens may also be used to treat (or complete treatment) at home for patients with uncomplicated IE.

Enterococci (*Enterococcus faecalis* and *Enterococcus faecium* [formerly *Streptococcus faecalis* and *S. faecium*]) and penicillin-resistant streptococci (MIC >0.1 μg per milliliter) must be treated with a synergistic combination of two drugs for 4 weeks (Table 3). Penicillin has been chosen over ampicillin because of its reduced risk of hypersensitivity reactions, especially delayed maculopapular rashes.

The choice of antibiotics for IE due to staphylococci (*S. aureus, S. epidermidis*) is determined by the sensitivities of the infecting organism (Table 4). The addition of low-dose gentamicin during the first week is recommended for its synergistic activity against *S. aureus*. Patients with staphylococcal IE are particularly at risk for metastatic suppurative infections requiring surgical drainage and antibiotic treatment for up to 6 weeks. Even in the absence of documented complications, patients with delayed response to therapy (as evidenced by bacteremia or fever beyond 1 week) should also receive 6 or more weeks of antibiotic therapy. The management of prosthetic valve endocarditis due to coagulase-negative staphylococci is discussed elsewhere (see the chapter *Prosthetic Valve Endocarditis*).

Antibiotic regimens for treating other less common organisms should be based on the MIC for the isolate (Table 5). If MICs are not available (e.g., fastidious organism), an attempt should be made to determine a serum bactericidal level (see later). Therapy for these organisms should generally be continued for 4 weeks (see exceptions in footnotes to Table 5).

TABLE 4 Antibiotic Treatment of IE Due to Staphylococci

S. aureus (penicillin-sensitive)
Penicillin G 4 × 10^6 U IV q4h × 4 wk* *plus* Gentamicin 1 mg/kg IV q8h (first week only)
S. aureus (methicillin-sensitive)
Nafcillin 2 g IV q4h × 4 wk* *plus* Gentamicin 1 mg/kg IV q8h (first week only)
S. aureus (methicillin-resistant or patient penicillin-allergic)
Vancomycin 1 g IV q12h × 4 wk*
S. epidermidis (4–6 wk)
Vancomycin 1 g IV q12h *plus* Gentamicin 1 mg/kg IV q8h *plus* Rifampin 300 mg PO q8h

* 4 wk sufficient for patients who respond within 1 wk; 6 wk recommended if course is complicated by fever or bacteremia >1 wk, metastatic *S. aureus* infection, or need for valve replacement.

TABLE 5 Antibiotic Treatment of IE: Other Organisms

Organism	Regimen
Haemophilus species	Ampicillin 2 g IV q4h *and* Gentamicin 1 mg/kg IV q8h
Actinobacillus actinomycetemcomitans	Ampicillin 2 g IV q4h *and* Gentamicin 1 mg/kg IV q8h
Cardiobacterium hominis	Ampicillin 2 g IV q4h *and* Gentamicin 1 mg/kg IV q8h
Eikenella corrodens	Ampicillin 2 g IV q4h *and* Gentamicin 1 mg/kg IV q8h
Kingella kingii	Ampicillin 2 g IV q4h *and* Gentamicin 1 mg/kg IV q8h
Brucella species	Doxycycline 100 mg PO b.i.d. *and* Gentamicin 1.5 mg/kg IV q8h
*Coxiella burnetii**	Doxycycline 100 mg PO b.i.d. *and* Trimethoprim 160 mg/sulfamethoxazole 800 mg PO b.i.d.
Diphtheroids	Vancomycin 1 g IV q12h
E. coli	Cefazolin 1 g IV q8h *and* Gentamicin 1.5 mg/kg IV q8h
Serratia marcescens†	Amikacin 7.5 mg/kg IV q12h *and* Piperacillin 2 g IV q4h
Pseudomonas aeruginosa†	Tobramycin 1.5 mg/kg IV q8h *and* Piperacillin 2 g IV q4h
Bacteroides fragilis	Metronidazole 7.5 mg/kg IV q6h
Fungi	Amphotericin B 0.7 mg/kg IV qd *and* 5-flucytosine 35 mg/kg PO q6h

* Treatment may need to be continued for 1 yr; valve replacement may be required.
† Treatment requires ≥6 wk of therapy and valve replacement.

Initial Treatment and Treatment of Culture-Negative IE

Antibiotics often must be started on the basis of organism morphology, before final identification is available. When gram-positive cocci are reported, the combination of vancomycin, 1 g intravenously every 12 hours, and gentamicin, 1 mg per kilogram intravenously every 8 hours, will offer initial coverage for viridans streptococci, staphylococci, and enterococci. When gram-negative rods are reported, ampicillin, 2 g intravenously every 4 hours, and gentamicin, 1.5 mg per kilogram intravenously every 8 hours, will provide initial coverage for most organisms.

Antibiotics may sometimes need to be initiated as soon as blood cultures are obtained. Prompt empiric treatment is recommended when IE is suspected and the patient is toxic or is in frank septic shock or congestive heart failure. In these situations, vancomycin and gentamicin should be started to cover the three most common organisms (viridans streptococci, enterococci, and staphylococci).

Culture-negative endocarditis (CNE) may be due to partial treatment of sensitive organisms such as viridans streptococci or fastidious gram-negative organisms such as the HACEK group (organisms 1 to 5 in Table 5). Combined treatment with ampicillin and gentamicin (as in Table 5) offers coverage of these possible etiologies. *S. aureus* is not covered with this regimen for CNE, so if antistaphylococcal coverage was given prior to blood cultures or if the history suggests a possible primary site of staphylococcal infection, nafcillin (or vancomycin) and gentamicin should be chosen (as in Table 4). Organisms 6 to 8 in Table 5 may also cause CNE and should be covered with the indicated regimen if the organism is suspected on the basis of epidemiology or serology.

MONITORING ANTIMICROBIAL EFFICACY

Since clinical expression of antibiotic failure may be insidious or delayed in recognition, an attempt should be made to determine whether the chosen antibiotic regimen and dose are producing bactericidal serum levels against the isolated organism. This is generally not necessary for evaluation of treatment of penicillin-sensitive streptococcal IE where standard regimens have a high success rate, but should be considered for all other organisms. Efficacy is determined by blood cultures while the patient is receiving treatment and by either comparing serum antibiotic levels to the MBC of the organism or determining a serum bactericidal titer (SBT).

Blood cultures should be repeated during the first few days after antibiotic treatment is instituted. Two blood samples should be obtained for culture at least 30 minutes apart at the expected trough antibiotic level. With penicillin-sensitive streptococcal IE, repeat blood cultures should be negative after 1 or 2 days of therapy. With *S. aureus* IE, blood cultures should become negative at approximately 1 week. With enterococcal IE and other organisms, blood cultures should become negative within a few days up to a week. Bacteremia that persists beyond the expected interval or fever that persists beyond 1 week suggests an inadequate antibiotic regimen, extensive infection of the valve ring, a metastatic focus of infection, or drug fever.

Bactericidal activity in serum should be assessed on the second day of treatment or on the second day after a significant change in dose or antibiotic. When the patient is receiving a single antibiotic and an MBC of the chosen antibiotic is available, bactericidal activity can be assessed by obtaining a peak serum level of the antibiotic. The peak serum level should be adjusted to a level four to eight times higher than the MBC (but not in excess of toxic levels, e.g., 10 to 12 μg per milliliter for gentamicin).

When a peak SBT is used to assess bactericidal activity, serum factors such as complement become part of the test system and enhance the apparent activity of the antibiotic. Thus, the SBT may provide a more biologic measure of antibacterial activity in vivo than the ratio of serum antibiotic level to MBC. The SBT will be the only feasible test of bactericidal activity when an MBC is unavailable and is the most practical test when multiple antibiotics are employed. A peak SBT of 1:8 or greater is advisable. The antibiotic dose should be raised or the drug(s) changed if the SBT is 1:8 or less and the patient is not responding clinically.

MONITORING FOR DEVELOPMENT OF COMPLICATIONS

Cardiac Dysfunction Requiring Valve Replacement

Approximately 20 to 30 percent of patients with active IE will require valve replacement (or debridement). All patients with IE should be seen by a cardiologist or a cardiac surgeon for a baseline evaluation. Indications for cardiac surgery in native valve IE are given in Table 6. Significant valvular incompetence in IE requires valve excision and replacement with a prosthesis. Obstruction from a vegetation requires debridement. Excision without replacement with a prosthesis may be successful when valvular complications occur in right-sided endocarditis. Bacteremia and fever that persist beyond a week and are not due to mycotic aneurysm or other extracardiac suppurative focus and cannot be eradicated with modification of the antibiotic regimen are other indications for valve replacement. Myocardial abscess cannot be confirmed without surgery but should be suspected in the patient with fever persisting beyond 1 week and/or with conduction defects; surgical drainage is required for cure. Fungal IE and some gram-negative bacillary IE requires valve excision for cure (see Table 5).

Indications for valve replacement in the face of systemic embolization are controversial. Surgery should be considered in the patient with two or more systemic emboli and a persistent vegetation by echocardiogram. The benefits and risks

TABLE 6 Indications for Cardiac Surgery in IE

Congestive heart failure due to valvular insufficiency or obstruction
Persistent bacteremia
Myocardial abscess
Fungal endocarditis
Systemic emboli (see text)

of surgery should be reviewed in patients with a single embolus.

Extracardiac Suppurative Foci Requiring Drainage

Embolization may result in extracardiac suppurative foci, including abscesses in brain, spleen, liver muscle, and soft tissue. Parenchymal abscesses are suggested by prolonged fever plus signs and symptoms in the affected organ and are usually documented by computed tomography. Surgical drainage is indicated if macroscopic abscesses fail to resolve on antibiotic therapy.

MONITORING FOR ANTIMICROBIAL SIDE EFFECTS

Prolonged parenteral antibiotic therapy is frequently complicated by drug hypersensitivity and other adverse effects. As a result, as many as 30 percent of patients will require a change in antibiotic during treatment for IE. Patients should be questioned and examined on a regular basis for evidence of antibiotic side effects. With some drugs, serum levels should be obtained to ensure that toxic concentrations are not exceeded. Standing orders are often advisable to follow for laboratory evidence of drug toxicity (Table 7).

TABLE 7 Monitoring for Adverse Effects of Antibiotics

Antibiotic	*Major Side Effects*	*Standing Orders (frequency)*
Penicillin Ampicillin	Neutropenia Hepatitis Interstitial nephritis	Complete blood count (2 ×/wk) Chemistry profile (1×/wk) Urinalysis (1×/wk)
Nafcillin	Phlebitis (*see* penicillin)	(*see* penicillin)
Piperacillin	(*see* penicillin)	(*see* penicillin)
Cefazolin Ceftriaxone	Neutropenia Interstitial nephritis Phlebitis	(*see* penicillin) (*see* penicillin)
Amikacin Gentamicin Tobramycin	Ototoxicity Nephrotoxicity	Peak and trough levels (1×/wk) Creatinine (3×/wk) Audiogram (1×/wk)
Vancomycin	Ototoxicity Nephrotoxicity	Peak and trough levels (1×/wk) Creatinine (3×/wk) Audiogram (1×/wk)
Erythromycin	Phlebitis Nausea/vomiting	None
Rifampin	Hepatitis	None*
Trimethoprim-sulfamethoxazole	Cytopenia Hemolytic anemia	Complete blood count (2×/wk)
Doxycycline	Gastrointestinal symptoms	None
Metronidazole	Antabuse effect Neurologic reactions	None
Amphotericin B	Renal insufficiency Hypokalemia	Creatinine (3×/wk) Potassium (1×/wk)
5-Fluorocytosine	Cytopenia	CBC (1×/wk)

Hypersensitivity and pseudomembranous colitis are possibilities for all drugs listed.
* Question for symptoms of hepatitis.

POSTTREATMENT EVALUATION AND COUNSELING

After completion of therapy, the patient should be evaluated to confirm cure. Two blood cultures should be obtained 3 to 7 days after antibiotics have been discontinued. Positive cultures for the original organism confirm the need for retreatment, usually with valve replacement. Cardiac evaluation should assess whether complications such as valvular insufficiency require further intervention. Patients with *Streptococcus bovis* IE should have barium studies or endoscopy of the entire gastrointestinal tract to exclude underlying tumor or other bowel pathology. Finally, all patients should be considered at risk for subsequent episodes of IE and should be given the standard American Heart Association guidelines for antibiotic prophylaxis during potentially bacteremic procedures.

MYCOTIC ANEURYSM

Infection of an artery with associated aneurysmal dilation of the vessel is known as mycotic aneurysm (MA). In the preantibiotic era, most cases of MA were the result of emboli in patients with underlying infective endocarditis (embolomycotic aneurysm). In recent years, as many as 50 percent of cases have other causes. These include bacteremic seeding of preexisting aneurysms, infection of traumatic pseudoaneurysms, and spread of contiguous foci of infection.

Mycotic aneurysm complicates approximately 5 to 10 percent of cases of IE. MA may be responsible for persistent fever in IE and may rupture or cause symptoms from progressive enlargement. As many as 80 percent of MAs are multiple, and many are asymptomatic. A ruptured MA may be the presenting feature of IE, but the peak incidence is 2 to 3 weeks after diagnosis, and symptomatic lesions may develop as late as 6 months after treatment. Because of their frequency, multiplicity, and potential for serious consequences, MAs should be sought with angiography in patients with IE who have suggestive focal symptoms, persistent fever, or one or more clinically apparent emboli.

The site of MA in patients with IE is cerebral in 50 percent and extracerebral in 50 percent (especially extremities, but also visceral and ascending aorta). Infecting organisms have a distribution similiar to that for all cases of IE, with a slight increase in frequency of *S. aureus*.

In MA complicating IE, antibiotic treatment is the same as for the underlying IE, but treatment should be extended to at least 6 weeks for all organisms. As an embolic event, MA becomes a factor in the decision to proceed with valve replacement in active infective endocarditis (see above). Intracranial aneurysm requires surgery for expansion or hemorrhage. Surgical management of asymptomatic cranial MA depends on the size and location of the aneurysm since small lesions may resolve with antibiotic therapy alone. Symptomatic extracranial aneurysm should also be managed with surgical excision. When revascularization is necessary, an autogenous graft is preferred, but a prosthesis may be required (and should be placed in an extra-anatomic location). Early removal of peripheral emboli will help prevent the development of mycotic aneurysms. Anticoagulation is contraindicated in cerebral mycotic aneurysm and has no proven value in other sites.

Other MAs (those not associated with IE) occur in various settings. In men over age 50 years with underlying vascular disease, bacteremic seeding of the abdominal aorta occurs with *Salmonella* species and with *Escherichia coli*. Intravenous drug abusers develop brachial or femoral infected pseudoaneurysms due to *S. aureus* at injection sites. Other types of trauma (e.g., penetrating injuries) and contiguous infection (e.g., cervical cellulitis, vertebral osteomyelitis) may cause MA with various organisms.

When MA occurs in the absence of IE, antibiotic therapy should be given for 6 weeks and should be based on sensitivity results. For *S. aureus*, treatment is with nafcillin (2 g intravenously every 4 hours). For *E. coli*, treatment should combine gentamicin (1.5 mg per kilogram intravenously every 8 hours) with either ampicillin (1 g intravenously every 4 hours) or cefazolin (1 g intravenously every 8 hours). For *Samonella*, sensitive strains should be treated with ampicillin (1 to 2 g intravenously every 4 hours), chloramphenicol (12.5 mg per kilogram intravenously every 6 hours), or trimethoprim-sulfamethoxazole (3.5 mg of TMP per kilogram intravenously every 8 hours). Surgical excision is always indicated, following the same principles for revascularization as for MA with IE.

Acknowledgment. The author wishes to thank Robert Arbeit, M.D., for reviewing the manuscript and Pauline Carter for secretarial assistance.

SUGGESTED READING

Dean RH, Meacham PW, Weaver FA, et al. Mycotic embolism and embolomycotic aneurysms: neglected lessons of the past. Ann Surg 1986; 204:300–307.

Douglas A, Moore-Gillon J, Eykyn S. Fever during treatment of infective endocarditis. Lancet 1986; 1:1341–1343.

Enzler MJ, Rouse MS, Henry NK, Geraci JE, Wilson WR. In vitro and in vivo studies of streptomycin-resistant, penicillin-susceptible streptococci from patients with infective endocarditis. J Infect Dis 1987; 155:954–958.

Sande MA, Kaye D, Root RK, eds. Endocarditis. New York: Churchill Livingstone, 1984.

Tuazon CU, Gill V, Gill F. Streptococcal endocarditis: single vs. combination antibiotic therapy and role of various species. Rev Infect Dis 1986; 8:54–60.

Wilson SE, et al, eds. Vascular surgery: principles and practices. New York: McGraw-Hill, 1987.

PROSTHETIC VALVE ENDOCARDITIS

PHILLIP I. LERNER, M.D.

The burgeoning use of prosthetic heart valves over the past quarter century produced an important new disease of medical progress, prosthetic valve endocarditis (PVE), a devastating complication estimated to follow 1 to 4 percent of all such operations. The unique characteristics of PVE demand recognition if the incidence, morbidity, and mortality of this infection are to be controlled. At major medical centers with active cardiac surgical programs, PVE currently accounts for 15 to 30 percent of all cases of endocarditis. Mortality rates ranged from 50 to 60 percent during the period 1965 through 1975. Although more recent experiences offer some encouragement, overall case-fatality rates remain discouragingly high, particularly for certain organisms. During the past 15 years, both the risk of infection and the types of infecting organisms have changed consequent to improved surgical techniques and equipment, a better understanding and application of antibiotic prophylaxis, and increased use of bioprosthetic devices (combining cloth-covered supporting struts with homologous or heterologous tissue, especially porcine valves) as opposed to completely mechanical valves.

INCIDENCE

Early PVE originally designated infections beginning within 60 days of surgery; in *late PVE*, endocarditis developed more than 60 days after valve insertion. Sixty days was chosen arbitrarily in the hope of separating those infections related to the operation from those not related to surgery and/or the immediate postoperative period. A recent modification, proposed by investigators at the Massachusetts General Hospital, argues for 12 months as the preferred breakpoint for defining nosocomial (early onset) PVE because of the very high incidence of methicillin resistance among coagulase-negative staphylococci isolated from patients with PVE in the first 12 months after surgery (approximately 85 percent), when compared to an incidence of only 22 percent methicillin resistance among coagulase-negative staphylococcal strains causing PVE beyond the first postoperative year. The spectrum of infecting organisms was similar throughout the first 12 months after surgery (Table 1), an observation suggesting that these cases probably share a similar pathogenesis and that the methicillin-resistant coagulase-negative staphylococci (MRCNS) may be a marker for hospi-

TABLE 1 Bacteriology of Prosthetic Valve Endocarditis

	Onset Following Surgery			
	*Cases Prior to 1975**		*Cases 1975–1983†*	
	<2 months	*>2 months*	*<12 months*	*>12 months*
Coagulase-negative staphylococci‡	41	36	41	10
S. aureus	30	22	5	5
Gram-negative bacilli; coccobacilli§	30	19§	4§	8§
Streptococci (viridans and other nonenterococci)	9	41	1	11
Enterococci	6	14	2	4
Pneumococci	2	0	0	1
Diphtheroids	12	6	4	1
Fungi	18	9	4	1
Others and mixed#	—	—	5	1
Culture-negative	3	7	6	2
Total	151	154	72	44

* From Karchmer AW, Swartz MN. Infective endocarditis in patients with prosthetic heart valves. In: Kaplan EL, Taranta AV, eds. Infective endocarditis. American Heart Association Symposium monograph no. 52. Dallas: American Heart Association, 1977.
† Calderwood SB, Swinski LA, Karchmer AW, et al. Prosthetic valve endocarditis. J Thorac Cardiovasc Surg 1986; 92:776–783; with permission.
‡ Mostly *S. epidermidis*.
§ Includes fastidious gram-negative coccobacilli (HACEK; see text).
# Includes two patients infected with coagulase-negative staphylococci plus a second organism.

tal acquisition of strains, and, thus, in turn, a marker for nosocomial infection. The attack rate of early PVE was considerably higher before 1969 (2.5 percent), compared with an average risk of 0.75 percent among reports published during 1969 through 1976. Before 1975 there were few good prospective studies of the risk of late PVE, which is now appreciated to be a time-related event, with a greater risk in the early months after surgery and a lower risk thereafter. Early estimates of the incidence of PVE overlooked the time-related nature of this infection and often failed to appreciate the importance of the comprehensiveness and duration of the follow-up.

Since 1975, prospective studies have provided a more detailed and accurate picture. A prospective analysis of 1,465 consecutive valve replacement survivors at the University of Alabama Medical Center (January 1975 through July 1979) found the cumulative actuarial risk per person to be 3.0 percent at 12 months and 4.1 percent at 48 months. The risk for PVE was greatest at 5 weeks but subsequently declined to a stable level 12 months after operation. Original surgery for native valve endocarditis (NVE) resulted in a fivefold incremental risk for subsequent PVE, whether the NVE was active or inactive at the time of valve replacement. PVE following NVE usually became evident within the first 6 months after surgery; organisms causing PVE in patients operated on for NVE were often different from those that caused the NVE. Black race was a risk factor (fourfold increment), and male gender doubled the risk, the latter also being more important in the first few months after surgery. Patients with a mechanical prosthesis had a threefold higher risk of PVE, especially in the early months after operation, than did persons with bioprostheses. There was no higher risk of PVE associated with aortic valve prostheses compared with mitral valve replacements. Thirty-four (64 percent) of the 53 patients with PVE died; most deaths occurred within 3 months of the onset of PVE.

An equally detailed analysis of risk factors for the development of PVE among 2,642 patients undergoing initial valve replacement at the Massachusetts General Hospital from 1975 through 1982 confirmed many of the findings in the Alabama survey; PVE developed in 116 patients (4.4 percent), with an actuarial risk for PVE of 3.1 percent at 12 months and 5.7 percent at 60 months (mean length of follow-up, 39.8 months). These investigators also found no overall difference between infection rates in patients with aortic and mitral prostheses and confirmed the higher early risk of PVE in recipients of mechanical prostheses vs. porcine prostheses ($p = .02$) in the first 3 months after surgery, but they uncovered a higher risk for porcine valve recipients 12 months or more after surgery ($p = .04$), although there was no significant difference in the cumulative risk of PVE by 5 years of follow-up between mechanical and porcine valve recipients. The Boston study confirmed that older patients had a higher risk of late PVE after multiple ($p = .04$) or mitral ($p = .08$) valve replacement but not after aortic valve replacement. Recipients of multiple valves had a higher risk of PVE than single valves ($p = .01$). Male gender was a risk factor for PVE on aortic prostheses in the 12 months after surgery ($p = .008$) but not thereafter, but gender did not influence the risk of infection on mitral valve prostheses.

MICROBIOLOGY

Microorganisms responsible for PVE differ considerably from those producing NVE, with clear-cut differences in the relative importance of certain pathogens in early and late PVE whether one uses the 2-month or the 12-month breakpoint for this designation (Table 1). *Staphylococcus epidermidis* is the single most common organism in both groups, accounting for 30 to 40 percent of all cases; in NVE, it is responsible only 1 to 3 percent of the time. Rarely, other coagulase-negative staphylococci are involved in PVE. *Staphylococcus aureus* is no longer a dominant organism, probably because of proper use of prophylactic antibiotics, but the case-fatality rate remains high. Streptococci currently cause few early infections. Gram-negative bacilli and fastidious gram-negative bacilli and coccobacilli, infrequent pathogens in NVE, account for 5 to 20 percent of early and 12 to 18 percent of late PVE cases. Case-fatality rates are high, especially in early PVE. The range of enteric and nonfermentative gram-negative bacilli associated with PVE is extensive and includes *Escherichia coli*, *Klebsiella* species, *Enterobacter* species, *Proteus* species, *Pseudomonas* species, *Serratia* species, and the *Mima/Herellea/Acinetobacter* complex. Increasingly, especially in late PVE, fastidious gram-negative coccobacilli, the so-called HACEK group (*Haemophilus* species, *Actinobacillus actinomycetemcomitans*, *Cardiobacterium hominis*, *Eikenella corrodens*, and *Kingella* species), are responsible, in addition to occasional anaerobic rods, such as *Bacteroides fragilis*.

Fungal PVE is not uncommon and is consistently associated with a poor prognosis. Early diagnosis may be difficult, due to minimal or nonspecific signs and symptoms; embolic events often herald the diagnosis and fungemia may be intermittent, with delayed growth in routine blood cultures not uncommon. *Candida* species are the most common isolates, followed by *Aspergillus* species, but *Histoplasma capsulatum*, *Cryptococcus neoformans*, *Mucorales*, and even saprophytes such as *Penicillium*, *Curvularia*, *Phialophora*, and *Paecilomyces* have been reported. *Trichosporon* species, normally strict cutaneous commensals or superficial pathogens, also on occasion attack prosthetic heart valves.

Contaminated gluteraldehyde-fixed porcine prostheses caused several cases of PVE with *Mycobacterium chelonei*. Other mycobacteria, *Corynebacterium diphtheriae*, *Listeria*, *Lactobacillus*, *Nocardia*, *Brucella*, *Neisseria*, *Rickettsia*, *Chlamydia*, and *Mycoplasma* have been implicated. Culture-negative cases account for 5 to 15 percent of cases in large series, particularly in patients recently exposed to antibiotics or in those with fungal PVE. The lysis centrifugation technique (DuPont Isolator system) may be more productive than conventional blood cultures (e.g., BACTEC system) for recovering fungi. Nutritionally variant (pyridoxal-dependent) streptococci may not grow in routine culture media. A deliberate search for *Legionella* species (*L. pneumophila* and *L. dumoffii*, nosocomially acquired) uncovered seven cases of late (3 to 19 months) PVE at Stanford University Medical Center since 1982; special culture methods directed at recovery of these organisms from blood cultures or valves at reoperation should not be neglected. *Legionella* species or other organisms with special growth requirements must be responsible for cases of unquestionable PVE with negative bacteriologic findings reported not uncommonly from a number of centers.

PATHOGENESIS AND DIAGNOSIS

It now seems evident that PVE developing in the first year after prosthetic valve surgery commonly derives from persistent and prolonged colonization with weakly pathogenic, perioperatively acquired organisms, probably suppressed by prophylactic and/or postoperative antibiotics. Small-colony variants, metabolically dormant and relatively immune to host defenses, may play a role in the prolonged, dormant course that often characterizes *S. epidermidis* PVE. Excluding *S. epidermidis* and the emerging occurrence of the HACEK group, the microbiology of late PVE beyond the first year increasingly resembles that seen in subacute NVE, with a predominance of streptococci, presumably from the transient bacteremias associated with dental, genitourinary, or gastrointestinal sources.

Cultures of valve prostheses and native cardiac tissues obtained during surgery often (70 percent) yield skin organisms (*S. epidermidis*, diphtheroids); the same bacteria may also be found in blood from the heart-lung machine and extracorporeal circulation and even from air in the operating room. Perioperative and postoperative sources of infection include arterial lines, intravenous catheters, cardiac pacing wires, chest tubes, urethral catheters, and endotracheal tubes—all vital but invasive elements in the intensive care setting. Pneumonia and/or an infected pleural space, sternal/mediastinal wound infections, phlebitis, urinary infections, and infected decubiti add to the risk of bacteremia in this vulnerable period.

The signs and symptoms of early PVE are neither sensitive nor specific, and the occurrence of fever and leukocytosis in the immediate postoperative period provokes a lengthy differential diagnosis. Splinter hemorrhages are of little diagnostic value in early PVE, as they occur commonly in uninfected patients following cardiopulmonary bypass. Pulmonary emboli and the postpericardiotomy syndrome readily mimic infectious complications. Some patients develop a febrile mononucleosis-like illness (postperfusion syndrome) 4 to 6 weeks after surgery, probably due to blood transfusions that transmit cytomegalovirus, or rarely Epstein-Barr virus.

Although bacteremia is its hallmark, fortunately not all early bacteremias in prosthetic valve recipients result in PVE. Some patients, in the early postoperative period, have obvious extracardiac sources of bacteremia without signs of endocarditis; provided that no such signs develop during treatment, such patients can be managed with short (2 to 3 weeks) courses of antibiotic therapy. Others have persistent bacteremia (often with gram-negative organisms) even after elimination of the extracardiac sources of infection. Bacteremia that persists for 24 or more hours suggests PVE when there is no proven extracardiac source or after extracardiac sources have been eliminated. Bacteremia associated with murmurs of prosthetic incompetence or stenosis, evidence of excessive or abnormal prosthetic motion, systemic embolization (particularly to large vessels), and new or progressive atrioventricular or bundle branch conduction disturbances usually poses no diagnostic problem.

Splenomegaly is often absent in early PVE, and 40 percent of patients may have a normal white blood cell count. Petechiae, particularly conjunctival, are the most common peripheral manifestations of PVE and occur in 30 to 60 percent of patients. Roth's spots, Osler nodes, and Janeway lesions, common peripheral stigmata of subacute NVE, are more likely to be found in late PVE than in early PVE. Anemia, microscopic hematuria, and an elevated erythrocyte sedimentation rate are useful findings, although obviously much less so in the early postoperative period; increased concentrations of circulating immune complexes may offer additional support to the diagnosis of PVE, regardless of the timing. Systemic emboli to the central nervous system, kidneys, spleen, and major peripheral vessels occur in 7 to 28 percent of patients, and splenomegaly occurs in approximately one-third of later cases.

Daily auscultation of the heart is essential to detect new or changing murmurs (particularly those of a regurgitant nature), changes in valve sounds in patients with a mechanical prosthesis, and the appearance of new sounds such as gallops or friction rubs. In contrast to NVE, where infection is usually confined primarily to the valve leaflet(s), PVE more commonly occurs at the interface of the sewing ring of the prosthesis and the valve annulus, with extension to adjacent cardiac tissues occurring in up to 60 percent of cases, and frank intraseptal aortic root or myocardial abscess, in almost 40 percent of cases. The murmurs of mitral and/or aortic insufficiency often indicate paravalvular leaks from dehiscence of the seat of the prosthesis from the periannular tissue. The absence of a regurgitant murmur unfortunately does not exclude the presence of a paravalvular leak. Infections primarily involving the central structures of the mechanical valve (i.e., the disk or ball) produce obstruction and thus muffle or obliterate the prosthetic heart sounds or cause other new or unusual murmurs.

Purulent pericarditis occurs in approximately 10 percent of autopsy cases (more commonly in staphylococcal infections); mycotic aneurysms and diffuse myocarditis are less common complications. In patients with aortic valve PVE, pulse pressure changes usually herald important developments; narrowing of the pulse pressure may accompany worsening heart failure or signal valve obstruction or thrombosis due to vegetations. Serial electrocardiograms may detect heart block or other arrhythmias, indicating conduction system involvement by an intraseptal abscess extending from paravalvular infection. New murmurs or congestive heart failure also can result purely from mechanical complications, such as tears along the annular suture line, without PVE. Beyond the first several months, the clinical and laboratory features of PVE more closely resemble the picture of NVE.

Late PVE caused by *S. epidermidis* may be indolent, with few classic signs. Valve dysfunction, arrhythmia, or a major embolus may be the first clue. Not all blood cultures yield the organism, and it may be difficult to differentiate infection from contamination. *S. epidermidis* PVE with annulus involvement or valve dehiscence or obstruction is more likely to involve a methicillin-resistant organism and will require surgery for cure. Uncomplicated cases more nearly resemble NVE with this organism: a higher percentage of methicillin-sensitive organisms and a 55 percent cure rate with antibiotics alone.

Early reports suggested that infection involving porcine bioprosthetic valves was usually confined to the central leaflets and was not notably invasive; subsequent experiences document invasion of paravalvular tissues in up to 50 percent of such cases, particularly when infection begins during the initial postoperative year, less so when porcine PVE begins more than a year after valve implantation. Occasionally, the tissue leaflets themselves are destroyed by the infection, producing significant valvular incompetence.

M-mode echocardiography is not always useful in the diagnosis of PVE, since intense echoes generated by mechanical prostheses can distort images and subtle changes indicative of a vegetation or abnormal valve motion. Two-dimensional studies are more helpful in detecting vegetations, documenting prosthetic dehiscence and paravalvular leaks and abscesses (aortic root, annular or intramyocardial), and assessing left ventricular function. Cinefluoroscopy may demonstrate abnormal rocking motion of the valve from disruption of the suture line, but unless a vegetation is demonstrated, it is difficult to distinguish infectious complications from purely mechanical difficulties. Finding decreased excursion of radiopaque elements of the prosthetic valve may suggest invasion by clot or vegetation, whereas excessive rocking motion may signal an aortic root or annular abscess. Cardiac catheterization and angiography have also been employed to assess prosthetic function and left ventricular performance, detect dysfunction of a second valve, examine the coronary circulation, and detect fistulae, aneurysms, and/or filling defects. Although there is some concern about dislodging thrombi and vegetations at the time of catheterization and angiography in patients with PVE, the risk is extremely small. Whether patients with PVE should have preoperative cardiac catheterization and angiography is a matter of some debate, despite its reported relative safety. Angiography is less sensitive than echocardiography for identifying vegetations. Currently, cross-sectional echocardiography provides an excellent method for visualizing intracardiac masses and vegetations, assessing valvular and myocardial status, and even detecting sinus of Valsalva aneurysms, fistulae, and aortic ring abscesses, although it is less helpful in detecting a myocardial abscess. Intraoperative (epicardial) echocardiography, performed just prior to cardiopulmonary bypass, may offer yet a further dimension to this technique in the preoperative assessment of PVE patients.

ANTIMICROBIAL THERAPY

The same principles guiding successful antimicrobial treatment of NVE pertain, including the use of parenteral bactericidal antibiotics, singly or in combination, given over extended periods. Precise in vitro susceptibility testing of the infecting organism (including studies for possible synergy) and assessment of the in vivo effectiveness of the antibiotics selected (serum bactericidal levels) are, with a few exceptions, essential. Most patients with PVE receive at least 6 weeks of antibiotic therapy, but infection with more virulent or resistant organisms occasionally extends treatment to 8 weeks.

Withholding antimicrobial therapy pending isolation and identification of an etiologic agent in a suspected case of PVE can pose a therapeutic dilemma. The clinical status of the patient will dictate the degree of urgency regarding the initiation of therapy, but since the range of pathogens is so great in the presence of an intravascular foreign body, every effort must be made to recover and identify the infecting organism before initiating therapy to insure optimal antimicrobial treatment and monitoring. When signs and symptoms suggest acute PVE, especially in the early postoperative period, empiric therapy (as described below for culture-negative PVE) should be instituted immediately after a series of blood samples is drawn. Likewise, when the patient is critically ill with congestive heart failure secondary to a recent onset of valvular insufficiency or a paravalvular leak with suspected valve ring abscesses, immediate empiric antimicrobial therapy is necessary. When the history suggests a more indolent process without evidence of hemodynamic deterioration, antibiotics may be withheld for 24 to 48 hours, either pending recovery of an organism from the blood cultures or simply to provide a longer antibiotic-free interval to obtain multiple blood samples for subsequent incubation. In the early postoperative period, when prophylactic or other antibiotics (employed for the treatment of specific extracardiac infections) are being used, blood samples should also be inoculated into culture media containing antibiotic-binding resins. Organisms normally considered contaminants, such as *S. epidermidis*, *Micrococcus*, and diphtheroids, should raise one's suspicion for PVE and always prompt the drawing of multiple additional samples for culture. Diphtheroids and other fastidious bacteria often do not provoke a high-grade bacteremia; consequently not all blood cultures will be positive, and many days may elapse before a blood culture is recognized as positive.

A combination of vancomycin, gentamicin, and ampicillin usually initiates presumptive treatment for suspected or culture-negative PVE. Ampicillin (2 g intravenously every 4 hours) is included because of the increasingly prominent role of fastidious gram-negative coccobacilli (HACEK group). Doses for vancomycin and gentamicin are similar to those given for proven *S. aureus* PVE (see below). Blood cultures are often negative (or delayed in turning positive) in fungal endocarditis, especially those not due to candida species (e.g., *Aspergillus*), and this possibility must be carefully considered when undertaking antibiotic therapy for "culture-negative" PVE. In selected patients with negative blood cultures, careful bacteriologic and histologic study of surgically extracted peripheral arterial emboli may yield an etiologic diagnosis. A search for *Legionella* species should also not be neglected.

Antibiotic therapy is usually initiated with two bactericidal antibiotics potentially synergistic for the suspected or proven pathogen (a penicillin or cephalosporin plus an aminoglycoside). A trough serum bactericidal level of 1:8 should be the minimum goal of therapy in these patients. In experimental animal models of endocarditis, antibiotics exhibiting in vitro synergy (checkerboard technique) sterilize vegetations more rapidly than do single-drug regimens. While the in vivo benefits of this phenomenon remain controversial in the treatment of NVE, most investigators generally employ such combinations when treating PVE.

In all cases of suspected or proven PVE due to *S. aureus*, therapy should be initiated with a penicillinase-resistant penicillin, provided that the patient has no history of penicillin allergy. Parenteral nafcillin or oxacillin (2 g every 4 hours) given for at least 6 weeks is generally recommended. High-dose penicillin G therapy, in the range of 20 to 30 million units per day, can be substituted if the MIC of the organism is less than 0.1 μg per milliliter. Gentamicin or tobramycin (1.5 mg per kilogram every 8 hours) is usually combined with the penicillinase-resistant penicillin or penicillin G in the treatment of *S. aureus* PVE, at least for the first 2 to 4 weeks of therapy, with careful renal functional monitoring. In patients with a history of penicillin allergy, either a first-generation cephalosporin (e.g., cefazolin 1 g every 8 hours) or vancomycin alone (1 g every 12 hours) can be substituted. In patients with PVE caused by methicillin-resistant strains of *S. aureus*, vancomycin is the antibiotic of choice; an aminoglycoside (gentamicin preferred or tobramycin) is added only with extreme caution if the response is incomplete or the blood culture remains positive. Vancomycin or a combination of nafcillin (or oxacillin) plus gentamicin (or tobramycin) has been advocated for patients whose *S. aureus* isolate is determined to be "tolerant" in vitro (as indicated by serum bactericidal studies). For patients failing conventional therapy, or in those where bacteremia persists, adding rifampin (300 mg orally every 8 hours in adults; 18 mg per kilogram per day in three divided doses in children) may produce a striking clinical and laboratory response.

The literature suggests that the prognosis for HACEK PVE is reasonably good for both clinical and bacteriologic cure; 80 percent of cases are cured by antibiotics (penicillin or ampicillin with or without an aminoglycoside) alone without the need for valve replacement; β-lactamase-producing strains of *Haemophilus influenzae* would require use of a β-lactamase-resistant cephalosporin, such as cefuroxime, ceftazidime, or ceftriaxone, until susceptibility test results are available.

Antimicrobial therapy for *S. epidermidis* and diphtheroid PVE requires a more detailed discussion. To treat *S. epidermidis* PVE properly, methicillin-resistant strains, which are very common, must not be overlooked. The microbiology laboratory can easily and mistakenly designate *S. epidermidis* strains methicillin-susceptible when they are actually methicillin-resistant, since only a small portion of the total bacterial population (one resistant cell in 10^5 to 10^7 susceptible cells) expresses resistance in the absence of exposure to that antibiotic. While every cell in the methicillin-resistant subpopulation is genetically capable of expressing resistance, only a small number do so under nonselective growth conditions (i.e., absence of methicillin). When exposed to methicillin, the resistant subpopulation declares phenotypic resistance, but takes 48 to 72 hours to do so. Therefore, standard antibiotic susceptibility test systems employing low inocula (10^5 colony-forming units per milliliter), such as agar dilution or microtiter broth or tube dilution, automated turbidimetric systems or those requiring rapid confluent growth around a paper disk (agar diffusion), usually fail to detect the cryptic, slow-growing, resistant subpopulation.

Methicillin-resistance is most reliably identified (Table 2) by testing higher inocula (10^7 colony-forming units per milliliter) incubated for 72 hours, easily performed by the properly alerted laboratory. Kirby-Bauer plates containing a methicillin disk incubated for 24 hours at 30°C may isolate resistant colonies in the clear zone around the disk, but the preferred method is described in Table 2. For clinical purposes, strains resistant to methicillin are considered resistant to all β-lactam antibiotics but are susceptible to vancomycin and usually to rifampin and gentamicin.

A prospective, randomized multicenter trial compared two 6-week regimens: (1) vancomycin, 7.5 mg per kilogram intravenously every 6 hours, plus rifampin, 300 mg orally every 8 hours; or (2) vancomycin and rifampin, as noted, plus gentamicin, 1 mg per kilogram intravenously every 8 hours during the initial 2 weeks of therapy. There was a 75 to 80 percent cure rate with either regimen (combined with surgical intervention in 64 percent of cases), but rifampin-resistant *S. epidermidis* strains were isolated from surgical specimens or blood cultures at the time of relapse in 40 percent of patients receiving the first regimen, whereas none were recovered from the group that received 2 weeks of gentamicin therapy. Therefore, the three-drug regimen, which minimizes the risk of nephrotoxicity by utilizing only 2 weeks of gentamicin, appears to be the current regimen of choice. When PVE is due to a methicillin-susceptible strain of coagulase-negative staphylococcus (*S. epidermidis* or otherwise), a semisynthetic penicillin or a first-generation cephalosporin is appropriate therapy; many investigators add either gentamicin and/or rifampin as second or third drugs. The addition of a second or third drug must always be monitored by in vitro studies documenting enhanced serum bactericidal activity, since not all such additions are enhancing.

Determining appropriate antimicrobial therapy for diphtheroid PVE may pose a problem, as these fastidious gram-positive coccobacilli may be difficult to isolate and maintain in culture and the microbiology laboratory may have difficulty performing MICs, MBCs, and serum bactericidal studies. When the isolate is sensitive to penicillin, a combination of penicillin G (4 million units every 4 hours) plus gentamicin (1.5 mg per kilogram every 8 hours) is administered for 6 weeks, because 90 percent of diphtheroid strains from PVE patients are synergistically killed by this combination. Isolates with MICs for penicillin as high as 256 μg per milliliter will yield to the synergistic influence of gentamicin, so long as the isolate is susceptible to gentamicin. Others recommend vancomycin in this situation. For patients allergic to penicillin or for those whose diphtheroid isolates are resistant to gentamicin, vancomycin, 7.5 mg per kilogram every 6 hours for 6 weeks, is recommended, alone or with the addition of gentamicin and rifampin. Renal function must be monitored closely.

TABLE 2 *Staphylococcus epidermidis*: Tests for Methicillin Susceptibility

Pick four or five colonies of strain and grow overnight in brain heart infusion broth (organisms = 5×10^8 cfu/ml)
Inoculate with 0.1 ml (5×10^7 cfu) by spreading on surface: Mueller-Hinton agar with 20 μg methicillin/ml; Mueller-Hinton agar with 12.5 μg methicillin/ml
Incubate agar plates 72 hours at 37°C
Read: Colonies on agar with 20 μg methicillin/ml = methicillin-resistant strain; No colonies on agar with 20 μg or 12.5 μg methicillin/ml = methicillin-susceptible strain

Modified from Archer GL. Antimicrobial susceptibility and selection of resistance among *Staphylococcus epidermidis* isolates recovered from patients with infections of indwelling foreign devices. Antimicrob Agents Chemother 1978; 14:353–359.
cfu = colony forming unit

Fungal PVE always requires combined medical and early surgical treatment. For candidal endocarditis, intravenous amphotericin B (up to 1 mg per kilogram per day) is combined with oral flucytosine (5-fluorocytosine; 200 mg per kilogram in four divided doses for as long as amphotericin B is given), with the dose adjusted for renal function, which is closely monitored. A total dose of 2 g of amphotericin B is usually the goal of postvalve replacement therapy. Oral imidazole compounds under current investigation (e.g., fluconazole, itraconazole) may offer future alternative approaches to the current need for long-term therapy with intravenous amphotericin B; ketoconazole has no current role in therapy of fungal PVE.

Prolonged parenteral therapy is the optimal way to treat PVE. Oral therapy has little or no role here, certainly not during the early stages of treatment. The average duration of treatment is 5 weeks, but patients infected with staphylococci or enteric and nonfermentative gram-negative bacilli or fungi often receive 6 or 8 weeks of therapy, respectively, because of the severe consequences of relapse in these patients. Serial (weekly) monitoring of C-reactive protein levels and the erythrocyte sedimentation rate may help determine how long a time antibiotic therapy must be continued; measurement of circulating immune complexes is probably just a more expensive way of accomplishing the same goal. Streptococcal infections (particularly those occurring after the first year) often respond to shorter courses of therapy (4 weeks), with intravenous penicillin (18 to 30 million units per day in six divided doses), with (my preference) or without the addition of gentamicin (1 mg per kilogram every 8 hours for the first 2 weeks, at least). Patients cured with antibiotic therapy alone are usually those developing PVE a year or more after surgery who are infected with relatively avirulent organisms highly susceptible to antibiotics: streptococci, fastidious gram-negative coccobacilli (HACEK), and methicillin-susceptible *S. epidermidis*. Such patients are usually hemodynamically stable with no evidence of an invasive infection.

Although more in vitro data and many more human studies remain to be done, teichoplanin, an experimental glycopeptide antibiotic structurally related to vancomycin and bactericidal for most gram-positive bacteria (except enterococci), has a much longer serum half-life than vancomycin (up to 40 or more hours), permitting once-daily injections (either intramuscular or intravenous) after an initial series of three 12-hourly doses. A more favorable toxicity profile (less thrombophlebitis, less nephrotoxicity) and the possibility of once-daily intramuscular injections suggest a possible future role in PVE patients infected with gram-positive pathogens. However, intravenous drug abusers display a significantly shorter serum half-life, and some bacteremic patients fail to respond; optimal doses remain to be determined.

The availability of oral ciprofloxacin, a new oral quinolone compound, provides at last an oral agent highly active against methicillin-resistant staphylococci, both MRSA and MRCNS, and *Pseudomonas aeruginosa*. If encouraging results in animal model experimental endocarditis are borne out in clinical practice, this compound (and possibly other new quinolones on the horizon, such as enoxacin and pefloxacin) may prove to be useful (adjuncts) for the oral or parenteral therapy of MRSA or MRCNS PVE and perhaps also in the treatment of resistant gram-negative rod PVE, including infections with *P. aeruginosa*.

SURGERY

Surgery plays an increasingly important role in managing these patients since it is now possible, with aggressive debridement and prolonged postoperative antibiotic therapy, to replace an infected prosthesis during active endocarditis without contaminating the new prosthesis or developing recurrent infection. During the past 10 to 15 years, debridement of infected tissues and restoring valvular function by placing a new prosthesis has become standard therapy for some 50 to 75 percent of patients during their initial period of antibiotic therapy. Some even consider early surgery the primary treatment for PVE, preferring not to wait for complications, since despite prolonged bactericidal antibiotic therapy, cultures of valves at surgery or autopsy are often positive and valve dehiscence is so common a complication, occurring in some 50 percent of patients at surgery or autopsy. Earlier intervention may lower the incidence of dehiscence, according to some investigators. One would ideally like to suppress the infection with appropriate antibiotic therapy for at least 10 to 14 days prior to surgery, but, as is true in NVE, survival is inversely related to the severity of heart failure at the time of surgery, so it is essential to operate before hemodynamic deterioration becomes severe and irreversible.

Surgical intervention must be considered an option in all patients with PVE, since complex surgical techniques, including aortic root reconstructions, are often required due to extensive annular infection and extraannular abscesses. When left ventricular–aortic discontinuity is present, a homograft aortic valve and ascending aorta (as conduit) may rescue an otherwise hopeless situation, illustrating some of the extraordinary surgical techniques possible. The question of if and when has been difficult to resolve. Earlier concerns that reoperation posed formidable technical problems have largely been allayed as cardiac surgical expertise has improved dramatically, and fatality rates for patients treated only medically remain substantial, in the range of 60 to 80 percent. In patients who undergo valve replacement, this figure drops to 15 to 40 percent. Circumstances warranting possible or definite surgical intervention are listed in Table 3.

Investigators at the Massachusetts General Hospital further analyzed the 116 patients with PVE they treated between 1975 and 1983, employing multivariate analysis to identify risk factors for in-hospital mortality and bad outcome during post-hospital follow-up. Complicated PVE (new or changing murmur, new or worsening heart failure, new or progressive cardiac conduction abnormalities, or prolonged fever during therapy) was present in 64 percent of patients, conditioned primarily by aortic valve infection (odds ratio 4.3, $p = .002$) and onset within 12 months of surgery (odds ratio 5.5, $p = .0001$). In-hospital mortality was 23 percent; complicated PVE patients had a higher mortality than uncomplicated PVE patients (odds ratio 6.4, $p = .0009$). Combined medical-surgical therapy was used in 39 percent of patients, more commonly in patients with complicated PVE (odds ratio 16, $p < .0001$) and in patients infected with coagulase-negative staphylococci (odds ratio 3.9, $p = .0003$). Survival after initially successful therapy was adversely affected by the presence of moderate or severe congestive heart failure at the time of discharge ($p = .03$). Bad outcome during follow-up (death, relapse, or further cardiac surgery) was more common in the medical-therapy-only group ($p = .02$). The presence of complicated PVE is thus a central variable in assessing prognosis and planning therapy, and these patients, for the most part, are best treated with combined medical-surgical therapy. Patients not treated surgically during

TABLE 3 Indications for Considering Surgical Intervention in PVE

Hemodynamic complications
Moderate to severe or rapidly progressive heart failure (N.Y. Heart Association Class III or IV) caused by valvular insufficiency (tissue valves) or valve dehiscence with paravalvular leak (mechanical valves)
Acute decrease in cardiac output, caused by valve obstruction
Evidence of extending valve infection (annular abscess, myocardial abscess, mycotic aneurysm) suggested by new or progressing conduction system disturbances, or purulent pericarditis; fever persisting >10 days in the face of appropriate antibiotic therapy
Antibiotic failure
Persistent fever and/or bacteremia, relapse following apparently "successful" antibiotic therapy, or ineffective or unavailable antimicrobial therapy
Selected organisms associated with increased mortality
Fungi (definitely)
S. aureus (debated; consider case by case)
S. epidermidis (with any feature[s] noted above)
Emboli
Recurrent or single major (e.g., coronary, cerebral) or new echocardiographic evidence of vegetations
Emboli associated with any of the features noted above

Adapted from Dismukes WE. Management of infective endocarditis. In: Cardiovascular clinics, 11/3, critical care cardiology. Philadelphia: FA Davis, 1981:189.

their initial hospitalization are at high risk for progressive prosthesis dysfunction and require careful follow-up.

The goals of prompt valve replacement are to curtail the extension of infection into vital or inaccessible cardiac structures, prevent or minimize abscess formation, and diminish the possibility of paravalvular leaks, dehiscence, or thrombotic (occlusive) stenosis. In general, I favor an aggressive approach to surgery in almost all patients who develop PVE in the first postoperative year and all patients with fungal endocarditis irrespective of the time interval. However, patients who develop PVE after the initial postoperative year and who are infected with antibiotic-sensitive organisms, such as streptococci and members of the HACEK group (the latter an increasingly important group) quite often respond to antibiotic therapy alone, so strict surgical indications (see Table 3) should be applied in this setting. In general, aortic PVE carries a worse prognosis than mitral PVE, porcine heterografts fare better than mechanical valves, and early PVE consistently demonstrates more risk factors than does late PVE. When the tissues removed at surgery harbor viable organisms or evidence of active inflammation, an additional 6 weeks of antibiotic therapy (dating from the time of surgery) is usually recommended; otherwise 4 additional weeks of therapy is sufficient, at least for more antibiotic-sensitive organisms.

Some investigators urge a careful survey for and repair (if possible) of cerebral mycotic aneurysms before undertaking prosthetic valve insertion, but cardiopulmonary bypass does not appear to exacerbate or provoke neurologic deficits associated with cerebral mycotic aneurysms in most reported medical center experiences. Magnetic resonance imaging (MRI) of the head may prove a useful screening test for those who wish to investigate this possibility.

Anticoagulation

Systemic emboli occur in 15 to 30 percent of patients with infected mechanical or porcine prosthetic valves. Hemorrhagic central nervous system events also complicate PVE, particularly when anticoagulation has been excessive. The role of anticoagulation in patients with PVE is thus highly controversial. In one study, mortality was similar for patients maintained on careful warfarin anticoagulation and those not anticoagulated, but morbidity due to systemic emboli, particularly to the central nervous system, was increased in the non-anticoagulated group. Current guidelines suggest continuing very closely monitored anticoagulation (1.5 times control) during treatment of PVE, but discontinuing warfarin if any cerebrovascular event occurs. If there is no evidence of hemorrhage or a hemorrhagic infarct, cautious anticoagulation can be resumed after 72 hours. Some investigators believe heparin achieves a more stable anticoagulation state than warfarin and prefer it during antibiotic therapy of PVE.

Prophylaxis

Since the infecting organism in most cases of early PVE gains access to the prosthesis during surgery, perioperative antibiotic prophylaxis is employed routinely and is directed against staphylococci, since it is not possible to provide prophylaxis against all potential pathogens. To date there is no well-designed prospective, double-blinded study conclusively proving the benefits of this practice. However, several properly designed studies have demonstrated that short-term (48 hours) use of prophylactic antibiotic during the perioperative period is as effective in preventing PVE as is the use of a prophylactic antibiotic given for a longer period. First-generation cephalosporins (cefazolin, 1 g) or penicillinase-resistant penicillins (oxacillin or nafcillin, 1 to 2 g) should be started just before surgery and continued every 6 hours for no more than 48 hours. However, since most nosocomial *S. epidermidis* strains are methicillin (and cephalosporin)-resistant, the empiric recommendation that substitutes vancomycin (15 mg per kilogram initially preoperatively, followed by 10 mg per kilogram immediately after cardiopulmonary bypass) seems not unreasonable. Some also favor adding gentamicin, 1.7 mg per kilogram intravenously, just before surgery and repeating this dose once 8 hours later.

Persons with prosthetic heart valves are an easily identified population that remains forever at risk for colonization of their prostheses during the transient bacteremias that accompany certain procedures, particularly dental treatments, gastrointestinal and genitourinary manipulations, and gynecologic procedures. The danger of bacteremia from a barium enema is commonly ignored in this setting. Prophylactic regimens derived from in vitro data and the rabbit model of experimental endocarditis suggest that bactericidal antibiotics (penicillin[s], cephalosporin[s], vancomycin) administered prior to the induction of bacteremia can prevent or suppress bacteremia and thus avoid prosthetic infection. A British solution for the problem of prophylaxis for oral procedures, a single 3-g dose of oral amoxicillin 1 hour before the procedure, provides bactericidal blood levels for most oral streptococci for at least 10 hours, almost certainly an adequate margin of safety, since experimental animal models of endocarditis suggest that 9 hours is the critical time following a bacterial challenge in this setting. Although no trials in humans as yet document the efficacy of any prophylactic antibiotic regimen in patients with prosthetic valves who undergo bacteremia-associated procedures, their use is justified on theoretical grounds and carries minimal risk. Prophylaxis should be employed according to the guidelines of the American Heart Association; unfortunately, recent studies indicate very poor physician compliance with these guidelines despite the easy recognizability of this group of high-risk patients. Radiologic departments are notably not aware of these recommendations, particularly in relation to barium enemas, genitourinary instrumentation (e.g., voiding cystogram), or gynecologic procedures (e.g., hysterosalpingogram). The use of an antiseptic mouthwash (such as Betadine; povidone-iodine; 10 to 20 ml for 30 seconds, twice, 2 minutes apart) just before a dental procedure can decrease the frequency of subsequent bacteremia, and should not be neglected, although gingival "degerming" by mouthwash is not a substitute for antimicrobial prophylaxis.

SUGGESTED READING

Calderwood SB, Swinski LA, Karchmer AW, et al. Prosthetic valve endocarditis. Analysis of factors affecting outcome of therapy. J Thorac Cardiovasc Surg 1986; 92:776–783.

Calderwood SB, Swinski LA, Waternaux CM, et al. Risk factors for the development of prosthetic valve endocarditis. Circulation 1985; 72:31–37.
Cowgill LD, Addonizio VP, Hopeman AR, et al. A practical approach to prosthetic valve endocarditis. Ann Thorac Surg 1987; 43:450–457.
Karp RB. Role of surgery in infective endocarditis. Cardiovasc Clin 1987; 17:141–162.
Kotler MN, Goldman A, Parry WR. Noninvasive evaluation of cardiac valve prostheses. Cardiovasc Clin 1986; 17:201–241.

BACTERIAL OSTEOMYELITIS

JACK L. LEFROCK, M.D.
BRUCE R. SMITH, Pharm. D.
ABDOLGHADER MOLAVI, M.D.

Osteomyelitis continues to pose both diagnostic and therapeutic dilemmas for the clinician, despite recent advances in radionuclide imaging, surgical techniques, and antimicrobial therapy. Intravenous drug abuse, radiation therapy for cancer, and newer orthopaedic procedures, such as total joint replacements, bone grafting, and reconstructive surgery, have broadened the scope of this disease.

Osteomyelitis is an inflammatory process in bone and bone marrow. It is caused most often by pyogenic bacteria but may be caused by other microorganisms including mycobacteria and fungi. Osteomyelitis may be classified on the basis of its pathogenesis as of either hematogenous origin or contiguous focus (with or without peripheral vascular disease) (Table 1). These in turn may be classified as either acute or chronic forms of the disease.

In the past, osteomyelitis usually resulted from hematogenous spread of bacteria to bone and was mostly seen in children with *Staphylococcus aureus* as the causative agent in 80 to 90 percent of the cases. However, in recent years the disease has changed. Hematogenous osteomyelitis is decreasing in frequency while contiguous osteomyelitis and osteomyelitis in association with peripheral vascular disease is increasing. In addition to these changes, there also has been a shift in the age distribution to older patients as well as increasing frequency of unusual bacterial causes, including gram-negative bacilli, anaerobes, and mixed organisms.

HEMATOGENOUS OSTEOMYELITIS

Hematogenous osteomyelitis is generally caused by a single organism, *S. aureus* being responsible for the majority of cases. However, the type of organism may vary with the age of the patient (Table 2). This disease generally occurs in children younger than 12 years, teenagers, and young adults who participate in strenuous physical activities. Bone infection follows bacteremia. The metaphyseal ends of long bones are the most frequent sites of involvement in children and the diaphysis of the long bones in adults.

S. aureus may also cause spinal osteomyelitis with paravertebral abscess formation. This syndrome generally occurs in older men who have had urinary tract manipulation and infection and in drug addicts.

Gram-negative enteric bacteria, *Staphylococcus epidermidis*, may also cause vertebral osteomyelitis secondary to urinary tract infection. Gram-negative bacilli are now isolated more frequently from cases of acute hematogenous osteomyelitis. *Pseudomonas aeruginosa* may cause vertebral, pubic, and clavicular infections in drug addicts, and *Salmonella* species are important in sickle cell disease. Polymicrobial osteomyelitis occurs in 5 percent of patients and is mostly due to *S. aureus* and a streptococcus.

CONTIGUOUS OSTEOMYELITIS

Contiguous osteomyelitis is secondary to an adjacent area of infection, as in postoperative infections, direct inoculation from trauma, or extension from an area of soft

TABLE 1 Classification of Osteomyelitis and Associated Features

	Hematogenous	*Secondary to Contiguous Focus of Infection*	*Due to Vascular Insufficiency*
Age distribution	1–20 and >50 years	25–50 years	≥50 years
Usual bones involved	Long bones, vertebrae	Long bones	Small bones of feet
Microbiology	Usually monomicrobial: *Staphylococcus aureus*, *Streptococcus* (group B)	Usually mixed infections: *Staphylococcus aureus* and *epidermidis*, gram-negative bacilli	Usually polymicrobial: *Staphylococcus aureus* and *epidermidis*, gram-negative bacilli
	Gram-negative bacilli (*Haemophilus influenzae*)		Anaerobes
Associated factors	Trauma, bacteremia, IV drug abuse	Trauma and surgery, soft tissue infections, radiation therapy	Diabetes mellitus, peripheral vascular disease
Clinical features	Fever, local tension and swelling	Fever, swelling and erythema	Fever, swelling, ulceration and drainage

TABLE 2 Osteomyelitis: Commonly Isolated Organisms

Hematogenous osteomyelitis
Infants <1 year
Group B *Streptococcus*
Staphylococcus aureus
Escherichia coli
Children 1-16 years
Staphylococcus aureus
Group A *Streptococcus*
Haemophilus influenzae
Adults >16 years
Staphylococcus aureus
Staphylococcus epidermidis
Gram-negative bacilli
Pseudomonas aeruginosa
Serratia marcescens
Escherichia coli
Contiguous focus osteomyelitis (polymicrobic infection), all ages
Staphylococcus aureus
Staphylococcus epidermidis
Group A *Streptococcus*
Enterococcus
Gram-negative bacilli
Anaerobes

tissue infection. In contrast to hematogenous osteomyelitis, more than one pathogen is often isolated from the infected bone. *S. aureus* is the most commonly isolated pathogen, but aerobic gram-negative rods and anaerobes also are often isolated. In this form of osteomyelitis, one often finds bone necrosis, compromised soft tissue, and loss of bone stability, which make this type more difficult to treat than acute hematogenous osteomyelitis.

OSTEOMYELITIS ASSOCIATED WITH VASCULAR INSUFFICIENCY

This infection usually develops in diabetic persons as an extension of a local infection either from cellulitis or a trophic skin ulcer. The small bones of the feet, generally the metatarsals and phalanges, are involved. These patients have impaired local inflammatory response that predisposes the involved tissues to infection and necrosis. Multiple aerobic and/or anaerobic pathogens often can be isolated from the infected bone.

CHRONIC OSTEOMYELITIS

Both of the above types of osteomyelitis can become chronic. There are no exact criteria as to when acute osteomyelitis becomes chronic.

DIAGNOSIS

In addition to the historical data and physical findings, cultures of infected material and hematologic and radiographic studies are helpful in making a clinical and etiologic diagnosis.

Blood cultures should be performed for all patients with suspected osteomyelitis. Approximately 50 percent of patients with acute hematogenous osteomyelitis have positive blood cultures. Leukocytosis may occur with white blood cell (WBC) counts exceeding 20,000 per cubic millimeter. However, normal or only slightly elevated WBC counts are not uncommon. The erythrocyte sedimentation rate may be normal early in the disease, but usually increases with the duration of illness.

Radiographic changes are often difficult to interpret. Bone density must change at least 50 percent to be detected radiologically. Thus, there may be no definable radiologic changes in osteomyelitis for the first 10 to 14 days in spite of bone destruction or periosteal new bone formation. The initial radiologic findings may be simply soft tissue swelling and/or subperiosteal elevation. Roentgenograms may give misleading information in up to 16 percent of patients and are of no diagnostic value in an additional 23 percent of patients with osteomyelitis. Lytic changes are not seen until 2 to 6 weeks after the onset of disease. Sclerotic changes of periosteal new bone formation (involucrum) denote a more chronic process.

On the other hand, changes are seen on bone scintigraphy as early as 24 hours after the onset of symptoms because of increased bone blood flow and early bone reaction. However, not all patients with acute osteomyelitis have abnormal bone scans. There are reports of normal bone scans, or "subtle" or "cold" defects. In some situations gallium scan shows increased uptake in areas of polymorphonuclear leukocyte infiltration. However, gallium scan does not show bone detail well so it is often difficult to distinguish between bone and soft tissue inflammation. Scanning the infected area with gallium 48 hours after injection and comparing with a ^{99m}Tc bone scan helps resolve this problem. Computed tomography (CT) is useful in identifying areas of dead bone (sequestrum). However, CT cannot be utilized when metal is present in or near the area of bone infection because of the scatter effect, with resultant loss of image resolution. Radiographic follow-up is important in assessing the effectiveness of drug therapy and the need for surgical intervention.

The bacteriologic diagnosis of osteomyelitis rests on isolation of the pathogenic bacteria from the bone or the blood. In chronic osteomyelitis, sinus tract cultures are not reliable in predicting which organism(s) will be isolated from the infected bone because there is a poor correlation between these cultures and those done on bone biopsy material. Bone biopsy specimens should be carefully cultured and stained for aerobes, anaerobes, mycobacteria, and fungi. The biopsied material should also be submitted for histopathologic evaluation.

THERAPY FOR HEMATOGENOUS OSTEOMYELITIS

In acute hematogenous osteomyelitis, a prolonged course of antimicrobial therapy (4 to 6 weeks), with a bactericidal agent, should be directed toward specific causative bacteria isolated by bone biopsy and culture. Therapy based on wound swab cultures of skin and skin structures above the infected bone is often inappropriate. These cultures usually reflect bacterial colonization without accurately identifying the organism in the underlying bone itself. Only the isolation of *S. aureus* from deep wound culture has correlated with its presence in bone.

Oral therapy has been used successfully after 2 weeks of parenteral therapy in the treatment of pediatric osteomyelitis. This method of therapy should be entertained where there is good laboratory backup and close patient monitoring to ensure compliance. Patients casually treated with oral antibiotics often receive inadequate dosage and inadequate monitoring, resulting in a failure rate of 19 percent. For successful therapy, the orally administered antibiotic should be monitored by the measurement of serum bactericidal activity against the causative pathogen. A peak bactericidal dilution of at least 1:8 or greater should be maintained. In children, this form of therapy offers advantages in convenience, comfort, and cost. We treat adults with 6 weeks of intravenous therapy and children with 3 weeks of intravenous therapy followed by 3 weeks of oral therapy.

THERAPY FOR CHRONIC OSTEOMYELITIS

Chronic osteomyelitis secondary to surgery, trauma, or contiguous focal infection must be approached with combined medical and surgical therapy. Debridement should be done as soon as possible to remove all necrotic bone and sequestra. Abscesses or fistulous tracts must be eliminated. Material obtained at the time of surgery should be cultured for aerobes and anaerobes. Internal fixation devices, plates, pins, and screws should be removed. If bone stabilization is required, an external fixation device can be utilized. The wound may have to be debrided every 48 to 72 hours until all nonviable tissue has been removed.

Antimicrobial therapy should be initiated as early as possible, should be directed specifically against the offending pathogen(s), and should be administered intravenously in high doses for 6 weeks after the last debridement. Antimicrobial therapy prior to the time when debridement cultures are obtained should consist of broad-spectrum antibiotics to cover both aerobes and anaerobes. It is advisable to give antibiotics prior to debridement in order to reduce cellulitis or soft tissue swelling and reduce the risk of bacteremia.

There is no good evidence that regional antibiotic perfusion of an extremity or wound irrigation with antibiotics confers an advantage, and irrigation may introduce superinfections with resistant organisms.

THERAPY IN GENERAL

The consequences of inadequate therapy can be grave and lifelong. Knowing the types of organisms producing the osteomyelitis should lead to the use of a specific bactericidal agent except when multiple organisms are involved. Blind therapy is dangerous. Empiric choice of a narrow-spectrum agent not effective against the organism(s) within the bone may lead to treatment failure and chronic relapses. On the other hand, empiric broad-spectrum therapy may unnecessarily expose the patient to excessive or potentially toxic antimicrobial therapy and also inflate the cost of treatment.

The agents chosen for use should be demonstrated to be effective against the organism isolated from bone by in vitro sensitivity tests, such as the minimum inhibitory concentration (MIC) and minimum bactericidal concentration (MBC). Disk sensitivities have been used as the basis of therapy, but disks contain concentrations of drugs in excess of those achievable in bone, and results may not be directly applicable to the clinical situation. The antimicrobial agent chosen should penetrate the involved bone in concentrations greater than those required to be active against the organisms.

We think that serum bactericidal testing should be done to predict the outcome of infection. In patients with acute osteomyelitis, peak serum bactericidal titers have no predictive value; however, trough titers of 1:2 or greater accurately predict cure, whereas trough titers of less than 1:2 predict therapeutic failure. In patients with chronic osteomyelitis, peak serum bactericidal titers of 1:16 or greater and trough titers of 1:4 or greater accurately predict cure, whereas peak titers of less than 1:16 and trough titers of less than 1:2 accurately predict failure.

Hyperbaric oxygen has been used as adjunctive therapy in chronic osteomyelitis, but the value of adding hyperbaric oxygen to conventional surgical and medical management remains debatable.

Soft tissue swelling, periosteal thickening, and periosteal elevation are the earliest changes but are subtle and may be missed. Lytic changes are not seen until 2 to 6 weeks after the onset of disease. Sclerotic changes of periosteal new bone formation (involvarum) denotes a longer process. Radionucleotide scanning (technetium plus gallium or indium) is most helpful in the course of acute disease prior to the development of radiologic changes. Positive scans may be seen as early as 24 hours after the onset of symptoms. CT is useful to identify areas of dead bone (sequestrum).

The bacteriologic diagnosis of osteomyelitis rests on the isolation of the pathogenic bacteria from the bone or the blood. In chronic osteomyelitis, sinus tract cultures are not reliable for predicting which organism(s) will be isolated from the infected bone. There is a poor correlation between sinus tract cultures and bone biopsy cultures. Bone biopsy material should be carefully cultured and stained for aerobes, anaerobes, mycobacterium, and fungus. The bone should also be submitted for histopathologic evaluation.

Antimicrobial therapy should be initiated as early as possible, should be directed specifically against the offending pathogen(s), and should be administered intravenously in high doses for 4 to 6 weeks. Surgical intervention, in the form of bone debridement, is usually required in addition to antibiotics in the therapy of osteomyelitis arising from a contiguous focus of infection, diabetic ulcers, and peripheral vascular disease. In addition, combination intravenous and oral antimicrobial therapy may need to be given for 3 to 6 months in forms of osteomyelitis where extensive bony changes and tissue damage have occurred.

The antimicrobial agent(s) chosen for use should be demonstrated effective against the organism isolated from bone by in vitro sensitivity tests—MIC and MBC. It is best to choose an antibiotic or antibiotic combination that has a low ratio of MIC to MBC relative to its expected serum concentration. We prefer the antibiotic chosen to be able to obtain serum levels at least eight times the MIC. Table 3

TABLE 3 Antibiotic Therapy for Osteomyelitis in Adults

Organism	*Antibiotics of First Choice**	*Alternative Antibiotics**
Staphylococcus aureus	Nafcillin or oxacillin 2 g q6h	Clindamycin 900 mg q8h, vancomycin 500 mg q6h, cefazolin 1 g q8h
Staphylococcus epidermidis	Nafcillin or oxacillin 2 g q6h	Vancomycin 500 mg q6h, cefazolin 1 g q8h
Nonenterococcal *Streptococcus*	Penicillin G 3 million units q6h	Clindamycin 900 mg q8h, cefazolin 1 g q8h
Enterococcal *Streptococcus*	Ampicillin 2 g q6h *plus* gentamicin 5 mg/kg per day q8h	Vancomycin 500 mg q6h *plus* gentamicin 5 mg/kg per day q12h
Enterobacter species	Cefotaxime 2 g q8h *plus* gentamicin 5 mg/kg per day q8h	Ceftazidime *or* ceftizoxime 2 g q8h *plus* gentamicin 5 mg/kg per day q12h
Escherichia coli	Ampicillin 2 g q6h	Cefazolin 1 g q8h, cefuroxime 1.5 g q8h
Proteus mirabilis	Ampicillin 2 g q6h	Cefazolin 1 g q8h, cefuroxime 1 g q8h
Proteus vulgaris	Cefotaxime 2 g q8h	Cefuroxime 1.5 g q8h, ceftizoxime 2 g q8h
Providencia rettgeri	Ceftazidime 2 g q8h	
Morganella morganii	Ceftazidime 2 g q8h	
Serratia marcescens	Cefotaxime 2 g q8h	Ceftazidime *or* ceftizoxime 2 g q8h, mezlocillin *or* piperacillin 4 g q6h, *plus* gentamicin 5 mg/kg per day q12h
Pseudomonas aeruginosa	Azlocillin 4 g q6h *or* piperacillin 3 g q4h *plus* tobramycin 5 mg/kg per day q8h (in order of choice)	Ceftazidime 2 g q8h *plus* tobramycin 5 mg/kg per day q12h
Bacteroides species	Clindamycin 900 mg q8h IV	Metronidazole 500 mg q8h, cefoxitin 2 g q6h Timentum 3.1 g q8h

* Administered intravenously.

outlines the choice of antibiotics for the therapy of bacterial osteomyelitis in adults.

On the basis of presently limited available data, ciprofloxacin appears to be useful for bone infections due to susceptible strains of the family Enterobacteriaceae and may be an important alternative for pseudomonal infections. Ciprofloxacin may prove useful as an oral extension of initial parenteral therapy or in patients who are not candidates for intravenous therapy. Careful monitoring for emergence of resistance is advised when treating infections due to *P. aeruginosa*.

SUGGESTED READING

Cierny G, Mader JT, Penninck JJ. A clinical staging system of adult osteomyelitis. Contemp Orthop 1985; 10:17.

Gentry LO. Approach to the patient with chronic osteomyelitis. In: Remington JS, Swartz MN, eds. Current clinical topics in infectious diseases. Number 8. 1987:62.

Raff MJ, Melo JC. Anaerobic osteomyelitis. Medicine (Balt) 1978; 57:279.

Wheat J. Diagnostic strategies in osteomyelitis. Am J Med 1978; 78 (Suppl 6B):218.

Wood MB, et al. Vascularized bone segment transfers for management of chronic osteomyelitis. Orthop Clin North Am 1982; 15:461.

BACTERIAL ARTHRITIS

RALPH TOMPSETT, M.D.

Bacterial arthritis is an infection of the joint space and involves all of the joint structures, including the synovium and the articular cartilage. The joint generally becomes involved by hematogenous infection, through trauma, following joint surgery, or after intra-articular injection of medications. In unusual circumstances the joint may become infected as a result of adjacent disease, such as in fungal or mycobacterial infection. The joint itself may basically be normal, as is usually the case in younger individuals, or it may have underlying structural disease, often rheumatoid arthritis, in older patients.

The possible causative microorganisms are numerous, but the majority of cases are due to just a few species. *Staphylococcus aureus*, *Neisseria gonorrhoeae*, *Haemophilus*, and streptococci of groups A and B are the most commonly encountered organisms. Staphylococcal infections occur at all ages but usually in individuals older than 45 years. Gonococci are found in younger, sexually active patients. *Haemophilus* is almost always encountered in children less than 2 years of age but is also seen occasionally in adults, especially in patients with underlying disease.

The knees are the most commonly involved joints, with fewer cases involving hips, elbows, shoulders, and ankles. The sternoclavicular joints are sometimes involved, particularly in drug addicts. Usually just one joint is affected. In gonococcal infections multiple joints and tendons may become involved, but even in this case the major involvement is frequently restricted to one joint.

DIAGNOSIS

The diagnosis is suspected on the basis of the clinical findings of pain on motion, tenderness about the joint, and signs of acute inflammatory reaction involving the joint. Radiologic examination may be helpful, especially in infants. Fever is usually present. Temporally related infections, such as staphylococcal skin and soft tissue infections or gonococcal urethritis, may give important clues as to the etiology of the arthritis. The diagnosis of septic arthritis may generally be made by examination of the joint fluid. Specific etiology is established by examination of stained smears of joint fluid and by culturing blood and joint fluids. Infected joint fluids usually contain more than 50,000 white blood cells, of which 90 percent or more are neutrophils. The total white blood cell count is a valuable diagnostic laboratory test. Occasionally, in acutely inflamed joints of rheumatoid arthritis or in crystal-induced arthropathy, the cell count reaches this level, but this is not the rule. Glucose concentrations are less than 50 percent of the blood glucose. Gram stains are positive in 40 to 50 percent of the patients and cultures are positive in most. Early diagnosis and initiation of therapy are extremely important in order to prevent joint damage due to the increased pressure in the joint from excessive exudate and to remove fluids containing leukocyte enzymes, which may cause destruction of cartilage.

TREATMENT

The treatment of bacterial arthritis consists of administration of antibiotics and appropriate drainage. If a reasonably certain etiology is established on the basis of the initial examination, including Gram stain of the joint fluid, the most appropriate antibiotic may be chosen from Table 1. If there are no clues as to the probable infecting organism, therapy may be initiated on the first day with intravenous nafcillin and gentamicin. If cultures prove negative and if the clinical response is good, this treatment may be continued. Once the active inflammatory process is under control, therapy may be simplified by changing to ceftriaxone or ciprofloxacin, in that order of preference.

TABLE 1 Antibiotics for Treatment of Bacterial Arthritis

Organism	*First-Line Drug*	*Alternative Drugs*
Neisseria gonorrhoeae	Penicillin G 4 million units IV q6h × 3 days, then penicillin V orally 500 mg q.i.d. × 4 days	Ceftriaxone 2 g IV q24h
		Cefoxitin 1 g IV q6h
	Amoxicillin 500 mg orally 4 times daily × 1 week	
Haemophilus influenzae		
Beta-lactamase-negative	Ampicillin 1.5 g IV q6h	Cefuroxime 1.5 g IV q8h
		Cefotaxime 2 g IV q6h
Beta-lactamase-positive	Cefuroxime 1.5 g IV q6h	Cefotaxime 2 g IV q6h
Staphylococcus aureus (coagulase-positive)	Nafcillin 2 g IV q4h	Cefazolin 1 g IV q8h
		Vancomycin 1 g IV ql2h
Streptococci, groups A and B, *Streptococcus pneumoniae*	Penicillin 4 million units IV q6h	Cefazolin 1 g IV q8h
		Vancomycin 1 g IV ql2h
Pseudomonas aeruginosa	Ticarcillin 3 g IV q4h *plus* gentamicin 1.5 mg/kg IV q8h	Ceftazidime 2 g IV q8h
		Ciprofloxacin 750 mg PO ql2h
Organism unknown	Nafcillin 2 g IV q4h *plus* gentamicin 1.5 mg/kg IV q8h	Ceftriaxone 1.5 g IV q8h
		Ciprofloxacin 750 mg PO ql2h
Staphylococcus, coagulase-negative	If methicillin sensitive: nafcillin 2 g IV q4h	Cefazolin 750 mg q8h *or*
	If methicillin resistant: vancomycin 1 g IV ql2h	Trimethoprim-sulfamethoxazole, 2 double-strength tablets b.i.d.
		Ciprofloxacin
Other organisms	Choice of drug dependent on species of microorganism and sensitivity tests	

General guidelines for duration of therapy in patients without prostheses and with good clinical response: *Neisseria gonorrhoeae*, 1 week; *Haemophilus*, streptococci, and *Streptococcus pneumoniae*, 2 weeks; remainder of organisms, 4 weeks. In patients with a prosthesis, therapy continues for 3 weeks after removal of the prosthetic device. In patients with prompt clinical response and for whom a good oral antibiotic is available, the latter portion of therapy may be accomplished with oral drug.

Repeated aspiration, daily if necessary, should be done over a period as long as a week if the clinical course requires it. If the course is unsatisfactory due to loculation of fluid, irrigation of the joint is appropriate. Irrigation of the knee through the arthroscope may be an excellent means of removing exudate. Open drainage is always required in infections of the hip. It is also required in other joints when despite aspiration and irrigation there is persistent purulent drainage, a persistent positive culture, or continued swelling and tenderness.

In addition to these measures the joints should be rested but not immobilized. Active weight-bearing may be begun early after subsidence of pain and the severe acute inflammatory reaction. Only rarely is synovectomy required.

INFECTION OF PROSTHETIC JOINTS

4/21/92

The problem of infection in prosthetic joints is quite different from that in native joints. A wide variety of microorganisms are found, the most common being coagulase-negative staphylococci, usually *Staphylococcus epidermidis*. Gram-negative rods, particularly *Serratia* and *Pseudomonas*, are common.

Treatment of infection of prosthetic joints usually requires removal of the prosthesis. With this done, appropriate antimicrobial therapy chosen on the basis of sensitivity tests is required for only a relatively short period, that is, for about 2 to 3 weeks. A waiting period thereafter of 3 to 6 months—if this is otherwise feasible—is generally advised before the joint is replaced.

In some patients with prosthetic joint infections, it is impossible to remove the prosthesis (e.g., because of other disease or refusal by the patient). Here, long-term suppressive therapy may be undertaken, and although drainage almost always continues, acute inflammatory episodes may be reduced to a minimum and overt sepsis avoided.

SUGGESTED READING

Carnesdale PG. Infectious arthritis. In: Crenshaw AW, ed. Campbell's operative orthopaedics. 7th ed. St. Louis: CV Mosby, 1987:677.

Smith JW. Infectious arthritis. In: Mandell GL, Douglas RG Jr, Bennett JE, eds. Principles and practice of infectious diseases. New York: John Wiley & Sons, 1985:700.

LYME DISEASE

GARY P. WORMSER, M.D.

Lyme disease, also known as Lyme borreliosis, is a newly recognized infectious disease caused by the spirochetal organism, *Borrelia burgdorferi*. It is spread by the bite of *Ixodes* ticks, and rodents are the principal reservoir of infection in nature. Lyme disease is the most common tick-borne disease in North America as well as the most common borrelial infection. Although infection is widespread, having been reported from at least 43 states of the United States and from much of Europe, most cases are clustered geographically and temporally, mirroring both the regional and seasonal prevalence and the activity of the vector tick species. For example, over 90 percent of reported cases in the United States occur in just nine states—New York, Connecticut, New Jersey, Pennsylvania, Massachusetts, Wisconsin, Minnesota, Rhode Island, and California—and the overwhelming majority of acute cases occur during the months of June and July, when the nymphal stage of *Ixodes dammini* is most abundant.

NATURAL HISTORY OF LYME DISEASE

Lyme disease, like the spirochetal diseases syphilis and relapsing fever, has protean clinical manifestations typically expressed in a pattern of acute exacerbations and spontaneous remissions, with variable periods of latency. Like syphilis, certain manifestations may first appear many months to years after infection.

The most specific clinical feature of Lyme disease is the characteristic skin rash, erythema migrans, which occurs approximately 7 days after the tick bite (3 days to a month or more). Beginning as an erythematous macule or papule, it may rapidly expand over the course of several days to an annular lesion, with diameters varying from as little as 2 cm to well in excess of 20 cm. The lesion is surprisingly asymptomatic, but a diagnostic hallmark is the presence of central clearing. However, erythema migrans may be completely homogeneous or may have a wide variety of other appearances including a pattern of concentric rings or target-like lesions (Fig. 1). On occasion, the center of the lesion may be vesicular, necrotic, or more intensely erythematous, or it may have a bluish cast. In some patients, erythema migrans is indistinguishable from ordinary bacterial cellulitis, although some of the favored anatomic locations such as the upper arm, axillary area, neck, groin, chest, or abdomen would be unusual for staphylococcal or streptococcal infections.

The pathogenesis of erythema migrans is local cutaneous infection with *B. burgdorferi* at the site of inoculation by the tick. In 15 to 25 percent of patients in the United States and in a lesser number in Europe, one or more secondary erythema migrans lesions will develop at sites remote from the tick bite, thought to be due to hematogenous dissemination of *B. burgdorferi* to other areas of the skin.

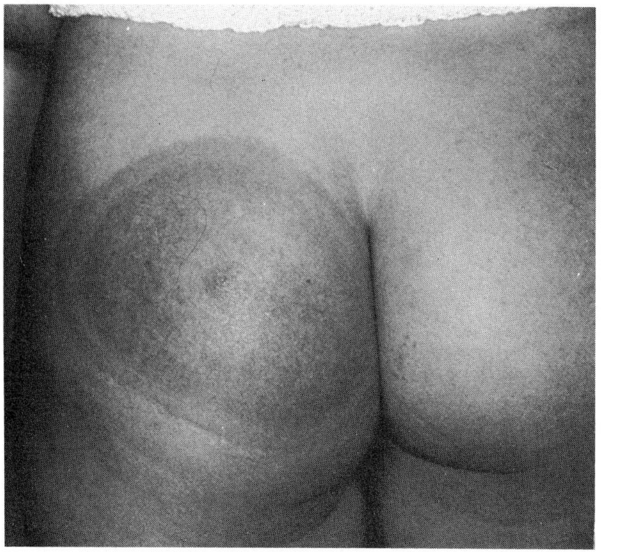

Figure 1 Erythema migrans on left buttock with a target-like appearance.

Flu-like symptoms including headaches and fever occur concomitantly with erythema migrans in 60 to 80 percent of cases. Other nonspecific symptoms are also common (Table 1). An unknown percentage of patients do not have a rash and only manifest a flu-like illness. Available data indeed suggest that subclinical infection associated with seroconversion is at least as common as recognized erythema migrans.

If the patient is untreated, erythema migrans will spontaneously resolve in about 3 weeks (longer in the European experience) but may recur later. Only approximately 20 percent of untreated patients, however, will remain completely well over a mean follow-up period of 6 years. Instead, 80 percent develop neurologic, cardiac, rheumatologic, or other manifestations of Lyme disease (see Table 1).

Typically, within a few weeks to several months after infection, approximately 15 percent of untreated patients manifest neurologic complications, most commonly facial nerve palsy (which may be bilateral), aseptic meningitis, or radiculopathy. Without therapy, spontaneous resolution will usually take place over the course of several months, but some complications may become chronic and, on occasion, irreversible despite antimicrobial treatment. It has also been recently recognized that certain neurologic manifestations may first appear several years after infection.

Approximately 8 percent of untreated patients (with or without neurologic complaints) are recognized to have cardiac involvement. Cardiac complications occur early after infection, within weeks to several months, and are self-limited. Myocarditis is the principal cardiac manifestation of Lyme disease, potentially resulting in varying degrees of heart block, arrhythmias, syncope, or in rare instances, death. In contrast to rheumatic fever, endocardial involvement and valvular lesions are not a recognized feature of Lyme disease.

The most common sequelae of Lyme disease are rheumatologic, with up to 80 percent of untreated erythema migrans patients developing either frank arthritis (60 percent) or arthralgias without arthritis (20 percent). Arthritis is typically a late manifestation appearing for the first time an average of 6 months after infection, although the range of time intervals when these symptoms may arise is broad (4 days to 2 or more years). Episodic monoarticular or asymmetric oligoarticular arthritis is the most common pattern of joint involvement. The joint most frequently involved is the knee. Temporomandibular joint arthritis is also relatively common, while involvement of the sacroiliac joints is distinctly unusual. Except for cases in children, most Lyme patients with arthritis do not have fever or the classic "hot joint" more typically associated with other bacterial causes of arthritis. A small percent of patients will develop a chronic synovitis lasting continuously for a year or more, possibly resulting in loss of articular cartilage and erosions of the articular cortex. Like most other complications of Lyme disease, spontaneous resolution of joint symptoms can occur without antibiotic treatment.

DIAGNOSIS

The three keys to diagnosis of Lyme disease are clinical suspicion, recognition of the characteristic signs and symptoms, and appropriate utilization of tests for antibody to *B. burgdorferi*. The vast majority of cases of early Lyme disease occur in the summer months among residents of, or travelers to, endemic areas. Recollection of a recent tick bite is a useful historical clue, but the absence of that history should never exclude the diagnosis, since only 20 to 30 percent of patients with confirmed cases recall such bites. The presence of erythema migrans (or its occurrence within the immediate past) is diagnostic of early Lyme disease. Serologic testing is neither necessary nor helpful at this stage since there is up to a 50 percent false negativity rate. Thus, early Lyme disease in the absence of erythema migrans, for example with a flu-like syndrome only, can be extremely difficult to diagnose. In addition, prompt antibiotic therapy may prevent a rise in antibody titer between tests done on acute and convalescent sera.

In endemic areas patients who develop facial nerve palsy, aseptic meningitis, radiculopathy in the absence of intervertebral disk disease, unexplained heart block, or an arthritis of any type should be carefully evaluated for Lyme disease (see Table 1). Fortunately, the majority of patients with these later manifestations of Lyme disease have a positive antibody test for *B. burgdorferi*. Culturing of clinical material for this organism has too low a yield and is too labor intensive and slow to serve as a practical diagnostic tool for Lyme disease. Other laboratory studies are only useful for the purpose of excluding alternative diagnoses.

A few caveats should be remembered in regard to optimal use of Lyme disease serology. First, early in the course of disease, specific tests for IgM antibody to *B. burgdorferi* are more sensitive than IgG tests. Second, because of lack of standardization of testing and interlaboratory variability of test results, a single negative antibody test result should never be interpreted as excluding Lyme disease in clinically suspicious cases. In these instances, repeat serologic testing

TABLE 1 Clinical Manifestations of Lyme Disease

Cutaneous	*Cardiologic*	*Neurologic*	*Rheumatologic*	*Miscellaneous*
Erythema migrans	Heart block	Cranial nerve palsy (esp. facial nerve)	Arthralgias	Fever
Lymphocytoma	Myocarditis	Radiculopathy	Arthritis	Fatigue
Acrodermatitis chronica atrophicans	Pericarditis	Meningitis	Myalgias	Sore throat
Malar rash	Arrhythmia	Encephalitis	Myositis	Conjunctivitis
Urticaria	Cardiomegaly	Peripheral neuropathy	Enthesopathy	Hepatitis
Septal panniculitis	Syncope	Plexopathy	Baker's cyst	Lymphadenopathy
	Dizziness	Chorea	Tendinitis	Splenomegaly
	Shortness of breath	Multineuritis multiplex		Hepatomegaly
	Chest pain	Transverse myelitis		Testicular swelling
	Palpitations	Cerebellar ataxia		Nausea, vomiting
	Gallops	Pseudotumor cerebri		Iritis
	Friction rubs	Guillain-Barré like syndrome		Panophthalmitis
		Optic neuritis		Cough
		Multiple sclerosis-like illness		Hoarseness
		Seizures		
		Dementia		
		Cranial arteritis		
		Arygyll Robertson pupil		
		Psychosis		
		Anorexia nervosa-like illness		
		Headaches		
		Photophobia		
		Stiff neck		
		Dysesthesias		
		Paresthesias		
		Diplopia		
		Irritability		
		Poor concentration		
		Hearing loss		
		Sleep disturbances		
		Hemiparesis		
		Paraparesis		
		Emotional lability		

should be performed, ideally by a second laboratory using a different testing methodology. In some patients with neurologic manifestations, specific antibodies are present in cerebrospinal fluid selectively and are absent in serum.

Immunoblotting or an antibody-capture enzyme immunoassays are more sensitive antibody assays than standard enzyme-linked immunosorbent assays (ELISA) or indirect immunofluorescent assays (IFA) but at present are available only in research facilities. Therefore, in selected patients who are seronegative, a strongly compatible clinical picture may nevertheless justify an empiric trial of antimicrobial therapy.

False-positive tests for antibody to *B. burgdorferi* may occur in other spirochetal diseases, particularly syphilis. Usually the clinical picture is sufficiently distinctive to avoid diagnostic confusion. If not, the diagnosis of syphilis is supported by a positive VDRL test (or other anticardiolipin antibody test), since this test is usually negative in Lyme disease.

TREATMENT

Optimal treatment for Lyme disease is unknown. A comparison of antimicrobial efficacy based on studies done in vitro, in infected laboratory animals, and in humans is shown in Table 2. Results of in vitro testing of antimicrobial agents against *B. burgdorferi* should be viewed cautiously as there is no standardized method of testing and no proven correlation with clinical effectiveness. For example, erythromycin is consistently among the most active drugs in vitro, but studies in laboratory animals and clinical trials in humans have suggested a relatively lower degree of activity. Studies comparing antibiotic efficacy in infected laboratory animals are limited by the failure to demonstrate comparability of dosing regimens on the basis of pharmacokinetic parameters and antibiotic blood levels.

Accumulating data based on recovery of *B. burgdorferi* from culture of clinical specimens suggest that most objec-

TABLE 2 Antimicrobial Activity in Vitro, in Laboratory Animal Models, and in Clinical Lyme Disease from Published Studies

	Activity		
Antimicrobial Agent	*In Vitro*	*Animal Models*	*Human Disease*
Amikacin	0	NA	NA
Ampicillin	++	NA	NA*
Amoxicillin	++	++	++
Amoxicillin–clavulanic acid	++	++	++
Cefotaxime	+++	++	NA*
Ceftriaxone	+++	++	++
Ciprofloxacin	+	NA	NA
Chloramphenicol	+	NA	NA*
Doxycycline	++	NA	NA*
Erythromycin	+++	+	+
Gentamicin	0	NA	NA
Imipenem	++	++	NA
Mezlocillin	++	NA	NA
Minocycline	+++	NA	++
Ofloxacin	+	NA	NA
Oxacillin	++	NA	NA
Penicillin	+	+	++
Rifampin	0	NA	NA
Tetracycline	++	++	++
Trimethoprim-sulfamethoxazole	0	NA	NA

NA = not available; 0 = not active; +, ++, +++ = degrees of activity, from least to most.
* Effective in anecdotal cases.

tive manifestations of Lyme disease are associated with viable organisms, underscoring the importance of defining exactly what constitutes curative antimicrobial therapy. The author's approach to treatment according to disease manifestation is found in Table 3.

Studies in adult patients with erythema migrans suggest that oral dosing regimens, consisting of 10-day treatment courses of 1 g daily doses of either penicillin preparations or tetracycline, are effective in shortening the course of the skin infection and in reducing the frequency of later manifestations of disease. Approximately 15 percent of patients treated in this manner develop a Jarisch-Herxheimer-like response with an intensification of symptoms during the first 24 hours of therapy. Because erythromycin (given as a 1-g daily dose) was significantly less effective in clearing erythema migrans than either penicillin or tetracycline at the same dosage, and because the latter two therapies were themselves associated with a failure rate of about 15 percent based on the need for retreatment or development of later sequelae, the author empirically recommends that standard oral therapy with all three drugs be increased to 2 g per day. Whether other oral antibiotics, such as ampicillin, amoxicillin, amoxicillin–clavulanic acid, cephalosporins, doxycycline, minocycline, or the addition of probenecid to a β-lactam regimen, are equally satisfactory or possibly superior therapies is not known. The optimal duration of therapy has not been established, although in one study of adult patients with erythema migrans, a 20-day course of tetracycline was no better than a 10-day treatment regimen.

The role of oral therapy for other manifestations of Lyme disease is less clear and less well studied. Patients with facial nerve palsy without overt signs of meningitis or other neurologic involvement may be treated orally and in almost all patients the palsy will completely resolve, with an average time to resolution of 24 days. However, this rate of resolution is no faster than has been seen in similar patients with Lyme disease who did not receive any antibiotic treatment. Thus, prevention of later sequelae of Lyme disease is the main reason to give antimicrobial therapy for patients with facial nerve palsy.

Higher-dose intravenous therapy with penicillin or the third-generation cephalosporin ceftriaxone, given for 10 to 14 days, has been successfully used in patients with other neurologic complications such as meningitis or encephalitis. Headache, stiff neck, and radicular pain improve rapidly with these therapies but motor deficits resolve much more slowly.

High-dose therapy with either penicillin or ceftriaxone is also effective for the majority of patients with Lyme arthritis, although it is possible that some of these patients would respond just as well to an oral antibiotic regimen. Lyme arthritis typically resolves slowly over the course of several weeks, and prolonged follow-up is necessary to evaluate outcome accurately because of the potential for late relapses. The relative efficacy of high-dose penicillin versus ceftriaxone is not established, but it is clear that some patients will respond to ceftriaxone who have previously failed a course of intravenous penicillin.

Few data are available to guide antibiotic therapy specifically for patients with cardiac involvement. Parenteral therapy, as for neurologic or rheumatologic disease, would seem appropriate. Perhaps the most important measure to

TABLE 3 Author's Approach to the Therapy of Lyme Disease

Manifestation of Lyme Disease	*Recommended Treatment Regimen*
Skin	
Erythema migrans	Regimen A
Lymphocytoma	Regimen A
Acrodermatitis chronica atrophicans	Regimen A or B
Neurologic	
Cranial nerve palsy, e.g., facial nerve palsy	Regimen A
Meningitis	Regimen B
Encephalitis	Regimen B
Radiculopathy	Regimen A or B
Cardiac	
Pericarditis/myocarditis	Regimen B
Heart block	Regimen B, insertion of temporary pacemaker to be considered
Rheumatologic	
Arthralgias	Regimen A
Arthritis	Regimen B
Miscellaneous	
Flu-like illness	Regimen A
Asymptomatic, seropositive; never previously treated	Regimen A (or observation)
Tick bite in endemic area, asymptomatic	Observation
Tick bite in a pregnant woman, asymptomatic	Regimen A (do not give tetracycline)
Lyme disease during pregnancy, any manifestation	Regimen B (do not give tetracycline)
Interstitial keratitis	Topical corticosteroids

Regimen A

Adults	Children	
Preferred	Preferred	
Tetracycline 500 mg PO q.i.d. x 10–14 days *or* Phenoxymethyl penicillin 500 mg PO q.i.d. x 10–14 days	*>8 yr* Tetracycline 12.5 mg/kg PO q6h x 10–14 days (up to 2 g/day)	*<8 yr* Phenoxymethyl penicillin 12.5 mg/kg PO q6h x 10–14 days (up to 2 g/day)
	or Phenoxymethyl penicillin 12.5 mg/kg PO q6h x 10–14 days (up to 2 g/day)	
Alternative	Alternative	
Erythromycin 500 mg PO q.i.d. x 10–14 days	Erythromycin 12.5 mg/kg PO q6h x 10–14 days (up to 2 g/day)	

Regimen B

Adult	Children	
Preferred	Preferred	
Penicillin G 3–4 x 10^6 U IV q4h x 10–14 days *or* Ceftriaxone 2 g IV/day x 10–14 days	Penicillin G 4 x 10^4 U/kg IV q4h x 10–14 days (up to 24 x 10^6U/day) *or* Ceftriaxone 37.5 mg/kg–50 mg/kg q12h IV/day x 10–14 days (up to 2 g/day)	
Alternative	Alternative	
Tetracycline 500 mg PO q6h x 30 days	*>8 yr* Tetracycline 12.5 mg/kg PO q6h x 30 days (up to 2 g/day)	*<8 yr* Erythromycin 12.5 mg/kg PO q6h x 30 days (up to 2 g/day)

be taken on behalf of these patients is the placement of a temporary cardiac pacemaker for patients with advanced heart block.

Benzathine-Penicillin Preparations

Benzathine-penicillin G, which gives prolonged but very low blood levels of penicillin after intramuscular administration, has been successfully used to treat both early and late manifestations of Lyme disease. As penicillin blood levels are actually higher with oral therapy, this preparation cannot be recommended.

PREGNANCY

The precise risk to the developing fetus of maternal Lyme disease during pregnancy is unknown, although it is well established that fetal infection can occur and may have serious outcomes, including malformations and death. Since anecdotal experience has suggested that oral antibiotic therapy does not invariably protect the fetus, this author prefers high-dose intravenous penicillin for pregnant women with active Lyme disease.

ASSESSMENT OF RESPONSE TO THERAPY

Assessing the adequacy of treatment for Lyme disease poses special problems because of the organism's latency and the intermittent pattern of exacerbations and remissions in the natural history of untreated infection. Furthermore, approximately 50 percent of patients with erythema migrans who apparently respond to antibiotic therapy based on prompt resolution of the skin manifestations and the absence of serious late complications over a several year follow-up nevertheless remain unwell, complaining of intermittent arthralgias, myalgias, headaches, or fatigue that may last from a few months to several years. Anecdotal observations of retreatment with high-dose intravenous penicillin did not show improvement in these complaints. Furthermore, there is no established laboratory test to follow, such as the VDRL in syphilis, to judge the adequacy of therapy in Lyme disease.

Two additional concerns arise in determining the response to therapy. First, reinfection with *B. burgdorferi*, leading to recurrence of clinical disease, is well documented. Reinfection in a recently treated patient could easily be misinterpreted as a treatment failure. Secondly, the tick vector of Lyme disease may simultaneously transmit other infectious agents, such as *Babesia* in the United States or tick-borne encephalitis virus in Europe. These agents cause illnesses with symptoms that may overlap with those of Lyme disease but which would not respond to the standard antibiotic therapies used for Lyme disease.

ADJUNCTIVE THERAPY

Nonsteroidal anti-inflammatory medications are useful adjuncts for controlling muscle or joint pains in Lyme disease. Previously, systemic corticosteroids were widely used to treat various neurologic, rheumatologic, or cardiac manifestations of Lyme disease. Evidence now exists, however, that these drugs may have a deleterious effect on the outcome of Lyme disease for some patients, and thus they should be used cautiously, if at all.

Arthroscopic synovectomy may sometimes be useful for arthritic patients in whom antibiotic treatment has not given relief, especially for those with knee involvement.

PREVENTION

Prevention of Lyme disease is a challenging problem in areas where infected ticks are abundant. Various methods of reducing tick numbers in the environment are under intensive investigation. Useful advice for individuals living in these areas is to wear light-colored protective clothing during outdoor activities, to consider spraying the surface of pants' legs and socks with an insect repellent containing either diethyltoluamide (DEET) or permethrin, and to inspect carefully the entire body surface and scalp at the end of each day for ticks. Household pets should be similarly scrutinized. As is the case with Rocky Mountain spotted fever, transmission of *B. burgdorferi* from tick to host is not immediate and can be prevented if ticks are promptly removed.

SUGGESTED READING

Anonymous. Treatment of Lyme disease. Med Lett 1988; 30:65–66.

Dattwyler RJ, Halperin JJ, Volkman DJ, Luft BJ. Treatment of late Lyme borreliosis—randomized comparison of ceftriaxone and penicillin. Lancet 1988; 1:1191–1194.

Duffy J. Lyme disease. Infect Dis Clin North Am 1987; 1:511–527.

Steere AC, Schoen RT, Taylor E. The clinical evolution of Lyme arthritis. Ann Intern Med 1987; 107:725–731.

Wormser GP. Treatment of Lyme disease—state of the art. N York Med Q 1985; 5:110–115.

HERPES SIMPLEX VIRUS INFECTIONS

MARY ALICE HARBISON, M.D.
SCOTT M. HAMMER, M.D.

Infections with herpes viruses are among the most common of human infections. The herpes simplex viruses (HSV) can cause a wide range of illness, from minor but irritating fever blisters and painful, recurrent genital ulcers to severe encephalitis and disseminated infections in neonates and immunocompromised hosts. Fortunately, treatment of HSV infections has been an area of signal medical progress in the last 10 years, and indeed, HSV has been the primary target of the first truly successful systemic antiviral agents, vidarabine and acyclovir.

MECHANISMS AND PHARMACOKINETICS

Vidarabine is an analogue of adenine and, following intravenous administration, is rapidly deaminated by adenosine deaminase to arabinosyl hypoxanthine. The latter possesses antiviral activity, but it is severalfold less active than the parent compound. Vidarabine is converted to its active form, vidarabine triphosphate, by cellular kinases. This compound then acts as a competitive inhibitor of the viral DNA polymerase. Incorporation into the growing viral DNA chain and DNA chain termination may both occur. The hypoxanthine metabolite, which is the measurable drug in serum, has a half-life of 3.5 hours and can accumulate in renal failure. Thus, dosage adjustments are necessary when there is renal insufficiency.

Acyclovir is an analogue of guanine that possesses an acyclic side chain instead of an intact ribose moiety. Antiviral specificity is conferred by the fact that it is selectively taken up by HSV-infected cells, and the first step in its activation (conversion to acyclovir monophosphate) is catalyzed by the virally specified enzyme, thymidine kinase. Subsequent conversion to the active form of the drug, acyclovir triphosphate, is completed by cellular enzymes. The triphosphate, in turn, inhibits the viral DNA polymerase and may also act as a viral DNA chain terminator. The much greater affinity of this agent for the HSV DNA polymerase than for the cellular α-polymerase confers further targeting specificity. The half-life of acyclovir is 2.5 to 3.9 hours following intravenous or oral administration. Oral bioavailability is low, however, being approximately 20 percent. Levels in cerebrospinal fluid (CSF) are approximately 50 percent of those in serum, and the drug is hemodialyzable. Acyclovir is largely excreted by renal mechanisms, and thus dosage adjustments are indicated when the creatinine clearance falls below 50 ml per minute. For creatinine clearances of 25 to 50 and 10 to 25 ml per minute, the normal intravenous dosing interval should be increased from 8 to 12 and 24 hours, respectively. Under 10 ml per minute, half of a single dose can be given every 24 hours. Redosing after hemodialysis is indicated.

MUCOCUTANEOUS HERPES SIMPLEX INFECTIONS IN NORMAL HOSTS

HSV syndromes may be divided into initial and recurrent episodes. Initial disease may be further subdivided into primary and nonprimary infections. Primary infections are those that occur in individuals who are seronegative for both type 1 and type 2. Nonprimary, initial infections are those that represent the first clinical episode of herpes in a patient who is seropositive at the outset. This is most commonly seen clinically in two settings: the individual with a past history of herpes labialis who acquires genital herpes and the individual who has not recognized mild earlier episodes of the disease. The differentiation is important, as true primary disease is typically more severe, often with systemic signs of fever, malaise, and myalgias, and with more local pain, more lesions, greater adenopathy, and a longer time to healing.

Oral herpes infections are usually caused by HSV type 1 and genital infections by type 2 virus strains, although 10 to 15 percent of cases at either anatomic site will be caused by the opposite virus type. Typing of virus isolates can be done simply by monoclonal antibody staining or by more involved techniques such as restriction endonuclease mapping. The latter can be used to compare individual virus strains for epidemiologic purposes. Typing of the isolate is of clinical relevance with regard to providing prognostic advice to patients concerning the pattern of recurrences. HSV type 1 recurs with greater frequency when it infects oropharyngeal sites, and HSV type 2 tends to recur more frequently when it infects the genital region. The reason for this difference in biologic behavior is unexplained.

The diagnosis of mucocutaneous HSV infection can usually be made on clinical grounds from the history and the presence of typical vesicular or ulcerated lesions on an erythematous base. Diagnosis should always be confirmed by culture of the lesions and/or by cytologic smear, using the Tzanck technique or direct immunofluorescent staining with monoclonal antibodies. The cytologic methods have the advantage of making an immediate diagnosis, whereas cell cultures may take from 24 to 72 hours to show typical cytopathic effects. When specimens are properly prepared and testing is done by experienced personnel, the immunofluorescent staining method approaches cell culture in diagnostic sensitivity and specificity for genital lesions. Because antibodies to HSV are prevalent, serologic testing is not generally useful diagnostically except to document primary episodes. However, new antibody tests are under development that may reliably distinguish between type 1 and type 2 infections.

Treatment of genital herpes infections continues to be the subject of active research, and recommendations are consequently still evolving. Initial studies focused on primary episodes and demonstrated that intravenous acyclovir was highly effective in shortening the period of viral shedding, the formation of new lesions, and the healing time, although it had no effect on the establishment of latency or the rate of subsequent recurrences. Oral acyclovir has also been shown to be similarly effective, and is now in general the drug of choice for both primary and recurrent attacks.

Because of their tendency to be more severe and prolonged, virtually all primary episodes of genital herpes should be treated with acyclovir, and the duration of therapy should be longer than for recurrent episodes. The usual dose of oral acyclovir for primary attacks is 200 mg every 4 hours (five times a day) for 10 days. Topical acyclovir ointment (5 percent) has some proven efficacy in the treatment of primary genital infection but has been largely supplanted by the oral preparation. Other more convenient oral dosing regimens are currently being tested. Severe cases with neurologic involvement (i.e., urinary retention or aseptic meningitis) may require hospitalization, and intravenous therapy (5 mg per kilogram every 8 hours) should then be considered until improvement occurs.

Recurrent episodes of genital herpes can be effectively treated with a 5-day course of oral acyclovir. Recently 800 mg twice a day has been found to be as effective as the more standard course of 200 mg five times daily for treatment of recurrent attacks. Many studies have shown that treatment of recurrences is most effective when initiated by the patient at the first prodromal symptoms; education of patients about their disease and its management is therefore a crucial part of therapy. Certainly not every recurrent episode requires drug treatment; in deciding upon a treatment protocol the clinician must take into account the frequency and severity of recurrences, the degree of inconvenience and discomfort to the patient, and psychosocial factors.

For patients with fewer than six recurrences per year, each attack is probably best managed individually. Patients with a higher number of recurrences should be considered potential candidates for chronic suppressive acyclovir treatment. Several studies have now shown that continuous administration of oral acyclovir can markedly decrease the rate of genital herpes recurrences for up to 2 years, with about 50 percent of patients experiencing no recurrences at all in any given year and about 30 percent remaining disease free for 2 years. Breakthrough episodes can occur but tend to be mild attacks. A total daily dose of 600 to 800 mg as a single or divided dose appears most effective for long-term suppression; lower daily doses and intermittent dosing (i.e., "weekend" therapy) have not proved satisfactory.

Minimal drug toxicity has been noted in these studies, and routine laboratory monitoring of patients does not appear necessary. However, patients should be advised about the cost of therapy ($2 to $3 per day), and female patients must be cautioned to use strict birth control measures for the duration of suppressive treatment. No congenital defects due to inadvertent acyclovir administration in pregnancy have been reported, but the long-term genetic effects of this nucleoside analogue remain to be determined. In two small studies, no effects were seen on white cell chromosomes or on sperm count and morphology after several months of continuous acyclovir. The current U.S. Food and Drug Administration recommendations for suppression with acyclovir extend only for 6 months, but in light of the accumulating data on the safety and continued efficacy of longer treatment, these recommendations are likely to change. Most authors still recommend interrupting suppressive therapy after 6 to 9 months to determine whether the natural frequency of recurrences has diminished.

In contrast to genital herpes, attempts to develop effective treatment for oral HSV infections in normal hosts have been mostly disappointing. One trial of oral acyclovir suspension in children with primary herpes stomatitis has been reported, in which an antiviral effect was documented but little clinical benefit obtained. Acyclovir is therefore not generally recommended for treatment of primary gingivostomatitis in otherwise healthy children, although the occasional severe case which might require hospitalization and intravenous hydration may warrant a trial of intravenous acyclovir therapy.

While other controlled trials have shown that continuous use of topical or oral acyclovir was helpful in preventing and minimizing the severity of recurrences of herpes labialis in adults who suffer frequent attacks, neither form of the drug was helpful in decreasing pain or duration of lesions when used for treatment of individual episodes. Again, therefore, for most patients with infrequent, uncomplicated attacks of herpes labialis, acyclovir treatment is not indicated. However, recent studies have shown that short-term oral acyclovir therapy with 400 mg twice daily can prevent recurrences of herpes labialis in patients with predictable recurrences, such as skiers with sun-related attacks, or patients undergoing trigeminal ganglion surgery or dermabrasion.

Acyclovir is also proving useful for treatment of other cutaneous HSV infections, and the list of indications will undoubtedly continue to expand as more experience is gained. For example, the hand is a common site of inoculation with both HSV 1 and 2, and oral acyclovir when taken in the prodrome has been shown to shorten the duration of primary episodes and to prevent recurrences. Individuals with atopic eczema and other skin conditions can develop a widespread cutaneous HSV infection known as eczema herpeticum. In children the condition can be severe, resulting in large areas of erosion, dehydration, secondary infection, and even death. Intravenous acyclovir, 5 mg per kilogram every 8 hours for 5 days, has been anecdotally successful and should be used in children and severely ill adults. Milder cases in adults have also responded to some degree to oral acyclovir 200 mg five times a day; 400 mg five times a day may be a more prudent dose to employ. Erythema multiforme is another rare but potentially serious complication of HSV infection. Oral acyclovir can abort recurrent attacks when started with the first prodromal symptoms, and some individuals with extremely frequent attacks have benefitted from chronic suppressive therapy for up to 6 months.

OCULAR HSV INFECTIONS

Superficial and deep structures of the eye can be involved in both primary and recurrent HSV infections. The cornea is by far the most commonly involved site, and recurrent HSV keratitis is the most common cause of infectious blindness in the United States. Treatment of ocular HSV infections should always be undertaken with qualified ophthalmologic consultation. However, it is important for all practitioners to consider HSV infection in patients with eye pain or corneal lesions, since delay in treatment or incorrect management (e.g., steroid treatment in superficial HSV keratitis) can have devastating consequences. Currently two topical antiviral agents are licensed for use in ocular HSV infections: vidarabine and trifluorothymidine. Trifluorothymidine is the more potent and more soluble agent with better penetration into the cornea and is therefore usually the drug of choice. Topical acyclovir has been used extensively in Europe with some success but is not yet licensed for ocular use in the United States. Anecdotal reports also indicate that oral and intravenous acyclovir may be useful in treating deep ocular infections.

HERPES SIMPLEX ENCEPHALITIS

Herpes simplex encephalitis (HSE) is certainly one of the most devastating forms of HSV infection and virtually the only life-threatening form to occur regularly in normal hosts beyond the neonatal period. HSV is the most frequent cause of fatal, sporadic encephalitis in the United States today, with an estimated annual incidence of 1,000 to 2,000 cases, or one case per 250,000 to 500,000 population. HSE must be differentiated from the aseptic meningitis seen in association with genital herpes, which is a benign and self-limited condition.

Patients with HSE generally have abrupt onset of fever, headache, altered behavior and mentation, and focal neurologic deficits, reflecting the common involvement of the temporal lobes. CSF profiles usually show elevated protein levels and a lymphocytic pleocytosis, but the formulas are not diagnostic. The availability of effective treatment for HSE, first with vidarabine and now with acyclovir, has dramatically escalated the debate over whether to perform a brain biopsy for diagnosis. Proponents of early biopsy argue that it is crucial to establish a firm diagnosis early, in order to be confident of the need for antiviral therapy and to rule out other treatable causes of encephalitis, which may be present in up to 20 to 30 percent of cases. Opponents argue that there is little harm in overtreating with acyclovir; that brain biopsy cannot possibly be done in every patient in whom HSE is considered; that the procedure itself may add morbidity; and that effective treatment may be delayed, especially in smaller institutions, while waiting for biopsy to be done. Rapid laboratory methods of diagnosis, such as measuring herpes simplex antigen in the CSF, are under development but not generally available. An elevated ratio of CSF to serum antibody or a fourfold rise in CSF HSV antibody titers correlates well with proven HSE, but these cannot be helpful diagnostically until at least the second week of illness. Recently, magnetic resonance imaging (MRI) has proven capable of identifying extremely early focal anatomic lesions in HSE; computed tomograms (CT) generally do not show defects before the fourth to fifth day of illness.

In the double-blind, placebo-controlled trial of vidarabine published in 1977 by the National Institute of Allergy and Infectious Disease (NIAID) Collaborative Antiviral Study Group, mortality in untreated cases of HSE was 70 percent at 6 months, with only 11 percent of survivors returning to a normal neurologic status. Vidarabine was proven to reduce mortality to 40 percent at 6 months and to increase the fraction of normal survivors to 20 percent. However, subsequent trials of acyclovir versus vidarabine have clearly established acyclovir as the drug of choice for HSE, reducing the 6-month mortality rate to 20 percent and further benefitting the survivors, with 30 to 60 percent regaining normal function. Age, Glasgow coma score, and duration of illness were important determinants of outcome; patients who were comatose when treatment started had no better prognosis than placebo-treated controls. Hence prompt diagnosis and treatment remain essential to ensure optimal results.

A prudent course to take with patients presenting with a febrile, focal encephalitis compatible with HSE is as follows: (1) MRI or CT should be done immediately, followed by a lumbar puncture if threatening cerebral edema is not seen. If focality is not demonstrated initially, an electroencephalogram, technetium brain scan, and early follow-up MRI or CT should be considered to see if focality develops. (2) In patients with a strongly suggestive presentation, acyclovir should be immediately administered intravenously at a dose of 10 mg per kilogram every 8 hours (if renal function is normal). (3) If a focal abnormality is demonstrated by one of the above techniques, a brain biopsy to confirm the diagnosis and exclude other treatable etiologies should be strongly considered in centers with appropriate neurosurgical and virologic support. Transfer to regional centers with such expertise is often appropriate. However, it should be reiterated that treatment should not be delayed pending either a diagnostic work-up or transfer of the patient, if an acceptable neurologic outcome is to be expected. Administration of acyclovir for 24 to 48 hours will not affect the diagnostic yield of biopsy if viral antigen testing in addition to viral culture is included. If HSE is confirmed, acyclovir treatment should continue for at least 10 to 14 days and possibly longer, depending on the clinical course. Rare cases of relapsing infection after acyclovir therapy have been reported, which may respond to a second course of treatment. A demyelinating postinfectious encephalomyelitis has also been recognized, which has a characteristic appearance on brain biopsy; partial responses to steroid treatment have been reported.

HSV INFECTIONS IN IMMUNOCOMPROMISED PATIENTS

In contrast to the situation in normal hosts, endogenous reactivation of HSV causes severe morbidity and mortality in patients with many forms of immune suppression. Sixty to eighty percent of seropositive transplant recipients and patients undergoing chemotherapy for hematologic malignancies will reactivate HSV, usually within the first 6 weeks of treatment. Oral HSV mucositis can be difficult to distinguish from (or may coexist with) candidiasis or drug-induced mucositis in such settings, so the clinician must be alert to this possibility. Individuals with the acquired immunodeficiency syndrome (AIDS) also suffer a high rate of HSV recurrences, which can be chronic, indolent, and difficult to manage. All such episodes can be prolonged and painful, with lesions taking twice as long to heal as in normal hosts, and relapses are frequent when therapy is stopped. HSV can also disseminate viscerally in immunosuppressed patients, causing hepatitis and pneumonia, and, by interrupting the normal skin barriers, can pose a risk of secondary infection.

It is now well established that intravenous and oral acyclovir are both effective treatments for HSV reactivations of all types in immunocompromised patients. The choice of drug route should depend on the overall condition of the patient and the ability to tolerate oral medications. The usual intravenous doses used are 250 mg per square meter (5 mg per kilogram) every 8 hours. Effective oral doses are somewhat higher than necessary in normal hosts, usually 400 mg five times a day. Length of treatment may depend somewhat on the response of lesions, but should be for at least 7 to 10 days.

Since HSV reactivation occurs commonly and often predictably in immunocompromised patients, acyclovir can also be used successfully as prophylaxis against recurrences. Several controlled studies have shown reactivation rates of 0 to 10 percent in acyclovir-treated patients compared to 60 to 80 percent in controls, with breakthrough episodes frequently being mild or consisting of asymptomatic viral shedding. Acyclovir prophylaxis is therefore now routine practice in many centers for seropositive patients undergoing bone marrow transplantation, induction therapy for leukemia, and solid organ transplantation. Both 250 mg per square meter (5 mg per kilogram) intravenously every 8 hours and 200 mg orally every 6 hours are generally effective, and treatment should continue from the day of conditioning, induction, or transplantation for 4 to 6 weeks. Indications for prophylaxis in patients with AIDS are not as well defined. Anecdotal experience has shown that higher oral doses may be required to maintain suppression in AIDS patients, i.e., 400 mg three to four times daily.

NEONATAL HSV INFECTIONS

Most neonatal HSV infections are acquired perinatally from infected genital secretions of the mother and are consequently caused by HSV type 2. It is estimated that 10 to 40 percent of exposed infants will become infected, but methods for identifying precisely which mothers and infants will be at risk at the time of delivery have not been perfected. The annual incidence in the United States is approximately one case per 2,500 to 5,000 live births.

HSV infection must be suspected in neonates with rash, with sepsis or meningoencephalitis without a bacterial source, and especially in those with a maternal history of genital herpes or cultures positive for HSV. Seventy to eighty percent of affected infants will have a vesicular rash from which virus can be isolated; the rest may have virus cultured from the oropharynx, eyes, or buffy coat. Three patterns of neonatal infection are seen: mucocutaneous disease limited to the skin, eyes, and oropharynx; disseminated infection with visceral involvement; and encephalomyelitis. Mortality rates in the latter two forms range from 50 to 80 percent without treatment, and even those infants with "only" mucocutaneous disease have a 30-percent incidence of subsequent neurologic deficits. Progression from mucocutaneous disease to disseminated infection and/or encephalitis can occur in up to 80 percent of infants; therefore, a major goal of therapy is prompt recognition and treatment to halt further progression. Hence, all neonates with any form of HSV infection should be treated.

Preliminary data from the most recent comparative trial from the NIAID Collaborative Antiviral Study Group has shown that vidarabine and acyclovir at doses of 30 mg per kilogram per day are probably equally efficacious in neonatal HSV infections. Mortality was decreased from 60 to 80 percent in untreated cases to 20 percent, and the fraction of normal survivors increased from 20 to 55 percent overall. As in the encephalitis trials, the duration of illness before institution of therapy had a major impact on outcome. No differences in short-term side effects or drug toxicities were noted, but the long-term follow-up from this latest comparative trial remains incomplete as yet.

Current recommendations are therefore to treat all neonates with any form of HSV infection with either acyclovir 10 mg per kilogram intravenously every 8 hours, or vidarabine 30 mg per kilogram administered intravenously over 12 hours at a concentration of 0.5 mg per milliliter. Duration of treatment with either drug is 10 days. Many children will develop recurrent skin vesicles within several months of treatment, but these do not require repeat therapy unless signs of systemic involvement are present.

Rapid identification of women at risk of transmitting HSV at delivery is a major area of ongoing research. Classic practice has been to perform caesarean section in all women with genital lesions or positive viral cultures at delivery, as well as in any woman with primary genital infection during the last trimester, provided that surgery was feasible before or within 12 hours of rupture of membranes. No controlled trials of acyclovir prophylaxis in peripartum mothers or in exposed neonates have yet been conducted because of ongoing concern over the possibility of long-term adverse effects. When more experience is gained with acyclovir in children, the potentially considerable benefits of prophylaxis in certain infants may eventually be realized.

ADVERSE EFFECTS

Vidarabine has numerous potential side effects. Its relative insolubility makes fluid management difficult in individuals with HSE and concomitant cerebral edema. Gastrointestinal and hematologic toxicities are not uncommon. Further, it possesses a significant neurotoxic potential, especially in individuals with preexisting neurologic insults, renal compromise (with subsequent drug accumulation), and concomitant allopurinol therapy.

Acyclovir is a much better tolerated agent. The most common side effects are minor: headache and nausea. More significant toxicities have been reported and include reversible renal dysfunction secondary to crystalluria, if the drug is too rapidly infused, and occasional neurotoxicity. High doses, preexisting neurologic disease, or concomitant therapies all may predispose to acyclovir-associated neurotoxic reactions.

ACYCLOVIR RESISTANCE

As with antibacterial therapy, there is much interest and concern whether resistance to antiviral agents will occur as they become widely used. Resistance of HSV strains to acyclovir is known to occur, but its precise frequency and its ultimate clinical importance are not fully defined. The most common mechanism of resistance demonstrated by HSV isolates is diminished thymidine kinase activity, but these strains are inherently less pathogenic and have a diminished capacity to establish latency in animal models. Other mechanisms of resistance include an intact viral thymidine kinase with an altered substrate specificity, so that the drug is not phosphorylated, and strains with an altered DNA polymerase that is no longer inhibited by acyclovir triphosphate.

In normal patients on chronic suppressive therapy for recurrent genital herpes, no overall increase in resistance of the HSV isolates has been observed. In immunocompromised patients, resistant isolates have been reported with increasing frequency in patients with AIDS, and this has correlated with a lack of clinical response. The situation is complex, however, as some lesions may heal despite the isolation of a resistant strain. Also, lack of response may not always indicate resistance to the antiviral agent, as host immune factors may be more crucial to the outcome. As a practical matter, one should use acyclovir prudently, but widespread resistance has not yet emerged as a major problem since its licensure. However, in a serious clinical situation, if a patient is not responding to adequate doses of acyclovir, resistance should be considered. Isolates can be tested for resistance in a number of research laboratories, and alternative treatment with vidarabine or foscarnet (an experimental agent) should be considered.

TABLE 1 Therapy of HSV Infections

Host/Syndrome	*Treatment*	*Alternatives*	*Comments*
Immunocompetent hosts			
Primary herpes genitalis	Acyclovir (ACV) 200 mg PO 5 ×/day ×10 days	ACV 400 mg PO b.i.d. × 10 days *or* ACV 5 mg/kg IV q8h (if severe) *or* ACV 5% ointment (topical)	
Recurrent herpes genitalis	ACV 200 mg PO 5 ×/day × 5 days	ACV 400 mg PO b.i.d. × 5 days	Consider chronic suppression if ≥ 6 recurrences/yr
Primary herpes gingivostomatitis	Supportive in most cases	ACV 200 mg PO 5 ×/day *or* ACV 400 mg PO b.i.d. *or* ACV 5 mg/kg IV q8h (if severe)	
Recurrent herpes labialis	Supportive		Short-term prophylaxis for specific indications can be considered
Cutaneous syndromes:			
Herpetic whitlow	ACV 200 mg PO 5×/day × 5 days	ACV 400 mg PO b.i.d. × 5 days	
Eczema herpeticum	ACV 5 mg/kg IV q8h	ACV 400 mg PO 5 ×/day (if mild)	
HSV-associated erythema multiforme	ACV 400 mg PO 5 ×/day (if mild)		Chronic suppressive therapy may be indicated
Keratitis	1% trifluorothymidine solution (topical)	3% vidarabine (VDB) ointment (topical)	Ophthalmologic consultation advised
Encephalitis	ACV 10 mg/kg IV q8h × 10–14 days	VDB 15 mg/kg IV qd × 10–14 days	
Immunocompromised hosts			
Mucocutaneous disease	ACV 5 mg/kg IV q8h × 7–10 days (if severe)	ACV 200–400 mg PO 5×/day × 7–10 days (as follow up to IV treatment or if less severe)	Higher oral doses indicated for patients with AIDS
Visceral involvement (pneumonia, hepatitis, meningoencephalitis, etc.)	ACV 10 mg/kg IV q8h × 10–14 days	VDB 15 mg/kg IV qd × 10–14 days	
Neonatal disease	ACV 10 mg/kg IV q8h × 10–14 days	VDB 30 mg/kg IV qd × 10–14 days	Superiority of ACV not yet established

Oral doses given are for adults. Doses recommended are for individuals with normal renal function; adjustments for renal insufficiency are necessary (see text). See text for discussion of prophylaxis/chronic suppression.

CONCLUSIONS

A summary of treatment recommendations for the major forms of HSV infection is shown in Table 1. In the past 5 years the availability of oral acyclovir has revolutionized the treatment of many mucocutaneous HSV infections. While treatment of primary HSV episodes with acyclovir does not prevent the establishment of latent infection and does not affect the rate of subsequent recurrences, alleviation of individual attacks and long-term prevention of many forms of recurrent infection are now feasible both in normal and immunocompromised individuals. Additionally, intravenous acyclovir remains the treatment of choice for all severe forms of HSV infection, including encephalitis and neonatal infections. Rapid diagnosis and prompt initiation of treatment are the cornerstones of successful therapy.

It is likely that acyclovir will remain the drug of choice for HSV for the foreseeable future. Meanwhile, the development of therapies that can prevent the establishment of viral latency, eradicate latent virus from neural tissue, or prevent reactivation of latent genomes are important and formidable goals for future investigation. Active research in HSV vaccine development continues and has been encouraging, but this form of preventive therapy remains a more long-term objective.

SUGGESTED READING

Dorsky DI, Crumpacker CS. Drugs 5 years later: acyclovir. Ann Intern Med 1987;107:859–874.

Gold D, Corey L. Acyclovir prophylaxis for herpes simplex virus infection. Antimicrob Agents Chemother 1987;31:361–367.

Liesegang TJ. Ocular herpes simplex infection: pathogenesis and current therapy. Mayo Clin Proc 1988;63:1092–1105.

Lietman PS, Fiddian P, Chapman SK, eds. The Wellcome International Antiviral Symposium. Am J Med 1988;85(no. 2A).

TUBERCULOSIS

ASIM K. DUTT, M.D.
WILLIAM W. STEAD, M.D.

With the dramatic decline of tuberculosis in Western countries, physicians often fail to consider the disease in the differential diagnosis, sometimes with tragic results. The index of suspicion should be especially high when persons in certain groups manifest cough with persistent fever or loss of weight: the elderly, disadvantaged persons, immigrants from developing countries, or immunosuppressed persons (e.g., on corticosteroid therapy or with human immunodeficiency virus [HIV] infection). The clinical presentation may vary over a wide spectrum from virtually no symptoms through symptoms such as mild, persistent fever and loss of weight to severe symptoms including cough, malaise, fever, and even hemoptysis. Isolation of *Mycobacterium tuberculosis* is essential for a firm diagnosis, but a strong clinical suspicion may suffice as an indication for specific chemotherapy.

Once the possibility of tuberculosis is considered, the steps for diagnosis are rather simple. Most important is the collection of secretions and/or biopsy materials for microscopy and culture. Radiologic examination and tuberculin testing are also of importance, but are not diagnostic. A classic roentgenogram of the chest may strongly suggest the disease, but all too often the radiographic presentation is quite atypical, especially when the infection has been acquired recently.

A positive tuberculin reaction by Mantoux test (10 or more millimeters' induration) indicates infection with tubercle bacilli. A compatible clinical presentation and radiographic abnormality increase the possibility of the disease. However, a negative tuberculin test does not necessarily rule out the diagnosis, as 20 to 25 percent of patients who are clinically ill may have an initial negative test. A repeat of the test 2 weeks later may be positive. Some patients are anergic and may not be able to show enough T-cell activity to develop a positive tuberculin reaction. Persons over age 12 years and under 60 years who react to tuberculin should be tested for HIV infection because its presence affects the risk of tuberculosis and the length of therapy.

DIAGNOSIS

Pulmonary Tuberculosis

Spontaneously produced sputum provides necessary material for smear and culture in diagnosis of pulmonary tuberculosis. At least three early-morning sputum specimens should be examined by microscopy (Fig. 1). If one of these is positive, no further collection is necessary. When all are negative on microscopy, at least five specimens should be submitted for culture.

If a patient is unable to produce sputum or is uncooperative, an alternative method is to induce sputum by inhalation of heated aerosol of saline. Other methods are early-morning gastric lavage and laryngeal swab or aspiration; these are not quite as productive.

When microscopy of sputum is negative on at least three specimens, bronchial washing through a fiberoptic bronchoscope may be indicated. In addition, postbronchoscopy sputum specimens should be collected because they often yield positive result. Transtracheal puncture may be necessary as a last resort in unconscious patients with a life-threatening illness. In occasional patients, transthoracic needle aspirate

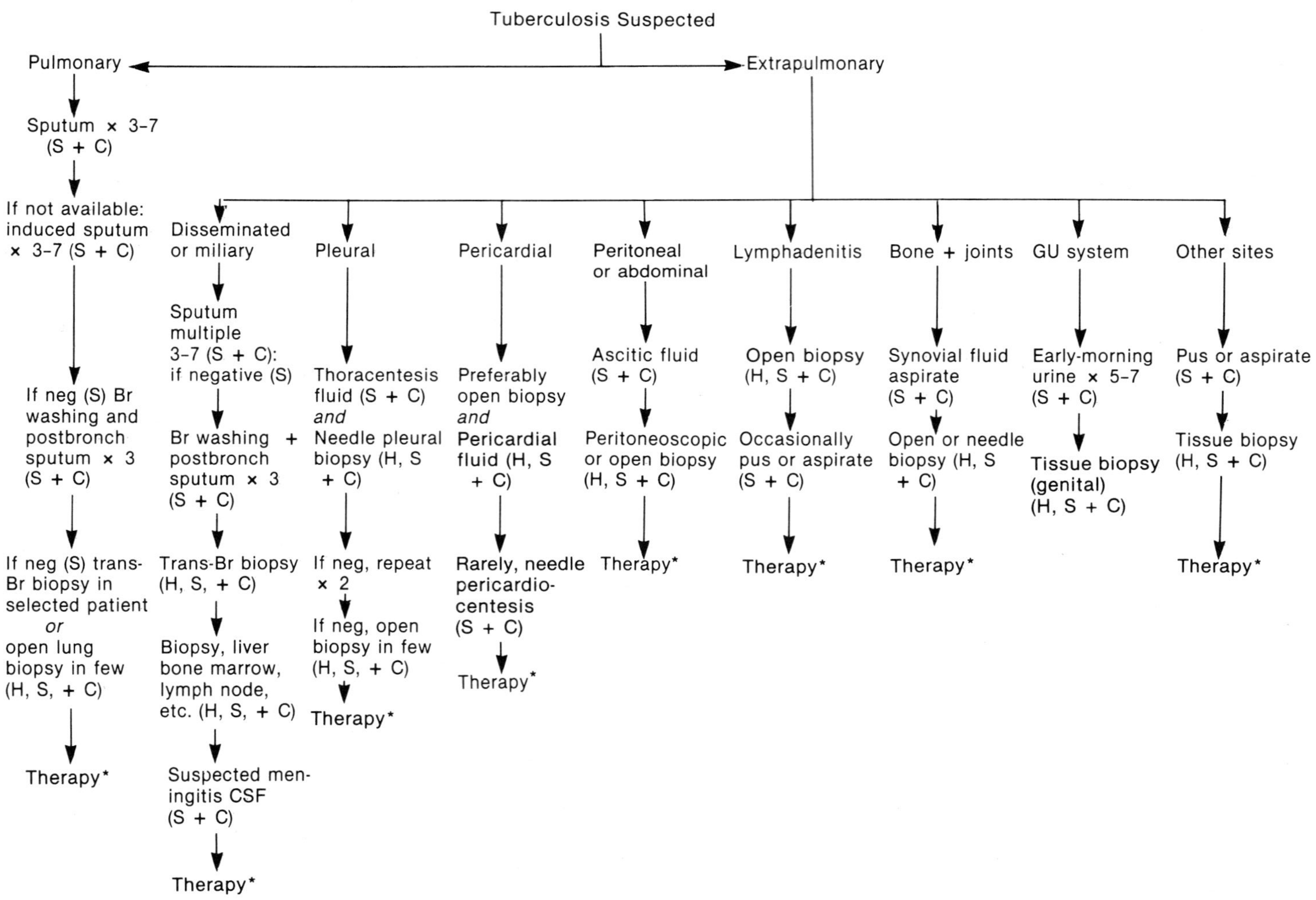

Figure 1 Diagnosis of suspected tuberculosis. Abbreviations: S = smear, C = culture for mycobacteria, H = histology, Br = bronchial, Bronch = bronchoscopy, CSF = cerebrospinal fluid, Bx = biopsy, neg = negative, GU = genitourinary; * therapy started in suspected cases, awaiting cultural results and/or clinical response.

of the lung may be indicated for obtaining necessary material for bacteriology. In rare circumstances the diagnosis is made only by open lung biopsy.

Although fluorescent microscopy is much more sensitive, it is quite nonspecific and must be confirmed by Ziehl-Neelsen or Kenyoun staining. Positive microscopy never confirms the presence of *M. tuberculosis* because other mycobacteria may be present. Therefore, cultural examination is necessary for isolation and identification of *M. tuberculosis*. Furthermore, testing for susceptibility to antituberculosis drugs is useful for identifying the occasional case of primary drug resistance.

Extrapulmonary Tuberculosis

For the diagnosis of tuberculosis in extrapulmonary sites, secretions and/or biopsy material should be obtained for examination (Fig. 1). In the case of pleural and pericardial effusion, biopsy and/or fluid should be examined and cultured. The yield from culture of pleural fluid is small, presumably because of the relatively small population of organisms present. Cerebrospinal fluid smear and cultural examination are necessary in meningitis, but positive results are found in only 20 to 40 percent of the cases of tuberculous meningitis. Cultural examination of ascitic fluid in tuberculous peritonitis may confirm the diagnosis, but microscopy and culture of a percutaneous biopsy specimen is preferred.

The definitive diagnosis of genitourinary tuberculosis requires the isolation of *M. tuberculosis* by urine culture. An acid-fast stain of an early-morning specimen should be performed on 3 to 5 separate days.

In tuberculosis of joints, bacteriologic examination of synovial fluid is important. Positive synovial fluid culture may be found in approximately 80 percent of cases, and about one-fourth may show the organism in the smear examination. Pus and fluids from discharging sinuses from any site should be submitted for microscopy and culture.

If the microscopic examination of fluid is negative, a definitive diagnosis is delayed for 6 to 8 weeks while cultural results are awaited. Hence, biopsy of the involved tissue, either by needle or exploratory surgery, is often required for early diagnosis.

In cases of the pleural effusion, closed-needle biopsy should be performed to obtain three to four pieces of pleura to submit for both microscopy and culture. The tissue sections should also be stained for acid-fact bacilli. It is common to find a typical granulomatous pleuritis in which no organisms can be found by special staining. Culture of one or two tissue fragments greatly increases the diagnostic yield of the procedure. It is a common error to place all tissue fragments into formalin, which precludes culture. If the first set of biopsies is not diagnostic, at least one more attempt should be made before considering the results negative. Repeated biopsies increase the yield of positive results by 15 to 20 percent. In rare circumstances, surgical biopsy of pleura may be indicated.

Surgical biopsy is preferred for pericardial disease because it is usually a safer procedure and gives enough tissue for examination, while providing drainage of the fluid through a pericardial "window." In disseminated or miliary tuberculosis, needle biopsy of liver and bone marrow is recommended. Hepatic biopsy is positive in more than 80 percent of cases and bone marrow, in more than 50 percent if examined by both microscopy and culture. Miliary pulmonary disease with negative sputum smears is best approached by transbronchial biopsy through a fiberoptic bronchoscope. Rarely, open lung biopsy may be necessary for the diagnosis. Percutaneous biopsy of the peritoneum is generally productive, but open biopsy may be obtained at exploratory laparotomy. Lymph nodes generally require excision biopsy. A Craig-needle biopsy of bone, joint, or vertebra is quite productive if specimens are examined both by microscopy and culture. If results are unsatisfactory, an open surgical biopsy is the next step.

Clinical Diagnosis

A diagnosis of tuberculosis may be justified despite negative bacteriologic results when the clinical picture is strongly suggestive and the clinical situation calls for therapy. Patients with a positive tuberculin test, with compatible abnormal radiographs with or without symptoms, and in whom other possible causes have been reasonably excluded should be given a trial of chemotherapy.

Chemotherapy is initiated only after necessary materials have been submitted for bacteriological studies.

Such patients are observed for the clinical response to therapy. If there is prompt improvement over a few weeks the diagnosis of tuberculosis is likely correct and therapy should be continued to completion. If there is no improvement or worsening over a few weeks, diagnostic efforts to find the correct diagnosis should be undertaken, because tuberculosis is not likely in those circumstances.

CHEMOTHERAPY

Until a few years ago, the standard therapy for tuberculosis consisted of isoniazid (INH) and ethambutol (EMB) with a supplement of 1 to 3 months of streptomycin (SM) in cavitary smear-positive cases. The therapy was effective provided that the drugs were taken for 18 to 24 months. During the past decade, the availability of another oral bactericidal agent, rifampin (RIF), has made it possible to complete therapy much more quickly. By using INH and RIF together, the duration of treatment has been reduced to 9 months. It can even be shortened to 6 months if SM plus pyrazinamide (PZA) or EMB plus PZA are added to the regimen for the first two months.

Bacteriologic Concept of Drug Therapy

Many in vitro and in vivo studies in animals have increased our understanding of the bacterial population in tuberculous lesions and the action of drugs on them. Tubercle bacilli are obligate aerobes and thrive best in an environment with high oxygen tension. There are at least three distinct bacterial populations in a tuberculous lesion: (1) the largest population (ranging from 10^7 to 10^9 organisms) is actively replicating in a neutral or slightly alkaline medium in cavitary lesions; (2) a much smaller population (ranging from 10^2 to 10^5 organisms) exists in a neutral or slightly alkaline milieu of closed caseous and noncaseous lesions where it is metabolically less active or even dormant; (3) a similar small population (ranging from 10^2 to 10^5 organisms) is slowly replicating in the acid medium inside macrophages.

The size and metabolic activity of these bacterial populations is important because tubercle bacilli mutate to drug-resistant forms at a predictable rate irrespective of the presence or absence of antituberculous drug. Mutants resistant to each drug develop independently of other mutations and at a rate of approximately one per 10^{-5} to 10^{-6} replications. Those resistant to two drugs develop rarely, approximately once per 10^{-10} to 10^{-12} replications. Hence, a cavitary lung disease with a bacterial population of 10^7 to 10^9 organisms may contain 100 to 10,000 mutants resistant to any effective drug, and small populations in closed caseous or noncaseous lesions and in macrophages may have few or none. Thus, all cavitary tuberculous lesions harbor a mixture of drug-sensitive and -resistant bacilli, making at least two drugs essential to success.

Tubercle bacilli replicate rather slowly, about every 16 to 20 hours. The antituberculous drugs are effective in killing tubercle bacilli only when the organisms are replicating. Hence, antituberculous drugs are best given in a single daily dose, but must be given for a prolonged period to allow time to kill the entire population, including those that are semidormant and divide only intermittently.

Rapid elimination of the actively multiplying large population of bacilli is essential to prevent emergence of drug-resistant mutants, a process that results in treatment failure. Elimination of smaller populations of intermittently multiplying organisms by extended therapy is necessary to prevent late relapse due to replication of the "persisters."

Drug Action on the Bacilli

The antituberculous drugs are generally classified as bactericidal and bacteriostatic. SM, capreomycin (CAP), RIF, INH, and PZA are considered bactericidal. The bacteriostatic drugs are EMB, ethionamide (ETA), cycloserine (CS), and *para*-aminosalicylic acid (PAS). EMB in a dosage of 25 mg per kilogram is considered by some to be bactericidal and certainly is more effective in eliminating bacilli than in the usually prescribed dose of 15 mg per kilogram.

Among the bactericidal drugs, SM, INH, and RIF are highly active against actively multiplying extracellular bacilli (Fig. 2). With intensive daily therapy, these organisms can be eliminated rapidly. Selection of drug-resistant mutants is avoided and conversion of sputum smears to negative is prompt. Inadequate dosage or irregular ingestion may lead to treatment failure, with emergence of drug resistance.

RIF, INH, and PZA are active against slowly replicating organisms located inside the macrophages or extracellularly (Fig. 2). PZA is particularly effective in the acid environment inside macrophages. RIF is capable of killing bacilli that show even the slightest metabolic activity and, hence, is a useful drug during the continuation phase. With adequate duration of therapy, even the persisters are eliminated, resulting in a permanent cure. Inadequate length of treatment may permit a late relapse due to late replication of the persisters. Such a relapse is usually due to drug-sensitive organisms. It has been shown that most antituberculous drugs are effective when given twice weekly after the initial period of intensive daily administration. The addition of SM or PZA is not generally necessary, but the bactericidal activity of RIF and INH can be intensified by a supplement of SM and PZA to the regimen for the first 2 months. Such a regimen can further reduce the total duration of therapy to 6 months, with an added advantage of being effective even in the presence of INH resistance.

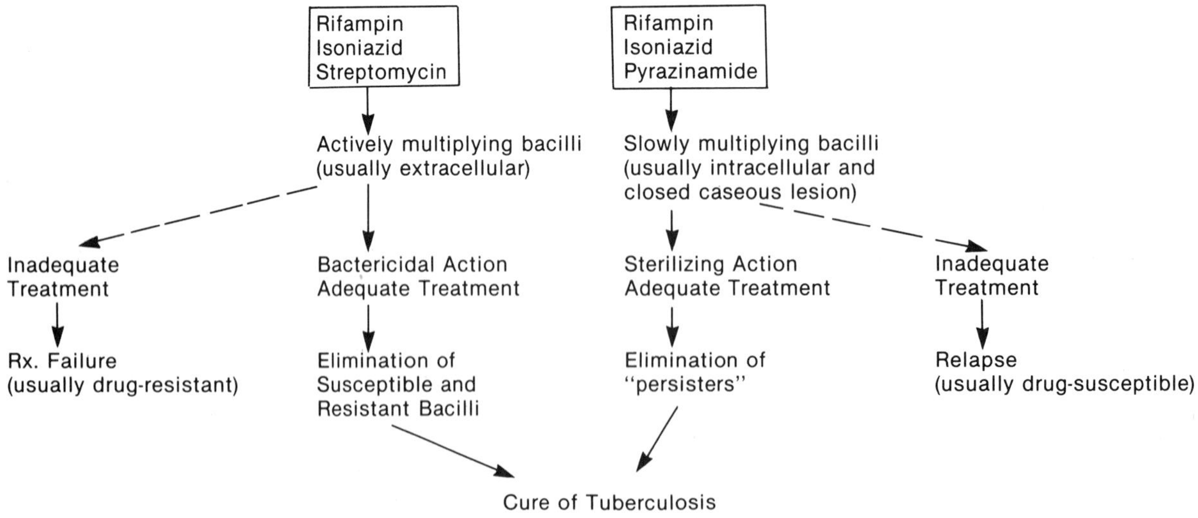

Figure 2 Current principles of tuberculosis chemotherapy.

Treatment of Newly Diagnosed Tuberculosis

Before initiation of therapy, four possible clues to the probability of INH resistance should be sought (Fig. 3): (1) Has the patient received antituberculous drugs anytime in the past? (2) Is the patient from a country with a high prevalence of disease and drug resistance, e.g., Southeast Asia, Africa, or Latin America? (3) Is it likely the patient acquired the infection from an individual with a drug-resistant case? (4) Does the patient live in an area where INH resistance is common (more than 5 percent)?

If the answers to all of these inquiries are "no," therapy may safely be initiated with INH, 300 mg, and RIF, 600 mg, daily. In the United States, the incidence of initial drug resistance is low except for a few areas—the Mexican border, large cities, parts of California—where the addition of SM/CAP and PZA should almost be routine. Drug susceptibility should be determined on the initial sputum specimen in each case. We recommend that the drugs be given as combination capsules, e.g., Rifamate (Merrell-Dow) or Rimactizide (Ciba). Each capsule contains INH, 150 mg, and RIF, 300 mg, and thus, two capsules a day in the early morning furnishes the total daily dose. In addition to the convenience of the combination capsule, the patient is precluded from taking only one of the drugs. Both drugs are given daily for 9 months or daily for 1 month followed by INH, 900 mg, and RIF, 600 mg twice weekly, for another 8 months, i.e., two combination capsules and two INH 300-mg tablets twice a week.

Our experience in more than 3,500 patients with the latter regimen has proved successful in more than 95 percent of cases now followed up to 12 years. We have also treated more than 500 patients with various forms of extrapulmonary tuberculosis with similar results and less than 1 percent relapse. Our experience also indicates that the regimen is effective in patients whose tuberculosis is associated with various medical disorders, e.g., diabetes, alcoholism, corticosteroid therapy, malignancy, and cytotoxic chemotherapy.

The addition of a third drug, e.g., EMB or SM, does not add significantly to the bactericidal action of INH and RIF. Such a supplement is recommended by some to ensure against failure in the event of initial INH resistance. We do not routinely add a third drug to our regimen, but add both SM and PZA if we have a clue that there may be INH resistance (see above). Several recent studies have shown that initial intensive treatment with SM (0.5 to 0.75 g, or about 20 mg per kilogram); INH, 300 mg; RIF, 600 mg; and PZA, 25 to 30 mg per kilogram daily for 2 months, followed by INH, 300 mg, and RIF, 600 mg daily or twice weekly for another 4 months (i.e., total, 6 months), produces similar results. The regimen considerably reduces the duration of therapy.

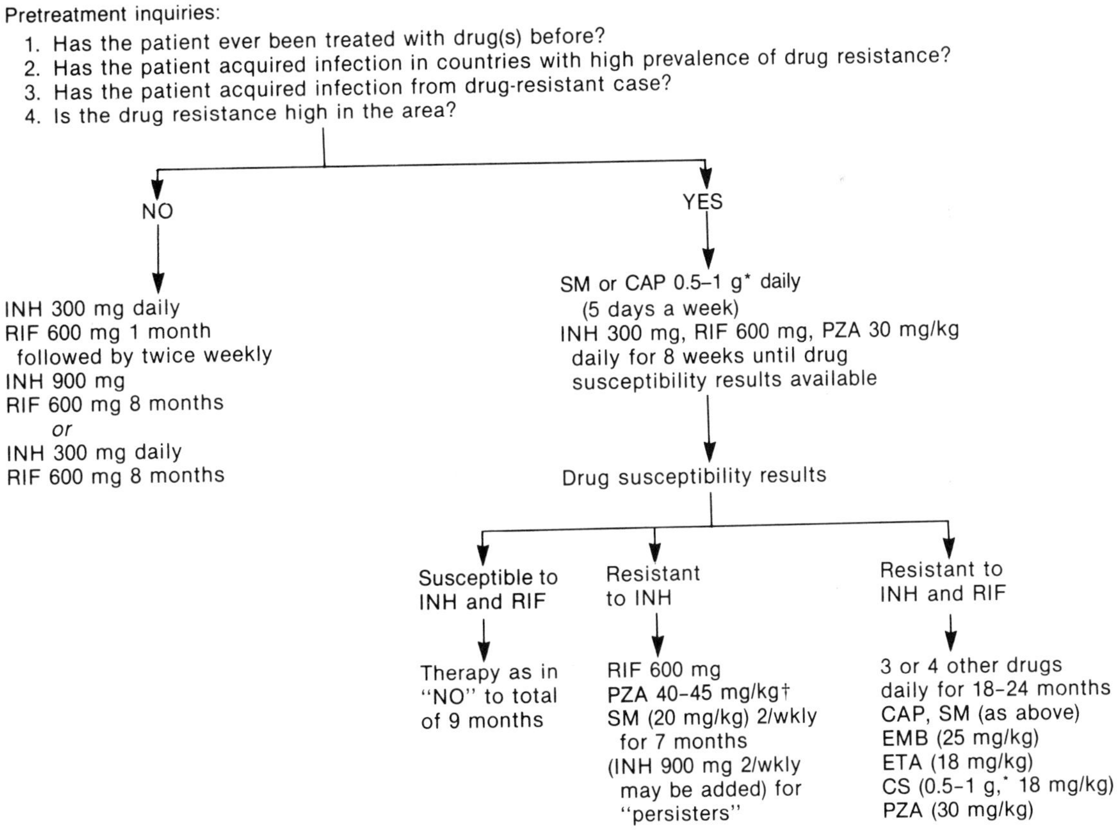

Figure 3 Chemotherapy of tuberculosis. * One gram is preferred; however, in patients who are elderly or weigh less than 100 pounds or have impaired renal function, the dose is revised downward. † Round off dose to tablet size.

Drug Therapy in Suspected or Proven INH Resistance

If drug resistance (to INH) is suspected, therapy should be initiated with SM, INH, RIF, and PZA in the dosages mentioned above until the drug susceptibility results are known (usually 2 months) (Fig. 3). Therapy is then changed according to the results. If the organisms prove to be sensitive to INH and RIF, the treatment may be completed with INH, 300 mg, and RIF, 600 mg daily, or INH, 900 mg, and RIF, 600 mg, twice weekly for the remainder of the 9 months. When INH or RIF resistance is found, the therapy is changed to SM (1.0 to 1.5 g; approximately 20 mg per kilogram); PZA, 40 to 45 mg per kilogram; and INH, 900 mg, or RIF, 600 mg (depending on susceptibility) twice weekly for the remainder of the 9 months. INH, 900 mg, is given even in the presence of acquired INH resistance because of its action on the persisters, which generally remain drug susceptible. This regimen ensures effectiveness of at least two bactericidal drugs against the resistant bacilli, i.e., SM and RIF on extracellular rapidly multiplying bacilli and RIF and PZA on the slowly replicating organisms.

In the presence of resistance to both INH and RIF, all drugs are discontinued, and therapy is instituted with three or four other antituberculous drugs. SM or CAP (if SM resistant) is given 5 days a week initially for 3 months along with two other drugs daily from the following: EMB, 25 mg per kilogram; PZA, 25 to 30 mg per kilogram; ETA, 500 to 750 mg (depending on tolerance; 750 mg is preferred, but this drug causes nausea); CS, about 18 mg per kilogram per day, accompanied by pyridoxine, 100 mg twice a day. The latter two are given in divided doses. As these drugs are not bactericidal, the total duration of therapy must be 18 to 24 months.

Preventive Therapy

Persons infected with tubercle bacilli (tuberculin reaction $\geq$10 mm) carry some risk of developing disease that may be prevented with INH preventive therapy. Since infected persons are not all at equal risk and since INH therapy may occasionally cause side effects, the risk and benefit of therapy must be assessed before prescribing preventive therapy. The American Thoracic Society and the Centers for Disease Control recommend the following groups for preventive therapy:

1. Household members and other close contacts of patients with infectious tuberculosis with positive tuberculin test and no previous history of reaction in the past. Contacts under age 4 years with negative tuberculin test should be given preventive therapy for 3 months and assessed again after 3 months with tuberculin test. If negative, the therapy is discontinued; otherwise, the full course is completed.
2. Newly infected persons (tuberculin converters).
3. Persons with a history of inadequately treated tuberculosis
4. Persons with a significant reaction and a stable abnormal chest roentgenogram
5. Positive tuberculin reaction and associated "risk" factors—silicosis, diabetes mellitus, prolonged therapy with costcosteroids, immunosuppressive therapy, hematologic and reticuloendothelial malignancy, acquired immunodeficiency syndrome, end-stage renal disease, and clinical conditions leading to rapid weight loss and chronic undernutrition.
6. Tuberculin skin test reactors under 35 years of age.

Although INH is generally safe, the adverse effect of hepatitis remains a major concern for clinicians. Before initiation of INH therapy, individuals must be screened for the risk factors. Preventive INH therapy of 300 mg daily for adults and 10 to 14 mg per kilogram, not exceeding 300 mg, in children is recommended for 6 to 12 months. Monitoring of preventive therapy for toxicity is no different than for treatment of clinical tuberculosis. Clinical monitoring for symptoms is adequate, obtaining liver function tests only when symptoms indicate. The supply of medication to the patient should not exceed one month's at a time. The patient must be informed of the symptoms of side effects and advised to discontinue therapy on development of symptoms and report immediately to the physician for evaluation.

At present, there is no preventive therapy that has been studied by clinical trial for persons infected with INH-resistant organisms. RIF, 600 mg daily, may be used for 12 months under the almost certain assumption that it would be effective. Similarly, in persons unable to tolerate INH therapy, RIF may be substituted if preventive therapy is strongly indicated.

Preventive therapy with INH has been shown to be 98.6 percent effective among tuberculin converters, both among children and elderly nursing home residents. However, in the treatment of incidentally discovered tuberculin reactors, the efficiency was only about 85 percent and the advantage of therapy more difficult to demonstrate.

Monitoring Adverse Effects of Drugs

The major adverse effect of both INH and RIF is hepatotoxicity, with an incidence of 2 to 4 percent. There is no detectable increase when PZA, another potentially hepatotoxic drug, is included in the regimen. We have encountered hepatotoxicity in 2.5 percent of more than 3,500 patients treated with INH and RIF, even though the majority were elderly and there were many alcoholics. However, prudence dictates that two hepatotoxic drugs should not be used together in patients with active hepatitis. For such persons, we recommend starting treatment with INH and EMB with a supplement of SM if the sputum smear is positive. When the hepatitis subsides, RIF may safely be exchanged for EMB to obtain the advantage of short-course therapy.

Beyond routine baseline biochemical tests for hepatic function, regular biochemical monitoring leads to more confusion than enlightenment, since transient benign elevation of hepatic enzymes is common during therapy. We advise each patient to stop therapy immediately upon development of suspicious symptoms—e.g., anorexia, nausea, vomiting, or scleral icterus—and to report to the clinic for hepatic enzyme estimation. If symptoms are accompanied by elevation of hepatic enzymes of more than five times the base level, drug toxicity is likely. After symptoms have abated and the hepatic enzymes have returned to base line, drugs are reintroduced one at a time, starting with half dosage and monitoring of hepatic enzymes. In this manner, the offending drug can be identified and therapy changed appropriately. It is not uncommon that both drugs can be reintroduced without further adverse effect.

Twice weekly therapy with RIF may give rise to immunologic and hematologic side effects of petechiae and thrombocytopenia. This rarely occurs with a dosage of 600 mg RIF, but was a problem when the dosage 900 to 1,200 mg was used, particularly when the interval between doses was prolonged beyond twice weekly. Petechiae with or without thrombocytopenia has occurred in only 0.5 percent of our patients. The patients should be advised to watch for bruised spots on the legs. RIF should be discontinued if this reaction develops. Twice weekly administration of RIF may also give rise to flu-like syndrome, associated with chills and fever and with considerable aches and pains over the body on the day the medication is taken. This has occurred in 2.5 percent of our patients. The incidence of these adverse effects also increases with the use of higher dosage of RIF (900 to 1,200 mg). The side effect may be eliminated by changing to daily therapy. Other major adverse effects reported in the literature are hemolytic anemia, acute renal failure, and "shock syndrome," but we have not encountered any in our 13 years' experience.

The other side effects are minor, e.g., drug fever, allergies, skin rashes, and gastrointestinal intolerance—these occur in approximately 5 percent of patients. These reactions subside on temporary withdrawal of the drug, which can often be reintroduced slowly without recurrence of symptoms.

SM may cause vestibular damage, but only rarely hearing loss. This adverse effect is dose related and may be reduced by injecting the drug only 5 days a week. Also, the dose of the drug should be cut to 0.5 g for persons older than 60 years of age and for patients with renal failure. Inquiry about dizziness and staggering may detect early toxicity. The drug may also cause allergic rashes and fever, which subside on withdrawal.

EMB is a well-tolerated drug and free from major adverse effects, but is of little value in short-course chemotherapy. The major side effect is optic neuritis (visual disturbances), which rarely occurs with the dose of 15 mg per kilogram, but may occur in 1 to 3 percent of patients receiving the more effective dose of 25 mg per kilogram. Monitoring of the side effect requires regular testing with reading and color charts and referral to an ophthalmologist for opinion in persons in whom toxicity is suspected.

PZA commonly causes flushing and, rarely, a skin rash. Hyperuricemia regularly occurs with PZA therapy, but rarely precipitates clinical gout. This is commoner during daily than during intermittent therapy. Arthralgia is frequent and occurs more often with daily treatment (7 percent) than with twice weekly administration (1 to 3 percent). Arthralgia is usually self-limiting and responds well to analgesics.

During therapy the health care team must remain in close contact with the patients because they may report suspicious symptoms. The patients should be informed about the symptoms of adverse effects and instructed to discontinue therapy if a problem is suspected and to report to the clinic promptly for clinical and laboratory assessment.

Surveillance of Patients During Therapy

Bacteriologic monitoring of patients during therapy is an important aspect in the management of tuberculosis. We suggest that three to five specimens of sputum be submitted for bacteriologic examination initially and that a drug susceptibility test be included. Then a sputum specimen should be submitted every 2 weeks until three specimens are reported to be negative. Thereafter, one specimen a month is adequate for the duration of therapy and for 6 months after completion. During follow-up one specimen every 3 months for another 6 months should be cultured after which the patient is discharged from supervision with the advice to return if symptoms recur.

A satisfactory response to treatment is observed by the gradual decline in the bacterial population of the sputum. Prolonged persistence of organisms in the sputum (more than 5 months) or reversion to positive bacteriology after conversion to negative should raise suspicion of treatment failure. Reevaluation of the patient's compliance and a repeat drug susceptibility test are then indicated in order to make the best choice of a retreatment four-drug regimen.

Frequent roentgenograms of chest are not indicated if bacteriologic studies are done as suggested. The health care team must evaluate whether the patient is taking the medications regularly as prescribed. This is carried out by frequent interviews with the patient, by checking attendance at clinic appointments and picking up of drugs, by surprise pill counts, and by random examination of urine for the color of RIF and for excretion of INH. In patients thought to be noncompliant, direct ingestion of drugs under supervision must be carried out. Twice weekly administration of drugs facilitates direct supervision.

Support by the Health Department

Most health departments provide facilities for collection of sputum specimens and bacteriologic examination. Monitoring of adverse effects of drugs and compliance of patients is provided through the able assistance of public health nurses. Expert advice is also provided by the personnel for difficult problems that may arise during management.

The public health nurses perform contact evaluation, with tuberculin testing and radiography when indicated, after receiving notification of an active case. Delay in notification of the health department may be catastrophic, particularly for children in whom the disease may progress rapidly with fatal results. Busy physicians who undertake to treat tuberculosis are well advised to take advantage of the facilities provided by local health departments in keeping up with patients for the 9 months of therapy.

MALARIA

SUSAN J. JACOBSON, M.D.
DAVID J. WYLER, M.D.

Human malaria is caused by four species of the genus *Plasmodium (P. falciparum, P. vivax, P. malariae,* and *P. ovale). P. falciparum* malaria can be fatal, and strains from many parts of the world have developed resistance to certain antimalarial drugs, such as chloroquine. Recognizing malaria and instituting appropriate therapy may be challenging but can be life saving.

LIFE CYCLE

The life cycle of the malaria parasite is important in understanding treatment and prevention. Malaria is transmitted by the bite of infected female anopheline mosquitoes or by inoculation of infected blood (e.g., transfusion malaria or congenital malaria). Mosquitoes inject sporozoites, which enter the liver within minutes of inoculation. In the liver, the parasites multiply as hepatic exoerythrocytic forms (schizonts). After 1 to 2 weeks of development, the hepatic schizonts rupture, releasing thousands of merozoites, which enter the circulation and invade erythrocytes. Some of the exoerythrocytic forms of *P. vivax* and *P. ovale* persist in the liver and remain as latent exoerythrocytic forms (or hypnozoites). These may remain latent in the liver for months or years, resulting in relapses of erythrocytic infection. Once malaria parasites invade the erythrocytes, they never reinvade the liver. Hence, transfusion malaria never results in development of exoerythrocytic forms. There are no latent exoerythrocytic forms in *P. falciparum* or *P. malariae* infections.

Merozoites invade erythrocytes by a complex interaction between specific receptors on merozoites and those on the surface of erythrocytes. Persons whose erythrocytes lack all Duffy blood-group determinants (a common phenotype in most of Africa) are not susceptible to *P. vivax* infection. *P. vivax* and *P. ovale* parasitize young erythrocytes, and *P. malariae* infects older erythrocytes, limiting the magnitude of parasitemia. *P. falciparum* can develop in erythrocytes of all ages, and parasitemia can reach very high levels. The magnitude of parasitemia is an important determinant of morbidity and mortality in malaria.

After entering erythrocytes, merozoites of three of the species mature and cause erythrocyte rupture within 48 hours (tertian malaria), while *P. malariae* requires 72 hours (quartan malaria). Maturation involves the development from ring forms through the trophozoite stage to the schizont stage (defined by evidence of nuclear division). Mature schizonts rupture and release many merozoites, which rapidly invade other erythrocytes, continuing the erythrocytic cycle of infection. The sexual cycle begins with some merozoites differentiating into gametocytes. These circulate in the blood and when ingested by an appropriate mosquito can initiate the sporogonic cycle that culminates in the development of sporozoites in about 10 days. At this time, transmission can occur. Only the asexual blood stages cause illness. Gametocytes can persist even after asexual blood stages have been eliminated.

EPIDEMIOLOGY

Malaria transmission occurs in large areas of Central and South America, sub-Saharan Africa, and Indian subcontinent, Southeast Asia, some areas of the Middle East, and Oceania, with an estimated 100 to 200 million cases occurring yearly worldwide. Species distribution varies in different parts of the world: *P. falciparum* predominates in Africa, Haiti, and New Guinea. *P. ovale* occurs primarily in Africa, while *P. vivax* is rarely encountered there. *P. falciparum* and *P. vivax* malaria are both prevalent in Southeast Asia, South America, and Oceania. *P. vivax* predominates on the Indian subcontinent, where infection with *P. falciparum* is infrequent. *P. malariae* distribution is relatively cosmopolitan.

In the United States malaria is generally imported, although occasional small epidemics due to local transmission occur, like that which involved 27 cases of *P. vivax* malaria in San Diego County in 1986. The number of reported cases of malaria in the United States has been stable over the last decade, with approximately 1,000 cases yearly.

Resistance of *P. falciparum* to chloroquine has been reported from all countries with known transmission except the Dominican Republic, Haiti, Central America, the Middle East, and the following countries in West Africa: Chad, Equatorial Guinea, Guinea, Guinea-Bissau, Liberia, Senegal, and Sierra Leone. Resistance to pyrimethamine and sulfonamides (e.g., Fansidar) as well as chloroquine is widespread in Thailand, Burma, and Kampuchea and exists in some areas of Brazil, Kenya, and elsewhere.

DIAGNOSIS

The malarial paroxysm—characterized by high fever, chills, rigor—is the hallmark of acute malaria. Sometimes there is a prodromal period of one to several days. Patients may complain of nonspecific symptoms, such as malaise, headache, myalgia, and fatigue, or have more localized complaints, such as chest pain, abdominal pain, or arthralgias, that may obscure the correct diagnosis. The malarial fever is rarely periodic or regular when it initially occurs in a nonimmune host. Absence of a 48- or 72-hour fever cycle does not exclude a diagnosis of malaria. Prompt diagnosis of malaria by physicians practicing in nonendemic areas requires a high index of suspicion for malaria in travelers in endemic countries. Malaria may occur as early as 9 days following exposure or may present months after the endemic area is left. Chloroquine prophylaxis may delay presentation of chloroquine-resistant *P. falciparum* malaria. Immune individuals may have relapses (emergence from latent exoerythrocytic stage) or recrudescences (rising wave of intraerythrocytic parasitemia from a persistent low level) years after exposure.

Diagnosis is made by demonstration of the malarial parasites on either thick or thin blood smears that have been stained with Giemsa. Since symptoms may appear a few days before parasites can be detected by blood smear, it is important to continue to obtain blood smears for several days before excluding the diagnosis. Thick smears are primarily used to identify the presence of parasites, and thin smears are used to make species differentiation. The extent of parasitemia should be quantified, either according to percent of parasitized erythrocytes, or—in settings of low-grade parasitemia—by numbers of infected erythrocytes per leukocyte and relating the latter ratio to the leukocyte count.

Clues to *P. falciparum* infection include multiply infected erythrocytes, a high-grade parasitemia (greater than 5 percent), the presence of only ring forms, and the banana-shaped gametocyte (rarely seen). Differentiation of other malaria species is less urgent, because malaria due to the three other species are all initially treated with chloroquine. The choice of therapy for *P. falciparum* infection is more complicated since it depends on the probability that the patient has been infected with a chloroquine-resistant strain and considers the presence of complications.

THERAPY

Prompt diagnosis and appropriate therapy are keys to a rapid recovery from malaria. The initial objectives of therapy are rapid reduction of parasitemia and prevention of complications of malaria, such as renal failure or cerebral malaria. The critical factors determining therapy include the clinical status of the patient, the presence of *P. falciparum* malaria parasites, and the potential for drug resistance if the infecting species is *P. falciparum*. Subsequent objectives of therapy may include elimination of dormant hepatic hypnozoites to prevent relapses of *P. vivax* or *P. ovale* malaria.

Drugs used clinically are primarily directed against the asexual parasite within the erythrocyte. These include the 4-aminoquinolines (chloroquine), the cinchona alkaloids (quinine, quinidine), antimetabolities (pyrimethamine, sulfadoxine), and tetracyclines. The 4-aminoquinolines are preferred unless drug resistance is suspected. There are also new drugs, currently not available in the United States, that are effective against chloroquine-resistant malaria. These include mefloquine (an amino alcohol), which is in use in Southeast Asia, is sold in France and Switzerland, and is pending licensing in the United States. Derivatives of a Chinese herbal compound, *quinhaosu*, are currently under study for treatment of multidrug-resistant *P. falciparum* infection.

Drugs of choice for therapy of malaria are indicated in Table 1. Uncomplicated infection with a nonresistant parasite is treated with oral chloroquine. When the patient is infected with *P. falciparum* acquired in areas where chloroquine resistance is a problem and has an uncomplicated infection, oral quinine sulfate should be used in conjunction with another drug. The additional drug can be a combination of pyrimethamine and a sulfonamide (such as Fansidar) in patients not allergic to sulfa drugs. For persons who acquire chloroquine-resistant *P. falciparum* malaria in Southeast Asia, tetracycline or doxycycline should be used with quinine, as Fansidar-resistant strains are widespread in this region. Children less than 8 years old and pregnant women should be administered tetracyclines only for life-threatening infection in which Fansidar resistance is anticipated.

Intravenous quinine or quinidine therapy should be begun in the patient who cannot take medications by mouth or has one or more of the following complications: more than 5 percent parasitized erythrocytes; evidence of organ dysfunction (such as cerebral malaria); or severe anemia. Quinine dihydrochloride (used for intravenous administration) is available in the United States from the Malaria Branch, Centers for Disease Control, Atlanta, Georgia 30333; telephone 404-488-4046 (404-639-2888 nights, weekends). A controlled clinical trial in Thailand showed that intravenous quinidine is as effective (perhaps more so) than quinine. Since intravenous quinidine is available in hospitals in the United States, its immediate use can be life saving. Administration of intravenous quinine or quinidine should be slow and accompanied by continuous cardiac monitoring. The patient can be switched subsequently to quinine administered orally. Pyrimethamine-sulfadoxine (Fansidar) or a tetracycline should be given with quinine once a patient is taking oral medication, as for uncomplicated chloroquine-resistant *P. falciparum* malaria.

For the patient with very high degree of parasitemia (more than 20 percent of erythrocytes infected), exchange transfusions should be considered. There are several anecdotal reports of patients, likely destined to die of malaria with 20 to 70 percent parasitized erythrocytes, recovering without significant sequelae when prompt exchange transfusions were used in conjunction with appropriate intravenous antimalarial therapy. Between 4 and 10 units of whole blood or component therapy (packed erythrocytes and fresh frozen plasma) has been given over a period of up to a day, preceded by venesection. The percent parasitemia is determined frequently (every 4 to 6 hours), and exchange transfusions are usually discontinued once parasitemia is less than 1 to 10 percent.

During the initial treatment of *P. falciparum* malaria, the parasitemia should be determined twice daily for the first 2 or 3 days. For other forms of malaria, a daily determination during the first few days of treatment is adequate. With severe malaria, the clinical status, hemoglobin, platelet count, glucose and electrolyte levels, renal function, and clotting parameters should all be followed.

COMPLICATIONS OF MALARIA

Patients with severe malaria are at risk for hypovolemia, due to salt and water loss from high fever, sweating, and poor fluid intake. Fluid and electrolyte replacement should be carefully undertaken to prevent precipitating noncardiogenic pulmonary edema. Hypoglycemia has been observed as a complication of severe, e.g., cerebral, malaria, often associated with intravenous quinine and particularly in pregnant women. Renal dysfunction occurs through multiple causes: tissue hypoxia, hypovolemia, hemoglobinemia, and disseminated intravascular coagulation (DIC). Correct-

TABLE 1 Drugs of Choice for Therapy of Malaria

Indication	Drug/Route	Dose: Adult	Dose: Pediatric
Uncomplicated infection with all species except chloroquine-resistant *P. falciparum*	Chloroquine, PO (Aralen)	600 mg base, then 300 mg base in 6 h, then 300 mg base/day × 2 days	10 mg/kg base to maximum of 600 mg, 1/2 in 6 h, then qd × 3 days
Uncomplicated infection with *P. falciparum* acquired in areas of chloroquine resistance	Quinine sulfate, PO	650 mg q8h × 7–10 days	25 mg/kg/day in 3 doses for 10 days
	plus Pyrimethamine 25 mg/sulfadoxine 500 mg (Fansidar)	3 tab single dose	2–11 mo: 1/4 tab 1–3 yr: 1/2 tab 4–8 yr: 1 tab 9–14 yr: 2 tab > 14 yr: 3 tab
	or Doxycyline*	100 mg b.i.d. × 7 days	Tetracyclines are not recommended in children < 8 yr
	or Tetracycline	250 mg q.i.d. × 7 days	
Severe (complicated) *P. falciparum* infection† Patient unable to take PO meds Parasitemia > 5% Presence of organ dysfunction (such as cerebral malaria)	Quinine, IV‡	25 mg/kg/day: 1/2 dose in 250–500 ml D5 1/2NS over 4-h infusion. Repeat in 6–8 h if oral therapy cannot be used. Give in same volume over same time, max 1,800 mg/day × 3 days. Adjust fluids for pediatric patients	
	or Quinidine gluconate IV§	15 mg/kg base loading dose in 250 ml NS, infused over 4 h. Subsequent doses 7.5 mg/kg base every 8 h × 7 days either IV or as oral quinidine sulfate or gluconate	
	plus Fansidar or tetracycline	Dose as above	
Prevention of relapses due to *P. vivax* and *P. ovale*	Primaquine, PO#	15 mg base/day × 14 days	0.3 mg base/kg/day × 14 days

* When given in combination with quinine, tetracycline has been shown to be an effective drug in the treatment of *P. falciparum* strains resistant to Fansidar and acquired in Southeast Asia.
† Consider exchange transfusions. See text for further details.
‡ Quinine hydrochloride can be obtained in the U.S. from the Centers for Disease Control, Malaria Branch, Atlanta, GA 30333 (404-488-4046 days; 404-639-2888 nights and weekends). Experts are also available for information regarding alternative regimens.
§ Frequent vital signs and continuous electrocardiographic monitoring should be performed.
# G6PD deficiency should be excluded before administration.

ing the abnormalities and a rapid reduction in parasitemia are the major goals to reducing renal dysfunction.

Hematologic abnormalities—anemia, thrombocytopenia, and rarely DIC—can all occur. If the anemia is severe, transfusions should be administered. Platelet transfusions are not generally necessary, as spontaneous bleeding is rare and the platelet count rapidly returns to normal with appropriate therapy. Heparin should not be used for DIC, although fresh frozen plasma—in conjunction with exchange transfusions—may be appropriate in some settings of DIC.

Cerebral malaria is the most feared complication of malaria. Controlled clinical trials have failed to show any benefit of corticosteroid use in cerebral malaria, which may actually be deleterious; hence, corticosteroids should not be used. With cerebral malaria, as with any coma, maintenance and protection of the airway is critical. If patients survive cerebral malaria, there is usually no major neurologic dysfunction, so supportive care during a malarial coma is important.

RADICAL CURE OF MALARIA

If a patient has had *P. vivax* or *P. ovale* malaria or has had a mixed infection in association with *P. falciparum* malaria, then the patient should receive primaquine therapy to prevent a relapse of *P. vivax* or *P. ovale* at a later time. There is a risk, however, of severe hemolysis if primaquine is given to a person with G6PD deficiency, particularly those of Mediterranean or Oriental background. Hence, G6PD level should be determined prior to the initiation of treatment with primaquine. Occasionally, patients will relapse with *P. vivax* or *P. ovale* malaria despite primaquine therapy and may require repeated therapy.

MALARIA IN PREGNANCY

Malaria during pregnancy poses dangers to the mother and the developing fetus. It can impair fetal growth and increases the risk of spontaneous abortion and stillbirth. Chloroquine therapy during pregnancy is safe, but most of the other antimalarial drugs used to treat chloroquine-resistant malaria are hazardous; hence, all efforts should be exerted to avoid acquiring malaria during pregnancy. Fansidar (pyrimethamine and sulfadoxine), with folinic acid supplementation, should be used in combination with quinine for the pregnant woman with chloroquine-resistant malaria. Relapses of malaria during pregnancy should be treated with the appropriate drugs for the acute episode, with primaquine administered only postpartum to prevent further relapses.

Mefloquine, one of the newer drugs not yet available in the United States, is safe during pregnancy.

PREVENTION

Prevention of malaria in travelers to malarious areas is becoming increasingly difficult. The spread of chloroquine-resistant and multidrug-resistant strains of *P. falciparum* malaria has forced use of drugs in addition to chloroquine. Adverse effects from some of these drugs have limited their safety. New drugs, under development for multidrug resistant malaria, may have a role in prophylaxis, but there are limited studies of efficacy and safety.

All travelers to malaria-endemic areas should be advised to use an appropriate drug regimen and personal protection measures to avoid mosquitoes. The most effective mosquito repellents contain N,N-diethylmetatoluamide (DEET). A pyrethrum-containing flying-insect spray should also be used in living and sleeping areas during evening and nighttime hours. Despite appropriate personal protection measures and use of an appropriate drug prophylaxis, travelers should be advised that they may still contract malaria. They should be instructed to seek prompt medical advise for symptoms of malaria during, or in the months subsequent to, travel to an area endemic for malaria.

There is some controversy concerning the most effective drug regimens for preventing symptoms of malaria, with differing opinions among experts in the field. There are limited studies of efficacy of prophylactic regimens among nonimmune travelers; hence, reliance is frequently placed on studies of suppression of malaria among semiimmune long-term residents in endemic areas. Recommendations for prophylactic regimens may change, depending on the distribution of drug-resistant strains of malaria. The following specific recommendations are accurate as of 1989 and based on the Centers for Disease Control's advice. For updated information consult the *Morbidity and Mortality Weekly Report* or *Health Information for International Travel*. The latter publication, revised annually, is available as DHHS publication no. (CDC)88-8280 from the Superintendent of Documents, U.S. Government Printing Office, Washington, D.C. 20402; telephone 202-783-3238. The Malaria Branch of the Centers for Disease Control has a computerized telephone service. Malaria Information for Travelers, 404-639-1610, which will provide specific advice to travelers to various areas of the world, is suitable for both travelers and their physicians, with frequent updates planned.

Table 2 outlines the drugs used in prophylaxis and the presumptive treatment of malaria. Preferably, malaria chemoprophylaxis should begin 1 to 2 weeks before travel to malarious areas and should continue throughout travel in a malaria endemic area and for 4 weeks after departure from these areas. The exception is doxycycline; because of its short half-life, its use should begin 1 to 2 days prior to entering a malarious area.

For travel to areas where risk of chloroquine-resistant *P. falciparum* malaria has not been reported or is low level or focal, chloroquine alone, once weekly, is recommended. Chloroquine is usually well tolerated. It can be taken with food. The related compound hydroxychloroquine may be better tolerated. Occasionally minor adverse effects such as gastrointestinal disturbance, headache, dizziness, blurred vision, and pruritis occur, but these do not generally require discontinuation of the drug. The retinopathy associated with chronic administration of chloroquine in the treatment of rheumatoid arthritis seems not to occur when chloroquine is taken in the doses used for malaria prophylaxis.

For travel to areas where chloroquine-resistant *P. falciparum* malaria is endemic, once-weekly use of chloroquine alone is recommended. In addition, travelers should be given a treatment dose of Fansidar to be carried during travel. They should be instructed to take the Fansidar promptly in the event of a febrile illness during travel when medical care is not promptly available. This presumptive self-treatment of malaria should be understood by a traveler as a temporary measure; prompt medical evaluation is still important. They should continue their weekly chloroquine prophylaxis after presumptive treatment with Fansidar.

Fansidar, taken once weekly in combination with chloroquine, may be considered in certain circumstances involving prolonged exposure in areas with intense transmission

TABLE 2 Drugs Used in Prophylaxis and Presumptive Treatment of Malaria

	Prophylaxis	
Drug	*Adult Dose*	*Pediatric Dose*
Chloroquine phosphate (Aralen)	300 mg base (500 mg salt), PO once/wk	5 mg/kg base (8.3 mg/kg salt) PO once/wk, up to maximum adult dose
Hydroxychloroquine sulfate (Plaquenil)	310 mg base (400 mg salt) PO once/wk	5 mg/kg base (6.5 mg/kg salt) PO once/wk, up to maximum adult dose
Doxycycline	100 mg PO once/day	>8 yr: 2 mg/kg PO once/day, up to adult dose
Proguanil (Paludrine)	1 tab (200 mg PO once/day combined with weekly chloroquine	<2 yr: 50 mg/day 2–6 yr: 100 mg/day 7–10 yr: 150 mg/day >10 yr: 200 mg/day
Pyrimethamine-sulfadoxine (Fansidar)	1 tab (25 mg pyrimethamine and 500 mg sulfadoxine) PO once/wk	2–11 mo: 1/8 tab/wk 1–3 yr: 1/4 tab/wk 4–8 yr: 1/2 tab/wk 9–14 yr: 3/4 tab/wk >14 yr: 1 tab/wk
Primaquine	See Table 1	See Table 1
	Presumptive Treatment of Malaria for Travelers to Areas of Chloroquine Resistance	
Pyrimethamine-sulfadoxine (Fansidar)	3 tabs (75 mg pyrimethamine and 1,500 mg sulfadoxine) PO as a single dose	2–11 mo: 1/4 tab 1–3 yr: 1/2 tab 4–8 yr: 1 tab 9–14 yr: 2 tabs >14 yr: 3 tabs

of chloroquine-resistant *P. falciparum* malaria. If weekly Fansidar is prescribed, the traveler should be cautioned about the risk of a severe, and possibly fatal, skin reaction. Between 1982 and 1985, there were 24 cases reported (seven fatal) of erythema multiforme, Stevens-Johnson syndrome, and toxic epidermal necrolysis among American travelers using Fansidar. These severe reactions were associated with Fansidar when used as once-weekly prophylaxis. Fansidar also is associated with serum sickness–type reactions, urticaria, and hepatitis. The estimated risk of a fatal, cutaneous reaction among Americans using Fansidar is from 1 in 11,000 to 1 in 25,000 users. If once-weekly Fansidar is prescribed, the traveler should be advised to discontinue it immediately if he or she develops a possible ill effect, especially any skin or mucous membrane irritation, such as itching, redness, rash, mouth or genital lesions, or sore throat. Fansidar should not be given to persons with a history of sulfonamide intolerance or to infants under 2 months of age.

Doxycycline alone, taken daily, is an alternative regimen for the short-term traveler to areas with risk of chloroquine-resistant *P. falciparum* malaria, particularly to areas where chloroquine-resistant and Fansidar-resistant strains are known to occur, such as forested areas of Thailand, Burma, and Kampuchea. It is also appropriate for an individual with a history of sulfonamide intolerance. Doxycycline prophylaxis can begin 1 to 2 days before travel to malarious areas and should be continued daily during travel in malarious areas and for 4 weeks after departure from these areas. Adverse effects of this drug include photosensitivity reactions (usually exaggerated sunburn reaction), and it may be associated with an increased frequency of monilial vaginitis. It is contraindicated in pregnancy and for children under 8 years of age.

Proguanil (Paludrine) is a dihydrofolate reductase inhibitor that is not available commercially in the United States but is widely available elsewhere. Resistance of *P. falciparum* to proguanil is present in some endemic regions such as Southeast Asia, where resistance to Fansidar exists, but the distribution is not well delineated. Travelers using proguanil should take a daily 200-mg dose (adult) in combination with a weekly regimen of chloroquine.

Amodiaquine, a 4-aminoquinoline similar to chloroquine, has been used as an alternative prophylactic drug in areas where chloroquine-resistant *P. falciparum* malaria is endemic. Amodiaquine-associated agranulocytosis has been reported, and hence this drug is NOT recommended for malaria prophylaxis.

Primaquine is used to prevent relapses of *P. vivax* and *P. ovale*. Prophylaxis with primaquine is generally indicated for persons who have had prolonged exposure in malaria-endemic areas, and the dose is as indicated in Table 1. G6PD deficiency should be excluded by appropriate laboratory testing. Primaquine should not be used during pregnancy because the drug may be passed transplacentally to a G6PD deficient fetus and cause life-threatening hemolytic anemia in utero. Chloroquine prophylaxis should be continued weekly through pregnancy and primaquine given after delivery.

Malaria prophylaxis during pregnancy is important to reduce the risk of acute malaria precipitating miscarriage, premature delivery, or stillbirth. Chloroquine or hydroxychloroquine are safe during pregnancy. Fansidar safety during pregnancy has not been completely determined but this drug is recommended to treat chloroquine-resistant *P. falciparum* malaria. Neither doxycycline nor primaquine should be used prophylactically during pregnancy.

Infants and children can contract malaria and should receive prophylaxis. Breast-fed infants do not receive sufficient antimalarial therapy through breast milk and should receive recommended doses of antimalarial agents. Children under the age of 8 years should not receive tetracyclines, and Fansidar is contraindicated in infants younger than 2 months. Chloroquine phosphate is manufactured in the United States only in tablet form and is quite bitter. Pediatric doses should be calculated carefully according to body weight, with pharmacists preparing capsules of calculated pediatric doses. Alternatively, chloroquine in suspension is widely available overseas.

SUGGESTED READING

Centers for Disease Control. Recommendations for the prevention of malaria in travelers. MMWR 1988; 37:277–284.

Chiodini PL, Somerville M, Salam I, et al. Exchange transfusion in severe falciparum malaria. Trans R Soc Trop Med Hyg 1985; 79:865–866.

Lobel HO, Roberts JM, Somaini B, Steffen R. Efficacy of malaria prophylaxis in American and Swiss travelers to Kenya. J Infect Dis 1987; 155:1205–1209.

Phillips RE, Warrell DA, White NJ, et al. Intravenous quinidine for the treatment of severe falciparum malaria. N Engl J Med 1985; 312:1273–1278.

Warhurst DC. Antimalarial drugs: an update. Drugs 1987; 33:50–65.

Wyler DJ. *Plasmodium* species (malaria). In: Mandell GL, Douglas RG Jr, Bennett JE, eds. Principles and practice of infectious diseases. 2nd ed. New York: John Wiley & Sons, 1985:1514.

AMEBIASIS AND GIARDIASIS

JONATHAN I. RAVDIN, M.D.

AMEBIASIS

Entamoeba histolytica is an enteric protozoan that infects 10 percent of the world's population, resulting in 50 to 100 million cases of invasive colitis or liver abscess per year and up to 100,000 deaths. The prevalence is highest in developing countries with poor levels of sanitation; however, modern travel and rates of emigration and the existence of high-risk groups require that physicians throughout the world be familiar with the diverse clinical disease syndromes due to *E. histolytica* and the varied agents used for treatment. The key to diagnosis and treatment of amebiasis is knowledge of the epidemiologic risk factors and clinical manifestations, a rational diagnostic approach, and an understanding of the sites of action of antiamebic drugs.

Epidemiologic Risk Factors

Highly endemic areas include Mexico, India, West and South Africa, and areas of Central and South America. Immigrants from or travelers to these areas are at risk (Table 1); amebic liver abscess occurs within 5 months after leaving an endemic area. An increased incidence of invasive amebiasis in the southwestern United States is solely due to disease in immigrants from Mexico. Institutionalized individuals, especially the mentally retarded, and those living in a communal setting are at particular risk. The oral-anal practices of sexually promiscuous male homosexuals result in a high prevalence of amebic infection. Severe invasive amebiasis can occur in the very young (under age 2 years), pregnant women, malnourished individuals, and those given corticosteroids, the latter often for an incorrect diagnosis of idiopathic inflammatory bowel disease.

Clinical Syndromes and Manifestations

E. histolytica infection has diverse clinical presentations (Table 2). Most common is asymptomatic intestinal luminal infection without evidence of tissue invasion (absence of serum antiamebic antibodies, blood in the stool, and mucosal alterations on colonoscopy). Nonspecific symptoms such as bloating, cramps, or decreased appetite have been reported in individuals with noninvasive *E. histolytica* infection; however, the etiologic association of such symptoms is unclear. Amebic colitis (Table 3) has a subacute onset characterized by dysenteric stools; fever occurs in only one-third of individuals. Despite the presence of mucosal ulceration and heme-positive stools, fecal leukocytes may be absent due to the parasite's ability to lyse host neutrophils. Fulminant colitis often results in perforation with peritonitis and has a poor prognosis. Chronic amebic colitis is clinically indistinguishable from idiopathic inflammatory bowel disease presenting with low-grade disease and recurrent episodes of bloody diarrhea. Ameboma is a localized chronic amebic

TABLE 2 Clinical Syndromes Due to Infection by *Entamoeba histolytica*

Asymptomatic cyst passers (colonization)
Symptomatic cyst passers
Acute rectocolitis
Fulminant colitis
Toxic megacolon
Perforation with peritonitis
Chronic nondysenteric colitis
Ameboma
Liver abscess
Peritonitis
Lung abscess, empyema
Pericarditis
Brain abscess
Venereal disease
Cutaneous disease

TABLE 1 Epidemiologic Risk Factors That Apparently Predispose to *Entamoeba histolytica* Infection and Increased Severity of Disease

Prevalence	*Increased Severity*
Lower socioeconomic status in an endemic area including:	Children, especially neonates
Crowding	Pregnancy and postpartum states
No indoor plumbing	Corticosteroid use
Immigrants from endemic area	Malignancy
Institutionalized population; especially mentally retarded	Malnutrition
Communal living	
Promiscuous male homosexuals	

Reprinted with permission from Amebiasis: human infection by *Entamoeba histolytica*. Ravdin JI, ed. New York: John Wiley & Sons, 1988:496.

TABLE 3 Clinical Manifestations of Acute Amebic Colitis

Bloody mucoid diarrhea of 1–4 weeks' duration
Abdominal pain, weight loss
Bloating, tenesmus, cramps
Fever (in only one-third of individuals)
Diffuse abdominal and right upper-quadrant tenderness
Heme-positive stools (in 100%)
Fecal leukocytes variably present

infection commonly occurring in the cecum or ascending colon that presents as a painful abdominal mass often mistaken on barium enema for a carcinoma.

Amebic liver abscess classically presents with right upper-quadrant pain, fever, and point tenderness over the liver (Table 4). Patients usually present acutely but may exhibit a chronic syndrome in which weight loss and pain predominate. Nonspecific laboratory abnormalities include leukocytosis, elevation of alkaline phosphatase and transaminase, decreased serum albumin and cholesterol, and proteinuria. Elevated bilirubin with jaundice is unusual. Left lobe abscesses are more likely to rupture, with resultant peritonitis or extension to the pericardium, resulting in cardiac tamponade. Pulmonary disease can result from direct extension from a liver abscess or less commonly by hematogeneous spread. Brain abscess is very uncommon; genital infection has been reported in India and can be confused with penile or cervical carcinoma.

Differential Diagnosis and Approach to the Patient

Diagnosis of intestinal amebiasis rests on examination of the stool or mucosal tissue by a skilled microscopist (Fig. 1). Virtually all patients test positive for occult blood; this is a useful, inexpensive screening test. As discussed, the absence or presence of fecal leukocytes is noncontributory. Three separate stool examinations are required to detect 90 percent of infected individuals; interfering substances such as barium, laxatives, antibiotics, and soap enemas should be avoided. Handling of samples and preparation of stained slides are detailed in the Suggested Reading (see below). Barium x-ray films do not differentiate amebiasis from other types of colonic ulceration. Serum antiamebic antibodies are detected in more than 85 percent of patients with invasive colitis; however, as antiamebic antibodies persist for years in a highly endemic area, these titers may not differentiate acute from remote infection. This is especially true with the indirect hemagglutination assay; gel diffusion, counterimmunoelectrophoresis, or latex agglutination often become negative 6 months after cure of invasive disease and may be useful in differentiating acute from remote infection.

TABLE 4 Clinical Manifestations of Amebic Liver Abscess

Fever
Right upper-quadrant pain
Weight loss
Diarrhea (in 20–40% of individuals)
Exquisite point tenderness over the liver
Hepatomegaly (in <50%)
Elevated white blood cell count, alkaline phosphatase, transaminases, sedimentation rate
Decreased cholesterol and serum albumin levels
Abnormal urinalysis

Total colonoscopy with scraping or biopsy of the ulcer edge is definitive. The diagnostic yield is very high and allows for evaluation of patients with ascending colon disease,

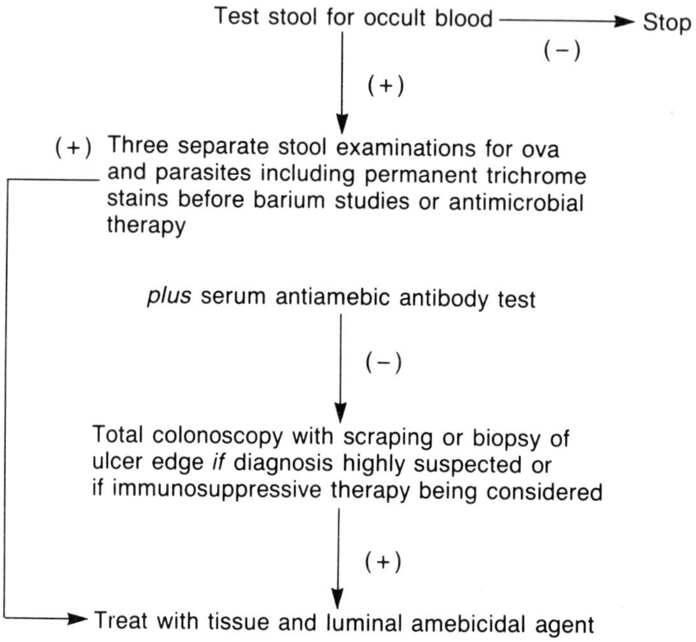

Figure 1 Diagnostic evaluation for acute amebic rectocolitis in a patient with suggestive epidemiology and clinical manifestations.

who often have negative stool examinations. If there is a strong suspicion or a need for immediate diagnosis, colonoscopy should be performed even if the stool examination is negative. Colonoscopy must be performed with care because of the risk of perforation. A tissue diagnosis is especially indicated if corticosteroid therapy is being considered for inflammatory bowel disease. The differential diagnosis for acute rectocolitis includes shigellosis, salmonellosis, campylobacteriosis, yersinia infection, invasive *Escherichia coli*, or other less common etiologies of inflammatory diarrhea.

The first step in approaching patients with possible amebic liver abscess (Fig. 2) is to perform an ultrasound examination of the liver and biliary tract. This sensitive nontoxic method detects cavities in the liver or stones and obstruction in the biliary tract. Abdominal computed tomography (CT) may be slightly more sensitive in detecting and delineating a liver abscess but should be reserved for patients with an equivocal nondiagnostic ultrasound examination. Serum antiamebic antibodies are eventually present in 99 percent of patients with amebic liver abscess; however, individuals presenting with fewer than 7 days of symptoms often lack serum antiamebic antibody. In the latter case, a study should be repeated 7 days after presentation.

The differential diagnosis of amebic liver abscess includes pyogenic abscess, echinococcal cyst, and hepatoma. Patients with bacterial abscesses are usually older and have biliary tract disease or abdominal malignancy or have had recent surgery. If the epidemiologic history, clinical profile, and serologic studies are nondiagnostic, a fine-needle aspirate under ultrasound or CT guidance can be performed to rule out bacterial disease. The yield for detection of *E. histolytica* trophozoites is low, especially after initiation of antiamebic therapy. Specific serologic studies must be performed prior to aspiration if there is any clinical suspicion of an echinococcal cyst because of the risk of peritoneal spillage and resultant prophylaxis or seeding.

Therapy and Management

It is uncertain whether noninvasive *E. histolytica* luminal infection requires treatment. Because individuals so infected may develop invasive disease or put others at risk for transmission, I favor eradicating the parasite. Such patients also frequently develop nonspecific gastrointestinal complaints that are difficult to differentiate from the onset of invasive amebiasis. However, I would not routinely screen asymptomatic individuals for amebic infection, nor has mass therapy of institutionalized individuals proved useful.

Agents that successfully eradicate intraluminal infection (Table 5) cannot be relied upon for treatment of deep tissue invasion. For patients with no evidence of invasive amebiasis, diloxanide furoate is the drug of choice. Unfortunately, in the United States this is available only from the Parasite Disease Drug Service of the Centers for Disease Control (CDC), Atlanta, Georgia (telephone 404–329–3670). Intestinal esterases hydrolyze the ester, diloxanide furoate, to the absorbable product, diloxanide. Delayed absorption accounts for high concentrations of diloxanide furoate in the large bowel lumen; adverse effects are uncommon and include flatulence or other mild gastrointestinal complaints. Paromomycin is a highly efficacious nonabsorbable aminoglycoside that is especially advantageous for use in pregnant women or children. Its main adverse effect is increased frequency of stools; in patients with amebic colitis, renal failure or other signs of aminoglycoside toxicity have not been noted. Diiodohydroxyquin is lowest on the list because of the long duration of therapy required, gastrointestinal toxicity, and other less common adverse effects such as fever, headache, generalized furunculosis, and interference with thyroid function tests due to its high iodine content (63 percent).

Metronidazole is the mainstay for treatment of invasive amebiasis. Outside of the United States, an efficacious and less-toxic nitroimidazole, tinidazole, is available and preferred (dose, 2 or 50 mg per kilogram orally once daily for 3 days).

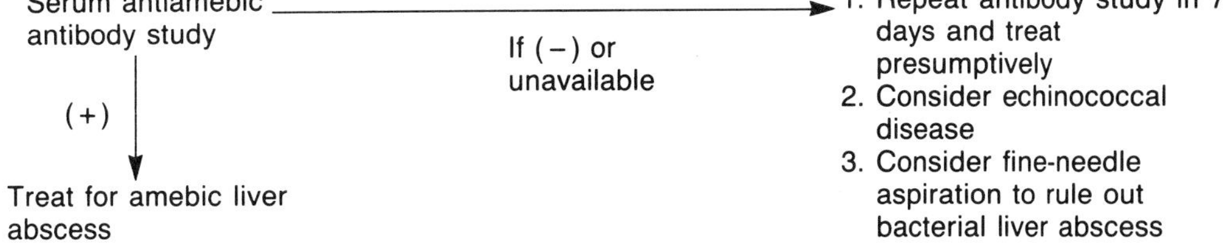

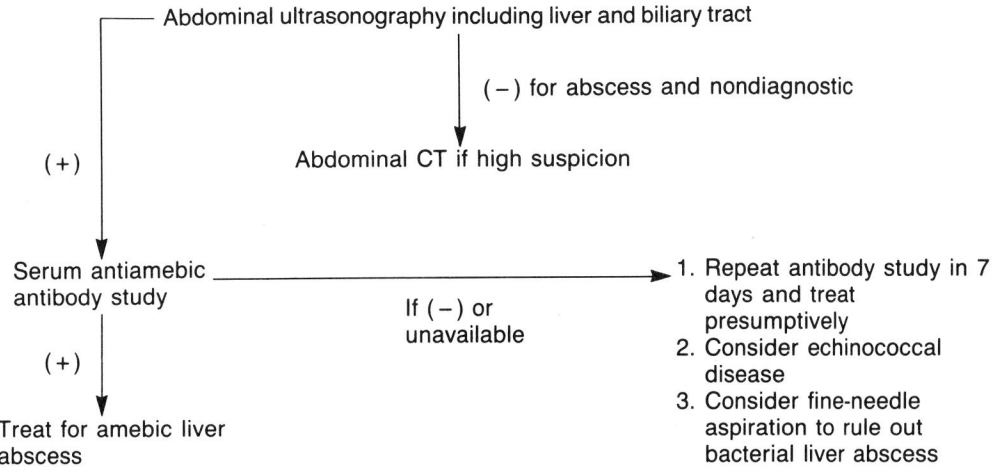

Figure 2 Diagnostic evaluation for amebic liver abscess in a patient with suggestive epidemiology and clinical manifestations.

TABLE 5 Therapy for Amebiasis

Presentation, Agent	*Adult Dose*	*Pediatric Dose*
Intraluminal infection		
Diloxanide furoate	500 mg orally t.i.d. × 10 days	20 mg/kg/day in 3 divided doses × 10 days
Paromomycin	30 mg/kg/day in 3 divided doses for 10 days	25 mg/kg/day in 3 divided doses × 7 days
Diiodohydroxyquin	650 mg orally t.i.d. × 20 days	30 mg/kg/day in 3 divided doses × 20 days
Invasive colitis		
Metronidazole*	750 mg orally t.i.d. or 500 mg IV q6h × 10 days	35 mg/kg/day in 3 divided doses × 10 days
Metronidazole*	2.4 g PO, single dose	
Tetracycline*†	250 mg orally t.i.d. × 10 days	Adults only
Erythromycin*†	500 mg orally q.i.d. × 10 days	Adults only
Dehydroemetine*	1 mg/kg/day (maximum 90 mg/day) IM in 2 divided doses × 5 days in hospital	Same as in adults, maximum of 60 mg/day
Liver abscess‡		
Metronidazole*†	750 mg PO t.i.d. or 500 mg IV q6h × 10 days	35 mg/kg/day in 3 divided doses × 10 days
Dehydroemetine*†	1 mg/kg/day IM × 5 days in hospital	Same as in adults

* Followed by a drug for luminal infection.
† Chloroquine (base) 600 mg orally per day for 2 days and 300 mg base orally per day for adults and 10 mg base/kg/day for children for 14–21 days is added by some clinicians for severe disease.
‡ Liver abscess needle aspiration only if no response to therapy for 5–7 days or high risk of abscess rupture.

Metronidazole distributes throughout the tissues and is metabolized mainly in the liver. Limiting factors for clinical use include its potential carcinogenicity, substantial frequency of gastrointestinal intolerance, disulfiram (Antabuse) effect, and rare neurologic toxicities. The short-course regimens cited (Table 5) may be better tolerated. Urine from patients receiving metronidazole causes genetic changes in bacteria; studies of humans do not reveal a carcinogenic effect, but large-scale, long-term follow-up is lacking. Ten days of metronidazole will also eliminate intraluminal infection in up to 90 percent of patients; therefore, use of a second agent may not be needed in individuals who complete the whole 10-day course of metronidazole. All patients treated for amebic colitis require careful follow-up stool examinations or colonoscopy to document cure; relapse occurs in 10 percent or more.

In patients who cannot tolerate metronidazoles, tetracycline or erythromycin followed by an intraluminal agent can be used for treatment of colitis, but this therapy will not eradicate amebae in the liver. Chloroquine is active only in the liver and can be added as a third agent; I prefer to avoid its use and carefully follow patients for evidence of hepatic involvement. Dehydroemetine is also available from the Parasite Disease Drug Service of the CDC; emetines have multiple adverse effects including gastrointestinal toxicity in up to 50 percent of patients; neuromuscular complaints including muscle weakness, tenderness, and stiffness; and most importantly, cardiovascular complications such as hypotension, chest pain, electrocardiogram abnormalities (T-wave inversion and prolonged QT interval in 25 to 50 percent), and tachycardia, which may be followed by congestive cardiomyopathy. Patients receiving emetines must be hospitalized and subject to continual monitoring of their cardiac status.

Amebic colitis can be fulminant in pregnant women; metronidazole did not cause untoward effects in one uncontrolled study of 216 pregnant women and should be used for severe amebic disease in this setting. Mild disease can be treated with paromomycin; pregnant women with asymptomatic colonization should be observed or treated with paromomycin. Intestinal perforation during amebic colitis is usually best managed conservatively with antiamebic and antibacterial therapy; attempts at surgical resection should be avoided. Only patients with toxic megacolon require surgery, usually a total colectomy.

Metronidazole alone is adequate initial therapy for amebic liver abscess. Some clinicians add chloroquine or dehydroemetine; however, there are no controlled studies indicating this improves the outcome, and I do not recommend it. Most patients will respond gradually over 3 to 5 days with a decrease in fever, right upper-quadrant pain, and other constitutional complaints. In patients who show no response by 5 to 7 days, aspiration of the abscess may be beneficial. One should also reconsider other diagnostic possibilities. An occasional patient may require open drainage or the addition of a second agent after aspiration, but this is unusual. Therapeutic aspiration of the abscess on presentation is indicated only if the abscess is very large and appears to be at high risk for rupture. Risks of needle aspiration include bacterial suprainfection. Resolution of the abscess cavity is a long-term process, requiring a median of 7 months. Patients should be followed clinically; persistence of a cavity in an asymptomatic individual is not an indication for invasive procedures. Up to one-fifth of patients will have a permanent hepatic cyst.

Avoiding fecal-oral contamination is the only effective means of preventing *E. histolytica* infection. A vaccine is not available; chemoprophylaxis has not been studied nor is it recommended. Boiling is the only certain means of eradicating *E. histolytica* cysts in water. Precautions such as avoidance of uncooked vegetables, salads, fruits that cannot be peeled, and ice cubes are advisable for travelers.

GIARDIASIS

Giardia lamblia, the most common parasitic cause of diarrhea worldwide, produces appreciable discomfort but not significant mortality. Giardiasis is generally a disease of the very young and presents in nonimmune adults who travel to an endemic area or interface with intense foci of infection in the developed world. The clinical syndrome resulting from *G. lamblia* infection is highly characteristic, easily recognized, and often treated even if the parasite cannot be demonstrated (but one should try). It is unclear whether asymptomatic infection in an endemic area or day care setting merits therapy.

Epidemiologic Risk Factors

At least 23 waterborne outbreaks of giardiasis have been reported; sporadic waterborne acquisition also clearly occurs, with beavers as well as humans implicated. Person-to-person spread in day care centers or among children in the developing world and among sexually promiscuous male homosexuals is also significant. Infection rates in the day care setting can approach 50 percent (Table 6); symptomatic disease occurs in a portion of infected individuals as well as frequent spread of infection to contacts in the home. *Giardia* cysts survive for weeks in surface water, especially at low temperatures. Institutionalized populations are at risk; as mentioned, foreign travel is also important. In addition to a high prevalence in developing countries, areas of the Soviet Union are notorious sites for the acquisition of giardiasis. The majority of infected individuals spontaneously clear the infection and are resistant to rechallenge; however, recent studies of antigenic variation in *G. lamblia* raise the possibility that the parasite can escape from host immune surveillance.

Clinical Manifestations

Up to 70 percent of individuals infected with *G. lamblia* have no manifestations of infection and spontaneously clear the parasite. This is especially so in the very young. Recent studies of experimental infection in volunteers suggest that pathogenicity is strain rather than host specific. After an incubation period of 1 to 2 weeks, infection can manifest as an acute diarrheal syndrome, with watery stools progressing to foul, greasy, malodorous diarrhea (Table 7). Bloating, flatulence, and abdominal cramps are characteristic. Although symptoms may resolve in 3 or 4 days, most patients have persistent complaints for weeks. The stool is heme-negative, and fecal leukocytes are absent. Given appropriate epidemiologic risk factors, the characteristic symptoms and duration of illness are pathognomonic for giardiasis. A minority of these patients have persistent complaints of diarrhea, malaise, headache, and weight loss lasting months (Table 7). Symptoms can be intermittent; lactose intolerance is common and may persist for weeks after therapy.

Differential Diagnosis and Approach to the Patient

There are few infectious etiologies that produce the prolonged noninflammatory diarrhea seen in giardiasis. In patients just returned from foreign travel, or others with fewer than 5 days of symptoms, enterotoxigenic *E. coli* or rotavirus is most likely. I begin diagnostic evaluation (Fig. 3) when symptoms persist for more than 5 to 7 days or when the incubation period and risk factors suggest *G. lamblia* infection. Careful examination of three separate stool samples provides a diagnostic yield of up to 90 percent. In a patient with suggestive risk factors and clinical syndrome, if the stool examinations are negative, examination of duodenal contents by a string test may be helpful. Although this is suggested

TABLE 6 Epidemiologic Risk Factors That Apparently Predispose to *Giardia lamblia* Infection and Increased Severity of Disease

Prevalence	*Increased Severity*
Day care center exposure	Hypogammaglobulinemia
Institutionalization	Common variable type
Foreign travel	X-linked agammaglobulinemia
Ingestion of untreated surface water	? IgA deficiency
Promiscuous male homosexual behavior	Malnutrition

TABLE 7 Clinical Manifestations of Giardiasis

Acute diarrhea (days to weeks in duration)
- Diarrhea progresses from watery to greasy and foul-smelling
- Weight loss
- Bloating, flatulence
- Abdominal cramps
- Heme (−), no fecal leukocytes

Chronic diarrhea (>3 weeks in duration)
- Diarrhea: small volume, high frequency, greasy, foul-smelling
- Malaise, lassitude
- Headache
- Diffuse abdominal cramps
- Weight loss

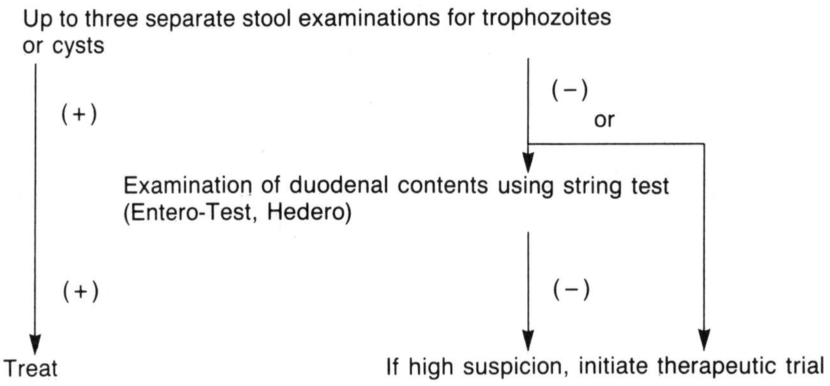

Figure 3 Diagnostic evaluation for giardiasis in a patient with suggestive epidemiology and clinical manifestations.

by some studies, in practice one rarely finds a positive string test in a patient with three negative stool examinations. A therapeutic trial, if there are no contraindications, is certainly reasonable and preferable, in my opinion, to performing a duodenal aspirate or biopsy. Patients infected with *G. lamblia* do develop a serum antibody response, but such studies are not yet available for routine clinical use.

Therapy

Many authorities consider quinacrine (Atabrine) the drug of choice for treatment of giardiasis (Table 8). However, given the occasional severe side effect of toxic psychosis as well as other toxicities, including yellow staining of sclerae and skin, gastrointestinal upset, and rarely exfoliative dermatitis, I and many other clinicians prefer to use metronidazole as initial therapy. The toxicities and carcinogenic potential of metronidazole are discussed in the section on amebiasis. Metronidazole, 250 mg orally three times daily for 10 days, has been reported to cure up to 90 percent of individuals, but many adult patients may require the higher dose (750 mg three times daily) for eradication of the parasite. Although metronidazole is better tolerated than quinacrine in children, the U.S. Food and Drug Administration has not officially approved metronidazole for the treatment of giardiasis; its potential risks should be carefully considered before its use. Shorter courses of other nitroimidazoles, such as tinidazole (single dose of 2 g), have been found to be highly efficacious, but these agents are not available in the United States. Furazolidone, a nitrofuran available in a liquid suspension, is useful for treatment of young children, with approximately 80 percent efficacy in the doses described (Table 8). Although it too has gastrointestinal toxicity, can turn urine brown, and can cause mild hemolysis in G6PD-deficient individuals, furazolidone is usually better tolerated than quinacrine. Paromomycin is a reasonable alternative agent, especially for use in pregnant patients for whom a nonabsorbable agent is ideal.

TABLE 8 Therapy for Giardiasis

Agent	*Adult Dose*	*Pediatric Dose*
Metronidazole	750 mg PO t.i.d. × 10 days	15 mg/kg/day PO in 3 divided doses × 7–10 days
Quinacrine	100 mg orally t.i.d. × 7 days	6 mg/kg/day PO in 3 divided doses × 7 days
Furazolidone		8 mg/kg/day PO in 4 divided doses × 10 days
Paromomycin	30 mg/kg/day PO in 3 divided doses × 10 days, especially for pregnant women	Same as adult dose

Prevention of giardiasis requires avoidance of person-to-person fecal-oral contact and proper handling and treatment of community water supplies. All backcountry surface water should be considered infectious. Boiling water is the most effective means of eradication of cysts; efficacy of added halogens may depend on water temperature and the level of proteinaceous sediment present. Rigorous hand-washing practices in highly endemic foci, such as day care centers, and avoidance of sexual activities that result in fecal-oral contact should be advised.

SUGGESTED READING

Davidson RA. Issues in clinical parasitology: the treatment of giardiasis. Am J Gastroenterol 1984; 79:256–261.

Drugs for parasitic infections. Med Lett Drugs Ther 1986; 28(issue 706): January 31.

Ravdin JI. Intestinal disease caused by *Entamoeba histolytica*. In: Ravdin JI, ed. Amebiasis: human infection by *Entamoeba histolytica*. New York: John Wiley and Sons, 1988:495.

Ravdin JI, Guerrant RL. Current problems in diagnosis and treatment of amebic infections. In: Remington JS, Swartz MN, eds. Current clinical topics in infectious diseases 7. New York: McGraw-Hill, 1980:82.

Reed SL, Braude AI. Extraintestinal disease: clinical syndromes, diagnostic profile, and therapy. In: Ravdin JI, ed. Amebiasis: human infection by *Entamoeba histolytica*. New York: John Wiley and Sons, 1988:511.

TOXOPLASMOSIS

GREGORY A. FILICE, M.D.

Toxoplasma gondii is an ubiquitous protozoan parasite that infects about half of all humans during their lifetimes. Infections in healthy people are usually mild or asymptomatic. In contrast, primary infection or reactivation of latent infection can be devastating in immunosuppressed people, and treatment is necessary to arrest the process. Women who become infected during pregnancy and who choose not to interrupt the pregnancy should be treated to prevent congenital infection or lessen its severity. Congenitally infected neonates should be treated to prevent progression of the infection and the appearance of sequelae.

Since severe disease is infrequent and often not recognized, there are few systematic studies of therapy. Recommendations are based on clinical experience, anecdotes, and uncontrolled series of treated patients. Clinicians should be prepared to modify their approach in particular clinical circumstances based on the growing knowledge of the pathogenesis *T. gondii* infection. Important facts and principles underlying therapy will be presented in this chapter to allow for rational implementation of the recommendations.

TOXOPLASMA GONDII

T. gondii is a coccidian protozoan parasite of worldwide distribution that infects a wide variety of birds, mammals, and probably reptiles. After an animal ingests an infective form of the parasite, tachyzoites are formed in the intestine and cross the intestinal wall to enter the circulation. They disseminate throughout the body, and after a brief proliferative phase, they give rise to tissue cysts containing up to several hundred, single-celled bradyzoites. Tissue cysts often persist for the life of the host. After the death of the host, the cysts are infectious if ingested along with the tissues by another animal.

Members of the cat family are the definitive hosts for *T. gondii* and support a sexual cycle. The parasite forms oocysts in the intestine that are shed in the feces from 7 to 20 days after acute infection. The oocysts sporulate in the next 2 to 5 days and become infectious. Sporulated oocysts remain infectious for months.

Like other animals, humans become infected by ingesting oocysts or by eating raw or lightly cooked meat. Since oocysts are hardy, it is thought that many infections occur through ingestion of contaminated vegetables or through contact with soil contaminated with cat feces. The prevalence of infection in adults varies throughout the world from 15 to 85 percent. It tends to be higher in the tropics and lower in colder climates, but there are exceptions.

DIAGNOSIS

Serology

Serologic study is the means of diagnosis in most patients suspected of having toxoplasmosis. A discussion of the most helpful serologic tests will enable the reader to understand the present recommendations for therapy.

Tests can be divided into those that measure IgG antibody and those that measure IgM. The Sabin-Feldman dye test (DT) is the standard for measurement of IgG antibodies. Other useful tests for IgG antibodies that usually produce similar results are the agglutination test for IgG antibody (performed with 2-mercaptoethanol to inactivate IgM) and the indirect fluorescent antibody (IFA) test for IgG. Titers rise rapidly after infection, usually before the onset of symptoms and typically to 1,000 or more. High titers persist for months to years and then gradually fall, but IgG antibodies rarely disappear.

There are three useful tests for IgM antibody. The double-sandwich IgM enzyme-linked immunosorbent assay (DS-IgM-ELISA) and IgM immunosorbent assay (IgM-ISA) are similar. They become positive soon after infection in most infected people and persist for several months to 2 or 3 years. The IgM-IFA test, the original test for IgM antibodies, is less sensitive and remains positive for a shorter time, usually a few months.

The indirect hemagglutination test (IHA) usually becomes positive several weeks after infection and after the IgG tests mentioned above become positive. Since the test is often negative early in infection, it is not useful for screening pregnant women. IHA titers may still rise after other titers have stabilized or are falling.

The behavior of the complement fixation test (CF) depends on the nature of the antigen, and there is no widely accepted standard. With cytoplasmic antigens, the test behaves like the IHA. With cell-membrane antigens, the test behaves more like the DT.

Demonstration of Organisms in Tissues

Tachyzoites in areas of inflammation are indicative of active replication and disease. They are rarely found in the lymph nodes of healthy people with acute lymphadenopathic toxoplasmosis. Cysts can be found in tissues of latently infected people, especially muscle, heart, and brain, but they do not indicate active replication and cannot be taken as evidence of active *T. gondii* infection.

Mouse Inoculation

T. gondii is isolated by inoculation into mice. Material should be triturated if necessary and injected intraperitoneally. If mice sicken or die, peritoneal fluid should be examined for tachyzoites. Unfortunately, many strains are not pathogenic for mice. Such strains are detected by testing serum from the mice for IgG antibody to *T. gondii*.

CLINICAL ILLNESS

Acute Acquired Infection in Immunocompetent People

Most immunocompetent people who become infected with *T. gondii* are asymptomatic. Between 10 and 20 percent have a mild, self-limited illness 1 to 3 weeks after infection, which is usually characterized by fever and lymphadenopathy. Rarely, manifestations of acute acquired toxoplasmosis include encephalitis, myocarditis, hepatitis, pneumonitis, polymyositis, or persistent fevers. The diagnosis is often suggested by the characteristic lymph node histologic findings, characterized by (1) reactive follicular hyperplasia with irregular clusters of epithelioid histiocytes that encroach upon and blur the margins of germinal centers and (2) focal distention of sinuses with monocytoid cells.

The syndrome is not specific, and the diagnosis is usually made by serologic studies. IgG antibody is common in the population, often with relatively high titers. A single positive test for IgG antibody is not sufficient for the diagnosis, although a very high titer ($\geq$16,000) is suggestive. Usually the titer of IgG antibody has peaked by the time symptoms bring the patient to a physician, and rising titers are seldom documented. IgM antibody should be measured in all patients suspected of having acute toxoplasmosis. A high ($\geq$1:2,000) titer of IgG antibody with a positive IgM test in a patient with a compatible clinical syndrome is diagnostic. Exact timing of recent infections can be difficult because IgG titers typically remain 1:2,000 or higher for months to years and the sensitive DS-IgM-ELISA or IgM-ISA tests often remain positive for 2 to 3 years.

Retinochoroiditis

Retinochoroiditis without other manifestations of active disease is usually a late manifestation of congenital infection. In this case it is usually bilateral. Retinochoroiditis occurs in fewer than 1 percent of cases of acute acquired toxoplasmosis, usually only in one eye. Retinochoroiditis is common in infants with generalized congenital toxoplasmosis and in immunocompromised people with reactivated toxoplasmosis.

The diagnosis is suggested by its characteristic ophthalmoscopic appearance. When the process is localized to the eye, serum IgG antibody titers are usually low and may be detectable only in undiluted serum. If antibody is not detected in undiluted serum, eye disease is unlikely to be caused by *T. gondii*. In patients in whom the retinal appearance is equivocal, the likelihood of the diagnosis is increased if local antibody production can be demonstrated (the ratio of IgG antibody to *T. gondii*/total IgG in aqueous humor is greater than the ratio of IgG antibody to *T. gondii*/total IgG in serum.

Toxoplasmosis in Immunosuppressed Patients

People with profound T lymphocyte deficits are unusually susceptible to severe toxoplasmosis, generally from reactivation of latent infection. Common associated conditions include lymphoid malignancies, organ transplantation, and the acquired immunodeficiency syndrome (AIDS). When seronegative organ transplant recipients receive an organ from a seropositive donor, severe toxoplasmosis may occur. Seropositive recipients frequently have increases in antibody to *T. gondii* during immunosuppressive therapy, but severe toxoplasmosis in these recipients is uncommon.

The most commonly recognized manifestation is encephalitis, which often progresses to necrosis of brain tissue. Computed tomography typically shows low-density masses with ring enhancement and mass effects, but a variety of patterns can occur. Toxoplasmosis of the central nervous system (CNS) should be considered in any AIDS patient with a focal or diffuse CNS lesion. Other common manifestations include pneumonitis, myocarditis, and fever without focal findings. Diagnosis and management are complicated by the fact that these severely immunosuppressed people often have concurrent opportunistic infections.

Recent attention has been focused on disease in AIDS patients. From 15 to 50 percent of adults in the United States are seropositive for *T. gondii* infection, depending on the region. Approximately 30 percent of seropositive AIDS patients will develop clinical toxoplasmosis. Nearly all AIDS patients with active toxoplasmosis have IgG antibody; the absence of IgG antibody makes the diagnosis unlikely. However, IgG titers are usually low and stable, and IgM antibody to *T. gondii* is usually undetectable.

A recent retrospective study indicated that IgG antibody produced locally in CNS toxoplasmosis was secreted into the cerebrospinal fluid (CSF) in sufficient quantitities to help with the diagnosis. In patients with CNS toxoplasmosis, the ratio of specific IgG antibody to total IgG was usually greater in the CSF than in the serum:

$$\frac{\text{CSF DT}^{-1}}{[\text{CSF IgG}]} > \frac{\text{serum DT}^{-1}}{[\text{serum IgG}]}.$$

This was not the case in patients with other CNS diseases. Further prospective experience will be necessary to determine the reliability of the detection of local production of specific IgG.

A definitive diagnosis can be made by obtaining brain tissue for histopathologic study. In cases in which the diagnosis is not apparent from traditional stains, the more sensitive immunochemical staining should be performed. Alternatively, when the clinical presentation is suggestive of *T. gondii* infection, patients and clinicians may decide to avoid the risk and discomfort associated with brain biopsy and undertake a therapeutic trial directed against *T. gondii*.

Infection During Pregnancy

The major risk from toxoplasmosis in pregnant women is congenital infection. The risk of transmission to babies born to mothers with primary infection occurring during the first, second, or third trimester is 15, 20, and 60 percent, respectively. In contrast, congenital transmission from mothers who were infected before conception is exceedingly rare; for practical purposes, infants born to women who were seropositive before conception are not at risk for congenital toxoplasmosis.

A major problem is that pregnant women with acute toxoplasmosis, like other healthy adults, are symptomatic only 10 to 20 percent of the time. Screening of women for antibodies to *T. gondii* should be undertaken before pregnancy and at monthly intervals during pregnancy to detect asymptomatic or mild infections.

For screening, IgG antibody to *T. gondii* should be measured by DT, agglutination, or IFA. If women are seropositive before pregnancy, further testing is not necessary. If the first test is done after conception, a positive titer should be followed by a test for IgM antibody.

The interpretation of positive serology when the first titer was obtained during pregnancy can be difficult. In the first 6 to 8 weeks after infection, IgG titers are usually unstable; a stable IgG titer in the first 2 months of pregnancy usually signifies infection acquired before pregnancy. After the second month, if the IgG titer is 2,000 or greater or there is IgM antibody, there is a substantial likelihood that infection was acquired during pregnancy.

Diagnosis of Fetal Infection

If infection is suspected in a woman during pregnancy, attempts at fetal diagnosis should be made. Between 20 and 28 weeks of gestation, fetal blood should be obtained and tested for the titer of IgM antibodies against *T. gondii* and for concentrations of total IgM antibodies, γ-glutamyl transpeptidase, lactate dehydrogenase, white blood cells, platelets, and eosinophils. A portion should be inoculated into mice for culture. Every 2 weeks ultrasound examinations should be performed to determine the size of the cerebral ventricles and the thickness of the placenta and to seek evidence for fetal ascites, hepatomegaly, or intracranial calcification. The likelihood that congenital infection has occurred should be estimated from these specific and nonspecific indicators (Table 1), and a decision should be made by the woman and her physician. One of three options can be offered: therapy for the mother to arrest fetal infection, termination of the pregnancy, or no treatment.

Congenital Infection

Infection acquired in utero can result in abortion, prematurity, stillbirth, or congenital infection. Only a minority of children with congenital infections are symptomatic at birth. Manifestations include fever, hydrocephalus, microcephalus, hepatosplenomegaly, jaundice, convulsions, chorioretinitis, cerebral calcifications, rash, abnormal CSF (mononuclear pleocytosis and xanthochromia), myocarditis, pneumonitis, deafness, erythroblastosis-like syndrome, thrombocytopenia, lymphocytosis, monocytosis, and nephrotic syndrome. Symptoms are more common at birth in those whose mothers were infected earlier during pregnancy. If those who are asymptomatic are not treated, the majority will develop neurologic, ocular, or other abnormalities later in life. Treatment appears to reduce the risk of sequelae, and all congenitally infected children should be treated.

In cases of suspected congenital toxoplasmosis, portions of the placenta should be inoculated into mice. Infants should have IgG and IgM titers performed at birth and periodically afterwards. IgM antibody is strongly suggestive of the diagnosis. IgM can be of maternal origin if there has been a leak in the placental barrier, but IgM has a half-life of only 8 days, and the titer in such cases should quickly disappear. If IgM antibody persists or increases in titer, the diagnosis

TABLE 1 Specificity, Sensitivity, and Predictive Value of Nonspecific Tests for Congenital Toxoplasmosis in 746 Pregnancies with Maternal Toxoplasmosis

			Predictive value	
Test	*Specificity (%)*	*Sensitivity (%)*	*Positive Test (%)*	*Negative Test (%)*
Ultrasound findings	99.8	45	95	97
Biologic tests				
White blood cell count	97	38	42	96
Eosinophil count	94	19	17	95
Platelet count	98	28	52	96
Total IgM antibody	97	52	49	97
IgM antibody to *T. gondii*	100	21	100	96
γ-Glutamyl transferase	97	57	52	97
Lactate dehydrogenase	98	17	33	95
Total IgM + white blood cell count	99.8	21	90	96
Total IgM + platelet count	100	21	100	96
γ-Glutamyl transferase + white blood cell count	99.8	26	91	96
γ-Glutamyl transferase + total IgM	99	38	64	96

Adapted from Daffos et al. Prenatal management of 746 pregnancies at risk for congenital toxoplasmosis. N Engl J Med 1988; 318:271–275.

is confirmed. One-fourth of congenitally infected infants will have IgM detectable by IgM-IFA and three-fourths will have IgM detectable by DS-IgM-ELISA. IgG crosses the placenta, and its half-life in the infant is approximately 30 days, which makes early diagnosis difficult. Titers should be followed monthly. If they do not decrease or if they begin to increase, the diagnosis is confirmed. An earlier diagnosis can sometimes be made by calculating "antibody load," the ratio of IgG antibody against *T. gondii* to total IgG. Ordinarily, by the second or third month the ratio falls in uninfected infants with passively acquired maternal antibody. In congenitally infected infants, the ratio levels off and begins to increase as the infant begins to make specific antibody against *T. gondii*.

THERAPEUTIC APPROACH

Chemotherapy

The combination of pyramethamine and sulfadiazine is the standard therapy for toxoplasmosis. The combination has been used extensively in humans, and it is synergistic in experimental infections in mice. Some other agents have activity in vitro or in experimental animals, but they have generally been less active in the laboratory than the combination of pyrimethamine and sulfadiazine. Several new agents are under active investigation, and these recommendations may be superseded over the next few years. When ranges of dosages are recommended, the exact dose should depend on severity of infection and the occurrence of any toxicity.

Pyrimethamine

Pyrimethamine (Daraprim, Chloridin, Malocide), a substituted phenylpyrimidine, inhibits folic acid production in *T. gondii* by interfering with dihydrofolate reductase. It is orally absorbed and has a half-life of 4.5 days in adults. I usually use 1 mg per kilogram per day, up to a maximum of 50 mg for the first 2 days and 25 mg thereafter. Daily doses of 50 mg for prolonged periods have been required in some AIDS patients. After a few weeks of therapy, I give pyrimethamine every 2 or 3 days because of its long half-life. For newborns being treated for congenital infection, I use 0.5 to 1 mg per kilogram per day.

The major toxicity of pyrimethamine is reversible dose-related bone marrow depression. Platelets are most commonly depressed, although leukopenia and anemia also occur. Pyrimethamine can also cause headache, gastrointestinal discomfort, and a bad taste in the mouth. Patients should have complete blood counts performed once or twice a week while taking pyrimethamine. Folinic acid can be absorbed by mammalian cells, but not by *T. gondii*, and it has been suggested that hematologic toxicity may be prevented or treated with folinic acid (citrovorum factor, leucovorin), 5 to 15 mg per day, but there is no good evidence that this is the case in humans.

Large doses of pyrimethamine are teratogenic in animals. Teratogenicity in humans has not been documented, but the drug should be avoided in the first 16 weeks of pregnancy. I recommend its use for documented fetal infection after 20 weeks of gestation (see below) because I believe that the potential benefits outweigh the potential risks in the latter half of pregnancy.

Sulfonamides

Sulfonamides inhibit *T. gondii* by preventing normal use of *p*-aminobenzoic acid in folate metabolism. Sulfadiazine and trisulfapyrimidines (sulfapyrazine, sulfadimidine, and sulfamerazine) are most active; all other sulfonamides are much less active. The half-life of sulfadiazine is 11 hours. I give a loading dose of 75 mg per kilogram (maximum, 4 g) followed by 100 to 150 mg per kilogram per day (maximum, 6 to 8 g per day). For newborns with congenital infection, I use 50 to 100 mg per kilogram per day. The exact dose depends upon the severity of infection and the occurrence of any toxicity.

A wide variety of toxicities have been associated with sulfonamides, including hemolytic anemia, aplastic anemia, agranulocytosis, thrombocytopenia, crystalluria, hepatitis, nephritis, neuritis, anorexia, nausea, vomiting, and reactions due to sensitization. Manifestations of sensitization include rash, arteritis, erythema multiforme, photosensitivity, serum sickness, and drug fever.

Spiramycin

Spiramycin, a macrolide antibiotic, is active against *T. gondii* in experimental animals, and there is clinical, uncontrolled evidence that it is effective in humans. The usual dose is 100 mg per kilogram per day in two to four divided doses.

Because spiramycin is a macrolide, its toxicity resembles that of erythromycin, but it is less toxic than erythromycin. Spiramycin is approved for use in Canada, Mexico, and Europe, but not in the United States. It can be obtained on an investigational basis for treatment of toxoplasmosis by contacting the Division of Antiviral Drug Products, U.S. Food and Drug Administration, Washington, D.C. (telephone, 301-443-0263).

Clindamycin

Clindamycin has activity against *T. gondii* in experimental animals, but its efficacy in humans is unproved. It is concentrated in the choroid, iris, and retina and has been used to treat retinochoroiditis. The usual dose is 15 to 30 mg per kilogram per day in four divided doses (maximum, 2,400 mg per day). Experience with such high doses in children is limited, and the maximal recommended dose for children is 20 mg per kilogram per day.

The most important toxic effect of clindamycin is diarrhea, especially from *Clostridium difficile* colitis. Other untoward effects include rashes, elevations of transaminase levels, granulocytopenia, thrombopenia, and anaphylaxis. Clindamycin has been administered locally through subconjunctival injection, but the toxicity of local therapy appears to outweigh the potential benefits.

Corticosteroids

Corticosteroids have been used to reduce inflammation in toxoplasmosis, especially for sight-threatening ocular disease or encephalitis. There is anecdotal evidence that they are effective in ocular disease, but they should always be used in conjunction with antimicrobial agents against *T. gondii*. I use prednisone, 1 to 2 mg per kilogram per day up to 75 mg per day maximum, or the equivalent. There is no good evidence that corticosteroids are effective for inflammation elsewhere in the body, including the CNS.

Therapy in Specific Clinical Circumstances

Acute Acquired Infection in Immunocompetent People

Most immunocompetent people with acute toxoplasmosis do not require specific therapy. Fevers may require treatment with antipyretics. If symptoms are unusually severe or prolonged, I use pyrimethamine and sulfadiazine. Where spiramycin is available, it may be used as a less-toxic, though probably less-effective, alternative. In the unusual cases when organs other than lymph nodes are clinically involved, I use antimicrobial therapy to prevent significant organ dysfunction.

Retinochoroiditis

Peripheral lesions that do not noticeably affect vision can be observed without the patient's receiving chemotherapy. If lesions progress, affect vision, or threaten important structures (i.e., macula, maculopapillary bundle, or optic nerve), pyrimethamine and sulfadiazine should be administered for 1 month. By 10 days, the borders of retinal lesions should sharpen, and vitreous haze should disappear. Steroids should be used in cases involving the macula, maculopapillary bundle, or optic nerve, always in conjunction with antiparasitic chemotherapy. Clindamycin appears to be an alternative for patients who cannot be treated with pyrimethamine and sulfadiazine.

Disease in Immunosuppressed Patients

Symptomatic toxoplasmosis in patients with severe T cell dysfunction should be treated with pyrimethamine and sulfonamides. The response is often slow and incomplete, and prolonged courses with high doses are often necessary.

Toxoplasmosis is common and particularly difficult to control in AIDS patients, and experiences with AIDS patients are redefining our approach to treatment. AIDS patients frequently become sensitized to sulfonamides and require nonstandard approaches. A few have been treated successfully with clindamycin and pyrimethamine. Others have been treated with 50 mg of pyrimethamine per day alone. The results are anecdotal and difficult to interpret because diagnoses are not always unequivocally established and because the underlying immunosuppression is progressive. At least three groups are studying therapy for toxoplasmosis in persons with AIDS, and further advances should be forthcoming.

Toxoplasmosis relapses in 50 percent or more of AIDS patients after therapy has been discontinued. I maintain AIDS patients on antimicrobial therapy with pyrimethamine and sulfadiazine for life to prevent relapse. I tailor the dose to avoid toxicity and still maintain effective blood levels. Other drugs, alone or in combination, have been used to prevent relapse, but none have emerged as effective substitutes for continual therapy with pyrimethamine and sulfadiazine.

Infection During Pregnancy

If toxoplasmosis is acquired during pregnancy, the parents and physician must decide between termination of the pregnancy and chemotherapy. If chemotherapy is chosen, I use 1 g of spiramycin three times daily, which appears to decrease the risk of fetal infection. Attempts to diagnose fetal infection should be made (see above). If fetal infection occurs and the decision is made to continue with the pregnancy, I prescribe pryimethamine, sulfadiazine, and folinic acid for the rest of the pregnancy.

Congenital Infection

I treat newborns having documented toxoplasmosis with courses of pyrimethamine, sulfadiazine, and folinic acid for 21 days and alternate this with courses of spiramycin for the balance of 2 months (38 to 41 days). If a newborn appears healthy and testing has not yet confirmed or excluded the possibility of congenital toxoplasmosis, I prescribe one course of pryimethamine and sulfadiazine followed by one course of spiramycin.

SUGGESTED READING

Daffos F, Forestier F, Capella-Pavlovsky M, et al. Prenatal management of 746 pregnancies at risk for congenital toxoplasmosis. N Engl J Med 1988; 318:271–275.

Hakes TB, Armstrong D. Toxoplasmosis. Problems in diagnosis and treatment. Cancer 1983; 52:1535–1540.

Luft BJ, Naot Y, Araujo F, Stinson EB, Remington JS. Primary and reactivated toxoplasma infection in patients with cardiac transplants. Clinical spectrum and problems in diagnosis in a defined population. Ann Intern Med 1983; 99:27–31.

McCabe RE, Remington JS. The diagnosis and treatment of toxoplasmosis. Eur J Clin Microbiol 1983; 2:95–104.

Navia BA, Petito CK, Gold JWM, et al. Cerebral toxoplasmosis complicating the acquired immune deficiency syndrome: clinical and neuropathological findings in 27 patients. Ann Neurol 1986; 19:224–238.

Potasman I, Resnick L, Luft BJ, Remington JS. Intrathecal production of antibodies against *Toxoplasma gondii* in patients with toxoplasmic encephalitis and the acquired immunodeficiency syndrome (AIDS). Ann Intern Med 1988; 108:49–51.

Wilson CB, Remington JS, Stagno S, Reynolds DW. Development of adverse sequelae in children born with subclinical congenital *Toxoplasma* infection. Pediatrics 1980; 66:767–774.

CANDIDOSIS

JOHN P. UTZ, M.D., F.A.C.P.

In the fifth century before Christ (circa 410 BC) Hippocrates described in his *Epidemics* a disease that was unequivocally thrush, and in his diary entry of 17 June 1665, Samuel Pepys introduced the word and disease, *thrush*, into the English language. In the early 1800s, Gruby established the *Candida* species as the cause of thrush.

A simple, but not necessarily the most helpful, approach to this disease is to classify it as superficial (of the skin, especially intertriginous sites; nails; and mucous membranes, especially the mouth, pharynx, esophagus, other gastrointestinal tract sites, vagina, and even the lower respiratory tract); and systemic (by hematogenous dissemination to such internal organs as the heart, kidneys, and brain; or by direct inoculation, for example, in the process of peritoneal dialysis, ocular surgery, or total parenteral nutrition). Not embraced by such a simplistic division are such notable and striking manifestations as chronic-mucocutaneous, allergic (uveitis and asthma), or even "intoxication" disease.

ETIOLOGY

Candida spp. are frequently described, even in classic mycology texts, as "pathogenic yeasts," which is not a helpful description. It is of even less relevance to physicians to know that, taxonomically, *Candida* spp. are in the phylum Deuteromycota, in the class blastomycetes, and even more confusing, in the family Cryptococcaceae. Specification by the mycologist is always of interest, but evidence of tissue invasion (pathogenesis) is more relevant, regardless of species. For the taxonomically oriented, *Candida* spp. multiply by pinching-off of rounded spores (blastoconidia), form both branching and nonbranching elongated forms (true and pseudo-hyphae), do not have polysaccharide capsules (as do *Cryptococcus* spp.), do not produce urease (as do *Cryptococcus* spp.), are not pigmented, and do not assimilate inositol.

Another troublesome aspect is their commensal status. *Candida* spp. are among the normal flora of the human oral cavity, gastrointestinal tract, vagina, and sometimes skin. Hence, in one limited sense, fungi are not "pathogens" in the way that *Histoplasma capsulatum* and *Coccidioides immitis* are pathogens. Rather, *Candida* spp. are "opportunists" that cause disease almost exclusively in the immunocompromised host. Hence, etiology is twofold and embraces more than just the fungus.

The eight species of *Candida* associated with systemic disease in humans are *C. albicans*, *C.* (formerly *Torulopsis*) *glabrata*, *C. guilliermondii*, *C. krusei*, *C. parapsilosis*, *C. pseudotropicalis*, *C. stellatoidea*, and *C. tropicalis*.

EPIDEMIOLOGY

Because *Candida* spp. are human commensals, their locus in nature has not seemed important. The fungus has rarely been recovered from soil, but since almost all mammals and birds have the fungus in their alimentary tracts, their excreta seem a likely source of *Candida* spp. in soil. It is not surprising, then, that the fungus can also be isolated from vegetation or even food. Despite the fact that this fungus is known to cause infective endocarditis, attempts to isolate it from "street drugs" used intravenously have had variable success. Geographic differences in incidence are not known.

PATHOGENESIS

Factors that predispose to disease from *Candida* are well understood, but are also increasing in numbers if not complexity.

1. Age is a predisposing factor; thrush occurs in 1 to 18 percent of infants in newborn nurseries, often in outbreaks.
2. Physiologic changes, notably pregnancy, can increase the incidence of *Candida* spp. in the vagina from a low of about 5 percent in nonpregnant women to 30 percent in pregnant women. This subject has recently had an excellent review by Ryley, and studies have implicated binding of the estrogen, estradiol, by a specific binding protein in the cytosol of *C. albicans*. The increased frequency of vaginitis has also been attributed to the increased vaginal carbohydrate content.
3. Antibacterial therapy has been associated with an increased incidence of fungal disease, especially since the introduction of tetracycline. The earliest explanation was the "vacuum," in which, if the substrate (food) stays roughly the same, antibacterial-resistant *Candida* spp. increase as bacterial populations fall. Recently, more sophisticated studies have shown that the indigenous intestinal bacterial flora inhibit both colonization and dissemination of *C. albicans* by outcompeting them for adhesion sites.
4. Candidosis is "a disease of the diseased." Patients with leukemia, terminal cancer, or diabetes mellitus are predisposed.
5. Physicians, deliberately or otherwise, produce an immunocompromised state by "breaking barriers" (e.g., surgical incision) or by administering drugs to prevent or to delay host-versus-graft (e.g., heart and kidney transplantation) or graft-versus-host (e.g., bone marrow transplantation) reactions. This immunocompromise may be effectuated, as in the last case, by suppression of specific lymphocytes or of polymorphonuclear cells in the leukopenic state. Corticosteroids are probably less important than other immunosuppressive drugs, e.g., other antileukemic agents or azathioprine.

From such primary sites and under conditions such as the foregoing, infection disseminates not by way of the lymphatics or into contiguous tissue, but hematogenously. A common mode of dissemination in nosocomial infections is through an intravenous catheter. Fungi usually enter around such catheters when there is total (or partial) parenteral nutrition or when the complex hyperalimentation solutions are contaminated. Organisms also may enter through the peritoneum after particularly prolonged surgery and antibacterial prophylaxis, during active treatment of bacterial peritonitis, or during peritoneal dialysis, particularly when given by long-term ambulatory or home administration. A third type of dissemination occurs in leukopenic patients. Normally, when fungi pass through the oral or gastrointestinal mucosa by a process termed *persorption*, they are promptly phagocytosed by polymorphonuclear leukocytes. However, this defense may be fatally impaired in the leukopenic patient. Thereafter, the intermediate step is fungal multiplication in the submucosa, which becomes necrotic. Since the submucosa is the best vascularized layer of the gastrointestinal tract, fungi are able to gain access to blood vessels. *Candida* spp. are only slightly less able or likely than *Aspergillus* spp. to produce active vasculitis. When invasion is from the gastrointestinal tract, the liver and spleen are involved more frequently than when invasion occurs through an intravenous catheter. In the latter event, ocular, pulmonary, central nervous system, and thyroid disease are more commonly seen. The kidney is involved with equal frequency by either route. A fourth mechanism by which pulmonary damage can occur is through aspiration of upper airway or stomach contents containing, among other things, *Candida* spp.

PATHOLOGY

In the patient who dies of disseminated disease, the gross pathology at the primary site (oral cavity, gastrointestinal tract, or vagina) is a multitude of superficial ulcers.

The microscopic pathology is usually an intense, suppurative, acute inflammation with microabscesses. However, this inflammation may be absent in the leukopenic patient; instead, there may be coagulation necrosis and, if the patient is also thrombocytopenic, hemorrhage. In chronic mucocutaneous candidosis, granulomas are almost always seen, but they are almost never seen in the otherwise immunocompromised patient. In other patients, such as those with *Candida* endocarditis or those being treated with antimycotics, granulomas may be present (e.g., in the myocardium, about hyphal forms).

In primary pulmonary disease, Myerowitz wrote, "It is not possible to ... describe accurately the macroscopic appearance of primary endobronchial (disease) ... Microscopically, endobronchial (disease) is characterized by *endobronchial proliferation of yeasts and pseudohyphae, which may or may not extend for a limited distance into the peribronchial pulmonary parenchyma*" (my emphasis added). "The tissue reaction may be one of necrosis with little or no cellular infiltration."

In hematogenously disseminated pulmonary involvement, the gross pathology is the classic target lesion: a nodular, round, well-circumscribed lesion, 2 to 4 mm in diameter, with a white-yellow center, and a hemorrhagic rim. Lesions are bilaterally distributed in a miliary fashion. Microscopically, the lesion consists of a central core of conidia (blastospores), germ tubes, and pseudohyphae in a necrotic area suffused and surrounded by intra-alveolar hemorrhage. In this site the most specific features are intravascular conidia (blastospores), germ tubes, and pseudohyphae. Fungal forms can be seen readily as hematoxophyl bodies with hematoxylin and eosin staining, but they stand out more vividly with such special stains as Gomori's methenamine silver, Gridley, or periodic acid–Schiff.

CLINICAL ASPECTS

A number of problems immediately emerge:

1. Despite the long history of both the disease (thrush) and the fungus, the pulmonary form has not been characterized, nor has its nosology been satisfactorily defined.
2. Because *Candida* spp. are commensals, their culture from sputum, bronchial washings, bronchoalveolar lavage fluid, or even mucosal biopsy material does not establish etiology.
3. When evidence of tissue invasion is necessary for diagnosis, biopsy may be dangerous or even precluded by the underlying disease or condition, e.g., thrombocytopenia.
4. When the pulmonary tissue is studied in the pathology laboratory, aspiration, endobronchial, or hematogenous dissemination (from another primary site) must be separated, defined, and established.
5. In as many as 50 percent of patients, it may not be possible to culture *Candida* spp. from blood when hematogenous dissemination occurs.
6. There is no specific roentgenographic appearance; according to Beff and colleagues, "chest roentgenograms fail to detect 73 to 96 percent of significant pulmonary...lesions, and 100 percent of small infiltrates," and other pulmonary diseases are invariably present.
7. Claims for diagnostic value of such tests as (1) transtracheal aspiration, (2) predominance of hyphal forms, (3) quantitative sputum cultures, (4) differences in *Candida* spp, (5) presence of complement-fixing, agglutinating, precipitin, agar gel double diffusion, or counter-immunoelectrophoresis antibodies in serum, or (6) presence of mannan, proteinase, and other antigens in serum have not been correlated with anatomic pathology findings.
8. Pleural disease and pleural effusion, which are so helpful in diagnosing tuberculosis or gram-negative bac-

terial rod pneumonias, are rarely present in diseases caused by *Candida* spp.

9. Autopsy findings show no diagnostic difference between persons with *Candida* spp. pulmonary disease and neoplastic disease and other persons with neoplastic disease alone.
10. Hematogenous spread rarely, if ever, occurs from a primary endobronchial site, even when blood vessel invasion can be demonstrated.
11. Although in consecutive, unselected autopsies, *Candida* spp. can be cultured from the lungs, histologic evidence of *Candida* spp. is seen in only 5 percent of these cases.

In the landmark report by Masur and associates, 30 patients were reported to have "significant," "contributory," or "insignificant" pulmonary involvement. The analysis was retrospective; the degree of involvement was based on the quantity of fungi present and the amount of lung involved, and it was discounted on the basis of other factors, e.g., tumor, hemorrhage, gastric aspiration, and other infection that compromised lung function. Disease was judged "significant" if more than 75 percent of at least two lobes were affected by *Candida* spp., and if the effect of *Candida* was "considerably greater" than that of hemorrhage, tumor, gastric aspiration, or "other factors" (presumably other microorganisms). "Contributory" classification applied when *Candida* spp. and other factors were more equally contributory, and "insignificant" applied when only a few microscopic foci (never more than four) were found.

By these criteria, the authors judged *Candida* spp. involvement to be significant in three and contributory in four of the 30 patients. All of the significant and one of the contributory cases resulted from aspiration; the other three contributory cases were caused by hematogenous spread. In only one of the seven was the cause of death disseminated candidosis.

In 10 patients the fungus was judged to have reached the lungs from hematogenous dissemination. Sixteen patients acquired disease from aspiration, and in four the route was "not obvious."

No roentgenographic pattern was observed that distinguished the route of *Candida* spp. infection from that of other disease or infection.

Candida organisms were cultured from the blood of only seven patients, but from none of the seven who were judged to have significant or contributory disease.

Candida spp. were cultured from the sputum of only nine patients (of 24 patients so tested), and from none of the five (so tested) who were judged to have significant or contributory disease.

Although no data were given, the authors believed that infection rarely compromised function. Moreover, infection usually occurred in areas previously damaged by hemorrhage, chemical pneumonitis, tumor, or other infection.

DIAGNOSIS

The difficulties of diagnosis by symptoms, physical findings, roentgenographic examination, sputum cultures, blood cultures, or serologic studies have already been documented.

One additional technique, lung biopsy, merits mention, even though it has not been helpful. In a study by Masur and colleagues, diagnosis by this means was documented in only one patient. In a larger study over a 5-year period, another group again uncovered only a single case. Other experience has confirmed this lack of utility.

MANAGEMENT

How can one treat a disease that is so infrequently significant and if that can be diagnosed so rarely and so imperfectly?

It has been customary in many institutions confronted with the problem of patients who are febrile and immunocompromised, especially by leukopenia, to begin prophylactic antifungal therapy. Regimens have included oral nystatin, oral and intravenous amphotericin B, oral flucytosine, oral clotrimazole, oral ketoconazole, or a combination of the aforementioned drugs. With intravenous amphotericin B, oral flucytosine, oral ketoconazole, and oral clotrimazole, serum levels of drug and systemic treatment can be expected, although only for a few days with the last agent.

Guidelines for the institution and discontinuation of such therapy have not evolved, and the opinion is pervasive that more treatment than necessary is being given. When controlled studies have been done, infection has occurred as frequently in systemically treated subjects as in those given a placebo. In less well controlled studies, some response (i.e., defervescence) has been seen after a few days of intravenous amphotericin B.

At some point, such prophylaxis becomes active treatment. For the most part, such active treatment is directed at hematogenously disseminated disease rather than disease localized to lung parenchyma.

Various options exist, but there is little unanimity as to which is best. Intravenous amphotericin B is probably still the gold standard. A minimal total dose should be 500 mg, and 1,000 to 1,500 mg, when the disease is confirmed by culture from the blood. It is not clear how the determination is derived, but combination with flucytosine is recommended when a rapidly fatal outcome is anticipated. Ketoconazole, though active in other forms of disease caused by *Candida* spp. is not generally used, since its oral route of administration leaves doubts as to absorption in the critically ill patient. Hence, there is a lack of data on experience and efficacy. When the patient cannot tolerate amphotericin B, which in my experience is rare considering the urgency of treatment and the dire results of no treatment, intravenous miconazole has been given.

Even less information about its use is available than for ketoconazole.

SUGGESTED READING

Anderson HA, Fontana RS. Transbronchial lung biopsy for diffuse pulmonary diseases. Techniques and results in 450 cases. Chest 1972; 62:125–128.

Beff SJ, McLelland R, Gallis HA, Mathay R, Pittman CE. *Candida albicans* pneumonia: radiographic appearance. Am J Roentgenol 1982; 138:645–648.

Brinker H. Prevention of mycosis in granulocytopenic patients with prophylactic ketoconazole treatment. A controlled study. Mykosen 1983; 26:242–247.

Emmons CW, Binford CH, Utz JP, Kwon-Chung KJ. Medical mycology. 3rd ed. Philadelphia: Lea & Febiger, 1977.

Hewitt CJ, Hull D, Keeling JW. Open lung biopsy in children with diffuse lung disease. Arch Dis Child 1974; 49:27–35.

Masur H, Rosen PP, Armstrong D. Pulmonary disease caused by *Candida* species. Am J Med 1977; 63:914–925.

Myerowitz RL. The pathology of opportunistic infections. New York: Raven Press, 1983.

Pagani JJ, Lifshitz HI. Opportunistic fungal pneumonias in cancer patients. Am J Roentgenol 1981; 137:1033–1039.

Pizzo PA, Robichaud KJ, Simon RM, Gill FA, Witebsky FG. Empiric antibiotic and antifungal therapy for cancer patients with prolonged fever and granulocytopenia. Am J Med 1982; 72:101–110.

Rippon JW. Medical mycology. 2nd ed. Philadelphia: WB Saunders, 1982.

Ryley JF. Pathogenicity of *Candida albicans* with particular reference to the vagina. J Med Vet Mycol 1986; 24:5–22.

Seelig MS, Kozin N. Clinical manifestations and management of candidosis in the immunocompromised patient. In: Warnock DW, Richardson MD, eds. Fungal infection in the compromised patient. Chichester: John Wiley & Sons, 1982:49.

INFECTION COMPLICATING IMMUNOSUPPRESSION

LOWELL S. YOUNG, M.D.

Patients may become immunosuppressed by two mechanisms: first, they may have an underlying condition with a defect in immune recognition or response. Secondly, they may receive medication or treatment such as x-rays which suppresses the immune system. Often both mechanisms contribute to a patient's susceptibility to infection. One may have a disorder such as a lymphoma or a leukemia and then receive treatment consisting of cytotoxic agents, anti-inflammatory agents such as corticosteroids, or radiation therapy, each of which can have a deleterious effect on the host immune response.

Table 1 lists examples of immunosuppressed states. This list is by no means all-inclusive, but it summarizes the major disorders associated with a blunted immune response and risk of developing opportunistic infection. It should be emphasized that increasing numbers of patients are receiving some type of medication that will impair humoral antibody synthesis, cellular immunity, or even the function of granulocytes. Many steroidal and non-steroidal anti-inflammatory agents will inhibit white cell mobilization; this defect is prominent in some of the collagen vascular disorders as well as in advanced alcoholic liver disease. Among the most commonly used medications that impair host defenses are adrenal corticosteroids. Their effect, fortunately, is dose dependent, and the risk of infection is small with doses equivalent to 100 mg of hydrocortisone per day or less.

CLINICAL SYNDROMES AND TYPES OF INFECTING ORGANISMS

Not surprisingly, microorganisms that cause serious infection in normal subjects, such as pneumococci, staphylococci, *Haemophilus influenzae*, and *Neisseria* species, can cause fulminant disease in immunosuppressed patients. Patients who are functionally asplenic or who are splenectomized (individuals, for instance, with Hodgkin's disease) are particularly susceptible to pneumococcal infections. Organisms of low intrinsic virulence, such as *Staphylococcus epidermidis*, may cause serious disease in immunosuppressed patients when associated with a foreign body such as an indwelling vascular catheter. Thus, the pathogenesis of disease in immunosuppressed patients is related to the intrinsic virulence of a potential pathogen and the degree to which host defenses are compromised. In the highly immunosuppressed patient, we see infections, such as disseminated aspergillosis and intestinal cryptosporidiosis, that are rarely if ever encountered in individuals with normal immune responses. In contrast, other processes that are quite common in the nor-

TABLE 1 Examples of Immunosuppressed States

Collagen vascular disease
Congenital immunodeficiency
Medications
Corticosteroids
Cyclosporine
Azathioprine
Alkylating agents
Antimetabolites
Neoplastic disease
Recipients of organ transplants

mal population, such as mycoplasmal pneumonia, are a rather infrequent problem in immunosuppressed subjects.

Clinical observations over the last two decades suggest that certain organisms are more likely to cause serious infections in immunosuppressed patients, and a background knowledge of the link between a clinical syndrome and a specific pathogen may be of some help in the early stages of clinical decision making. Table 2 summarizes some of these associations, but the list is not intended to be comprehensive.

Central nervous system infections result from bloodstream spread or by direct extension from infected sites adjacent to the brain, such as sinus cavities or the middle ear. The usual causes of meningitis in the normal population are group B streptococci, *Escherichia coli*, meningococci, and *H. influenzae* (often depending on age). In contrast, *Listeria monocytogenes* is the most common cause of bacterial meningitis in the immunosuppressed patient, and *Cryptococcus neoformans* is the most common fungal pathogen isolated from the spinal fluid. This is not to exclude a wide variety of other bacterial and fungal processes that usually result from bloodstream seeding, but these are rather less common than listeriosis and cryptococcosis. Among the most common causes of infection around the oropharynx in immunosuppressed patients are *Candida* species. Oral thrush is common but it may progress to a severe esophagitis that may necessitate systemic therapy. The association between esophagitis and *Candida* infections is well known, but two other organisms are gaining increasing prominence as causes of esophagitis: *Herpes simplex* virus and the cytomegalovirus.

One of the most dramatic clinical presentations in immunosuppressed patients is the sudden appearance of necrotizing vasculitis or cutaneous lesions that represent septic emboli. Perhaps best known are the cutaneous lesions of *Pseudomonas aeruginosa* septicemia, so-called ecthyma gangrenosum. Similar appearing lesions, however, may be caused by other gram-negative rods, particularly two other groups of organisms, the *Aeromonas* species and noncholera vibrios. *Staphylococcus aureus* has classically been associated with peripheral embolization, in which case one should strongly suspect an underlying bacterial endocarditis. Additionally, septic emboli and macronodular skin lesions are now well recognized as manifestations of the dissemination of *Candida* infections. *Aspergillus* species and other filamented fungi (*Mucor* species) can cause peripheral embolic lesions.

TABLE 2 Suggested Pathogens in Immunosuppressed Patients by Site of Involvement

Meningitis	*Listeria monocytogenes, Cryptococcus neoformans*
Esophagitis	*Candida sp., Herpes simplex,* cytomegalovirus
Necrotizing vasculitis	*Pseudomonas aeruginosa, Aeromonas* sp., noncholera vibrios
Septic emboli	*Candida* sp., *Aspergillus* sp., *Staphylococcus aureus*
Pneumonia	
Diffuse	*Pneumocystis carinii,* cytomegalovirus
Segmental, lobar	*Legionella pneumophila,* pneumococcus
Cavitary	*Aspergillus* sp., *Nocardia, Mucor* sp.
Diarrhea	*Salmonella*
	Giardia lamblia
	Antibiotic side effects
	Cryptosporidia
	Isospora belli

One of the greatest challenges in managing infectious complications in immunosuppressed subjects is the diagnosis and treatment of pneumonia. Although radiographs may readily identify lung infiltrates and the presence of pneumonia is further corroborated by physical findings, it is often difficult to establish the nature of a parenchymal lung abnormality without an invasive procedure. Sputum examination may be helpful in the patients who can cough and produce good material, but frequently contamination of respiratory secretions with oropharyngeal flora makes interpretation of culture results difficult. Two very important pulmonary pathogens in the immunosuppressed host, *Pneumocystis carinii* and *Legionella pneumophila*, may not be diagnosed by examination of expectorated sputum. The pattern of lung abnormality as suggested in Table 2 may occasionally be helpful in pointing toward diagnostic possibilities, but "pattern recognition" should not be relied on too heavily. *P. carinii* and cytomegalovirus are among the best appreciated causes of diffuse interstitial pneumonia, although technically *Pneumocystis* infection is usually a dense intra-alveolar inflammatory process. Lobar consolidation should still lead one to suspect pneumococcal disease, but *L. pneumophila* should now be high on the list of causes of a consolidative pulmonary process that develops in an immunosuppressed subject. The appearance of cavitary pneumonia in a patient who is severely neutropenic should lead to the suspicion of infection caused by a filamented fungus, such as one of the *Aspergillus* species. However, other fungi besides *Aspergillus* can cause an identical picture. These fungi belong to the *Mucor* group or are *Petriellidium boydii*. As organism now classified as a higher bacterium, *Nocardia asteroides*, can cause lung abscess plus multiple abscesses elsewhere in the body, such as in subcutaneous regions and the brain.

A wide variety of bacterial pathogens that cause diarrhea in normal hosts must be considered in evaluating diarrhea in immunosuppressed hosts. Outbreaks of salmonellosis have occurred among hospitalized immunosuppressed patients exposed to a common food source. Parasitic pathogens are increasingly recognized, including *Strongyloides stercoralis*, *Giardia lamblia*, and most recently, cryptosporidiosis or *Isospora* infection (the latter two now strikingly associated with the acquired immunodeficiency syndrome). Clinicians should not overlook the fact that diarrhea in immunosuppressed subjects is commonly a complication of antimicrobial therapy. The diarrhea and possible associated colitis may be the results of a toxin-producing *Clostridium* species.

DIAGNOSTIC APPROACHES

One of the cardinal errors in the management of immunosuppressed patients is the hasty administration of antimicrobial agents before appropriate diagnostic studies, including cultures, are done. Aggressive intervention with antibiotics may be lifesaving, but careful sampling of blood and body fluids prior to antibiotic intervention should be strongly emphasized. In the case of lung infections, premature or hasty intervention with antimicrobial agents may interfere with ability to diagnose an intrapulmonary process such as *Pneumocystis* infection. The care of immunosuppressed patients requires a well-organized team effort. The team should include specialists of many disciplines, including surgery. Invasive operation procedures such as organ biopsy sampling may be necessary to obtain a definitive diagnosis. Skilled laboratory workers are also required to perform special studies on any material obtained by an invasive procedure.

THERAPEUTIC SELECTIONS

While I have emphasized the need for appropriate diagnostic studies, the decision to initiate antimicrobial therapy may have to be made very rapidly. Those factors that must be considered are the patient's underlying disease and stage of underlying disease, physical findings, blood pressure, magnitude of body temperature, respiratory rate, and any clue to a rapidly progressing infectious process. If sepsis, meningitis, or severe pneumonia is diagnosed, therapeutic intervention should be considered within a matter of minutes.

Table 3 lists suggested choices for the initial therapy of suspected bacterial septicemia, meningitis, pneumonia, and intra-abdominal infection. The choices are conventional, and the reader should consult more detailed sources for further information on dosages and dose adjustments. For the neutropenic patient, my preference is to give an aminoglycoside such as gentamicin or tobramycin (5 mg per kilogram per day) or amikacin (15 mg per kilogram per day) combined with an antipseudomonal penicillin such as mezlocillin (16 g per day) or piperacillin (12 g per day). Alternatively, ceftazidime (6 g per day) plus an aminoglycoside may be used. The neutropenic patient is defined as an individual with a white count of 1,000 normal neutrophils per cubic millimeter or less, or one whose white count is progressively falling by a factor of ½ on successive days as a result of immunosuppressive and/or cytotoxic chemotherapy. For the non-neutropenic patient in whom staphylococci may be a stronger consideration, the combination of an aminoglycoside plus a first-generation cephalosporin or vancomycin is preferred. Alternative antistaphylococcal medications include first-generation cephalosporins and vancomycin.

TABLE 3 Recommended Antimicrobial Therapy for Infection Developing During Immunosuppression

Bacterial Sepsis
Neutropenic patient (neutrophil count < 1000 mm^3): anti pseudomonal penicillin plus aminoglycoside or antipseudomonal cephalosporin plus aminoglycoside
Non-neutropenic patient third-generation cephalosporin or imipenem
Meningitis
Ampicillin plus third generation* cephalosporin
Pneumonia
Same for bacterial sepsis unless *Staphylococcus aureus* isolated (then use oxacillin)
Trimethoprim-sulfamethoxazole for *Pneumocystis carinii* infection
Erythromycin for *Legionella* infection
Intra-abdominal Infection
Aminoglycoside plus clindamycin, metronidazole, cefoxitin, or broad-spectrum penicillin
Fungal Infection
Amphotericin B ± flucytosine

* Cefotaxime or ceftriaxone

Any immunosuppressed patient who develops evidence of meningitis but in whom spinal fluid examination fails to identify the cause should be empirically treated with a regimen that includes ampicillin, 12 g per day, until results of cultures are known. Ampicillin will be effective against *L. monocytogenes* and pneumococci but is now less reliable against *H. influenzae*. Suspicion of *H. influenzae* should lead to a prescription of a third-generation cephalosporin such as cefotaxime in a dose of 12 g per day; alternatively, ceftriaxone in a dose of 2 g intravenously every 12 hours one day, followed by 2 g per day, may be substituted. If *P. aeruginosa* is the central nervous system pathogen, ceftazidime in a dose of 4 g every 8 hours (12 g total) should be combined with an intravenous aminoglycoside. Although chloramphenicol has traditionally been cited as an effective agent against gram-negative bacillary infections of the central nervous system, the activity of the newer cephalosporins and related compounds is broader.

Treatment of pneumonia is a complex subject that is covered in other chapters of this book. In the immunosuppressed patient, the likelihood of gram-negative infection is high. Combination therapy with an aminoglycoside and a beta-lactam agent is recommended. Choices include an antipseudomonal penicillin or one of the newer cephalosporins such as ceftazidime that is active against *Pseudomonas*, *Klebsiella*, and *Serratia* species. Trimethoprim-sulfamethoxazole is the initial agent of choice for the treatment of *P. carinii* pneumonia. It is also effective against a wide variety of bacteria, including most of the gram-negative bacilli except *P. aeruginosa*. This agent should be used at an initial dose of 10 to 15 mg per kilogram per day (calculated in terms of trimethoprim).

Intra-abdominal infections are not particularly common in immunosuppressed patients unless there is trauma, tumor, or some other "mechanical" disruption that results in sudden soilage of the abdominal or pelvic cavities with fecal contents. Therapeutic regimens should include an aminoglycoside for the gram-negative rods and clindamycin, chloramphenicol, metronidazole, or one of the newer penicillins or cephalosporins that are active against the abundant anaerobes in bowel flora.

The choice of agents for treatment of fungal infection is extremely limited. Amphotericin B is the only broadly active antifungal agent that might be used for empiric therapy, and there are serious untoward effects associated with use of the compound. Amphotericin B is usually recommended in a dosage of 1 mg per kilogram per day, but this dosage can rarely be tolerated for a long period of time; a more realistic dosage is 0.7 mg per kilogram per day. The latter target dosage cannot be used initially, but a daily dosage is achieved by successive incremental doses of 5 mg of intravenous amphotericin (for example, a test dose of 1 mg followed daily by 5, 10, 15 mg, and so on until the target dosage is reached). The total recommended dose of amphotericin B for systemic infection if often given as 2 g, but patients with hematologic malignancies who achieve remission can be treated with less. The addition of flucytosine may be beneficial in cases of yeast infection, such as those caused by *Candida* species and *C. neoformans*. A new azole, fluconazole, appears effective against central nervous system cryptococcis and other systemic yeast infections; the maximal dose may be up to 400 mg per day orally. Some viral infections, such as those due to *Herpes simplex* or varicella-zoster, may be treated with acyclovir or adenine arabinoside.

Preventive regimens vary from the well accepted to the controversial. Any immunosuppressed patient who has a history of old tuberculosis (untreated) or a positive tuberculin test and Ghon complex on chest x-ray film should be a candidate for isoniazid prophylaxis. Trimethoprim-sulfamethoxazole is effective prophylactically against *P. carinii* in leukemics. There have been many studies of the use of trimethoprim-sulfamethoxazole for the prevention of bacterial infection in neutropenic patients. The results have been quite variable, and the agent could not be expected to prevent *P. aeruginosa* infection. In institutions where the incidence of resistance to trimethoprim-sulfamethoxazole is low and relatively few *P. aeruginosa* infections occur, prophylactic use may be efficacious. The usual adult dosage is 160 to 320 mg of trimethoprim (with a comparable five times that amount of sulfamethoxazole) given twice daily. Alternatively, a quinolone such as ciprofloxacin, 500 mg orally trice a day, or norfloxacin, 400 orally twice daily, provides effective suppression of the gastrointestinal flora and can minimize the development of bacterial infection. Topical nystatin is often used to prevent localized (upper gastrointestinal tract) and vaginal candidal colonization, but patient compliance may be poor. Ketoconazole is a systemically absorbed oral agent that is fungistatic and exerts a satisfactory long-term suppressive effect in patients with chronic mucocutaneous candidiasis (in a dosage of 200 to 600 mg daily). Its efficacy when used prophylactically in severely immunosuppressed patients is unclear.

A small proportion of patients who are immunosuppressed have quantitative or qualitative defects in circulating immunoglobulins. Patients with congenital hypogammaglobulinemia or acquired hypogammaglobulinemia have benefited from routine monthly or twice monthly injections of intramuscular gammaglobulins. Preparations of IgG that have been modified for intravenous use have become available, but their prophylactic role has been best established in a limited number of diseases such as chronic lymphatic leukemia where hypogammaglobulinemia is to be expected.

OTHER ASPECTS OF THE PROBLEM

This short review cannot provide an adequate discussion of the role of "protected environments" in preventing infections, nor the use of therapeutic or prophylactic granulocyte transfusions in immunosuppressed patients. In summary, it can be stated that both are rarely indicated in the management of immunosuppressed patients. In the case of prophylactic granulocyte transfusions, the evidence suggests that the complications far outweigh the anticipated benefits. Use of granulocyte transfusions does not appear to be indicated in the neutropenic patient unless there is a documented bacterial infection that fails to respond to appropriate antimicrobial therapy. Recombinant cytokines, such as the granulocyte or granulocyte-macrophage colony-stimulating factors may be more effective in restoring circulating neutrophil counts. "Protected environments" may be defined in many ways, but most are designed as strict isolation units with filtered air. Although it is associated with reduced rates of infection, patient management in a protected environment seems to have had little impact on treatment of the underlying disease.

A final point for emphasis is that the outcome of the management of infection in immunosuppressed patients is critically related to control of the underlying disease. Thus, the onset of infection in cancer patients should not deter appropriately designed antineoplastic therapy as long as adequate treatment of the infectious complication is also given. On the other hand, a documented infection complicating therapeutic immunosuppression, such as that given to a renal transplant recipient to prevent graft rejection, is the signal for temporary reduction in the immunosuppressive treatment.

SUGGESTED READING

EORTC International Antimicrobial Therapy Cooperative Group. Ceftazidime combined with a short or long course of amikacin for empirical therapy of gram-negative bacteremia in cancer patients with granulocytopenia. N Engl J Med 1987; 317:1692.

Rubin RH, Young LS. Clinical approach to infections in the compromised host. 2nd ed. New York: Plenum, 1988.

Young LS. Empirical antimicrobial therapy in the neutropenic host. N Engl J Med 1986; 315:580–581.

INTRAVASCULAR CATHETER-ASSOCIATED INFECTION

CYRUS C. HOPKINS, M.D.

Infection associated with intravascular catheters can involve several different parts of the system: the entry site of the catheter into the skin, the subcutaneous tissue between the skin entry site and the vessel, the intravascular portion of the catheter, or the intraluminal fluid within the catheter, tubing, bottle or bag, or pressure transducers.

Infection at each of these sites has its own likely organisms and may appear with different clinical presentations. The skin entry site is probably the most common site of entry of the organism. Clinically significant infection at this site may present as a purulent cellulitis centered around the entry site. Colonization of this site and extension through the subcutaneum to the intravascular catheter segment can occur without signs of infection. In the case of a "tunneled" catheter with a long subcutaneous segment, tunnel infection alone may occur, in which case a red streak of apparent cellulitis is often visible. Infection may involve the intravascular segment alone, either serving as a focus of origin or as a nidus for adherence of organisms hematogenously disseminated to it from another source. Finally, some species will grow readily within the fluid itself, which provides logarithmic growth, yielding a high inoculum of organisms (usually gram-negative bacilli) or a source of endotoxin.

DIAGNOSIS

Appropriate treatment rests on clinical suspicion, for most primary clinical diagnoses of catheter-associated infections are diagnoses of exclusion, except for the few catheter entry-site or tunnel infections, which are clinically manifest at the site. Fevers—or septic signs occurring in hospital in a patient with intravascular catheters—should always raise the question of a catheter-associated infection but are statistically far more likely to be caused by infections at other common sites of nosocomial infection, such as the catheterized urinary tract, the surgical wound, or the lower respiratory tract. Initial evaluation, then, rests on a complete history, focusing on recent in-hospital events, and physical and laboratory examination of the most commonly infected sites. During this initial evaluation, the catheter site should be examined and inquiries made into the duration of use of any indwelling catheter; the frequency of change of fluids, tranducers, and tubings; and any recent manipulation of the catheter.

TREATMENT

The general principle of therapy involves: (1) search for the organism by blood culture, Gram stain, and culture of drainage (if any) and, in some instances, culture of the intravenous fluids; (2) in general, removal of the catheter; (3) then, but before waiting for culture results, initiation of broad-spectrum antibiotics, especially covering for *Staphylococcus aureus* unless otherwise guided by the results of the above; and finally, (4) simplification of the antibiotics when culture results become available.

If erythema and purulence are found, the catheter is removed whenever possible. Peripheral or non-tunneled catheters should always be removed, and purulent drainage should be Gram stained and cultured. Occasionally, a trial of therapy can be successful for tunneled, hard-to-replace catheters (Hickman, Broviac). Blood cultures should also be obtained before treatment is begun (Fig. 1).

If only local signs of erythema and tenderness are found without any signs of systemic sepsis, a non-tunneled catheter should be removed, and a short course of oral antibiotics, such as dicloxacillin, 500 mg orally four times a day, can be used.

If no local signs of catheter-related infection are found, the search for other unrelated sites should continue. Physical examination, chest roentgenogram, urinalysis, and inspection of wound sites should be performed to exclude other sites. Blood cultures should be obtained. If another focus is found, Gram stain and culture of material reflecting this site should be performed and treatment of this focus begun.

If blood cultures are positive for the same organism found in another infected site (urine, wound, sputum), and if the clinical course is favorable with appropriately directed therapy, the catheter need not be removed, unless the bacteremia-causing organisms are staphylococci (either coagulase-positive or coagulase-negative). If so, the catheter should then be removed and cultured. If not, the underlying infection should be treated and the catheter and catheter changes handled in a routine manner and then reevaluated. Catheters removed for documented sepsis should not be changed over a guidewire, as infection of the new catheter remains a risk.

If the catheter remains in place, treatment should generally begin with vancomycin, until *Staphylococcus epidermidis,* or even methicillin-resistant *S. aureus* (MRSA) has been excluded by culture results.

If the initial evaluation reveals signs of severe sepsis of sudden onset, such as septic shock, the intravenous fluid should be immediately suspected. In that case, all intravascular lines, tubing, and fluid sources should be removed and saved intact for culture and identification. Treatment must include both vancomycin (in case of MRSA) and an aminoglycoside, since there is little margin for error.

Antibiotic Selection

Always begin with antistaphylococcal therapy (nafcillin 1 g intravenously every 4 hours or cefazolin 1 g intravenously every 8 hours), then revise or add aminoglycosides (gentamicin, 1.5 mg per kg per dose) if gram-negative rods are found on Gram stain or culture of drainage of blood. If MRSA is known to be present in the institution, or if the catheter must be retained, treatment is better begun with vancomycin (2 g per day, for an adult with normal renal func-

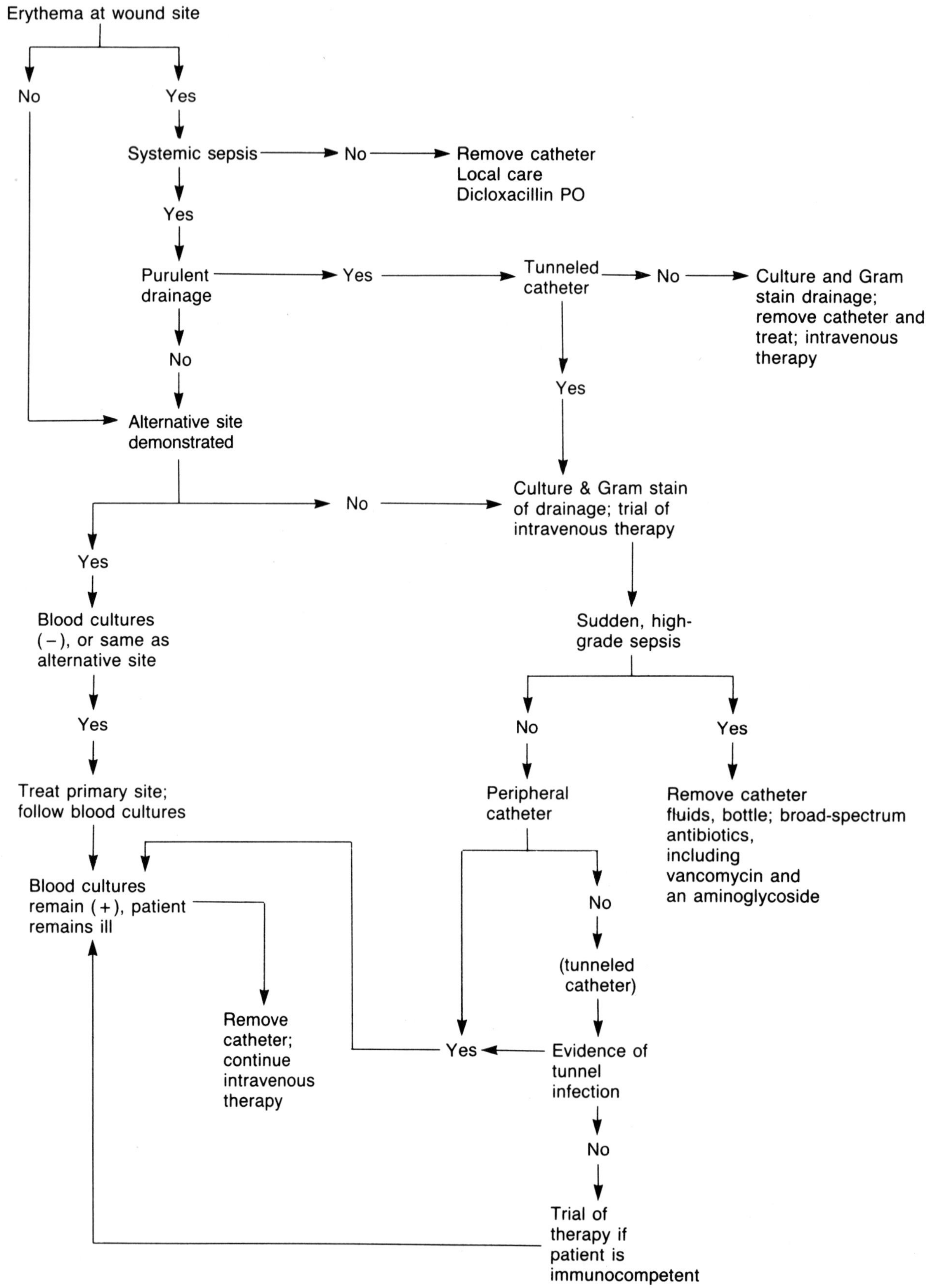

Figure 1 Possible infection in a patient with indwelling intravascular catheter.

tion). If yeasts are found in blood cultures, amphotericin B is the drug of choice.

Duration

The duration of therapy is not well defined. Prolonged *Staphylococcus aureus* bacteremia requires 4 weeks of intravenous therapy with a penicillinase-resistant semisynthetic penicillin (oxacillin, nafcillin), a first-generation cephalosporin (cefazolin), or vancomycin. If the infection has been detected promptly and the offending catheter is immediately removed, and if no hardware is present, many experts recommend only 2 weeks of therapy, assuming that the patient responds promptly (bacteremia with a removable focus). In this era of increasing use of home delivery of intravenous antibiotics, I use this shorter course only infrequently. Coagulase-negative staphylococci will require 4 weeks of treatment only if other indwelling hardware is present (e.g., prosthetic cardiac valves). Gram-negative bacteremia usually requires up to 3 weeks of therapy, depending on the response of the patient. Management of fungal sepsis is also unclear: fundoscopic examination should be performed initially and later in the course. If the fundi show no evidence of candidal infection, 500 mg (total dose) of amphotericin B will suffice for an immunocompetent patient, but there are no good data to guide us on this at this time.

Failure of Treatment

Failure to respond to appropriate therapy requires reevaluation of several clinical issues, especially the certainty of the diagnosis, the exclusion of other sites, and whether secondary endocarditis or septic phlebitis is likely. Reexamination of the site is critical; persistent pain and induration over the involved vein and signs of impaired venous drainage (especially for central catheters) prompt consideration of septic phlebitis. "Milking" the involved vein toward the insertion will occasionally produce purulent drainage. Persistent purulence, induration, and lack of response necessitate surgical involvement.

SPECIAL PROBLEMS

Hyperalimentation solutions provide a source (presumably because they provide a special growth medium) for organisms not often associated with septicemia, such as *Candida albicans* or similar yeasts, or, especially in infants, *Malassezia furfur*. In both cases, initial conventional blood cultures may be negative. The catheter should be removed and blood cultures performed with special techniques, such as lysis-centrifugation, which may have a higher yield. Comparing colony counts on specimens obtained through the catheter versus peripheral specimens may allow some prediction of whether the catheter is the source. If fungal infection is a possibility, Gram stain of the catheter may be helpful, since it may be positive even though blood cultures are negative.

Hickman, Broviac, and other central tunneled catheters become infected much less frequently than do peripheral catheters or other centrally inserted catheters. There is increasing evidence that treatment of an intravascular site, or even of the entry site alone, may often be successfully completed even if the catheter is left in place. Infections along the track of the tunneled catheter, however, particularly if caused by gram-negative bacilli, are unlikely to respond, and the catheter will have to be removed. Bacteremia in children with a Hickman catheter in place will often be cured without removing the catheter. There are inadequate data to guide us in adults.

Immunocompromised patients may develop catheter-associated sepsis with a wide variety of organisms. Positive blood cultures, or even fever of unclear origin in a catheterized patient, should be followed by removal of the catheter. New skin lesions, especially at the entry site, but even peripherally, should be biopsied.

SUGGESTED READING

Allo MD, Miller J, Townsend T, et al. Primary cutaneous aspergillosis associated with Hickman intravenous catheters. N Engl J Med 1987; 317:1105–1108.

Benezra D, Kiehn TE, Gold JWM, et al. Prospective study of infections in indwelling central venous catheters using quantitative blood cultures. Am J Med 1988; 85:495–498.

Bernhardt LL, Antopol SC, Simberkoff MS, et al. Association of teichoic acid antibody with metastatic sequelae of catheter-associated Staphylococcus aureus bacteremia. A failure of the two-week antibiotic treatment. Am J Med 1979; 66:355–357.

Pettigrew RA, Lang SDR, Haydock DA, et al. Catheter-related sepsis in patients on intravenous nutrition: a prospective study of quantitative catheter cultures and guidewire changes for suspected sepsis. Br J Surg 1985; 72:52–55.

Raucher HS, Hyatt AC, Barzilai A, et al. Quantitative blood cultures in the evaluation of septicemia in children with Broviac catheters. J Pediatr 1984; 104:29–33.

Walsh TJ, Bustamente CI, Vlahov D, et al. Candidal suppurative peripheral thrombophlebitis: recognition, prevention, and management. Infect Control 1986; 7:16–32.

CARDIOVASCULAR DISEASES

ACUTE PULMONARY EDEMA

DAVID T. KAWANISHI, M.D.
SHAHBUDIN H. RAHIMTOOLA, M.B., F.R.C.P.

Acute pulmonary edema is the abrupt accumulation of fluid in the lungs resulting either from high intravascular pressure (cardiogenic pulmonary edema) or from increased permeability of the alveolar-capillary membrane, which allows rapid fluid extravasation (noncardiogenic pulmonary edema). In the clinical setting many forms of pulmonary edema will have some component of both because it is difficult to affect vessel permeability without affecting pressures at the microvascular level and vice versa. However, it is important to determine the nature of the predominant underlying disorder to guide the direction of therapy.

THERAPEUTIC ALTERNATIVES

Treatment of acute pulmonary edema may range from use of simple general measures to extremely invasive and costly interventional maneuvers or mechanical support (Table 1). General measures that may be employed quickly may produce a rapid improvement in comfort and in the condition of the patient and include placement of the patient in a semi-upright position, application of supplemental oxygen, careful use of intravenous morphine, and titration of intravenous aminophylline, particularly if the patient is wheezing. Simple nonpharmacologic measures for reduction of venous return to the heart, such as rotating tourniquets or phlebotomy, are used less often in the modern medical setting owing to the improved effectiveness of medications. Failure to respond to these general measures usually requires that the patient be intubated, suctioned vigorously to aid in clearing the copious secretions, and mechanically ventilated.

Subsequent specific therapy should be directed at the underlying cause of the acute pulmonary edema and any aggravating factors. Alternatives directed at improving cardiovascular hemodynamics include administration of positive inotropic medications, preload reducing agents, and afterload reducing agents. Proper selection and adjustment of dosage usually requires measurement of pulmonary vascular pressure and cardiac output using a thermodilution pulmonary artery catheter. The potential of calcium entry blockers to improve diastolic compliance may be of added benefit and may be considered as a therapeutic adjunct when they are employed for vasodilation or for heart rate control. When the underlying cardiac disorder is extreme, the pulmonary edema may not respond or may improve incompletely until definitive correction of the disorder can be achieved. In these cases, identification of the underlying disorder becomes of paramount importance. Intervention with temporary artificial pacing for bradyarrhythmias or intra-aortic balloon pumping for ischemic heart disease, for example, may help to stabilize the patient's condition temporarily. Definitive correction of such cardiac disorders, however, often requires additional maneuvers, such as implantation of a permanent pacemaker or coronary reperfusion with percutaneous coronary angioplasty or bypass surgery, respectively, unless the acute pulmonary edema was precipitated by a correctable aggravating condition. Other examples of therapy for specific disorders include surgical valve reconstruction or implantation of a prosthesis for acute regurgitant valve lesions and pericardiocentesis and pericardial window or pericardiectomy for tamponade.

TABLE 1 General Therapeutic Measures in Acute Pulmonary Edema

Semi-upright position
Supplemental oxygen
Intravenous morphine
Intravenous aminophylline
Rotating tourniquets
Phlebotomy
Intubation, mechanical ventilation

PREFERRED APPROACH

Medical Treatment

Initial therapy of acute pulmonary edema is directed toward improving pulmonary gas exchange. Once the condition of acute pulmonary edema is recognized, immediate implementation of general supportive measures using semi-upright positioning of the patient and administration of supplemental oxygen is indicated. Measurement of blood pressure and assessment of peripheral perfusion should be made at the earliest opportunity because associated hypotension or hypoperfusion or both suggests the need for a more global cardiovascular approach to therapy as in the case of cardiogenic shock. In the early stages of pulmonary edema, arterial oxygen saturation is depressed with an associated hyperventilation that may decrease carbon dioxide; therefore, supplemental 50 percent oxygen administered via nasal prongs at rates of 6 to 8 liters per minute may suffice. Use of Venturi masks or reservoir bag masks may improve delivery. With progression of the condition, the patient may become cyanotic, increasingly dyspneic, and tachypneic, and pulmonary rales become more prominent. When available, measurement of blood gases should be used to guide therapy, although advanced therapy should not be delayed in the presence of clinical deterioration. Inability to maintain a PaO_2 at 60 mm Hg or better, even at high supplemental oxygen concentrations and flow rates; evidence of carbon dioxide retention; clinical evidence of hypoventilation; or inability to clear the edema fluid and secretions adequately suggests the need for endotracheal intubation, suctioning, and mechanical ventilation.

If the pulmonary edema is secondary to damage to the alveolar-capillary membranes, further medical treatment may include use of positive end-expiratory pressure (PEEP) to maintain or improve arterial blood oxygen concentrations. Use of PEEP may reduce venous return and increase the afterload of the right ventricle, with a resultant decrease of cardiac output. An even more pronounced depression of cardiac output may occur in the presence of some cardiac disorders. Monitoring of pulmonary artery and wedge pressures along with cardiac output is essential in these patients. Another potential complication of PEEP is barotrauma resulting in pneumomediastinum, pneumothorax, and subcutaneous emphysema. The patient may also benefit by maintenance of pulmonary artery wedge pressures at as low a pressure as possible, to decrease the rate of pulmonary edema fluid extravasation, as long as cardiac output is not compromised. Finally, treatment of any reversible causes of alveolar-capillary membrane injury, such as pneumonia, may hasten the healing process.

If the cause of the acute pulmonary edema is a cardiac disorder, additional measures to improve hemodynamics may be essential (Table 2). Intravenous morphine sulfate is in general very helpful as a supportive measure for cardiogenic pulmonary edema. In addition to improving patient comfort, reduction of central sympathetic activity may result in venous and arteriolar dilation. An initial dose of 3 to 5 mg repeated approximately every 15 minutes to a total of 15 mg is generally effective. Reduction of dosages is advisable in the elderly and in individuals with very small body habitus. For persons with large body habitus or for young or extremely agitated individuals, larger doses may be needed to effect improvement. Morphine sulfate may produce depression of respiratory effort and should be used cautiously or avoided entirely when ventilation may be compromised, as in patients with altered consciousness, intracranial hemorrhage, or bronchial or chronic pulmonary disease or when there is carbon dioxide retention.

If the patient with pulmonary edema has associated bronchospasm and is wheezing, intravenous aminophylline should be considered as part of the initial treatment regimen. Because of its bronchodilating action, it is indicated particularly if there is uncertainty whether the breathlessness is due to an attack of bronchial asthma or is a result of cardiogenic pulmonary edema. In patients with the latter, aminophylline also has the beneficial effects of stimulation of myocardial systolic function, venodilation, and production of a mild diuresis. The initial intravenous dose of aminophylline is 5 mg per kilogram given over 10 to 15 minutes, followed by an infusion of 0.9 mg per kilogram per hour in a patient not previously given aminophylline or related preparations. In patients already taking theophylline, for example, the infusion rate should be reduced to approximately 0.5 mg per kilogram per hour. The latter infusion rate, or occasionally even slower rates, may be indicated in the elderly and in those with hepatic or renal dysfunction. Agitation, marked tachycardia and arrhythmias, nausea and vomiting, hypotension, headaches, and seizures occur when aminophylline levels rise toward toxicity. With maintenance of infusion beyond 12 hours, aminophylline dosage should be adjusted according to measured blood levels of the drug.

Reduction of preload is a desirable therapeutic objective in cardiogenic pulmonary edema and can be accomplished initially by employing rotating tourniquets. Wide rubber tourniquets or, preferably, blood pressure cuffs should be used, with the objective being to inflate to just below the arterial diastolic pressure and thus to allow arterial inflow but restrict venous outflow. Placed proximally at three of the four limbs, the tourniquets should be released every 15 to 20 minutes, and one of the tourniquets should be rotated to the free extremity at that time. Although in most cases drug therapy alone may produce satisfactory improvement, rotating tourniquets

TABLE 2 Measures for Improvement of Cardiac Function in Cardiogenic Pulmonary Edema

Functional Derangement	*Medical*	*Interventional/Surgical*
Heart rate/rhythm		
Tachyarrhythmia	Digitalis, calcium entry blockers, cardioversion, antiarrhythmics	
Bradyarrhythmia	Isoproterenol	Artificial pacemaker
Loss of A-V synchrony	Cardioversion	A-V sequential pacemaker
Myocardial systolic function		
Inadequate	Digitalis, aminophylline, isoproterenol, epinephrine, norepinephrine, dopamine, dobutamine, amrinone	Intra-aortic balloon pump, coronary reperfusion via CABG
Excessive (as in hypertrophic cardiomyopathy)	Propranolol, disopyramide	
Myocardial diastolic function	Anti-ischemic, antianginal therapy; calcium-entry blockers	Intra-aortic balloon pump, coronary reperfusion via PTCA or CABG, pericardiocentesis, pericardiectomy
Volume excess or maldistribution	Diuretics, digitalis, aminophylline, nitrates, nitroprusside, angiotensin converting enzyme inhibitors, rotating tourniquets, morphine	Valve surgery, catheter balloon valvuloplasty
Hypertension or excessive resistance to ventricular outflow	Nitroprusside, phentolamine, trimethaphan, hydralazine, angiotensin converting enzyme inhibitors, morphine	Intra-aortic balloon pump, valve surgery, catheter balloon valvuloplasty
Regional wall motion abnormality due to myocardial ischemia	Improve arterial Po_2; reduce MVO_2 by: slowing tachycardia, preload reduction, afterload reduction; increase cardiac output and correct hypotension	Intra-aortic balloon pump, PTCA, CABG

A-V = Atrioventricular, CABG = coronary artery bypass graft, PTCA = percutaneous transluminal coronary angioplasty.

may occasionally hasten or be a helpful adjunct in helping to resolve the pulmonary edema.

A potent loop diuretic such as furosemide may be very useful in treatment of most cases of cardiogenic pulmonary edema, and its initial beneficial effect is probably also preload reduction through venodilation. As a general rule, drugs should be administered intravenously in these patients because there may be significant constriction of many vascular beds, making absorption via oral, subcutaneous, or intramuscular routes less reliable or predictable. An initial dose of 40 to 60 mg should be given, and improvement resulting from its vasoactive property may be expected even before the onset of diuresis. Diuresis may begin as rapidly as 5 minutes. In some patients, the diuresis may be massive, with several liters of urine being produced over 0.5 to 2 hours. In others, especially when renal function is compromised, repeated incrementally doubled doses of 80 and 160 mg of furosemide may be given until diuresis is initiated. Alternatively, intravenous ethacrynic acid at an initial dose of 50 mg or bumetanide 0.5 to 1.0 mg may occasionally produce diuresis when there is no response to furosemide. In some cases, as in frank renal failure, the only way to effect reduction of fluid volume may be dialysis. An early potential complication of diuretic treatment is a marked reduction of intravascular volume, resulting in a catastrophic fall of cardiac output, especially when ventricular function is depressed and is unusually preload dependent. Later, hypokalemia, hyponatremia, alkalosis, and hyperuricemia may occur. The elderly, dehydrated, or malnourished patient or those on chronic diuretic regimens may be particularly susceptible to such complications.

If diuresis is inadequate to produce a resolution or a satisfactorily rapid improvement of the pulmonary edema, or as an added initial maneuver when a rapid response is desired, additional reduction of preload may be achieved using nitrates to produce venodilation. Nitroglycerin 0.4 mg sublingually has a rapid onset of action of 2 minutes or less and may produce a reduction in pulmonary artery wedge pressure within 5 to 10 minutes. It has the advantage of not requiring vascular access for administration, but it has the disadvantage of a short (approximately 15 minutes) duration of effect. When venous access becomes available, titration of intravenous nitroglycerin as an infusion beginning at 10 μg per minute may be used to maintain venodilation. Tolerance to nitroglycerin may develop rapidly, within 24 hours, and infusion rates should be adjusted according to measured pulmonary artery wedge pressure if sustained nitrate therapy is indicated. Nitrates are very potent venodilators and may lead to excessive reduction of cardiac output when ventricular function is unusually preload dependent, as in acute myocardial infarction, especially with large infarctions of the left ventricle or when the right ventricle is involved.

When there is evidence of depressed cardiac output, and especially when systemic vascular resistance is known to be increased in the patient with pulmonary edema, intravenous nitroprusside should be used to obtain arterial dilation as well as venodilation. As a result, both systemic and pulmonary artery pressures may be lowered quickly. Preferably, arterial pressure should be directly monitored through an indwelling arterial catheter along with pulmonary pressures and cardiac output through a thermodilution pulmonary artery catheter when using nitroprusside. However, if the patient is frankly hypertensive, nitroprusside should be initiated immediately as arrangements for monitoring are being made. In such a hypertensive patient, initial sublingual nitroglycerin immediately followed by intravenous nitroprusside may be the preferred sequence of therapy. An initial infusion of 8 to 10 μg per minute should be increased by increments of 5 to 10 μg per minute at intervals as short as 5 minutes, until the desired pulmonary artery wedge pressure, cardiac output, systemic resistance, or systemic arterial pressure is achieved. Individuals with underlying systemic hypertension may require larger doses, whereas patients with diminutive stature, the elderly, or those with severely depressed ventricular function may require very precise and careful titration of relatively small doses of nitroprusside. Although the usual maximum dose of nitroprusside is in the range of 500 μg per minute, it may be considerably less in the latter types of patients as well as in those with renal failure, in whom the thiocyanate metabolites of nitroprusside may accumulate to toxic levels.

The angiotensin converting enzyme inhibitors captopril, enalapril, and possibly lisinopril appear to have an increasingly valuable role in treatment of chronic heart failure. In addition to blockade of the renin-angiotensin system, they may also act by increasing the level of vasodilating prostaglandins. Their role, if any, in the treatment of acute pulmonary edema has not been established. They may be significant, however, as a potential aggravating factor in patients with chronic underlying cardiac disease who are under chronic therapy with these agents because their use may be associated with a deterioration of renal function.

Intravenous administration of a short-acting cardiac glycoside is still a mainstay of treatment in patients with cardiogenic pulmonary edema. It should be a part of the initial regimen, particularly when the pulmonary edema is associated with atrial fibrillation or other supraventricular tachyarrhythmias in patients in whom the pulmonary vascular pressures are increased as a result of a shortened diastole and elevation of left atrial pressure. The patient with mitral stenosis is the prototypical example of this situation. Digoxin acts by increasing the effective refractory period and reducing the ventricular response rate. Occasionally, it may result in conversion to sinus rhythm. Digoxin may also be considered as initial therapy in patients with pulmonary edema and impaired systolic left ventricular function, especially when cardiomegaly is present. Such patients will benefit from the positive inotropic effect and mild diuretic effect of digoxin. If the patient has not previously been receiving digoxin, an intravenous loading dose of 0.5 mg should be given over 15 minutes to avoid the possibility of systemic or coronary arterial vasoconstriction with a too-rapid infusion. Subsequently, 0.25 mg may be given every 6 hours to a total of 1.0 to 1.5 mg, depending on the adequacy of the clinical response. In general, even those patients previously receiving digoxin may benefit from additional drug when they develop acute pulmonary edema, as long as there is no evidence of toxicity, and especially when the deterioration is due to supraventricular tachyarrhythmias with accelerated ventricular response. However, such patients should be examined carefully prior to administration of additional digoxin for manifestations of digitalis toxicity, such as nausea and vomiting, accelerated nonparoxysmal junctional tachycardia, atrial tachycardia with intermittent atrioventricular nodal block, premature ventricular complexes, ventricular tachycardia, bradycardia, and heart block. In the presence of hypokalemia, severe renal failure, or both, extreme caution should be used when giving intravenous digitalis preparations, or it may be avoided entirely. Oral diltiazem in doses of 30 to 90 mg may provide additional blockade of the atrioventricular node and may be a useful adjunct to the digoxin regimen if additional rate-slowing is needed.

If the aforementioned regimens are ineffective, use of the positive inotropic agents dopamine or dobutamine may be considered. Intravenous dopamine infused at 2 to 5 μg per kilogram per minute improves myocardial contractility, and by decreasing peripheral resistance and improving renal blood flow, it may help to initiate diuresis when previous efforts have failed. However, at higher rates of infusion, tachycardia and vasoconstriction with resultant increase of peripheral resistance may be produced. Dobutamine at intravenous infusion rates of 2 to 10 μg per kilogram per minute may have a positive inotropic effect on cardiac function, with either a small increase or a reduction of left ventricular end-diastolic pressure. Both are sympathomimetic amines and should be used with caution when the pulmonary edema is associated with ischemic coronary disease, especially acute myocardial infarction, because their use may result in an increase in myocardial oxygen demand or production of ventricular arrhythmias.

All the aforementioned therapeutic agents are generally useful, within the guidelines described in each discussion, regardless of the nature of the underlying cardiac disorder. However, the importance of an early, accurate diagnosis cannot be overemphasized. For some cardiac causes of acute pulmonary edema, specific therapy is urgently indicated. Acute pulmonary edema coincident with onset of atrial fibrillation may be quickly reversed with a minimum of pharmacotherapeutics in patients known to have disorders that are critically dependent on coordinated atrial systole, such as mitral stenosis, aortic stenosis with left ventricular hypertrophy, acute myocardial infarction, or hypertrophic cardiomyopathy, if rapid electrical cardioversion can be performed. Similarly, acute pulmonary edema associated with a bradyarrhythmia that fails to respond to isoproterenol may show minimal response to medical treatment until artificial pacing can be instituted. Pericardial tamponade may be dramatically relieved by pericardiocentesis when the response to medications is minimal. Other cardiac conditions may actually be exacerbated by some of the usual therapies. For example, in hypertrophic cardiomyopathy, the patient condition may be severely aggravated by overdiuresis or use of positive inotropic agents or arteriolar dilation. In addition to attempting to make a precise cardiac diagnosis, effort should be directed at identifying and correcting any precipitating or aggravating medical conditions while the above supportive measures are being applied. Appropriate and early treatment of acute infection, hyperthyroidism, renal failure, or pulmonary embolism, as examples, may greatly facilitate patient response to medical treatment of acute pulmonary edema.

Surgical Treatment

In most cases, medical treatment of acute pulmonary edema can result in satisfactory recovery of the patient. However, there are some cardiac conditions that can result in acute pulmonary edema and that are unlikely to result in more than a modest improvement, if any, with the aforementioned supportive medical approach. These usually involve a major structural alteration of some part of the cardiovascular system. Examples include acute and severe valvar insufficiency of the aortic or mitral valve and, in some cases, severe aortic or mitral stenosis or rupture of the ventricular septum or free wall. In such cases, medical treatment should be instituted as arrangements for corrective surgery are being made. In some cases of chronic heart failure, pulmonary edema may be relatively refractory to medical treatment even after identification and correction of any precipitating or aggravating factors. In such cases, the episode of pulmonary edema may be indicative of progression of the chronic disorder to a critical state. Although emergent or urgent surgery in a patient with incompletely resolved pulmonary edema may be associated with increased risk, undue delay may be associated with an equally poor prognosis. The timing and nature of the cardiac surgery and preparation of the patient should then be based on the nature and severity of the underlying disorder.

SUGGESTED READING

Chatterjee K, Parmley WW. The role of vasodilator therapy in heart failure. Prog Cardiovasc Dis 1976; 19:301.

DeMots H, Rahimtoola SH, McAnulty JH, Murphy ES. Acute pulmonary edema. In: Mason DT, ed. Cardiac emergencies. Baltimore: Williams & Wilkins, 1978:173.

Nishimura H, Kubo S, Ueyama M, et al. Peripheral hemodynamic effects of captopril in patients with congestive heart failure. Am Heart J 1989; 117:100.

Spann JF, Hurst JW. Recognition and management of heart failure. In: Hurst JW, ed. The heart, 6th ed. New York: McGraw-Hill, 1986:345.

Szidon JP. Pathophysiology of the congested lung. Cardiol Clin 1989; 7:39.

CARDIOGENIC SHOCK

DAVID W. FERGUSON, M.D.

Cardiogenic shock is a pathophysiologic state arising from a variety of underlying etiologies, in which the common denominator is marked inadequacy of tissue perfusion due to a primary myocardial defect. Peripheral tissue perfusion is dependent on both arterial pressure and regional vascular resistance, with systemic arterial pressure being determined by cardiac output and systemic vascular resistance. Cardiac output is the product of heart rate and stroke volume. Stroke volume is determined by three major factors: ventricular preload, ventricular afterload, and the inotropic state of the myocardium.

In common clinical usage, cardiogenic shock describes clinical conditions in which forward cardiac output is inadequate to meet peripheral metabolic demands, usually as a result of inadequate forward stroke volume rather than a primary disorder of heart rate. A strict hemodynamic definition, requiring invasive hemodynamic monitoring, is essential for defining this pathophysiologic state and for excluding nonmyocardial etiologies (e.g., hypovolemia) as the cause of the reduced stroke volume. The clinical hemodynamic definition of cardiogenic shock is summarized in Table 1.

ETIOLOGY AND PATHOGENESIS

Cardiogenic shock most commonly occurs as an acute deterioration of myocardial function, although this may be superimposed on chronic impairment of cardiac function. In the majority of cases, cardiogenic shock results from acute myocardial infarction, with shock complicating the clinical course in 5 to 15 percent of patients with myocardial infarction. Shock is seen more commonly following anterior wall infarctions than following inferior wall infarctions. Detailed postmortem studies have demonstrated that patients sustaining a myocardial infarction complicated by cardiogenic shock, in the absence of a mechanical lesion, usually have infarct involvement of at least 35 percent of their functioning left ventricular mass. However, large inferoposterior infarctions and inferior wall infarctions with significant involvement of the right ventricle may also be complicated by cardiogenic shock. Mechanical defects resulting in regurgitant lesions (e.g., ventricular septal rupture and mitral insufficiency) may produce cardiogenic shock in the setting of an acute infarction and occur with similar frequency in inferior and anterior infarctions. Other noninfarct etiologies of cardiogenic shock are summarized in Table 2.

DIAGNOSIS

A high index of clinical suspicion and early diagnosis are essential for effective management of the patient in cardiogenic shock. The prognosis of these patients varies both with the underlying myocardial insult and with the rapidity with which secondary consequences of the shock state develop (e.g., acidosis, multiorgan system failure). Early clinical recognition, rapid hemodynamic assessment, initiation of supportive therapy as soon as possible, and expeditious anatomic diagnosis are the keys to successful management. The major goals of therapy are to stabilize the patient hemodynamically and metabolically and to reverse the shock state prior to the development of irreversible end-stage cellular shock.

Cardiogenic shock following myocardial infarction may occur in one of three general patterns: (1)

TABLE 1 Hemodynamic and Clinical Essentials for Defining Cardiogenic Shock

- Arterial hypotension (intra-arterial catheter)
  - Absolute: systolic arterial ≤90 mm Hg
  - Relative: systolic arterial pressure ≥60 mm Hg below baseline
- Impaired forward cardiac output (thermodilution pulmonary arterial catheter)
  - Cardiac index ≤22.1/min/m^2
  - Widened arterial mixed-venous (preshunt) oxygen content difference
- Adequate ventricular preload (pulmonary arterial catheter)
  - Left ventricular filling pressure ≥12–15 mm Hg
- Clinical end-organ hypoperfusion
  - Depressed or altered mentation
  - Oliguria (urine output <30 ml/h) or anuria
  - Peripheral vasoconstriction and/or cyanosis
- Presence of primary myocardial insult

TABLE 2 Differential Diagnosis of Cardiogenic Shock

Acute Myocardial Infarction

- Impairment of critical muscle mass
  - Large anterior left ventricular infarction
  - Large inferoposterior left ventricular infarction
  - Massive right ventricular infarction
  - "Global" subendocardial infarction
- Acute mechanical (regurgitant) lesions
  - Ventricular septal rupture
  - Acute mitral insufficiency
    - Severe papillary muscle dysfunction
    - Rupture of mitral valvular apparatus
  - Left ventricular free wall rupture
  - Left ventricular aneurysm

Valvular Heart Disease

- Critical valvular stenosis
- Severe valvular insufficiency

Obstructive Nonvalvular Cardiac Lesions

- Cardiac tamponade
- Hypertrophic cardiomyopathy with ventricular outflow obstruction
- Constrictive pericardial disorders
- Atrial myxoma with ventricular inflow obstruction
- Massive pulmonary embolism
- Severe restrictive cardiomyopathy

Infectious Cardiac Lesions

- Infective endocarditis with valvular involvement
- Fulminant myocarditis

Pharmacologic or Physiologic Myocardial Depression

- Pharmacologic depressants
  - Beta-adrenergic blocking agents
  - Calcium channel blocking agents
  - Antiarrhythmic agents
  - Cardiotoxic chemotherapeutic agents
  - Anesthetic agents
- Physiologic depressants
  - Severe hypoxemia
  - Severe acidosis
  - Severe alkalosis

Miscellaneous

- End-stage cardiomyopathy
- Post–cardiopulmonary bypass myocardial depression
- Myocardial depression complicating nonmyocardial disease process
  - Acute pancreatitis
  - Septicemia

rapid onset of fulminant cardiovascular collapse within the early hours following myocardial insult, usually as a result of massive myocardial involvement or rupture of the left ventricular free wall; (2) abrupt onset of shock with pulmonary edema remote in time from the initial insult, accompanied by a new systolic murmur (papillary muscle dysfunction or rupture with mitral insufficiency or ventricular septal rupture) (Fig. 1); or (3) gradual onset of a low-flow state, culminating in low cardiac output failure and shock over many days, as a result of recurrent "piecemeal" myocardial necrosis. The presentation of other forms of cardiogenic shock varies with the underlying disease processes involved.

The physical examination of the patient with cardiogenic shock also varies with the underlying etiology. Special attention should be directed at determining the presence or absence of tachycardia, hypotension, narrowed pulse pressure, neck vein engorgement, Kussmaul's sign, pulmonary edema, ventricular gallops, murmurs of valvular stenosis or insufficiency, peripheral signs of low output, and stigmata of disease etiologies (e.g., splinter hemorrhages in the setting of endocarditis). The clinician needs to remember, however, that many auscultatory signs of cardiac pathology (e.g., murmurs) are dependent on the forward flow state and may therefore be minimal or absent in patients with severe impairment of cardiac output.

Noninvasive diagnostic studies that may be of benefit include chest roentgenogram, electrocardiogram, two-dimensional echocardiogram with Doppler flow measurement, and radionuclide angiography for assessment of both right and left ventricular function.

Certain physiologic measurements are essential in the management of patients with cardiogenic shock and are outlined in Table 3.

PREFERRED APPROACH

Management of the patient with cardiogenic shock needs to be directed simultaneously at correction (if possible) of the underlying myocardial insult and at reversal of the secondary consequences of the shock state. Management can be conceptualized in seven phases (Fig. 2). In reality, all seven phases of management need to overlap and to be implemented in close succession. The exact order of management varies with the condition of the patient. These phases of management include clinical suspicion, initial stabilization, invasive hemodynamic assessment, tailored pharmacologic therapy, anatomic diagnosis, mechanical circulatory support, and definitive therapy.

Initial Assessment and Stabilization

Once the clinical suspicion of cardiogenic shock is entertained, prompt initiation of invasive hemodynamic monitoring is essential. This is because the

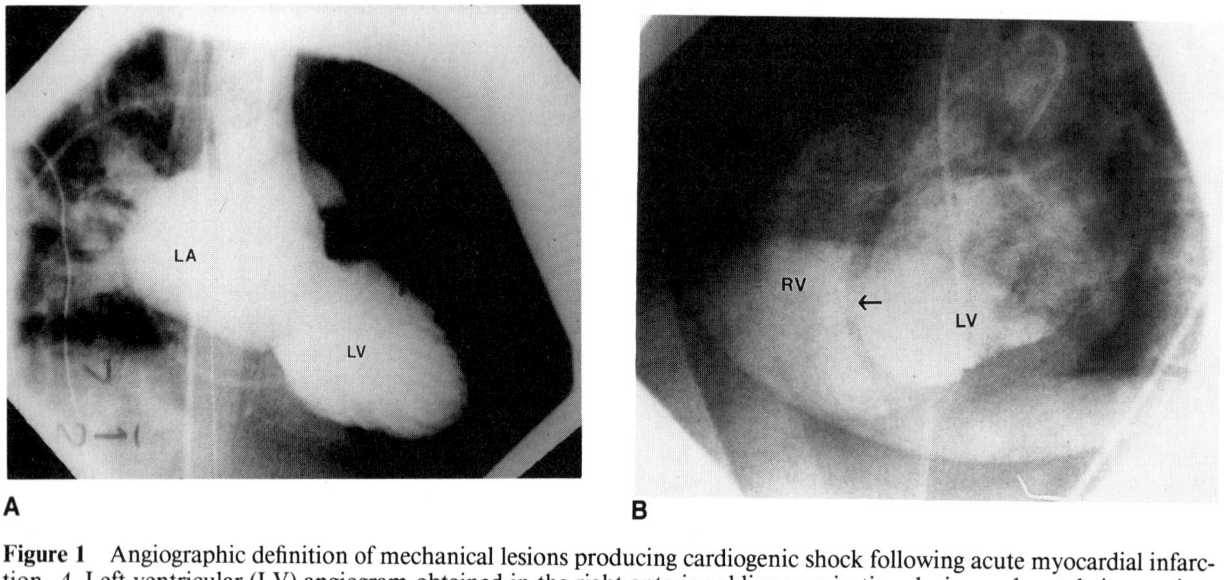

A B

Figure 1 Angiographic definition of mechanical lesions producing cardiogenic shock following acute myocardial infarction. *A*, Left ventricular (LV) angiogram obtained in the right anterior oblique projection during end-systole in a patient with cardiogenic shock and new systolic murmur following an acute inferior wall myocardial infarction. Left ventriculography demonstrates severe mitral insufficiency, with opacification of the entire left atrium (LA) and all four pulmonary veins. *B*, Left ventricular angiogram obtained in the left anterior oblique projection with cranial angulation in a patient with cardiogenic shock and a new systolic murmur occurring 48 hours after acute anterior wall myocardial infarction. A large ventricular septal defect is visualized in the midseptal region (*arrow*) with left-to-right opacification of the left (LV) and right (RV) ventricles.

TABLE 3 Essential Physiologic Monitoring in Cardiogenic Shock

Electrocardiographic monitoring (continuous)
Intra-arterial pressure monitoring (continuous)
Pulmonary artery pressure monitoring
Balloon flotation catheter
Thermodilution cardiac output capability
Serial (or on-line) oxygen saturation capability
Indwelling Foley catheter with hourly urimetrics
Serial physiochemical assessment
Arterial blood gases: pH, Pco_2, Po_2, O_2 saturation
Arterial-mixed venous oxygen content difference (preshunt)
Alveolar-arterial oxygen tension gradient
Serum electrolytes, blood urea nitrogen, creatinine
Hemoglobin and hematocrit

bedside physical examination is not sensitive enough to predict reliably and serially cardiac filling pressures and forward cardiac output. In addition, these patients require administration of potent pharmacologic agents, with the titration of these agents being dependent on close attention to the patient's hemodynamic response.

Initial assessment of the patient's airway patency and adequacy of ventilation is of paramount importance. The patient should be intubated if unable to protect the airway and should be ventilated mechanically if there is failure of ventilation or severe failure of oxygenation. Intubation and mechanical ventilation should also be considered in select patients in whom

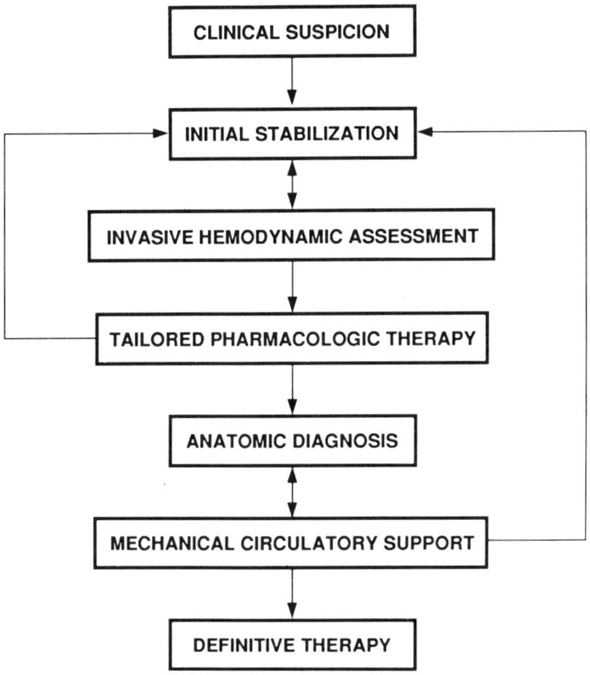

Figure 2 Therapeutic schema for the management of patients with cardiogenic shock.

the work of breathing may be too great in view of minimal or no cardiac reserve. Nonintubated patients who have either confirmed hypoxemia (increased alveolar-arterial oxygen gradient) or suspected tissue hypoxia should be maintained on a high-flow oxygen delivery system in which a continuous and known FIO_2 can be administered and carefully titrated (e.g., with a venti-mask). Adequacy of systemic circulation should be assessed rapidly by the level of patient consciousness, palpation of large peripheral pulses, presence of peripheral cyanosis, and assessment of arterial pressure. Cardiopulmonary resuscitation should be implemented if adequate peripheral perfusion cannot be achieved pharmacologically.

At least two large-bore intravenous catheters ($\geq$16 gauge) should be inserted as soon as possible, with one preferably placed centrally under optimal sterile conditions. Ideally, the central catheter should be a venous sheath with sidearm attachment (for drug administration into central circulation), which permits subsequent passage of a pulmonary artery monitoring catheter.

An indwelling arterial line, preferably in a central artery (e.g., femoral), should be inserted as rapidly as possible for accurate measurement of core blood pressure in the patient with profound shock. Accurate assessment of blood pressure in these patients requires the continuous monitoring of blood pressure from a large central artery (e.g., femoral) rather than that from a smaller distal artery (e.g., radial). This is related to the presence of intense intrinsic or pharmacologically induced vasoconstriction in these patients, which results in inaccurate pressure waveforms for analysis. A rapid but complete right heart catheterization should be performed with assessment of right atrial, right ventricular, pulmonary arterial, and pulmonary capillary wedge pressures. Careful attention should be paid to obtaining reliable pressure tracings during end-expiration. Visual examination of the waveforms should be performed to assess for diastolic equilibration of right heart pressures (e.g., cardiac tamponade), correlation of pulmonary arterial diastolic and mean pulmonary capillary wedge pressures, ratio of mean right atrial to mean pulmonary capillary wedge pressures (e.g., elevated in right ventricular infarction), and magnitude of atrial and ventricular waveforms in the pulmonary capillary wedge tracing (large *v* waves with slow upslope in the wedge position suggest mitral insufficiency). In addition, initial oximetric assessment should be performed at the time of insertion of the pulmonary arterial catheter, with duplicate blood samples obtained from the superior vena cava, right atrium, pulmonary artery, and systemic artery.

Initial assessment of cardiac output should be performed directly by the thermodilution technique and indirectly by assessment of arterial-mixed venous oxygen content difference. In the presence of a left-to-right intracardiac shunt (e.g., ventricular septal rupture), thermodilution cardiac output will not reflect true forward left heart output, and the repeated bedside determination of an accurate preshunt mixed venous oxygen content sample is impractical. The most important information obtained from this initial hemodynamic assessment is to confirm the true systemic arterial pressure, exclude (or correct) inadequate ventricular preload (e.g., pulmonary capillary wedge pressure < 12 mm Hg) as the etiology of the low stroke volume, assess for intracardiac left-to-right shunt (oxygen step-up), and provide a baseline hemodynamic profile on which to base pharmacologic therapy. If the patient is hypovolemic, rapid fluid resuscitation with isotonic saline should be administered initially to maintain the pulmonary capillary wedge pressure in the 15 to 18 mm Hg range.

This initial assessment of the patient in cardiogenic shock should be completed within the first hour of presentation. Other features of initial stabilization include correction of acidosis (or alkalosis), correction of hypoxemia (alveolar-arterial oxygen gradient ≥ 20 torr), and control of hemodynamically significant cardiac arrhythmias.

Pharmacologic Therapy

All pharmacologic therapy administered to patients in cardiogenic shock must be delivered through secure intravenous lines, preferably via centrally placed catheters where the risk of extravasation is minimized. Pain relief and control of anxiety can be achieved by judicious titration of a reversible narcotic agent such as morphine sulfate. Close monitoring of ventilation (arterial Pco_2), blood pressure, cardiac rate and rhythm, and cardiac filling pressures is essential following administration of morphine. Antiarrhythmic agents should be administered only in the presence of hemodynamically significant cardiac arrhythmias because most of these agents have myocardial depressant actions. The use of lidocaine solely as a prophylactic agent is contraindicated in the presence of cardiogenic shock.

As noted previously, adequate ventricular preload should be maintained by volume administration with normal saline to maintain cardiac filling pressures at 12 to 15 mm Hg or greater. Sequential performance of in vivo Starling curves with assessment of forward cardiac output at various levels of preload will be required to determine optimal preload in these patients because ventricular compliance is usually decreased and may change rapidly.

On the basis of assessment of arterial pressure, cardiac output, and cardiac filling pressure, patients can be categorized hemodynamically, and appropriate pharmacologic treatment can be tailored to the patient's hemodynamic state. In the presence of cardiogenic shock due to inotropic failure (impaired stroke volume with adequate preload) without severe hypotension, the preferred agent is the synthetic ($beta_1$ and $beta_2$) adrenergic agonist dobutamine. Dobutamine can be titrated (2 to 15 μg per kilogram per minute intravenously) to achieve the desired inotropic effect on the basis of serial measurements of cardiac output, arteriovenous oxygen content difference, and clinical effect (e.g., mentation, urine output). An alternative agent would be the phosphodiesterase inhibitor amrinone administered as an intravenous bolus of 0.75 mg per kilogram over 3 to 5 minutes, followed by an infusion of 5 to 10 μg per kilogram per minute.

In patients with cardiogenic shock manifested by marked inotropic impairment *and* arterial hypotension of more than moderate degree, the administration of dopamine would be the preferred agent. At low doses (0.5 to 2.0 μg per kilogram per minute intravenously), dopamine selectively stimulates dopaminergic receptors primarily in the kidney, with resultant renal arterial dilation and increased urine flow. At intermediate doses (2 to 10 μg per kilogram per minute intravenously), cardiac beta-adrenergic effects predominate, with increases in cardiac output and small increases in heart rate and blood pressure. At higher doses (10 to 20 μg per kilogram per minute intravenously), dopamine produces mixed beta-adrenergic effects and alpha-adrenergic–mediated vasoconstriction, with further increases in cardiac output and heart rate as well as an increase in blood pressure. At very high doses ($> 20 \mu g$ per kilogram per minute intravenously), dopamine acts essentially as an alpha-adrenergic agent with marked peripheral vasoconstriction. The selective dopaminergic renal vasodilating effects of dopamine achieved at low infusion rates are overcome and negated by alpha-vasoconstricting effects of the agent at the upper dose ranges.

Cardiogenic shock complicated by profound hypotension initially may require the use of more potent vasopressor agents such as norepinephrine. Because coronary artery perfusion occurs primarily during diastole, norepinephrine may be required in some patients to maintain diastolic arterial pressure within acceptable ranges to ensure adequate coronary blood flow. Norepinephrine has both beta-adrenergic inotropic and chronotropic effects, but its most profound effect is alpha-adrenergic–mediated vasoconstriction. Norepinephrine should be titrated (2 to 20 μg per minute intravenously) to achieve desired hemodynamic effects. However, as soon as possible an attempt should be made to wean the patient to either dopamine or dobutamine.

Adverse side effects can be encountered with all the vasopressor and inotropic agents. Potential side effects include cardiac arrhythmias (both atrial and ventricular), nausea, aggravation of ischemia, ventilatory depression, and profound vasoconstriction. Care must be taken to monitor the patient's cardiac rhythm closely and to ensure the stability of the infusion site during the use of these agents.

Vasodilator therapy may be of significant benefit in patients with cardiogenic shock, especially when used in combination with an intravenous inotrope such as dobutamine or dopamine. However, essential hemodynamic features that must be present to permit effective utilization of vasodilators include adequate ventricular preload and absence of fixed obstruction to ventricular outflow (e.g., critical aortic stenosis). Vasodilators are of particular benefit in the management of regurgitant lesions such as ventricular septal defects and acute aortic or mitral insufficiency. The most appropriate commercially available agent for afterload reduction in the setting of cardiogenic shock is the direct-acting arteriolar vasodilator sodium nitroprusside. Nitroprusside should be administered with close monitoring of arterial pressure and can be titrated every 1 to 3 minutes from an initial intravenous infusion rate of 0.4 μg per kilogram per minute to achieve the desired hemodynamic effect. The major risks associated with nitroprusside infusion are hypotension, adverse reflex tachycardia, arterial hypoxemia due to increase in pulmonary ventilation-perfusion mismatch, and thiocyanate toxicity following prolonged administration. Intravenous nitroglycerine may be of some benefit in patients with low output state, pulmonary congestion, and ongoing myocardial ischemia as the basis for inotropic impairment. The agent is administered via intravenous infusion beginning at approximately 10 μg per minute and is titrated to achieve the desired hemodynamic and clinical effect.

Every effort should be made to stabilize the patient in cardiogenic shock rapidly within the first 2 to 3 hours of presentation. If the patient can be stabilized, further diagnostic studies should be performed to define the precise nature of the cardiac impairment as a guide to definitive therapy. If the patient cannot be stabilized, these additional studies should still be performed, although preceded by placement of mechanical circulatory support devices.

Specialized Diagnostic Studies and Support Procedures

The decision to proceed with specialized studies and mechanical support procedures is one that must be made as rapidly as possible in the course of managing the patient with cardiogenic shock, preferably within the first 4 to 6 hours following initial assessment and stabilization. The decision to proceed with these invasive procedures must be based on a number of factors, including the overall condition of the patient prior to development of cardiogenic shock, the expressed wishes of the patient and the patient's family, and the potential for reversible pathology. It must be remembered, however, that in the setting of cardiogenic shock following myocardial infarction, a survival rate of 50 to 60 percent is the best that can be achieved, even under optimal conditions and with the utilization of the most advanced support procedures. In general, in the absence of definite medical contraindications or wishes expressed by the patient or family to the contrary, it is desirable to proceed with anatomic definition as a guide to both short-term and long-term therapeutic options.

In most cases, definitive and comprehensive anatomic diagnosis requires invasive cardiac catheterization. Noninvasive studies such as echocardiography and nuclear angiography may be of benefit in directing the cardiac catheterization, but they rarely provide all the information required to guide management. The cardiac catheterization should include a comprehensive right heart hemodynamic study with assessment of oxygen saturations via sampling from the superior and inferior vena cava, right atrium, pulmonary artery, and left ventricle. A biplane left ventricular angiogram should be performed if at all possible, followed by selective coronary arteriography. Additional angiographic studies depend on the underlying disease processes being considered (e.g., aortic root angiography for suspected acute aortic insufficiency in a patient with endocarditis). A minimal but appropriate amount of the least toxic angiographic contrast agent should be used to ensure an adequate angiographic study.

Mechanical circulatory support may be required before, during, or after the cardiac catheterization. From a technical standpoint, the cardiac catheterization suite is probably the preferred locale for placement of such devices via the percutaneous approach. The most frequently used mode of mechanical circulatory support is the intra-aortic balloon pump (IABP). The potential clinical indications for IABP support include (1) cardiogenic shock refractory to maximal medical therapy, (2) mechanical regurgitant lesions for which the IABP may be the preferred therapeutic approach (e.g., acute severe mitral insufficiency or ventricular septal rupture), (3) perioperative support of the high-risk patient with cardiogenic shock who is to undergo surgical intervention, and (4) management of medically refractory myocardial ischemia producing ventricular dysfunction in patients with high-grade coronary lesions.

The IABP can be placed percutaneously over a guidewire from the femoral artery and can be positioned in the thoracic aorta just distal to the left subclavian artery. Under ideal operation, the IABP functions to increase coronary artery diastolic pressure (increase myocardial oxygen delivery), reduce mechanically impedance to left ventricular ejection and lower ventricular preload (reduce myocardial oxygen demand), and reduce the magnitude of regurgitant lesions, thereby improving forward ejection fraction. These effects are achieved without increasing heart rate, as would likely occur if pharmacologic means were employed to achieve the same objectives. Major complications occur in 10 to 30 percent of patients undergoing IABP support and include vascular insufficiency and trauma, infection, and bleeding. Definite contraindications to IABP include severe atherosclerotic peripheral vascular disease, aortic insufficiency, or systemic anticoagulation. Other types of temporary mechanical support devices that can be considered for percutaneous placement include portable cardiopulmonary bypass apparatus. In addition to percutaneous support devices, left and right ventricular assist devices and mechanical heart devices are available but require surgical replacement via thoracotomy.

All these mechanical support devices should be considered for use only as temporizing therapy in patients who have correctable or reversible disorders of cardiac function. Every attempt should be made to proceed with definitive therapy and subsequent removal of these devices as soon as possible because complications increase with the duration of use.

Definitive Therapy

Various acute medical and surgical interventional therapies have been described for the treatment of patients with cardiogenic shock. Not unexpectedly, most of these therapeutic approaches have not undergone careful prospective, randomized, controlled trials to assess their efficacy in comparison to conventional noninvasive medical therapy in large numbers of patients with cardiogenic shock. Historical controls emphasizing a mortality rate of 80 to 90 percent in large series of patients treated with medical therapy alone for cardiogenic shock following acute myocardial infarction have been used as justification for these alternative therapies. The individual clinician should consider these alternative therapies but cannot rely on well-designed comparative studies for guidance.

Medical interventions for cardiogenic shock following myocardial infarction include thrombolytic therapy and emergent coronary angioplasty. Successful thrombolytic reperfusion has been shown clearly to improve survival following anterior myocardial infarction and has been described as effective therapy for cardiogenic shock in selected patients. Recently, emergent coronary angioplasty has been reported to offer significant benefit over medical therapy alone when compared retrospectively in a moderate-sized group of patients with acute myocardial infarction complicated by cardiogenic shock. Finally, aortic balloon valvuloplasty has been described recently as a potentially effective therapy for patients with cardiogenic shock resulting from end-stage critical aortic stenosis.

Surgical revascularization for ischemic left ventricular dysfunction and shock has been described but remains controversial. Surgical interventions for mechanical complications of acute myocardial infarction has been the best described approach for the care of the patient with severe mitral insufficiency or large ventricular septal rupture following acute myocardial infarction. The timing of surgery remains controversial, although recent data suggest that early intervention is probably better than delayed intervention. Whether or not surgical repair of the defect should be accompanied by myocardial revascularization remains unclear.

Certain forms of cardiogenic shock, such as cardiac tamponade, are reversed readily by definitive intervention (e.g., pericardiocentesis). Surgical valvular replacement has been described as effective therapy in patients with severe regurgitant valvular lesions complicating endocarditis, and in patients with cardiogenic shock due to severe valvular stenosis. Mechanical circulatory support may be a useful temporizing measure in the management of patients with fulminant myocarditis and cardiogenic shock.

The role of urgent cardiac transplantation for younger patients with refractory cardiogenic shock of any etiology is being evaluated. Obviously, the keys to the use of this mode of definitive therapy include adequate donor availability and timing of the transplantation. One would not wish to consider transplantation before it is clear that conventional modes of therapy are not sufficient. Yet, one would like to proceed with transplantation before secondary organ failure or complications of shock management (e.g., infection, pulmonary embolism, stress ulceration, adult respiratory distress syndrome) develop and prohibit transplantation.

SUGGESTED READING

Barbour DJ, Roberts WC. Rupture of a left ventricular papillary muscle during acute myocardial infarction: analysis of 22 necropsy patients. J Am Coll Cardiol 1986; 8:558.

Chatterjee K. Myocardial infarction shock. Crit Care Clin 1985; 1:563.

Ferguson DW, Abboud FM. The pathophysiology, recognition, and management of shock. In: Hurst WJ, ed. The heart. 7th ed. New York: McGraw-Hill, 1990:442.

Joyce LD, Johnson KE, Toninato CJ, et al. Results of the first 100 patients who received symbion total artificial hearts as a bridge to cardiac transplantation. Circulation 1989; 80(Suppl III):192.

Lee L, Bates ER, Pitt B, et al. Percutaneous transluminal coronary angioplasty improves survival in acute myocardial infarction complicated by cardiogenic shock. Circulation 1988; 78:1345.

Moore CA, Nygaard TW, Kaiser DL, et al. Postinfarction ventricular septal rupture: the importance of location of infarction and right ventricular function in determining survival. Circulation 1986; 74:45.

Pennington DG, Kanter KR, McBride LR, et al. Seven years' experience with the Pierce-Donachy ventricular assist device. J Thorac Cardiovasc Surg 1988; 96:901.

Schreiber TL, Miller DH, Zola B: Management of myocardial infarction shock: current status. Am Heart J 1989; 117:435.

Stone PH, Raabe DS, Jaffe AS, et al for the MILIS GROUP. Prognostic significance of location and type of myocardial infarction: independent adverse outcome associated with anterior location. J Am Coll Cardiol 1988; 11:453.

Thanavaro S, Kleiger RE, Province MA, et al. Effect of infarct location on the in-hospital prognosis of patients with first transmural myocardial infarction. Circulation 1982; 66:742.

CARDIAC ARREST AND RESUSCITATION FROM SUDDEN DEATH

COREY M. SLOVIS, M.D., F.A.C.P., F.A.C.E.P.
STEVEN L. BRODY, M.D.

Sudden death has been defined by various authors as death occurring instantaneously, 1, 2, or 24 hours after the onset of acute symptoms. Most sudden deaths that occur within 2 hours of the acute onset of symptoms are due to a malignant rhythm disturbance in patients with underlying coronary atherosclerotic heart disease (CASHD) or cardiomyopathy. Approximately 60 to 70 percent of these arrhythmia-induced sudden death victims have ventricular fibrillation (VF), whereas asystole or brady-asystole, electromechanical dissociation, and ventricular tachycardia (VT) each account for about 10 percent. Only one-half of patients have a known history of coronary artery disease. Pathologic evidence of an acute myocardial infarction as the terminal event is seen in only a minority of cardiac sudden death victims. The other major noncardiac causes of sudden death are ruptured aortic aneurysm, pulmonary embolism, and cerebrovascular accident.

RISK FACTORS

Risk factors for sudden cardiac death include a history of CASHD, especially in association with abnormal ventricular function or aneurysm; hypertension; hypercholesterolemia; diabetes mellitus; cigarette smoking; family history; male sex; black race; history of prior malignant arrhythmias, especially primary VF; hereditary prolongation of the Q-T interval; and use of any medication that has significant effects on the electrocardiogram (ECG), such as quinidine and other oral antiarrhythmic agents.

SURVIVAL

In general, resuscitation rates from cardiac arrest are dismal. Only 8 to 15 percent of all patients who suffer a cardiac arrest will survive to hospital discharge, and up to one-half of these patients will have a significant degree of functional impairment, intellectual impairment, or both. Survival of cardiac arrests in hospitalized patients is similarly poor.

Factors that favor a successful resuscitation from cardiac arrest include a witnessed arrest, bystander cardiopulmonary resuscitation (CPR), advanced life support in under 4 to 8 minutes, VF as the underlying arrest rhythm, rapid defibrillation, and quick return of a perfusing rhythm. Additional favorable factors include a primary cardiac etiology for the arrest, no functional impairment prior to the arrest, and less than two major organ system diseases in hospitalized patients. Based on the results of multiple studies and the Brain Resuscitation Clinical Trials, functional survival after 10 to 15 minutes of pulselessness is highly unlikely.

Successful resuscitation from cardiac arrest requires an organized and rapid response by any or all of the following: the victim's family, prehospital care providers, and hospital workers from all areas of the hospital, particularly the emergency department and coronary care unit. Sudden death usually occurs out of the hospital, and most cases are witnessed, often by relatives. Thus, the learning of basic cardiac life support (BCLS) is imperative for the entire family of patients with CASHD.

BASIC CARDIAC LIFE SUPPORT

Many of the recent changes in BCLS reflect a better understanding of the biomechanics involved with manual chest compression. Because of the possible co-existence of cervical spine injury, the airway should be opened with a chin lift or jaw thrust and not by hyperextending the neck. Foreign bodies in the airway should be cleared by the Heimlich maneuver and not via back slaps. After an arrest state has been established, two slow breaths, rather than the previously recommended four rapid breaths, should be provided. Chest compressions for adults should be at a depth of 1½ to 2 inches and given at the increased rate of 100 per minute.

ADVANCED CARDIAC LIFE SUPPORT

The American Heart Association's advanced cardiac life support (ACLS) recommendations serve as the basis for resuscitating patients in cardiac arrest. The ACLS guidelines are not inviolate standards of care; they are merely recommendations that should be modified, based on the most current available information. The use of high-dose epinephrine, multiple antiarrhythmic agents for VF, or other therapies is not inconsistent with the philosophies of the ACLS national faculty.

Isoproterenol, a potent beta-agonist, has long been used to treat asystole and electromechanical dissociation. It is no longer recommended, however, because it lacks the alpha-adrenergic agonist properties necessary for coronary artery and cerebral perfusion. Calcium chloride was also commonly used in cardiac arrests. It is no longer routinely used because of a lack of proven efficacy. Calcium administration may also increase the likelihood of post-arrest ischemic neuronal damage and cerebral hypoperfusion.

PREFERRED APPROACH

Asystole

The cornerstone of treatment of asystole is the rapid administration of an effective amount of epinephrine. A 1.0-mg dose of epinephrine was used in the landmark studies of Redding and Pearson during the 1960s, using small mongrel dogs. Unfortunately, this 1.0-mg dose has long been used for adult humans weighing 70 to 100 kg. It has only recently been appreciated that this amount of epinephrine is ineffective in raising aortic diastolic pressures above 25 to 27 mm Hg, the minimum pressure required to perfuse coronary and cerebral blood vessels during manual CPR.

Recent studies have established that 0.2 mg per kilogram of epinephrine is required to obtain the coronary and cerebral blood flow necessary to allow successful resuscitation from a pulseless state. This dose equals 10 to 20 mg of epinephrine, a dose unfamiliar to most clinicians. Norepinephrine (0.16 mg per kilogram) may also prove to be beneficial in treating asystole. Pure alpha-agonists, such as phenylephrine and methoxamine, have not shown similar benefits.

Table 1 outlines a five-step protocol that uses an escalating dosage of epinephrine in an effort to maximize survival from asystole. Because epinephrine works in 30 to 60 seconds, this time interval is chosen as the interval between escalating doses of this potent alpha- and beta-agonist. Patients who respond to low-dose or moderate-dose epinephrine are spared the potential complications of high-dose drug administration, yet needed time is not wasted assessing epinephrine's success.

TABLE 1 Five-Step Protocol for Treating Asystole

Step 1
Confirm asystole
Check monitor and lead connections
Switch to 2 or more leads
Step 2
Oxygenate
Intubate, oxygenate, and hyperventilate with 100% oxygen
Step 3
Begin therapy
Epinephrine 1 mg
Atropine 1 mg
Defibrillate at 360 ws
Step 4
Epinephrine titration
Epinephrine 2 mg
Epinephrine 5 mg
Epinephrine 10 mg
Step 5
Treat acidosis
Check and correct arterial blood gas abnormalities*

*Give sodium bicarbonate if the pH is below 7.1. If arterial blood gas analysis is unavailable, give 2 ampules (88 to 100 mEq) of sodium bicarbonate 10 minutes into the arrest. Repeat 1 ampule every 10 minutes.

1 mg of epinephrine = 1 ml of 1:1,000 *or* 10 ml of 1:10,000.

Modified from Brody SL, Slovis CM. The technique of managing asystole. J Crit Illness 1989; 4:86. Reproduced by permission of the authors and publisher.

The treatment of asystole begins with confirming the diagnosis of a pulseless, electrically silent rhythm. Loss of a monitor lead, failure to increase the ECG's gain, or fine ventricular fibrillation may all simulate asystole, and all these should be ruled out rapidly. The patient's airway should then be secured, and the patient should be oxygenated and hyperventilated. Endotracheal intubation is the optimal way to secure an airway and also allows endotracheal drug administration of the patient's initial medications if a large-bore intravenous line is not yet functional (Table 2). Epinephrine, atropine, and lidocaine may all be given via the endotracheal route; calcium and bicarbonate should never be given endotracheally.

As the patient is being hyperventilated, 1.0 mg of epinephrine and 1.0 mg of atropine should be administered rapidly. Atropine is especially useful in primary bradycardiac arrests. One 360-watt-second shock may also be administered in the hope of reversing fine VF or VF in which positive deflection is parallel to the sensing lead, resulting in a flat ECG line. An epinephrine titration is indicated in patients who do not respond. Epinephrine should be administered every 30 to 60 seconds in amounts of 2, 5, and 10 mg (or 2, 4, 8, and 10 mg). The exact amount of each dose is not important; the key to therapy is the administration 0.2 mg per kilogram (10 to 20 mg) of epinephrine in 2 to 3 minutes.

The role of pH correction by bicarbonate administration in cardiac arrest victims is not yet clearly established. Based on data from Weil and co-workers, limited use of bicarbonate appears to be most appropriate for pulseless patients in asystole, electromechanical dissociation, and VF. This is because the acidosis seen early in cardiac arrest is predominantly a respiratory acidosis that should be treated by hyperventilation. Because bicarbonate and carbon dioxide ions attempt to equilibrate ($HCO_3 \leftrightarrow HCO_3 \leftrightarrow H_2O + CO_2$), bicarbonate administration has the potential

TABLE 2 Guidelines for Endotracheal Medications Given in Cardiac Arrests

Use the maximum recommended drug dosage
Either dilute to 10 to 20 ml or flush the medication with 5 to 10 ml of saline
Inject the medication into the distal portion of the endotracheal tube using a plastic intravenous catheter (not a needle) affixed to the syringe
Stop manual cardiac compressions for 5 sec postadministration
Hyperventilate the patient

From Slovis CM, Brody SL. The technique of reversing ventricular fibrillation. J Crit Illness 1988; 3:93. Reproduced by permission of the authors and publisher.

of paradoxically lowering the pH as a result of a cellular increase in carbon dioxide. At present, bicarbonate administration (1 mEq per kilogram) should be reserved for those patients who have an arterial pH below 7.1 or after 10 minutes of unsuccessful advanced life support, when no arterial blood gas values or pH measurements are available.

The survival rate for victims of asystole is approximately 1 to 2 percent. Pacemaker insertion, calcium chloride administration, and isoproterenol infusion have proved to be ineffective. It seems morally and ethically justified to discontinue CPR in these arrest victims after 10 to 15 minutes of advanced life support that has included optimal oxygenation, appropriate doses of epinephrine, and attempts at pH correction.

Ventricular Fibrillation

The successful treatment of VF is based on rapid defibrillation. All other therapy rendered for VF is merely an attempt to make the myocardium more responsive to electrical reversion. Patients found in VF should be immediately shocked at 200 watt-seconds. Time should not be wasted attempting to secure the airway or administering medications. It is easiest to remember the treatment of VF by using a four-phase protocol (Table 3).

Phase I of the VF protocol is the electrical reversion phase. Patients are successively shocked at 200, 300, and 360 watt-seconds if VF continues. A 200-watt-second initial shock maximizes the chance for a successful defibrillation without increasing the likelihood of electrically induced myocardial damage. Firm paddle pressure should be applied (25 lb per square inch) as the patient is defibrillated, and it is imperative that no one be in contact with the patient or stretcher-bed at the time the shock is delivered.

Phase II is the reversible causes phase. Potentially reversible causes of VF, including hypoxia, acidosis, vasodilation, and coronary hypoperfusion, are treated by intubation, oxygenation, hyperventilation, and administration of at least 1 mg of epinephrine (10 ml of 1 : 10,000). This phase, like all others, ends with a 360-watt-second shock.

Phase III in the management of VF is the antiarrhythmic phase. One or two antiarrhythmic agents should be administered rapidly and briefly allowed to circulate, and the patient should be reshocked with 360 watt-seconds. A bolus dose of lidocaine (1 mg per kilogram) and bretylium (500 mg) are currently the two best initial antiarrhythmic choices. Lidocaine has a long history of use in malignant ventricular arrhythmias, although its use in ischemic VF is not well studied. It works by depressing excitability and normalizing conduction in ischemic myocardial cells. Bretylium, which works via a poorly understood mechanism as an antifibrillant, seems to have similar efficacy in VF. The combined use of these two agents may have additive or synergistic effects in VF.

TABLE 3 Treatment of Ventricular Fibrillation (and Pulseless Ventricular Tachycardia)

Phase I
Electrical reversion phase
Shock 200 ws
Reshock 300 ws
Reshock 360 ws
Phase II
Correctable causes phase
Intubate, oxygenate, and hyperventilate with 100% oxygen
10 ml of epinephrine 1 : 10,000
Shock at 360 ws
Phase III
Antiarrhythmic phase
1 mg/kg lidocaine (75–100 mg IV push)
One ampule bretylium (500 mg IV push)
Shock at 360 ws
Phase IV
Refractory phase
Electrical
Reshock at 360 ws every 1 min
Correctable
Check and correct arterial blood gas abnormalities*
Repeat epinephrine 10 ml 1 : 10,000 every 5 min
Antiarrhythmic
1 mg IV propranolol every 1 min
and/or
2 g of magnesium sulfate (4 ml of 50%) and 1 g (2 ml) every 1 min
20 mg/min procainamide
and/or
Double dose—two ampules bretylium (100 mg IV push)†
and/or
Repeat 1 mg/kg lidocaine (75–100 mg IV push)

*Administer sodium bicarbonate ($NaHCO_3$) if pH below 7.1. If no arterial blood gases are available, administer two ampules (88–100 mg) sodium bicarbonate 10 minutes into the arrest. Repeat one ampule every 10 minutes.

†Wait at least 5 minutes from initial dose.

In phase IV, refractory VF is treated by attempts at defibrillation at least every 60 seconds, checking for and correcting arterial blood gas abnormalities, repeating epinephrine, and trying additional antiarrhythmic agents. Although repeat doses of lidocaine and bretylium may be tried, administering additional antiarrhythmic agents is more prudent. Magnesium sulfate (2 g intravenous, push), propranolol (1 mg), or both should be administered every minute for at least three doses. Magnesium, which speeds repolarization and decreases spontaneous depolarization, has had empiric successes in numerous patients with refractory VF. Beta-blockers such as propranolol increase the relative refractory period of ischemic myocardium and have membrane stabilizing effects when given intravenously.

Survival rates in VF may approach 50 percent in patients who are rapidly defibrillated, and most survivors usually respond to the first few shocks. Patients with prolonged VF rarely survive and may convert to asystole or electromechanical dissociation after defibrillation. Pulseless idioventricular rhythms after defibrillation should be observed for 30 seconds to allow for spontaneous reversion to a perfusing rhythm.

Ventricular Tachycardia

The therapy of VT is determined by patient stability. It is most helpful to think of the treatment of VT along a continuum that ranges from the administration of antiarrhythmic medications to immediate electrical conversion (Table 4). Patients who are pulseless are treated exactly like those patients in VF (see Table 3). Patients who are unstable as evidenced by hypotension, chest pain, or alterations in mental status should be electrically converted with 50 watt-seconds. Although VT is electrically responsive and may respond with as little as 5 to 10 watt-seconds, a 50-watt-second shock will maximize the likelihood of a one-shock conversion.

Progressively lower electrical energy settings should be used in patients who revert back to VT after a prior 50-watt-second shock. There is a question regarding the use of the synchronized mode when electrically converting VT. There is no clear answer, and unless a separate and distinct T wave is apparent, the unsynchronized mode is probably most appropriate.

Stable patients in VT should be treated initially with antiarrhythmic agents. Lidocaine in an intravenous dose of 1 mg per kilogram (75 to 100 mg) is the best initial choice. It has a very high safety profile in single-dose administration, works rapidly, and is very effective in VT associated with acute myocardial infarction. Lidocaine is not as effective in cases of torsades de pointes VT or in VT that is recurrent or chronic. Patients who respond to a bolus of lidocaine should be placed on a lidocaine drip at 2 to 3 mg per minute. A rebolus of lidocaine at one-half the initial loading dose has been recommended 8 to 10 minutes after the first administration. This dose must be slowly administered over 1 to 2 minutes to avoid lidocaine toxicity.

Many of the side effects of lidocaine have occurred at the time of the rebolus or when the patient is left on a drip for more than 6 to 12 hours. Patients with heart failure, liver failure, or renal failure; who are over age 74; and who are taking medications that decrease the hepatic metabolism of lidocaine, such as erythromycin, cimetidine, and propranolol, are at highest risk for lidocaine toxicity. Clinicians must make a risk-benefit analysis before choosing to rebolus stable patients.

Patients who do not respond to a single dose of lidocaine should receive a second agent or be cardioverted (Table 5). The use of a concurrent lidocaine drip is at the physician's discretion. The efficacy of a continued lidocaine infusion is minimal in the patient who has failed to respond to a bolus dose.

Procainamide and magnesium sulfate are the two second-line agents that are most likely to be effective in patients with VT in the acute setting. Procainamide is an electrically stabilizing agent that works by decreasing rates of conduction through the conducting system and ventricular tissue. It is administered at a dose of 20 mg per minute until the VT abates. It must be discontinued temporarily if hypotension or QRS widening (of 50 percent or more) occurs. A slow intravenous infusion of bretylium (25 to 50 mg per minute) may also be tried. The side effects of nausea, vomiting, and hypotension make this drug less attractive.

Magnesium sulfate has begun to receive considerable attention as a ventricular antiarrhythmic. It has calcium blocking effects, speeds repolarization, and stimulates the sodium-potassium adenosine triphosphatase (ATPase)–mediated pump. It shortens the duration of phase II and increases the negativity of the resting membrane potential (phase IV), thus making spontaneous depolarization less likely.

Magnesium is the drug of choice for the torsade de pointe variant of VT. It works immediately and has reversed torsades in patients who had been previously unresponsive to treatment with multiple agents. Magnesium is also very effective in patients

TABLE 4 Initial Treatment of Ventricular Tachycardia

Stable	*Borderline*	*Unstable*	*Arrest*
(No chest pain, normal blood pressure) Lidocaine 1 mg/kg over 1–2 min	(Chest pain, borderline blood pressure, elderly) Lidocaine 1 mg/kg over 1–2 min and Shock at 50 ws if no response to lidocaine (premedicate with IV diazepam)	(Hypotensive, unconscious, pulmonary edema) Shock at 50 ws and Administer lidocaine 1 mg/kg over 2 min	Treat as ventricular fibrillation
Once Converted			
Maintain patient on antiarrhythmic(s) (i.e., lidocaine 3 mg/min *and/or* magnesium 1–2 g/hour)			

TABLE 5 Treatment of Refractory Ventricular Tachycardia

Stable	*Antiarrhythmics*		*Borderline or Unstable*
Antiarrhythmic(s) and consider shock	Magnesium sulfate	2 g (4 ml of 50%) over 1–5 min and/or	Reshock at 100 ws (if unsuccessful) Reshock at 200 ws and Begin antiarrhythmic(s)
	Procainamide	20 mg/min and/or	
	Propranolol	0.5–1 mg every 1–5 min and/or	
	Bretylium	25–50 mg/min and/or	
	Lidocaine	0.5 mg/kg over 2 min (if 1.0 mg/kg given 10 min previously)	

with VT associated with hypokalemia, cyclic antidepressant overdose, or digitalis toxicity or in patients with prolonged Q-T intervals. Its efficacy in the VT of acute ischemia is being evaluated. Magnesium should be given as a 2.0-g rapid infusion. It may be pushed as a bolus in less stable patients or infused over 1 to 20 minutes in relatively stable patients. An infusion of 2.0 g per hour should be started in any patient who initially responds to magnesium. Flushing or dysphoria may be experienced temporarily by patients, but serious side effects of magnesium at these doses are nearly nonexistent in patients with normal renal function.

Beta-blocking agents, including propranolol or esmolol, may be used in the acute setting of VT. These agents work by decreasing sympathetic tone and decreasing rate of impulse conduction. Patients with VT associated with cocaine overdose or VT after epinephrine use are most likely to benefit from propranolol (0.5 to 1 mg every 1 minute) or esmolol (0.5 mg per kilogram intravenous push).

A brief attempt at pharmacologic control of VT prior to a 50-watt-second shock seems most appropriate in patients who border on instability. A single bolus of lidocaine and a brief trial of procainamide or magnesium sulfate may be appropriate for this group of patients. In general, stable patients should be sedated with low doses of an intravenous benzodiazepine prior to electrical reversion. The risks of sedation prior to elective cardioversion and possible intubation must be weighed against delaying cardioversion.

Patients who have recurrent ventricular ectopy or VT must have reversible causes of ventricular instability ruled out. These include hypoxia, hypokalemia, hypomagnesemia, profound acidosis or alkalosis, and concurrent arrhythmogenic medication administration or device insertion (e.g., isoproterenol or theophylline administration or pacemaker or Swan-Ganz catheter insertion).

Electromechanical Dissociation

The treatment of electromechanical dissociation focuses on finding and treating reversible causes of this often agonal rhythm. There are numerous irreversible causes of electromechanical dissociation, including aortic dissection, free wall rupture, and massive pulmonary embolus. The reversible causes fall into five categories (Table 6). Therapy is directed toward ruling out each category in an orderly fashion (Table 7). An epinephrine titration should be administered rapidly if no reversible cause can be established.

Patients in electromechanical dissociation should be rapidly intubated, oxygenated, and hyperventilated. This will correct both hypoxia and acidosis; it will also allow assessment of breath sounds and ease of Ambu-bag compressions, two keys in identifying a tension pneumothorax. Electromechanical dissociation in a patient with asthma or chronic obstructive pulmonary disease should be considered due to a tension pneumothorax until proved otherwise. After intubation for electromechanical dissociation in patients with an increased risk for pneumothorax, a 14-gauge needle should be inserted in the second intercostal space of each midclavicular line in an attempt to relieve the pneumothorax.

TABLE 6 Reversible Causes of Electrical Mechanical Dissociation

Hypoxia
Tension pneumothorax
Hypotension
Cardiac tamponade
Toxic metabolic causes

TABLE 7 Treatment of Electrical Mechanical Dissociation

Intubate, oxygenate, and hyperventilate with 100% oxygen
Evaluate ECG for hyperkalemia* and bradycardia†
Evaluate neck veins for hypovolemia, tension pneumothorax, and tamponade
Consider toxic metabolic disorders
Begin pressor therapy
- IV normal saline solution run wide open
- Epinephrine in increasing doses every 30–60 sec

1 mg epinephrine	(1 ml of 1 : 1,000 or 10 ml of 1 : 10,000)
2 mg epinephrine	(2 ml of 1 : 1,000)
5 mg epinephrine	(5 ml of 1 : 1,000)
10 mg epinephrine	(10 ml of 1 : 1,000)

- Check and correct arterial blood gas abnormalities‡

*If hyperkalemia is suspected, give 5 ml of 10% calcium chloride IV push.
†If heart rate is below 60, begin drug protocol with 1 mg atropine IV or via endotracheal tube.
‡Administer sodium bicarbonate if the pH is below 7.1. If arterial blood gas analysis is unavailable, give 2 ampules (88–100 mEq) of sodium bicarbonate 10 minutes into the arrest. Repeat 1 ampule every 10 minutes.

Once the patient in electromechanical dissociation is intubated, the ECG should be evaluated closely for evidence of hyperkalemia and bradycardia. Hyperkalemia should be strongly suspected in patients with renal failure or in others at risk for hyperkalemia. Calcium at a starting dose of 5 ml of 10 percent calcium chloride should be administered to patients with wide complex electromechanical dissociation and suspected hyperkalemia as evidenced by tall-peaked T waves. It should be followed immediately by glucose (100 ml of 50 percent) and insulin (10 units intravenous push). Atropine (1 mg intravenous push) should be given to patients in electromechanical dissociation with a rate of less than 60.

The patient's neck veins should also be evaluated rapidly. Hypovolemia is assumed if the neck veins are not prominent and should be treated by aggressive volume repletion (two large-bore intravenous lines of crystalloid, run wide open). Pericardial tamponade should be suspected in patients with electromechanical dissociation and elevated neck veins. Tamponade is a relatively rare cause of electromechanical dissociation but should be strongly suspected in patients with a history of renal failure, lymphoma, tuberculosis, recent myocardial infarction, or after chest trauma. Pericardiocentesis is required in these patients. A palpable pulse will return when as little as 10 to 30 ml of blood is removed from the pericardium.

If the patient continues in electromechanical dissociation, toxic metabolic causes other than hyperkalemia should be considered. An arterial blood gas sample should be sent for arterial pH determination, and bicarbonate should be administered if the pH is below 7.1. Other potentially toxic metabolic reversible causes of electromechanical dissociation include drug overdoses with digitalis, cyclic antidepressants, beta-blockers, and calcium blockers; hypothermia; and hyperthermia (see below).

If no reversible cause of electromechanical dissociation is identified, a rapid epinephrine titration to a total dose of 0.2 mg per kilogram should be attempted. If no return of circulation is obtained after all reversible causes have been ruled out and epinephrine in appropriate doses has been administered, the resuscitation should be terminated. The survival rate of patients with electromechanical dissociation is similar to the 1 to 2 percent survival rate reported in patients with asystole.

Special Cardiac Arrest Situations

Drowning

Drowning victims who suffer cardiac arrest should be evaluated for concomitant hypothermia, cervical spine injury, head trauma, other occult injuries, tension pneumothorax, and profound acidosis. Early bicarbonate administration is usually indicated owing to the likelihood of a combined metabolic and respiratory acidosis.

Drug Overdose

Cardiac arrest from an overdose of digitalis, cyclic antidepressant, calcium channel blocker, or beta-blocker should be treated by attempting to reverse the pharmacologic actions of the offending agent. Digitalis-induced arrests should be treated by Fab fragment antibodies, magnesium, and evaluation for digitalis-induced hyperkalemia. Magnesium stimulates the sodium-potassium ATPase pump, which digitalis poisons. Phenytoin's efficacy in ventricular arrhythmia associated with digitalis toxicity is predominantly anecdotal, and its role in life-threatening overdoses is unclear.

Cyclic antidepressant overdose should be treated by attempting to alkalinize the patient to an arterial pH of 7.5 to 7.55 via both sodium bicarbonate administration and hypoventilation. Sodium bicarbonate helps normalize conduction in poisoned sodium channels, and alkalinization increases the percentage of protein bound inactive drug. Magnesium is very effective in ventricular arrhythmia due to cyclic toxicity because of its ability to shorten the prolonged Q-T interval (phase 2 prolongation) associated with the antidepressants.

Beta-blockers and calcium blocking agents may cause arrests by inducing bradycardias and hypotension. Both may be treated by an epinephrine drip (1 mg in 250 ml D_5W). Calcium blocker toxicity should also be treated by immediate calcium chloride infusion (1 to 20 ml of 10 percent calcium chloride). Beta-blocker toxicity may also respond to calcium. Glucagon (2 to 5 mg intravenously) has been effective in refractory cases of beta-blocker and calcium blocker overdose. Its mechanism of action appears to be via the stimulation of non-alpha, nonbeta myocardial receptors. If readily available, cardiopulmonary bypass may be lifesaving. Isoproterenol is of little value in these overdoses.

Hypothermia and Hyperthermia

Cardiac arrests due to hypothermia should be treated by aggressive core rewarming techniques, including heated mist and heated peritoneal, orogastric, or rectal lavage. If readily available, cardiopulmonary bypass provides the highest likelihood for successful resuscitation from hypothermia. Cardiac arrests due to hyperthermia may respond to aggressive volume resuscitation in association with rapid cooling, using evaporative heat loss. A fan should be directed onto the hyperthermic patient, and the skin should be kept constantly wet.

Traumatic Arrests

Patients suffering traumatic cardiac arrests should be rapidly intubated and evaluated for tension pneumothorax and pericardial tamponade. Thoracotomy and open chest compressions are indicated for penetrating chest injuries that result in cardiac arrest. Patients who suffer a cardiac arrest after penetrating chest injuries may be successfully resuscitated neurologically intact if they have early open chest CPR and thoracic exploration for aortic cross-clamping and ventricular repair. Patients rarely survive cardiac arrest due to blunt trauma; open thoracotomy in these patients is rarely beneficial.

Post-arrest Management

Attention should be focused on optimizing oxygenation, ventilation, and hemodynamic status while minimizing metabolic demands following the successful resuscitation from cardiac arrest. A constant infusion of 2 to 3 mg per minute of lidocaine should be maintained if VT or VF was the arrest rhythm. Serum levels of magnesium and potassium along with arterial blood gases should be evaluated in surviving patients. Unstable patients, especially those with a depressed level of consciousness, should remain intubated and fully supported by mechanical ventilation. Ventilator settings that provide an FIO_2 of 90 percent, a tidal volume of 12 ml per kilogram, and a rate of 12 are appropriate for most patients immediately following arrest. Mean arterial pressures should be tightly controlled within the 100 to 200 mm Hg range to maximize cerebral and coronary artery perfusion. An arterial catheter should be placed for continuous blood pressure monitoring and arterial blood gas sampling. Hypotension should be treated with crystalloid infusion or, if unsuccessful, with dopamine infusion (starting at 5 μg per kilogram per minute). Hypertension should be treated with nitroprusside or nitroglycerine infusion, rapidly titrating upward from 5 to 10 μg per minute. A pulmonary artery catheter may be useful in the unstable patient. Metabolic demands should be minimized by providing sedation, controlling temperature, maintaining normoglycemia, providing nutrition, and aggressively treating seizures with a benzodiazepine and phenytoin.

Careful serial examination of neurologic status is mandatory in post-arrest patients. To date, no specific drug has been found to improve cerebral outcome. The deeply comatose patient with minimal brainstem function after 3 to 4 days is unlikely to have a normal outcome, and consideration of further life support should be discussed with the patient's family.

SUGGESTED READING

Brown CG, Wesman HA. Adrenergic agonists during cardiopulmonary resuscitation. Resuscitation 1990; 19:1.

Eisenberg MS. Sudden cardiac death and resuscitation: the results. In: Cerra FB, ed. Critical care state of the art. Fullerton, CA: Society of Critical Care Medicine, 1987:133.

Paraskos JA. Cardiovascular pharmacology III: atropine, calcium, calcium blockers, and beta blockers. Circulation 1986; 74(suppl IV):86.

Robinson LA, Brown CG, Jenkins J, Van Ligten PF, et al. The effect of norepinephrine versus epinephrine on myocardial hemodynamics during CPR. Ann Emerg Med 1989; 18:336.

Weil MH, Rackow EC, Trevino R, et al. Difference in acid base state between venous and arterial blood during cardiopulmonary resuscitation. N Engl J Med 1986; 315:153.

SINOATRIAL BLOCK: BRADYCARDIA–TACHYCARDIA SYNDROME

SCOTT E. HESSEN, M.D.
LEONARD S. DREIFUS, M.D.

Dysfunction of the sinoatrial node is a common cardiovascular disorder and is responsible for a galaxy of symptoms including lightheadedness, syncope, drop attacks, fatigue, shortness of breath, and periods of rapid heart action alternating with sinus arrest or bradycardia. Lown first used the term sick sinus syndrome to describe certain post-cardioversion arrhythmias as well as pacemaker activity in subsidiary pacemakers following cardioversion. He also recognized the association of asystolic periods with tachycardia.

Sinus node dysfunction, sometimes described as sick sinus syndrome, consists of (1) persistent, severe, and unexpected sinus bradycardia; (2) sinus arrest, brief or sustained, with escape atrial or atrioventricular (AV) junctional rhythm; (3) prolonged sinus arrest with failure of a subsidiary pacemaker, resulting in total cardiac asystole; (4) chronic atrial fibrillation with slow ventricular responses not caused by drug therapy; (5) inability of the heart to resume sinus rhythm following an electroconversion for atrial fibrillation; and (6) alternating bradyarrhythmias and tachyarrhythmias. The carotid sinus syndrome includes marked slowing of the sinus rate or arrest greater than 3 seconds, fall in systemic blood pressure of more than 50 mm Hg with carotid sinus stimulation, or both.

Three types of carotid sinus syndrome are recognized: a cardioinhibitory type with bradycardia or asystole, a vasodepressive type with hypotension but minimal change in the sinus rate, and a primarily cerebral type. The disease is usually seen in elderly individuals, although rarely it may occur in childhood or adolescence. The majority of patients in the older age groups also suffer from hypertensive or coronary heart disease. Sinus dysfunction may result from abnormal autonomic tone, particularly increased vagal activity. It can be associated with acute myocardial infarction or coronary ischemia. A sclerodegenerative process has been observed to result in sinus node dysfunction. Sinus node dysfunction may also result from surgical trauma, active myocardial or pericardial disease, drug excess with agents such as digitalis, sensitivity to beta-adrenergic and calcium channel blocking agents, electrolyte imbalance, and other metabolic diseases.

Systemic embolization may occur in up to 16 percent of patients with the sick sinus syndrome, especially in those individuals with the bradycardia-tachycardia syndrome.

Sinus node dysfunction may be due to either failure of impulse formation within the sinus node or exit block from the sinus node to perinodal atrial tissue as a result of conduction abnormalities. The fact that conduction disturbances from the sinus node to the perinodal cells can lead to sinus node reentry and tachycardia as seen in Figure 1 suggests that the bradycardia tachycardia syndrome may be related to conduction abnormalities in and near the sinus node. In addition, supraventricular tachycardias that suppress sinus node function due to so-called overdrive suppression may result in long periods of sinus arrest, which also characterize the bradycardia-tachycardia syndrome (Fig. 2).

DIAGNOSIS

The diagnosis of sinus node dysfunction should be suspected when neurologic symptoms of lightheadedness, dizziness, or frank syncope occur. In

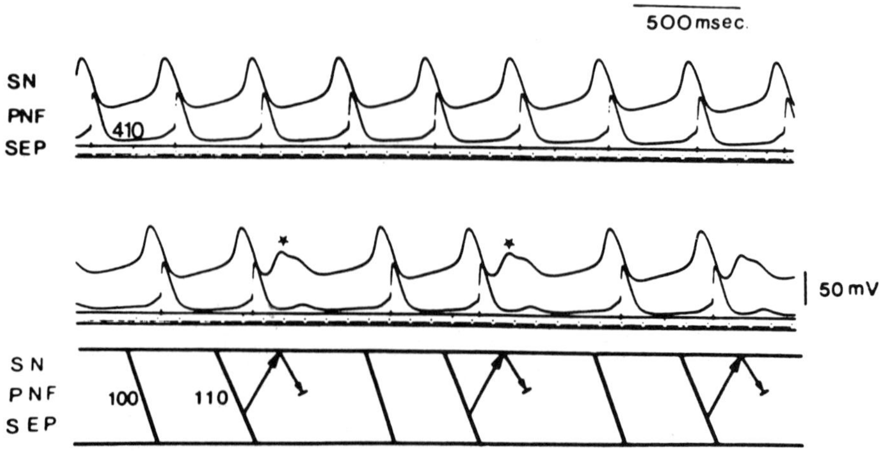

Figure 1 Concealed reentry from the perinodal to the sinus nodal fibers causing periods of sinus node arrest. SN = Sinus node intracellular electrogram, PNF = perinodal cell intracellular electrogram, SEP = atrial septal electrogram.

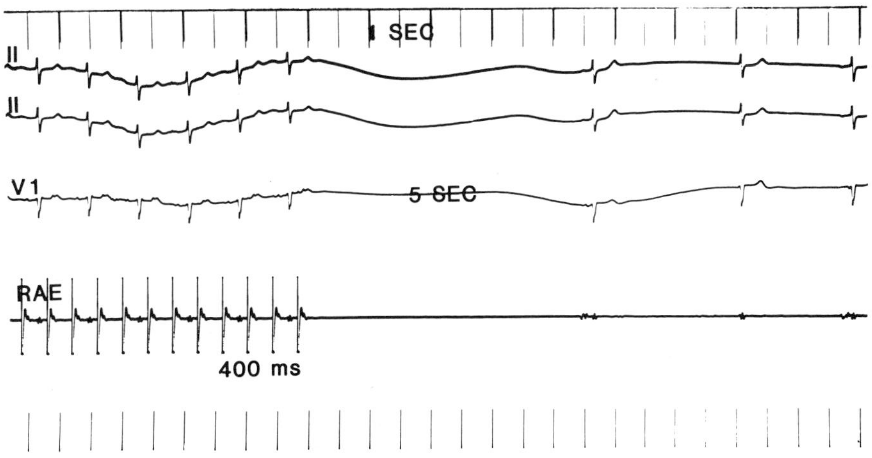

Figure 2 Atrial pacing at 400 milliseconds (150 beats per minute) with 2:1 atrioventricular conduction. There is a 5-second pause following cessation of pacing (sinus node recovery time = 5,000 msec, basic sinus cycle length = 900 msec, corrected sinus node recovery time = 4,100 msec). A secondary pause is also seen.

addition, the association of resting heart rates below 50 beats per minute, atrial tachyarrhythmias, and neurologic symptoms often alerts the clinician to the presence of sinus node disease. Existent and unexplained sinus bradycardia and an inability to increase the heart rate with exercise may also be clues to the presence of sinus node dysfunction. It is important to emphasize that asymptomatic individuals with sinus bradycardia at rest, especially if young, generally will not have sick sinus syndrome. The presence of long periods of cardiac asystole either following the termination of tachycardia in the bradycardia-tachycardia syndrome or due to sinus node dysfunction or exit block implies failure of a subsidiary pacemaker as well (Fig. 3).

Although it is possible to record electrograms directly from the region of the sinus node using closely spaced bipolar catheters, diagnosis of sinus node dysfunction is often apparent from the surface electrocardiogram, Holter monitor, or rhythm strips in many cases (Fig. 4). Because most episodes of syncope or dizziness are paroxysmal, a 24-hour or longer Holter monitor may be necessary to document the arrhythmia. However, unexplained sinus bradycardia in the presence of an exaggerated response to carotid sinus pressure or the presence of various degrees of sinoatrial exit block can be diagnostic (Fig. 5). The asystolic periods associated with symptoms can obviate the need for expensive invasive electrophysiologic studies (see Figs. 3 and 4). The inability to increase the heart rate above 90 beats per minute with moderate exercise can also lead the clinician to suspect the presence of sinus node dysfunction. Because symptoms resulting from sinus node dysfunction are unpredictable and often difficult to document, specific electrophysiologic studies can be used to aid the clinician in the diagnosis of this disorder. In addition, in patients suspected of having sinus node dysfunction, electrophysiologic testing may document other etiologies for clinical symptoms, such as transient AV block or ventricular tachyarrhythmias.

The following electrophysiologic tests of sinus node function may be performed on patients suspected of having symptomatic sick sinus syndrome when the diagnosis is not apparent from long-term electrocardiographic monitoring, particularly when a decision regarding pacemaker implantation is entertained (Table 1).

Electrophysiologic Testing

The most useful test of sinus node function is the measurement of the sinus node recovery time

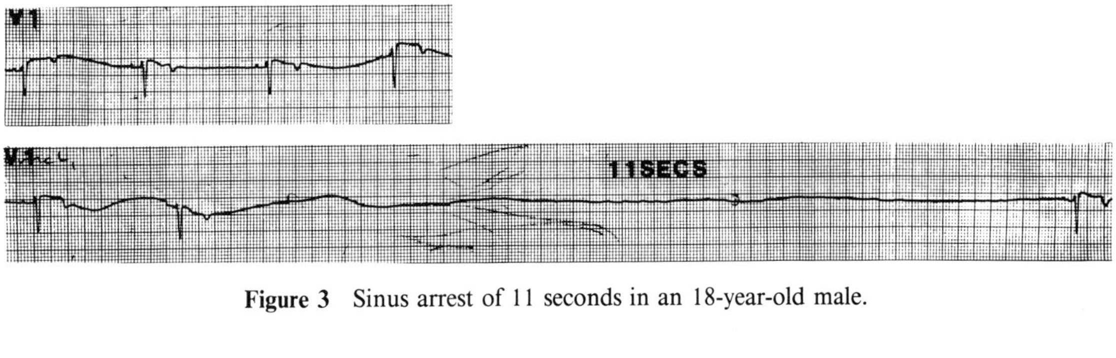

Figure 3 Sinus arrest of 11 seconds in an 18-year-old male.

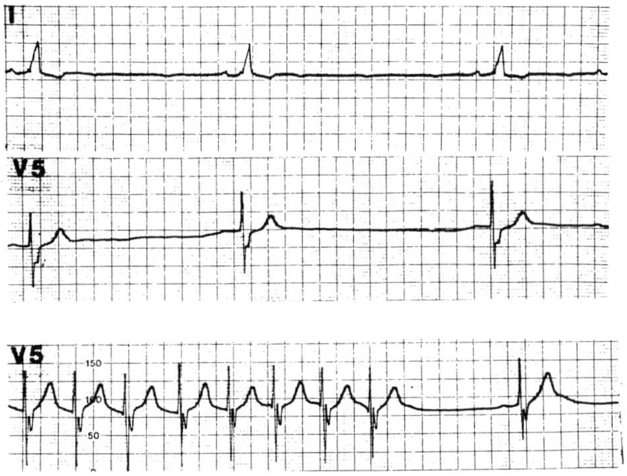

Figure 4 Sinus node dysfunction in a 70-year-old man, demonstrated by periods of sinus tachycardia alternating with sinus bradycardia.

TABLE 1 Sinus Node Function Tests

Automaticity	
SNRT	A pace near SN for 1 min at incremental rates: "overdrive suppression" (normal = 1300 to 1500 msec or 130–150% of BCL)
CSNRT	SNRT − BCL (normal < 550 msec)
TRT	5 beats < 5 sec total
CSP	Normal < 3-second pause
IHR	117.2 − (0.53 × age in years)
Conduction	
SACT	A pace minimally faster than BCL for 8 beats (method of Narula), or atrial extrastimulus method: $\frac{\text{A2A3} - \text{A1A1 (BCL)}}{2} < 125$ msec
CSP	SA exit block
SN reentry	Atrial extrastimulus method

A = Atrial, BCL = basic sinus cycle length, CSNRT = corrected sinus node recovery time, CSP = carotid sinus pressure, IHR = intrinsic heart rate, SA = sinoatrial, SACT = sinoatrial conduction time, SN = sinus node, SNRT = sinus node recovery time, TRT = total recovery time.

(SNRT) (Fig. 6). Atrial pacing is performed near the sinus node at rates above the sinus rate to approximately 150 to 200 beats per minute. Pacing should be performed for 30 seconds to 1 minute at each cycle length, with at least 1 minute of recovery time between paced drives. The interval from the last paced atrial complex to the first sinus node escape beat is the SNRT. Subtracting the basic sinus cycle length from the SNRT yields an SNRT corrected for the prevailing sinus rate, the corrected SNRT (CSNRT). The CSNRT should be measured at several different paced cycle lengths. Normally the maximal CSNRT is less than or equal to 550 milliseconds. An abnormal CSNRT has been found in 35 to 93 percent of patients suspected of having sinus node dysfunction. Abnormal responses are commonly seen in patients with symptomatic tachycardia-bradycardia syndrome. Another measure of sinus node recovery is the time required to return to basic sinus cycle length after pacing, the total recovery time. Normally, this is less than 5 seconds and occurs between the fourth to sixth recovery beat.

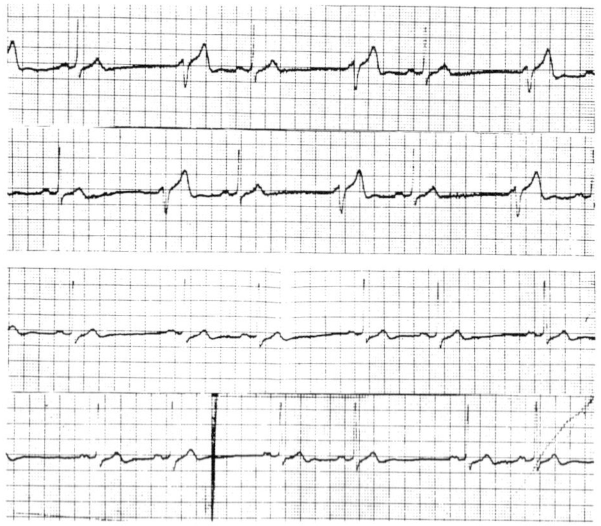

Figure 5 Escape capture bigeminy. Lower two tracings demonstrate a bigeminal rhythm due to 3:2 sinoatrial (SA) exit block. Sinus cycle length = 780 milliseconds. This accounts for 2:1 SA exit block seen in the upper two tracings. Ventricular escape complexes are also noted.

The sinoatrial conduction time (SACT) may be measured either directly or indirectly by several techniques. One indirect method involves pacing the atria minimally faster than the basic sinus rate for eight beats and measuring the interval from the last paced atrial beat to the first sinus escape beat as shown in Figure 7*A* (method of Narula). When subtracted from the prevailing sinus cycle length, this measurement approximates two times the SACT. Another indirect method involves scanning the diastolic period with atrial extrastimuli as shown in Figure 7*B* (method of Strauss). The intervals from the extrastimulus to the return sinus beat are measured. Four patterns of behavior are seen: collision, reset, interpolation, and reentry. During the reset zone, the return cycle interval minus the prevailing sinus cycle interval approximates two times the SACT. Atrial extrastimulation may also initiate sinus node reentry tachycardia in some patients. Normal SACT intervals range from 50 to 125 milliseconds. Measurement of the SACT is not a sensitive test for sinus node dysfunction because only 40 percent of patients with clinical sinus node dysfunction will have abnormal SACTs.

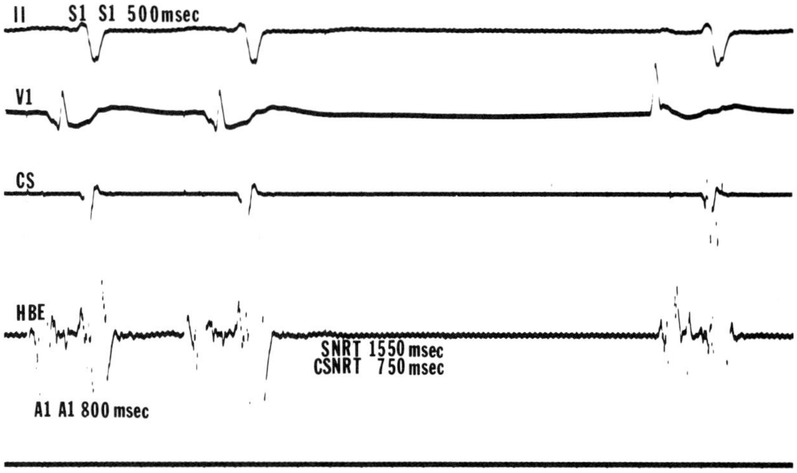

Figure 6 Sinus node recovery time (SNRT) and corrected sinus node recovery time (CSNRT).

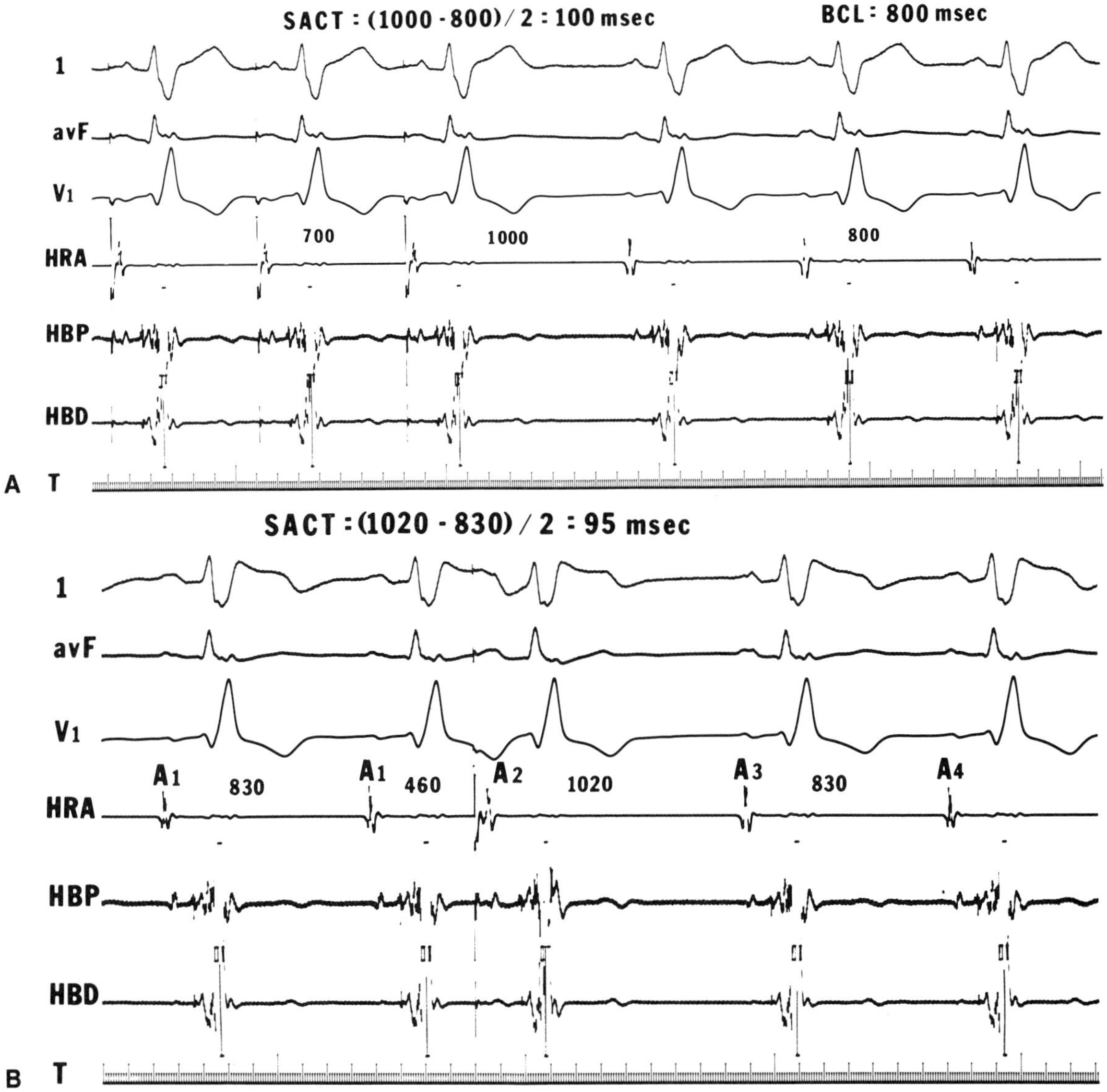

Figure 7 *A*, Sinus node conduction time as measured by the method of Narula. *B*, Sinus node conduction time as measured by the atrial extrastimulus method (Strauss) in the same patient. HRA = High right atrium, HBP = proximal His bundle electrogram, HBD = distal His bundle electrogram.

Autonomic control of sinus node function may be measured by the effect of intravenous atropine (1 to 3 mg) to assess parasympathetic tone. The heart rate should increase to greater than 90 beats per minute or at least 20 to 50 percent above the control rate following injection of atropine. To assess sympathetic responsiveness, isoproterenol may be infused at a rate of 1 to 3 μg per minute; the heart rate should accelerate by at least 25 percent. An absent or blunted response to atropine or isoproterenol suggests sinus node dysfunction.

Pharmacologic denervation using atropine 0.04 mg per kilogram and propranolol 0.2 mg per kilogram allows measurement of the sinus rate unaffected by autonomic tone. Between the ages of 15 and 70 years, this basic or intrinsic heart rate (IHR) normally decreases with age according to the regression equation IHR = 117.2 − (0.53 × age in years). A depressed IHR correlates well with other abnormalities of sinus node function and can differentiate patients with isolated sinus bradycardia due to increased vagal tone from those with true sinus node dysfunction.

The use of sinus node function testing can be important in patient management. Clearly if the symptoms are associated with electrophysiologic abnormalities reproduced during testing, it can be of extreme importance for further management. Notably, patients presenting with syncope and an abnormality in the sinus node during electrophysiologic studies are usually rendered free of syncope following the implantation of a cardiac pacemaker. Unfortunately, electrophysiologic testing of sinus node function is not always predictive of outcome. Even considering the battery of studies discussed, an exact prognostic implication cannot always be ascertained.

Recommendations for electrophysiologic studies have been published recently by the Joint Task Force of the American Heart Association and the American College of Cardiology (ACC/AHA Task Force Report, 1989).

PREFERRED APPROACH

Medical Treatment

A meticulous drug history must be obtained in patients suspected of sinus node dysfunction. Drugs such as digitalis, beta-adrenergic blocking agents, calcium channel antagonists, and antiarrhythmic agents such as quinidine, procainamide, disopyramide, flecainide, encainide, propafenone, and amiodarone can be potent suppressors of sinus node automaticity in patients with sinus node dysfunction. Patients receiving beta-blocking eye drops for glaucoma may have sufficient systemic absorption to provoke sinus node dysfunction. Drugs known to depress sinus node function should be discontinued in patients with sick sinus syndrome unless a permanent pacemaker is present. Patients with the tachycardia-bradycardia syndrome may benefit from antiarrhythmic agents if tachyarrhythmias can be suppressed and if bradyarrhythmias are not significantly worsened.

In general, pharmacologic therapy usually fails to control symptoms and can never be absolutely depended on to manage patients with sinus node disease.

Commonly, patients will develop atrial flutter or fibrillation in the presence of sinus node dysfunction, which may alleviate symptoms related to bradycardia or pauses, but patients will require AV nodal blocking agents for control of ventricular rate and may be at increased risk of systemic embolization. At least one-half of patients experiencing symptoms from sinus node dysfunction will require permanent cardiac pacing.

Surgical Treatment

A majority of initial permanent pacemakers are implanted in the United States for the treatment of sinus node dysfunction. Although ventricular demand (VVI) pacemakers have been used in the past for the treatment of sinus node dysfunction, other pacing modes, including atrial demand (AAI), AV sequential pacing, and rate adaptive modes, have become increasingly common.

Natural history studies have shown that there is a high incidence of atrial fibrillation and systemic embolization in patients with sinus node dysfunction. Although ventricular demand pacing may alleviate symptoms in many patients with sick sinus syndrome, retrospective studies have shown that the rate of atrial fibrillation and systemic embolization may be decreased using either pacemakers that both stimulate and sense in the atria (AAI) or AV sequential pacing modes. In a review of previous studies encompassing 1,171 patients followed for a mean of 38 months, 3.9 percent of patients treated with AAI pacing developed atrial fibrillation compared with 22.3 percent treated with pacemakers pacing and sensing only in the ventricles (VVI). A similar low incidence has been reported using AV sequential pacing modes. Similarly, the incidence of systemic embolization was 1.3 percent with AAI pacing compared with 13 percent with VVI pacing.

Several retrospective studies have suggested decreased mortality among patients with sinus node dysfunction when treated with AAI or AV sequential pacing. Although these patients were similar with regard to baseline characteristics as patients treated with VVI pacing, these results must be interpreted cautiously, since the studies are retrospective and an implantation bias cannot be excluded.

Atrial demand pacing offers the advantages of a simple pacing system, decreased cost, and maintenance of AV synchrony, and it allows a normal sequence of ventricular conduction and contraction. The development of atrial fibrillation and advanced grade AV block may limit the usefulness of this modality, however. Atrial demand pacemakers should not be implanted in patients with sustained or frequent paroxysms of atrial fibrillation or in those patients whose AV nodal Wenckebach point is reached at pacing rates less than 120 beats per minute.

Dual chamber AV sequential pacing alleviates concern about the future development of AV block and maintains AV synchrony, but these devices are more complicated and more expensive than single chamber pacemakers. In addition, universal AV sequential pacemakers, devices that pace and sense in both the atria and ventricles (DDD), may track atrial tachyarrhythmias and may produce pacemaker medicated tachycardias, resulting in rapid ventricular pacing. Dual chamber inhibited (DDI) mode pacemakers are perhaps ideal for patients with sinus node dysfunction, since AV synchrony is maintained but atrial tachyarrhythmias are not sensed and pacemaker medicated tachycardias cannot occur.

More recently, electrophysiologists have recognized the importance of chronotropic incompetence among patients with sinus node dysfunction. In these individuals, there is a failure to increase the sinus rate appropriately for the patient's metabolic needs. These patients, especially younger individuals, may not be capable of increasing their physical activity. Consequently, rate adaptive single and dual chamber pacing using a physiologic sensor such as vibration (activity), temperature, pH, bioimpedance, ventricular gradient, and Po_2 have become available.

Patients with sick sinus syndrome should be considered candidates for permanent pacing if they have symptoms related to sinus bradycardia or sinus pauses that are unrelated to medications. In view of the studies showing a decreased incidence of atrial fibrillation and systemic embolization, and possibly increased survival with atrial (AAI) or AV sequential pacing modalities, these pacemakers should be used whenever possible. Patients with documented chronotropic incompetence should have atrial or AV sequential rate adaptive systems implanted (AAIR, DDIR, or DDDR). In carefully selected patients without evidence of significant AV nodal disease, AAI or AAIR pacing may be modalities of choice.

Complications of cardiac pacing are relatively uncommon and are related mainly to premature battery failure, infection, lead displacement or fracture, or problems associated with the physiologic sensing mechanism of rate responsive pacemakers.

SUGGESTED READING

ACC/AHA Task Force Report. Guidelines for clinical electrophysiologic studies: a report of the American College of Cardiology/American Heart Association Task Force on assessment of diagnostic and therapeutic cardiovascular procedures (subcommittee to assess clinical intracardiac electrophysiologic studies). J Am Coll Cardiol 1989; 14:1827.

Bigger JT, Reiffel JA. Sick sinus syndrome. Am Rev Med 1979; 30:91.

Dhingra RC. Sinus node dysfunction. PACE 1983; 6:1062.

Hatano K, Kato R, Hayashi H, et al. Usefulness of rate responsive atrial pacing in patients with sick sinus syndrome. PACE 1989; 12:16.

Mazgalev T, Dreifus LS, Michelson EL. Modulation of the effects of postganglionic nasal stimulation in the sinus and atrioventricular nodes by cardioactive agents and electrolytes. In: Mazgalev T, Dreifus LS, Michelson EL, eds. Electrophysiology of the sinoatrial and atrioventricular nodes. New York: Alan R. Liss, 1988:207.

Reiffel JA, Bigger JT Jr. Current status of direct recordings of the sinus node electrogram in man. PACE 1983; 6:1143.

Reiffel JA, Livelli F, Gliklide J, Bigger JT Jr. Indirectly estimated sinoatrial conduction time by the atrial premature stimulus technique: patterns of error and the degree of associated inaccuracy as assessed by direct sinus node electrography. Am Heart J 1983; 106:459.

Rosenqvist M, Brandt J, Schuller H. Long-term pacing in sinus node disease: effects of stimulation mode on cardiovascular morbidity and mortality. Am Heart J 1988; 116:16.

Strauss HC, Saroff AL, Bigger JT Jr, Grardina EGV. Premature atrial stimulation as a key to the understanding of sinoatrial conduction in man. Presentation of data and critical review of the literature. Circulation 1973; 47:86.

Sutton R, Kenny RA. The natural history of sick sinus syndrome. PACE 1986; 9:1110.

ATRIAL PREMATURE DEPOLARIZATION, ATRIAL TACHYCARDIA, ATRIAL FLUTTER, AND ATRIAL FIBRILLATION

YOSHIO WATANABE, M.D.
TAKAKAZU KATOH, M.D.

ATRIAL PREMATURE DEPOLARIZATION

Atrial premature depolarization (or atrial premature systole) is defined as an ectopic impulse formation in the atria occurring earlier than an expected sinus node discharge. An enhanced physiologic automaticity (phase 4 depolarization), the development of abnormal automaticity (including triggered activity), and reentry have been suggested as possible electrophysiologic mechanisms underlying this arrhythmia. The premature depolarization may occur either singly or in pairs (couplets).

Therapeutic Alternatives

Atrial premature depolarizations usually do not require treatment regardless of their number, unless the patient is markedly symptomatic. However, underlying cardiac, pulmonary, or other systemic diseases must be treated because they may predispose the patients to ectopic impulse formation. Similarly, when certain predisposing factors such as smoking, alcohol, caffeine, or emotional stress can be identified, an attempt must be made to reduce those factors. The therapeutic approach to symptomatic patients should begin with reassurance and a full explanation of the benign nature of this arrhythmia. If the patients still complain of severe palpitation and chest discomfort, administration of minor tranquilizers or beta-adrenergic blocking agents often successfully ameliorates these symptoms. An antiarrhythmic drug should be administered only when all these measures have failed. Although sporadic appearance of atrial premature depolarizations would not cause significant hemodynamic derangements, nonconducted premature depolarizations occurring in bigeminal pattern could sometimes produce lightheadedness or even syncope and must be treated.

Preferred Approach

Table 1 shows the commonly accepted classification and dosage of antiarrhythmic agents. Generally, class II agents (beta-adrenergic blockers) are effective in suppressing a majority of atrial premature depolarizations. Class I (sodium channel blocker) and class III (potassium channel blocker) drugs may exert a potent inhibitory action on atrial premature depolarizations as they directly block ionic channels of the cardiac cell membrane. Conversely, class IV drugs (calcium channel blockers) appear to be less effective in suppressing atrial premature depolarizations. These antiarrhythmic agents should be administered when atrial premature depolarizations are responsible for the initiation of supraventricular tachyarrhythmias such as atrial tachycardia, atrial flutter and fibrillation, and paroxysmal supraventricular tachycardia. In other words, the management of atrial premature depolarizations should be directed at (1) reducing the associated symptoms and (2) preventing the induction of more serious tachyarrhythmias.

ATRIAL TACHYCARDIA

Atrial tachycardia is usually defined as a consecutive appearance of three or more atrial premature depolarizations. Its electrophysiologic mechanism is either sinus node or intra-atrial reentry, enhanced physiologic automaticity, or abnormal automaticity due to a triggered activity occurring in an ectopic focus within the atria. Infrequently occurring atrial tachycardias of a short duration (10 seconds or less) are usually asymptomatic and do not require medical treatment. Indeed, many patients in whom brief periods of atrial tachycardia were recorded on 24-hour ambulatory electrocardiograms failed to note such episodes.

Ectopic Atrial Tachycardia

Ectopic atrial tachycardias of either persistent or incessant type should be treated. To make a correct diagnosis, one must distinguish this entity from so-called paroxysmal supraventricular tachycardias involving the atrioventricular node in their reentry circuit. Because vagotonic maneuvers such as breath-holding, eyeball pressure, and carotid sinus massage depress conduction through the atrioventricular node, paroxysmal supraventricular tachycardias can be interrupted by these maneuvers, whereas atrial tachycardia usually is not terminated despite the development of atrioventricular block. However, it is possible that paroxysmal atrial tachycardia due to sinus node reentry is terminated by vagal stimulation because its reentry circuit is richly innervated by vagal nerve fibers.

Preferred Approach

To treat atrial tachycardia pharmacologically, intravenous administration of digoxin or deslanoside may be indicated, especially in patients with congestive heart failure. Although this therapy may

TABLE 1 Classification, Dosage, and Side Effects of Antiarrhythmic Agents

Class	*Agent*	*Oral Dosage*	*Intravenous Dosage*	*Side Effects*
IA	Quinidine sulfate	200–400 mg q 6 h		Prolongation of Q-T interval, ventricular tachycardia (torsade de pointes), conduction block, enhanced AV nodal conduction due to anticholinergic action, hypotension, diarrhea, vomiting, thrombocytopenia
	Procainamide	250–500 mg q 6–8 h	25–50 mg/min up to 15 mg/kg	Ventricular tachycardia (torsade de pointes), conduction block, lupus-like syndrome (arthralgia, positive antinuclear antibodies), agranulocytosis
	Disopyramide	100–200 mg q 6–8 h	10–15 mg/min up to 3 mg/kg	Congestive heart failure, anticholinergic action (urinary retention, constipation)
IB	Lidocaine		20–50 mg/min up to 1–3 mg/kg, then infusion at a rate of 2–4 mg/min	Central nervous system symptoms (seizures, drowsiness, dysarthria, paresthesia)
	Mexiletine	200–400 mg q 8 h		Neurologic symptoms (tremor, blurred vision, dizziness), rash, thrombocytopenia, bradycardia
	Tocainide	400–600 mg q 8–12 h	10–20 mg/min up to 10 mg/kg	Hypotension, congestive heart failure, nausea, vomiting, paresthesia, tremor, dizziness
IC	Flecainide	100–200 mg q 12 h	10–15 mg/min up to 2 mg/kg	Conduction block, congestive heart failure, aggravation of arrhythmia, increased pacing threshold, hypotension, paresthesia, visual disturbance, tremor, insomnia, blurred vision
	Encainide	25–50 mg q 8 h	5–10 mg/min up to 1 mg/kg	Ventricular tachycardia, conduction block, worsened arrhythmia, congestive heart failure, increase in defibrillation threshold, dizziness, blurred vision, ataxia, slurred speech
	Propafenone	100–300 mg q 8 h	10–20 mg/min up to 2 mg/kg	Hypotension, conduction block, nausea, vomiting, headache, tremor
II	Propranolol	10–60 mg q 6 h	1 mg/min up to 0.1 mg/kg	Bronchial asthma, congestive heart failure, sinus bradycardia, SA and AV block, hypotension, hypoglycemia, Raynaud's phenomenon, carcinogenesis, oculomucocutaneous reaction
	Metoprolol	50–100 mg q 12 h	2 mg/min up to 0.2 mg/kg	Identical to those with propranolol, but lesser adverse effects on bronchial and vascular β-adrenoceptors
III	Amiodarone	800–1600 mg/day for 2 wks, then 200–600 mg/day	3–5 mg/kg over 30 min	Hypotension, interstitial pneumonitis, hyperthyroidism or hypothyroidism, corneal microdeposits, photosensitivity of the skin
IV	Verapamil	80-120 mg q 8 h	0.075–0.15 mg/kg over 1–2 min. If unsuccessful, repeat IV 10 min later	Sinus bradycardia, SA and AV block, hypotension, congestive heart failure, constipation

Continued

TABLE 1 Classification, Dosage, and Side Effects of Antiarrhythmic Agents *Continued*

Class	*Agent*	*Oral Dosage*	*Intravenous Dosage*	*Side Effects*
	Diltiazem	30–90 mg q 6–8 h	0.15–0.30 mg/kg over 3 min. If unsuccessful, repeat IV 10 min later	Sinus bradycardia, SA and AV block, hypotension, congestive heart failure, headache
Others	Digoxin	0.25–0.5 mg q 24 h	0.75–1.0 mg over 3 min	Atrial and ventricular premature depolarizations, nonparoxysmal atrial, AV junctional and ventricular tachycardias, AV block, enhanced conduction in the accessory pathway, nausea, vomiting, diarrhea, gynecomastia
	Deslanoside	—	0.4–0.8 mg over 3 min	Similar to those with digoxin
	ATP	—	10 mg in less than 1 sec. If unsuccessful, 20 mg IV 2 min later	Transient nausea, headache, dyspnea, flushing, sinus bradycardia, AV block, atrial and ventricular premature depolarizations and tachycardias
	Adenosine	—	5 mg in less than 1 sec. If unsuccessful, 10 mg IV 2 min later	Similar to those with ATP
	Coumarin	15 mg for 3 days, then 2–10 mg daily depending on prothrombin time		Systemic hemorrhage

ATP = Adenosine triphosphate, AV = atrioventricular, IV = intravenous, SA = sinoatrial.

not always terminate the tachycardia, its beneficial effects on co-existing heart failure can be expected. If atrial tachycardia is accompanied by atrioventricular block, cardiac glycosides should not be administered because such an arrhythmia most often results from digitalis overdosage. The initial treatment for digitalis-induced atrial tachycardia is to discontinue the drug and correct serum electrolyte imbalance (especially hypopotassemia) if such a condition exists. When the aforementioned treatment does not convert the tachycardia to sinus rhythm, an antiarrhythmic drug therapy should be considered.

It is well known that atrial tachycardias are often refractory to drug treatment. Indeed, most of the class IA and IB antiarrhythmic drugs are usually ineffective against this arrhythmia. Quinidine and procainamide (class IA) may even accelerate the tachycardia probably as a result of their anticholinergic action. For an acute termination of persistent or incessant atrial tachycardia, intravenous administration of propranolol (class II) is probably the first choice (Table 1). This drug is successful in approximately half the patients but cannot be applied to patients with lung disease. Intravenous amiodarone (class III) is also quite effective in terminating the tachycardia without significant adverse effects. We have observed a permanent suppression of chronic ectopic atrial tachycardia in a young, postmyocarditic patient with oral amiodarone treatment (Fig. 1). Intravenous flecainide or encainide (class IC drugs) has been reported to be as potent as amiodarone, but further clinical evaluation may be necessary before these drugs can be considered as first-line agents. Among class IB agents, ethmozin appears to be the only drug that suppresses atrial tachycardia, but its clinical efficacy has not yet been established. Because all these class I drugs more or less cause conduction disturbances in both the atria and the ventricles and lower the blood pressure, continuous electrocardiographic monitoring and frequent blood pressure measurements are mandatory during their intravenous administration. If QRS complexes in sinus beats become widened to 0.12 seconds or longer, of if arrhythmogenic side effects (either the development of a new tachyarrhythmia or aggravation of the initial arrhythmia) are observed, the drug injection should be discontinued immediately. If the patient has a preexisting intraventricular conduction disturbance, class I drugs are contraindicated for the same reason. Verapamil (class IV) also should not be used because this agent seldom terminates the tachycardia and may even accelerate it after an intravenous administration.

Following a successful termination of the episode of atrial tachycardia, long-term pharmacologic therapy is often required to prevent its recurrence. In most instances, an acute intravenous drug test is helpful in predicting the clinical response to long-term oral drug therapy. Hence, oral administration of those intravenously effective drugs can be initi-

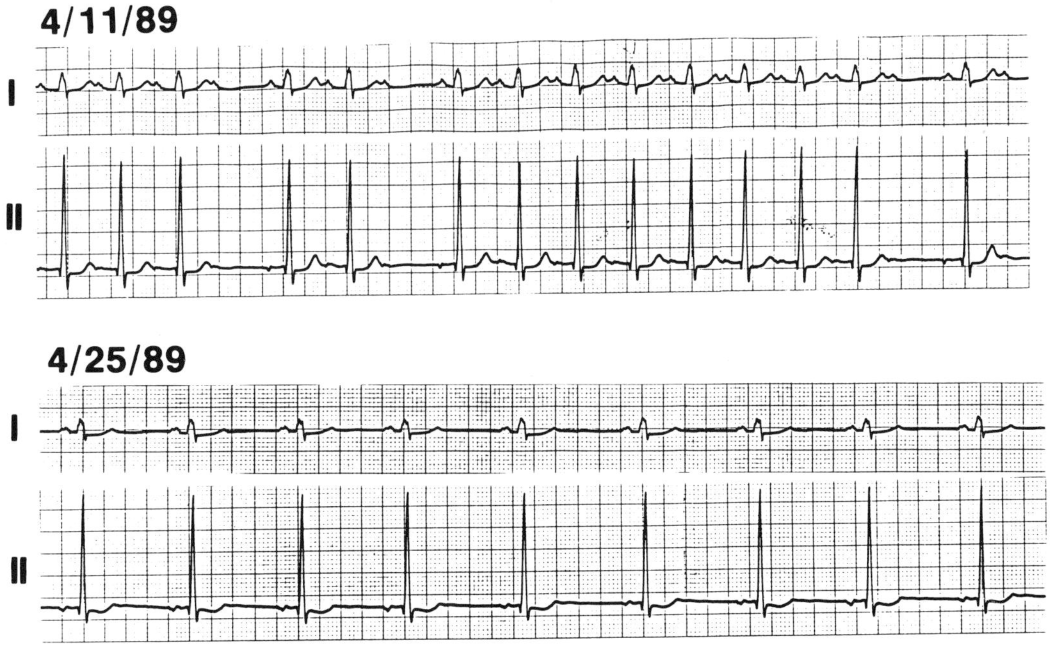

Figure 1 Treatment of persistent atrial tachycardia with oral amiodarone. This 19-year-old male student developed a rapid heart action 6 months after suffering from acute myocarditis. The tachycardia had rates ranging from 110 to 140 beats per minute and was diagnosed as an ectopic atrial tachycardia. It was resistant to various antiarrhythmic drugs, including quinidine, disopyramide, propranolol, and verapamil, and persisted for more than 2 years before these electrocardiograms were recorded. Simultaneous records of leads I and II in the upper panel (4/11/89) reveal an atrial tachycardia at the rate of 115 beats per minute associated with a Wenckebach type second-degree atrioventricular (AV) block. Such an AV block was observed only in the supine position. Oral administration of 200 mg per day of amiodarone was started on this day, and the tachycardia was completely suppressed in 2 weeks as shown in the bottom panel (4/25/89).

ated. Such a drug may well be taken in combination with oral digoxin because the latter agent is beneficial in the management of heart failure. Adverse effects that might be observed on long-term administration of these drugs are listed in Table 1.

For those ectopic atrial tachycardias entirely refractory to these pharmacologic approaches, surgical resection of the arrhythmogenic atrial foci may provide a complete cure. The operative risk of this procedure is low, but the recurrence of tachycardia has been observed in 30 to 50 percent of the cases. Thus, surgical ablation should be considered for patients whose ectopic atrial tachycardia proves refractory to antiarrhythmic drug therapy and in whom the rapid heart action causes hemodynamic deterioration. Recently, new techniques such as cryoablation and catheter electroablation of the arrhythmogenic foci have been reported to abolish the tachycardia successfully. However, further experience is needed to establish their feasibility and clinical values. In fact, serious complications such as perforation of the heart, thromboembolism, and sudden death have been reported with the latter procedure. Electrical treatments such as atrial or ventricular pacing and direct current cardioversion are generally not indicated against ectopic atrial tachycardia.

Multifocal (or Chaotic) Atrial Tachycardia

Multifocal or chaotic atrial tachycardia is another form of atrial tachycardia often resistant to medical treatment. This arrhythmia is characterized by a relatively slow atrial rate of 100 to 150 beats per minute, three or more P wave morphologies, and varying P-P and P-R intervals. Triggered activity caused by an increased intracellular calcium concentration has been suggested as a possible electrophysiologic mechanism. Endogenous or exogenous catecholamines are likely to facilitate the development of this arrhythmia by increasing the calcium current in the atria.

Preferred Approach

Multifocal atrial tachycardia is associated most often with chronic obstructive pulmonary disease, followed by congestive heart failure and coronary artery disease. Hence, the initial treatment should be focused on the correction of these precipitating factors. For instance, improved ventilation with better oxygenation of the blood, correction of serum electrolyte imbalance, and amelioration of congestive heart failure must be attempted. If multifocal atrial tachycardia persists despite such measures, pharmacologic therapy should be instituted because the prognosis of patients with this arrhythmia is quite grave as evidenced by the average in-hospital mortality rate of 38 to 62 percent. As in the case of persistent or incessant ectopic atrial tachycardia, class IA and IB drugs and digitalis glycosides are usually ineffective, whereas intravenous injection of up to 0.2 mg per kilogram metoprolol (a cardioselective $beta_1$-adrenergic receptor blocking agent) has been shown to terminate the tachycardia without significant adverse effects, even in patients with pulmonary disease. However, utmost caution should be exercised when metoprolol is administered to such patients. Intravenous propranolol is also effective against this arrhythmia, but this drug should not be used in the presence of chronic pulmonary disease because of its adverse action on the respiratory function. Hypotension constitutes another serious side effect of class II agents. Hence, one must be careful in administering these agents to patients with congestive heart failure.

The drug of second choice against multifocal atrial tachycardia is either verapamil (class IV) or amiodarone (class III). Intravenous administration of verapamil may convert the tachycardia to sinus rhythm without major complications. Although this agent appears less potent than metoprolol in terminating the tachycardia, it has an additional benefit of slowing the ventricular response when the tachycardia persists. Hence, verapamil may be selected for patients who are resistant to class II agents. Intravenous amiodarone is also known to terminate multifocal atrial tachycardia. Because an acute administration of this drug usually does not cause any adverse side effects, amiodarone may be used for any patient regardless of underlying disease. However, amiodarone therapy against this arrhythmia has not yet been widely accepted, and we should await further clinical investigation to establish its usefulness.

Long-term management of multifocal atrial tachycardia should be directed primarily at the correction of underlying disease. This must be supplemented by the oral administration of drugs initially proved to be effective in terminating the tachycardia with intravenous injection. As has been described above, metoprolol, verapamil, and amiodarone are the drugs of choice. Because the former two drugs may sometimes show adverse effects, including hypotension, aggravation of preexisting pulmonary disease, and congestive heart failure, careful patient selection is mandatory. It is true that chronic amiodarone therapy may cause asymptomatic corneal microdeposits, thyroid dysfunction, pulmonary fibrosis, or congestive heart failure. However, these changes can usually be reversed by discontinuation of the drug therapy.

There is a report that an overdrive ventricular pacing was successful in suppressing this arrhythmia in some cases, but this treatment is probably not feasible against multifocal atrial tachycardia with high rates. Electrical cardioversion has been associated with rather poor results in terminating the tachycardia. Surgical resection of arrhythmogenic atrial foci has not yet been successful, probably because of the widespread pathologic changes in the entire atrial tissue.

ATRIAL FLUTTER

Atrial flutter is rapid, regular, and repetitive atrial depolarizations at rates ranging from 250 to 400 beats per minute. Electrocardiographically, it is characterized by "saw-tooth" undulations of the baseline without being separated by a horizontal isoelectric segment in typical cases (Fig. 2). This arrhythmia is usually initiated by an atrial premature depolarization. A macroreentry movement involving the bulk of the atrial tissue is generally considered responsible for the maintenance of atrial flutter.

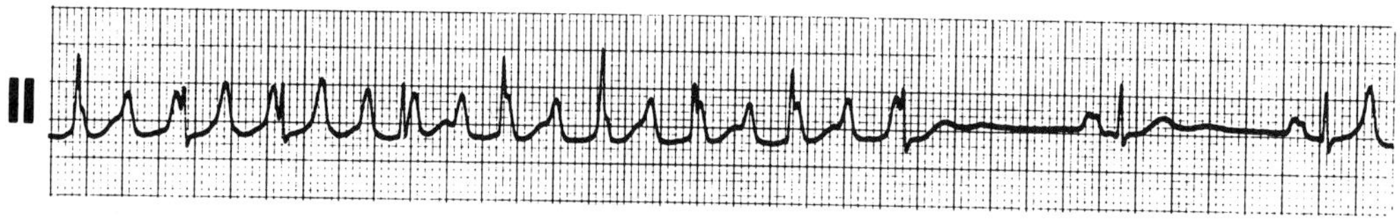

Figure 2 Treatment of paroxysmal atrial flutter with intravenous disopyramide. The patient was a 57-year-old woman who complained of severe palpitation for more than 5 hours. The patient initially showed large "saw-tooth" undulations of the baseline, with their amplitude almost equaling the QRS complexes. After an intravenous injection of 100 mg of disopyramide over 5 minutes, the flutter rate was slowed from 282 to 228 beats per minute, with the maintenance of a 2:1 AV conduction ratio. Sinus rhythm was reestablished 2 minutes after the injection was over, although a single atrial premature depolarization occurred on the T wave of the last beat.

Paroxysmal and Persistent Atrial Flutter

Paroxysmal and persistent atrial flutter should be treated, although it is frequently resistant to pharmacologic treatment. When atrial flutter is associated with an atrioventricular conduction ratio of 1 : 1, an Adams-Stokes attack may develop because the rapid ventricular rate of more than 250 beats per minute can compromise the cardiac output. Even in the presence of a more common atrioventricular conduction ratio of 2 : 1, the ventricular rate can be too high to maintain adequate cardiac hemodynamics. Hence, the treatment must be aimed initially at slowing the ventricular response by depressing atrioventricular conduction.

Preferred Approach

Although intravenous injection of cardiac glycosides (digoxin or deslanoside) is a classic approach for this purpose, the drug action is not sufficiently rapid. Therefore, when the ventricular rate is higher than 150 beats per minute and the patient is symptomatic, intravenous injection of verapamil or diltiazem should be given promptly to prevent the development of hypotension, congestive heart failure, and ventricular fibrillation. Although these calcium antagonists are not potent in converting atrial flutter to sinus rhythm, they can immediately decrease the ventricular rate.

Following this treatment or when the ventricular rate is relatively slow without any medication, antiarrhythmic agents can be used to restore a sinus rhythm. Class IA drugs are considered the first choice, and oral quinidine has been used most frequently to achieve this goal. More recently, however, quinidine has been replaced by newer antiarrhythmic agents because (1) it takes more than several hours or even a few days to convert flutter to sinus rhythm, (2) there is a possibility of quinidine toxicity causing more serious ventricular arrhythmias, and (3) its anticholinergic action may cause an atrioventricular conduction ratio of 1 : 1. Hence, class IA drugs currently recommended include intravenous disopyramide and procainamide. Because these two agents also possess an anticholinergic action, the patients should always be pretreated with digitalis glycosides or calcium antagonists to prevent the acceleration of ventricular response. Reversion of atrial flutter to sinus rhythm with these drugs is often preceded by a period of atrial fibrillation. Although atrial fibrillation may persist in some instances, the ventricular response can be controlled much more easily in atrial fibrillation than in atrial flutter. Intravenous administration of class IC drugs (flecainide, encainide, or propafenone) may be more potent than class IA drugs in terminating atrial flutter, whereas class IB drugs are usually ineffective against this arrhythmia. However, some investigators pointed out a possible risk of class IA and IC drugs in treating this arrhythmia because theoretically these agents may shorten the wavelength in the reentry circuit (determined as the product of conduction velocity and refractory period), may widen the excitable gap, and may make the reentry movement more stable. If this assumption turns out to be valid, intravenous amiodarone (potassium channel blocker) may be considered a drug of choice in restoring sinus rhythm because this drug markedly prolongs the refractory period. However, its clinical efficacy has not yet been established, and another class III agent, sotalol, and class II and IV agents appear generally ineffective in terminating atrial flutter.

The most effective way to convert atrial flutter to sinus rhythm is electrical cardioversion. If the patient is in the state of circulatory failure because of an extremely rapid ventricular rate, synchronized direct current shock of 5 to 10 joules should be applied immediately. If unsuccessful, the energy is increased stepwise to 50 joules. In this way, almost 95 percent of patients can be converted to sinus rhythm. When the patient is fully digitalized, withhold the glycoside before cardioversion. In the absence of such an emergency, rapid atrial pacing can also be used to convert atrial flutter to either sinus rhythm or atrial fibrillation. For this purpose, transesophageal atrial pacing is recommended because it is a noninvasive procedure and still shows the same success rate as transvenous right atrial pacing. As has been pointed out above, class IA and IC agents may widen the excitable gap in the reentry circuit. It can then be suggested that, in the presence of these agents, electrical stimuli would more easily enter the excitable gap and interrupt the reentry movement. Indeed, successful conversion of refractory atrial flutter to sinus rhythm with a combination of intravenous procainamide and rapid atrial pacing has been reported recently.

Prophylactic treatment of paroxysmal and persistent atrial flutter is different from that aimed at their termination. If the arrhythmia develops in the presence of either valvular heart disease, cardiomyopathy, coronary artery disease, pulmonary embolism, or hyperthyroidism, such an underlying disease must be treated intensively. Because atrial flutter is initiated by atrial premature depolarizations, oral administration of class IA, IC, II, or III drugs is recommended to reduce the number of premature depolarizations. Oral digitalis or a class IV agent such as verapamil or diltiazem may be added to the aforementioned antiarrhythmic drugs in the hope that the former would effectively control the ventricular rate by depressing atrioventricular conduction even when atrial flutter does develop. Electrical or surgical treatment is not indicated for prophylaxis.

Chronic Atrial Flutter

Preferred Approach

In certain cases, atrial flutter is quite refractory to pharmacologic treatment and tends to recur shortly after an electrical cardioversion. The term chronic atrial flutter is applied to those cases, and no further attempts should be made to terminate this arrhythmia. The only therapy is to control the ventricular rate by depressing atrioventricular conduction with a maintenance oral dose of either digitalis glycosides, beta-adrenergic blockers, or calcium antagonists, and an optimal ventricular rate of 60 to 80 beats per minute can be obtained by producing an atrioventricular conduction ratio of 4 : 1. Drug selection should be based on the underlying disease. For instance, if chronic atrial flutter is associated with congestive heart failure, digitalis is the drug of choice and calcium antagonists are contraindicated. In the presence of a pulmonary disease, digitalis or calcium antagonists should be administered but not beta-blockers. For this type of atrial flutter, class IA drugs with an anticholinergic action as well as class IC drugs are not desirable because a resultant slowing of the flutter rate may permit a better atrioventricular conduction and increase the ventricular rate.

There is no indication for rapid atrial pacing. However, catheter ablation or surgical section of either the atrioventricular node or the His bundle may have to be considered in patients in whom a good atrioventricular conduction is maintained despite the aforementioned drug therapies. Because these ablative procedures cause a complete atrioventricular block, a permanent artificial pacemaker must be implanted to provide a stable ventricular rhythm.

Anticoagulation therapy is not needed for chronic atrial flutter.

ATRIAL FIBRILLATION

Atrial fibrillation is a completely disorganized, rapid atrial excitation. Electrocardiographically, the isoelectric line is replaced by rapid, irregular undulations called f waves usually having rates higher than 400 beats per minute. Because of the filtering action of the atrioventricular node, many atrial impulses are blocked in this node, and only some of the depolarization waves are conducted to the ventricles, causing an entirely irregular ventricular response. Atrial fibrillation is initiated usually by an atrial premature depolarization occurring in the vulnerable period of atrial excitability. Numerous microreentry circuits are considered to sustain this arrhythmia.

Paroxysmal and Persistent Atrial Fibrillation

Preferred Approach

An attempt must be made to convert paroxysmal and persistent atrial fibrillation to sinus rhythm. If the patient has an underlying disorder such as valvular heart disease, coronary heart disease, cardiomyopathy, or thyrotoxicosis, its treatment is necessary. However, regardless of the type of underlying diseases (except for Wolff-Parkinson-White [WPW] syndrome), the initial treatment for atrial fibrillation is generally intravenous digitalis. This drug is expected to slow the ventricular response by depressing atrioventricular conduction and often successfully converts paroxysmal atrial fibrillation to sinus rhythm. If paroxysmal atrial fibrillation is not terminated, intravenous disopyramide or procainamide (class IA drugs) should be given. Although not mandatory, combination with digitalis is recommended to prevent the occurrence of a rapid ventricular response before the restoration of sinus rhythm. Oral quinidine is also very potent to convert atrial fibrillation to sinus rhythm, but this treatment is not encouraged for the reason described in the treatment of atrial flutter. If this mode of treatment is chosen, the patient should be pretreated with digitalis. It has been reported recently that intravenous flecainide, encainide, propafenone (class IC), or amiodarone (class III) is successful in restoring sinus rhythm without significant adverse effects. The success rate for chemical cardioversion with these drugs (60 to 80 percent) is equal to or slightly better than that with class IA drugs, although individual success rates largely depend on the duration of atrial fibrillation, the atrial size, and the underlying heart diseases. Propranolol (class II) and verapamil (class IV) are not effective in terminating atrial fibrillation and are used mainly to control the ventricular response. When atrial fibrillation is accompanied by WPW syndrome, cardiac glycosides and, to lesser extent, verapamil are contraindicated because they tend to enhance conduction in the accessory pathway and may induce ventricular fibrillation. In such cases, class IA, IC, or III drugs should be administered intravenously to depress conduction or prolong refractoriness in the accessory pathway and to restore a sinus rhythm.

Another excellent way of treating this arrhythmia is electrical cardioversion. This treatment is indicated for any type of atrial fibrillation. Above all, atrial fibrillation with a rapid ventricular response due to accessory atrioventricular conduction (WPW syndrome) or with congestive heart failure is best treated with this method. A synchronized, direct current shock of 50 joules should be applied initially. If the current is not sufficient to terminate fibrillation, its energy is increased stepwise to 200 joules, and a normal sinus rhythm can be established in 95 percent of cases. Conversely, electrical pacing is useless to terminate atrial fibrillation or to control the ventricular rate during fibrillation. No surgical treatment is indicated for this arrhythmia. Recently, however, catheter ablation of the atrioventricular junction has been used in cases of refractory paroxysmal atrial fibrillation. Although this procedure does not cure atrial fibrillation and permanent ventricular pacing is required, the patient's quality of life and exercise capacity appear to be improved significantly.

After a successful conversion of atrial fibrillation to sinus rhythm, treatment of underlying diseases should be maintained. Efforts must also be made to reduce the precipitating factors such as smoking, alcohol, caffeine, mental stress, or fatigue. If atrial fibrillation recurs in spite of these measures, the patients should be treated pharmacologically. Because atrial fibrillation is initiated by atrial premature depolarizations in most of the cases, and occasionally by ventricular premature systoles in cases of WPW syndrome, prophylactic therapy should be focused on the prevention of these premature systoles. In general, class IA drugs (especially disopyramide) are recommended for these purposes. Although class IC and class III drugs may be more potent, they should be used only when class IA drugs fail to maintain sinus rhythm because their long-term administration may cause adverse side effects as listed in Table 1.

Patients with atrial fibrillation have a 5 to 10 times higher risk of systemic embolization compared with patients with a regular sinus rhythm. Hence, even when thrombus formation is not demonstrated by echocardiography, anticoagulation therapy must be used in cases of persistent and recurrent atrial fibrillation associated with valvular heart disease, cardiomyopathy, prosthetic valves, or a history of embolism. Although it has been said classically that atrial fibrillation in the absence of underlying heart diseases (so-called lone atrial fibrillation) would not cause thromboembolism, systemic embolization does occasionally develop in those cases as well. Coumarin is usually administered for 3 weeks prior to pharmacologic or electrical cardioversion. Its dosage should be determined according to the prothrombin time. Because hemorrhagic complications may develop when the prothrombin time is prolonged to more than twice the control, it should be maintained at approximately 1.5 times the control level. After cardioversion, anticoagulation therapy should be continued for another week or two, including those patients who were not pretreated with coumarin because of an emergency cardioversion. No convincing evidence has been presented so far that aspirin or dipyridamole provides sufficient protection against thromboembolism.

Chronic Atrial Fibrillation

Preferred Approach

Chronic atrial fibrillation is defined as atrial fibrillation that cannot be converted to sinus rhythm nor prevented from recurrence by any means. Hence, its treatment should be focused on controlling the ventricular rate. Drugs to be used are those that depress atrioventricular conduction, including digitalis, beta-adrenoceptor blockers (class II), and calcium antagonists (class IV). They should be administered depending on the types of underlying diseases. There is no way to treat chronic atrial fibrillation with electrical measures. Recently, it has been reported that surgical isolation of a conducting pathway between the sinus and atrioventricular nodes by multiple incisions to and suturing of the atrial tissue could produce a slower and stable "sinus" rhythm in certain instances. However, more extensive studies are definitely needed before this procedure is accepted as an effective treatment against chronic atrial fibrillation. Anticoagulant therapy should be applied to those patients as discussed above. However, care should be taken when coumarin is administered to hypertensive or elderly patients because they have a greater risk of developing cerebral hemorrhage.

SUGGESTED READING

Bianconi L, Boccadamo R, Pappalardo A, et al. Effectiveness of intravenous propafenone for conversion of atrial fibrillation and flutter of recent onset. Am J Cardiol 1989; 64:335.

McGuire MA, Johnson DC, Nunn GR, et al. Surgical therapy for atrial tachycardia in adults. J Am Coll Cardiol 1989; 14:1777.

Moak JP, Smith RT, Garson A Jr. Newer antiarrhythmic drugs in children. Am Heart J 1987; 113:179.

Scher DL, Arsura EL. Multifocal atrial tachycardia: mechanisms, clinical correlates, and treatment. Am Heart J 1989; 118:574.

Van Gelder IC, Crijns HJGM, Van Gilst WH, et al. Efficacy and safety of flecainide acetate in the maintenance of sinus rhythm after electrical cardioversion of chronic atrial fibrillation or atrial flutter. Am J Cardiol 1989; 64:1317.

Watanabe Y, Dreifus LS. Cardiac arrhythmias. Electrophysiologic basis for clinical interpretation. New York: Grune & Stratton, 1977.

VENTRICULAR PREMATURE DEPOLARIZATIONS AND VENTRICULAR TACHYCARDIA

ALFRED E. BUXTON, M.D.

The approach to the evaluation and therapy of patients with ventricular premature depolarizations (VPD) and ventricular tachycardia (VT) varies widely. This undoubtedly reflects the fact that much is unknown regarding the relative risks versus benefits of available therapies for certain of these arrhythmias. Furthermore, a range of techniques has been used to evaluate therapy for these arrhythmias, including noninvasive methods (e.g., ambulatory electrocardiographic monitoring, exercise testing) and invasive methods (e.g., programmed stimulation), none of which has proved to be superior to the others. The arrhythmias considered in this chapter include VPD, nonsustained VT (defined as three or more sequential premature depolarizations at rates of 110 beats per minute or more and terminating spontaneously within 30 seconds), and sustained VT (defined as tachycardias lasting more than 30 seconds).

There are two primary reasons why we treat patients with ventricular arrhythmias: (1) to make the patient feel better when the arrhythmia causes annoying or disabling symptoms and (2) to prolong the patient's life in the case of arrhythmias that result in severe hemodynamic compromise or cardiac arrest. Many have advocated the treatment of asymptomatic narrhythmias (VPD and nonsustained VT) on the theory that treatment will prevent sustained tachyarrhythmias causing cardiac arrest. To date, there is no evidence to suggest that there is a cause and effect relationship between VPDs and sustained ventricular tachyarrhythmias, nor do data exist demonstrating that eradication of asymptomatic arrhythmias will prevent sudden death. Because all available antiarrhythmic therapies carry significant toxicity, both cardiac and noncardiac, it is imperative before initiating antiarrhythmic therapy to be certain that the risks of the arrhythmia to the patient far exceed the risks of therapy.

THERAPEUTIC ALTERNATIVES

Before initiating specific antiarrhythmic therapy, the physician must be certain that the arrhythmia to be treated represents a primary electrophysiologic abnormality and is not occurring secondary to other factors. A number of pharmacologic agents may precipitate isolated VPDs and VT. These include both cardiovascular drugs (e.g., all antiarrhythmic agents, digitalis preparations) and noncardiac drugs (e.g., phenothiazines, certain antibiotics). Secondly, one should determine whether a metabolic disturbance such as an electrolyte abnormality or myocardial ischemia could be responsible for precipitating the ventricular arrhythmia. Finally, ventricular arrhythmias may occur in patients with severe ventricular dysfunction. It is unlikely that arrhythmias precipitated by any of these factors will respond favorably to specific antiarrhythmic therapy without correcting the underlying primary abnormality: withdrawing the responsible pharmacologic agent, correcting myocardial ischemia or electrolyte abnormalities, or optimizing the hemodynamic state.

The next decision that the physician must make prior to initiating specific antiarrhythmic therapy is how to assess the efficacy of therapy. Therapeutic efficacy may be assessed directly by observing the effects of treatment on the actual spontaneous arrhythmia. This empiric method, expectantly observing the patient for spontaneous recurrence, is satisfactory in the case of arrhythmias that do not cause severe hemodynamic compromise, such as cardiac arrest or syncope. It is less than satisfactory when failure of therapy is revealed by a life-threatening arrhythmic event. This method is also less than optimal in patients whose arrhythmias occur infrequently, with spontaneous events separated by months to years.

Two general techniques have evolved to evaluate efficacy of therapy. *Indirect methods* of assessing antiarrhythmic efficacy include ambulatory electrocardiographic monitoring to observe the effect of drugs on spontaneous ventricular ectopy. This method has a number of disadvantages, including the fact that there is often enormous spontaneous variation in the frequency of spontaneous ventricular depolarizations and nonsustained ventricular tachycardias that may mimic changes in arrhythmia frequency caused by antiarrhythmic therapy. Furthermore, in many patients there is a dissociation between the effects of antiarrhythmic drugs on spontaneous ectopy and symptomatic sustained arrhythmias. Finally, there is no proof that the effect of a drug on spontaneous ectopy will mimic its effect, both beneficial and potentially harmful, on spontaneous sustained tachyarrhythmias, which are the primary reason to treat.

Direct, provocative methods have been developed in an attempt to circumvent the limitations of passive electrocardiographic monitoring. These include exercise testing, infusion of sympathomimetic amines such as isoproterenol, and programmed stimulation. Exercise testing works well for some patients whose arrhythmias are precipitated by exercise. Unfortunately, most sustained ventricular tachyarrhythmias are not precipitated by exercise, and in those cases associated with exercise, the provocation with exercise is often not reproducible. Isoproterenol infusion also precipitates only a minority of sustained ventricular tachyarrhythmias but may be useful in certain patients. Programmed stimulation uses pacing techniques to induce and reproduce a patient's spontaneous arrhythmia. The sensitivity and specificity of this technique vary depending on the type of arrhythmia, anatomic substrate, and skill of the operator. To interpret the results of programmed stimulation appropriately, one must demonstrate that the arrhythmia can be induced reproducibly first in the absence of antiarrhythmic drugs. The patient is then treated with an antiarrhythmic agent, and programmed stimulation is repeated, the endpoint being absence of induction of the same arrhythmia. A number of studies have demonstrated that eradication of inducibility following an antiarrhythmic agent correlates well with prevention of spontaneous recurrent arrhythmias. Some have suggested that an alteration in the mode of induction by an antiarrhythmic agent may also be a favorable endpoint, but no systematic data exist to support this.

PREFERRED APPROACH

Medical Treatment

Having arrived at a decision to initiate treatment, one must decide among several available modes of antiarrhythmic therapy, including pharmacologic agents, implanted antiarrhythmic devices, or ablative, potentially curative therapy such as surgery. Some general statements about each of the modes of antiarrhythmic therapy are warranted.

Pharmacologic therapy for ventricular arrhythmias is palliative, as the substrate for the arrhythmia remains. Thus, the patient is always subject to recurrences if levels of the antiarrhythmic drug drop below those that are therapeutic for the individual patient. In addition, in some cases, the antiarrhythmic effect may be overridden by changes in autonomic nervous system tone. In spite of numerous laboratory studies demonstrating the effects of antiarrhythmic drugs on various measurable electrophysiologic parameters, the mechanism(s) by which these drugs act in humans is unknown. Thus, although many of these drugs slow conduction and prolong refractoriness, it has not yet been determined which, if either, of these effects accounts for antiarrhythmic efficacy. Furthermore, many of these agents have direct or indirect effects on the autonomic nervous system, which may account in part for antiarrhythmic actions. A further caveat is the observation that under the proper circumstances, the actions of pharmacologic agents to slow conduction and prolong refractoriness may facilitate the development of arrhythmias. These effects may or may not be predictable.

Unfortunately, the efficacy of antiarrhythmic drugs is frequently limited in the patients who are most dependent on them. Several studies have documented that patients with increasingly severe underlying heart disease are progressively less likely to respond to drug therapy. The overall response rates of patients with recurrent sustained VT to pharmacologic therapy have been between 30 and 40 percent. Moreover, the chance of cardiac side effects, especially "paradoxical" facilitation of arrhythmias (or "proarrhythmia") may be increased in patients with severe cardiac disease. As a general principle, whatever method is used to judge antiarrhythmic efficacy, when serum drug levels are available these should be checked at the time that the antiarrhythmic effect is noted, and these levels should be maintained chronically in each patient to ensure continued efficacy. Published "therapeutic" and "toxic" drug levels are useful only as a general guide and may be totally irrelevant in an individual patient. The physician treating a patient can judge what drug level is therapeutic only by correlating the serum level with the desired effect. Likewise, the toxic level for an individual patient is any level that results in an undesired side effect. Our lack of understanding of the mechanisms by which antiarrhythmic agents exert beneficial and harmful actions means that pharmacologic therapy of ventricular arrhythmias remains largely empiric, with no antiarrhythmic agent superior to any others, and no specific antiarrhythmic agent or group of agents can be specifically recommended for any given type of ventricular arrhythmia.

Surgical Treatment

A second type of palliative therapy is the *implantable electrical device* (see the next chapter, *Automatic Implantable Cardioverter Defibrillator*). Currently there are two types of antitachycardia devices available: antitachycardia pacemakers and implantable automatic cardioverter defibrillators. Both types of devices may be useful in selected patients with sustained ventricular tachyarrhythmias. The use of pacemakers is based on observations suggesting intraventricular reentry as the mechanism of most sustained VT in humans; delivery of premature impulses may produce block in a reentrant circuit, resulting in tachycardia termination. Although antitachycardia pacemakers are available that are capable of automatically sensing the onset of a tachycardia, these devices should not be used alone in patients because of the propensity for pacing to accelerate and destabilize a previously stable tachycardia. Externally activated antitachycardia pacemakers, which are activated by a physician with the capability to defibrillate immediately, may be useful in selected patients. These devices may be used in patients with tachycardias that do not cause loss of consciousness, thereby allowing the patient time to reach a medical facility.

Patients whose tachyarrhythmias result in cardiac arrest may be candidates for implantable automatic cardioverter defibrillators. These devices have the capability of automatically sensing the onset of VT or fibrillation and deliver a direct current shock that may terminate the arrhythmia. Limitations to the use of these devices include the fact that they do not prevent the onset of tachyarrhythmias but merely terminate them. Therefore, they may not prevent loss of consciousness associated with tachyarrhythmia. Furthermore, patients with frequent episodes of tachycardia often will require concomitant pharmacologic therapy to decrease the frequency of spontaneous episodes. Pharmacologic therapy is also often required with currently available devices to suppress brief runs of asymptomatic tachycardia, which would trigger the device. A further limitation to current devices is the usual requirement for a thoracotomy or median sternotomy for implantation.

The only therapy that offers the chance for cure of VT is *surgery*. Several approaches to surgical care of VT have been developed. All are based on the evidence supporting reentry as the mechanism underlying sustained VT and are dependent on the ability to initiate VT using programmed stimulation in the catheterization laboratory or operating room. The ability to initiate and terminate reproducible VT permits one to map the sequence of ventricular excitation during a single cycle of VT. On the basis of these observations, a critical portion of the circuit may be identified. Once identified, this area may be ablated using cryosurgical techniques, resected mechanically (the subendocardial resection), or isolated from the remaining viable myocardium using a procedure called encircling ventriculotomy. The most successful of these procedures has been subendocardial resection, combined in some cases with supplementary cryoablation. This approach is limited to patients having a uniform tachycardia morphology. Polymorphic tachycardias, in general, have not been amenable to this approach. Limitations to the surgical approach are the obvious requirements for open heart surgery, with an operative mortality of 10 to 15 percent. Cure rates have been as high as 75 percent in the absence of further antiarrhythmic therapy.

APPROACH TO THERAPY OF SPECIFIC VENTRICULAR ARRHYTHMIAS

Ventricular Premature Depolarizations

The vast majority of patients with VPDs are unaware of them. Therefore, I do not treat such patients, regardless of the presence or absence of structural heart disease. Patients complaining of palpitations are discovered frequently to have VPDs; most often the symptoms do not correlate with the occurrence of VPD. In patients in whom VPDs cause annoying symptoms, I make every effort to treat with reassurance. When reassurance does not suffice, my next line of therapy, regardless of the presence or absence of structural heart disease, is to institute therapy with beta-adrenergic blocking agents. I believe that these agents work as often by decreasing the patient's awareness of the VPD as by actually suppressing the VPD. Only as a last resort would I institute therapy with specific antiarrhythmic drugs. The reasoning behind this is that regardless of the presence, absence, or severity of underlying heart disease, the potential risks of antiarrhythmic therapy outweigh its benefits in these patients.

Nonsustained Ventricular Tachycardia

Nonsustained VT is not often found in patients without structural heart disease. Most commonly when it does occur in patients without structural heart disease, it appears as a syndrome called repetitive monomorphic VT, which consists of frequent paroxysms of uniform VT usually arising from the right ventricular outflow tract. This appears electrocardiographically as a left bundle branch block pattern with a normal (inferior) frontal plane QRS axis. In most cases, nonsustained VT is discovered fortuitously during a routine physical examination or electrocardiogram and is not associated with symptoms. In such cases, I reassure the patient and do not institute antiarrhythmic therapy. We have seen occasional patients having disabling symptoms associated with nonsustained VT in the absence of structural heart disease. In such cases, pharmacologic therapy may suppress these arrhythmias. Frequently, patients with repetitive monomorphic VT arising from the right ventricular outflow tract have the arrhythmia provoked with exercise or isoproterenol. These patients constitute one of the rare cases in which beta-adrenergic blocking therapy may actually suppress the arrhythmia. Other specific antiarrhythmic agents may also suppress VT in such patients. These patients often have such frequent spontaneous arrhythmias that the efficacy of therapy may be judged from the ambulatory electrocardiogram. Repetitive monomorphic VT from the right ventricular outflow tract is usually not inducible by programmed stimulation, although bursts of ventricular pacing will initiate the arrhythmia in approximately one-third of cases. In these patients, the pacing induction of VT may be used to assess antiarrhythmic efficacy. Because repetitive monomorphic VT most often is not associated with symptoms and does not place patients at risk for sudden death, I make every effort to avoid antiarrhythmic therapy in these patients.

Nonsustained VT is frequently found in patients with severe ventricular dysfunction due to noncoronary heart disease. Twenty-four-hour Holter monitors in patients with valvular disease and with both hypertrophic and dilated cardiomyopathies have shown nonsustained VT in at least 50 percent of cases. Most often these arrhythmias are not associated with symptoms. In such patients, they may indicate a higher risk for sudden death, but their utility as a specific marker for sudden (rather than nonsudden) cardiac death is unproven. There are no data to suggest that prophylactic antiarrhythmic therapy in such patients is beneficial. Programmed stimulation in such patients induces sustained uniform VT in 10 percent of patients and appears to be of no utility to predict sudden death at present. I do not treat patients who are asymptomatic with nonsustained VT in the setting of noncoronary heart disease with ventricular dysfunction.

Patients with coronary artery disease are found not infrequently to have nonsustained VT remote from an acute infarction. Although nonsustained VT discovered late after myocardial infarction is associated with an increased risk for sudden death, these patients are at a similarly increased risk for nonsudden cardiac death. A number of studies suggest that when nonsustained VT is found in patients with coronary artery disease and with ejection fractions greater than 40 percent, the risk for sudden death is very low. Therefore, I do not evaluate such patients, nor do I treat them. Patients with nonsustained VT and ejection fractions of 40 percent or less present a difficult problem. Even when asymptomatic with regard to the arrhythmia, some of these patients are at increased risk for sudden death. A number of studies have suggested that programmed stimulation in these patients may be useful in stratifying risk for sudden death. About 45 percent of such patients will have sustained VT inducible by programmed stimulation. Those without inducible VT appear to be at low risk for sudden death and do not warrant therapy with antiarrhythmic agents. It is unclear at present whether antiarrhythmic treatment will benefit asymptomatic patients with inducible sustained VT.

Patients who have nonsustained VT that is clearly documented to cause symptoms such as syncope should receive antiarrhythmic therapy. The manner in which to guide therapy depends in large part on the frequency of spontaneous episodes of nonsustained VT and on the anatomic substrate associated with the VT. Patients with syncope and nonsustained VT associated with chronic coronary artery disease should undergo electrophysiologic studies. These studies frequently reveal inducible sustained VT, and the results of these studies may be used to guide antiarrhythmic therapy. Patients with severe symptoms due to nonsustained VT not associated with chronic coronary artery disease are less likely to have inducible VT when subjected to programmed stimulation. Approximately 10 percent of patients with dilated cardiomyopathies and nonsustained VT will have inducible sustained uniform VT, and in these patients programmed stimulation may help to identify appropriate antiarrhythmic therapy. Patients with frequent (more than 20 to 30 daily) episodes of nonsustained VT associated with intolerable symptoms may undergo trials of pharmacologic therapy with assessment by continuous electrocardiographic monitoring, regardless of the presence, absence, or type of underlying heart disease.

Sustained Ventricular Tachycardia

The treatment of sustained VT must be based on the impact of the arrhythmia on the clinical state of the patient. Patients with VT who remain conscious without angina or severe congestive heart failure may be acutely treated pharmacologically, whereas those experiencing marked hypotension, severe heart failure, or angina should be cardioverted immediately. Our initial choice is usually procainamide, administered at a rate of 50 mg per minute to a total dose of 15 mg per kilogram. When administered at this rate, procainamide may cause hypotension, and the blood pressure must be monitored every 5 minutes. If hypotension occurs, the rate of infusion is slowed, usually to 25 mg per minute. If the arrhythmia terminates during the loading dose, it is not usually necessary to continue a maintenance infusion because most patients have discrete episodes of sustained VT; continued drug administration in certain cases may facilitate spontaneous development of the arrhythmias, converting paroxysmal tachycardias into incessant tachycardias. If continued antiarrhythmic medication is desired following the loading dose, procainamide must be administered at a rate of 0.11 mg per kilogram per minute to maintain levels that are likely to be therapeutic. Even when procainamide infusion fails to terminate VT, it usually slows the arrhythmia, stabilizing the hemodynamic status. If the tachycardia fails to convert to sinus rhythm following the loading dose of procainamide, cardioversion is performed.

Following restoration of sinus rhythm after an acute episode of sustained VT, several diagnostic and therapeutic avenues may be pursued. If the tachycardia did not result in severe symptoms and a stable hemodynamic state was maintained after the first episode of sustained VT, one may choose not to pursue further diagnostic studies nor to institute specific antiarrhythmic therapy. The natural history of paroxysmal sustained VT is extremely variable, with some patients experiencing gaps of many months or years between spontaneous episodes even in the absence of treatment. In some cases, institution of empiric therapy may increase the frequency of episodes of spontaneous tachycardia. If a patient has had more than one episode, or the initial episode caused severe hemodynamic embarrassment, the optimal method to guide therapy is electrophysiologic study, because I believe this permits the most objective evaluation of the effects of pharmacologic and other therapy. A baseline electrophysiologic study in the absence of antiarrhythmic drugs is likely to induce sustained VT in over 90 percent of patients with spontaneous sustained VT. If antiarrhythmic drugs are then administered, programmed stimulation may be repeated, with the endpoint being eradication of inducible sustained VT. In some patients who have either failed multiple trials of antiarrhythmic drugs, or in whom curative therapy appears preferable, surgical attempts at ablation of the arrhythmia may be undertaken after performing activation mapping of spontaneous or induced VT in the electrophysiology laboratory. If surgical therapy is not desired or accepted, patients are generally given pharmacologic therapy that results in the greatest degree of hemodynamic stability during the tachycardia. Usually this means the drug or combination of drugs that results in the greatest slowing of the tachycardia when induced by programmed stimulation. In some cases, no drug regimen can be found that produces an acceptable hemodynamic state during tachycardia. These patients are then usually offered an antitachycardia device such as an implantable defibrillator in combination with pharmacologic therapy.

The choice of pharmacologic therapy for recurrent sustained VT is entirely empiric. For chronic therapy, our usual initial choice is either quinidine, disopyramide, or procainamide. We avoid disopyramide in patients with left ventricular ejection fractions of less than 30 percent or with a history of congestive heart failure due to systolic ventricular dysfunction. We usually initiate therapy with a standard, short-acting preparation of one of these agents, aiming for plasma concentrations of 3.5 to 5 mg per liter for quinidine, 8 to 10 mg per liter for procainamide, and 2 to 5 mg per liter for disopyramide. We avoid the long-acting preparation initially because attainment of adequate serum drug levels is often delayed with these preparations. We avoid the use of disopyramide in older men because of frequent side effects of bladder outlet obstruction. Quinidine administration is limited in some patients by gastrointestinal side effects and the occasional development of anemia or thrombocytopenia. The utility of quinidine is frequently limited in patients who require phenytoin because an interaction between the two drugs limits attainment of adequate serum quinidine levels. Chronic procainamide administration is usually limited by development of the systemic lupus-like syndrome. Patients may also complain of insomnia. Although serum procainamide levels of 10 to 20 mg per liter may occasionally be necessary to suppress spontaneous and inducible sustained tachycardias, levels greater than 10 mg are rarely tolerated on a long-term basis.

If trials of quinidine, disopyramide, or procainamide fail to control tachycardias, our next step is to combine one of these agents with mexiletine at a dose of 150 to 200 mg every 8 hours. Mexiletine rarely suppresses sustained tachycardia by itself, but the combination of mexiletine with one of the aforementioned agents is often useful. Administration of mexiletine is usually limited by gastrointestinal side effects such as nausea and vomiting, the development of skin rash, or neurologic toxicity such as lightheadedness, tremor, or ataxia. If the combination of quinidine, procainamide, or disopyramide plus mexiletine fails to control VT, the next step is to consider either an agent such as encainide, flecainide, propafenone, or amiodarone or surgical therapy as outlined previously. In general, although individual patients may respond to encainide, flecainide, or propafenone, these agents often fail to control VT when the other agents are not successful.

Amiodarone may be useful in selected patients, although it too has many limitations. Amiodarone is not available in an intravenous form, and when given orally it requires several days to attain therapeutic effects. Therefore, it is not usually useful for acute control of VT, although recently some investigators have shown an accelerated effect with very large oral doses. When a decision is made to give amiodarone for chronic recurrent VT, we usually administer it as a single dose of 1400 mg per day for 1 week, followed by a maintenance dose of 400 mg per day. Occasionally, patients experience marked symptomatic sinus slowing on the loading dose, requiring a lower loading dose. The utility of electrophysiologic studies to judge the efficacy of amiodarone therapy is controversial, but the weight of evidence suggests that suppression of induction of tachycardia by amiodarone is meaningful in most cases, whereas failure to suppress induction by programmed stimulation correlates with eventual recurrence of tachycardias. Patients in our laboratory are studied with programmed stimulation after 2 to 4 weeks of amiodarone therapy. The hemodynamic stability of induced tachycardias may be predictive of the hemodynamic stability of spontaneous recurrences should they occur. Amiodarone therapy is limited by side effects of hypothyroidism or hyperthyroidism, symptomatic hepatitis (and frequent asymptomatic elevations in liver enzymes), and pulmonary fibrosis. We follow thyroid and liver studies and chest roentgenograms three to four times yearly in patients on amiodarone. Serial pulmonary function studies may also be useful in predicting amiodarone pulmonary toxicity. Chronic amiodarone therapy frequently causes corneal microdeposits visible on slit lamp examination, but these rarely cause symptoms. Occasionally patients appear to benefit from a combination of mexiletine and amiodarone when VT recurs in the presence of amiodarone alone. However, other combinations of antiarrhythmic drugs plus amiodarone have not been very useful and seem only to increase the chance of drug toxicity.

SUGGESTED READING

Buxton AE, Waxman HL, Marchlinski FE, et al. Right ventricular tachycardia: clinical and electrophysiologic characteristics. Circulation 1983; 68:917.

Kadish AH, Buxton AE, Waxman HL, et al. Usefulness of electrophysiology study to determine the clinical tolerance of arrhythmia recurrences during amiodarone therapy. J Am Coll Cardiol 1987; 10:90.

Kuchar DL, Rottman J, Berger E, et al. Prediction of success of sustained ventricular tachyarrhythmias by serial drug testing from data derived at the initial electrophysiologic study. J Am Coll Cardiol 1988; 12:982.

Marchlinski FE. Ventricular tachycardia associated with coronary artery disease. Prog Cardiol 1988; 1(1):231.

Mitchell LB, Duff HJ, Manyari DE, Wyse DG. A randomized clinical trial of the noninvasive and invasive approaches to drug therapy of ventricular tachycardia. N Engl J Med 1987; 317: 1681.

Pratt CM, Thornton BC, Magro SA, Wyndham CR: Spontaneous arrhythmia detected on ambulatory electrocardiographic recordings lacks precision in predicting inducibility of ventricular tachycardia during electrophysiologic study. J Am Coll Cardiol 1987; 10:97.

The Cardiac Arrhythmia Suppression Trial (CAST) Investigators. Increased mortality due to encainide or flecainide in a randomized trial of arrhythmia suppression after myocardial infarction. N Engl J Med 1989; 321:406.

Wilber DJ, Garan H, Finkelstein D, et al. Out-of-hospital cardiac arrest: use of electrophysiologic testing in the prediction of long-term outcome. N Engl J Med 1988; 318:19.

AUTOMATIC IMPLANTABLE CARDIOVERTER DEFIBRILLATOR

THOMAS GUARNIERI, M.D.
MICHEL MIROWSKI, M.D.

Transthoracic cardioversion became an important reality in the practice of medicine in the 1950s following the work of Kouwenhoven and later of Lown and colleagues. It was not until the early 1970s that reports began to appear in the literature about the feasibility of automatic internal defibrillation. Mirowski and colleagues demonstrated over a 10-year period that an implanted automatic defibrillator was feasible. Some of the important principles for internal cardioversion were tested in the cardiac operating room, where coronary bypass surgery was often performed with the heart fibrillating. A chronically implanted unit was first tested in a canine model in 1978. After more than a decade of preliminary investigation, the first automatic defibrillator was implanted in a patient at the Johns Hopkins Hospital in 1980. The device then underwent intense experimentation in clinical trials between 1980 and 1986, after which it was released for general use. The defibrillator became widely available and entered the clinical realm in the late 1980s.

The first decade of clinical research on automatic internal defibrillation has demonstrated one important principle: automatic internal defibrillation is feasible. The design principles of early cardioverter defibrillators were based on simplicity of detection and delivery of a high-energy cardioverting shock. It became apparent that algorithms for detection should be kept simple. In the original clinical trials, the first device tested was an automatic internal defibrillator (AID). With this device, the method of detecting the arrhythmia was exclusively a probability density function. It was the purpose of this algorithm to detect ventricular fibrillation. This method of detection compared the detected rhythm with a sinusoidal waveform. The algorithm was satisfied when the rhythm lost its isoelectric segments (became sinusoidal). It was clear in the early phases of the clinical trials that many forms of ventricular tachycardia would retain parts of an isoelectric baseline (and not satisfy the algorithm) but would produce significant hemodynamic compromise before the rhythm became fibrillatory. Therefore, simple rate detection was added to the sensing algorithm. In the early generators, the sensing was either rate detection only or rate detection and probability density function. In these early models, however, the defibrillator acted primarily as a rate detector and as such was a very sensitive, yet not specific, detector of ventricular tachycardia/fibrillation. It was the design intent of these early defibrillators to achieve nearly 100 percent sensitivity at the expense of specificity.

Although early experiments suggested that a transvenous cardioverter system was feasible, the early units used at least one epicardial patch. In the first generation of devices, an epicardial patch served as the cathode while a large coil placed at the junction of the superior vena cava–right atrium served as the anode. Shortly thereafter, two epicardial patches became the system of choice.

Various waveforms for delivery of energy were available in the 1970s. The data suggested that different waveforms for cardioversion had different degrees of success. However, size constraints prevailed, and a truncated exponential waveform was used. With this form of energy, a 30-joule shock is delivered over approximately 6 milliseconds. The peak current is 5 to 6 amperes, and the peak voltage is 1 kilovolt. Early measurements suggested that the impedance across the lead system was on the order of 50 ohms. In the early generations, a shocking sequence of a lowenergy (25 to 28 joules) discharge was followed, if unsuccessful, by a sequence of high-energy (29 to 32 joules) shocks. Later generations of machines delivered 30-joule shocks for all arrhythmia sequences. In fact, the ability of the automatic defibrillator to deliver a sequence of high-energy shocks should the first shock fail, or to accelerate the arrhythmia, was a major reason for its success.

CLINICAL PERFORMANCE

In retrospect the success of the automatic defibrillator seems to have been a very straightforward and predictable event. The automatic defibrillator performs according to its name: it defibrillates the patient when other modes of therapy have been unsuccessful. To date there have been no clinical trials comparing an automatic defibrillator with other forms of therapy in a randomized fashion. Performance characteristics of the defibrillator have been compared with historically derived controls or with data from ongoing medical trials. Throughout the world, approximately 8,000 devices have been implanted (Table 1). The vast majority of these individuals are in their fifth or sixth decades of life and suffer from coronary artery disease. The left ventricular ejection fraction is approximately 30 percent. In most series published to date, approximately 75 percent of the patients had coronary artery disease (Table 2). The other 25 percent of patients are generally individuals with cardiomyopathy and other less common forms of heart disease.

TABLE 1 Clinical Diagnosis for Patients Using Automatic Implantable Cardioverter Defibrillators

Coronary artery disease	75.1%
Nonischemic cardiomyopathy	12.0%
Other: long Q-T interval, valvular, primary electrical, congenital	12.9%

Data from A. Thomas, CPI, St. Paul, MN.

TABLE 2 Characteristics of Patients Using Automatic Implantable Cardioverter Defibrillators

Total patients	7,788
Percentage of male/female	80.5/19.5
Average age	60.5
Mean ejection fraction	33%

Data from A. Thomas, CPI, St. Paul, MN.

In general, performance of the automatic implantable cardioverter defibrillator (AICD) has been described in terms of Kaplan-Meier survival curves (Fig. 1). The survival statistics are generally discussed in the context of mortality from sudden death versus mortality from underlying heart disease, or total mortality. Mortality from cardiac arrest appears to be approximately 5 percent or less at 5 years. Total mortality is approximately 20 percent. In general, total cardiac mortality continues to reflect the severity of the underlying disease process, generally expressed as the ejection fraction. Nonetheless, when data have been subdivided according to ejection fraction, impressive increases in survival have been seen.

PREFERRED APPROACH

Indications

Indications for implantation have become somewhat more liberal since the original requirement of multiple cardiac arrests In general, the indi-

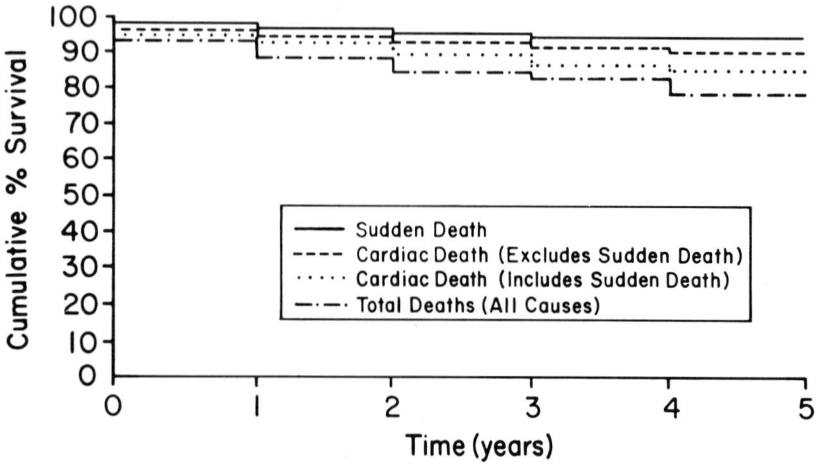

Figure 1 Cumulative survival of patients using automatic implantable cardioverter defibrillators worldwide (approximately 8,000) versus time from implant. Survival is described in terms of sudden death, cardiac death, and total death. (Data from A. Thomas, CPI, St. Paul, MN.)

cation for implantation of the device is a history of at least one episode of ventricular tachycardia or fibrillation, which is not controlled by antiarrhythmic therapy or surgery. Although this indication is simple, it is clear that the inherent definitions may be complex. For example, what constitutes control of the ventricular arrhythmia is subject to a great deal of variation. In addition, the choice between an automatic defibrillator and antiarrhythmic surgery may be made on the basis of comparative mortality and morbidity of the two procedures. The device is thought to be contraindicated in those individuals whose survival from noncardiac sources is less than 2 years. In the current generation of devices, a second contraindication is the presence of incessant or frequent tachycardia, which will repetitively trigger the defibrillator.

Surgical Treatment

The primary morbidity of the AICD rests in the surgical approach for insertion. For AICD insertion only, the mortality is 1 to 3 percent. Mortality increases as the complexity of the cardiac surgery increases, including coronary artery bypass, valve replacement, or aneurysmectomy and subendocardial resection. Morbidity is directly related to the surgical approach and includes bleeding, pulmonary complications, and infection. Infection of the generator system can be a particularly devastating phenomenon, and in most circumstances mandates extirpation of the entire device system. Infection rates vary but range between 0 and 5 percent. It remains to be seen whether this higher infection rate, as compared with that for pacemakers, is secondary to the surgical approaches or to the size of the hardware.

As noted previously, the design of the device was predicated on sensitivity and not specificity of detection. As such, when the rate criterion of the AICD was met for any reason, a shock would be given. Evaluation of the success or failure of the device became problematic because of the frequency of asymptomatic shocks. Since the device has no memory loop, the exact mechanism for triggering any shock is unknown but is particularly more bothersome with shocks preceded by no symptoms. The issue of all asymptomatic shocks being inappropriate became even more problematic when it was described that approximately 20 percent of all asymptomatic shocks are due to ventricular tachycardia. Other reasons for asymptomatic shocks include inappropriate sensing of pacemaker artifact and T waves.

Two other important shortcomings of the device are its longevity and cost. Longevity is directly related to the interaction between energy delivered and the batteries and capacitors currently available. Current battery life allows for approximately 24 to 30 months of patient use. The cost in 1990 dollars for the device alone is approximately $15,000. As such, this represents expensive technology. Studies are underway to determine whether increasing battery life may allow for more cost-effective technology.

Future

There are two major trends in the future of automatic defibrillators: (1) nonthoracotomy approach and (2) a much more sophisticated programmable antitachycardia unit.

Mirowski and colleagues (1972) knew early on that a nonthoracotomy approach using an array of catheters in the heart was feasible. This observation has been reconfirmed by Winkle and co-workers (1988), who demonstrated that approximately 60 percent of individuals could be successfully defibrillated with a nonthoracotomy system. Initial clinical trials using a nonthoracotomy system are currently underway.

Because much of the sensing and energy delivery are based on the logic of programmable computer software, it comes as no surprise that the AICD of the future will have a variety of programming techniques to terminate tachycardia. Trials are underway for devices that are antitachycardia pacemakers, cardioverters, defibrillators, and back-up pacers. The potential array for electrical therapy that may be delivered to terminate ventricular tachycardia is astonishing. In addition, advances in the memory of microprocessors will allow for the implanted device to record the arrhythmias prior to shock.

Perhaps one of the most intriguing aspects of future automatic defibrillation is the potential for altering the way in which energy is delivered to the heart. The current generation device delivers a truncated exponential waveform. However, and as was well known in the 1950s and 1960s, other waveforms may be more efficacious in defibrillation. Currently, biphasic waveforms are under experimentation. These waveforms may be successful enough to allow for making the defibrillator even smaller than its current size. Additionally, the manner and direction in which energy may be delivered across various parts of a patient's heart may be varied, allowing for more successful defibrillation.

SUGGESTED READING

Chapman PD, Troup P: The automatic implantable cardioverter-defibrillator: evaluating suspected inappropriate shocks. J Am Coll Cardiol 1986; 7:1075.

Echt DS, Armstrong K, Schmidt P, et al. Clinical experience, complications, and survival in 70 patients with the automatic implantable cardioverter-defibrillator. Circulation 1985; 71: 289.

Guarnieri T, Strickberger A, Magiros E, et al. Is an asymptomatic implantable cardioverter defibrillator discharge a false positive? International Conference on the Management of Cardiac Arrhythmias. PACE 1987; 10:II–982.

Marchlinski FE, Flores BT, Buxton AE, et al. The automatic im-

plantable cardioverter defibrillator: efficacy, complications, and device failures. Ann Intern Med 1986; 104:481.
Mirowski M, Mower MM, Staewen WS, et al. The development of the transvenous automatic defibrillator. Arch Intern Med 1972; 129:773.
Reid PR, Mirowski M, Mower MM, et al. Clinical evaluation of the internal automatic cardioverter-defibrillator in survivors of sudden cardiac death. Am J Cardiol 1983; 51:1608.
Winkle RA, Bach SM, Mead RH, et al. Comparison of defibrillator efficacy in humans using a new catheter and superior vena cava spring and left ventricular patch. J Am Coll Cardiol 1988; 11:365.

ATRIOVENTRICULAR BLOCK

DAVID P. RARDON, M.D.
CHARLES FISCH, M.D.

Atrioventricular (AV) block occurs when atrial impulse transmission to the ventricle is delayed or blocked secondary to pathologic refractoriness or interruption of AV pathways. The normal cardiac impulse originates in the sinus node and conducts through the atrium, AV node, and His-Purkinje system to the ventricle. The sinus node discharge is not recorded on the surface electrocardiogram but is inferred from the presence of upright P waves in electrocardiographic leads II, III, and aVF. The P-R interval, therefore, represents conduction through the atrium, AV node, and His-Purkinje system. Atrioventricular block may result from conduction delay or block at one or more of these sites.

His bundle recordings allow delineation of three anatomic sites of AV block: (1) proximal (above the His bundle), representing delay or block in the AV node; (2) intra-Hisian, representing delay within the His bundle; and (3) infra-Hisian or distal to the His bundle, representing block or delay distal to the His bundle either in the distal His bundle or in the bundle branches. Although the His bundle potential is not recorded on the surface electrocardiogram, the electrocardiographic patterns of AV block correlate with the anatomic site of block. In general, the prognosis of patients with AV block is dependent on the site of block. Block within the AV node proximal to the His bundle implies a favorable prognosis, whereas block distal to the His bundle implies a more onerous prognosis. In most cases the electrocardiogram, without need for electrophysiologic testing, provides enough information to make appropriate decisions concerning the prognosis and management of patients with AV block.

PREFERRED APPROACH

First-Degree Atrioventricular Block

By definition, AV block is classified as first, second, or third degree. First-degree AV block is present when the P-R interval exceeds 0.20 or 0.22 second. When first-degree AV block occurs with a QRS of normal duration, the site of delay is most often within the AV node and only rarely within the atrium, His bundle, or bundle branches. In the presence of a bundle branch block, the site of conduction delay can be localized to the AV node with less certainty. Regardless of the site of conduction delay, the prognosis of patients with first-degree AV block is excellent, and no specific therapy is indicated. Even when first-degree AV block is associated with chronic bifascicular block, the rate of progression to complete or third-degree AV block is slow, and prophylactic ventricular pacing is not indicated in the asymptomatic patient.

Second-Degree Atrioventricular Block

Second-degree AV block is divided into two types: Type I (Mobitz I or Wenckebach AV block) and Type II (Mobitz II AV block). Type I Wenckebach AV block is characterized typically by a progressive prolongation of the P-R interval, with the largest increment following the second conducted P wave. The gradual prolongation of the P-R interval is at progressively decreasing increments, and thus the R-R intervals gradually shorten. The pause that follows the blocked P wave is less than the sum of two basic sinus cycles (Fig. 1). In Type I second-degree AV block with a QRS of normal duration, block is usually within the AV node and only rarely within or distal to the His bundle. When the QRS duration is prolonged, block may be within the AV node or below the His bundle.

The prognosis and management of Type I second-degree AV block are dependent on the clinical setting and the presence of associated organic heart disease. Ambulatory electrocardiographic monitoring has demonstrated that Type I second-degree AV block occurs in a small percentage of normal persons during sleep and with some increased frequency in well-trained athletes. In asymptomatic individuals without organic heart disease, Type I second-degree AV block has an excellent prognosis and no therapy is required.

Second-degree Type I AV block occurs in 4 to 10 percent of all patients admitted to the coronary care unit with acute myocardial infarction. Type I

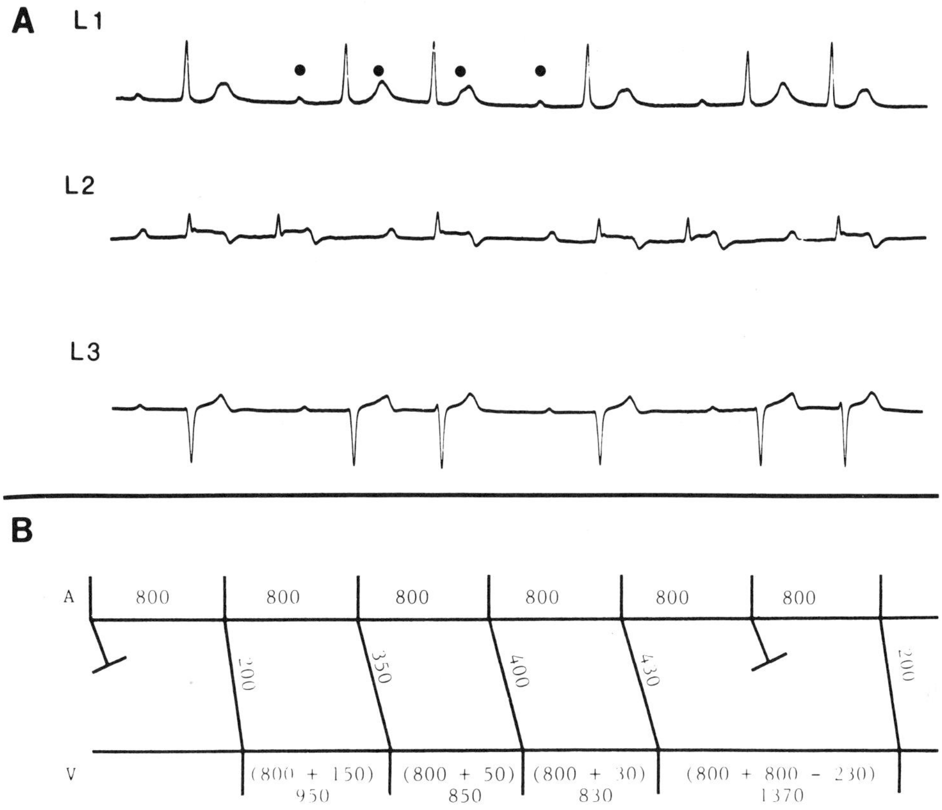

Figure 1 Type I second-degree atrioventricular (AV) block. *A*, Type I second-degree AV block in a patient with an acute inferior myocardial infarction. The P waves are denoted by bullets. Both 3 : 2 and 2 : 1 Wenckebach cycles are present in this record. *B*, The structure of a "typical" Wenckebach cycle. The P-P interval is constant at 800 msec. The P-R interval progressively lengthens, with the greatest prolongation occurring with the second conducted P wave. Therefore, the R-R intervals progressively shorten. The pause encompassing the blocked P wave is less than the sum of two basic cycles by an amount equal to the total delay at the AV node (800 + 800 − 150 − 50 − 30 = 1,370 msec).

block occurs more commonly in association with inferior versus anterior myocardial infarctions. In the setting of an acute inferior myocardial infarction, the QRS duration is usually normal, and the block occurs within the AV node. Type I block in this setting is usually transient and commonly resolves within the first 48 to 72 hours after the infarction. Most patients are asymptomatic, and rarely does Type I AV block progress to advanced second-degree or third-degree block. Therefore, no specific therapy is warranted. Rarely, because of "symptomatic" bradycardia or hypotension, therapy is required. Symptomatic bradycardia includes conditions in which absolute or relative bradycardia is associated with hypotension, ventricular ectopy, or myocardial ischemia. Because Type I second-degree AV block is often secondary to increased vagal tone in the setting of an acute inferior infarction, patients may respond to atropine. Atropine is given in 0.5-mg aliquots intravenously every 5 minutes until the desired response is achieved (i.e., an increased heart rate of usually ≥60 beats per minute or abatement of signs and symptoms). Two milligrams of intravenous atropine is a fully vagolytic dose in most patients. Doses of atropine smaller than 0.5 mg can produce a paradoxical bradycardia as a result of the central or peripheral parasympathomimetic effects of low doses. Rarely, temporary transvenous ventricular pacing is required for persistent bradycardia or hypotension that fails to respond to atropine.

Although Type I second-degree AV block in general is associated with a good prognosis, occasional patients with organic heart disease and elderly patients have a worse prognosis. When Type I AV block complicates organic heart disease, the clinical course tends to be more malignant, but the worsened clinical course is secondary to the extent and severity of the organic heart disease and not to the presence of AV nodal block. Currently routine prophylactic pacing is not recommended in patients with AV nodal Wenckebach block and organic heart disease, unless they have recurrent syncope or bradycardia that exacerbates congestive heart failure. Occasionally, Type I second-degree AV block is present in patients with syncope. The QRS is usually widened, and either block occurs below the His bundle or delay occurs both within the AV node and distal to the His bundle. In these patients, permanent ventricular or atrioventricular sequential pacing is indicated.

Type II second-degree AV block (Mobitz II) is characterized by constant P-R intervals preceding the nonconducted P wave (Fig. 2). Type II AV block is seen most frequently in association with a bundle branch block, and the anatomic site of block is almost always within or below the His bundle. Type II AV block often progresses to complete AV block and Adam-Stokes attacks. Therefore, prophylactic ventricular or atrioventricular sequential pacing is indicated in most patients.

Type II second-degree AV block occurs in less than 1 percent of patients with acute myocardial infarction. In contrast to Type I block, Type II second-degree AV block occurs more commonly with anterior as opposed to inferior myocardial infarctions. There is usually an associated bundle branch block, and the anatomic site of block is distal to the His bundle. Because of the potential for progression to complete heart block, patients with Type II second-degree AV block should be treated with temporary transvenous ventricular demand pacemakers set at approximately 60 beats per minute.

A 2 : 1 AV block may be either Type I or Type II, and the differential diagnosis may be difficult or impossible to determine. Although the P-R interval is not helpful in differentiating the type of AV block, the QRS duration may be. A 2 : 1 block with a normal QRS duration supports the diagnosis of Type I block, and a prolonged QRS favors, but is not diagnostic of, Type II AV block. More prolonged electrocardiographic recording will help at times to delineate 2 : 1 AV block as Type I or II. In general, the management does not differ from that outlined for Type I or Type II AV block, respectively, as outlined here.

Third-Degree Atrioventricular Block

Third-degree or complete AV block is characterized by the failure of all the P waves to conduct, resulting in complete dissociation of P waves and QRS complexes. The rate of the subsidiary pacemaker is slow, approximately 40 to 60 beats per minute, in the presence of a junctional pacemaker (narrow complex QRS in the absence of a preexisting bundle branch block) and is approximately 30

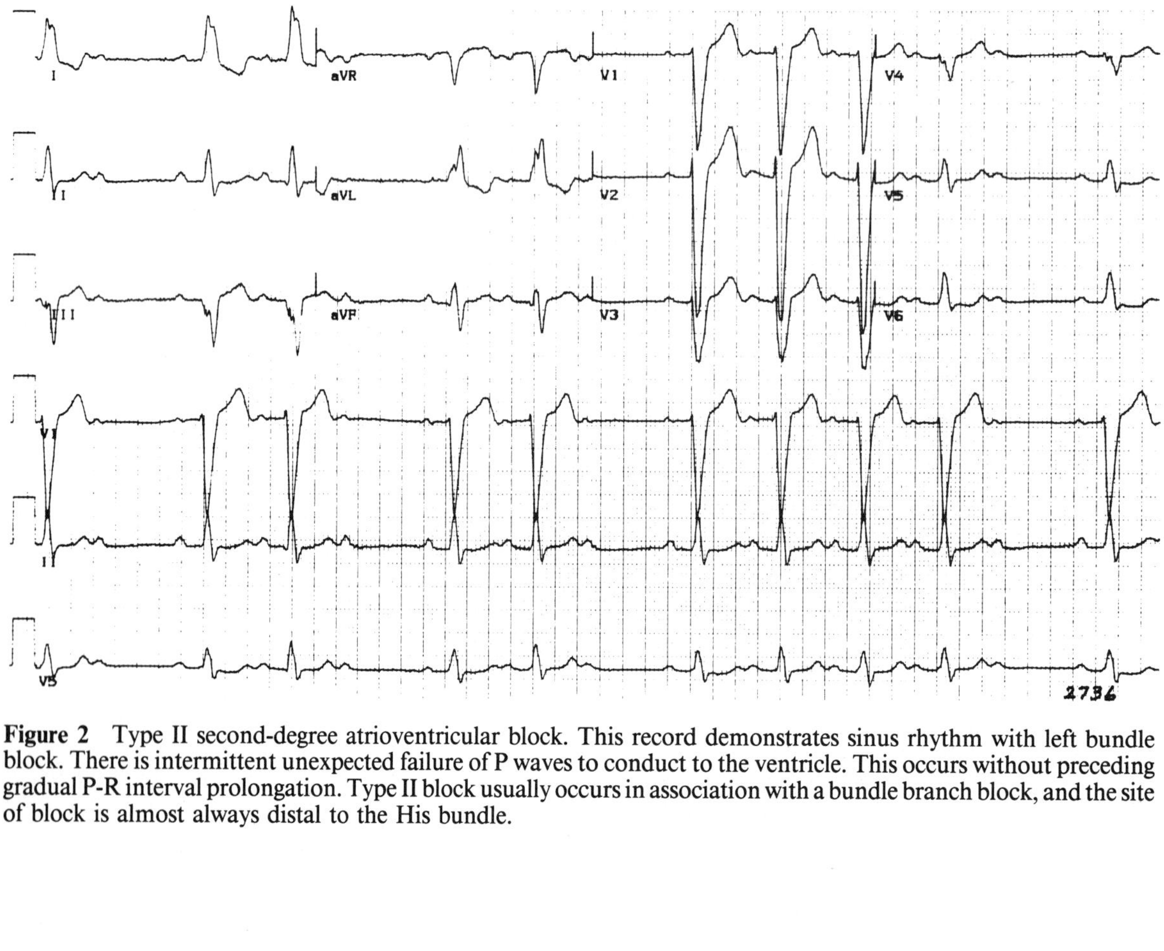

Figure 2 Type II second-degree atrioventricular block. This record demonstrates sinus rhythm with left bundle block. There is intermittent unexpected failure of P waves to conduct to the ventricle. This occurs without preceding gradual P-R interval prolongation. Type II block usually occurs in association with a bundle branch block, and the site of block is almost always distal to the His bundle.

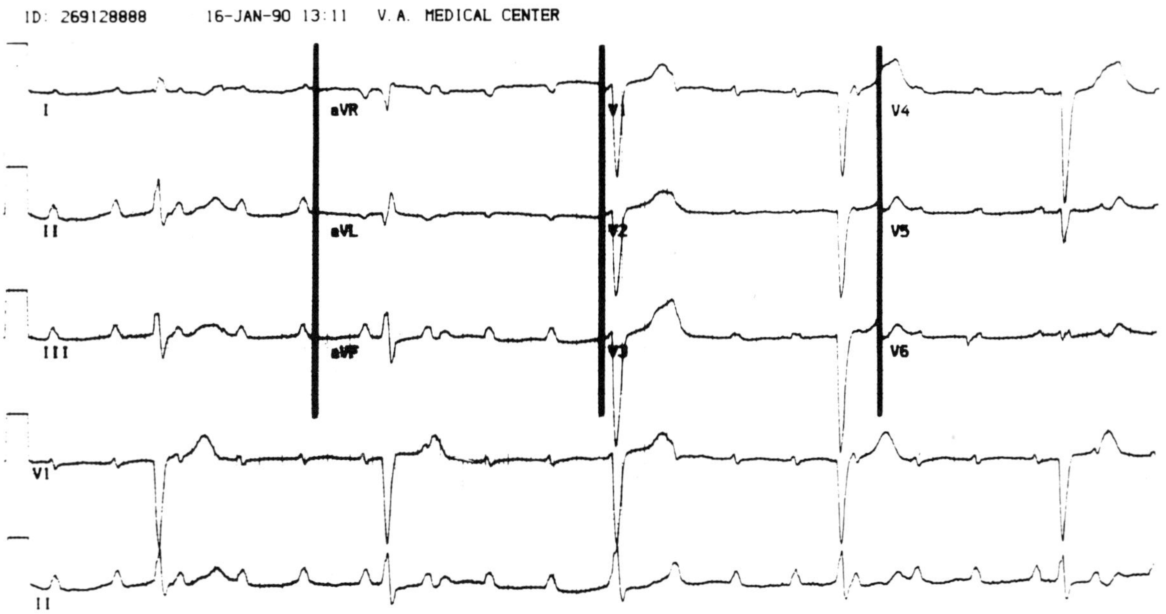

Figure 3 Third-degree atrioventricular block. There is sinus tachycardia at a rate of 107 beats per minute. There is no relationship between the P waves and the QRS complexes. The ventricular rate is 30 beats per minute, and the QRS has a left bundle branch block morphology. This suggests that the ventricular focus arises in the Purkinje system.

beats per minute if the impulse originates in the Purkinje fibers (wide complex QRS) (Fig. 3). Complete AV block may result from block within the AV node (usually congenital), block within the bundle of His, or block distal to the His bundle in the Purkinje system (usually acquired).

Acquired third-degree AV block is usually due to drug intoxication, coronary artery disease, or sclerotic degeneration of the AV conduction system. Sclerotic degeneration produces partial or complete anatomic or electrical disruption within the AV node, the His bundle, or both bundle branches. In patients in whom sclerosis of the conduction system produces third-degree AV block, there is general agreement that permanent pacing is indicated, with symptomatic bradycardia manifest as transient dizziness, light-headedness, near syncope, or frank syncope or more generalized symptoms such as marked exercise intolerance or frank congestive heart failure. Even in asymptomatic patients with complete heart block and ventricular rates greater than 40 beats per minute, the natural history appears to be one of progression to the point of symptoms, and prophylactic ventricular or atrioventricular pacing is recommended.

The choice of the appropriate permanent pacing modality for patients with either Type II second-degree AV block or third-degree AV block should be considered on a case-by-case basis. Ventricular (VVI) pacing provides symptomatic improvement in the majority of patients with impaired AV conduction by establishing a basal ventricular rate that ensures an adequate cardiac output. However, ventricular pacing has several disadvantages. This pacing mode does not allow physiologic increases in heart rate and cardiac output to meet the demands of normal daily living. Inappropriately timed atrial systole may impair cardiac output, and consistent ventriculoatrial activation may produce significant hemodynamic compromise. Atrioventricular pacing has been shown to increase cardiac output and work capacity substantially compared with ventricular pacing. Table 1 summarizes current recommendations regarding preferred pacing modes for patients with AV block. One must emphasize that a patient's overall physical and mental state, including the presence of associated diseases that might result in a limited prognosis for life, should influence both the decision to pace and the pacing modality selected.

Complete heart block develops in 5 to 8 percent of patients with acute myocardial infarction. Complete heart block can occur in patients with both inferior and anterior myocardial infarctions. With inferior infarctions, complete heart block usually develops secondary to AV nodal block. The escape rhythm is often junctional with a rate exceeding 40 beats per minute and a narrow QRS complex. It is generally agreed that temporary ventricular demand pacing is indicated in most patients with acute inferior myocardial infarctions and complete AV block,

TABLE 1 Preferred Pacing Modalities for Atrioventricular Block

	Atrial Rhythm		
AV Conduction	*Normal*	*Bradycardia*	*Bradycardia/ Tachycardia*
AV block without prolonged retrograde VA conduction time	DDD	DDD or VVI-RR	VVI-RR or DDI
AV block with prolonged retrograde VA conduction time	VVI-RR or DVI	VVI-RR or DVI	VVI-RR or DDD

DDD = AV universal pacemaker with dual chamber pacing and inhibited on channel sensed and triggered on alternate channel, DDI = AV sequential pacemaker with dual chamber pacing and dual chamber inhibited sensing, DVI = AV sequential pacemaker with dual chamber pacing and ventricular inhibited sensing, VVI-RR = rate-responsive ventricular demand pacemaker.

Modified from Zipes DP, Duffin EG. Cardiac pacemakers. In: Braunwald E, ed. Heart disease: A textbook of cardiovascular medicine. 3rd ed. Philadelphia: WB Saunders, 1988:717. Reproduced with permission of the publisher and author.

particularly if the ventricular rate is slow (less than 45 beats per minute) or if there is associated hypotension. Atropine may be used in this setting but is rarely of value. In patients with anterior myocardial infarction, complete AV block is often preceded by intraventricular block or Type II AV block. The escape rhythm is often ventricular with rates less than 40 beats per minute. The block is usually distal to the His bundle. Temporary transvenous ventricular demand pacing is indicated in all patients with anterior infarctions and complete heart block. This patient population has a high mortality secondary to large infarctions and impaired left ventricular function.

The need for permanent pacing in the small group of patients with anterior myocardial infarction complicated by conduction defects and transient complete heart block is controversial. These patients have a high incidence of sudden death due to either ventricular fibrillation or complete heart block. A retrospective study suggests that this incidence may be reduced by a permanent ventricular demand pacemaker, suggesting a role for prophylactic permanent pacing in patients with acute myocardial infarction and bundle branch block with transient third-degree AV block.

Congenital complete heart block is secondary to discontinuity between the atrial musculature and the AV node or the His bundle, if the AV node is absent. No known etiology exists for the majority of cases, but fetal myocarditis, idiopathic hemorrhage, and necrosis of the conduction tissue and transplacental passage of immune complexes from mothers with systemic lupus erythematosus are all entities capable of causing congenital heart block. Treatment is not required for the asymptomatic infant. Patients usually remain asymptomatic during childhood and adolescence, with some patients developing symptoms later in life. Pacing is indicated for patients with congenital second-degree or third-degree AV block with symptomatic bradycardia. It is difficult to predict which children will develop symptoms; therefore, pacing has been recommended for congenital AV block with a wide QRS escape rhythm or for asymptomatic patients with a ventricular rate of less than 45 beats per minute. Additionally, pacing has been recommended for patients with documented infra-Hisian block. Pacing is not recommended for asymptomatic congenital heart block without profound bradycardia in relation to age.

SUGGESTED READING

Fisch C. Electrocardiography of arrhythmias. Philadelphia, Lea and Febiger, 1990:354.

Frye RL, Collins JJ, DeSanctis RW, et al. Guidelines for permanent cardiac pacemaker implantation, May 1984. J Am Coll Cardiol 1984; 4:434.

Hindman MC, Wagner GS, JaFo M, et al. The clinical significance of bundle branch block complicating acute myocardial infarction. 2. Indications for temporary and permanent pacemaker insertion. Circulation 1978; 58:689.

Kugler JD, Danford DA. Pacemakers in children: An update. Am Heart J 1989; 117:665.

Langendorf R, Pick A. Atrioventricular block, type II (Mobitz). Its nature and clinical significance. Circulation 1968; 38:819.

Mullins CB, Atkins JM. Prognosis and management of ventricular conduction blocks in acute myocardial infarction. Mod Concepts Cardiovasc Dis 1976; 45:129.

CHRONIC CONGESTIVE HEART FAILURE

KANU CHATTERJEE, M.B., FRCP

Chronic congestive heart failure, a common clinical syndrome, results from various etiologies, including valvular heart disease, hypertension, ischemic heart disease, and primary myocardial and pericardial diseases. The presenting symptoms, such as dyspnea, fatigue, and edema, and the hemodynamic abnormalities, such as systemic and pulmonary venous hypertension and decreased cardiac output, may be similar, regardless of the etiology of chronic congestive heart failure. During the initial evaluation, it is imperative to exclude primary valvular disorders and pericardial diseases as the potential cause for chronic heart failure. Myocardial dysfunction, however, is the most frequent cause of chronic congestive heart failure, and assessment of myocardial function is necessary before a rational therapeutic approach is considered.

Both abnormal ventricular systolic and diastolic function can be the predominant mechanism of the hemodynamic abnormalities and symptoms of heart failure. Impaired systolic function, the most frequent cause of chronic heart failure, is recognized by the presence of reduced (40 percent or less) left ventricular ejection fraction, which can be assessed noninvasively by echocardiography or radionuclide ventriculography or invasively by contrast ventriculography. In ischemic or idiopathic dilated cardiomyopathy, ventricular end-systolic and end-diastolic volumes are also increased, and there is only a slight-to-modest increase in left ventricular wall thickness. Once dilated cardiomyopathy is diagnosed, it is desirable to investigate the presence of myocardial ischemia due to obstructive coronary artery disease (exercise testing or dipyridamole thallium scintigraphy). Pharmacologic therapy, nonpharmacologic therapy, or both for the relief of ischemia may be necessary and of benefit, in addition to antifailure treatment, for optimal management of such patients. If left ventricular ejection fraction is normal, abnormal diastolic function due to hypertrophic cardiomyopathy, hypertensive heart disease, or restrictive cardiomyopathy should be suspected as the cause of chronic heart failure, and appropriate investigations are required to establish the diagnosis. Because impaired systolic function is the principal cause of chronic heart failure in the majority of patients with this syndrome, therapy for chronic heart failure resulting from depressed systolic function, as in patients with dilated cardiomyopathy, is emphasized.

The objectives of pharmacotherapy in chronic heart failure are to relieve symptoms, to improve cardiac performance and exercise tolerance, and, if possible, to achieve a better prognosis. During the last two decades, several therapeutic options have been explored to achieve these goals (Table 1). Based on the results of many investigations, it is now possible to adapt a rational therapeutic approach for the management of patients with chronic congestive heart failure.

PREFERRED APPROACH

Medical Treatment

Diuretics

Diuretics, in general, are effective in relieving congestive symptoms. They decrease pulmonary and systemic venous pressures, principally by decreasing intracardiac volumes resulting from diuresis and decreased intravascular volume. Diuretics, however, do not usually increase cardiac output or improve ventricular performance. In patients with heart failure, ventricular function curve shifts downward and to the right compared with that in patients with normal ventricular function (Fig. 1). Most patients with chronic heart failure and congestive symptoms have elevated systemic and pulmonary venous pressures and lie on the flat portion of the ventricular function curve. A modest reduction of ventricular preload in these patients is associated with little or no decrease in cardiac output, although systemic venous and pulmonary capillary wedge pressures are likely to decrease. With excessive diuretic therapy, however, cardiac output may decrease as a result of a marked decrease in ventricular preload. Hypotension and impaired renal function may also result. Furthermore, aggressive diuretic therapy alone may activate renin-angiotensin-aldosterone systems, which may produce adverse effects on cardiac and renal function. *Thus, diuretic therapy alone is not recommended for treatment of chronic heart failure, and diuretics should be used in conjunction with other drugs that have the potential to increase cardiac output.*

TABLE 1 Therapeutic Options in Chronic Heart Failure

Pharmacotherapy
Diuretics
Digitalis
Vasodilators
Beta-adrenergic antagonists
New inotropic drugs
Antiarrhythmic drugs
Cytotoxic drugs
Surgical Therapy
Cardiac transplantation
Cardiomyoplexy
Coronary artery bypass surgery
Artificial heart

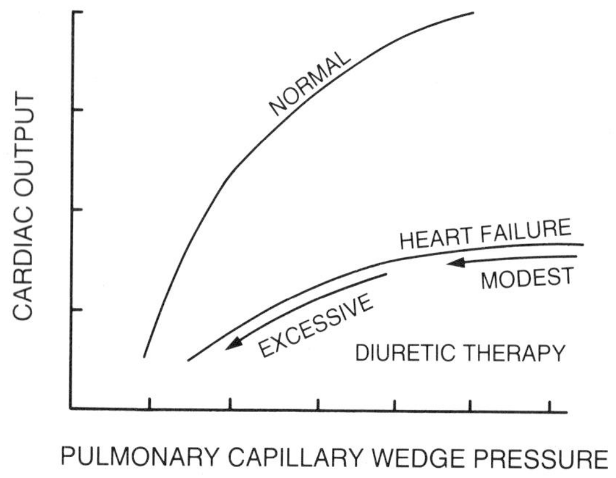

Figure 1 Diuretic therapy in chronic heart failure and expected changes in systemic hemodynamics. During diuretic therapy, with a modest reduction in pulmonary capillary wedge pressure, there is little or no decrease in cardiac output; with excessive reduction in pulmonary capillary wedge pressure, however, cardiac output will fall.

As a guide to diuretic therapy, monitoring of renal function is helpful, and the doses of the diuretics should be reduced when there is a significant increase in blood urea nitrogen (BUN) and creatinine levels. For patients with severe resistant heart failure, with markedly elevated systemic venous pressures and peripheral edema, a combination of diuretics (e.g., furosemide and metolazone) is frequently employed. Intravenous diuretic therapy may be more effective than oral therapy in these patients. It should be emphasized, however, that concomitant vasodilator therapy, inotropic therapy, or both should always be considered to maintain adequate cardiac output.

Digitalis

The role of maintenance digitalis therapy in the management of patients with chronic heart failure in sinus rhythm remains somewhat controversial, although many recent studies have demonstrated its usefulness in improving clinical status and left ventricular function. Withdrawal of digoxin therapy is associated with an increase in pulmonary capillary wedge pressure and a decrease in left ventricular stroke work index, indicating a deterioration of left ventricular function; reinstitution of digoxin therapy increases stroke work index and decreases pulmonary capillary wedge pressure. Compared with placebo, long-term digitalis therapy results in clinical improvement in patients with heart failure with depressed ejection fraction and S3 gallop. In patients with mild-to-moderate heart failure, digoxin has the greater potential to increase left ventricular ejection fraction compared with captopril, although the improvement in exercise tolerance with digoxin is less than that with captopril. In patients with more severe heart failure (New York Heart Association [NYHA] class III and IV), the magnitude of increase in exercise tolerance with digoxin is comparable to that with milrinone, a peak III phosphodiesterase inhibitor. In patients with very mild heart failure, digoxin is less effective than xamoterol, a partial $beta_1$-adrenergic agonist, in improving exercise tolerance. *Thus, except in patients with no or minimal symptoms, digoxin therapy is indicated provided that impaired left ventricular systolic function is the principal mechanism for heart failure.*

Digoxin is also indicated to control ventricular response in the presence of atrial fibrillation complicating chronic heart failure. Digoxin should be avoided in patients with severe renal failure because of the propensity to develop toxicity. Digoxin is also contraindicated in patients with sinoatrial or atrioventricular nodal disease because it may induce unacceptable bradycardia. The prognosis of patients with chronic heart failure treated conventionally with digitalis and diuretics alone has been determined by prospective, controlled studies. In patients with mild-to-moderately severe heart failure, 1-year mortality is approximately 20 percent; in patients with more severe heart failure, mortality is approximately 50 percent. The addition of certain vasodilators or angiotensin converting enzyme inhibitors has been shown to improve the prognosis of such patients. *Thus, combination therapy with vasodilators or angiotensin converting enzyme inhibitors and digitalis and diuretics (triple therapy) should always be considered until specific contraindications exist and such therapy is tolerated without adverse effects.*

Vasodilators and Angiotensin Converting Enzyme Inhibitors

The rationale for the use of vasodilators is to reduce afterload and preload and thereby improve cardiac performance (Fig. 2). A large number of vasodilators with different mechanisms of action have been evaluated for the management of chronic heart failure. The systemic hemodynamic effects of some of the commonly used vasodilator agents and their mechanisms of action are summarized in Table 2. The systemic hemodynamic effects of vasodilators are determined primarily by their principal site of action on the peripheral vascular bed. Drugs with predominantly arterial dilating effects, such as hydralazine and calcium entry blocking agents, increase cardiac output by decreasing systemic vascular resistance and may not cause any significant decrease in systemic and pulmonary venous pressures. Predominant venodilators such as nitrates and nitroglycerin decrease systemic and pulmonary venous pressures with little or no increase in cardiac output. With the combination of an arterial dilator and a venodilator, a significant increase in cardiac output and a decrease in systemic and pulmonary

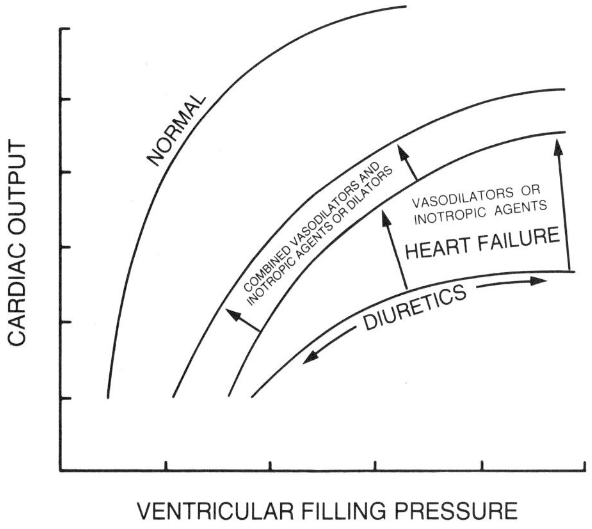

Figure 2 Effects of diuretics, vasodilators, inotropic agents, and combined vasodilators and inotropic agents in ventricular function curve. Ventricular function curves are constructed by relating changes in cardiac output to changes in ventricular filling pressure. Compared with normal values, in heart failure, ventricular function curve is shifted downward. With diuretics, there is no shift in ventricular function curve. With vasodilator or inotropic agents, ventricular function curve moves toward normal; cardiac output increases with a fall in ventricular filling pressures. With combined vasodilator and inotropic therapy, there is further upward and leftward shift of ventricular function curve, with a further increase in cardiac output and decrease in ventricular filling pressure.

venous pressures are expected. Drugs with both arterial and venodilating properties, such as angiotensin converting enzyme inhibitors and alpha-adrenergic blocking drugs, produce similar hemodynamic effects.

Although systemic hemodynamic effects of various vasodilators are qualitatively similar, their effects on regional hemodynamics may differ. Angiotensin converting enzyme inhibitors and nitrates decrease myocardial oxygen consumption, whereas hydralazine and prazosin may increase oxygen consumption. Dihydropyridine, a class of calcium entry blocking agents, may increase coronary blood flow due to primary coronary vasodilation. Renal function tends to improve with hydralazine and angiotensin converting enzyme inhibitors and remains unchanged with nitrates and prazosin. Long-term efficacy in maintaining improved clinical status and exercise tolerance has not been demonstrated with all vasodilators. In general, angiotensin converting enzyme inhibitors and nitrates have been shown to cause sustained improvement in exercise tolerance; hydralazine, prazosin, and calcium channel blocking agents usually do not cause sustained improvement in clinical status or exercise tolerance. Improved prognosis of patients with chronic heart failure has been documented only with the use of certain vasodilators. Combined hydralazine and nitrate therapy, in addition to digitalis and diuretics, decreases mortality significantly in patients with mild-to-moderately severe chronic heart failure. The angiotensin

TABLE 2 Expected Hemodynamic Effects of Vasodilators in Chronic Heart Failure

Agents	*Principal Mechanism of Action*	*Principal Sites of Action on Peripheral Vascular Bed*	*Cardiac Output*	*Pulmonary Capillary Wedge Pressure*	*Systematic Venous Pressure*	*Mean Blood Pressure*	*Heart Rate*
Hydralazine	Direct acting	Arterial	Increase	No change or slight decrease	No change or slight decrease	No change or decrease	No change or decrease
Nitrates and nitroglycerin	Direct acting	Venous	No change or slight increase	Decrease	Decrease	No change or decrease	No change or increase
Angiotensin converting enzyme inhibitors*	Angiotensin II inhibition	Arterial and venous	Increase	Decrease	Decrease	Decrease	Decrease or no change
Alpha-adrenergic antagonists†	Alpha-receptor blockage	Arterial and venous	Increase	Decrease	Decrease	Decrease	No change or decrease
Calcium channel blocking agents‡	Calcium antagonism	Arterial	Increase or no change	No change or decrease	No change or decrease	Decrease or no change	Increase or no change

*Captopril, enalapril, lisinopril.
†Prazosin, trimazosin, terazosin.
‡Nifedipine, nicardipine, diltiazem.

converting enzyme inhibitors captopril and enalapril decrease mortality not only in patients with mild-to-moderately severe heart failure, but also in patients with severe chronic heart failure (NYHA class IV). *Thus, the addition of hydralazine, isosorbide dinitrate, or angiotensin converting enzyme inhibitors should be considered in all symptomatic patients with chronic heart failure regardless of its severity—mild, moderate, or severe.*

Angiotensin converting enzyme inhibitors are preferred over hydralazine-nitrates for a number of reasons. The potential benefits of angiotensin converting enzyme inhibitors are (1) consistent decrease in myocardial oxygen consumption, (2) reduction of aldosterone levels, (3) decrease in norepinephrine levels, (4) increase in prostaglandins and bradykinins, (5) improved renal function, (6) decreased ventricular arrhythmias, and (7) better tolerance.

Approximately 30 percent of patients cannot tolerate the doses of hydralazine and nitrates that are effective in improving hemodynamics. Tachycardia, recurrence of angina, gastrointestinal intolerance, arthralgia, and lupus-like syndrome are important adverse effects. Angiotensin converting enzyme inhibitors may also not be tolerated by some patients. Hypotension, deterioration of renal function, cough, skin rash, and dysgeusia (associated with captopril) are important side effects. In patients with bilateral renal artery stenosis or even in hypotensive patients with a low cardiac output, angiotensin converting enzyme inhibitors may cause severe renal failure. In patients with hypotension, particularly in those with hyponatremia, angiotensin converting enzyme inhibitors may induce further hypotension and renal failure; in such patients, angiotensin converting enzyme inhibitor therapy should be initiated with a very small dose (captopril, 6.25 mg, enalapril or lisinopril, 2.5 mg) after hypotension and low output states are partially corrected with inotropic therapy. Frequently, a combination of angiotensin converting enzyme inhibitors or vasodilators and newer inotropic agents are required along with digitalis and diuretics in the management of such patients.

Calcium entry blocking agents should not be used as the principal agent for vasodilator therapy for chronic heart failure. Verapamil is contraindicated in patients with overt heart failure resulting from depressed systolic function because of its pronounced negative inotropic effect. Dihydropyridines, such as nifedipine, nicardipine, and felodipine, may improve cardiac performance in some patients; however, their long-term benefits have not been demonstrated. Diltiazem also improves left ventricular function in some patients; its long-term effect in improving exercise tolerance and prognosis has not been established. In patients with coronary artery disease and evidence of myocardial ischemia, calcium entry blocking agents such as nifedipine or diltiazem can be added to hydralazine-nitrates or angiotensin converting enzyme inhibitors in an attempt to relieve myocardial ischemia, provided that significant hypotension does not result.

Alpha-adrenergic blocking agents such as prazosin, trimazosin, and terazosin produce short-term beneficial hemodynamic and clinical effects in patients with chronic heart failure; hemodynamic and clinical tolerance develops rather rapidly in response to these agents. Thus, these agents alone should not be used for the treatment of chronic heart failure. However, in some patients who cannot tolerate adequate doses of hydralazine-nitrates or angiotensin converting enzyme inhibitors, alpha-adrenergic agents may be used along with lower doses of angiotensin converting enzyme inhibitors, particularly in relatively hypertensive patients. However, long-term benefit of such combination therapy has not been determined.

The role of newer vasodilator agents such nicorandil, flosequinan, and atrial natriuretic peptide in the management of chronic congestive heart failure remains unclear.

Nondigitalis Inotropic Drugs

Several adrenergic and nonadrenergic agents with positive inotropic effects have been evaluated. The adrenergic agents dobutamine and dopamine and the nonadrenergic peak III phosphodiesterase inhibitor amrinone are available only for short-term intravenous use. Of many nonparenteral adrenergic agents—pirbuterol, xamoterol, ibopamine, and levodopa—currently levodopa is the only drug available that can be used for long-term management of patients with chronic heart failure. Many nonparenteral peak III phosphodiesterase inhibitors—milrinone, enoximone, piroximone, pimobendan, and others—are currently undergoing clinical trials and are not available for clinical use. Intermittent intravenous infusion of dobutamine (5 to 10 μg per kilogram per minute) can cause sustained hemodynamic and clinical improvement for a few days to a few weeks in some patients. However, the duration of sustained improvement is variable, and the more severe the heart failure and hypotension, the shorter the duration of benefit. Furthermore, improvement in prognosis has not been documented with intermittent dobutamine infusion. Similarly, although intermittent amrinone infusion improves hemodynamics and clinical status of patients with refractory failure, it does not improve prognosis in these patients.

Levodopa (1.5 to 2 g three to four times daily) is converted to dopamine by dopa-decarboxylase, and the hemodynamic effects of levodopa are similar to those of low-dose (2 to 4 μg per kilogram per minute) dopamine infusion. Usually there is a modest increase in cardiac output with little or no change in mean arterial, right atrial, and pulmonary capillary wedge pressures. Approximately 30 percent of patients do not tolerate levodopa, particularly large doses that are required to produce beneficial effects; gastrointestinal intolerance and central nervous system side effects prohibit its use in many patients. Long-term hemodynamic or clinical benefit of other nonparenteral adrenergic agents, pirbuterol, xamoterol, and ibopamine, has not been demonstrated in patients with moderately severe or severe heart failure.

The peak III phosphodiesterase inhibitors milrinone, enoximone, and others exert direct positive inotropic and vasodilatory effects and thus are called inodilators. Following their acute administration, cardiac output increases markedly along with a substantial decrease in systemic and pulmonary venous pressures, a slight decrease in mean arterial pressure, and a slight increase in heart rate. However, clinical deterioration occurs in a significant proportion of patients during the long-term administration of these agents, and larger doses of diuretics frequently need to be added to prevent fluid retention. Prospective, controlled studies have reported that the phosphodiesterase inhibitors enoximone and milrinone can improve clinical status and exercise tolerance in patients with moderately severe and severe heart failure during 3 months of follow-up. However, in the study in which effects of milrinone and digoxin were compared, more patients treated with milrinone had clinical deterioration and died compared with those treated with digoxin during the 3 months of follow-up. Thus, indications for the use of nonglycosidic inotropic agents or inodilators are limited for those patients who fail to respond to vasodilators or angiotensin converting enzyme inhibitors. These agents are also used in patients awaiting cardiac transplantation as "pharmacologic bridge" therapy. Frequently, combination therapy using vasodilators, angiotensin converting enzyme inhibitors, and newer inotropic agents in addition to conventional therapy is required in prospective cardiac transplant recipients.

Beta-adrenergic Blocking Agents

In patients with idiopathic dilated cardiomyopathy, beta-blocker therapy has been shown to improve clinical status and left ventricular function, presumably resulting from upregulation of myocardial beta-adrenergic receptors. However, the precise role of beta-blocker therapy in patients with chronic heart failure remains to be established.

When beta-blocker therapy is initiated, deterioration in clinical status and hemodynamics such as decreased cardiac output and arterial pressure and increased pulmonary capillary wedge pressure may occur. Following maintenance therapy for 6 to 8 weeks, clinical and hemodynamic improvement may be apparent. Hemodynamic improvement is characterized by an increase in cardiac output and systolic blood pressure, decreased left ventricular end-diastolic pressure, and deceased left ventricular end-systolic volume, with little or no change in end-diastolic volume. Although the precise mechanism for the hemodynamic improvement with chronic beta-blocker therapy remains unclear, upregulation of myocardial beta-adrenoreceptors and enhanced contractile response are likely to be contributory. A few uncontrolled studies have claimed improved prognosis with long-term beta-blocker therapy; however, controlled studies have not substantiated this claim. Uncontrolled studies have also demonstrated decreased incidence of sudden death with beta-blocker therapy. *Clinical experience suggests that certain subsets of patients with dilated cardiomyopathy with tachycardia, gallop rhythm, relatively preserved cardiac output, and elevated pulmonary capillary wedge pressure are more likely to benefit from chronic beta-blocker therapy, particularly in combination with angiotensin converting enzyme inhibitors.* To avoid initial clinical deterioration, the starting dose of beta-adrenergic blocking agent should be very low (e.g., metoprolol, 5 mg once or twice daily), and the dose should be increased slowly until the resting heart rate decreases by 10 to 15 beats per minute. The potential benefit or hazard of beta-blocker therapy has not been established.

Cytotoxic Drugs and Corticosteroids

In a few patients with active myocarditis proved by myocardial biopsy, cytotoxic drugs (azathioprine) and corticosteroids have been reported to improve left ventricular function. However, controlled studies suggest that the potential benefit of corticosteroid treatment is too little compared with the risk of developing serious side effects. *Thus, corticosteroid therapy is not recommended for the treatment of chronic heart failure.*

Amiodarone and Other Antiarrhythmic Drugs

Approximately 50 percent of patients with moderately severe or severe chronic heart failure die suddenly, and it is generally accepted that the majority of these deaths result from ventricular arrhythmias and occasionally from bradyarrhythmias. As a result, antiarrhythmic drug therapy has been postulated to decrease the incidence of sudden death in these patients. However, type IA antiarrhythmic drugs have not been found to be particularly effective in patients with heart failure and asymptomatic ventricular arrhythmias. Furthermore, type IA and IB antiarrhythmic drugs may cause significant deterioration of ventricular function in patients with overt heart failure. Type IC antiarrhythmic drugs such as flecainide and encainide may enhance mortality of patients with depressed left ventricular function, presumably owing to increased incidence of drug-induced proarrhythmia in these patients. Thus, type I antiarrhythmic drugs should not be used for suppression of asymptomatic ventricular arrhythmias in patients with chronic heart failure. A few uncontrolled studies have reported that amiodarone, a type III antiarrhythmic drug, can potentially decrease the incidence of ventricular arrhythmias and mortality of patients with severe chronic congestive heart failure without causing deterioration in left ventricular function. Indeed, the addition of amiodarone to conventional therapy and angiotensin converting enzyme inhibitors can increase left ventricular ejection fraction. *Thus, it is reasonable to consider the addition of a low dose of amiodarone (200 mg per day after initial loading dose) to conventional treatment in selected patients with severe heart failure and with asymptomatic complex ventricular arrhythmias or nonsustained ventricular tachycardia.* There are several undesirable side effects of amiodarone, of which pulmonary toxicity is the most serious. *Development of pulmonary toxicity may preclude cardiac transplantation in potential candidates, and thus in such patients amiodarone should be used cautiously, if at all.*

TABLE 3 Therapeutic Approach in Chronic Heart Failure

1. To exclude valvular heart disease and pericardial disease
2. To determine whether heart failure is primarily due to abnormal ventricular diastolic function or due to systolic dysfunction
3. Symptomatic chronic heart failure due to diastolic dysfunction associated with ventricular hypertrophy. Cautious use of diuretics, nitrates, and a trial of calcium entry blocking agents; cardiac transplantation in appropriate subsets who remain unresponsive to medical therapy
4. Chronic heart failure due to systolic dysfunction (reduced ejection fraction, mild-to-severe dilation of ventricular cavity with or without increased wall thickness)
   A. Totally asymptomatic—observe or use angiotensin converting enzyme inhibitors
   B. Mild-to-moderately severe heart failure—diuretics, digitalis, and angiotensin converting enzyme inhibitors or hydralazine, nitrates, diuretics, and digitalis (when angiotensin converting enzyme inhibitors produce adverse effects or are not tolerated). Continues to be symptomatic or deterioration—consider cardiac transplant in appropriate subsets and intermittent dobutamine or amrinone therapy or newer inotropic drugs for patients awaiting cardiac transplantation or for those who are not candidates for cardiac transplantation
   C. Severe chronic heart failure—digitalis, diuretics, and angiotensin converting enzyme inhibitors. Consider cardiac transplant for patients who fail to respond quickly; intermittent dobutamine or amrinone infusion or newer inotropic agents for patients awaiting cardiac transplantation or for patients considered not suitable for cardiac transplantation; consider low-dose beta-blocker or amiodarone therapy in selected patients

Surgical Treatment

Cardiac Transplantation and Other Surgical Therapy

Cardiac transplantation is the most effective treatment to improve the prognosis in patients with severe refractory heart failure. Two-year survival with medical therapy in such patients is, at best, 25 percent; in contrast, 5-year survival rate following cardiac transplantation may exceed 60 percent. *Thus, patients who remain significantly symptomatic despite aggressive medical therapy or those who fail to respond to conventional therapy including vasodilators and converting enzyme inhibitors should be considered for cardiac transplantation, provided that there are no contraindications for transplantation.* However, the very limited availability of donor hearts does not allow such treatment for the vast majority of potential candidates. Cardiomyoplexy, a surgical technique to wrap skeletal muscle such as latissimus dorsi around the heart to improve cardiac mechanical performance, is now undergoing clinical trials, and the role of such surgery in the management of severe chronic heart failure needs to be established

Stepwise Therapeutic Approach

Therapy of chronic congestive heart failure includes use of diuretics, digitalis, vasodilators, angiotensin converting enzyme inhibitors, newer inotropic drugs, and cardiac transplantation. However, based on available information, a stepwise therapeutic approach should be undertaken as outlined in Table 3.

SUGGESTED READING

Chatterjee K, Parmley WW. Vasodilator therapy for acute myocardial infarction and chronic congestive heart failure. J Am Coll Cardiol 1983; 1:133.

Chatterjee K. Digitalis, catecholamines and other positive inotropic agents. In: Parmley WW, Chatterjee K, eds. Cardiology. Philadelphia: JB Lippincott, 1988:1.

Chatterjee K. Digitalis and non-ACE inhibitors in heart failure. Cardiol Clin 1989;7:99.

Dzau VJ, Creager MA. Progress in angiotensin-converting enzyme inhibition in heart failure. Cardiol Clin 1989;7:119.

Lee HR, O'Connell JB, Mason JW. Immunosuppression and beta blockade in heart failure. Cardiol Clin 1989; 7:171.

DIGITALIS TOXICITY

ELLIOTT M. ANTMAN, M.D.
THOMAS W. SMITH, M.D.

Because digitalis glycosides have a relatively narrow therapeutic index, clinicians must determine which individual patients have a favorable risk : benefit ratio for digitalis use and promptly identify signs and symptoms of digitalis toxicity. Fortunately, the incidence of digitalis toxicity has dropped compared with that in the 1960s and early 1970s, probably as a result of enhanced understanding of pharmacokinetics, more widespread use of radioimmunoassays of serum digoxin levels, increased appreciation of the multitude of drug interactions that may predispose a patient to digitalis toxicity, and an appropriate tendency to use lower doses of digoxin as alternative drugs have become available for treatment of cardiovascular conditions in which digoxin was traditionally employed. Among these new drugs are verapamil (for paroxysmal supraventricular tachycardia and control of the ventricular rate in atrial fibrillation), beta-adrenergic blocking agents (for control of the ventricular rate in atrial fibrillation), and angiotensin converting enzyme inhibitors (for a balanced vasodilator effect in congestive heart failure).

No specific serum digoxin level can be relied on to differentiate clearly between toxic and nontoxic states; rather, such data must be interpreted in the broader clinical context, with appropriate attention to the multitude of factors that may predispose to digitalis toxicity. Electrocardiographic manifestations of digitalis toxicity are characterized by disturbances of impulse formation or conduction (at atrial, atrioventricular [AV] junctional, or ventricular levels) or a combination of both types of phenomena. Clinical symptoms of digitalis toxicity typically include anorexia, nausea and vomiting, and visual symptoms as well as a variety of nonspecific complaints such as weakness, fatigue, headache, dizziness, and psychiatric disturbances ("digitalis delirium").

THERAPEUTIC ALTERNATIVES

In addition to withholding further cardiac glycoside administration, therapeutic options in the management of digitalis toxicity range from simple observation of the patient for infrequent, asymptomatic non–life-threatening arrhythmias to administration of the recently marketed digoxin-specific Fab fragments for potentially life-threatening arrhythmias (ventricular tachycardia, ventricular fibrillation, high-grade AV block with a slow escape rhythm not responsive to atropine), hyperkalemia (>5 mEq per liter), or both.

Between these extremes are found patients with mild digitalis toxicity (non–life-threatening but symptomatic cardiac arrhythmias) and those in whom the etiology of the arrhythmia is not certain but in whom the question of digitalis toxicity arises. Because clinical experience remains relatively limited and the potential hazards of repeated exposure have not been fully defined, digoxin-specific Fab fragment treatment is not indicated for mild digitalis toxicity, and conventional antiarrhythmic therapy remains appropriate in such cases. Similarly, the use of Fab fragments as both a diagnostic and potentially a therapeutic tool in cases in which the diagnosis of digitalis toxicity is uncertain remains investigational at this time. As additional experience is accumulated with digoxin-specific Fab fragments, it is possible that the indications for their use may be extended beyond overtly life-threatening cases in the future. Provided safety is borne out in further experience, broader use of Fab fragments may have useful cost-effectiveness implications by decreasing intensive care unit requirements and overall length of hospital stay.

PREFERRED APPROACH

Prompt identification of digitalis-toxic arrhythmias is vital to successful clinical management. We advocate the following general therapeutic measures for all patients with clinically evident digitalis toxicity.

- Cardiac glycoside administration should be discontinued, and the use of catecholamines should be avoided if possible.
- The arrhythmia and its potential impact on the patient should be evaluated. Serious rhythm disturbances (e.g., complex ventricular arrhythmias) necessitate admission to an intensive care unit, whereas less hazardous arrhythmias may be adequately treated on a general hospital floor, assuming that adequate electrocardiographic monitoring is available.
- Unless the serum potassium level is elevated when the patient is first seen (e.g., >5.0 mEq per liter), renal insufficiency is present, AV block is present or conduction is prolonged (P-R interval >0.26 second), or the patient has taken a large overdose of digitalis (in which case serum potassium may rise to dangerously high levels), potassium repletion should be considered.
- Bradyarrhythmias that cause hypotension or a significant reduction in cardiac output may be treated initially with intravenous atropine (typically 0.5 to 1.0 mg in adults). We insert a temporary demand ventricular pacemaker if atropine fails to resolve the problem in less than 5 minutes. Infusion of beta-adrenergic

agonists such as isoproterenol is best avoided in view of the potential for provoking more serious arrhythmias.

- Cardiac arrhythmias due to enhanced automaticity that are not overtly life threatening (e.g., paroxysms of nonsustained ventricular tachycardia) may require suppression with conventional antiarrhythmic therapy (intravenous lidocaine or phenytoin) in addition to potassium supplementation.
- Cases involving large accidental or suicidal cardiac glycoside ingestions and those with potentially life-threatening arrhythmias, hyperkalemia, or both are treated with digoxin-specific antibody (Fab) therapy.

Potassium Repletion

Potassium repletion should be undertaken only under closely monitored conditions because of the risk of provoking more troublesome arrhythmias, marked hyperkalemia, and even death. Either the intravenous or the oral route of administration may be used. We prefer the latter when the rhythm disturbance is not immediately life threatening. The rate of intravenous infusion of potassium should be limited to less than 0.5 to 1.0 mEq per minute. Potassium solutions are mixed in either normal saline or D5W but should not exceed a concentration of 120 to 160 mEq per liter. When oral potassium repletion is used, doses of 40 mEq every 1 to 4 hours are given, provided that acidosis is not present (pH >7.30) and renal function is adequate (creatinine <2.0 mg per deciliter). Regardless of the potassium administration route employed, we review the 12-lead electrocardiogram every 15 minutes to detect early evidence of impending potassium excess, and serum potassium levels are measured every 30 to 60 minutes. Because of the possibility of paradoxical worsening of hypokalemia when D5W is used, we prefer to use normal saline in cases of severe potassium depletion (<3.5 mEq per liter).

Conventional Antiarrhythmic Agents

Clinical reports of lidocaine use in cases of digitalis toxicity suggest that this classic antiarrhythmic drug is of value for the management of digitalis-related arrhythmias, and we continue to employ it in cases of tachyarrhythmias of less than life-threatening severity. Lidocaine is administered as serial intravenous 100-mg boluses every 3 to 5 minutes (to a total dose of 300 mg) until either a therapeutic effect or lidocaine toxicity develops. This may then be followed by continuous infusion of 15 to 50 μg per kilogram of body weight per minute if further suppression of the arrhythmia is needed. Adverse reactions to lidocaine usually involve the central nervous system and may range from feelings of dissociation to agitation or frank seizures. Several reports have indicated that the slow intravenous infusion of phenytoin 100 mg every 5 minutes (not to exceed a total dose of 1,000 mg) is also useful for digitalis-toxic arrhythmias (e.g., ectopic automatic atrial tachycardia).

Clinical experience with beta-blockers, quinidine, or procainamide has been less favorable than that with lidocaine. Because of the greater risk of cardiac toxicity (both electrophysiologic and hemodynamic) with these drugs, we do not consider them to be initial pharmacologic agents of choice to suppress non-life-threatening digitalis-induced arrhythmias. Clinical experience with newer antiarrhythmic agents (tocainide, mexiletine, amiodarone) is insufficient to evaluate their safety and efficacy in comparison with the standard agents, and we do not advocate their use of digitalis-toxic arrhythmias at the present time. However, of potential interest is verapamil, for which there are abundant experimental data indicating that it is useful for treating a specific electrophysiologic abnormality referred to as triggered automaticity. Triggered automaticity appears to be related to oscillations of the membrane potential during the terminal phase of repolarization known as delayed after depolarizations; the oscillatory activity is believed to be caused by release of calcium from overloaded intracellular stores. Verapamil has been shown to prevent or abort such triggered activity in experimental preparations and in scattered clinical reports. Available experience is too limited at present to permit any statement of appropriate clinical guidelines.

Cardioversion

A common clinical problem centers around direct current (DC) cardioversion in the patient receiving a digitalis preparation. It is a widely held belief that DC cardioversion can be hazardous in individuals receiving cardiac glycosides. However, this is based on earlier studies reporting that the electrical shock provoked serious ventricular arrhythmias (refractory ventricular tachycardia or fibrillation). Although near-toxic levels of digitalis can lower the threshold for post-shock ventricular arrhythmias, clinical studies have shown that therapeutic digoxin levels do not increase the risk of serious post-shock ventricular arrhythmias. Thus, an increased risk of arrhythmias does not appear to be present when transthoracic shocks are delivered in the absence of digitalis toxicity. We use the following approach when considering DC cardioversion in digitalized individuals.

- Electrolyte imbalances are corrected, fever is suppressed, and hypoxia and anxiety are treated before DC cardioversion is undertaken.

- When there is overt electrocardiographic evidence of digitalis toxicity (e.g., atrial fibrillation with very slow ventricular rate, accelerated AV junctional rhythm, multifocal ventricular premature depolarizations), elective DC cardioversion is not performed.
- Under all circumstances, the smallest amount of energy that is likely to be effective is used. Our usual schedule of energy titration starts with 25 to 50 watt-seconds, with subsequent increments of 25 to 50 watt-seconds as needed. Ventricular tachycardia can often be abolished with as little as 10 watt-seconds or less.

Digoxin-Specific Antibody (Fab Fragments) for Life-Threatening Toxicity

Hemodialysis or hemoperfusion is of limited value for prompt reversal of life-threatening toxicity because of the widespread tissue binding of digoxin. Advanced digitalis intoxication should now be treated with purified digoxin-specific polyclonal antibody fragments (Fab) obtained from sheep immunized with digoxin coupled as a hapten to a carrier protein to render it antigenic. The advantages of the smaller size of the Fab fragment (molecular weight 50,000) as compared with the whole IgG molecule (molecular weight 150,000) include a more rapid onset of action due to enhanced diffusion into the interstitial space and, in patients with normal renal function, relatively rapid renal clearance of digoxin bound to Fab fragments (with a half-life of about 16 hours). The enhanced rate of clearance by renal mechanisms minimizes the chance of late release of bound digoxin and reemergence of toxicity. Although the average affinity constant for digoxin is 30-fold to 100-fold higher than that for digitoxin in typical preparations, the affinity for the latter is still high enough to permit digoxin-specific Fab antibody fragments to be used effectively for life-threatening intoxication with digitoxin as well as digoxin.

We recommend the following protocol for administration of Fab fragments.

- The dose of Fab fragments is calculated to be equal on a mole-for-mole basis to the amount of digoxin or digitoxin in the patient's body, estimated from the medical history, determinations of serum digoxin or digitoxin concentrations, or both (Table 1). Examples of the calculation of the body load of digoxin to be neutralized are shown in Table 2.
- Screening for hypersensitivity was performed during clinical trials with digoxin-specific antibody fragments, and only 1 of 150 patients developed erythema at the site of skin testing, but without a wheal reaction. In view of this statistic and because such hypersensitivity testing can delay treatment in urgent cases, we restrict skin testing to high-risk individuals, such as those with a history of allergy to sheep products and those who have previously received a course of treatment with Fab fragments. The skin test is performed by reconstituting 0.1 ml of a 10 mg per milliliter solution of Fab fragments in 10 ml of isotonic saline. Subsequently 0.1 ml of the above 1 : 100 dilution (10 μg) is injected intradermally, and the patient is observed for an urticarial wheal over the next 20 minutes.
- The Fab fragments should be administered intravenously through a 0.22-μm membrane filter over 15 to 30 minutes, unless the gravity of the clinical situation demands more rapid infusion.
- It is important to note that in states of advanced digitalis toxicity, potassium excretion through renal mechanisms coupled with efforts to reduce hyperkalemia using potassium binding resins can deplete total body potassium even though the serum potassium may be normal or even elevated. A dramatic fall in serum potassium concentration can occur after Fab administration, since reversal of NaK-ATPase inhibition tends to restore the normal transmembrane potassium gradient rapidly. For this reason, serum potassium should be monitored at least every hour for the first 4 to 6 hours after Fab treatment. The decline in serum potassium (which can occur even if supplemental potassium is given) is usually complete by 4 hours.
- The sequence of events that takes place following injection of digoxin-specific Fab fragments includes prompt binding of intravascular digoxin, followed by diffusion of the Fab frag-

TABLE 1 Calculation of Equimolar Dose of Digoxin-Specific Fab Fragments

Calculation of Body Load of Digoxin

Ingested amount (mg) × bioavailability of digoxin tablets = mg × 0.8

$$\frac{\text{Serum digoxin concentration ng/ml)} \times 5.6^{*} \times \text{weight in kg}}{1{,}000}$$

Calculation of Fab Fragment Dose

$$\frac{\text{MW Fab} = 50{,}000}{\text{MW Digoxin} = 781} = 64 \times \text{body load (mg)} = \text{Fab dose (in mg)}$$

$$\frac{\text{Body load of digoxin (mg)}}{0.6 \text{ mg neutralized/40-mg vial}} = \text{Number of vials of Fab fragments}$$

*Volume of distribution of digoxin in average adult (liters per kilogram). For digitoxin, use 0.56 rather than 5.6.

MW = Molecular weight.

Modified from Antman EM, Wenger TL, Butler VP, et al. Treatment of 150 cases of life-threatening digitalis intoxication with digoxin-specific Fab antibody fragments: Final report of a multicenter study. Circulation 1990; 81:1744; by permission of the American Heart Association, Inc.

TABLE 2 Examples of Calculation of Equimolar Dose of Digoxin-Specific Fab Fragments

Case 1

75-year-old man (weight 70 kg) with chronic coronary heart disease and atrial fibrillation receiving maintenance therapy with digoxin 0.25 mg daily. He becomes confused and takes two of his digoxin tablets daily for 2 weeks and presents with complaints of weakness and palpitations. ECG shows sustained ventricular tachycardia at 150 beats/min. SDC = 3.0 ng/ml

$$\text{Body load of digoxin} = \frac{\text{SDC} \times 5.6 \times 70}{1{,}000} = \frac{3.0 \times 5.6 \times 70}{1{,}000} = 1.176 \text{ mg} \approx 1.2 \text{ mg}$$

$$\text{Dose of Fab fragments} = \frac{1.2 \text{ mg}}{0.6 \text{ mg neutralized/40-mg vial}} = 2 \text{ vials}$$

Case 2

40-year-old woman (weight 70 kg) with no history of heart disease ingests 100 tablets of digoxin 0.25 mg in a suicide attempt. She presents 8 hours later with nausea, vomiting, hypotension, complete heart block, and an idioventricular escape rhythm at 35 beats/min. Serum digoxin concentration result not yet returned from laboratory (and not needed for Fab dose determination). Serum potassium = 6.1 mEq/liter.

$$\text{Body load} = [\text{ingested amount} \times 0.8] = 25 \text{ mg} \times 0.8 = 20 \text{ mg}$$

$$\text{Dose of Fab fragments} = \frac{20 \text{ mg}}{0.6 \text{ mg neutralized/40-mg vial}} \approx 34 \text{ vials}$$

Case 3

60-year-old woman (weight 65 kg) with chronic rheumatic heart disease and mitral regurgitation maintained on digoxin 0.25 mg daily for control of the ventricular rate in atrial fibrillation. SDC = 2 ng/ml on maintenance therapy. She ingests 75 tablets of digoxin 0.25 mg during a period of depression and presents 36 hours later with fascicular tachycardia, an unusual form of ventricular tachycardia originating in or near the left anterior fascicle. Serum potassium = 5.9 mEq/liter.

Ingested amount ≈ 18 mg digoxin (tablets)

$$\text{Body load} = [\text{ingested amount} \times 0.8] + \left[\frac{\text{SDC} \times 5.6 \times 65}{1{,}000}\right] = 14.4 + 0.728 \approx 15 \text{ mg}$$

$$\text{Dose of Fab fragments} = \frac{15}{0.6 \text{ neutralized/40-mg vial}} = 25 \text{ vials}$$

SDC = Serum digoxin concentration.

ments into the interstitial space and binding of free digoxin. The decrease in free digoxin in the extracellular space to near-zero levels creates a concentration gradient promoting egress of tissue stores of digoxin into the extracellular space, where it is also rapidly bound by Fab fragments. Free digoxin molecules freshly dissociated from membrane receptors are rapidly bound and cannot reassociate with the digoxin binding (inhibitory) site on the alpha subunit of NaK-ATPase. This dissociation event and the subsequent step of binding to Fab are critically important rate-limiting events in the reversal of digitalis toxicity. Typically, the total extracellular digoxin concentration rises dramatically but such digoxin is pharmacologically inactive, since only the unbound form can associate with the inhibitory site on the alpha subunit of NaK-ATPase. For this reason as well as technical problems imposed on assay systems by the presence of high-affinity Fab fragments, measurements of serum digoxin concentration are not reliable indicators of the state of digitalization for about 1 to 2 weeks after Fab administration. We have not found this to be a noteworthy clinical problem. In those uncommon cases in which loss of the inotropic support or rate-slowing action previously provided by digitalis results in hemodynamic compromise, it is possible in principle to "back titrate" with digoxin. We have not found this necessary and do not recommend attempting it for at last 7 days after Fab administration.

We have recently reported the results of the initial multicenter study of 150 patients treated with purified digoxin-specific Fab fragments. These patients all had actual or potentially life-threatening cardiac rhythm disturbances or hyperkalemia (or both) caused by digitalis intoxication and were considered clinically refractory to or likely to be refractory to treatment with conventional therapeutic modalities. On the basis of the results of that trial, it can be anticipated that an initial response to Fab will be seen within 60 minutes in most patients suffering from digitalis toxicity, and complete reversal of glycoside effects will be evident within 4 hours of administration of an adequate dose of Fab fragments. Approximately 80 percent of the 150 individuals treated showed resolution of all signs and symptoms, 10 percent were definitely improved (partial resolution), and 10 percent showed no response. Only one patient was judged to have a clinical course suggesting a true lack of response; a lack of response should thus raise the suspicion that too low a dose of Fab fragments was given, or alternatively, that the clinical signs and symptoms were not the result of digitalis toxicity. In two of the 150 patients, a recrudescence of digitalis toxicity was observed after an initial response. Neither patient had renal failure, and both appeared to have received inadequate doses of Fab to neutralize the calculated body load of digoxin.

In this multicenter trial, no acute allergic reactions or illnesses suggesting serum sickness occurred in conjunction with Fab fragment treatment. The expected adverse reactions caused by prompt reversal of digitalis effects (rapid ventricular response to atrial fibrillation, deterioration of the level of left ventricular systolic function, or hypokalemia) were seen in less than 10 percent of patients and were generally manageable using conventional approaches.

Previous reports of survival in patients with life-threatening digitalis toxicity who received conventional treatment measures are strongly indicative of therapeutic efficacy of purified digoxin-specific Fab fragments. Thus, despite the absence of a concurrent control group, the outcome with emergency use of Fab fragments in the 150 patients enrolled in the multicenter trial (12.5 percent mortality in patients with digitalis toxicity and a serum potassium > 6.4 mEq per liter) appears to be substantially better than that reported in similarly ill patients with advanced toxicity and hyperkalemia treated conventionally. Furthermore, the mortality rate was 46 percent in those patients in whom a cardiac arrest occurred as a consequence of digitalis toxicity; this result includes several patients treated only after relatively prolonged cardiopulmonary resuscitative efforts and compares favorably with the near 100 percent mortality reported in other series when conventional therapy alone was used.

Clinical Implications

On the basis of the results of the multicenter trial completed in 1986, the United States Food and Drug Administration approved the marketing of purified ovine digoxin-specific Fab fragments (Digibind, Burroughs Wellcome Co.) as an orphan drug for treatment of potentially life-threatening digitalis toxicity. A post-marketing surveillance study will provide additional data on more than 700 patients treated (for the most part in community hospitals) with Digibind. Preliminary review of data from post-marketing clinical experience supports the observations in the 150-patient multicenter trial discussed previously. The rate of allergic reactions has remained low (< 1 percent, clustered mainly in patients with an atopic history), and the rapid time course of resolution of toxicity over 1 to 4 hours after digoxin-specific Fab fragment treatment instead of several days substantially facilitated patient care.

Future clinical applications under consideration include expansion of the indications of digoxin-specific Fab fragment treatment to less overtly life-threatening cases, production of even smaller immunoglobulin fragments with reduced immunogenicity in humans, possible diagnostic as well as therapeutic use, and extension of this immunotherapeutic approach to antibody reversal of toxicity from other drugs or endogenous substances.

SUGGESTED READING

Antman EM, Wenger TL, Butler VP, et al. Treatment of 150 cases of life-threatening digitalis intoxication with digoxin-specific Fab antibody fragments: final report of a multicenter study. Circulation 1990; 81:1744.

Smith TW, Antman EM, Friedman PL, et al. Digitalis glycosides: mechanisms and manifestations of toxicity (part I). Prog Cardiovasc Dis 1984; 26:413.

Smith TW, Antman EM, Friedman PL, et al. Digitalis glycosides: mechanisms and manifestations of toxicity (part II). Prog Cardiovasc Dis 1984; 26:495.

Smith TW, Antman EM, Friedman PL, et al. Digitalis glycosides: mechanisms and manifestations of toxicity (part III). Prog Cardiovasc Dis 1984; 27:21.

ANGINA PECTORIS: STABLE

MICHAEL A. KUTCHER, M.D., F.A.C.C.

Stable angina pectoris may be defined as a chest pain syndrome, usually precipitated by exertion, the pattern of which is essentially unchanged for 60 days or more.

Obstructive coronary atherosclerotic heart disease is the etiology in the great majority of patients with stable angina. The pathophysiologic mechanism is based on a directly proportionate relationship between an increase in myocardial oxygen demand and the development of myocardial ischemia. Significant fixed obstructive coronary lesions provide the anatomic basis, in that the mechanical impediment to coronary blood flow prevents adequate delivery of oxygen to the myocardium at predictable levels of exertion.

THERAPEUTIC ALTERNATIVES

Symptoms, signs, physiologic data, and anatomic data should be used to identify coronary atherosclerotic heart disease. Once the extent of disease has been quantitated, the three major goals to which therapy for stable angina must be directed are

- Relief of angina
- Prevention of myocardial infarction
- Promotion of longevity

The three major therapeutic "weapons" available are

- Medical therapy
- Coronary angioplasty
- Coronary bypass surgery

Each therapeutic option must address the supply and demand problem of stable angina. Ideally, the best therapy for each individual patient is that which can most effectively achieve the three goals with the minimum of risk.

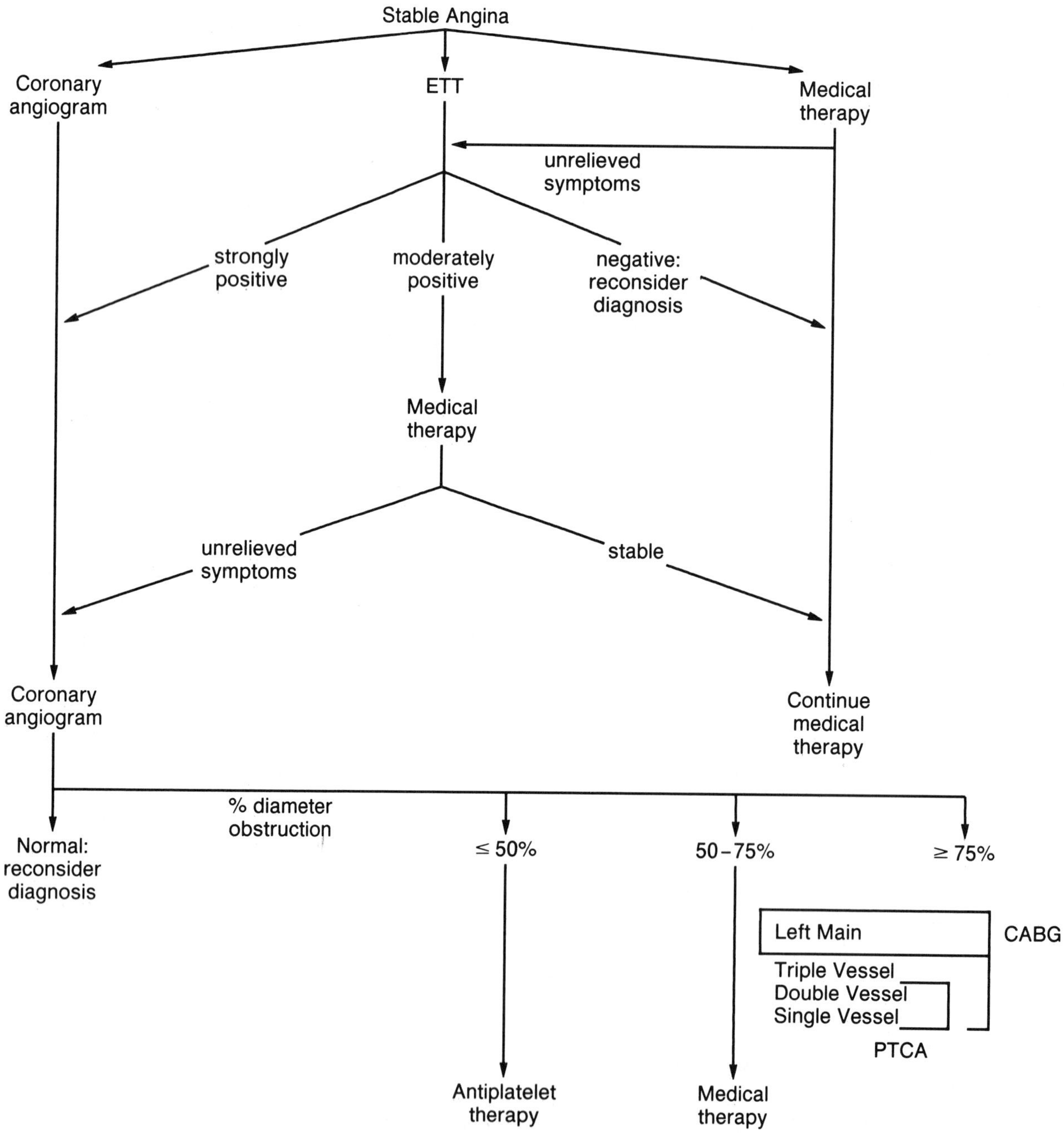

Figure 1 Schema for stable angina pectoris. CABG = Coronary artery bypass graft, ETT = exercise tolerance test, PTCA = percutaneous transluminal coronary angioplasty.

PREFERRED APPROACH

Figure 1 is a flow diagram representing a diagnostic strategy to select therapy for patients with stable angina pectoris.

Medical Treatment

Most patients with stable angina should be managed at least initially with medical therapy directed toward reducing myocardial oxygen demand and improving coronary blood flow. Long-term medical therapy is acceptable in patients with a low Canadian Classification angina score, good exercise tolerance test, and moderately obstructive coronaries in the range of 50 to 75 percent diameter reduction. The more elderly the patient, the more acceptable a medical regimen may be for the goal of promoting longevity with the disease stabilized. Patients who have poor vessels for revascularization or prohibitive left ventricular function may have no alternative but medication.

The three major antianginal pharmacologic groups are listed in Table 1. Individual agents, dosage, routes, and frequency of administration are provided.

Nitrates

Long-acting nitrates in oral, sublingual, or patch form represent the first line of therapy in stable angina. They primarily work by dilating coronary arteries and thus improving blood flow. A moderate preload reduction and a minor afterload reduction effect may also be beneficial by reducing demands made on the myocardium.

In view of the controversy regarding nitrate tolerance, it may be better to prescribe a long-acting oral or sublingual preparation and skip the nighttime dose. On the other hand, most patients find the patches more convenient. If patches are prescribed, removal at nighttime and reinstitution of a new patch in the morning would be an appropriate approach.

Nitrates may cause flushing, headache, dizziness, hypotension, and tinnitus. A lower dose may be better tolerated but less effective.

Short-acting sublingual nitroglycerin may be used to dissipate or to forestall periodic anginal attacks. The patient should be cautioned to sit or recline after administration of a dose (usually 0.4 mg sublingually) to obviate the potential hypotensive and orthostatic effects. If a protracted episode of angina lasts longer than 45 minutes and is unrelieved by three nitroglycerin tablets, the patient should be instructed to report to the nearest emergency room for evaluation.

Quantification of the amount and frequency of nitroglycerin administration by the patient may be used as a barometer to indicate effectiveness of the therapeutic plan or to alert the physician that additions to the pharmacologic regimen may be necessary.

Beta-blockers

Beta-blockers work by blocking the beta-adrenergic pathway. This results in a reduction of heart rate, myocardial contractility, and blood pressure—all favorable maneuvers to decrease myocardial oxygen demand.

In patients with stable angina and relatively good left ventricular function, the combination of beta-blocker with nitrates is a logical step. Beta-blockers are a particularly good choice in patients who also have hypertension, tachycardia, ventricular arrhythmias, or a combination of these disorders. In individuals who have had a previous history of myo-

TABLE 1 Antianginal Pharmacologic Groups

Generic Name	*Total Daily Dose (mg)*	*Route*	*Dosing Frequency*
Long-acting nitrates			
Isosorbide dinitrate	40–240	SL or PO	qid
Pentaerythritol tetranitrate	40–160	SL or PO	qid
Nitroglycerin patch	5–20	Topically	qd
Beta-blockers			
Propranolol	40–360	PO	tid/qid
Metoprolol	50–200	PO	bid
Timolol	10–60	PO	bid
Atenolol	25–100	PO	qd
Nadolol	40–240	PO	qd
Calcium channel blockers			
Nifedipine	30–120	PO	tid/qid
Diltiazem	90–360	PO	tid/qid
Verapamil	120–480	PO	tid/qid

SL = Sublingually, PO = orally, qid = four times per day, qd = every day, tid = three times per day, bid = twice a day.

cardial infarction but who now have stable angina, beta-blockers are the treatment of choice in view of the impressive mortality and morbidity results in several randomized post-infarction trials.

Congestive heart failure, hypotension, bradycardia, and asthma are contraindications to beta-blocker therapy. Side effects of therapy may include worsening of heart failure, hypotension, bradycardia, advanced atrioventricular block, impotency, insomnia, nightmares, and excessive tiredness. Beta-blocker therapy may also mask the hypoglycemic response of insulin-dependent diabetes. These side effects may be less likely with the more cardioselective agents such as metoprolol or atenolol.

It is a better strategy to start with a basic beta-blocker in divided doses, titrate the effect, and then observe the long-term anginal response before trying the patient on a single or reduced frequency beta-blocker agent.

Calcium Channel Blockers

This biochemically disparate group of agents acts by interfering with the calcium channel kinetics of smooth muscle and specialized cells. In stable angina, they work by dilating coronary arteries and preventing spasm, thus improving coronary blood flow. To different degrees, the individual calcium channel blockers may also reduce blood pressure, afterload, and contractility to relieve myocardial oxygen demand.

Nifedipine is the best direct coronary and vasodilating agent of the group. It may also have benefit as an afterload reducing agent in patients with impaired left ventricular function, but used alone it may cause a reflex tachycardia and a paradoxical increase in angina. If possible, it could be combined with a beta-blocker to counteract these side effects.

Diltiazem has a good multidimensional capacity to vasodilate, reduce heart rate, and to some extent reduce contractility. It is the best "stand alone" calcium channel blocker agent. If necessary, it may be combined with a beta-blocker, but this should be done with caution in view of the potential cumulative effects on the heart rate and atrioventricular node.

Verapamil has the least vasodilatory action and the greatest effects on the atrioventricular node. It is an appropriate agent in stable angina patients who have atrial tachyarrhythmias as a component of their presentation. Patients with congestive heart failure and borderline left ventricular function may be worsened by the reduced contractility effects of verapamil. Verapamil should be used with extreme caution, or not at all, with beta-blockers owing to potential profound conduction disturbances.

Side effects of calcium channel blockers in general include flushing, pedal edema, dizziness, hypotension, increased atrioventricular block, nausea, and vomiting. Pedal edema and flushing are particular problems with nifedipine as this reflects its strong vasodilatory action.

As with beta-blockers, it is better to use a basic calcium channel blocker agent in divided doses, titrate therapy, and observe response before committing the patient to the newer long-acting calcium channel blocker preparations.

Antiplatelet Therapy

In view of recent studies documenting improved mortality and morbidity in patients with unstable angina or myocardial infarction treated with aspirin, it is appropriate to consider long-term aspirin therapy as a prophylactic strategy in patients with stable angina. If no contraindications exist, a dose of 80 mg every day or 325 mg every day or every other day may be used. Therapy should be discontinued if gastrointestinal intolerance, bleeding, or other side effects occur.

Coronary Angioplasty

In patients with stable angina, coronary angioplasty should be considered in those who are significantly symptomatic in spite of optimal therapy, who continue to have a strongly positive exercise test or limited functional status, and who have lesions amenable to balloon dilation.

Mildly symptomatic patients who have critical stenoses (>90 percent diameter reduction) in a very proximal major artery or arteries, with a great deal of myocardium at jeopardy, should be considered for coronary angioplasty. However, the goals of preventing myocardial infarction and promoting longevity have not been substantiated as yet by large-scale randomized trials comparing this approach with either medical therapy or coronary bypass surgery.

Although coronary angioplasty has a high primary success rate (90 to 95 percent) and a low morbidity (2 to 3 percent myocardial infarction or emergency bypass surgery, less than 1 percent mortality), it must be weighed against the high restenosis rate (25 to 35 percent).

Several hours prior to coronary angioplasty, patients should receive aspirin (650 mg) to prevent acute platelet activation. Long-acting nitrates and a calcium channel blocker (diltiazem if the patient has had no previous therapy, or nifedipine if the patient is already on a beta-blocker) should be started prior to and continued for at least 1 month after angioplasty to obviate the problem of reactive coronary artery spasm. Recent studies have indicated that an antiplatelet regimen after angioplasty does not reduce the long-term restenosis rate. However, if there are no contraindications, aspirin (325 mg every day) is reasonable to continue for 6 months after angioplasty, especially if the patient has had a previous myocardial infarction or an unstable anginal pattern in the past. In these cases, indefinite use may be warranted. Controversy exists over the benefits of dipyridamole.

Successful coronary angioplasty should be followed up with an exercise tolerance test within a week after the procedure. This will serve as a baseline if questions of restenosis arise in the future. A negative exercise test 6 months after angioplasty may be an indirect prognostic sign that long-term patency of the dilated vessel has persisted. Thereafter, yearly evaluation and exercise testing are appropriate to rule out progression of disease elsewhere or late restenosis.

Coronary Bypass Surgery

Both randomized and observational trials have documented the effectiveness of coronary bypass surgery over medical therapy in either completely alleviating or at least significantly relieving the frequency and severity of angina. Assuming acceptable coronary anatomy and reasonable left ventricular function, coronary bypass surgery is an appropriate alternative if a stable anginal pattern does not respond to medical therapy or if it interferes with a patient's life-style and expectations. However, in patients with mild anginal symptoms and single, double, or triple vessel disease with good left ventricular function, randomized trials have not shown a benefit of improved mortality rates with surgery over medicine.

Randomized trials have shown definite advantage of coronary bypass surgery over medical therapy in reducing mortality in mildly symptomatic patients with significant left main or with significant triple vessel disease and reduced left ventricular function.

The risks of coronary bypass surgery must be weighed against the expected benefits and the three major goals of therapy. Complications of surgery include mortality, 1 percent; myocardial infarction, 4 percent; reoperation for postoperative bleeding, 2 percent; infection, 1 percent; cerebrovascular accident, 1 percent; and postoperative arrhythmia, 10 percent. The one-year patency rate of internal mammary grafts is 90 percent, that of saphenous vein grafts is 75 percent. Internal mammary grafts have a 10-year patency rate of 85 percent compared with a 50 percent patency rate with saphenous vein grafts.

Preoperative and postoperative care of patients undergoing coronary bypass graft surgery are discussed in other chapters of this textbook.

Risk Factor Reduction

A strong attempt at risk factor reduction is imperative to ensure success of the overall therapeutic plan. Patients should be encouraged to stop smoking, maintain reasonable body weight, control blood pressure, and achieve acceptable blood lipid levels. An individualized exercise program is an essential component of any long-range patient strategy. A strong physician-patient relationship and mutual awareness of risk factor control are just as important as the vast pharmacopeia and high-technology to treat individuals with stable angina pectoris effectively.

SUGGESTED READING

Abrams J. Nitroglycerin and long-acting nitrates in clinical practice. Am J Med 1983; 74:85.

CASS principal investigators and their associates. Coronary artery surgery study: a randomized trial of coronary artery bypass surgery; survival data. Circulation 1983; 68:939.

DeMots H, Glasser SP. Intermittent transdermal nitroglycerin therapy in the treatment of chronic stable angina. J Am Coll Cardiol 1989; 13:786.

Mabin TA, Holmes DR, Smith HC, et al. Follow-up clinical results in patients undergoing percutaneous transluminal coronary angioplasty. Circulation 1985; 71:754.

Petru MA, Crawford MH, Sorensen SG, et al. Short- and long-term efficacy of high-dose diltiazem for angina due to coronary artery disease: a placebo-controlled, randomized, double-blind crossover study. Circulation 1983; 68:139.

Sherman LG, Liang C. Nifedipine in chronic stable angina: a double-blind placebo-controlled crossover trial. Am J Cardiol 1983; 51:706.

Thadani U, Davidson C, Chir B, et al. Comparison of the immediate effects of five beta-adrenoreceptor-blocking drugs with different ancillary properties in angina pectoris. N Engl J Med 1979; 300:750.

ANGINA PECTORIS: UNSTABLE

CRAIG M. PRATT, M.D.
ROBERT ROBERTS, M.D.

Unstable angina has been defined in a variety of ways and encompasses a wide spectrum of patients with coronary artery disease. The unstable angina syndrome describes the clinical features of patients presenting with a symptom complex intermediate to that of chronic stable angina and acute myocardial infarction. But the distinction is more than semantic because patients presenting with unstable angina have a severalfold higher incidence of myocardial infarction and death than patients with chronic stable angina. A reasonable estimate of the 1-year mortality of patients presenting with unstable angina is 5 percent, and a larger number will develop an acute myocardial infarction within weeks after the clinical presentation. The syndrome of unstable angina, therefore, represents a state of increasing myocardial ischemia. The various presentations in Table 1 have common temporal and prognostic elements and represent high-risk patients who should be targets for intensive diagnostic evaluation and aggressive medical management.

In the purest sense, unstable angina occurs in the absence of recent myocardial infarction and without the presence of other noncardiac conditions that might precipitate or heighten myocardial ischemia. Post-infarction angina is presented as a separate category because of differences in pathophysiology and treatment. Unstable angina includes patients presenting with new onset of severe and prolonged episodes of angina or patients with previous stable exertional angina pectoris who developed more prolonged, intense chest pains at lower levels of activity. Patients may also present with either new onset or heightened episodes of chest pain that occur at rest or that wake the patient out of sleep (nocturnal angina). In general, the clinical situation is more urgent if the patient has documented transient ischemia as evidenced by electrocardiographic (ECG) changes (transient ST-segment shifts or T-wave changes) during the anginal episode, which normalize after the cessation of pain. Likewise, the clinical situation is more severe if the patient develops unstable angina while already taking conventional doses of pharmacologic agents for ischemia.

TABLE 1 Clinical Presentations of Unstable Angina Syndrome

New onset of angina pectoris*
As first manifestation of coronary artery disease
Worsened prognosis with:
Rest angina/nocturnal angina
With evidence of reversible electrocardiographic changes (T-wave and ST-segment changes)
Recent exacerbation of frequency, duration, or severity of angina pectoris*
Less responsive to sublingual nitroglycerin/anti-ischemic therapy
New rest or nocturnal angina
With evidence of reversible electrocardiographic changes
Angina within days/weeks of acute myocardial infarction*
With evidence of reversible electrocardiographic changes

*May be exacerbated by noncardiac disorders (see text).

A reasonable question to ask is how do these clinical presentations differ from acute myocardial infarction? In fact, there is considerable overlap, such that the working diagnosis of unstable angina rests on the premise that the diagnosis of acute myocardial infarction has been ruled out by obtaining serial ECGs and serial CK-MB enzymatic assays. In addition, these definitions assume that the chest pain is due to structural or functional abnormalities in the coronary arteries, either from fixed atherosclerotic coronary stenosis or altered vasomotor tone or coronary thrombus. However, even with a careful clinical history, at least 10 percent of patients who present with "unstable angina" will turn out to have angiographically normal coronary arteries, most of which will not have demonstrable coronary spasm during provocative ergonovine testing. Also, some of the patients presenting initially with unstable angina will develop an acute non-Q-wave myocardial infarction within the first 24 to 48 hours of observation. The overlap of patients with normal coronary arteries and patients developing non-Q-wave infarction is inevitable because of the heterogeneity of the clinical presentations characterizing the unstable angina syndrome.

ETIOLOGY AND PATHOGENESIS OF UNSTABLE ANGINA

Unstable angina occurs in the clinical setting of significant atherosclerotic coronary artery disease. In most cases, the coronary stenosis involves 50 percent or greater stenosis of the intraluminal diameter of the involved coronary artery. At times, in patients with multivessel disease it is unclear as to which coronary artery represents the "culprit lesion." Pathophysiologic mechanisms implicated in the unstable angina syndrome include rapid progression of fixed coronary atherosclerosis, the contribution of increased vasomotor tone in the area of a fixed coronary stenosis, and subtotal or partially occlusive thrombus in the area of a fixed coronary stenosis. Intracoronary thrombus has been documented to play a role in certain patients with unstable angina, although the observed frequency of reported thrombus has been highly variable, ranging from 30 to 50 percent of patients. Coronary angioscopy has revealed that intraluminal coronary lesions frequently have a pattern described as eccentric and irregular with fissured plaques, often containing visible thrombus. The activation of platelets and of the clotting system is also likely to be of importance in the pathogenesis of unstable angina. Coronary spasm in the presence of angiographically normal coronary arteries is often accompanied by transient ST-segment elevation and is covered as part of the variant angina or Prinzmetal's angina syndrome. Given the variety of contributing factors believed involved in the pathogenesis of unstable angina, it should not be surprising that the therapeutic approaches are myriad.

THERAPEUTIC ALTERNATIVES

Patients fitting the aforementioned clinical descriptions should be hospitalized in a coronary care unit for monitoring and definitive therapy. The wide variety of therapeutic alternatives reflects the large number of potentially contributory pathophysiologic mechanisms involved in unstable angina. Therapeutic options include antiplatelet therapy, especially aspirin; intravenous heparin; elimination of myocardial ischemia with nitrates, calcium channel blockers, and beta-blockers; the use of intravenous thrombolytic agents such as tissue plasminogen activator (rt-PA) and streptokinase; and, in some instances, the necessity for coronary artery angioplasty, coronary artery bypass surgery, or both. A presentation of our preferred approach is followed by a discussion of each of the medical and invasive alternatives in the treatment of unstable angina.

PREFERRED APPROACH

Unstable angina should be considered a medical emergency, and the patient should be put in a monitored bed in a coronary care unit as expeditiously as possible. A number of general issues should be addressed immediately. First, the patient should be in a calm environment and, if necessary, sedated. The therapeutic goal is to render the patient free of chest pain with pharmacologic therapy as soon as possible. A rapid screen for noncardiac contributions to myocardial ischemia should be made. This should include a search for anemia, thyrotoxicosis, hypotension or dehydration, tachyarrhythmias, hypoxemia, fever, and infection. Appropriate tests should be performed to confirm the presence or absence of these contributing factors and, if found, corrected. Even if an ECG were obtained in the emergency room, a repeat 12-lead ECG should be obtained immediately. This will expeditiously identify a few patients whose ECG will evolve rapidly, revealing ST-segment elevation signifying acute myocardial infarction. These patients merit immediate consideration of thrombolytic therapy if no contraindications exist. Serial CK-MB enzymes should be obtained every 4 to 6 hours for 24 hours.

Medical therapy should begin immediately. First and most important is the administration of oral aspirin, one 325-mg tablet. Aspirin should be continued daily on an indefinite basis. Although the aspirin may seem a trivial part of this regimen, it is the mainstay of therapy for unstable angina, as demonstrated in large American and Canadian trials in which aspirin reduced the incidence of myocardial infarction and mortality by 50 percent. Administration of intravenous heparin is a reasonable alternative and, in comparative trials, is nearly as effective as aspirin but not more effective, nor is the combination more effective. Therefore, we prefer aspirin alone. It is easier to administer, has less potential side effects, and will be one of the medications that the patient will be discharged on regardless of the initial therapy.

In addition, pharmacologic therapy should be initiated immediately and aimed to render the patient free of angina and eliminate objective evidence of myocardial ischemia. A combination of nitrates, calcium channel blockers, and beta-blockers may be necessary and administered as described subsequently. Because a majority of these patients have a critical stenosis in at least one of the major coronary arteries, the goal should be a "cooling off" phase in which the patient is rendered free of angina for 24 to 48 hours, after which coronary angiography should be performed. It is our belief that coronary angiography is mandatory; however, ideally the timing should be on an elective basis before hospital discharge. In some cases, the patient cannot be rendered free of angina or ischemia, mandating immediate cardiac catheterization and coronary angiography, with the alternatives of angioplasty and bypass surgery ultimately considered. We consider the role of intravenous thrombolytic therapy such as rt-PA and streptokinase to be applicable only in selected patients rather than "routine" at this time and describe their roles later.

Medical Therapy of Unstable Angina and Post-Infarction Angina

The therapeutic goal of medical therapy is to alleviate all episodes of clinical angina pectoris as well as to eliminate objective evidence of myocardial ischemia as rapidly as possible. Therefore, intravenous therapy is frequently chosen initially. Intravenous nitroglycerin is a mainstay of therapy for patients with unstable angina. As an initial therapy, we recommend intravenous nitroglycerin to be administered in doses ranging from 10 to 200 μg per minute, with the endpoint being the elimination of all episodes of chest pain. In general, the dose should be sufficient to lower the observed intra-arterial pressure by 10 or 15 mm Hg, with care not to lower the systolic blood pressure below 100 to 110 mm Hg. Obviously, there is more

TABLE 2 Intravenous Pharmacologic Therapy for Unstable Angina

Drug	*Dose*	*Monitoring*	*Contraindications*
Nitroglycerin*	10–200 μg/min IV	Dose sufficient to lower arterial pressure 10–15 mm Hg, not <100 mm Hg systolic	Hypotension
Beta-Blockers*			
Metoprolol†	5 mg IV every 5 min for 3 doses, reevaluating patient after each dose	Dose not to exceed 10 mm Hg. Fall in systolic BP or <100 mm Hg or heart rate <55	Hypotension, bradycardia, heart block, congestive heart failure, asthma
Propranolol†	0.025–0.05 mg/kg IV over 15–30 min reevaluating patient after each dose	Dose not to exceed 10 mm Hg. Fall in systolic BP or <100 mm Hg or heart rate <55	Hypotension, bradycardia, heart block, congestive heart failure, asthma

*Must be individually tailored with frequent and careful clinical evaluation (see text).
† Dosing interval will vary with individual patients. Transition to oral therapy recommended in first 6 to 12 h.

flexibility in patients who are hypertensive. Also, attention must be given to the heart rate during intravenous nitroglycerin therapy because patients with low filling pressures may develop a tachycardia that would increase myocardial oxygen consumption. A summary of the dose and administration information for intravenous nitroglycerin as well as for intravenous beta-blockers is included in Table 2.

Intravenous beta-blockers may make an important contribution to the therapy of individual patients with unstable angina, especially in patients presenting with hypertension and tachycardia. In such patients, the initial therapy with beta-blockers should be either intravenous metoprolol or intravenous propranolol (see Table 2), with the goal of transition to oral beta-blockers within 12 hours. However, in most patients with unstable angina, we initially use an oral beta-blocker because we do not believe that there are clear-cut demonstrated advantages of administering intravenous beta-blockers in most patients. The use of intravenous beta-blockers is more complicated than intravenous nitroglycerin, requiring close attention to contraindications (Table 2) and careful administration. The resting heart rate represents a reliable index to follow, and repeat examination for signs of congestive heart failure is mandatory.

After the patient has been stabilized and rendered free of chest pain for 12 to 24 hours, transition to oral therapy is recommended. The dose ranges of oral beta-blockers, calcium channel blockers, and long-acting nitrates are presented in Table 3. We believe that calcium channel blockers play a useful role in the oral therapy of the unstable angina syndrome as a result of the important pathophysiologic contribution of increased vasomotor tone. The disadvantage of oral nitrates is that there must be a nitrate-free interval during long-term therapy to avoid the development of nitrate tolerance. The implications of using oral nitrates with a nitrate-free dosing interval in a clinical syndrome that is unstable are unknown. Frequently, intravenous nitroglycerin is maintained for 1 to 3 days until coronary angiography is performed for decisions regarding definitive therapy.

With regard to the calcium channel blockers, nifedipine (or nicardipine) may not be preferable because the dihydropyridine calcium blockers increase heart rate as a result of their vasodilatory effects. A number of clinical trials using nifedipine in patients with unstable angina have failed to demonstrate a

TABLE 3 Oral Pharmacologic Therapy for Unstable Angina

Pharmacologic Class	*Generic/ Brand Name(s)*	*Total Daily Dose (mg)*	*Dosing Frequency*
Selected beta-blockers	Propranolol (Inderal)	120–360	tid/qid
	Metoprolol (Lopressor)	100–200	bid
	Timolol (Blocadren)	20–60	bid
	Atenolol (Tenormin)	50–100	qd
	Nadolol (Corgard)	40–240	qd
Selected calcium blockers	Nifedipine (Procardia)	30–120	tid/qid
	Diltiazem (Cardizem)	90–360	tid/qid
	Verapamil (Isoptin, Calan)	240–480	tid/qid
Selected long-acting nitrates*	Isosorbide dinitrate (Isordil, Sorbitrate)	40–240	q 4–6 h*
	Nitroglycerin (Nitro-bid)	10–50	q 4–6 h*
	Pentaerythritol tetranitrate (Peritrate)	40–160	q 4–6 h*

*With long-term use, tolerance may develop without a nitrate-free interval (see text).
tid = Three times per day, qid = four times per day, bid = twice a day, qd = every day.

therapeutic benefit. If nifedipine is the selected calcium channel blocker, it should be used in combination with a beta-blocker. Nifedipine, verapamil, and diltiazem should be used with caution in patients with left ventricular dysfunction. Verapamil should not be used with beta-blockers. Diltiazem is effective alone or in combination with beta-blockers and is well tolerated and does not result in a reflex tachycardia. Diltiazem is our preferred calcium channel blocker for use in the treatment of the unstable angina syndrome.

Oral beta-blocker therapy should be considered, especially in patients with hypertension, tachycardia, and preserved left ventricular function. The doses of selected oral beta-blockers are presented in Table 3. The heart rate at rest, during normal activity, and with peak exercise all serve as good clinical indices of adequate beta-blockade. We believe that the shorter acting nonselective beta-blockers are preferable in this clinical situation.

Other Pharmacologic Approaches to Unstable Angina

A number of clinical trials have addressed the issue of the administration of intravenous thrombolytic therapy to patients with unstable angina. The majority of these trials have used intravenous rt-PA and have failed to demonstrate a clinical benefit. As previously mentioned, it appears that the majority of patients presenting with unstable angina do not have objective evidence of a partial or totally occluding thrombus at the time of coronary angiography. Thus, although administration of thrombolytic agents appears a promising approach in this syndrome, we do not recommend it as routine therapy. Thrombolytic agents should be administered to any patient who has objective evidence of coronary thrombus at the time of coronary angiography. It may be that the failure to show a clinical benefit of thrombolytic agents is due to the small number of patients in clinical trials reported. A definitive trial of more than 1,500 patients with unstable angina will be completed in 1991.

Although presented separately, *post-infarction angina* occurring in the initial days or weeks following acute myocardial infarction has prognostic similarities to other types of unstable angina. Post-infarction angina is more common in patients incurring a non-Q-wave infarction than in those with a Q-wave infarction; likewise the incidence of recurrent infarction is at least fourfold higher in non-Q-wave infarction. In these patients, it is important to obtain a 12-lead ECG during chest pain. It has been demonstrated that the combination of post-infarction angina and transient ECG changes identifies high-risk patients in whom aggressive therapy and coronary angiography are mandatory. In the largest trial reported studying non-Q-wave infarcts, prophylactic diltiazem was effective in reducing both the incidence of post-infarction angina and the incidence of recurrent acute myocardial infarction by approximately 50 percent. We believe that effectiveness of diltiazem in this clinical setting is consistent with the hypothesis that patients with non-Q-wave infarction have a larger component of increased vasomotor tone than do those with Q-wave infarcts, in whom thrombosis is the primary pathophysiologic mechanism.

The management of post-infarction angina is quite similar to other unstable angina syndromes. However, we routinely recommend oral diltiazem because it has documented effectiveness in this clinical situation. Also, coronary angiography is recommended in all cases when transient ECG changes are documented during the anginal episode or objective ischemia is documented during predischarge exercise testing or thallium imaging.

Coronary Angioplasty

We believe that all patients who present with the unstable angina syndrome should have coronary angiography performed prior to hospital discharge. This is because of the relatively high incidence of myocardial infarction and death within the first few weeks after this clinical presentation. Thus, coronary angiography is performed to identify those patients with left main coronary artery disease or multivessel disease prior to hospital discharge. Continued chest pain, especially with ECG changes despite aggressive medical therapy, is an indication for immediate coronary angiography.

A number of high-risk subgroups may be considered candidates for coronary artery angioplasty (Table 4). One such subgroup is patients not responding to aggressive medical therapy who have coronary angiographic evidence of a single critical coronary stenosis appropriate to an approach with angioplasty

TABLE 4 Indications for Angioplasty/Bypass Surgery for Unstable Angina

Continued angina despite aggressive medical therapy (emergency)
Angioplasty considered for a single critical coronary stenosis meeting generally accepted anatomic criteria. Consideration of multivessel angioplasty instead of coronary artery bypass surgery in this clinical setting made on an individual case basis*
Coronary artery bypass surgery for single vessel coronary stenoses not amenable to angioplasty and multivessel disease, left main coronary artery disease, or its equivalent
Patients responding to initial pharmacologic management (elective)
Angioplasty considered for single critical coronary stenoses, especially for proximal left anterior descending lesions and proximal dominant right lesions†
Coronary artery bypass surgery considered for multivessel disease, especially with some left ventricular dysfunction; triple vessel disease or left main coronary stenosis†

*See text for discussion.
†Decision usually based on demonstration of objective evidence of ischemia rather than anatomy alone.

as judged by accepted anatomic criteria. In addition to unstable patients, certain patients who are rendered asymptomatic by aggressive medical therapy may also be considered as candidates for elective coronary angioplasty prior to hospital discharge. We should emphasize that there are no well-controlled clinical trials establishing the superiority of angioplasty over conventional anti-ischemic therapy in such patients, but the following patients should be considered: patients with critical lesions in the proximal left anterior descending artery, which are considered anatomically appropriate for coronary angioplasty. Although we would recommend angioplasty in most cases involving the proximal left anterior descending coronary artery, single vessel stenoses of either the right coronary artery or the circumflex coronary artery represent more difficult and nebulous decisions. In these cases, we rely heavily on an assessment of the extent of myocardial ischemia by SPECT thallium, during treadmill exercise or with intravenous adenosine administration. Asymptomatic patients with large perfusion defects, despite optimal medical therapy, are reasonable candidates for coronary angioplasty. The choice of angioplasty for patients with unstable angina and multivessel critical stenoses is more controversial. Although we do not believe that angioplasty should be considered routinely, it may be considered in individual institutions that have the appropriate skill and experience.

Coronary Bypass Surgery

In general, we select patients with unstable angina for coronary artery bypass surgery who are in one of the following categories. First, there are patients who do not respond to aggressive medical management and who continue to have significant angina, especially with transient ECG changes. In such cases, we recommend bypass surgery for patients with multivessel coronary artery disease, especially if they have some degree of left ventricular dysfunction (Table 4). In cases in which ischemia is pharmacologically controlled, coronary artery bypass surgery should be limited primarily to patients with left ventricular dysfunction and multivessel disease and patients with left main coronary artery stenosis. In selected cases, patients with single or multiple critical stenoses who have normal left ventricular function are selected for bypass surgery, especially if the lesions are in such a location or severity that angioplasty cannot be considered. As is the case with decisions regarding angioplasty, objective assessment of the extent of myocardial ischemia with quantitative SPECT thallium imaging is useful in patient selection.

SUGGESTED READING

Ambrose JA, Alexopoulos D. Thrombolysis in unstable angina: Will the beneficial effects of thrombolytic therapy in myocardial infarction apply to patients with unstable angina? J Am Coll Cardiol 1989; 13:1666.

Braunwald E. Unstable angina. Circulation 1989; 80:410.

Cairns JA, Gent M, Singer J, et al. Aspirin, sulfinpyrazone, or both in unstable angina: Results of a Canadian multicenter trial. N Engl J Med 1985; 313:1369.

Lewis HD, Davis JW, Archibald DG, et al. Protective effects of aspirin against acute myocardial infarction and death in men with unstable angina. N Engl J Med 1983; 309:396.

Theroux P, Quimet H, McCan J, et al. Aspirin, heparin or both to treat acute unstable angina. N Engl J Med 1988; 319:1105.

Yusuf S, Wittes J, Friedman L. Overview of results of randomized clinical trials in heart disease. II. Unstable angina, heart failure, primary prevention with aspirin and risk factor modification. JAMA 1988; 260:2259.

EARLY MYOCARDIAL INFARCTION: THROMBOLYTIC THERAPY

ALAN D. GUERCI, M.D.

The administration of thrombolytic therapy early in the course of transmural myocardial infarction may preserve left ventricular function and reduce mortality. These benefits are particularly striking among patients with anterior infarctions and among those treated very early, in which cases mortality risk may be reduced by as much as 50 percent. At the same time, thrombolytic therapy causes intracranial hemorrhage in as many as 0.5 percent of patients without any recognized risk of bleeding. Although the risk of intracranial hemorrhage is offset by a corresponding reduction of the incidence of embolic stroke in patients with large myocardial infarctions, the risk of intracranial hemorrhage is not balanced by a reduction in embolic stroke in patients with smaller infarctions. These observations necessitate the timely and careful administration of thrombolytic therapy. This chapter reviews patient selection criteria, adjunctive therapy, and selection of a thrombolytic agent.

PREFERRED APPROACH

Patient Selection

Inferior Myocardial Infarction

GISSI (Gruppo Italiano per lo Studio della Streptochinasi nell' Infarto Miocardico [GISSI], 1986) and ISIS-2 (ISIS-2 [Second International Study of Infarct Survival], 1988), the two largest placebo-controlled trials of thrombolytic therapy, reported a mortality rate of 8 percent for patients with inferior infarction not receiving thrombolytic agents and 7 percent for patients treated with streptokinase. Although this difference is not statistically significant ($P = 0.09$), it would be premature to conclude that thrombolytic therapy cannot reduce morbidity and mortality in patients with inferior infarction. GISSI and ISIS-2 reported mortality rates according to time to treatment and infarct location but not both. Thus, the aforementioned figures include large numbers of patients treated at 6 to 24 hours, in which case benefit was probably marginal. In addition, the benefit of thrombolytic therapy is related more closely to the size of an ischemic region than to its location. Thus, in GISSI and ISIS-2 the beneficial effect of streptokinase was almost certainly diluted by the inclusion of large numbers of patients with small inferior infarcts and patients presenting more than 6 hours after the onset of symptoms.

It is likely that thrombolytic therapy will improve ventricular function and reduce mortality among patients with large ischemic regions in patients treated very early. Efforts should be made to identify and treat such patients as rapidly as possible (Table 1). This would include patients with inferior infarction and hemodynamic compromise unresponsive to atropine because such patients are usually in the throes of larger rather than smaller infarctions. Widespread ST-segment deviation, defined as ST-segment elevation in leads V5 and V6 (as well as in the inferior leads), or, alternatively, inferior ST-segment elevation and precordial ST-segment depression is another sign of larger rather than smaller inferior infarction. In general, patients with widespread ST-segment deviation should be treated.

In the absence of specific contraindications, patients with previous anterior infarction should probably also be treated. Even when hemodynamically compensated, such patients usually have fair or even poor left ventricular function. Small amounts of myocardial salvage may substantially improve these patients' functional status and prognosis for survival.

Patients presenting very early in the course of inferior infarction, within 2 to 3 hours, are treated usually because treatment at this early time interval can preserve ventricular function. Finally, even in the absence of the above criteria, young patients with inferior infarction are treated usually with thrombolytic therapy, provided that such therapy can be initiated within 4 hours of the onset of symptoms. The justification for this practice is that most young patients with acute myocardial infarction have one or more risk factors that place them in danger of sustaining a second myocardial infarction over the next 5 to 10 years. It is widely believed that these patients will have a better chance of surviving a second infarction if the inferior wall is hypokinetic rather than akinetic.

Emergency two-dimensional echocardiography may clarify ambiguous situations, particularly when the size of the inferior wall ischemic region is in question. Ischemia severe enough to cause ST-segment elevations usually causes akinesis or even dyskinesis. As a rule, if the quality of a two-dimensional echocardiogram is good, and if an ischemic segment cannot be seen in the inferior wall of the left ventricle, the ischemic segment is probably too small to justify treatment. If echocardiography is employed in patient selection, it should be remembered that most hypotension occurring in the setting of inferior infarction is due to activation of the Bezold-Jarisch reflex or to widespread right ventricular ischemia rather than to ischemia of a large portion of the inferior wall of the left ventricle. Hypotension caused by the Bezold-Jarisch reflex is accompanied usually by bradycardia; both respond to atropine. Hypotension as a result of widespread ischemia of the right ventricle does not respond to atropine and is frequently undetectable in the acute phase by echocardiography. Thus, a patient with acute inferior infarction, hypotension unresponsive to atropine, and well-preserved motion of the inferior wall of the left ventricle is assumed to have massive right ventricular infarction and is considered a good candidate for thrombolytic therapy.

TABLE 1 Inferior Infarction Candidates for Thrombolytic Therapy

Hemodynamic compromise unresponsive to atropine
Widespread ST-segment deviation
Previous anterior myocardial infarction
Very early presentation
Young age

The Elderly

The exclusion of patients over the age of 75 years from American trials of angioplasty following thrombolytic therapy has led to the widespread misconception that elderly patients are not suitable candidates for thrombolytic therapy. This misconception may have tragic consequences because age, along with infarct size, is one of the two most powerful determinants of the mortality risk of myocardial infarction.

There is abundant evidence of reduction in all-cause mortality with thrombolytic therapy in patients up to the age of 75, and there are good reasons to believe that thrombolytic therapy reduces mortality in patients over the age of 75. Highly significant reductions in all-cause mortality were observed in the AIMS trial of acylated plasminogen streptokinase activator complex (APSAC) among patients aged 65 to 70 (AIMS Trial Study Group, 1988) and in the ASSET study of tissue plasminogen activator (tPA) among patients aged 65 to 75 years (Table 2). Although the reduction in mortality among patients over the age of 75 years was not quite significant in GISSI ($P = 0.12$), this failure to achieve significant reduction in mortality may be attributable to inadequate sample size and the inclusion in the GISSI trial of substantial numbers of patients now known not to benefit from thrombolytic therapy (GISSI, 1986). The ISIS-2 results probably bridge this gap. More than 3,400 patients over the age of 70 were entered into ISIS-2, with a reduction in mortality from 22 percent in the control group to 18 percent among patients treated with streptokinase ($P < 0.02$). The ISIS-2 experience includes more than 400 patients aged 80 years or older, in whom there was no increased incidence of bleeding (ISIS-2, 1988).

There is some evidence of increased risk of intracranial hemorrhage with tPA in elderly patients. The most prudent interpretation of these data would admit the possibility of a small increase in the risk of serious hemorrhage among elderly patients treated with thrombolytic agents. In quantitative terms, this risk does not appear to be prohibitive. Therefore, advanced age should probably be regarded as a relative and minor contraindication to thrombolytic therapy. Emphasis should be placed on early treatment of larger rather than smaller infarcts, and the patients should be in good overall health.

TABLE 2 All-Cause Mortality Among Elderly Patients Given Thrombolytic Therapy for Acute Myocardial Infarction

		Mortality (%)		
Drug/Study	*Age*	*Control*	*Treatment*	P *value*
APSAC				
AIMS	65–70	30	12	0.005
tPA				
ASSET	65–75	16	11	0.001
SK				
ISIS-2	>70	22	18	<0.02
GISSI	>75	33	29	0.12

APSAC = acylated plasminogen streptokinase activator complex, tPA = tissue plasminogen activator, SK = streptokinase.

Non-ST-Segment Elevation Infarction

GISSI and ISIS-2 reported no reduction in mortality in patients with ischemic myocardial pain and ST-segment depression who were treated with streptokinase. Insofar as most patients with ST-segment depression infarcts do not have total thrombotic occlusion of the infarct-related artery, this result is not surprising. These data do not support the widespread application of thrombolytic therapy to patients with ST-segment depression infarcts. There are several exceptions to this rule. The first includes patients with known high-grade circumflex disease and normal or relatively normal anterior descending coronary arteries. In such patients, ST-segment depression in the precordial leads could reasonably be attributed to posterior transmural ischemia. A second group deserving of thrombolytic therapy includes patients with widespread ST-segment depression and hemodynamic compromise, in whom thrombolytic therapy would be applied as a temporizing measure until aortic balloon counterpulsation, coronary arteriography, or both could be performed. Acute myocardial infarction characterized clinically and electrocardiographically by hemodynamic compromise and widespread ST-segment depression is usually due to subtotal occlusion of the left main coronary artery, its equivalent, or high-grade proximal left anterior descending coronary artery disease. The very high mortality rate associated with this presentation seems to justify thrombolytic therapy on the grounds that it may help stabilize the patient until more definitive therapy can be provided.

Patients with ischemic myocardial pain and new left bundle-branch block or left bundle-branch block not known to be old should be regarded as having an acute anterior myocardial infarction until proven otherwise. These patients have very high mortality rates, and mortality risk can be reduced with timely thrombolytic therapy. Emergency echocardiography, looking for akinesis of the anterior portion of the interventricular septum and the anterior free wall, may be useful in supporting the diagnosis of acute myocardial infarction in such cases.

Late Treatment

ISIS-2 reported a significant reduction in mortality when patients were treated with streptokinase 6 to 24 hours after the onset of infarction (ISIS-2, 1988), but GISSI reported no reduction in mortality when streptokinase was given 6 to 12 hours after the onset of infarction (GISSI, 1986). Pooling the data from these two studies yields fairly strong but ultimately nonsignificant trends toward reduced mortality with streptokinase (Table 3). It is unknown whether this failure to achieve statistical significance is due to inadequate sample size, insufficient quantities of viable myocardium, or other factors.

TABLE 3 Time to Treatment and Mortality

	Mortality (%)		
Time	*Control*	*SK-treated Patients*	P *value*
6–12 hours	12.9	11.5	0.12
12–24 hours	10.8	8.7	0.08

SK = Streptokinase.

Information from other sources may help to resolve the dilemma of late treatment. In experimental myocardial infarction, late reperfusion, i.e., reperfusion too late to salvage ischemic myocardium, has consistently accelerated scar formation and reduced aneurysm formation. Because aneurysm formation is strongly associated with congestive heart failure and sudden cardiac death, late reperfusion might prevent these unfavorable outcomes.

There is some indirect evidence in humans that this may actually be the case. In the Western Washington trial of intracoronary streptokinase, reperfusion at a mean of 5.8 hours after the onset of symptoms had no effect on ejection fraction but reduced the 30-day mortality rate from 11 percent to 4 percent ($P = 0.02$). The results of long-term follow-up were also consistent with the hypothesis that late reperfusion exerts beneficial effects, not by salvage of ischemic myocardium but by acceleration of scar formation. When patients with anterior myocardial infarction treated with intracoronary streptokinase were classified according to whether the treatment succeeded in opening the infarct-related artery or failed to open the infarct-related artery, a huge mortality difference emerged. Among the 68 percent in whom treatment was successful, the mortality rate at one year was 5 percent. Among the 32 percent in whom intracoronary streptokinase failed to open the infarct artery, one-year mortality was 35 percent.

In considering late treatment, the physician must have a clear objective in mind. If the patient has ongoing ischemic myocardial pain and well-preserved R waves, it is reasonable to believe that thrombolytic therapy will preserve left ventricular function and reduce mortality. On the other hand, if ischemic myocardial pain has already subsided spontaneously, and if Q waves are already established, it is highly unlikely that thrombolytic therapy will salvage ischemic myocardium. However, thrombolytic therapy may still prevent aneurysm formation. This is a worthy goal of therapy, but it should be understood that aneurysm formation occurs most often in patients with large infarcts. For practical purposes, aneurysm formation is a problem associated with anterior myocardial infarction, and, in the main, it is these patients who should be considered for thrombolytic therapy. Patients with inferior infarction and hemodynamic compromise may also benefit. Patients with hemodynamically uncomplicated inferior infarction and those with small anterior infarctions probably should not be treated. This point of view is also supported by the Western Washington trial of intracoronary streptokinase, in which the benefit of reperfusion was limited to patients with anterior infarction.

An important and unanswered question concerns the period of time in which thrombolytic therapy can prevent infarct expansion. The answer to this question is largely unknown, although some data indicate benefit with treatment as late as 24 hours after the onset of infarction. This benefit is probably not large enough to justify treatment of patients with known risk of hemorrhage.

Contraindications

Active bleeding or recent bleeding, which, if exacerbated, would be life threatening, constitutes an absolute contraindication to thrombolytic therapy. Similarly, recent surgery or trauma in an incompressible and vital location is a contraindication to thrombolytic therapy. Primary angioplasty should be considered in these cases.

Advanced age, hypertension, cardiopulmonary resuscitation, and menstruation are frequently cited as contraindications to thrombolytic therapy. In fact, the published record does not lend a great deal of support to these restrictions of therapy. As discussed previously, advanced age may be a minor relative contraindication to thrombolytic therapy, but by itself advanced age is not associated with a prohibitive risk of bleeding. Similarly, available evidence does not support the widely held belief that hypertension is associated with a prohibitive risk of intracranial hemorrhage among patients given thrombolytic therapy. In ISIS-2, among more than 1,000 patients with systolic blood pressure greater than 175 mm Hg, all-cause mortality was 5.7 percent among patients given streptokinase and 8.7 percent among patients receiving placebo (ISIS-2, 1988). The authors commented that there was no excess bleeding "among the 178 with a systolic blood pressure of 200 mm Hg or more." As in the case of treatment of elderly patients, there is some evidence of an increased risk of intracranial hemorrhage among hypertensive patients treated with tPA. As with advanced age, therefore, hypertension may be a minor and relative contraindication to thrombolytic therapy, but is not an absolute contraindication.

The TAMI investigators reported on their experience with 62 patients who received less than 10 minutes of cardiopulmonary resuscitation, who awoke immediately after the cardiopulmonary resuscitation, and who did not have obvious chest wall trauma. These patients were enrolled in trials of thrombolytic therapy and represented 9 percent of the population of these studies. Among the 62 patients with pretreatment cardiac arrest and cardiopulmonary resuscitation (CPR), there were no cases of cardiac tamponade or hemothorax. Blood loss and transfusion requirements were similar for patients with or without CPR. Predischarge ejection fraction was lower in patients requiring pretreatment CPR and mortality was higher, but these adverse outcomes were a consequence of large infarctions rather than the combination of CPR and thrombolytic therapy. It is likely that the outcome would have been even worse had these patients not been treated with thrombolytic agents.

Premenopausal women infrequently sustain acute myocardial infarction. Nevertheless, the question as to whether menstruating women can safely be given thrombolytic agents does arise from time to time. Experience with the use of thrombolytic agents for pulmonary embolism indicates that menstruation is also a minor and relative contraindication to thrombolytic therapy. This observation is consistent with the fact that menstrual bleeding is regulated more by vasospasm than by protein-mediated hemostasis.

As in the case of patients with recent surgery or major trauma, when doubt exists in the above-mentioned situations, primary angioplasty should be considered.

Adjunctive Therapy

The decision to treat a patient with thrombolytic therapy for acute myocardial infarction should include consideration of adjunctive mechanical therapy to maximize reperfusion and adjunctive medical therapy to minimize reocclusion.

Although salvage angioplasty, that is, angioplasty of infarct-related arteries that remain occluded despite thrombolytic therapy, has not been proved beneficial, it should be considered in patients who present early in the course of large myocardial infarctions. This recommendation is based on two lines of reasoning. First, 15 to 20 percent of patients treated with tPA will have persistent total occlusion of the infarct-related artery 90 to 120 minutes after the initiation of therapy, and most of these vessels will not be recanalized over the next 24 hours. With streptokinase, 35 to 40 percent of infarct-related arteries remain totally occluded 90 to 120 minutes after the initiation of therapy. Although as many as half of these vessels will recanalize over the next 24 to 48 hours, the time course and benefit of this late reperfusion are undefined. In view of the morbidity and mortality risks associated with nonreperfusion among patients who present to hospitals early in the course of large infarcts, these nonreperfusion rates may be considered unacceptable. Second, the conclusion that salvage angioplasty is not routinely beneficial is an inference derived from a European cooperative study of emergency angioplasty for patent and occluded infarct-related arteries, rather than a direct result of a randomized trial of salvage angioplasty. It is possible that the benefit of salvage angioplasty in this study was obscured by adverse effects of emergency angioplasty of patent infarct-related arteries, high reocclusion rates when salvage angioplasty is applied to patients treated with tPA as a single thrombolytic agent, and the relatively small penalty associated with nonreperfusion or reocclusion in patients with small-to-intermediate sized myocardial infarctions treated with thrombolytic agents at 3 and 4 hours.

On the basis of these considerations and in view of the overwhelming evidence of benefit of reperfusion in large infarcts, it seems advisable to screen all patients with large infarcts for emergency angiography and, if necessary, salvage angioplasty. Large infarct may be defined as any myocardial infarction with hemodynamic compromise unresponsive to atropine or any anterior infarction with widespread ST-segment elevation. Given the frequent difficulty of distinguishing reperfusion from nonreperfusion on the basis of clinical or electrocardiographic criteria, and in recognition of the opportunity for salvage of ischemic myocardium which may be lost by 1 or 2 hours of observation, it is probably best to begin to make arrangements for emergency angiography and, if necessary, salvage angioplasty immediately after initiation of thrombolytic therapy in such patients. These plans may be changed later if there is evidence of reperfusion.

In conjunction with streptokinase, aspirin has been shown to reduce the incidence of nonfatal and fatal recurrent infarction. Heparin also reduces mortality after treatment with streptokinase, and the magnitude of reduction of mortality is similar to that obtained with aspirin. Thus, one of these drugs should be given to all patients treated with streptokinase. Optimal duration of therapy is not known. Current practice usually involves either indefinite treatment with aspirin or several days of heparin followed by indefinite treatment with aspirin. Whether the combination of aspirin and heparin is preferable to either agent alone is unknown.

Heparin is known to reduce the incidence of reocclusion following treatment with intravenous tPA. Low-dose aspirin, 80 mg daily, is not as effective as heparin for this purpose on the first hospital day. However, higher doses of aspirin (325 mg daily) may be substituted for heparin on the second hospital day and seem to be as effective as continued heparin therapy. As in the case of treatment with streptokinase, it is not known whether the combination of aspirin and heparin is more effective than either drug alone.

Drug of Choice

The twelvefold higher price of tPA has generated a lively controversy over the thrombolytic drug of choice. What is known about these two agents and thrombolytic therapy generally can be summarized in a few statements. Infarct-related artery patency 90 to

120 minutes after the initiation of treatment with tPA is 80 to 85 percent, whereas infarct-related artery patency 90 to 120 minutes after initiation of therapy with streptokinase is only 60 to 65 percent. Infarct artery patency at these points in time correlates with preservation of ventricular function and reduced mortality. When heparin and aspirin are used to prevent reocclusion, infarct-related artery patency rates 24 to 48 hours after the initiation of therapy are similar for both drugs, approximately 85 percent. Whether reperfusion 2 or more hours after the initiation of therapy is beneficial to the "typical" patient receiving thrombolytic therapy (intermediate-sized infarct treated at 3 to 4 hours) is unknown. Likewise, optimal infusion regimens for each of these drugs remain undefined. There is substantial evidence that the Food and Drug Administration (FDA)–approved regimens, for streptokinase 1.5 million units given over 1 hour, and for tPA 100 mg given over 3 hours, do not lead to the best clinical or angiographic results. The best clinical results achieved with streptokinase in large randomized trials have been obtained in connection with an accelerated infusion (1.5 million units over 30 minutes). Angiography was deferred for 3 weeks in both of these studies, and the reperfusion rate associated with this regimen is unknown.

There is also evidence that front-loaded, accelerated regimens of tPA lead to better angiographic results than the FDA-approved regimen. These newer regimens include a 15- or 20-mg bolus and infusion of the remaining 80 to 85 mg over 90 to 120 minutes. Typically, most of the dose is given during the first 30 to 60 minutes of the infusion, so that only 20 or 30 mg are given during the final hour of the infusion. Patency rates in excess of 90 percent at 90 minutes have been reported with these accelerated regimens. It is possible that combination therapy with an initial bolus of tPA followed by an infusion of tPA or a nonfibrin specific agent, such as streptokinase or urokinase, will lead to high initial patency rates and reduced risk of reocclusion.

SUGGESTED READING

AIMS Trial Study Group. Effect of intravenous APSAC on mortality after acute myocardial infarction: preliminary report of a placebo-controlled clinical trial. Lancet 1988; 1:545.

Gruppo Italiano per lo Studio della Streptochinasi nell' Infarto Miocardico (GISSI). Effectiveness of intravenous thrombolytic treatment in acute myocardial infarction. Lancet 1986; 1:397.

Guerci AD, Ross RS. TIMI II and the role of angioplasty in acute myocardial infarction (editorial). N Engl J Med 1989; 320:663.

ISIS-2 (Second International Study of Infarct Survival) Collaborative Group. Randomised trial of intravenous streptokinase, oral aspirin, both, or neither among 17,187 cases of suspected acute myocardial infarction: ISIS-2. Lancet 1988; 2:349.

Mauri F, Gasparini M, Barbonaglia L, et al. Prognostic significance of the extent of myocardial injury in acute myocardial infarction treated by streptokinase (the GISSI trial). Am J Cardiol 1989; 63:1291.

Neuhaus KL, Femerer W, Jeep-Tebbe S, et al. Improved thrombolysis with a modified dose regimen of recombinant tissue-type plasminogen activator. J Am Coll Cardiol 1989; 14:1566.

Van de Werf F, Arnold AER. Intravenous tissue plasminogen activator and size of infarct, left ventricular function, and survival in acute myocardial infarction. Br Med J 1988; 297:1374.

MYOCARDIAL INFARCTION: UNCOMPLICATED

GERMANO DISCIASCIO, M.D.
GEORGE W. VETROVEC, M.D.

The management of transmural myocardial infarction has changed dramatically with the advent of thrombolytic therapy, resulting in an increase in the frequency of uncomplicated infarctions. Uncomplicated infarction refers to no severe pump failure, cardiogenic shock, or life-threatening arrhythmias. Likewise, the recognition that a nontransmural (non-Q) infarction is not a "small event" but is a warning of worse short-term risk prompting more aggressive drug and invasive therapy has led to a further reduction in short-term adverse outcomes. Thus, although management strategies may be more complex, the overall outcome results in a higher proportion of uncomplicated infarctions.

THERAPEUTIC ALTERNATIVES

The therapy of uncomplicated myocardial infarction involves the use of certain drugs and, after coronary arteriography, a consideration of angioplasty or surgery.

PREFERRED APPROACH

Medical Treatment

Myocardial Infarction in the Era of Thrombolytic Therapy

The efficacy of acute thrombolytic therapy during evolving myocardial infarction is well established, and in future years thrombolysis will be primary treatment for most infarct patients without major contraindications. Therefore, the subacute and late management of myocardial infarction of the 1990s will largely involve patients after thrombolytic therapy. Clinical recognition of reperfusion is somewhat limited, making the definition of patients who fail to reperfuse difficult. Although acute invasive intervention may be appropriate for patients who fail to reperfuse, those who have strong clinical suspicion of reperfusion, such as improvement of chest pain (although chest pain frequently may not disappear completely and may sometimes be difficult to differentiate from pericardial pain), abatement of ST-segment elevation, and early (< 16 hours) peak of creatine kinase, may be treated expectantly. Risk is stratified according to the outline described subsequently. However, successful thrombolysis is also associated with recurrent in-hospital ischemic events and the possibility of in-hospital, infarction-related artery reclosure, which occurs most frequently after heparin is discontinued (usually after 3 to 4 days) or if heparinization is subtherapeutic (activated partial thromboplastin time more than twice that of control). Those patients with acute reclosure comprise 5 to 20 percent of successfully reperfused patients. However, because of recurrent infarction, such patients often are candidates for urgent angiography, for retreatment with thrombolytic therapy potentially to salvage the benefits of initial early reperfusion, or both.

Risk Stratifications and Prognosis

Several factors are associated with increased mortality risk after myocardial infarction, and their recognition is of paramount importance in optimal management post-infarction. Patients at increased risk may account for up to 55 percent of the population under 75 years of age experiencing myocardial infarction. Ischemia during the hospital phase beyond the initial 24-hour period after infarction is associated with a 18 percent mortality between day 6 and 1 year. Patients with a previous myocardial infarction and evidence of congestive heart failure carry a 25 percent 1-year mortality after discharge; patients with left ventricular ejection fraction between 20 and 44 percent have a 12 percent 1-year mortality. Predischarge exercise testing may further characterize higher risk groups; ability to achieve 4 Mets without ischemic changes is associated with a 1 to 3 percent 1-year mortality; a positive test or inability to achieve a 4-Met workload identifies a subgroup with higher risk (11 percent 1-year mortality). In all the above-mentioned groups, coronary angiography is indicated vis-à-vis possible revascularization and improvement in mortality rate.

Coronary Care Unit

The original goal of coronary care units was to provide arrhythmia monitoring and treatment before catastrophic events occur. In addition, the ability to observe patients closely and to monitor hemodynamic status is a continuously evolving use of the coronary care unit, with availability of invasive hemodynamic monitoring and intra-aortic balloon pump support.

Practical considerations in the coronary care unit include appropriate patient sedation when necessary for anxiety. Likewise, pain management for the completed, uncomplicated myocardial infarction often requires utilization of nonsteroidal analgesics for the moderate discomfort that patients may continue to experience for the first 24 to 48 hours. In some instances, this discomfort may be associated with a pericardial rub.

Decisions about transfer from the coronary care unit are made relative to the stability of the patient. In general, patients with successful reperfusion and no evidence of life-threatening arrhythmia once antiarrhythmic therapy has been discontinued are candidates for transfer by 72 hours. The risk of serious arrhythmia is decreased substantially by this time, even for patients who have failed to reperfuse but who are otherwise uncomplicated.

Cardiovascular Drug Therapy

Anticoagulants. Following infarction all patients, even those receiving heparin, should be maintained on aspirin, unless it is contraindicated, such as in the case of adult asthma and nasal polyps. Although recommended dosages are variable, we favor using one adult enteric-coated aspirin daily for dosing convenience, which is maintained indefinitely.

Patients receiving thrombolytic therapy should be started and maintained on intravenous heparin therapy, unless this is contraindicated by risk or occurrence of bleeding, with dosage titrated to a partial thromboplastin time of twice control. Our practice is to maintain heparin for at least 48 hours or longer if ischemic symptoms recur or until coronary angiography if an early angiogram is anticipated. Longer heparinization may be warranted for documented intracoronary thrombus, or following angioplasty for persistent, severe congestive failure, or because of prolonged bed rest, systemic embolic events, or echo-documented left ventricular thrombus. Heparin in the latter conditions is maintained until oral sodium warfarin (Coumadin) anticoagulation is therapeutic.

Dipyridamole (Persantine) is not currently thought to be superior to or additive to aspirin in ischemic and infarction syndromes, and thus it is not routinely used except in patients unable to take aspirin. A dose of 75 mg twice daily is believed to be sufficient in such circumstances.

Indications for sodium warfarin (Coumadin) are limited to documented left ventricular thrombus, systemic embolization, and severe congestive failure. The risk:benefit ratio of chronic anticoagulation with

Coumadin must always be considered. Recent evidence is emerging that less stringent Coumadin anticoagulation may be equally effective with a lower risk of bleeding complications. A prothrombin time of 1.5 times control is usually quite satisfactory and is safer than higher levels. Coumadin is begun at 5 mg daily without loading. Heparin needs to be maintained until therapeutic effects from Coumadin administration are seen, usually by 5 days. Early, once or twice weekly, out-patient observation is necessary to assess any significant variation in prothrombin level. Patient education regarding increased bleeding tendency, especially from trauma or changes in associated drug therapy including nonprescription agents, is imperative.

Beta-Blockers. Prior to the era of thrombolytic therapy, beta-blockers in significant dosages (e.g., propranolol 120 mg per day) were demonstrated to reduce the risk of subsequent mortality and reinfarction with beneficial effects decreasing over time, such that the efficacy abated 18 to 24 months following transmural infarction. Such beneficial effects of beta-blockers are unknown following thrombolytic therapy. The TIMI IIB Trial demonstrated the efficacy of intravenous beta-blockers followed by oral beta-blockers in reducing the incidence of early recurrent ischemic events in the first 6 weeks without effect on mortality. Oral beta-blockers had no effect on short-term outcome.

Our current bias is to maintain beta-blockers in patients begun acutely on intravenous beta-blocker therapy and to institute subsequent oral beta-blockers only in patients not receiving thrombolytic therapy, particularly in patients with large or anterior infarction without contraindications. Alternatively, beta-blockers may be used as an anti-ischemic agent in patients having continued anginal symptoms, persistent hypertension, or both.

Contraindications to beta-blockers include a history of asthma and severe congestive failure. Common side effects include fatigue, lethargy, bad dreams, and impotence. Because of frequent troublesome side effects, the popularity of routine beta-blocker treatment after thrombolysis in an uncomplicated infarction seems to be waning.

Calcium Blockers. Routine administration of calcium blockers following transmural infarction has not proved useful in preventing major ischemic events. Although in one study patients without congestive failure receiving diltiazem had fewer recurrent adverse ischemic events, patients with congestive failure had an overall worse survival. Likewise nifedipine has not been shown to have preventive properties following transmural infarction. Thus, use of calcium blockers after transmural infarction is limited to the treatment of hypertension or ischemia.

Nifedipine is particularly effective for rapidly reducing severe hypertension, which is useful in the face of ongoing ischemia, anticoagulation, or thrombolytic therapy. Likewise, nifedipine's marked vasodilation potentially produces the least depression of left ventricular function. Nifedipine GITS is now the only calcium blocker available for once-daily therapy of ischemia or hypertension, with a reduced side effect profile enhancing patient convenience and compliance during chronic therapy.

Diltiazem has been demonstrated to reduce the risk of subsequent ischemic events in patients following nontransmural infarction. Because many of these patients undergo coronary angiography and subsequent intervention owing to known increased short-term risk of an adverse outcome, there is no evidence that continued calcium blocker therapy after intervention has any benefit. Thus, calcium blocker treatment seems prudent for most nontransmural infarctions, at least until angiographic documentation of limited extent or revascularization of underlying coronary disease is completed. Subsequent therapy should be indicated for continuing ischemia; if revascularization is complete, however, calcium blockers are not necessary except for blood pressure control. The usual effective dose of diltiazem is 240 to 360 mg every 24 hours. Side effects include nausea, headache, and edema. Occasional patients develop marked bradycardia, sinus node block, or atrioventricular node block which may be exacerbated by digoxin.

Angiotensin Converting Enzyme Inhibitors. Recent evidence suggests a beneficial effect for angiotensin converting enzyme (ACE) inhibitors following infarction for reducing subsequent morbidity and mortality, presumably by supporting more favorable ventricular remodeling. The impact of ACE inhibitors seems greatest in patients with the most severe ventricular impairment. Although hypotension may be an acute side effect of these agents, subsequent subacute effects on kidney function of white blood counts are of concern. Although not life-threatening, a persistent dry cough limits therapy in over 10 percent of patients.

Antiarrhythmic Drugs. Lidocaine is frequently begun routinely on admission to the coronary care unit. If not administered routinely, lidocaine is given later for increasing frequency of ventricular premature beats ($>$ 8 per minute, couplets, R on T phenomena, nonsustained ventricular tachycardia), maintained for 48 hours, and then discontinued while monitoring is available. Elderly patients and patients with hepatic disease are at increased risk of toxicity. Seizures, and mental confusion, or both should prompt discontinuing lidocaine and obtaining a blood level. Lidocaine is instituted with a 50 to 75-mg bolus and is followed by a 2 mg per minute drip. If by blood level or clinical efficacy the dosage needs to be increased, an increase in the drip rate to 3 to 4 mg per minute should be preceded by an additional bolus of 50 to 75 mg. Further antiarrhythmic management is discussed in a subsequent chapter.

Patient Education

The reality of coronary artery disease manifested by myocardial infarction produces significant psychological effects in most patients, whether expressed or not. Education and discussion regarding feelings are important to allay anxiety. Simply reassuring a patient that feelings of anxiety or depression are common is often helpful.

Patients should be given basic explanations for the anatomic causes of coronary disease and myocardial infarction. Patient concerns regarding prevention of future coronary events are probably greatest at this time. Thus, education of risk factors should be instituted early and continued throughout hospitalization.

The anxiety of future activity and life expectancy are common concerns. Early discussion of the potential rehabilitation of most patients back to a normal life-style is helpful in allaying anxiety and limiting early concerns regarding disability.

Prior to discharge, patient education should be directed to understanding prescribed medications, including actions and potential side effects.

Following hospitalization, patient education should persist, reinforcing earlier teaching, which may have been forgotten perhaps as a result of distraction from anxiety during hospitalization. The potential for and timing of return to work should be clearly based on the patient's progress. Likewise, reinforcement of risk factor modification remains a lifetime goal.

Lipid Screening

The importance of cholesterol as a potentially reversible risk factor is now well documented and recognized by many patients. Questions regarding cholesterol are common, and we therefore always discuss cholesterol and diet with patients. However, it is important to point out that cholesterol levels drawn at the time of a major illness such as myocardial infarction do not represent baseline values. Thus, early therapy is directed toward diet, with plans for lipid evaluation following hospitalization. Conversely, for patients with extraordinarily high or known lipid abnormalities, drug treatment should be initiated during hospitalization.

Activity

Early mobilization decreases the disability of bed rest and reduces the risk of thrombophlebitis. Following myocardial infarction patients should be mobilized as rapidly as possible. Sitting is easier on myocardial function even early, and thus patients may sit up within the first 24 hours if they are stable. Sitting in a chair is appropriate beyond 24 hours following infarction.

For the successfully reperfused patient, ambulation in the hospital can be quite brisk. Conversely, patients with marked congestive failure or large infarction even with successful reperfusion have to be mobilized somewhat more slowly. Because the major time frame of myocardial rupture is in the first 7 days, only moderate activity should be considered reasonable until at least 2 weeks after the event.

Hospital Discharge

Timing of hospital discharge should be based on the complexity of the infarction. Preliminary studies have demonstrated safety in discharge as early as 5 days following successfully reperfused infarctions without residual significant coronary artery disease. Conversely, patients with more extensive left ventricular dysfunction, and residual ischemia, or both should be observed longer, with discharge at approximately 12 days.

Management Following Hospitalization

In those patients who leave the hospital without evidence of residual ischemia or need for early revascularization, continued out-patient follow-up remains important to recognize subsequent ischemia, which may develop with increasing activities. Four to 6 weeks after an uncomplicated myocardial infarction, a full-level exercise test is warranted for evidence of ischemia. If there is no evidence, the patient can resume normal activities within the context of his or her cardiac and general medical history. Conversely, if there is evidence of ischemia, we recommend angiography for those patients not undergoing catheterization during hospitalization to assess the extent of myocardium in jeopardy. Patients having undergone angioplasty should have a baseline stress test performed early, with a follow-up study at 6 months to document any evidence of asymptomatic restenosis. Furthermore, effective rehabilitation, risk factor modification, and patient education are important aspects of management following hospitalization.

Surgical Treatment

Coronary Angiography and Revascularization

Coronary angiography is recommended for the higher risk subgroups outlined previously because coronary bypass surgery may enhance survival in patients with depressed left ventricular function, three-vessel coronary artery disease, or post-infarction angina. Furthermore, coronary angiography following nontransmural infarction is important to document extent of disease and need for intervention. Coronary angiography after successful thrombolysis is more controversial. The TIMI IIB Trial indicates that for patients who sustain a myocardial infarction there is generally no significant benefit to urgent angiography and angioplasty. Thus, the recommendations from that study are that patients be considered for angiography and possible intervention only if there is evidence of recurrent ischemia in the hospital, a positive low-level exercise treadmill before discharge, or both. However, in hospitals with available catheterization laboratories, early angiography may be the most efficient and useful method to assess patients fully following thrombolytic therapy. Benefits include identifying patients with nonsevere residual occlusions, which require no further interventions, and patients with limited coronary artery disease who may, on the basis of this anatomic information, be returned safely to earlier activity and hospital discharge. Conversely, patients with multivessel disease and depressed left ventricular function may be more readily triaged to revascularization. Although angiography may be an acceptable alternative screening technique, the recognition of a lesion is not an automatic indication for angioplasty without evidence of ischemia. The potential benefits of nonacute reopening of occluded arteries to enhance recovery of "stunned" myocardium or to enhance ventricular remodeling are under investigation.

SUGGESTED READING

Ross J, et al. A decision schema for coronary angiography after acute myocardial infarction. Circulation 1989; 79:292.

TIMI Study Group. Results of the Thrombolysis in Myocardial Infarction (TIMI) Phase II Trial. N Engl J Med 1989; 320:618.

CARDIAC ARRHYTHMIAS FOLLOWING MYOCARDIAL INFARCTION

KENNETH M. KESSLER, M.D.

Cardiac arrhythmias are common following acute myocardial infarction (Table 1). Mechanisms include increased automaticity, reentry related to focal conduction slowing, and enhanced sympathetic and parasympathetic tone. Approaches to therapy depend on the presence or absence of symptoms and whether the arrhythmia occurs in the early phase (first 72 hours) or recovery phase of the infarction process. The acute goal of therapy is usually hemodynamic stabilization, whereas long-range therapy often relates to the more elusive endpoint of improving survival.

THERAPEUTIC ALTERNATIVES

Symptomatic arrhythmias deserve prompt treatment (Fig. 1). Symptoms may be overt and include syncope, hypotension, angina, and heart failure. However, symptoms of hypoperfusion may be more occult and include clouding of the sensorium, coolness of the skin, and decreased urinary output. An arrhythmia must not be considered to be well tolerated simply because the patient has normal blood pressure. The arrhythmia per se, the signs of tissue perfusion, and the general condition of the patient must be considered when determining the need for, and urgency of, treatment. Symptomatic tachyarrhythmias almost always deserve prompt electrical conversion (alternative initial strategies may be indicated in the rare cases of digitalis toxicity). Symptomatic bradyarrhythmias require rate support and are best approached in a logical sequence: atropine, external pacemaker, and temporary transvenous pacemaker. The goal of therapy of early symptomatic arrhythmias is the restoration of normal circulatory function. In treating chronic asymptomatic arrhythmias, the direction of therapy is often preventive, and solid therapeutic information is often lacking. In general, the treatment of arrhythmias can be approached using a hierarchy of therapies (Table 2). In each case the physician should be thoroughly aware of the indications, dosage, and contraindications of therapy. The following sections may serve as a guide to such treatment.

TABLE 1 Cardiac Arrhythmias

Persistent, early tachyarrhythmias
Sinus tachycardia
Atrial flutter and fibrillation
Ventricular tachycardia and fibrillation
Persistent, early bradycardias
Sinus bradycardia
Atrioventricular conduction disturbances and block
Transient, early arrhythmias
Atrial arrhythmias
Accelerated atrioventricular junctional rhythms
Accelerated idioventricular rhythm
Torsade de pointes
Ventricular premature complexes
Reperfusion arrhythmias
Late arrhythmias
Ventricular tachycardia and fibrillation
Nonsustained ventricular tachycardia
Premature ventricular complexes

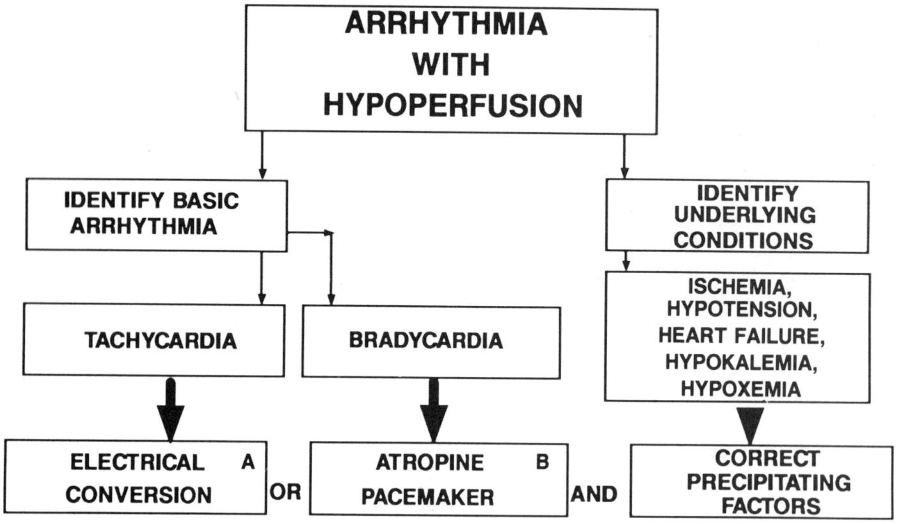

Figure 1 Simplified approach to the treatment of arrhythmias associated with signs of hypoperfusion (see text for details). *A*, Electrical conversion should be avoided in arrhythmias associated with digitalis toxicity. *B*, Underdosing with atropine may induce a paradoxical bradycardia.

PREFERRED APPROACH

Persistent, Early Tachyarrhythmias

In general, acute tachyarrhythmias are best treated by prompt cardioversion or defibrillation. Hemodynamic instability caused by such arrhythmias is not tolerated in the acute ischemic setting. Hesitation is justified only in the case of digoxin toxicity, in which correction of hypokalemia and other metabolic factors and the use of intravenous lidocaine, intravenous phenytoin, digitalis antibodies, or a combination of therapies are preferred. Cardioversion in the clinical setting of digitalis toxicity may lead to irreversible ventricular fibrillation.

Sinus tachycardia often accompanies acute myocardial infarction. Therapy must first address aggravating conditions, including hypoperfusion, heart failure, pain, fever, anxiety, pericarditis, and pulmonary embolus. When the sinus rate is increased disproportionally and is not compensatory to a low cardiac output, beta-adrenergic blocking agents can lower heart rate and improve myocardial oxygen utilization. Metroprolol in standard dosage is often adequate (Table 3). Esmolol has the advantage of being short-acting (Table 3), although if heart failure or bronchospasm is precipitated, it may persist beyond the half-life of the drug. Beta-adrenergic blocking agents should be avoided in patients with overt heart failure or bronchospasm or in those in whom sympathetic support is required to maintain perfusion. When fever is a contributory factor to sinus tachycardia, suppression of fever with an antipyretic such as acetaminophen is indicated after the possibility of infection is evaluated. Drugs with positive chronotropic effects, e.g., theophylline or vasodilators, which promote reflex tachycardia, should be avoided when possible (Table 4).

Atrial flutter and atrial fibrillation may occur as the consequences of atrial hypertension, sinus node ischemia, or pericarditis. The ventricular response is often uncontrolled, and an increase in myocardial oxygen demand resulting in further hemodynamic impairment may occur. Atrial flutter is often drug resistant and is usually best treated with cardioversion using as little as 25 to 50 joules (increasing energies are used, with caution, as needed). Digitalis, beta-adrenergic blocking agents, and verapamil may all be used to increase atrioventricular block and thereby slow the ventricular response in less urgent cases or if repeated cardioversion fails. Digitalis has the disadvantage of a relatively slow onset of action, and atrial flutter is often resistant to digitalis. Beta-adrenergic blocking agents should be used cautiously and avoided in overt heart failure because they will worsen the failure if the dysrhythmia is not controlled adequately. Esmolol has the advantage of a rapid onset and offset of action. Verapamil can slow the rate and at times aid in the maintenance of sinus rhythm; how-

TABLE 2 Hierarchy of Treatment Modalities*

No treatment: Preferred whenever medically sound
Alleviate aggravating factors: Treat ischemia, hypotension, heart failure, hypoxemia, hypokalemia, anemia, drug side effects, and other conditions
Modulate sympathetic or parasympathetic tone: Beta-adrenergic blocking agents or atropine are simple and relatively safe
Electrons: Pacing, cardioversion, and defibrillation are relatively safe and potentially life-saving procedures
Antiarrhythmic drugs: Because of the side effects and proarrhythmic potential of all the group I, III, and IV antiarrhythmic agents, they should be used with caution
Implantable devices and antiarrhythmic surgery: Because of the necessity for invasion, these are listed last, although in given circumstances these modalities may become the approach of choice

*Least to most potential for side effects.

TABLE 3 Antiarrhythmic Drug Dosage and Kinetics*

	Usual Dosing Range	*Half-life (h)*	*Therapeutic Range (μg/ml)*	*Major Route of Excretion*
Class IA				
Quinidine (Quinaglute, Quinidex)	Oral sulfate: 200–600 mg q6h Oral long-acting: 330–660 mg q8h or q6h	5–7	2.3–5	H
Procainamide (Pronestyl, Procan SR)	Oral: 250–750 mg q4h or q6h Oral long-acting: 500–1500 q8h or q6h IV: 10–15 mg/kg at 25 mg/min; then 1–6 mg/min	3–5	4–10	R
Disopyramide (Norpace)	Oral: 100–200 mg q8h or q6h	8–9	2–5	H/R
Class IB				
Lidocaine (Xylocaine)	IV: 1–3 mg/kg at 20–50 mg/min; then 1–4 mg/min	1–2	1–5	H
Tocainide (Tonocard)	Oral: 400–600 q8–12h	15	4–10	H
Mexiletine (Mexitil)	Oral: 200–400 mg q8h	10–12	0.5–2.0	H
Class IC				
Flecainide (Tambocor)	Oral 100–200 mg ql2h	20	0.2–1.0	H
Encainide (Enkaid)	Oral: 25–50 mg q8h	3–4†	.5–1.0†	H
Propafenone (Rythmol)	Oral: 150–300 mg q8h	2–10†		H
Class II				
Propranolol (Inderal)	Oral: 10–100 mg q6h IV: 0.1 mg/kg in divided 1-mg doses	4–6	0.04–0.10	H
Esmolol (Brevibloc)	IV: 500 mg/kg/min for 1 min, followed by 50 mg/kg/min for 4 min. Repeat with 50-mg increments to maintenance dose of 200 mg/kg/min	9 min	—	H
Metoprolol (Lopressor)	Oral: 50–200 mg bid IV: (dosing for acute MI with careful monitoring) 5 mg q 2 min × 3; if tolerated 50 mg q 6 × 48 h then 100 mg bid	3–4	0.5–0.10	H
Class III				
Amiodarone (Cordarone)	Oral: 800–1600 mg/day × 1–3 weeks; then 600–800/d × 2–4 weeks; then 200–400 mg/d	50 days	1–2.5	H
Bretylium (Bretylol)	IV: 5–10 mg/kg at 1–2 mg/kg/min; then 0.5–2.0 mg/min	8–14	0.5–1.5	R
Class IV				
Verapamil (Isoptin, Calan)	Oral: 80–120 mg q6–8h IV: 5–10 mg in 1–2 min	3–8	0.1–0.15	H
Digoxin (Lanoxin)	Oral: 1.25–1.5 mg in divided doses over 24 hours, followed by 0.125–0.375 mg/d IV: approximately 70% of oral dose	36	0.8–1.4 (ng/ml)	R

*All dosing should follow Food and Drug Administration approved guidelines as outlined in package insert or Physician's Desk Reference.
†Active metabolites and genetic differences in metabolic rates limit the significance of these measurements.
H = Hepatic, R = renal, MI = myocardial infarction.
Modified from Myerburg RJ, Kessler KM. Clinical assessment and management of arrhythmias and conduction disturbances. In: Hurst JW, ed. The heart. 7th ed. New York: McGraw-Hill, 1990:1803. Reproduced by permission of the publisher and editor.

ever, its negative inotropic and peripheral vasodilatory effects may be disadvantageous. Drugs that enhance atrioventricular conduction, such as lidocaine and quinidine, are contraindicated in initial management.

Atrial fibrillation is not uncommon in the early phases of acute myocardial infarction. Heart failure that may be independent of the arrhythmia may be evident and must be addressed separately. Drugs that block the atrioventricular node such as digitalis, beta-adrenergic blocking agents, or verapamil are more efficacious for treatment of atrial fibrillation than for atrial flutter. However, the same cautions hold (see above), and the unstable patient should be cardioverted. Cardioversion should commence with low energy levels, e.g., 25 to 50 joules; however, higher levels are often needed. Care should be taken to avoid cardioversion in patients with digitalis excess. Atrial fibrillation with a wide QRS complex may be confused with ventricular tachycardia. If lidocaine is administered to such patients, an alarming increase in ventricular response due to enhanced

TABLE 4 Antiarrhythmic Drug Interactions and Side Effects

	Selected Drug Interactions	*Selected Side Effects*	*Cautions*		
			QTc	*CHF*	*SN/AVN*
Class IA					
Quinidine	Amiodarone, cimetidine, coumarin anticoagulants, digoxin, verapamil	Nausea, diarrhea, cinchonism, thrombocytopenia, hemolytic anemia	***		
Procainamide	Cimetidine, trimethoprim-sulfamethoxazole	Rash, fever, lupus syndrome	**		
Disopyramide	Cimetidine, hepatic enzyme inducers	Blurred vision, dry mouth, constipation, urinary retention	**	***	
Class IB					
Lidocaine	Cimetidine, halothane, propranolol	Drowsiness, hallucinations, seizures, hypotension, respiratory arrest			
Tocainide	—	Paresthesias, ataxia, tremor, hematologic abnormalities			
Mexiletine	Hepatic enzyme inducers	Gastrointestinal upset, liver dysfunction			
Class IC					
Flecainide	Amiodarone, cimetidine			***	**
Encainide	—			*	**
Propafenone	Digoxin				**
Class II					
Propranolol	Cimetidine, lidocaine, indomethacin, NSAID	Depression, fatigue, bronchospasm, heart failure, bradycardia		***	***
Esmolol	—	Depression, fatigue, bronchospasm, heart failure, bradycardia		***	***
Metoprolol	Verapamil, cimetidine	Depression, fatigue, bronchospasm, heart failure, bradycardia		***	***
Class III					
Amiodarone	Quinidine, procainamide		**		
Bretylium	—	Transient hypertension, postural hypotension, nausea			
Class IV					
Verapamil	Cimetidine, digoxin, prazosin, quinidine, theophylline	Constipation, bradycardia, heart failure		***	***
Digoxin	Antacids, erythromycin, tetracycline, cholestryamine, amiodarone, captopril, diltiazem, nifedipine, prazosin, propafenone, quinidine, verapamil	Anorexia, nausea, vomiting, neurologic symptoms, cardiac arrhythmias, gynecomastia			**

QTc = Avoid or use cautiously with other agents that prolong QTc.
CHF (congestive heart failure) = Negative inotrope, use with caution, if at all, in combination with other negative inotropic agents.
SN/AVN (sinus node/atrioventricular node) = Negative chronotrope, use with caution with other drugs that depress sinoatrial or atrioventricular nodal activity.
*, **, *** denote increasing need for caution.
NSAID = Nonsteroidal anti-inflammatory drug.

atrioventricular conduction may occur. Verapamil and beta-adrenergic blocking agents have additive negative chronotropic and negative inotropic actions; their simultaneous intravenous use is discouraged.

Ventricular tachycardia and ventricular fibrillation occur commonly in the acute phase of myocardial infarction, in which they are life-threatening, may be accompanied by an increased in-hospital mortality, but parodoxically do not necessarily indicate an increased risk of mortality after hospital discharge. Ventricular tachycardia may occur intermittently, in which *control of ischemia* including the use of beta-adrenergic blocking agents and *antiarrhythmic therapy* using lidocaine, procainamide, bretylium or a combination of agents (see below) are addressed simultaneously. In rare cases, intermittent arrhythmias are related to spasm associated with ST-segment elevation; this situation is treated with nitrates and cautious administration of calcium channel blocking agents. Symptomatic, sustained ventricular tachycardia is best treated with cardioversion beginning at low energy levels, e.g., 25 joules; increased energies are used as needed. Lidocaine can be considered as primary therapy for ventricular tachycardia in awake patients who are hemodynamically stable. Ischemia and contributory factors, especially hypokalemia, are meticulously explored and corrected. Ventricular fibrillation requires immediate electrical defibrillation: 300 to 400 joules may be needed, although repeated lower energy shocks (e.g., 100 to 200 joules) may be effective and are preferred by some to prevent the adverse effects of high energies.

Recurrences are common; close monitoring and antiarrhythmic medications are indicated to prevent further events. Antiarrhythmic medications often begin with lidocaine; a variety of regimens have been recommended. Lidocaine may be administered as a 75-mg bolus over 3 to 5 minutes, followed by a 50-mg bolus over 2 to 3 minutes at 15 minutes, and if needed 50 mg is administered again at 30 minutes. A 2 to 4 mg per minute drip is initiated after the first bolus. A decreased loading dose, given more slowly, is recommended in elderly patients or when the volume of distribution of lidocaine is known to be decreased, as in patients with heart failure or shock. Both lidocaine levels and lidocaine binding increase during acute myocardial infarction, probably rendering free drug form constant and obviating the need to taper dosing routinely for this reason alone. If lidocaine is ineffective, procainamide can be given intravenously. A commonly used regimen is a loading dose of 750 to 1,000 mg administered at 25 mg per minute, followed by a 3 to 4 mg per minute drip. Hypotension may occur but most often responds to leg-up positioning and fluids. If symptomatic ventricular arrhythmias remain troublesome, 5 to 10 mg per kilogram of bretylium is given intravenously at a rate of 1 to 2 mg per kilogram per minute and may be followed with a drip at 0.5 to 2.0 mg per minute. These three drugs have additive vasodilatory effects; hypotension caused by these drugs may be accentuated by other antiarrhythmic and anti-ischemic therapies and by volume depletion, especially that associated with chronic diuretic therapy. The decision to discontinue bretylium after 24 hours of rhythm control may be appropriate, but the patient should be carefully monitored for the return of aggressive arrhythmias. Both beta-adrenergic blocking agents and overdrive pacing have roles in patients with resistant ventricular arrhythmias. Verapamil is to be avoided in wide complex tachycardias: it is not generally efficacious for ventricular tachycardia, it can cause hemodynamic instability, and deaths have been reported.

Persistent, Early Bradyarrhythmias

Sinus bradycardia may be related to enhanced vagal tone, ischemia, and medications (including beta-adrenergic blocking agents and calcium channel blocking agents). Although bradycardia is relatively protective in the ischemic setting, overt and occult signs of hypoperfusion may occur especially when rates fall into the 40s. Slower rates with hemodynamic impairment may also foster ventricular ectopy or allow the expression of accelerated idioventricular rhythms (see subsequently). Although most episodes of sinus bradycardia are asymptomatic, symptoms of hypoperfusion and the emergence of significant ventricular ectopy are indications for treatment. Atropine sulfate 0.4 to 0.6 mg may be given intravenously and repeated. Doses above 1.5 to 2 mg rarely add to the effectiveness. Small doses of atropine, 0.1 to 0.3 mg, should be avoided because these doses parodoxically may slow the heart rate. Atropine may be ineffective or, at times, too effective, with unacceptable increases in heart rate. Its effects are of uncertain duration. Most often, more reliable, longer term rate control is needed, and a temporary transvenous pacemaker is inserted. In borderline situations a bedside external pacing unit on standby is helpful. It is important to identify the fact that the primary rhythm problem is a bradycardia and to treat it as such because treatment of bradycardia-aggravated ventricular ectopy with antiarrhythmic agents may slow the underlying rhythm and may actually worsen the problem. Finally, if the sinus rate returns to near normal but hemodynamic impairment persists, volume and mechanical issues should be addressed promptly.

Atrioventricular conduction disturbances and block are noted commonly during the course of acute myocardial infarction, and the treatment varies as a function of the site of infarction. Progressive conduction disturbances may occur with inferior wall infarction, and when symptomatic, the institution of atropine, external pacing, temporary transvenous pacing, or a combination of modalities is indicated. Most often the escape pacemaker shows a relatively normal QRS complex at a rate of 40 to 60 beats per minute, and the patient remains asymptomatic. Block often improves in hours to days, and permanent pacing is rarely needed. With anterior wall infarction, heart block usually denotes extensive necrosis. Escape pacemakers are often lower and consequently slower, with resultant symptoms. Treatment with atropine is often less successful for block associated with anterior wall infarction than for block associated with inferior wall infarction, and temporary transvenous pacing and meticulous attention to mechanical factors are indicated. Because of the rapid progression to complete heart block, prophylactic pacing has been advocated for new right bundle branch block associated with hemiblock. The indication for pacing new right bundle branch block with first-degree atrioventricular block, alternating bundle branch block or preexisting left bundle branch block, is debatable. Permanent pacing is recommended for those patients with anteroseptal myocardial infarction who manifest complete heart block or Mobitz Type II block, even if these conduction disturbances are transient. The benefits of these pacing recommendations are clouded by the high mortality of such patients as a result of pump failure.

Transient, Early Arrhythmias

Atrial arrhythmias including premature atrial depolarizations, sinus node dysfunction, and atrial tachycardias are often transient and are best treated by optimizing the hemodynamic and metabolic milieu. When a dominant symptomatic rhythm is noted, therapy is indicated. Rapid supraventricular tachycardias are best treated with cardioversion (carotid sinus massage may precipitate untoward bradycardia on conversion in the acute infarction setting). Tachycardia-bradycardia symptoms are best treated by the combined use of pacing (to treat underlying and drug-induced bradycardia) and antiarrhythmic drugs (directed to the treatment of the atrial tachyarrhythmias).

Accelerated atrioventricular junctional rhythms generally are noted in inferior wall infarction when sinus node depression is coupled with increased automaticity of the junction. The patient is often asymptomatic, since the rate is often at the lower side of the 60 to 100 beats per minute range. Occasionally symptoms are noted because of inadequate rate or loss of synchronized atrial contraction. In such cases, atropine or the more reliable approach of temporary transvenous pacing (including the option of dual chamber pacing) may be helpful. If symptoms are due to an increased rate (especially in anterior infarction in which this rhythm is associated with an excess mortality), class I antiarrhythmic drugs may be tried, but their efficacy may be marginal and caution should be used. Digitalis, propranolol, and verapamil are other options. Elements of left and right ventricular dysfunction should be addressed, and digitalis toxicity, another cause for this dysrhythmia, should be excluded.

Accelerated idioventricular rhythms, or so-called slow ventricular tachycardia, may appear intermittently during the early course of myocardial infarction particularly involving the inferior wall. Most often the rate is controlled, the rhythm transiently appears and disappears often as a function of the underlying sinus bradycardia and sinus arrhythmia, and the patient is asymptomatic. Such rhythms are best carefully observed but left untreated. In fact, treatment with antiarrhythmic agents may further suppress pacemaker function and lead to potentially deleterious vasodilation and left ventricular dysfunction. Most often when symptoms occur they relate to a slow rate or lack of synchronized atrial contraction. Treatment is directed to speeding the heart rate by the use of atropine or transvenous pacing (including the option of dual chamber pacing). The rhythm may become faster and symptomatic; at such times it is treated as any other ventricular tachycardia.

Torsade de pointes may occur rarely as a direct result of ischemia per se and also as a side effect of many of the agents used to treat arrhythmias. Hypokalemia, bradycardia, and other factors that prolong the Q-T interval should be eliminated. Treatment using isoproterenol, which is advised in some cases of torsade de pointes, is contraindicated in the setting of ischemia. Lidocaine, acute cardioversion, and overdrive pacing have roles in therapy. However, correction of underlying causes, including ischemia, is the primary direction of therapy.

Premature ventricular complexes occur in the majority of patients early in the course of acute myocardial infarction. Premature ventricular complexes have been considered a warning sign for more malignant ventricular arrhythmias. However, ventricular tachycardia and ventricular fibrillation may occur without warning, and not all patients with premature ventricular complexes go on to develop life-threatening forms. The R-on-T phenomenon, particularly in the early acute ischemic setting, may initiate ventricular fibrillation, but this relationship does not have as strong a predictive value as once thought. Premature ventricular complexes may reflect automatic foci and are aggravated by hemodynamic instability and hypokalemia, such that primary therapy should correct underlying abnormalities. Lidocaine can prevent ventricular tachycardia and ventricular fibrillation. Because of the lack of a one-to-one relationship between warning arrhythmias and life-threatening arrhythmias and because of the failure of lidocaine regimens to change hospital mortality (when patients are in the equivalent of a coronary care unit setting), the routine use of prophylactic therapy for premature ventricular complexes, although customary, should be individualized. Prophylactic therapy seems prudent early in the course of the therapy of patients with acute myocardial infarction (e.g., within 6 hours), when the incidence of primary ventricular fibrillation is highest, and for those with evident, especially symptomatic, advanced forms (e.g., R-on-T phenomenon, multiform, couplets, salvos). Prophylactic therapy may not be warranted when the risk of adverse effects is high such as in the elderly and in patients with shock, hypotension, moderate-to-severe heart failure, or primary liver disease. Dosing should be decreased in patients with hypotension or heart failure or in those patients receiving cimetidine. Low- to moderate-grade ectopy is often preferable to drug side effects. Careful dosing and monitoring are required.

Spontaneous and therapeutically induced *reperfusion* is commonly recognized to be associated with arrhythmias, although the relatively high frequency of arrhythmias in early infarction often makes a cause and effect relationship uncertain. Arrhythmias associated with reperfusion include premature ventricular complexes, couplets, and runs of accelerated idioventricular rhythm. At times ventricular tachycardia or ventricular fibrillation is seen. Treatment guidelines are as previously mentioned; the potential transient nature of the disturbance should be recognized.

Chronic Arrhythmias

In general, the tachyarrhythmias and bradyarrhythmias of the acute infarction period resolve over the first 24 to 72 hours. Heart block associated with anterior infarction is an indication for permanent pacemaker placement (see previously). Symptomatic ventricular tachyarrhythmias and bundle branch block that appear after the first 72 hours of infarction portend a poor prognosis and are approached aggressively. The most vexing problem is how to evaluate and treat low- and moderate-grade ventricular arrhythmias that occur after the initial 72 hours of acute myocardial infarction. Such arrhythmias appear to be associated with risk, but guidelines for therapy are scarce and conflicting. Because of the beneficial effects of beta-blocking agents, their use should be considered routine except when specifically contraindicated.

Late ventricular tachycardia or ventricular fibrillation occurs rarely but is associated with a substantial excess mortality. A logical stepwise approach is useful. Noncardiac causes are identified and corrected. Cardiac anatomy, hemodynamics, and electrophysiology are defined. Therapy guided by electrophysiologic study is preferred. The hierarchy of therapies is the alleviation of ischemic potential including revascularization, antiarrhythmic drugs, and antiarrhythmic surgery and implantable devices. Ambulatory monitoring to guide therapy is an alternative in those patients (about one-third) who show adequate baseline ectopy both as a reflection of risk and as an adequate endpoint for therapy. Suppression is recommended for 90 percent or greater of repetitive forms and more than 50 to 70 percent of premature ventricular complexes. Patients with bundle branch block and anterior myocardial infarction have a high rate of ventricular fibrillation independent of warning arrhythmias. This risk window is of about 6 weeks' duration. Antiarrhythmic therapy in this unique subgroup should be individualized, and its empiric nature must be noted.

Nonsustained ventricular tachycardia is unusual but appears to be associated with an excess mortality. Symptomatic patients may undergo electrophysiologic testing when risk (inducibility into sustained ventricular tachycardia) and therapy can be addressed. The benefits of therapy are not as clear as in patients with sustained ventricular tachycardia. In patients at lower risk, those found not to be inducible, cautious therapy may still be warranted to address symptoms. Late potentials detected by signal-averaged electrocardiography appear to predict risk but are not directly affected by antiarrhythmic therapy and therefore cannot serve yet as an endpoint to guide treatment.

Premature ventricular contractions are seen in about 20 percent of patients in the recovery phase of acute myocardial infarction. This is a particularly confusing area in which risk appears defined, and proof of the benefit of therapy has eluded investigators for decades. Risk relates independently to both ventricular function, for which patients with the greatest impairment of ventricular function have the highest risk, and ventricular ectopy. Risk increases virtually with the appearance of premature ventricular complexes, becomes significant at 6 to 10 premature ventricular complexes per hour, and then abruptly plateaus. This risk occurs independently of form, although symptomatic nonsustained ventricular tachycardia is considered a more important form when it is noted.

Ambulatory monitoring of patients following acute myocardial infarction to identify ventricular ectopy followed by suppression of such ectopy by antiarrhythmic drugs has been common. Although there is some consensus on the degree of suppression of premature ventricular complexes required for statistical significance (70 to 85 percent comparing a 24-hour pre-drug to a 24-hour post-drug monitoring period), the grade of ectopy that needs treatment is unclear. Clinical trials focusing on the use of specific antiarrhythmic agents or the suppression of premature ventricular complexes have been disappointing. The preliminary results of the Cardiac Arrhythmia Suppression Trial (CAST) (CAST Coordinating Center, 1989) suggest that high-grade suppression of ventricular ectopy by the class IC agents flecainide and encainide may actually be deleterious. A single drug, moricicine remains to be evaluated in CAST. Most efforts are now being concentrated on the treatment of nonsustained forms, leaving the issue of the treatment of premature ventricular complexes more unclear than ever. It would seem prudent to monitor patients, especially when symptomatic, but controlled data denoting the efficacy of antiarrhythmic therapy are nonexistent. Some investigators suggest the treatment of complex forms, especially in patients with low ejection fractions, but this is empiric. Type 1A agents may be used with caution. Type 1B agents are less effective against premature ventricular complexes but at times are effective; mexiletine particularly may be combined with other agents. Type 1C agents should be avoided for anything less than well-documented, resistant, symptomatic, nonsustained, and sustained ventricular tachyarrhythmias until further guidelines are available. *First-line therapy is beta-adrenergic blocking agents, but all eligible patients should be receiving these drugs.*

SUGGESTED READING

CAST Coordinating Center. The cardiac arrhythmia suppression trial (CAST) investigators. Preliminary report: effects of en-

cainide and flecainide on mortality in a randomized trial of arrhythmia suppression after myocardial infarction. N Engl J Med 1989; 6:406.
Lie KL, Wellens HJ, Van Capelli FJ. Lidocaine in the prevention of primary ventricular fibrillation. A double blind randomized study of 212 consecutive patients. N Engl J Med 1974; 291:1324.
Myerburg RJ, Kessler KM. Clinical assessment and management of arrhythmias and conduction disturbances. In: Hurst JW, ed. The heart. 7th ed. New York: McGraw-Hill, 1990:535.
Myerburg RJ, Kessler KM. Management of patients who survive cardiac arrest. Mod Conc Cardiovasc Dis 1986; 55:61.
Opie LH. Adverse cardiovascular drug interactions. In: Hurst JW, ed. The heart. 7th ed. New York: McGraw-Hill, 1990:1803.
Stewart RB, Bardy GH, Greene LH. Wide complex tachycardia: misdiagnosis and outcome after emergent therapy. Ann Intern Med 1986; 104:766.
Velebit V, Podrid P, Lown B, et al. Aggravation and provocation of ventricular arrhythmia by antiarrhythmic drugs. Circulation 1982; 65:886.
Woosley RL. Antiarrhythmic agents. In: Hurst JW, ed. The heart. 7th ed. New York: McGraw-Hill, 1990:1682.

VENTRICULAR ANEURYSM DUE TO MYOCARDIAL INFARCTION

ANDRÉ L. CHURCHWELL, M.D.

Ventricular aneurysm occurs in 12 to 15 percent of patients surviving myocardial infarctions. It is considered to be one of the mechanical complications of an acute infarction and is believed to occur as part of the spectrum of infarction expansion. There are many definitions for a ventricular aneurysm, but the most widely accepted definition is based on the appearance of systolic dyskinesis and diastolic deformation noted on left ventriculography or on a radionuclide ventriculogram. In this chapter, current medical and surgical treatment strategies for ventricular aneurysms are discussed.

The clinical expression of a left ventricular aneurysm is related to a number of factors: (1) the extent to which the aneurysm "steals" a portion of the stroke volume, leading to a low output state; (2) diastolic volume overload of the left ventricle, which may lead to an elevated left ventricular end-diastolic pressure and therefore symptoms of pulmonary congestion; (3) associated coronary disease, which may lead to angina, aggravated by increased wall stress in the myocardium adjacent to the distending aneurysm; (4) scar formation in the aneurysm itself, leading to reentrant ventricular tachycardia and syncope or sudden death; and (5) thrombi in the aneurysm pouch, leading to thromboembolic events. Therefore, our therapeutic choices must address each of the cardinal manifestations of ventricular aneurysms: congestive heart failure, ventricular tachycardia, left ventricular thrombus, and recurrent angina pectoris.

THERAPEUTIC ALTERNATIVES

The mainstay of treatment for the mechanical complications of a myocardial infarct is surgical repair. This is often the case for a ventricular aneurysm that manifests the cardinal symptoms. Problems with surgery include the facts that (1) the ventricular aneurysm may occupy such a large portion of the left ventricular body that there will be no effective left ventricular cavity for an adequate end-diastolic volume and, therefore, an adequate stroke volume and (2) the nonaneurysmal portion of the left ventricle may not manifest normal contractility. Thus, when the aneurysm is removed, the patient's congestive heart failure symptoms may persist. The nonaneurysmal portion of the left ventricle may be hypocontractile owing to coexistent critical coronary artery disease or some unexpected myopathic process. There have been many studies to determine if the nonaneurysmal ventricle possesses normal or supernormal contractile indices and if the ventricle is sufficiently large enough to produce a normal stroke volume. Many cardiologists use radionuclide ventriculography and make use of the ability to use a "region-of-interest" approach to calculate the nonaneurysmal left ventricle ejection fraction and estimate its volume. Medical therapy is used for those patients who are not surgical candidates because of noncardiac factors, for patients whose aneurysm is "too large," or for patients whose normal portion of the left ventricle is sufficiently hypocontractile. It is also the treatment of choice in the asymptomatic patient.

PREFERRED APPROACH

There are no firm rules concerning medical versus surgical therapy because neither one offers the chance for an absolute cure. Following aneurysectomy, many patients require continued anticoagulation (owing to the likelihood of either continued blood stasis *or* injured endocardium, which serves as a catalyst for further thrombogenesis). In addition, despite the use of aneurysectomy and endocardial resection for ventricular tachycardia, many patients require antiarrhythmic drugs (probably due to other sites for ventricular tachycardia that were not resected or suture line [ventriculotomy]-related arrhythmias). Therefore, surgery offers no panacea, and many patients require continued medical therapy. We review the current medical and surgical treatment of the cardinal manifestations of ventricular aneurysm.

Medical Treatment

Congestive Heart Failure

The pathophysiology of heart failure in patients with a ventricular aneurysm is based on two factors: (1) the aneurysm may steal a significant portion of the forward stroke volume, leading to a decreased forward cardiac output and therefore symptoms of weakness and fatigue; (2) because the aneurysm serves as a diastolic volume overload lesion of the left ventricle, there is an increase in the end-diastolic volume and, depending on the overall compliance of the heart, an increase in the end-diastolic pressure. The elevated end-diastolic pressure leads to symptoms of pulmonary congestion (i.e., dyspnea, orthopnea, and paroxysmal nocturnal dyspnea).

I believe, as do others, that left ventricular aneurysectomy should not be performed for mild or easily controlled congestive heart failure but rather for heart failure that fails maximum outpatient medical therapy. Treatment is designed initially along the lines of standard therapy for congestive heart failure. This would involve the following:

- *Digoxin* blocks the quabain-inhibited sodium potassium adenosine triphosphatase membrane pump. It is given once a day as either 0.125 mg or 0.25 mg in a patient with normal renal function. In patients with abnormal renal function, digoxin levels are mandatory to avoid digoxin toxicity. The side effects of digoxin are noted primarily in patients with digoxin toxicity or sensitivity. Patients may become sensitized to digoxin in the presence of a normal blood level. These include patients with hypomagnesemia, hypokalemia, hypoxia, and hypocalcemia and patients with chronic obstructive pulmonary disease and hypothyroidism. The main symptoms of digoxin sensitivity or toxicity are primarily gastrointestinal in origin, i.e., nausea and vomiting. There may be increased atrioventricular node block leading to atrial tachycardia and block, accelerated junctional rhythm, and increased ventricular automaticity. This may lead to increased premature ventricular contractions, ventricular bigeminy, and bidirectional ventricular tachycardia.
- *Furosemide* (Lasix), a loop diuretic blocking the active chloride pump in the thick ascending limb of the nephron, is indicated for patients with pulmonary congestive symptoms. With normal renal function a dosage of 20 mg orally each day may be instituted. One would then increase the dosage by 20-mg increments to achieve the desired diuresis, depending on the level of the serum creatinine. In that furosemide lasts 6 to 8 hours, one often uses a twice-a-day schedule. The main side effects and complications of chronic furosemide use center around the development of intravascular volume depletion (one should use orthostatic blood pressure to monitor this), hypokalemia (leading to the increased tendency for ventricular arrhythmias), and hypochloremic alkalosis metabolic alkalosis (which leads to poorer oxygen delivery through its effect on the hemoglobin oxygen-saturation curve). The therapeutic response of furosemide is judged clinically as the loss of symptoms of pulmonary congestion and rales on the physical examination or the resolution of pulmonary edema on the plain chest roentgenogram.
- *Captopril*, a competitive inhibitor of angiotensin I converting enzymes, is also a useful medication in the treatment of patients with heart failure. It holds some theoretical value in any state of heart failure with elevated angiotensin II levels. I know of no studies that specifically address the role of captopril in patients with congestive heart failure due to ventricular aneurysm. The lack of studies does not negate the known effectiveness of captopril in improving cardiac output and diminishing pulmonary capillary wedge pressure in patients with poor left ventricular function. In that the aneurysm is a cardiac lesion associated with a "lower pressure leak," as in the case of ventricular septal defect and mitral regurgitation, one could view afterload reduction with captopril working in a similar vein. Specifically, captopril serves to diminish the arterial resistance and thus aortic impedance, such that more blood passes through the aortic valve and less into the aneurysm, thus diminishing the diastolic left ventricular volume overload state. The preload reduction features of captopril also serve to diminish pulmonary congestion.

Captopril should be considered in any patient with a left ventricular aneurysm in congestive heart failure. In patients with preexisting moderate renal impairment, captopril should be used cautiously. Patients with known bilateral renal artery stenosis have developed acute renal failure when given captopril and thus should avoid this medication. Marked hypotension has been noted in patients with intravascular volume depletion or moderate hyponatremia. A hypotensive response is not a reason to disallow use of the drug. One may replete the volume in these patients and use a smaller initial dose. We often use 3.125 mg as a starting dose in patients who have an initial systolic blood pressure between 100 and 110 mm Hg.

The total white blood count needs to be followed in patients on captopril. Leukopenia appears to occur more often in patients with renal impairment. It does appear to be reversible in the majority of cases. Lastly, we have noted a captopril-associated rash, which is often an erythematous macular eruption on the trunk and legs in elderly patients. The rash may be pruritic and resolves with discontinuation of the medication.

One may assess the therapeutic response to captopril on multiple levels: (1) follow resolution of symptoms; (2) resolution of chest roentgenogram findings of increased lung water; (3) radionuclide ventriculogram revealing an increase in the left ventricular ejection fraction.

Ventricular Tachycardia

Ventricular premature contractions are commonly associated with ventricular aneurysm. The management of isolated ventricular premature contractions is an open question given our increasing understanding of the proarrhythmic tendencies of virtually all antiarrhythmic medications. It is easier to recommend treatment of sustained ventricular tachycardia in the setting of a ventricular aneurysm. We know that such a rhythm is potentially lethal in this group of patients. The current climate is such that we offer surgical therapy to patients with malignant ventricular arrhythmias who are unresponsive to conventional antiarrhythmia therapy. Ventricular tachycardia is a more common indication for ventricular aneurysectomy than is heart failure. It is my belief that for patients who are at poor surgical risk for aneurysm/endocardial resection surgery, an automatic internal defibrillator is strongly recommended once antiarrhythmia therapy has failed.

I should hasten to add that, compared with 5 to 10 years ago, we tend to be more aggressive with surgical therapy (for those who are candidates) in the treatment of malignant ventricular arrhythmias (sustained ventricular tachycardias and ventricular fibrillation). This practice has been influenced by the poor success rate of antiarrhythmic agents in this setting.

Programmed ventricular stimulation is used to assess drug efficacy in the suppression of ventricular tachycardia. Owing to the lethal nature of these arrhythmias, drug combinations such as mexiletine and quinidine or mexiletine and procainamide may be used. If surgery again is not an option, amiodarone may also be considered. The following is a review of a brief list (not complete) of the antiarrhythmic agents noted above, which I would use in the medical treatment of sustained ventricular tachycardia in the setting of a ventricular aneurysm.

Procainamide and Quinidine. Procainamide and quinidine are both Class IA antiarrhythmic agents. They slow His-Purkinje, ventricular, and bypass tract effective refractory periods. Procainamide on a chronic basis is administered usually in the more convenient slow-release or "SR" form. This is administered to achieve a 50 mg per kilogram per day dose. Dosage guidelines for procainamide are provided in Table 1. I should note that individual drug clearance and renal function must be included in dosage considerations. As a rule, drug levels need to be used (after five half-lives of administration) to set the correct dosage for each patient.

Quinidine comes in two tablet forms. Quinidine sulfate is administered in the average adult as 200 mg orally four times a day as a starting schedule. The long-acting form, quinidine gluconate extended-release tablets, is administered typically as 324 mg orally three times a day. As opposed to procainamide, there are no schedule guidelines based on body weight. The drug dosage is adjusted again based on blood levels.

Both drugs may cause gastrointestinal distress (in the case of quinidine up to one-third of patients experience this side effect). The major concern with quinidine is its known rare risk of quinidine syncope. This is an idiosyncratic reaction to quinidine that leads to first-dose markedly prolonged Q-T interval and polymorphic ventricular tachycardia. Furthermore, during chronic use there is the concern of quinidine toxicity, resulting in a markedly prolonged Q-T interval and torsades de pointes, a very rapid form of ventricular tachycardia. Proarrhythmia noted in 10 to 20 percent in some series may occur with any antiarrhythmia medication and leads to the induction of increased ventricular premature contractions progressing to ventricular tachycardia.

Procainamide may lead to unexplained fever and to a drug-induced lupus disorder. In patients on chronic procainamide, 50 to 75 percent may develop a positive test for antinuclear antibodies. Of those that develop a positive test, approximately 25 percent will develop a clinical lupus syndrome with fever, serositis, and so forth. The lupus syndrome usually re-

TABLE 1 Dosage Guidelines for Procainamide SR

Patient Weight (kg)	*Dosage**
40–50	500 mg
60–70	750 mg
80–90	1 g
>100	1.25 g

*Given by mouth every 6 hours.
From Physicians' Desk Reference. 44th ed. Oradell, NJ: Medical Economics, 1990.

solves with discontinuation of therapy. These are the major highlights of drug-related problems; many more are discussed in more complete reviews.

Mexiletine. Mexiletine is an orally active class IB antiarrhythmic agent that is functionally analogous to lidocaine. I believe that it has small merit by itself in the suppression of lethal ventricular arrhythmias but is most efficacious when combined with quinidine or procainamide. The drug inhibits the inward sodium current, thus reducing phase 0 of the action potential. Mexiletine decreases the effective refractory period (ERP) in Purkinje fibers but with a lesser decrease in action potential duration (APD), thus leading to an increase in the ERP/APD ratio. The drug therapy is usually begun with a loading dose of approximately 400 mg, followed by 300 to 1200 mg per day in three divided daily doses. One should wait a minimum of 2 hours after the loading dose before beginning maintenance therapy. Blood levels are available to adjust the dosage schedule. The dosage should be decreased in patients with liver disease. Its main side effects—mental confusion, lethargy, dizziness, paresthesias—are a result of the drug's local anesthetic properties. The drug clinically appears to have a narrow therapeutic-toxic ratio.

Amiodarone. Amiodarone is a class III antiarrhythmic agent. Its main electrophysiologic action is the slowing of conduction diffusely and uniformly throughout the heart. It has been touted as the most effective single agent for a host of arrhythmias ranging from refractory atrial flutter to recurrent ventricular tachycardia. It does appear to be highly effective but unfortunately at a cost. Specifically, in over 10 percent of patients on chronic therapy, a severe pneumonitis develops (in some cases analogous to acute respiratory distress syndrome). We have seen high morbidity and fatality associated with this condition in our hospital, and the literature confirms this experience. There are no sure tests to predict a priori in whom this will occur, and stopping the medication and initiating steroid therapy has not lead to a uniform cure. Other complications or side effects include hyperthyroidism and hypothyroidism (owing to its similar structure to thyroid hormone). Less serious side effects include blue discoloration of the skin and corneal deposits. The drug requires a prolonged loading dose period before it reaches therapeutic blood levels and antiarrhythmic efficacy. I usually begin with 400 mg orally three times a day for 7 to 10 days and then move to a maintenance dose of 400 mg a day. One may see an onset of action after 10 to 14 days of therapy.

Left Ventricular Thrombus

The occurrence of thrombi in left ventricular aneurysms is quite high. In some autopsy reports, thrombi occur in over 90 percent of aneurysms. The presence of a thrombus in an aneurysm is related primarily to blood stasis and resultant clotting. There are no strong recommendations based on randomized series regarding the role of chronic anticoagulation in patients with left ventricular aneurysms. I adhere to the conceptual approach recently outlined by Stein and Fuster (1989). The prevalence of clinical thromboembolism for chronic aneurysm is lower than for a fresh acute anterior myocardial infarction. The incidence of embolism for chronic aneurysm has been cited to be as low as 0.35 percent per year. The fresh infarct with its injured endothelium is more likely to develop a protruding, mobile thrombus. These thrombi have been reported by echocardiography studies to be more prone to embolism. In the case of a chronic left ventricular aneurysm, the thrombus is laminated and more attached to the endocardium and thus is less likely to embolize. Consequently, Stein and Fuster do not recommend anticoagulation for chronic left ventricular aneurysm if the thrombus appears laminated and is *not* protruding into the lumen. This is a sound recommendation, but I reserve the right to use sodium warfarin (Coumadin) in those cases with mobile/protruding thrombi, for patients with *one* embolic event off Coumadin therapy, and for patients with severe globally impaired left ventricular function (including the nonaneurysmal segment).

Warfarin is used for long-term anticoagulation. The protime is adjusted to 1.2 to 1.5 times that of control. Warfarin inhibits vitamin K–dependent clotting factors. The major complication of warfarin therapy is bleeding, with major bleeding occurring at a risk of 1 percent per year. Any patient with previous bleeding history, ulcer, or recent surgery is not a candidate for warfarin therapy. Careful follow-up of stool guaiacs and hematocrits is necessary in the outpatient setting. Aspirin and other antiplatelet agents are not adequate prophylaxis against thromboembolism in this setting.

Recurrent Angina

Recurrent angina in a patient with a known left ventricular aneurysm implies that the patient has been on standard antianginal medical therapy of nitrates, calcium blockers, or beta-blockers. These patients require coronary revascularization; this is discussed later.

It is my belief that recurrent angina in a patient with left ventricular aneurysm is not due to the *aneurysm* but due to coexistent critical coronary disease. Therefore, aneurysectomy often is performed as an aside in patients undergoing coronary bypass surgery for refractory or recurrent angina.

Surgical Treatment

In most patients presenting for left ventricular aneurysectomy, the usual indications are congestive heart failure, followed by aneurysectomy taking place in the setting of a primary need for coronary bypass surgery for severe recurrent/refractory angina. Less common indications include systemic emboli (on anticoagulant therapy) and ventricular tachycardia.

In general, patients should be considered for primary aneurysectomy if they have either congestive heart failure not easily controlled by medical therapy or ventricular tachycardia resistant to traditional antiarrhythmia therapy. However, patients who have suffered sudden death or shock owing to malignant ventricular arrhythmias should probably be considered for urgent surgery rather than a trial of medication.

For patients presenting for aneurysectomy with conditions other than ventricular tachycardia, some cardiologists advocate signal-averaged electrocardiograms to determine if these patients should undergo programmed ventricular stimulation and endocardial resection at the time of surgery. This is not yet sorted out.

For patients with congestive heart failure, the only preoperative preparation includes maximal medical therapy to optimize left ventricular function as much as possible before surgery. If the patient is taking warfarin, the drug should be discontinued days before surgery to allow the vitamin K-dependent factors to become effective and therefore to decrease the postoperative coagulopathy seen after bypass surgery. The choice of operation is somewhat dependent on the location of the aneurysm. A small apical aneurysm may be plicated; however, in general, aneurysectomy involving scar tissue resection and ventriculotomy is required. Inferoposterior aneurysms are less common than apical aneurysms and are more difficult to approach surgically because of the location. Furthermore, the infarction may involve the papillary muscle of the mitral valve, and mitral valve replacement may be required for severe mitral regurgitation. This may be best determined intraoperatively with transesophageal echocardiography. One must be careful when removing the aneurysm not to dislodge the thrombus. The exposed ends of the ventricle are closed with Teflon felt and heavy sutures.

The specific problems noted in the postoperative setting relate to congestive heart failure, low output state, and new ventricular tachycardia. Congestive heart failure may persist in the postoperative state because the remaining nonaneurysmal segment was not as vigorous as expected. It may have lost its vigor because of inadequate vascularization. A low output state may result because the remaining nonaneurysmal segment is not of sufficient size to accommodate the patient's normal end-diastolic volume. Consequently, the stroke volume drops, leading to poor tissue perfusion. In addition, patients return from surgery for heart failure and in the early postoperative period may develop malignant ventricular tachyarrhythmias. It is unclear why this occurs, but it is speculated that a ventriculotomy scar or new ischemia from poor revascularization is involved. Most patients will take months to show marked improvement in function (even in uncomplicated cases), but it does occur and surgery increases their lifespan.

The approach to surgery for ventricular tachycardia has undergone major changes over the past decade. Simple aneurysectomy was not universal in its cure for ventricular tachycardia, and most patients were relegated to chronic antiarrhythmia treatment. Work by teams in Boston and Philadelphia has shown the way for endocardial mapping of ventricular tachycardia in the operating room. In an attempt to determine origin of the ventricular tachycardia, one maps the aneurysm and its adjoining endocardium in the operating room using specific programmed stimuli. Once the site of the tachycardia has been established, the aneurysectomy is performed and the adjoining endocardium that participates in the lethal rhythm is also resected. No controlled randomized trials have been performed comparing routine aneurysm resection with map-directed surgery, but data from Mason et al (1982) show that there is a 50 percent ventricular tachycardia relapse rate in the postoperative period for routine operation versus 13 percent relapse rate for the map-directed patients at Stanford. Thus, endocardial map-directed approach is considered state-of-the-art for surgery for refractory ventricular tachycardia due to a left ventricular aneurysm. The biggest concern in the postoperative period for the map-directed patients is recurrent ventricular tachycardia from *another site* not detected in the operating room. This is one of the reasons for continued postoperative need for antiarrhythmic therapy. It is interesting to note that in some series the mortality rate for elective aneurysectomy is 8 to 10 percent. If one combines the endocardial resection, the Massachusetts General Hospital surgical mortality is increased to 17 percent.

Lastly, surgical reviews reveal that demographics in our patient population are changing. Patients are becoming older, and increasing numbers of bypass grafts are being performed on patients with poorer left ventricular function. This more difficult population has been approached with minimal increase in surgical mortality owing to better surgical techniques.

SUGGESTED READING

Cohn LH. Surgical management of acute and chronic cardiac complications due to myocardial infarction. Am Heart J 1981; 102:1049.

Cosgrove DM, Lytle BW, Taylor PC, et al. Ventricular aneurysm resection—trends in surgical risk. Circulation 1989; 79(Suppl I):97.

Garan R. Perioperative and long-term results after electrophysiologically directed ventricular surgery for recurrent ventricular tachycardia. J Am Coll Cardiol 1986; 8:201.

Magovern GJ, Sakert T, Simpson K, et al. Surgical therapy for left ventricular aneurysms—a ten year experience. Circulation 1989; 79(Suppl I):102.

Mason JW, et al. Surgery for ventricular tachycardia: efficacy of left

ventricular aneurysm resection compared with operation guided by electrical activation mapping. Circulating 1982; 65:1148.
Singh BN, Opie LH, Harrison DC, Marcus FI. Antiarrhythmic agents. In: Opie LH, ed. Drugs for the heart. Orlando: Grune & Stratton, 1987.
Stein B, Fuster V, Halperin JL, Cheesboro JH. An antithrombotic therapy in cardiac disease: an emerging approach based on pathogenesis and risk. Circulation 1989; 80:1501.

CORONARY ANGIOPLASTY

JOHN S. DOUGLAS JR., M.D., F.A.C.C.

Percutaneous transluminal coronary angioplasty (PTCA) was first performed by Gruentzig in 1977 to relieve myocardial ischemia in a patient with discrete single-vessel coronary artery disease. During the subsequent decade, improvements in PTCA technology, radiographic imaging systems, and operator experience permitted a substantial broadening of indications for the technique, which today is a revascularization alternative for many patients with symptomatic coronary artery stenosis in one or more coronary arteries.

THERAPEUTIC ALTERNATIVES

The risk of angioplasty, along with its ability to relieve symptoms and favorably influence a patient's quality of life, are important issues that help to determine the place of this technique compared with that of bypass surgery and, in some patients, compared with medical therapy. Results of randomized trials comparing PTCA with coronary artery bypass grafting (CABG) and medical therapy are, unfortunately, not available. However, long-term observational studies of patients undergoing PTCA in Zurich and Atlanta have indicated an acceptable degree of safety and efficacy in the patients treated. Of Gruentzig's initial 169 patients, 133 were treated successfully with no procedural deaths and with follow-up of up to 8 years; 68 percent of the successful patients were asymptomatic and only five cardiac deaths were recorded. Restenosis occurred in 30 percent of patients, leading to CABG in 19 patients and PTCA in 27 patients. Of 427 patients who underwent PTCA at Emory University Hospital in 1981, 5-year cardiac survival was 98 percent, and 85 percent were asymptomatic at last follow-up. Repeat PTCA was required in 20 percent and CABG in 15 percent of patients. Actuarial event-free survival (freedom from cardiac death, myocardial infarction, and CABG) at 5 years was 79 percent. Single-vessel disease was present in a majority of patients in both series (58 percent and 86 percent).

In recent years, PTCA has been applied increasingly in multivessel disease. In the 1985 National Heart, Lung, and Blood Institute (NHLBI) PTCA Registry, twice as many multivessel disease patients were entered compared with those in the 1982 registry (53 percent versus 25 percent), with a higher procedural success and fewer complications. However, long-term follow-up studies of patients with multivessel disease analyzing the impact of incomplete revascularization and restenosis are limited. In over 1,000 patients with multivessel disease who underwent PTCA at Emory University Hospital, 77 percent of patients were asymptomatic at last follow-up, and freedom from cardiac death, myocardial infarction, and bypass surgery at 5 years was 95 percent, 90 percent, and 76 percent, respectively. In the 1985 NHLBI Registry, 75 percent of 402 multivessel patients were free of cardiac events (death, myocardial infarction, or CABG) at 1-year follow-up.

Because PTCA is applied most often as an alternative to CABG, the excellent symptomatic relief and long-term outlook following surgery must be considered. Operative mortality in most active centers is approximately 1 percent for the most favorable candidates, and symptomatic benefit is maintained for 5 years in approximately 70 percent of patients. However, up to 5 to 10 percent of patients require reoperation at 5 years, and the risk of in-hospital death and myocardial infarction is at least twice that encountered with the first operation. Symptomatic benefit and long-term survival following reoperation are also less favorable than with primary procedures. These facts have fostered a strategy of delaying surgery when adequate palliation can be achieved with less invasive methods.

PREFERRED APPROACH

The decision to offer PTCA to an individual patient must be made with the knowledge of the potential impact of multiple clinical variables on procedural success, risk, and long-term benefit. The risk associated with PTCA should be equal to or less than that encountered with bypass surgery or medical therapy during early and long-term follow-up. Initial results of PTCA in the first 7,254 patients at Emory University Hospital are shown in Table 1. Factors favoring success of PTCA are age less than 65 years, male gender, single-vessel disease, single-lesion PTCA, subtotal occlusion, absence of calcification, accessibility of the lesion, and normal left ventricular function.

Because acute coronary occlusion is the most common serious complication of PTCA, accounting for most of the in-hospital morbidity and mortality, the risk of the procedure is related closely to the probability of acute occlusion and the adverse consequences if this should occur. The following factors are associated with an increased risk of acute occlusion: lesion length, female gender, bend point or branch point stenosis, thrombus in situ, multiple stenoses in the vessel dilated, and multivessel disease. After completion of angioplasty, the presence of an intimal tear or dissection and a high residual translesional pressure gradient are predictors of acute closure. For patients who experience acute occlusion, the clinical variables associated with an increased mortality include age greater than 65 years, female gender, hypertension, diabetes, prior myocardial infarction, previous bypass surgery, multivessel disease, left main coronary disease, a large area of myocardium at risk, poor left ventricular function, and collaterals originating from the vessel to be dilated.

Restenosis following PTCA, observed in approximately 30 percent of patients within 3 months, is a fibrocellular proliferative reaction that is more common in the presence of certain clinical variables. These variables include unstable angina, diabetes, variant angina, multivessel disease, ostial lesions, stenoses in a proximal or midsaphenous vein graft, total occlusions, intracoronary thrombus, and suboptimal angioplasty results as indicated by a residual stenosis greater than 30 percent or a residual pressure gradient greater than 15 to 20 mm Hg.

TABLE 1 Results of the First 7,254 Consecutive Coronary Angioplasty Procedures at Emory University Hospital*

	Number	*Percentage*
Patients	7,254	—
Arterial segments dilated	8,893	—
Initial success†	6,706	93
Complication-free success‡	6,467	89
Single-vessel disease	4,772	66
Multivessel disease§	2,482	34
Multivessel PTCA‖	594	8.2
Emergency CABG	240	3.3
Q-wave acute myocardial infarction	103	1.4
In-hospital death	15	0.2

*Patients with evolving infarction are excluded.
†<50% residual stenosis.
‡<50% residual stenosis and freedom from complications.
§>50% stenosis of LAD + RCA, LAD + CIRC, CIRC + RCA, or LAD + CIRC + RCA.
‖Dilation of LAD + RCA, LAD + CIRC, CIRC + RCA, or LAD + CIRC + RCA.
PTCA = Percutaneous transluminal coronary angioplasty, CABG = coronary artery bypass grafting.

As with any treatment, selection of PTCA involves an analysis of risk and benefits for the individual patient, incorporating clinical and anatomic factors known to influence outcome. Estimates must be made of the likelihood of successful dilation, acute closure with consequent morbidity and mortality, and restenosis. The skill of the angioplasty operator and of the backup surgical and anesthesia teams must also be considered.

Recognizing the critical importance of lesion morphology in predicting procedural success or failure, the American College of Cardiology/American Heart Association (ACC/AHA) Task Force subcommittee developed a risk-stratified classification of coronary artery lesions (Ryan et al, 1988) (Table 2).

Type A lesions have characteristics that permit an anticipated procedural success rate of 85 percent or greater and a low risk of acute closure.

Type B lesions have characteristics that predict a lower success rate (60 to 85 percent), a moderate risk of acute closure, or both. Because the presence of multiple adverse lesion features increases the probability of procedural failure and acute closure, the term *complex B lesions* is used to describe a lesion with two or more adverse features.

Type C lesions have characteristics that result in a low success rate (less than 60 percent), that have a high risk of acute closure, or both.

This lesion classification may be modified as new insights are gained, but analysis of results at Emory University Hospital suggests that such a classification is useful and will stand the test of time. It should be recognized in certain instances that the likelihood of acute closure may be high, but the risk to the patient is low; examples include total occlusions and well-collateralized vessels.

Currently, the level of angioplasty experience and skill is not uniform. A patient with relatively complex anatomy selected for PTCA in an experienced angioplasty center may receive a more effective surgical revascularization if he or she were in a strong surgical center without extensive angioplasty experience. In centers with excellent PTCA and surgical skills, most patients with proximal single-vessel disease who require revascularization are treated initially with PTCA; patients with triple-vessel disease who are suitable for surgery undergo bypass grafting. Between these extremes, there is little standardization of therapy. Strategies recommended in the following patient subgroups reflect current practices at Emory Univer-

TABLE 2 Lesion-Specific Characteristics of Type A, B, and C Lesions

Type A Lesions	
Discrete (<10 mm in length)	Little or no calcification
Concentric	Less than totally occlusive
Readily accessible	Nonostial in location
Nonangulated segment, <45°	No major branch involvement
Smooth contour	Absence of thrombus
Type B Lesions	
Tubular (10 to 20 mm in length)	Moderate to heavy calcification
Eccentric	Total occlusions <3 mo old
Moderate tortuosity of proximal segment	Ostial in location
Moderately angulated segment >45°, <90°	Bifurcation lesions requiring double-guide wires
Irregular contour	Some thrombus present
Type C Lesions	
Diffuse (>2 cm in length)	Total occlusion >3 mo old
Excessive tortuosity of proximal segment	Inability to protect major side branches
Extremely angulated segments >90°	Degenerated vein grafts with friable lesion

From the ACC/AHA Task Force Report: Guidelines for percutaneous transluminal coronary angioplasty. J Am Coll Cardiol 1988; 12:529. Reproduced by permission of the publisher and authors.

sity Hospital and guidelines of the ACC/AHA Task Force Report on angioplasty.

Single-Vessel Disease: Asymptomatic or Mildly Symptomatic

Percutaneous transluminal coronary angioplasty has become the treatment of choice for many minimally symptomatic patients with significant stenosis (≥50 percent diameter reduction) in a major coronary artery that serves at least a moderate-sized area of viable myocardium. These patients should (1) have objective evidence of myocardial ischemia; (2) have been resuscitated from cardiac arrest or sustained ventricular tachycardia in the absence of acute myocardial infarction; or (3) must undergo noncardiac surgery such as repair of aortic aneurysm, iliofemoral bypass, or carotid artery surgery. Patients with little or no symptoms should have a lesion that would predict a high probability of angioplasty success and a low risk for morbidity (acute closure probability less than 5 percent) and mortality (less than 0.5 percent), i.e., a Type A or Type B lesion with favorable features. An example of a favorable Type B lesion is one with a single negative feature, such as eccentricity or irregular contour or a bifurcation lesion. In some cases, occupation or life-style may influence the selection process in favor of PTCA over medical therapy, especially if the safety of others is involved (e.g., pilots, air traffic controllers, firefighters, policemen, athletes).

Patients with symptomatic or mildly symptomatic single-vessel disease who should not undergo PTCA include those who (1) have only a small area of viable myocardium at risk, (2) do not have objective evidence of myocardial ischemia, (3) have lesions of less than 50 percent diameter reduction, (4) have Type C lesions, or (5) are in a moderate-risk or high-risk group for morbidity or mortality.

Single Vessel Disease: Symptomatic

Among the most ideal patients for PTCA are those with angina pectoris (functional Classes II to IV and unstable angina) and those with single-vessel disease who have one or more significant lesions in a major epicardial artery that subtends at least a moderate-sized area of viable myocardium. These patients (1) have objective evidence of myocardial ischemia, (2) have angina pectoris that is inadequately controlled on medical therapy, or (3) are intolerant to the side effects of medical therapy. These patients have a high likelihood for success and low risk of procedure-related morbidity and mortality, i.e., they have Type A or more favorable Type B lesions.

Patients with single-vessel disease in whom there is some divergence of opinion with respect to indications for PTCA include those who have a significant stenosis in a major coronary artery that supplies at least a moderate area of viable myocardium and those who have objective evidence of ischemia or disabling symptoms on medical therapy. Disease in these patients has the following characteristics: (1) one or more lesions predicted to have a moderate risk of morbidity (acute closure less than 8 percent) and mortality (less than 1 percent), i.e., a complex Type B, or a favorable Type C lesion; (2) disabling symptoms and a small area of viable myocardium at risk and at least a moderate likelihood for successful PTCA with low procedural risk predicted, i.e., a Type A or Type B lesion; or (3) despite significant angina, no objective evidence of myocardial ischemia and at least a moderate likelihood for PTCA success and low procedure risk, i.e., Type A or B lesions.

Patients with symptomatic single-vessel disease in whom PTCA is not indicated include those who (1) have only a small area of viable myocardium at risk in the absence of disabling symptoms, (2) have clinical symptoms not likely indicating ischemia, (3) have unfavorable lesions for PTCA, or (4) are in a high-risk group for morbidity and mortality.

Because of the excellent prognosis of single-vessel disease treated medically, it is important that the risk/benefit ratio of a PTCA procedure be carefully analyzed and that the symptoms are indeed due to the lesion targeted for dilation.

Multivessel Coronary Artery Disease: Asymptomatic or Mildly Symptomatic (Functional Class I)

The most clear-cut indication for PTCA in this patient subgroup is in the individual with one significant lesion in a major coronary artery, the successful dilation of which would result in a nearly complete revascularization because other lesions subtend small or nonviable areas of myocardium. For PTCA to be indicated, patients must (1) have a large area of viable myocardium at risk, and (2) have objective evidence of ischemia, or (3) have been resuscitated from cardiac arrest or sustained ventricular tachycardia in the absence of myocardial infarction, or (4) need to undergo high-risk noncardiac surgery. All patients in this category should have Type A or favorable Type B lesions and be in a low-risk group for morbidity and mortality.

Indications for PTCA are more controversial when patient characteristics are similar to those previously described. However, these patients have (1) moderate-sized (rather than large) areas of myocardium at risk; or (2) significant lesions in two or more major epicardial coronary arteries, each supplying at least a moderate-sized area of viable myocardium. These patients should have objective evidence of myocardial ischemia and one or more Type A or favorable Type B lesions, the dilation of which would relieve ischemia. They should be in a low-risk group for morbidity and mortality.

Patients with asymptomatic or mildly symptomatic multivessel disease in whom PTCA is not indicated include those who (1) have only a small amount of myocardium at risk; (2) have a PTCA-targeted vessel, the occlusion of which would result in cardiogenic shock; (3) have two or more major arteries with complex Type B lesions; (4) have Type C lesions in a major coronary artery supplying a moderate or large area of viable myocardium; or (5) are in a high-risk group owing to extreme left ventricular dysfunction or diffuse coronary atherosclerosis.

Multivessel Coronary Artery Disease: Symptomatic

Patients with symptomatic multivessel disease in whom PTCA is indicated include those with one dilatable lesion in a major coronary artery, which would result in nearly complete revascularization, and those with significant stenoses in each of two major coronary arteries, both subtending at least moderate-sized areas of viable myocardium. These patients with symptomatic disease should (1) have objective evidence of myocardial ischemia, (2) have angina pectoris that is poorly responsive to medical therapy, (3) have intolerable side effects on medical therapy, or (4) are judged by their attending cardiologist to need revascularization. These patients should have Type A and B lesions, for which successful dilatation would provide complete or nearly complete relief of ischemia, and should be in a low-risk to moderate-risk group for morbidity (less than 10 percent risk of acute occlusion) and mortality (less than 1 percent).

An increasing number of symptomatic patients are referred for PTCA because they are considered poor candidates for bypass surgery as a result of advanced physiologic age, coexisting medical problems, multiple prior cardiac operations, or extremely poor left ventricular function. These so-called salvage patients should have one or more Type A or B lesions that could be dilated, with resultant complete or partial relief of ischemia. Lesions selected for PTCA should have a low risk of acute closure because surgical intervention may be impossible or may carry a high risk. Many patients in this category present ethical dilemmas to the PTCA operator because of the high risk if PTCA fails.

In general, patients with multivessel disease require more intensive scrutiny prior to PTCA, with the goal of achieving symptomatic and ischemia relief at an acceptable risk. Morphologic characteristics of each lesion must be considered relative to all other lesions and to the amount of myocardium subtended. An estimate must be made of the likelihood of acute closure and the consequences likely to ensue if any or all of the dilated segments closed. For example, Type B lesions with multiple adverse features in major coronary arteries supplying a large proportion of the remaining viable myocardium may be inappropriate targets if surgery is feasible.

Patients with symptomatic multivessel disease who are not suitable for PTCA include those who (1) have only a small area of myocardium at risk in the absence of disabling symptoms, or (2) have a Type C lesion in a major coronary artery serving moderate or large areas of viable myocardium, or (3) are in an unacceptably high-risk group for morbidity and mortality.

Acute Myocardial Infarction

There is overwhelming evidence of the benefit of intravenous thrombolytic therapy in acute myocardial infarction. Because improved survival has been documented using this strategy, intravenous thrombolytic therapy has become the treatment of choice for most patients with acute myocardial infarction. The place of angioplasty in the treatment of acute myocardial infarction has been studied for the past decade, and many questions remain. Although direct PTCA appears to be extremely effective ($\geq$ 90 percent patency rate) in skilled hands, the procedure cannot often be implemented immediately, and a more common question is when to intervene with angiography and angioplasty after thrombolytic therapy has been administered. Randomized trials (European, TAMI, TIMI-2A) have shown that thrombolysis and immediate PTCA were associated with increased mortality, acute closure, emergency bypass surgery, and bleeding complications, with no improvement in left ventricular function when compared with thrombolysis and deferred PTCA. More recently, the TIMI-2B trial indicated that thrombolytic therapy and watchful waiting with utilization of angiography and PTCA only for recurrent or inducible ischemia may be a satisfactory approach.

Unfortunately, the most effective intravenous thrombolytic agents fail to reestablish flow in approximately 25 percent of patients, and reocclusion following thrombolytic therapy occurs in about 15 percent of patients with severe consequences (a twofold increase in mortality and a decrement in left ventricular function). Selection of patients for angiography and PTCA, therefore, should be carried out in a way that would include patients in whom thrombolytic therapy has failed, those who are not candidates for thrombolytic therapy (patients with hypertension, active peptic ulcer disease, recent surgery), and patients with successful thrombolytic therapy but with ischemia producing atherosclerotic lesions. In general, PTCA in the setting of acute myocardial infarction should be confined to the infarct-related artery.

Patients referred for angiography and PTCA in our practice include those who (1) have severe, persisting angina in spite of thrombolytic therapy (reperfusion failures), recurrent ischemia following thrombolytic therapy (reocclusion), or inducible ischemia by stress testing at 5 to 7 days following thrombolytic therapy; (2) present in cardiogenic shock; (3) have symptoms compatible with acute myocardial infarction but have conditions that prevent a definitive diagnosis (permanent pacemaker or left bundle branch block); (4) present at a time when immediate angiography and direct PTCA would be possible; (5) have recurrent ventricular tachycardia or ventricular fibrillation or both in spite of antiarrhythmic therapy; (6) experience non-Q-wave infarction; or (7) are relatively young or have physically demanding jobs or life-styles.

Patients in whom angioplasty is not performed are those who (1) have residual stenosis less than 50 percent, (2) have Type C lesions, (3) have high-risk lesions for PTCA (for which bypass surgery or medical therapy would be a better option), or (4) have PTCA targets in vessels other than the infarct-related artery.

Angioplasty Procedure

Patients undergoing elective PTCA may be admitted to the hospital the day of the procedure in a fasting state. Aspirin 160 to 325 mg and diltiazem 60 mg are administered orally prior to angioplasty. In patients with very unstable angina and in those with lesion-associated thrombus or recent infarction, attempts are made to stabilize the patient on intravenous heparin, aspirin, and intensive medical treatment for 3 to 7 days before the PTCA. There is an increased risk of acute occlusion in patients who cannot be stabilized and in whom emergency PTCA is required. Patients generally receive 10,000 units of heparin intravenously after vascular access is achieved and 5,000 units of heparin per hour during the procedure. Intravascular sheaths are usually removed 3 hours after the angioplasty in elective patients, and patients with ideal angioplasty results are discharged the next morning. Many patients receive overnight heparinization when intracoronary thrombus is recognized, if a very unstable lesion necessitates emergency PTCA, or if considerable intimal disruption or dissection is induced. In multivessel PTCA, dilation of one or more lesions may be deferred to the following day, if the initial PTCA results are not optimal, if procedural time or the amount of contrast media administered is excessive, or if acute closure of all dilated sites would result in cardiogenic shock. Following PTCA, patients receive aspirin 160 to 325 mg daily, diltiazem 60 mg four times a day, and topical nitrates during their hospitalization. Prior to discharge, patients receive instructions regarding a low-fat diet, exercise, cessation of smoking, and a follow-up procedure plan. In some patients, a stress evaluation may be appropriate before discharge to assess the results of angioplasty. Following discharge, patients take aspirin 160 to 325 mg once daily. If all areas of myocardial ischemia have been relieved by angioplasty, antiangina medications may be discontinued.

SUGGESTED READING

Anderson HV, Talley JD, Black AJR, et al. Usefulness of coronary angioplasty in asymptomatic patients. J Am Coll Cardiol 1990; 65:35.

Gruentzig AR, King SB, Schlumpf M, Siegenthaler W. Long-term follow-up after percutaneous transluminal coronary angioplasty, the early Zurich experience. N Engl J Med 1987; 316:1127.

Gruentzig AR, Senning A, Siegenthaler WE. Nonoperative dilation of coronary-artery stenosis: percutaneous transluminal coronary angioplasty. N Engl J Med 1979; 301:61.

Ryan TJ, Faxon DP, Gunnar RM, et al. ACC/AHA Task Force Report Guidelines for percutaneous transluminal coronary angioplasty. J Am Coll Cardiol 1988; 12:529.

Talley JD, Hurst JW, King SB, et al. Clinical outcome 5 years after attempted percutaneous coronary angioplasty in 427 patients. Circulation 1988; 77:372.

Weintraub WS, Jones EL, King SB III, et al. Changing use of coronary angioplasty and coronary bypass surgery in the treatment of chronic coronary artery disease. J Am Coll Cardiol 1990; 65:183.

CORONARY BYPASS SURGERY

MICHAEL A. KUTCHER, M.D., F.A.C.C.

Coronary bypass surgery is a therapeutic alternative to treat significant obstructive coronary atherosclerotic heart disease by improving coronary blood flow via surgically placed bypass conduits.

In 1967, Favaloro et al reported the successful use of aortocoronary artery saphenous vein grafts in patients with severe obstructive coronary disease. The successful utilization of the internal mammary artery as a conduit to bypass coronary obstructions was described by Green in 1970. Since that time, improvements in anesthesia, cardiopulmonary bypass, myocardial preservation, preparation of graft material, surgical technique, and postoperative care have made coronary bypass surgery acceptable, safe, and effective in appropriate patients.

THERAPEUTIC ALTERNATIVES

Once coronary atherosclerotic heart disease has been identified and the extent of disease has been documented by physiologic and anatomic parameters, the three major goals of therapy are

- Relief of angina
- Prevention of myocardial infarction
- Promotion of longevity

To determine which modality may best achieve the three goals in an individual patient—the safest, most effective way—coronary bypass surgery must be compared with medical therapy and coronary angioplasty.

PREFERRED APPROACH

Appropriate clinical settings for the application of coronary bypass surgery are outlined in Table 1.

Assessment

Key technical issues to consider in assessing patients for bypass surgery include the suitability of distal coronary vessels for grafting, the degree of anticipated revascularization (complete versus incomplete), and a reasonable left ventricular function to permit successful disengagement of cardiopulmonary bypass. Additional clinical factors include age, body habitus, functional state, and presence of other major medical problems, which may preclude the benefits of the procedure by increasing the risk of complications.

Results of Trials

As a result of several randomized and observational trials, coronary bypass surgery is accepted as being superior to medical therapy in eliminating or improving the quantity and quality of angina. Furthermore, successful surgery results in improved objective indices of functional capacity and myocardial ischemia. However, patients with significant single-vessel disease may be served as well by percutaneous transluminal coronary angioplasty as by revascularization, but subsets of significant double-vessel and triple-vessel disease may be served with either coronary angioplasty or coronary bypass surgery. The results of several major randomized trials comparing angioplasty with surgery for angina relief, morbidity, mortality, and long-term patency will be available by the mid 1990s. The major American trials in progress include the Emory Angioplasty and Surgery Trial (EAST) and the Bypass Angioplasty Revascularization Investigation (BARI). Until definitive recommendations come from these trials, the indications, risks, and benefits of the two revascularization alternatives must be weighed for each individual patient.

Coronary bypass surgery is definitely superior to medical therapy for mildly symptomatic or even asymptomatic patients with significant obstructive left main disease. In addition, recent reports of the long-term follow-up of randomized trials indicate a beneficial effect of surgery on mortality in mildly symptomatic patients with triple-vessel disease and with reduced left ventricular function. However, these same trials have not detected a reduction in mortality in surgically treated patients with single-

TABLE 1 Indications for Coronary Bypass Surgery

Assume: —acceptable coronary anatomy for grafting
— not amenable to coronary angioplasty
— ejection fraction >20%
Angina unresponsive to optimal medical therapy
Significant single-, double-, or triple-vessel disease
—moderate to severe symptoms
—strongly positive exercise test
—major amount of myocardium at jeopardy
Significant triple-vessel disease
—mild symptoms
—compromised left ventricular function
Significant left main disease
—regardless of symptoms or signs
Acute myocardial infarction
—onset of chest pain within 6 hours
—thrombolytic therapy contraindicated or failed
Failed coronary angioplasty attempt
—acute or threatened vessel closure
Second restenosis of coronary angioplasty site
Adjunctive to valve or aortic surgery
—significant single-, double-, or triple-vessel disease
—regardless of symptoms or signs

vessel or double-vessel disease. The subset of patients with stable angina, critical three-vessel obstructions, and excellent left ventricular function is still controversial, but coronary bypass surgery may be acceptable in this setting, depending on individual factors.

Benefit/Risk

The benefits of coronary bypass surgery, compared with medical therapy and coronary angioplasty, are that surgery provides a more direct approach to improve coronary blood flow and a more effective or complete revascularization.

The percentages of risks and complications of a "standard" coronary bypass procedure are as follows: mortality 1 percent, myocardial infarction 4 percent, reoperation for bleeding 2 percent, infection 1 percent, cerebrovascular accident 1 percent, and arrhythmia 10 percent. The more complex and unstable the case, the higher the risk. Risk for an individual patient must be carefully assessed.

The incidence of graft closure at 1 year is 10 percent with an internal mammary graft and 25 percent with a saphenous vein graft. At 10 years, the internal mammary has an 85 percent patency rate compared with only a 50 percent patency rate with saphenous vein grafts. Obviously, if at all possible, at least one internal mammary graft should be used in a coronary bypass procedure to ensure the best chances of long-term patency.

Preoperative Preparation

The patient should be continued on an antianginal regimen up to the time of surgery. Some surgeons have expressed concern about intraoperative and postoperative variations in systemic vascular resistance in patients treated with high-dose nifedipine. It might be well to reduce nifedipine or eliminate it if possible before coronary bypass surgery.

If surgery is elective, aspirin should be discontinued approximately 7 to 10 days before the procedure. This obviates the increased bleeding tendencies during surgery in patients on chronic aspirin therapy. It is still debatable whether pretreatment with dipyridamole offers any benefit in reducing platelet adhesiveness and thus improving chances of long-term graft patency without increasing the bleeding time during surgery. Continuation of a postoperative antiplatelet regimen of at least 325 mg of aspirin every day is an acceptable practice. Another acceptable option is to add dipyridamole 75 mg three times a day to the regimen.

Risk Factor Reduction

The long-term benefits of revascularization surgery are improved with attention paid to reduction of risk factors. Patients should stop smoking, maintain reasonable body weight, control blood pressure, and lower blood lipids. An exercise rehabilitation program after surgery is a key element in recovery. Regular exercise should be continued in the long-term.

SUGGESTED READING

Califf RM, Harrell FE, Lee KL, et al. The evolution of medical and surgical therapy for coronary artery disease: a 15 year perspective. JAMA 1989; 261:2077.

CASS Principal Investigators and Their Associates. Coronary artery surgery study: a randomized trial of coronary artery bypass surgery; survival data. Circulation 1983; 68:939.

Detre K, Peduzzi P, Murphy M, et al and the Veterans Administration Cooperative Study for Surgery for Coronary Arterial Occlusive Disease. Effect of bypass surgery on survival in patients in low- and high-risk subgroups delineated by the use of simple clinical variables. Circulation 1981; 63:1329.

European Coronary Surgery Study Group. Long term results of prospective randomized study of coronary artery bypass surgery in stable angina pectoris. Lancet 1982; 2:1173.

Favaloro RG, Effler DB, Groves LK. Severe segmental obstruction of the left main artery and its divisions: surgical treatment by the saphenous vein graft technic. J Thorac Cardiovasc Surg 1970; 60:469.

Hultgren HN, Peduzzi P, Detre K, et al. The five-year effect of bypass surgery on relief of angina and exercise performance. Circulation 1985; 72 (Suppl V):79.

MITRAL STENOSIS

ROBERT C. SCHLANT, M.D.

Mitral stenosis is narrowing or obstruction of the mitral valve orifice. The normal mitral valve circumference is approximately 10 cm, and the mitral valve area is approximately 4 to 6 cm^2.

Mitral stenosis almost always results from postinflammatory reactions to acute rheumatic fever, although a history of rheumatic fever is seldom obtained in more than 50 to 60 percent of patients. Rarely, mitral stenosis can be the result of congenital valve defects, infective endocarditis with a large vegetation, left atrial myxoma, calcified mitral annulus, malignant carcinoid, systemic lupus erythematosus, or methysergide therapy. A viral etiology has not been established.

THERAPEUTIC ALTERNATIVES

Medical therapy can lessen the symptoms in patients with mild to moderate mitral stenosis, but medical therapy is only slightly effective when the stenosis is very severe. Basic medical therapy consists of the following: advice regarding the avoidance of occupations associated with significant physical exertion, a decrease in physical activity, limited sodium intake (2 g sodium or 5 g sodium chloride per day), and diuretics to decrease pulmonary congestion or peripheral edema. If atrial fibrillation is present (either paroxysmally or chronically), it is important to avoid rapid heart rates and to control the ventricular response rate with the use of digoxin, at times in combination with a beta-blocker, diltiazem, or verapamil. Two types of prophylaxis are important: prophylaxis to prevent recurrence of streptococcal infection and prophylaxis to prevent infective endocarditis during procedures potentially associated with bacteremia. When the stenosis becomes moderately severe (1.0 to 1.5 cm^2) or severe (less than 1.0 cm^2), medical therapy is no longer sufficient and it is necessary to increase the mitral orifice, either by surgery or by catheter balloon valvuloplasty (CBV). In general, medical therapy for patients with moderate or severe mitral stenosis is of limited value in the relief of symptoms in view of the fixed, mechanical obstruction.

PREFERRED APPROACH

Medical Treatment

The normal mitral valve orifice in the adult is 4 to 6 cm^2. As the orifice becomes progressively narrowed, it produces no significant hemodynamic obstruction until it is rather markedly narrowed. The narrowing is probably hemodynamically insignificant down to 2.6 cm^2; when it is between 2.1 and 2.5 cm^2 (very mild mitral stenosis), it is usually responsible for symptoms only with marked exertion, pregnancy, tachycardia, or marked anemia. Narrowing between 1.6 and 2.0 cm^2 (mild mitral stenosis) is associated with symptoms with moderate exertion but not with light exertion, unless this is associated with marked tachycardia, pregnancy, thyrotoxicosis, or mitral regurgitation (Fig. 1). When the valve area is narrowed to between 1.0 and 1.5 cm^2 (moderately severe mitral stenosis), most patients will experience symptoms with light exertion. Symptoms and signs of pulmonary congestion are especially likely to occur when the area is 1.2 cm^2 or less. When the mitral valve area is reduced to the critical area of 1.0 cm^2 or less, symptoms occur with very mild exertion. A mitral valve area of 0.3 to 0.4 cm^2 is about the smallest area compatible with life.

At any orifice size, the patient's symptoms are influenced by the patient's total body size or body surface area, activity, heart rate and the total duration for diastolic flow per minute, and conditions (e.g., anemia, exertion, fever, emotional stress, associated mitral regurgitation) that increase flow across the mitral orifice. In some patients, mitral stenosis is very slowly progressive; in other patients, the disease is more rapid, progressive, and severe. In some areas of the world, severe mitral stenosis is not uncommonly encountered in teenage patients.

Approximately 10 to 20 percent of patients with mitral stenosis develop pulmonary vascular disease and disproportionate pulmonary hypertension. In these patients, symptoms of right heart failure (e.g., hepatomegaly, ascites, peripheral edema) may become prominent. The pulmonary hypertension, which in part is due to pulmonary arteriolar vasoconstriction, may be improved significantly with the relief of the mitral stenosis.

Although most patients with mitral stenosis have progressively severe dyspnea and fatigue with exertion, a few, very rare patients unconsciously decrease their physical activity and assume that their exertional fatigue and dyspnea are normal consequences of aging. These rare, nearly asymptomatic patients must be evaluated on the basis of objective data. Exercise testing is often useful in these patients to assess the duration of exercise and to observe the patient during the exercise.

Some patients with mild or moderate mitral stenosis have episodic symptoms of pulmonary congestion only during conditions that cause an increase in cardiac output and heart rate, such as pregnancy, fever, exertion, emotional stress, anemia, or paroxysmal atrial fibrillation or flutter. Some of these patients have only mild symptoms once the precipitating event has passed and can be managed successfully medically, although the recurrence or

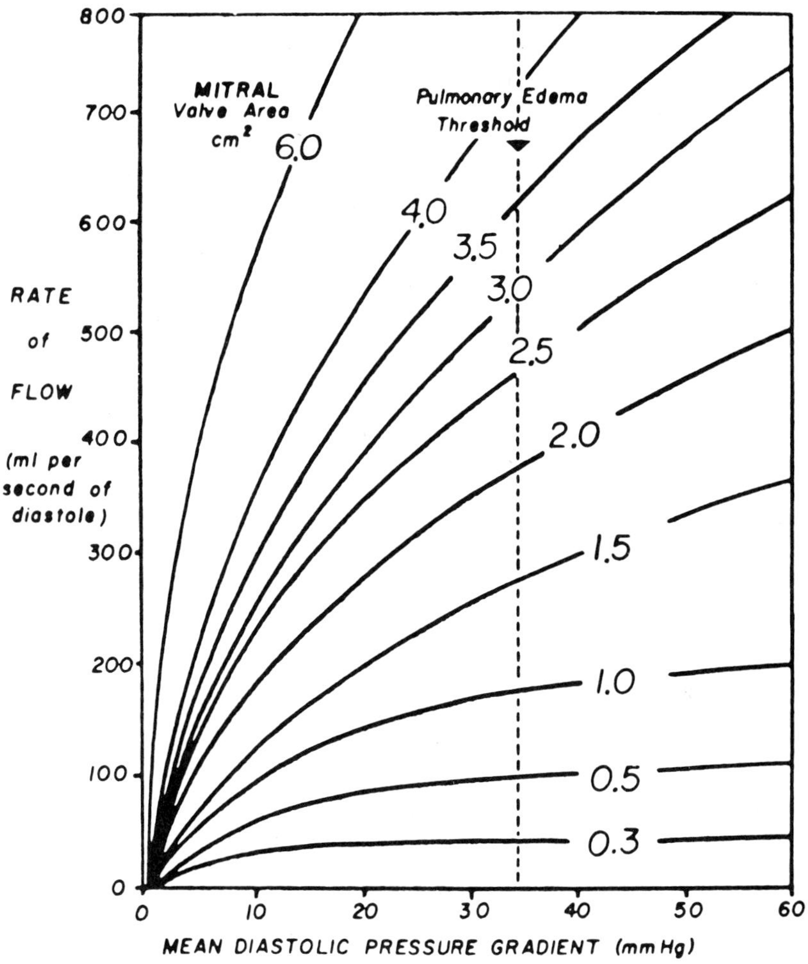

Figure 1 Diagram illustrating the relationship between mean diastolic gradient across the mitral valve and rate of flow across the mitral valve per second of diastole, as predicted by the Gorlin and Gorlin formula. Note that when the mitral valve area is 1.0 cm^2 or less, very little additional flow can be achieved by an increased pressure gradient. Transudation of fluid from the pulmonary capillaries and the development of pulmonary edema begins when pulmonary capillary pressure exceeds the oncotic pressure of plasma, which is about 25 to 35 mm Hg. It is also apparent that severe mitral regurgitation is incompatible with very tight mitral stenosis. (Reproduced from Schlant RC. Altered cardiovascular function in rheumatic heart disease. In: Hurst JW, Logue RB, eds. The heart. New York: McGraw-Hill, 1966:505; with permission of the publisher and editor.)

persistence of symptoms may require surgery (or balloon valvuloplasty) for alleviation.

As the stenosis becomes more severe, most patients unconsciously will decrease their physical activity to avoid major symptoms of dyspnea and fatigue on exertion. The progressive development of moderately severe dyspnea on exertion, decreased exercise tolerance, paroxysmal nocturnal dyspnea, peripheral edema, and acute pulmonary congestion are generally signs for the initiation of diuretic therapy, low salt diet, and the possibility of mechanical enlargement of mitral orifice.

Prophylaxis Against Rheumatic Fever and Infective Endocarditis

It is important to diagnose mitral stenosis even when the patient is asymptomatic to initiate appropriate prophylaxis against recurrent streptococcal infection. Once the diagnosis is established, I prefer to maintain the patients on prophylaxis against recurrent streptococcal infection with daily oral penicillin V 250 mg twice daily. Alternatively, one can use sulfadiazine (0.5 g twice a day) or monthly intramuscular injections of 1.2 m units of benzathine penicillin G. The latter, however, is associated with some discomfort and may also elevate the sedimentation rate. Oral erythromycin 250 mg twice daily is used for individuals allergic to penicillin and sulfadiazine. In most patients, prophylaxis is continued indefinitely; the only exceptions are the few patients older than 40 years who have very few contacts with other individuals.

Prophylaxis against infective endocarditis during dental or respiratory tract procedures is accomplished by using either penicillin V (2 g orally 1 hour before the procedure and 1 g 6 hours later) or amoxicillin (3 g orally 1 hour before, then 1.5 g 6 hours later). For genitourinary or gastrointestinal surgery or instrumentation, a combination can be used of ampicillin (2 g intramuscularly or intravenously) and gentamicin (1.5 mg per kilogram intramuscularly or intravenously) 30 minutes to 1 hour before the procedure and repeated 8 hours later.

Diet

A low-sodium diet (2 g sodium or 5 g sodium chloride) is fundamental to therapy and should be initiated early. In most instances it is also appropriate to have the patient follow a low-fat, low-cholesterol phase I American Heart Association diet. All patients should not use tobacco.

Diuretics

For most patients with any symptoms of inappropriate dyspnea on exertion, the use of a thiazide diuretic is appropriate. This can be given in doses equivalent to 25 mg of hydrochlorothiazide once a day. If patients are able to take adequate orange juice, bananas, and other fruits, potassium supplementation may not be necessary; however, serum potassium levels should be monitored to avoid hypokalemia. Some patients require the addition of a supplement of potassium chloride. In a few patients, a combination of thiazide with triamterene or amiloride to avoid hypokalemia may be useful. If the congestion does not respond to therapy with thiazide, the use of furosemide (20 to 80 mg daily) may be necessary. For severe failure, combination diuretic therapy with furosemide and either a thiazide diuretic or metolazone may be instituted. Patients on diuretics should weigh themselves each morning. This often allows patients to detect an asymptomatic weight gain and to take an extra diuretic to prevent more severe symptoms.

Heart Rate and Rhythm

An increase in heart rate results in a decreased time for diastolic flow across the mitral orifice. This, in turn, results in an increase in pressure in the left atrium and pulmonary veins and capillaries. Accordingly, an excessive heart rate both at rest and during exercise should be avoided. If the patient has normal sinus rhythm, it may be necessary to employ a beta-blocker to slow the heart rate and to prevent excessive heart rate increases during exercise. If the patient develops atrial fibrillation, digoxin should be employed to control the ventricular response rate, both at rest and during moderate exercise. An average dose of digoxin is 0.25 mg daily, with a range from 0.125 to 0.75 mg daily. In most patients, the ventricular response rate at rest and during moderate exercise (up two flights of stairs or walking a long hallway rapidly) can be used as an index of the appropriate dosage. Rare patients with atrial fibrillation treated with digoxin therapy once a day have an increase in their ventricular response rate in the early morning hours. In such patients, the institution of twice-daily therapy may provide a more uniform control of heart rate. If the ventricular response rate during exercise is not well controlled with digoxin, the addition of diltiazem, verapamil, or a beta-blocker often permits better control. The development of chronic atrial fibrillation usually signifies the presence of severe mitral stenosis.

Acute paroxysmal atrial fibrillation may precipitate acute pulmonary edema. It usually can be controlled satisfactorily with intravenous digoxin. Alternately, intravenous verapamil can be used. Many patients have recurrent paroxysmal atrial fibrillation before the fibrillation becomes chronic. These patients should be maintained on therapy both with digoxin to ensure reasonable control of the ventricular response during the paroxysms and with quinidine (or procainamide) to lessen the likelihood of recurrence.

Because most patients with severe mitral stenosis who have atrial fibrillation will have recurrence of the atrial fibrillation if it is converted back to sinus rhythm (unless the severe stenosis is mechanically relieved), it is seldom appropriate to repeatedly convert atrial fibrillation either pharmacologically or electrically. The risk of systemic embolization may increase with cardioversion even for patients who are on warfarin anticoagulation for 4 to 6 weeks. Whenever cardioversion (electrical or pharmacologic) is performed on a patient with mitral stenosis, there is a small but real risk of systemic embolization. In general, patients with mitral stenosis undergoing cardioversion of atrial fibrillation that may have been present for more than 24 hours should be on warfarin anticoagulation for 4 to 6 weeks before cardioversion. Quinidine is usually started 24 to 48 hours before electrical cardioversion. If the cardioversion is successful, quinidine (or procainamide) and digoxin are continued indefinitely, as long as the patient is in normal sinus rhythm, to lessen the likelihood of recurrence of atrial fibrillation and to control the ventricular response rate if it does recur. The potential for systemic embolism each time cardioversion is performed decreases the appropriateness of conversion in patients who have recurrent episodes of atrial fibrillation despite adequate quinidine. Such patients are better left in chronic atrial fibrillation until the severe stenosis is relieved. Conversely, for patients with only mild or moderate mitral stenosis and atrial fibrillation of less than a few days' or months' duration, a trial of electrical cardioversion after anticoagulation with warfarin for 4 to 6 weeks may be successful for a number of months or years and may improve symptoms significantly.

Arterial Vasodilators

Arterial vasodilators are of limited value in patients with isolated mitral stenosis and may occasionally increase cardiac output and worsen the symptoms of pulmonary congestion.

Anticoagulation

Patients with moderately severe or severe mitral stenosis have an increased risk of left atrial thrombus and systemic embolization even if they are in normal sinus rhythm. This risk is much greater with the onset of atrial fibrillation. The preferred medical therapy to decrease the risk of arterial embolization consists of the use of warfarin (Coumadin) in dosage to prolong the prothrombin time to 1.3 to 1.5 times normal using North American rabbit brain thromboplastin, which corresponds to an international normalized ratio (INR) prothrombin time suppression of 2.0 to 3.0. The relative risks of therapy with warfarin must be balanced against potential side effects, such as gastrointestinal bleeding or bruising, and consideration of patient characteristics, especially the likelihood of falling, chronic alcoholism, or noncompliance with medications. For patients in whom warfarin therapy is not appropriate, aspirin (325 mg enteric-coated daily) may be used with only a slight hazard of gastritis.

Whenever possible, thromboembolism during episodes of paroxysmal atrial fibrillation should be prevented by the prompt initiation of intravenous heparin therapy and the subsequent conversion to warfarin therapy. It is usually well to maintain the warfarin therapy for about 1 month after the reversion to normal sinus rhythm. Patients with very frequent episodes of paroxysmal atrial fibrillation or chronic atrial fibrillation should be maintained on long-term warfarin anticoagulation indefinitely.

Complications

Hoarseness may develop from enlargement of the left pulmonary artery and tension on the recurrent laryngeal nerve. *Chest pain* resembling angina pectoris can be caused by right ventricular hypertension, coronary embolism, or associated coronary atherosclerosis. *Hemoptysis* should be treated with intravenous furosemide, control of the ventricular heart rate (by using a beta-blocker if there is normal sinus rhythm and by using intravenous digoxin and occasionally a beta-blocker if the rhythm is atrial fibrillation), sedation, and the upright position. Blood transfusion may be necessary.

Patients who have a *systemic or cerebral embolus* often require long-term rehabilitation. Patients who sustain a systemic embolus should be evaluated for mitral valve surgery, although some patients have systemic embolization in association with mild mitral stenosis that is no more severe than that produced by a prosthetic valve. Most patients with mitral stenosis who have had a systemic embolus should be maintained on long-term warfarin anticoagulation sufficiently to prolong the prothrombin time to 1.5 to 2.0 times control using North American rabbit brain thromboplastin (standardized INR = 3.0 to 4.5) for at least one year, following which the prothrombin time may be reduced to 1.3 to 1.5 times control to lessen the risk of bleeding.

Side Effects of Therapy

The major side effects of diuretic therapies are the development of dehydration, hypotension, hypokalemia, and hypomagnesemia and the precipitation of digitalis toxicity. The major side effects of digoxin include anorexia, nausea, and cardiac arrhythmias, particularly premature ventricular complexes, especially in a bigeminal rhythm, and atrial tachycardia, especially with atrioventricular block. In fact, virtually any cardiac rhythm disturbance can be produced by excess digitalis. One should always consider digitalis toxicity when the patient's rhythm changes either from regular to irregular or from irregular to regular.

Interventional or Surgical Treatment

The development of progressively severe symptoms and progressively decreased exertional tolerance despite medical therapy is usually an indication for mechanical relief of the mitral stenosis, by either surgery or CBV in highly selected patients. Surgical treatment consists of "closed" or "open" commissurotomy, "open" valvuloplasty, or mitral valve replacement. All such therapies should be considered to be palliative.

As noted previously, most patients have minimal, if any, symptoms if the mitral orifice is greater than 2.5 cm². Symptoms usually develop and become progressively severe as the stenosis decreases from 2.5 cm² to 1.5 cm², which is often considered the valve orifice below which surgery or CBV may be indicated. Mechanical relief of the stenosis is indicated in virtually all patients with an orifice of 1.0 cm² or less. The development of severe mitral stenosis may be clinically apparent by the progressive decrease in exercise tolerance with an increase in severity of dyspnea and fatigue on exertion, the occurrence of hemoptysis, the development of pulmonary congestion on chest roentgenogram, or evidence of progressive increase in the severity of the mitral stenosis on Doppler echocardiography.

Doppler echocardiography is usually the best objective test with which to follow patients who have mitral stenosis. When the stenosis is mild and slowly progressive, this can be performed at 5-year intervals; when the stenosis becomes more severe, echocardiography should be performed at 1-year or 2-year intervals or even more frequently. It is important not only to assess the estimated pressure difference across the mitral valve but also to evaluate the degree of mobility of the valve leaflets, the amount of thickening of the valve leaflets, the amount of valve calcification, the status of the subvalvular apparatus, and the presence or absence of left atrial thrombus and mitral regurgitation. These variables help determine whether CBV or commissurotomy is likely to be effective.

In symptomatic younger patients who have mitral valves that are not very thickened or heavily calcified, who are still mobile, and who do not have evidence of significant subvalvular fusion of chordae tendineae or significant mitral regurgitation, CBV is an effective modality of therapy, but only if this can be performed by a very skilled team. In most other patients, surgery is usually preferred. *Surgery* may be either closed or open mitral commissurotomy, open valvuloplasty, or valve replacement. In general, commissurotomy is used for patients with valvular characteristics that are similar to those desired for patients undergoing CBV. In general, mitral commissurotomy or CBV is effective in decreasing symptoms for 5 to 20 years, after which it may be necessary to implant an artificial valve, although occasionally a second commissurotomy or valvuloplasty can be performed. The long-term results of CBV are not yet available but are likely to be similar to the results of closed mitral commissurotomy.

In young patients with classic symptoms and signs and excellent Doppler and echocardiographic evidence of tight mitral stenosis, *cardiac catheterization* prior to surgery may not be necessary. In patients in whom there are any significant differences between the clinical and echocardiographic estimates of severity, cardiac catheterization is advisable. Catheterization is also advisable to evaluate the coronary arteries in older or middle-aged patients with risk factors for coronary artery disease.

Prosthetic Valve Selection

In a young female patient who wishes to become pregnant, it is advisable to implant a bioprosthesis. It is not necessary to employ chronic warfarin anticoagulant therapy, which is teratogenic, if there is normal sinus rhythm. On the other hand, it is useful to employ routine warfarin anticoagulation for 3 months after implantation in such patients to decrease thromboembolic events. If a patient with a mechanical ball or disk valve prosthesis, all of which require life-long warfarin anticoagulation to prevent thromboembolism, wishes to become pregnant, it is necessary to convert the warfarin therapy to subcutaneous heparin two or three times a day. This should be accomplished before the patient becomes pregnant and should be maintained at least during the first trimester and the last few weeks of pregnancy.

In other patients, the choice of a prosthetic heart valve is often determined locally based upon many variables. The major advantage of bioprostheses is the lack of need for chronic warfarin anticoagulation unless there is chronic atrial fibrillation. Bioprostheses tend to have accelerated fibrosis and calcification when inserted in young patients (up to 30 to 35 years of age) or in patients with chronic renal insufficiency. Mechanical bioprostheses may have an advantage in durability, but all require life-long anticoagulation.

Postoperative Care

Some patients with normal sinus rhythm develop atrial fibrillation at the time of mitral valve surgery. These patients should undergo cardioversion to restore the rhythm to normal either before leaving the hospital or within the 4 to 8 weeks following hospitalization. If reversion is accomplished, patients should be maintained on quinidine sulfate or procainamide for 6 months following reversion to normal sinus rhythm to lessen the likelihood of reversion of atrial fibrillation. In those patients who have chronic atrial fibrillation prior to mitral valve surgery, there is less likelihood of postoperative reversion. Such patients should be maintained on long-term warfarin anticoagulation, and an attempt at electrical cardioversion should be made several months postoperatively. If cardioversion is successful, the patient should be maintained on both digoxin and either quinidine sulfate or procainamide. If normal sinus rhythm cannot be maintained after one or two conversions, the patient should be maintained on digoxin to control the ventricular rate and on chronic warfarin anticoagulation; however, quinidine or procainamide should be discontinued.

Warfarin anticoagulation should be maintained routinely for at least 3 months following closed or open mitral commissurotomy, open valvuloplasty, insertion of a mitral bioprosthesis, or CBV. In most patients the prothrombin time should be prolonged to 1.3 to 1.5 times control using North American thromboplastin (INR = 2.0 to 3.0) after commissurotomy, valvuloplasty, or implantation of a bioprosthesis for the first 3 months. The prothrombin time should be prolonged to a level of 1.5 to 2.0 times control (INR = 3.0 to 4.5) in patients with a history of systemic embolization, evidence of thrombus at surgery, or chronic atrial fibrillation treated with long-term warfarin therapy. After 3 months, warfarin may be discontinued in the former patients if the results of the procedure were thought to be satisfactory and if the rhythm is normal sinus. For patients in the latter group, the dosage of warfarin is adjusted after 3 months to maintain the prothrombin time prolongation to 1.3 to 1.5 times control (INR = 2.0 to 3.0).

Patients who have a mechanical prosthetic heart valve should be treated with long-term warfarin sufficiently to prolong the prothrombin time to 1.5 to

2.0 times control (standardized INR = 3.0 to 4.5), starting soon after surgery. These patients should also be considered for long-term therapy with dipyridamole (400 mg per day), particularly if there is a history of systemic embolism. Indefinite warfarin anticoagulation is indicated in all patients with mechanical bioprostheses, in patients with chronic atrial fibrillation with a dilated left atrium, and in many patients with a history of systemic embolization.

It is especially important to use appropriate postoperative prophylaxis against infective endocarditis whenever patients are in situations likely to be associated with bacteremia.

The postpericardiotomy syndrome is manifest by symptoms and signs of pericarditis, at times with fever, pleural effusion, and pleurisy. Most patients respond well to nonsteroidal anti-inflammatory agents, although occasional patients require corticosteroids.

SUGGESTED READING

Bansal RC, Shah PM. Usefulness of echo-Doppler in management of patients with valvular heart disease. Curr Probl Cardiol 1989; 14:281.

Cheitlin MD. The timing of surgery in mitral and aortic valve disease. Curr Probl Cardiol 1987; 12:69.

Committee on the Prevention of Rheumatic Fever and Bacterial Endocarditis of the American Heart Association. Prevention of bacterial endocarditis. Circulation 1984; 70:1123A.

Cosgrove, Stewart WJ. Mitral valvuloplasty. Curr Probl Cardiol 1989; 14:353.

Dalen JE, Hirsch J, eds. Second ACCP Conference on Antithrombotic Therapy, Chest 1989; 95(Suppl):1S.

Kaye D. Prophylaxis for infective endocarditis: an update. Ann Intern Med 1986; 104:419.

Kulick DL, Kawanishi DT, Reid CL, Rahimtoola SH. Catheter balloon valvuloplasty in adults. Curr Probl Cardiol 1990; 15:500.

Nishimura RA, Holmes DR Jr, Reeder GS. Percutaneous balloon valvuloplasty. Mayo Clin Proc 1990; 65:198.

Rahimtoola SH. Perspective on valvular heart disease: an update. J Am Coll Cardiol 1989; 14:1.

Schlant RC, Nutter DO. Heart failure in valvular heart disease. Medicine 1971; 50:421.

Wood P. An appreciation of mitral stenosis. Br Med J 1954; 1:1051.

MITRAL VALVE BILLOWING AND PROLAPSE

JOHN B. BARLOW, M.D.
WENDY A. POCOCK, M.B.

As a result of their cineangiographic observations of abnormal bulging of the bodies of mitral leaflets, Criley et al introduced in 1966 the term *prolapse of the mitral valve.* Few cardiologists or cardiac surgeons have not addressed this conundrum, and many have contributed to the scientific literature. Attempts to assess so-called mitral valve prolapse based principally on variable echocardiographic criteria and with ongoing use of Criley's terminology are misleading and compound the present confusion. Webster's dictionary defines prolapse as "the slipping out of place or falling of some internal organ." Prolapse, whether intermittent or permanent, implies disease and is abnormal (e.g., hemorrhoids or prolapse of the rectum, the uterus, or the lens of the eye). It is thus regrettable that the term is used even when the valve anomaly is mild, clinically silent, and functionally normal.

In accord with the morphologic observations of cardiac surgeons, such as Carpentier, Duran, and Yacoub in Europe, Cosgrove, Kay, and Spencer in the United States, and Antunes in our surgical unit, who have had to evaluate anatomy and function before attempting a reconstructive procedure, we define mitral valve prolapse as failure of leaflet coaptation, resulting in displacement of an involved leaflet's *edge* toward the left atrium. Unless a leaflet is fibrosed, shortened, or retracted or has a cleft or hole in it, a mitral valve is competent throughout systole because of sustained coaptation of leaflets (Fig. 1 *A* through *D*). If leaflets are normal in size, or larger, failure of sustained apposition must result in prolapse of a leaflet edge and mitral regurgitation (Fig. 1 *E* through *H*).

The terms *billowing*, *floppy*, and *flail* also require definition in the context of correlating the clinical evaluation with mitral valve functional anatomy. Normal mitral leaflets bulge slightly, after closure, into the left atrial cavity. When this physiologic bulging is exaggerated, the term billowing is appropriate. Billowing, and its more advanced form floppy, are *anatomic* terms that describe the leaflet *bodies*. There is a gradation of mild billowing of near-normal leaflet bodies toward the left atrium during ventricular systole to marked displacement when the leaflets are voluminous, or floppy, and the chordae are elongated. A floppy mitral valve, albeit anatomically pathologic, may also remain functionally competent throughout systole. Prolapse, and its more advanced form flail, reflect failure of leaflet *edge* apposition and therefore essentially describe valve *function*. Two-dimensional echocardiography contributes to the evaluation of both the rheumatic

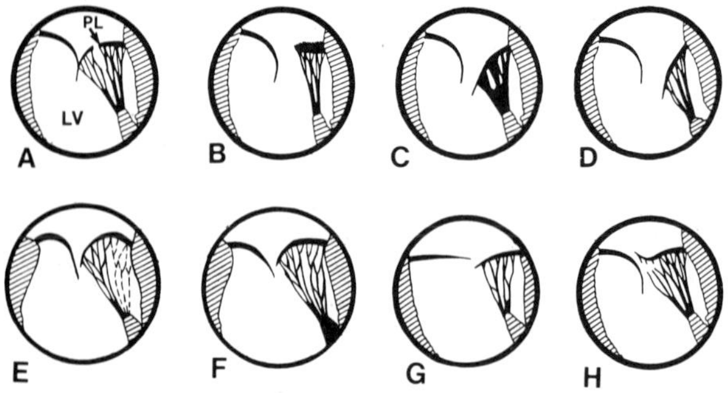

Figure 1 The mechanisms of mitral regurgitation. Some possible causes are mentioned. *A*, Perforation or cleft in a leaflet. *B*, Scarred and shortened leaflet due to chronic rheumatic heart disease or mitral annular calcification. *C*, Retracted and tethered leaflet, the result of shortened chordae tendineae in chronic rheumatic carditis. *D*, Failure of leaflet apposition because of papillary muscle retraction by a left ventricular aneurysm. *E*, Primary degeneration of mitral valve resulting in leaflet billowing, lengthened chordae tendineae, annular dilatation and failure of leaflet edge apposition (Barlow's syndrome). *F*, Failure of leaflet apposition due to papillary muscle dysfunction secondary to occlusive coronary artery disease. *G*, Marked annular dilatation causing anterior leaflet prolapse in acute rheumatic carditis. *H*, Flail leaflet with ruptured chordae due to infective endocarditis, trauma, or of unknown cause. PL = Posterior leaflet, LV = left ventricle.

and degenerative processes that may involve the complex mitral valve mechanism and result in functional prolapse, but the echocardiographic appearances are essentially different because functional anatomy is different (Fig. 2). The degenerative condition, widely and often inappropriately referred to as primary mitral valve "prolapse," affects principally the leaflet bodies. However, in our environment, where fulminant acute rheumatic carditis is prevalent, we have observed both echocardiographically and at surgery that the markedly dilated annulus allows lengthening of chordae tendineae with consequent supervention of true prolapse of the relatively normal anterior leaflet and thus mitral regurgitation. Redundancy and billowing of the leaflet bodies are seldom associated features.

In the degenerative nonrheumatic condition that provokes widespread interest in developed countries, billowing of the leaflet bodies, which has been the principal echocardiographic criterion for the prolapse misnomer, can range from a variant of normal to clearly pathologic floppy leaflets (Fig. 3). With markedly billowing or floppy leaflets, failure of leaflet edge apposition (prolapse) may indeed ensue, but the prolapse is seldom demonstrable on echocardiography until it becomes severe or manifests as a flail leaflet. Clinical auscultation for the appropriate apical regurgitant murmur, particularly if it is late or pansystolic, remains the most reliable and practical method for evaluating mitral regurgitation. Doppler techniques continue to have pitfalls, and the color Doppler criteria for mild mitral insufficiency that has pathologic significance still require clarification.

In addition to rheumatic carditis, which remains prevalent in Third World countries, there are many pathologic conditions affecting the papillary muscles, chordae tendineae, annulus, leaflets, or the size and shape of the left ventricular cavity that may result in a billowing mitral leaflet (BML) and mitral valve prolapse (MVP). When such BML and MVP is secondary or is an associated entity, the prognosis is determined as much or more by the underlying or coexisting condition. This is well exemplified in Western countries by a BML or MVP secondary to hypertrophic cardiomyopathy or occlusive coronary artery disease.

Discussion is confined in the remainder of this section to management of the degenerative condition, which still provokes so much interest and which, in its severe form, is now recognized as the most frequent cause of pure mitral regurgitation requiring surgery in developed countries.

THERAPEUTIC ALTERNATIVES

Preferred Approach

Medical Treatment

The Syndrome. We use the term BML syndrome for what is also variously called primary MVP, floppy valve, myxomatous leaflet, click-murmur, or Barlow's syndrome. Idiopathic or primary MVP syndrome is a misnomer in the many patients who have no evidence, principally on auscultation, of mitral insufficiency. A distinction between BML syndrome alone and that with MVP is crucial in formulating a management policy. The physician has to decide whether repeated auscultation, vasoactive maneuvers, echocardiography, or Doppler ultrasonography will help to determine whether regurgitation is present. As already intimated, echocardiographic criteria for BML are suspect, but the demonstration of advanced billowing, or floppy, bodies of leaflets would be compatible with clinically suspected mitral regurgitation.

The importance of making the diagnosis of primary BML syndrome, particularly in symptomatic patients, lies in the knowledge that in the large majority of cases reassurance can and should be given that significant heart disease is not present and that the prognosis for life is excellent. The BML may be focal, involving only a portion of one scallop, usually the middle scallop of the posterior leaflet, or it may be more advanced and diffuse. A constant or intermittent nonejection systolic click may be heard. Depending on the criteria used, two-dimensional

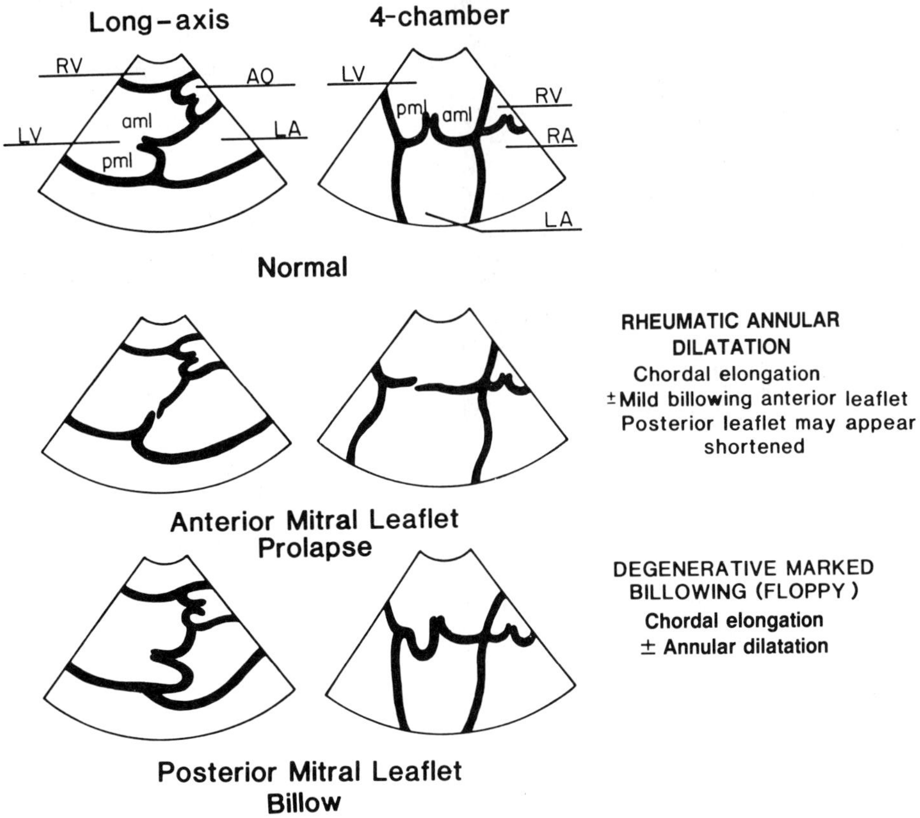

Figure 2 Two-dimensional echocardiographic appearance during systole of normal, prolapsed, and billowing mitral valves in the parasternal long axis and apical four-chamber views. In the normal valve the leaflets coapt. In rheumatic mitral prolapse, the annulus is dilated and the free edge of the prolapsing anterior leaflet is displaced beyond the line of valve closure. In degenerative mitral billow, the body of the posterior leaflet bulges into the left atrium (LA), but the leaflet margins usually appear coapted. Principal functional anatomic features are listed in the right column. Ao = Aorta, LV = left ventricle, pml = posterior mitral leaflet, RA = right atrium, RV = right ventricle. (From Barlow JB, et al. Mechanisms and management of heart failure in active rheumatic carditis. S Afr Med J 1990; in press. Reproduced by permission of publisher and authors.)

echocardiography may indicate part of a leaflet body on the left atrial side of the annulus. The valve is competent and a "normal variant." Nonetheless, if the patient is symptomatic owing to chest pain or palpitations, he or she should seek assistance and the medical adviser should be wary before concluding that the symptoms are not causally related to the valve anomaly. It is now acknowledged—and this complication is addressed later in more detail—that ventricular arrhythmias may supervene when mitral leaflets are markedly billowing or floppy. It has yet to be demonstrated that a BML does not indeed cause chest pain, albeit by an unknown mechanism or mechanisms.

Many symptomatic patients are anxious. Reasons for anxiety in patients with primary BML are not always apparent, and the role of a causally related autonomic disorder requires confirmation. Anxiety supervenes in some patients after an incorrect diagnosis of occlusive coronary artery disease has been made or when no interpretation of the chest pain, sometimes allegedly severe, has been offered. An explanation that there is "a very mild but also very common anomaly of a heart valve which sometimes causes ill-understood symptoms of nuisance value only," is a comprehensible explanation from which the patient can derive reassurance. Excessively anxious patients with chest pain who fail to respond to reassurance may often improve on a small dose of a beta-adrenergic blocking drug such as propranolol (Inderal). Chest pain and an abnormal electrocardiogram are prominent features of both the primary BML syndrome and occlusive coronary artery disease; thus the differentiation of these two conditions is a prevalent problem in clinical practice. Although this differentiation is clearly more

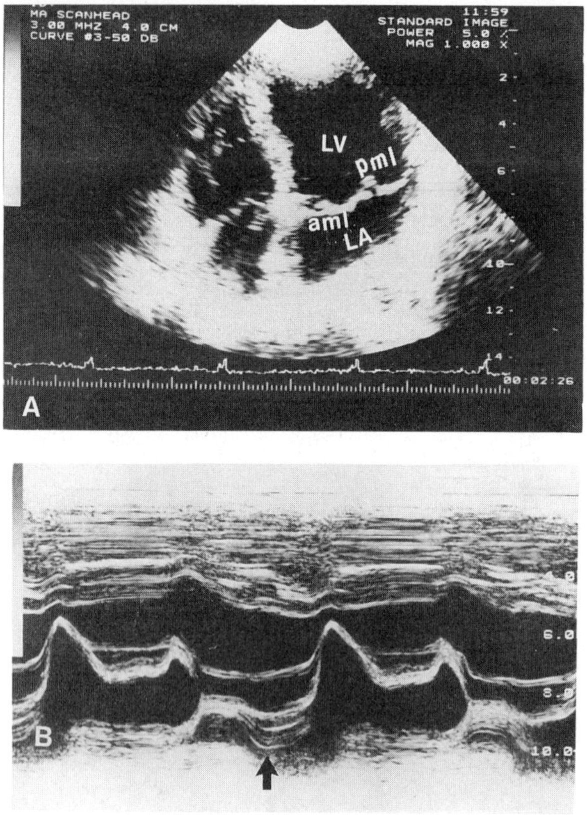

Figure 3 *A*, Two-dimensional echocardiogram, apical four-chamber view, demonstrates moderate billow of the anterior (aml) and posterior (pml) mitral leaflets. Both leaflets are thickened. Although the edges coapt on the ventricular side of the mitral annulus, a grade 3/6 late systolic murmur (indicative of prolapse) is present. (From Barlow JB, Pocock WA. Mitral leaflet billowing and prolapse. Implications for management. Cardiovasc Drugs Ther 1988; 1:543. Reproduced by permission of publisher and authors.) *B*, M-mode echocardiogram of the same patient illustrates marked late systolic billow of the posterior mitral leaflet. LA = Left atrium, LV = left ventricle.

difficult in a middle-aged man than in a young woman, careful history taking and stress electrocardiography should resolve the problem. The widely held belief that the postexercise ST-segment and T-wave changes of MVP are indistinguishable from those of myocardial ischemia, and hence are a cause of a false-positive stress test, is no longer valid. These electrocardiographic abnormalities can be reliably differentiated according to their time-course patterns after cessation of exercise. Radionuclide studies or selective coronary arteriography seldom should be necessary.

Most patients with the BML syndrome follow a benign course, but complications may sometimes ensue. In addition to the auscultatory, electrocardiographic, and anatomic features of the syndrome originally identified in 1965, other components include skeletal abnormalities, arrhythmias, conduction defects, systemic emboli, hereditary factors, and possibly autonomic disorders and myocardial dysfunction. A major contribution of two-dimensional echocardiography is that it can demonstrate whether the leaflet bodies are floppy and thickened (see Fig. 3). Patients with such leaflets do indeed make up a subgroup in that a majority of them have associated true MVP, with consequent mitral regurgitation, and are thus at increased risk for important complications such as infective endocarditis, spontaneous progression of the mitral regurgitation, and systemic emboli. Moreover, voluminous leaflets and lax chordae predispose some patients to life-threatening ventricular arrhythmias.

Infective Endocarditis and Progression of Mitral Regurgitation. Whether symptomatic or not, patients with MVP will invariably have a more marked BML, and both prophylaxis against infective endocarditis and observation for progression of the mitral regurgitation are mandatory. Most nonpansystolic murmurs, whether confined to early or late systole, do not change over many years. Nonetheless, rapid progression of MVP, even in the absence of infective endocarditis, may occur unpredictably. However, unequivocal billowing on echocardiography or a loud nonejection systolic click on auscultation do not imply that MVP, let alone severe MVP, will inevitably ensue.

Systemic Emboli. Bland emboli manifested as transient ischemic attacks or partial strokes are a recognized but rare complication of a prominent BML. Deposits of fibrin and platelet thrombi on the atrial surface of a floppy posterior leaflet may be the site of origin. We suggest that coronary embolism with coronary artery spasm is a possible mechanism for unexplained myocardial infarction in some cases of marked BML. A purported association of MVP and migraine requires confirmation and clarification, as does a possible common role of increased platelet aggregability in both conditions. We recommend antithrombotic therapy only in patients who have had emboli. We have had good results with aspirin (150 to 300 mg daily) plus dipyridamole (Persantin) (100 mg three times daily), although the effectiveness of dipyridamole as an antithrombotic agent has been challenged recently. When systemic emboli are recurrent or large or if an underlying supraventricular tachyarrhythmia is suspected, warfarin (Coumadin) therapy should be added.

Arrhythmias and Sudden Death. Palpitations, lightheadedness, or dizziness suggest the presence of arrhythmias, but exercise electrocardiography or ambulatory monitoring is advisable for evaluation. Arrhythmias may occur without symptoms, and, conversely, dizziness and palpitations have been prominent complaints at times when electrocardiographic monitoring and clinical examination provide no objective confirmation. Orthostatic hypotension should be excluded in all patients with these symptoms. A wide variety of arrhythmias has been encountered with the primary BML syndrome and includes supraventricular tachycardia, atrial fibrillation and flutter, atrial ectopic beats, ventricular tachycardia, and ventricular fibrillation. Ventricular extrasystoles are the most prevalent rhythm disturbance, may be unifocal or multifocal, may occur with or without an abnormal resting electrocardiogram, and occasionally display the R-on-T phenomenon. They are often precipitated or aggravated by emotion and exercise. If symptoms are troublesome, even if the arrhythmias are not potentially dangerous, patients should be given the benefit of treatment with antiarrhythmic drugs, preferably verapamil (Isoptin) (if supraventricular) or beta-blocking agents.

A reliable history of syncope, provided that it occurs outside of a context of probable vasovagal syncope, is cause for major concern. Ambulatory monitoring and stress testing are then mandatory to detect multiform ventricular extrasystoles, the R-on-T phenomenon, or ventricular tachycardia. Although any antiarrhythmic drug or beta-receptor blocking agent may contribute to therapy, we have had favorable experience with the unique beta-receptor blocking agent sotalol (usual dose range 80 to 320 mg daily). Because of its important class III activity, sotalol has the potential to precipitate ventricular tachycardias of the torsade de pointes variety and should be used with caution in high dosage or in the presence of hypokalemia. Amiodarone (Cordarone), 200 to 400 mg daily after a loading dose, is effective in the treatment of refractory ventricular tachyarrhythmias, but serious side effects militate against its long-term use, especially in young patients. The management of potentially lethal arrhythmias, in accordance with electrophysiologic drug testing, by overdrive pacing or with implantable defibrillator devices are approaches that require further study.

Approximately 100 patients with the BML syndrome and unexpected sudden death have been reported. Identification of patients at higher risk is crucial. A prominent BML, demonstrable on M-mode or two-dimensional echocardiography, and indisputable MVP, evaluated clinically by a constant apical late systolic murmur that becomes louder and longer on standing, are pertinent features. Abnormal T waves and ventricular ectopy detected on the resting electrocardiogram, multiform ventricular ectopy on exercise or ambulatory monitoring, and, most importantly, a history of unexpected syncope are other risk factors. Should patients continue to exhibit dangerous arrhythmias despite therapy with sotalol, amiodarone, or other antiarrhythmic measures, the question of mitral valve surgery arises, which is discussed next.

Surgical Treatment

Severe Mitral Regurgitation. Largely because of imprecise terminology, the frequency of progressive mitral regurgitation requiring surgery in patients with BML or MVP remains unknown. Studies undertaken retrospectively or based principally on suspect echocardiographic criteria suggest that the overall frequency is approximately 5 percent, that at least two-thirds are male, and that the majority are older than 50 years. Neither we nor, to our knowledge, other investigators have followed prospectively for 10 or more years a meaningful number of unselected patients with constant late or early systolic murmurs, intermittent systolic murmurs judged mitral in origin, or isolated nonejection clicks. The follow-up study by Düren et al in Amsterdam (1988) of symptomatic patients with MVP and late or pansystolic murmurs suggests that progression to severe mitral regurgitation requiring surgery may occur in at least 10 percent. This high figure relates to a selected group of patients with established mitral regurgitation and does not provide data that dispute an anticipated excellent prognosis for patients with clinical and echocardiographic signs of a BML alone. It does confirm, however, that prognosis should be more guarded and regular observation more important in patients with MVP and constant apical late systolic murmur.

Indications for surgery in patients with severe MVP and hemodynamically important mitral regurgitation may be modified by whether or not valve repair is judged feasible. If clinical, echocardiographic, and sometimes cineangiocardiographic evaluation indicate rupture of chordae to the middle scallop of the posterior leaflet, a McGoon type valvuloplasty is reasonably certain to be successful and should be attempted. In such instances, we are more aggressive regarding earlier surgery and have operated on patients with class II symptoms, especially when relatively young (under about 60 years of age). When both leaflets are shown echocardiographically to be floppy and thickened, the annulus dilated, and a number of chordae elongated or ruptured, there is more difficulty in deciding on the timing of surgery. A few surgeons claim that mitral valve repair can be performed successfully in at least 80 percent of such cases. However, the prospects of a failed valvuloplasty, a long period on cardiopulmonary bypass, and obligatory valve replacement with its enhanced valve-related morbidity and mortality risks still influence a large majority of cardiologists and cardiac surgeons toward both postponing surgery until the patient is significantly symptomatic and insisting that the patient leave the hospital with a "normal" mitral valve, hence settling for valve replacement. We encourage relatively early surgery with Carpentier ring valvuloplasty, but decisions inevitably depend much on the surgeon's ability and experience of this procedure.

Potentially Fatal Arrhythmias. A policy of surgical valvuloplasty for ventricular arrhythmias in patients with the BML syndrome without significant MVP and hemodynamically important mitral regurgitation may seem unduly aggressive. On the other hand, technically difficult valvuloplastic procedures for severe mitral regurgitation are generally successful, and similar operations in patients with mild mitral regurgitation are relatively easy. Although only about 100 instances of unexpected sudden death due to a markedly BML are known to us, it is likely that the valve abnormality is not always recognized at necropsy and that many cases are not reported. High-grade ventricular tachyarrhythmias have been documented in some patients prior to the fatal event, and ventricular fibrillation probably accounts for the sudden death. The mechanisms proposed to explain the enhanced ventricular irritability in MVP include tugging on the papillary muscles, asynchronism of myocardial relaxation, endocardial friction, coronary embolism, and "diastolic dumping." Virtually all these are dependent on voluminous and excessively mobile mitral leaflets. Successful surgical results obtained by reduction in leaflet size and shortening of the chordae favor the operation of one or more of these mechanisms. Provided that a surgeon experienced in valvuloplastic procedures is available, we regard the combination of an advanced BML demonstrated echocardiographically, a reliable history of syncope, and potentially lethal ventricular arrhythmias as indications for mitral valve repair. Mitral valve replacement, however, with its need for anticoagulation and attendant risks of thromboembolism or hemorrhage, is probably not justified in these patients in whom surgery is essentially prophylactic.

SUGGESTED READING

Barlow JB, Bosman CK, Pocock WA, Marchand P. Late systolic murmurs and non-ejection ("mid-late") systolic clicks. An analysis of 90 patients. Br Heart J 1968; 30:203.

Barlow JB, Pocock WA. Billowing, floppy, prolapsed or flail mitral valves? Am J Cardiol 1985; 55:501.

Barlow JB, Pocock WA. Mitral leaflet billowing and prolapse. In: Barlow JB, ed. Perspectives on the mitral valve. Philadelphia: FA Davis Co, 1987:45.

Boudoulas H, Kolibash AJ, Baker P, et al. Mitral valve prolapse and the mitral valve prolapse syndrome: a diagnostic classification and pathogenesis of symptoms. Am Heart J 1989; 118:796.

Carpentier A. Cardiac valve surgery—the "French correction." J Thorac Cardiovasc Surg 1983; 86:323.

Düren DR, Becker AE, Dunning AJ. Long-term follow-up of idiopathic mitral valve prolapse in 300 patients: a prospective study. J Am Coll Cardiol 1988; 11:42.

Marcus RH, Sareli P, Pocock WA, et al. Functional anatomy of severe mitral regurgitation in active rheumatic carditis. Am J Cardiol 1989; 63:577.

Marks AR, Choong CY, Sanfillipo AJ, et al. Identification of high-risk and low-risk subgroups of patients with mitral-valve prolapse. N Engl J Med 1989; 320:1031.

Pini R, Greppi B, Kramer-Fox R, et al. Mitral valve dimensions and motion and familial transmission of mitral valve prolapse with and without leaflet billowing. J Am Coll Cardiol 1988; 12:1423.

MITRAL REGURGITATION

ALBERT E. RAIZNER, M.D.
CRAIG O. SIEGEL, M.D.

Mitral regurgitation may result from acute or chronic damage to any component of the mitral valve apparatus, including the valve annulus, leaflets, chordae tendineae, and papillary muscles. Mitral regurgitation may be acute or chronic. The most common etiologies of acute mitral regurgitation are ischemic heart disease, infective endocarditis, and rupture of the chordae tendineae. The most common causes of chronic mitral regurgitation are myxomatous degeneration of the leaflets, rheumatic heart disease, ischemic heart disease, and calcification of the mitral annulus. Mitral regurgitation may also be secondary to left ventricular enlargement from any cause. The diagnosis is usually suggested by an apical systolic murmur on physical examination. Doppler echocardiography has become the mainstay of noninvasive diagnosis. Additionally, Doppler and two-dimensional echocardiography are used to estimate the severity of valvular dysfunction and left ventricular chamber size and function and thereby to follow the course of the disease and the response to treatment.

Understanding the pathophysiology of mitral regurgitation is vital to the rational management of patients with the disorder. Acutely, volume overload of the left ventricle with regurgitation into a noncompliant left atrium produces pulmonary venous congestion and pulmonary hypertension. Congestive heart failure symptoms occur abruptly and are often severe. Further, the acutely volume-overloaded left ventricle cannot immediately compensate, and a low output state is often seen. In chronic mitral regurgitation, progressive dilation of the left ventricle and atrium occurs. The dilated and compliant left atrium provides a low impedance for regurgitant flow across the mitral valve. Symptoms of congestive heart failure occur late in the course of the disease and are often insidious in origin. Despite a marked increase in preload, indices of left ventricular systolic function often remain normal until late in the course of the disease. The timing of surgical intervention remains an important and challenging part of the management of patients with mitral regurgitation.

THERAPEUTIC ALTERNATIVES

Asymptomatic patients with mild degrees of mitral regurgitation may require little if any specific therapy. However, medical management is appropriate for the symptomatic patient with more severe degrees of regurgitation. Vasodilators, specifically those agents that reduce systemic arterial pressure, or afterload, are the cornerstones of treatment and may be administered intravenously in the acute setting or orally in the chronic setting. Digitalis glycosides and diuretics are used frequently as well. Arrhythmias, particularly atrial flutter and fibrillation, are encountered commonly and are treated with specific antiarrhythmic medications. In acute mitral regurgitation, intravenously administered inotropic agents and, in some cases, insertion of an intra-aortic balloon may be necessary. Patients with ischemic mitral regurgitation may be candidates for revascularization with coronary angioplasty or coronary artery bypass surgery. Surgical options include repair of the mitral valve apparatus or valve replacement using either a bioprosthetic or mechanical prosthetic valve.

PREFERRED APPROACH

To establish appropriate therapy, several critical questions must be addressed. (1) Is the mitral regurgitation acute or chronic? (2) Is it primary or secondary? What is the likely etiology? (3) Is the patient symptomatic? (4) What is the severity of valvular dysfunction? (5) What is the status of left ventricular function? A generalized schema of management is shown in Figure 1.

Medical Treatment

Acute Mitral Regurgitation

The patient presenting with acute mitral regurgitation should be evaluated by two-dimensional and Doppler echocardiography. By so doing, the diagnosis of mitral regurgitation can be confirmed. This is particularly important in patients with acute myocardial infarction in whom the traditional hallmark of clinical diagnosis, the systolic murmur, is often absent. Echocardiography may help to establish a specific etiology of mitral regurgitation. Additionally, the severity of valvular dysfunction, including measurement of regurgitant fraction, and qualitative and quantitative assessment of left ventricular function may be ascertained. Patients who are hemodynamically unstable require Swan-Ganz catheter insertion to monitor pulmonary artery and pulmonary capillary wedge pressure as well as to measure cardiac output. Although many of these patients will require surgical intervention, initial stabilization with aggressive medical therapy is generally advisable. Central to this approach is the use of vasodilator therapy. By reducing left ventricular afterload, the regurgitant flow into the left atrium is reduced and forward cardiac output is enhanced. Additionally, left ventricular volume may decrease, thereby reducing the size of the mitral annulus and the regurgitant orifice. This latter effect may be of particular benefit in patients with secondary forms of acute mitral regurgitation.

The drug of choice for afterload reduction in the acute setting is sodium nitroprusside. A balanced vasodilator, nitroprusside relaxes both arterial and venous vascular smooth muscle. The drug is administered via a continuous intravenous infusion. It must be protected from light to prevent degradation. The initial dose is 0.5 μg per kilogram per minute. The infusion is titrated for the desired hemodynamic effect to a maximum dose of 10 μg per kilogram per minute. A fall in systemic vascular resistance, a decrease in pulmonary capillary wedge pressure, and a rise in cardiac output indicate a satisfactory hemodynamic response. Cyanide toxicity, manifested as headache, vomiting, depressed mentation, or coma, is a major concern with the use of nitroprusside, occurring more frequently in the setting of renal insufficiency. Thiocyanate levels should be monitored during prolonged infusion and should not exceed 6 mg per deciliter.

In patients who are intolerant to nitroprusside, intravenous nitroglycerin may be used to achieve afterload reduction. The drug is particularly useful in the setting of underlying ischemic heart disease. The infusion is started at 10 μg per minute and is titrated to achieve an optimal hemodynamic effect. It is imperative to monitor cardiac output frequently when intravenous nitroglycerin is used; because nitroglycerin is a more potent venodilator, a fall in pulmonary capillary wedge pressure may occur with no change or even a decrease in cardiac output.

If the cardiac output is low or if other parameters of left ventricular systolic function are abnormal, the addition of an inotropic agent is beneficial. Dobutamine, a synthetic sympathomimetic amine that stimulates predominantly beta$_1$-receptors, is administered by continuous intravenous infusion. The usual starting dose is 2.5 μg per kilogram per minute and may be titrated up to 15 μg per kilogram per minute. Therapeutic doses range from 5 to 10 μg per kilogram per minute. Hemodynamically, one sees a rise in cardiac output coupled with a mild to modest fall in systemic vascular resistance; heart rate is minimally changed, and arrhythmogenic potential is negligible.

Dopamine, the catecholamine precursor of norepinephrine, is a sympathomimetic amine with multiple hemodynamic effects mediated through its binding to alpha, beta, dopaminergic, and serotonin receptors. Its hemodynamic effects depend on the dose used. In doses of 2 to 5 μg per kilogram per minute, the predominant effect is one of improved renal blood flow; cardiac contractility is only mildly enhanced. In doses ranging from 5 to 10 μg per kilogram per minute, cardiac contractility is increased with little effect on peripheral vascular resistance. Consequently, this dose range is most efficacious in patients with mitral regurgitation. Doses above 10 μg per kilogram per minute may produce a significant

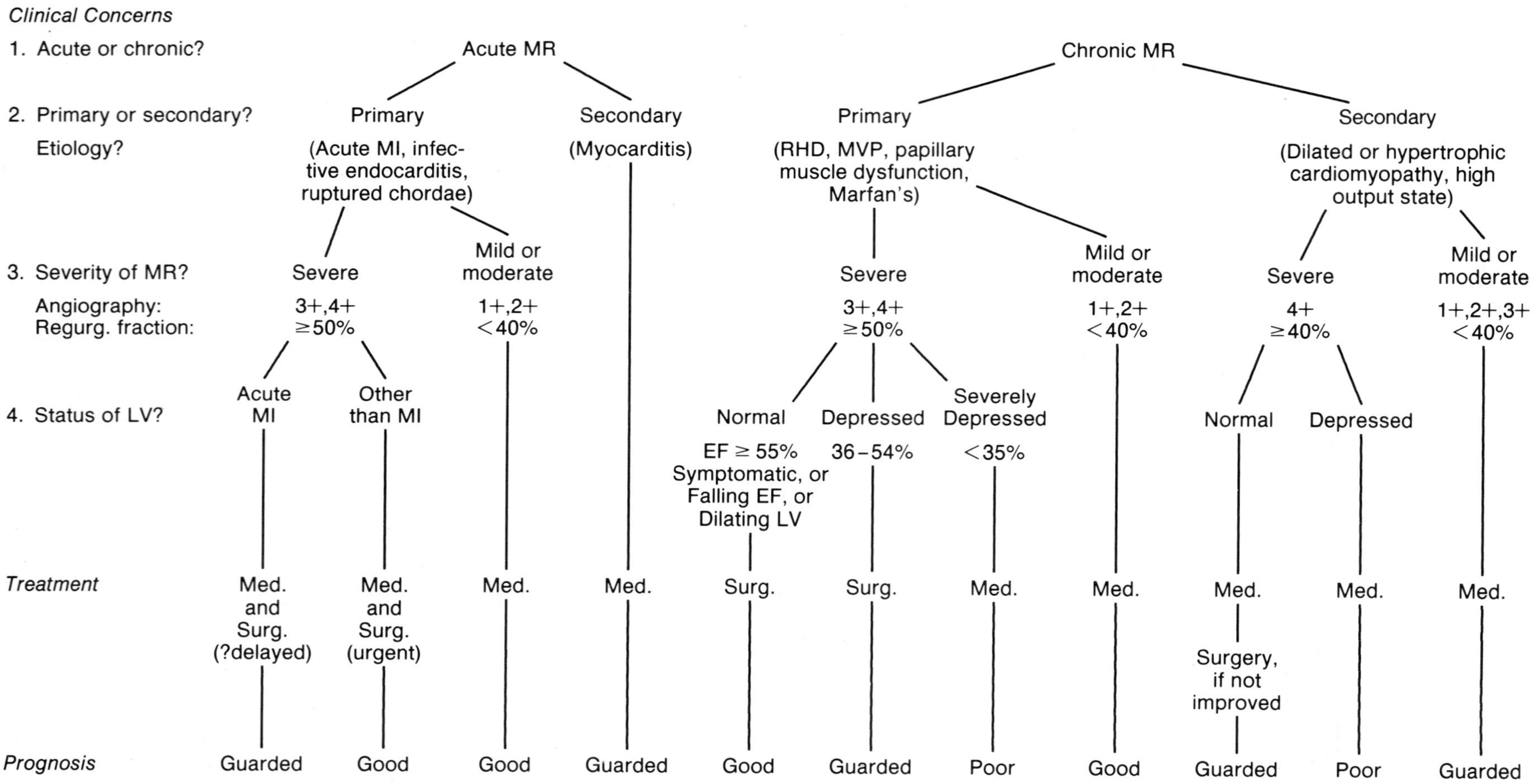

Figure 1 Management of patients with mitral regurgitation. EF = Ejection fraction, LV = left ventricle, MI = myocardial infarction, MR = mitral regurgitation, MVP = mitral valve prolapse, RHD = rheumatic heart disease.

increase in systemic vascular resistance, an effect that may worsen mitral regurgitation. Tachyarrhythmias and increased ventricular ectopy may occur with dopamine administration and limit its usefulness.

Patients presenting with evidence of cardiogenic shock, including low cardiac output, elevated pulmonary capillary wedge pressure, and systemic hypotension, may require more aggressive management. In this setting, insertion of an intra-aortic balloon pump may be life saving, permitting stabilization while preparations are made for surgical interventions. Deflation of the intra-aortic balloon during systole provides effective afterload reduction while diastolic balloon expansion enhances coronary blood flow. Intra-aortic balloon counterpulsation is contraindicated in patients with concomitant aortic valve regurgitation.

Acute ischemic mitral regurgitation occurring in the setting of myocardial infarction most commonly results from papillary muscle dysfunction. Complete or partial rupture of a papillary muscle occurs less frequently. In patients with acute ischemic mitral regurgitation, consideration should be given to reperfusion therapy using a thrombolytic agent or coronary angioplasty because this approach may restore valve competence in addition to salvaging viable myocardium. Thrombolytic therapy with tissue plasminogen activator, streptokinase, or anisoylated plasminogen streptokinase activator complex (APSAC) is indicated in the first 4 to 6 hours after the onset of infarction. Its effectiveness in establishing reperfusion beyond this early time frame has not been firmly established. Because the onset of clinically apparent ischemic mitral regurgitation may be delayed by several hours or days following infarction, the applicability of thrombolysis to such patients is limited. Coronary angioplasty, however, may be performed at any time during the course of acute myocardial infarction if the clinical need becomes manifest. It must be noted that patients with rupture of the papillary muscle are not expected to benefit from reperfusion therapy; in such patients, rapid deterioration and death often will occur within 24 hours unless mitral valve replacement is performed immediately. In contrast, patients with ischemic dysfunction of the papillary muscle may be stabilized hemodynamically with intravenous vasodilators and inotropic agents in conjunction with coronary angioplasty when anatomically appropriate. This may allow temporization of these otherwise precarious patients until definitive surgical therapy can be carried out more safely.

Patients with acute mitral regurgitation secondary to infective endocarditis are particularly troublesome. Depending on the virulence of the organism isolated and the degree of valvular dysfunction, early surgical intervention may be necessary. Although it is advantageous to eradicate the infection preoperatively with an appropriate course of antibiotics, this is not always possible. Urgent surgical intervention, regardless of the length of antibiotic treatment, should be performed if left ventricular function deteriorates.

Chronic Mitral Regurgitation

Medical treatment for chronic mitral regurgitation is prescribed usually for those patients with milder degrees of mitral regurgitation, for those with severely depressed left ventricular function who are believed to be poor surgical candidates, and for those with secondary forms of valvular dysfunction.

Vasodilator therapy plays a key role in managing patients with chronic mitral regurgitation. Orally administered angiotensin converting enzyme (ACE) inhibitors such as enalapril and captopril are preferred. Enalapril should be started at 2.5 mg twice a day and may be increased to 10 mg twice a day. Important side effects include orthostatic hypotension and renal dysfunction manifested as an increase in blood urea nitrogen and creatinine. This latter effect is more likely to occur when diuretics are used concomitantly. A particularly bothersome and subtle side effect is the development of a chronic, nonproductive cough. It is sometimes difficult to distinguish the cough associated with congestive heart failure from that attributed to enalapril. Discontinuation of the drug for several days should clarify the etiology; amelioration of the cough indicates a drug effect. Captopril may be started at 6.25 to 12.5 mg three times a day and should be titrated to a maximum dose of 50 mg three times a day. Its side effect profile is similar to that of enalapril.

Patients with preexisting renal dysfunction or those who develop renal dysfunction during the course of therapy with an ACE inhibitor may be treated with hydralazine, a peripheral vasodilator that directly relaxes vascular smooth muscle. The usual initial dose is 25 mg four times a day; this may be increased to a maximum of 100 mg four times a day. Side effects include palpitations due to reflex tachycardia and hypersensitivity reactions such as arthralgias and fever. A lupus-like syndrome may occur when higher doses are used.

Digitalis glycosides and diuretics are indicated if there is evidence of left ventricular dysfunction or pulmonary venous congestion. A loading dose of digoxin, 0.75 to 1.0 mg, should be given over 7 to 8 hours and followed by daily maintenance therapy. Diuretics may be administered intravenously or orally, depending on the clinical circumstance. A loop diuretic such as furosemide is preferred. If an inadequate diuretic response is achieved, the addition of metolazone, which inhibits sodium reabsorption in the proximal convoluted tubule and enhances the effectiveness of loop diuretics, may be useful. It is most effective when given 1 hour before administration of furosemide. Hypokalemia, sometimes to a profound degree, may occur when this diuretic combination is used. Importantly, the hemodynamic effect of diuretics in patients with chronic mitral regurgitation must be monitored closely. Because left ventricular dilation is a compensatory mechanism to maintain cardiac output in a chronically volume-overloaded state, volume depletion resulting from diuretic usage may result in a fall in forward cardiac output manifested as fatigue, orthostatic hypotension, or progressive renal dysfunction.

Arrhythmias, particularly atrial fibrillation and atrial flutter, are encountered commonly and may herald impending hemodynamic deterioration. Attempts to control the heart rate and restore sinus rhythm should be pursued vigorously. Digoxin is the drug of choice to initiate therapy. It slows the ventricular rate and may convert the patient to sinus rhythm in some instances. Verapamil may be used concomitantly with digoxin; 5 to 10 mg intravenously over 10 to 15 minutes is usually effective in quickly slowing the ventricular rate. Oral maintenance therapy in dosages of 120 to 360 mg daily generally is required. Because verapamil is a vasodilator and has only minimal negative inotropic effects, it is particularly useful in patients with chronic mitral regurgitation. Beta-blocking drugs are also effective in slowing the ventricular rate and in converting some patients back to sinus rhythm. The negative inotropic effects of most of the drugs in this category dictate their cautious use.

Despite the effectiveness of digoxin, verapamil, and beta-blockers in slowing the ventricular rate in patients with atrial fibrillation and flutter, the ultimate goal of antiarrhythmic treatment should be the conversion to sinus rhythm if the arrhythmia has been present for less than 6 months. The most effective drug in this regard is quinidine. Initial doses of 400 mg every 4 hours to a total of 2 g is generally effective in establishing sinus rhythm. Quinidine gluconate, 325 to 650 mg every 8 hours, is used for maintenance therapy. Drug levels of digoxin and quinidine should be checked periodically, particularly when changes in drugs and dosages are made, because these agents have important and potentially dangerous interactions. Gastrointestinal side effects are common with quinidine and may be severe enough to prevent its continued use. Procainamide can be substituted as a second-line drug.

Patients with rheumatic mitral regurgitation should be maintained on an antibiotic regimen to prevent recurrent rheumatic fever (discussed on page 426). Additionally, prophylaxis for infective endocarditis should be prescribed for patients with mitral regurgitation from any cause or for those with a prosthetic heart valve.

Surgical Treatment

The timing of surgical intervention remains one of the most difficult decisions in managing patients with mitral regurgitation. Many considerations must be taken into account, including the patient's hemodynamic and clinical status, the function of the left ventricle, the presence of other noncardiac disease, and the experience and skill of the surgical team.

In patients with severe acute mitral regurgitation, surgical intervention must be considered early in the course of the illness because deterioration of left ventricular function may occur rapidly. Initial stabilization with intravenous vasodilator and inotropic agents along with hemodynamic monitoring are necessary to optimize the patient's hemodynamic status in preparation for surgery. This period of stabilization may not be possible in patients with papillary muscle rupture who require immediate surgical intervention. Papillary muscle dysfunction in the setting of myocardial infarction demands surgical consideration. However, the operative mortality when performed within the first week following acute myocardial infarction is substantially higher than when performed 4 to 6 weeks later. Therefore, temporizing with aggressive medical therapy, as outlined previously, is advantageous. Some patients may even respond with a reduction in the degree of mitral regurgitation, obviating the need for surgical intervention. It must be emphasized, however, that hemodynamic parameters must be monitored attentively and surgery should be delayed only if a good hemodynamic response is achieved. Otherwise, further left ventricular deterioration and even higher operative risk result. In patients with ruptured chordae presenting with acute mitral regurgitation, surgery should be performed as soon as hemodynamic stabilization is achieved. There is little benefit to delaying surgery under these circumstances.

In patients with chronic mitral regurgitation, the timing of surgical intervention is more difficult. Hemodynamic deterioration may develop insidiously over many years. Consequently, the patient tends to adjust his or her life-style and activities, and the gradual development of symptoms may go unnoticed by the patient and physician. Symptoms that are noticeably limiting generally indicate an advanced stage of the disease. Operation is indicated in symptomatic patients provided that left ventricular function is not severely depressed (ejection fraction below 35 percent) because left ventricular function tends to deteriorate after mitral valve surgery as the low impedence route of ventricular ejection is eliminated. Consequently, such patients often continue to deteriorate despite surgical correction.

In patients with severe regurgitation who are asymptomatic or who have only minimal symptoms, mitral valve surgery should be performed in an effort to preserve further deterioration of left ventricular function if sequential echocardiograms show (1) decreasing ejection fraction (approximately 5 units or more) or (2) enlarging left ventricular size, with end-systolic diameter approaching 50 mm or 26 mm per square meter of body surface area or end-systolic volume approaching 60 per square meter. Angiography is used to confirm the severity of the regurgitation, to further assess the degree of left ventricular dilation or dysfunction, and to define coronary anatomy.

Surgical options include mitral valve repair (valvuloplasty or annuloplasty) or replacement with either a bioprosthetic or a mechanical prosthetic valve. Valve repair or reconstruction should be considered in patients with noncalcific mitral regurgitation or annular dilation or in some patients with ruptured chordae. Repair should not be attempted in patients with severe valve scarring or marked chordal thickening or in those with severe myxomatous degeneration of the valve apparatus. Advantages of repairing rather than replacing the valve are the avoidance of long-term anticoagulation and the preservation of left ventricular geometry, which favorably affects left ventricular function postoperatively. However, a note of caution is warranted: An inadequate or poor surgical repair is worse than no repair because a second operation to replace the inadequately repaired valve carries a higher surgical risk. Surgical expertise in repairing mitral valves varies widely depending on the skill and experience of the surgeon. Proper selection of the surgeon is as important as appropriate selection of the patient.

In choosing between a bioprosthetic or a mechanical prosthetic valve, consideration should be given to the patient's age, the presence of atrial fibrillation, and any contraindications to oral anticoagulant therapy. The older patient at increased risk for bleeding complications or the female patient of child-bearing age in whom oral anticoagulants are undesirable should be considered for a bioprosthetic valve. In most other patients in whom chronic anticoagulation is feasible, we favor a mechanical prosthesis, such as the St. Jude's valve, because of long-term durability and favorable hemodynamic properties. In experienced centers, an operative mortality of less than 5 percent should be anticipated.

Postoperatively, patients should be followed for evidence of left ventricular deterioration as manifested by a reduction in ejection fraction. A reduction in ejection fraction does not necessarily imply clinical deterioration because stabilization at this level is the general rule as long as severe left ventricular dysfunction was not present preoperatively. Long-term anticoagulation with sodium warfarin should be monitored on a regular basis, with prothrombin times obtained no less often than every 2 months. Although previous recommendations suggested that a prothrombin time of 2 times that of control was needed, more current data show that 1.5 times control provides equally satisfactory prophylaxis against thromboembolic events with a lower risk of serious bleeding.

SUGGESTED READING

O'Rourke RA, Crawford MN. Mitral valve regurgitation. Curr Probl Cardiol 1984; 9:1.

Perloff JK, Roberts WC. The mitral apparatus: functional anatomy of mitral regurgitation. Circulation 1972; 46:227.

Rankin JS, Hickey MStJ, Smith LR, et al. Ischemic mitral regurgitation. Circulation 1989; 79 (Supp I):116.

Ross J. Afterload mismatch in aortic and mitral valve disease: implications for surgical therapy. J Am Coll Cardiol 1985; 5:811.

AORTIC STENOSIS

JAMES A. RONAN JR., M.D.

Patients with aortic stenosis usually first become aware of it when the characteristic murmur is detected, typically on a routine examination. There is then a long asymptomatic period followed by a much shorter symptomatic period, which usually begins in mid or late life. After the onset of symptoms, most patients have surgical replacement of the aortic valve but continue active life-styles for many more years. Proper management throughout the patient's lifetime includes not only determining when and if the aortic valve needs to be replaced, but also carefully attending to many other details both before and after the valve replacement.

During the many asymptomatic years, the aortic valve, although partially stenotic, has not yet reached a critical degree of narrowing. The normal aortic valve has an area of 3 to 5 cm^2. In aortic stenosis the area becomes progressively smaller over a period of many years, and it is not until it reaches about 1.5 cm^2 that a transvalvular pressure gradient is first produced. Symptoms do not usually begin until the valve narrows even further and a high pressure gradient has been present for many years. Critical aortic stenosis is often defined as a valve area of less than 0.7 cm^2, and it is usually associated with a transvalvular pressure gradient of more than 50 to 75 mm Hg.

THERAPEUTIC ALTERNATIVES

Medical therapy of some sort, such as the treatment of heart failure or arrhythmias, is often required. The major problem, however, is to determine if and when surgery is to be performed. Percutaneous aortic valvuloplasty is also available but has significant limitations.

PREFERRED APPROACH

Medical Treatment

Asymptomatic Period

The medical and surgical treatment of aortic stenosis are not merely alternative forms of therapy, but rather they are therapies used to address different goals at various stages in the natural history of the disease. During the long asymptomatic period, the patient should be educated about the aortic stenosis and its natural history and the patient should have a clear understanding that aortic valve replacement may be needed in the future. The patient should be encouraged to remain physically active, but once a critical degree of stenosis has been reached, extreme physical activities such as overly competitive sports should be avoided. To prevent endocarditis the patient should be instructed carefully in the use of prophylactic antibiotics at the time of dental work or whenever there is possible exposure to a bacteremia. For dental work 2 g penicillin VK orally 30 to 60 minutes before the procedure and 1 g 6 hours later is advised. If the patient has had rheumatic fever, continuous prophylaxis against beta streptococcal infections is indicated to avoid subsequent episodes of rheumatic fever. The prophylaxis should be given in the form of 200,000 units of penicillin G orally twice daily or 1.2 million units of benzathine penicillin intramuscularly each month. This should be continued until the risk of rheumatic fever is minimal, typically at about 40 years of age.

Whenever the diagnosis of aortic stenosis is established for the first time, baseline data about its severity should be obtained by a careful cardiac physical examination, a chest roentgenogram, an electrocardiogram, and an echocardiogram with Doppler studies. Cardiac catheterization is not necessary, particularly if a modern, reliable echocardiography laboratory is available. Estimate of the severity of aortic stenosis is usually as accurate by echocardiography as by heart catheterization. Furthermore, the echocardiogram provides additional useful information, such as the anatomy and pathology of the valve (congenital, rheumatic, or degenerative), the size and function of the left ventricle and other chambers, and the presence of additional lesions such as hypertrophic subaortic stenosis, aortic regurgitation, and mitral regurgitation. There should be a regularly scheduled longitudinal follow-up for each patient; physical examination should be repeated every 2 years and the other studies should be repeated every 3 to 5 years.

As long as the patient remains asymptomatic, aortic valve replacement is not indicated, even when the valve becomes critically stenotic, because evidence shows that mortality from aortic stenosis is extremely rare in truly asymptomatic individuals. However, asymptomatic patients who develop critical aortic stenosis should be seen more frequently (every 4 to 6 months) so that decisions about surgery can be made as soon as symptoms appear. The course may accelerate after the onset of symptoms. Then, too, it must be remembered that occasionally patients with severe aortic stenosis remain asymptomatic simply because they are inactive.

Symptomatic Phase

The symptoms of aortic stenosis are dyspnea, syncope, and angina. By the time the symptoms appear, the aortic stenosis either is already at or is approaching the critical level of narrowing, and the prognosis for survival is about 2 to 5 years. Aortic valve replacement is recommended soon after symptom-onset because medical treatment provides only mild and temporary improvement in symptoms and has little effect on survival. However, during the interval before surgery, or if a patient refuses surgery, medical treatment may help temporarily. Dyspnea is the most common symptom of heart failure; it is due to left atrial pressure elevation, secondary to either systolic or diastolic dysfunction of the left ventricle. The distinction between these two types of ventricular dysfunction can be made easily by echocardiography, and it will help in the choice of the correct medical treatment. In systolic dysfunction the left ventricle is dilated and contracts poorly; in diastolic dysfunction the cavity size is normal or small and contractility is normal. In both types there is ventricular hypertrophy and left atrial enlargement. Systolic dysfunction may also be recognized by low ejection fraction whether measured by angiography, echocardiography, or nuclear studies. In both types of dysfunction, reduction of left atrial pressure with diuretics is usually helpful, but diuretics should be given cautiously in patients with diastolic dysfunction to avoid hypovolemia and hypotension. Inotropic agents such as digoxin may be helpful if there is left ventricular dilation and systolic dysfunction, but it will be of no value in diastolic dysfunction. Vasodilator therapy may be of limited benefit in systolic dysfunction, if used, it should be administered in low doses (such as captopril 12.5 mg 1 to 2 times daily) to avoid hypotension. It is not expected to help in diastolic dysfunction and should be avoided.

Syncope or lightheadedness may be provoked by sudden physical activity or abrupt postural change. However, when syncope occurs at rest, it is often due to cardiac arrhythmia, which can be evaluated best by a 24-hour ambulatory electrocardiogram and treated accordingly. If atrial fibrillation occurs, heart failure usually follows. In such cases the rhythm should be converted back to a sinus rhythm, either by electrical cardioversion or medications depending on the seriousness of the clinical presentation.

Angina pectoris may be due either to excessive wall tension from the high intraventricular pressure of aortic stenosis or to coexisting coronary artery disease. Coronary angiography is the optimal method for making that distinction. A thallium-201 myocardial perfusion scan and exercise electrocardiography are of some value in that assessment. Exercise treadmill testing carries a small risk in symptomatic patients with aortic stenosis, so it should always be done very carefully, avoiding hypotension and never exercising to maximum tolerance. The decision to operate can be made on clinical grounds, including echocardiography, and does not require heart catheterization. However, all patients going to surgery who are older than 35 to 40 years should have coronary angiography to ensure the absence of significant coronary artery disease.

Surgical Treatment

Critical aortic stenosis is a mechanical obstruction to left ventricular outflow, and the optimal treatment is surgical relief by aortic valve replacement; no medical therapy can relieve or overcome that obstruction. Because the prognosis is poor once symptoms begin and improves after aortic valve replacement, there is no advantage to delaying surgery. Severe congestive heart failure is not a contraindication to aortic valve replacement because in almost all cases there will be improvement in systolic ventricular function after valve replacement. The congestive heart failure in aortic stenosis is usually due to an "afterload mismatch," i.e., the obstructed valve produces a resistance to ejection that is just too great for the contractile strength of the myocardium (a mismatch). But it is a relative, not an absolute, myocardial weakness, and the solution is to relieve the obstruction, allow the ventricle to perform to its capacity, and improve the ejection fraction. There are a very few patients with critical aortic stenosis who have a serious primary myocardial contractile dysfunction (e.g., as a result of large myocardial infarction or after many years of heart failure); in these patients, replacing the valve is not likely to improve ventricular function. Identifying patients with that primary dysfunction is often difficult, but they characteristically have the findings of critical aortic stenosis plus left ventricular dilation, diminished contractility, and a low transvalvular aortic gradient (less than 20 mm Hg). Because all aortic prosthetic valves, regardless of design, are partially obstructing and have inherent pressure gradients of 10 to 25 mm Hg, it is not likely that substituting a prosthetic valve for the native valve in this situation would effect any significant improvement. These patients should not have surgery; instead they should continue on a medical regimen although their prognosis is poor. Fortunately this occurs in only a very small percentage of patients with aortic stenosis.

Age alone is not a contraindication to surgery. Because aortic stenosis is more common in older age, many patients are in their 70s and 80s, and many can have successful valve replacement. However, the patient's overall situation should be considered carefully before advising surgery. If there are coexisting serious diseases, which are so common in the elderly (e.g., cancer, respiratory failure, renal failure, stroke) and which by themselves severely limit life expectancy, or if the patient has so many other limitations that improving the aortic valve would not allow any improvement in overall quality of life, then the risk, stress, and discomfort that accompany aortic valve surgery may not be worthwhile. These patients should be given medical management, and it is likely that survival will be determined by other, noncardiac problems.

Choice of Prosthetic Valve

The aortic valve may be replaced with either a mechanical (nontissue) valve or a bioprosthetic (tissue) valve. However, there are no perfect prosthetic valves; all of them are more obstructive than the normal native valve, so all patients with prosthetic valves should be viewed as still having mild or moderate aortic stenosis. In general, the mechanical valve is preferred in aortic stenosis because it is more durable than the tissue valve, there is no difference in hemodynamic characteristics or risk of thromboembolism, and the risk of complications from anticoagulation is small. Tissue valves are advised over mechanical valves whenever long-term anticoagulation with warfarin is inadvisable, such as when a pregnancy is planned, if the patient has a bleeding tendency, or if there is a contraindication to anticoagulation, including the likelihood of unreliability or poor compliance.

Management of the Patient Following Aortic Valve Replacement

To provide careful long-term management there should be a definite schedule of annual clinical evaluations, including a cardiovascular physical examination, a battery of laboratory tests, an electrocardiogram, a chest roentgenogram each year, and a two-dimensional echocardiogram with Doppler studies about every 2 years.

Anticoagulation. All mechanical valves need long-term anticoagulation with warfarin, but anticoagulation is not necessary for tissue aortic valves. The prothrombin time should be checked at least monthly and maintained at 1.5 to 2 times the control value. Antiplatelet agents have not been as effective as warfarin; however, if warfarin cannot be used, dipyridamole in a dose of 100 mg four times a day offers some benefit and is clearly better than no anticoagulation at all. The major complication in patients on anticoagulation is bleeding rather than thrombosis. Minor bleeding occurs in about 2 to 4 percent of patients per year and major bleeding in about 1 to 2 percent of patients per year.

Thrombosis. When thrombosis occurs in a prosthetic valve, there is great risk of death from valvular obstruction. There is also a very high risk if surgical valve replacement is attempted. A new alternative to surgery is thrombolytic therapy with streptokinase or urokinase, and it has been effective in lysing the thrombus in the prosthetic valve. A loading dose of 250,000 to 500,000 units of streptokinase can be given over 30 to 60 minutes and then followed by an infusion of 100,000 units per hour for 24 to 72 hours. When urokinase is used, a loading dose of 150,000 units is given over 30 minutes and is followed by 75,000 to 150,000 units per hour for 24 to 48 hours. The majority of cases have been successful in that they become asymptomatic and have not required surgery. Complications include fever, which resolves when the drug infusion is stopped, hemorrhage, and embolization of thrombotic material. Fortunately, permanent neurologic or circulatory deficit is rare.

Prophylaxis Against Endocarditis. Whenever the patient is exposed to a bacteremia, such as with dental work, genitourinary surgery, or gastrointestinal surgery, prophylactic antibiotics should be taken according to American Heart Association recommendations. Because the danger of endocarditis is greater in a prosthetic valve than it is in a native valve, the intensity of the prophylaxis is increased for prosthetic valves. For dental work that recommendation is 1 to 2 g of ampicillin plus 1.5 mg per kilogram of gentamicin intramuscularly or intravenously 30 minutes before dental work followed by 1 g of oral penicillin V 6 hours later.

Endocarditis. Prosthetic valve endocarditis is a complication with high morbidity and mortality and may lead to persistent sepsis and valvular dehiscence if treatment is unsuccessful. Medical treatment alone is usually unsuccessful but should be attempted if the organism is very sensitive to an antibiotic and if the patient does not have congestive heart failure or emboli. However, if these complications occur, the prognosis is grave and the patient should have surgical replacement of the valve immediately.

Hemolysis. All normally functioning mechanical valves cause at least a small amount of hemolysis, but the normal bioprosthetic valve causes none. However, if a perivalvular leak or prosthetic valve obstruction occurs, the rate of hemolysis may become unusually high, regardless of the type of valve. The serum lactate dehydrogenase (LDH) level is a good index of the amount of hemolysis, so the routine annual postoperative evaluation should include a complete blood count and serum LDH. In most patients with hemolysis, replacement therapy with folic acid and iron is adequate to maintain normal hemoglobin levels. Occasionally refractory cases occur and valve replacement is required.

Pregnancy. If pregnancy should occur while a mechanical valve is in place, the risk of the effect of warfarin on the fetus can be minimized by switching to subcutaneous heparin every 12 hours for the first trimester and for the last 3 weeks of pregnancy. The heparin dose is adjusted to maintain a partial thromboplastin time at 1.5 times the control valve. Warfarin can be used fairly safely during the remainder of the pregnancy. Some cases of warfarin embryopathy may still appear, but the risk is reduced if it is not given in the first trimester. The prothrombin time should be kept at 1.5 times the control. Another method of anticoagulation has been to use subcutaneous heparin every 12 hours throughout the pregnancy. Neither method is without risks, but both are reasonable approaches to the problem.

Percutaneous Aortic Valvuloplasty

Since 1985 aortic valvuloplasty has been used in the treatment of selected adult patients with aortic steonosis, primarily in very elderly or debilitated patients who are considered to have prohibitive cardiac surgical risk either because of heart failure or some severe noncardiac disability. Aortic valvuloplasty clearly is not equivalent to aortic valve replacement for the treatment of severe aortic stenosis, and patients should be made aware of this so that they do not have false expectations for the procedure. Percutaneous aortic valvuloplasty is performed by passing a balloon-tipped catheter retrograde from the femoral artery into the aortic valve orifice. The balloon (which may have a diameter of 15 to 25 mm) is inflated and dilates the valve, usually by cracking the nodular calcific plaques in the leaflets or occasionally by separating commissural fusion. In most cases there has been an improvement in symptoms, a small increase in the aortic valve area (e.g., from 0.5 to 0.9 cm^2), and a reduction in the transvalvular aortic gradient (e.g., from 75 to 30 mm Hg). These results have been considered successful even though severe aortic stenosis persists. Unfortunately, the immediate improvement is often not sustained, and the stenosis may return to the previous degree of severity in weeks or months. Other complications may be aortic regurgitation, sepsis, nonfatal cardiac tamponade, transient ischemic attacks, and trauma to the artery requiring surgical repair.

Although many patients have had improvement for 1 year after valvuloplasty, symptoms have returned in over 40 percent of patients within 9 months and restenosis rates range from 40 to 80 percent. The risk of mortality from the valvuloplasty is less than the risk of aortic valve replacement in the perioperative period, but the mortality at 1 year generally ranges from 24 to 45 percent. A randomized, prospective trial comparing valvuloplasty with valve replacement and with nonoperative (medical) treatment for this select group of very sick patients has not yet been undertaken. The procedure's main usefulness may be to improve heart failure temporarily so that a patient might be better prepared for definitive aortic valve replacement. More experience is needed in order to make a final judgment about the long-term benefits of valvuloplasty, but the initial impression is disappointing. However, aortic valve replacement has been proven to be an effective method of therapy and has a prolonged effect.

SUGGESTED READING

Berland J, Cribier A, Savin T, et al. Percutaneous balloon valvuloplasty in patients with severe aortic stenosis and low ejection fraction; immediate results and 1-year follow-up. Circulation 1989; 79:1189.

Committee on Rheumatic Fever and Infective Endocarditis of the Council of Cardiovascular Disease in the Young: Prevention of bacterial endocarditis. Circulation 1984; 70:1123A.

Dalen JE. Valvular heart disease, infected valves and prosthetic heart valves. Am J Cardiol 1990; 65:29C.

Kelly TA, Rothbart RM, Cooper CM, et al. Comparison of outcome of asymptomatic to symptomatic patients older than 20 years of age with valvular aortic stenosis. Am J Cardiol 1988; 61:123.

Rahimtoola SH. Valvular heart disease: a perspective. J Am Coll Cardiol 1983; 1:199.

Ross J, Braunwald E. Aortic stenosis. Circulation 1968; 38(Suppl 5):61.

Stein PD, Kantrowitz A. Antithrombotic therapy in mechanical and biologic prosthetic heart valves and saphenous vein bypass grafts. Chest 1989; 95(Suppl 2):107S.

AORTIC REGURGITATION

CHARLES B. TREASURE, M.D.

Aortic regurgitation is manifested in acute and chronic forms. Infective endocarditis, dissection of the aortic root, and trauma are the most common causes of acute aortic regurgitation. Chronic aortic regurgitation occurs in patients with rheumatic heart disease or congenitally bicuspid aortic valves. The timing and approach to therapy depend largely on etiology and disease progression. If the valve lesion is chronic and stable, etiology becomes less important. The clinical course then depends on the left ventricle's ability to handle a progressive volume overload. Acute aortic regurgitation may demand immediate surgical intervention, whereas chronic aortic regurgitation may be managed conservatively for years before surgical intervention is considered.

The diagnosis of aortic regurgitation is made readily by history, physical examination, electrocardiography, and chest roentgenogram. Acute aortic regurgitation typically occurs with acute pulmonary edema and depressed forward cardiac output. Physical examination usually reveals tachycardia, a minimally widened aortic pulse pressure, and a medium-pitched early diastolic murmur. The first heart sound may be soft or absent. A third heart sound and a low-grade aortic systolic murmur may be present. The dramatic peripheral manifestations seen in chronic aortic regurgitation are absent. Pulmonary congestion with a normal cardiothoracic ratio is seen on chest roentgenogram. Electrocardiography may show nonspecific ST-T wave changes and P-R prolongation (in infective endocarditis).

Advances in echocardiography have allowed us to diagnose rapidly acute aortic regurgitation noninvasively. The left ventricle is hyperdynamic, and chamber dimensions are usually normal. Aortic valve vegetations or an ascending aortic dissection may be seen. Premature closure and delayed opening of the mitral valve are compatible with markedly elevated left ventricle diastolic pressures. Doppler echocardiography demonstrates a regurgitant jet below the aortic valve.

Chronic aortic regurgitation often appears as an asymptomatic diastolic murmur. Exertional dyspnea may be present. Chest pain is a less common presentation. Pulses are bounding (Corrigan's pulse), and the pulse pressure is widened. The classic peripheral manifestations of chronic aortic regurgitation (Quincke's, Hill's, and Duroziez's signs among others) may be present. The chest roentgenogram may show an increased cardiothoracic ratio. Although the electrocardiogram may be normal, left ventricular hypertrophy is usually present in long-standing aortic regurgitation. Doppler and two-dimensional echocardiography confirm the diagnosis of aortic regurgitation, grades its severity, characterizes valve morphology, and allows accurate assessment of left ventricular geometry and function. The left ventricular walls may be thickened.

If aortic regurgitation is rheumatic in origin, concomitant mitral valve disease should be sought. Rheumatic mitral stenosis may mask the severity of aortic regurgitation. A combination of aortic regurgitation and mitral regurgitation may occur in endocarditis or connective tissue disease (such as Marfan's syndrome) and portends a worse prognosis than either lesion alone.

PREFERRED APPROACH

Management of Acute Aortic Regurgitation

Patients who present with acute aortic regurgitation and *hemodynamic instability* should be prepared for urgent aortic valve replacement (Fig. 1). Treatment with inotropic and afterload reduction therapy may stabilize the patient temporarily and allow time for a limited evaluation (e.g., echocardiography to define aortic valve and root anatomy, aortography in aortic root dissection). Other indications for urgent surgery include P-R prolongation or multiple emboli in patients with endocarditis. A nonstreptococcal etiology of endocarditis and large-valve vegetations or early mitral valve closure seen on echocardiography are relative indications for urgent aortic valve replacement. Intra-aortic balloon counterpulsation is contraindicated in patients with aortic regurgitation.

In acute aortic regurgitation associated with *hemodynamic stability*, close observation with afterload reduction therapy may be indicated to allow further evaluation and therapy. Ten to 14 days of antibiotic treatment for endocarditis will improve operative outcome and survival. Syphilitic aortitis should be treated with penicillin. Aortography may provide the surgeon a better definition of anatomy in aortic root dissection.

Better surgical results are seen in those patients with acute aortic regurgitation whose clinical condition will allow appropriate medical therapy and evaluation and subsequent elective aortic valve replacement. Close preoperative observation is mandatory, including daily clinical evaluation, physical examination, and electrocardiography. Serial echocardiography may be helpful to assess for a perivalvular abscess or worsening left ventricular function. Aortic valve replacement should be performed for any evidence of hemodynamic deterioration.

Management of Chronic Aortic Regurgitation

The management of chronic aortic regurgitation presents the clinician with one of the most interesting challenges in cardiology. Substantial clinical judgment and judicious use of invasive and noninvasive tests are required to manage these patients (Fig. 2). Chronic aortic regurgitation is a relentless progression of worsening regurgitation and left ventricular dysfunction. Severe aortic regurgitation may remain asymptomatic for decades. Symptoms often will not be manifest until left ventricular decompensation has occurred. Careful serial assessment of left ventricular function is critical.

The course of aortic regurgitation is marked by progressive left ventricular volume overload. With aortic regurgitation, the left ventricle must eject a large stroke volume to maintain normal forward cardiac output. The left ventricle, by dilating to increase preload, is able to maintain this large stroke volume. Cavity dilation increases left ventricular wall stress (force per unit area), and increased wall stress stimulates left ventricular hypertrophy. This myocardial adaptive response normalizes wall stress and allows systolic function to be maintained.

Eventually, the left ventricle cannot compensate (by further hypertrophy) to accommodate the large stroke volume necessary to maintain forward cardiac output. Systolic wall stress increases and left ventricular decompensation ensues as systolic function deteriorates. This turning point of left ventricular function (when elevated afterload overcomes the left ventricle's ability to compensate) has been termed *afterload mismatch.*

Because the disease progresses slowly over decades, symptoms may not appear until late in the course and may be preceded by irreversible left ventricular decompensation. Often, sedentary patients are unaware of their limitations. Standard treadmill exercise testing provides objective evidence of the patient's symptomatic status, and exercise capacity correlates significantly with survival. Undoubtedly, exercise testing is superior to the more subjective assessments of functional status (New York Heart Association and Canadian Classifications). Achieve-

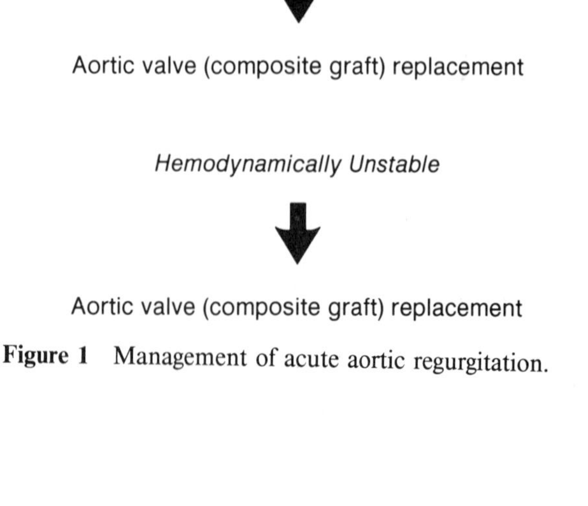

Figure 1 Management of acute aortic regurgitation.

Asymptomatic with Normal LV Function

↓

Annual examination, echocardiogram, exercise test for LVESD <50 mm, FS >25%, and no symptoms

↓

Biannual examination, echocardiogram, exercise test for LVESD 50–55 mm, FS >25%, and no symptoms

Asymptomatic with Depressed LV Function

↓

Biannual examination, echocardiogram, exercise test for LVESD 50–55 mm and/or FS 25–30%

↓

Repeat echocardiogram in 2–4 weeks for LVESD >55 mm, FS <25%

↓

Catheterization to assess severity, other lesions

↓

AVR on individual basis

Symptomatic with Depressed LV Function

↓

Echocardiogram, catherization to assess severity, other lesions

↓

AVR on individual basis

Figure 2 Management of chronic aortic regurgitation. AVR = Aortic valve replacement, FS = fractional shortening, LV = left ventricular, LVESD = left ventricular end-systolic dimension.

ment of 60 percent of functional aerobic capacity on the exercise treadmill is good objective evidence of an asymptomatic status.

After diagnosing aortic regurgitation, and coincident with assessment of the patient's symptomatic status, one must evaluate left ventricular contractile function. Numerous parameters derived from invasive and noninvasive tests have been used to assess left ventricular contractile function and to predict postoperative left ventricular function and survival. The most useful and accepted index is derived from M-mode echocardiography. Henry et al have identified left ventricular end-systolic dimension (LVESD) and fractional shortening (FS) as important determinants of postoperative left ventricular function and prognosis. A LVESD of greater than 55 mm and an FS of less than 25 percent correlate with a worse postoperative prognosis. However, Carabello et al suggest that, even in the symptomatic patient with noninvasive evidence of depressed left ventricular function, postoperative outcome is not significantly worse. This improved outcome is attributed to better surgical techniques and better intraoperative techniques of myocardial preservation in the modern era. These echocardiographic parameters are probably better predictors of postoperative left ventricular function than postoperative mortality and should be used as loose guidelines for managing these patients.

Exercise radionuclide ventriculography has been touted as a predictor of postoperative outcome. A preoperative exercise ejection fraction of less than 40 percent is said to be a sensitive predictor of poor postoperative left ventricular function. However, this has not been confirmed in subsequent studies. The limited usefulness of exercise radionuclide ventriculography is, in part, related to the complex circulatory changes associated with exercise. Exercise ejection fraction depends on many factors (e.g., systemic vascular resistance, heart rate, venous capacitance) other than the left ventricular contractile state. Clearly, patients with an abnormal response to exercise can have an excellent prognosis provided that the resting ejection fraction is normal.

Other end-systolic indices hold promise as predictors of postoperative left ventricular function and survival. The end-systolic pressure volume relationship is an excellent indicator of the left ventricular contractile state. Unfortunately, the many assumptions necessary to make this parameter clinically useful detract from its accuracy. Because end-systolic wall stress is not completely afterload independent, its usefulness alone is limited. However, a promising contractility index is the relationship of end-systolic wall stress and the rate-corrected velocity of circumferential fiber shortening. This noninvasively determined index is preload and heart rate independent and incorporates afterload. Indices of regurgitation severity (regurgitant volume or regurgitant fraction) and preload (end-diastolic pressure, end-diastolic dimension, or end-diastolic wall stress) are unreliable predictors of surgical outcome.

Asymptomatic Patients with Good Left Ventricular Function

In addition to the initial history and physical examination, electrocardiogram, chest roentgenogram, and echocardiogram, asymptomatic patients should undergo annual examination and echocardiography to assess changes in left ventricular function and dimensions. The LVESD should increase no more than 7 mm per year in chronic aortic regurgitation. Therefore, provided that LVESD remains less than 50 mm, annual echocardiograms are adequate. When LVESD is 50 to 55 mm or FS is 25 to 30 percent, examination and echocardiography on a biannual basis are warranted. Close observation is sufficient provided that the patient remains truly asymptomatic and left ventricular systolic function is preserved.

Medical therapy of chronic aortic regurgitation with inotropic agents and vasodilators appears to be of no proven benefit for increasing survival or deferring surgery, although adequate randomized trials have yet to be performed. Hydralazine, however, does improve systolic function and volume overload. Unfortunately, left ventricular hypertrophy, the degree of regurgitation, and left ventricular size are unaffected by this drug. Of potential benefit are other untested vasodilators (e.g., angiotensin converting enzyme inhibitors). All patients with aortic regurgitation should receive antibiotic prophylaxis.

Asymptomatic or Minimally Symptomatic Patients with Depressed Left Ventricular Function

Asymptomatic or minimally symptomatic patients pose a significant management dilemma for clinicians. The goal is to intervene with aortic valve replacement when the immediate and late risks of aortic valve replacement are less than the risk of irreversible damage to left ventricular contractility.

Currently, there are no objective data on the optimal level of left ventricular dysfunction at which to intervene with aortic valve replacement in asymptomatic patients. Because recent data indicate that asymptomatic patients with moderate left ventricular dysfunction do well after aortic valve replacement, careful observation may be appropriate. If severe left ventricular dysfunction exists, however, aortic valve replacement should be considered. Ultimately, management decisions for these patients must be made on an individual basis.

Annual exercise testing should be performed in these patients to assess symptom status and to maintain an objective yardstick on functional capacity. Biannual echocardiography (assuming LVESD is greater than 50 mm and FS is less than 30 percent) should be performed to assess LVESD, FS, and rate of change of these parameters. When LVESD and FS are confirmed at greater than 55 mm and less than 25 percent, respectively, a cardiac catheterization should be performed. If all data confirm aortic regurgitation with severe left ventricular dysfunction, aortic valve replacement should be considered. Each surgical decision must be individualized. Factors such as life-style, surgeon's experience, age, coexisting coronary artery disease, or other co-morbidities must be taken into account. A decision to operate on an asymptomatic patient is difficult for both the patient and the physician, but in those patients with moderate to severe left ventricular dysfunction it is an appropriate one.

As in the asymptomatic patient with normal left ventricular function, medical therapy offers no proven survival benefit. However, vasodilators may provide symptomatic relief and some improvement of systolic function. Likewise, limitation of physical activity has not been shown to affect survival.

Symptomatic Patients with Severe Aortic Regurgitation

In general, symptomatic patients should receive aortic valve replacement. Aortic valve replacement will provide symptom relief and prevent further left ventricular damage for the majority of patients. Many will experience improved left ventricular function and survival postoperatively. Although patients with severe left ventricular dysfunction are at higher risk of persistent left ventricular dysfunction and death postoperatively, it is probably never "too late" to operate on patients with aortic regurgitation. Currently, no clinical criteria identify precisely who within this subset of patients with symptoms and severe left ventricular dysfunction will suffer from persistent left ventricular failure postoperatively. Again, each patient must be evaluated individually. Age, other severe illnesses, coexisting coronary artery disease, and other factors that make operative risk higher or increased survival irrelevant must be taken into consideration. Digoxin, diuretics, and afterload reduction agents (hydralazine, nifedipine) will provide symptomatic relief and hemodynamic benefit in preparation for aortic valve replacement. All patients should undergo cardiac catheterization to confirm lesion severity and to assess other valvular or coronary lesions prior to surgery. As for any patient facing prosthetic valve implantation, possible sources of infection (e.g., dental caries, urinary tract infection) should be treated prior to surgery.

Survival

One must consider the natural history of aortic regurgitation when making management decisions. Seventy-five percent of patients with moderate to severe chronic aortic regurgitation treated medically survive 5 years, and 50 percent survive 10 years after diagnosis. However, when symptoms develop, the prognosis with medical therapy worsens. Angina and heart failure portend death within 4 years and 2 years, respectively. Acute hemodynamically significant aortic regurgitation treated medically has an in-hospital mortality rate of 50 to 90 percent.

The available survival data for patients with surgically treated chronic aortic regurgitation are from the late 1970s and early 1980s. These data may not reflect recent benefits gained from improved surgical techniques. Operative mortality for elective aortic valve replacement is 2 to 6 percent. Emergency surgery for acute aortic regurgitation secondary to endocarditis or aortic root dissection increases this operative risk to 10 percent. Increased age, preoperative heart failure, and decreased exercise capacity have been associated with increased operative and long-term mortality. Five-year survival after aortic valve replacement varies from 50 to 86 percent, reflecting differences in etiology of aortic regurgitation, left ventricular function, and anticoagulation. Approximately 80 percent of patients experience symptom improvement, and in those patients with preoperative depression of left ventricular function (ejection fraction 25 to 50 percent), 50 percent experience improvement of left ventricular function.

Types of Aortic Valve Replacements

Although the 10-year failure rate for porcine valves is approximately 15 to 20 percent, these valves do not require long-term anticoagulation. In general, porcine valves are appropriate for the elderly, females of child-bearing age, and patients with contraindications to anticoagulation. The cryopreserved homograft may be the most suitable valve for patients with active endocarditis. Its lack of struts and ability to be custom-fit in the left ventricular outflow tract and aortic root allow complete debridement of infection and provide resistance to reinfection. Patients with ascending aortic dissection may require a composite graft-valve consisting of an aortic valve prosthesis sewn into a Dacron graft.

The more durable mechanical prosthesis is the best choice for most other patients. Currently, the St. Jude medical prosthetic valve has the best hemodynamic performance of the mechanical valves. Its durability is probably equal to that of other mechanical prostheses, although adequate data are not yet available. The risk of bleeding and thromboembolic complications related to the mechanical valve is approximately 2 to 3 percent per year. Bleeding complications are minimized with warfarin anticoagulation, maintaining the prothrombin time approximately 1.5 times control. This moderate intensity regimen does not increase the risk of thromboembolism. Prosthetic valve endocarditis occurs in approximately 1 to 2 percent of cases. Both mechanical and biologic valves are equally susceptible to endocarditis, although bioprostheses may be more easily sterilized once infected.

SUGGESTED READING

Carabello BA, Usher BW, Hendrix GH, et al. Predictors of outcome for aortic valve replacement in patients with aortic regurgitation and left ventricular dysfunction: a change in the measuring stick. J Am Coll Cardiol 1987; 10:991.

Frankl WS, Brest AN. Valvular heart disease: Comprehensive evaluation and management. Philadelphia: F.A. Davis, 1986:281–312, 335–358, 361–374, 399–426.

Goldschlager N, Pfeifer J, Cohn K, et al. The natural history of

aortic regurgitation: a clinical and hemodynamic study. Am J Med 1973; 54:577.
Henry WL, Bonow RO, Borer IS, et al. Observations on the optimum time for operative intervention for aortic regurgitation. I. Evaluation of the results of aortic valve replacement in symptomatic patients. Circulation 1980; 61:471.
Nishimura RA, McGoon MD, Schaff HV, Giuliani ER. Chronic aortic regurgitation: indications for operation—1988. Mayo Clin Proc 1988; 63:270.
Saour JN, Sieck JO, Mamo LAR, Gallus AS: Trial of different intensities of anticoagulation on patients with prosthetic heart valves. N Engl J Med 1990; 332:428.
Zwischenberger JB, Sahalaby TZ, Conti VR: Viable cryopreserved aortic homograft for aortic valve endocarditis and annular abscesses. Ann Thorac Surg 1989; 48:365.

ACUTE AND RECURRENT PERICARDITIS

NOBLE O. FOWLER, M.D., F.A.C.C.

The therapy of acute pericarditis depends on its presenting features, its etiology, its complications, and its clinical course. In some instances, symptom relief and observation for complications are enough; in others, pericarditis is a clue to a major systemic illness, such as septicemia, connective tissue disease, or cancer, which requires specific therapy. Perhaps the most common variety of pericarditis in outpatients is acute idiopathic or nonspecific pericarditis. Although most instances of this disease require only symptomatic relief and observation, cardiac tamponade requiring pericardial drainage develops in some, and approximately 15 to 32 percent have recurrences that are usually painful and often difficult to manage.

The presenting features of acute pericarditis are listed in Table 1. Chest pain, aggravated by lying, turning, or deep breathing, may be excruciating and may require urgent relief. Pain is common in idiopathic pericarditis, occurring in as many as 90 percent of instances; on the other hand, pain is less common in uremic pericarditis and is often absent in neoplastic pericarditis.

In hospital practice, no more than 10 to 15 percent of patients with acute pericarditis have nonspecific pericarditis. In many patients the cause is obvious, e.g., neoplasm, pneumonia, septicemia, or end-stage renal disease. Conversely, the discovery of pericarditis may be the first clue to previously unrecognized septicemia, neoplasm, myocardial infarction, or connective tissue disease. Because pericarditis has so many causes, a discussion of its treatment cannot be undertaken without discussion of the many possible etiologies toward which treatment may be directed. In some instances, no specific therapy is required; in others, specific treatment for infection, renal failure, or connective tissue disease must be carried out. In still others, treatment may consist of withdrawing a causative drug, e.g., procainamide, phenytoin, or anticoagulants. A list of the major causes of acute pericarditis is given in Table 2. In our hospital, metastatic neoplasm or lymphoma is the most common etiology. Idiopathic pericarditis, infections, and end-stage renal disease make up the next most common group. In hospital practice, these four etiologic groups comprise approximately 50 percent of patients with acute pericarditis.

THERAPEUTIC ALTERNATIVES

Generally speaking, the treatment of acute pericarditis is medical. Surgical removal of the pericardium may be used occasionally for recurrent pericarditis, and surgical drainage may be necessary for cardiac tamponade or purulent pericarditis.

PREFERRED APPROACH

Medical Treatment of Acute Pericarditis

The patient should be hospitalized in order to relieve pain, to observe for complications (e.g., myocarditis or cardiac tamponade), and to perform a diagnostic evaluation.

Observation

Initially, if there is no evidence of cardiac tamponade (e.g., elevated systemic venous pressure, paradoxical arterial pulse, falling arterial blood pressure,

TABLE 1 Presenting Features of Acute Pericarditis

Chest pain
Precordial oppression
Dyspnea
Cardiac tamponade
Fever
Pericardial friction rib
Systemic illness (tumor, infection, connective tissue disease)
Radiologic changes
Electrocardiographic changes

From Fowler NO. The pericardium in health and disease. Mt. Kisco, NY: Futura, 1985. Reproduced by permission of the publisher and author.

TABLE 2 Etiology of Acute Pericarditis

Neoplastic disease
Idiopathic (nonspecific)
Uremia (especially during hemodialysis)
Infections: bacterial, viral, fungal, tuberculosis, protozoal, and miscellaneous
Drugs: anticoagulants, procainamide, hydralazine, diphenylhydantoin, and so forth
Dissecting aortic aneurysm
Connective tissue diseases, arteritis, rheumatoid arthritis, lupus, rheumatic fever
Radiation
Trauma: blunt or penetrating chest injury, pacemaker placement, heart catheterization, placement of central venous lines, diagnostic cardiac puncture, injection of esophageal varices with sclerosing agents
Delayed myocardial injury syndromes: Dressler's syndrome, trauma, cardiac operations, postinfectious syndromes
Chylopericardium
Other: sarcoidosis, myxedema, amyloidosis, hypereosinophilic syndrome

the patient may be observed at bed rest in an ordinary hospital room. Observation for the development of these signs should be carried out every 6 hours for the first few days. When the patient has the aforementioned signs of tamponade, transfer to an intensive care unit, insertion of a Swan-Ganz catheter, and cardiac or thoracic surgical consultation should be made for the possibility of pericardiocentesis or open pericardial drainage. Persistent fever, especially with chills, and elevated white blood cell count, especially above 20,000 per cubic millimeter, suggest the need to investigate for purulent pericarditis by means of pericardial drainage. Persistent fever or increasing effusion after a week or so suggest the need for diagnostic pericardiocentesis when the cause of pericarditis is not obvious from the diagnostic evaluation.

Pain Relief

Initial chest pain may be excruciating and may resemble that of acute myocardial infarction. Aspirin 650 mg every 4 hours orally, ibuprofen 400 to 800 mg every 6 hours, or indomethacin 25 to 50 mg three times a day may provide pain relief. In the beginning, severe pain may require meperidine 50 to 100 mg intramuscularly or morphine 8 to 15 mg intramuscularly every 4 hours. Persistent pain in idiopathic and certain other varieties of pericarditis may require therapy with adrenal steroids (e.g., prednisone) as described subsequently. Ibuprofen may cause nausea, gastrointestinal ulceration, dizziness, headache, skin rash, tinnitus, pancytopenia, fluid retention, aggravation of congestive heart failure, bronchospasm, or acute renal failure. Hepatitis occurs rarely. Indomethacin may cause esophageal, gastric or duodenal ulcer, fluid retention, gastrointestinal bleeding, headache, dizziness, somnolence, tinnitus, mental confusion, corneal deposits, retinal disturbances, and hepatitis. Drug-related dementia is a common problem in patients over 65 years.

Diagnostic Evaluation

The history should evaluate the possibility of pericarditis related to trauma, neoplasm, cardiac surgery, x-irradiation, renal failure, or medication. When the cause of acute pericarditis is not evident, certain tests should be carried out routinely. These include chest radiogram, electrocardiogram, blood culture, antistreptozyme titer, viral neutralizing antibody titers, especially for Coxsackie B virus, complete blood count, intermediate purified protein derivative skin test, renal profile, histoplasma complement fixation test (in endemic areas), and test for antinuclear antibodies. A two-dimensional echocardiogram may show evidence of lymphoma or metastatic neoplasm. Serum myocardial enzyme determinations (creatine phosphokinase [CPK] and CPK-MB) performed at 6-hour intervals during the first 24 hours of pain will aid in excluding the possibility of acute myocardial infarction, although minor elevations may occur with pericarditis due to associated epicarditis or myocarditis.

Pericardiocentesis

There are generally three indications for pericardiocentesis:

- To relieve cardiac tamponade (see the chapter *Cardiac Tamponade*)
- To evaluate suspected purulent pericarditis
- To make an etiologic diagnosis when fever, persistent or progressive effusion, or both are present after 1 to 3 weeks (perhaps sooner)

Pericardiocentesis is a major procedure, with a mortality risk of 1 to 3 percent. It should be carried out only by a skilled physician, e.g., a cardiac surgeon or a cardiologist, unless there is a life-threatening emergency due to cardiac tamponade. The procedure should be carried out after demonstration of fluid location by echocardiography and under hemodynamic and electrocardiographic monitoring. In our institution, agitated saline is injected after the aspirating needle is placed under two-dimensional echocardiographic visualization. This provides assurance that the needle tip lies within the pericardial fluid and increases the safety of aspiration. Resuscitation equipment should be at hand, and a thoracic surgeon should be available in the event of cardiac laceration by the pericardiocentesis needle. Laceration of a cardiac chamber or a coronary artery may occur. Callahan et al (1985) reported no deaths among 117 consecutive patients when pericardiocentesis was guided by two-dimensional echocardiography at Mayo Clinic. As an alternative, open pericardial drainage permits pericardial biopsy as well as evaluation of the pericardial fluid and may be a safer and more definitive procedure. The pericardial fluid should be examined for infectious agents and tumor cells.

Treatment of Specific Varieties of Pericarditis

Idiopathic (Nonspecific) Pericarditis. When pain, fever, and pericardial effusion do not respond to aspirin, ibuprofen, or indomethacin as described above, therapy with adrenal steroids may be necessary. The initial dose in adults is 60 mg of prednisone daily, given orally in a dose of 20 mg three times daily. After 5 days the dosage is reduced to 20 mg twice daily. Some patients respond to an initial dose of 20 mg twice daily; others require a total dose of 90 to 120 mg per day. After 5 days at 20 mg twice daily, the dosage is reduced to 10 mg daily for 5 days, and then to 5 mg daily for 5 days. The drug is then discontinued. Some patients have a recurrence of symptoms when the dosage is reduced below 15 to 20 mg a day. In such cases, the dose of 15 mg per day is resumed for 1 to 3 weeks, and the daily dose is reduced more slowly at a rate of 2.5 mg each week. Occasionally the prednisone may have to be continued at reduced dosages for a number of months.

Certain other varieties of acute pericarditis are treated in the same way as acute nonspecific pericarditis. These may include post-traumatic pericarditis and post-pericardiotomy syndrome.

Pericarditis associated with an infection may persist after the infection has been controlled, e.g., in meningococcemia, histoplasmosis, and tuberculosis. In such cases prednisone may be useful. Prednisone is indicated in the pericarditis of rheumatic fever, but the patient should also receive benzathine penicillin 1,200,000 units intramuscularly. Patients with Dressler's post-infarction pericarditis may respond to indomethacin or prednisone. Although these agents may delay healing in experimental myocardial infarction, this does not seem to be a practical problem in the clinical setting.

Infectious Pericarditis. Infectious pericarditis is treated with the appropriate antibiotic. Infectious pericarditis may be associated with trauma, surgical procedures, septicemia, infective endocarditis, pneumonia, or liver abscess, including amebic abscess. Attention should be given to the primary source. Purulent pericarditis requires open pericardial drainage in addition to the appropriate antibiotics. Pericardial resection will be necessary when adequate drainage cannot be obtained. Purulent pericarditis is especially common in patients who have burns, who are immunocompromised, who have pneumonia, or who have had thoracic surgical procedures.

Uremic Pericarditis. Uremic pericarditis is primarily a problem in patients with end-stage renal disease who are on a hemodialysis program. The condition may respond to more frequent hemodialysis or to a change to peritoneal dialysis. Some authorities find intrapericardial instillation of triamcinolone to be useful. When there is cardiac tamponade, pericardiocentesis is needed, and persistent or recurrent effusion may require pericardial resection.

Withdrawal of Offending Agents. The patient's medication history should be reviewed for the possibility that therapeutic agents may be responsible for the pericarditis. Most common among these are procainamide, phenytoin, and anticoagulants. Antineoplastic agents, especially doxorubicin and daunorubicin, may be responsible. Hydralazine and isoniazid may cause a lupus-like syndrome that includes pericarditis. Anticoagulants, especially following myocardial infarction or in excessive dosage, can cause pericarditis and even tamponade of the heart. The offending drug should be withdrawn when pericarditis complicates its use.

Tuberculous Pericarditis. Tuberculous pericarditis usually requires triple-drug therapy for at least 9 months. Isoniazid 300 mg daily orally and pyridoxine 50 mg daily orally together constitute the first therapeutic agent. Rifampin 600 mg daily is the preferred second agent. Ethambutol 15 mg per kilogram of body weight daily is the third agent. Some authorities prefer 18 months of therapy, with isoniazid and pyridoxine being discontinued after a few months. Isoniazid may produce peripheral neuropathy, and pyridoxine is given to prevent this. Isoniazid also may produce hepatitis, drug fever and rash, encephalopathy, and a lupus-like syndrome. Rifampin may cause hepatitis in approximately 19 percent of patients. Ethambutol may cause optic neuritis. In some cases, where there is considerable pericardial thickening resulting in constrictive or constrictive-effusive pericarditis, pericardial resection is necessary also. Adrenal corticosteroid therapy may be useful in patients who continue to have large effusions or mild effusive-constrictive pericarditis following several weeks of chemotherapy. Strang et al (1988) made a controlled study of 240 patients with active tuberculous pericardial effusion. Their study found that therapy with prednisolone for 11 weeks in addition to antituberculous drugs for 6 months reduced the death rate and the need for repeat pericardiocentesis, but did not lessen the need for later operation for constrictive pericarditis.

AIDS-Related Pericarditis. Pericarditis occurs in 5 to 15 percent of patients with acquired immunodeficiency syndrome (AIDS). Its cause should be determined. The cause of pericarditis associated with AIDS may be viral disease, tuberculosis, neoplasm, or fungal disease. When pericarditis is due to *Mycobacterium avium-intracellulare*, *Mycobacterium tuberculosis*, or fungal infection, specific antibiotics are indicated. Lymphoma or Kaposi's sarcoma may be responsible. When the cause is a neoplasm, antineoplastic therapy is indicated. Patients with AIDS with tuberculous pericarditis often present with cardiac tamponade and then require surgical drainage of the pericardial sac.

Fungal Pericarditis. Histoplasma pericarditis usually pursues a course similar to that of idiopathic pericarditis and then does not require specific therapy. However, pericarditis associated with disseminated histoplasmosis requires therapy with amphotericin B or keotoconazole. Similar therapy will be needed for pericarditis due to disseminated *Candida* or other fungal infections. Cryptococcosis may respond to amphotericin B; flucytosine may be used as additional therapy.

Neoplastic Pericarditis. When metastatic neoplastic disease is responsible for acute pericarditis, appropriate chemotherapy is indicated. Lung cancer, breast cancer, lymphoma, and leukemia are the most common varieties of neoplastic disease leading to pericarditis. Intrapericardial instillation of tetracycline 500 to 1000 mg in 20 ml normal saline, repeated if necessary, often prevents recurrent effusions in malignant pericardial disease. Atrial arrhythmias, pain, and fever may complicate this treatment. Cardiac tamponade is an indication for pericardiocentesis, and recurrent tamponade may be an indication for pericardial resection. Pericardial windows may be used instead of pericardial resection, but these may be ineffective owing to sealing off or widespread pericardial involvement by neoplasm.

Dissecting Aneurysm. Pericarditis associated with dissecting aneurysm results from leakage or rupture from the intrapericardial portion of the ascending aorta. The treatment is immediate surgical repair of the dissection.

Radiation. Effusive or fibrinous pericarditis may follow mediastinal irradiation after a period of months or years. Ten to 50 percent of patients develop pericarditis, depending on the amount of radiation directed toward the heart. Prednisone therapy as outlined under the treatment of idiopathic pericarditis is often useful. Constrictive or effusive-constrictive pericarditis may develop eventually. Pericardial resection may be necessary, but the results may be disappointing if there is associated myocardial fibrosis resulting from radiation.

Medical Treatment of Recurrent (Relapsing) Pericarditis

Recurrent pericarditis may follow idiopathic pericarditis (15 to 32 percent of instances), Dressler's post–myocardial infarction pericarditis, post-pericardiotomy syndrome, intrapericardial bleeding, or traumatic pericarditis. This discussion of its treatment does not include recurrent attacks of pericarditis associated with a chronic systemic disease, such as cancer or connective tissue disease. Recurrent pericarditis may be a minor problem, with one or two relapses, which may respond to indomethacin, ibuprofen, or a brief course of prednisone. However, recurrences may be numerous and may, in our experience, take place over a period as long as 15 years. Complications after the original attack, such as cardiac tamponade, myocarditis, arrhythmias, or constrictive pericarditis, are uncommon. Treatment therefore is directed toward relief of pain, malaise, and apprehension.

Early attacks of relapsing pericarditis should be managed as described under idiopathic pericarditis, including observation in hospital for complications. Because complications are unlikely after the first few attacks, we manage most patients without hospitalization for later spells. Attacks should be managed without prednisone whenever possible. In some cases, patients are already receiving long-term adrenal steroids when first seen. Others may require long-term adrenal steroids because of almost immediate recurrences, when prednisone dosage is reduced below 15 to 20 mg per day. In such cases, we reduce prednisone gradually, at a rate of 2.5 mg daily per week. Flare-ups of pericarditis are treated with codeine or oxycodone rather than by increasing prednisone dosage. Because prednisone has undesirable side effects and may actually prolong the course of the illness, our ultimate goal is to withdraw the agent completely. Complete withdrawal may require as much as 1 year. The long-term dose of prednisone should be kept at a minimum, preferably 7.5 mg per day or less to minimize complications.

Adrenal steroid therapy may be complicated by infections, hypokalemia, alkalosis, fluid retention, decreased glucose tolerance, hypertension, moon facies, hirsutism, buffalo hump, peptic ulcer, poor wound healing, skeletal myopathy, osteoporosis, and aseptic necrosis of the femoral head. Emotional disorders are common. Glaucoma and cataracts may occur.

Surgical Treatment of Prolonged or Recurrent Pericarditis

Pericardiectomy may be considered in patients with prolonged and numerous attacks of pericarditis. The success rate may vary from 80 percent to under 50 percent. Because of its frequent failure and because major complications of recurrent pericarditis are uncommon, we reserve pericardiectomy for patients with prolonged disabling attacks of painful pericarditis who do not respond to anti-inflammatory agents or adrenal steroids or who develop complications with prednisone therapy.

In difficult cases, other possibilities may be considered. Although azathioprine has been reported to be successful in a few instances, it was not helpful in two patients whom we treated. Guindo et al described improvement in relapsing pericarditis with oral colchicine, 1 mg daily. This report is encouraging but needs confirmation.

SUGGESTED READING

Acierno LJ. Cardiac complications in acquired immunodeficiency syndrome (AIDS): a review. J Am Coll Cardiol 1989; 13:1144.

Callahan JA, Seward JB, Nishimura RA, et al. Two dimensional echocardiographically guided pericardiocentesis: experience in 117 consecutive patients. Am J Cardiol 1985; 55:476.

Connolly DC, Burchell HB. Pericarditis: a ten year survey. Am J Cardiol 1961; 7:7.

Fowler NO. The pericardium in health and disease. Mount Kisco, NY: Futura Publishing Co., 1985.

Fowler NO, Harbin AD III: Recurrent acute pericarditis: follow-up study of 31 patients. J Am Coll Cardiol 1986; 7:300.

Guindo J, de la Serna AR, Ramió J, et al. Recurrent pericarditis: relief with colchicine. Circulation (in press).

Strang JIG, Gibson DG, Mitchison DA, et al. Controlled clinical trial of complete open surgical drainage and of prednisolone in treatment of tuberculous pericardial effusion in Transkei. Lancet 1988; 2:759.

CARDIAC TAMPONADE

E. WILLIAM HANCOCK, M.D.

Cardiac tamponade is a condition in which the function of the heart or circulation is compromised by the presence of fluid under increased pressure in the pericardial space. More specific definitions vary. Some use the term tamponade only for those critical situations in which the arterial blood pressure has dropped to a definitely low level, perhaps only when cardiogenic shock is considered to be present. Others require the presence of a fall in cardiac output, to a definitely low level, as part of the definition. I prefer a broader definition, in which milder forms of compromise, such as a rise in central venous pressure, with normal arterial pressure and cardiac output, are considered to represent cardiac tamponade. Under this definition, cardiac tamponade can be mild, moderate, or severe. The severe forms can be regarded as decompensated, or critical tamponade. The importance of such a definition is to indicate that the appropriate time to relieve cardiac tamponade by removing the fluid is usually when the condition is mild or moderate. Waiting until the crisis state of decompensated or critical tamponade increases the possibilities of an unsatisfactory outcome.

ETIOLOGY AND PATHOGENESIS

Cardiac tamponade can occur in any of the conditions in which pericardial effusion occurs. The etiology thus includes a wide variety of medical and surgical conditions and diverse clinical settings. The pericardial fluid may be pure blood, or it may be serosanguinous, serous, or purulent fluid. The pericardial effusion may develop rapidly or slowly. The amount of pericardial fluid is less important than the speed of its accumulation, since the pericardium is resistant to sudden stretch but does stretch markedly over the course of weeks or months.

DIAGNOSIS

The diagnosis of cardiac tamponade requires two elements. It must be demonstrated that pericardial effusion is present, and it must be demonstrated that there are hemodynamic abnormalities that can be attributed to pericardial fluid under increased pressure. Ultimately, a proven diagnosis of cardiac tamponade requires the demonstration of reversal of such hemodynamic abnormalities by removal of the pericardial fluid.

Evidence from the history, physical examination, electrocardiogram, and plain chest roentgenogram can only be suspicious, at most, of the diagnosis of pericardial effusion. An objective method of imaging is required to establish this point. Echocardiography is the most useful method of imaging because it is highly accurate and can be applied easily in almost any clinical setting. Computed tomography (CT) and magnetic resonance imaging (MRI) are also highly reliable and provide better definition of some anatomical details; they should be used as supplementary methods when echocardiography is inconclusive.

Imaging methods, on the other hand, should not be relied on to demonstrate that hemodynamic signs of compression of the heart are necessarily present or absent. The history and physical examination are the prime methods for determining this. Patients with cardiac tamponade usually have dyspnea and other symptoms. The jugular venous pressure can virtually always be seen to be elevated if the circumstances of the examination are adequate. Paradoxical pulse is usually present, although it is often difficult to assess by examination or by sphygmomanometry alone. Echocardiography does provide useful signs of compression of the heart. These include a reduced diameter of the right ventricle, inward movement of the right atrial and right ventricular walls in early systole ("systolic collapse"), persistent full distention of the inferior vena cava throughout the respiratory cycle, and exaggerated respiratory variation in the velocity of blood flow through the mitral and tricuspid valves. In questionable cases, direct measurements of right atrial pressure and arterial pressure should be used to confirm the presence of hemodynamic signs of tamponade.

THERAPEUTIC ALTERNATIVES

The treatment may be divided into conservative medical approach, pericardiocentesis, and surgical pericardiostomy. No one of these approaches is the most appropriate for all cases. The choice of therapy depends on many considerations. Some of the questions that should be raised in making a choice are listed in Tables 1 and 2.

PREFERRED APPROACH

Conservative Medical Approach

In moderate or severe cardiac tamponade the conservative medical approach is at best an interim and short-term approach because removal of the fluid is the only therapy that can be expected to be successful quickly and dependably. In milder forms, however, the conservative medical approach may be appropriate. Patients who are selected for this approach should have only mild elevation of jugular venous pressure, to a level equivalent to approximately 8 to 10 mm Hg (elevated to less than the angle of the jaw in the sitting upright position). They should have no symptoms attributable to the tamponade itself and should have no evidence of hypotension, pulmonary congestion, or impaired renal or cerebral perfusion. There should be confidence either that a diagnosis is known, such as neoplasm, dialysis, or a rheumatic disease, or that a diagnosis is highly unlikely to be established by studies on the pericardial fluid, e.g., the clinical picture is that of idiopathic acute pericarditis or idiopathic chronic pericardial effusion. The decision for a conservative medical approach is also supported if the natural history of the patient's illness is believed to be benign and self-limited, as in idiopathic acute pericarditis. It is also supported if the pericardial effusion is believed to be part of a systemic disorder that is responsive to systemic therapy, such as breast cancer, rheumatic disease, or uremia. Employing a conservative medical approach also implies that the patient will remain under close observation during a follow-up period, usually as a hospital inpatient initially. Thus, the conservative medical approach to mild cardiac tamponade consists of close observation of the patient for evidence of increasing tamponade, while the basic condition is treated systemically or allowed to resolve spontaneously.

TABLE 1 Should a Pericardial Effusion Be Drained?

Is cardiac tamponade of more than a mild degree present?
Is the amount of pericardial effusion increasing?
How important is the cytologic study of the pericardial fluid?
How important is the bacteriologic study of the pericardial fluid?
Does the natural history of the underlying condition predict spontaneous resolution?
Is there an effective systemic treatment for the underlying condition?
Will draining the pericardial effusion permit a less intense level of in-hospital care?
Will draining the pericardial effusion shorten the hospital stay?

TABLE 2 Should Pericardial Fluid Be Drained by Pericardiocentesis or Surgery?

How quickly are a skilled cardiologist and cardiac catheterization laboratory available?
How quickly are a skilled surgeon and operating room available?
How readily accessible is the fluid to a needle approach?
Is the fluid likely to be blood that is partially clotted?
How likely is there to be associated constrictive pericarditis?
How likely is there to be associated superior vena caval obstruction?
How likely is there to be associated congestive heart failure/fluid overload?
Does the patient have a coagulopathy?
How important is a pericardial biopsy?
How likely is there to be a site of bleeding from the heart that requires surgical control?

Supportive Therapy in Critical Tamponade

Patients who are hypotensive because of critical cardiac tamponade may benefit from supportive therapy while the diagnosis of tamponade is being confirmed, or while the preparations for the drainage procedure are being carried out. Such supportive therapy should not be regarded as more than an interim temporizing approach. The administration of fluid intravenously is the most important measure. Fluid should be administered even when the central venous pressure is considerably elevated, remembering that the right atrial pressure and the intrapericardial pressures are virtually equilibrated in tamponade. It is necessary for the right atrial pressure to exceed the intrapericardial pressure at least slightly in order that the right ventricular transmural pressure be positive and therefore the appropriate stimulus to right ventricular contraction be present. Blood, plasma, or dextran may be used for intravenous fluid administration, but simple saline solution is equally acceptable in most situations.

The systemic arterial pressure and cardiac output may be supported by the infusion of drugs such as dopamine, dobutamine, or isoproterenol. A drug that tends to reduce the size of the heart, by a combination of inotropic action and systemic vasodilation, is optimal, remembering that if the heart is made smaller it will be compromised less by a given amount of fluid in the pericardial space. The more potent vasodilating agents such as sodium nitroprusside should generally not be used in critical cardiac tamponade because the maintenance of an adequate systemic arterial pressure is critically dependent on a reasonable level of systemic vascular tone. Support of the systemic circulation with drug infusions in cardiac tamponade does little to favor the renal, cerebral, or splanchnic circulations; its greatest importance is in supporting the coronary arterial filling pressure when the arterial pressure is markedly reduced.

Pericardiocentesis

Selection of Patients

If a skilled invasive cardiologist and a cardiac catheterization laboratory are readily available, pericardiocentesis is the preferred approach to most cases of cardiac tamponade that are seen in the medical setting. Such cases include most of those resulting from idiopathic pericarditis, tuberculous infection, neoplasm, radiotherapy, rheumatic diseases, and uremia/dialysis. Demonstration of the presence of pericardial effusion, usually by echocardiography, is a prerequisite. Furthermore, the fluid should be present in significant amount over the inferior or anterolateral regions of the pericardial cavity.

Timing

Pericardiocentesis should be carried out when the jugular venous pressure has risen to approximately 10 mm Hg or higher. The procedure should be scheduled urgently, within a few hours of the time that the diagnosis has been made. It should not be carried out as an emergency, under less than optimal conditions, unless the patient is in cardiogenic shock or severe respiratory distress. Even under such emergency conditions, it is usually preferable to transfer the patient to the cardiac catheterization laboratory.

Preparation

The intravascular volume should be repleted if it is thought to be relatively or absolutely deficient. Atropine should be given as premedication, to aid in avoiding the vasodepressor response that may accompany either the insertion of the needle or the withdrawal of pericardial fluid. The apparatus for hemodynamic monitoring should be assembled, as appears appropriate for the clinical problem. At a minimum, the central venous pressure should be monitored. In many cases the direct arterial pressure should be monitored, and in some the right heart pressures, left heart pressures, and cardiac output should also be monitored.

Procedure

In most instances the optimal site for the insertion of the needle is in the subxiphoid area just to the left of the midline. However, it is helpful to use echocardiography in selecting the site; when this is done, an apical or parasternal site may prove to be better. A local anesthetic agent should be instilled, using a long thin needle. The local anesthesia should be carried out to the pericardium itself; entering the pericardial space and withdrawing a few milliliters of fluid into the local anesthetic syringe identify the depth and direction for the subsequent insertion of the larger bore pericardiocentesis needle. A long No. 16 or No. 18 needle is then passed into the pericardial space. The needle may be attached to a unipolar exploring electrocardiogram electrode, to provide an indication of contact of the needle with the myocardium. However, the experienced operator will note a characteristic sensation as the needle penetrates the pericardium.

When the needle enters the pericardial space, a pressure measurement should be made within the pericardial space. In cardiac tamponade the value is nearly equivalent to the central venous pressure, and the waveform shows a monomorphic fall in systole and rise in diastole, with only minor variation with respiration. A flexible j-tipped guide wire should then be passed, the needle withdrawn, and a No. 7 pigtail catheter placed in the pericardial space over the guide wire. The pericardial fluid can then be withdrawn gradually through the catheter. At the end of the procedure, the pericardial pressure should again be measured, along with the right atrial pressure. The catheter is then secured to the skin and left indwelling with a heparin lock.

Post-Procedure Course

The pigtail catheter should be left in place for up to 4 days, or until there is no further pericardial fluid accumulation. The central venous pressure should be monitored especially closely during the first 24 hours after the procedure; it may not drop fully to normal immediately after the procedure but should do so by the next day as the patient has a diuresis. Persistence of an elevated central venous pressure, when the intrapericardial pressure has been restored to normal, indicates the presence of a further cardiac abnormality, often an associated visceral constrictive pericarditis.

Complications

The most important complication of pericardiocentesis is an aggravation of cardiac tamponade due to bleeding from an inadvertent puncture of the heart. The risk can be minimized by reserving the procedure for experienced operators in optimal conditions, using echocardiographic guidance and thoughtful selection of patients. Other complications include the vasodepressor responses that are minimized by atropine premedication and infection associated with the indwelling catheter in the pericardial space. Although not strictly a complication, perhaps the most frequent adverse sequelae of pericardiocentesis stem from a false sense of security about its efficacy; there must be a clear documentation of how successful the procedure was and also a careful observation of the patient following the procedure, so that clinical deterioration due to persistent or recurrent tamponade can be recognized and dealt with, usually by surgical pericardiostomy.

Surgical Pericardiostomy

Selection of Patients

The prime indication for surgical pericardiostomy is acute traumatic hemopericardium, as seen in the emergency room. Not only do the acuteness and severity of the condition require very quick action, but also the likelihood of the presence of clotted blood and of a bleeding site in the heart that requires surgical control make pericardiocentesis a temporary delaying action at best in this situation. Postoperative cardiac tamponade after cardiac surgery and tamponade due to rupture of the heart in acute myocardial infarction or rupture of an acute dissection of the aorta into the pericardial space also call for a surgical approach. Purulent bacterial pericarditis is best managed with surgical pericardiostomy to provide adequate drainage and to prevent the development of acute constriction of the heart; however, this diagnosis is usually established first by pericardiocentesis. A surgical approach may be preferred when tuberculous pericarditis is a prominent possibility because in this condition the pericardial biopsy is superior to the fluid alone for bacteriologic diagnosis. Finally, patients with cardiac tamponade of various etiologies may require surgery if the tamponade recurs after pericardiocentesis or if the fluid is inaccessible because of location or loculation.

Timing and Preparation

Timing and preparation are similar to that of pericardiocentesis.

Procedure

The surgical approach is usually subxiphoid, which permits resection of a small area of the inferior pericardium and digital exploration of the pericardial space. A limited left thoractomy may also be used; this permits resection of a larger area of anterolateral parietal pericardium and the establishment of a drainage pathway into the left pleural space.

Postoperative Course

The surgical drainage tubes are left in place for several days and then removed. Recurrent pericardial effusion after such procedures occurs only rarely. Complications and adverse sequelae are rare after surgical pericardiostomy. Wound infection, as in thoracotomy, is the most serious complication.

SUGGESTED READING

Krikorian JG, Hancock EW. Pericardiocentesis. Am J Med 1978; 65:808.

Callaham ML. Pericardiocentesis in traumatic and nontraumatic cardiac tamponade. Ann Emerg Med 1984; 13:924.

Callahan JA, Seward JB, Nishimura RA, et al. Two-dimensional echocardiographically guided pericardiocentesis: Experience in 117 consecutive patients. Am J Cardiol 1985; 55:476.

Palatianos GM, Thurer RJ, Kaiser GA: Comparison of effectiveness and safety of operations on the pericardium. Chest 1985; 88:30.

Burstow DJ, Oh JK, Bailey KR, et al: Cardiac tamponade: Characteristic Doppler observations. Mayo Clin Proc 1989; 64:312.

CONSTRICTIVE PERICARDITIS

JAMES J. FERGUSON III, M.D.
JAMES T. WILLERSON, M.D.

Constrictive pericarditis is a disorder in which there is limitation of diastolic filling of the heart as a result of the relatively fixed volume of a thickened, fibrotic pericardium. There is usually uniform restriction of filling of all heart chambers by the rigid and nondistensible pericardium, although in very unusual circumstances there can be localized pericardial thickening.

ETIOLOGY AND PATHOPHYSIOLOGY

Constrictive pericarditis is most frequently the result of a previous episode of acute pericarditis that subsequently progresses to a stage of chronic scarring, fibrosis, and thickening. Basically, any process that can cause acute pericarditis may ultimately result in constrictive pericarditis. The most common causes of constrictive pericarditis include neoplastic disease (especially lung cancer, breast cancer, and lymphoma), mediastinal irradiation, and chest trauma (including surgery). Other less frequent causes include chronic renal failure and dialysis, connective tissue disorders (such as rheumatoid arthritis and systemic lupus erythematosus), and bacterial pericardial infections. Tuberculosis was at one time a leading cause of constrictive pericarditis, but today it is a major cause only in underdeveloped countries. Constrictive pericarditis is also increasingly recognized as a complication of cardiac surgery.

The fundamental physiologic abnormality in constrictive pericarditis is a rigid nondistensible pericardium that limits late diastolic filling of the ventricles. Early rapid diastolic filling is abruptly halted when it reaches the limiting volume of the rigid pericardium. The net result is impaired overall cardiac diastolic function with associated systemic and pulmonary congestion, reduced cardiac output, and hypotension. Systolic function usually remains relatively unaffected. It must be remembered that the pericardium itself has a fundamental curvilinear pressure–volume relationship, and when taken to its limits, even normal pericardium will limit the filling of the ventricle (as occurs in acute right heart failure or right ventricular infarction). The point at which limitation of filling occurs depends on the compliance (change in volume per unit change in pressure) of the pericardium, as shown in Figure 1. An understanding of this relationship serves as a basis for distinguishing so-called "rigid" from "elastic" constriction.

PERICARDIAL PRESSURE - VOLUME RELATIONSHIP

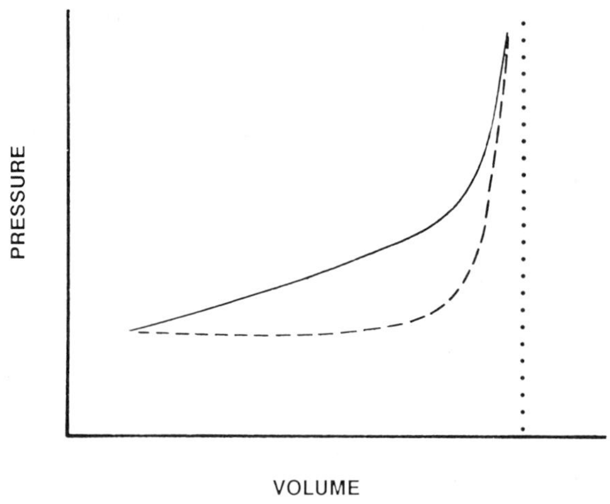

Figure 1 A schematic diagram of the curvilinear pressure–volume relationship of the pericardium. The solid line shows a curve for a rigid, calcified, nondistensible pericardium that limits further expansion as it approaches its limiting volume. The dotted line represents the absolute upper limit of pericardial volume. The dashed line shows a normal pericardium, which is more distensible but also has a limiting volume.

DIAGNOSIS

On physical examination, the single most striking finding in constrictive pericarditis is elevation of the jugular venous pressure, which usually has a prominent y-descent, coincident with the prominent early rapid filling of the ventricle. Patients in sinus rhythm may also have a prominent x-descent coincident with filling of the atrium as the ventricle is ejecting. Peripheral edema, hepatomegaly, and ascites are common. Kussmaul's sign (an inspiratory increase in jugular venous pressure) may be present, but pulsus paradoxus is only occasionally found with constrictive pericarditis. An early diastolic pericardial knock (high frequency diastolic sound) coincident with the cessation of rapid ventricular filling may be noted on auscultation.

The size of the cardiac silhouette on chest film is not particularly helpful, although pericardial calcification may be seen (especially with a previous history of tuberculous pericarditis). The electrocardiogram usually demonstrates nonspecific ST-segment and T wave changes, low QRS voltages, and left atrial enlargement. The presence of ventricular hypertrophy, conduction disturbances, or Q waves suggests the presence of underlying myocardial disease, and possible coronary artery involvement.

M-mode and two-dimensional echocardiography may be useful in documenting the increased pericardial thickness and abnormal ventricular diastolic function in the setting of normal systolic function. However, the sensitivity of echo images in identifying thickened pericardium is limited unless calcium is present, and with the advent of newer imaging modalities, echo images are much less useful. Doppler echocardiography may show impaired late diastolic flow across the mitral or tricuspid valves and prominent respiratory variations in left ventricular isovolumic relaxation time and peak mitral flow velocity. The sensitivity of this technique is, as yet, untested, and these findings will probably not be specific for constrictive pericarditis. Both gated cardiac magnetic resonance imaging (MRI) and ultrafast cine-computed tomography (CT) have emerged as useful techniques that allow direct measurements of pericardial thickness. Both techniques can also identify dilation of the vena cavae and hepatic veins and pericardial impingement on the right ventricle (Figs. 2 and 3).

Cardiac catheterization is the definitive technique for documenting the elevation and equalization of right and left ventricular diastolic pressures observed in constrictive pericarditis (Fig. 4). Early ventricular filling is unimpaired, but as the rapid fill-

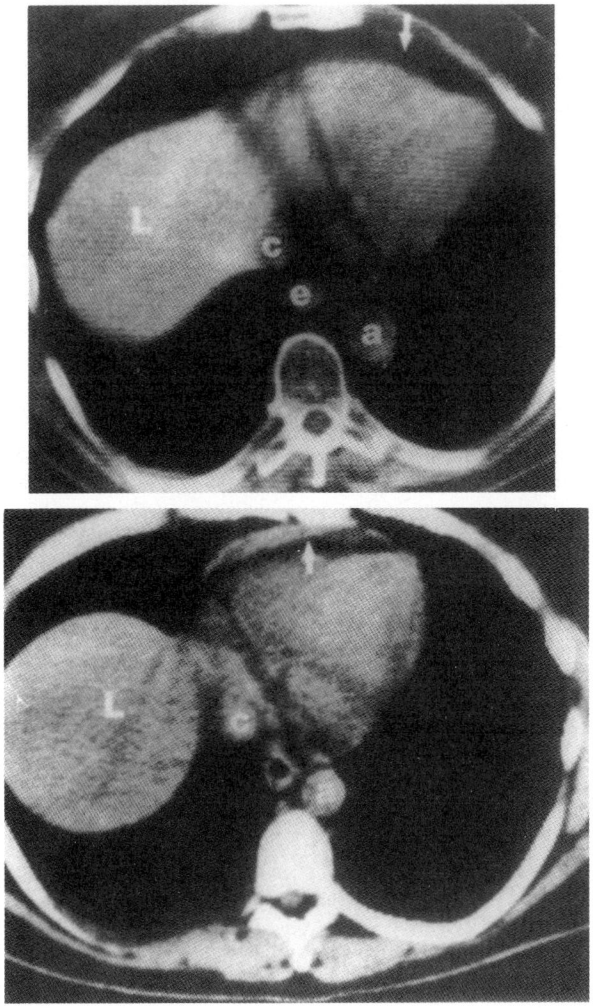

Figure 2 Ultrafast computed tomographic scans at the level of the right hemidiaphragm from a normal adult (*top*) and from a patient with constrictive pericarditis (*bottom*). In contrast to the normal pericardium, which appears as a thin line (*arrow*), the pericardium in constrictive pericarditis appears thickened. Other structures visualized include liver (L), inferior vena cava (c), esophagus (e), and descending aorta (a). (From Sutton FJ, et al. The role of echocardiography and computed tomography in the evaluation of constrictive pericarditis. Am Heart J 1985; 109:350. Reproduced by permission of the publisher and author.)

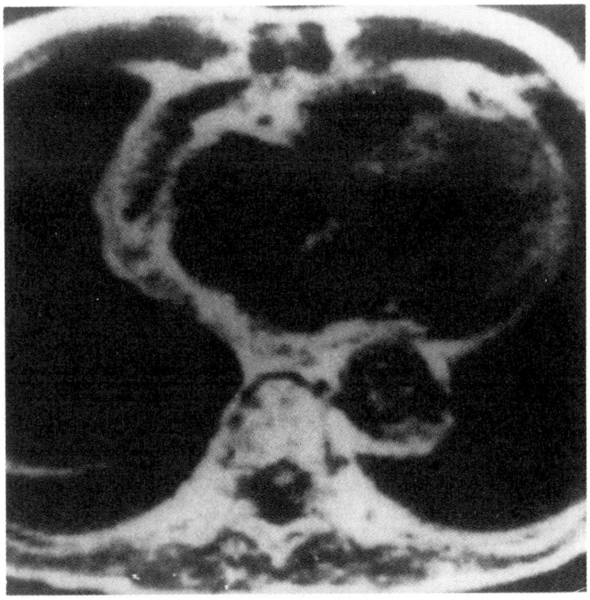

Figure 3 Magnetic resonance image from a patient with constrictive pericarditis. There is thickening of both the visceral and the parietal pericardium, with some fluid noted as well as hypertrophy of the left ventricle. (From Soulen RD, et al. Magnetic resonance imaging of constrictive pericardial disease. Am J Cardiol 1985; 55:480. Reproduced by permission of the publisher and author.)

ing phase progresses and the ventricle reaches the limits imposed by the pericardium, filling will abruptly slow, resulting in the characteristic "dip-and-plateau" or "square root" sign that may be evident on right and left ventricular diastolic pressure recordings. Because the pericardium limits both left and right ventricular filling, there will be equalization of the left and right ventricular pressures throughout diastole until the onset of systole. After the rapid filling phase, very little filling takes place (the diastolic plateau). In the presence of tachycardia, however, these features are difficult to identify (see Fig. 4). Recordings of right atrial pressure usually show a prominent y-descent and preservation of the x-descent (Fig. 5). Right atrial pressure may also fail to decrease (or may even increase) with inspiration, the hemodynamic counterpart to Kussmaul's sign. Rapid administration of intravenous saline, exercise, or both may help bring out equalization of diastolic pressures and a dip-and-plateau contour to the ventricular pressure waveform if resting hemodynamics are nondiagnostic. The converse is also true: volume depletion may mask the characteristic equalization of diastolic pressures.

There are a number of relatively unique diagnostic features that may help to distinguish constrictive pericarditis from other similar clinical syndromes, and they are listed below.

Cirrhosis

Some of the clinical features of constrictive pericarditis (ascites, hepatomegaly, and abnormal liver function tests) may suggest the presence of cirrhosis. The high central venous pressures of pericardial constriction can also cause hepatic congestion and a clinical picture indistinguishable from cirrhosis. The obvious factors distinguishing cirrhosis from constrictive pericarditis are the level of central venous

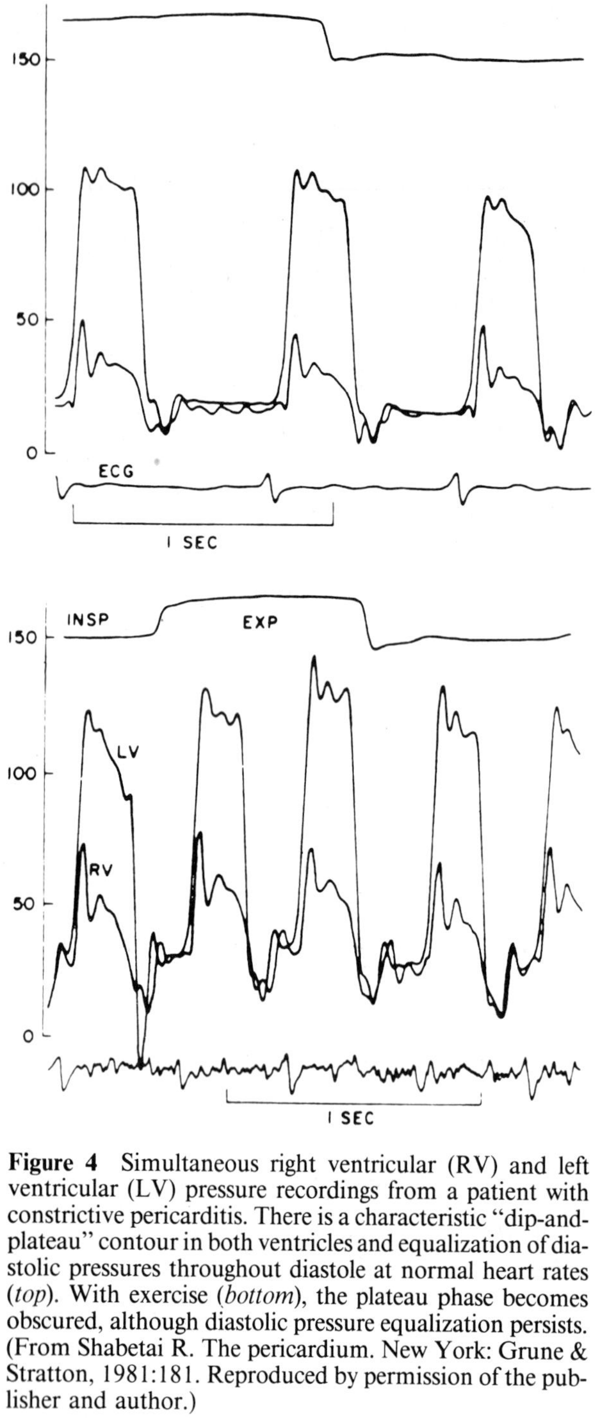

Figure 4 Simultaneous right ventricular (RV) and left ventricular (LV) pressure recordings from a patient with constrictive pericarditis. There is a characteristic "dip-and-plateau" contour in both ventricles and equalization of diastolic pressures throughout diastole at normal heart rates (*top*). With exercise (*bottom*), the plateau phase becomes obscured, although diastolic pressure equalization persists. (From Shabetai R. The pericardium. New York: Grune & Stratton, 1981:181. Reproduced by permission of the publisher and author.)

pressures (usually normal in cirrhosis, elevated in constriction) and the status of ventricular diastolic function (normal in cirrhosis, impaired in constriction).

Right-Sided Chronic Heart Failure

Some of the clinical features of constrictive pericarditis (i.e., elevated jugular venous pressure, edema,

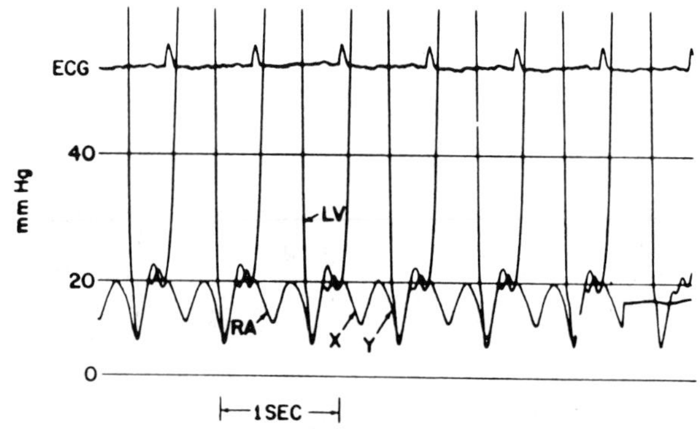

Figure 5 Simultaneous right atrial (RA) and left ventricular (LV) pressure tracings from a patient with constrictive pericarditis. There is a prominent y-descent on the RA waveform, indicating intact rapid filling and normal early diastolic ventricular function. Right atrial and left ventricular diastolic pressures are both elevated and equal throughout diastole. (From Lorell BH, Grossman W. Profile in constrictive pericarditis, restrictive cardiomyopathy, and cardiac tamponade. In: Grossman W, ed. Cardiac catheterization and angiography. 4th ed. Philadelphia: Lea & Febiger, 1991. Reproduced by permission of the publisher and authors.)

Kussmaul's sign, hepatomegaly, ascites) may also mimic chronic right heart failure. In general, differentiating between the two is relatively simple by considering pulmonary artery pressures (often elevated in right-sided failure, usually normal to slightly elevated in constriction), equalization of right and left ventricular diastolic pressures (usually absent in right-sided failure, present in constriction), rapidity of the jugular venous or right atrial y-descent (normal to attenuated in right-sided failure, accentuated in constriction), "dip-and-plateau" or "square-root" sign (usually absent in right-sided failure, present in constriction), and left ventricular diastolic function (usually normal in right-sided failure, abnormal in constriction). However, acute right heart failure (as with massive pulmonary embolus or right ventricular infarction) may cause abrupt right ventricular dilation leading to a constrictive pericarditis-like hemodynamic picture. Acute right-heart failure is also usually abrupt in onset, without any of the historical factors suggestive of pericardial constriction.

Right Ventricular Infarction

Right ventricular infarction may present a constrictive-like hemodynamic pattern. The presumptive mechanism is that sudden right ventricular dilation within the pericardium and constraint by the normal pericardium leads to the hemodynamic abnormalities that are also found with constrictive pericarditis. The hemodynamic profile may be indistinguishable from classic pericardial constriction, but the clinical setting of acute right ventricular infarction is usually obvious, with chest pain, inferior or posterior electrocardiographic changes, and hypotension as well as changes on right-precordial chest leads (ST-segment elevation in V4R-V6R), or impairment of right ventricular function on echocardiogaphy or gated radionuclide ventriculography.

Cardiac Tamponade

It is usually not difficult to differentiate pericardial constriction and cardiac tamponade. Among the clinical data that favor a diagnosis of constrictive pericarditis over cardiac tamponade are pulsus paradoxus (often absent in constriction, usually present in tamponade), Kussmaul's sign (usually absent in tamponade, often present in constriction), a "dip-and-plateau" or "square root" sign on ventricular pressure tracing (absent in tamponade, present in constriction), a prominent y-descent of the jugular venous or right atrial pressure (absent in tamponade, present in constriction), timing of impaired diastolic function (occurring throughout diastole in tamponade but only in the latter part of diastole in constriction) and the absolute level of pericardial pressure (high in tamponade, normal in constriction).

Restrictive Cardiomyopathy

The clinical picture of constrictive pericarditis may be extremely difficult to distinguish from restrictive cardiomyopathy. Restrictive cardiomyopathy is usually the result of some infiltrative process of the myocardium that results in diastolic dysfunction. The most important restrictive cardiomyopathies are amyloidosis, hemachromatosis, and endomyocardial fibroelastosis. Extensive radiation to the mediastinum may also lead to restrictive cardiomyopathy. Diastolic dysfunction usually occurs throughout diastole, but depending on the degree of ventricular involvement and the slope of the diastolic pressure–volume relationship, it may occur early or late in diastole. The hemodynamic picture may be indistinguishable from constrictive pericarditis. Both syndromes can exhibit equilibration of right and left ventricular diastolic pressure with a "dip-and-plateau" or "square root" sign. There may be a disparity between right ventricular and left ventricular end-diastolic pressures in restriction (that is not present in constriction), which may be brought out by exercise or fluid loading. The disparity between ventricular pressures is, to a large extent, dependent on the degree of left ventricular involvement; the more involved the left ventricle with the infiltrative process, the greater the disparity. Other data that may differentiate pericardial constriction from restrictive cardiomyopathy include RV systolic hypertension (absent in constriction, present in restriction), prominent respiratory variation in left ventricular isovolumic relaxation time and peak mitral flow velocity (present in constriction, absent in restriction), timing of impaired diastolic function (occurring throughout diastole in restriction, only in the latter part of diastole in constriction), and the surface electrocardiogram (depolarization and conduction abnormalities in restriction, repolarization abnormalities in constriction). Involvement of other systems with amyloidosis (renal, gastrointestinal) and hemochromatosis (liver, skin, diabetes) may help to identify an underlying systemic cause of restrictive cardiomyopathy. Endomyocardial biopsy may also be helpful in identifying causes (amyloidosis, hemochromatosis, endomyocardial fibroelastosis) of restrictive cardiomyopathy. Ultrafast cine-CT and MRI are particularly useful in distinguishing between constrictive pericarditis and restrictive cardiomyopathy.

Effusive-Constrictive Disease

Effusive-constrictive disease is a disorder in which there is a combination of pericardial tamponade and constrictive physiology. The causes of effusive-constrictive disease are generally the same as those of constrictive pericarditis (neoplasm, previous radiation, acute pericarditis, tuberculosis). Effusive-constrictive physiology may, in fact, be an early stage in the development of chronic constrictive pericarditis. The hemodynamic features of effusive-constrictive disease are most consistent with cardiac tamponade, and the diagnosis is confirmed with the documentation of persistently elevated right atrial pressure and equilibration of right and left ventricular diastolic pressures after pericardiocentesis and return of intrapericardial pressure to zero. Pericardiocentesis may provide temporary relief, but as with constrictive pericarditis, the definitive therapy for effusive-constrictive disease is surgical resection.

THERAPEUTIC ALTERNATIVES

Once the diagnosis is established, efforts should be directed toward avoiding further hemodynamic compromise prior to surgery. As with the management of acute right ventricular failure or right ventricular infarction, maintenance of an adequate preload without causing worsening constriction and further hemodynamic deterioration is crucial. Drugs that decrease preload (venodilators, nitrates, diuretics) ordinarily are not used. Drugs that decrease heart rate and increase ventricular filling (such as beta blockers and some calcium blockers) may have theoretical disadvantages and should also be used with caution. It should be emphasized that constrictive pericarditis is not a reversible phenomenon, and the underlying problem requires surgical correction. Without surgical correction, there are no pharmacologic or hemodynamic manipulations that will reverse the underlying problem, although stabilization prior to surgery is important to minimize the risks of the operative procedure. Surgical outcome is unfavorably influenced by severe clinical disability, and surgical intervention should be undertaken early in the course of symptomatic patients.

PREFERRED APPROACH

Surgical Treatment

Constrictive pericarditis is a progressive disorder, and the majority of patients who come to medical attention because of symptoms will, over time, become more symptomatic. The definitive therapeutic procedure for the treatment of constrictive pericarditis is surgical resection of the pericardium. This can be best accomplished with a midline thoracotomy and cardiopulmonary bypass, which allows better mobilization of the heart and total removal of the pericardium, which can be densely adherent.

Operative mortality is low, on the order of 5 percent, and the majority of patients will have complete relief of symptoms. In some patients, symptomatic and hemodynamic improvement will be immediately apparent; whereas in others there will be more gradual improvement over days to weeks. An inadequate response to pericardiectomy is usually due to an incomplete surgical resection, especially with densely adherent pericardium and involvement of the visceral pericardium. A small number of patients will have refractory and progressive cardiac failure following surgery, ending in death. In these patients, there is usually underlying myocardial disease (or atrophy) or persistent constriction of the left ventricle (due to incomplete resection). In these patients, left ventricular performance is inadequate to handle the increased pulmonary blood flow after relief of constriction of the right ventricle.

Given the fact that there is one basic treatment—surgery—for patients with constrictive pericarditis, the primary management problem lies in establishing the diagnosis and distinguishing constrictive pericarditis from the other pericardial compressive syndromes, namely cardiac tamponade and restrictive cardiomyopathy. Other disorders involving right-sided failure may also be confused with constrictive pericarditis and must also be excluded (Table 1).

TABLE 1 Clinical Syndromes That Mimic Pericardial Constriction

Cirrhosis
Right-sided congestive heart failure
Right ventricular infarction
Cardiac tamponade
Restrictive cardiomyopathy
Effusive-constrictive disease

TABLE 2 Historical and Physical Examination Features of Constrictive Pericarditis

History
Previous history of pericarditis
Tuberculosis
Renal failure
Neoplastic disease
Mediastinal irradiation
Chest trauma
Prior cardiac surgery
Physical Examination
Elevated jugular venous pressure
Prominent y-descent
Peripheral edema, ascites, hepatomegaly
Kussmaul's sign
Pericardial knock
Absence of pulsus paradoxus

Factors in the history and physical examination that support a diagnosis of constrictive pericarditis are summarized in Table 2. Elevated jugular venous pressure with a prominent y-descent is strongly suggestive of either pericardial constriction or restrictive cardiomyopathy. An early diastolic pericardial knock, if present and clearly distinguishable from an S_3, is virtually diagnostic. A pericardial knock is usually best heard along the left sternal border and occurs 0.09 to 0.12 second following A_2. It corresponds to the abrupt cessation of ventricular filling by the limiting pericardium. It is usually higher in pitch than a typical S_3, occurs somewhat earlier than S_3, and may be confused with the opening snap of mitral stenosis.

The data available from other diagnostic modalities have been previously discussed and are sum-

TABLE 3 Diagnostic Modalities Useful in the Clinical Recognition of Constrictive Pericarditis

Chest film	Pericardial calcification
	Left atrial enlargement
Electrocardiography	Usually nonspecific ST and T changes
	Low QRS voltages and left atrial abnormality may be present
Echocardiography	Increased pericardial thickness
	Rapid early diastolic filling
	Attenuated late diastolic filling
	Accentuated respiratory variation in isovolumic relaxation time and peak mitral flow velocity
Ultrafast cine-CT and MRI	Thickening of pericardium
	Dilated venae cavae or hepatic veins
	Impingement on right ventricle
Cardiac catheterization	Equalization of right and left ventricular diastolic pressures
	"Square root" sign
	Prominent y-descent
	Endomyocardial biopsy
Surgery	Pericardial histology

CT = Computed tomography, MRI = magnetic resonance imaging.

marized in Table 3. Electrocardiography and chest roentgenogram provide suggestive, but not definitive, diagnostic information. Echocardiography may document pericardial thickening and abnormal diastolic function, but it is relatively insensitive. Other new noninvasive diagnostic techniques for imaging the pericardium appear to be more useful, including ultrafast cine-CT and MRI. Cardiac catheterization provides the definitive hemodynamic data as well as an opportunity for endomyocardial biopsy to exclude restrictive cardiomyopathy (such as with amyloidosis, endomyocardial fibroelastosis, hemochromatosis) as a diagnostic possibility. There are still isolated cases in which a definitive diagnosis cannot be made until surgery, but fortunately with the advent of ultrafast cine-CT and MRI, they are becoming increasingly rare.

SUGGESTED READING

Fowler NO. Constrictive Pericarditis: New Aspects. Am J Cardiol 1982; 50:1014.

Hatle LK, Appleton CP, Popp RL. Differentiation of constrictive pericarditis and restrictive cardiomyopathy by Doppler echocardiography. Circulation 1989; 79:357.

Hirschmann JV. Pericardial Constriction. Am Heart J 1978; 96:110.

Reddy PS, Leon DF, Shavers JA (eds). Pericardial disease. New York: Raven Press, 1982.

Shabetai R. The pericardium. New York: Grune & Stratton, 1981.

Shabetai R, Fowler NO, Guntheroth WG. The hemodynamics of cardiac tamponade and constrictive pericarditis. Am J Cardiol 1970; 26:480.

Soulen RD, Stark DD, Higgins CB, et al. Magnetic resonance imaging of constrictive pericardial disease. Am J Cardiol 1985; 55:480.

Sutton FJ, Whitley NO, Applefeld MM, et al. The role of echocardiography and computed tomography in evaluation of constrictive pericarditis. Am Heart J 1985; 109:350.

MYOCARDITIS

CANDACE MIKLOZEK McNULTY, M.D.

Myocarditis has been implicated as a significant contributing factor in the pathogenesis of dilated cardiomyopathy, a major cause of congestive heart failure. Experimental and clinical studies suggest that, if diagnosed early, it is a potentially reversible cause of myocardial dysfunction. It is initiated by viruses (most often enteroviruses) and has both an acute and a chronic stage. During the acute stage, virus-induced myocyte degeneration occurs in the absence of a cellular infiltrate. Key pathologic features of the chronic or autoimmune stage are an inflammatory infiltrate (primarily lymphocytes and monocyte-macrophages) and necrotic myocytes; virus is absent. Destruction of myocytes, both infected and uninfected, is mediated through the immune response with activation of natural killer cells, helper cells, suppressor T cells, or a combination of these. Myosin, released from virus-damaged myocytes, can also induce autoimmune myocarditis. The virus type and genetic makeup of the host determine the immune mechanism of myocyte destruction. Failure to culture virus from the myocardium in patients with biopsy-proven myocarditis suggests that most patients are in the chronic or autoimmune stage of the disease at the time of diagnosis. In the future, therapeutic strategies and drugs specific for the stage of disease and mechanism of immunologic dysfunction will be developed. At present, in the majority of patients, the therapy of myocarditis is supportive and directed to the symptoms resulting from structural cardiac damage.

PREFERRED APPROACH

General Considerations

A high index of suspicion of myocarditis and clinical recognition of the disease are the first steps in treatment. Myocarditis is a focal disease; the area involved may be extensive or small. One or both ventricles, the conduction system, or pericardium may be involved. The size and location of the infiltrate and necrotic myocytes determine clinical manifestations. The spectrum of abnormalities is diverse, ranging from an absence of findings to congestive heart failure and sudden death. It not uncommonly mimics other types of heart disease such as acute myocardial infarction and dilated cardiomyopathy. Myocarditis should be considered in any patient with new cardiac symptoms or abnormalities that develop during a viral prodrome and, particularly, in the patient with recent onset dilated cardiomyopathy.

The diagnosis is supported by positive hot spot cardiac scans, using Tc pyrophosphate or gallium-67 radioisotopes and endomyocardial biopsy. The specificity of the gallium-67 scan is greater than that of the Tc pyrophosphate scan in myocarditis; a scan should be obtained in all patients. An endomyocardial biopsy should be performed in patients with severe cardiac dysfunction such as congestive heart failure, new onset dilated cardiomyopathy, acute myocardial infarction, ventricular tachycardia, sudden death, and cardiogenic shock. A negative biopsy does not exclude the diagnosis; biopsies are more likely to be positive if performed early (i.e., within 1 month of onset of symptoms). All patients should undergo noninvasive assessment of ventricular function by two-dimensional echocardiography and radionuclide ventriculography and ambulatory electrocardiographic monitoring for detection of conduction disturbances and arrhythmias. Serial electrocardiograms and cardiac enzymes should be obtained to determine the extent of acute myocardial damage. These test results, by determining the extent of structural cardiac damage, will focus symptomatic treatment and serve as a baseline in assessing response to therapy. The goal of treatment is to preserve or salvage myocardium so that systolic ventricular function can be maintained or improved. This is attempted through restriction of physical activity, use of antiviral and immunosuppressive agents in selected cases, use of conventional cardiac therapy for symptoms related to structural damage, and avoidance of recurrent episodes.

Although not all patients are ill enough to require admission to the hospital, patients should be observed and monitored in the hospital if certain symptoms or findings are present. These include a history of syncope, acute myocardial infarction, ventricular or atrial arrhythmias, sudden death, conduction disturbances, congestive heart failure, shock, a pericardial friction rub, enlargement of the cardiac silhouette by chest film, or an unreliable patient. The length of hospital stay is determined by the extent of structural damage and the clinical response of the patient; it does not usually exceed 5 to 7 days.

Restriction of Physical Activity

Animal studies have shown convincingly that exercise during acute viral myocarditis increases myocardial viral titers, inflammation, myocyte necrosis, heart size, and mortality. These suggest that restriction of physical activity with bed rest at the time of diagnosis and sedentary activity during convalescence is the most effective measure available in the treatment of myocarditis. Rest leads to a reduction in cardiac work by a decrease in blood pressure and heart rate. The optimal duration has not been ascertained. At the time of diagnosis, bed rest or sedentary activity is recommended for 2 weeks. The period of restriction is increased (in some cases, 6 months to a year) in patients with extensive structural abnormalities, i.e., those with low ejection fractions, ventricular dilation, high-grade ventricular ectopy, or significant wall motion abnormalities. After the initial 2 weeks, and in the absence of heart failure or high-grade ventricular ectopy, the degree of physical activity is progressively liberalized; patients may return to the work force if it does not involve heavy physical labor. Other activities such as swimming, weight lifting, aerobics, cycling, jogging, housework, and carrying heavy objects should be avoided for 6 months. The American College of Cardiology has recommended that the athlete not return to competitive sports for 6 months. Participation should be allowed only when ventricular function and the electrocardiogram have returned to normal and clinically significant arrhythmias are not present by ambulatory electrocardiographic monitoring. An exercise test, preferably with radionuclide ventriculography, should be performed 6 months from the time of diagnosis for the reassurance of both the patient and physician.

A possible alternative is the use of competitive beta-receptor blocking agents. These drugs, which decrease heart rate, reduce contractility, and lower blood pressure, could provide a chemical means of resting the heart. Although beneficial effects have been shown in patients with dilated cardiomyopathy, myocardial necrosis and mortality were increased in mice with early myocarditis treated with metoprolol. Further studies are needed to confirm this.

Antiviral Agents

A search for a specific viral etiology and other causes of myocarditis should be made. This helps to date the onset and stage of infection and may identify other treatable causes of myocarditis such as lupus erythematosus, mycoplasma, and *Borrelia burgdorferi* (Lyme disease) infections. Antibody levels of Epstein-Barr virus, cytomegalovirus, and hepatitis should be measured and body fluids (stool, urine, and throat swab samples) cultured in continuous cell lines in a virology laboratory. A titer for human immunodeficiency virus (HIV) should be obtained if there is a past history of blood transfusion or high risk sexual behavior.

Amantadine, acyclovir, vidarabine, and ganciclovir have been approved for treatment of selected, usually life-threatening, viral infections but not for myocarditis. Ribavirin (a broad-spectrum antiviral agent) treatment of mice with early myocarditis is associated with less inflammation and necrosis. This positive effect, as with other antiviral agents, occurs only when the drug is administered just before or at the onset of infection. The methodologic time delay in identifying virus and failure to isolate virus from a substantial number currently limits their use in most myocarditis patients.

Immunosuppressive Therapy

The prognosis of patients with dilated cardiomyopathy, congestive heart failure, and decreased systolic function is poor; the majority of patients are dead within 5 years. Twenty-three to 67 percent of patients with recent onset dilated cardiomyopathy have myocarditis by endomyocardial biopsy. The biopsy findings in patients with myocarditis resemble those of patients with cardiac transplant rejection. For this reason, many were enthusiastic that treat-

TABLE 1 Summary of Clinical Studies of Myocarditis Treated with Immunosuppressive Drugs

Author	*CHF/DCM*	*+MYO*	*Immunosuppressive Agent(s)*			*Control Group*		
	N	*N*	*N*	*Improvement*	*Death*	*N*	*Improvement*	*Death*
Mason (1980)	10	7	10	5	3			
O'Connell (1981)	39	19	15	6	3	20	—	5
Edwards (1982)	10	10	5	3	1	5	3	1
Fenoglio (1983)	34	34	19	5	4	15	2	—
Daly (1984)	12	12	9	7	0	3	—	
Dec (1985)	27	18	9	4	2	18	6	8
Hosenpud (1985)	6	6	6	0	0			
Latham (1989)	52	1	23	?	7	29	?	5

CHF = Congestive heart failure, DCM = dilated cardiomyopathy, Improvement = in left ventricular function, +MYO = myocarditis by biopsy in all except O'Connell (gallium scan), N = number.

ment with immunosuppressive agents of patients with myocarditis and dilated cardiomyopathy would be effective in restoring myocardial function. Since 1980, eight such clinical studies have been published (Table 1). A corticosteroid agent alone or in combination with azathioprine was used; dosages and duration of therapy varied among studies. Patient numbers were small, and sometimes a control group was not used. Results have been conflicting. In spite of resolution of both infiltrate and muscle damage by follow-up biopsy in most cases, improvement in ventricular function did not always occur. Moreover, spontaneous improvement occurred in as many as 33 to 60 percent of untreated patients. Effectiveness was suggested in some patients with initial improvement because clinical features worsened when the immunosuppressive agent(s) were discontinued.

Patients with biopsy-proven myocarditis, intact ventricular function, and ventricular tachycardia, or sudden death have also been treated with prednisone and azathioprine. Following therapy, the arrhythmia resolved. However, numbers of patients were small, and a control group was not used.

Increased myocardial viral titers, inflammation, and necrosis as well as greater mortality occur in mice with early acute myocarditis treated with corticosteroid agents. These agents inhibit migration of macrophages to the site of infection. Because one function of macrophages is to limit virus replication, inhibition results in increased virus and myocyte damage. Corticosteroids do not have this effect when given after clearance of virus. Immunosuppressive agents have significant risks. Corticosteroid agents increase susceptibility to bacterial infections and the incidence of osteoporosis, aseptic necrosis of the hip, systemic arterial hypertension, glucose intolerance, and psychosis. Jaundice, alopecia, and bone marrow suppression with leukopenia and thrombocytopenia can result from azathioprine.

Until the efficacy of immunosuppressive therapy in the treatment of myocarditis is resolved by a large controlled series of patients, its use should be limited to research protocols. It should only be considered when congestive heart failure and a low ejection fraction are present because of the association of the latter with a poor prognosis and mortality. The only exception would be the patient with a rapidly deteriorating cardiac picture and cardiogenic shock.

Precautions prior to administration of these agents include exclusion of active viral infection with viral cultures and titers and performance of an endomyocardial biopsy. The latter is done to ensure that histologic criteria of myocarditis are present and to provide tissue as a comparison with follow-up biopsies for assessment of response to therapy.

Conventional Therapy for Symptoms Due to Myocardial Damage

Symptoms resulting from structural cardiac damage in myocarditis include left ventricular systolic dysfunction with congestive heart failure, (myo)pericarditis, conduction disturbances, ventricular ectopy, and sudden death. Therapy for these has been well defined but except for congestive heart failure has not been specifically studied in myocarditis. Nonetheless, conventional therapy is used and is discussed in this section.

Congestive Heart Failure

An angiotensin converting enzyme inhibitor agent such as captopril should be given if the left ventricular ejection fraction is less than 35 percent and congestive heart failure is present. Captopril improves the symptoms of heart failure and lowers mortality by improving cardiac performance via a reduction in afterload by lowering blood pressure; the major side effect is acute renal failure precipitated by hypotension. Caution in increasing the dose and in using diuretic and other vasodilator agents minimizes this risk.

Digitalis should be added only if left ventricular dilation or supraventricular arrhythmias are present. Digoxin levels should be periodically measured because myocarditis patients are thought to be prone to digoxin toxicity.

Systemic and pulmonary congestion are treated with diuretic agents such as furosemide. Regardless of the path of administration, the initial dose should be small to avoid excessive intravascular volume depletion; later doses are determined by the patient's response and volume of urine output. The serum potassium level should be followed closely because the reabsorption of potassium is blocked by furosemide, and hypokalemia may result.

Systemic anticoagulation is recommended because of the increased risk of arterial emboli in patients with a low ejection fraction (less than 25 percent) or with a thrombus by echocardiography. Initially, this is accomplished by intravenous heparin followed by oral warfarin. Bleeding is the major complication of anticoagulation but can be minimized if the partial thromboplastin time (in the case of heparin) and the prothrombin time (in the case of warfarin) are maintained at 1.5 times the control value. The dose of warfarin should be reduced in the presence of hepatic congestion since the latter potentiates the anticoagulant effect. The effects of heparin can be reversed by protamine sulfate and warfarin by fresh frozen plasma and vitamin K. Anticoagulation should not be instituted if a pericardial effusion is present because of the risk of bleeding.

Sympathomimetic agents (epinephrine, norepinephrine, and dobutamine) may produce toxic myocarditis and should not be given. Low-dose intravenous dopamine (the immediate precursor of norepinephrine) may be used if a vasopressor agent is needed. Larger doses are to be avoided because of the risk of myocardial necrosis.

Cardiac transplantation is considered in the patient with symptoms of congestive heart failure at rest, ejection fraction response less than 20 percent, and no response to medical therapy.

Pericarditis

Anti-inflammatory nonsteroidal agents are effective in the relief of pericarditic pain probably through inhibition of the cyclo-oxygenase enzyme system and prostaglandin formation. In early acute myocarditis, nonsteroidal agents are associated with increased myocardial necrosis in mice but not when given later. Because most myocarditis patients are no longer excreting virus at the time of presentation, it appears safe to administer this drug. Potential adverse effects include occult bleeding due to a reversible antiplatelet effect, gastritis due to inhibition of prostaglandin E_2, renal toxicity, and reduction in diuretic effectiveness. Its use is not contraindicated in patients with a pericardial effusion. There are a variety of acceptable agents available; toxicity is less common with the oxicam and proprionic acid compounds. Most patients have difficulty tolerating indomethacin for prolonged periods of time because of dizziness and epigastric discomfort due to gastritis. Dosages employed should be those recommended by the manufacturer. After 2 weeks of therapy, the dosage should be tapered and discontinued over the ensuing 2 weeks. Pain may recur in some patients; the medication should be continued in this group. It is worthwhile to try a different compound if there is no relief of pain. Corticosteroid agents, although effective in the relief of pain, should be avoided for reasons already discussed.

Patients should be observed closely for tamponade physiology, but this occurrence is unusual. If hemodynamic compromise develops, pericardiocentesis should be performed.

Ventricular Arrhythmias

Electric d.c. cardioversion should be promptly applied to the patient with sustained ventricular tachycardia and associated hemodynamic findings such as syncope, sudden death, and shock. Asymptomatic patients with sustained ventricular tachycardia (longer than 30 seconds) can be treated with intravenous lidocaine.

After electrolyte abnormalities and hypoxia have been corrected, quantification of ventricular ectopy is determined by extended ambulatory monitoring; the initial study serves as a baseline in assessing the response to therapy. Chronic oral antiarrhythmic therapy is recommended in patients with sustained ventricular tachycardia with or without symptoms. Programmed stimulation may be helpful in patients with witnessed sudden death caused by ventricular tachycardia and negative follow-up electrocardiographic monitoring. Treatment is also recommended in patients without symptoms and high-grade ectopy (frequent multifocal premature beats > 30 per hour, R-on-T phenomenon, couplets, and triplets) if left ventricular systolic dysfunction is present because of the increased risk of sudden death.

A variety of antiarrhythmic agents are available. Quinidine should be avoided because it may produce toxic myocarditis. Regardless of which agent is selected, oral therapy should be instituted in a monitored hospital setting because all agents have some degree of proarrhythmic effect. All agents require a loading dose for therapeutic effect. The maintenance dose should be determined by trough and peak levels. Treatment is continued for a minimum of 6 months. When scans and biopsy findings have reverted to negative, the medication is discontinued while the patient is monitored in the hospital. It is not uncommon for the arrhythmia to resolve.

Conduction Disturbances

Conduction disturbances are common and include first-degree block, Mobitz types I and II AV block, bundle-branch blocks, and complete heart block. During the acute illness, patients should be monitored in either a coronary care or a telemetry unit where insertion of a temporary pacemaker can be easily performed. First degree block, Mobitz type I (Wenckebach) AV block, and bundle-branch blocks are usually asymptomatic and do not require therapy. A temporary pacemaker should be inserted when either Mobitz type II AV block or complete heart block is present. Some of these patients may require placement of a permanent pacemaker.

Acute Myocardial Infarction

During the acute illness, treatment of the myocarditis patient and the patient with atherosclerotic coronary artery disease and acute infarction is the same with one exception. The efficacy of coronary artery reperfusion with thrombolytic therapy has been established in atherosclerotic disease. Because the mechanism of infarction in myocarditis is not known, thrombolytic therapy should not be employed in myocarditis patients. Patients should be monitored in the coronary care unit. Hypoxia should be treated with oxygen. Initial chest pain is treated with intravenous morphine in doses of 2 to 4 mg at 5-minute increments; recurrent chest pain should be treated as angina pectoris with nitrates until diagnostic procedures are performed. If congestive heart failure is present, it should be managed with the previously described medications. Measurement of intracardiac pressures by insertion of a central line may be required for optimal management of shock and heart failure. Because atherosclerotic coronary artery disease remains the most common cause of acute infarction, it is essential that coronary angiography be performed to exclude fixed coronary artery lesions because the long-term therapy and prognosis for each disease is different. Exercise testing prior to catheterization should not be performed if myocarditis is suspected, for the reasons discussed earlier.

Recurrences of Myocarditis

Recurrences are common. Patients should be instructed to avoid factors that increase susceptibility to myocarditis especially during symptoms of an acute viral prodrome. These include exercise and the use of alcohol. Cocaine, amphetamines, and sympathomimetic agents (contained in diet pills, cough syrups and nasal decongestants) have the potential to produce myocarditis and should be avoided. Medications known to produce toxic myocarditis should not be prescribed; these include theophylline, phenothiazines, lithium carbonate, and anthracycline agents.

SUGGESTED READING

Abelmann WH. Myocarditis as a cause of dilated cardiomyopathy. In: O'Connell (ed): Drug therapy in dilated cardiomyopathy and myocarditis. New York: Marcel Dekker, 1988:221–231.

Daly K, Richardson PJ, Olsen EGJ, et al. Acute myocarditis. Role of histological and virological examination in the diagnosis and assessment of immunosuppressive treatment. Br Heart J 1984; 51:30.

Dec QW Jr, Palacios IF, Fallon JT, et al. Active myocarditis in the spectrum of acute dilated cardiomyopathies, clinical features, histologic correlates and clinical outcome. N Engl J Med 1985; 312:885.

Edwards WD, Holmes Jr DR, Reeder GS. Diagnosis of active lymphocytic myocarditis by endomyocardial biopsy, quantitative criteria for light microscopy. Mayo Clin Proc 1982; 57:419.

Fenoglio JJ, Ursell PC, Kellogg CF, et al. Diagnosis and classification of myocarditis by endomyocardial biopsy. N Engl J Med 1983; 308:12.

Hosenpud JD, McAnulty JH, Niles NR. Lack of objective improvement in ventricular systolic function in patients with myocarditis treated with azathioprine and prednisone. J Am Coll Cardiol 1985; 6:797.

Latham RD, Mulrow JP, Virmani R, et al. Recently diagnosed idiopathic dilated cardiomyopathy: Incidence of myocarditis and efficacy of prednisone therapy. Am Heart J 1989; 117:876.

Lerner AM, Wilson FM. Virus myocardiopathy. Prog Med Virol 1973; 15:63.

Leslie K, Blay R, Haisch C, et al. Clinical and experimental aspects of viral myocarditis. Clin Microbiol Rev 1989; 2:191.

Mason JW, Billingham ME, Ricci DR. Treatment of acute inflammatory myocarditis assisted by endomyocardial biopsy. Am J Cardiol 1980; 45:1037.

O'Connell JB, Robinson JA, Henkin RE, Gunnar RM. Immunosuppressive therapy in patients with congestive cardiomyopathy and myocardial uptake of gallium-67. Circulation 1981; 64:780.

Woodruff JF. Viral myocarditis. Am J Pathol 1980; 1:427.

CARDIOMYOPATHY: DILATED

CELIA M. OAKLEY, M.D., F.R.C.P., F.A.C.C., F.E.S.C.

Dilated cardiomyopathy is characterized by reduction in contractile force of the left ventricle not caused by limitation of blood flow through the extramural coronary arteries and unassociated with specific pathology. The left ventricle is dilated, and the ejection fraction is usually less than 0.40 but may be much lower. Left ventricular failure is usually the first clinical event. The right ventricle may also be dilated, and rarely the dilation affects the right ventricle alone. Disturbances of atrial and ventricular rhythm are common, and in the right ventricular form recurrent ventricular tachycardia may dominate the clinical scene, leading to the descriptive title of "arrhythmogenic right ventricular dysplasia."

THERAPEUTIC ALTERNATIVES

Dilated cardiomyopathy is a condition of unknown etiology, so that advances in treatment are largely a result of improvement in the management of cardiac failure. The possibility of an enterovirus etiology for some cases has followed the development of molecular cloning techniques for viruses, but until more is known neither antiviral agents nor immunosuppressive therapy is appropriate.

Therapy is therefore directed toward alleviating heart failure, improving exercise tolerance, preventing thromboembolism, treating symptomatic arrhythmias, and preventing sudden death and progressive heart failure. Despite this, cardiac transplantation offers the only hope of restoration to full activity in some patients.

PREFERRED APPROACH

Medical Treatment

Most patients are not seen until after their first episode of left ventricular failure. Only a few are recognized because of a third heart sound or mitral regurgitant murmur, left bundle-branch block, or otherwise abnormal electrogram or cardiac enlargement on chest film. Systemic embolism is occasionally the first event. In others, the onset of atrial fibrillation or the observation of frequent ventricular ectopic beats or even ventricular tachycardia may bring the underlying disease to notice.

Left Ventricular Dysfunction

Diuretics. It is rational to try to unload and to shrink the size of the left ventricle. Although prognostic benefit is hard to prove, many patients in this category either improve or remain unchanged for years. An angiotensin converting enzyme (ACE) inhibitor alone may suffice or be combined with a thiazide diuretic, especially if the blood pressure is high.

Diuretics, ACE inhibitors, and inotropes are introduced in that order according to severity (Fig. 1). After the first episode of left ventricular failure, a diuretic usually removes evidence of failure and improves exercise tolerance. Some patients are rendered asymptomatic, although the left ventricle remains abnormal. When fluid retention is mild, a thiazide drug is first choice coupled with moderate dietary sodium restriction. These drugs inhibit sodium transport proximal to the distal tubule where sodium is reabsorbed without water. Salt excretion is affected for about 8 hours, with the exception of chlorthalidone, which has an effect lasting for over 24 hours. All thiazide drugs increase urinary potassium loss, and the diet should be high in potassium-containing fruits such as oranges and bananas. This may be sufficient, but since it is desirable to maintain potassium levels at between 4 and 5 mmols per liter, the addition of a potassium-sparing agent such as amiloride is preferable to potassium supplements that do more good to the manufacturer than to the patient. Bendrofluazide 5 mg plus amiloride 5 or 10 mg daily may be sufficient. Spironolactone is an alternative to amiloride in women but in men has a high incidence of causing painful gynecomastia. Treatment will lower blood pressure, but the aim should be to keep it low, around 100 to 110 systolic if the patient is younger and a little higher in older patients.

More resistant fluid retention requires a loop diuretic such as bumetanide or furosemide. These act by inhibiting sodium and chloride transport in the ascending limb of Henle's loop and promote a greater chloride than sodium diuresis. They also increase urinary potassium loss leading to hypokalemic alkalosis. Secondary aldosteronism increases potassium depletion.

Bumetanide and furosemide have an action that peaks in about 4 hours and is complete at 6 hours, allowing the patient to choose a convenient time of day for the dose. When heart failure is more severe, the drug may need to be given twice or even three times a day, although it is usually still possible to arrange for undisturbed nights. There is a widespread tendency to use excessive doses of diuretics. This leads to hypovolemia with postural hypotension, increased fatigability and uremia. It is often not realized that fatigue and breathlessness are symptoms of an inadequate cardiac output response to exercise and not an indication for increasing the dose of diuretic that normally should not exceed 4 mg of bumetanide or 120

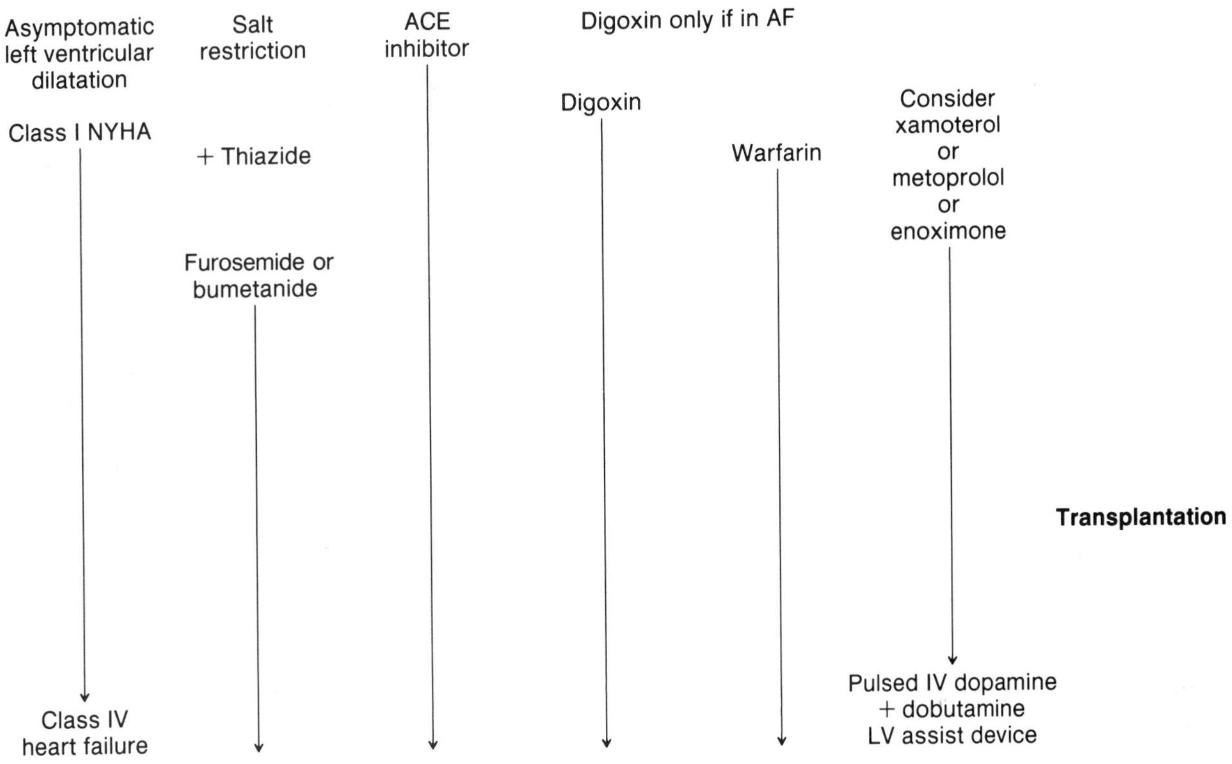

Figure 1 Management of dilated cardiomyopathy.

mg of furosemide in patients with normal renal function and frequently may be much less.

The natriuretic effect of loop diuretics is increased by the addition of amiloride or spironolactone and potassium loss reduced, but the effect of ACE inhibitors introduced at an early stage is to bring the potassium levels up and usually render potassium-sparing agents unnecessary.

Both loop diuretics and thiazides can induce hyperuricemia and precipitate gout. Thiazides may cause hyperglycemia, slight hyperlipidemia, and hypercalcemia. Skin rashes may be caused by amiloride but occasionally also by thiazides.

Hyponatremia follows use of these potent drugs and is due to relative water overload or, rarely if ever, to genuine sodium depletion. Mild hyponatremia needs no treatment, but more severe hyponatremia is a bad prognostic omen. Water restriction, although often advocated, can be intolerable to patients as well as not being very effective. The hyponatremia reflects a shift of sodium into cells due to magnesium depletion that inhibits membrane sodium/potassium adenosine triphosphatase (ATPase). Magnesium depletion has recently come back into prominence as a problem in heart failure patients. It contributes to depression and muscular weakness and is often associated with refractory hypokalemia and rhythm disturbances.

Hypomagnesemia can be treated with magnesium glycerophosphate in doses of 3 to 6 g daily orally.

Angiotensin Converting Enzyme Inhibitors. Angiotensin converting enzyme inhibitors act as vasodilators by reducing the circulating level of angiotensin II, by inhibiting the breakdown of bradykinin, and by interacting with the sympathetic nervous system to reduce its activity. They reduce "afterload" and also lower "preload," with largely secondary effects on the heart resulting in an increase in cardiac output and some redistribution of regional blood flow.

Angiotensin converting enzyme inhibitors have rendered direct acting vasodilators obsolete except for occasional patients who cannot tolerate them because of hypotension, renal failure, or intractable cough. In contrast to direct-acting vasodilators, alpha-blockers, and calcium entry blocking agents, ACE inhibitors diminish aldosterone secretion, reduce sodium and water retention, increase potassium retention, antagonize angiotensin-induced vasoconstriction, reduce raised circulating spillover catecholamine levels, and reduce myocardial oxygen consumption. Coronary vasodilation may occur, subendocardial blood flow may increase, and improved ventricular function is associated with some decrease in ventricular arrhythmia.

The effect of diuresis is to stimulate aldosterone secretion, which opposes this, so diuretic dosage should be kept as low as possible and ACE inhibitors introduced early with the objective of reducing this secondary aldosteronism and improving left ventricular output. It is best to start with a short-acting drug such as captopril 6.25 mg. If starting the drug in the hospital, the first dose should be given in the morning so that the blood pressure response can be observed. If starting the drug at home, the first dose should be taken after retiring at night so that any hypotensive response is minimized. The dose can then be increased quite quickly to a maximum of 25 mg three times a day. In some patients a maximum effect is achieved with a dose even lower than this. Once established on a short-acting ACE inhibitor, patients can be changed onto a long-acting, once-a-day ACE inhibitor such as lisinopril in a dose of up to 20 mg per day. The blood pressure is always reduced by ACE inhibitors and in some patients, hypotension, which is itself a poor prognostic omen in heart failure, may make it impossible to get the patients onto effective doses.

Hypotension is the most common and most worrisome side effect. It can be obviated to some extent by reducing the dose of diuretic or omitting it altogether for 24 hours before starting the ACE inhibitor, thus rendering it relatively ineffective so that the onset of action is gradual. Patients who are most likely to suffer a severe first dose hypotensive response are predictable. These are patients who are on high doses of diuretics, who already have low blood pressure, and who are hyponatremic and may also have impaired renal function. Great caution should be exercised in such patients in whom the first dose should be even lower than 6.25 mg. If it occurs, hypotension should be countered by posture. Saline infusion or vasoconstrictors are undesirable and rarely necessary after captopril, but hypotension after enalopril can be severe and prolonged.

Renal function may deteriorate in the first few days following the introduction of an ACE inhibitor. This is not only in patients with renal artery stenosis or occult bilateral renal artery stenosis who are thrown into profound renal failure, but also in patients with severe heart failure and reduced renal blood flow whose glomerular filtration is dependent, as in renal artery stenosis, on constriction of the efferent arterioles. In most such patients renal function gradually returns to normal after some days, but the rise in urea and creatinine can be worrying and renal failure may be precipitated by x-ray contrast agents.

Angiotensin converting enzyme inhibitors increase plasma levels of potassium, and this may contribute to reduction of ventricular arrhythmias, but hyperkalemia may reach dangerous levels if potassium-sparing diuretics or potassium supplements are not stopped, particularly as the levels may continue to rise. Despite this, some patients remain hypokalemic while on ACE inhibitors and these patients still need a carefully titrated dose of amiloride. It follows that potassium levels need to be checked frequently, particularly at first and in patients with advanced failure.

"Captopril cough" is recognized early. All the ACE inhibitors can increase the sensitivity of the cough reflex and cause a dry, irritating, repetitive cough in 10 to 15 percent of patients. Many patients tolerate the cough because of the benefit they gain once the cause of the cough is explained. This avoids unnecessary investigations.

Skin rashes may occur. Thrombocytopenia and membranous nephritis were seen in the early days of captopril when doses of 200 mg per day and more were given. They do not seem to occur with the low doses now used.

Digitalis. Digitalis has been used in the treatment of heart failure ever since William Withering discovered that foxglove leaves were valuable in the treatment of dropsy. It is probable that most of these early patients had rheumatic heart disease and that their heart failure was precipitated by the onset of atrial fibrillation with a fast ventricular rate. The efficacy of digitalis in the treatment of heart failure with sinus rhythm has been fiercely debated of recent years, but it now seems clear that digitalis is effective as a weak inotrope in some but not all patients with heart failure. Digitalis is ineffective in mainly diastolic heart failure as occurs in the elderly, in some cases of coronary heart failure, and in hypertrophied hearts. Digitalis is most effective in thin-walled, volume-loaded dilated left ventricles. The inotropic effect of digoxin was shown to be linear in acute studies with ouabain so that the greatest inotropic effect occurs close to the toxic dose. The problem is that in patients with sinus rhythm there is no endpoint as in atrial fibrillation, so the tendency is to be conservative and to use low and relatively ineffective doses. Therapy is not helped by the rather variable correlation between plasma levels and toxicity, which is enhanced in hypokalemic patients and through interaction with certain antiarrhythmic drugs including quinidine and amiodarone. Plasma levels should usually be between 1 and 3 nmol per liter.

Diet and Exercise. Obese patients should be counseled to lose weight, and the diet should be moderately low in salt and high in potassium-containing foods such as bananas and oranges. Avoidance of table salt and obviously salty foods cuts the intake to about 100 mmol per day. Patients with acute heart failure or exacerbations need bed rest, but the stable treated heart failure patient should be encouraged to take regular frequent walking exercise. This is in direct contrast to the conventional advice of only a few years ago when heart failure patients were advised to rest as much as possible. It has been shown that exercise tolerance is slowly and steadily improved by regular exercise training with an increase in stroke volume and peak oxygen consumption and a fall in heart rate and noradrenaline. The beneficial effect can be significant. Serial exercise testing in placebo-controlled drug trials was the way in which the benefits of training were first observed. This led to studies that proved benefit in trained compared with nonexercising patients.

Other Inotropes. No other orally active inotropes apart from digoxin have been shown to be either effective or safe. The so-called "inodilators," amrinone and milrinone, which are phosphodiesterase inhibitors, act only as vasodilators in long-term use with little evidence, if any, of continued beneficial effect on myocardial function and much concern about toxicity because of an excess of deaths in placebo-controlled trials of oral dosage. More recent drugs in this category, such as enoximone, have still to prove themselves.

Acute use of intravenous inotropes can be effective in the short term, and a combination of dopamine in renal doses with dobutamine can result in a rise in cardiac output with a fall in filling pressure, but the effects are usually only short term because of tachyphylaxis through down regulation of myocardial beta-receptors. Nevertheless, they may help to keep a patient going while awaiting transplantation. Pulsed doses for 48 hours every 2 weeks can be effective. Occasionally, substitution of adrenaline for dobutamine may bring about short-term further improvement, but arrhythmias may be precipitated.

Patients who require parenteral use of inotropes on account of hypotension, unresponsiveness to diuretics, or deteriorating renal function are in class IV failure with a prognosis measuring days, weeks, or months, and all should be considered for urgent transplantation unless there are contraindications.

Beta-Adrenergic Blocking Drugs. The acute use of beta-blocking drugs in patients with heart failure can cause profound loss of output with bradycardia and hypotension. There was therefore considerable incredulity and opposition when in 1975 the Swedes introduced the idea of using beta-blockers in heart failure. They started metoprolol in very small doses of 10 mg daily increasing only very slowly to not exceed 50 mg twice a day. Benefit was first seen in patients with coronary heart failure and tachycardia but then was found also when the treatment was extended to patients with dilated cardiomyopathy. Benefit was confined to about half of the patients and is sometimes delayed, even following early deterioration. The Swedish work has been confirmed and extended by more recent studies in Germany, in which starting dosage was even lower, and it was suggested that benefit may not be seen for several months.

The rationale for using beta-blocking drugs remains controversial. A fall in heart rate will reduce metabolic demand as well as improve coronary blood flow, and up regulation of myocardial beta-receptors may render the heart again sensitive to endogenous inotropes, particularly if they have prevented calcium overload from excessive beta stimulation.

An interesting new beta-blocker with considerable partial agonist action, xamoterol, showed promising results in early trials but an excess of deaths in a later trial of the drug in class III and IV heart failure. Benefit in the earlier trials may have been because of inclusion of a majority of patients with coronary heart failure because xamoterol is a useful antianginal agent. In milder heart failure xamoterol caused an increase in stroke volume and cardiac index with a fall in filling pressure that was maintained without tachyphylaxis. The excess of deaths in severe heart failure is still unexplained but may have to do with the drug working as a beta-blocker during waking hours but causing tachycardia during sleep.

Xamoterol may be useful in a few patients with mild heart failure in whom low blood pressure prevents the use of ACE inhibitors. A pure beta-blocker without partial agonist action such as metoprolol may be useful in occasional patients with heart failure and persistent tachycardia. The results of a multicenter placebo controlled trial of metoprolol in dilated cardiomyopathy are still awaited.

Antiarrhythmic Drugs. Ventricular ectopic activity is common in patients with a risk of sudden death in dilated cardiomyopathy as it is also in patients with advanced coronary disease, in hypertrophic cardiomyopathy, and in severe hypertensive heart disease, but it is now seen as a marker of a poor myocardium rather than as an independent prognostic indicator. In the CAST study of patients with asymptomatic ventricular ectopic activity following myocardial infarction, the membrane stabilizing antiarrhythmic effect of the class IC drugs effectively suppressed asymptomatic ventricular ectopic activity. The same effect depresses myocardial contractile activity, and it is the latter that may have been responsible for the increased deaths in this study. Although the results of CAST cannot necessarily be transferred to patients with dilated cardiomyopathy, there is no reason to believe that they would be different. Patients with dilated cardiomyopathy have ventricular ectopic activity whose frequency and complexity can be related to the severity of the myocardial dysfunction. Sudden death accounts for approximately half of the deaths of patients with dilated cardiomyopathy compared with about 70 percent of deaths in coronary heart failure. It has been assumed that they are caused by ventricular fibrillation precipitated by the ventricular ectopic activity, but it now seems that ventricular ectopic activity is simply a marker of a bad heart with a bad prognosis. Suppression of arrhythmia may follow improvement in left ventricular function, as was hinted at in a study of captopril. Certainly there is no present indication for seeking and suppressing asymptomatic ventricular arrhythmias in dilated cardiomyopathy. All the class I antiarrhythmic drugs have a myocardial depressant effect, and the results of two large trials of the class III drug, amiodarone, are still awaited. Only if it is believed that ventricular ectopic activity is so frequent that it is having a deleterious hemodynamic effect would there be an indication for amiodarone. There is some interest in the possibility that sudden death in patients being treated with class I antiarrhythmic drugs may be caused by the development of electromechanical dissociation rather than ventricular fibrillation.

In our own natural history study of dilated cardiomyopathy, sudden death was confined to patients with class III and IV heart failure.

There has been a revival of interest in sotalol for its combined class II and weak class III antiarrhythmic action.

Anticoagulants. There has been no controlled trial of anticoagulants in dilated cardiomyopathy. My own practice is to use anticoagulants in all patients who are in atrial fibrillation and in most patients with more than mild failure who are in sinus rhythm. This is because of a considerable incidence of systemic embolism. The source is probably the small thrombi that form in the trabecular crevices of the dilated left ventricle.

Cardiomyopathy Associated with Pregnancy and Parturition

Ventricular dilation and heart failure usually follow parturition but occasionally develop in late pregnancy. Because it is rare, the literature is muddled by anecdotal cases, reviews, and heterogeneous cases.

Heart failure may be sudden and catastrophic or more insidious. Treatment is for the heart failure. An immunologic interaction between mother and fetus can be postulated and short-term immunosuppressive therapy given. Genuine improvement can occur from severe hypokinetic left ventricular and congestive failure with reduction in left ventricular size. Although this usually has started within weeks of delivery and is complete by 6 months, a few patients may only start to improve after more than a year. Prognosis is therefore difficult, and transplantation should be avoided if at all possible while there may still be improvement. Not all patients relapse in future pregnancies, although further childbearing is inadvisable in any patient whose left ventricular function remains significantly abnormal.

Right Ventricular Dilated Cardiomyopathy and Arrhythmogenic Right Ventricular Dysplasia

This is probably a heterogeneous group of conditions in which right ventricular dysfunction varies from subclinical to severe but the left ventricle is apparently spared. Most common are patients with ventricular tachycardia originating from the right ventricle and showing a leftward axis and left bundle-branch block pattern. These cases are sometimes familial and may show adipose replacement of myocardial tissue in the right ventricular wall. Many of these patients have excellent hemodynamic function and are asymptomatic apart from the arrhythmias, whereas others develop profound low output failure with marked systemic congestion. Apart from control of heart rate and rhythm, right ventricular failure is exceedingly difficult to treat. A very high venous pressure can often be lowered without loss of output to reduce hepatic discomfort and edema, but no attempt should be made to lower venous pressure to normal, particularly if there is evidence of tricuspid regurgitation. Normally the pulmonary artery pressure is low and there is then no possibility of reducing right ventricular afterload, although balloon pumping of the pulmonary artery has been used in congestive heart failure with raised pulmonary vascular resistance.

Patients with arrhythmogenic right ventricular dysplasia have a high tendency to sudden death. Their symptomatic ventricular tachycardias are seen to degenerate into ventricular fibrillation and need to be treated vigorously. We have found amiodarone to be the most effective drug for this purpose and have followed some patients for up to 10 years while they remained symptom-free on a low dosage of 200 mg daily. A few of these patients have shown evidence of progressive right ventricular failure.

Cardiac Toxins

Alcohol. All patients with dilated cardiomyopathy should be asked about their alcohol consumption. Macrocytosis is a useful indicator of chronically high consumption even in the absence of abnormal liver function tests. A raised gamma glutamyltransferase may be an indicator only of recent rather than long-term intake, whereas raised levels for other liver enzymes may be due to a chronic alcohol hepatitis. There seems to be individual susceptibility to the adverse effects of alcohol on the myocardium because the heart only rarely shows dramatic improvement in function after a patient has stopped drinking. Individual susceptibility to the effects of alcohol may be shown by the finding of immunoglobulin A on the sarcolemma and in small blood vessels on biopsy of patients with alcoholic heart disease. A gratifying improvement may be an indicator of an important role for alcohol in an individual patient or of a still reversible state of myocardial depression. It seems that alcohol plays only a subsidiary role in the majority of patient with dilated cardiomyopathy who enjoy social drinking. In such patients it is still worthwhile to advise abstinence because of alcohol's adverse though mild pharmacologic effects.

Patients with alcoholic cardiomyopathy tend to be male and beer drinkers. This is despite the removal of cobalt, a myocardial toxin that was included in the secret formula of certain breweries until the 1960s, when there was an outbreak of cobalt-induced heart failure in Canadian and Belgium beer drinkers, all of whom were taking most of their calories in the form of beer.

Cocaine addiction can cause both coronary thrombosis and myocardial depression.

Other Toxins. Anthracyclines given as doxorubicin have important toxic subcellular effects that eventually lead to intracellular calcium overload and depressed cardiac function.

Surgical Treatment

Indications for Transplantation

It is obviously of great importance to be able to predict prognosis with some accuracy in patients with dilated cardiomyopathy. We have found that this is not invariably a relentlessly progressive disease with an invariably fatal outcome as has been suggested. Many patients with NYHA class I or II symptoms remain stable for many years. A few patients show unexplained and remarkable improvement. Most of these have had only moderate left ventricular dilation, but occasionally patients with greater degrees of impairment improve and become asymptomatic with good exercise tolerance, although rarely with entirely normal left ventricular function.

Patients with advanced dilated cardiomyopathy in NYHA classes III or IV usually have left ventricles measuring between 8 and 10 cm in diameter on echo with ejection fractions below 15 percent on multigated angiogram scanning. These patients have less than a 50 percent chance of surviving 1 year and should be considered for transplantation. Sudden death is very uncommon in patients who are stable with mild symptoms, but it accounts for about 50 percent of the deaths in patients with advanced failure. Patients with dilated cardiomyopathy do not need to be considered for transplantation until their quality of life has become considerably impaired. Because dilated cardiomyopathy behaves as though the impairment in function follows a single insult and has not shown itself to be a progressive disease, consideration for transplantation frequently needs to be given very soon after the patient is first referred. Such patients may have had only weeks or a few months of a downhill course. Only very rarely is the patient with dilated cardiomyopathy an "emergency" because the need for transplantation can usually be predicted. This is in contrast to coronary heart failure, in which deterioration is often abrupt owing to further myocardial necrosis, and the prognosis is unpredictable because of interruption by sudden death at almost any stage and accounting for 70 percent of the deaths in patients who reach the stage of heart failure.

Contraindications to transplantation include diseases of other organ systems that seriously limit prognosis, although multiorgan transplantation is sometimes practiced for combined cardiac and renal or cardiopulmonary and liver disease. More commonly, it is infection, usually in the lungs or thromboembolism with pulmonary infarction that can preclude cardiac transplantation. Anticoagulant treatment, although arguable in milder heart failure, is mandatory in advanced heart failure patients.

Relative contraindications to cardiac transplantation include severe reactive pulmonary hypertension. These patients may be successfully treated in the domino procedure, whereby patients with primary pulmonary hypertension receiving heart/lung transplants donate their good hearts to patients who need a hypertrophied right ventricle in case pulmonary vascular resistance fails to fall to normal after cardiac transplantation. Both are linked up in parallel. This procedure also allows removal of the donor heart, which can act as an assist device in patients who may have remedial heart disease. Theoretically this might include patients with a severe postpartum cardiomyopathy or patients with a severe life-threatening acute myocarditis.

Most patients with dilated cardiomyopathy inquire about transplantation before the subject is broached by the physician, and this is always helpful. It is obvious that patients need to be highly motivated, compliant to sometimes arduous treatment regimens, and possessed of determination and confidence in success. The good results of transplantation justify their confidence, but some patients still have a difficult early postoperative course if there are complications, and of course hearts are in short supply so that it is improper to refer patients whose prognosis may still be relatively open ended.

Other surgical procedures such as training the serratus anterior muscle by pacing it and then wrapping it around the heart and pacing it to augment left ventricular output are still in an experimental stage.

The wholly implanted permanent artificial heart is still some distance away, but temporary implantation has been used as a bridge to cardiac transplantation when a heart has not been available in a patient who seemed otherwise unlikely to survive. These hearts are still highly subject to thromboembolism, and survival of such patients is inversely proportional to the duration of time that the implant is used.

Left ventricular assist devices are gaining ground for the temporary support of patients who are awaiting a heart. The use of such devices is of course undesirable because of the risk of infection and thromboembolism.

SUGGESTED READING

Bouhour JB, Helias J, De Lajartre AY. Detection of myocarditis during the first year after discovery of a dilated cardiomyopathy by endomyocardial biopsy and gallium 67 myocardial scintigraphy: prospective multi-centre French study of 91 patients. Eur Heart J 1988; 9:520.

Diaz RA, Obasohan A, Oakley CM: Prediction of outcome in dilated cardiomyopathy. Br Heart J 1987; 58:393.

Keogh AM, Freund J, Baron DW, Hickie JB: Timing of cardiac transplantation in idiopathic dilated cardiomyopathy. Am J Cardiol 1988; 61:418.

Neri R, Mestroni L, Salvi A, et al. Ventricular arrhythmias in dilated cardiomyopathy: efficacy of amiodarone. Am Heart J 1987; 113:707.

Oakley CM: The cardiomyopathies. In: Weatherall D, Ledingham J, and Warrell D, eds. Oxford textbook of medicine. 2nd ed. Oxford: Oxford University Press, 1987: 209–229.

Stewart RAH, McKenna WJ, Oakley CM: A good prognosis in dilated cardiomyopathy. Q J Med 1990; 74:309.

AORTIC DISSECTION

JOSEPH LINDSAY Jr., M.D.

The term *aortic dissection* denotes a disease process characterized by the separation of the elastic fibers of the aortic media by a column of blood. The cleavage plane may extend for only a few centimeters or, not uncommonly, for the entire length of the aorta. Rarely, in some segments the dissection involves the entire circumference of the aorta. More often 40 to 60 percent of the cross section is "dissected."

This process jeopardizes the patient's life in three major ways. The aortic wall, weakened by the medial cleavage, frequently ruptures. Further, major aortic branches may be occluded if their origins and adjacent aortic segments become involved in the dissection. Finally, severe aortic regurgitation may result from involvement of the aortic root. Thus, successful therapy must prevent rupture and retard extension of the medial cleavage.

Aortic dissection should not be confused with expansion or rupture of a preexisting atherosclerotic, luetic, or mycotic aneurysm. Although the clinical picture of such a complication may mimic aortic dissection, the pathogenetic process and the therapeutic approach differ.

Aortic dissection is encountered most commonly in the sixth decade of life or later as a complication of hypertension. Younger or normotensive victims of aortic dissection have, as a rule, underlying congenital weakness of the aortic media associated with entities such as Marfan's syndrome, coarctation of the aorta, Turner's syndrome, anuloaortic ectasia, or bicuspid aortic valve.

THERAPEUTIC ALTERNATIVES

In as much as aortic dissection is a structural problem, surgical repair constitutes the most logical long-term remedy. Thus, the assessment in each patient of the risks and benefits of operative therapy becomes the central management decision. Teamed with a cardiovascular surgeon, the attending physician must decide whether the patient should undergo operation at once, whether it should be delayed and reconsidered at a later time, or whether operative repair can never be an option because of the patient's age, the presence of complicating illnesses, or of severe neurologic injury consequent to the dissection (Table 1). Unfortunately, a substantial number of patients fall into the last of these three categories.

Prior to operation and when surgery is not recommended, vigorous antihypertensive therapy is indicated to reduce stress on the aortic wall and thereby to provide protection against rupture of the wall and extension of the dissection. Such therapy has unfortunately failed to meet earlier expectations for long-term effectiveness.

PREFERRED APPROACH

Having said that operative repair is potentially the most desirable treatment for all patients with aortic dissection, it follows that the operative risk must in each case be weighed against the immediacy of the threat posed by the disease.

Before a discussion of the threat to the patient can be undertaken, the most frequently encountered anatomic variations of its aortic involvement must be described. The most common pattern (type I of DeBakey) accounts for about two-thirds of all dissections. The proximal limit of a type I dissection lies just above the aortic valve, and an intimal ("entrance") tear is typically located near this proximal end. Type II of DeBakey is a subgroup of type I. Patients whose

TABLE 1 Management of Patient Subsets in Aortic Dissection

Subset A: Those with Syncope or Hypotension
Assessment of prognosis: External rupture is likely present
Management: Emergency surgery

Subset B: Hypertensive Patients with Dissection Involving the Ascending Aorta
Assessment of prognosis: External rupture is likely within hours or days despite aggressive antihypertensive treatment
Management: Urgent surgery. Aggressive antihypertensive treatment preoperatively

Subset C: Hypertensive Patients with Dissection Sparing the Ascending Aorta
Assessment of prognosis: With aggressive antihypertensive treatment, the risk of rupture is no greater than risk of operation
Management: Aggressive antihypertensive treatment. Elective operative repair in younger individuals, those in good general health, and those with large aneurysms

Subset D: Complicated Patients with Severe Aortic Regurgitation or Ischemia of a Limb, the Heart, the Kidney, or the Central Nervous System
Assessment of prognosis: Prospect for survival and recovery limited unless defect can be corrected
Management: Urgent surgery in those in whom there is a reasonable expectation of correction of the problem

Subset E: Patients with Advanced Comorbid Disease or Severe Ischemic Complication of the Dissection that Preclude Reasonable Chance for Surgical Success
Assessment of prognosis: Patient will not survive operation or will not benefit from it
Management: Antihypertensive therapy and/or supportive care

dissection is limited to the ascending aorta may be so categorized. Absent surgical correction and despite aggressive antihypertensive treatment, patients in these categories have an exceedingly high mortality in the acute phase, most often the consequence of external rupture into the pericardial space. In the only other common pattern (type III of DeBakey), the medial dissection is limited to the distal arch and descending aorta. The "entrance" tear is characteristically found just distal to the left subclavian artery. This type, accounting for about one-fourth of all aortic dissections, carries a far more favorable acute prognosis than do those involving the ascending aorta. Surgery may safely be delayed in these cases unless a life-threatening complication has occurred. The choice is less clearly defined for the small number of dissections not falling into these readily identifiable types.

In addition to the identification of the anatomic type of aortic dissection, recognition of the existence of external rupture is crucial to the choice of therapy. As is the case with any disruption of the continuity of the aortic wall, only operative management can be expected to be successful. External rupture has almost always occurred when the patient presents with syncope or when he or she is hypotensive on admission (Doroghazi and Slater, 1983). About one-fifth of all dissections involving the ascending aorta will appear in this way. External rupture most often occurs in the region of the entrance tear (Lindsay, 1979). Inasmuch as this tear is located in the proximal aorta in two-thirds of instances (types I and II), the rupture communicates most often with the pericardial space, hence a presentation of syncope or hypotension in the absence of appreciable blood loss. In another one-fourth of cases (type III) the intimal tear is situated just beyond the left subclavian artery. In such cases rupture will occur into the left pleural space, producing a left hemothorax.

Patients with anuloaortic ectasia, many of whom have ocular or musculoskeletal manifestations of Marfan's syndrome, constitute a discrete group. The medial dissection in such instances is usually, but not invariably, only a few centimeters in length and appears to represent a complication of the progressive dilation of the aortic root that is characteristic of this disorder. These limited dissections are usually asymptomatic until the onset of rupture.

Infrequently, aneurysmal dilation of the aorta that has developed in an aortic segment weakened by a clinically unrecognized acute dissection will be the presenting evidence of this process. Most such "chronic" dissections are of the type III variety, since unrecognized and untreated dissections involving the ascending aorta are usually fatal during the acute phase. In such aneurysms the risk of rupture must be weighed against operative risk in a manner not very different from that employed in the assessment of patients with aortic aneurysm of any etiology.

Medical Treatment

General Treatment of Acute Dissection

Sudden, life-threatening complications, such as very severe hypertension, cardiac tamponade, massive hemorrhage, acute aortic regurgitation, or ischemic injury to the heart, kidneys, or central nervous system, threaten patients with acute dissection. Optimal management includes careful monitoring of vital functions in an intensive care unit. Aggressive reduction of the blood pressure, often an important part of therapy, may necessitate an intra-arterial line and careful monitoring of the urine output by means of an indwelling urinary catheter. Any uncertainty as to the status of the intravascular volume should be resolved by means of bedside right heart catheterization.

Specific Therapy in Acute Dissection

Wheat and Palmer and associates provided an experimental and clinical foundation for the aggressive administration of antihypertensive medications to reduce the hemodynamic stress on the aortic wall and thus to avert progression of the medial cleavage and external rupture of the weakened aortic wall (DeSanctis et a!, 1987). Their data emphasize the importance of reducing not only the aortic pressure but also its rate of rise. According to this construct, drugs that reduce arterial pressure but result in reflex augmentation of left ventricular contractility and rate of rise of aortic pressure are not useful. This approach was received with great enthusiasm at the time of its introduction in 1965, but greatly improved surgical results and disappointing clinical experience in type I patients have tempered the early enthusiasm. It is now reserved for the preoperative preparation of patients and is employed long-term only in those for whom surgical treatment cannot be recommended.

The ability of intravenous nitroprusside to reduce arterial pressure promptly and consistently and the ease with which its hypotensive effects can be titrated certify it as the current drug of choice for the hypertensive patient with acute dissection. Its infusion rate is adjusted to attain a systolic blood pressure of 100 to 120 mm Hg. As little as 0.5 μg per kilogram per minute may produce the desired result. Occasionally as much as 10 μg per kilogram per minute will be necessary. Infrequently the pain of the dissection, and by inference its progression, will not be relieved unless arterial pressure is lowered even further. On the other hand, optimal blood pressure reduction may not be possible if oliguria (less than 25 ml per hour) or mental confusion appears.

Animal data suggest that nitroprusside does not reduce, and may enhance the rate of rise of aortic pressure. Because of this possibility, its use in conjunction with a beta-blocking drug enjoys wide clinical acceptance. Propranolol can be administered in 0.5 mg increments at 1- to 5-minute intervals until the pulse rate slows or until 1.5 mg per 10 kg of body weight has been given. This procedure should be repeated at 4- to 6-hour intervals, and medication may be given orally once the proper amount is identified.

Trimethaphan, the intravenous agent first employed by Wheat and Palmer, can be substituted for nitroprusside in patients who cannot be given beta-blocking drugs because this agent reduces the rate of rise of aortic pressure. Infused at an initial rate of 1 to 2 mg per minute, this ganglionic blocker can be titrated to the same therapeutic goals as for nitroprusside. When compared with nitroprusside in clinical use, this agent does not as reliably reduce the blood pressure, especially after 24 to 48 hours when tachyphylaxis frequently appears. Because it is a ganglionic blocker, it more often than nitroprusside produces side effects such as ileus.

Other occasionally useful substitutes for nitroprusside include intravenous methyldopa and intramuscular reserpine.

As has been stated, exclusion of external rupture is the therapist's primary concern in those patients who present with a systolic blood pressure already at or below the target level for aggressive antihypertensive therapy. When rupture can be confidently excluded, intravenous beta blockage may be indicated.

Once the patient has been stabilized and a decision has been made that surgical therapy will not at once be undertaken, a plan must be developed for shifting to intramuscular and to oral medications for subacute or chronic blood pressure control. Beta-blocking drugs, sympatholytic agents, and diuretics are useful, but direct vasodilators such as hydralazine, diazoxide, and minoxidil should be avoided because of the reflex sympathetic stimulation that attends their use. Little or no experience with the angiotensin converting enzyme inhibitors or with calcium-entry blockers is available to guide their use in this context.

Treatment of Subacute and Chronic Dissection

Once several days or weeks have elapsed, the target for control of the arterial pressure may be relaxed. Blood pressure goals similar to those of any hypertensive patient are usually appropriate for long-term management.

Side Effects of Drug Therapy

Problems may arise from the therapeutic effects of the agents previously described. Oliguria, mental confusion, and postural hypotension may result from diminished perfusion pressure. The goals of treatment may have to be altered in response and the dose of the agent adjusted accordingly.

Nitroprusside possesses a specific, potentially toxic characteristic. Its metabolism produces cyanide ions that are converted to thiocyanate. Cyanide toxicity can result from overdosage. For this reason the dose of 10 μg per kilogram per minute should not be exceeded. In patients with thiosulfate depletion, lower doses may be toxic. The appearance of metabolic acidosis is a useful early sign of cyanide toxicity. Blood pH and acid-base balance should therefore be monitored. Plasma thiocyanate levels are not useful for the detection of cyanide toxicity.

Surgical Treatment

Selection for and Timing of Surgery

When a decision has been reached that the patient has no limiting comorbid conditions or complications of the dissection that preclude operative treatment, the information contained in the section "Preferred Approach" provides guidance for the appropriate timing of surgical intervention. Clearly the individual with evidence of external rupture must be operated on an emergency basis. Those with involvement of the ascending aorta are at high risk of rupture, and surgery should be delayed only long enough to stabilize the patient and to obtain adequate diagnostic information regarding the extent of the dissection and the location of the proximal intimal tear. Surgery may be deferred in those whose dissection is limited to the descending aorta because medical management has proved to be as efficacious as operation during the acute phase. Evidence of external rupture or of progression of the dissection during drug therapy may require reconsideration of this decision. A decision with regard to operation in patients who have survived for 2 weeks or more or for those who present with chronic dissection will of necessity be individualized. Factors such as the age of the patient, the state of general health, and the size of the residual aneurysm must be considered.

Operative Treatment

Resection of the aorta containing the "entrance tear" (the intimal laceration at the proximal limit of the dissection that allows communication between the true lumen of the aorta and the false lumen created by the dissecting hematoma) is the primary objective. Reapproximation of the transected ends after closure of the false channel may be done directly or, more commonly, with a graft. In some instances revascularization of vital structures, repair of the aortic valve, or other reconstructive procedures may also be required.

Modern surgical techniques have changed such surgery from a risky, problematic enterprise to one in which success may be expected even in gravely ill individuals such as those with dissection. Better means have evolved for the preservation of vital tissue, such as the myocardium, the brain, and the spinal cord, during manipulations that might result in ischemia of these structures. Moreover, improvements in the vascular prostheses available for reapproximation of the aorta now reduce the likelihood of anastomotic leaks, formerly a major hazard of repairing the fragile aortic tissue encountered at the site of dissection.

Preoperative Preparation

For patients who present with hypotension or syncope and in whom external rupture is probable, little time is available for preoperative preparation. Restoration of blood volume and emergency treatment of other physiologic derangements should be carried out concomitantly with those diagnostic procedures essential to the surgeon for his or her decisions as to the operative approach.

The evaluation and correction of physiologic derangements may be a bit more deliberate for other patients with type I or type II dissection, although the presence of severe aortic regurgitation or of acute myocardial ischemia from obstruction of a coronary artery may dictate haste. Aggressive reduction of any elevation of the blood pressure (see "Medical Treatment") is an important preoperative step.

For patients with type III dissections who do not have life-threatening complications, operative therapy may be delayed. The measures described under "Medical Treatment" should be implemented until the chosen time for operation.

Postoperative Course and Potential Complications

Postoperatively the patient is at risk for all the neurologic, pulmonary, and renal complications of major cardiovascular surgery. Dyfunction of any organ system damaged as a result of preoperative shock, dissection-related arterial occlusion, or aortic valve damage may have to be reckoned with. Management of these patients will challenge the skills of an experienced specialist in intensive care.

Two complications of the operation are of significance. Rupture of the suture line is perhaps the most feared. The tissue that must be repaired after resection of the aortic segment is extremely friable. Creation of a firm suture line can be extraordinarily difficult even for the most experienced cardiovascular surgeon. Secondly, paraplegia, a consequence of interruption of the blood supply to the spinal cord, complicates repair of type III dissections in a significant percentage of patients. Fear of this outcome may play a leading part in forming a decision to avoid operation in some patients with type III dissection.

SUGGESTED READING

DeSanctis RW, Doroghazi RM, Austen WG, Buckley MJ. Aortic dissection. N Engl J Med 1987; 317:1060.

Doroghazi RM, Slater EE, eds. Aortic dissection. McGraw-Hill: New York, 1983.

Ergin MA, Galla JD, Lansman S, Griepp B. Acute dissections of the aorta: Current surgical treatment. Surg Clin North Am 1985; 65:721.

Hirst AE Jr, Johns VJ Jr, Kime SW Jr. Dissecting aneurysm of the aorta: A review of 505 cases. Medicine (Baltimore) 1958; 37:217.

Lindsay J Jr, Hurst JW. Clinical features and prognosis in dissecting aneurysm of the aorta: A re-appraisal. Circulation 1967; 35:880.

Lindsay J Jr: Aortic dissection. In Lindsay J Jr, Hurst JW, eds. The aorta. New York: Grune & Stratton, 1979:239–262.

AORTIC ANEURYSM: NONDISSECTING THORACIC

E. STANLEY CRAWFORD, M.D.
JOSEPH S. COSELLI, M.D.

Aneurysm of the thoracic aorta is a serious form of disease. Death occurs in 75 percent of untreated patients within 2 years and 90 percent within 5 years. The cause of death in over half the patients is rupture, either by spontaneous laceration (simple bursting) or by superimposed dissection. This complication tends to be size dependent. In our series of 101 patients treated for rupture, the external aortic diameter at the site of rupture was 5 to 6 cm (15 percent), 7 to 10 cm (69 percent) and greater than 10 cm (19 percent). The diameter of the ruptured aneurysm in all cases was more than twice the diameter of the adjacent uninvolved aorta.

ETIOLOGY

The etiologies of aneurysms of the thoracic aorta include congenital malformations (coarctation of aorta, persistent arch abnormalities, and abnormalities of fusion of aortic root with aortic annulus), infection (mycotic), trauma, autoimmune disturbances (giant cell aortitis, Takayasu's disease, Bechet's disease), connective tissue disorders (Marfan's syndrome, Turner's syndrome, Ehlers-Danlos syndrome), atherosclerosis, aortic dissection, and medial degenerative disease. The latter two conditions are the most frequent disorders. Contrary to popular thinking, atherosclerosis is a rare etiology. To be sure, atheromatous lesions are frequently superimposed on the other diseases; however, this is a rare cause of thoracic aortic aneurysm. Aortic dissection is discussed elsewhere; this presentation concerns those aneurysms of other origins.

CLINICAL MANIFESTATIONS

The ages of our patients ranged from 15 months to 87 years. The younger patients have disease as a result of infection, trauma, congenital abnormalities, autoimmune disorders, and heritable connective tissue defects. The remaining patients (the majority), whose median age was 66 years, had aneurysms due to nonspecific medial degenerative change. Thus, aneurysmal disease of degenerative origin occurs most frequently in older patients.

Some of our patients referred for treatment were asymptomatic. Thoracic aortic aneurysm was discovered in these cases by routine chest film or computed tomographic scan that showed an abnormal mediastinal mass. Most patients were symptomatic at the time of admission. Symptoms were due to pressure of the expanding aneurysm on adjacent structures and the presence of superimposed dissection or rupture. These symptoms varied with the aortic segment involved and are discussed accordingly.

ASCENDING AND ARCH

The aortic annulus is dilated in 75 to 80 percent of patients with aneurysms of the ascending and transverse aortic arch. These patients have varying degrees of aortic valve insufficiency, and many have symptoms of heart failure. The aneurysmal mass may cause obstruction of the superior vena cava, pulmonary artery, airway, and esophagus. In rare neglected cases, the aneurysm may erode through the anterior chest wall.

Rupture occurs either by spontaneous laceration or dissection of aneurysmal wall into pericardium, heart chamber, or mediastinum. These terminal events produce serious symptoms of hemorrhage, great vein and myocardial compression, or large left to right cardiac shunts.

DESCENDING AND THORACOABDOMINAL AORTA

Aneurysms of the descending thoracic and thoracoabdominal aorta produce symptoms of compression of adjacent structures including left recurrent laryngeal nerve, esophagus, chest wall, and bronchus. These include hoarseness, dysphagia, and chest wall pain. Rupture at these levels occurs into the mediastinum, lung, bronchus, esophagus, and left chest cavity. This stage of the disease may be manifested by hypotension, increase in pain, hemoptysis, or hematemesis.

PREFERRED APPROACH

Diagnosis

Initial chest film may show a left sided mediastinal shadow adjacent to the cardiac silhouette suggestive of an aneurysm involving the descending thoracic aorta. A right-sided anterior upper mediastinal shadow suggests an aneurysm of the ascending aorta or aortic arch. Unfortunately, even large aneurysms of the ascending aorta are frequently not visualized by this method of examination because the aneurysm is located within the normal cardiac shadow. Thus, special studies are necessary for the diagnosis in these cases and should be routinely performed when evaluating the heart in patients with high risk of aneurysms, i.e., those with connective tissue defects, valve pathology, coronary artery disease, and others that are to be treated by operation. The logic of this approach lies in the concept that the aortic root is part of the heart based on the fact that the aortic valve arises at its base and the coronary arteries that supply blood to the heart arise from it. Thus, a complete examination of the heart includes evaluation of the aortic root.

Echocardiography is an excellent method for this purpose as well as for evaluation of myocardial and valve function. The aortic root should also be routinely visualized during left-sided heart catheterization. Traditionally echocardiography is not effective in evaluating the transverse aortic arch and descending thoracic aorta. Transesophageal echocardiography is a satisfactory method for evaluating the distal arch and descending thoracic aorta. Prototypes of equipment are now available in a few centers for evaluation of both ascending, transverse, and descending thoracic aortic disease, and the method may be useful in the future in the evaluation of these cases.

The best screening methods for the diagnosis and localization of aortic aneurysms is computed tomography and magnetic resonance imaging. Computed tomographic scanning with contrast enhancement is preferable because of its general availability, ease of performance, safety, reproducibility, cost effectiveness, and most reliable method of determining aortic diameter. Magnetic resonance imaging is time-consuming, unpleasant to the patient, expensive, and not applicable to patients with support systems that cannot be subjected to the magnetic field.

Total aortography in three projections is the preferred method of examination in patients who are to be treated by operation. This method allows evaluation of the entire aorta, aortic valve function, the location and condition of branch vessels, the presence of fistulas and sites of perforation or rupture. Approximately 15 percent of patients have branch vessel occlusive disease, which is best identified and evaluated by aortography. Patients with symptoms of coronary artery disease should have separate cardiac catheterization and selective coronary artery angiography with consideration for concurrent myocardial revascularization. Thus, minimal studies in our cases include computed tomographic scanning for diagnosis and estimation of aneurysmal size and total aortography for evaluation of valve function, branch vessel disease, and relationship of aneurysm position to brachiocephalic arterial origin.

Assessment of Associated Disease

Cardiac evaluation includes an estimate of myocardial and valve function with echocardiography and Doppler examination. These are usually augmented with 24-hour Holter monitor to detect cardiac arrhythmias. Patients with coronary artery disease are catheterized and selective coronary artery studies performed. Aortic valve replacement, coronary artery bypass, or both are performed at the time of ascending and arch replacement. Patients with ejection fractions of 30 percent are considered suitable for operation. Pulmonary function is assessed clinically, with room air arterial blood gases and spirometry testing. Patients whose pulmonary function is 50 percent of normal are suitable for operation. Renal function is determined by blood creatinine levels. Patients with substantial chronic reduction in renal function may be candidates for operation. In fact, over 75 percent of patients receiving chronic hemodialysis survive operation. However, operation is reserved for such patients who have symptoms or large aneurysms.

Surgical Treatment

Graft replacement is the only treatment of thoracic aortic aneurysm that relieves the complication of the disease and prevents dissection and rupture. This operation is recommended in good risk asymptomatic patients in whom the aneurysm is twice the size of the uninvolved aorta (5 to 6 cm). Operation is performed in patients with limiting risks for symptoms or larger aneurysms.

Aortic Grafts

Tubular Dacron fabric grafts are employed to replace aneurysms of the thoracic aorta. All such grafts commercially available for use at this level are porous. To prevent bleeding through their interstices during operation, the graft walls are saturated with 25 percent human serum albumin solution and steam autoclaved at 250°F for 3 minutes. Two pretreated grafts have been approved for use in the human on an experimental basis, and both are likely to be approved for general use in the near future. One is a knitted graft pretreated with human serum albumin solution, and the other is a woven graft pretreated with bovine collagen.

We prefer the St. Jude valve for separate valve graft replacement because of its flow characteristics and the St. Jude composite valve graft because of the matching relationship between graft diameter and valve size.

Techniques of Operation

The method of operation varies with the location and extent of aneurysm and is discussed accordingly.

Ascending Aorta and Transverse Aortic Arch. Cardiopulmonary bypass is employed to maintain circulation in patients during aortic cross-clamping for replacement of aneurysms of the ascending aorta and transverse arch. Myocardial protection is achieved with intermittent coronary artery perfusion with cold (5°C) hyperkalemic dilute blood solution maintaining myocardial temperature less than 15°C. Using a heat exchanger in the extracorporeal circulation circuit, moderate hypothermia (25 to 28°C) is maintained during the period of aortic clamping for reconstruction of the ascending aorta. Profound hypothermia sufficient to produce electrocerebral silence (isoelectric electroencephalogram) is achieved for complete circulatory arrest during the period of graft replacement of the transverse aortic arch. After completion of the reconstruction, rewarming to 38°C (rectal) is accomplished using cardiopulmonary bypass.

Aortic Reconstruction. The method and extent of graft replacement is dependent on the location and extent of aneurysm. Aneurysms that involve the tubular segment of ascending aorta (that segment extending from innominate artery to the insertion of the aortic valvular commissures) are replaced with a tube graft (Fig. 1). Associated aortic valvular disease in such cases is replaced by separate prosthetic aortic valve (Fig. 2), and patients with coronary artery disease are treated with bypass graft (Fig. 3). Aneurysms that extend down to involve the sinus segment of ascending aorta (the segment containing the coronary artery origins extending from the level of commissural attachment to the aortic valvular annulus) require replacement of both tubular and sinus segments to prevent progressive sinus enlargement and rupture into the right-sided heart chambers. The method of this operation is dependent on the distance between coronary artery origins and aortic annulus. The Wheat operation may be performed in cases in which the coronary arteries arise near the aortic annulus (< 2 cm) (Fig. 4). The aortic valve is usually replaced, and the ascending aorta is excised except for a tongue of aortic tissue containing the origins of the coronary arteries. The proximal end of the graft is then sutured to the aortic valve sewing ring, annulus, or residual

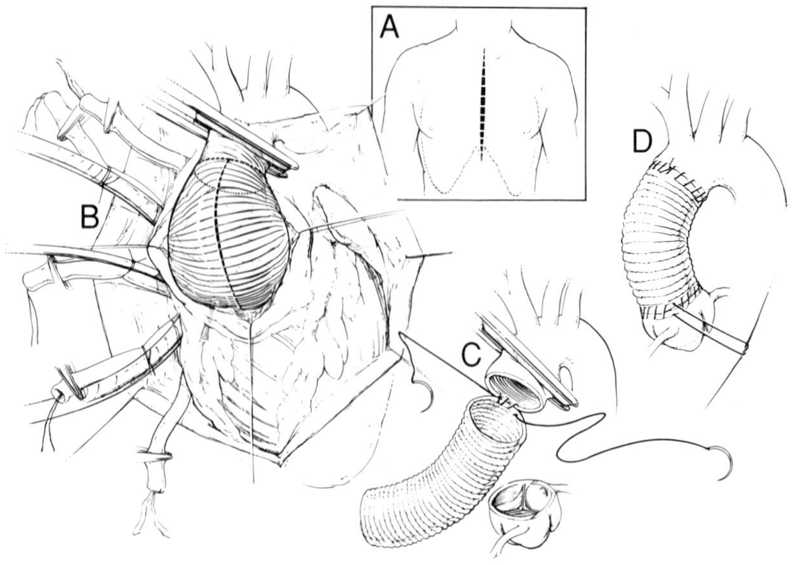

Figure 1 Graft replacement of aneurysm involving tubular segment of ascending aorta. *A*, Midsternal incision, *B*, location of aneurysm, *C*, excised aortic segment and distal anastomosis, *D*, completed reconstruction. (Copyright 1990 by Baylor College of Medicine.)

aorta except at the tongue of aortic tissue containing the coronary arteries. The end of the graft is sutured to the aorta distal to the coronary arteries at these sites. The operation is then completed as previously described.

The other method for replacing aneurysms that involve both the sinus and tubular segments of ascending aorta is replacement of aortic valve and ascending aorta with a composite valve graft. The aortic leaflets are removed, and the valve end of the graft is attached to the aortic annulus by interrupted sutures (Figs. 5 and 6). The other end of the graft is sutured end to end to the distal transected uninvolved aorta. Coronary artery circulation may be restored by insertion of separate coronary artery bypass grafts (see Fig. 3), by direct reattachment of coronary origins to openings made in the graft (see Fig. 5), by use of a smaller Dacron tube graft (see Fig. 6), or by reattaching a button of aorta from which the coronary arteries arise directly to openings made in the graft. The as-

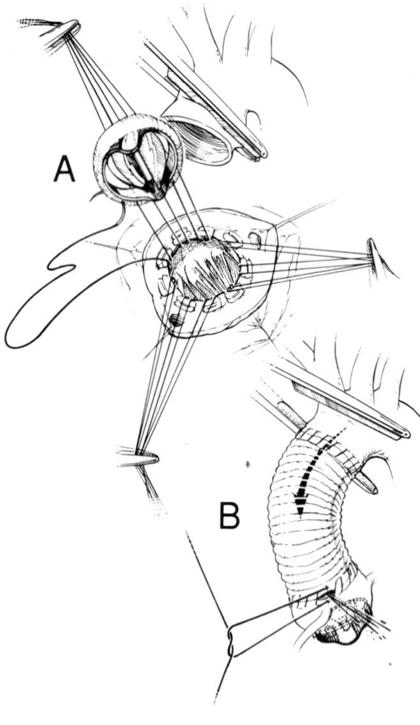

Figure 2 Separate valve-graft replacement of the ascending aorta. *A*, Tubular segment of aorta is excised and St. Jude valve is inserted. *B*, Operation is completed by graft insertion. (Copyright 1990 by Baylor College of Medicine.)

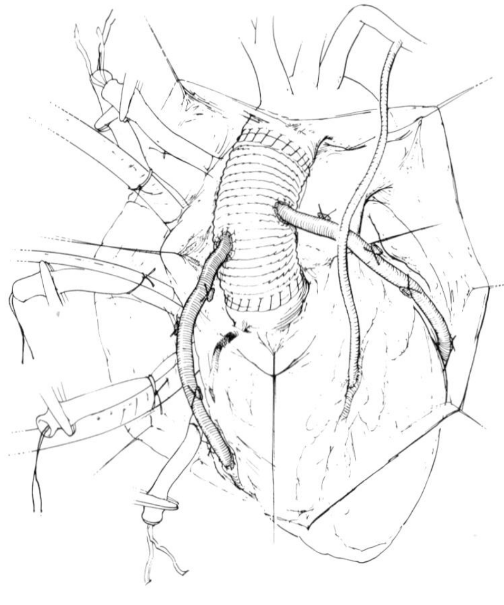

Figure 3 Position of coronary bypass grafts inserted in a patient at time of ascending aortic replacement. (Copyright 1990 by Baylor College of Medicine.)

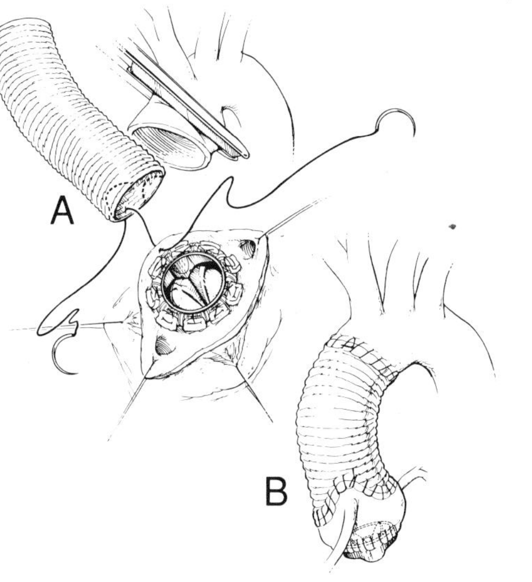

Figure 4 Separate valve graft replacement of the aortic valve and ascending aorta after removal of most of the aorta except that from which the coronary arteries arise in a patient with sinus segment involvement and coronary artery origins located near the aortic annulus. (Copyright 1990 by Baylor College of Medicine.)

cending aorta is completely excised in the latter operation except for buttons from which the coronary arteries arise. The coronary arteries are mobilized to their first branch to obtain length and then reattached. Although we use all these methods in the replacement of diffuse aneurysms, we prefer the radical excision and separate graft replacement in patients with low lying coronary ostia and reattachment by graft. We use smaller dacron tube in other patients because coronary artery circulation can be restored without tension that avoids operative bleeding and postoperative false aneurysm formation. The incidence and results of the various methods of ascending aortic reconstruction in our patients with nondissection aneurysms of the ascending aorta and transverse aortic arch are shown in Table 1.

Aortic Arch. With circulation arrested, the aneurysm is opened and the aorta transected proximally and distally and frequently excised except for an island from which the brachiocephalic vessels arise (Fig. 7). One end of the aortic graft is attached to the uninvolved distal end of the aorta. An opening is made in the side of the graft opposite the origins of the brachiocephalic vessels and the island of aortic tissue from which the brachiocephalic vessels arise is attached to the graft. Cardiopulmonary bypass is restarted and air removed from the aorta and graft. The graft is cross-clamped proximal to the innominate artery and full bypass and rewarming begun. About two-thirds of patients with arch aneurysms have involvement of the ascending aorta (Table 1), and this segment is then reconstructed according to the principles outlined previously for ascending aortic aneurysms to complete the operation.

One-third of patients with aneurysm of the aortic arch have *diffuse aneurysms that also involve the descending thoracic aorta* or *descending thoracic aorta and abdominal aorta.* Operation is staged in these cases with the ascending aorta and arch being replaced first in most cases; the distal aneurysm is then

Figure 5 *A–D* The steps of composite valve graft replacement of the aortic valve and ascending aorta in which the coronary arteries are attached directly to openings made in the graft. (Copyright 1990 by Baylor College of Medicine.)

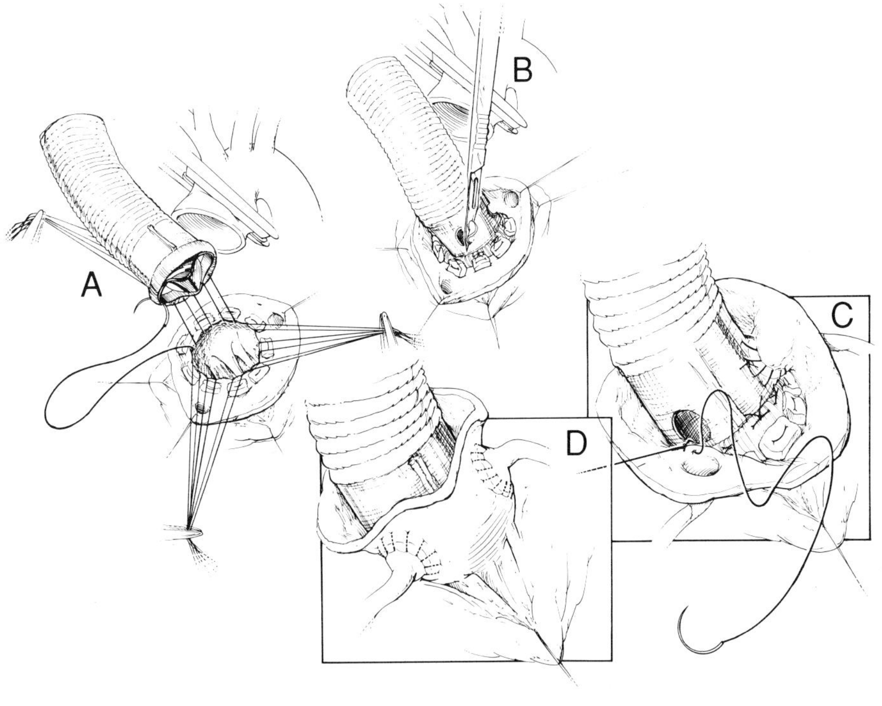

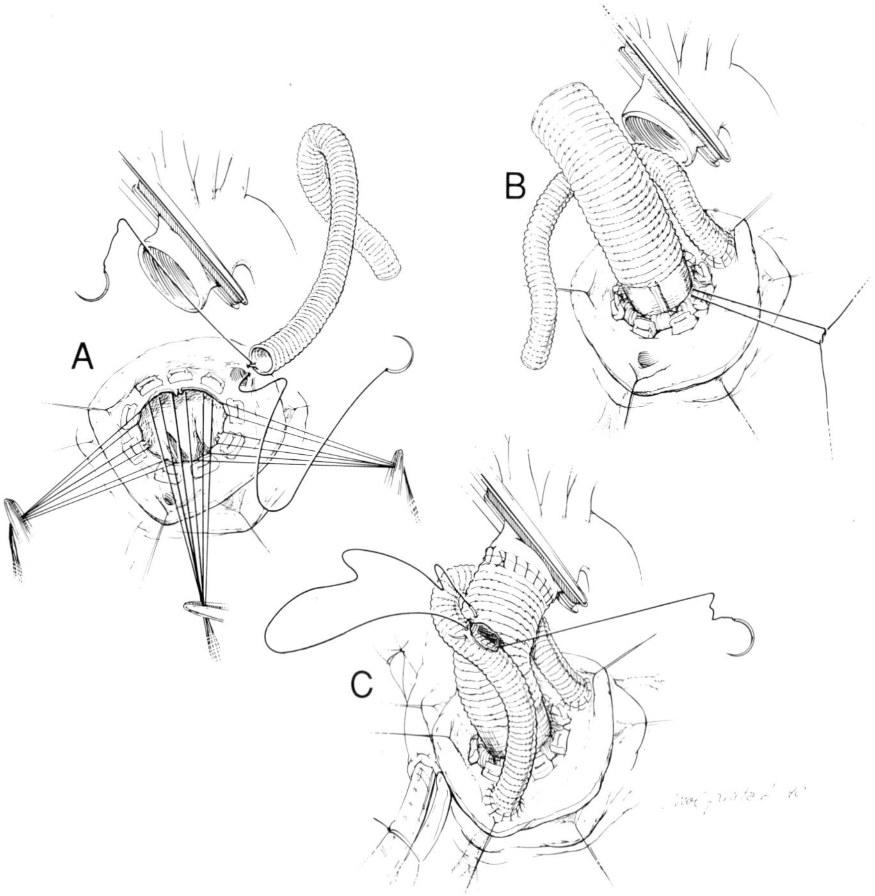

Figure 6 *A–C*, The steps of composite valve graft replacement showing attachment of coronary arteries using a smaller (10-cm) Dacron tube graft. (Copyright 1990 by Baylor College of Medicine.)

replaced at a second operation 6 to 8 weeks later. The ascending aorta and arch are replaced as described previously except that a segment of free graft is left extending into the distal aneurysm to attach the proximal end of the second graft at the second operation (Fig. 8). The free end of graft is easily exposed inside the aneurysm and does not require the tedious exposure needed using conventional techniques (Fig. 8*F*).

Descending Thoracic and Thoracoabdominal Aortic Aneurysm. Although varying aortic lengths may be involved in each entity, aneurysms of the descending thoracic aorta are confined to the chest and thoracoabdominal aortic aneurysms involve both the descending thoracic aorta and abdominal aorta. Both types of aneurysms require left posterolateral thoracic chest wall incisions for exposure (Figs. 9 and 10). Exposure of thoracoabdominal aneurysms requires extension of the incision into the abdomen made by crossing the costal arch and extending downward in the midline of the abdomen. The abdominal aorta, in the latter cases, is exposed retroperitoneally first by mobilizing the peritoneum from dia-

TABLE 1 Method of Ascending Aortic Replacement According to Extent of Proximal Involvement

	Ascending Aorta		*Aortic Arch*		*Ascending and Arch*	
Method	*No. Patients*	*30-Day Survival*	*No. Patients*	*30-Day Survival*	*No. Patients*	*30-Day Survival*
CVG	153	143 (93%)	0	—	38	35 (92%)
SVR	49	41 (84%)	0	—	80	80 (74%)
GFT	21	18 (86%)	54	48 (89%)	100	95 (95%)
Other	18	14 (78%)	62	57 (92%)	2	2 (100%)
Totals	241	216 (90%)	116	105 (91%)	220	212 (96%)

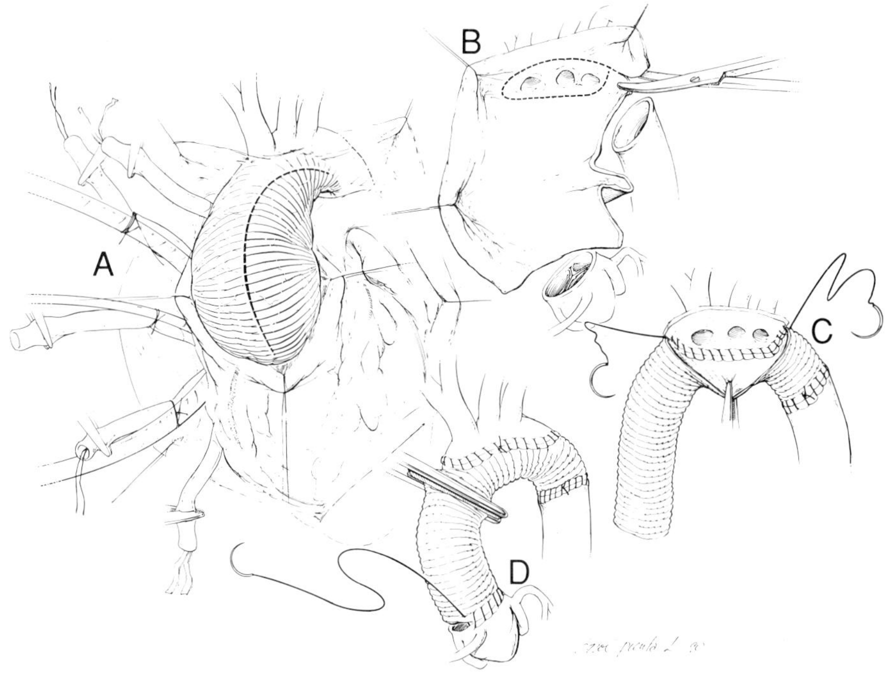

Figure 7 The common method of graft replacement of the ascending aorta and transverse aortic arch for aneurysm. *A*, The aneurysm is incised longitudinally and (*B*) excised except for a button containing the origins of the brachiocephalic arteries. *C*, The distal end of the graft is inserted by end-to-end anastomosis, and the button containing the brachiocephalic vessels is attached to an opening made in the graft. *D*, The reconstruction is completed by proximal anastomosis. (Copyright 1990 by Baylor College of Medicine.)

phragm and abdominal wall, cutting the diaphragm, and displacing the viscera upward and to the right.

The aorta is clamped proximally and distally. To prevent heart strain with aortic clamping, proximal blood pressure is controlled with pharmacologic agents in the usual case and by temporary left atrial-left common femoral artery centrifugal pump bypass in patients with heart disease. With the aorta clamped, the aneurysm is opened (Fig. 9*B*), the contained blood retrieved by cell saver, and the upper intercostal arteries are ligated at their origins. The aorta is transected proximally and separated from the esophagus. The proximal anastomosis is made by the continuous suture avoiding the esophagus and recurrent laryngeal nerve (Fig. 9*C*). A similar type of exposure and distal anastomosis is made in the chest in patients with aneurysm limited to the descending thoracic aorta (Fig. 9*D*). The abdominal segment of aneurysm is opened behind the left renal artery in patients with thoracoabdominal aortic aneurysms (Fig. 10*C*). An opening made in the side of graft is sutured around the origins of the lower intercostal and upper lumbar arteries to preserve spinal cord blood supply (Fig. 10*D*). Another opening is made in the side of the graft and sutured around the origins of the celiac axis and superior mesenteric and right renal arteries (Fig. 10*D,E*). The distal end of the graft is sutured to the uninvolved distal aorta. The origin of the left renal artery is mobilized from the aneurysm and adjacent tissues saving a button of aorta (Fig. 10*D*). The artery is then reattached by suturing the aortic button to a third opening made in the graft (Fig. 10*E*). In both types of cases, air is removed from the graft to prevent cerebral embolization. This is accomplished by slowly removing the clamp in the head-down position prior to completing the last anastomosis and by aspirating the uppermost segment of graft using needle and syringe.

RESULTS

The results of operation according to aortic segment replaced in 2,141 cases treated since January 1, 1980, are shown in Table 2. The 30-day survival varied from 90 to 95 percent depending on segment replaced. Survival at 1 year varied from 76 to 86 percent and at 5 years, 60 to 69 percent. The causes of both early and late death were heart, lung, stroke, kidney disease, and rupture of other aneurysms listed in order of frequency. These results are deemed very satisfactory considering the condition of patients at time of operation, including the fact that the median age of all patients was 64 years.

The most disabling complication that occurred in patients with distal aortic reconstruction (descending thoracic aorta and thoracoabdominal aorta) was neurologic disturbances in the lower extremities. This complication varied with extent of operation and varied from 5 percent in patients with descending thoracic aortic reconstruction to 10 percent in those with thoracoabdominal aortic operation. The deficit was mild to moderate in half of these cases and permanently crippling in the other half.

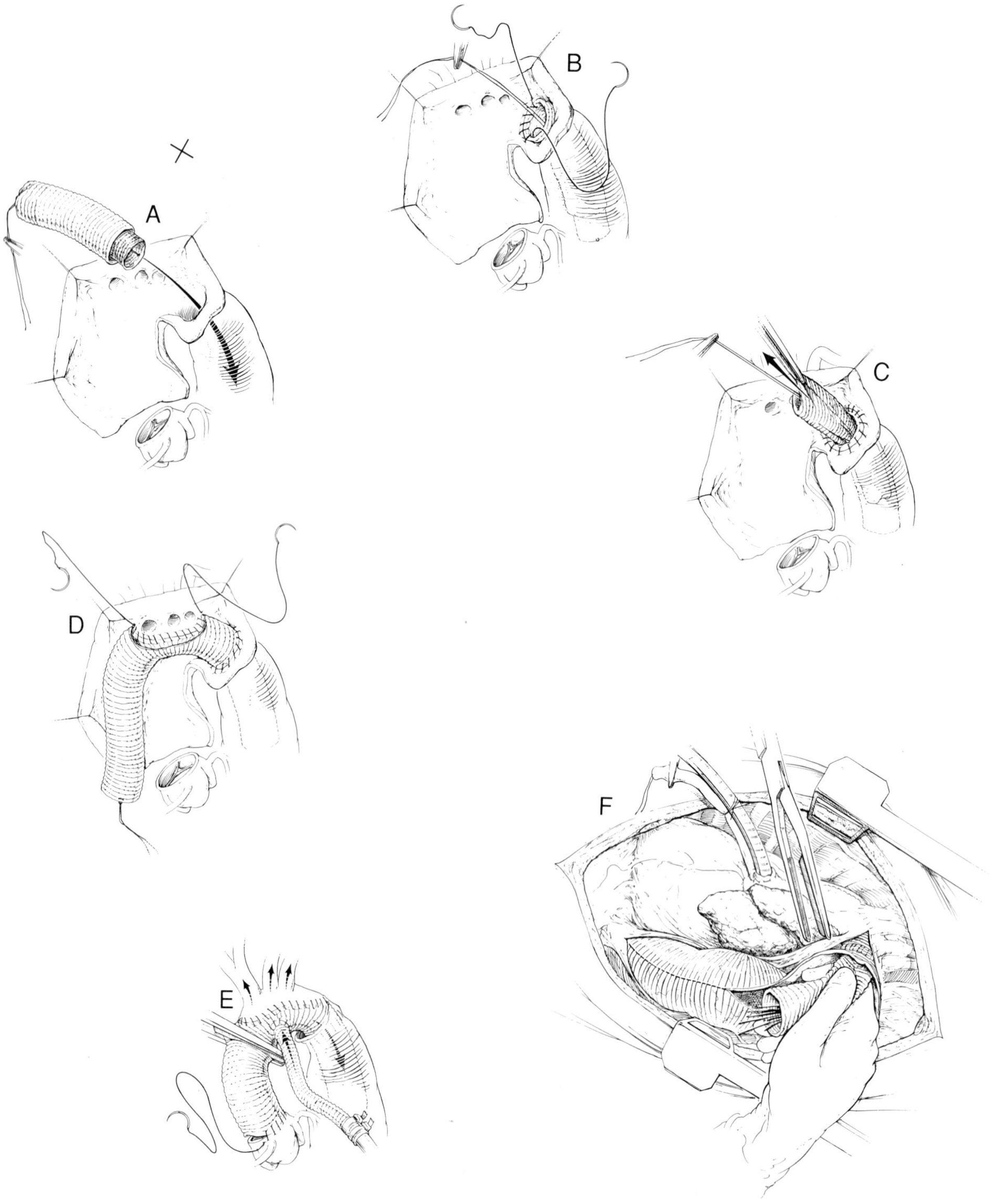

Figure 8 Elephant trunk technique, leaving a free segment of graft extending down into residual aneurysm to facilitate later graft replacement of the segment. *A*, An invaginated graft is inserted into the descending thoracic aortic aneurysm, and (*B*) the proximal end of this graft is sutured circumferentially to the aorta distal to the origin of the left subclavian artery. *C*, The invaginated segment of graft is withdrawn, and (*D*) an opening in the graft is sutured around the origins of the brachiocephalic arteries. *E*, Antegrade circulation to prevent cerebral emboli from the distal aorta is restored by changing femoral bypass perfusion to arch perfusion using a separate arterial perfusion line through a small graft. *F*, The free end of the graft is exposed for operations shown in Figures 9 and 10 by making a small proximal incision in the aneurysm, inserting a finger, controlling graft flow, extending aneurysm incision, and clamping of graft. (Copyright 1990 by Baylor College of Medicine.)

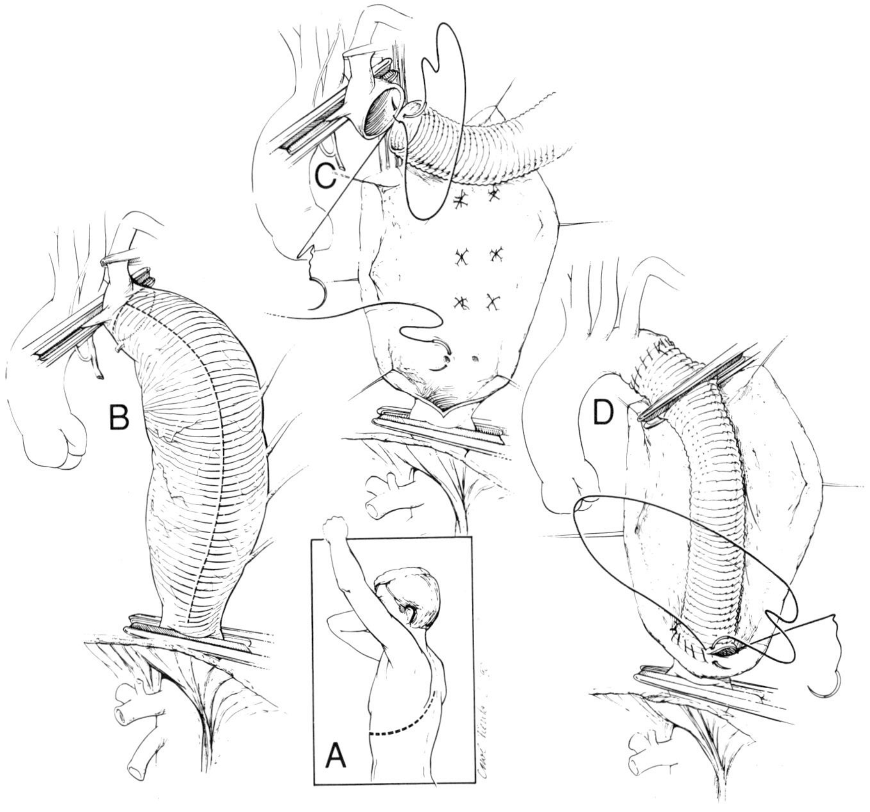

Figure 9 Graft replacement of aneurysm involving the descending thoracic aorta. For details, see text. (Copyright 1990 by Baylor College of Medicine.)

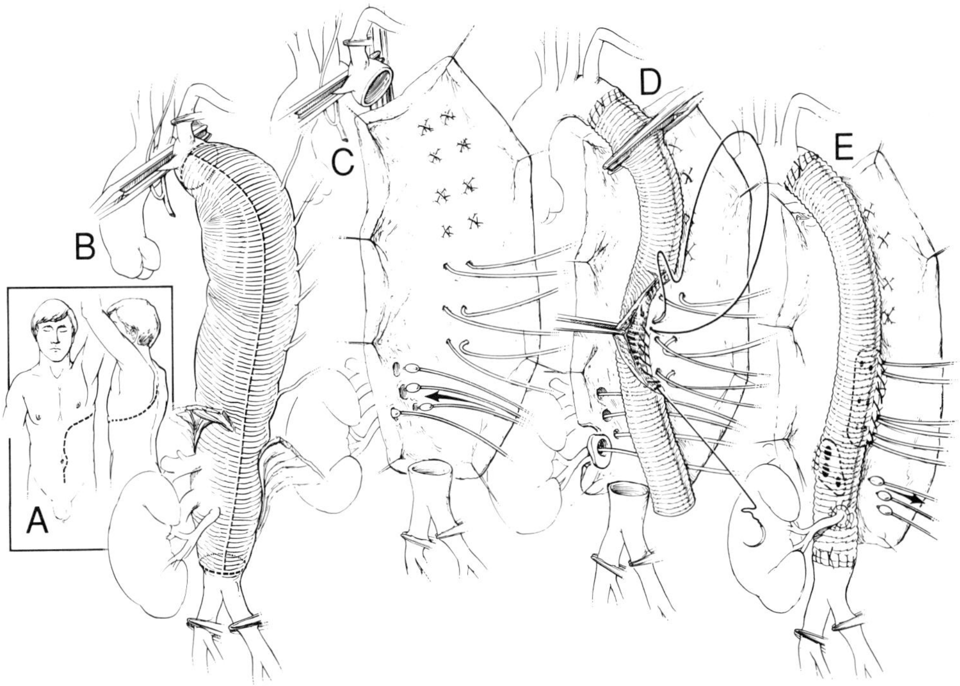

Figure 10 The author's technique for graft replacement of thoracoabdominal aortic aneurysms. For details, see text. (Copyright 1990 by Baylor College of Medicine.)

TABLE 2 Results According to Segment (Nondissection)

Segment	No. Patients	Survival 30-Day	1-Yr	5-Yr
Ascending	241	216 (90%)	86%	69%
Arch	116	105 (95%)	79%	67%
Ascending and Arch	220	206 (94%)	76%	60%
Descending	467	432 (94%)	82%	60%
Thoracoabdominal	1,097	1,007 (92%)	79%	60%
Totals	2,141	1,966 (92%)		

We have employed various methods recommended to prevent the complication. These include temporary bypass, surface hypothermia, profound hypothermia, spinal fluid drainage, somatosensory evoked potential monitoring, steroids, mannitol, and barbiturates. These methods have not proved to be useful. Our recent studies using hydrogen injection of intercostal and lumbar arteries monitored by intraspinous platinum electrodes indicate that the source of cord blood supply can be determined at operation and paraplegia avoided by reattachment. It is hoped that continued studies of this method will prove its usefulness in reducing the incidence of this complication.

SUGGESTED READING

Bentall H, DeBono A. A technique for complete replacement of the ascending aorta. Thorax 1968; 23:338.

Borst HG, Frank G, Schaps D. Treatment of extensive aortic aneurysms by a new multiple-stage approach. J Thorac Cardiovasc Surg 1988; 95:11.

Cabrol C, Pavie A, Mesnildrey P, et al. Long-term results with total replacement of the ascending aorta and reimplantation of the coronary arteries. J Thorac Cardiovasc Surg 1986; 91:17.

Coselli JS, Crawford ES. Composite valve graft replacement of aortic root using separate dacron tube for coronary artery reattachment. Ann Thorac Surg 1989; 47:558.

Crawford ES, Saleh SA. Transverse aortic arch aneurysm: Improved results of treatment employing new modifications of aortic reconstruction and hypothermia cerebral circulatory arrest. Ann Surg 1981; 194:180.

Crawford ES, Crawford JL, Safi HJ, et al. Thoracoabdominal aortic aneurysms: preoperative and intraoperative factors determining immediate and long-term results of operation in 605 patients. J Vasc Surg 1986; 3:389.

Crawford ES, DeNatale RW: Thoracoabdominal aortic aneurysm: Observations regarding the natural course of the disease. J Vasc Surg 1986; 3:578.

Crawford ES, Svensson LG, Coselli JS, et al. Surgical treatment aneurysm and/or dissection of the ascending aorta, transverse aortic arch, and ascending aorta and transverse aortic arch: Factors influencing survival in 717 patients. J Thorac Cardiovasc Surg 1989; 98:659.

Crawford ES, Coselli JS, Svensson LG, et al. Diffuse aneurysmal disease (chronic aortic dissection, Marfan and mega aorta syndromes) and multiple aneurysm: Treatment by subtotal and total aortic replacement emphasizing the elephant trunk technique. Ann Surg 1990; 211.

Wheat MN Jr, Wilson JR, Bartley TD: Successful replacement of the entire aorta and aortic valve. JAMA 1964; 188:717.

AORTIC ANEURYSM: ABDOMINAL

ROBERT B. HOLTZMAN, M.D.
ARTHUR C. BEALL Jr., M.D.

Arteriosclerosis accounts for over 90 percent of aneurysms of the abdominal aorta. Causes for aneurysmal dilation other than atherosclerosis are syphilis, trauma, infection, congenital conditions, prior vascular procedures with anastomotic leak or dehiscence, and pregnancy. The vast majority of aneurysms are confined to the infrarenal aorta and extend to the aortic bifurcation or below into the iliac arteries. Lesions that extend up to the orifice of the renal arteries, leaving no normal infrarenal aorta, are considered juxtarenal aneurysms and are less common. Suprarenal aneurysms that involve the renal arteries, the superior mesenteric artery, and the celiac artery and can extend up to or beyond the diaphragm are classified with thoracoabdominal aneurysms. Fortunately, this type of aneurysm constitutes only 2 percent of aortic aneurysms; operative intervention in these patients carries a considerably higher morbidity and mortality rate than the routine infrarenal variety.

Although the pathogenesis of aneurysm formation is a combination of atherosclerotic, familial, mechanical, hemodynamic, and enzymatic factors, the most recent research has focused on the biochemical abnormalities in the weakened aortic wall. This degenerative process is related to a mechanical failure of the major structural proteins of the aorta, namely elastin and collagen. In experimental studies of human iliac arteries, failure of elastin by treatment with the enzyme elastase results in aneurysmal dilation but a stiffer, less compliant vessel. This shifts the load of the distending effects of blood pressure from elastin to collagen. Subsequent treatment of these elastase-treated vessels with collagenase resulted in rupture in all instances. In contrast, when treated with collagenase first, the vessel dilated and promptly ruptured. In vitro analyses of the abdominal aorta in patients with aneurysms have shown a degradation of the aortic media, a loss of elastin and smooth muscle cells, and an increase in the enzymes elastase and collagenase. Perhaps contrary to traditional teaching, atherosclerosis is not the most important factor in aneurysmal disease. Aneurysms do occur in the absence of atherosclerosis in younger patients with connective tissue disorders. Some of these patients exhibit an abnormality of factors, such as copper, that may affect elastin and collagen cross-linking.

In 1988, over 30,000 aortic aneurysmorrhaphies were performed at a cost of at least 400 million dollars in medical care. Thirty years ago the diagnostic capabilities were much less than today, and most aneurysms were discovered because they were large or symptomatic. Today, most abdominal aortic aneurysms are asymptomatic; however, on occasion patients will complain that they can feel their heart in their abdomen. Sometimes patients present with a chronic back pain because the aneurysm abuts the vertebral bodies; however, they can grow to dangerous sizes without symptoms. The first clue to the presence of aneurysmal disease comes from a thorough history and physical examination. In many patients the aorta is easily palpated through the abdominal wall, and a determination of its size and whether it is normal or dilated can be made. This can be difficult in obese or muscular patients. At least 25 percent of abdominal aortic aneurysms are undetected on physical examination.

Routine x-ray films of the abdomen, lumbosacral spine, gastrointestinal tract, or urinary tract can result in the incidental finding of an aneurysm, and in the past the radiologist accounted for many of the referrals to the vascular surgeon. Still more than 50 percent of aneurysms do not contain enough calcium to be seen on plain film examination.

Ultrasonography provides an accurate, noninvasive, widely available, and relatively inexpensive technique to determine aorta size. Because there is no risk or discomfort to the patient, it is valuable for serial examinations to evaluate growth in aneurysmal size. Increased use of ultrasonography is undoubtedly one of the reasons the incidence of abdominal aortic aneurysms has increased from 8.7 new aneurysms per 100,000 person years from 1950 to 1960, to 36.5 from 1970 to 1980. As more people are living longer and remaining in better health, a true increase is also expected. Current mortality rates from elective aneurysm repair is 1 to 5 percent, which compares quite favorably with the 60 to 90 percent mortality rate quoted for ruptured aneurysms. Clearly, if lives are to be saved and costs reduced, abdominal aortic aneurysms must be diagnosed and treated before rupture occurs. This has led to consideration of screening programs for the detection of abdominal aortic aneurysms using ultrasonography. Although mass screening of the population is unlikely to be implemented, the astute physician should screen those patients who are at high risk, namely those patients with first degree relatives with aneurysms, and patients over 50 years of age with hypertension and other vascular disease.

Although sonography is an excellent means for detecting an aneurysm, for mass screening, and for surveillance to detect expansion, it fails to provide reliable anatomic information needed for preoperative evaluation. Although resecting an aneurysm with ultrasonographic evaluation only may be good for cost containment, we doubt that it is good for the patient. Computed tomography (CT), unlike ultrasonography, is less operator dependent and provides more information about the abdominal aorta, its branches, and any other intraabdominal pathology. For this reason, we almost routinely obtain a preoperative CT scan and an angiogram. By combining these two modalities, all the following anatomic information can be obtained: the size and extent of the aneurysm (thoracoabdominal component, involvement of the iliac arteries), the relationship of the aneurysm to surrounding structures (inferior vena cava, retroaortic left renal vein, ureters, horseshoe kidneys), the status of the visceral vessels and peripheral circulation (renal artery stenosis, a meandering artery, iliac occlusion), unusual presentation (inflammatory aneurysms, infected aneurysms, erosion of vertebral bodies, aortocaval fistula) and other concomitant pathology (retroperitoneal fibrosis, lymphoma, cholelithiasis, nephrolithiasis, and pancreatic abnormalities). Preoperative knowledge of potential difficulties can aid the surgeon in formulating the operative approach and can make for a smoother and safer intraoperative and postoperative course.

Preoperative evaluation is not limited to determining the characteristics of the aneurysm. Coronary artery disease accounts for the majority of postoperative complications. As many as 20 percent of these patients can have severe correctable coronary disease with no clinical or electrocardiographic evidence of cardiac ischemia. We favor the liberal use of preoperative coronary angiography and revascularization. Those patients who maintain an active life-style and have no electrocardiographic abnormalities, no history of cardiac symptoms, and no significant family history of cardiac disease should be allowed to undergo aneurysm repair without further cardiac workup. Patients with diabetes, mild or stable angina, history of cardiac disease, or no symptoms with a sedentary life-style should undergo noninvasive stress testing. The dipyridamole thallium stress test has been shown to be the most accurate of the noninvasive techniques to assess a patient with known or suspected ischemic heart disease. Patients with regional wall abnormalities or hypoperfusion defect during stress testing should undergo cardiac catheterization and coronary revascularization, if indicated. Likewise, patients with significant cardiac symptoms should go directly to cardiac catheterization and surgery as needed.

There are some patients with abdominal aortic aneurysms in whom preoperative coronary revascularization is not justified, owing to their high risk for this procedure. Included in this group are patients more than 85 years of age, patients with left ventricular ejection fraction less than 20 percent, patients after multiple failed coronary bypass operations, and patients with severe diffuse unreconstructable disease. Observation of small aneurysms is recommended in these people.

THERAPEUTIC ALTERNATIVES

Unlike obstructive lesions, in which balloon dilation or laser can be offered as a nonsurgical alternative, there is no satisfactory nonsurgical treatment for aneurysmal disease. Alternatives to aneurysm resection for the highest risk patients involve some mechanism of thrombosis of the aneurysm, by proximal and distal ligation, percutaneous embolization with coils, detachable balloons, or thrombotic materials and extra-anatomic bypass. Because these patients have an increased risk even for these lesser procedures, and still have a chance to rupture, we prefer to perform a standard resection and accept a higher mortality rate. Of interest in the future may be the development of percutaneously placed intraluminal stents across aortic aneurysms in nonoperative candidates.

PREFERRED APPROACH

Surgical Treatment

Selection of Patients

The surgical treatment of abdominal aortic aneurysms has improved during the past 3 decades, so that the mortality rates from an elective aneurysm resection have fallen from 15 to 20 percent to 1 to 3 percent. Much of the decrease in mortality rate occurred within the first decade of surgical therapy from refinements in surgical technique, such as use of the endoaneurysmal approach rather than total excision of the aneurysm. Improvements during the next decade were seen in the intraoperative care of the patients by the anesthesiologist and in the postoperative care of the patient by better monitoring and technology in the intensive care unit. More recently, a further reduction in mortality rate has come from more accurately assessing the preoperative medical condition of the patient. As previously noted, we perform cardiac catheterization in any patient with symptoms suggestive of coronary artery disease. Other factors affecting the mortality rate are similar to those of any major abdominal procedure and includes cerebrovascular disease, renal disease, chronic obstructive pulmonary disease, and cirrhosis.

The selection and timing of operation in patients with aneurysms traditionally has been a balancing act between the risk of operation and the chance of rupture. However, operation also is advised for patients with distal emboli (blue toe syndrome), with associated gastrointestinal hemorrhage, with pain or tenderness on palpation, and with ureteral or visceral obstruction. Since the early 1960s, physicians have recommended that abdominal aortic aneurysms larger than 6 cm be repaired as the risk of rupture was great, and those less than 6 cm be observed. It soon became apparent that as many as 30 percent of patients followed with small aneurysms (less than 6 cm) died of rupture. Further, an autopsy series found that 18 percent of 182 ruptured abdominal aortic aneurysms were less than 5 cm in size. Since current mortality rates for aneurysm repair are kept below 5 percent, all good risk patients with the diagnosis of an aneurysm should undergo surgery. For this purpose an aneurysm is present when the diameter of the infrarenal aortic segment is at least one and one-half times the diameter of the aorta measured at the renal arteries. In general, patients over age 50 years have an aortic diameter on the average of 2.5 cm (range 2 to 3 cm); we would recommend surgery when the diameter is greater than 4 cm in the low-risk patient and greater than 6 cm in the high-risk patient. The risk of rupture plotted against aneurysm diameter forms a sigmoid-shaped curve similar to the oxyhemoglobin dissociation curve where the risk of rupture increases almost exponentially beyond a diameter of 6 cm. At 4 cm, the 5-year risk of rupture is 15 percent, whereas at 8 cm it is more than 75 percent. There are several other factors that contribute to the risk of rupture besides size. Diastolic blood pressure and obstructive pulmonary disease have been found to be independent predictors of rupture. A patient with a 4-cm aneurysm, a diastolic pressure greater than 90 mm Hg, and pulmonary disease with an FEV_1 greater than 50 percent but less than 75 percent predicted has a 5-year risk of rupture of 52 percent, not 15 percent. If the diastolic pressure is increased to 105 mm Hg and the FEV_1 is reduced to less than 50 percent predicted, the 5-year risk of rupture is greater than 90 percent for the same size aneurysm. Thus, the timing of surgery in aneurysmal disease is more complex than a matter of size versus rupture.

The high-risk patient further complicates the decision-making process. Criteria for high risk include age greater than 85 years, home oxygen, arterial Po_2 less than 50 mm Hg, class III to IV angina, recent or recurrent congestive heart failure, complex ventricular ectopy, severe valvular disease, nonreconstructable coronary artery disease, large left ventricular aneurysm, recurrent angina after coronary artery bypass, cirrhosis with ascites, retroperitoneal fibrosis, and morbid obesity. The rate of enlargement of aneurysms is generally accepted at 0.4 cm per year; however, the rate is quite variable, and the rate of expansion has been reported as low as 0.13 cm per year to as high as 1.5 cm per year. Some aneurysms do not change for years, whereas others undergo rapid enlargement. Therefore, it is reasonable to follow 4 cm aneurysms with serial ultrasonography in the poor-risk patient. As many as 50 percent of patients will die from the underlying medical problem first. Evidence of rapid enlargement (0.5 cm between sequential studies) or on reaching a diameter of 6 cm, should alert the surgeon to operate. These factors increase the likelihood of rupture and place the patient in a precarious position. Mortality rates from elective aneurysm resection even in a high-risk group can be held to 10 percent or less.

This can be done by maximizing their preoperative and postoperative care. For patients with severe pulmonary disease, we recommend cessation of smoking, preoperative respiratory therapy including instruction in incentive spirometry, chest physiotherapy, bronchodilators, and antibiotics. Patients who are dialysis dependent can undergo operation with only a slight increase in morbidity and mortality. Those patients who have borderline renal function but do not require dialysis also fall into a high risk group. Meticulous attention to hydration status, fluid balance, and, if necessary, temporary dialysis in the early postoperative period can avoid serious complications. As many as one-third of patients with cardiac disease not amenable to myocardial revascularization and large aneurysms will die from their aneurysm. With careful perioperative monitoring to maintain optimal cardiac function, operative repair can be accomplished with an acceptable mortality. The use of dopamine and dobutamine along with sodium nitroprusside and nitroglycerin is clearly helpful in these patients. Rarely, postoperative intra-aortic balloon counterpulsation is required.

Operative Technique

Preoperatively the patient is hydrated and given prophylactic antibiotics; however, we do not routinely use a bowel preparation. A Swan-Ganz catheter is placed immediately preoperatively by the anesthesiologist. Intraoperatively, we do not routinely use systemic heparin when cross-clamping the aorta. With vigorous flushing of the graft and vessels, we have not seen an increased incidence of graft or distal thrombosis. In patients with occlusive disease, such as occlusion of the superficial femoral artery, we will use heparin.

Although many of the details of the operation are beyond the scope of this chapter, there have been several important developments that have decreased the morbidity and mortality of the procedure. Recognition of the fact that the aneurysm need not be excised led to a substantial decrease in the difficulty of the operation. Use of this endoaneurysmorrhaphy technique, where the posterior wall of the aneurysm remains in its bed in the retroperitoneum, has minimized the massive blood loss encountered in the early years of aneurysm surgery when complete removal of the aneurysm was performed. Using this technique the aorta is opened longitudinally down the anterior surface. Back bleeding from lumbar arteries and the inferior mesenteric artery is controlled with suture ligatures from within the aneurysm sac. The upper and lower ends of the aneurysm are cut laterally, however, the posterior half of the aneurysm wall is left undivided. A graft then is placed inside the aneurysm and sutured proximally to the native aorta and distally to the aortic bifurcation, common iliac bifurcations, or femoral arteries, depending on the extent of the disease. The aneurysm wall then is closed around the graft to prevent graft erosion into the duodenum and subsequent aortoduodenal fistula.

A more recent development is that of rapid blood collection, processing, and retransfusion in a short period of time (5 minutes). This has minimized the need for homologous blood transfusion. Use of intraoperative blood salvage has enabled approximately 50 percent of elective aneurysm surgery to be performed without transfusion and has significantly reduced the volume of banked blood required in cases of ruptured aneurysms.

The key to treatment of a ruptured abdominal aortic aneurysm is rapid diagnosis and expeditious transport to the operating room. Any delay can literally mean the difference between success and failure. The diagnosis should be suspected in any patient with the classic triad of hypotension or syncope, sudden onset of abdominal or back pain, and a pulsatile abdominal mass. The unstable, hypotensive patient has probably ruptured anteriorly into the peritoneal cavity and should be taken directly to the operating room after establishing intravenous access, electrocardiogram, and type and crossmatch in the emergency room. Rupture can occur laterally or posteriorly into the retroperitoneum, which may contain blood loss. However, a patient with a ruptured aneurysm can present as normotensive with complaints of sudden onset of back pain. In up to 80 percent of patients with ruptured aneurysms a pulsatile mass can be found, and in this patient we would proceed to the operating room without further diagnostic tests. If the patient is obese or a good abdominal examination is not possible and the patient is completely stable, we would proceed to CT scan for diagnosis. Aneurysms most commonly rupture to the left of the base of the mesentery and dissect downward. The presence or absence of distal pulses has no diagnostic significance when evaluating a patient with a ruptured aneurysm.

Patients who present as normotensive with a small contained periaortic hematoma have an operative mortality of about 20 percent. Patients presenting as hypotensive but who respond quickly to resuscitation have a more extensive retroperitoneal hematoma and a mortality rate closer to 40 percent. If hypotension persists or recurs at the time of induction, mortality rate is nearer to 60 percent, and if in addition to being unstable the patient has had no urine output by the time of operation, the mortality rate is closer to 80 percent.

Intraoperatively, the speed of proximal control may determine the ultimate outcome. Blood is ready and hanging, but we do not start transfusing until the proximal aortic clamp has been applied. An experienced vascular surgeon can gain control of the aorta in less than 5 minutes, either at the level of the diaphragm or suprarenal aorta. After the hemorrhage has been controlled, the clamp is moved to the infrarenal aorta and the operation is continued in the routine fashion.

Unusual Presentations

Although most patients with abdominal aortic aneurysms, if left untreated, will develop the typical complications of rupture, embolization, or thrombosis, a few patients will present with unusual manifestations of the aneurysm. One of the more frequent unusual presentations, occurring in 2.5 percent of cases, is an inflammatory aneurysm. Most of the time this type of aneurysm is not identified prior to operation. There is a marked inflammatory response involving the aneurysm wall and adjacent structures (ureters, duodenum, inferior vena cava), making dissection difficult. Operative mortality is increased to 10 percent. Sometimes preoperative diagnosis is made if the patient has an elevated sedimentation rate, weight loss, or a thickened aneurysmal wall and perianeurysmal fibrosis on CT scan.

Rupture or compression of the aneurysm into adjacent structures can occur. Aortocaval or aortorenal vein fistula results from spontaneous rupture on the aneurysm into those structures. As a result of the fistula, these patients develop high output failure, cardiomegaly, a continuous abdominal bruit, hypotension, and abdominal pain. Repair is accomplished from within the aneurysmal sac and care taken to prevent embolization of air or debris into the venous circulation.

A small group of patients have a chronic contained rupture that is diagnosed on CT scan for back pain. Usually these aneurysms rupture posteriorly onto the vertebral bodies and are contained by the prevertebral fascia. Survival beyond 6 weeks with this condition is unlikely, and operation is indicated within 24 hours of diagnosis.

If rupture occurs into the duodenum, gastrointestinal hemorrhage ensues. A primary aortoenteric fistula occurs when an untreated aneurysm erodes into the third or fourth portion of the duodenum. Only rarely does an exsanguinating hemorrhage happen initially. More often the patient presents with a sentinel or herald bleed and may have only minor hemorrhage prior to operation. A secondary aortoenteric fistula refers to a connection between a prosthetic graft and the gastrointestinal tract. This is usually associated with a graft infection or suture line failure with false aneurysm formation. This is the most dreaded complication of aortic surgery and results in a mortality rate of at least 50 percent. The diagnosis of aortoenteric fistula is difficult to determine preoperatively and a high index of suspicion is required. Often the diagnosis is only made after exclusion of other causes or the time of exploration. Treatment is by graft excision and replacement or by ligating the aorta with interposition of viable tissue between the aortic stump and the bowel and extra-anatomic bypass.

The management of patients with abdominal aortic aneurysm and concomitant intra-abdominal pathology poses a problem for the surgeon. Operation of the more symptomatic lesion is the basis of our approach to this problem. Thus, if a patient with an asymptomatic aneurysm develops acute cholecystitis, active peptic ulcer disease requiring surgery, or an obstructing colon lesion, we would operate on the gastrointestinal tract first. If the aneurysm is large, we would repair it during the same admission. We have not had an increase in mortality by performing simultaneous cholecystectomy or parietal cell vagotomy with aneurysm resection in patients who have given a history of biliary tract or peptic ulcer disease. To the contrary, these problems seem to be aggravated in the postoperative period if not treated. Patients who are symptomatic from both the gastrointestinal tract and the aneurysm require synchronous procedures. It is important to close the retroperitoneum prior to the intraperitoneal portion of the operation to minimize the risk of graft contamination and infection.

Complications

Postoperatively, the patients remain in the intensive care unit, where they can be monitored closely, because these patients are among the most critically ill in the unit. Barring any complications, the patient is moved to the floor on the second or third postoperative day, and discharge can be expected in 7 to 10 days. Although most deaths are of myocardial origin, other serious complications can cause loss of limb, paralysis, and organ failure. Most serious complications can be averted by good technique and sound operative judgment. Intraoperative problems can occur from exsanguinating hemorrhage, atheroembolism (trash foot), and declamping hypotension. In the early postoperative period, complications can arise from acute renal failure by ischemic or toxic injury, from ureteral injury, and from varying degrees of colonic ischemia causing mucosal lesions to transmural infarction. Paralysis is extremely rare (0.23 percent) but can occur from an anomalously positioned artery of Adamkiewicz. Late complications that involve graft infection may present as an aortoenteric fistula or graft thrombosis.

SUGGESTED READING

Bernstein EF, Chan EL. Abdominal aortic aneurysm in high risk patients: Outcome of selective management based on size and expansion rate. Ann Surg 1984; 200:255.

Crawford ES, Saleh SA, Babb JW, et al. Infrarenal abdominal aortic aneurysm: Factors influencing survival after operation performed over a 25 year period. Ann Surg 1981; 193:699.

Crawford ES, Hess KR. Abdominal aortic aneurysm, editorial. N Engl J Med 1989; 321:1040.

Cronenwett JL, Murphy TF, Zelenock GB, et al. Actuarial analysis of variables associated with rupture of small abdominal aortic aneurysms. Surgery 1985; 98:472.

Lawrie GM, Morris GC Jr, Crawford ES, et al. Improved results of operation for ruptured abdominal aortic aneurysms. Surgery 1979; 85:483.

Tilson MD. Histochemistry of aortic elastin in patients with nonspecific abdominal aortic aneurysmal disease. Arch Surg 1988; 123:503.

RAYNAUD'S SYNDROME

J. TIMOTHY FULENWIDER, M.D.

Of the clinical vasospastic disorders, none incites more patient anxiety, encompasses a broader clinical disease spectrum, and invokes more etiologic and therapeutic controversy than Raynaud's syndrome (RS). Raynaud's syndrome is characterized by episodic digital arteriospasm resulting in pathognomonic biphasic or triphasic digital cutaneous color changes. Most patients with RS (70 to 90 percent) are women between the ages of 25 to 40 years with cold-induced or emotion-induced symmetrical finger pallor that persists in cold exposure. With rewarming, digit pallor changes to cyanosis (sluggish reperfusion) and occasionally to intense rubor (reactive hyperemia). The color changes may extend into the distal palm and may be frequently accompanied by transient, reversible digital hypothermia, mild pain, and hypesthesia. The fingers and hands are most commonly involved, although the toes, cheeks, and ears may demonstrate typical evanescent color changes. Raynaud's syndrome is often seasonal and geographic; episodes are more common and severe in northern climates during the winter months.

The clinical spectrum of RS includes "Raynaud's disease": patients with normal extremity arterial anatomy and supraphysiologic vasoconstrictor responses hypothetically due to a "local vascular fault" or exaggerated adrenergic neuroeffector activity and increased $alpha_2$ adrenergic receptors of digital arteries are included in this group. "Raynaud's phenomenon" includes those patients with fixed, pressure-reducing, organic obstructive arteriopathies of the digital, palmar, or proximal extremity arteries whose superimposed normal vasoconstrictor responses effect critical arterial closure, cessation of blood flow, and the ischemic event. Although Raynaud's disease classically occurs in the absence of an identifiable clinical systemic disease, Raynaud's phenomenon is associated with a myriad of disease states (Table 1). Unfortunately, precise initial stratification of patients into such clinical subsets is arbitrary because of the well-documented long latency intervals between the onset of RS and the evolution of an associated systemic disease state. To avoid confusion, many have suggested the abandonment of the labels "Raynaud's disease" and "Raynaud's phenomenon" for the more inclusive category "Raynaud's syndrome." Raynaud's syndrome can then be pathophysiologically segregated into "vasospastic" and "obstructive" subsets.

THERAPEUTIC ALTERNATIVES

All therapeutic plans for RS are palliative and are directed toward a reduction in the frequency and severity of digital ischemia attacks. The majority (70 to 80 percent) of patients with RS are effectively managed by explaining the involved pathophysiology of the syndrome to them and reassuring them of the favorable prognosis of RS of the purely vasospastic variety. Digital gangrene never occurs as a consequence of vasospasm alone. Preventive measures to minimize cold exposure by wearing mittens to maintain hand warmth is an important mainstay of therapy. Additional preventive measures include proper attire for cold weather exposure to maintain central body core temperature at near-normal levels. The use of multilayered insulated garments (polypropylene, Gore-tex, down, or Thinsulate) and battery-heated socks and gloves have proved indispensable in main-

TABLE 1 Conditions Associated with Raynaud's Syndrome

Immunologic and collagen vascular diseases
Scleroderma
CREST syndrome
Systemic lupus erythematosus
Rheumatoid arthritis
Mixed connective tissue disease
Undifferentiated connective tissue disease
Dermatomyositis
Polymyositis
Hepatitis B–associated vasculitis
Drug-induced vasculitis
Sjögren's syndrome
Schönlein-Henoch purpura
Polyarteritis nodosa
Reiter's syndrome
Hypersensitivity vasculitis
Obstructive arteriopathies
Arteriosclerosis obliterans
Thromboangiitis obliterans (Buerger's disease)
Post-thromboembolic arterial obstruction
Thoracic outlet compression syndrome
Takayasu's disease
Other arteritides (giant cell, syphilitic)
Occupational or environmental trauma
Hypothenar-hammer syndrome
Vibratory tool exposure
Direct large or small arterial trauma
Cold injury, frostbite
Neurologic diseases
Central or peripheral neuropathy
Reflex sympathetic dystrophy
Carpal tunnel syndrome
Endocrinopathy
Myxedema
Graves' disease
Hypopituitarism
Addison's disease
Cushing's disease
Drug-associated conditions
Ergot alkaloids
Beta-adrenergic blockers
Oral contraceptives
Cytotoxic therapy
Nicotine
Caffeine
Sympathomimetics
Methysergide
Miscellaneous conditions
Fabry's disease
Paroxysmal hemoglobinuria
Primary pulmonary hypertension
Pheochromocytoma
Vinyl chloride exposure
Chronic renal failure
Cold agglutinins
Cryoglobulinemia
Hyperviscosity states
Malignant neoplasms
Myeloproliferative disorders (leukemia, myeloid metaplasia, polycythemia rubra vera, thrombocytosis)
Macroglobulinemia
Disseminated intravascular coagulation
Heavy metals

taining normal active life-styles for patients with RS. Tobacco, in all forms, must be avoided. Alkaloids, beta-blockers, oral contraceptives, and sympathomimetic medications are also relatively contraindicated. A physical measure that is alleged to be capable of aborting a prolonged episode of digital ischemia is the whirling arm maneuver. In this maneuver, the patient, while standing, rapidly whirls the affected upper extremity in a 360-degree arc for 1 to 2 minutes or for a shorter interval should the digital ischemia subside. The avoidance of vibratory machinery (drills, sanders, chainsaws, jackhammers, grinders) is preferable; however, oscillatory trauma can be minimized by grasping the tools as lightly as possible; reducing motor speed, and the wearing of heavy gloves (especially those with antivibrational properties). Several investigators have reported salutary responses to stress modification instruction and biofeedback training; however, most investigators also concur that these measures should be reserved for highly motivated individuals.

A minority (20 to 30 percent) of patients with RS will require pharmacologic therapy, often only during the colder months. That no single drug or combination of drugs has achieved universal acceptance as the regimen of choice is shown by the multiplicity of medications either formerly or presently endorsed as effective (Table 2.) Pharmacologic investigations of patients with RS have been hampered by the paucity of objective tests that accurately quantitate the effects of medications on digital arterial flow. Accordingly, investigators have relied on subjective end responses in the majority of trials, most of which are not randomized, blinded, or placebo controlled. Nonetheless, the consensus is that pharmacotherapy does play a vital role for many patients with RS, and that those with the purely vasospastic etiology respond far more favorably than those with fixed organic arterial obstructions. Medications reported to be effective in patients with RS are listed in Table 2. Favorable anecdotal responses to plasmapheresis have also been reported and are presumably related to the reduction of whole blood viscosity with improvement of red blood cell membrane deformability during microcirculatory transit.

Contemporary surgical management of RS is primarily directed toward arterial reconstruction of pressure-significant stenoses or complete occlusions because operative cervicothoracic and lumbar sympathetic denervations have been virtually abandoned. Although microsurgical palmar digital arterial sympathectomy is technically feasible, its propriety for RS is obviously dubious because of the well-documented, short-lived favorable results following conventional sympathetic denervations. Technically incomplete sympathetic denervation, post-denervation receptor hypersensitivity, and sympathetic neural fiber regeneration have been incriminated in the late clinical failures following sympathectomy.

TABLE 2 Medications Used in Raynaud's Syndrome

Class	*Dose/Route*	*Response Rate (%)*	*Major Adverse Effects*
Calcium channel blockers			
Nifedipine	30–60 mg/d; PO	60–70	Vasomotor flushing, edema, headaches, giddiness, hypotension, late tachyphylaxis (?)
Diltiazem	90–180 mg/d; PO	60–70	Edema, hypotension, prolongation AV node conduction palpitations, syncope, vasomotor flushing
Nicardipine	60–120 mg/d; PO	60–70	Edema, headache, dizziness, asthenia, palpitations
Sympatholytics			
Reserpine	0.25–1.0 mg/d; PO	40–50	Depression, orthostatic hypotension, peptic ulcer disease, diarrhea, impotence, asthenia, nasal congestion
Guanethidine	10–40 mg/d; PO	40–50	Orthostatic hypotension, impotence, diarrhea, bradycardia, edema
Methyldopa	250–1,000 mg/d; PO	40–50	Impotence, orthostatic hypotension, sedation, asthenia; Coombs positive anemia, hepatitis, systemic lupus erythematous syndrome
Alpha-adrenergic blockers			
Prazosin	2–20 mg/d; PO	50	Dizziness, headache, asthenia, somnolence, nausea, palpitations, orthostatic hypotension
Phenoxybenzamine	20–80 mg/d; PO	40–50	Orthostatic hypotension, tachycardia, fatigue
Vasodilators			
Griseofulvin	250–1,000 mg/d; PO	30–40 (?)	Photosensitivity, nausea, vomiting, diarrhea, mental confusion, paresthesias
Nicotine acid	250–2,000 mg/d; PO	40	Flushing, pruritus, diarrhea, postural hypotension, headache, hyperuricemia
Papaverine	150–450 mg/d; PO	30–40	Nausea, headache, malaise, abdominal distress, vertigo, sweating
Captopril	37.5–75 mg/d; PO	30	Hypotension, angioedema, dysgeusia, tachycardia
Nitrates	5–10 mg/d; topical 0.04 mg; sublingual	20–30	Headaches, palpitations, flushing, nausea, hypotension
Iloprost	Investigational; IV	30	Hypotension, flushing, headache, nausea, vomiting
Prostacyclin (PGI_2)	Investigational; IV	Indeterminate	Hypertenison, flushing, tachycardia, nausea, vomiting
Prostaglandin E_1 (PGE_1) Alprostadil	Investigational; IV	Indeterminate	Hypotension, flushing, tachycardia, nausea, vomiting
Serotonin H_2 Receptor antagonist			
Ketanserin	10 mg IV; 60–120 mg/d PO	Indeterminate	Hypotension
Beta receptor agonists			
Terbutaline sulfate	7.5–15 mg/d; PO	Minimal	Headache, tremor, palpitations, nausea, vomiting, sweating
Nylidrin	9–48 mg/d; PO	Minimal	Tremor, palpitations, nausea, asthenia
Isoproterenol, isoxuprine*			
Fibrinolytic agents			
Stanozolol†		Indeterminate	Malaise, fluid retention, amenorrhea, acne, hirsutism, elevated liver enzymes
Miscellaneous drugs of marginal benefit			
Triiodothyronine*			
Dextran (low molecular weight)*			
Pentoxifylline*			

*No dose/route and response rate published.
†No dose/route published.

PREFERRED APPROACH

The history of episodic biphasic or triphasic digital cutaneous color changes lasting 20 to 60 minutes provoked by cold exposure or emotional stimuli is sufficient to establish the diagnosis of RS. Not infrequently, the patient's sympathoadrenal response during the initial introduction in a cool office environment is sufficient to demonstrate a typical episode of digital ischemia. Having established the historical diagnosis of RS, a detailed medical history is obtained, as at least 60 to 70 percent of individuals with symptoms and signs of the severity necessary to consult a physician will prove to have an associated illness (see Table 1). Specific questions regarding medications are warranted and should include nonprescription remedies such as nasal aerosols and oral decongestants which, if taken in sufficient quantities, have potent vasoconstrictor activities. A history of Prinzmetal's angina, migraine headaches, or abdominal migraine is important because of presumed similar "local vascular faults" creating regional episodic vasospasm. Occupational history assumes critical importance, exemplified by data suggesting that from 40 to 90 percent of loggers and 50 percent of miners using vibratory equipment experience RS. Additionally, the history of malignancy, neurologic disorder, blood and clotting dyscrasias, endocrinopathy, or claudication may assume etiologic significance. Approximately 30 to 40 percent of patients with RS have evidence of some associated illness and small artery obliterative disease (see Table 1). Approximately one-half of these RS-associated illnesses are autoimmune connective tissue disorders, most frequently either scleroderma or a CREST variant; therefore, the examination should include questioning for special evidence of connective tissue disease: myalgias, arthralgias, cutaneous edema or induration, dermatitis, cutaneous photosensitivity or tightening, atrophy and pigment changes, sicca complex symptoms, and dysphagia.

The complete physical examination should emphasize the integument and peripheral arterial tree. Important features include qualitative assessment of all peripheral pulses, including an attempt to palpate digital arteries of the hands. The Allen test is performed to determine patency of the palmar arches. A Doppler ultrasonographic arterial survey using a portable 10 MHz pencil transducer provides a rapid, qualitative assessment of arterial velocimetry; a method of determining patency of small arteries; and flow detection to assess segmental limb systolic pressures. The presence of digital skin ulcerations or pitted scars of healed ulcerations suggests the presence of an underlying obstructive etiology of RS because pure vasospasm of normal arterial anatomy never causes cutaneous infarction or ulceration. In the presence of chronic digital ulceration, widespread palmar and digital obliterative arteriopathy will usually be present and is most likely due to vasculitis of scleroderma or CREST syndrome, hypersensitivity angiitis, or atherosclerosis obliterans, in this order of frequency.

Other physical examination clues of importance include skin eruptions, telangiectasias, and atrophy and tightening as well as joint deformities or other manifestations of connective tissue disease.

The extent of laboratory investigation is guided by clinical suspicions aroused by the history and physical evaluations; however, certain basic tests are routinely performed: complete blood count, erythrocyte sedimentation rate, chemistry profile, urinalysis, and antinuclear antibody. Additional investigations include the following: serum protein electrophoresis, quantitative serum immunoglobulin and complement levels, antibody to DNA, antiextractable nuclear antigens, HEP-2 ANA assay, anticentromere antibody, serum cryoglobulin and cryofibrinogen levels, hepatitis B surface antigen and antibody, chest film, nerve conduction velocities and electromyography, pulmonary function studies, and cine-esophagography.

Although the noninvasive vascular laboratory is not essential for the diagnosis of RS, its adjunctive roles include validation of the diagnosis of suspected RS patients who do not manifest typical digital color changes and the assessment of medical and surgical therapeutic efficacy. The ice water immersion test with serial fingertip thermistor probe temperature measurements is a simple and specific test for the diagnosis of RS; however, this examination suffers from low sensitivity. Digital photoplethysmography and waveform analysis has been frequently used because 70 percent of patients with RS are said to exhibit a characteristic "peak waveform." The digital photoplethysmography also provides excellent specificity but low sensitivity. The most accurate (97 percent), yet complex, RS diagnostic test is the occlusive digital hypothermic challenge described by Nielsen and Lassen (1977). This test is performed using a double inlet cuff, for local cooling, over the proximal phalanx of the test finger. Using a mercury-in-rubber strain gauge distal to the cuff, baseline pressures are determined and repeated after 5 minutes of ischemic hypothermic perfusion until pressure recovery occurs. The results are expressed as the percentage of decrease in the cool finger systolic pressure upon reperfusion compared with the reference finger. A decrease in digital pressure of 20 percent or greater is positive. I prefer simple digital plethysmography with waveform analysis and digital arterial pressures after ice bath immersion. These tests combined with extremity segmental air plethysmography and segmental arterial pressure determinations provide accurate, objective measurements of digital arterial flow; allow distinction between vasospastic and obstructive RS; and provide accurate, objective information regarding proximal arterial flow. Normally, the brachial-to-finger systolic pressure gradient is 10 to 15 torr. A brachial-to-finger pressure gradient of greater than 15 torr, absolute digital arterial pressure less than 70 torr, or pressure difference of more than 15 torr between any two fingers suggests the presence of significant palmar or digital arterial obstruction.

Contrast arteriography is warranted in selected patients with RS whose medical comorbidity would not contraindicate a major arterial reconstruction if remedial situations are discovered. Virtually all patients with ischemic digital ulcers should undergo complete extremity arteriography primarily to detect proximal arterial lesions (e.g., subclavian artery aneurysm) responsible for distal palmar and digital arterial occlusion (e.g., arterioarterial emboli). Magnified hand views are requested because microsurgical reconstruction techniques presently allow vein interposition grafting of small arteries, in carefully selected patients. Severely symptomatic individuals whose clinical or noninvasive laboratory investigations suggest significant proximal arterial obstruction should also undergo arteriography because revascularization in this group will frequently result in the most gratifying and durable relief of RS symptoms.

The use of digital subtraction arteriographic techniques and nonionic contrast media has greatly improved small artery resolution, minimized contrast load, injection pain, hypersensitivity reactions, and nephrotoxicity. However, preangiographic crystalloid hydration and intravenous mannitol are believed to be useful in preventing risks of postangiographic small artery thrombosis and acute renal insufficiency, especially in the diabetic population.

Medical Treatment

Pharmacologic therapy is indicated in the small minority of patients for whom a 6 to 8 week trial of preventive measures provides incomplete palliation. The physician's decision to institute pharmacotherapy depends on the patient's severity of complaints, the underlying pathology of RS, and the complete understanding of potential adverse effects of medications. Numerous medications, both single and in combinations, have been used with reasonable success; however, all the sympatholytics, alpha-adrenergic blockers, beta-receptor agonists, vasodilators, and calcium channel blockers may create intolerable systemic reactions (see Table 2).

At present, most agree that the newer calcium channel blockers have yielded the greatest palliation with least toxicity when compared with previous medications. The pharmacologic action of the slow channel blockers is smooth muscle relaxation by the selective inhibition of calcium influx into the cell. Nifedipine, having the most potent peripheral action, is presently considered the single agent of choice. The recommended starting dose of nifedipine is 10 mg orally three times a day increasing to 20 mg orally three times a day in stepwise fashion as dictated by clinical response. The RS experience with the long-acting nifedipine preparation is presently limited; however, similarly favorable results with dosage convenience are anticipated. Diltiazem in oral doses of 90 to 180 mg per day is another leading choice of monotherapy with clinical responses that parallel those using nifedipine. Patients who remain refractory to nifedipine or diltiazem alone may benefit from the addition of prazosin, a specific alpha-adrenergic blocker; however, prazosin must be titrated in 1 mg increments every 7 to 10 days because of well-documented side effects of hypotension, palpitations, headache, dizziness, nausea, and fatigue. Another useful oral drug combination, which will rarely be required, is guanethidine (10 mg per day) with prazosin (1 to 3 mg per day). In general, palliative doses of either guanethidine or prazosin used alone are associated with intolerable side effects of impotence, fatigue, and orthostatic hypotension; therefore, these drugs are presently believed to be unsatisfactory single-agent choices for RS. Similarly, phenoxybenzamine has been followed by frequent orthostatic hypotension and has been abandoned as monotherapy for the treatment of RS.

Therapeutic responses to all medication regimens are judged clinically with the aim of reducing frequency and severity of RS attacks to tolerable levels without superimposing significant adverse effects. I have had no experience with the other proposed RS regimens listed in Table 2 but have included these medications for reader awareness of their possible effectiveness in RS patients.

Conservative management of digital ulcerations is usually successful in achieving complete secondary healing, despite the presence of underlying small vessel occlusive disease. Limited surgical debridement of necrotic tissue with twice daily gentle soap cleansing followed by topical antimicrobial application (1% silver sulfadiazine [Silvadene]) is a regimen that has proved successful.

Surgical Treatment

Arterial reconstruction should be reserved for those with angiographically documented large vessel occlusive disease whose ischemic ulcers fail to heal with maximal conservative efforts or for those who suffer life-style–limiting claudication of the extremity. Rarely will reconstruction of remote radial, ulnar, or palmar arteries be necessary. Although cervicothoracic or lumbar sympathectomies are occasionally endorsed for medically refractory vasospastic RS, these procedures are virtually never indicated, particularly with the evolution and effectiveness of the slow channel calcium blockers.

SUGGESTED READING

Cardelli MB, Kleinsmith DM. Raynaud's phenomenon and disease. Med Cl N Am 1989; 73:1127.

Fitzgerald O, Hess EV, O'Connor GT. Prospective study of the evolution of Raynaud's phenomenon. Am J Med 1988; 84:718.

Jamieson GG, Ludbrook J, Wilson A. Cold hypersensitivity in Raynaud's phenomenon. Circulation 1971; 44:254.

Nielson SL, Lassen NA. Measurement of digital blood pressure after local cooling. J Appl Physiol 1977; 43:907.

Porter JM, Friedman EI, Mills JL. Occlusive and vasospastic diseases involving distal upper extremity arteries - Raynaud's syndrome. In: Rutherford RB, ed. Vascular Surgery. Philadelphia: WB Saunders, 1989: 844.

Priollet P, Vayssairat M, Housset E. How to classify Raynaud's phenomenon. Long-term follow-up study of 73 cases. Am J Med 1987; 83:494.

Raynaud M. On local asphyxia and symmetrical gangrene of the extremities (1862). New researchers on the nature and treatment of local asphyxia of the extremities (1884). Translated by T. Barlow. In: Selected Monographs, Vol 121. London: The New Syndenham Society, 1988; 1.

Rivers SP, Porter JM. Raynaud's syndrome, upper extremity vasospastic disorders, and small artery occlusive disease. In: Wilson SE, et al, eds. Vascular Surgery. Principles and Practice. New York: McGraw-Hill, 1987: 696.

Sumner DS, Strandness DE. An abnormal finger pulse associated with cold sensitivity. Ann Surg 1972; 175:294.

ACUTE THROMBOPHLEBITIS

JOSEPH D. ANSLEY, M.D.

Acute thrombophlebitis is the clinical syndrome of venous thrombosis with or frequently without symptomatic inflammation of the superficial or deep venous systems of the extremities, neck, or occasionally the trunk. Etiologic mechanisms involve any physical or physiologic state that results in stasis of venous blood, injury to the vein wall, or hypercoagulability. The inflammatory reaction is most often noninfectious, but septic thrombophlebitis does occur secondary to intravenous lines, access procedures, or intravenous drug abuse.

The diagnosis of acute thrombophlebitis relies on the demonstration of occlusion of the venous system or inflammation of the vein and surrounding tissue. Swelling of the extremity, tenderness along the vein, or palpable venous cords may be noted on physical examination, but often symptoms are minimal particularly in deep venous thrombosis. Clinical examination alone is not completely reliable, particularly for deep venous thrombosis; the examination should be augmented with tests for venous thrombosis including Doppler flow studies, venous plethysmography, venous duplex imaging, and radioisotope or contrast venography. Contrast venography remains the most definitive test and is recommended when placing the patient on a course of anticoagulation therapy for 3 to 6 months for deep venous thrombosis.

Therapeutic alternatives for nonseptic superficial thrombophlebitis include local warm compresses, elevation of the extremity for improved venous drainage, and nonsteroidal anti-inflammatory agents for symptomatic control in most cases. Surgical excision and ligation of the superficial venous system may be required for recurrent episodes of superficial thrombophlebitis associated with varicosities. Septic thrombophlebitis may require surgical excision and drainage when purulence is present; local warm compresses, elevation, removal of intravenous lines, and antibiotics are usually sufficient for nonpurulent cases. Deep venous thrombosis requires therapeutic anticoagulation, bed rest, and elevation of the involved extremities for 7 to 10 days combined with oral anticoagulation therapy for 3 to 6 months in most cases. Some patients may be candidates for thrombolytic therapy in addition to anticoagulation therapy, and on rare occasions venous thrombectomy may be indicated.

THERAPEUTIC ALTERNATIVES

Medical and surgical treatments are available for the treatment of acute thrombophlebitis.

PREFERRED APPROACH

Medical Treatment

Management of acute thrombophlebitis is primarily medical; surgical intervention is required infrequently. Superficial thrombophlebitis not related to intravenous lines is managed by local warm compresses over the involved vein, elevation of the extremity if swelling is present, and the use of anti-inflammatory agents such as aspirin or ibuprofen if not contraindicated by a history of allergy or gastric irritation. Active exercise to increase venous flow is recommended if it does not increase discomfort. It is important to rule out concomitant deep venous thrombosis, which may be present in 10 to 15 percent of these patients, because the therapy for deep venous thrombosis requires more aggressive management with anticoagulation therapy and bed rest to decrease the risk of pulmonary embolization.

Septic thrombophlebitis requires the removal of intravenous lines when present, local warm compresses for comfort, elevation of the extremity, and antibiotics if the patient is febrile or has other evidence of sepsis. If purulence is present in the venous system, surgical consultation is necessary for consideration of excision and drainage of the involved vein.

Deep venous thrombosis is the most significant form of acute thrombophlebitis because of the associated complications of pulmonary thromboembolism, subsequent chronic venous insufficiency of the post-phlebotic syndrome, and the possibility of venous gangrene with phlegmasia cerulea dolens (iliofemoral vein thrombosis) if early therapy with anticoagulation and elevation to reduce venous pressure is not effective.

Deep venous thrombosis of the lower extremities should be treated initially with full heparin anticoagulation therapy and bed rest with elevation of the lower extremities to increase venous drainage. Heparin should be given by continuous intravenous infusion after an initial bolus of 5,000 to 10,000 units. Adequate anticoagulation is obtained by prolonging the partial thromboplastin time (PTT) to 1.5 to 2.0 times the control value; for the average patient approximately 1,000 to 1,200 units per hour is required, but must be monitored by frequent PTT laboratory examinations and adjusted accordingly. Bed rest with elevation of the extremities by approximately 30 degrees should be continued until swelling and pain is controlled, which may take 7 to 10 days. Contraindications to anticoagulation therapy such as active gastrointestinal bleeding, recent intracranial or eye surgery, or bleeding disorders will require individualized treatment with elevation of the extremity continued but consideration for prophylactic inferior vena cava interruption for thrombosis extending into the vena cava or the occurrence of pulmonary embolism.

Oral anticoagulation therapy with warfarin for 3 to 6 months is indicated for most patients with deep venous thrombosis to decrease the incidence of recurrence. The length of time will vary depending on the response to therapy and factors predisposing to recurrence such as immobility or associated disease. Warfarin therapy should be begun while the patient is on heparin therapy with a 5 to 7 day overlap to allow the protime to come into range and to preclude the potential thrombotic state that may occur due to the initial warfarin effect on protein C. Warfarin is begun at 10 mg per day and adjusted after several days when the protime is prolonged appropriately. The protime is used to control and monitor therapy with prolongations of 1.3 to 1.5 the control value (15 to 18 seconds) being effective in preventing the recurrence of thrombosis and less likely to be complicated by the bleeding that has been associated with the higher levels used in the past.

Heparin therapy is associated with bleeding complications due to overcoagulation and to heparin-associated thrombocytopenia so that close monitoring is imperative. The PTT levels should be followed every 6 to 8 hours until stable and then daily after initial stabilization. Platelet counts should be obtained every other day and if it falls below 100,000 cells per μL, heparin should be discontinued and platelet aggregation test for heparin-associated antibodies performed. With positive test platelet inhibition, aspirin at 300 mg twice a day or dextran solution at 20 ml per hour may be given until adequate oral anticoagulation is obtained.

Warfarin therapy is associated with bleeding if excessive prolongation of the protime occurs; therefore, proper monitoring is necessary, daily while hospitalized and then on a weekly basis as an outpatient. Skin necrosis secondary to warfarin therapy occurs in some patients and may require excision of involved areas and discontinuation of oral anticoagulation therapy. Adjusted dose subcutaneous heparin may then be used to prevent thrombophlebitis recurrence with 10,000 to 15,000 units administered twice a day with monitoring to prolong the PTT by 15 seconds 6 hours following administration.

Surgical Treatment

Surgical treatment for acute deep vein thrombosis is only necessary when appropriate anticoagulation therapy is not effective or is contraindicated by a bleeding diathesis. Recurrent superficial thrombophlebitis may require vein ligation and stripping or excision. Septic thrombophlebitis may require excision and drainage when purulence is present or if sepsis persists despite antibiotic therapy. Ileofemoral venous thrombectomy may be indicated when impending venous gangrene occurs despite adequate anticoagulation and proper elevation of the extremity to reduce venous pressure. This procedure is associated with an increased morbidity and mortality and therefore is not widely accepted as appropriate therapy but may be indicated in selective patients.

SUGGESTED READING

Comerota AJ, Katz ML, Greenwald LL, et al. Venous duplex imaging: Should it replace hemodynamic test for deep venous thrombosis? J Vasc Surg 1990; 11:53.

Dalen JE, Paraskos JA, Ockene IS, et al. Venous thromboembolism: Scope of the problem. Chest 1986; 89:370S.

Lofgren EP, Lofgren KA. The surgical treatment of superficial thrombophlebitis. Surgery 1981; 90:49.

Schafer AI. The hypercoagulable states. Ann Intern Med 1985; 102:814.

Sidorov J. Streptokinase vs heparin for deep venous thrombosis: Can lytic therapy be justified? Arch Intern Med 1989; 149:1841.

Silver D: Heparin induced thrombocytopenia and thrombosis. Semin Vasc Surg 1988; 1:228.

Wessler S, Gitel SN. Warfarin from bedside to bench. N Engl J Med 1984; 311:645.

PULMONARY EMBOLISM

ADAM N. HUREWITZ, M.D.
EDWARD H. BERGOFSKY, M.D.

Few diseases pose greater risks to otherwise healthy patients than pulmonary emboli. It is one of few rapidly fatal conditions of previously healthy young adults, it is a major cause of perioperative mortality, and it is at present the major cause of peripartum maternal death.

Despite extensive efforts to control this disease, death remains an unacceptably common consequence of pulmonary embolism. Of the more than 500,000 cases of pulmonary embolism estimated to occur in the United States, approximately 10 percent die within 1 hour of the embolic event. In these 50,000 patients, preventive therapy is the only means of reducing the recognized mortality. An additional 20 percent of all patients with pulmonary emboli survive beyond the first hour, but eventually succumb without receiving a correct diagnosis or appropriate therapy. Mortality in this group clearly depends on improved diagnostic techniques. Of the patients who survive the initial event and in whom a diagnosis is made and therapy is instituted, 8 percent still die from causes related to pulmonary emboli. Although this represents an unacceptably high mortality in treated patients, it does compare favorably with the 33 percent fatality rate in patients who survive the first hour but are never correctly recognized as having pulmonary emboli. This 15 percent reduction in mortality is largely attributable to the success of anticoagulation therapy. Attempts to further improve survival by thrombolysis have recently been recommended. Unfortunately, the benefits of thrombolytic therapy have, so far, been minimal.

We focus this review upon diagnostic and therapeutic decisions, with an emphasis on establishing clinically useful algorithms. The initial focus is on prevention, including recognition of patients at risk and selection of appropriate therapy. The second focus is on early and accurate diagnosis, so that effective prophylactic therapy can be instituted to prevent recurrent episodes. The final focus is on thrombolysis for pulmonary emboli causing hemodynamic compromise.

VENOUS THROMBOPHLEBITIS

Pathogenesis of Venous Thrombosis

Most pulmonary emboli originate from thrombophlebitis of the lower extremities. The incidence of emboli originating in the lower limb has been estimated at 80 to 90 percent. In both autopsy studies and noninvasive leg vein scans of populations at risk for pulmonary embolism, calf vein thrombi are more common than proximal vein thrombi. However, the most common source of clinically significant pulmonary embolism is felt to be the proximal leg veins, including the iliofemoral and popliteal systems. Whether calf vein thrombi can ever embolize directly to the lung is uncertain and actively debated. What seems clear is that approximately 20 percent of calf vein thrombi propagate into the more proximal venous tree and from there pose a threat to embolize to the lung. Superficial venous disease of the legs poses essentially no risk of emboli. Thrombi in the pelvis and mural thrombi of the heart account for only a small portion of emboli, perhaps 10 percent.

Clinical Detection of Thrombophlebitis

Clinical examination is an insensitive and nonspecific method of detecting thrombophlebitis of the legs. More than 50 percent of deep venous thrombi are clinically silent. Thus, a normal clinical examination of the leg veins does not exclude underlying thrombophlebitis. When apparently positive clinical signs are present, confirmatory evidence of deep venous thrombosis is absent in up to 75 percent. As shown in Table 1, several other relatively common clinical conditions simulate venous thrombophlebitis. For these reasons, patients suspected of having deep venous disease should undergo a confirmatory study by one of several objective tests now available (see Methods of Detection of Thrombophlebitis, later in this chapter).

TABLE 1 Clinical Simulators of Deep Venous Disease

Superficial phlebitis
Muscle strain of the calf or thigh muscles
Cellulitis
Popliteal (Baker's) cyst
Stasis swelling of the leg

Risk Factors for Thrombophlebitis

Three key pathogenetic factors underlie most instances of thrombophlebitis and pulmonary embolism. These factors, known collectively as Virchow's triad, are *stasis, hypercoagulability*, and *endothelial injury*. For each component of Virchow's triad, a list of associated clinical risk factors can be compiled (Table 2). This list can help estimate a patient's risk of developing thrombophlebitis.

Of these clinical risk factors, previous deep venous thrombosis is one of the most important predictors of recurrent thrombophlebitis. This predictive value magnifies the importance of documenting all diagnoses of either deep venous thrombophlebitis or pulmonary emboli. Surgery is another common and extremely important risk factor, not simply because of stasis produced during the intraoperative and postoperative periods, but also because of a hypercoagulable state induced during many prolonged surgical procedures. Within this surgical risk group, patients with pelvic, knee, or hip procedures are particularly susceptible to venous thrombosis. Calf vein thrombi occur in 50 percent of patients undergoing elective hip or major knee surgery. The incidence of proximal vein thrombi with these procedures is about 10 percent, and the incidence of pulmonary embolism is 1 to 2 percent. With fractures of the hip, the incidence of pulmonary embolism approaches 5 percent in some series.

For some nonsurgical patients, estimates of risk have been given numeric values; for others, the alteration of risk is not as well known. For example, pregnant women have five to six times the risk of developing venous thrombophlebitis as do their nonpregnant counterparts. Patients with cancer of the pancreas or lung may have a two- to six-fold greater risk of thrombophlebitis.

Iliofemoral Thrombosis

Two striking clinical syndromes of iliofemoral thromboses have been described. These are phlegmasia cerulea dolens and phlegmasia alba dolens. Phlegmasia cerulea dolens refers to a severe ileofemoral thrombophlebitis with total occlusion of the deep venous circulation and absence of adequate collaterals. The leg is swollen, tense, and painful and takes on a blue color as a result of massive vascular congestion. Occasionally, a gangrenous extremity results from the nearly complete cessation of blood flow that has been produced by the venous obstruction. Because of the peripheral gangrene, this condition is often misdiagnosed as arterial occlusive disease. If blood flow does not improve after administration of heparin, thrombectomy may be necessary to save the gangrenous limb.

TABLE 2 Risk Factors for Deep Venous Disease*

Stasis	Hypercoagulation state	Local endothelial injury
Prolonged bed rest	Certain malignancies (2–6)	Prior deep venous disease (4)
Prolonged travel	Postoperative hyper-coagulation	Trauma
Orthopaedic leg cast	Birth control pill (4–7)	Extensive pelvic surgery
Congestive heart failure	Deficiency of anti-thrombin III	Burns
Pregnancy (5–6)	Deficiency of protein S or C	Endotoxic sepsis
Obesity (1.5–2)	Acquired platelet-induced thromboses	

* Some estimates of relative increase in risk compared with normal persons are shown in parentheses.

A second striking clinical presentation of patients with iliofemoral thrombosis is phlegmasia alba dolens, the ''milk leg.'' In this instance, the leg is white rather than blue, perhaps because of obstruction to lymphatic as well as venous drainage. This condition is more common in the left leg because of compression of the left common iliac vein by the right common iliac artery.

Some clinicians have suggested that phlegmasia alba dolens and phlegmasia cerulea dolens are less likely to cause pulmonary emboli because the clot is more firmly attached to the vascular endothelium; however, it is not clear that this hypothesis has ever been substantiated. Although these are striking examples of how thrombophlebitis can manifest to the clinician, they are rarely seen and, as noted previously, are a far less common mode of presentation than is the normal-appearing leg.

Methods of Detecting Thrombophlebitis

The proliferation of noninvasive tests for venous thrombosis has remarkably improved the capacity to diagnose both venous thrombosis and pulmonary embolism. These tests are briefly reviewed in the subsequent paragraphs.

One of the most useful tests for detecting deep venous disease above the calf is *impedance plethysmography (IPG)*. An extensive literature is available, citing excellent sensitivity (95 percent) and specificity (96 percent). IPG measures venous obstruction rather than active thrombogenesis. Following obstruction to venous flow by an inflated pneumatic cuff, electrical impedance is monitored as a measure of venous flow. When cuff inflation is rapidly released, changes in electrical impedance correlate with changes of flow and can be compared with predicted normal values. IPG is applicable for disease in the femoral, iliac, and popliteal systems, but is far less accurate for detecting disease of the calf veins. The pneumatic cuff IPG technique is readily mastered, painless, free of risk, and relatively inexpensive. As a consequence of these properties, IPG can be safely repeated on consecutive days if desired. Occasional false positive results are due to nonthrombotic obstruction of leg veins (i.e., muscle contraction) or reduced venous filling caused by associated arterial obstruction.

A second choice of noninvasive test to detect proximal deep venous disease is *Doppler ultrasonography*. Like the IPG, ultrasonography has an excellent record of sensitivity and specificity for venous disease above the calf. One disadvantage is that considerably greater skill is needed to carry out this test properly; however, it shares with IPG the advantages of being free of risk or pain and low in cost. It, too, is a poor test for detecting calf vein disease.

To document calf vein thrombophlebitis, the *^{125}I-fibrinogen leg scan* is recognized as the best noninvasive test presently available. Rather than testing for patency of venous flow, the leg scan reflects active deposition of fibrin within a clot. Thrombus formation below the knee is detected with an accuracy of 90 percent, thrombi in the proximal veins are detected only 60 to 80 percent of the time. The major limitations are reduced sensitivity for thrombi in the thigh or pelvis, a modest radiation exposure, and a delay of 24 to 72 hours between isotope administration and scanning. Its value lies in its excellent detection of lower leg thrombi, which can then be monitored by IPG for extension into the proximal veins.

In our practice, we initially rely on IPG to evaluate patients with pulmonary emboli or signs of lower extremity thrombophlebitis. If IPG is normal, we proceed with radionuclide leg scanning if a suspicion of deep venous disease in the calf exists. Because of our uncertainty about the relationship between thrombi in the calf and direct embolization to the lung, we still recommend prophylactic anticoagulation on the basis of a positive leg scan.

Contrast venograms have long been used to confirm a diagnosis of venous thrombosis. With the advent of noninvasive techniques, the indications for contrast venography have diminished. Its sensitivity is not appreciably superior to that of IPG or leg scans, and the side effects include reactions to contrast agents and induction of a reactive phlebitis that, in itself, can produce thromboembolic complications.

PULMONARY EMBOLISM

Methods of Detecting Pulmonary Embolism

Clinical signs and symptoms of pulmonary embolism have been extensively described in multiple internal medicine and pulmonary medicine texts and are not covered in this review. However, it should be emphasized that many clinical findings, such as pleuritic pain, hypoxemia, and unexplained dyspnea, are valuable when present, but are frequently absent. None of these findings is specific and certainly not sufficient to justify therapy in the absence of confirmatory testing. An algorithmic approach to diagnosis, combining both noninvasive and relatively invasive tests, should yield the highest sensitivity and specificity for decision making. This algorithm is shown in Figure 1.

Noninvasive methods are obviously preferred initially to evaluate patients suspected of having pulmonary embolism or deep venous disease. Since prophylaxis or therapy are identical for both diseases, a positive finding for venous thrombosis is sufficient to begin therapy and avoid further invasive testing for pulmonary embolism. If noninvasive tests are not diagnostic, we proceed to pulmonary angiography for suspected cases of pulmonary embolism.

As Figure 1 indicates, in suspected cases of pulmonary embolism, a radionuclide lung perfusion scan (^{99m}Tc MAA) and IPG should be requested. In general, four levels of specificity have been defined for lung radionuclide scans: (1) *high probability*—multiple segmental or lobar defects, with a normal chest radiograph or with fewer than half of these defects matched by ventilation defects; (2) *indeterminate probability*—multiple perfusion defects accompanied by radiographic or ventilation matching defects; (3) *low probability*—single defects of perfusion scans with or without matching radiographic or ventilation abnormalities; and (4) *normal*—no perfusion defects whatsoever.

From the practical standpoint, clinical decisions are largely based on only three categories of lung radionuclide scan: high probability, normal, and a combined group including indeterminate and low probability. The high probability perfusion scan has been regarded as having a high degree of specificity (greater than 70 percent) with a high positive predictive value. Recent results from the National Heart, Lung and Blood Institute–sponsored Prospective Investigation of Pulmonary Embolism Diagnosis (PIOPED) has confirmed this confidence in the high probability perfusion scan. For instance, a high probability radionuclide study has a 95 percent predictive value (i.e., truly reflects the presence of pulmonary embolism) when the clinical suspicion of embolism is high, and its positive predictive value is only slightly reduced (i.e., to 83 percent) when clinical suspicion is low.

The normal radionuclide lung scan also is useful as a definitive test; it generally excludes the diagnosis of pulmonary embolism. However, the PIOPED study demonstrated that the low probability (normal) scan had a positive predictive value of 4 percent. In other words, 4 percent of such scans might have emboli by contrast angiography.

Indeterminate and low probability radionuclide scans are the most troublesome. The PIOPED study showed that 41 to 73 percent of these had positive predictive value of pulmonary emboli by angiography when clinical suspicion was high, but only 4 to 14 percent had positive predictive value when clinical suspicion was low.

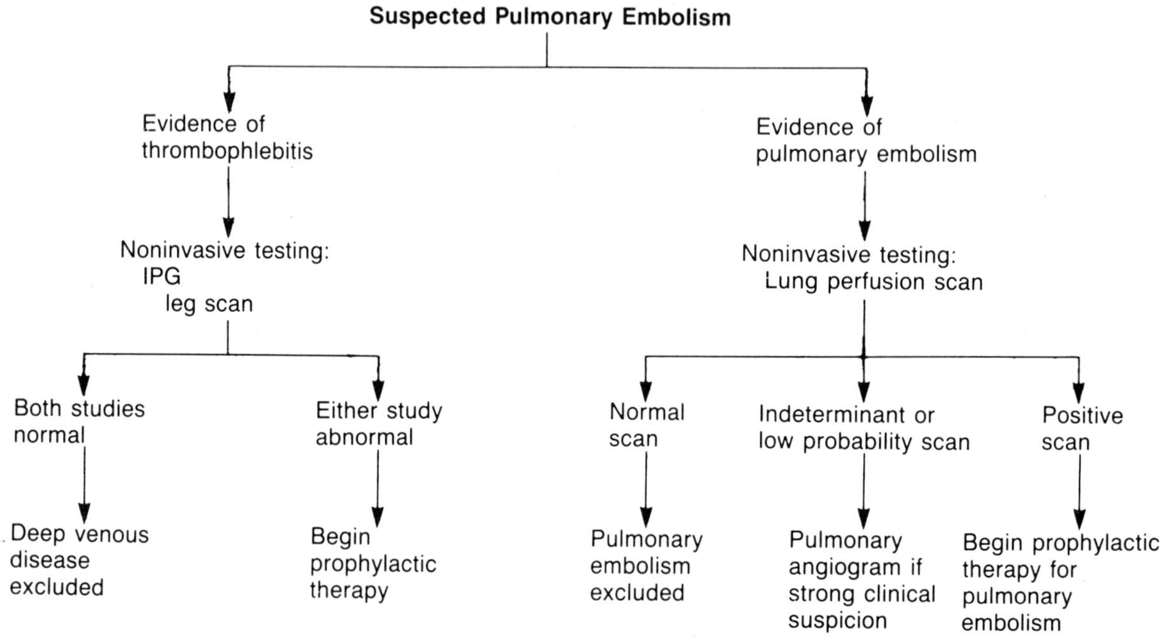

Figure 1 An algorithmic approach to the diagnosis of pulmonary embolism.

With indeterminate scans, a search for venous thrombophlebitis using noninvasive methods (IPG) is often used. If the findings of these are positive, we begin anticoagulation therapy. If the findings are either negative or nondiagnostic, the next step is pulmonary angiography. In some instances, the clinical suspicion of pulmonary embolism is so low that the risks of angiography are not warranted. However, in most instances, the clinical suspicion that warranted the perfusion scan in the first place cannot be readily dismissed. To some extent, decisions to proceed with angiography also depend on the expertise of the angiographer.

Some centers do not routinely obtain ventilation scans despite reports that the specificity of perfusion scans is improved by the addition of ventilation studies. The added specificity is small, and the interpretation may be confused in instances of infarction or hypoxic bronchoconstriction associated with pulmonary emboli. A recent study by Hull et al showed 86 percent of patients with ventilation-perfusion ($\dot{V}/\dot{Q}$) mismatch had pulmonary emboli, but three of 13 patients with $\dot{V}/\dot{Q}$ matches also had emboli.

THERAPY OF VENOUS THROMBOSIS AND PULMONARY EMBOLISM

The therapy of venous thrombosis and pulmonary embolism can be broken down into three broad categories: preventive, prophylactic, and thrombolytic. Important modifications have recently been proposed for each of these categories, and these are discussed in the following sections. Each mode of therapy can be thought of as altering the balance between thrombus formation and ongoing endogenous fibrinolysis. When treatment permits the balance of forces promoting fibrinolysis to exceed those favoring thrombosis, the benefits include an improvement of regional blood flow and a reduction of the risk of recurrent pulmonary embolism or deep venous thrombophlebitis.

Preventive Therapy

Preventive therapy is one that is instituted in the absence of established deep venous thrombosis or pulmonary embolism. It is the only therapy that can conceivably diminish the early 10 percent incidence of death associated with pulmonary emboli. Before initiating preventive therapy, the risk factors are evaluated using the same criteria used for venous thrombosis (see Table 2). Since these risks are magnified in the perioperative period, we have described an approach for predicting thromboembolism in the perioperative patient (Table 3). On the basis of this approach (see Tables 2 and 3) specific preventive modalities for perioperative patients in a particular risk category can be recommended.

Defining Perioperative Risk. Patients with the least risk of thromboembolism are those who are young (less than 40 years of age), have none of the recognized predisposing factors (see Table 2), and will be anesthetized for only a brief period. Venous thromboembolism is rare in these patients, as indicated in Table 3. A moderate risk group is defined as those patients who are older (over 40 years of age) and undergoing more prolonged surgery. These patients are at even greater risk if other factors such as obesity or recent use of oral contraceptives can be documented. The high risk group consists of those patients undergoing prolonged surgery and having either a prior history of thrombophlebitis or pulmonary embolism or those who are undergoing high risk surgery such as hip replacement or repair of the knee.

TABLE 3 Predicted Perioperative Risk for Thromboembolism*

	Distal Vein Thrombosis	*Proximal Vein Thrombosis*	*Fatal Pulmonary Embolism*
Low risk	5%	1%	0.1%
Moderate risk	25%	5%	0.5%
High risk	50%	10%	1.0%

* See text for definitions of relative risk categories.

Using these general guidelines, predictions of perioperative risk can be established (see Table 3). These predictions are largely extracted from data compiled by Hull and colleagues.

Selection of Therapy. Low risk patients can be treated with conservative measures, such as early ambulation, range of motion exercises of the legs, and graduated elastic stockings. Elastic stockings, if applied preoperatively, are low in cost and reasonably effective. These modalities reduce stasis as a risk factor. Since the probability of pulmonary embolism is less than 1 percent in the low risk patient, conservative intervention is appropriate.

Moderate risk patients have a 5 to 10 percent incidence of proximal vein thrombosis and should be offered pharmacologic therapy in addition to the conservative measures described previously. The substitution of intermittent pneumatic compression stockings (IPCS) for the elastic stockings lowers the risks of thromboembolism in these patients. In patients for whom anticoagulation is contraindicated, IPCS are an extremely effective and low risk mode of protection. This applies to high risk neurosurgical patients, patients with hip fractures, and those undergoing total hip replacement. IPCS should be applied preoperatively and continued for about 3 days into the postoperative period.

If the patient's risk falls somewhere between moderate and high risk and if anticoagulation can be tolerated, a low dose heparin regimen should be added. A commonly used dosage is 5,000 units given subcutaneously 2 hours preoperatively and repeated every 8 to 12 hours. An adjusted dose regimen has been recommended to improve effectiveness without increasing bleeding complications. Using this regimen, the dose of heparin is adjusted until the activated partial thromboplastin time (APTT) is between 32 and 36 seconds; this generally requires a dose of 18,000 units per day.

In high risk patients, a combination of IPCS and limited anticoagulation is an excellent preventive regimen. Anticoagulation can be achieved by either a low dose heparin regimen or by using a two-stage warfarin protocol. In the warfarin protocol, therapy is started 2 weeks prior to surgery at a dose of warfarin that prolongs the prothrombin time to 1.5 to 3 *seconds* above the control time. Postoperatively, the dose is raised until the prothrombin time is 1.5 to 2 *times* the control time. This regimen reduces the risk of deep venous disease by about 50 percent.

Prophylactic Therapy

Prophylaxis refers to anticoagulation therapy of patients with established deep venous thromboses or recent pulmonary emboli. It is prophylactic because the goal is prevention of future episodes. Benefit accrues from reduced thrombogenesis, allowing spontaneous fibrinolysis to proceed uninhibited. As noted in the introduction to this chapter, prophylaxis does not benefit the 10 percent of patients who die within the first hour after embolization. This therapy also does not benefit the additional 20 percent of patients who die before a correct diagnosis is made. Clearly, the success of prophylactic therapy depends on a timely and accurate diagnosis. Since the approach to prophylactic therapy has not undergone significant changes in the past few years, this section briefly summarizes the common usage of heparin and warfarin in patients with deep venous thrombophlebitis and pulmonary embolism. Table 4 summarizes a recommended approach to prophylactic therapy. Some of the important studies that justify this approach are summarized in the following paragraphs.

Heparin

Heparin prophylaxis is the standard therapy for acute pulmonary embolism and deep venous thrombophlebitis. Only a few studies have demonstrated a reduction of mortality when heparin is used to treat pulmonary embolism as compared with patients receiving no treatment. Heparin acts by inducing conformational changes of antithrombin III (AT III), allowing this inhibitor to bind thrombin and other clotting factors more effectively. In the absence of AT III, heparin does not work; a deficiency of AT III is a rare but recognized cause of impaired response to heparin.

Heparin is effective only by parenteral administration. Intravenous heparin is more effective than subcutaneous boluses, and a constant intravenous infusion regimen causes less bleeding complications than intermittent infusion regimens. Bleeding complications, however, are high, averaging 5 to 10 percent in most studies.

The dose of heparin is adjusted by monitoring the APTT. The APTT should be prolonged to 1.5 to 2 times the control time. Lower levels fail to prevent recurrent emboli, higher levels may increase the risk of bleeding, though this is not certain. A typical regimen is 5,000 units given as an initial bolus followed by a constant infusion of 1,000 units per hour. The infusion rate is adjusted after checking an APTT in 4 to 6 hours.

Because of the risks of bleeding, heparin is contraindicated in patients susceptible to central nervous system hemorrhage (post–neurosurgical procedures, intracranial aneurysm) and in those with active internal bleeding (i.e., peptic ulcer). Other than bleeding complications, thrombocytopenia is the second most frequent complication of heparin therapy. The reduction of the platelet count probably occurs on an immune basis with aggregation of platelets. The consequences include not only increased bleeding due to reduced circulating platelets, but also regional thrombosis due to the platelet aggregates. Therefore, platelet counts should be monitored during heparin therapy, and heparin should be discontinued if the platelet count falls.

Warfarin

Warfarin is the standard of therapy for chronic anticoagulation of patients with thrombophlebitis or pulmonary embolism. It has proven benefit in reducing the risk of recurrent thromboembolism. It derives its anticoagulation effect from the inhibition of hepatic synthesis of the vitamin K–dependent clotting factors (II, VII, IX, and X). Concurrent liver disease increases the antiprothrombin effect of these agents. Although other diseases and congenital conditions may also alter drug responsiveness, the most common cause of altered warfarin metabolism is drug interaction. Some of these interactions are listed in Table 5.

The appropriate time to start administering warfarin is controversial. Acute therapy begins with heparin since the prophylactic value of warfarin is not as clearly established. Since heparin is usually continued for 10 days to permit stabilization of the thrombus, warfarin is usually started several days after hospitalization. Patients typically remain in the hospital for an additional week or more until the prothrombin time can be regulated with warfarin to a value that is 1.5 to 2 times the control time.

Recent trials have compared this delayed warfarin schedule to one in which warfarin therapy begins 24 hours after heparin is started. The rate of recurrence of venous

TABLE 4 Guidelines for Prophylactic Therapy

Prothrombin time, APTT, and platelet count prior to therapy
Heparin (IV infusion) starting with 5,000 U bolus and 1,000 U/hour. APTT in 4 hours. Goal: Raise APTT to 1.5 to 2 times control.
Monitor APTT and platelet count daily (while patient is on heparin)
Warfarin after 24 to 48 hours of heparin. Start with 10 mg in PM. Check prothrombin time each AM. Aim for prothrombin time 1.25 times control.
Discontinue heparin after 7 days and continue warfarin

TABLE 5 **Medications that Interact with Warfarin**

Increased Prothrombin Time	*Decreased Prothrombin Time*
Acetylsalicylic acid (aspirin)	Barbiturates
Nonsteroidal anti-inflammatory drugs	Rifampin
Metronidazole (Flagyl)	Cholestyramine (Questran)
Trimethoprim-sulfamethoxazole (Bactrim)	Diuretics
Cimetidine (Tagamet)	Oral contraceptives
Quinidine	Griseofulvin

thrombosis or pulmonary embolism remains unchanged, as do bleeding complications. However, the duration of heparin is reduced by 50 percent to a total of 4 to 5 days. As a result, the duration of hospitalization is reduced by 4 days.

Warfarin is given in an initial dose of 5 to 15 mg, depending on body size. Although previously published guidelines recommended raising the prothrombin time to 1.5 to 2 times the control time, recent evidence suggests that a prothrombin time of 1.25 times the control time is equally effective in preventing recurrent thrombophlebitis or pulmonary embolism. Furthermore, bleeding complications are reduced when compared with doses of warfarin, which prolong the prothrombin time to 1.5 to 2 times the control time.

During the initial 72 hours of warfarin therapy, coagulation factors with the shortest half-lives are depleted first. With rapid depletion of factor VII, the prothrombin time is increased prior to the onset of effective anticoagulation (i.e., depletion of the factors with a longer half-life such as II, IX, and X). This is the major reason not to give larger doses of warfarin in an attempt to increase the prothrombin time more rapidly. This approach exacerbates bleeding risks and does not effectively shorten the onset of the anticoagulant state.

Warfarin also rapidly depletes protein C, which like factor VII, has a short half-life. When this occurs, a paradoxic hypercoagulable state may develop and be associated with thrombogenesis and skin necrosis. Heparin administration will prevent these thrombotic complications; this is a second reason to begin heparin before administering warfarin.

Duration of Therapy

The duration of long-term anticoagulation therapy is presently under discussion. Previous guidelines were to continue warfarin for 6 months in all patients with pulmonary embolism and to continue the therapy longer if the risks of recurrence persisted. We recommend a modified duration, depending on a given patient's risk of recurrence. Patients with acute thrombophlebitis caused by acute and nonpersistent factors need warfarin for only 3 months. For example, a healthy person in whom a pulmonary embolism developed following an automobile accident need not take warfarin beyond 3 months if IPG findings return to normal. One might even consider therapy of less than 3 months in this instance. Alternatively, a quadriplegic patient with recurrent thrombophlebitis warrants warfarin prophylaxis indefinitely. In cases in which duration of therapy is uncertain, IPG is useful for predicting risk of recurrence and for monitoring for the later development of thrombophlebitis.

Therapeutic Failures

Recurrent thrombophlebitis or pulmonary embolism develops in a small percentage of patients with proven thromboembolic disease despite institution of prophylactic therapy. These instances of treatment failures can be divided into three categories. The first is due to physician error when adequate anticoagulation is not rapidly established. Inadequate anticoagulation during the initial 24 hours (i.e., APTT of less than 1.5 times control) is associated with a substantially greater risk of recurrent emboli.

The second group of patients who fail to respond to treatment are biochemically resistant to heparin. AT III deficiency is the most common cause of this resistance; patients with protein S or protein C deficiencies respond to warfarin. A patient who is resistant to heparin (i.e., adequate doses and inadequate prolongation of APTT) should be tested for AT III deficiency. Deficiencies of protein S and protein C should be considered in patients who are susceptible to deep venous thromboses while not receiving therapy.

The third group with treatment failure includes those patients with significant bleeding complications during prophylactic therapy. This is the most common group; up to 20 percent of patients receiving heparin or warfarin have been reported to experience either major or minor bleeding. Unless the bleeding is due to excessive doses of medication, most instances warrant discontinuation of medication and consideration of venous interruption if the risk of thromboembolism remains significant.

Venous Interruption

Patients for whom prophylactic therapy fails should be evaluated for a venous interruption procedure. The most common form of venous interruption now in use is the Greenfield filter. This device is inserted percutaneously, usually via a right internal jugular cutdown. The filter is positioned distal to the renal veins and proximal to the iliac veins and prevents most thrombus material from embolizing to the lung. These devices have been constructed so as to permit caval patency to be sustained, thus averting the stimulus to formation of large collateral vessels, which could permit embolization to occur. Although this patency might be improved with concurrent anticoagulation, this is possible in only patients for whom the filter is placed as a supplementary protection, not in those for whom anticoagulants are contraindicated. Since most patients respond to prophylactic anticoagulation, vena caval filters are rarely necessary. The major indications in our hands are failure of prophylaxis (usually because of bleeding) and persistent pulmonary hypertension in a patient with acute pulmonary embolism.

Complications of these filters are relatively few. Complications during insertion are unusual, and only rarely is the attempt at insertion unsuccessful. Subsequent migration of the filter is exceedingly rare. Exacerbation of venous stasis has been reported, but it usually responds to elastic stockings.

Thrombolytic Therapy

Indications for Thrombolysis

The third therapeutic option is thrombolysis. Although some investigators recommend thrombolytic therapy in nearly all instances of thromboembolism or deep venous thrombosis, the only widely adopted clinical indication for thrombolytic therapy is hemodynamic compromise secondary to pulmonary embolism. This condition comprises approximately 10 percent of angiographically proven pulmonary emboli. These patients have both systemic hypotension and pulmonary hypertension and are estimated to have a 33 percent mortality rate.

Although a more rapid clot lysis with thrombolytic medication has been documented, improved survival when compared with heparin therapy has not been shown. Some indications of improved long-term function of the pulmonary capillary bed and of venous valve function have been recognized, but it is not clear whether these benefits are sufficient to justify the increased risks associated with thrombolytic therapy. We presently use thrombolytic therapy in patients with hemodynamic compromise, but not in other patients with pulmonary emboli or thrombophlebitis.

Mode of Administration. Three thrombolytic agents are presently available: streptokinase (SK), urokinase (UK), and tissue plasminogen activator (tPA). SK is the most widely used because of availability and reduced cost. The complex of SK and plasminogen converts residual free plasminogen into plasmin. Plasmin binds to fibrin and promotes a more rapid dissolution of the fibrin clot.

An initial dose of 250,000 units of SK diluted in saline or dextrose solution is given over 30 minutes, and a maintenance dose of 100,000 units is given hourly for 24 hours. Although various regimens of monitoring therapeutic efficacy have been proposed, the production of a lytic state is readily documented by a thrombin time of 2 to 5 times the control time. Low thrombin times indicate either resistance to SK or inadequate levels of free plasminogen. If the thrombin time exceeds 5 times the control, discontinuation of therapy until the level reaches the desired range is recommended, followed by a reduction of the constant infusion to 50,000 units per hour. If thrombin times are difficult to obtain, a prolongation of the APTT to 2 to 5 times the control is a reasonable alternative.

UK can be substituted for SK when resistance or allergic reaction to the latter is suspected. This occurs in 5 percent of patients taking SK. Attempts to develop a clot-specific thrombolytic agent have not been as successful as originally suspected. tPA was synthesized with expectations that only the plasminogen within clots would be activated, thereby minimizing undesired effects on the circulating coagulation cascade. Unfortunately, recent studies have indicated that tPA does not significantly reduce the bleeding complications when compared with SK or UK.

Absolute contraindications to thrombolytic therapy include active internal bleeding, central nervous system diseases or procedures performed within the past 2 months, and major surgery, trauma, or obstetric delivery within the past 10 days. Relative contraindications include coagulopathies or gastrointestinal lesions that are prone to bleeding, such as inflammatory bowel diseases. Bleeding with thrombolytic agents can be reduced to less than 5 percent with careful patient selection. Patients who have received arteriotomies and central vein lines for monitoring must be carefully evaluated for risks of bleeding; if insertion of the lines was associated with more than minimal trauma to the vessel, the risks of bleeding may contraindicate thrombolytic therapy.

After 24 hours, SK is discontinued and heparin is started without a loading dose when the thrombin time has fallen below 2 times the baseline. During the infusion, these patients must be carefully monitored for evidence of bleeding, and all invasive procedures should be avoided.

SUGGESTED READING

Barritt DW, Jordan SC. Anticoagulant drugs in the treatment of pulmonary embolism Lancet 1960; 1:1309–1312.

Dalen JE, Alpert JS. Natural history of pulmonary embolism. Prog Cardiovasc Dis 1975; 17:259–269.

Gallus A, Jackaman J, Tillett J, Mills W, et al. Safety and efficacy of warfarin started early after submassive venous thrombosis or pulmonary embolism. Lancet 1986; 2:1293–1296.

Havig O. Deep vein thrombosis and pulmonary embolism. Acta Chir Scand [Suppl] 1977; 478:1–93.

Hull R, Delmore T, Genton E, et al. Warfarin sodium versus low-dose heparin in the long-term treatment of venous thrombosis. N Engl J Med 1979; 301:855–858.

Hull RD, Hirsh J, Carter CJ, et al. Pulmonary angiography, ventilation lung scanning, and venography for clinically suspected pulmonary embolism with abnormal perfusion lung scan. Ann Intern Med 1983; 98:891–899.

Hull R, Hirsh J, Jay R, et al. Different intensities of oral anticoagulant therapy in the treatment of proximal-vein thrombosis. N Engl J Med 1982; 307:1676–1681.

Hull RD, Raskob GE, LeClerc JR, et al. Diagnosis of clinically suspected venous thrombosis. Clin Chest North Am 1984; 5:439–456.

Kanter B, Moser KM. The Greenfield vena cava filter. Chest 1988; 93:170–175.

Leyvraz PF, Richard J, Bachmann F, et al. Adjusted versus fixed dose subcutaneous heparin in the prevention of deep-vein thrombosis after total hip replacement. N Engl J Med 1983; 309:954–958.

Moser KM, LeMoine JR. Is embolic risk conditioned by location of deep venous thrombosis? Ann Intern Med 1981; 94:439–444.

NHLBI–DLD National Prospective Study. Prospective investigation of pulmonary embolism diagnosis. Presented at annual meeting, American Thoracic Society, May 1988.

Wheeler HB, Anderson FA, Cardullo PA, et al. Suspected deep vein thrombosis: management by impedance plethysmography. Arch Surg 1982; 117:1206–1209.

CHRONIC VENOUS INSUFFICIENCY

ENRIQUE CRIADO, M.D.
GEORGE JOHNSON Jr., M.D.

Chronic venous insufficiency (CVI) of the lower extremities is characterized by sustained venous hypertension that results from inadequate drainage of the venous system of the legs. This physiologic disturbance produces venous dilation, edema, and soft tissue infiltration that eventually leads to tissue damage.

The clinical relevance of CVI spans from a simple disorder in which the patient complains of mild subjective symptoms or undesirable leg appearance to a disease state in which the symptoms are severe, the signs are prominent, and the morbidity and disability are stunning. Leg swelling can vary from minimal to massive. Subjective symptoms range from heaviness, aching, itching or discomfort, to severe pain or even venous claudication. The degree of venous dilation upgrades from small telangiectasias to large tortuous subcutaneous varices. Cutaneous changes progress from hyperpigmentation to brawny edema and eventually ulceration.

Chronic venous insufficiency to different degrees afflicts a significant proportion of the adult population. It constitutes a major health problem in terms of disability, producing an immense loss of work days.

The etiology of venous insufficiency remains largely unknown. Valvular incompetence of the deep venous sytem, in many instances, is secondary to deep venous thrombosis (DVT). Thrombus organization, lysis, and recanalization following DVT destroys the delicate valve leaflets to a variable extent, rendering the valves incompetent. However, there is a substantial number of patients with valvular incompetence of the deep veins without a history of DVT. The term *postphlebitic syndrome* applied to all patients with CVI is inappropriate because it implies that the pathogenesis of this disorder is always secondary to the consequences of DVT.

Primary varicose veins resulting from structural weakness in their wall or valvular incompetence of the perforating veins are the most common form of venous disease, and they rarely lead to CVI. Valvular incompetence most frequently progresses from the sapheno-femoral junction distally. They differentiate from secondary varicose veins by the absence of deep vein valvular incompetence or obstruction.

As a result of the fact that a large proportion of patients with primary varicose veins have a family history of this problem, they are considered an inherited condition. Yet, there are many patients with primary varicose veins without a family history of the condition. Therefore, heredity cannot be universally claimed. There are other factors that seem to contribute to the development of varicose veins. Among them are occupational habits that require protracted standing, hormonal influence during pregnancy or the progestational phase of the menstrual cycle, and advanced age.

Congenital venous valvular aplasia of the lower extremities and congenital aplasia of the deep veins of the legs are two well-recognized diseases that normally manifest at an early age and rarely are the cause of CVI in adults.

Advances in noninvasive vascular diagnosis and phlebography have greatly contributed to the understanding of venous disease. Surgical procedures developed during the last two decades have achieved encouraging results and have now found definite indications in the treatment of CVI of the lower extremities. These two facts allow better selection of those patients that may benefit from surgery for venous disease. Nevertheless, the management of CVI remains primarily nonoperative.

PATIENT EVALUATION

In most patients the history, physical examination, and noninvasive functional studies are sufficient to establish the diagnosis and to confirm that the signs and symptoms present are secondary to venous insufficiency rather than to other leg problems.

In selecting the appropriate treatment for patients with venous insufficiency of the lower extremities, it is important to understand the underlying physiologic defect. Current concepts suggest that valvular incompetence, the degree of venous obstruction, and the anatomic distribution of the disease are the most important determining component in the pathophysiology of CVI. Impairment of the pumping action of the lower extremity muscles may also be an important contributing element. Chronically elevated venous pressure produces an imbalance in the capillary pressure equilibrium, thereby increasing the accumulation of interstitial fluid until the interstitial pressure rises to a new equilibrium. The flow of fluid into the interstitium carries proteins and red cells into the subcutaneous tissues. Red cells are lysed and proteins become organized, producing subcutaneous hyperpigmentation and fibrosis, a condition known as lipodermatosclerosis.

Patients with venous ulcerations show defective fibrinolysis and elevated plasma fibrinogen levels. The accumulation of fibrin around the capillaries causes impairment of oxygen diffusion into the tissues, producing local hypoxia and inadequate nutrient supply. In this substrate, minor trauma is able to produce chronic skin ulceration. The incidence of stasis changes and ulceration correlates well with the ambulatory venous pressure. High venous pressures are associated with frequent ulceration, while limbs with low pressure seldom ulcerate. It becomes obvious that reduction of ambulatory venous pressure should be the treatment goal in patients with CVI.

From the anatomical stand point CVI can aggrieve the superficial, the deep, or the communicating (perforators) venous systems, individually or in combination.

Preoperative evaluation should assess whether there is an obstructive component at any level of the venous sytem, and more importantly the presence of valve incompetence in the superficial, deep, or communicating system.

Objective evaluation of valve incompetence and venous obstruction is best done by functional noninvasive vascular testing. There is a multitude of noninvasive tests currently available for the diagnosis of venous insufficiency. Ambulatory venous pressure measurement is considered the gold standard for the determination of venous hypertension. It appraises both venous reflux and calf muscle pump action and when used in conjunction with tourniquets may be able to identify the level of valvular incompetence. Although reliable and minimally invasive, measurement of ambulatory venous pressure is cumbersome and impractical in patients with severe leg swelling.

The most practical and useful functional tests are directional Doppler ultrasonic blood flow detection, photoplethysmography, and venous duplex scanning.

Directional Doppler ultrasonography is a simple and versatile method to detect obstruction or valvular incompetence in the deep and superficial venous systems of the lower extremities. However, this technique demands great experience on the part of the examiner, it is subjective, it may not identify partial venous obstruction, and it is unable to differentiate between profunda and superficial femoral vein incompetence at a proximal level. Duplex scanning combines Doppler directional flow velocity detection and real time B-mode ultrasonographic imaging. It has the advantage that it can identify nonocclusive venous thrombi and allows individual assessment of the veins at different levels.

Photoplethysmography detects changes in skin blood content during active or passive calf muscle exercise. Evaluation of the venous recovery time (VRT) following calf exercise with photoplethysmography appraises the capability of the calf muscle pump to empty the veins and the valvular competence of the venous system. When used with tourniquets (50 to 60 mm Hg) compressing at different levels, it can differentiate superficial from deep valvular incompetence (Fig. 1). Normal venous recovery time is over 22 seconds. When the venous recovery time is accelerated it means that there is valvular incompetence at some level of the venous sytem. If the VRT normalizes with a tourniquet placed above the knee, great saphenous vein incompetence is diagnosed. If it corrects with a tourniquet at calf level, lesser saphenous or above the knee perforator incompetence is likely. And if the VRT normalizes only after tourniquet placement at the ankle level it suggests that there is perforator valvular incompetence in the calf. Lack of prolongation of an accelerated refill time with placement of tourniquets at any level implies the presence of deep venous valvular incompetence. If the plethysmograph shows that there is actual increase, rather than decrease, in blood volume after calf muscle exercise, it reveals poor venous emptying, strongly suggesting deep venous outflow obstruction.

Noninvasive functional studies have greatly reduced the need for venography. Yet, phlebographic studies still are the reference anatomical examination for the assessment of CVI. They should be reserved for those patients in which functional noninvasive testing is unable to diagnose the presence of valvular incompetence or venous obstruction adequately or for those patients in whom surgical valvular reconstruction or venous bypass is considered.

Ascending phlebography evaluates the patency and anatomy of the deep and superficial venous systems from ankle to pelvis; it identifies the presence of incompetent perforators, venous anomalies, and collateral venous pathways.

Descending phlebography is the best method to evaluate valvular anatomy and competence of the

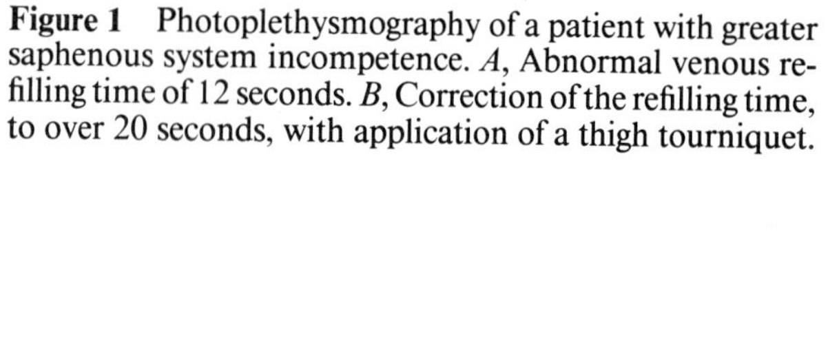

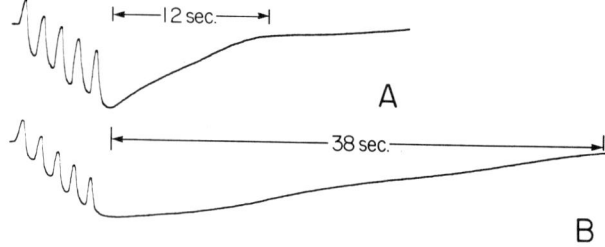

Figure 1 Photoplethysmography of a patient with greater saphenous system incompetence. *A*, Abnormal venous refilling time of 12 seconds. *B*, Correction of the refilling time, to over 20 seconds, with application of a thigh tourniquet.

saphenofemoral system. It is mandatory for the planning of valvular reconstruction. Descending venography also offers a quantitative assessment by grading valvular incompetence from minimal to severe depending on the level that reflux reaches distally. It is important to know that 10 to 15 percent of normal individuals present a small degree of valvular reflux.

THERAPEUTIC ALTERNATIVES

The nonoperative management of CVI is very important and is often carried out in conjunction with surgical treatment.

PREFERRED APPROACH

Nonoperative Management of Chronic Venous Insufficiency

Nonoperative therapy of CVI includes skin care, leg elevation, compression therapy, and sclerotherapy. Currently in the United States there is no approved pharmacologic agent effective for the treatment of venous insufficiency. Most patients with mild to moderate CVI will improve their symptoms by using these measures.

Skin Care

To prevent cutaneous ulceration, patients with CVI should be instructed to pay special attention to the care of the skin of their lower extremities. They should wash them frequently with neutral soap and dry them well without rubbing. Lanolin lotions are recommended to keep the skin hydrated and well lubricated. Special caution to avoid skin trauma should be advised, and if skin damage does occur, medical attention should be sought immediately.

Postural Measures

Avoiding prolonged immobility in the standing position and frequent leg elevation are important behavior routines for patients with venous insufficiency. During elevation the limbs should be above the right atrium, and the legs should maintain a slight 15 degree flexion at the knee level to avoid popliteal vein compression that may occur with full knee extension. Surprisingly, patients comply very poorly with these simple measures as a result of discomfort, inconvenience, and interference with sleeping habits or other daily activities. Some commercial lower extremity elevators are advisable because they seem to improve patient comfort and increase compliance with elevation.

Compression Therapy

Lower extremity external compression for venous disease has been used for many centuries. Compressive therapy in patients with venous insufficiency restores the pressure balance between the interstitium and the capillaries and decreases venous pressure, thus reversing the physiologic disturbance that accompanies valvular incompetence.

There are several different methods of external compression available. Among them are elastic bandages, adhesive elastic bandages, rigid zinc oxide impregnated rolls (Unna boot), custom-made velcro wraps, and elastic stockings. Our preferred method of compressive therapy is the use of calf length graded high-compression hosiery (40 mm Hg gradient). Elastic stockings constitute a constant pressure, variable volume dressing. The greater the compression gradient between ankle and calf exerted by the stocking, the greater the decrease in ambulatory venous pressure of the limb.

Elastic stockings that exert a high gradient compression (30 to 40 mm Hg at ankle level) between ankle and calf have been shown to increase deep venous flow and to decrease the caliber of superficial veins. They also reduce ambulatory venous pressure and normalize accelerated photoplethysmographic venous recovery time in patients with deep valvular incompetence. On the other hand, low gradient compression stockings (20 mm Hg) have been shown not to improve venous recovery time in patients with CVI. There is no evidence that thigh-length or pantyhose stockings provide any benefits superior to those from calf-length hosiery.

The circumferential pressure applied by a stocking on a limb depends both on the limb contour at different levels and the tension produced by the stocking at each level. When there is calf-ankle disproportion, that is, narrow ankles and large calves, elastic stockings can actually produce a tourniquet effect at the calf level that traps blood distally, thus producing further physiologic impairment. Therefore, custom-fit garments should be used in these patients. This situation illustrates the need for individual attention when prescribing elastic stockings.

Venous outflow obstruction may be a contraindication for the use of elastic compressive therapy. In some patients it may increase the ambulatory venous pressure, thereby worsening symptoms. Patients with significant lower extremity arterial insufficiency may experience exacerbation of symptoms with compression therapy. In our experience 30 to 40 mm Hg gradient compression is well tolerated by patients with moderate ischemia.

Wrapping with elastic bandages is an easy and inexpensive alternative form of compressive therapy most suitable for those patients who require frequent ulcer wound care, or for those who do not tolerate stockings. There are two techniques of elastic leg wrapping, spiral and figure-of-eight. Although figure-of-eight wrapping requires higher skill levels from the caregiver, it has been shown that is more effective in reducing leg swelling, and it seems to stay longer in place when compared with spiral wrapping.

The Unna boot bandage provides a constant volume, variable pressure dressing. The advantage of the Unna boot is that during dependency it produces maximal pressure support, which is precisely when it is most needed. The Unna boot is an excellent option for patients with ulcerations because it allows drainage through the wrap, while maintaining a moist environment at the ulcer-dressing interface that favors epithelial growth. The Unna boot can be changed on a weekly basis, maintaining good compression during this interval.

Sclerotherapy

Sclerotherapy should be considered as a complement to surgery in the treatment of varicose veins. In some situations sclerotherapy and surgery can be used interchangeably with comparable results. However, to avoid therapeutic failures it is important to recognize those patients who will not benefit from sclerotherapy and who should be treated by other methods.

Failure of sclerotherapy is due to vein recanalization secondary to persistent proximal valvular incompetence. Inadequate technique is also a common source of unsatisfactory results.

In the presence of saphenofemoral valvular incompetence, treatment of varicose veins with sclerotherapy carries an extremely high long-term recurrence rate; therefore, surgery should be the choice in this situation.

Some simple principles apply to the use of injection sclerosis for the treatment of varicose veins. In general, the smaller the vein, the better results with sclerotherapy; the larger the vein, the better results with surgery; thus, injection of large varicose veins is not advisable. Whenever treating veins over 1 mm in diameter, injection sclerotherapy should always be followed by compression therapy. The duration of compression therapy following injection should be proportional to the size of the veins. Small veins should be wrapped for a few days, while large varicosities for several weeks. Because of the difficulty in bandaging, very fat thighs should not be injected.

Sclerotherapy is best suited to and offers best results in the treatment of superficial venular dilatation, teleangectasias, venous spiders, and other small caliber vascular lesions without underlying hemodynamic derangement. These lesions are rarely symptomatic and the indication for sclerosis in most cases is cosmetic concern. Another acceptable indication for sclerotherapy is in patients with varicose veins without incompetence of the long saphenous or perforating veins. Although others advocate the use of sclerotherapy for varicose veins with incompetent perforators, it is our practice to recommend surgery in these patients, if treatment is needed. Sclerotherapy is a reasonable option in patients who are at very high risk for surgery and warrant or demand some kind of treatment. In patients with a large number of varices who undergo surgical excision, sclerotherapy is an excellent choice for the treatment of residual varicosities to avoid excessive number of skin incisions and to reduce operative time.

The technical execution of the injection of the sclerosing agent is very important and demands careful attention. The treatment goal of sclerotherapy is to inject a small volume of the sclerosing agent in the lumen of the vein, to immediately apply adequate compression to allow fibrosis of the collapsed vein, and to avoid formation of thrombi. There are multiple sclerosing agents available in the market; our preference is the use of three percent sodium tetradecyl sulfate.

The veins that are being sclerosed should be marked with the patient in the standing position, and injected with the patient supine. To prevent extravasation, injection is done only when it is certain that the needle tip is located in the vein lumen. Small volumes (0.25 to 0.5 ml) of sclerosing solution should be used at each injection site to avoid extended venous damage. After each injection, a small soft cotton ball or other fluffy material is taped under pressure over the injection site. Once all the injections are completed, a compressive wrap is applied and ambulation allowed immediately. The bandage should be replaced as needed to maintain adequate compression during the prescribed period of time. After a few days of wearing elastic wraps, these can be substituted by graded high compression stockings.

There are several contraindications to sclerotherapy; in general, any patient with a high risk for deep venous thrombosis should not be a candidate. Pregnant women and patients on oral contraceptives fall in such a group. Hypercoagulable states such as protein C, protein S, and antithrombin III deficiencies are absolute contraindications for sclerotherapy.

Complications of sclerotherapy are generally minor and in experienced hands infrequent. Allergic reaction to the sclerosing agent is unusual; it more commonly occurs as a local phenomenon than as a systemic reaction. It is also more likely to occur after several injections. Toxic reactions are related to an excessive volume of sclerosing agent. Strict limitation of the volume in each individual injection and of the maximal number of injection sites should prevent this problem. In general, not more than 20 to 25 veins should be injected in a single session. When a substantial volume of the sclerosing agent extravasates, subcutaneous and skin necrosis occurs, leading to a small but permanent scar. Extreme caution and use of small volumes should prevent this complication. Intra-arterial injection, although very unusual, can produce extensive distal necrosis. Stabilization of the needle and backdrawing blood from the vessel before injecting will avoid this complication. Variceal thrombosis without obliteration is generally a consequence of inadequate compression. If it occurs, a small venupuncture suffices to evacuate the clot. The bandage is then replaced to allow completion of the sclerosing process.

Deep venous thrombosis is a rare complication of sclerotherapy. It is best prevented by limiting the injection volume and by good compression therapy.

Long-term sequelae of sclerotherapy are hyperpigmentation and persistent tenderness at the injection site and recurrence.

Surgical Treatment of Chronic Venous Insufficiency

Most operations done for CVI involve the superficial system. Varicose veins constitute the most common indication. Direct surgery of the deep venous system is less frequently performed. The indications, procedures, and results of surgical intervention in these two systems are distinctively different. For this reason we consider surgery of the superficial and the deep system separately.

Surgery of the Superficial Venous System

Surgery for varicose veins is indicated for relief of symptoms, for treatment of complications such as ulceration or bleeding, or for cosmetic reasons. With appropriate patient selection, attention to detail in preoperative marking, meticulous surgery, and adequate postoperative elastic support, the results will be predictably satisfactory for the patient and surgeon.

The tributaries to the long saphenous vein are most commonly affected with varicose transformation. The main saphenous trunk is often spared from dilation, probably because it has a thick medial layer and a fibrous attachment to the deep fascia. This anatomic distribution of the disease suggests that treatment of varicose veins should be directed toward the venous tributaries rather than to the main saphenous trunk itself. Preservation of the long saphenous vein as a potential vascular graft should also be a concern when considering patients for surgery.

The most suitable candidate for an operation for varicose veins is that patient with a patent deep system and competent valves in the deep and perforator veins. When the long saphenous vein trunk has incompetent valves or is dilated, high ligation and stripping alone offers excellent long-term results. When incompetent perforators are present, the procedure should include their ligation or excision. Subfascial ligation of incompetent perforators and ulcer excision, with or without skin grafting, has been advocated in patients with chronic skin ulcers but has been shown to have a high recurrence rate. Nevertheless, it can result in ulcer healing in some patients.

Patients with deep valvular incompetence or obstruction are not good candidates for superficial vein procedures, because recurrent or worsening venous hypertension will most likely ensue. Prior to surgery, resolution of leg edema and ulcer healing should be attempted with conservative therapy.

Perioperative anticoagulation is only indicated in those patients with a history of DVT or pulmonary embolism. Prophylactic antibiotics are not necessary.

Key to the success of the procedure is the preoperative marking of the dilated veins to be removed. It should be done by the operating surgeon, with the patient standing and with good illumination for optimal visualization.

During surgery, high ligation of the greater saphenous vein and all its early branches, and thorough avulsion of all the varicose tributaries are important technical factors that will prevent recurrent or residual varices. Minimal size skin incisions and subcuticular closure provides optimal cosmetic results. To prevent hematoma formation, the operated leg is wrapped with elastic bandages while the patient is still on the table. The patient is allowed to ambulate on the first postoperative day and is discharged home the same or following day. On the first office visit the elastic wraps are substituted by graded stockings, and compressive therapy is continued for several weeks.

Complications of surgery for varicose veins are infrequent. Hematoma formation is probably the most common. Saphenous nerve injury may occur during stripping; it can be avoided by stripping from the ankle incision rather than from the groin. Deep venous thrombosis is a rare event following surgery for varicose veins.

Surgery of the Deep Venous System

During the last decade the results of surgical procedures for the treatment of deep venous insufficiency have been encouraging. However, most of these procedures are still fraught with a significant incidence of early failure, and their long-term results remain uncertain. Given the fact that most patients with venous insufficiency improve with conservative therapy, caution should be exercised when indicating surgery for deep venous insufficiency. Only patients with severe disease who have failed to improve with nonoperative therapy should be considered for surgical intervention.

The goal of surgery in CVI is to reduce venous hypertension. The majority of patients with deep venous insufficiency have valvular incompetence as the underlying problem. This group of patients may benefit from procedures directed to reestablish valvular competence (Table 1). Less than 10 percent of the cases of deep venous insufficiency are secondary to venous obstruction; these patients are seldom candidates for venous bypass procedures (Table 2).

Heparin administered during surgery followed by long-term oral anticoagulation therapy and postoperative elastic support is our practice for direct deep venous surgery. The postoperative evaluation and follow-up of direct venous surgery should include

TABLE 1 Surgical Procedures for Deep Valvular Incompetence

Valvuloplasty
Vein transposition
Valve autotransplantation
Homologous valve transplant
Xenograph monocusp valve transplant
External valvular support

clinical assessment, functional noninvasive testing, and phlebography.

Surgery for Valvular Incompetence

The concept that valvular incompetence plays a key role in the pathophysiology of venous insufficiency prompted enthusiasm in the development of valvular reconstructive surgery. However, if a multitude of deep venous valves are incompetent, it seems questionable that the reconstruction of a single one would correct the physiologic valvular deficit. This idea is reinforced by the fact that correction of physiologic abnormalities following valvular reconstruction, in terms of reduced ambulatory venous pressure or normalization of venous refill time, has not been conclusively documented. However, symptomatic improvement following valve reconstruction has been satisfactory.

Valve reconstruction would be indicated in patients with severe symptoms, or ulceration, with very shortened venous refill times, and with severe valvular reflux documented by descending phlebography, in whom conservative therapy has failed.

Valvuloplasty is suitable for those patients with incompetent valves due to cusp elongation; it is not always feasible because valves may be severely damaged or destroyed by previous episodes of thrombosis. When valvuloplasty is not practical, autotransplantation of a valve containing venous segment is a good alternative. External support of the transplanted venous segment may prevent subsequent dilation and incompetence. Preoperatively, the presence and competence of brachial vein valves has to be ascertained by phlebography. It is important to know that there is a substantial percentage of the population with incompetent brachial veins.

In patients in whom the superficial femoral vein is incompetent and the profunda femoral or greater saphenous vein remain competent, transposition of the superficial femoral into the profunda or saphenous vein can achieve good clinical and hemodynamic results.

Correction of valve reflux without correction of perforator incompetence has been associated with a high recurrence rate of ulceration. For this reason, valvular reconstruction procedures are frequently combined with communicating vein ligation; thereby, it is difficult to elucidate which individual procedure is responsible for the results. Femoral or popliteal vein ligation has not been used with much success and is currently in disuse, whereas homologous and heterologous valve transplantation remain as experimental techniques.

The most common complications of direct valvular surgery are thrombosis, wound hematoma, seroma, and infection.

TABLE 2 Surgical Procedures for Deep Venous Obstruction

Femorofemoral crossover saphenous vein bypass
Femorofemoral crossover reinforced PTFE bypass
Saphenopopliteal bypass
Free venous bypass
Prosthetic caval reconstruction
Isolated or adjunctive arteriovenous fistula
Resection of venous webs

PTFE = Polytetrafluoroethylene.

Surgery for Venous Obstruction

The physiologic impairment produced by venous obstruction is sustained venous hypertension and poor venous emptying. In the preoperative evaluation of patients with venous obstruction, ascending venography is able to delineate the anatomy of the obstruction and collateral venous pathways. Impedance plethysmography offers a quantitative evaluation of venous outflow. Bilateral direct venous pressure measurement is the most reliable method to ascertain the hemodynamic significance of an obstruction lesion and may be warranted in some cases.

Indication for surgery is found in those patients with severe swelling and pain, with phlebographic demonstration of proximal vein obstruction.

The results of bypass procedures for venous obstruction are best when an autogenous vein is used. Construction of a distal arteriovenous fistula seems to improve the patency of venous bypass grafting consistently, and this is even more important when prosthetic material is used. Best results with venous bypass have been attained in patients with venous claudication. It also seems that patients who undergo venous bypass for extrinsic obstruction obtain better results than those with intralumenal thrombosis.

Femorofemoral crossover venous bypass using saphenous vein or ring supported polytetrafluoroethylene graft is indicated in patients with femoral or iliac vein obstruction. The saphenopopliteal vein bypass is used in cases of superficial femoral vein occlusion. Free saphenous vein grafts can be used to bypass any obstructed venous segment. Reconstruction of the inferior vena cava, if ever indicated, can be accomplished with externally supported polytetrafluoroethylene graft. Isolated arteriovenous fistulas can be used to increase venous return but are more effective when used in conjunction with bypass procedures because they increase bypass flow and thereby improve bypass patency. Yet, patency of venous by-pass procedures remains to be the limiting factor for their success, and the thrombogenicity of prosthetic grafts further enhances this problem.

Despite all recent advances, the management of CVI continues to be a challenge for the vascular surgeon. To improve the treatment of this frustrating disease, we should encourage the development of new diagnostic and therapeutic techniques and the appropriate evaluation of the ones available.

SUGGESTED READING

Abramowitz HB, Queral LA, Flinn WR, et al. The use of photoplethysmography in the assessment of venous insufficiency: A comparison to venous pressure measurement. Surgery 1979; 86:434.

Bergan JJ, Yao JST, Flinn WR, McCarthy WJ. Surgical treatment of venous obstruction and insufficiency. J Vasc Surg 1986; 3:174.

Johnson Jr, G, ed. The management of venous disorders. In: Rutherford RB, ed. Vascular Surgery, 3rd ed. Philadelphia: WB Saunders, 1989:1480.

Kistner RL. Surgical repair of the incompetent femoral vein valve. Arch Surg 1975; 110:1336.

Linton RR. The communicating veins of the lower leg and the operative technic for their ligation. Ann Surg 1938; 107:582.

Palma EC, Esperon R. Vein transplants and grafts in the surgical treatment of the postphlebitic syndrome. J Cardiovasc Surg 1960; 1:94

Queral LA, Whitehouse Jr, WM, Flinn WR, et al. Surgical correction of chronic venous insufficiency by valvular transposition. Surgery 1980; 87:688.

Raju S, Fredericks R. Valve reconstruction procedures for nonobstructive venous insufficiency: Rationale, techniques, and results in 107 procedures with two- to eight-year follow-up. J Vasc Surg 1988; 7:301.

CHRONIC ANTICOAGULATION

PEDER M. SHEA, M.D., F.A.C.C., F.A.C.P.

Long-term anticoagulation is indicated in a widening range of illnesses. With the advent of thrombolytic therapy in ischemic syndromes and the recognition of the rate of thromboemboli in atrial fibrillation, an increasing number of patients are prescribed "chronic anticoagulation" implying at least 3 months of therapy. Even the intensity of anticoagulation has been modified in recent years. This chapter considers these changes in the indications for therapy and the level of anticoagulation in specific clinical settings.

PREFERRED APPROACH

Drugs Used for Anticoagulation

Several classes of medications are used for chronic anticoagulation. The drugs themselves and their use are discussed below.

Warfarin

The principal oral anticoagulants are antagonists of vitamin K, the most common of which is warfarin. Warfarin prevents vitamin K–dependent carboxylation of Factors II, VII, IX, and X, thus depleting the bulk of procoagulants. The onset of activity depends on the half-life of the remaining, circulating levels of these same factors, of which Factor II is the shortest.

Other vitamin K–dependent and warfarin-sensitive proteins are natural anticoagulants known as protein C and S. As the half-life of protein C is shorter even than Factor II, for the "first day" the effect of warfarin may be paradoxical and shift the balance of hemostasis towards coagulation. Clinically such as hypercoagulable state is manifested as skin and fat necrosis. For this reason a loading dose of warfarin is not advisable.

The hepatic effects of warfarin and vitamin K are in strict competition, thus warfarin can be "reversed" by loading with vitamin K, usually given intravenously. There appears to be little or no evidence of a hypercoagulable state with such vitamin K administration. Likewise patients with low levels of vitamin K, as seen in severe fasting states or with antibiotic suppression of vitamin K absorption, will require lower doses of warfarin.

Warfarin therapy is best monitored with the prothrombin time (PT) usually expressed as a ratio of the patient's PT to that of normal for that laboratory. The PT is obtained daily while initiating warfarin therapy. Once stabilized and therapeutic, the PT is monitored every 2 to 4 weeks. Home PT monitoring, akin to home glucose monitoring, is currently in clinical trials and promises to increase the safety and reduce the cost of warfarin therapy.

The intensity of anticoagulation with warfarin as reflected by the PT has recently been clarified. The PT utilizes a reagent thromboplastin to stimulate in vitro coagulation. Thromboplastin is extracted from tissues, usually lung, brain, or placenta, each having a different "responsiveness." A "more responsive" thromboplastin will result in a greater prolongation of the PT than a "less responsive" thromboplastin on the same sample. The thromboplastins used in North America today are less responsive than those used between 1940 and 1960 and those used in Europe. Using the same recommended target range for the PT established in the 1960s would result today in a significantly increased level of anticoagulation because of today's "less responsive" thromboplastin.

The World Health Organization has provided a standard thromboplastin, and current manufacturers provide a comparison with this standard called the International Sensitivity Index for each batch of thromboplastin. Using the International Sensitivity Index, a standard PT ratio, called the International Normalized Ratio, can be obtained. Reviewing recommended levels of anticoagulation expressed in comparable terms of the International Normalized Ratio has resulted in a less intense level of anticoagulation, fewer bleeding complications, and more accurately reflects the intentions of the original investigators.

Heparin

Heparin is a true anticoagulant in that it inhibits coagulation by its action on antithrombin III, a natural inhibitor of Factors XIIa, XIa, Xa, IXa, thrombin (IIa), and plasmin. At least some of its effect is due to the strong negative charge of heparin and can be reversed by the strong positive charge of protamine. Heparin has an immediate onset of action and it's half-life is less than one hour. Besides bleeding, the most significant side effect is thrombocytopenia. The most common variety occurs in approximately 10 percent of patients, is mild and not progressive, and is not associated with thrombosis. A second, severe, and progressive variety occurs with thrombosis. Fortunately both will resolve if recognized and if the heparin is stopped completely, including that in flush solutions of indwelling catheters.

The activated partial thromboplastin time (aPTT) is used to monitor heparin therapy. A therapeutic range for full anticoagulation with heparin is achieved when the aPTT is between one and a half and two times the control. As an initial estimate of the dose required for full anticoagulation with heparin, 10 units per kilogram per hour is given intravenously. A clinical observation has been that when there is a large "clot burden," a larger dose of heparin will be required to reach a therapeutic aPTT than will be required toward the end of a therapeutic intervention. It is not uncommon for the aPTT to be significantly prolonged with the addition of warfarin to a stable dose of heparin while switching to oral therapy. Monitoring the aPTT in unstable situations treated with intermittent injections may not reduce the risk of bleeding, thus the emphasis on a continuous infusion in the hospitalized patient. In the outpatient setting heparin is administered by subcutaneous injection usually in a dose of 12,000 to 15,000 units every 12 hours. The aPTT is sampled 6 hours after injection and if therapeutic, will remain above the target range during the entire 12 hours.

Platelet-Inhibitory Drugs

Aspirin irreversibly inhibits the enzyme cyclooxygenase thereby inhibiting platelet aggregation, platelet synthesis of vasoactive substances such as thromboxane A_2, and endothelial prostacyclin synthesis. This enzymatic inactivation lasts for the entire platelet lifespan. Aspirin dosages remain unclear as experimental results show a variety of effects at differing doses and clinical results use a wide range of doses. Ibuprofen and other nonsteroidal antinflammatory agents also inhibit cyclooxygenase.

Dipyridamole inhibits phosphodiesterase, which reduces the availability of calcium and decreases platelet aggregation. Its effects are additive to those of aspirin in theory and in some clinical experience. There is evidence that some of these effects are mediated by endothelial prostacyclin.

Anticoagulation Problems During Pregnancy

Because warfarin crosses the placental barrier and is teratogenic, a change in anticoagulant therapy is required with the onset of pregnancy. Warfarin is particularly dangerous in the first trimester as it causes central nervous sytem abnormalities. Later in pregnancy, hemorrhage threatens the fetus as well as the mother. Thus, women of child-bearing age must take precautions to prevent pregnancy while on warfarin. Once pregnancy is planned or confirmed, a switch to heparin is required.

Heparin does not cross the placental barrier nor is it teratogenic. The safest time for changing to heparin is before conception but certainly in the first trimester. Intermittent, subcutaneous injection is continued throughout pregnancy, keeping the aPTT in the therapeutic range. Elective induction is ideal in allowing the heparin to be stopped early in labor to allow full coagulant potential during this vulnerable time. Heparin is restarted after hemostasis is achieved and continued until a therapeutic warfarin dose is achieved. Fortunately heparin does not cross into breast milk and warfarin does so at such a low level as to not effect the child's coagulation potential. An alternate approach is to prescribe heparin in the first trimester and during the last 2 weeks of the pregnancy but allowing oral warfarin during the rest of the pregnancy. If labor should begin before stopping warfarin, fresh frozen plasma should be given to normalize the PT.

INDICATIONS FOR ANTICOAGULATION THERAPY

Venous Thromboembolic Disease

Long-term anticoagulation is essential in the management of venous thromboembolic disease (see also *Acute Thrombophlebitis*) as short-term heparin therapy, even up to 14 days, does not prevent recurrent thrombophlebitis. Warfarin is started, without a loading dose, at day 5 of heparin therapy. The two are continued simultaneously until the PT is in the therapeutic range; the heparin is then stopped. It is not uncommon for the subsequent PT values to be slightly shorter due to the combined effect of warfarin and heparin on some of the clotting factors reflected by the PT. Hospitalized patients are usually kept 1 to 2 days further to establish a stable dose of warfarin. In those patients with massive pulmonary emboli in which thrombolytic therapy (streptokinase, urokinase, or tissue plasminogen activator [tPA]) has been used, the duration of heparin therapy and the timing of warfarin initiation is still not clear.

The intensity of long-term warfarin therapy has recently been adjusted downward (Table 1). If transient or reversible etiologies of the venous disease such as immobilization or estrogen use are present, then 3 months of therapy should be sufficient. When venous thrombosis is documented at the time of initial presentation, a repeat study is indicated just before discontinuation of warfarin. Venous patency shown by Doppler echo with both visible flow and venous compression is a reassuring result although its predictive value is not known. For long-term immobilization, severe heart failure, tumors, antithrombin III or protein C deficiencies, life-threatening pulmonary emboli, or recurrent venous thromboembolism, treatment should be lifelong.

Long-term subcutaneous heparin is an alternate therapeutic approach although it suffers from problems of repeated injections and patient compliance, as well as severe osteopenia. The dose should prolong the aPTT to at least 1.5 to 2 times the control time. If the aPTT is prolonged to 2.9 times the control time, the risk of bleeding is increased threefold. For aPTTs greater than 3 times the control time, the risk of bleeding increases eightfold.

Valvular Heart Disease

Rheumatic Mitral Valve Disease

Both rheumatic mitral stenosis and mitral regurgitation can be complicated by arterial emboli at a rate of 1.5 to 4.7 percent per patient year. Atrial fibrillation dramatically increases the risk of emboli sevenfold. After the first embolus, a recurrent event is likely (30 to 60 percent) with the majority occurring in the first 6 months. Although never subjected to a randomized trial, the value of anticoagulation has been shown by a recurrent emboli rate of 9.4 percent per patient year without anticoagulation which is reduced to 3.4 percent per patient year with warfarin therapy.

Warfarin therapy (PT ratio = 1.3 to 1.5) is indicated prophylactically for patients with mitral valve disease in both paroxysmal and chronic atrial fibrillation as well as those in sinus rhythm with a left atrium of 5.5 cm or larger. More intense therapy (PT ratio = 1.5 to 2.0) is required if documented emboli have occurred. Dipyridamole (225 mg to 400 mg daily) may reduce further emboli if they should occur in spite of the more intense regimen.

Aortic Valve Disease

Thromboemboli from isolated aortic valve disease is uncommon although calcific emboli may occur in as many as 19 percent of patients. Likewise, in the absence of mitral valve disease, atrial fibrillation is uncommon in aortic valve disease. Thus, prophylactic anticoagulant therapy is not recommended.

Mitral Valve Prolapse

In recent years clinicians have recognized transient ischemic attacks (TIA) in patients with mitral

TABLE 1 Intensity of Anticoagulation and Risk of Hemorrhage in Major Disease Categories

	Level of Warfarin			
Indication	*PT Ratio*	*INR*	*Bleeds (%)*	*Major Bleed/100 Patient-Years*
Thromboembolism	1.3–1.5	2–3	4–22	–
Bioprosthetic valves	1.3–1.5	2–3	5–7	–
Ischemic heart	1.3–1.5	2–3	17–36	0–4.8
Cerebrovascular	1.3–1.5	2–3	11–28	2–22
Atrial fibrillation	1.3–1.5	2–3	15	–
Mechanical valve	1.5–2.0	3–4.5	8–13	0.7–0.8
Recurrent emboli	1.5–2.0	3–4.5	–	–

PT = Prothrombin time, INR = International Normalized Ratio.

Modified from Hirsh J, et al. Optimal therapeutic range for oral anticoagulants. Chest 1989; 95:5S; and Levine MN, et al. Hemorrhagic complications of long-term anticoagulant therapy. Chest 1989; 95:26S.

valve prolapse and no other identifiable etiology. One estimate of the risk of stroke in young adults with prolapse is 1 per 6,000 adults per year. In the absence of atrial fibrillation or documented stroke, prophylactic anticoagulant therapy is not indicated at such a low incidence. Patients with documented TIAs but with no other diagnosis than prolapse are given aspirin (325 mg to 1 g daily). Patients with recurrent emboli events despite aspirin therapy require warfarin (PT ratio = 1.3 to 1.5) for life. Patients with mitral valve prolapse and atrial fibrillation have not been studied but experience with other mitral valve disease would suggest that chronic warfarin therapy is likely to prevent thromboemboli.

Mitral Annular Calcification

Mitral annular calcification is an increasingly recognized source of embolic events due to both calcific spicules and thromboemboli. There are no studies on the use of anticoagulant therapy in uncomplicated mitral annular calcification; however, in the setting of mitral annular calcification associated with mitral stenosis or regurgitation, with or without atrial fibrillation, thromboembolic events are likely and anticoagulation is rational. There is no information on the usefulness of antiplatelet drugs in this disease.

Cardiomyopathy

Atrial fibrillation complicates both the hypertrophic and dilated forms of cardiomyopathy when there is left atrial enlargement and mitral regurgitation. Prompt cardioversion is usually necessary to improve cardiac symptoms. This is best performed after full anticoagulation with heparin for as long as the patient's clinical status will allow. Lifelong warfarin therapy (PT ratio = 1.3 to 1.5) is initiated before discontinuing heparin, whether or not the cardioversion is successful. In patients with the end-stage dilated cardiomyopathy, venous thromboembolism is very frequently a cause of clinical deterioration and is preventable with chronic warfarin therapy.

Mechanical Prosthetic Valves

With warfarin anticoagulation, the rate of thromboembolic events in mechanical valve prostheses such as the Starr-Edwards, Lillehei-Kaster, and Bjork-Shiley valves is reduced from approximately 23 episodes per 100 patients per year to 2.5 episodes per 100 patients per year with a wide range of results in multiple studies. With the addition of aspirin (1 g per day) or dipyridamole (400 mg per day) a further reduction of embolic events to 1.8 percent per year can be achieved. Unfortunately, aspirin also increases the risk of bleeding. The intensity of warfarin therapy is increased with these prostheses (see Table 1). For patients with bleeding on the full dose of warfarin therapy, lower doses (PT ratio = 1.3 to 1.5) often with dipyridamole (400 mg per day) have been used with success.

The St. Jude valve, especially in the aortic position, has been studied with antiplatelet therapy alone. Yet the short-term incidence of emboli may be as high as 12.5 percent in 4 years. Until this is further clarified, full anticoagulant therapy is still prescribed for St. Jude valves even in the aortic position.

Bioprosthetic Valves

After implantation, the risk of thromboembolism ranges from 10 percent for patients in sinus rhythm to 16 percent for those in atrial fibrillation followed over 36 months. Although patients with a prosthetic mitral valve are more likely to embolize than those with valves in the aortic position, warfarin for 6 to 12 weeks (PT ratio = 1.3 to 1.5) is prescribed for both. Longer courses of warfarin are under study for prevention of calcific degeneration by blocking the vitamin K–dependent binding of calcium to prosthesis.

Ischemic Cerebrovascular Disease

Cerebral Emboli

In several studies on ischemic cerebral events, approximately 15 percent had a cardiac source of cerebral emboli. Symptoms of a TIA and amaurosis fugax can occur with cardiac emboli as well as the more common hemispheric and hemorrhagic infarction. Prophylactic anticoagulant recommendations with warfarin have been outlined in Table 1; however, once a cerebral embolus has occurred, the timing of anticoagulant therapy is difficult. The risk of extending the area of damage by hemorrhage must be balanced with the risk of recurrent embolic events occurring at a rate of roughly 1 percent per day. At this time no clear parameters other than the presence of hemorrhage and the size of the infarct on computed tomographic scan will predict the risk of hemorrhage. In the presence of large infarctions, anticoagulation is delayed 5 to 7 days to reduce the risk of delayed hemorrhage. If hemorrhage is already present the anticoagulation is delayed at least 10 days in hopes of reducing the risk of extension.

In the setting of infective endocarditis and septic emboli, anticoagulant therapy is not indicated.

For patients presenting with TIAs or minor strokes there is very good evidence that antiplatelet agents, particularly aspirin (1 g per day), will reduce the rate of recurrent, nonfatal stroke by 25 percent. However in a completed stroke, antiplatelet therapy is not conclusively shown to alter recurrence rates. Finally in primary prevention studies in patients free of cerebrovascular disease, strokes were uncommon yet the risk of disabling and fatal strokes was increased fivefold with aspirin therapy. Thus, antiplatelet therapy is limited to TIAs and incompleted strokes. Dipyridamole has not been shown to add safety or benefit to aspirin therapy.

Ischemic Coronary Heart Disease

Angina Pectoris

Recent research has focused attention on the thrombotic process in the progression from stable to unstable angina and to myocardial infarction (see also the chapters *Angina Pectoris: Stable* and *Angina Pectoris: Unstable*).

As a means of preventing the initial development of ischemic syndromes, aspirin (325 mg per day) is shown to reduce the risk of myocardial infarction in previously healthy individuals by 47 percent. There was however a concomitant 15 percent increase in strokes. Thus, enthusiasm is tempered for broad recommendations for aspirin therapy to the general population. It remains useful to recommended aspirin to high-risk individuals particularly smokers and patients with significant hyperlipidemia. In patients with hypertension even this recommendation includes a discussion with the patient of the increased risk of hemorrhagic stroke.

When results of five major, randomized trials of antiplatelet agents after a myocardial infarction are pooled, the risk of cardiovascular death is reduced 16 percent and the risk of subsequent myocardial infarction is reduced by 21 percent. Dipyridamole does not increase the benefits seen with aspirin and is not routinely prescribed. No benefit has been shown with sulfinpyrazone in this population. Likewise long-term anticoagulation with warfarin or heparin is not supported in the current literature.

Myocardial Infarction

Significant reductions, ranging from 39 to 55 percent, in the rate of recurrent myocardial infarction with warfarin therapy have reopened the discussion of long-term, anticoagulation following a myocardial infarction (see the chapter *Early Myocardial Infarction: Thrombolytic Therapy*). Although not yet "standard therapy" for all survivors, in certain subgroups of patients warfarin is recommended. Patients with large anterior myocardial infarctions have a risk of embolic stroke of 2 to 6 percent, usually in the presence of a mural thrombus. Thus, early heparinization followed by warfarin therapy (PT ratio = 1.3 to 1.5) for at least 3 months is justified. Longer term anticoagulation is not necessary because once the thrombus is well incorporated into the chamber wall the risk of embolic episodes is so low as to not justify the risk of significant hemorrhage due to warfarin.

Atrial Fibrillation

The Framingham study has focused attention on the risks of cerebral thromboembolic events in the setting of atrial fibrillation even in the absence of valvular heart disease. The incidence of stroke in patients 60 to 69 years of age without atrial fibrillation is 9 per 1,000 and 43 per 1,000 when atrial fibrillation is present; increasing further with age. Unfortunately 17 percent die and many have severe permanent neurologic deficits with the first embolus. Clearly one must take an aggressive, prophylactic approach to anticoagulation to reduce these risks. The intensity of anticoagulant therapy is kept in the low range (PT ratio = 1.3 to 1.5) particularly in light of the largely elderly patient population. Once undertaken, the risk of anticoagulant-induced intracranial hemorrhage is one half the risk of stroke in untreated patients with atrial fibrillation. There is no evidence that antiplatelet agents are of any benefit in preventing stroke in the setting of atrial fibrillation.

Thyrotoxicosis is associated with atrial fibrillation in as many as 30 percent of patients and one third of these will have a cerebral embolus. This can occur early in the course of this disease as well as weeks after conversion to sinus rhythm, even in the euthyroid state. Consequently early warfarin therapy is recommended and therapy continued at least 4 weeks after achieving both a euthyroid state and sinus rhythm.

"Lone" atrial fibrillation occurs in young patients with no identifiable heart disease. Thromboemboli are thought to be rare in this setting and anticoagulant therapy is not required in the absence of documented emboli.

Cardioversion

Because the risk of an embolic complication with direct current cardioversion for atrial fibrillation is 5 percent, anticoagulant therapy has been recommended to reduce this risk. Although there are no controlled trials, an incidence of emboli as low as 0.8 percent has been reported for cardioversion while anticoagulated and supports this recommendation. On theoretical grounds alone, patients with atrial fibrillation of less than 3 days duration, in the absence of valvular heart disease or documented emboli, have not been anticoagulated. For elective direct current cardioversion of more sustained atrial fibrillation, 2 to 3 weeks of adequate warfarin therapy (PT ratio = 1.3 to 1.5) is recommended prior to cardioversion followed by 4 weeks of therapy after successful cardioversion. This is prophylactic for those patients who will quickly return to atrial fibrillation as well as the rare patients with "late" emboli.

SUGGESTED READING

Kitchens CS, Mehta JL. Pharmacology of platelet-inhibitory drugs, anticoagulants, and thrombolytic agents. Cardiovas Clin 1987; 18:195.

O'Reilly A. Vitamin K antagonists. In: Colman RW, et al, eds. Hemostasis and thrombosis: Basic principles and clinical practice. Philadelphia: JB Lippincott, 1987: 1367–1372.

Wolf PA, Abbott RD, Kannel WB. Atrial fibrillation: A major contributor to stroke in the elderly. The Framingham Study. Arch Intern Med 1987; 147:1561.

HEART DISEASE AND PREGNANCY

JOHN H. MCANULTY, M.D.

A woman may first develop heart disease as a result of pregnancy, but most cardiovascular abnormalities exist before conception. Treatment should preferably begin at that time. Therapy before and during pregnancy is unique because it so directly affects the health of two individuals. When treating all pregnant women with heart disease, it is essential to address the following issues: establish health priorities, provide counseling, and balance the potential benefits and risks of diagnostic procedures.

Maternal safety is the highest priority. The well-being of the fetus should be considered when treating maternal heart disease, but procedures and medications necessary to protect the mother should be used.

The woman and her family should understand the heart disease. In selected cases the risk of pregnancy to the woman is so great that avoidance is recommended, or if pregnancy has occurred, interruption is advisable (Table 1). The parents should understand the potential for fetal loss and the potential for abnormalities in the newborn infant. Parents with congenital heart disease should be advised that their offspring have an increased chance of being born with a cardiac abnormality (Table 2).

Desirable activity levels should be reviewed in each case. In healthy women, the heart is able to meet maternal needs as well as those of the fetus. In the woman with heart disease, however, uterine blood flow may be compromised, even at rest. Although the effects of exercise have not been well studied, pregnant women with heart disease should be advised to keep their exercise level below that which causes symptoms.

The electrocardiogram and echocardiogram are safe for the mother and fetus, but interpretation should be done by an individual who recognizes the changes of a normal pregnancy. Radiographic procedures are best deferred until after pregnancy or to as late in pregnancy as possible, when fetal development is complete. Optimal shielding of the fetus is required. Radionuclide studies should be avoided unless absolutely essential for maternal safety.

USE OF CARDIOVASCULAR MEDICATIONS DURING PREGNANCY

Cardiovascular drugs may be essential for maternal safety. However, in addition to causing side effects in the mother, they may adversely affect the fetus. They may depress uterine blood and may adversely affect labor and delivery. Most cardiovascular drugs cross the placenta. Some are potential teratogens. Many drugs are secreted in breast milk, thereby continuing to expose nursing infants to potential problems. Information about drug use during pregnancy is incomplete, but recommendations for use of selected cardiovascular drugs are presented in Table 3. Doses used should be similar to those in nonpregnant women. If a desired effect is not achieved, blood levels should be evaluated.

TABLE 1 Cardiovascular Abnormalities Placing a Mother and Fetus at Extremely High Risk

Advise avoidance or interruption of pregnancy
Pulmonary hypertension
Dilated cardiomyopathy with congestive failure
Marfan's syndrome with dilated aortic root
Cyanotic congenital heart disease
Symptomatic obstruction lesions
Prepregnancy counseling and close clinical follow-up required
Prosthetic valve
Coarctation of the aorta
Marfan's syndrome
Dilated cardiomyopathy in asymptomatic women
Obstructive lesions

From McAnulty JH, Morton MJ, Ueland K. The heart and pregnancy. Curr Prob Cardiol 1988; 13:595. Reproduced by permission of the publisher and author.

TABLE 2 Congenital Heart Disease in the Offspring of a Parent with Congenital Heart Disease

Congenital Heart Defect in Parent	*Risk of Congenital Heart Disease in Offspring if One Parent is Affected (%)*
Intracardiac shunts	
ASD	3–11
VSD	4–22
PDA	4–11
Obstruction to flow	
Left-sided obstruction*	3–26
Right-sided obstruction	3–22
Complex abnormalities	
Tetralogy of Fallot	4–15
Ebstein's anomaly	Uncertain
Transposition of the great arteries	Uncertain

NOTE. The higher number in each range comes from one large series. The incidence of congenital heart disease in the offspring tends to be closer to the lower numbers for most other reported series.

The risk in obstructive lesions is decreased by corrective surgery prior to pregnancy.

*Includes coarctation, aortic stenosis, discrete subaortic stenosis, supravalvular stenosis. It does not include IHSS; with this the child has a 50 percent chance of having IHSS.

From McAnulty JH, Mecalfe J, Ueland K. Cardiovascular disease. In: Burrow GN, Ferris TF, eds: Medical Complications during Pregnancy. Philadelphia: WB Saunders 1988. Reproduced by permission of the publisher and authors.

TABLE 3 Cardiovascular Drugs Used During Pregnancy

Drug Group	*Use During Pregnancy*	*Adverse Effects*
Diuretics	Use as in nonpregnant women. Should not be used prophylactically or to treat pedal edema unless there is associated pulmonary vascular congestion	May exacerbate preeclampsia by reducing uterine blood flow
Inotropic agents	Pregnancy does not alter the indications for digitalis therapy. An increased dose may be required to achieve acceptable serum levels. Digitalis crosses the placenta and is excreted in breast milk but fetal or infant toxicity is unusual	Labor potentially earlier and shorter in women on digitalis
	Beta-stimulation or dopaminergic agents should be reserved for life-threatening situations	May decrease uterine blood flow
Vasodilator agents	Afterload-reducing agents: adverse fetal effects not reported with hydralazine. There is little experience during pregnancy with captopril, enalapril, clonidine, diazoxide.	Hypotension may jeopardize uterine blood flow
	Preload reducing agents; nitrates indicated as in nonpregnant state. Nitroprusside justified in life-threatening situations. There is little experience with prazosin	Concern about but no documentation of cyanide toxicity with nitroprusside
Antiarrhythmic agents	Indications for use as in nonpregnant state. Greatest experience with quinidine but procainamide and disopyramide not clearly inferior. Lidocaine crosses placenta but no teratogenic effects reported. Little information is available on tocainide, mexiletine, flecainide, encainide, propafanone, or amiodarone	Potential fetal dysrhythmias Phenytoin can cause fetal abnormalities and should be avoided
Beta-blocking agents	May be used to treat hypertension, angina, and supraventricular tachyarrhythmias when there are no reasonable alternatives. Close fetal and neonate monitoring required	May depress intrauterine growth Newborn bradycardia, hypotension, hypoglycemia, and respiratory depression
	Selective beta-1 blockers may result in fewer adverse fetal effects	
Calcium channel blockers	Verapamil use as in a nonpregnant state. There is little information on nifedipine, diltiazem hydrochloride, or nicardipine	
Anticoagulants	Warfarin is *contraindicated* at time of conception and during pregnancy because of teratogenic effects and placental and fetal bleeding	10–20% teratogenic effect in first trimester
	When anticoagulation is required, heparin via subcutaneous administration at home is preferred. It does not cross the placenta	Maternal, placenta bleeding
	Acetylsalicylic acid may be used but there is some increased risk of bleeding	Maternal plus fetal bleeding. Potential premature closure of ductus arteriosus by prostaglandin inhibition
	There is no reported experience with dipyridamole or sulfinpyrazone	

Modified from McAnulty JH, Metcalfe, J, Ueland K. Pregnancy in the cardiac patient. In Parmley WW, Chatterjee K (eds). Cardiology. Philadelphia: JB Lippincott, 1987. Reproduced with permission from the publisher and author.

MANAGEMENT OF CARDIOVASCULAR SYNDROMES DURING PREGNANCY

Congestive Heart Failure

Pulmonary edema is as much an emergency during pregnancy as at other times. Therapy with oxygen, diuretics, morphine sulphate, or preload and afterload reducing agents should be initiated. Arrhythmias should be controlled with drugs if necessary.

Chronic congestive heart failure should also be treated in a standard fashion by limiting sodium intake, restricting activity, and, if necessary, medication. If chronic congestive heart failure cannot be controlled and the condition is due to a potentially correctable anatomic lesion, surgery (or potentially a balloon valvuloplasty if a valve is involved) should be performed.

Low Cardiac Output Syndromes

Traditionally volume excess is a cautionary symptom but, in pregnancy, it is sudden loss or depletion of intravascular volume that is more dangerous. This is true in all pregnant women with heart disease, but it is of particular concern in those with pulmonary artery hypertension, right and left ventricular outflow tract obstructive lesions, or mitral stenosis. Support stockings should be used when the woman stands, and leg elevation should be encouraged when she is sitting. Dehydration should be avoided. Diuretics and vasodilator agents should be used cautiously. Bleeding should be avoided, with rapid repletion if it occurs. In mid to late pregnancy, the enlarged uterus compresses the inferior vena cava. In some women, especially when they are in the supine position, this compression is not followed by a compensatory increase in heart rate and vascular tone. Syncope may therefore occur. Resting on the side, particularly the left side, can prevent this syndrome.

If hypotension occurs, err on the side of the volume repletion. At the time of labor and delivery, administer 1,000 to 1,500 ml of saline just prior to the administration of anesthesia. The anesthesia should be selected with the aim of minimizing venous pooling. In women with a high risk cardiovascular condition, pulmonary capillary wedge and arterial pressure monitoring lines should be inserted at the beginning of labor and pressures should be followed during labor, and for 24 to 48 hours after delivery.

Systemic Arterial Hypertension

Hypertension during pregnancy is defined as a systolic blood pressure exceeding 130 mm Hg or a diastolic pressure greater than 80 mm Hg. The condition may precede pregnancy. When present, women have a five-fold greater risk of developing toxemia (preeclampsia or eclampsia) during pregnancy than do normotensive women. Treatment should include limitation of sodium intake in the diet to less than 2 g daily. If the blood pressure does not normalize, atenolol (50 to 100 mg), hydrochlorothiazide (50 to 100 mg), or both should be given daily. Hydralazine 25 to 50 mg four times daily should be added if control is not achieved. The safety of angiotensin converting enzymes has not been established.

Preeclampsia (hypertension associated with proteinuria and with mild central nervous system instability) makes blood pressure control even more essential. Limitation of activity is required, and diuretics should be stopped as they may worsen the syndrome. If hypertension is associated with visual disturbances, pulmonary edema, convulsions, or vascular accidents (i.e., the syndrome of eclampsia), immediate hospitalization is required. Magnesium sulfate (1 g intravenously each hour) may effectively treat both the hypertension and the symptoms. If they persist, nitroprusside should be started and titrated to the level of blood pressure control. Intravenous diazepam (5 to 20 mg) should be given for convulsions. When blood pressure control has been achieved and the patient is stable, delivery, which is the ultimate treatment, should be performed as soon as the fetus is considered mature.

Arrhythmias

Pregnancy should not significantly alter the approach to arrhythmia treatment. The urgency of therapy for symptomatic arrhythmias should increase slightly since they are likely to be causing hemodynamic embarrassment to the fetus. If an arrhythmia is recognized, it is essential to determine whether treatment is worth any hoped-for benefits. No treatment should be given until the rhythm abnormality is documented and defined.

Tachyarrhythmias

Treatment for the tachyarrhythmia should be the same as in the nonpregnant woman. If at all possible, drugs should be avoided since all cross the placenta. If the woman is in significant distress, cardioversion can be used without adverse effects to the fetus.

Sinus tachycardia is a reason to search for a cause (the heart rate at rest should not exceed 100 beats per minute, even at term, in the normal pregnancy), but treatment of the rhythm itself is not appropriate. Premature atrial and ventricular beats do not require treatment, no matter what their frequency, unless they cause intolerable symptoms.

Paroxysmal supraventricular tachycardia can be treated with a vagal maneuver. If this is unsuccessful, intravenous verapamil (5 to 10 mg) or adenosine (6 to 12 mg) can quickly convert the rhythm without compromise to the fetus. A rare arrhythmic event does not justify daily medication. Some women can use oral verapamil (120 to 160 mg) on an as-needed basis if the rhythm recurs (with warnings about hypotension). If there are frequent recurrences, daily drug therapy with digoxin (0.25 to 0.5 mg) is appropriate. Sustained-release verapamil preparations (240 to 480 mg) or the selective $beta_1$ blocking agents (atenolol 50 to 100 mg) are reasonable alternatives. Suspicion of an accessory atrioventricular pathway would make the beta-blocker the preferred drug. Intolerable recurrent rhythms justify the use of a class I agent. Quinidine (900 to 1,800 mg daily in three divided doses) has been used most often without adverse effects on the fetus.

Atrial fibrillation and flutter suggest the presence of underlying heart disease. It is appropriate to consider other explanations (particularly drugs or hyperthyroidism). If ventricular rate control is required, intravenous verapamil or digoxin can be given or cardioversion performed. If fibrillation or flutter persists after rate control, one attempt at DC cardioversion is indicated. Persistence or recurrence is a reason to institute daily digoxin therapy for rate control. Thromboembolic complications are of concern, but the risk in women of this age is low. Still the consequences are high enough to recommend one aspirin tablet (325 mg) daily.

Treatment of ventricular tachyarrhythmias should be no different than in the nonpregnant woman. Recurrent symptomatic nonsustained ventricular tachycardia or sustained ventricular tachycardias justify antiarrhythmic drug therapy. Quinidine therapy, beta-blocker therapy, or both should be used first. If they are ineffective, use of agents less thoroughly evaluated during pregnancy is necessary.

Bradyarrhythmias

Therapeutic therapy for treatment of these arrhythmias should not be influenced by pregnancy. If a reversible cause of arrhythmias cannot be found and if the rhythms are symptomatic, pacemaker insertion is required. If this is necessary early in pregnancy, efforts to shield the fetus from radiation during pacemaker insertion are essential.

Endocarditis

Prevention of endocarditis is preferable to treatment. Although ineffective endocarditis occurs in less than 0.1 percent of deliveries, bacteremia is estimated to occur in 5 percent of women with normal labor and delivery and in up to 20 percent of patients undergoing cesarean section. Because of this, and because endocarditis continues to be associated with a high morbidity and mortality, antibiotic prophylaxis with penicillin (vancomycin if patient is penicillin allergic) and an aminoglycoside should be initiated at the onset of labor and continued for 24 hours after delivery. A false labor will make this recommendation difficult in some select cases, but in most it can be applied. If endocarditis occurs during pregnancy, evaluation and treatment should be treated as aggressively as at other times. If urgent surgery is required, it too should be performed. Depending on fetal maturity, cesarean section can be performed in concurrence with the cardiac surgery.

Pulmonary Hypertension

Primary or secondary pulmonary artery hypertension is a contraindication to pregnancy. When first documented during pregnancy, interruption should be recommended. Maternal mortality approaches 50 percent, with many of the deaths occurring at the time of interruption of the pregnancy or labor and delivery. If pregnancy occurs and interruption is not accepted by the mother, close clinical follow-up is essential. Activity should be kept at an absolute minimum. Hypovolemic states should be avoided. Capillary wedge pressure and arterial monitoring lines are appropriate during labor and for 24 to 48 hours after delivery. The anesthesiologist should take all measures to avoid venous pooling.

CONGENITAL HEART DISEASE

Effective surgery is making maternal congenital heart disease more common. Because these women have children with an increased chance of congenital heart disease, this trend will continue (see Table 2).

Intracardiac Shunts

Whether due to an atrial septal defect, a ventricular septal defect, or a patent ductus arteriosus, left to right shunts are generally well tolerated by the mother. This is probably because the fall in vascular resistance during pregnancy is similar in the pulmonary and systemic beds and there is no significant alteration in shunting. Surgical closure of the defects is generally preferable before delivery but this does not decrease the chance that the offspring will have heart disease. In the rare case when heart failure or symptomatic arrhythmias develop, they should be treated as described earlier.

Whether they are due to right ventricular outflow obstruction with normal pulmonary vascular resistance or to elevated pulmonary vascular resistance syndromes, right to left shunts are associated with high maternal and fetal morbidity and mortality. They are often associated with complex heart disease and associated cyanosis. Until corrected, it is advised that pregnancy should be avoided and, if pregnancy occurs, interruption is recommended. Tetralogy of Fallot is the most common cause of shunting caused by obstruction to pulmonary outflow. Once surgical correction has been performed, pregnancy can be completed with almost no maternal mortality and a small (10 to 20 percent) incidence of spontaneous abortions. Ebstein's anomaly may occasionally be associated with severe right to left shunting. Milder forms of the syndromes, with little shunting, are associated with a well-tolerated pregnancy.

Obstructive Lesions to Ventricular Outflow Tracts

Right and left ventricular outflow tract obstructions are associated with increased maternal and fetal mortality and with an increased chance of congenital heart disease in the offspring. Surgical correction before pregnancy will alleviate each of these problems. If pregnancy occurs and these lesions are recognized, activity should be limited to the level below which symptoms occur and, if symptoms accelerate despite this curtailment, surgical intervention may be necessary to protect the mother.

One syndrome of left outflow tract obstruction, coarctation of the aorta, is associated with a 3 to 9 percent maternal mortality rate. Surgical correction before pregnancy is advisable. If severe coarctation is noted when a patient is pregnant, interruption is recommended. If the woman does not wish to accept this recommendation, strict limitation of activity and control of systemic hypertension is indicated.

Another cause of outflow tract obstruction is idiopathic hypertrophic subaortic stenosis. Affected women may have increased symptoms during pregnancy; there has been only one reported death. Treatment of the symptoms is as difficult as at any other time but if they are severe, beta-blocker therapy (atenolol 50 to 100 mg daily) should be instituted.

Marfan's Syndrome

Complications of Marfan's syndrome frequently occur at the time of pregnancy with reported maternal mortality rates varying from 4 to 50 percent. Because of this and because long-term survival is uncommon and the offspring have a 50 percent chance of having the same abnormality, avoidance of pregnancy is recommended. Interruption should be considered if the syndrome is recognized after a woman is pregnant. This recommendation should be made more strongly if there is evidence of aortic root dilation (greater than 40 mm by echocardiography). If this advice is unacceptable to the mother, activity should be strictly limited, blood pressure well controlled, and a $beta_1$ selective blocking agent should be instituted. Cesarean section is preferable to labor and vaginal delivery.

Valve Disease

Management of valve disease addressing the issues of endocarditis prophylaxis, prophylaxis against rheumatic fever, the need for anticoagulation, and treatment of complications should be the same during pregnancy as at other times.

Mitral Stenosis

Recognition and mechanical correction of mitral stenosis before pregnancy is the preferred approach. The more severe the hemodynamic abnormality, the greater the risk of pregnancy. Mitral commissurotomy is preferable to prosthesis insertion (see prosthetic valve disease below). If a woman with mitral stenosis becomes pregnant, symptoms and complications should be treated in the standard fashion. Prophylactic digoxin should be given to minimize the fast ventricular response if she develops atrial fibrillation. If severe symptoms persist despite limitation of activity and use of medications, mitral commissurotomy or balloon valvuloplasty is required.

Mitral Regurgitation

This lesion is generally well tolerated during pregnancy. Arrhythmias or congestive heart failure should be treated in the standard fashion.

Mital valve prolapse is common in women of child-bearing age. The incidence of symptoms, arrhythmias, endocarditis, or emboli does not alter during pregnancy. Antibiotic prophylaxis at the time of labor and delivery is recommended for those women with a murmur.

Aortic Stenosis

Maternal mortality as high as 10 percent make surgical correction (preferably a valvotomy) before pregnancy desirable. No treatment is necessary for women with aortic stenosis who become pregnant and are asymptomatic. Symptomatic women should limit activity; again, it is important to avoid hypovolemia. If congestive heart failure occurs and cannot be controlled, surgical or balloon valvuloplasty should be considered.

Aortic Regurgitation

This lesion is well tolerated during pregnancy. In those who do develop congestive heart failure or arrhythmias, standard treatment should be used. If acute aortic regurgitation occurs owing to bacterial endocarditis or to aortic dissection, emergency treatment, even surgery, is required despite the pregnancy.

Pulmonic Valve Disease

Pulmonic stenosis should be corrected before conception. If first recognized during pregnancy, hypovolemia should be avoided. Pulmonic insufficiency is uncommon except after previous heart surgery. No specific treatment is needed during pregnancy.

Tricuspid Valve Disease

Isolated tricuspid valve stenosis is rare and treatment should be individualized. The incidence of regurgitation is increasing (because of illicit drug use), but the lesion is well tolerated during pregnancy and no specific therapy is required.

Prosthetic Heart Valves

Insertion of a prosthetic heart valve commits an individual to a 3 to 6 percent chance per year of a major complication. Pregnancy may increase this risk and a prosthetic valve is a relative contraindication to pregnancy. Complications occurring in pregnant women with a prosthetic valve require standard urgent therapy.

Selecting a prosthesis for a woman who desires subsequent pregnancies is difficult. A tissue valve lessens the need for anticoagulation therapy, but pregnancy may accelerate the already high incidence of early valve degeneration, making early reoperation likely. A mechanical prosthesis mandates the need for anticoagulation therapy. Since warfarin is contraindicated (see drugs above) this means the woman must administer heparin subcutaneously throughout the pregnancy. The choice of prosthesis must be individualized, but, in balance, the long-term durability makes a mechanical prosthesis the preferable choice despite the issue of anticoagulation therapy.

Myocardial Disease

A woman with dilated cardiomyopathy has a 30 percent chance of congestive heart failure and an increased mortality rate with pregnancy. These and her guarded long-term prognosis make the diagnosis a relative contraindication to pregnancy. If pregnancy occurs, interruption is advisable. If the woman chooses to proceed with pregnancy, heart failure, arrhythmias, and thromboembolic complications require treatment.

If dilated cardiomyopathy develops late in pregnancy or in the first 6 weeks after delivery, the pregnancy itself is considered the cause. This is a peripartum cardiomyopathy. Treatment for myocarditis as a cause is reasonable if the disease is rapidly progressive and the diagnosis is proved by biopsy.

Coronary Artery Disease

Coronary artery obstruction occurs on rare occasions during pregnancy. Spasms, dissection, thromboemboli, and, rarely, atherosclerosis are the presumed causes. Complications of a myocardial infarction require standard treatment. The risk of thrombolytic therapy has not been defined, and it should be reserved for those likely to get the very highest benefit.

Pericardial Disease

Pregnancy should not alter the treatment of pericardial disease syndromes.

SUGGESTED READING

McAnulty JH, Metcalfe J, Ueland K. The heart and certain physiological conditions. In: Hurst JW, Rackley CE, Schlant RC, Sonnenblick EH, Wenger NK, eds. The Heart, 7th ed. New York: McGraw-Hill, 1990; 1465–1478.

McAnulty JH, Morton MJ, Ueland K. The heart and pregnancy. Curr Prob Cardiol 1988; 13:595.

Whittemore R, Hobbins JC, Engle MA. Pregnancy and its outcome in women with and without surgical treatment of congenital heart disease. Am J Cardiol 1982; 50:641.

GASTROINTESTINAL DISEASES

GASTROESOPHAGEAL REFLUX: MEDICAL TREATMENT

ROY C. ORLANDO, M.D.

Gastroesophageal reflux is a frequent daily occurrence in everyone. When it occurs without symptoms or evidence of mucosal injury, it has been designated "physiologic reflux." This distinguishes it from "pathologic reflux," which is commonly associated with esophageal symptoms (heartburn) or esophageal mucosal damage. However, "pathologic reflux" may also produce symptoms and signs of oropharyngeal and respiratory disease. For this reason, the term "gastroesophageal reflux disease" (GERD) has been coined to encompass the constellation of problems accompanying this process.

As noted, the most common features of GERD are symptoms (heartburn) and evidence of esophageal mucosal injury, the latter ranging from inflammation to ulceration. This occurs primarily from the prolonged contact of refluxed gastric acid with esophageal epithelium. In healthy individuals, the esophagus is protected from prolonged contact with gastric acid by a two-tiered defensive system: antireflux barriers (primarily the lower esophageal sphincter) and acid clearance mechanisms (peristalsis, gravity, and saliva); there is also a third defensive system, epithelial resistance, that minimizes damage during actual contact with acid (Fig. 1).

Conceptually, GERD occurs when the offense (gastric acid) overruns the three-tiered esophageal defense: antireflux barriers, acid clearance mechanisms, and epithelial resistance. This usually takes a great deal of time, and consequently GERD is characteristically only a slowly progressive mucosal disorder, in which acute life-threatening events are rare. For this reason, most patients deserve a trial of medical rather than surgical therapy.

MEDICAL TREATMENT

Medical management can be conveniently divided into two types: (1) lifestyle modification and (2) drug therapy. Both of these work to improve GERD by either reducing the offense (acid) or enhancing the defense (antireflux barriers. clearance mechanisms, epithelial resistance).

Lifestyle Modification

Lifestyle modification should be part of the initial management in all patients (Table 1). This has several valuable features. First the price is right. It costs almost nothing since there are no additional medications, merely the procurement of two blocks or bricks to elevate the head of the bed. Second, the potential benefits are great, both short and long term. Short-term benefits include a reduction in symptoms and healing of esophageal lesions. Long-term benefits include the prevention of recurrence of GERD and the development of other serious nongastrointestinal disorders (e.g., ischemic heart disease, cirrhosis, emphysema, and cancer). Thus, lifestyle modifications provide an opportunity for the physician to focus patients on the habits that ad-

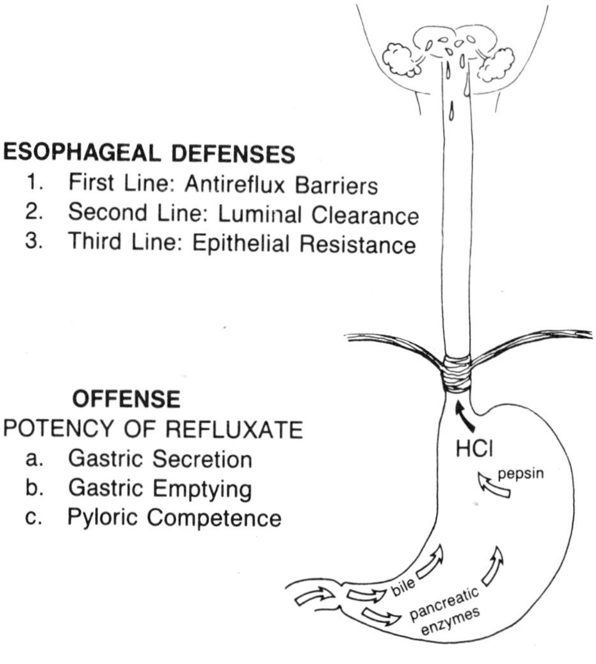

Figure 1 Determinants of reflux injury. (Modified from Orlando RC. Oesophageal defences. CML Gastroenterol J [in press].)

versely affect their health and to emphasize that by altering these habits, they can improve their chances of a favorable treatment outcome.

The bases for recommending the lifestyle modifications listed in Table 1 are as follows. Elevation of the head of the bed or (for patients for whom this is intolerable) sleeping on a 10-inch wedge enhances, through gravity, the rate of acid clearance at bedtime. Cessation of smoking and alcohol are valuable because both increase reflux frequency by lowering lower esophageal sphincter (LES) pressure, prolong acid contact with epithelium by reducing acid clearance, and have direct toxic effects on squamous epithelium. Reduction of meal size and the intake of fat, carminatives, and chocolate, should reduce the frequency of reflux: the first by reducing gastric distention, which increases the frequency of transient LES relaxations, and the others by avoiding foods that favor reflux by lowering LES pressure. Other foods to be avoided are coffee (both caffeinated and decaffeinated) and tea and cola beverages, which both stimulate acid secretion and (along with tomato juice, orange juice, and other citrus products) may produce symptoms by their acidity or osmolality. Finally, avoidance, when possible, of any drug that lowers LES pressure may reduce the frequency of reflux. These agents are listed in Table 1. Obviously, medications that can injure the mucosa (e.g., tetracyclines, aspirin, or nonsteroidal anti-inflammatory drugs should be used judiciously or avoided altogether.

TABLE 1 Lifestyle Modifications for Reflux Esophagitis

Elevate the head of the bed 6 inches
Stop smoking*
Stop excessive alcohol consumption*
Reduce dietary fat†*
Reduce meal size
Avoid bedtime snacks
Reduce weight (if overweight)
Avoid these foods:
- Chocolate
- Carminatives (spearmint, peppermint)
- Coffee (caffeinated and decaffeinated)
- Tea
- Cola beverages
- Tomato juice
- Citrus fruit juices

Avoid, when possible, these drugs:
- Anticholinergics
- Theophylline
- Diazepam
- Narcotics
- Calcium channel blockers
- Beta-adrenergic agonists (isoproterenol)
- Progesterone (some contraceptives)
- Alpha-adrenergic antagonists (phentolamine)
- Nonsteroidal anti-inflammatory drugs

* These measures have major long-term gastrointestinal and nongastrointestinal health benefits.

† Fat intake should be reduced to $<30\%$ of calories, which is equivalent to 67 g fat per day on a 2,000-calorie diet.

Drug Therapy

Drug therapy is important in the medical management of GERD and, like lifestyle modification, either reduces the offense (acid) or enhances the defense (antireflux barriers, clearance mechanisms, epithelial resistance). A list of drugs and their mechanisms of action is provided in Table 2.

Antacids

Antacids on an as-needed basis, are the mainstay for rapid, safe, effective relief of symptoms. The liquid forms are preferable to tablets, although form is not as important as patient satisfaction with response. Antacids may also be effective in healing esophageal lesions but, even in well-motivated patients, compliance with a regimen rigorous enough to accomplish this is limited. Problems with compliance arise because of poor palatability and major side effects that affect bowel habits (magnesium-containing agents producing diarrhea and aluminum-containing agents producing constipation). The potential for magnesium or aluminum toxicity further limits their use in patients with significant renal disease, and low-sodium antacids (e.g, magaldrate [Riopan]) are preferable for individuals on salt-restricted diets.

Gaviscon

Gaviscon, an antacid-alginate combination, can be used empirically, like antacids, for symptom relief or as an adjunct to therapy in patients with more severe disease. Although Gaviscon is safe, it contains aluminum, magnesium, and sodium; therefore, the same precautions listed for antacids apply.

H_2-Receptor Antagonists

Just as antacids are the mainstay for immediate symptom relief, the H_2 antagonists are the mainstay for continuous treatment of GERD; they are generally both safe and effective. Their capacity for inhibiting acid secretion renders the refluxate less noxious to the epithelium, providing protection against the development of symptoms during reflux and increasing the chances for lesions to heal. Although the dosages and frequency of administration vary, all H_2 antagonists can reduce acid secretion, and as such may be effective in chronic treatment of GERD. However, to date ranitidine is the only agent with Food and Drug Administration approval for use in this condition. Although effective, ranitidine has not proved to be a panacea for all patients with GERD. In particular, patients with gross (erosive) esophagitis do moderately better with full-dose therapy (150 mg twice a day) than those on placebo, but relapse is common when dosage is reduced for maintenance (150 mg at bedtime). The safety and efficacy of ranitidine at higher doses and for longer periods in GERD are actively under study.

In the choice between H_2 antagonists, aside from efficacy, consideration should be given to cost, frequency of administration, and possible side effects. Reduced cost and

TABLE 2 Drug Therapy for Reflux Esophagitis

	Dose	*Mechanism(s) of Action*
Antacid: liquid		
e.g., Mylanta II/Maalox TC (HCl neutralizing capacity 25 mEq/5 ml)*	15 ml/qid 1 hr pc & qhs	Buffer HCl ↑ LESP
Gaviscon		
(Aluminum hydroxide, magnesium trisilicate, $NaHCO_3$, alginic acid)	2–4 tabs qid pc & qhs	↓ reflux by viscous mechanical barrier Buffer HCl in esophagus
H_2-receptor antagonists		
Cimetidine (Tagamet)	300 mg qid pc & qhs	↓ HCl secretion, ↓ gastric volume } by inhibiting H_2 receptor
Ranitidine (Zantac)	150 mg bid pc & qhs	Same as cimetidine
Famotidine (Pepcid)	40 mg qhs	Same as cimetidine
Nizatidine (Axid)	300 mg qhs	Same as cimetidine
Bethanechol (Urecholine)	25 mg qid ½ hr ac & qhs	↑ LESP ↑ esophageal acid clearance
Metoclopramide (Reglan)	10 mg qid ½ hr ac & qhs	↑ LESP ↑ gastric emptying
Sucralfate (Carafate)	1 g qid 1 hr pc & qhs	↑ tissue resistance Buffer HCl in esophagus Bind pepsin-bile salts
Agents under investigation		
Inhibitors of H^+-K^+ ATPase		
Omeprazole	20–60 mg/day	↓ HCl secretion ↓ gastric volume
Cisapride	10 mg tid–qid	↑ LESP, ↑ gastric emptying
Domperidone	10–20 mg tid–qid	↑ LESP, ↑ gastric emptying

* Patients with reflux are not known to be hypersecretors of gastric acid. Therefore, therapeutic doses of antacids are based on the capacity to buffer basal HCl secretion of about 1–7 mEq/hr (mean 2 mEq/hr) and peak meal-stimulated HCl secretion of about 10–60 mEq/hr (mean 30 mEq/hr).

LESP = lower esophageal sphincter pressure; pc = after meals; ac = before meals; qhs = at bedtime.

↑ = increase, ↓ = decrease.

less frequent administration may improve patient compliance. Side effects, although infrequent, differ among agents. Cimetidine may cause gynecomastia, impotence, hypospermia, mental confusion, nephritis, and drug-drug interactions. Ranitidine, generally free of the antiandrogenic and central nervous system (CNS) effects and drug-drug interactions associated with cimetidine, may produce a higher incidence of hepatic injury than cimetidine. Famotidine and nizatidine are the newest members of the H_2-antagonist category, and both appear to have side-effect profiles closer to that of ranitidine than to cimetidine.

Bethanechol

Bethanechol is a cholinergic agonist that has been shown to be effective in reducing symptoms and healing lesions in some, but not all, trials. Its usefulness is limited because of troublesome side effects including flushing, blurry vision, headaches, abdominal cramps, and urinary frequency. It is also contraindicated in a number of common conditions, such as asthma, peptic ulcer disease, ischemic heart disease, and obstructive disease of the intestine or urinary tract. Many experts prefer to use bethanechol as an adjunct to H_2-antagonist therapy at bedtime only when the risk from reflux is greatest and side effects are less bothersome.

Metoclopramide

Metoclopramide is a dopamine antagonist that has limited efficacy in reducing symptoms. It also does not appear to heal esophageal lesions except when used in combination with H_2 antagonists. Metoclopramide crosses the blood-brain barrier, and consequently CNS side effects such as drowsiness, insomnia, agitation, tremor, and dyskinesias are frequent and often severe enough to require cessation of treatment. Tardive dyskinesia that does not reverse with drug withdrawal has been reported.

Sucralfate

Sucralfate is the basic aluminum salt of sucrose octasulfate. It has been shown in a European trial to be more effective than placebo in reducing symptoms and healing lesions in GERD. American trials have shown only marginal benefits with sucralfate, although, interestingly, patients with the more severe (erosive) disease appeared to benefit most from its use. This inconsistency may reflect the greater retention of sucralfate within the esophagus of patients with larger epithelial defects (erosions, ulcers). Sucralfate acts topically and, because it has limited systemic absorption, it appears to be extremely safe. The most common side effect reported is constipation, a reflection of its aluminum content. This content, which can be absorbed, requires that it be used cautiously and at reduced dosage in patients with renal disease. (Sucralfate can be used as an adjunct to therapy with H_2 antagonists because, at standard doses, H_2 antagonists do not raise gastric pH high enough to prevent the acidic refluxate from activating sucralfate.)

Investigational Agents

Domperidone. Domperidone, a dopamine antagonist, has few side effects because it crosses the blood-brain barrier less readily than metoclopramide. However, domperidone has had little documented success in reducing symptoms or healing lesions in GERD. This may be due to its limited ability to increase LES pressure when given orally.

Cisapride. Cisapride is a prokinetic agent that increases gastric emptying and LES pressure by enhancing the release of acetylcholine from the myenteric plexus. Trials in GERD have been limited but the preliminary results are encouraging. In at least one report, cisapride has been shown to be superior to placebo in reducing symptoms and healing lesions. Side effects have been minimal but a wider experience with this agent is needed.

Omeprazole. Omeprazole, a substituted benzimidazole, is a potent inhibitor of acid secretion. In once-per-day dosing it is capable of producing complete achlorhydria. This is because it irreversibly blocks the parietal cell H^+-K^+ adenosine triphosphatase, which is the final common pathway for acid secretion. (After omeprazole is stopped, the enzyme can be restored through renewed synthesis in 3 days.) Its superiority over H_2 antagonists in inhibiting acid secretion appears to be responsible for reports of dramatic improvement in symptoms and rapid rates of lesion healing in GERD. Although the effectiveness of omeprazole for acute treatment in GERD has not been challenged, relapse rates are high (greater than 80 percent in 6 months) and concern has been expressed about its safety for long-term use. Thus, complete acid suppression, presumably by enhancement of gastrin release, has been shown to produce enterochromaffin tumors (carcinoids) in experimental animals. Complete acid suppression, by removing the acid barrier to ingested organisms, also increases the potential for complications such as gastrointestinal and systemic infections or gastric carcinoma due to bacterial overgrowth converting food components into carcinogens. Studies attempting to resolve these concerns are ongoing.

TREATMENT STRATEGY

All patients with symptomatic reflux who have failed initial empiric therapy in the primary care setting should undergo upper endoscopy. This procedure is indicated at this time to (1) rule out other diagnoses, (2) assess the type and extent of esophageal mucosal damage, and (3) guide treatment. Esophageal biopsy at the time of endoscopy is useful for confirmation of diagnosis but has little influence on treatment strategy.

Endoscopy permits patients with symptomatic reflux to be subdivided into two groups, depending on the presence or absence of gross (endoscopic) esophagitis. In this regard it should be emphasized that symptoms do not predict endoscopic findings, so patients with severe heartburn may have little or no mucosal damage, and patients with minimal to no heartburn may have severe erosive disease. Those with symptoms but no gross evidence of esophageal damage can be considered at *low risk* for complications, whereas those with (or without) symptoms and gross esophagitis (i.e., erosions or ulcers but not erythema) are at *high risk* for complications. The basis for this separation is that the mucosal complications accounting for the major morbidity and, in some cases, mortality from GERD are strictures and Barrett's esophagus, lesions unlikely to develop in the absence of necrosis extending to the basement membrane. Patients found endoscopically to already have either a stricture or Barrett's esophagus are managed as high-risk patients.

Since patients with symptoms and no (or microscopic) mucosal disease are at low risk for complications, the primary goal of therapy is control of symptoms. Endoscopic follow-up in these cases is generally unnecessary. In contrast, patients with mucosal destruction (erosions, ulcers) with or without symptoms are at high risk for complications, and thus the primary goal of therapy is healing of lesions. This requires endoscopic follow-up irrespective of symptoms.

Initial therapy for both groups is based on lifestyle modification as outlined in Table 1, and selective use of the drugs listed in Table 2. Drug therapy starts with an H_2 antagonist and antacids. H_2 antagonists should be taken at bedtime, because this period carries the greatest risk of prolonged contact of refluxed acid with epithelium; one or two additional doses during the day are also desirable to prolong the time that gastric pH is less acid. Therapy with antacids is recommended on an as-needed basis for immediate symptom relief. A therapeutic trial can be as short as a few weeks if the goal is symptom relief, but should be considerably longer (e.g., 3 months) if the goal is lesion healing.

If this regimen fails to accomplish the necessary goal, i.e., symptom relief in low-risk patients (no endoscopy) or endoscopic healing in high-risk patients, the program should be modified. Modifications include (1) higher or more frequent dosages of the H_2 antagonist, (2) switching to another H_2 antagonist, or (3) adding a second agent. If a second agent is chosen, its mechanism of action should complement, not duplicate, that of the H_2 antagonist. Second agents in this case would include bethanechol, sucralfate, or metoclopramide. Bethanechol, because of side effects, is best given as a single bedtime (25-mg) dose. Sucralfate should be taken as a suspension (1-g tablet suspended in 30 ml of water or glycerol) four times per day; metoclopramide, if not limited by side effects, should be taken in 10-mg doses four times per day. The modified regimen, as before, can be short (a few weeks) if used for symptomatic relief, or long (3 months) if used for lesion healing. If this fails, an optimumably tolerable drug regimen might include all of the following: an H_2 antagonist, antacids or gaviscon as needed, bethanechol at bedtime, and sucralfate, 1 g four times per day. This regimen, even if successful and not limited by side effects, may be difficult to maintain because of cost and inconvenience.

Failure of lesions to heal on this regimen or failure to maintain the healed state mandates that high-risk patients be considered for surgery. (Patients who for reasons of age or health are not candidates for surgery may qualify for treatment with omeprazole on a compassionate-use basis.) In contrast, failure of this regimen to control symptoms in low-risk patients should prompt repeat endoscopy. If endoscopy shows progression to gross disease, surgical consultation is recommended. If endoscopy reaffirms the absence of gross disease, surgical consultation is not recommended; the patient is better served by a Bernstein test, 24-hour pH monitoring, and an in-depth history (medical and personal). The Bernstein test and pH monitoring are useful for defining the relationship between symptoms and esophageal acidification, and the history is useful for identifying areas of stress that may affect the patient's capacity for coping with symptoms. A lack of correlation between symptoms and esophageal acidification on Bernstein and 24-hour pH testing can add further support for the failure of treatment being due to factors other than reflux (e.g., stress).

In general, the same medical regimens described above are applicable in the treatment of the mucosal complications of GERD (i.e., strictures and Barrett's esophagus). In addition, strictures, when severe, require dilatation. Barrett's esophagus, because of the cancer risk, requires routine endoscopy and biopsy at intervals of 1 to 2 years. Another major complication of GERD is aspiration. This nonmucosal complication, when severe enough, can lead to pneumonia or respiratory compromise. Although studies are generally lacking, medical therapy has little to offer under these circumstances and surgery is the treatment of choice.

SUGGESTED READING

Dent J, Dodds WJ, Friedman RH, et al. Mechanisms of gastroesophageal reflux in recumbent asymptomatic human subjects. J Clin Invest 1980; 65:256–257.

Hamilton JW, Boisen RJ, Yamamoto MD, et al. Sleeping on a wedge diminishes exposure of the esophagus to refluxed acid. Dig Dis Sci 1988; 33:518–522.

Helm JF, Dodds WJ, Reidel DR, et al. Determinants of esophageal acid clearance in normal subjects. Gastroenterology 1983; 85:607–612.

Hetzel DJ, Dent J, Reed WD, et al. Healing and relapse of severe peptic esophagitis after treatment with omeprazole. Gastroenterology 1988; 95:903–912.

Koelz HR, Birchler R, Bretholz A, et al. Healing and relapse of reflux esophagitis during treatment with ranitidine. Gastroenterology 1986; 91:1198–1205.

Richter JE, Castell DO. Gastroesophageal reflux: pathogenesis diagnosis and therapy. Ann Intern Med 1982; 97:93–103.

ESOPHAGEAL MOTOR DISORDERS AND CHEST PAIN

JOEL E. RICHTER, M.D.

Recurring, angina-like chest pain is an important clinical problem, causing anxiety for both patients and physicians. Despite the excellent medical prognosis, many patients for whom cardiac disease has been reasonably excluded continue to use medical facilities and have compromised lifestyles. Just how common is this problem of noncardiac chest pain? A recent nationwide survey estimated that approximately 600,000 new patients per year undergo cardiac catheterization. Normal coronary arteries are found in up to 30 percent of patients with anginal syndromes. Of these, studies suggest that approximately 50 percent can be expected to show demonstrable esophageal abnormalities; therefore, an estimated 90,000 new cases could be diagnosed yearly. These figures are probably underestimations, however, since many patients do not undergo cardiac catheterization, particularly if they are under the age of 40 years.

The specific mechanisms producing esophageal chest pain are not well understood. Traditionally, esophageal pain has been attributed to acid reflux or esophageal "spasm." Studies suggest that gastroesophageal reflux disease is by far the most common cause of esophageal chest pain. Most patients have concomitant heartburn, but 10 to 20 percent have only chest pain. In my experience, approximately 30 percent of patients with noncardiac chest pain are found to have esophageal motility disorders identified during routine manometric testing. High-amplitude peristaltic contractions (the nutcracker esophagus) and a grab bag of nonspecific motility changes are most commonly found, whereas classic diffuse esophageal spasm is an infrequent finding (Table 1). However, despite this common association, patients rarely have spontaneous pain during motility testing. Therefore, provocative agents such as edrophonium chloride, balloon distention, and more recently, ambulatory 24-hour pH and pressure monitoring are needed to define better the relationship between chest pain and abnormal esophageal motility. These studies suggest that esophageal chest pain is less commonly associated with motility disorders than previously

TABLE 1 Manometric Criteria for Painful Esophageal Motor Disorders*

Diffuse Esophageal Spasm
Simultaneous contractions (>10% of wet swallows)
Intermittent normal peristalsis
Minor criteria:
Repetitive contractions (>2 peaks)
Prolonged duration (>6 sec)
High amplitude
Spontaneous contractions
Incomplete LES relaxation
Nutcracker Esophagus
High-amplitude contractions (mean >180 mm Hg)
Normal peristalsis
Possible contractions of prolonged duration
Hypertensive LES
Elevated LES pressure (>45 mm Hg)
Normal LES relaxation
Normal peristalsis
Nonspecific Motor Disorders
Increased nontransmitted contractions (>20%)
Prolonged duration
Triple peaked contractions
Retrograde contractions
Low-amplitude peristalsis
Incomplete LES relaxation with normal peristalsis

* Criteria developed after defining normal motility patterns and pressures in 95 healthy individuals (ages 17–81 years).
LES = lower esophageal sphincter.

thought. For example, prolonged ambulatory monitoring has identified abnormal motility as the cause of chest pain in only 15 to 30 percent of patients.

Although disappointing, these experimental results suggest that other factors may contribute to esophageal chest pain. We have found that these patients frequently note replication of their pain with smaller volumes of esophageal balloon distention than required to produce pain in asymptomatic individuals. Thus, lower visceral pain thresholds may also be a contributing factor. To further confuse the issue, patients with noncardiac chest pain have a high prevalence of psychiatric conditions including anxiety, depression, somatization, and panic disorders. Whether these emotional problems cause chest pain, or vice versa, remains unclear. Nevertheless, many aspects of painful esophageal motility disorders parallel the characteristic features of the irritable bowel syndrome. Overall, both groups seem to have increased gut sensitivity to a number of stimuli, many of which do not cause pain in healthy individuals. The complex nature of these patients' chest pain may account for their frequent poor response to conventional medical therapies.

CLINICAL MANIFESTATIONS

The cardinal symptoms of esophageal dysfunction are dysphagia and chest pain. Patients with motility disorders frequently present with a combination of these symptoms.

Dysphagia

Typical esophageal dysphagia associated with motility disorders is usually slowly progressive, is noted with both liquids and solids, and may be associated with weight loss. It is often relieved with repeated swallowing, by a Valsalva maneuver, or by throwing the arms over the head. In patients with painful esophageal motility disorders, dysphagia is more likely to be intermittent in nature, interspersed by many periods of relatively normal swallowing. It also may be related to swallowing specific substances, such as large boluses of food, medications, or liquids of extreme temperatures. In contrast, patients with achalasia generally have more persistent dysphagia, often with every meal.

The symptoms of dysphagia result from interference in the orderly transport of liquids or solids down the esophagus into the stomach. Therefore, radiographic studies and esophageal manometry frequently show abnormal results. In my experience, more than 50 percent of patients have esophageal motility disorders when their primary complaint is dysphagia with a normal barium esophagram. In contrast to patients with chest pain, achalasia is the most commonly found motility disorder and the nutcracker esophagus is infrequent.

Chest Pain

Intermittent anterior chest discomfort is the most frequent complaint of patients with painful esophageal motility disorders. Chest pain is usually described as squeezing and substernal in location, and may radiate into the back, neck, jaw, or arms, making it sometimes indistinguishable from angina-like pain. Some features suggesting esophageal rather than cardiac pain include (1) pain that is nonexertional and continues for hours; (2) pain that interrupts sleep or is meal related; (3) pain that is relieved with antacids; or (4) the presence of associated esophageal symptoms including heartburn, dysphagia, or regurgitation. Unfortunately, none of these features applies exclusively to esophageal chest pain. Therefore, the initial evaluation of chest pain should always be directed toward the exclusion of cardiac disease, because of its potential morbidity and mortality.

DIAGNOSIS

The diagnostic evaluation of patients with suspected esophageal motility disorders should be guided by the primary complaint of either dysphagia or chest pain (Fig. 1). All patients with dysphagia should initially be evaluated by a barium esophagram with fluoroscopic observation or videotape recording of the swallowing mechanism. Identification of an anatomic cause of dysphagia generally is followed by endoscopy. The presence of a normal esophagram or aberrant bolus activity should suggest a functional disorder. Esophageal manometry is required to define precisely the presence of an esophageal motility disorder. Radionuclide scintigraphic studies may be needed to assess the impact of abnormal esophageal pressures on bolus movement or esophageal emptying. If chest pain is the predominant symptom, the diagnostic approach should differ somewhat. Because of the potentially more serious prognosis, coronary artery disease must be ruled out initially. An upper gastrointestinal (GI) series with barium esophagraphy (or perhaps

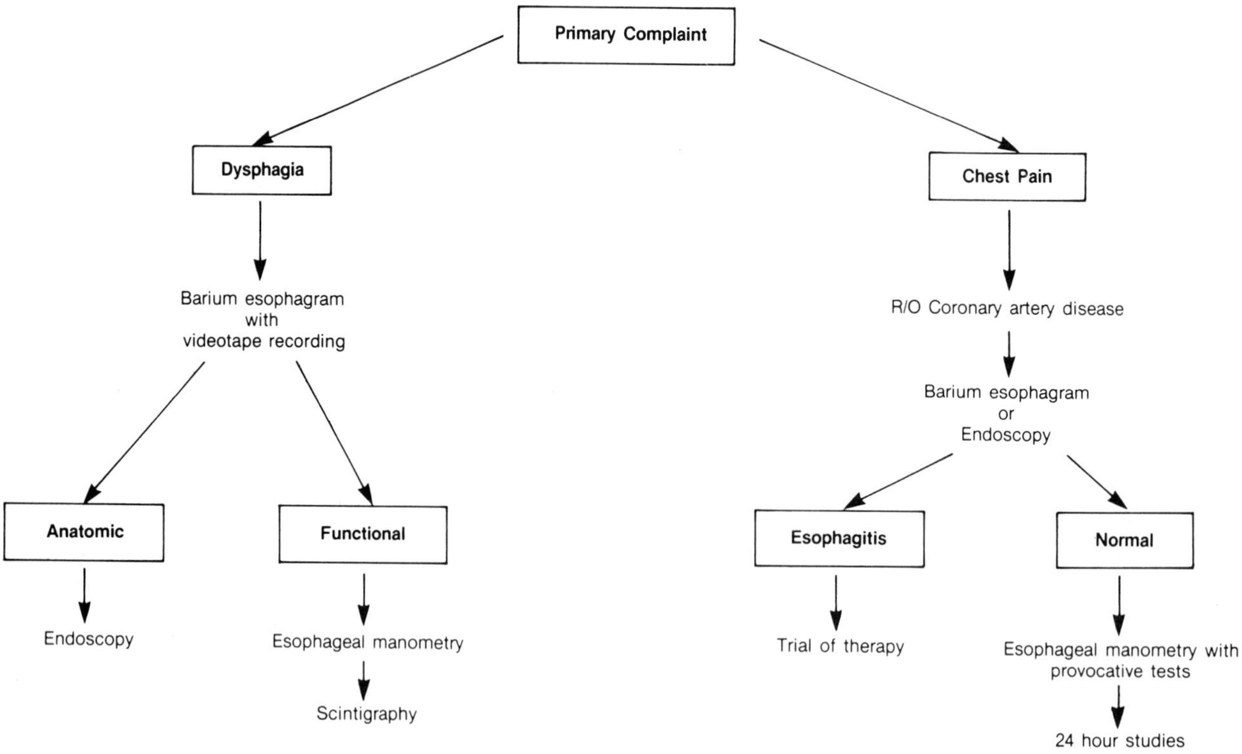

Figure 1 Approach to patients with suspected esophageal motility disorder.

endoscopy) should follow to identify peptic ulcer disease and esophagitis as the possible cause of chest pain. If these studies are unrevealing, an esophageal manometry with provocative tests (Bernstein, edrophonium chloride [Tensilon], balloon distention) is performed. Prolonged ambulatory pH or pressure studies also may be performed to define better the presence of gastroesophageal reflux, and the relationship between esophageal motility disorders and chest pain.

TREATMENT

The treatment of painful esophageal motility disorders is quite variable, no single agent being totally effective for any group of patients (Table 2). Since we do not understand the cause of most of these disorders, current therapies are often empiric. A good patient-physician relationship and confident reassurance are the cornerstone of management. In most patients, my experience suggests that pain related to esophageal motility disorders decreases with time regardless of the intervention. This must be kept in mind when considering dangerous or invasive therapeutic approaches.

Exclusion of Gastroesophageal Reflux

Since chest pain and dysphagia produced by gastroesophageal reflux may mimic esophageal motility disorders, it is important to exclude this diagnosis. Traditionally, this has been done with the acid perfusion (Bernstein) test. However, increasing evidence suggests that 24-hour ambulatory esophageal pH monitoring is more sensitive and specific in defining abnormal acid reflux and correlating symptoms with acid exposure. Since this instrumentation is now widely available, I would use it routinely in the evaluation of difficult cases of noncardiac chest pain. Only after reflux disease has been excluded is it appropriate to proceed with other therapy for primary esophageal motility disorders.

Nitrates

These are usually my first choice of drugs when symptoms are mild and intermittent. Sublingual nitroglycerin may be used before meals if symptoms are closely associated with eating. More intermittent chest pain or dysphagia may respond to either isosorbide dinitrate (Isordil), 10 to 30 mg four times a day, or erythrityl tetranitrate (Cardilate), 10 to 15 mg four times a day, orally. Dosage is often limited by headache, which is the major side effect of the nitrates.

The rationale for using nitrates to treat esophageal motility disorders relates to their ability to relax smooth muscle. Early reports found both symptomatic improvement and manometric response to nitroglycerin and long-acting nitrates in patients with esophageal spasm. More recent studies, however, suggest that the effects of nitrates on esophageal pressures are minimal. No control studies have been reported in patients with esophageal chest pain. Nevertheless, the nitrates should be tried empirically, since they are successful in some patients.

TABLE 2 Therapy for Painful Esophageal Motor Disorders

Treatment	*Dose*	*Mode of Administration*	*Side Effects*
Nitrates			
Nitroglycerin	0.4 mg sublingually	Before meals	Headaches
Isosorbide dinitrate	10–30 mg PO	qid	
Erythrityl tetranitrate	10–15 mg PO	qid	
Anticholinergics			
Dicyclomine	10–20 mg PO	qid	Dry mouth; blurred vision
Antidepressants			
Trazodone	50–100 mg PO	tid	Drowsiness, lightheadedness
Amitriptyline	50–150 mg PO	At bedtime	Drowsiness, dry mouth
Calcium Channel Blockers			
Nifedipine	10–30 mg PO	qid	Dizziness, headaches, edema
Diltiazem	90 mg PO	qid	
Smooth Muscle Relaxants			
Hydralazine	25–50 mg	tid	Lupus-like reaction
Bougienage			
Pneumatic dilatation	8–12 psi for 1 min	prn	Perforation
Esophageal myotomy			Gastroesophageal reflux

Anticholinergics

Some authorities use anticholinergic agents as initial therapy for esophageal motility disorders, but I have been reluctant because of their frequent side effects. As do the nitrates, anticholinergics relax smooth muscle. It has been shown that intravenous atropine sulfate can temporarily relieve painful esophageal contraction in patients with diffuse esophageal spasm. Studies with oral anticholinergics have also demonstrated decreased esophageal pressures in healthy adults, but reports are lacking in patients with painful esophageal motility disorders. There is no evidence to suggest that any one of the anticholinergics is preferable.

Psychotropic Drugs

Patients frequently recognize stress as precipitating their esophageal symptoms. These factors should be explored early in the course rather than waiting until all diagnostic tests and therapies have failed. A simple discussion about the relationship between emotional factors and the symptoms may be helpful. Some patients may need referral to a psychiatrist or psychologist, but most can be helped best by their primary physician.

Anecdotal reports suggest that anxiolytic or antidepressant agents may help some patients with painful esophageal motility disorders. A placebo controlled study supports these observations. Clouse and associates found that low-dose trazodone (Desyrel), 100 to 150 mg per day decreased symptoms associated with esophageal motility disorders without changing esophageal pressures. Behavioral modification programs and biofeedback may also be beneficial.

Calcium Channel Blockers

Calcium is intimately involved in the genesis of esophageal contractions and lower esophageal sphincter (LES) function. Blockade of calcium receptors, in an effort to reduce esophageal pressures and control pain, is an attractive hypothetical solution, but therapeutic results have been variable and generally disappointing.

High-dose *diltiazem* (150 mg orally) reduces contraction amplitude and duration in patients with the nutcracker esophagus, but not in control subjects. An open-labeled study in patients with nutcracker esophagus led to a reduction in the frequency and severity of chest pain. Preliminary results of a subsequent double-blind crossover study with diltiazem, 90 mg four times a day, found similar symptomatic results, associated with a trend toward reducing esophageal amplitude and duration. However, another group, studying patients with diffuse esophageal spasm and nutcracker esophagus, was unable to replicate these beneficial findings with diltiazem therapy.

Nifedipine produces a predictable dose-dependent reduction in LES and distal esophageal contraction pressures in normal individuals and patients with esophageal motility disorders. Nifedipine (10 to 30 mg orally three times a day) has been compared with placebo in a double-blind crossover study of patients with nutcracker esophagus and persistent chest pain. It significantly reduced distal esophageal contraction amplitude and duration and LES pressures as compared with placebo. However, chest pain significantly diminished during *both* placebo and nifedipine treatment periods, suggesting that symptom improvement was unrelated to the decline in esophageal pressures. The only placebo controlled trial of nifedipine in patients with diffuse esophageal spasm also revealed no benefit from active treatment.

Calcium channel blockers may be useful in patients with esophageal motility disorders, but they probably need to be combined with other therapies, or used when pain episodes show a clear relationship with simultaneously recorded abnormal esophageal contractions. Until these subsets can be easily defined, I recommend a trial of a calcium channel blocker in patients with more severe, recurrent chest pain. I prefer to start with nifedipine, 10 mg before meals and at bedtime. The dosage can be increased as needed, although side effects (headaches and dizziness) are common.

Hydralazine

One study investigated the effects of the smooth muscle-relaxing agent hydralazine (Apresoline) on esophageal contractions. Although this drug did not affect the resting contraction pressures in the esophageal body, it did diminish the pressure response to cholinergic stimulation with bethanechol. Further studies in three patients with esophageal spasm who were given hydralazine, 25 to 50 mg orally three times a day, appeared to produce a meaningful degree of symptom improvement. Unfortunately, this study was not placebo controlled, and therefore true efficacy is uncertain. My experience with this drug has been limited, but it appears to be less useful than the previously mentioned smooth muscle relaxants.

Esophageal Dilation

If the medical regimens described above fail to alleviate most of the symptoms, esophageal dilation may be necessary. Anecdotally, many physicians find that the passage of a mercury-filled dilator temporarily relieves dysphagia and chest pain in some patients with esophageal motility disorders. However, the available studies demonstrate conflicting results from bougienage. One preliminary report from the Ochsner Clinic suggested that some degree of relief can be obtained following dilation in up to 83 percent of patients. However, studies from my laboratory found that bougie dilation produces some relief of symptoms, but similar responses can be obtained with either a large dilator (54 French) or a much smaller one (24 French). Hence, the therapeutic effect of dilation is likely a placebo response. At any rate, some patients do experience symptomatic improvement for variable periods of time after dilation. In these patients, my approach is to repeat the procedure as often as needed, the frequency being dictated by the symptoms.

Pneumatic dilation has been used in severely symptomatic patients with diffuse esophageal spasm, especially when dysphagia is the dominant symptom. In this situation, one may be treating an early transitional phase of diffuse esophageal spasm into achalasia. I suggest reserving this therapy for patients with intractable symptoms in whom a delay in distal esophageal emptying can be documented. I have seen dramatic relief of dysphagia but not of chest pain after pneumatic dilation. However, one must consider the morbidity and risks involved in this procedure. Esophageal perforation may occur after 2 to 10 percent of pneumatic dilations.

Esophageal Myotomy

In my experience, refractory esophageal chest pain is exceedingly rare. Only an occasional patient with severe symptoms and a compromised lifestyle requires a long esophageal myotomy. This procedure involves a left thoracotomy, which exposes the distal two-thirds of the esophagus and the LES. The myotomy is carried out with an incision beginning just proximal to the LES and extending toward the mouth to include the manometrically defined area of dysmotility. The procedure is based on the premise that abnormal motility is directly leading to the patient's symptoms, particularly chest pain. However, this simplistic hypothesis is not generally supported by the available data. Ellis, who has published on this subject for over 30 years, recently reviewed his experience with painful esophageal motility disorders treated by esophageal myotomy and followed for 5 years. Seventy percent of patients were improved, but only 50 percent had complete relief of pain. Unfortunately, these patients may develop postoperative acid reflux and subsequent acid-induced pain. Therefore, some authors advocate an antireflux procedure with the myotomy, which may add to the morbidity of the operation. The difficulties associated with surgical treatment of esophageal motility disorders other than achalasia has been emphasized by DeMeester: "The creation of a defect to correct a defect can never restore the function of an organ to normal."

Reassurance

Despite the major technical and pharmacologic advancements in medicine, it is disturbing that beneficial therapies for painful esophageal motility disorders have been slow in evolving. Nevertheless, we should not despair, because clinical experience and long-term follow-up studies suggest that most of these patients do well. However, it may be that a strong patient-physician relationship based on careful diagnostic studies offers patients the most help. Many patients improve after learning that their symptoms are not due to cardiac disease but are caused by an esophageal condition. My group has observed that this supportive approach results in better patient acceptance of their symptoms, less limitation in lifestyle, and frequently a decrease or resolution of chest pain. Considering that other therapies are often less than satisfactory, with frequent side effects, reassurance during office visits and telephone conversations may be the simplest, safest, and most cost-effective approach to these patients. In our zeal to diagnose and treat esophageal motility disorders, we must always remember to see the patient, not just the esophagus.

SUGGESTED READING

Clouse RE, Lustman PJ, Eckert TC, et al. Low-dose trazodone for symptomatic patients with esophageal contraction abnormalities. A double-blind, placebo-controlled trial. Gastroenterology 1987; 92:1027–1036.

Ellis FH, Crozier RE, Shea JA. Long esophagomyotomy for diffuse esophageal spasm and related disorders. In: Siewert JR, Holscher AH, eds. Diseases of the esophagus: pathophysiology, diagnosis, conservative and surgical treatment. New York: Springer-Verlag, 1988: 913.

DeMeester TR. Surgery for esophageal motor disorders. Ann Thorac Surg 1982:34:225–226.

Richter JE, Castell DO. Esophageal disease as a cause of noncardiac chest pain. Adv Intern Med 1988; 33:311–336.

Richter JE, Dalton CB, Bradley LA, Castell DO. Oral nifedipine in the treatment of non-cardiac chest pain in patients with the nutcracker esophagus. Gastroenterology 1987; 93:21–28.

GASTRIC ULCER

WALTER P. DYCK, M.D.

The precise pathogenetic mechanisms responsible for gastric ulcer disease remain unknown. "Aggressive" factors (such as acid and pepsin) and a disturbance of "protective" factors (such as gastric mucus, secreted bicarbonate, and an intact microvasculature) undoubtedly both play a role in the pathogenesis of duodenal as well as gastric ulcer disease. However, evidence suggests that aggressive factors play a more prominent role in the causation of duodenal ulcers, whereas impaired defense mechanisms are of greater importance in gastric ulcer formation. Such evidence includes (1) the demonstration that patients with duodenal ulcer exhibit higher mean basal and stimulated acid secretory values than do demographically matched healthy control subjects, while patients with gastric ulcer have lower mean secretory values than do healthy controls; and (2) the observation that agents that disrupt gastric epithelial integrity, such as nonsteroidal anti-inflammatory drugs (NSAIDs) and salicylates, play a significant role in the production of gastric ulcers, but are of relatively little importance in duodenal ulcer disease.

CLINICAL PRESENTATION

The symptoms and signs of gastric ulcer disease are usually quite similar to those ascribed to duodenal ulcers. The most common initial complaint is upper abdominal pain, which may lack the periodicity and pain–food–relief pattern so common in duodenal ulcer disease. Bleeding is a less common presenting event. In contrast to patients with duodenal ulcer disease, patients with gastric ulcer may experience anorexia, exacerbation of symptoms with food ingestion, and weight loss. Thus, the nature of the symptoms alone does not permit a confident differentiation between a benign gastric ulcer and a gastric neoplasm.

EVALUATION

Peptic ulcers are usually first identified radiographically, although endoscopy is increasingly being used as the initial diagnostic procedure for the assessment of "dyspepsia." Radiographic identification of a duodenal ulcer does not require endoscopic assessment, but endoscopic evaluation of a gastric ulcer has come to be considered the standard approach. It is important, however, to recognize the complementary nature of these two diagnostic modalities in defining a cost-effective approach to the diagnosis and follow-up of gastric ulcers. In a retrospective study at the University of Utah, a 3-year experience was reviewed in which endoscopy was used as the initial method of evaluation in 96 percent of patients, but follow-up was performed by either a combination of endoscopy and double-contrast upper gastrointestinal (GI) series or endoscopy alone. In this limited experience, the authors found that selection of one diagnostic and follow-up modality over the other had no effect on survival. They then constructed an algorithm in which endoscopy would be used only when an upper GI series yielded equivocal or suspicious results, or when inadequate healing followed a therapeutic trial. Retrospective application of such an algorithm to their cases resulted in a theoretical net savings of 55 percent. On the basis of such a cost efficacy analysis, it is difficult to justify the stance of many that x-ray studies no longer have a place in the assessment and follow-up of gastric ulcer disease. Conversely, few would question that endoscopy is a more precise and accurate method for the evaluation of gastric ulcers. It is for this reason that I, like many others, consider endoscopy to be the preferable approach except for relatively young patients who have been on ulcerogenic drugs and whose upper GI series yield an unequivocally benign radiographic interpretation. For such patients I consider it acceptable to treat them for 6 to 8 weeks and follow this with an x-ray examiniation or endoscopy to ensure complete healing. All other gastric ulcers deserve initial endoscopic assessment to include multiple biopsies of the ulcer margin (and base) with follow-up endoscopy at 6- to 8-week intervals until complete healing has occurred. My suspicion is that socioeconomic trends will have the effect of bringing endoscopy fees closer to x-ray fees in the near future, and this will probably result in endoscopy being appropriately used almost exclusively in the assessment and follow-up of gastric ulcer disease.

TREATMENT

Drug therapy for gastric ulcer disease is similar to that for duodenal ulcers. On theoretical grounds, one would expect agents that promote mucosal protection to be most useful in the treatment of gastric ulcers, while therapeutic approaches directed against acid and pepsin might be expected to be less effective than for the treatment of duodenal ulcers. In reality, however, H_2-receptor antagonists have been shown to be highly effective in promoting gastric ulcer healing, and currently represent the most popular form of therapy for both duodenal and gastric ulcers. Because of better patient compliance and dosing convenience, I usually recommend one of these agents in preference to antacids; the latter, however, remains an acceptable and effective alternative form of therapy.

Antacids

On the basis of the studies of Fordtran in the 1960s, the concept developed that in order for antacids to promote ulcer healing effectively, they must be given seven times daily in doses adequate to neutralize 120 mEq of HCl. Such a regimen, in which a potent antacid such as Maalox or Mylanta is given in doses of 30 ml 1 and 3 hours after meals and at bedtime, continues to be the accepted form of antacid therapy for both duodenal and gastric ulcer disease. Such doses of antacids have been proved effective in promoting duodenal ulcer healing and in preventing relapse. Similar data are not available for gastric ulcer disease. Emerging evidence suggests that much smaller doses of antacid may be equally effective in promoting duodenal ulcer healing, and it might be anticipated that this would be particularly applicable to gastric ulcer disease where hyperacidity does not exist.

Side Effects

A large variety of potent, low-sodium antacids exist, and the clinician should become familiar with a few agents and be aware of their side effects. Magnesium preparations such as Maalox and Mylanta may cause diarrhea; aluminum antacids such as Amphojel tend to produce constipation. Both magnesium and aluminum preparations may cause phosphorus depletion with hypophosphatemia, weakness, and malaise. The same antacids can interfere with the absorption of drugs such as tetracycline through adsorption; also, by increasing the gastric pH, they can alter drug solubility and thereby interfere with the absorption of a variety of drugs, including salicylates and barbiturates, while enhancing the absorption of others. A very low-sodium preparation such as Riopan may be used in patients in whom sodium retention might be expected to present problems.

Antacids are effective for both ulcer healing and pain relief, but no good correlation exists between the two responses. Furthermore, antacids and placebo have been shown to produce similar pain relief in patients with duodenal ulcer, which suggests that factors other than acid neutralization or ulcer healing are responsible for the relief of ulcer pain obtained by antacid use.

Parietal Cell Inhibitors

Drugs may interfere with parietal cell secretion of acid by (1) blocking the parietal cell receptor site for a secretory agonist (e.g., H_2-receptor antagonists, anticholinergics, antigastrin analogues); (2) interfering with intracellular transport processes; or (3) inhibiting the hydrogen-potassium ATPase "pump" enzyme that facilitates the exit of hydrogen ion from the parietal cell to the gastric lumen.

H_2-Receptor Blockers

Of the inhibitors of parietal cell function, H_2-receptor antagonists have been by far the most extensively studied and have gained wide clinical use. The oldest of these agents, cimetidine, has been shown to be effective in healing gastric ulcers in several large studies, with healing rates approaching 85 percent by 8 weeks of treatment. The initial recommended dosage was 300 mg four times daily, but subsequent studies in duodenal ulcer disease suggested that 400 mg twice daily or 800 mg once daily as a nighttime dose was equally effective. It now appears that the suppression of nocturnal acid secretion is the most important factor in promoting ulcer healing, and therefore the single nighttime dose of 800 mg is usually given.

Newer, more potent H_2-receptor antagonists have been developed and approved, including ranitidine (150 mg twice a day or 300 mg at bedtime), famotidine (40 mg at bedtime), and nizatidine (300 mg at bedtime). There is no convincing evidence that these newer and more potent H_2 blockers are more effective than the earlier agents, and I do not have a clear preference for one over another except in patients who require multiple other medicines. For these I prefer to use a drug that has less effect on the hepatic cytochrome P-450 enzyme system (ranitidine, famotidine, or nizatidine) than does cimetidine.

Substituted Benzimidazoles

This group of drugs can effectively block parietal cell function and produce achlorhydria by inhibiting the hydrogen-potassium ATPase "proton pump." Omeprazole, the prototype that has been studied extensively, has proved highly effective in promoting duodenal ulcer healing, particularly in hypersecretory states such as the Zollinger-Ellison syndrome. The development of carcinoid tumors in a large number of experimental animals may limit the future application of this drug. It is not likely to be promoted for use in the treatment of gastric ulcer disease.

Drugs That Promote Mucosal Protection

Sucralfate

For patients in whom gastric ulcer disease is accompanied by evidence of a more diffuse mucosal inflammation such as bile or drug-associated gastritis, I tend to use sucralfate, a chemical complex of aluminum hydroxide and sulfated sucrose, in an attempt to promote epithelial regeneration. In a Swedish multicenter double-blind trial comparing a 12-week course of cimetidine with sucralfate, healing rates of 92 percent and 87 percent, respectively, were achieved. Symptom relief and ulcer recurrence did not differ for the two treatment groups. This agent was formerly thought to exert its beneficial effect by "coating" the ulcer base and thus forming a protective barrier, but it now appears that the mechanism of action may involve the stimulation of factors such as prostaglandins, which in turn promote improved mucosal integrity and enhance epithelial regeneration.

Prostaglandin Analogues

The availability of prostaglandin analogues for clinical testing was greeted with great enthusiasm in view of their efficacy in preventing gastric ulceration in a variety of experimental settings. Overall, these agents proved disappointing, largely because of the unacceptable side effects encountered with their use. However, one such agent, misoprostil (Cytotec), has now been examined in several multicenter trials and found to possess efficacy similar to that of cimetidine in dosages of 300 mg four times a day to treat gastric ulcer. It has also proved relatively free of side effects and has been approved for clinical use in the United States to prevent erosions and ulcerations due to the use of NSAIDs. The recommended dosage for this purpose is 200 mcg four times a day. Starting slowly and dosing with meals appears to lessen the main side effects of cramps and diarrhea.

Other Factors

An important point to emphasize is the need to advise patients to avoid the further use of NSAIDs, particularly in the elderly patients in whom there is a strong association between the use of these agents and gastric ulcer disease. When the continued use of potentially ulcerogenic drugs is unavoidable, I favor maintenance therapy with an agent such as sucralfate. At the moment, misoprostil has just been approved by the Food and Drug Administration for this purpose. Since many older women with NSAID-associated gastric ulcers have no GI symptoms before presenting with hemorrhage, it is difficult to know which patients on NSAIDs, besides those with a history of peptic ulcer, should receive "prophylactic" medications (sucralfate or misoprostil).

Smoking has been shown to interfere with the healing of duodenal ulcers and to increase the risk of recurrence. It appears that smoking exerts a similar adverse effect on gastric ulcer healing and recurrence rates, although this has been less well documented. Small to modest amounts of alcoholic beverage consumption do not appear to have an adverse effect on ulcer healing or recurrence rate.

ASSESSMENT OF THERAPEUTIC RESPONSE

A point that cannot be emphasized too strongly is that *all gastric ulcers must be followed to complete healing* in order to be sure of their benign nature. My approach is to treat with a therapeutic agent such as an H_2-receptor antagonist for 6 to 8 weeks and then assess healing endoscopically. If the patient has responded with symptomatic relief, but the ulcer is incompletely healed although still benign appearing and of smaller size, treatment is continued and endoscopic reevaluation scheduled after 6 to 8 more weeks. If there appears to have been no decrease in ulcer size after the initial 8 weeks of treatment or if there is incomplete healing after an additional 8 weeks of treatment, and there are no obvious contributing factors such as the use of ulcerogenic drugs, surgical intervention is usually called for.

In giant gastric ulcers and chronic recurrent ulcers, there is a higher incidence of complications, including perforation and bleeding. These are particularly prone to show a poor response to drug therapy and are more likely to require surgery.

Editor's Note: NSAID-associated erosions and ulcerations in the stomach are reaching epidemic proportions as increasing numbers of the population grow older and take these agents. It is estimated that there is a yearly bleeding or perforation rate of 2 to 4 percent among patients with rheumatoid arthritis. Half of the bleeders had a history of peptic ulcer disease and half had a history of GI bleeding. Other risk factors included age (patients over 60), smoking, and female gender. It is important to note that most patients with erosions or ulcerations had no GI symptoms. To date, only misoprostil has been approved by the FDA for prevention of NSAID-induced erosions or ulcerations. However, some physicians are prescribing sucralfate in an attempt to prevent erosions and ulcerations, even with a minimum of supporting data.

SUGGESTED READING

Adkins RB, DeLozier JB, Scott HW, et al. The management of gastric ulcers: a current review. Ann Surg 1985; 201:741–751.

Armington WG, Mann FA, Nelson JA. Cost-effective means of diagnosing and following benign and malignant gastric ulcers. Invest Radiol 1985; 20:171–176.

Glise H, Carlings L, Hallerback B, et al. Treatment of peptic ulcers—acid reduction or cytoprotection? Scand J Gastroenterol (Suppl) 1987; 140:39–47.

Graham DY, Akdamar K, Dyck WP, et al. Healing of benign gastric ulcer: comparison of cimetidine and placebo in the United States. Ann Intern Med 1985; 102:573–576.

Howden CW, Jones DB, Peacke KE, et al. The treatment of gastric ulcer with antisecretory drugs. Relationship of pharmacological effect to healing rates. Dig Dis Sci 1988; 33:619–624.

Rachmilewitz D. Efficacy of prostanoids in the treatment of gastric ulcer. Clin Invest Med 1987; 10:238–242.

Rydning A, Weberg R, Lange O, et al. Healing of benign gastric ulcer with low-dose antacids and fiber diet. Gastroenterology 1986; 91:56–61.

DUODENAL ULCER

CHARLES T. RICHARDSON, M.D.

Duodenal ulcer disease is a relatively common disorder. Estimates indicate that approximately 200,000 to 400,000 new patients are diagnosed each year with duodenal ulcers in the United States. Duodenal ulcers were originally believed to be caused exclusively by the aggressive action of hydrochloric acid and pepsin on the duodenal mucosa, but only 30 to 40 percent of patients with duodenal ulcer disease have acid secretion rates above the upper limits of normal. The remainder have acid secretion rates in the normal range. Although this does not prove that these patients develop ulcers because of factors other than increased acid secretion, it suggests that there may be other causes. Currently, it is believed that duodenal ulcers represent a heterogeneous group of disorders. Most patients develop a duodenal ulcer because of either too much acid and pepsin secretion or decreased mucosal defense, but other mechanisms such as emotional stress, hereditary factors, or perhaps *Campylobacter pylori* may play a role.

Pain, usually localized to the epigastric region, is the most common symptom of duodenal ulcers. Some patients do not experience pain even though they have an active ulcer crater, and bleeding from a duodenal ulcer occurs occasionally in patients who are asymptomatic. Elderly individuals are more prone to asymptomatic active duodenal ulcers. The physical examination is usually normal in patients with duodenal ulcer disease.

Patients rarely have a single occurrence of duodenal ulcer. Controlled clinical trials in which patients with duodenal ulcers have been treated with an active medication or a placebo, and endoscoped before and after therapy, have added greatly to our knowledge of the natural history of duodenal ulcer disease. The results of these studies demonstrate that once an ulcer is healed by therapy, it recurs in 50 to 80 percent of patients during the 6 to 12 months after initial healing. Some of these patients may require maintenance medical therapy to prevent recurrence (see below).

TREATMENT

The goals of ulcer therapy are to relieve symptoms, heal craters, prevent recurrences, and prevent complications. Even though there may be different causes of duodenal ulcers in individual patients, medical therapy is the same for most. It includes treatment with one or a combination of the following: (1) a drug that reduces gastric acidity by either inhibiting acid secretion or neutralizing acid; (2) a drug that coats ulcer craters and prevents acid and pepsin from reaching the ulcer base; (3) a prostaglandin analogue; (4) removal of environmental factors, such as nonsteroidal anti-inflammatory drugs (NSAIDs) and cigarette smoking; and (5) reduction in emotional stress in some patients.

Drugs That Reduce Gastric Acidity

Drugs reduce gastric acidity either by inhibiting acid secretion or by neutralizing acid. Drugs that inhibit acid secretion include H_2-receptor antagonists; anticholinergic or antimuscarinic drugs that block the muscarinic receptor on parietal cells; and the experimental compound omeprazole, which inhibits the hydrogen-potassium ATPase enzyme (proton pump) located on the luminal surface of parietal cells.

H_2-Receptor Antagonists

Histamine causes acid secretion by acting on a receptor on the gastric parietal cell. H_2-receptor antagonists block the action of histamine on this receptor and reduce acid secretion. Presently, four H_2-receptor antagonists are available for use in treating patients with duodenal ulcer disease (Table 1). Acid secretion is decreased effectively by each of these compounds, although they differ in structure and potency. Cimetidine contains an imidazole ring, ranitidine contains a furan ring, and famotidine and nizatidine contain a thiazole ring. Famotidine is the most potent of the four drugs on a molar basis. Ranitidine and nizatidine are equally potent and are approximately five to six times more potent than cimetidine. Side effects have occurred more frequently with cimetidine than with the other H_2-receptor antagonists. However, each of these agents is relatively safe, and the possibility of side effects should not be a factor in choosing between H_2-receptor antagonists. The *Physicians' Desk*

TABLE 1 Drugs Commonly Used to Treat Patients With Duodenal Ulcer Disease

		Treatment of Active Ulcers		*Maintenance Therapy*	
Generic Name	*Trade Name*	*Dosages for Adults (mg, ml, or g/day)*	*Frequency of Administration (times/day)*	*Dosages for Adults (mg, ml, or g/day)*	*Frequency of Administration (times/day)*
Drugs That Inhibit Acid Secretion					
H_2-Receptor Antagonists					
Cimetidine	Tagamet	300 mg	With each meal and at bedtime (four times daily)	400 mg	At bedtime
		400 mg	Twice daily, in morning and at bedtime		
		800 mg	Once daily at bedtime		
Ranitidine	Zantac	150 mg	Twice daily, in morning and at bedtime	150 mg	At bedtime
		300 mg	Once daily at bedtime		
Famotidine	Pepcid	40 mg	Once daily at bedtime	20 mg	At bedtime
Nizatidine	Axid	300 mg	Once daily at bedtime	150 mg	At bedtime
Drugs That Coat Ulcer Craters					
Sucralfate	Carafate	1 g	Four times daily		
Drugs That Neutralize Acid					
Antacids	*	30 ml	1 and 3 hr after meals and at bedtime		

* A number of antacids are available. See Peterson and Richardson (Suggested Reading) for the relative potencies of some antacids.

Reference or the drug package insert should be consulted for a complete list of side effects from each compound.

The effect of each of the four H_2-receptor antagonists on healing of duodenal ulcers has been evaluated and compared with placebo therapy in a number of controlled clinical trials. In most of these studies the active compound has been shown to be more effective than placebo in healing duodenal ulcers. For cimetidine, there are three dosages from which to choose; for ranitidine, there are two (Table 1). For famotidine and nizatidine, one regimen each is available.

With any of the four drugs or any of the dosage regimens, the incidence of duodenal ulcer healing is approximately the same. Bedtime dosages are desirable in treating most patients because patient compliance is probably better with single, daily-dose therapy than with multiple-doses. In choosing one of the four drugs or dosage regimens, the cost is one of the most important factors; it often differs among pharmacies or hospitals. Thus, physicians should determine the cost of the drugs in their particular area and select the most cost-effective regimen.

Pain from ulcer disease usually subsides within 1 or 2 weeks of the initiation of therapy. However, patients with active ulcers should be treated for 4 to 6 weeks. If at the end of 6 weeks of therapy a particular patient is asymptomatic, treatment should be stopped. No repeat barium x-ray study or upper gastrointestinal (GI) endoscopy is necessary to document healing of duodenal ulcers. Some patients require maintenance medical therapy (see below) to prevent recurrent ulcer disease.

Anticholinergic (Antimuscarinic) Drugs

These compounds reduce acid secretion by blocking the acetylcholine receptor on gastric parietal cells. The drugs also block muscarinic receptors in other parts of the body, and as a result cause side effects such as dry mouth, blurred vision, and urinary retention, which limit the amount of drug that can be given to humans. Consequently, the dosages that can be prescribed are not enough to reduce gastric acid secretion effectively. Thus, these agents are not recommended as first-line treatment for patients with ulcers. They sometimes are used in combination with an H_2-receptor antagonist in treating refractory ulcer disease or markedly elevated gastric acid secretion. The dosage is usually one tablet of a compound such as propantheline bromide (Pro-Banthine) or glycopyrrolate (Robinul) with meals and at bedtime.

Omeprazole

This compound is a member of a family of drugs called "substituted benzimidazoles," which inactivate a hydrogen-potassium ATPase enzyme located on the luminal surface of parietal cells. This enzyme is a proton pump that is the final step in hydrogen ion secretion from parietal cells. Acid secretion is markedly reduced when this enzyme is inactivated. Omeprazole is undergoing clinical evaluation in the United States and Europe and has been shown to be very effective in healing duodenal ulcers. Because of its ability to dramatically inhibit acid secretion, the drug is useful in treating patients with the Zollinger-Ellison syndrome. One daily dose is often adequate to treat this disease, even though there may be very high rates of acid secretion. See also the chapter *Gastric Cancer.*

Enterochromaffin-like cell hyperplasia and carcinoid tumors have developed in the stomachs of female rats treated with omeprazole. This was likely related to markedly elevated serum gastrin concentrations that occurred as a result of prolonged achlorhydria caused by the doses of omeprazole given. Whether this observation in rats will apply to humans is not known; if so, the usefulness of the drug in humans may be limited.

Antacids

These compounds reduce gastric acidity (increase intragastric pH) because of a chemical reaction between the ingredients of antacids and hydrochloric acid. Various antacids differ in their ability to neutralize acid, owing to the relative proportions of chemical constituents and differences in manufacturing techniques.

A liquid antacid in doses of 30 ml 1 and 3 hours after meals and at bedtime (Table 1) has been shown to be more effective than placebo in healing duodenal ulcers. In another controlled clinical trial, liquid antacid was demonstrated to be as effective as cimetidine in healing duodenal ulcers. Even though results of these studies have shown liquid antacid to be effective in healing ulcers, the amount of antacid necessary to achieve healing was relatively large. Also, the doses were given seven times daily. Because of the large amount of antacid and the frequency of administration believed necessary to heal ulcers, antacids are not recommended as first-line medication in treating most duodenal ulcers. Antacids are recommended in combination with an H_2-receptor antagonist or sucralfate in patients with persistent ulcers that do not heal with either of the above medications given alone.

Diarrhea is the major side effect of antacids and is caused by magnesium hydroxide, which most antacids contain. It can be prevented by alternating an antacid containing only aluminum hydroxide with one that contains both aluminum and magnesium hydroxides.

Drugs That Coat Ulcer Craters

Sucralfate (Carafate)

The exact mechanism of action of this drug is uncertain. The compound is believed to coat ulcer craters and form a shield that protects the crater from acid and pepsin. Results of studies performed in animals suggest that sucralfate may stimulate prostaglandin synthesis from gastric mucosa, and thus enhance mucosal defense. Sucralfate is significantly more effective than placebo and as effective as cimetidine in healing duodenal ulcers. The usual dose is 1 g four times daily (Table 1). Patients should be treated for 4 to 6 weeks.

Since sucralfate is absorbed poorly from the GI tract, systemic side effects are rare. Constipation occurs in some patients treated with sucralfate.

Bismuth Compounds

De-Nol (tripotassium dicitratobismuthate) is a bismuth compound which is not available in the United States but is obtainable in other countries. De-Nol coats ulcer craters and protects craters from acid and pepsin. Results of controlled clinical trials indicate that De-Nol is effective in healing duodenal ulcers. It has been suggested that bismuth compounds such as De-Nol may lead to ulcer healing in some patients because of their bactericidal effect on *Campylobacter pylori*. Additional studies are needed to prove or disprove this hypothesis.

Prostaglandin Analogues

These compounds probably lead to ulcer healing by two mechanisms. They enhance mucosal defense in the stomach and duodenum, and also inhibit acid secretion. Several prostaglandin analogues are currently being evaluated for treating duodenal ulcers. One compound, misoprostol, has been approved for use in the United States.*

Combination Drug Therapy

More than one drug is required in some patients to heal ulcers or relieve the symptoms. A second drug is usually added if symptoms persist after 2 to 3 weeks of therapy with a single drug. If a patient is treated initially with an H_2-receptor antagonist or sucralfate, the addition of an antacid or an antimuscarinic drug may be indicated. The inhibitory effect on acid secretion of H_2-receptor antagonists can be enhanced and prolonged by giving an antimuscarinic drug. This presumably occurs because both the histamine and muscarinic (acetylcholine) receptors on parietal cells are blocked simultaneously. Combining an H_2-receptor antagonist and an antimuscarinic drug can be useful in treating patients with basal acid hypersecretory states such as the Zollinger-Ellison syndrome or systemic mastocytosis.

INDICATIONS FOR MAINTENANCE MEDICAL THERAPY

Some patients require chronic therapy with an H_2-receptor antagonist, although chronic therapy is not indicated in all cases of duodenal ulcer disease. Prolonged therapy is indicated for patients with two to three recurrences of duodenal ulcer per year and those who have had a complication of ulcer disease, such as bleeding, perforation, penetration, or obstruction. Patients who are elderly and have a medical condition such as severe coronary artery disease, pulmonary disease, renal disease, or arthritis in addition to ulcer disease should also be considered candidates for maintenance medical therapy with an H_2-receptor antagonist. Duodenal ulcer patients with severe, debilitating arthritis who must take NSAIDs may also be candidates for maintenance medical therapy with an H_2-receptor antagonist or sucralfate. Some data support the use of H_2-receptor antagonists, sucralfate, or prostaglandin analogues to prevent recurrent ulceration in patients with severe arthritis who must continue to take NSAIDs. However, additional information is needed to evaluate adequately the role of H_2-receptor antagonists, sucralfate, or prostaglandin analogues in the long-term (prophylactic) therapy of patients requiring NSAIDs.†

When an H_2-receptor antagonist is prescribed for chronic maintenance therapy, lower dosages than those used in treating patients with active disease should be given. For example, 400 mg of cimetidine, 150 mg of ranitidine, 20 mg of famotidine, or 150 mg of nizatidine are usually taken at bedtime. Once maintenance therapy is initiated, there are no data to indicate how long it should be continued. In elderly patients the drug probably should be continued for life. In younger patients the drug should be taken for several years and then discontinued. Patients can then be observed for recurrence, and maintenance therapy reinstituted if ulcers develop again. This is a suggested approach and is not based on results of controlled clinical trials.

OTHER FACTORS TO CONSIDER IN TREATING DUODENAL ULCER PATIENTS

Nonsteroidal Anti-inflammatory Drugs

There is no convincing data to indicate that these compounds cause duodenal ulcers. However, since NSAIDs are known to inhibit prostaglandin synthesis and cause damage to the gastric mucosa, it seems reasonable to assume that they also may damage the duodenal mucosa. Additionally, there is a possibility that these drugs may contribute to complications such as bleeding or perforation in a few patients. For these reasons I recommend that patients discontinue NSAIDs, especially while an active ulcer is present. Some ulcer patients have such debilitating arthritis that they must continue to take NSAIDs. As stated previously, these patients probably should be treated with maintenance medical therapy with an H_2-receptor antagonist, sucralfate, or a prostaglandin analogue.

Alcohol and Caffeine-Containing Beverages

There is no evidence that alcohol intake contributes to the pathogenesis of duodenal ulcer disease. However, it seems reasonable to advise patients with duodenal ulcer to drink in moderation, especially while an ulcer is active. There also are no data to support eliminating the intake of caffeine-containing beverages, especially since coffee without caffeine stimulates acid secretion to approximately the same extent as caffeine-containing coffee.

---

* **Editor's Note:** Misoprostol has been approved by the FDA as prophylactic and therapeutic for NSAID-associated gastric erosions and ulcerations.

† **Editor's Note:** At present, such "prophylactic" therapy with NSAIDs would cost about $1,000 per year.

Cigarette Smoking

This has not been shown to be important in the pathogenesis of duodenal ulcer disease, but there is an epidemiologic association between smoking and ulceration. For example, patients with ulcers smoke more frequently than do patients without ulcers or normal individuals. Also, duodenal ulcers heal less well in patients who smoke than in nonsmokers, and recur more commonly in patients who smoke than in those who do not smoke. The death rate is higher among patients who smoke than among nonsmokers. Thus, patients with duodenal ulcer disease should be advised to stop smoking cigarettes.

Reduction of Emotional Stress

The exact role of emotional stress in the pathogenesis of duodenal ulcer disease is uncertain. Some data indicate that ulcer patients react to stress differently from control patients. For example, the results of one study showed that hospitalized duodenal ulcer patients perceived life events more negatively than control patients who were admitted to the hospital with gallstones or kidney stones. The results of another study indicated that the level of anxiety in some ulcer patients may affect their response to medical therapy. In this study, 17 of the patients who had moderate to severe anxiety, as determined by an interview, had persistent ulcer pain 6 months after treatment for an active ulcer. Only four of 36 patients without anxiety at the time of acute ulceration had persistent ulcer pain 6 months after therapy.

Reduction of emotional stress in patients with duodenal ulcer disease is a reasonable therapeutic goal. This can be accomplished best by establishing a good relationship between the patient and the personal physician. The physician should be willing to establish such a relationship and to talk with patients about their anxieties. There is no evidence that psychotherapy with a psychiatrist is useful in treating patients with ulcers.

Diet

There is no evidence that special diets reduce gastric acidity to a greater extent than does a regular diet. Several controlled clinical trials have shown that bland food and regular food have similar effects on the clinical course of peptic ulcers. Patients should be told to eat three meals a day from a diet of their own choosing. If certain foods cause symptoms, they should be avoided.

COMPLICATIONS

Bleeding from a duodenal ulcer occurs in 15 to 20 percent of patients and is the most common complication of duodenal ulcer disease. Initially, bleeding from an ulcer should be treated medically, although surgery may be indicated in patients who continue to bleed, or those who are hospitalized for bleeding and rebleed in the hospital.

Perforation into the abdominal cavity is another complication of duodenal ulcer disease. Perforation of an ulcer causes severe abdominal pain; the diagnosis can be suspected by the finding of free air under the diaphragm on an upright chest film. Usually, perforation is an indication for immediate surgery.

Ulcers can also penetrate into other organs such as the pancreas, liver, biliary tract, or colon. Patients with penetrating ulcers sometimes develop persistent or intractable pain, either as a result of the ulcer per se, or from pancreatitis that has developed because of the penetration. Penetration is treated medically at first with an H_2-receptor antagonist and antacid. The usual dosage of H_2-receptor antagonist is prescribed, and antacids are given every hour while the patient is awake. Nasogastric suction may be helpful in some patients.

If a duodenal ulcer occurs near the pylorus, it may cause edema and scarring of the pylorus. This leads to gastric outlet obstruction, which in turn may result in nausea and vomiting. Patients usually vomit food that they have eaten 10 to 12 hours before the vomiting episode. Weight loss may be the earliest sign of pyloric obstruction. Obstruction is treated by decompressing the stomach with nasogastric suction and prescribing an H_2-receptor antagonist to be given intravenously. Endoscopy should be performed after the nasogastric tube has been in place for several days. It is important to differentiate between pyloric obstruction and a motility disorder of the stomach as the cause of delayed gastric emptying. It also is important to determine whether a benign process such as duodenal ulcer disease is causing obstruction, or whether gastric cancer in the prepyloric region is the cause of outlet obstruction. In some patients with outlet obstruction secondary to ulcer disease, the obstruction resolves with medical therapy. Anticholinergic (antimuscarinic) drugs may theoretically worsen gastric outlet obstruction. Surgery is necessary in patients who do not respond to medical therapy.

SUGGESTED READING

Grossman MI, ed. Peptic ulcer. A guide for the practicing physician. Chicago: Year Book, 1981.

Hawkey CJ, Ramptom DS. Prostaglandins and the gastrointestinal mucosa: are they important in its function, disease, or treatment? Gastroenterology 1985; 89:1162–1188.

Lauritsen K, Rune SJ, Bytzer P, et al. Effect of omeprazole and cimetidine on duodenal ulcer. N Engl J Med 1985; 312:958–961.

Peterson WL, Richardson CT. Pharmacology and side effects of drugs used to treat peptic ulcer. In: Sleisenger MH, Fordtran JS, eds. Gastrointestinal disease: pathophysiology, diagnosis, management. 3rd ed. Philadelphia: WB Saunders, 1983:708.

Soll AH. Duodenal ulcer disease. In: Sleisenger MH, Fordtran JS, eds. Gastrointestinal disease. 4th ed. Philadelphia: WB Saunders, 1988:814.

UPPER GASTROINTESTINAL BLEEDING

MICHAEL V. SIVAK Jr., M.D., F.A.C.P., F.A.C.G.

CLINICAL PROBLEM

The mortality rate for upper gastrointestinal (UGI) bleeding has remained constant at about 10 percent over the past 4 decades. However, the patient population with UGI hemorrhage now includes more individuals over 60 years of age and more with coexistent diseases, so that our methods of diagnosis and treatment may be more satisfactory than is immediately evident from the statistical data.

GI bleeding is becoming less frequent as a primary reason for hospitalization. Treatment methods appear to be altering the natural history of certain common disorders. For example, the acute onset of bleeding from a peptic ulcer in an otherwise healthy individual may be less common. Although uncomplicated UGI bleeding is a less frequent clinical problem, bleeding in association with other unrelated disorders, and especially the treatment of such disorders, is becoming more familiar.

UGI bleeding can occur after virtually any complex surgical procedure of either an elective or an emergency nature. Bleeding from the upper digestive tract may occur in association with extensive trauma. Certain therapeutic measures, such as anticoagulation, may facilitate bleeding. Patients with UGI bleeding associated with another serious condition often have only a limited ability to withstand hemodynamic stress and its effects on cardiovascular and renal function. Prompt control of the bleeding is always desirable in such patients, but the therapeutic options for achieving hemostasis may be restricted if the risks of general anesthesia and surgery are prohibitive.

UGI bleeding is a secondary manifestation of diverse GI disorders. Despite the heterogeneous nature of the lesions that are responsible for bleeding, blood loss stops spontaneously in about 75 to 85 percent of episodes. Approximately one-quarter of patients do not require transfusion. Therefore, general supportive measures are sufficient for most patients. However, there is a smaller subset of patients in whom bleeding is persistent, severe, and apt to be recurrent.

About 15 to 20 percent of patients with UGI bleeding require transfusion of 6 or more units of blood; the mortality rate increases in parallel with increasing numbers of units transfused. Approximately one-third of patients who receive 10 or more units die, and one-third sustain serious complications. Surgery is performed on approximately 15 percent of patients with UGI bleeding, the mortality rate for emergency operation being about 15 percent. However, patients with severe bleeding are more likely to require surgery, and as a group they have increased morbidity and mortality rates compared with the group of patients in whom bleeding ceases spontaneously.

INITIAL HEMODYNAMIC EVALUATION AND RESUSCITATION

Treatment of the abnormality that is the source of UGI bleeding is usually of secondary importance in the immediate management of patients who are bleeding. The initial treatment steps are therefore the same no matter what the cause of the bleeding.

It is usually difficult to determine accurately the seriousness of UGI hemorrhage at its onset. Since the exact level of risk to the patient is unknown, the bleeding must always be regarded as momentous. UGI bleeding is always an emergency until the clinical circumstances prove otherwise.

It is essential to deal with this problem in an orderly manner. This process is described below as a logical progression, but in practice effective action must be directed simultaneously toward several objectives. Usually a number of physicians, nurses, and other support personnel are involved in the management, and it is essential that the attending physician direct, coordinate, and prioritize these efforts.

The first priority is an assessment of the patient's hemodynamic status. Heart rate and blood pressure determinations are the first and most objective measures of hypovolemia, although the experienced physician will note the more subtle signs of inadequate vascular volume at a glance: tachypnea, pallor, evidence of peripheral vasoconstriction, a rapid and thready pulse to palpation, and apprehension. If there is hypotension when the patient is supine, at least 25 percent of the usual intravascular volume has been lost. If pulse and blood pressure are within acceptable ranges, these parameters should be determined again with the patient in the sitting or head-up position. A decline in diastolic pressure of more than 10 to 15 mm Hg and an increase in heart rate of 20 or more beats per minute indicate hypovolemia. This initial evaluation of the patient may also be misleading if the onset of hemorrhage is relatively recent. The intravascular volume may still be adequate despite a substantial rate of blood loss.

As vascular volume is being estimated, resuscitative measures should be initiated. Elevation of the patient's feet and legs is a very simple and effective measure to counteract shock, albeit one that is often forgotten. The most important steps, however, are to establish a large-bore intravenous line and begin fluid replacement. There are several possible approaches to intravenous access, including the placement of central lines. The choice depends on circumstances and experience, although one or more peripheral lines are almost always adequate initially. Repeated and hurried attempts at insertion of a central line may consume precious time and lead to a complication that the patient can ill afford.

Rapid volume replacement should begin as soon as the intravenous line is secure. In general, glucose infusions should not be used, but there are several solutions suitable for the initial expansion of the intravascular volume, including isotonic saline and Ringer's lactate. The latter is preferred if there is metabolic acidosis. However, the initial choice is one of personal preference, since there will be little or no information to guide selection. The infusion should be changed to whole blood or packed red cells and isotonic saline as soon as possible, with the aim of restoring and maintaining the hematocrit at a level of at least 30 percent.

It is necessary to monitor urinary volume, but the insertion of a catheter into the bladder is not without risk. The decision to do this should be based on circumstances. If the condition of the patient warrants close attention to the volume of urine produced, an indwelling bladder catheter is indicated.

PATIENT HISTORY

Estimates by the patient or relatives of the quantity of blood lost are almost always inaccurate. However, certain inferences can be drawn about the location of the bleeding lesion from an exact description of the symptoms. Some speculation is also possible as to the seriousness of bleeding, although it is unwise to presume too much about the rate of bleeding from the patient's history. UGI bleeding is more often intermittent than sustained, and there should be no assumption as to the patient's subsequent course based on the nature of the presenting symptoms. There are three symptoms to be concerned with: melena, hematemesis, and hematochezia.

A distinction should be made between black stool (as a result of bleeding) and true melena. Black stools can result from the introduction of as little as 100 to 200 ml of blood into the GI tract at any location proximal to the hepatic flexure. The term "melena" refers to the passage of stools that are jet black and of a consistency similar to tar. This analogy is so accurate that almost all patients with melena understand the inquiry about "tarry stools." The transition from red blood to melena is initiated by the action of acid and pepsin in the stomach, and the process is completed by bacterial action. The latter requires some time, and blood must remain in the gut for up to 8 hours if melena is to occur. Therefore, intestinal transit time has a direct bearing on the development of melena. True melena usually indicates a source of bleeding proximal to the ligament of Treitz, although this is not axiomatic. Because of the several factors that contribute to the development of melena, no firm conclusions can be made concerning the status of the bleeding or the volume of blood lost based on this symptom alone. Melena may persist for several days after bleeding has stopped, or it may be the result of persistent or recurrent bleeding at a relatively slow rate.

Hematemesis may be defined as the vomiting of either fresh red blood or blood clots. Blood changes color rapidly in the acid-pepsin environment of the stomach, so that hematemesis always indicates active or very recent bleeding. If hematemesis has occurred, the lesion responsible for the bleeding is almost always proximal to the ligament of Treitz. However, this symptom does not indicate that the bleeding is necessarily serious or persistent, and in fact the bleeding may stop as suddenly as it occurred. If hematemesis is to occur, the patient must vomit. The latter is a complex process that may not occur in all patients with serious UGI bleeding. Since the action of gastric acid on blood is rapid, the vomitus may contain small flecks of brown material. This is usually described as "coffee-ground" vomitus, and it should not be regarded as evidence that the bleeding is minor or that it has stopped.

The combination of melena with hematemesis implies not only that bleeding is active or recent but also that it has been present or recurrent over some time. The development of hematochezia subsequent to the onset of melena in the absence of hematemesis may indicate a source of bleeding in the small bowel, such as a Meckel's diverticulum, or colon. However, the combination of hematemesis and hematochezia is especially ominous, since this can be explained only by the presence of substantial and ongoing bleeding in the UGI tract.

The source of UGI bleeding cannot be determined with any degree of certitude from the patient's symptoms or past history. Even a history of a specific GI disorder has no special relevance in terms of predicting the source of bleeding. This does not mean that the history is unimportant to the overall care of the patient. For example, the knowledge that a patient has cirrhosis and portal hypertension has a bearing on management and outcome, but an established diagnosis of cirrhosis cannot be taken as a priori evidence of variceal bleeding.

Death by exsanguination is a relatively rare result of UGI bleeding. However, virtually all organs and tissues have a common need for blood, so that the lack of it will have serious consequences, especially for organs already compromised by other diseases. Although this is obvious, the importance of disorders in organ systems other than the gut is often overlooked in the initial evaluation and management of patients with UGI bleeding. In most cases, the bleeding is ultimately controlled, but the adverse effects of hypotension on other organ systems may lead to serious complications or even death. For this reason, it is essential that any associated disorders be identified as quickly as possible. With respect to the immediate resuscitation of the patient, a history of congestive heart failure, cardiac arrhythmia, renal or pulmonary insufficiency, hypertension, or diabetes is more important to successful management than a detailed history of GI disorders.

The evaluation and treatment of patients with serious UGI bleeding can be chaotic and stressful, so that there is a tendency to become disorganized and ineffective. Confusion can be avoided by adopting a standardized approach with an established set of steps and rules. This is clearly valuable, but the approach must not become excessively mechanical. It is necessary to remain a reasoning physician rather than a technician; a reasonable amount of attention must be devoted to the history as the clinical situation becomes more stable.

The medical history of any patient with UGI bleeding may contain information that is vital to successful management even though it is of limited value in predicting the source of bleeding. It is impossible to list every fact that might be of importance. Previous surgery on the UGI tract may have a bearing on diagnosis and treatment. A partial gastric resection with vagotomy eliminates certain types of lesions as candidates for the source of bleeding and has significance with respect to endoscopic examination. Previous surgery for repair of an abdominal aortic aneurysm should always raise the question of an aortoenteric fistula. This possibility always increases the urgency of diagnosis and therapy, and it is usually wise to proceed as if a fistula is actually present. Thus, additional units of blood should be cross-matched, and the patient should undergo endoscopy in the operating room as soon as possible and while preparations are being made for surgery. A history of blood dyscrasia or other hematologic disorders may require special measures. Recent sclerotherapy for esophageal varices raises the possibility of additional sources and types of bleeding.

Accurate information should be obtained about the use of medication. It will be necessary to continue certain essential medications, and the list of drugs may draw attention to potential problems with other organ systems. The use of aspirin or aspirin-containing compounds may indicate a potential source of bleeding. However, aspirin is not the only agent that disrupts the normal hemostatic mechanisms. All patients (and a reliable relative or friend if possible) should be questioned concerning the ingestion of alcohol. The existence of any drug allergies should be defined.

PHYSICAL EXAMINATION

One of the most important steps in the initial evaluation of the patient, after attending to hemodynamic status, is examination of the stool. Even though an accurate description of melena or the passage of blood or clots per rectum is obtained, a digital rectal examination must be performed and the contents of the rectum noted.

A large-bore tube should be inserted into the stomach in virtually all cases of UGI bleeding. The inner diameter of the tube should be at least 10 mm. It serves to aspirate the gastric contents and to clear the stomach of blood, clots, and debris. A small-diameter nasogastric tube is inadequate for these purposes and serves only to increase the patient's suffering. The aspiration of blood, clots, or coffee-ground material verifies the diagnosis of GI bleeding proximal to the ligament of Treitz. However, a negative aspirate does not eliminate the presence of UGI bleeding. In about 10 to 15 percent of patients with a duodenal source of bleeding, the gastric aspirate does not contain blood.

The remainder of the physical examination should be focused on the major organ systems that are most directly affected by hypotension. With experience, this can be accomplished while the patient is being questioned about other diseases. With respect to the digestive organs, evidence of portal hypertension should be noted. The abdomen should be examined in the usual manner. Although evidence of enlarged organs, tenderness, or masses usually does not contribute directly to the diagnosis of the source of bleeding, such findings are important to the subsequent treatment of the patient. However, signs of GI obstruction or peritoneal irritation may be of immediate importance to the management and must not be overlooked.

LABORATORY AND OTHER STUDIES

Laboratory studies should be obtained as soon as resuscitation is under way. A single venipuncture can be performed to obtain a specimen for laboratory studies as well as the type and cross-match. Studies should include a complete blood count, prothrombin time, partial thromboplastin time, blood urea nitrogen, creatinine, electrolytes, blood glucose, and liver function tests. Since the ongoing evaluation of the patient may disclose the need for further laboratory tests, it may be efficient to set aside a small excess quantity of blood for additional studies. For example, a serum amylase may be useful if the history or physical examination suggests the presence of acute pancreatitis, as distinguished from a penetrating duodenal ulcer. Urinalysis should be performed, although it may be difficult to obtain a specimen.

The decision to undertake studies such as a chest x-ray, a plain x-ray of the abdomen, or an electrocardiogram should be based on the clinical circumstances, history, and physical examination. If the patient's age, status, or history justify electrocardiography, it should be performed as early as possible. It may disclose previously unrecognized heart disease, and silent myocardial ischemia or infarction is a well-known complication of shock due to bleeding.

DIAGNOSIS AND TREATMENT

Endoscopy is the essential element in the diagnosis and treatment of UGI bleeding. However, the hemodynamic status of the patient should be stable if at all possible before endoscopy is performed. Rarely, bleeding may be so profuse that endoscopic treatment must be attempted in the absence of complete hemodynamic control, and on occasion endoscopy may not be possible because of very heavy bleeding. Prompt surgery is often required in such cases.

Gastric Lavage

Gastric lavage should be performed with a large-bore gastric tube to remove blood and clots. The solution used for this is debatable, but the choice is probably of little importance. About 200 to 300 ml of lavage solution should be forcefully injected via the tube so that clots are disrupted. The gastric contents should then be siphoned by placing the end of the tube at a level below that of the stomach (off the side of the bed and into a large container). If the lavage fluid is forcefully aspirated with a syringe, trauma to the gastric mucosa is inevitable. This is not harmful to the patient, but the resultant red marks on the gastric mucosa may be misinterpreted at endoscopy as hemorrhagic erosions or vascular lesions. Gravity drainage is less traumatic and more effective. Slight adjustments in the position of the tube by moving it in and out help to maintain flow.

Every health care professional should be aware that blood can be a vehicle for infection. The attending physician has a responsibility toward all who participate in the care of the bleeding patient and should insist that all personnel be properly gowned and gloved.

Infusion of large quantities of an iced lavage solution into the UGI tract has been performed for many years to induce hemostasis. This practice is largely empiric, and there is no proof that it is either effective or ineffective. However, there is growing evidence that endoscopic methods for control of bleeding are effective, so that any debate on the merits of gastric lavage with cold solutions is irrelevant. Endoscopic diagnosis and therapy should not be delayed by a prolonged effort to control bleeding with lavage.

Endoscopic Diagnosis

Endoscopy should be performed as soon as gastric aspiration yields clear or pink-tinged fluid.

The accuracy of endoscopic diagnosis in UGI hemorrhage is greater than 90 percent with respect to actual and potential sources of bleeding. This greatly exceeds the accuracy obtained from UGI x-rays. However, there are no data to indicate that diagnostic endoscopy alone has significantly altered the overall morbidity and mortality rates for GI hemorrhage. Conversely, much of the available evidence is flawed, and it cannot be said that endoscopy does *not* have a positive influence on outcome.

The fact that UGI bleeding stops spontaneously in most patients explains much of the difficulty in substantiating the efficacy of diagnostic endoscopy. For example, to demonstrate a 1.2 percent reduction in mortality, assuming an expected mortality of 10 percent, about 6,000 patients would have to be enrolled in a randomized trial. Erickson and Glick calculated that only 1,948 patients had been enrolled in all the prospective trials of diagnostic endoscopy as of 1986. As an issue, however, the benefit of diagnostic endoscopy is no longer relevant because of increasing evidence that endoscopic methods of hemostasis are effective.

The complication rate for diagnostic endoscopy in UGI bleeding, according to Gilbert and colleagues, is about 0.9 percent, with a mortality rate of 0.13 percent. Katon found a mortality rate of 0.02 percent in a review of 26 published reports. These figures are approximately the same as those for routine diagnostic UGI endoscopy. However, there is a decided tendency for complications and death to occur in the more seriously ill patients who undergo endoscopy. For example, Noel and colleagues found that the complication rate in patients aged 65 and older was 5 percent, with a mortality rate of 2 percent. Complications of emergency endoscopy include perforation, precipitation of hemorrhage, pulmonary aspiration, various cardiovascular problems, and problems stemming from premedication. The most common of these is probably aspiration.

Endoscopic findings in patients with UGI bleeding can have prognostic significance. For some lesions, simple conservative measures are appropriate, whereas in others the most aggressive steps are dictated by the endoscopic findings. Bleeding from lesions such as hemorrhagic-erosive gastritis can be relied on to be self-limiting, while others such as an aortoenteric fistula carry a mortality rate that approaches 100 percent without proper treatment. One of the most important aspects of diagnostic endoscopy is the recognition of esophageal varices as the cause of bleeding, since there are substantial differences in the treatment (and outcome) of bleeding varices compared with other causes of bleeding. Endoscopic sclerotherapy, for example, has substantially altered the management of bleeding varices.

The first objective of endoscopic diagnosis should be to localize the site of hemorrhage. This usually is not difficult if gastric lavage has been adequate. Even if bleeding is profuse, if the precise nature of the responsible lesion cannot be determined, and if endoscopic treatment is impossible or ineffective, accurate localization of the source saves valuable time for the surgeon. Even if the lesion cannot be visualized adequately, certain diagnoses can be inferred from the location: bleeding in the region of the cardia in the absence of varices suggests a Mallory-Weiss laceration. Bleeding within the duodenal bulb is most likely due to an ulcer.

The endoscopist should be familiar with all potential causes of UGI bleeding. As a practical matter, I divide these into three categories: varices, peptic ulcer disease, and other causes.

Since there are substantial differences between the management of bleeding from varices and the treatment of that from other causes, the presence or absence of varices should be considered first. However, varices cannot be implicated as the source of bleeding by their presence alone, and patients with established portal hypertension are often found to be bleeding from another lesion. Therefore, careful examination of the entire UGI tract is essential. In about 45 percent of cases of variceal hemorrhage, there is evidence of variceal bleeding at endoscopy. Active bleeding from a varix may be seen, but it is more common to find a clot protruding from a varix near the distal end of the esophagus. The presence of esophageal varices, plus the existence of a second potential source of bleeding without active bleeding or signs of hemorrhage, poses a difficult problem. Careful endoscopic assessment may reveal some feature that implicates one or the other lesion, e.g., a visible vessel in an ulcer crater. If it appears that the bleeding has stopped, it is sometimes prudent to defer endoscopic treatment. If bleeding recurs, prompt endoscopic evaluation usually resolves the issue.

Other focal lesions should be sought once varices are eliminated as the source of bleeding. The area of the UGI tract containing the most fresh blood may draw attention to a specific lesion, although the endoscopic examination should be performed in the same systematic manner as a routine diagnostic procedure. The location of the lesion may present certain problems in terms of endoscopic visualization, such as an ulcer in the region of the apex of the duodenal bulb. Profuse hemorrhage may make it difficult to obtain an adequate view. Sometimes this can be overcome by changing the patient's position, but frequent turning of an unstable patient from side to side may also be difficult because of the various monitoring devices, intravenous lines, and catheters. I believe that the risk of aspiration is increased when the patient is completely supine. However, slight shifts in position from the usual left decubitus toward a semiprone or semisupine position may be of assistance.

Endoscopy

There are no specific rules with regard to the timing of endoscopy. An issue can be made of this, but in practice the timing of the procedure is determined by the individual case. According to one view, diagnostic accuracy is improved by prompt endoscopy; others hold that there is no difference in outcome if the examination is performed within 6 to 8 hours of hospital admission. Either approach may be correct or incorrect. If there is any indication, based on the initial evaluation and response to treatment, that the bleeding is serious, endoscopy should be performed promptly. In less urgent circumstances, some delay in the procedure does not compromise the care of the patient. However, the value of accurate diagnosis is a tenet of modern medicine, and to reject this possibility simply because treatment measures may be inadequate strikes me as absurd. Patients with less serious UGI bleeding should also undergo endoscopy within a reasonable time, usually within 6 hours of admission.

Ongoing hemorrhage or evidence of recent bleeding can be observed in about one-third of patients if endoscopy is performed within 6 hours of the onset of bleeding. These findings are associated with a significant increase in mortality and morbidity rates, transfusion requirements, and the number of patients undergoing emergency surgery. Although all actively bleeding lesions are suitable for endoscopic treatment, bleeding stops spontaneously in most patients. This creates problems with regard to the selection of patients for endoscopic treatment if bleeding is less than active.

Certain aspects of the endoscopic appearance of a peptic ulcer can be used to predict the clinical course and outcome. These features are usually referred to as stigmata of hemorrhage (SH). The decision for endoscopic treatment in patients who have stopped bleeding is based primarily on these findings.

The definition of SH is imprecise, but generally the term encompasses the presence of adherent fresh or altered clot within an ulcer crater or a "visible vessel." The latter term refers to an elevated red, purplish, yellow-white, or black spot in an ulcer crater. In most cases, the visible vessel is probably a clot protruding from an arterial vessel. SH associated with an ulcer generally indicates an increased risk of further bleeding that is likely to be severe or protracted, and is more likely to require surgical treatment. Ulcers without SH may be expected to remain quiescent in terms of further bleeding and do not require endoscopic treatment.

The relative importance of the various SH with respect to the potential for bleeding is of considerable importance. The most important of the SH as detailed by Bornman and colleagues, is the visible vessel. Although some investigators found this to be unreliable as a predictor of recurrent bleeding, most studies emphasize its value as an indicator of further hemorrhage. On the basis of current knowledge, treatment of a visible vessel is justified.

Clot adherent to an ulcer is somewhat problematic. Removal of the clot may reveal a visible vessel, or may precipitate active bleeding. Conversely, clot removal may reveal a crater with a smooth base and little or no bleeding. Whether removal of a clot is acceptable as a method of determining which lesions to treat is also unclear. In trials of therapy, removal of an adherent clot is probably indicated. In the individual case, it may not be justified if the endoscopist is inexperienced or unprepared to deal with the active bleeding that may result.

There are considerable technical problems related to the application of any hemostatic technique. It may be impossible to obtain an adequate view of the lesion because of heavy bleeding or an inaccessible location. Actual contact with tissue is necessary with some devices, which also allows use of the most fundamental method of achieving hemostasis, i.e., mechanical pressure on the bleeding vessel. However, removal of a contact device after coagulation of the bleeding point occasionally disrupts the coagulum and causes resumption of bleeding. Precise placement of contact devices greatly increases their effectiveness. To achieve this, it is usually necessary that blood, clots, and debris be cleared from the lesion before the application of the hemostatic mechanism. Most, but not all, devices incorporate some method of washing the lesion, usually by irrigation with a fluid or insufflation of a gas.

The currently available endoscopic methods for control of gastrointestinal hemorrhage can be divided into four categories (Table 1): thermal, chemical/injection, topical, and mechanical. Except for sclerotherapy for esophageal varices as a chemical/injection technique, the most widely used methods of endoscopic hemostasis are thermal in nature. All of these employ tissue heating as a means of hemostasis, but their mechanisms for delivery of thermal energy differ. Each of the four general types of thermal hemostatic devices has advantages and disadvantages.

TABLE 1 Endoscopic Methods for Control of UGI Hemorrhage

Thermal
Electrocoagulation
Monopolar
Multipolar
Laser photocoagulation
Heater probe coagulation
Electrohydrothermal coagulation
Microwave coagulation
Chemical/Injection
Injection sclerotherapy
Injection hemostasis
Topical
Tissue adhesives
Ferromagnetic tamponade
Clotting factors
Mechanical
Hemoclip

Electrocoagulation may be either monopolar or bipolar. Monopolar electrocoagulation, in which a high frequency electrosurgical current is caused to flow from a small active electrode through the patient to a larger indifferent electrode and then back to an electrosurgical generator, is a well-established method of hemostasis. Although it is widely available and relatively inexpensive, the use of monopolar electrocoagulation for endoscopic hemostasis has been virtually abandoned because it produces a depth of tissue injury greater than that caused by other methods. In animal studies the depth of tissue injury produced is equal to that of the Nd:YAG laser. Perforations have been reported from monopolar electrocoagulation.

The fundamental difference between bipolar and monopolar electrocoagulation is the absence of current flow through the patient. Rather, the current travels between two (or more) active electrodes at the end of the probe. This results in a very high current density in the tissue near the electrode, and limitation of the depth of tissue injury. Other desirable features of bipolar electrocoagulation include the ability to irrigate, effective application at various angles, and compression of the bleeding point. The device is portable and relatively inexpensive. The efficacy of the bipolar probe has been demonstrated in some but not all controlled trials.

The heat probe consists of a heating coil within an aluminum cylinder, the outer aspect of the cylinder being coated with polytef (Teflon) to circumvent sticking to the tissue after coagulation. Although the inner coil is heated electrically, there is no flow of current through the patient. The heat probe delivers a precise quantity of energy, permits irrigation of the bleeding site, may be applied at various angles, has a limited depth of tissue injury, and may be used to compress the bleeding point. The device is portable and relatively inexpensive. In theory, the heat probe is ideal for endoscopic hemostasis, but prospective data on its use are limited.

Electrohydrothermal coagulation is designed to circumvent the problem of disruption of coagulated tissue by hemostatic devices that require contact with the tissue. The electrohydrothermal probe induces coagulation through a liquid interface between the probe and the tissue. Published experience with this type of device is almost exclusively European in origin.

Nd:YAG and argon lasers have been used for endoscopic control of GI hemorrhage. Each has certain technical problems and advantages. For endoscopic treatment of GI bleeding, lasers are being supplanted by devices that are more portable and less expensive.

Laser photocoagulation may be performed without touching the tissue to be treated, so that there is no problem with disruption of the coagulum after the bleeding has been controlled. As with the other devices, the bleeding point can be approached from different angles. With argon laser photocoagulation, the depth of tissue damage is limited because the wavelength of light produced by this machine is readily absorbed by tissues that are red. However, this also makes it necessary to clear blood and clots from the area to be treated, a formidable technical problem in some cases.

The Nd:YAG laser has all the advantages of the argon laser, but is the most expensive device used for endoscopic hemostasis. It also has a greater potential for deep tissue injury, and is not portable for practical purposes. There are a relatively large number of controlled trials of Nd:YAG laser therapy for endoscopic hemostasis. Several of these studies, albeit not all, have shown this form of treatment to be effective for endoscopic control of bleeding ulcers.

Other approaches to the endoscopic control of bleeding have been devised, including microwave coagulation, application of various substances (tissue adhesives, clotting factors), ferromagnetic tamponade, placement of various types of clips on bleeding vessels, and injection of chemical agents. Most of these have not been investigated extensively, some have been discarded for technical and other reasons, and most should be considered experimental at present. The most promising of these novel methods is the injection of small volumes of a chemical agent around or directly into a bleeding point. A variety of agents have been used, including alcohol, epinephrine, and sclerotherapy agents. The obvious advantages of this method are that it is simple and inexpensive. There is considerable interest in injection methods of hemostasis, but the data on this form of treatment are limited, and it must be considered experimental except for sclerotherapy. The latter is the treatment of choice for bleeding esophageal varices and is discussed in another chapter.

The diversity of endoscopic techniques that have been proposed or are available for treatment of UGI bleeding increases the difficulty of critical evaluation. Although there is some evidence that several methods may be effective in certain clinical circumstances, data comparing the various techniques and methods are extremely limited. Except for injection therapy for variceal bleeding, it is difficult, probably impossible, to identify the best overall method for endoscopic control of bleeding.

Practical Considerations

Endoscopic diagnosis of and therapy for UGI bleeding is a difficult procedure when bleeding is profuse. A successful outcome depends on skill, training, and especially practical experience.

Almost any endoscope can be used for the diagnosis and treatment of UGI bleeding. I prefer a double-channel instrument. This type may be slightly less maneuverable than a large single-channel instrument. However, significant improvements have been made in the design of two-channel models, and any slight compromise in handling is more than compensated for by the ability to use one channel for suction and the other for a hemostatic device. Furthermore, switching the device from one to the other channel sometimes improves the angle of approach with the probe. One channel can also be used to wash the lesion, by means of a large plastic syringe with a large-bore, blunt-ended needle inserted through the accessory port. Many models also have an extra wash channel for washing.

The use of sedative drugs for endoscopy may be problematic in unstable patients, but, I generally use small intravenous doses of meperidine (25 to 75 mg). The major reason for preferring this drug to all others is that its effects are readily reversed with naloxone. Meperidine blunts the patient's anxiety and usually provides enough sedation for the patient to cooperate with the procedure.

The heat probe is the hemostatic device that I favor in most circumstances. These probes are available in two diameters; the larger (3.2-mm) probe appears to be more effective. If heat probe coagulation fails and there is persistent bleeding, I also inject small volumes (0.2 ml) of absolute alcohol around the bleeding point to a maximum of 1.5 ml. However, when one treatment method has failed to stop the bleeding, a second method also is frequently ineffective.

Measures to Counteract Acid-Peptic Effects

There is no evidence that the usual medications for treatment of acid-peptic disease are effective in controlling UGI bleeding. However, if endoscopy reveals a lesion that is amenable to such therapy, e.g., an ulcer, such treatment should be started. Although this has no immediate effect on bleeding, it promotes healing and may reduce the risk of recurrent bleeding. I prefer an intravenous route for this treatment so that the stomach remains empty if further endoscopic therapy becomes necessary.

Surgical Consultation

It is always prudent to involve an experienced surgeon in the care of every patient with UGI bleeding. Since most bleeding episodes stop spontaneously, a formal consultation is not necessary for most patients. However, the seriousness of the bleeding and subsequent course cannot be forecast at initial evaluation, and the simple step of notifying the surgical service of the patient's admission may save valuable time and effort if surgery is required. If the bleeding proves to be serious and persistent, a surgeon should see the patient. A team effort then becomes essential, although the final responsibility for the care of the patient must always reside with the attending physician.

Persistent or Recurrent Bleeding

UGI hemorrhage may recur despite initial control of bleeding by endoscopic means. Further endoscopic therapy may be performed in such cases, although the decision depends largely on the clinical circumstances. It is difficult to offer any fixed rules for the number of times a patient should undergo endoscopic treatment. If bleeding is recurrent after a second endoscopic treatment, I usually recommend surgery, since in my experience further endoscopic therapy is unlikely to be of permanent benefit. However, this rule should not be absolute, since there are always a few patients who are not candidates for surgery under any circumstances.

The decision for surgery must also be based on the clinical status and a multitude of other factors. With serious bleeding, there is frequently a point in the patient's course at which surgery becomes conservative therapy. As a general rule, this possibility should be weighed against other clinical parameters of the patient's condition when the number of transfusions exceeds six. Surgery is highly effective for the control of UGI bleeding. When there is persistent or serious hemorrhage, the risk to the patient is usually increased by prolonged and ineffective efforts to control bleeding with endoscopic methods.

Angiotherapy

Selective and subselective angiography may be used to demonstrate the vessel that supplies a bleeding lesion. Angiographic methods may also be employed to control bleeding, usually by infusion of vasoconstrictive agents or embolization of clot and other substances. Although there are few data from controlled studies, these techniques appear to be effective for some types of bleeding. However, angiotherapy is not without complications, and high levels of experience and skill are required, as for other forms of therapy. When this expertise is available, angiotherapy may be an option for patients in whom endoscopic therapy has failed.

SUGGESTED READING

Bornman PC, Theodorou NA, Shuttleworth RD, et al. Importance of hypovolaemic shock and endoscopic signs in predicting recurrent hemorrhage from peptic ulceration: a prospective evaluation. Br Med J 1985; 291:245–247.

Erickson RA, Glick ME. Why have controlled trials failed to demonstrate a benefit of esophagogastroduodenoscopy in acute upper gastrointestinal bleeding? A probability model analysis. Dig Dis Sci 1986: 31:760–768.

Escourrou J. Nd:YAG laser therapy for acute gastrointestinal hemorrhage. In: Atsumi K, Nimsakul N, eds. Laser Tokyo 1981. Tokyo: Intergroup Corp, 1981.

Fleischer D. Endoscopic Nd:YAG laser therapy for active esophageal variceal bleeding. A randomized controlled study. Gastrointest Endosc 1985; 31:4–9.

Foster DN, Miloszewski KJ, Losowsky MS. Stigmata of recent haemorrhage in diagnosis and prognosis of upper gastrointestinal bleeding. Br Med J 1978; 1:1173–1177.

Freitas D, Donato A, Monteiro JG. Controlled trial of liquid monopolar electrocoagulation in bleeding peptic ulcers. Am J Gasteroenterol 1985; 80:853–857.

Gilbert DA, Silverstein FE, Tedesco FJ, et al. National ASGE survey on upper gastrointestinal bleeding. Complications of endoscopy. Dig Dis Sci 1981; 26(Suppl):55s–59s.

Griffiths WJ, Neumann DA, Welsh JD. The visible vessel as an indicator of uncontrolled or recurrent gastrointestinal hemorrhage. N Engl J Med 1979; 300:1411–1413.

Harris DC, Heap TR. Significance of signs of recent hemorrhage at endoscopy Med J Aust 1982; 2:35–37.

Ihre T, Johansson C, Seligsson U, et al. Endoscopic YAG laser treatment in massive UGI bleeding. Scand J Gastroenterol 1981; 16:633–640.

Katon RM. Complications of upper gastrointestinal endoscopy in the gastrointestinal bleeder. Dig Dis Sci 1981; 26(Suppl):47s–54s.

Kernohan RM, Anderson JR, McKelvey ST, Kennedy TL. A controlled trial of bipolar electrocoagulation in patients with upper gastrointestinal bleeding. Br J Surg 1984; 71:889–891.

Laine L. Multipolar electrocoagulation in the treatment of active upper gastrointestinal tract hemorrhage. A prospective controlled trial. N Engl J Med 1987; 316:1613–1617.

MacLeod I, Mills PR, MacKenzie JF. Nd:YAG laser photocoagulation for major acute upper gastrointestinal haemorrhage. Gut 1982: 23:905.

Matek W, Fruhmorgen P, Kaduk P, et al. Modified electrocoagulation and its possibilities in the control of gastrointestinal bleeding. Endoscopy 1979: 4:253–258.

Noel D, Deloge Y, Liguory C, et al. Upper gastrointestinal hemorrhage in patients aged over 65 years: the contribution of endoscopy. Nouv Presse Med 1979: 8:589–591.

Rutgeerts P, Van Trappen G, Broebaert L, et al. Controlled trial of YAG laser treatment of upper digestive hemorrhage. Gastroenterology 1982; 83:410–416.

Storey DW, Bown SG, Swain CP, et al. Endoscopic prediction of recurrent bleeding in peptic ulcers. N Engl J Med 1981; 305:915–916.

Swain CP, Bown SG, Salmon PR, et al. Controlled trial of Nd:YAG laser photocoagulation in bleeding peptic ulcers. Gastrointest Endosc (abstr) 1984; 30:137.

Swain CP, Storey DW, Bown SG, et al. Nature of the bleeding vessel in recurrently bleeding gastric ulcers. Gastroenterology 1986; 90:595–608.

Wara P, Hojsgaard A, Amdrup E. Endoscopic electrocoagulation: an alternative to operative hemostasis in active gastroduodenal bleeding. Endoscopy 1980; 12:237–240.

STRESS ULCER AND ACUTE EROSIVE GASTRITIS

CRAIG E. CHAMBERLAIN, M.D., Maj. MC
DAVID A. PEURA, M.D., F.A.C.P., Col. MC

Stress-related mucosal damage (SRMD) to the upper gastrointestinal (GI) tract is a well-recognized cause of significant morbidity and mortality in critically ill patients. Endoscopic studies show that the mucosal injury can develop within hours of admission to an intensive care unit (ICU) and occurs in over 70 percent of patients at risk. Approximately 20 percent of patients with mucosal lesions develop GI bleeding, which when severe can be associated with a mortality in excess of 50 percent. It therefore behooves the physician who cares for critically ill patients to be keenly aware of the mechanisms and approaches to prophylaxis of and therapy for this clinical condition.

Most patients in an ICU setting are at risk of SRMD, but those who are most susceptible to mucosal injury are severely traumatized or burned patients: those with central nervous system (CNS) injury, multiple organ failure, sepsis, or shock. Risk is relatively less for patients with renal failure on dialysis, less extensive burns (less than 35 percent of body surface), intracranial lesions without coma, isolated soft tissue injury, and uncomplicated cardiac disease (myocardial infarction, dysrhythmias, or congestive heart failure). The condition usually is not recognized until upper GI bleeding occurs, because most patients are asymptomatic. Endoscopy is the best method to diagnose and monitor mucosal damage and should be considered the "gold standard" for clinical studies. The macroscopically visible abnormalities are located predominantly in the body and fundus of the stomach. Submucosal petechiae and hemorrhages appear first, followed initially by erosions and later by superficial ulcers. These lesions tend to ooze blood; because of their relatively superficial nature, massive bleeding and perforation are uncommon.

The opinions or assertions contained herein are those of the authors and are not to be construed as reflecting the views of the Department of the Air Force, the Department of the Army, or the Department of Defense.

The precise pathogenesis of SRMD is not known. It is useful, however, to think of it as resulting from an imbalance between aggressive (destructive) and defensive (protective) mucosal factors. The most important aggressive mucosal factor is gastric acid, without which SRMD does not occur. This dependence on the presence of acid for mucosal damage is the basis for therapy with antacids and H_2-receptor antagonists (discussed below). The amount of acid necessary for the development of SRMD is variable and largely dependent on the influences of mucosal blood flow, acid-base balance, and the effectiveness of the other endogenous protective mechanisms of the stomach. Additional aggressive mucosal factors include pepsin and bile acids, agents that enhance gastric epithelial damage in the presence of acid.

The disruption of mucosal protective factors is probably as important in the pathogenesis of SRMD as are the aggressive factors just mentioned. Gastric epithelium is normally protected from intraluminal acid and other noxious stimuli by the "mucosal barrier," a constellation of mucosal protective mechanisms that permit the existence of a high hydrogen ion gradient between lumen and tissue without damage to the latter. Stress-induced changes in gastric mucosal blood flow, mucus production, bicarbonate secretion, prostaglandin synthesis, and epithelial cell renewal have all been implicated in the disruption of the integrity of the gastric mucosal barrier. Barrier breakdown leads to back diffusion of hydrogen ions, which promotes the actual mucosal damage.

MEDICAL TREATMENT

Treatment of Underlying Disease

Both the risk of bleeding and the mortality in critically ill patients with SRMD are more closely correlated with the status of the underlying disease than with the mucosal damage itself. Therefore, treatment for this condition must first be directed at the underlying cause of physiologic stress. Gastric mucosal improvement generally parallels overall clinical improvement. Consequently, it is important that the clinician be aggressive in efforts to reverse metabolic and physiologic abnormalities, thereby maintaining an adequate mucosal blood flow to prevent mucosal ischemia. Prompt and aggressive treatment of sepsis, hypovolemia, systemic acidosis, respiratory failure, and inadequate nutrition are probably as important as therapeutic interventions aimed at treating the SRMD itself.

Antacids

Because gastric acid is strongly implicated in the pathogenesis of SRMD, much of the effort in treating this disorder is aimed at reducing intraluminal acid content. An intensive antacid regimen has been demonstrated in numerous studies to be effective in preventing and treating stress-induced bleeding of the upper GI tract, and remains the standard therapy with which alternative treatments are compared. The effectiveness of antacid therapy depends on maintenance of an intraluminal pH of 3.5 or greater. This necessitates that nursing personnel periodically determine the pH of a gastric aspirate and administer the antacids frequently. The dosage we use is 30 ml of a combination aluminum hydroxide and magnesium hydroxide liquid antacid such as Mylanta or Maalox, given on a 1- to 2-hour schedule. Gastric residuals should be checked before each subsequent dose to assess stasis and retention. The high dose of antacids required may cause diarrhea, metabolic abnormalities, and even aspiration pneumonia in patients with delayed gastric emptying. Because of these problems, we favor H_2-receptor antagonists over an intensive antacid regimen.

H_2-Receptor Antagonists

Numerous studies using either GI bleeding or endoscopic changes as therapeutic end points have demonstrated that H_2-receptor antagonists are effective in treating and preventing SRMD and are virtually equivalent to therapy with an intensive antacid regimen. Although the beneficial effects of the H_2 blockers are most likely related to their ability to inhibit acid secretion, they are effective even when no attempt is made to ensure gastric pH values greater than 3.5. Cimetidine has been shown to preserve gastric mucosal blood flow and stimulate endogenous prostaglandin production during stress, two mechanisms that may contribute significantly to its therapeutic efficacy. H_2-receptor antagonists can be given either parenterally or orally, but parenteral administration is preferred in the ICU setting. We favor a continuous intravenous infusion over intravenous bolus dosing. Therapeutic blood levels are more effectively maintained and a favorable intragastric pH more evenly controlled by the continuous infusion technique. An additional benefit of a more constant blood level may be a decreased incidence of adverse reactions and easier dosage adjustment of potentially interacting drugs such as theophylline, warfarin, and phenytoin. A typical regimen is a 300-mg bolus injection of cimetidine followed by a 37.5 to 100 mg per hour continuous infusion, or a 50-mg bolus of ranitidine followed by a 6 to 10 mg per hour continuous infusion. Appropriate dosage adjustments must be made for patients with underlying renal or hepatic insufficiency.

In high-risk patients this therapy is begun on admission to the ICU and can be added to standard total parenteral nutrition solutions, since these solutions are administered at a constant infusion rate. With this regimen, we are usually able to maintain intraluminal pH above 3.5. If this is verified early, routine checks of intragastric pH beyond the initial 6 to 8 hours are generally unnecessary. Adjunctive administration of antacids can be used in the rare patient whose intraluminal pH remains low despite full-dose H_2-antagonist therapy. If bolus therapy is utilized, the dosage of cimetidine we recommend is 300 mg every 6 to 8 hours over at least a 5-minute infusion time. Slow administration is recommended to minimize the risk of cardiac dysrhythmias or hypotension, which have been rarely reported following rapid infusion. Ranitidine and famotidine can also be administered by bolus infusion: 50 mg every 6 to 8 hours for ranitidine and 20 mg every 8 to 12 hours for famotidine.

Sucralfate

Since sucralfate has proved an effective substance in therapy for peptic ulcer disease, it was inevitable that it would be evaluated as an alternative to acid manipulative therapy for SRMD. Initial studies using macroscopic evidence of bleeding as a measure of mucosal damage support its efficacy. The dosage we recommend is 1 g in a liquid slurry given through a nasogastric tube every 4 to 6 hours. The tube must be flushed with water or saline to prevent clogging. The overall reported clinical experience with sucralfate in this setting is relatively limited compared with that with antacid or H_2-receptor antagonist therapy. It is not, therefore, our current recommendation for ICU prophylaxis.

The incidence of nosocomial pneumonia in ICU patients treated with sucralfate has been reported to be less than in patients treated with antacids or H_2-receptor antagonists. The postulated mechanism for this difference is an increase in bacterial colonization in the nonacidic gastric lumen that results from therapy with antacids and antisecretory agents. A multiplicity of other endogenous and exogenous variables, however, have an effect on the potential for nosocomial pneumonia, and complicate the interpretation of data. Variables such as intragastric volumes, gastric emptying, patient posture, other pharmacologic agents, underlying neurologic disorders, and the types of intubation and ventilator systems must be considered. Further studies will perhaps help to clarify whether sucralfate does indeed have a therapeutic advantage over acid manipulative therapy on this basis.

Newer Agents

Prostaglandins

A variety of other therapeutic modalities have been postulated to be effective in the prevention and treatment of SRMD, and may have a role in the future management of this clinical condition. Exogenous prostaglandins are known to protect the gastric mucosa from a variety of insults, probably by augmenting the effects of endogenous prostaglandins. They have been demonstrated to be antisecretory, to enhance and maintain mucosal blood flow, and to stimulate gastric mucus and bicarbonate secretion. Most clinical trials, however, have utilized antisecretory dosages of the prostaglandins, making it difficult to separate this effect from their other potentially beneficial effects. Because they are not yet widely available for clinical use, few studies have been conducted to assess their efficacy in SRMD. At least one clinical trial, however, has shown that misoprostol, a prostaglandin E_1 analogue, is effective in preventing stress ulceration in postoperative ICU patients. Further studies are needed to determine whether prostaglandins will have a role in the future management of SRMD. Recent Food and Drug Administration approval of misoprostol may enhance clinical trials.

Omeprazole

Omeprazole is the newest of an expanding group of drugs that inhibit gastric acid secretion, and has been shown to be a very effective agent for the healing of peptic ulcers. To date, there has been little investigation of its efficacy in preventing or treating SRMD. In theory, it may be a useful agent for this purpose, but clinical trials are needed to confirm its utility as a therapeutic agent in this clinical condition.

Potential New Approaches

On the basis of animal studies, several additional agents may be considered as future therapies for stress ulceration. These include glucagon, lithium chloride, and epidermal growth factor, all of which have been shown to decrease mucosal damage in animals subjected to various types of experimental stress or noxious mucosal agents. The administration of oxygen radical scavengers and inhibitors of xanthine oxidase, such as allopurinol, has also been postulated to be clinically useful in the management of SRMD. Their potential benefit is based on the hypothesis that SRMD may be caused in part by the injurious effects of reactive oxygen metabolites generated by mucosal xanthine oxidase when normal blood flow to a previously ischemic mucosa is restored. No clinical data evaluating these agents are available.

Enteral Feeding

One final potential prophylactic therapy for stress ulceration is nonpharmacologic. Retrospective data have demonstrated that the incidence of GI bleeding in mechanically ventilated patients receiving enteral alimentation is very low, suggesting a potentially protective effect of enteral feeding on the gastric mucosa. No prospective studies, however, have been made to evaluate directly the efficacy of enteral feeding in the prevention of SRMD or to confirm its potential utility.

NONMEDICAL TREATMENT

The best treatment of SRMD is prevention. The key to prevention at this time appears to be the maintenance of an intraluminal pH of 3.5 or more. Most patients who develop bleeding respond to conservative measures consisting of aggressive treatment of the underlying medical problems and acid neutralization. Patients who show evidence of ongoing bleeding despite therapy, or who present with massive upper GI tract bleeding, require prompt resuscitation and stabilization. Adequate intravascular volume replacement with blood is essential. Underlying coagulopathies or thrombocytopenia should be excluded or treated. Endoscopy is mandatory to confirm that stress ulceration is indeed the source of bleeding and to define the bleeding site or sites precisely. Further, endoscopic therapeutic steps, including electrocoagulation, heater probe coagulation, or intramucosal vasoconstrictor injection, can favorably alter the bleeding course. As with bleeding from classic peptic ulcer disease, if endoscopic therapy fails, more invasive techniques may be necessary. Arteriography for localization and embolization of the bleeding site, or infusion of intra-arterial vasopressin, has proved effective in some patients; the dose of vasopressin is 0.2 to 0.4 U per minute infused through the intra-arterial catheter, which is left in place by the invasive radiologist in the celiac or left gastric artery. Contraindications to the use of vasopressin (water intoxication, congestive heart failure, and angina) should be excluded before this therapy is begun.

Surgical intervention is indicated for patients in whom bleeding continues despite other therapeutic measures, or in whom perforation has occurred. Because of other underlying medical problems that have predisposed them to SRMD, these patients are poor operative candidates. As might be expected, the operative mortality is very high—up to 70 percent in some series. The ideal operation is one that controls the bleeding with the lowest operative mortality and rebleeding rates. There are few prospective clinical trials to substantiate the superiority of one surgical approach over another. The choice of surgery, therefore, must be individualized for each patient, based on the experience of the surgeon, the condition of the patient, and the extent of gastric ulceration present at endoscopy. Rebleeding rates for vagotomy and pyloroplasty are higher than those for vagotomy and gastric resection, but extensive gastric resection carries a higher mortality rate. The procedure of gastric devascularization has been advocated by some and offers an alternative to total gastrectomy in patients with extensive ulceration. Rebleeding rates with this procedure are low, but the operative mortality remains high. In general, total gastrectomy is infrequently performed for SRMD because of the high mortality associated with this procedure.

SUGGESTED READING

Chamberlain CE, Peura DA. Stress ulceration and prevention. In: DiPalma JA, ed. Problems in critical care. Philadelphia: JB Lippincott (in press).
Cheung LY. Treatment of established stress ulcer disease. World J Surg 1981; 5:235–240.
Hillman K. Acute stress ulceration. Anaesth Intens Care 1985; 13:230–240.
Shuman RB, Schuster DP, Zuckerman GR. Prophylactic therapy for stress ulcer bleeding: a reappraisal. Ann Intern Med 1987; 106:562–567.

FUNCTIONAL DISORDERS OF THE UPPER GASTROINTESTINAL TRACT

WILLIAM V. HARFORD Jr., M.D.
MARK FELDMAN, M.D.

A functional gastrointestinal (GI) disorder can be defined as a disturbance of GI function in the absence of an objectively demonstrable pathologic condition. As diagnostic techniques improve, disorders currently believed to be functional may be shown to have an organic basis. For example, some patients with chronic diarrhea and "negative" tests (stool microbiology, barium enema, colonoscopy), once thought to have functional diarrhea, have now been found to have microscopic colitis.

Physician attitudes play an important role in the treatment of functional GI disorders. Many physicians prefer to treat specific biochemical, infectious, or structural abnormalities, and lack the patience to assess functional disorders. They may assume that the symptoms are due to psychopathology or hypochondriasis, and patients may be told that nothing can be found. In these circumstances, patients remain distressed and may feel that the evaluation was incomplete, or that the physician did not believe them. Confidence in the physician may be therapeutic. This does not necessarily require repeated or exhaustive clinical investigations, but rather a thoughtful evaluation, along with empathy, reassurance, and a clear explanation of the diagnosis and prognosis. In general, this approach is satisfactory for both physician and patient. There are only a few instances in which the efficacy of medications, beyond the placebo effect, has been demonstrated in functional GI disease.

NONULCER DYSPEPSIA

Clinical Features

There is a large and heterogeneous group of patients with symptoms of epigastric discomfort or burning, early satiety, fullness, and nausea for which no cause can be found. These patients are often said to have nonulcer dyspepsia (NUD). Some patients have pain virtually identical to that of peptic ulcer disease, but no ulcer. Others have symptoms suggestive of disturbances of gastric emptying, and some have an overlap of symptoms. This variability in presentation, along with our incomplete understanding of the pathophysiology, accounts for the variety of terms used for this syndrome, such as functional dyspepsia, nervous dyspepsia, pyloroduodenal irritability, pseudoulcer syndrome, and gastritis. NUD is a common problem found in perhaps 30 to 60 percent of patients presenting with upper abdominal symptoms, and 30 percent of those presenting for gastroscopy. It is at least two to five times as common as peptic ulcer disease (PUD).

In making a diagnosis of NUD it is important to exclude esophagitis, PUD, biliary tract disease, pancreatitis, and small bowel mucosal disease. Symptoms of gastroesophageal reflux or irritable bowel syndrome (IBS) are associated with NUD in about 30 percent of patients, but this is also true of a control population. Heartburn from GER or the disordered bowel habits of IBS should be considered as separate from NUD. Gallstones occur in 5 percent of patients with NUD, about the same as in control populations. One must be cautious in attributing symptoms of nausea, vague abdominal pain, and flatulence to gallstones, as this may lead to unnecessary cholecystectomies.

Pathophysiology

There is no evidence of acid hypersecretion in NUD. It has been proposed that acid back-diffusion causes pain in NUD, but intragastric acid infusion does not consistently reproduce the pain, and acid suppression (with H_2-receptor antagonists) has been of only marginal benefit compared with placebo (see below).

Gastritis occurs in 50 percent of patients with NUD, but also in 50 percent of asymptomatic individuals above the age of 40. The discovery of the association of *Campylobacter pylori* with gastritis has caused interest in the role of this organism in NUD. *Campylobacter* occurs in 30 to 50 percent of patients with NUD, but again this is not much different from asymptomatic, age-matched controls.

Analgesic use has not been shown to be increased in NUD. However, it is recommended that patients with NUD who are taking aspirin or other nonsteroidal anti-inflammatory drugs (NSAIDs) discontinue these drugs if possible; if not, a trial of another NSAID is warranted.

Duodenogastric reflux has been proposed as a mechanism of NUD, but seems to occur as often in controls as in symptomatic patients. About 20 percent of patients have endoscopic duodenitis, with redness, erosions, and microscopic inflammation on biopsy. These patients may have typical ulcer symptoms, in the absence of an ulcer. The gross and histologic findings are not consistently related to symptoms, and the mechanism of pain in these patients is not clear. Some authors believe that duodenitis is part of a spectrum that includes duodenal ulcer disease, but the natural history of duodenitis is not clear.

Another group of patients with NUD (as many as 50 percent) have symptoms primarily suggestive of a gastric motility disorder, including epigastric discomfort, bloating, fullness, nausea, and belching after meals. Some studies have suggested abnormalities of antral motility and delayed gastric emptying of solids. Other patients have been shown to have abnormalities of gastric electrical activity. In such patients, it is important to exclude identifiable causes of delayed gastric emptying, such as diabetes mellitus and pyloric stenosis.

Treatment

Most studies have shown no appreciable benefit from antacids or H_2-receptor antagonists compared with placebo. A few have demonstrated a small benefit from cimetidine in patients with more typical ulcer symptoms, or associated heartburn. One study suggested that sucralfate in a dosage of 1 g, 30 minutes before meals, was better than placebo in relief of mild to moderate symptoms, but this remains to be confirmed.

At this time, there is no convincing evidence to support the use of therapy directed against *C. pylori* in patients with NUD. Side effects from the therapy (bismuth and antibiotics) may be worse than the original problem. *C. pylori* is also discussed in the chapter *Chronic Gastritis*.

In the subset of patients with symptoms suggestive of delayed gastric emptying, metoclopramide, cisapride, and domperidone have all been tried (Table 1). These agents are prokinetic and improve gastric emptying. In addition, metoclopramide, and to a lesser extent domperidone, have central antiemetic effects, which may be as important as their prokinetic effects for relief of symptoms. Metoclopramide has been found to be better than placebo in relieving dyspeptic symptoms. However, it has up to a 20 percent incidence of side effects, and we are reluctant to recommend it for chronic use in NUD. Domperidone and cisapride have fewer side effects, and both have been shown to relieve postprandial discomfort in NUD. Cisapride seems to accelerate distal bowel transit, and may be of benefit in NUD patients with constipation. However, cisapride and domperidone are not yet available in the United States.

Standard antimuscarinic agents have not been helpful in NUD. Pirenzepine, an M_1 receptor–specific antimuscarinic, in a dosage of 25 to 50 mg twice daily, was beneficial in two studies, but not in a third. Pirenzepine reduces gastric acid secretion and may modulate migrating motor complexes. It has little effect on gastric emptying.

Therapeutic Approach

In patients with primarily "peptic" symptoms or who have associated heartburn, aggravating factors such as analgesics, alcohol, and tobacco should be eliminated. If this fails to relieve symptoms, a trial of low-dose antacid, sucralfate, or cimetidine (400 mg twice daily) is warranted. In patients with symptoms suggestive of a gastric motility disturbance, metoclopramide may be tried, but the dosage should be as low as possible to avoid adverse effects, and the duration of therapy should be as short as feasible. When domperidone or cisapride become available for use in the United States, these agents may be useful alternatives, with fewer side effects.*

NAUSEA AND VOMITING

Vomiting is coordinated by a center in the lateral reticular formation of the medulla. This center receives afferent input from the vagus nerves, from GI sympathetic nerves, from the chemoreceptor trigger zone in the area postrema of the fourth ventricle, and from other brain centers. The chemoreceptor trigger zone has receptors for dopamine and opiate neurotransmitters.

Some known causes of nausea and vomiting are outlined in Table 2. Even after extensive evaluation, there remains a group of patients with nausea and vomiting of unknown cause. Some of these patients may have psychophysiologic disturbances, and others may have idiopathic disturbances of gastric emptying, which may be documented by radionuclide gastric emptying studies or gastric electrophysiologic testing.

* **Editor's Note:** Some authors advocate treating *C. pylori* with bismuth and antibiotics if it is proved to be present in patients with NUD.

TABLE 1 Gastrointestinal Prokinetic Agents

Agent	*Mechanism of Action*	*Dose*	*Adverse Effects*
Metoclopramide	Central antiemetic Prokinetic (dopamine receptor antagonist and cholinergic agonist)	5–20 mg PO ½-hr before meals 10 mg IV q6h	Drowsiness, anxiety, restlessness: 20%; extrapyramidal symptoms: 1%; hyperprolactinemia, breast enlargement and tenderness, galactorrhea, menstrual irregularities
Domperidone	Prokinetic (dopamine antagonist)	20–30 mg PO tid (suppository form available)	Hyperprolactinemia, etc., as above; dry mouth, headache, diarrhea, rash, itching
Cisapride	Prokinetic (increased acetylcholine release)	4–8 mg PO tid 10 mg IV	Loose stool

TABLE 2 Causes of Nausea and Vomiting

Acute

Gastroenteritis, enterotoxins
Drugs, including chemotherapeutic agents, NSAIDs
Acute mechanical obstruction
Anesthesia and surgery
Vestibular disorders
Visceral pain
Metabolic disturbances
Hepatitis
Motor sickness

Chronic

Gastric outlet obstruction
- Duodenal, pyloric, or gastric ulcer
- Gastric carcinoma
- Pancreatic disease

Motility disorders
- Diabetic gastroparesis
- Gastric dysrhythmias
- Drug-induced stasis
- Postgastric surgery
- Chronic intestinal pseudoobstruction
- Idiopathic gastric stasis

Metabolic disorders

Pregnancy

Increased intracranial pressure

Eating disorders
- Anorexia nervosa
- Bulimia

Psychogenic

TABLE 3 Examples of Phenothiazines Used for Nausea and Vomiting

Prochlorperazine maleate (Compazine)	5–10 mg IM q3–4h 25-mg suppository bid 5–10 mg PO q3–4h
Promethazine hydrochloride (Phenergan)	12.5–25 mg IM q4h 12.5–25-mg suppository q4–6h 25 mg PO bid
Perphenazine (Trilafon)	5 mg IM q6h 2–4 mg PO q6h
Chlorpromazine hydrochloride (Thorazine)	25–50 mg IM q4h 10–25 mg PO q4–6h

Treatment

In the treatment of nausea and vomiting, it is of obvious importance to exclude underlying organic conditions that can be corrected. This may require very careful history taking, including review of all medications; physical examination, including neurologic evaluation; laboratory studies, including tests for metabolic and endocrine disorders; endoscopy; and GI x-ray studies. In any woman of childbearing age, it is critical to exclude pregnancy before proceeding with radiologic studies or with treatment.

Phenothiazines

When it is not possible to correct the underlying condition, the most commonly used medications are the phenothiazines, which act as dopamine antagonists in the central nervous system (CNS). Examples of these agents, with suggested dosages, are given in Table 3. Drowsiness and extrapyramidal reactions are the most common adverse effects.

Metoclopramide

In patients who appear to have a disturbance of gastric emptying, prokinetic agents such as metoclopramide or domperidone may be helpful (see Table 1). In the treatment of gastric stasis, absorption of medication may be delayed, so it may be necessary to "prime" patients with intravenous or intramuscular medication. The dosage of metoclopramide should be reduced in older patients to 5 mg four times a day, because of the high frequency of extrapyramidal side effects. Contraindications to the use of metoclopramide include evidence of GI obstruction, Parkinson's disease, or the use of other dopamine antagonists, such as phenothiazines. Anticholinergics partially antagonize the effect of metoclopramide.

Metoclopramide is also useful for the nausea and vomiting associated with cancer chemotherapy. Up to 2 mg per kilogram can be given by slow intravenous infusion 30 minutes before beginning chemotherapy; this can be repeated every 2 hours for two doses, and then every 3 hours for three additional doses.

Tetrahydrocannabinol

An oral form of tetrahydrocannabinol has been released under the name dronabinol or Marinol for use in cancer chemotherapy. It has been shown to be superior to placebo and phenothiazines in preventing nausea and vomiting after cancer chemotherapy. It can cause side effects of drowsiness, orthostatic hypotension, dry mouth, and tachycardia, as well as CNS effects of anxiety, manic psychosis, visual hallucinations, and depression.

Nausea and vomiting associated with motion sickness can be treated with meclizine (Antivert) in an oral dose of 25 to 50 mg, taken 1 hour before embarkation, or similarly with transdermal scopolamine (Transderm-Scop) applied 4 hours before embarkation. Both drugs can cause drowsiness and anticholinergic side effects.

Postgastric Surgery Symptoms

After vagotomy or partial gastrectomy, some patients develop nausea and vomiting that may be due to delayed gastric emptying, but may also be caused by reflux of bile and duodenal contents into the stomach. A variety of agents have been tried for this latter condition, such as cholestyramine, aluminum hydroxide–containing antacids, sucralfate, and metoclopramide, but none with any uniform success. In severe and unresponsive cases, it may be necessary to revise the gastroenterotomy, forming a Roux-en-Y jejunal limb to prevent bile reflux, but this should be done cautiously, since if the disturbance is primarily one of delayed gastric emptying the patient may not improve.

RUMINATION

Rumination is the repeated and involuntary regurgitation of food, usually one mouthful at a time, after a meal. Part of the material may be ejected, and part chewed and swallowed again. It usually occurs within 15 minutes of eating, and may last several hours. It characteristically ceases when the food becomes acid to the taste. There is no associated abdominal discomfort, heartburn, or nausea, and it should be distinguished from GER reflux and vomiting. Certain personality disturbances, such as hypochondriasis and depression, appear to be common in rumination. The problem often occurs in young people, for whom it may be a source of considerable embarrassment. Aside from its social consequences, rumination does not pose a threat to health, although in children it may be associated with weight loss and failure to thrive. There is sometimes a family history of rumination.

Motility studies have shown that esophageal, gastric, and upper small bowel motility are normal. Lower esophageal sphincter (LES) pressure is also normal. The episodes of rumination are associated with spike waves seen simultaneously in the esophagus and stomach, which appear to be due to sudden increases in intra-abdominal pressure.

Reassurance, and a careful explanation of the pathophysiology, are probably the most important form of therapy. Certain forms of behavior modification have been found helpful. One such method consists of having the patient eat in the presence of the therapist, while being encouraged to refrain from regurgitation. The quantity of food is increased in gradual fashion. Biofeedback, including a technique of relaxing the abdominal muscles during and after eating, has also been successful. Neither drug therapy nor surgery is indicated.

GLOBUS PHARYNGEUS

Globus pharyngeus (or globus hystericus) is a continuous sensation of a lump in the throat. It is not true dysphagia, in that it is not associated with difficulty in swallowing; in fact, it may be transiently relieved by swallowing. Globus pharyngeus is common: up to 45 percent of normal individuals have experienced it at one time. Typically, a careful examination does not disclose an organic cause for this symptom; hence, the term globus hystericus, implying that the symptom is hysterical or psychoneurotic. In point of fact, surveys of patients with this condition have not disclosed any significant psychopathology. Patients are often referred from specialist to specialist, and are told by each that there is nothing to be found. They may then become desperate, convinced that a cancer or other serious problem has been missed, or that the physicians believe them to be mentally ill. A minority of patients have conditions such as sinusitis, pharyngitis, dental infection, a vallecular polyp or cyst, a pharyngeal pouch, a goiter, or (importantly) squamous cell carcinoma. In a rare patient, globus is the first symptom of a motor neuron disease. Although there is no increase in symptoms of heartburn among patients with globus pharyngeus, several studies have suggested that there may be an increased incidence of gastroesophageal reflux.

Treatment

Our approach to globus pharyngeus is as follows. In young patients with a short history, reassurance and possibly a brief trial of antacids are indicated. In older patients, or those with a longer history of globus or with risk factors for pharyngeal carcinoma, a careful oropharyngeal examination, laryngoscopy, and fiberoptic esophagoscopy are indicated. When evidence of esophagitis is found, a trial of H_2 blockers may improve symptoms. In other patients, sympathetic reassurance and follow-up suffice.

HICCUPS

Hiccups are usually short-lived and constitute only an embarrassment or an inconvenience. Occasionally, they can be chronic and unremitting, causing fatigue, sleeplessness, and difficulty with eating.

A hiccup is a sudden contraction of the inspiratory muscles, terminated by abrupt closure of the glottis. The hiccup center is located in the cervical spinal cord between C3 and C7. Afferent impulses are transmitted via the vagus nerves, phrenic nerves, and sympathetic chain of the sixth to the twelfth thoracic segments. Phrenic efferents innervate the glottis and the accessory muscles of respiration. Hiccups may be caused by a wide variety of metabolic disorders, drugs, or conditions affecting some part of the reflex arc, including the CNS, chest, diaphragm, or abdomen (Table 4).

In treating hiccups, it is most important to search carefully for an underlying cause and correct it, if possible. If no cause is found, or if the underlying cause cannot be treated, simple physical maneuvers should be tried. Some examples are listed in Table 5. These maneuvers have in common an attempt to disrupt the hiccup reflex arc. When physical maneuvers fail, pharmacologic agents may be required. There are scores of anecdotal reports of different drugs, which reflects the inconsistent success of pharmacotherapy; some of the most commonly used are listed in Table 5. Several authors have reported successful use of hypnosis, and acupuncture has been used in the Far East. When hiccups are refractory to all the above therapies, phrenic nerve block can be considered. Fluoroscopy should first be performed to determine which diaphragmatic leaflet is contracting. A temporary block should be done before a phrenic nerve crush or transection is attempted. We would exhaust all conservative measures, including hypnosis and acupuncture, before proceeding to phrenic block.

TABLE 4 Causes of Hiccups

Transient Hiccups

Gastric distention
Alcohol ingestion
Sudden excitement, emotional stress
Sudden change in temperature
Esophageal obstruction

Chronic Hiccups

Metabolic/toxic: uremia, diabetes, hyperventilation, hypokalemia, hypocalcemia, hyponatremia, gout, fever

Drugs: barbiturates, alpha-methyldopa, diazepam, chlordiazepoxide, dexamethasone

General anesthesia

Postoperative state

Diaphragmatic irritation

Gastroesophageal reflux

Irritation of vagus nerve (meningeal, auricular, pharyngeal, thoracic, or abdominal branches or recurrent laryngeal branch)

Central nervous system disorder: traumatic, infectious, vascular, or structural lesions

Psychogenic

Idiopathic

AEROPHAGIA AND BELCHING

Normally, 2 or 3 ml of air reaches the stomach with every swallow. Upon eating a gastric air bubble accumulates, and under the appropriate circumstances relaxation of the lower and upper esophageal sphincters allows us to belch. Anxiety, and certain activities such as chewing gum and smoking, increase the amount of air swallowed. Carbonated beverages obviously add to the gastric air bubble. Some patients who complain of belching can simply be given an explanation of their symptom and reassured.

TABLE 5 Methods of Treating Hiccups

Nonpharmacologic Methods	*Examples*
Irritation of uvula or nasopharynx	Tongue traction, lifting the uvula, swabbing the pharynx
Counterirritation of vagal nerve	Carotid sinus massage
Interruption of respiratory rhythm	Breath holding
Respiratory center stimulants	Hyperventilation
Counterirritation of diaphragm	Pulling knees up to chest
Relief of gastric distention	Nasogastric aspiration
Pharmacologic Methods (Agents)	*Dosages*
Chlorpromazine	25–50 mg IV q6h 25–50 mg PO q6h
Metoclopramide	10 mg IV q4h 10 mg PO q6h
Quinidine sulfate	200 mg PO qid
Diphenylhydantoin	200 mg IV 100 mg PO qid
Valproic acid	15 mg/kg PO daily

However, belching can be a much more distressing and dramatic symptom. It is possible to learn how to take large amounts of air into the esophagus and the stomach. Some patients have been observed to swallow up to 250 ml of air in a fraction of a second. They can be seen to elevate the chin and extend the neck, which holds open the esophagus, while making an inspiratory effort with the glottis closed. In these circumstances, the ingested air does not always go into the stomach, but may stay in the esophagus, and is then forced out by a contraction of the chest wall and the diaphragm. In some patients a substantial fraction of air enters the stomach, and from there, the small bowel. Belching may be a learned response or a "bad habit." Initially, the patient may have learned to associate relief of certain symptoms with belching. These initial symptoms may include dyspepsia from peptic ulcer, gastroesophageal reflux, IBS, biliary tract disease, or even angina pectoris. Nausea or psychological stress may increase the swallowing rate, and thus lead to accumulation of gas in the stomach. Occasionally, treatment of the underlying condition decreases the stimulus to the learned reflex, and the belching stops. However, this learned reflex may persist even if the initial inciting disorder resolves, and the vicious cycle of belching, relief, and air swallowing will be perpetuated subconsciously.

Some patients with aerophagia may retain a significant amount of gastric air without belching, causing the "gas bloat syndrome," or may pass a significant amount of gas into the small intestine, causing additional distention and discomfort. Symptoms in these patients are usually aggravated by meals, especially large meals.

It is irrational, given the pathophysiology of belching, to use antacids, simethicone, charcoal, or pancreatic enzymes, unless these are aimed at some underlying condition. If belching persists once the underlying condition is treated, careful explanation and reassurance may be all that is required. Patients with a strong psychoneurotic overlay are difficult to reassure. Some physicians have learned to demonstrate belching at will, and this may be an effective technique for reassuring the patient that belching does not indicate serious organic pathology. Unfortunately, not all of us have been able to master this technique.

SUGGESTED READING

Amarnath RP, Abell TL, Malagelada J-R. The rumination syndrome in adults. A characteristic manometric pattern. Ann Intern Med 1986; 105:513–518.

Batch AJ. Globus pharyngeus. Parts I and II. A discussion. J Laryngol Otol 1988; 102:156–158, 227–230.

Hanson JS, McCallum RW. The diagnosis and management of nausea and vomiting. A review. Am J Gastroenterol 1985; 80:210–218.

Kahn KL, Greenfield S. The efficacy of endoscopy in the evaluation of dyspepsia. A review of the literature and development of a sound strategy. J Clin Gastroenterol 1986; 3:346–358.

Lewis JH. Hiccups: cause and cures. J Clin Gastroenterol 1985; 7:539–552.

Roth JL, Bockus HL. Aerophagia: its etiology, syndromes, and management. Med Clin North Am 1957; 141:1673–1696.

Talley NJ, Phillips SF. Nonulcer dyspepsia: potential causes and pathophysiology. Ann Intern Med 1988; 108:865–879.

IRRITABLE BOWEL SYNDROME

DOUGLAS A. DROSSMAN, M.D.

The irritable bowel syndrome (IBS) is an extremely common disorder of intestinal motility seen in about 15 percent of the population. It accounts for 25 to 50 percent of referrals to gastroenterologists and makes up 28 percent of their practice. Despite its high prevalence and general benignity, physicians often regard IBS as one of the most difficult conditions to treat. There is no "gold standard" to validate the diagnosis; the patient's functional state and illness behaviors may be out of proportion to the degree of physiologic dysfunction; treatment is nonspecific; and the clinical responses may be unpredictable and unrewarding.

DIAGNOSIS

IBS is diagnosed by patient complaints of altered bowel function, usually with abdominal pain, and a negative medical evaluation. These nonspecific symptoms, coupled with the absence of clearly defined pathologic or laboratory findings, can make it difficult to be confident of a diagnosis of IBS. No physician is comfortable with diagnostic uncertainty, and the persistence of this feeling affects the physician-patient interaction and the patient's clinical response. For these reasons, a five-man international working team presented consensus guidelines for the diagnosis of IBS (Table 1). The emphasis on using positive symptom criteria and a minimal diagnostic assessment is supported by at least five prospective studies that show a rediagnosis rate averaging only 3.5 percent for patients initially diagnosed as IBS and followed for up to 6 years. Therefore, unless there is objective evidence of a change in the clinical picture, an initial diagnosis of IBS using these guidelines should not require extensive or repeated diagnostic evaluation.

PATHOGENESIS

Physiologic studies show that patients with IBS, compared with normal persons, have an exaggerated behavioral and motility response to environmental stimuli including diet, hormones, and physical and psychological stress. It is likely that IBS is a biologically heterogeneous disorder, and for any given patient there may be one or several factors contributing to the clinical picture (e.g., abnormal myoelectric pattern, altered sensation threshold, abnormalities in neurotransmitters or their receptors, psychological factors). When a specific cause is found to explain the symptom complex (e.g., lactase deficiency, collagenous colitis), the person is no longer considered to have IBS. However, given the high prevalence of IBS symptoms in the population, it is also likely that IBS may coexist with other disorders. This latter concept is reinforced in the chapters *Carbohydrate Malabsorption* and *Ulcerative Colitis*.

Biologic factors underlie the exaggerated physiologic response, but psychosocial factors affect how the disorder is experienced and acted upon. In one study, my colleagues and I confirmed that compared with normals, IBS patients exhibit more abnormal psychological features. However, when we controlled for symptom severity, these abnormal psychological features were not seen to the same degree in patients with IBS who had never visited a physician. In fact, nonpatients with IBS were not psychologically different from normals. I concluded that the abnormal psychological features previously attributed to IBS relate not to the disorder per se, but to the subset of individuals who see physicians. The important implication is that treatment directed solely toward ameliorating the bowel disturbance is insufficient to achieve an optimal clinical response; attention must also be paid to the psychosocial factors influencing the patient's decision to see a doctor.

GENERAL APPROACH TO TREATMENT

Once the diagnosis is established, treatment should be directed toward amelioration of symptoms, identification and modification of factors that aggravate the disorder, and helping the patient adapt to the condition. Some recommendations follow.

Develop a Therapeutic Relationship

Whether you see the patient as a consultant or in a primary care role, the establishment of a good physician-patient relationship is the foundation of therapeutic response.

TABLE 1 Guidelines for Diagnosis of Irritable Bowel Syndrome*

Symptom Criteria
Continuous or recurrent symptoms of:
Abdominal pain, relieved by defecation or associated with change in frequency or consistency of stool
and/or
Disturbed defecation (two or more of)
Altered stool frequency
Altered stool form (hard or loose/watery)
Altered stool passage (straining or urgency, feeling of incomplete evacuation)
Passage of mucus
usually with
Bloating or feeling of abdominal distention
Physical Examination
Excludes other disorders causing bowel symptoms
No diagnostic physical signs
Appropriate Investigation
Complete history and physical examination
Sigmoidoscopy once (rigid or flexible)
Complete blood count
Sedimentation rate
Stool testing as clinically indicated (Hemoccult, ova and parasites, culture)
Additional diagnostic studies only if clinically indicated

* Presented at The International Congress of Gastroenterology, Rome, September 6, 1988.

In my experience, it is not what you do, but *how* you do it that makes the difference in treatment. This may explain why patients with IBS are found to be such high responders to placebo, ranging from 30 to 80 percent. To establish a therapeutic relationship, the physician must (1) obtain the history through a nondirective, patient-centered interview; (2) be nonjudgmental; (3) determine the patient's understanding of the illness ("What do you think is causing your symptoms?") and his or her concerns; (4) identify and respond realistically to the patient's expectations for improvement ("How do you feel I can be helpful to you?"); (5) set consistent limits ("I appreciate how bad the pain is, but narcotic medication is not medically indicated"); and (6) involve the patient in the treatment approach. For example, it is helpful to give the patient treatment options to choose from: to indulge individual preferences in increasing dietary fiber, and to decide on the type and timing of prescribed medication.

Establish Continuity of Care

Because patients with IBS may have chronic or recurring symptoms, it is important that they visit a primary care physician on a regular basis. Frequent brief visits may be needed initially and during exacerbations to reduce discomfort and allay anxiety. During quiescent periods, one or two visits each year suffice. Regular visits assure patients of physicians' long-term commitment, and patients make fewer late night calls or "emergency" visits when they know their doctor is familiar with the problem.

Educate

The physician should help the patient develop a realistic understanding of the illness and the factors contributing to its exacerbation, the goal being to modify these factors or the patient's attitude toward them. It is usually helpful to explain that IBS is a very real disorder in which the intestine is oversensitive to a variety of stimuli such as food, hormonal changes (e.g., menses), and stress. The relationship between altered bowel response (e.g., segmental spasm of the colon) and clinical symptoms should be illustrated. Patients may be relieved to learn that the condition is not associated with malignancy or shortened life expectancy, and does not require surgery. It is important to emphasize that both physiologic and psychological factors interact in the illness; IBS is not solely *psychological* or *organic*. Any implication that the problem is all "emotional" will be interpreted by the patient as a rejection.

Don't Just Do Something: Stand There!

Although the physician should respond empathetically to patients' needs, this does not mean "going along" with them when it would not be in their best interest. Polypharmacy, polyprocedure, narcotics, and disability are examples of possible physician responses to the demanding patient even when the responses are against the physician's better judgment ("furor medicus").

Determine and Respond to Why the Patient is Coming

On the basis of my observations, clinical improvement is best obtained when the physician addresses not only the symptoms, but also the factors contributing to the patient's decision to seek health care. The reasons for the visit may not be stated voluntarily, but this type of information can be elicited by careful questioning ("What led you to see me at this time?") and by observing the patient's verbal and nonverbal behavior during the visit. Table 2 lists some factors that may contribute to the patient's decision to see the doctor.

DIETARY AND PHARMACOLOGIC TREATMENTS

For the reasons mentioned, it is understandable that no pharmacologic agent or behavioral intervention has been shown to be effective for IBS. There have also been methodologic problems in determining drug efficacy in IBS: (1) previous studies did not use consistent patient selection criteria; (2) the placebo response is high and sample sizes are small, thereby raising the potential for type II error; (3) there are no objective markers for improvement; (4) treatment periods have tended to be short in a disorder with unpredictable periods of exacerbation and remission; and (5) compliance is difficult to assess, particularly when many drugs produce undesirable side effects.

Diet

The first approach is to determine whether certain food items (particularly lactose, caffeine, fatty foods, alcohol, sorbitol gum, and gas-producing foods, such as beans and cabbage) exacerbate the symptoms. If a food item is identified (I prefer this be determined by a food diary), the patient should monitor the symptoms first by eliminating that item and then by rechallenging. This approach minimizes the tendency of some patients to overgeneralize the effects of diet. The items mentioned may bring about reproducible physiologic effects on intestinal function, but the possibility of immunologically mediated food hypersensitivity in IBS remains more controversial, and is likely to play only a minor role, or none. It has been suggested that several food items (e.g., milk, wheat, and tea) may produce prostaglandin E_2-mediated diarrhea.

I generally recommend that patients increase the amount of fiber consumed, either through the diet or with supplements (e.g., Metamucil). Dietary fiber of 15 to 20 g per day increases stool weight and decreases intestinal transit time. It is effective for constipation, but the results are mixed with regard to its benefit for diarrhea and bowel-related pain. Patients seen in primary care settings seem to achieve some benefit, and it is a moot point whether this is accomplished via a therapeutic effect, by placebo response, or because the patient is allowed an active role in the treatment. I recommend fiber for all my patients since it is safe and inexpen-

TABLE 2 Why is The Patient Coming to the Doctor?

Reason	*Treatment Approach*
Recent symptom exacerbation	1. Identify exacerbating factors (e.g., use a patient diary) 2. Help patient modify exacerbating factors (e.g., diet change, medication)
Fear of serious disease	1. Determine underlying concerns (e.g., recent family death or GI illness, prodding by spouse, recent media exposure) 2. Offer counseling and reassurance to address concerns 3. Avoid reassurance that is premature or that undermines the legitimacy of the complaints ("There's nothing wrong . . . it's nerves")
Environmental stressor(s)	1. Identify stressor(s) 2. Establish patient's ability and willingness to acknowledge stressor and work toward change 3. Develop treatment approach based on #2 a. Wait expectantly for resolution or b. Counsel patient c. Suggest stress reduction techniques (exercise, relaxation training, hypnosis) d. Refer for psychological counseling
Psychological distress	1. Make a psychological diagnosis a. Anxiety b. Depression c. Somatization d. Abnormal illness behavior 2. Consider pharmacologic intervention a. Antidepressants b. Brief trial of antianxiety agent 3. Obtain psychiatric consultation if needed
Functional impairment (physical/psychosocial)	1. Determine change in functional status 2. Set treatment outcome to be improved function, rather than relief of symptoms
"Hidden agenda"	1. Identify hidden agenda a. Narcotics b. Laxative abuse c. Disability d. Keep sick role privileges at work and/or home 2. Articulate agenda and clarify your role and limits of treatment

sive. One anticipated side effect is increased bloating and gaseousness due to colonic metabolism of nondigestible fiber. If this occurs, I encourage patients to reduce the dosage and "stick with it" for at least 3 to 4 weeks before deciding that it is not helpful.

Anticholinergics

Anticholinergics ("antispasmodics") are the most frequently used pharmacologic agents to treat IBS. The rationale for their use relates to their effects on reducing stimulated colonic motor activity in patients with IBS. However, a clear relationship between symptoms and gut motility has not been established. Clinical trials for IBS have shown mixed results, and most were methodoiogically flawed. I tend to prescribe these drugs (dicyclomine, 10 to 20 mg, glycopyrrolate, 1 to 2 mg, 30 minutes before meals and at bedtime) as a second line of treatment when pain symptoms are episodic, particularly if they occur in response to meals. Side effects of dry mouth and blurred vision tend to occur when optimal dosage levels are achieved. There is little, if any, value in combination anticholinergic and antianxiety drugs.

Antidepressants

Antidepressants have a theoretical role in the control of IBS symptoms, either through their effects on pain perception, through their anticholinergic action, or as therapy for an associated depression. Data from randomized clinical trials of various chronic pain syndromes (migraine headache, low back pain, herpetic neuralgia, diabetic neuropathy) show clinical benefit. However, the few trials done in IBS had methodologic limitations and had variable results. I use antidepressants for patients with IBS who (1) have symptoms of major or atypical depression (e.g., weight loss, fatigue, sleep disturbance, crying spells, past history of depression); (2) have panic attacks or agoraphobia (episodes of anxiety, feelings of doom, loss of control, severe restriction of daily function); or (3) who are physically or psychosocially disabled by their condition (e.g., unable to work or engage in usual social activities). The tertiary amine tricyclic antidepressants (e.g., doxepin, amitriptyline, 50 to 150 mg at bedtime) have theoretical advantages in controlling pain by virtue of their serotonin-enhancing effect in the central nervous system (CNS). Patients must agree to stay on medication for 3 to 4 weeks before discontinuing, and then commit themselves to continuous treatment for 3 to 6 months. If side effects develop, I prefer to reduce the medication rather than temporarily discontinue it.

Anxiolytics

Benzodiazepines have not been shown to be effective in improving IBS symptoms, but may have a role in the short term (less than 2 weeks) treatment of patients who are temporarily dysfunctional as a result of situational anxiety. These agents should not be chronically used because of their sedative effects, and their risk of habituation and interaction with other drugs and alcohol. A newer anxiolytic agent, buspirone (5 to 10 mg four times a day), has a theoretical advantage since it does not act upon the benzodiazepine receptor.

Opioid Agents

Opioid-like drugs act via peripheral receptors in the gut. Loperamide (2 to 4 mg four times a day) decreases intestinal motility, enhances intestinal water and ion absorption, and may strengthen rectal sphincter tone. It has been proved effective in treating the diarrhea and urgency of IBS and may also help patients with fecal soiling. Dextromethorphan (15 to 30 mg four times a day), the D-isomer of a narcotic, levomethorphan, was found in one multicenter study to be better than placebo in improving the pain of patients with IBS. Oral naloxone, an opiate antagonist, was shown to increase stool weight and frequency in patients with constipation and to alter colonic motility in patients with IBS, but it is expensive and its use is still experimental. These drugs appear to be safer than narcotics since they do not cross the blood-brain barrier. There is no role for narcotics in IBS.

Peppermint Oil

Used primarily in Great Britain, peppermint oil acts on the smooth muscle as an antispasmodic and may reduce abnormal gut motor activity in patients with IBS. Clinical trials show mixed benefit, but since the side effects are minimal, the drug can be safely used if available.

Dopamine Antagonists

Metoclopramide (10 to 20 mg four times a day) and domperidone may benefit IBS patients with symptoms of delayed gastric emptying, but treatment trials show mixed results. These agents may be considered for patients with early satiety and functional vomiting.

PSYCHOSOCIAL AND BEHAVIORAL TREATMENTS

Patients vary in the degree of physiologic and psychosocial factors influencing their illness and in their response to treatment. For example, people with IBS who do not visit physicians have more normal psychological profiles, and may either have minimal physiologic disturbance or not recognize their symptoms as problematic. Little if any treatment is needed. Patients seen in primary care settings often have minimal or moderate treatment requirements, and often respond to education, dietary modifications, and occasional prescribed medication. On the other hand, patients who often visit the referral gastroenterologist's office and who are psychosocially disabled are refractory to simple treatments and symptomatic drugs. For this group, behavioral interventions that identify and modify stressors and help them cope with their illness are also required. The following suggestions may be applied to all patients, but have particular value for IBS patients with refractory illness and impaired function.

Reset Treatment Goals

IBS is a chronic disorder, and even more refractory patients may maintain the prospect of cure. Once the physician elicits this expectation, treatment can be refocused to accomplish reasonable goals. Patients should be informed that (1) the illness is incurable, (2) it is unrealistic to expect quick improvement, (3) all chronic disorders have their ups and downs—the physician will offer symptomatic treatment during difficult times and help the patient maintain health during good times, and (4) improvement needs to be gauged more by return of previous function (e.g., return to work and social activities) than by amelioration of symptoms.

Modify Abnormal Illness Behaviors

Despite patients' intent to be well, there can be hidden benefits (increased family attention, privileges at work, financial compensation, or a dependent relationship with a physician) that tend to maintain the illness. These "sick role" benefits are appropriate for patients with acute illness, but are detrimental for those with chronic illness. Patients who over many years continue to focus attention on the illness and maintain a passive and dependent relationship with others relating to the illness are considered to have abnormal illness behavior. When this occurs in IBS, the physician should attend more to patients' ability to function autonomously in the face of the illness, rather than to patients' needs for attention as exhibited by physical complaints (thereby maintaining a sick role behavior). Examples include (1) limiting discussions about patients' symptoms to no more than is needed to satisfy medical considerations, (2) not responding to each new complaint with studies or prescriptive medication, (3) encouraging patients to take more active responsibility in their health care, and (4) prescribing and positively reinforcing patients' increased activities at home and work.

Psychotherapy

A goal of psychotherapy is to elucidate and modify stressors or patients' attitudes toward them. This can be accomplished through (1) sharing and working through personal thoughts, conflicts, and perceptions (insight therapy); (2)

identifying relationships between symptoms and the stressors that exacerbate them, and attempting to change previously established maladaptive behaviors that occur in this setting (cognitive-behavioral therapy); or (3) improving interpersonal relationships (family or group therapy). In one study, 3 months of weekly insight and cognitive psychotherapy led to greater improvement in IBS symptoms and psychological scores than in a matched control group receiving standard medical therapy. The differences were even more pronounced after 1 year. This study highlighted the potential benefit of psychotherapy in improve patients' ability to cope with the everyday stresses producing the symptoms.

Since many refractory patients with IBS are reluctant to see therapists, or do so to prove that "nothing is wrong," treatment should be recommended only if patients believe that it will be personally beneficial. One recommended approach is to present the treatment as a means to help patients develop coping strategies to function better. Therefore, psychotherapy should also be considered if patients are physically or psychosocially impaired.

Behavior Therapy

Since the association of stress with exacerbation of IBS symptoms is well documented, stress reduction is a reasonable treatment approach. Behavioral techniques seek to modify the physical and emotional consequences of stress without addressing the psychological determinants. They are of particular benefit for patients seeking stress reduction who do not want to "dig into the past." Relaxation training, meditation, and biofeedback work best when patients can perceive muscular tension and other physiologic responses to stress. Biofeedback enhances this response. Hypnotherapy was shown in one study to be comparable with psychotherapy in reducing pain and abdominal distention and enhancing general well-being. These approaches are oriented toward general stress reduction; there is no evidence that more specific techniques, such as biofeedback to relax colonic motor activity, are clinically beneficial.

SUGGESTED READING

Drossman DA. Psychosocial treatment of the refractory patient with irritable bowel syndrome. J Clin Gastroenterol 1987; 9:253–355.

Drossman DA, McKee DC, Sandler RS, et al. Psychosocial factors in the irritable bowel syndrome: a multivariate study of patients and nonpatients with irritable bowel. Gastroenterology 1988; 95:701–708.

Klein KB. Controlled treatment trials in the irritable bowel syndrome: a critique. Gastroenterology 1988; 95:232–241.

Mitchell CM, Drossman DA. The irritable bowel syndrome: understanding and treating a biopsychosocial illness disorder. Ann Behav Med 1987; 9:13–18.

CARBOHYDRATE MALABSORPTION

JEFFREY S. HYAMS, M.D.

It is quite common for children and adults to experience occasional or even frequent nonspecific gastrointestinal (GI) distress such as gassiness, cramps, bloating, or loose stools. Such individuals are often thought to have functional bowel disease and are given diagnoses such as irritable bowel, spastic colon, or colic. These problems often cause much suffering and usually require considerable time and effort from health professionals. All too often both patient and physician regard the outcome as less than optimal despite extensive diagnostic evaluation and pharmacologic intervention. My view is that many of these individuals are suffering discomfort resulting from the incomplete absorption of dietary carbohydrate.

When ingested carbohydrate escapes complete absorption by the small bowel, it enters the colon, where fermentation by fecal bacteria results in the production of gas and short-chain organic acids. The osmotic load generated by the malabsorbed carbohydrate and organic acids may cause diarrhea. Gut distention and increased peristalsis result in cramps, bloating, and borborygmi. Increased flatus may be noted. Whether the carbohydrate malabsorption is primary or secondary, relief of symptoms depends on identification and then removal or restriction of the offending carbohydrate.

LACTOSE

In patients who appear to develop GI symptoms after ingesting milk-containing products, it is crucial to differentiate among milk allergy, lactose malabsorption, and lactose intolerance. Milk allergy represents a sensitivity to cow's milk protein. It generally requires total elimination of milk-containing products from the diet. Extraintestinal symptoms (e.g., eczema, wheezing) are not necessarily found in milk allergy. Lactose malabsorption connotes incomplete intestinal absorption of a lactose load, as documented by a standard technique such as breath hydrogen testing. Lactose malabsorption does not necessarily imply that GI symptoms are present, but if they are the patient is said to have lactose intolerance. This distinction is important, since the presence of lactose malabsorption (as evidenced by the very sensitive method of breath hydrogen testing) does not necessarily mean that lactose malabsorption is the cause of the problem. It does suggest, however, that lactose malabsorption may be a contributing factor. I rely heavily on the breath hydrogen test as a diagnostic tool, since my experience has been that even a detailed history concerning the relationship of symptoms to milk ingestion may be misleading.

If I find evidence of lactose malabsorption, my approach to patients depends heavily on their age. In Caucasian children under the age of 5 years, and in blacks or Hispanics under the age of 3 to 4 years, lactose malabsorption is virtually always a secondary disorder. In other words, there have been events such as viral infection, parasitic infection (e.g., *Giardia*), celiac disease, or protein-sensitive enteropathy that

TABLE 1 Lactose-Free Diet

This diet is for the patient who must eliminate *all* sources of lactose from the diet. Lactose is the sugar found in milk, so all foods containing milk are to be excluded from the diet.

Read the label carefully. Avoid any food containing milk, nonfat milk solids, skim milk, butter, cream, and lactose.

	Foods Allowed	*Foods Avoided*
Milk	None	All milk, milk drinks— including whole, skim, low fat, dried, evaporated, and condensed milk, human breast milk Yogurt, any type Cream, sweet or sour Infant formulas other than those permitted Frappes, ice cream sodas
Beverages	Powdered, fruit-flavored drinks, ginger ale, carbonated beverages, cocoa without added milk, solids, coffee, tea	Any made with milk, such as frappes, eggnog, hot chocolate
Meats	Any baked, broiled, roasted, and boiled, except those to be avoided	Creamed or breaded meat, fish, or poultry, and prepared meats that may contain dried milk solids, including bologna and cold cuts, frankfurters, salami, commercially prepared fish sticks, and some sausage
Eggs	As desired	Any made with milk—use specific formula; do not prepare with butter
Cheese	None	
Breads	Breads made without milk only, such as French bread, Italian bread, water bagels, or "pareve" breads; saltines, graham, oyster, and soda crackers, Triscuits	Made with any form of milk; any baked product made with milk (muffins, biscuits, waffles, pancakes, donuts, sweet rolls); commercial mixes
Cereal	Any made without milk, cooked or ready to eat (read labels); macaroni, spaghetti, pasta, rice, all prepared without milk or cheese	Any prepared cereal that contains dry milk solids
Vegetables and Potatoes:	All—cooked, canned, frozen, or fresh	Any vegetable prepared with milk, butter, milk solids, bread or bread crumbs; no cheese or cream sauces
Fruit	All	
Desserts	Any made without milk or milk products, such as gelatin desserts, fruit crisp, snow puddings, fruit and water sherberts, pie with fruit filling, angel cake, milk-free cookies (fig bars, ginger snaps, lemon snaps), tofu ice cream	All commercial cake and cookie mixes, ice cream, custard puddings, junket, ice milk, or sherberts that contain milk; frostings made with milk or butter, dessert sauces, cheese cakes
Soup	All prepared without milk or milk products; homemade or canned, e.g., chicken rice	All creamed soups, chowders; no cheese
Fats	Milk-free margarine or "pareve" margarine; oils, nuts, peanut butter	Butter, margarine, some commercial salad dressings (check labels)
Sugar and Seasonings	Sugar, honey, molasses, maple syrup, corn syrup, jelly and jam, hard candy, gum drops, marshmallows, hard peppermints, fondant; salt, pepper, spices, herbs, condiments, vinegar, catsup, relish, pickles, olives, tomato sauce, coconut, wheat germ; artificial flavoring and extracts	Any product made from milk, butter, cream, chocolate, toffee, cream mints, caramel candy, candy with cream centers, butterscotch
Miscellaneous	Coffee Rich, Coffee Mate	Medications that may contain lactose as filler or bulk agents; party dips, nonprescription vitamins, spice blends, Easter egg dyes; dietetic foods and foods advertised as "high protein" sometimes contain lactose or dry milk solids *Check all labels carefully*

From Perman JA. Carbohydrate malabsorption. In: Bayless T, ed. Current therapy in gastroenterology and liver disease. Toronto: BC Decker. 1986:150. Reprinted with permission.

have caused mucosal damage and secondary lactase deficiency. It is imperative that diagnostic studies be conducted for these underlying conditions. Appropriate therapy for these problems will result in mucosal healing and eventual return of lactose absorption.

In older children, adolescents, and adults, lactose malabsorption usually is the result of constitutional lactase deficiency. Unless accompanied by other signs or symptoms suggesting systemic illness (e.g., fever, weight loss, edema), the finding of lactose malabsorption may be considered a primary diagnosis. It should be emphasized to patients that they do not have a disease, but rather a condition associated with the aging process (even if they are still quite young). Although this is an area of some controversy in the literature, I have found lactose intolerance to be a common cause of recurrent abdominal pain in adolescents.

Once I have identified lactose malabsorption, whether primary or secondary, diet modification is attempted in order to determine whether the symptoms may be associated with the malabsorption. Initially, I suggest a 3 to 4-week period of strict avoidance of lactose-containing products (Table 1). Although many patients may be able to tolerate small amounts of lactose without difficulty, this is not known at the start of intervention. If all symptoms abate on the strict lactose-free diet, I ask that small amounts of lactose-containing products be added back to the diet consistent with control of symptoms (Table 2). I emphasize to the patient that a dietary indiscretion such as an ice cream sundae will not cause significant harm beyond the temporary suffering it may cause. Only the patient can decide if it was worth the price.

Information should also be provided about lactose-reduced products. Beta-galactosidases obtained from yeasts and fungi have been isolated, and can be added to milk or ingested immediately before its consumption. LactAid (Lact-Aid, Inc., Pleasantville, NJ) may be added to milk, which is then refrigerated for at least 24 hours before it is used in order to provide time for effective hydrolysis (70 to 90 percent lactose reduction, depending on the dose added and the length of incubation). The milk may be noticeably sweeter after enzymatic treatment. Alternatively, capsules containing lactase (Lactrase, Kremers-Urban Co., Milwaukee, WI)

TABLE 2 Lactose Content of Selected Milk, Milk Products, and Substitutes

Product	*Unit*	*Lactose (Approx. g/unit)*
Milk	1 cup—244 g	11
Low-fat milk, 2% fat	1 cup—244 g	9–13
Skim milk	1 cup—244 g	12–14
Chocolate milk	1 cup—244 g	10–12
Sweet acidophilus	1 cup—244 g	9–10
Sweetened condensed whole milk	1 cup—244 g	35
Dried whole milk	1 cup—128 g	48
Nonfat dry milk, instant	1½ cup—91 g	46
Buttermilk fluid	1 cup—245 g	9–11
Whipped cream topping	1 tbs—3 g	0.4
Light cream	1 tbs—15 g	0.6
Low-fat yogurts	8 oz	8–15
Cheese		
Blue	1 oz—28 g	0.7
Camembert	1 oz—28 g	0.1
Cheddar	1 oz—28 g	0.4–0.6
Colby	1 oz—28 g	0.7
Cream	1 oz—28 g	0.8
Gouda	1 oz—28 g	0.6
Limberger	1 oz—28 g	0.1
Parmesan, grated	1 oz—28 g	0.8
Cheese, pasteurized, processed		
American	1 oz—28 g	0.5
Pimento	1 oz—28 g	0.5–1.7
Swiss	1 oz—28 g	0.4–0.6
Cottage cheese	1 cup—210 g	5–6
Cottage cheese, low-fat (2% fat)	1 cup—226 g	7–8
Butter	2 pats—10 g	0.1
Oleomargarine	2 pats—10 g	0
Ice cream		
Vanilla, regular	1 cup—133 g	9
French, soft	1 cup—173 g	9
Ice milk, vanilla	1 cup—131 g	10
Sherbert, orange	1 cup—193 g	4
Ice, orange	100 g	0

From Welsh JD. Carbohydrate malabsorption. In: Bayless T, ed. Current therapy in gastroenterology and liver disease. Toronto: BC Decker, 1984:136. Reprinted with permission.

can be taken orally at the time lactose is ingested. The number of capsules required varies from person to person according to the intrinsic degree of lactose malabsorption, tolerance of symptoms, and quantity of lactose ingested. Unpasteurized yogurt retains some bacterial lactase activity ("autodigesting") and may be well tolerated by some lactose-intolerant individuals. Interestingly, even pasteurized yogurt with minimal lactase activity is associated with few symptoms in lactose-intolerant patients. Conventional sweet acidophilus milk is not well tolerated by many lactose-intolerant people.

A prolonged restriction of dairy products significantly diminishes calcium intake and may pose a long-term problem. An inexpensive calcium supplement is Tums (Norcliff Thayer, Inc., Tarrytown, NY); each tablet contains 200 mg of elemental calcium. Suggested daily calcium intakes are 1200 mg per day for teenagers and 800 mg per day for children and adults. I generally recommend that at least 75 percent of the recommended daily calcium allotment be supplemented in individuals on strict lactose-free diets, with the remainder coming from other dietary sources.

SUCROSE

Sucrose malabsorption is a relatively uncommon problem in children and adults. It may be secondary to severe mucosal disease or short gut, or associated with congenital sucrase-isomaltase deficiency. Diagnosis may be suggested by breath hydrogen testing and confirmed by evaluation of sucrase-isomaltase activity on intestinal tissue. Restriction of dietary sucrose is needed to control symptoms. Increasing tolerance to ingested sucrose is frequently observed in children with sucrase-isomaltase deficiency as they get older. Recently there has been evidence that exogenous sucrase activity can be obtained by the ingestion of viable yeast cells (*Saccharomyces cerevisiae*). When taken on a full stomach, a suspension of these yeast cells may greatly decrease the symptoms associated with sucrose ingestion in children with congenital sucrase-isomaltase deficiency.

MONOSACCHARIDES

Congenital glucose-galactose malabsorption is an extremely rare disorder in which there is an inability to digest and absorb any carbohydrate other than fructose. Presenting at birth and associated with severe diarrhea, it is treated with commercially available carbohydrate-free formulas to which fructose is added. Acquired glucose malabsorption may be observed in the setting of severe villous atrophy associated with intractable diarrhea of infancy from a variety of causes. Central venous hyperalimentation is invariably required in these infants, and only after prolonged periods of nutritional support are small amounts of carbohydrate (glucose polymers, fructose) given by mouth. I sometimes use Mead-Johnson formula 3232A (hydrolyzed casein, medium- and long-chain fat) to which I add increasing amounts of sugar as tolerated.

Although fructose has been traditionally thought of as an efficiently absorbed carbohydrate, we now know that excessive amounts present in certain foods may be incompletely absorbed (Table 3). Ingestion of as little as 10 to 25 g of fructose has been associated with increased breath hydrogen excretion and GI symptoms in children and adults. If a careful dietary history reveals the ingestion of foods high in fructose, empiric fructose restriction and subsequent observation may be useful.

TABLE 3 Fructose Content of Foods

Figs*	30.9†
Dates*	23.9†
Prunes*	15.0†
Grapes*	8.0†
Soft drinks containing high-fructose syrup	37.5‡

* Dried.
† Per 100-g edible portion.
‡ Per 18–19 oz of soda.
From Ravich WJ, Bayless TM, et al. Fructose: incomplete intestinal absorption in humans. Gastroenterology 1983; 84:26. Reprinted with permission.

SORBITOL

Several reports have now clearly documented that the sugar alcohol sorbitol is poorly absorbed by the small bowel, and its passage into the colon is associated with the development of GI symptoms in some individuals. Sorbitol is an endogenous component in a variety of fruits and fruit juices, and is used as a sweetener in "sugar-free" or dietetic products (Table 4). Particularly in young children, a careful inquiry should be made concerning the ingestion of these products. I suggest that fruit juices be restricted in young children who appear otherwise to have chronic nonspecific diarrhea. A restriction of sorbitol should also be suggested in adults with nonspecific GI distress. As little as 5 g may be associated with increased gas and bloating. I also inquire whether any medications the patient may be taking are compounded in a sorbitol-containing base.

TABLE 4 Sorbitol Content of "Sugar-Free" Products and Various Foods

"Sugar-free" gum	1.3–2.2 g/piece
"Sugar-free" mints	1.7–2.0 g/piece
Pears	4.6*
Prunes	2.4*
Peaches	1.0*
Apple juice	0.5*
Pear juice	2.0*

* Grams of sorbitol per 100 g dry matter or 100 g juice. Dry weight equals 15% of fresh weight.
From Hyams JS. Sorbitol intolerance: an unappreciated cause of functional gastrointestinal complaints. Gastroenterology 1983; 84:30; and Hyams JS, et al. Carbohydrate malabsorption following fruit juice ingestion in young children. Pediatrics 1988; 82:64. Reprinted with permission.

COMPLEX CARBOHYDRATES

It is not uncommon to see patients who have symptoms consistent with carbohydrate malabsorption but in whom extensive evaluation for malabsorption of lactose, sucrose, fructose, and sorbitol proves unrewarding. Until recently, it has been assumed that starch is absorbed completely by the small bowel. However, breath hydrogen testing after ingestion of various complex carbohydrates by normal volunteers has shown that this is not true for most individuals. The starch in white bread and macaroni is incompletely absorbed by the small bowel. Similarly, the carbohydrate in oat bread, corn bread, potatoes, and navy beans may escape full intestinal absorption. Low-gluten flour and gluten-free flour (rice flour) appear to be completely absorbed. Gluten-free diets have been of benefit in a few carefully selected patients of mine experiencing bloating, cramps, and diarrhea, even though celiac disease was excluded by biopsy. With interventions such as these, the aid of a dietitian is invaluable in making sure that the dietary restrictions are appropriate.

GASSY PATIENTS

Given this background, how do I approach the patient who primarily complains of gassiness? If the problem is increased belching, this is usually secondary to increased air swallowing. The air swallowing may be habitual, or may be associated with excessive gum chewing or the ingestion of large quantities of carbonated beverages. Some patients with giardiasis complain of a sulfur-like quality in their eructation.

If the patient complains of increased flatus, an initial evaluation for a history of carbohydrate malabsorption should be made. Empiric restriction of potential offending carbohydrates can be attempted, although breath hydrogen testing may be required to identify specific problem sugars. Some individuals may be ingesting large amounts of fiber, which may also contribute to colonic gas production. Appropriate dietary counseling can be given. My experience with the use of "antigas" agents such as simethicone has been that they are harmless but generally disappointing.

SUGGESTED READING

Barr RG, Levine MD, Watkins JB. Recurrent abdominal pain of childhood due to lactose intolerance: a prospective study. N Engl J Med 1979; 300:1449–1452.

Corazza GR, Strocchi A, Rossi R, et al. Sorbitol malabsorption in normal volunteers and in patients with coeliac disease. Gut 1988; 29:44–48.

Harms HK, Bertele-Harms RM, Bruer-Kleis D. Enzyme-substitution therapy with the yeast *Saccharomyces cerevisiae* in congenital sucrase-isomaltase deficiency. N Engl J Med 1987; 316:1306–1309.

Levitt MD, Hirsh P, Fetzer CA, et al. H_2 excretion after ingestion of complex carbohydrates. Gastroenterology 1987; 92:383–389.

Rosado JL, Solomons NW, Lisker R, et al. Enzyme replacement therapy for primary adult lactase deficiency. Effective reduction of lactose malabsorption and milk intolerance by direct addition of beta-galactosidase to milk at mealtime. Gastroenterology 1984; 87:1072–1082.

Wald A, Chandra R, Fisher SE, et al. Lactose malabsorption in recurrent abdominal pain of childhood. J Pediatr 1982; 100:65–68.

CELIAC SPRUE AND RELATED PROBLEMS

PARVEEN J. KUMAR, B.Sc., M.D., F.R.C.P.

Celiac disease is a condition characterized by abnormalities of small intestinal structure and function that result in malabsorption.

ETIOLOGIC FACTORS

It is over 40 years since Dicke (see Selected References) in Holland discovered that dietary gluten withdrawal clinically improved children who had what was then known as "idiopathic steatorrhea." The role of gluten in the treatment of these patients has now become firmly established, but the exact mechanism by which gluten causes mucosal damage in the small intestine remains unknown. Several theories have been suggested. These include an enzyme deficiency in which the gluten cannot be detoxified and therefore damages the mucosa. An immunologic reaction to the gluten does seem to occur. Another hypothesis suggests a damaged cell membrane whereby gluten (acting as a lectin) can react with a glycoprotein previously not exposed, and thus set in motion a series of reactions leading to damage. A recent intriguing hypothesis suggests that celiac disease may be related to a previous viral infection, as a sequence homology has been found between the structure of amino acids in A-gliadin (a component of gluten) and the adenovirus 12.

There is no doubt that certain patients have a genetic susceptibility. The HLA haplotype of HLA, B8, DR3, DR7, and DQW2 appears to be present in over 90 percent of patients with celiac disease. However, equally interesting is the reason why normal individuals with this haplotype do not develop celiac disease, and why patients without this haplotype also have this condition.

CLINICAL PICTURE

Patients present with a very wide range of symptoms. There may be gross malabsorption with steatorrhea or minor symptoms related to nutritional deficiency. Children may present with failure to thrive or occasionally shortness of stature. The variation in symptoms is probably due to individual susceptibility, but also to the fact that gluten-sensitive enteropathy is a proximal enteropathy and only affects the upper gut to a variable degree; the remaining normal distal bowel takes over the function of the proximal end. Currently we suspect the diagnosis of celiac disease on the basis of a raised mean corpuscular volume or a low red cell folate, often in patients with very few other symptoms. This therefore casts a doubt over the treatment we offer to patients with virtually no symptoms.

DIAGNOSIS

There are no easy screening tests for celiac disease. The serum antireticulin and antigliadin antibodies are not 100 percent positive. The only definitive way to diagnose the condition is by a jejunal biopsy. Histologically the mucosa shows a characteristic subtotal villous atrophy, crypt hyperplasia, a chronic inflammatory cell infiltrate of the lamina propria, and flattening of the surface epithelial cells. Between these epithelial cells there are increased numbers of intraepithelial lymphocytes.

This is the usual histologic appearance of celiac disease. However, there are other causes of a flattened jejunal mucosa, and these are different in children and adults (Table 1). I find that confusion over the diagnosis usually results if the mucosa shows only partial villous atrophy; in this event the only way to confirm the diagnosis is often to start treatment and assess the clinical and histologic response on follow-up.

The diagnosis must be firmly established by a jejunal biopsy before treatment is initiated. Other nonspecific conditions can cause diarrhea and malabsorption, and some of these may even show an initial response to gluten withdrawal.

TREATMENT

By definition, patients with a gluten-sensitive enteropathy must respond to a strict gluten-free diet. A very small percentage of patients do not respond to this diet, and the most common reason is noncompliance. Theoretically, nonresponsive patients who have never responded to the diet should not be defined as having celiac disease; they are considered below.

Once the diagnosis has been established, I always have a long discussion with patients explaining the condition and stressing that it is not a grave illness. There is no reason why they should not lead a normal, active, healthy life provided that they comply reasonably with the treatment. Drawing a simple schematic diagram of the gastrointestinal (GI) tract and the jejunual mucosa for patients in the consulting room often helps them understand the nature of the problem. They then usually have an interview with the dietitian, who explains the diet in detail and discusses the practicalities of how to obtain the appropriate flour or bread. Often the patient or spouse makes another visit to the dietetic kitchen for a demonstration of how to make bread, but this is now less necessary with the instant gluten-free bread mixes and frozen loaves currently available. Patients are given a diet sheet with specimen diets as examples (Table 2). They are also given the address of the Coeliac Society (London), which distributes literature, and an extensive list of commercial items of food that are gluten free. The Society has local branches that hold regular meetings, and it also holds national meetings once a year in the United Kingdom, as in the United States and Canada.

Gluten-Free Diet

In principle a gluten-free diet is very simple to follow, although in practice, because gluten is so widely used in different foods, patients often find it difficult to follow a strict diet. The diet implies withdrawal of wheat, rye, oats, and barley. Corn and rice are not normally harmful and therefore can be eaten and used as thickening in soups or gravies. Essentially the diet means avoiding bread, cakes, cookies, and pasta and these items are usually easy to avoid. "Hidden" items containing gluten such as soups and canned foods (e.g., sausages) are perhaps more difficult to remember. Patients also are often asked to avoid mustard, white pepper, or gravies, although the amount of gluten contained in these items is negligible.

Occasionally, on diagnosis, some patients cannot tolerate milk and dairy products owing to a secondary lactase deficiency. However, a few weeks after the introduction of a gluten-free diet, these items can often be eaten safely; diarrhea is not then a problem because the jejunal

TABLE 1 Some Causes of a Flattened Jejunal Mucosa

<table>
<tr><th>Children</th><th>Adults</th></tr>
<tr><td colspan="2">Celiac disease
Dermatitis herpetiformis
Giardiasis
Tropical sprue</td></tr>
<tr><td>Cow's milk sensitive enteropathy
Soy protein intolerance
Gastroenteritis/postgastroenteritis syndrome</td><td>Zollinger-Ellison syndrome</td></tr>
</table>

TABLE 2 Gluten-Free Diet

	Foods Allowed	*Foods Forbidden*
Bread	Gluten-free bread Gluten-free crispbread	All other types of bread and crispbread
Flour	Gluten-free flour, soya flour, potato flour, pea flour, rice flour	Wheat flour Rye flour Barley flour
	Soya bran, rice bran	Wheat bran
Pasta	Gluten-free pasta	Ordinary pasta, e.g., macaroni, spaghetti, ravioli, noodles
Biscuits and Cakes	Gluten-free biscuits and cakes (made with gluten-free baking powder)	Ordinary cakes and biscuits
Breakfast cereals	Cornflakes Rice Krispies	Other breakfast cereals Porridge oats
Other cereals	Rice, tapioca, sago, arrowroot, buckwheat, millet, maize	Barley, oatmeal, semolina
Meat	Fresh or frozen meat, including poultry, game, liver, sweetbreads, tripe, kidneys	Meat pies, meat cooked with flour, beefburgers, most sausages
Fish	Plain fresh fish, plain frozen fish, fish canned in plain oil	Fish with breadcrumbs or batter, fishcakes, fish in sauce
Eggs and cheese	Eggs Plain cheese, cottage cheese, cream cheese, curd cheese	
Milk	Fresh, canned, dried or sterilized milk	
Cream and fats	Fresh and canned cream, butter, margarine, dripping, lard, oil	
Soups and sauces	Home-made soups and sauces (made with gluten-free thickening)	
Vegetables Potatoes	Fresh or frozen Canned (in salt and water), plain dried	Potato croquettes
Fruits and nuts	Canned fruit in syrup or natural juice, fresh or frozen fruits, nuts	Fruit pies
Beverages	Tea and coffee, fruit juice, fruit squash, "fizzy drinks"	Horlicks, Ovaltine, barley water
Miscellaneous	Sugar, glucose, boiled sweets, syrup, honey, jam, marmalade, molasses, treacle, jelly, and gelatine	Sweets and chocolate containing "biscuits," e.g., Kit Kat, ice cream gateaux, ice cream wafers and cornets
	Pure pepper and salt, pure mustard and vinegar, pure herbs and spices, monosodium glutamate	Bisto, Oxo cubes
Alcohol	Wine, beers, spirits, liqueurs	Use care with real ales, home-brewed beers

List compiled by the Dietetic Department at St. Bartholomew's Hospital, London, England.

mucosa has improved morphologically. Thus, parents and relatives can be told that the patients may eat relatively normal meals with meats, potatoes, green vegetables, salads, rice, and corn, which constitute the major items in our diet. Unfortunately our Western diet contains a large proportion of processed and junk foods to which gluten is added, and it is this part of the diet that is difficult to follow. The Coeliac Society has a symbol of a "crossed grain" that many manufacturers now use on their labels; e.g., many baby foods are now gluten free and carry the label.

One question patients often ask is whether beer is gluten free. Most processed beer is allowed because most of the gluten is destroyed during its manufacture. However, there is some doubt about home-made beers. Some years ago there was a case reported in the literature of a patient who failed to respond because of taking Holy Communion at church. A communion wafer contains minuscule amounts of gluten, and a communicant taking this sacrament three or four times a week should suffer no ill effects.

Initial Progress

A gluten-free diet is usually recommended for life. With this treatment, patients' well-being improves and their jejunal morphologic abnormalities return toward a more normal pattern. It has always been arguable whether older, asymptomatic patients presenting with minor nutritional abnormalities require a gluten-free diet when these abnormalities can be treated with the requisite hematinic. However, many people are unaware of the extent of their ill health and only notice the difference after treatment has started.

Ill patients often begin to feel better within 1 to 2 weeks of starting a gluten-free diet. The diarrhea is lessened, abdominal distention decreases, and they gain in energy and weight. Hematologic and biochemical parameters start improving over a few weeks. If there are gross nutritional abnormalities, I prescribe iron, folic acid, and vitamin D if necessary.

Severely ill patients with dehydration due to diarrhea, hypokalemia, hypocalcemia, or hypomagnesemia require correction of these deficiencies. Patients with severe steatorrhea can be put on a low-fat diet, calories being replaced with medium-chain triglycerides and a calorie-rich liquid. If diarrhea is still troublesome, antidiarrheal agents may be used for a while. Very rarely there may be a deficiency due to malabsorption of vitamin B_{12}; this requires few injections of hydroxocobalamin over some months.

How Strict a Gluten-Free Diet?

Compliance with a strict, 100 percent gluten-free diet is seldom possible, since even a gluten-free diet contains small amounts of gluten. Nevertheless, there is a feeling among many physicians who treat celiac disease that their patients often cheat on their diets and eat items of gluten, having discovered that these have no immediate harmful side effects. Patient and physicians enact a well-worn script within the confines of the clinic whereby patients pretend to be sticking to a strict gluten-free diet although knowing that the doctor is well aware that they are not telling the truth.

In a recent survey conducted at our hospital of 102 teenage patients who had been told to adhere to a strict gluten-free diet, we found that approximately 50 percent were in fact eating gluten, and 9 percent, once their parents were out of the consulting room, admitted to eating a normal diet. Most of these patients were keeping to a strict gluten-free diet at home, but when out for lunch during school hours were visiting the local hamburger bars. Teenage patients often find it difficult to comply with the diet because of their life style. They also feel shy in admitting to their friends that they are on a special diet; boys in particular feel that they are the "odd one out."

Interestingly, we conducted a similar study in about 100 adults using a visual analogue scale for assessment of the strictness of their diet, and found very similar results. Most patients had previously experimented to discover whether small amounts of gluten upset them, and had gone on to eat more gluten. In view of this we have recently been giving patients a low-gluten diet prospectively, and have carefully followed their progress both clinically and by the use of biochemical and hematologic parameters as well as jejunal biopsies. For this research project our dietitian has listed items of food containing 2.5 g of gluten, and patients can choose one item per day, rather like exchangeable portions in a diabetic diet. Some patients have proved to be intolerant of this small amount of gluten, but most of our patients on 2.5 g of gluten per day can lead normal healthy lives without the constraints of a very strict diet. We hope that in the future patients may be allowed items with a low gluten content, such as gravies or pie crusts, while avoiding items of high gluten content, such as bread. Although there is no doubt that a strict gluten-free diet is the optimal treatment for these patients, the actual amount of gluten that these patients can tolerate has never really been assessed. Whether a gluten-free diet protects against malignancy is discussed later. I always explain to each patient that malignancy may be a risk, but that in our present state of knowledge there is little evidence that small amounts of gluten are harmful.

TABLE 3 Suppliers of Gluten-free Products*

Anglo-Dietetics, Ltd., 641 Lancaster Pike, Fraser, PA 19335
Chicago Dietetic Supply, Inc., 405 Shawmut Avenue, La Grange, IL 60525
El Molino Mills, 345 N. Baldwin Park Blvd., City of Industry, CA 91746
Ener-G Foods, Inc., P.O. Box 24723, Seattle, WA 98124
General Mills Chemicals, Inc., 4620 W. 77th Street, Minneapolis, MN 55435.
Giusto's Specialty Foods, Inc., San Francisco, CA 94080
Shiloh Farms, P.O. box 97, Sulphur Springs, AK 72768
Vita Wheat Baked Products, Inc., 11839 Hilton Road, Frendale, MI 48220
Walnut Acres, Penns Creek, PA 17862
White Oaks Farms, 13 Lake Street, Sherborn, MA 01770

* Health food stores remain the best source of specialized gluten-free items.

From Douglas AP. Celiac sprue and related diseases. In: Bayless TM, eds. Current therapy in gastroenterology and liver disease—2. Philadelphia: BC Decker, 1986.

Follow-up

The continued follow-up of patients is important. After the initial diagnosis I usually see patients after 3 to 4 weeks to assess clinical problems and dietary compliance. Children are assessed on their weight and height percentile charts, and adults on their weight gain. Continuing assessment with blood tests to measure serum and red cell folate levels and serum alkaline phosphatase and albumin levels is made. Once the gluten-free diet is begun, a jejunal biopsy is usually performed at about 3 months, and then repeated either after 1 year or earlier if there are problems or if the biopsy has not "grown." The jejunal mucosa usually shows an increase in villus and enterocyte height, a decrease in intraepithelial lymphocyte count, and a decrease of inflammatory cells in the lamina propria. Once patients are clinically well and the jejunal mucosa has reverted toward a more normal pattern, I usually see them about once a year.

All patients diagnosed in childhood, and especially those under the age of 7 years, should have a gluten challenge to confirm the diagnosis. This is because a transient gluten intolerance can occur, for example, after gastroenteritis. A challenge can be performed in many ways, but the easiest for the patient is to undergo an initial jejunal biopsy before starting on a normal diet containing at least four slices of ordinary bread per day. A repeat biopsy can then be performed either when symptoms develop or at 3 months. In children and teenaged patients, abnormalities of the mucosa on gluten reintroduction often take a long time to appear. Originally it was suggested that these patients should be followed up for 4 years before the diagnosis is discounted, but recent evidence suggests that they may maintain a normal jejunal mucosa for up to 9 years before abnormalities return. In adults a gluten challenge is less necessary unless there has been an atypical presentation or unless the diagnosis has not been differentiated from tropical sprue or giardiasis. Again, it can take the same form as that followed for children. A gluten challenge can also be performed by means of intubation studies in which different fractions of gluten are instilled directly into the duodenum; however, this requires a lot of the doctor's time and also involves measurements of finer parameters of mucosal damage produced by gluten.

PROGNOSIS

The prognosis is excellent and most patients lead normal lives on a gluten-free diet. Even in patients who do not adhere to a very strict diet, very few abnormalities in hemotologic or biochemical parameters are found. Many years ago it was suggested that children "grew out of their disease" after puberty, but this is not the case. All patients who have been correctly diagnosed have lifelong celiac disease.

If the diagnosis is not made until after puberty, patients may give a history of delayed menarche, and a few may be short in stature. The rare patient with infertility may well become pregnant soon after the diet is started. Severely ill patients may have hepatic and neurologic abnormalities. The hepatic abnormality usually takes the form of a raised serum alkaline phosphatase level; this is common in grossly malnourished patients and improves on treatment. A liver biopsy may well show a fatty change. Neurologic abnormalities have also been described in extremely ill patients, and these include peripheral neuropathies, epileptiform attacks, paresthesia, Wernicke's encephalopathy, and a central pontine demyelination that has been described in association with malabsorption. Once these abnormalities become established, they do not improve with gluten restriction.

UNRESPONSIVE MALABSORPTION SYNDROMES

These syndromes constitute a heterogeneous group of conditions having in common a flattened intestinal mucosa. On treatment with a gluten-free diet however, these patients fail to respond either clinically or histologically. The unresponsiveness has three main causes. First, and most common is noncompliance with a strict gluten-free diet; these patients often improve after the diet has been rechecked by a dietitian. Second, the original diagnosis may have been incorrect and here the histology and x-ray studies should be reviewed and the case carefully reevaluated. Third, a group of patients are "true nonresponders"; for these the management is difficult and the prognosis often poor. The incidence of unresponsive patients has been reported as between 10 and 20 percent of all patients with a flattened mucosa. These figures are high because the reports of many tertiary referral centers are included. However, in our hands the incidence of true unresponsiveness is much nearer 2 percent.

Having initially excluded compliance as a cause of nonresponsiveness, it is important to rule out other causes of flattened mucosal lesion, as shown in Table 1. Patients with tropical sprue give a history of recent or remote travel to an affected area, and in these the histologic lesion is usually partial villous atrophy, which is present throughout the whole length of the small bowel. *Giardia lamblia* should be excluded on jejunal biopsies and stool examinations. A few patients with the Zollinger-Ellison syndrome may have a flattened jejunal mucosa owing to the effects of hyperacidity on the small bowel. Finally, there is the possibility that a patient may have developed small bowel ulceration or a malignancy, such as a lymphoma or carcinoma, in addition to the celiac disease.

In a small group, despite a strict gluten-free diet, the clinical and morphologic abnormalities do not improve. These patients may benefit from a short course of prednisolone, starting with 45 mg per day. Originally it was thought that this unresponsive group had peculiar histologic abnormalities such as a layer of collagen below the basement membrane; subsequent studies have shown that, although this may well be present in patients with unresponsive celiac disease, collagen is also seen in patients who respond adequately.

Patients who continue to lose weight, have persistent low sodium and low albumin levels, have severe steatorrhea and diarrhea, and are generally very ill should have a repeat small bowel follow-through or a small bowel enema to exclude ulceration of the jejunum and stricture formation. This is a rare condition, and opinion is still divided as to whether these patients in fact have an underlying lymphoma.

Having ruled out ulceration and, if possible, lymphoma, in a very ill patient with a presumed diagnosis of celiac disease, I usually commence with prednisolone 45 mg per day, and reduce this to a maintenance dose of 10 to 15 mg. A few of these patients improve and are eventually weaned off steroids. In the very rare patient who still does not respond, we have over the years prescribed azathioprine in addition to steroids, and have found that with this combination patients have eventually improved. If neither of these measures is successful, we have tried taking patients off all antigens in foods and prescribed an enteral diet. In the severely ill, total parenteral nutrition may eventually be required, but in these patients treatment is usually unsuccessful.

Some patients may have bacterial overgrowth; if this is proved either by a breath test or by direct intubation studies, it is worthwhile trying a broad-spectrum antibiotic. Pancreatic insufficiency has also been found in a small number of patients. This generally is not a severe problem, but about 4 percent of these patients may require pancreatic supplements. However, once the mucosa has grown, the intraluminal stimulus for pancreatic secretion returns.

MALIGNANCY

Over the years evidence has accumulated that patients with celiac disease are more at risk for developing lymphomas and carcinomas. In a recent nationwide study in the United Kingdom, 259 histologically confirmed malignancies were found in 235 patients with histologically proven celiac disease. A total of 133 of those with malignant lymphomas had a predominant histologic type of malignant histocytosis, with the common site of the lesion being in the small intestine.

Patients with celiac disease also have a greatly increased risk for development of small intestinal adenocarcinoma. Among 116 invasive nonlymphomatous malignancies, there were 19 small intestinal adenocarcinomas; this compares with an expected incidence of 0.2 from the National Cancer Register, adjusted for age and sex. Surprisingly, there appears to be an increased incidence of carcinoma, particularly of the esophagus; the reason is unknown. A lymphoma or a carcinoma should be suspected in any patient with celiac disease who fails to respond to a strict gluten-free diet, or in a previously well patient who suddenly deteriorates despite the diet. These patients continue to lose weight and have diarrhea, steatorrea, and hypoalbuminemia. They are often anemic and may well present with continuous abdominal pain, bleeding, perforation, or (very rarely) bowel obstruction. The diagnosis is often difficult; but computed tomographic (CT) scanning of the abdomen has been of some help. (Occasional uncomplicated patients with celiac disease will have reversible lymphadenopathy on CT.) These patients may need surgery, radiotherapy, or chemotherapy, depending on the type of tumor and its site; the prognosis is usually grim.

DERMATITIS HERPETIFORMIS

Patients with this subepidermal blistering skin eruption also have an associated gluten-sensitive enteropathy. I have usually followed the practice of biopsying most patients with dermatitis herpetiformis, although patients very rarely present with gross malabsorption. It has been shown that if sufficient biopsies are taken and the correct measurements made, most of these patients show an abnormal jejunal mucosa. If the mucosa is flat and the skin lesion difficult to control, a gluten-free diet will help the skin lesion as well as the GI abnormalities. However, a glutenfreen diet may well take a mean of 3.5 years before its effect on the skin is determined. Usually the skin lesion is treated with dapsone, which itself has no effect on the enteropathy.

SUGGESTED READING

Cooke WT, Holmes GKT. Coeliac disease. New York: Churchill Livingstone, 1984.

Dawson AM, Kumar PJ. Coeliac disease. In: Booth CC, Neale G, eds. Disorders of the small intestine. Blackwell Scientific Publications, 1985.

Dicke WK, Weijers HA, van de Kamer JH. Coeliac disease, presence in wheat of a factor having deleterious effect in cases of coeliac disease. Acta Paediatr Scand, 1953; 42:34–42.

Swinson C, Slavin G, Coles EC, Booth CC. Coeliac disease and malignancy. Lancet 1983; 1:111–114.

SHORT BOWEL SYNDROME

JON A. VANDERHOOF, M.D.

The term "short bowel syndrome" refers to the malabsorptive state that occurs after removal of a substantial segment of small intestine. Most patients can tolerate resection of a small segment of jejunum or ileum with little or no symptoms. However, depending on the extent and location of the segment resected, significant malabsorption may occur and massive resection may commit the patient to life-long dependence on parenteral nutrition.

THE ADAPTATION RESPONSE

Patients with surprisingly massive degrees of small bowel resection may eventually develop the ability to live without parenteral nutrition as a result of a compensatory increase in mucosal surface known as the adaptation response. Up to a fourfold increase in absorptive area is possible. This compensatory growth is dominated by villous hyperplasia, although some dilatation and lengthening of the small intestine does occur, especially in small infants. As RNA to DNA ratios remain largely unchanged, the response is characterized by an increase in cell number as well as cell mass, and therefore is described as hyperplasia rather than hypertrophy. The number of villus cells per column increases as a function of the percentage of the small bowel resected. As villus length is much less in the ileum than in the jejunum, the potential for further adaptation in the ileum is much greater after jejunal resection than is the potential for adaptation in the jejunum after ileal resection.

As one might expect, the increase in villus length and absorptive surface results in a gradual increase in absorption of nearly all nutrients. Water, electrolytes, mono- and disaccharides, calcium, and bile acids may all be absorbed more rapidly after a period of adaptation than immediately following bowel resection. This increase in absorption occurs primarily as a result of an increase in absorptive surface rather than an increase in the absorptive capacity of new enterocytes. In fact, some data suggest that the efficiency for absorption per gram of mucosa may actually be decreased after intestinal resection. Digestive enzyme content such as dipeptidase and disaccharidase activity may be decreased in the adaptive epithelium per gram of mucosa. The net effect, however, is increased absorption due to the much greater positive change in intestinal mass.

STIMULATION OF THE ADAPTATION PROCESS

In addition to ensuring adequate nutritional rehabilitation and maintenance, stimulation of the adaptation response becomes a primary goal of therapy in the treatment of patients with the short bowel syndrome. The importance of intraluminal nutrition in stimulation of this process has been well documented by many studies. Studies in animals suggest that parenteral nutrition alone results in actual atrophic changes in the remaining bowel if no concurrent enteral feedings are given. Provision of a comparable amount of enteral nutrition, however, results in increased mucosal mass within a very short time. Supplemental intravenous nutrition is nearly always necessary after massive intestinal resection; in addition to maintaining the nutritional status of the patient, it ensures the structural and functional integrity of the small intestine.

How intraluminal nutrients stimulate intestinal adaptation is not known. Certain trophic hormones appear to be involved in this response, most likely produced and released from enterocytes. These substances probably stimulate both the reproduction and longevity of new epithelial cells through a variety of second messengers, including polyamines and possibly prostaglandins. Many investigators have likened the intestinal epithelium to that of a muscle, in that stimulating it to fulfill its biologic function increases its capacity and to do so effectively, and the lack of stimulation results in atrophic changes.

EARLY MANAGEMENT AND INTRODUCTION OF ENTERAL NUTRITION

Clinical management of patients with the short bowel syndrome is a multistage process. Most clinicians consider there to be three phases: phase I consists of nutritional repletion with total parenteral nutrition (TPN); phase II includes gradual introduction of enteral nutrition, usually by continuous infusion: and during phase III, continuous enteral infusion is incrementally reduced as patients are gradually weaned over to oral feedings.

Central Venous Catheter

During phase I, repleting nutritional deficiency states and stabilizing fluid and electrolyte balances are the major goals of therapy. Because many patients with massive bowel resections will be on parenteral nutrition for an extended time, early consideration of the likelihood of home parenteral nutrition is necessary. It is therefore reasonable to place a permanent indwelling central venous catheter such as a Broviac or Hickman in anticipation of home care. This also simplifies hospital care and reduces the risk of catheter-related complications. The decision whether or not long-term TPN will be necessary may be obvious in the case of massive small bowel resection, but a trial of postoperative enteral nutrition after a brief period of central parenteral nutrition may be required before that decision can be made.

Fluid and Electrolyte Requirements

The major difficulties in phase I of patient management primarily relate to fluid and electrolyte considerations. Standardized parenteral nutrition solutions with typical electrolyte concentrations are usually possible provided that abnormal losses are appropriately replaced. It is generally preferable to hang an additional intravenous solution for replacement of abnormal losses and replace losses on an every-2-hour basis than to constantly adjust and alter parenteral nutrition solutions. Output from nasogastric tubes, gastrostomy tubes, or ostomies can be replaced milliliter for milliliter with electrolyte concentrations similar to that present in the fluid lost. Typical electrolyte concentrations of such fluid are listed in Table 1. As long as this simple rule is followed, standardized parenteral nutrition solutions can be used on a daily basis with little change in electrolyte concentrations. Examples of such solutions are listed in Table 2. One must remember that postoperative patients often have poor gastrointestinal (GI) motility with substantial reflux of duodenal fluid into the stomach. If the nasogastric contents are bilious in appearance, it is likely that the sodium content in the solution is much higher than in typical gastric fluid. Sending a sample of the fluid lost from the ostomy or from the nasogastric tube for electrolyte determination permits more specific formulation of the replacement solution.

TABLE 1 Electrolyte Concentrations in Fluid Commonly Lost in Patients with the Short Bowel Syndrome

	Na (mEq/L)	*K (mEq/L)*
Nasogastric tube	70	10–15
Stool	70–120	5–10
Ostomy	120–140	5–10

TABLE 2 Standard Adult and Pediatric TPN* Solutions†

	Adult	*Pediatric*
Dextrose (%)	25	20
Amino acids (%)	3.3	2.5
Sodium chloride (mEq Na/L)	30	20
Sodium acetate (mEq Na/L)	20	10
Potassium chloride (mEq K/L)	20	
Potassium phosphate (mEq K/L)	20	20
Calcium gluconate (mEq Ca/L)	5	10
Magnesium sulfate (mEq Mg/L)	8	5

* TPN = total parenteral nutrition.
† Must also add vitamins, trace elements, and heparin, if desired.

Parenteral Nutrition

Parenteral nutrition is usually initiated at a 10 percent dextrose, 3.3 percent crystalline amino acid solution infused continuously at a rate equal to 1 to 1.3 times the maintenance fluid rate for the individual patient. This rule applies to pediatric patients as well as adults, but children may require extra free water and a lower concentration of amino acids. The concentration of dextrose can then be gradually increased up to 25 percent on a daily basis by 5 percent increments. Maintenance quantities of parenteral vitamins and trace metals are added to the parenteral nutrition solution, usually via commercial preparations available for this purpose. Patients with high-output proximal fistulae may require extra zinc supplementation, as may small preterm infants. Twenty percent intravenous lipid solution should be used to provide a minimum of 8 percent of the total caloric intake as fat if substantial enteral feedings are not administered early. Although the primary purpose of intravenous lipid is to prevent essential fatty acid deficiency, daily use of lipid solution may allow the provision of additional calories if needed. This may be given as a separate infusion or given intermittently mixed in the TPN solution. Essential fatty acid deficiency may impair the adaptation process, so that administration of essential fatty acid becomes even more important in the management of patients with the short bowel syndrome.

Gastric Hypersecretion

A large percentage of patients with the short bowel syndrome develop hypergastrinemia and as a consequence have gastric hypersecretion. Patients are therefore at risk of gastric and duodenal ulceration as well as excess fluid loss, and H_2-blocker therapy is often initiated. It is perhaps easiest to administer the H_2 blocker through the parenteral solution, since most are compatible with TPN solutions and can be given by continuous infusion.

Laboratory Monitoring

During early phases of therapy, electrolyte, BUN, and glucose levels should be measured daily. Periodic determinations of calcium, magnesium, phosphorus, liver enzymes, and occasionally trace element and vitamin levels are also required. After the patient stabilizes on parenteral nutrition, the monitoring intervals can gradually be increased, often to as few as every 1 to 3 months in patients undergoing long-term TPN.

Home Hyperalimentation

Parenteral nutrition can now be safely administered at home. All day-to-day care can be done by most patients themselves, provided that they are adequately instructed before discharge by physicians and nurses skilled in home care management. Pharmaceutical supplies may be supplied by hospital-based or corporate-based programs, and supplementary nursing care is often available. The key to success with home management is continued long-term contact and supervision by medical teams with special expertise in home TPN.

Enteral Nutrition

Once the patient has been stabilized on parenteral nutrition, fluid and electrolyte losses have been brought under control, and GI motility has returned to normal, phase II begins with a gradual introduction of enteral nutrition, preferably by continuous infusion. This can usually be accomplished either by a soft silicone rubber nasogastric tube or, if long-term infusion is contemplated, through a feeding gastrostomy, which can be placed either intraoperatively or percutaneously by means by endoscopic techniques. Initially, only a small percentage of the total daily intake is administered in this fashion, usually 3 to 5 percent, and the remainder of the calories are administered intravenously. A marked increase in stool or ostomy volume necessitates reduction of the rate of infusion.

Selection of an appropriate liquid diet for continuous enteral feeding is controversial. Protein hydrolysates or crystalline amino acids are typically used for a protein source. Protein hydrolysates have the advantage of being more rapidly absorbed than nonhydrolyzed protein, and because protein is mainly absorbed in the form of dipeptides and tripeptides, the use of individual amino acids may be unnecessary. Carbohydrate is generally provided in the form of either glucose polymers or sucrose. Glucose polymers are readily hydrolyzed by pancreatic and mucosal enzymes and have the advantage of reducing the osmolality of the formula. Lactose is poorly tolerated and should be avoided. Most elemental diets contain either very low fat or a substantial percentage of the fat in the form of medium-chain triglycerides. Research suggests however that long-chain fats may be important in stimulating the adaptation process and should be included in the liquid diets in significant concentrations. Contrary to popular belief, high-fat diets do not result in increased fluid loss in patients with the short bowel syndrome. They may increase loss of divalent cations but may significantly increase the amount of calories absorbed. Medium-chain triglycerides are more rapidly absorbed, especially in the absence of bile acids, and an isocaloric substitution of medium-chain triglycerides for long-chain fats may significantly improve absorption and decrease fecal fluid loss. As fat absorption is not carrier mediated, administration of additional fat often results in increased caloric absorption in spite of significant steatorrhea. Fat malabsorption usually causes little symptoms, so selection of an elemental diet containing a significant portion of fat appears quite appropriate.

Substitution of Enteral for Parenteral Feedings

As greater concentrations of enteral feedings are tolerated, the amount of parenteral nutrition given each day can be reduced. It is preferable to wean patients gradually from parenteral nutrition during the daytime, giving them all their parenteral nutrients over an 8- to 12-hour infusion at night. This can be done by gradually increasing the rate and reducing the duration of infusion each day. On day 1, the central venous catheter can be capped and heparinized with 3 to 5 ml of a 100 units per milliliter heparin-saline solution. The volume of TPN previously given over 24 hours can then be given over 22 hours, and the line capped for 2 hours. The duration off TPN can subsequently be increased by 2-hour increments each day until the patient is finally off TPN for 12 to 16 hours per day. This obviously necessitates giving not only the TPN but also the ostomy replacement solutions over a shorter interval, and very large infusion rates may be required. Some patients with the short bowel syndrome may have ostomy output in the 2- to 3-liter range, but as patients stabilize it is often possible to predict their losses, discontinue constant replacement, and give the extra 2 to 3 liters of replacement solution along with the TPN over an 8- to 12-hour period at night. Eventually, it may be possible to total the parenteral nutrition solution concentrations and extra free water and electrolytes from the replacement solutions, and place this all in one solution to be administered over 8 to 12 hours. This step should be delayed until the patient is relatively stable on a combination of enteral and parenteral feedings. If enteral feedings are advanced too rapidly, large increases in ostomy output may occur, predisposing the patient to dehydration and electrolyte imbalance.

Oral Feedings

During phase III of therapy, oral feedings are initiated. This can actually occur relatively early in the course of therapy during phase II, provided that feedings are given in relatively small quantities as a supplement to both the continuous enteral and parenteral administration. Oral feedings can be given adequately around either an indwelling nasogastric catheter or with a gastrostomy tube in place. Enteral calories, parenteral calories, and oral calories, as well as other nutrients, must all be considered in maintaining adequate balance for the patient. Patients with very short bowel syndrome and relatively high ostomies are often very sensitive to the osmotic load of orally administered nutrients. Continuous enteral infusion has the advantage of reducing the likelihood of dumping large quantities of nutrients into the small bowel at one time. A large meal, especially one high in carbohydrate, often results in an influx of fluid into the small bowel lumen, with a marked increase in ostomy output. During the oral feeding phase, it is important to monitor ostomy output carefully and adjust replacement accordingly. A slow, gradual introduction is important during this phase.

Avoidance of Nutritional Deficiencies

As patients are gradually weaned off parenteral nutrition and maintain appropriate weight on the combination of oral and continuous enteral feeding, attention must be paid to potential nutritional deficiency states, which are likely to develop as a consequence of their malabsorptive state. Patients may absorb adequate calories through the carbohydrate, protein, and fat intake, but certain vitamins, minerals, and trace elements are likely to be absorbed less effectively. Calcium, magnesium, and zinc deficiency states are commonly observed. Poor absorption of vitamin D and calcium may result in symptoms of vitamin D deficiency, and after ileal resection, bile acid and vitamin B_{12} malabsorption may be major problems. Bile acid deficiency may compound the malabsorption of fat and fat-soluble vitamins. Additional vitamin D may be required in such patients as aqueous suspension, as may vitamin A. Parenteral administration of vitamin K may occasionally be necessary. Vitamin E deficiency has been described in adults with the short bowel syndrome, resulting in ataxia and visual field defects. Neurologic disorders consisting of sensory and motor deficits have also been associated with depletion of omega 3 essential fatty acids in children with the short bowel syndrome. Because zinc is important in cell replication, zinc deficiency may further exacerbate the malnourished state by impairing mucosal adaptation; thus, zinc stores should be carefully maintained. Biotin deficiency has been observed in an adult patient with the short bowel syndrome, resulting in complete hair loss, eczema, dermatitis, waxy palate, lethargy, and hyperesthesia. Intravenous biotin was successful in correcting the condition in that patient.

Malabsorption of Medications

In addition to nutritional deficiency states, one must consider the likelihood that medications administered orally will be absorbed at less than desired levels. This becomes important in treating patients who develop common infectious disorders; 10 to 90 percent of commonly used antibiotics may be malabsorbed in patients with the short bowel syndrome, often resulting in unpredictable therapeutic outcomes. If the patient is on home parenteral nutrition, intravenous antibiotic therapy may be utilized.

LONG-TERM PROBLEMS IN THE SHORT BOWEL SYNDROME

Bile Acid Malabsorption

Bile acid malabsorption is a problem unique to patients with terminal ileal resection. In adults it is usually problematic when more than 100 cm of ileum is removed. Malabsorption of bile acids into the colon can result in cholerhoeic diarrhea, a secretory state that results from stimulation of fluid secretion in the colon. Resins such as cholestyramine, which bind bile salts, are frequently helpful in controlling diarrhea in such patients. The dosage should be 4 g per day in adults, subsequently titrated downward.

Fat-Soluble Vitamins

Patients with extensive ileal resection often lose great quantities of bile salts, resulting in decreased intraluminal bile acids and a reduced bile salt pool. These individuals develop an exacerbation of steatorrhea, weight loss, and significant loss of fat-soluble vitamins. Cholestyramine usually does not improve their diarrheal state, and may actually exacerbate the steatorrhea by binding up the few bile salts remaining for solubilizing intraluminal fat. Careful monitoring of fat-soluble vitamin deficiency, including vitamins A, D, E, and K, is essential in such patients, and supplements are often required. Measurement of serum 25-hydroxy vitamin D levels, vitamin A and E levels, and prothrombin time should periodically be undertaken.

Vitamin B_{12} Malabsorption

An additional problem in terminal ileal resection is loss of vitamin B_{12} absorption. This function cannot be assumed by the jejunum, and life-long administration of parenteral vitamin B_{12} will be required in the form of monthly injections. Monitoring of serum vitamin B_{12} levels after ileal resection enables one to determine whether such supplementation is necessary.

Large-Volume Ostomy Output or Diarrhea

Certain patients with the short bowel syndrome continue to have large-volume ostomy output or substantial diarrhea; in some instances the administration of potent antimotility agents may be helpful. Loperamide is perhaps most useful, and may improve caloric retention as well as fluid absorption. Recent data suggest that some actions of such agents may occur through actual changes in fluid transport in addition to alteration in intestinal motility.

Chronic Bacterial Overgrowth

One of the most common chronic complications of small bowel resection is chronic bacterial overgrowth. Bacterial overgrowth is likely to occur when the ileocecal valve is absent, when a tight anastomosis or partial obstruction is present, or when there is a dilated segment of bowel with poor motility. Such patients may respond to intermittent broad-spectrum antimicrobial therapy, such as a combination of metronidazole and trimethoprim-sulfamethoxazole, or clindamycin. In some instances, continuous administration of cyclical antibiotics is required to control the bacterial overgrowth, usually for 5 to 7 days each month, or they can be given only when needed. Resecting a tight anastomosis or performing an intestinal tapering procedure in patients with widely dilated segments of bowel may be useful in alleviating the bacterial overgrowth; despite the fact that some of the mucosal surface area may be lost, this often results in marked improvement of absorption. Bacterial overgrowth should be suspected in patients who are vitamin B_{12} deficient as well as patients with elevated fasting breath-hydrogen levels. Utilization of the lactulose breath hydrogen test may be useful in diagnosing bacterial overgrowth, especially when an early "small bowel" peak is observed after administration of lactulose.

Liver Disease

Liver disease due to long-term TPN is now a major cause of high morbidity and mortality rates in very short bowel syndrome. After several months to years on TPN, many patients develop severe cholestatic liver disease, which ultimately may progress to cirrhosis. It is commonly thought that provision of a significant portion, perhaps 20 to 30 percent of total calories, enterally may offer significant protection from severe liver disease. The exact mechanism of this liver injury is unknown. It occurs more commonly in small infants than in adults. Combined liver-bowel transplantation has been proposed by some authors as a therapeutic alternative for these patients.

D-Lactic Acidosis

Some patients, especially children, have developed metabolic acidoses due to production of excessive D-lactate by intestinal bacteria. Although both D- and L-lactate are produced by intestinal bacteria, only the L form can be metabolized in humans. D-Lactic acidosis is correctable by elimination of bacterial overgrowth, and should be considered in patients with the short bowel syndrome who demonstrate repeated attacks of dyspnea and drowsiness.

SURGICAL CONSIDERATION

A number of surgical procedures have been devised to improve absorption in patients with the short bowel syndrome. Most involve slowing intestinal transit. The most direct approach is construction of a valve or sphincter that functions in the same way as the ileocecal valve, causing constriction of the lumen and creating a partial mechanical obstruction. The intention is also to prevent retrograde reflux of bacterial contents into the small intestine. Creation of intestinal valves can lengthen transit time two- to threefold and can significantly increase absorptive capacity in experimental animals. Recent clinical experience has been less than satisfactory in humans, so the technique is not often used. Antiperistaltic segments of small intestine have also been employed for the same purpose, as has colonic interposition, but results are frequently unsatisfactory.

Intestinal Tapering Procedures

Perhaps the main mechanism by which surgery can benefit patients with the short bowel syndrome is through either intestinal tapering or lengthening procedures. Patients often develop a markedly dilated intestine secondary to both chronic partial obstruction and adaptation. This may result in bacterial overgrowth, which contributes to malabsorption because of injury to the intestinal mucosa induced by bacteria and by deconjugation of bile acids. Tapering dilated segments reduces stasis and bacterial content, and improves intestinal function, while preserving intestinal length. Tapering procedures have proved a valuable adjunct in patients with dilated segments of bowel who are responding poorly to standard therapy for bacterial overgrowth.

Intestinal Lengthening Procedures

An intestinal lengthening procedure has been described in children. Blood vessels are dissected longitudinally at the mesenteric border of the intestine and allocated to either side of the bowel wall. The intestine can then be transected longitudinally, and two parallel intestinal segments can be created and anastomosed end to end so that the original dilated segment becomes a narrower segment of twice that length. Long-term patency and function has been good in our patients; we have had the opportunity to explore two patients surgically 1 year after this procedure, and visually observed normal motility through a lengthened segment of bowel.

Intestinal Transplantation

The ultimate cure for the short bowel syndrome probably rests with intestinal transplantation. Recent improvements in immunosuppression with cyclosporin therapy suggests that this procedure may ultimately be possible. Some experience has been gained in performing intestinal transplant in experimental animals, but less experience in humans. Major problems in humans have included diarrhea with severe mucosal injury and mesenteric lymphomas.

PROGNOSIS

The prognosis for the short bowel syndrome has been markedly altered through the use of parenteral nutrition. Recent advances in parenteral therapy, including changes in catheters and solutions, understanding of the importance of intraluminal nutrition, and finally the use of parenteral nutrition in the home have markedly altered the management of the short bowel syndrome. Patients almost never succumb to malnutrition, and death from sepsis is rare. Liver disease associated with long-term parenteral nutrition remains a major cause of morbidity and mortality.

SUGGESTED READING

Dorney SF, Ament ME, Berquist WE, et al. Improved survival in very short small bowel of infancy with use of long-term parenteral nutrition. J Pediatr 1985; 107:521–525.

Grey VL, Garofalo C, Greenberg GR, Morin CL. The adaptation of the small intestine after resection in response to free fatty acids. Am J Clin Nutr 1984; 40:1235–1242.

Simko V, McCarroll M, Goodman S, et al. High-fat diet in a short bowel syndrome. Intestinal absorption and gastroenteropancreatic hormone responses. Dig Dis Sci 1980; 25:333–339.

Thompson JS, Rikkers LF. Surgical alternatives for the short bowel syndrome. Am J Gastroenterol 1987; 82:97–106.

Thompson JS, Vanderhoof JA, Antonson DL. Intestinal tapering and lengthening for the short bowel syndrome. J Pediatr Gastroenterol 1985; 4:495–497.

Vanderhoof JA, Grandjean CJ, Burkley KT, et al. Effect of high-percentage medium-chain triglyceride diet on mucosal adaptation following massive bowel resection in rats. JPEN 1984; 8:685–689.

CROHN'S DISEASE OF THE SMALL BOWEL

DANIEL H. PRESENT, M.D.

Current treatment of Crohn's disease is as variable as the disease itself. To treat this chronic gastrointestinal (GI) disorder adequately, the clinician must be familiar with its natural history, the exact extent of the inflammatory process, the presence or absence of complications (fistulization and obstruction), the recurrence rate, and the patterns of recurrence after surgical resection.

Illustrative Cases

A presentation of a recently encountered case will set the background for my recommendations as to therapy for Crohn's disease of the small bowel. A 16-year-old white female with "no" GI symptoms developed secondary amenorrhea. A gynecologic examination was normal, and an endocrinologic consultant found normal growth, secondary sexual development, and no abnormal physical findings other than clubbing of the fingernails. Hormonal levels were normal, but the sedimentation rate was elevated to 32 mm per hour and the hemoglobin and albumin levels were lowered to 11.8 and 3.1 g, respectively. The astute clinician ordered GI x-rays, which showed Crohn's disease involving 5 inches of jejunum as well as 8 inches of the terminal ileum and the cecal tip. The questions then arose, is it possible to treat clinically asymptomatic Crohn's disease and to alter the future course by any dietary change or medicinal administration? I polled ten experts in inflammatory bowel disease (IBD) and was given six different therapeutic approaches.

There are no controlled trials in the literature to answer these questions, and unfortunately very few controlled clinical trials showing efficacy of the currently available medications in the treatment of Crohn's disease. With this limited data in mind, I would like to present my personal experience of treating about 1,000 patients with small bowel Crohn's disease. Many of the lessons I have learned are contrary to what is espoused in the literature as standard treatment, and some of my recommendations will be controversial or unorthodox.

The most important advice I can give the clinician is to listen to the patient. I often "hear" what the patient tells us but fail to "listen" to the specifics and their meaning. Another clinical story will demonstrate this point. A 38-year-old female with Crohn's disease was seen who had 8 inches of ileitis for approximately 10 years. The symptoms were predominantly those of recurrent obstruction with limitation of food intake and subsequent weight loss. The patient had taken steroids on several occasions with good results, but she experienced significant emotional lability and relapsed on stopping oral prednisone. Treatment with sulfasalazine had failed and her gastroenterologist recommended a resection. I agreed that surgery was a reasonable alternative, but the patient asked if there was "any" medication that she had not taken that might be effective. I suggested that broad-spectrum antibiotics were effective in some patients with Crohn's disease but usually not when there was obstruction. She requested a trial and was treated with ampicillin, 500 mg, four times daily. The patient's symptoms abated and she called 3 months later to ask for a renewal of ampicillin. I advised that she visit her primary gastroenterologist but she informed me he would not renew the prescription since "antibiotics did not work in Crohn's disease." I contacted her physician and tried to convince him to continue the medication, but he refused since there was no literature to support this treatment. I renewed the ampicillin and the patient has at this time been well for approximately 3 years while taking intermittent ampicillin. Clearly, the physician was not "listening" to this patient. I learned of the efficacy for antibiotics from many patients who told me of clinical improvement of their Crohn's disease while receiving antibiotics for other indications.

Information Required Before Institution of Therapy

In order to treat the patient with Crohn's disease a basic set of information is required. Most important is the history of patterns of exacerbations and remissions as well as the type of symptoms (inflammatory or obstructive). The finding of a tender mass on physical examination is crucial to therapeutic decisions. Diagnostic studies must be performed for stool culture, ova and parasites, and *Clostridium difficile* to exclude other concurrent problems. Also indicated are blood studies to gauge the degree of inflammation (sedimentation rate, C-reactive protein, orosomucoid) and basic blood studies (complete blood count, SMA 6 and 12) to indicate malabsorption or chronicity.

A complete set of bowel x-rays is mandatory to define the extent of the disease (colon and/or small bowel) and any complications. A single contrast barium enema is the first procedure of choice; a double contrast enema is often very uncomfortable for the patient and is not absolutely required. I feel strongly that a barium enema is of greater value than a colonoscopy; the latter gives no extra information, and minimal findings such as scattered aphthous ulcers are of little value in the management of the patient. Crohn's disease affects the entire wall of the colon, and a look at the mucosa through the colonoscope does not add valuable data. GI series and small bowel follow-through with "spotting" of the terminal ileum or other disease sites is essential. Fistulization, shortening, and strictures as well as dilatation of the bowel proximal to the stricture are best seen with barium studies.

Severity of disease does not necessarily correlate with severity of the inflammatory process as seen on x-ray or colonoscopy. More important is the presence of a fistula on x-ray, which suggests a different therapeutic approach from that appropriate for patients without fistulization.

MEDICAL TREATMENT

General

The goal is to control the disease process while maintaining the patient's normal life style as closely as possible. I therefore do not place major restrictions on the patient unless it is essential. I do not routinely advise dropping out of school to "rest" or taking off from work for long periods. Patients with small bowel Crohn's disease should try if possible to exercise routinely, maintain a normal social life, and not be confined to home or hospital unless absolutely essential.

Nutrition

A dietary history should be obtained, but I consider that the role of diet has been overemphasized to most patients. If physicians "listen" carefully, they will hear that most patients when feeling well can eat almost all foods, and that when they are going through an active phase, many foods increase symptoms. In my experience there is no increase in bowel symptomatology with the ingestion of spicy or seasoned food in comparing patients with and without Crohn's disease. Patients, without their physician's advice, usually discover which foods increase the symptoms. Rather than ordering an expensive lactose tolerance test, I advise 7 to 10 days with no milk or milk products, and then a return to these foods; the patient should note any change in symptoms while on or off lactose.

A nutritional profile of blood studies may be a good academic approach, but for most patients is often expensive and unrewarding. A simple measurement of weight and height (especially in children) plus a complete blood count and check of sedimentation rate and serum albumin, will reveal as much about the nutritional status as tests of vitamin B_{12} serum iron, serum folate, serum magnesium, and blood levels of trace minerals. If the patient is underweight, a complete history of the amounts and types of food being consumed is important. It is also important to determine whether there are audible bowel sounds suggesting obstruction. If the patient has obstructive symptoms, the diet must be modified to avoid roughage (raw fruits, raw vegetables, nuts, chinese food vegetables, popcorn, and so forth) while maintaining adequate caloric intake. If there is malabsorption a diet adequate in calories while low in fat, supplemented with medium-chain triglycerides, is indicated. Vitamin supplements are indicated for patients with inadequate nutritional intake.

Elemental Diets

Elemental diets have been shown to be as effective as steroids in inducing remission in acute Crohn's disease. They are more effective in small bowel disease than in Crohn's colitis. However, there are major drawbacks to their use. Frequently, potential patients are systemically ill and too anorectic to drink these preparations. Most patients relapse after returning to normal diets, and the currently available oral preparations are not palatable for long periods. In my experience, adult patients do not follow this form of therapy for any prolonged period, and since this disorder is a chronic one, elemental diets play only a small therapeutic role in Crohn's disease of the small bowel. However, in active patients I often supplement oral intake with formulas such as Ensure or Ensure Plus, to maintain adequate caloric intake while I am treating with other medications.

Parenteral Nutrition

Parenteral nutrition, on the other hand, can play a major role in small bowel Crohn's disease if used for the appropriate indications. It must be strongly emphasized that parenteral nutrition is not a primary therapy of the bowel disease, but rather an adjunctive modality. It can be used in patients with:

1. Active Crohn's disease plus poor nutrition.
2. Major internal fistulae such as ileocolic or ileocutaneous fistulae, before treatment with immunosuppressive agents.
3. Preoperatively and postoperatively in patients with major nutritional depletion.
4. Growth retardation.
5. Short bowel syndrome.

In my experience, parenteral nutrition seems to restore the patient's responsiveness to other medications that may have failed, such as steroids and immunosuppressives, and if an extensive small bowel resection is the only alternative, a trial with parenteral nutrition plus the previously failed medications is warranted before surgery. Parenteral nutrition is not indicated:

1. For chronic stenotic obstruction of the small bowel.
2. Postoperatively as a routine if the patient's nutritional status is adequate.

Recently it has been shown that total parenteral nutrition (TPN) with nothing by mouth and bowel rest is no more effective than parenteral nutrition plus added oral feedings. In fact, many patients with Crohn's disease develop worse diarrhea when they are NPO than when they are allowed one or two small feedings daily. I therefore do not stop oral intake when prescribing parenteral nutrition except when there are major enterocutaneous fistulae.

Children and adolescents are a special case in whom adequate energy intake is crucial for growth, and enteral diets and nasogastric supplements are better tolerated. These patients are best managed by a pediatrician with experience in both nutritional therapy and the standard oral medications.

Symptomatic Medications

It is not unusual for me to evaluate patients who are taking steroids for protracted periods, sulfasalazine, immunosuppressives and even parenteral nutrition who are having diarrhea and have not been given adequate doses of antidiarrheal agents. The currently available medications for diarrhea include diphenoxylate in dosages of 2.5 to 5 mg, loperamide, 2 to 4 mg; codeine, 15 to 30 mg; and deodorized tincture of opium, 8 to 15 drops. All of these medications are given up to four times daily depending on the severity of the process, preferentially one-half hour before meals and before sleep if the diarrhea is nocturnal. Patients should be allowed to take these medications as needed depending on their symptoms. Some patients with Crohn's disease of the small bowel may also respond to anticholinergics such as propantheline bromide (Pro-Banthine), 7.5 to 15 mg; dicyclomine (Bentyl), 10 to 20 mg; and hyoscyamine sulfate (Levsin), 0.125 to 0.25 mg. All these medications again are given one-half hour before meals and sleep as needed. None of the above agents should be given if there are signs of clinical obstruction, and patients should be advised as to the early symptoms of intestinal obstruction when they are taking these medications.

Approximately 6 percent of the population have addictive personalities, and since patients with Crohn's disease invariably have pain, the use of narcotic agents such as meperidine (Demerol), Percodan, and Percocet should be restricted and used only for short periods (1 to 2 weeks). Injectable narcotics should almost never be given to patients at home. Likewise, sedatives and tranquilizers, which are often required during high-dose steroid usage, should be carefully monitored by the physician, especially in patients who have demonstrated addictive tendencies.

Cholestyramine, often used in patients who have undergone previous ileal resection and have significant diarrhea, is presumed to counter the diarrheal effect of bile salts on the colon. The medication is available in 4-g packets and should be administered in as low a dose as will control the diarrhea: often half a packet one to three times daily, or one packet once or twice daily. Many patients have difficulty taking this medication since it does not dissolve easily in citrus juices. My personal experience is that dissolution occurs easily in natural apple juice and that this combination is quite palatable.

Psychosocial Support

The early literature described an inflammatory bowel disease type personality. These judgments were made by physicians who saw patients mostly during hospitalizations and after they had been ill for a long time. Recent studies have not suggested an IBD personality, although it has recently been reported that depression is more common in Crohn's patients even after taking into account the chronicity and severity of the illness. My experience does not agree with this published report, and I find Crohn's patients to be no different than others with a chronic illness. I rarely refer patients to psychiatrists for help with this illness, but rather rely on mutual self-help groups. The National Foundation for Ileitis and Colitis, 444 Park Avenue South, New York, NY 10016 (phone 212-685-3440) can provide supportive literature as well as referring patients to local areas that have mutual support groups. If the patient does need psychotherapy, I often rely on a family therapist, since this illness is chronic and requires support of all family members.

SPECIFIC DRUG THERAPY

Sulfasalazine

There is disagreement among physicians as to the value of sulfasalazine in the management of Crohn's disease confined to the small bowel. Three controlled trials are available for review and none have shown statistically significant efficacy when only the ileum is involved. In contrast, two of the three studies have demonstrated efficacy in comparison with placebo when there is involvement of both small and large bowel. Other experienced clinicians have reported not only the clinical effectiveness of sulfasalazine in the treatment of small bowel Crohn's disease but also radiologic improvement and healing.

These discrepancies arise, first, from the fact that in few of the patients who were entered into these controlled trials was the disease limited to the small bowel and second, due to the metabolism of sulfasalazine. Although sulfapyradine and 5-aminosalicylic acid (5-ASA) are azo linked to produce sulfasalazine, it is only the 5-ASA that is the active therapeutic moiety. Sulfasalazine is split in the terminal ileum and right colon by bacteria, which then release the 5-ASA. Transit times through the intestine are uncertain, and narrowing of the small bowel may build up bacteria and delay transit. It is therefore possible that in different patients 5-ASA may be released in greater amounts in the small bowel, whereas in others sulfasalazine may have left the small bowel before significant cleavage occurs. The newer 5-ASA agents in which more of the 5-ASA is released through the small bowel may resolve this controversial issue.

My experience agrees with that of many clinicians rather than with the controlled trials, and indicates that sulfasalazine is an effective agent and the initial drug of choice for mild to moderate Crohn's disease. The dosage is increased slowly to 2 to 4 g daily in divided doses to be administered with food. In patients who develop upper GI symptoms with sulfasalazine, this is a strong clue to duodenal involvement with Crohn's disease or peptic disease of the antrum or duodenum. A change to coated sulfasalazine may overcome this problem. I also maintain sulfasalazine in preventive doses of 2 g doses daily after a clinical remission has been obtained. My patients usually stay on this drug for approximately 6 to 12 months. If the disease exacerbates, I increase the dose to 4 g daily. Although controlled trials indicate that the combination of sulfasalazine and steroids is not of value, my experience suggests that sulfasalazine may function in a steroid-sparing role in many patients. I therefore introduce sulfasalazine to patients who have been brought under control with steroids, and at the same time attempt to decrease and discontinue the oral steroid agent.

The toxicity of sulfasalazine includes symptoms such as nausea, indigestion, and heartburn. Also noted are headache (especially in patients who are slow acetylators), allergic skin rashes, arthritis, low-grade hemolysis, and a decreased sperm count. It is rare to observe severe allergic reactions such as agranulocytosis, sulfasalazine lung, and hepatitis. Clinicians tend to treat all patients who receive sulfasalazine with folic acid since there is competitive inhibition for this vitamin. I do not prescribe folic acid supplements to all patients, but instead monitor blood counts every few months; if macrocytic anemia develops, I treat with 1 mg of folic acid two to three times daily until the anemia comes under control, and then maintain a preventive dose of 1 mg daily.

Steroids

If physicians were polled as to the drug of choice for active Crohn's disease of the small intestine, they would certainly select corticosteroids. Two multicenter-controlled trials confirmed the short-term efficacy of these agents. The National Cooperative Crohn's Disease Study (NCCDS) achieved control of active disease in approximately 60 percent of patients, usually within 6 weeks. A somewhat disconcerting factor regarding the accuracy of the study was the lack of response in patients with colonic Crohn's disease, since most clinicians have seen a short-term dramatic response in patients with Crohn's colitis. The European Cooperative Crohn's Disease Study (ECCDS) demonstrated the efficacy of steroids in both colonic and small bowel Crohn's disease, although only 24 patients with small bowel disease were entered into the study. It was rather disturbing that 80 percent of the deaths in the ECCDS were of patients treated with steroids, especially those with abdominal masses. Also of concern was the inability of patients to stop steroids once having started them. In the NCCDS, over 50 percent of patients could not withdraw without clinical relapse.

These factors might have been expected to cause many objections to the use of steroids in a chronic lifetime illness such as small bowel Crohn's disease. However, this has not occurred, and as noted above, corticosteroids are used by most physicians as first-line treatment. I will suggest an alternative approach later.

If steroids are initiated, they should be administered in adequate dosage, 30 to 60 mg of prednisone daily. Physicians disagree as to whether this should be given in a single dosage in the morning or spread through the day. In my clinical experience, three or four times daily dosing works more quickly and effectively than a single administration; however, spreading the dose also produces more side effects. I prefer rapid control of the inflammatory process with a high initial dose and then quick lowering of the steroids, which is preferable to "creeping" up to higher doses. In my experience the latter technique often results in the patient's inability to stop steroids. I have tried alternate-day dosing in moderate to severe disease and have found it ineffective. Although many physicians use alternate-day dosing to reduce side effects, I believe that it is not effective in active disease. For inactive disease my goal is to stop steroids not "maintain" low alternate-day dosing. I therefore reject alternate-day administration of the drug until there is controlled evidence to support its use. I do not consider that prednisolone, methylprednisolone, or triamcinolone is preferable to prednisone.

When the patient has improved, steroids can be decreased rapidly from the initial 40-mg to 60-mg daily dosage. I usually decrease the dosage by 5 to 10 mg weekly until a dose of 20 mg is reached. Flare-ups invariably occur between 20 and 10 mg of daily prednisone. Therefore, at 20 mg I slow the reduction to a rate of 2.5 mg per week or 2.5 mg every other week, until the patient is able to stop steroids. Close clinical observation for an exacerbation is required at this crucial stage of management.

Should sulfasalazine be added while steroids are being reduced? The NCCDS suggests that this carries no advantage, but many experienced clinicians believe that some patients will benefit with this combination. Should other agents be added to steroids during withdrawal? The role of antibiotics and immunosuppressives will be discussed later. In my experience there is a role for combined therapy (steroids plus antibiotics, steroids plus sulfasalazine, steroids plus antibiotics and sulfasalazine), in selected subsets. In addition, numerous trials have shown that immunosuppressive agents are specifically steroid sparing in Crohn's disease.

Patients who are severely ill with active small bowel Crohn's disease should be admitted to the hospital for parenteral medications. Although there are no controlled data regarding the use of intravenous steroids in the management of Crohn's disease, most clinicians consider them more effective than oral steroids. Patients to be considered for intravenous steroids include those with obstruction, severe weight loss, malnutrition, or systemic manifestations such as fever. I prefer hydrocortisone sodium succinate (Solu-Cortef), 300 mg daily, given by continuous intravenous infusion. In my clinical experience, the drug works more quickly and with better response when given continuously as compared to pulse administration. Intravenous adrenocorticotropic hormone (ACTH) has been shown to be more effective than intravenous Solu-Cortef in acutely ill ulcerative colitis patients who have not been taking steroids before admission to the hospital. Although the same controlled trial has not been performed for active Crohn's disease, experience and common sense suggest the use of ACTH (120 units intravenously over 24 hours) rather than Solu-Cortef if the patient has not been taking steroids previously.

I often use ACTH gel injections in outpatients for control of active small bowel Crohn's disease. I find it as effective as oral prednisone (possibly more effective in patients with malabsorption) and when administered in the following regimen it produces fewer steroid side effects. I administer 40 units of ACTH gel daily for 4 days and then on alternate days for another 2 weeks. Further tapering depends on the clinical response, but usually the drug is lowered to three times weekly and stopped in most patients in about 6 to 8 weeks. Despite the annoyance of injections, most patients report equal effectiveness and fewer steroid side effects with intermittent ACTH injections than with continuous oral prednisone. The long-term use of steroids (more than 4 to 6 months) is to be avoided if at all possible. There are no controlled data to support a long-term benefit of steroids for maintenance, prevention of relapse, or prevention of recurrence after surgical resection. The ECCDS suggests low-dose steroids for up to 2 to 3 years if remission has been obtained with steroids in some patients. This vague suggestion has not been confirmed in trials and my clinical experience suggests that this is a foolhardy approach. Steroid toxicity such as cosmetic side effects (especially in adolescents and young adults), thinning of the skin with easy bruisability, hypertension, diabetes, failure to grow, cataracts, aseptic necrosis of the hips, and bone collapse outweigh the unsubstantiated efficacy of long-term corticosteroids for small bowel Crohn's disease.

As regards intestinal obstruction, steroids are of limited value. Small bowel obstruction may be related to dietary indiscretion in a patient with a narrowed lumen secondary to Crohn's disease. This may be triggered by the ingestion of high-residue foods, especially raw fruits and raw vegetables. If these obstructed patients are treated with intravenous fluids and nothing by mouth (occasionally a nasogastric or Cantor tube is required for vomiting), most improve within 24 hours without the addition of intravenous steroids. I therefore do not administer steroids if I can obtain a history of dietary indiscretion and *no* history or signs of an inflammatory process (e.g., fever, aphthous ulcers, elevated erythroycte sedimentation rate).

Conversely, in patients in whom inflammation has preceded obstruction, steroids are usually beneficial in decreasing mucosal edema and ulceration, and can be given in the form of ACTH or Solu-Cortef, depending on previous medications.

The third factor in obstruction is a fibrous stricture of the lumen. In my experience, steroids offer no "long-term" benefit (although sometimes a temporary benefit) with this type of obstruction. I believe that in this clinical situation surgical resection is inevitable. Fixed fibrotic stricture is diagnosed when there is no superimposed evidence of active inflammation and when the proximal small bowel is becoming increasingly dilated.

Active small bowel Crohn's disease with a tender abdominal mass is a special situation that requires important clinical decisions. Steroids given alone to patients with an inflammatory mass is not only contraindicated but may be deleterious. In these patients who have usually fistulized (into the mesentery, to other bowel loops, to internal organs such as bladder and vaginal), many may already have an abscess or go on to develop one. As noted above, three deaths were seen in the ECCDS study in clinically active patients who received steroids in the face of an abdominal mass. I believe that steroids should be avoided until a computed tomographic (CT) scan is performed, and even if an abscess is not detected on CT scan, I rarely administer steroids to these patients. I prefer to treat with triple antibiotics (aminoglycosides, ampicillin, and metronidazole) through the entire course of the hospitalization. Most patients improve, and I add ACTH to the antibiotic regimen only in an occasional patient. After improvement, I discharge these patients on oral antibiotics alone, or antibiotics plus rapidly tapering intramuscular ACTH gel. If steroids are thought to be essential when a mass is present, antibiotics should be initiated at the same time.

Since (1) there is no evidence for long-term efficacy of steroids in Crohn's disease (2) over 50 percent of patients cannot stop steroids after they are initiated, and (3) corticosteroids involve major toxicity. I try never to use steroids for small bowel Crohn's disease.

Antibiotics

Despite inadequate controlled data to justify the use of antibiotics in Crohn's disease, a vast underground group of clinicians are using these agents as first- or second-line therapy. A variety of antibiotic agents have been tried, with anecdotal reports on symptomatic efficacy and radiographic improvement. In one uncontrolled study, antibiotics were administered singly or in combination for over 6 months with success. In one controlled trial, a nonabsorbable antibiotic plus elemental diet was compared with steroids plus a normal diet with equal results; this trial is too confusing to draw conclusions from it. Likewise, a trial of three antibiotic regimens, trimethoprim-isoxazole, metronidazole, and a combination of both, compared with placebo showed no long-term benefit of any group. Sites of disease (large or small bowel) were not mentioned in this study and early response was seen in both groups taking metronidazole.

On the other hand, metronidazole alone has shown efficacy in both uncontrolled and several controlled trials. A European trial showed metronidazole to be more effective than sulfasalazine in small bowel disease. Metronidazole has also been demonstrated to be clearly effective in patients with perianal fistulae complicating both small and large bowel Crohn's disease. Metronidazole alone has never proved effective in closing internal fistulae in Crohn's disease, although as noted above it may help prevent abscess formation in patients with tender inflammatory masses that have fistulized into the mesentery.

With this conflicting data, should the clinician use antibiotics for small bowel Crohn's disease? I prefer antibiotics to steroids for short and long-term use and prescribe ampicillin or cephexalin (Keflex), 500 mg four times daily, for signs of mild activity. My patients take the antibiotic for a minimum of 6 weeks, and some have continued for up to 2 years. I have not seen major superinfections in these long-term users. If the patient becomes quiescent I gradually withdraw the antibiotics over 2 to 4 weeks; if there is a flare-up, I reintroduce or raise the dosage. If a patient becomes active while taking ampicillin, I often rotate to cephexalin and vice versa. Broad-spectrum antibiotics are my drugs of choice if there is radiographic evidence of internal fistulae, a secondary suppurative process, or evidence of an inflammatory mass.

If the patient presents with moderately active disease, I often use metronidazole as the initial drug of choice; it appears to be more effective when there is colonic involvement. However, I have had success in patients who have ileocolitis and/or small bowel disease alone. The standard dosage in adults is 750 to 1,500 mg of metronidazole daily. The higher dose often is not well tolerated (causing nausea and loss of appetite, and having a metallic taste) and must be reduced as soon as the disease is under control. Peripheral neuropathy is a frequent complication with high doses, and patients must be forewarned to be alert to symptoms of numbness and tingling, which necessitate stopping or lowering the dose. The drug usually has to be completely discontinued when neuropathy appears. It may take over 6 to 12 months for the symptoms to reverse and I have seen tingling, albeit mild persist for over 1 year.

Patients are usually cautioned by pharmacists and physicians not to drink alcohol while taking metronidazole because of an Antabuse-type effect. In fact, this reaction occurs in about one in 100 people, and I advise patients who are taking the drug for a long period, and would like to have an occasional drink, to try alcohol. This should be done at home to prevent embarrassment if vomiting should occur, but most patients experience no reaction.

Animal studies have shown an increase in tumor production with metronidazole (particularly liver and lung), although short-term administration of metronidazole has demonstrated no predisposition to neoplasm in large numbers of women who received the drug for vaginitis. There are no data showing that long-term administration of metronidazole is safe in humans. Isolated case reports of neoplasm with long-term usage suggest maintenance of low doses of 500 to 750 mg daily. Although a 6 to 8 week course of metronidazole is preferred for treatment of active small bowel disease, the condition of many patients is exacerbated with early discontinuation of the drug. The clinician must carefully weigh the need for long-term usage and try to substitute other antibiotics (broad spectrum) in patients who have continued low-grade activity or who worsen when metronidazole is lowered or stopped.

Broad-spectrum antibiotics are of value in patients with jejunoileitis with stricture, low-grade obstruction, and bacterial overgrowth. Tetracycline in doses of 250 mg twice daily helps malabsorption and often decreases symptoms of bloating, diarrhea, and abdominal discomfort.

Combination antibiotics can be used in more seriously ill hospitalized patients with inflammatory masses. For patients on chronic steroids whose condition worsens with lowered dosages, I add single or double antibiotics to the regimen prior to another attempt to withdraw prednisone. I have had some success in substituting antibiotics for steroids, especially in patients with internal fistulization.

Immunosuppressive Agents

Both 6-mercaptopurine (6-MP) and azathioprine have been studied in uncontrolled and controlled trials of patients with Crohn's disease. The uncontrolled data are convincing, showing efficacy in approximately 70 to 75 percent of cases. These studies do not specifically emphasize small or large bowel involvement, and with a wide clinical spectrum of Crohn's disease it is difficult to determine the indications for use of these agents in isolated small bowel disease. Controlled studies have shown effectiveness in four of eight trials, including those with involvement of large bowel or small bowel and/or ileocolitis. Immunosuppressives have shown healing of fistulae and prevention of exacerbation. However, in the NCCDS they were used in 49 patients with only small bowel involvement; statistical significance was "not seen but there was a trend in favor of azathioprine." The failure to show efficacy in this study was due to the design of the trial, which was prejudiced against a slow-acting drug such as azathioprine. The duration of the trial was only 4 months, and patients were taken off all other agents and randomized to azathioprine alone, which did not have enough time to show efficacy before exacerbation occurred.

In our 6-MP study, we demonstrated that the mean time to respond was 3.1 months, with 68 percent response at 3 months and 80 percent at 4 months; some patients took as long as 6 to 7 months to respond. Efficacy was seen in both small bowel and colonic disease, although the quality of the response was better in patients with Crohn's colitis and ileocolitis than in those with ileitis or ileojejunitis. We have demonstrated success in closing and improving fistulae both from the large and small bowel, including ileovesical, ileosigmoid, ileocutaneous, and perineal fistulae. Steroid sparing is seen in 70 percent of patients, and it was possible to stop prednisone completely in 50 to 60 percent of patients while maintaining clinical improvement.

In our controlled trial, we used 1.5 mg per kilogram daily as the initial dosage. When administering 6-MP I now start with a lower dosage; I give 50 mg daily and closely monitor the white blood cell (WBC) count (weekly for 1 month, every other week for 1 month, and then monthly). If the WBC count is maintained above 5,000, the dose can be slowly raised to 75 to 100 mg daily. A lower dose is associated with a longer time to respond, but rarely produces leukopenia. Since the drug takes a long time to act, I maintain all other medications (steroids, antibiotics, and 5-ASA agents) until the 6-MP has had an opportunity to be effective. When improvement is seen, steroids are gradually reduced.

When should immunosuppressives be used in patients with small bowel Crohn's disease? They should be considered in patients who have already undergone resection and in whom further resection might compromise nutritional status. This also applies to patients in whom the initial resection is so extensive that it might produce a short bowel syndrome. 6-MP is indicated in patients with major internal fistulization or fistulization to the skin or bladder. 6-MP should not be introduced in these patients in the face of an active secondary infection or abscess until antibiotics have quieted the process or drainage has occurred. Immunosuppressives are indicated in patients with active small bowel disease and active perianal fistulae. They should be considered in patients on chronic steroids (for 6 months or longer) in whom at least two attempts have been made to stop the corticosteroids. They should also be used in patients suffering from steroid toxicity and in whom surgical resection would be extensive.

I have seen marked healing of pyoderma gangrenosum in almost all patients treated with 6-MP. I have had less success with other extraintestinal manifestations such as arthritis and erythema nodosum, but my colleagues who also use 6-MP think differently and have reported success in treating these latter complications.

I do not use 6-MP in the face of obstruction due to a fibrous stricture, but it may be effective when the obstruction is due to inflammatory swelling. There has been an excellent response to recurrent ileitis, in ileostomies after colectomy. Response has also been observed in internal and/or stomal fistulae with an ileostomy.

I do not administer 6-MP to patients who have limited disease in the terminal ileum and in whom a simple resection would lead to rapid recovery without the long-term close observation required with 6-MP. We are now administering 6-MP to patients who have required two to three resections within a short time (5 years or less). We hope to prevent recurrence by giving 6-MP, but at this time no data are available to assist therapeutic conclusions. I have not seen dramatic effects on growth in children, even when the 6-MP has quieted the inflammatory process. In such cases, we use 6-MP plus nutritional supplementation (elemental or parenteral feedings).

Side Effects

There has been great fear of the long-term toxicity in IBD patients treated with 6-MP. Our studies of 396 patients (with ulcerative colitis and Crohn's disease) with a mean follow-up of over 5 years have shown few serious side effects. Allergic reactions (pancreatitis, rash or fever, hepatitis) occur in 6 percent of patients and rapidly disappear when the drug is stopped. Leukopenia is seen rarely when the drug is administered as advised. Care must be taken when giving 6-MP or azathioprine to patients taking allopurinol: in this situation, one-quarter to one-third the usual dosage is given.

We have seen few severe infections that might be related to 6-MP (1.8 percent), and no deaths attributable to an infectious complication.

We have observed a number of tumors in patients taking 6-MP, but apart from one histiocytic lymphoma of the brain, these neoplasms are not associated with immunosuppressive drugs. Considering the increased risk of lymphoma in IBD (especially Crohn's disease), this single case may be a chance occurrence.

Since 6-MP and azathioprine have shown efficacy in prevention, and since discontinuing the drug within 1 year often results in exacerbation, I advise administration for at least 2 to 3 years before the drug is stopped. Many patients have taken the drug for more than 10 years without any major secondary complication. There have been no abnormalities in children born to patients who are taking 6-MP or had taken it prior to conception, but I still advise stopping the drug 2 to 3 months before attempting pregnancy. A recent United Kingdom study has confirmed the lack of abnormalities in children conceived on 6-MP; physicians did not stop the drug during pregnancy.

Cyclosporine

Cyclosporine has shown efficacy in about 60 to 70 percent of patients with Crohn's disease, but thus far the experience is limited to approximately 150 patients, mostly in uncontrolled studies with one double-blind controlled trial. In many of these studies, information on the extent of disease and whether it is limited to the small bowel is not available. Short-term toxicity is minimal with careful administration of cyclosporine, but long-term toxicity data are not available.

A recent uncontrolled trial has also shown intramuscular methotrexate to be effective in both chronic ulcerative colitis and Crohn's disease. The Crohn's data is limited to 14 chronic patients of whom five had small bowel disease alone, six colonic, and three ileocolonic. Four of the five patients with small bowel disease responded clinically, with good steroid sparing in three of the four.

The role of both cyclosporine and methotrexate in small bowel Crohn's disease is uncertain and will require further trials and greater experience.

T-lymphocyte apheresis is also being studied in Crohn's disease in combination with TPN. A report of 54 patients treated with this modality showed a high rate of remission (15 of 54). This study also needs controlled trials.

INDICATIONS FOR SURGERY

The main indications for surgery are:

1. Obstruction with fibrous stricture of the small bowel.
2. Intra-abdominal abscess.
3. Massive bleeding.
4. Intractability.
5. Perianal abscess.

As noted, surgery is indicated for obstruction due to fibrous stricture but not for inflammatory spastic obstruction. Although an abscess has been considered an indication for surgery, some medical centers are performing percutaneous needle drainage of abscesses. This modality should be pursued but only in patients who can then be managed medically without surgical resection. Percutaneous drainage appears to have no value if surgery is still required after drainage. The surgeon in these situations can drain and resect at the same time.

Massive bleeding is rare (5 percent) and usually stops with intravenous steroids and transfusions.

The definition of intractability should be determined by the patient. The physician must be a partner in helping patients define their disability, and the physician must explain the risks of surgery and of recurrence. Also to be clarified are the chronic need for medications and their side effects versus patients' ability to function normally with and without resection. Patients who select surgery will usually be gratified with their postoperative status.

Postoperative diarrhea usually responds to cholestyramine or antidiarrheals agents. Vitamin B_{12} is rarely required after surgery, and there should be few dietary restrictions unless there has been substantial resection (over 50 cm). In these cases, if the patient has excessive diarrhea, malabsorption should be documented with fecal fat collection and a Schilling test. Patients often undergo elective surgery to rid themselves of medications and permit a liberal diet; therefore, the fewer restrictions and the fewer medications the better for patients' emotional well-being.

TABLE 1 Therapy for Crohn's Disease of the Small Bowel

Indication	*Preferred Treatment of Choice*
Mild activity	Symptomatic drugs Sulfasalazine or oral 5-ASA agent Broad-spectrum antibiotics Metronidazole Combinations of above
Moderate activity	Symptomatic drugs Sulfasalazine Metronidazole Broad-spectrum antibiotics ACTH gel intramuscular Combinations of above Hospitalization with IV antibiotics with or without ACTH Oral steroids
Severe activity	Metronidazole + broad-spectrum antibiotics Hospitalization with intravenous triple antibiotics with or without ACTH Metronidazole + broad-spectrum antibiotics + oral prednisone
Obstruction:	
inflammatory	Hospitalization with IV antibiotics with or without ACTH
stricture	Surgery
Internal fistula with tender mass and/or fever	IV triple antibiotics IV triple antibiotics + IV ACTH Addition of TPN
Chronic steriods after failure of antibiotics and 5-ASA agents:	
Short segment	Surgery
Extensive segment	6-MP
Perianal disease:	
Mild	Metronidazole: stop steroids
moderate to severe	6-MP: stop steroids

THERAPY FOR COMPLICATIONS: SPECIAL SITUATIONS

Aphthous Ulcerations. These are usually treated symptomatically with topical diphenhydramine (Benadryl) or triamcinolone Kenalog in Orabase: some physicians have had success with topical sucralfate (Carafate). I have had little success with any therapy for these painful lesions.

Gastroduodenal Crohn's Disease. Crohn's disease involving the distal antrum or first portions of the duodenum is common (over 25 percent of patients), behaves like peptic disease, and usually responds to H_2 blockers in adequate doses. Occasionally a higher than normal dosage of H_2 blockers is required for a few weeks to control these upper GI symptoms. I have rarely had to use steroids to control symptoms. A recent abstract described the use of Omeprazole.

Erythema Nodosum. This complication usually is not associated with small bowel disease alone, but with colonic or ileocolonic involvement. If the bowel disease is inactive or minimal, I treat erythema nodosum with oral aspirin, two tablets 3 to 4 times daily. If the Crohn's disease is mild, I add aspirin to current therapy such as 5-ASA agent and/or an antibiotic. I try never to use oral steroids for this self-limiting complication. Some of my colleagues report success with colchicine in patients with erythema nodosum. If the condition is refractory, injections of ACTH gel, 40-units given intramuscularly two to three times a week for 1 to 4 weeks will help to quiet this process.

Pyoderma Gangrenosum. Pyoderma is not treated like erythema nodosum and requires more intensive medical management, even though the bowel disease is quiescent or mild in over 50 percent of cases. Pyoderma gangrenosum often occurs soon after withdrawal of sulfasalazine and especially after local trauma. The patient should be restarted on sulfasalazine or the dosage should be raised, and intralesional steroids should also be given. If there is no response, a course of high-dose steroids is indicated to close the wound rapidly. I have also had success with hyperbaric oxygenation and with 6-MP. Most recently there have been excellent results from cyclosporin, with closures seen in 1 to 2 weeks. Resection of the bowel is not indicated for pyoderma gangrenosum.

Peripheral Arthritis. Arthritis should be treated in a similar manner to erythema nodosum, with aspirin, and if the bowel disease is active, with an oral 5-ASA agent or antibiotics. Oral steroids should be avoided, although ACTH may be helpful in refractory cases. Effusion into the knee may require drainage with injection of steroids. Nonsteroidal anti-inflammatory drugs (NSAIDs) such as sulindac, 200 mg twice daily, may be helpful, but may also upset the upper GI tract and may trigger activity of the Crohn's disease.

Ankylosing Spondylitis. This should be treated with NSAIDs; in my experience the best is indomethocin, 25 to 50 mg three to four times daily. The activity of the spondylitis does not correlate with the activity of the IBD and therefore does not require a change in therapy for the latter.

Ocular Manifestations. Eye complications such as episcleritis and uveitis are best treated by an ophthalmologist with topical steroids. Systemic steroids are rarely required for these complications.

Cholelithiasis and Urolithiasis. These are treated in the same manner as in patients without Crohn's disease. If an ileal resection is required and the gallbladder is known to be diseased, it can be resected at the same time, if there is no complicating intra-abdominal abscess.

Sclerosing Cholangitis. There is no indication for bowel resection for this complication. The patient should be continuously monitored and a liver transplant performed for major hepatic deterioration.

Hydronephrosis. This complication per se does not require surgery since it simply indicates extension of the inflammatory process by fistulization to the retroperitoneum. Secondary pyelonephritis does not occur unless the patient undergoes cystoscopy. The ileal disease should be treated as described in previous sections, especially with antibiotics.

Pregnancy. Patients do well if they become pregnant while quiescent; however, there is often an early flare-up if pregnancy occurs when the disease is clinically active. I treat these patients with sulfasalazine and broad-spectrum antibiotics, trying to avoid metronidazole. Usually the process will be subdued during the second and third trimester; there is an increased risk of exacerbation post partum. Steroids may be used safely if the process is severe. The fetus is at little risk when the mother has IBD, and fortunately in most women IBD remains under control during pregnancy.

Perianal Disease. This is generally treated in a conservative manner with topical skin therapy, sitz baths, and soaking in order to obtain adequate drainage. Metronidazole or 6-MP is administered for active perianal fistulae. If an abscess occurs and does not drain spontaneously, the surgeon may have to perform incision and drainage. Internal sphincterotomy and drainage (Park's procedure) may be required if there is severe perianal pain associated with an internal collection. Although this procedure is quite successful in alleviating symptoms, some sphincter muscle is lost and disability may result. In my experience, it should be used primarily for younger patients and should not be performed repeatedly.

There are many forms of therapy for Crohn's disease of the small bowel. A summary of the drugs of choice for mild, moderate, and severe disease given in Table 1. Each patient must be individualized; the problem is challenging, but the rewards for the clinician are great. There are few circumstances more satisfying in medicine than to have a long-term partnership with an appreciative patient with Crohn's disease.

SUGGESTED READING

Bicks RO, Groshart KD, Luther RW. Total parenteral nutrition (TPN) plus T-lymphocyte apheresis (TLA) in the treatment of severe chronic active Crohn's disease. Gastroenterology 1988; 94:A34.

European Cooperative Crohn's Disease Study; Results of drug treatment. Gastroenterology 1984; 86:249–266.

Goldstein F, Farquhar S, Thornton JJ, et al. Favorable effects of sulfasalazine on small bowel Crohn's disease: a long-term study. Am J Gastroenterol 1987; 82:848–853.

Greenberg GR, Fleming CR, Jeejeebhoy KN, et al. Controlled trial of bowel rest and nutritional support in the management of Crohn's disease. Gut 1988; 29:1309–1315.

Korelitz BI, Present DH. Favorable effect of 6-mercaptopurine in fistulas of Crohn's disease. Dig Dis Sci 1985; 30:58–64.

Kozarek RA, Patterson DJ, Gelfand MD, et al. Methotrexate induces clinical and histologic remissions in refractory inflammatory bowel disease. Ann Intern Med 1989; 110:353–356.

National Cooperative Crohn's Disease Study: results of drug treatment. Gastroenterology 1979; 77:847–869.

O'Donaghue DP, Dawson AW, Powell-Tuck J, et al. Double-blind withdrawal trial of azathioprine as maintenance treatment of Crohn's disease. Lancet 1978; 2:955–957.

Present DH, Korelitz BI, Wisch N, et al. Treatment of Crohn's disease with 6-MP. N Engl J Med 1980; 302:981–987.

Present DH. 6-Mercaptopurine and other immunosuppressive agents in the treatment of Crohn's disease and ulcerative colitis. Gastro Clin North Am 1989; 18:57–71.

Rasmussen SN, Lauritsen K, Tage-Jensen U, et al. 5-aminosalicylic acid in the treatment of Crohn's disease. Scand J Gastroenterol 1987.

Saverymuttu SH, Gupta S, Keshavarzian A, et al. Effect of a slow-release 5-aminosalicylic acid preparation on disease activity in Crohn's disease. Digestion 1986; 33:89–96.

Ursing B, Alm T, Barany F, et al. A comparative study of metronidazole and sulfasalazine for active Crohn's disease. Gastroenterology 1982; 83:550–562.

MESENTERIC ISCHEMIA

DESMOND J. LEDDIN, M.B., B.Ch., FRCPC, M.R.C.P.(I.)
JAMES A. BARROWMAN, Ph.D., M.B.Ch.B., F.R.C.P., FRCPC, F.A.C.P.

The frequency with which the diagnosis of mesenteric ischemia is made may be increasing. A greater proportion of the general population is in the older age groups and thus at risk for atherosclerotic disease including the splanchnic circulation. The increasing frequency of diagnosis of these syndromes may also be due to the increased awareness of physicians of the manifestations of splanchinic ischemia. On the other hand, the development of an aggressive approach to cardiogenic and other forms of shock during the last decade may actually be decreasing the incidence of nonocclusive mesenteric ischemia, a condition primarily associated with systemic hypotension.

In this chapter, the normal vascular anatomy, the physiology of intestinal oxygenation, and the physiologic consequences of tissue ischemia are reviewed. The management of these syndromes is approached from the point of view of the clinical diagnosis.

VASCULAR ANATOMY

The vascular anatomy is shown in Figure 1. Note that there are two important anastomotic arcades between the splanchnic vessels and one area of anastomosis between the splanchnic and systemic circulations. The pancreaticoduodenal arcade links the celiac artery with the superior mesenteric artery. The superior mesenteric artery, in turn, is joined to the inferior mesenteric artery by the arch of Riolan and by the marginal artery of Drummond. The inferior mesenteric artery is linked to the systemic circulation via its anastomoses in the rectum with the rectal branches of the internal iliac artery.

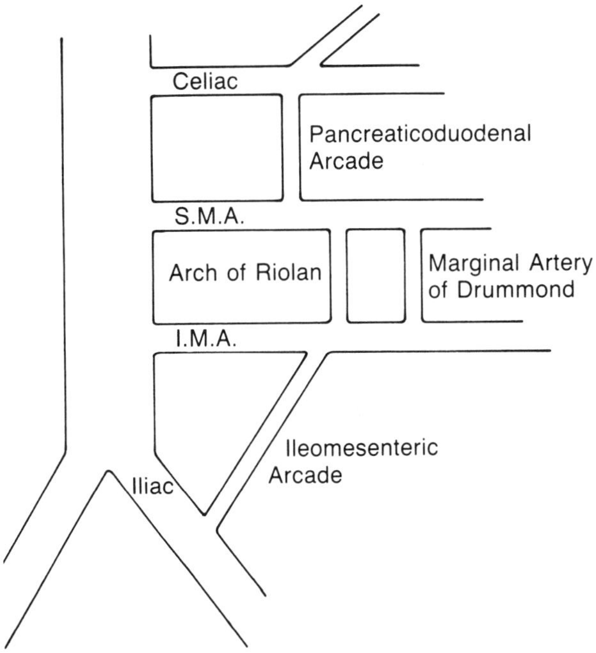

Figure 1 The splanchnic circulation and the major anastomoses of the vessels supplying the intestine.

The venous drainage of the splanchnic organs closely follows the arterial supply and ultimately drains into the portal vein. The major branches joining to form the portal vein are the splenic, superior mesenteric, and inferior mesenteric veins.

Splanchnic Blood Flow and Oxygenation

The splanchnic branches of the aorta receive approximately 30 percent of cardiac output. Small intestinal blood flow per unit of tissue is approximately five times that of the stomach and twice that of the colon. Mucosal blood flow is generally believed to account for 70 percent of total gut blood flow.

Oxygen delivery to the splanchnic organs is determined by arterial oxygen tension and by the relationship between mesenteric blood flow, vascular resistance, and vascular pressure. Mesenteric flow is directly proportional to mesenteric pressure and inversely related to changes in mesenteric resistance. Splanchnic pressure and resistance are in part dependent on systemic pressure and resistance, but local regulation also occurs by both extrinsic and intrinsic mechanisms. Electrical stimulation of sympathetic efferents has been shown to cause splanchnic vasoconstriction. The parasympathetic system appears to have little effect on the vasculature of the proximal gut, but stimulation of the sacral parasympathetic nerves produces vasodilatation. The intrinsic regulation is similar to that seen in other tissues. Both local metabolic factors and myogenic responses to changes in vascular wall tension regulate local blood flow.

The oxygen uptake of the intestine and stomach is constant over a wide range of blood flows, indicating the existence of a considerable margin of safety against hypoxic damage. It is the mucosal fraction of the intestine that is most metabolically active and therefore most sensitive to hypoxia. During the postprandial period, blood flow to the small intestine increases by 30 to 130 percent, with a redistribution in favor of the mucosal and submucosal layers.

Ischemic Injury and Vascular Spasm

The normal control mechanisms of splanchnic vessel flow are deranged after vessel occlusion. It has been found that vasoconstriction occurs in the splanchnic vasculature during ischemic events. However, despite relief of an arterial obstruction or restoration of systemic pressure, vasoconstriction may persist. An appreciation of this phenomenon has been of critical importance in determining the management of mesenteric ischemic syndromes. Although the mechanism of this vasoconstriction is not clear, it does not appear to be related to alpha-adrenergic stimulation and may be related to the abnormalities in the release of renin and angiotensin.

Reperfusion Injury

The second important experimental observation is that the damage in ischemic segments of intestine is made worse by reperfusion. This appears to be caused in part by the formation of reactive oxygen metabolites during reperfusion. These are generated by oxidases of mucosal epithelium and vascular endothelium. These free radicals, in addition to causing microvascular and parenchymal injury, attract polymorphonuclear leukocytes that also generate oxygen free radicals through the activity of neutrophilic NADPH oxidase.

An etiologic classification of mesenteric ischemia is shown in Table 1. These etiologic categories are not necessarily exclusive. A low flow state, for example, may give rise to nonocclusive ischemia or may precipitate mesenteric thrombosis.

Vasculitis may produce infarction but more often presents as mucosal ulceration alone. The management is primarily directed toward control of the vasculitic process. It is increasingly recognized that oral contraceptives may produce acute mesenteric ischemia, and there is some suspicion that these agents may produce a more subacute illness resembling regional enteritis. Use of oral contraceptives should be discontinued; acute infarction should be managed as described below.

DIAGNOSIS AND MANAGEMENT OF INTESTINAL ISCHEMIA

The management of ischemic intestinal syndromes is largely determined by the clinical diagnosis. In superior mesenteric ischemia, for example, urgent angiographic examination of the vascular supply is indicated, but in ischemic colitis, angiography is rarely required. The management of these syndromes is therefore approached from the point of view of the clinical presentation. The major clinical entities are shown in Table 2.

TABLE 1 The Etiology of Mesenteric Ischemia

Arterial occlusion
Atheromatous
Embolic
Miscellaneous (vasculitis, dissection, oral contraceptives)
Nonocclusive ischemia
Systemic hypotension
Digitalis
Idiopathic
Venous thrombosis
Hypercoagulable states
Oral contraceptives
Anti-thrombin-3 deficiency
Protein C deficiency

TABLE 2 Classification of Ischemic Intestinal Syndromes

Acute
Superior mesenteric ischemia
Mesenteric venous thrombosis
Acute ischemic colitis
Chronic
Celiac axis compression syndrome
Mesenteric angina
Chronic ischemic colitis

Acute Ischemic Syndromes

Acute Superior Mesenteric Ischemia

Clinical Presentation. The typical patient with acute mesenteric ischemia is elderly and often has a history of cardiac or peripheral vascular disease. Not infrequently these patients are seen in the intensive care unit or coronary care unit.

In cases of mesenteric artery thrombosis, the patient may complain of epigastric or periumbilical pain. The severity of the pain is variable; the pain may be constant or cramping, and initially may be intermittent. There may be a history suggestive of mesenteric angina preceding the acute attack. Pain due to mesenteric embolization characteristically begins abruptly and is often located periumbilically or in the right upper quadrant. In patients with nonocclusive mesenteric ischemia, the pattern of abdominal pain is variable, and the abdominal complaints may be overshadowed by the associated illness.

There may be associated symtoms of nausea, vomiting, and diarrhea. Passage of large amounts of blood is not common, but the vomitus and stool may be positive for occult blood. When mucosal ulceration occurs grossly, bloody diarrhea may be passed. A history of digitalis use may be obtained. In the obtunded patient, the presentation may mimic that of systemic sepsis with hypotension and rapid deterioration.

On examination, hypotension may be found. Fever, at least during the early stages, is uncommon. Cardiovascular examination may reveal congestive heart failure, arrhythmias, or evidence of valvular heart disease. Abdominal examination reveals variable signs; there may be no abnormal abdominal physical signs whatsoever. Indeed, the finding of a patient in severe pain with a paucity of signs on abdominal examination should raise the possibility of mesenteric ischemia. An epigastric bruit may be heard, but this is neither specific nor sensitive for the presence of mesenteric ischemia. There may be tenderness, guarding, and obvious peritoneal signs. Bowel sounds may be either diminished or increased, depending on the stage of the ischemic damage. Rectal examination may reveal occult blood in the stool or grossly bloody stool if tissue infarction has occurred.

Investigations. Investigations must be made with extreme urgency. There are no specific diagnostic laboratory findings. Hemoconcentration and an elevated white blood cell count are common but entirely nonspecific. The serum alkaline phosphatase and amylase levels may be elevated. The serum phosphate level may be elevated if there is extensive tissue necrosis. Arterial blood gas measurement may reveal evidence of acidosis, but this is a late finding.

Radiologic Diagnosis. The radiologic appearance of the bowel in superior mesenteric ischemia may range from the unremarkable to a pattern of ileus with gas in the bowel wall or mesenteric venous circulation.

Management. In general we favor the schema presented by Brandt and Boley in 1981. It is not always possible to follow this scheme of management, but it has the advantage of offering an organized and rational approach (Fig. 2).

Resuscitation. This is critical to both the management and the investigation of patients with mesenteric ischemia. In the presence of hypovolemia, intravascular volume should be replaced as rapidly as possible without precipitating cardiac failure. In patients suffering from low cardiac output states secondary to myocardial dysfunction, measurement of central pressures via a Swan-Ganz catheter and optimization of cardiac output is necessary. Judicious use of systemic vasodilators to decrease afterload may be indicated, but excessive dilatation of the systemic circulation should be avoided, since this may lead to stealing of blood from the splanchnic circulation. Frequent measurement of systemic vascular resistance and cardiac output may be necessary.

General Measures. A nasogastric tube is inserted and the patient is fasted. A urinary catheter is placed in order to monitor urine output. Arterial blood gas measurements should be made and oxygen started if indicated.

Antibiotics should be administered. Ampicillin, an aminoglycoside such as tobramycin, and metronidazole are administered intravenously. There is a high incidence of positive blood cultures in patients with mesenteric ischemia, and prophylactic antibiotics are indicated.

The indications for anticoagulation, the optimal dosage of heparin infusion, and the timing of initiation of therapy are somewhat controversial. We treat patients with superior mesenteric artery thrombosis and those with superior mesenteric artery embolization with heparin administered intravenously and begin therapy preoperatively. We administer 10,000 units of heparin as a bolus, which is followed by an infusion of 1,000 units per hour. Therapy is monitored by measurement of the partial thromboplastin time. If excessive bleeding occurs, anticoagulation can be quickly reversed. In the rare circumstance of a patient presenting with superior mesenteric ischemia and gross hematochezia, anticoagulants are not started.

Angiography. Angiograms should be performed after adequate resuscitation. There is little point in performing an angiogram on a patient in shock; the risk of the precedure is increased and renal tubular damage is made more likely. In addition, hypotension may cause spasm of the splanchnic vasculature making adequate visualization difficult.

1. *Normal angiogram.* If the angiogram is normal and the patient is stable with no peritoneal signs, observation is indicated and a search for an alternative diagnosis commenced. In the presence of peritoneal signs, even if the angiogram is normal, a laparotomy is usually indicated.

2. *Thrombotic arterial occlusion.* If there are no peritoneal signs, the patient is stable, and the angiogram shows the presence of developed collaterals and the absence of splanchnic vasoconstriction, management is conservative with frequent reassessment.
ischemic event has developed rapidly. The absence of collaterals makes infarction more likely. Splanchnic vasoconstriction will usually be present, and a papaverine infusion should be started if it is possible to catheterize the occluded vessel. The patient should then be managed in the same manner as for patients with peritoneal signs, and surgery should be undertaken as soon as possible.

If the occlusion is relatively minor with no peritoneal signs, a period of cautious observation may be appropriate. If vasoconstriction is present, the patient should be-

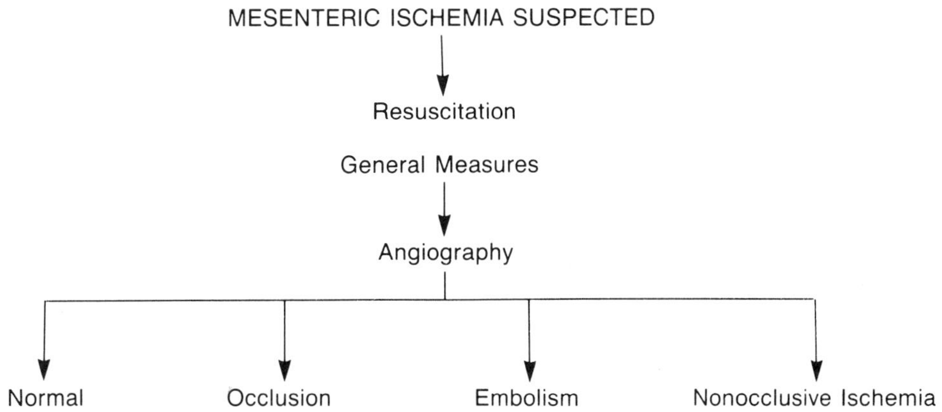

Figure 2 The management of mesenteric ischemia. See text for rationale and details.

gin receiving papaverine. If persistent peritoneal signs are present, the patient should be managed as described for major occlusive events.

3. *Embolism.* The management of embolism is somewhat different from that of thrombotic occlusion, since collateral circulation is unlikely to have developed. The management is essentially surgical, with preoperative and postoperative papaverine infusion. The papaverine infusion is managed as in nonocclusive mesenteric disease.

For patients who are unlikely to withstand surgery, or those with a minor embolism, a papaverine infusion alone may be administered in the hope that clot retraction may occur with opening of the occluded vessel. The angiogram should be repeated after 24 hours of therapy.

4. *Nonocclusive mesenteric ischia.* If the angiogram shows vasospasm but no evidence of obstruction and the patient is stable, a papaverine infusion may be started and the angiogram repeated 24 hours later.

If there are persistent peritoneal signs, surgery is indicated. Postoperatively, the papaverine should be continued and managed as described below.

Management of Papaverine Infusion. Papaverine is an opium alkaloid. It is a nonspecific dilator of the vascular tree and may work through cyclic nucleotide phosphodiesterase inhibition. When administered systemically, papaverine nonspecifically dilates all vascular systems, but when administered intra-arterially, few systemic effects occur.

Dosage. The infusion is made up in normal saline to a concentration of 1 mg per milliliter of papaverine hydrochloride. The infusion is begun at 30 mg per hour and may be increased to 60 mg per hour. Heparin need not be added to the infusion solution, since catheter occlusion by clot is uncommon; however, heparin can be infused via the arterial catheter, if necessary—provided that the heparin and papaverine are injected separately into 1 liter of the infusate. If the heparin and papaverine are mixed together directly, they will crystallize.

After 24 hours, the papaverine is discontinued and normal saline is infused into the artery. An angiogram is repeated, and if persistent spasm is present, the papaverine is restarted. It can be continued in this manner for as long as 5 days.

Unwanted Effects. The unwanted effects of papaverine include decreased arterioventricular (AV) conduction and cardiac arrhythmias. Patients who receive papaverine infusion should therefore be monitored for these effects. Papaverine is quickly metabolized by the liver, and systemic effects during arterial infusion are uncommon. Derangements in liver function have been reported.

The major risk of papaverine infusion relates to the complications of persistent catheterization. Leakage may occur at the arterial puncture site, as may dislodgement of the catheter. The patient should be monitored closely and the catheter stitched to the skin at the arterial puncture site.

Mesenteric Venous Thrombosis

Clinical Presentation. This entity used to be seen in association with intra-abdominal sepsis. It is now more commonly seen in patients with portal hypertension and hypercoagulable states, and in association with the use of oral contraceptives and vasoconstrictor drugs. Neoplasia, trauma, and bowel obstruction may also cause venous thrombosis.

Patients may present with abdominal pain located in the epigastrium or in the periumbilical area. The onset may be insidious, and there may be associated nausea, vomiting, and diarrhea. As is the case with arterial ischemia, gross bleeding is not common in the initial stages.

The physical examination reveals variable signs, depending on the stage of bowel ischemia. Earlier in the evolution of the disease, physical findings may be unremarkable. In the advanced case, hypotension and obvious peritoneal signs may be present.

Investigations. There are no specific blood tests. Leukocytosis is common, and acidosis may be found if bowel infarction has occurred. Not infrequently, the diagnosis is made at laparotomy.

Angiography is useful in the exclusion of arterial ischemia, and may permit diagnosis of venous thrombosis. Spasm of the arterial vessels may be seen with delayed or markedly impaired venous filling.

Management. The patient should be resuscitated, and the general measures used in the management of arterial ischemia should be initiated. Anticoagulation should be started preoperatively and continued indefinitely during the postoperative period. During surgery, nonviable bowel is resected. Although it is generally believed that a thrombectomy should be performed, this is not usually possible and at our institution is not routinely carried out. A "second-look" laparotomy is generally advisable.

Surgery and the Assessment of Bowel Viability. As indicated above, the timing of surgical intervention may be difficult. A second problem facing the surgeon is the assessment of bowel viability. Clearly it is desirable to keep the extent of resection to a minimum. A number of intraoperative techniques, such as Doppler flow measurements, and fluorescein dye injection, have been used to aid the clinical assessment of viability. Doppler ultrasonography allows the detection of arterial and venous blood flow. If an arterial pulse is detected, the bowel is presumed to be viable. Unfortunately, it is necessary to examine the bowel at intervals of few centimeters. If extensive ischemia is suspected, the time required to examine the entire bowel is a disadvantage of this technique. Fluorescein dye injection, on the other hand, allows rapid assessment of large segments of intestine. One gram of dye is injected intravenously. The bowel is examined under an ultraviolet light for fluorescence. If fluorescence occurs, the tissue is presumed to be viable. Problems may arise in interpretation of nonhomogenous staining patterns, but localized areas of questionable viability may be examined by Doppler.

At our center, we undertake a "second-look" operation at 24 hours after the initial surgery for all patients undergoing surgery for superior mesenteric ischemia. This practice is, however, somewhat controversial.

Acute Ischemic Colitis

Clinical Presentation. Patients with acute ischemic colitis are usually elderly and frequently have many of the same features as patients with superior mesenteric ischemia. Patients typically present with crampy suprapubic or left lower quadrant pain. Diarrhea is common and may be grossly bloody. Physical examination may reveal tenderness over the descending and sigmoid colon. An abdominal bruit and evidence of peripheral vascular disease may be found. The patient may present after undergoing aortofemoral bypass or after abdominal aneurysm repair in which the inferior mesenteric artery has been sacrificed.

Investigations. A moderate leukocytosis is common. The plain abdominal radiograph may reveal evidence of submucosal edema with "thumb-printing" in the colon.

We have found flexible sigmoidoscopy to be a useful investigation. Air insufflation should be kept to a minimum. The presentation of an acute colitic illness with a normal rectum and inflammation beginning in the proximal rectum or sigmoid colon is highly suggestive of ischemic colitis. Enteric pathogens should be excluded by stool culture.

Angiography. We do not perform mesenteric angiography in patients with ischemic colitis unless there is a question as to whether the ischemia is superior mesenteric in origin. Angiographic assessment of the superior mesenteric and celiac vessels is favored by some surgeons if surgical intervention is required.

Management. Management of ischemic colitis consists of keeping the patient fasted and administering intravenous fluids. Precipitating factors such as congestive heart failure should be corrected and digitalis discontinued, if possible. The patient should begin receiving ampicillin, metronidazole, and an aminoglycoside, and should be carefully followed for the development of peritoneal signs indicating the need for surgery. Massive hemorrhage will rarely necessitate surgical intervention. Anticoagulation is not required.

In our experience, very few patients with acute ischemic colitis need emergency surgery. After the acute episode of colitis, patients should be followed up, since approximately 10 percent will develop a colonic stricture.

Chronic Ischemic Syndromes

The classification of these syndromes is shown in Table 2. In our experience, they are encountered far less frequently than acute mesenteric vascular disease.

Celiac Axis Compression Syndrome

The major symptom of celiac axis compression syndrome is recurrent epigastric pain. Nausea and vomiting are not commonly associated. Physical examination may reveal an epigastric bruit, although this may also be heard in asymptomatic individuals. Angiography may show the presence of partial occlusion of the celiac artery close to its take-off from the aorta. The superior mesenteric artery is usually patent. The management is surgical.

It should be noted that there is considerable debate as to whether celiac axis compression syndrome exists. Although incidental findings of celiac artery stenosis at autopsy have been reported, the response to surgery is variable, and the entity is difficult to understand pathophysiologically since the superior mesenteric artery is usually patent and the collateral circulation should be adequate for tissue perfusion.

Chronic Mesenteric Ischemia (Mesenteric Angina)

Clinical Presentation. The patient usually presents with recurrent epigastric or periumbilical pain. Initially, the pain may not be clearly related to meals, but as the disease progresses an association is recognized. The patient will frequently decrease the size of his meals and characteristically will lose a great deal of weight. The pain usually begins within 15 to 30 minutes after eating and lasts for 2 to 3 hours. Some relief may be obtained by squatting or drawing up the knees. There may be associated diarrhea or steatorrhea.

Physical examination generally reveals signs of peripheral vascular disease. An abdominal bruit may be heard, but this is not specific or sensitive for the presence of mesenteric ischemia.

Mesenteric Steal Syndrome. In a variant of this presentation known as the "**mesenteric steal syndrome**," the abdominal pain is precipitated by exercise. Significant lower limb ischemia is present, and the primary vascular supply of the lower limbs is derived from the splanchnic circulation via collaterals. The metabolic work of walking may lead to stealing of blood from the splanchnic circulation with subsequent abdominal pain.

Investigations. The diagnosis is based on the exclusion of other causes of abdominal pain such as cholelithiasis, peptic ulceration, neoplasia, or inflammatory bowel disease. Routine blood work may be normal or it may reflect the patient's poor dietary intake. In some instances, steatorrhea has been reported.

Angiography may reveal the presence of significant atherosclerotic disease. It is generally believed that a significant lesion must be present in two of the three major splanchnic vessels before this syndrome develops. Rarely will other causes of vascular occlusion or arteriovenous fistulae be seen. It should be noted that 10 to 20 percent of asymptomatic elderly patients have significant lesions on mesenteric angiography. A diagnosis of this syndrome is therefore based on clinical grounds; at present, there are no specific tests for mesenteric ischemia.

Endoscopic evaluation of the colon and stomach should be performed, although there are usually revealed to be normal. At endoscopy, we have seen transient antral and duodenal erosions in association with mesenteric angina; however, these have been reported only rarely.

Management. The patient with mesenteric angina should discontinue smoking and digitalis should not be prescribed and should be discontinued, if possible. If the angiogram shows a significant lesion, consideration should be given to relieving the obstruction by means of percutaneous transluminal angioplasty.

Unfortunately, the atherosclerotic lesions frequently occur at the origins of the splanchnic vessels and tend to be an extension of aortic plaques. Because of the association with aortic disease, proximal orifice lesions and multiple vessel involvement, transluminal angioplasty is difficult to perform, is not always successful, and has significant complications. A surgical revascularization procedure is required if transluminal angioplasty fails or is deemed inadvisable.

Chronic Ischemic Colitis

Clinical Presentation. In the majority of cases, acute ischemic colitis resolves without difficulty. However, a percentage of patients with acute ischemic colitis go on to develop colonic stricture or persistent ischemic colitis. The development of chronic colitis after an episode of acute ischemia is poorly documented in the literature.

Investigations. Colonoscopy is very useful in the diagnosis of this condition. In those patients whom we believe have developed this condition, the ulceration is patchy and deep with clearly demarcated margins. The radiologic appearance is similar to that of Crohn's disease. Biopsies show nonspecific inflammation. Enteric infections should be excluded.

Management. Although chronic ischemic colitis closely resembles Crohn's colitis, in our experience it is resistant to standard medical management. The colonic ulceration may improve, but not infrequently surgery may have to be considered. Patients with chronic ischemic colitis are generally elderly and poor surgical candidates. In our experience, this condition does not carry a good prognosis.

FUTURE DEVELOPMENTS

Diagnosis

Intraperitoneal Xenon Washout

This technique may be used to estimate intestinal blood flow and to provide an image of ischemic segments of intestine. After an intraperitoneal injection of xenon-133 has been administered, the gas is cleared from the peritoneum by diffusion into the splanchnic circulation. It is then transported to the lungs and excreted. If a segment of intestine is ischemic, the gas will diffuse into the tissue but will not be cleared as rapidly as from normally perfused intestine. This delay in clearance may be detected by counting the isotope emissions and plotting the clearance against time. Alternatively, the retained isotope may be imaged using a gamma camera. The role of this technique in the management of intestinal ischemia is currently under evaluation.

Treatment

Urotensin 1

This is one of three structurally related peptides that have the ability to selectively dilate the mesenteric vasculature when administered intravenously. In experimental animals they have been shown to produce a minimal fall in systemic pressure that can be accounted for by splanchnic vasodilatation. When administered intravenously, these agents may be as effective as intra-arterial papaverine. Clearly this would represent a major advance in the management of mesenteric vasospasm. These drugs are currently undergoing evaluation; at present they are not recommended for the treatment of human disease.

Pentoxifylline

This orally administered agent is a xanthine derivative. It is a vasodilator and improves the flexibility of red cells, thus improving arterial flow. Pentoxifylline also causes platelet deaggregation. It has been used for treatment of peripheral vascular disorders and conceivably could be of benefit in the management of chronic mesenteric ischemia. As yet there have been no reported clinical trials of its use in mesenteric ischemia.

Allopurinol

The inhibition of xanthine oxidase–generated free radicals during reperfusion is theoretically beneficial in ischemic injury of any tissue. No clinical trials of the use of allopurinol in this situation have been reported.

SUGGESTED READING

Brandt LJ, Boley SJ. Ischemic intestinal syndromes. Adv Surg 1981; 15:1–42.

Marston A. Vascular disease of the gastrointestinal tract: pathophysiology, recognition and management. Baltimore: Williams & Wilkins, 1986.

Parks DA, Jacobson ED. Intestinal ischemia. In: Kvietys PR, Barrowman JA, Granger DN, eds. Pathophysiology of the splanchnic circulation. Vol I. Boca Raton, FL: CRC Press, 1987:125–140.

SECRETORY DIARRHEA

KIERTISIN DHARMSATHAPHORN, M.D.

Secretory diarrhea results from the stimulation of water and electrolyte secretion in the intestine. In most cases, secretion of chloride ions is the primary driving force for water secretion by the epithelial cells. Inhibition of electrolyte absorption may also result in secretory diarrhea, but is probably a less frequent cause. The clinical features of secretory diarrhea include excessive watery stool, more than 225 g per day (most patients with severe secretory diarrhea have a stool volume greater than 1,000 g per day); and a stool osmolarity essentially equal to the concentrations of its ions, i.e., stool ($Na^+ + K^+$) × 2 approximately equals stool osmolarity. This chapter omits the discussion of acute infectious diarrhea and chronic secretory diarrhea induced by bile salts or fatty acids (see other chapters). Diarrhea associated with inflammatory bowel disease (IBD) is also discussed in other chapters. This leaves us with chronic secretory diarrhea due to endocrine tumors and laxative abuse, and secretory diarrhea of unknown cause. The profile of chronic secretory diarrhea has changed with the increased numbers of patients who have acquired immunodeficiency syndrome (AIDS). Until now, it was the general rule that infections did not lead to chronic secretory diarrhea, but the unusual infections associated with AIDS have changed this rule.

Therapy for secretory diarrhea focuses on fluid and electrolyte replacement, along with treatment of the specific cause, if the latter is feasible. For example, exclusion of fat in the diet is essential for treatment of diarrhea associated with fat malabsorption, and cholestyramine is useful for diarrhea induced by bile salts, as are gluten-free diets for celiac sprue and proper antimicrobial agents for infectious diarrhea. In many cases of chronic secretory diarrhea, however, specific treatment may not be available or possible. Such patients may benefit from antidiarrheal drug therapy in addition to fluid and electrolyte replacement.

FLUID AND ELECTROLYTE REPLACEMENT

Fluid and electrolyte management is most critical when stool volume exceeds 1 to 2 liters per day. Dehydration, acid-base disorder, and potassium, sodium, and chloride depletion in these patients usually requires immediate attention. First, it must be emphasized that the absorptive and secretory mechanisms of the intestine are two separate and unrelated processes. When the secretory process is stimulated by exogenous toxin or endogenous secretagogues, the intestinal cells can still absorb glucose, sodium, and water normally. Second, glucose, together with sodium, is avidly and actively absorbed by the intestinal epithelial cells via the sodium glucose cotransport mechanism. Therefore, in the presence of glucose (sugar or starch), electrolytes and water are absorbed at an accelerated rate. Sustaining the absorptive mechanism for water and electrolytes should improve the water-electrolyte balance and prevent dehydration. Despite the ability to restore fluid and electrolyte balance, carbohydrate-electrolytic solutions usually do not decrease stool output, and may even make the diarrheal symptoms worse.

The composition of oral replacement solutions varies from one institution to another. Balanced salt-carbohydrate solutions containing potassium are generally used. The World Health Organization recommends a replacement solution containing the following (in g per liter): glucose, 20; sodium chloride, 4; potassium chloride, 2; sodium bicarbonate, 2. This results in a solution containing (in mmol per liter): glucose, 111; sodium chloride, 60; potassium chloride, 20, and sodium bicarbonate, 30; with an osmolarity of about 331. The electrolyte content of the different replacement solutions varies mainly in the sodium concentration, which does not appear to be critical in patients with normal kidney function. In patients with impaired kidney function, however, the composition of electrolytes should be modified accordingly, depending on their fluid and electrolyte status. For these patients, a lower sodium concentration in the replacement fluid may be needed. On the other hand, patients with the short bowel syndrome may need a replacement solution with a higher sodium content. When a higher sodium content is necessary, glucose is best given as glucose polymer to prevent hypertonicity of the solution. Glucose polymers are available commercially as Polycose (Ross Laboratories, Columbus, OH), Moducal (Mean Johnson, Evansville, IN), or Caloreen (Roussell Ltd., Wembley Park, England). A solution containing (in g per liter) glucose polymer, 20; sodium chloride, 7; and potassium chloride, 1, is recommended.

Some patients may not be able to tolerate the excessive amount of oral intake required to keep up with the diarrhea. If may be necessary to use a feeding jejunostomy tube or total parenteral nutrition (TPN) in these patients. At our institution, TPN has proved to be a very useful way to compensate for severe loss in diarrheal fluid. This technique should be considered at an early stage in patients with AIDS whose diarrhea does not respond to conventional management.

PHARMACOLOGIC INTERVENTION IN SECRETORY DIARRHEA

Reversal of excessive electrolyte secretion, either by stimulation of a receptor-mediated process that increases electrolyte absorption, or by interruption of the cellular signal transduction events (secondary messengers) leading to secretion, is the key to pharmacologic intervention. Knowledge regarding the regulation of water and electrolyte transport by peptides and neurotransmitters can be applied to the treatment of diarrhea: opiates, alpha-adrenergic agents, and somatostatin interfere effectively at the receptor sites; chlorpromazine, and its derivative trifluoperazine, interferes with the cellular signal transduction events. Alternative approaches that may be possible in the future include prevention of the

TABLE 1 Summary of Pharmacologic Options

Drug	*Effectiveness*	*High Doses Tolerated?*	*Side Effects*	*Comments*
Opiates	Quite effective	Usually	Drowsiness, nausea	First-choice drug
Alpha-adrenergic agonists	Good	Usually not	Postural hypotension, drowsiness	Combined with an opiate and/or verapamil
Prostaglandin synthetase inhibitors	Good in selected patients	Follow manufacturer's recommended dose	Vary with drug	Need testing, still not widely used
Chlorpromazine and trifluoperazine	Good	Yes but not commonly used	Retinopathy, movement disorders, blood dyscrasias, abnormal liver function tests	Monitor all patients closely
Verapamil	Not good as a single drug	Follow manufacturer's recommended dose	Cardiovascular	Combine with an opiate and/or an alpha-adrenergic agonist (use only if no heart disease)
Lithium	Good	Yes	Cardiovascular, neuromuscular, CNS	Relatively safe
Glucocorticoids	Good in selected patients with VIPoma	Not well	Many side effects of steroid, particularly at high dosage	Decrease dose to smallest effective dose
Somatostatin	Good	Usually	Steatorrhea, abnormal glucose tolerance	Must be given subcutaneously

binding of toxin to the receptor and blockage of the chloride channels. Chloride channels serve as the chloride exit pathway on the luminal membrane of the intestinal epithelial cells. Table 1 lists pharmacologic options.

Opiate Agents

Since ancient times, opiates have been the mainstay in the treatment of diarrhea. Endogenous opiates both inhibit water and electrolyte secretion and stimulate water and electrolyte absorption by intestinal epithelial cells. These compounds also stimulate contraction of the circular smooth muscle to delay gastrointestinal (GI) transit. Although the high doses of synthetic opiates normally used in clinical practice can stimulate water and electrolyte absorption, the efficiency of synthetic opiates is mainly due to their effects on intestinal motility. Opiates currently commercially available include diphenoxylate with atropine (Lomotil), loperamide (Imodium), and codeine. These compounds are quite effective, but their clinical utility is limited by the possible side effects at high doses, specifically the central nervous system (CNS) side effects. Most notable among these is a depressed mental status; other CNS side effects include nausea, vomiting, respiratory depression, and the possibility of development of physical dependence with prolonged use. The toxicity of atropine is a limiting factor when a high dose of Lomotil is needed. Imodium is more expensive than codeine or Lomotil. Because Imodium does not cross the blood-brain barrier well, it produces much fewer CNS side effects than the other opiates and can be administered safely in high doses; it also does not cause physical dependence. Few, if any, reports suggest that codeine or Lomotil causes physical dependence. The usual dosage of Lomotil is one to two tablets (each containing 2.5 mg diphenoxylate) four times a day; of Imodium, one to two capsules (each containing 2 mg) twice a day; and of codeine, 30 to 60 mg four times a day.

It is worthwhile to try Imodium at a very high dosage in patients who fail to improve after treatment with the usual doses of synthetic opiates. In our clinic these patients are started on 16 capsules (32 mg) of Imodium per day. Dosages of up to 64 mg per day have been given without significant side effects, but patients who do not respond to 32 mg of Imodium per day generally do not respond to a higher dose.

Alpha-Adrenergic Agents

Alpha-adrenergic agonists represent a new class of antidiarrheal agents. They inhibit water and electrolyte secretion and slow GI transit. Clonidine is a readily available alpha-adrenergic agent, but it crosses the blood-brain barrier easily and has many side effects. The cardiovascular side effects, in particular, limit its clinical application to relatively mild disorders such as diarrhea. In the future, newer alpha-adrenergic agonists developed for their intestinal action may produce fewer side effects. At the present time, alpha-adrenergic agents should be used to control diarrhea only in patients who either are unresponsive to synthetic opiates or are unable to use the opiate compounds because of the side effects. Electrocardiography (ECG) should be performed; patients who have significant cardiac disease should be excluded.

Clonidine should be given in combination with loperamide, starting with 0.1 mg per day and slowly increasing the dosage every 4 to 5 days. When clonidine is used alone it is usually effective at a dose of 0.3 to 0.4 mg or more per day. Postural hypotension is invariably detected at these effective doses and may be very troublesome, although it usually becomes more tolerable as time passes. About half of all patients are able to tolerate the drug after being on it for approximately 1 week; the other half unfortunately experience no significant decrease in this side effect. Some patients with diabetic diarrhea tolerate the medication well, and dosages of up to 1.2 mg per day have been used without significant side effects. Patients' diabetic neuropathy may cause them to have less or no postural hypotension. However, some patients with diabetic diarrhea are sensitive to the medication and may not be able to tolerate a dose of clonidine as small as 0.1 mg per day. Therefore, patients are started on 0.1 mg per day for at least a couple of days before the dosage is gradually increased. To avoid troublesome withdrawal symptoms, the medication should not be discontinued abruptly. A gradual tapering off over 4 to 5 days is recommended, even when the side effect is the reason for discontinuing the medication.

Inhibitors of Prostaglandin Synthesis

Interest in these agents stems from the fact that prostaglandins stimulate water and electrolyte secretion and that many immune mediators cause intestinal secretion by increasing prostaglandin synthesis. Therefore, inhibition of prostaglandin synthesis may result in less water and electrolyte secretion. Indomethacin has proved useful in some selected patients with secretory diarrhea who have an increased prostaglandin production. Salicylates may also be effective: bismuth subsalicylate (Pepto-Bismol) can prevent traveler's diarrhea, and 5-aminosalicylic acid is effective in IBD. The manufacturer's recommended dose should be given.

Chlorpromazine Derivatives and Verapamil

Alteration of the cellular signal transduction events that lead to intestinal secretion is another approach to the effective treatment of diarrhea. After binding of the hormone or toxin to the receptor, the critical signal transduction events involve an increase in either cellular cyclic adenosine monophosphate, cyclic guanosine monophosphate, or calcium and calcium-dependent effectors. Chlorpromazine derivatives inhibit water secretion and reduce diarrhea, possibly by binding to and inactivating the calcium-calmodulin complex. Clinically, trifluoperazine has been used successfully in patients with watery diarrhea due to VIPoma. Adverse effects are relatively common, however, and trifluoperazine should therefore be started at a small dosage, 2 or 4 mg per day, and increased to 30 mg per day over a period of about 1 week while the patient is monitored closely. An eye examination is recommended, because retinopathy has been reported as a side effect of phenothiazines. The medication should be discontinued if the patient develops any movement disorder (e.g., parkinsonism, tardive dyskinesia), abnormal blood count, or abnormal liver function. The effectiveness of chlorpromazine has been observed at 1 to 4 mg per kilogram of body weight in patients with cholera. The precautions outlined for trifluoperazine also apply to chlorpromazine.

Verapamil, a calcium channel blocker, inhibits calcium entry into the cells, inhibits water secretion, and causes constipation. Little or no information is available regarding its effectiveness in diarrheal diseases. However, because the drug is reasonably safe, I usually combine verapamil, 80 mg three times a day, with loperamide and clonidine in patients with severe secretory diarrhea who have no cardiac disease.

Other Medications

Lithium carbonate, glucocorticoids, and somatostatin are effective in patients with VIPoma and chronic idiopathic secretory diarrhea. The mechanism of action of lithium is not well understood. At the usual dose, 300 mg twice a day, the medication appears to be relatively safe. Troublesome side effects may involve the cardiovascular, neuromuscular, and central nervous systems.

Glucocorticoids stimulate the absorption of water and electrolytes, and may improve diarrhea in some patients with pancreatic cholera. Prednisone should be started at 60 mg per day. If it is effective, the dosage can be gradually decreased and the patient kept on the smallest dose possible to maintain effectiveness.

Somatostatin is a peptide hormone that inhibits water and electrolyte secretion in the intestine. A long-acting somatostatin analogue (Sandostatin) has been used successfully to treat diarrhea in patients with endocrine tumors such as carcinoid tumors and VIPoma, as well as other diarrheal syndromes. The side effects are relatively few and mild, despite the concern that somatostatin affects many organ systems. Abnormal glucose tolerance and steatorrhea are the major side effects, and theoretically gallstones may develop with prolonged use. However, the medications are currently available only the injectable form. The lack of oral drugs makes somatostatin an impractical medication for diarrheal diseases, except in the most severely affected patients who are unresponsive to other medications. The dosage of Sandostatin is 50 to 500 μg subcutaneously two to four times a day.

SPECIAL CONSIDERATIONS

Pancreatic Cholera Syndrome

Pancreatic cholera syndrome is also known as watery diarrhea, hypokalemia, achlorhydria syndrome (WDHA); VIPoma; or Verner Morrison syndrome. The large volume of watery diarrhea results from intestinal secretion secondary to the high circulating levels of vasoactive intestinal polypeptide (VIP) or other endogenous secretagogues that may be secreted along with the VIP. The tumor usually originates in the pancreas, but can also arise from the stomach or upper duodenum. Bronchogenic carcinoma, ganglioneuroma, or ganglioneuroblastoma can also secrete VIP and cause this syndrome.

Despite the fact that about one-third of these patients have metastases at the time of diagnosis, total excision of the tumor should be the objective if it proves to be feasible. When complete resection is not possible, the surgeon may decide to excise some tumor mass to reduce the source of endogenous secretagogues. Hepatic artery embolization has also been attempted. Chemotherapy with streptozocin or 5-fluorouracil is effective in some patients. When resection is not possible, a therapeutic trial of antidiarrheal agents should be carried out. Normally, patients with advanced disease do not respond adequately to a single drug. If a high dose of Imodium (16 mg twice a day) is not effective, or if the patient is unable to tolerate the side effects of the medication, a trial of other drugs such as lithium carbonate (300 mg twice a day), trifluoperazine (gradually increasing the dose to 30 mg per day), or indomethacin (25 to 50 mg three times a day) is indicated. Finally, if oral medications fail, one should try Sandostatin, which is usually quite effective but has to be administered as subcutaneous injections. The combination of two partially effective medications may result in better control than the use of either drug alone.

Malignant Carcinoid Syndrome

Diarrhea in this syndrome results from excessive secretion of serotonin and other peptides or neurotransmitters that are secreted along with it. Surgery should be considered, but is not feasible in most patients because of the advanced, although slow-growing, metastases. For medical therapy, the same guidelines as those outlined for pancreatic cholera syndrome apply to the carcinoid syndrome. Most patients show some response to opiates or other medications, particularly somatostatin. In addition, serotonin antagonists such as methylsergide, cyproheptadine, or ketanserin, a selective $5HT_2$-antagonist (Janssen Pharmaceuticals, New Brunswick, NJ) are useful. Chemotherapy with 5-fluorouracil, streptozocin, and doxorubicin may result in some objective responses, but the side effects generally outweigh the benefits of these drugs.

Zollinger-Ellison Syndrome and Medullary Carcinoma of the Thyroid

Diarrhea in the Zollinger-Ellison syndrome results from excessive delivery of acidic gastric fluid to the small bowel as a result of a gastrin-secreting tumor. If tumor resection is not feasible, an H_2 blocker such as cimetidine or ranitidine is usually effective in controlling the diarrhea. If the H_2 blocker proves inadequate, other medications can be added as outlined for the pancreatic cholera syndrome. Medullary carcinoma of the thyroid leads to excessive release of calcitonin, a hormone that causes intestinal secretion. Again, resection of the tumor is the primary treatment; if this is neither adequate nor feasible, the treatment is that outlined for the pancreatic cholera syndrome. Debulking the tumor theoretically should lessen the amount of circulating secretagogue.

Editor's Note: There are several published reports of control of diarrhea with somatostatin in several patients with AIDS. Some have *Cryptosporidium* or other infectious agent while others have no recognizable agent, either viral or parasitic. However, this latter group has also responded to somatostatin.

SUGGESTED READING

Cook DJ, Kelton JG, Stanisz AM, Collins SM. Somatostatin treatment for cryptosporidial diarrhea in a patient with the acquired immunodeficiency syndrome (AIDS). Ann Intern Med 1988; 108:708–709.

Dharmsathaphorn K. Intestinal water and electrolyte transport. In: Kelley WN, ed. Textbook of internal medicine. Philadelphia: JB Lippincott, 1989:442–452.

Dobbins J. approach to the patient with diarrhea. In: Kelley WN, ed. Textbook of internal medicine. Philadelphia: JB Lippincott, 1989:669–680.

Gillin JS, Shike M, Alcock N, et al. Malabsorption and mucosal abnormalities of the small intestine in the acquired immunodeficiency syndrome. Ann Intern Med. 1985; 102:619–622.

Gorden P, Comi RJ, Maton PN, Go VLW. Somatostatin and somatostatin analog (SMS 201-995) in treatment of hormone-secreting tumors of the pituitary and gastrointestinal tract and non-neoplastic diseases of the gut. Ann Intern Med 1989; 110:35–50.

Schiller LR, Davis GR, Santa Ana CA, et al. Studies of the mechanism of the antidiarrheal effect of codeine. J Clin Invest 1982; 70:999–1008.

Schiller LR, Santa Ana CA, Morawski SG, Fordtran JS. Studies of the antidiarrheal action of clonidine: Effects on motility and intestinal absorption. Gastroenterology 1985; 89:982–988.

CONSTIPATION

NICHOLAS W. READ, M.D., F.R.C.P.

Constipation is a symptom, not a disease. It is a feature of a large number of diseases, and a side effect of many drugs (Table 1). It may occur in normal people as a result of changes in diet, fluid intake, physical exercise, or emotional tension.

STRATEGY FOR MANAGEMENT OF CONSTIPATION

As for many other symptoms, the effective management of constipation depends on identifying the cause of the problem. Treatment cannot be separated from investigation. My strategy for managing patients with constipation is indicated in Figure 1.

Initial Consultation

At the patient's first visit it is important to determine whether the onset of the condition was related to any

TABLE 1 Chemicals and Drugs That May Cause Constipation

Analgesics
Anesthetic agents
Antacids (calcium and aluminum compounds)
Anticholinergic agents
Anticonvulsant agents
Antidepressive agents
Barium sulfate
Bismuth
Diuretics
Drugs for parkinsonism
Ganglionic blockers
Hematinics (iron especially)
Hypotensives
Monoamine oxidase inhibitors
Metallic intoxication: Arsenic, lead, mercury, phosphorus
Muscle paralyzers
Opiates
Psychotherapeutic drugs
Laxative addiction?

changes in diet, drug treatment, exercise, or social circumstances, and to carry out a few simple screening tests for other diseases. It is particularly important to rule out hypothyroidism and electrolyte disturbances such as hypokalemia and hypercalcemia, and to note whether there is a history of injury or disease involving the nervous system. I usually carry out a sigmoidoscopy to identify local lesions that may obstruct defecation, such as hemorrhoids, anterior mucosal prolapse, or tumor. If patients are over 40 years old, if the change in bowel habit is of recent onset, or if there are stigmata of neoplastic disease, such as weight loss or bloody stools, I order a barium enema study or colonoscopy. I also ask patients to increase their intake of dietary fiber, prescribing a bulk laxative such as ispaghula (Metamucil) three times a day, and I instruct them to keep a careful diary of the frequency of defecation.

When patients return a month later, I have excluded colon cancer and other common diseases, modified drug therapy that may be causing the condition, gained some insight into the severity and the nature of the constipation, and tested whether it is likely to respond to a high-fiber diet. Often the condition has resolved, and patients can be reassured and discharged at this stage. If the constipation is no better and increasing the dose of Metamucil does not help, I perform some more specific investigations.

The aims of these investigations are to determine whether the condition is related to a disorder of defecation or to one of colonic motility, or both, and to identify the nature of the disorder.

Is the Condition Related to a Disorder of Defecation?

Tests are clinically useful only inasmuch as they indicate the appropriate therapeutic option. Constipation can be caused by several different anorectal disorders, each of which requires a specific treatment. Two tests are particularly useful: (1) combined anorectal manometry and electrophysiology and (2) defecography.

Anorectal Manometry and Electrophysiology

Anorectal manometry and electrophysiology are used to obtain an index of rectal and external and internal anal sphincter activity under provocative conditions that are appropriate to defecation.

In the procedure used in my laboratory, anorectal pressures are recorded by means of a multilumen anorectal probe, which includes a rectal balloon. Perfused side holes are sited in the rectum, sigmoid colon, and anal canal. The electrical activities of the internal and external sphincters are recorded at the same time via a simple bipolar wire electrode inserted into the groove between the two sphincters.

Anorectal manometry is perhaps the most useful means of identifying patients with short-segment Hirschsprung's disease, although it is not the only cause of failure of internal anal sphincter relaxation in response to rectal distention. Internal sphincter relaxation can be masked by concomitant contraction of the external anal sphincter, or by the vascular pressure in patients with hemorrhoids. The internal sphincter may fail to relax because its resting tone is absent or extremely low, or because the patient has a megarectum, which requires abnormally large volumes of distention to induce internal sphincter relaxation. In fact, I have never diagnosed short-segment Hirschsprung's disease in manometric recordings from over 500 constipated patients. Hirschsprung's disease is normally treated by internal sphincterotomy and the same procedure has been advocated for other causes of constipation, especially when the depth and duration of internal sphincter relaxation are attenuated. The success of this procedure in non-Hirschsprung's patients varies from center to center, and most surgeons have abandoned it.

Irritable Bowel Syndrome. Assessment of the anorectal responses to rectal distention is, in my opinion, the single most useful test for the irritable bowel syndrome (IBS), which can often present with constipation. The rectum in IBS is sensitive to distention; the feeling of a desire to defecate is generated by very small volumes. It contracts more vigorously in response to rectal distention, and it has a reduced compliance. These features are shared by inflammatory conditions, such as ulcerative colitis and the solitary rectal ulcer syndrome, which make the rectum irritable. The treatment of IBS is unsatisfactory and beyond the scope of this article. Increasing the bulk of the stools with Metamucil may produce a more satisfactory bowel action and ameliorates the feeling of incomplete evacuation that most patients describe. Simple psychotherapy and dietary adjustment are often very helpful, and bile acid binding agents can be useful in some patients, even those who complain of constipation.

Nervous System Lesions. Patients with diseases of the spinal cord and brain often have great difficulty in voiding feces, and constipation may be the only indication of

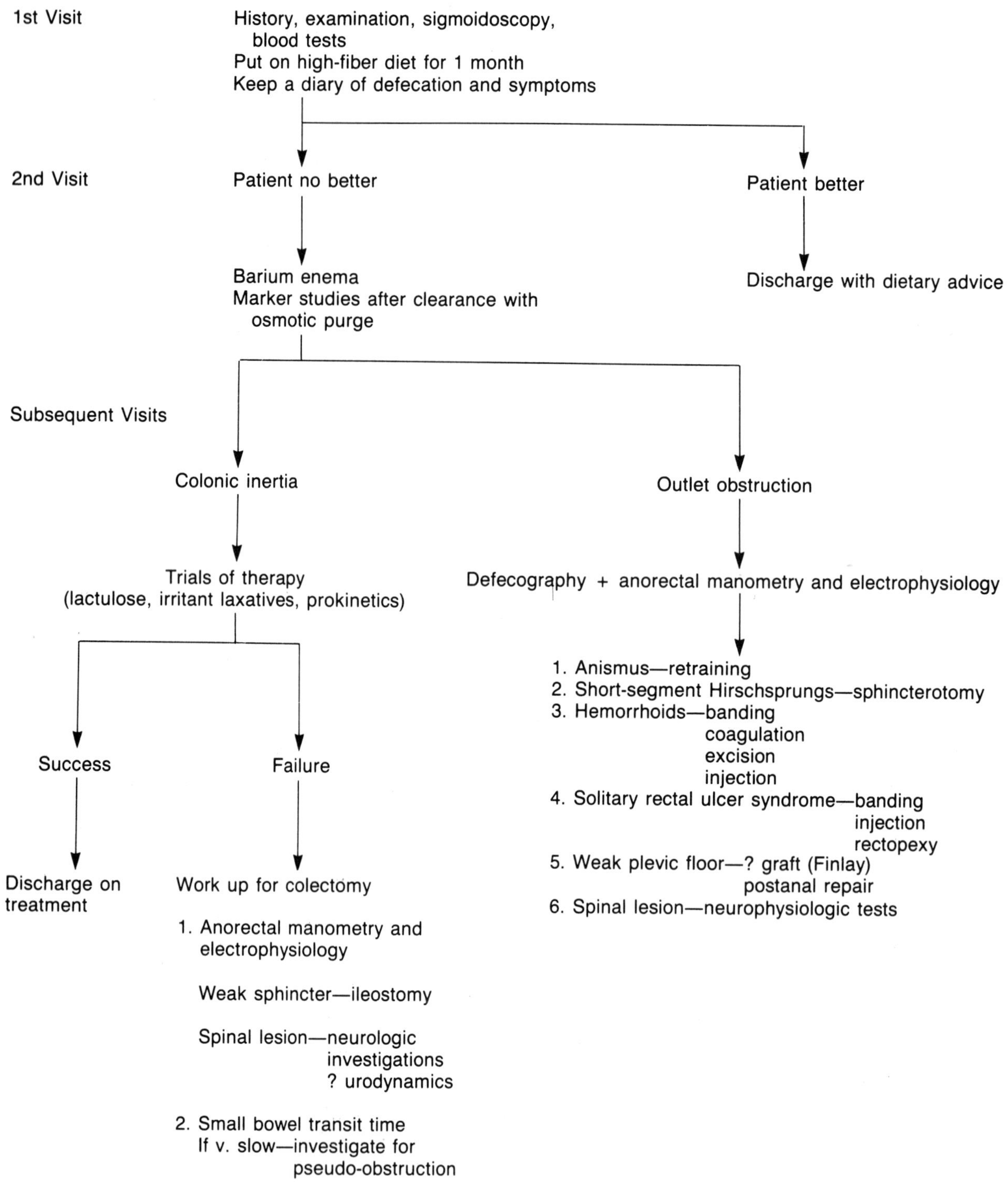

Figure 1 An algorithm for the investigation of the constipated patient.

a problem in the central nervous system. Patients with a lesion in the sacral cord or the cauda equina often have low anal pressures and a capacious, hypercompliant, and insensitive rectum and distal colon that does not exhibit any propagative response to local infusion of bisacodyl. The presence of these features in a patient who has no history of spinal disease would make me seek a neurologic opinion or carry out more complicated neurophysiologic tests. The disorder of defecation in patients with a low spinal lesion is difficult to manage; most patients use a combination of bulk laxatives, enemas, and digital evacuation, but some find it easier to cope with an ileostomy or proximal colostomy. Patients with a lesion in the high spinal cord exhibit no conscious contraction of the external anal sphincter, no rectal sensation, and no gastrocolonic response to a meal. Reflex responses to rectal distention are present and may be enhanced. Defecation is less of a problem in these patients; many can defecate in response to bulk laxatives or self-digitation of the anus, but enemas and suppositories may be necessary in some.

Hemorrhoids Versus Anterior Mucosal Prolapse. Surprisingly, it can be difficult to distinguish between patients with hemorrhoids and those with an anterior mucosal prolapse on clinical examination alone, in that both can cause symptoms of constipation and a feeling of incomplete evacuation. However, the manometric features are quite distinct. Patients with anterior mucosal prolapse have low anal pressures, the rectum is abnormally sensitive and reactive to low volumes of distention, and increases in intra-abdominal pressure often cause the rectal pressure to rise above that recorded in the sphincter. In patients with hemorrhoids the pressures in the outermost anal canal are abnormally high, show ultraslow waves, and do not relax during rectal distention. Both conditions may respond to treatment with bulk laxatives, such as Metamucil, but if conservative treatment fails, specific surgical measures may be necessary.

Tests of Defecation and Defecography

Recordings of rectal pressure and the electrical activity of the sphincter, during attempted defecation of either simulated solid stools or pastes mimicking the consistency of feces, can identify paradoxical contraction of the external anal sphincter (anismus) or insufficient abdominal effort. The existence of anismus in some normal individuals, studied under the same conditions as the patients, and the observation that most adult patients with anismus have no stools in the rectum on examination and may show abnormal colonic motility, challenge the significance of anismus as a cause of constipation. Nevertheless, impressive results have been claimed for biofeedback techniques, aimed at training patients to relax the sphincter during attempts at defecation. Performed correctly, these techniques occupy a great deal of technician time. Failure to devote sufficient time and effort may account for the disappointing experience of most investigators. Greater success for biofeedback training has been claimed in children who present with fecal impaction and anismus.

Defecography is radiographic visualization of the dynamics of evacuation of radiopaque pastes. This technique can identify obstruction to defecation caused by hemorrhoids, prolapsing anterior rectal mucosa, and inappropriate contraction of the puborectalis muscle. It is also possible with this technique to demonstrate impaired contraction of the levatores ani, which normally lift the pelvic floor during defecation. Patients with this condition are almost all women who either have had several children or have undergone pelvic surgery. The anorectal angle does not open up when they attempt to defecate; instead, they demonstrate excessive perineal descent on straining, and appear to be trying to force feces through the pelvic floor behind the anus. This problem has been managed by strengthening the pelvic floor with a postanal repair and a connective tissue graft. Defecography may also identify patients with vaginal rectocele; this can be repaired surgically, but rectocele often occurs in association with paradoxical contraction of the puborectalis muscle and impaired contraction of the levators, and may not by itself be a significant cause of obstructed defecation.

Is the Condition Related to a Disorder of Colonic Motility?

Having eliminated those patients who are easily treated with bulking agents and those who have a treatable anorectal problem, we are left with a "hard core" whom we suspect of having a primary defect in colonic motility. A barium enema will demonstrate an abnormally long or abnormally dilated colon, and reveal the presence of diverticular disease or any obstructing lesion, but it provides little insight into disturbances of colonic propulsion.

The simplest way to investigate colonic motility in such patients is to perform marker transit studies. The aims of these tests are to establish whether the patient has a disturbance of colonic propulsion, and to identify the site of any hold-up. A number of radiopaque markers are ingested together with a meal, and the results of each bowel movement are collected over the next 5 days in individual containers. These are then x-rayed to determine the rate of expulsion of the markers. Normal individuals tend to pass over 50 percent of markers in about 3 days and over 80 percent of markers in 5 days. Information about the site of hold-up of markers may be revealed by an abdominal x-ray, taken 48 to 72 hours after ingestion of the markers. If the markers are all in the rectum, the problem is rectal dyschezia or fecal impaction. Most of these patients are elderly and have impaired rectal sensation and motility. Disimpaction with enemas and manual evacuation is necessary, but provided that the problem is not secondary to an obvious outlet obstruction or a low spinal lesion, recurrence may be prevented by keeping the motions soft with ispaghula, while instructing patients to attempt to defecate every day. Severe megarectum in a young person that is resistant to simple training programs may be effectively treated by distal colonic resection.

Abnormally slow transit, with markers spread throughout the colon, suggests a global disturbance in colonic propulsion, but could be secondary to severe obstruction downstream. When there is a doubt, we find it helpful to repeat tests after completely clearing out the colon with an osmotic purgative, such as Picolax or Golytley. A single measure of colonic transit may give misleading information because of day-to-day variations, related to diet, exercise, and the menstrual cycle. This problem can be overcome by administering a standard number of markers every day for 2 weeks, estimating a running transit time by dividing the number of markers present in the abdominal cavity by the number ingested each day. Having established that the patient has severe slow-transit constipation or colonic inertia, it is important to decide whether this is secondary to a disturbance in the extrinsic or intrinsic nerve supply. Patients who have a dilated colon or segment of colon, and who fail to show any propulsive response to bisacodyl, probably have a neuropathic colonic condition. Since the pelvic paraympathetic nerves have such a dominant control over colonic motility, the problem may be secondary to a lesion involving the sacral cord or cauda equina, or to damage sustained during pelvic surgery, or may be related to a widespread autonomic neuropathy. Prolonged ingestion of irritant laxatives has also been implicated in the pathogenesis of colonic neuropathy. In most patients these distinctions may be of only academic interest, since there is no way of reversing longstanding nerve damage. However, colonic paralysis secondary to ongoing demyelinating disorders, cauda equina compression, and metabolic nerve damage (as in diabetes mellitus) may respond to specific treatment. In most cases, neuropathic disease of the colon is extremely difficult to manage. Such patients do not respond well to any laxative agent, and the only effective method of treatment may be a total colectomy. The question then is whether the surgeon should attempt an anastomosis or go straight for an ileostomy. The decision rests on whether the sphincter tone and squeeze pressure are normal, and whether the sphincter responds normally to increases in intra-abdominal pressure. If the sphincter is normal, an ileorectal or cecorectal anastomosis may be effective; if not, the patient needs an ileostomy.

Tests of gastric emptying and small bowel transit should be carried out in patients suspected of having a colonic neuropathy, in order to rule out a widespread intestinal pseudo-obstruction, caused by disturbances of the nerve supply to many areas of the GI tract. This knowledge may influence the surgeon's decision, since resection of the colon in patients with chronic intestinal pseudo-obstruction may be unsuccessful.

Other patients are found to have a long redundant colon that has no dilated segments and responds normally to stimulation with bisacodyl. Some may have an occult high spinal or cerebral lesion, and should undergo a full neurologic examination. This usually reveals nothing, and it is difficult to persuade neurologists to investigate the patient further. Patients are usually managed by a judicious combination of bulk laxatives, osmotic agents such as lactulose; and when these measures are ineffective, by irritant laxatives such as bisacodyl.

The new prokinetic agent cisapride is worth trying, since it stimulates colonic propulsion in paraplegic patients, and can be surprisingly effective in some patients with constipation who do not respond to irritant laxatives. Finally, everyone who treats constipation is impressed by the occasional patient whose problem of severe slow transit constipation, which may have resisted all forms of treatment for several years, suddenly improves. This happened to one of my patients a month after she divorced her husband. While I would not recommend a divorce for most patients with severe constipation, the time spent gaining patients' confidence and encouraging them to talk about the frustrations and depressions in their lives can lead to quite spectacular remissions when investigations do not reveal an obvious lesion.

SUGGESTED READING

Bartram CI, Mahieu PHG. Radiology of the pelvic floor. In: Henry MM, Swash M, eds. Coloproctology and the pelvic floor. London: Butterworth, 1985:151–186.

Devroede G. Constipation. In: Kumar D, Gustavsson S, eds. An illustrated guide to gastrointestinal motility. New York: John Wiley & Sons, 1988:412–445.

Henry MM, Swash M. Coloproctology and the pelvic floor. In: Pathophysiology and management. London: Butterworth, 1985.

Kamm MA, Hawley PR, Lennard Jones JE. Outcome of colectomy for severe idiopathic constipation. Gut 1988; 29:969–973.

Krishnamurthy S, Schuffler MD. Severe idiopathic constipation is caused by an obstructive abnormality of the colonic myenteric plexus. Gastroenterology 1983; 84:1218.

Lubowski DZ, Swash M, Henry MM. Neural mechanisms in disorders of defaecation. In: Read NW, Grundy D, eds. Gastrointestinal neurophysiology. Baillieres Clinical Gastroenterology, 1988; 2:201–224.

Read NW, Timms JM. Defecation and the pathophysiology of constipation. Clin Gastroenterol 1986; 15:937–965.

ULCERATIVE PROCTITIS AND LEFT-SIDED COLITIS

STEPHEN B. HANAUER, M.D.

Ulcerative colitis limited to the left colon is a common syndrome confronting gastroenterologic specialists and primary care physicians. Indeed, more than 70 percent of patients with ulcerative colitis have disease that is limited distal to the splenic flexure (left-sided colitis), and half of these have colitis limited to the rectum (ulcerative proctitis). Proctosigmoiditis is an intermediate variant, with inflammation distal to the descending colon. These definitions assume the exclusion of more proximal disease, as recent endoscopic studies have revealed minor macro- and microscopic inflammation of the right colon in many patients initially thought to have had disease limited to the distal colon. Hence, a complete colonoscopic evaluation is warranted at an early point in the patient's initial evaluation, both for therapeutic and prognostic reasons. Patients with subclinical right-sided colitis may develop active inflammation if topical therapy is limited to the distal colon, and these individuals may be at greater risk for colonic neoplasms, even in the absence of symptomatic or macroscopic right-sided colonic disease. Biopsies of the more proximal areas will allow histologic confirmation of the true extent of colitis, which typically remains constant in the majority of patients. Approximately 10 percent of patients will develop a proximal spread of their initial disease, usually early in the course of their illness.

Ulcerative colitis confined to the left side of the colon affords the opportunity for oral and/or topical (rectal) therapy. Many of the early clinical studies of ulcerative colitis did not define the proximal extent of colonic inflammation. Therefore, most therapeutic practices must be extrapolated from the experience of treating pancolitis. More recent studies of topical therapy in distal ulcerative colitis have excluded more proximal disease, while there remains little available controlled experience with oral therapy of left-sided colitis. Additionally, there are few studies comparing available approaches (oral versus rectal therapy, steroids versus salicylates, or combination therapy) to define optimal treatment. Therefore, there is a significant variation in practices based on the preferences of physician and patients instead of on guidance from controlled clinical trials.

THERAPEUTIC ALTERNATIVES

Sulfasalazine

Sulfasalazine remains the standard for oral therapy of mild to moderate ulcerative colitis against which all alternatives must be measured. Sulfasalazine has been used safely for more than four decades for ulcerative colitis, independent of extent, with well-recognized short-term side effects, including intolerance (e.g., nausea, headache, and malaise), allergy (skin rash, fever, exacerbation of colitis), and toxicity (hepatitis, bone marrow suppression, sperm abnormalities). When tolerated, sulfasalazine can be taken safely for decades without recognized long-term sequelae. Patients with mild intolerance or minor allergic manifestations (rash or fever) can be safely desensitized by a slowly progressive introduction of sulfasalazine tablets or suspension.

Recently, 5-aminosalicylic acid (5-ASA, mesalamine) has been shown to be an equally effective therapy for ulcerative colitis when compared with sulfasalazine. Although it appears that sulfasalazine is merely a delivery system for 5-ASA into the colon, an independent activity of the intact sulfasalazine compound has not been disproven. A dose-response for both acute ulcerative colitis and for maintenance of remissions has been identified such that patients who do not respond or who actually relapse with low doses (2 to 3 g per day) should be given higher doses (4 to 6 g per day), if tolerated. A gradual introduction of increasing doses may prevent many of the minor symptoms of intolerance.

New Salicylates

Oral Preparations

With the recognition that 5-ASA is as effective as sulfasalazine in the therapy of ulcerative colitis, a large number of 5-ASA preparations are being developed (Tables 1 and 2). Because 5-ASA in an unprotected form is rapidly absorbed from the proximal small bowel, it is necessary to protect 5-ASA with either slow or delayed-release formulations or via attachment to an alternative carrier molecule. Additionally, proximal release of 5-ASA in the

TABLE 1 New Salicylates (Oral)

Product	*Preparation*	*Dose*	*Delivery*
Pentasa (Marion, US) (Ferring, Denmark)	Mesalamine encapsulated in ethylcellulose microgranules	250 mg	Time/pH release 30–55 percent urinary recovery
Asacol (Norwich-Eaton, US) (Tillots, UK)	Mesalamine coated with Eudragit-S	400 mg	Release at pH > 7 20–35 percent urinary recovery
Claversal/Salofalk (SmithKline/Falk)	Mesalamine in sodium/glycine buffer coated with Eudragit-L	250–500 mg	Release at pH > 6 25–45 percent urinary recovery
ROWASA (Reid-Rowell)	Mesalamine in enteric-coated compress, coated with coteric opadry	250–500 mg	Release at pH >4.5 ≃60 percent urinary recovery
	Mesalamine in enteric-coated tablet coated with Eudragit-L100	250–500 mg	Release at pH >5 ≃30 percent urinary recovery
4-ASA (Reed and Carnrick)	Enteric coated with Eudragit compound	500 mg	Time/pH release
Dipentum (Pharmacia)	Olsalazine (azodisalicylate)	250 mg	Two molecules of 5-ASA released into colon ≃25 percent 5-ASA urinary recovery
Balsalazide (Brorek)	4-aminobenzoyl-B-alanine-5-ASA	500 mg	Inert carrier delivers 5-ASA into colon

TABLE 2 Rectal Preparations

Product	*Preparation*
ROWASA/Salofalk/Claversal (Reid-Rowell, US) (Interfalk, Canada) (SmithKline, International)	Enemas (4 g/60 ml buffered suspension pH 4.5) Suppository (0.5 g/1 g)
Pentasa (Marion, US) (Ferring, Denmark)	Enema (1, 2, 4 g/100 ml) Buffered suspension pH 4.8
4-ASA	Enema (2 g Na-4-ASA— requires reconstitution)

small bowel or right colon may reduce the amount available for local activity in the distal colon. In most clinical trials, doses of 5-ASA comparable to that administered with sulfasalazine have demonstrated equal efficacy to the parent compound, although there is limited defined experience with distal ulcerative colitis. One must extrapolate data from unspecified ulcerative colitis, assuming no difference between distal and pancolonic disease. It is hoped that specific dose-response studies will be performed in strata of proctitis or proctosigmoiditis patients.

In sulfasalazine-intolerant patients, Asacol, Salofalk/Mesasal/Claversal, Pentasa, and Dipentum have been shown to have an improved side-effect profile. It is yet to be proven that these compounds have a benefit as first-line therapy for previously untreated patients or for sulfasalazine-tolerant individuals. Nevertheless, there remains a theoretical benefit for initial treatment with compounds without the sulfa moiety, especially in males who are susceptible to the sperm abnormalities caused by sulfasalazine. Cost may also become an issue, however, if these new sulfa-free preparations are much more expensive than generic sulfasalazine. As each new preparation becomes available, these cost-benefit decisions must be analyzed.

Topical Preparations

Numerous clinical trials have now confirmed the efficacy of topically applied 5-ASA to the distal colon via enemas or suppositories. Although less well-studied than 5-ASA, 4-ASA also seems to be effective in treating left-sided colitis. There does not seem to be a dose-response with 1 to 4 g delivered locally, as long as the delivery system allows application to the inflamed mucosa. Suppositories have been shown to be effective in treating proctitis when administered in doses as low as 500 mg twice per day for acute disease, while enemas of 60 to 100 ml reliably deliver medication to the splenic flexure in active ulcerative colitis. Less than 20 percent of 5-ASA is absorbed, and serum levels of 5-ASA and metabolites do not accumulate with long-term treatment.

High-dose (4-g) 5-ASA enemas are more effective than currently available steroid enemas as monotherapy for distal colitis. The 4-g 5-ASA (Rowasa) enemas can be effective in about 75 percent of refractory patients who have not previously responded to sulfasalazine or local or systemic steroids.

As with sulfasalazine, maintenance therapy is also necessary. It remains uncertain whether patients who have achieved remission with local 5-ASA can be maintained with oral preparations. Clinical trials have demonstrated that nightly therapy with 1-g 5-ASA enemas can maintain remissions for as long as 1 year and intermittent therapy (nightly for 1 week each month) may also be useful. At present, the only commercially available product is the Rowasa 4-g, 60-ml suspension. From a practical standpoint, most patients should continue with nightly therapy until remission (usually 2 to 8 weeks), after which the enema administration can be gradually tapered to every other night or every third or fourth night, as long as remission is maintained. It may be reasonable to maintain refractory patients or patients with more extensive disease with adjuvant oral sulfasalazine or a 5-ASA preparation in conjunction with topically delivered rectal 5-ASA.

5-ASA enemas have been well tolerated by the majority of patients. Perianal irritation may occur rarely, and hair loss has been reported to be caused by 5-ASA, although this has not been confirmed. Very rarely, patients who are sensitive to salicylates may develop an exacerbation of colitis with either oral or topical 5-ASA. The main target organ for 5-ASA toxicity is the kidney; however, in doses prescribed for humans, no significant nephrotoxicity has, as yet, been recognized.*

Corticosteroids

Both topical and systemic steroids are useful for the treatment of distal colitis, and rectally administered steroid enemas remain the preferred initial therapy in many centers. Hydrocortisone enemas have been of benefit even for patients with more severe disease who are receiving

* **Editor's Note:** Some patients who are unable to retain an entero-enema may be more comfortable using half of an enema or taking a warm bath before administering the enema.

oral steroids concurrently. Unlike 5-ASA products, steroids are useful for acute disease and generally are not used for maintenance therapy. In controlled clinical trials, high-dose 5-ASA enemas have been more effective than 100-mg hydrocortisone enemas for distal colitis; however, 2-g 5-ASA enemas were equal to 40-mg prednisolone enemas. Systematic steroids, on the other hand, are probably more effective than sulfasalazine alone for acute ulcertive colitis, although a direct comparison of these therapies in distal colitis has not been performed.

At present in the United States, the only topical preparations commercially available are hydrocortisone (Cortenema) (100 mg in 60 ml of solution) and hydrocortisone acetate (Cortifoam) (80 mg per dose in a foam). In patients with severe tenesmus or those requiring more than a single daily application, Cortifoam may be better tolerated than enemas. Preparations of more potent steroids such as methylprednisolone powder can be administered as a rectal drip, and some physicians use hydrocortisone in safflower oil as an enema. Steroid suppositories in the United States are generally of insufficient dose to be useful in all but the mildest cases of distal proctitis or anal cryptitis. Significant systemic absorption (up to 50 to 80 percent) does occur with topical steroids, producing dose- and duration-related adverse effects. These undesirable consequences have led to the development of a number of nonsystemic steroid preparations that are not yet available.

Immunosuppressants

Immunosuppressants are rarely necessary or indicated for patients with left-sided ulcerative colitis. However, a few individuals with steroid-dependent colitis benefit from the addition of either 6-mercaptopurine (Purinethol) or azathioprine (Imuran) to taper steroids. These agents appear to be equally effective in treating ulcerative colitis and Crohn's disease. As always, the risk-benefit factor must be considered in individual patients with limited disease before one prescribes potent therapy for colitis that is potentially curable by colectomy.

Miscellaneous Agents

Sodium cromoglycate enemas have been used in Europe for patients with "allergic proctitis" and may be beneficial for a few patients with prominent mucosal eosinophilic infiltrates, although they have not been superior to placebo in controlled trials of patients with ulcerative proctitis. Similarly, case reports have suggested benefit from sucralfate enemas; however, in controlled trials using enemas of up to 10 g, sucralfate has not been shown to be superior to placebo. Investigational therapies including prostaglandin enemas, nicotine gum, resumption of cigarette smoking in smokers who have developed colitis after quitting, and leukotriene inhibitors and antagonists are currently being studied. Antibiotics have never been proven to be useful in ulcerative colitis, although a few reports have suggested that metronidazole may be useful as a long-term therapy in refractory, distal ulcerative colitis. One must always be cautious that these were not examples of "mimicking" Crohn's disease.

APPROACH TO THERAPY

First Attacks

Patients presenting with newly diagnosed ulcerative colitis deserve complete colonoscopic evaluations of the extent of colonic disease, with biopsies to determine both the macro- and microscopic extent. This is useful both to develop a treatment plan and to assess the long-term prognosis. In addition, a few patients may be found, by histologic study, to have Crohn's disease initially presenting as proctitis. In addition, stool cultures for enteric pathogens, ova and parasites, and *Clostridium difficile* should be obtained to rule out mimicking or superimposed infections. Homosexuals should also be evaluated for potential anorectal infections including syphilis, gonorrhea, *Chlamydia*, and herpes.

Proctitis

Patients with newly diagnosed proctitis have several options for either oral or local therapy. Most patients with mild symptoms of tenesmus, blood, and mucus coating the stool with minimal urgency will tolerate 2 to 4 g of sulfasalazine, daily. Presumably, oral 5-ASA alternatives will provide similar efficacy. If symptoms do not improve within a few weeks, either 4-g 5-ASA enemas or a steroid enema can be added to the oral therapy. Some clinicians still prefer initial treatment with topical steroids (enemas or foam), and initial treatment with 5-ASA enemas will certainly be effective, although somewhat more expensive. The patient should be advised to eat only bland, low-residue foods to reduce the symptoms of diarrhea or to eat high-roughage foods and take fiber supplements or stool softeners to reduce the symptoms of constipation; antidiarrheals or antispasmodics can also alleviate many of the uncomfortable symptoms until the mucosa begins to heal. Once the acute inflammation has resolved, one must decide whether to continue with maintenance therapy with sulfasalazine, to begin a gradual reduction in the frequency of 5-ASA enemas, or discontinue therapy, with the contingency of reinstituting treatment if the colitis flares.

Proctosigmoiditis

The higher the extent of colitis, the more likely I am to add an oral delivery system for 5-ASA. Many patients will respond to sulfasalazine alone or, if symptoms are more severe, combined with steroid or 5-ASA enemas. With the advent of 5-ASA enemas, oral steroids are necessary only in rare patients presenting with prolonged or severe symptoms when rapid symptom control is a priority. If either oral or local steroids are used, sulfasalazine should be introduced at doses of 2 to 4 daily to maintain remissions in most patients. Sulfasalazine has been a successful maintenance therapy regardless of whether steroids were required to induce the initial remission. Maintenance therapy after the use of 5-ASA enemas may be instituted either by gradually reducing the frequency of enemas or by replacing them with sulfasalazine or oral 5-ASA. Many patients who respond only to 5-ASA enemas will require continuous treatment with the local therapy.

Recurrent Disease

Patients who respond initially to therapy but then relapse should be reevaluated to confirm the proximal extent of disease and to exclude exacerbating features such as intercurrent infections. If previously discontinued, therapy should be resumed with 5-ASA enemas, sulfasalazine, or local steroids, then maintained indefinitely with sulfasalazine or 5-ASA enemas at the lowest dosage that prevents relapse. If patients have relapsed while receiving sulfasalazine, the dose can be increased and maintained at the highest tolerated dose. If necessary, 5-ASA or steroid enemas can be added and then tapered once the mucosa has healed.

It is uncertain whether high doses of oral 5-ASA (e.g., up to 4.8 g) will be more successful than the standard doses of 2 to 4 g of sulfasalazine (providing 800 mg to 1.6 g of 5-ASA).

Refractory Disease

Individuals who do not respond to sulfasalazine and/or local steroids will usually improve with the addition of high-dose (4-g) 5-ASA enemas. Because these patients may take longer to respond to initiation of the 5-ASA enemas, treatment should be continued for as long as 3 to 4 months before it is considered a failure. If symptoms are severe, oral steroids can be added and then tapered with maintenance of sulfasalazine and/or 5-ASA enemas. As many as 75 percent of these "refractory patients" can be controlled without steroids; however, it may be necessary to maintain nightly or alternate-night 5-ASA enemas indefinitely. Our patients have required an average of two enemas per week after 1 year of initial treatment.

A small proportion of newly treated patients and about one-quarter of patients unresponsive to sulfasalazine and/or steroids will not respond to 5-ASA enemas. These are the most challenging patients, requiring a great deal of patience, perseverance, and creativity to treat. Again, it is necessary to exclude more proximal disease, even if an apparent cut-off is seen in the distal bowel. If topical 5-ASA alone is not effective for confirmed left-sided disease, the addition of oral prednisone usually will induce a remission that can be maintained with sulfasalazine and/or topical 5-ASA. Sometimes the addition of topical steroids, either by enema or foam, to 5-ASA enemas will recruit additional responders. The combination can be alternated in a twice-daily schedule (e.g., steroid foam in the morning, 5-ASA enemas can night) or on an every-other-day schedule. A change to a more potent steroid enema (e.g., hydrocortisone to methylprednisolone) sometimes can be of benefit.

A few patients with documented distal colitis will remain refractory to outpatient management despite steroids, sulfasalazine, and topical 5-ASA. In this situation, admission to the hospital for intensive intravenous management, similar to that employed for acute, severe colitis will induce mucosal healing and allow subsequent adoption of a maintenance program.

Alternatively, some patients respond to oral steroids but repeatedly experience flare-ups with tapering, despite maintenance with sulfasalazine and/or 5-ASA enemas. Alternatives for medical mangement include (1) maintenance and more gradual tapering of steroids in conjunction with all of the approaches previously mentioned, (2) attempts at high doses of 5-ASA (up to 4.8 g of oral 5-ASA in conjunction with rectal therapy), (3) resumption of cigarette smoking for patients in whom smoking cessation induced a relapse, or (4) the addition of an immunosuppressant. Colectomy, of course, is a final option that can afford a permanent solution for long-standing symptoms or complications of continued medical therapy. Approximately 5 percent of colectomies for ulcerative colitis are performed for limited disease. Because none of these options is ideal, intense discussion with the individual patient and family members will be important for the long-term planning of patients who are difficult to control.

It has become apparent that immunosuppressants can be used successfully in the tapering of steroids, but there has been reluctance to use potentially carcinogenic therapy for patients who are already disposed to colonic cancers and lymphomas. Nevertheless, 6-mercaptopurine or azathioprine, in doses of 50 to 150 mg daily, allows steroid tapering in approximately 75 percent of refractory patients. As with immunosuppressants in the treatment of Crohn's disease, it may take as long as 6 months to achieve a response with immunosuppressives. If steroid tapering is not accomplished by 6 months, the approach should be considered a failure and be abandoned. Immunosuppressives will need to be continued indefinitely to prevent flare-ups, although the dose can gradually be tapered to the minimum level at which the response is maintained (generally 25 to 75 mg per day).

Long-Term Therapy

It is well-known that ulcerative colitis is a risk factor for colonic cancer. The risk of developing cancer is related to the chronicity of disease and the extent of bowel involved, and therefore patients with left-sided colitis are at less risk than those with panulcerative colitis. However, after several decades, their risk of colonic cancer does increase. Therefore, individuals with left-sided colitis do need to be under some form of surveillance, although a less vigorous form than that for patients with extensive colitis. Other long-term sequelae include sperm abnormalities in males receiving long-term sulfasalazine and metabolic bone disease in patients receiving steroids for a prolonged period. The effect of immunosuppressants on bone marrow must be closely monitored.

Although distal colitis often is more troublesome than severe for the patient, the condition presents the physician and patient with challenging decisions. Both are reluctant to embark on potent, complicated medical therapy for limited colitis, and most gastroenterologists hesitate to recommend colectomy for proctitis or proctosigmoiditis. Fortunately, most patients now can be treated successfully and maintained symptom-free, and even patients who previously had been refractory to treatment are likely to respond to high-dose 5-ASA enemas. In the future, nonsystemic steroids will add another option in our therapeutic armamentarium. We can be optimistic that newer therapies will continue to evolve, enabling us to treat the majority of patients effectively without the troublesome side effects that have often plagued patients as much as or more than the disease itself.

Editor's Note: Considering the possibility of coexistent irritable bowel syndrome may also provide the physician with therapeutic ideas regarding the treatment of patients with persistent pain or altered bowel habits.

SUGGESTED READING

Campieri M, Lanfranchi GA, Bazzocchi G. Treatment of ulcerative colitis with high dose 5-aminosalicylic acid enemas. Lancet 1981; 2:270–271.

Farmer RG. Long-term prognosis for patients with ulcerative proctosigmoiditis (ulcerative colitis confined to the rectum and sigmoid colon. J Clin Gastroenterol 1979; 1:47–50.

Jarnerot G, Rolny P, Sandberg-Gertzen H. Intensive intravenous treatment of ulcerative colitis. Gastroenterology 1985; 89:1005–1013.

Sutherland LR, Martin F, Greer S, et al. 5-aminosalicylic acid enema in the treatment of distal ulcerative colitis, proctosigmoiditis, and proctitis. Gastroenterology 1987; 92:1894–1898.

ULCERATIVE COLITIS

ROBERT BURAKOFF, M.D.

This chapter focuses on the current medical management of ulcerative colitis and toxic megacolon, excluding a discussion of ulcerative proctitis. A few introductory comments regarding the etiology, pathogenesis, and diagnosis are warranted. The etiology of this inflammatory disease that involves the mucosa and submucosa in a continuous pattern in the colon is still unknown. However, some advancement has been made regarding the pathogenesis of the inflammatory process in ulcerative colitis, specifically the observation that lipoxygenase pathway metabolites of arachidonic acid metabolism (i.e., leukotrienes) are increased in the colonic mucosa of patients with ulcerative colitis. This chapter also discusses the therapeutic implications of these observations and future directions in medical management. The disease, with a peak incidence at 20 to 40 years of age, is characterized by recurrent episodes of bloody diarrhea and abdominal pain. However, the initial presentation of the disease is indistinguishable from other forms of acute colitis, clinically as well as sigmoidoscopically. I do not believe a diagnosis of ulcerative colitis should be made until all infectious causes of colitis (including amebiasis and *Clostridium difficile*) are ruled out and symptoms have persisted for at least 2 weeks. Once a diagnosis has been made by exclusion and it is known that the disease is more extensive than proctosigmoiditis, one can begin treatment without performing a barium enema.

MEDICAL MANAGEMENT OF ULCERATIVE COLITIS

General Comments

Since publication of the last edition of this book there is, as usual, good news and bad news regarding the medical management of ulcerative colitis. The bad news is that there is still no specific drug therapy for ulcerative colitis, and the new oral salicylate preparations and topical, rapidly metabolized steroid preparations have not yet appeared on the market. The good news is that recent studies have shown the new oral 5-aminosalicylate (5-ASA) preparations to be as effective as sulfasalazine, and they should be on the market soon. More good news is that a topical 5-ASA has become available.

Therefore, the drug armamentarium for treating ulcerative colitis is gradually increasing, although the mainstays of therapy remain sulfasalazine and corticosteroids. Other therapeutic options include immunosuppressive therapy, metronidazole, antibiotics, and antidiarrheal agents. There is nothing new regarding nutrition, psychotherapy, or behavioral therapy in the treatment of ulcerative colitis. Finally, progress has been made with the new anal sphincter-sparing operations.

Once the diagnosis has been made, the decision regarding treatment will depend on the severity of symptoms. The only diagnostic procedure necessary is a flexible sigmoidoscopy to determine if the patient has proctosigmoiditis as opposed to more extensive disease.

Treatment of Mild Ulcerative Colitis

In treating mild ulcerative colitis (i.e., patients who have fewer than five bloody bowel movements per day with minimal abdominal pain and no anorexia or fever), the first line of drug therapy will be sulfasalazine.

Sulfasalazine

Sulfasalazine has been used to treat mild to moderate ulcerative colitis for the past 50 years. It consists of sulfapyridine linked to 5-ASA by an azo bond. Investigations into the pharmacology of the drug have revealed that sulfasalazine is partially absorbed as a whole compound and excreted unchanged into the urine. The remainder of the drug is excreted unchanged into the bile and then split into its two moieties by intestinal bacteria in the distal ileum and colon. The sulfapyridine is absorbed and excreted in the urine essentially unchanged, and the 5-ASA remains unabsorbed and in contact with the colonic mucosa. It was initially believed that the sulfapyridine moiety played as important a role as the 5-ASA in decreasing the symptoms of ulcerative colitis. However, during the past 10 years it has been observed that the 5-ASA component of the drug inhibited the synthesis of prostaglandins from the mucosa of colitic colons significantly more than did sulfapyridine. Because prostaglandins lead to increased secretion and diarrhea, it was concluded that the 5-ASA was the active moiety of the drug. This of course has led to the recent development of 5- and 4-ASA oral and topical preparations, which I discuss later in this chapter.

Sulfasalazine has been found to be effective in treating mild to moderate disease in 75 to 80 percent of patients. I begin treatment by prescribing 500 mg twice a day and have the patient add one pill, every 1 to 2 days, until a dose of 3 to 4 g is reached. If there is no improvement after 2 to 3 weeks, I try to increase the dose to 4 to 5 g, but usually with little success. Some patients tend to improve after 4 to 8 weeks, but these may be spontaneous remissions.

After the patient's symptoms have resolved and there is gross sigmoidoscopic improvement of the disease, I continue to prescribe the above-mentioned dosage for at least 1 month to be sure the patient does not relapse. The drug should then be tapered to 2 g per day. At 2 g per day, 75 percent of patients will remain in remission for at least 1 year. However, even with no therapy, 35 percent of patients will remain well.

The major issue that is raised is, should the patient continue to receive maintenance sulfasalazine indefinitely? If this is the initial episode of colitis, I stop administering the drug after 3 to 6 months and determine if the symptoms recur. If a relapse occurs and the patient responds to sulfasalazine, I have the patient take the drug indefinitely, but review the situation yearly.

The biggest problem with sulfasalazine is its side effects. Approximately 25 to 30 percent of patients experience headaches, nausea, anorexia, and dyspepsia. People allergic to sulfa drugs develop fever and rash. Less common side effects include hemolysis and neutropenia, which are related to serum sulfapyridine levels. More rare idiosyncratic reactions include pancreatitis, hepatitis, serum sickness–like illness, and alveolitis.

More recently, it has been found that sulfasalazine may actually cause an exacerbation of the disease. This may be due to a rebound phenomenon in which there is an increase in arachidonic acid metabolites such as prostaglandins and leukotrienes, resulting in diarrhea and an inflammatory response. Another complication is an increase in infertility in males, resulting from decrease in sperm count and motility. This can be reversed within a few weeks after discontinuation of the drug. Finally, sulfasalazine does cross the placenta, but has been found to be safe to use during pregnancy.

There are several maneuvers one can use to avoid side effects. The first is to initiate the drug slowly, as discussed above. If a patient has persistent dyspepsia, I use enteric-coated tablets and can avoid the upper gastrointestinal side effects in approximately 50 percent of patients. For the remaining 50 percent, one must lower the dose. For patients who experience mild allergic reactions (i.e., fever and rash), one can follow a desensitization regimen. The simplest regimen is to discontinue the drug for 2 weeks, then give the patient increments of 250 mg per day until a dosage of 2 to 4 g per day is reached. However, it is hoped that this will all be unnecessary with the soon-to-be-released oral 5-ASA preparations. Finally, mention should be made of the fact that sulfasalazine interferes with dietary folate absorption. Because many patients with chronic ulcerative colitis are mildly anemic, I prefer to administer 1 mg of folate per day while the patient remains on sulfasalazine to avoid the confusion of the contribution of a macrocytic anemia to the overall anemia picture.

What other treatment options are available for mild ulcerative colitis? How good are topical treatments? Clearly, one does not want to escalate treatment by using systemic steroids, and one should also remember that minimal symptoms are best left untreated or treated symptomatically. Fortunately, the discovery that 5-ASA is the active moiety of sulfasalazine has led to the development and testing of new 5-ASA compounds.

5-ASA Preparations

Several oral preparations of 5-ASA and 4-ASA have been studied. The basic concept is to protect the molecule before it is absorbed in the proximal bowel. This has been accomplished by coating the tablet so that it will only dissolve at alkaline pH of 6 or 7, corresponding to the pH in the terminal ileum and colon. These preparations include Asacol, Claversal, Salofalk, and Pentasa. One other preparation (Dipentum) uses the azo bond to link two 5-ASA molecules together, which is broken by bacterial azo reductase activity. In all studies to date, these compounds have been shown to be as efficacious as sulfasalazine in treating acute ulcerative colitis as well as in preventing relapses. Approximately 20 percent of the 5-ASA is absorbed, and although there are far fewer side effects than with sulfasalazine, the person who is salicylate-sensitive will experience worsening of diarrhea. Various preparations may be available by the time this edition goes to press.

Topical Agents

The other therapeutic modality is the use of topical steroids. Although extremely good for proctitis and proctosigmoiditis, I have been disappointed in their performance in patients with left-sided disease to the splenic flexure, despite the studies showing that steroids sometimes reach the distal transverse colon. However, because it is impossible to know who will respond to topical steroids, it is always worth a trial for patients with mild to moderate disease.

What's new in topical agents? This year the topical 5-ASA Rowasa has been released. It is 4 g of 5-ASA in a 60-ml suspension given as a once-nightly enema, and it has been shown to be highly effective in treating left-sided colitis. In one study, 75 percent of patients had a complete remission and even improved, despite failure to respond to sulfasalazine. However, once the drug is withdrawn, the majority of patients experience a relapse. Studies are ongoing and show good results with 1 g of 5-ASA enemas nightly to prevent relapse. Obviously, the drawback is that most patients prefer oral therapy versus enemas, and the major adverse effects, although uncommon, are perianal irritation and an increase in colitis symptoms due to sensitivity to salicylates.

Nutritional Management

Initially I withdraw patients from lactose-containing products, but I have the patient undergo a hydrogen breath test for lactose intolerance to determine if long-term withdrawal of lactose-containing products is necessary.

In addition to ruling out lactose intolerance, I encourage my patients to eat a normal, well-balanced diet and to avoid specific foods that may bother a given individual. I recommend a limitation on caffeine to decrease diarrhea and avoiding significant ingestion of fruits and vegetables that may lead to increased gas and cramps.

There are no data at present that indicate that there is a food allergy component in exacerbation of ulcerative colitis symptoms.

Treatment of Moderate Ulcerative Colitis

Patients with moderate disease, whether left-sided or universal, have six to ten bloody bowel movements per day, abdominal pain, usually no fever (certainly a temperature of less than 100° F), are often slightly anemic with an increased sedimentation rate, and usually have an adequate nutritional status.

These patients always require some form of systemic therapy. My approach is an additive one. I try sulfasalazine (up to 4 g per day), and if there is not significant improvement within approximately 2 weeks, I add topical steroids in the form of enemas, suppositories, or foam. These various preparations contain 100 mg of hydrocortisone and will reach beyond the splenic flexure. I recommend the foam or suppositories when a patient has difficulty retaining enemas. For moderate disease, I recommend morning and evening enemas for 2 weeks. Patients with universal and left-sided disease have a variable response, with response rates of 40 to 80 percent with left-sided disease and 40 to 50 percent with universal colitis. If there is no improvement after 1 week, I add a 5-ASA enema at bedtime. If there is no significant improvement of symptoms after 2 to 4 weeks, the patient will not respond to this regimen and will need systemic corticosteroids.

Whether steroid enemas are effective because of their systemic versus local effect has been debated. Controlled studies have shown that the effectiveness of rectal instillation of steroids is definitely related to its local activity and depends on many factors including dose, duration of retention, volume administered, and bacterial degradation.

Tixocortol Pivalate

In an attempt to avoid systemic effects of steroid enemas, tixocortol pivalate was developed. It is a nonsystemic steroid that has been synthesized by adding a thiol ester group at position 21 on the hydrocortisone molecule, which results in rapid metabolism. To date, in trials with left-sided colitis, tixocortol pivalate has resulted in a statistically significant reduction in clinical symptoms and sigmoidoscopic findings within 2 weeks. The only complication was perianal irritation in 5 percent of patients. In the one open study involving patients whose symptoms were refractory to sulfasalazine and hydrocortisone enemas, the patients received 250 or 500 mg of tixocortol pivalate nightly as an enema, and all had improvement in clinical symptoms and sigmoidoscopic findings by 2 weeks. Tixocortol pivalate has not yet been released commercially, but it is hoped that it will find its way to the market in a timely fashion.

Prednisone

If the patient with moderate ulcerative colitis does not respond to the conservative regimen discussed, oral corticosteroids must be introduced. Although there are many preparations of corticosteroids, there is no evidence that one particular preparation is better than another. Most of my experience has been with prednisone. Approximately 75 to 80 percent of patients will have a clinical remission with prednisone with the initial course. In patients with moderate disease, the usual dose is 30 to 60 mg per day, depending on the severity and duration of symptoms. If there has been no improvement with sulfasalazine and topical steroids, I usually begin administering prednisone to the patient in doses of 20 mg taken orally twice per day.

If the patient's clinical symptoms and sigmoidoscopic findings improve, one can start to taper the dosage after 2 weeks. Although there have been no controlled studies on the effects of rapid tapering of prednisone, there is no question that clinical experience has shown that this is often associated with relapse of symptoms. A general recommendation is to decrease the dosage by no more than 5 mg per week.

At dosages of 15 mg or less, I suggest tapering by no more than 2.5 mg per week. Once a remission has been achieved, it is reasonable to restart sulfasalazine at 2 g per day in an attempt to preserve that remission. Although there are no data supporting the use of low-dose prednisone (10 mg or less) in maintaining a remission there is no question that 10 to 15 percent of patients with ulcerative colitis will remain only relatively symptom-free with the use of low-dose prednisone. If one must maintain a patient on low-dose steroids for a prolonged period, the patient should be checked frequently for high blood pressure and hyperglycemia. In addition, the patient should have an opthalmology evaluation at least once a year to rule out formation of posterior cataracts. Finally, the patient should receive calcium and vitamin D supplements to avoid osteoporosis and osteomalacia secondary to long-term steroids.

Treatment of Severe or Fulminant Ulcerative Colitis

Approximately 10 to 20 percent of patients have a more severe course with ulcerative colitis and usually require hospitalization. These patients generally have more than ten bloody bowel movements per day, abdominal pain, fever (< 102° F), anorexia, anemia, and a low albumin level.

As a result of their poor nutritional status and anemia, these patients must be hospitalized and be given supportive nutritional therapy with hyperalimentation. Initially, the patient should be given complete bowel rest to diminish the episodes of diarrhea and lessen the abdominal cramping.

The use of a given corticosteroid parenterally will vary from center to center depending on one's bias. For patients who have been receiving oral steroids, I favor prednisolone (60 to 80 mg per day) or methylprednisolone (48 to 60 mg per day) in three divided doses or administered as a continuous infusion, rather than hydrocortisone (300 mg per day) because there is less salt retention with the former drugs. For the minority of patients who have not been receiving oral steroids, adrenocorticotropic hormone (ACTH) given as a continuous infusion in a dosage of 120 units per day may be at least as effective as hydrocortisone. Although prednisolone and methylprednisolone have not been compared with ACTH, I have found them to be more effective steroids than hydrocortisone. In addition, occasionally there are patients who will respond to higher doses of prednisolone (100 to 120 mg per day) when symptoms have not improved on 60 to 80 mg per day. The role of total parenteral nutrition (TPN) in helping manage the patient with severe ulcerative colitis who is responding slowly to parenteral steroids should not be understated. TPN has enabled us to treat our patients with steroids for a longer period in the hope of achieving a remission as well as providing the needed caloric intake to achieve a positive nitrogen balance. Of course, TPN plays no role in ameliorating the inflammatory response in ulcerative colitis, but with TPN I believe that a patient can and should, if possible, be given at least a 3- to 4-week course of parenteral steroids before surgery is contemplated.

During the acute episode of severe colitis, pain medications and antidiarrheals should be avoided to prevent provocation of toxic megacolon.

Once the patient has responded clinically, to avoid changing two variables at once, I begin administering oral fluids to the patient. If the patient tolerates fluids without a significant increase in bowel movements or abdominal pain, the patient then begins receiving prednisone (30 mg twice per day, taken orally), and the same slow tapering of prednisone will begin.

TOXIC MEGACOLON

What is toxic megacolon? As the term has always implied, one is dealing with a clinical syndrome. Obviously there are degrees of toxicity and distention of the colon. For purposes of discussion, a reasonable definition of toxic megacolon is that a syndrome in which a patient has significant bloody diarrhea, usually more than ten times each day, severe abdominal pain, usually a fever of more than 101° F, and a supine abdominal film demonstrating accumulation of air predominantly in the transverse colon with distention of the transverse colon diameter of more than 5 to 6 cm.

In approximately one-third of patients who develop toxic megacolon, toxic megacolon is the initial presentation of their ulcerative colitis. In this group of patients, one must therefore be sure to rule out other infectious causes of colitis such as *Campylobacter, Shigella, Salmonella*, and certainly *Clostridium difficile* colitis secondary to antibiotics. It should be kept in mind that *Clostridium difficile* colitis may occur for as long as 3 to 4 weeks after discontinuing an antibiotic. Additionally, stool should be screened for *Entamoeba histolytica*. A simple test to insure against recent exposure to *Entamoeba histolytica* is a serum complement fixation test. For the other two-thirds of patients with established ulcerative colitis, stool examination and cultures should also be performed.

After a surgery consult is called and a central line is placed for monitoring volume status and for parenteral alimentation, a careful flexible sigmoidoscopy should be performed to confirm this clinical impression. There is no need to pass the simoidoscope beyond the distal sigmoid, and of course no air should be instilled.

Antibiotics

Unfortunately, there are no data to support the use of antibiotics in toxic megacolon, but since one is treating a patient who may perforate, the use of antibiotics to cover gram-negative organisms and anaerobes would be considered prudent. Despite the fact that third-generation cephalosporins have a broad spectrum, I still prefer an aminoglycoside and metronidazole.

Corticosteroids

If the patient is receiving steroids at the time of admission, I use methylprednisolone, 60 to 80 mg given intravenously in divided doses every 8 hours or as a continuous infusion. If a patient has not been receiving steroids, 40 units of ACTH every 8 hours, administered intravenously, has been shown to be as effective as other steroid preparations.

During the initial phase of the illness, all pain medications should be avoided and, of course, no antidiarrheal medications should be used. Included in the initial management is the decision of whether or not to use a long tube. In my experience, the use of an nasogastric tube and rectal tube has been just as effective. In many institutions, the problem with a long tube is that too much attention is placed in watching the long tube and not the clinical status of the patient.

Surgery

Once the initial management has been instituted, the critical decision regarding surgery will usually be made within the next 48 to 72 hours. The patient must be examined several times each day and have an abdominal film done at least daily. The abdominal film becomes paramount, since the patient's initial pain is often masked by the intravenous steroids. There are two findings on the abdominal film that will be good indicators of the need for surgery. First is increasing distention of the transverse colon in the supine position. Second, and most important, is the presence of "thumbprinting" or "scalloping" of the outline of the colonic air shadow. This finding has been associated with a high incidence of some degree of perforation of the colon. With this finding, as well as with the lack of significant clinical improvement within 72 hours, surgery should be performed.

As has been previously shown, the reason for the distention of the transverse colon is that the air accumulates in the transverse colon in the supine position. Therefore, it is reasonable to have the patient change position in bed every 2 to 3 hours to redistribute the colonic air.

With the above medical regimen, at least 50 percent of patients should be able to avoid surgery. Of course, every effort should be made to treat the patient medically, since long-term follow-up has shown that only one-third of patients who are treated successfully for toxic megacolon will eventually require a colectomy for chronically active ulcerative colitis.

Obviously, in making the decision to operate, one must individualize each case. Besides the obvious signs of deterioration secondary to sepsis and peritonitis, the decision about the timing of surgery becomes much more difficult. Patients who have persistent low-grade fevers of 100 to 101° F and who have a significant shift to the left on the complete blood count (CBC) differential after 4 to 5 days will usually require surgery. But certainly with an aggressive medical regimen as outlined above, many patients can be treated up to a week before a decision to operate is made.

If surgery is performed, the patient will almost inevitably have a subtotal colectomy either in consideration of a future ileoanal anastomosis operation or because the patient is too unwell to have a proctectomy.

For the 50 percent of the patients who are successfully treated for toxic megacolon, at least 10 days of the initial high-dose steroids and 7 to 10 days of antibiotics will usually be required. I usually prefer to continue administering intravenous steroids until the patient can start oral feedings without relapse of symptoms. Once oral intake has been tolerated, I recommend that the patient start oral prednisone, 60 mg daily, divided into two or three doses.

Support Systems

A final comment should be made about the emotional support that the patient's family needs. This is obviously a traumatic time for the patient and family, and frequent conversations regarding the treatment plan and how it works are most helpful. Certainly, discussing the possibility of surgery is warranted, but the patient must feel that he or she is included in the decision on the timing of surgery. Because acute psychosis may occur with high-dose steroids, the patient should be informed of these side effects, and minor tranquilizers can be prescribed. Finally, the National Foundation for Ileitis and Colitis (444 Park Avenue South, New York, NY 10016; (212) 685-3440) has started hospital visitor programs where patients who have had similar experiences can provide much needed support to the patient and family. (The United Ostomy Association also has hospital visitor programs in many cities.)

ALTERNATIVE DRUG THERAPIES FOR ULCERATIVE COLITIS

Immunosuppressive Drugs

Is there a role for azathioprine or 6-mercaptopurine in the treatment of ulcerative colitis? Yes, albeit a limited role. Most controlled studies have not shown either drug to have a beneficial effect in treating ulcerative colitis. Furthermore, because these drugs do not produce a clinical response for at least 3 to 4 weeks, they have no role in acute ulcerative colitis.

Recently, in an uncontrolled study, two-thirds of patients with chronic ulcerative colitis who had responded poorly to steroids showed a significant improvement when receiving 6-mercaptopurine, resulting in either their discontinuing steroids or a significant reduction in dose while remaining in a clinical remission. While receiving 6-mercaptopurine, approximately 75 percent of the responder group remained in remission over a 2-year period. However, when 6-mercaptopurine was stopped after 1 year of clinical remission, approximately 75 percent of the patients relapsed.

The major side effects of 6-mercaptopurine, although infrequent, are neutropenia, pancreatitis, fever, and rash.

Although these data need to be confirmed in a controlled study, I believe that for patients who continue to have exacerbations of symptoms each time prednisone is decreased below 40 to 20 mg per day, a trial of 1.5 mg per kilogram per day of 6-mercaptopurine is reasonable before a colectomy is performed. Obviously, the major questions and concerns are how long one should continue 6-mercaptopurine and what is the true risk of malignancy with long-term use. My opinion regarding the former question is that if long-term use of 6-mercaptopurine is required to maintain a remission, one should encourage the patient to consider strongly a colectomy, except for older patients with ulcerative colitis. The latter question cannot be answered as yet, except to note that the 15-year experience to date with 6-mercaptopurine reveals a very low incidence of malignancy.

Metronidazole

To date, there are still no good controlled data demonstrating a beneficial effect of metronidazole in treating patients with ulcerative colitis. However, just as sulfasalazine can definitely benefit patients with small bowel Crohn's disease, despite controlled studies not demonstrating a statistically significant improvement, one can make the same argument for the use of metronidazole in ulcerative colitis. In the small group of patients who do not respond well to sulfasalazine but are not unwell enough to start taking steroids, a trial with 250 mg of metronidazole four times per day may be helpful. However, the major problem with metronidazole is patient intolerance secondary to side effects such as metallic taste and paresthesias. At present there are no data on the long-term use of metronidazole in ulcerative colitis, and therefore its long-term use cannot be recommended.

Antidiarrheal Agents

Antidiarrheal agents (e.g., diphenoxylate with atropine, loperamide, deodorized tincture of opium and codeine) should not be used in acute ulcerative colitis, but certainly have an important role in chronic ulcerative colitis.

I find the major use for these agents to be bedtime administration for patients with nocturnal diarrheal symptoms. It is important to educate the patient emphatically to keep the use of these agents to a minimum to avoid colonic distention and, if symptoms of ulcerative colitis are worsening, to avoid precipitating toxic megacolon.

SURGERY

A brief comment on the role of surgery in ulcerative colitis. The decision to recommend surgery for a patient with ulcerative colitis will obviously result in a cure, and most gastroenterologists will agree that there are certain circumstances that mandate surgery. In addition to the patient with toxic megacolon who is not responding to medical management, patients who have severe dysplasia on colonoscopy are strong candidates for colectomy. However, the largest group of patients who will require surgery are those with significant chronic symptoms who cannot be weaned from steroids. In the end, the gastroenterologist should never allow the patient to incur significant long-term side effects of steroids (such as diabetes, progressive bone disease, or chronic hypertension) when a colectomy can be performed.

FUTURE DIRECTIONS FOR THE MEDICAL MANAGEMENT OF ULCERATIVE COLITIS

As understanding of the mechanisms of inflammation in ulcerative colitis increases, more specific drugs can be developed to treat the disease. It is already known that metabolites of arachidonic acid metabolism of both the cyclo-oxygenase pathway (prostaglandins) and lipoxygenase pathway (leukotrienes) are increased in the colonic mucosa of patients with ulcerative colitis. We know that 5-ASA will inhibit to some extent the formation of prostaglandins and leukotrienes. Research is taking an exciting course in developing specific inhibitors of leukotrienes. With the knowledge that leukotrienes, specifically leukotriene B_4, are powerful neutrophil chemoattractants, a multicenter study is ongoing to determine if eicosapentanoic acid (EPA), which itself is known to have effects on neutrophil function by inhibiting arachidonic acid metabolism, is of benefit in treating ulcerative colitis. In one small open trial, 2 to 4 g of EPA given once a day resulted in a significant clinical improvement in ulcerative colitis.

One would hope by the next writing of this chapter that specific inhibitors of inflammation will have proved safe and effective in the treatment of ulcerative colitis.

SUGGESTED READING

Dissanayake AS, Truelove CS. A controlled therapeutic trial of long term maintenance treatment of ulcerative colitis with sulfasalazine (salazopyrine). Gut 1973; 14:923–926.

Fazio VF. Toxic megacolon in ulcerative colitis and Crohn's disease. Clin Gastroenterol 1980; 9:389–407.

Hanauer SB, Kirsner JB, Barrett WE. The treatment of left-sided ulcerative colitis with tixocortol pivalate (TP). Gastroenterology 1986; 90:1449.
Meyers S, Sachar DB, Goldberg JD, Janowitz HD. Corticotropin versus hydrocortisone in the intravenous treatment of ulcerative colitis. Gastroenterology 1983; 85:351–357.
Peppercorn MA. Sulfasalazine: pharmacology, clinical use, toxicity, and related new drug development. Ann Intern Med 1984; 3:337.
Schroeder KW, Tremaine WJ, Ilstrup DM. Coated oral 5-aminosalicylic acid therapy for mildly to moderately active ulcerative colitis: a randomized study. N Engl J Med 1987; 317:1625–1629.

CROHN'S DISEASE OF THE COLON

THEODORE M. BAYLESS, M.D.
MARY L. HARRIS, M.D.
JOHN O'BRIEN, M.D.

USEFUL BUT IMPRECISE GENERALIZATIONS

The following are useful but imprecise generalizations regarding Crohn's disease of the colon:

1. In contrast to Crohn's disease in the ileum, in which scarring and obstruction lead to surgery in two-thirds to three-fourths of patients, Crohn's disease of the colon is mainly characterized by varying degrees of active, often deeply ulcerating, disease activity.
2. If Crohn's disease of the colon is going to exhibit aggressive characteristics including fistulization, perforation, or abscess formation, this usually begins to manifest itself in the first 5 or 6 years of the illness, or after suppressive medications such as azathioprine are withdrawn.
3. Likewise, if resective surgery for active Crohn's disease of the colon is necessary, this is generally in the first 5 to 6 years of known illness. Lennard-Jones and colleagues (Elliot and Ritchie, 1985) in London described 57 patients with predominantly colonic disease, of whom 25 underwent bowel resection, 10 within a year of first being seen. The cumulative probability of surgery was 35 percent at 5 years and 39 percent at 10 years.
4. After the initial 5 or 6 years, medical therapy usually suppresses disease activity. Seven of the 28 patients treated medically in the London series were off all medications at the time of the 1985 report. Eight were on sulfasalazine and three were on systemic steroids, including one person on azathioprine as well. Earlier in their course 20 patients were taking azathioprine but it was possible to withdraw this agent.
5. After total colectomy, Crohn's disease that is seemingly localized to the colon, i.e., in which the ileum (preoperatively) is clearly normal radiographically, will probably (in 80 percent of patients) not recur in the small bowel.
6. Prednisone therapy is sometimes, but not always, able to suppress disease activity in the colon. Corticosteroid therapy alone is usually inadequate or even deleterious once complications such as perforation or abscess have occurred.
7. Sulfasalazine exerts anti-inflammatory effects in mild to moderate Crohn's colitis. In terms of continuous disease suppression with sulfasalazine, there have not been uniformly positive reports in control trials. However, we and other physicians believe that, as in ulcerative colitis, long-term sulfasalazine therapy, 3 g per day, may help to sustain remissions in mild to moderate Crohn's colitis.
8. Metronidazole in doses of 1,000 mg per day or less seems to have anti-inflammatory effects in some patients with Crohn's colitis even in the absence of perianal disease.
9. About two-thirds of patients with severe but uncomplicated Crohn's colitis who would otherwise be considered for colectomy go into remission on prolonged bowel rest. This may be achieved via a double-barreled ileostomy as used by Kettlewell and Jewell, who reported a 93 percent initial response rate with defunctionalizing surgery. After 12 to 18 months, they were able to reanastomose two-thirds of these patients. The remissions lasted for several years in many patients.

Another method of obtaining bowel rest is by total parenteral nutrition (TPN). We have studied 17 consecutive patients with Crohn's colitis referred to us for surgery, who were treated with bowel rest and intensive medical therapy. Only one of the 17 required colectomy. The previous literature on TPN and Crohn's colitis shows a 76 percent response rate in 36 patients treated with TPN. It is also likely that complete bowel rest is not absolutely essential, since there are reports that elemental diets and defined liquid diets, such as Ensure and Sustacal, may also be helpful. Levi and colleagues, studying patients with colonic disease, reported that the 32 percent prolonged response rate with elemental diet therapy was not as favorable as the 72 percent response rate in patients with ileitis. The patients with Crohn's colitis also seemed to relapse rather quickly despite medical therapy. Again, it was clear that there is a need for effective anti-inflammatory medical therapy to sustain the remission obtained with any type of bowel rest.

10. Azathioprine or 6-mercaptopurine (6-MP) administration are associated with improvement in over 65 percent of patients with nonobstructed, nonperforated Crohn's colitis who either have been resistant to medical therapy or have been dependent on daily steroid therapy to maintain control of their disease.
11. There may be an as yet unobserved enhanced risk of nonintestinal malignant neoplasms in Crohn's disease. However, the added risk from the relatively low doses of azathioprine or 6-MP currently in vogue (maximum, 1.5 mg per kilogram) must be small and has not yet become obvious.
12. There is an increased risk of colon cancer in patients with Crohn's colitis, even in bypassed rectal stumps. Most patients with Crohn's disease and colon cancer have dysplasia at some site in the colon, which may be detectable by some type of surveillance program. Other patients develop squamous carcinoma in long-standing fistulae.

GOALS OF THERAPY

In selecting therapeutic options, it is important to determine the stage of the illness, whether it be (1) active inflammation with diarrhea, cramps, hypoalbuminemia, subtle bleeding and anemia; (2) deep ulceration with massive hemorrhage secondary to erosion into a sizable vessel; (3) fissure, fistula, or perforation with or without abscess formation; or (4) fixed obstruction due to scarring of the colon (not common).

The principles of management of active disease are the same as for small bowel disease, except that the outcome from medical therapy is often unpredictable. Some patients with rather extensive disease respond quickly, while others continue to be symptomatic despite multiple therapies.

Our goal, based on the assumptions listed above, is to suppress disease activity for as long as possible while still trying to avoid steroid side effects and other drug-related adverse effects. Other physicians, basing their decisions only on control trial results, may be less aggressive in treating this disease once a remission has been achieved. As stated, we are impressed by the concepts that fistulizing or perforating complications usually occur in the first 5 to 6 years of known disease activity. In an effort to suppress disease activity throughout this period, multi-drug therapy and one or more periods of bowel rest may be needed. Since we began to use azathioprine for unremitting or steroid-dependent disease, colon resection has seldom been needed. We currently refer patients for surgery mainly for complications such as persistent hemorrhage, perforation, fistulization into important organs or sites, symptomatic obstruction (unusual in the colon, in contrast to small bowel Crohn's disease), severe and progressive perianal disease, dysplasia, or carcinoma.

ACTIVE DISEASE

Sulfasalazine

Sulfasalazine has been shown in controlled trials to be effective for mild to moderate Crohn's disease of the colon. The usual dosage is 3 to 4 g per day in divided doses; some clinicians use even higher doses. Larger doses of 5-aminosalicylic acid (5-ASA) compounds, equivalent to 12 g of sulfasalazine, can be delivered by the new oral 5-ASA compounds. Thus, theoretically, some patients with only moderate Crohn's colitis who do not respond to 3 g of sulfasalazine may respond to large amounts of oral 5-ASA, such as 4.8 g of mesalamine (Asacol), which is equivalent to 12 g of sulfasalazine. In addition, the availability of oral 5-ASA compounds will make it possible to treat most patients who are intolerant of the sulfapyridine component of sulfasalazine. Individuals whose diarrhea gets worse on sulfasalazine or who are allergic to aspirin may also be sensitive to the 5-ASA products.

Once a remission is obtained, 2 or 3 g per day of sulfasalazine or 1.2 to 2.4 g of oral 5-ASA is continued indefinitely. As stated, there are no controlled trial data to support this approach, but experienced students of this disease believe that long-term suppression is possible, as in ulcerative colitis.

Adrenocortical Steroids

For more active disease, often with systemic symptoms, prednisone given initially as 30 to 60 mg per day has been shown by both clinical trial (National Cooperative Crohn's Disease Study [NCCDS]) and experience to be an effective method of suppressing mild, moderate, and even severe disease activity. The lower dose range is used for mild to moderate relapses; the larger doses are employed for highly active disease in an adult. Dosages of less than 20 mg per day of prednisone are generally ineffective in ameliorating active, previously untreated disease in adults. Severely ill patients may require hospitalization, bowel rest, and parenteral adrenocortical steroids.

Combination Therapy

We almost always link prednisone therapy with an antibiotic such as metronidazole or the combination drug sulfasalazine. Before metronidazole was known to suppress bowel inflammation as well as provide antianaerobic effects, we used tetracycline. We thought we might be lessening some of the effects of secondary bacterial invasion of inflamed and deeply ulcerated tissues. These multiple therapies were also employed in an effort to lessen the amount of prednisone needed to continuously suppress clinical manifestations of disease activity. However, most controlled trials have not shown combination therapy to be more effective then prednisone. Our own experience suggests that using multiple agents is helpful. Work by Stenson and others has demonstrated that sulfasalazine and 5-ASA affect several different steps in the arachidonic acid–inflammatory mediator cascade that are beyond the site of action of prednisone. In addition, sulfasalazine and 5-ASA are capable of binding oxygen-free radicals, perhaps another phase in their therapeutic action.

There are very few guidelines as to the optimal duration of steroid therapy, especially in the form of alternate-day medications. We are concerned about osteoporosis as well as ischemic necrosis. We discuss the seriousness of these complications with patients before, and again regularly during, prolonged therapy.

Metronidazole

Metronidazole, 250 mg four times a day, has been shown in controlled studies to diminish bowel symptoms and to be helpful for perianal disease and fistulae. Nausea, a metallic taste, or "hairy tongue" has somewhat limited the use of metronidazole, but most patients can tolerate 250 mg at least three times a day. They are warned about alcohol intolerance, seizure induction, and peripheral neuropathy. We rarely encounter neuropathy if the total dosage is kept at 1,000 mg per day or less. At higher dosages, almost all our patients develop peripheral neuropathy after 6 to 8 weeks. The neuropathy is usually, but not always, reversible if the dosage is lowered or the medication discontinued. Patients are informed that the peripheral neuropathy, although usually not incapacitating, may resolve very slowly or perhaps not completely. They are also told about serious concerns regarding mutagenicity in bacterial systems and carcinogenesis in animals. Women are urged not to become pregnant while taking metronidazole. The unknown potential of malignant transformation in humans after prolonged usage is also stressed. As for prednisone, azathioprine, and 6-MP, the pros and cons of long-term metronidazole use are clearly delineated initially and at least every 6 months to the patient, and if possible to the family. Postantibiotic diarrhea, including *Clostridium difficile* toxin–induced colitis, can be an aggravating factor in some relapses of Crohn's colitis. Since metronidazole has occasionally been associated with pseudomembranous colitis, one or two stool assays for *Clostridium difficle* toxin are indicated at the time of flare-up in a patient who has been or is on antibiotics.

Broad-Spectrum Antibiotics

Broad-spectrum antibiotics, including tetracycline, ampicillin, or sulfamethoxazole-trimethoprim (Bactrim), have been used continuously or intermittently, usually as an additive to prednisone in some patients with persistent or unresponsive but moderate Crohn's colitis. Presumably, these drugs are decreasing the usual bacterial flora, which is acting as a secondary factor and helping perpetuate the chronic inflammation. In an attempt to maintain effectiveness for prolonged periods, some investigators recommend alternating antibiotics every 4 to 6 weeks.

Topical Anti-Inflammatory Therapy

Topical steroid enemas, such as Cortenema, and topical 5-ASA enemas, such as Rowasa, can be used if there are prominent rectal symptoms, such as urgency and tenesmus. Since these products have been shown to reach well up into the left colon, they can sometimes be useful even when there is more extensive disease that is also being treated with oral medications.

Bowel Rest

Patients with moderate or severe disease including cramps and diarrhea often feel better on some form of bowel rest, as an adjunct to medical therapy. Switching to liquid formula diets such a Ensure or Sustacal as the main source of nutrition may be helpful. If the patient is moderately or severely ill or if there is painful perianal disease, an elemental diet may help for the several weeks until azathioprine or 6-MP begin to take effect.

If patients on an elemental diet can get past the first 3 days, perhaps in the hospital with a nasogastric feeding tube, they can usually tolerate 4 weeks of elemental diet, such as Vivonex or Vital, as the main source of nutrition. Some patients can also tolerate an additional 16 to 32 oz of clear liquid per day. Unfortunately, the results in colonic Crohn's disease do not seem to be as predictable as in uncomplicated small bowel disease. In this latter group a 60 to 70 percent response rate can be expected. It is now clear that prolonged medical therapy is usually needed to sustain these remissions. However, the British literature suggests that a carefully constructed, severely restricted diet may keep some fraction of these patients in remission. Further investigation of the role of restricted diets for long-term maintenance of remissions is needed. We have not had experience with this approach.

Total parenteral nutrition, perhaps with small amounts of clear liquids, appears the most reliable method of achieving a remission in severe but uncomplicated Crohn's colitis. As stated earlier, 16 of 17 patients with recent-onset (2.9 years) refractory but uncomplicated colitis referred to Johns Hopkins for surgery went into remission on intensive medical therapy combined with prolonged parenteral nutrition, including several weeks of home TPN. Only one of 17 required a colectomy. Sepsis, or thrombosis necessitating removal of the indwelling catheter, did not occur in any of these patients but has been a problem in others on long-term TPN. The average duration of TPN was 6 weeks. In six patients this rest period was used to start azathioprine. Subsequently, all 16 responders were left on some form of medical therapy to maintain the remission.

Immunomodulators

In the United States, the use of the immunomodulators azathioprine and 6-MP has been championed by a few groups, but there is still a general reluctance to use these medications. This attitude persists even though at least five controlled trials show that azathioprine or 6-MP help patients with chronic uncomplicated Crohn's colitis refractory to other therapy, usually including steroids. It is now clear that the NCCDS tested a heterogenous group of patients, including some with very acute disease and others with complications such as obstruction. For this and other reasons, such as the limited duration of the study, the NCCDS could not confirm the usefulness of azathioprine. Several factors, including lack of confirmation of effectiveness; the early toxicity, including pancreatitis and bone marrow suppression; and the concern about the long-term cancer risk have kept many gastroenterologists from using immunosuppressives.

We have given azathioprine or 6-MP (1 to 1.5 mg per kilogram) to 13 percent of 500 patients with inflammatory bowel disease (IBD) seen over the last 10 years. Interestingly, Present and colleagues used 6-MP in 14 percent of their 700 patients. All our patients were on other anti-inflammatory agents at the onset of immunomodulator therapy. Several studies confirm that a 70 percent response rate can be expected in patients with chronic Crohn's disease who either have been refractory to prednisone therapy or cannot be kept in remission without daily prednisone usage. As a group, patients with Crohn's colitis respond somewhat less often than those with ileocolitis. All nine of our 70 patients who worsened on azathioprine had some colonic involvement. Steroid sparing was achieved in over two-thirds of patients with an average decrease in prednisone dosage of 15 mg per day. Perianal disease and single perianal fistula improved in 80 percent of those for whom this was the indication for azathioprine or 6-MP.

The dosage schedule we employed was usually 50 mg once a day for 2 to 3 weeks. If no side effects occurred, the dosage was increased to 1 or 1.5 mg per kilogram, usually a total of 75 or 100 mg. In some unresponsive patients the dosage was later raised to 125 mg. We have monitored blood counts, differentials, liver function tests, and amylase levels at 2, 4, and 6 weeks and then every 4 to 6 weeks.

Short-term toxicity necessitating discontinuation of azathioprine or 6-MP occurred in 10 percent of our patients. The same percentage was reported in other series. Only one patient in our series had pancreatitis. Other series reported five or six patients with pancreatitis in the first 4 weeks of therapy. As mentioned, most of our patients were also on prednisone. Whether concomitantly administered prednisone protects some patients from pancreatitis and other side effects while starting azathioprine is not known. The dosage of azathioprine or 6-MP had to be lowered temporarily because of possible side effects in another 10 percent of our patients. Only one patient had transient leukopenia; she and the others were able to resume their previous dosage.

Concern over lymphoma and other malignancies arises because of the experience with renal transplant patients on azathioprine. Fortunately, to date there is no evidence of an increased occurrence of lymphoma in patients with Crohn's disease on long-term immunosuppressive medications. However, the longest duration of therapy in most studies is less than 10 years. If there *is* an increased risk in patients with Crohn's disease receiving azathioprine or 6-MP at the dosage of 1 to 1.5 mg per kilogram, the risk seems to be relatively low. Since most patients on immunosuppressive medications, even at this lowered dosage, require long-term therapy, a detailed discussion of the benefits and drawbacks of such therapy should precede the onset of treatment. Some physicians obtain informed consent before the use of azathioprine or 6-MP. We explain the potential side effects very clearly and provide printed material from The National Foundation for Ileitis and Colitis (NFIC).

Beneficial effects are not usually noted before 6 to 8 weeks. Our series and those of others report an average of 3 months before a therapeutic response is established. However, by 4 months at least 80 percent of our patients who were going to respond had done so. Some individuals demonstrated progressive improvement over a 12- to 18-month period. We have not usually raised the dose beyond 125 mg per day (1.5 mg per kilogram per day), although there are reports of larger doses leading to a response in some patients. Obviously this is at the potential price of some degree of bone marrow suppression.

Most patients (perhaps 75 percent) who require azathioprine or 6-MP to achieve a remission or as a means of lowering the prednisone dosage experience a return of signs or symptoms at variable intervals when the immunomodulator is discontinued. We therefore lower the dosage very gradually over many months or even years. In a few patients with Crohn's colitis it was finally possible to withdraw the dosage completely after several attempts. The data from Lennard-Jones and colleagues suggested that this might be possible after 5 to 7 years of Crohn's colitis, but those authors did not study this issue directly.

Cyclosporine

Cyclosporine, a powerful suppressor of cell-mediated immunity, has been associated with a few dramatic responses in a small number of highly selected patients with IBD. In one trial of patients refractory to other therapies, improvement was noted in 10 of 15; the beneficial effect was sustained in seven. There are other open trials that also show a rapid clinical response in severely ill patients. A placebo-controlled trial is under way that may provide information to help balance any beneficial effects against the potential renal and hepatic toxicity. It is possible that new agents along the same line may be developed that have less toxicity. Theoretically, cyclosporine may be a useful drug for acute treatment of patients with severe and aggressive Crohn's colitis who are not responding to bowel rest and adrenocortical steroids. It may prove possible to use this relatively fast-acting drug in these highly selected patients and then later reduce it as azathioprine or 6-MP is added. Again, this is still theoretical and as yet untested. There was preliminary report at the 1989 American Gastroenterology Association (AGA) meeting of the use of cyclosporin enemas for refractory proctosigmoiditis.

Methotrexate

A recent open trial of methotrexate, 25 mg intramuscularly once a week for 12 weeks included 14 patients with Crohn's disease. Five had chronic rectal fistulae, and six had Crohn's disease in the colon. Five patients, all with colonic disease alone, went into endoscopic remission, and four went into histologic remission. If improvement was evident by 12 weeks, as it was in five of eight Crohn's colitis patients, the 25-mg dose was followed by a tapering oral dose down to a minimum of 7.5 mg per week. Four of the five patients were left on oral methotrexate for a total follow-up period of 22 to 40 weeks (an average of 31 weeks). The average prednisone dosage in the four responders who were on steroids fell from 16.5 mg per day to 3.1 mg per day. Two of the three patients with both small bowel and colonic disease also responded.

Some patients improved dramatically in 2 weeks, while most of the responders improved markedly after 8 to 10 weeks. Side effects of methotrexate in the 21 patients included transient postinjection nausea and diarrhea in two; a 1.5-fold increase in amino-aspartate transferase (AST) in two; and leukopenia and brittle nails in one. The long-term concern will be the development of hepatotoxicity with fibrosis and cirrhosis. Reportedly, this problem is expected to be less common with weekly dosing. Accumulated doses of methotrate in excess of 3 g may also be toxic. Kozarek and colleagues recommended follow-up liver function tests and possibly serial liver biopsies.

Further studies are needed to confirm effectiveness and then to define the ideal patient and chronic dosage regimen. Ten of the total 21 patients with IBD had failed previous therapy with azathioprine. Since, in our 70-patient series, all nine of the patients whose condition worsened on azathioprine or 6-MP had some colonic involvement, methotrexate theoretically might be the next agent to consider for such individuals.

T-Lymphocyte Apheresis

T-lymphocyte apheresis following a TPN-induced remission has been utilized by Bicks and colleagues to treat 21 patients with chronic and severe Crohn's disease. All patients were considered treatment failures from conventional forms of therapy. These authors performed eight to 26 three- hour apheresis procedures removing 80 to 100 billion cells. All 21 patients had a sustained remission for 10 to 36 months. It was noted that T-lymphocyte apheresis following TPN did not heal internal or perianal fistulae, abscesses, or obstruction. Later, 52 patients were reviewed. There were no deaths and no indication of immunosuppression This interesting approach to achieve prolonged remissions is clearly worthy of further study for specially selected patients unable to respond to azathioprine, 6-MP, and perhaps methotrexate. The report of James of chronic Crohn's disease activity decreasing as a patient developed AIDS also focused attention on the important role of helper T cells in active Crohn's disease.

PERIANAL DISEASE

Perineal fistulae and abscesses may occur with gross colonic involvement or with only small bowel disease. Rarely, perianal disease may be the only manifestation of what seems to be Crohn's disease. This latter situation usually presents as a prolonged diagnostic dilemma.

Local Care

If the active disease process is confined primarily to the perianal area, the goal of management is often palliation of symptoms and prevention of progression. Local care, including sitz baths and control of diarrhea, is an important aspect of reducing drainage, inflammation, and discomfort. Intractable pain is usually due to a perianal abscess that may drain spontaneously or require surgical drainage. Surgical drainage of abscesses is usually done in a conservative fashion. Some surgeons use curettage; others use setons plus occasional curettage. Others, and presumably the minority, lay fistula tracks open but only when Crohn's disease activity is well controlled. Preservation of anal sphincter musculature should be one of the prime concerns of the surgeon treating intersphincteric fistulae. In general, local surgery is used for relief of pain.

Medical Therapy

Diarrhea control usually requires adequate suppression of disease activity, as outlined earlier. If there is extensive bowel disease, steroids and antibiotics, including metronidazole, azathioprine, or 6-MP, are often helpful. If the perianal area is painful, bowel rest with elemental diets, formula diets such as Ensure or Sustacal, or TPN can be very helpful. This initial medical treatment period may also allow azathioprine or 6-MP to become active. Without additional medical therapy, most of the improvement observed with bowel rest will be quickly dissipated with refeedings. Prednisone alone adds little to the treatment of perianal disease except to control active small bowel or colonic disease. Although metronidazole seems to help control perianal disease for long periods in some patients, prolonged administration in patients already on azathioprine does not seem to be helpful.

Bowel Diversion

Diversion of the fecal stream by colostomy or perhaps ileostomy, often with resection of the most obviously diseased bowel, can help perianal disease. If the rectum is severely inflamed and the perineal disease is complex and progressive, a temporary colostomy may not be sufficient and total proctectomy may be necessary. We have been able to reanastomose a few selected patients with a long segment of very quiescent or uninvolved rectosigmoid who also demonstrated narrowing or closure of the fistulae as determined by colonoscopy, rectal biopsies, and computed tomography (CT). We have generally waited 1 or 2 years, usually in association with azathioprine therapy, before attempting a reanastomosis. Our data are too meager to provide information on how often reanastomosis is successful.

COLON RESECTION

Results

The recurrence rate after total colectomy and ileostomy is relatively low, especially if the ileum was normal radiographically before surgery. The literature suggests that 80 or 85 percent of such patients remain free of gross disease in the ileum for many years. Even in patients with ileal disease at the time of colectomy, the recurrence rate is lower than with ileocolonic resection.

Sequential resections are most successful when anastomoses are made in areas that are grossly normal. At Johns Hopkins our surgical service has found that an ileosigmoid resection in a patient with a normal or easily distensible rectosigmoid can usually be well tolerated for years. In contrast, connecting the ileum to a diseased and contracted rectum is usually doomed to failure. Most of these patients have needed an ileostomy, often with removal of the rectum.

As regards the number of bowel movements to be expected after ileorectal anastomoses, it is estimated that this will be double the number of times that patients need to empty their ileostomy appliance.

Indications

Colectomy has previously been recommended for patients with intractable disease that is unresponsive to maximal medical treatment. However, since we have become comfortable with azathioprine therapy as well as the use of prolonged periods of bowel rest, we rarely have to resort to colon resection or colectomy for refractory uncomplicated disease.

Complications, including fulminant colitis, hemorrhage, perforation abscesses, obstruction, and cancer, are still valid indications for partial or complete removal of the colon.

Dysplasia that is found repeatedly in one area, in several areas of the colon, or on an obvious mass or obstruction is usually considered an indication for total colectomy. As with ulcerative colitis, our pathologists, despite years of experience with dysplasia identification, still exchange "problem" slides with other pathologists to confirm the presence of dysplasia before recommending colectomy. Adenomatous polyps (which are a form of dysplasia) are usually regarded as another site of dysplasia when considering colectomy, but this remains controversial if there is no dysplasia on the stalk or base of the polyp and no dysplasia elsewhere in the colon.

SURVEILLANCE FOR DYSPLASIA

The patient with Crohn's disease of the colon is at a four- to 20-fold increased risk of developing colon cancer. These cancers develop in grossly involved areas in two-thirds of instances, but one-third of the malignancies appear in apparently uninvolved segments. The average patient with colon cancer has had Crohn's disease of the colon for 20 years. These patients are on the average, 10 years younger than the typical patient with "standard" colon cancer.

Hamilton found that all ten patients with colon cancer and Crohn's disease whom he reviewed had dysplasia at some site or sites in the colon. However, there were several hindrances to a potential surveillance program. Two patients were found to have cancer before the diagnosis of Crohn's disease was made. Another had had symptoms related to Crohn's disease for only 4 years. Two patients had retained but strictured rectal stumps that could not be examined. Two others had squamous carcinomas in long-standing fistulae. Thus, it would have been difficult to describe a cost-effective surveillance program for these ten patients.

As a compromise, we perform colonoscopy with multiple biopsies from eight areas of the colon (if possible) in patients who have had Crohn's disease of the colon for over 12 to 15 years. We have no recommendations on how often to repeat the studies if these have been negative for 1 or 2 consecutive years. In practice, we may skip a year or two if the pathologists find no evidence of possible dysplasia.

We try to avoid leaving rectal stumps after colon resection. However, some young men, especially physicians, wish to defer proctectomy to avoid any risk of impotence. If the rectum becomes so scarred that surveillance is not possible, serious consideration should be given to its removal.

SUPPORT SYSTEMS

The National Foundation for Ileitis and Colitis (NFIC) has been both a national source of literature, books, and other information and a local source of support groups and patient education. In addition to providing priceless information to patients and to their doctors, the NFIC raises over $1.5 million per year for basic research in Crohn's disease and ulcerative colitis. Their national offices are at 444, Park Avenue South, New York, NY 10016 (telephone 1-800-343-3637); local chapters are active in over 70 cities.

OUTLOOK FOR PATIENTS WITH CROHN'S DISEASE

We believe guarded optimism is justified in managing patients with Crohn's colitis. Medical therapy is clearly a long-term commitment that challenges both physician and patient. The current era of therapy has been aided by the recognition of the role of bowel rest and better understanding of the role of steroids, metronidazole, sulfasalazine, oral 5-ASA products, and azathioprine and 6-MP. Medical-nutritional therapy is often able to achieve a prolonged and seemingly permanent remission. Methotrexate or cyclosporine may prove helpful in patients with disease resistant to other therapy. The role of surgery has also been better defined. Colonoscopy and surveillance for dysplasia may help identify some individuals at greater risk for colon cancer development. Thus, the outlook for the average patient with Crohn's disease of the colon is better today then ever before.

SUGGESTED READING

Bicks RO, Groshart KW. A progress report—five years of treating Crohn's disease with T-lymphocyte apheresis (TLA). Gastroenterology 1989; 96:A43.

Brandt LJ, Bernstein LH, Boley SJ, Frank MS. Metronidazole therapy for perineal Crohn's disease: a follow-up study. Gastroenterology 1982; 83:383–387.

Elliott PR, Ritchie JK, Lennard-Jones JE. Progress of colonic Crohn's disease. Br Med J 1985; 291:178.

Hamilton SR. Colorectal carcinoma in patients with Crohn's disease. Gastroenterology 1985; 89:398–407.

James SP. Remission of Crohn's disease after human immunodeficiency virus infection. Gastroenterology 1988; 95:1667–1669.

Kozarek RA, Patterson DJ, Gelfand MO, et al. Methotrexate induces clinical and histologic remissions in refractory inflammatory bowel disease. Ann Intern Med 1989; 110:353–356.

Present DH, Korelitz BI, Wisch N, et al. Treatment of Crohn's disease with 6-mercaptopurine. A longterm, randomized double blind study. N Engl J Med 1980; 302:981–987.

Teahon K, Levi J. Dietary management. In: Bayless TM, ed. Current management of inflammatory bowel disease. Toronto: BC Decker, 223–230, 1989.

Ursing B, Alm T, Barany F, et al. A comparative study of metronidazole and sulfasalazine for active Crohn's disease: the cooperative Crohn's disease study in Sweden. Gastroenterology 1982; 83:550–562.

LOWER GASTROINTESTINAL BLEEDING

VALERIE J. JAGIELLA, M.D.
FRANCIS J. TEDESCO, M.D., F.A.C.P., F.A.C.G.

Bleeding from the lower gastrointestinal (GI) tract, or more specifically, the lower intestinal tract, may be defined as that which occurs distal to the ligament of Treitz. It can range from occult to massive hemorrhage. Even occult blood loss can be life-threatening unless dealt with in an efficient and timely manner with accurate detection and treatment of the bleeding sites(s). Although endoscopy plays a major role in diagnosis and therapy, lower GI bleeding remains a complex issue, often requiring a multidisciplinary team approach (Fig. 1). Because management depends on the acuteness and severity of blood loss, bleeding should be classified as acute when there is massive hemorrhage and as chronic when there are Hemoccult-positive stools or passage of small amounts of bright red blood through the rectum. Melena generally indicates an upper GI lesion, whereas hematochezia suggests a rectal or lower intestinal source. However, acute massive bleeding with passage of large amounts of bright red blood or maroon stools with clots can reflect either lower or upper GI lesions. With upper GI lesions, bleeding is more likely to be accompanied by significant orthostatic changes, cardiovascular compromise, or even shock.

ACUTE LOWER GASTROINTESTINAL BLEEDING

Clinical Evaluation

Major acute hemorrhage is a medical emergency requiring resuscitative measures. At presentation, the patient should be rapidly assessed and stabilized. Vital signs should be observed with the patient in the supine and upright positions. If significantly hypotensive when supine, the patient is considered unstable with large volume depletion. In the upright position, a 10 to 20 mm Hg decrease in systolic blood pressure or an increase in resting heart rate of 20 beats per minute reflects approximately 1 L of blood loss. Factitious changes from autonomic nervous system blockade by medications should be ruled out. Hypovolemia must be corrected rapidly with intravenous fluid and/or transfusions, and a coagulation profile must be checked and managed accordingly.

Clinical manifestations will depend on the myriad of causes that can present with lower intestinal bleeding (Table 1). The initial evaluation should include a careful history and physical examination. Because an upper GI tract lesion may be the culprit in massive rectal bleeding, the history is of prime importance. The patient should be questioned as to the nature, rapidity, and duration of bleeding, abdominal pain, weight loss, and change in bowel habits. A past history of similar bleeding, diverticulosis, peptic ulcer disease, alcoholism, cirrhosis, inflammatory bowel disease, or radiation therapy should also be considered when deciding on a treatment method.

The physical examination can provide valuable information. Cutaneous changes may point to a specific disorder (Table 2). Abdominal examination may demonstrate hepatosplenomegaly, ascites, a mass, or lymphadenopa-

TABLE 1 Causes of Lower Gastrointestinal Bleeding

- Nonvascular causes
  - Diverticulosis
  - Neoplasms
    - Adenomas
    - Carcinoma
    - Kaposi's sarcoma
  - Inflammatory bowel disease
  - Ischemic colitis, radiation colitis
  - Meckel's diverticulum (in infants and older children)
  - Uncommon
    - Infectious colitis
    - Drug-induced cecal ulceration
    - Small intestinal lesions
      - Leiomyomas
      - Carcinoids
  - Postpolypectomy
- Vascular Causes
  - Angiodysplasia of the colon or small intestine
  - Uncommon
    - Colonic varices
    - Hereditary hemorrhagic telangiectasias
    - Cavernous hemangiomas
    - Vasculitis of the colon

thy. Inspection of the perianal region and digital rectal examination may uncover possible masses, fistulas, strictures, hemorrhoids, or blood.

Diagnostic Methods

While the patient is being stabilized, an upper GI source of bleeding must be excluded. Nasogastric aspiration for blood is a simple preliminary screening test for patients with hematochezia and hypotension requiring transfusion. Rarely (in less than 10 percent of cases) do patients with a negative gastric aspirate have an upper gastrointestinal source of bleeding, but when this does occur, the site is most commonly duodenal. In clinical settings suggestive of ulcer disease, even if the aspirate is negative, esophagogastroduodenoscopy should be performed before evaluation of the lower intestinal tract.

TABLE 2 Mucocutaneous Lesions Associated With Gastrointestinal Bleeding

Lesion	*Disease/Disorder*
Spider angiomas	Cirrhosis
Purpura	Thrombocytopenia
	Henoch-Schönlein purpura
Telangiectasias	Osler-Weber-Rendu
Mucocutaneous pigmentation	Peutz-Jeghers syndrome
	Cronkhite-Canada syndrome
Dark blue papules, macules	Kaposi's sarcoma
Pink papules → scars	Degos' disease
Acanthosis nigricans	Malignancy, especially gastric
Fragile skin, bruising	Ehlers-Danlos syndrome
Epidermal inclusion cysts	Gardner's syndrome
Pyoderma gangrenosum	Inflammatory bowel disease
Erythema nodosum	

Bright red blood is most commonly associated with lesions distal to the splenic flexure, whereas patients with right-sided lesions generally present with chronic blood loss and Hemoccult-positive stools or, less frequently, melena. Approximately two-thirds of colonic lesions are within reach of a 60-cm flexible sigmoidoscope. Hence, proctosigmoidoscopy should be the first procedure performed for patients with significant lower GI hemorrhage. Using a flexible instrument, preferably with a large suction channel, proctosigmoidoscopy can be done at the bedside in the intensive care unit. We generally use a colonoscope, which enables us to advance beyond 60 cm if visualization is adequate. Bowel preparation is not necessary, but tap water enemas can be helpful in removing the large clots, thereby allowing better visualization of the bowel lumen. This procedure creates little discomfort or risk to the patient and may pinpoint the site of bleeding, or at least provide important clues to its etiology. Such indicators include characteristics of inflammatory, infectious, or ischemic colitis. If a rectosigmoid lesion is identified, a second, more proximal one may be bleeding simultaneously. For example, a distal polyp does not exclude right-sided angiodysplasia or cancer. There have also been rare instances of bleeding from two different diverticula. If active bleeding is noted from the rectum and no blood is detected proximally, the site of hemorrhage is most likely in the rectum. Careful evaluation of this area cannot be overemphasized. Severe hemorrhage can occur with hemorrhoidal bleeding in cirrhotic patients who have portal hypertension, whereas small rectal ulcers with arterial bleeding can sometimes lead to cardiovascular compromise in patients with inflammatory bowel disease or fecal impactions. In those cases in which no source can be identified and blood is noted more proximally beyond the reach of the instrument, the work-up must be pursued further.

Arteriography

At this point, the approach one should take in treating the patient with acute lower GI bleeding will depend on the rate of blood loss. If the patient is bleeding, actively and significantly, immediate investigation is warranted. Colonoscopy is often technically difficult and offers only a limited view of the lumen because of the blood and clots. Selective mesenteric arteriography becomes the procedure of choice, especially for patients in whom an upper GI lesion has been ruled out and who continue to bleed at a rate of at least 0.5 to 1.0 ml per minute. In 40 to 80 percent of patients, the site and type of lesion can be demonstrated.

Vasopressin Infusion

Intra-arterial infusion of vasopressin (up to 0.4 unit per minute) can be administered if extravasation is observed. This will stop the bleeding at least temporarily in 80 to 90 percent of patients and allow better preparation for colonoscopy or surgery. Vasopressin should be continued for 24 hours, and then slowly tapered. During this period, the bowel can be prepped with polyethylene glycol electrolyte solution (Colyte or GoLYTELY) administered orally or by nasogastric tube. Unfortunately, as soon as the infusion is discontinued, bleeding recurs in approximately half of the patients. For those lesions not amenable to endoscopic treatment, or if bleeding does not abate, surgical intervention is indicated. Transcatheter embolization of bleeding arteries widely used in the upper GI tract has been successful in a small number of patients with lower GI bleeding. However, because of the complications with colonic infarction and delayed strictures that have been observed after this form of therapy, its place in routine management of lower intestinal bleeding remains unclear.

Arteriography can also successfully identify a lesion with bleeding potential in 20 to 40 percent of those patients who are not actively bleeding at the time of the procedure. When extravasation is not present, particularly when the bleeding is intermittent (e.g., in bleeding from vascular ectasias and diverticula), other signs highly suggestive of a source of hemorrhage may point to the diagnosis and therapeutic approach. These signs include a densely opacified, slowly emptying vein, a vascular tuft, or an early filling vein. Nevertheless, certain technical aspects, such as the availability of a radiologic team on short notice and the need to transport the patient to the procedure room, limit the use of arteriography. Other factors to be considered include the risks involved in using contrast material in patients with hypovolemia, underlying renal disease, or known allergy to the contrast, and the possibility of arterial trauma and bleeding in those patients with coagulopathies.

Colonoscopy

In situations where arteriography is not feasible or in patients who are not bleeding heavily, colonoscopy should be attempted before radionuclide scanning. The blood has usually acted as a cathartic, and with some enemas and/or oral electrolyte preparation, visualization of the bowel lumen may be sufficient to localize and eventually treat the bleeding site. Although colonoscopy during active major hemorrhage is technically difficult to perform, it may provide valuable information and may benefit those patients with lesions amenable to endoscopic treatment with injection sclerotherapy, electrocautery, or photocoagulation.

Radionuclide Scanning

Radionuclide scanning can be useful in patients with less significant, active bleeding that does not require urgent therapeutic measures. Scintigraphy, although less precise, may detect and localize the source of bleeding. The major disadvantage of scintigraphy is that it cannot reveal the type of lesion. Moreover, the patient must be actively bleeding (at a rate of at least 0.05 to 0.1 ml per minute) for the few minutes during which the radiopharmaceutical is in the blood stream. Although most positive scans will occur within the first 90 minutes, the study may take longer to complete, and false localization can occur when an insufficient number of delayed views are taken. The certainty of diagnosis increases as the interval between negative and positive scans decreases.

CHRONIC OR INTERMITTENT GASTROINTESTINAL BLEEDING

Diagnostic Evaluation

The urgency and extent of the diagnostic work-up will depend on the patient's clinical condition. Assessment of stabilized patients who are not actively bleeding or who have chronic occult blood loss should begin with colonoscopy after oral preparation and, if necessary, enemas. If a bleeding source is detected, treatment will depend on the type of lesion identified. Endoscopy will occasionally reveal a sentinel clot or active bleeding from a diverticulum or specific area of the colon known to have diverticula. The presence of bright red blood can be from back-wash and does not necessarily mean the origin of bleeding is in that area.

Diverticular Bleeding

Treatment of diverticular bleeding consists of supportive care and transfusions as needed. Intravenous vasopressin has not been shown to be effective in stopping this type of hemorrhage, and because of the risks of myocardial and mesenteric ischemia, intravenous infusion of vasopressin should not be used. However, if profuse bleeding persists or recurs, arteriography and selective intra-arterial administration of vasopressin should be attempted before surgical intervention is carried out.

Colonic Angiodysplasia

Electrocautery or photocoagulation can be used to ablate angiodyplasia that has caused significant bleeding. Unlike other vascular lesions, angiodysplasia of the colon is not associated with vascular abnormalities in other parts of the body. These vascular ectasias are acquired, of unknown etiology, and occur primarily in the elderly. Generally they are numerous and small (1 to 10 mm in size), and are situated in the cecum and ascending colon. The bleeding is painless, intermittent, and can range from minimal to massive. The patients are otherwise asymptomatic. A presumptive diagnosis of bleeding from colonic angiodysplasia cannot be made unless additional lesions have been excluded. An estimated 25 percent of these patients have other potential sites of bleeding. Therefore, before endoscopic ablation of the vascular ectasias, complete colonoscopy should be performed. Hemostatic methods include monopolar electrocoagulation (by applying the "hot biopsy forcep"), bipolar electrocoagulation (BICAP), thermal cautery with the heater probe, and laser photocoagulation. Injection sclerotherapy requires special sclerosing catheters that are long enough to pass through the colonoscope. The technique is not without risk of delayed perforation from the formation of an ulcer at the site of injection therapy. Few attempts have been made to use this method for angiodysplasia. However, it is useful in halting delayed hemorrhage from postpolypectomy sites, which generally occurs within the first 24 hours but has been reported up to 21 days after the procedure.

In general, we use either electrocoagulation or thermal cautery for angiodysplasia. The probe is first applied circumferentially on the periphery of the vascular ectasia to fulgurate the "feeders," and is then applied to the center of the lesion. Precise guidelines for safe and effective energy limits are difficult to define. Coagulation should be sufficient to reach the submucosa without creating a full-thickness burn. The main risks include delayed hemorrhage and perforation. Acute perforation can be prevented by decompressing the thin-walled cecum and ascending colon before using a Teflon-coated contact probe, and by avoiding excessive power intensity with the laser. Generally, it is better to undertreat initially and follow up with a repeat colonoscopy a few months later. Surgical resection is usually reserved for patients with large, diffuse angiodysplastic lesions whose hemoglobin cannot be maintained with iron therapy or who have had life-threatening hemorrhage.

Other Studies

If the colonoscopist cannot locate the source of bleeding, esophagogastroduodenoscopy (EGD) should be performed to exclude an upper GI lesion. If this too does not reveal a bleeding site, a barium contrast study of the small bowel may reveal a lesion beyond the reach of the endoscope. In certain instances, a sterilized colonoscope has been used to evaluate the duodenum and proximal jejunum. This has occasionally revealed a potential bleeding site. Small bowel enteroscopy, an investigational tool available in certain centers, allows visualization of the small intestinal mucosa, and may in the future become a standard procedure in cases of obscure bleeding.

If these procedures do not demonstate the source of bleeding, the next steps to be taken should be radionuclide scanning, celiac arteriography, and if necessary, further barium contrast studies. During the acute phase of bleeding, the barium studies have limited indications in that they cannot demonstrate actual bleeding, they have no therapeutic applications, and they make subsequent arteriography

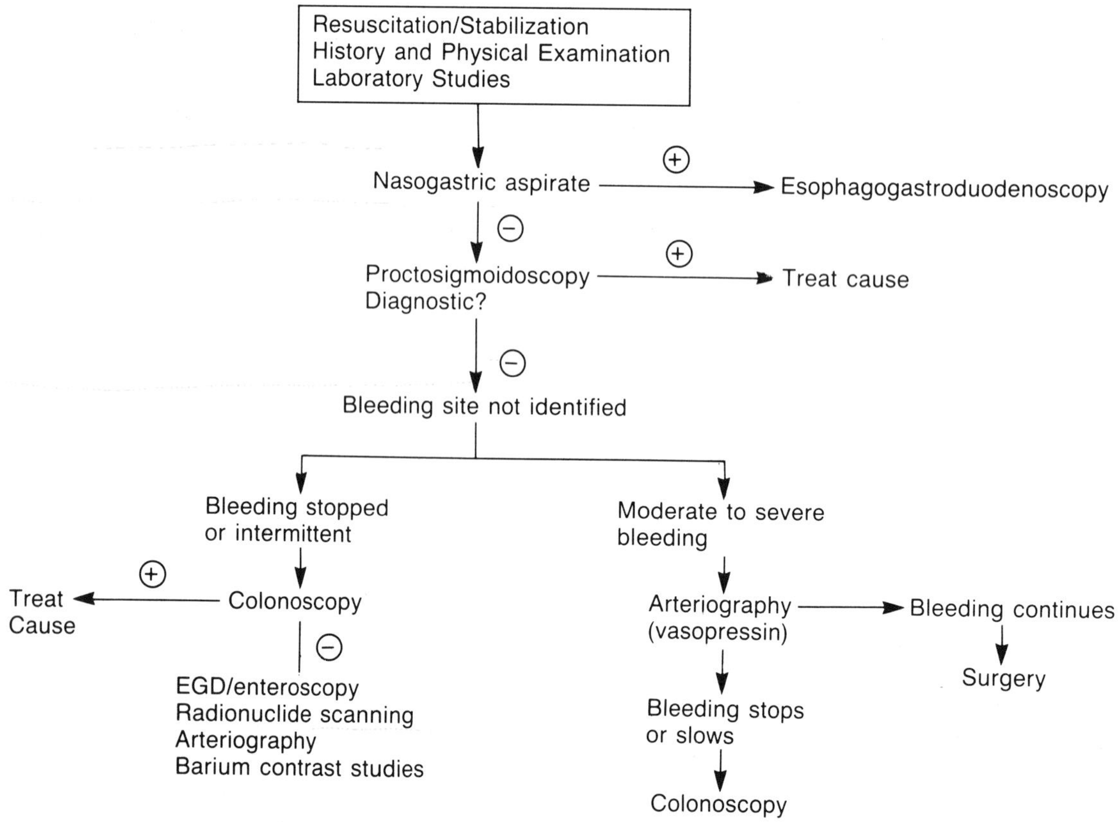

Figure 1 Management of lower gastrointestinal bleeding.

TABLE 3 Management of the Most Common Causes of Lower Gastrointestinal Bleeding

Causes	*Proctosigmoidoscopy*	*Treatment*
Diverticulosis	Outpouching in colon wall Normal mucosa ± Sentinel clot	Supportive (transfusions if necessary) Bulk laxatives
Angiodysplasia	Flat, fernlike red vascular lesions	Colonoscopic fulguration
Inflammatory bowel disease		
Ulcerative colitis (blood loss rarely massive)	Hyperemic, friable mucosa Mucosa may bleed spontaneously ± Pseudopolyps	Corticosteroids Sulfasalazine Metronidazole Colectomy
Crohn's disease (blood loss may be massive)	Linear, "punched-out" ulcers May resemble ulcerative colitis	Corticosteroids Metronidazole Bowel rest
Ischemic colitis	Acute Alternating hyperemic and pale mucosa with edema, submucosal hemorrhage Subacute Mimics inflammatory bowel disease	Conservative treatment Avoid digitalis, vasopressin
Hemorrhoids/anal fissures	Blood in rectal vault Adherent clot overlying hemorrhoid or fissure	Bulk laxative Anal suppositories

impossible or insensitive. Nonetheless, despite its limitations and potential false-negative results, barium examinations may be helpful when other methods cannot be performed or do not reveal the source of bleeding.

TREATMENT

Diagnosing or at least localizing the bleeding site is generally possible in over 90 percent of patients. Thus "blind" partial or total colectomies are reserved for a very small number of cases. The therapeutic approach will depend on the cause of lower gastrointestinal bleeding (Fig. 1 and Table 3). Occasionally, however, emergency exploratory laparotomy is indicated. Intraoperative endoscopy should be attempted, but in patients with massive bleeding with an unidentified or uncontrolled site of hemorrhage, surgery must be performed. The role of elective surgery for patients in whom bleeding cannot be localized remains controversial. The risks—particularly the likelihood of significant recurrent hemorrhage—must be weighed against the benefits.

In a few patients the source of gastrointestinal bleeding remains obscure. If bleeding is occult and not significant and a malignant lesion has been excluded, it may be adequate to merely follow the patient. On the other hand, if bleeding is significant (requiring hospitalization and transfusions), localization of the site may be as important as diagnosing a specific bleeding lesion. A radionuclide scan should precede arteriography and both should be attempted before exploratory laparotomy is performed. Once the site is documented, appropriate therapy can be rendered. In those cases where a colon source is suspected but no specific site has been identified, it appears to be better, although controversial, to perform a subtotal colectomy rather than a blind hemicolectomy.

SUGGESTED READING

Boley SJ, Brandt LJ, Frank MS. Severe lower intestinal bleeding: diagnosis and treatment. Clin Gastroenterol 1981; 10:65–91.

Caos A, Benner KG, Manier J, et al. Colonoscopy after GoLYTELY preparation in acute rectal bleeding. J Clin Gastroenterol 1986; 8:46–49.

Gianfrancisco JA, Abcarian H. Pitfalls in the treatment of massive lower gastrointestinal bleeding with "blind" subtotal colectomy. Dis Colon Rectum 1982; 25:441–445.

Lewis BS, Waye JD. Chronic gastrointestinal bleeding of obscure origin: role of small bowel enteroscopy. Gastroenterology 1988; 94:1117–1120.

Markisz JA, Front D, Royal HD, et al. An evaluation of ^{99m}Tc-labeled red blood cell scintigraphy for the detection and localization of gastrointestinal sites. Gastroenterology 1982;83:394–398.

Peery WH. Clinical spectrum of hereditary hemorrhagic telangiectasia (Osler-Weber-Rendu disease). Am J Med 1987; 82:989–997.

Peterson WL. Obscure gastrointestinal bleeding. Med Clin North Am 1988; 72:1169–1177.

Protell RL, Morgan TR, Kogan FJ, et al. Endoscopic heater probe coagulation improves patient outcome in hereditary hemorrhagic telangiectasias. Gastrointest Endosc 1985; 3:135.

Tedesco FJ, Griffin JW, Khan AQ, et al. Vascular ectasia of the colon: clinical, colonoscopic, and radiographic features. J Clin Gastroenterol 1980; 2:233–238.

DIVERTICULAR DISEASE OF THE COLON

PATRICIA L. ROBERTS, M.D.
MALCOLM C. VEIDENHEIMER, M.D., C.M., FRCSC, F.A.C.S.

Diverticular disease is predominantly a disease of the 20th century. In North America, diverticulosis is estimated to occur in one-third of all persons older than 45 years of age and in two-thirds of all persons older than 85 years of age. The incidence of inflammatory changes associated with diverticulosis is 10 to 25 percent. Although diverticular disease was initially reported to occur with equal frequency in men and women, an increasing female preponderance (2:3) has been suggested in most recent series. The sigmoid colon, the most frequent site of diverticular disease, is involved in as many as 95 percent of patients, with cecal involvement accounting for 5 percent of patients. This discussion is confined to the surgical treatment of diverticular disease, since the etiology, physiologic changes of the bowel, and role of fiber are well known to most physicians. (The chapter *Irritable Bowel Syndrome* provides useful information on these topics.)

INITIAL TREATMENT

The patient who presents with signs and symptoms of acute diverticulitis should be treated initially with bowel rest, intravenous hydration, and broad-spectrum antibiotics. We prefer a second-generation antibiotic (cefoxitin), but an aminoglycoside (gentamicin) and an antibiotic with good anaerobic coverage (metronidazole, clindamycin) are reasonable alternatives. Nasogastric tubes are not used routinely unless the patient is vomiting or has some degree of obstruction. Resolution of abdominal tenderness, fever, and leukocytosis usually occurs progressively over 24 to 48 hours. Antibiotics are continued for 7 days, and oral intake is resumed gradually and advanced to a low-residue diet. When signs of peritoneal inflammation have resolved, a low-pressure enema with water-soluble contrast medium is performed. Radiologic findings associated with (but not necessarily pathognomonic of) diverticulitis include spasm, spiculation of the bowel, localized perforation, and intramural fistulization. Some institutions have found abdominal and pelvic computed tomography (CT) helpful. Sigmoidoscopy with minimal insufflation of air is useful in excluding other diseases, such as inflammatory bowel disease. Spasm frequently precludes examination proximal to the rectosigmoid and is indirect evidence of the presence of diverticulitis. After completing a 1-week course of intravenous antibiotics, the patient is observed for 24 to 48 hours after discontinuing antibiotics and is discharged home, where he or she will be maintained on a low-residue diet for 6 to 8 weeks. For the patient who is less than 55 years old and in otherwise good health, we recommend that an elective sigmoid resection be performed in 6 to 8 weeks.

Immediate laparotomy is indicated for the patient in whom generalized peritonitis develops. Time-consuming and unnecessary radiologic tests are not required. If the patient remains febrile with localized peritoneal signs despite maximal medical therapy, further radiologic and laboratory tests should be performed both to evaluate and treat the acute episode and to exclude another disease process. Continued spiking fever is suggestive of a pericolic abscess; CT may not only confirm the presence of the abscess, but may also afford the opportunity for percutaneous drainage and obviate the need for urgent laparotomy. CT may also confirm the diagnosis of acute diverticulitis or suggest such unsuspected diagnoses as acute appendicitis or pelvic inflammatory disease.

Patients with extremely mild abdominal tenderness and no systemic signs may be treated on an outpatient basis. A low-residue diet is advised and an oral antibiotic (metronidazole, tetracycline, or ampicillin) is prescribed. Close follow-up is necessary. Patients who improve with this regimen may be investigated further at a later date. Development of fever, systemic toxicity, or peritoneal signs warrants hospitalization.

SURGICAL INTERVENTION

Surgical intervention is mandatory for complications of diverticulitis, including perforation, abscess, fistula, obstruction, and often, massive hemorrhage. However, surgical intervention is frequently associated with appreciable morbidity and mortality. Ideally, patients should undergo operation electively, before complications ensue.

A variety of operative approaches have been advocated for treatment of diverticulitis (Table 1). A one-stage procedure is the procedure of choice for patients who undergo an elective operation for diverticular disease. Two-stage procedures, consisting of an initial resection of the involved segment of colon followed by colostomy closure at a later date, are commonly used for management of complicated diverticular disease. Three-stage procedures, consisting of initial transverse colostomy and pelvic drainage, sigmoid resection, and finally, colostomy closure, are rarely performed today but were considered the treatment of choice for complicated diverticular disease as recently as 10 to 15 years ago.

TABLE 1 Operations for Diverticular Disease

One-stage procedures
Resection with primary anastomosis
Two-stage procedures
Resection with primary anastomosis and proximal colostomy
Hartmann's resection
Resection with proximal end colostomy and distal mucous fistula
Mikulicz's operation
Three-stage procedures
Transverse colostomy and drainage

Elective Resection

We take an aggressive approach for treatment of young patients with diverticular disease. Indeed, diverticulitis in young persons is associated with a more virulent course with frequent recurrent episodes and complications. We advocate elective resection for patients under 55 years of age who fulfill the following criteria: (1) have had one or more attacks of proved diverticulitis associated with abdominal pain, fever, mass, or leukocytosis; (2) have had an attack of diverticulitis associated with barium leakage at the time of barium or water-soluble enema examination, obstructive symptoms, urinary symptoms, or inability to differentiate between diverticulitis and carcinoma. In older patients (older than 55 years), we advocate a sigmoid colectomy after two attacks of diverticulitis. We generally wait 6 to 8 weeks after the initial episode to allow the inflammatory process to resolve; waiting any longer increases the possibility of another episode of diverticulitis. We have seen no deaths after elective sigmoid resection for diverticular disease.

Surgery for Complicated Diverticular Disease

Abscess and Phlegmon

Abscess and phlegmon are the most common complications of diverticulitis and have been reported to occur in 10 to 57 percent of patients treated surgically. Localized abscesses develop slowly as a result of pericolitis and may affect epiploic appendices, omentum, small bowel, bladder, and uterus. Abscesses may also penetrate into the pelvis, retroperitoneum, and extraperitoneally and become manifest in such unusual locations as the hip and thigh.

Operative intervention is indicated for patients who do not resolve the acute process while receiving maximal medical therapy. On occasion, percutaneous drainage of an abscess may be accomplished. A later single-stage resection with anastomosis may then be performed without the need for a colostomy. A single-stage sigmoid resection with primary anastomosis may be performed safely for patients with a localized pericolic, pelvic, or intra-abdominal abscess. Patients with purulent or fecal peritonitis as a result of free rupture of an abscess require sigmoid resection with proximal diversion. This procedure may be performed as a Hartmann operation or with left transverse colostomy after colorectal anastomosis to the rectosigmoid colon.

Obstruction

Most series report a 10 percent incidence of colonic obstruction associated with diverticular disease. Obstruction may be caused by repeated episodes of acute diverticulitis resulting in fibrosis or scarring, by pericolic abscess, phlegmon, or extrinsic compression from adjacent loops of the small bowel.

Obstruction on the basis of diverticular disease is usually incomplete and is resolved in many patients by bowel rest, nasogastric suction, and intravenous hydration. The cause of the obstruction can be investigated further by contrast studies, CT, and endoscopy. The distinction between obstructing diverticular disease and carcinoma can pose a problem for the clinician.

For patients in whom the obstruction is resolved by conservative measures, a primary resection and anastomosis of the involved segment (usually the sigmoid colon) may be performed in an elective time frame. If the obstruction does not resolve, a sigmoid resection with descending colon end colostomy and either distal mucous fistula or a Hartmann closure of the rectum is indicated. An alternative procedure, if the colon viability is not compromised, is resection with anastomosis and proximal diverting colostomy.

Fistula

Fistulas associated with diverticular disease result from perforation of pericolic abscesses and may involve the bladder, uterus, vagina, small intestine, and abdominal wall. Fistulae have been found in 10 to 24 percent of patients undergoing operation for diverticular disease. The diagnosis of Crohn's disease should be considered and carefully excluded.

Colovesical fistulas account for 50 percent of fistulae associated with diverticular disease. They are more common in men because of the protective effect of the intervening uterus in women. Because the higher pressure colonic side has decompressed into the lower pressure bladder, patients generally present with urinary tract signs and symptoms, such as pneumaturia and recurrent urinary tract infections. Colovesical fistulas are seen infrequently on barium enema examination, intravenous pyelography, or cystography. CT may be the only positive study. Cystoscopy may demonstrate an area of edema or erythema at the site of the fistula. Treatment consists of sigmoid resection with excision of the fistula and simple closure of the bladder. After the operation, a Foley catheter is left in place for 7 to 10 days.

Colovaginal fistulas are rare and occur almost exclusively in women who have previously undergone a hysterectomy. Treatment consists of sigmoid resection with excision of the fistula.

Colocutaneous fistulas rarely occur spontaneously. Rather, they are a complication found in patients who have undergone prior operation for diverticular disease (often in the setting of acute inflammation), and they often represent anastomotic leak.

Free Perforation

Free perforation is uncommon because the slowly developing inflammatory process associated with diverticulitis usually allows for sealing of the peritoneal cavity. Free perforation accounts for appreciable morbidity and mortality and may be the most common presenting complication in immunocompromised patients, especially those receiving steroid therapy.

Patients who present with this complication are acutely ill and require a brief period of volume replenishment and broad-spectrum antibiotics followed by immediate laparotomy. The aim of operative intervention is to remove the septic process. Expeditious sigmoid resection with end colostomy and a Hartmann closure of the rectum is the procedure of choice. Alternatively, we have also performed sigmoid resection, primary anastomosis, and proximal diversion with the same morbidity and mortality rates as with the Hartmann procedure. Three-stage procedures, consisting of initial transverse colostomy followed by sigmoid resection and colostomy closure as the final stage, are mentioned only to be condemned; they do not fulfill the primary goal of operative intervention—that is, to remove the septic process at the initial operation.

Hemorrhage

It has been estimated that as many as 30 percent of patients with diverticulosis bleed at some point. Diverticular bleeding is rarely associated with inflammatory changes (diverticulitis). Although bleeding manifested by guaiac-positive stools may be investigated leisurely, the evaluation and treatment of the massively bleeding patient must progress in a logical and orderly fashion. Diverticular disease and vascular ectasias, two of the most common causes of lower gastrointestinal tract bleeding in elderly patients, may coexist in the same patient.

Initial volume replenishment with large-bore intravenous catheters and blood products as indicated are administered. A bilious nasogastric aspirate excludes bleeding proximal to the ligament of Treitz in 90 percent of patients. Sigmoidoscopy, although rarely revealing, should be performed to rule out an anorectal source of bleeding. A radionuclide scan is then performed; this procedure is simple, fast, and noninvasive. Bleeding as slow as 0.1 ml per minute may be detected as well as intermittent bleeding. If the scan is positive for bleeding, superior and inferior mesenteric angiography is performed. The angiographer can focus on the approximate site determined by radionuclide scan. If angiography demonstrates extravasation consistent with a diagnosis of diverticulosis, administration of vasopressin is begun through the angiography catheter at a dose of 0.2 unit per minute and is gradually increased to a dose of 0.4 unit per minute. If the bleeding stops, the patient is slowly weaned off vasopressin over 24 hours. Vasopressin may cause hypertension, arrhythmia, and depressed cardiac output and should be used with caution in patients with cardiovascular diseases. All patients having vasopressin infusion should be monitored in an intensive care unit. If the patient continues to bleed, an emergency segmental colectomy is performed. If the bleeding site is located before operation, this operation has a mortality rate and rate of recurrent bleeding of approximately 5 percent. We have not advocated angiographic embolization because this technique is associated with an appreciable incidence of infarction of the colon.

Patients who continue to bleed without the bleeding site having been localized pose a particular challenge to the surgeon. As the incidence of bleeding diverticula on the right is equal to that on the left side of the colon, resecting only the area with the predominance of diverticula is doomed to failure. Blind segmental resection has been associated with a mortality rate of 30 to 40 percent and a rate of recurrent bleeding of 33 percent. If the bleeding site cannot be located before operation, subtotal colectomy is the procedure of choice. On occasion, intraoperative colonoscopy may be helpful in identifying the bleeding site. Colonoscopy is difficult if not impossible in the massively bleeding patient, but is very useful in the patient whose bleeding has stopped. (See the chapter *Lower Gastrointestinal Bleeding*.)

Cecal Diverticulitis

Cecal diverticulitis is rare; patients present with signs and symptoms identical to those of acute appendicitis. The age at presentation tends to be older (mean age of 40 years) than for patients with acute appendicitis, but this can by no means be used as a way to distinguish the two conditions. Radiographic signs may include a paracolic mass, calcified fecalith, and localized ileus. Recently, improved diagnostic accuracy with CT has been reported.

A diagnosis is made before operation in less than one-third of patients. Treatment is dictated by intraoperative findings. If a solitary diverticulum with a small area of inflammation is encountered, simple diverticulectomy may be performed. More often, a large adherent inflammatory mass is encountered and differentiation from cecal carcinoma is impossible; in these patients, right hemicolectomy is indicated.

SUGGESTED READING

Almy TP, Howell DA. Medical progress: diverticular disease of the colon. N Engl J Med 1980; 302:324–331.

Hackford AW, Schoetz DJ Jr, Coller JA, Veidenheimer MC. Surgical management of complicated diverticulitis: the Lahey Clinic experience, 1967 to 1982. Dis Colon Rectum 1985; 28:317–321.

Hackford AW, Veidenheimer MC. Diverticular disease of the colon: current concepts and management. Surg Clin North Am 1985; 65:347–363.

Parks TG. Natural history of diverticular disease of the colon: a review of 521 cases. Br Med J 1969; 4:639–642.

Pillari G, Greenspan B, Vernace FM, Rosenblum G. Computed tomography of diverticulitis. Gastrointest Radiol 1984; 9:263–268.

Rodkey GV, Welch CE. Changing patterns in the surgical treatment of diverticular disease. Ann Surg 1984; 200:466–478.

FECAL INCONTINENCE

PHILIP B. MINER Jr., M.D.

Urinary and fecal continence are some of the first areas of independence children have over their world. By managing their bowels they can control both their own activities and the response of family members to their behavior. It may be expected that loss of this control produces profound psychological changes in incontinent patients. Because of the psychological issues and the social stigma associated with a loss of bowel control, patients often hide this symptom and become increasingly isolated and drawn on a short tether toward the toilet. The extent of the problem of incontinence is masked by the social stigma attached to admitting incontinence. Leigh and Turnberg showed that over half the patients they interviewed who had diarrhea of more than 2 weeks' duration had incontinence. Fewer than half of those patients volunteered that symptom to their physician. Most lay people, and many physicians, believe fecal incontinence to be a disease of old, disabled individuals who are either too senile to recognize impending fecal incontinence or unable to move fast enough to reach the toilet. In most studies, if specific questions about incontinence are asked, the average patient with fecal incontinence is in the middle-age range. Leigh and Turnberg concluded that patients often suffer silently while compensating for their fecal incontinence with an increasingly withdrawn life style. Unfortunately, physicians unwittingly contribute to these feelings of despair because they do not believe that anything useful can be done to manage fecal incontinence, apart from use of antimotility agents.

ASSESSMENT

The initial assessment includes a history and physical examination, with specific attention directed toward those factors that precipitate fecal incontinence. Episodic severe diarrhea and the consistency of the stool associated with incontinent episodes are important features of the history. Incontinence of solid stool is far worse than incontinence of liquid stool or flatus. If there is incontinence of solid stool, management with antimotility agents may increase the symptoms by causing severe constipation without altering anorectal function. The level of assessment is dependent on the facilities available. Examination of the perineum, anal canal, and rectum can be conducted by all physicians. Chemical dermatitis around the anus suggests mucus leakage or loss of liquid stool. Anatomic lesions of the perineum and anal canal from trauma or surgery are often suspected by visual examination, and should be carefully assessed by the examining finger to determine any interruption in the circular continuity of the anal canal. A "springlike" surgical repair suggests a reconstruction of the sphincter that did not properly approximate the ends of the muscle, leaving a noncontracting tissue channel between the leaves of the spring.

Digital assessment of the strength of the internal and external anal sphincters is a notoriously poor test when correlated with manometric measurements, but appropriate contraction can be determined by asking the patient to squeeze and to attempt defecation (pseudodefecation) during the examination. Table 1 outlines the findings that should be assessed by a rectal examination. Anoscopic evaluation of the anal canal and the rectum will demonstrate lesions suspected by digital examination. Instances of minor degrees of anterior mucosal prolapse may be suspected by the presence of edematous or ulcerative changes in rectal mucosa descending into the anal canal. Generally, results of visual inspection of the anal canal are normal, since most incontinence is due to physiologic abnormalities of (1) sensation, (2) sigmoid colon or rectal contraction, or (3) dysfunction of the pelvic floor or anal canal muscles. Optimal evaluation of these factors depends on specific anorectal tests.

Radiographic tests and electromyography of the pelvic floor are important investigative tools in the understanding of problems with defecation, but in individual patients they provide limited useful information. Rectal infusion of 1,500 ml of 37° C saline at a rate of 60 ml per minute has been utilized as a retraining technique, and is an excellent functional stress test of the competence of pelvic floor musculature. It evaluates important features of the continence mechanism. First, it assesses the ability of the rectum to move saline from the rectum into the sigmoid colon. If the rectum moves saline proximally and the sigmoid colon can accommodate the contents of the rectum, incontinence can be avoided because the rectum is empty. Second, it compares the pressure generated by rectal contraction against the pressure barrier created by the pelvic floor and anal canal. The saline infusion test is an excellent predictor of fecal incontinence, but it has limited effectiveness for retraining purposes, although it can be used. Anorectal manometry is important, but has not been a popular evaluation tool for patients with incontinence because the procedure is time consuming and interpretation requires considerable experience. I will outline some of the important manometric findings, but detailed discussion of the technique was made by Read and Bannister. I will focus on management techniques not dependent on anorectal manometry.

OBJECTIVE FINDINGS

The findings associated with fecal incontinence include low basal pressure, low squeeze pressure, an obtuse anorectal angle, perineal descent, impaired sensation, spontaneous unrecognized relaxation, low rectal compliance, and high-volume diarrhea. Often, the anorectal findings in a particular patient are a combination of a number of these abnormal measurements. For example, Schiller and colleagues found that diabetes mellitus patients with fecal incontinence have low basal and squeeze pressures.

TABLE 1 Anorectal Examination in Patients with Fecal Incontinence

Examination	*Abnormal Finding*	*Significance*
Perineal skin	Chemical dermatitis	Incontinence of liquid stool or mucus causing skin injury
Perineal descent	Anus descending below imaginary line between ischial tuberosities with straining	Weakness of pelvic floor, usually implying damage to pudendal nerve
Stroking perianal skin	Loss of external anal sphincter contraction	Absence of cutaneoanal reflex; suggests sacral nerve injury
	No sensory awareness	Absence of sensation can indicate either sacral nerve root or suprasacral injury
Length of anal canal	Less than 2.5 cm	Loss of muscle mass
Deformity of anal canal	Loss of smooth circular muscular ring; focal, constrictive scarring; "keyhole" scarring	Obstetric, surgical, or traumatic changes in anal canal
Anorectal angle	Resting angle normally orients finger toward umbilicus	Loss of muscle mass or tone usually signifying a neurologic injury such as obstetrically related pudendal nerve injury
Resting pressure	Relatively weak	Gives impression of weakness, but does not correlate well with manometric findings
Squeeze pressure	Puborectalis normally moves toward symphysis pubis; it should be symmetric and smooth; external anal sphincter pressure is very distal, symmetric, and without defect	Anatomic and neurologic defects give clues to origin of injury (e.g., nerve root injury, poor alignment after perineal tear)
Pseudodefecation	Puborectalis does not move posteriorly and down with attempts to expel examining finger	Paradoxical contraction of pelvic floor (a cause of constipation) or failure to move due to neurologic injury

More important, however, the saline incontinence test is markedly impaired, with the first leak of 10 ml of saline occurring at less than 500 ml of infused saline, and the total volume retained being around 700 ml. Wald and Tunuguntla demonstrated that the ability to sense an inflated balloon in the rectum is also abnormal in incontinent patients; about 40 percent more volume is needed before the balloon can be sensed. The interrelationship between these findings provides important information regarding the etiology and management of fecal incontinence in diabetes mellitus. Improving rectal sensation decreases the number of incontinent episodes, suggesting that the factors that impair saline continence and low basal pressures may not be significant in maintaining continence. The control of incontinence by improving sensation has important implications in many other types of incontinence. Another example of complex findings associated with fecal incontinence is in ischemic or radiation proctitis. In these patients, there is decreased compliance of the rectum related to scar tissue or radiation changes. This is manifest clinically by frequent passage of small formed stools, and manometrically by very sharp change in rectal pressure with the increased volume of balloon distention. Although decreased compliance appears to be the most important factor in the incontinence of these patients, there are numerous other abnormalities. The rectoinhibitory reflex has a low-amplitude relaxation and a prolonged relaxation phase. The rectoanal contractility reflex has a short duration but a normal amplitude, and there are abnormalities of anal canal relaxation after puborectalis pressure.

The complex observations in incontinence allow us to consider many management protocols. Table 2 lists five major approaches to therapeutic intervention.

TABLE 2 Theoretical Points of Intervention in Treatment of Fecal Incontinence

Goal	*Physiology*	*Example*
Alter colonic function	Decrease stool water	Bulk laxatives, antimotility drugs, cholestyramine
	Decrease motility	Antimotility drugs
	Slow sigmoid emptying	Antimotility drugs, retraining
	Decrease rectal contractility by decreasing inflammation	Rectal or oral anti-inflammatory drugs (sulfasalazine, 5-aminosalicylic acid, glucocorticoids)
	Decrease pelvic floor muscle spasm (e.g., stiff man syndrome)	Striated muscle relaxants
Change anorectal anatomy	Repair "keyhole" scar	Surgery
	Correct anorectal angle	Surgery
	Eliminate prolapse	Postanal repair
	Decrease size of anal outlet	Thiersch ring
	Add voluntary muscle mass	Muscle transposition
Enhance external anal sphincter pressure	Correct disrupted sphincter	Surgical repair
	Increase muscle strength	Exercise; electrical stimulation of external anal sphincter
	Improve "automatic" contraction associated with rectal filling	Retraining
Control internal anal sphincter pressure and relaxation	Enhance basal pressure	Loperamide
	Control spontaneous relaxation and excessive relaxation to a small volume	Retraining; antimotility agents, antihistamines
	Postsqueeze relaxation	Retraining
Change anorectal sensation	Decrease rectal sensitivity	Treat inflammation with glucocorticoids or 5-aminosalicylic acid
	Improve sensation of rectal filling so that sensory threshold is smaller than volume causing relaxation	Retraining
	Sense internal and sphincter relaxation	Retraining

MANAGEMENT

Chemical Dermatitis

Even minor degrees of fecal incontinence can damage the perineal skin. The colonic contents remove the protective oils from the skin, cause chemical injury, and result in physical damage when patients try to clean the perineum. Steps should be taken to educate patients regarding the cause of injury and to instruct them in appropriate techniques of hygiene that avoid physical trauma. In addition, the skin needs to be protected with a lotion or cream. Cholestyramine plus lanolin paste may help if there is incontinence of bile salts, as in patients with ileocecal pouches or after ileal bypass.

Alteration of Colonic Function

Pharmaceuticals are available that alter colonic motility, colonic absorption, the amount of fluid contents in the colon, and rectal sensitivity. These drugs have been useful in controlling fecal incontinence in patients with diarrhea of diverse etiologies. Primary management of the diarrhea (e.g., metronidazole for giardiasis, glucocorticoids for inflammatory bowel disease) can be important in controlling incontinence regardless of the function of the anorectum. Patients with fecal incontinence may have diarrhea that defies an explanation. Many eventually are classified as having the irritable bowel syndrome (IBS). The episodic incontinence and diarrhea can often be controlled with bulk laxatives that absorb fluid from the colon, preventing accumulation of liquid stool in the rectum. Most of the patients referred to me have already failed treatment for IBS with bulk laxatives and anticholinergics.

The second important area of colonic function is motility. Although the colonic motility disorders are rare causes of fecal incontinence, managing motility with codeine, diphenoxylate, or loperamide has been documented to be useful in improving the number of stools per day as well as the incontinence. These drugs have complex effects on the colon, but it is most likely the decrease in colonic motility that benefits the patients. I favor the use of loperamide because it is long-acting, and management with low doses has been very effective. Dependable colonic activity is the therapeutic goal that can be achieved by a regular loperamide schedule, rather than following diarrhea stools. Although 16 mg a day is considered an acceptable dose, 2 to 4 mg at night controls incontinence in many patients. This low dosage may be effective because of the long half-life of loperamide and the fact that many patients need only a minor delay in motility to regain control. A dose of 16 mg a day is rarely used, and in fact may complicate the patient's problems, inducing severe constipation that may require cathartic treatment.

The classic article by Thaysen and Pedersen describing idiopathic bile salt catharsis discusses three patients, two of whom have certain and the other probable fecal incontinence. Idiopathic bile salt catharsis is a rare disease, but, bile salts can influence patients with a number of different disorders. There is excellent evidence that in patients with radiation to the pelvis, bile acid malabsorption is the sole cause of their diarrhea 50 percent of the time. In addition, urgency and incontinence in Crohn's disease are often associated with isolated small-bowel Crohn's disease, suggesting that failure of bile salt absorption by a diseased ileum could cause incontinence in these patients. In addition, patients with IBS have been shown to be more sensitive to bile acids than age-matched controls. In each of these patient groups, fecal incontinence could be related to changes in anorectal motility due to bile acids. Cholestyramine is remarkably effective in the management of many patients with fecal incontinence. Although it changes the consistency of the stool by the nature of its resin, the marked improvement in patients with IBS, choleretic enteropathy, or radiation enteritis suggests an important role for bile acid–sequestering agents in managing incontinent patients. In patients in whom there is no obvious cause of the incontinence, I begin a treatment trial with a dose of 4 g of cholestyramine at night in patients who have had a cholecystectomy or a single dose in the morning if they have not had a cholecystectomy. Some patients have paradoxical diarrhea with cholestyramine resin (Questran), probably owing to the dye. By changing to colestipol hydrochloride (Colestid), which binds bile acid but does not contain dye, this unexpected diarrhea can be avoided.

Rectal inflammation induces muscular spasm of the rectum that is exacerbated by distention. Treating proctitis with glucocorticoid enemas or foam, or 5-aminosalicylic acid enemas decreases rectal inflammation and hypersensitivity of the rectum, improving urgency and reducing incontinence. Since inflammatory disease of the rectum and sigmoid colon impairs motility in the proximal colon, I avoid the use of antimotility agents to control the incontinence, since this may result in severe constipation proximal to the inflamed rectum.

Electrical stimulation of the pelvic floor is a nonsurgical approach to fecal incontinence intended to strengthen the external anal sphincter muscle. Although the devices do stimulate muscle contraction of the pelvic floor, I have been disappointed in objective measures of muscle strength or improvement in fecal incontinence.

Using the manometric techniques designed to analyze anorectal function, training protocols for incontinence have evolved. The success of these protocols is phenomenal considering the severity of the problem and the relative failure of other methods to control fecal incontinence. Most series find about a 70 percent success rate with retraining in all groups of patients except those with spinal cord injury. There are many possible ways by which retraining techniques can improve continence. Training can improve muscle activity to give greater strength to the muscular barrier; sensation can be improved to provide an earlier warning of stool in the rectum; sensation can be improved to a level where the internal anal sphincter does not relax prior to sensation; or net pressure of the anal canal (the sum of internal and external anal sphincter components) can be altered by better regulation of the external anal sphincter. I began retraining patients on the premise that continence would improve if the level of sensation was trained to be lower than the level that caused internal anal sphincter relaxation. If this were to occur, the competence of the muscular barrier would be intact with the first sensation of rectal filling. While evaluating the success of this approach to retraining, I found that one-quarter of my patients had delayed perception of balloon distention in the rectum. Obviously, if internal and sphincter relaxation occurs 4 to 8 seconds after balloon distention, the process of automatic defecation can begin without patient awareness. Arresting incontinence after automatic defecation begins is extraordinarily difficult. In a controlled trial of feedback for improving sensory perception, I found that an active training program is essential to correct the sensory delay.

The first step in retraining is to teach patients to sense large volumes in the rectum immediately. Once they can sense the balloon at the time of inflation, smaller volumes are introduced with the objective of maintaining immediate sensation at lower balloon volumes. In our published study (Buser and Miner) and in my subsequent observations, nearly all patients with delay can be corrected to normal. In several patients, correcting the delayed sensation was sufficient to eliminate the incontinence despite the failure to achieve the philosophical objective that the volume should be decreased below the level at which relaxation occurred.

Once the delay is corrected, I attempt to improve the sensory threshold by specific retraining. This is done by inflating the balloon to a volume that is easily recognized by the patient. The next balloon inflation volume is 50 percent less. If this is not sensed, the new volume is repeated, with a warning to the patient 3 seconds before the balloon is inflated. If the patient recognizes the balloon distention, the volume is repeated without warning. If the patient fails to recognize the distention, the last sensory volume is used and a smaller differential volume (e.g., 75 percent of the sensed volume) used. The larger the volume required for sensation, the shorter is the necessary retraining session, since sensory recognition diminishes quickly at large volumes. No training session exceeds 15 minutes.

After eliminating the delay and attempting to establish a sensory threshold below 15 ml, the next step is to have sensory-squeeze sequences. During these sequences patients are requested to squeeze the muscles of the pelvic floor, as if they were trying to delay defecation, as soon as they perceive balloon distention. The goal is to have patients squeeze quickly and appropriately during a random sequence of inflations. The character of the squeeze is studied on a monitor in order to modify the squeeze pressure profile. The squeeze should be brisk so that the upstroke from the basal pressure to maximal pressure occurs in less than two-thirds of a second. The squeezes during this part of the retraining are very brief (less than 5 seconds) to avoid muscle fatigue. Once a prompt response has been established, patients are instructed to maintain a strong plateau of pressure for the 10 to 15 seconds of balloon distention. The best effort is expected, although often it is difficult for patients to maintain maximal pressure for the entire 12 to 13 seconds. When patients are asked to relax, postsqueeze relaxation should be noted (Fig. 1). If present, it should be eliminated by retraining. This is done by asking patients to gradually relax while informing them of the proper level of the resting pressure. A relaxation period of 5 seconds is usually sufficient to avoid postsqueeze relaxation.

Generally, three to five training sessions are sufficient to change an adult from an abnormal sensation to normal sensation with good sensory squeeze responses. If management by anorectal manometry alone is insufficient to improve the incontinence, I add a low dose of loperamide or cholestyramine for long-term management. Success of retraining is around 70 percent, with excellent long-term results.

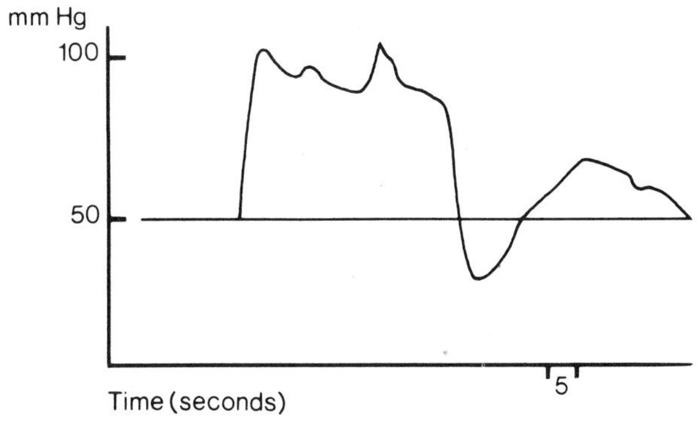

Figure 1 Postsqueeze relaxation manometric finding.

MANAGEMENT OF PATIENTS WITH SPINAL CORD INJURY

Spinal cord injuries can be divided into suprasacral or sacral injuries. The differences in anorectal manometry findings are listed in Table 3. These differences have important implications with regard to management (Table 4). Suprasacral injuries, although more neurologically severe, can usually be managed by puborectalis stimulation and planned defecation. Since the sensory deficit is usually quite severe, attempts to train these patients are often frustrating; however, retraining should be attempted at least once. The prognosis for successful retraining is generally dependent on the amount of neurologic impairment. Management includes education about the early warning signs of impending defecation (sympathetic outflow with piloerection or dizziness). If patients can use these signals, they may be able to anticipate defecation. Unfortunately, the physical disability that accompanies suprasacral spinal cord injury is usually so severe that insufficient time is available to prepare properly for defecation. An appropriate protocol for planned defecation with suprasacral lesions is listed in Table 4.

TABLE 3 Anorectal Findings in Patients With Spinal Cord Injuries

	Sacral Lesions	*Suprasacral Lesions*
Sensation of rectal filling	Usually absent	Absent
Basal anal canal pressure	Normal or low	Normal
Voluntary squeeze pressure	Probably absent	Absent
Reflex defecation	Usually absent	Present
Warning of impending defecation	No warning, but occasionally abdominal pain is present	Often there is no warning, but autonomic signs (e.g., piloerection, dizziness) are present

TABLE 4 Management of Defecation in Patients With Spinal Cord Injuries

Suprasacral Lesions

1. Control diet or use nonstimulating osmotic agents (e.g., magnesium antacids, lactulose) to keep stool consistency predictable
2. Respond to autonomic warning of impending defecation if possible
3. Planned defecation: attempt to identify a consistent time
   A. Transfer to toilet or position on bed
   B. Manual check for stool and stimulation of anal canal (puborectalis)
   C. Glycerin suppository if needed
   D. Stimulant laxative if needed (in order of preference):
      1. Rectal liquid
      2. Rectal suppository
      3. Oral agent
   E. Manual recheck

Sacral Lesions

1. Prevent hard stools that may damage anal canal, but avoid bulk laxatives (use diet, stool softeners, osmotic agents that can be tightly controlled (e.g., occasionally this is successful)
2. Trial of digital stimulation or glycerin suppositories (occasionally this is successful)
3. Manual evacuation twice a day

Sacral lesions are more difficult to manage owing to the impaired contractility of the rectum and sigmoid colon. Patients with sacral lesions usually require manual evacuation and stimulating suppositories (bisacodyl) or enemas as part of the treatment. Because the manual evacuation is such an important part of managing sacral lesions, bulk laxatives are best avoided, since they increase the time and effort needed to clear the rectum. Non–bulk-forming stool softeners are preferable in order to avoid the injury associated with hard stools. To be continent, patients may need to employ manual evacuation on a twice-daily basis.

SUGGESTED READING

Buser WD, Miner PB. Delayed rectal sensation with fecal incontinence: successful treatment using anorectal manometry. Gastroenterology 1986; 91:1186–1191.

Leigh RJ, Turnberg LA. Faecal incontinence: the unvoiced symptom. Lancet 1982; 1:1349–1351.

Read NW, Bannister JJ. Anorectal manometry: techniques in health and anorectal disease. In: Henry MM, Swash M, eds. Coloproctology and the pelvic floor—pathophysiology and management. London: Butterworths, 1985:65.

Schiller LR, SantaAna CA, Schulen AC, et al. Pathogenesis of fecal incontinence in diabetes mellitus: evidence for internal anal sphincter dysfunction. N Engl J Med 1982; 307:1666–1671.

Thaysen EH, Pedersen L. Idiopathic bile acid catharsis. Gut 1976; 17:965–970.

Wald A, Tunuguntla AK. Anorectal sensorimotor dysfunction in fecal incontinence and diabetes mellitus. N Engl J Med 1984; 310:1282–1287.

ALCOHOLISM

DONALD M. GALLANT, M.D.

An unprecedented government-supported study by the National Institute of Mental Health (NIMH) on the lifetime prevalence of specific psychiatric disorders in approximately 17,000 respondents 18 years of age or older showed that alcohol abuse or dependence affects 11 to 16 percent of the population. The enormity of this medical problem is further emphasized by the high incidence of alcoholism seen in hospital walk-in clinics (28 percent), emergency rooms (38 percent), and general hospital wards (32 percent in males and 8 percent in females). Objective research data by Petersson et al show that alcohol abuse is the major cause of death in middle-aged males and that alcoholics have a suicide rate 300 to 600 times higher than that of nonalcoholics. These data should convince us of the need for intervention in the early or middle phases of this illness.

INTERVENTION TECHNIQUE

All physicians involved in the treatment of alcoholics should be exposed to the techniques of early intervention, since a delay of treatment could easily result in tragedy. Early intervention may save years of hardship for the family and friends of the patient, as well as for the patient himself. With the alcoholic, early intervention compresses the past crises caused by the misuse of alcohol into one dramatic confrontation, in order to brush aside the denial mechanism and get the patient to agree to seek help. It is a therapeutic maneuver designed to offer immediate help to the patient, an alternative to waiting interminably for the alcoholic to "hit bottom," to lose or destroy his or her family, health, or job. If we wait, it may be too late. Details of this technique are described elsewhere (Gallant, 1987).

MANAGEMENT OF THE ACUTE WITHDRAWAL SYNDROMES

Alcohol withdrawal is defined in DSM-III-R as cessation of or reduction in prolonged (several days or longer) heavy ingestion of alcohol, followed within several hours by coarse tremor of the hands, tongue, and eyelids, and at least one of the following: (1) nausea and vomiting, (2) malaise or weakness, (3) autonomic hyperactivity (e.g., tachycardia, sweating, elevated blood pressure), (4) anxiety, (5) depressed mood or irritability, and (6) orthostatic hypotension.

Mild to Moderate Alcohol Withdrawal

For the majority of patients displaying the syndrome of alcohol withdrawal, outpatient office treatment may be sufficient and one need not resort to hospitalization. The blood alcohol level can be used as one of the more reliable guidelines for making a decision about whether to place the patient in a social alcohol detoxification unit with specialized care, to refer him to a medical ward for more intensive treatment of severe withdrawal symptoms, or to follow the patient at home with proper supervision. For example, if the blood alcohol level is 250 to 300 mg per deciliter and the patient appears to be alert and not dysarthric, the physician should be on guard for the possible appearance of withdrawal symptoms as the blood alcohol level decreases. In this type of patient, the tolerance for alcohol is too high and suggests chronic alcohol abuse with an increased predisposition to develop withdrawal symptoms upon cessation of alcohol use.

In one study, only 45 of 564 acute alcohol outpatient admissions (8 percent) required hospitalization. In another extensive study of alcohol detoxification, fewer than 10 percent required medical detoxification; the remainder of the 1,024 patients in the study received nondrug detoxification. Seizures occurred in only 1 percent, hallucinations in 3.7 percent, and delirium tremens in fewer than 1 percent. However, 8 percent of the original sample did require medical referral to a hospital emergency room for further evaluation. Thus, the use of benzodiazepines was required in less than 10 percent of the entire patient population. Many physicians refer patients to inpatient facilities where they are automatically placed on medication; this step makes it difficult to withdraw them later from the sedative hypnotics. The majority of alcoholic patients should be able to withdraw from alcohol without the use of habituating minor tranquilizers.

One may help the patient to decrease the intake of alcohol with family aid and the use of a short-acting hypnotic (e.g., chloral hydrate) for sleep for the next 5 to 7 days. Other relaxation techniques, including the use of mild, pleasurable sensory stimulations such as music, the company of friends and relatives, attempts to keep the patient active, and reassurance may also help the patient during this uncomfortable phase. In this way, it may be possible to substitute psychological management for the automatic pharmacologic approach used by some detoxification units.

Thiamine, 50 to 100 mg per day, in addition to multivitamins and folic acid, 1 to 3 mg per day, should be given to all patients experiencing mild to severe alcohol withdrawal, orally for patients in the mild to moderate stages, and intramuscularly or intravenously for hospitalized patients with poor gastrointestinal absorption or those who are in a severe stage of withdrawal. Short-term administration of a high dosage of vitamins should not result in any serious side effects. Shortly after the patient's blood alcohol level reaches zero, disulfiram (Antabuse) should be seriously considered unless there are definite medical contraindications. It is not unusual for us to have patients come to the clinic on a daily basis when they begin taking disulfiram. We may give them only enough tranquilizers to last until they return to the clinic the next day. Dependency-producing medications such as benzodiazepines should not be used for more than 1 to 2 weeks, because patients with problems of alcohol abuse are more likely to misuse these tranquilizers as well.

Among the safer agents to use on a temporary basis for sleep are sedative antihistamines, paraldehyde, and benzodiazepines. If emesis occurs, prochlorperazine, 10 mg intramuscularly, can be used to control it temporarily. The oral dosage of chlordiazepoxide for the outpatient management of withdrawal symptoms should not exceed 150 mg daily, or not more than 30 mg of diazepam per day. If higher dosages are necessary, this usually means that the withdrawal symptoms are worsening and that the patient may have to be placed on a detoxification unit or hospitalized.

If the patient continues to drink sporadically during this outpatient treatment, it may be necessary to institute inpatient detoxification even though the patient may not be experiencing severe withdrawal symptoms. From a therapeutic viewpoint, it may be necessary to interrupt the self-destructive cycle of heavy drinking followed by withdrawal symptoms, which are then relieved through resumption of alcohol intake.

Severe Alcohol Withdrawal (Alcohol Withdrawal Delirium)

Diagnostic criteria for alcohol withdrawal delirium include a clouding of consciousness, difficulty in sustaining attention, disorientation to present circumstances, and autonomic hyperactivity associated with tachycardia, sweating, and elevated blood pressure. These symptoms occur within 1 week after the cessation of or reduction in heavy alcohol ingestion. With adequate treatment, these symptoms should disappear by the end of the first week and certainly by no later than the beginning of the second week. If such patients are left untreated, the mortality rate may be as high as 15 percent. A diagnostic problem may occur with the emergency room patient if the history of alcohol intake is unknown and there is no family available to give information. Diagnoses such as schizophrenia, schizophreniform disorder, other psychotic disorders, or dementia can be confused with alcohol withdrawal delirium if the history of alcohol intake is lacking.

If the diagnosis of alcohol withdrawal delirium is correct, immediate hospitalization is indicated, since the diagnosis implies that the patient is unable to care for himself and is seriously ill.

Because benzodiazepines possess anticonvulsant activity as well as sedative properties, the temporary use of these compounds may be of considerable help to alcoholics who have experienced recent alcohol withdrawal convulsions. If the patient is suspected of having a moderate amount of liver damage, the most appropriate benzodiazepine to use may be oxazepam or lorazepam, since they do not require hydroxylation by the liver and therefore do not accumulate. Chlordiazepoxide, diazepam, and chlorazepate are all metabolized in the liver and can accumulate in the patient who has a fair degree of liver damage, particularly because these agents have relatively long half-lives. Hydroxyzine is the safest sedative as regards drug-dependency, but its anticholinergic activity may confuse the patient if the drug is administered in high dosages. Unlike the benzodiazepines, it has no anticonvulsant properties. Sedative-hypnotic therapy for severe withdrawal symptoms, good nursing care, absence of restraint, a well-lighted room, and use of thiamine and multivitamins can help to alleviate the symptoms.

In another study of acute alcohol withdrawal, the effects of clonidine, administered in doses as great as 0.2 mg three times per day, versus chlordiazepoxide, administered in doses as great as 50 mg three times per day, were compared in a 60-hour treatment period of acute alcohol withdrawal. Clonidine was more effective than chlordiazepoxide in reducing alcohol withdrawal symptoms and maintaining stable systolic blood pressures and heart rates over the entire study period. The adverse drug reactions reported by patients of each group was similar, although there was less nausea and vomiting than in the clonidine group. Of course, clonidine is not a controlled substance and has not shown abuse or addiction potential when used only for alcohol withdrawal. However, because clonidine does not have any anticonvulsant properties, the combination of clonidine plus a benzodiazepine may be more safe for patients with a previous history of postalcohol withdrawal seizures.

The use of antipsychotic agents or neuroleptics for the withdrawal syndrome is questionable, since these agents can lower the convulsive threshold, potentiate orthostatic hypotension, and cause uncomfortable atropine-like side effects. Some alcoholic patients receiving neuroleptics have been reported to develop prolonged unconsciousness.

The dosage range for benzodiazepines should vary with the duration and intensity of the alcohol consumption that preceded withdrawal, the weight of the patient, and other pharmacokinetic variables for which data are available. Although patients who present with high blood alcohol levels usually experience more severe withdrawal symptoms than patients with relatively low blood levels, these observations are not consistent. Exceptions may include patients who have experienced severe withdrawal symptoms after previous drinking episodes and those who have developed intercurrent illnesses during the present withdrawal stage. In mild to moderate cases of the alcohol withdrawal syndrome without delirium, the dosage of oxazepam may vary from 15 mg four times per day to 30 mg four times per day; the dosage of chlordiazepoxide, from 25 mg four times per day to 50 mg four times per day; and the dosage of diazepam, from 5 mg four times per day to 15 mg four times per day. In severe cases of the alcohol withdrawal syndrome with delirium, a dosage of oxazepam as high as 45 mg four times per day may be needed; the dosage of chlordiazepoxide may have to be as great as 100 mg four times per day; and the dosage of diazepam as high as 25 mg four times per day may be required.

In one double-blind comparison of lorazepam and diazepam in the treatment of patients displaying mild to moderate alcohol withdrawal symptoms, 6 mg of lorazepam showed no significant differences in efficacy compared with 30 mg of diazepam, except for a significant drop in blood pressure in the diazepam-treated patients. Lorazepam is a benzodiazepine with a relatively short half-life compared with diazepam; thus, it may be simpler and more predictable in its pharmacologic effects for patients with the alcohol withdrawal syndrome.

It is extremely important to decrease and then discontinue the use of benzodiazepine before the patient's discharge from the hospital. It appears that those patients who are discharged while receiving benzodiazepine are more likely either to become habituated to the medication or to return to drinking alcohol. An interesting analogy of this experience comes from a report on mice. After chronic involuntary administration of alcohol, mice have been shown to have an increased tendency toward self-administration of the alcohol when offered free choice between alcohol and tap water. Diazepam administered during the period of withdrawal served to maintain the self-administration of alcohol. Without diazepam, the tendency toward self-administration of alcohol returned to control levels. The similarity between the examples of mice and human subjects concerning the return to alcohol consumption after using diazepam as a means of withdrawal is noteworthy.

Concerning the subcutaneous or intramuscular use of benzodiazepines, the clinician should be aware that compounds such as chlordiazepoxide and diazepam are poorly absorbed. For example, within 2 hours after oral ingestion of 50 mg of chlordiazepoxide, plasma levels are significantly higher than those after a 50-mg intramuscular dose administered to an abstinent patient. If the patient is vomiting profusely and unable to tolerate oral medication, then the use of intramuscularly administered lorazepam or prochlorperazine is indicated, along with possible use of 25 mg of prochlorperazine as suppository. It should be stressed that intravenous infusions should be used only in patients who are definitely dehydrated from excessive vomiting or diarrhea. Even in these cases, the clinician has to be cautious with glycogen-depleted patients who may be thiamine deficient, since the patient may be converted to Wernicke's encephalopathy by a glucose infusion that would require additional use of thiamine. These patients should be *weighed daily* in order to evaluate their hydration state.

MANAGEMENT OF ALCOHOLICS WITH MULTIPLE DRUG ABUSE PROBLEMS

Increasing numbers of patients abuse habituating drugs in association with alcohol. The combined alcohol-barbiturate patient presents an additional medical problem in the treatment of withdrawal, since he or she is more likely to have seizures. A fairly reliable method of calculating the dosage of medication to be used during withdrawal in this type of patient is a substitution of 15 mg of phenobarbital for 1 oz of 100-proof alcohol. Administration of 200 mg of pentobarbital may help the physician determine the extent of physical dependence. The appearance of ataxia with slurred speech at this dose suggests that the patient is not severely physically dependent and should not require a large dosage of the long-acting barbiturate for withdrawal purposes. If the patient is addicted, a relatively safe procedure for treating barbiturate addiction has been detailed by Robinson et al. Phenobarbital is administered in a dose of 120 mg per hour until the patient develops three of the five following symptoms: dysarthria, ataxia, nystagmus, confusion, and drowsiness. The urine is maintained at a pH of less than 6.5, which slows the excretion of phenobarbital, allowing the patient to follow a "smooth" withdrawal from the combination alcohol-barbiturate drug addiction. In a series of 54 cases, not one convulsion developed with the use of this technique.

When combined with alcohol, stimulants or euphorigenic agents, such as cocaine or amphetamines, may result in a facilitation of withdrawal seizures if their use continues during the first few days of withdrawal from alcohol. Routine urine drug screens of these patients should enable the physician to clarify the confusing symptoms.

DISULFIRAM (ANTABUSE)

A great deal of misinformation exists about the use of psychopharmacologic medications in treating alcoholic patients. Over the years, I have heard patients make such statements as, "One of my alcoholic friends tells me that Antabuse can kill you even if you don't take a drink." Having been medically responsible for administering Antabuse to more than 20,000 patients during the past 27 years, I have no doubt that the benefits of Antabuse far outweigh the risks of taking this medication.

Antabuse does inhibit liver aldehyde dehydrogenase as well as dopamine beta-hydroxylase. The former metabolic action appears to be associated with the Antabuse-alcohol reaction (disulfiram-ethanol reaction, or DER). This DER apparently results in an increase of blood acetaldehyde, which is associated with hypothermia and hypotension occurring during the DER.

The DER is associated with some unpleasant symptoms, which include flushing, increased heart rate, palpitations, and hypotension. In addition, some patients may feel an uncomfortable tightness in the chest, become nauseated, and vomit. This type of reaction makes it extremely difficult for most patients to become intoxicated, because they must wait 4 to 14 days after taking the last Antabuse tablet before they may have a drink; this period provides ample time for them to stop and think before they act.

Risks of Antabuse

I have found Antabuse, when given in a dosage of 250 mg at bedtime and when the patient has full information about potential side effects and the medications and foods to avoid, to be one of the safest compounds to administer. In addition to having patients read to *Physicians' Desk Reference* (PDR), I have them review the controlled studies that have compared Antabuse with placebo. I strongly believe that educating patients not only decreases their anxieties about various medications but also enhances their compliance with the treatment regimen. In a placebo-Antabuse, double-blind controlled study of alcoholic patients by Christensen et al, the evaluation of side effects in 158 patients who completed the study showed no statistically significant differences between the two groups, except for a greater number of complaints of sexual problems in the placebo group. Surprisingly, fatigue, itching, unpleasant taste, and skin reactions were no more common in the Antabuse group than in the placebo group. However, complaints of "bad breath" did occur more frequently in the Antabuse group. The dosage of Antabuse used in the study was *250 mg*, dissolved in plain soda water, taken daily for 6 weeks under staff supervision. The investigators emphasized the importance of using this dosage of Antabuse when performing this type of controlled evaluation.

Peripheral nerve damage, including optic neuritis, has been described, usually in association with daily doses of 500 mg of Antabuse, which is an unnecessarily high dosage.

In the study of Christensen et al, which specifically evaluated the potential liver toxicity of Antabuse, 453 alcoholism patients were randomly assigned to receive either Antabuse or placebo for a 12-month period. The evaluation of drinking status included analyses of blood and urine samples, subject interviews, and contact with household members at regular intervals. Liver tests were performed every 2 months. The results showed that there was no relation between liver enzyme elevation and Antabuse treatment, but there was a correlation between elevated liver enzymes and drinking status. These results point out that there is frequent drinking by alcoholic patients that goes undetected by the physician and is denied by the patient; 76 percent of the patients were found to have been drinking at some time during the study. The authors concluded that patients receiving Antabuse who show liver test abnormalities are usually drinking.

In my clinical experience, the most important contraindication to the use of Antabuse has been an associated diagnosis of schizophrenia. I have seen a number of schizophrenic patients who have been convicted of driving while intoxicated (DWI) and placed in a court-referred treatment program including administration of Antabuse without an adequate psychiatric evaluation. In these particular patients, the initiation of a dosage of Antabuse of 500 mg daily resulted in a number of psychotic reactions. Because one of the metabolic functions of Antabuse is to inhibit dopamine-beta-hydroxylase with a subsequent increase of dopamine in the brain, large doses of Antabuse (500 mg per day) or perhaps even low doses (250 mg daily) can exacerbate schizophrenic psychoses. Therefore, it is best not to use Antabuse in this patient population, or to use a placebo dose of only 62.5 mg as a reminder for the patients.

The most serious side effects I have ever seen in alcoholic patients were three cases of mild peripheral neuropathies that appeared to be Antabuse-related and that disappeared when the medication was discontinued, and one possible case of optic neuritis that showed no further progression after the cessation of Antabuse use. Approximately 2 to 3 percent of my patients develop a slight skin rash, usually a mild, acne-type rash on the trunk or forehead and, at other times, an erythematous rash on the trunk. This rash is responsive to hydrocortisone cream and usually does not reappear if the routine daily dosage of 250 mg of Antabuse is reduced to 125 mg.

Occasionally, the patient may complain of a bad taste in the mouth or mild tension headaches. Approximately 5 to 8 percent of our patients develop daytime lethargy even though the medication is administered at night before sleep. With these patients, we reduce the dosage to 125 mg administered at bedtime.

Drug interactions with Antabuse may occur when patients are receiving concurrent treatment with several compounds. Antabuse can inhibit the metabolism of phenytoin and coumarin, resulting in higher levels of both these compounds. The simultaneous administration of Antabuse and metronidazole (Flagyl) can result in confusional states. At present, there is no definite proof of teratogenic or carcinogenic activity associated with Antabuse administration.

Benefits of Antabuse

During my 27 years of experience as medical director of two alcoholism inpatient treatment programs and of the state substance-abuse clinic in New Orleans, I have been extremely impressed by the value of Antabuse. On innumerable occasions, patients who have undergone some discouraging experience have said to me, "If it were not for Antabuse, I would have drunk that day." On other occasions, after having achieved some goal and wanting to celebrate, patients have often told me, "We were all having such a great time that evening that I would have drunk with my friends if it were not for Antabuse." The former case occurs more frequently and has made me realize what an invaluable help Antabuse has been to many of my patients.

There are some excellent, well-controlled scientific investigations showing the effectiveness of Antabuse and objectively confirming my subjective experiences. The efficacy of Antabuse has been demonstrated in a number of studies, including one by Fuller and Williford. In this study, 128 alcoholic males were assigned randomly to one of three treatment groups: (1) 500 mg of disulfiram (Antabuse) daily for 1 week, followed by 250 mg daily for 1 year; (2) 1 mg Antabuse daily as a control for the implied threat of illness from the Antabuse-alcohol reaction (DER); and (3) nondrug medical care. Patients in all three groups received counseling. Motivation was equal among the groups, since all patients in the study had requested Antabuse. The results showed statistically significant therapeutic gains for both medical groups (the 500/250 mg Antabuse group and the 1 mg Antabuse group) as compared with the control group. Fuller and Williford used a life-table analysis through which they evaluated the effects of alcoholism treatment over time. This method provides information about the number of additional months of abstinence (as compared to end-point analysis) that may delay or even prevent occurrence of tissue damage to various organs. This study also showed that the threat of taking Antabuse may be more therapeutic than the action of the drug itself.

The efficacy of an outpatient program involving mandatory, supervised Antabuse therapy for patients who wish to remain "connected" to the clinic was shown in another study. Of those patients who had previously continued to drink while attending the clinic, approximately 60 percent who agreed to this mandatory regimen achieved significant periods of sobriety. It is clear, then, that Antabuse increases the therapeutic success rates of patients who are very difficult cases, as well as the average alcoholic patients who are treated in an outpatient setting. Compliance can be determined by testing the urine for diethylamine, a metabolite of Antabuse.

Before giving a patient a medication such as Antabuse, it is important to be certain that the following three essentials of informed consent are fulfilled: (1) the patient understands the information, (2) the patient's use of the medication is voluntary, and (3) complete information about the major risks and benefits has been given. It is particularly important to explain to patients that individuals prone toward schizophrenic or psychotic reactions are more likely to develop adverse psychological reactions to Antabuse.

VITAMINS

Alcoholism produces multiple nutritional deficiencies. When an alcoholic population is evaluated for specific types of nutritional deficiencies, such as zinc, magnesium, and various vitamin deficiencies, it is not unusual to find a sizable proportion with one or more of the nutritional deficits. Most researchers and clinicians in the field agree that supplemental thiamine (vitamin B_1) should be administered to all patients who have a history of chronic alcoholism. Although a considerable percentage of normal subjects have low tissue thiamine status, alcoholics with poor diets are even more likely to be lacking in adequate thiamine tissue levels. In severe alcoholics, immediate treatment with 100 mg of thiamine daily can be of some help and definitely is of no harm to the patient.

Thiamine treatment is the specific treatment of Wernicke's encephalopathy, a rapidly deteriorating organic mental syndrome secondary to alcoholism. This alcohol-related brain damage appears to be associated with progressive neuronal degeneration, particularly in the periventricular area of the brain. Unfortunately, it is frequently not diagnosed until death. Of 51 patients with this disease first diagnosed at autopsy, 45 were alcoholics, only seven of whom had been diagnosed as such before death. Many of the patients died of hemorrhage into the brain stem, involving the cardiac and respiratory nuclei. Cerebral and ventricular atrophy was commonly found at autopsy. One major recommendation resulting from this study was the routine use of large doses of prophylactic thiamine in alcoholic patients, particularly those with clinical evidence of cerebral damage.

Research into the etiology of the Wernicke-Korsakoff syndrome has indicated that thiamine pyrophosphatase (TPP)–dependence transketolase activity may be decreased in patients who develop the syndrome. It is suggested that some alcoholics may have a greater genetic-metabolic tendency than others for the development of the Wernicke-Korsakoff syndrome.

The use of 1 to 3 mg of folic acid daily is also recommended by some clinicians. In one study, a folate deficiency was found in the erythrocytes of 35 percent of the patients, in the liver of 31 percent, and in the serum of 28 percent. Enlargement of the red blood cells may be caused by a direct toxic effect of alcohol on the developing erythrocytes as well as by a folate deficiency. It is interesting to note that alcoholics frequently show a relative macrocytosis without a significant anemia (38 percent in one study) and without abnormal folic acid and vitamin B_{12} levels. Only 2 percent of the nonalcoholic population displays this type of hemogram. Thus, a patient with a relative macrocytosis without an anemia and without a folic acid and B_{12} deficiency would have only a 5 percent chance of being misdiagnosed as an alcoholic. The complete blood count to determine macrocytosis is one of the better screening tests for chronic alcoholism.

A significant percentage of alcoholics have peripheral neuropathies with symmetrical symptoms of numbness, tingling sensations, burning sensations, and sometimes weakness in both legs. It may be that chronic thiamine deficiency, as well as pantothenic acid and pyridoxine deficiency, may be responsible for the development of this syndrome. However, because we are not sure whether one or several of these vitamin deficiencies are specific causes of development of this syndrome and because we are uncertain as to what part direct alcohol toxicity plays in producing this pathology, multiple mega-B therapy is recommended for these patients.

Other diseases that may be treated with supplemental thiamine therapy include alcoholic amblyopia, characterized by blurring of vision due to central scotomas, which can develop into optic atrophy if untreated. Improvement has been reported in association with vitamin B supplements, but there are no controlled studies in this area; controlled data are similarly lacking in most of the other areas involving vitamin therapy of alcohol-related diseases. In many cases, it is difficult to delineate the damage that is produced by alcohol and that which is produced by vitamin deficiencies secondary to chronic alcohol intake with malnutrition. However, vitamin and mineral supplements will seldom be harmful to alcoholic patients. Because of the occasional episodes of night blindness and reports of alcoholic amblyopia, vitamin A therapy and zinc supplements have been recommended by some clinicians. On our alcohol and drug abuse (ADU) service, the routine orders include daily thiamine (100 mg), mega-B vitamins, and a multivitamin supplement. This vitamin therapy is continued throughout the patient's stay on the unit and is then maintained for several weeks in the clinic. Although there is no scientific basis for this duration of vitamin therapy, this type of short-term vitamin supplementation can do no harm and may be of some slight value in patients who are still undergoing the protracted withdrawal syndrome or subacute organic mental disorder for several weeks or months after the cessation of alcohol use.

All personnel involved in the treatment of alcoholic patients should be aware of the various indications for the use of psychopharmacologic medications as well as the value of appropriate vitamin and mineral therapy. I believe that there are few contraindications for the use of Antabuse, and the research data indicate the significant benefits that occur when an alcoholic takes this medication daily. In patients who present dual diagnoses, such as major depression or bipolar disorder or severe generalized anxiety disorder in association with the illness of alcoholism, correct use of an anti-depressant, lithium, or a nonhabituating anxiolytic agent may not only enable the patient to remain abstinent but enhance the quality of his sober life.

SUGGESTED READING

Christensen JK, Ronstead P, Vaag UH. Side effects after disulfiram. Acta Psychiatr Scand 1984; 69:265–273.

Fuller RK, Williford WO. Life-table analysis of abstinence in a study evaluating the efficacy of disulfiram. Alcoholism 1981; 4:298–301.

Gallant DM. Alcoholism: a guide to diagnosis, intervention, and treatment. New York: WW Norton, 1987.

Perry PP, Wilding DC, Fowler RC. Absorption of oral and intramuscular chlordiazepoxide by alcoholics. Clin Pharmacol Ther 1978; 23:535–541.

Petersson B, Kristenson H, Krantz P, et al. Alcohol-related death: a major contributor to mortality in urban middle-aged men. Lancet 1982; 2:1088–1090.

Robinson GN, Sellers EM, Janacek E. Barbiturate and hypnosedative withdrawal by oral pentobarbital loading dose techniques. Clin Pharmacol Ther 1981; 28:71–76.

ALCOHOLIC LIVER DISEASE

MACK C. MITCHELL, M.D.

Alcoholic liver disease remains the major cause of cirrhosis in the United States and other Western countries. Within the last decade, per capita consumption of alcoholic beverages plateaued and declined slightly after consistent increases between 1960 and 1980. The mortality rates for alcoholic cirrhosis have not been measured specifically, but it is estimated that one-half to two-thirds of all cases of cirrhosis are attributable to excessive alcohol consumption. The mortality rate from all causes of cirrhosis has declined since 1975.

RISK FACTORS IN DEVELOPMENT

Several studies have attempted to define the lower limits of alcohol consumption required to produce serious liver damage. In some, there were small increases in relative risk after consumption of a daily average of 60 g of ethanol, although most reports found increased risk with consumption exceeding 80 g per day in men. This amount of ethanol is contained in roughly half a pint of 80 proof spirits, six 12-oz cans of beer, or one 750 ml bottle of table wine (11 percent ethanol). Women are more susceptible than men to the development of liver injury from alcohol, even after the lower average body weight of women is taken into account, but the causes of the increased toxicity are not well understood. There is an increased risk of alcoholic liver disease in women who drink more than 40 g per day.

The dose and duration of excessive alcohol consumption have emerged as the most important factors in the pathogenesis of alcoholic cirrhosis. The observation that serious alcoholic liver injury occurs in only 20 to 30 percent of alcoholics drinking more than 80 g per day suggests that other factors may modulate the risk of liver disease from alcohol. There is evidence that heredity may influence risk, although the genetic basis for this is unknown. Advances in molecular biology now being used to study patients with alcoholic liver disease may elucidate the specific genes that increase susceptibility. The role of nutrition and other environmental variables has been studied extensively. Later in this chapter, nutrition is discussed both as a risk factor (nutritional deficiency) and as treatment for alcoholic liver disease.

DIFFERENTIAL DIAGNOSIS

In managing alcoholics showing clinical or laboratory evidence of liver disease, the clinician must remember that although most have alcoholic liver injury, other diseases may also occur. Furthermore, alcohol may contribute to damage from other agents independently of direct injury to the liver from ethanol itself. In particular, the risk of hepatotoxicity from other drugs is greatly increased in alcoholics, despite the absence of specific alcohol-related damage. Acetaminophen is clinically the most important drug with increased hepatotoxicity in alcoholics. Numerous cases of severe, even fatal hepatic necrosis have been observed in alcoholics ingesting therapeutic doses of acetaminophen. Characteristically, these individuals have extraordinarily high serum aminotransferase levels, often exceeding 10,000 IU per liter. Such values do not occur in alcoholic liver disease and are rarely seen in patients with acute viral hepatitis. Because acetaminophen is a widely used analgesic contained in many over-the-counter medications, acetaminophen hepatotoxicity is most often an inadvertent complication in alcoholics, in contrast to the intentional overdose that causes hepatotoxicity in otherwise healthy individuals. Chronic alcohol consumption enhances the hepatotoxicity of acetaminophen and other drugs by increasing the formation of its toxic metabolites (cytochrome P-450) and decreasing its subsequent detoxification by altering glutathione metabolism. Several other drugs, including cocaine and perhaps halothane and isoniazid, appear to be more hepatotoxic in alcoholic patients for similar reasons.

Alcoholics may be more susceptible to viral hepatitis because of altered immune function and possibly increased exposure. Persistence of hepatitis B infection may also be more frequent in alcoholics. Inherited diseases such as alpha$_1$-antitrypsin deficiency and hemochromatosis are possibly exacerbated by heavy alcohol consumption. Furthermore, the frequency of alcoholism appears to be higher in patients with hereditary hemochromatosis. It is important not to overlook this condition in evaluating alcoholics with liver disease, since treatment of hemochromatosis requires phlebotomy or iron chelation. Liver biopsy with quantitation of hepatic iron content is the only satisfactory method of distinguishing hemochromatosis from hepatic iron overload due to alcohol.

Liver biopsy should be strongly considered in the evaluation of all alcoholics with liver disease in order to exclude nonalcoholic causes. In one study, in 20 percent of patients presumed to have alcoholic liver disease on the basis of clinical, biochemical, and radiographic tests, another cause was found on liver biopsies. Liver biopsy provides an index of severity of disease and is useful for determining the prognosis in patients with alcohol-related liver damage.

SPECTRUM OF ALCOHOL-RELATED DAMAGE

Alcohol consumption may cause fatty infiltration of the liver (steatosis), necroinflammatory disease (alcoholic hepatitis), fibrosis, or cirrhosis. Intracellular fat accumulation is a reversible condition that results from changes in hepatic redox state occurring with metabolism of ethanol. During oxidation of ethanol by alcohol dehydrogenase, the pyridine nucleotide NAD^+ is reduced to NADH. These redox shifts favor increased synthesis of triglycerides and decreased oxidation of fatty acids. Since the molecular weight of ethanol is 46 (three drinks = one mole), a large amount of NAD^+ is reduced even with "social drinking." Increases in hepatic triglyceride content occur within a short time after excessive ethanol ingestion both in experimental animals and in humans.

Alcoholic hepatitis is characterized clinically by jaundice, tender hepatomegaly, abdominal pain, nausea, and anorexia. Hepatocytic necrosis, polymorphonuclear leukocyte infiltration, and Mallory's hyaline (intracellular eosinophilic deposits) are found on liver biopsy. In most cases, active fibrosis is also present. Numerous studies have documented the importance of alcoholic hepatitis in the progression of alcoholic liver disease. In patients with alcoholic hepatitis proved on liver biopsy there is a significantly higher mortality rate than in those without, even if cirrhosis is already present. For this reason, most therapy for alcoholic liver disease has focused on treating alcoholic hepatitis.

Clinical parameters are also useful in determining the severity of alcoholic liver disease. The development of hepatic encephalopathy in the absence of gastrointestinal (GI) bleeding, infection, or other precipitating events, deep jaundice (bilirubin level greater than 20 mg per deciliter) and persistent coagulopathy (prothrombin time greater than 17 sec despite vitamin K administration) are all associated with a high mortality rate in the first 3 months after presentation. These criteria have been used in combination to select patients at greatest risk of dying in order to evaluate appropriate therapy.

TREATMENT OF FATTY LIVER

Abstinence is the cornerstone of therapy for all stages of alcoholic liver disease and is almost universally effective in reversing fatty liver. A high-calorie, high-protein diet with vitamin B supplementation is recommended. Although inpatient management may not be required, I find initial hospitalization to be beneficial for several reasons. Diagnostic tests such as liver biopsy, to confirm the diagnosis and establish the prognosis, can be performed with greater safety and comfort for the patient. Hospitalization may help in initial detoxification and initiation of treatment of alcoholism. Furthermore, hospitalization conveys the potential seriousness of the disease. Too often, patients report that they did not understand the importance of strict abstinence when this was recommended in an outpatient setting. In most patients with fatty liver alone, marked improvement or full resolution occurs within 1 month. A few patients may die suddenly with fatty liver, although the cause of death in these instances is unknown.

TREATMENT OF ALCOHOLIC HEPATITIS

Jaundiced patients with symptoms and clinical signs of alcoholic hepatitis should be hospitalized, since it is vital that abstinence begin as soon as possible in this group. Paradoxically, a significant number actually worsen in the first week of hospitalization, although such deterioration may have occurred in the natural progression of the illness. In patients with a prolonged prothrombin time and elevated bilirubin level, there is very high mortality in the first 30 days after hospitalization. Maddrey and colleagues formulated a discriminate function based on prothrombin time and bilirubin level that I find useful in assessing the severity of alcoholic hepatitis. The algebraic function 4.6 (prothrombin time in seconds) + bilirubin $<$ 85 defines a subgroup of patients with a high short-term mortality rate (30 to 50 percent).

Nutritional Therapy

Anecdotal reports from the 1950s and 1960s suggested that symptoms and clinical signs of alcoholic liver disease improved in patients after institution of a nutritious diet *even* if these individuals continued to drink more than 50 g of ethanol daily. These early observations have encouraged the routine use of high-calorie, high-protein diets for treatment of alcoholic liver disease, although continued drinking must be discouraged. Nutritional status correlates well with the short-term prognosis for alcoholic hepatitis, and may be assessed by anthropometric measurements and routine biochemical and hematologic tests, including serum albumin, transferrin, lymphocyte counts, and delayed hypersensitivity skin tests. Body fat stores can be assessed by the thickness of the abdominal wall and the triceps skin fold, which are easily measured at the bedside. Even qualitative determinations reflect the extent of malnutrition.

As mentioned above, nutritious diets supplemented with water-soluble vitamins, magnesium, and zinc are recommended. Anorexia often limits caloric intake, particularly in the most severely ill patients. For this reason, calorie counts should be monitored daily in hospitalized alcoholics with liver disease, since even overnight fasts have been shown to accelerate protein catabolism in patients with liver disease. Presumably, this occurs because of limited glycogen reserves in the alcohol-damaged liver.

The extent of nutritional deficiencies in severely ill patients, combined with their poor voluntary intake, provides a rationale for enteral or parenteral hyperalimentation. In general, this approach is supported by evidence from randomized trials of nutritional supplementation in patients with alcoholic hepatitis. In one study, mortality was reduced in patients receiving parenteral amino acids as compared with those on high-calorie, high-protein diets alone. Although other randomized trials have not confirmed the reduction in the mortality rate, the trend is toward more rapid improvement in patients managed with aggressive nutritional support. More rapid improvement may help reduce the length of hospitalization in the severely ill group.

Steroids

Recognition of the inflammatory character of alcoholic hepatitis has provided the rationale for numerous studies of the efficacy of corticosteroids in treating alcoholic hepatitis. One universal conclusion of these studies is that patients with mild or moderate alcoholic hepatitis do *not* benefit from steroids. The short-term efficacy of corticosteroids is controversial: most studies have not found steroids to be beneficial, but a few carefully conducted trials have. One characteristic that distinguishes those trials in which steroids have been beneficial is the higher percentage of women studied. Most of the clinical research on alcoholic liver disease has been carried out in Veterans Administration hospitals and unfortunately does not provide data on how women may respond to treatment differently from men. Women with a predominantly cholestatic form of alcoholic hepatitis appear to benefit most from 40 mg of prednisolone daily for 1 month. The incidence of serious infections does not seem to be higher in patients treated with steroids. In one study, anabolic steroids improved long-term, but not short-term, survival of patients with both moderate and severe alcoholic hepatitis. Because of their potential complications, anabolic steroids have not been widely prescribed to treat alcoholic hepatitis or cirrhosis.

Propylthiouracil (PTU)

Several investigators have reported increased hepatic oxygen consumption during ethanol metabolism. This increased oxygen demand has led to a hypothesis of a hypermetabolic state that contributes to hepatic injury in alcoholic liver disease. A recently published trial found improved survival in patients with alcoholic hepatitis who were treated with 300 mg daily of PTU. Patients receiving PTU were given placebo one month in four to avoid serious hypothyroidism. In analyzing the results, the authors noted that beneficial effects were seen only in patients who did not continue drinking heavily. The group with continued alcohol intake did not benefit, a somewhat surprising finding in light of the original hypothesis, but reflective of the importance of abstinence in any successful treatment of alcoholic liver disease. These results are intriguing, but confirmation is needed before this therapy is widely recommended. Although very few patients suffered serious side effects, they were carefully monitored in order to avoid severe hypothyroidism.

Colchicine

For over a decade, it has been postulated that colchicine prevents the progression of fibrosis because of its capacity to prevent the cross-linking of collagen. It is also an anti-inflammatory agent. Impressive improvement has been reported in the 5-year survival rate (75 percent versus 34 percent) in patients with Child's class A and B cirrhosis from a variety of causes who were treated with 1 mg of colchicine daily. Abstinence from alcohol was not examined in the 45 patients with alcoholic liver disease. All patients had cirrhosis, but the frequency of alcoholic hepatitis was not reported. Surprisingly few side effects, primarily diarrhea, nausea, and abdominal pain, were noted. The absence of serious side effects has persuaded me to use this medication in selected patients, although much remains to be learned about the setting in which it is most efficacious.

LONG-TERM FOLLOW-UP

In almost every instance in which the long-term outcome has been measured, abstinence is the most vital factor ensuring success. Furthermore, regular and uninterrupted drinking results in the worst prognosis. In addition to managing the liver disease, the clinician must institute specific supportive treatment for alcoholism. There is a separate chapter on Alcoholism. Laboratory tests such as those for gamma-glutamyltranspeptidase, the red cell mean cell volume, uric acid, and aspartate aminotransferase may be helpful in monitoring compliance, as can the checking of urine specimens for ethanol.

The clinician should also watch for signs of other unprescribed drug use in patients. The widespread availability and use of benzodiazepines and cocaine has made it necessary to monitor blood and urine for these substances as well as for continued alcohol abuse.

SUGGESTED READING

Kershenobich D, Vargas F, Garcia-Tsao G, et al. Colchicine in the treatment of cirrhosis of the liver. N Engl J Med 318:1709–1713, 1988.
Maddrey WC, Boitnott JK, Bedine MS, et al. Corticosteroid therapy of alcoholic hepatitis. Gastroenterology 75:193–199, 1978.
Mendenhall CL, Anderson S, Garcia-Pont P, et al. Short-term and long-term survival in patients with alcoholic hepatitis treated with oxandrolone and prednisolone. N Engl J Med 311:1464–1470, 1984.
Mendenhall CL, Tosch T, Weesner RE, et al. VA cooperative study on alcoholic hepatitis II: prognostic significance of protein-calorie malnutrition. Am J Clin Nutr 43:213–218, 1986.
Mitchell MC, Herlong HF. Alcohol and nutrition: caloric value, bioenergetics, and relationship to liver damage. Annu Rev Nutr 6:457–474, 1986.
Orrego H, Blake JE, Blendis LM, et al. Long-term treatment of alcoholic liver disease with propylthiouracil. N Engl J Med 317:1421–1427, 1987.
Orrego H, Blake E, Blendis M, Medline A. Prognosis of alcoholic cirrhosis in the presence and absence of alcoholic hepatitis. Gastroenterology 92:208–214, 1987.

PORTAL HYPERTENSION

NORMAN D. GRACE, M.D.

Portal venous pressure is a function of portal venous flow and hepatic resistance. The normal portal pressure range in humans is 4 to 10 mm Hg, and the normal gradient between the portal vein and inferior vena cava pressures (PVP − IVC = PVPG) is less than 6 mm Hg. These measurements can be obtained by direct percutaneous or operative catheterization of the portal vein and inferior vena cava. They can also be approximated by catheterization of the hepatic vein. With a balloon catheter to occlude the hepatic vein, the difference between the occluded or wedged hepatic vein pressure (WHVP) and the free hepatic vein pressure (FHVP) yields the hepatic venous pressure gradient (HVPG), which, under normal conditions, correlates well with the PVPG. Portal hypertension is defined as an increase in the PVPG and can result from a variety of conditions. The lesion can be prehepatic (portal vein thrombosis), presinusoidal (schistosomiasis), postsinusoidal (cirrhosis), or posthepatic (Budd-Chiari syndrome). The most common cause of portal hypertension is cirrhosis, and the remainder of this discussion will concentrate on this entity.

In patients with cirrhosis, there are both an increase in portal venous flow as a result of a hyperdynamic splanchnic and systemic circulation, and an increase in hepatic resistance from compression of hepatic sinusoids. Clinically, portal hypertension results in several of the most serious complications of cirrhosis, including the development of esophagogastric varices, ascites, and hypersplenism. From the time of diagnosis of esophagogastric varices, preferably by endoscopy, patients carry a 25 to 30 percent risk of significant hemorrhage; most bleeding episodes occur within 1 year of the time of diagnosis. With each bleeding episode, the risk of death approaches 50 percent. Even with initial control, the rebleeding rate averages 25 to 35 percent within 6 weeks. Therefore, attention needs to be directed not only to control of the acute bleeding episode but also to prevention of recurrent variceal bleeding, and, ideally, prevention of the initial episode of variceal hemorrhage.

DIAGNOSIS OF ESOPHAGOGASTRIC VARICEAL HEMORRHAGE

The diagnosis of bleeding from esophageal or gastric varices can be made only by endoscopy. A gastrointestinal (GI) series is of little value since the presence of varices does not establish them as the source of bleeding. In some studies, up to half the patients with cirrhosis and esophageal varices are found to have another source of bleeding, such as duodenal or gastric ulcers or portal hypertensive gastropathy. Since the treatment will vary, depending on the source of bleeding, accurate diagnosis is of utmost importance. In the experience of most endoscopists, varices can be seen actually bleeding in only 10 to 15 percent of patients. The diagnosis is made in the remaining patients by the presence of endoscopic signs of bleeding such as fresh erosions over the varices, or signs associated with a high risk of bleeding such as red color signs or blue varices, and (most important) the absence of any other source of bleeding. If there is doubt about varices as the source of bleeding, measurements of the PVPG or HPVG may be helpful when the patient is hemodynamically stable. In my experience, all patients in whom varices are the source of hemorrhage have had a pressure gradient of at least 11 mm Hg. In individuals with alcoholic cirrhosis (postsinusoidal block), the HVPG is approximately equal to the PVPG. However, in those with primary biliary cirrhosis or posthepatitic cirrhosis, when there is a significant presinusoidal component, measurements of HVPG may underestimate the PVPG. In addition, patients with large varices, i.e., varices measuring at least 5 to 6 mm in greatest diameter and partially occluding the esophageal lumen, are at much greater risk of bleeding than those with small varices.

CONTROL OF ACUTE VARICEAL HEMORRHAGE

General Measures

As with GI bleeding from any source, resuscitative measures are important. There are separate chapters on Gastrointestinal Bleeding. Adequate access lines for blood replacement need to be established, and the activity of bleeding must be closely monitored by nasogastric intubation and lavage with frequent hematocrits. Placement of a central venous line or Swan-Ganz catheter can be very helpful in determining the need for volume replacement. In general, it is best to keep patients with variceal bleeding slightly undertransfused, since an increase in portal pressure from overreplacement may aggravate the bleeding episode. Because patients with cirrhosis usually are deficient in coagulation factors, replacement should include one unit of fresh frozen plasma for every 2 to 3 units of packed red blood cells. Patients are often given 5 to 10 mg of vitamin K intramuscularly, although its value is questionable because of the impairment of hepatic synthetic function. One needs to be judicious about the use of saline so as not to aggravate ascites formation. If tense ascites is present, a 2- to 3-liter paracentesis can transiently lower portal pressure and occasionally may be helpful. The use of antacids and H_2-receptor antagonists is controversial. There is no evidence that esophagitis related to gastric acid reflux plays any role in the initiation of variceal hemorrhage. In spite of this, most patients with esophageal variceal hemorrhage are given intravenous H_2-receptor antagonists during the course of the acute bleeding episode. In order to prevent the development of hepatic encephalopathy, they are usually given lactulose or cathartics to minimize the absorption of ammonia from blood in the gastrointestinal tract. All acute variceal bleeders should be managed in an intensive care unit.

A classification proposed by Turcotte and Child remains the gold standard for estimating operative risk and prognosis for patients with cirrhosis and portal hypertension. This scheme makes use of serum bilirubin and albumin levels and the clinical assessment of ascites, portasystemic encephalopathy, and nutritional status; this was modified by Pugh, who substituted prothrombin time for nutritional state. Conn recommended a point system for each of these features, which should be used to standardize the classification for comparison purposes (Table 1).

Specific Measures

Pharmacologic Agents

Pharmacologic agents can lower portal pressure either by decreasing portal venous flow or by decreasing hepatic resistance. Among the agents that have been used for controlling acute variceal hemorrhage, vasopressin, somatostatin, and terlipressin act by causing a splanchnic arterial vasoconstriction, resulting in a decrease in portal venous flow. Nitroglycerin causes a more modest decrease in portal venous flow and some decrease in hepatic resistance. Of these, somatostatin and terlipressin are investigational drugs and are not available for routine use. Results have been mixed from controlled trials of their efficacy.

Lysine vasopressin continues to be the mainstay for pharmacologic control of acute variceal hemorrhage. Although an initial bolus of 20 units given over 15 to 20 minutes intravenously is still used in many centers, there are no data available as to whether this form of treatment improves the efficacy of vasopressin. My preference is to start with an intravenous dose by continuous infusion of 0.4 unit per minute. The dosage is adjusted according to response with cessation of bleeding and the development of side effects. Once bleeding is controlled, the dose is lowered by 0.1 unit every 6 to 12 hours until treatment can be discontinued. Treatment with vasopressin is associated with a number of side effects including hypertension, bradycardia, peripheral vasoconstriction, myocardial ischemia and infarction, mesenteric ischemia, cerebrovascular accidents, diarrhea, and hyponatremia with fluid retention. Data from controlled trials show that vasopressin is effective in control of variceal bleeding in half the patients, but this control is often transient, and one-third to one-half of the patients experience recurrent bleeding. Although the use of vasopressin has not been shown to influence survival favorably, neither has any other type of therapy for the acute control of variceal bleeding altered long-term outcome. Improvement in survival is probably more dependent on therapy instituted to prevent recurrent bleeding once the acute episode is under control.

Recent studies have shown nitroglycerin, when used in combination with vasopressin, to be superior to vasopressin alone in controlling variceal bleeding. Although nitroglycerin has a modest effect on lowering portal pressure, its major advantage is the amelioration of many of the more serious side effects of vasopressin by producing a systemic vasodilation. The use of nitroglycerin allows for the occasional need for higher doses of vasopressin (in some studies, up to 0.9 units per minute) to be used with reasonable safety. Nitroglycerin is given intravenously by continuous infusion, starting with a dose of 40 μg per minute and adjusted to maintain the systolic blood pressure greater than 90 mm Hg, with a maximal dose of 400 μg per minute. The mean dose is between 200 and 300 μg per minute. Alternatively, nitroglycerin can be given sublingually in a dosage of 0.6 mg per 30 minutes and adjusted to the arterial blood pressure. The variable absorption and blood levels obtained from use of transdermal nitroglycerin preclude use of this route of administration for the control of acute variceal bleeding.

Future therapy may involve drugs that increase lower esophageal sphincter pressure, thereby decreasing variceal blood flow and pressure. Studies using metoclopramide or cisapride are in progress, but these drugs should not be used in clinical practice at the present time. However, because of the relatively modest success of vasopressin in controlling hemorrhage and the significant complication rate associated with its use, a search for better agents seems warranted.

TABLE 1 Child's Classification Criteria

Criterion				*Score*
Serum bilirubin (mg/dl)	A	<2.0	= 1	
	B	2.0–3.0	= 2	
	C	>3.0	= 3	______
Serum albumin (g/dl)	A	>3.5	= 1	
	B	3.0–3.5	= 2	
	C	<3.0	= 3	______
Ascites	A	None	= 1	
	B	Easily controlled	= 2	
	C	Poorly controlled	= 3	______
Neurologic disorder	A	None	= 1	
	B	Minimal	= 2	
	C	Advanced, "coma"	= 3	______
Nutrition	A	Excellent	= 1	
	B	Good	= 2	
	C	Poor, "wasting"	= 3	______
	Total Score			______

Child's classification: A, total score 5–7; B, total score 8–11; C, total score 12–15.

Sclerotherapy

On the basis of data from controlled trials, sclerotherapy is successful in controlling hemorrhage from esophageal varices in 75 to 90 percent of patients and should be considered the current treatment of choice. The sclerosants commonly used in the United States are sodium tetradecylsulfate or sodium morrhuate; ethanolamine and polidocinol are more popular in Europe. Sclerotherapy, which is discussed in a separate chapter, is also associated with a significant rebleeding rate, and further long-term measures are needed to prevent recurrent variceal hemorrhage. Sclerotherapy is of little to no value for control of bleeding from gastric varices.

Balloon Tamponade

Once the mainstay of treatment for the control of variceal bleeding, balloon tamponade is now reserved for patients who fail vasopressin and sclerotherapy, and for whom emergency surgical intervention is not deemed advisable. The success and complication rates are directly related to the experience of the medical team. I prefer to use the Minnesota tube, which has an esophageal suction lumen in addition to the esophageal and gastric balloons and the gastric suction lumen. After passage into the stomach, the gastric balloon should be inflated with 350 to 400 ml of air and its placement verified by a flat film of the upper abdomen. I prefer traction with a pulley system and a 500-g weight to maintain compression of the esophagogastric junction by the balloon. Use of a helmet to anchor the tube is unreliable; in 90 percent of patients the gastric balloon suffices. If the esophageal balloon is needed, it should be attached to a manometer and maintained at a pressure of 35 mm Hg. It is very important to keep scissors at the bedside and to give instructions to cut the tube before trying to remove it if any sign of respiratory distress develops. Ideally, the balloons should not be inflated for more than 24 hours, because the complications of mucosal ulceration and necrosis rise dramatically after this time.

Surgery

Emergency portasystemic shunt surgery has been associated with high morbidity and mortality rates, but this may be a function of patient selection, with only medical failures going to surgery. In at least one center, a portacaval shunt is performed within 12 hours of the diagnosis of variceal hemorrhage, with excellent results reported. However, until controlled trials verify this course of action, shunt surgery is not recommended as the initial treatment of variceal bleeding. Selective shunts (distal splenorenal) have no role in the management of acute variceal bleeding.

On the basis of recent reports from Europe, esophageal transection followed by repair with a staple gun appears to be a reasonable alternative to sclerotherapy, and is associated with a lower transfusion requirement and rebleeding rate.

PREVENTION OF RECURRENT VARICEAL HEMORRHAGE

Despite successful initial control of variceal bleeding, as many as 60 to 70 percent of patients experience recurrence of variceal hemorrhage, most occurring within 6 months of the initial episode. Because of the high mortality associated with recurrent bleeding, therapy to prevent recurrence is needed.

Pharmacologic Agents

Although a number of drugs are currently under investigation, the only group of agents for which there are reasonable data are the beta-adrenergic blockers propranolol and nadolol. These nonselective beta-blockers act by decreasing cardiac output and producing splanchnic vasoconstriction, which leads to a decrease in portal venous blood flow and pressure. They are more effective than the selective beta-blockers. Data from controlled clinical trials are mixed; some studies indicate marked superiority to placebo in preventing recurrent bleeding, while others report no difference. These drugs have little if any effect upon survival.

Data from the Boston-West Haven Liver Study Group show that 20 percent of patients with cirrhosis do not have a decrease in portal pressure with increasing doses of propranolol. However, in most studies the dosage of propranolol or nadolol is adjusted to obtain a 25 percent decrease in resting heart rate. Unfortunately, the Boston-West Haven Liver Study Group data reveal no correlation between the decrease in resting heart rate and a decrease in HVPG. Ideally, the dosage of beta-blockers should be determined by obtaining at least a 20 percent decrease in HVPG. Using this technique, data suggest that a dose of propranolol somewhat lower than reported in the literature may be effective in lowering portal pressure. Since the availability of portal pressure measurements is limited, propranolol can be given, starting with a dose of 40 mg twice daily and adjusted to achieve a 25 percent decrease in resting heart rate. Using this method, the mean dosage is between 160 and 200 mg per day. Because of the need for daily dosing, compliance can be a problem. The side effects of beta-adrenergic blockers are well known, and a significant number of patients may need to have the dosage lowered or the drug discontinued for this reason. Although there are scattered case reports of precipitation of hepatic encephalopathy or renal failure, this has not been a problem in the controlled clinical trials. Sudden cessation of the beta-blocker carries the theoretical risk of producing a rebound increase in portal pressure, but this has not been a major problem in the reported clinical trials. Nadolol has a theoretical advantage over propranolol in that it is not metabolized by the liver, it does not cross the blood-brain barrier, and there is less effect on renal blood flow. However, there are no studies comparing nadolol with propranolol in the prevention of recurrent variceal hemorrhage.

Sclerotherapy

Most studies comparing sclerotherapy given over several sessions to obliterate esophageal varices with standard treatment report that the former has significant benefit in preventing recurrent esophageal variceal bleeding, and at least one of these reports a significant survival benefit. Some trials have compared sclerotherapy with propranolol for the prevention of recurrent variceal hemorrhage. Half have reported sclerotherapy to be superior to propranolol, while the other half have found the two therapies comparable. Data on survival are comparable for the two therapies. In one study comparing sclerotherapy with portacaval shunt surgery, there was an early advantage for sclerotherapy in terms of lower transfusion requirement and cost, but this advantage disappeared with longer follow-up. In that study, follow-up of patients successfully discharged from the hospital after the initial variceal bleed revealed a readmission rate of 75 percent for recurrent variceal hemorrhage in the sclerotherapy group, compared with none in the surgical group. There were no long-term survival differences. Sclerotherapy should not be used to prevent recurrent bleeding from gastric varices.

Surgery

A portacaval shunt to prevent recurrent variceal hemorrhage has a dramatic advantage over supportive medical therapy in the prevention of recurrent variceal bleeding and a slight advantage in enhancing survival. However, the prevalence of postshunt hepatic encephalopathy is high. The distal splenorenal shunt was designed to preserve portal venous blood flow to the liver while allowing for decompression of esophagogastric varices. Several studies have compared distal splenorenal and portasystemic shunts. Half reported less hepatic encephalopathy with the distal splenorenal shunt; half reported no difference. None of the studies reported a survival advantage for either operation. The distal splenorenal shunt has been compared with sclerotherapy for long-term prevention of recurrent variceal bleeding. One study concluded that sclerotherapy was preferable for the initial management of these patients, the distal splenorenal shunt being reserved for sclerotherapy failures. Another study could discern no advantage for either treatment.

CONCLUSION

With the available data, it is difficult to favor one of these therapies for prevention of recurrent variceal hemorrhage, although all appear to be somewhat better than supportive treatment. The best approach is probably to tailor the treatment to the individual patient. For the initial episode of variceal bleeding that is readily controlled by acute therapy, I would prefer medical therapy, either a beta-blocker or sclerotherapy, to surgery. For patients with relatively minor hemorrhage in whom there are no contraindications to beta-blockers and who are deemed reasonably compliant, I would favor propranolol or nadolol. For patients with a more significant bleeding episode, and especially those in whom compliance may be a problem, sclerotherapy is a reasonable course to follow, although compliance may be an issue in sclerotherapy as well. Shunt surgery should be reserved for patients who fail medical therapy.

Since many of these patients may eventually be candidates for liver transplantation, surgery involving the portal vein should be avoided. For transplant candidates, I favor a beta-blocker as the treatment with the least likelihood of interfering with future surgery. Reports of portal vein thrombosis as a complication of chronic sclerotherapy make this approach somewhat more risky. The distal splenorenal shunt would be the preferable procedure, not because it is a better shunt but because it spares the portal vein for the transplant surgeon.

Prophylaxis Against Initial Variceal Hemorrhage

As mentioned earlier, the ideal therapy is one that prevents the initial episode of variceal hemorrhage.

Pharmacologic Agents

Several studies have shown beta-adrenergic blockers to have significant benefit in preventing the initial episode of variceal hemorrhage, compared with a placebo, and one study demonstrated a survival advantage. Determination of dosage is as described for prevention of recurrent variceal hemorrhage. For compliant patients in whom there are no medical contraindications, propranolol appears to be the treatment of choice. The ideal duration of therapy is unclear from the literature. Since most variceal bleeding occurs within the first year after the diagnosis of varices, it appears reasonable to treat for at least 1 year. Whether cessation of treatment at this point would prevent variceal bleeding or simply delay the risk period is unknown.

Sclerotherapy

Early enthusiasm for the role of sclerotherapy in the prevention of initial variceal hemorrhage has been tempered by more recent reports in which there was a high incidence of variceal bleeding in the sclerotherapy group compared with controls. At the present time, sclerotherapy should not be used for this group of patients.

Surgery

There is no role for shunt surgery in the prevention of initial variceal hemorrhage.

Portal Hypertensive Gastropathy

Portal hypertensive gastropathy is a newly recognized condition with a distinct pathologic picture that may be associated with significant GI hemorrhage. Acute control of bleeding from this entity involves the pharmacologic agents for esophagogastric varices previously discussed. Sclerotherapy has no role. In rare circumstances a portasystemic shunt, with or without a gastrectomy, may be necessary. For the prevention of recurrent bleeding, the data are limited, but propranolol is a reasonable therapeutic option.

SUGGESTED READING

Garcia-Tsao G, Grace ND, Groszmann RJ, et al. Short-term effects of propranolol on portal venous pressure. Hepatology 1986; 6:101–106.
Grace ND, Conn HO, Resnick RH, et al. Distal splenorenal vs. portal-systemic shunts after hemorrhage from varices: a randomized controlled trial. Hepatology 1988; 8:1475–1481.
Graham D, Smith JL. The course of patients after variceal hemorrhage. Gastroenterology 1981; 80:800–809.
Lebrec D, Paynard T, Bernuau J, et al. A randomized controlled study of propranolol for prevention of recurrent gastrointestinal bleeding in patients with cirrhosis: a final report. Hepatology 1984; 4:355–358.
Polio J, Groszmann RJ. Hemodynamic factors involved in the development and rupture of esophageal varices: a pathophysiologic approach to treatment. Semin Liv Dis 1986; 6:318–331.
Terblanche J, Burroughs AK, Hobbs KEF. Controversies in the management of bleeding esophageal varices. Part 1. N Engl J Med 1989; 320:1393–1398.

SCLEROTHERAPY OF ESOPHAGEAL VARICES

ANTHONY N. KALLOO, M.D.

Hemorrhage from esophageal varices is a major cause of morbidity and mortality in patients with chronic liver disease. After an initial variceal hemorrhage, approximately one-third of patients experience rebleeding by 6 weeks. The mortality rate as reported by Graham and Smith is approximately 40 percent in these patients at 6 weeks.

Endoscopic sclerotherapy was originally introduced in 1939. Its use declined owing to the popularity of portal decompressive surgery, but there has been a resurgence since the late 1950s.

INDICATIONS

The accepted indications for endoscopic sclerotherapy include the control of acute variceal hemorrhage and the prevention of recurrent variceal hemorrhage. Controversies concerning prophylactic sclerotherapy are discussed later in this chapter and in the chapter on Portal Hypertension.

TECHNIQUES OF ENDOSCOPIC SCLEROTHERAPY

There has been a lack of standardization with respect to the method of sclerotherapy. The use of different types of endoscopes and sclerosing agents and different sites of injection, the use of balloons and overtubes, and the timing of sclerotherapy make critical comparisons of studies difficult.

Types of Endoscopes

In one study, Bornman and colleagues evaluated patients randomized to either fiberoptic or rigid endoscopy for endoscopic sclerosis of varices. Flexible endoscopy was found to be safe, did not require general anesthesia, and could be performed on an outpatient basis. However, rigid injection sclerotherapy was recommended for recurrent acute bleeding where endoscopy under general anesthesia would provide safer and more effective sclerotherapy.

A double-channel fiberoptic endoscope is probably the ideal instrument for most patients. One channel can be used for insertion of the sclerotherapy device and the second for suction to maintain a clear field, especially when there is active bleeding.

Site of Injection

There has been controversy over whether the sclerosing agent should be injected directly into the lumen of the varix (intravariceal), or into the mucosa adjacent to the varix (paravariceal). Most endoscopists tend to favor the intravariceal technique, but it is technically difficult to make either purely intravariceal or purely paravariceal injections. Sarin and colleagues attempted to compare the two techniques and found the intravariceal technique superior for controlling bleeding and obliterating varices.

Type of Sclerosing Agent

Several types of sclerosing agents are currently used, including morrhuate sodium, sodium tetradecyl sulfate, ethanolamine oleate, thrombin in dextrose, and alcohol. These agents are all capable of causing sclerosis of varices by initially producing venous thrombosis with necroinflammation and subsequent fibrous obliteration of the vessel. The lack of randomized controlled trials comparing these agents precludes the recommendation of any particular agent as the ideal one. At the Johns Hopkins Hospital, 5 percent morrhuate sodium is the agent routinely used.

Endoscopic Technique

As with any acute gastrointestinal (GI) hemorrhage, an attempt should be made to establish hemodynamic stability with fluid and blood product replacement and correction of any coagulopathies. Some authors have advocated a stabilization period prior to sclerotherapy after esophageal varices have been endoscopically established to be the source of bleeding. During this period, intravenous vasopressin and balloon tamponade may be used to control the bleeding. In addition, the patient's intravascular volume deficit, coagulopathy, or any other medical condition can be corrected. However, a study by Prindwille and Trudeau showed that lower rates of rebleeding, complications, and death from exsanguination were obtained if sclerotherapy was performed early. However, there was no difference in longevity.

It may be advisable to perform airway intubation in some patients to decrease the risk of aspiration and thereby have immediate airway access in the event of a cardiorespiratory problem.

Once esophageal varices have been established as the source of bleeding, the endoscope should first be used to suction the stomach to reduce gastric distention, patient discomfort, and the risk of aspiration. Intravariceal injection should be performed beginning at the level of the gastroesophageal junction. At this point, all columns are injected with a volume of 0.5 to 2 ml; the actual volume injected depends on the size of the varix, the end point being an apparent maximal distention of the varix. Care should be taken not to have the needle exposed unnecessarily except during injection of the sclerosing region. This reduces unnecessary trauma to the esophageal mucosa.

After all columns have been injected at the site of the gastroesophageal junction, the scope is withdrawn approximately 2 cm and the columns at this level are injected. This is repeated for every 2 cm until the full length of the variceal columns is treated. At each level the scope should be reintroduced into the stomach to suction blood and air.

TREATMENT OF ACTIVE BLEEDING

Treatment of patients who are actively bleeding, either spontaneously or as a result of sclerotherapy, is made difficult because of the inability to visualize the varices clearly. In patients who are hemodynamically stable, elevating the head of the bed slightly causes the blood to drain into the dependent stomach and therefore improves visualization. It is important that patients be carefully monitored while the head of the bed is elevated.

Once a bleeding point is identified, the injection should be made at about 1 to 2 cm just proximal to this site on the same column. In addition, paravariceal injections placed adjacent to the bleeding point may be helpful. If a bleeding point cannot be located, injection should begin at the gastroesophageal junction and be continued proximally. In actively bleeding patients, an infusion of vasopressin at the time of the procedure may assist in reducing blood flow and facilitate sclerotherapy.

A clot that is seen protruding from the varix should be treated in the same way as an actively bleeding spot.

TIMING OF SCLEROTHERAPY SESSIONS

There are no set time schedules in which repeat sclerotherapy sessions should be performed. The first 6 weeks after an initial bleed represent a high-risk period in which rebleeding may occur. During this phase, repeat endoscopy with or without sclerotherapy should be performed at frequent intervals, the intervals lengthening as the varices are obliterated. However, the urge to perform repeat sclerotherapy early after the initial bleed should be tempered with the knowledge that the maximal inflammatory response of the sclerotherapy may not be endoscopically apparent until 4 days after injection. Therefore, injecting the sclerosing agent into an area that does not endoscopically appear to be inflamed, but is undergoing an acute inflammatory process, increases the risk of hemorrhage and perforation. Often, at the time of endoscopy, one may encounter significant ulcerations with esophageal inflammation resulting from sclerotherapy. Sclerotherapy should be avoided at this time and be deferred until the inflammatory process has resolved. After the patient is clinically stable, subsequent treatments can be given on an outpatient basis.

The aim of long-term endoscopic injection therapy is the endoscopic obliteration of varices. The number of sessions may vary from patient to patient, but up to 13 may be required, for complete obliteration. At this point, the mucosa may appear irregular, and small irregular vessels that may represent vessel regeneration or remnants of the vaso vasorum of the varices may be seen. These small veins are not likely to bleed.

Even after endoscopically complete obliteration, patients should be followed endoscopically at 6-month to yearly intervals, because recurrence of varices has been noted.

OUTCOME OF SCLEROTHERAPY

Endoscopic sclerotherapy can effectively control acute GI bleeding in 75 to 90 percent of patients. Sclerotherapy reduces the blood transfusion requirements, but may not affect long-term survival.

Sclerotherapy is most commonly used to prevent recurrent variceal hemorrhage. Several clinical trials showed that it is more effective in reducing the rate of rebleeding than medical therapy or portocaval shunts.

Recent studies have shown no benefit from prophylactic sclerotherapy in patients who have not had variceal bleeding. In fact, the complications of sclerotherapy may increase the morbidity and mortality risks in patients who have never previously had variceal bleeding. A subgroup of patients may benefit from prophylactic sclerotherapy, but at present its use should be restricted to clinical trials.

COMPLICATIONS

Fortunately, the most common complications of esophageal variceal sclerotherapy are benign and self-limiting, but occasionally they can be life-threatening. (Table 1). Some authors state that complications may occur in up to 40 percent of patients. However, esophageal ulcerations have often been included in many studies as

TABLE 1 Complications of Sclerotherapy

Minor	*Major*
Chest pain	Perforation
Fever	Bleeding
Esophageal dysmotility	Necrosis of esophagus
Small pleural effusions	Acute respiratory distress
	Aspiration pneumonitis

a complication of esophageal variceal sclerotherapy. If endoscopy is performed early enough after variceal sclerotherapy, Singal and coworkers have shown that almost all patients will be found to have ulcerations. Therefore, ulceration alone should not be considered a complication, but more properly a side effect.

Major complications such as esophageal perforation and severe bleeding may occur in up to 3 percent of patients. Esophageal perforations after sclerotherapy usually have a more benign course than perforation from other causes. Most of these perforations are walled off and are usually discovered days or weeks after a procedure. The highest incidence of complications have been found with the use of the paravariceal injection technique.

Postinjection fever may occur in up to 50 percent of patients. It usually subsides within 48 hours and has not been associated with bacteremia. However, spiking temperatures or persistent fever may suggest a bacterial origin and should be investigated as such.

Substernal chest pain may also be noted in about 25 percent of patients. The pain is usually mild, and may be burning in nature and associated with odynophagia; it usually subsides in 48 to 72 hours and is probably related to esophageal spasm.

SUGGESTED READING

Ayres SJ, Goff JS, Warren GH. Endoscopic sclerotherapy for bleeding esophageal varices: effects and complications. Ann Intern Med 1983; 98:900–903.

Bornman PC, Kahn D, Terblanche J, et al. Rigid versus fiberoptic endoscopic injection sclerotherapy. A prospective randomized control trial in patients with bleeding esophageal varices. Ann Surg 1988; 208:175–178.

Cello JP, Grendell JH, Crass RA, et al. Endoscopic sclerotherapy versus portocaval shunt in patients with severe cirrhosis and variceal hemorrhage. N Engl J Med 1984; 311:1594–1600.

The Copenhagen Varices Sclerotherapy Projects. Sclerotherapy after first variceal hemorrhage in cirrhosis. N Engl J Med 1984; 311:1589–1594.

Galambos JT. Endoscopic sclerotherapy. Ann Intern Med 1983; 98:1009–1011.

Graham DY, Smith JL. The course of patients after variceal hemorrhage. Gastroenterology 1981; 80:800–809.

Gregory P, Hartigan P, Amodeo D, et al. Prophylactic sclerotherapy for esophageal varices in alcoholic liver disease: results of VA cooperative randomized trial. Gastroenterology 1987; 92:1414.

Prindwille T, Trudeau W. A comparison of immediate versus delayed endoscopic injection sclerosis of bleeding esophageal varices. Gastrointest Endosc 1986; 32:385–388.

Santangelo WC, Dueno ML, Estes BL, Krejs GJ. Prophylactic sclerotherapy of large esophageal varices. N Engl J Med 1988; 318:814–818.

Sarin SK, Nanda R, Sachda G, et al. Intravariceal versus paravariceal sclerotherapy: a prospective, controlled randomized trial. Gut 1987; 28:657–662.

Sauerbruch T, Wotza R, Kopchke W, et al. Prophylactic sclerotherapy before the first episode of variceal hemorrhage in patients with cirrhosis. N Engl J Med 1988; 319:8–15.

Singal AK, Sarin SK, Misra SP, Broar SL. Ulceration after esophageal and gastric variceal sclerotherapy. Influence of sucralfate and other factors on healing. Endoscopy 1988; 20:238–240.

Snady H. The role of sclerotherapy in the treatment of esophageal varices: personal experience and review of the randomized trials. Am J Gastroenterol 1987; 82:813–822.

Soehendra N, Deheer K, Kempeneers I, Frommelt L. Morphological alterations of the esophagus after endoscopic sclerotherapy of varices. Endoscopy 1983; 15:291–296.

Terblanche J, Bornman PC, Kain D, et al. Failure of repeated injections sclerotherapy to improve long-term survival after oesophageal variceal bleeding. A five-year prospective control clinical trial. Lancet 1983; 2:1328–1332.

HEPATORENAL SYNDROME AND ASCITES

GIORGIO LA VILLA, M.D.
PERE GINÈS, M.D.
VICENTE ARROYO, M.D.

ASCITES IN CIRRHOSIS

Ascites may develop as a consequence of several disorders, such as tuberculosis, neoplasms, congestive heart failure, nephrosis, and noncirrhotic liver diseases, but in most cases it indicates the presence of advanced cirrhosis. This chapter deals with the management of ascites in patients with cirrhosis of the liver. Treatment of noncirrhotic ascites and the differential diagnosis of ascites are not discussed.

In patients with cirrhosis, the onset of ascites indicates a severe impairment of systemic and splanchnic hemodynamics, secondary to sinusoidal portal hypertension. This leads to a reduction in effective arterial blood volume, probably as a consequence of a marked generalized splanchnic arterial vasodilation, and thus to arterial hypotension, overactivity of the renin-angiotensin-aldosterone and sympathetic nervous systems, nonosmotic hypersecretion of antidiuretic hormone (ADH), and alterations of renal function (sodium and water retention and functional renal failure [FRF], also called the hepatorenal syndrome).

It is not surprising, therefore, that the onset of ascites markedly worsens the prognosis of these patients. In a series of 139 cirrhotic patients admitted to our liver unit for the treatment of an episode of ascites, the survival rate was 62 percent, 56 percent, and 49 percent at 6, 12, and 24 months, respectively. The main causes of death were gastrointestinal (GI) bleeding and liver failure. In cirrhotic individuals with ascites, variables estimating systemic hemodynamics and renal function (portal pressure, mean arterial pressure, plasma renin activity, plasma norepinephrine concentration, glomerular filtration rate [GFR], and urinary sodium excretion) are better predictors of prognosis than those currently used to evaluate liver function.

Management of Ascites in Cirrhosis

Bed Rest and Low-Sodium Diet

In patients with cirrhosis and ascites, the assumption of upright posture is associated with a marked activation of the renin-angiotensin-aldosterone and sympathetic nervous systems and a reduction of GFR, sodium excretion, and the natriuretic response to intravenous furosemide. Therefore, bed rest may be of value in the treatment of ascites, especially in patients who do not respond satisfactorily to diuretics.

A low-sodium diet (40 mmol per day) is another useful measure to treat ascites. In about 20 percent of cirrhotic patients with ascites who spontaneously show a relatively high urinary sodium excretion, a reduction of sodium intake leads to the disappearance of ascites. Moreover, in the remaining patients, a negative sodium balance, which is the purpose of the medical treatment of ascites, is better achieved by reducing dietary sodium than by increasing the dosage of diuretics. An inadequate sodium restriction is a frequent cause of diuretic-resistant ascites. This should be suspected when body weight and ascites volume do not decrease despite an appropriate natriuresis. After the disappearance of ascites, a moderate to strict low-sodium diet is usually required in order to avoid fluid reaccumulation.

Diuretics

Loop diuretics, mainly furosemide, and distal diuretics, especially spironolactone, are the drugs most commonly used to treat patients with cirrhosis and ascites. Loop diuretics are the most effective diuretics available today. They interfere with the binding of chloride to a specific site on the Na:K:2Cl cotransport system located on the luminal surface of the ascending limb cells, thus inhibiting sodium uptake in this segment of the nephron where between 20 and 50 percent of filtered sodium is reabsorbed. Loop diuretics also increase renal prostaglandin synthesis. Prostaglandins are potent natriuretic compounds and are probably involved in the renal response to loop diuretics and spironolactone. As a consequence, the administration of nonsteroidal anti-inflammatory drugs (NSAIDs), which inhibit cyclo-oxygenase activity, impairs the renal response to these drugs.

Spironolactone and the other "distal" diuretics have a much lower natriuretic potency than loop diuretics. They can increase sodium excretion up to only 2 percent of the filtered sodium. Spironolactone antagonizes the sodium-retaining effects of aldosterone by competitively inhibiting its binding to a specific receptor protein in the cytoplasm of cortical and medullary collecting duct cells. The standard therapeutic dosage of spironolactone is 100 to 200 mg per day; however an even higher dosage, up to 500 mg per day, may be necessary in patients with very high plasma aldosterone levels.

Despite the extensive use of diuretics in the treatment of ascites during the last 30 years, few studies have been published analyzing the effectiveness of these drugs. The results of these investigations clearly indicate that, contrary to what might be expected on the basis of their respective natriuretic potency, spironolactone is more effective than loop diuretics. The administration of furosemide alone to nonazotemic cirrhotic patients with ascites resulted in an adequate natriuresis in about 50 percent of patients, whereas spironolactone was able to relieve ascites in more than 90 percent. Moreover, many patients not responding to furosemide were later found to respond to spironolactone. These apparently paradoxical results can be explained on the basis of the marked activity of the renin-angiotensin-aldosterone system that usually occurs in these patients. Since loop diuretics inhibit sodium reabsorption in the ascending limb of the loop of Henle, but not in the distal and collecting tubules, it is possible that most sodium escaping reabsorption in the loop of Henle is subsequently taken up along the collecting duct because of hyperaldosteronism. This is consistent with the observation that patients failing to respond to furosemide are those with the highest plasma aldosterone levels. The possibility that altered pharmacokinetics of furosemide may contribute to the reduced effectiveness of this drug has also been considered, but this has not been confirmed in most investigations. The diuretic treatment of ascites, therefore, should always include spironolactone. The simultaneous use of furosemide and spironolactone increases the natriuretic effectiveness of both agents, without major changes in plasma potassium levels. Therapy is usually started at low dosages (25 to 50 mg of furosemide and 100 mg of spironolactone per day). In patients not responding satisfactorily, the dosage is increased stepwise up to 150 mg per day of furosemide and 400 mg per day of spironolactone. Patients not showing an adequate natriuresis despite these high doses of diuretics should be considered as having diuretic-resistant ("refractory") ascites.

The response to diuretics in patients with cirrhosis and ascites can be predicted on the basis of renal function: the finding of a reduced GFR usually indicates that the patient will require high doses of diuretics or will not respond at all. This is probably due to changes in intrarenal sodium handling. In cirrhotic individuals with renal failure, sodium retention is mainly due to a decrease in filtered sodium load associated with increased proximal sodium reabsorption, thus leading to a reduced fluid delivery to the loop of Henle and distal nephron. Another mechanism contributing to the diuretic resistance of these patients may be a reduced access of drugs to their effective site as a consequence of the impaired renal perfusion.

Complications. The use of diuretics in cirrhosis with ascites is frequently associated with complications, the incidence of which has been reported to range between 11 and 71 percent, depending on the characteristics of the patients studied and the types and dosages of diuretics. Diuretic administration to edematous patients results in a net loss of body fluids. These fluids initially come from the intravascular compartment, leading to a decrease in circulating blood volume. In patients with peripheral edema, this is easily compensated by the passage of fluids from the interstitial to the intravascular compartment. However, this may not be the case in cirrhotic individuals in whom edema is localized within the abdominal cavity. In these patients the reabsorption of ascites has been shown to be a rate-limited process, ranging from 100 to 900 ml per day. Any fluid loss above this upper limit therefore results in a reduction of effective arterial blood volume and impaired renal perfusion.

Azotemia is one of the most frequent side effects of diuretics in cirrhosis with ascites. It is usually moderate and, contrary to spontaneous FRF, is always reversible after diuretic withdrawal. As expected, azotemia is less frequent in cirrhotic patients with ascites and peripheral edema than in those having only ascites. Hyponatremia is another common complication of diuretics in patients with cirrhosis and ascites. It is also related to diuretic-induced reduction in plasma volume, which triggers a baroreceptor-mediated hypersecretion of ADH, thus impairing renal water handling. The inhibition by loop diuretics of sodium reabsorption in the loop of Henle (a critical event in the generation of hypotonic urine) and a reduced fluid delivery to this segment of the nephron, caused by hypovolemia, may play a contributory role.

Diuretic treatment is generally considered a precipitating factor of hepatic encephalopathy. Proposed mechanisms for this condition are an increased renal production of ammonia and alterations in amino acid metabolism. Hyperkalemia is commonly observed when high-dose distal diuretics are given, especially in patients with renal impairment. Finally, spironolactone, because of its antiandrogenic activity, often leads to sexual disturbances, such as gynecomastia, impotence, and reduced libido.

Therapeutic Paracentesis

For many centuries, paracentesis was the only effective way to relieve ascites. However, it was abandoned after the introduction of modern diuretics because of some reports describing serious complications associated with this procedure. During the last 4 years three randomized controlled trials have been published reevaluating the usefulness of therapeutic paracentesis in the treatment of cirrhosis with ascites. This first trial compared therapeutic paracentesis plus intravenous albumin infusion with standard diuretic therapy in 117 patients with tense ascites and avid sodium retention who were admitted to several hospitals in the Barcelona area. Patients with severe liver impairment (hepatic encephalopathy, serum bilirubin over 10 mg per deciliter, and prothrombin activity less than 40 percent) or renal failure (serum creatinine over 3 mg per deciliter) were not included in the study. Fifty-eight patients were treated with large-volume paracentesis (4 to 6 L per day until the disappearance of ascites) plus intravenous human serum albumin (40 g per day); the remaining 59 patients received diuretics.

The results of this study, later confirmed by a similar trial performed in Milano, showed that (1) paracentesis was more effective than diuretics in eliminating ascites (96.5 percent versus 72.8 percent, respectively); (2) paracentesis plus intravenous albumin did not induce significant changes in hepatic and renal function, serum electrolyte levels, cardiac output, plasma volume, plasma renin activity, and plasma concentration of norepinephrine and ADH; (3) the incidence of hyponatremia, azotemia, and hepatic encephalopathy was remarkably lower in patients treated with paracentesis than in those receiving diuretics; (4) the duration of hospital stay and the cost of treatment were also lower in patients treated with paracentesis; and (5) no significant differences in the probability of readmission to the hospital during the follow-up, the causes of readmission, the probability of survival, and the causes of death were observed between the two groups of patients.

The third controlled trial, also performed by the Barcelona group, aimed to establish whether intravenous albumin should be administered to patients with ascites treated with paracentesis. The group treated with paracentesis without intravenous albumin (53 patients) showed a higher incidence of hyponatremia (17 percent versus 2 percent of the 52 patients receiving albumin) and renal impairment (11 percent versus 0 percent, respectively), together with a significant increase in blood urea nitrogen, plasma renin activity, and plasma aldosterone concentration; this indicates that paracentesis without intravenous albumin impairs systemic and renal hemodynamics.

Finally, a recent study has shown that total paracentesis (complete removal of ascites in a single paracentesis session) plus intravenous albumin (6 g per liter of ascites removed) is also a safe form of therapy for ascites in cirrhosis, thus suggesting that tense ascites in cirrhosis can be treated in a single-day hospitalization regimen. Therapeutic paracentesis plus intravenous albumin administration is therefore a rapid, effective, and safe therapy for ascites in patients with cirrhosis of the liver, and at present is probably the first-choice treatment for patients with tense ascites. Nevertheless, further studies are required to assess the role of therapeutic paracentesis in the management of patients with severe liver failure or renal impairment. The possible usefulness of other less expensive plasma expanders instead of human serum albumin should also be investigated.

Peritoneovenous Shunt

The LeVeen peritoneovenous shunt (PVS) consists of a perforated intra-abdominal tube connected through a one-way pressure-sensitive valve to a silicone tube that traverses the subcutaneous tissue up to the neck, where it enters one of the jugular veins (usually the internal jugular). The tip of the intravenous tube is positioned in the superior vena cava near the right atrium or the right atrium itself. When intraperitoneal pressure exceeds venous pressure by 3 to 5 cm H_2O, the valve opens and ascitic fluid flows into the vascular bed. Mobilization of ascitic fluid by PVS is thus associated with continuous expansion of the intravascular compartment. The Denver shunt, another commonly used PVS, has a valve system with a manual pumping mechanism. This valve opens at a lower pressure gradient than the LeVeen shunt, or when the pumping chamber is externally pressed. The Denver shunt was designed to create turbulence within the valve, thus reducing the likelihood of valve obstruction, frequently observed with the LeVeen shunt. However, the incidence of shunt obstruction with the Denver and LeVeen shunts is probably similar. PVS has been shown to relieve ascites while simultaneously correcting most of the hemodynamic and renal alterations occurring in these patients. PVS increases plasma volume and the cardiac index; reduces plasma renin activity and plasma levels of aldosterone, norepinephrine, and ADH; increases sodium excretion and free water clearance and improves renal function in patients with ascites and FRF. Furthermore, PVS markedly reduces portal pressure, as estimated by the hepatic venous pressure gradient. In most cases, these hemodynamic and hormonal changes persist as long as the shunt is patent.

Complications. Unfortunately, PVS is associated with a high rate of complications. Early complications include bacterial infection, coagulopathy, pulmonary edema, and GI bleeding. This high incidence, reported in the initial series of patients, has been now considerably reduced by adequate preventive measures, such as prophylactic antibiotics and removal of most ascitic fluid before PVS insertion. Nevertheless, PVS is still associated with a perioperative mortality rate ranging between 10 and 26 percent. At present, shunt obstruction is the most common complication of PVS, occurring in more than 30 percent of patients. Shunt failure may be observed in the early postoperative period, but it usually takes place several months later and can be due to deposition of fibrin within the valve or around the intravenous catheter, thrombosis of the venous limb of the prosthesis, or thrombosis of the superior vena cava or right atrium. Vascular thrombosis may result in pulmonary embolism.

Shunt obstruction is often followed by ascites reaccumulation. In these cases, Doppler ultrasonography or scintigraphy after the intraperitoneal injection of radioactive technetium (^{99m}Tc) will show the absence of flow through the shunt. When shunt obstruction is confirmed by these techniques, a shuntogram after the injection of contrast media into the proximal subcutaneous limb of the shunt should be performed in order to identify the site of obstruction. Patients with obstruction at the venous limb of the shunt usually require venography or digital angiography to rule out vascular thrombosis. Recent data suggest that the insertion of a 3-cm-long titanium tip into the venous limb of the LeVeen shunt is of value in preventing the development of superior vena cava thrombosis. A new heparin-coated Denver shunt has also been marketed with similar purposes. Peritoneal fibrosis, which may be followed by intestinal obstruction, is another late complication of PVS.

Despite the extensive use of PVS during the last 10 years, its role in the treatment of ascites is still unclear, owing to the small number of controlled trials comparing PVS with other treatments. Furthermore, a critical analysis of these studies is often difficult, since most of them have been published as abstracts and include a very small number of patients. Because of the high incidence of complications related to the shunt, most authors agree that PVS should be restricted to patients with refractory ascites. These patients, however, often have end-stage liver disease and an extremely poor prognosis, which cannot be modified by a successful treatment of ascites. In fact, an overall analysis of the three prospective randomized trials comparing PVS with conventional medical treatment in patients with refractory ascites does not disclose any benefit for PVS in terms of readmission to the hospital and survival. The role of PVS in the management of patients with FRF is also unclear; a beneficial effect of PVS has been observed in single cases, but the results obtained in the only two randomized trials published so far seem to indicate that PVS, although preventing the progression of FRF, does not improve the chances of survival.

Complications of Ascites and Their Management

Spontaneous Bacterial Peritonitis

Spontaneous bacterial peritonitis (SBP) is a frequent and severe complication of cirrhosis with ascites; it occurs in about 15 percent of hospitalized patients and carries a mortality rate of about 50 percent. The infection of ascitic fluid is usually due to enteric gram-negative aerobic bacteria of probable intestinal origin; however, in about 30 percent of cases other organisms, including gram-positive cocci, are the responsible agents. The pathogenesis of SBP has been recently clarified. The first step consists of the passage of bacteria from the intestinal lumen or an extra-intestinal infectious focus, such as the urinary tract, to the bloodstream. In healthy individuals, organisms reaching general circulation are rapidly cleared by the defensive mechanisms against infection. In patients with cirrhosis, however, these mechanisms are markedly impaired, because of depressed reticuloendothelial system phagocytic activity, impaired leukocyte function, and reduced serum complement and fibronectin levels, so that bacteremia frequently occurs. The second step is the colonization of ascitic fluid. This depends on the antibacterial activity of ascitic fluid, which varies markedly from one cirrhotic individual to another. The antibacterial activity of the ascitic fluid is related to the concentration of defensive factors, such as immunoglobulins, fibronectin, and complement, and can be easily assessed by measuring the total protein concentration in the ascitic fluid.

Diagnosis and Treatment. Since early diagnosis and prompt administration of antibiotics dramatically decrease mortality due to SBP, this condition should be recognized before the development of the classic signs of peritonitis. The occurrence of abdominal discomfort, fever, hepatic encephalopathy, renal failure, or an otherwise unexplained deterioration of the clinical status must prompt the attending physician to perform a diagnostic paracentesis. The presence of more than 500 polymorphonuclear leukocytes per milliliter in the ascitic fluid will confirm the diagnosis of SBP. Treatment should be started with an active drug against gram-positive cocci and enteric gram-negative organisms, until culture results are available. A third-generation cephalosporin, such as cefotaxime, is at present considered the first-choice antibiotic, since it has been shown to be more effective than the combination of ampicillin and tobramycin. Furthermore, third-generation cephalosporins are not nephrotoxic, while the incidence of aminoglycoside nephrotoxicity in cirrhotics with SBP is remarkably higher than in the general population.

Risk Factors. At present, three groups of cirrhotic patients with ascites have been recognized as having a high risk of developing SBP: (1) those with acute upper GI bleeding, (2) those with a history of a previous episode of SBP, and (3) those with a low total protein concentration in the ascitic fluid (less than 1 g per deciliter). In the first of these groups, oral administration of nonabsorbable antibiotics active against gram-negative aerobic bacteria has been proved to reduce the incidence of SBP significantly. The clinical value of selective intestinal decontamination in the other two groups of patients needs to be assessed in prospective controlled trials.

Hyponatremia

In patients with cirrhosis, ascites, and hyponatremia, total body sodium is increased, indicating that the reduced serum sodium concentration is due to a dilution of body fluids, because of an impaired water excretion. Treatment of hyponatremia should thus be directed toward a reduction of total body water. The classic treatment of dilutional hyponatremia in cirrhosis consists of water restriction. However, this is very difficult to accomplish and is rarely effective. Demeclocycline, a tetracycline that antagonizes the renal effects of ADH, corrects the impaired water excretion in these patients, yet frequently induces renal failure. Recent data from our laboratory have shown that in rats with carbon tetrachloride-induced cirrhosis, the administration of a drug that inhibits the binding of ADH to its renal (V_2) receptors normalizes the renal ability to excrete a water load. No antagonist of V_2 receptors, however, is at present available in humans.

Hepatorenal Syndrome

The hepatorenal syndrome (FRF of cirrhosis) is the most severe alteration of renal function that occurs in patients with cirrhosis and ascites. It is defined as the development of azotemia and oliguria in the absence of any known cause of renal failure. The kidneys are histologically normal, or show minimal changes, insufficient to justify the reduction of renal function. Retrospective studies indicate that FRF is present in more than 15 percent of patients with cirrhosis and ascites admitted to the hospital. FRF of cirrhosis is associated with a very poor prognosis.

This condition is secondary to an active renal vasoconstriction that impairs renal perfusion and GFR. Recent studies suggest that this phenomenon could be related to an inappropriately low renal synthesis of vasodilating prostaglandins in the presence of a marked activation of the renal vasoconstrictor systems.

Up to now, all attempts to improve renal function in patients with FRF of cirrhosis have been unsuccessful. The infusion of renal vasodilators, such as dopamine, produces a moderate increase in renal plasma flow, but does not modify GFR and sodium excretion. Linoleic acid, an essential fatty acid that is able to markedly increase renal prostaglandin synthesis in healthy individuals, was unable to modify urinary prostaglandin excretion and renal function when infused into patients with FRF. PVS may improve renal function and sodium excretion, but has no effect on survival. Patients with FRF should therefore be considered candidates for liver transplantation, although there may be a high postoperative mortality rate.

Approach to Patients With Cirrhosis and Ascites

At the Liver Unit in Barcelona, cirrhotic patients with mild to moderate ascites are treated on an outpatient basis. In these patients, the first therapeutic measure is the prescription of a low-sodium diet (40 mmol per day). We then obtain routine liver function tests; check BUN, serum creatinine, and serum and urinary electrolyte levels; and perform abdominal ultrasonography and diagnostic paracentesis. These investigations allow us to (1) confirm the diagnosis, since even in patients with known cirrhosis, ascites may be the expression of an unrelated disorder or the development of complications (e.g., hepatocellular carcinoma); (2) establish the prognosis; and (3) obtain data of therapeutic usefulness. Patients are also carefully interviewed about their use of NSAIDs. If sodium excretion is less than 40 mEq per day, or if body weight does not decrease with sodium restriction, spironolactone (100 mg per day) and furosemide (40 mg per day) are given. Patients are then reevaluated at a 5- to 7-day interval, and the dosage of diuretics is increased stepwise until a satisfactory diuretic response is achieved. After the disappearance of ascites, the dosage of diuretics is gradually reduced, depending on the individual ability to maintain sodium balance. Bed rest, which greatly reduces social and working life, is recommended only in patients requiring high-dose diuretics.

Patients with tense ascites are admitted to the hospital and treated with total paracentesis plus intravenous albumin. In these cases the use of diuretics, even if effective, is excessively expensive and time-consuming, since only about 500 ml of fluids can be safely mobilized every day. Paracentesis is performed in the left lower abdominal quadrant after local anesthesia and under strict sterile conditions. The needle used is a modification of the Kuss needle, which is a sharp-pointed blind metal needle inside a 7-cm long, 17-gauge metal, blunt-edged cannula with side holes. Once the needle enters the peritoneal cavity, the inner part is removed and ascites is mobilized with the aid of a large-volume capacity suction pump. The attending physician remains at the patient's bedside during the entire procedure, which takes about 1 hour. After ascites has been eliminated, the patient is given diuretics in order to avoid reaccumulation.

In practical terms, no patient with ascites is "resistant" to paracentesis; with this treatment, ascites can be considered "refractory" when it rapidly reaccumulates after each paracentesis session despite the administration of high-dose diuretics, so that the patient requires frequent readmissions to the hospital for the treatment of tense ascites. In this group of patients, PVS is the only available alternative to therapeutic paracentesis. A randomized, controlled trial is necessary to assess which of these two approaches is better.

Progressive FRF occurring in the setting of cirrhosis with ascites may be considered a terminal event. Since the prognosis for renal failure due to intrinsic renal disease is usually better than that for FRF, every effort should be made to achieve a correct diagnosis. In these patients, the relief of the offending condition, together with appropriate supportive measures, such as hemodialysis, can lead to a recovery of renal function. Renal failure in cirrhosis is often related to the use of diuretics, nephrotoxic antibiotics, and NSAIDs. All these drugs must be discontinued. Intravascular volume depletion due to bleeding or nonrenal fluid losses must also be carefully identified and corrected. Obstructive uropathy can be easily recognized by abdominal ultrasonography. When no known cause of renal failure is recognized, PVS or liver transplantation, if not contraindicated, are the last therapeutic resources, even though their clinical value is still unsettled.

Acknowledgment. This work was supported by grant PA86-0405 from the "Secretaría de Estado de Universidades e Investigación," Spain. Giorgio La Villa is a visiting investigator from the Clinica Medica II, University of Florence School of Medicine, Florence, Italy.

SUGGESTED READING

Epstein M, ed. The kidney in liver disease. 3rd ed. Baltimore: Williams & Wilkins, 1988.

Ginés P, Arroyo V, Quintero E, et al. Comparison of paracentesis and diuretics in the treatment of cirrhosis with tense ascites. Results of a randomized study. Gastroenterology 1987; 93:234–241.

Pérez-Ayuso RM, Arroyo V, Planas R, et al. Randomized comparative study of efficacy of furosemide versus spironolactone in nonazotemic cirrhosis with ascites. Gastroenterology 1984; 84:961–968.

Schrier RW, Arroyo V, Bernardi M, et al. Peripheral arterial vasodilation hypothesis: a proposal for the initiation of renal sodium and water retention in cirrhosis. Hepatology 1988; 8:1151–1157.

ACUTE HEPATITIS: MANAGEMENT AND PREVENTION

TALLEY PARKER, M.D.
EUGENE R. SCHIFF, M.D.

Patients with viral hepatitis are often anicteric, asymptomatic, and not brought to the attention of a physician. Therefore, patients who do present for medical care tend to be more sick and are frequently icteric. The physician must establish the diagnosis of viral hepatitis, determine the severity of the illness, render the appropriate treatment, and initiate prophylactic measures for the patient's family and contacts.

DIAGNOSIS

Initial evaluation is aimed at determining the severity of the illness and its etiology. A decision has to be made whether to hospitalize the patient for intensive support. The history, physical findings, and standard liver chemistries will quickly characterize the nature of the hepatobiliary disorder.

Most patients with viral hepatitis have a suggestive epidemiologic background. The typical prodrome is one of a flu-like illness followed by anorexia, nausea, vomiting, dark urine, light stools, and jaundice. Right upper quadrant pain is minimal but rarely may be severe. Pruritus is more prominent if a cholestatic phase evolves.

On physical examination, particular attention should be paid to mental status, signs of chronic liver disease, and the presence of ascites or peripheral edema and hepatosplenomegaly. Tattoos or "tracks" associated with parenteral drug abuse are sought. Kayser-Fleischer rings or dysarthria are indicative of Wilson's disease.

The liver profile conforms to a hepatitis-like picture with striking elevation, more than 1,000 IU, of the aminotransferase levels. The white blood cell count is normal or slightly depressed with a relative lymphocytosis, and the prothrombin time is 0 to 2 seconds greater than controls. The best indicators of severity are prothrombin time greater than 3 seconds over controls, a bilirubin level greater than 20 mg per deciliter, and leukocytosis. Hypoglycemia and renal insufficiency are particularly ominous.

There are at least five hepatitis viruses: types A, B, delta (D), C (and possibly another non-A, non-B), and E (epidemic non-A enteric hepatitis). Consideration of the mode of transmission of each of these viruses facilitates the history taking. Type A is almost exclusively transmitted by fecal-oral routes; types B and D sexually, parenterally and perinatally; type C parenterally and possibly sexually; and type E by fecal-oral routes outside the United States. Serologic tests are commercially available for types A, B, and D and establish the diagnosis of viral hepatitis. A blood sample should be sent for IgM anti-HAV, HBsAg, and IgM anti-HBc. Depending on the results, additional serologic parameters may be necessary. Table 1 describes the serologic patterns of acute hepatitis A, B, and D and the serologic patterns in immunity to hepatitis A or B.

Once the type of hepatitis is established, prophylactic measures should be initiated and the health department notified; this is a reportable disease. In the absence of a serologic diagnosis, acute non-A, non-B (?C) hepatitis is a possibility, but other viral and nonviral illnesses must be considered. Epstein-Barr virus (EBV) and cytomegalovirus (CMV) infections can be associated with a clinical picture of hepatitis. The presence of a high serum gamma globulin and antinuclear antibodies should raise the suspicion of chronic active autoimmune hepatitis presenting as acute hepatitis. In such patients a liver biopsy should be performed to establish the diagnosis before treatment with corticosteroids. Delay in the recognition of this entity presenting as acute hepatitis can be tragic. Drug-induced hepatitis (e.g., from isoniazid or halothane) can mimic viral hepatitis clinically and histologically. Other conditions to be considered in the differential diagnosis are toxic hepatitis, Wilson's disease, ischemia or hypotensive liver injury, hepatic vein thrombosis, biliary tract disease, and sepsis. If drug-induced hepatitis is considered, the physician should ask family members or roommates to bring in every medicine, both prescribed and over-the-counter, that can be found in the patient's home.

If any of the initial tests indicate severe hepatic failure, additional diagnostic work-ups should be initiated immediately and tailored to the patient's particular presentation. Young patients should be evaluated for Wilson's disease (serum copper and ceruloplasmin, 24-hour urine for copper, and slit-lamp examination for Kayser-Fleischer rings), and autoimmune hepatitis (antinuclear antibodies, anti-smooth muscle antibodies, and quantitative serum immunoglobulin levels), and a toxicology screen should be sent. In the presence of ascites or an enlarged painful liver, the Budd-Chiari syndrome should be considered. Reye's syndrome is most often seen in young patients who show evidence of hepatic failure without markedly elevated transaminase levels. When abdominal pain is prominent, ultrasonography or computed tomography (CT) may be indicated. Cases of necrosing hepatic tumors with high aminotransferase levels have been misdiagnosed as viral hepatitis. Doppler ultrasonography has proved very useful to rule out portal and hepatic vein thrombosis. Once hepatitis B has been diagnosed, superimposition or co-infection with delta virus is a possibility, and delta antibody should be sent.

TREATMENT

Most patients with viral hepatitis have an uncomplicated course characterized by fatigue, anorexia, nausea, and often jaundice but do not require hospitalization, and the infection resolves without sequelae. Some patients, with an otherwise uncomplicated course, may require

TABLE 1 Serologic Patterns of Acute Hepatitis

Acute Hepatitis	*IgM Anti-HAV*	*Anti-HAV*	*HBsAg*	*IgM Anti-HBc*	*Anti-HBc*	*Anti-HBs*	*Anti-delta*
Acute hepatitis A	+	+	−	−	−	−	−
Acute hepatitis B	−	−	+	+	+	−	−
Acute hepatitis B	−	−	−	+	+	−	−
Acute hepatitis B with delta coinfection	−	−	+	+	+	−	+
Chronic hepatitis B with delta superinfection	−	−	+	−	+	−	+
Chronic hepatitis B with reactivation	−	−	+	+/−	+	−	−
Acute non-A, non-B or another etiology	−	−	−	−	−	−	−
Immune Status							
To hepatitis A	−	+	−	−	−	−	−
To hepatitis B	−	−	−	−	+	+	−

hospitalization because of lack of support at home (someone to cook, perform necessary tasks, and observe the patient for changes in mental status). Others require hospitalization for intravenous therapy, for nutrition, and to correct volume depletion secondary to intractable vomiting. At this point patients should be closely observed for signs for worsening mental status, hypoglycemia, coagulopathy, volume depletion, or renal insufficiency. Once it is apparent that there is fulminant hepatic failure, plans for possible liver transplantation should be made. Elderly patients and those with other significant medical problems should be hospitalized.

CARE OF THE HOSPITALIZED PATIENT

There is little new in the specific treatment of acute hepatitis. Antiviral therapy remains investigational. Care is supportive with emphasis on volume repletion, maintenance of adequate calorie intake, rest, and close observation for progression to subacute fulminant or fulminant hepatitis.

Diet

Patients with hepatitis are anorectic and have altered dietary preferences, often favoring "junk" foods and colas. Dietary restriction should not be imposed and intake should supply at least 4 g of glucose per kilogram of body weight. Patients requiring hospitalization because of severe hepatitis or impending fulminant failure are treated with a 10 percent glucose infusion. Blood sugar is checked by fingerstick every 6 hours. Hypoglycemia may be profound, necessitating hyperalimentation via a central venous catheter with a 25 percent dextrose infusion. If encephalopathy is present, hepatic formula with a high percentage of branched chain amino acids may be helpful, although the efficacy of modified amino acid supplements in acute hepatitis has not been adequately studied. Patients who have difficulty consuming adequate calories are fed liquid supplements high in branched chain amino acids. In general, patients tolerate frequent small feedings better than three large meals a day. Some patients are able to consume more calories at breakfast than at other meals.

Activity

The fatigue associated with acute hepatitis naturally limits patients' activities, but those who feel well enough to ambulate and perform their usual activities should be permitted to do so. Early ambulation is no longer thought to be detrimental, although previously believed to increase the frequency of relapse. The optimal time for return to work will depend on the level of fatigue, the presence of other symptoms, and the degree of jaundice.

Treatment

No antiviral drugs have been licensed for use in acute viral hepatitis, although many have been tested including ribavirin, cyanidanol, acyclovir, anti-HBs hyperimmune globulin, and alpha-interferon. Of these, perhaps the most promising is alpha-interferon.* An effective antiviral drug is ideally used in cases of acute viral hepatitis in an attempt to shorten the course and ameliorate the severity of the illness. There is no place for corticosteroids in the treatment of "garden variety" or fulminant viral hepatitis. However, corticosteroids may hasten the resolution of cholestatic hepatitis A (prednisone, 40 mg per day for 4 days with tapering over 2 weeks). The use of steroids in cholestatic type B or non-A, non-B hepatitis cannot be advocated because of their potential for enhancing the evolution into chronic hepatitis.

Therapy is directed at correcting the various manifestations and symptoms of acute hepatitis. The patient is observed closely for signs of encephalopathy. If encephalopathy is detected, lactulose should be prescribed, 30 ml every 6 hours with the dosage adjusted to achieve two to three soft stools per day. If the patient is unable to take therapeutic doses of lactulose by mouth and there is no evidence of renal failure, neomycin can be added, 500 mg orally every 8 hours, or the lactulose can be given by enema (300 ml lactulose and 700 ml water as a retention enema).

Hypoprothrombinemia is treated with vitamin K, 10 mg per day subcutaneously for 3 days, and is particularly efficacious in cholestatic patients. Fresh frozen plasma should be given only if patients are bleeding. H_2 blockers reduce the risk of gastrointestinal (GI) bleeding in severely ill patients. Ascites may develop, but paracentesis should be reserved for those with respiratory distress or marked abdominal distention.

For moderate ascites, low doses of spironolactone or furosemide can be given with close monitoring of electrolytes, BUN, and creatinine. Nausea and vomiting are common and impair adequate calorie intake. Effective treatment includes metoclopramide, 10 mg intravenously or intramuscularly before meals. Phenothiazines should be avoided. Pruritus can be treated with hydroxyzine, 50 mg every 6 hours. Cholestyramine may be used and is effective, but is frequently not well tolerated. Severe abdominal pain due to hepatomegaly and stretching of Glisson's capsule is uncommon but may require meperidine. Symptomatic fever can be treated with acetaminophen (total dosage less than 2.5 g per day). Salicylates are contraindicated because of their tendency to precipitate bleeding. Hypnotics should be avoided, but if sedation is necessary, oxazepam is preferred.

Evaluation

Outpatients should have complete blood count (CBC), prothrombin time, aminotransferases, bilirubin, serum electrolytes, BUN, and creatinine checked twice weekly. As the hepatitis resolves, testing can be done less frequent-

---

***Editor's Note**: Additional information on the use of interferon for hepatitis should be available in the near future.

ly; monitoring should continue until values return to normal or chronic hepatitis is established. If chronic hepatitis is suspected at 6 months, liver biopsy is considered. After the initial serologic diagnosis is made, patients with hepatitis B should undergo serial testing of HBsAg. Seroconversion to anti-HBs may take as long as 6 months.

PREVENTION AND PROPHYLAXIS

Safe and effective prophylactic measures are now available for viral hepatitis.

Hepatitis A

Household and intimate contacts should be given standard immune globulin (IG) as soon as possible (2 milliliters intramuscularly in adults; 0.02 ml per kilogram in children). The percentage of susceptible persons is high in the U.S., and determination of anti-HAV before administration of IG only serves to delay prophylaxis. Family members and housemates should be advised against sharing food or utensils; disposable utensils are recommended. Strict handwashing should be observed and intimate contact avoided for 2 weeks. If the index case is a child who attends a day care facility or has siblings who do so, all day care employees and other children attending should receive IG. In the case of a common source outbreak, all those exposed should receive IG, but often it may be too late. No licensed active HAV vaccines are available, but heat inactivated, attenuated, and recombinant prototypes are being studied. Once available, universal vaccination is anticipated, particularly in underdeveloped countries. Recommendations for travelers to Central and South America, North Africa, and the Middle East are for prophylaxis with IG, 0.06 ml per kilogram intramuscularly every 4 to 6 months or 0.02 ml per kilogram once if traveling for less than 3 months.

Hepatitis B

There are now safe and effective vaccines for active immunization against hepatitis B, which ideally would be given universally if the cost were not prohibitive. Certain groups at high risk of exposure should receive pre-exposure vaccination regardless of cost: health care workers exposed to human blood, secretions, and tissue, as well as those who handle hospital waste; intimate and household contacts of HBV carriers; hemodialysis patients; recipients of frequent blood products; the institutionalized mentally impaired and the staff who care for them; homosexually active men; and parenteral drug abusers. Serologic screening for susceptibility to hepatitis B with anti-HBs or anti-HBc is controversial. The significance of isolated low titer anti-HBs or anti-HBc in persons at moderate risk of exposure is not clear. Therefore, it is most reasonable to reserve pre-vaccination screening for those at highest risk: spouses of chronic HBV carriers, persons who have received many transfusions, male homosexuals, parenteral drug abusers, and the institutionalized mentally retarded. The recommended screening parameter is anti-HBs. The vaccine should be given if the titer of anti-HBs is less than 10 (S/N—sample to negative cutoff ratio) or mIU per milliliter. Others who might be considered for

TABLE 2 CDC Recommendations for Postexposure Immunoprophylaxis

Source	*Exposed Person Unvaccinated*	*Exposed Person Vaccinated*
Parental: Known HBsAg (plus)	One dose of HBIG 0.06 ml/kg immediately Initiate hepatitis B vaccine series	Test exposed person for anti-HBs. If inadequate antibody (less than 10 sample ratio units by radioimmunoassay or negative by EIA), give one dose of HBIG immediately plus hepatitis B vaccine booster dose
Known source high risk of HBsAg (plus)	Initiate hepatitis B vaccine series Test source for HBsAg; if positive, give one dose of HBIG immediately	Test source for HBsAg only if exposed person is vaccine nonresponder; if soure is HBsAg positive, give one dose of HTSIG immediately plus hepatitis B vaccine booster dose
Known source* low risk of HBsAg (plus)	Initiate hepatitis B vaccine series Consider IG 0.06 ml/kg†	Consider IG 0.06 ml/kg†
Unknown source†	Initiate hepatitis B vaccine series Consider IG 0.06 ml/kg†	Consider IG 0.06 ml/kg†
Sexual‡ Known HBsAg (+)	HBIG 0.06 ml/kg IM, single dose within 14 days of exposure	Test exposed person for anti-HBs. If inadequate antibody, treat as if unvaccinated
Perinatal HBsAg (+) mother	HBIG 0.5 ml IM and vaccine series, 0.5 ml within 12 hours of birth and repeat at 1 and 6 months	N/A

* Authors recommend testing source even though less cost effective; if HBsAg (+), give HBIG rather than IG.
† Authors recommend.
‡ Vaccine is recommended for homosexual men and regular sexual contacts of HBV carriers, and is optional for heterosexual contacts of persons with acute HBV.

vaccination are inmates of long-term correctional facilities, heterosexually active persons with multiple partners, and travelers to endemic areas.

The practicing physician is most frequently confronted with questions about postexposure prophylaxis. Typically, a spouse or sexual partner has been diagnosed with acute or chronic hepatitis B, or a health care worker has had accidental needlestick exposure. Because it will be several months before protective levels of antibody can be achieved after the initial vaccination, hyperimmune hepatitis B globulin (HBIG) should be given with the vaccine (using separate syringes and separate injection sites) to provide passive immunity until active immunity develops. Both initial vaccination and HBIG should be given within 48 hours of exposure if possible. In the case of acute hepatitis B, the spouse or sexual partner should be given vaccine and HBIG without waiting for results of anti-HBs, because the likelihood of long-term previous exposure and natural immunization is low. If HBIG is given without active vaccination, it should be repeated in 1 month. Isolated sexual exposure may be treated with a single dose of HBIG within 14 days, according to Centers for Disease Control (CDC) recommendations.

It is now recommended by CDC that all pregnant women be screened early in prenatal care for HBsAg. If HBsAg is positive, liver tests including AST, ALT, alkaline phosphatase, and bilirubin should be performed and prothrombin time checked to assess for active hepatitis. At birth, the infant receives HBIG 0.5 ml intramuscularly and 0.5 ml of vaccine within 12 hours; active vaccination is repeated at 1 and 6 months as with adult vaccination.

Table 2 lists CDC recommendations for postexposure immunoprophylaxis. Some authors have recommended screening for anti-HBs 1 month after vaccination is completed to assess the immune status. Long-term booster vaccinations may be necessary for those with continued exposure.

Both recombinant hepatitis B vaccines and the first-generation plasma-derived vaccine have been shown to be effective in most recipients unless factors such as obesity, immunosuppression, or use of an improper injection site are present. Failure to respond to active vaccination increases with age. Patients with these risk factors should be checked for anti-HBs on a regular long-term basis and should receive a booster vaccine if anti-HBs S/N is less than 10. It is noteworthy that neither vaccine nor IG preparations have ever been demonstrated to transmit HIV infection.

SUGGESTED READING

Centers for Disease Control. Update on hepatitis B prevention. Recommendations for the Immunization Practices Advisory Committee. Ann Intern Med 1978; 107:353–357.

Centers for Disease Control. Prevention of perinatal transmission of hepatitis B virus; prenatal screening of all pregnant women for hepatitis B surface antigen. MMWR 1988; 37:341–351.

Koff RS, Galambos JT. Viral hepatitis. In: Schiff L, Schiff ER, eds. Diseases of the liver, 6th ed. Philadelphia: JB Lippincott, 1987:457–581.

Schiff E. Immunoprophylaxis of viral hepatitis: a practical guide. Am J Gastroenterol 1987; 82:287–291.

FULMINANT HEPATIC FAILURE

DANIEL F. SCHAFER, M.D.
JEREMIAH P. DONOVAN, M.D.

Treating a patient with an acutely failing liver is among the most challenging tasks in clinical medicine. Even with the best of supportive care, only 5 to 30 percent of such patients can be expected to survive. Liver transplantation appears to be the only therapy currently available that may significantly change this grim prognosis. This chapter outlines the elements of the best supportive care. Also, the anticipation, recognition, and treatment of complications are stressed and suggestions are made as to the role of the referring physician in hepatic transplantation.

CLINICAL FEATURES

Etiology

Viruses, drugs, and toxins all regularly contribute to fulminant hepatic failure. Inherited diseases such as Wilson's disease and tyrosinemia affect children and infants, whereas vascular causes such as heat stroke, shock, and pericarditis are usually restricted to adults. In all age groups there is a certain number of patients in whom no cause can be ascertained. Such patients are usually regarded as having non-A, non-B hepatitis, but might be classified more correctly as indeterminate.

Determining the etiology of fulminant hepatic failure is important because it may influence survival. No patient with fulminant Wilson's disease is known to have survived without transplantation. On the other end of the scale is acetaminophen toxicity; in a recently reported large series, more than half of the patients with acetaminophen toxicity have survived with good supportive care. Our own experience reflects this relatively more optimistic prognosis for patients with acetaminophen-induced fulminant hepatic failure. During the last 2 years, we have seen five such patients in a grade III or IV coma, all of whom survived without transplantation. This contrasts sharply with our experience with patients with virus-induced disease, all of whom either required transplantation or died before a transplant could be performed.

Liver Biopsy

Because the etiology of fulminant hepatic failure has prognostic significance, it should be investigated by history and laboratory screening for types A and B hepatitis viruses, serum copper level, and drug levels, including acetaminophen. Often, the cause of fulminant hepatic failure is not immediately obvious, and therefore some consideration is given to the usefulness of biopsy. The low probability that histologic findings will contribute to therapeutic decisions, combined with the risk of performing this procedure in a patient with coagulopathy, has led us to reject diagnostic percutaneous biopsy in almost all patients. Transvenous biopsies have been touted as a method by which liver tissue can be safely obtained for diagnostic and prognostic purposes. Unfortunately, the samples are usually small and may be insufficient for making judgments about the degree of hepatic regeneration. We prefer serial ultrasonic determinations of liver size for this purpose.

Coagulopathy

The failure of the damaged liver to synthesize clotting factors results in a progressive coagulopathy. In the presence of adequate vitamin K, the prolongation of the prothrombin time is related to the severity of the hepatic lesion. Thrombocytopenia is also a common finding in fulminant hepatic failure and may be due to marrow failure, increased consumption, or both. It is probable that clotting factors with short half-lives, such as factor VII, are the first factors to decrease to critically low levels. In some centers, the measurement of individual clotting factors, such as factor V, is used for prognostic significance. If panels of clotting studies are performed, they sometimes suggest that patients with fulminant hepatic failure have disseminated intravascular coagulation. This is not an indication for heparin therapy. It is a common observation that patients may present with abnormal clotting studies and yet have no physical signs of hemorrhage. This is a grace period and not a pardon. At the least provocation, such patients can and will hemorrhage massively.

Attempts at Correction

Should attempts be made to correct the coagulopathy of fulminant hepatic failure? In certain situations, the answer is yes. As a general rule, it is not profitable to attempt this prophylactically. Large volume loads are not well tolerated in patients at risk for adult respiratory distress syndrome, renal insufficiency, ascites, pleural effusions, and cerebral edema. However, if the patient is actively bleeding, or if correction is needed for the performance of some procedure such as the placement of an epidural pressure monitor, the administration of platelets and fresh frozen plasma is helpful. The volume status of patients with renal failure may preclude the administration of several units of plasma. Recently, the combination of fresh frozen plasma and exchange plasmapheresis has been used to help correct the clotting state of such patients.

Vitamin K

Patients with fulminant hepatic failure should receive at least three daily doses of 10 mg of vitamin K. Some authors recommend that this drug be given intravenously rather than intramuscularly to avoid bleeding. Unfortunately, intravenous vitamin K may precipitate shock. Therefore, reasoning that bruises are easier to care for than shock, we prefer the shots.

Gastrointestinal Hemorrhage

Gastrointestinal hemorrhage deserves special mention because of its frequency. Over 50 percent of patients with fulminant hepatic failure develop upper gastrointestinal bleeding if not given prophylaxis with an H_2 antagonist. Controlled trials have shown that patients treated in this manner require fewer units of blood. We give sufficient medication to maintain the pH of gastric fluid above 5.0. Reduced dosages are required for patients with renal failure. Antacids may cause electrolyte disturbances and may not be as effective. No studies using sucralfate have been reported, but the use of this agent in patients with endoscopically verified gastritis seems justified. If hemorrhage occurs despite prophylaxis, patients are treated according to standard regimens of endoscopic diagnosis and therapy.

Neurologic Complications

The neurologic complications of fulminant hepatic failure can be divided into metabolic and structural causes. The metabolic causes of neurologic deterioration include hypoglycemia, electrolyte imbalance, drugs, and hepatic coma. The structural causes include intracranial hemorrhage and cerebral edema. Accurate diagnosis of the etiology of altered mental status in these patients is vital for therapeutic and prognostic reasons.

By definition, all patients with fulminant hepatic failure have an altered mental status that can be attributed to their liver disease. This syndrome, hepatic encephalopathy, may differ in acute and chronic liver disease. Clinically, the most important definable feature is the excited delirium that may precede coma in acute cases. This may present as a paranoid psychosis that makes medical management difficult. The temptation is to treat this phase of the illness with sedatives or tranquilizing drugs. If at all possible, this should not be done. Because the natural history of the syndrome is for the patient to become progressively obtunded, all one has to do is apply physical restraint until coma supervenes. A quiet environment and a minimum of stimulation also helps to calm such patients.

Coma

Once the patient lapses into coma, simple bedside tests of mental function such as the Glasgow Coma Score can be used to monitor neurologic function. We have provided such a scale in Table 1. This scale does not contain tests of oculovestibular or oculocephalic function. These tests require movement of the head which, when sudden, can have dramatic effects on intracranial pressure (ICP). Therefore, despite the undoubted prognostic significance of these tests, we do not advocate their use. We also recommend an electroencephalogram (EEG) and a computed tomographic (CT) scan as early as possible. These will be useful for comparative purposes if other neurologic problems develop. Treatment of the coma is a controversial area. There is no good evidence that lactulose, neomycin, or other agents alter the course of fulminant hepatic failure, where survival depends more on the recovery of the liver than on the level of consciousness. Also, some transplant surgeons prefer that lactulose not be given to patients because of the large amount of gas that forms in the colon.

Cerebral Edema

Cerebral edema is a regular consequence of fulminant hepatic failure and a leading cause of death. The problem of cerebral edema is twofold: recognition and treatment. If monitoring of ICP is not performed directly, one must rely on physical and radiologic signs to assess the probability that a rapid change in neurologic function is the result of increased ICP. Patients who develop focal neurologic abnormalities (anisocoria, decerebrate posturing, abnormal oculovestibular reflexes, myoclonus) are at definite risk, as are patients who develop seizures. CT may reveal loss of gray-white matter definition, a sign of cerebral edema which is preceded by pressure increases.

TABLE 1 Bedside Coma Profile

Verbal ability	Motor response
None	None
Incomprehensible	Abnormal extensor
Normal	Abnormal flexor
	Withdrawal
Eye opening	Pattern of respiration
None	None (ventilated)
To painful stimuli only	Irregular
To noise	Regular >22/min
Spontaneous	Regular <22/min
Pupillary light reflex	Deep tendon reflexes
Absent	Absent
Present	Increased
	Normal or decreased
Corneal reflex	Skeletal muscle tone
Absent	None (flaccid)
Present	Abnormal
	Normal
Spontaneous eye movements	
None	
Dysconjugate	
Roving conjugate	
Orienting	

Intracranial Pressure Measurement

ICP can be measured directly by a number of methods, including both subdural and epidural pressure sensors. All of these require surgical placement with attendant risk of hemorrhage. We believe that for epidural monitors to be used most safely, they must be placed by a neurosurgeon in the operating room where the maximal control of a possibly delirious patient can be attained. Placement of monitors in the intensive care unit reduces this control. An important result of pressure monitoring is the added information used to make the decision not to perform a transplant. Prolonged periods of intracranial hypertension have been associated with patients who survive transplant surgery but do not recover neurologically. Finally, ICP monitoring assists anesthesiologists with volume and blood pressure control during surgery. Timing of the placement of the monitor is an important consideration. If the patient is a transplant candidate, this procedure should probably be performed at the transplant center. If the patient is not a transplant candidate, the onset of stage III coma might be an appropriate time, but there is too little information on this point to be dogmatic. In general, such maneuvers should probably not be attempted by teams of physicians who are inexperienced in the care of patients with hepatic failure.

Management of Cerebral Edema

Once cerebral edema is strongly suspected or confirmed, a series of therapies can be instituted. These include elevation of the head to at least 30 degrees (reverse Trendelenburg) and hyperventilation to a P_{CO_2} of 30 mm Hg. Positive end-expiratory pressure should be avoided because it directly raises ICP. Next, mannitol can be given in a dose of up to 1 g per kilogram by intravenous bolus. This should not be done in patients with renal failure or in those whose measured serum osmolality is greater than 315 mOsm. Repeated doses should not be given without evidence of a good diuretic response or before repeating a measurement of serum osmolality. Decreasing mean arterial pressure will reduce ICP. Unfortunately, this may also reduce cerebral perfusion pressure (CPP). The CPP is obtained by subtracting the ICP from the mean arterial pressure. The CPP should not be allowed to fall below 60 mm Hg. As a goal, the ICP should be maintained below 25 mm Hg and ideally below 20 mm Hg. If a patient is stable or improving and an abrupt increase in ICP occurs, a repeat CT scan should be performed to look for structural lesions.

Renal Failure

Renal failure is known to occur from several causes in fulminant hepatic failure. These include acute tubular necrosis, hepatorenal syndrome, and glomerulonephritis. Renal failure of any cause worsens the prognosis of fulminant hepatic failure.

Tests of renal function are not reliable in the face of liver failure. The liver is the major site of urea production in the body, and the blood urea nitrogen is often low in patients presenting with fulminant hepatic failure. Also, the serum creatinine may be falsely decreased as a result of increased tubular secretion of creatinine. Therefore, the actual renal function of most patients with fulminant hepatic failure is probably worse than one might expect from routine studies.

Dialysis

Regardless of the cause of renal insufficiency, dialysis must be considered. Renal physicians may be reluctant to provide this service for patients with hepatic failure because of cardiovascular instability and coagulopathy. These are valid concerns, and the goal of the dialysis must be clearly defined. Because symptomatic uremia is rarely a problem in fulminant hepatic failure, the reasons for intervention are usually hyperkalemia or volume overload. This is a special problem in patients with increasing ICP. Ultrafiltration rather than routine dialysis should be considered. Venous access is optimal through a double-lumen tube in the subclavian vein. If femoral vessels are used, we prefer the right side, since this preserves the left vessels for venovenous bypass during transplantation. The use of heparin during dialysis significantly increases the risk of major hemorrhage. Heparin-free dialysis is the preferred method in these patients. We do not expect dialysis to have any influence on the course of functional renal failure (hepatorenal syndrome). This is reversed by transplantation. The goal of the dialysis is temporization.

Ventilation

Hyperventilation is a hallmark of early fulminant hepatic failure. This is not pernicious and no attempt should be made to correct it. As the patient slips into deeper stages of coma, cough reflexes diminish and the patient becomes progressively unable to protect his airway. This threat is compounded by ileus and delayed gastric emptying. In order to prevent repeated aspiration, the stomach should be decompressed with a nasogastric tube connected to low suction. Also, the patient should be placed in reverse Trendelenburg position. We routinely intubate all patients in grade III coma. Whenever possible this should be done by the oral endotracheal route with a tube large enough to permit bronchoscopy (7.5 F or larger). Intubation not only helps prevent aspiration, but also permits ventilator support to decrease the work of breathing and improve pulmonary toilet. As discussed below, mechanical hyperventilation assists in the management of increased ICP. Surgical tracheostomy is discouraged.

Hypoglycemia

Loss of hepatocellular function deprives the body of most gluconeogenic and glycolytic capability. Thus, hypoglycemia can occur at any time during the course of fulminant hepatic failure. The amount of glucose required to insure euglycemia in these patients is almost always 300 g per day in adults. Some patients may require a good deal more; it has been reported that one patient had a daily requirement of 2,000 g. This amount of glucose cannot be safely administered through a peripheral vein. To avoid volume overload, a 20 percent solution of glucose must be supplied centrally. Either the subclavian or the jugular route is preferred over femoral or "cut-down" sites.

The institution of glucose therapy should mark an increase in the frequency of glucose monitoring. Every 2 hours is not too often to monitor glucose. Maintenance of blood glucose between 60 and 200 mg per deciliter is a reasonable goal for therapy.

Electrolyte Imbalances

Every sort of electrolyte imbalance has been reported in patients with fulminant hepatic failure. As a rule of thumb it is best not to overtreat these disturbances.

Hyponatremia is usually due to a combination of altered free-water clearance and fluid treatment. Total body sodium is normal to increased in fulminant hepatic failure. Hypernatremia is usually iatrogenic. Sudden changes in sodium concentrations, whether by intravenous therapy or by dialysis, should be avoided, since these are causally associated with central pontine myelinolysis, an irreversible and preventable catastrophe.

Potassium balance in fulminant hepatic failure is altered by several factors, including renal wasting, vomiting, nasogastric suction, and diuretic therapy. We are careful not to begin treatment of hypokalemia until the serum potassium falls below 2.5 mEq per deciliter, and if treatment is required, the level is not raised above 4.0 mEq per deciliter. This is especially true when acidosis or renal failure is present. If transplantation remains an option for the patient, this point must be stressed, since life-threatening hyperkalemia may occur during graft reperfusion.

Hypocalcemia and hypomagnesemia have been reported in fulminant hepatic failure, and periodic monitoring is advisable.

Cardiac Complications

Hypotension (systolic blood pressure of less than 80 mm Hg) occurs in most cases of fulminant hepatic failure. The causes of the hypotension include hemorrhage, sepsis, arrhythmias, respiratory failure, and probably liver failure itself. About 40 percent of hypotension seen in fulminant hepatic failure can be attributed to a specific cause other than liver failure. Proper diagnosis hinges on timely measurement of the hemodynamic state.

At the first sign of any cardiac instability, regardless of depth of coma, we begin cardiovascular monitoring. A Swan-Ganz catheter is placed for pressure and cardiac output determinations, and an arterial line is installed in the radial artery for continuous blood pressure monitoring and nontraumatic phlebotomies. A Foley catheter is passed for accurate urine output determinations. Low central pressures in the presence of decreased urine output or hypotension are treated with packed red blood cells, albumin, fresh-frozen plasma, or crystalline solutions in order to achieve a wedged pressure of 12 mm Hg or higher.

The response to low systemic vascular resistance is volume expansion, along with an investigation for sepsis. If the volume expansion raises the wedge pressure but does not alter the systemic resistance, pressor agents are used. We begin with dopamine and hold dobutamine and phenylephrine hydrochloride (Neo-Synephrine) for use as second-line agents. The choice between these two agents depends on heart rate. If the patient is tachycardic we use Neo-Synephrine.

Systemic hypertension occurs in fulminant hepatic failure and may be the result of increased ICP. Therefore, a CT scan is performed to investigate structural abnormalities, and the treatments described above are employed. Direct treatment of the hypertension is begun using continuous intravenous infusions of nitroprusside, nitroglycerin, or trimethaphan camsylate (Arfoned). All of these agents have significant drawbacks. Nitroprusside may lower CPP and is associated with thiocyanate toxicity if used long-term. Nitroglycerin is made up in alcohol, which has independent pharmacologic and neurotropic effects. Arfoned exhibits tachyphylaxis. Because of its familiarity and safety, we usually start with nitroprusside. Such treatment is performed only in patients with continuously recorded systemic and intracranial pressures.

Infections

Patients with fulminant hepatic failure become infected because their defenses are down and their exposures increased. Their polymorphonuclear leukocytes are less effective than normal and decreased complement levels impede opsonization. Line sepsis will occur, and as discussed above, these patients are predisposed to pulmonary infections. Some patients may have received corticosteroids, and these drugs promote both bacterial and fungal diseases. Despite this, we do not encourage the use of empiric, broad-spectrum antibiosis. Patients who appear septic should receive adequate coverage, but what type they should receive depends largely on local effects. In general, nephrotoxic drugs such as aminoglycosides should be avoided. Involvement of infectious disease consultants seems most appropriate in these circumstances. Just to stay ahead of the game, we perform screening blood cultures twice per day in all patients. Viral diseases are seen most often in these patients after transplantation. In anticipation of this, we screen for cytomegalovirus (CMV) titers early on, and if the results are negative, attempt to give only CMV-negative blood products.

Pancreatitis

Hemorrhagic pancreatitis is a mercifully rare complication of fulminant hepatic failure for which there is no standard interventional therapy.

THERAPY

Nutritional Support

There has been little scientific attention paid to the nutritional support of patients with fulminant hepatic failure. We use "special formulas" such as Hepatic Aid not because they have any proven effects on coma or survival, but because some of them contain essentially no sodium or potassium. Some patients hospitalized with fulminant hepatic failure will have prolonged hospital stays, making it seem reasonable to have them in positive nitrogen balance as soon as possible. Parenteral nutrition is begun if the bowel cannot be used for such reasons as pancreatitis or ileus.

Fulminant hepatic failure is a desperate disease to which desperate remedies have been applied, most of them useless or deleterious. Exchange transfusion, charcoal hemoperfusion and hepatic B immune globulin (HBIG) infusion have all failed trials. "Total body wash-out," pig-liver perfusion, and human cross-circulation did not receive adequate trials and probably do not warrant them. The most recent desperate therapy to receive attention is orthotopic liver transplantation. In modest-sized series reported to date, survival has been reported in the 50 to 70 percent range. If these figures are confirmed, this would represent a significant therapeutic advance. We doubt that a randomized trial of transplantation will occur in the near future, and therefore physicians must decide for themselves if this therapy is worth pursuing.

Discussions with hepatologists at several transplant centers have resulted in some of the recommendations mentioned above, and a special plea concerning early communication and referral was a frequent theme. If transplantation is not an option, we believe that meticulous supportive care offers the best chance for survival. Time is very important in the care of these patients and decisions must be made rapidly. At a large center in France, over half of those patients referred for treatment of fulminant hepatic failure who died did so within 24 hours of admission.

Treatment Summary

This is not an algorithm, but an incomplete checklist.

1. Admit patient to intensive care unit.
2. Notify blood bank, laboratory, and consultants (pulmonology, nephrology, neurology, hematology, neurosurgery) of patient condition and projected needs.
3. If the patient is a transplant candidate, call a transplant center and discuss the case.
4. Draw blood for diagnostic serologic and drug testing. Include CMV titers and blood gases.
5. Order routine phlebotomies, liver profile and blood cultures every 12 hours, and blood count and electrolytes every 6 hours.
6. Institute a bedside profile of neurologic status.
7. Obtain EEG and CT scan of the head.
8. Avoid corticosteroids and sedative-hypnotic drugs.

9. Give vitamin K and sufficient H_2 blocker to maintain gastric pH above 5.0.
10. Be alert for signs of increased ICP.

ASSESSMENT OF THERAPEUTIC RESPONSE

It is not hard to tell if things are going well or things are going poorly for patients with fulminant hepatic failure. Depth of coma, coagulopathy, and size of the liver are all of prognostic significance. One must remember that fulminant hepatic failure is a severe, but not hopeless, clinical challenge. Best supportive care is important even when the outlook is bleak. We have seen young patients recover to normal after days of decerebrate posturing. Such cases make one stay the course.

SUGGESTED READING

Bismuth H, Samuel D, Gugenheim J, et al. Emergency liver transplantation for fulminant hepatitis. Ann Intern Med 1987; 107:337–341.

Canalese J, Gimson AES, Davis C, et al. Controlled trial of dexamethasone and mannitol for the cerebral edema of fulminant hepatic failure. Gut 1982; 23:625–629.

Jones EA, Schafer DF. Fulminant hepatic failure. In: Zakim D, Boyer TD, eds. Hepatology. Philadelphia: WB Saunders, 1982; 415.

O'Grady JG, Gimson AES, O'Brien DJ, et al. Controlled trials of charcoal hemoperfusion and prognostic factors in fulminant hepatic failure. Gastroenterology 1988; 94:1186–1192.

DRUG-INDUCED LIVER DISEASE

GEOFFREY C. FARRELL, M.D., F.R.A.C.P.

Although drugs are a relatively uncommon cause of liver disease, accounting for approximately 5 to 10 percent of hospital cases of jaundice and hepatitis, the diversity of potential reactions spans the entire spectrum of hepatobiliary disorders. Moreover, the number of therapeutic agents recognized to be potentially toxic is not only vast but continues to grow rapidly. Some hepatic drug reactions are severe, and patients require the type of intensive supportive management described in the chapter on Fulminant Hepatic Failure. More usually, however, the hepatobiliary disorder resolves promptly upon withdrawal of the offending agent. Hence, recognition that a drug etiology is possible and identification of the responsible agent are the crux of management. Mechanisms of hepatic drug reactions will not be discussed, except in relation to acetaminophen poisoning. In this instance, precise knowledge about the pathogenesis of hepatic necrosis has led to specific and effective therapy.

RECOGNITION OF HEPATIC DRUG REACTIONS

Frequently Implicated Drugs

With the exception of acetaminophen poisoning (see below), many of the best known examples of drug-induced liver disease are now less common owing to declining use or more appropriate dosing of the incriminated agents. For example, oxyphenisatin hepatitis, tetracycline fatty liver, alpha- methyldopa hepatitis, and erythromycin estolate cholestatic hepatitis are mainly of historic interest. The use of halothane, until recently the most common cause of fatal hepatic drug reactions, is declining in most countries. Thus, agents such as psychotropic drugs, nonsteroidal anti-inflammatory drugs (NSAIDs), cardiotropic agents, antibiotics, H_2-receptor blockers, and antimitotic agents, each individually rare causes of hepatic drug reactions, are those most likely to be seen by today's physicians. Some representative examples are given in Table 1. Ideally, physicians should apprise themselves of the possible hepatotoxicity of any agent they prescribe and be especially alert to this possibility from new and nonproprietary drugs. In practice, reference to a deskside compendium of known hepatic drug reactions is most helpful, and many local health authorities can provide such information. The toxicity of many compounds was not appreciated until several years after widespread introduction of their use. Every practicing physician has a responsible role in postmarketing surveillance to report adverse drug reactions to the relevant authority.* Workplace toxins, usually ketone-based solvents or haloalkane herbicides and pesticides, should be considered, but in practice seem to be extremely rare causes of significant hepatotoxicity.

Classification of Hepatic Drug Reactions

In my view, the so-called mechanistic classification into direct ("predictable") hepatotoxins and indirect ("unpredictable" or idiosyncratic) is misleading. For carbon tetrachloride and acetaminophen (both classic predictable hepatotoxins) the parent compound is not directly toxic, and thus toxicity also depends on other factors such as metabolism, while for several idiosyncratic reactions occult dose dependency is now evident. Of more use to phy-

* In the United States, physicians are encouraged to report documented adverse drug effects to the Washington Registry for Drug-induced Liver Injury, Veteran's Administration Medical Center, 50 Irving Street, NW, Washington, DC 20422.

TABLE 1 A Classification of Drug-Induced Liver Disease

Clinicopathologic Type	*Typical Agents*	*Comment*
Cytotoxic		
Zonal necrosis	Acetaminophen, halothane,	Often dose-dependent toxins
Fatty change	aspirin, tetracycline	Microvesicular fat
Lobular hepatitis (viral hepatitis–like)	Isoniazid, halothane, sulfonamides, penicillins	Subacute or massive hepatic necrosis occurs in severe reactions; overlaps with zonal necrosis
Cholangiolytic hepatitis	Chlorpromazine, tricyclic antidepressants, azathioprine	Varying degree of parenchymal involvement
Cholestasis (without hepatitis)	Anabolic steroids	
Granulomatous hepatitis	Carbamazepine, hydralazine, allopurinol	Often some lobular hepatitis and/or cholestasis
Chronic liver disease		
Chronic active hepatitis	Alpha-methyldopa, nitrofurantoin	
Steatohepatitis	Perhexiline maleate	Resembles alcoholic hepatitis
Fibrosis-hepatitis	Hypervitaminosis A, methotrexate	Often normal liver function tests
Vascular abnormalities		
Sinusoidal dilatation	Oral contraceptives	
Peliosis hepatitis	Anabolic androgenic steroids	
Hepatic venous obstruction	Thioguanine (veno-occlusive disease)	
	Oral contraceptives (Budd-Chiari syndrome)	
Neoplasms		
Focal nodular hyperplasia	Oral contraceptives	Increased vascularity, size
Adenoma	Oral contraceptives	True etiologic association
Hepatocellular carcinoma	Oral contraceptives, anabolic androgenic steroids,	Possible etiologic association
Angiosarcoma	arsenic	

sicians is a clinicopathologic classification, such as the simplified version set out in Table 1. Almost all reactions are unpredictable; i.e., they occur rarely after a variable but prolonged latent period (days to months), appear to be independent of dose (many exceptions are now known, e.g., tetracycline, cyclophosphamide, methotrexate, and perhexiline maleate), and cause a diversity of histologic and clinical features. It must be emphasized that this kind of classification is only a guide to the more usual agents. In the field of hepatic drug reactions the unusual rules, there is overlap between syndromes (especially in the spectrum from "hepatitis" to "cholestasis"), and several agents are known to cause more than one type of picture, e.g., carbamazepine typically is associated with granulomatous hepatitis, but occasionally causes cholestasis and, rarely, severe hepatocellular necrosis.

Aids to Diagnosis

Clearly a drug etiology is most likely when the patient has been exposed during the previous 3 months to one or more agents known to cause drug-induced liver damage. Even when such a history is not obtained, one should always suspect a drug cause if confronted by unexplained cholestasis (when biliary disease has been carefully excluded) and seronegative hepatitis in the absence of risk factors for parenterally transmitted non-A, non-B hepatitis and autoantibodies suggestive of autoimmune disease. The presence of extrahepatic features of drug hypersensitivity may heighten the suspicion that a drug is responsible. Fever, rash, eosinophilia, the pseudomononucleosis syndrome, vasculitis, and the involvement of bone marrow, kidney, or pancreas indicate systemic allergy, as occurs in reactions to phenytoin, sulfonamide (usually in co-trimoxazole), penicillin (typically an oxypenicillin), and allopurinol. However, such features are unusual in hepatic reactions to halothane, chlorpromazine, erythromycin estolate, and isoniazid, so that the absence of, say, eosinophilia is of no value in the individual case.

Liver biopsy may be helpful in individual and especially difficult cases but is not mandatory when the diagnosis seems obvious. Unfortunately few if any histologic features are unique to hepatic drug reactions, but some patterns are typical enough to suggest a possible drug cause. These include zonal patterns of necrosis, or necrosis of a severity that is disproportionate to the clinical picture; microvesicular fatty change; a predominance of eosinophils in an inflammatory infiltrate; periportal cholestasis early in the course of an illness; and damage to bile duct epithelium.

Rechallenge remains the only conclusive method by which an individual drug can be proved to be the cause of an hepatic reaction. It should be considered when the continued use of that drug is highly desirable or when accurate documentation of a newly observed hepatic drug reaction is required for reporting purposes. It should not be performed when the reaction has been severe; fatal hepatic necrosis has followed deliberate or inadvertent rechallenge with halothane, isoniazid, phenytoin, alpha-methyldopa, or sulfonamides. Low- or single-dose challenge is usually recommended but can give a false-negative response, or even a false-positive one if minor serum aminotransferase elevation is the end point. The author has a conservative approach to rechallenge because of the hazards to the patient and the potential pitfalls in interpretation. When used, it has been under stringent conditions of close monitoring (usually in the hospital) for the earliest signs of a positive response. In vitro tests are much needed for confirmation of hepatic drug reactions, but at this stage of their development they are not available to the practicing physician.

PREVENTION

Prevention is highly desirable but difficult to accomplish. Some measures to minimize the incidence of hepatic drug reactions include appropriate selection of therapeutic agents, awareness of toxic dose thresholds, and avoidance of potential drug-drug interactions relevant to the pathogenesis of liver injury. Predisposing factors for hepatic drug reactions include the age and sex of the patient; most drugs, such as isoniazid and halothane, are much more likely to cause liver injury in females and in those over the age of 40 years, while sodium valproate is unusual in that it causes hepatotoxicity in children only. A history of any adverse drug reaction is a risk factor for hepatic drug reactions, as may be a family history of a similar reaction (e.g., to halothane) or of drug allergy. Special risk categories exist for some drugs and should be borne in mind when prescribing. Examples include aspirin hepatotoxicity, which is common among patients with systemic lupus erythematosus, the juvenile form of rheumatoid arthritis, and sulfonamide allergy (usually to cotrimoxazole), which is common in patients with AIDS. Although no purely hepatic drug reactions are involved, avoidance of aspirin for febrile disorders in young children because of its likely role in Reye's syndrome, and the possible exacerbation of acute viral hepatitis by NSAIDs, are noted here for their relevance to prescription and the risk of hepatic necrosis.

Relationships between the total or daily dosage of pharmacologic agents and drug-induced liver injury are increasingly recognized. The risk of toxicity appears dependent on the dosage of the follow drugs: acetaminophen (see below); tetracycline (more than 2 g per day, especially in pregnancy); methotrexate (total dose more than 2 g over 3 years); perhexiline (total dose more than 45 g in 6 months); cyclophosphamide (daily dose more than 400 mg per square meter), and oral contraceptive steroids (the incidence of hepatic adenoma increased 500-fold after 7 years of use). Further examples will come to light as more is learned about pharmacogenetics, i.e., the genetically determined variability in rates of drug metabolism.

Some drug combinations also increase the toxicity of potential hepatotoxins, usually because induction of drug metabolizing enzymes by one agent enhances metabolism of the second drug to a reactive intermediate. Known examples are chronic heavy alcohol ingestion, which increases the risk and severity of acetaminophen, isoniazid, and possibly halothane toxicity; and phenytoin, which may predispose to valproate- and halothane-induced hepatotoxicity.

Early detection of hepatic drug reactions also centers around physician awareness. Fatalities from hepatotoxicity due to isoniazid, halothane, valproate, allopurinol, alpha- methyldopa, nitrofurantoin, and perhexiline have often occurred when patients have continued or resumed exposure to the agent after the onset of symptoms. Patients should be warned about the possible significance of nonspecific symptoms (typically malaise, nausea, fever, and right upper abdominal quadrant discomfort) during supervision of a new form of therapy. If any abnormality of liver biochemistry accompanies such symptoms, medication should be suspended or altered. When the agent is vital and difficult to find a substitute for, liver biopsy may be helpful in resolving whether the symptoms are attributable to hepatotoxicity.

A priori, one might expect routine monitoring of liver enzymes to be a useful way to detect early toxicity, but this approach is probably unhelpful. Many drugs that potentially cause severe reactions are associated with elevated serum aminotransferase levels during the first few weeks of therapy in 10 to 50 percent of patients. Such abnormalities rarely forecast progression to clinically significant hepatitis, and toxicity often is not preceded by asymptomatic liver enzyme abnormalities. For medicolegal considerations, it is difficult to recommend abolition of routine screening by liver function tests when prescribing agents such as isoniazid for which routine screening is common practice. However, there are few data that allow one to recommend guidelines as to what level of biochemical abnormality contraindicates continued use of the drug. On an empirical basis, I recommend stopping an agent if the serum alanine aminotransferase level exceeds 250 U per liter. Disturbances of serum albumin concentration, prothrombin time, and serum bilirubin concentration are usually of much greater importance, and any symptoms or clinical features of liver disease or extrahepatic manifestations of allergy mandate immediate drug withdrawal. Conversely, a raised serum gamma-glutamyltranspeptidase level and (in the absence of symptoms and other abnormalities) concomitant minor elevation of alkaline phosphatase are usually manifestations of hepatic enzyme induction, and in this context usually do not indicate hepatobiliary disease.

Liver biopsy is not generally indicated as an "early detection" measure for hepatic drug reactions, except in the case of equivocal reactions to vital therapy (see below). One exception may be methotrexate, which can cause progressive fibrosis leading to cirrhosis; this may occur even with normal liver function test results. Since preexistent liver disease appears to be a risk factor for methotrexate-induced fibrosis, pretreatment liver biopsy has been recommended, and 6-monthly or annual biopsy to assess progressive toxicity. However, more recent studies suggest that the most critical determinant of methotrexate toxicity is the dosage; with lower doses (less than 25 mg once weekly, and less than 2 g over 3 years), monitoring by liver biopsy may be unnecessary.

TREATMENT

Acetaminophen

The biochemical basis of hepatotoxicity produced by acetaminophen, and the clinical and laboratory features resulting from the hepatic necrosis that follows acetaminophen poisoning, are well described elsewhere. They are summarized only briefly here. In therapeutic dosages (1 to 4 g per day), acetaminophen does not cause liver injury, although extremely rare cases have been described of chronic liver disease in patients consuming 2 to 5 g per day for many months or years. Acetaminophen, itself inert, is extensively conjugated to sulfate and glucuronide metabolites, which are also nontoxic. However, about 5 percent of acetaminophen is oxidized by cytochrome P-450 (principally by the ethanol- inducible form, cytochrome P-450 HLj) to a highly reactive oxy-intermediate, *N*-acetyl-*p*-benzoquinoneimine (NAPQI). Glutathione (GSH), an abundant cellular nucleophile, protects cell macromolecules from "attack" by NAPQI, principally by formation of the GSH conjugate. It follows that cell damage occurs only when available GSH is consumed. In turn, this depends on the total dose of acetaminophen, the rate of NAPQI formation (enhanced by chronic alcoholism and some other drugs) and the amount of GSH (decreased in malnutrition and alcoholism). Conversely, if given within 12 hours of acetaminophen ingestion, sulfhydryl donors such as *N*-acetylcysteine stimulate GSH synthesis and prevent or substantially ameliorate liver injury. The timing of *N*-acetylcysteine administration is critical; the elimination half-life of acetaminophen is 3 to 4 hours (although this becomes prolonged during severe hepatotoxicity) and the processes leading to hepatocellular necrosis are probably irreversible after 12 hours.

The following is a recommended management plan for suspected acetaminophen poisoning, which usually occurs in the setting of suicidal or parasuicidal overdosage.

Early Assessment and Monitoring

The use of plasma drug screening is helpful in mixed overdoses when the ingested medication is not known. The risk of liver injury from acetaminophen may be accurately predicted from nomograms of plasma acetaminophen levels in relation to the time after drug ingestion. Further management depends entirely on this predicted risk, since the onset of clinical or biochemical features of liver injury is delayed for 2 to 3 days.

Removal of Unabsorbed Drug

Induction of vomiting in the conscious patient, and gastric lavage with a large-bore stomach tube in the drowsy or unconscious individual, are useful ways to empty the stomach. Activated charcoal or cholestyramine is often administered in an attempt to adsorb unabsorbed intestinal drug or to facilitate removal of unmetabolized acetaminophen from the extracellular fluid space; it is unlikely to play an important role when used more than 1 hour after acetaminophen ingestion.

Administration of N-Acetylcysteine

In all suspected overdoses of 10 g or more, and when plasma acetaminophen levels are in the range predictive of moderate or severe liver injury (this is greater than 1,300 μmol per liter at 4 hours or greater than 300 μmol per liter at 12 hours), *N*-acetylcysteine should be administered intravenously in an initial dose of 150 mg per kilogram in 200 ml of 5 percent dextrose over 15 minutes. A second dose of 50 mg per kilogram can be given 4 hours later when the risk of hepatotoxicity is considerable, and up to a total of 300 mg per kilogram can be used over 20 hours. I prefer the intravenous route for *N*-acetylcysteine administration, since gastric emptying is often impaired after self-poisoning, thus making absorption from the oral route unreliable. Physicians should be aware of a possible risk of hypersensitivity reactions, which sometimes can be severe.

Continued Observation for Evidence of Hepatotoxicity for up to 72 Hours

Late presentation is a difficult problem, particularly in alcoholics in whom the risk of hepatotoxicity is increased. Acute tubular necrosis occurs in 25 percent of such cases and cardiac toxicity may also occur. After 12 hours there is evidence that *N*-acetylcysteine does not ameliorate liver injury, and this is unlikely on theoretical grounds. In patients with established hepatic necrosis, *N*-acetylcysteine may precipitate hepatic encephalopathy and thus should not be given. Management of acute hepatic failure is along usual lines (see the chapter *Fulminant Hepatic Failure*) except that hypoglycemia is often profound and should be prevented by intravenous dextrose infusion. In cases progressing to encephalopathy, hepatic transplantation should be considered, but psychosocial assessment is obviously crucial in the selection of appropriate candidates. The author's view is that extracorporeal perfusion of blood through charcoal columns is not of value in management of late acetaminophen overdose.

Experimental work in laboratory animals has led some writers to suggest that cimetidine, by virtue of an inhibitory effect on cytochrome P-450–mediated metabolism of acetaminophen to NAPQI, may be of value in managing acetaminophen overdose. However, I believe that cimetidine should not be used. This drug is itself cleared by hepatic metabolism and renal elimination, so that the very large doses required to inhibit cytochrome P-450 would be likely to result in drug accumulation, with resultant mental confusion. Ranitidine should also be avoided, since it has been shown in experimental animals to exacerbate liver damage produced by acetaminophen administration. It is worth stressing that intravenous *N*-acetylcysteine, when given within 12 hours of acetaminophen ingestion, is so effective in abrogating liver injury that it is inappropriate to consider alternative therapeutic approaches.

Drug Hepatitis

Immediate and permanent cessation of exposure to the causative agent is critical. This may be reinforced by use of a Medic-Alert bracelet or similar notification carried on the patient's person (especially in the case of reactions to anesthetic agents). There is no specific therapy. Symptomatic and supportive therapy is along the lines for viral hepatitis. Progressive deterioration of liver function is an ominous sign. There is no place for corticosteroids or "heroic" measures to remove residual drug from the body, but liver transplantation is an option that should be considered as soon as it is evident that a favorable outcome is unlikely. These considerations also apply to chronic active hepatitis due to drugs, a disorder that fortunately usually responds to drug withdrawal. Corticosteroids are not indicated.

Nonalcoholic steatohepatitis or cirrhosis due to perhexiline maleate or amiodarone is treated by cessation of the toxic agent and supportive management of the patient, who is often in liver failure. There is no specific therapy and the prognosis is often poor.

Cholestasis

Cholestasis, whether resulting from impairment of bile secretion (e.g., by estrogens) or from a "cholestatic hepatitis," usually resolves promptly after the agent is stopped. Cholestyramine is effective for relieving pruritus, usually the most unpleasant symptom. In my experience, other drugs such as phenobarbitone, antihistamines, and cimetidine are ineffective antipruritic agents in drug-induced cholestasis. Refractory cases occasionally occur. When estrogens are responsible, the patient may have an inherited predisposition to estrogen-induced cholestasis and have had previous episodes of cholestasis of pregnancy. Intractable pruritus may respond to plasmapheresis. Cholestatic hepatitis triggered by phenothiazines or tricyclic antidepressants may sometimes progress to a primary biliary cirrhosis–like syndrome (without antimitochondrial antibodies). This eventually leads to liver failure and the possible need for liver transplantation.

Granulomatous Hepatitis

This is probably the most common type of hepatic drug reaction and at least 40 agents have been incriminated. In a febrile patient with abnormal liver function tests and a liver biopsy showing granulomas, a drug etiology should be considered and any possible offending agent suspended. Prompt improvement is usual (1 to 4 days). A notable exception is when hepatic involvement is part of a severe systemic drug reaction with small vessel vasculitis. Allopurinol can cause this syndrome, usually with prominent vasculitic rash and renal involvement; there is a high mortality rate. Such a patient should be started on prednisolone, 60 mg daily, as there is some uncontrolled evidence that corticosteroids improve the outcome.

Drugs as a Cause of Hepatic Fibrosis

Among the known causes of hepatic fibrosis and noncirrhotic portal hypertension, methotrexate, hypervitaminosis A, vinyl chloride, and arsenic figure prominently. The last two have also been associated with rare cases of angiosar coma of the liver. Prevention and recognition of the relevant environmental agent are the important issues here. The several factors that have been suggested as increasing the risk of methotrexate-induced hepatic fibrosis and cirrhosis include pretreatment abnormality of liver morphology, heavy alcohol ingestion, frequency of dosing, and total cumulative dose. A once-weekly dose schedule (maximal dose 25 mg) and total dose of less than 2 g is probably safe. Standard liver function tests are of no value in predicting liver damage. Despite some views to the contrary, I still prefer pretreatment and annual liver biopsy for patients requiring long-term treatment with methotrexate (usually for psoriasis). Vitamin A intoxication can occur with as little as 25,000 to 40,000 IU per day for several years; a careful dietary history should be elicited to clarify the cause. The liver biopsy appearances of Ito cell hypertrophy and fluorescence of fresh specimens under ultraviolet light are characteristic. The disease may slowly improve after vitamin A ingestion is stopped.

Vascular Lesions

Sinusoidal dilatation should be managed by withdrawal of sex steroids. Pregnancy is contraindicated because of the concern that this could be a precursor lesion for peliosis hepatis (blood lakes). Patients with peliosis hepatis should be observed for the onset of the life-threatening complications of spontaneous rupture of the liver with hemoperitoneum, or hepatic failure. Any future exposure to sex steroids should be carefully avoided. A surgical approach is best avoided (except in the case of associated tumors, or in response to bleeding), because there is a risk of uncontrollable hemorrhage.

Hepatic venous outflow obstruction (the Budd-Chiari syndrome) is associated with use of oral contraceptive steroids, most often in association with an underlying hypercoagulable state. Thrombolytic therapy may be attempted in the very early stages but is usually ineffective; anticoagulants are indicated for a persisting thrombotic tendency. Rapid deterioration of hepatic function or complications of portal hypertension may be relieved by a side-to-side portacaval shunt, but this procedure is undesirable in patients who may eventually be candidates for liver transplantation. Hence, a transplantation team should be consulted before deciding about surgical intervention in this disorder.

Hepatic Tumors

Focal nodular hyperplasia may be left untreated in asymptomatic patients if the diagnosis is confirmed by imaging and fine needle aspiration biopsy. In patients taking oral contraceptives, symptoms may indicate an expanding size or hypervascularity of the lesion. Tumor size may decrease after cessation of contraceptive steroids, but surgical resection is available if symptoms persist, or if the tumor is found incidentally during laparotomy.

Hepatic adenomas may also regress after oral contraceptive steroids are stopped. However, surgical resection of large lesions is more important for this entity because of the high risk of hemorrhage. Oral contraceptives and pregnancy should be avoided, since there is a 10 to 15 percent recurrence rate.

Hepatocellular carcinomas occurring during treatment with oral contraceptive or anabolic androgenic steroids are usually well differentiated. Serum alpha-fetoprotein is negative and tumors are present in a noncirrhotic liver. Despite the observation in some patients of considerable tumor regression after steroid withdrawal, it is recommended that surgical resection be attempted, since eventual spread is a more likely outcome. In patients with very extensive tumor replacement of the liver but without metastases or invasion of contiguous structures, hepatic transplantation may be considered, although long-term cures are uncommon.

SUGGESTED READING

Farrell GC. The hepatic side-effects of drugs. Med J Aust 1986; 145:600–604.

Ishak KG. Hepatic lesions caused by anabolic and contraceptive steroids. Semin Liver Dis 1981; 1:116–128.

Ludwig J, Axelsen R. Drug effects on the liver. An updated tabular compilation of drugs and drug-related hepatic diseases. Dig Dis Sci 1983; 28:651–666.

Prescott LF, Critchley JA. The treatment of acetaminophen poisoning. Annu Rev Pharmacol Toxicol 1983; 23:87–101.

Zimmerman HJ. Drug-induced liver disease: an overview. Semin Liver Dis 1981; 1:93–103.

CHRONIC HEPATITIS

FREDRIC G. REGENSTEIN, M.D.
ROBERT P. PERRILLO, M.D.

The term "chronic hepatitis" refers to a group of disorders associated with ongoing hepatic inflammation and necrosis. The diagnosis is suspected when aminotransferase elevations persist for longer than 6 months, and is established when the characteristic histologic abnormalities are identified on liver biopsy. On the basis of the histologic features, chronic hepatitis can be further classified into chronic active hepatitis, chronic persistent hepatitis, or chronic lobular hepatitis. The prognosis, and particularly the risk of progression to cirrhosis, appear related to the histologic findings.

In chronic persistent hepatitis (CPH), the inflammatory infiltrate is limited to the portal tract; there is little or no periportal hepatocyte necrosis, and little if any fibrosis. Chronic persistent hepatitis is generally considered a benign disorder that rarely progresses to cirrhosis or liver failure. In some patients, however, the initial identification of CPH on liver biopsy may be associated with the development of progressive liver disease. In particular, the CPH seen after treatment of idiopathic or autoimmune chronic active hepatitis, and the CPH observed in some patients with inactive hepatitis B or chronic non-A, non-B virus infections, may be associated with the transition to chronic active hepatitis.

The hallmark histologic feature of chronic active hepatitis (CAH) is the presence of hepatocyte necrosis extending into the periportal area, leading to areas of focal or "piecemeal necrosis". In more severe cases, destruction of periportal parenchymal leads to "bridging necrosis" between adjacent portal tracts or between portal tracts and central veins. Fibrosis develops as a consequence of the destruction and collapse of the liver architecture. While CAH is a variably progressive disorder, progression to cirrhosis and eventual hepatic failure is most apt to occur in individuals with the more severe histologic forms of this disease (e.g., bridging necrosis).

Chronic lobular hepatitis (CLH) is uncommon and is characterized by histologic features resembling an acute hepatitis. CLH is associated with cycles of remissions and relapses over a period of years, and is generally thought to carry a benign prognosis.

With the exception of hepatitis A virus, chronic hepatitis can be caused by all the hepatitis viruses (i.e., hepatitis B; hepatitis non-A, non-B; hepatitis D), by a variety of different medications, by several metabolic diseases, and by certain disorders of the immune system. In some patients no apparent etiology can be identified.

CHRONIC VIRAL HEPATITIS

Hepatitis A Virus (HAV)

Hepatitis A is a self-limiting illness. Although in rare cases HAV can result in a relapsing illness associated with recurrent viral shedding, chronic infection does not occur.

Hepatitis B Virus (HBV)

Chronic hepatitis B infection occurs in approximately 5 to 10 percent of adults after an acute infection. However, the age and immunologic status of the affected individual are critical factors in determining the outcome of infection. Thus, chronic infection occurs in 20 to 30 percent of young children infected, and in almost all neonates exposed to HBV. Likewise, the incidence of chronic infection is much greater than 5 to 10 percent in adults with underlying immunologic disorders (e.g., patients on chronic hemodialysis). There are estimated to be 200 to 300 million carriers of the hepatitis B virus throughout the world, with 1 to 1.5 million carriers in the United States alone.

There appear to be two stages in the natural history of chronic HBV infection. The early, or replicative phase is characterized by an active hepatitis associated with elevated aminotransferase values and expression of markers of active viral replication, hepatitis B e antigen (HBeAg), HBV, DNA, and HBV DNA polymerase. After a highly variable period, there is evolution to the late, or nonreplicative phase of infection. This transition occurs in 10 to 20 percent of carriers per year, and is often heralded by a sudden, but usually asymptomatic exacerbation in aminotransferase values. After the exacerbation, there is improvement in aminotransferase values and loss of active viral replication markers. Evolution to the nonreplicative phase of infection is usually associated with loss of detectable levels of circulating HBeAg, HBV DNA, and DNA polymerase; acquisition of antibody to the HBeAg (anti-HBe); and integration of HBV DNA into the host cell genome. Typically, during the nonreplicative phase of infection, there is a reduction or resolution of the hepatic inflammatory activity seen on liver biopsy. In many patients, cirrhosis has already developed by the time of transition to a nonreplicative phase of infection. In addition, hepatocellular carcinoma can be a late sequela of chronic HBV infection.

Non-A, Non-B Hepatitis (NANB)

Isolation and characterization of the agents responsible for non-A, non-B hepatitis remains elusive. On the basis of transmission experiments in chimpanzees, there appear to be at least two NANB agents that can result in chronic infections. Recently, however, a putative NANB viral agent has been characterized as a single-stranded RNA virus. An apparent virus-related protein has been isolated that appears to react with antibodies from patients with post-transfusion NANB hepatitis. This development may lead to the availability of a marker for at least one type of NANB hepatitis in the near future.

After an acute infection, approximately 40 to 60 percent of individuals with post-transfusion hepatitis develop a chronic infection. A substantially lower percentage of those with sporadic NANB develop chronic infection. On the basis of the NANB attack rates in recipients of transfused blood, it is estimated that 1 to 2 percent of the volunteer blood donor population are carriers, and 2 to 4 million Americans suffer from chronic NANB hepatitis.

The natural history of chronic NANB infection remains to be determined, but substantial evidence has accumulated to indicate that chronic infection with this agent is frequently severe and progressive. In studies of patients who have undergone liver biopsy, as many as 50 percent of those with chronic NANB infections have either chronic active hepatitis or cirrhosis.

Hepatitis D Virus (HDV)

HDV infection is caused by a novel virus that afflicts only individuals already infected with the hepatitis B virus. Chronic hepatitis D infection usually occurs in HBV carriers during the nonreplicative phase of the infection. HDV infection is endemic in certain areas of the Mediterranean basin, Middle East, Africa, and South America. Infection is infrequent in North America and western Europe, where most cases occur in illicit drug users and recipients of multiple blood products.

Chronic HDV infection is frequently associated with a severe chronic active hepatitis. Superimposed on a liver previously damaged by HBV, HDV infection can rapidly lead to the development of cirrhosis and liver failure.

Clinical and Laboratory Features

Most patients with chronic viral hepatitis are asymptomatic. Fatigue is the most common complaint in symptomatic individuals; abdominal pain, anorexia, nausea, weight loss, and arthralgias occur less often. Patients with cirrhosis, and those with very active disease (e.g., aminotransferase values elevated more than fivefold), more often have symptoms.

Physical examination is usually unremarkable. Hepatomegaly, splenomegaly, and right upper quadrant tenderness are the abnormalities most often detected. Scleral icterus, stigmata of chronic liver disease, and signs of portal hypertension are usually present only in patients with severe chronic active hepatitis, cirrhosis, or hepatocellular carcinoma.

Aminotransferase activity is almost always elevated in this disease. Alanine aminotransferase (ALT) is usually elevated to a greater extent than aspartate aminotransferase (AST), but once cirrhosis ensues, AST elevations may predominate. Although there is incomplete correlation between the magnitude of the aminotransferase elevation and the severity of the liver disease, individuals with persistent, moderate elevations (more than three times above normal) usually have CAH on biopsy. Elevation of serum bilirubin, decreased serum albumin, and prolongation of the prothrombin time do not usually occur until there is evolution to cirrhosis.

Treatment

Hepatitis B Virus

Currently, there is no clearly effective form of therapy for chronic type B hepatitis, and a variety of antiviral and immunomodulatory agents have been tried or are currently under investigation (see Table 1). Adenine arabinoside (ara-A), its more soluble monophosphate derivative (ara-AMP), and interferon (IFN) are the most active single agents against the HBV. Recent studies have shown ara-AMP to be minimally effective and associated with significant toxicity; it has therefore been withdrawn from investigative use in the U.S. and Europe. At the present time,

TABLE 1 Agents Currently Under Investigation for Treatment of Chronic Hepatitis B

Agents	*Comments*
Single Agents	
Interferons	
Alpha (α)	Most promising single agent
Beta (β)	Questionable activity when used as a single agent; perhaps more useful in combination with other interferons*
Gamma (γ)	Perhaps more useful in combination with other interferons*
Adenine arabinoside (ara-A, ara-AMP)	Toxic, low clinical efficacy, withdrawn from clinical trials in Europe and U.S.
Acyclovir or deoxyacyclovir	Minimal efficacy alone, ? more useful in combination with interferon*
Interleukin-2	Toxic, minimal efficacy alone*
Zidovudine (AZT)	Toxic, ? useful in patients with coincidental HIV-1 infections*
Suramin	Toxic, minimal efficacy alone*
Ganciclovir (DHPG)	Some antiviral activity based on studies in animals*
Foscarnet	Very limited information in humans
Phyllanthus niruri	Animal studies only*
Combination therapy	
Prednisone + adenine arabinoside	More effective than either agent alone, but ara-AMP has been withdrawn from clinical trials
Prednisone + α-interferon (α-IFN)	Promising combination for patients with well-compensated liver disease; prednisone withdrawal is potentially dangerous in patients with advanced liver disease
Interferon + adenine arabinoside	Toxic, limited efficacy
Acyclovir or deoxyacyclovir + interferon	Preliminary data appears promising; unclear whether combination therapy is more effective than treatment with α-IFN alone*
Combined interferons (α + β, α + γ, β + γ)	Limited information available; unclear whether combination therapy is more effective than treatment with α-IFN alone

* Indicates information is based on limited data.

IFN appears to be the most promising agent. The effectiveness of α-IFN for patients with chronic HBV infection and active viral replication has been demonstrated in several clinical trials, but combination therapy may prove to be even more effective than treatment with any single agent. In particular, combination therapy consisting of a short course of corticosteroids followed by a course of IFN appears especially promising. The short course of corticosteroids appears to promote viral replication and increased expression of viral antigens on liver cells. Once corticosteroids are tapered and withdrawn, the immune system seems better able to target and destroy HBV-infected hepatocytes. Corticosteroid withdrawal alone has minimal effect, but combined with the antiviral and immunomodulatory activity of IFN, eradication of HBV is possible in some cases. Application of this type of therapy appears to be restricted to patients with well-compensated liver disease, because those with advanced liver disease may undergo clinical deterioration and decompensation during corticosteroid withdrawal.

On the basis of currently available information, by employing a regimen of α-IFN, 5 to 10 million units administered daily or three times a week for 3 to 4 months, approximately 30 to 40 percent of IFN-treated patients respond to therapy with a sustained loss of viral replicative markers (i.e., HBeAg, HBV DNA), and a much smaller percentage lose hepatitis B surface antigen. While IFN is likely to be licensed in the near future by the U.S. Food and Drug Administration for the treatment of chronic type B hepatitis, optimal drug dosages and the duration of IFN therapy remain to be determined in future studies. Long-term treatment with corticosteroids or corticosteroids combined with immunosuppressive medication (e.g. azathioprine) does not appear to be useful and may be deleterious.

Non-A, Non-B Hepatitis

Therapeutic trials for NANB hepatitis have been seriously hindered by the failure, to date, to identify an etiologic agent. Preliminary data from several studies indicates that α-IFN has some beneficial activity in patients with post-transfusion NANB hepatitis. Unfortunately, the improvement in aminotransferase values seen during IFN therapy appears to be transient, and relapse occurs in most patients once IFN therapy is discontinued. Additional trials currently under way should help determine the role of IFN for patients with chronic NANB hepatitis. Corticosteroid therapy, with or without azathioprine, does not appear to be of benefit in the management of this disease.

Hepatitis D Virus

No form of therapy has been clearly shown to be effective for chronic HDV infection. Corticosteroid and immunosuppressive therapy has been ineffective, and several current trials are evaluating treatment with α-IFN. Preliminary information has demonstrated that α-IFN reduces HDV replication and improves the results of liver function tests; unfortunately, there appears to be a high relapse rate once therapy is discontinued.

IDIOPATHIC CHRONIC HEPATITIS

Idiopathic chronic hepatitis is a form of chronic hepatitis in which evidence of either a viral, metabolic, drug, or toxin related etiology cannot be identified. Many of these patients demonstrate immunologic abnormalities, and are thus designated as having autoimmune chronic hepatitis. The association between autoimmune chronic hepatitis and the major histocompatibility antigens HLA-B8 and HLA-DR3 provides additional evidence for the immunologic basis of this disease.

Clinical and Laboratory Features

The clinical features of autoimmune hepatitis are similar to those in chronic viral hepatitis, but patients with autoimmune chronic hepatitis appear to present more frequently with symptoms than their counterparts with chronic viral hepatitis. Fatigue and malaise are often present, but in severe cases fever, anorexia, weight loss, jaundice, and extrahepatic manifestations (e.g., rash, arthritis, thyroiditis, glomerulonephritis) may predominate. Women are affected more often than men (4:1), the typical patient being a woman in the third to fifth decades of life. In symptomatic cases, the physical examination is often remarkable for the presence of hepatosplenomegaly, spider angiomata, and palmar erythema. As in chronic viral hepatitis, the aminotransferase activity is elevated, but patients with autoimmune hepatitis are more likely to present with elevated serum bilirubin and immunoglobulin levels and depressed serum albumin. The presence of significant titers of antinuclear or anti–smooth muscle antibodies are a characteristic feature in patients with autoimmune hepatitis, and is a key factor in distinguishing autoimmune hepatitis from chronic NANB hepatitis.

Treatment

Therapy with corticosteroids alone or in combination with azathioprine leads to clinical and biochemical remission in most cases. In addition, corticosteroid therapy has been demonstrated to improve the survival rate in patients with severe disease. The natural history of patients with milder forms of disease has not been well defined. Furthermore, the efficacy versus the risk of long-term immunosuppressive therapy in this population has not been established in controlled trials. Thus, therapeutic decisions are made on an individual, case by case basis, taking into account the constellation of clinical, laboratory, and histologic features. Our approach has been to treat those patients with symptomatic disease, and those with severe biochemical abnormalities (e.g., elevated bilirubin, aminotransferase activity elevated more than four times, hypoalbuminemia, marked hyperglobulinemia) or severe histologic changes (i.e., bridging necrosis or fibrosis, multilobular necrosis). Asymptomatic patients, the elderly, and individuals with mild aminotransferase elevations or mild histologic abnormalities are generally observed without therapy. In difficult cases, a repeat biopsy 6 to 12 months after the initial one can be helpful in deciding whether or not to initiate therapy. Alternatively, a 3 to 6 month therapeutic trial can indicate whether the disease is responsive to treatment. Individuals not demonstrating either clinical, biochemical, or histologic improvement during this trial period are unlikely to benefit from continued therapy.

The goals of therapy are (1) to control symptoms, (2) to reduce aminotransferase values to less than twice the upper limit of normal and the gamma globulin level to less than 2.0 g per deciliter, and (3) to improve hepatic histology from a chronic active hepatitis to a chronic persistent hepatitis, mild nonspecific hepatitis, or ideally to a normal-appearing liver. We usually begin therapy with prednisone at dosages ranging from 20 to 60 mg per day and taper the dose to 20 mg per day over a 2 to 6 week period. Since combination therapy with prednisone and azathioprine appears to be equally effective as treatment with prednisone alone and is associated with fewer steroid-related side effects, we treat most of our patients with azathioprine and prednisone. Our approach is to begin prednisone therapy alone and to add azathioprine, 50 mg per day, within the first 2 months of therapy, once clinical and biochemical improvement has been demonstrated. The prednisone can usually be tapered to 10 mg per day or less when used in combination with azathioprine. In occasional patients, especially those weighing more than 70 kg, higher doses of prednisone (up to 20 mg per day) and azathioprine (up to 1.5 mg per kilogram or 150 mg per day) may be needed to induce and maintain a biochemical remission. In patients who respond to immunosuppressive therapy with improvement in liver function test results, symptoms, and liver histology, treatment is generally continued for 6 to 12 months. An attempt is then made to taper and ultimately to discontinue medication. Patients experiencing marked improvements in symptoms and histologic appearance on therapy, but who relapse upon drug withdrawal, may require lifelong treatment. In these individuals, the benefits of continued treatment need to be weighed against the risks of long-term immunosuppressive therapy and reevaluated on a continuing basis.

Relapse is common and probably is noted in more than 50 percent of cases. In patients requiring long-term treatment, reduction of the corticosteroid dosage to the lowest dose that is capable of controlling the symptomatic, biochemical, and histologic manifestations of the disease is desirable. In many patients, remission can be maintained with azathioprine alone, thus allowing for the eventual discontinuation of corticosteroids. Initial therapy with azathioprine alone and treatment with alternate-day corticosteroids appear to be ineffective.

Patients need to be closely followed during the initial months of treatment. Blood pressure, serum electrolytes, blood glucose, and (for patients receiving azathioprine) complete blood counts are monitored biweekly during the first 3 to 4 months, and then monthly for the remainder of the first 6-month period. Particular attention is paid to individuals with histories of glucose intolerance, hypertension, fluid retention, and peptic ulcer disease. Liver chemistries are followed monthly for the first 4 to 6 months, and at intervals of 3 to 4 months thereafter.

HEPATIC TRANSPLANTATION

Liver transplantation is reserved for patients with advanced, symptomatic, and irreversible liver disease. Individuals with complications related to chronic hepatitis or cirrhosis should be referred to medical centers specializing in liver transplantation for evaluation. Optimally, transplant referrals should be obtained before the onset of the terminal phase of liver disease (hepatorenal syndrome, hepatic coma). Transplantation can prolong and dramatically improve the quality of life in patients with advanced and otherwise untreatable forms of liver disease.

Differential Diagnosis

Chronic hepatitis needs to be differentiated from other disorders associated with hepatocellular injury. Occasionally, primary biliary cirrhosis and primary sclerosing cholangitis can be confused with chronic hepatitis. It is essential, however, that chronic hepatitis be distinguished from Wilson's disease, hemochromatosis, drug-induced hepatitis, alcoholic liver disease, and $alpha_1$-antitrypsin deficiency. There are individual chapters on these entities (except $alpha_1$-antitrypsin deficiency) in this text.

SUGGESTED READING

Bonino F, Smedile A. Delta agent (type D) hepatitis. Semin Liver Dis 1986; 6:28.

Dienstag JL, Alter HJ. Non-A, non-B hepatitis: evolving epidemiologic and clinical perspective. Semin Liver Dis 1986; 6:67.

Payne JA. Chronic hepatitis: pathogenesis and treatment. DM 1988; 34:110.

Perrillo RP. Antiviral therapy of chronic viral hepatitis. Curr Opinion Gastroenterol 1988; 4:420.

Schaffner F. Autoimmune chronic active hepatitis: three decades of progress. In: Popper H, Schaffner F, eds. Progress in liver diseases. New York: Grune & Stratton, 1986.

LIVER DISEASE IN PREGNANCY

WILLIAM M. STRAIN, M.D.
CAROLINE A. RIELY, M.D.

A review of the obstetric and medical history of a pregnant patient with liver disease narrows the differential diagnosis considerably. One should be aware of the normal changes that occur during pregnancy. It is important to determine the gestational age of the fetus, and whether there are severe nausea and vomiting or weight loss. There may be a history of (1) similar episodes during previous pregnancies, or during the taking of oral contraceptives, (2) a similar condition in a family member, or (3) severe pruritus. The presence of seizures and peripheral edema in combination with liver disease should also be noted. These data help to determine whether the condition is a liver disease unique to pregnancy, one intercurrent with pregnancy, or one that antedates the pregnancy, i.e., is preexistent (Table 1).

NORMAL PHYSIOLOGIC CHANGES

With uncomplicated pregnancy there are few, if any, alterations related to hepatic function. The marked increase in blood volume is not accompanied by an increase in hepatic blood flow; there is no increase in liver size. Because the enlarging uterus displaces the liver superiorly and posteriorly, the liver usually is not palpable. Therefore, a palpable liver may be pathologically enlarged. The gallbladder has an increased volume at rest as well as increased residual volume after contractions, giving rise to the term "sluggish gallbladder of pregnancy." Two-thirds of normal women may develop palmar erythema or spider angiomata, and it is reported that esophageal varices may transiently develop in normal pregnant women. Routine laboratory test results may become abnormal during pregnancy. The serum alkaline phosphatase level may increase two- to threefold owing to the production of placental alka-

TABLE 1 Liver Disease and Pregnancy

Unique to Pregnancy
- Hyperemesis gravidarum
- Cholestasis of pregnancy
- Toxemia—associated
- Acute fatty liver of pregnancy

Intercurrent Liver Disease
- Viral hepatitis
  - Hepatitis A
  - Hepatitis B
  - Delta hepatitis
  - Non-A non-B hepatitis
    - Sporadic
    - Epidemic
  - Other
    - Herpes simplex
    - Cytomegalovirus
    - Epstein-Barr virus
- Cholelithiasis
- Benign hepatic tumors
  - Focal nodular hyperplasia
  - Hepatic adenoma
- Drug-induced
- Budd-Chiari

Preexisting Liver Disease with Pregnancy
- Portal hypertension
- Chronic viral hepatitis
- Alcoholic liver disease
- Familial hyperbilirubinemia
- Wilson's disease
- Autoimmune chronic active hepatitis

line phosphatase. Other laboratory values that may change are listed in Table 2.

LIVER DISEASE UNIQUE TO PREGNANCY

Hyperemesis Gravidarum

Vomiting during early pregnancy is very common, occurring in approximately 50 percent of all pregnancies. When vomiting becomes marked and results in dehydration, weight loss, and ketonuria, it is defined as hyperemesis gravidarum. The etiology is unknown, but may be related to hormones such as estradiol and to sex hormone binding-globulin binding capacity. Hyperemesis may also be accompanied by transient hyperthyroidism. In one report, 40 percent of patients with hyperemesis gravidarum had an abnormally blunted response of thyroid stimulating hormone (TSH) to thyrotropin releasing hormone (TRH). This "hyperthyroidism" resolves with resolution of the hyperemesis. Liver dysfunction with hyperemesis usually consists of a mild hyperbilirubinemia and modest elevations of the transaminase and alkaline phosphatase levels. The prothrombin time usually is within 2 seconds of normal. Liver biopsy is rarely indicated; results either are normal or show mild cholestasis with occasional liver cell necrosis.

TABLE 2 Clinical Findings According to Type of Liver Disorder Occurring During Pregnancy

Type of Clinical Findings	*Normal Range for Pregnancy*	*Hyperemesis Gravidarum*	*Cholestasis*	*Cholelithiasis*	*Viral Hepatitis*	*Toxemia*	*AFLP*
Symptoms/signs	—	Vomiting	Pruritus	Abdominal pain, nausea, vomiting	Jaundice, nausea, vomiting	Hypertension, proteinuria, edema, ± seizures	Nausea, vomiting, pain, confusion, ± toxemia
Trimester	—	I	II–III	II, III	Any	III	III
Aminotransferases, U/L	Normal	Normal to 150	Normal to 500	Normal to 100	500–2,000	Normal to 250, may be >1,000	Normal to 500
Alkaline phosphatase	2×↑	Normal	10×↑	2–10×↑	2–3×↑	2–3×↑	3×↑
Bilirubin, mg/dl	Normal	Normal to 3.5	1–5	Variable	1–5	Sl↑ to 10	1–10
Prothrombin time	Normal	Normal	Normal to 2 sec prolonged	Normal	Normal to 5 sec prolonged	Normal early, >5 sec prolonged late	Normal to >5 sec prolonged
Percentage decrease in albumin	20%	Normal	Normal	Normal to 20%	Normal to 20%	Normal	20%
WBC	Slight increase	Normal	Normal	Normal or ↑	Normal	Normal to slight increase	↑ 20–30K
Bile acids	Normal	Normal	10–100×↑		Normal	Normal	Normal
Biopsy	Normal	Normal	Cholestasis, centrilobular	↑ Cholestasis	Typical hepatitis	Sinusoidal fibrin deposition, periportal hemorrhage	Centrilobular, microvesicular fat
Radiology	Normal	Normal	Normal	Ultrasonography—gallstones, dilated bile ducts	Normal	CT—infarcts	CT ? Fat

"Normal" means within the normal range for pregnancy.

Cholestasis of Pregnancy

Cholestasis of pregnancy encompasses a spectrum of cholestatic disease, ranging from pruritus gravidarum to the more severe jaundice of pregnancy. It is the most common liver disease unique to pregnancy. Isolated populations have been identified that demonstrate an extraordinarily high frequency of cholestasis, particularly among Scandinavians and Chilean Indians. Pruritus is usually the initial and most prominent complaint, beginning typically during the second or third trimester and intensifying as the pregnancy progresses. Frequently there is a history of similar episodes during previous pregnancies (about 70 percent) or with oral contraceptive use, and there may be a positive family history. The pruritus is usually associated with excoriations, and when the cholestasis is severe, jaundice may develop.

Laboratory evaluation shows cholestasis with a marked elevation in the serum bile acids, alkaline phosphatase, gamma guanosine triphosphate, and 5′-nucleotidase, with absent or mild hyperbilirubinemia. Although the transaminase levels are usually only mildly elevated, they may occasionally be extremely high (700 to 1,000 units). Liver biopsy demonstrates pure cholestasis in the centrilobular region and minimal, if any, cellular infiltrates.

Therapy should be directed toward relief of pruritus and prevention of peripartum hemorrhage. Cholestyramine in divided doses of 16 to 20 g per day is frequently given and may provide symptomatic relief of pruritus. Ultraviolet light and phenobarbital have also been used, but no treatment, short of delivery, has been predictably successful. It is important to recognize the risks, especially with severe cholestasis, during the perinatal period. Vitamin K deficiency may develop because of fat-soluble vitamin malabsorption due to a decrease in bile acid secretion, but this deficiency may be corrected with subcutaneous vitamin K before the delivery. A fourfold increase in fetal mortality has been reported. Fetal distress may develop in as many as 40 percent of patients, and 30 to 60 percent of infants are born prematurely. As with most pregnant patients with liver disease, management by a team specializing in maternal-fetal medicine is suggested. Long-term follow-up in these women has shown an increased incidence of cholelithiasis but no other liver dysfunction.

The cholestasis is clearly related to estrogenic hormones and may be reproduced in these patients by exogenous estrogen administration. Affected families have been identified, and males may transmit this susceptibility to their daughters. The exact cellular and molecular basis has not been identified, but may be related to changes in the permeability of biliary epithelium, decreased membrane Na^+-K^+-ATPase activity, changes in membrane fluidity, or a change in bile acid receptors. Recently, S-adenosyl-L-methionine (SAM), which may alter membrane fluidity or bile acid metabolism, has been used to reverse cholestasis during pregnancy, but this observation has not yet been reproduced.

Liver Disease Accompanying Preeclampsia

In order to understand and define liver disease in the setting of preeclampsia, we must first review what is meant by preeclampsia. Preeclampsia usually occurs during the third trimester of pregnancy and includes proteinuria, elevated blood pressures, and peripheral edema. It is important to note that the blood pressure is expected to fall in pregnancy, and a diastolic blood pressure of greater than 80 to 90 mm Hg may well be abnormal. Often the patient is a primagravida; if not there may be a history of preeclampsia with previous pregnancies. Preeclampsia is more common with multiple gestations than single ones. Frequently the serum uric acid level is elevated. Preeclampsia becomes eclampsia with the development of a major complication, the most frequent being seizures. This is an obstetric emergency requiring immediate delivery to avoid substantial maternal-fetal morbidity and mortality.

The most common liver disease associated with preeclampsia is the HELLP syndrome: *h*emolysis, *e*levated *l*iver enzymes, and *l*ow *p*latelets. These patients may present with epigastric pain without more conventional signs of severe preeclampsia. The blood pressure may be elevated and the liver tender. The peripheral smear shows evidence of microangiopathy and thrombocytopenia. Disseminated intravascular coagulation (DIC) usually is not present initially, and the prothrombin time and partial thromboplastin time and fibrinogen levels are normal in early stages. The aminotransferase levels are moderately to markedly elevated, the bilirubin level is elevated but not markedly so (less than 10), and proteinuria and hyperuricemia are frequently present. On liver biopsy, fibrin and fibrinogen may be found in periportal areas, sinusoids may be dilated, and there may be periportal necrosis and hemorrhage. Periportal hemorrhage has been called the "classic" lesion of preeclampsia but is seen less often now, presumably because of earlier diagnosis and treatment. Therapy for preeclampsia-associated liver disease is straightforward. After correction of any underlying coagulopathy, delivery should be accomplished. After delivery the liver disease improves and returns to its previous function without residual damage.

An extreme presentation of preeclampsia-associated liver disease is hepatic rupture. This occurs more often in older, multiparous patients and is suggested by a history of acute onset of abdominal pain. These patients frequently have a tender right upper quadrant and extremely high transaminase levels. If the hemorrhage is not confined by the hepatic capsule, hemoperitoneum with cardiovascular collapse may result. Conceptually this results from the coalescence of periportal hemorrhages causing a subcapsular hematoma, which may rupture through the hepatic capsule. The most common location of the rupture is reported to be the anterior superior segment of the right lobe. Computed tomography (CT) may demonstrate the hematoma clearly and is the imaging procedure of choice. There are case reports of successful angiographic embolization of the hematoma followed by delivery.

Acute Fatty Liver of Pregnancy

The incidence of acute fatty liver of pregnancy seems to be increasing owing to an increased index of suspicion and the detection of milder cases. It is a third-trimester liver disease and may be part of a "family" of liver disease that accompanies preeclampsia. Classically, acute fatty liver of pregnancy presents as hepatic failure associated with microvesicular fat deposition in the liver. Reportedly, primigravidas, especially those with twins or male offspring, are more commonly affected. Presenting symptoms include nausea, vomiting, abdominal pain, malaise, headache, fatigue, and restlessness, which may progress to altered mental status or hepatic encephalopathy. Hypertension, peripheral edema, jaundice, asterixis, or encephalopathy may be present. There is frequently an associated leukocytosis, with white blood cell (WBC) counts of between 15,000 and 30,000. Hyperamylasemia, hyperuricemia, thrombocytopenia, DIC, azotemia, hyperammonemia, hypoglycemia, and diabetes insipidus may also be present. The serum bilirubin level is normal early but may become markedly elevated. Imaging techniques of the liver may possibly be helpful if abdominal ultrasonography shows a diffuse increase in echogenicity and if CT shows decreased attenuation of the liver, but liver biopsy is the diagnostic procedure of choice. Lobular disarray is common, with patchy hepatocellular necrosis and pale, swollen centrizonal hepatocytes. The demonstration of microvesicular fat is the key diagnostic point. This requires cooperation between the gastroenterologist and pathologist. Immediately after biopsy, the fresh liver biopsy should be delivered to the pathologist for frozen section and the preparation of special stains for fat, such as the oil red O stain. Paraffin imbedding results in dissolution of the fat with loss of staining. In correctly processed tissue, small red fat droplets are seen, concentrated in the central zones.

Acute fatty liver of pregnancy historically has been viewed as involving a high incidence of maternal and fetal death. As late as the 1970s, an 85 percent mortality rate was mentioned, but more recently a significant reduction in morbidity and mortality has been achieved. This is partly due to earlier recognition of the disorder and the institution of prompt therapy and intensive support. Recently, morbidity and mortality have been decreased to 22 percent with early cesarean section. Postpartum management often requires intensive care, because there may be continued liver failure with hypoglycemia-hypoprothrombinemia that may persist for weeks. Mothers who survive have become pregnant again without recurrence of the disease.

Management of acute fatty liver of pregnancy involves supportive care and delivery. Because this disease involves a spectrum of clinical presentations, it may be divided into two broad groups.

Early Acute Fatty Liver of Pregnancy. In this phase hepatic failure is absent and the coagulation profile is acceptable for percutaneous liver biopsy. Special stains such as the oil red O should be done on fresh tissue to demonstrate microvesicular fat. If the biopsy is consistent with acute fatty liver of pregnancy, the baby should be delivered. Serum glucose levels, coagulation profiles, and fetal well-being should be closely monitored.

Late Acute Fatty Liver of Pregnancy. This phase presents with hepatic failure and encephalopathy. Percutaneous liver biopsy is contraindicated and an emergency cesarean section should be performed. Liver biopsy with the TruCut needle (Travenol) may then be carried out under direct visualization. Postoperative management may be complicated by liver failure, which may take up to 2 or 3 weeks to resolve and requires intensive supportive care.

A relationship between acute fatty liver of pregnancy and preeclampsia-eclampsia has been suggested by several authors. These diseases have overlapping features on both clinical and cellular levels. In a 1987 report, all nine patients with acute fatty liver of pregnancy met the criteria for preeclampsia: elevated blood pressure, proteinuria, and hyperuricemia. It appears that acute fatty liver of pregnancy and the liver disease associated with preeclampsia may be related.

INTERCURRENT LIVER DISEASE

Viral Hepatitis

The incidence and severity of viral hepatitis during pregnancy has been debated. Initially it was thought that pregnant women were at increased risk for fulminant hepatitis, but studies in the United States have not demonstrated this. Recently, epidemic non-A, non-B (NANB) hepatitis has been reported to involve an increased mortality risk for pregnant women. Hepatitis B is endemic in high-risk groups and remains an important cause of maternal-fetal morbidity. With the advent of vaccines directed against hepatitis B, there is an opportunity to limit perinatal transmission and prevent long-term complications of hepatitis B (Table 3).

Hepatitis A

The incidence of hepatitis A (HA) has decreased over the past 25 years in the U.S. The HA virus (HAV) does not appear to have increased virulence during pregnancy and, as in nonpregnant patients, no long-term carrier state has been described. There is no increased risk of perinatal transmission to the fetus unless the mother is infectious at the time of delivery. Treatment of infants is warranted if the mother was infected during the third trimester, and consists of 0.5 ml immune serum globulin (ISG) given intramuscularly. Household contacts should be treated with 0.02 ml per kilogram of ISG.

Hepatitis B

Hepatitis B (HB) continues to be a major health problem worldwide. Although there is no increased morbidity risk to the mother, the infant is in danger of becoming infected at the time of delivery (Table 3). Perinatal

TABLE 3 Vertical Transmission of Viral Hepatitis

	HA	*HB*	*Delta*	*NANB*	*Herpes Simplex*
Transmission risk	If perinatal infection	HB_eAg+ >90% HB_eAg- >50%	Rare	Low, but incidence unknown	Rare
Infant disease					
Acute	Hepatitis in ~30 days	None Mild hepatitis	Severe hepatitis	None Mild hepatitis	Disseminated HSV
Late	None	80% carriers 35% Late complications	Unknown	Unknown ?? chronic carrier	None
Prophylaxis	ISG 0.5 ml	HBIG 0.5 ml; begin HB vaccine	HBIG 0.5 ml; begin HB vaccine	ISG 0.5 ml	Acyclovir

HB_eAg = hepatitis B e antigen; HSV = herpes simplex virus; ISG = immune serum globulin; HBIG = hepatitis B immune globulin.

transmission of the HB virus (HBV) is a very efficient means of viral transfer. If the mother is positive for both hepatitis B surface antigen (HB_sAg) and hepatitis B_e antigen (HB_eAg), the infant has a greater than 90 percent chance of becoming infected. Acute hepatitis in the infant is rare, although fulminant hepatitis may occur. Most infected newborns show no disease. Unfortunately, of those infected, 80 to 90 percent become carriers of HBV, with an approximately 35 percent risk of dying from the disease, notably because of portal hypertension or hepatoma.Among women with chronic HB, the following subsets have been identified as having an especially high incidence of transmission: (1) those with active disease, (2) those with positive HBeAg, and (3) Oriental people.

Because of the serious nature of neonatal transmission and the potential for disastrous long-term consequences, the Centers for Disease Control in 1988 recommended screening of all pregnant women to exclude HB. If the patient is positive for HBsAG, hepatitis B immune globulin (HBIG) should be administered as soon after birth as possible, certainly within 24 hours; it may be given at the same time as the HBV vaccine, but in separate sites. Guidelines for prophylaxis of viral hepatitis are listed in Table 3. Infants should be tested at 12 months of age for HBsAb. If they are immunized, there is no reported risk of transmission of HBV via breast milk.

Delta Hepatitis

Delta hepatitis is a recently described incomplete virus that requires the presence of HBsAg for replication. By definition, this requires either preexisting infection with hepatitis B or a simultaneous inoculation of HB and the delta agent. Vaccination against HB prevents delta infection if adequate titers of antibody against HBsAg are achieved. Vertical transmission of delta hepatitis has been reported to occur but the incidence is unknown. Appropriate active and passive immunization directed against HBV should be successful in more than 80 percent of cases.

Non-A, Non-B Hepatitis

Non-A, non-B hepatitis (HNANB) is assumed to have a viral etiology, and is most likely due to at least two separate viruses. The more common presentation in the United States involves blood products and may be either "cholestatic" or "hepatitic." As long as portal hypertension is not present, the course of pregnancy and the disease is unchanged. The risk of vertical transmission is unknown but is believed to be low. Treatment of the infant with 0.5 ml of ISG has been recommended, but there are no data indicating whether this is helpful.

The second form of HNANB is a waterborne hepatitis that acts and even looks like HA. this has been reported in India, Nepal, and Mexico and recently has been isolated from stool and photographed by electron microscopy. This virus is similar in size and shape to true HAV, but does not have similar nucleic acids as determined by DNA probes, and infection is not reflected by a rise in anti-HAV IgG or IgM. Epidemics were first noted in India during the monsoon season or when water supplies were contaminated with raw sewage. Young adults were affected most frequently and there was a high case-fatality ratio in pregnant women (about 10 percent). This has yet to be reported in the United States.

Other Viruses

Other viruses have been reported during pregnancy. Herpes simplex virus (HSV) appears to have an increased incidence during the third trimester and may be confused with pregnancy-associated liver disease. Of the 37 reported cases, 23 percent were noted during pregnancy. Frequently there is evidence of HSV infection elsewhere, e.g., cervical or skin lesions. The hepatitis may be accompanied by a marked increase in transaminase levels and mild hyperbilirubinemia, usually without clinical jaundice. It is important to make this diagnosis before delivery and to institute prompt therapy with acyclovir. Liver biopsy demonstrates HSV inclusion bodies.

Cholelithiasis

Cholelithiasis is more common during pregnancy, presumably because of alterations in the physiology of bile formation and excretion. There is an increased volume of the gallbladder at rest, an increased residual post-contraction, and alterations in bile flow. Characteristic biliary colic may be present, and abdominal ultrasound examination may demonstrate gallstones and possibly dilated intrahepatic bile ducts. Surgery remains the treatment of choice for acute cholecystitis.

Benign Hepatic Tumors

Hepatic adenomas have been reported to enlarge and even rupture, perhaps owing to the increased circulating estrogens that occur during pregnancy. Focal nodular hyperplasia may enlarge, but it is rare for this to rupture.

Drugs-Related Disease

Fortunately most drugs are avoided during pregnancy. There is some debate over the relative hepatotoxicity of drugs during pregnancy, and some authors have speculated that there is an increased incidence of drug-induced hepatitis. The latter can occur during pregnancy and should always be considered.

Budd-Chiari Syndrome

The Budd-Chiari syndrome, or thrombosis of the hepatic veins, may be seen either during pregnancy or in the postpartum period. The cause is unknown, but may relate to changes in the coagulation system that occur at term. Management usually consists of surgical construction of a decompressive shunt, one of several types, depending on the individual anatomy.

PREEXISTING LIVER DISEASE

Portal Hypertension

The most important determinants of the outcome of pregnancy in patients with preexisting liver disease are the severity of the liver disease and the presence or absence of portal hypertension. The prognosis for patients with cirrhosis, portal hypertension, ascites, and progressive jaundice is poor if they become pregnant. Fortunately, pregnancy in such a setting is rare. The cirrhosis-induced changes in estrogen metabolism result in secondary amenorrhea and anovulation, with few pregnancies. In addition, alcoholic liver disease, the most severe liver disorder, usually occurs in an older population. Patients with severe liver disease have an increased incidence of stillbirths and fetal wastage, but no apparent increase in congenital malformations.

The most life-threatening and feared complication of pregnancy in the setting of portal hypertension is gastrointestinal (GI) hemorrhage. Most commonly this results from esophageal varices, especially in women with a history of variceal bleeding. In this group, a prophylactic decompressive shunt has been suggested on the basis of one study. Esophageal variceal sclerotherapy, with injection of agents designed to obliterate varices, may be helpful, but no studies have been reported to date. Another cause of life-threatening hemorrhage is the rupture of a splenic artery aneurysm, which is more common in the setting of portal hypertension and cirrhosis.

Familial Hyperbilirubinemia

Patients with Gilbert's syndrome have an increase in indirect bilirubin, especially with stress or infection. Pregnancy in this condition is uneventful and should be uncomplicated. In Rotor's syndrome, direct bilirubin is increased but there is no increased morbidity with pregnancy. The Dubin-Johnson syndrome may become apparent during pregnancy, when a rise in direct bilirubin may occur especially in the third trimester. The hyperbilirubinemia returns to normal in the postpartum period.

Wilson's Disease

Wilson's disease is an important but rare cause of liver disease in young people. The basic defect is a failure to excrete copper into bile. Recently the gene for Wilson's disease was found to be on chromosome 13. Clinically, Wilson's disease may present as acute or subacute hepatitis, with Kayser-Fleischer rings, low ceruloplasm, high 24-hour copper urinary excretion, and increased copper content on liver biopsy. The prognosis of Wilson's disease changed dramatically with the introduction of D-penicillamine, and there is now some experience of this treatment during pregnancy (Table 4). There does not appear to be any increased risk of congenital malformations if D-penicillamine is used. The dosage should be 750 mg to 1 g per day during the first and second trimesters, reduced to 250 mg per day during the third trimester. It is important to reduce the dosage rather than stop the medicine. Wilson's disease may develop into fulminant hepatitis if D-penicillamine is stopped, and there is an increase in "allergic" reactions if D-penicillamine is stopped and restarted; this may be avoided by giving daily low doses of the medication. In addition, lowering the dosage helps to prevent postpartum wound complications, which a higher dose of D-penicillamine may induce. Recently, trientine has been found to be effective in treating Wilson's disease. Experience with pregnancy is limited, but there have been successful uncomplicated pregnancies when trientine was given. This may decrease iron absorption from the GI tract, so it should not be taken at the same time as oral iron. It is also important to remember that the degree of underlying liver disease and portal hypertension are very important determinants of outcome, as with all chronic liver diseases.

TABLE 4 Management of "Treatable" Liver Disease During Pregnancy

	Rx
Wilson's disease	750 mg—1 g/day until 3rd trimester, then 250 mg/day
Steroid-responsive chronic active hepatitis	If possible, decrease prednisone to 15–20 mg/day, azathioprine to 50 mg/day

Hemochromatosis

Although hemochromatosis is the most common genetic disease, it is not a problem during pregnancy. In all likelihood this reflects a lower hepatic iron content in young women; normal, uncomplicated pregnancies are the rule in women who are found to have hemochromatosis at a later age.

Chronic Autoimmune Hepatitis

Chronic autoimmune, or "steroid-responsive," hepatitis usually occurs in young women. This disease characteristically shows a high gamma-globulin level; serologic abnormalities, including positive antinuclear antibody and rheumatoid factor; and a dramatic response to prednisone. Reportedly there is an increased risk of preeclampsia and fetal wastage in pregnant patients with chronic autoimmune hepatitis. Treatment with prednisone, 15 to 25 mg per day, and low-dose azathioprine, 50 mg per day, has been reported to produce no complications (Table 4). The risk of pregnancy with chronic autoimmune hepatitis is related largely to the degree of underlying liver disease. There is clearly an increased incidence of fetal wastage if cirrhosis is present.

Other Preexisting Liver Diseases

The familial intrahepatic cholestasis syndromes, including Alagille's syndrome, are reported to be associated with increased cholestasis during pregnancy, which may return to baseline after delivery. Increased cholestasis may also be seen with primary biliary cirrhosis, but interestingly, pruritus may not increase. The hepatic porphyrias may appear during pregnancy, but seem to have no effect on the course of the pregnancy.

SUGGESTED READING

Khuroo MS, Teli MR, Skidmore S, et al. Incidence and severity of viral hepatitis in pregnancy. Am J Med 1981; 70:252–255.
Larrey D, Rueff B, Feldman G, et al. Recurrent jaundice caused by recurrent hyperemesis gravidarum. Gut 1984; 25:1414–1415.
Reyes H. The enigma of intrahepatic cholestasis of pregnancy: lessons from Chile. Hepatology 1982; 2:87–96.
Riely CA. Case studies in jaundice of pregnancy. Semin Liver Dis 1988; 8:191–199.
Riely CA, Latham PS, Romero R, et al. Acute fatty liver of pregnancy: a reassessment based on observations in 9 patients. Ann Intern Med 1987; 106:703–706.
Weinstein L. Syndrome of hemolysis, elevated liver enzymes, and low platelet count: a severe consequence of hypertension in pregnancy. Am J Obstet Gynecol 1982; 142:159–167.

ACUTE CHOLECYSTITIS

MELODY O'CONNOR ALLEN, M.D., F.A.C.S.

Acute cholecystitis is still one of the most common problems faced by today's general surgeon. Of the 500,000 cholecystectomies performed in the United States each year, nearly 20 percent are for acute cholecystitis. The majority of cases of cholecystitis are related to impaction of a stone in the cystic duct, causing late necrosis of the gallbladder wall. Acalculous cholecystitis represents about 5 percent of all cases of acute cholecystitis, occurring during the early postoperative or post-trauma period. The first portion of this chapter deals primarily with calculous cholecystitis, while a separate discussion of acalculous cholecystitis is given at the end.

DIAGNOSIS

Acute cholecystitis is a clinical diagnosis based on historical data and physical findings. Laboratory and radiographic tests provide confirmatory data, but the surgeon's clinical impression is usually the most accurate. The classic history of a patient with acute calculous cholecystitis includes a past history of biliary colic (nearly 75 percent of patients) and the recent acute onset of right upper quadrant pain, fever, nausea, and emesis. Physical findings of subcostal tenderness, diminished or absent bowel sounds, and occasionally a right upper quadrant mass suggest acute gallbladder disease. Most patients with acute cholecystitis have a leukocytosis (over 10,000 cells per cubic millimeter) with a left shift, and as many as 30 percent have an abnormality of liver function tests.

Radiographic evaluation of the patient with suspected cholecystitis begins with plain abdominal radiographs, which may show a small bowel ileus pattern localized to the right upper quadrant, and in a few patients (less than 15 percent), a calcified gallstone will be visible. Air in the gallbladder wall or the biliary tree suggests emphysematous cholecystitis or a biliary intestinal fistula.

Right upper quadrant ultrasonography and technetium-99m biliary scintigraphy are the most reliable studies for confirming the diagnosis of acute cholecystitis. Ultrasonographic findings of stones within the lumen of the gallbladder, thickening of the gallbladder wall, and distension of the gallbladder are all consistent with the diagnosis of acute cholecystitis. A reliable sign of acute cholecystitis is pain experienced when pressure is exerted directly over the region of the gallbladder when localized by the ultrasonographic probe. Nonfilling of the gallbladder on scintigraphy (HIDA, PIPIDA) establishes the diagnosis of acute cholecystitis in as many as 95 percent of patients. Caution is necessary since false-positive test (nonfilling) results are obtained in patients who have not received oral alimentation for a long time. Oral cholecystography is of no value in the diagnosis of acute cholecystitis, since these acutely ill patients are unable to take the necessary test substances by mouth.

DIFFERENTIAL DIAGNOSIS

The most challenging aspect in the treatment of patients with acute biliary tract disease is differentiation of uncomplicated acute cholecystitis from complicated (gangrenous or perforated) cholecystitis, pancreatitis, acute cholangitis, or hepatitis. Differentiating these diseases is critical to planning medical or surgical therapy and requires a well reasoned assessment of the "big picture," including clinical presentation and diagnostic laboratory and radiographic tests. A history of high fever and shaking chills, physical findings of jaundice and significant elevations of serum bilirubin (greater than 4.5 mg per deciliter) and alkaline phosphatase (more than twice the normal levels) suggest acute cholangitis. That diagnosis of acute cholangitis may be confirmed by ultrasonographic findings of cholelithiasis and dilation of the intrahepatic bile ducts. Pancreatitis is suspected in patients with hyperamylasemia and a history of excessive alcohol or certain medication use (alcoholic or drug-induced pancreatitis) or ultrasonographic findings of cholelithiasis and dilated intrahepatic bile ducts (gallstone pancreatitis). A palpable right upper quadrant mass with generalized peritonitis and/or ileus suggests complicated cholecystitis. Air in the gallbladder wall or lumen suggest gangrene or empyema of the gallbladder, and a pericholecystic fluid collection suggests gallbladder perforation. Jaundice with elevation of serum glutamic-oxaloacetic transaminase (SGOT) or serum glutamic-pyruvic transaminase (SGPT) and no increase in alkaline phosphatase suggest hepatocellular disease. The diagnosis of drug-related cholestasis and alcoholic or infectious hepatitis should be considered. A careful history of drug use or alcohol intake and exposure to other infected individuals is helpful.

THERAPEUTIC ALTERNATIVES

Acute cholecystitis may be prevented by early cholecystectomy in patients with asymptomatic gallstones or biliary colic. Potential alternative preventive modalities include dissolution therapy with cheno- or ursodeoxycholic acid and biliary lithotripsy. Although these methods may ultimately prove useful in the treatment of patients with biliary colic and hence prevent the disease, they are of no use in the treatment of the patient with acute cholecystitis. (Options for managing cholelithiasis are described in the chapter *Cholelithiasis: Medical and Surgical Aspects*.)

Operative cholecystectomy is the "gold standard" in treatment of acute cholecystitis, against which all other forms of therapy must be compared. Successful removal of the gallbladder not only treats the acute illness but prevents its recurrence. Alternative therapies for acute cholecystitis include medical therapy and operative and percutaneous cholecystostomy. Many patients with acute cholecystitis respond to 3 to 5 days of "conservative therapy" including intravenous hydration, bowel rest, and broad-spectrum antibiotics. The major drawback of "conservative therapy" as definitive treatment is that nearly 25 percent of patients will experience a recurrence of acute cholecystitis within 3 months.

Recent advances in interventional radiography have led to the use of fluoroscopic or ultrasound-guided percutaneous drainage of the gallbladder, most often in patients who are at high risk for surgery. This method carries some risk in that, because it does not allow direct visualization of the diseased gallbladder, necrosis or perforation can be missed. Both operative and percutaneous cholecystostomy leave the diseased gallbladder in situ, and the patient is at risk for redeveloping stones and having further episodes of cholecystitis. These techniques are occasionally useful as temporizing measures, with cholecystectomy planned as a second stage. Ablation of the gallbladder by injection of sclerosing agents via the tube tract may eventually obviate the need for cholecystectomy after cholecystostomy, but as yet remains experimental.

PREFERRED APPROACH

Timing of Cholecystectomy

The most controversial aspect of the management of acute cholecystitis is the timing of cholecystectomy. In my practice, the patient's clinical presentation dictates the urgent or "semielective" nature of the operation. Most patients with acute cholecystitis are clinically stable with mild to moderate symptoms and should undergo "early" cholecystectomy (on the next scheduled OR day). If at any time the patient shows deterioration of clinical status, cholecystectomy must be performed immediately. If the patient shows clinical improvement with conservative treatment (intravenous fluids, antibiotics), it is possible to postpone the operation for a few days to allow time for concomitant medical problems to be diagnosed and treated. This approach is not justified as a routine, since it increases the duration of hospitalization without diminishing the incidence of perioperative complications of cholecystectomy.

Patients presenting with high fever or chills, a very high white blood cell count, and signs of sepsis or generalized peritonitis require urgent cholecystectomy (within 4 to 6 hours of presentation) since they are very likely to have gangrenous or perforating cholecystitis. The final decision as to the timing of surgery for these critically ill patients should be made by balancing the potential benefit of urgent cholecystectomy (i.e., removal of the septic focus) against the benefit of brief delay in operation to permit optimization of general conditions.

Preoperative Preparation

Preoperative management of the patient with acute cholecystitis is based on the severity of clinical findings when the diagnosis is made. Patients with mild symptoms should be given intravenous fluids, receive nothing by mouth, and require only a short course of perioperative antibiotics for wound prophylaxis 30 minutes before the operation is begun. Many patients present with a history of prolonged emesis and should undergo careful assessment of fluid balance with aggressive fluid resuscitation and replacement of electrolytes. These patients are likely to have a significant ileus and require nasogastric suction to prevent further emesis.

Patients with obvious sepsis (high white blood cell counts, fever and chills, hypotension) require careful monitoring of cardiorespiratory status with replacement of intravascular volume to optimize cardiac output. Broad-spectrum antibiotics should begin immediately to provide coverage against biliary contaminants. There is debate in the literature regarding the efficacy of third-generation cephalosporins in this clinical situation. I believe that it is safest to institute more aggressive antibiotic therapy using an aminoglycoside to provide coverage against likely aerobic pathogens (*Escherichia coli*, *Klebsiella*, *Proteus*) and clindamycin or metronidazole to provide coverage against anaerobic pathogens (*Bacteroides*). If enterococcal infection is suspected, ampicillin should be included, providing so-called triple antibiotic therapy. Antibiotics should be modified during the postoperative course according to the results of intraoperative bile cultures and should be continued until the patient has a normal white blood cell count and temperature for 24 hours.

Choice of Procedure

Optimal surgical therapy for acute cholecystitis is total removal of the gallbladder. Severe inflammation with distortion of normal tissue planes make removal of the acutely diseased gallbladder more difficult than elective cholecystectomy for chronic cholecystitis. The gallbladder is often firm and distended, with bile further obscuring surgical anatomy. I use several techniques to facilitate removal of the acutely inflamed gallbladder while protecting extrahepatic ductal structures from inadvertent injury. I aspirate as much bile as possible from the gallbladder to decompress the biliary tree, sending a specimen for Gram stain and culture. Before performing extensive dissection, I perform cholangiography via the gallbladder (through the same site used to aspirate bile) to clarify the location of structures within the triangle of Calot. I remove the gallbladder "fundus first" and delay irrigation of the cystic duct until the anatomy is clear. When severe inflammation makes total resection hazardous, it is wise to perform a partial cholecystectomy, leaving a portion of the gallbladder wall in the liver bed. This technique is also helpful as a means of minimizing blood loss in patients with alcoholic cirrhosis and portal hypertension. Many surgeons advocate cholecystostomy in patients with acute cholecystitis who are gravely ill and clinically unstable. I have found that a combination of epidural and local anesthesia provides adequate analgesia to allow cholecystectomy in even the most difficult cases, and find that cholecystostomy is rarely indicated.

Common Bile Duct Stones

Ten to 25 percent of patients operated on for acute cholecystitis have concomitant common bile duct stones. One should perform judicious common bile duct exploration at the time of cholecystectomy, recognizing that inflammation and edema may make this procedure extremely hazardous. If on cholangiography the common duct is less than 1 cm in diameter, it may be wise to defer duct exploration and plan to perform endoscopic sphincterotomy with stone removal during the postoperative period. Attempts at choledochotomy and T-tube placement or choledochoenterostomy in a patient with a small common duct can result in damage to the duct with late stricture formation.

Wound Management

Wound management is based on operative findings. In cases where infected bile is spilled in the operative field, I close the fascia of the wound, packing the skin and subcutaneous tissues open with saline-soaked gauze. I also pack wounds open if the presence of *Clostridium* is suspected on Gram smear. I do not use drains unless I strongly suspect a bile leak at the time of closure. Routine use of drains in the subhepatic space after uncomplicated cholecystectomy has not been shown to reduce the incidence of postoperative complications and may in fact increase the rate of infection.

POSTOPERATIVE COURSE

The majority of patients who undergo uncomplicated cholecystectomy for acute cholecystitis recover and leave the hospital within 7 to 10 days. Nasogastric suction and intravenous hydration should be maintained until bowel function has returned. Patients who presented initially with mild symptoms should receive a short course of perioperative antibiotics. Severely ill patients presenting with clinical signs of sepsis should continue to receive antibiotics (appropriate to organisms and sensitivities from intraoperative bile culture) during the postoperative period until they are afebrile and their white blood cell counts have been normal for 24 hours.

Complications

Major postoperative complications after cholecystectomy occur in as many as 6 percent of patients. The most common complication after cholecystectomy is wound infection, occurring in approximately 5 percent of cases. This complication should be anticipated and prevented in the operating room by packing wounds open in patients at high risk for infections. Abnormal bile leakage occurs in 1 percent of patients, presenting as bile peritonitis, bile ascites, or external biliary fistula. Bile leakage is usually related to cystic duct leak or to intraoperative damage to common or hepatic bile ducts. Basic principles of treatment of bile leaks include drainage of bile collection, antibiotic therapy when biliary sepsis is present, and delineation of the nature and site of leak by cholangiography (T-tube or endoscopic retrograde cholangiopancreatography). Major ductal disruptions or transections require reoperation with restoration of ductal continuity, usually by choledochoenterostomy. Regardless of therapy for bile leak, there is a high incidence of late ductal stricture that is probably related to periductal inflammation and fibrosis. Retained common bile duct stones occur in as many as 5 percent of patients, and should be suspected in any patient with postoperative jaundice, biliary sepsis, high output of bile through T-tube or drains, or bile leakage from the wound. Retained stones should be extracted either via the T-tube tract (Burhenne technique) or at endoscopic sphincterotomy. (These techniques are described in other chapters of this book.) Other complications include pancreatitis, intra-abdominal abscess, upper gastrointestinal hemorrhage, and various infectious complications (pneumonia, urinary tract infection, septicemia).

Overall mortality after cholecystectomy for acute cholecystitis is 5 percent. The most common causes of death are cardiorespiratory failure, sepsis, or hepatic failure. In a careful study of patients undergoing biliary tract surgery of all types, Pitt et al determined that the preoperative factors most often related to death included the following:

1. Age more than 60 years
2. Albumin less than 3.0 g per dl
3. Hematocrit less than 30 percent
4. White blood cell count more than 10,000 per cubic millimeter
5. Total bilirubin more than 10 mg per dl
6. Alkaline phosphatase more than 100 International Units
7. Creatinine more than 1.3 mg per dl

In addition to these risk factors, the presence of established hepatic cirrhosis and portal hypertension significantly increases the risk of complications and death in acute cholecystitis. Although diabetes mellitus has long been considered to increase the risk of death in patients with acute cholecystitis, the most recent studies indicate that with modern surgical and perioperative care there is no increase in mortality over nondiabetic patients.

SPECIFIC COMPLICATIONS OF UNTREATED ACUTE CHOLECYSTITIS

Acute cholecystitis can rapidly progress to gangrene, empyema, or perforation if treatment is delayed. Patients with gangrenous or perforated cholecystitis may present with severe right upper quadrant pain, peritoneal signs, high white blood cell count, spiking fevers, or even septic shock. Unfortunately, the patients in whom these complications are most common (i.e., the elderly, diabetic, or immunosuppressed patient) may not manifest any of these clinical findings and present with rather mild symptoms.

The diagnosis of gangrenous, empyematous, or perforated cholecystitis is rarely made preoperatively, but should be suspected in any high-risk patient. Abdominal radiographic or computed tomography studies show air in the gallbladder wall or lumen or a pericholecystic fluid collection. Although gram-negative organisms are present in the majority of patients with complicated cholecystitis, *Clostridium* is also found in as many as 50 percent of patients. If gangrenous cholecystitis is suspected or if gram-positive rods are noted on intraoperative Gram smear, high-dose penicillin therapy should be initiated immediately. Because the mortality of complicated cholecystitis approaches 40 percent, the surgeon should be willing to operate early in the clinical course of high-risk patients who have acute cholecystitis despite other medical problems. In these cases, the adage that a patient is "too sick to operate" is more appropriately stated "too sick *not* to operate."

ACALCULOUS CHOLECYSTITIS

Acalculous cholecystitis occurs in patients who have a history of trauma, burns, serious bacterial infections, or recent operations. In these patients, inflammation of an otherwise normal gallbladder is thought to be caused by vascular insufficiency (hypovolemia, shock, or vasoactive drugs) in combination with prolonged bile stasis (fasting, total parenteral nutrition, ileus, and narcotic analgesics). Patients with acalculous cholecystitis may have a rapidly progressive course, with almost 50 percent developing gangrene and 10 percent developing perforation of the gallbladder. Presenting symptoms are often mild and difficult to identify, leading to frequent delays in diagnosis. Failure of the gallbladder to fill on cholescintigraphy is diagnostic of acalculous cholecystitis. As in complicated calculous cholecystitis, the best results are obtained when the diagnosis is made early and expedient cholecystectomy is performed. Mortality for acute acalculous cholecystitis has been reported to range from 8 to 20 percent. A high level of suspicion must be maintained concerning patients known to be at risk for the disease, and the diagnosis should be ruled out by cholescintigraphy.

GALLBLADDER INFARCTION

Gallbladder infarction is a rare disorder occurring spontaneously in hypertensive patients, patients with endocarditis, or in the extremely rare case of gallbladder torsion. Most often, infarction occurs as a postoperative complication of hepatic artery ligation or intra-arterial infusion of chemotherapeutic agents. For this reason, prophylactic cholecystectomy should be performed at the initial operation.

SUGGESTED READING

Addison NV, Finan PJ. Urgent and early cholecystectomy for acute gallbladder disease. Br J Surg 1988; 75:141–143.

Geenen JE, Hogan WJ, Dodds WT, et al. The efficacy of endoscopic sphincterotomy after cholecystectomy in patients with sphincter of Oddi dysfunction. N Engl J Med 1989; 320:82–87.

Glenn F. Acute cholecystitis: an increasing entity. Ann Surg 1982; 195:131–136.

Lewis RT, Goodall RG, Marien B, et al. Biliary bacteria, antibiotic use, and wound infection in surgery of the gallbladder and common bile duct. Arch Surg 1987; 122:44–47.

McSherry CK, Glenn F. The incidence and causes of death following surgery for nonmalignant biliary tract disease. Ann Surg 1980; 191:271–275.

Pitt HA, Cameron JL, Postier RG, Gadacz TR. Factors affecting mortality in biliary tract surgery. Am J Surg 1981; 141:66–71.

CHOLELITHIASIS: MEDICAL AND SURGICAL ASPECTS

DAVID F. RANSOHOFF, M.D.

The management of gallstone disease has been affected greatly in the last 10 years by new methods of diagnosis, new nonsurgical therapies, and new understanding of natural history. Although this chapter is concerned primarily with choices of therapy, it is written in light of recent advances in treatment and in our understanding of natural history.

ISSUES IN DIAGNOSIS

The diagnosis of the presence of gallstones is no longer difficult, because the sensitivity of ultrasonography is very high. However, while it has become easy to diagnose the presence of stones in the gallbladder, it still may be a challenge to determine whether symptoms are caused by gallstones. The issue of attribution becomes critically important in deciding whether gallstones need treatment because, as discussed later, the natural history of symptomatic gallstone disease appears to be much different from that of asymptomatic gallstone disease. (Attributing to gallstones such complications as acute cholecystitis and pancreatitis is relatively easy, and this will not be discussed further; acute cholecystitis and pancreatitis are covered in other chapters.)

A good rule of thumb is that biliary pain is characterized by infrequent episodes, and the patient feels well between episodes. These may occur a few times a year or even less often. Exceptions do occur, but they appear to be uncommon; for example, some persons may have very frequent pain episodes over the course of 1 or 2 weeks caused by a gallstone in the common bile duct. Internists should be cautious over blaming the gallbladder for pain that is continuous over days or weeks or that occurs frequently over months and years. If such patients undergo a cholecystectomy, the "postcholecystectomy syndrome" may occur; i.e., pain may return because gallstones were not the cause of pain in the first place.

AVAILABLE THERAPIES FOR GALLSTONES

Cholecystectomy

Cholecystectomy has been the primary mode of therapy for persons who need treatment of gallstones. The advantage of cholecystectomy is that gallstones are removed promptly and, with rare exception, do not recur. The main disadvantage is the operative mortality, although this is low. Rarely, there are important complications such as bile duct stricture. Also, of course, some patients simply do not want an abdominal operation. The advantages and disadvantages of cholecystectomy must be compared with those of other available therapies.

Oral Bile Acid Dissolution

For patients with cholesterol gallstones, bile acid dissolution with chenodeoxycholic acid (cheno) or ursodeoxycholic acid (urso) may be an option. Most, however, are not candidates for oral dissolution. Proper patient selection is the key to therapeutic efficacy. Oral dissolution agents work best in persons with radiolucent, small (under 1.7 cm), and floating gallstones. The gallbladder must be functioning, as indicated by oral cholecystography. The length of treatment required varies from about 6 to 24 months. Once stones are dissolved, they may recur in over 5 years in about 50 percent of patients. This should not be surprising because the gallbladder is left intact. The side effects of cheno include diarrhea (in 40 percent of patients at a dosage of 750 mg per day), which is often transient; slight increases in serum cholesterol; and slight elevations of serum glutamic oxaloacetic transaminase (SGOT) (clinically significant in about 3 percent). To monitor patients on therapy, serum cholesterol should be measured every 6 months and SGOT monthly for 3 months, and ultrasonography or oral cholecystography should be performed yearly. Urso appears not to have these adverse effects. If therapy is to be successful, gallstones will be fully or partially dissolved at 1 year.

The important advantage of oral dissolution therapy is that surgery may be avoided. There are several disadvantages: not every patient is a candidate, there may be a lengthy initial treatment period before gallstone dissolution, stones may recur, and the costs are not inconsiderable. A 2-year treatment program may be less expensive than a cholecystectomy, but the possible requirement for repeated ultrasound monitoring and retreatment may make a total program very expensive. On the other hand, for patients who do require some form of treatment, who are candidates, who want to avoid surgery, and who are willing to undertake a possibly chronic treatment program, oral dissolution may be an appropriate choice. Oral bile acid dissolution therapy is likely to be most appropriate for some persons with symptomatic (i.e., painful) stones. It is not prompt enough in action to treat patients who have had complications such as acute cholecystitis.

MTBE (Methyl-tert-butyl-ether)

MTBE is a dissolution agent administered directly into the gallbladder after access has been obtained by a catheter, placed percutaneously through the liver. Over the course of about 8 hours, a solvent ether can be used to dissolve single or multiple cholesterol gallstones. The technique requires special catheters (i.e., ones that will not be dissolved by the ether) and a special pump to prevent overflow into the common duct and the duodenum where ether may be absorbed. This is currently an experimental therapy. In experienced hands it may be safe and have minimal side effects. A disadvantage is that it requires invasive access. Further, the rate of recurrence may be expected to be as high as after dissolution with bile acid therapy, because the gallbladder is left intact.

Extracorporeal Shock-Wave Lithotripsy (ESWL)

In the last 5 years two generations of shock-wave lithotripsy machines have been developed, and lithotripsy is becoming increasingly simple to use. The basic principle of therapy is to focus acoustic shock waves onto stones to fragment them into small pieces that will pass through the common duct and into the duodenum. Adjuvant dissolution therapy appears to be necessary to dissolve residual fragments, to prevent their becoming multiple niduses for new stones. The earliest model of lithotripsy machine required general anesthesia and immersion of the patient's torso into a water bath to provide a path for the acoustic shock wave. More recent lithotripsy machines have a self-contained water bath. Furthermore, they deliver lower-power shock waves, thus obviating the need for general anesthesia. Therapy requires about 1,500 shock pulses administered over about 1 hour, and multiple sessions may be required. Patients are currently considered eligible if they have three or fewer stones in the gallbladder, stones with no calcified rim or nidus, and a patent cystic duct. The success rate in early reports appears promising: there is a 60 to 90 percent rate of dissolution when accompanied by 3 to 24 months of chemotherapy. The complication rate appears to be relatively low, only 1 to 2 percent developing acute pancreatitis and 3 to 5 percent developing gross hematuria. There is a detailed chapter, *Biliary Lithotripsy.*

This procedure is currently experimental in the United States. The results in Europe have been promising, but there are some unanswered questions about lithotripsy that will affect its appeal to patients and physicians. One disadvantage of ESWL is that months of bile acid chemotherapy appear to be necessary for initial dissolution. Furthermore, the recurrence rate appears to be as high as after oral bile acid therapy and may be associated with symptoms. Two outstanding questions will affect the potential usefulness of lithotripsy (as well as chemotherapy): (1) can recurrent stones be prevented? and (2) must recurrent stones be managed as "symptomatic" stones, or may they be considered as asymptomatic stones (i.e., that may be ignored until symptoms occur)? If the natural history of recurrent stones is not as benign as that of asymptomatic stones, patients who have received lithotripsy may require periodic ultrasound monitoring and retreatment if stones recur. Such a requirement would probably be considered an important disadvantage by both patients and physicians. On the other hand, for those who do not want surgery and who are candidates for lithotripsy, lithotripsy appears to be a highly promising approach.

Expectant Management

Expectant management consists of watchful waiting until pain or a complication occurs. Whether such a strategy is acceptable depends, in large part, on the natural history of untreated gallstones.

Choices of Therapy In Patients With Gallstone Disease

The choice of whether to institute *any* therapy depends primarily on the patient's symptom state, because each has a different natural history. Once a decision about *whether* to treat has been made, the type of treatment may be somewhat discretionary, as desired by the patient.

Asymptomatic Gallstones

In the past, persons with asymptomatic gallstone disease were advised to have prophylactic cholecystectomy because it was believed that they had a high risk of developing biliary pain and complications (25 to 50 percent over 10 to 20 years). However, recent evidence about natural history suggests that such an aggressive therapeutic strategy is not necessary, because natural history appears to be relatively benign, with a 15 to 20 percent rate of pain over 15 years and few biliary complications. Even nonsurgical therapy is unlikely to be attractive to patients with asymptomatic gallstones, because the natural history appears to be so benign.

Asymptomatic Gallstones In Diabetics

Diabetics have been considered different from nondiabetics because of a very high mortality rate (up to 22 percent) when acute cholecystitis occurs. This rate, reported decades ago, appears to have decreased over recent years. Diabetics currently carry an operative mortality rate about twice as high as that of nondiabetics (about 7 percent compared with 3 percent in an age-adjusted comparison group of nondiabetics). This rate is markedly lower that the rate of 22 percent reported in the past. More important, only a few diabetics with gallstones ever get acute cholecystitis. For these reasons, it does not appear worthwhile to treat asymptomatic gallstones in diabetics any differently from those in nondiabetics. However, it must be remembered that when diabetics develop acute cholecystitis, they may have a worse clinical course than nondiabetics.

Symptomatic (Painful) Gallstones

An important area of controversy and research concerns the management of patients who have had an episode of biliary pain. It is clear that persons with biliary pain have a very different natural history from that of persons with asymptomatic gallstone disease. The choice of treatment is clinically important, because pain is by far the most common problem that demands a decision about treatment of gallstone disease. There are few data about the long-term natural history of persons with symptomatic gallstones, but some good short-term evidence about natural history comes from the placebo group of the National Cooperative Gallstone Study. Persons with pain had a high incidence of recurrent biliary pain (about 70 percent over 2 years) and a modest rate of biliary complications (about 6 percent over 2 years). Interestingly, most of the recurrent pain episodes were isolated.

Most authorities currently recommend prompt treatment for persons who have had an episode of biliary pain. In the past, this meant cholecystectomy. It now seems reasonable also to offer chemotherapy (cheno or urso) for those who are candidates and, as it becomes available, lithotripsy. At the same time, however, it may be worthwhile to reconsider whether any therapy is needed for symptomatic gallstones, and whether expectant management may be acceptable for some patients. At issue is whether the natural history of symptomatic stones is ominous enough to warrant preventive intervention, or whether it may be acceptable for a person with symptoms to be managed expectantly until symptoms recur or a complication arises. While a strategy of watchful waiting involves some risk, the possible benefit is avoidance of therapy altogether. The concept is to manage biliary pain as a "chronic disease," which is treated when symptoms become severe enough or when a complication develops.

COMMON DUCT STONES

Common duct stones require treatment because they may cause pain, biliary tract infection, or acute pancreatitis. A detailed discussion of the management of common duct stones is beyond the scope of this chapter, but is covered in several other chapters. In the past, cholecystectomy with common bile duct exploration was the only treatment available. Now, ERCP with papillotomy is an available initial therapy, and may be the only therapy necessary for patients who are not good surgical candidates. Also, for common duct stones ESWL may be used, in combination with ERCP, to fragment large stones that otherwise will not pass through a papillotomy. Oral dissolution agents have no use because they act too slowly, and MTBE cannot be used because of limited surface contact with stones in the common duct. Monooctanoin, a vegetable oil contact solvent, can be used in some cases of intrahepatic stones, but dissolution may take days.

SUGGESTED READING

Allen MJ, Borody TJ, Bugliosi TF, et al. Rapid dissolution of gallstones in humans using methyl-tert-butyl-ether. N Engl J Med 1985; 312:217–20.

Friedman LS, Roberts MS, Brett AS, Marton KI. Management of asymptomatic gallstones in the diabetic patient. Ann Intern Med 1988; 109:913–919.

Gracie WA, Ransohoff DF. The natural history of silent gallstones: the innocent gallstone is not a myth. N Engl J Med 1982; 307:798–800.

Ransohoff DF, Gracie WA, Wolfenson LB, Neuhauser D. Prophylactic cholecystectomy or expectant management of silent gallstones: a decision analysis to assess survival. Ann Intern Med 1983; 99:199–204.

Ransohoff DF, Miller GL, Forsythe SB, Hermann RE. Outcome of acute cholecystitis in patients with diabetes mellitus. Ann Intern Med 1987; 106:829–832.

Sackmann M, Weber W, Delius M, et al. Extracorporeal shock-wave lithotripsy of gallstones without general anesthesia: first clinical experience. Ann Intern Med 1987; 107:347–348.

Schoenfield LJ, Lachin JM, and Steering Committee, National Cooperative Gallstone Study. A controlled trial of efficacy and safety of chenodeoxycholic acid for dissolution of gallstones. Ann Intern Med 1981; 95:257–282.

Thistle JL, Cleary PA, Lachin JM, et al. The natural history of cholelithiasis: the National Cooperative Gallstone Study. Ann Intern Med 1984; 101:171–175.

BILIARY LITHOTRIPSY

TILMAN SAUERBRUCH, M.D.
MICHAEL SACKMANN, M.D.
JOSEPH HOLL, M.D.
GUSTAV PAUMGARTNER, M.D.

Shock waves are high-pressure waves. At present, a variety of shock wave generation techniques is employed. In all of the techniques, the shock waves are generated in water outside the body. Using various systems, such as reflectors, acoustic lenses, or certain arrangements of the acoustic sources, they are directed to a focal area (Fig. 1). Because most human tissue has an acoustic impedance approximately equal to that of water, the shock wave energy can be transmitted into the body with little attenuation. If a stone is located in the focal area of the shock waves, where rapidly changing pressures of approximately 1,000 bar occur, disintegration of the calculus can be achieved after repeated shock wave application. This is due to compressive and tensile wave forces and due to cavitation phenomena. Placement of the stone in the focal area of the shock waves is achieved by a biplanar x-ray system for the treatment of bile duct stones and by ultrasonography for location and treatment of gallbladder stones.

The currently available extracorporeal shock wave lithotripsy (ESWL) machines differ from each other with respect to the energy source (spark gap, piezoelectric array, or electromagnetic membrane movement) the focusing system (ellipsoidal reflector, shaped array, or lens), and location systems (x-ray, ultrasonography). At present, no controlled clinical trials have been published allowing a direct comparison of these different systems and machines.

The principle of focused shock waves is to create a limited area of high pressure, while keeping the pressure in the surrounding tissue relatively low. This allows tissue damage outside the focal area to be kept to a minimum, provided that the total shock wave energy is not too high. Nevertheless, the patients should have normal coagulation parameters to avoid the risk of hematomas, and the shock wave energy should not pass through lung tissue, which is very sensitive to shock wave damage. Previous experience with kidney stone lithotripsy and initial clinical trials with gallstone lithotripsy suggest that with this novel therapeutic approach, tissue damage directly attributable to shock waves is a minor problem. Shock wave lithotripsy may induce a dull pain, the degree of which probably depends on the shock wave pressure and focal

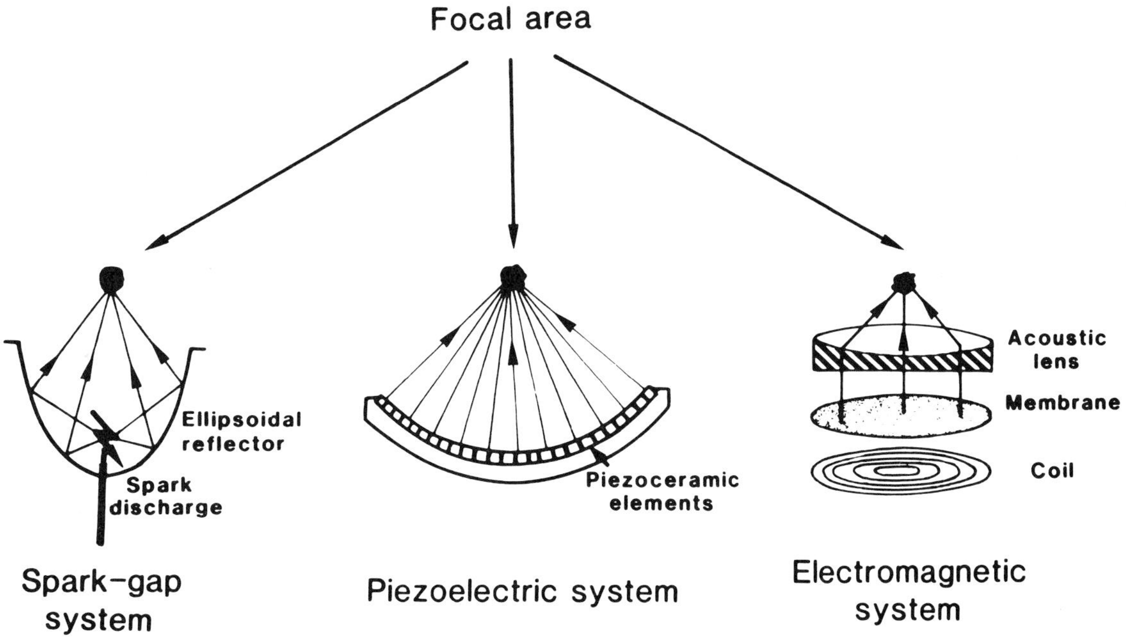

Figure 1 Schematic drawing of different systems for extracorporeal generation of shock waves in water. Shock waves are generated by spark discharge (Dornier System), piezoelectric elements (Wolf System) or electromagnetic deflection of a metal membrane (Siemens' System). Focusing of the shock waves is achieved by reflection of the primary wave (Dornier), by arraying the piezoceramic elements on a hemispherical "dish" (Wolf), or by an acoustic lens (Siemens). Coupling of the shock waves into the body is achieved by a water cushion or a water basin. The stone must be located within the focal area where pressures of approximately 1,000 bar occur and where disintegration is achieved after about 500 to several thousand shocks, depending on the machine and stone characteristics. (Republished with permission from Sauerbruch T, Holl J, Sackmann M, Paumgartner G. The role of extracorporeal lithotripsy (ESWL) in the treatment of gallstones. Endoscopy 1988; 20:285.)

volume. Because of the development of newer systems with a smaller focal volume and with increasing experience of physicians using the method, general anesthesia is usually not required for the treatment of gallbladder stones. Indeed, the procedure is increasingly performed on outpatients. However, pain may necessitate either sedation or analgesia.

RATIONALE OF ESWL

Disintegration of biliary stones into fragments may allow for the spontaneous passage of particles from the biliary tract into the intestine. Because of the anatomic structure of the cystic duct and the papilla of Vater, only small fragments not larger than 2 to 3 mm will leave the gallbladder spontaneously. However, even small fragments may remain in the gallbladder when contraction is incomplete. In addition, shock waves often produce fragments too large to pass the biliary tract spontaneously. Therefore, treatment of gallbladder stones is combined with oral administration of bile acids, which cause cholesterol desaturation of the bile and thus allow dissolution of the remaining stone fragments, provided these are mainly composed of cholesterol. (See article by Sauerbruch et al, published in *New England Journal of Medicine.*) It may be assumed that shock wave disintegration of stones enhances cholesterol stone dissolution by increasing the surface area to volume ratio and by disrupting noncholesterol stone layers. In the case of bile duct stones, fragmentation of calculi in the biliary tree may obviate the necessity for open surgery in patients in whom anatomy of the bile duct or size and location of the stones hinder successful endoscopic extraction of the calculi.

ESWL OF GALLBLADDER STONES

Machines

The bulk of clinical data for lithotripsy of gallstones is based on treatment with electrohydraulic shock wave generation (spark gap—Dornier system, Fig. 2). However, initial reports with other devices using piezoelectric or electromagnetic shock wave generation have now been published (see Fig. 1). The effect of different shock wave sources on stone fragmentation is at present ill-defined. For the treatment of gallbladder stones, it is important that the machines be equipped with high-resolution real-time ultrasonographic facilities mounted in the shock wave axis for detection and location of the stones in the shock wave focus and for monitoring the disintegration process. Enlargement of the aperture of the shock wave source, together with a smaller focal volume and the option to reduce pressures in the focal area, have led to pain-free treatment for many patients. However, the optimal relationship between shock wave energy, pain, and efficacy still needs to be defined for different stone types, stone sizes, and machines.

Adjuvant Therapy

To date, we have no data from controlled trials showing that lithotripsy of gallbladder stones is successful

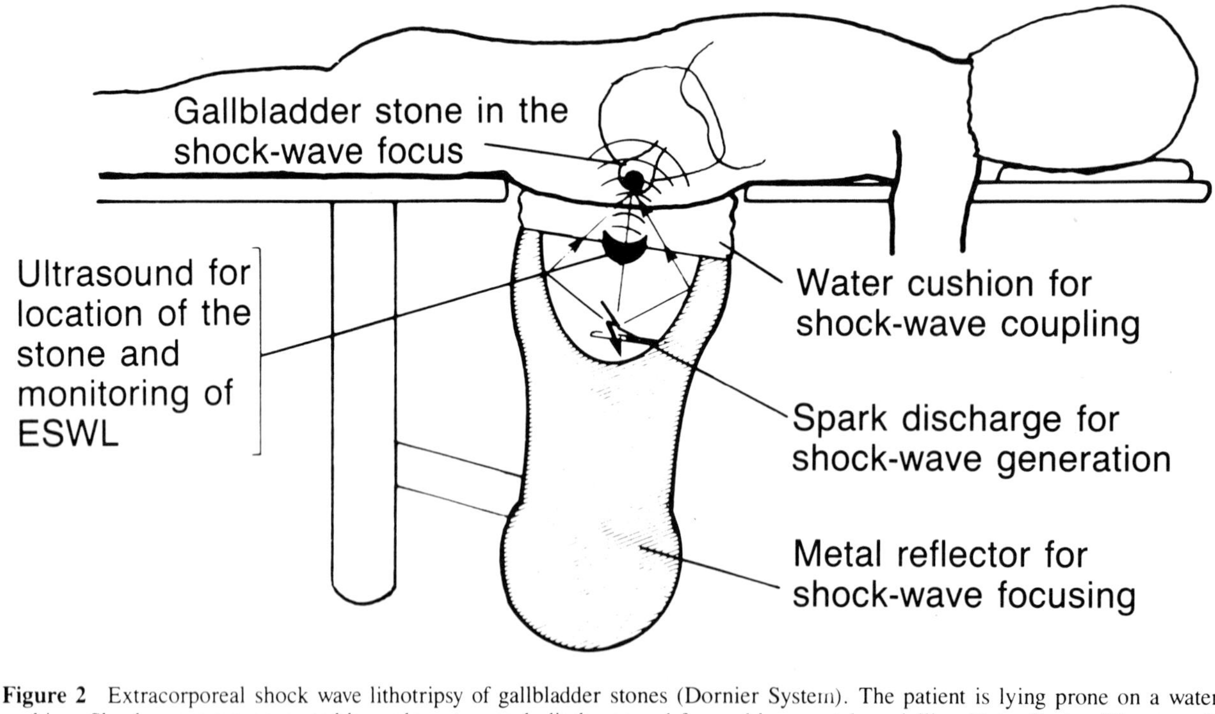

Figure 2 Extracorporeal shock wave lithotripsy of gallbladder stones (Dornier System). The patient is lying prone on a water cushion. Shock waves are generated by underwater spark discharge and focused by a metal semiellipsoidal reflector. The stone is located within the focus, and disintegration is monitored by inline ultrasonography.

without adjuvant treatment. We therefore administer chenodeoxycholic acid and ursodeoxycholic acid to obtain dissolution of remaining fragments. Given the slightly different mechanisms of action of the two bile acids and a possible synergistic effect of the combined treatment, we administer 7 to 8 mg of chenodeoxycholic acid and 7 to 8 mg of ursodeoxycholic acid daily as a single bedtime dosage. It is currently being evaluated whether monotherapy with ursodeoxycholic acid is equally efficacious. This treatment should be started about 2 weeks before lithotripsy and continued for as long as 3 months after sonographic disappearance of the stone to dissolve very small particles that are no longer detectable by ultrasonography.

Inclusion Criteria for ESWL of Gallbladder Stones

Table 1 summarizes the inclusion and exclusion criteria for ESWL of gallbladder stones. Because the prognosis for silent gallstones is favorable in most patients, ESWL is probably not appropriate for treatment of patients without biliary symptoms. Very large stones and multiple stones are more difficult to treat than solitary stones up to 20 mm in diameter. Seventy to 80 percent of radiolucent stones are composed of cholesterol. A positive oral cholecystogram documents a patent cystic duct, a prerequisite for adjuvant bile acid therapy and for spontaneous passage of the fragments. Lung tissue may be damaged by shock waves and bone, or air-filled bowel loops may absorb or reflect the shock wave energy. Patients with complications of gallbladder stone disease, such as acute cholecystitis or gallbladder empyema, represent a contraindication for lithotripsy.

Patients should be meticulously evaluated to be sure that extrabiliary diseases such as gastroduodenal ulcers or pancreatitis are not the cause of their symptoms.

Patients with spontaneous or drug-induced coagulopathy may develop a hematoma when they undergo ESWL. It is still unclear whether vascular aneurysms, which come into the shock wave path, might rupture, especially if they are calcified. These patients should therefore be excluded. Pregnancy is a contraindication for ESWL as well as for bile acid therapy. Taking into account these criteria of eligibility and contraindications, probably no more than 20 percent of all symptomatic gallbladder stone patients are suitable candidates for ESWL in its present form.

Adverse Effects

To date, no fatal complications directly attributable to shock wave lithotripsy have been reported. It may be assumed that ESWL of gallbladder stones is at least as safe as surgery. Relevant tissue damage caused by shock waves is extremely rare, provided that the total dosage is limited to 1,600 shocks when the electrohydraulic system is used.

Symptoms and complications caused by the passing of fragments may be of a more serious nature. In our series, 35 percent of the patients experienced biliary pain, especially within the first 2 months after undergoing ESWL. These symptoms are most probably caused by spontaneous passage of fragments. Although these symptoms can be easily treated by spasmolytic therapy, impaction of particles is a more serious problem. Occlusion of the cystic duct occurred in 5 percent of the patients. However, it was in no instance accompanied by acute cholecystitis. In half of these patients, the obstruction resolved spontaneously; however, few of these patients became stone-free. Obstruction of the common bile duct is a very rare occurrence. It was seen in only one of 175 patients.

The most important complication is probably acute biliary pancreatitis. In our series, 1 percent of the patients developed mild pancreatitis, and of these, only one out of 175 patients required endoscopic sphincterotomy.

Success Rate

In our most favorable study (see article by Sackmann et al, published in New England Journal of Medicine, 1988), we reported a stone clearance rate of about 85 percent 8 to 12 months after ESWL of gallbladder stones. This rate had been achieved in patients with solitary stones who had received adjuvant bile salt therapy after fragmentation. The average time to stone clearance in these patients was 4 months, at which point all patients without stones were free of symptoms. In patients with two or three

TABLE 1 Criteria for Extracorporeal Shock-wave Lithotripsy of Gallbladder Stones

Inclusion Criteria	*Exclusion Criteria*
History of biliary pain	Gallbladder stones with symptoms and signs of complications (e.g., acute cholecystitis, empyema, acute biliary pancreatitis)
Radiolucent stones (preferably solitary) up to 30 mm in diameter or	Concomitant bile duct stones
Up to three radiolucent stones not larger than 2 cm	Symptoms attributable to extrabiliary gastrointestinal diseases (e.g., peptic ulcers, pancreatitis)
Visualization of the gallbladder on oral cholecystography	Vascular aneurysms, large bones, or air-filled tissue in the shock wave path
	Coagulopathy or current medications with drugs inhibiting platelet aggregation
	Pregnancy

stones, the 8- to 12-month clearance rate was 40 percent, and in patients with stones with a calcified rim, it was 50 percent. It is therefore obvious that in its present form, ESWL of gallstones can compete with surgery only if patients are carefully selected.

Long-Term Follow-Up

In our series, elective surgery has been necessary in only 1 percent of the patients. This rate may increase slightly, given that some symptomatic patients who do not clear the fragments from the gallbladder will need surgery in the long run.

Recurrence of stones is a major problem in every nonsurgical procedure for the treatment of gallstones. From the postdissolution studies, it is known that the rate of recurrence of gallstones increases to about 50 percent within 5 years after discontinuation of bile acid therapy, after which time it appears to level off. Studies from our group show that the recurrence after ESWL of gallbladder stones is similar (about 10 percent within the first year).

Summary of Findings

For patients with symptomatic radiolucent solitary gallbladder stones who have a positive cholecystogram, ESWL is efficient, safe, relatively painless, and highly acceptable. In these selected patients (probably no more than 10 to 20 percent of all candidates with symptomatic stones), it may become the treatment of choice.

ESWL OF BILE DUCT STONES

Machines

In contrast to gallbladder stones, bile duct stones may be shadowed by gas-filled intestine if shock waves enter the body from the ventral side. Therefore, we have chosen shock wave entry from the back for shattering bile duct stones (Fig. 3). In addition, location of the stones in the shock wave focus requires x-ray examination. This requirement is best fulfilled with the older kidney machines (e.g., HM3, Dornier Medizintechnik GmbH), which can also be used for disintegration of bile duct stones. These machines have a relatively high focal volume and often necessitate general anesthesia. It remains to be seen whether similar results can be achieved by shock wave devices with less energy that do not necessitate anesthesia.

Inclusion Criteria

All patients with stones primarily not amenable to endoscopic measures are eligible for this treatment, provided that they have normal coagulation parameters and no aneurysms or lung tissue in the shock wave path, and provided that the stone can be located in the focal area.

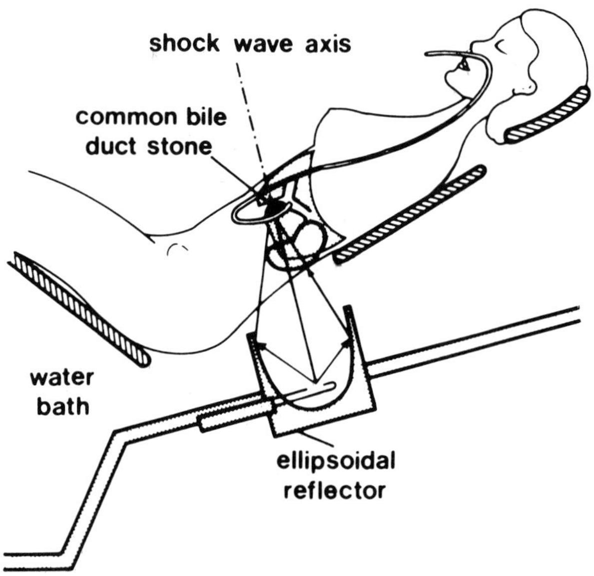

Figure 3 Extracorporeal shock wave lithotripsy of bile duct stones (Dornier System). In the supine position, the patient is immersed in a water bath and the shock waves enter the body from the rear. An endoscopically placed nasobiliary catheter allows injection of contrast medium to visualize the stone. Positioning and disintegration of the stone are monitored by fluoroscopy using a two-dimensional x-ray system. (Republished with permission from Sauerbruch T, Holl J, Sackmann M, et al. Treatment of bile duct stones by extracorporeal shock waves. Semin Ultrasound CT MR 1986; 8:155.)

Adverse Effects

In a multicenter prospective trial reported in 1989, severe adverse effects (primarily fever) occurred in 8 percent of the patients after ESWL. This may have been caused by introduction of micro-organisms into the blood stream during the treatment and might have been prevented by prophylactic administration of antibiotics. The 30-day mortality rate in these high-risk patients was 1 percent, which compares favorably with open surgery.

Success Rate

Using the older kidney machines (Dornier HM3 with a capacity of 80 nF), the stone clearance rate is within the range of 80 to 90 percent. These figures may be lower when less powerful machines with a smaller focal volume are used. About three-fourths of the patients require endoscopic extraction of the fragments after ESWL. Fragmentation of the stones in the biliary tree is more coarse than in the gallbladder for various reasons (larger stone volume, more impacted stones, and less crystalline stones).

Summary of Findings

ESWL of bile duct stones is an adjuvant procedure to interventional endoscopic measures for extraction of stones from the biliary tree. The number of patients who require adjuvant ESWL is small, but in this group the treatment is highly beneficial.

SUGGESTED READING

Paumgartner G. Fragmentation of gallstones by extracorporeal shock waves. Semin Liver Disease 1987; 7:317–321.
Sackmann M, Delius M, Sauerbruch T, et al. Shock wave lithotripsy of gallbladder stones: the first 175 patients. N Engl J Med 1988; 318:393–397.
Sackmann M, Ippisch E, Sauerbruch T, Holl J, Paumgartner G. Early gallstone recurrence after successful shock-wave therapy (abstract). Hepatology 1988; 8:1221.
Sackmann M, Sauerbruch T, Holl J, et al. Results of ESWL in gallbladder stones with radiopaque rim compared to radiolucent calculi (abstract). J Hepatol 7 (suppl):S74.
Sauerbruch T, Delius M, Paumgartner G, et al. Fragmentation of gallstones by extracorporeal shock waves. N Engl J Med 1986; 314:818–822.
Sauerbruch T, Holl J, Sackmann M, et al. Treatment of bile duct stones by extracorporeal shock waves. Semin Ultrasound CT MR 1986; 8:818.
Sauerbruch T, Holl J, Sackmann M, Paumgartner G. The role of extracorporeal lithotripsy (ESWL) in the treatment of gallstones. Endoscopy 1988; 6:305–308.
Sauerbruch T, Stern M, and the Study Group for Shock Wave Lithotripsy of Bile Duct Stones. Fragmentation of bile duct stones by extracorporeal shock waves: a new approach to biliary calculi after failure of routine endoscopic measures. Gastroenterology 1989; 96:146–152.

ACUTE PANCREATITIS

JAMIE S. BARKIN, M.D., F.A.C.P., F.A.C.G.
SHAKIR A. HYDER, M.D.

Approximately 5,000 new cases of acute pancreatitis are diagnosed in the United States each year. Seventy to 85 percent can be classified as mild to moderate in severity. These patients respond to supportive management and carry a low morbidity rate. The remaining 15 to 30 percent develop a severe illness within 24 to 72 hours of admission to the hospital and may develop one or more complications of pancreatitis. These patients require vigorous supportive measures and occasionally surgical intervention. The mortality rate in this group is approximately 25 to 50 percent, although there is a better prognosis for patients who have alcohol-related pancreatitis.

ETIOLOGY

The exact pathogenesis of acute pancreatitis remains uncertain, but various etiologies have been identified (Table 1), the most common being biliary tract disease and alcohol abuse. Their respective prevalence varies, depending on the population studies.

Gallstones

In private hospitals the incidence of gallstone-associated pancreatitis is 55 percent, whereas in city hospitals it is 30 percent. The association of gallstones with pancreatitis is well established, especially with stones less than three mm in diameter. In addition, 50 percent of patients who have episodes of biliary pancreatitis and who do not undergo cholecystectomy have recurrent episodes of pancreatitis.

Alcohol Related Pancreatitis

Most patients seen in large public hospitals have alcohol-related pancreatitis, which carries a lesser mortality rate than gallstone pancreatitis. This may be because these patients are younger and have underlying chronic pancreatitis. These factors may be important, since age over 55 years has been shown by Ranson to be a variable that portends a poorer prognosis. Also, an underlying chronic pancreatitis reduces pancreatic secretory ability and may protect the gland from autodigestion.

Hypertriglyceridemia

Clinical and experimental studies have demonstrated that acute pancreatitis may be initiated by hyper-

TABLE 1 Conditions Associated With Acute Pancreatitis

90% of all cases
Gallstones (No. 1 in private hospitals)
Alcoholism (No. 1 in public hospitals)
Idiopathic (up to 30%)
Other 10%
Medications (especially sulfonamides and antimetabolites)
Postoperative (abdominal, cardiac surgery)
Trauma (No. 1 in young people)
Post-ERP (1% of ERCPs)
Hyperlipidemia (types I, IV, and V)
Hypercalcemia (hyperparathyroidism, myeloma, TPN)
Pancreas divisum
Renal transplantation
Cardiac transplantation
Infectious agents
Pregnancy (90% gallstone associated, third trimester)
Scorpion bite (Trinidad, West Indies)
Ampullary disease
Hereditary
Penetrating duodenal ulcer
Connective tissue disorders with vasculitis
Eating disorders (anorexia nervosa, bulimia)

Adapted from Fayne SD, Barkin JS. Acute pancreatitis: update 1986. Mt Sinai J Med 1986; 53:396–403.

triglyceridemia. This usually occurs with levels greater than 1,700 mg per deciliter. The exact mechanism of this association is unknown, but it is postulated that the total release of cytototic free fatty acids by pancreatic lipase may be the initiating factor. The hyperlipidemia may be primary, as in Frederickson types I, IV, or V, or secondary to estrogen therapy.

Medications

Multiple medications have been associated with acute pancreatitis. The drugs known to have a definite causal relationship include azathioprine, thiazides, furosemide, sulfonamides, estrogen, tetracycline, and valproic acid. Other drugs such as chlorthalidone, ethacrynic acid, L-asparaginase, phenformin, and methyldopa (Aldomet) should be added to the list. The association of steroids with acute pancreatitis remains controversial. Recently, corticosteroid- induced pancreatitis was demonstrated and recurrence noted when a patient was rechallenged with this medication. Acute pancreatitis after cutaneous exposure to an organophosphate insecticide has also been reported.

ERCP

Acute pancreatitis develops within 24 hours in approximately one percent of patients, following endoscopic retrograde cholangiopancreatography (ERCP). The factors that may be implicated include the speed, volume, and pressure of injection as well as the amount of contrast material used and the underlying pancreatic anatomy. We have also shown that the type of contrast material affects the incidence of chemical acute pancreatitis. The use of nonionic agents is associated with a decreased incidence of pancreatitis.

Hypercalcemia

Hypercalcemia from any cause may lead to acute pancreatitis. This should often be considered in patients receiving total parenteral nutrition (TPN) who are predisposed to the development of hypercalcemia in association with pancreatitis.

Pancreas Divisum

Pancreas divisum was previously considered to be a cause of acute pancreatitis. Recent evidence suggests that pancreas divisum should be regarded not as an etiologic factor, but as a coincidental anatomic variant, encountered in 10 percent of the population. If pancreatic divisum is found at ERCP in a patient who has had an episode of acute pancreatitis, cannulation of the minor ampulla to visualize the dorsal pancreatic duct is vital. This will detect a subgroup of patients in whom pancreatic divisum is a pathologic condition.

Viral Infections

Viral infections may be the most frequently overlooked cause of acute pancreatitis. Those most commonly encountered include mumps and hepatitis B.

Postoperative Pancreatitis

Postoperative pancreatitis may develop after a variety of intra-abdominal surgical procedures. The mechanism of injury is thought to be secondary to direct operative trauma or to vascular compromise with development of ischemic pancreatitis. Pancreatitis following cardiac surgery has previously been described as severe and associated with a mortality rate up to 63 percent despite aggressive therapy. We prospectively reviewed the incidence and severity of postcardiopulmonary pancreatitis and found an incidence of 46 percent. Overall, it was not associated with an increase in mortality. An explanation for this discrepancy could be that previous studies consisted of either retrospective or autopsy series, whereas ours was prospective. In the retrospective studies, only seriously ill patients were reported; our study included a wide spectrum of diseases. The possible etiologic factors postulated included prolonged cardiopulmonary bypass with low cardiac output, which leads to hypoperfusion and ischemia of the pancreas. However, we did not find this association of pancreatitis with hypotension.

Renal Transplantation

Renal transplantation is associated with a two to seven percent incidence of acute pancreatitis. Contributing causes include the use of immunosuppressive agents such as azathioprine and L-asparaginase, secondary hyperparathyroidism, vasculitis, and superimposed viral infection.

PROGNOSIS

The purpose of the many protocols developed to assess the prognosis is to facilitate the early recognition of those patients who will pursue a "malignant" course. The most frequently used prognostic signs are the Ranson criteria (Table 2). The overall mortality rate was reported to be approximately one percent in patients with fewer than three signs, 15 percent if three or four signs are positive, 40 percent if five or six signs are positive, and 100 percent is seven or more signs are positive. These criteria suffer from the fact that they are assessed at 48 hours and can be altered by the therapy received. Hypoxemia, for example, may be induced by overhydration with subsequent pulmonary edema. Therefore, the criteria have been simplified by Bank and colleagues, who found that in patients with acute or acute-relapsing pancreatitis, if one or more organ system in addition to the pancreas was affected, the mortality rate was 56 percent; if no other organ system was affected, mortality was only two percent. The degree of amylase elevation has no prognostic significance.

TABLE 2 Signs for Classification of Severity of Acute Pancreatitis

At time of admission or diagnosis	
	Age >55 yr
	White blood cell count >16,000/mm
	Blood glucose >200 mg/dl
	Serum lactate dehydrogenase more than twice normal
	Serum glutamic-oxaloacetic transaminase more than six times normal
During initial 48 hours	
	Decrease in hematocrit of >10%
	Serum calcium <8 mg/dl
	Increase in blood urea nitrogen of >5 mg/dl
	Arterial Po_2 <60 mm Hg
	Base deficit >4 mEq/liter
	Estimated fluid sequestration >6,000 ml

Adapted from Ranson JH, Rifkind KM, Turner JW. Prognostic signs and non-operative peritoneal lavage in acute pancreatitis. Surg Gynecol Obstet 1976; 143:209–219.

TREATMENT: GENERAL GUIDELINES

Supportive Measures

The initial approach to the management of patients with acute pancreatitis should be to assess its severity and establish its etiology, since both of these influence the therapeutic approach. The initial phase of management includes supportive measures to ensure the maintenance of an adequate circulating blood volume and oxygenation, as well as relief of pain. These alone lead to rapid clinical improvement in most patients. A nasogastric tube should be inserted to reduce the abdominal distention of an associated ileus or reduce vomiting and retching. It has limited value in patients with mild to moderate pancreatitis not complicated by ileus.

Drug Therapy

We were once able, with some confidence, to conclude that a variety of drug therapies were ineffective for patients with acute pancreatitis. However, this was challenged by Steinberg and Schlesselman, who compared the outcome of 25 studies utilizing animals with experimentally induced pancreatitis with 13 studies of humans with acute pancreatitis in whom the same therapies were used. These included aprotinin, glucagon, 5-fluorouracil (5-FU), somatostatin, and peritoneal lavage. Interestingly, 81 percent of animal studies showed an improvement in the survival rate, whereas only 7.7 percent of human studies demonstrated a positive effect on survival. Of the 12 human studies that showed no effect of treatment on survival, none had sufficient statistical power for the investigators to have confidence in the negative outcome. This was because the studies covered too few patients or because the event rates in the untreated populations were too low. Overall, only five of the human studies reported the complication rates of acute pancreatitis in patients who did not die of their disease. Therefore, although we are restudying these agents, their therapeutic effectiveness, or lack thereof, remains undetermined.

The guiding principle to most treatment methods is "to put the pancreas at rest" and, although various methods of suppressing pancreatic secretion have been devised, their therapeutic value, as reviewed by Ettien and Webster, has not been established. Cimetidine theoretically could suppress pancreatic secretion because of its effect of decreasing acid secretion. It was prospectively evaluated in two randomized trials, both of which found no beneficial effect. The lack of effective neutralization of intragastric acid with antacids for the treatment of acute pancreatitis has also been shown.

Nutritional Needs

It is important to consider the nutritional needs of the patient early in the course of acute pancreatitis. In patients who do not show rapid resolution of symptoms or who are intolerant of oral alimentation within a few days of hospitalization, peripheral or total parenteral nutrition should be considered. In theory this should be beneficial, but no prospective studies have been performed. Conversely, concern has been raised that the infusion of lipids along with the hyperalimentation may cause an exacerbation of pancreatitis, but no studies support this objection.

Peritoneal Dialysis

Peritoneal dialysis has been used in patients with necrotizing pancreatitis in an attempt to remove vasoactive substances from the peritoneal cavity before their absorption. Initial noncontrolled studies suggested the efficacy of this procedure, but a multicenter randomized controlled trial by Mayer and colleagues showed no benefit. Peritoneal lavage might be of benefit in the subgroup of patients with necrotizing pancreatitis who develop ascites in the course of their disease. This is based on the concept that removal of toxin-rich peritoneal fluid, and not the lavage itself, may be important.

Fluid Resuscitation

In patients with acute pancreatitis, large quantities of fluid collect within the retroperitoneal spaces and within the peritoneal cavity as a result of chemical burn. This causes a significant decrease in circulating blood volume. If intravenous fluid replacement is insufficient to compensate for these third space losses, systemic hypotension may lead to stasis within the microcirculation of the pancreas, causing intensification of pancreatic inflammation. Therefore, a high priority should be placed on fluid resuscitation with central venous monitoring or Swan-Ganz catheter insertion.

Respiratory Monitoring

Respiratory complications are well-recognized sequelae of acute pancreatitis and occur in 15 to 55 percent of cases. Arterial hypoxemia as well as early adult respiratory distress syndrome (ARDS) in patients with acute pancreatitis may be difficult to recognize by physical examination and chest radiography. Therefore, arterial blood gases should be measured every 12 hours during the initial 48 to 72 hours of treatment in severely ill patients. With appropriate therapy, the ARDS may be totally, functionally, and histologically reversible.

Hypocalcemia

Hypocalcemia is commonly seen in patients with acute pancreatitis, but the low serum calcium level is usually a reflection of low albumin with a normal ionized calcium. Thus, in many patients calcium replacement is not needed until clinical evidence of hypocalcemia is seen.

The newer therapeutic agents that are being evaluated include beta-adrenergic agonist receptors such as isoproterenol and terbutaline sulfate. These drugs inhibit the increase in microvascular permeability induced by histamine and related vascoactive substances. These are the inflammatory mediators released during the course of experimental and human pancreatitis. Harvey and colleagues investigated the effects of isoproterenol and terbutaline sulfate on the development of acute edematous pancreatitis (AEP) and acute hemorrhagic pancreatitis (AHP) in cats. They administered these agents 12 hours after the onset of acute edematous pancreatitis and found that it reduced the pancreatic inflammation; however, neither drug was effective in treating established acute hemorrhagic pancreatitis. It remains to be seen, therefore, whether early administration in humans can prevent the progression from acute edematous pancreatitis to acute hemorrhagic pancreatitis.

TREATMENT OF SEVERE PANCREATITIS

This entity was formerly referred to as "hemorrhagic pancreatitis," but we now know that the prognostic variable is the amount of tissue necrosis. The newer terminology applied to this subgroup of patients with a high mortality rate is "necrotizing pancreatitis." The mortality rate is initially related to release and absorption of pancreatic enzymes and vasoactive material that result in progressive organ damage, respiratory failure, and subsequently secondary infection of the devitalized tissue and the possible development of generalized sepsis.

The indications for surgery in patients with necrotizing pancreatitis are evolving. The uncertainty of the diagnosis was once the major reason for exploration. However, pancreatic visualization via computed tomography (CT) enables us to determine whether pancreatitis is present. In our prospective study, we found that no patient with normal CT scan results had necrotizing pancreatitis. In patients with suspected acute pancreatitis, an abnormal CT scan is supportive, whereas a normal pancreatic area precludes (or should at least make us search diligently for) another diagnosis. Contrast-enhanced CT can be used to visualize areas of pancreatic necrosis; these areas are not well perfused and therefore do not enhance. They appear as a nonhomogenous density of the pancreas. Chronic pancreatitis, neoplasm, and fatty degenerative change can appear quite similar on CT without enhancement. However, after intravenous contrast material injection, a phasic change of density can be observed, delineating necrotic tissue as nonperfused areas that retain their original density. A correct diagnosis of pancreatic necrosis was reported by Block and colleagues in 85 percent of their patients with acute pancreatitis and even in 90 percent of those with extensive pancreatic necrosis.

Surgery

Our increasing ability to confirm the diagnosis of acute pancreatitis noninvasively has modified the indications for surgery. Previously, uncertainty of diagnosis was a leading indication, whereas now surgery in acute pancreatitis is most commonly employed (1) for clinical deterioration despite maximal medical support, (2) to treat the complications of acute pancreatitis, and (3) to provide definitive treatment of biliary pancreatitis.

Clinical Deterioration

The questions of if and when to perform a laparotomy in the presence of clinical deterioration is undergoing evolution. If such worsening continues beyond 72 hours despite maximal supportive measures, and especially if there is at least 50 percent of pancreatic necrosis as determined by contrast-enhanced CT, laparotomy may be indicated. This is based on studies showing that the greater the extent of pancreatic necrosis, the worse is the prognosis. The prognosis is also affected by whether the pancreatic necrosis has become colonized with bacteria.

One cannot use clinical parameters to distinguish sterile from infected pancreatic necrosis. Therefore, in patients with suspected infected pancreatic necrosis (e.g., with a temperature higher than 101° F or a fulminant course), percutaneous needle aspiration of the pancreatic area should be performed. The aspirant should be Gram stained and cultured. If the colon was avoided during insertion of the needle and the Gram stain reveals bacteria, infected necrosis is almost certain.

Necrosectomy is the surgical procedure used for these findings. It includes careful debridement of the demarcated, nonviable pancreatic and peripancreatic tissue and debris. When necrosectomy alone and necrosectomy with local continuous lavage were compared in a group of patients in whom the surgical indication was clinical deterioration, the group who underwent necrosectomy and local lavage showed a significantly lower mortality rate than that of the group treated solely with necrosectomy (8 percent versus 27 percent).

Complications

The local complications of acute pancreatitis are best classified by (1) the time of their occurrence: less than 2 weeks or more than 2 weeks; (2) the characteristics of the pancreatic mass on CT, solid or cystic; and (3) whether they are septic or sterile (Table 3). Pancreatic necrosis as described above occurs in close proximity to the initial episode and may be sterile or become infected.

Pancreatic abscess develops 3 to 5 weeks after an attack of acute pancreatitis. Ranson found that the mortality rate from pancreatic abscesses is related to the severity of the underlying pancreatic inflammation, ranging from 14 percent in patients with mild pancreatitis to 100 percent in those with severe forms of the disease. The pathogenesis of pancreatic abscess formation involves the secondary infection of necrotic pancreatic and peripancreatic tissue. The primary organism involved is gut bacteria, including *Escherichia coli*, *Klebsiella*, *Proteus*, *Enterobacter*, *Pseudomonas*, and *Enterococcus*. Clinically, abdominal pain, distention, and tenderness are present in most patients. An abdominal mass may be palpable in approximately 50 percent, but its significance is questionable.

Computed tomography is the most accurate diagnostic procedure for demonstrating abscesses. Predominantly, it shows a solid mass that may have one or more fluid densities. These collections are indistinguishable from noninfected fluid collections. The presence of air bubbles is highly suggestive of pancreatic necrosis, although it is not pathognomonic, since rupture of a pseudocyst into the gut may result in a similar appearance. CT or ultrasonographic percutaneous guided needle aspiration with Gram stain and culture has been described for the diagnosis of pancreatic abscess. This technique allows us to differentiate sterile from infected collections. The predominantly solid characteristics of the pancreatic abscess do not allow adequate catheter drainage, so that the appropriate treatment is surgical drainage and antibiotic coverage. Repeat surgery for recurrent abscesses is required in 30 percent of patients. In an attempt to overcome this need, Bradley and Fulenwider spearheaded the concept of open drainage, which allows daily debridement under local anesthesia, or occasionally at the bedside. The mortality rate after standard surgical drainage has ranged from 20 percent to 50 percent, whereas it was 15 percent after use of open drainage in Bradley's series.

TABLE 3 Local Complications of Acute Pancreatitis

Type	*Predominant CT Characteristic*	*Time of Onset From Episode*	*Septic vs. Sterile*
Phlegmon necrosis	Solid	<2 wks	Sterile
Infected necrosis	Solid	<2 wks	Infected
Pancreatic abscess	Solid	>2 wks	Infected
Pancreatic pseudocyst	Cystic	Either	Sterile
Infected pancreatic pseudocyst	Cystic	Either	Infected

Pseudocysts occur in approximately 25 percent of patients with acute pancreatitis. Overall, approximately 85 percent of these resolve within the first few weeks after diagnosis. They are especially likely to occur if there has been a recent history of an episode of acute pancreatitis and if the pseudocyst wall neither is thick nor contains calcium. Therapy should be withheld for 6 weeks in asymptomatic patients unless the pseudocyst is increasing in size.

The complications directly related to pseudocysts include (1) spontaneous rupture, which occurs into the peritoneum, resulting in pancreatic ascites, or into the pleural cavity, with resultant effusion; (2) obstruction of contiguous organs, the most commonly involved being the common bile duct and the stomach; and (3) erosion into the vascular tree or gastrointestinal tract, which may result in bleeding if a pseudoaneurysm is created or the spleen is invaded. Conversely, spontaneous resolution may occur if there is erosion into a hollow viscus.

Our initial approach to a pseudocyst that has been present for 6 weeks is percutaneous aspiration in combination with prolonged catheter drainage. This is successful in up to 75 percent of patients. If the pseudocyst is impinging upon the lumen of the stomach or duodenum, endoscopic cystogastrostomy or duodenostomy may become an alternative initial approach, but at present only a few studies have been reported. Surgical decompression is used as a back-up if the above procedures are readily available, or as the initial procedure if they are unavailable. The surgical procedures most often used include cystogastrostomy and Roux-en-Y drainage.

Definitive Therapy for Biliary Pancreatitis

The concept of immediate surgery for biliary pancreatitis was initially proposed by Acosta and associates, who reported that 63 percent of patients had stones impacted at the ampulla when their surgery was performed within the first 48 hours of gallstone-induced pancreatitis. Early common duct exploration or, if needed, transduodenal sphincteroplasty appeared to reduce mortality rates from 16 to 2 percent. Importantly, this was not a prospective controlled series. The purpose of early surgery is to relieve the obstruction and therefore halt the progression from edematous to necrotizing pancreatitis. Conversely, many investigators have found a higher rate of complications and an increased mortality rate among patients subjected to early biliary surgery. Ranson noted a 23 percent mortality rate among 22 patients with gallstone pancreatitis who underwent laparotomy during the first week; there were no deaths among 58 patients who were treated nonoperatively until the pancreatitis had subsided, and then underwent cholecystectomy and common duct exploration. This initial increased early mortality was confirmed by Kelly, who reported on 172 patients with acute gallstone pancreatitis; a 12 percent mortality rate was noted when patients were operated on immediately, whereas there were no deaths when surgery was delayed for 5 to 7 days.

The sole randomized prospective study comparing immediate with delayed surgery was reported by Stone and colleagues in 65 patients. Thirty-six were randomized to undergo cholecystectomy, transduodenal sphincteroplasty, and pancreatic duct septotomy within 72 hours of admission. The remaining 29 patients were managed conservatively during initial hospitalization and were readmitted 3 to 6 months later to undergo the same operative procedure. Common duct stones were present in 75 percent of patients treated with immediate surgery, compared with 28 percent in those managed by elective surgery. These authors found that although immediate surgery may be performed safely in patients with gallstone pancreatitis, it is of no benefit in altering the clinical course of the illness. Thus, most surgeons currently favor initial supportive management followed by elective biliary surgery during the same hospitalization. This expectant approach allows most common duct stones to pass spontaneously and early enough to prevent a recurrent bout of pancreatitis.

ERCP may be safely performed in up to 90 percent of patients with gallstone pancreatitis. Even in series containing a large proportion of elderly and high-risk patients, the complication rate can be as low as six percent and the mortality rate below one percent. These figures are considerably lower than those for surgical exploration of common bile duct. ERCP can be utilized in patients with biliary pancreatitis who fail to improve with supportive therapy. If an impacted stone is demonstrated, endoscopic sphincterotomy with stone removal should be attempted. Neoptolemos and colleagues reported a randomized controlled trial of ERCP and endoscopic sphincterotomy versus conventional therapy in patients with gallstone pancreatitis. This showed that urgent ERCP and sphincterotomy is not hazardous in the presence of acute gallstone pancreatitis. It resulted in a reduced mortality rate in the group of patients with severe pancreatitis who were treated with ERCP and sphincterotomy within 72 hours of admission: two percent as opposed to eight percent in the conventionally treated group. This mortality rate was not significantly different, but the incidence of overall complications was significantly reduced in the group that underwent endoscopic sphincterotomy.

In summary, the pendulum has returned to a more aggressive interventional approach to patients who fail to respond readily to early supportive therapy.

Editor's Note: A 66-item bibliography is available by request to Dr. Barkin.

SUGGESTED READING

Acosta JM, Pellegrini CA, Skinner DA. Etiology and pathogenesis of acute biliary pancreatitis. Surgery 1980; 88:118–125.

Bank S, Wise L, Gersten M. Risk factors in acute pancreatitis. Am J Gastroenterol 1983; 78:637–640.

Barkin JS, Smith FR, Pereiras R, et al. Therapeutic percutaneous aspiration of pancreatic pseudocysts. Dig Dis Sci 1981; 26:585–587.

Block WM, Bittner R, Buchler M, et al. Identification of pancreas necrosis in severe acute pancreatitis: imaging procedure versus clinical staging. Gut 1986; 27:1035–1042.

Bradley EL, Fulenwider JJ. Open treatment of pancreatic abscess. Surg Gynecol Obstet 1984; 159:509–513.

Ettien JT, Webster PD. The management of acute pancreatitis. Adv Intern Med 1980; 25:169–198.

Fayne SD, Barkin JS. Acute pancreatitis: update 1986. Mount Sinai Med 1986; 53:396–403.

Geokas MC, Baltaxe HA, Banks PA, et al. Acute pancreatitis. Ann Intern Med 1985; 103:86–100.

Harvey MH, Wedgwood KR, Reber HA. Treatment of acute pancreatitis with β-adrenergic drugs. Surgery 1987; 102:229–234.

Hill MC, Dach JL, Barkin JS, et al. The role of percutaneous aspiration in the diagnosis of pancreatic abscesses. Am J Roentgenol 1984; 141:1305–1308.

Karlson KB, Martin EC, Fankuchen EI, et al. Percutaneous drainage of pancreatic pseudocysts and abscesses. Radiology 1982; 142:619–624.

Kelly TR. Gallstone pancreatitis. The timing of surgery. Surgery 1980; 88:345–350.

Mallory A, Kern F, Jr. Drug-induced pancreatitis. A critical review. Gastroenterology 1980; 78:813–820.

Mayer D, McMahon MJ, Corfield AP, et al. Controlled clinical trial of peritoneal lavage for the treatment of severe acute pancreatitis. N Engl J Med 1985; 312:399–404.

Neoptolemos JP, Carr-Locke DL, London NJ, et al. Controlled trial of urgent endoscopic retrograde cholangiopancreatography and endoscopic sphincterotomy versus conservative treatment for acute pancreatitis due to gallstones. Lancet 1988; 2:979–983.

Ranson JH. The timing of biliary surgery in acute pancreatitis. Ann Surg 1979; 189:654–663.

Ranson JH. Acute pancreatitis. Where are we? Surg Clin North Am 1981; 61:55–70.

Ranson JH. Etiological and prognostic factors in human acute pancreatitis. A review. Am J Gastroenterol 1982; 77:633–638.

Steinberg WM, Schlesselman SE. Treatment of acute pancreatitis: comparison of animal and human studies. Gastroenterology 1987; 93:1420–1427.

Stone HH, Fabian TC, Dunlop WE. Gallstone pancreatitis. Biliary tract pathology in relation to time of operation. Ann Surg 1981; 194:305–312.

CHRONIC PANCREATITIS: EXOCRINE AND ENDOCRINE INSUFFICIENCY

SUDHIR K. DUTTA, M.D.

DIAGNOSIS

The diagnosis of chronic pancreatitis is generally considered in patients who present with upper abdominal pain, chronic diarrhea, or significant weight loss. In a given case, any combination of these symptoms may be present. Furthermore, in many cases, recurrent attacks of acute pancreatitis may precede the onset of chronic pancreatitis. However, 10 to 15 percent of patients with chronic pancreatitis present initially with only diarrhea or weight loss or both. The development of malabsorption in a patient with chronic pancreatitis indicates more than 90 percent loss of exocrine pancreatic function.

The abdominal pain associated with chronic pancreatitis is characterized by a midepigastric location, a dull and continuous nature, and radiation to the back that is relieved by forward bending. Diarrhea in these patients is chronic, with a frequency ranging from only one bowel movement per day to as many as six or more per day. Weight loss is often significant (10 lb or more) and frequently associated with clinical manifestations of uncontrolled diabetes mellitus. As a result of weight loss, protein energy malnutrition of the marasmus type is initially present in 30 to 50 percent of cases of chronic pancreatitis. It is important to assess the extent of malnutrition carefully in order to determine the response to pancreatic enzyme or nutritional therapy. It is equally important to record the symptoms in detail, because the response to medical therapy is generally evaluated in relation to the presenting symptoms.

Irreversible Structural Damage

The diagnosis of chronic pancreatitis is often difficult to establish in clinical situations. This is particularly true for patients with early disease associated with only mild to moderate pancreatic dysfunction. Evidence of irreversible structural damage or permanent functional impairment of the pancreatic gland should be obtained by various clinical tests available to the physician. Clinical evidence of irreversible structural damage generally includes (1) pancreatic calcification, (2) pancreatic duct strictures, and (3) chronic inflammation on histologic views of the pancreatic gland. Pancreatic calcification is noted on plain radiographs of the abdomen or on computed tomographic (CT) scans. Pancreatic duct abnormality is delineated by pancreatography, which can be obtained endoscopically and occasionally at the time of surgery. Pancreatic histologic findings are available in a few patients who undergo pancreatic biopsy or resection. In clinical practice, the presence of chronic pancreatitis is frequently diagnosed on the basis of calcification and/or abnormal pancreatographic results.

Permanent Functional Impairment

The presence of permanent functional impairment of the pancreatic gland can be determined by traditional tests such as the secretin stimulation test or one of the newer tests of pancreatic function, such as the bentiromide (NBT-PABA) test. It should be emphasized that although the secretin stimulation test is tedious and inconvenient because of the need for duodenal intubation, it is still the most sensitive test for diagnosing early pancreatic disease in patients who have not yet developed malabsorption. Among a large number of "tubeless" pancreatic function tests, the bentiromide test appears to be the one that is most convenient, inexpensive, and easily available for diagnosing advanced chronic pancreatitis. Because of these features, sequential bentiromide tests are being used to evaluate the response to pancreatic enzyme therapy in patients with exocrine pancreatic insufficiency. However, the bentiromide test and similar "tubeless" pancreatic function tests have low sensitivity for diagnosing *early* or mild pancreatic gland dysfunction. Furthermore, it is essentially a urine test, which requires normal renal function, sufficient diuresis, and proper intestinal absorption. Bentiromide is a synthetic tripeptide that is specifically cleaved by pancreatic chymotrypsin. The cleavage of this molecule by chymotrypsin in the duodenum releases *para*-aminobenzoic acid (PABA), which is rapidly absorbed, conjugated in the liver, and excreted in the urine. Patients with chronic pancreatitis consistently excrete less PABA in the urine than healthy controls, because of impaired chymotrypsin secretion.

TREATMENT

Treatment of patients with chronic pancreatitis is generally directed toward (1) relief of upper abdominal pain and (2) correction of diarrhea, weight loss, and malnutrition.

Treatment of Abdominal Pain Due To Chronic Pancreatitis

Abdominal pain is the most difficult problem to treat in the management of chronic pancreatitis for several reasons. First, pain is a subjective sensation without any available objective parameter to document or monitor its occurrence. Second, alcoholism is often an underlying problem in many of these patients, and alcoholics are well known to be drug dependent. Not infrequently, alcoholic patients feign abdominal pain in order to obtain analgesics, sedatives, and narcotics. Consequently, it is sometimes difficult to determine whether the abdominal pain is truly due to an underlying organic disease. Abstinence from alcohol is obviously desirable. In the management of ab-

TABLE 1 Five Important Steps in Evaluation of Patients With Abdominal Pain Associated With Chronic Pancreatitis

Step 1	Seeking evidence of active pancreatic inflammation during painful periods (elevation of serum amylase, lipase, or urinary amylase activity)
Step 2	Seeking evidence of complications of pancreatitis (pancreatic pseudocyst or phlegmon)
Step 3	Ruling out other upper gastrointestinal diseases (peptic ulcer disease, gastritis, and gallstone disease)
Step 4	Reevaluation of evidence of irreversible structural abnormality or permanent functional impairment of exocrine pancreatic gland
Step 5	Close follow-up of patient's abdominal pain for 4–6 months

TABLE 2 Important Steps in Management of Abdominal Pain From Chronic Pancreatitis

1. Patient education (about natural history of chronic pancreatitis, risk of prolonged analgesic abuse, and need for alcohol abstinence)
2. Administration of non-narcotic analgesics (acetaminophen, ibuprofen, and nonsteroidal analgesics)
3. Exogenous pancreatic enzyme therapy
4. Periodic administration of narcotic analgesics (acetaminophen with codeine)
5. Celiac ganglionectomy
6. Surgical intervention
   a. Pancreaticojejunostomy
   b. Pancreatectomy

dominal pain from chronic pancreatitis, I have found a five-step strategy exceedingly helpful (Table 1). The first step is documentation of the presence of pancreatic inflammation. Biochemical or radiologic evidence of pancreatic inflammation tends to suggest a pancreatic origin for such pain. Elevated serum amylase or lipase activity or evidence of an abnormal pancreatic gland suggests active pancreatic inflammation. However, patients with chronic pancreatitis sometimes have normal serum amylase and lipase levels and a fibrotic calcified pancreatic gland without any evidence of edema. The second step in management of pancreatic pain involves careful evaluation of complications such as pseudocyst or phlegmon. Again, pancreatic gland imaging helps to confirm or rule out these complications. The third step is to rule out other gastrointestinal (GI) lesions that can present clinically with upper abdominal pain. These include peptic ulcer disease, penetrating ulcer, gastritis, and cholelithiasis. Upper endoscopy, ultrasonography, and a profile of liver function tests can help the differential diagnosis. The fourth step includes careful reevaluation of the diagnosis of chronic pancreatitis in terms of irreversible structural damage or permanent impairment of pancreatic gland function; this often involves repeat pancreatography or CT scan. The fifth and final step in the management of chronic pancreatic pain is a close follow-up, monitoring the severity of pain and the analgesic needs of the patient for 4 to 6 months. Again, abstinence from alcohol is essential. Alcoholism is the subject of a separate chapter.

After a thorough evaluation of pancreatic pain, a number of treatment measures can be instituted (Table 2).

Patient Education

The first step is educating patients about the natural history of this chronic ailment, its associated complications, and its likely long-term outcome. Each patient with chronic pancreatitis should understand that after 5 to 10 years the episodes of pancreatic pain generally diminish in frequency and often disappear altogether. However, at about the time that abdominal pain diminishes, most patients with chronic pancreatitis also develop hyperglycemia and malabsorption.

Analgesics

The second step involves generous use of non-narcotic analgesics (e.g., acetaminophen, ibuprofen, and nonsteroidal analgesics) to control abdominal pain. In my experience, a large percentage of patients with chronic pancreatic pain can be managed for a long time with these two measures. Limited prescription of narcotic analgesics such as acetaminophen with codeine is also reasonable during episodes of severe abdominal pain. Patients should always be reminded that long-term use of narcotic analgesics can frequently result in drug dependence. If a patient's requirements for narcotic analgesic appear to be gradually increasing, strong consideration should be given to possible enrollment in a pain relief program and the use of pain control by other means. Pain due to chronic pancreatitis is frequently intermittent and postprandial, but when abdominal pain becomes more frequent and persistent, affecting the lifestyle of the patient, relief of pain becomes the most crucial part of the overall management. In these situations, celiac ganglionectomy and surgical intervention should be considered.

Pancreatic Enzyme Therapy

The third measure in the control of chronic pancreatitis–related pain is the ingestion of exocrine pancreatic enzymes. In patients with idiopathic chronic pancreatitis, the control of pancreatic pain by exogenous pancreatic enzyme therapy has been reported in two studies. In one, ingestion of pancreatic enzymes (four to eight tablets) with meals along with sodium bicarbonate (1,300 mg) was associated with a significant reduction in abdominal pain. Most patients who respond to this treatment were middle-aged females. However, in my experience the use of oral pancreatic enzymes has not been effective in patients with alcohol-related pancreatitis. To examine this issue more definitively, a double-blind, placebo-controlled clinical trial is needed in a carefully selected group of patients with alcoholic pancreatitis. The goal of pancreatic enzyme therapy in the treatment of chronic pancreatic pain is pharmacologic suppression of exocrine pancreatic secretion, which is presumably responsible for abdominal pain in a small subset of these patients. Exogenous pancreatic enzymes have been demonstrated to modulate endogenous pancreatic secretion both in healthy individuals and in those with chronic pancreatitis. Since pancreatic enzyme therapy is relatively innocuous and inexpensive, a 4-week trial is frequently employed. If pain is relieved, pancreatic enzyme therapy is continued on a long-term basis for idiopathic chronic pancreatitis.

Celiac Ganglionectomy

If medical treatment fails to control abdominal pain and the patient continues to consume narcotic analgesics frequently, invasive measures such as surgical intervention or celiac ganglionectomy should be considered. Local anesthetic agents such as lidocaine have been injected in the celiac ganglion under fluoroscopic guidance to reduce abdominal pain in patients with chronic pancreatitis. If pain relief is significant, the celiac ganglion can be destroyed by injecting alcohol at the same site (celiac ganglionectomy). Alternatively, complete destruction of celiac ganglion can be achieved surgically. The duration of pain relief after celiac ganglion destruction is approximately 6 months in about 50 percent of patients who respond to this treatment. In view of the limited benefits from and clinical experience with this procedure, it should be used with caution in the management of chronic pancreatitis-related abdominal pain.

Surgery

The fifth and final measure used to control pancreatic pain is surgical intervention. However, a decision for surgery is often difficult because the clinical course of this disease is unpredictable, and pain frequently disappears spontaneously after a few years in a subgroup of patients. Patients should be advised of this possible outcome and encouraged to avoid surgery whenever possible.

Patients with chronic pancreatitis who have a dilated main pancreatic duct due to fibrotic strictures are generally treated by surgical drainage of the duct. Although a dilated, abnormal pancreatic duct and pancreatic pain are not well correlated, pain relief for a significant length of time has been well documented in some patients after a pancreatic drainage procedure. The choice of operation for abdominal pain from chronic pancreatitis includes (1) caudal pancreaticojejunostomy (DuVal procedure), (2) longitudinal pancreaticojejunostomy (Puestow procedure), and (3) subtotal pancreatectomy. The Puestow is the most popularly used drainage procedure in patients with chronic pancreatitis associated with a dilated main pancreatic duct. The entire main duct is opened in a longitudinal manner and all the pancreatic stones are extracted. A loop of jejunum is then opened longitudinally and sewn over the open duct so that the pancreatic juice can empty into the lumen of the jejunum. The results of surgery are generally better in patients who are neither alcoholic nor drug dependent. The surgical mortality rate from longitudinal pancreaticojejunostomy is less than 4 percent. As many as 50 percent of patients with chronic pancreatitis have been reported to obtain relief from pain for 5 years. In those who do not respond favorably to this operation, an endoscopic pancreatogram should be obtained to verify the patency of pancreaticojejunal anastomosis. Anastomotic revision or pancreatic resection may provide pain relief in a subgroup of these patients. There is a chapter on Pancreatitis: Surgical Considerations.

Treatment of Diarrhea and Weight Loss

Pancreatic enzyme therapy is the cornerstone of management of pancreatic malabsorption. Symptomatic diarrhea is significantly improved with oral pancreatic enzyme therapy, but complete correction of steatorrhea is exceedingly difficult even with large amounts of pancreatic enzyme supplementation. Before pancreatic enzyme therapy is prescribed the following information should be kept in mind (Table 3).

Type of Enzyme Preparation

Many pancreatic enzyme preparations are commercially available; only those with a significant amount of lipase should be used. Well-known preparations include Ilozyme, Cotazym, Viokase, and Ku-Zyme HP. The pH-sensitive, enteric-coated preparations include Pancrease and Cotazym-S. There should be at least 4,000 or more units of lipase per capsule or tablet. In general, capsules are preferable to tablets because there is no unpalatable flavor and smell in the encapsulated preparation. The powder form of pancreatic enzyme preparation should not be used because of extensive inactivation by the acidity in the food articles and the stomach. Low-potency enzyme preparations do not provide adequate concentrations of pancreatic enzymes in the upper small intestine. In my experience, prescription of a few potent capsules of pancreatic enzyme preparation results in better patient compliance.

Amount of Pancreatic Enzyme

The dosage of the pancreatic enzyme preparation should be adequate to reduce steatorrhea significantly and improve symptoms satisfactorily. Large amounts of these

TABLE 3 Selection of Exogenous Pancreatic Enzyme Therapy

1. Type of preparation: any potent preparation that contains 4,000–8,000 units of lipase activity per capsule or more (e.g., Cotazym, Viokase, Ilozyme) can be used
2. Amount of preparation: Approximately 30,000 units of lipase per meal (6–8 capsules or tablets per meal)
3. Form of preparation: Capsules are preferable to tablets; powder form is of dubious value
4. Time of administration: With meal; total dose distributed evenly during ingestion of meal (two capsules in beginning, two in middle, and two at end)
5. Adjuvant therapy (H_2-receptor antagonists, antacids)
6. pH-sensitive, enteric-coated pancreatic enzyme preparations (Pancrease, Cotazym)

enzyme preparations are inactivated in the stomach and only 5 to 10 percent of the orally ingested enzymes reach the upper small intestine. It has been estimated that about 30,000 units of lipase are necessary with a standard meal to provide a significant reduction in steatorrhea. Once ingested, lipase activity is inactivated below pH of 4.0 and trypsin is inactivated below pH of 3.0. These pH values are frequently reached in the stomach and in the upper small intestine during the postprandial period in this group of patients. Clinical studies have shown that as many as 6 to 8 tablets or capsules (24,000 to 32,000 units of lipase) of potent pancreatic enzyme preparations can provide a significant concentration of pancreatic enzymes in the upper GI tract. These amounts of pancreatic enzymes are generally able to reduce steatorrhea by 60 percent and stool nitrogen loss by 75 percent.

In order to improve the efficacy of pancreatic enzyme preparations, antacids and sodium bicarbonate have also been used. It has been reported that antacids such as aluminum hydroxide and sodium bicarbonate are effective as adjuvant therapy. However, magnesium- and calcium-containing antacids should not be used, because they precipitate fatty acids and bile acids. H_2-receptor antagonists (H_2 blockers) as adjuncts to pancreatic enzyme supplementation have been shown by clinical studies to reduce steatorrhea significantly. H_2 blockers are likely to be more helpful in patients with hyperchlorhydria than in patients with low gastric acid secretion. H_2-blocker therapy should be added only in patients with an inadequate response to conventional pancreatic enzyme therapy alone.

Enteric-Coated Products

In order to protect pancreatic enzymes from the hostile acidic environment of the gastric acid, pH-sensitive, enteric-coated pancreatic enzyme preparations have become available on the market. These preparations have pancreatic enzymes rolled into microspheres 1.5 to 2.5 mm in diameter, packed in a capsular form. The pH-sensitive enzyme coatings dissolve only at pH of 5.5 to 6.0 and release pancreatic enzymes into the environment. The enteric-coated preparations have been shown to be effective in reducing steatorrhea, but have not proved more effective than potent conventional enzyme preparations in alcoholic patients with pancreatic insufficiency. However, patients with cystic fibrosis seem to do better with enteric-coated preparations than with conventional preparations. The different responses of cystic fibrosis and alcoholic pancreatitis patients to enteric-coated preparation may be related to higher gastric acid secretion and gastric emptying in young patients with cystic fibrosis. The enteric-coated preparations are generally more expensive than conventional ones.

Hyperuricemia

There are no significant side effects from pancreatic enzyme therapy. Pancreatic extracts contain large amount of nucleic acid, and large doses have been reported to lead to hyperuricemia in some patients.

Poor Compliance

Compliance with pancreatic supplements is generally poor because of the large number of tablets or capsules that a patient with exocrine pancreatic insufficiency has to take with each meal. The preparations also have an unpleasant taste, so that capsules are much better tolerated by patients than the tablets.

Therapeutic Goals

The goal of pancreatic enzyme therapy is generally to help patients control diarrhea and gain body weight. A number of objective parameters can be used to evaluate the efficacy of pancreatic enzyme therapy in patients with exocrine pancreatic insufficiency (Table 4). With adequate pancreatic enzyme therapy, patients should gain 1 or 2 lb of weight each week and stabilize at about 10 percent below ideal body weight. In addition, anthropometric and biochemical parameters of nutritional assessment generally show improvement. Patients who do not respond well to pancreatic enzyme therapy should be carefully evaluated for noncompliance or for the presence of other associated disorders such as celiac sprue, altered gastric emptying, or bacterial overgrowth (Table 5). Specific steps to diagnose and treat each of these disorders are necessary in such individuals.

Treatment of Protein Energy Malnutrition

Nutritional support is also of paramount importance in patients with exocrine pancreatic insufficiency. Malnutrition is a frequent abnormality in patients with chronic pancreatitis, as many as 40 percent of whom have clinically significant protein energy malnutrition.

These patients generally have diminished muscle mass as demonstrated by anthropometric and biochemical parameters of nutrition evaluation. The salient factors responsible for the development of protein energy malnutrition include diminished caloric intake and malabsorption due to impaired pancreatic enzyme secretion by the pancreatic gland. Not infrequently, uncontrolled diabetes mellitus and protein loss from a fistula also contribute significantly to protein energy malnutrition.

Besides generalized protein energy malnutrition due to maldigestion and malabsorption of fat, proteins, and carbohydrates, specific nutrient depletion can occur in these patients. Depletion of fat-soluble vitamins (particu-

TABLE 4 Parameters for Evaluation of Clinical Response to Pancreatic Enzyme Therapy in Exocrine Pancreatic Insufficiency

1. Weight gain and growth (in children)
2. Reduction in frequency and volume of bowel movements
3. Improvement in intestinal absorption
   a. Decrease in fecal fat excretion
   b. Increase in bentiromide excretion
4. Nutritional improvement
   a. Height-weight relationship
   b. Midarm muscle circumference
   c. Serum albumin
   d. Creatinine height index

TABLE 5 Management of Patients with Poor Response to Pancreatic Enzyme Therapy

1. Increase pancreatic enzyme therapy
2. Add adjuvant therapy
   a. H_2-blocker therapy
   b. Antacid therapy
   c. Sodium bicarbonate
3. Switch to pH-sensitive, enteric-coated pancreatic enzyme therapy
4. Check for noncompliance
5. Search for other associated disorders
   a. Celiac sprue
   b. Altered gastric emptying (status post gastric surgery)
   c. Uncontrolled diabetes mellitus
   d. Bacterial overgrowth
   e. Ileal disease or resection
   f. Pancreatic cancer

larly vitamins A and E) has been described in children with exocrine pancreatic insufficiency due to cystic fibrosis, and in adult patients with chronic alcoholic pancreatitis. Zinc deficiency manifesting as perioral and perianal eczematous rash has also been reported in patients with alcoholic pancreatitis. Vitamin B_{12} malabsorption can be documented in 40 to 50 percent of patients with untreated exocrine pancreatic insufficiency, but severe vitamin B_{12} deficiency and related anemia are rare in this group of patients. The physician should be aware of potential nutritional problems and should treat them appropriately when indicated. I do not routinely screen or treat patients with chronic pancreatitis for these specific nutrient deficiencies. However, patients with poor response to pancreatic enzyme therapy or with recurrent attacks of pancreatitis are carefully evaluated for deficiencies of fat-soluble vitamins and minerals.

Management of protein energy malnutrition due to exocrine pancreatic insufficiency requires not only correction of malabsorption but also administration of a high-protein high-calorie diet. Poor caloric intake is a significant problem in some of these patients, and is generally related to postprandial pain, dietary restrictions due to a recurrent flare-up of pancreatitis, and anorexia. Nutritional supplementation in this type of clinical setting entails (1) assessment of the most appropriate nutritional support (e.g., total parenteral nutrition [TPN] or an elemental diet), (2) assessment of the duration of anticipated nutritional support, and (3) identification of the underlying problem contributing to the severe malnutrition.

If patient with chronic pancreatitis is severely malnourished, early TPN may be the treatment of choice. The pancreatic gland is very nutrition sensitive, and severe malnutrition has been reported to lead to atrophy and fibrosis. Nutritional repletion in these patients is associated with an improvement in pancreatic gland function.

In patients with mild to moderately severe malnutrition, elemental diets, protein hydrolysate preparations, or other supplemental diet therapies should be carefully considered. Medium chain triglyceride (MCT) preparations are attractive sources of lipid calories in this group of patients. Most such preparations contain primary fatty acids with 8 to 10 carbon chains as an energy source, and do not require lipase activity for absorption; they are derived mainly from coconut oil. However, poor taste and the development of nausea frequently limit the use of MCT in the treatment of severe malnutrition due to pancreatic insufficiency. MCT is available in a formula diet (Portagen) and also as a pure oil preparation for food. A specific nutrition supplemental therapy should be given to each patient in consultation with the dietitian and nutrition support team of the hospital.

Management of Diabetes Mellitus

The principal steps in the management of diabetes mellitus associated with chronic pancreatitis consist of correction of irregular food intake, malabsorption, and malnutrition and elimination of alcohol intake. Most patients require low doses of insulin, 5 to 15 units per day, to correct the hyperglycemia. The insulin requirement fluctuates between 10 and 40 units on a daily basis. Because of erratic and partial absorption of carbohydrates, these patients have a propensity to develop hypoglycemia; this may also be related to impaired glucagon secretion in chronic pancreatitis. Episodes of hypoglycemia have been reported in as many as one-third of patients being treated with insulin. The most prudent course to avoid hypoglycemia in this group of patients is to achieve higher-than-normal blood glucose levels, using the minimal doses of insulin necessary to avoid significant glucosuria. This approach appears to be reasonable, since the development of ketoacidosis and microvascular complications is relatively uncommon in these patients, and hypoglycemic episodes are frequent. Once the malabsorption is corrected with an appropriate diet plus pancreatic enzyme supplements, and after the body weight is stabilized, finer adjustment of blood glucose should be made. The importance of patient education about insulin administration and the management of its potential complications, cannot be overemphasized.

SUGGESTED READING

Adsor MA, McIlrath DC. Surgical treatment of chronic pancreatitis. In: Go VLW, et al, eds. The exocrine pancrease: biology, pathobiology and diseases. New York: Raven Press, 1986:587–599.

DiMagno EP, Go VLW, Summerskill WHJ. Relations between pancreatic enzyme outputs and malabsorption in severe pancreatic insufficiency. N Engl J Med 1973; 288:813–815.

DiMagno EP, Malajelada JR, Go VLW, Moertel CG. Fate of orally ingested enzymes in pancreatic insufficiency. N Engl J Med 1977; 296:1318–1322.

Dutta SK, Hubbard VS, Appler M. Critical examination of therapeutic efficacy of a pH-sensitive enteric-coated pancreatic enzyme preparation in the treatment of exocrine pancreatic insufficiency secondary to cystic fibrosis. Dig Dis Sci 1988; 33:1237–1244.

Dutta SK, Rubin J, Harvey J. Comparative evaluation of the therapeutic efficacy of a pH-sensitive coated pancreatic enzyme preparation with conventional pancreatic enzyme therapy in the treatment of exocrine pancreatic insufficiency. Gastroenterology 1983; 84:476–482.

Graham DY. Enzyme replacement therapy of exocrine pancreatic insufficiency in man. N Engl J Med 1977; 296:1314–1317.

Regan PT, Malagelada JR, DiMagno EP, et al. Comparative effects of antacids, cimetidine, and enteric coating on the therapeutic response to oral enzymes in severe pancreatic insufficiency. N Engl J Med 1977; 297:854–858.

RESPIRATORY DISEASES

ADULT RESPIRATORY DISTRESS SYNDROME

JOHN J. MARINI, M.D.

The term *adult respiratory distress syndrome* (ARDS) is often applied to any fulminant, diffuse parenchymal infiltrative process associated with severe hypoxemia and not clearly attributable to hydrostatic pulmonary edema. However, this designation is most helpful when restricted to problems with characteristic features, such as (1) discernible delay between precipitating event and the onset of dyspnea, (2) diminished lung compliance, (3) reduced lung volume, (4) hypoxemia refractory to supplemental oxygen but improved by restoration of lung volume, and (5) delayed resolution. As most clinicians realize, the precise pathogenesis of permeability edema remains unsettled and is almost certain to vary with the precipitating event. The numerous synonyms previously applied to this syndrome (shock lung, post-pump lung, and so forth) reflect the diversity of its potential causes. Yet despite this multitude of potential inciting events, the pathophysiology is sufficiently similar to warrant a common treatment approach.

BIOCHEMICAL MECHANISMS

A prominent feature of all forms of ARDS is injury to the gas-exchanging membrane, either from the alveolar side (e.g., inhalation of toxic fumes or smoke, aspiration) or the capillary side (e.g., sepsis, fat embolism). Increased permeability allows seepage of protein-rich fluid into the interstitial and alveolar spaces. Surfactant function and production are inhibited, contributing to widespread microatelectasis. Although pulmonary arterial occlusion (wedge) pressure usually remains normal, increased pulmonary vascular resistance and pulmonary hypertension are invariable in the latter stages of the disease. Indeed, heart failure contributes to the adverse outcome in many fatal cases. Apart from hydrostatic pressure (measured by the wedge), permeability edema differs from hydrostatic pulmonary edema (HPE) in that it resolves more slowly, resists clearance by diuretic therapy, and produces cellular infiltrate as well as proteinaceous edema fluid. From a roentgenographic viewpoint, the infiltrates of ARDS are less likely to follow a gravitational distribution and are distributed in more patchy fashion than those of HPE. Air bronchograms and reluctance of the infiltrates to vary with position are other roentgenographic features of ARDS that differ from HPE. Such distinctions are important to make because similar patterns of diffuse pulmonary infiltration with normal wedge pressure can be seen not only in ARDS, but also in such problems as rapidly resolving HPE (''flash'' pulmonary edema), diastolic dysfunction, and partially treated congestive heart failure.

A few disorders that fall loosely under the heading of ARDS are worth noting because of their fundamentally different pathophysiology and clinical course. Transient disruption in the barrier function of the pulmonary capillary can occur without overt endothelial damage. For example, neurogenic and heroin-induced pulmonary edema are two conditions in which transient elevations of pulmonary venous pressure are believed to open endothelial tight junctions, forcing a self-limited extravasation of proteinaceous fluid. However, resealing and resolution tend to occur promptly, without widespread endothelial damage. A similar process may be seen during severe metabolic acidosis, immediately following cardiopulmonary resuscitation, and perhaps during use of high levels of end-expiratory pressure.

In recent years, our understanding of ARDS has dramatically improved with recognition that ARDS is often but one manifestation of multiple organ injury, particularly when caused by sepsis or trauma. In multiple organ failure, mortality roughly parallels the number of failing organs, and pulmonary or abdominal infection (overt or hidden) is frequently the underlying event that culminates in death. The clinical risk factors for development of ARDS are (in descending order of frequency):

1. The sepsis syndrome (evidence of serious infection accompanied by a deleterious systemic response).
2. Aspiration of gastric contents (directly observed or documented by airway suctioning).
3. Drug overdosage that leads to depressed consciousness and need for monitoring in the intensive care unit.

4. Near drowning (immersion accident requiring endotracheal intubation and intensive care).
5. Pulmonary contusion (blunt thoracic trauma resulting in a localized parenchymal infiltrate on the chest film within 6 hours of the event).
6. Multiple major fractures.
7. Multiple emergency transfusions (more than 15 units of blood over a 24-hour period for emergent resuscitation).
8. Head injury (traumatic head injury resulting in sustained loss of consciousness, intracranial hemorrhage, lateralizing neurologic signs, or evidence of an increased intracranial pressure).

When two or more risk factors are present, the likelihood of ARDS approximately doubles.

A great deal of exciting work is currently underway in the attempt to define the biochemical pathogenesis of organ injury in this syndrome. A broad spectrum of ARDS-related circulating factors, both humoral and cellular, has been described. However, despite many positive reports of associations between ARDS and high or low levels of various blood-borne mediators, only a few studies have been properly controlled. Thus, the hope of identifying an easily measured final common mediator of ARDS has not yet been realized. Of the plasma markers reported in the literature, Factor VIII antigen, lactoferrin, and phospholipase A_2 perhaps show the greatest promise as predictors of risk of ARDS.

If the search for a key circulating factor has been unrewarding, experimental work probing the interaction of macrophages and endothelial cells now promises to explain some of the metabolic effects of multiple organ injury and raises new possibilities for therapeutic intervention (Table 1). The patient with multiple organ failure is often febrile, catabolic, and acidemic, as well as having obvious derangements of the inflammatory and coagulation mechanisms. Although our current understanding is far from complete, it appears that activation of circulating monocytes and tissue macrophages by circulating endotoxin or other biochemical irritant could explain how distant organs can be injured by a focal infection, injury, or inflammatory process. As the pathogenetic scheme is currently visualized, the favorite target organs of injury in this disease—the kidney, liver, lung, and gut—have high blood flows and unusually large resident populations of macrophages and phagocytic cells capable of releasing potent biochemical mediators, such as interleukin-1, tumor necrosis factor (cachectin), platelet activating factor, leukotrienes, and other products that cause direct cellular injury or activation of the inflammatory system. It is still too early to state with certainty the relative importance or activation sequence of these mediators. Furthermore, the role for specific subcellular products and processes may well vary with the inciting stimulus. Nonetheless, the identification of such mediators encourages innovation in the treatment approach. The potent effects of platelet activating factor, interleukin-1, cachectin, and other biomolecules may, in theory, be opposed by drugs that interfere with their ability to fix to receptors or by antibodies developed specifically against them. Indeed, direct blockage of endotoxin using polyclonal antibodies to core glycolipid has shown promise in gram-negative sepsis, and monoclonal antibodies to endotoxin may soon be available for clinical use. Use of such selective measures would seem a more hopeful approach than general suppression of inflammatory cell function. Indeed, glucocorticoids and prostaglandin E_1 have proved disappointing in early controlled trials. For the moment, the basic principle of treatment in ARDS is to reverse any underlying stimulus for the continuation of tissue injury while compensating for gross deficits in cardiopulmonary function consequent to the syndrome.

TABLE 1 Selected Mediators of Acute Lung Injury

Interleukin 1
Tumor necrosis factor
Platelet activating factor
Leukotrienes
Prostaglandins
Complement
Granulocyte colony stimulating factor
Plasminogen activator

PATHOPHYSIOLOGIC DERANGEMENTS IN ARDS

The major physiologic problems caused by ARDS are arterial hypoxemia, impaired CO_2 elimination, and cardiovascular compromise. Scientific management of patients with ARDS requires a sophisticated understanding of the derangements it produces in the overall process of cellular respiration. Respiratory failure may be thought of as a problem in one or more of the steps necessary to sustain energy production at the mitochondrial level. Dysfunction may occur in ventilation (the bidirectional movement of gases between the environment and the lungs), in intrapulmonary gas exchange (the process in which mixed venous blood releases CO_2 and becomes oxygenated), in gas transport (the delivery of adequate quantities of oxygenated blood to the metabolizing tissue), or in tissue gas exchange (the ability of peripheral tissues to extract or to utilize oxygen and release CO_2). The latter two steps in this process may fail independently of the performance of the lung or the ventilatory pump. Tissue oxygen delivery depends not only on arterial oxygen tension (PaO_2), but also on nonpulmonary factors such as cardiac output, hemoglobin concentration, and the ability of hemoglobin to release oxygen.

Arterial Hypoxemia

Each of the major mechanistic categories of hypoxemia contributes to the arterial desaturation of ARDS: hypoventilation, impaired alveolar diffusion of oxygen, ventilation-perfusion ($\dot{V}/\dot{Q}$) mismatching, and shunting of abnormally desaturated venous blood to the systemic arterial circuit. Damage to the small airways and to the alveolar-capillary membrane seriously impairs the normal matchup of ventilation to perfusion and increases the diffusion distance between air space and blood. Many lung units flood or collapse, thereby contributing to true shunt. Ventilation inefficiency is reflected in the very high fraction of wasted ventilation (deadspace, V_D/V_T). Consequently, the minute ventilation ($\dot{V}_E$) required to maintain alveolar carbon dioxide tension (P_ACO_2) at its normal level is often enormous, even beyond the ability of a mechanical ventilator to provide it. Thus, in the end stage of ARDS, a rising P_ACO_2 contributes a minor, but still significant, amount to the impairment in oxygen exchange. In far advanced ARDS, ventricular dysfunction and reduced cardiac output can develop in response to disturbances of the biochemical environment and gross afterloading of the right ventricle, reducing the oxygen saturation and content of mixed venous blood.

Mixed venous oxygen saturation ($S\bar{v}O_2$) is influenced by hemoglobin concentration (Hgb), cardiac output ($\dot{Q}$), arterial oxygen saturation (SaO_2), and oxygen consumption ($\dot{V}o_2$):

$$S\bar{v}O_2 \propto SaO_2 - \dot{V}o_2/(Hgb^*\dot{Q})$$

It is clear from this equation that $S\bar{v}O_2$ is directly influenced by any imbalance between oxygen consumption and oxygen delivery. Thus, anemia and inappropriate reductions in cardiac output can both cause $S\bar{v}O_2$ to fall. If shunt fraction remains unchanged, PaO_2 also declines. The impact of a falling $S\bar{v}O_2$ is attenuated if hypoxic vasoconstrictive mechanisms remain intact. Thus, fluctuations in $S\bar{v}O_2$ tend to influence PaO_2 more profoundly when the shunt fraction is fixed, as in regional lung disease (e.g., atelectasis), than when shunt varies with changing cardiac output (as in many forms of diffuse lung injury).

Lactic acidosis and reduced oxygen saturation of mixed venous blood characterize oxygen transport failure, even in the face of adequate arterial oxygenation. Failure of O_2 uptake refers to the inability of tissue to extract and utilize oxygen for aerobic metabolism. Although the clearest clinical examples of derangements in this terminal phase of the oxygen transport chain are cyanide poisoning and septic shock, there is some evidence that an extraction deficit, whether caused by a maldistribution of perfusion or by an inherent defect in cellular metabolism, may occur in ARDS as well. As in failure of oxygen transport, lactic acidosis also occurs when tissues fail to take up oxygen. However, the latter process is distinguished by normal or high values for mixed venous oxygen tension, saturation, and content. For this reason, many indices that are so helpful in monitoring other forms of oxygenation failure (cardiac output, arterial oxygen tension, and mixed venous oxygen saturation), may be misleading when impaired uptake is the cause.

The patient with severe ARDS presents a major therapeutic challenge on several fronts. First, the disease is a multi-system disorder, and therapy directed at one organ may compromise the function of another. Second, although ARDS is often equated with noncardiogenic pulmonary edema, pathologic processes other than atelectasis and alveolar flooding contribute to abnormal gas exchange. For example, as pulmonary vascular resistance rises, intracardiac right-to-left shunts may open through a patent foramen ovale. In similar fashion, emboli and thrombi may clog the pulmonary vascular system, retained secretions and airway edema can impair ventilation-perfusion matching, and reduced cardiac output can impede oxygen transport as well as reduce arterial oxygen tension. Third, the primary therapies available to treat the pulmonary consequences of ARDS—positive pressure ventilation and high concentrations of inspired oxygen—themselves have toxic consequences that may overshadow the natural clinical problem. Thus, barotrauma-induced cystic changes and pneumothorax impair ventilation, compromise oxygenation, and pose a lethal threat. Iatrogenic pulmonary infections are a frequent cause of death.

Impaired Carbon Dioxide Elimination

Fluid restriction, positive end-expiratory pressure, and parenchymal injury give rise to ventilation-perfusion mismatching and deadspace formation. Ventilator-related barotrauma enlarges ventilated airspaces at the expense of perfusion, which helps to account for failure to eliminate CO_2 despite the enormous minute ventilation requirements of advanced disease.

Cardiovascular Compromise

Because the oxygen delivery mechanism depends so closely on perfusion adequacy, any derangement of cardiovascular function presented by ARDS amplifies the crisis of tissue oxygenation. An increasing body of evidence indicates that biventricular dysfunction during ARDS is often accompanied by maldistribution of blood flow in the peripheral tissues. Right ventricular strain is expected to develop as this chamber is afterloaded by vessel destruction, hypoxic vasoconstriction, and arterial plugging. Reduced apparent compliance of the left ventricle is also explicable on this basis, via the interdependence mechanism. However, a few studies have shown overt myocardial dysfunction as well, presumably mediated on a humoral basis. Finally, the delivery dependence of oxygen consumption suggested by several careful studies of this disorder points to a generalized oxygen extraction defect or dysregulation of perfusion.

BASIC THERAPEUTIC PRINCIPLES

The multiplicity of precipitating factors and pathophysiologic derangements of ARDS demand an individualized approach to the treatment of this disorder. It is axiomatic that the underlying pathology must be reversed, and whenever there is a clear possibility of ongoing injury (e.g., recurrent aspiration or occult infection), such problems must be aggressively sought and treated. Thus, it is important to decompress the stomach of aspiration-prone patients and to place the upper body in an upright position. Furthermore, it is now known that many patients with ARDS harbor occult infections in the lungs, abdomen, and sinuses that may perpetuate the tissue-injury process. On this basis, I believe that the aggressive use of broad-spectrum antibiotics is justified in the setting of fever and ARDS, even when a precise focus of infection cannot be identified.

Although atelectasis, fluid overload, and infection may yield to specific measures, the treatment of diffuse lung injury remains largely supportive. The primary therapeutic aims are to maintain oxygen delivery, to support the breathing workload, to establish electrolyte balance, and to maintain nutrition while preventing further damage from oxygen toxicity, barotrauma, infection, and other complications. To these ends, the clinician should bear in mind a few fundamental principles.

1. Deliver adequate quantities of oxygen to vital tissues, but minimize the risk of iatrogenic damage to the lungs. As is often true in clinical medicine, practice is based more on intuition and physiologic rationale than on hard empiric or scientific evidence. In attempting to optimize the quantity of oxygen delivered to tissues, the practitioner should be aware that this keystone of treatment strategy has never been shown to favorably affect the outcome of this disease. On the other hand, the tools with which improved tissue oxygen delivery is achieved—positive end-expiratory pressure (PEEP), high fractions of oxygen, fluid deprivation, and vasopressors—are all potentially hazardous.

2. Frequent reassessment of the need for PEEP, the current level of ventilator support, and the FIO_2 is essential. Toxic levels of FIO_2 and PEEP may not always be necessary or effective; an oxygen saturation of 85 percent may be acceptable if the patient has adequate oxygen carrying capacity, a strong heart, good cardiovascular reflexes, and shows no signs of critical oxygen deprivation (e.g., lactic acidosis). Similarly, allowing $PaCO_2$ to climb (buffering pH as needed with infused sodium bicarbonate) may minimize the ventilatory requirement and reduce the risk of barotrauma. At shunt fractions of more than 30 percent, lowering the FIO_2 out of the upper (exponentially toxic) range may greatly reduce the hazard with little change in arterial saturation. Although dyspneic patients must receive full support, mean intrathoracic pressure can usually be reduced by allowing the patient to provide as much ventilatory power as possible, compatible with capability and comfort.

3. Keep patients under strict observation at all times and closely monitor for adverse developments. The hands must be restrained in disoriented patients who receive mechanical ventilation because abrupt ventilator disconnections and extubations can produce lethal bradyarrhythmias, hypoxemia, asphyxia, or aspiration. Paralyzed patients must be watched with special care since ventilation is totally machine dependent. In the initial phase of pulmonary edema, the interruption of PEEP for even brief periods (suctioning, tubing changes) may cause profound and slowly reversing oxygen desaturation as lung volume falls and the airways rapidly flood with alveolar edema fluid. Because air swallowing and ileus are common, the stomach should be decompressed in most recently intubated patients. The clinician must be ready to intervene immediately to decompress a tension pneumothorax. Prophylactic chest tubes may be indicated for patients who demonstrate tension cyst formation.

4. Remember that oxygenation failure is often a multisystem disease. Severe fluid restriction may reduce lung water and improve oxygen exchange but simultaneously compromise the perfusion of gut and kidney. (Parenthetically, there is no convincing evidence that reducing lung water speeds recovery or improves survival.) The routine use of corticosteroids is not justified; systemic changes in metabolism and protein wastage in conjunction with the increased risk of infection overshadow any potential therapeutic benefit, except perhaps in the setting of proven vasculitis, bronchospasm, allergic reaction, or fat embolism. Appropriate levels of nutritional support and prophylaxis against gastrointestinal hemorrhage are important adjunctive measures.

RE-ESTABLISHING THE BALANCE BETWEEN OXYGEN DELIVERY AND DEMAND

Once the underlying pathogenetic process has been identified and treated, most clinicians focus their therapeutic attention on maintaining the balance between oxygen delivery and demand (Table 2). Adequacy of oxygen delivery is determined by tissue oxygen needs and by the availability of oxygen.

Improving Tissue Oxygen Delivery

Increasing Cardiac Output

Oxygen delivery is the product of cardiac output and the oxygen content of each unit volume of blood. Cardiac output can be improved by increasing preload, decreasing afterload, or enhancing cardiac contractility. However, increasing the filling pressure of the left ventricle is problematic in that any increase in pulmonary venous pressure may cause alveolar flooding and the need

TABLE 2 Principles of Physiologic Support During ARDS

Maintain adequate oxygen delivery
Hgb > 12 g/dl
SaO_2 > 85% (FIO_2, PEEP)
Maintain adequate cardiac output
Reduce oxygen demands
Avoid barotrauma
Secretion clearance
Minimize V_T, $\dot{V}_E$ and PEEP
Treat infection aggressively

for higher FiO_2 or PEEP. Therefore, fluid manipulations must be cautious; too much fluid contributes to the impairment of oxygen exchange, whereas too little fluid may compromise preload, cardiac output, and oxygen delivery. Although invaluable in the management of difficult cases, a pulmonary artery catheter is not always required. Patients who can be oxygenated at PEEP levels of less than 10 cm H_2O, with adequate urine output and blood pressure, can often be managed safely without one. Patients with hemodynamic compromise (as manifested by end organ dysfunction or lactic acidosis) and those who require high levels of PEEP usually benefit from invasive monitoring.

The Swan-Ganz catheter provides three essential types of information: cardiac output, wedge pressure, and mixed venous oxygen saturation. All three are important when gauging the impact of such therapeutic interventions as fluid administration, PEEP application, or vasopressor usage. Except when the wedge pressure is very high or very low, it is often difficult to judge the adequacy of a given filling pressure, especially when high levels of PEEP are needed. Not only is the transmural filling pressure of the left ventricle influenced by pleural pressure, but also the effective compliance of the left ventricle is affected unpredictably by fluctuations in right ventricle swelling, hypoxemia, ischemia, or circulating catecholamines. For these reasons, it is wise to challenge the wedge pressure with a modest fluid bolus (e.g., 250 to 500 ml over 10 minutes) when serious doubt exists regarding preload adequacy. Significantly improved cardiac output and blood pressure with minimal increase of wedge pressure is consistent with the need for liberalizing fluids.

Afterload reduction of the right ventricle is difficult to achieve unless hypoxemia and the underlying pathologic process can be corrected. Vasodilators may be of benefit in selected cases, but their beneficial effect is often outweighed by adverse side effects. For example, pulmonary vasodilation may be achieved at the expense of reversing hypoxic vasoconstriction. On the left side, vasodilators are usually ineffectual or overtly detrimental.

On the other hand, inotropic agents such as dobutamine often help. Dopamine is the agent of choice when both vasopressor and inotropic effects are desired. However, the clinician should be aware that dopamine can, on occasion, exacerbate venous admixture. Reversal of acidosis can improve cardiac contractility response to inotropes and peripheral vascular tone. Continuous hemofiltration may allow removal of the sodium and water load that accompanies bicarbonate infusion.

Optimizing Hemoglobin

Oxygen delivery also can be improved by optimizing the concentration and the dissociation characteristics of hemoglobin. Both factors can be important, for example, hemoglobin performance is enhanced by reversing alkalemia to facilitate O_2 off loading. As hemoglobin concentration rises, blood viscosity increases, retarding passage of erythrocytes through capillary networks. Thus, actual O_2 delivery can be impaired as hematocrit is boosted higher than 50 percent. Although the optimal hemoglobin concentration in patients suffering an oxygenation crisis is not known with certainty, it makes sense to restore hemoglobin to the normal range (approximately 13 g per deciliter, or a hematocrit of 35 to 40 percent). More aggressive supplementation increases transfusion related risks without proven benefit.

Improving Arterial Oxygenation

Oxygen content is the product of Hgb concentration and saturation (SaO_2). Because of the sigmoidal shape of the oxyhemoglobin dissociation curve, a PaO_2 of 50 to 60 mm Hg achieves 85 to 90 percent of maximal saturation. Two basic interventions are available to help compensate for impaired pulmonary oxygen exchange: (1) supplemental oxygen and (2) PEEP to recruit alveoli and redistribute lung liquid. Unfortunately, both may engender additional lung injury.

Oxygen Therapy

Increasing the FiO_2 improves PaO_2 in all instances in which true shunt is not the primary mechanism of hypoxemia. The goal is to increase the saturation of hemoglobin to 85 to 90 percent, without risking O_2 toxicity. It should be noted that the response to oxygen may not be linear across the spectrum of FiO_2—on occasion, very high concentrations of O_2 may be needed to elicit evidence of brisk O_2 ($F_2O_2>0.6$) responsiveness. Changes in PEEP often affect the slope of the FiO_2–PaO_2 relationship.

The incidence of O_2 toxicity is both concentration and time dependent. As a general rule, very high inspired fractions of oxygen can be safely used for brief periods (less than 24 to 48 hours) as simultaneous efforts are made to reverse the underlying pathogenetic process. Such a strategy can often avoid the need for intubation and machine support. However, because sustained elevations in FiO_2 may cause inflammatory changes, alveolar infiltration, and eventual fibrosis, every effort should be made to keep the FiO_2 less than 0.6 during the support phase of illness.

Positive End-Expiratory Pressure

PEEP and newer specialized modes of ventilation designed to increase mean alveolar pressure (e.g., inverse ratio ventilation) often succeed in recruiting lung volume and redistributing lung water from the alveolar spaces to the interstitium. Reversal of atelectasis not only improves oxygenation, but also reduces the work of breathing. Virtually all critically ill patients benefit from low levels of PEEP (3 to 5 cm H_2O), regardless of lung pathology, and it is my practice to prescribe such levels to all intubated patients. Low-level PEEP helps to compensate for the loss of volume that accompanies the supine posture and translaryngeal intubation. At the same time, there is no evidence that PEEP offers prophylaxis against the onset of ARDS in high risk patients.

The volume recruiting effects of PEEP can be negated by the vigorous efforts of a dyspneic patient if expiratory muscle action forces the chest to a lung volume at end-expiration lower than the equilibrium position. When this happens, as it commonly does during the initial phase of ventilator support,sedation or paralysis can be helpful. Paralysis relieves the work of breathing, thereby releasing the obligate perfusion of the respiratory musculature to other organs. Lung volume also increases as compliance improves.

PEEP applied to the common airway may prove ineffective or hazardous if the compliant or necrotic lung units of a nonhomogeneous infiltrate are forced to overdistend during tidal inflation. Tidal volume should be reduced to keep peak distending pressures from rising when high levels of PEEP are needed.

It is important to select the minimum level of PEEP that achieves the therapeutic goals of volume recruitment, adequate oxygenation, and optimal oxygen delivery. The potentially adverse effects of PEEP include reduced cardiac output, diminished blood flow to vital organs, increased intracranial pressure, and increased risk of barotrauma. Many approaches for adjusting PEEP are in use. One approach is to increase PEEP until the static chest compliance, calculated oxygen delivery, or oxygen consumption is maximal, or until the calculated shunt fraction falls to some arbitrary level (e.g., less than 15 percent). Perhaps the most common approach (and the one that I use) is to titrate PEEP to a level that allows appropriate hemoglobin saturation with a reduction of the FIO_2 to a safe level. When PEEP trials are conducted, PEEP is added in increments (usually 5 cm H_2O) at specified intervals, commonly every 20 to 30 minutes. Although ear and pulse oximetry are helpful adjuncts in gauging arterial oxygen saturation, a 20 gauge Teflon catheter inserted into a radial artery facilitates blood sampling and arterial pressure monitoring. The combination of a pulse oximeter and a fiberoptic Swan-Ganz catheter can facilitate PEEP adjustment. During the PEEP trial, clinical evaluation and measurement of arterial blood gases are undertaken after each incremental increase. Arterial and mixed venous gases, thermodilution cardiac output, central venous pressure, pulmonary arterial wedge pressure, and systemic arterial pressure are commonly measured at each increment of PEEP above 10 to 12 cm H_2O. (I do not routinely place a pulmonary artery catheter for titrating low levels of PEEP unless there are other indications or unless there is evidence of PEEP-related cardiovascular dysfunction.) The trial is terminated when sufficient improvement in oxygen exchange occurs to allow a decrease in FIO_2 to 0.6 or less with an SaO_2 of 85 percent or more. The PEEP trial is also terminated when the proposed increment of PEEP causes a significant decrease in cardiac output, end-organ dysfunction, a drop in mixed venous oxygen tension ($P\bar{v}O_2$), widening of the arteriovenous content difference, falling blood pressure, or a reproducible drop in thoracic compliance.

Positioning

When one lung is differentially affected, oxygenation may improve dramatically with the good lung dependent. However, care should be taken to ensure that secretions from the infiltrated lung are not aspirated into the airway of the dependent, viable lung during this process. When disease is highly unilateral, selective intubation and independent lung ventilation can allow individual tailoring of the pattern of lung inflation, FIO_2 and PEEP, thereby improving oxygenation and reducing the risk of barotrauma.

Lung infection, secretion retention, and barotrauma must be avoided at all costs. To these ends, maintenance of excellent bronchial hygiene should be a clinical priority. The patient should remain as upright as possible to preserve the maximal functional lung volume, and recumbent patients should be turned frequently. Alternating lateral decubitus positions puts different regions of the lung on maximal stretch and improves secretion drainage. Position changes are especially important in comatose or paralyzed patients, in whom secretions pooled in dependent regions add to the tendency for lung collapse and hypoxemia. Intermittent shifts of the patient from the supine to prone position may occasionally help dramatically in reversing the hypoxemia of ARDS.

Secretion Management and Bronchodilation

Although ARDS is often regarded mainly as a problem of parenchymal injury, airway edema, bronchospasm, and secretion retention frequently contribute to hypoxemia. This is especially true in cases of ARDS caused or complicated by aspiration, bronchopneumonia, coma, or paralysis. Retained secretions pose a generally overlooked problem that encourages both maldistribution of ventilation and barotrauma. In some patients with diffuse lung injury, profound bradycardia develops during ventilator disconnections, discouraging airway hygiene. Although hypoxemia occasionally contributes, this "disconnection bradycardia" is usually reflex in nature and responds to prophylactic intramuscular atropine.

Oral tubes or tracheostomies are preferable to nasal tubes in the long-term treatment of ARDS for several reasons, the most important of which are that the nasal tubes tend to kink and are smaller in diameter than tubes placed orally in the same patient. Nasal tubes also tend to incite purulent sinusitis.

The Role of Barotrauma in Recovery from Lung Injury

In recent years there has been growing suspicion that high levels of positive pressure routinely produce lung damage that perpetuates ventilator dependence and plays a vital role in deciding the eventual outcome, even when pneumothorax fails to surface as a clinical problem. On a microscopic level, ARDS is a disease characterized by patchy involvement. When high mean and peak cycling pressures are required to accomplish adequate alveolar ventilation, compliant and necrotic alveoli tend to rupture and coalesce, causing cystic changes and expanding the deadspace. In a high percentage of patients ventilated for longer than 10 to 14 days, barotrauma in the form of tension pneumothorax or bronchopleural fistula often results. Recent studies indicate that such developments strongly predict a fatal outcome. Interstitial emphysema and subpleural cystic changes so commonly precede tension pneumothorax that a strong argument can be made for inserting prophylactic chest tubes when these changes appear.

It is interesting to note that the salvage of patients with ARDS has been reported to improve dramatically when extracorporeal CO_2 removal reduces the need for positive pressure ventilation. It is also interesting to note that the reported success in the treatment of the infant respiratory distress syndrome (IRDS) has also been enhanced by these techniques. Controlled objective data must be gathered before this aggressive strategy can be generally recommended. Nonetheless, on the strength of such information, I currently make every effort to reduce the minute ventilation requirement and peak cycling pressure during routine management and consider the early removal of mechanical support to be an urgent priority.

Reducing Oxygen Requirements

Reducing the tissue oxygen demand can be as effective as improving oxygen delivery in re-establishing appropriate balance. Because fever, agitation, overfeeding, vigorous respiratory activity, shivering, sepsis, and a host of other commonly observed clinical conditions can markedly increase the rate of oxygen consumption and the need for ventilation, steps should be taken to eliminate these stimuli. Although fever reduction is a rational therapeutic goal, shivering must be prevented in the cooling process. Sedation and the use of antipyretics (rather than cooling blankets) make good therapeutic sense.

As already noted, paralysis is a valuable means by which to reduce $\dot{V}O_2$ and to improve PaO_2 in patients who remain agitated or fight the ventilator despite more conservative measures. (In this setting, $\dot{V}O_2$ may double during periods of vigorous breathing.) Although often helpful in the first hours of machine support, extended periods of paralysis must be avoided. Paralysis places the entire responsibility for achieving adequate oxygenation and ventilation with the medical team—the patient is defenseless during an unobserved ventilator disconnection. Paralysis also silences the coughing mechanism and creates a monotonous breathing pattern that encourages secretion retention and collapse in dependent lung regions.

Specialized Forms of Ventilatory Support

In recent years, a number of interesting approaches have been undertaken in an attempt to establish adequate ventilation and reverse hypoxemia. Inverse ratio ventilation is a technique in which pressure controlled ventilation is applied for an inspiratory time fraction (t_i/t_{tot}) that exceeds 0.5. In this way, dynamic end-expiratory and mean alveolar pressures rise, placing sustained tethering forces on the lung tissue without exposing well-ventilated units to high peak cycling pressures. Although there are encouraging anecdotal reports in the literature, to my knowledge there are no prospective, controlled data that confirm its efficacy in adults. Inverse ratio ventilation generally requires deep sedation or paralysis.

Some physicians attempt to minimize the levels of positive pressure applied to the airway by supporting oxygenation with continuous positive airway pressure while allowing the patient to bear the entire ventilatory workload. Whereas this technique is attractive in reducing barotrauma and preserving cardiac output, the ventilatory workload of patients with full-blown ARDS is often too great to permit its use. (In my practice, I generally support respirations fully for the first 24 to 48 hours of acute illness, withdrawing positive pressure as soon as feasible, consistent with patient comfort.) Recently it has been suggested that intermittent release of continuous positive airway pressure may boost ventilation sufficiently to allow spontaneous ventilation without compromising oxygenation. This theory appears sound physiologically, but must be proven before it can be suggested for widespread clinical use.

SUGGESTED READING

Bone RC, ed. Adult respiratory distress syndrome. Clin Chest Med 1982; 3:1–213.

Fallat RJ, Luce JM, ed. Cardiopulmonary critical care management. Clin Crit Care Med 1988; 14:1–215.

Maunder RJ, Hudson LD. The adult respiratory distress syndrome. In: Simmons DH, ed. Current Pulmonology. Chicago: Year Book Medical Publishers, 1986:97.

Pepe PE, Hudson LD, Carrico CJ. Early application of positive end-expiratory pressure in patients at risk for the adult respiratory distress syndrome. N Engl J Med 1984; 311:281–286.

Rinaldo JE, Rogers RM. Adult respiratory distress syndrome. N Engl J Med 1986; 310:578–580.

Wiedemann HP, Matthay MA, Matthay RA, eds. Acute lung injury. Crit Care Clin 1986; 2:377–667.

ACUTE UPPER AIRWAY INFECTION

HANS PASTERKAMP, M.D., FRCPC
VICTOR CHERNICK, M.D., FRCPC

Acute upper airway infection in association with severe increase in *inspiratory* airflow obstruction is a common occurrence in young infants and children, but may occur in the adult. In the United States, approximately 20,000 children per year are hospitalized with viral croup for an average length of stay of about 3 days. About 3,000 children per year are hospitalized with epiglottitis for an average length of stay of 6 days. The susceptibility to upper airway obstruction with infection in infants and children is related to the small size of the triangular glottic inlet (7 × 4 mm in an infant) and the narrow diameter of the subglottic area (5 to 6 mm in an infant). Reduction of these diameters results in increased turbulent flow and production of a harsh whistling sound (stridor) during inspiration (negative intraluminal pressure). Obstruction is less severe during expiration because of the positive intraluminal pressure (dilating effect) and is not associated with sound production in these conditions. Therapy is aimed at relieving obstruction and reducing the inspiratory work of breathing.

The major cause of croup used to be diphtheria, but several distinct clinical entities are currently recognized: laryngotracheobronchitis (viral croup), spasmodic croup, epiglottitis, and bacterial tracheitis. The management of each is different, and a precise diagnosis is important to avoid such complications as severe hypoxia and death.

VIRAL CROUP (LARYNGOTRACHEOBRONCHITIS)

The major cause of this condition is the parainfluenza virus (usually type 1), but it may be caused by influenza, respiratory syncytial virus, adenovirus, and rarely, *Mycoplasma pneumoniae*. Infection results in inflammation, swelling, and edema of the subglottic area of the trachea. The condition usually occurs in children under 3 years of age, during the fall or winter. It is characterized by signs and symptoms of an upper respiratory tract infection including coryza, followed after several days by an onset of inspiratory stridor, a barking cough, and a mild tachypnea.

The diagnosis is confirmed by the typical clinical course and by the absence of epiglottitis noted on *gentle* direct examination of the pharynx. If this examination is not possible, a lateral roentgenographic study of the neck may demonstrate subglottic swelling and a normal-sized epiglottis. The disease is usually self-limited (3 to 5 days), and treatment is largely symptomatic.

Management

Mist Therapy

The mainstay of therapy for patients with croup is the provision of high humidity (running the shower in the bathroom) or mist (home mist generator or mist or croup tent in the hospital). Rigid scientific documentation of the efficacy of this therapy has not been done, but most clinicians and nurses attest to its effectiveness. Precisely how mist or high humidity works is unclear. It is thought that increased airflow through a narrowed trachea may have a local drying effect, may stimulate irritant receptors, and may cause local smooth muscle constriction. Alternatively, large-particle mist that rains out in the upper airway may reflexively slow respiration, resulting in a decrease of inspiratory flow rate, a lesser decrease in intraluminal pressure during inspiration, and a decrease in inspiratory work.

Oxygen

Since most patients with croup that is severe enough to require hospitalization have some degree of hypoxemia, the mist tent is a convenient way of providing supplemental oxygen (30 to 35 percent), which is sufficient to relieve the hypoxemia.

Racemic Epinephrine

The administration of aerosolized 2.25 percent racemic epinephrine (0.25 ml in 1.5 ml saline for patients 5 kg of body weight or less; 0.5 ml in 1.5 ml saline for patients of more than 5 kg of body weight) by simple face mask is effective in relieving obstruction in patients with viral croup within a few minutes. We do not believe that there is a "rebound" phenomenon with this therapy, but some patients may require this treatment as often as every hour. Usually the therapy is effective for 2 to 4 hours. If a child has obstruction severe enough to warrant this therapy, hospitalization and close observation are mandatory.

Sedation

Although many clinicians prescribe sedation with phenobarbital or chloral hydrate in the treatment of this condition, we believe that this practice is dangerous to a patient with severe obstruction. We do not recommend the use of sedatives since anxiety is a sign of severe obstruction and hypoxemia, and sedation may hasten sudden respiratory arrest.

Steroids

The use of steroids in the treatment of children with viral croup is becoming more widely accepted. Current evidence suggests that an intramuscular dose (0.6 mg/kg) of dexamethasone should be given when patients are admitted to hospital. If croup persists for several days, one should also consider other causes for the prolonged obstruction, such as tracheomalacia, subglottic tumor, or a foreign body.

Helium and Oxygen Breathing

Theoretically, breathing a mixture of 80 percent helium and 20 percent oxygen—a mixture that is one-third as dense as air—should greatly reduce the resistance to turbulent airflow that characterizes upper airway obstruction. This therapy has not been extensively studied in children with croup, but theoretical considerations and a few case reports indicate that it is effective in relieving the inspiratory work of breathing. The lowest effective concentration of helium is contained in a mixture of 60 percent helium and 40 percent oxygen (about one-half the density of air). This therapy is expensive and unlikely to be widely adopted.

Intubation

Intubation for the relief of obstruction from viral croup is required in only a small percentage of patients. Prior to the use of racemic epinephrine, about 6 percent of children with viral croup were intubated or had a tracheotomy. In more recent years, and in association with the use of aerosolized epinephrine, this rate has dropped to less than 1 percent. We do not recommend tracheotomy. Nasotracheal intubation under anesthesia by a skilled anesthesiologist or surgeon is our preferred method of therapy in the vast majority of patients since the artificial airway is rarely required for more than 4 or 5 days. This subject is considered in greater detail under Epiglottitis.

Follow-up Studies

Long-term follow-up studies of patients with viral croup indicate that 35 percent have increased bronchial reactivity to inhaled methacholine and 50 percent have exercise-induced bronchospasm. Baseline pulmonary function may be normal, and enhanced bronchial reactivity is not related to allergies. The reason for this long-term effect is not known, but some of these patients may require an inhaled bronchodilator.

SPASMODIC CROUP

Spasmodic or recurrent croup is a poorly understood clinical entity that usually occurs in children, but may occur in adults. It presents as recurrent attacks of croup with a sudden onset, usually at night, without signs of upper respiratory tract infection or fever. Acute adductor spasm of the vocal cords has been considered the major cause of the obstruction, but a pale edema of the subglottic area has been noted at laryngoscopy. These children have a distinct response to histamine challenge, which affects both the inspiratory and the expiratory portion of the flow-volume loop, suggesting the presence of both extrathoracic and intrathoracic airway hyperactivity.

Management

One study reports that although dexamethasone (0.6 mg per kilogram given intramuscularly in a single dose) was ineffective in viral croup, it was effective in relieving spasmodic croup. Adults have been successfully treated with intermittent positive pressure breathing (IPPB) or continuous positive airway pressure (CPAP). Aerosolized racemic epinephrine also may be effective.

EPIGLOTTITIS

In contrast to viral croup, epiglottitis is an acute fulminating infection of the epiglottis, the aryepiglottic folds, and the surrounding tissues. It has a sudden onset with fever, sore throat, inspiratory stridor, and progressive toxicity. The patients are usually between 2 and 6 years of age, but the condition may occur at any age, even in adults. As the obstruction worsens, stridor may disappear, and the patient has slow, deep breathing, a muffled voice, and drooling. The condition is diagnosed by the typical clinical course as well as visualization of a cherry-red, swollen epiglottis. Examination of the pharynx *must* be done *gently*. Vigorous attempts that make the child cry may cause sudden, complete airway obstruction. In no case should the pharynx be examined unless the physician is in a facility that is prepared for an emergency intubation. If the pharynx cannot be visualized, a lateral roentgenographic study of the neck demonstrates the swollen epiglottis ("thumb-print" sign) and aryepiglottic folds. The causative organism in the majority of cases is *Haemophilus influenzae* type B, but in rare instances, it may be *Streptococcus* or *Staphylococcus*. *Candida* epiglottitis should be considered in immunocompromised patients who have symptoms of refractory pharyngitis. Epiglottitis constitutes a medical emergency and must be treated promptly in order to avoid the significant morbidity and mortality associated with severe hypoxemia. Pulse oximetry may be helpful as adjunctive monitoring in the emergency room.

Management

Intubation

The mainstay of therapy in patients of any age is provision of an adequate airway for 36 to 48 hours. In our institution, we have abandoned tracheotomy, and all children with epiglottitis are intubated immediately on admission without waiting for signs of worsening obstruction. Nasotracheal intubation should be done in the operating room under anesthesia administered by a skilled anesthesiologist or surgeon. A rigid bronchoscope should be available if intubation is difficult. We have used nasotracheal intubation for this condition for a decade, have not had any failed intubations, have zero mortality, and have had no significant complications. In the majority of cases, it is possible to remove the endotracheal tube after 48 hours of antibiotic therapy. Extubation should be done in the operating room where a staff is prepared to reintubate if necessary.

Antibiotics

Because of the emergence of resistant strains of *H influenzae*, most clinicians now use cefuroxime, 150 mg per kilogram per day in three divided doses. Alternatively, some use a combination of ampicillin, 200 mg per kilogram per day in four to six divided doses, and chloramphenicol, 50 to 100 mg per kilogram per day every 6 hours; the total adult dose of chloramphenicol is 2 to 4 g per day. Once culture and sensitivity results are known, the inappropriate antibiotic may be discontinued. Antibiotics are given intravenously for the first 3 or 4 days and then continued orally for a total of 10 days. If an ampicillin resistant organism is being treated, intravenous cefuroxime may be changed to oral trimethoprim/sulfa, Clavulin or cephalosporin.

BACTERIAL TRACHEITIS

This condition, also known as pseudomembranous croup, membranous laryngotracheobronchitis, or bacterial tracheobronchitis, was well recognized in the early third of this century. It has recently re-emerged with a number of reports from various centers across North America. Bacterial tracheitis is an infection of the trachea and bronchi by either *Staphylococcus aureus* or *H. influenzae* and is associated with the formation of thick purulent secretions in the large airways. Symptoms resemble those of viral croup, i.e., croupy cough and inspiratory stridor. The patients affected may be 1 month to 7 or 8 years of age. The illness is more progressive than viral croup, but less acute than epiglottitis. It is associated with fever and leukocytosis. The hallmark is the presence of thick purulent secretions. In practice, the condition may be difficult to distinguish from viral croup or epiglottitis. The latter is ruled out when the normal epiglottis is seen on direct examination or on the lateral roentgenographic study of the neck. Subglottic swelling is usually absent, but secretions may be seen as a vague density or as a "dripping candle" effect on the tracheal mucosa. The diagnosis is confirmed by smear and subsequent culture of tracheal secretions.

Management

Intubation and Pulmonary Toilet

Patients with bacterial tracheitis cannot handle the copious purulent secretions and are in danger of sudden complete obstruction with large plugs of material. The hallmark of therapy is nasotracheal intubation (as described for epiglottitis). Patients must be managed in an intensive care unit, where frequent and vigorous pulmonary toilet is mandatory. Saline solution should be instilled into the endotracheal tube prior to suctioning. In only one instance of 14 cases that we have seen, that of a 3-year-old child, was intubation unnecessary since he was able to cough out the secretions. Extubation may be accomplished 5 to 6 days after beginning antibiotic therapy, but we have seen cases in which prolonged (7 to 10 days) intubation was required.

Antibiotics

Appropriate antibiotics (antistaphylococcal or anti-*H. influenzae* as for epiglottitis) are required for 10 to 14 days. They are given intravenously for the first 4 to 6 days and then orally.

SUGGESTED READING

Cramblett HG. Croup. In: Kendig EE, Chernick V, eds. Disorders of the respiratory tract in children. 4th ed. Philadelphia: WB Saunders, 1983:268.

Gussack GS, Tacchi EJ. Pulse oximetry in the management of pediatric airway disorders. South Med J 1987; 80:1381–1384.

Loughlin GM, Taussig LM. Upper airway obstruction. Semin Resp Med 1979; 1:131–146.

Newth JJL, Levison H, Bryan AC. The respiratory status of children with croup. J Pediatr 1972; 81:1068–1073.

Skolnik NS. Treatment of croup—a critical review. Am J Dis Child 1989; 143:1045–1049.

Sofer S, Duncan PD, Chernick V. Bacterial tracheitis, an old disease rediscovered. Clin Pediatr 1983; 22:407–411.

AEROBIC GRAM-POSITIVE PNEUMONIA

OSWALD VAN CUTSEM, M.D.
WILLIAM W. MERRILL, M.D.

The organisms that stain positively with Gram's technique are a large and diverse group with varying potential to cause human disease. In the following paragraphs we discuss those members of this group that commonly cause pneumonia.

An important consideration in the bacterial etiology of pneumonia is the clinical status of the host prior to infection. Pneumonias that arise in subjects living in the community (community acquired pneumonia [CAP]) are caused by a different group of organisms than pneumonias that complicate the illnesses of persons who are hospitalized for another reason (nosocomial pneumonia [NP]). For example, the most common cause of CAP is *Streptococcus pneumoniae*, which is incriminated in 36 to 76 percent of these pneumonias. Among gram-positive bacteria, *Staphylococcus aureus* follows far behind, with an estimated frequency of 1 to 6 percent. From one study to another, a wide variation of the percentage of the different etiologic pathogens can be seen. The factors influencing these variations in incidence include the precise diagnostic criteria and the presence of epidemic spread of mycoplasmas, viruses, and *Legionella* organisms. Moreover, different results are found if investigators study all CAPs or only those necessitating hospitalization. By contrast, in NP, *Str. pneumoniae* is still frequent (30 percent), but the incidence of *Staph. aureus* rises dramatically (25 percent).

Uncommon gram-positive pathogens responsible for respiratory tract infections are other streptococci (e.g., *Str. pyogenes* and *Str. faecalis*), *Bacillus anthracis*, *Nocardia* species, *Actinomyces* species, and the mycobacteria. We have limited our discussion to the more common causes.

EPIDEMIOLOGY

The majority of bacterial pneumonias arise because of contamination of the lower respiratory tract by organisms present in the pharynx. Usually, this implies aspiration of upper airway material during periods of diminished consciousness (e.g., sleep, seizure, or alcoholic debauch). Therefore, the context in which pneumonia appears is very important in establishing the suspicion of certain etiologic pathogens. Because *Str. pneumoniae* may be among the normal flora, everyone is susceptible to pneumococcal pneumonia. *Str. pneumoniae* (and *Haemophilus influenzae*) also may colonize the lower respiratory tract of patients with chronic obstructive lung disease or bronchiectasis. This explains the high incidence of pneumococcal pneumonia in this population. Splenectomized patients are particularly likely to develop more severe infections with encapsulated species such as *Pneumococcus*.

CAP caused by *Staph. aureus* is seen in young children, especially in the first 6 months of life, and in patients with underlying disease (diabetes mellitus, alcoholism, chronic lung and heart disease, bronchial carcinoma, early infections of cystic fibrosis, bronchiectasis). At times, distant foci of staphylococcal infection also can be responsible for hematogenous pneumonia, such as in right-sided endocarditis of intravenous drug addicts, in soft tissue infection, and in osteomyelitis.

Viral infection is a well-known predisposing factor for bacterial pneumonia. During an influenza epidemic, *Pneumococcus* remains the most common agent of bacterial pneumonia, but in CAP, *Staph. aureus* rises from 6 to 20 percent.

In hospital acquired lower respiratory tract infection, the incidence of *Staph. aureus* and gram-negative bacteria rises because of many factors, including suppression of physiologic defenses with drugs (steroids, cytotoxic therapy), intubation, catheterization, skin damage due to extensive burns, and altered nutritional status.

DIAGNOSIS

Clinical signs of gram-positive pneumonia are not specific. They are the signs of bacterial pneumonia and may include herpes labialis, chills, fever, cough, purulent sputum, pleurodynia, dyspnea, cyanosis, dullness on percussion, crackles, or bronchial breath sounds.

Radiologic signs of gram-positive pneumonia also are not specific. As in other bacterial pneumonias, there are parenchymal infiltrates and lobar consolidation. Multiple and bilateral infiltrates are more often encountered in hematogenous staphylococcal pneumonia. Staphylococcal pneumonia also more commonly gives rise to abscesses and pneumatoceles, which are rapidly growing thin-walled cavities.

The results of direct sputum examination are useful when many white cells (infection) and few epithelial cells (low oropharyngeal contamination) are found. In this case, the presence of gram-positive cocci or lancet-shaped diplococci (especially intracellular organisms) is suggestive of lower respiratory tract infection with these bacteria. Unfortunately, the specificity of this observation is only about 50 percent. The results of the sputum culture may be falsely positive because of oropharyngeal contamination with *Pneumococcus* or *Staphylococcus*. Even the lower respiratory tract secretions of chronic obstructive lung disease may contain *Str. pneumoniae* without this organism being necessarily responsible for the infiltrate. The same has to be said about these organisms in bronchiectasis. Furthermore, pneumococcus culture is difficult and may yield false negative results. By contrast, *Staph. aureus* grows easily. Its absence from cultures of purulent sputum has a good negative predictive value if antimicrobial therapy has not been prescribed.

When a representative sputum sample cannot be obtained and when potential severity of the infection justifies an aggressive approach, we suggest that bronchofibroscopy with a protected brush be done. Recent reports suggest that quantitative culture of a small wedged bronchoalveolar lavage specimen may be more sensitive than protected brush samples. However, the clinical role of this technique is uncertain. We prefer this approach to transtracheal aspiration, which gives only a sample of central airways secretions, is not free of complications (e.g., hemorrhage), and may itself induce aspiration.

The estimated incidence of positive blood cultures in pneumococcal pneumonia is only 10 to 20 percent. Blood cultures are more frequently positive in staphylococcal pneumonia and nearly always so in hematogenous pneumonias. Because of their great specificity, blood cultures should always be obtained.

If pleural effusion is present, we perform thoracentesis to obtain cultures and to differentiate parapneumonic effusion from empyema, which is characterized by the presence of gram-positive pathogens on direct examination or positive culture, low glucose levels, and low pH (less than 7.20) corresponding to high lactic acid levels (more than 6 mmol per liter).

We do not have personal experience with antigen detection of pneumococcal capsular antigen (PCA) by countercurrent immunoelectrophoresis (CIE) or by latex agglutination (LA) of different body fluids (blood, urine, pleural fluid) or secretions. The main use for these techniques seems to be rapid diagnosis and the possibility of identifying *Str. pneumoniae* after the initiation of antimicrobial therapy. In most instances, PCA is said to be positive in the blood and urine of patients with bacteremic pneumonia and is therefore a factor of a poor prognosis. Antigenemia may be present for several days. Different authors find a good sensitivity of CIE and LA (about 80 percent) in the detection of PCA in the sputum of patients with pneumococcal pneumonia, but false-positive results exist. In the sputum of patients with chronic bronchitis, PCA frequently is found independently from eventual coexisting pneumonia. Thus, positivity of this test result has to be interpreted with caution, especially in sputum.

COMPLICATIONS

In pneumococcal pneumonia, the infectious complications, in their order of incidence, include meningitis, empyema (1 to 3.6 percent), endocarditis, arthritis, peritonitis, and pericarditis. These extrapulmonary foci develop in bacteremic pneumonia. They are unusual after the institution of antimicrobial therapy, which drastically reduces their emergence. For example, in the preantibiotic era, *Str. pneumoniae* and *Str. pyogenes* were common causes of culture-positive empyema. Now, *Staph. aureus*, gram-negative bacilli, and anaerobic bacteria are the most common.

Noninfectious complications of pneumococcal pneumonia include delayed resolution (the pneumonia may take as long as a few months to disappear), sterile effusion in 25 percent of patients, and other nonspecific problems of severely ill patients.

Staphylococcal pneumonia may evolve to cavitation and cause pulmonary abscess in 25 percent of the patients. Empyema is another frequent phenomenon (10 percent). Many extrapulmonary foci of infection, including endocarditis, meningitis, and osteomyelitis, may be encountered. A peculiar evolution of staphylococcal pneumonia is the development of pneumatoceles, thin-walled cysts that appear during the first week of evolution and are more frequent in children. They may even be responsible for respiratory distress caused by parenchymal compression. Rupture into the pleural space may cause pyopneumothorax. With antibiotics, pneumatoceles generally disappear in a few weeks.

MANAGEMENT

Antimicrobial Therapy

The usual antimicrobial therapy for *Str. pneumoniae* is penicillin. We prescribe this antibiotic as the sole therapy only when the diagnosis of the etiologic pathogen is certain or when the presumption is very high and the lower respiratory tract infection is not life-threatening. Previously healthy subjects who are mildly to moderately ill may be treated as outpatients with oral phenoxymethyl penicillin (250 mg every 6 hours). Otherwise, we prescribe intramuscular injections of procaine penicillin G (600,000 U every 12 hours). When hospitalization is necessary, we administer penicillin G intravenously (1 million U every 6 hours). Higher doses of penicillin (20 million U every 24 hours) have not shown superiority in the treatment of severe pneumococcal pneumonia. In fact, some authors have suggested that colonization with resistant pathogens, superinfection, and adverse reactions are more common with high dosages.

There are, however, two indications for high dose penicillin G (20 million units per day by infusion): extrapulmonary foci (meningitis, empyema, endocarditis, arthritis) and infection with intermediate sensitive *Str. pneumoniae*.

The emergence of strains resistant to penicillin G is a relatively new problem first described in South Africa and later found in many other countries. Resistance is not due to beta-lactamase production, but is the result of modification of the concentration and affinity of the penicillin-binding protein.

Sensitivity of *Pneumococcus* is tested in vitro by disk diffusion with 1 μg of oxacillin. If the diameter of the inhibitory zone is more than 20 mm, the organism is said to be sensitive. If it is less than 20 mm, intermediately sensitive or resistant *Str. pneumoniae* should be suspected. Laboratories that determine minimal inhibitory concentration (MIC) are able to differentiate two degrees of resistance. If MIC is higher than 1 μg per milliliter, *Pneumococcus* is resistant. If MIC is between 0.1 and 1 μg per milliliter, it is said to be of intermediate sensitivity. Resistant *Str. pneumoniae* is rare in North America, but the estimated frequency of intermediate sensitive pathogen is between 2 and 15 percent.

Pneumonia with resistant *Pneumococcus* should be feared when (1) the patient presents with a nosocomial lower respiratory tract infection, (2) he has been recently hospitalized or treated with beta-lactam antibiotics, (3) it is the second episode of pneumonia during the last year, or (4) the initial presentation is severe.

In the case of resistant *Pneumococcus*, the recommended dosage of penicillin G is 150,000 to 250,000 U per kilogram every 24 hours (and even higher in the presence of extrapulmonary foci). The problem is the degree of resistance and the site of infection. Despite a high blood level of penicillin, meningitis due to intermediately sensitive *Pneumococcus* may not respond because of low diffusion of this antibiotic in cerebrospinal fluid. Penicillin-resistant *Pneumococcus* often shows multiple antibiotic resistance. Alternative treatment should be guided by the antibiogram and, in the case of meningitis, by the diffusion of the antibiotic in cerebrospinal fluid. Considering these conditions, the antimicrobial therapy of resistant *Pneumococcus* may include chloramphenicol, ampicillin, recent generation cephalosporins, rifampin, vancomycin, or clindamycin.

In the patient who is allergic to penicillin, erythromycin is used. Other beta-lactam antibiotics also may be prescribed, but with caution because cross reaction is present in about 10 percent of the cases.

Respiratory infections caused by *Staph. aureus* are treated by penicillinase-resistant penicillin-like oxacillin. In mild cases, as in infected bronchiectasis, the oral route of medication may be used (500 mg of dicloxacillin every 6 hours). In other situations, 2 g of oxacillin is given intravenously every 4 hours.

In life-threatening lower respiratory tract infections, we recommend the addition of an aminoglycoside for the first few days (e.g., gentamicin, 5 mg per kilogram per day given in three doses) if there is no relative contraindication (dehydration, renal insufficiency, diabetes mellitus). Aminoglycosides have a high bactericidal activity against *Staph. aureus*, and tolerant strains to beta-lactam antibiotics have been described. Tolerance is defined as the dissociation of the MIC and the minimal bactericidal concentration (MBC), which in this case may be eight to 100 times higher. Although the clinical significance of this phenomenon is not yet clear, the killing rate of the antibiotic between MIC and MBC is slower and might be responsible for delayed resolution. If there are risk factors for prescription of aminoglycosides, rifampin may be added in severe infections.

In nosocomial pneumonia, methicillin-resistant *Staph. aureus* is frequently encountered. Currently, vancomycin is employed at the dose of 1 g by slow infusion (over 30 minutes) two times a day.

If the patient is allergic to penicillin, other antibiotics than oxacillin may be used according to the antibiogram, either erythromycin (1 gr every 6 hours) or clindamycin (600 mg every 6 hours). The fluoroquinolones (ciprofloxacin, ofloxacin) achieve reasonable tissue levels and have excellent antistaphylococcal activity at usual serum levels. This spectrum of activity includes methicillin-resistant strains. Ciprofloxacin, 500 mg every 8 hours, may be an excellent alternative to the agents listed above.

Infections caused by streptococci other than *Str. pneumoniae* (*Str. pyogenes* and others), are treated with high doses of penicillin G (20 million U per day). *S. faecalis* infections of the respiratory tract may be treated with ampicillin 1 g every 4 to 6 hours.

Side Effects

Not all side effects of the aforementioned antibiotics are described, but a few should be stressed. For beta-lactam antibiotics, the main problem is allergic reactions, which can be severe. We prefer to use oxacillin rather than methicillin in staphylococcal infections because allergic nephropathy is less frequent. In cases of hypersensitivity to penicillin, cross reaction with cephalosporins is seen in 10 percent of the cases. Alternative therapy in allergic patients has been discussed previously. We recommend measurement of serum concentration of aminoglycosides before and after administration of the third infusion to make sure the therapeutic range has been reached and to limit ototoxicity and renal toxicity. For gentamicin, the peak serum level after infusion should be 5 to 8 μg per milliliter in severe infections and 1.5 μg per milliliter before the next administration. Special care in monitoring these concentrations and renal function has to be taken when vancomycin, another ototoxic and nephrotoxic antibiotic, is associated. The desired serum peak level of vancomycin is 35 μg per milliliter, and the trough is 5 to 10 μg per milliliter. Pseudomembranous colitis, caused by proliferation of *Clostridium difficile* and toxin liberation, may be the result of almost any antibiotic therapy, but is frequently seen with clindamycin.

Other Therapy

The patient suffering from pneumonia is febrile, polypneic, and may be confused. Fluid administration must be sufficient to avoid dehydration. Arterial blood gases must be monitored to adjust oxygen supply (PaO_2 greater than 60 mm Hg) and to detect hypoventilation. Otherwise, acute respiratory failure requires mechanical ventilation.

One controlled trial has shown that chest physiotherapy has no place in the treatment of uncomplicated pneumonia. We reserve its use for cases associated with profuse bronchial secretions (e.g., bronchiectasis). However, we do encourage patients to cough to clear their own secretions.

If possible, antipyretic drugs should be avoided as persistent or recurrent fever is a sign of inadequate antimicrobial therapy or the emergence of complications.

Besides antibiotics, treatment of lower respiratory tract infection must include appropriate management of eventual associated empyema. First, we proceed with thoracentesis to establish the diagnosis. In mild cases, this procedure alone may be sufficient. We closely follow the chest roentgenogram, and if significant effusion reappears after the second thoracentesis, we drain the pleural space with a large chest tube. Some authors recommend irrigation and injection of lytic enzymes if the liquid is thick or multiloculated. We have no experience of such therapy. In case of failure, a surgical procedure is necessary (thoracotomy, pleural debridement, decortication).

PROGNOSIS

Despite antimicrobial therapy, the pneumococcal pneumonia mortality rate remains between 10 and 20 percent. Significantly, antibiotics, although important to reduce complications and total mortality, do not reduce early mortality. Currently, the majority of deaths occur in this period.

Different factors indicating a poor prognosis have been identified, including bacteremia (and therefore antigenemia), coexisting extrapulmonary sites of infection, infection caused by certain serotypes of *Str. pneumoniae* (type III), involvement of more than one pulmonary lobe, leukocyte count lower than 10,000 or higher than 25,000 per cubic millimeter, and a patient older than 60 years or with underlying disease.

Staphylococcal pneumonia has severe morbidity and mortality rates, especially if hospital acquired. In this setting, the pneumonia tends to infect subjects with severe underlying disease. Moreover, the emergence of methicillin-resistant strains further complicates therapy in this patient group.

PREVENTION

We recommend yearly influenza vaccination for all patients aged 65 years or older or for anyone with chronic disease (pulmonary, renal, or cardiovascular disease, diabetes mellitus). We have already said that influenza is responsible for a higher incidence of pneumococcal and staphylococcal pneumonia, which have a high rate of morbidity and mortality in chronically ill patients.

Pneumococcal vaccine contains polysaccharides of the main serotypes of *Str. pneumoniae* responsible for pneumonia (14 in 1977, 23 since 1983). It has proven efficacy among young healthy adults, but recent studies made in high risk populations failed to confirm the protection against pneumococcal pneumonia and bacteremia found in earlier studies. These conflicting data have caused controversy among physicians about the value of this vaccine. However, because pneumococcal vaccination has no important side effect, we recommend its use in high risk populations.

SUGGESTED READING

Bartlett JG, O'Keere P, Tally FP, Loviet J, et al. Bacteriology of hospital-acquired pneumonia. Arch Intern Med 1986; 146:868–871.

Musher DM, Franco M. Staphylococcal pneumonia. Chest 1981; 79:172–173.

Pallares R, Gudiol F, Linares J, Ariza J, et al. Risk factors and response to antibiotic therapy in adults with bacteremic pneumonia by penicillin-resistant pneumococci. N Engl J Med 1987; 317:18–22.

Woodhead MA, Macfarlane JT, McCracken JS, Rose DH, Finch RG. Prospective study of aetiology and outcome of pneumonia in the community. Lancet 1987; 1:671–674.

AEROBIC GRAM-NEGATIVE PNEUMONIA

GUSTAVE A. LAURENZI, M.D.
MARK S. DRAPKIN, M.D.

Aerobic gram-negative pneumonia has become a major threat in hospitalized patients. Successful treatment depends on early recognition of the problem and identification of the causative bacteria. The sputum Gram stain allows the timely administration of appropriate antibiotics, and modification of antibiotic regimens is made after culture results are available.

TYPICAL CLINICAL PROBLEM

A 65-year-old man with a history of arteriosclerotic heart disease and chronic bronchitis was admitted to the intensive care unit with severe respiratory insufficiency. He required tracheal intubation, mechanical ventilation, and blood pressure support. After 4 days, a fever developed. A right lower lobe infiltrate was identified on the chest film, and the white blood cell count rose to 16,500 per cubic millimeter with 8 percent band forms. The sputum was thick and mucopurulent. Gram stain showed many polymorphonuclear leukocytes and gram-negative bacilli. The approach to this patient's problem requires familiarity with the epidemiology, pathogenesis, and treatment of gram-negative pneumonia.

EPIDEMIOLOGY

Aerobic gram-negative pneumonias are predominantly nosocomial infections; however, *Klebsiella pneumoniae*, *Haemophilus influenzae*, and *Pseudomonas aeruginosa* continue to be important pathogens in community-acquired disease, especially in the elderly and chronically ill. Nonencapsulated strains of *Haemophilus*, which cause 5 percent of community-acquired pneumonias, are common inhabitants of the upper respiratory tracts of healthy individuals and chronically colonize the bronchi of patients with chronic bronchitis. *P. aeruginosa* may colonize the oropharynges of diabetics and alcoholics, and mucoid forms are found in the bronchial secretions of patients with fibrocystic disease. These patients are at higher risk for the development of pneumonia.

Gram-negative bacteria account for more than half the cases of hospital acquired pneumonia and for 60 percent of deaths attributable to nosocomial infections. In that setting, *Klebsiella* and *Pseudomonas* pneumonias are the most common, but a wide spectrum of gram-negative pathogens, including *Enterobacter*, *Acinetobacter*, *Serratia*, and *Proteus*, have emerged. These factors correlate directly with the high incidence of oropharyngeal colonization in severely ill patients, and local epidemiology often dictates which organisms predominate in a particular institution.

PATHOGENESIS

Bacterial colonization of the upper respiratory tract is the major source of contamination and infection of the bronchopulmonary tree because the aspiration of oropharyngeal secretions is a common and almost inevitable occurrence. However, pulmonary defenses are effective against infection, so that the normal lower respiratory tract is free of bacteria. These mechanisms break down in the damaged bronchial tree in which chronic bacterial colonization may exist.

The highest incidence of gram-negative pneumonia is found in intensive care units, where oropharyngeal colonization occurs rapidly in the severely ill patient. In addition, artificial airways, inhalation therapy equipment, and suctioning maneuvers serve to introduce organisms into the lower respiratory tract. Retrograde pharyngeal colonization by organisms from the stomach may also contribute to the pathogenesis of pneumonia, and it has been demonstrated that H_2-histamine blockade and antacids increase gastric colonization. Mechanical defenses, such as cough and gag reflexes, are depressed by altered levels of consciousness, and the cleansing action of the mucociliary stream is impaired by viscid mucus, viral infections, trauma, and the inhalation of enriched oxygen mixtures. Cellular defenses at the alveolar macrophage level are adversely affected by many of the same conditions. The spread of gram-negative organisms from intravenous lines is often responsible for hematogenous pulmonary infection. Cancer victims, burn patients, and patients receiving chemotherapeutic agents, corticosteroids, and antibiotics are at great risk. The combination of contaminated hospital surroundings, oropharyngeal colonization, and susceptible patients provides circumstances especially conducive to the opportunistic characteristics and hardy nature of gram-negative bacteria. The interplay of bacterial virulence and the immune state of the host determines the progression from inoculation to bronchopulmonary colonization and pneumonia.

CLINICAL FEATURES

Most clinical findings are not specific in differentiating gram-negative infections from other types of pneumonia. The hallmarks of pulmonary infection are common: fever, cough, sputum, chills, and chest pain. Physical findings of percussion dullness, bronchial breathing, and rales depend on the site and the extent of parenchymal involvement. Bacteremia with its serious consequences is sometimes heralded by marked tachypnea, respiratory alkalosis, and metabolic acidosis; and a fulminant course can occur with hypotension, severe respiratory insufficiency, and anuria. Radiologic patterns are nonspecific, although gram-negative infection has a predilection for the lower lobes. Patchy infiltrates are seen most often; coalescence and lobar involvement occur, and air bronchograms are the rule. The characteristic lobar consolidation with bowing fissures and abscess formation of *Klebsiella* pneumonia is worthy of mention, although it is seen much less often now than in the past. Nonhematogenous and hematogenous *Pseudomonas* pneumonia often causes multiple lower lobe nodular densities, which may cavitate, and *Escherichia coli* may show the same pattern. A difficult clinical problem is the identification of pulmonary infection in patients who show diffuse alveolar filling patterns on a chest roentgenogram.

LABORATORY EVALUATION

Leukocytosis with a shift to the left is usually present, and blood cultures may be positive in one-third to one-half of the cases. Once pneumonia is suspected, the next step is to establish the specific microbial etiology as rapidly as possible. Initially, this information is best provided by the sputum Gram stain. Cultures of sputum and blood may not give helpful data for days. Newer techniques of culturing blood, which employ the Bactec automated system or the Isolator lysis-centrifugation system, can shorten this time lag, but immediate therapeutic guidance is lacking. Pleural fluid Gram stain may be diagnostic if empyema is present. Unfortunately, information from sputum Gram stain and culture is compromised by the unavoidable contamination of expectorated sputum by secretions of the upper respiratory tract. Multiple specimens of bronchial mucus should be obtained by exaggerated cough maneuvers, and deep sputum specimens may be induced by moistened aerosols, positive pressure breathing, and endotracheal suctioning techniques. Sputum washing is not helpful in removing surface contamination. Transtracheal aspiration became a popular technique whereby the upper respiratory tract could be avoided; however, we rarely use this method because oropharyngeal organisms contaminate the respiratory tract to the level of the carina and there is significant risk of hemorrhage, subcutaneous emphysema, and airway obstruction. Needle aspiration of a pulmonary infiltrate should be avoided because of complications of hemorrhage, pneumothorax, and, rarely, air embolus. Bronchoalveolar lavage, transtracheal biopsy, and open lung biopsy are usually reserved for patients who are immunocompromised by chemotherapy or the acquired immunodeficiency syndrome.

The Gram stain should be carefully evaluated before the culture is planted. The presence of at least 25 granulocytes and the absence of more than 10 oral epithelial cells per high-dry lens field are criteria widely accepted as indicative of an adequate specimen. In most instances, if these criteria are not met, the specimen should be discarded. An exception to this rule is the granulocytopenic patient, in whom white cells may be absent. If the smear is of adequate quality, the morphology of bacteria seen under oil immersion can be invaluable in dictating initial treatment. Sometimes, despite valiant attempts, organisms are not seen on smear, but grow in abundance from multiple specimens. In our opinion, these hidden organisms probably warrant attention as long as the smear is adequate.

AEROBIC GRAM-NEGATIVE BACTERIA

K. pneumoniae is the most common pathogen in hospital-acquired gram-negative pneumonia. This large bacterium is suspected on Gram stain because of its prominent capsule, a structure that may help confer virulence. Of the species of *Klebsiella*, *K. pneumoniae* predominates, but *K. oxytoca* is also seen; *K. ozaenae* is uncommon. The characteristic settings of alcoholism, diabetes, or nursing home residence may not be present. Thick, bloody sputum is seen in about one-third of the cases.

H. influenzae is often suggested, but sometimes overlooked, on Gram stain because of its pleomorphism and wispy quality. It is usually community acquired but can emerge in the hospital, especially in patients treated with aminoglycosides. Encapsulated strains, such as type B, are important pathogens in serious pediatric infection, but they may cause pneumonia in adults as well. Nonencapsulated strains also are important potential pathogens. *H. influenzae* may cause adult febrile purulent tracheobronchitis. Sputum must be cultured on appropriate media such as chocolate agar incubated in a carbon dioxide-enhanced environment.

P. aeruginosa is well adapted to the hospital environment, especially special care units. *P. cepacia* and *P. maltophilia*, which are resistant to many of the newer antibiotic agents, emerge as nosocomial respiratory pathogens. The first intensive care patient that we treated with imipenem developed *P. cepacia* pneumonia. *P. aeruginosa* may be suggested by green-tinted sputum and long, thin organisms on Gram stain. In hematologic disorders, bacteremic *P. aeruginosa* pneumonia is more common than in other settings. Reversal of the usual diurnal fever pattern has been observed.

E. coli is a cause of hematogenous infection and of aspiration pneumonia. Gram stain shows ordinary boxy bacilli. *Acinetobacter* occasionally causes community acquired bacteremic pneumonia, but it is more commonly encountered as a nosocomial pathogen, especially in patients receiving antibiotics to which the pathogen is resistant. On Gram stain, the organism has a stubby shape and bipolar staining and resembles *Neisseria* and *Branhamella catarrhalis*.

MANAGEMENT

The effective management of gram-negative pneumonia depends on the prompt administration of appropriate antibiotic therapy. Since most patients are severely ill, supportive therapy may already be in place, but it is worthy of emphasis. The treatment of respiratory insufficiency is critical; hypoxemia should be corrected by the inhalation of safe concentrations of oxygen, and severe ventilatory failure requires assisted ventilation through an established airway. Control of bronchial secretions is essential; chest physiotherapy may facilitate drainage in patients with chronic bronchitis and bronchiectasis. Any accompanying bronchospasm can be controlled by aerosolized or intravenous bronchodilators. Other general measures include blood transfusion, blood pressure support, correction of electrolyte and metabolic imbalance, and maintenance of adequate nutrition. In the case of empyema, chest tube drainage is necessary. The use of large doses of corticosteroids to treat bacteremic shock remains controversial, but recent studies suggest no benefit.

THERAPY

General Principles

When deciding which antibiotics to employ, one must bear the following principles in mind:

1. Gram stains of sputa are immeasurably more helpful than sputum cultures. Ordering a culture and waiting for the result is not sufficient; the culture may take a few days to be finalized, and then, if not interpreted in light of the Gram stain, it may be misleading. The morphology of organisms on Gram stain may permit appropriate treatment to be started early.
2. Local epidemiology must be considered. In large teaching hospitals, gentamicin resistance may be common among gram-negative bacilli, whereas in other hospitals, gentamicin resistance may be rare. If aminoglycoside therapy is selected before complete culture data are available, amikacin should be chosen in the former setting; in the latter, gentamicin is acceptable.
3. Therapy should be broad in its coverage initially and then narrowed down. In many instances, there is no single regimen of choice, many options exist, and drug toxicity as well as efficacy must be considered. Initially, the use of one or more than one antibiotic may depend on whether the Gram stain suggests polymicrobic infection; two or more pathogens are found in half of the cases. If only one organism is present in a severely ill patient, two drugs may still be preferable.

Initial Therapy

With these principles in mind, let us return to the patient described previously and explore our therapeutic options (Tables 1, 2, and 3). The sputum Gram stain showed gram-negative bacilli. A third generation cephalosporin is a reasonable choice for initial treatment. These antibiotics have a broad spectrum of activity against gram-negative bacteria, possess improved resistance to beta-lactamase, and have relatively low toxicity. Among these agents, cefotaxime, ceftizoxime, and ceftriaxone have virtually identical spectra of activity, and the long half-life of ceftriaxone makes it particularly attractive as a once-daily agent. Ceftazidime has especially good activity against *Pseudomonas*; cefoperazone is less active than ceftazidime against gram-negative bacilli, including *Pseudomonas*, and occupies no particular therapeutic niche.

If the patient is severely ill, one of the aminoglycosides (gentamicin, tobramycin, or amikacin) is added for enhanced bactericidal activity, although a recent randomized trial suggests it may not be necessary. Gentamicin and tobramycin are virtually interchangeable; the former is much less expensive ($.10 versus $5.00 per dose in our hospital); previous reports that tobramycin is less nephrotoxic have not been confirmed. Tobramycin is more active in vitro against *P. aeruginosa*, but whether or not this translates into greater clinical efficacy against that pathogen is not known. As indicated previously, amikacin is the agent of choice if gentamicin or tobramycin resistance is common in the particular institution. With any aminoglycoside, serum drug levels must be monitored. If levels are too low (a peak of less than 7 μg per milliliter for gentamicin or tobramycin), treatment is less likely to be effective. This ineffectiveness may be a result of the drug's decreased activity at the low pH of bronchoalveolar secretions. If levels are too high, toxicity is more likely, especially if other potentially toxic agents such as vancomycin are given concurrently. In patients with renal insufficiency, a major reduction in dose or a lengthening of the interval between doses is required; we prefer the latter approach, and we aim for peak levels of 7 to 10 μg per milliliter, with trough levels of less than 2 μg per milliliter.

If Gram stain suggests mixed aspirational aerobic and anaerobic flora in addition to gram-negative bacilli, penicillin, ampicillin, or clindamycin should be added. Another approach to both gram-negative bacilli and anaerobes is to use imipenem alone. This drug is actually a thienamycin, but it is conveniently considered along with the cephalosporins. Imipenem is combined with cilastatin, which is an agent that inhibits its renal tubular degradation. The combination, Primaxin, has a broad spectrum of activity. Resistance during treatment can also appear in other pathogens. If the Gram stain suggests *Hae-*

TABLE 1 The Etiologic Agents of Aerobic Gram-Negative Pneumonia

Class	*Agents*
Enterobacteriaceae	*Escherichia coli* *Klebsiella* *Enterobacter* *Serratia* *Proteus*
Pseudo-monadaceae	*Pseudomonas aeruginosa* *P. capacia* *P. maltophilia*
Other	*Acinetobacter* *Haemophilus* *Branhamella*

TABLE 2 Approach to the Treatment of Aerobic Gram-Negative Pneumonias

Sputum Gram Stain	*Initial Action*	*Adjusted Action*
Poor specimen	Discard; try again If adequate specimen not forthcoming, treat as below	
Adequate specimen (less than 10 epithelial cells, more than 15 polymorphonuclear neutrophil leukocytes per high power field)		
Gram-negative bacilli only	Third generation cephalosporin; add aminoglycoside if patient is very ill or if *Pseudomonas* is suspected	Based on culture and sensitivity data No change if *E. coli*, *Klebsiella, proteus* If *P. aeruginosa*, two effective drugs
Gram-negative bacilli plus mixed mouth flora	As above plus penicillin, ampicillin, or clindamycin	Based on culture, but retain penicillin, ampicillin, or clindamycin

TABLE 3 Antibiotics for Gram-Negative Pneumonias

Class	*Drug*	*Daily Dosage*	*Comment*
Third generation cephalosporins	Cefotaxime Ceftriaxone Ceftizoxime	4 to 12 g 1 to 4 g 4 to 12 g	All have broad gram-negative activity, moderate gram-positive activity, low toxicity
	Ceftazidime	3 to 6 g	Added activity against *P. aeruginosa*
Aminoglycosides	Gentamicin, tobramycin Amikacin	5 to 7 mg/kg 15 mg/kg	All have broad gram-negative activity and significant toxicity
Thienamycins	Imipenem/cilastatin	1 to 4 g	Extremely broad aerobic and anaerobic spectrum
Monobactams	Aztreonam	1 to 8 g	Gram-negative activity only; low toxicity; alternative to aminoglycosides
Quinolones	Ciprofloxacin	1 to 1.5 g	Oral; broad spectrum
Antipseudomonal penicillins	Carbenicillin Ticarcillin Mezlocillin Azlocillin Piperacillin	30 to 40 g 6 to 18 g 6 to 18 g 8 to 18 g 12 to 24 g	Used with aminoglycoside; carbenicillin least desirable
Other	Trimethoprim-sulfamethoxazole	8 to 20 mg/kg (trimeth)	Fairly broad spectrum; not active against *P. aeruginosa*
	Ampicillin, sulbactam	6 to 12 g	Broad aerobic and anaerobic, not *P. aeruginosa*
	Ticarcillin, clavulanate	9 to 12 g	As above plus *P. aeruginosa*

mophilus, any second or third generation cephalosporin except cefoxitin or cefotetan may be employed. In case our patient had acquired his gram-negative pneumonia at home rather than nosocomially, a second generation cephalosporin, such as cefuroxime, which has effective activity against *Klebsiella* and *Haemophilus*, is a reasonable choice.

Adjustments in Therapy Based on Culture Data

Several days later, culture data are available. If *P. aeruginosa* is isolated, standard treatment consists of an aminoglycoside along with an antipseudomonal penicillin such as carbenicillin, ticarcillin, mezlocillin, azlocillin, or piperacillin. Of these agents, carbenicillin has the disadvantages of a lower specific activity and a high sodium content. Ceftazidime or imipenem may be substituted for the antipseudomonal penicillin, and aztreonam might replace the aminoglycoside, especially in a patient with preexisting renal insufficiency. In the event that the culture yields *Klebsiella* or *Proteus*, the initial cephalosporin can be retained. If *Serratia* or *Enterobacter* is identified, two drugs effective in vitro against the particular strain can be used. Although duration of treatment is not well defined, 10 to 14 days of antibiotics usually suffices.

Newer Approaches

Aztreonam, a monobactam, is active only against gram-negative organisms. Several studies have compared this agent with aminoglycosides in patients with well-documented gram-negative pneumonia; the results were comparable. Aztreonam may come to occupy an important place in therapy, but it is too soon to be certain. The tissue-active quinolones, of which only oral ciprofloxacin is available in the United States, are particularly promising. This agent's broad gram-negative activity, along with some effectiveness against gram-positive organisms, make it useful for follow-up treatment after parenteral therapy with other agents. Once it is available for intravenous administration, initial treatment may also prove effective. In cystic fibrosis, it appears to be effective for exacerbations associated with *Pseudomonas*, even if resistance tends to develop during treatment. Ampicillin, ticarcillin, clavulanate, and sulbactam also combine broad-spectrum aerobic and anaerobic activity. Fortunately, such resistance tends to dissipate after the drug is stopped. Trimethoprim/sulfamethoxazole has also been used to advantage in gram-negative pneumonia. Indeed, some organisms, such as *P. cepacia*, are particularly sensitive to this combination.

PROGNOSIS

Despite prompt and appropriate antibiotic treatment, mortality is as high as 50 percent. This outcome reflects as much the underlying debility of patients with gram-negative pneumonia as the severity of the infection itself. Therefore, one must be wary of reports that claim 90 percent or greater cure rates; the patients in these series probably have colonization rather than true pneumonia. In an ill, hospitalized population with pulmonary infiltrates, the adult respiratory distress syndrome or congestive heart failure can mimic pneumonia, and gram-negative bacilli may be cultured from "sputa" that are really mouth or tracheal specimens. Eradication of organisms from such patients does not represent a therapeutic triumph.

SUGGESTED READING

Lerner AM. The gram negative bacillary pneumonias. DM 1980; 27:1–56.
Levison ME, Kaye D. Pneumonia caused by gram negative bacilli: an overview. Rev Infect Dis 1985; 7(Suppl 4):S656–S665.
Macfarlane JT. Treatment of lower respiratory infections. Lancet 1987; 2:1446–1449.
Moore RD, Smith CR, Lietman PS. Association of aminoglycoside plasma levels with therapeutic outcome in gram-negative pneumonia. Am J Med 1984; 77:657–662.
Phair JP, Bassaris HP, Williams JE, Metzger E. Bacteremic pneumonia due to gram-negative bacilli. Arch Intern Med 1983; 143:2147–2151.
Pierce AK, Sanford JP. Aerobic gram-negative bacillary pneumonias. Am Rev Respir Dis 1974; 110:647–658.

ANAEROBIC BACTERIAL PLEUROPULMONARY INFECTIONS

DAVID L. LONGWORTH, M.D.
MARTIN C. McHENRY, M.D., M.S.

Over the past 15 years, numerous studies have emphasized the importance of anaerobic bacteria in lower respiratory tract infections. The major clinical syndromes of anaerobic pleuropulmonary infection include uncomplicated pneumonia, necrotizing pneumonitis, lung abscess, and empyema. The epidemiology, pathogenesis, and microbiology of these syndromes have been thoroughly elucidated. However, controversy continues regarding the need to establish a precise microbiologic diagnosis, the optimal method of specimen collection, and the choice of antimicrobial agents in the therapy of anaerobic pulmonary infections. In this chapter we briefly review the epidemiology, pathogenesis, microbiology, and clinical manifestations of these syndromes and summarize our diagnostic and therapeutic approach.

EPIDEMIOLOGY AND PATHOGENESIS

Anaerobic pleuropulmonary infections may result from aspiration of oropharyngeal secretions, contiguous spread from subdiaphragmatic abscesses, or hematogenous seeding from distant sites of infection, such as septic thrombophlebitis of the pelvic or jugular veins. By far the most common pathogenetic mechanism is aspiration. Since as many as 50 percent of normal individuals aspirate during sleep, host factors and inoculum size are of critical importance in determining whether aspiration leads to anaerobic pleuropulmonary infection. Factors that impede protection of the airway, such as obtundation, seizures, dysphagia, or neuromuscular weakness of the pharyngeal musculature, may predispose to aspiration of larger volumes of infected secretions. Focal anatomic abnormalities of the tracheobronchial tree, such as obstructing neoplasms or bronchiectasis, may serve as a nidus for infection or impair normal clearance of aspirated secretions. Gingivitis and pyorrhea have been cited as predisposing factors for anaerobic pulmonary infections. The presence of up to 10^{12} organisms per gram of tissue in the gingival crevice of patients with poor dentition provides a concentrated inoculum of organisms when aspirated. A common clinical dictum suggests that anaerobic pleuropulmonary infections rarely occur in edentulous individuals. Numerous exceptions to this observation have been reported; however, the incidence appears to be substantially lower than in patients with intact dentition.

MICROBIOLOGY

The microbiology of aspiration pneumonia, necrotizing anaerobic pneumonitis, lung abscess, and associated anaerobic empyema is similar and has been extensively studied. These are typically polymicrobial infections, and the most common isolates include *Bacteroides melaninogenicus*, peptostreptococci, and *Fusobacterium* species. On the average, two or three anaerobes are isolated per case. *Bacteroides fragilis* has been recovered in 15 to 20 percent of these infections, which is of interest because of its resistance to penicillin. The source of this organism is often unclear, since *Bacteroides fragilis* is not part of the normal oral flora. Although multiple anaerobes are usually present in these infections, aerobic organisms such as gram-negative bacilli, *Staphylococcus aureus*, or pneumococci may also be recovered in up to 40 percent of cases. Hospitalized patients and individuals who have recently received antimicrobial chemotherapy are especially likely to have mixed infections with aerobic gram-negative bacilli. These organisms can be isolated from up to two-thirds of patients with hospital acquired aspiration pneumonia.

CLINICAL MANIFESTATIONS

The clinical presentation of anaerobic pneumonitis is usually acute, and most patients present with an illness of only several days' duration. Fever, cough, and production of purulent sputum are common. In those without a history to suggest aspiration, the differential diagnosis often includes common causes of community acquired pneumonia. True rigors occur infrequently in patients with anaerobic pneumonitis, and their presence suggests more common causes of community acquired pneumonia, such as the pneumococcus. On occasion, subacute or chronic anaerobic pneumonia occurs and may be confused with pulmonary tuberculosis or bronchogenic carcinoma.

A predisposing epidemiologic factor can be identified in up to 90 percent of patients with anaerobic pneumonitis. Since aspiration of oropharyngeal secretions is the most common precipitating event, it is not surprising that anaerobic pneumonia is more common on the right side than on the left and typically occurs in those areas of the lung that are gravitationally dependent—namely, the posterior segments of the upper lobes and the superior segments of the lower lobes when aspiration occurs in the supine position, and the basilar segments of the lower lobes when aspiration occurs in the upright position. Production of putrid sputum is a helpful finding and suggests the presence of anaerobic infection. Unfortunately, it is present in only about 5 percent of patients with anaerobic pneumonitis; therefore, the absence of this finding does not exclude the diagnosis.

Necrotizing anaerobic pneumonitis, termed pulmonary gangrene in the older literature, is defined by the roentgenographic presence of multiple small cavities with diameters of less than 1 cm. Necrotizing pneumonitis most frequently results from the progression of uncomplicated anaerobic pneumonia. Although the presentation may be acute, patients more typically present with an illness of greater than 1 week's duration. Putrid sputum is produced by about 60 percent of patients, and weight loss and anemia are present in about half, reflecting the more chronic nature of the illness. Involvement of multiple lobes is more common than in uncomplicated anaerobic pneumonia and occurs in about 50 percent of cases. Necrotizing anaerobic pneumonitis must be distinguished from other causes of cavitary bacterial pneumonia such as *Staphylococcus aureus* and aerobic gram-negative bacilli.

Lung abscess is another complication of untreated anaerobic pneumonia and requires 1 to 3 weeks to develop. As in the case of necrotizing pneumonitis, patients usually present with a subacute or chronic illness. Many patients have symptoms of several weeks' duration prior to seeking medical care. Fever, cough, anemia, and weight loss are common. Putrid sputum is produced by about 50 percent of patients and is a helpful clinical clue. In patients with suspected lung abscess, the major differential diagnostic considerations usually include cavitating neoplasm, an infected emphysematous bleb, and other infectious causes of chronic cavitary pneumonias, such as tuberculosis and histoplasmosis.

Anaerobic empyema is usually seen in association with pneumonitis or lung abscess, although it may occasionally be an isolated finding in patients with subdiaphragmatic abscess. The right pleural space is involved in approximately two-thirds of cases, reflecting the propensity of aspirated secretions to drain dependently to the right lung. Fever, pleuritic chest pain, cough, and associated sputum production are common, and most patients present with an illness of greater than 1 week's duration. Purulent pleural fluid is present in about 90 percent of cases and is frequently loculated. A putrid odor is detectable in the majority and provides a compelling clinical clue to the diagnosis before definitive microbiologic data are available.

DIAGNOSIS

Establishing a microbiologic diagnosis in patients with anaerobic pleuropulmonary infections may be difficult. Expectorated sputum is an inadequate specimen for culture since contamination with oropharyngeal flora cannot be reliably distinguished from true infection. Sputum Gram stain is principally useful in patients with acute pneumonitis in whom other organisms such as pneumococcus, *Staphylococcus aureus*, *Haemophilus influenzae*, or gram-negative bacilli are in the differential diagnosis. A compelling sputum Gram stain with numerous polymorphonuclear leukocytes and a predominance of one of these other organisms may provide a useful clue to the diagnosis and aid in the selection of initial antibiotic therapy. However, sputum Gram stain may occasionally be helpful in the diagnosis of lung abscess. Gopalakrishna and Lerner have described characteristic findings on Gram-stained smears of fresh sputum in some patients with necrotizing anaerobic pneumonitis and lung abscess. These findings include numerous polymorphonuclear leukocytes, necrotic debris, and an abundance of bacteria, including gram-positive cocci, pleomorphic gram-negative bacilli, and spirochetes.

Adequate specimens for anaerobic culture include transtracheal aspirates, blood, pleural fluid, material collected via transthoracic needle aspiration or thoracotomy, and quantitative cultures obtained bronchoscopically utilizing the protected specimen brush. Blood cultures should be obtained, but are infrequently positive. In Bartlett's series of 193 patients with anaerobic pleuropulmonary infections, only five had positive blood cultures. Thoracentesis should be performed in patients with pleural effusion, since a putrid odor establishes the diagnosis of anaerobic infection and definitive microbiologic information may be obtained with appropriate cultures. It is imperative that specimens be expeditiously transported under anaerobic conditions to the microbiology laboratory and inoculated into appropriate media without delay so as to maximize the yield from culture.

The major controversy in the diagnosis of anaerobic pleuropulmonary infection relates to the necessity for and the timing of more invasive diagnostic procedures to identify responsible pathogens. Recommendations must be tailored to the individual clinical setting. Transtracheal aspiration is an acceptable means of obtaining culture material, since the trachea is sterile in about 80 percent of individuals and harbors small quantities of anaerobes in the remaining 20 percent. However, transtracheal aspiration is not without risk and should be performed only by individuals who are experienced with the procedure. Because of occasional reports of significant morbidity and mortality with transtracheal aspiration, this procedure has fallen out of favor in many centers. We do not routinely employ it and advocate other diagnostic modalities such as bronchoscopy with the protected specimen brush or transthoracic needle aspiration in individuals in whom invasive procedures are felt to be warranted.

The majority of patients encountered with anaerobic pleuropulmonary infections do not have an associated empyema or bacteremia. The risks and benefits of invasive techniques in order to obtain material for definitive microbiologic diagnosis in such individuals must be carefully weighed. In patients with uncomplicated pneumonia and a history suggestive of aspiration, we favor instituting empiric antimicrobial therapy, and we reserve sampling for those patients who fail to respond to appropriate antibiotics. In critically ill patients with community acquired pneumonia who may have anaerobic pneumonitis, but in whom the diagnosis is uncertain, we favor bronchoscopy with the protected specimen brush to obtain material for microbiologic diagnosis.

Patients presenting from the community with putrid sputum, a cavitary lesion on chest roentgenogram with an air fluid level, and a compatible clinical history and sputum Gram smear are presumptively treated for lung abscess. If the sputum is not malodorous, or if neoplasm or tuberculosis are differential diagnostic considerations, we advocate bronchoscopy for culture, cytology, and exclusion of an endobronchial lesion. Patients with anaerobic or mixed aerobic-anaerobic lung abscess usually improve clinically within 4 to 7 days after appropriate antimicrobial therapy is begun. In patients who remain febrile beyond 10 days, we consider transthoracic needle aspiration of the cavitary lesion in order to establish a microbiologic diagnosis.

Patients with community acquired necrotizing pneumonitis with a definitive or suspicious history for aspiration and a compatible sputum Gram smear are treated empirically with appropriate antibiotics. Invasive procedures are reserved for critically ill patients in whom the diagnosis is uncertain or for those who fail to respond to initial therapy.

MANAGEMENT

Anaerobic Pneumonia

The selection of antimicrobial agents for the treatment of anaerobic pleuropulmonary infections is controversial. For patients with community acquired anaerobic pneumonitis or lung abscess, several regimens have been advocated by different authorities (Table 1). These include penicillin G, clindamycin, or penicillin G combined with metronidazole. In these infections, metronidazole alone has an unacceptably high failure rate of up to 40 percent, which is most likely attributable to its marginal activity against aerobic and microaerophilic streptococci. In the therapy of uncomplicated pneumonitis, there is no good evidence to suggest that penicillin G plus metronidazole is superior to penicillin alone. Several studies in the 1960s and 1970s established the efficacy of parenteral penicillin G in the therapy of anaerobic pneumonitis and lung abscess. However, over the past 15 years up to 25 percent of anaerobes isolated from patients with these infections have been resistant to penicillin G. Clindamycin has remained highly active against these isolates and is a superior anaerobic drug in vitro. This has led some investigators to recommend clindamycin for these infections. The issue remains unsettled as to whether all penicillin-resistant isolates must be covered in these polymicrobial infections in order to achieve cure. We are aware of no recent data directly comparing the utility of penicillin G versus clindamycin in the therapy of uncomplicated or necrotizing anaerobic pneumonia. In the absence of such data, we favor penicillin G for patients with uncomplicated community acquired aspiration pneumonia or for patients with necrotizing anaerobic pneumonitis who are clinically stable. Clindamycin is reserved for

TABLE 1 Therapeutic Recommendations for Anaerobic Bacterial Pulmonary Infections

Infection	*Community Acquired*	*Hospital Acquired*	*Usual Duration of Therapy*
Uncomplicated pneumonia	Penicillin 2 million U IV q4h or clindamycin 600 mg IV q6h	Clindamycin 600 mg IV q6h plus aminoglycoside or 3rd generation cephalosporin	7 to 14 days
Necrotizing pneumonia	Penicillin 2 million U IV q4h or clindamycin 600 mg IV q6h	Clindamycin 600 mg IV q6h plus aminoglycoside or 3rd generation cephalosporin	14 to 21 days
Empyema*	Penicillin 2 million U IV q4h or clindamycin 600 mg IV q6h	Clindamycin 600 mg IV q6h plus aminoglycoside or 3rd generation cephalosporin	4 weeks
Lung Abscess	Penicillin 2 million U IV q4h or clindamycin 600 mg IV q6h followed by oral therapy	Clindamycin 600 mg IV q6h plus 3rd generation cephalosporin or aminoglycoside. Complete course with oral cephalosporin and clindamycin if possible	6 to 12 weeks

* Drainage is essential. Select clindamycin if infection originates below the diaphragm.

those who are critically ill at the time of initial presentation, who fail to respond to penicillin therapy, or who are allergic to penicillins.

Patients with hospital acquired aspiration pneumonia generally require antimicrobial drug therapy directed against both anaerobes and aerobic gram-negative bacilli. Since patients are often more ill in this setting, we prefer to give clindamycin conjointly with an aminoglycoside or third generation cephalosporin. The selection of an aminoglycoside or a third generation cephalosporin is governed by several factors, including the status of the patient's renal function, the prevalence and susceptibility patterns of various nosocomial gram-negative bacilli within the institution, and the cost. Monotherapy with the carbapenem antibiotic imipenem provides a broad spectrum of activity against anaerobes and aerobic gram-negative bacilli and is thus a potential alternative. We feel, however, that this agent should be reserved for patients with serious nosocomial infections with gram-negative bacilli resistant to cephalopsorins in whom aminoglycoside therapy is contraindicated. Hospitalized patients who aspirate and are known to be colonized with *Staphylococcus aureus* or resistant gram-negative bacilli, such as *Pseudomonas aeruginosa*, may require alternative regimens with agents active against these pathogens.

The duration of antimicrobial therapy in patients with uncomplicated anaerobic pneumonitis and necrotizing pneumonia is dictated by the clinical course. Most patients with uncomplicated anaerobic pneumonia respond to a 7- to 14-day course of parenteral therapy, whereas those with necrotizing infections usually require a 14- to 21-day course or more.

Anaerobic Lung Abscess

Several studies in the 1960s and 1970s demonstrated the utility of penicillin G in the therapy of anaerobic lung abscess, and until recently, penicillin G was considered the unequivocal drug of choice in this setting. A recent randomized prospective study published by Levison et al challenged this dogma and compared the efficacy of clindamycin versus penicillin in the treatment of lung abscess. Patients were treated with clindamycin 600 mg intravenously every 8 hours or penicillin G 1,000,000 units intravenously every 4 hours for 3 to 10 days and subsequently switched to oral therapy with these respective agents. Clindamycin recipients had a significantly higher cure rate and a shorter time to defervescence than patients who received penicillin. The authors concluded that clindamycin was the agent of choice for the treatment of anaerobic lung abscess. However, this study has been criticized for several reasons. Nearly one-third of patients were lost to follow-up, and the criteria for failure may have been too stringent. In addition, outpatient compliance was not strictly monitored.

Because of its proven track record, we advocate penicillin G for the initial treatment of anaerobic lung abscess in patients who present with a subacute illness and who are clinically stable. We reserve clindamycin for patients who are seriously ill at the time of presentation, allergic to penicillin, or who fail to respond to a 5- to 7-day course of penicillin. We administer penicillin or clindamycin intravenously to individuals at the time of presentation and continue therapy by that route for several days beyond defervescence and clinical improvement. Thereafter, the patient is continued on oral therapy, and the radiographic progress of the abscess is monitored. Therapy is continued until the abscess resolves or until a small, stable lesion remains. Since cavity closure is a slow process, most patients require 6 to 12 weeks of antibiotic therapy.

Patients with lung abscess usually become afebrile within the first week of parenteral antibiotic therapy. Failure to respond to antibiotics may be attributable to several factors, including the presence of an undrained empyema, an unrecognized pathogen such as an aerobic gram-negative bacillus, or to the presence of an obstructing endobronchial lesion that prevents adequate drainage. One should consider fiberoptic bronchoscopy to exclude airway obstruction and transthoracic needle aspiration of the cavity to obtain material for culture in patients who remain febrile after 10 days of therapy.

In the preantibiotic era, surgical drainage or resection was the mainstay in the therapy of anaerobic lung abscess. The vast majority of patients in the antibiotic era respond to conservative antimicrobial therapy alone. Surgery should be reserved for those with rapidly progressive infection, pulmonary hemorrhage, or documented neoplasm.

Anaerobic Empyema

Anaerobic empyema is not amenable to conservative antibiotic therapy, and drainage is essential for cure. Anaerobic infections of the pleural space have a propensity to form loculations. Closed tube thoracostomy is a reasonable first approach, although some patients may require open thoracotomy with rib resection or pleural decortication to effect cure. In several recent studies, up to 75 percent of patients with anaerobic empyema ultimately required an open surgical procedure for adequate drainage. The importance of early diagnosis of anaerobic empyema cannot be overemphasized. Patients with suspected lung abscess or anaerobic pneumonitis should undergo prompt diagnostic thoracentesis if a pleural effusion is present. In patients with anaerobic empyema in association with pneumonia or lung abscess, penicillin G or clindamycin is the agent of choice. If the infection is hospital acquired, coverage against aerobic gram-negative bacilli should be provided pending results of cultures. Empyemas associated with subdiaphragmatic abscesses require a regimen that covers bowel anaerobes (including *Bacteroides fragilis*) and enteric gram-negative bacilli. We favor clindamycin together with an aminoglycoside or third generation cephalosporin. Anaerobic empyema usually requires a minimum of 4 weeks of parenteral antibiotic therapy, even in the face of prompt and adequate drainage.

SUGGESTED READING

Bartlett JG. Anaerobic bacterial infections of the lung. Chest 1987; 91:901–909.

Bartlett JG, Finegold SM. Anaerobic infections of the lung and pleural space. Am Rev Respir Dis 1974; 110:56–77.

Bartlett JG, Finegold SM. Anaerobic pleuropulmonary infections. Medicine 1972; 51:413–450.

Bartlett JG, Gorbach SL, Finegold SM. The bacteriology of aspiration pneumonia. Am J Med 1974; 56:202–207.

Bartlett JG, Gorbach SL, Tally FP, Finegold SM. Bacteriology and treatment of primary lung abscess. Am Rev Respir Dis 1974; 109:510–518.

Bartlett JG, Thadepalli H, Gorbach SL, Finegold SM. Bacteriology of empyema. Lancet 1974; 1:338–340.

Finegold SM. Anaerobic pleuropulmonary infection. Chest 1990; 97:1–2.

Finegold SM, George WL, Mulligan ME. Anaerobic infections: part 1. Disease-a-Month 1985; 31:1–76.

Gopalakrishna KV, Lerner PI. Primary lung abscess: analysis of 66 cases. Cleve Clin Q 1975; 42:3–13.

Levison ME, Mangura CT, Lorber B, et al. Clindamycin compared with penicillin for the treatment of anaerobic lung abscess. Ann Intern Med 1983; 98:466–471.

NOSOCOMIAL RESPIRATORY INFECTIONS

WALDEMAR G. JOHANSON Jr., M.D.

The great majority of nosocomial respiratory infections are caused by bacteria. The principal exceptions occur in markedly immunosuppressed patients, including those with acquired immunodeficiency syndrome (AIDS). Nosocomial infections in these patients can be caused by virtually anything—bacteria, fungi, viruses, or parasites. This chapter concentrates on the treatment of bacterial infections that develop during the hospitalization of nonimmunocompromised patients.

Nosocomial infections most often develop in seriously ill patients who require invasive procedures or devices as part of their care; however, it is the serious, underlying illness that is the root cause of the infection, not the hospital environment care. This truism is often unappreciated by the lay press, resulting in articles with titles such as "Our Hospitals Are Killing Us." Nevertheless, it is important for physicians and other hospital workers to fully appreciate the various risks to which patients are exposed in the hospital and to minimize or eliminate them if at all possible. Infection by highly virulent, multiply resistant bacterial "superbugs" does occur, usually in confined outbreaks. However, most nosocomial respiratory infections are caused by much more ordinary pathogens that colonize the respiratory tracts of many hospitalized patients. The latter leads to one of the vexing problems in this area, distinguishing colonization from infection, with the presumption that one requires treatment, while the other does not.

It may be useful to consider briefly a few aspects of bacterial virulence before discussing common patient presentations. *Virulence* refers to the propensity of an organism to cause infection, which is an abnormal condition associated with host responses, tissue damage, or both. A highly virulent organism commonly produces clinically recognized infections, whereas an organism of low virulence does not. Customarily, virulence is defined in terms of normal hosts, so an organism said to be of low virulence in normal hosts may not be so when acquired by persons with impaired defenses. Similarly, a highly virulent organism is often catastrophic for individuals with impaired defenses. Bacterial pathogens that commonly cause respiratory tract infections in normal people, such as *Streptococcus pneumoniae* or *S. pyogenes*, are highly virulent in the respiratory tract. Other organisms, particularly gram-negative bacilli, that cause many nosocomial infections possess little virulence in healthy people. In nosocomial infections, the prominence of the latter organisms is due not to their virulence but to the fact that more virulent organisms are not present, usually as a result of antimicrobial therapy.

Within any particular hospital and often on particular services, certain gram-negative bacilli tend to predominate in clinical specimens. Antimicrobial susceptibilities of given species vary from hospital to hospital, often reflecting antibiotic usage patterns. It is helpful for clinicians to be informed of these patterns on a regular basis so the antibiotics for initial therapy can be selected on a rational basis.

PATIENT PRESENTATIONS

Sinusitis

Sinusitis is included here not because it is a common nosocomial infection but because it is relatively unknown by many physicians. Risk factors obviously include all those that predispose people to sinus infections when they are out of the hospital. However, tubes that traverse the nose, nasogastric suction or feeding tubes, and nasotracheal tubes place the patient at additional risk because of obstruction of the sinus orifices. In conscious patients, the typical symptoms include headache, facial pain, fever, and occasionally purulent drainage from the nose. The larger problem arises in patients with impaired levels of consciousness who cannot report localizing symptoms.

In these patients, the presentation is that of "fever of unknown origin." A part of the evaluation of such patients, especially if nasal tubes are or have been in place recently, must be a careful inspection of the nasal passages and the posterior pharynx to look for signs of infection. Presence of a purulent exudate in the nose, particularly if confined to one side, is highly suggestive of sinusitis. Confirmation can be obtained by roentgenograms or computed tomographic (CT) scan of the head in which there is a demonstration of fluid retention in a paranasal sinus. The inconvenience of performing these tests on patients in an intensive care unit is often considerable, and one can usually obtain sufficient information from a bedside roentgenogram. Causative organisms include *Haemophilus influenzae*, *S. pneumoniae*, *Staphylococcus aureus*, anaerobes, and occasionally gram-negative bacilli.

Management

Treatment must include efforts to promote sinus drainage. The offending tube should be removed or transferred to the other nostril if continued use is necessary. Decongestant nasal drops should be used; in seriously ill patients, oral agents for this purpose are generally avoided. The antibiotics selected for initial therapy should provide coverage against the organisms listed; ampicillin, cefoxitin, or sulfamethoxazole-pyrimethamine are good choices unless ampicillin-resistant *Haemophilus* is common in your area.

If clinical improvement does not occur promptly, consultation with regard to surgical drainage should be obtained. Good temporizing results usually ensue from needle drainage of an involved maxillary sinus; the need for a more definitive drainage procedure is best assessed at a later date.

Pneumonia

Clinical criteria that have reasonable accuracy for diagnosing pneumonia in other contexts do not work well in seriously ill, hospitalized patients. In these patients, new roentgenographic infiltrates may be caused by atelectasis, pulmonary embolism, or pulmonary edema. Fever may be caused by any of a variety of inflammatory conditions, as may leukocytosis. Within a few days, colonization of the oropharynx and the upper airways by pathogenic bacteria, usually gram-negative bacilli, occurs in most seriously ill patients. Small volumes of contaminated oropharyngeal secretions are aspirated into the lungs, even in the presence of a cuffed endotracheal tube. Thus, the respiratory tract secretions of hospitalized, seriously ill patients usually contain pathogenic bacteria, whether suctioned from the trachea or expectorated by the patient. Experienced clinicians attempting to diagnose whether or not pneumonia was present at the time of a patient's death during treatment of adult respiratory distress syndrome (ARDS) were wrong in 30 percent of cases, as determined by autopsy findings. This observation indicates that the diagnosis of nosocomial pneumonia requires care and judgment and is an educated guess at best.

Certain findings may be helpful. The patient's course must be considered. The discovery of new gram-negative bacilli in the sputum of someone who is improving generally should not be cause for action. On the other hand, a change in respiratory symptoms or physiology in a patient who appears to be deteriorating should arouse suspicions of pneumonia, even in the absence of new infiltrates or pathogens in the sputum. Purulence of sputum and Gram stain findings are useful; numerous polymorphonuclear neutrophil leukocytes (PMNs) and an abundant bacterial flora are likely to indicate infection, and both correlate well with quantitative cultures of the sputum. New roentgenographic infiltrates may or may not be present, but a chest film always should be obtained in a patient suspected of having a nosocomial pneumonia. A thoracentesis should be strongly considered if pleural effusion is present, especially if it was not present on previous films. Even though the results are usually negative, the finding of bacteria in smears or cultures of pleural fluid affords a precise diagnosis. Blood cultures also should be obtained, but they are positive in only 8 to 15 percent of patients with nosocomial pneumonia for reasons that are not well understood. In fact, if blood cultures are positive in a hospitalized patient with fever, new roentgenographic infiltrates, and respiratory symptoms, the most likely diagnosis is diffuse lung injury (ARDS) due to sepsis from a nonpulmonary source, not bacteremic pneumonia. Elastin fibers may be found in the sputum of patients with gram-negative bacillary pneumonias; this finding appears to be highly specific for pneumonia, although it is present in only about 50 percent of cases.

Invasive sampling techniques may be indicated if the patient's illness appears rapidly life-threatening and if noninvasive approaches have not been helpful. Fiberoptic bronchoscopy is a surprisingly safe technique for seriously ill patients. Samples should be collected with both the protected specimen brush (PSB) and bronchoalveolar lavage (BAL) techniques. Stains of the BAL specimen are useful for promptly identifying intracellular bacteria as well as other organisms and cytologic features. Recovery of more than 10^3 bacteria by PSB is highly predictive of clinically significant distal lung infection. Patients whose PSB samples contain fewer than 10^3 bacteria usually do not require antimicrobial therapy despite the presence of clinical signs that suggest lung infection. Falsely negative PSB samples occur in perhaps 10 percent of cases, especially in the presence of current antibiotic therapy, and close patient observation is required if antimicrobial therapy is withheld. However, recent data suggest that most episodes of fever, new pulmonary infiltrates, and leukocytosis among intubated, intensive care patients are not caused by bacterial pneumonia, as evidenced by improvement without administration of antibiotics. The approach outlined allows the clinician to avoid unnecessary therapy and the risks of toxicity, selection of resistant strains, and expense.

Management

The choice of initial antimicrobial agents depends on the length of the patient's hospitalization, the prior antibiotic therapy, the Gram-stain findings, and other features of the patient's illness. Pneumonias developing during the first 72 hours of hospitalization are usually caused by oropharyngeal organisms, the same ones that cause community acquired infections. Such infections are likely to arise in victims of trauma or in patients who have had a seizure, a drug overdose, or any sudden illness associated with impaired consciousness or emergency endotracheal intubation. Treatment with penicillin alone is probably sufficient for most patients. A first- or second-generation cephalosporin is suitable as well.

Most nosocomial pneumonias that develop after 72 hours or during antimicrobial therapy are due to gram-negative bacilli or staphylococci. The latter can be readily identified in smears of tracheal secretions. If *S. aureus* is suspected from the smear, treatment with nafcillin, 8 to 10 g per day intravenously, should be started. Vancomycin, 2 g per day, should be used for penicillin-allergic patients. An aminoglycoside is usually given concurrently until the culture results are known.

In most patients, initial therapy for nosocomial pneumonia should include coverage of gram-negative bacilli. Combination therapy with an aminoglycoside plus a third-generation cephalosporin such as ceftazidime or cefotaxime is a good first choice. A broad-spectrum penicillin, such as ticarcillin or azlocillin, may be substituted for the latter if *Pseudomonas* infection is suspected. Monotherapy with broad-spectrum agents such as aztreonam or imipenem has been recommended by some investigators. I prefer combination therapy. It should be recognized that the outcome of nosocomial pneumonia is strongly influenced by underlying lost factors that are difficult to quantitate. Clinical studies purporting to demonstrate greater efficacy of one regimen over another must be interpreted with this consideration in mind.

Bronchopneumonia

This is an interesting syndrome, which I believe to be fairly common. Typically, the patient has had a period of impaired consciousness or has been intubated. After seeming to do well for several days, the patient's white blood cell count rises, low-grade fever develops, and the volume of respiratory secretions increases; mental confusion is often present in older patients. Chest roentgenograms reveal either nothing or nondiagnostic prominence of interstitial markings. Sputum smears show PMNs and a mixed bacterial flora, and blood cultures are always negative. Sputum cultures usually show a multitude of organisms, often including one or more gram-negative bacilli.

This constellation of findings is caused by the aspiration of oropharyngeal secretions with a resulting bronchopneumonia. The illness is mild, at least initially, and its presence is often overlooked. Before beginning therapy, it is wise to be certain that the patient is not aspirating gastric contents, especially if nasogastric feedings are being given. Checking for glucose in secretions is generally sufficient; a positive test means aspiration, since the normal glucose concentration of secretions is low.

Management

Therapy should consist primarily of physiotherapy, bronchial toilet, and bronchodilators. Antibiotic therapy should be started promptly and continued for at least 5 to 7 days or until the patient's symptoms are improved. A reduction in the volume of secretions is a particularly good indicator of a favorable response to treatment. Failure to treat this syndrome in its early stages often results in a more seriously ill patient and in a disease that responds less well to treatment. The initial selection of antibiotics should be based on a Gram stain of respiratory secretions. In particular, look for clusters of a plump gram-negative cocci suggesting *S. aureus* or numerous small pleomorphic gram-negative organisms suggesting *Haemophilus.* Most often, multiple bacterial species are present. Coverage for *S. aureus* should be provided if that organism is present. *H. influenzae* is an important pathogen in this syndrome; treatment with ampicillin or amoxicillin, or even oral trimethoprim-sulfamethoxazole if the illness is mild, is often sufficient. The question for the clinician is whether to attempt to treat all of the organisms present. My approach is usually to treat only the more virulent organisms, coupled with physical therapy and bronchodilators, and to avoid the use of multiple antimicrobial agents unless the patient fails to respond. Third-generation cephalosporins, such as cefotaxime, or agents with enhanced anti-*Pseudomonas* activity, such as ceftazidime, are excellent single agent choices for patients in whom gram-negative bacilli predominate.

From time to time, enthusiasm arises for treatment of this condition with topical antibiotics, which are delivered into the airways by aerosol or in a liquid bolus. There is excellent evidence that the topical use of potent antibiotics in the respiratory tract promotes the emergence of drug-resistant strains; the evidence that this type of therapy is substantially better than parenteral dosing is much less impressive. Therefore, use of topical drugs should be avoided, particularly if the drug in question is one that might be used systemically, such as gentamicin.

SUGGESTED READING

Fagon JY, Chastre J, Hance AJ, et al. Detection of nosocomial lung infection in ventilated patients. Am Rev Respir Dis 1988; 138:110–116.

Haley R, Hooton T, Culver D, et al. Nosocomial infections in U.S. hospitals, 1975–1976. Estimated frequency by selected characteristics of patients. Am J Med 1981; 70:947–959.

Johanson WG Jr, Pierce AK, Sanford JP, Thomas GD. Nosocomial respiratory infections with gram-negative bacilli: Significance of colonization of the respiratory tract. Ann Intern Med 1972; 77:701–706.

Levison ME, Kaye D. Pneumonia caused by gram-negative bacilli: An overview. Rev Infect Dis 1985; 7:S656–S665.

Moore RD, Smith CR, Lietman PS. Association of aminoglycoside plasma levels with therapeutic outcome in gram-negative pneumonia. Am J Med 1984; 77:657–662.

Salata R, Lederman M, Shlaes D, et al. Diagnosis of nosocomial pneumonia in intubated, intensive care unit patients. Am Rev Respir Dis 1987; 135:426–432.

MYCOPLASMAL PULMONARY INFECTIONS

THEODORE C. EICKHOFF, M.D.

Pulmonary infection caused by *Mycoplasma pneumoniae* is the single largest component of that entity known as "primary atypical pneumonia" or, more recently, the atypical pneumonia syndrome. The term "primary atypical pneumonia" was first used in 1938 by Reimann to denote a form of pneumonia with generally mild symptoms and less toxicity and not productive of the obviously purulent sputum that characterized most bacterial pneumonias. Furthermore, it became apparent that patients with primary atypical pneumonia did not respond to sulfonamides or penicillin in the dramatic way that most patients with bacterial pneumonia responded.

The major contribution of *M. pneumoniae* infection to the atypical pneumonia syndrome was not fully defined until the early 1960s. Although it is now possible to identify most, but not all, of the organisms that cause the atypical pneumonia syndrome, the concept remains a clinically useful one in patients whose condition is less severely toxic, whose sputum is not typically purulent, and in whom the Gram stain of expectorated sputum fails to reveal bacterial pathogens. In addition to *M. pneumoniae* infection, the atypical pneumonia syndrome includes pulmonary infection caused by a rickettsial organism (Q fever); a chlamydial organism (psittacosis), viral infection (such as adenovirus or influenza virus pneumonia), and, in more recent years, *Pneumocystis carinii* pneumonia and legionnaires' disease.

None of the specific entities that comprise the atypical pneumonia syndrome are readily diagnosable by the usual techniques of examination of sputum. Consequently, the epidemiologic setting must be relied upon to suggest possible etiologies and often reveals useful clues. Thus, an atypical pneumonia in a patient whose occupation provides exposure to cattle, sheep, or goats should suggest the possibility of Q fever. Patients with pet birds at home may be at risk of psittacosis. During a major outbreak of influenza, patients with atypical pneumonia may have influenza virus pneumonia. In the hospital setting and increasingly in some communities in the United States, legionnaires' disease occurs as a community acquired atypical pneumonia and frequently is accompanied by gastrointestinal distress and/or diarrhea. In the immunocompromised host, as in patients with acquired immunodeficiency syndrome (AIDS), *P. carinii* is the major cause of the atypical pneumonia syndrome. In mycoplasmal pulmonary infection, the epidemiologic setting is not specific, and it is really the absence of other risk factors that suggests the clinical diagnosis.

Infection rates with *M. pneumoniae* are highest in school-age children, and although rates decrease substantially thereafter, they remain elevated through young adulthood and in adults through the age of 50 to 60 years. Although infection rates subside in the older adult, it is important to recognize that *M. pneumoniae* infections do occur in the elderly, albeit infrequently.

The principal recognized infection caused by *M. pneumoniae* is, of course, pneumonia. In many patients, however, its clinical expression is varied and includes bronchitis and bronchiolitis (especially in infants and older children), tracheobronchitis, pharyngitis, rhinitis, and myringitis. In fact, nonpneumonic respiratory tract infections caused by *M. pneumoniae* are believed to outnumber pneumonic infections by about 10 to 1. Nonetheless, this organism is the most common cause of pneumonia in adolescents and through adulthood and into the 50th year.

Specific etiologic diagnosis is possible, but in most patients with relatively mild disease (walking pneumonia), the benefit is probably not worth the cost. It is possible to isolate the organism from expectorated sputum, but most clinical microbiology laboratories are not equipped to do so. Furthermore, definitive identification of the organism may take several weeks. Serologic diagnosis is established by complement fixation, fluorescent antibody, indirect hemagglutination, and growth inhibition tests, which demonstrate a fourfold or greater increase in specific antibodies to *M. pneumoniae* between acute and convalescent sera. These tests are positive in the majority of patients with *M. pneumoniae* pneumonia, but the diagnosis is again retrospective in nature, since most patients have either fully recovered or are recovering from their disease by the time the diagnosis is confirmed. Contemporary techniques of genetic analysis using DNA probes are expected to provide much more rapid etiologic diagnosis in future years.

Cold agglutinin titers may be helpful, but the test is neither highly specific nor sensitive. Cold agglutinin titers of 1:128 or higher correlate well with infections caused by *M. pneumoniae*, but at least half the patients with mycoplasmal pulmonary infection may not demonstrate elevated cold agglutinin titers.

Thus, if a patient with the atypical pneumonia syndrome is suspected of having mycoplasmal pulmonary infection, the physician must rely on the clinical and epidemiologic setting to exclude or to minimize the other possible causes and manage the patient on the basis of a working clinical diagnosis.

SPECTRUM AND COMPLICATIONS

Many patients with mycoplasmal pulmonary infection never consult a physician, and only a minority become ill enough to require hospitalization. The onset of the disease is typically gradual, with headache, malaise, and fever. Headache is generally more pronounced in adults than in children. After several days, cough begins and usually becomes such a predominant complaint that its absence should make the diagnosis of *M. pneumoniae* infection highly unlikely. Typically, the cough is nonproductive, although occasional flecks of purulent material or blood may be seen. A general soreness in the substernal area is common, but frank pleuritic pain is rare. Typically, fever varies, with a temperature, between 38° and 39.5° C. Chilly sensations are common, but frank shaking chills are rare. Marked dyspnea and cyanosis are similarly rare. The disease is generally benign, and death is rare. In untreated patients the disease usually runs a course of 2 to 4 weeks, with slow, gradual improvement. Cough and roentgenographic abnormalities may persist for as long as 6 weeks. Small pleural effusions may be seen in as many as 25 percent of patients, but large pleural effusions are infrequent.

Occasionally, patients develop extensive and severe disease, accompanied by marked tachypnea, dyspnea, and hypoxemia. A few such patients develop respiratory failure, requiring intubation, ventilatory assistance, and even positive end-expiratory pressure. Infants in particular, should they acquire *M. pneumoniae* infection, are at increased risk of developing severe respiratory distress, requiring intubation and ventilatory support. In addition, patients with sickle cell disease appear to have an increased risk of developing large multilobar pneumonias and major pleural effusions with mycoplasmal pulmonary infection.

Complications of mycoplasmal pulmonary infection are relatively infrequent and include respiratory insufficiency (as previously noted), clinical relapse in as many as 10 percent of patients, maculopapular rashes, urticaria, and erythema multiforme. *M. pneumoniae* infection appears to be one of the major antecedent infections causing erythema multiforme major, or the Stevens-Johnson syndrome. Other complications include intravascular hemolysis in association with high titers of circulating cold hemagglutinins, Raynaud's phenomenon, and in rare instances, disseminated intravascular coagulation. Myocardial and pericardial involvement have been reported, and although arthralgia is a common complaint, frank arthritis is rare.

A variety of neurologic complications have been associated with mycoplasmal pulmonary infection, including meningoencephalitis, mono- or polyneuritis, transverse myelitis, and the Guillain-Barré syndrome. It has not been established whether such neurologic complications are immunologically mediated or result from direct spread of the organism to the central nervous system or possibly both.

MANAGEMENT

Antibiotics

Only two classes of drugs are known to be clinically effective in the treatment of mycoplasmal pulmonary infection: the tetracyclines and erythromycin. Clindamycin has been reported to be active against *M. pneumoniae* in vitro, but has not been found to be clinically effective. Both the tetracyclines and erythromycin act by inhibiting protein synthesis in *M. pneumoniae* and thus are primarily mycoplasmastatic in nature, rather than mycoplasmacidal. This is supported by the observation that *M. pneumoniae* can continue to be recovered from the sputum of many patients being treated with either tetracycline or erythromycin and may indeed be recoverable for several weeks after chemotherapy has been discontinued. Since mycoplasmas lack a rigid cell wall, none of the cell-wall-active antibiotics, such as the beta-lactam drugs, are effective against them.

The decision whether to treat with erythromycin or tetracycline must be made purely on clinical grounds and based on the severity of illness and similar risk-benefit considerations. Since the costs and adverse reaction risks with either drug are relatively modest, I would suggest treating any patient with significant symptomatic pneumonia in whom mycoplasmal infection was suspected.

Several clinical considerations should influence the choice of antibiotic. The tetracyclines have been proved effective in the treatment of psittacosis and Q fever, in addition to mycoplasmal infections; thus, if either psittacosis or Q fever is significant in the differential diagnosis, tetracycline obviously is the preferred drug. Because of its particular binding and staining qualities, however, it is not generally used in children under the age of 10 years.

Erythromycin, on the other hand, is known to be effective in legionnaires' disease, as well as in pneumococcal pneumonia. Thus, particularly in adults in whom legionnaires' disease cannot be confidently ruled out, or in communities in which legionnaires' disease is known to be a relatively frequent community acquired infection, or in settings in which pneumococcal pneumonia cannot confidently be ruled out, erythromycin logically is the drug of choice. All of the aforementioned considerations relative to the choice between tetracycline or erythromycin point to erythromycin as the preferred drug in most clinical settings.

The dosage of erythromycin for adults is 20 to 25 mg per kilogram per day, given in three equal doses every 8 hours; for children, the dosage is 35 to 50 mg per kilogram per day, also in three equal doses, given every 8 hours. The adult dosage should be used in children who weigh more than 25 kg. For tetracycline, the adult dosage is 15 to 30 mg per kilogram per day in four equal doses, given every 6 hours. For children, the dosage is 25 mg per kilogram per day, also in four equally divided doses given every 6 hours. The usual dosage for adults is 500 mg of erythromycin every 8 hours or 250 to 500 mg of tetracycline every 6 hours, given orally.

At the clinical level, the tetracyclines and erythromycin appear to be equally effective. Among the various erythromycin preparations available, none is documented to be superior to any other. Erythromycin estolate has been associated with infrequent hepatotoxicity, estimated to be on the order of 1 per 1,000 treatment courses, consisting of reversible cholestatic jaundice; this complication has been only rarely observed with other erythromycin preparations. Consequently, lacking any evidence of superiority of erythromycin estolate over other erythromycin preparations, it would be prudent to avoid erythromycin estolate. Similarly, no tetracycline congener has been found to be superior to tetracycline hydrochloride in treating patients with mycoplasmal pulmonary infection; if drugs other than tetracycline HCl or oxytetracycline are used (e.g., doxycycline), the dosage should be adjusted as appropriate.

Patients who are too severely ill to take medication by mouth may be safely treated with either of the intravenous preparations of erythromycin or with intravenous tetracycline; erythromycin is preferred.

Adverse reactions commonly encountered with erythromycin include gastrointestinal intolerance, occasional rashes, and rare hepatotoxicity. Similarly, adverse reactions encountered with tetracycline therapy include gastrointestinal intolerance, occasional rashes, mottling of tooth enamel, and photosensitivity. Vertigo, ataxia, nausea, and vomiting have been uniquely associated with minocycline therapy, and therefore, it is prudent to avoid the use of that drug.

Most patients begin to show some symptomatic improvement after 72 hours of therapy with either erythromycin or tetracycline. However, the clinical response is not dramatic, and the patient should not be expected to become afebrile and generally improved after 48 hours of therapy, as may often happen in treated cases of pneumococcal pneumonia. The effect of antibiotic therapy in mycoplasmal pulmonary infections consists simply of a decrease in the duration of fever, other clinical manifestations, and infiltrates on chest film, as compared with patients who are not treated or are treated with ineffective drugs.

In most patients, however, some degree of clinical improvement is apparent after 72 hours of therapy. The patient might not yet be afebrile, however, and it is not at all unusual for the roentgenographic findings to worsen somewhat, even during the first several days of antibiotic therapy.

Treatment for 7 to 10 days usually results in significant improvement. However, there is a relapse rate of 5 to 10 percent, and therapy should probably continue for 2 weeks or, in patients with extensive disease, as long as 3 weeks. As a working rule of thumb, 2 weeks of therapy appears appropriate.

Other Therapeutic Measures

The mild-to-moderate degree of hypoxemia that almost invariably is seen in patients ill enough to require hospitalization usually can be managed satisfactorily with oxygen delivered by nasal cannulae, at flow rates of 1 to 3 liters per minute. As previously indicated, however, only rarely do patients with extensive disease develop frank respiratory failure, requiring intubation, ventilatory support, and occasionally positive end-expiratory pressure as well. Fortunately, such severe illness is rarely caused by *M. pneumoniae*.

Cough or headache is sometimes so severe and incapacitating as to merit therapy with judicious amounts of codeine, 16 to 32 mg by mouth every 4 to 6 hours. There is little reason to use antipyretic drugs. In particular, external cooling should be avoided in severely ill patients who have high titers of circulating cold hemaglutinins since a hemolytic crisis may be precipitated.

SUGGESTED READING

Cassell GH, Cole BC. Mycoplasmas as agents of human disease. N Engl J Med 1981; 304:80.

Couch RB. Mycoplasma diseases. In: Mandell G, Doulas RG, Bennett JE, eds. Principles and practice of infectious diseases. 2nd ed. New York: John Wiley & Sons, 1985:1064.

Foy HM, Nolan CM, Allan ID. Epidemiologic aspects of *M. pneumoniae* disease complications: a review. Yale J Biol Med 1983; 56:469.

Lind K. Manifestations and complications of *Mycoplasma pneumoniae*: a review. Yale J Biol Med 1983; 56:461.

Reimann HA. An acute infection of the respiratory tract with atypical pneumonia. A disease entity probably caused by a filterable virus. JAMA 1938; 111:2377–2384.

LEGIONELLOSIS

LOUIS S. LIBBY, M.D., F.C.C.P.

In 1976, a devastating epidemic of pneumonia occurred in members of the Pennsylvania American Legion who were attending a state convention in Philadelphia. Within months, an etiologic agent had been identified, and in retrospect, numerous other outbreaks of febrile respiratory illness were confirmed to have been caused by this agent. The species that caused "legionnaires' disease" has been named *Legionella pneumophila* because it is truly "lung loving." Since then, many serogroups of *L. pneumophila* have been defined, and 12 other species of *Legionella* have been named. Table 1 lists the known *Legionella* species that have caused human disease.

The clinical syndromes caused by *Legionella* organisms are known as legionellosis. Legionnaires' disease refers to pneumonia caused by *L. pneumophila*. Other *Legionella* species can cause pneumonia indistinguishable from legionnaires' disease. *L. pneumophila* also has been implicated in an acute influenza-like febrile illness without pneumonia, commonly called Pontiac fever. Most of this presentation is directed at legionnaires' disease because it is the most common, serious illness caused by *Legionella*.

PATHOGENESIS

Legionella are aerobic gram-negative bacilli with fastidious growth requirements. They cannot be grown on standard bacteriologic media, but will grow on charcoal yeast extract media. These organisms only rarely are detected with standard Gram stain.

The *Legionella* species appear to be nearly ubiquitous water microorganisms and seem to grow best in stagnant, warm water. The organisms are easily isolated from lakes and ponds and are occasionally found in potable water, including drinking water and plumbing fixtures. Large buildings are more likely to harbor *Legionella* species because of the lower temperature of the hot water circulating in them.

Airborne spread of *Legionella* from environmental sources is thought to be the major means of spread. Direct inhalation of the organism appears most likely, though aspiration of colonized oral flora has not been completely eliminated as a mode of pneumonic infection. Once the organism enters the lungs, an acute inflammatory response occurs in the terminal bronchioles and in the alveoli. *Legionella* are intracellular parasites that neutralize monocytic intracellular defense mechanisms, including the alveolar macrophage. Thus cell-mediated immunity is important in control, and antibiotics that do not penetrate intracellularly are not effective.

Clearly, immunosuppressed patients are most susceptible to *Legionella* infections, especially renal transplant patients. Table 2 lists some predisposing conditions. It is rare in children, and person-to-person transmission does not occur.

TABLE 1 ***Legionella*** **Species Associated with Human Disease**

L. pneumophila
L. micdadei
L. bozemanii
L. dumoffii
L. gormanii
L. longbeachae
L. jordanis
L. wadsworthii
L. oakridgensis
L. feeleii
L. sainthelensi
L. hackeliae
L. maceachernii

CLINICAL FEATURES

Epidemiologic studies using serologic techniques suggest that mild or even asymptomatic infections are quite common. Two distinct forms of infection caused by *L. pneumophila* have been described: the highly publicized legionnaires' disease and an acute self-limited febrile illness of the upper respiratory tract called Pontiac fever. Extrapulmonary disease clearly occurs, although rarely. Pneumonias caused by species of *Legionella* other than *L. pneumophila* are essentially indistinguishable from legionnaires' disease.

Legionnaires' Disease

The most common form of legionellosis that leads to a diagnosis is *L. pneumophila* pneumonia. It can occur sporadically or in epidemics. Community acquired and nosocomial modes of infection are seen. The incubation period varies from 2 to 10 days and can be affected by concomitant antibiotic usage and level of immunosuppression. No specific clinical feature can be used to differentiate legionnaires' disease reliably from other forms of

TABLE 2 Host Factors in ***Legionella*** **Infections**

Elderly
Cigarette smokers
Chronic cardiopulmonary disease
Chronic renal failure
Diabetes mellitus
Steroids
Other medications that affect cell-mediated immunity
Alcoholism
Malignancy

pneumonia. However, a constellation of features help the clinician direct diagnostic efforts toward legionnaires' disease. These include the host factors outlined in Table 2. Additionally, a knowledge of local experience with *Legionella* infections is important. Some communities have reported 20 percent of pneumonias to be caused by *L. pneumophila*. Other areas note only 2 to 3 percent of all pneumonias to be caused by *L. pneumophila*.

Typically, the onset begins gradually over 1 to 2 days with malaise, anorexia, and lethargy. The lack of upper respiratory tract symptoms is notable. A nonproductive, mild cough appears in the early stages. Within 48 hours, chills occur along with the development of more impressive symptoms, which include dyspnea, pleuritic pain, and a more prominent cough. In one-half of the patients, the cough becomes mildly productive, and in about one-quarter of the patients, slight hemoptysis occurs. Diarrhea occurs in one-half of the patients and was originally thought to be a differentiating clinical feature. Headache is common, as are other central nervous system symptoms, including confusion and lethargy.

About 95 percent of the patients have fever, and generally, the fever is impressive. The onset of the fever is abrupt, and chills are common. Temperatures higher than 40°C are seen in nearly 50 percent of patients and are difficult to control with antipyretics. Relative bradycardia is seen in relation to the fever.

Generally, patients appear acutely ill and in a toxic condition after a few days of illness. Scattered crackles might be heard, but complete consolidative abnormalities are rarely detected early in the course of the disease.

Roentgenographically, a patchy unilateral pneumonitis is seen early. Progression to multilobar and/or bilateral consolidative involvement is common, even with prompt initiation of appropriate antibiotics. Occasionally, small pleural effusions have been seen. Rarely, documented empyemas have been reported. Cavitation occurs in a few cases and is more common in the more severely immunocompromised. In the majority of patients, roentgenographic resolution lags far behind clinical improvement. Only one-third of patients have clear chest roentgenograms within 1 month.

Leukocytosis is common and exceeds 20,000 cells per cubic millimeter in 10 percent of patients. Urinary abnormalities are common, as are abnormalities of liver function tests. Hyponatremia is the most commonly reported laboratory abnormality and is likely caused by inappropriate secretion of the antidiuretic hormone. It is significantly more common in legionnaires' disease than other pneumonias but is not diagnostic. Hypophosphatemia is also common, though also nonspecific. Hypoxemia is common and can be associated with hypocarbia or hypercarbia, depending on the presence of underlying lung disease.

Numerous associated conditions have been seen with legionnaires' disease, including pericarditis, myocarditis, encephalitis, rash, pleuritis, renal failure, rhabdomyolysis, and bronchospasm. The exact pathogenesis is not known, and *Legionella* organisms are not usually found in these tissues.

Pneumonia Caused by Other Legionella Species

Much less is known about these organisms and their associated diseases than is known about *L. pneumophila*. It is assumed that infection occurs by direct inhalation of contaminated aerosols, presumably from water sources. No information is available about incubation periods, partly because these organisms cause nosocomial infections in a sporadic manner.

The clinical presentations of pneumonia caused by these agents appear to be indistinguishable from legionnaires' disease. It appears that hospital environments are the common source of these infections, they occur sporadically, and underlying chronic illness or immunosuppression is required for the infection to occur. Laboratory and roentgenographic abnormalities are similar to those of legionnaires' disease.

Pontiac Fever

Pontiac fever is an acute, self-limited febrile illness, which is named for an epidemic of an influenza-like illness that occurred in employees and visitors in a health department building in Pontiac, Michigan. It is characterized by fever, chills, myalgias, and headache, which develop rapidly over 6 to 12 hours. Some patients also develop a mild dry cough, sore throat, or coryza. Vague neurologic symptoms, including dizziness, photophobia, and confusion are also commonly seen. Body temperature of 39 to 40° C is common, but generally there are no other significant physical findings. Routine laboratory tests and chest roentgenograms are normal.

Pontiac fever usually lasts for 3 to 5 days, and antibiotics do not seem to affect the course of the illness. When an outbreak occurs, the diagnosis is usually confirmed serologically. Although most reported cases have been epidemic in nature, it is likely that sporadic cases do occur but are difficult to distinguish from influenza and influenza-like illnesses. Hot tubs and whirlpools have been reported to be common environmental sources, and such exposure might provide an important clue to the diagnosis.

DIFFERENTIAL DIAGNOSIS

Pneumonia caused by *Legionella* can be difficult to diagnose. The clinical presentation overlaps with other pneumonias, which are usually called atypical pneumonias. These pneumonias are characterized by a cough and scant sputum production that is devoid of a prominent organism on a Gram stain examination. The common atypical pneumonias include mycoplasmal pneumonia, psittacosis, and Q fever as well as *Legionella* infection. Diagnosis is suspected best by the presence of certain risks and generally is confirmed serologically. Table 3 defines populations at risk for each atypical pneumonia, the mode of infection, and the means of laboratory diagnosis. *Legionella* infection should be suspected during known outbreaks. It should also be suspected when multisystem abnormalities are seen with a pneumonia that appears to

TABLE 3 Atypical Pneumonias

Pneumonia	*Cause*	*Population at Risk*	*Transmission of Infection*	*Laboratory Diagnosis*
Mycoplasma	*Mycoplasma pneumoniae*	Children and young adults	Person to person	DNA probe Serology
Psittacosis	*Chlamydia psittaci*	Bird handlers	Bird contact	Serology
Q fever	*Coxiella burnetti*	Farmers, livestock handlers	Dust inhalation	Serology
Legionnaires' disease	*Legionella*	Older people with chronic disease	Airborne from water	See text

be resistant to beta-lactam antibiotics and to aminoglycosides.

Certain *Legionella* infections can overlap with common community acquired pneumonias and nosocomial infections. Sputum Gram stain can help point toward these bacterial pneumonias, but a subgroup have scanty or no sputum production in spite of the standard bacterial origin. *Legionella* infections also have been documented to coexist with other pyogenic organisms. A poor clinical response to appropriate antibiotics should raise the clinician's suspicion for this unusual occurrence.

Pulmonary emboli with infarction can also simulate *Legionella* pneumonia. The hypoxia, pleurisy, and bloody sputum can all lead to consideration of a pulmonary embolic phenomenon. In addition, the host factors predisposing to *Legionella* pneumonia overlap with risk factors for thromboemboli. The prodrome of malaise, anorexia, and lethargy seen in *Legionella* infections is uncommon in pulmonary thromboemboli, and fever is usually higher with *Legionella* infections than it is with thromboemboli.

DIAGNOSIS

The diagnosis of *Legionella* infections remains difficult in spite of the many tests that are now available. Usually, multiple methods are used in combination to make the diagnosis. Table 4 reviews the available methods, the various advantages and disadvantages, and the costs of diagnostic tests.

Cultures are now mandatory in the evaluation of suspected *Legionella* infections and appear to be both the most sensitive and the most specific means of confirming

TABLE 4 Diagnostic Methods for *Legionella*

Method	*Advantages*	*Disadvantages*	*Cost**
Culture	Gold standard with high specificity (100%), high sensitivity (80%) Good for all species and serogroups	Need special media Takes 2 to 7 days Negative test does not exclude the diagnosis	$70
Direct fluorescent antibody	Rapidly performed (1 to 3 hrs)	Sensitivity only about 60 to 80% Need different antibody for each serogroup, species	$35
Serologic testing	Epidemiologic testing Need blood only	Takes weeks for paired serum samples Not helpful with initial diagnosis Lower specificity	$60
DNA probe	Rapidly performed (3 to 4 hrs) High specificity	Limited clinical experience	$50
Urine antigen detection	Easy to collect Rapidly performed (3 to 4 hrs)	Limited clinical experience May detect remote infection (i.e. false positive)	Not available

* Cost based on published material at single community hospital.

Legionella infection. However, cultures can take 2 to 7 days to become positive, and a negative test does not fully exclude the diagnosis.

Gram stain of clinical specimens very rarely detects *Legionella*. A direct immunofluorescent examination of clinical specimens is now available and can be rapidly performed in most clinical laboratories. Unfortunately, a different antibody must be used for each serogroup, which makes sensitivity less than optimal.

Serologic testing of paired samples of serum is probably still the most common means of confirming *Legionella* infections. Unfortunately it can take 3 to 6 weeks to see the four-fold rise in antibody titer required to make the diagnosis. A single titer of greater than 1:256 is compatible with *Legionella* infection, but is quite uncommon. Occasional cross reactions with other bacteria have been reported, which leads to false positive testing. In spite of that, antibody detection is vital in epidemiologic testing and in confirming the possibility of *Legionella* infections in local communities.

The most exciting and potentially revolutionary test for *Legionella* is the new deoxyribonucleic acid (DNA) probe test. This test depends on the known specificity of the DNA sequence of each bacterial species. A *Legionella*-specific radiolabeled single-stranded DNA is used to probe respiratory secretions (including expectorated sputum) for complementary ribosomal ribonucleic acid (RNA). Detection can be confirmed within hours. A positive test is highly specific and likely has a sensitivity of approximately 80 percent. This test is now commercially available, and further clinical evaluation should be available soon.

Tests for soluble antigen of *Legionella* in the urine are now becoming available. This test generally can be performed rapidly and is quite specific. Rare false positives have been reported, and prolonged antigen excretion has been reported after a remote infection. This potentially negates the diagnostic value of this rapidly performed test. Sensitivity appears to be approximately 75 to 80 percent.

In my experience, respiratory tract secretions are best evaluated by culture and by DNA probe, if available, or by direct immunofluorescent testing if the DNA probe is not available. Serologic testing is reserved for epidemiologic purposes, primarily to know whether *Legionella* is a problem in the local community.

When faced with a patient with pneumonia, *Legionella* infection is just one of many possibilities. Given the myriad of tests available, the most reasonable approach is usually based on the clinical setting. Specifically, whether the pneumonia is community acquired or nosocomial is important, as are the patient's age and the presence of underlying illnesses. I favor initial cultures of blood, Gram stain analysis of expectorated sputum, and empiric antibiotics for most patients based on initial sputum analysis. Seriously ill patients and patients who deteriorate in spite of appropriate initial therapy require further aggressive investigation. In these settings, flexible fiberoptic bronchoscopy is valuable in order to evaluate airway protection and patency and to obtain optimal respiratory tract secretions. Bronchoalveolar lavage, triple lumen plugged brushes, and if necessary, transbronchial biopsies can be obtained to clarify the etiology of a serious pneumonia or a pneumonia not responding to initial empiric treatment. Samples must be obtained carefully, and contamination with lidocaine, which can inhibit growth of some microorganisms, must be avoided. Some investigators have suggested that transtracheal aspirates offer major advantages in diagnosing *Legionella* infections. My experience suggests that bronchoscopy can be equally effective in obtaining respiratory tract secretions and offers other advantages in regard to other difficult-to-diagnose pulmonary infections.

MANAGEMENT

Treatment of pneumonia caused by *Legionella* species starts with general supportive measures. These include oxygen, intravenous fluids when necessary, antipyretics, and occasionally, nutritional support. Corticosteroids and other immunosuppressives should be withheld, if at all possible, or certainly reduced to the lowest possible dose to control the underlying disease process.

Erythromycin is the antimicrobial agent of choice for the treatment of *Legionella* infections. The initial epidemiologic investigation of the Philadelphia outbreak suggested erythromycin's effectiveness, and clinical studies and experience have repeatedly confirmed this. Mild illness with no respiratory compromise can be treated with oral erythromycin, 500 mg four times daily for 2 weeks. Moderately serious infections, especially when associated with respiratory compromise, are best treated with intravenous erythromycin, 750 to 1,000 mg every 6 hours. Intravenous therapy usually should be used for 1 week or until the patient has been afebrile for 48 hours. Completion of a 2- to 3-week course with oral erythromycin, 500 mg four times a day, is then indicated. Relapses occur infrequently, generally respond to erythromycin, and probably can be prevented by using a full 3-week course of treatment for patients with serious infections and those who are immunosuppressed.

Doxycycline and other tetracyclines are advocated by some as an alternative treatment, but failures appear to be more frequent than with erythromycin. Thus, tetracyclines should be reserved for the rare patient who has well-documented erythromycin allergies. Experimental infections in animal models appear to be successfully treated with erythromycin, doxycycline, trimethoprim-sulfamethoxazole, and rifampin. Additionally, the new quinolone derivative ciprofloxacin also appears effective in experimental *L. pneumophila* infections. Limited data suggest the new carbapenem beta-lactam antibiotic imipenem also is effective. Treatment with these newer agents must be considered experimental and should not be used until more extensive clinical trials are reported. A common characteristic that appears necessary for successful treatment is the ability of an antibiotic to penetrate alveolar macrophages.

Limited data and some clinical experience support the addition of rifampin to intravenous erythromycin when patients are critically ill or do not respond to erythromycin in the first 96 hours. This may be especially important in patients who are significantly immunosuppressed.

Most patients respond to treatment within 2 to 3 days, but a significant minority may continue to have fever for up to a week. As discussed previously, the chest roentgenogram may show significant deterioration even though the patient is clinically improving, and it may not clear completely for 6 weeks. Pulmonary fibrosis develops in some patients as a result of *Legionella* infections. This appears to be relatively uncommon and usually occurs in the setting of severe infections. Bronchiolitis also has been reported.

The original Philadelphia outbreak of *Legionella* pneumonia had a mortality of 16 percent. Most outbreaks reported since then have had a similar mortality. Immunosuppressed patients who are not treated with erythromycin have a mortality of 80 percent, whereas appropriately treated non-immunocompromised patients have a low mortality of approximately 5 percent.

Cases of Pontiac fever generally have been diagnosed retrospectively and do not require antibiotics for successful cure. Antibiotics do not appear to affect the course of the illness.

Pneumonia caused by species other than *L. pneumophila* usually respond to erythromycin, although the prognosis appears less favorable than with legionnaires' disease. Most patients with these infections are immunocompromised, and most infections appear to be hospital acquired. These two factors certainly contribute to the occasional failures of appropriate treatment and the high mortality reported.

Prevention of *Legionella* infections is dependent on identifying environmental depositories. When a local outbreak occurs, water supplies are the most likely source. Hyperchlorination of contaminated water supplies or keeping the water temperature above 60°C can eradicate *Legionella* species. Vaccines may be developed in the future and might be useful for immunocompromised hosts in susceptible environments.

SUGGESTED READING

Edelstein PH, Meyer RD. Legionnaires' disease: a review. Chest 1984; 85:114–120.

Fraser DW, Tsai TR, Orenstein W, Parkin WE, et al. Legionnaires' disease: description of an epidemic of pneumonia. N Engl J Med 1977; 297:1189–1197.

McDade JE, Shepard CC, Fraser DW, Tsai TR, et al. Legionnaires' disease: isolation of a bacterium and demonstration of its role in other respiratory disease. N Engl J Med 1977; 297:1197–1203.

Yu VL, Kroboth FJ, Shonnard JW, Brown A, et al. Legionnaires' disease: new clinical perspective from a prospective pneumonia study. Am J Med 1982; 73:357–361.

Zuravleff JJ, Yu VL, Shonnard JW, Davis BK, et al. Diagnosis of legionnaires' disease. JAMA 1983; 250:1981–1985.

VIRAL RESPIRATORY INFECTIONS

ROLAND A. LEVANDOWSKI, M.D.
MARY RUBENIS, B.S.
GEORGE G. JACKSON, M.D.

Viral respiratory infections are caused by many different viruses, each of which can produce a variety of clinical syndromes that overlap in clinical manifestations from one viral cause to another. Each infection is further modified by the age, constitution, and prior experience of the host. With so many variables affecting the resultant clinical illness, the diagnosis, evaluation, and treatment of viral respiratory infections are resolved by different means for different purposes depending on the epidemiology, the anatomic site of the major symptoms, and the detection of the specific viral etiology. Each of these approaches provides understanding of a part of the clinical problems, the likely cause, the possible treatment, and the expected course of the disease. Only identification of the virus permits an accurate etiologic diagnosis and offers the possibility of specific antiviral therapy. Other treatments, including most of those in common practice, are nonspecific and consist mostly of symptomatic and supportive care.

SEASONAL EPIDEMIOLOGY OF RESPIRATORY VIRUSES

The epidemiologic patterns of occurrence of the different taxonomic groups of viruses that cause most of the acute clinical illnesses have contributed to the factual biology of the viruses. The seasonality of occurrence tends to be consistent, and the prevalence of infection may be endemic (parainfluenza 3) or epidemic with twice yearly (rhinoviruses), annual (respiratory syncytial virus, influenza A), biannual (parainfluenza 1, 2), or sporadic (influenza B, pandemic influenza A) episodes of occurrence. In the northern temperate climates, the season in which most of the viral respiratory disease occurs is from September to May. The biology of the viruses regulates this pattern to some degree, but it is augmented to a large extent by climatologic and sociologic modalities.

The respiratory disease season starts with an epidemic

of acute rhinovirus infections from September through November. In the beginning, the etiology of the outbreak may be pure, but in October and November, the epidemic spread of parainfluenza viruses type 1 or 2 occurs with an increase in the baseline occurrence of parainfluenza type 3. Annually, a sharp outbreak of respiratory syncytial virus (RSV) infections occurs alternately in the fall and in the spring. This mixed group of respiratory viruses continues to cause infections through the early winter months.

Rhinovirus infections almost disappear after the occurrence of severe cold weather, and influenza viruses make a sharply inserted midwinter appearance, with some displacement of the paramyxoviruses. The peak of epidemic influenza may occur any time between early December and late February and affects school children, parents, working adults, and shut-ins, sometimes in discernible successive waves. About 80 percent of the time, the epidemic strain is influenza A; on average, once in 5 years, the cause is influenza B. A continual drift in the surface antigens, hemagglutinin (HA) and neuraminidase (NA), characterizes influenza viruses. Pandemics tend to occur in 10- to 15-year cycles, based on the emergence of a strain with a major antigenic shift; the last major antigenic shift in influenza A virus was H_3N_2 in 1968. In the years when RSV does not appear in November, the epidemic occurs in the following February. These myxoviruses (influenza A and B) and paramyxoviruses (parainfluenza and RSV) continue to cause sporadic infections into the spring.

By March or April, influenza has disappeared, and in April or May, a second wave of rhinovirus infections occurs. Infectious summer colds are usually caused by a rhinovirus or parainfluenza 3. Adenoviruses types 3, 4, 7, 14, and 21 cause up to 5 percent of acute respiratory infections in civilian populations. During the summer these infections may be asymptomatic. Occasional outbreaks of adenoviral disease occur in school dormitories. In military recruit camps, adenovirus infections become endemic, infect almost all recruits, and account for a large amount of acute respiratory disease.

Some types of Coxsackie A and B and ECHO viruses cause respiratory infections, usually in the summer months. Coronaviruses and influenza C can be related to outbreaks of common colds in the winter. Reoviruses and perhaps several other viruses cause asymptomatic infections of the respiratory tract. Herpesviruses are commonly recovered from respiratory secretions during an acute infection, but they are not considered to be primary in the cause of disease other than ulcerative stomatitis. Viral respiratory infections with systemic manifestations, such as Epstein-Barr virus (EBV), measles, varicella, and others, replicate in the mucosal cells of the respiratory tract and cause local as well as systemic symptoms. They can be clinically differentiated from the common causes of acute respiratory infections. Mycoplasmal pneumonia must be differentiated from pneumonia of viral origin, and *Chlamydia* can cause bronchiolitis of newborns resembling viral infections.

SYNDROMES BY ANATOMIC SITES

The anatomic site of the main symptoms of infection has a correlation with the viral etiology, but the site of infection does not permit a reliable etiologic diagnosis. The exception is that during an epidemic in which the viral cause has been demonstrated, the clinical diagnosis can be specific with about 70 percent accuracy. The clinical description of common infections is divided into categoric anatomic diagnoses as upper respiratory tract infection, including the common cold with coryza and nasopharyngitis, acute laryngitis (croup), bronchitis or bronchiolitis, pneumonia, and febrile respiratory disease with respiratory and systemic symptoms (flu). The relation of these syndromes to the most common respiratory viruses is illustrated in Figure 1. Each syndrome represents an acute infection with a short incubation period of 1 to 3 days. During this time and preceding the onset of symptoms, infectious virus can be found in the respiratory tract secretions. With influenza, viremia may occur, but it is of short duration and usually disappears before the abrupt onset of clinical disease.

The virus replicates in permissive cells of the respiratory tract and involves an increasing area of the airway. The difference in temperature between the anterior nares (33 °C) and the distal bronchioles (37 °C), and perhaps also the density and the histologic arrangement of virus-susceptible cells, influence the locality in which viral replication occurs most rapidly and achieves the highest titers. The amount of virus collected in washings of respiratory secretions usually is between 10^2 and 10^5 tissue culture infectious doses. In the normal respiratory tract, the secretions contain no plasma proteins except albumin and no cellular or humoral products of inflammation. In the initial asymptomatic phase of infection, serum globulins begin to appear in the secretions followed transiently by polymorphonuclear leukocytes, and then with increasing symptoms, all components of the serum, lymphocytes, interferon, secretory mucus, antibody, and other immunoreactive products appear along with exfoliated cells of the respiratory mucosa. Sometimes, especially with influenza, there is hemorrhagic denudation at the site of infection. The time relation of some of these events, as observed in influenza in volunteers, is shown in Figure 2.

In the peripheral blood there is transient lymphopenia with specific reduction of T-helper cells. In influenza and perhaps other respiratory viral infections, a reversal of cell-mediated delayed dermal hypersensitivity occurs. The cause and effect relation between the symptoms and the sequence of virologic and immunologic manifestation is not entirely clear. The replication of virus that initiates the process is initially asymptomatic, and the virus titer, although usually related to the severity of disease, does not uniformly parallel the symptomatology. Interferon is delayed in appearance following the onset of symptoms and declines following the decrease of symptoms. From these temporal relations, its production could cause, reflect, or ameliorate the symptoms. Clinical improvement has almost always occurred before a demonstrable

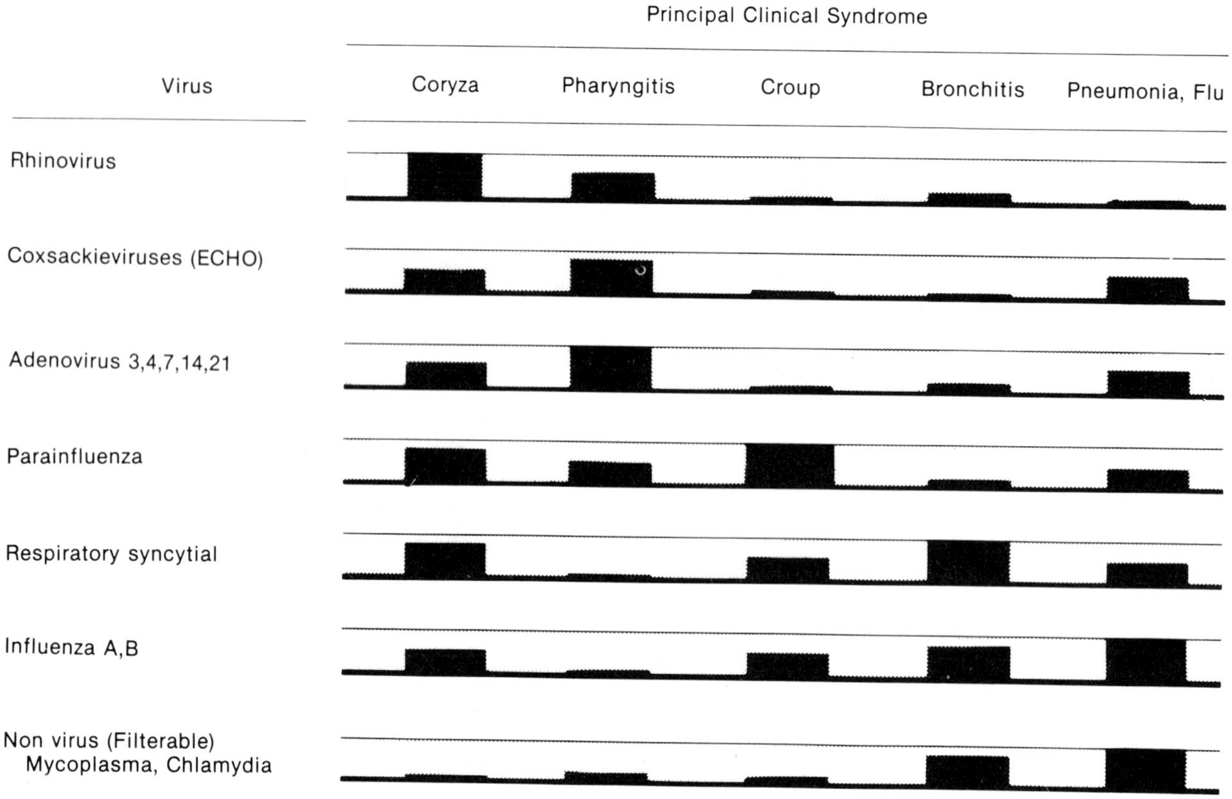

Figure 1 Schematic representation of the relative frequency of different clinical manifestations of respiratory infection with particular viruses.

rise of antibody in the secretions or in the serum. The antibody in the secretions may be secretory IgA, IgM, or IgG. The appearance of antibody is correlated with the termination of virus shedding.

Laryngeal stridor (croup) and bronchiolitis are dangerous pathophysiologic consequences of infection with parainfluenza viruses 1 and 2 and RSV, respectively. Respiratory insufficiency and pneumonia of viral and/or bacterial cause complicate influenza. Infection with parainfluenza 3 is a common cause of "walking pneumonia." Although rhinoviruses infrequently cause systemic manifestations, they can provoke asthma and produce altered ciliary function of the lower respiratory tree. The latter is most disturbed in influenza. The nature and effect of the disruption in the numbers and functions of immunoreactive cells that occurs during the acute viral infection is still mostly in the descriptive phase of investigation. The early changes may be pathogenic in producing symptoms, and the later changes may be components of the curative immune response. What relation, if any, the immune responses have to the apparent increased susceptibility to bacterial infections in the convalescent phase is unknown. If the transient acquired immune insufficiency persists into the convalescent period, reactivation of latent infections (e.g., herpes and tuberculosis) can be observed in some persons.

DIAGNOSIS

Most of the viral respiratory infections cause only a brief period of acute morbidity with a benign outcome. Thus, the justification for more than a categoric diagnosis and nonspecific symptomatic treatment, except for influenza and RSV, has not been compelling or cost effective. Heretofore, the specific viral diagnosis has been made mostly for research and epidemiologic purposes. Surveillance of influenza is done by the United States Public Health Service and the World Health Organization. Different research groups have provided data about the prevalence and the specific etiology of some of the other types of respiratory infections. Now, the increasing availability of virology laboratories, the accomplishment of a rather complete classification of the respiratory viruses, the standardization and simplification of viral diagnostic methods, and the development of useful virus-specific antiviral drugs all promise increasing need and application of rapid specific viral diagnosis of patients with acute viral respiratory infections.

Classically, specific diagnosis is made by recovery of the virus from respiratory secretions in tissue cultures or in embryonated eggs and demonstration of a fourfold or greater rise in the titer of specific antibody in the convalescent phase serum. Virus isolation permits characteri-

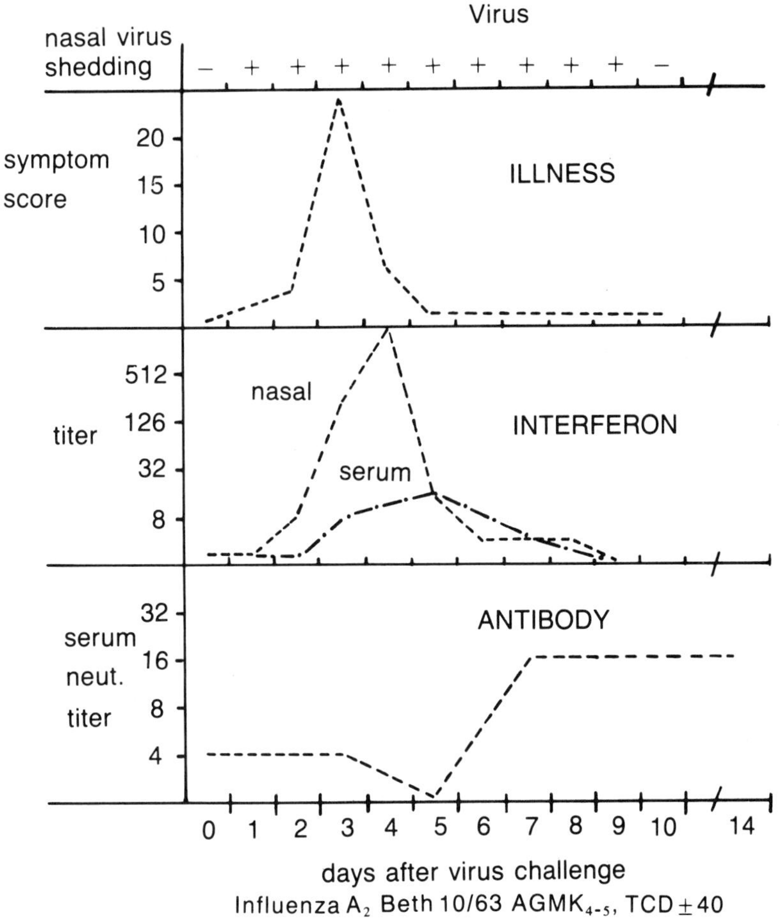

Figure 2 Characteristics of viral respiratory infection in volunteers.

zation of the strain, including recognition of antigenic drift and drug resistance. Therefore, it remains the fundamental standard for an etiologic diagnosis. However, classic virologic and serologic methods do not satisfy the clinical need for rapid diagnosis with a high level of sensitivity as well as selectivity. To satisfy the need for rapid specific diagnosis, methods using the technology of fluorescent antibody, biotin-avidin conjugation of specific antisera, and enzyme-linked immunoabsorbent antigen-antibody reactions are being developed and are available for RSV and influenza. In addition to early detection, these methods approach the sensitivity of virus isolation with high specificity. Methods that further increase the sensitivity of antigen detection are desirable and necessary for early diagnosis in one-third of the patients. Hybridization blots using labeled specific probes and kinetic assays for enzyme-specific products have the promise of meeting this need. Whether or not we will see wide application of molecular diagnostic technology for the rapid specific viral diagnosis of respiratory viruses will depend on the cost and utility of the information gained and on the capability for specific treatment.

MANAGEMENT

Nonspecific Treatment

Most of the experience with the treatment of viral respiratory infections is nonspecific, testimonial, uncontrolled, and, in a scientific sense, unevaluable—partly because of the nature of the problem. The variability in the number and virulence of the viruses, the sites and pathologic manifestations of different syndromes, and the effects of specific host modification make trials of therapeutic measures difficult and rife with artifacts as the basis for conclusion. The only animal model for controlled therapeutic studies that has been useful is for influenza. Proper moral, ethical, and economic considerations prevent many controlled observations in humans. It is also difficult to disprove treatment regimens that are ineffective. In this milieu there is much room for opinion and individual experience that is meaningful in limited application, but much effort has gone into the proclamation of ideas or products with inconclusive data and of doubtful value with the hope of fame or profit. Topical inactivators of viruses (e.g., treated tissues, sprays), products for increased host resistance (e.g., vitamins, including ascorbic acid), various host remedial measures (e.g., antihistamines and minerals), and symptomatic remedies (e.g., aspirin, decongestants, mucolytics, secretion inhibitors, antitussive agents, expectorants) have been developed or recommended and may be applicable at particular times for special persons and specific symptoms, but they are without any general value in the prevention and management of viral respiratory infections. Zinc gluconate, specific amino acids, and other substances are sometimes claimed by faddists to have an antiviral effect. Even if this is true, they have no clinical value. The short benign course of most of these illnesses requires absolute assurance that the treatment will "do no harm." In spite of the difficult constraints on the treatment of viral respiratory infections and the unavailability or deficient use of immunoprophylaxis (for influenza), the prevalence of the infections in all ages and classes of people and their severity with life-threatening or fatal effects in some demand a continued effort for improved specific management. The increasing availability of selective, safe, and effective prophylactic and treatment measures marks progress in this direction with a promise of increasing success.

Supportive Treatment

Recognizing the need for and maintaining an adequate patent airway and minimizing anoxia are the paramount objectives of nonspecific treatment of acute viral respiratory infections. In infants and children, the problem is far greater than in adults. The physician must be alert to the potential need and prepare for intubation or tracheotomy to bypass laryngeal obstruction and to decrease dead space in the airway. Specific measures for other pathophysiologic manifestations, such as excessive fever and dehydration, may be necessary, and attention to supportive measures to provide rest and promote the comfort of the patient is desirable. High humidity created by a cold water vaporizer has generally been considered useful in decreasing laryngeal spasm and in liquefying secretions in croup.

Specific Treatment

The control and management of specific viral respiratory infections should be considered in terms of immunoprophylaxis, chemoprophylaxis, and therapy.

Immunoprophylaxis for Influenza

Inactivated influenza virus vaccine is effective in preventing the currently circulating strains of influenza A, H_1N_1, H_3N_2, and influenza B. After 17 years without a major antigenic shift in the H_3 hemagglutinin and 28 years for the N_2 neuraminidase of influenza A viruses, most persons have been exposed to these antigens. Influenza A, H_1N_1 was prevalent prior to 1957 and then reappeared in 1977. People over 25 years of age had a prior primary exposure, but in younger persons who have not been vaccinated or have not had the natural infection since 1977, successive primary and booster doses of the vaccine are indicated. Annual immunization is recommended to produce a booster response and heighten protection. The vaccines can be used with a high degree of confidence that they will be at least 70 percent effective in preventing influenza of the present types.

The formulation of the vaccine is reviewed annually, and changes are made to match the antigenic character of the prevalent strains. Inactivated trivalent vaccines contain 15 μg of each of three hemagglutinin antigens, H_1, H_3, and B per 0.5-ml dose. A single subcutaneous or intramuscular dose elicits an adequate antibody response in 90 percent of vaccine recipients. Intradermal injection of 0.1 ml has sometimes been used as a booster, but it has no advantages and some drawbacks. The present inactivated vaccines have limitations imposed by (1) the number and amount of antigens that can be included without eliciting an unacceptable reaction and (2) the short duration of a strain-specific response. The character of the antibody elicited is affected by the prior immunologic experience of the person vaccinated. These conditions require annual or nearly annual reimmunization. Attenuated live virus vaccines have been developed and are expected to bring about a broader longer-lasting response, easy modification of the antigens, and acceptable reimmunization, but they are not approved for widespread use. The purity of the present vaccines has greatly diminished the occurrence of adverse local and systemic reactions. With the recommended dose, only 10 to 15 percent of recipients have a noticeable local reaction, and about 1 percent of adults have fever and systemic symptoms. For children who are more prone to significant febrile reactions, split-hemagglutinin vaccine is recommended. The Guillain-Barré syndrome, which may have been associated with the swine flu antigen, has not been associated with the vaccine preparations used since 1976 and is not considered to be a risk with currently recommended vaccines. The vaccines are prepared from viruses grown in embryonated eggs,and a high degree of hypersensitivity to eggs is a contraindication to vaccination.

The use of influenza vaccine is predominantly directed toward protection of the individual recipient and not as a general public health measure to decrease transmission of influenza. However, persons who may nosocomially transmit infection (doctors, nurses, other health care providers) to high risk individuals are also being targeted. People who are recognized to be at high risk of acquiring severe influenza are categorized in Table 1. In the high risk groups, immunization with influenza vaccine not only decreases the rate of influenza infection, but also appears to reduce the number of hospitalizations for any cause, including decompensation of the underlying disease during the influenza season. Although there are occasional paradoxical failures in the protective effect of influenza vaccines, the principal problem in the application of immunoprophylaxis for influenza lies in the atti-

TABLE 1 Conditions Placing Patients at High Risk from Influenza

Acquired or congenital heart disease with altered hemodynamic flow, including valvular heart disease, congestive failure, and pulmonary edema or excessive vascular load.

Chronic pulmonary disease of any type accompanied by compromised ventilation or respiration, bronchial secretions, or a history of lung infection. Pregnancy in the third trimester may place women in this category.

Chronic metabolic disease associated with renal failure, diabetes or severe anemia.

Immunodeficiency resulting from disease, certain malignant tumors, or immunosuppressive therapy.

Advanced age, especially over 65 years; the risk of excessive mortality begins after 45 years and is significant after age 65.

Exposure while providing essential community services.

tudes and practices of physicians. Most physicians accept the effectiveness of influenza vaccine, but they fail to make specific recommendations to their patients and do not prepare for and accomplish their immunization. Surveys show that most patients who are hospitalized for influenza have been seen by a physician in the preceding 3 months. Adult patients dislike having "shots," and only about 15 percent of selected populations who are eligible for free vaccination seek and take it. However, mailed reminders appear effective in increasing vaccine usage. In America, implementation of the vaccine policy rests with individual physicians, with only education as a prod to performance and personal awareness as a basis for evaluation of the practice adopted.

Chemoprophylaxis

Amantadine. The most effective use of amantadine is for prophylaxis against influenza A. The recommended dose is 100 mg twice daily for 3 days, then once or twice daily for the duration of prophylaxis. Under defined conditions, amantadine or rimantadine can prevent influenza A infection in 70 percent or more of exposed persons and has been highly successful in preventing the occurrence of illness. Results from some prospective double-blind controlled studies of this effect in representative groups are given in Table 2.

Fear of drug intoxication has diminished as experience and further definition of its occurrence have been developed. Mild central nervous system side effects occur in about 7 percent of persons taking the recommended dose of 100 mg twice a day. The effects may disappear with subsequent doses and do so quickly with no sequelae after discontinuation of the drug. It is recommended that vaccine be given simultaneously with chemoprophylaxis, which is continued as protective cover for 10 days thereafter. Otherwise, chemoprophylaxis must be continued for the entire period of risk as there is no posttreatment protection.

Interferon. Inducers of interferon in situ, interferon derived from leukocytes, and alpha-interferon produced by a cloned gene in bacteria have all been shown to be capable of reducing the frequency and severity of rhinovirus infections. The last product has been available for field trials in which rhinovirus infections, but not other viral respiratory infections, were decreased. Although the original description of interferon showed protection of mice against influenza, controlled trials against influenza in humans have given equivocal results, partly because of problems of dosage. When given topically in the repeated mega-unit doses that are necessary for prophylaxis, cloned alpha$_2$-interferon commonly produces congestion and bleeding of the nasal turbinates. Some preparations of alpha$_2$-interferon produce myalgia and other systemic symptoms that are similar to the "flu syndrome," At this time, the biology of interferon and its potential prophylactic and therapeutic role in viral

TABLE 2 Studies of Amantadine Prophylaxis of Influenza A

		Clinical and Serologic Influenza		*Serologic Antibody Rise Only*		*Not Infected*	
	No.	*No.*	*(%)*	*No.*	*(%)*	*No.*	*(%)*
Families (H_2N_2)*							
Amantadine	48	0	(0)	7	(15)	41	(85)
Placebo	69	10	(15)	27	(39)	32	(46)
Hospital ward (H_2N_2)†							
Amantadine	50	0	(0)	2	(4)	48	(96)
Placebo	61	7	(12)	5	(8)	49	(80)
Students							
Amantadine (H_1N_1)‡	136	8	(6)	18	(13)	110	(81)
Placebo	139	28	(20)	14	(10)	97	(70)
Amantadine (H_3N_2)§	113	2	(2)	5	(4)	106	(94)
Placebo	132	27	(20)	5	(4)	100	(76)

* Galbraith, 1969.
† O'Donahue, 1973.
‡ Monto, 1979.
§ Dolin, 1984.

respiratory infections remain questions of investigative interest, but temporarily cannot be beneficially applied.

Chemotherapy

Amantadine. This drug has a therapeutic effect on influenza A when given early in the course of illness. It has no effect on influenza B. The effect is more subtle than with prophylaxis and can be shown best when the illness (as determined from untreated control patients) is destined to be severe, with fever and symptoms lasting for several days. This is most likely to occur with certain strains of virus and in people in the designated high risk groups. In young, healthy, ambulatory patients, the disease can be of too short a duration to demonstrate a significant difference between treated and untreated patients. Whenever objective measures are available for evaluation, such as fever or increased terminal airway resistance, the effect of amantadine has been beneficial. In other cases, the benefit may be reflected by a more rapid return to usual duties, but the difference has not been documented to have statistical significance.

The approved dose of amantadine or rimantadine is 100 mg twice a day. However, much remains unknown about the optimal therapeutic dose. Amantadine and its congener, rimantadine, have different pharmacokinetics. Oral administration of rimantadine gives a lower plasma level and, on this basis, causes somewhat fewer side effects at equivalent doses than amantadine, presumably because of a larger volume of distribution. If confirmed to have equal absorption, these characteristics of rimantadine would appear to be favorable for therapy. Both compounds have a long half-life (±16 hours), are not biodegraded, and are excreted almost completely in the urine. There is progressive accumulation of drug even in people with normal kidney function, but the dose does not need to be adjusted for short courses of therapy or in the absence of severe renal insufficiency. The therapeutic activity should be enhanced by an initial loading and a sequential decrease in the amount and frequency of drug given. The use of this strategy is handicapped by the direct relation between the amount of the individual dose and the symptoms of acute intoxication. A personal recommendation for therapy is that 100 to 200 mg be given initially, and a dose of 100 mg given at 6 and 12 hours, then twice daily for 3 days, then once daily for 3 days. Prophylactic administration of amantadine should be considered for the household or ward contacts of the case and for nonimmunized health care personnel with close exposure (Table 3).

TABLE 3 Indications for Amantadine

Prophylaxis
Household contacts of an index case of influenza A.
Hospital patients at risk for nosocomial spread when patients with influenza A are admitted.
Elderly patients in semiclosed institutions when influenza A is causing disease
Unvaccinated adults with a serious underlying disease during epidemic influenza A
Vaccinated adults who are at high risk of serious consequences from influenza A
Well university and boarding school students during periods of epidemic influenza A
Specialized health care workers during periods of pandemic influenza A
Therapy
Patients with acute influenza A within 48 hours of onset and/or manifestations of severe influenza A.

Ribavirin. The administration of ribavirin in a monodispersed, small-particle aerosol has had a significant beneficial effect on severe influenza A or B in adults and on infants hospitalized with bronchiolitis from RSV infection. In both instances, the benefit was demonstrated by objective physiologic measurements, rapidity of defervescence, and a faster rate of improvement of impaired oxygenation, respectively, and by a more rapid disappearance of virus from respiratory secretions. Various dosage regimens have been used. The initial equilibration of the tissues with the drug concentration in the aerosol is rapid, and the dose delivered to the patient depends on the duration of aerosol administration. In prior studies, the concentration of ribavirin in the liquid reservoir was 20 mg per milliliter. The aerosol that is generated with compressed air at 50 p.s.i. had particles with a median diameter of 1.6 μm, of which 95 percent were less than 5.0 μm and contained an average of 190 μg of ribavirin per liter. The dose deposited in the lungs was calculated to be 55 mg per hour. The small particle aerosol is administered for several hours or continuously each day, usually for 2 to 5 days, but to infants for as long as 22 days. The average dose given the patients treated for influenza was 3.0 g, but the optimal dose and regimen must still be determined. No adverse local responses have been observed, nor any apparent systemic toxicity. Although small-particle aerosol has been used to show the applicability and the effectiveness of ribavirin treatment against severe influenza A or B and RSV, only the treatment of RSV bronchiolitis is currently approved. The need for aerosol rather than oral administration of the drug in the treatment of adults has yet to be established.

Investigational Drugs. Several new drugs with activity against rhinoviruses, paramyxoviruses, or myxoviruses are under investigation and some of them have had preliminary clinical trials. Inhibition of viral replication usually is not the limiting factor; rather, the difficulties pertain to the pharmacokinetics of in vivo drug delivery to the target tissue, adverse reactions which—although mild—disqualify the compound from general applicability, or drug activity that is virustatic without a lasting effect. A novel approach under study is the blockade of specific viral receptors on the surface of susceptible cells in the respiratory tract. The full investigation and development of new drugs with specific antiviral action against the respiratory viruses is a difficult, laborious, and expensive process, but it is proceeding with experience and skill that will yield products for more effective and specific treatment of viral respiratory infections.

SUGGESTED READING

ACIP. Prevention and control of influenza. MMWR 1987; 36:373–387.
Dolin R, Reichman RC, Madore HP, Maynard R, et al. A controlled trial of amantadine and rimantadine in the prophylaxis of influenza A infection. N Engl J Med 1982; 307:580–585.
Hall CB, McBride JR, Walsh EE, Bell DM, et al. Aerosolized ribavirin treatment of infants with respiratory syncytial viral infection. N Engl J Med 1983; 308:1443–1447.
McClung HW, Knight V, Gilbert BE, Wilson SZ, et al. Ribavirin aerosol treatment of influenza B virus infection. JAMA 1983; 249:2671–2674.

CRYPTOCOCCAL PULMONARY INFECTIONS

JOHN R. PERFECT, M.D.

The management of pulmonary infections with *Cryptococcus neoformans* requires an understanding of the pathophysiology of this infection. *C. neoformans* is a ubiquitous encapsulated yeast with worldwide distribution. Small capsular or unencapsulated yeasts measuring less than 10 μm are likely aerosolized from an environmental source and are inhaled by the host. Once the yeast is deposited in the respiratory tract and is under the influence of higher carbon dioxide concentrations, it forms a prominent polysaccharide capsule to protect itself from the onslaught of host defenses. With our present knowledge of host responses, it appears reasonable to suggest that, in most cases, the initial clinical infection with *C. neoformans* mimics mycobacterial or histoplasmal infections. A primary hilar lymph node–pulmonary complex is established. The majority of initial infections do not induce symptoms. With a loss of certain immune functions, the yeast infection can progress or reactivate, producing a pneumonia and/or spreading to the meninges. The lung and the subarachnoid space represent the most common sites of infection with *C. neoformans*.

CLINICAL PRESENTATION

In the diagnosis of cryptococcal lung infection, there is simply no definite clinical presentation. Patients may present with a chronic cough and fever. However, patients without symptoms also reach medical attention as a result of solitary chest nodule(s) or masses on a chest roentgenogram. In extreme cases with severe immune depression, patients can develop the adult respiratory distress syndrome. Despite claims that pulmonary cryptococcosis may have characteristic roentgenographic presentations, my experience suggests that any type of infiltrate, nodule, or effusion located in any lobe of the lung may occur. Recently, a more common presentation in patients infected with the human immunodeficiency virus (HIV) has been an interstitial infiltrate that appears to mimic *Pneumocystis carinii* infections. Pulmonary cryptococcosis also may be superimposed on another pulmonary disease process. Unlike in coccidioidal or histoplasmal infections, a history of certain geographic exposures is not helpful, and skin testing is not routinely available.

Despite the pleomorphic presentation of pulmonary cryptococcosis, the astute clinician with careful microbiologic and pathologic support should not find it difficult to establish the presence of *C. neoformans* in the lung. Sputum, bronchial lavage fluids, or lung biopsy specimens generally reveal the yeast on appropriate culture media in 4 to 7 days. Histopathologic study of tissue or cytologic examination of fluids demonstrates the encapsulated yeast with stains such as methenamine silver, alcian blue, or mucicarmine. The most common mistake made when attempting to diagnose a cryptococcal lung infection is failing to send specimens for culture. A culture of specimens is generally a more sensitive method of detecting infection than is histopathologic study. However, histologic examination of biopsy specimens may occasionally reveal organisms that are not viable on culture. This could have therapeutic implications. Serologic studies may help document a cryptococcal pulmonary infection. Although there is no commercially available antibody test, an excellent latex agglutination antigen test can reliably detect circulating cryptococcal polysaccharide antigen in serum or in cerebrospinal fluid (CSF). With appropriate controls, this test has few false-positive results. However, most patients with infection limited to the lung have no detectable polysaccharide antigen circulating in the serum; when serum antigen is found, one must seriously consider the possibility that the infection has disseminated. The recent use of lysis-centrifugation methods for blood cultures increases the sensitivity of detecting fungemia and might be helpful in the diagnosis of certain cases of pulmonary cryptococcosis.

MANAGEMENT

The basic theme of this discussion is the management of pulmonary cryptococcosis. Unfortunately, there are no absolute guidelines for the treatment of this infection. Although cryptococcal meningitis is one of the best-studied fungal infections, there is no standard prescription for the management of cryptococci in the respiratory tract. However, there are several important management principles to consider. First, a lumbar puncture to obtain specimens for CSF culture, cell count, and antigen testing should be performed on any patient from whose respiratory tract *C. neoformans* has been isolated. This includes patients without symptoms or underlying disease. Second, it appears essential that patients with evidence of immune compromise, either from chemotherapeutic agents such as corticosteroids or from an underlying disease such as the acquired immunodeficiency syndrome (AIDS), receive antifungal treatment. The risk of dissemination or progression of disease is too high in the immunocompromised population not to treat even the asymptomatic patient. These two statements are reasonable general guidelines with which few experts would disagree, but application to individual cases and to specific drug regimens can be controversial. In this discussion I present my personal opinion regarding the appropriate treatment and use of antifungal regimens.

I treat the apparently normal host who has *C. neoformans* isolated in culture from the respiratory tract with antifungal agent(s) if there is evidence of parenchymal lung involvement on the chest film. However, there is a group of patients who may have only cryptococcal colonization of the tracheobronchial tree without evidence of lung invasion. Commonly, these patients have chronic obstructive pulmonary disease, and their risk for progression or dissemination is small. If such a patient with colonization only is asymptomatic, I do not treat but continue with careful follow-up. There also are patients who are apparently normal hosts with lung nodules or masses removed surgically. Cryptococci may be seen on pathologic examination but do not grow when properly cultured. This situation suggests that few, if any, organisms are replicating in the host. For these patients it may be reasonable to withhold therapy but schedule periodic follow-up visits. I treat all other apparently normal hosts. However, it should be understood that a large portion of these patients would have a self-limiting infection without treatment, and yet a small portion would experience dissemination to the subarachnoid space or perhaps harbor the yeasts for reactivation during a future illness. In most cases, I believe the side effects and the expense of the antifungal agents do not outweigh the serious complications that can occur when meningitis develops. Also, if cryptococcal polysaccharide antigen can be detected in the serum of a patient with cryptococcal pneumonia despite normal results of lumbar puncture, disseminated disease must be considered and therapy started.

In immunocompromised hosts, the risk of dissemination from a pulmonary focus is substantial, and therapy should be started even in patients with negative CSF tests. AIDS patients represent a new group of immunocompromised hosts who are particularly susceptible to *C. neoformans* infections. Cryptococcal pneumonia can be severe in these patients, and dissemination to the central nervous system is frequent. When a patient presents with cryptococcal pneumonia or meningitis, coinfection with HIV should be considered and appropriate serologic tests performed. A simultaneous infection with these two organisms has prognostic and therapeutic importance in the management of cryptococcal meningitis, and even infection limited to the chest on presentation would probably alter my therapy.

Antifungal Agents

Basically, there are four antifungal agents available for the treatment of cryptococcosis. Amphotericin B remains the most thoroughly tested agent in the treatment of pulmonary cryptococcosis. A regimen of amphotericin B at 0.4 to 0.5 mg per kilogram per day for 5 to 6 weeks adequately treats most cases of cryptococcal pneumonia. The use of amphotericin B has many drawbacks, including toxicity and the requirement for intravenous administration. However, with careful monitoring of blood counts, electrolyte levels, and renal functions, combined with the lower doses of amphotericin B now being used, this agent can be administered with minimal problems. It also can be given on an outpatient basis through indwelling catheters, using every other day administration.

My personal choice of therapy for invasive cryptococcosis in an immunocompromised host is the combination of amphotericin B and flucytosine. Amphotericin B, 0.3 mg per kilogram per day, plus flucytosine, 100 mg per kilogram per day, for 4 weeks has been shown to be effective in treating meningitis and should be successful for invasive pulmonary disease. It should be mentioned that duration of therapy is arbitrary, and some patients may need longer treatment. Flucytosine has been criticized for its ability to produce life-threatening bone marrow suppression and diarrhea. Side effects of this agent are serious, but with careful dosing, it is a relatively safe drug. In most patients, 100 mg per kilogram per day in four divided doses provides adequate drug levels. In patients who receive the drug for more than 2 weeks or who have reduced renal function, flucytosine serum levels should be measured. A drug level between 30 and 100 μg per milliliter 2 hours after a dose is optimal. Levels higher than 100 μg per milliliter should be avoided, to reduce the possibility of bone marrow toxicity. All patients with renal impairment should receive a reduced dose. Guidelines for dosage reduction have been published and should be followed.

Despite the effective use of amphotericin B or its combination with flucytosine for cryptococcal pneumonia, there are many patients, in particular asymptomatic normal hosts, for whom an oral regimen is desirable. My regimen for these patients has been flucytosine alone for approximately 3 months. One drawback to flucytosine treatment by itself is the development of drug resistance during treatment and later relapse with a resistant isolate. I generally do not use it alone in severely immunocompromised hosts or in those with a large burden of organisms. Also, on occasion, a symptomatic patient does not respond to flucytosine alone but improves after the addition of amphotericin B.

Another antifungal agent currently available is ketoconazole. This oral imidazole has been found effective in the treatment of pulmonary histoplasmosis and blastomycosis, but there are few published reports of its use in pulmonary cryptococcosis. Ketoconazole has not been effective in cryptococcal meningitis because, with standard doses, it penetrates poorly into the central nervous system. My limited experience suggests that ketoconazole may be an adequate alternative regimen in some patients with pulmonary cryptococcosis. However, it is essential to rule out central nervous system involvement before this drug is used. I would administer doses of 400 to 600 mg per day for at least 3 months. Periodic checks of liver function in order to identify a serious drug-induced hepatitis are reasonable during therapy.

There are other azole compounds with anticryptococcal activity. Experience with miconazole is too limited to recommend it for general use in cryptococcosis. New agents such as itraconazole and fluconazole are now in clinical trials. Both have been used successfully in treatment of cryptococcal meningitis and will likely be effective in cryptococcal pneumonia.

A final comment on treatment of cryptococcal pneumonia in AIDS patients is warranted. Relapses of cryptococcal meningitis and prostate and pulmonary infections occur frequently in this group of patients. At present, it appears reasonable to continue suppressive antifungal regimens after initial treatment indefinitely.

Surgery

The importance of surgery in pulmonary cryptococcosis requires a short review. There have been some suggestions in the literature that operating on a patient with pulmonary cryptococcal infection may promote its dissemination. I am not convinced that surgery influences dissemination. On the other hand, it is also unlikely that complete removal of a cryptococcal nodule or mass in the lung eliminates infection. A clinician should consider antifungal therapy if the organism is cultured from the lesion. Pleural cryptococcal effusions occasionally occur and in most cases can be managed with antifungal chemotherapy without surgical drainage.

Immunosuppression

Immunosuppressed patients remain the most difficult management problems in cryptococcosis. Control of the underlying disease such as malignancy with chemotherapy and AIDS with antiretroviral agents and reduction of immunosuppressive agents to minimal doses will be essential parts of the successful treatment of lung infections. It is hoped that in the future, immune modulators will be available for treatment of HIV infection.

SUGGESTED READING

Baker RD. The primary pulmonary lymph node complex of cryptococcosis. Am J Clin Pathol 1976; 65:83–92.

Campbell DG. Primary pulmonary cryptococcosis. Am Rev Respir Dis 1966; 94:236–243.

Duperval R, Hermans PE, Brewer NS, et al. Cryptococcosis with emphasis on the significance of isolation of *Cryptococcus neoformans* from the respiratory tract. Chest 1977; 72:13–19.

Hammerman KJ, Powell KE, Christianson CS, et al. Pulmonary cryptococcosis: Clinical forms and treatment. Am Rev Respir Dis 1973; 108:1116–1123.

Kerkering TM, Duma RJ, Shadomy S. The evolution of pulmonary cryptococcosis. Ann Intern Med 1981; 94:611–616.

Tynes B, Mason KN, Jennings AE, et al. Variant forms of pulmonary cryptococcosis. Ann Intern Med 1968; 69:1117–1125.

Warr W, Bates JH, Stove A. The spectrum of pulmonary cryptococcosis. Ann Intern Med 1968; 69:1109–1116.

Young EJ, Hirsch DD, Fainstein V, et al. Pleural effusions due to *Cryptococcus neoformans*: A review of the literature and report of two cases with cryptococcal antigen determination. Am Rev Respir Dis 1980; 121:743–747.

PROTOZOAN AND HELMINTHIC PULMONARY INFECTIONS

ROBERT A. SALATA, M.D.
ADEL A. F. MAHMOUD, M.D., Ph.D

Protozoa and helminths represent a major group of infectious agents that cause considerable pulmonary morbidity and mortality. Although their prevalence in developed and developing countries has always been considerable, the increasing proportion of patients with suppressed immune responses has added significantly to the clinical spectrum of protozoan and helminthic infections in the lungs. In this chapter, we concentrate on the clinically significant diseases; less important infections are briefly mentioned.

The approach to a patient with protozoan or helminthic pulmonary infection must be planned with particular care. Most of these infections result in clinical syndromes not dissimilar from those caused by other infectious or noninfectious processes. A thorough geographic history, knowledge of the immune status of the individual patient, and a high index of suspicion are the three critical elements. In addition, requesting the appropriate diagnostic test may save a lot of unnecessary procedures and provides a sound basis for initiating appropriate therapeutic modalities.

PROTOZOAN INFECTIONS

Pneumocystis carinii Pneumonia

Although most authors have favored a protozoan classification for *Pneumocystis carinii*, recent analysis of *P. carinii* ribosomal RNA suggests a close relationship to fungi. Nevertheless, *Pneumocystis carinii* pneumonia is still discussed here in the context of protozoan pulmonary infection.

Recently, the prevalence of *Pneumocystis carinii* infection has increased dramatically and has become distressingly familiar in the setting of the acquired immunodeficiency syndrome (AIDS). *P. carinii* has been found in the lungs of humans and in many animal species. The source of human infection is unknown but presumably occurs through the respiratory route. Latent infection is common; 65 percent of healthy individuals are found to have specific antibody responses by the age of 4 years. *P. carinii* pneumonia (PCP) is probably the result of a reactivation of latent infection. Depression of cell-mediated immunity is the most important factor leading to reactivation. Before the recognition of AIDS, children with acute lymphocytic leukemia were at highest risk for developing PCP. Patients with other lymphocytic leukemias and lymphomas, organ transplant recipients, and those receiving high doses of corticosteroids are also at high risk. For unclear reasons, the incidence of PCP in patients with AIDS has been higher than in any other group.

Clinically, PCP is characterized by dyspnea, nonproductive cough, and fever; symptoms in AIDS patients are usually more insidious and prolonged. There is hypoxemia and an increased alveolar to arterial (A-a) gradient, although these findings may be mild or absent in patients with AIDS. Chest roentgenograms demonstrate bilateral diffuse infiltrates, which may be interstitial or alveolar in nature; localized infiltrates or nodules are observed infrequently. Pleural disease has been reported rarely. Normal chest films are seen in 5 to 20 percent of patients with AIDS who have a parasitologically proven diagnosis. PCP can progress to cause severe respiratory failure and the adult respiratory distress syndrome. In this setting, prognosis is grave.

Bronchoscopy is the procedure of choice for diagnosis. Cytologic examination of induced sputum is positive in approximately 25 percent of patients with AIDS and should always be attempted. Bronchoalveolar lavage has a 90 percent sensitivity in the diagnosis of PCP in patients with AIDS; the yield is increased if transbronchial biopsy is performed. Bronchoscopy is of lower diagnostic yield in patients without AIDS; occasionally open lung biopsy is necessary to confirm the diagnosis in these patients. Gallium-67 scanning is sensitive, but not specific, and it is sometimes used to determine the need for an invasive procedure. Definitive diagnosis should always be sought in patients with AIDS, since coexistent pathogens occur commonly and frequent adverse effects from therapeutic agents are seen.

Trimethoprim-sulfamethoxazole (TMP/SMZ) is the treatment of choice for PCP in patients without AIDS because it is equally effective as and less toxic than pentamidine (Table 1). Patients with AIDS have a greater than 60 percent incidence of adverse effects to TMP/SMZ or pentamidine. Since efficacy between these two drugs is similar in patients with AIDS, neither has emerged as the drug of choice. Preliminary experience with trimethoprim–dapsone in patients with AIDS suggests that this drug combination may be as effective and better tolerated than standard therapy in mild to moderately ill individuals. In patients unable to tolerate any of these regimens, experimental treatment with aerosolized pentamidine, trimetrexate, or difluoromethylornithine has been attempted. A short course of corticosteroids may be beneficial adjunctively in the patient with impending respiratory failure.

Prophylaxis against PCP is advisable in patients at high risk. In patients without AIDS, long-term ad-

TABLE 1 Commonly Used Drugs for Protozoan and Helminthic Pulmonary Infections

Infection	*Drug*	*Dosage*	*Side Effects*	*Comments*
Pneumocystis carinii pneumonia	*Drugs of choice:* Trimethoprim-sulfamethoxazole	TMP 20 mg/kg/day SMZ 100 mg/kg/day IV or PO in 4 doses × 14 to 21 days*	Fever, hypersensitivity reactions, hematologic abnormalities	Increased adverse effects in patients with AIDS
	Alternatives: Pentamidine isethionate	4 mg/kg/day IV or IM × 14 to 21 days*	Hypotension, hypoglycemia, azotemia, transaminitis, neutropenia, pancreatitis	Side effects more frequent in patients with AIDS. Chronic glucose intolerance occasionally seen.
	Trimethoprim-dapsone	TMP 20 kg/day in 4 doses IV or PO, dapsone 100 mg/day × 14 to 21 days*	GI toxicity, rash, agranulocytosis, and other blood dyscrasias, hemolysis in G6PD deficiency	Fewer side effects vs TMP/SMZ or pentamidine in patients with AIDS
Pleuropulmonary amebiasis	Metronidazole	750 mg t.i.d. orally × 10 days	GI toxicity, headache, occasional rash, or neutropenia	Drug has an Antabuse-like effect
	followed by Dilozanide furoate†	500 mg t.i.d. orally × 10 days		
Plasmodium falciparum malaria (pulmonary edema)				
Chloroquine-sensitive *P. falciparum*	*Drug of choice:* Chloroquine phosphate	600 mg base, then 300 mg base 6 h later, then 300 mg bases/day × 2 days	Occasional GI and CNS disturbances, retinopathy only with chronic dosing	Parenteral (IM) chloroquine can be given to those unable to take oral medications
Chloroquine-resistant *P. falciparum*	*Drugs of choice:* Quinine sulfate‡ *plus*	650 mg t.i.d. IV or orally × 3 days	Cinchonism (tinnitus, headache, nausea, visual disturbances) with oral dosing, arrhythmias with parenteral form	ECG monitoring with parenteral therapy is advisable
	Pyrimethamine	25 mg b.i.d. × 3 days	Rash, hematologic abnormalities, folic acid deficiency	Supportive therapy also is essential. In fulminant cases, exchange transfusion may be considered.
	plus Sulfadiazine	500 mg q.i.d. × 5 days	See sulfamethoxazole	
	Alternatives: Quinine sulfate *plus* Tetracycline§	500 mg q.i.d. × 7 days	GI toxicity, sun sensitivity, permanent discoloration of teeth in children	For infection acquired in Thailand, quinine should be given × 7 days. Quinine plus tetracycline may be regimen of choice for infection acquired in Thailand.
Toxoplasma Pneumonitis	*Drugs of choice:* Pyrimethamine	25 mg/days orally for 4 to 6 weeks after resolution of symptoms	Rash, hematologic abnormalities, folic acid deficiency	

Table continues

TABLE 1 Commonly Used Drugs for Protozoan and Helminthic Pulmonary Infections (Continued)

Infection	*Drug*	*Dosage*	*Side Effects*	*Comments*
	plus Sulfadiazine	2 to 6 g/days orally for 4 to 6 weeks after resolution of symptoms	See sulfamethoxazole	
Ascariasis or hookworms	*Drugs of choice for treatment of adult worms:* Mebendazole	100 mg b.i.d. × 3 days	Transient GI toxicity	
Strongyloidiasis	Thiabendazole	25 mg/kg b.i.d. × 2 days	GI toxicity, CNS disturbances, occasional rash	In immunocompromised patients, therapy should be continued for 10 to 15 days
Tropical pulmonary eosinophilia	Diethylcarbamazine	2 mg/kg t.i.d. × 7 to 21 days	Fever, headache, GI toxicity, arthralgias, chills within first 24 to 36 h of therapy	Intensity of side effects related to degree of microfilaremia
Lung hydatid disease	See text			
Schistosomiasis	*Drug of Choice:* Praziquantel	40 mg/kg once for *S. mansoni, S. haematobium* and *S. intercalatum* and 20 mg/kg t.i.d. × 1 day for *S. japonicum* and *S. mekongi*	Mild GI toxicity, malaise and transient headache occur rarely	
Paragonimiasis	*Drug of Choice:* Praziquantel	25 mg/kg t.i.d. × 2 days		Considered an experimental drug by the US Food and Drug administration

* Three weeks of therapy for *Pneumocystis carinii* pneumonia has been necessary in patients with AIDS.
† To be obtained from the Centers for Disease Control.
‡ Therapy with parenteral quinidine gluconate can be substituted in adults if parenteral quinine is not readily available.
§ Contraindicated in pregnancy and in children less than 8 years old.
GI = gastrointestinal, CNS = central nervous system, GGPD = glucose-6-phosphate dehydrogenase, ECG = electrocardiographic

ministration of TMP/SMZ has been well tolerated and has proved highly effective. Long-term administration of TMP/SMZ generally has not been tolerated by patients with AIDS. Currently prophylaxis for PCP with aerosolized pentamidine (300 mg dose every 4 weeks via the Respirgard II jet nebulizer) is recommended for adult HIV-infected patients who have had an episode of PCP or if their CD4+ cell count is less than 200 per cubic millimeter or if their CD4+ cells are less than 20 percent of total lymphocytes.

Pleuropulmonary Complications of Amebiasis

Entamoeba histolytica, which infects 10 percent of the world's population, occurs in the United States in high-risk groups including the chronically institutionalized, homosexual males, and travelers to and immigrants from endemic areas. Infection is transmitted by the ingestion of cysts in contaminated food or water or less frequently through fecal-oral routes. Invasive disease usually manifests as amebic dysentery or liver abscess. Intrathoracic complications most commonly arise from liver infection, with rupture of the abscess into the pleural cavity and empyema formation. Direct or hematogenous amebic invasion of the thorax may result rarely in lung abscess. Patients with pleuropulmonary amebiasis are in toxic condition and present with cough, dyspnea, and chest pain. Right upper quadrant abdominal pain is frequent. Hemoptysis may be prominent. Diarrhea and dysentery may or may not be present.

A chest roentgenogram may be a helpful but nondiagnostic clue to the development of pleuropulmonary complications of amebic liver abscesses. Imaging studies of the liver and pleural space may be extremely useful in demonstrating the process and its extent. Examination of stool for *E. histolytica* trophozoites and cysts is often negative. Diagnostically, 90 to 95 percent of cases of tissue-invasive amebiasis are associated with positive serologic findings. Management of intrathoracic amebiasis requires the administration of metronidazole, followed by a course of diloxanide furoate (see Table 1). Closed tube drainage may be needed, and open surgical procedures occasionally may be necessary.

Pulmonary Edema in Malaria

Plasmodium falciparum malaria is the leading parasitic cause of death worldwide. The incidence of pulmonary complications in falciparum malaria has been estimated to be between 3 and 10 percent and has been viewed as a major determinant of mortality in infected individuals. The mechanism of lung injury in falciparum malaria is not known but may be due to tissue hypoxia, abnormal autonomic effects on the lung, immunologic injury to alveolocapillary structures, or pulmonary damage resulting from morphologic changes on the surface of infected erythrocytes. Both high-grade parasitemia and delay in institution of appropriate antimalarial therapy appear to increase the risk of pulmonary involvement in falciparum malaria.

Diagnosis must be rapid and relies on blood smear examination to document parasitemia, its degree, and species differentiation. Therapy must be prompt and, most important, consider the potential for chloroquine-resistant strains of *P. falciparum* (see Table 1). For respiratory insufficiency and pulmonary edema, aggressive supportive care is necessary to maintain oxygenation while awaiting resolution of the pulmonary process.

Toxoplasma Pneumonitis

Toxoplasma gondii can infect both normal and immunocompromised individuals. Infection most commonly occurs through the ingestion of contaminated food. Immunocompromised individuals at risk for toxoplasmosis include those receiving steroids or cytotoxic agents, those with lymphoreticular malignancy, organ transplant recipients, and those with AIDS. These persons may have primary or, more usually, reactivation disease. The majority have encephalitis, meningoencephalitis, or brain mass lesions. Pneumonitis or myocarditis may develop in this setting. Rarely has *T. gondii* been considered a cause of atypical pneumonia in normal individuals.

Diagnostically, finding *T. gondii* in blood, body fluids, or histologic sections establishes acute infection. Serologic testing for specific antibodies is the primary means of diagnosis, but may be limited in immunocompromised hosts because of depressed antibody responses. More invasive procedures are frequently performed to establish the etiology of pulmonary infiltrates in compromised hosts, even if toxoplasmosis is a possibility. The most efficacious drugs for toxoplasmosis are pyrimethamine and the sulfonamides (see Table 1). Alternative agents have included spiramycin, clindamycin, and trimetrexate. No widespread experience with these agents in compromised hosts with cerebral and pulmonary involvement has been reported.

Respiratory Cryptosporidiosis

Recently, cryptosporidiosis has been recognized as a cause of severe, protracted diarrhea in immunocompromised patients and of self-limited diarrhea in normal persons. This coccidian has a complicated life cycle and appears to be capable of reinitiating recurrent infection.

In compromised hosts, *Cryptosporidium* causes severe diarrheal illness characterized by frequent, voluminous, watery bowel movements, cramping abdominal pain, malabsorption, and severe weight loss. Extraintestinal sites of involvement that have been reported in patients with AIDS include the tracheobronchial tree and the pulmonary parenchyma. It is thought that respiratory involvement results from aspiration of gastrointestinal contents.

The diagnosis of cryptosporidiosis is most often established by the identification of oocysts in stool; intestinal biopsy occasionally may be necessary. Successful therapy of cryptosporidiosis in immunocompromised individuals has been achieved only when the underlying immune defect can be reversed. Multiple drugs have been attempted in patients with AIDS without consistent success.

HELMINTHIC INFECTIONS

Nematode-Induced Löffler's Syndrome

Human infection with *Ascaris lumbricoides*, *Ancylostoma duodenale*, *Necator americanus*, and *Strongyloides stercoralis* produces a characteristic Löffler's-like syndrome in immunocompetent individuals. In contrast, the hyperinfection syndrome with *S. stercoralis* is a specific clinical entity noted in immunocompromised patients. All of the adult stages of these nematode agents infect the human gastrointestinal tract; they pass eggs (*A. lumbricoides*, *A. duodenale*, and *N. americanus*) or larvae (*S. stercoralis*), which undergo maturation in soil. Human infection results from the ingestion of mature *A. lumbricoides* eggs or from penetration of intact skin by the infective larvae of other species. Ascaris larvae emerge from hatched eggs and penetrate the gastrointestinal wall. This larval species, as well as those of hookworms or *S. stercoralis*, begin a migratory pathway via venous blood to the right side of the heart and eventually to the lungs. It is this pulmonary migratory phase of the nematode larvae that is associated with transient lung disease; larvae usually proceed from the vascular to the alveolar spaces and ascend toward the trachea to be swallowed to reach their final habitat.

Significant clinical lung disease occurs in ascariasis in immunocompetent individuals; less severe disease has been described in those with hookworm or *Strongyloides* infection. In ascariasis, pulmonary symptoms usually begin 1 to 2 weeks after infection, which coincides with larval migration in the lungs. Symptoms include persistent nonproductive cough, substernal pain, and occasionally hemoptysis and dyspnea. Eosinophilia and patchy pulmonary infiltrate may be seen. Symptoms usually subside within 2 to 4 weeks. In some areas of the world, a recurrent syndrome known as seasonal pneumonitis has been observed to coincide with the known seasonal transmission of ascariasis, suggesting a hypersensitivity element in the pathogenesis of this syndrome.

In the immunosuppressed, *S. stercoralis* hyperinfection results in massive invasion of the lungs with parasite larvae. Clinically, these patients present with either asthma or chronic cough associated with multiple lung opacities, consolidation, and sometimes cavitation. Most of these individuals present with secondary infection from invasion by bowel flora.

Diagnosis of pulmonary disease caused by ascariasis or hookworms is usually difficult. One has to wait until adult worms in the gut start egg production (4 to 8 weeks) to be able to detect parasite ova in stools. In patients suspected of having the strongyloidiasis hyperinfection syndrome, examination of sputum, bronchial lavage fluid, or stools demonstrates the infective filariform larvae. Management of patients with pulmonary ascariasis is symptomatic; antiparasitic drugs have not been shown to be effective against the pulmonary larval stage. Once the worms reach maturity in the gastrointestinal tract, mebendazole is the drug of choice for ascariasis and hookworms (see Table 1). It is given orally, 100 mg twice a day for 3 days. In the immunocompetent host, treatment of strongyloidiasis can be accomplished by the oral administration of thiabendazole, 25 mg per kilogram of body weight twice a day for 2 days. In the immunocompromised patient, the drug should be started as early as possible and should be continued for 10 to 15 days (see Table 1).

Tropical Pulmonary Eosinophilia

This is a clinically distinct disease entity seen in individuals living or who have lived in areas endemic for *Wuchereria bancrofti* and *Brugia malayi*. The main clinical manifestations are chronic nocturnal cough, eosinophilia, and a remarkable improvement following diethylcarbamazine therapy. Although the etiology and pathogenesis of this syndrome are still unclear, tropical pulmonary eosinophilia is now recognized as one of the amicrofilaremic syndromes. In these individuals, high levels of specific IgG and IgE antibodies have been demonstrated in the absence of peripheral blood microfilariae.

Tropical pulmonary eosinophilia usually occurs in young males. Nocturnal episodes of dry cough are frequently associated with low-grade fever and fatigue. Pulmonary function tests may show restrictive defects, and reticulonodular opacities may be seen on chest films. Besides the characteristic clinical and serologic features, diagnosis is confirmed by a favorable therapeutic response. Diethylcarbamazine is administered orally, 5 mg per kilogram of body weight per day in divided doses for 2 to 3 weeks (see Table 1).

Human dirofilariasis has been reported infrequently. Individuals infected with the dog heartworm *Dirofilaria immitis* may present with diffuse lung infiltrate or solitary nodules. Diagnosis is difficult and necessitates examination of biopsy material.

Visceral Larva Migrans (Toxocariasis)

Human infection with dog or cat ascarids results in tissue invasion with the larval stages of the parasite that are unable to reach maturity. The syndrome is more common in children. Human infection is initiated by ingestion of mature parasite eggs, which are found in soil or may contaminate food or drinks. Eggs hatch in the stomach, liberating larvae that migrate throughout the host tissues, which induces pathology in the liver, lungs, and eyes.

Pulmonary complaints, including cough and wheezing, and lung infiltrates may be seen in approximately one-third of infected children. The syndrome is usually associated with considerable peripheral blood eosinophilia. Diagnosis may be confirmed serologically. Since visceral larva migrans is usually self-limiting, no specific chemotherapy is recommended. Patients with extensive pulmonary function impairment may benefit from a short course of corticosteroids.

Hydatid Disease (Echinococcosis)

Accidental infection of humans with the larval stage of the dog tapeworm *Echinococcus granulosus* results in the development of hydatid cysts in tissues. Infection is acquired through the ingestion of parasite eggs that contaminate soil, food, or drink. These cysts are found mainly in the liver (50 percent) and the lungs (20 percent). Pulmonary hydatid is found more frequently in children. The space-occupying cysts usually do not cause symptoms. In contrast, symptomatic patients usually complain of cough, dyspnea, or chest pain. Chest roentgenograms show the smooth, thin-walled cyst with air-fluid levels, the water lily sign, or rarely, calcification. Multiple cysts also may occur.

Diagnosis of the hydatid nature of a pulmonary

cyst is based on serologic testing for antibodies against defined parasite antigen (arc-5). Management depends on the number and size of cysts. Solitary large cysts are usually removed surgically. Albendazole, a new anti-*Echinococcus* agent, may be used in patients with multiple or disseminated pulmonary cysts (see Table 1). The efficacy of the drug and its optimal dosage are not yet uniformly accepted.

Schistosomal Cor Pulmonale

Five species of schistosomes infect humans: *Schistosoma haematobium*, *S. mansoni*, *S. japonicum*, *S. mekongi*, and *S. intercalatum*. Only the first three have been reported to result in significant pulmonary disease. Human infection is initiated by penetration of intact skin by the freshwater infective stage, called cercaria. Upon penetration, these organisms change into migrating schistosomula that go through the host lungs and, in 2 to 4 weeks, settle in the liver to mature into adult worms, which establish their final habitat in defined areas of the abdominal venous vasculature.

Mature worms begin oviposition inside the host vasculature; some of these eggs migrate toward the lumen of the gut or urinary tract to be carried with excreta to the outside environment for completion of the parasite life cycle. A varying proportion of these ova are retained in the host and impact at the point of deposition, whereas others are carried by blood flow to lodge eventually at the smaller venous branches in the liver and other organs. Pulmonary schistosomiasis is the result of egg deposition and subsequent granuloma formation and fibrosis. Eggs reach the pulmonary vasculature either directly through the inferior vena cava, as in *S. haematobium* infection, or indirectly via anastomotic collaterals between the portal and systemic venous circulations, as in *S. mansoni* or *S. japonicum* infection.

The most significant clinical sequelae in the lungs of individuals infected with any of the schistosome species relate to cor pulmonale. Pulmonary hypertension results from the presence of *Schistosoma* ova within the pulmonary arteries or arterioles. Clinically, patients with schistosomal cor pulmonale are indistinguishable from others with the same syndrome due to other causes. Diagnosis is based on geographic history and the presence of parasite eggs in urine or stool. When active schistosomal infection is found, treatment with praziquantel is indicated. The drug is administered orally as a single dose of 40 mg per kilogram of body weight for *S. mansoni*, *S. haematobium*, and *S. intercalatum* infection and as 20 mg per kilogram of body weight three times a day for *S. japonicum* or *S. mekongi* infection (see Table 1). Eradication of schistosome infection prevents further egg deposition and may reduce subsequent pulmonary lesions. It is not known, however, whether antischistosomal chemotherapy has an effect on existing lung pathology. In these cases, symptomatic treatment of cor pulmonale also is indicated.

Paragonimiasis

The lung fluke *Paragonimus* is endemic in many areas of the Far East, Africa, and South and Central America. Infection is acquired by eating raw or poorly salted freshwater crayfish or crabs in an endemic area. The infective metacercariae are liberated in the gastrointestinal tract, penetrate the intestinal wall, and migrate to the lungs where they mature into encapsulated adult worms. During the migratory phase of the adults in the lungs, they are located in tunnels surrounded by mixed eosinophil and neutrophil infiltrates. In established infection, adult worms are usually enclosed within cystic lesions.

Clinical features of established pulmonary paragonimiasis include cough productive of rusty, blood-stained sputum. Parasite eggs, necrotic material, and Charcot-Leyden crystals may be seen in sputum. Massive hemoptysis also has been reported. Chest films may be normal or may show infiltrate, cavitation, or fibrosis. The characteristic ring shadow with a crescent corona has not been consistently seen. Diagnosis of paragonimiasis is based on demonstration of parasite eggs in sputum or stool. Praziquantel is the first effective chemotherapeutic agent. It is administered orally in a dosage of 75 mg per kilogram of body weight per day for 2 days (see Table 1).

SUGGESTED READING

Abdel-Wahab AF, Mahmoud SS. *Schistosomiasis mansoni* in Egypt. In: Mahmoud AAF, ed. Clinical medicine and communicable diseases. Vol 2. Philadelphia: WB Saunders, 1987:371.

Adams EB, MacLeod IN. Invasive amebiasis. I. Amebic dysentery and its complications. Medicine 1977; 56:315–324.

Adams EB, MacLeod IN. Invasive amebiasis. II. Amebic liver abscess and its complications. Medicine 1977; 56:315–324.

Adkins RB, Dao AH. Pulmonary dirofilariasis: A diagnostic challenge. South Med J 1984; 77:372–374.

Aytak A, Yurdakul Y, Ikizlen C, et al. Pulmonary hydatid disease: Report of 100 patients. Ann Thorac Surg 1977; 23:145–151.

Feldman RM, Singer C. Noncardiogenic pulmonary edema and pulmonary fibrosis in falciparum malaria. Rev Infect Dis 1987; 9:134–139.

Igra-Siegman Y, Kapila R, Sen P, et al. Syndrome of hyperinfection with *Strongyloides stercoralis*. Rev Infect Dis 1981; 3:397–407.

Johnson RE, Jong EC, Dunning SB, et al. Paragonimiasis: Diagnosis and the use of praziquantel in treatment. Rev Infect Dis 1985; 7:200–206.

Kovacs JA, Hiemenz JW, Macher AM, et al. *Pneumocystis carinii* pneumonia: A comparison between patients with the acquired immunodeficiency syndrome and patients with other immunodeficiencies. Ann Intern Med 1984; 100:663–671.

Mahmoud AAF. Praziquantel for the treatment of helminthic infections. Adv Intern Med 1987; 32:193–206.

McCabe RE, Remington JS. *Toxoplasma gondii*. In: Mandell GL, Douglas RG, Bennett JE, eds. Principles and practice of infectious disease. New York: John Wiley & Sons, 1985:1540.

Miller TA. Hookworm infection in man. Adv Parasitol 1979; 17:315–383.

Ottesen EA. Filariasis and tropical eosinophilia. In: Warren KS, Mahmoud AAF, eds. Tropical and geographical medicine. 2nd ed. New York: McGraw-Hill, 1990.
Pavlowski ZS. Ascariasis: Host-pathogen biology. Rev Infect Dis 1982; 4:806–814.
Prata A. Schistosomiasis in Brazil. In: Mahmoud AAF, ed. Clinical tropical medicine and communicable diseases. Vol 2. Philadelphia: WB Saunders, 1987:349.
Schantz PM, Okelo GBA. Echinococcus. In: Warren KS, Mahmoud AAF, eds. Tropical and geographical medicine. 2nd ed. New York: McGraw-Hill, 1990.
Soave R, Armstrong D. *Cryptosporidium* and cryptosporidiosis. Rev Infect Dis 1986: 8:1012–1023.

ASPIRATION OF GASTRIC CONTENTS

JOHN K. JENKINS, M.D.
ALPHA A. FOWLER III, M.D.

Pulmonary aspiration of gastric contents is one of the most frequent causes of admission to intensive care units and is among the leading causes of death related to anesthesia and obstetric procedures. It is encountered by clinicians of virtually all specialties and continues to be a significant cause of morbidity and mortality despite their best efforts at medical management. Although the dangers of aspiration have been recognized since the time of Hippocrates, it was not until 1946 that Mendelson described the syndrome of respiratory failure due to aspiration of gastric contents in a series of obstetric patients. Significant advances in our understanding of the pathophysiology of gastric aspiration have occurred in the ensuing four decades.

The spectrum of clinical syndromes resulting from gastric aspiration ranges from acute life-threatening respiratory distress to chronic pulmonary disease due to recurrent aspiration. Recent studies show that aspiration of small volumes of gastric contents or oropharyngeal secretions is a common event in normal individuals. This phenomenon usually goes unnoticed and produces no adverse effects. However, certain patient groups are at risk for aspiration of larger quantities of gastric contents and may develop pulmonary disease. Disorders that predispose patients to gastric aspiration are listed in Table 1. In general, any patient with altered gastrointestinal motility, an abnormal swallowing mechanism, or altered level of consciousness should be considered at risk for aspiration. Massive aspiration is most often seen in patients undergoing cardiopulmonary resuscitation or emergency anesthesia for surgical or obstetric procedures.

PATHOPHYSIOLOGY

The clinical syndrome that develops in response to gastric aspiration is related to the nature, volume, and distribution of the aspirate as well as the frequency of aspiration. Several syndromes of aspiration have been described; however, the syndromes may overlap in individual patients.

Aspiration of solid particles leads to variable degrees of airway obstruction. In this setting, obstruction may produce acute asphyxiation and death due to tracheal obstruction or may simply result in lobar or segmental atelectasis following bronchial obstruction. Hypoxemia frequently occurs in association with atelectasis due to altered ventilation:perfusion (V/Q) relationships. Secondary bacterial infections such as pneumonia, lung abscess, or empyema are common if the obstructing particle is not removed.

Aspiration of nontoxic liquids, such as isotonic saline solution, blood, barium, or neutralized gastric secretions, produces no direct injury to the lung; however, respiratory distress and hypoxemia occur because of flooding of the airways and V/Q mismatching. Secondary bacterial infection is rare, and patients usually recover quickly.

Aspiration of toxic liquids, such as gastric acid, bile, hydrocarbons, or alcohol, leads to direct lung injury and chemical pneumonitis. This is the most severe of the aspiration syndromes. Once gastric acid is aspirated into the trachea, it is rapidly distributed to the distal airways and alveoli, and a chemical burn to the alveolocapillary membrane results. The extent and severity of the resulting lung injury are related to the pH and volume of the aspirate entering the lungs. Laboratory experiments using animal models of aspiration lung injury indicate that a critical pH of 2.5 or less and a volume of 30 to 50 ml are required to produce significant chemical airway and alveolar "burns." Acid injury results in necrosis of alveolar epithelial cells and a loss of integrity of the alveolocapillary membrane. As a result, focal areas of alveolar hemorrhage are observed, and the alveoli are flooded by exudative edema fluid. Polymorphonuclear leukocytes migrate into the airways in large numbers and are speculated to contribute to the lung injury by re-

TABLE 1 Factors That Predispose to Aspiration

Decreased Level of Consciousness
Cerebrovascular accident
Head trauma
Seizures
Drug overdose
Alcohol intoxication
Sepsis
Hepatic encephalopathy
Hypothermia
Malignant hyperthermia
Metabolic encephalopathy
Other causes of coma
Altered Pharyngeal Motility
Cerebrovascular accident with diminished gag reflex
Neuromuscular diseases (myasthenia gravis, Guillain-Barré syndrome, multiple sclerosis, amyotrophic lateral sclerosis)
Tumor of pharynx or larynx
Altered Esophageal Function
Gastroesophageal reflux
Motility disorders (achalasia, scleroderma, diffuse esophageal spasm, tumor)
Tracheoesophageal fistula (congenital or neoplastic)
Altered Gastrointestinal Motility
Gastric dilatation (autonomic dysfunction, electrolyte imbalances, outlet obstruction)
Adynamic ileus
Intestinal obstruction
Iatrogenic
General anesthesia
Cardiopulmonary resuscitation
Emergency tracheal intubation
Endotracheal tubes and tracheostomies
Nasogastric tubes
Tube feedings
Esophageal balloon tamponade
Miscellaneous
Upper gastrointestinal hemorrhage
Labor and delivery
Trauma

lease of proteolytic enzymes, receive oxygen intermediates, and proinflammatory mediators, such as prostaglandins or leukotrienes. The aspirated acid is rapidly buffered by proteins and soluble buffers in the edema fluid. It is well established that bacterial infection plays no role in the initial pathophysiology of acid aspiration.

Hypoxemia following acid aspiration is sudden and profound and develops before there is histologic evidence of alveolar edema. The early onset of hypoxemia may be due to mechanical airway obstruction that is secondary to the aspirate or to reflex airway closure. Systemic hypotension frequently develops following high volume aspiration and may be secondary to intravascular volume depletion owing to a massive flux of fluid into the alveolar spaces.

CLINICAL PRESENTATION

The clinical presentation of patients following gastric aspiration ranges from mild respiratory distress to acute respiratory failure. The onset of symptoms is rapid, usually occurring within 1 hour after aspiration. Clinical signs include tachypnea, tachycardia, hypotension, cough, cyanosis, fever, rales, rhonchi, and wheezes. Fever is the most consistent finding and is related to the physiologic response to the aspiration, not to infection. The laboratory examination usually reveals an elevated white blood cell count, an elevated hematocrit owing to hemoconcentration, variable degrees of hypoxemia, widened alveolar-arterial $P(A\text{-}a)O_2$ gradient, and a normal to low $PaCO_2$. The degree of $P(A\text{-}a)O_2$ gradient widening correlates with the severity and the prognosis of the lung injury.

Within several hours, chest roentgenograms usually show alveolar infiltrates that may be localized or diffuse. Areas of atelectasis may be present if the airway has been obstructed by a solid particle. Localization of the roentgenographic findings correlates with a patient's position at the time of the aspiration. In patients who are in the upright or the semirecumbent position, the right lower and right middle lobes are most affected. In patients who are supine, the right upper lobe is most frequently affected. In general, progression of roentgenographic findings that are solely due to aspiration ceases within 24 to 36 hours. The extent or type of initial roentgenographic findings does not correlate with prognosis or mortality.

The clinical course of aspiration-induced lung disease generally follows one of three patterns: (1) 10 to 15 percent of patients exhibit rapid progression of respiratory failure and die within 24 hours after aspiration; (2) approximately 60 percent manifest initial respiratory distress followed by rapid clinical and roentgenographic improvement within 4 to 5 days; and (3) 25 percent have initial improvement followed by clinical worsening associated with bacterial pleuropulmonary infection. Patients in whom infection develops have a mortality rate of up to 60 percent. The overall mortality from aspiration of gastric contents has been reported as 30 to 60 percent.

PREVENTION

In most patients, aspiration of gastric contents is preventable if proper precautions are taken. During an episode of witnessed vomiting, the patient should be turned on the right side with the head down to minimize the risk of aspiration. The head of the bed should be elevated for any patient with known gastroesophageal reflux. Tube feedings should be performed with care in patients who have altered mental status or diminished gag reflex. Optimally, tube feedings should be administered via small duodenal tubes by constant small-volume infusion.

Patients who are unable to protect their airways are at high risk of aspiration and should undergo elective endotracheal intubation. The stomach should be emptied by a nasogastric tube before intubation is attempted. Use of external cricoid cartilage pressure to occlude the esophagus may help prevent aspiration during intubation.

Efforts to decrease gastric volume and increase gastric pH before anesthesia is induced may reduce the risk of aspiration and minimize the severity of lung damage if aspiration occurs. Prior to elective surgery, patients should fast for 8 to 12 hours. In emergency cases, the stomach should be emptied by nasogastric tube. The role of pharmacologic agents in this setting is unclear and controversial. Orally administered antacids are effective in raising gastric pH. However, these agents do not prevent further acid secretion, have a short duration of efficacy, increase gastric volume, and produce acid rebound. Particulate antacids (e.g., magnesium-containing antacids) cause severe pulmonary inflammatory reactions if aspirated and should not be used. Sodium citrate solution is the oral antacid of choice.

Anticholinergic agents, such as atropine and glycopyrrolate, are generally not effective in raising gastric pH or lowering gastric volume. Histamine$_2$ (H_2) receptor antagonists, such as cimetidine, ranitidine, and famotidine, effectively raise gastric pH by blocking acid secretion, but fail to reduce gastric volume. When administered orally or parenterally, these agents have a long duration of action; however, the onset of action is slow, and the potential for systemic side effects exists. Metoclopramide, a dopamine antagonist, stimulates gastric emptying and increases lower esophageal sphincter pressure. Therefore, in selected patients, metoclopramide may be useful in reducing gastric volumes and the risk of reflux.

The combination of an H_2 receptor antagonist administered 2 hours preoperatively and an oral antacid given 30 minutes preoperatively is effective in raising the gastric pH above 3.5. In theory, this regimen reduces the risk of serious lung damage should aspiration occur during anesthesia. However, the efficacy of such a regimen has not been proved in clinical studies.

MANAGEMENT

Once aspiration of gastric contents occurs and lung damage is produced, there is no specific curative therapy. Medical management is supportive and consists of (1) mechanical maneuvers to clear and protect the airways, (2) ventilatory and hemodynamic support, and (3) treatment of secondary bacterial infection should it occur.

Mechanical Maneuvers

In the event of witnessed aspiration, the patient should immediately be placed on the right side in a head-down position. This maneuver may help prevent further aspiration and also may localize aspirated material, thereby reducing the severity of lung injury. Immediate tracheal suctioning should be performed to clear the airways of aspirated material. The stomach should then be emptied of residual contents by nasogastric tube. Should aspiration continue despite these maneuvers, or if the patient appears to be at high risk for repeat aspiration (e.g., altered mental status), the trachea should be intubated with a high-volume, low-pressure cuffed endotracheal tube. This helps protect the airway and facilitates tracheal suctioning.

In certain patients, emergency fiberoptic bronchoscopy may play an important role as an adjunct to routine tracheal suctioning. Patients in whom solid particle aspiration is strongly suspected and who show persistent evidence of airway obstruction despite tracheal suctioning may benefit from diagnostic fiberoptic bronchoscopy. If impacted solid particles are seen, they often can be removed by the use of a retrieval basket during bronchoscopy. A rigid bronchoscope may be needed for removal of larger particles.

Lung lavage with saline or bicarbonate solutions was employed in the past in an effort to reduce lung injury. This procedure has been shown to be ineffective because of the rapidity with which acid-induced lung injury occurs. This, lung lavage plays no role in the modern management of aspiration and is potentially hazardous to the patient.

Ventilatory and Hemodynamic Support

Hypoxemia develops rapidly after significant aspiration. Therefore, all patients should receive supplemental oxygen. Supplemental oxygen should be delivered by face mask at a concentration of 40 to 50 percent. An arterial blood gas reading should be obtained after 10 to 15 minutes of oxygen administration to ensure adequate oxygenation. The PaO_2 should be maintained above 60 mm Hg. In most cases, this level provides adequate tissue oxygenation.

Patients sustaining massive aspiration may experience severe respiratory distress and require endotracheal intubation and mechanical ventilation. Indications to begin mechanical ventilation include (1) hypoxemia (i.e., $PaCO_2$ less than 55 mm Hg) that is unresponsive to nontoxic levels of oxygen (i.e., FIO_2 of less than 0.6); (2) hypercapnea (i.e., $PaCO_2$ greater than 45 mm Hg) with respiratory acidosis (i.e., pH less than 7.32); (3) inability of the patient to protect the upper airway; (4) apnea or a respiratory rate of more than 30 to 35 breaths per minute; (5) severe bronchospasm unresponsive to inhaled bronchodilators or intravenous aminophylline; and (6) hypotension unresponsive to intravenous fluid infusion. In this setting, prompt institution of mechanical ventilatory support is critical. A delay in instituting appropriate supportive measures increases the risk of death.

The patient should be placed on a volume ventilator with a tidal volume of 10 to 15 ml per kilogram of body weight. Synchronized intermittent mandatory ventilation with initial ventilatory rates of 12 to 16 breaths per minute and an initial FIO_2 of 0.5 to 0.6 should be selected. Periodic readings of arterial blood gases should be obtained to assure the adequacy of oxygenation and ventilation. One initial goal in ventilation is to obtain a PaO_2 of greater than 60 mm Hg with an FIO_2 of less than 0.6. This diminishes the risk of pulmonary oxygen toxicity.

Positive end-expiratory pressure (PEEP) is indicated in patients requiring high FIO_2 to maintain adequate oxygenation. PEEP helps to reduce alveolar collapse, thus providing improved oxygenation by the normalization of $V/\dot{Q}$ relationships. The optimal amount of PEEP is that level which produces maximal reduction in venous admixture without substantially reducing cardiac output. The pulmonary capillary wedge pressure and the cardiac output should be monitored by pulmonary artery catheterization if more than 10 cm water pressure of PEEP is required. PEEP increases mean airway pressures and therefore predisposes the patient to barotrauma. Careful observation for the development of pneumothorax or subcutaneous and mediastinal emphysema is critical because these can be life-threatening.

Systemic arterial hypotension may develop following massive aspiration. This is hypothesized to occur because of intravascular volume depletion which results from a shift of intravascular fluid into the air spaces of the lungs. Aggressive intravascular volume repletion with crystalloid (normal saline or Ringer's lactate solution) or colloid (fresh frozen plasma or albumin) solutions is indicated in hypotensive patients. Fluid balance is critical in seriously ill patients and often difficult to assess adequately on clinical grounds. Pulmonary artery catheterization may be indicated to guide fluid therapy and to avoid volume overload.

Antimicrobial Therapy

Bacterial infection plays no role in the initial pathophysiology of gastric aspiration. However, the aspiration injury damages the lung's normal defense mechanisms and greatly increases susceptibility to infection. Secondary bacterial infection is common following aspiration and usually develops 48 to 72 hours after the aspiration episode. Prophylactic antibiotic administration before there is evidence of bacterial infection should be avoided. Antibiotics have not been shown to alter the risk, severity, or outcome of subsequent infections and may select out resistant organisms.

Patients should be monitored closely for signs of development of bacterial pneumonia. These signs include (1) onset or exacerbation of fever, (2) new or expanding infiltrates observed on chest films more than 36 to 48 hours after aspiration, (3) new or increasing leukocytosis with a shift toward immature granulocytes, (4) development of purulent sputum, (5) sputum cultures positive for pathogenic bacteria, (6) a positive Gram stain of sputum smear, (7) progressive hypoxemia, or (8) unexplained clinical deterioration. Because of the high rate of contamination of sputum cultures by oral flora and the frequent bacterial colonization of the trachea in intubated patients, the Gram stain of the sputum is more helpful in detecting bacterial infection than sputum cultures.

Once signs of bacterial infection have developed, appropriate antibiotics should be administered promptly after obtaining appropriate material (e.g., blood, sputum) for culture. Selection of antibiotics should be based initially upon the appearance of the sputum Gram stain and knowledge of the most common causative organisms.

Most community-acquired postaspiration bacterial pleuropulmonary infections are oropharyngeal anaerobes and aerobic gram-positive cocci. Hospital-acquired infections and infections in debilitated or immunosuppressed patients are usually produced by oropharyngeal anaerobes, *Staphylococcus aureus*, and gram-negative aerobic bacilli. Mixed infections are common and occur more often than single pathogen infections. Community-acquired infections are more likely to be indolent in their presentation and are associated with a higher incidence of lung abscess and empyema than hospital-acquired infections.

Community-acquired infections should be treated initially with high-dose intravenous penicillin G (4 to 12 million U per day). Penicillin-allergic patients can be treated with intravenous clindamycin (1 to 2 g per day). After 5 to 10 days of intravenous therapy, most patients can be converted to oral antibiotics to complete a 14- to 21-day course. Patients with lung abscesses or empyema may require 6 to 8 weeks of therapy. Appropriate oral antibiotics include penicillin V, clindamycin, and amoxicillin-clavulanate.

Hospital-acquired infections require treatment with high-dose intravenous penicillin G or clindamycin for anaerobes as well as an aminoglycoside or third-generation cephalosporin for aerobic gram-negative bacilli. If the Gram stain or culture of the sputum shows the presence of staphylococci, the addition of nafcillin or vancomycin may be indicated. The combination of ticarcillin and clavulanate also is effective as a single agent in the treatment of hospital-acquired infections. Patients with hospital-acquired infections are more likely to develop pneumonia than lung abscess or empyema, and treatment should continue for 14 to 21 days. In all cases, initial antibiotic choices may have to be modified on the basis of culture results and the patient's clinical response.

Steroids

Intravenous administration of high doses of corticosteroids has been recommended in the past by many physicians for the treatment of aspiration pneumonitis. The rationale for steroid use was based on the potent anti-inflammatory properties of these agents. However, there have been no conclusive laboratory or clinical studies showing the efficacy of steroids either in reducing lung injury after aspiration or in improving clinical outcome. High doses of steroids may induce serious fluid and electrolyte abnormalities and may place the patient at a higher risk for bacterial infection. Therefore, high doses of steroids should not be used to treat aspiration pneumonitis.

CHRONIC ASPIRATION

Recurrent aspiration of small volumes of oropharyngeal secretions or gastric contents can occur in patients who have esophageal motility disorders, gastroesophageal reflux, abnormal pharyngeal motility due to neuromuscular diseases or tumors, or tracheoesophageal fistulas. Chronic aspiration can lead to recurrent episodes of laryngitis, bronchitis, bronchospasm, and pneumonia, and over time to restrictive or obstructive lung disease.

In many instances, the diagnosis of recurrent aspiration can be easily suspected on the basis of the patient's history. Other patients may present with vague symptoms of chronic cough, wheezing, or shortness of breath. In these patients, the chest roentgenogram may show interstitial infiltrates in dependent lung zones. The diagnosis often may be made by barium esophagogram or esophagoscopy. The possibility of chronic aspiration should be considered in patients with recurrent bronchitis or pneumonia, bronchiectasis, chronic cough, or recurrent episodes of bronchospasm, since it represents a treatable cause of lung disease.

Treatment should be aimed at correcting the underlying cause of aspiration. This may range from medical management of gastroesophageal reflux to tracheostomy or, in more difficult cases, surgical isolation of the airway or percutaneous gastric or jejunal feeding tube placement. Appropriate antibiotic therapy, as previously described, should be utilized when indicated.

SUGGESTED READING

Bartlett JG, Gorbach SL. The triple threat of aspiration pneumonia. Chest 1975; 68:560–566.
Bartlett JG, Gorbach SL, Finegold SM. The bacteriology of aspiration pneumonia. Am J Med 1974; 56:202–207.
Bynum LJ, Pierce AK. Pulmonary aspiration of gastric contents. Am Rev Respir Dis 1978; 114:1129–1136.
Mendelson CL. The aspiration of stomach contents into the lungs during obstetric anesthesia. Am J Obstet Gynecol 1946; 52:191.
Wynne JW. Aspiration pneumonitis: Correlation of experimental models with clinical disease. Clin Chest Med 1982; 3:25–34.

CHRONIC BRONCHITIS AND EMPHYSEMA

NICHOLAS J. GROSS, M.D., Ph.D., F.A.C.P., F.R.C.P.(Lond)

The pathophysiology of chronic bronchitis and emphysema (collectively called chronic obstructive pulmonary disease [COPD]) is complicated and still not fully understood. In pure bronchitis, the major pathologic changes are in the walls of the airways where mucosal inflammation and edema are found together with enlargement of the submucosal glands, sometimes massive enlargement. The goblet cells, which account for a minor portion of mucus secretion, are hyperplastic and extend down to lower levels of the respiratory tract than usual. Chronic colonization of the airways with saprophytes is invariably present, but may be secondary to mucus hypersecretion. These changes, together with variable amounts of mucus within the lumen of the airway, account for the airway obstruction that is present in all forms except "simple bronchitis." Cough and sputum production are their most obvious manifestations. Smooth muscle hypertrophy, so common in asthmatic airways, is absent or minor. The obstruction involves airways of all sizes, although the small airway changes probably result in most of the physiologic disturbances.

The typical bronchitic patient has moderate to severe increases in airways resistance, but less dramatic increases in lung volumes or decreases in gas transfer capacity. There is moderate to severe hypoxemia, sometimes with hypercapnia (i.e., hypoventilation), in addition to the ventilation-perfusion inequality found universally in patients with COPD. Largely because of this combination of blood gas abnormalities, bronchitic patients have a propensity for cor pulmonale and a poor prognosis.

Pure emphysema represents the other end of the spectrum. In this disease, the primary abnormality is thought to be in the parenchyma, where destruction and disappearance of alveolar septa lead to the coalescence of adjacent alveoli into enlarged terminal airspaces—the cardinal histologic feature of emphysema. The loss of alveolar septa also results in a loss of radial traction on small airways. The small, untethered airways tend to collapse; they close prematurely during expiration and trap air in the more distal airspaces they serve. Lung volume increases, particularly residual volume, both as a consequence of premature airway closure and to compensate for the loss of lung recoil by tending to maintain radial traction on the small airways. The intrinsic structure of the airway walls is otherwise relatively normal.

Because breathing is carried out at high lung volumes and there is an increase in wasted ventilation, dyspnea is a prominent symptom. Gas exchange is impaired partly because of a reduction in the surface area of the gas exchange membrane. This reduction is a result of the destruction of alveoli. Ventilation-perfusion inequality is marked, but hypoventilation is uncommon. Typically, arterial hypoxemia is not as severe as in the pure bronchitic patient, so complications such as cor pulmonale are absent, at least until the terminal period of the disease.

It is important to recognize that most patients have features of both disorders. Although chronic irritation of the airways, caused by air pollution or, more importantly, smoking, is almost a sine qua non of these conditions, the precise mechanisms are not clear. Nor is it understood why some smokers predominantly develop chronic bronchitis, some predominantly develop emphysema, and some develop neither.

CLINICAL PRESENTATION

A combination of cough, sputum production, and dyspnea in a chronic cigarette smoker, aged about 50 years or older, is usually all one needs to make the diagnosis of COPD in the absence of other specific causes, such as pulmonary tuberculosis or lung cancer. The major differential diagnosis is bronchial asthma, but in my view this is largely an academic question, because the management of both asthma and COPD is essentially empirical and differs only in emphasis. The distinction becomes important mainly when one is considering basic mechanisms or epidemiology.

A chest roentgenogram and spirometry (forced expiratory volume in 1 second [FEV_1] and forced vital capacity [FVC] before and after use of an inhaled bronchodilator) constitute an essential and minimal data base. More detailed pulmonary function tests (lung volumes, diffusion capacity, and so forth) add to the evaluation of functional disturbance, but the FEV_1 provides the most useful index of disease severity, prognosis, and response to therapy. Arterial blood gas measurements obtained when the patient is relatively well are most helpful if complications occur later. Gross examination of the sputum, both its amount and quality, provides useful clues to the presence of infection. I perform microscopic examination of a smear only when the sputum is visibly abnormal. There are almost always numerous white blood cells and organisms consistent in appearance with *Streptococcus pneumoniae* and *Haemophilus* species, but the major purpose of microscopy is identification of other pathogens, such as *Staphylococcus* species or coliform gram-negative organisms. Sputum culture is misleading and unnecessary unless other microorganisms have been seen on the Gram stain. Other laboratory tests that are occasionally indicated are the $alpha_1$-antitrypsin level and phenotype and the sweat chloride tests.

MANAGEMENT

Smoking

Smoking is not only the most important etiologic factor; more important, it is responsible for much of the patient's current symptoms and continued deterioration. Patients who are still smoking are those who can be helped the most, because no therapy is as beneficial as cessation of smoking. Not only does this usually ameliorate the present symptoms; it reduces the rate of future decline in pulmonary function. In this sense, the stable door has never shut for the smoker. One should not assume that patients are fully aware of the health hazards of continued smoking.

For those who have difficulty stopping, smoking cessation can be aided by smoking cessation programs. Most regional chapters of the American Lung Association have such programs or can provide referral to a local smoking cessation clinic. Many can provide kits that include nicotine chewing gum to aid the patient through the initial weeks. A clonidine patch may also help in smoking cessation.

Other Irritants

Other forms of air pollution, such as in the workplace, may be important, particularly for those who work or live close to heavy industrial plants in the Rust Belt. One should inquire and counsel patients about these irritants, but one must not allow consideration of environmental factors to deflect the patient from the need to stop smoking. However polluted the environment, smoking is a far more potent etiologic factor.

Bronchodilators

Although patients with COPD do not respond to bronchodilators as dramatically as do asthmatic patients, some increase in the FEV_1 and a reduction in dyspnea are nearly always achieved by the administration of bronchodilator agents, which, except in relatively mild cases, are best given as regular maintenance therapy.

A word concerning the route of administration: the metered-dose inhaler (MDI) form is convenient, inexpensive, and therapeutically appropriate because it delivers the agent directly to the site where its action is needed. This route minimizes the dose, the time preceding onset of action, and the systemic side effects, and it is the preferred route. If this method is chosen, it is important to ensure that the patient uses the MDI correctly. Briefly, the MDI should be shaken, held a few inches in front of the mouth with a spacer (if available), and actuated at the beginning of inspiration. Inspiration should be slow and start at about the functional residual capacity ("a normal breathing position" is what I say to my patients). Inspiration should continue to the total lung capacity, at which point the breath is held for a few seconds before slow expiration. It is helpful to rehearse the patient through the maneuver and to observe him or her from time to time during follow-up because many patients do not use their MDI correctly. The clinic nurse can be invaluable for this purpose.

Solutions of many bronchodilators are also available for nebulization. Their main use is for patients with acute dyspnea or for those who lack coordination. Oral forms ensure intake of the drug, may be longer acting, and may have effects on small airways, which inhaled medication may not reach.

Drugs

The three drug options now available are adrenergic agents, methylxanthines, and anticholinergic agents. Each has its advantages and drawbacks (Table 1).

Anticholinergic Agents

My own preference is first to administer an anticholinergic MDI for regular maintenance use; ipratropium bromide is the only such agent currently available. Studies indicate that it is more effective and longer lasting as a bronchodilator in patients with COPD than is an adrenergic agent in conventional dosage. Because it is poorly absorbed, ipratropium has almost no systemic side effects and has a large therapeutic margin; there is no tachyphylaxis. However, it is quite slow in its onset of action, so it is best taken on a regular basis. I feel the recommended dose of ipratropium (2 actuations three or four times daily) is probably too low for patients with severe airway obstruction, and I often advise 4 rather than 2 actuations of the MDI at each use.

TABLE 1 Comparative Aspects of Bronchodilators in COPD

	Adrenergics	*Methylxanthines*	*Anticholinergics*
Onset of action	Rapid	Rapid	Slow
Potency in COPD	Good	Fair	Good
Duration	Good	Excellent	Good
Ease of use*	Good	Poor	Good
Danger of side effects	Small	Great	Negligible
Tachyphylaxis	Yes	No	No
Other beneficial actions†	Yes	Yes	No
Availability by MDI	Yes	No	Yes

* Includes therapeutic margin; blood levels need to be monitored; risks of abuse
† Includes inhibition of release of inflammatory mediators, stimulation of mucociliary clearance, inotropic effect on respiratory muscles.

Beta-adrenergic Agents

I use inhaled beta-selective adrenergic agents by MDI as an adjunct to inhaled anticholinergic therapy, either on a regular basis in patients who are still symptomatic despite ipratropium administration or on an as-needed basis in those patients who experience acute dyspnea from time to time. There is little to choose between the various options for MDI beta-adrenergic therapy. Albuterol, metaproterenol, terbutaline, and bitolterol are similar in their actions, selectivity, side effects, and potency. I tend to use one of the first two.

A number of patients take both classes of agents by MDI on a regular basis. There is little evidence that using both provides greater bronchodilatation than either given in sufficient dosage. However, the combination provides the rapid onset of action of the adrenergic agent with the prolonged action of the anticholinergic. In these cases, I advise the patient to take the adrenergic agent first and the anticholinergic agent 5 to 10 minutes later. This may improve penetration of the second agent into the airways.

Methylxanthines

Methylxanthines have enjoyed enormous popularity in the treatment of COPD in the last 2 decades. Although useful, they have limitations and require great care and supervision. Their principal advantage is that the many long-acting oral forms available provide bronchodilatation for at least 12 hours. Methylxanthines also may have beneficial effects on the diaphragm and are mild respiratory stimulants, the latter two effects being demonstrable in the laboratory but of unknown clinical significance. On the other hand, they are not potent bronchodilators and have a narrow therapeutic margin together with serious toxic effects if not used with care. Adverse effects include ventricular arrhythmias and, most important, epileptiform convulsions, which can be fatal. Recently, subtle changes in mood, short-term memory, and sleep pattern also have been described. Large individual differences in metabolism exist; genetic differences in metabolism of methylxanthines divide the population into two groups, slow and rapid eliminators. Metabolism is slower in older persons, in nonsmokers, and in those who use any of a number of other commonly administered drugs, especially cimetidine, erythromycin, and quinolone antibiotics. Metabolism also is delayed when the patient develops cardiac or hepatic failure or an acute respiratory tract infection. Consequently, even when the dose has been stabilized, a change in the patient's clinical status or in the concomitant therapy can lead to toxicity. Therefore, administration should be monitored by blood levels.

In spite of these drawbacks, methylxanthines have at least two important roles in the maintenance therapy of COPD. First, a number of patients seem to derive from them a subjective benefit for which other bronchodilators cannot substitute. In such cases I administer a long-acting preparation in a dose that keeps the blood level at about 10 μg per milliliter. Because of the logarithmic nature of the dose response, this level provides nearly all of the bronchodilatation achievable at the maximal permissible blood level (20 μg per milliliter), yet provides some margin for changes in theophylline metabolism. The dose that results in a blood level of 10 μg per milliliter should be based on feedback from the laboratory, but is usually achieved by a maintenance dosage of a long-acting preparation of about 10 mg per kilogram per day, which is given in two divided doses per day. Blood levels should be checked 2 and 5 days after institution of long-acting methylxanthines, and at 1- to 2-month intervals thereafter, as well as whenever the patient's clinical status changes.

A second role of these agents is in the control of nocturnal symptoms. A single dose of 250 to 500 mg of a long-acting preparation at bedtime minimizes the diurnal fluctuation in airflow that causes many patients with COPD to experience their worst dyspnea in the early hours of the morning.

Many more-or-less equivalent long-acting theophylline preparations are available. I almost never use short-acting preparations except in acute exacerbations, nor do I usually institute therapy with a loading dose.

My usual bronchodilator strategy is outlined in Table 2.

Corticosteroids

The use of corticosteroids in COPD is somewhat controversial, yet many pulmonologists feel that there are some patients who derive unequivocal benefit from them. This feeling is supported by objective trials. Such patients experience not only subjective benefit but also an increase in airflow that is occasionally remarkable. It is not possible to predict which patients will benefit on the basis of any tests other than a clinical trial. Therefore, patients who are not well controlled on other therapy should be given a therapeutic trial. I start with 40 mg per day of prednisone for 2 weeks and monitor the FEV_1 and FVC as well as the patient's account of effort tolerance. If there is no convincing evidence of improvement (i.e., an improvement in FEV_1), steroids can be rapidly curtailed. Otherwise, I attempt to switch to inhaled steroids, of which several equivalent options are available. Three puffs three to four times daily are prescribed, and then oral steroids are tapered over the next 1 to 2 weeks.

It is very important that the patient not use oral corticosteroids on a long-term basis because of their many side effects. Osteoporosis, sometimes leading to vertebral body collapse, is perhaps the most troublesome of these effects, but peptic ulceration, weight gain, fluid retention, hypertension, cataracts, glucose intolerance, and psychiatric disturbances all occur with some frequency in this older, more susceptible population who continue to need corticosteroids for years. Thus, every attempt should be made to stabilize the patient on inhaled steroids. When these attempts are unsuccessful, a daily oral dose of 10 mg of prednisone (or 20 mg every other day) together with inhaled steroids usually controls symptoms and avoids serious side effects.

In spite of these efforts, a few patients require larger doses of oral steroids, sometimes 20 to 25 mg per day. It may be possible to minimize osteoporosis in these patients by the regular administration of calcium supplements (500 to 1,000 mg per day) and by recommending as much physical activity as possible.

TABLE 2 Bronchodilator Strategy in COPD

Step 1	Ipratropium MDI, 2 actuations q6h
Step 2	Double-check correct MDI use, increase dose to 4 actuations q6h
Step 3	Add an adrenergic MDI, 2 actuations prn or q6h
Step 4	Add a long-acting theophylline, 10 mg/kg/day in two doses, and adjust daily dosage to a blood level of 10 μg/ml
Step 5	Consider a trial of corticosteroids, switching to MDI if beneficial
Step 6	Add or substitute an oral adrenergic agent instead of MDI

Antibiotics

One assumes that the airways of patients with COPD are chronically colonized with relatively nonpathogenic organisms—typically nonpneumonic strains of *S. pneumoniae* and *H. influenzae*. These commensal organisms become more abundant when exacerbations occur, the latter presumably as a consequence of viral infections, which we all experience from time to time. They can be eradicated from the respiratory tract, but only at the risk of substituting more pathogenic organisms, such as *Staphylococcus* species or gram-negative rods. This situation is undesirable. The commensals are, in a sense, beneficial in that they tend to exclude other, more dangerous microorganisms. A rational antibiotic policy, therefore, aims to control their numbers in exacerbations without eliminating them.

Many clinical trials in the 1960s showed that long-term administration of broad-spectrum antibiotics offered no benefit to the stable patient, but that these antibiotics tended to diminish the severity and duration of acute exacerbations. An appropriate policy, therefore, is to administer antibiotics only at the first sign of respiratory tract infection, and to continue them for 7 to 10 days. Suitable antibiotics for this purpose include ampicillin or amoxicillin (2 g per day), erythromycin (2 g per day), or trimethoprim-sulfamethoxazole (one double-strength capsule twice per day). Tetracycline (2 g per day) is used less often than in the past because of the emergence of organisms resistant to it. When these antibiotics fail to render the sputum clear, I favor chloramphenicol (2 g per day), which penetrates well into respiratory tract secretions and has an excellent spectrum of activity. Its major complication, aplastic anemia, is quite rare, and when other antibiotics fail I consider the risk-benefit ratio to be acceptable.

To ensure that the patient receives antibiotics at the first sign of infection, I provide him or her with a 10-day course to be kept in the refrigerator and to be used at the first indication of symptoms. If the amount of sputum increases, if it becomes discolored, or if the patient or someone else in the household contracts a cold, the patient should start using the antibiotic and complete the 10-day course. The prescription should then be refilled and kept on hand as before. I am less concerned about unnecessary use of antibiotics than about a delay in their use when they are necessary. From the foregoing it is clear that antibiotic policy is much more liberal in COPD than in the treatment of other infections.

Measures for Cor Pulmonale

The patient most at risk for cor pulmonale is the "blue bloater" who typically has features of chronic bronchitis rather than emphysema. Sputum production, a tendency to be overweight, and a history of frequent and severe respiratory tract infections alert one to the risk of cor pulmonale. Blood gas abnormalities tend to be more severe and may include chronic CO_2 retention. Polycythemia, clinical and electrocardiographic evidence of right-sided cardiac abnormalities, and an enlarged heart with fullness of the hilar vessels suggest that cor pulmonale is already present.

Oxygen

Long-term oxygen therapy should be prescribed for these patients. Strictly speaking, oxygen is given only to those whose arterial oxygen pressure (PaO_2) is persistently below 55 mm Hg. In practice, if a patient is polycythemic, there is evidence of sufficient hypoxemia over the long-term to stimulate the renal-hematopoietic axis, and this warrants oxygen therapy to prevent overt cor pulmonale. Roentgenographic or electrocardiographic evidence of right atrial or right ventricular abnormalities might also persuade one to prescribe long-term oxygen.

Long-term administration of oxygen is probably the most effective therapy for the prevention and treatment of cor pulmonale. However, if given, it must be undertaken as a carefully instituted program, not as occasional therapy when the patient is dyspneic. It should be taken indefinitely for at least 18 hours every day, including the sleeping hours. Even 12 hours per day is insufficient to provide optimal benefit. The delivery rate is less important provided it is kept low; 1 to 2 L per minute by nasal prongs or catheter is generally adequate. An oxygen concentrator is the most economical source of oxygen over the long term, but large "H" tanks are an alternative. Small "E" tanks or a "walker" unit containing a liquid oxygen source can be used outside the home, enabling patients to continue working or at least be ambulant. The cost of these ancillary sources is substantial. "Transtracheal oxygen," which delivers oxygen at a very low flow rate directly into the trachea through a small-gauge plastic cannula, is an alternative modality that is being employed in several centers.

Additional therapy for cor pulmonale includes administration of a thiazide or loop diuretic and salt restriction. Digitalis and other pharmacologic agents are of limited benefit in cor pulmonale.

Exercise and Rehabilitation

Many rehabilitation protocols have been explored for patients with COPD. Without doubt, patients have a tendency to limit their dyspnea by decreasing their activity. Many have the notion that effort to the point of dyspnea may be harmful to their health and consequently become unfit. This is a misconception that should be dispelled. These patients need to be reassured that no harm will result from exercise or dyspnea. Patients, other than those in heart failure, should be encouraged to indulge in as much activity as they can tolerate by frequent exertion to the limit of their effort tolerance. This will increase their capability over time and improve their sense of well-being and morale. The type of activity to be encouraged is not important. Walking is acceptable to most patients, but routine household activities, such as climbing stairs and cleaning, can be beneficial as well as personally rewarding to patients. Reassurance about sexual activity can be included in this context.

Rehabilitation programs provide a structured approach to the same end, to maximize physiologic fitness. Patients may perceive the setting as being more "medical" and supervised and therefore may be more willing to comply. The evidence from such programs is that pulmonary functions, including blood gases, do not change as a result of the program. However, effort tolerance improves, presumably as a result of physiologic training, and psychological benefits accrue.

"Breathing exercises," which were advocated 2 to 3 decades ago, have not been shown to be of objective benefit. However, there is some current interest in inspiratory resistance training, which aims to improve the strength of the inspiratory muscles.

Other Modalities

Cough medications are of limited efficacy. Adequate hydration is important in liquefying secretions, and patients should be encouraged to drink plenty of fluids. Expectorants have not shown objective benefit, and cough suppressants should be avoided except in selected short-term situations. Humidification of the household environment, particularly the bedroom, may help to limit water loss from the respiratory tract and is probably desirable in cold, dry climates, although this has not been documented.

Surgical procedures for COPD itself, such as bullectomy, are almost never clinically indicated or worthwhile. Occasionally a patient presents with rapidly progressive dyspnea that can be correlated with roentgenographic evidence of enlarging bullae in a single lobe of a lung. Because a rapidly expanding bulla may compromise the function of adjacent lung tissue, its surgical removal may be warranted, but this is rare. The temptation to remove multiple bullae in more than one lobe should be resisted because they always recur rapidly and the surgery is fraught with danger.

ACUTE EXACERBATIONS OF BRONCHITIS AND EMPHYSEMA

Increases in dyspnea, cough, and sputum production, associated with a change in the character and volume of sputum, signify an acute exacerbation. Sometimes, patients also experience fever and have leukocytosis with a "left shift" in the differential count, but this is not universal. Likewise, spirometry and arterial blood gases may show deterioration as compared with "baseline" levels, but they may be unchanged. The symptoms and general condition of the patient are more relevant.

The management of exacerbations, although usually requiring hospitalization, differs from the therapy outlined previously only in the intensity with which it is applied. Complete rest, hydration, antibiotics, and bronchodilators should always be given, although the choice of bronchodilator is not crucial. Some physicians, myself included, always institute short-term corticosteroid therapy; others rarely do. Low-flow oxygen is almost always given unless the PaO_2 is well above the critical range of 55 to 60 mm Hg. Attention should be given to the presence of heart failure, because patients with cor pulmonale usually develop overt signs of failure during acute exacerbations. Management of failure is essentially the same as outlined previously with the possible addition of load-reducing agents. I routinely give such patients low-dose heparin, 5,000 U two to three times daily, by subcutaneous injection while in the hospital to reduce the risk of venous thrombosis and embolism, which is known to be high in this population. Tranquilizers and sedatives must be strenuously avoided

Mechanical Ventilation

The major question in exacerbations concerns the decision to intubate and mechanically ventilate a patient who is in frank or incipient respiratory failure. The decision carries the risk of a long-term stay in an intensive care unit and possibly chronic ventilator dependence. It is among the most crucial decisions one makes, because the financial consequences can be disastrous both to the patient and to the family. The considerations involved in such decisions deserve more space than is available here, but basically revolve around one's assessment of the degree of reversible pathology in the patient. A patient who has moderately severe COPD and develops an acute but reversible complication (such as pneumococcal pneumonia, rib fracture, or pneumothorax) that precipitates respiratory failure would be a candidate for intubation and mechanical ventilation. One who has advanced disease and is approaching the terminal stage of their natural history without another acute cause for respiratory failure would not. Between these extremes there is much uncertainty, hesitation, and reluctance to intubate. The decision calls for one's most thoughtful clinical judgement and is not made lightly.

SUGGESTED READING

American Thoracic Society. Standards for the diagnosis and care of patients with chronic obstructive pulmonary disease (COPD) and asthma. Am Rev Respir Dis 1987; 136:225–244.

Bergofsky EH, ed. Cholinergic pathway in obstructive airways disease. Am J Med 1986; 81(Suppl 5A): 1–102.

Nocturnal Oxygen Therapy Trial Group. Continuous or nocturnal oxygen therapy in hypoxemic chronic obstructive lung disease: A clinical trial. Ann Intern Med 1980; 93:391–397.

Rebuck AS, Chapman KR, Abboud R, Pare PD, et al. Nebulized anticholinergic and sympathomimetic treatment of asthma and chronic obstructive airways disease in the emergency room. Am J Med 1987; 82:59–64.

Sackner MA, ed. Recent advances in the management of obstructive airways disease. Chest 1985; 88(Suppl): 77S–170S.

ACUTE RESPIRATORY FAILURE IN CHRONIC OBSTRUCTIVE PULMONARY DISEASE

ASHOK M. FULAMBARKER, M.D.
ERIC C. RACKOW, M.D.
MAX HARRY WEIL M.D., Ph.D.

When acute respiratory failure occurs in patients with chronic obstructive pulmonary disease (COPD), it is usually caused by an acute complication that compromises the gas exchange. The most frequent cause is respiratory infection. Other precipitating causes are pulmonary thromboembolism, left ventricular failure, spontaneous pneumothorax, respiratory depression due to sedative hypnotic and narcotic analgesic drugs, the administration of high concentrations of inspired oxygen to the patient with chronic hypercapnia, and surgical operations on the abdomen and/or chest. The onset of acute respiratory failure may be suspected on the basis of clinical manifestations (Table 1). Analysis of arterial blood gases confirms the diagnosis.

PATHOPHYSIOLOGY

The pathophysiologic defects of COPD are typically exacerbated. Accordingly, airflow is constrained by bronchospasm, mucosal edema, and airway secretions. The

TABLE 1 Clinical Manifestations of Impending Respiratory Failure in COPD

Symptoms
Unusual change in the amount, consistency, and viscosity of sputum
Change in the color of sputum to yellow, green, or brown
Hemoptysis
Unusual increase in the severity of shortness of breath
Increase in orthopnea
Increased use of metered-dose inhalers
Lack of energy, malaise, and fatigue
Headaches and dizziness
Insomnia
Lack of sexual drive
Signs
Tachypnea and tachycardia
Wheezing or silent chest
Paradoxical breathing
Increase in pedal edema and weight gain
Restlessness and apprehension
Confusion and disorientation
Impaired judgment
Motor instability and slurred speech
Drowsiness and stupor

work of breathing is increased, and this is associated with increased CO_2 production and acute respiratory acidosis. Ventilation-perfusion mismatching also is increased and results in hypoxemia. When sedatives or narcotic drugs are administered to alleviate agitation, dyspnea, and insomnia, the respiratory drive is blunted so that both hypercapnia and hypoxemia progress. Respiratory muscle fatigue also is likely to be present. In the hyperinflated chest, the flat diaphragm and shortened muscle fibers preclude the generation of maximal transdiaphragmatic pressure. This, together with increased inspiratory resistance (load) and hypoxia, increases the likelihood of diaphragmatic fatigue.

The alveolar CO_2 pressure (P_ACO_2) is related to CO_2 production ($\dot{V}CO_2$) and CO_2 elimination, which is contingent on alveolar ventilation ($\dot{V}A$), given by the relationship $P_ACO_2 = K\dot{V}CO_2/\dot{V}A$. Accordingly, increases in $\dot{V}CO_2$ in the setting of decreased $\dot{V}A$ would account for increases in P_ACO_2 and, therefore, arterial CO_2 pressure ($PaCO_2$).

Since renal compensation for chronic hypercapnia results in an adjustment of blood pH at or near normal levels, an acute increase in $PaCO_2$ can often be judged by the pH of arterial blood unless there is associated metabolic acidosis. From a practical standpoint, when the pH of arterial blood declines to less than 7.3 with any level of hypercapnia, this constitutes acute respiratory (or ventilatory) failure. This is typically associated with an acute decrease in arterial oxygen pressure (PaO_2) of 10 mm Hg or more from baseline values prior to the clinical onset of acute respiratory failure.

MANAGEMENT

The primary principles of management include (1) the prompt recognition and early treatment of the precipitating causes of the acute exacerbation, (2) the treatment of reversible elements of the underlying disease, (3) the maintenance of acceptable levels of oxygenation and ventilation, and (4) the avoidance of endotracheal intubation and mechanical ventilation.

Recognition and Treatment of Causes of Exacerbation

Although acute respiratory infection, which is the most common precipitating event, is readily recognized clinically (see Table 1), other precipitating events such as pulmonary thromboembolism and left ventricular failure should be specifically excluded. Left ventricular failure should be considered in patients who present without exacerbation of cough or sputum production. In patients with COPD and underlying heart disease, even mild episodes of left ventricular dysfunction may precipitate acute respiratory failure. A change in left ventricular size and roentgenographically identified redistribution of blood flow to the upper lung fields in an upright position as compared with previous chest films may be helpful for diagnosis. Echocardiographic or radionuclide imaging also may be of aid in the assessment of left ventricular dimensions and function.

Digitalis is best employed only after secure evidence of left ventricular failure has been obtained. Hypoxemia and respiratory acidosis should be reversed before digitalis therapy is begun. Diuretic agents should be used with caution to avoid the risk of hypokalemia and metabolic alkalosis.

Pulmonary embolism is suspect when the onset is hyperacute and associated with a decline in both $PaCO_2$ and PaO_2. Perfusion scans alone are not likely to have adequate sensitivity or specificity for diagnosis. However, a high probability ventilation-perfusion scan, together with evidence of deep venous thrombosis from venous ultrasonography (Doppler) or impedance plethysmography, may be sufficiently diagnostic of venous thromboembolism to justify anticoagulant therapy for control of progressive embolization. When there is a relative contraindication to the use of conventional anticoagulants, pulmonary angiography should be performed to confirm the diagnosis.

When the sensorium is unusually impaired, the use of sedative, hypnotic, and narcotic analgesic drugs should be suspected. A thorough preoperative evaluation and management of COPD patients prior to elective abdominal and thoracic surgery may reduce the risk of acute postoperative respiratory failure.

Treatment of Infection

When acute bronchitis complicates COPD, sputum culture typically yields multiple microorganisms, including *Streptococcus pneumoniae* and *Haemophilus influenzae*. These usually reflect colonization rather than true infection. Although controversial, clinical experience suggests that broad-spectrum antibiotics may ameliorate the acute exacerbation. The oral administration of 250 to 500 mg of ampicillin at intervals of 6 hours, or of trimethoprim-sulfamethoxazole in amounts of 160 mg and 800 mg, respectively, at intervals of 12 hours, is an acceptable empirical intervention. If the exacerbation is due to pneumonia, every effort should be made to identify a specific pathogen. Initial antibiotic therapy should be selected on the basis of the predominant organism observed on the Gram stain of sputum. The antibiotic regimen is appropriately modified, if necessary, when the results of sputum culture become available.

Control of Retained Secretions

Retained secretions are controlled by treatment of infection and adequate (but not forced) hydration. The secretions are mobilized by training the patient to cough after maximal inspiration and by frequent changes in the patient's position. Nasotracheal suctioning may be required for voluminous and troublesome secretions. Chest physical therapy and postural drainage after aerosol inhalation of a beta-2 agonist often helps to improve tracheobronchial clearance. The effectiveness of these interventions may be assessed by the extent to which sputum volume is increased and dyspnea is relieved. Nebulized acetylcysteine and other mucolytic agents are not effective and may induce bronchospasm.

Treatment of Bronchospasm

Vigorous therapy aimed at producing bronchodilatation should be instituted even though the predominant mechanism of increased airway resistance is difficult to determine during the acute episode. Bronchodilator therapy may initially decrease PaO_2 because improved ventilation is not necessarily accompanied by parallel changes in pulmonary blood flow, which results in regional ventilation-perfusion inequalities. Since oxygen is always administered concomitantly, this effect is unlikely to have any significant clinical impact. Bronchodilator drugs, such as aminophylline, beta-2 agonists, atropine, and glucocorticoids, are most commonly used in this acute setting.

Intravenous aminophylline and a nebulized beta-2 agonist are initially administered. The intravenous loading dose of aminophylline is 6 mg per kilogram over 20 minutes. If the patient is already taking a theophylline preparation and the theophylline level is unknown, the loading dose is halved. The maintenance dose of aminophylline is 0.5 mg per kilogram per hour in nonsmokers, and 0.8 mg per kilogram per hour in smokers. The maintenance dose should be reduced to 0.2 mg per kilogram per hour in case of congestive heart failure, pneumonia, or liver dysfunction. The theophylline level should be determined 12 to 36 hours after starting initial infusion to ensure that the value is in the therapeutic range (10 to 20 μg per milliliter) to avoid toxicity. Acutely dyspneic and confused patients may not effectively use metered-dose inhalers. Therefore, hand-held compressor-driven or compressed air-driven nebulizers are used to deliver selective beta-2 agonist aerosols. Albuterol sulfate, 0.5 ml of 0.5 percent solution diluted in 3 ml of sterile normal saline solution every 6 hours, or metaproterenol, 0.3 ml of 5 percent solution diluted in 2.5 ml of normal saline solution every 4 hours, are preferred beta-2 agents. Isoetherine, 0.5 ml of 1 percent solution diluted in 2.5 ml of normal saline solution every 4 hours, also can be used. Atropine sulfate, 0.02 mg per kilogram, aerosolized in a fluid volume of 2 to 3 ml every 4 to 6 hours, can reverse bronchospasm in some patients who do not improve with the combination of aminophylline and beta-2 agonist aerosol. Although data regarding usefulness of corticosteroids in the treatment of an acute exacerbation are conflicting, intravenous corticosteroids are recommended because faster improvement is demonstrated when they are used along with oxygen, bronchodilators, and antibiotics. Methylprednisolone, 0.5 mg per kilogram every 6 hours, or hydrocortisone, 2.5 mg per kilogram every 6 hours, is given intravenously for 72 hours. Once the patient is stabilized, aminophylline and corticosteroids can be given orally, and use of metered-dose inhalers can be resumed instead of compressor-driven nebulizers.

Oxygen Therapy

Severe hypoxemia is potentially fatal and must be corrected by supplemental oxygen. Oxygen therapy is tailored to keep the PaO_2 in the mid-50 mm Hg range, since a further increase above PaO_2 of 65 mm Hg removes the hypoxic respiratory stimulus. Oxygen is administered beginning with a fraction of inspired oxygen (FIO_2) of 0.24 from a Venturi mask or, alternatively, although less precisely, from nasal prongs at a flow rate of 1 to 2 liters per minute. Nasal prongs are often preferred because the patient can eat or talk without removing the oxygen therapy. Further increases in FIO_2 should be based on the PaO_2. Even a small improvement in PaO_2 results in a significant increase in arterial oxygen content because of the shape of the oxygen-hemoglobin dissociation curve. The concomitant rise in $PaCO_2$ during oxygen therapy is due to both removal of the hypoxic drive and worsening of ventilation-perfusion relationships. Some increase in $PaCO_2$ is expected and should not be worrisome as long as the patient is alert and the arterial pH is greater than 7.3. If significant hypercapnia and a pH of less than 7.3 are noted, the FIO_2 should be cautiously lowered to achieve a PaO_2 in the mid-50 mm Hg range. Oxygen should never be removed to correct hypercapnia since fatal arrhythmias and death may ensue as a result of severe hypoxemia.

Mechanical Ventilation

Most patients with acute respiratory failure secondary to an acute exacerbation of COPD can be managed successfully without intubation or mechanical ventilation. Intubation impairs patients' ability to clear secretions. The complications from intubation and mechanical ventilation are frequent. Prolonged mechanical ventilation often becomes necessary because of the difficulty in weaning. An awake and alert patient seldom needs to be ventilated. However, a severely hypoxemic and acidotic patient with altered sensorium should be intubated and mechanically ventilated. Nasotracheal intubation is generally preferred because it is more comfortable and easier to secure than orotracheal tubes. A high-compliance low-pressure cuffed endotracheal tube is always used.

Mechanical ventilation is initiated with a tidal volume of 12 to 15 ml per kilogram and a respiratory rate of 10 to 20 breaths per minute. Full ventilatory support is recommended for the first 24 to 48 hours of intubation in order to facilitate recovery of fatigued respiratory muscles while measures to reduce workload (bronchodilation, control of secretions) are underway. We recommend the assist-control mode, with the trigger sensitivity adjusted to the least effort possible without autocycling.

The ventilator rate and tidal volume are adjusted to gradually decrease the $PaCO_2$ to the patient's usual $PaCO_2$ level. Since the patient's usual $PaCO_2$ is frequently unknown, arterial pH is monitored to guide ventilator settings. The pH should be maintained between 7.35 and 7.45. The $PaCO_2$ should not be lowered too rapidly, because doing so may induce metabolic alkalosis, in a patient with chronic hypercarbia. The FIO_2 is adjusted to keep the PaO_2 between 50 and 65 mm Hg. Ventilation to poorly ventilated regions can be improved by increasing the inspiratory flow rate to 70 to 100 L per minute, thereby lengthening the time of exhalation. Positive end-expiratory pressure (PEEP) should be avoided because of the likelihood of hemodynamic compromise and barotrauma.

Careful monitoring during mechanical ventilation is essential. Arterial blood gases are measured frequently until the patient is stable. Once gas exchange is adequately established, the intervals between arterial blood gas determination can be prolonged. Changes in peak and plateau inspiratory pressures at a given tidal volume may help identify changes in the effective compliance of the respiratory system. The patient's weight, electrolyte level, and daily fluid intake and output should be watched carefully, since fluid overload and electrolyte abnormalities are quite common. Atelectasis, nosocomial pneumonia, pulmonary barotrauma, and gastrointestinal bleeding caused by stress ulceration are well-known complications. Early "routine" tracheostomy for airway maintenance is not recommended. The decision to perform tracheostomy should be based not on an arbitrary number of days of endotracheal intubation, but rather on a thoughtful consideration of multiple factors related to the individual patient. Some patients can tolerate endotracheal intubation well for up to 3 weeks.

Weaning

Weaning from mechanical ventilation should begin as soon as the patient appears alert and responsive and there is evidence of improved gas exchange and lung mechanics. Measurable physiologic parameters, such as maximal inspiratory mouth pressure greater than −25 cm H_2O, vital capacity greater than 10 ml per kilogram of body weight, and spontaneous minute ventilation less than 10 liters, are reassuring. However, many patients can be removed from ventilatory support with values less than these. We prefer the intermittent T-piece method of weaning, in which intermittent periods of independent breathing are progressively lengthened according to patient tolerance. This method offers low resistance, stress periods alternating with periods of total rest (endurance), and ability to test a patient's responsibility to assume the ventilatory work load. Pressure support, a recently introduced weaning mode that provides a set level of airway pressure throughout inspiration, appears promising.

It is usually possible to wean the patient if the precipitating events and complications are successfully managed. Patients receiving long-term mechanical ventilation (more than 30 days) are often difficult to wean. When faced with weaning a difficult patient, careful attention to the checklist provided in Table 2 often leads to successful weaning. Ventilatory muscle fatigue is a common cause of weaning failure. It is identified by clinical observation of paradoxical indrawing of the abdominal wall and rib cage during inspiration. Inductive plethysmography offers useful continuous monitoring of abdominal paradox, irregular breathing pattern, and tachypnea during weaning. Fatigued muscles should be rested to regain strength. The assist-control mode with trigger sensitivity adjusted to minimize triggering effort and inspiratory flow rate adjusted to exceed patient effort are important interventions that allow respiratory muscles to rest. In general, the duration of assisted mechanical ventilation should be as short as possible.

TABLE 2 Checklist for Difficult-to-Wean Patients

Minimize work of breathing
Control secretions and bronchospasm
Ensure low resistance circuitry
Identify ventilatory muscle fatigue (paradoxical breathing)
Ensure cardiovascular stability
Eliminate sepsis
Control fever, shivering, agitation, and pain
Provide adequate nutrition
Correct anemia
Correct thyroid deficiency
Correct pH; treat metabolic alkalosis
Correct hypokalemia, hyponatremia, and hypophosphatemia
Ensure adequate rest and sleep
Withdraw sedatives and tranquilizers
Reassure patient and alleviate anxiety
Convey therapeutic plan to patient
Encourage normal activity

SUGGESTED READING

Block ER. Oxygen therapy. In: Fishman AP, ed. Pulmonary diseases and disorders. New York: McGraw-Hill, 1988:2317.

Cherniack RM. Management of acute respiratory failure in chronic obstructive pulmonary disease. Semin Respir Med 1986; 8:158–164.

Marini JJ. The physiologic determinants of ventilator dependance. Respir Care 1986; 31:271–282.

Roussos C, Macklem PT. The respiratory muscles. N Engl J Med 1982; 307:786–796.

BRONCHIECTASIS

JOHN G. KIRBY, M.B., M.R.C.P.I., FRCPC
MICHAEL T. NEWHOUSE, M.D., M.Sc., FRCPC, F.A.C.P.

Bronchiectasis is a dilatation of the bronchial tree, usually with severe injury or destruction of the mucosal elements and cartilage within its wall. It may be congenital or acquired. In acquired bronchiectasis, the ectasia is thought to be caused by extramural traction phenomena due to adjacent pneumonitis and atelectasis, acting on severely damaged airway walls. Bronchiectasis is almost always caused by a failure of normal lung defenses in association with infection (pneumonia) and a failure to clear bronchial secretions. This may be due to primary or secondary ciliary dysfunction, gastric acid or foreign body aspiration, bronchial obstruction by tumor, or the abnormal mucus clearance of cystic fibrosis or allergic aspergillosis. Failure of the immune system (cell mediated, humoral, or both) may also predispose to infection leading to bronchiectasis. These various factors often coexist and are more likely to cause severe, chronic airway and pulmonary injury in the developing bronchial tree of the child. We have displayed the most important interrelationships in Figure 1.

DIAGNOSIS

The diagnosis of bronchiectasis is primarily clinical, and the features of the history and physical examination are well known. Pulmonary function abnormalities are nonspecific and are frequently a combination of obstructive and nonobstructive abnormalities.

We usually perform spirometry, assess lung volumes and diffusing capacity, and in many cases, perform a stan-

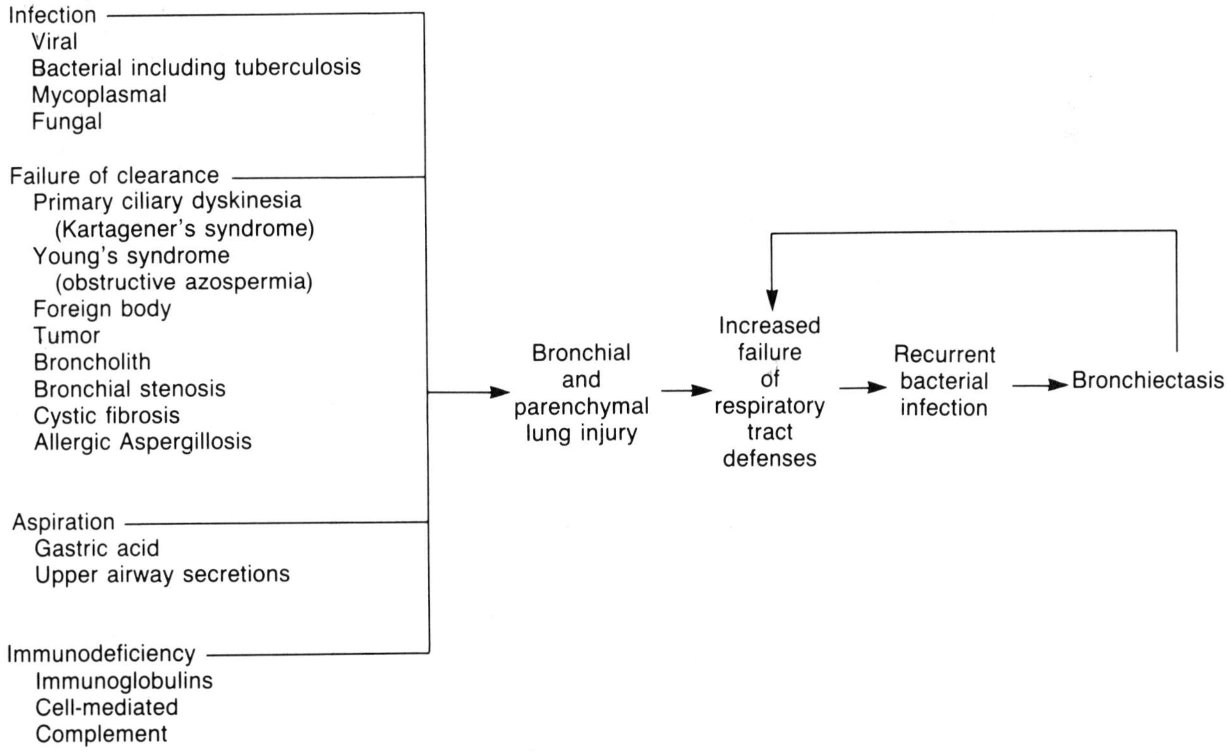

Figure 1 Etiology and pathogenesis of bronchiectasis.

dard maximum exercise study to determine if desaturation develops. The purpose of these tests is to document existing pulmonary function as a baseline for future comparison, detect patterns of pulmonary function abnormality (obstructive, restrictive, or mixed ventilatory defect), and assess whether there is reversible airflow obstruction by the response to an inhaled adrenoceptor agonist or anticholinergic bronchodilator.

The chest film may show signs (ring shadows or "tram lines") that are typical of or consistent with bronchiectasis. However, roentgenographic changes also may be nonspecific or absent. This, once again, points to the importance of the clinical diagnosis of bronchiectasis. Sinus films are obtained to evaluate the presence of fluid. Rubbery brown mucus plugs, blood eosinophilia, and proximal upper zone finger-like shadows on the chest film characterize allergic aspergillosis. The diagnosis can be confirmed with skin prick tests and serum precipitins as well as fungus cultures.

There have been suggestions that computed tomography (CT) of the lung may be useful in assessing the presence and extent of bronchiectasis, although another view is that the bronchiectasis that is detected by CT is also obvious on a plain chest film. At this time, we are just beginning to employ CT in the diagnosis of bronchiectasis, and its use in this condition requires further validation.

Bronchography is the gold standard for confirming the clinical diagnosis and assessing the extent of disease. It is our usual practice to defer this procedure until patients are considered for surgical resection of diseased lung on clinical grounds. We then obtain bilateral bronchograms by means of a transcricothyroid instillation of contrast medium, although some bronchoscopists are now instilling contrast medium through the bronchoscope.

MANAGEMENT

Prevention

Bronchiectasis is often a sequel of severe bacterial (including mycobacterial), mycoplasmal, or viral pulmonary infection, particularly in childhood. The decline of bronchiectasis in developed countries is probably due to better nutrition and living conditions, use of antibiotics early in the treatment of pulmonary infection, and immunization against childhood infections, particularly pertussis and measles. It is a matter for concern that the decline of full immunization because of fear of adverse reactions appears to have resulted in resurgence of pertussis, especially in some developed countries. We strongly recommend full immunization of all children, except the relative few who have the definite contraindications of a severe systemic reaction to previous injection with the same vaccine, ongoing neurologic disorders, or immunodeficiency states.

General Measures

Causes of continuing lung damage or failure of lung defense should be treated, if possible. If indicated by the history, we do skin tests for atopic disease. We also may monitor IgE levels in patients with bronchopulmonary aspergillosis, because these levels may fall in response to effective therapy. We refer patients with recurrent sinusitis and persistent purulent drainage to an otolaryngologist for evaluation and a possible drainage procedure, if chronic aspiration of purulent sinus secretions seems to be a significant factor. After investigation, which includes an upper gastrointestinal series and sometimes pH and motility studies, we vigorously treat patients who have gastroesophageal reflux and aspiration with H_2 agonists, such as famotidine (40 to 80 mg, 1 hr before the evening meal) and peripheral dopamine antagonists (e.g., domperidone, 10 mg 30 minutes before the evening meal), and an alginate-antacid combination, such as Algicon (2 tablets before meals and 4 tablets at bedtime). We also advise that the head of the bed be elevated 6 to 8 inches on blocks; we recommend a light meal before 7 PM and no coffee, tea, cola, alcohol, or bedtime snack afterward. The minority who fail to respond to this regimen are referred for surgical correction unless other contraindications are present. We perform a bronchoscopic examination initially on patients who have hemoptysis, recurrent infection, or persistent atelectasis in one lobe or segment to detect the presence of a foreign body, tumor, broncholith, or bronchial stenosis. We advise an annual vaccination against influenza, pneumococcal vaccine once, and the cessation of smoking.

Patients whose bronchiectasis is a result of recurrent bacterial infection due to IgG deficiency have in the past been treated with intramuscular (IM) injections of 0.6 ml per kilogram of a 16.5 percent solution of gamma globulin, up to a maximum of 20 ml per dose, every 2 to 4 weeks (maximum 5 ml per IM site). Treatment usually starts in childhood and continues indefinitely. Recently, the intravenous (IV) route has been shown to be more effective than the IM route. Currently, gamma globulin is given intravenously at 3- to 4-weekly intervals in a dose of 600 mg per kilogram. The serum gamma globulin is measured before the next infusion. The uncommon reactions can be treated with hydrocortisone, 100 mg IV, with pretreatment on subsequent occasions. However, treatment of specific mucosal IgA deficiency is not possible in this way.

Antibiotics

The most important feature of antibiotic use is individualization of treatment, which remains an art, rather than a science, in the treatment of bronchiectasis (Table 1). Most patients with bronchiectasis have large amounts of chronically infected sputum, usually caused by mixed aerobic and anaerobic "normal" respiratory flora or by *Haemophilus influenzae*, *Pseudomonas aeruginosa*, or much less frequently, *Staphylococcus aureus*. Complete eradication of the airway infection is rarely possible for more than a short period even with large doses of intravenous antibiotic and optimal physical therapy. We use antibiotics for an alteration of the sputum character (puru-

TABLE 1 Antibiotic Therapy

Infection Severity	*Initial Treatment*	*Continuing Treatment*
Mild to Moderate	Tetracycline, 0.5 to 1 g q.i.d., *or* amoxicillin 0.5 to 2 g t.i.d., *or* cotrimoxazole, 2 to 4 tablets b.i.d. PO for 14 to 21 days	Continued for recurrent infection in minimum maintenance doses
Severe	Ampicillin 2 g IV q.i.d.	Continued for recurrent infection in minimum maintenance doses PO
Pseudomonas	Ticarcillin 3 g IV q.i.d. + Tobramycin 1.5 mg/kg IV q8h (normal renal function) *or* ceftazidime 30 mg/kg IV q8h, + Tobramycin as above, *or* ciprofloxacin 3 mg/kg IV q12h for approximately 5 days, followed by 7 to 10 mg/kg PO q12h for 7 to 10 days	Nebulized tobramycin, 160 mg t.i.d.
S. aureus	Cloxacillin 1 g IV q.i.d.	
Anaerobes	Penicillin G 2 to 3 million units IV q4h *or* metronidazole 500 mg IV or PO t.i.d.	

lence, increased volume, or tenacity) together with a change in symptoms, especially increase in dyspnea or hemoptysis. We treat episodes of deterioration individually unless they follow one another at short intervals. Continuous antibiotic therapy then may be tried, and this frequently results in improved well-being, decreased exacerbations, and fewer hospitalizations.

Some recent work has suggested that even patients who appear clinically stable may have an increased amount of neutrophil-derived elastase in their sputum, which damages epithelium, inhibits normal ciliary function, and can be cleared by antibiotics. If confirmed, this would be a useful marker for continuous antibiotic therapy, although it is our practice, at present, to start treatment based on clinical deterioration.

We use amoxicillin, 0.5 to 2 g three times a day; tetracycline, 0.5 to 1 g four times a day; or cotrimoxazole (trimethoprim, 160 mg, and sulfamethoxazole, 800 mg) twice a day orally (PO) for 14 to 21 days. However, the response of the frequently present *Pseudomonas* organisms is negligible. Recently, we have tended to use larger doses of antibiotics because studies suggest that lower doses may not produce adequate tissue levels of antibiotic, whereas high doses result in a higher response rate and a longer period before clinical relapse. Others have cautioned against these high doses because of their effect on the gut flora and the possibility of selecting out resistant organisms. This controversy must await further work on the benefits and hazards of such treatment.

Patients with cystic fibrosis, those who fail to respond to a couple of antibiotic courses, or those who have a more severe initial infection with systemic features usually have a *Pseudomonas* infection. For many years we treated this with a combination of ticarcillin, 3 g IV every 4 hours, and tobramycin, 1.5 mg per kilogram IV every 8 hours (normal renal function), for 10 to 14 days, but more recently we have started using ceftazidime, 30 mg per kilogram IV daily in three divided doses together with tobramycin as above, which has been shown to be more efficacious. The recently introduced quinolone analogue, ciprofloxacin, has excellent anti-*Pseudomonas* activity and is available for intravenous administration in a dose of 6 mg per kilogram per day or for oral administration in a dose of 14 to 20 mg per kilogram per day in divided doses. Some investigators have reported multiple drug resistances associated with the use of this antibiotic, particularly in patients who are immunocompromised and those with cystic fibrosis. The nature of this resistance is not yet fully understood. Infection with *S. aureus* is usually treated with cloxacillin, 1 g IV four times a day for 10 to 14 days, unless the organism is resistant to this antibiotic, in which case we use vancomycin, 500 mg IV four times a day (normal renal function). Sometimes a patient with mixed respiratory flora continues to produce large amounts of purulent sputum with troublesome symptoms. In this situation, anaerobic infection may be responsible, and we use penicillin G, 2 to 3 million units IV every 4 hours, or metronidazole, 500 mg PO three times a day for 14 days.

Previously, intravenous administration of antibiotics necessitated hospitalization, but patients can be taught to administer all or part of an antibiotic course themselves through an intravenous cannula. Recently, another approach in the maintenance therapy of cystic fibrosis has been to use antibiotics inhaled as an aerosol from a nebulizer to reduce the total lung burden of *Pseudomonas* infection. We nebulize tobramycin, 160 mg three times a day, with a Devilbiss D646 nebulizer, but carbenicillin, 1 g, and gentamicin, 80 mg, both nebulized twice a day, have been used by others for prolonged periods of 6 weeks to several months. The poor systemic absorption of aminoglycosides has been confirmed by measuring blood levels, and this approach is likely to be free of the renal complications of the systemically administered drug.

Bronchodilators

There is some evidence that many patients with bronchiectasis may have increased airway hyper-reactivity, although the mechanism by which this might occur is unclear, and in the presence of a component of fixed airflow obstruction, measurements of airway responsiveness, such as by methacholine inhalation, may be unreliable. We rely on the demonstration of an increase in the forced expiratory volume in 1 second (FEV_1) of more than 15 percent after an inhaled bronchodilator. We have found salbutamol, 200 to 400 μg every 4 to 6 hours, and/or ipratropium bromide (Atrovent), 40 to 80 μg every 6 hours, to be useful. In rare instances, we use long-acting theophylline preparations for maintenance, and then only if we have been able to demonstrate additonal bronchodilatation after the maximum effect has been achieved with individualized and sometimes relatively large doses of inhaled bronchodilators. The additional small benefit to airflow, if any, is often outweighed by frequent side effects, especially gastrointestinal symptoms of nausea and gastric acid reflux, which are obviously undesirable because of the risk of further aspirational pulmonary injury. The starting dose of long-acting theophylline (Theo-Dur) is 200 mg every 12 hours; this is increased after a few days to 300 mg every 12 hours or more. We check the serum theophylline level to confirm a therapeutic serum level and to help minimize possible side effects.

We often find that a patient who gives a good history of variable airflow obstruction demonstrates a response to bronchodilator therapy both subjectively and by spirometric criteria. However, if we cannot demonstrate some objective evidence of reversibility after a reasonable clinical trial over 3 to 4 weeks, when the patient's condition is relatively stable, bronchodilator therapy is discontinued or used only intermittently. Nevertheless, there may be an indication for bronchodilator therapy along with antibiotics and occasionally systemic steroids in such patients during infective exacerbations.

Physical Therapy

For raising moderate amounts of secretions, vigorous and frequent self-directed coughing has been shown to be as effective in most patients as formal physiotherapy programs, which include percussion and postural drainage. There is still some controversy regarding the best type of cough maneuver, and vigorous end-expiratory cough (huffing) is thought by some investigators to be more effective than cough initiated at high lung volumes.

However, there may be situations in which a patient becomes ill with an infection and cannot cough effectively. In this setting we suggest that, in association with rehydration, postural drainage supplemented by percussion and vigorous cough may help to clear secretions, particularly if these are copious. The relative merits of manual percussion versus mechanical vibration have been reviewed by Wanner.

We are not convinced that there is evidence to justify the use of oral or inhaled mucolytic agents, and we do not use them.

Allergic Aspergillosis

Bronchiectasis caused by allergic bronchopulmonary aspergillosis occurs almost invariably in asthmatics of long standing whose clinical features of airflow obstruction, mucus plugging, and mainly upper lobe patchy atelectasis respond to therapy with systemic steroids, but in whom antifungal agents are of no value. We usually start such patients on prednisone, 0.5 mg per kilogram, and continue this until symptoms, spirometry, lung volumes, and the roentgenogram approach normal or plateau. Prednisone then is gradually decreased by 5 mg a week until a minimum maintenance dose is achieved. To minimize adrenal suppression, alternate-day therapy is used for maintenance whenever possible. Although beclomethasone aerosol has not previously been effective, the newer high-dose formulations in dosages of up to 2 mg per day might provide a useful systemic steroid-sparing strategy. Such large doses should always be given via an add-on device, such as the Aerochamber, which reduces the total body dose of steroid by 75 percent and greatly decreases local side effects such as hoarseness and oral candidiasis.

Surgery and Other Measures

The clinical criteria for removing the bronchiectatic area of lung have changed somewhat in the last 20 years. We recommend surgery if bronchiectasis is confined to one lobe and the patient experiences recurrent severe infection, frequent severe cough and sputum that impairs the quality of life, or frequent major hemoptysis of 100 ml or more that is not readily controlled by antibiotic therapy. We would advise lobectomy for profound or life-threatening hemorrhage, even if disease is not confined to one lobe, provided the patient has sufficient reserve of pulmonary function to avoid becoming a respiratory invalid (assuming that one lung might have to be removed). If pulmonary function is thought to be marginal, an isotope ventilation-perfusion scan might be helpful preoperatively to predict adequate residual function after the planned resection. It should be remembered that the area being removed is usually nonfunctioning, and its removal should not further decrease functional reserve. As a general guide, an FEV_1 less than 50 percent of predicted and a PaO_2 of less than 60 mm Hg at sea level while room air is breathed are relative contraindications to pulmonary resection.

When hemorrhage is profuse or life-threatening, it is

best managed by a thoracic surgeon with measures such as rigid bronchoscopy to identify and isolate the uninvolved lung and to achieve tamponade of a bleeding segmental or subsegmental bronchus with a Fogarty catheter. In the face of massive hemorrhage threatening to cause asphyxiation (greater than 200 ml per 24 hours), selective intubation and ventilation of the unaffected lung is often a prelude to emergency lobectomy or pneumonectomy due to persistent bleeding.

For patients with severe or life-threatening hemorrhage who are not surgical candidates because of severely impaired pulmonary function, the technique of therapeutic embolization by selective bronchial arterial catheterization usually arrests bleeding with relatively little risk, unless the arteries feeding the spinal cord are inadvertently embolized, resulting in neurologic damage from spinal cord ischemia or infarction. It is essential that this risk be explained to the patient before hand and that written consent be obtained. The risk of cord injury can be minimized by injecting a small bolus of contrast material to visualize the vessels before Gelfoam is injected.

On occasion, we have had some success using irradiation to an area of lung from which recurrent severe hemorrhage originated, but where bronchial artery catheterization could not be achieved. The dose of radiation we used was 2,000 rad in two divided doses one week apart, but we would suggest discussion with a radiotherapist to assess the needs of an individual patient.

Frequently, foreign bodies can be removed transbronchoscopically, unless they have gone undetected for long periods and are completely encased in granulation tissue. An open surgical procedure may then be needed to resect the involved area of bronchus or the entire lobe if, as is often the case, there is marked destruction of the parenchyma distal to the obstruction.

SUGGESTED READING

Cole PJ. Inflammation: a two-edged sword–the model of bronchiectasis. Eur J Respir Dis 1986; 69(147S):6–15.

Hodson ME, Penketh ARL, Batten JC. Aerosol carbenicillin and gentamicin treatment of *Pseudomonas aeruginosa* infection in patients with cystic fibrosis. Lancet 1981; 2:1137–1139.

Rossman C, Waldes R, Sampson D, Newhouse MT. Effect of chest physiotherapy on the removal of mucus in patients with cystic fibrosis. Am Rev Respir Dis 1982; 126:131–135.

Sanders CD, Sanders WE Jr, Goering RV, Werner V. Selection of multiple antibiotic resistance by quinolones, β-lactams and aminoglycosides with special reference to cross resistance among drug classes. Antimicrob Agents Chemother 1984; 26:797–801.

Stockley RA, Hill SL, Morrison HM. Effect of antibiotic treatment on sputum elastase in bronchiectatic outpatients in a stable clinical state. Thorax 1984; 39:416–419.

Wanner A. Does chest physical therapy move airway secretions? Am Rev Respir Dis 1984; 130:701–702.

CYSTIC FIBROSIS

ERNEST K. COTTON, M.D.

Cystic fibrosis (CF) was discovered in 1938 by Dorothy Anderson, who reported the clinicopathologic findings in a series of 49 cases, all children. In 1944, Farber linked the pancreatic abnormality described by Anderson to abnormalities of the lung, upper respiratory tract, liver, gallbladder, and upper alimentary tract. Theorized in the 1950s to be a genetic disease, CF has been shown to be inherited as an autosomal recessive disease. Its incidence is 1 in 2,000 live births among whites, 1 in 17,000 blacks, and 1 in 50,000 Asians.

Over the past decade there have been major advances in our understanding of the mechanisms underlying this disorder. It is hoped that this increased knowledge will bring about specific changes in therapy.

MECHANISMS UNDERLYING CYSTIC FIBROSIS

Genetics

Localization of the CF gene to the seventh chromosome was reported in the fall of 1986. The specific gene has not been isolated as yet (late 1988). A gene thought to be the CF gene was sequenced in late 1987, but was found to be normal. Fragments of chromosomes obtained by flanking-marker assay have been shown to have the CF gene and have become commercially available. More than 60 restriction-fragment-length polymorphisms have been located, some very close to the CF gene on chromosome 7. Because of the many probes with close approximation to the CF gene, CF can be identified with 99 percent accuracy in a fetus of 8 to 10 weeks' gestation through chorionic villus sampling. These probes also can identify the carrier state in siblings and close relatives of affected individuals. When the gene is isolated and cloned, it will be possible to diagnose the homozygote and heterozygote state without the need of a relative with CF.

Ion Transport and the Cystic Fibrosis Cell Defect

The electrical potential difference between the skin surface and the respiratory epithelium is greater in CF patients than in normal subjects. Ductal transport and reabsorption of ions, specifically Na^+ and Cl^-, have been known to be different in patients with CF, and the defect has been located to the Cl^- channel. This channel has been found to be patent. Through patch clamping, the alteration in movement of Cl^- in and out of the cell is localized to a possible protein-like gate which may be tied to Ca^{++} cyclic adenosine monophosphate, and possible other biochemical mediators. Evidence now seems to indicate that the chloride channel "gate" defect is the basic defect in CF. The high concentration of Na^+ and Cl^- in the sweat of CF homozygotes results from the impermeability of Cl^- reabsorptionin the sweat duct. The Cl^- impermeability malfunction in the respiratory tissue leads to an increase in electrical potential. All of these effects may be a direct consequence of the genetic abnormality that causes CF.

Biochemical Alteration of Mucus

Recent evidence indicates that mucus from a patient with CF differs from normal mucus only in its lower water and electrolyte content.

Immunocomplexes

The evaluation of 4- to 6-week old infants (see the following section on newborn screening) indicates the presence of interstitial lung disease, as evidenced by perihilar infiltrates without hyperexpansion on chest roentgenogram, and a decrease in specific lung compliance. Auerbach has shown that the prognosis of a patient with CF worsens when the serum gamma globulin is elevated, and there may be improvement in these individuals when steroids are used. Immunoglobulin-G subclasses do not seem to be elevated in the absence of *Pseudomonas* infection, and in the newborn with CF, circulating immune complexes (CIC) and leukotrienes are abnormal.

Newborn Screening

Trypsinogen has been found to leak from the pancreas into the blood of the fetus if the pancreas has been shocked or if its duct has been obstructed. Since 99 percent of all 34-week or older homozygous fetuses with CF have pancreatic obstruction, the trypsinogen, which is detected by radioimmunologic techniques, is utilized to diagnose CF in the neonate. Continued elevation of immunoreactive trypsinogen (IRT) levels during the first 4 weeks after birth suggests the possibility of CF, and a sweat test should be done. Since the IRT test can be performed on the blood spot taken at birth and used to screen for other diseases, the test can be done at birth and repeated at 3 to 6 weeks of age.

For the past 6 years, the state of Colorado has been screening newborns for CF so that it has been possible to establish the diagnosis prior to the development of any clinical manifestations. More than 75 infants have been diagnosed and followed on a 3- to 6-month basis. This study has demonstrated several important insights into nutritional, metabolic, and pulmonary status.

Growth is abnormal at birth and remains so even when administration of pancreatic enzymes has been started immediately.

Early abnormalities are present on the chest roentgenogram and pulmonary function tests before bacterial colonization is present.

Staphylococcus aureus and *Hemophilus influenzae* remain the most frequent early isolates, but *Pseudomonas aeruginosa* has been found as early as 3 months. Genetic typing has revealed that each patient has a specific persistent strain of *Pseudomonas*.

Respiratory syncytial virus (RSV) has been the most important cause of morbidity in the infant with CF.

Infants with low serum albumin levels at diagnosis, despite early correction, are more likely to require admission for treatment of respiratory exacerbations and have a greater frequency of lobar atelectasis.

CLINICAL INFORMATION

Table 1 presents the major symptoms and signs of CF for each age range, although all of these findings are rarely seen in any one person. Clinically, CF has a variable expression, which ranges from the asymptomatic person with only abnormal sweat to the individual who develops lung disease in infancy and is associated with a majority of the gastrointestinal (GI) aspects. Most patients lie somewhere in between.

The basic pathologic lesion is duct or airway obstruction caused by abnormally thick mucus. If the duct of an organ is obstructed, then that system malfunctions; e.g., if the pancreas fails to get the proper enzymes to the GI tract, fat and protein malabsorption results. As can be seen in Table 1, many of these malfunctions start in the fetus, and the significant pulmonary pathology starts after birth.

PATHOPHYSIOLOGY

To date it appears that CF could be the result of three defects:

1. Exocrine cell dysfunction resulting in a thickened mucus, which leads to organ-ductal, and airway obstruction.
2. Inflammation, which exists prior to bacterial or viral insults.
3. Autonomic nervous system imbalance.

Whether these defects are interrelated is not known, and will not be known until the gene is isolated. It will then be possible to insert the isolated CF gene into normal cells and observe the mechanism of the malfunction.

Figure 1 presents a scheme for looking at the progression of the disease.

DIAGNOSIS

The diagnosis of this disease has not changed since the 1950s. The sweat test originally described by di Sant'agnese and refined by Cook and Gibson (stimulation with pilocarpine) remains the only way a suspected diagnosis can be confirmed. However, the test cannot determine carrier state.

The test is simple on paper, but is fraught with errors in collection and analysis. Therefore, it should be

TABLE 1 Symptoms, Signs, and Pathology of Cystic Fibrosis

Age	*Organ system*	*Clinical expression*
34 wks' gestation	Pancreatic duct	Enzyme leak (trypsinogen)
	Testis–seminiferous tubules	None until adult
	Small intestine	Thick meconium, intestinal obstruction
	Sweat gland	Increased low of Na^+ and Cl^-
Newborn	Pancreas and GI tract	Low birth weight, malabsorption of fat and protein, serum albumin loss, increased appetite, meconium ileus
	Biliary tract	Non remarkable
	Airway and lung interstitium	Few clinical signs, abnormal chest film and pulmonary function, possible early colonization with *S. aureus* and *H. influenzae*
Infant	Pancreas and GI tract	Poor weight gain, bulky fatty stools, increased appetite, failure to thrive, albuminemia, decreased serum vitamine E, kwashiorkor, rectal prolapse
	Small airways	Airway obstruction, reactive airway disease, segmental atelectasis. Colonization with *Pseudomonas aeruginosa*, CIC prominent, viral infection a disaster–especially RSV, bronchopneumonia
	Sinuses	Poor or no aeration–rarely infected
	Biliary tract	Large liver
Childhood	Pancreas and GI tract	Same as for the infant, but with the following added: prominent abdomen, poor appetite, occasional intestinal obstruction (intussusception.)
	Biliary tract	Large liver (biliary cirrhosis), increased splenic size with signs of hypersplenism, roentgenographic evidence of esophageal varices
	Small and large airways, pulmonary vascular bed	Obstructive airway disease (60 to 80% have a hyperreactive component), thick tenacious sputum, atelectasis in upper lung fields, segmental bronchiectasis, decreased oxygenation, pulmonary hypertension (hypoxic vasoconstriction), recurrent bronchopneumonia
	Sinonasal tract	Same as for infant, nasal polyps
	Sweat gland	Hyponatremia–heat prostration
	Combined systems	Vitamin deficiency coagulopathy, clubbing, rheumatoid-like arthritis
Adolescence	Pancreas and GI tract	Same as in childhood, with the addition of recurrent abdominal pain (meconium ileus equivalent)
	Biliary system	Same as in childhood, but esophageal bleeding can now occur from varices, fatty live infiltration
	Airway and pulmonary vascular bed	Same as in childhood, but more pronounced: exaggerated ventilation-perfusion mismatch, right ventricular failure from pulmonary vascular bed hypoxic constriction (cor pulmonale), allergic bronchopulmonary aspergillosis
	Sinuses and Sweat Glands	Same as in childhood
	Combined systems	Same as in childhood, plus delayed puberty, poor exercise tolerance, glucose intolerance
Adult	The disease is now similar to that in childhood and adolescence, but has numerous variations that can be explained by the continued insults to the organ involved or by the late expression of the disease. Some of these manifestations that occur more frequently in the adult age range are as follows:	Pneumothorax Hemoptysis Recurrent acute pancreatitis Appendicitis, periappendiceal abscess Cholelithiasis, cholecystitis Obstructive azoospermia Thickened cervical mucus Pregnancy complications Hypertrophic osteoarthropathy

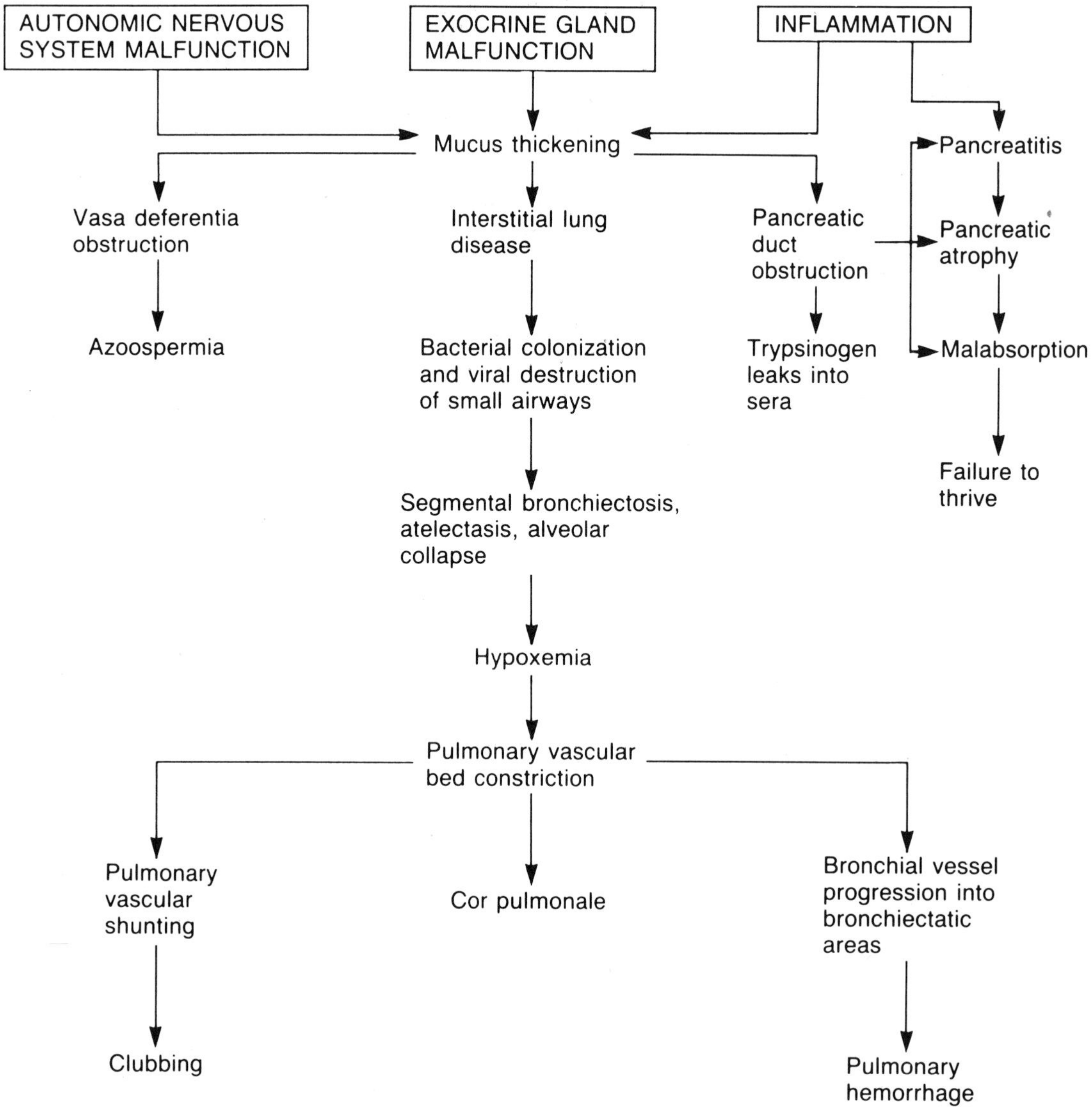

Figure 1 Progression of cystic fibrosis.

performed in laboratories where many tests are done by a specified technician, such as in the CF clinical-research centers. In a positive test, the Cl^- value is above 60 mEq per liter and the Na^+ value is above 70 mEq per liter. When the Na^+ and Cl^- in the sweat of a patient with CF are assessed together, the Cl^- is always higher than the Na^+, which is not the case in the normal subject. The basic criterion for accuracy is collection of more than 50 μl of sweat; 100 μl is preferred. Newer screening sweat tests, such as the disk developed by Medtronics Inc. of Minneapolis, should be considered screening tools, and the diagnosis should be confirmed using the standard sweat test.

Fetal diagnosis now can be made by analyzing gene markers from chorionic villus tissue. These markers are dependent upon having an informative relative. This test is performed on pregnant women who have had a previous child with CF and who are considering abortion. The test is complicated because of the tissue collection, which should be performed only by an experienced obstetrician. There are several genetic laboratories that can analyze the tissue. The results yield homozygote and heterozygote information.

As indicated earlier, the disease can be suspected in the newborn by analysis of the serum IRT, a test that can be performed in many laboratories throughout the United States, Canada, Australia, and Europe. Two tests must be done. An elevated IRT level at birth can be due to pancreatic stress or to CF. If the second test, done at 3 to 6 weeks of age, shows an elevated IRT level, a confirmatory sweat test must done.

MANAGEMENT

No specific therapy exists for this disease. Present treatment consists of replacement of enzymes and nutrients, clearance of abnormal mucus from airways, and treatment of inflammation and infections. Success of this therapy depends upon the degree of pathologic destruction and the intensity and perseverance of the therapy. Frustration exists for both the caregiver and the patient, but treatment, even though nonspecific, has resulted in a definite increase in life expectancy.

In this section treatment is discussed from three standpoints: nutritional and gastrointestinal, pulmonary, and other. Controversial treatments such as mist, mucolytics, and tents are not discussed since they are rarely used by most centers. The reader is referred to the two standard texts (see Suggested Reading) for discussions of their use and for the pros and cons.

Nutritional and Gastrointestinal Management

Pancreatic Enzyme-Replacement

Pancreatic enzyme replacement is the most important therapy offered for the treatment of the malabsorption of fat and protein. The material has changed in the last several years. Originally, the powder obtained from porcine pancreases was placed in a semiacid-resistant capsule, and most of the enzyme was destroyed. The newer material is packaged in wax pellets, which dissolve in an alkaline medium, and the pellets are placed in a semiacid-resistant capsule. With this type of enzyme packaging, the therapy for malabsorption has become more effective. The number of stools per day have decreased, weight has increased, and abdominal pain has been diminished. The number of capsules needed also has decreased. Recently, the amount of lipase has been increased in two preparations, and this has decreased the number of enzymes needed by some patients. The three preparations most commonly used are Pancrease, Cotazym S., and Creon. The dosage is based on the number of capsules needed to obtain near-normal bowel pattern. Capsules are usually taken before meals, but this varies with the individual.

Surgery

Intestinal obstruction exists in about 10 percent of all newborns with CF. The majority of these infants have to be treated by surgery, but occasionally nonsurgical treatment, such as enemas, oral mucolytics, and hydrophobic agents, is successful.

Nutritional Management

In the last 5 years, the nutritional management of patients with CF has changed from a low fat diet without emphasis on calories to one with normal or high fat content and a caloric intake of 1.5 to 2 times the normal requirement. The increase in fat worsens the malabsorption, but this can be corrected by increasing the enzymes. Multivitamins with minerals and vitamin E are used daily. All vitamins have to be water soluble.

Pulmonary Therapy

Pulmonary therapy consists of maximizing an effective cough by chest percussion and drainage, reversing bronchoconstriction by inhaled bronchodilators, and minimizing infection and inflammation with antibiotics.

Physiotherapy

Percussion and drainage (PD) is the best foundation for pulmonary therapy. Twelve positions are used. Percussion is carried out by a cupped hand or by a mechanical percussor. PD is done once to twice daily for outpatients and every 4 hours for hospitalized patients.

Bronchodilators

The airways of patients with CF have been found to be more reactive than normal. Whether this reactivity is related to inflammation, to an abnormal autonomic nervous system, or to allergens is not known. Bronchodilators are effective in reversing the bronchospasm. Inhaled beta-2 agents (albuterol, Alupent) are used prior to PD and exercise. The primary rationale for their use is to dilate the airways so clearance can be maximized. Patients who are older than 5 to 6 years and their parents can be taught to use the metered-dose inhalers. In children under the age of 5 years, the agent is delivered by a compressor-nebulizer. The agents used and their doses are shown in Table 2.

Some patients with CF have associated mild to severe reactive airway disease (RAD). The treatment is the same for anyone with RAD. Theophylline is used, but the dose has been found to be variable because the majority of patients with CF are rapid metabolizers of this drug. As with the treatment of RAD, I prefer to use inhaled bronchodilators.

Antibiotics

The antibiotic treatment for the airway infections that occur with CF is carried out by three routes: oral, intravenous, and inhaled. The respiratory flora in persons with CF generally include *Staphylococcus aureus, Haemophilus influenzae*, and *Pseudomonas aeruginosa; P. aeruginosa* occurs later in the course of the disease. Oral antibiotics basically are effective against *S. aureus* and *H. influenzae* but not *Pseudomonas*. Sputum cultures are important to establish what flora are present, but they do

TABLE 2 Bronchodilators

Agent	*Dosage*
Alupent solution	0.1 to 0.5 ml in 2 ml water
Terbutaline (IV solution—1 mg/ml	0.03 to 0.05 mg/kg in 2 ml water
Albuterol (0.5% solution)	0.02 to 0.03 ml/kg in 2 ml water

TABLE 3 Antibiotics in Cystic Fibrosis

Antibiotic	*Route*	*Dosage*
Tobramycin	IV	6 to 10.8 mg/kg/day
Ticarcillin	IV	200 to 400 mg/kg/day
Ceftazidime	IV	200 mg/kg/day
Ciprofloxacin	Oral	250 to 750 mg q 12 h
Gentamicin	Aerosol	80 mg into 1.5 ml water t.i.d.
Carbenicillin	Aerosol	1 g diluted to 2 ml with water t.i.d.

not indicate what specific organism is causing the symptoms. Whether antibiotics should be used on a continual basis has not been established. I tend not to use them except with clinical signs of infection; however, when patients have chronic symptoms I use continuous oral therapy. Intravenous therapy usually starts in the hospital, but more patients are receiving this type of therapy in the home. The antibiotics used for intravenous treatment are usually directed against the three organisms, even when they have not been isolated. Peak and trough levels are important, especially for the aminoglycosides. The duration of the hospital stay is geared to maximal improvement of the pulmonary functions, which is usually about 2 weeks. Inhaled antibiotics are being evaluated. I have used them in selected cases, such as in patients with repeated hospitalizations or when intravenous access is difficult. The antibiotics used in these patients, with doses and route of administration, are listed in Table 3.

The oral antibiotics that we have found useful are trimethoprim-sulfamethoxazole, chloramphenicol, or a second generation cephalosporin. Usually, the sulfa drug is used first. If symptoms worsen, oral chloramphenicol is tried for several days in hopes of preventing hospitalization.

If hospitalization is necessary, antibiotics are not the only reason for the admission. Vigorous PD, increased nutrition, and oxygen (if indicated) are important in the treatment. No study has shown that one specific treatment is the answer; however, the combined therapy has resulted in a significant increase in life expectancy of the patient with CF.

Other Therapies

Anti-Inflammatory Agents

Anti-inflammatory agents such as steroids have not been proved effective, but are warranted if reversal is not seen in a reasonable period, usually by 14 days. I usually try a 3- to 5-day course of oral prednisone (2 to 5 mg per kilogram per day) and see if a clinical or pulmonary function improvement has occurred. It is possible that effective inhaled agents similar to cromolyn may be available in the future.

Exercise

Exercise seems to be extremely effective in clearing the airways. No specific study has proven it to be a panacea, but most centers are emphasizing some form of exercise in the management of the patient with CF. The best form of exercise seems to be one that uses both the arms and the legs for a period of 20 minutes every other day. Swimming and cross country skiing are excellent, but limited in availability. I encourage any type of activity in which the heart rate and breathing are increased. Coughing usually starts during the activity, and of course this is to be encouraged.

Oxygen

Oxygen therapy is essential to prevent cor pulmonale. I start nasal O_2 when the oxygen saturation falls below 89 percent. If fatigue, weight loss, and headache cannot be explained, then an evaluation of arterial oxygen saturation (SaO_2) during sleep is indicated. Enough supplemental O_2 is given so that the SaO_2 reaches 92 percent.

SUGGESTED READING

Auerbach HS, Kirkpatrick JA, Williams M, Colten MR. Alternate-day prednisone reduces morbidity and improves pulmonary function in cystic fibrosis. Lancet 1985; 2:686–688.

Gerber MJ, Adult cystic fibrosis. Respir Med Pract 1987; 1:1–8.

Lloyd-Still JD, ed. Textbook of cystic fibrosis. Boston: John Wright PSG, 1983.

Taussig LM, ed. Cystic fibrosis. New York: Thieme-Stratton, 1984.

Thomassen MJ, Demko CA, Doershuk CF. Cystic fibrosis: a review of pulmonary infections and interventions. Pediatr Pulmonol 1987; 3:334–351.

LUNG ABSCESS

RICHARD B. BYRD, M.D.

Since the advent of antibiotics, lung abscesses have become both less common and more amenable to therapy. However, in the subgroups of the population who are predisposed to aspiration, especially alcoholics, the problem remains significant. As a further challenge, most of these patients have a history of heavy tobacco use as well, so that the differential diagnosis of bronchogenic carcinoma is often present. A variety of other pulmonary conditions, such as the necrotizing pneumonias, tuberculosis, and fungal diseases, may also have to be considered. Although effective treatment can be expected to cure up to 80 percent of the patients, it may prove a formidable challenge in the chronically ill patient with limited pulmonary reserve. In those who fail with the usual medical therapy, percutaneous drainage with a small bore catheter is often effective and does not carry the risk of resectional surgery.

PATHOPHYSIOLOGY

Aspiration and embolization are the two primary mechanisms by which the lungs become infected to form lung abscesses. It has been shown that scrapings from infected human gums induce lung abscesses when placed into animal tracheas. The bacteria in such scrapings and in aspiration pneumonia with associated lung abscess are primarily anaerobic. This is not surprising since the anaerobic flora of the mouth outnumber the aerobic or facultative bacteria by about ten to one. The predominant anaerobic organisms present are *Bacteroides melaninogenicus*, *Fusobacterium nucleatum*, *Peptostreptococcus*, *Peptococcus*, and *Eubacterium*. All these organisms are penicillin sensitive. However, *Bacteroides fragilis*, which is present in about 20 percent of lung abscesses, is penicillin resistant. Anaerobic organisms are more readily isolated from bronchoscopic or transtracheal aspirate specimens than from sputum cultures.

Embolic lung abscesses are often multiple and account for only a small percentage of those with the problem. Causes that should be considered when embolic abscess occurs are septic abortion, surgical manipulation of the genitourinary or gastrointestinal tract,and heroin addiction with associated right-sided endocarditis.

CLINICAL PRESENTATION

Most patients with lung abscess complain of having had a cough and a fever for a week or even several weeks; an insidious progressive course is the usual presentation. Copious, foul-smelling sputum is eventually produced, with the occasional occurrence of hemoptysis. However, should the bronchus in the area be obstructed, relatively little sputum is expectorated. Pleuritic pain reflecting the usual peripheral location of the abscess is also common. Certain clinical clues should suggest that one is dealing with an abscess (Table 1).Most often, a history of a period of unconsciousness, often resulting from an excess of alcohol or from a neurologic problem such as seizures or a cerebrovascular accident, is obtained. However, the patient may not be able to or may choose not to reveal these facets of the history.

On physical examination, the patient often appears chronically ill with the stigmata of alcoholism and has poor dental and gingival hygiene. Signs of consolidation over the involved area of the lung with associated inspiratory crackles on auscultation is most often noted. Clubbing of the digits is unusual during this antibiotic era, although it can occur after only 3 to 4 weeks of symptoms.

DIAGNOSIS

The diagnosis is established primarily by chest roentgenograms. Although a number of conditions may present with similar roentgenographic findings (Table 2), the diagnosis is usually not difficult when the entire clinical picture is considered. If the films are done early enough in the course of the disease, only the infiltrate of a necrotizing pneumonia is seen. However, for practical purposes, when the lesion is first documented roentgenographically, it usually shows cavitation. An air fluid level, if present, indicates that the abscess is communicating with a bronchus. The walls of the abscess are usually thick and irregular. The most common locations for primary lung abscess are the superior segments of the lower lobes and the posterior segments of the upper lobes, because these segmental bronchi come off directly posteriorly and are thus the most dependent segments when the patient is supine. The right lung is more frequently involved than the left because the less acute angle of the right bronchial main stem takeoff favors aspiration into that side. Although involvement of other segments of the lung may occur with primary lung abscess, the suspicion of other cavitary lung disease should be increased in such circumstances. In any event, it should be remembered that re-exacerbation pulmonary tuberculosis also primarily involves the posterior (and apical) segments of the upper lobes and the

TABLE 1 Pathogenic Factors in Primary Lung Abscess

Factors leading to aspiration
Alcoholism
Anesthesia
Seizures
Neurologic disorders including coma
Esophageal disease
Drug overdosage
Poor oral and dental hygiene
Endobronchial obstruction
Foreign body
Benign or malignant tumor

TABLE 2 Lesions Simulating Primary Lung Abscess

Cavitating carcinoma of the lung, primarily squamous cell
Tuberculosis
Infected pulmonary cysts
Fungal infection
Pneumonia
Staphylococcal
Necrotizing gram-negative pneumonia
Hematogenous septic embolic disease
Pulmonary infarction
Infected bullae or cyst
Vasculitis including Wegener's
Necrotic rheumatoid nodule
Bronchostenosis
Pulmonary sequestration

TABLE 3 Indications for Bronchoscopy in Lung Abscess

Need for adequate bacteriologic specimens from abscess
Roentgenographic clues suggesting underlying carcinoma
Central obstructing lesion
Minimal inflammation surrounding abscess
Hilar or mediastinal adenopathy
Bone destruction
Edentulous patient
Patient without identifiable predisposition who has
Minimal fever
Minimal systemic symptoms
Nonelevated white blood cell count
History or chest film suggestive of foreign body
History or chest film suggestive of specific infections, but which can't be confirmed
Failure to drain with antibiotics and physical therapy

superior segments of the lower lobes and thus may mimic lung abscess.

Sputum smears and cultures should be obtained from all patients. In those with primary lung abscess, the Gram stain shows abundant mixed flora with many polymorphonuclear leukocytes, whereas the culture grows only normal oral flora. If the patient appears likely to have primary lung abscess, no further invasive procedures, such as transtracheal aspiration or bronchoscopy, are necessary to confirm the presence of anaerobic bacteria. Should other pathogens known to produce cavitation, such as *Staphylococcus* or *Klebsiella*, be isolated from the sputum, consideration should be given to treating these if the clinical presentation is compatible with a pyogenic pneumonia of that type.

THE ROLE OF BRONCHOSCOPY

In the past, it was the usual standard of care to do bronchoscopic examination of all patients with lung abscesses to rule out underlying lung cancer. Fortunately, specific radiographic and clinical clues suggesting malignancy are present in most patients who have underlying cancer; therefore, bronchoscopy can be used selectively (Table 3).

Chest roentgenographic abnormalities suggesting an obstructing lesion central to the abscess, mediastinal or hilar adenopathy, or bone destruction are all indications for the procedure. Another important radiographic clue suggesting cancer is a limited, rather than extensive, infiltrate surrounding the abscess. By contrast, the size of the abscess or the presence of thick, irregular walls is not helpful in identifying malignant lesions. Bronchoscopy also should be done on those with no recognizable risk for aspiration as well as those who have low grade fever (less than 38° C orally), low white blood cell counts (less than 11×10^3 per cubic millimeter), and minimal systemic complaints. The procedure also should generally be done in all edentulous patients, because even when aspiration does occur in such patients, primary lung abscess is unusual due to the small inoculum of anaerobic material.

If it is suspected that foreign body aspiration might be the cause of the abscess, bronchoscopy is also indicated. If available, rigid bronchoscopy is the preferred method in this situation because many foreign bodies cannot be removed with the fiberoptic instrument. Another indication for bronchoscopy is the situation in which the clinical presentation suggests mycobacterial or fungal disease, but sputum studies are negative for these organisms. Brushing, washing, and biopsies under fluoroscopic control of the abscess area often are diagnostic when these conditions are present. Reliable anaerobic cultures can be obtained at the same time.

Another less frequent indication for bronchoscopy is the patient with primary lung abscess who fails to drain properly with the usual medical therapy. In these individuals, one may be able to open the bronchus leading to the cavity by inserting an instrument into the area under fluoroscopic control. A coronary angiocatheter threaded through the bronchoscope is useful in this respect. However, the procedure is not without hazard; sudden flooding of the entire lung may occur and can asphyxiate the patient. For this reasons, in most instances, the procedure should be done under local anesthesia and should be approached with extreme caution in the patient who is unable to cough effectively. Another measure of safety is to do the fiberoptic bronchoscopy through an endotracheal tube, which enables the operator to introduce quickly a large regular suction catheter to help remove the large quantity of secretions that may be delivered. In the patient whose level of consciousness is depressed or who has no cough reflex, the drainage procedure should be done through a double-lumen endotracheal tube, which protects the uninvolved lung.

MANAGEMENT

Patients with lung abscesses generally should be admitted to the hospital for treatment. The infection itself is a serious one, and in addition, these patients often are unreliable and have other major medical problems. Hospitalization allows for intravenous administration of high-dose antibiotics, respiratory and physical therapy, and close monitoring for the complications that may occur (Table 4).

Antibiotics

If the abscess is secondary to a specific pathogen, such as *Staphylococcus aureus* or *Mycobacterium tuberculosis*, specific antibacterial therapy for that organism should be employed. However, for the primary lung abscess characterized by mixed oral flora, penicillin is the antibiotic of choice, given intravenously in a dosage of 1 million units every 4 hours. After 7 to 10 days, if the patient has improved and is no longer in a toxic condition, a switch to oral penicillin, in a dosage of 750 mg four times a day, should be made. It is of interest that although these abscesses often contain penicillin-resistant *B. fragilis* organisms, the patients nevertheless usually respond favorably. This is explained by the fact that these are synergistic infections, and therefore not all the organisms must be killed to achieve a cure. In those who fail to improve or in those who are allergic to penicillin, clindamycin is the alternative drug of choice. It is initially given intravenously in a dose of 600 mg every 8 hours. After improvement occurs, it is changed to the oral route at 300 mg every 6 hours.

In addition to the antibiotic, it is important that these patients have postural drainage with chest percussion four times daily. The position required for drainage varies with the location of the abscess. The treatment should continue for 20 minutes or until drainage has ceased. Because of the associated bronchiectasis in the area of the abscess, postural drainage may be of continued benefit even after the air fluid level has resolved.

The course of resolution is often slow; therapy is usually required for several weeks. Chest films need to be obtained no more often than weekly in the patient who appears to be doing satisfactorily. Improvement is first noted in the pneumonia surrounding the cavity; later, a decrease in cavity size is seen. About 50 percent of the lesions resolve roentgenographically in 4 weeks, and 70 percent by 3 months. Not surprisingly, the rate of resolution is slower in those with large cavities. Also, abscesses in the right upper lobe seem to respond more slowly than those in other locations. Antibiotic therapy should be continued for as long as roentgenographic improvement continues to occur. Re-exacerbation of the disease may occur if therapy is stopped prematurely. In some cases, the lesion never resolves completely, but rather evolves into a cyst-like residuum, at which time antibiotic therapy may be discontinued. These cysts do not require surgical removal as they rarely become reinfected.

Drainage

In a small percentage of primary lung abscesses, medical therapy proves ineffective, and the patient remains septic. In this situation, percutaneous catheter drainage of the abscess cavity should be considered. However, one must remember that there is a risk of pneumothorax, bronchopleural fistula, and empyema if a tube or catheter is inserted through a free pleural space into the cavity. Fortunately, pleural symphysis most often is present between the visceral and the parietal pleura in the area of the abscess. If one cannot be certain whether pleural symphysis is present on chest films, computed tomography cuts of the area usually clarify the situation. If pleural symphysis is not present, it should be created, if time permits. This can be done by removing a portion of the rib overlying the abscess and placing a strip of gauze into the area to induce scarring between the two pleural areas. In about 4 days, one can then safely insert the catheter. A No. 10 French catheter is usually adequate in size and appears to produce fewer problems than using standard size chest tubes. The catheter can be left in place until

TABLE 4 Therapy of Lung Abscess

Type	Therapy
Medical	Penicillin
	Initially 1 million units q4h IV
	After therapeutic response, 750 mg PO q6h
	Clindamycin
	Initially 600 mg q8h IV
	After therapeutic response, 300 mg PO q6h
	Continue therapy until clinically well and roentgenographically stable
Surgical	Percutaneous catheter drainage in nonresolving abscess
	Resection
	Uncontrolled hemoptysis
	Abscess not responsive to catheter drainage

the abscess cavity is dry and healing. Patients who are doing well otherwise may even be sent home with the device in place with an attached drainage bag or gauze dressing.

Surgery

In certain circumstances, resection of the abscess may be a more attractive alternative than catheter drainage. The duration of the illness may be shortened by resecting the lesion as compared to catheter drainage. However, this is considered only if the patient's pulmonary function is adequate enough to tolerate resection of lung tissue and if his health is otherwise strong enough to undergo anesthesia. However, if this operation is carried out, it is critically important that a double-lumen anesthesia tube be used to avoid spillage of the abscess into the good lung. Lobectomy, rather than segmental resection, is the procedure of choice because the chance of spillage of abscess contents into the pleural space is less with this procedure. The empyema that results from cutting through the abscess cavity and causing spillage is associated with a high mortality.

Other indications for surgery include persistent massive hemoptysis. In this situation, the danger primarily relates to death from asphyxiation caused by flooding of the tracheobronchial tree with blood. With sudden, massive hemoptysis, the placement of a double-lumen tube may be life-saving by protecting the good lung from flooding and allowing it to be ventilated. With less severe hemoptysis, one may temporize by watching the patient carefully and making some modifications in the treatment. The patient is kept as quiet as possible and given cough suppressants with codeine to avoid excessive coughing. Chest percussion is stopped, and if the patient appears to be actively bleeding, he is kept with the abscess side down. The quantity of blood expectorated should be calibrated on an 8-hour basis, and the bleeding monitored with regular chest films as well to see if the fluid level in the abscess cavity is changing. Close and continued consultation between the medical physician and the thoracic surgery consultant is essential to determine when and if surgical intervention is necessary. In those who are unsuitable candidates for surgery, endobronchial balloon tamponade or iced saline lavage may be tried through the rigid bronchoscope if bleeding persists. Transcatheter bronchial artery embolization also may be considered.

SUGGESTED READING

Bartlett JG, Finegold SM. Anaerobic infections of the lung and pleural space. Am Rev Respir Dis 1974; 110:57–77.

Estrera AS, Platt MR, Mills LJ, Shaw RR. Primary lung abscess. J Thorac Cardiovasc Surg 1980; 79:275–282.

Levinson ME, Mangura CT, Lorber B, Abrutyn E, et al. Clindamycin compared with penicillin for the treatment of anaerobic lung abscess. Ann Intern Med 1983; 98:466–471.

Parker LA, Melton JW, Delany DJ, Yankaskas BC. Percutaneous small bore catheter drainage in the management of lung abscesses. Chest 1987: 92:213–218.

Sosenko A, Glassroth J. Fiberoptic bronchoscopy in the evaluation of lung abscesses. Chest 1985; 87:489–494.

PLEURAL EFFUSION AND EMPYEMA

MAURICE A. MUFSON, M.D.

Invasion of the pleural space by fluid (pleural effusion) and pus (empyema) as a complication of infection occurs in 40 to 50 percent of bacterial pneumonias, but much less often in mycoplasmal or viral pneumonias. It occurs with varying frequency in other infections such as pulmonary tuberculosis and fungal infections, in noninfectious conditions including carcinoma of the lung, cirrhosis, congestive heart failure, pancreatitis, and in collagen vascular diseases (Fig. 1). The initial step in the diagnosis and treatment of pleural effusion is to decide whether fluid invasion is a transudate associated with a noninfectious disease, an exudate complicating pneumonia (a parapneumonic effusion) or other infection, or an empyema (frankly purulent pleural fluid). Early recognition and therapeutic intervention are essential to achieve complete resolution of parapneumonic effusions and empyemas.

ETIOLOGY

Pleural effusions accompanying pneumonia develop most commonly in the course of bacterial pneumonias—mainly those due to *Staphylococcus aureus*, pneumococcus (*Streptococcus pneumoniae*), *Haemophilus influenzae*, hemolytic streptococci, anaerobic bacteria, and gram-negative bacteria—as well as in pulmonary tuberculosis. Pleural effusion, but not empyema, occurs occasionally in *Mycoplasma pneumoniae*, but rarely in viral pneumonias. The predominant bacterial pathogens of empyema are *S. aureus* and various gram-negative bacteria, such as *Klebsiella*, Enterobacteriaceae, *Pseudomonas*, and the anaerobic bacteria.

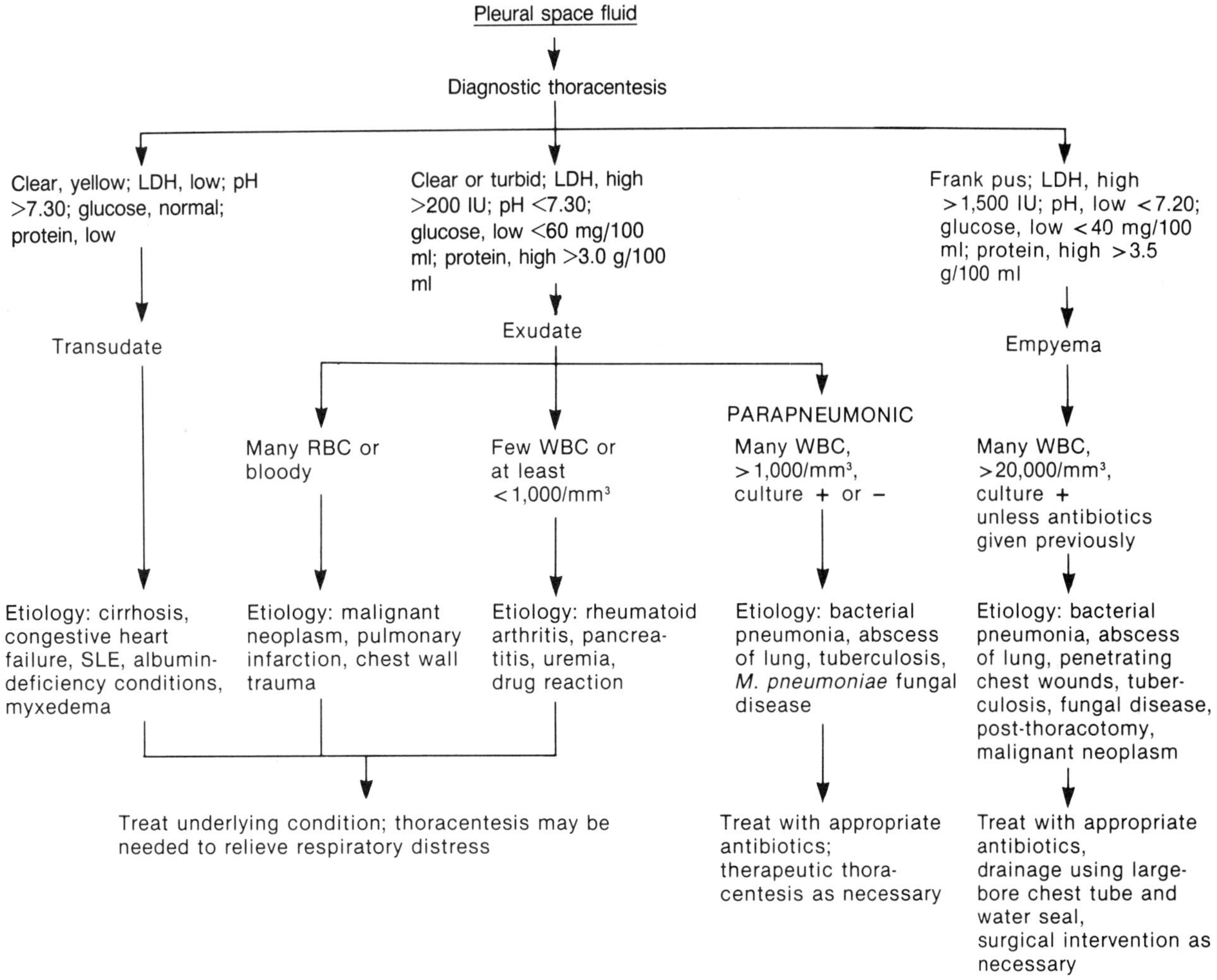

Figure 1 Evaluation, common etiologies, and management of pleural effusion and empyema.

DIAGNOSIS

Physical examination and the upright chest radiograph can detect accumulations of fluid in the pleural space of at least 300 to 500 ml. The characteristic physical findings of pleural effusion and empyema are decreased chest wall expansion; diminished, markedly decreased, or absent breath sounds and a flat percussion note; and, in the presence of large amounts of pleural fluid, a contralateral mediastinal shift. Fever, rapid respirations, shallow breathing, and involuntary or voluntary splinting of the affected side of the chest accompany parapneumonic effusions and empyema. Large effusions can be detected by physical examination alone. Small pleural effusions may be overlooked, however, without the aid of radiographic examination. If the patient is asymptomatic and an effusion is suspected to be small, further diagnostic tests would not be warranted to confirm its presence. However, if the patient has symptoms, e.g., fever, malaise, for which no other cause is apparent, then a thorough diagnostic work-up should follow. Small effusions may be recognized by comparing radiographs (lateral and anterior-posterior films) of the chest that are taken upright with the lateral decubitus radiograph with the affected lung inferiorly. Small effusions should be suspected when the costophrenic angle is blunted or one hemidiaphragm is obscured. However, when an effusion or empyema is loculated, little, if any, change occurs in its configuration in the lateral decubitus position. Small or loculated effusions may need to be confirmed by diagnostic thoracentesis, by ultrasound, or by computed tomography.

A diagnostic thoracentesis should be done in all cases and 50 to 100 ml withdrawn. The tests usually done on pleural fluid include determination of lactic dehydrogenase (LDH), total protein, glucose, and pH; culture for bacteria and other microorganisms as appropriate; Gram stain of smear; total white blood cell and differential counts; a total red blood cell count; and, when available, determination of adenosine deaminase (ADA). The selection of tests should appropriately reflect the list of diagnostic possibilities. Exudative pleural effusions contain high levels of LDH, usually greater than 200 IU (or a level more than 60% of the serum LDH level), total protein values of at least 50 percent of the serum protein (usually 3.0 g per 100 ml or greater in the effusion), glucose levels of less than 60 mg per 100 ml, pH less than 7.30, and a total white blood cell count of more than 1,000 to 2,000 per cubic centimeter. Polymorphonuclear leukocytes predominate in parapneumonic effusions of bacterial origin, and lymphocytes, in tuberculous effusions. The combination of an ADA value of more than 40 IU per liter and a polymorphonuclear leukocyte exudate strongly suggests a parapneumonic effusion. When pulmonary tuberculosis is suspected, a pleural biopsy should be done for identification of the organism by histologic examination and culture. Grossly bloody effusions, however, are unusual as part of infections and usually indicate malignant neoplasms, pulmonary infarction, or trauma to the chest.

TREATMENT

The basic approach to the treatment of parapneumonic pleural effusions and empyema involves therapy directed both at eradication of the infection and removal of the accumulated fluid. The appropriate choice of antibiotics demands that the infecting organism be identified. In the treatment of parapneumonic effusions (except those caused by *Mycoplasma pneumoniae*), antibiotics should be used intravenously and in adequate doses. The selection of antibiotics for the treatment of parapneumonic effusions and empyema follows these guidelines: for *S. pneumoniae* and hemolytic streptococci, aqueous penicillin (2.4 to 6.0 million units daily in divided doses IV), ampicillin (200 to 400 mg per kilogram per day IV), or for the penicillin-allergic patient, vancomycin (0.5 g every 6 hours IV); for *S. aureus*, penicillin for appropriately sensitive strains—otherwise, nafcillin (2 g every 4 hours IV; for *H. influenzae*, chloramphenicol (50 mg per kilogram per day IV); for anaerobic bacteria (except *Bacteroides fragilis*), penicillin G; for *B. fragilis*, clindamycin (300 to 900 mg every 6 hours IV); for gram-negative bacteria, tobramycin (3 to 5 mg per kilogram per day in divided doses IV) alone or in combination with piperacillin, especially for *Pseudomonas* species (3.0 g every 4 hours IV); and for *Mycoplasma pneumoniae*, erythromycin (1 g every 6 hours PO).

Parapneumonic effusions usually clear without drainage procedures. However, a few of these patients may require one or more therapeutic thoracenteses. When the fluid has a pH of less than 7.00 and/or a glucose level below 40 mg per 100 ml, consideration should be given to immediate closed-tube thoracostomy. Complicated parapneumonic effusions and empyema require complete drainage using a large-bore thoracostomy tube. The tube is positioned in the most dependent portion and connected to underwater-seal drainage with continuous suction. As the volume of drainage diminishes to less than 50 ml daily or ceases, the chest tube is gradually withdrawn. Adhesions or a "lung peel" require surgical intervention. When the lung does not reexpand or when a "pleural peel" forms, thoracotomy and a decortication procedure must be performed. Such procedures are necessary in relatively few cases of empyema.

COLLAGEN VASCULAR LUNG DISORDERS

JOHN I. KENNEDY Jr., M.D.
JACK D. FULMER, M.D.

The collagen vascular disorders are a diverse collection of diseases that are grouped together because of common clinical and pathologic features. All are systemic diseases and may involve multiple organs, including the musculoskeletal, cardiovascular, respiratory, and digestive systems. The major pathology of these diseases is inflammation of blood vessels and connective tissue.

Thoracic involvement by specific connective tissue diseases is varied and ranges from chest wall diseases to parenchymal disease. Although the thoracic pathology of some of these diseases is unique (i.e., the rheumatoid nodule), most exhibit a nonspecific acute or chronic inflammatory pattern, and the diagnosis of each can be made only by the clinical features in concert with serologic studies.

In the discussion to follow, an overview of the thoracic complications of each of the collagen vascular diseases and specific treatment regimens are presented, as well as an overview of the general principles of management of the thoracic complications of these diseases.

RHEUMATOID ARTHRITIS

Rheumatoid arthritis (RA) is a chronic inflammatory disease of unknown etiology that mainly affects synovial joints but has a variety of extra-articular manifestations. Six types of thoracic diseases have been associated with RA: (1) pleural disease, (2) necrobiotic nodules, (3) diffuse interstitial fibrosis, (4) Caplan's syndrome, (5) pulmonary arteritis, and (6) chronic airways disease. In general, the thoracic manifestations of RA follow the development of classic or definite RA. In many cases, however, the thoracic manifestations precede the development of clinical joint disease.

Pleural Disease

Pleural disease, with or without effusion, is the most common thoracic manifestation of RA. Necropsy studies indicate that half of these patients have pleural disease, but in practice, it is noted in 7 to 9 percent of men and 2 percent of women. Effusions may be unilateral or bilateral and are generally small and recurrent, although they may be persistent. The pleural fluid is almost always exudative with a high protein level and low pH, and typically it has a low glucose level (less than 30 mg per deciliter).

Management

Most patients with pleural disease may require no therapy. Pain can almost always be managed with nonsteroidal anti-inflammatory agents. If salicylates fail, indomethacin, 25 to 50 mg three times a day, is usually effective. Ibuprofen and sulindac, given in standard dosages, do not appear to be as effective as indomethacin. Large symptomatic pleural effusions should be drained by needle aspiration. If the effusion recurs, a course of prednisone, 35 mg daily for 3 days followed by a rapid taper over 10 days to 2 weeks, is generally effective. Failure to respond or rapid recurrence of the effusion should alert one to the possibility of another underlying disease, such as an infection, neoplasia, or heart failure.

For the rare refractory rheumatoid effusion, tube thoracostomy and obliteration of the pleural space by a sclerosing agent is indicated. Chemical sclerosis can be accomplished by instilling 500 mg of tetracycline with 100 to 150 mg of lidocaine by tube thoracostomy. We recommend premedication with 0.6 to 0.8 mg of atropine. Once the sclerosing agent is instilled, the tube is clamped and the patient is turned every 20 to 30 minutes for approximately 3 hours. The chest tube is then attached to waterseal drainage and, if the drainage stops, removed after 24 hours.

Necrobiotic Nodules

Usually appearing as multiple well-circumscribed lesions, necrobiotic nodules range from a few millimeters to several centimeters in diameter. Necrobiotic nodules are usually pleura-based, but can be deep in the lung parenchyma. Generally, the person with necrobiotic nodules is asymptomatic, but the nodules can pose a diagnostic dilemma in a middle-aged smoker in whom carcinoma must be excluded. Excisional biopsy may be required in these patients.

Management

Once a diagnosis of necrobiotic nodules is established, treatment is rarely required; the nodules generally wax and wane with the activity of the underlying RA. Excision may be required if they cavitate, become infected, or rupture into the pleural space to form a bronchopleural fistula. Large nodules that compromise ventilation or obstruct airways generally respond to moderate-dose prednisone (35 mg daily) for 1 to 2 months, followed by a rapid taper over 3 to 4 weeks.

Diffuse Interstitial Lung Disease

Often termed "rheumatoid lung," diffuse interstitial disease is a well-described feature of RA. Clinically, diffuse interstitial disease associated with RA is similar to idiopathic pulmonary fibrosis (IPF), but it may not be as aggressive. The decision to treat patients with interstitial disease can be made on the basis of objective evidence of progression. Physiologic and radiologic data are preferable. We generally recommend open lung biopsy to exclude more treatable causes of interstitial disease, to exclude more aggressive types of interstitial disease (e.g., pulmonary vasculitis), and to stage the disease accurately. Bronchoalveolar lavage and gallium lung scans have been recommended for initial staging and follow-up, but their effectiveness has not been proved and they remain research procedures.

Management

Once the decision is made to treat the patient, the initial treatment of choice is prednisone, 1 mg per kilogram of ideal body weight per day, or up to 80 mg daily. Treatment is continued for 6 to 8 weeks at that dosage; then the dose of prednisone is slowly tapered (5 to 10 mg per week) to a maintenance dose of 15 to 20 mg daily. Repeat physiologic testing is performed at 6-month intervals; if the patient's data indicate continued progression of the disease, high-dose corticosteroids are reinstituted along with cyclophosphamide, 1.0 to 1.5 mg per kilogram of ideal weight per day. The dosage of cyclophosphamide is adjusted to maintain the white blood cell count at about 3,000 cells per cubic millimeter. Corticosteroid dosage is tapered, as already described, and then maintained at 15 to 20 mg daily. Azathioprine, 2.0 to 2.5 mg per kilogram of ideal body weight per day, is a useful alternative drug. Treatment is generally maintained until pulmonary function has been stable for 1 year, and then both drugs are slowly tapered.

Caplan's Syndrome

Pneumoconiosis associated with RA and pulmonary nodules is termed Caplan's syndrome. Initially described in soft-coal workers in South Wales, this syndrome has been observed in persons with silicosis and other pneumoconioses. Multiple peripheral well-defined nodules that range from 0.5 to 5 cm in diameter are most typical. The nodules develop rapidly and are often associated with subcutaneous nodules. Their appearance often signals exacerbation of the RA.

Management

Generally, treatment is not indicated, although compromise of ventilatory function or cavitation and rupture of the nodules may necessitate surgical excision.

Pulmonary Arteritis

A rare complication of RA is pulmonary arteritis which can occur with or without pulmonary hypertension. In general, pulmonary arteritis occurs as part of a disseminated vasculitis in RA. Several clinical presentations of rheumatoid vasculitis have been described. The clinical and laboratory manifestations of pulmonary arteritis can be identical to those of idiopathic pulmonary hypertension. In these patients, arteritis should be considered because of the underlying connective tissue disease. In rare cases, acute pulmonary arteritis can result in localized infiltrates that mimic pneumonia or pulmonary infarction. Lung biopsy is necessary to confirm the diagnosis, however.

Management

In patients with necrotizing vasculitis, we recommend a combination of corticosteroids and cyclophosphamide in the dosages already described.

Airways Disease

Patients with RA can have chronic obstructive disease of small airways. Pathologic studies have described both bronchiolitis and peribronchiolar fibrosis with narrowing of small airways. Some studies have shown bronchiolitis obliterans with intraluminal polyps of granulation tissue in respiratory bronchioles. In some patients, presumably those with bronchiolitis, airflow may improve with corticosteroid therapy when the drug is prescribed as for rheumatoid lung.

Management

We generally treat these patients with standard-dosages of a long-acting oral theophylline preparation, but we rarely can document physiologic improvement. However, improved mucociliary clearance with therapeutic theophylline could be an added benefit.

There also appears to be a small subgroup of patients with RA who develop progressive small airways emphysema. The etiology of the bronchiolitis obliterans in this disease is unclear, but it may be part of the autoimmune process affecting pulmonary interstitium. However, limited pathologic studies have not shown parenchymal lung disease or mucous gland hypertrophy. Treatment with bronchodilators and corticosteroids is recommended, but often is not effective. We add cyclophosphamide in dosages as described for progressive disease. A severe obstructive defect with ventilatory insufficiency may result.

Drug-Induced Lung Disease

Patients with RA are treated with a wide variety of drugs, many of which have been associated with lung disease. Gold salt therapy has been associated with acute pneumonitis and characterized by dyspnea, fever, and malaise. Rechallenge with parenteral gold salts can precipitate life-threatening respiratory insufficiency. High-dose, short-term corticosteroids generally reverse the acute disease. Uncommonly, gold salts can cause progressive interstitial disease. Lung biopsy in most patients with gold salt-induced chronic interstitial disease is of little value, and a trial without gold and corticosteroids is indicated. We generally use a dose similar to that prescribed for rheumatoid lung. Chest roentgenograms and pulmonary function studies should be used to monitor the response to treatment. If the patient is to improve on corticosteroids and without the gold salts, a 6-week trial generally suffices.

Pulmonary infiltrates, with or without eosinophilia, have resulted from treatment with several nonsteroidal anti-inflammatory drugs (e.g., naproxen, sulindac) and with penicillamine. Corticosteroids may be useful if discontinuance of the agent fails to improve the roentgenograms or pulmonary function. There is at least one report of association between penicillamine and bronchiolitis obliterans in RA; however, the relationship has not been established.

SYSTEMIC LUPUS ERYTHEMATOSUS

Systemic lupus erythematosus (SLE) is a chronic inflammatory disease of unknown etiology that mainly affects skin, joints, and kidneys, although thoracic disease is relatively common. Six thoracic manifestations of SLE are described: (1) pleural disease, (2) atelectasis, (3) acute pneumonitis, (4) pulmonary hemorrhage, (5) diffuse interstitial disease, and (6) respiratory muscle dysfunction.

Pleural Disease

Pleural disease is the most frequent thoracic abnormality associated with SLE. Generally, the pleuritis is symptomatic and coincides with a clinical exacerbation of the disease. Effusions are usually small and bilateral and rarely need therapeutic drainage or sclerosis. Diagnostic tap is indicated because of the high incidence of infection in these patients. Persistent effusions and pain should be managed as in RA.

Atelectasis

Usually basilar and peripheral, atelectasis is a common roentgenographic finding in SLE. Respiratory muscle dysfunction probably contributes to recurrent atelectasis, although multiple causes such as pneumonitis and impaired perfusion of parenchyma also exist. The treatment consists of managing the infections or the respiratory muscle dysfunction (to be discussed).

Acute Lupus Pneumonitis

Generally presenting with high fever, tachypnea, hypoxemia, and diffuse or patchy infiltrates on the chest roentgenogram, acute lupus pneumonitis is a well-described entity. Careful evaluation to exclude an infectious etiology must be undertaken in these patients.

Management

Until an infectious agent is excluded, we frequently treat with a first generation cephalosporin in concert with erythromycin and an aminoglycoside. Simultaneously, high-dose corticosteroids (methylprednisolone succinate, 80 mg every 6 hours) are given. Patients typically improve in 48 to 72 hours, but for the rare patient who does not, we add cyclophosphamide, 1.5 to 2.0 mg per kilogram of ideal body weight per day. Alternatively, azathioprine, 2.5 to 3.0 mg per kilogram of ideal body weight per day, may be used. For the rare patient with aggressive lupus pneumonitis that progresses to an ARDS-like picture, we recommend 3 days of intravenous high-dose cyclophosphamide (5 mg per kilogram of ideal body weight per day) followed by oral (enteric) cyclophosphamide at previously stated dosages.

Pulmonary Hemorrhage

Pulmonary hemorrhage with glomerulonephritis is a recognized manifestation of lung involvement in SLE. Patients generally present with dyspnea, cough, hemoptysis, and bilateral lower lobe alveolar infiltrates. However, hemoptysis may be absent even with massive intra-alveolar hemorrhage. In patients with nephritis, renal biopsy with immunofluorescent and ultrastructural studies is the initial procedure of choice to exclude Goodpasture's syndrome. Once the diagnosis of SLE pulmonary hemorrhage is made, the objectives are to control the alveolar hemorrhage and to prevent irreversible damage to the kidneys.

Management

We use high-dose pulse corticosteroid therapy in dosages of 1 to 2 g per day of methylprednisolone succinate for 3 days, followed by a maintenance dose of prednisone at 1 to 2 mg per kilogram of ideal body weight per day. Plasmapheresis is recommended for Goodpasture's syndrome, but generally is not used in other forms of alveolar hemorrhage. High-dose pulse methylprednisolone appears to be effective in pulmonary hemorrhage associated with SLE, but cyclophosphamide may be used to treat the refractory patient.

Diffuse Interstitial Lung Disease

Interstitial lung disease in SLE is much less common than diffuse interstitial disease in RA; most patients with diffuse disease have had SLE for years. Clinically, these patients mimic those with rheumatoid lung or IPF. Whether therapy can alter the natural history of this disease is unclear. However, we manage patients with progressive disease just as we do patients who have rheumatoid lung.

Respiratory Muscle Dysfunction

A recently recognized complication of SLE is respiratory muscle dysfunction, which may present as lower lobe atelectasis, a restrictive ventilatory defect without parenchymal disease, or as hypoxic-hypercarbic respiratory failure. Diaphragmatic dysfunction may occur alone or in combination with chest wall dysfunction. Efforts should be made to document an active myositis with biochemical, electromyographic, or histologic studies.

Management

Myositis can respond to large or medium dosages of corticosteroids (prednisone at a dosage of 0.5 to 1.0 mg per kilogram per day). Patients may initially present with dyspnea in the supine position. A permanent tracheostomy with nocturnal ventilation may suffice in these cases, but ultimately, continuous home ventilatory support may be needed. In rare cases, we have seen phrenic nerve neuritis in association with small vessel vasculitis produce diaphragmatic dysfunction. Corticosteroids in dosages similar to those used in diffuse interstitial lung disease may be helpful.

ADULT STILL'S DISEASE

Patients with adult Still's disease may develop pleuritis and an effusion. In rare cases, mild interstitial disease may coexist.

Management

Most patients can be managed easily with aspirin or nonsteroidal anti-inflammatory drugs, as described for lupus pleuritis. If there is progressive interstitial disease, its management is the same as that of rheumatoid lung.

PROGRESSIVE SYSTEMIC SCLEROSIS

Physiologic or roentgenographic evidence of diffuse interstitial disease is present in most patients with progressive systemic sclerosis (PSS). Additional thoracic diseases include pulmonary vascular disease, aspiration pneumonia due to esophageal dysfunction, and chest wall restriction due to sclerosis of thoracic skin.

Management

Usually, the interstitial disease of PSS is not responsive to steroids. However, there are some reported cases of steroid-responsive disease, and a trial of prednisone at the dosages used in rheumatoid lung may be indicated.

Most patients have pulmonary hypertension by catheter study; approximately one-third have clinical pulmonary hypertension with cor pulmonale. There have been reports of response of the pulmonary hypertension to vasodilator agents such as hydralazine and nifedipine. Such treatment must be viewed as experimental, but if attempted, should be performed with pulmonary artery pressure and cardiac output monitoring in the intensive care unit.

Aspiration pneumonitis is a potential problem in all patients with esophageal disease. We routinely recommend an elevation of the head of the bed and a delay of bedtime until 3 or 4 hours after the ingestion of food.

POLYMYOSITIS-DERMATOMYOSITIS

Thoracic diseases in polymyositis-dermatomyositis (PM-DM) include interstitial lung disease, aspiration pneumonia, and ventilatory failure secondary to respiratory muscle weakness. The development of interstitial disease appears to be unrelated to the severity or duration of the myopathy and may precede the muscle disease. Clinically and roentgenographically, the interstitial disease mimics IPF.

Management

Generally, corticosteroid therapy is effective in reversing or delaying progression of the disease. When corticosteroid therapy fails, we recommend cyclophosphamide in doses similar to those prescribed for rheumatoid lung.

Pharyngeal muscle disease with aspiration pneumonia constitutes a major problem in patients with PM-DM. Aggressive treatment of the myositis is indicated; therapy with cyclophosphamide may be indicated, but alternative agents such as methotrexate do not appear to be more effective than corticosteroids alone.

In the uncommon case, respiratory muscle myositis can result in respiratory insufficiency with hypoxemia and hypercarbia. Corticosteroid therapy with prednisone, 1.0 mg per kilogram per day, is generally effective.

SJÖGREN'S SYNDROME

Sjögren's syndrome consists of a triad of keratoconjunctivitis sicca, xerostomia, and recurrent parotid gland swelling. Glandular dysfunction appears to result from infiltration with lymphocytes.

Pleuropulmonary involvement occurs in as many as 50 percent of patients and includes tracheobronchitis, chronic nonspecific pneumonitis-fibrosis, lymphocytic interstitial pneumonitis (LIP), recurrent pneumonitis, pleural effusions, pseudolymphoma, and malignant lymphoma. Only the lymphoid diseases and xerotracheobronchitis are specific for Sjögren's syndrome. Lymphoid infiltration of tracheal and bronchial mucous glands results in drying of airways with tracheobronchitis and recurrent pulmonary infections.

Management

Management of this problem involves treatment of infections, bronchodilator therapy, artificial humidification of airways, and corticosteroids. Expectorants are not helpful, but ingestion of spicy foods is said to increase production of mucus.

Lymphoid lung disease can range from LIP to malignant lymphoma or lymphocytic infiltration of pleura with pleural effusion. Benign lesions have been known to progress to malignant tumors. Early benign lymphoid disease is generally steroid-responsive and can be managed with prednisone in the same dosage prescribed for rheumatoid lung. Untreated LIP has been known to progress to end-stage "honeycomb" lung. Nonspecific pneumonitis and fibrosis are managed in the same manner as rheumatoid lung. Malignant lung disease should be treated according to the cell type and the biologic behavior of the disease with the aid of a medical oncologist.

MIXED CONNECTIVE TISSUE DISEASE

Mixed connective tissue disease (MCTD) is a syndrome characterized by an admixture of clinical features found in SLE, PSS, and PM-DM. However, pleural effusions, interstitial disease, and pulmonary vascular disease are dominant.

Management

In general, the interstitial disease is responsive to corticosteroids when treated in the same way as the interstitial disease of RA and SLE. However, there is a small group of patients with severe, rapidly progressive interstitial disease who respond poorly to corticosteroids; for these patients, a combination of corticosteroids and cyclophosphamide or chlorambucil (8 to 10 mg per day) has been recommended.

RELAPSING POLYCHONDRITIS

Relapsing polychondritis (RP) is an uncommon disease characterized by (1) destruction of articular and nonarticular cartilage and (2) inflammation of eyes and ears. The pulmonary manifestations of RP occur as a result of involvement of laryngeal, tracheal, or bronchial cartilage. Laryngeal or tracheal flaccidity can result in severe airflow obstruction with suffocation. Bronchial involvement can result in recurrent bronchitis and pneumonitis with bronchiectasis.

Management

Treatment consists of permanent tracheostomy, if indicated, and bronchodilators with broad-spectrum antimicrobials for bronchitis or pneumonitis. Corticosteroids improve acute episodes and reduce the frequency and severity of recurrences, but may not stop the progression of the disease. Acute episodes may require as much as 200 mg of prednisone daily, but most patients can be maintained on 15 to 20 mg per day of prednisone. Resistant disease may respond to immunosuppressive drugs. Dapsone has been used in doses of 25 to 200 mg per day and compares favorably to prednisone.

ANKYLOSING SPONDYLITIS

Ankylosing spondylitis is characterized by progressive inflammation and sclerosis with ankylosis of sacroiliac joints, spine, costovertebral joints, and occasionally hips and shoulders. Fixation of costovertebral joints can occur, but rarely causes disability. Pulmonary function testing reveals an increase in the functional residual capacity and the residual volume, with a reduction in vital capacity. One of the most common pulmonary findings is upper lobe fibrobullous disease of indeterminate etiology. These bullae are susceptible to the development of aspergillomas.

Management

There is no therapy for the fibrobullous disease. Although amphotericin and, more recently, ketoconazole have been prescribed, their efficacy in treating aspergillomas has not been established. In rare instances, invasive aspergillosis can result and is responsive to amphotericin. Resection or embolization may be necessary for the control of massive hemoptysis.

GENERAL MANAGEMENT

Certain general principles of management apply to all the pulmonary manifestations of the collagen vascular disorders. Current concepts of the pathogenesis of the interstitial diseases are that there is some type of injury to the alveoli that results in alveolitis. Unchecked, the alveolitis progresses to destruction of the alveoli and to fibrosis. The overall objectives of treatment are to suppress the alveolitis to prevent progression of the disease, to treat the complications of the disease (i.e., infection,

TABLE 1 Complications of Corticosteroid Therapy

Side Effects	*Monitoring*	*Precautionary Measures*
Sodium retention (edema, hypertension, CHF)	Weekly weights, physical examination	Sodium restriction to 2 to 4 g
Hyperglycemia	History (e.g., polydipsia), serum glucose level	Weight reduction, Vanderbilt diet
Gastric ulceration	History of gastrointestinal upset, stool for occult blood	Antacids in patients with history of peptic ulcer
Adrenal suppression	Blood pressure, serum electrolyte level	Slow withdrawal of steroids
Osteoporosis	—	Shortest possible duration of therapy
Posterior subcapsular cataracts	Slit lamp examination for visual symptoms	—
Mood alteration or psychosis	—	Use lowest effective dosage
Increased appetite or weight gain	Weekly weights	Caloric restriction (Vanderbilt diet)

TABLE 2 Complications of Cytotoxic Agents

Agent	*Side Effects*	*Monitoring*	*Precautionary Measures*
Cyclophosphamide			
	Bone marrow suppression	Weekly WBC count and differential	Adjust dose to maintain WBC $\geq$ 3,000 cells/mm^3
	Hemorrhagic cystitis	History of hematuria, monthly urinalysis	Force fluids (10 to 12 glasses H_2O daily)
	Nausea and vomiting	—	Antiemetics (e.g., metoclopramide)
	Alopecia	—	—
	Gonadal suppression	—	—
	Potential carcinogenesis	—	—
Azathioprine			
	Bone marrow suppression	Weekly WBC count and differential	Adjust dose to maintain WBC $\geq$ 3,000 cells/mm^3
	Nausea and vomiting	—	Antiemetics
	Oral ulcers	—	—

hypoxemia), and to try to restore activity. Corticosteroids are the mainstay of therapy, but immunosuppressive or cytotoxic therapy is indicated in the more aggressive diseases. Therapy may not restore ventilatory function, but may prevent progression of the disease. The side effects of corticosteroids and cytotoxic agents are formidable, but can be easily controlled if drugs are given under close supervision (Tables 1 and 2).

Preventive and supportive measures are also important in the management of thoracic manifestations of the collagen vascular diseases. Airways disease and interstitial disease constitute an important host defense problem. Influenza and pneumococcal vaccines are recommended, and acute bronchitis should be treated aggressively with antimicrobials, using sputum cultures as a guide. Supplemental oxygen is appropriate in acute conditions when there is documentation of a PaO_2 below 60 mm Hg or an arterial saturation below 90 percent. Long-term oxygen therapy is indicated for patients who have a PaO_2 below 55 mm Hg after being on an optimal medical regimen for at least 30 days. Long-term oxygen therapy should be considered if there is evidence of hypoxic organ dysfunction such as secondary pulmonary hypertension, cor pulmonale, secondary erythrocytosis, or central nervous system dysfunction. Patients who demonstrate PaO_2 values of 55 mm Hg or less during exercise, and in whom O_2 administration improves exercise duration, performance, or capacity should be considered for long-term O_2 therapy. Oxygen should be given at the lowest dosage that alleviates the hypoxemia (e.g., increase the PaO_2 to 60 to 80 mm Hg) or the hypoxic organ dysfunction.

Depending on the type of lung disease, patients are generally tapered off corticosteroids after the disease has been stable for at least 1 year. There are recorded cases in which exacerbations occurred during the tapering of corticosteroids, and for this reason, close clinical and physiologic monitoring must be maintained. In our experience, ventilatory function lost during the tapering of corticosteroids is often not regained once a high dose is reinstituted.

SUGGESTED READING

Eisenberg H, Dubois EL, Sherwin RP, Balchum OJ. Diffuse interstitial lung disease in systemic lupus erythematosus. Ann Intern Med 1973; 79:37–45.

Hunninghake GW, Fauci AS. State of the art: pulmonary involvement in the collagen vascular diseases. Am Rev Respir Dis 1979;119:471–503.

Matthay RA, Schwarz MI, Petty TL, et al. Pulmonary manifestations of systemic lupus erythematosus: review of twelve cases of acute lupus pneumonitis. Medicine 1974; 54:397–409.

Peters-Golden M, Wise RA, Schneider P, et al. Clinical and demographic predictors of loss of pulmonary function in systemic sclerosis. Medicine 1984; 63:221–231.

Schwarz MI, Matthay RA, Sahn SA, et al. Interstitial lung disease in polymyositis and dermatomyositis: analysis of six cases and review of the literature. Medicine 1976; 55:89–104.

Sullivan WD, Hurst DJ, Harmon CE, et al. A prospective evaluation emphasizing pulmonary involvement in patients with mixed connective tissue disease. Medicine 1984; 63:92–107.

DRUG-INDUCED LUNG DISEASE

JOE H. DWEK, M.B., F.A.C.P., F.R.C.P.(E)

More than 40 drugs have been implicated as a cause of lung injury since the first reported case of gold-associated toxic alveolitis in 1945. The extent of the problem is difficult to determine for a number of reasons.

There is difficulty in establishing a diagnosis. Drug-induced syndromes simulate other disease patterns. They do not have characteristic clinical features or diagnostic pathologic criteria. There are no specific markers. The diagnosis depends on temporal relationships of drug use with a clinical syndrome and may be tenuous. It is often difficult to separate an adverse drug reaction from the underlying disease process. The problem is compounded by the use of multiple drugs and other therapies, such as gamma irradiation and high concentrations of oxygen. It has become clear that such agents can be at least additive in producing lung toxicity. Patients receiving many of these agents are susceptible to a variety of infections that can produce findings similar to those seen with drug-induced injury. In one study of pulmonary syndromes in immunologically deficient patients, spread of the underlying disease, superinfection, and adverse drug reactions accounted for 90 percent of the cases. Almost one-quarter of the patients were believed to have evidence of lung toxicity. Twenty percent had two or more separate processes contributing to their lung disease, and 15 percent had no definitive diagnosis even after lung biopsy.

There is limited information on the incidence of disease. The literature is based on case reports and occasional surveys. Reactions may be idiosyncratic or may be dose-dependent. There is virtually no epidemiologic data on the true frequency of adverse reactions.

The lung may be the sole target of injury or part of a systemic reaction, such as vasculitis or lupus erythematosus. The primary impact may be on the lung parenchyma or on the airways. This review concentrates on the direct effects of drugs on the lung parenchyma itself.

Alveolar reactions range from acute pulmonary edema or adult respiratory distress syndrome at one extreme to an insidiously developing pulmonary fibrosis at the other extreme. The chief clinical forms of drug-induced disease are noncardiogenic pulmonary edema, diffuse pneumonitis, and hypersensitivity reactions. Less common patterns include bronchiolitis obliterans and pulmonary hemorrhage. Although these entities are reviewed as well-defined syndromes, there may be considerable overlap within the individual case. Host response to many of these agents seems to vary in certain clinical situations, and there may be histologic evidence of more than one type of reaction in the same patient.

MECHANISM OF INJURY

The mechanism by which drugs cause widespread alveolar damage and propagate injury is complex and not clearly understood. Most of the evidence is circumstantial. Some drugs, such as bleomycin and amiodarone, are selectively concentrated in the lung and may predispose patients to pulmonary toxicity. In the case of bleomycin, individual susceptibility has been ascribed to an inherent lack of detoxifying enzyme.

Alteration of the normal balance between oxidants and antioxidants may play a role. There is evidence that nitrofurantoin, bleomycin, and amiodarone produce tissue-damaging oxygen radicals. These radicals are directly toxic to epithelial and endothelial cells and trigger other inflammatory reactions. Carmustine alters tissue concentrations of glutathione, which is a molecule important in the antioxidant defenses of the lung. These mechanisms provide a link with the known toxicity of oxygen itself and the established synergistic effects of high oxygen concentrations with some cytotoxic agents. It has been suggested that some persons are more susceptible to oxygen toxicity because of a lack of antioxidant defense enzymes.

Injury may occur from the recruitment of inflammatory cells, particularly neutrophils, and the subsequent release of a number of proteolytic enzymes and toxic mediators.

A number of drug reactions appear to be caused, at least in part, by cell-mediated immune reactions. The T lymphocyte is the major effector cell in this reaction. Bronchoalveolar lavage analysis has demonstrated a predominance of T-suppressor cells in patients with pneumonitis associated with gold, nitrofurantoin, methotrexate, and amiodarone. Similar findings have been reported in patients with hypersensitivity pneumonitis caused by organic dusts and seem to indicate an alteration of the normal pulmonary immune parameters. Lymphocytes obtained from patients with gold- and nitrofurantoin-induced lung disease have shown in vitro blastogenesis in the presence of the drug. Humoral mechanisms also may be operative. Specific antibodies to both cytotoxic and noncytotoxic agents have been documented. Circulating immune complexes have been demonstrated in nitrofurantoin-treated patients.

It is likely that a number of different mechanisms contribute to the resulting parenchymal injury, and certain drugs may result in a different form of injury (Table 1). The clinical presentations, the radio-

TABLE 1 Drugs Associated with Pulmonary Reactions

Reaction	*Drug*
Acute noncardiogenic pulmonary edema	*Overdose*
	Heroin
	Propoxyphene
	Salicylates
	Methadone
	Tricyclic antidepressants
	Oxygen
	Idiosyncratic
	Hydrochlorothiazide
	Colchicine
	Cocaine
	Methotrexate
	Cytosine arabinoside
	Mitomycin
	Cyclophosphamide
	Cyclosporine
	Temiposide
	Intravenous contrast agents
	Protamine sulfate
	Blood products
	Amphotercin B
Diffuse pneumonitis	*Cytotoxic Agents*
	Bleomycin
	Busulfan
	Carmustine (BCNU)
	Lomustine (CCNU)
	Cyclophosphamide
	Mitomycin
	Melphalan
	Azathioprine
	Cytosine arabinoside
	Other Agents
	Amiodarone
	Nitrofurantoin
	Methotrexate
	Sulfasalazine
	Gold salts
	Tocainide
	Oxygen
Hypersensitivity reactions	Nitrofurantoin
	Methotrexate
	Procarbazine
	Gold salts
	Sulfonamides
	Cromolyn
	Isoniazid
	Bleomycin
	Phenytoin
	Ampicillin
	Penicillin
	Naproxen
	Hydralazine
	Cocaine

logic features, and the course of the drug-induced syndromes are summarized in Table 2.

NONCARDIOGENIC PULMONARY EDEMA

This syndrome is characterized by severe dyspnea, fever, hypoxemia, and bilateral diffuse infiltrates. The edema occurs within minutes to hours after administration of the drug. There is leakage of the pulmonary capillaries and accumulation of a protein-rich fluid in the alveoli.

Noncardiogenic pulmonary edema should be differentiated from cardiac pulmonary edema, especially in patients who may have an anthracycline-associated cardiomyopathy or in those with preexisting heart disease who are taking beta-adrenergic blocking agents. Portable roentgenograms are rarely helpful and are difficult to evaluate. Pulmonary artery catheterization reveals normal left ventricular pressures. A trial of diuretics may provide the answer.

The most common cause of noncardiogenic pulmonary edema is an overdose of narcotic drugs or sedative hypnotic agents, which leads to depressed levels of consciousness. Patients are usually obtunded, have pinpoint pupils, and show evidence of carbon dioxide retention. High doses of salicylates can produce acute noncardiogenic pulmonary edema. It is more commonly associated with an acute aspirin overdose but has been reported in chronic ingestors of aspirin who unintentionally exceed the therapeutic range. Serum salicylate levels are usually higher than 35 mg per deciliter. Findings of a metabolic acidosis associated with hyperventilation and hypoxemia should alert the clinician to this diagnosis.

Pulmonary edema, attributable to idiosyncratic reactions, occurs in isolated cases with a large number of drugs, including the hydroradical of chlorothiazide, colchicine, and ampicillin. Edema that occurs following the use of beta-adrenergic drugs as tocolytic agents to arrest premature labor is probably due to fluid overload rather than to an increase in capillary permeability, as was originally thought.

Transfusion of blood and blood products, particularly granulocytes, may induce noncardiogenic pulmonary edema more often than is commonly believed. The diagnosis should always be considered in patients who experience severe dyspnea within 4 hours after transfusion. Associated manifestations often include hypotension, urticaria, and fever. The mechanism appears to be a reaction of leukoagglutinin antibodies from the donor's blood with the recipient's white blood cells. This results in sequestration of the white blood cells in the pulmonary capillary bed and release of proteolytic enzymes.

The prognosis generally is good. Most patients rapidly respond to withdrawal of the agent and rarely require further diagnostic evaluation. Amphotericin B has been thought to increase the toxicity of leukocyte infusion. Although this observation has not been corroborated, it would be wise to exercise caution and to separate the infusions of amphotericin B and transfusion of white blood cells or platelets, which are rich in leukocytes.

A few cases may progress to a fully developed adult respiratory distress syndrome and pulmonary fibrosis. A number of fatal outcomes from noncardiogenic pulmonary edema (50 percent) have been

TABLE 2 Drug-Induced Syndromes

Reaction	*Onset*	*Systemic Manifestation*	*Chest Roentgenogram*	*BAL**	*Histology*	*Response to Steroids*	*Prognosis*
Noncardiogenic pulmonary edema	Acute	Minimal	Diffuse alveolar pattern	No information	Fibrinous edema	None	Good
Diffuse pneumonitis	Chronic Rarely acute	Minimal	Alveolar and interstitial pattern or interstitial fibrosis	Variable cellular infiltrate Dysplastic cells	Dysplastic cells Alveolitis with fibrosis	Poor	Acute—poor chronic disability
Hypersensitivity reactions	Subacute	Severe eosinophilia†	Alveolar and interstitial pattern Pleural effusions	May be lymphocytic	Alveolitis Eosinophilia	Good	Good to excellent
Bronchiolitis obliterans	Chronic	None	Normal	No information	Peribronchiolar inflammation with obliteration	None	Poor
Intrapulmonary hemorrhage	Acute to subacute	None	Diffuse alveolar pattern	Macrophages laden with hemosiderin	Pulmonary hemorrhage	None	Poor

*BAL = Bronchoalveolar lavage.
†Not consistent.

reported in association with cytosine arabinoside and in patients with hemolytic uremic syndrome due to mitomycin C.

DIFFUSE PNEUMONITIS

Patients may have an acute presentation, with cough, fever, shortness of breath, and occasionally a systemic upset. A more common presentation is a much more insidious syndrome extending over several weeks to months. Typical features are cough, dyspnea, and fatigue. Moderate fever is usually present but not invariable. Bibasilar end-inspiratory crackles can often be heard at both lung bases. Initially, chest roentgenograms may be normal or may show a fine interstitial process in the lower lung zones, which advances to a diffuse alveolar pattern and eventually to pulmonary fibrosis. Pleural effusions are rare. Lung scanning with gallium-67 citrate may be positive.

Pulmonary function tests in these patients are nonspecific and show a restrictive pattern and a diffusion defect. Histologic examination of the lung tissue reveals a spectrum of diffuse alveolar damage. There is destruction of the lining cells, proliferation of type 2 pneumocytes with dysplastic features, and a variable and patchy inflammatory exudate and fibrosis. In many cases it is not clear whether the effects are due to direct toxicity or to hypersensitivity. The onset usually occurs 1 to 6 months after initiation of therapy but has been reported after 4 years of treatment with busulfan. With many drugs, particularly bleomycin, amiodarone, and busulfan, there is evidence of a dose relationship. The prognosis is variable. Most patients respond to discontinuation of the drug but show residual impairment. In others the condition may be progressive and irreversible, leading to respiratory failure and death. In general, corticosteroids are not helpful. There is some anecdotal data that corticosteroids may be valuable for treatment of pneumonitis associated with amiodarone, gold, and mitomycin.

HYPERSENSITIVITY REACTIONS

A number of drugs have been associated with a subacute clinical syndrome consistent with a pulmonary hypersensitivity reaction, Nitrofurantoin and sulfonamides are the drugs most frequently reported. The reactions are usually idiosyncratic, occur shortly after the administration of the drug, and do not appear to be dose-related. Patients present with cough, fever, shortness of breath, and systemic symptoms such as arthralgias, myalgias, and headaches. Rash and peripheral eosinophilia may be present. The roentgenologic appearance is that of a diffuse reticulonodular or an alveolar process reminiscent of pulmonary edema. Pleural effusions are common. Tissue samples of the lung reveal a patchy inflammatory cell reaction of predominantly mononuclear cells, often with tissue eosinophilia. Fibrosis is uncommon. A lymphocytic alveolitis by bronchoalveolar lavage has been documented in a few patients with pulmonary disease due to gold salts, nitrofurantoin, and methotrexate. The prognosis is almost invariably good, with complete resolution following withdrawal of the drug. Corticosteroids appear to hasten recovery.

BRONCHIOLITIS OBLITERANS

Bronchiolitis obliterans occurs when the pathologic process extends to the terminal bronchioles. This is a rare complication of exposure to three drugs: gold, sulfasalazine, and penicillamine. Clinical presentation is similar to that of a chronic alveolitis. Chest roentgenograms may be normal or may show localized infiltrates. Pulmonary function testing may be helpful and may demonstrate both an obstructive and a restrictive defect. The diagnosis is based on the histologic findings of areas of inflammation involving the bronchioles and causing obliteration. Prognosis in the few reported cases is poor. Fifty percent of patients develop progressive disease, and the remainder have residual defects despite discontinuation of the drug and the institution of corticosteroid therapy.

INTRAPULMONARY HEMORRHAGE

Intrapulmonary hemorrhage may complicate excessive systemic anticoagulation with heparin, warfarin, or thrombolytic therapy. There are isolated case reports in association with nitrofurantoin, methotrexate, penicillamine, and cocaine. Clinical manifestations include respiratory difficulty, hemoptysis, and anemia. Chest roentgenograms reveal bilateral diffuse air space consolidation. Absence of cardiomegaly and pleural effusions helps differentiate this condition from congestive heart failure. Changes may occur from day to day as a result of recurrent bleeding. The diagnosis can be confirmed by analysis of bronchial fluid and identification of hemosiderin-containing macrophages. The four cases associated with penicillamine had evidence of renal failure and the manifestations resembled those of Goodpasture's syndrome, although antibodies to the basement membrane component were not found. The only survivor had been treated with immunosuppressive agents and plasmapheresis.

CYTOTOXIC AND IMMUNOSUPPRESSIVE DRUGS

The majority of these agents are potentially toxic to the lungs. Bleomycin, methotrexate, and busulfan appear to cause the most frequent problems. Cyclophosphamide and azathioprine, the most widely used agents, only rarely produce reactions.

Methotrexate-induced pneumonitis can occur in both acute and chronic forms. It is most commonly associated with the clinical syndrome of hypersensitivity pneumonitis. There are reports, however, of the pulmonary disease subsiding despite continuation of therapy. Repeat challenge with the drug may not cause recurrent pneumonitis. Although most patients improve, deaths from an acute progressive alveolitis have been reported in up to 10 percent of patients.

Bleomycin occasionally causes hypersensitivity reactions in the lung, but more commonly it produces a chronic pneumonitis. The incidence has been reported as 4 to 6 percent of all treated patients. Hypersensitivity is rare with cumulative doses of less than 150 U. Severe pulmonary fibrosis has occurred in approximately 10 percent of patients receiving more than 500 U.

Among the alkylating agents, busulfan is considered the prototype for drug-induced pulmonary fibrosis and produces severe cytologic dysplasia in most organs. Changes mimicking neoplasia can be seen in the alveolar cells of sputum or bronchial washings in 40 percent of cases, although the nuclear cytoplasmic ratio remains normal. Prognosis generally is poor.

Mitomycin usually produces chronic pneumonitis. The outlook for these patients seems to be somewhat better than for those with chronic pneumonitis caused by other cytotoxic agents. This may be because of a more frequent response to corticosteroids.

Many of these agents cause the pneumonitis in a dose-dependent manner. Estimation of frequency is more predictable at higher doses. Busulfan toxicity occurs only above a critical dose of 500 mg. Carmustine toxicity seems more linearly related to the total dose. The incidence can be predicted with 80 percent accuracy when the patient's age, number of cycles, and cumulative dose and presence of lung disease are taken into account. It is important to recognize that the incidence of toxicity varied greatly among reports and that pulmonary toxicity from any of these agents may occur several years after cessation of therapy.

SYNERGISTIC EFFECTS

Synergistic effects occur as a result of combining radiation therapy or high concentrations of oxygen with many of the agents causing pulmonary toxicity. This has been shown clearly with the use of bleomycin. Radiation reactions may precipitate a pneumonitis in patients who have completed treatment with bleomycin. Bleomycin has been reported to produce rapidly progressive fibrosis 3 years after a patient received radiotherapy. It is not known how long this synergistic effect persists.

Bleomycin and alkylating agents have been associated with well-documented cases of pneumonitis precipitated by the use of oxygen. Most often, the setting has been the administration of oxygen during surgery or in the postoperative period. Clinicians who are unaware of oxygen-induced toxicity may give supplemental oxygen to patients in distress, which further aggravates the condition. The use of a forced inspiratory oxygen (FIO_2) of approximately 30 percent appears to be safe. Caution should be exercised for at least 6 months after the use of bleomycin or an alkylating agent.

Other factors that may increase the toxicity of a given drug are the tapering or withdrawal of corticosteroids (which may exacerbate or unmask a drug reaction), advanced age, and the use of chemotherapeutic agents in combination

AMIODARONE

Amiodarone is a very effective antiarrhythmic drug associated with an estimated 6 percent incidence of pulmonary toxicity. Complications appear to be greater in the United States, where a daily dose of more than 400 mg is often prescribed. Toxicity is rare in the first 2 months of therapy. The reaction may be acute and may mimic an infectious pneumonitis or congestive heart failure. More commonly, the reaction progresses slowly over 2 to 3 months, with cough and low-grade fever. The roentgenographic lesions may be localized (at least initially) or diffuse. There is poor correlation between drug levels in the serum and adverse pulmonary reactions.

Bronchoalveolar lavage yields neutrophils, lymphocytes, and foamy alveolar macrophages resulting from the accumulation of phospholipids within lysosomes. Phospholipid accumulation is not diagnostic and may be found in asymptomatic patients being treated with a drug. Uptake of gallium-67 has been seen in patients with amiodarone pneumonitis and may help differentiate such patients from those with cardiac failure. Prognosis is good if toxicity is recognized early and the drug is discontinued. Corticosteroids seem to be helpful in some patients and should be used for at least 6 months because of the long half-life of the drug, which is 30 days. A number of patients who need amiodarone to control ventricular arrhythmias and who would be in danger if the drug were withdrawn have been maintained successfully with the lowest effective dose of amiodarone in combination with corticosteroids. As many as 10 to 20 percent of patients ultimately die of the complication. Prognosis seems to be worse in the more rapidly progressive form of the disease.

COCAINE

Free-base cocaine, also known as "crack" or "rock," is the alkaloid form sufficiently heat-stable to be smoked and retain its pharmacologic properties.

Pulmonary reactions associated with its use appear to be rare phenomena despite the drug's current popularity. A wide spectrum of pulmonary complications has been reported: noncardiogenic pulmonary edema, hypersensitivity pneumonitis, bronchiolitis obliterans, and pulmonary hemorrhage. It is not known whether these varied effects are associated with different modes of administration or are caused by the toxic effects of contaminants being volatilized. The long-term effects of smoking free-base cocaine are not yet determined. Persistent reduction of the diffusion capacity of the lung has been observed.

Such barotraumatic effects as pneumothorax, pneumomediastinum, and pneumopericardium may occur and have been ascribed to Valsalva maneuvers during the inhalation of the drug. These are usually self-limiting and resolve spontaneously. Similar complications have been observed following the use of marihuana and nitric oxide.

DIAGNOSIS

The diagnosis of a drug-induced syndrome is difficult because of the lack of specific clinical, roentgenologic, or pathologic findings. Diagnosis requires a high index of clinical awareness of the potential toxicity of drug therapy, a careful drug history, and the exclusion of other possible etiologic factors. The drug history should include the unit dose, the cumulative dose, the relation of onset of symptoms to the initiation of therapy, and details of concomitant or previous treatments.

Roentgenograms of the chest are neither sensitive nor specific. They may be normal, particularly in the early phases of the disease. A combined alveolar and interstitial pattern may alert the radiologist to the possibility of drug-induced injury, but it is not characteristic and can be caused by many other disease processes.

Physiologic testing of the lungs provides a more sensitive method of detecting early toxicity than the chest roentgenogram. Impairment of diffusion capacity is, however, neither predictive nor specific for drug-induced injury but may be a useful parameter for monitoring progress.

There is evidence that chest computed tomography (CT) may in fact be more sensitive than chest roentgenograms in predicting the development of pulmonary disease. CT is valuable in differentiating air space disease from interstitial disease. High-resolution CT scans may be useful in differentiating lymphangitic carcinomatosis from interstitial fibrosis. A mesh of irregularly thickened lines that have a pearly appearance and correspond to the boundaries of the secondary lobule enclosing a central vessel is highly suggestive of lymphangitic carcinomatosis.

Accumulation of gallium-67 within the lung has been demonstrated with pneumonitis associated with bleomycin, methotrexate, amiodarone, and some alkylating agents. The scan cannot differentiate lung toxicity from other inflammatory diseases. Its potential value may be in the identification of pulmonary disease in patients who are symptomatic but have normal chest roentgenograms.

Currently, bronchoalveolar lavage cellular analysis must be viewed as a research tool. The findings of a lymphocytosis composed of predominantly T-suppressor cells is highly suggestive of drug-induced injury. The principal value of fluid analysis, often combined with intrabronchial brushing, is for evidence of superinfection or extension of tumor.

Transbronchial biopsy may demonstrate the cytotoxic changes, but frequently a larger sample with open lung biopsy is required. Histologically, most cytotoxic drugs produce evidence of diffuse alveolar damage with destruction of lining cells, formation of hyaline membranes, and a variable inflammatory infiltrate and degree of fibrosis. With certain drugs, eosinophilia may be a prominent part of this alveolar reaction. The finding of atypical type 2 pneumocytes may be misinterpreted as being of indeterminate cause unless the possibility of a drug reaction is kept in mind. They are characteristic but not diagnostic of drug-induced disease.

MANAGEMENT

Withdrawal of the drug usually results in clinical improvement. The efficacy of corticosteroids is unclear. They seem to speed recovery from drug-induced hypersensitivity pneumonitis. Corticosteroids are ineffective in the rapidly progressive form of acute pneumonitis and have not proved useful in the more chronic syndromes, except for individual case reports indicating their value in pneumonitis caused by mitomycin, amiodarone, and possibly gold salts.

Early detection of lung toxicity offers the greatest chance of reversibility. Failure to implicate the drug can result in progressive respiratory impairment and possibly death. Challenge with the drug can precipitate life-threatening emergencies.

The problem of drug-induced pulmonary toxicity is becoming more significant every year. To date, there are no adequate tests for early detection of pulmonary damage by drugs. Physicians may be presented with the dilemma of placing the patient at risk by withdrawing an effective mode of therapy because of possible undesirable pulmonary reactions or of risking progressive pulmonary disease due to drug toxicity.

It is hoped that an awareness of the factors that predispose the patient to drug toxicity and a familiarity with the common clinical syndromes prove helpful in the prevention and diagnosis of drug-induced pulmonary disease.

SUGGESTED READING

Cooper JAD Jr, White DA, Matthay RA. Drug-induced pulmonary disease. Part 1. Cytotoxic drugs. Am Rev Respir Dis 1986; 133:321–340.

Cooper JAD Jr, White DA, Matthay RA. Drug-induced pulmonary disease. Part 2. Noncytotoxic drugs. Am Rev Respir Dis 1986; 133:488–505.

Ettinger NA, Albin PJ. A review of the respiratory effects of smoking cocaine. Am J Med 1989; 87:664–668.

Mason JW. Amiodarone. N Engl J Med 1987; 316:455–466.

Rosenow EC, Wilson WR, Cockerill FR. Pulmonary disease in the immunocompromised host (first of two parts). Mayo Clin Proc 1985; 60:473–487.

SARCOIDOSIS

JACK LIEBERMAN, M.D.

It is difficult to define sarcoidosis completely because the exact etiology of the disease remains unknown. Sarcoidosis is a multisystem disease marked by the formation of noncaseating epithelioid cell granulomas in multiple organs or tissues. These granulomas may resolve totally, or they may progress to a fibrotic state, causing permanent tissue damage and dysfunction. The presence of noncaseating granulomas in any one tissue is not necessarily diagnostic of sarcoidosis unless there is histologic or clinical evidence of multiple organ or tissue involvement; noncaseating granulomas may be seen in conditions such as mycobacterial disease, neoplasms, (especially lymph node draining tumors), allergic alveolitis, chemical reactions to beryllium or zirconium, primary biliary cirrhosis, Wegener's granulomatosis, regional ileitis, and systemic lupus erythematosus. Sarcoidosis may be distinguished from these diseases by the pattern of organ involvement, the usual presence of bilateral hilar lymphadenopathy and/or lung infiltrates, and, less frequently, involvement of the eyes, parotid glands, skin, spleen, central nervous system (CNS), bone, or other lymph nodes.

The immunologic nature of sarcoidosis has long been suspected because of the presence of anergy to skin test antigens, the marked reduction in circulating T lymphocytes, the occasional presence of hypergammaglobulinemia, and of course, the occurrence of granulomas. Noncaseating granulomas were thought to be a manifestation of cell-mediated immunology, but their presence did not seem to agree with the reduced number of circulating T lymphocytes or with the anergic state. However, with the advent of bronchoalveolar lavage techniques, it was discovered that sarcoidosis is characterized by enhanced cellular immunologic processes, but only at the sites of involvement. Thus, T lymphocytes may be reduced in number in blood, but present in large numbers in bronchoalveolar lavage fluid and in biopsy specimens from tissue into which Kveim antigen has been injected. It is now recognized that sarcoidosis is an unusual cell-mediated immunologic response to a number of unknown antigens. Whether this type of immunologic response is specific for these antigens, or whether some individuals inherit the tendency to respond in this manner, is uncertain.

CLINICAL PRESENTATION

Sarcoidosis presents clinically most often because of chest involvement, either with symptoms of dyspnea, cough, or chest pains or with chest roentgenographic evidence of bilateral hilar adenopathy or lung infiltrates (70 percent of patients). Approximately one-quarter of the patients may present with generalized symptoms of fever, weight loss, anorexia, or arthralgias, whereas approximately 7 percent present with complaints resulting from specific, nonpulmonary organ involvement, such as the skin, CNS, eyes, joints, heart, spleen, and liver.

The clinical manifestations of sarcoidosis seem to differ between blacks and whites. It has been stated that sarcoidosis is 10 times more frequent in blacks than in whites in the United States, but it now appears that the disease is more severe and chronic in blacks. The disease is more progressive, less stable, and has a lower remission rate and a higher death rate in blacks. Therefore, the expected response to treatment is poorer in blacks than in whites. Because sarcoidosis may resolve spontaneously and be associated only with some respiratory discomfort and transient, undetected, hilar adenopathy, many cases of the disease probably go unrecognized in whites. In countries other than the United States, sarcoidosis is seen mostly in the white population, although the disease tends to be less severe than in American blacks, and the higher incidence of erythema nodosum reflects a better prognosis and a milder disease.

DIAGNOSTIC PROCEDURES

Clinical Studies

A chest roentgenogram and pulmonary function tests (PFTs) are useful in revealing chest pathology (bilateral hilar adenopathy and/or lung infiltrates) and the presence of restrictive lung disease (with reduced diffusion capacity or hypoxemia with exercise) or obstruction resulting from airway deformity. Serial chest roentgenograms and PFTs can assist in the longitudinal evaluation of treatment or in looking for spontaneous regression of the disease. PFTs can be normal in these patients.

Tissue Biopsy and Kveim Test

The pathologic demonstration of noncaseating granulomas is almost always necessary to confirm the diagnosis of sarcoidosis. The most rewarding site for obtaining a positive biopsy result is a skin nodule or plaque; 100 percent of such lesions show the typical granulomas, which indicates that a careful examination of the skin is warranted. The skin is involved in approximately 25 percent of patients with sarcoidosis. On the other hand erythema nodosum or multiforme does not contain granulomas, and a biopsy should not be performed if these skin conditions are recognized; these skin changes may occur in sarcoidosis as a secondary reflection of the disease. Transbronchial biopsy of the lung is the procedure of choice in most patients for obtaining a useful biopsy specimen; the high success rate for detecting granulomas in lung tissue is probably related to the tendency of granulomas to form along the bronchial tree, which makes them accessible to transbronchial biopsy. Biopsy of a palpable lymph node (e.g., a scalene node) can be useful, although node drainage of tumors can make the results less specific. The conjunctival sac and the lacrimal glands, when grossly nodular, are other available biopsy sites. Liver biopsy specimens also may show granulomas; however, since these are seen commonly in other diseases the liver is not a recommended biopsy site unless significant liver disease is present.

A Kveim test involves preparation of an antigen-containing suspension of sarcoid spleen, intracutaneous injection, and a 4- to 6-week wait, followed by a biopsy of the injection site to determine whether noncaseating granulomas have developed. Kveim antigen has not been approved by the Food and Drug Administration for general use, and is available only in selected institutions. If the test is available, a positive result is equivalent to a positive tissue biopsy.

Serum Angiotensin Converting Enzyme Level

An elevated level of serum angiotensin converting enzyme (SACE) is diagnostically helpful and has approximately a 75 percent sensitivity for detecting active sarcoidosis, although it is not entirely specific for sarcoidosis. SACE levels also may be elevated in patients with Gaucher's disease, hyperthyroidism, leprosy, cirrhosis of the liver, diabetes mellitus (especially in those diabetic patients who have retinopathy), and silicosis. However, in an appropriate clinical setting, an elevated SACE level strongly supports a diagnosis of sarcoidosis. Serial testing of SACE levels is of great value in evaluating the clinical course of such patients; a falling SACE level indicates an improving clinical state, whereas a rising SACE level reflects worsening or impending relapse.

Gallium 67 Scan

The major value of a gallium scan is to reveal the multiple organ involvement in a patient with sarcoidosis. Thus, a scan should be ordered to cover the patient from head to pelvis, and not be limited only to the chest. A characteristic pattern with ocular, parotid, hilar, lung parenchymal, and possibly splenic gallium uptake is highly characteristic, if not diagnostic, of sarcoidosis. Response to therapy is reflected by a reduction of gallium uptake at these sites. The frequency with which gallium scans may be performed is limited because of the radiation load involved.

Skin Tests for Anergy

The detection of anergy in a patient suspected of having sarcoidosis is extremely valuable for supporting the initial diagnosis. A panel of skin tests should include the purified protein derivative (PPD) (5 units), cocci, mumps, and *Candida* skin tests. A positive PPD in a patient with other characteristics of sarcoidosis should be an indication for anti-tuberculosis medication (isoniazid).

Bronchoalveolar Lavage

Bronchoalveolar lavage (BAL) is still primarily a research tool and is not indicated for routine evaluation of patients. BAL may be of value for detecting the earliest stage of alveolitis, when granulomas have not yet formed and the SACE level is not yet elevated. The value of and necessity for detecting this stage of the disease is uncertain.

Serum Calcium Level

Detection of hypercalcemia is important as an indicator for immediate treatment of sarcoidosis. Hypercalcemia can cause serious symptoms and renal damage. Measurement of urine calcium excretion also may be of value in this regard, but this is not generally agreed upon.

MANAGEMENT

Corticosteroids

The major treatment of sarcoidosis is through the use of corticosteroids, usually given systemically, but occasionally applied topically. The goals of therapy are to suppress the initial inflammatory (alveolitis-like) stage, to suppress and resolve the granulomatous stage, and to prevent the formation of fibrous scar tissue. It appears that sarcoid inflammation and granulomas may be totally reversible, but that the stage of fibrosis is not; treatment begun before fibrosis takes place should be more effective than treatment begun after fibrosis has occurred.

There is disagreement about whether treatment with corticosteroids actually modifies the long-term outcome of patients with sarcoidosis, in spite of an initial benefit. Review of published reports has suggested that the conflict may have arisen because of late and inadequate dosages of medication, which resulted in poor control of the underlying disease. Interpretation of these publications also must take into account the racial distribution of the patients involved, since, as mentioned previously, blacks have a poorer prognosis than do whites. In addition, the stage of the disease on chest roentgenography affects the expected result; patients in stage I (bilateral hilar adenopathy alone) have a better prognosis (71 percent chance of spontaneous remission) than do patients in stage II (hilar adenopathy with infiltrates) or stage III (lung infiltrates without adenopathy), who remit spontaneously only 50 percent of the time. With the advent of the SACE test, adequacy of initial treatment and of maintenance treatment now can be objectively evaluated. A return of the SACE level to normal suggests good control of the disease process; a reduction to a still elevated level suggests incomplete resolution and a poorer prognosis; a rise in SACE level implies reactivation of the disease and a need for increased corticosteroid dosage.

Indications for Treatment

Indications for treatment of patients with sarcoidosis are listed in Table 1. Most of the indecisiveness about a need for therapy involves the treatment of the respiratory component of the disease. The tendency now is to treat early in the course of the disease, i.e., if a patient has chest symptoms or has evidence of lung infiltration on chest roentgenograms. Too long a period of observation may reduce the chance of obtaining complete remission before irreversible fibrosis occurs.

There is less disagreement about the extrapulmonary indications for treatment. Any delay in treating hypercalcemia may result in renal damage; cardiac involvement may result in sudden death from arrhythmia; ocular involvement may result in blindness; CNS involvement can result in nerve damage, paralysis, or both; skin lesions can cause permanent disfigurement; hypersplenism can result in blood dyscrasias or splenic rupture; and progressive liver involvement may result in cirrhosis.

TABLE 1 Indications for Treatment of Sarcoidosis with Corticosteroids

Pulmonary

- Stage II or III disease, when symptomatic (dyspnea) or when there is no evidence of improvement on chest film or pulmonary function tests
- Stage I disease, only with severe obstructive ventilatory impairment; otherwise do not treat Stage I disease

Extrapulmonary

- Hypercalcemia
- Cardiac (myopathy or conduction disturbances)
- Ocular (uveitis; anterior or posterior)
- Central nervous system involvement
- Disfiguring skin lesions
- Hypersplenism
- Xerophthalmia or xerostomia
- Persistent systemic disease (fever, weight loss)
- Progressive liver involvement

Method of Treatment

When initiating a treatment program with corticosteroids, one must plan to treat a patient for at least 1 year, and possibly for the remainder of the patient's life. To avoid the undesirable side effects of corticosteroids (prednisone), I use an every-other-day program of 40 mg of prednisone in the morning, which has had excellent results. The response to therapy is judged clinically as well as by SACE assays weekly during the first month, then monthly. If improvement takes place, the prednisone dosage is reduced by 10 mg at 3-month intervals. If a therapeutic response is initially deemed inadequate, the starting dosage may be increased to 60 mg every other day, or 40 to 60 mg daily, depending on the severity of the symptoms. A monthly reduction of these higher dosages should be attempted until the 40 mg every other day dosage is again tried as described. Should worsening of the condition take place at any dosage, the preceding higher, effective dose should be reinstituted for 3 months, at which time the dosage reduction should again be attempted. Many patients require a maintenance dosage of 10 to 20 mg of prednisone every other day for an indefinite period to maintain the therapeutic response, whereas others are able to discontinue medication in a year's time.

Mechanism of Action

Corticosteroids are thought to block the production of interleukin 1 and 2 by macrophages and T lymphocytes, thereby reducing the recruitment of additional T cells. In addition, corticosteroids reduce the response of macrophages to other lymphokines, thereby reducing the number of cells available to form granulomas and reducing the inflammatory response.

Topical Use of Corticosteroids

Topical corticosteroids may be used to treat anterior uveitis (steroid eye drops) and deforming skin lesions (triamcinolone acetonide, diluted with 1 percent procaine to a concentration of 2 to 5 mg per milliliter, injected directly into the lesions) at weekly intervals.

Other Drugs

In the rare instance when steroid therapy is absolutely contraindicated, treatment with other drugs may be necessary. This may occur in patients with steroid psychosis or in those whose diabetes mellitus is difficult to control. The drugs that have been used on occasion are listed in Table 2, but most cannot be used for any prolonged intervals (i.e., more than 4 months), and side effects are more common than with corticosteroids.

TABLE 2 Other Drugs Used for Treatment of Sarcoidosis

Drug	*Dosage*	*Duration*	*Specific Use*
Chloroquine	250 mg b.i.d.–q.o.d.	9 mo	Hypercalcemia; cutaneous; lupus pernio
Methotrexate	5 mg weekly	3 mo	
Azathioprine	50 mg t.i.d.	6 mo	
Chlorambucil	4 mg q.d.; may increase by 2 mg weekly to max of 12 mg		
Oxyphenbutazone	100 mg q.i.d.	6 mo	
Levamisole	150 mg q.o.d.	2 wk on, 1 wk off, ×6 mo.	
Cyclosporin A	10–15 mg/kg daily		Intraocular sarcoid; pulmonary
Cyclophosphamide	150 mg daily; 900 mg IV bolus q24h ×2 doses	5 mo	
Allopurinol	100 mg q.i.d.	3 mo	
Isotretinoin	40 mg daily (0.67 mg/kg/day)	30 wk	Cutaneous
Potassium iodide	300 mg t.i.d.		Erythema nodosum; arthritis
Thymopoietin 32–36	50 mg IV t.i.w.	6 wk	Cutaneous

SUGGESTED READING

Crystal RG, Bitterman PB, Rennard SI, et al. Interstitial lung diseases of unknown cause. N Eng J Med 1984; 310:154–166, 235–244.

James DG, Williams WJ. Sarcoidosis and other granulomatoses. Philadelphia: WB Saunders, 1985.

Lieberman J, ed. Sarcoidosis. Orlando: Grune & Stratton, 1985.

Sharma OP. Sarcoidosis; clinical management. Boston: Butterworth, 1984.

IDIOPATHIC PULMONARY FIBROSIS

GERALD S. DAVIS, M.D.

Idiopathic pulmonary fibrosis (IPF) usually leads to severe respiratory impairment and often to death over several years if left without treatment. Most patients are older than 45 years of age, the peak incidence being about age 65 years. IPF is a disease of unknown cause, and it produces diffuse interstitial inflammation and fibrosis, which results in progressive disorganization of pulmonary architecture, stiff lungs with a high work of breathing, and impaired gas exchange. IPF is characterized by dyspnea with exertion, dry cough, basilar crackles, digital clubbing, diffuse small irregular shadows on chest roentgenogram, and restrictive lung function tests with hypoxemia that worsens with exercise. Surgical open lung biopsy is usually required in order to accurately establish the diagnosis and to indicate the choice of therapy.

It is believed that IPF develops through the mechanism of a chronic immune-inflammatory reaction mediated by activated macrophages with the participation of lymphocytes, neutrophils, and fibroblasts. The inciting cause for initiating and perpetuating this response is unknown. Initial inflammation, secondary tissue injury, and finally fibrosis are believed to occur in sequence, but these processes may all take place simultaneously in nearby alveolar units. Anti-inflammatory and immunosuppressive drug therapy is aimed at controlling inflammation before tissue injury and fibrosis take place.

In most cases, treatment is only partially effective, but at times disease progression may be arrested even if lung function does not return to normal. Many patients deteriorate despite the best available therapy. The median survival is about 9 years for patients who respond to therapy, and 2 years for those who do not respond. Overall, approximately half the patients with IPF remain alive 5 years after initial diagnosis. The drugs used to treat IPF are toxic, and most patients experience at least minor side effects during therapy. There are many similarities between cancer and IPF in both course and management. These features all highlight IPF as a serious illness that requires definitive and detailed diagnosis, aggressive therapy, and skilled management.

CLINICAL PRESENTATION

Patients with IPF complain of gradually progressive shortness of breath on exertion. About three-quarters of patients are bothered by dry cough. These symptoms usually have been present for several months, and sometimes for several years, before medical attention is sought. Climbing stairs or hills, carrying packages, or moderate exercise usually brings on dyspnea. Constitutional symptoms are common, and most patients report general fatigue, malaise, lack of energy, and reduced endurance that are out of proportion to their measured impairment in pulmonary function. Sputum production, chest pains, episodes of paroxysmal coughing, and wheezing are usually absent. Symptom levels remain stable from day to day. Table 1 summarizes the clinical features of IPF.

The most striking physical finding in IPF is the presence of high-pitched end-inspiratory crackles (dry or "Velcro" rales) over the lower one-third or two-thirds of both lung fields. Breath sounds may be enhanced, and tactile fremitus is often increased. In late disease, findings of cor pulmonale may appear. Digital clubbing is common and occurs in two-thirds of patients, but without the other features of symptomatic hypertrophic pulmonary osteoarthropathy.

The chest roentgenogram typically shows a diffuse symmetrical pattern of small irregular shadows predominantly in the lower lung zones. The fine vascular markings and the adjacent heart borders and pleural surfaces become blurred. A definite fraction of patients, perhaps 5 to 10 percent, appear with symptoms and physiological abnormalities before the chest roentgenogram becomes abnormal. Both the extent (profusion) and coarseness of the infiltrate noted on roentgenogram increase as the disease progresses. A destructive "honeycomb" pattern, with small airspaces surrounded by dense linear shadows, may be seen in advanced disease. Generally, pleural effusion is not part of IPF, and hilar lymph node enlargement is not seen.

A more detailed view of lung parenchyma can be obtained with thin section high-resolution computed tomography (CT) of the chest. Initial reports indicate a good correlation between this specialized CT technique and lung biopsy histopathologic features in IPF. At this time, it is not clear exactly how thin section CT will aid management decisions for individual patients, but it appears to be a promising refinement on the information provided by the conventional chest roentgenogram.

In IPF, pulmonary function testing documents the nature and the extent of abnormality and provides important benchmarks for measuring the effect of treatment. A pattern typical of "restrictive" disease is seen. The vital capacity and the total lung capacity are reduced. Pulmonary compliance is decreased, with the pressure-volume curve shifted down and to the right, which evidences stiff lungs that are hard to inflate. Air flow rates are normal or even super-normal, and thus the FEV_1/FVC ratio is preserved or increased. Abnormalities of oxygenation and gas transfer are present in most patients at rest and in virtually all patients during exercise. The single-breath diffusing capacity for carbon monoxide (D_LCO) is usually decreased to 50 percent of predicted or less. Hypoxemia with normal or slightly reduced arterial blood carbon dioxide tension is usually found. Hypercarbia is almost never present until late disease with end-stage respiratory failure. The arterial blood oxygen tension (Po_2) is often normal or nearly normal at rest, but falls dramatically with moderate treadmill or bicycle exercise. Arterial Po_2 levels of 45 to 55 torr during exercise are common in patients who may have normal or nearly normal lung volumes and resting arterial blood gas values. Exercise testing is usually essential to bring out the degree of abnormality and to follow the impact of treatment.

Laboratory tests are not helpful in IPF. The erythrocyte sedimentation rate is often moderately elevated; antinuclear antibodies are frequently present in low titer. Neither of these findings seems to be of particular diagnostic or prognostic value. Obviously, laboratory tests may be useful in excluding other diseases and before administering drugs whose side effects might change test results.

These various clinical features can be drawn together to estimate a composite index of severity of IPF for an individual patient at the time of evaluation, the Clinical-Radiographic-Physiologic (CRP) score. Semiquantitative estimates of dyspnea, profusion of radiographic opacities, and pulmonary physiologic impairment are weighted and summed to produce a CRP score. Changes in this score over time can be used to help determine whether a patient has improved, remained stable, or deteriorated, and the score may assist the physician in making decisions about therapy.

TABLE 1 Clinical Features of Idiopathic Pulmonary Fibrosis

Symptoms
Dyspnea with exertion
Dry cough
Malaise, reduced energy and endurance
Lack of occupational exposure
Physical findings
Bibasilar dry end-inspiratory rales
Digital clubbing
Laboratory tests
Elevated erythrocyte sedimentation rate
Positive antinuclear antibodies
Chest roentgenogram
Small irregular shadows
Diffuse symmetrical pattern
Lower lung zone predominance
High diaphragms
Pulmonary function
Reduced vital capacity
Normal airflow rates
Small lung volumes
Reduced diffusing capacity
Hypoxemia without hypercarbia
Hypoxemia worse with exercise
Reduced lung compliance
Lung biopsy tissue
Interstitial lymphocytes and macrophages
Alveolar inflammatory cells
Alveolary exudates
Interstitial collagen deposition
Hyperplasia of fibroblasts
Hyperplasia of interstitial contractile cells
Obliteration of small blood vessels
Distortion of alveolar architecture

ESTABLISHING THE DIAGNOSIS

Before beginning therapy, it is essential to establish with certainty the diagnosis of IPF in order to estimate the likelihood of response to treatment and to document the severity of impairment. The clinical picture already described makes IPF likely if features of other diseases are absent. Unfortunately, these features alone do not make the diagnosis certain, and lung tissue biopsy is required in almost all cases. We have found that as many as 20 percent of patients with suspected IPF proved to have other diseases upon open lung biopsy. Sarcoidosis, hypersensitivity pneumonitis, eosinophilic granuloma, lymphangitic carcinomatosis, environmental dust diseases, and other causes can all be mistaken for IPF without tissue proof.

I obtain an open lung biopsy on almost all patients with suspected IPF. A limited thoracotomy, with a small anterior submammary intercostal incision, is performed under general anesthesia. Small portions from the margins of two lobes are obtained; the tip of the lingula is avoided since it may be scarred in normal individuals. A thoracostomy tube is left to suction drainage for about 24 hours. Most patients leave the hospital 4 to 6 days after surgery. Some centers perform outpatient lung biopsy in this manner. The safety record for open biopsy is good, with little morbidity and less than 1 percent mortality in the reported series. Patients are excluded from open biopsy if they are elderly or have serious cardiovascular disease, severe pulmonary impairment, or other major operative risk factors. Patients who are poor candidates for open lung biopsy may still undergo bronchoscopic transbronchial biopsy in an attempt to confirm the diagnosis and particularly to exclude other diseases.

Bronchoalveolar Lavage

Over the past 15 years, bronchoalveolar lavage (BAL) has provided a powerful research tool for investigating the pathogenesis of IPF; its role as a clinical technique for the evaluation of individual patients remains controversial. BAL is performed through the channel of a flexible fiberoptic bronchoscope; the tip is gently wedged in a bronchopulmonary subsegment of matching size. A small volume (20 to 60 ml) of sterile isotonic saline solution is instilled and immediately withdrawn, and the washing is repeated 4 to 6 times with fresh volumes of saline. A lavage totaling 240 ml (4 × 60 ml) is the most widely used method, but volumes from 100 to 300 ml are reported commonly. The free airspace cells are separated from the soluble epithelial lining fluid in saline by low speed centrifugation. The cell population is enumerated and characterized. Cytocentrifuge cell spreads are used to differentially count alveolar macrophages (85 to 95 percent of cells in normal subjects), lymphocytes (5 to 15 percent), neutrophils (0 to 2 percent), eosinophils (0 to 1 percent), and basophils-mast cells (0 percent). The surface antigen phenotypes and the functions of the lymphocytes can be characterized. The secretion of cytokines and other substances by BAL alveolar macrophages has been studied extensively. The supernatant BAL fluid can be analyzed for its soluble proteins, surfactant lipids, and other biologically active materials.

Analysis of BAL cells and fluid from patients with IPF demonstrates a spectrum of results as summarized in Table 2. Many, but not all, patients with IPF exhibit each of these features, and there is great variability among subjects. BAL reveals a population of immune-inflammatory cells that have been recruited into the airspaces and that are accompanied by increased local production of immunoglobulins, decreased surfactant phospholipids, and the presence of many mediators and biologically active substances.

BAL results from small series of patients with IPF (5 to 35) studied in many centers in several countries generally support the findings listed in Table 2. Valiant efforts at relating BAL abnormalities to clinical status, prognosis, and response to therapy have only been partially successful. Increased BAL lymphocytes have been identified as a marker of active disease by several centers and appear to correlate with the degree of histopathologic alveolar septal inflammation and with a favorable response to therapy. The percentage of neutrophils does not appear to be a sensitive index of disease activity. In most patients with IPF, neutrophils are increased in BAL; they may remain elevated despite a good therapeutic response, or they may decrease without clinical improvement. Eosinophils in BAL have been linked to severe disease and a poor prognosis by some, but not all, investigators. Decreased total phospholipids may correlate with a worse prognosis. Serial BAL analyses in the same patients over several years show slight, but quite variable correla-

TABLE 2 Bronchoalveolar Lavage Features of Idiopathic Pulmonary Fibrosis

Increased free lung cells:	
Alveolar macrophage number	[moderate, usual]
Lymphocyte number and percentage	[moderate, variable]
Neutrophil number and percentage	[moderate, usual]
Eosinophil number and percentage	[slight, variable]
Increased in BAL fluid:	
Total protein	
Immunoglobulins (IgG, IgA, IgM)	
Immune complexes (variable)	
Type III procollagen peptides	
Fibronectin	
Collagenase	
Histamine	
Decreased in BAL fluid:	
Total phospholipids	
Increased secretion by alveolar macrophages:	
Platelet-derived growth factor (competence)	
Macrophage-derived growth factor (progression)	
Fibronectin	
Neutrophil chemotactic activity	
Reactive oxygen species	

tions, between clinical improvement and a return towards normal of the BAL parameters.

Functional studies of the immune-inflammatory cells recovered by BAL from patients with IPF have provided important insights into the mechanisms of this disease. The macrophage is clearly implicated as a central modulator of alveolar and interstitial inflammation, injury, and connective tissue remodeling in IPF. Results from many different laboratories suggest that the macrophage in IPF is activated and produces cytokines that attract and activate lymphocytes, attract neutrophils, and particularly induce fibroblast proliferation. The inciting events that trigger initial injury and inflammation remain obscure, although immune complexes have been implicated by some authors.

Unfortunately, the generalities derived from groups of subjects are difficult to apply to individual patients with IPF. Great variations in BAL results from person to person are common, and many patients seem to be exceptions to the average "rules" derived from series. Multifactorial analysis gives promise of improving the diagnostic and predictive value of BAL results, but this approach has not yet been applied extensively. At this time, I do not use BAL results as a major guide for making treatment decisions in IPF.

MANAGEMENT

The therapy of IPF is aimed at suppression and elimination of the chronic immune-inflammatory response. The agents that have proved useful in the treatment of IPF are believed to work by "quieting down" the proinflammatory actions of activated macrophages and lymphocytes, by reducing neutrophil chemotaxis and adherence, and by selectively reducing the number of these cells in the lung and the circulation.

Diagnosis should be established as early as possible, and treatment should be instituted in order to intervene before tissue destruction and fibrosis become extensive. Treatment should be aimed at suppressing the immune-inflammatory response and ideally should be monitored by observing the activity of this response. Future treatments should modulate and normalize fibroblast replication and collagen production (Table 3).

TABLE 3 Current Therapy of Idiopathic Pulmonary Fibrosis

Drug therapy
Corticosteroids
Cyclophosphamide
Azathioprine
Supportive treatment
Home exercise program
Diet counseling
Stationary home oxygen therapy
Portable oxygen for exertion
Cough suppressants
Lung transplantation
Compassionate health professionals

Corticosteroids

Corticosteroids are the major drugs used for the treatment of IPF. Oral prednisone or methylprednisolone, taken in moderate to high doses on a daily or alternate-day basis, is the most common regimen. The glucocorticoids are believed to work in IPF by suppressing inflammation, by impairing activated lymphocyte function, and by their lympholytic effects. Alveolar macrophages recovered from IPF patients have cell membrane receptors for glucocorticoids, but steroid therapy of patients does not diminish the exaggerated in vitro production of fibronectin and growth factors by their cells. Although steroids have been used in almost every case series of IPF that has been reported, the dosage, schedule, and end-points for success have varied widely within most series as well as between them. A few patients achieved impressive improvement, whereas most had slight or no objective improvement and only partial relief of symptoms. Unfortunately, most authors do not distinguish the patients who stopped getting worse (arrested disease) from those who continued to deteriorate (progressive disease). Higher doses appear to have somewhat greater effectiveness than lower doses. At 6 weeks, a small Norwegian trial showed no difference between high doses of intravenous steroids (methylprednisolone, 1 g, alternate days) and more conventional daily oral therapy (prednisolone, 30 mg). The incidence of complications usually is not described, but anecdotal experience suggests that minor side effects are usual and significant ones are not rare. As a crude estimate, 20 to 30 percent of patients with IPF achieve stabilization of disease or improvement with steroid therapy alone.

Cyclophosphamide

Cyclophosphamide (Cytoxan) has been used to treat IPF in several published trials and has demonstrated apparent effectiveness in preliminary results from an ongoing randomized study in Great Britain. Anecdotal clinical experience supports its effectiveness in some patients. In a recent short-term study, steroids alone did not suppress BAL neutrophils, whereas cyclophosphamide with or without steroids induced a significant reduction in neutrophil alveolitis. The importance of this BAL finding for the long-term outcome of patients with IPF is not clear. Curiously, cyclophosphamide also can cause pulmonary fibrosis in patients treated for cancer with this agent. Cyclophosphamide is an alkylating agent of the nitrogen mustard group. It is well absorbed orally and is activated in the liver to several cytotoxic compounds. It is believed that the drug works by depleting lymphocyte numbers and by suppressing the function of those that remain. Cyclophosphamide is usually administered in a daily oral maintenance dosage (to be discussed). Weekly or monthly high-dose pulse therapy with cyclophosphamide has been successful in systemic lupus erythematosus with renal disease and in other chronic immune-inflammatory conditions. This treatment scheme has not been reported for IPF, but may hold the promise for greater or equal efficacy with fewer side effects than the daily dosage scheme. Cyclophosphamide is usually reserved for use in patients in whom steroid therapy has proved unsuccessful. An additional 20 to 30 percent of patients may achieve stabilization or improvement with this drug. Preliminary results of the use of cyclophosphamide as initial primary therapy for IPF look encouraging. It must be emphasized that cyclophosphamide has not been approved by the Food and Drug Administration for use in the treatment of this particular disease.

Azathioprine

In several small trials, azathioprine (Imuran) has been reported to have some effectiveness in the treatment of IPF. Azathioprine is a purine analogue that is slowly converted to mercaptopurine in body tissues. It appears to act both by substitution for purines in DNA synthesis and, perhaps more importantly, as an inhibitor of adenine deaminase. Lymphocytes are particularly susceptible to adenine deaminase deficiency which results in impairment of both cellular and humoral immunity. This action might explain the particular sensitivity of T-lymphocytes to azathioprine and its utility as an immunosuppressive drug. It is usually given daily by mouth. Azathioprine, like cyclophosphamide, has been used mainly for patients who have already failed to respond to steroid therapy. Several small studies suggest that an additional 20 to 30 percent of patients respond to this agent. These may be the same patients who respond to cyclophosphamide, and there is no direct evidence that patients who fail to respond to one cyctotoxic drug will respond to another. Azathioprine was no more effective than steroids in the preliminary results of one recent randomized study. It has not been approved by the Food and Drug Administration for use in the treatment of IPF.

D-Penicillamine

Because of its effectiveness in the treatment of several of the rheumatologic diseases, D-penicillamine has been considered for use in IPF. Although the trials have been small and generally not randomized or controlled, the results are not encouraging. The use of D-penicillamine for treatment of IPF is not warranted until further evidence supports its effectiveness.

The drug treatment programs available for IPF do not work in all patients, and most only achieve a partial response at best. Although most clinicians use steroids as the first line of treatment, in many cases the patient's condition not only does not improve, but continues to worsen during therapy. Since the disease progresses to disability and death, attempts to achieve remission through the use of drugs that are not yet fully approved seems justified and appropriate. Cyclophosphamide and azathioprine are used for this reason. Available therapies may effect improvement or stabilization in 50 to 60 percent of patients. Large-scale multicenter treatment trials with proper randomization are needed; multiple-drug schedules as well as single-drug treatments should be considered. The models developed for the conduct of multicenter treatment programs in oncology should be applicable to the treatment of IPF. The treatment schedules that follow are clearly not an ideal drug therapy program for IPF, but they are believed to be the best available therapy at present.

Selection of Patients for Therapy

The course of IPF is highly variable among patients. Whether to treat at all, and if so, what program to use, must be individualized for each patient. Factors that predict advancement of the disease are listed in Table 4; these factors also seem to predict a more likely response to therapy. Patients who exhibit these features deserve aggressive therapy. Acceptance of a higher rate of side effects and complications seems justified by the greater likelihood of a favorable result.

Some patients appear to have disease that is not likely to respond to therapy (see Table 4). These patients deserve a more conservative approach. Treatment is probably still indicated since our ability to anticipate precisely response and outcome is limited. Treatment should be closely monitored, secondary drugs may not be justified, and therapy probably should be reduced or discontinued if significant or uncomfortable side effects develop. We do not wish to make the cure worse than the disease.

Patients with severe complicating diseases may not be candidates for aggressive therapy. Mild IPF that appears to be progressing slowly may not warrant treatment if the patient is aged or infirm.

Occasionally, patients may not require therapy at the time of presentation. These individuals usually have few or no symptoms and normal or nearly normal pulmonary function. Most importantly, they fail to show evidence of disease progression over time. These patients may be young, in contrast to the middle-aged predominance for IPF. Typically, these patients are referred for evaluation because of an abnormal chest roentgenogram that demon-

TABLE 4 Prognostic Factors in Idiopathic Pulmonary Fibrosis

Favorable predictors
Cellular lung biopsy
Immune complexes in lung and serum
Lymphocytes in bronchoalveolar lavage (?)
Early disease
Mild lung function abnormalities
Younger age at presentation
Female sex
Unfavorable predictors
Fibrotic biopsy without inflammation
Neutrophils and eosinophils in lavage (?)
Late disease
Honeycomb pattern on chest roentgenogram
Severe function impairment
Older age at presentation
Male sex

strates a diffuse pattern of small irregular shadows in low profusion. When they are available, old films often show that the same pattern has been present for years. Lung biopsy shows minimal fibrosis with no cellularity or inflammation. Perhaps these individuals carry an inactive scar that is the evidence of some previous infection, inhaled insult, or self-limited inflammatory process.

Drug Treatment Program

Patients who present with suspected IPF undergo a defined initial evaluation and follow a specific treatment algorithm. This treatment plan, which is shown schematically in Figure 1, is similar to that used for a recent multicenter study of bronchoalveolar lavage. The initial evaluation is designed to establish the diagnosis, to assess the prognosis and likelihood of response to therapy, and to provide baselines against which future progress can be measured. It must be emphasized that this treatment program is empiric and somewhat arbitrary in dose and schedule. These choices need to be validated by proper randomized and controlled trials.

Patients are interviewed for a careful medical and occupational history, with emphasis on precise description of their current level of dyspnea, any complicating medical conditions, and any occupational or environmental exposures that might provide an explanation for their respiratory disease. Current body weight and blood pressure are recorded. Physical examination documents current findings and focuses on detecting complicating illnesses. The eyes are carefully examined for cataracts and glaucoma. Excellent quality 72-inch posteroanterior

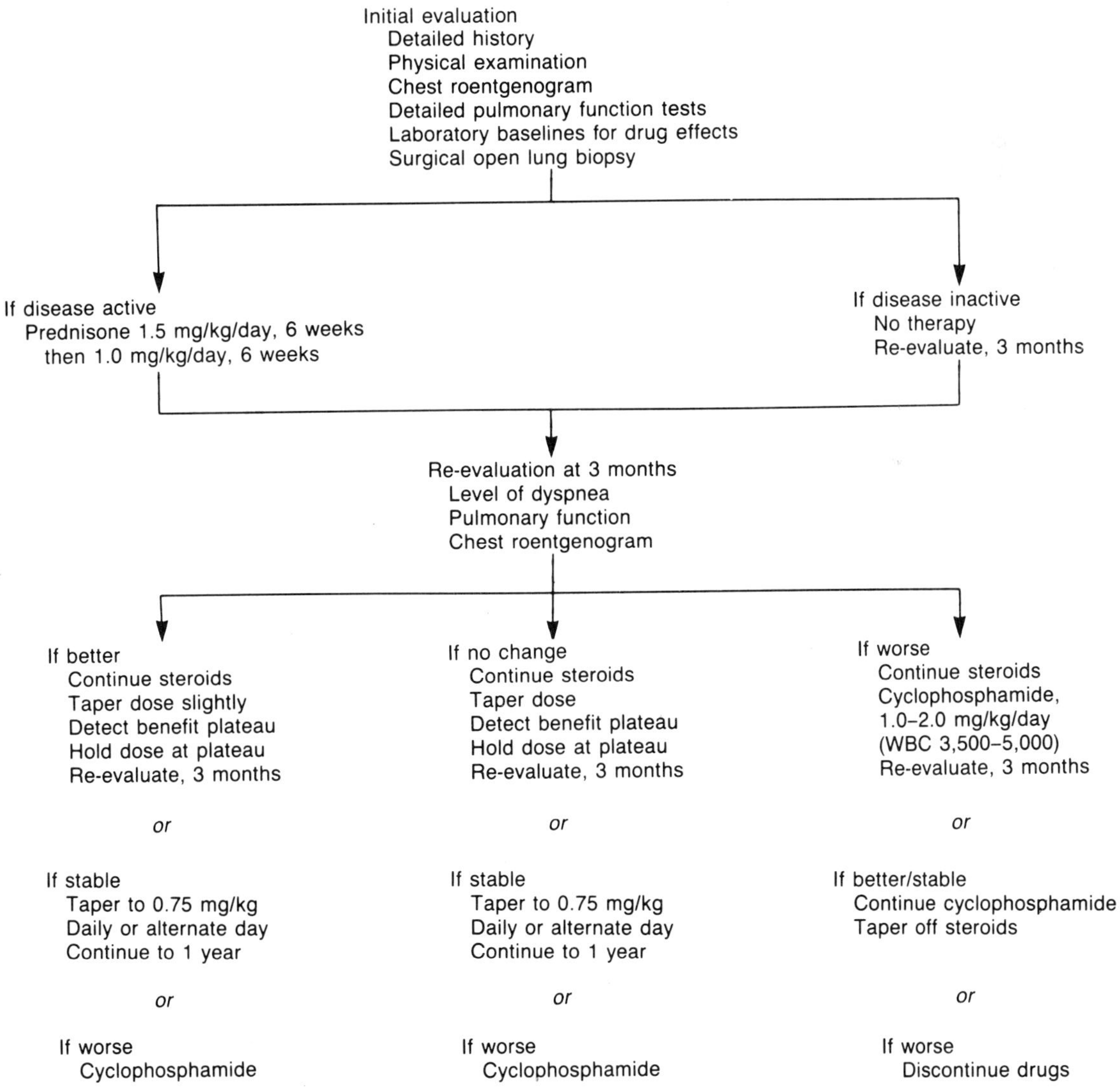

Figure 1 Drug treatment algorithm for idiopathic pulmonary fibrosis.

and lateral chest films, made with a small focal spot and high kilovoltage technique, are essential for proper definition of small irregular shadows. Laboratory tests include a complete blood count, a sedimentation rate, an antinuclear antibody determination, measurement of electrolytes, renal function tests, fasting glucose test, and a urinalysis. These measurements are important primarily to establish normality before possible drug toxicities appear. Pulmonary function testing must be meticulous, including measurement of lung volumes, flow rates, single breath diffusing capacity for carbon monoxide, and measurements of arterial blood gases and oxygen consumption at rest and during exercise. As already discussed, an open surgical lung biopsy is obtained in almost all patients.

Patients who have progressive disease, as evidenced by a cellular biopsy and other features shown in Table 4, should receive full therapy. They are treated with high daily doses of corticosteroids for 3 months. The high initial dose is prescribed so that failure of the patient to respond can be attributed to lack of sensitivity to the drug, rather than too low a dose of the drug. Patients are allowed 2 or 3 weeks to recover from their biopsy surgery before treatment is begun. Treatment is started with prednisone, 1.5 mg per kilogram body weight, taken as a single oral dose each morning. Total dose is not to exceed 100 mg per day, even if body weight exceeds 70 kg. Methylprednisolone is used in equipotent doses (1.2 mg per kilogram) for patients in whom sodium retention, preexisting congestive heart failure, or hypertension is a problem.

The many side effects of steroid therapy must be discussed with each patient before treatment is started. I warn all patients beginning this high-dose steroid program that they can expect a change in their body habitus and self-image; cushingoid changes are universal. They have to fight hard against increased appetite and weight gain. Their face becomes rounded, often red and flushed. Body hair may become coarser. They bruise easily as their skin becomes more delicate, and acne may develop. Many patients feel emotionally labile or irritable. I assure them that all of these changes are fully reversible and are related to the dose of the drug. These side effects disappear as dosage is reduced or stopped. Somewhat more serious side effects are common as well: mild glucose intolerance, mild hypertension, obesity, frequent urinary tract infections, vaginitis, or bronchitis are often seen. The risk of peptic ulcer disease and gastrointestinal bleeding may be increased, but this remains controversial. Loss of bone density, osteoporosis of the spine, and vertebral compression fractures are a particular problem in older women. Some physicians recommend supplemental calcium and vitamin D for women who are receiving steroid therapy.

Fortunately, the most serious side effects of steroid treatment are rare. Although host defenses against infection are theoretically (and measurably) impaired, serious infections are uncommon, and opportunistic pathogens are almost never involved in IPF patients. The clinician must remain alert for early signs of infection since symptoms are suppressed by the anti-inflammatory drug effects. Myopathy may occur. Posterior subcapsular cataracts develop rarely, and then only in patients who have been treated for a long time.

Patients receiving high-dose steroid therapy must be cautioned not to stop treatment abruptly under any circumstances. The risk of adrenal insufficiency is real, particularly under stress. Steroids must be tapered gradually once dosage is below the level of estimated normal endogenous production. These patients require supplemental steroids at times of physical stress, surgery, or trauma for as long as one year after this treatment course. It may be helpful for patients to enroll in the Medic Alert program and to carry a warning bracelet or other identification that states that they are receiving steroid therapy.

The patient returns for brief follow-up 7 to 14 days after steroid therapy has been started. The purpose of this visit is solely to monitor drug side effects; no impact on IPF is expected. Blood pressure, urine glucose, and possibly blood glucose and potassium are checked. Most patients have many questions, and this visit is a good time for teaching and reassurance.

Prednisone dosage is reduced to 1.0 mg per kilogram per day after 6 weeks of therapy. Limited re-evaluation is carried out at this time, which includes measurement of vital capacity and of arterial blood gases at rest and a chest roentgenogram. Some early treatment response or deterioration may be seen. These interval tests help to indicate the extent of day-to-day variability in these measurements. Evidence of adverse steroid side effects should be sought at each visit; the patient is checked for diabetes, hypertension, excessive potassium loss, infections, and other common complications.

A detailed re-evaluation is performed after 3 months of steroid therapy to determine whether treatment is succeeding. A symptom history is obtained in an attempt to quantitate the level of dyspnea as precisely as possible. Complete lung function testing is performed, which includes studies of gas exchange at rest and during exercise. Chest roentgenograms and laboratory blood tests are repeated.

The next step in therapy depends on whether the patient's condition can be classified as better, worse, or unchanged. For some patients, the changes over 3 months are so obvious that classification is easy, but for many it may be difficult. Each test variable should be assessed independently and as objectively as possible. Vague symptoms related to energy, endurance, and general well-being are important with regard to the patient's quality of life; however, they are nearly impossible to quantitate and are susceptible to placebo effects and the euphoria of steroids. Semiquantitative assessment of dyspnea is useful, as measured by the ability to perform routine activities that are repeated frequently. Roentgenographic changes are important, but these are often minimal or evolve more slowly than other variables. Pulmonary function tests should receive the most weight; changes for better or worse that are greater than 5 to 10 percent are probably significant. I have found that exercise arterial blood oxygen tensions are often the most sensitive reflection of improvement or deterioration and may change significantly when lung volumes do not. The clinician should attempt to develop a composite assessment based on a synthesis of all of these factors. The CRP score may be useful for this purpose.

Patients whose condition is improved on steroid therapy should continue on this treatment with re-evaluations at frequent intervals until a plateau is reached. The dose may be reduced slightly, and gradual transition toward alternate-day treatment should keep side effects to a minimum. Doses in the range of 0.75 to 1.0 mg per kilogram every other day might be reached in another 2 or 3 months and then maintained until repeat evaluations no longer show interval improvement. Evaluation, as just described, should be repeated every 2 or 3 months. When maximal beneficial effect is achieved, steroids may be tapered further and re-evaluations stretched to 4- or 6-month intervals. Maintenance prednisone dosage at 20 to 30 mg every other day may be reached about 6 to 8 months after treatment is begun and should be continued empirically for a total course of about 1 year. Patients should be re-evaluated frequently as therapy is withdrawn so that recrudescence can be detected. In many cases, after a year of treatment, drug therapy can be tapered without a reappearance of active disease.

Patients whose condition deteriorates despite high-dose steroid therapy are candidates for cytotoxic drug treatment. The decision to use agents in which the side effects can be serious or life-threatening and in which the effectiveness is not yet fully proved must be based on firm evidence that the patient is experiencing a progressive downhill course expected to result in respiratory insufficiency and death. Both a secure tissue-proven diagnosis and clear objective evidence of active disease are required. Cyclophosphamide appears somewhat more effective than azathioprine in the limited studies available to date. Initially, the cytotoxic drug is added to a moderate dose of steroids.

I begin with cyclophosphamide in a dose of about 1.5 mg per kilogram body weight per day and increase to 2.0 mg per kilogram per day if tolerated and needed. Doses greater than 150 mg per day are rarely required. The target for proper dosage is a total peripheral white blood cell count (WBC) between 3,500 and 5,000 cells per cubic millimeter. The dose should be increased up to 2.0 mg per kilogram per day until this slight-to-moderate WBC depression is achieved. Dosage should be reduced if the WBC falls below 3,500. Patients should be cautioned to drink liquids aggressively and to void frequently in order to minimize the concentration and residence time of the drug in the bladder, and thus reduce the risk of hemorrhagic cystitis. Some patients experience nausea and anorexia. Most patients experience hair thinning, and women may wish to purchase a wig before alopecia becomes apparent. Once again, patients should be assured that this bothersome cosmetic change can be reversed in almost every case when treatment is completed. The WBC and the urinalysis should be monitored every several weeks as treatment is begun and dosage is adjusted. The frequency of these tests can be decreased somewhat once a stable dosage is obtained, but frequent re-evaluation is still necessary. With these moderate doses of cyclophosphamide, and with close observation for toxicity, severe side effects are uncommon. Dosage often has to be reduced as treatment progresses in order to avoid excessive WBC depression. High-dose intermittent pulse therapy may prove useful in the future.

Clinical progress and detailed pulmonary function testing should be reassessed after 3 months of combined prednisone-cyclophosphamide treatment. The techniques and the criteria already described are used to determine whether patients are better, worse, or unchanged. Patients who show definite improvement on cyclophosphamide, and probably those whose condition worsened during steroid therapy but stabilized with cyclophosphamide treatment, should continue on this drug for 1 year of therapy. The concomitant steroid treatment can be discontinued by tapering over the next 2 or 3 months, and cyclophosphamide continued as a single drug for the last 6 months. It can be stopped without tapering when treatment is completed or if intolerable side effects appear. If pulmonary function tests continue to deteriorate despite the combination of cyclophosphamide and prednisone, the former drug should be stopped and the latter drug tapered off as quickly as possible. No alternative drug treatments have been shown to be effective for those unfortunate patients.

Azathioprine is an alternative cytoxic drug that could be used in place of cyclophosphamide. Preliminary results suggest it may be less effective than cyclophosphamide, but its side effects are probably more manageable as well. Hair loss is not a problem, and WBC depression is less pronounced. A dose of 1 to 3 mg per kilogram of body weight as a single dose each day is standard. This drug may be useful for patients who are unable to tolerate cyclophosphamide, but who appear to be good candidates for aggressive therapy. If patients fail to respond to full doses of prednisone and cyclophosphamide, I would not expect azathioprine to be useful.

The cytotoxic agents, cyclophosphamide and azathioprine, theoretically increase the risk of neoplasia in patients who receive them. Data supporting this risk come from relatively young patients whose malignant disease developed a number of years after drug treatment. This risk may be of less concern in the older age group of patients with IPF. These drugs are also teratogenic, but most IPF patients are beyond the childbearing years. The cytotoxic agents are generally much better tolerated than are high-dose steroids, and patients seem much less aware of their day-to-day side effects.

The patient whose symptoms, pulmonary function, and chest roentgenogram remain unchanged during treatment presents a difficult problem. On the one hand, such a patient may have had inactive and nonprogressive disease all along. Drug therapy would have no effect in that case, and the side effects would be incurred with no benefit to counterbalance them. Alternatively, an active and progressive inflammatory process may have been arrested successfully, and a downhill course may have been stopped. The residual, but now stable, pulmonary dysfunction may represent irreversible lung scarring. This frequent therapeutic dilemma emphasizes the need for careful documentation of the degree of disease activity before treatment is begun. If definite activity and progressive disease have been documented previously, treatment should be considered a success and should be continued. We may not have been able to make this patient better, but we have stopped him or her from getting worse. I would manage this patient in the same way as a patient who shows clear improvement.

Supportive Care

Patients with IPF require considerable supportive care in addition to specific drug therapy. Of greatest importance is their need and their family's need for supportive and compassionate physicians and other health care providers. These patients have a serious and often progressively disabling disease, which may impair their quality of life and constrain their activities as it progresses. The drugs used to treat this disease produce unsightly and sometimes uncomfortable side effects. These patients need encouragment and understanding, advice regarding ways to accomplish their activities of daily living, and clear explanations about their illness. Hospice care or home nursing is recommended to help family members if dyspnea becomes severe and if patients are bedridden.

Exercise programs for IPF patients can help to maintain muscle strength and ambulation. Daily walks are excellent. A stationary bicycle used with supplemental oxygen can help most patients to get daily exercise. Diet counseling should help patients to avoid excessive weight gain while on steroids and to maximize nutrition when dyspnea makes eating difficult.

Oxygen therapy is needed by many IPF patients, particularly during exertion. Exercise tolerance in IPF is often limited by hypoxia as well as by the high work of breathing; the hypoxia can be effectively relieved by portable supplemental oxygen. A number of my IPF patients have been able to resume shopping, light housework, socializing, and full-time sedentary jobs after portable oxygen therapy was begun. Portable oxygen for use while walking or otherwise exercising is probably helpful if the Po_2 level during exercise measures less than 55 torr or if the saturation level measures less than 88 to 90 percent. I believe that both the need for portable oxygen and the efficacy of supplemental oxygen during exercise should be documented by testing with a treadmill or bicycle. A transcutaneous ear or digital oximeter is particularly useful for this type of testing. Oxygen dosage can be adjusted during moderate steady-state exercise until a saturation greater than 90 percent is achieved. Oxygen during exercise usually provides a higher saturation, greater exercise endurance, greater comfort, a lower pulse rate, and a shorter recovery time after exercise stops. Many patients with severe IPF require high oxygen flow rates by nasal cannulae to reach these goals. Oxygen therapy should be continued for 5 to 10 minutes after exertion.

Small portable aluminum or stainless steel oxygen tanks weigh about 6 pounds, carry enough oxygen for about 1 hour of use, and can be refilled by patients from a large reservoir cylinder at home. Liquid oxygen systems also provide convenient portable units; they can be refilled by patients from reservoirs at home, and each provides several hours of oxygen. They may be more suitable for patients who require extremely high flow rates. The liquid units weigh 8 to 11 pounds, and thus are somewhat more difficult for frail or elderly patients to carry while walking.

With more advanced disease, supplemental oxygen may also be required to relieve hypoxia at rest. Arterial blood gas levels that show a Po_2 of less than 55 torr (or less than 60 torr with evidence of heart failure) at rest indicate likely benefit from continuous home oxygen therapy at flow rates adequate to raise the Po_2 to about 65 to 70 torr or the saturation to about 92 to 94 percent. Oxygen concentrators, which operate on home electric power and concentrate oxygen from room air, are useful for patients who require continuous oxygen therapy. They are reliable, relatively quiet, unobtrusive, and cost-effective. They can be transported from room to room as activities change during the normal day. Liquid oxygen systems for continuous stationary use may be a good choice for IPF patients who are active and also require oxygen with exercise.

Cough is a troublesome manifestation of IPF, it interrupts sleep and meals and often makes conversation difficult and embarrassing. Codeine cough suppressants work for a few days at a time, but tolerance soon appears. They are best reserved for occasional use at night and for patients with terminal disease and intractable cough.

Ventilatory support usually is not appropriate for IPF patients who slide gradually into progressive respiratory failure. These patients typically have run a course of several years of progressive disease and already have been treated aggressively with the drugs that are available. Unfortunately, there is little hope of reversing the disease in these patients, and they are dependent on a ventilator for the remainder of their lives. Conversely, ventilatory support usually is indicated for the patient with IPF who has not yet received definitive diagnosis or therapy. The mortality rate is high, but some of these patients can achieve a remarkable reversal of their disease.

Lung transplantation remains an experimental procedure, but it holds great promise for some patients with IPF. Only a few centers throughout the world have undertaken lung transplantation, but IPF patients have enjoyed some of the most successful outcomes in several of these programs. The Toronto Lung Transplant Group has achieved remarkable success, with better than 60 percent long term survival in a small but growing series of IPF patients. The technique of wrapping the bronchial anastomosis with omentum to improve blood supply and to reduce dehiscence, cyclosporine and other immunosuppressives, better management of rejection and infection, and an aggressive pre- and post-operative rehabilitation program have contributed to their dramatic progress. Single lung transplantation, rather than combined heart-lung transplantation seems to be particularly well suited to patients with IPF. Transplantation is becoming a realistic option for patients with end-stage IPF. Patients who are relatively young, who do not have any other complicating medical illnesses, and who have severe progressive IPF that has been resistant to other forms of therapy should be considered for referral.

This work was supported in part by grant HL-14212 (SCOR) from the National Heart, Lung and Blood Institute and by grant RR-109 from the General Clinical Research Centers Program of the National Institutes of Health.

SUGGESTED READING

Crystal RG, Bitterman PB, Rennard SI, Hance AJ, Keogh BA. Interstitial lung diseases of unknown cause: disorders characterized by chronic inflammation of the lower respiratory tract. N Engl J Med 1984; 310:154–166 and 235–244.

Reynolds HY. Bronchoalveolar lavage: state of the art. Am Rev Respir Dis 1987; 135:250–263.

The Toronto Lung Transplant Group. Experience with single-lung transplantation for pulmonary fibrosis. JAMA 1988; 259:2258–2262.

Turner-Warwick M, Burrows B, Johnson A. Cryptogenic fibrosing alveolitis: clinical features and their influence on survival. Thorax 1980; 35:171–180.

Turner-Warwick M, Burrows G, Johnson A. Cryptogenic fibrosing alveolitis: corticosteroid treatment and its effect on survival. Thorax 1980; 35:593–599.

Watters LC, King TE, Schwarz MI, Waldron JA, Stanford RM, Cherniack RM. A clinical, radiographic, and physiologic scoring system for the longitudinal assessment of patients with idiopathic pulmonary fibrosis. Am Rev Respir Dis 1986; 133:97–103.

Winterbauer RH, et al. Diffuse interstitial pneumonitis: clinicopathological correlations in 20 patients treated with prednisone/azathioprine. Am J Med 1978; 65:661–672.

WEGENER'S GRANULOMATOSIS

GAIL LEVEE, M.D.
DANIEL H. SIMMONS, M.D., Ph.D.

Wegener's granulomatosis is a disease characterized by necrotizing vasculitis involving both small arteries and veins with granulomas; it potentially affects any organ system (Table 1). Patients usually present with necrotizing lesions in the upper and/or lower respiratory tract and with glomerulonephritis. If untreated, less than 20 percent of patients survive more than 1 year and less than 10 percent, 2 years. However, there are a few untreated long-term survivors among the 10 to 15 percent of patients without glomerulitis. Renal failure causes over 80 percent of the deaths; respiratory complications cause most of the rest. Immunosuppressive therapy dramatically improves survival. Cyclophosphamide is the drug of choice; it induces long-term complete remission in about 90 percent of cases and, in the one-third that relapse, induces a second remission about 95 percent of the time. Rapid institution of treatment is critical to prevent irreversible renal damage.

CLINICAL MANIFESTATIONS

Organ Involvement

Presenting symptoms most often involve the upper respiratory tract; they include rhinorrhea and paranasal sinus pain or discharge, often associated with nasopharyngeal mucosal ulceration or tissue necrosis.

Lung involvement, present in over 80 percent of patients, is usually associated with cough, dyspnea, or hemoptysis; however, it may be asymptomatic. The trachea is involved in 10 percent of cases. Chest roentgenograms typically show round cavitating nodules greater than 1 cm in diameter, most often in the lower lobes. Transient infiltrates may occur. Pleural effusions are present in 20 percent of patients. Hilar adenopathy is not seen, and calcification is rare.

Renal involvement typically follows respiratory tract involvement. Ten percent of patients have azotemia when first seen. Thirty percent develop end-stage renal failure in spite of therapy, usually if irreversible changes occur before diagnosis or if exacerbations are undetected and untreated. Proteinuria, hematuria, or red blood cell casts are often present before overt renal failure. Renal biopsy is usually nonspecific; although glomerulonephritis is present, parenchymal granulomas or true renal arteritis is rare.

Fever, weight loss, malaise, and other constitutional symptoms are common, but are unfortunately nonspecific and, in themselves, do not usually lead to the diagnosis.

Symptomatic disease may occur in many other organs (see Table 1). Joint involvement may manifest as either arthralgia or nondeforming arthritis. Angiitis of dermal vessels usually results in ulceration; papules, vesicles, palpable purpura, and subcutaneous nodules also occur. The severity of skin lesions typically parallels disease activity. Proptosis is the most frequent ocular manifestation. Conjunctivitis, episcleritis, scleritis, uveitis, optic nerve vasculitis, retinal artery occlusion, and nasolacrimal duct obstruction occur. Eustachian tube blockage frequently causes otitis media. Sensorineural deafness may occur. Pericarditis and coronary vasculitis are the most common cardiac complications. Nervous system disease may manifest as cranial neuritis or mononeuritis multiplex, either from invasion by granulomas in

TABLE 1 Organ System Involvement in Wegener's Granulomatosis

Organ System	*Frequency (%)*	*Clinical Manifestations*
Nasopharynx	75	Sore throat, epistaxis, "saddle-nose deformity"
Paranasal sinuses	90	Sinusitis, secondary bacterial infection
Eyes	60	Keratoconjunctivitis, sclerouveitis, proptosis, orbital mass lesions
Ears	35	Hearing loss, serous otitis media, secondary bacterial infection
Lungs	95	Cough, dyspnea, hemoptysis, multiple nodular cavitary infiltrates
Kidneys	85	Proteinuria, red blood cell casts, focal glomerulitis, fulminant glomerulonephritis in advanced cases
Heart	15	Pericarditis, coronary vasculitis
Nervous system	20	Mononeuritis multiplex, cranial nerve palsies, diabetes insipidus
Skin	40	Palpable purpura, cutaneous nodules, ulcerations
Constitutional symptoms	70	Fever, weight loss, malaise, fatique

paranasal sinuses or from vasculitis. The spleen and male adnexal organs frequently contain necrotizing granulomas.

LABORATORY DIAGNOSIS

Although laboratory findings are not specific for Wegener's granulomatosis, they are useful for detecting changes in disease activity, which is critical to therapy. Normochromic normocytic anemia, leukocytosis, and thrombocytosis frequently occur. Over 90 percent of patients have an elevated sedimentation rate during active disease. C-reactive protein levels may be useful because their half-life is hours compared with weeks for the sedimentation rate, allowing changes to be detected sooner; further, it may be a more specific marker of activity. Nearly 50 percent of patients have circulating immune complexes; immunoglobulin deposition in the kidney and lung have frequently been described. Mild hyperglobulinemia, particularly of IgA, is common. Rheumatoid factor is present in 50 percent of cases; delayed hypersensitivity cutaneous reactions are preserved, and antinuclear antibody is negative. Recent studies suggest that a specific diagnostic test may soon be available; antineutrophil-cytoplasm antibodies are almost always present and are highly specific for Wegener's granulomatosis. The test has been reported to increase the frequency of diagnosis threefold and to hasten detection of exacerbations and remissions.

Pulmonary function tests show an obstructive or restrictive pattern. Obstructive defects are usually associated with focal large airway lesions and narrowing, which occasionally results in tracheal obstruction or lobar collapse.

TISSUE DIAGNOSIS

Diagnosing Wegener's granulomatosis requires a biopsy of the involved tissue. Open lung biopsies of masses seen on chest roentgenograms typically show classic arteritis, consequent necrosis and hemorrhagic infarcts, and adjacent granulomas. Endobronchial biopsies are usually nondiagnostic. Similarly, 50 percent of upper airway biopsies are nonspecific, since they rarely detect both granulomas and vasculitis.

MANAGEMENT

Careful monitoring of the activity of Wegener's granulomatosis is an extremely important part of treatment. Exacerbations must be detected as rapidly as possible because renal function and the function of other critical organs can deteriorate rapidly and irreversibly with inadequate therapy. Apparent remissions must be monitored to avoid decreasing the intensity of therapy and permitting irreversible changes while the disease is still active. Since about one-third of patients in apparently complete remission eventually relapse, they must be carefully monitored indefinitely.

Unfortunately, evaluating activity can be difficult. Many criteria for activity are also affected by infection, a common confounding variable during immunosuppressive therapy. This may result in treating the disease when infection is the main problem—often worsening the infection—or treating the infection when dangerous increased activity is the main problem. For example, patients who have serious sinus or nasal disease develop secondary infections, typically caused by *Staphylococcus aureus*; worsening symptoms may require antibiotics rather than increased immunosuppressive therapy.

Disease activity is an indicator of drug effectiveness; it should be assessed frequently by constitutional or other symptoms, lesions on chest roentgenogram or in easily examined areas such as skin and eye, serum creatinine levels, urinalysis, and sedimentation rate. C-reactive protein also can be used, but unfortunately both markers increase with infections as well as with disease activity and therefore cannot differentiate between them. Finally, changes in serum antineutrophil-cytoplasm antibody concentrations may be extremely useful.

Drug Therapy

Immunosuppressive agents are the only therapy proven almost universally successful.

Cyclophosphamide

Cyclophosphamide is the drug of choice because it induces complete remission in more than 90 percent of patients, unless irreversible changes have occurred in the kidney. The mechanism by which cyclophosphamide works is uncertain. Blocking of an immune-mediated mechanism is suggested by the presence of serum immune complexes in nearly half of patients and by the presence of antineutrophil-cytoplasm antibodies. Cyclophosphamide may work through its actions on lymphocytes, since it reverses hyperglobulinemia and causes leukopenia.

The dose of cyclophosphamide is determined by the severity of disease and its rate of progression. If a patient's disease is stable or has progressed only slowly over months, oral administration of cyclophosphamide should be started at 1 to 2 mg per kilogram per day. If no improvement is evident after 2 weeks of therapy, the daily dose should be increased by 25 mg and the patient reevaluated in 2 weeks. This cycle should be repeated until either improvement occurs or side effects become limiting.

Because cyclophosphamide administration takes 1 to 2 weeks to achieve maximum effect, corticosteroids may be started simultaneously for their immediate anti-inflammatory and immunologic effects; they are tapered as the cyclophosphamide takes full effect.

Fulminant disease, such as rapidly progressive glomerulonephritis or other life-threatening situations, requires higher doses of cyclophosphamide and steroids. Cyclophosphamide dosage is 4 to 5 mg per kilogram per day by mouth or intravenously for 3 days before tapering to conventional doses over another 3 days. Prednisone dosage is at least 1 mg per kilogram per day for 1 to 2 weeks until the cyclophosphamide takes effect; it should then be tapered to an alternate-day schedule over 1 to 2 months to 1 mg per kilogram every other day and slowly tapered off completely over 6 to 12 months.

Cyclophosphamide should be continued for at least 1 year after complete remission to minimize the likelihood of relapse. The dosage can then be gradually tapered by 25 mg every 2 to 3 months or the drug can be discontinued abruptly. The tapering schedule is preferable because recurring activity can usually be detected earlier as the drug is tapered; dosage should then be returned to the usual level.

It has been suggested that 500-mg boluses of cyclophosphamide given weekly are equally as effective as the usual daily dosages and might cause fewer side effects.

The most common complications of cyclophosphamide therapy are bone marrow suppression (almost 100 percent) and hemorrhagic cystitis (about 30 percent). Because leukopenia is common with the recommended dosage and leads to the usual infections, the leukocyte count should be checked every other day during induction and the dosage reduced to keep the leukocyte count above 3,000 to 3,500 per cubic millimeter and neutrophils above 1,000 to 1,500. Once the leukocyte count is stable, it can be checked every 1 to 2 weeks. If the patient becomes leukopenic on a dose that allows the disease to flare, corticosteroids can be added in an attempt to increase the leukocyte count, or the cyclophosphamide can be decreased or discontinued and administration of azathioprine started.

Since hemorrhagic cystitis occurs in one-third of patients taking cyclophosphamide, any patient with microscopic hematuria who is in apparent remission should be evaluated with cystoscopy and biopsy. If the cystitis is severe, cyclophosphamide may need to be discontinued, although no long-term sequelae are reported. Most patients experience mild hair loss. Patients should be warned of possible gonadal dysfunction, which is manifested in women by oligomenorrhea or amenorrhea and in men by impotence or loss of libido.

Cyclophosphamide is oncogenic, but leukemias have been reported rarely with its use in Wegener's granulomatosis. However, many types of tumors have been reported following cyclophosphamide treatment for other diseases. Preceding pancytopenia is thought to be a factor in drug-related leukemias. Cardiomyopathy has been reported during chronic cyclophosphamide administration. Deaths caused by drug-induced pulmonary fibrosis have been reported when cyclophosphamide has been given for other conditions.

Steroids

Corticosteroids are not required in all patients. Indications for their use, usually in combination with cyclophosphamide or azathioprine, include fulminant renal or pulmonary disease, severe skin vasculitis, cerebral vasculitis, progressive neuropathy, deep eye involvement, and severe serosal inflammation, e.g., pericarditis. Superficial eye involvement responds to topical steroids. The usual side effects that occur with steroids can develop, but are uncommon because, in most instances, steroids are tapered rapidly.

Other Therapies

When cyclophosphamide is not tolerated, azathioprine is the best alternative; it should be given in similar dosages as cyclophosphamide. However, uncontrolled trials suggest that azathioprine alone induces remissions only occasionally; yet it maintains remissions induced by cyclophosphamide successfully and is useful in other situations, such as following renal transplantation.

Other therapeutic modalities have been tried in refractory cases. There are case reports of the successful use of cyclosporin when conventional therapy failed. Trimethoprim-sulfamethoxazole was given to 12 patients who either had indolent disease when they were taking no drugs or showed no improvement on standard therapy; 11 clearly improved clinically, although relapse was usual when the drug was withdrawn. It was suggested that infection might have precipitated the immunologic abnormalities leading to Wegener's granulomatosis.

Plasma exchange has been used in selected cases; however, no controlled studies have documented its effectiveness, and failures of this therapy in fulminant disease have been reported.

Surgical Treatment

Surgical treatment may be required for complications of Wegener's granulomatosis. Sudden proptosis caused by ocular granulomatous vasculitis may require rapid orbital decompression. Otitis media, a common complication, often requires drainage through the tympanic membrane. Surgical treatment of nasolacrimal duct obstruction may be required to prevent recurrent conjunctivitis and episcleritis. Serious sinus disease complicated by infection requires antibiotics and possibly surgical drainage. Severe large airway obstruction, if not responding to medical therapy, may require surgical dilation or tracheostomy. Endobronchial lesions in mainstem bronchi progressing to stenosis may require sleeve resection to preserve pulmonary function. Renal transplantation should be considered for patients who have developed irreversible renal failure and who are in remission; it is as successful as in other forms of glomerulonephritis. The usual immunosuppressive therapy is recommended.

INFECTIOUS COMPLICATIONS

Infections of the leukopenic or immunocompromised host, particularly sepsis, are a major problem, both by their own threat to the patient and by making it difficult to tell whether new symptoms require a more aggressive Wegener's granulomatosis therapy or a treatment of the infection. However, infection is usually not a problem if the leukocyte count is kept above the recommended minimum. Cutaneous herpes zoster occurs about twice as often as in the general population and is more likely caused by treatment rather than by the disease; yet it does not disseminate more often.

Relapses are frequently associated with infection at the site of disease activity. The infection cannot be eradicated unless the underlying disease is treated. Conversely, before immunosuppressive therapy is increased or restarted for an exacerbation, infection should be looked for and treated as a possible cause of the apparent flare-up.

Gram-negative sepsis, cytomegalic virus pneumonia, and *Pneumocystis carinii* pneumonia are uncommon when steroids and cyclophosphamide are given for Wegener's granulomatosis if leukopenia is avoided.

SUGGESTED READING

DeRemee RA, McDonald TJ, Weiland LH. Wegener's granulomatosis: observations on treatment with antimocrobial agents. Mayo Clin Proc 1985; 60:27–32.

Fauci AS, Haynes BF, Katz P, Wolff SM. Wegener's granulomatosis: prospective clinical and therapeutic experience with 85 patients for 21 years. Ann Intern Med 1983; 98:76–85.

Flye MW, Mundinger GH, Fauci AS. Diagnostic and therapeutic aspects of the surgical approach to Wegener's granulomatosis. J Thorac Cardiovasc Surg 1979; 77:331–337.

Landman S, Burgener F. Pulmonary manifestations of Wegener's granulomatosis. AJR 1974; 122:750–757.

Leavitt RV, Fauci AS. Pulmonary vasculitis. Am Rev Respir Dis 1986; 134:149–166.

Littlejohn GO, Ryan PJ, Holdsworth SR. Wegener's granulomatosis: clinical features and outcome in seventeen patients. Aust NZ J Med 1985; 15:241–245.

Van der Woude FJ, Rassmussen N, Lobatto S, Wiik A, et al. Autoantibodies against neutrophils and monocytes; tool for diagnosis and marker of disease activity in Wegener's granulomatosis. Lancet 1985; Feb. 23:425–429.

COR PULMONALE

STUART RICH, M.D.

Cor pulmonale, pulmonary hypertension caused by changes in the pulmonary vascular bed resulting from advanced heart and lung disease, is a common clinical entity. When mild, cor pulmonale is often overlooked because of the relatively small influence it has on the patient's clinical state. When advanced, however, cor pulmonale can be responsible for the majority of the patient's symptoms and ultimately can lead to death. The management of cor pulmonale requires an accurate diagnosis of the etiology, and treatments are often frustrating and ineffective. Because considerable confusion exists regarding therapeutic options, it is important that some principles regarding cor pulmonale be understood.

PATHOPHYSIOLOGY OF PULMONARY HYPERTENSION AND RIGHT VENTRICULAR FAILURE

It is not uncommon for patients with cor pulmonale to present with extreme pulmonary hypertension, which may even seem out of proportion to the severity of the underlying cardiac or pulmonary disease. It is erroneous to conclude that a patient can have both primary and secondary pulmonary hypertension, since primary pulmonary hypertension is a diagnosis of exclusion. However, the pulmonary vascular bed may be hyper-reactive because considerable heterogeneity in the response of the pulmonary vascular bed to a variety of stimuli exists. A typical example is high-altitude pulmonary edema, which can develop in people who appear to be normal and healthy from all other parameters. Physicians frequently encounter patients with mitral stenosis who have similar valve areas but different levels of pulmonary hypertension (Table 1), which demonstrates that the degree of pulmonary vasoconstriction in response to high filling pressures of the left ventricle also can vary considerably from patient to patient.

The prognosis of patients with cor pulmonale is closely related to right ventricular function. Although the right ventricular ejection fraction is directly related to the level of pulmonary artery pressure, some patients adapt to the pulmonary hypertensive state better than others. An important contributor to right ventricular failure in pulmonary hypertension is chronic ischemia. The right ventricle has a poor native blood supply, but compensates by receiving coronary artery blood flow during both systole and diastole. Normally, a substantial gradient exists between aortic and right ventricular systolic and diastolic pressures. In the presence of pulmonary hypertension, however, the systolic gradient for right coronary blood flow becomes reduced and can even be eliminated, making the right ventricular myocardium diastolic flow dependent. Thus the hypertrophied right ventricle is in a chronic state of increasing metabolic demands with a relatively limited blood supply. Once the right ventricle becomes ischemic, a vicious cycle can develop in which right ventricular systolic function becomes impaired with reduced-cardiac output, resulting in an increased heart rate, which further diminishes diastolic filling. Systemic hypotension and elevated right ventricular end-diastolic pressures also reduce the diastolic flow gradient. For these reasons, vasodilators can be particularly hazardous if they reduce systemic blood pressure without significantly affecting the pulmonary artery pressure.

TABLE 1 Hemodynamics in Mitral Stenosis

Test	*Patient A**	*Patient B*
Pulmonary artery pressure (mm Hg)	54/26	86/48
Pulmonary wedge pressure (mm Hg)	25	26
Mitral value area (cm^2)	1.1	1.0

* Data from two patients with mitral stenosis of similar severity are presented. Patient B, however, has reactive pulmonary vasoconstriction in addition to high pulmonary wedge pressures, which contributes to the level of pulmonary hypertension.

EVALUATION OF THE PATIENT WITH PULMONARY HYPERTENSION

Because the etiology may not always be apparent from the patient's clinical presentation, it is mandatory that a systematic evaluation be performed on every patient who presents with unexplained pulmonary hypertension. The evaluation should begin with a high quality upright posterior-anterior and lateral chest roentgenogram. If hyperinflation and emphysematous changes are apparent, it may be reasonable to assume that the pulmonary hypertension is secondary to chronic obstructive pulmonary disease (COPD). If diffuse interstitial markings predominate the lung fields, it is likely secondary to interstitial lung disease. If the chest film shows cardiomegaly with clear lung fields, a number of causes remain possible, although it should be kept in mind that having clear lung fields does not necessarily exclude parenchymal lung disease as the underlying etiology.

Although pulmonary function tests are necessary to evaluate lung flow and volumes, there is no minimal level of obstructive airways disease necessary to produce cor pulmonale. Restrictive changes are somewhat more difficult to interpret because the presence of pulmonary hypertension in the absence of lung disease results in a reduction in lung volumes of approximately 15 to 20 percent of the predicted value, and changes of twice that amount can be related to the pulmonary hypertension alone. In these patients, the constellation of findings based on the chest roentgenogram, the pulmonary function tests, and the history would be most important in directing the physician toward a correct etiology. Sleep apnea also can cause pulmonary hypertension, and since its management is so different from that of other pulmonary disease, it should be pursued whenever the clinical diagnosis appears possible. Reductions in arterial oxygen saturation can occur from underlying lung disease or as a manifestation of low cardiac output and may be magnified by the presence of ventilation: perfusion inequalities within the lung. An abnormality in the diffusing capacity for carbon monoxide has been observed in the presence of pulmonary hypertension from most any cause and, by itself, is not diagnostic of any particular condition.

I have found the perfusion lung scan a most informative test in the evaluation of the patient with pulmonary hypertension, and it is mandatory to identify pulmonary thromboembolic disease as a cause. It should be noted that the patient who has pulmonary hypertension from chronic thromboembolic disease often does not give a history of previous or recurrent pulmonary embolism. A perfectly normal perfusion lung scan virtually eliminates thromboembolic causes, whereas the presence of a diffuse mottled appearance suggests underlying pulmonary thrombotic arteriopathy, which is seen in primary pulmonary hypertension and in pulmonary hypertension secondary to congenital heart disease. Patients with pulmonary veno-occlusive disease may also have a mottled lung scan pattern, although this entity is quite rare.

If the perfusion lung scan suggests segmental or subsegmental filling defects, a pulmonary angiogram must be done. To reduce the morbidity of the procedure, it should be performed selectively on the basis of the perfusion lung scan pattern. In the instance of chronic pulmonary thromboembolism, large proximal vascular cutoffs often are noted, coexistent with changes in the uninvolved pulmonary vascular bed showing vascular enlargement, tortuosity, and tapering toward the periphery. Although physicians have been cautioned about performing perfusion lung scans and pulmonary angiograms in the setting of pulmonary hypertension, these procedures remain relatively safe in experienced hands as long as adequate precautions are taken. In patients with right ventricular failure, I routinely administer 1 mg of atropine intravenously prior to the angiogram, use low-osmolar, nonionic contrast agents, and monitor systemic blood pressure directly through an arterial line.

Echocardiography and Doppler studies are particularly helpful in determining the presence of valvular or myocardial disease. As stated previously, any abnormality of left ventricular filling, whether from chronic essential hypertension, coronary heart disease, or valvular heart disease, is a potential cause for the development of extreme levels of pulmonary hypertension. The echocardiogram also allows for the noninvasive assessment of underlying congenital heart disease. The patient with cor pulmonale generally has a left ventricle that is either normal or small in size, with an abnormal septal curvature, which is the chronic adaptive response to elevated pulmonary artery pressures. The appearance of the two-dimensional echocardiogram is often one of a large right ventricle that is compressing the left ventricle. This is not actually the case, since there is adequate room in the thorax to accommodate an enlarged right and left ventricle together. With severe pulmonary hypertension however, a markedly reduced cardiac output and a high pulmonary arterial pressure results in dilatation of the right ventricle and relative underfilling of the left ventricle, which gives it a compressed appearance. Pulmonary hypertension also reduces the compliance of the left ventricle, which may make the left ventricle extraordinarily dependent on effective atrial systole. Because of this, the development of atrial fibrillation or atrial tachycardias can have catastrophic hemodynamic consequences.

The definitive evaluation of the patient with pulmonary hypertension requires cardiac catheterization. The physician must exclude congenital heart disease, even if the patient denies any knowledge of its existence. In addition, it is necessary to determine the pulmonary wedge pressure, which, if elevated, implies either mitral stenosis or left ventricular dysfunction. Finally, the hemodynamics help establish the prognosis of these patients, which is closely linked to right ventricular performance. Right atrial pressure and cardiac output measurements appear to be better predictors of the clinical course of patients with cor pulmonale than the level of pulmonary artery pressure. Systemic and pulmonary artery oxygen saturations should be measured because they provide physiologic information about cardiac output and any underlying lung disease.

MANAGEMENT OF COR PULMONALE

The treatment of pulmonary hypertension has been problematic because of the difficulty in detecting mildly elevated pulmonary artery pressure in a noninvasive manner, and because of the lack of drugs that are specific for the pulmonary vascular bed. Although there has been a tendency to apply similar strategies to the treatment of pulmonary hypertension irrespective of the etiology, a review of the literature shows that the most effective therapies are those that are directed toward the underlying cause.

The use of digitalis and diuretics has been a general measure applied to cor pulmonale of any etiology associated with right ventricular dysfunction. Because it is difficult to show beneficial effects of digitalis in patients with left ventricular failure, data are lacking that prove efficacy in patients with right ventricular dysfunction. On the other hand, there is nothing unique about the right ventricular myocardium that would make it unresponsive to digitalis. Diuretics, which do not directly influence right ventricular performance, may help relieve much of the dyspnea and the venous congestion associated with cor pulmonale. In addition, diuretics reduce right ventricular wall stress in a right ventricle that is volume and pressure overloaded. In my experience, systemic hypotension has not been a problem with the use of diuretics in patients who have elevated right atrial pressures, thus I initiate diuretic therapy in the patient with dyspnea and elevated jugular venous pressure, and I titrate the dose to the patient's symptoms. The physician should monitor closely for the development of prerenal azotemia, which would suggest intravascular volume contraction.

Primary Pulmonary Hypertension

Primary pulmonary hypertension (PPH) is an example of relatively "pure" cor pulmonale caused by pulmonary vascular disease. In the last decade, the therapeutic approach has been toward the use of vasodilator drugs, which has remained controversial. For every article describing the beneficial effect of a vasodilator, another seems to appear describing adverse effects. Thus, it has been difficult to establish any consistent benefit from the use of tolazoline, acetylcholine, isoproterenol, the alpha-adrenergic blockers, diazoxide, nitroprusside or other nitrate preparations, hydralazine, or the converting-enzyme inhibitors. The calcium channel blocking drugs appear to hold the most promise for the treatment of PPH, although the literature is also equivocal on their long-term effectiveness in conventional doses. Recently, however, I have started a new regimen using high doses of calcium blocking drugs as therapy for PPH; in eight of 13 patients initially evaluated, I have achieved a reduction of 48 percent in pulmonary artery pressure and 60 percent in pulmonary vascular resistance. When restudied a year later, each of the patients showed a sustained reduction in pulmonary artery pressure associated with regression of right ventricular hypertrophy based on chest roentgenogram, electrocardiogram, and echocardiogram. Thus, at the preset time, the use of high-dose calcium channel blocking drugs appears to be the most effective established long-term treatment in some patients with PPH. Although systemic hypotension, the major concern about the use of calcium blockers, has not been a problem in the management of these patients, I still advocate central hemodynamic monitoring during initial treatment. Patients may require unusually high doses—as much as 240 mg per day of nifedipine or 1,020 mg per day of diltiazem. In my experience, side effects of flushing, headache, dizzy spells, and leg edema have not been problematic in the patients who respond to this drug regimen. Since I have not had a patient who failed to respond to a calcium blocker respond to a different class of drug, it is not my practice to test different classes of drugs in the patients who fail the high dose calcium channel blocker regimen.

Histologically, there is a subset of patients with PPH who have a thrombotic arteriopathy, which can be suggested by the mottled appearance on perfusion lung scan. In this subset of patients, I also advocate the use of anticoagulant therapy, which, although it may not affect pulmonary hemodynamics, may lead to improved survival over time.

Pulmonary Hypertension Secondary to Chronic Obstructive Pulmonary Disease

The development of pulmonary hypertension in patients with COPD results in an increased mortality, with the assumption that pulmonary hypertension develops from chronic alveolar hypoxia, although destruction of the pulmonary vascular bed from emphysematous changes may also be a contributory factor. The only established effective treatment of pulmonary hypertension in patients with COPD has been long-term oxygen therapy. Although it rarely causes an acute reduction in pulmonary artery pressure, oxygen has been shown in several trials to improve survival and to retard the progression of the pulmonary hypertension. The effectiveness of oxygen appears to be proportional to the number of hours per day the patient uses the treatment.

Vasodilators have been widely tested in patients with pulmonary hypertension from COPD, but there is little documentation of their long-term effectiveness. Experimental findings showing that hypoxia-induced pulmonary vasoconstriction can be inhibited by calcium blockers provides a rationale for the use of these drugs. However, in clinical trials, pulmonary artery pressure is minimally reduced by calcium blockers or by any class of vasodilator drugs. More important, however, is that there may be a pronounced effect on gas exchange with the development of a marked reduction in arterial oxygen saturation, believed to be caused by pulmonary vasodilatation in regions of abnormal ventilation, which results in increased intrapulmonary shunting. Thus, in these patients, the measurement of systemic arterial blood gases before and after a challenge of vasodilator drugs is mandatory.

Pulmonary Hypertension Secondary to Collagen Vascular Disease

Pulmonary hypertension complicating collagen vascular disease is becoming increasingly recognized and is likely to be multifactorial in etiology. Some patients present with marked interstitial lung disease, which is highlighted by infiltrates on chest roentgenogram and by restrictive changes on pulmonary function tests. Coexisting hypoxemia also is common, but patients with collagen vascular disease who present with moderate to severe pulmonary hypertension is the absence of any clinical parameters of restrictive lung disease also have been identified.

Unfortunately, these patients probably represent the group that is the most resistant to any form of treatment. Although the use of immunosuppressive therapy may make intuitive sense, there is no documentation in the literature that it is effective in treating pulmonary hypertension in these patients. My personal experience with vasodilator drugs is that they have never been effective and more often than not lead to hypotension or hypoxemia, making their chronic use hazardous.

Pulmonary Hypertension from Chronic Thrombotic Obstruction of the Major Pulmonary Arteries

Acute pulmonary embolism can produce transient mild pulmonary hypertension, which usually abates as the embolism lyses. There also are patients who develop severe cor pulmonale as a result of thromboembolic obstruction of the major pulmonary arteries. Although it has been presumed to result from recurrent pulmonary emboli, most of these patients have no clinical history of recurrent embolization and often no identifiable source of venous thrombosis. These patients usually present with chronic pulmonary hypertension and a markedly abnormal lung scan that is highly suggestive of pulmonary embolism. Heparin and thrombolytic agents are of no value because the thrombus is organized, endothelialized, and resistant to lysis. If pulmonary angiography documents the proximal extent of the clot to be at the level of the lobar arteries, surgical thromboendarterectomy is the procedure of choice. In patients deemed inoperable, warfarin (Coumadin) anticoagulant therapy should be instituted as prophylaxis against further thrombus formation.

Pulmonary Hypertension Secondary to Mitral Stenosis

Pulmonary hypertension is an expected complication of mitral stenosis due to increased left atrial pressure transmitted back into the pulmonary vascular bed. As stated previously, some patients with mitral stenosis develop severe pulmonary vasoconstriction in addition to the passive pulmonary hypertension from increased left atrial pressure. The obvious treatment for these patients is mitral valve surgery. Although the operative mortality increases in patients who have extreme levels of pulmonary hypertension, there is no level of pulmonary artery pressure that would preclude mitral valve replacement or valvotomy, since the pulmonary artery pressure usually regresses by 50 percent even with extreme levels of pulmonary hypertension.

Pulmonary artery pressure may fail to lower in some patients in the early postoperative period following mitral valve replacement because of reactive pulmonary vasoconstriction. In this setting, nitroglycerin infusions and prostaglandin E_1 have been used to lower the gradient between the pulmonary wedge and left atrial pressures. If the patient can be supported hemodynamically until the pulmonary hypertension regresses, a sustained reduction in pulmonary artery pressure is the rule following mitral valve replacement.

Pulmonary Hypertension Secondary to Congenital Heart Disease

Pulmonary vascular disease secondary to congenital heart disease is well recognized in infants and children and is seen occasionally in adults. The fundamental principle in the management of congenital heart disease with pulmonary hypertension is surgical correction. However, patients who present with pulmonary hypertension and reversed shunting (Eisenmenger's syndrome) are considered inoperable. Vasodilators have been administered to these patients without success. In the presence of a patent intracardiac shunt, any reduction in systemic vascular resistance is associated with a worsening of the right-to-left shunting, which worsens systemic hypoxemia and could potentially lead to acidosis and hypotension. On the other hand, if the vasodilator is successful in reducing the pulmonary vascular resistance, it would promote increased left-to-right shunting, which would increase pulmonary blood flow and pulmonary artery pressure. At present, heart-lung transplantation is considered the best therapeutic option for the patient with congenital heart disease and Eisenmenger's syndrome.

SUGGESTED READING

Rich S, Brundage BH. High dose calcium channel blocking therapy for primary pulmonary hypertension: evidence for long-term reduction in pulmonary artery pressure and regression of right ventricular hypertrophy. Circulation 1987; 76:135–141.

Rich S, Dantzker DR, Ayres SM, et al. Primary pulmonary hypertension: a national prospective study. Ann Intern Med 1987; 107:216–223.

Rich S, Levitsky S, Brundage BH. Pulmonary hypertension from chronic pulmonary thromboembolism. Ann Intern Med 1988; 108:425–434.

Timms RM, Khaja FU, Williams GW, et al. Hemodynamic response to oxygen therapy in chronic obstructive pulmonary disease. Ann Intern Med 1985; 103:29–36

Zener JC, Hancock EW, Shumway NE, et al. Regression of extreme pulmonary hypertension and mitral valve surgery. Am J Cardiol 1972; 30:820–826.

SLEEP DISORDERED BREATHING

DAVID W. HUDGEL, M.D.
NEIL S. CHERNIACK, M.D.

Sleep disordered breathing is a general term that incorporates the following patterns: (1) repetitive episodes of cessation of breathing (apnea) or (2) intermittent or continuous hypoventilation. Sleep disordered breathing results from conditions such as sleep apnea, obesity-hypoventilation syndrome, and obstructive lung disease complicated by sleep hypoxemia. Although definitive epidemiologic studies are not available, it is estimated that as much as 5 percent of the adult population has sleep disordered breathing. Convenient diagnostic tests and a number of therapeutic options are available for the evaluation and treatment of disorders of ventilation during sleep. However, the mere presence of sleep disordered breathing does not dictate that treatment is necessary, especially if the therapeutic interventions carry significant potential risks and costs. Since complete information about the natural history of sleep disordered breathing syndromes is not available at present, there is little justification for treating persons who have these disorders prior to the development of recognizable complications known to result in morbidity. In the following discussion, we focus on diagnostic tests, the current indications for treatment, and the therapeutic options available for patients with different types of sleep disordered breathing.

OBSTRUCTIVE SLEEP APNEA

Obstructive sleep apnea is characterized by intermittent, repetitive inspiratory collapse of the pharyngeal airway that prevents airflow into the lungs and results in hypoxemia and sleep disruption. Subjects who snore excessively and experience inappropriate daytime sleepiness, may have obstructive apneas during sleep. Although other symptoms and systemic hypertension may be present in these patients, without the presence of snoring and sleepiness, the diagnosis is very unlikely.

Clinical Presentation

Identification of the person with sleep apnea is most often made by the bed partner or another family member who becomes sufficiently disturbed by, or concerned about, the loud snoring to encourage the patient to seek medical attention. Characteristically, the snoring varies in intensity and is not present continually. The snoring is usually worse when the patient is lying in the supine position. The snoring is loudest between apneas, when the patient is taking large tidal volume breaths; it often has a medium pitch and tends to have a "gasping" character, unlike the low-pitched rumbling noise generated by snorers without sleep apnea. In fighting to break the inspiratory airway occlusion, the person with sleep apnea sleeps very restlessly. This restlessness is often more bothersome to the bed partner than is the snoring.

A number of complications of sleep apnea are responsible for the morbidity of this syndrome (Table 1). Sleep hypoxemia may lead to dangerous cardiac arrhythmias, such as ventricular tachycardia, or to pulmonary hypertension and cor pulmonale. Occasionally, patients with sleep apnea present in florid right ventricular failure, which is usually unresponsive to diuretic agents alone. Secondary erythrocytosis and the associated complications of increased blood viscosity can also appear in these patients.

Neurologic complications of sleep apnea are more frequently seen than cardiovascular complications. The most common of these complications is excessive daytime sleepiness. Symptoms associated with this hypersomnolence may vary in severity. For instance, patients can fall asleep while driving, during conversations, or while working—especially at a desk, but even during physical labor. There is also a group of patients with obstructive sleep apnea who have less obvious hypersomnolence, but who are definitely impaired by their disease. These patients are usually productive workers who struggle through the day fighting their sleepiness. They compensate by drinking large quantities of caffeine-containing beverages, by staying on their feet at work, by playing the radio loudly and so forth. These patients are at particular risk of falling asleep when driving, especially when traveling home from work. They consume their evening meal and typically collapse in their easy-chair and sleep the evening hours away. These patients often have to be awakened to go to bed, and are "out-like-a-light" once there, leaving the bed partner feeling neglected, angry, and frustrated. The restlessness and snoring of the patient disturbs the healthy bed partner's sleep. In the morning, the bed partner has to pry the still sleepy patient out of bed. Both individuals are anxious and pessimistic about facing another day of fighting somnolence. With this picture, it

TABLE 1 Indications for Treatment of Obstructive Sleep Apnea

Cardiovascular
Cor pulmonale not secondary to lung disease
Right ventricular failure
Secondary erythrocytosis
Dangerous cardiac arrhythmia
Atrial flutter or fibrillation
Frequent multifocal premature ventricular contractions
Ventricular tachycardia
Neuropsychiatric
Daytime hypersomnolence that interferes with function
Memory loss
Diminished cognitive function
Impotence

is easy to understand why mental depression, cognitive dysfunction, decreased libido, physiologic impotence, and other functional disorders are often encountered in these patients. If the couple goes "out-on-the-town" for an evening to relieve some stress, any alcohol consumed by the patient only worsens the sleep apnea. Obviously, such a situation puts considerable strain on a marriage, which for these reasons can end in divorce.

Diagnosis

The vivid history just described, or some facsimile thereof, is most important in making a tentative diagnosis of obstructive sleep apnea. Family members should be interviewed to determine the true sleep pattern of the patient. Obviously, the patient knows this information only indirectly. Hypothyroidism can be associated with obstructive sleep apnea and should be considered in patients suspected of having obstructive sleep apnea. The pharynx needs to be inspected for obvious anatomic narrowing or mass lesions. Pharyngeal roentgenograms are usually not helpful in making a definitive diagnosis. A sleep study performed during the patient's usual bedtime hours is the crucial examination needed to make the diagnosis and to determine the severity of hypoxemia. Tests performed during wakefulness, such as electrocardiogram, chest roentgenogram, and red blood cell mass, establish whether cardiovascular and/or hematologic consequences of sleep apnea are present. Pulmonary function tests are useful in diagnosing lung diseases, which might produce the same hypoxic complications as sleep apnea.

Variables measured during a sleep study should include sleep stages (determined by monitoring the electroencephalogram, electro-oculogram, and submental electromyogram), airflow measured at the nose *and* mouth with thermistors, thoracic inspiratory muscle effort, arterial oxygen saturation measured by oximetry, and cardiac rhythm. When properly applied, the electrodes and the sensors required for these measurements do not inhibit sleep, especially in hypersomnolent subjects.

Of all the measurements, respiratory effort is the most technically difficult. Least-to-most reliable methods are (1) a single strain gauge placed around or applied to the abdomen, (2) strain gauges on both the abdomen and the chest, (3) inductance vest, (4) chest wall electromyogram, and (5) esophageal balloon. In our hands, the chest wall electromyogram recorded from the costal margin in the anterior axillary line is the best compromise for patient comfort, technical ease, and accuracy. In extremely obese subjects, the positioning of these surface electrodes may be difficult, and perspiration often interferes with good electrode contact. Another drawback to this technique is that the signal is dampened if the patient lies on electrodes. An esophageal balloon is the most sensitive method for detecting ventilatory effort. After a local anesthetic is sprayed in the nose and pharynx, the balloon can be easily swallowed and placed in the midesophagus, at the site of least cardiac artifact, so that pleural pressure swings, which indicate inspiratory muscle activity, can be recorded.

A sleep study may be misleading. First of all, the patient is asked to sleep in an unfamiliar environment, under observation, while attached to a machine. However, when studies are conducted during a patient's usual sleeping hours, adequate sleep is almost always obtained. If a patient with symptoms suggestive of obstructive sleep apnea cannot sleep in the laboratory, he or she probably is not hypersomnolent enough to warrant treatment. In research studies, subjects are often asked to undergo two sleep studies on consecutive nights in order to minimize the effects of the unfamiliar environment and the test itself. For clinical evaluations, this first night effect usually is not important to consider. However, if rapid eye movement (REM) sleep is not obtained during a study and if significant hypoxemia has not been observed in a patient with signs of hypoxic complications, the study should be repeated since the lowest arterial oxygen desaturation is commonly seen during this sleep stage.

Technical problems can arise with equipment used for a sleep study. Good arterial perfusion to the site being sampled for arterial oxygen saturation is important for accurate oximeter recordings. If the thermistors detecting nasal and oral flow become dislodged, the flow signal may be absent and, therefore, it appears as though an apnea is present when it is not. If an apnea is not accompanied by some decrease in arterial oxygen saturation, the apnea is either very short and inconsequential, or the thermistors are displaced. If the measurement of inspiratory effort is too insensitive, obstructive apneas may be mistakenly called central apneas, which are characterized by absence of respiratory effort. Technicians should be instructed to make direct visual observations of the patient's respiratory activity, body position, body movements, and snoring pattern in order to be certain that there is consistency between the visual observations and the events being recorded. Technicians performing these evaluations need to be sufficiently trained to recognize technical problems, to trouble-shoot malfunctions in the recording equipment, and to make simple repairs of equipment during a study.

We do not believe that oximetry alone is adequate for a sleep study. This question has been debated by workers in the field, and most agree that a record of respiratory effort, airflow, and sleep stages should be obtained simultaneously with oximetry. Without such an evaluation, one is uncertain whether the patient entered REM sleep, when oxygenation might be substantially lower than during non-REM sleep, and is unable to distinguish obstructive from central apneas, a distinction that has therapeutic implications.

Oximetry can be used as a screening test if one is not sure that sleep apnea is likely from the clinical findings. However, if a sawtooth pattern consistent with sleep apnea is not seen on the oximetry tracing, the screening should be repeated to increase the chances of obtaining REM sleep.

Usually, a daytime nap study is not adequate. During a nap study, patients frequently do not enter REM sleep. However, some laboratories perform daytime nap studies after sleep deprivation the night before. To accomplish sleep deprivation, it is not enough to instruct a patient to stay awake at night. We surely cannot rely on a hypersomnolent patient to remain awake without supervision! It is also well known that sleep deprivation disturbs normal distribution of sleep stages during the sleep following the deprivation period. Therefore, sleep studies are best conducted during the patient's usual sleeping hours.

TABLE 2 Treatment Options for Obstructive Sleep Apnea

Change in sleeping body position
Weight loss
Supplemental oxygen
Respiratory stimulants
Medroxyprogesterone
Protriptyline
Nasal continuous positive airway pressure (CPAP)
Uvulopalatopharyngoplasty, tonsillectomy
Tracheostomy

Management

Once patients are appropriately diagnosed, treatment should be started if any of the cardiovascular or neurologic complications of sleep apnea listed in Table 1 are present. Therapeutic options are listed in Table 2. Our preference is to begin therapy with the simplest, safest treatment demonstrated to be effective in the laboratory. A therapeutic regimen can be developed by progressing from simple to more involved treatment, assuming the patient is not at acute risk because of a significant cardiac arrhythmia or because of obtundation caused by severe somnolence. Individual patient characteristics help in the design of the therapeutic plan. Examples of these characteristics and how they influence therapy are as follows:

1. Obesity dictates that a weight loss program should be part of the therapy.
2. Large tonsils and/or adenoids probably should be removed.
3. Respiratory stimulants should be tried if alveolar hypoventilation is present during wakefulness.

In order for the physician to begin with a simple, progressive treatment program, patients must be willing to comply with trials of various regimens. With this approach, one member of the health-care team needs to track the patient to assure that he or she returns for follow-up. If the patient becomes discouraged with this approach, the predictably most successful form of therapy should be instituted without delay.

Posture

The simplest therapy is a change in sleeping posture, such as either sleeping laterally or with the head and torso elevated. Such elevation should be designed so that head flexion is not increased, since head flexion narrows the upper airway. If significant improvement in arterial oxygen saturation is demonstrated with a change in body position, the patient should be instructed to sleep in that position. Only with the help of the bed partner can this approach be successful, and even then this approach is often not reliable. If improvement is not observed, another form of treatment is indicated. Evening alcohol and sedative-hypnotic medication use should be eliminated.

Weight Reduction

A weight reduction of approximately 10 percent of the body weight can have a substantial impact on the occurrence of apneas and the extent of arterial oxygen desaturation. Patients should be encouraged to engage in weight loss group therapy—one that does not just teach dietary restriction, but that also retrains the patient and the spouse in food selection, cooking, and portion size. Of course, the adverse impact of snacking and drinking alcoholic beverages on a weight loss diet and on sleep apnea should be emphasized. If there are no contraindications, patients should be encouraged to exercise regularly.

Oxygen

Oxygen administration may improve the hypoxemia in patients with obstructive apnea enough to prevent or to resolve pulmonary hypertension and significantly improve daytime hypersomnolence. However, oxygen may prolong apneas so that the nadir of oxygen saturation is not improved. Therefore, it is important to evaluate the response to oxygen in the sleep laboratory. Oxygen may be added to nasal continuous positive pressure (see below) when patients have persistent, usually continuous, hypoxemia secondary to alveolar hypoventilation. Often, alveolar hypoventilation spontaneously resolves after a period of good oxygenation, so that oxygen supplementation is no longer needed. Weight loss also may contribute to improvement of alveolar ventilation.

Ventilatory Stimulants

Ventilatory stimulants can be useful in some patients; usually we try these medications in those without anatomic abnormalities of the upper airways. Protriptyline, a tricyclic antidepressant with minimal sedation, is useful in some patients. Protriptyline works by two mechanisms. First, it decreases the REM sleep time, during which the most severe arterial oxygen desaturation often occurs. Second, protriptyline has been shown to stimulate inspiratory activity of upper airway muscles, thereby dilating the upper airway. Protriptyline is usually prescribed at an initial dose of 10 mg at bedtime. If this dose does not cause significant anticholinergic side effects, such as constipation, symptoms of bladder neck obstruction, impotence, tremor, blurred vision, or cardiac arrhythmia, the dose should be increased by 10 mg increments to 30 mg, depending on the presence of side effects. A sleep study should be repeated after the patient has the protriptyline for 2 to 4 weeks in order to determine whether or not improvement has occurred.

Medroxyprogesterone can be helpful, especially for the obstructive sleep apnea patient who has obesity-hypoventilation. Medroxyprogesterone may improve ventilation during wakefulness as well as during sleep, probably by increasing the ventilatory response to CO_2 and hypoxia. Again, verification of a beneficial effect should be obtained with a repeat sleep study 2 to 4 weeks after therapy is begun. Medroxyprogesterone is contraindicated in patients with a recent history of deep vein thrombophlebitis, transient ischemic attacks, hypercoagulable state, and in those males who cannot accept some diminution in their libido.

Continuous Positive Airway Pressure

Nasal continuous positive airway pressure (CPAP) is delivered via a nasal mask from a high-flow air compressor. A threshold pressure valve is placed in the system to establish a given degree of positive pressure within the system. This system is effective in resolving the majority of obstructive apneas in nearly every patient. Nasal CPAP acts as a pressure splint to the upper airway, thereby counterbalancing the collapsing pressure applied to the upper airway during inspiration by chest wall inspiratory muscle contraction. Adequate nasal CPAP equipment is available commercially through medical supply outlets. The instruction given to the patient and the patient's initial encounter with the nasal CPAP apparatus are crucial to the patient's acceptance of the system and willingness to continue its use. One helpful training technique is to set the threshold pressure valve at a low level (for example, at 5 cm H_2O pressure), even though this level of pressure is not likely to resolve the apneas, so that the patient can adapt to the sensation of breathing with this positive pressure in place. The pressure can be increased over the sleep period until the apneas are eliminated or until the arterial oxygen saturation improves. The goal of this treatment should be to keep the arterial oxygen saturation above 85 percent. The nasal CPAP may cause or aggravate rhinitis. Of course, the nasal CPAP is not effective when nasal congestion is present. Long-acting nasal decongestant sprays or drops help resolve this problem. Occasionally, intranasal corticosteroid administration is necessary to resolve the nasal congestion. The other complication of nasal CPAP is skin irritation from the plastic mask seal. Padding or changing the mask size usually alleviates this problem. Some patients report that their symptoms of daytime somnolence are controlled satisfactorily even if the nasal CPAP is not always used nightly. As long as the patient does not have a cardiac arrhythmia associated with apnea, this pattern of nasal CPAP use is satisfactory.

We do not assume that nasal CPAP is a definitive treatment for sleep apnea. Most patients do not tolerate wearing the nasal CPAP mask for more than a few months. By improving alertness, attention span, and mood, CPAP treatment aids compliance with weight loss programs by obese patients. Once significant weight loss has been accomplished, a repeat sleep study without nasal CPAP should be performed to assess the impact of weight loss. If the arterial oxygen saturation stays above 85 percent, except for rare, brief dips below this level, the nasal CPAP can be stopped.

Surgery

Uvulopalatopharyngoplasty (UPP), during which the soft palate, excess lymphoid tissue, and redundant pharyngeal tissue are resected, was designed to increase upper airway caliber and thus prevent upper airway inspiratory collapse during sleep. Most studies have demonstrated that approximately 50 percent of patients improve after this procedure. Two explanations are usually given for surgical failure: (1) the wrong anatomic site was resected, or (2) abnormal compliance of the upper airway tissue exists and was not corrected by surgery, so apneas continue. We have demonstrated that about one-half of apnea patients obstruct primarily in the hypopharynx, below the site of surgical resection. Therefore, it is hypothesized that these patients may not benefit from surgery. Because of the possibility of failure of UPP, it is important to do a follow-up sleep study 3 to 4 weeks postoperatively to objectively document improvement in the patient's sleep pattern. Patients who do not respond to surgery can be given nasal CPAP. Although there are some case reports that nasal CPAP is ineffective after the soft palate has been resected, this has not been our experience.

Other more radical surgical procedures that have been proposed for treatment of obstructive sleep apnea, such as mandibular or hyoid advancement or facial reconstruction, have not been well investigated and are not routinely considered as therapeutic options.

Tracheostomy

Tracheostomy should be reserved for those patients who are critically ill on presentation (although nasal CPAP also may be used in this setting) or for those in whom UPP fails and nasal CPAP is not beneficial. Some surgeons prefer to do a tracheostomy at the time of UPP to preserve the airway in the immediate postoperative period, when pharyngeal edema might result in airway compromise. In our experience, parenterally administered corticosteroids during surgery and postoperatively sufficiently reduce the risk of edema and/or inflammation at the operative site so that a tracheostomy is not routinely required. In addition, the endotracheal tube can be left in place for 12 to 24 hours postoperatively to eliminate the postoperative risk of upper airway closure. Other than bleeding or infection, there are two complications of tracheostomy that are infrequently appreciated. In obese individuals, there may be enough adipose tissue between the trachea and the skin so that it becomes nearly impossible to fit a tracheostomy tube properly. Tissue necrosis with infection and/or hemorrhage can occur when this subcutaneous tissue is externally compressed. In addition, submental adipose tissue (double chin) may obstruct the tracheostomy orifice externally when the patient is in a supine position, especially if he or she lies on a pillow that produces some degree of neck flexion. A wide collar around or an extension placed on the tracheostomy tube will resolve this problem.

CENTRAL SLEEP APNEA

Apneas characterized by absence of respiratory effort are termed central apneas. Essentially, patients with central apnea have periodic breathing, with the apneas occurring at the nadir of respiratory activity. Snoring is often present during the hyperpneic portion of the periodic breathing cycle because of rapid inspiratory airflow. Therefore, these patients may present with a history of snoring and mild daytime sleepiness or fatigue. Symptoms are usually less severe than in patients with obstructive sleep apnea, probably because these patients usually do not experience as much sleep hypoxemia as do those with obstructive apnea. Fatigue reported by these patients may be due to the apneic arousals that may occur on resumption of ventilation following the central apnea.

Management

The indications for treatment for patients with central apnea are the same as for obstructive sleep apnea: hypoxic cardiovascular or neurologic complications. Treatment is based on the principle that metabolic acidosis eliminates periodic breathing during sleep and thereby eliminates the central apneas. Carbonic anhydrase inhibitors, such as acetazolamide or dichlorphenamide, are often useful in these patients. However, patients may decide that the digital paresthesia they may experience with either of these medications is more bothersome than the mild fatigue associated with the central apnea. One should be aware that there are reports of patients who develop obstructive apnea while receiving carbonic anhydrase inhibitor treatment for central apneas.

OBESITY-HYPOVENTILATION SYNDROME

If lung function is relatively normal, persistent hypoxemia during sleep is usually an indication of alveolar hypoventilation. Obese patients are especially susceptible to this problem. The primary etiology of sleep-related alveolar hypoventilation is likely related to a combination of factors. Obesity places a large mechanical elastic load on the respiratory system. During sleep, the respiratory muscles do not fully compensate for this added load to breathing, and hypoventilation occurs. Hypoventilation results in hypoxemia and hypercapnia. Either because ventilatory drive is innately low or because there is adaptation to repetitive intermittent hypoxemia and hypercapnia, reducing ventilatory drive responses, there is no effort to correct the hypoventilation. In addition, hypoxemia itself may suppress central ventilatory activity. Since obesity is a predisposing factor for obstructive sleep apnea, patients with obesity-hypoventilation can also have obstructive apnea. In these patients, resolution of the sleep apnea may relieve, or improve, the hypoventilation.

Management

Treatment of obesity-hypoventilation syndrome is based on principles of mechanical load reduction, normalization of oxygenation, and stimulation of ventilation. Administration of medroxyprogesterone and weight reduction are the initial treatments recommended. Theophylline usually is not a good respiratory stimulant in adults, although it can be useful in children with hypoventilation. Oxygen administered by nasal prongs may be needed. Interestingly, high levels of nasal CPAP, such as 15 cm H_2O pressure, recently have been reported to improve alveolar hypoventilation during sleep, probably by reducing the mechanical load to breathing.

SLEEP HYPOXEMIA IN PATIENTS WITH OBSTRUCTIVE AIRWAYS DISEASE

Patients with bronchial asthma or chronic obstructive pulmonary disease (COPD) may develop periodic breathing or increased ventilation-perfusion mismatch during sleep, precipitating sleep hypoxemia. In addition, ventilatory responses to hypercapnia and hypoxia may be suppressed for similar reasons or exist in obesity-hypoventilation patients. Although these patients are usually not obese, they have a mechanical load to breathing, but it is a resistive load, not an elastic one. Ventilatory drives also can be suppressed by chronic hypoxemia and hypercapnia in these patients. In asthmatic persons, nocturnal worsening of bronchoconstriction is not related to a specific sleep stage, but usually occurs toward the early morning hours, often between 4 and 6 A.M. This worsening may occur whether or not the patient actually sleeps at night and, therefore, is at least partially due to diurnal fluctuations of bronchomotor tone. Administration of long-acting oral and/or inhaled bronchodilators at bedtime helps prevent nocturnal asthma.

Usually, arterial oxygen desaturation in COPD patients occurs in REM sleep and is associated with periodic breathing. It is important to recognize that such nocturnal hypoxemia may occur in COPD patients, especially in those whose awake arterial oxygen tension is below 65 mm Hg. Because of the shape of the oxygen dissociation curve, the lower the awake arterial oxygenation, the lower the sleep arterial oxygen saturation may fall. This nocturnal hypoxemia can be the cause of cor pulmonale in COPD patients with an awake arterial oxygen tension in the range not thought to precipitate chronic pulmonary hypertension. Oxygen supplementation usually compensates for this sleep-related hypoxemia and thereby prevents cardiovascular complications.

SUGGESTED READING

Brouillette RT, Thach BT. A neuromuscular mechanism maintaining extrathoracic airway patency. J Appl Physiol 1979; 46:272–279.

Fletcher EC, ed. Abnormalities of respiration during sleep. Orlando: Grune and Stratton, 1986.

Fujita S, Conway WA, Sicklesteel JM, et al. Evaluation of the effectiveness of uvulopalatopharyngoplasty. Laryngoscope 1985; 95:70–74.

Hudgel DW. Variable site of airway narrowing among obstructive sleep apnea patients. J Appl Physiol 1986; 61:1403–1409.

Longobardo GS, Gothe B, Goldman MD, Cherniack NS. Sleep apnea considered as a control system instability. Respir Physiol 1982; 50:311–333.

Mathew OP, Sant'Ambrogio G. Respiratory function of the upper airway. Lung Biology. In: Lenfant C, ed. Health & Disease. Vol. 35. New York: Marcel Dekker, 1988.

Remmers JE, deGroot WJ, Sauerland EK, Arch AM. Pathogenesis of upper airway occlusion during sleep. J Appl Physiol 1978; 44:931–938.

Smith PL, Haponik FG, Allen RP, et al. The effects of protriptyline in sleep-disordered breathing. Am Rev Respir Dis 1983; 127:8–13.

Strohl KP, Cherniack NS, Gothe B. Physiologic basis of therapy for sleep apnea. Am Rev Respir Dis 1986; 134:291–802.

CARDIOPULMONARY SYNDROME OF OBESITY

MICHAEL MANDEL, M.D.
NORMAN H. EDELMAN, M.D.

Our concept of the cardiopulmonary syndrome of obesity has evolved significantly over the past generation. Initial attention and therapy were focused on cardiac failure, which was assumed to be the primary defect. With the discovery of the central role of general hypoventilation and elucidation of the secondary nature of cor pulmonale, attention was focused on overall gas exchange and relief of the cause of its impairment. More recently, we have discovered that hypoventilation is not uniformly distributed over the day but, in the majority of patients, is far more severe during sleeping hours because of intermittent occlusion of the upper airway—the obstructive sleep apnea syndrome.

None of the aforementioned concepts is wrong, nor are they mutually exclusive. This discussion takes the point of view that there are cardiopulmonary effects of obesity even in the absence of general hypoventilation or obstructive sleep apnea. These are generally not of major import, but may become so in situations of stress, such as surgery. Obese patients, predominantly males, frequently display the manifestations of the obstructive sleep apnea syndrome (OSA); only a subset of these develop general hypoventilation (continual hypercapnia) and thereby manifest the obesity hypoventilation syndrome (OHS). A small subset of patients with OHS do not have obstructive sleep apnea.

CIRCULATORY EFFECTS OF OBESITY

Obese patients have increases in total blood volume and cardiac output that parallel excesses in body fat and weight. Pulmonary blood volume also increases and remains a constant proportion of total circulating volume. Pulmonary hypertension may develop in obese patients. One study of 40 obese patients who were twice their predicted ideal weights described resting pulmonary hypertension in 10 patients and exercise-induced pulmonary hypertension in another 20 patients. Systemic hypertension is common. Thus, the left ventricle faces both high preload and afterload. The left ventricle responds by hypertrophy and eventually by dilatation and failure. The usual therapy for hypertension and left ventricular failure is given, but weight loss is required to reverse the causative factors.

In patients with OHS hypoxia and hypercapnia cause pulmonary vasoconstriction and pulmonary hypertension. The right ventricle enlarges and ultimately fails. Initially, pulmonary hypertension may be confined to sleep when desaturation occurs. Anatomic narrowing of pulmonary arterioles and occasional thromboembolic disease contribute to persistent pulmonary hypertension in the awake state. Hypoxia stimulates production of red blood cells, which adds to the circulatory load and increases blood viscosity. When the right ventricle fails, the usual signs of venous distention, peripheral edema, and hepatic congestion are present.

RESPIRATORY EFFECTS OF OBESITY

In obesity, mass loading of the chest wall and abdomen leads to lower functional residual capacity (FRC), expiratory reserve volume, and chest wall compliance. In simple obesity, chest wall compliance decreases by 20 percent; in OHS, it may fall 60 percent and may not improve when weight is lost. Although distribution of pulmonary perfusion is normal in the absence of pulmonary hypertension, low FRC diminishes dependent ventilation and promotes ventilation-perfusion ($\dot{V}/\dot{Q}$) mismatch. Arteriovenous (AV) shunting past closed alveoli results in arterial hypoxemia. Diaphragm displacement in the supine position exaggerates these abnormalities, as does the significant loss of diaphragm function that accompanies upper abdominal surgery.

Lung compliance is reduced by the increased pulmonary blood volume, pulmonary hypertension, and excess extravascular lung water from congestive heart failure. This may be a contributing factor in the pathogenesis of alveolar hypoventilation.

Thus, respiratory muscles must overcome this decreased compliance and increased inertness. The work of breathing and respiratory muscle oxygen consumption increase. Change in body configuration due to obesity causes these muscles to function at low efficiency with poor mechanical advantage at an unfavorable part of their length-tension curve. Patients with OHS have only 60 to 70 percent of the predicted inspiratory muscle strength. In response to CO_2 stimulation, patients with OHS have difficulty overcoming the excessive respiratory impedance of the mass-loaded thorax. Acidosis and hypoxemia seen in OHS are thought to further depress respiratory muscle function.

Patients with OHS have abnormalities in the control of breathing. Most often, a severely depressed ventilatory response to CO_2 is observed, which does not return to normal with weight loss or simple relief of airway obstruction. Chronic hypoxia may depress carotid body ventilatory response to acute hypoxia. Abnormal respiratory muscle function, increased O_2 cost of breathing, mass loading of the chest wall, and circulatory abnormalities contribute to the pathogenesis of alveolar hypoventilation.

OBSTRUCTIVE SLEEP APNEA

Sleep disordered breathing in the form of OSA is more commonly found in obese males, post menopausal females, and the elderly. However, in our laboratory, we have documented OHS (the Pickwickian syndrome) in seven premenopausal females. Patients with OHS usually have nocturnal airway occlusion. Snoring, which is a common complaint of these patients and their bed partners, is caused by palatal or uvular vibration during partial airway occlusion. At the termination of complete occlusive episodes snoring volume magnifies in intensity as the patient takes large breaths while awaking from sleep.

Inspiratory muscle contraction creates a negative collapsing pressure in the supraglottic airway. Normally, airway patency is maintained by a phasic inspiratory increase in neural input and by the resultant tone of the genioglossus muscle and the pharyngeal dilator muscles. During OSA, neural input and muscle tone are decreased. This decrease permits the pharyngeal lumen to collapse against the negative inspiratory pressure and allows the tongue to occlude against the soft palate and the posterior pharyngeal wall while respiratory efforts continue. Anatomic abnormalities, including tonsillar hypertrophy, micrognathia, nasal septal deviation, long soft palate, and macroglossia, narrow the airway and predispose to increased intraluminal negative pressures and inspiratory obstruction.

Episodes of obstruction usually last 20 to 40 seconds and may occur several hundred times each night. Periodic breathing and brief apneas occur in normal persons during the transition from wakefulness to sleep. Occlusive episodes and gas exchange abnormalities are exaggerated in patients with OSA and OHS. During rapid eye movement (REM) sleep, breathing pattern abnormalities are more marked.

With cessation of breathing, alveolar and arterial CO_2 increases and O_2 decreases. The degree of fall in oxyhemoglobin saturation depends on three factors: (1) the awake arterial oxygen pressure (PaO_2), which determines the starting position on the sigmoid oxyhemoglobin dissociation curve and most profoundly affects the fall in saturation; (2) the duration of apnea; and (3) the lung volume, which provides an oxygen reserve for gas exchange during apnea. The effects of obesity on $\dot{V}/\dot{Q}$ mismatch and low FRC predispose to desaturation during apnea. Therefore, patients with OHS are at greater risk for desaturation.

With recurrent nocturnal hypoxemia, pulmonary hypoxic vasoconstriction may lead to pulmonary hypertension. Right ventricular hypertrophy and failure usually require sustained daytime hypoxemia and hypercapnia, thus leading the OHS. Hypoxic carotid body stimulation causes bradycardia and sinus pauses. Catecholamine release from systemic hypoxemia results in systemic hypertension, which may persist during wakefulness. Ventricular ectopy and transient heart block develop in some patients. Nocturnal deaths from apnea-related arrhythmias constitute one of the most serious complications of this syndrome.

Apneas are terminated by arousals that involve increased activity of upper airway muscles. Hypercapnia is a stronger arousal stimulus than hypoxia, but hypoxia will lower the arousal threshold for any degree of hypercapnia. Breathing resumes with deep, rapid inspirations and often with extremely loud snoring. These hundreds of nocturnal arousals fragment sleep, decrease slow wave and REM sleep, and lead to daytime hypersomnolence, intellectual deterioration, and adverse personality and behavioral effects.

DIAGNOSIS

Patients with OSA (and OHS) usually present with complaints of daytime hypersomnolence, morning headache, personality and cognitive deterioration, and anamnestic automatic behavior. Bed partners complain of loud snoring, excessive tossing during sleep, and respiratory pauses.

We compile a profile of the patient's nocturnal and daytime sleep habits, alcohol use, and other drug history. Coexisting lung disease, such as chronic obstructive pulmonary disease or bronchospasm, is identified and assessed for independent therapy. Symptoms and history related to the nose, sinuses, mouth, and pharynx are reviewed. We explore relationships between symptoms and changes in weight.

The physical examination focuses on anatomic conditions that may predispose to airway obstruction, including micrognathia, tonsillar hypertrophy, acromegaly, uvular enlargement, nasal polyps, septal deviation, carcinoma, cysts, and rhinitis. Indirect laryngoscopy is performed to exclude laryngeal obstruction. Cephalometric roentgenograms may complement physical findings in patients with suspected skeletal deformities. Cardiac and respiratory examinations seek evidence of right or left ventricular failure, hypertension, adequate tissue perfusion, extrapulmonary restriction (kyphoscoliosis), and abnormalities in upright and supine airflow. Signs of hypothyroidism and hyperandrogen states are sought, as they predispose to OSA.

Laboratory

Polycythemia may indicate occult nocturnal or persistent daytime hypoxemia and desaturation. Hypoxemia with normal arterial carbon dioxide pressure ($PaCO_2$) is the most common arterial blood gas finding in severe obesity. Carbon dioxide retention defines alveolar hypoventilation in patients with OHS. To determine whether patients hypoventilate because of muscle weakness (can't breathe) or because of abnormal central control (won't breathe), we have them perform voluntary hyperventilation, and we repeat the blood gas measurements to determine if they can lower their $PaCO_2$ by at least 5 mm Hg. Pulmonary function testing (PFT) of obese patients demonstrates normal residual volume to total lung capacity ratio and decreased expiratory reserve volume and FRC. Airflow obstruction and bronchodilator responsiveness evidenced on PFTs warrant therapeutic intervention. A flow volume loop with a saw-tooth pattern suggests variable extrathoracic airway obstruction. Flat inspiratory and expiratory limbs of the flow volume loop indicate fixed extrathoracic airway obstruction. Maximum minute ventilation is reduced in obese patients.

Polysomnography

All patients with suspected OSA or OHS are studied in the sleep laboratory. Full nocturnal studies are preferred to sleep-deprived nap studies. We monitor sleep stage, respiratory effort, and airflow at the nose and mouth, oxygen saturation (SaO_2), and the electrocardiographic findings. These variables are monitored for a minimum of 3 hours during the diagnostic part of the sleep study. An apnea is defined as cessation of airflow at the nose and mouth for 10 or more seconds. If 30 or more apneas are present during 360 minutes of nocturnal recording (or proportionate amounts for shorter studies), sleep apnea syndrome is diagnosed. Patients with observed apneas and desaturation during the diagnostic part of the study are given nasal continuous positive airway pressure (CPAP) (see the following section) at 5 cm H_2O. Sleep parameters are monitored with CPAP. The level of CPAP is increased progressively to 12.5 cm H_2O or until resolution of apneas. If O_2 desaturation persists during administration of CPAP, supplemental low flow oxygen given by nasal cannula is added.

MANAGEMENT

Many forms of medical and surgical treatment have been developed for OSA and OHS as understanding of their genesis has progressed. Some patients require more than one intervention from the menu of therapeutic options. Individualization of therapy depends on (1) the patient's physical characteristics, including anatomic obstruction and degree of obesity; (2) sex; (3) acuity of physiologic abnormalities; and (4) patient preference and tolerance.

In the following section, we discuss the advantages and disadvantages of the various treatment modalities and present our approach to their use.

Avoidance of Inciting Agents

Alcohol has been shown to increase arousal threshold, which allows greater oxyhemoglobin desaturation. Alcohol also increases the frequency and duration of apneas. Benzodiazepines, such as flurazepam, increase duration and desaturation of obstructive episodes without increasing the number of episodes in patients with OSA. Although narcotic analgesics have not been directly shown to worsen sleep physiology in patients with OSA, narcotic antagonists (e.g., naloxone) have had a beneficial effect in some patients with OSA. Therefore, we strictly recommend avoidance of alcohol, hypnotics, and narcotics in these patients.

Weight Control

Normal adults demonstrate increasing episodes of abnormal breathing with increased weight. A weight gain of as little as 20 to 30 pounds may unmask the full syndrome of OSA in predisposed patients. Studies have demonstrated improvement in apnea, hypopnea index, daytime and nocturnal desaturation, and daytime hypersomnolence in obese patients after weight reduction. Weight loss also reduces the oxygen cost of breathing, decreases airway resistance, and increases FRC, which leads to less $\dot{V}/\dot{Q}$ mismatch and improved PaO_2.

In patients with weight gain of recent onset and nondebilitating symptoms, a diet and exercise program to sustain weight loss to the level at which they were symptom-free may be the only intervention necessary. Often these patients cycle between weight loss with relief of symptoms and weight gain with redevelopment of the full spectrum of symptoms. Markedly symptomatic and morbidly obese patients with OSA require initiation of other therapeutic measures concomitant with aggressive efforts at weight reduction. We have referred select morbidly obese patients for hypocaloric diets or for surgical approaches to weight loss.

Oxygen Supplementation

Hypoxemic patients are at great risk for cardiac and pulmonary vascular complications. Low flow O_2 supplementation by nasal cannula increases baseline SaO_2 and shifts the patient to the flat portion of the oxyhemoglobin dissociation curve. It was once feared that a decrease in hypoxic ventilatory drive with supplemental O_2 would prolong apneas. However, hypoxemia proves a poor arousal stimulus, and the O_2 related increase in apnea duration is offset by decreased desaturation during apneic periods. In non-REM sleep, baseline SaO_2 increases, the peak fall in SaO_2 decreases, and the rate of sleep disordered breathing decreases. In REM sleep, the rate of disordered sleep decreases, although the baseline and peak falls in saturation do not change (probably because of atelectasis, $\dot{V}/\dot{Q}$ mismatch, and shunting).

Supplemental oxygen delivered by low flow nasal cannula is initiated in the sleep laboratory during polysomnography in patients with documented desaturation despite CPAP. Indwelling arterial lines are placed in hypercapnic patients for blood gas monitoring and detection of further CO_2 retention. Decreased apnea time and desaturation are indications for continued oxygen therapy. Blood gas measurements are repeated in hypoventilating patients in 1 week. With correction of sleep disordered breathing by CPAP or other interventions and with improvement in physiologic consequences of nocturnal desaturation, we expect resolution of hypercapnia and elevation of PaO_2. Periodic monitoring of blood gases will guide the decision about whether to discontinue supplemental O_2. Established cor pulmonale and daytime hypoxemia require 24 hour-per-day administration of oxygen.

Continuous Positive Airway Pressure

Nasal CPAP is the mainstay of our nonsurgical therapy of moderate and severe obstructive sleep apnea with and without OHS. It is the one definitive therapy of airway obstruction that can be tested and directly adjusted within the sleep laboratory at the time of initial polysomnography. CPAP works by pneumatically "splinting" the airway open when inspiratory muscle activity collapses the pharynx. Increased airflow and pressure in the nares also reflexly stimulate upper airway muscle tone to maintain patency. During CPAP, FRC increases and provides a larger oxygen reservoir to prevent desaturation and to improve $\dot{V}/\dot{Q}$ matching. The CPAP mask fits comfortably over the patient's nose and is secured with straps around the head. An air-filled plastic cuff around the mask provides a seal to prevent air leakage and corneal ulceration. A low-resistance tubing delivers humidified air from a compressor to the mask, and an expiratory valve allows adjustment of resistance. In the sleep laboratory, the mask is modified to contain a pressure transducer for measuring mask pressures and a capnograph to measure end-tidal CO_2.

During polysomnography, CPAP is applied to patients who demonstrate obstructive apnea. The level of CPAP is increased incrementally (2.5, 5.0, 7.5, 10.0, and 12.5 cm H_2O) to the level that abolishes apneas. The minimum effective pressure is prescribed for continued home use. We generally aim to completely abolish obstructive episodes. However, if this requires 12.5 cm or more of CPAP, we may use a lower level of pressure that precludes desaturation and eliminates apneas, but allows hypopneas to persist. Risks of CPAP include decreased cardiac output and renal function, sinusitis, middle ear infections, and barotrauma leading to pneumomediastinum. We have also noted increased CO_2 retention during CPAP trials in three already hypercapnic patients.

CPAP has been well tolerated and accepted by approximately 80 percent of our patients with moderate to severe OSA and 50 percent of our patients with OHS. Consistent with published reports, we have found rapid improvement in daytime hypersomnolence and neuropsychiatric manifestations. Improved cardiovascular status facilitates diuresis and initial weight loss. In patients with hypoventilation caused by OSA, $PaCO_2$ returns toward normal as ventilation and chemoreceptor function progressively improve. However, hypercapnia due to obstructive lung disease may worsen during administration of nasal CPAP. Patients who maintain weight loss or who undergo corrective surgical procedures may no longer require CPAP therapy. The majority of patients will require continued therapy, and upper airway obstruction will resume as therapy is withdrawn.

Drug Therapy

Progesterone

Medroxyprogesterone and related compounds centrally stimulate respiration to increase minute ventilation and tidal volume. The central drive to hyperventilate in response to hypercapnia is restored. However, nocturnal obstruction, arterial desaturation, and cardiac arrhythmias remain unchanged. Medroxyprogesterone is not indicated for treatment of upper airway obstruction, but may be effective therapy for decreased respiratory drive. We have found it to be effective in half of our hypercapnic patients.

The major side effect is impotence. We have not observed thrombogenic complications despite the well-established risk with these compounds. The treatment dose of medroxyprogesterone is 20 mg three to four time daily. Maximal effects on respiratory function are seen in 1 week. At this dose, the drug has been well tolerated in our patients.

Acetazolamide

Acetazolamide, a carbonic anhydrase inhibitor, causes bicarbonate wasting and acidification of pH. As acidosis shifts the hypercapnic ventilatory response curve to the left with a parallel slope, respiratory drive in response to CO_2 increases. Acetazolamide may have a direct respiratory stimulating effect independent of pH. In patients with central apnea, acetazolamide decreases nocturnal desaturation and apneic events.

We prescribe acetazolamide, 250 mg orally, approximately three times a day, to patients with alveolar hypoventilation in order to decrease pH to a minimum of 7.33 and to stimulate ventilatory drive. We prefer acetazolamide to progesterone in male patients because of the relative lack of significant side effects. Patients may complain of paresthesias, but tolerate the drug well.

For rare patients with OHS, acetazolamide and progesterone are prescribed together. However, adding acetazolamide rarely produces clinical benefit in patients who have failed to respond to medroxyprogesterone.

Protriptyline

Protriptyline, a nonsedating tricyclic antidepressant, is variably effective in treating obstructive apneas. Protriptyline alters sleep architecture and decreases REM sleep, during which time apneas are most frequent and most severe. This improves the overall nocturnal oxygen saturation. Protriptyline may also increase upper airway muscle activity to promote airway patency during inspiration. Protriptyline does not affect ventilatory drive and is not effective for alveolar hypoventilation syndromes. Some patients with mild OSA have decreased daytime hypersomnolence after a short period of therapy.

We begin treatment with 5 mg prior to sleep and increase the dose to 10 mg after 1 to 2 weeks, as indicated by symptom relief (decreased hypersomnolence and snoring). Side effects of urinary retention in elderly men and dry mouth limit dose and patient acceptance. Cardiac side effects, including tachyarrhythmias, restrict the maximal dose to 15 mg.

Vasodilators

There is some evidence that vasodilator therapy is beneficial in OHS. We have had occasional success in patients who are very sensitive to oxygen (that is, they experience inordinate hypercapnia with even a modest flow of nasal oxygen). Vasodilator therapy is not an important part of our regimen.

Anticoagulants

Pulmonary embolism is an important cause of death in OHS. We use prophylactic anticoagulation when the manifestations of right ventricular failure are severe. When pulmonary embolism has been demonstrated, we continue anticoagulation for 3 to 6 months, and longer if right ventricular failure persists.

Surgical Therapy

Uvulopalatopharyngoplasty

Uvulopalatopharyngoplasty (UPPP) involves excision of the uvula, soft palate, tonsils, and redundant posterior pharyngeal mucosa to relieve upper airway obstruction. Patients with oropharyngeal sites of obstruction demonstrate greater benefit than those with hypopharyngeal obstruction. Although cine-computed tomography and supine and seated fiberoptic endoscopy have been utilized, selection of appropriate patients remains difficult. Those with a low arched soft palate, large tonsils, or excessive pharyngeal folds are considered appropriate candidates. Since UPPP does not address abnormal control of breathing, hypoventilating patients referred for UPPP require other therapy, such as progesterone or acetazolamide.

Preoperative weight of more than 125 percent of the ideal body weight has been recommended as a necessary, but not sufficient, criterion for response to UPPP (defined as a greater than 50 percent decrease in apnea index). However, the significance of preoperative weight has varied in published series, and UPPP has had variable success in producing weight loss.

Complications of the procedure include nasopharyngeal-palatal stenosis and palatal incompetence with air leak or nasal regurgitation. We restudy patients 6 to 8 weeks after UPPP to measure effectiveness on OSA.

Most patients undergoing UPPP report subjective improvement, although only about half have more than a 50 percent reduction in apnea index. Nonresponders, by the apnea index criteria, may have improvement in oxygen saturation during sleep.

Among responders, benefits of UPPP decrease with time, although prediction of clinical course is not possible. Periodic re-evaluation of symptoms will indicate a need for repeat polysomnography and additional treatment. Weight gain may exacerbate symptoms of OSA in patients who have undergone UPPP.

Tracheostomy

By bypassing the site of airway occlusion, tracheostomy assures patency and provides definitive relief of obstructive symptoms. Patients with OSA experience immediate relief of daytime hypersomnolence. Cardiac arrhythmias, pulmonary hypertension, and oxygen desaturation are controlled. Sleep architecture normalizes. Sustained periods of Stages 3 and 4 sleep ensue, and the time in Stage 1 diminishes as awakenings abate.

Tracheostomy is indicated as emergency therapy in patients with life-threatening arrhythmias, cardiac decompensation, severe desaturation, and markedly excessive daytime somnolence. With relief of symptoms and stabilization of the patient, other medical and surgical therapies may be employed in an effort to wean the patient from the tracheostomy. Effectiveness of other therapies should be evaluated with the tracheostomy site plugged prior to pulling the tracheostomy tube. Tracheostomy may be necessary as a procedure of last resort in patients with OHS who have failed other weight loss, medical, or surgical interventions. These patients may require nocturnal mechanical ventilation to control refractory hypoventilation. Some patients require temporary tracheostomy during UPPP because of perioperative oropharyngeal edema.

Tracheostomy is technically difficult in obese, short-necked patients who have large amounts of adipose tissue. Complications of long-term tracheostomy include granuloma, stricture, bleeding, and respiratory infections.

Patient acceptance is poor, and difficult psychosocial problems are anticipated.

SUGGESTED READING

Edelman NH, Santiago TV, eds. Breathing disorders of sleep. New York: Churchill Livingstone, 1986.

Fletcher EC, ed. Abnormalities of respiration during sleep. Orlando: Grune and Stratton, 1986.

Guilleminault C, Dement WC, eds. Sleep apnea syndromes. New York: Alan R. Liss, 1978.

Thawley SE, ed. Symposium on sleep apnea disorders. Med Clin North Am 1985; 69:1123-1412.

PNEUMOTHORAX

DAVID N. OSTROW, B.Sc.(Med), M.D., M.A., FRCPC, F.C.C.P., F.A.C.P.
BILL NELEMS, B.A.Sc., M.D., FRCSC

Pneumothorax can be classified as spontaneous or traumatic. The vast majority of spontaneous pneumothoraces occur in healthy hosts, but there are a number of lung conditions that can predispose to spontaneous pneumothorax. These include (1) eosinophilic granuloma, (2) emphysema, (3) necrotizing pneumonia, including tuberculosis, (4) usual interstitial pneumonia (in the honeycomb or end-stage phase), and (5) asthma. Traumatic pneumothorax may be iatrogenic or related to chest wall trauma. Iatrogenic pneumothoraces are most commonly related to diagnostic aspiration needle biopsies or to complications of intermittent positive pressure ventilation. Thoracentesis and subclavian vein catheterization also cause this problem. Chest wall trauma may be due either to nonpenetrating blunt damage to the ribs, which in turn penetrate the lung, or to penetration of the chest wall by foreign objects.

SPONTANEOUS PNEUMOTHORAX

Pathogenesis

Spontaneous pneumothorax occurs most commonly in tall, thin, healthy males. Males are said to be between four and eight times more susceptible to the condition than females. There are a number of cases of familial pneumothorax also described. The pathogenic mechanism is related to rupture of subpleural blebs, which are thought to be congenital in nature. Usually these subpleural blebs are on the surface of the lung, and their rupture causes air to enter the pleural cavity. Although the onset of pneumothorax in most patients is unrelated to any type of respiratory or physical activity, a significant number of patients describe a cough or sneeze as the initiating event. Persons with asthma or chronic bronchitis may have excessive mucus within their medium and small airways. This and excessive inflammation around these airways may lead to the development of check valves, which in turn may cause communicating blebs within the lungs to enlarge and subsequently to rupture. Catamenial pneumothorax occurs coincident with menses and may be related to ectopic endometrial tissue or to fenestrations in the diaphragm.

Mediastinal emphysema is presumably caused by the alveolar air tracking along the vascular bundle into the mediastinum. It may lead to pneumopericardium and subcutaneous emphysema without any clear-cut clinical evidence of pneumothorax.

Clinical Presentation

Nearly 90 percent of patients with spontaneous pneumothorax complain of sharp, pleuritic chest pain. The precise cause of this problem has never been adequately explained. Since the parietal pleura has the most exquisite pain sensation, it is tempting to attribute the pain to tension on adhesions between the parietal and visceral pleura. Since these adhesions are not usually present in well persons, one is tempted to draw the conclusion that many symptomatic pneumothoraces are preceded by small asymptomatic leaks that lead to the development of pleural adhesions. It is interesting that even patients who are treated conservatively, without a chest tube, notice that the pain tends to disappear within 48 to 72 hours. The reason for this is not clear. Dyspnea is present in approximately 80 percent of patients and is particularly noticeable during exercise. Cough is present in 50 percent of patients.

The physical findings are fairly classical and include tachypnea, tachycardia, shift of the trachea to the side without the pneumothorax, and decrease in tactile fremitus over the affected side. There is hyper-resonance and decreased air entry on auscultation. The cardiac apex may be shifted to the unaffected side. Occasionally, with the presence of mediastinal air, one can hear a crunch, which is synchronous with the cardiac cycle.

A tension pneumothorax is due to a check-valve phenomenon within the ruptured bleb, such that each inspiration allows more air into the pleura, and with each expiration the check-valve closes. The mediastinum is markedly shifted over to the unaffected side, and the lung is increasingly collapsed. In such patients the heart rate may exceed 150 beats per minute, and the characteristic feature on examination is cardiovascular collapse, with a rapid fall in blood pressure. It is incorrect to believe that only a tension pneumothorax has positive intrapleural pressure within the pleural cavity. All pneumothoraces have positive pressure in relation to the unaffected lung. With tension pneumothorax, the pressure is of a sufficient degree to impede venous return to the heart.

Study of arterial blood gases reveals an initial hypoxemia, because some time must elapse before there is hypoxic vasoconstriction and a leveling out of ventilation-perfusion ratios. The electrocardiogram may demonstrate a shift of the QRS axis, especially with left-sided pneumothoraces.

The diagnosis is usually fairly easily confirmed on a chest roentgenogram. Occasionally, when there is some doubt, it is useful to obtain inspiratory and expiratory films. Since the air within the pneumothorax cavity does not easily communicate with the bronchi, the volume of the cavity does not decrease during expiration. This causes a relative increase in the size of the intrapleural air in an expiratory film.

Estimating the size of the pneumothorax is an important step in clinical decision-making. The geometry of the collapsing lung is complex, somewhat like a cylinder tethered on one side to the mediastinum. One useful way of estimating the volume of the pneumothorax is to determine the ratio of the distance from the medial aspect of the lung at the hilum to the edge of the collapsed lung (D_2) and from the hilum to the edge of the thoracic cavity (D_1). The expression

$$\frac{D_1^3 - D_2^3}{D_1^3} \times 100$$

is a fairly accurate assessment of the pneumothorax size (expressed as a percentage).

Management

The decision regarding the approach to treatment of-spontaneous pneumothorax depends on the size of the pneumothorax and on the presence of symptoms. Generally, it is estimated that a pneumothorax absorbs at the rate of approximately 1.25 percent per day (50 to 75 ml). This means that a 20 percent pneumothorax is likely to take about 2 weeks to resolve completely. The use of 100 percent oxygen denitrogenates the blood and increases the gradient for nitrogen from the air within the pneumothorax to the gas within pleural tissues, which speeds up recovery. However, this exposes the patient to high concentrations of oxygen and is not a practical means of therapy. It is generally accepted that pneumothoraces of less than 20 percent, especially in an asymptomatic patient, can be treated by observation. There is some evidence from Britain that larger pneumothoraces also may be treated in that fashion without any serious complications. The concern about observation as a mode of therapy is that it still leaves the patient at risk for the development of a tension pneumothorax as well as for the development of pneumonia in the atelectatic lung. Thus, we do not believe that observation as a mode of therapy is indicated if the pneumothorax is greater than 20 percent. Whatever the size of the pneumothorax, if it is secondary to an underlying pulmonary condition or associated with severe pain, we attempt to drain the air.

Needle Aspiration

Needle aspiration of the thoracic cavity with a small plastic catheter can be used to partially drain the pleural cavity. Air can be removed manually through a stopcock and syringe, or the catheter can be attached to a vacuum bottle. Our experience has been that polyethelene air-filled catheters attached to suction bottles tend to collapse from the negative pressure. Teflon catheters have been introduced and these have the advantage of rigid walls as well as the convenience of a narrow diameter. Needle aspiration of the pleural cavity is not a particularly successful technique. We have used it only in instances where the pneumothorax is related to trauma from the needle aspiration biopsy of a lung lesion.

Tube Thoracostomy

Tube thoracostomy is the most common technique employed to drain a large pneumothorax or a pneumothorax associated with persisting symptoms or underlying lung disease. Generally, we place the tube in the sixth intercostal space in the midaxillary line rather than in the anterior chest wall. This placement allows the patient some mobility of the limbs without leaving a scar in a cosmetically obvious place. We tend to use the technique of blunt dissection down to the pleura and penetration of the pleura with the dissecting clamp, rather than inserting the plastic chest tube with a trocar. This technique minimizes the chance of trauma to the lung, especially if there is evidence that part of the lung is tethered to the chest wall by adhesions. The chest tube is directed toward the apex of the lung. In a simple pneumothorax, we generally use a No. 20 French catheter. If there is evidence of fluid or blood in the chest cavity, a No. 28 to No. 32 French catheter should be used.

The chest tube must be attached to a one-way valve to allow the egress of air from the pleura. The most commonly used valve is a tube connected to an underwater seal. Most units have the capability of providing negative suction to the pleural cavity, although for uncomplicated spontaneous pneumothoraces this tends not to be necessary. Generally, expansion of the lung can be accomplished by having the patient cough three or four times. The patency of the tube can be monitored by watching fluctuations of the fluid level in the tube leading into the bottle. Although this system has been used for many years, it has the disadvantage of keeping the patient relatively immobile.

A one-way rubber valve within a plastic cylinder (Heimlich valve) has the advantage of being extremely light and easily portable. There are two disadvantages of the Heimlich valve: (1) the collapsible rubber, which acts as a one-way valve, can become stuck if there is a significant amount of fluid or blood within the pleural cavity, and (2) it is difficult to monitor whether or not there is a continuing leak from the pneumothorax. We overcome this problem by attaching to the distal end of the valve a collapsible urine drainage system, which acts somewhat like a highly compliant balloon. During a fixed period of time (perhaps over 4 hours), the urine drainage system is observed by the nursing staff. If air enters the "balloon," a slow continuous leak from the lung is indicated. The method must be used only when the patient is being observed. If the urine draining system becomes completely full of air, it inactivates the one-way valve. Nevertheless, we find this system useful, especially because of the mobility it offers patients. The chest tube is usually left in place for 24 hours after the air leak has ceased.

Suction

The two most important complications of pneumothorax are persisting leak and recurrence. If a pneumothorax continues to leak air beyond 24 hours, we attach the one-way valve to suction. Generally, 20 cm of water pressure suction is applied to the chest tube in a continuous manner. If the leak persists for more than 10 days to 2 weeks, we consider that the tube thoracostomy has failed, and surgery is recommended.

The rate of recurrence of a pneumothorax varies but is approximately 30 percent. A second pneumothorax has approximately an 80 percent chance of recurrence. Because of this, it is recommended that a second recurrence of pneumothorax should be treated surgically.

Surgery

The surgical treatment is to oversew or staple the apical bleb through a limited third interspace transaxillary incision. To prevent further leaks from blebs that are not clearly apparent at the time of surgery, a pleuritis may be induced by vigorous abrasion of the parietal pleura with gauze to stimulate the formation of adhesions between the lung and the chest wall. Alternatively, an apical pleurectomy is performed, which separates the parietal pleura from the endothoracic fascia over the apex of the thorax. This procedure induces an even better fusion of lung to apical chest wall and further minimizes the possibility of recurrence.

Pleurodesis

Medical pleurodesis with tetracycline is recommended by some, although we tend to avoid this technique. Generally, 20 to 30 mg per kilogram of tetracycline is instilled into the pleural cavity through the chest tube. A solution of 60 to 100 ml must be used to displace the dead space of the pleural catheter. This procedure initiates an extremely severe pleuritis and causes very severe pain. Some recommend the administration of lidocaine before the tetracycline to avoid pain, but we have not found this particularly helpful. The pain is difficult to control with opiates and actually is best controlled with aspirin or nonsteroidal anti-inflammatory agents. However, these agents are not recommended because they lessen the inflammatory process. Recently, the concomitant use of fentanyl, a short-acting anesthetic, has been recommended to avoid the severe pain. When tetracycline is used for pleurodesis, we usually pretreat the patient with atropine. This prevents a vasovagal episode due to the pain. Besides the problem of pain, medical treatment also has the disadvantage of not addressing the primary problem of removing the blebs.

TRAUMATIC PNEUMOTHORAX

Traumatic pneumothorax may be iatrogenic or related to chest wall trauma. In our experience, needle aspiration biopsy, which is now a popular method of obtaining tissue from peripheral pulmonary lesions, is the most common cause of this condition. Intermittent positive pressure ventilation, especially for patients with emphysema or patients with end-stage honey-comb lung, is associated with a relatively high incidence of pneumothorax. If performed carefully, thoracentesis and pleural biopsy should not allow air to enter the pleural cavity. Bronchoscopy and biopsies, both transbronchial and brush biopsies, can be associated with pneumothorax. This is especially true in patients with diffuse inflammatory lung disease, such as *Pneumocystis carinii* pneumonia or other diffuse alveolar processes. The insertion of subclavian vein catheters may be associated with both air and fluid within the chest. It has been demonstrated that after cardiopulmonary resuscitation a significant number of rib fractures may occur, with subsequent pneumothorax.

Management

Tube Thoracostomy

A tube thoracostomy is the treatment of choice for traumatic pneumothorax. For pneumothorax caused by needle aspiration biopsy, we have occasionally attempted to use a small noncollapsible catheter inserted in the second anterior intercostal space and attached to a vacuum bottle.

Chest wall trauma may be associated with penetrating injuries to the chest wall or with blunt trauma to the ribs. Blunt trauma may cause fractured ribs to penetrate the pleural surface. In such traumatic pneumothoraces, the presence of coexistent fluid and blood requires the placement of a large bore catheter (No. 28 to No. 32 French). An important complication of blunt trauma to the chest may be the rupture of a bronchus. This usually occurs within a few centimeters of the carina and is clinically manifested by a persisting air leak despite adequate placement of chest tubes. All trauma patients who have pneumothoraces that fail to expand should be explored with a fiberoptic bronchoscope to ascertain whether damage has occurred to the mainstem bronchi.

SUGGESTED READING

Green R, McLeod RC, Stark P. Pneumothorax. Semin Reontgenol 1977; 12:312.
Jenkinson SG. Pneumothorax. Clin Chest Med 1985; 6:153–161.
Seremetis MG. The management of spontaneous pneumothorax. Chest 1970; 57:65–68.
Stradling P, Pool G. Conservative management of spontaneous pneumothorax. Thorax 1966; 21:145.

DROWNING AND NEAR DROWNING

MICHAEL J. CICALE, M.D.
A. JAY BLOCK, M.D.

Drowning and near drowning are becoming more frequent causes of mortality and morbidity in the young population throughout the United States. Recent reports from the United States indicate that drowning accounts for 9,000 deaths annually and that there are 80,000 near drowning accidents annually. Although these accidents are more common in areas where outdoor water activities are popular, submersion accidents can occur in drainage ditches, shallow ponds, bathtubs, toilet bowls, and ice chests. The definition of drowning is a submersion accident resulting in asphyxia and death while submerged or within 24 hours after being submerged. Near drowning is defined as a submersion accident resulting in the victim being transferred to a hospital, but not resulting in death within the first 24 hours.

CLINICAL AND PATHOPHYSIOLOGIC FEATURES

The pathophysiology of near drowning is initiated after the subject's face becomes submerged. There is an initial period of panic, which is followed by a violent struggle and a period of breath holding. During this time, the subject may swallow large quantities of water and subsequently vomit and aspirate water, food, and particulate matter. When breath holding ceases, the subject may then gasp for air and directly aspirate additional quantities of water into the tracheobronchial tree. This water aspiration results in asphyxia. After the subject loses consciousness, passive aspiration of additional fluid occurs. Prolonged asphyxia results in severe hypoxemia, hypoventilation, and acidosis, all leading to cardiorespiratory arrest. Approximately 10 to 20 percent of patients who are victims of submersion accidents have prolonged laryngospasm without any evidence of aspiration. In these subjects, it appears that asphyxia alone results in loss of consciousness and, subsequently, hypoxemia, hypoventilation, acidosis, and cardiorespiratory arrest. Therefore, the major problems encountered in treating victims of submersion accidents include acute respiratory failure and pulmonary aspiration as well as the effects of prolonged hypoxemia on the central nervous system.

The diving reflex is a neurogenic reflex independent of baroreceptors and chemoreceptors that, in some animals, appears to provide protection from drowning. This reflex results in the shunting of blood away from the nonessential organs to the heart and brain. The diving reflex is triggered by submersion of the face and is associated with variable degrees of bradycardia. It is not known whether the diving reflex plays a significant role in human drowning. This reflex may be more active in young children than in adults, especially when drowning is associated with a water temperature of less than 20° C. In addition, cold water immersion results in a rapid fall in body temperature. The degree of hypothermia induced by cold water immersion is more pronounced in children than in adults because of their relatively larger surface area and lack of insulation. Hypothermia occurring at the onset of a submersion accident may have a protective effect on the central nervous system because of decreased metabolic requirements at lower body temperatures.

A variety of laboratory abnormalities are associated with near drowning. Theoretically, in subjects who are submerged in fresh water, hypotonic fluid enters the tracheobronchial tree, alveoli, and, subsequently, the systemic circulation. The absorption of this hypotonic fluid results in a decrease in hemoglobin, hematocrit, serum sodium, and serum chloride. There may be an associated increase in serum potassium due to red blood cell hemolysis. In addition, there may be an increase in blood volume and central venous pressure. The pathophysiology of near drowning in salt water may result in different laboratory abnormalities. When subjects are submerged in salt water, hypertonic fluid enters the tracheobronchial tree and alveoli, and this hypertonic fluid draws free water from the pulmonary circulation into the alveoli. This movement of water from the circulation into the alveoli results in hemoconcentration manifested by a decrease in circulating blood volume and an increase in hemoglobin, hematocrit, serum sodium, and serum chloride. The laboratory abnormalities associated with near drowning in fresh and salt water may be mostly theoretical because, experimentally and clinically, changes in hemoglobin, hematocrit, and serum electrolytes are very small in magnitude. The explanation for the discrepancy between the theoretical laboratory abnormalities and the actual laboratory abnormalities seen experimentally and clinically is that only a small volume of fluid may be aspirated into the tracheobronchial tree. Systemic acidosis is common after submersion accidents and is initially thought to be a combined metabolic and respiratory acidosis. Once resuscitative efforts are initiated and mechanical ventilation is established, the persistent acidosis is the result of a metabolic acidosis induced by hypoxemia and hypoperfusion with resultant lactic acidosis.

Respiratory failure occurs commonly during and after submersion accidents. The pathophysiology of respiratory failure resulting from fresh water submersion is slightly different from that due to salt water submersion. When fresh water is aspirated into the tracheobronchial tree and alveoli, pulmonary surfactant is washed out of the alveoli. This decrease in surfactant changes the surface tension properties of the alveoli, resulting in alveolar collapse and atelectasis. Although these atelectatic areas are not being ventilated, they continue to be perfused by pulmonary arterial blood, resulting in an intrapulmonary right-to-left shunt and the development of hypoxemia. In addition, the aspirated fluid within the alveoli results in ventilation-perfusion abnormalities that cause further intrapulmonary shunting and hypoxemia. In experimental studies of near drowning in fresh water, a precipitous decline in arterial oxygen tension, an increase in arterial carbon dioxide tension, and a decline in pH have been documented within 5 minutes after aspiration. Although the hypercarbia and acidosis resolve within 105 minutes, the amount of intrapulmonary shunting and related hypoxemia persist for a much longer period. With salt water submersion accidents, there is no disruption of pulmonary surfactant. The pathophysiology of respiratory failure associated with near drowning in salt water is due to the fluid-filled and poorly ventilated alveoli continuing to be perfused by pulmonary arterial blood, which causes intrapulmonary shunting of blood and hypoxemia. In addition, many victims of near drowning inhale a variety of particulate matter, including gastric contents, sand, or mud. Aspiration of these materials may result in the development of a superimposed bacterial or aspiration pneumonia, which also may contribute to the development of respiratory failure.

The other major consequence of submersion accidents is the development of neurologic dysfunction. The pathophysiology of neurologic injury induced by near drowning is related to the effect of asphyxia and hypoxemia on the central nervous system. Asphyxia and cerebral hypoxemia lasting longer than 4 to 5 minutes generally results in irreversible brain damage. However, there are many anecdotal reports of near drowning victims surviving after being submerged for up to 40 minutes in fresh water and 17 minutes in salt water. Many of these reported events occurred in very cold water, which may have protected the central nervous system by causing marked hypothermia. These anecdotal reports of survival after prolonged submersion indicate that there is tremendous individual variation in ability to tolerate submersion.

A neurologic classification system proposed jointly by Conn and Modell in 1980 categorized patients, on admission to the emergency room, depending on their level of neurologic function. The purpose of this classification system is to group victims of near drowning accidents into different categories in order to better predict their outcome and choose the most appropriate form of therapy. There are three categories in this neurologic classification system. Patients are classified according to their initial neurologic evaluation in the emergency room. Category A includes all patients who are awake, alert, and oriented. Category B represents patients with a blunted level of consciousness and includes patients who are lethargic, semicomatose, combative, agitated, and disoriented. Category C includes all patients who are comatose. Comatose patients are subclassified as C_1 (patients with decorticate posturing, that is, flexor response to painful stimuli), C_2 (patients with decerebrate posturing, that is, extensor response to painful stimuli, hyperventilation, and fixed and dilated pupils), and C_3 (patients exhibiting a flaccid comatose state with systemic hypotension and no spontaneous respirations). In a large study of victims of submersion accidents, 100 percent of patients in category A survived with normal brain function. In category B, 89 percent of adults and 92 percent of children survived, all with normal brain function. All the deaths in this category were attributed to respiratory failure. In category C, 73 percent of adults and 44 percent of children survived with normal brain function. In this category, an additional 17 percent of children survived, but with incapacitating brain injury.

Chest roentgenographic abnormalities of near drowning victims are quite variable. Patients who have aspirated little or no water may have normal chest films. However, in one- to two-thirds of patients, chest roentgenograms are abnormal, with most showing varying degrees of pulmonary edema. In uncomplicated cases, these roentgenographic abnormalities may clear after approximately 3 to 5 days. In cases complicated by the development of the adult respiratory distress syndrome or superimposed bacterial pneumonia, these roentgenographic infiltrates may persist for more prolonged periods.

COMPLICATIONS

A wide range of complications can occur in victims of near drowning. Water inhalation results in the development of pulmonary edema with subsequent hypoxemia. In addition, water swallowing and subsequent regurgitation and aspiration contribute to the development of severe hypoxemia. Hypoxemia is the direct cause of further lung, central nervous system, kidney, heart, and liver injury. In the lung, leaky alveolar capillary membranes may result in the adult respiratory distress syndrome. In the central nervous system, hypoxemia causes hypoxic encephalopathy with associated brain edema, intracranial hypertension, and seizures. The effects of hypoxemia on the myocardium include arrhythmias, left ventricular failure, and myocardial infarction. The effect of hypoxemia on the kidneys may lead to the development of acute tubular necrosis, and the effect of hypoxemia on the liver may result in massive hepatic necrosis.

PROGNOSTIC FACTORS

Many studies of near drowning have attempted to evaluate the effects of a variety of physiologic parameters on subsequent morbidity and mortality. Modell and colleagues, in a study of 91 near drowning victims, reported that those subjects who had a normal chest roentgenogram on admission to the hospital survived regardless of the initial arterial oxygen tension. In addition, all near drowning victims who were alert on admission survived, whereas all patients who were comatose with fixed and dilated pupils subsequently died. However, it is more difficult to predict the outcome of near drowning victims if, neurologically, they are functioning somewhere between these two extremes. Fandel and associates, in a study of 34 children who were victims of submersion accidents, reported that severe neurologic sequelae occurred in approximately 12 percent of subjects. All patients who suffered severe neurologic sequelae had a pH of less than 7.0, were comatose, and required cardiopulmonary resuscitation while in the emergency room.

Jacobsen and co-workers, in a report of 26 children who were victims of near drowning in warm water, evaluated a variety of prognostic factors. Specifically, they analyzed the adequacy and duration of cardiopulmonary resuscitation, need for cardiopulmonary support, immersion time, water temperature, level of consciousness on admission, serum pH, and use of therapy directed at cerebral protection. They concluded that neurologic complications were inevitable if spontaneous ventilation was not present after cardiopulmonary resuscitation.

Another study categorized patients according to the Glasgow coma scale and attempted to document a relationship between the initial neurologic evaluation and morbidity and mortality. However, no prognostic factors were identified that would allow the emergency room physician to predict with certainty those subjects who were going to die or suffer permanent neurologic sequelae. Studies suggest that near drowning victims who arrive in the emergency room deeply comatose with severe acidosis and require cardiopulmonary resuscitation and mechanical ventilation may suffer significant morbidity and mortality. However, some of these severely injured patients may survive with little or no evidence of neurologic sequelae, so there is no justification for making a decision not to resuscitate any near drowning victim.

MANAGEMENT

The primary objective in treating victims of near drowning should be to reverse the hypoxemia and acidosis as soon as possible. At the scene of the accident, therapy should include artificial ventilation and circulatory support, even in the water, if possible. If cardiopulmonary resuscitation cannot be performed adequately in the water, the patient should be transported as soon as possible to a hospital emergency room. On route to the emergency room, it is important to continue cardiopulmonary resuscitation if necessary, and to administer supplemental oxygen by mask or nasal cannula in spontaneously breathing patients. If possible, inadequately ventilated patients should be endotracheally intubated and mechanically ventilated with supplemental oxygen.

At the scene of the accident, if there is evidence or strong clinical suspicion of upper airway obstruction by foreign particulate matter, the obstruction should be removed manually or by performing a subdiaphragmatic abdominal thrust (Heimlich maneuver). There is no scientific evidence that warrants performing a subdiaphragmatic abdominal thrust in all victims of submersion accidents. Performing a Heimlich maneuver on a near drowning victim without evidence of upper airway obstruction results in removal of an insignificant amount of fluid from the tracheobronchial tree and may predispose the subject to gastric regurgitation and subsequent pulmonary aspiration.

Once admitted to the hospital emergency room, patients should be evaluated quickly with a history, physical examination including a detailed neurologic examination, complete blood count, serum electrolyte levels, chest roentgenogram, electrocardiogram, and arterial blood gas analysis. Patients who are awake, asymptomatic, and have no laboratory abnormalities can safely be discharged after a brief period of observation. Patients with minimal symptoms or signs of pulmonary or neurologic abnormalities should be monitored for at least 24 hours and treated with supplemental oxygen.

Patients with more severe pulmonary and neurologic impairment should be admitted to the intensive care unit for further monitoring and therapy. While in the intensive care unit, the patient should be monitored with frequent checking of vital signs, neurologic examinations, complete blood count and analysis of serum chemistry as indicated by the clinical situation, daily chest roentgenograms, and frequent arterial blood gas analyses. Comatose patients or patients with hypoxemic or hypercapneic respiratory failure should be treated with tracheal intubation and mechanical ventilation. Noncardiogenic pulmonary edema and hypoxemia can be treated successfully with positive end-expiratory pressure (PEEP) or continuous positive airway pressure (CPAP). PEEP opens atelectatic alveoli and increases functional residual capacity, which results in improved ventilation: perfusion ratios and improved arterial oxygenation. Victims of near drowning in fresh water are best treated with a combination of mechanical ventilation and PEEP. As previously noted, such patients have a decrease in pulmonary surfactant resulting in microatelectasis. These microatelectatic areas can be easily inflated with positive pressure mechanical ventilation, and PEEP can then maintain these alveoli in an inflated state. In victims of salt water aspiration, surfactant is normal, so spontaneous respiratory efforts may be adequate to inflate the alveoli, and PEEP can be used to maintain the alveoli in an inflated state. Therefore, after near drowning in salt water, PEEP with either mechanical ventilation or spontaneous ventilation should be utilized. In experimental near drowning in pigs, delaying the initiation of 5 cm of PEEP for 20 minutes still resulted in beneficial effects on hypoxemia, thus providing experimental evidence to suggest that PEEP applied after successful cardiopulmonary resuscitation in the field may be beneficial.

The second major therapeutic objective is reversal of central nervous system injury and protection of the central nervous system from further insult. In an attempt to achieve this therapeutic objective, vigorous supportive therapy and stabilization of cardiopulmonary function should be initiated. Cardiovascular stabilization should be achieved by maintaining an adequate intravascular volume to maintain an acceptable blood pressure and by treating any serious arrhythmias. The arterial oxygen tension should be maintained at approximately 100 mm Hg by the addition of supplemental oxygen, PEEP, or mechanical ventilation. Mechanical ventilation is indicated to maintain a normal arterial carbon dioxide tension and pH.

In 1978 Conn and associates popularized a specific form of cerebral salvage therapy designated by the acronym HYPER. This therapy was designed to combat hyperHydration, hYperventilation, hyperPyrexia, hyperExcitability, and hyperRigidity, clinical features associated with near drowning that may effect brain recovery. Hyperhydration, due to water ingestion and aspiration as well as fluid administration during aggressive resuscitative efforts, should be treated with fluid restriction. Hyperventilation, a result of reduced pulmonary compliance and direct central nervous system injury, is treated with sedation, intubation, and mechanical ventilation. Hyperpyrexia, a result of central nervous system injury, causes deleterious effects on the already injured central nervous system and should be treated with hypothermia, which reduces the metabolic demand for oxygen. Hyperexcitability, a result of acute central nervous system injury, results in further increases in intracranial pressure, which may cause additional central nervous system injury, and is best treated with barbiturate sedation. Hyperrigidity, which occurs in patients with decerebrate or decorticate posturing, may further increase intracranial pressure and can be treated with muscle paralysis. Significant complications can result from inducing barbiturate coma, muscle paralysis, and hypothermia. There is good evidence that hypothermia results in a reduction in circulating polymorphonuclear leukocytes and an increased incidence of bacterial infection. In a recent retrospective study of several aspects of HYPER therapy on morbidity and mortality after near drowning, Conn and associates concluded that hypothermia and barbiturates are not beneficial because severe cerebral edema after submersion accidents generally is associated with irreversible brain damage. Until prospective and randomized clinical studies confirm the benefit of HYPER therapy, this form of cerebral salvage therapy should not be used routinely.

Intracranial pressure monitoring in near drowning victims is controversial. Nussbaum and colleagues, in a study of 21 pediatric near drowning victims, continuously monitored intracranial pressure and cerebral perfusion pressure (mean systemic arterial pressure minus intracranial pressure). All of these patients were in a deep coma with flaccid paralysis, hypotension, and no spontaneous respirations. An intracranial pressure of greater than 20 mm Hg and a cerebral perfusion pressure of less than 50 mm Hg was universally associated with death. An intracranial pressure of less than 20 mm Hg and a cerebral perfusion pressure of greater than 50 mm Hg was associated with survival. However, the levels of intracranial pressure and cerebral perfusion pressure could not distinguish between survival with normal neurologic function and survival with severe neurologic sequelae. Therefore, in this subgroup of patients, intracranial pressure and cerebral perfusion pressure monitoring may be good predictors of mortality, but are not good predictors of central nervous system morbidity. Therefore, the routine use of intracranial pressure monitoring in comatose near drowning victims is not indicated.

Antibiotics are not useful empirically in near drowning victims. Antibiotics are indicated when superimposed infection is clearly documented. The use of systemic steroids in victims of submersion accidents has not been shown to be beneficial. In a prospective controlled experiment, methylprednisolone was administered to dogs after near drowning in fresh water, and there was no difference in arterial oxygenation, shunt fraction, or survival in the steroid-treated dogs.

SUGGESTED READING

Bohn DJ, Biggar WD, Smith CR, Conn AW, Barker GA. Influence of hypothermia, barbiturate therapy, and intracranial pressure monitoring on morbidity and mortality after near-drowning. Crit Care Med 1986; 14:529–534.

Conn AW, Edmonds JF, Barker GA. Near drowning in cold fresh water: current treatment regimen. Can Anaesth Soc J 1978; 25:259–265.

Fandel I, Bancalari E. Near-drowning in children: clinical aspects. Pediatrics 1976; 58:573–579.

Jacobsen WK, Mason LJ, Briggs BA, Schneider S, Thompson JC. Correlation of spontaneous respiration and neurologic damage in near-drowning. Crit Care Med 1983; 11:487–489.

Modell JH, Graves SA, Kuck EJ. Near drowning: correlation of level of consciousness and survival. Can Anaesth Soc J 1980; 27:211–215.

Modell JH, Graves SA, Ketover A. Clinical course of 91 consecutive near-drowning victims. Chest 1976; 70:231–238.

Nussbaum E, Galant SP. Intracranial pressure monitoring as a guide to prognosis in the nearly drowned, severely comatose child. J Pediatr 1983; 102:215–218.

HIGH ALTITUDE DISEASE

TIMOTHY C. KENNEDY, M.D., F.C.C.P.
JACK ECK, M.D.
ALAN SALLIMAN, M.D.

In recent years the spectrum of high altitude illnesses has been more frequently encountered because of greater numbers of people seeking recreation at high altitudes (over 8,000 feet) and because of improved transportation, which allows more abrupt ascents and disables important adaptive mechanisms. The incidence and severity of high altitude illnesses vary widely with different circumstances, including absolute altitude and the rapidity of ascent. Acute altitude illnesses are reported in the Andes, the Alps, the North American Rockies, Alaska, the African peaks, and of course, the Himalayas. Although the different syndromes probably share a common pathophysiologic basis, differences in individual susceptibility, irreproducibility, and failure to find reliable animal models have confounded our understanding and management of these syndromes.

DEFINITION OF SYNDROMES

Acute Mountain Sickness

Acute mountain sickness (AMS), the most commonly encountered syndrome, occurs in the unacclimatized person who is above 8,000 feet. Symptoms include headache (most common), anorexia and vomiting, malaise, occasionally a stiff neck, and disturbed sleep. It is probable that most of these symptoms are accounted for by hypoxia, respiratory alkalosis, sleep-disordered breathing, and increased intracranial pressure. Supporting this hypothesis is the fact that acetazolamide is effective in preventing and treating most cases and is capable of improving hypoxia, respiratory alkalosis, and sleep-disordered breathing and in reducing production of cerebrospinal fluid (CSF). By definition, AMS is self-limited, resolving in 1 to 5 days as a result of increased renal bicarbonate excretion. This excretion corrects symptoms associated with alkalemia and also improves respiratory drive and minute ventilation, which is blunted by the alkalosis, thereby improving oxygenation. AMS occurs in more than half of unacclimatized visitors at 14,000 feet.

High Altitude Pulmonary and Cerebral Edema

Additional, less well understood mechanisms produce the more disabling and life-threatening syndromes of high altitude pulmonary edema (HAPE) and high altitude cerebral edema (HACE). These syndromes, less common than AMS, occur unpredictably at high altitudes and rarely below 9,500 feet.

HAPE, a noncardiogenic pulmonary edema progressing on the heels of AMS, is recognized by dyspnea and tachypnea at rest, rales, and a cough that is usually nonproductive; however, bloody or pink frothy sputum is seen in the more fulminant cases. Cyanosis is variable. Low grade fever (temperature of 37.5 to 38.5 ° C), leukocytosis (12,000 to 18,000 per cu mm), and elevated noncardiac creatine phosphokinase levels are common. Evidence of volume overload is usually absent. The pulmonic valve closure sound may be accentuated. Both cardiogenic pulmonary edema and atypical pneumonia are considered in the differential diagnosis. Confusion, lethargy, ataxia, and coma also are seen as a result of severe hypoxia and/or concomitant HACE. HAPE is reported in one visitor out of 10,000 to Summit County, Colorado (8,000 to 10,000 feet is the average resident altitude), but the incidence climbs to 15 percent when the altitude is abruptly attained and sustained at 14,500 feet. More than half of climbers over 16,000 feet have rales on auscultation but are often asymptomatic.

HACE also is far less common than simple AMS, but may be subclinical and initially perceived as AMS. Overt symptoms include a progressively severe headache, ataxia, emotional lability, poor judgment, memory loss, hallucination, and confusion that can progress to coma and death. Meningeal signs, papilledema, plantar extension, and "hand flap" are all described. CSF pressures are usually high, and CSF may be hemorrhagic or reveal leukocytosis. An unpredictable, heterogeneous pattern of CNS involvement is the rule.

High Altitude Retinal Hemorrhages

High altitude retinal hemorrhages (HARH) are probably biologically identical to HACE and can be visualized with the ophthalmoscope. Mild changes are common, occurring in 50 percent of visitors at 14,000 feet, and include dilated retinal veins and arteries and flame-shaped preretinal hemorrhages that are usually peripheral but occasionally are found in the macula. Macular involvement may result in blurred vision, scotomata, and sometimes persistent visual disturbances. More serious findings include vitreous hemorrhages, papillary hemorrhages, and papilledema; the last sign suggests significant cerebral edema.

Though histopathologic studies, physiologic observations, hormonal measurements, and bronchoalveolar lavage have led to many insights concerning the biologic mechanisms of HAPE, HACE, and HARH, the precise mechanisms remain unknown. A poor hypoxic drive and relative hypoventilation appear common in susceptible individuals. Patients studied subsequent to the development of HAPE demonstrate decreased hypoxic drives and an exaggerated hypoxic pulmonary vasoconstrictor response. Some have hypothesized that pulmonary capillary damage results from shear forces associated with the combination of increased pulmonary blood flow from exercise and the underlying vasoconstriction, resulting in endothelial damage and interstitial, then alveolar, flooding of proteinaceous fluid typical of other forms of noncardiogenic pulmonary edema. Platelet aggregates and sludged erythrocytes are seen in histologic samples in both HAPE and HACE. Leukotrienes, complement fragments, and inhibitors of neutrophil chemotactic factor are found in these severe syndromes, but these observations are also generally seen in the adult respiratory distress syndrome, sepsis, and other conditions of diffuse tissue injury or generalized activation of the immune system and are not specific. However, Schoene and Hackett observed less intense neutrophil accumulations than in other forms of acute lung injury. The rapid recovery of persons with HAPE differs from the sluggish rate of recovery in most other forms of increased permeability pulmonary edema. Others have speculated that derangements of the adenosine triphosphate-dependent sodium pump lead to interstitial edema.

MANAGEMENT

Strategies to reduce the likelihood of HAPE or HACE are of great interest to the vacationer, the trekker, the climber, and even the military strategist.

Prevention

When feasible, slow ascent is probably the most important method of prevention. A day of rest at 8,000 feet, then ascents of 1,000 feet per day until 10,000 feet, appears to reduce the incidence and severity of these disorders by allowing time for adaptive mechanisms to be effective. Thereafter, limiting the ascent to 500 feet per day and, whenever possible, sleeping at a lower altitude at night is recommended. Travel capabilities, time constraints, and emergencies often are compelling, and thus normal adaptive mechanisms cannot be effected.

Carbonic Anhydrase Inhibitors

Acetazolamide (Diamox) has been advocated to accelerate renal bicarbonate excretion. Although there is now good evidence that this drug ameliorates AMS, there are several concerns with its use. Diuretics aggravate dehydration, thus reducing performance and increasing the risk of frostbite. Hypokalemia is an additional risk. Paresthesias, nausea, and drowsiness are common side effects of acetazolamide; the drug also ruins the taste of carbonated beverages. Climbers with sulfa allergy should avoid acetazolamide. We advocate using a low dose (250 mg per day) only on the day prior to and the day of a significantly abrupt ascent, in association with adequate fluid and potassium replacement. Continuous treatment while sustaining an altitude is probably unwarranted.

The use of other diuretics, though advocated, have not been of proven value and may be deleterious.

Corticosteroids

Dexamethasone, 4 mg every 6 hours before and during ascents, has been shown to reduce the incidence and the established symptoms of slight or moderate AMS, perhaps by reducing intracranial pressure and/or cerebral edema. Interestingly, hypoxia also was ameliorated and pulmonary function tests improved. Spontaneous diuresis was observed with administration. Lower doses that were capable of suppressing inflammatory responses but not vasogenic cerebral edema failed to work. It may be that the short-term use of dexamethasone has fewer potential side effects than acetazolamide. However, experience in high altitude clinics suggests that mild HACE is common and frequently mistaken for AMS. Theoretically, the routine use of dexamethasone may mask the onset of HACE, which could delay treatment (descent) until extensive brain dysfunction occurs. There is no evidence that dexamethasone prevents HAPE or HACE.

Because sleep-disordered breathing, Cheyne-Stokes respirations, or aggravation of underlying sleep apnea is common, sleep at high altitudes probably is a period of higher risk than wakefulness. Acetazolamide has been shown to improve nocturnal hypoxia. More important, it may be wise to adhere to the adage, "Climb high; sleep low." Experienced climbing teams attempt to retreat to lower altitudes for sleep during periods of adaptation. A recent effort to address this idea in an innovative way was the development of a portable hyperbaric shell for mountainside slumbering.

Since it is clear that sleep-disordered breathing is considerably worsened by use of alcohol and sedative drugs, visitors to altitude should be cautioned against the temptation to treat insomnia with these agents. This is particularly true in persons with a history of snoring. We have discovered anecdotal accounts of a number of patients with previously unrecognized sleep apnea who had experienced HAPE or HACE, though the epidemiologic significance of this phenomenon is unknown.

Acetylsalicylic Acid

Because hypercoagulability may play a role in the pathogenesis of HAPE and HACE, and because headache is common in persons with these syndromes, the use of aspirin is tempting. Although acetylsalicylic acid reduces headache, the hemorrhagic aspects of HACE associated with a significant incidence of subarachnoid and intracerebral hemorrhage suggest the need to avoid this strategy. Sheep studies also suggest that salicylates cause increased fluid transudation into the pulmonary interstitium. Naproxen also failed to prevent illness, again suggesting that an inflammatory etiology is unlikely.

Hydration

Hydration is recommended. There is no evidence that overhydration is a risk factor for HAPE or HACE, even though Hackett showed that fluid retention was common in symptomatic patients and spontaneous diuresis was associated with recovery; we suspect that this is a cytotoxic or vasogenic third spacing effect. Elevated central venous pressures in the absence of cardiac dysfunction, have not been found in HAPE or HACE. Low filling pressures in the face of hypoxia and exercise may aggravate mixed venous desaturation and, in the presence of any right-to-left shunting, may aggravate arterial hypoxia as well.

Cigarette or cannabis smoking carries the striking disadvantage of adding 5 to 15 percent carboxyhemoglobin level to the effective hypoxic burden.

Phenytoin

Phenytoin (Dilantin) was recently reported to reduce symptoms of AMS and the incidence of HARH, although the sample studied was small. No side effects were reported, which is in contradistinction to experience with acetazolamide.

Immediate Care and Management Strategies

Lower Altitude

Prompt descent is the most important step in the therapy of HACE, HAPE, or severe HARH. First, the condition must be recognized. Many reported tragedies were not avoided because of the competitive desire to "get to the top," and impaired judgment resulting from hypoxia compounds this issue. Rest also may help by reducing cardiac output and hypertension.

Oxygen

Oxygen, delivered by mask and preferably by continuous positive pressure to improve lung volume and reduce shunt effects, is desirable when available.

Fluids

Fluid management is controversial. We favor a careful clinical estimation of volume status, noting difficulties in estimating effective preload in the setting of pulmonary hypertension, pulmonary edema, cerebral edema, and peripheral edema all of which may be seen in the presence of underlying central hypovolemia. Generally, patients are somewhat dehydrated when first seen, and cautious volume expansion is helpful. In the past, the use of furosemide resulted in greater mortality and overt hypotension.

Corticosteroids

Dexamethasone is helpful in mild HACE, and although it does not appear useful in severe HAPE or HACE, it may help some persons and the risk of use is low. Findings that lung volumes and hypoxia improved in persons with mild AMS after administration of dexamethasone support this use.

Other Drugs

Acetazolamide also has not been shown to help patients with severe HAPE or HACE. However, since it may ameliorate some of the components of the underlying pathophysiology, its potential benefits may outweigh the risk of use.

Narcan also has been proposed as a temporizing measure, presumably to increase respiratory drive. Risks of use include excessive increase in sympathetic discharge and tachyarrhythmias.

A recent anecdote suggested a head down–buttocks up postural drainage tactic with abdominal support by a companion to enhance periodic forceful coughing. This procedure may help mobilize edema fluid from dependent areas of the lung and then temporarily clear edema from the large airways.

Calcium channel blockers and nitrates have been tried and may help reduce pulmonary vascular resistance. However, the potential for worsening of ventilation-perfusion mismatch and hypotension suggest that this tactic should be reserved for the acute-care hospital setting where these effects can be managed should they occur.

We also avoid the use of morphine sulfate because of the risk of respiratory drive depression and of the decrease in preload by increasing venous capacitance.

None of these drug strategies replaces descent and oxygen therapy.

OTHER HIGH ALTITUDE DISORDERS

Thromboembolism and hypercoagulability are reported sporadically in visitors to high altitude. Increases in platelet factor 2 and platelet adhesiveness have been demonstrated. Recurrent atrial fibrillation has been described in some individuals as an irritating consequence of visiting 8,000 feet. Sickle-cell crisis should be considered in black visitors to high altitude who show symptoms of high altitude disease, even if they were not previously known to have sickle-cell trait.

Chronic mountain sickness is seen by virtually all practitioners at high altitude. When first seen, persons with this condition have cor pulmonale, minimal dyspnea, and either no intrinsic lung disorder or unexpectedly little lung disease considering the presence of cor pulmonale. Carefully evaluated patients have depressed hypoxic drive and sleep-disordered breathing. Higher than expected PCO_2 levels are noted in the face of hypoxia. Alveolar to arterial pressure may be normal or high, reflecting the degree (if any) of lung dysfunction. Nocturnal hypoxia is usually profound. All-night pulse oximetry with a strip chart recorder is an excellent screening tool. Patterns seen include periodic (10 to 40 minutes) hypoxia, which represents hypoventilation and decreased functional residual capacity in rapid eye movement sleep, or rhythmic spikes of hypoxia, which usually represents obstructive sleep apnea. Nocturnal oxygen, acetazolamide, methylprogesterone, and nasal continuous positive pressure all have been used to reduce pulmonary hypertension and other consequences of chronic hypoxia.

SUGGESTED READING

Hackett PH, Roach RC. Medical therapy of altitude illness. Ann Emerg Med 1987; 16:980–986.

Hamilton AJ, Cymmerman A, Black PM. High altitude cerebral edema. Neurosurgery 1986; 19:841–849.

Schoene RB. High altitude pulmonary edema: pathophysiology and clinical review. Ann Emerg Med 1987; 16:987–992.

Sophocles AS. High-altitude pulmonary edema in Vail, Colorado 1975–1982. West J Med 1986; 144:569–573.

Sutton JR, Jones NL, Houston CS. Hypoxia: man at altitude. New York: Thieme-Stratton, 1982.

Wiedman M, Tabin G. High altitude retinal hemorrhage as a prognostic indicator in altitude illness. Int Ophthalmol Clin 1986; 26:175–186.

HEMATOLOGIC DISEASES

APLASTIC ANEMIA

NEAL S. YOUNG, M.D.

The infrequency of aplastic anemia (incidence = 2 to 6/10^6) does not allow most hematologists to have comfortable familiarity with its treatment. Aplastic anemia is often fatal, but more than half of patients with severe bone marrow failure can be cured. All forms of definitive therapy require adequate supportive care; these are the subject of this chapter.

Before a therapeutic strategy is decided on, the diagnosis must be exactly established and an estimate made of the patient's prognosis.

Differential Diagnosis. Despite the clarity of the clinical presentation of aplastic anemia—pancytopenia with an "empty" bone marrow—many patients with low blood counts are misdiagnosed because of inadequate tissue sampling, mistaken pathologic interpretation, or ignorance of pathophysiologic mechanisms. Careful examination of the aspirate smear and judgment of cellularity from a 1-cm core biopsy are the minimal diagnostic requirements. Idiopathic aplastic anemia should be especially distinguished from (1) Fanconi's anemia or congenital aplastic anemia (by cytogenetic analysis of peripheral blood mononuclear cells cultured in the presence of mitomycin C or diepoxybutane); (2) paroxysmal nocturnal hemoglobinuria, which may develop from or into aplastic anemia (by Ham's test); (3) aleukemic acute leukemia and lymphoma restricted to the bone marrow (by attention to blast cells that can be nestled close to spicules in an otherwise hypocellular specimen); (4) myelofibrosis (by remembering that failure to aspirate marrow, or a dry tap, is unusual in aplasia); and (5) dysmyelopoietic syndromes, which may be hypocellular and associated with chromosomal abnormalities restricted to marrow cells.

Prognosis. Blood counts at presentation are the major determinants of survival, whereas age, sex, toxic exposures, and other historical features have had no important prognostic role in patient populations analyzed retrospectively. Patients with aplastic anemia re generally categorized as having severe disease if at clinical presentation they fulfill two of three blood count criteria: polymorphonuclear cell number less than 500 per cubic millimeter; platelets less than 20,000 per cubic millimeter; reticulocytes less than 1 percent (corrected) or less than 60,000 per cubic millimeter (absolute). Very low neutrophil counts have a particularly dire significance. Severity implies a poor prognosis, with mortality for disease untreated at 1 year of 80 to 90 percent; patients with moderate disease have a better outlook. Although many ultimately die of the complications of pancytopenia or transfusional hemosiderosis. Unfortunately, blood count criteria are not infallible. Some patients with virtually absent granulocytes or platelets survive for years. Conversely, a patient's blood count may fall following presentation, refractoriness to platelet transfusions may permit fatal hemorrhage, or a trivial untreated infection may become established. Nevertheless, patients with severe aplastic anemia require immediate definitive therapy, usually either bone marrow transplantation or horse antikaymecyte globulin therapy.

Initial Evaluation. The rapidity of the initial clinical and laboratory evaluation is intrinsic to the appropriate care of the aplastic anemia patient. Severely pancytopenic patients can deteriorate rapidly as a result of sepsis or bleeding, and the initiation of curative therapy is then postponed in order to treat cascading complications. These complications and their treatments can further diminish the probability of success of the definitive treatment. For example, avoidance of transfusions enhances the survival of the patient undergoing bone marrow transplantation. For either replacement therapy in the form of transplantation or immunologic therapy with horse antiserum to human lymphocytes, the patient in good general medical condition has the best opportunity of immediate survival and ultimate recovery. Table 1 summarizes the crucial laboratory studies that should be completed within the first several days of presentation.

TABLE 1 Initial Evaluation

Complete blood counts, with differential, reticulocytes × 2
Bone marrow aspiration and 1-cm biopsy
If < 30 years old, cytogenetics of peripheral blood leukocytes
Ham's test
Liver enzymes
HLA typing

BONE MARROW TRANSPLANTATION

Transplantation in the form of bone marrow infusion can restore normal blood counts and can decrease acute mortality in aplastic anemia. The procedure itself carries a significant risk of death, acute and delayed morbidity, and expense. Patients with histocompatible family members (four identical human leukocyte antigens [HLA] plus absence of mixed lymphocyte reactivity), almost always siblings, should always be considered for bone marrow transplantation. Although occasional patients have successfully received transplants across HLA barriers from relatives or from HLA-identical unrelated donors, the overall success rate using nonidentical or unrelated donors is very low. Fewer than half of patients have identical sibling donors.

The major factors that contribute to the outcome of bone marrow transplantation in bone marrow failure are: (1) patient age, (2) transfusion history, and (3) infection at time of transplant. The incidence of graft-versus-host disease (GVHD), one of the major complications of bone marrow transplantation, increases with age and is more than 90 percent in patients over 30 years of age. Untransfused (actually meaning no transfusions within 72 hours before conditioning therapy begins) patients have a lower incidence of graft rejection because their lymphocytes have not been sensitized by prior antigen exposure.

Good candidates—young, untransfused, and uninfected—have an excellent prospect of hematopoietic recovery when undergoing transplants at experienced centers, as high as 75 percent long-term survival with hematopoietic engraftment. Statistics almost as good for transfused patients have been reported in some studies, although survival rates of 40 to 65 percent are more common. Death immediately following transplantation usually results from acute GVHD or interstitial pneumonitis. Chronic GVHD, even if not fatal, can be a serious multisystem disease and is not always responsive to immunosuppressive therapy. There is a roughly inverse relationship between graft rejection and GVHD. Success at reducing the rejection rate to about 10 percent by intensifying immunosuppression preconditioning has been accompanied by an increased incidence of GVHD, and efforts, at least to date, to reduce GVHD by in vitro T-cell depletion of donor bone marrow have resulted in higher rates of graft rejection.

Delayed complications of marrow transplantation for any indication result from the effects of irradiation and chemotherapy: diminished pulmonary function, endocrine dysfunction and infertility, cognitive disorders and leukoencephalopathy, and secondary malignancies. Patients with Fanconi's anemia have undergone successful transplants using a necessary reduced conditioning regimen; already at risk for malignancy, they have exaggerated long-term effects.

Patients with aplastic anemia may experience graft rejection because of the underlying pathophysiology of bone marrow failure. Simple infusions of marrow from syngeneic twins, without immunosuppressive therapy of the host, fail about half the time. Recurrence of aplasia in identical twins who were immunosuppressed prior to transplantation is further evidence of an inhospitable environment for stem cells in some patients with bone marrow failure.

ANTITHYMOCYTE GLOBULIN

Mathé, who first noted recovery of autologous bone marrow function in some patients in whom rejection of marrow grafts had occurred, suggested that aplastic anemia might be immunologically mediated. This clinical demonstration of functionally quiescent stem cells in aplastic patients indicated that the empty bone marrow contains cells capable of rescue with nonreplacement therapy. Laboratory experiments in general have supported the hypothesis of suppression of hematopoiesis by T cells and their soluble products, but when applied to individual patients, these tests have been inadequate to predict clinical response to immunologic therapy. The decision to employ antilymphocyte sera is therefore clinical.

Two types of horse serum preparations are in wide use. Antithoracic duct lymphocyte globulin (ALG or ATDLG) is European and is manufactured by the Swiss Serum Institute or Institut Merieux of Lyons; despite extensive experience with these agents, they have not been approved for use in the United States. Antithymocyte globulin (ATG, ATGAM), manufactured by Upjohn, is commercially available. Although it is a controversial subject, there is little convincing laboratory or clinical evidence of important differences between ATG and ALG preparations or among lots. Regimens have also varied, ALG usually being administered in higher doses over shorter periods of time than ATG. Because the foreign proteins are rapidly cleared once the patient produces antihorse IgG antibodies at about 1 week, briefer treatment is probably more rational. We currently administer ATG, 40 mg per kilogram per day for 4 days.

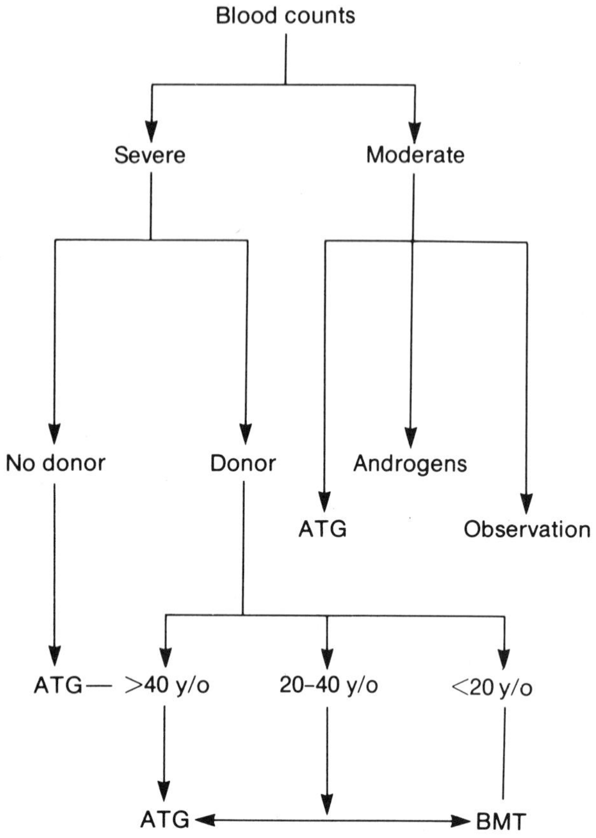

Figure 1 Treatment alternatives in aplastic anemia. BMT = bone marrow transplant.

About half of patients treated with ATG recover hematopoiesis, often not to completely normal blood counts but sufficient to be free of infection and the need for transfusion of red cells and platelets. Hematopoietic recovery rates in different studies have ranged from 25 to 85 percent; this is possibly related to differences among centers in patient selection and supportive care. Recovery rates are not apparently related to age, sex, or the etiology of bone marrow failure. Patients with very severe neutropenia (<200 neutrophils per cubic millimeter) may not survive to benefit from ATG. Hematopoietic improvement is usually apparent within a few months of ATG therapy. Later improvement can occur, although specific therapeutic benefit due to ATG is then harder to distinguish from the effects of subsequent therapy and spontaneous late remission in well-supported aplastic anemic patients. No more than 10 percent of patients who have remissions with ATG subsequently relapse, and they may respond to a second course of ATG.

The complications of ATG therapy are best managed by a hematologist experienced in its use; however, patients do not require routine transfer to intensive care units for ATG therapy. Although rare, anaphylaxis due to horse protein allergy is the most serious consequence and has been fatal. Skin testing may predict susceptible patients. We currently test by epicutaneous prick testing with undiluted ATG. A wheal and flare reaction would indicate the need for desensitization before ATG administration. More common allergic symptoms are fever, chills, and urticaria with the first few infusions. Serum sickness at about day 10 of therapy is also common and manifests usually as a flu-like illness with a characteristic maculopapular eruption, fever, arthralgia and myalgia, and gastrointestinal symptoms. Serum transaminase and creatinine levels may be transiently increased and the albumin value may be depressed. Although it is generally tolerated when corticosteroids are administered at high doses (60 to 80 mg methylprednisolone in divided daily doses), serum sickness can be temporarily incapacitating; myositis and myocarditis have been observed. Finally, as ATG binds to circulating blood elements as well as lymphocytes, lower platelet and granulocyte counts during ATG therapy should be expected and may necessitate increased numbers of transfusions or antibiotic administration; Coombs' test may become positive during ATG therapy.

CYCLOSPORINE

Cyclosporine, which interferes with T-cell function more specifically than ATG, is effective in about 40 percent of patients who have failed conventional immunosuppressive therapy; preliminary European data suggest that cyclosporine added to ALG may increase the initial response rate in severe disease. We administer cyclosporine at 12 mg per kilogram per day in adults and 15 mg per kilogram per day in children and adjust dosage for nephrotoxicity and blood levels (tests obtained every 2 weeks). Aplastic anemia patients receiving cyclosporine can resemble patients with acquired immunodeficiency syndrome and are susceptible to infection with unusual agents such as *Pneumocystis carinii.*

ANDROGENS

Often disparaged but often used, androgens have a mixed reputation, mainly because only trials from Europe have supported their use. Nonetheless, most hematologists have had at least one aplastic patient who has clearly responded to hormone therapy. Androgens may work best in patients with some residual hematopoiesis. Dosage is also probably important. Choice of androgen is largely individual: oxymetholone, fluoxymesterone, and nandrolone decanoate are among the more popular formulations. We employ nandrolone decanoate at 5 mg per kilogram per week, given intramuscularly (injection is well tolerated even in thrombocytopenic patients if followed by 15 minutes of pressure); parenteral androgens avoid the hepatotoxicity associated with oral preparations. With any androgen, a fair clinical trial is 3 to 6 months.

HEMATOPOIETIC GROWTH FACTORS

A few patients have been reported to respond to granulocyte macrophage colony-stimulating factor (GM-CSF) and interleukin-3 in early trials, usually with neutrophil improvement but occasionally with increased platelets and reticulocytes. In general, the best responses have been in cases with residual hematopoiesis or chronic disease; GM-CSF has not been shown to be helpful in severe neutropenia associated with serious infection. Cytokine flu and a capillary leak syndrome are the major toxicities of GM-CSF. Interleukin-3 and also GM-CSF appear to be much less toxic. Future trials will test factors that act at the primitive hematopoietic stem cell level (interleukin-1 and interleukin-3) and combinations of growth factors.

SUPPORTIVE THERAPY

Infections

Febrile episodes and serious infections are common in severely affected patients and represent the major cause of death in aplastic anemia. Fever, local infections, and even vague symptoms such as generalized malaise suggestive of early sepsis must be regarded with extreme seriousness in the setting of neutropenia. Suspicion of sepsis should initiate administration of broad-spectrum, full-dose parenteral antibiotic therapy (ceftazidime or a combination of a cephalosporin, semisynthetic penicillin, and an aminoglycoside). Unless a nonbacterial cause of fever becomes obvious (e.g., serum sickness, viral infection), therapy should be continued for 10 to 14 days, even with negative blood cultures. More important is the prompt institution of antibiotics rather than the precise choice of agents prescribed.

With the first episodes of infection, neutropenic patients defervesce and improve symptomatically within a few days of treatment. Persistent or recurrent fever despite antibiotics occasionally responds to addition of a more specific drug that broadens bacterial coverage, such as vancomycin (for resistant *Staphylococcus*) or clindamycin (for anaerobes). More usually, persistent fever in the repeatedly treated patient signifies fungal infection and demands amphotericin B therapy; empiric antifungal therapy should be started in a patient who has fever after 7 days of antibacterial antibiotics. Infections caused by resistant organisms, rare bacterial species, and *Pneumocystis* are uncommon in aplastic anemia patients.

Delaying administration of antibiotics may lead to seeding of organisms, a virtually intractable problem in aplastic patients. Surgical approaches tend to spread infection across fascial planes, and concentrated collections of bacteria, even sensitive *Escherichia coli* and *Pseudomonas*, may not be eradicated even with prolonged antibiotic treatment. The role of granulocyte transfusions, which may be employed in the deteriorating patient with a seated infection, is uncertain.

Bleeding and Platelet Transfusions

Bleeding is common in bone marrow failure but is rarely fatal. Thrombocytopenia alone usually results in mucocutaneous hemorrhage and manifests as petechiae, ecchymoses, and gingival oozing. Spontaneous intracranial hemorrhage is the most feared complication; it is often, but not invariably, fatal. Major gastrointestinal, genitourinary, or pulmonary bleeding is not usually due to diminished platelet numbers alone but occurs in the setting of infection, stress, and corticosteroid therapy.

Serious bleeding is treated by platelet transfusions administered as often as required for clinical effect. Four units of platelets or the donation from a single cytophoresed donor may raise the platelet count above 30,000 to 40,000 and may stem hemorrhage; transfusions as often as three times daily may be required in other circumstances. Life-threatening hemorrhage is customarily treated with platelet transfusions even in the absence of satisfactory increments in peripheral blood platelet numbers in the hope of homing to bleeding sites.

Platelets administered prophylactically can prevent hemorrhage, although there are no data indicating improved survival as a result of prophylaxis as compared with platelets on demand. A convenient goal is to maintain platelet counts at over 5,000 per cubic millimeter. There is no rationale for prophylactic transfusion in patients whose disease has become refractory because of alloantibody formation. Bleeding in these patients may respond to Amicar, an oral antifibrinolytic agent. Patients should, of course, be advised not to take aspirin or aspirin-like drugs, and abnormalities of coagulation factors, induced by inanition and antibiotic therapy, must be corrected.

Erythrocytes and Hemochromatosis

Blood should be transfused regularly to permit comfortable physical activity, usually achieved with a normal cardiovascular state at a hemoglobin concentration of over 7 to 8 g per deciliter and in the presence of coronary disease at a hemoglobin concentration over 9 g per deciliter. Complete replacement of erythropoiesis in an adult requires transfusion of about 1 unit per week of packed red blood cells. Hemochromatotic damage to the heart, liver, and endocrine glands can be expected once the transfusion burden exceeds 100 U, a good point at which to start desferrioxamine chelation in patients with chronic disease.

ALTERNATE, EXPERIMENTAL, AND FUTURE THERAPIES

Immunosuppression

Very high dose corticosteroid therapy has had success rates comparable to those of ALG in Europe, although it probably is most effective in patients treated within a few weeks of diagnosis. Methylprednisolone therapy has aimed at infusion of 100 mg per kilogram during the first week, 50 mg per kilogram during the second week, and gradual tapering of the dose over 30 to 40 days. Toxic effects are common, including salt and water retention, hypertension, diabetes, electrolyte imbalance, occult infection, and aseptic joint necrosis. High-dose corticosteroids should be reserved for treatment of patients when and where ATG is unavailable.

Antiviral Therapy

Some cases of aplastic anemia follow infectious mononucleosis, and in other patients, Epstein-Barr virus can be found in the bone marrow despite a negative clinical history. Remissions have followed acyclovir therapy. Acyclovir is not very toxic and can be given to patients with herpesvirus associated with aplasia at 15 mg per kilogram per day in three divided, intravenous doses.

SUGGESTED READING

Hathorn JW, Pizzo PA. Infectious complications in the pediatric cancer patient. In: Pizzo PA, Poplack DG, eds. Pediatric oncology. Philadelphia: JB Lippincott, 1989.

Kurtzman G, Young N. Aplastic anemia. In: Masur H, Parrillo J, eds. The critically ill immunosuppressed patient. Rockville, MD: Aspen, 1987.

Leonard EM, Raefsky E, Griffith P, et al. Cyclosporine therapy of aplastic anaemia, congenital and acquired aplastic anemia. Br J Haematol 1989; 72:278–284.

O'Reilly RJ. Allogeneic bone marrow transplantation: Current status and future directions. Blood 1983; 62:941–964.

Young NS, Alter BA. Bone marrow failure. In: Handin RI, Lux SE, Stossel TP, eds. Blood: Principles and practice of hematology. Philadelphia: JB Lippincott, in press.

Young N, Speck B. Antithymocyte and antilymphocyte globulins: Clinical trials and mechanism of action: In: Young N. Levine A, Humphries PK, eds. Aplastic anemia: Stem cell biology and advances in treatment. New York: Alan R. Liss, 1984:221.

MEGALOBLASTIC ANEMIA

BERNARD A. COOPER, M.D.

Megaloblastic anemia is characterized by megaloblastic morphology in bone marrow smears, caused by either (1) relatively specific and undefined defects in nucleotide metabolism induced by antimetabolites or deficiency of certain coenzymes, or (2) equally undefined metabolic abnormalities in erythroid precursors in some clonal hematologic diseases, such as the leukemias. Although morphologic features in peripheral blood (such as macrocytosis or multilobed neutrophils) and some biochemical abnormalities (such as elevations of levels of iron or LDH in serum, abnormal deoxyuridine suppression test in stimulated lymphocytes, methylmalonate excretion in urine, or low levels of folate or vitamin B_{12} in serum or blood) correlate with megaloblastic morphology. They do not invariably predict it.

DIAGNOSIS

The effectiveness of therapy is often determined by how effectively diagnostic procedures are selected when the patient is first seen. Initial examination should include detailed history for evidence of nutritional deficiency, intestinal disease, dysphagia, ingestion of antimetabolic drugs, alcohol, or other medications which might predispose to deficiency, and previous episodes of anemia and their response to therapy. Careful examination may reveal evidence of weight loss, hepatic cirrhosis, reflex changes, loss of vibration sense, glossitis, or petechiae and/or ecchymosis. Blood samples should be taken for determinations of levels of vitamin B_{12} and folate in serum and of erythrocyte folate. The former utilizes serum from clotted blood, and commercially available vacutainers (red top) are appropriate. The latter requires unclotted blood and should be taken into either citrate (blue top) or EDTA (purple top) vacutainers. It is recommended that 5 ml of serum be provided to the laboratory so that the remaining unclotted specimen can be sent for determination of plasma methylmalonic acid and total homocysteine if this is required. Routine hematologic studies including reticulocyte count, platelet count, and peripheral smear are required, and prothrombin time determination may aid in recognition of intestinal malabsorption.

Bone marrow aspiration should be performed before therapy is instituted. For most cases, aspiration and smear are adequate, and biopsy is not required.

GENERAL THERAPY

Anemia. If life-threatening, anemia should be treated by blood transfusion sufficient to provide adequate peripheral oxygenation and cardiac function.

Patients seeking medical aid because of anemia often do so because the reflex increase of cardiac output caused by the anemia exceeds the capacity of their myocardium. In such cases, cardiac failure responds to transfusion of a single unit of packed erythrocytes, together with appropriate therapy for cardiac failure. Cardiac failure responds to diuretic therapy, and so in the uncomplicated patient, furosamide, 20 mg, should be injected as transfusion is begun or as soon as the patient is seen. Further diuretic therapy should be selected on the basis of central venous pressure observation and standard clinical criteria.

Leukopenia. Seldom is leukopenia of sufficient degree to cause susceptibility to infection.

Thrombocytopenia. Occasionally thrombocytopenia may cause life-threatening hemorrhage: Although in uncomplicated megaloblastic anemia, it usually is associated with severe anemia, thrombocytopenia may appear without anemia, and its cause may thus be obscure. Severe thrombocytopenia with evidence of petechiae and ecchymoses or bleeding should be treated with platelet transfusion.

Other Somatic Manifestations. These include glossitis, dysphagia, anorexia, diminished levels of circulating immunoglobulins, and decreased lymphocyte reactivity; they are probably never dangerous and require no specific therapy.

Severe Psychologic Depression. This has been described in association with pernicious anemia and possibly with folate deficiency. There is evidence that the depressive features are corrected when diagnosis is made and may thus be reactive. Specific therapy is thus not required. For serious depression, sedation and antidepressive therapy are identical with those used in depressive disorders of other etiologies. The organic brain syndrome and loss of intellectual function associated with deficiency of vitamin B_{12} respond only to replacement therapy with vitamin B_{12}.

SPECIFIC THERAPY

Clinical Situation I

In this case, bone marrow is megaloblastic, with macrogranulocytes present, and clinical examination is consistent with nutritional megaloblastic anemia. Based on clinical information and the presence or absence of neurologic signs or symptoms, a presumptive diagnosis of deficiency of vitamin B_{12} or folate is made.

If the anemia is presumed to be the result of vitamin B_{12} deficiency, treatment consists of subcutaneous injections of vitamin B_{12} (cyanocobalamin), 5 μg per day for 2 days, followed by 100 μg per day if patient is in hospital, or weekly if not.

If the presumption is that the anemia is due to folate deficiency, treatment consists of oral folic acid as follows: 200 μg per day for 2 days followed by 2 mg per day for 1 week.

Monitoring Response

The classic *reticulocyte response* to therapy may be monitored, and some response will be observed, even if anemia is partially corrected by transfusion. *Neutrophil count* increases by the third or fourth day following initiation of therapy, simultaneously with the earliest increase of reticulocytes. *Serum iron*, if elevated, decreases to deficient levels within 24 hours of initiation of specific therapy, and erythropoiesis in the *bone marrow* becomes morphologically normoblastic within 48 hours of initiation of appropriate therapy (macrogranulocytosis persists for 10 to 14 days). With this recommended dosage schedule for vitamin B_{12}, serum iron may not decrease to very low levels before 72 hours after therapy. If response is not observed in the peripheral blood, demonstration of conversion to normoblastic bone marrow morphology confirms the selection of correct therapy. It is well established that infection and iron deficiency obscure response to therapy in the peripheral blood, but do not prevent conversion of bone marrow to normoblastic.

Follow-Up Therapy

One week after the first injection of 100 μg of vitamin B_{12}, vitamin B_{12} absorption should be tested by the *Schilling test* if deficiency of vitamin B_{12} has been confirmed. If deficiency of vitamin B_{12} is confirmed by serum level and malabsorption of the vitamin confirmed by the Schilling test, therapy should be continued for life with 100 μg of vitamin B_{12} monthly. If vitamin B_{12} malabsorption is shown to be caused by a lack of intrinsic factor by correction of absorption with a source of intrinsic factor, no further investigation is required. If intestinal malabsorption is suggested by the Schilling test, and the reliability of the test used is confirmed, further investigation is required, but therapy should be continued as above. If blind loop syndrome is recognized, surgical correction is required if vitamin B_{12} injections are to be discontinued. Antibiotic therapy produces only a transient improvement in malabsorption of vitamin B_{12} caused by bacterial infestation of segments of the small bowel.

Variant of Clinical Situation I

In this case, neurologic manifestations strongly suggestive of those caused by deficiency of vitamin B_{12} (subacute combined degeneration of the spinal cord, or dementia) are present without macrocytosis, anemia, or serum vitamin B_{12} level that is diagnostic of deficiency. There is now increasing awareness that such patients may comprise 30 to 40 percent of all patients with symptomatic deficiency of vitamin B_{12}, and in 5 percent serum B_{12} level may be within the normal range. In most of these, bone marrow is megaloblastic and the investigation described in Clinical Situation I will suffice. In such patients, serum should be analyzed for total homocysteine and for methylmalonic acid, which if elevated will diagnose deficiency of vitamin B_{12} and if absent will exclude it as a cause of the patient's symptoms. After treatment with vitamin B_{12}, changes should be recorded in lab parameters listed under Clinical Situation I, and the elevated homocysteine and methylmalonic acid levels will disappear.

Clinical Situation II

In this case bone marrow is megaloblastoid, and macrogranulocytes usually are not observed. Deficiency of vitamin B_{12} or folate is clinically improbable.

Atypical morphology in bone marrow usually is not caused by nutritional deficiency, and so specific therapy may be withheld until investigation suggests the presence of deficiency of vitamin B_{12} or folate. A few cases of sideroblastic anemia with megaloblastic changes have responded to large doses of pyridoxine (100 mg per day by mouth) or other nutrients (viz, thiamine); a few cases have been corrected by discontinuing drugs usually considered innocuous (e.g., analgesics), but most of these are caused either by antimetabolic drugs or by stem cell defects, some of which terminate as acute leukemia.

General therapy should be instituted depending on the clinical situation. Anemia and thrombocytopenia, which may threaten survival, should be treated as already described. In the absence of exposure to antimetabolites, no effective therapy is available for these conditions. Diagnosis must thus be precise and nutritional causes must be excluded. Most observers verify that the cause is not nutritional deficiency by *therapeutic trial* of vitamin B_{12} and folate over several weeks. Although it is possible that treatment with these vitamins may augment the development of early neoplastic disease, the evidence for this is weak, and thus such therapeutic trials should not be withheld. A normal *deoxyuridine suppression test* on cells obtained from a bone marrow aspirate also may be used as strong evidence against nutritional deficiency as cause of the megaloblastic morphology.

Treatment consists of the following:

1. Manage life-threatening anemia or thrombocytopenia as above.
2. Exclude nutritional deficiency by either (a) treating with vitamin B_{12} and folate in the doses listed above, and verifying the persistence of megaloblastoid morphology in bone marrow after 3 days, or of failure of hematocytopenias to improve over 2 to 3 weeks, or (b) doing a deoxyuridine suppression test on cells obtained from a bone marrow aspirate and demonstrating that this is normal.
3. Exclude the taking of antimetabolic drugs, especially those with antifolate activity.

If evidence is obtained that the patient has taken a drug known to interfere with intracellular metabolism, this usually should be discontinued. Following discontinuation of some antimetabolites such as 6-mercaptopurine, megaloblastoid features may persist for several weeks with only very slow correction of hematocytopenia. There is no evidence that administration of purines, amino acids, or other nutrients accelerate the correction of these drug-related diseases except that megaloblastic features and hematocytopenia induced by folate antagonists respond to administration of folates. Included in this category are: methotrexate, trimethoprim (often administered with sulfonamide), pyrazinamide and certain other antimalarials, triampterin, and a variety of antineoplastic agents that are modifications of methotrexate.

Treatment includes discontinuation of the drug and treatment with either folic acid, 5 mg per day by mouth, or a reduced (tetrahydro-) folate (folinic acid), which may be administered orally at 3 mg per day or by injection at similar dose. It is apparent that in patients receiving large doses of antifols for treatment of neoplastic disease, the usual therapeutic considerations for these are required, including monitoring of plasma methotrexate level and therapy with folinic acid until plasma level approaches 0.1 micromolar (10^{-6} M). In situations in which antifol therapy should not be discontinued (e.g., high-dose trimethoprim-sulfonamide treatment of *Pneumocystis* infection), treatment with folic acid, 5 mg per day for 3 to 4 days, should revert the megaloblastic change without neutralizing the beneficial effects of the antimicrobial therapy because most organisms inhibited by this type of preparation do not effectively accumulate folate. However, following initial therapy of the anemia, it probably is prudent to limit daily folic acid intake to 200 to 500 μg per day—a dose that should prevent megaloblastic anemia without affecting antimicrobial activity.

Most megaloblastoid anemias without macrogranulocytes in the bone marrow and in which bone marrow morphology is not typical of megaloblastic change are due to clonal diseases of the bone marrow and may terminate as acute leukemia. Megaloblastic morphology is also observed in some congenital and acquired aplastic anemias. Macrocytosis in peripheral blood and neutropenia and thrombocytopenia often coexist. In a minority of these, bone marrow morphology is typically megaloblastic, and their differentiation from nutritional anemias is more difficult. Bone marrow biopsy in these cases often reveals hypoplasia with islands of erythroid hyperplasia in contrast to the generalized hyperplasia in classic megaloblastic anemia.

NUTRITIONAL MEGALOBLASTIC ANEMIA: ADDITIONAL OBSERVATIONS

Treatment with Large Doses of Vitamin B_{12} and Folate

Patients deficient in either vitamin respond to such therapy. The availability of assays for vitamin B_{12} and folate in blood make therapeutic trials rarely useful. Most patients with pure deficiency of folate do not respond to usual doses of vitamin B_{12}, although in some, reticulocytosis is observed. Although all patients with pure deficiency of vitamin B_{12} show some hematologic response to large doses of folic acid, conversion of the bone marrow to normoblastic by folic acid alone is probably not complete. Complete conversion of bone marrow to normoblastic after therapy with one or the other vitamin thus is reasonable evidence that deficiency was caused by that vitamin. The latter is little justification for single therapy, however, since second bone marrow aspirations, although useful, are rarely performed in practice.

The major justification for treating with small doses of a single vitamin relates to possible dangers of too rapid conversion of bone marrow to normoblastic. Sudden death has occurred during therapy of pernicious anemia—especially in patients with severe anemia. Some of these have been ascribed to severe hypokalemia, relatively refractory to prophylaxis with potassium supplements, and more severe in severely anemic patients with thrombocytopenia and neutropenia. Thrombotic and embolic episodes have also been reported in patients treated for megaloblastic anemia with large doses of vitamins. It is not known whether these catastrophic episodes during therapy are caused by abrupt conversion of megaloblastic to normoblastic bone marrow with arrest of potassium leak from cells, changes of lipids in the plasma, thrombocytosis, correction of platelet defects observed in megaloblastic anemia, or another cause.

It has been demonstrated that single doses of vitamin B_{12} in excess of 80 μg completely converts megaloblastic bone marrow to normoblastic with correction of the anemia, whereas single doses less than 15 μg never completely correct the abnormality.

Because of the possibility that abrupt conversion of megaloblastic to normoblastic maturation may be dangerous, and the observations that the rate of correction of anemia is not significantly decreased by treating with small doses of the deficient vitamin, it would seem prudent to initiate therapy with small doses of vitamin B_{12} or folate, which would convert megaloblastic to normoblastic maturation over 3 to 4 days. This can be accomplished with the treatment regimen recommended above, which is best applied using single nutrients for therapy. It must be emphasized, however, that the advantage of this approach has not been tested.

Vitamin B_{12} Absorption Test (Schilling Test) as Initial Therapy

Flushing radioactivity into the urine in this test requires injection of 1000 μg (1 mg) of vitamin B_{12}. As previously indicated, it is possible that this may be dangerous. Such an approach may also produce erroneous data with misdiagnosis and inappropriate duration of therapy. A proportion of patients with megaloblastic anemia due to deficiency of vitamin B_{12} or folate develop transient malabsorption of vitamin B_{12}, which is corrected after therapy. Although this correction may occasionally be delayed for several weeks, it probably is corrected in most subjects over one cycle of intestinal epithelial cells—about 3 days. A patient might thus have transient malabsorption of vitamin B_{12} secondary to folate deficiency, with malabsorption observed in the first stage of the test, and with apparent correction with intrinsic factor in a later test because of correction of the intestinal defect by therapy. In tests of vitamin B_{12} absorption using simultaneous administration of free and IF-bound vitamin B_{12}, an intestinal malabsorption pattern is observed. Thus, it is recommended that replacement therapy should be continued for at least 3 to 4 days before absorption of vitamin B_{12} is tested.

Repletion of Stores of the Deficient Vitamin

Vitamin B_{12} stores in the liver are repleted slowly following depletion and may require many months to reach normal levels. The anemia caused by deficiency of vitamin B_{12} does not respond to therapy more quickly when large doses are administered—maximum rate of hemoglobin rise being achieved by 2 to 5 μg of vitamin B_{12} per day. Patients treated with larger doses of vitamin B_{12} (e.g., 30 to 100 μg per month by injection) require longer to relapse when therapy is discontinued than do patients treated with smaller doses (e.g., 20 μg per month). The benefit of the slower relapse is unknown.

There is no evidence that injections given more frequently produce better health, although many patients insist that they feel fatigued immediately before their next injection. There is no evidence that this represents deficiency of vitamin B_{12}, as serum levels are not depleted, and stores remain high. It is the impression of most physicians that these symptoms are psychologic.

Folate stores are small and are depleted to levels associated with megaloblastic anemia within 4 months of stopping folate intake. Thus, there is no benefit to treating with more folate than is required to correct clinical and chemical manifestations of deficiency.

Treatment of Subacute Combined Degeneration of the Spinal Cord

Neurologic lesions similar to human subacute combined degeneration of the spinal cord have been produced in monkeys and bats made deficient in vitamin B_{12} or treated with nitrous oxide. In these animals, folate supplementation appears to aggravate the lesions, and methionine supplementation appears to prevent them. Clinical studies appear to indicate that small doses of vitamin B_{12} arrest neurologic disease in pernicious anemia, and neither clinical studies nor animal experiments have demonstrated benefit with larger doses of vitamin B_{12}. Single injections of vitamin B_{12} of less than 50 to 100 μg do not increase spinal fluid cobalamin level within a few hours of injection, and this might support use of large doses of vitamin B_{12} in neurologic disease. Despite this indirect evidence, treatment with standard doses of vitamin B_{12}, as described above, should be considered adequate.

Situations in which cyanocobalamin or folic acid, the standard vitamin B_{12} and folate preparations available commercially, are not the best forms of vitamin therapy.

In nutritional anemia in adults, the aforementioned commercial forms of vitamin B_{12} and folate are adequate and probably represent the preferred therapy because of their stability and purity. Although the frequency of injections of vitamin B_{12} required to maintain normal levels of serum vitamin B_{12} is less when hydroxocobalamin is used, the trivial clinical advantage is probably offset by the periodic development of antibodies against hydroxocobalamin during such therapy. Because reduced folates are transported 100 times better into most mammalian cells than is folic acid, reduced folate is preferable to folic acid when counteracting antifols, and so folinic acid is used routinely.

In infants and children with inherited intracellular defects of folate or cobalamin metabolism, the inherited defect may prevent optimal utilization of these forms of the vitamins. In children with intracellular defects of cobalamin metabolism, treatment with hydroxocobalamin is more effective than that with cyanocobalamin, and treatment usually requires large doses (500 to 1000 μg per day) of this material. In children with deficiency of transcobalamin 2, either cobalamin may be used, but because cyanocobalamin is more effectively absorbed when fed, these children usually are maintained on oral cyanocobalamin (500 μg, 2 to 7 times per week). In children with defective intracellular folate enzymes (e.g., 5 to 10 methylene tetrahydro folate reductase), folinic acid probably represents better therapy than does folic acid, but optimal therapy would be provided by injections of 5-methyl tetrahydrofolate, if available. Such children also should receive methionine supplements. Note that such children usually do not have megaloblastic anemia.

In inherited metabolic defects, efficacy of therapy should be monitored by disappearance of homocystinuria or methyl malonic aciduria, and by restoration of normal levels of plasma methionine.

SUGGESTED READING

Cooper BA, Rosenblatt DS. Inherited defects of vitamin B_{12} metabolism. Ann Rev Nutr 1987; 7:291–320.

Hall CA. Pernicious anemia: diagnosis and treatment. Geriatrics 1967; 22:109–118.

Reizenstein P, Ljunggren G, Drougge E. Quality of diagnosis and managing anemia in four countries. Biomed Pharmacother 1984; 38:194–198.

IRON DEFICIENCY ANEMIA

JAMES D. COOK, M.D., F.A.C.P.

There are three treatment modalities for the management of patients with iron deficiency anemia: oral iron, parenteral iron, and blood transfusion. In the vast majority of patients, repair of iron deficiency anemia is achieved readily with oral therapy. In a small subset of patients who are either intolerant of oral iron or unable to absorb iron from the gastrointestinal tract, parenteral therapy may be required. When managing patients with severe recurrent iron deficiency anemia, the primary objective is to eliminate the need for blood transfusions. This can usually be accomplished by developing effective therapeutic iron regimens tailored to meet the needs of the individual patient.

ORAL IRON THERAPY

In a patient with significant iron deficiency anemia, oral therapy should be initiated at a level that provides 150 to 200 mg elemental iron daily in divided doses. The form of iron is relatively unimportant providing that it is in the reduced state; most ferric iron preparations have been withdrawn from the market because absorption is markedly less than that of ferrous iron. In selecting one of the numerous forms of medicinal iron available, the most important consideration is the amount of elemental iron contained in each tablet. Ferrous sulfate tablets generally contain 60 to 65 mg elemental iron, whereas ferrous gluconate tablets contain about half this amount. Ferrous sulfate is the most widely prescribed form of oral iron at the present time because it is the most soluble and the least expensive, especially when calculated on the basis of administered iron. Percentage of absorption is maximal with ferrous sulfate, although many forms of ferrous iron are absorbed equally well.

A number of proprietary iron preparations are promoted on the basis of either superior absorption or reduced gastrointestinal side effects, but there is little convincing evidence that these offer any therapeutic advantages. For example, many pharmaceutical preparations contain ascorbic acid which facilitates iron absorption, but does so at the expense of more frequent gastrointestinal side effects. The higher amount of absorption from preparations containing ascorbic acid can be obtained less expensively by increasing the amount of iron in each dose.

Maximal absorption occurs when iron is taken

separately from main meals. The most rapid hematologic response occurs when iron tablets are taken 1 to 2 hours before each meal. Absorption is further increased by taking an additional dose at bedtime. Iron absorption from this regimen will approach 50 mg iron daily, or an amount that can offset blood loss in excess of 100 ml daily in chronically anemic patients. It should be noted that this absorption ceiling falls sharply as iron deficiency is corrected.

The major difficulty with oral iron therapy is that a significant proportion of patients develop gastrointestinal side effects on these maximal doses of oral iron. It is important to distinguish between upper and lower gastrointestinal symptoms. Many patients complain of an alteration in bowel habit, either diarrhea or constipation, but these symptoms are unrelated to the dosage of administered iron. Side effects of this type can usually be treated symptomatically and seldom require alteration or discontinuation of the oral regimen. Symptoms of the upper intestinal tract are more significant and troublesome. When mild, these include nausea, epigastric discomfort, and heartburn. When severe, they may be associated with vomiting and severe abdominal cramping. These symptoms usually occur within the first hour following iron administration and appear to be related to the concentration of ionized iron in the lumen of the stomach or upper small intestine. The frequency and severity of side effects increase progressively as the dosage of iron is increased.

In many patients, mild nausea or epigastric discomfort can be eliminated if the iron is taken with or immediately following meals, because food binds and insolubilizes a significant portion of medicinal iron. Administering iron with food also delays gastric emptying and reduces the concentration of unbound iron in the duodenum. When iron is taken with meals, there is a 50 to 75 percent reduction in absorbed iron. The magnitude of reduction varies with the nature of the diet and is much less marked when the meal contains ample quantities of meat or ascorbic acid. Since there is seldom an urgency to correct mild iron deficiency anemia, it is sometimes preferable to prescribe iron with meals initially and thereby avoid the development of gastrointestinal symptoms.

If nausea or epigastric discomfort persists when iron is taken with meals, the amount of iron prescribed in each dose should be reduced. This can be accomplished conveniently by switching to a preparation such as ferrous gluconate, which contains a much smaller amount of elemental iron. Further reductions in dosage can be accomplished by prescribing a liquid preparation of ferrous sulfate. Reducing the number of doses each day to eliminate side effects is usually less effective than decreasing the amount of iron contained in each dose. Another approach for patients with troublesome gastrointestinal side effects is to employ sustained-release forms of iron, which are aggressively promoted by many pharmaceutical firms. These preparations reduce side effects by delaying the release of iron within the gastrointestinal lumen until it is beyond the area of maximal iron assimilation in the upper small intestine. Not surprisingly, a decrease in symptoms is paralleled by a reduction in absorbed iron. With some preparations, such as enteric-coated tablets, the resulting impairment of iron absorption may be profound. However, with other proprietary preparations, absorption in the presence of food may be comparable to that obtained with ferrous sulfate. Sustained-release forms of iron deserve a trial in patients with intractable gastrointestinal symptoms. A major disadvantage with these preparations is their cost, which may be 20 to 30 times higher than ferrous sulfate containing the equivalent amount of iron. Sustained-release preparations should be reserved for patients who encounter side effects with conventional forms of iron, and should be given with the understanding that absorption may be substantially less than with standard tablets of ferrous sulfate.

RESPONSE TO IRON THERAPY

Because iron deficiency impairs proliferation of the erythroid marrow, it takes 7 to 10 days following initiation of iron therapy to achieve maximal reticulocyte response. Although the degree of reticulocytosis is never dramatic, the reticulocyte count should increase two to three times over basal level. In patients with an initial hemoglobin below 10 g per 100 ml, full therapeutic doses of oral iron should produce an increase in a circulating hemoglobin level of about 0.2 g per 100 ml whole blood daily after the first week of treatment. An increase of less than 0.1 g hemoglobin per 100 ml blood daily is a suboptimal response, although from a clinical standpoint this slower increase is usually acceptable. A therapeutic trial of iron must be considered a failure if full doses of a conventional form of oral iron do not result in a normal hemoglobin concentration within 6 weeks of initiating therapy.

By far the most common cause of failure to obtain a complete response to oral iron is poor compliance. Because of the wide distribution of iron in vitamin supplements and fortified foods, many patients regard iron as a nutritional supplement rather than a medication. The number of treatment failures can be significantly reduced if the physician takes time to explain to the patient the importance of taking the iron tablets regularly. A measure of compliance can be obtained by prescribing only enough iron to last until the next visit. Most patients will not ask for a refill of their prescription if they have an unused supply.

An inadequate response is commonly attributed to intestinal malabsorption, but this is an exceedingly uncommon cause of therapeutic failure. Patients who have had a partial gastrectomy absorb medicinal iron poorly when it is taken with food, but absorb medicinal iron well when it is taken between meals. Patients who have undergone a total gastrectomy or extensive resection of the upper small intestine have a more severe defect in iron assimilation and do not usually respond to oral therapy. Diseases of the upper small intestine such as celiac sprue may occasionally present as iron deficiency because of impaired assimilation of dietary iron. If there is any reason to suspect iron malabsorption, a convenient and simple test is to administer 100 mg elemental iron as liquid ferrous sulfate while the patient is fasting and measure the rise in serum iron level at 1 and 2 hours following administration. In iron deficient patients with a basal serum iron level below 50 μg per deciliter, an increase of 200 to 300 μg per deciliter is commonly seen. A rise of less than 100 μg per deciliter warrants a presumptive diagnosis of intestinal malabsorption and justifies a small bowel biopsy.

A more common cause of so-called refractory iron deficiency anemia is an error in the original diagnosis. The anemia of chronic disease is often mistaken for iron deficiency because of the associated low transferrin saturation, hypochromia, and microcytosis. In this situation, therapeutic failure can be avoided by establishing that the serum ferritin level is less than 20 μg per liter prior to initiating therapy. Higher pretreatment values suggest that the anemia is due, at least in part, to an underlying inflammatory process. In some patients, an inadequate response to oral iron is due to continuing blood loss. These patients can usually be detected by a sustained reticulocytosis or by positive tests of occult blood in the feces.

Iron therapy should be continued until iron stores are replenished. A reasonable target is to increase iron reserves to 500 mg, or the amount of iron contained in two units of whole blood. In the past, this has usually been obtained empirically by continuing oral iron for 4 to 6 months beyond the point that the hemoglobin deficit is fully corrected. However, the replenishment of iron stores can now be determined accurately by monitoring the rise in serum ferritin levels. Since 1 μg per liter serum ferritin corresponds to approximately 10 mg storage iron, oral iron should be continued until the serum ferritin is greater than 50 μg per liter. Ferritin measurements can subsequently be used to detect early relapse of iron deficiency.

PARENTERAL IRON THERAPY

A number of studies have established that repairing iron deficiency anemia with parenteral iron is no more rapid than with an optimal regimen of oral iron. Parenteral iron may be associated with serious and occasionally fatal anaphylactic reactions. In addition to being more hazardous than oral therapy, parenteral iron is more expensive because it must be administered under careful medical supervision. Therefore, parenteral iron therapy should never be undertaken to achieve a more dramatic hematologic response or as a matter of convenience to the patient or physician.

The three main indications for parenteral iron therapy are intractable gastrointestinal side effects, malabsorption, and severe recurrent iron deficiency due to uncontrollable blood loss. The most common indication is patients who are unable or unwilling to continue with oral therapy because of persistent side effects. The number of these individuals can be reduced by designing an oral regimen that minimizes gastrointestinal symptoms and by encouraging patients to continue with oral iron therapy despite minor symptoms. If iron requirements are not excessive, many patients with some degree of impaired absorption can absorb sufficient iron to correct iron deficiency or forestall its recurrence. On the other hand, repeated courses of parenteral iron are often justified when there is large, uncontrollable blood loss, as in patients with hereditary telangiectasia. However, a note of caution is in order if patients are given parenteral iron repeatedly. Parenteral iron should never be given without careful monitoring of the serum ferritin level. At one time, parenteral iron was used extensively in patients on chronic hemodialysis to offset their high requirements due to gastrointestinal bleeding, laboratory sampling, and dialyzer use. Some of these patients developed the clinical syndrome of hemochromatosis due to parenchymal iron-loading.

Iron dextran (Imferon) is now used almost exclusively for parenteral iron therapy in the United States. Iron dextran is a complex of ferric hydroxide and dextrans of molecular weights ranging between 5,000 and 8,000. It is supplied as a dark colloidal solution containing 50 mg iron per milliliter. Iron dextran may be given either intramuscularly or intravenously. When the intramuscular route is used, it is given in the upper outer buttock in doses of 50 to 250 mg iron per injection site. There are several drawbacks with intramuscular administration. Permanent skin staining may result, although this problem can be lessened by using the Z-technique of intramuscular administration. Another disadvantage is that a significant proportion of the administered iron may remain at the site of injection for weeks or even months. Some patients complain of persistent pain at the site of injection, which in some instances may be due to an immunologic reaction to the dextran moiety. On this basis, extensive local muscle necrosis has been described in some patients. Another potential concern with intramuscular administration relates to studies showing that sarcomas have developed in rats given massive injections of iron dextran. This prompted temporary withdrawal of iron dextran at one time, but extensive follow-up studies in humans have not provided convincing evidence of a carcinogenic risk.

Many of the problems with intramuscular use of iron dextran can be eliminated by giving the drug intravenously. In several early trials, the undiluted preparation was administered by direct intravenous infusion over 5 to 10 minutes. Injections of 500 to 1,000 mg are repeated at weekly intervals to achieve a total dose. A more convenient and less hazardous approach is to administer the total calculated dose in a single intravenous infusion. The amount of iron required is calculated from the deficit in circulating hemoglobin, assuming that 1 g hemoglobin per 100 ml whole blood corresponds to 150 mg iron in an average-sized adult.

An additional 500 to 1,000 mg iron is given to replenish iron stores. This amount of iron dextran is diluted in normal saline to a concentration not exceeding 5 percent, and administered slowly over 2 to 3 hours.

The most serious concern with total dose infusion is the occurrence of anaphylaxis. Iron dextran should be given intravenously only when resuscitative measures are immediately available. To safeguard against severe anaphylaxis, the rate of intravenous infusion should be kept to less than 10 drops per minute during the first 10 to 15 minutes of administration. If no reaction occurs, the rate can be increased to several hundred milliliters per hour. In patients who have not been given iron dextran previously, it is prudent to limit the total dose of administered iron to 1,000 mg on the first occasion. A variety of less serious side effects, such as skin rash, fever, arthralgias, and lymphadenopathy, have been reported. Although relatively uncommon, these side effects are important because they may herald the development of more serious reactions with subsequent therapy. Iron dextran administration is contraindicated in patients with rheumatoid arthritis because it is known to exacerbate synovitis.

SUGGESTED READING

Boggs DR. Fate of a ferrous sulfate prescription. Am J Med 1987; 82:124–128.

Bothwell TH, Charlton RW, Cook JD, Finch CA. Iron metabolism in man. Oxford: Blackwell Scientific, 1979: 69.

Brise H, Hallberg L. Absorbability of different iron compounds. Acta Med Scand 1962; 171 (Suppl 376):23–38.

Callender ST. Treatment of iron deficiency. Clin Haematol 1982; 11:327–338.

Hallberg L, Ryttinger L, Solvell L. Side effects of oral iron therapy. A double blind study of different iron compounds in tablet form. Acta Med Scand 1966; 180 (Suppl. 459):3–10.

SECONDARY ANEMIA IN RENAL FAILURE AND CHRONIC DISEASE

MICHAEL C. BRAIN, D.M., F.R.C.P., FRCPC

The secondary anemias are due to the impairment of erythropoiesis that accompanies certain nonhemopoietic diseases. This definition has to be qualified, as secondary anemia does not include anemia due to blood loss or deficiency of iron or of vitamins essential for hemopoiesis, such as vitamin B_{12} or folic acid, all of which can be brought about by disease of the gastrointestinal tract. Secondary anemia is an ill-defined group of disorders of erythropoiesis that poses a diagnostic problem once the more obvious causes of anemia have been ruled out. Thus, the diagnosis of secondary anemia necessitates precluding primary disorders of hemopoiesis, such as preleukemia; refractory anemia, with or without excess blast cells; thalassemia minor; the hypoplastic anemias; and infiltrative diseases of the bone marrow, such as the myeloproliferative disorders. Table 1 lists the disorders that can give rise to secondary anemia. The recognition that the anemia is secondary in etiology is dependent on (1) excluding a primary disorder of hemopoiesis of the types mentioned, and (2) recognizing the underlying cause. The latter may be obvious in patients with the symptoms, signs, and radiological or laboratory evidence of a chronic infective or inflammatory disease, such as active rheumatoid arthritis or of renal failure. On the other hand, recognizing the underlying cause may be difficult unless all possible causes are considered and appropriate investigations are carried out. It is also important to consider that secondary anemia may coexist with a primary disorder of erythropoiesis. Thus, patients with rheumatoid arthritis may also be iron deficient due to chronic intestinal blood loss due to treatment with nonsteroidal anti-inflammatory drugs. Blood loss or malabsorption may complicate chronic inflammatory bowel diseases, such as Crohn's disease or ulcerative colitis. However, in these cases, the anemia usually persists despite the correction of iron or vitamin deficiency.

TABLE 1 Causes of Secondary Anemia

Chronic bacterial infections
Pulmonary: tuberculosis, abscess, fungal
Cardiac: subacute bacterial endocarditis
Pelvic inflammatory disease
Bone: osteomyelitis
Infected ischemic disease: arteriosclerotic, diabetic, etc.
Chronic urinary tract infections
Noninfective inflammatory diseases
Rheumatoid arthritis
Systemic lupus erythematosus
Sjögren's syndrome
Crohn's disease
Ulcerative colitis
Sarcoidosis
Neoplastic diseases
Occult carcinoma: renal, gastrointestinal, pancreatic, ovarian, etc.
Hodgkin's and nonHodgkin's lymphoma
Multiple myeloma
Endocrine
Panhypopituitarism
Hypothyroidism
Chronic renal failure

DIAGNOSIS

Since the diagnosis of secondary anemia is usually made by excluding primary disorders of hemopoiesis, obtaining the blood count and examining the bone marrow by aspiration and by biopsy is important. The anemia is usually normochromic and normocytic, although hypochromic microcytic erythrocytes may be present. The absolute number of reticulocytes is normal or reduced, and is usually inappropriately low for the degree of anemia, thereby reflecting the inadequate erythropoietic response to the anemia. The white cell count is normal, or may be increased, with a normal differential count. The platelet count is normal or may be increased. The erythrocyte sedimentation rate is often raised. The level of serum iron and the total iron binding capacity is reduced, a finding that may be misinterpreted as indicating iron deficiency. The level of serum ferritin, a more accurate indicator of body iron stores, is normal or increased, thereby excluding iron deficiency as a cause of the anemia. The level of folic acid in the serum and red cells is usually normal, as is the serum vitamin B_{12} level. A bone marrow aspiration and biopsy should reveal normal cellularity. Erythropoiesis is reduced, with normal maturation, but may reveal poor hemoglobinization and the absence of iron granules in late erythroblasts, despite normal or increased amounts of iron in macrophages, as well as marrow fragments. The number and maturation of white cells are normal, as are megakaryocytes and platelet formation.

Having excluded a primary disorder of erythropoiesis and having demonstrated defective iron utilization by the presence of a normal serum ferritin level and by adequate bone marrow iron stores, the underlying cause for the secondary anemia must be sought, guided by such symptoms and signs that the patient may have. Laboratory tests of renal and hepatic function, the measurement of immunoglobulins, and the detection of autoantibodies, such as antinuclear antibodies, may be helpful. A radiograph of the chest must be obtained. An abdominal ultrasound examination may prove useful in detecting intra-abdominal disease, such as lymphadenopathy or, as in two recent cases I have seen, unsuspected symptomless renal carcinoma. The finding of pelvic inflammatory disease without obvious gynecologic cause may justify gastrointestinal investigation to exclude Crohn's disease of the small or large bowel. Endocrine causes of secondary anemia should be considered, such as hypothyroidism and pituitary adenoma, especially in younger patients in whom the more obvious features of these disorders may be difficult to recognize.

TREATMENT

Human Erythropoietin in Chronic Renal Failure

The treatment of secondary anemia has, until recently, been particularly frustrating unless the underlying cause of the anemia could be recognized and corrected, as in the case of reversal of the anemia due to erythropoietin deficiency of chronic renal failure by renal transplantation. The large scale preparation of human erythropoietin using recombinant human DNA techniques has made sufficient amounts of erythropoietin available for it to be used therapeutically in patients with chronic renal failure who are maintained on hemodialysis. The erythropoietin is given as an intravenous bolus injection at the end of dialysis, usually three times a week. The magnitude of the erythropoietic response is dose dependent and may vary from patient to patient. Preliminary studies suggest that a dose of between 50 and 150 IU three times a week results in a rise in the hematocrit from .20 to .30 to .40 in 8 to 10 weeks, with an accompanying reticulocyte response and a cessation of the previous requirement for regular red cell transfusions. Lessening of the anemia results in greater exercise tolerance and an improved sense of well-being.

However, there are certain risks and side effects associated with the expansion in blood volume and the increased blood viscosity that accompany the rise in the hematocrit. The blood pressure may rise to dangerous levels and may require careful monitoring and treatment. The time required for dialysis may be increased because of the reduced plasma volume. The risk of thrombosis in arteriovenous shunts may increase. Nevertheless, alleviating the symptoms of anemia and reducing the risks of transfusion transmitted diseases, such as hepatitis and acquired immunodeficiency syndrome (AIDS), are major benefits to the patient. Greater experience with the use of recombinant erythropoietin will assist in determining the optimal response that will maximize the benefit while minimizing the side effects. It seems unlikely that erythropoietin will be of benefit to patients other than those who have erythropoietin deficiency due to severe renal disease.

Other Treatment Concerns

Despite this exciting advance in the treatment of the anemia of chronic renal failure, there is still much to be learned about the mediators of the anemia of other chronic diseases. For many patients with chronic nonbacterial inflammatory diseases, such as active chronic rheumatoid arthritis, the only hope has been that the underlying disease would respond to treatment or gradually improve therefore the anemia would also improve. The therapeutic problem reflects our lack of understanding of the mechanism of the anemia and the means to correct the anemia, were the mechanism known. It seems likely that anemia is but one of the manifestations of a more general response to infectious, inflammatory, and neoplastic diseases.

Biological Response Modifiers

There have been important advances in our understanding of the role that cachetin plays in mediating the response to a variety of stimuli as well as the interrelationship between cachetin and interferons, especially as beta-2 interferon has recently been found to be the primary mediator of the acute phase response of the liver. Cachetin has been shown to modify hematopoiesis in vitro, but its in vivo effects have yet to be described—information that may provide insight into the mechanism of the anemia that accompanies chronic inflammatory diseases. Recognition of the role played by cachetin and other biological modifiers of cell responses might lead to more specific therapy than has been achieved by the administration of steroidal or nonsteroidal anti-inflammatory drugs. The specific neutralization of cachetin and related cytokines may provide new methods of treating the broad spectrum of diseases, one of the manifestations of these being secondary anemia.

General Treatment Guidelines

At present, one can only put forward some general guidelines for those patients in whom the underlying cause of the secondary anemia cannot be readily corrected. There is no benefit from the administration of oral or parenteral iron preparations unless iron deficiency is shown to be present by either a low serum ferritin level or by absence of bone marrow iron stores. A low serum iron, a common feature of secondary anemia, is not an indication for iron therapy. The gastrointestinal side effects of oral preparations and the risk of adverse allergic reactions to parenteral iron far outweigh the nonexistent benefit; furthermore, there is some evidence that iron compounds may mediate an inflammatory response and can thus exacerbate the symptoms of nonbacterial inflammatory diseases. Folic acid deficiency, if present, should be corrected after vitamin B_{12} deficiency has been excluded.

The transfusion of packed red cells should be restricted to situations where anemia is a major contributor to disability owing to cardiopulmonary disease or when surgical procedures are undertaken. In other circumstances, the benefits of transfusion are brief, and the risks of prolonged transfusion therapy in terms of antibody formation, and ultimately iron overload, are unacceptable. The limited exercise potential of patients with chronic rheumatoid arthritis is often more restricting than their chronic anemia. The potentially adverse side effects on hemopoiesis of many of the treatments for the chronic nonbacterial inflammatory diseases must always be borne in mind. An exacerbation of anemia in the absence of blood loss, especially when accompanied by a fall in the white cell or platelet count, should alert one to this possibility and should lead to an immediate cessation of the treatment. Unfortunately, the duration of these adverse reactions to many of the drugs used, such as gold preparations, may be prolonged and recovery may be slow and incomplete. These toxic side effects are usually accompanied by evidence of dyshemopoiesis on bone marrow aspiration and biopsy. In such circumstances, transfusions of red cells may be given to maintain an adequate level of hemoglobin until recovery of hemopoiesis takes place.

SUGGESTED READING

Beutler B, Cerami A. Cachetin: more than a tumour necrosis factor. N Engl J Med 1987; 316:379–385.

Eschbach JW, Egrie JC, Downing MR, et al. Correction of the anemia of end-stage renal disease with recombinant human erythropoietin: results of a combined phase I and II clinical trial. N Engl J Med 1987; 316:73.

Winearls CG, Oliver DO, Pippard MJ, et al. Effect of human erythropoietin derived from recombinant DNA on the anemia of patients maintained by chronic haemodialysis. Lancet 1986; 2:1175.

AUTOIMMUNE HEMOLYTIC ANEMIA

LAWRENCE D. PETZ, M.D.

Autoimmune hemolytic anemias (AIHA) are a diverse group of disorders that have in common the presence of a red cell autoantibody, which results in a shortened red cell life span as the major mechanism of the cause of the anemia. AIHA have a number of etiologies and result from a variety of pathogenetic mechanisms. They may be caused by warm autoantibodies, which are optimally reactive at 37°C and are usually of the IgG immunoglobulin class, or by cold autoantibodies, which are optimally reactive at 4°C and are usually IgM immunoglobulins. They are also classified as idiopathic or secondary, depending on whether or not an underlying disorder that is known to be associated with AIHA is present. In addition, an ever-increasing number of drugs have been shown to cause AIHA. These distinctions are important because appropriate management varies among the different diagnostic groups. Table 1 lists a classification of AIHA.

WARM ANTIBODY AUTOIMMUNE HEMOLYTIC ANEMIA

Corticosteroids

The initial therapy for patients with AIHA of warm antibody type should be corticosteroids. An appropriate regimen is prednisone in a dosage of 1 to 1.5 mg per kilogram per day orally. Comparable dosages

TABLE 1 Autoimmune Hemolytic Anemias (AIHA)

Warm antibody AIHA
- Idiopathic (unassociated with another disease)
- Secondary (associated with chronic lymphocytic leukemia, lymphomas, systemic lupus erythematosus, etc.)

Cold agglutinin disease (CAD)
- Idiopathic CAD
- Secondary CAD
  - Associated with *M. pneumoniae* infection or infectious mononucleosis (polyclonal cold agglutinin)
  - Associated with malignancies such as chronic lymphocytic leukemia, lymphomas, etc. (monoclonal cold agglutinin)

Paroxysmal cold hemoglobinuria (PCH)
- Idiopathic
- Secondary to syphilis (rare) or viral infection

Drug-induced AIHA
- α-methyldopa, procainamide, L-dopa, mefenamic acid, phenacetin, chlorpromazine, streptomycin

of other corticosteroid preparations are also effective, but offer no therapeutic advantage and often have more prominent side effects. The increased effectiveness of higher dosages or of parenteral administration has not been documented.

A great majority of patients manifest a clinical response within 2 weeks of initiation of treatment, and a complete lack of response at 21 days should be considered a steroid failure. A response is indicated by an increasing hematocrit, often with an increasing reticulocyte count, until the hematocrit nears normal levels. The direct antiglobulin (Coombs') test often remains positive, although weaker; the indirect antiglobulin test usually becomes negative.

For those patients who do respond to corticosteroids, a normal or stable hematocrit and reticulocyte count are found within 30 to 90 days. At this time, a progressive but slow reduction of dosage is indicated. The following schedule is recommended: a weekly reduction of the daily dosage of prednisone by 10 mg until a dosage of 30 mg per day is reached. Thereafter, a reduction of 5 mg of the daily dosage is made every week or 2 until a dosage of 15 mg per day is reached. Subsequently, the dosage should be reduced 2.5 mg every 2 weeks. If a relapse occurs, one should return to the last previous dosage unless the relapse has produced an abrupt fall in hematocrit, in which case it is preferable to return to a somewhat higher dosage to again establish a remission.

A majority of patients relapse as the corticosteroid dosage is reduced. Some of these patients can be maintained on acceptably low dosages of prednisone, but if more than 10 to 15 mg per day of prednisone is required to keep the hematocrit above 30 percent, the response should be considered inadequate and other therapies should be strongly considered. Indeed, alternative types of treatment are indicated for perhaps 50 percent of patients to try to avoid the adverse effects of long-term corticosteroid administration, which can be devastating. These include increased susceptiblity to infection, osteoporosis, myopathy, gastritis, peptic ulcer disease, emotional lability, exacerbation of diabetes, and hypertension. The decision regarding the use of therapies other than corticosteroids should be made within several months of diagnosis and not delayed until serious side effects become apparent.

Splenectomy

If the response to corticosteroids is inadequate according to the aforementioned criteria, splenectomy should be performed, unless surgery is strongly contraindicated. Approximately 50 to 75 percent of patients show marked improvement or complete hematologic remission after splenectomy. Remissions are not always permanent, however, and relapse can occur months or years after splenectomy. If an incomplete remission develops, or a relapse occurs following splenectomy, much lower dosages of corticosteroids may prove effective in controlling the disease activity.

The surgical morbidity and mortality associated with splenectomy for AIHA is low because the spleen is usually not massively enlarged, platelet levels are usually normal or only moderately reduced, and patients are often relatively young and in good general health. However, splenectomized patients have a risk of fulminant bacteremia, usually caused by *Streptococcus pneumoniae* or *H. influenzae*. This risk is greatest in young children, especially for the first 2 years after surgery. Immunization with Pneumovax some weeks before elective splenectomy is indicated in an effort to reduce this long-term complication. An additional potential complication is the development of postsplenectomy thrombocytosis, which is most common in patients with continuing anemia and active hematopoiesis. This is usually a benign abnormality, although in occasional patients hemorrhagic or thromboembolic phenomena occur.

Immunosuppressive Drugs

A number of cytotoxic drugs have been used in therapeutic trials of AIHA because of their demonstrated effects on the immune system. These drugs are indicated after both corticosteroids and splenectomy have failed to produce an adequate remission, and it is further demonstrated that an adequate remission is not possible using small doses of prednisone postsplenectomy. However, immunosuppressive drugs may be used instead of splenectomy if surgery is contraindicated.

Most patients have been treated with azathioprine or cyclophosphamide. Clinical benefit has been noted in about 50 percent of patients. Azathioprine, 100 to 150 mg per day, or cyclophosphamide, 50 to 100 mg per day, may be used to initiate cytotoxic drug therapy.

Immunosuppressive drugs work by decreasing the production of antibody, and they generally take at least 2 weeks to produce a response. In patients who do not respond after 4 weeks of therapy, the dosage may be increased by increments of 25 mg per day every 2 weeks until a response or limiting side effects occur. Particularly important adverse effects are gastrointestinal intolerance, hemorrhagic cystitis (with cyclophosphamide), and evidence of marrow depression as manifested by leukopenia. Drug dosage should be adjusted to maintain the granulocyte count above 1,000 per microliter and the platelet count above 100,000 per microliter. Blood counts should be obtained weekly during the first month of therapy, and for a similar period of time after each dosage increase. Thereafter, blood counts should be performed biweekly for several months and, if stable, monthly thereafter. Long-term administration results in some increase in risk of developing a malignancy or serious acute infections. Corticosteroids are usually administered in conjunction with immunosuppressive drugs, but should be reduced in dosage if possible and discontinued if remission occurs.

Other Therapies

A number of anecdotal reports describe beneficial effects of plasma exchange. Acute hemolytic episodes are reported to have stabilized after other therapies have been ineffective. I find it hard to be enthusiastic about the role of plasma exchange in the therapy of AIHA, however, because in almost all reports it has been difficult to separate the effects of the plasma exchange from those of other therapies given concomitantly. Furthermore, it seems a temporary measure at best, as it does not seem to have a fundamental effect on the pathogenesis of the disease. Nonetheless, in some cases of severe hemolysis, even temporary improvement may be worthwhile.

Danazol, a modified androgen with reduced masculinizing effects, may be used in dosages of 600 to 800 mg per day. Response may occur in unsplenectomized patients. Danazol has usually been used in conjunction with prednisone, either as initial therapy or after an inadequate response to corticosteroids alone. The drug frequently produces improvement, typically within 1 to 3 weeks. Thereafter, corticosteroids may be tapered to a low dose or discontinued. Once remission is sustained, the dosage of danazol may be reduced to 200 to 400 mg per day and may be discontinued ultimately, particularly if the direct antiglobulin test becomes negative.

AIHA has also responded to high-dosage intravenous immunoglobulin, although there are also numerous reports of its ineffectiveness in other patients. This treatment has usually been given in association with other therapies and, when effective, has produced only temporary benefit.

Transfusion Therapy

The most important point concerning transfusion therapy in patients with AIHA is that blood must never be considered contraindicated, even though the compatibility test may be strongly incompatible. The need for transfusion is determined on the basis of a clinical evaluation, the most critical aspects of which are the symptoms and signs resulting from the anemia. The hemoglobin and hematocrit values are significant, but are too often overemphasized as criteria for transfusion.

When life-threatening manifestations of anemia are present, transfusion is mandatory. These manifestations include progressively severe angina, cardiac decompensation, and neurologic signs, beginning as lethargy and weakness and progressing to somnolence, mental confusion, coma, and death. It is rare for such indications to be present if the hemoglobin is above 8 g per deciliter, unless the hemolysis is hyperacute in onset, usually with grossly evident hemoglobinuria and hemoglobinemia. Even at hemoglobin levels of 5 to 8 g per deciliter, most patients tolerate the anemia well if treated with bed rest, oxygen, and institution of high dosages of corticosteroids, as described previously.

Recently, improved pretransfusion compatibility testing in AIHA has been emphasized. The patient's autoantibody usually reacts with all red cells tested, thus making all crossmatch tests incompatible. Such broadly reactive autoantibodies make the detection of red cell alloantibodies, such as anti-D, anti-Kell, and anti-Kidd, more difficult. However, a number of methods are available for absorbing autoantibody from the serum, which can then be used to test for alloantibodies. If alloantibodies are found in the absorbed serum, it can be used for crossmatching, thus providing "alloantibody-compatible" blood and avoiding hemolytic transfusion reactions that could occur as a result of their presence. Thus, it is no longer justifiable to omit a search for alloantibodies in the serum of patients with AIHA before blood is transfused, and the use of "least-incompatible" units without more detailed compatibility testing should be considered obsolete.

In spite of in vitro incompatibility caused by the red cell autoantibody, hemolytic transfusion reactions are uncommon. The transfused erythrocytes survive about as well as the patient's own cells, thus affording temporary benefit until more definitive treatment becomes effective.

Consideration of the optimal volume of blood to be transfused is of particular importance. The kinetics of red cell destruction always describe an exponential curve of decay, indicating that the number of cells removed in a unit of time is a percentage of the number of cells present at the start of this time interval. Thus, the more cells present at zero time, the more cells in absolute number will be destroyed in the unit time span. A rapid rise in red cell volume by transfusion of several units of red cells therefore may result in the development of increased signs of hemolysis, such as hemoglobinemia and hemoglobinuria, even though the rate of hemolysis has not changed. This has been erroneously interpreted as an increased severity of the AIHA. Such a marked increase in the amount of hemolysis has the potential for precipitating intravascular coagulation, possibly as a result of procoagulant substances present in red cell lysates. This risk is best minimized by transfusion of relatively small volumes of (packed) red blood cells, with the aim of maintaining a tolerable level of hematocrit until other therapy becomes effective. A hematocrit above 20 is usually adequate for hospitalized patients, providing there are no manifestations of severe coronary artery disease.

COLD AGGLUTININ DISEASE (CAD)

Cold agglutinin disease (CAD) is frequently not severe and often results in chronic mild hemolytic anemia with a hemoglobin of 9 to 12 g per deciliter. Such patients require no therapy other than avoiding exposure to cold, which can precipitate more severe hemolytic episodes. Even with strict avoidance of cold, however, some hemolysis usually persists.

More severely anemic patients should be treated with chlorambucil, 4 mg per day. This dosage can be increased at monthly intervals by 2 mg per day until improvement in the anemia or limiting side effects occur. The latter are usually gastrointestinal intolerance or marrow depression. Maximum tolerated dosages are often in the range of 8 to 12 mg per day. Blood counts should be performed weekly until a maintenance dose is found. If no leukopenia or thrombocytopenia occurs after 6 weeks on a constant dose, blood counts may be performed every 2 to 4 weeks thereafter.

Only a minority of patients with CAD respond favorably to chlorambucil with an increase in hemoglobin and decrease in cold agglutinin titer. There are few reports of splenectomy having been performed for CAD, and it has generally been of little benefit. Similarly, corticosteroid drugs are generally ineffective in this syndrome in contrast with their documented benefit in patients with warm antibody AIHA. There are anecdotal reports of temporary benefit of plasma exchange.

PAROXYSMAL COLD HEMOGLOBINURIA (PCH)

Almost all recent reports of PCH describe an acute transient nonrecurring hemolytic anemia not related to exposure to cold. The red cell autoantibody, first described by Donath and Landsteiner, is known as a biphasic antibody because it attaches to red cells only in the cold, but it is best demonstrated by subsequent warming of the red cells to 37°C in the presence of complement, under which conditions the red cells are hemolyzed. Most patients are children, and the onset of hemolysis usually occurs during or soon after an infection, especially those caused by viruses. The hemolysis is usually abrupt in onset and often produces severe anemia. Corticosteroid therapy has been disappointing, although it is nevertheless still used empirically. Patients are best managed with avoidance of cold and, when necessary, with blood transfusion, usually for several weeks, by which time the disease resolves spontaneously.

The red cell autoantibody, in the vast majority of cases, has anti-P specificity. Since blood lacking the P antigen is extraordinarily rare and can be obtained only from rare donor files, P-positive red cells usually must be used for transfusion. It is logical and customary to warm the blood as it is infused by using an in-line blood warmer. Such transfusions usually produce an appropriate, although temporary, rise in hemoglobin. If transfusions of P-positive red cells provoke reactions, it is preferable to use cells of the rare blood group p (Tj^a negative), if available.

DRUG-INDUCED AUTOIMMUNE HEMOLYTIC ANEMIA

Most drugs that cause immune hemolytic anemia produce an antibody that has specificity for the drug or one of its metabolites and reacts in vitro with red blood cells only in the presence of the drug. The antibody has specificity for the drug and not for intrinsic red cell antigens. Thus, these drug-induced immune hemolytic anemias are not truly autoimmune. However, an ever-increasing number of drugs have been shown to result in the production of red cell autoantibodies that react with normal red cell antigens in the absence of the drug and demonstrate no specificity for drug-related antigens. The drugs can be implicated only by clinical observations because immunohematologic findings are indistinguishable from warm antibody autoimmune hemolytic anemia.

AIHA has most frequently been implicated as a result of the administration of procainamide and α-methyldopa (Aldomet). Other drugs that have rarely caused AIHA are L-dopa, mefenamic acid, phenacetin, chlorpromazine, and streptomycin. Recognition of these unusual disorders is important because the hemolysis can be life-threatening if the drug therapy is continued. Corticosteroids have also been used empirically when hemolysis is severe, and this is logical, although their efficacy is difficult to establish because the AIHA resolves after the causative drug is discontinued.

SUGGESTED READING

Chaplin H Jr, ed. Immune hemolytic anemias. Methods in hematology, Vol 12. New York: Churchill Livingstone, 1985.

Coon WW. Splenectomy in the treatment of hemolytic anemia. Arch Surg 1985; 120:625–628.

Petz LD, Garratty G. Acquired immune hemolytic anemias. New York: Churchill Livingstone, 1980.

SICKLE CELL ANEMIA

BERTRAM H. LUBIN, M.D.
ELLIOTT VICHINSKY, M.D.

Sickle cell anemia refers to the doubly heterozygote inheritance of the sickle gene, which gives rise to abnormal hemoglobin that polymerizes upon deoxygenation. This process is accelerated by cellular dehydration and acidosis. Sickle hemoglobin containing red blood cells has two abnormal properties that result in the clinical manifestations of this disease. These properties are (1) short survival and (2) adherence to vascular endothelium. These two properties result in anemia and vascular occlusion; the latter can eventually result in organ damage. Sickling disorders, such as sickle cell β° thalassemia, sickle β^{+} thalassemia, and sickle cell-hemoglobin C disease have similar clinical manifestations, although in most cases to a lesser degree than sickle cell anemia.

GENERAL GUIDELINES—DIAGNOSIS AND COMPREHENSIVE CARE

The treatment of sickle cell disease involves preventive, as well as interventive, techniques. Among the important recent advances in the treatment of this disease has been the ability to detect patients in the newborn period. This, combined with prophylactic use of antibiotics to prevent pneumococcal sepsis, has markedly diminished the incidence of death in the young child with sickle cell disease.

Proper identification of patients is very important as it enables appropriate counseling, enrollment in a comprehensive care program, and treatment of medical complications. Table 1 indicates the comprehensive care guidelines we use for all patients with sickle cell disease. Together with surveillance for infection and organ damage, education, counseling, and immunization are key factors.

Painful Crises

Analgesia

Of all the complications associated with sickle cell disease, painful crises are the most frequent and difficult to manage. The first and most important step in treating this complication is to identify the precise cause of the pain, and not simply to label it a "vaso-occlusive crisis." Surgical problems and infectious complications must be ruled out. The second step is to treat the pain properly. The reason for difficulty in pain crisis management often lies in the physician's inability to use appropriate analgesics, combined with an inadequate doctor-patient relationship. The notion that use of narcotic analgesics for sickle cell patients results in addiction is inaccurate. Although there are a small number of patients who may become addicted to narcotic analgesics, withholding adequate pain medication from the majority of sickle cell patients for fear of this problem will result in inadequate pain control, a feeling of distrust by the patient, a "pain-" dependent personality, and a patient who "shops around" from emergency room to emergency room in order to get pain relief.

We have developed a consistent approach to use of analgesic agents, which has decreased the number of emergency room visits, as well as hospital days for our patients. A mutually-agreed-upon contract is established between patient and health care provider, which describes the type of analgesics to be used, their dose, and duration. All medical staff involved in sickle cell

TABLE 1 Sickle Cell Comprehensive Care Outline

	Interval
Physical examination	
Under 6 months	Monthly
6 months–1 year	Every 2 months
1–5 years	Every 3 months
Over 5 years	Every 4 months
Social worker interview	Bi-annually
Social worker home visit	Annually
School assessment, job assessment	Annually
Genetic counseling services	
Family studies	Initial
Counseling and education	Annually
Hematology evaluation	
CBC, reticulocyte count	Quarterly
Hemoglobin electrophoresis	Initial
Quantitative hemoglobin F	Initial
Kleihauer-Betke stain	Initial
Alpha-Gene mapping, haplotypic analysis	Initial
Ferritin	Annually
Evaluation for red cell alloantibodies	Baseline, pre- and post-transfusion
Red cell phenotype	Initial
Liver-gallbladder evaluation	
Liver functions	Annually
Hepatitis antibody and antigen	Annually
Abdominal ultrasound	Annually, after age 10
Renal	
BUN, creatinine, uric acid, urinalysis	Annually
Cardiac	
ECG, echocardiogram	Annually
Pulmonary	
Chest x-ray, pulmonary function tests, blood gases	Annually, after age 5
Dental evaluation	Annually
Nutrition Assessment	Annually
Indirect opthalmologic exam	Annually, age 10 and up
Immunization schedules	
Standard OPV/DPT/MMR and booster	Standard intervals
Pneumococcal vaccine	Age 1, 2, 6 years
H. influenzae vaccine	Age 2 years
Hepatitis B vaccine series	Initiate at 1 year
Influenza vaccine	Annually
Prophylactic penicillin	125 mg b.i.d. 3 mos –3 years; 250 mg b.i.d. > 3 years

patient care are instructed in the proper use of analgesic agents. A list of analgesic agents and their dose schedules is given in Table 2. The medications are grouped according to pain severity. When given by the oral route, the dose of analgesics is considerably higher than when given intravenously. Non-narcotic agents should be used whenever possible. However, for severe pain, sufficient doses of narcotic agents should be promptly administered. Continuous intravenous infusion of narcotic agents provides excellent pain control, but should be performed only by institutions familiar with this technique.

The protocol we use for in-patient management of severe pain in sickle cell patients is indicated in Table 3. This program is effective in most patients. The dose of an individual analgesic may vary from patient to patient, and should be determined by patient response, not by a predetermined decision on the physician's part. Differences in drug metabolism, drug receptors, and pain threshold may contribute to the variability in analgesic requirements among patients. When patients are discharged from the hospital following a painful crisis, it is important that only small amounts of analgesics be prescribed. This is done in order to minimize the risk of drug abusive behavior.

TABLE 2 Recommended Initial Dose and Interval of Analgesics Necessary to Obtain Adequate Pain Control in Sickle Cell Disease

Severity of Pain	*Max Dose (mg)*	*Route*	*Interval*	*Comments*
Severe				
Morphine	0.15 mg/kg/dose (max 10mg)	SC,IM	q3h	Drug of choice
Merperidine	1.5 mg/kg/dose	IM	q3h	Increased incidence of seizures. Avoid in patients with renal or neurologic disease
Moderate				
Oxycodone (Percocet) (Percodan)	2 tabs/dose (1 tab = 5 mg)	PO	q4h	
Methadone	0.15 mg/kg/dose	PO	q6h	Effective in patients usually requiring parenteral narcotics. *Not for routine use*
Merperidine	1.5mg/kg/dose (max 100 mg/dose)	PO	q3-1/2h	
Mild				
Codeine	.75 mg/kg/dose	PO	q4h	May be effective up to 6 hours
Aspirin	1.5 $g/m^2/24$ h	PO	q4h	May be given with a narcotic for added analgesia
Acetaminophen	1.5 $g/m^2/24$ h	PO	q4h	May be given with a narcotic for added analgesia
Motrin (Ibuprofen)	300–600 mg/dose	PO	q8h	

TABLE 3 Analgesic Therapy for In-Patient Management of Severe Pain in Sickle Cell Disease

First 24 hours

- Morphine sulfate (IM or SQ) given on a fixed schedule (not prn) every 3 hours. Dose = 0.15 mg/kg. Young infants may require a lower dose (0.1 mg/kg).
- Aspirin PO every 4 hours

Usually after 24–48 hours, or when acute pain has diminished

- Taper parenteral dose by 10–20% daily; do not change administration interval
- Switch to oral medication when one-half the initial starting parenteral dose is achieved. Oral narcotic analgesics are given every 4 hours in an equivalent analgesic dose to the initial parenteral dose
- Change oral dose as needed to control pain, but do not revert to parenteral medication
- Discharge the patient on oral medication as soon as possible
- Write small discharge prescriptions

In addition to analgesic therapy, intravenous fluids should also be administered. Due to the hyposthenuria associated with sickle cell nephropathy, measurement of urine specific gravity does not help in determining intravenous fluid requirements. Measurement of the patients' daily weight is essential. Usually one-and-a-half to two times maintenance fluids given as D5 1/3 NS normal saline are adequate to maintain hydration and electrolyte balance. Potassium supplements should be given as required. Electrolytes should be obtained at baseline and monitored on a regular basis. Acidosis should be corrected, but we do not use alkali therapy in the absence of acidosis. Oxygen therapy has no place in the treatment of a vaso-occlusive crisis unless the crisis is associated with hypoxia, documented by low arterial blood gas.

Anemic Crises

Patients with sickle cell disease are anemic due to shortened *in vivo* red blood cell survival. Most patients compensate well for anemia with a shift in the oxygen dissociation curve to the right, and an increase in cardiac output. However, if erythroid production is suppressed, the hemoglobin level can fall precipitously, and the extent of anemia can be severe and life-threatening. Such aplastic crises are heralded by a drop in the reticulocyte count. The parvovirus has been implicated in a number of these aplastic crises.

Increased rate of hemolysis can also occur (hyperhemolytic crises), sometimes in association with glucose 6-phosphate dehydrogenase (G6-PD) deficiency and/or with infection. Increase in bilirubin levels is associated with this complication.

Acute sequestration crisis is common in infants with sickle cell anemia. In other hemoglobin variants, even in adults, chronic hypersplenism and occasionally acute sequestration may occur. In the acute condition, this complication is characterized by rapid onset of splenomegaly and a precipitous drop in hemoglobin level. Exchange transfusion is often required and splenectomy considered, as recurrent splenic sequestration crises are not uncommon.

Transfusion

The treatment of severe anemic crises requires red cell transfusions. Depending upon the clinical evaluation, including the degree of anemia and the underlying cardiac status, a decision to administer either a simple red cell transfusion or an exchange transfusion is made. Guidelines for performing transfusions in sickle cell patients are given in Table 4. The rate of transfusion should be determined by the cardiovascular status. Usually transfusions are given over 4 to 6 hours. If available, we prefer to use racially-matched donor blood to minimize the risk of alloimmunization. Blood matched for Kell, E, C, and Duffy in multiply-transfused patients may prevent hemolytic transfusion reactions. Washed cells should be used for chronically transfused patients.

There are several other indications for transfusion in sickle cell anemia (Table 5). In each case, the risk of transfusion is felt to be less than the risk of complications from transfusion. This is clearly true for splenic sequestration crises and stroke. In the case of stroke management, the duration of transfusion therapy has not been established. However, if cumulative transfusions are given for longer than 2 years, consideration should be given to chelation therapy to minimize iron overload.

Red cell transfusions are used by many physicians in the preoperative management of sickle cell patients. Correction of anemia, as well as improvement in blood viscosity, are the goals of such treatment. In addition to transfusion, the guidelines for preoperative management of sickle cell patients are listed in Table 4. Careful attention to hydration cannot be overemphasized, especially during the postoperative period. Monitoring the hemoglobin S levels to maintain a value below 30 percent is the therapeutic goal, while preventing the hemoglobin from exceeding 14 g per deciliter. Depending upon the urgency for surgery, the transfusion can either be a simple packed red cell transfusion or an exchange transfusion. Certain minor surgical procedures can be performed without preoperative transfusion, and in some sickle cell centers, even major surgical procedures such as cholecystectomy are performed without transfusion. However, in our hands, even with excellent anesthetic management, preoperative red cell transfusion is used in all major surgical cases.

Transfusion therapy during pregnancy should be individualized. We transfuse all pregnant sickle cell anemia patients during the last trimesters of pregnancy

TABLE 4 Protocol for Elective Surgery

LABORATORY TESTS

Baseline

CBC, reticulocytes, % HbS, % HbA, red cell phenotype, alloantibody status, creatinine, LFT, PT, PTT
Baseline pulse oximetery or arterial blood gas within 6 months
Cardiac examination—Echo or ECG within 6 months of surgery

Goal

A preoperative Hb $>$ 10 g/dl but not to exceed 13 g/dl with HbS $<$ 30%. Ideally, HbA to be 70% or greater

METHODS OF TRANSFUSION

Simple transfusion (tx)

Start 1 month prior to surgery, tx to Hb 12 g/dl
Repeat 2 weeks prior to surgery, if necessary, and preoperatively

Formula

Blood volume (BV) = 75 cc/kg for children, 65 cc/kg for adults

$$\text{cc of packed RBC} = \frac{\text{BV} \times (\text{Hb}_{\text{desired}} - \text{Hb}_{\text{observed}})}{23\ (\text{Hb of packed RBC})}$$

Obtain percent HbA, S (or C) prior to each transfusion

Exchange transfusion

Remove 0.8% of blood volume and replace volume removed using a (50/50) mixture of packed RBC and normal saline

ADMISSION GUIDELINES

Preoperative

Admit 24 hours prior to surgery
All patients seen by anesthesiologist 1 day prior to surgery
1 1/2 × maintenance fluids given intravenously at least 24 hours prior to surgery
Strict monitoring of intake and output, as well as weight

Intraoperative

Minimum 50% O_2 with anesthetic agent
Monitor blood O_2 by pulse oximetry

Postoperative

Provide O_2 until anesthetic agent wears off
Measure input and output and weight immediately postoperatively
Determine CBC and reticulocyte count day 1, 3, and 7
Continue 1 1/2 maintenance fluids intravenously until PO intake is sufficient to maintain stable weight

TABLE 5 Indications for Transfusion in Sickle Cell Anemia

Severe anemic crises (aplastic, sequestration, hemolytic)
Life-threatening events
Acute, impending, or suspected cerebrovascular accident
Acute progressive lung disease
Preparation for major surgery
Acute priapism with no response to intravenous hydration
Recalcitrant leg ulcers
Pregnancy
Chronic organ failure (cardiac, renal, pulmonary, hepatic)

to maintain Hb S levels below 30 percent. For patients who have recurrent vaso-occlusive complications, we may transfuse earlier. Not all sickle cell centers agree with this approach, and some have found that certain untransfused patients have no difficulty during pregnancy. In our experience, transfused patients have a feeling of well-being, as well as fewer crises.

Pulmonary complications frequently involve a combination of infection and infarction, and can lead to rapid compromise in pulmonary function and to extreme hypoxia. Since baseline pulmonary functions are below normal in most patients with sickle cell disease, the superimposition of vaso-occlusive complications and infection can lead to acute pulmonary decompensation. Treatment of this potentially fatal complication involves the use of red cell transfusions, fluid therapy, oxygen, and antibiotics. Therapeutic guidelines for management of patients with this complication are given in Table 6. A major factor in the management of pulmonary complications is careful monitoring of patients. It is not uncommon for decompensation to occur within hours during this type of complication. During the first 24 to 48 hours of hospitalization, we monitor these patients frequently to identify signs of pulmonary decompensation.

TABLE 6 Protocol for Acute Chest Syndrome

All patients with chest or lung symptoms must be examined immediately

Review medical record to determine patient's previous steady-state respiratory rate, arterial blood gas, chest x-ray, and VQ scan

Patients should undergo the following investigation
- Chest x-ray
- CBC, reticulocyte count
- Blood culture, sputum culture (if possible)
- Arterial blood gas in room air
- Mycoplasma titer (acute and follow-up)
- VQ scan (this scan is indicated when chest signs exist with a negative chest x-ray
- ECG (optional)
- Viral studies (optional)
- Type and hold (optional)

All patients with evidence of acute pulmonary pathology should be admitted to the hospital. IV hydration should be given. IV + PO should equal a minimum of one-and-a-half times maintenance fluids.

Oxygen should be administered if patient hypoxia ($PO_2 < 70$ mm Hg) demonstrated by arterial blood gas measurements

IV Cefuroxime (100 mg/kg/day) should be started immediately. Optional erythromycin dose can be added if mycoplasma is suspected

If pleural fluid is present on a chest x-ray and contributing to respiratory distress, thoracentesis is indicated

Arterial blood gas should be closely monitored

A partial exchange transfusion should be initiated for any of the following criteria:
- A PaO_2 below 70 mm Hg
- A 25% drop in the patient's baseline PaO_2
- Acute congestive heart failure or acute right heart strain
- Rapidly progressive pneumonia
- Marked dyspnea with tachypnea

Following recovery from an acute pulmonary event, patients should undergo baseline pulmonary function tests, arterial blood gas measurements, and a steady-state ventilation profusion scan to facilitate future evaluation for acute pulmonary disease.

Infections

We treat patients with sickle cell anemia as if they were immunocompromised hosts. The absence of splenic function, defects in the alternate complement pathway, and perhaps other, as yet to be defined, immunologic defects contribute to the increased risk of bacterial infections. In the younger patient in particular, death is often related to bacterial sepsis.

Sepsis, pneumonia, urinary tract infections, meningitis, and osteomyelitis are the most frequent sites. Bacterial infections caused by *Streptococcus pneumoniae, Haemophilus influenzae, Neisseria meningitis, Mycoplasma pneumoniae, Staphylococcus aureus, Streptococcus pyogenes,* and *Salmonella* are the most frequent.

The problem of bacterial infections in patients with sickle cell disease can best be addressed by immunization, patient education, awareness on the part of caretakers of the potential severity of bacterial infection, and prompt, aggressive intervention with antibiotics. Immunization guidelines are indicated in Table 1. It is important to recognize that immunization against *S. pneumococcus* and *H. influenzae* may not result in adequate antibody response, therefore affording limited protection.

Management of febrile patients should include extensive testing to identify the source of the infection, including studies of blood, urine, and chest roentgenogram. Cerebrospinal fluid (CSF) examination should be done when clinically indicated. When osteomyelitis is suspected, aspiration of the bone is useful to identify the organism, and coverage for salmonella and staphylococcus should be given. Since pneumococcal sepsis is the most rapidly fatal infection, antibiotics given to any febrile patient should cover this type of infection.

Sepsis due to gram negative infections is frequent in adults. The etiology is often renal or pelvic inflammatory disease.

Obstetrics-Gynecology

Proper counseling regarding pregnancy and birth control is important for sickle cell patients. Education should include discussions regarding available prenatal diagnosis by amniocentesis or chorionic villus sampling. Although there are many methods of birth control, use of diaphragm, spermicide, and condoms is recommended by many due to the theoretical risk of a hypercoagulable state. However, since there are few data to support this increased risk and since compliance with barrier methods is poor, we use low estrogen-containing birth control pills. Our patients have had no complications with this therapy.

Gallstones

Gallstones frequently develop in patients with sickle cell disease, and, for that reason, a regular surveillance program that employs abdominal ultrasound is recommended (see Table 1). This is especially so for patients who have abdominal painful crises. Although they are not necessarily the cause of the abdominal pain, detection of gallstones is sufficient to consider a causal relationship. If patients have both recurrent attacks of abdominal pain and gallstones, demonstrated on ultrasound, cholecystectomy is recommended. We transfuse such patients preoperatively and follow the guidelines indicated in Table 4.

Aseptic Necrosis of the Hip

Aseptic necrosis of the hip is a common problem in adolescents and adults with sickle cell disease. Early diagnosis can be made using bone scan and/or MRI. Preliminary data suggests that treatment with a decompression procedure, by removing a core of bone from the head of the femur, and transfusion for 3 months postoperatively, may be beneficial. If the diagnosis is not made until the necrosis has progressed to a late stage, hip prosthesis and physical therapy are options, but response to therapy is limited.

Leg Ulcers

Leg ulcers are treated by cleaning, debridement, topical oil, and, in selected chronic cases, transfusion. If infection is documented, topical and/or systemic antibiotics may be helpful. Recurrence is common. Since most skin ulcers are traumatic, proper selection of shoes, together with protective socks, are necessary.

NEW TREATMENT

Antisickling agents, attempts to increase fetal hemoglobin production, bone marrow transplantation, and drugs to decrease red cell vascular endothelial interactions are all experimental therapies for sickle cell disease, and some may hold promise for the future. Comprehensive care, counseling and education, and aggressive therapy of complications are the best currently-available methods for decreasing morbidity and mortality in sickle cell disease.

SUGGESTED READING

Charache S, Lubin B, Reid CD, eds. Management of therapy of sickle cell disease, 1985.
Serjeant G. Sickle cell disease. Oxford Univ Press, 1985.
Bunn HF, Forget BG. In: Hemoglobin: molecular, genetic and clinical aspects. Philadelphia: WB Saunders, 1986.

POLYCYTHEMIA RUBRA VERA

STEVEN M. FRUCHTMAN, M.D.
LOUIS R. WASSERMAN, M.D.
PAUL D. BERK, M.D.

The etiology of polycythemia vera is not known, and the optimal management to prevent complications and enhance well-being and longevity in patients with this disorder is controversial. However, as our conceptual understanding of this disease on a cellular level increases, our ability to manage these patients rationally is improving. Of utmost importance in caring for patients with polycythemia is careful attention to establishing the correct diagnosis and familiarity with the natural history of the disease.

Through the use of glucose-6-phosphate dehydrogenase isoenzyme analysis and cytogenetic data, polycythemia vera has been shown to be a hematologic malignancy involving an abnormal clone of the pluripotent marrow stem cell, leading to a panhyperplasia of the bone marrow that involves the erythroid, myeloid, and megakaryocytic series as well as B-lymphocytes. The hyperplastic marrow leads to elevation of the red cell mass, considered essential for the diagnosis of the disease, and varying degrees of leukocytosis and thrombocytosis. It is believed that the hemorrhagic and thrombotic complications of the disease, which our therapeutic armamentarium is aimed at minimizing, are secondary to the hyperplastic marrow and increased numbers of circulating elements, on a mechanical, vascular, and perhaps humoral basis.

Left untreated, patients with polycythemia do poorly; 50 percent are reported to die within 18 months after the onset of the first symptom or sign. Untreated polycythemia vera patients are at an especially high risk of developing both thrombotic and hemorrhagic complications, with death resulting from thrombosis of the cerebral, coronary, and pulmonary circulation. Occlusions at unusual sites for thrombosis, such as the hepatic veins, femoral artery or vein and mesenteric vein, are also seen.

The pathogenesis of the increased frequency of thrombosis in these patients is unclear. Although the increase in blood viscosity resulting from an elevated hematocrit no doubt plays an important role, other factors are also significant. Studies using xenon-133 have shown that cerebral blood flow decreases in individuals with hematocrits above 53 percent and returns to normal with hematocrit reduction to more typical normal levels. Cerebral function is also improved by reduction of the hematocrit to levels below 45 percent. The degree of hematocrit elevation may influence the size of a cerebral infarct in both animals and humans. Thus, the propensity for thrombosis and infarction in polycythemia may be related to a reversible impairment of blood flow.

Although blood fluidity is important in influencing the thrombotic and hemorrhagic tendencies seen in polycythemia vera, these patients are still prone to thrombotic and hemorrhagic complications even when the blood volume is normalized by phlebotomy. Therefore, in addition to whole blood viscosity, it is believed that qualitative abnormalities of the circulating elements and vascular endothelium may play a role. Typically, patients with polycythemia vera have elevated platelet counts and a multitude of in vitro abnormalities in platelet aggregation.

Because of the potentially malignant nature of polycythemia vera, close monitoring and appropriate therapy are of great importance. With therapy, a dramatic improvement in survival has been reported, with most recent studies citing median survivals of 8 to 15 years. However, before appropriate therapy can be started, one must be able to differentiate between the various clinical conditions that share an abnormally increased concentration of packed red cells per unit volume of peripheral blood. Relative or spurious polycythemia must be differentiated from absolute polycythemia, and secondary erythrocytosis from primary. Treatment designed to suppress the bone marrow would be harmful in situations in which increased erythropoietic activity reflects the marrow's physiologic response to a hypoxemic state. In the secondary polycythemias, one must find the underlying cause and attempt to correct it. It is therefore essential that the clinician understand the mechanism of erythrocytosis before initiating therapy.

The Polycythemia Vera Study Group (PVSG) was founded in 1967 to help determine the optimal treatment for polycythemia vera. The group recognized the importance of defining rigorous and widely available criteria before a diagnosis of polycythemia vera could be established. By using the criteria outlined in Table 1, the diagnosis can be made rapidly and with great confidence.

Measurement of the Cr^{51} erythrocyte mass is essential in confirming the existence of true erythrocytosis. A hematocrit above 60 percent almost invariably predicts an elevated erythrocyte mass, but at hematocrits below 60 percent the erythrocyte mass may be elevated, normal or even low, depending on the extent to which the

TABLE 1 Parameters for the Diagnosis of Polycythemia Vera*

A1. Increased red cell mass Males $\geq$ 36 ml/kg Females $\geq$ 32 ml/kg	B1. Thrombocytosis: platelet count >400,000/μl
A2. Normal arterial O_2 saturation ($\geq$92%)	B2. Leukocytosis: WBC > 12,000/μl (no fever or infection)
A3. Splenomegaly	B3. ↑Leukocyte alkaline phosphatase: >100 (no fever or infection)
	B4. ↑Serum B_{12}(>900 pg/ml) or unbound B_{12} binding capacity (>2,200 pg/ml)

* Diagnosis acceptable if following combinations are present: A1 + A2 + A3; A1 + A2 + any from category B.

TABLE 2 Principles in the Management of Patients with Polycythemia Rubra Vera

1. *Patient Status* Therapy should be tailored to suit the needs of the individual patient, taking into account the levels of cells in the blood, bone marrow morphology, and complications of hepatosplenomegaly. No single therapy is appropriate for all patients at all ages and stages of the disease.

2. *Blood Volume* This should be normalized by phlebotomy as rapidly as clinically possible (usually 250 to 500 cc every other day). Elderly patients and those with cardiovascular disease should be phlebotomized cautiously, and by reduced amounts.

3. *Age: The Older Patient* In all patients over the age of 70, panmyelosis should be suppressed with chemotherapy or P^{32}, in combination with phlebotomy, because of the increased risk of thrombosis.

4. *Age: The Younger Patient* Patients under the age of 50 years, especially women in the child-bearing age, are best treated by phlebotomy only, unless factors indicate an increased risk for thrombosis. Marrow suppression is advised in younger patients with (1) a thrombotic tendency despite a normal red cell volume following phlebotomy or (2) a high phlebotomy requirement and the development of thrombocythemia following phlebotomy.

5. *Age: Patients between 50 and 70* Although the choice of treatment is more controversial, we recommend phlebotomy for the physiologically young patient not at risk for thrombosis and myelosuppression for patients with a thrombotic tendency or a high phlebotomy requirement.

6. *Indications for Myelosuppression* Splenomegaly causing mechanical compromise, bone pain, excessive symptoms of hypermetabolism, intractable pruritus, and poor venous access may be additional reasons for myelosuppressive treatment.

7. *Choice of Myelosuppressive Agent* Hydroxyurea is the agent we recommend for patients under the age of 70 years. Alkylating agents are not recommended because of the increased risk of leukemia and of certain types of cancer associated with their long-term use.

8. *Avoiding Toxicity* Chemotherapy and/or radiation should be used judiciously, and supplemented with phlebotomy to control the hematocrit and avoid undue myelosuppression of the marrow.

9. *Hyperuricemia* Allopurinal (100 to 300 mg per day orally) should be given until remission has been achieved. Colchicine, or other anti-inflammatory agents are indicated for acute attacks of gout.

10. *Surgery* Elective surgery should be postponed until the long-term control of the disease has been established.

elevated hematocrit reflects a reduced plasma volume rather than an expanded erythron. By following the algorithm outlined in Figure 1, patients with an elevated hematocrit or hemoglobin concentration can be categorized as having relative, secondary, or primary polycythemia. In difficult cases specialized tools available mainly through large centers, such as determination of plasma and urinary erythropoietin levels and studies of the growth characteristics of erythroid precursors in tissue culture, can help. Once the diagnosis of polycythemia vera is established, attention must be given to the level of the circulating platelets and white cells, the degree of immaturity of the white cell series in the peripheral blood, the size of the spleen, the history of bleeding or thrombosis, and the performance status of the patient. Important clinical factors must be evaluated before the treatment modality is decided on, i.e., the age of the patient, the presence of diabetes, arteriosclerosis, cardiopulmonary disease, and venous access. Guidelines for managing patients with polycythemia vera are offered in Table 2.

PHLEBOTOMY

Once the diagnosis of polycythemia vera is established, relatively rapid, controlled reduction in the

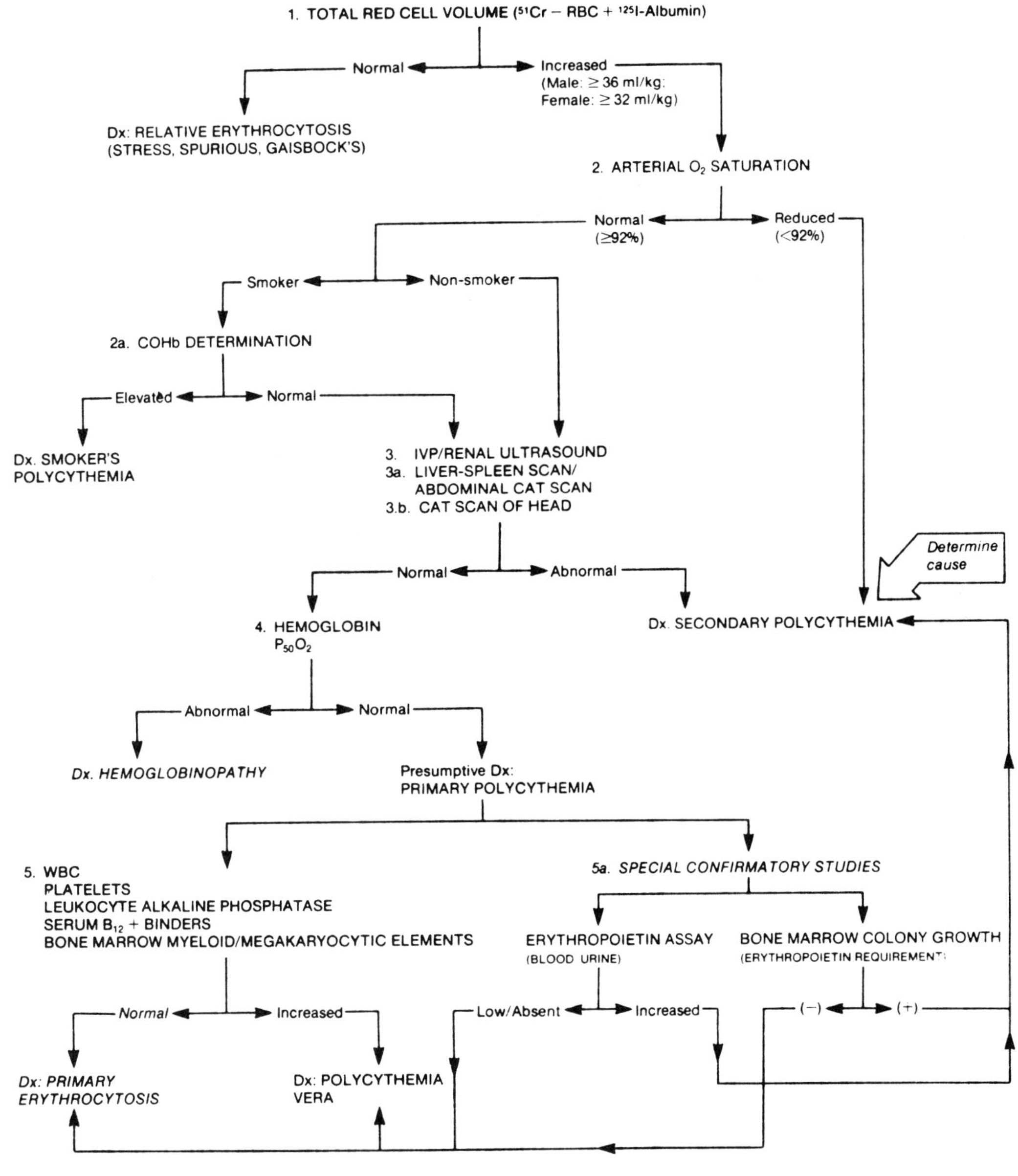

*Perform only where indicated.

Figure 1 Algorithm for evaluation of an elevated hematocrit, (modified from Berlin, NI. Diagnosis and classification of the polycythemias. Semin Hematol 1975; 12:343).

blood volume may prevent serious hemorrhagic and/or thrombotic complications in patients susceptible to such problems. Initially, phlebotomies of 250 to 500 cc should be performed every other day until a hematocrit of between 40 and 45 percent is obtained. In the elderly, or those with a compromised cardiovascular status, blood should be withdrawn only twice weekly. Phlebotomy therapy is particularly useful in indolent cases of polycythemia vera in which only occasional blood removal is sufficient to control the erythrocytosis. Once a normal hematocrit has been reached, blood counts at regular intervals (every 4–8 weeks) determine the frequency of future phlebotomies. Sufficient blood should be removed to maintain the hematocrit between 40 and 45 percent. Figure 2 outlines the management of polycythemia vera with phlebotomy. Iron supplements should be avoided because this may cause the hematocrit and red cell mass to increase rapidly. Although hypochromic, microcytic red cells have altered red cell deformability, these changes are believed to be insufficient to change whole blood viscosity at a given hematocrit. Iron deficiency is reported to produce symptoms that are unrelated to anemia, such as dysphagia, soreness or burning of the tongue, fissures at the corners of the mouth, koilonychia, and pica. Despite these potential problems, patients invariably feel better once adjustment to their lower red cell mass has occurred, and the rarity of the reported signs and symptoms of iron deficiency in clinical practice is noteworthy.

Phlebotomy is the treatment of choice in young patients because of the fear of neoplastic transformation associated with the long-term use of myelosuppressive therapy or radioactive agents. Patients below the age of 50 and all women in the child-bearing years should be managed with phlebotomy unless there are specific thrombosis-associated risk factors, as indicated earlier, in which case myelosuppression with hydroxyurea may be required. The rare patient with polycythemia vera who is pregnant should be treated with phlebotomy, although in such patients the hematocrit often declines to normal or anemic levels as a result of changes in blood volume and/or hormonal effects associated with pregnancy.

In the clinical management of polycythemia vera, the venous hematocrit should be maintained at or below the lower end of the normal range. Based on the observation that there are fewer vascular occlusive episodes in these patients when the hematocrit is maintained below 45 percent than when it is in the higher normal range, the value of 45 percent is the therapeutic objective. In patients who require myelosuppressive therapy, phlebotomy must be used initially to bring the hematocrit into the therapeutic range (40–45 percent), so that the morbidity and potential mortality of an elevated red cell mass can be avoided before the effects of bone marrow suppression become evident in the peripheral blood. In these patients, intermittent phlebotomy must be used as needed when the hematocrit is above 45 percent, to help minimize the amount of myelosuppression that is employed.

MYELOSUPPRESSION

Phlebotomy effectively reduces the blood volume to normal in patients with polycythemia vera. However, it will not control thrombocytosis, leukocytosis, the painfully enlarging spleen, hyperuricemia and its complications, or pruritus. Patients treated with phlebotomy alone, especially early in the course of their disease, have a higher incidence of thrombotic events that can be fatal or disabling. Thrombosis is the cause of 43 percent of deaths in patients treated with phlebotomy, compared to 23 percent in a chlorambucil-treated group and 29 percent in patients treated with radioactive phosphorus. Thrombosis is especially common in the elderly, in patients with a prior history of thrombosis, or those with a high phlebotomy requirement. Thus, although phlebotomy is the treatment of choice for many patients with polycythemia vera, it does not control all the ramifications of the disease; patients so treated, especially the elderly, remain susceptible to thrombotic complications. Myelosuppression with either P^{32} or cytostatic agents helps control the thrombocytosis, leukocytosis, painful splenomegaly, and hyperuricemia that can be found in association with this disorder. Patients so treated early in the course of their disease have fewer

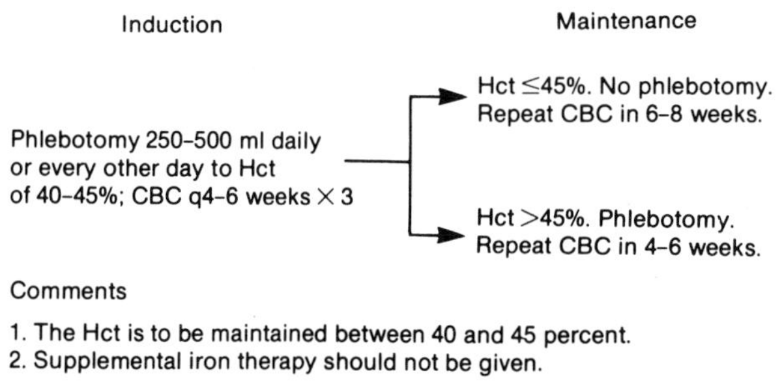
Induction
Maintenance
Hct ≤45%. No phlebotomy.
Repeat CBC in 6–8 weeks.
Phlebotomy 250–500 ml daily
or every other day to Hct
of 40–45%; CBC q4–6 weeks × 3
Hct >45%. Phlebotomy.
Repeat CBC in 4–6 weeks.
Comments
1. The Hct is to be maintained between 40 and 45 percent.
2. Supplemental iron therapy should not be given.

Figure 2 Management of polycythemia vera with phlebotomy.

thrombotic events. Control of hypermetabolism, weight gain, improved sense of well-being, and relief from pruritus can accompany marrow suppression and hematologic control. In a majority of cases the size of the liver and spleen is reduced. A standardized schema for assessing clinical response to myelosuppressive regimens is presented in Table 3.

Alkylating Agents

Chlorambucil (Leukeran) was a commonly used alkylating agent for the treatment of polycythemia vera. However, it has been shown that the risk of developing leukemia in patients given chlorambucil was 2 to 3 times that in patients given P^{32}, and 13 times that in patients treated with phlebotomy alone. Therefore, the Polycythemia Vera Study Group no longer recommends the use of chlorambucil in the treatment of polycythemia vera. Other groups have used melphalan, cyclophosphamide, and busulfan as cytostatic agents. These agents are effective in normalizing the numbers of peripheral blood cells. However, no alkylating agent has been absolved from leukemogenic potential, and there are numerous reports of the association of alkylating agent therapy and leukemia in both hematologic and nonhematologic disorders. The need for a safe myelosuppressive agent in patients with polycythemia vera in whom phlebotomy is not ideal therapy prompted the use of hydroxyurea.

Hydroxyurea

Hydroxyurea is a nonalkylating myelosuppressive agent specific for the inhibition of cells in the synthetic phase of the cell cycle. It decreases DNA synthesis by inhibiting ribonucleoside diphosphate reductase, and has been shown to control the hematocrit and platelet levels adequately in between 80 and 90 percent of patients within 12 weeks of initiation of therapy. Since it is a myelosuppressive agent, however, it must be used with caution and the peripheral blood count monitored closely. The dose requirements can vary widely and some patients are controlled with small doses of drug. Following normalization of the hematocrit with phlebotomy, if there is no urgency for profound bone marrow suppression, we recommend starting hydroxyurea at a low dose and increasing the dosage of drug if necessary. If these recommendations are followed, significant drug toxicity can be avoided. In this setting hydroxyurea is administered orally at a starting dosage of 15 mg per kilogram per day after the hematocrit has been normalized with phlebotomy. The patient must be followed with weekly blood counts. If at any time during therapy the white blood cell (WBC) count falls below 3,500 per cubic millimeter or the platelet count to less than 100,000 per cubic millimeter, hydroxyurea must be withheld and reinstituted at 50 percent of the prior dose when the blood count normalizes (Figure 3). When a steady state is achieved, the interval between

TABLE 3 Classification of Response to Therapy

Hematocrit (%)	*Platelets/mm*^{3}	*Classification**
42–47	≤600,000	CR I
<42	≤600,000	CR II
42–47	>600,000	PR I
<42	>600,000	PR II
>47	>600,000	NR

* Key to abbreviations: CR = complete remission; PR = partial remission; NR = no response.

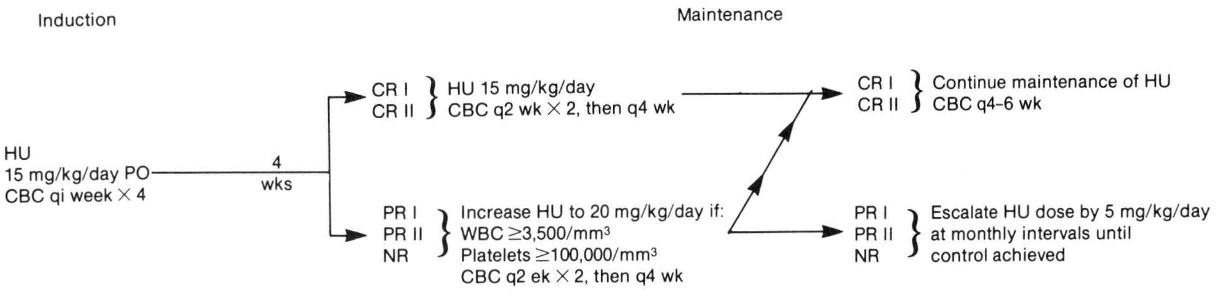

1. Hematocrit to be maintained between 40 and 45 percent by supplementary phlebotomy if necessary.
2. If WBC <3,500 per cubic millimeter and/or platelet count <100,000 per cubic millimeter stop therapy. Patient to be managed with phlebotomy alone. When WBC >3,500 per cubic millimeter and/or platelets >100,000 per cubic millimeter, HU can be restarted at 50 percent of maintenance dose.
3. After dose of HU is increased, obtain CBC every 2 weeks × 2, then every 4 to 6 weeks during maintenance.
4. Patients unable to achieve CR I or CR II despite escalation of HU dose because of WBC <3,500 per cubic millimeter or platelets <100,000 per cubic millimeter should be placed on optimum HU dose and phlebotomized.

Figure 3 Management of polycythemia vera with hydroxyurea (HU).

blood counts is lengthened to 2 weeks and then to 4 weeks. For poorly controlled patients who require frequent phlebotomies or are thrombocythemic (with platelet counts greater than 600,000 per cubic millimeter), the dosage can be increased by 5 mg per kilogram per day at monthly intervals, with frequent monitoring until control is achieved, or to a maximum dosage of 2 g per day of hydroxyurea. Most patients are controlled with dosages of between 500 and 1,000 mg per day, but in occasional patients as little as 500 mg, three times weekly, suffices. Supplemental phlebotomy in addition to hydroxyurea is preferable to excessive myelosuppression alone. In occasional patients, particularly those presenting with neurologic symptoms in the setting of marked thrombocytosis, more rapid control of the disease is essential. In this setting, phlebotomy to a hematocrit of 45 percent or less may be accompanied by the use of a loading dose of hydroxyurea of 30 mg per kilogram per day for 7 days, followed by 15 mg per kilogram per day. A fall in the platelet count is observed within 2 weeks in most patients on this regimen. However, approximately 55 percent may also experience transient, and usually clinically insignificant cytopenias. Hence, this regimen is recommended only when rapid onset of effective myelosuppression is urgent. Some investigators also recommend the use of platelet pheresis in urgent clinical settings where a rapid reduction in platelet count is desired, pending effective myelosuppression with hydroxyurea.

Besides the potential for bone marrow suppression, acute toxicity with hydroxyurea is rare; occasionally patients develop a rash, nausea, oral ulcerations, or fever. To date, hydroxyurea has not been shown to be leukemogenic, and the incidence of leukemic transformation in patients with polycythemia vera treated with hydroxyurea is no greater than in a large group of patients followed by PVSG and treated with phlebotomy alone.

Radioactive Phosphorus

P^{32} has been used for the treatment of polycythemia vera for almost 50 years. Since P^{32} emits beta-rays, which travel short distances, it offers a method of giving localized irradiation in diseases of the bone marrow. Bone has a high inorganic phosphorus content, and it takes up a significant amount of the radioactive isotope. Neoplastic tissue invariably takes up more phosphorus than does the same type of tissue in a normal state of growth, and since the radioactive isotope is built into nucleoprotein just as is naturally occurring P^{31}, cells multiplying at the fastest rate use proportionately more of the P^{32} than do cells that are produced more slowly. Therefore, relatively high concentrations of radioactivity are reached in the organs principally involved in polycythemia vera; the bone marrow and sites of extramedullary hematopoiesis. However, enough radioactive material is taken up by normal tissues and cells to limit the total dosage that can be given without the potential for toxic manifestations.

The beta-particle released by P^{32} produces sufficient radiation effects in the hyperplastic marrow, so that the peripheral blood is normalized in about 80 percent of all cases. Radioactive phosphorus is an effective agent for controlling the clinical symptoms of polycythemia vera, such as fatigability, headache, bone pain, weight loss, and pruritus. About two-thirds of enlarged spleens and livers shrink and many become nonpalpable after treatment.

Therapy with P^{32} is a very convenient method for the patient. Radiation sickness is not associated with its use, and the patient does not have to use a drug whose dosage must be constantly regulated or be subjected to the inconvenience of repeated phlebotomies. One intravenous injection may produce a remission without further therapy for many months or years. The dosage schedule (Figure 4) is as follows: 2.3 mCi per square meter of body surface area, administered intravenously, not to exceed 5 mCi for the first dose. This usually produces a satisfactory remission with normal peripheral blood counts, but if the response is found to be suboptimal in 3 months, a second injection is given, for which the dose may be increased by 25 percent. If, at the expiration of an additional 3 months, remission is still not satisfactory, a third injection at a further 25 percent increase in dose may be administered, not to exceed 7 mCi. Retreatment should be restricted to 6-month intervals thereafter (total yearly dosage of 15 mCi), and supplemental phlebotomies should be used as necessary before and during P^{32} therapy. Complete blood counts should be followed every 2 to 3 months. If there is no response or a minimal effect, other forms of therapy, such as hydorxyurea, must be used. Administering the same inadequate dose of P^{32} repeatedly is ineffective therapy.

Since P^{32} can be an effective therapy and is easy to administer, it would be the ideal therapy for polycythemia vera. However, like chlorambucil, this agent is leukemogenic. Of 134 patients managed with phlebotomy and followed by PVSG, 2 patients developed leukemia; of 141 patients managed with chlorambucil, 24 have developed leukemia or lymphoma; and of 156 patients managed with P^{32}, 18 have developed leukemia, although the peak incidence of acute leukemia in patients treated with P^{32} occurred several years later than that in those treated with chlorambucil. This leukemogenic potential markedly restricts the use of P^{32}, particularly in young patients with potentially long life spans.

GENERAL RECOMMENDATIONS

Based on the observations described here, we believe the best treatment for polycythemia vera in younger patients, with the fewest treatment-associated complications, is phlebotomy. In the elderly (patients over 70), the excessive risk of thrombotic complications

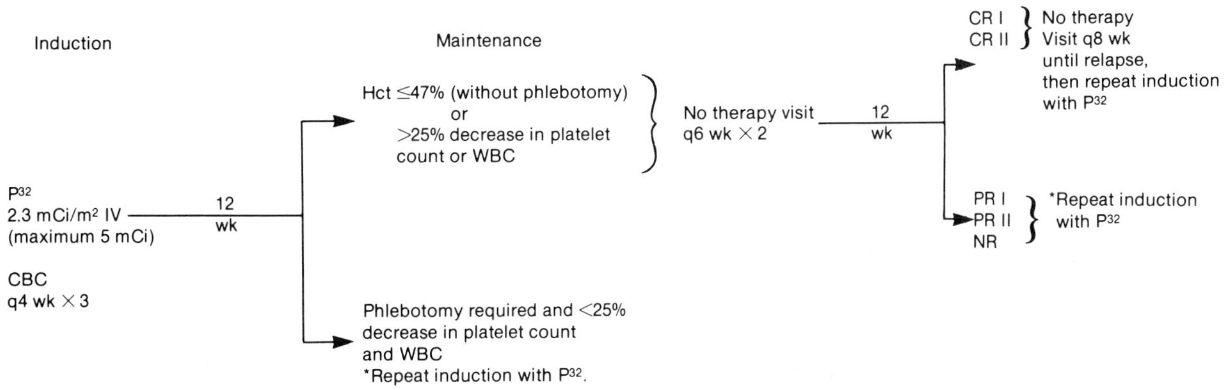

1. Hematocrit to be maintained between 40 and 45 percent by supplementary phlebotomy if necessary.
2. Minimum interval between P^{32} doses is 12 weeks.
3. Second and subsequent doses of P^{32} may be increased by 25 percent of the preceding dose (limit 7 mCi).
4. If after 1 year of incremental doses of P^{32}, response is inadequate, control with phlebotomy alone or hydroxyurea.

Figure 4 Management of polycythemia vera with radioactive phosphorus (P^{32}).

in patients treated with phlebotomy alone requires the addition of a myelosuppressive agent. Hydroxyurea, though effective in this age group, requires stringent monitoring and frequent follow-up, which, in the elderly, may lead to problems in compliance. Because P^{32} has no such compliance-associated problems, and because its mutagenic complications may be delayed a decade or more, P^{32} remains the myelosuppressive treatment of choice in this age group. The agent of choice in younger patients requiring myelosuppression —i.e., those with a history of thrombotic tendencies, high phlebotomy requirement, painful splenomegaly, or other indications for myelosuppression—is hydroxyurea. If the patient cannot be managed successfully with hydroxyurea, then P^{32} may have to be used.

ADJUVANT THERAPY

As part of the comprehensive care of the patient with polycythemia vera, it is necessary to provide treatment of symptoms associated with active disease.

Hyperuricemia

Complications of hyperuricemia, such as acute gout and nephrolithiasis, are a result of increased nucleoprotein breakdown secondary to the accelerated hematopoiesis and can usually be controlled by effective myelosuppressive therapy. However, if the patient is being managed by phlebotomy alone, allopurinol 300 mg per day given orally will control the hyperuricemia. Acute attacks of gout can be managed with colchicine or nonsteroidal anti-inflammatory agents such as naproxen, as required.

Pruritus

Present in about 50 percent of patients with polycythemia vera, pruritus can be generalized and may be made worse by bathing or showering and by brisk rubbing with a towel. It can be a very disturbing symptom in many patients with polycythemia vera. The skin should be patted gently to dry and not rubbed. If myelosuppressive therapy is used, itching frequently subsides as the peripheral blood normalizes. Antihistamines may prove helpful, and H_1 antagonists (cyproheptadine, 4 mg orally three times daily) alone or in combination with H_2 antagonists (cimetidine, 300 mg orally four times daily) have been used. The response to histamine antagonists in patients with pruritus has suggested a role for hyperhistaminemia or some other derangement of histamine metabolism in these patients.

Surgery

Since the majority of patients with polycythemia vera are middle aged or elderly, surgical and dental intervention in these patients frequently becomes necessary. However, such procedures can be dangerous and accompanied by excessively high morbidity and mortality. Because of the expanded blood volume and platelet abnormalities, the difficulties in obtaining effective hemostasis and avoiding thrombotic complications are understandable. A postoperative morbidity of almost 50 percent and a postoperative mortality of 16 percent have been reported in patients with polycythemia vera, compared to a mortality rate of between 2 and 5 percent for major surgery in an age-matched general population. The tendency for adverse complications is directly related to the level of elevation of the hematocrit. Postoperative mortality was seven times greater in uncontrolled patients than in those in whom hematocrit control was achieved. The duration of control is also important; patients had fewer complications when hematologic control was maintained for more than 4 months.

Therefore, in patients with polycythemia vera, elective surgery should not be contemplated unless hematologic control has been achieved for several months. If emergency surgery is necessary, the patient should be phlebotomized until a normal hematocrit is achieved. The intravascular volume should be maintained with intravenous fluids. As part of good postoperative care, these patients should be mobilized as rapidly as possible to avoid thrombotic complications. Dental extractions can also cause excessive bleeding and if possible should be delayed until hematologic control has been achieved.

SUGGESTED READING

Adamson JW, Fialkow PJ, Murphy S, et al. Polycythemia vera. Stem-cell and probable clonal origin of the disease. N Engl J Med 1976; 295:913–916.

Berk PD. In: JB Wyngaarden, LH Smith Jr, eds. Erythrocytosis and polycythemia in Cecil's textbook of medicine, 17th ed. New York: WB Saunders, 1985:963.

Berk PD, Goldberg JD, Donovan PB, et al. Therapeutic recommendations in polycythemia vera based on polycythemia vera study group protocols. Semin Hematol 1986; 23:132–143.

Berk PD, Goldberg JD, Silverstein MN, et al. Increased incidence of acute leukemia in polycythemia vera associated with chlorambucil therapy. N Engl J Med 1981; 304:441–447.

Berlin NI. Diagnosis and classification of the polycythemias. Semin Hematol 1975; 12:339–351.

Donovan PB, Kaplan ME, Goldberg JD, et al. Treatment of polycythemia vera with hydroxyurea. Am J Hematol 1984; 17:329–334.

Tohgi H, Yamanouchi H, Murakami M, et al. Importance of the hematocrit as a risk factor in cerebral infarction. Stroke 1978; 9:369–374.

Wasserman LR, Balcerzak SP, Berk PD, et al. Influence of therapy on causes of death in polycythemia vera. Trans Assoc Am Phys 1981; XCIV:30–38.

Wasserman LR, Gilbert HS. Surgical bleeding in polycythemia vera. Ann NY Acad Sci 1964; 115:122–138.

Willison JR, Thomas DJ, Boulay GH, et al. Effect of high hematocrit on alertness. Lancet 1980; 1:846–848.

Zanjani ED, Lutton JD, Hoffman R, et al. Erythroid colony formation by polycythemia vera bone marrow in vitro. J Clin Invest 1977; 59:841–848.

CHRONIC GRANULOCYTIC LEUKEMIA

ALEXANDER S. D. SPIERS, M.D., Ph.D., F.R.C.P.(E), F.R.A.C.P., F.R.C.Path.A., F.A.C.P.

Chronic granulocytic leukemia (CGL) is a disease of unknown etiology characterized by a pathognomonic peripheral blood picture and the replacement of normal hematopoietic tissue by a monoclonal proliferation of neoplastic cells that possess the Philadelphia (Ph) chromosome, an abnormally foreshortened No. 22 chromosome that results from an unequal but reciprocal translocation between the long arms of chromosomes 9 and 22. Recent major advances in understanding the molecular genetics of CGL have not yet explained its cause or indicated how its management might be improved.

The CGL clone suppresses normal hematopoietic tissue and expands to an extent not seen in the acute leukemias, so that massive splenomegaly and a great increase in the mass of the bone marrow are typical findings. In its initial or chronic phase, CGL behaves like a differentiated neoplasm of bone marrow, producing granulocytes, erythrocytes, and platelets that possess only minor abnormalities and function relatively well. As a result, the infections and hemorrhagic phenomena so typical of the acute leukemias are rarely encountered in the early stages of CGL. In the later stages, best described by the general term metamorphosis, the leukemic cells lose their capacity for differentiation, sometimes in a stepwise fashion, and the manifestations of severe bone marrow failure appear. As a rule, subsequent survival is short.

Conventional therapy for CGL does not result in true remissions of the type seen in the acute leukemias. The dividing cells in the bone marrow remain uniformly Philadelphia chromosome–positive and normal hematopoietic cells do not reappear, and in most instances the marrow remains markedly hypercellular. Treatment reduces the mass of leukemic tissue and corrects organomegaly, thrombocytosis, and anemia, but suppression of the leukemic clone is partial at best. Thus, it is not surprising that although therapy greatly enhances the quality of each patient's life, it produces only a modest increase in its duration. The treatment of CGL is unsatisfactory because it is only palliative, and with the exception of a few patients who undergo bone marrow transplantation, cures are not seen.

INITIAL EVALUATION OF THE PATIENT

The Diagnosis

Details are not discussed here, but it should be pointed out that the diagnosis must be firmly established. Various myeloproliferative disorders and myelodysplastic syndromes are occasionally confused with CGL. Their natural history, prognosis, treatment, and response to therapy are quite different and, in the best interest of the patients, such cases must be recognized at the outset.

Cytogenetic Evaluation

The bone marrow chromosomes should be studied in every patient. Demonstration of the Ph chromosome helps to confirm the diagnosis of CGL. Its absence does not absolutely exclude the diagnosis but mandates its careful review. Molecular genetic techniques are of assistance in further evaluation of the Ph-negative cases. The 9;22 translocation that produces the Ph chromosome results in the formation of an abnormal hybrid gene, *bcr/abl*. Demonstration that *bcr/abl* is present, even in the absence of a visible Ph chromosome, indicates that the leukemia is Ph-positive in genetic and biochemical terms, although not according to light microscopy. At diagnosis, the finding of chromosomal anamolies additional to the Ph chromosome furnishes a warning that the disease may be on the threshold of the refractory state. If cytogenetic studies are repeated at regular intervals after diagnosis, they may continue to serve as an early warning system for an alternation in the behavior of the disease and permit active intervention—for example, with intensive cytotoxic chemotherapy. The value of this latter approach has not yet been conclusively established.

Bone Marrow Biopsy

Biopsy of the bone marrow is not essential for the diagnosis of CGL but is an important part of the initial evaluation. Extensive fibrosis of the marrow generally indicates both a poorer response to therapy and a shorter prognosis. Occasionally, the biopsy indicates the onset of metamorphosis of the disease when this is not apparent from study of the marrow aspirate by revealing islets of proliferating myeloblasts within the more differentiated leukemic tissue.

Other Medical Problems

It is important to identify medical problems that are unrelated to CGL. Many of these (for example, angina, hypertension, rheumatoid arthritis, asthma) have already been diagnosed and are under treatment when the patient is first seen. Other unsuspected conditions may be disclosed in the initial evaluation. Examples I have encountered include diabetes mellitus, primary gout, chronic hepatitis, Crohn's disease, iron deficiency anemia, chronic renal insufficiency, and schizophrenia. These problems may affect both the details of management and the overall prognosis of each patient. Coexistent deficiency of folate or vitamin B_{12} may thoroughly confuse the picture of untreated CGL, tending to lessen the characteristic leukocytosis while aggravating the anemia. The classic hematologic findings may not appear until the hematinic deficiency has been corrected.

Bone Marrow Transplantation

Patients aged 45 years or younger who are without major medical problems other than CGL are potential candidates for bone marrow transplantation if they have a histocompatible sibling. Histocompatibility typing should be arranged for the patient, the siblings and, if possible, the parents. This possibility should be investigated early, since it may affect the subsequent course of management. As techniques and results improve, the potential for transplantation is increasing. Selected patients older than 45 years are candidates in some programs. Siblings who are only partial matches to the patient in terms of histocompatibility typing may sometimes serve as donors, and increasing numbers of transplants utilize matched but unrelated donors obtained through large donor registries. Some patients are clearly ineligible for a transplant, for example, because of advanced years or severe cardiac or pulmonary disease. For many or most other patients, a consultation at a bone marrow transplant center should be sought.

Assessment of Prognosis

Once CGL has entered its refractory phase, survival is uniformly short. As a result, the major determinant of overall survival in this disease is the time that elapses between diagnosis and the onset of the refractory state, i.e., the duration of the chronic phase. Therapy affects this time only to a minor degree. The duration of the chronic phase of CGL varies widely among patients, making accurate prognostication for the individual difficult. Recent studies have shown that certain presenting features of CGL are of prognostic importance. Marked splenomegaly or hepatomegaly, older age, high leukocyte count, a high proportion of immature cells in the blood or bone marrow, thrombocytosis, eosinophilia, and basophilia are all adverse features that may be used to divide patients into high, average, and low risk groups. The median survival rates of these groups are 2, 3.5, and 5 years, respectively. Patients in the high risk group may reasonably be offered marrow transplantation or other investigational therapy at an early stage in their disease.

Cell Harvesting

At presentation, patients with CGL possess large numbers of pluripotential hematopoietic stem cells circulating in the peripheral blood. At some centers, it is routine to collect large numbers of these cells by leukapheresis—a single 4-hour outpatient procedure—and cryopreserve them in liquid nitrogen. The stored stem cells may later be used in several ways, for example, to rescue the patient after rejection of a bone marrow transplant or as a component of treatment for the refractory phase of the disease. Since the procedure carries very little risk, it is a wise precaution.

TREATMENT

General

In the majority of patients, neither blood transfusion nor admission to a hospital is necessary. A complication of the disease, for example, angina or painful splenic infarction, occasionally necessitates inpatient treatment. Unrelated diseases of the cardiovascular system or kidneys require special attention because they may be exacerbated by the hematologic and biochemical abnormalities produced by CGL.

Hyperleukocytosis

In CGL, extreme leukocytosis rarely causes the major problems seen in acute leukemias with comparable leukocyte counts because *the absolute count of blast cells is much lower in CGL.* More mature cells are much less prone to occlude or invade blood vessels and cause complications. When leukocytosis leads to compromise of the cerebral, pulmonary, or retinal circulation, this is best treated by emergency leukapheresis. Such problems are usually associated with a leukocyte count of 600,000 per microliter or greater, whereas in acute myeloid leukemia the corresponding figure is 100,000 per microliter. Leukapheresis should be combined with hydroxyurea, 1 g every 4 hours by mouth, and allopurinol, 600 mg daily, together with hydration. If leukapheresis is not immediately available, the drug therapy alone is effective in 24 to 48 hours.

Hyperuricemia

Moderate hyperuricemia is frequently present at diagnosis of CGL. In patients with renal disease or a gouty diathesis, it may already be causing problems. When treatment is begun, particularly with the rapidly acting agent hydroxyurea, the lysis of leukemic tissue may produce severe hyperuricemia, urate nephropathy, and ureteric calculi. Treatment with allopurinol, 300 mg daily, should begin at the same time as chemotherapy and continue until the leukocyte count falls below 20,000 per microliter. For established hyperuricemia, intravenous hydration and alkalinization of the urine with intravenous bicarbonate and oral acetazolamide, 500 mg every 6 hours, should be combined with allopurinol, 600 mg daily. Hemodialysis is rarely necessary for the initial control of hyperuricemia, although it may be required in patients with preexisting renal disease.

Drug Therapy in Chronic Phase CGL

Although many alkylating agents and antimetabolite drugs are effective, no one is outstandingly better than the others. In particular, no agent consistently produces a median survival time markedly longer than that achieved with busulfan, which has been in use for almost 40 years. For reasons of less toxicity, greater flexibility, and a slightly improved survival, I prefer hydroxyurea for the majority of patients.

Hydroxyurea. The advantages of hydroxyurea are rapid control of the leukocyte count and relatively rapid reversal of the drug's effects, thus minimizing the hazards of overdose. Hydroxyurea also lacks the chronic toxic effects of busulfan (see below). If, at some later stage, aggressive therapy is necessary (for example, bone marrow transplantation or the grafting of cryopreserved autologous stem cells), it will be to the patient's advantage not to have been exposed to busulfan, which is radiomimetic, inflicts permanent tissue damage, and may enhance the sequelae of intensive therapy. In addition, there is evidence that the median survival of patients treated with hydroxyurea is a few months longer than that of patients who receive busulfan. Recent work indicates that treatment with intensive pulses of hydroxyurea is frequently followed by the emergence of Ph-negative (and presumably nonleukemic) cells in the bone marrow. Although there has been no instance of complete and permanent suppression of Ph-positive cells, this finding suggests that hydroxyurea might be used as a component in programs that aim for eradication, rather than mere palliation, of CGL. For example, hydroxyurea might be combined with interferon, which also selectively suppresses Ph-positive cells (see below).

The disadvantages of hydroxyurea include greater cost, the need for continuous therapy and frequent blood counts (every 3 to 4 weeks), and occasional difficulty in finding the dose that will maintain the leukocyte count in the desired range of 5,000 to 10,000 per microliter.

Hydroxyurea is begun at a dose of 1 g twice daily, with concurrent allopurinol and a blood count performed not less than once weekly; the leukocyte count begins to decline in 24 hours or less. The dose is halved when the leukocyte count reaches 20,000 per microliter, and adjustments are then made to secure a stable count below 10,000 per microliter. Most patients require between 1 and 1.5 g daily. Once stability has been secured, a blood count every 3 to 4 weeks is sufficient. Relative resistance to hydroxyurea may arise while CGL remains in its chronic phase, and this is countered by increasing the dose. When CGL enters a refractory phase, more pronounced resistance to hydroxyurea is common. Side effects are uncommon, but they include nausea and stomatitis, especially a painful tongue, and usually occur only at doses exceeding 2 g daily. Less frequent adverse effects are skin rashes, hyperkeratosis of the palms and soles, and disturbed liver function.

Busulfan. Busulfan is the least expensive and most convenient drug therapy for CGL. It is begun at a dose of 3 mg per square meter of body surface area daily, and it is rarely necessary (or wise) to exceed a daily dose of 6 mg. Because the drug has a delayed onset of action, there is no point in fractionating the daily dose. In fact, a single dose of 42 mg every 14 days has effects resembling those of 3 mg daily for 14 days.

When busulfan is administered daily, the leukocyte count may not fall until 10 to 14 days have elapsed and may not cease falling until 2 to 3 weeks after the drug is discontinued. This delay is believed to result from the action of busulfan at a stem cell level in the bone marrow, and for this reason it is wise to interrupt therapy when the leukocyte count falls to 20,000 per microliter and resume it when the count begins to rise once more. When the count stabilizes in the 5,000 to 10,000 range, busulfan is discontinued and the patient observed. Normal platelet count and hemoglobin concentration usually are attained 2 to 6 weeks after correction of the leukocytosis, but splenomegaly resolves more slowly. Resolution of massive splenic enlargement may require 6 or more months and more than one course of busulfan. The duration of response to an initial 4 to 8 week course of busulfan varies widely. Occasional patients require no more busulfan for 24 months, but most require retreatment within 6 to 12 months. It has been recently shown that a high requirement for busulfan (more than 500 mg) in the first year after diagnosis correlates with a shorter chronic phase and shorter overall survival.

The value of closely controlling the leukocyte count has not been proved, although there is some evidence that patients who are re-treated only when the count rises over 100,000 have a shorter survival time. Most physicians prefer to keep the count below 20,000 per microliter. Early in the course of CGL, this may be achieved by intermittent treatment. However, a later increasing requirement for busulfan leads to regular maintenance therapy, which may vary from as little as 4 mg once a week to 2 mg daily. Unlike hydroxyurea, resistance to busulfan is usually associated with a change in the course of CGL; often it is the earliest sign of the onset of metamorphosis. If the requirement for busulfan exceeds 2 mg daily in the long term, it is wise to change to another therapy, since the risk-to-benefit ratio is likely to become unacceptable.

Management of CGL with busulfan has the advantage of a high response rate (approximately 98 percent) and the possibility, in the early stages, of intermittent therapy with relatively few office visits and blood counts. These advantages are substantial when patients live in remote areas. Disadvantages of busulfan include a sustained duration of effect, so that overdose may produce prolonged, life-threatening pancytopenia. The physician should never authorize renewals of prescriptions for busulfan and should prescribe only the amount that the patient requires until the next office visit. Deaths have occurred as a result of failing to observe these simple precautions. Chronic administration of busulfan has numerous adverse effects, including amenorrhea, skin pigmentation, sterility, teratogenesis, and pulmonary fibrosis. Rarely, patients develop a wasting syndrome superficially resembling Addison's disease but without hypoadrenalism. In patients with solid tumors, busulfan therapy has induced acute myeloid leukemia. The risk of this hazard is virtually impossible to measure in patients with CGL because there is a high incidence of conversion to a more acute disorder even when no therapy is given. I prefer to use busulfan when control with hydroxyurea is poor; when no intensive form of therapy is contemplated later in the disease; or when age, infirmity, or geographical considerations dictate a treatment that causes minimal inconvenience for the patient.

Other Drugs in Chronic Phase CGL. Many other agents, including melphalan, cyclophosphamide, uracil mustard, dibromomannitol, desacetylmethyl-colchicine (Colcemid), mercaptopurine, and thioguanine are effective in chronic phase CGL but have no definite advantages over hydroxyurea or busulfan. Mercaptopurine is a useful substitute for hydroxyurea in the few patients who develop skin rashes with that drug. Allopurinol potentiates the action—and the toxic effects—of mercaptopurine by blocking its metabolism by xanthine oxidase, and these two drugs should not be administered together. If the patient must receive allopurinol, thioguanine may be administered because its metabolism is unaffected by the inhibition of xanthine oxidase.

Radiotherapy

Ionizing radiation, most frequently administered to the spleen, has been used since the beginning of this century to control CGL in its chronic phase. Although the clinical and hematologic results are satisfactory in the short term, the inconvenience to the patient and the expense of treatment are greater than those of drug therapy. Further, a randomized comparative study by the British Medical Research Council shows that patients treated by radiotherapy have a median survival rate approximately 1 year shorter than that of patients who receive busulfan. Splenic irradiation is rarely employed now. It can be useful if

CGL is diagnosed and requires treatment in the early stages of pregnancy. With careful shielding of the uterus, the spleen can be irradiated and the disease controlled without injury to the fetus and without recourse to cytotoxic drugs.

IMPROVING THE PROGNOSIS OF CGL

Curing the Disease

Only *bone marrow transplantation* has produced apparent cures of CGL. At present, this treatment is usually restricted to patients aged 45 years or less who have a well-matched sibling donor. Since such CGL patients are in the minority, even curing all of them would not alter the median survival in this disease. The situation will improve if transplantation can be made more available by overcoming some of its risks and complications.

Intensive chemotherapy with multiple drugs can temporarily suppress the Ph-positive leukemic clone, but permanent eradication of the clone and cure of the disease have not been demonstrated. The treatment programs are unpleasant and hazardous, and this approach to treating CGL remains purely investigative.

Prolonging the Chronic Phase

The prognosis of CGL would be improved if the length of its chronic phase could be increased. Controlled trials of *splenectomy* early in the chronic phase of CGL failed to demonstrate prolonged median duration of the chronic phase or prolonged survival. The same negative result follows the use, during the chronic phase, of *pulsed therapy* with drugs that are active in acute lymphocytic leukemia or acute myeloid leukemias. A more promising approach is regular *cytogenic monitoring* of the bone marrow, three to four times a year, and intervention with intensive drug therapy at the earliest sign of clonal evolution (a known harbinger of metamorphosis). This treatment program has not yet been evaluated in a controlled trial and its value is not proved. It would not be helpful in those cases in which metamorphosis (especially the lymphoid variety) is *not* preceded by cytogenetic evolution.

Although *intensive chemotherapy* does not appear to cure CGL, it may increase the duration of the chronic phase, particularly in those patients who possess an adverse prognosis at diagnosis. At present, the evidence to support this is based on historical controls, not on randomized controlled studies, and therefore it must be viewed with caution.

Unfortunately, the prognosis of CGL has improved very little, if at all, since the introduction of busulfan therapy in 1953. During the same period, advances in the management of the acute leukemias threaten to give CGL the worst prognosis of all the more common forms of leukemia.

TREATMENT OF CGL IN METAMORPHOSIS

The general term metamorphosis is used to encompass the wide spectrum of changes that may occur as CGL progresses beyond its chronic phase. Older terms—e.g., blastic crisis—describe only a limited part of that spectrum and are inadequate. The approach to treatment varies with the type of metamorphosis that occurs, the age and general medical status of the patient, and the patient's personal attitude regarding intensive therapy versus purely palliative care.

Accelerated Myeloproliferative Phase

This phase is characterized by the appearance of hematopoietic imbalances. The "cost" of treatment increases—for example, control of the leukocyte count can no longer be achieved without producing anemia or thrombocytopenia. In this phase, *hydroxyurea* or *mercaptopurine* are often of value, whereas busulfan tends to worsen the situation. Many patients require *blood transfusion*, which is rarely necessary when CGL is in its chronic phase. *Splenectomy* is helpful in carefully selected patients with refractory splenomegaly that is symptomatic and/or associated with hypersplenism. In this phase, CGL may mimic many of the characteristics of refractory anemia, myeloid metaplasia, or myelofibrosis. The role of intensive chemotherapy has not been evaluated, but both stem cell autografting and bone marrow transplantation have been successful in patients with CGL in the accelerated myeloproliferative phase. It should be noted that the results of allogeneic bone marrow transplantation are less effective when the procedure is carried out in the accelerated phase rather than the chronic phase of the disease. Administration of interferon is generally ineffective in the accelerated phase but may be useful for control of excessive thrombocytosis.

Metamorphosis to an Acute Leukemia-Like Process (Acute Transformation)

In the *lymphoid* type of acute transformation (identified by cell morphology and cytochemical, immunologic, and enzymatic [TdT] markers), a majority of patients respond to vincristine sulfate with prednisone, and this is the preferred initial therapy. Unfortunately, responses usually last for only a few weeks. Maintenance therapy has been ineffective in prolonging remission, and attempts to induce a further remission are generally unsuccessful. Other stratagems, including bone marrow transplantation, may be employed once a remission has been achieved with vincristine and prednisone. Although approximately 75 percent of patients with lymphoid transformation respond to this therapy, that is only 15 percent of all patients with CGL in acute transformation.

In *myeloid* acute transformation, which is approximately four times more frequent than the lymphoid variety, treatments that are efficacious in acute lymphocytic leukemia are ineffective. Responses to regimens that are highly effective in acute myeloid leukemias are infrequent, usually incomplete, and transient, even when the treatment is very intensive and highly toxic. Exceptions are the eight-drug TRAMPCOL regimen and the more recently studied combinations of high-dose cytosine arabinoside with amsacrine or with mitoxantrone. The TRAMPCOL regimen combines thioguanine, daunorubicin, cytosine arabinoside, methotrexate, prednisolone, cyclophosphamide, vincristine, and asparaginase. It has a 42 percent response rate in myeloid acute transformation of CGL. The median duration of response is only 26 weeks, so the regimen is far from ideal.

In 1986, it was reported that the antitumor antibiotic plicamycin (mithramycin) could control CGL in acute transformation. Low doses of plicamycin appeared to induce maturation of the leukemic blast cells rather than extensive cell killing. Unfortunately, studies at several institutions have failed to reproduce these results. Plicamycin remains of value when advanced CGL, with bone lesions, is complicated by hypercalcemia.

Autografting with Cryopreserved Stem Cells

In terms of patient survival, this palliative treatment is superior to intensive chemotherapy alone. Patients with CGL in metamorphosis receive high-dose chemotherapy, with or without total body irradiation, followed by the intravenous infusion of their own stem cells, harvested and frozen at the time of diagnosis. The aim of the program is to restore the disease to its chronic phase; cure is not a possible outcome. The procedure is of value in younger patients who would be candidates for bone marrow transplantation but who have no suitable donor. Experience with this technique may be summarized as follows: (1) adequate numbers of stem cells are readily obtained and can be stored for long periods without loss of viability; (2) successful engraftment is almost invariable; (3) the technique has been effective in all types of metamorphoses, including those predominantly characterized by myelofibrosis; (4) the procedure is less hazardous than intensive chemotherapy alone; (5) the major limitation has been the variable, but frequently short, duration of the second chronic phase after autografting. This appears to reflect the inadequacy of the ablative chemotherapy for eradicating transformed CGL cells. Recent studies indicate that a *second* autografting procedure, performed electively a few weeks after the first, may increase the duration of the second chronic phase. After an autografting procedure, some patients manifest *Ph-negative* metaphases in the bone marrow. These might originate from the harvested cells that are administered or from cells already in the bone marrow that have been released from homeostatic suppression by the intensive chemotherapy. It is uncertain whether the appearance of Ph-negative cells indicates an improved prognosis.

Palliative Care

The patient with CGL in acute transformation may be successfully palliated for a few weeks by outpatient transfusions of erythrocytes and platelets. Fever and night sweating, common symptoms, may respond to prednisone, but better results are usually obtained with indomethacin, 25 mg four times daily. In the presence of thrombocytopenia, the indomethacin should be accompanied by alkali or cimetidine. Some control of the leukocyte count is desirable to prevent hypermetabolic symptoms and bone pain. The combination of *mercaptopurine* (50 mg three times a day) with *hydroxyurea* (500 mg three times a day) is relatively innocuous and frequently is effective for a few weeks. Painful bone lesions, lymphadenopathy, and painful splenomegaly may benefit from the cautious application of local radiotherapy.

INTERFERON

Recently, it has been reported that alpha interferon, administered daily, will control CGL in its chronic phase. Organomegaly regresses and the blood count may become normal. Of greater interest, Ph-negative cells may appear in the bone marrow, and in some patients the Ph-negative clone becomes completely suppressed, although there is no evidence that it is eradicated. Interferon is not effective in controlling CGL in its refractory phase, and there is no evidence that it can prevent the onset of metamorphosis to a refractory state.

These findings are of great biologic interest, but it is uncertain whether they will be of practical importance. Interferon is an expensive and inconvenient treatment for CGL, especially when compared with a cheap, orally administered agent like busulfan. If the median duration of the chronic phase of CGL is significantly longer when using interferon—this information is not yet available—then the expense, inconvenience, and greater side effects of interferon may be justified. An important and as yet unanswered question is the potential role of interferon followed by intensive drug therapy. If the bone marrow can be rendered Ph-negative with interferon alone, might a multiple-drug regimen then eradicate the Ph-positive clone or reduce its size so substantially that CGL would go into remission for several years? Ongoing results from the first study of interferon in CGL suggest that there is a prolongation of time to metamorphosis and median survival time. If these results are confirmed in the several randomized studies of interferon versus chemotherapy currently in progress, the role of interferon in the management of CGL will require reassessment. The outcome of these studies is awaited with much interest.

CGL is easy to manage in its chronic phase, and the results of treatment are very good in the short term. A major problem is our inability to cure the disease other than in a minority of patients who can undergo bone marrow transplantation. A further problem is the lack of improvement in survival of patients with CGL despite the study of several new treatment strategies. The failure to improve survival is the result of our inability to postpone significantly the onset of the refractory phase of CGL or to prolong survival greatly once that phase has begun. Recent advances in understanding the molecular genetic basis of CGL have not yet produced a superior treatment, but that is a hope for the future.

SUGGESTED READING

Sokal JE, Cox EB, Baccarani M, et al. Prognostic discrimination in "good risk" chronic granulocytic leukemia. Blood 1984; 63:789–799.

Spiers ASD. The clinical features of chronic granulocytic leukaemia. Clin Haematol 1977; 6:77–94.

Spiers ASD. Metamorphosis of chronic granulocytic leukaemia: Diagnosis, classification and management. Br J Haematol 1979; 41:1–5.

Spiers ASD. The management of chronic myelocytic leukemia. In: Henderson ES, Lister TA, eds. Leukemia. Philadelphia: WB Saunders, 1990:515.

Spiers ASD, Goldman JM, Catovsky D, et al. Multiple-drug chemotherapy for acute leukemia. The TRAMPCOL regimen: Results in 86 patients. Cancer 1977; 40:20–28.

Talpaz M, Kantarjian HM, McCredie K, et al. Hematologic remission and cytogenetic improvement induced by recombinant human interferon alpha-A in chronic myelogenous leukemia. N Engl J Med 1986; 314:1065–1069.

CHRONIC LYMPHOCYTIC LEUKEMIA

KANTI R. RAI, M.D., F.A.C.P.

The most common type of leukemia found in a population aged 50 years and over is chronic lymphocytic leukemia (CLL). The classic form of CLL is the B-cell type (B-CLL); only about 5 percent of cases manifest as the T-cell type of CLL or as prolymphocytic leukemia. These latter two variants exhibit certain phenotypic and morphologic characteristics and they are generally not responsive to therapy. However, there are no therapeutic approaches for these variants that are distinct from those applied in B-CLL. This discussion focuses on management of patients with B-CLL. As is the case with many other malignancies, approach to treatment differs considerably in different centers. The treatment plan practiced in my clinic is detailed here.

OBSERVATION PHASE

It is our practice not to institute any cytotoxic therapy immediately upon making a diagnosis of CLL. A period of observation after diagnosis is advisable to determine if any treatment is indicated.

Clinical Staging of Chronic Lymphocytic Leukemia

It is first necessary to establish the clinical stage of a patient newly diagnosed as having CLL. The criteria of staging are as follows:

Stage 0. This stage manifests only with lymphocytosis in the peripheral blood and the bone marrow. Although an absolute lymphocyte count of 5,000 per cubic millimeter is an acceptable definition of lymphocytosis in peripheral blood, in most instances this count is over 15,000. Bone marrow aspirate must show 30 percent or more mature-appearing lymphocytes upon differential count of all nucleated cells, or a biopsy specimen must show lymphocytic infiltration.

Stage I. This stage exhibits lymphocytosis with evidence of enlarged lymph nodes.

Stage II. This stage exhibits lymphocytosis with evidence of enlargement of the spleen and/or the liver. Lymph nodes may or may not be enlarged.

Stage III. This stage is characterized by lymphocytosis with anemia (hemoglobin < 11 g per deciliter). The nodes, spleen, and liver may or may not be enlarged.

Stage IV. This stage exhibits lymphocytosis with thrombocytopenia (platelets $< 100{,}000$ per cubic millimeter). Anemia and enlargement of nodes, spleen, and liver may or may not be present.

When we examine the actuarial survival curves of patients with CLL, we recognize that there are three distinct patterns rather than five. Therefore, in accordance with the survival curves, I recently recommended that stage 0 be called low-risk group, stages I and II combined be called intermediate-risk group, and stages III and IV combined be called high-risk group. This modified Rai staging system is being used in all clinical trials in the United States.

After the clinical stage is determined, I try to find out if symptoms (e.g., weakness, weight loss, night sweats, fever, and increased susceptibility to infections) are present. In addition, blood counts are serially monitored at intervals of 2 to 4 weeks.

INDICATIONS FOR THERAPEUTIC INTERVENTION

After an observation period of about 4 to 6 months, during which time the patient is seen regularly in the clinic, a decision is made about whether therapeutic intervention is necessary. I use the following indications as guidelines and institute therapy if any one of these is present:

1. Progressive disease-related symptoms.
2. Evidence of progressive marrow failure (i.e., worsening anemia, thrombocytopenia, and recurrent sepsis associated with hypogammaglobulinemia).
3. Autoimmune hemolytic anemia or immune thrombocytopenia.
4. Massive splenomegaly with or without evidence of hypersplenism.
5. "Bulky" disease, as evidenced by large lymphoid masses.
6. Progressive hyperlymphocytosis. The rate of increase of blood lymphocyte count is a more persuasive indicator than the absolute number. I generally do not withhold therapy when the count is higher than 150,000 per cubic millimeter. Leukostasis, which is associated with a high leukocyte count in other leukemias, is seldom encountered in CLL, but complications from hyperviscosity syndrome from hyperleukocytosis have been reported in CLL.

On rare occasion, however, the patient is markedly symptomatic at the time of initial diagnosis of CLL. It may not be advisable to withhold therapy under such a circumstance. I do not go through an observation period but institute therapy immediately in these patients.

THERAPEUTIC PLAN FOR SPECIFIC INDICATIONS

Progressive Disease-Related Symptoms

Usually such symptoms are controlled with chlorambucil and prednisone. I prefer to give intermittent bursts of treatment at intervals of 3 to 4 weeks rather than to treat by continuous daily regimens throughout the month. Chlorambucil is given, 0.7 mg per kilogram by mouth in a single dose on day 1, day 28, and so forth. Prednisone is given, 0.5 mg per kilogram by mouth, in one dose or divided in two doses daily for 7 days (days 1 through 7) in each monthly cycle. Concomitantly, allopurinol, 300 mg daily by mouth, is prescribed for 7 days of each cycle. Usually, symptoms (e.g., weakness, night sweats, fever) are controlled within 6 to 8 months after institution of therapy, at which time such therapy may be discontinued and the observation phase resumed.

Evidence of Progressive Marrow Failure

Progressive marrow failure is treated in the same manner as detailed above, by intermittent chlorambucil and prednisone.

Autoimmune Hemolytic Anemia or Immune Thrombocytopenia

Prednisone alone is given for these complications. Prednisone is started at 0.8 mg per kilogram per day by mouth for 2 weeks, and if the anemia or the thrombocytopenia has started to improve, the prednisone dose is reduced by 50 percent at each 2-week interval for an overall continuous therapy time of 6 weeks' duration. Thereafter, prednisone may be given for 1 week every month at 0.5 mg per kilogram per day for an additional 4- to 6-month period.

It should be emphasized that patients with CLL are generally elderly people with a somewhat high incidence of diabetes mellitus. Therefore, special attention must be given to the control of hyperglycemia, which may be exaggerated with prednisone therapy.

Massive Splenomegaly With or Without Evidence of Hypersplenism

Radiation therapy of the spleen is our first choice of treatment. Usually total doses of between 250 and 1,000 rad, delivered in 5 to 10 fractions, are adequate to reduce spleen size and control hypersplenism. However, if there is inadequate control with radiation therapy or the spleen again enlarges to significant proportions or hypersplenism remains a major problem, splenectomy is advisable. Even elderly patients (with good cardiopulmonary status) withstand this surgery without undue morbidity. However, it should be noted that if massive splenomegaly is not a solitary feature of a patient's disease (i.e., if adenopathy of a significant degree is also present), chemotherapy should be the initial therapeutic choice. If hypersplenism and splenomegaly persist after an adequate trial, splenic irradiation or splenectomy should be considered.

"Bulky" Disease of Large Lymphoid Masses

Most often chlorambucil therapy (without prednisone) at the dosage already detailed is adequate to reduce the size of large lymphoid masses. Such therapy is usually necessary for a period of 1 to 2 years on an intermittent monthly schedule. However, if the lymphoid masses are not generalized but are present at only one or two sites, or such masses are causing or likely to cause symptoms by pressing on adjacent vital organs (e.g., on a bronchus or the superior vena cava), local irradiation therapy is recommended. The total dose necessary under these circumstances ranges between 500 and 1,500 rad delivered in 5 to 15 fractions.

Progressive Hyperlymphocytosis

Usually chlorambucil at the dosage already detailed is adequate to reduce the blood lymphocyte count. If resources are available, it is recommended that leukapheresis be the first step in therapy when the starting blood count is in excess of 600,000 per cubic millimeter; chlorambucil therapy is initiated immediately after three to four treatments on a cell-separator machine. Side effects of chlorambucil are usually mild nausea and minimal suppression of bone marrow function. Allopurinol should always be added while treating hyperlymphocytosis.

THERAPEUTIC GUIDELINES BASED ON CLINICAL STAGING

Low-Risk Group (Stage 0). Patients in this stage are generally without any symptoms, and no cytotoxic agent is prescribed. However, patients should be seen in the clinic at intervals of 1 to 3 months. Median life expectancy is in excess of 12 years.

Intermediate-Risk Group (Stages I and II) A. Asymptomatic. There is no evidence that cytotoxic therapy is necessary or beneficial in these patients. I continue to observe them at monthly intervals. The median life expectancy of these patients ranges between 6 and 8 years and is probably not changed with therapy.

Intermediate-Risk Group (Stages I and II) B. Symptomatic. I recommend chlorambucil on an intermittent, monthly schedule at the dosage already detailed. The median life expectancy of these patients is about 5 years. It is not yet known whether therapy increases life expectancy.

High-Risk Group (Stages III and IV). Patients in these stages have a median life expectancy of 1.5 years. I give chlorambucil and prednisone to these patients as per the dosage already detailed. The therapeutic objective is to achieve a partial or a complete remission (CR). Usually it takes 8 to 10 months of therapy to achieve a partial remission. Patients achieving either a CR or a partial remission have prolongation of median survival time to about 5 years, whereas those patients achieving less than a partial remission have a 1.5-year median survival.

Alternative to Chlorambucil

I use cyclophosphamide in lieu of chlorambucil if the patient cannot tolerate the latter drug or is no longer showing a satisfactory response to it. Cyclophosphamide is administered by mouth or by intravenous injection. The dose of cyclophosphamide, on intermittent schedule, is 200 mg per square meter per day by mouth for 5 days in cycles that repeat at 3-week intervals or 750 mg per square meter on day 1 by intravenous injection every 3 weeks. Toxicity of this drug consists of controllable nausea and vomiting, hair loss, bone marrow suppression, and chemical cystitis.

Second-Line Therapy

When single-agent therapy (chlorambucil or cyclophosphamide) with or without prednisone fails to control CLL-related problems, we resort to combination chemotherapy. These are combinations that are usually administered in treatment of non-Hodgkin's lymphoma or multiple myeloma, e.g., cyclophosphamide, vincristine, and prednisone (COP), COP with doxorubicin (CHOP) and COP with carmustine (BCNU), and melphalan (M-2 protocol). The dosages utilized in each drug combination are decided on after considering each patient's bone marrow reserve, previous exposure to and level of tolerance of cytotoxic therapy, and the overall medical status.

Assessment of Therapeutic Response

I define a CR when there are no symptoms and no abnormal findings on physical examination, and hemogram and bone marrow study reveal normal values. If all these criteria are fulfilled but serum immunoglobulin levels are still lower than normal or there is persistence of increased B lymphocytes, I would rate such a response as a CR. Achievement of even such a CR is a rather unusual occurrence in CLL, and it is my belief that our target must be to increase the incidence of CR according to this clinical definition before we can aim to achieve a CR that would include normalization of immune function and lymphocyte subpopulations ratios as well. A partial remission is defined as a 50 percent decrease in absolute lymphocyte count in peripheral blood, hemoglobin more than 11 g per deciliter, platelets more than 100,000 per cubic millimeter, or improvement in these values by 50 percent of their deviation from normal and decrease in palpable lymph nodes and spleen by at least 50 percent.

SUPPORTIVE THERAPY

In order to control signs and symptoms of anemia, transfusion of packed red cells is given as supportive therapy. Transfusions of platelets and granulocytes are rarely given in CLL. High-dose gamma globulin therapy by intravenous route, 400 mg per kilogram body weight every 21 days, is of benefit to those patients who have marked hypogammaglobulinemia or have recurrent bacterial infections. There are no contraindications to giving pneumococcal vaccine or flu vaccine, but the usefulness of such vaccines is in doubt in patients with CLL. Analogues of androgens have been effective on a few occasions by stimulating erythropoiesis in patients with significant anemia. However, such therapy may be associated with adverse side effects of hepatotoxicity, fluid retention, exacerbation of symptoms of prostatic hypertrophy in men, and masculinizing effects in women. I have observed beneficial responses to cyclosporine therapy in those patients with CLL whose severe anemia is found to be from pure red cell aplasia.

TERMINAL PHASE

In CLL, death occurs most often from infectious complications secondary to disease-induced or therapy-induced neutropenia and immunodeficiency. Complications are especially difficult to control in advanced stages of CLL. The next most common causes of morbidity and mortality are bleeding complications, hepatic failure, and inanition and wasting. On rare occasions, CLL is transformed into a large cell lymphoma (Richter's syndrome) or a prolymphocytoid cell leukemia. Such cases receive aggressive chemotherapy generally used in high-grade lymphoma, but there is little evidence that any regimen is effective in prolonging life. Even less frequently, CLL transforms into acute myelocytic leukemia, which is also refractory to intensive therapy that is currently used successfully in de novo acute leukemia.

Supported by grants from Aaron Diamond Foundation, Helena Rubinstein Foundation, Denis Klar Leukemia Fund, Rosenstiel Foundation, Doyle Dane Bernbach, National Leukemia Foundation, United Leukemia Fund, and Wayne Goldsmith Leukemia Fund.

ACUTE LYMPHOBLASTIC LEUKEMIA

ANDREW D. JACOBS, M.B., B.S.M.D., M.R.C.P.
ROBERT P. GALE, M.D., Ph.D.

Acute lymphoblastic leukemia (ALL) is a hematologic malignancy characterized by an uncontrolled proliferation of immature lymphocytes and their progenitors. Although ALL is most common in children, a substantial proportion of cases occur in adolescents and adults. Recently, there has been considerable progress in the treatment of children with the disease, with cure rates of 50 to 70 percent reported in several large studies. Progress in the treatment of adults with ALL has been more difficult to achieve, with recent studies reporting 30 to 40 percent disease-free survival at up to 5 years of follow-up.

CLASSIFICATION

Both morphologic and immune features are used to classify patients with ALL. The French-American-British (FAB) morphologic classification of ALL recognized three types of lymphoblasts termed L1, L2, and L3. Adults have a predominance of L2 lymphoblasts. Such cells are typically large, with an irregular nuclear outline; the nucleus may be clefted and contain one or more large nucleoli. The cytoplasm is deeply basophilic and may be abundant. The L3 morphology, resembling Burkitt's lymphoma, is occasionally present in adults with ALL.

A second approach to the classification of adult ALL is based on the immune features of the leukemic cells. Currently, subtypes include the common (50 percent), T (15 percent), B (5 percent), and null phenotypes (30 percent). Recent data suggest that in some cases of null cell ALL, the cells may represent mecloid or hybrid leukemias rather then typical ALL. If correct, this may explain the poor response of patients with this subtype to chemotherapy designed for ALL.

CHROMOSOMES

Recent data indicate that up to two-thirds of adults with ALL have chromosome abnormalities. Up to 25 percent of adults with ALL have the Philadelphia (Ph^1) chromosome [t(9;22) (q34;q11)]. Patients with the L3 form of ALL have a high frequency of the t(8;14) translocation. Less common translocations involving chromosomes 8 and either 2 or 22 are found t(2;8) and t(8;22). There have been several reports of the t(4;11) translocation in both patients with ALL and those with hybrid leukemias. Overall, patients with chromosomal abnormalities have a worse prognosis.

PROGNOSIS

Studies correlating FAB subtype with prognosis consistently indicate the poor prognosis of patients with the L3 subtype. However, data concerning the prognosis of patients with the L1 and L2 are less clear. The incidence of central nervous system (CNS) and intra-abdominal involvement is particularly high with the L3 subtype. Data from several studies of adults with ALL suggest that those with the common and T cell phenotypes have the best prognosis; the results of treatment in these patients have approached those in children receiving identical therapy. As already indicated, the results of cytogenetic studies suggest that adults with chromosome abnormalities have a worse prognosis. Over 70 percent of adults with a normal karyotype have remissions with conventional therapy compared to 45 percent of those with chromosomal abnormalities. More studies suggest that increasing age is associated with a worse prognosis, particularly for patients over the age of 35. Other factors reported to influence remission duration include white blood cell (WBC) count at presentation (over 30×10^9 per liter per millimeter cubed), time to achieve complete remission, (greater than 4 weeks) and initial presentation with central nervous system leukemia. Definitive conclusions about the prognostic value of those findings must await prospective data on similarly treated patients.

SUPPORTIVE THERAPY

Most adults with ALL present with some combination of anemia, granulocytopenia with fever, and thrombocytopenia with bleeding. Disseminated intravascular coagulation is unusual. Transfusions of packed red cells should be given to maintain the hematocrit at or near 30 percent. Physical examination should be performed, and chest x-ray studies and blood and urine cultures should be obtained. Intravenous broad spectrum antibiotics should be started immediately in granulocytopenic patients (granulocytes less than 0.5×10^9) with fever. A suitable combination is an aminoglycoside together with a synthetic penicillin. A third generation cephalosporin may be used in patients allergic to penicillin. Platelet transfusions are commonly recommended in patients with bleeding or for those with platelets less than 20×10^9 per liter.

Other commonly used supportive measures include use of antibacterial soaps and shampoos, careful attention to oral hygiene, and the use of antibiotics that modify or sterilize the gastrointestinal tract. Examples are co-trimoxazole or a combination of vancomycin, polymyxin B, and nystatin. Co-trimoxazole is also recommended for patients with ALL who are undergoing corticosteroid therapy and who are at increased risk of developing infection with *Pneumocystis carinii*. Patients presenting with a high WBC count (over 30×10^9 per liter) or organomegaly should also be treated with allopurinol, 300 mg per day, to prevent deposition of urate in the renal tubules during therapy. Allopurinol may be discontinued when the WBC count is reduced or organomegaly has resolved.

INDUCTION THERAPY

The optimal remission induction therapy in adult ALL is controversial. Three trials involving 103 patients treated with vincristine and prednisone reported response rates of 46 to 66 percent. Many studies have used vincristine, prednisone, an anthracycline (daunorubicin or doxorubicin), and sometimes L-asparaginase. Response rates of 70 to 79 percent are reported in most of these series. We favor a combination of prednisone, vincristine, and daunorubicin as shown in Table 1. Patients so treated have pancytopenia for 21 to 28 days and require intensive transfusions and antibiotics during this time. Response status should be evaluated by day 28. As indicated, 70 to 80 percent of patients are expected to achieve remission with this approach. For those patients who do not achieve remission, we repeat this treatment with the addition of L-asparaginase, 10,000 units every other day for 10 days.

CENTRAL NERVOUS SYSTEM PROPHYLAXIS

The incidence of CNS relapse in childhood ALL has been reduced from 50 percent to 5 percent with cranial irradiation (24 Gy) and intrathecal methotrexate. Uncontrolled studies show that this same regimen is effective in adults. We give intrathecal methotrexate in doses of 8 mg per meter squared twice weekly for six doses during the course of prophylactic cranial radiation. The latter usually consists of twelve 2-Gy fractions.

Two additional methods of prophylaxis have been reported for adults. In one study, intrathecal methotrexate alone was reported to be as effective as the combination of intrathecal methotrexate with cranial irradiation. In those patients with a high risk of developing CNS leukemia (those presenting with a WBC over 30×10^9 per liter), it has been recommended that intrathecal methotrexate be delivered via an Ommaya reservoir. This may result in higher cerebrospinal fluid methotrexate levels. Others have found high dose intravenous methotrexate (100 to 300 mg per kilogram) with folic acid rescue to be effective in preventing CNS relapse in adults with ALL. In view of the expense and potential toxicity of this approach and the reported high complication rate associated with the Ommaya reser-

TABLE 1 ALL Induction Therapy

Drug	*Dose*	*Days*
Prednisone	80 mg	1–28
Vincristine	0.75 mg/m^2	1, 8, 15, 22
Daunorubicin	40 mg/m^2	1, 2, 3

voir and those not accustomed to placing them, we recommend the more proven combination of cranial irradiation and intrathecal methotrexate by lumbar puncture. Use of high dose cytarabine systemically may also afford some benefit in preventing CNS leukemia.

POSTINDUCTION THERAPY

There are limited data available regarding the role of consolidation-intensification therapy in adults with ALL. The available data suggest that adults with ALL who receive intensive postinduction therapy, including consolidation-intensification and maintenance therapy, have the longest remissions. Approaches that have been used include a combination of teniposide and cytarabine, and the administration of high doses of cytarabine (6–12 doses of 2 g per meter squared 12 hourly). These approaches have not shown any benefit. Perhaps the best results are reported by Clarkson and co-workers at Memorial Hospital and by Hoelzer co-workers, who utilize complex combinations of drugs. A simpler approach is to repeat courses of vincristine and prednisone as in induction therapy, but with a lower dose of daunorubicin (25 mg per meter squared) given once weekly for 3 weeks instead of on 3 consecutive days. This is usually less myelosuppressive and may avoid life-threatening bone marrow failure. These courses may be given at 3-month intervals, with standard maintenance therapy consisting of methotrexate and 6-mercaptopurine between courses. This alternative approach is summarized in Table 2. It should be emphasized that the value of these interventions is, as yet, unproven in adults with ALL.

TABLE 2 ALL Postinduction Therapy

Drug	*Dose*	*Days*
Prednisone	80 mg	1–28
Vincristine	0.75 mg/m^2	1, 8, 15, 22
Daunorubicin	25 mg/m^2	1, 8, 15

Repeat these cycles every 3 months with 6-mercaptopurine 1.5 to 2.5 mg/kg/day by mouth and methotrexate 15 mg/m^2/week by mouth between cycles.

The optimal duration of chemotherapy in adult ALL is not yet known. Most relapses occur within the first 1 to 2 years following remission. Most data support continuing intensive therapy for at least 2 years. With this approach, 5-year disease-free survival rates of 35 to 45 percent may be achieved.

In view of the relatively low incidence of adult ALL and the paucity of data on therapeutic guidelines, we strongly recommend that such patients be entered into prospective studies wherever possible.

SUGGESTED READING

Hoelzer D, Thiel E, Loffler H, et al. Intensified therapy in acute lymphoblastic and acute undifferentiated leukemia in adults. Blood 1984; 64:38–47.

Omura G, Raney M. Long-term survival in adult acute lymphoblastic leukemia: follow-up of a Southwestern Cancer Study Group trial. J Clin Oncol 1985; 3:1053–1058.

Schauer P, Arlin ZA, Merkelsmann R, et al. Treatment of acute lymphoblastic leukemia in adults: results of the L-10 and L-10M protocols. J Clin Oncol 1983; 1:462–470.

ACUTE NONLYMPHOCYTIC LEUKEMIA

PETER H. WIERNIK, M.D.

Although acute nonlymphocytic leukemia (ANLL) is a fatal illness for most patients, more than 60 percent achieve a complete remission with appropriate therapy, and the median duration of the disease-free state in most studies varies from 1 to 2 years. Approximately 30 percent of complete remitters remain in first complete remission for 5 years or more. Late relapses, although uncommon, do occur.

Acute leukemia treatment requires an experienced team of clinicians supported by special laboratories and blood banks, and should not be attempted by those not fully versed in its ramifications.

PRETREATMENT CONSIDERATIONS

The patient with ANLL requires a complete physical and laboratory examination prior to chemotherapy. It is important to classify precisely the ANLL by routine examination of blood and bone marrow, by histochemical definition of the leukemic cells, by immunophenotyping of those cells, and by karyotypic analysis. Certain variants of ANLL have a poor prognosis, such as acute megakaryocytic leukemia; some have a relatively good prognosis, such as those associated with +(8;21) on inversion of chromosome 16; and some are often associated with complications that, if unrecognized, may lead to death before an adequate trial of chemotherapy can be given. For instance, acute promyelocytic leukemia, which has a characteristic translocation involving chromosomes 15 and 17, is often associated with a consumptive coagulopathy that may become lethal during treatment if unrecognized.

The cerebrospinal fluid must be examined by lumbar puncture in patients with acute myelomonocytic or monocytic leukemia, especially if the leukemia is associated with an inversion of chromosome 16. Such patients have a relatively high incidence of occult meningeal leukemia. Lumbar puncture should be performed only after a successful platelet transfusion in thrombocytopenic patients.

A coagulation profile must be obtained in any ANLL patient with the morphology of acute promyelocytic leukemia or acute monocytic leukemia, or a translocation involving chromosomes 15 and 17. In addition, if eccymoses are present, a clotting profile should be examined. Such patients may have a consumptive coagulopathy, the hallmarks of which are low fibrinogen and increased fibrin degradation products. If the fibrinogen concentration is 100 mg or less, the patient should receive low dose heparin therapy, even in the absence of clinical bleeding. Give heparin as a continuous infusion at the rate of 50 units per kilogram per day. Measure plasma fibrinogen every 12 hours, and double the rate of heparinization if the fibrinogen has fallen below the preheparinization level after 24 hours of treatment. Continue heparin until the bone marrow is hypocellular.

Patients who are dangerously thrombocytopenic (platelet count less than 20,000 per microliter) require prophylactic platelet transfusion. In general, previously untransfused patients respond to random donor platelets. However, previously pregnant women may not respond, despite the lack of a transfusion history. Such patients may require human leukocyte antigen (HLA) matched platelet transfusions obtained from a sibling, parent, child, or platelet donor registry. Patients with circulating lymphocytes should have HLA typing performed prior to treatment for immediate or future reference. Patients who may be considered for allogeneic bone marrow transplantation should not receive blood products from the potential donor(s) to minimize the possibility of marrow rejection.
assessed by determining the 1-hour post-transfusion corrected count increment (CCI) from the formula:

$$CCI = \frac{\text{absolute platelet count increment} \times \text{BSA}}{\text{no. platelets transfused} \times 10^{11}}$$

A CCI greater than 10 indicates a successful transfusion. A CCI of less than 10 usually indicates alloimmunization and requires that another donor source of platelets be obtained.

Approximately one-third of ANLL patients who achieve complete remission become alloimmunized to random donor platelets in the process. Those patients will not be able to undergo intensive postremission therapy safely without a source of platelet transfusion from other than random donor pools. The usual platelet source in such cases is an HLA compatible donor. However, less expensive and more reliable sources are the patients themselves. Once the platelet count has become normal, alloimmunized patients may be plateletpheresed on multiple occasions prior to and between postremission treatments. The pheresed platelets are banked in dimethyl sulfoxide (DMSO) at liquid nitrogen temperature. The platelets can then be reinfused during postremission therapy.

A febrile granulocytopenic patient must be considered infected until proven otherwise. Temperature should be monitored every 4 hours before and during treatment until the granulocyte count has risen above 1,500 per microliter. Any fever should trigger a careful examination for the source of infection, and cultures should be taken of blood, sputum, throat and the perianal area. Even if no source of infection is found, empiric antibiotic therapy should be started, after appropriate cultures have been taken. Cefaperazone plus an aminoglycoside antibiotic can be used for this purpose. The regimen provides excellent *Pseudomonas* coverage and provides adequate coverage for *Staphylococcus epidermidis*. The former is a frequent cause of septic death in leukemia patients, and the latter has become increasingly important as a cause of infection in leukemia patients with central venous access catheters. Empiric antibiotics should be continued until culture results warrant modification, or if there is no improvement after 4 days. If there is clinical improvement and the patient becomes afebrile, the regimen should be given for a full 10 days. If after 4 days, the patient is still febrile but does not clinically appear to have a progressive infection and cultures have been unhelpful, antibiotics should be stopped at midnight of the fourth day and cultures should be taken the next morning. Examine the patient for clinical deterioration and a source of infection every 2 to 4 hours throughout the fifth day. If there has been no response to the empiric antibiotic regimen by the fourth day and the patient appears ill, start empiric amphotericin B therapy and continue the antibacterial antibiotics. Empiric antifungal therapy is especially valid if there has been a prolonged period of granulocytopenia, which is the factor most associated with fungal infection in leukemia patients.

Oral prophylactic antibiotics are often used in an effort to prevent infection in ANLL, although not all authorities agree on their efficacy. Trimethoprim-sulfamethoxazole plus nystatin are commonly used for this purpose. The former is given as 160 mg trimethoprim plus 800 mg sulfamethoxazole twice daily, beginning before induction chemotherapy and continuing until the granulocyte count is greater than 1,500 per microliter. Nystatin oral suspension, 1 million units is given every 4 hours during the same period of time. The patient should swash the nystatin around the mouth for several minutes and then swallow it. Once oral antibiotic prophylaxis is begun, it must not be discontinued while the patient is granulocytopenic unless broad spectrum parenteral antibiotics have been administered. Discontinuation of oral prophylactic antibiotics prematurely in the absence of other antibiotic therapy will almost certainly result in sepsis.

Uric acid production must be controlled in order to prevent urate nephropathy. All ANLL patients should receive allopurinol, 300 mg per day, for at least 36 hours before starting chemotherapy, if possible. The treatment should continue until the bone marrow is normocellular or hypocellular. If it is not possible to delay induction therapy for 36 hours, or if the patient has extreme leukocytosis (WBC greater than 100,000 per microliter), or if the serum acid is elevated, the urine should be alkalinized during allopurinol administration. This can be accomplished by bicarbonate administration during the day and acetazolamide, 500 mg given orally, nightly.

INDUCTION CHEMOTHERAPY

The most widely used regimen for the initial treatment of previously untreated patients with ANLL is a combination of cytarabine and daunorubicin. The former is given as a continuous intravenous 7-day infusion at the rate of 100 mg per meter squared per day, and the latter is given as a bolus intravenous injection of 45 mg per meter squared daily on each of the first 3 days of the cytarabine infusion. Care must be taken not to extravasate daunorubicin, which is a strong vesicant that can cause profound soft tissue necrosis. Injecting the drug into a running infusion through an indwelling venous catheter maximizes safety.

Approximately 65 percent of adults with ANLL achieve a complete remission with this regimen. Most responders do so after one course of treatment, but a minority of patients require two courses. If a complete response is not achieved after two courses, switch to a regimen for refractory patients rather than give a third course of the same drugs, since success with the latter approach is rare.

There is an inverse relationship between patient age and success of induction therapy. Patients over the age of 65 have a higher death rate during treatment than do younger patients, probably due more to an inability of elderly patients to withstand the toxicity of treatment rather than an intrinsic difference in leukemic cell drug sensitivity. For this reason, some have advocated less intensive therapy with low dose cytarabine for remission induction in patients of advanced age. The complete response rate with this regimen is lower than that observed with standard therapy, and toxicity with the low dose regimen as measured by frequency of infectious complications, transfusion requirement, and duration of hospitalization is comparable to that of standard therapy. Therefore, elderly patients desiring treatment should be offered standard therapy.

Pancytopenia occurs 3 to 7 days after beginning standard induction therapy, and the marrow usually becomes severely hypoplastic 7 to 10 days later. Marrow recovery and subsequent blood count normalization generally occur during the third or fourth week. The platelet count usually rises before the granulocyte count, and anemia resolves last.

Rarely, complete remission occurs without bone marrow hypocellularity resulting from treatment. This is especially true in patients with acute promyelocytic leukemia.

After successful induction therapy, a normal marrow usually regenerates. Occasionally, the marrow may become repopulated with blasts before evidence of normal marrow differentiation is obtained. Such a marrow may be incorrectly interpreted as leukemic, and another induction course may be contemplated. It is of paramount importance to distinguish between a normally regenerating marrow and a regenerating leukemic marrow. If the marrow examination demonstrates blasts but is hypocellular and associated with a rising platelet count, the marrow is probably regenerating normally. This can be confirmed with another examination 2 to 3 days later when clear evidence of normal marrow maturation and differentiation should be seen. If the marrow is regenerating leukemia, a more cellular marrow devoid of normal maturation and differentiation will be evident. The first post-treatment marrow examination should occur after the platelet count has risen. Treatment decisions based on examining the marrow at some fixed time, such as post-treatment day 8, may lead to inappropriate and potentially lethal additional induction therapy.

The platelet count may begin to rise after induction therapy only to level off or fall over the next few days. This may represent unsuccessful induction therapy which can be confirmed by observing a frankly leukemic marrow. On the other hand, the marrow may suggest evolving remission. In that circumstance, folic acid administration, 1 to 5 mg per day intravenously, may result in a normal bone marrow and normal blood counts in 7 to 10 days. Some elderly acute leukemia patients become folate depleted during induction therapy due to poor food intake or trimethoprim administration. Delayed peripheral blood count recovery may also result from the administration of certain antibiotics such as amphotericin B or trimethoprim. When both of those agents are given, granulocyte recovery may be seriously delayed.

High dose cytarabine alone or in combination with such experimental agents as amsacrine may induce complete remission in 30 to 40 percent of patients who are refractory to initial treatment. In such regimens, cytarabine is given at a dose of 3 g per meter squared as a 1-hour intravenous infusion every 6 hours for a total of 12 doses. Recently, superior results in refractory patients have been reported with high dose cytarabine in combination with the experimental agent mitoxantrone. Those data need to be confirmed.

Relapsed patients have been treated in a variety of ways with varying success. Patients who have had an initial complete remission for at least a year have a 50 to 60 percent chance of obtaining a second complete remission when retreated with the regimen initially used to obtain the first remission. However, those patients are also candidates for other approaches, as are all patients with shorter initial remissions. High dose cytarabine treatment alone or with other agents results in a second complete remission rate of greater than 60 percent in patients under the age of 55, whereas older patients have a poorer result and sustain considerably more toxicity in the process. Standard dose cytarabine given as described above for initial induction therapy and combined with three daily doses of the experimental agent mitoxantrone (8 mg per meter squared daily) also results in a second complete remission rate of greater than 60 percent in younger relapsed patients. In addition, that treatment is almost as successful in older patients at a cost of much less toxicity than commonly observed with high dose cytarabine. This regimen results in less gastrointestinal toxicity and less alopecia than cytarabine-daunorubicin, but marrow recovery is somewhat delayed with the former compared with the latter. About 15 percent of patients who respond to reinduction therapy with cytarabine-mitoxantrone have second remissions significantly longer than the first. With most other chemotherapy regimens, second remissions are virtually always significantly shorter than the first.

Allogeneic bone marrow transplantation is infrequently successful when performed during relapse. However, as many as 20 percent of relapsed patients have achieved a second complete remission of significant duration by this method. The procedure requires the availability of an HLA compatible donor and is currently recommended only for relapsed patients less than 40 years old.

POSTREMISSION THERAPY

Most investigators agree that postremission therapy prolongs disease-free and overall survival in adult ANLL, although occasional reports to the contrary continue to appear. Three methods of postremission therapy are currently in use: (1) consolidation therapy employing high dose chemotherapy for a short period of time, usually months; (2) intermittent long-term maintenance therapy, which results in periodic marrow aplasia, given for several years; and (3) allogeneic bone marrow transplantation. The common thread among these methods is intensification of therapy. Postremission therapy designed to avoid hospitalization is of little or no value.

Most consolidation programs employ high dose cytarabine alone or in combination with amsacrine, L-asparaginase, daunorubicin, or other drugs. There is little evidence that multidrug regimens are superior to high dose cytarabine alone. The drug is usually given as soon as the marrow has completely recovered from the effects of induction therapy. Cytarabine, 3 g per meter squared, is given as a 1-hour infusion every 6 hours for a total of 12 doses. The regimen is repeated after full recovery from the first consolidation course, then no further therapy is given. This treatment is reasonably well tolerated in young patients, but severe toxicity to the mucous membranes, marrow, and cerebellum may occur in patients over the age of 50. The median duration of complete remission with this and similar treatments is 12 to 24 months, and 20 to 40 percent of patients have continued in first complete remission for at least 3 years. Five to 15 percent of patients have died from treatment-related toxicity while in complete remission.

An intermittent, long-term maintenance therapy consisting of cytarabine, 100 mg per meter squared, given subcutaneously every 12 hours, and oral 6-thioguanine at the same dose on the same schedule has been successful. The regimen is given for a variable number of days until severe marrow hypoplasia results. The treatment is begun after the patient has fully recovered from induction therapy and is repeated every 3 months for 3 years. An average of 10 days of treatment is required during the first year to produce the desired marrow effects, whereas 5 days or less may be required later. The treatment is begun in the clinic, and the patient is hospitalized when granulocytopenia occurs after the first course and is discharged when the granulocyte count rises to at least 500 per microliter. Bone marrow examinations must be used to monitor the treatment. When the blood granulocyte count falls to zero during therapy, the bone marrow should be examined. If it is more than 1+ cellular, give an additional 5 days of treatment and then stop. If the marrow is 1+ cellular or less, give an additional 2 days of treatment. If the marrow is essentially aplastic, stop treatment.

Patients who do not become infected during the first course are managed entirely as outpatients during subsequent courses if they are reliable and live closeby.

This treatment is reasonably well tolerated by patients up to age 65. Bone marrow toxicity is the principal untoward effect, and only 1 to 2 percent of patients have died from drug related toxicity while in complete remission. Patients who develop serious infection during the initial course tend to have recurrent infections with subsequent courses, while those who do not become infected initially tend to remain infection-free with further treatment. The tonsils are a frequent site of infection in younger patients, and tonsillectomy may allow them to sustain further therapy without infection.

Alloimmunized patients are not placed on this program unless autologous frozen platelets have been banked before the first maintenance course. Subsequent maintenance courses should be preceded by plateletpheresis when necessary, so that effective platelet transfusions are always available.

Results with this treatment are at least comparable with those of intensive consolidation therapy. Thirty percent of 86 patients with a median age of 46 have remained in continuous complete remission for 8 years, and most have had therapy discontinued at this time. Two women have conceived and delivered normal children after completing this treatment.

Allogeneic bone marrow transplantation has been extensively studied for postremission treatment of ANLL. The procedure is available only to approximately 20 percent of patients in complete remission because of the requirement for an HLA compatible donor and age limitations imposed by the toxicity of the procedure. Approximately 20 to 50 percent of patients who undergo transplantation experience fatal toxicity, usually manifested by interstitial pneumonitis and acute graft versus host disease (GVHD). However, a presumed cure rate of 20 to 50 percent, defined as leukemia-free survival for at least 3 years post-transplantation, has been reported from many centers, although some such patients manifest permanent evidence of chronic GVHD, such as dermatitis, hepatitis, or enteritis. There is evidence that chronic GVHD has an antileukemic effect in ANLL and may account for some of the success of transplantation. Most studies in which that complication has been modified by intervention have been associated with a greater leukemic relapse rate, and relapse in donor cells has rarely occurred.

Overall postremission survival rates after allogeneic transplantation do not differ significantly from those obtained with chemotherapy alone in most comparative studies, although disease-free survival is often superior after transplantation. In addition, results after allogeneic transplantation in first complete remission appear to be comparable to those obtained in early relapse or second complete remission. Therefore, most authorities now recommend reserving allogeneic marrow transplantation for eligible patients in the latter two situations. This avoids toxic deaths from transplantation in patients in first complete remission who may be long-term, disease-free survivors with less toxic therapy, and reserves the procedure for patients who have little chance of extended survival with other treatments.

SPECIAL CONSIDERATIONS

Central Nervous System (CNS) Leukemia

CNS leukemia is relatively uncommon in ANLL, except in certain subtypes, as discussed previously. About 5 percent develop this complication while in bone marrow remission. Patients usually complain of symptoms related to increased intracranial pressure, and the diagnosis is confirmed by examination of the cerebrospinal fluid (CSF) in most cases. However, the CSF may be normal if only cranial nerves are involved. A cranial nerve palsy in an acute leukemia patient should be considered as evidence of CNS leukemia. Cranial nerve palsy due to leukemic infiltration of the nerve sheath requires immediate radiotherapy if maximum return of function is to be obtained. The entire course of the nerve should be irradiated with curative intent. If there is no CSF pleocytosis, it is not necessary to administer intrathecal therapy. If there are leukemic cells in the CSF, intrathecal methotrexate or cytarabine should be administered every third day until the CSF is free of leukemia, and then monthly thereafter. Methotrexate, 12 mg total dose, or cytarabine, 40 mg total dose, in preservative-free diluent is administered through a lumbar puncture needle with vigorous mixing with CSF by withdrawing and injecting fluid over a 5-minute period. Alternatively, the medication can be instilled via a ventricular reservoir placed under the scalp. The reservoir allows the patient to avoid the discomfort of repeated lumbar puncture and of adhesive arachnoiditis that may rarely result from multiple instillations of chemotherapy into the lumbar subdural sac. Patients who have had multiple lumbar punctures sometimes have chronically low CSF pressure, which makes lumbar puncture difficult. The intraventricular reservoir avoids this problem also.

Radiotherapy is reserved for the rare patient with refractory meningeal or intracerebral leukemia in addition to those with cranial nerve involvement.

The Pregnant Patient

The pregnant leukemia patient poses special problems. If the patient is in the first trimester, abortion should be strongly considered before antileukemic therapy. If abortion is refused and induction therapy given, spontaneous abortion is likely. Since most such abortus have fetal abnormalities, one can assume that if the pregnancy were to have gone to term congenital abnormalities would be observed with a high frequency, although there is little actual data on this point. A large number of case reports suggest that the drugs most commonly used during induction therapy of ANLL, including cytarabine and daunorubicin, can frequently be given during the third trimester of pregnancy without apparent untoward effect on the fetus.

Granulocytic Sarcoma (Chloroma)

A rare patient may relapse with extramedullary disease at sites other than the CNS at a time when the bone marrow, peripheral blood, and remainder of the physical examination are normal. Radiation therapy and surgery are usually effective in resolving the local problem, but it is not yet clear whether such patients benefit from systemic chemotherapy. In general, systemic reinduction therapy is recommended if multiple granulocytic sarcomas are noted or if the disease-free interval has been less than 1 year. Patients who are long-term, disease-free survivors at the time a single granulocytic sarcoma develops are usually treated with local therapy. Limited results reported to date suggest that this approach is rational.

SUGGESTED READING

Wiernik PH. Acute leukemia in adults. In: DeVita VT Jr, Hellman S, Rosenberg SA, eds. Cancer: principles and practice of oncology, 3rd ed. Philadelphia: JB Lippincott, 1989:1809.

Wiernik PH. Diagnosis and treatment of acute nonlymphocytic leukemia. In: Wiernik PH, Canellos GP, Kyle RA, Schiffer CA, eds. Neoplastic diseases of the blood. 2nd ed. New York: Churchill Livingstone, 1990, in press.

Wiernik PH. The acute leukemias. In: Kelley WN, ed. Textbook of internal medicine. Philadelphia: JB Lippincott, 1989:1173, 1298.

IDIOPATHIC MYELOFIBROSIS AND MYELOPHTHISIC ANEMIA

SCOTT MURPHY, M.D.

Idiopathic myelofibrosis is one of the myeloproliferative diseases. Polycythemia vera, essential thrombocythemia, and chronic myelocytic leukemia are the other diseases that fall into this category. They all result from the proliferation of a clone of blood and bone marrow cells derived from a single hematopoietic stem cell that has gained a growth advantage over its normal counterparts. The syndrome of myelofibrosis may present originally or it may evolve in the later stages of the other myeloproliferative diseases, and the therapeutic approach is similar in both situations. There are three major pathophysiologic mechanisms, which may appear together or in an asynchronous fashion during the course of the disease. They are as follows:

1. Proliferation of fibrous tissue in the bone marrow with extension of hematopoietic marrow from its normal central location into the long bones. The fibrosis is reactive to the progeny of the abnormal stem cell and, at least in theory, can be reversed by replacing the abnormal stem cell with a normal one, as in allogeneic bone marrow transplantation. The fibrosis may be minimal and distributed throughout the marrow in a patchy fashion, so it is common for little or none to be present on initial biopsy.

2. Extramedullary hematopoiesis primarily in the spleen, but also in the liver, lymph nodes, and other organs. Enlargement of the spleen may be massive and may produce mechanical symptoms of pain and early satiety as well as cytopenias related to hypersplenic thrombocytopenia, leukopenia, and hemolysis. Since it is common for there to be relatively little marrow fibrosis and a great deal of extramedullary hematopoiesis with prominent splenomegaly, the syndrome of myelofibrosis has also been referred to as myeloid metaplasia (agnogenic if it develops originally or post polycythemic if it occurs during the course of polycythemia vera).

3. Ineffective hematopoiesis. The bone marrow biopsy may demonstrate many erythroid precursors and megakaryocytes, but anemia and thrombocytopenia may still result from failure to produce red cells and platelets.

This syndrome must be distinguished from acute myelofibrosis, which is really a form of acute leukemia. Fibrosis is present in the marrow, but the spleen is not enlarged, and leukemic blasts can be identified in the peripheral blood. The therapeutic approaches described below would be inappropriate for acute myelofibrosis.

Myelophthisic anemia refers to the syndrome produced by invasion of the bone marrow by malignancies such as carcinomas and lymphomas as well as tuberculosis or fungal infections, although these latter two are rare. Fibrous tissue is often present as a reaction to the invading cells. Primary management depends on treatment of the underlying disorder, which may be made more difficult by the impairment of bone marrow function.

THERAPY OF IDIOPATHIC MYELOFIBROSIS

Therapy for this condition is problem-oriented. The tempo of disease progression and problem development varies extremely from patient to patient, and many patients remain relatively free of symptoms for years or even decades. The only so-called cure is allogeneic bone marrow transplantation. Since complications from this procedure increase in frequency with increasing age above 20, and since the majority of these patients are over 40, bone marrow transplantation is generally a theoretical consideration. Therefore, it is best to follow the patient over time until one of the following treatable problems presents itself.

Proliferative Phase

Although the patient may have marrow fibrosis and marked splenomegaly, hematopoiesis throughout the skeleton may still be effective and hyperactive, thereby leading to polycythemia, thrombocytosis, or both. Management should be based on the principles outlined in the chapter on polycythemia vera. Intermittent phlebotomy of 500 ml of blood should be used to keep the hematocrit at 43 or below. Because of the splenomegaly, the platelet count rarely exceeds 1,000,000 per millimeter cubed, and there is generally no need to treat the thrombocytosis unless it is associated with microvascular symptoms such as transient cerebral ischemic attacks, peripheral arterial insufficiency, or erythromelalgia. The latter is characterized by intermittent, painful discoloration of the fingers and toes. For such symptoms during the proliferative phase, one should administer hydroxyurea, starting at 15 mg per kilogram of body weight per day by mouth, with dose adjustment to keep the platelet count under 600,000 per millmeter cubed and the leukocyte count over 3,000 per millmeter cubed. Complications of such treatment are rare if the blood count is carefully monitored, preferably weekly, at least initially. Aspirin, 300 to 600 mg by mouth daily, also relieves these symptoms, but it may predispose the patient to gastrointestinal hemorrhage. Therefore, myelosuppression is preferred. Approximately 10 to 20 percent of patients have an unsatisfactory response to hydroxyurea. In these cases, busulfan can be started at 2 mg by mouth daily. The dose should be adjusted according to therapeutic response and its effect on the blood count.

It is extremely important to recognize that the patient is still in the proliferative phase so that the dangers of splenectomy can be appreciated. When the platelet count is high prior to surgery, or even when it is normal, splenectomy can be followed by a massive thrombocytosis, which can be accompanied by life-threatening vascular manifestations. If splenomegaly produces mechanical symptoms during the proliferative phase, myelosuppressive therapy as described above is indicated.

Anemia

Anemia generally results from a combination of ineffective erythropoiesis and hemolysis secondary to hypersplenism. However, it is important to look for complicating iron deficiency, which is often residual from phlebotomy therapy for previous polycythemia. One should also look for deficiences of folic acid and vitamin B_{12}, which can be treated with appropriate replacement therapy. If such simple measures are not effective and the patient has significant symptoms from the anemia, two units of packed red cells should be transfused frequently enough to alleviate the symptoms.

Once iron and vitamin deficiencies have been corrected, one should try to distinguish between ineffective erythropoiesis and hemolysis by measuring the red cell survival time after labeling an aliquot of red cells with ^{51}chromium. The patient with ineffective erythropoiesis generally has a low reticulocyte count (less than 5 percent), a normal or nearly normal red cell survival time, and a transfusion requirement of no more than 2 to 3 units of red cells every 2 to 3 weeks. Patients with a major hemolytic component to their anemia have shortened red cell survival times and more frequent requirements for red cell transfusions.

In addition to transfusion as required, initial therapy should attempt to stimulate red cell production with androgenic steroids. In men, these can be testosterone enanthate or cypionate, 500 mg intramuscularly weekly. It is important to perform a careful rectal examination prior to therapy to exclude prostatic carcinoma that may be stimulated by testosterone. Otherwise, the major complication is fluid retention. Because of virilizing side effects, most women cannot tolerate testosterone injections at this high level. They can be started on a less virilizing compound such as nandrolone decanoate, 200 to 400 mg intramuscularly weekly. Approximately one-half of patients show an improvement in hematocrit as well as reduced transfusion requirements. If there is no response within 3 months, the therapy should be considered to have failed, and the medication should be discontinued. If there is an improvement in the hematocrit, the time between doses can be gradually extended until a maintenance program of once-monthly treatments is reached. In women, the extent of and tolerance to virilizing side effects must be considered in arriving at the final dosage schedule.

Splenectomy should be considered for patients who do not respond to androgenic steroids and who have a significant hemolytic component to their anemia. A careful risk-to-benefit analysis should be performed. Approximately one-half of such patients have an improvement in their transfusion requirements after splenectomy. On the other hand, most of these patients are beyond middle age, and the mortality risk with surgery is 1 to 5 percent, with a risk of surgical morbidity in the range of 5 to 15 percent. A high or even normal platelet count is a relative contraindication because of the risk of postsplenectomy thrombocytosis. The ideal candidate is the patient in relatively good health whose transfusion requirements approach 2 to 3 units every 1 to 2 weeks, and whose platelet count is less than 150,000 per millimeter cubed. Such a transfusion schedule often becomes psychologically intolerable, which helps to motivate the patient to accept the risks of surgery. In general, it is best to continue transfusion therapy until these criteria are met. The frequency of response has not been shown to be related to the size of the spleen or the extent of uptake of labeled red cells by organ scanning. Polyvalent pneumococcal vaccine, 0.5 ml, should be administered intramuscularly prior to surgery. Many surgeons find that embolizing the spleen just prior to surgery shrinks the organ, thereby facilitating its removal.

Thrombocytopenia

Platelet counts less than 100,000 per millimeter cubed result from the combination of ineffective thrombopoiesis and hypersplenism. The bleeding tendency and the prolongation of the bleeding time are often greater than predicted on the basis of the platelet count alone because of an associated defect in platelet function. Approximately 50 percent of patients have a significant improvement in both their platelet count and bleeding tendency after splenectomy. Again, a risk-to-benefit analysis has to be performed. Splenectomy should be performed in patients in good general health and significant hemorrhagic symptoms. In general, surgery should be deferred in a patient with asymptomatic thrombocytopenia unless benefits can also be expected in anemia or symptoms related to spleen size or hypermetabolism (see below).

Symptoms Related to Massive Spleen Size

Myelofibrosis produces a degree of splenic enlargement as great as any disease in clinical medicine. Shear size is not an indication for therapy. However, splenic enlargement can lead to pain when there is recurrent infarction, weight loss due to splenic hypermetabolism and interference with gastrointestinal function, and manifestations of portal hypertension related to a massive increase in portal blood flow from the spleen. If the patient is still in the proliferative phase of the disease, with normal or high granulocyte and platelet counts, myelosuppressive therapy as described above should be tried first. This may reduce splenic size and alleviate symptoms. The presence of granulocytopenia and/or thrombocytopenia contraindicates myelosuppressive therapy, therefore splenectomy should be done if the patient's general health allows.

Splenic radiotherapy can also be considered. Up to 250 rads in 50 rad fractions can shrink the spleen, but there is frequently dramatic and unpredictable suppression of the granulocyte and platelet counts with such treatment. Furthermore, the response is generally transient, and the patient is generally a poorer candidate for splenectomy when the spleen regrows. Therefore, splenectomy is preferred if the risks of surgery are not too great.

SUGGESTED READING

Besa EC, Nowell PC, Geller NL, Gardner FH. Analysis of the androgen response of 23 patients with agnogenic myeloid metaplasia. The value of chromosomal studies in predicting response and survival. Cancer 1982; 49(2):308–313.

Greenberger JS, Chaffey JT, Rosenthal DS, Moloney WC. Irradiation for control of hypersplenism and painful splenomegaly in myeloid metaplasia. Int J Radiat Oncol Biol Phys 1977; 2:1083.

Hocking WG, Machleder HI, Golde DW. Splenic artery embolization prior to splenectomy in end-stage polycythemia vera. Am J Hematol 1980; 8:123–127.

Silverstein MN, ReMine WH. Splenectomy in myeloid metaplasia. Blood 1979; 53:515–518.

ALLOGENEIC BONE MARROW TRANSPLANTATION

HANS A. MESSNER, M.D., Ph.D., FRCPC

Allogeneic bone marrow transplants (BMT) are performed with curative intent in a wide variety of hemopoietic disorders. These include severe aplastic anemia, immune deficiency disorders, acute leukemia, chronic myeloid leukemia, and other hemopoietic malignancies, as well as a number of genetic defects. The commonly used preparative regimens usually combine high dose chemotherapy with total body irradiation (TBI). The purpose of these pretreatment schedules is to suppress the immune system of the host to induce graft tolerance and to eliminate malignant cell populations in recipients with hemopoietic neoplasms. Chemotherapy and TBI are delivered at maximum dose as determined by the toxic influence on the next most sensitive organ or organ system. Complications of BMT may relate to toxicity of the preparative regimen or its failure to control immunologically active, or residual malignant cell populations of the host. The transplant procedure may also be associated with poor engraftment, slow reconstitution of the immune system, or the development of graft versus host disease.

PREPARATIVE REGIMENS

The majority of transplant centers have used regimens that combine one or more chemotherapeutic agents with TBI. Some centers have explored the use of high dose single or combination chemotherapy without radiation for various indications.

Total Body Irradiation

The classic regimen for hemopoietic malignancies combined cyclophosphamide (CTX) at a dose of 60 mg per kilogram per day for 2 days with 1,000 cGy TBI. At the different centers, TBI was delivered either by cobalt sources or linear accelerators at dose rates that varied from 2 to 85 cGy per minute. This schedule resulted in sustained engraftment and prolonged disease-free and relapse-free survival. However, it was also associated with radiation induced interstitial pneumonitis in a significant proportion of recipients when radiation was delivered in dose rates that exceeded 5 to 8 cGy per minute. Two changes in the delivery of radiation have nearly eliminated radiation induced interstitial pneumonitis:

The majority of transplant teams adopted fractionated total body irradiation (FTBI), where a cumulative dose of 1,200 to 1,350 cGy is given in six fractions at dose rates up to 30 cGy per minute.

Based on a large experience with palliative, wide field radiation, our own institution elected to reduce TBI to a single dose of 500 cGy delivered at 50 to 85 cGy per minute by a single cobalt source.

Both schedules appear to result in comparable disease-free survival rates as a measurement of their biologic effect on malignant cell populations.

Chemotherapy

Many centers have continued to use CTX as previously described. Other groups have added additional chemotherapeutic agents such as cytosine arabinoside at various doses, dimethylmyleran, Adriamycin, melphalan, and others. In some studies, particularly those of high risk patients, CTX was replaced by VP-16, high dose cytosine arabinoside, or high dose cytosine arabinoside combined with mitoxantrone. None of these variations have improved disease-free survival significantly, although the regimen combining VP-16 with FTBI shows some promise.

The combined use of high dose busulfan and CTX and the omission of TBI represents an alternative approach to the above mentioned regimens with similar long-term, disease-free survival in comparable patient populations.

CLINICAL RESULTS

Leukemia

Single institution studies and BMT registry reviews have identified a number of recipient related risk factors that contribute to the clinical outcome of BMT. These include recipient age, disease status at BMT, and history of exposure to cytomegalovirus (CMV). The observed clinical results in various analyses are generally in agreement. Patients transplanted in first remission acute myeloid leukemia (AML), acute lymphoblastic leukemia (ALL), or chronic phase chronic myeloid leukemia (CML) have a 50 to 65 percent long-term, disease-free and relapse-free survival. The results are less favorable when the procedure is performed in patients who have more advanced disease. The survival rates may vary from as low as 10 to 35 percent. The difference in long-term survival of both patient groups is related to an increased relapse rate in patients transplanted with more advanced disease.

Other Hemopoietic Malignancies

The benefit of BMT for other hemopoietic malignancies is less well defined. For instance, patients with myeloma and malignant lymphoma appear to have a very high relapse rate, and only 20 to 30 percent of transplant recipients demonstrate long-term, disease-free survival.

Aplastic Anemia

Until very recently, BMT was the treatment of choice for patients with severe aplastic anemia. A cure rate that exceeded 80 percent was observed for patients that were untransfused before receiving the transplant. The recent use of methotrexate (MTX) and cyclosporin A (CyA) as graft versus host disease (GVHD) prophylaxis appears to approach these results also for previously transfused patients. However, developments such as the availability of antithymocyte globulin (ATG), the effectiveness of CyA in the treatment of severe aplastic anemia, and the future use of recombinant hemopoietic growth factors such as erythropoietin and GM-CSF, G-CSF or IL3 may require reevaluation of BMT for this disease. Currently, the advantage of BMT is related to a more complete reestablishment of hemopoiesis. Disadvantages include graft rejection and transplant related complications such as GVHD and CMV pneumonitis. Patients treated with ATG or CyA respond slowly and often incompletely, however, they do not develop transplant related complications. This therapeutic approach may be preferable for older patients with severe aplastic anemia.

As an adult transplant center, we have performed a pilot study to test whether patients with severe aplastic anemia that have failed ATG can subsequently receive a successful bone marrow transplant. All patients with severe aplastic anemia presented to our institution were initially treated with ATG. Seventeen of these 21 are alive with improved or reestablished normal bone marrow function. The patient population included six patients with HLA identical donors. Four of these recovered with ATG therapy. Two failed to respond to ATG treatment and subsequently received a bone marrow transplant. Both patients had no difficulties with engraftment and have reestablished normal hemopoietic parameters.

Metabolic Disorders

The use of BMT in genetically determined metabolic disorders has been successful in approximately 36 reported indications with reversal of the disease causing enzyme defects.

FAILURE ANALYSIS AND THERAPEUTIC APPROACHES

Failure to achieve long-term, disease-free survival after BMT may relate to multiple problems. The three most commonly encountered problems are related to life-threatening infections, the development of GVHD, and relapse of the underlying hemopoietic malignancy.

SELECTED INFECTIOUS COMPLICATIONS

BMT recipients remain severely immunocompromised for weeks and months and may be exposed to a series of life-threatening infections of various etiology. A number of prophylactic and therapeutic approaches have shown promise in successfully controlling some of the problems.

Bacterial Infections

Bacterial infections are common during the neutropenic early postBMT period. The majority of these infections can be controlled with aggressive antibiotic therapy. Patients that have undergone a splenectomy or who are functionally asplenic are at risk of developing rapidly progressive diplococcal septicemia. Early therapy with penicillin or erythromycin is essential. In spite of timely administration of these antibiotics, patients may succumb to this infectious complication. The role of a pneumococcal vaccine has not been fully evaluated.

However, its use appears to be of limited effectiveness. Alternatively, patients may carry a supply of penicillin or erythromycin and initiate therapy at the earliest sign of an infection.

Pneumocystis carinii

The prophylactic use of trimethoprim-sulfamethoxazole during the early post-transplant period may prevent some of the gram-negative infections. However, attention should be drawn to the fact that its use may lead to the development of trimethoprim-sulfamethoxazole resistant indole-negative *Escherichia coli* related infections.

Trimethoprim-sulfamethoxazole is also effective in preventing *pneumocystis carinii* related pneumonias. For this purpose, it is sufficient to administer the drug on three consecutive days per week at a dose of two tablets orally every 12 hours. Therapy should likely be continued for 1 year.

The therapy of *pneumocystis carinii* related pneumonia may present a problem since it usually occurs in BMT recipients who have developed a hypersensitivity to trimethoprim-sulfamethoxazole and therefore had the drug stopped or where the drug had been discontinued because of low peripheral blood values and decreased bone marrow cellularity. The typical therapeutic dose for *pneumocystis carinii* is four ampules administered every 6 hours through a peripheral intravenous access; the drug has to be diluted in a large volume, for instance 500 cc of 5 percent dextrose in water. If administered through a central venous catheter, the drug can safely be given in smaller volumes. A full course requires therapy for 3 weeks. If no response is observed after 1 week, trimethoprim-sulfamethoxazole may be replaced by pentamidine, to be administered at a dose of 4 mg per kilogram per day intramuscularly or intravenously. The treatment should be maintained for 14 to 21 days.

Herpes Simplex and Zoster

The advent of antiviral agents such as acyclovir has changed the clinical course of herpes infections in BMT recipients. Herpes simplex, a common problem during the early postBMT period, can almost be eliminated if acyclovir is used prophylactically at a dose of 200 mg orally every 8 hours. Discontinuation of the drug, however, may rapidly lead to viral shedding and development of virally induced lesions. The disadvantage of a postBMT course of acyclovir is delayed engraftment.

Herpes zoster infections, a common occurrence even in BMT recipients with normal peripheral blood counts, also respond to therapy with acyclovir. Intravenous therapy at a dose of 10 mg per kilogram every 8 hours is recommended for patients with normal renal function when more than two dermatomes are involved or if dissemination has occurred. The therapy should be continued until the lesions have dried. Acyclovir may prevent further spreading and may reduce posthepetic neuralgia. The role of oral acyclovir in herpes zoster is not established. We have investigated its use in patients with lesions that are limited to one or two dermatomes. The examined patients did not demonstrate further spreading. However, further study is necessary.

Cytomegalovirus Induced Disease

The development of CMV related disease, in particular CMV induced pneumonitis, represents a life-threatening and often fatal complication of BMT. CMV disease may result from reactivation of CMV residing in the BMT recipient or by transmission through CMV containing blood products. Approaches to improve the clinical outcome focus on prevention as well as on the exploration of new therapeutic modalities.

Preventive measures include the administration of immunoglobulin preparations with high antiCMV titer. A series of studies suggest that symptomatic cytomegalovirus infections and interstitial pneumonia occur with lower frequency in patients who receive prophylactic immunoglobulins.

The exclusive use of CMV-negative blood products for CMV-negative recipients was also associated with a significantly reduced frequency of CMV disease. It will be necessary to combine both approaches and to evaluate critically if the influence of immunoglobulin is upheld when only CMV-negative blood products are given to all patients.

The availability of acyclovir and 9-(1,3 dihydroxy-2-propoxymethyl)guanine (DHPG) have added further opportunities to develop new prophylactic and therapeutic strategies. Caution with the use of these antiviral agents has to be applied, since both are toxic to bone marrow and may impair renal function.

It is difficult to influence the clinical course of established CMV disease, particularly CMV pneumonitis. Although both acyclovir and DHPG may have been effective in individual cases, larger studies do not show a significant improvement in survival when these drugs are used. DHPG was found to be effective in reducing or eliminating shedding of CMV in patients with biopsy proven, CMV induced disease when used at the recommended dose of 5 mg per kilogram every 12 hours for a total of 10 mg per kilogram per day. Unfortunately, if DHPG is introduced late into the treatment schedule, tissue damage may have progressed to an irreversible state. This appears to be of particular importance when CMV induced lung disease is treated.

Therefore, the use of DHPG early in the clinical course may be more effective. It will be necessary to conduct studies where patients are treated with DHPG at the moment when shedding of CMV is documented, without the development of CMV related disease. Under these conditions, it may also be feasible to reduce the usually administered dose of DHPG and to reduce the toxic effect on the newly established graft. In addition to the administration of DHPG alone, the drug may also be combined with immunoglobulins that contain high antiCMV titers. Preliminary studies show some promise.

GRAFT VERSUS HOST DISEASE

Prophylaxis and Treatment of Acute Graft Versus Host Disease

Acute and chronic graft versus host disease have plagued the prognosis of BMT recipients. The incidence of GVHD is age dependent and may vary from 50 to 75 percent in adults. Severe GVHD (grades II–IV) may occur in 25 to 50 percent of all patients. This frequency was similar when MTX or CyA was used prophylactically. More recently, the combination of MTX and CyA appears to have reduced the incidence and severity of graft versus host disease. Patients that develop GVHD in spite of MTX and CyA prophylaxis may benefit from steroid medications in a conventional dose of 40 mg per meter squared per day. This dose may be escalated in nonresponders. However, combined administration of CyA and high dose steroids may cause CNS side effects, including seizures.

Alternative methods to prevent GVHD include the use of procedures that eliminate or reduce the frequency of donor derived T-lymphocytes in the BMT inoculum. Centers that have performed these studies report a very low incidence of GVHD and a severity that usually does not exceed grade II. Unfortunately, the use of T cell depleted transplant inocula has resulted in graft rejections in 10 to 20 percent of recipients and is associated with a significantly increased relapse rate in patients with hemopoietic malignancies. The increased relapse rate may relate to the absence of a beneficial graft antileukemic effect observed in patients that display some GVHD. In particular, recent studies in chronic myeloid leukemia show a relapse rate that significantly exceeds the previous experience. The observation of increased relapse rates is not confirmed by all BMT teams that use T cell depleted bone marrows. Further studies will be necessary to determine whether the higher relapse rate and poor engraftment may be linked to the use of specific antibodies, to the completeness of T-cell removal, or to the additional use of other medications such as CyA.

Chronic GVHD

Chronic GVHD may result in syndromes that are reminiscent of rheumatoid disorders such as the sicca syndrome and progressive systemic sclerosis. Occasionally, prolonged liver dysfunction and jaundice can be observed. These disorders require intensive management with immunosuppressive agents. The disease process gradually decreases in some patients. However, other patients demonstrate a failure to thrive that is associated with progressive worsening of the symptoms and that may eventually lead to their death. Treatment approaches with steroids, azathioprine, CTX, and CyA, either alone or in combination, have shown some benefits. More recently, thalidomide is also being explored.

RELAPSE OF HEMOPOIETIC MALIGNANCIES

Unfortunately, a certain proportion of BMT recipients relapse with their underlying disease. The frequency of relapse varies from study to study and ranges from 10 to 40 percent for patients transplanted with AML in first remission. Recent experience in acute leukemia and CML has clearly demonstrated that this relapse rate may relate to the manipulation of the BMT inoculum prior to infusion.

A significantly higher relapse rate is universally observed for patients transplanted with more advanced disease. A study replacing the more conventionally used CTX and TBI with VP-16 (60 mg per kilogram total dose) and FTBI (1,350 cGy total dose) shows some promise and results in a 48 percent disease-free survival rate at 2 years. It will therefore be mandatory to develop novel approaches to eliminate the malignant disease in the host prior to transplantation and to consider further interventions after the transplant. The latter approach was examined for patients with previous CNS leukemia. Continuing intrathecal therapy with MTX after transplantation has lowered the CNS relapse rate. In addition to the administration of chemotherapy post-transplantation, one may consider the use of biologic response modifiers such as interferon as alternative interventions.

FUTURE DIRECTIONS

Some of the problems discussed above may relate to the fact that BMT recipients usually do not demonstrate a complete normalization of hemopoiesis when bone marrow function is assessed by the frequency of hemopoietic precursors. The reduced numbers suggest incomplete engraftment and a poor reserve. The availability of hemopoietic growth factors obtained by recombinant technology may provide additional means to increase the rate of engraftment and to enhance the probability of reestablishing a more complete reserve. Various hemopoietic growth factors may either be used to stimulate clonogenic precursors in the transplant inoculum or to be administered directly to the patient. The safety of these maneuvers may have to take into account that some malignant precursors may be receptors for the same growth factors.

In summary, BMT is a form of therapy that facilitates the increase of chemotherapy and radiation beyond the level of bone marrow tolerance. It allows us to determine whether or not escalated dose schedules are able to control proliferation of malignant hemopoietic cells. At the moment, it is not clear whether transplantation of allogeneic cells contributes to the disease control as suggested by the graft versus leukemia effect and by the increased relapse rate in T-cell depleted transplants. The putative benefit of these interactions between donor derived cell populations and residual malignant cell populations in the host has to be further explored. The use of hemopoietic growth factors may facilitate the administration of intensive courses of chemotherapy without the requirement for a bone marrow transplant. This approach may allow a direct comparison of the clinical outcome in patients receiving the same aggressive treatment protocol with and without transplantation.

SUGGESTED READING

Bowden RA, Sayers M, Flournoy N, et al. Cytomegalovirus immunoglobulin and seronegative blood products to prevent primary cytomegalovirus infection after marrow transplantation. N Engl J Med 1986; 314:1006–1010.
Champlin R. Bone marrow transplantation for acute leukemia: a preliminary report from the international bone marrow transplant registry. Transplant Proc 1987; XIX:2626–2628.
Champlin R. Bone marrow transplantation for leukemia: effects of T-lymphocyte depletion of donor bone marrow. Transplant Proc 1987; XIX:157–159.
Gratwohl A, Nissen C, Speck B. Severe aplastic anemia. In: Fairbanks VF, ed. Current hematology and oncology 1986. Vol 4. Chicago: Year Book Medical Publishers, 1986:91.
Herve P, Cahn JY, Flesch M, et al. Successful graft vs. host disease prevention without graft failure in 32 HLA-identical allogenic bone marrow transplantations with marrow depleted of T-cells by monoclonal antibodies and complement. Blood 1987; 69:388–393.
O'Reilly RJ, Reich L, Gold J, et al. A randomized trial of intravenous-hyperimmune globulin for the prevention of cytomegalovirus infections following marrow transplantation: preliminary results. Transplant Proc 1983; 15:1405–1411.
Prentice HG. T-cell depletion in allogenic bone marrow transplantation. Transplant Proc 1987; XIX:155–156.
Prentice HG, Blackloch HA, Janossy G, et al. Pretreatment of donor bone marrow with monoclonal antibody OKT 3 for prevention of acute graft vs. host disease in allogenic histocompatible bone marrow transplantation. Lancet 1982; 1:1266-1269.
Ringden O, Zwaan F, Hermans V, et al. European experience of bone marrow transplantation for leukemia. Transplant Proc 1987; XIX:2600–2604.
Storb R, Deeg HJ, Whitehead J, et al. Marrow transplantation for leukemia and aplastic anemia: two controlled trials of a combination of methotrexate and cyclosporin v. cyclosporin alone or methotrexate alone for prophylaxis of acute graft vs. host disease. Transplant Proc 1987; XIX:2608–2613.
Winston DJ, Ho WG, Lin CH, et al. Intravenous immunoglobulin for prevention of cytomegalovirus infection and interstitial pneumonia after bone marrow transplantation. Ann Intern Med 1987; 106:12–18.

AUTOLOGOUS BONE MARROW TRANSPLANTATION

ANDREW M. YEAGER, M.D.
GEORGE W. SANTOS, M.D.

Intensive chemoradiotherapy followed by allogeneic bone marrow transplantation (BMT) may be curative in some patients with lymphohematopoietic malignancies whose chances for cure are negligible with conventional therapy. Acute and chronic graft-versus-host disease and opportunistic infections, especially interstitial pneumonitis caused by cytomegalovirus, are the major causes of morbidity and mortality after allogeneic BMT, whereas leukemic relapses are uncommon. Since most allogeneic BMTs are carried out with healthy histocompatible (human leukocytic antigen–matched) related donors, 60 to 75 percent of patients who otherwise might be eligible for allogeneic transplantation cannot undergo the procedure because they lack a suitable donor.

A promising alternative to allogeneic BMT is to use the patient's own (autologous) marrow, collected when the patient is in remission and then cryopreserved, as the source of hematopoietic stem cells. The therapeutic efficacy of autologous BMT has been demonstrated in some patients with acute leukemias, Hodgkin's disease, and non-Hodgkin's lymphoma. Intensive therapy with autologous marrow rescue may also be applicable to the treatment of other neoplastic diseases, such as sarcomas and carcinomas. However, certain other conditions in which allogeneic BMT is therapeutic, e.g., aplastic anemia, selective cytopenias, and immunodeficiency states, cannot be effectively treated by autologous transplantation because of the lack of sufficient and/or competent stem cells in the patient's marrow.

LIMITATIONS AND PRACTICAL CONSIDERATIONS OF MARROW AUTOGRAFTING

The major limitation to the use of autologous BMT in patients with leukemias is the risk that viable occult tumor cells may be present in the marrow, even though the disease appears to be in remission according to microscopic examination of samples. This concern is also valid in lymphomas and in other neoplastic diseases (e.g., neuroblastoma) in which tumor involvement of the bone marrow may occur. One strategy to overcome this problem is the treatment ("purging") of the marrow cell suspension before cryopreservation and infusion into the recipient, in an attempt to eliminate residual tumor cells from the graft. Ideally, such ex vivo marrow treatment methods should eradicate all occult neoplastic cells and spare normal hematopoietic stem cells, thus allowing reasonably prompt hematologic reconstitution after intensive cytoreductive therapy and autologous BMT.

Evaluation of the therapeutic efficacy of autologous BMT must take into account two factors: the ability of the in vivo intensive cytoreductive regimen to eradicate residual tumor cells in the patient, and the ability of the ex vivo treatment to eliminate viable neoplastic cells from the autograft. Therefore, clinical trials of autologous BMT are most appropriately analyzed and compared with the results of syngeneic (identical twin) BMT in similar groups of patients, i.e., a situation in which both contamination of the marrow graft with neoplastic cells and allogeneic graft-versus-tumor effects are absent.

Several methods for ex vivo purging of autografts are being examined in laboratory studies and clinical trials (Table 1). Some of these treatment strategies are based on the physical, physicochemical, or immunologic differences between malignant and normal cells, whereas others rely on the differential sensitivity of neoplastic versus normal cells to cytotoxic agents. At The Johns Hopkins Oncology Center, pharmacologic purging of marrow autografts with 4-hydroperoxycyclophosphamide (4-HC) a congener of cyclophosphamide and an active alkylating agent in aqueous solution, has been studied. In current trials, autologous marrow cell suspensions are incubated with 100 μg per milliliter of 4-HC, a dose that in phase I studies did not impair normal hematopoietic repopulating ability.

TABLE 1 Methods for In Vitro/Ex Vivo Treatment of Marrow Autografts to Eliminate Tumor Cells

Physical
Albumin density gradient centrifugation*
Elutriation
Immunologic
Monoclonal antibodies (MoAbs) and complement*
Immunotoxin conjugates*
Tumor necrosis factor (TNF)
Pharmacologic
4-hydroperoxycyclophosphamide (4-HC)*
Mafosfamid (Asta Z-7557)*
4-HC and methylprednisolone*
Etoposide (VP-16)*
Etoposide and 4-HC*
Bleomycin
Photodynamic
Merocyanine 540*
Immunomagnetic microspheres*
Immunopharmacologic
4-HC and MoAbs
Mafosfamid and immunotoxins

*Evaluated in clinical trials as well as laboratory studies.

AUTOGRAFT COLLECTION, PROCESSING, AND INFUSION

Patients must have reasonable performance status and adequate cardiac, pulmonary, hepatic, and renal function to be eligible for autologous BMT regimens. Generally, patients should have adequate levels of platelets ($\geq 100 \times 10^9$ per liter) and neutrophils ($>0.5 \times 10^9$ per liter) at the time of marrow collection to ensure adequate levels of hematopoietic progenitor cells and to permit a safe and efficient marrow collection. The marrow should be in remission and/or without evidence of tumor involvement by microscopic techniques, and its cellularity should be at least 60 percent of normal. Multiple bone marrow aspirates are obtained from the iliac crests under general or spinal anesthesia, and the cells are collected and suspended in heparinized tissue culture medium (TC 199). The marrow buffy coat is obtained by centrifugation or Ficoll-Hypaque (diatrizoate meglumine and diatrizoate sodium) separation before ex vivo treatment. When marrow chemopurging regimens are used, the incubation hematocrit value should be standardized because erythrocytes act as a "sink" to inactivate 4-HC; in our marrow processing laboratory, the hematocrit value of the marrow buffy coat is adjusted to 6 to 7 percent. For our 4-HC treatment studies, approximately 2.5 to 3.0×10^8 nucleated marrow cells per kilogram of recipient weight are incubated at 37°C with 100 μg per milliliter of 4-HC for 30 minutes. After incubation, the nucleated marrow cells are centrifuged, resuspended in a mixture of 45 percent irradiated autologous plasma, 45 percent TC 199, and 10 percent dimethylsulfoxide, placed in 50-ml aliquots in polyolefin bags, and cryopreserved in liquid nitrogen. At the time of BMT, the marrow aliquots are rapidly thawed in a 37°C water bath and infused directly into a large-bore central venous catheter at a rate of 10 to 15 ml per minute. We have not observed any significant adverse reactions associated with infusion of the dimethylsulfoxide-containing cell suspension.

PREPARATIVE REGIMENS

The preparative regimens employed in autografting are generally similar to those used in allogeneic or syngeneic BMT. At The Johns Hopkins Oncology Center, patients with acute lymphocytic leukemia receive high-dose intravenous cyclophosphamide (50 mg per kilogram per day for 4 days) followed by total body irradiation (300 rad per day for 4 days, with the lungs shielded after 900 rad) (CY-TBI). Patients with acute nonlymphocytic leukemia are given high-dose combination alkylating agent chemotherapy without total body irradiation, consisting of oral busulfan (1 mg per kilogram per dose every 6 hours for 16 doses), followed by intravenous cyclophosphamide (50 mg per kilogram per day for 4 days) (BU-CY). The autologous marrow is infused 24 hours after the last dose of total body irradiation in the CY-TBI regimen and 48 hours after the last dose of cyclophosphamide in BU-CY recipients. In autologous BMT for Hodgkin's disease or non-Hodgkin's lymphoma, CY-TBI is used in patients who are in remission or have minimal residual disease, and BU-CY is given to patients who cannot receive total body irradiation because of previous extensive radiotherapy. Several centers are studying alternative polychemotherapy regimens with autologous marrow rescue to eradicate bulky and metastatic disease in patients with solid tumors. For example, we are using the BU-CY regimen and 4-HC-purged marrow autografts to treat children with refractory and relapsing solid tumors such as rhabdomyosarcoma, Ewing's sarcoma, and neuroblastoma. In addition, we are evaluating a combination of busulfan, cyclophosphamide, and etoposide (VP-16) as a preautograft conditioning regimen in patients with bulky (i.e., over 20 cm^2 of tumor) and refractory relapsed Hodgkin's disease or non-Hodgkin's lymphoma.

COMPLICATIONS OF AUTOLOGOUS BMT

All patients have a period of aplasia for several weeks after autologous BMT. For example, in patients with leukemias and lymphomas receiving 4-HC-treated marrow, the median times to attain an absolute neutrophil count greater than 0.5×10^9 per liter and to attain a platelet count greater than 50×10^9 per liter without transfusions are 30 and 60 days, respectively. Similar durations of neutropenia and thrombocytopenia have been described in patients with leukemia who have undergone autologous BMT with unpurged or monoclonal antibody–treated marrow. During aplasia, patients are at risk for both hemorrhagic complications and systemic infections (including gram-positive, gram-negative, and fungal pathogens). Although support with platelet transfusions has lessened the risks of life-threatening bleeding, there is a significant risk of death from bacterial or fungal sepsis in the immediate post-BMT period. Several studies have in fact suggested that the risk of fatal sepsis during aplasia is greater in autograft patients than in allograft recipients. Attention to surveillance cultures and development of appropriate empirical and specific antibiotic regimens to be employed during febrile episodes may help decrease the risks of this fatal complication.

Hepatic veno-occlusive disease is characterized by hepatomegaly, hyperbilirubinemia, profound elevation of transaminases, ascites, and shortened platelet survival time. This complication, which has been described in both autograft and allograft recipients, occurs 3 to 6 weeks after BMT. Patients with abnormal hepatic enzyme studies at the time of transplant and with a history of multiple relapses and extensive previous chemotherapy are especially at risk for developing veno-occlusive disease, which has approximately a 50 percent case-fatality rate. Interestingly, low-grade acute graft-versus-host disease has been described in a small number of autologous BMT recipients, in whom the response to steroid therapy was good; no patients subsequently developed chronic graft-versus-host disease syndromes. The mechanism by which autologous graft-versus-host disease occurs is not known. Interstitial pneumonitis caused by viral pathogens such as cytomegalovirus is uncommon after autologous BMT, although cases have been reported. In contrast, the risk of idiopathic interstitial pneumonitis is similar in both allogeneic and autologous BMT recipients. Sterility, a consequence of intensive cytoreductive therapy, is likely to occur in peri- and postpubertal autograft recipients.

RESULTS

Acute Lymphocytic Leukemia (ALL). Several centers have employed ex vivo immunologic or pharmacologic purging methods and high-dose myeloablative therapy to treat patients with ALL in second or subsequent remissions. Our center has studied autologous BMT with 4-HC-treated marrow and a CY-TBI preparative regimen in 24 patients (median age, 18 years) with ALL in second remission; the results of this trial were not encouraging (Table 2). One patient died in remission with necrotizing *Pseudomonas* pneumonitis 5.5 months after BMT. One patient had an isolated central nervous system relapse with no evidence for leukemia in the bone marrow at 9.5 months after autograft; he received both systemic and intrathecal induction and consolidation therapy and then died after a marrow relapse 40 months after the central nervous system relapse. Seventeen patients had isolated marrow relapses at a median time of 4 months (range, 2 to 17 months) after BMT, and all died as a consequence of leukemic relapse or its treatment. Five patients with ALL in second remission are still in unmaintained remission at a median of 13+ months (range, 4.5+ to 93+ months) after autologous BMT. Other groups have shown disease-free survival rates of 20 to 30 percent in ALL patients in second or subsequent remissions undergoing autografting with monoclonal antibody–treated marrow; the nature and timing of relapses in these series were similar to those seen in our chemopurged group.

Unlike the results with chemotherapy in childhood ALL, the prognosis for long-term survival in adults with ALL in first remission is poor. We have performed autologous BMT with CY-TBI preparation and 4-HC-treated marrow grafts in 15 adults with ALL in first remission (see Table 2). Two patients died in the immediate post-BMT period (one with bacterial sepsis, one with fulminant central nervous

TABLE 2 Autologous Transplantation with 4-HC-Treated Marrow in Patients with Acute Lymphocytic Leukemia

CR	*No. Patients*	*Median Age (Range) (Yr)*	*No. BMT-Related Deaths*	*No. Relapses*	*No. Disease-Free Survivors*	*Median Duration (Range) of Disease-Free Survival (Mo)*
1	15	31 (18–40)	2 (13%)	10 (67%)	3 (20%)	55+(9+–77+)
2	24	18 (3–39)	1 (4%)	18* (75%)	5 (21%)	13+(4.5+–93+)

*Includes one isolated central nervous system relapse and 17 marrow relapses.
Abbreviations: CR = Complete remission; 4-HC = 4-hydroperoxycyclophosphamide.
All patients received autologous marrow grafts treated with 100 μg per milliliter of 4-HC.

system leukemia). Ten patients relapsed at a median of 4 months (range, 1.5 to 25.5 months) after autografting. Three patients are in unmaintained first remission at a median of 55+ months (range, 9+ to 77+ months) after BMT. More experience is needed to determine the optimal regimens for both ex vivo autograft purging and in vivo pre-BMT conditioning and thus the therapeutic efficacy of autografts for adult ALL in first remission.

Acute Nonlymphocytic Leukemia (ANLL). The results of autologous BMT with chemopurged marrow in ANLL are encouraging (Table 3). One hundred fourteen patients with ANLL (29 in first remission, 71 in second remission, and 14 in third remission) received 4-HC-treated autografts after a BU-CY preparative regimen. Twenty-three patients (20 percent) died of transplant-related complications: 14 with bacterial or fungal sepsis, 2 with interstitial pneumonitis (1 cytomegalovirus, 1 idiopathic), and 7 with hepatic veno-occlusive disease. Forty-nine patients (43 percent) relapsed at a median of 6 months (range, 2 to 23 months) after BMT; 12 of these patients were in first remission, 32 were in second remission, and 5 were in third remission. Forty-two patients (37 percent) are in unmaintained remission at a median of 25+ months (range, 1+ to 106+ months) after autograft. The actuarial relapse rate in this series is 58 percent, comparable to what might be anticipated in syngeneic BMTs for ANLL. The lack of satisfactory monoclonal antibodies has hitherto limited the application of immunologic purging to autografts in ANLL. Recent reports of autologous BMT with monoclonal antibody-treated marrow in ANLL are encouraging, although the results are preliminary and the duration of follow-up is short.

The need for ex vivo purging of autologous marrow in patients with ANLL in first remission is controversial. Some investigators have shown that autografts with unpurged marrow in patients with ANLL in first remission is associated with a disease-free survival of at least 50 percent, whereas others have been unable to demonstrate any advantage of autologous BMT with unpurged marrow over conventional remission-induction therapy. One important variable is the duration of first remission at the time of autografting: patients with prolonged unmaintained first remission might already have been cured by per primam ANLL therapy at the time of BMT. In the 29 patients in our series undergoing autologous BMT for ANLL in first remission, the median duration of first remission at the time of autologous BMT was 2.5 months; although the period of follow-up is short, the disease-free survival is encouraging (13 of 29 patients or 45 percent). However, randomized prospective

TABLE 3 Autologous Transplantation with 4-HC-Treated Marrow in Patients with Acute Nonlymphocytic Leukemia

CR	*No. Patients*	*Median Age (Range) (Yr)*	*No. BMT-Related Deaths*	*No. Relapses*	*No. Disease-Free Survivors*	*Median Duration (Range) of Disease-Free Survival (Mo)*
1	29	17 (12–37)	4 (14%)	12 (41%)	13 (45%)	14+(1+–106+)
2	71	22 (2–54)	13 (18%)	32 (45%)	26 (37%)	25+(1+–79+)
3	14	31 (19–54)	6 (43%)	5 (36%)	3 (21%)	57+(56+–98+)

Abbreviations: CR = complete remission; 4-HC = 4-hydroperoxycyclophosphamide.
All patients received autologous grafts treated with 100 μg per milliliter of 4-HC.

TABLE 4 Autologous Transplantation with 4-HC-Treated Marrow in Patients with Relapsed Lymphoma*

Diagnosis	*No. Patients*	*Median Age (Range) (Yr)*	*No. BMT-Related Deaths*	*No. Disease-Free Survivors*	*Median Duration (Range) of Disease-Free Survival (Mo)*
HD	26	31 (11–51)	8 (31%)	13 (50%)	24+(4+–48+)
NHL	62	23 (3–53)	10 (16%)	34 (54%)	23+(1+–154+)

*Includes patients in second or subsequent remission and responding (sensitive) first or subsequent relapse.
Abbreviations: HD = Hodgkin's disease; NHL = non-Hodgkin's lymphoma; 4-HC = 4-hydroperoxycyclophosphamide.
All patients received autologous marrow grafts treated with 100 μg per milliliter of 4-HC.

trials of chemotherapy versus autografting and of autografting with treated versus unpurged marrow are warranted to address this issue in ANLL therapy.

Lymphoma. Patients with both Hodgkin's disease and non-Hodgkin's lymphoma who have relapsed after initial intensive therapy may benefit from autologous BMT. In our program, 26 patients with relapsed Hodgkin's disease and 62 patients with relapsed non-Hodgkin's lymphoma have received CY-TBI or BU-CY therapy followed by 4-HC-treated marrow autografts (Table 4). The disease-free survival is 50 percent in patients with Hodgkin's disease and 54 percent in those with non-Hodgkin's lymphoma, with median follow-up times of 24+ and 23+ months, respectively. Tumor response rates and prolonged disease-free survival were similar in both the CY-TBI and BU-CY treatment groups. Only patients with minimal residual disease or in complete remission at the time of BMT had prolonged disease-free survival in our series; no patients with bulky disease (< 20 cm^2 of tumor) and/or lymphoma that was not responding to salvage chemotherapy at the time of BMT (resistant relapse) demonstrated sustained relapse-free survival, despite therapy and marrow autografting. Other investigators have shown similar response and remission rates in Hodgkin's disease and non-Hodgkin's lymphoma with intensive myeloablative regimens and unpurged or monoclonal antibody–treated autografts.

Solid Tumors. In children with stage D neuroblastoma, treatment with high-dose L-phenylalanine mustard (L-PAM) and total body irradiation followed by autografts of immunomagnetically purged marrow to eliminate occult neuroblastoma cells have yielded encouraging results when applied in first remission patients. Intensive chemo(radio)therapeutic regimens and autologous marrow rescue are also being studied in patients with solid tumors that are not likely to be cured with conventional therapy, including high-risk sarcomas (e.g., rhabdomyosarcoma, Ewing's tumor), carcinomas (e.g., breast, small cell lung, testicular), and central nervous system tumors (gliomas). Some of these studies are preliminary, whereas others have not demonstrated any beneficial effect of autologous BMT in these conditions. At this time, with the exception of neuroblastoma, there are no definite indications for autograft therapy in non-lymphohematopoietic neoplasms.

SUGGESTED READING

Dicke KA, ed. Autologous bone marrow transplantation: Proceedings of the Third International Symposium. Houston: University of Texas M.D. Anderson Hospital and Tumor Institute at Houston, 1987.

Goldstone AH, ed. Autologous bone marrow transplantation. Clin Haematol 1986; 15(1).

Santos GW. Bone marrow transplantation in acute leukemia: Current status. Cancer 1984; 54:2732–2740.

Yeager AM, Kaizer H, Santos GW, et al. Autologous bone marrow transplantation in patients with acute nonlymphocytic leukemia, using *ex vivo* marrow treatment with 4-hydroperoxycyclophosphamide. N Engl J Med 1986; 315:141–147.

MULTIPLE MYELOMA AND RELATED MONOCLONAL GAMMOPATHIES

ANN M. BENGER, M.D., FRCPC
WILLIAM E. C. WILSON, M.D., C.M., FRCPC, F.A.C.P.

Individuals proven to have myeloma come to medical attention for a variety of reasons. Patients with overt disease present with symptoms that generally involve one or more of three pathogenetic mechanisms: skeletal destruction, bone marrow failure, and synthesis of an abnormal protein. The symptomatic consequences of cortical bone destruction may be bone pain, hypercalcemia, pathological fracture, and spinal cord compression. Bone marrow failure may manifest itself with the symptoms of anemia, susceptibility to infection related to leukopenia or a hemorrhagic diathesis consequent to thrombocytopenia. The dysproteinemia of multiple myeloma may become symptomatic as a consequence of renal failure, hyperviscosity, amyloid deposition, coagulation disturbance, and/or impaired humoral immunity. Finally, nonspecific symptoms of malignancy may accompany those related to these three pathogenetic mechanisms.

At the other extreme, a patient destined to die from myeloma may first be recognized by the presence of a small monoclonal protein identified during the investigation of an unrelated problem.

The challenge presented to the clinician by this range of immunoproliferative disease is to identify those patients whose prognosis is sufficiently poor to warrant the risks attendant upon any therapy. For those who do require treatment, the physician must devise a therapeutic strategy that provides the best chance for active productivity for the patient's remaining limited life.

ASSESSMENT OF PROGNOSIS

When a diagnosis of myeloma is established, several clinical and laboratory parameters have an adverse effect on prognosis. These are renal failure, hypercalcemia, anemia, leukopenia, thrombocytopenia, light chain disease, and poor performance status. The marked reduction in median survival associated with Bence Jones proteinuria, complicating IgG and IgA myeloma, is due to a strong association with uremia. For a given amount of paraprotein, patients with IgA myeloma fare worse than those whose tumor cells secrete IgG. It is clear that several of these factors relate well to tumor load.

In addition to clinical staging, more specialized laboratory techniques may assist in assessing prognosis. The tritiated thymidine labelling index of plasma cells is low in patients with indolent or smoldering myeloma. In patients who are not azotemic, the beta 2 microglobulin level correlates well with the tumor burden.

Current studies are exploring methods by which patients with a very poor prognosis might be identified for participation in trials of more radical therapy. Heavy marrow infiltration with malignant plasma cells is negatively associated with prognosis in patients with IgG and light chain myeloma. Immature morphology of tumor cells predicts a poor prognosis and is accompanied by preB cell phenotype and chromosomal abnormality. In vitro assays for melphalan sensitivity have demonstrated that these cells are drug resistant. In another study, determination of the RNA content of myeloma cells by flow cytometry revealed that a low level of RNA was associated with greater resistance to initial and salvage chemotherapy.

GENERAL PLANS OF MANAGEMENT

Monoclonal Gammopathy of Undetermined Significance

Because the term benign monoclonal gammopathy can only be used retrospectively with any certainty, a patient who presents with a small monoclonal protein that is identified incidentally must be considered a potential myeloma candidate. A history and physical examination to exclude the other causes of dysproteinemia should be recorded.

In the absence of contraindicating illness or infirmity, the initial investigation should include a bone marrow aspiration and biopsy, determination of the parameters of bone marrow function, evaluation of renal function, a serum calcium level, estimation of the serum levels of the three major classes of immune globulin, serum immunoelectrophoresis, a 24-hour urine collection for total protein measurement and electrophoresis, and a skeletal x-ray survey.

The individual least likely to develop overt myeloma is older and has no further abnormalities identified by the additional investigation.

A repeat serum protein electrophoresis should be obtained after 3 months. If the abnormality is stable, the interval may safely be increased to 6 months.

Indolent or Smoldering Myeloma

Not all patients with multiple myeloma have an overtly progressive malignancy. When a patient presents with multiple myeloma (more than 10 percent plasma cells in the bone marrow and an MCP in excess of 30 g per liter), who is asymptomatic and lacks hematologic, biochemical and radiologic evidence of overt myeloma, it is reasonable to withhold chemotherapy. Many patients of this type remain stable, and, therefore, are best protected from the complications that attend chemotherapy.

The interval for initial reassessment should be 2 months. If the protein abnormality remains stable, the follow-up interval can be lengthened progressively to 6 months. For patients in this group, treatment should be considered if the abnormal protein level increases by 50 percent or if the symptoms of complications become evident.

Overt Multiple Myeloma

Generally, patients with overt multiple myeloma have symptoms related to skeletal damage, renal failure, or compromised bone marrow function, and have a progressive disease. Historical data indicate a median survival of 7 months without treatment. Melphalan and prednisone therapy has extended the median survival to 30 months.

Whether initial therapy with intensive multidrug chemotherapy can improve the outlook for most patients with multiple myeloma remains controversial. Until this controversy is resolved, it is generally reasonable to institute therapy with melphalan, 9 mg per meter squared per day for 4 days, orally on an empty stomach every 4 weeks. The dose should be increased to 12 mg per meter squared for 4 days if the granulocyte nadir is over 500.

If the patient does not respond with a fall of MCP, the dose should be increased progressively to 15 mg per meter squared per day for 4 days, 18 mg per meter squared per day for 4 days, etc., until clear evidence of hematologic toxicity is observed, thereby indicating adequate absorption of melphalan. Prednisone, 100 mg orally, should accompany each day of melphalan.

An expected 70 percent of patients demonstrate a drop in the MCP to 50 percent of the pretreatment value. A slow, progressive diminution in the level of abnormal protein signifies a better prognosis than a rapid fall.

The duration of chemotherapy is controversial. Cessation results in earlier relapse, but not necessarily a shortening of median survival. Continued therapy might increase the likelihood of refractory anemia and acute leukemia. Until more data are available, it is reasonable to discontinue therapy at 2 years in those patients who have had a good response.

A trial is currently underway to determine if the addition of alpha interferon might increase the duration of remissions induced with melphalan and prednisone.

Cyclophosphamide is a reasonable substitute for patients who are allergic to melphalan or are intolerant to melphalan in other ways.

Advanced Myeloma

Some patients present with manifestations of disease that warrant aggressive therapeutic intervention if major morbidity or immediate mortality is to be avoided. Examples of this include patients with serious hypercalcemia and those with critical neurologic complications. For those in this category who seem otherwise fit, consideration should be given to one of the multiagent regimes. In an uncontrolled study of 46 previously untreated patients, the M-2 protocol produced objective responses in 87 percent. Other multiagent regimes may be superior to melphalan and prednisone in this setting.

SPECIFIC CLINICAL PROBLEMS

Solitary Myeloma

An occasional patient presents with an apparently isolated bone lesion. This is generally symptomatic. After the diagnosis is established by biopsy, the initial assessment parameters outlined previously should be obtained. If these reveal no abnormality or only a small monoclonal protein peak, the patient may have a localized malignancy and may possibly be cured by intense radiotherapy. Most patients who present with apparently localized disease manifest progressive disease within 2 years. If a monoclonal protein is present and does not disappear with radiation, overt multiple myeloma can be anticipated.

Extramedullary Plasmacytoma

Plasma cell tumors presenting outside bone are generally found within the respiratory tract. The lymph nodes and the gastrointestinal tract are less frequent sites. They are generally single, but may be multiple. Therapy has included resection and/or radiation, depending on location. While local recurrence or metastases to soft tissues (lymph nodes) or bone can be anticipated, the prognosis is generally better than that of overt multiple myeloma.

Nonsecretory Myeloma

Less than 5 percent of patients with multiple myeloma have tumor cells that do not secrete clinically measureable amounts of abnormal protein into the serum or urine. Nonsecretory tumors generally are identified because of bone lesions. The tumor cell mass tends to be less and the levels of hemoglobin and normal immune globulin tend to be preserved. The prognosis of these patients is better than that seen in patients with overt multiple myeloma.

Pathologic Fractures

Pathologic fracture is a frequently presenting manifestation of overt disease. In non-weight bearing areas, therapy for the systemic disease is generally followed by relief from the local symptoms. When fracture of a major long bone occurs, internal fixation followed by local irradiation is recommended.

Patients with a pathologic vertebral collapse must be immediately assessed with respect to spinal cord compression. If no evidence of cord compromise is present, urgent local radiotherapy should be initiated and be accompanied by high dose dexamethasone therapy. The patient must be reassessed during the first few days of radiotherapy for signs of spinal cord compression. Patients with evidence of compromised spinal cord function should be considered for immediate decompression laminectomy followed by local radiotherapy. Because the ultimate outlook for the patient depends on their tolerance for chemotherapy, the volume of active bone marrow irradiated should be as conservative as is reasonable.

Spinal Cord Compression

Spinal cord compression that is identified and treated early because of an accompanying pathological fracture generally has a good prognosis. Occasional patients with myeloma have spinal cord compression from an extradural deposit that is not associated with overt bone destruction. These patients are often not diagnosed until major impairment of spinal cord function has been present for some time. The tumor is usually identified by the neurosurgeon. Once the diagnosis is established, the patient should receive local radiation while being assessed for systemic chemotherapy. As permanent neurologic sequelae are all too frequent, active rehabilitation therapy should be instituted as soon as the postoperative state allows.

Renal Failure

The most common renal lesion to complicate multiple myeloma is tubular atrophy and degeneration. Dimers of light chains filtered by the glomerulus are reabsorbed and catabolized in the tubular cells. Patients who excrete light chains are more likely to have impaired renal function.

Other possible mechanisms of deterioration in renal function include interstitial tumor cell infiltration, dehydration, hypercalcemic nephropathy, pyelonephritis, and amyloid deposition in the glomeruli.

Management of the renal failure should include prompt correction of any recognized complicating factors (i.e., hypercalcemia, dehydration, and infection) and aggressive treatment of the myeloma. The patient may require the support of dialysis. Acute renal failure may reverse with forced alkaline diuresis and dialysis. Occasional reports suggest an added benefit from plasmapheresis.

Bone Marrow Failure

Some manifestation of impaired bone marrow function can be anticipated in most patients being treated for multiple myeloma. The degree of marrow failure usually worsens temporarily with initiation of treatment, and the patient may require transfusions.

Disproportionate neutropenia often complicates chemotherapy in patients with advanced myeloma. When this is associated with major marrow infiltration, chemotherapy sometimes has to be cautiously continued in the hope that a reduction of the tumor burden will be followed by increased granulopoiesis.

Plasma cell leukemia is a rare and particularly malignant form of marrow failure. These patients typically have a high tumor burden, disproportionate tissue and organ involvement, and a median survival of 2 months in one series.

Acute leukemia, often preceded by a period of refractory anemia, is a recognized complication of melphalan therapy. In one series, the incidence of acute leukemia in patients with multiple myeloma after alkylator therapy was 1.9 percent (actuarial 2.8 percent at 5 years, 10.1 percent at 10 years). When a refractory anemia develops, alkylating therapy should be stopped. Patients who develop acute myeloid leukemia and who are otherwise fit may respond to intense chemotherapy.

Hyperviscosity

The hyperviscosity syndrome is not a common manifestation of multiple myeloma, since it is more frequently found in Waldenström's macroglobulinemia. However, certain IgA proteins and some monoclonal IgG molecules of the IgG 1 and IgG 3 subclasses may aggregate in vivo, thereby resulting in increased serum viscosity. Prompt reversal of the manifestations of the hyperviscosity syndrome can be anticipated from plasmapheresis. Long-term control, however, depends on response to chemotherapy.

Hypercalcemia

Hypercalcemia is present at the time of diagnosis in 30 percent of patients with multiple myeloma. It is generally not severe and responds to treatment of the underlying malignancy. Symptomatic hypercalcemia can usually be ameliorated temporarily by hydration and diuretic administration while the chemotherapy exerts its effect. Occasional severe cases may benefit from mithramycin, calcitonin, or oral phosphate solutions.

Amyloid Deposition

Myeloma patients with significant amyloid deposition in vital organs have a dismal prognosis, with a median survival of 5 months in one series. In the absence of cardiac amyloid, some patients respond to chemotherapy. The responsive patients have a median survival in excess of 2 years.

Myeloma in the Elderly

The incidence of multiple myeloma rises with age from 7 per 100,000 at age 50 to more than 20 per 100,000 at age 80. Because of increased longevity, elderly patients are coming more frequently to medical attention for treatment of myeloma. In a large, multi-institutional study of myeloma therapy, patients over 80 years seemed to be underrepresented when compared with a broader epidemiologic survey. This possibly reflected referral bias and investigator bias with exclusion of those considered too frail or otherwise unable to tolerate chemotherapy. However, for those elderly patients who were included in the study group, the prognostic risk factor representation was the same as that of younger patients. The older patients had responses and survival rates equivalent to the younger patients. Hematologic toxicity was no greater in the older group. The older patients did experience greater gastrointestinal toxicity in the treatment arm employing melphalan and prednisone. The authors conclude that myeloma treated without bone marrow ablation has a similar outcome when young patients were compared to the elderly.

RELAPSED OR RESISTANT MYELOMA

If treatment is discontinued, myeloma relapses in patients who have responded well to therapy with melphalan and prednisone. Relapse in this setting is best treated by reinstitution of melphalan and prednisone.

The outlook is poor for most patients when their disease progresses despite therapy with melphalan and prednisone. In addition to the manifestations of advancing disease, which may include impaired mobility related to bone pain and/or pathologic fractures, the clinical problem is often complicated by impaired tolerance to chemotherapy because of previous treatment and recurrent infection. For the subset of patients judged to be preterminal, the judicious but liberal use of narcotics may constitute the best therapy. Prednisone pulse therapy may provide some palliation for patients unable to tolerate more toxic regimes.

Four-day infusions of vincristine and doxorubicin combined with dexamethasone pulse therapy has produced a 70 percent response rate in patients whose myeloma was resistant to alkylating therapy. This observation requires confirmation in a larger group of patients. The regime involves an indwelling catheter, the need for hospitalization for the chemotherapy infusion each month, and admission for treatment of the infectious complications.

Bone marrow transplantation is currently under investigation. When the donor is an identical twin, response is seen, but progression of the myeloma generally supervenes. The results of allogeneic transplantation have not been encouraging. Autologous bone marrow transplantation studies demonstrate that dosage escalation can overcome drug resistance to some extent. The clinical benefits observed to date have been disappointing, perhaps because the patients were in a state of advanced disease and marrow purging had not been carried out.

The treatment of patients with plasma cell dyscrasias has been improved by the recognition that chemotherapy can be safely withheld from some.

A combination of melphalan and prednisone is the mainstay of therapy for overt disease. For those whose disease becomes progressive and required therapy, most die of multiple myeloma within 3 or 4 years of initial diagnosis.

Physicians who accept responsibility for the care of patients with myeloma should attempt to align themselves with a myeloma study group in the hope that expanded clinical research will improve the reults of therapy.

SUGGESTED READING

Alexanian R. Localized indolent myeloma. Blood 1980; 56:521.

Barlogie B, Smith L, Alexanian R. Effective treatment of advanced multiple myeloma refractory to akylating agents. N Engl J Med 1984; 310:1353.

Corwin J, Lindberg RD. Solitary plasmacytoma and their relationship to multiple myeloma. Cancer 1979; 43:1007.

Durie BGM, Salmon SE. A clinical staging system for multiple myeloma: correlation of measured myeloma cell mass with presenting clinical features, response to treatment, and survival. Cancer 1975; 36:842.

Durie BGM, Salmon SE. The current status and future prospects of treatment for multiple myeloma. Clin Haematol 1982; 11:181.

Greipp PR, Kyle RAP. Clinical, morphological, and cell kinetic differences among multiple myeloma, monoclonal gammopathy of undetermined significance and smouldering multiple myeloma. Blood 1983; 62:166.

IMMUNE NEUTROPENIA AND HYPERSPLENISM

JAMES B. BUSSEL, M.D.
JOSEPH HAIMI, M.D.

IMMUNE NEUTROPENIA

For the purposes of this discussion, autoimmune neutropenia is defined as neutropenia (absolute neutrophil count <1,000/μl) mediated either by antibodies or by cells (i.e., lymphocytes). This definition extends the scope of autoimmunity beyond a restricted definition such an antibody-mediated neutropenia, and therefore it permits a more comprehensive view of the treatment. Unlike isolated thrombocytopenia (ITP), which is a common problem usually caused by antiplatelet antibodies the occurrence of "pure" autoantibody-mediated neutropenia in adults is relatively uncommon.

The majority of patients with "immune" neutropenia probably have a cell-mediated process in which the pathophysiology is not well characterized and the treatment is not well established, e.g., Felty syndrome. This uncertainty is caused by the complicated nature of the interactions among different subpopulations of cells and the difficulties involved not only in identifying pathophysiologically significant but numerically small subsets of the total cell population, but also in defining their function. Another difficulty is that neutrophil antibody testing is considerably more complicated than red-cell and even platelet-antibody testing because of the tendency of neutrophils to agglutinate in vitro, and very few centers in the United States (Lalezari, Logue, Madyastha, Boxer, for example) are capable of providing reliable testing. A complicating factor in this is that neutrophils cannot be shipped overnight and experience with the results of neutrophil antibody testing in different clinical settings is limited. Consequently, the implications of a positive or negative test for the patient's clinical course, long-term outcome, and pathophysiology of the neutropenia are often uncertain. Nonetheless, recent advances have allowed a clearer understanding of pathophysiology and treatment in many cases of neutropenia.

Immune neutropenia has been divided into the following categories (1) autoantibody-mediated neutropenia including (a) idiopathic in both children and adults, (b) associated with immune deficiency, (c) with human immunodeficiency virus infection, (d) with lymphoproliferative disorders, (e) after bone marrow transplantation, and (f) with systemic lupus erythematosus (SLE); (2) cell-mediated neutropenia syndromes including (a) Felty syndrome and (b) large-granular lymphocytosis; (3) other causes of immune neutropenia, including autoantibodies directed against neutrophil precursors; and (4) hypersplenism.

DIAGNOSIS

Immune neutropenia should be suspected, especially in the setting of *persistent selective* neutropenia; if leukopenia is also present, antibody-mediated immune neutropenia is less likely. An acute *increase* in the neutrophil count in association with an infection and/or the presence of other autoantibodies (positive Coombs test, positive antinuclear antibody [ANA]) also suggest neutropenia mediated by an immune process. Other laboratory findings suggesting an autoimmune etiology of the neutropenia include coexistent humoral immune deficiency and/or very high levels of IgM. Other clinical features consistent with immune neutropenia (which may also be found in chronic benign nonimmune neutropenia) include a relatively benign course, a lack of septic episodes, and a relatively unimpaired quality of life.

If reliable neutrophil antibody testing is available, then ideally, testing in a suspect patient would reveal both neutrophil-associated and circulating neutrophil-binding antibody. A diagnostic problem involves the patient who has a negative test for neutrophil-associated antibodies but a positive test for a circulating antineutrophil antibody. If the patient has been either transfused or pregnant in the past, it is uncertain whether one should attribute these findings to auto- or alloantibodies. If a specificity of the antibody can be identified (i.e., directed at neutrophil antigen NA 1), it may be more likely a result of an alloantibody, but autoantibodies have, on occasion, been characterized by specificity. In addition, certain authors have reported antibodies that cross-react with neutrophils. These may also create confusion regarding evaluation of the etiology of neutropenia. In these uncertain settings, a response to therapy—whether steroids, intravenous gammaglobulin (IVGG), or splenectomy—may be of diagnostic use.

Neutropenia per se is not a reason to initiate treatment. Many work-ups are initiated to exclude malignancy and to define the etiology of the neutropenia, *not* because treatment is urgently needed. With the exception of newborn infants, in whom the risk of sepsis may be great enough to warrant therapy even in an asymptomatic patient, the critical determinant for the initiation of therapy (of any kind) is the history of infection. A patient with a very low absolute neutrophil count (ANC), but no past history of serious infections, rarely requires any treatment. Fortunately, most cases of neutropenia, immune or not, are relatively benign. Unlike severe anemia, which leads to heart failure, or severe thrombocytopenia, which may result in serious hemorrhage, severe neutropenia may have no adverse clinical consequences. In addition the patients' condition usually does not worsen with the passage of time, so that observation may be all that is required, with judicious use of antibiotics as appropriate. Vitamin C has no proven usefulness.

If therapy is required, however, several agents are available (Table 1). Among the newer therapies,

TABLE 1 Available Agents for Treatment of Neutropenia

Treatment	*Mechanism of Effects*	*Side Effects*	*Use*
Prednisone*	Shift in granulocyte pool out of marrow Immunosuppressive effect	Increased susceptibility to infection Other: myopathy, diabetes, osteoporosis, hypertension	SLE Felty syndrome Any neutropenia
IVGG	RES Fc receptor blockade decrease in autoantibody synthesis	Headache Cost	Autoantibody-mediated neutropenia: immune deficiency, SLE
Splenectomy	Eliminate filtration function Decrease autoantibody production	Increased susceptiblity to infection Venous thrombosis Operative morbidity	HIV-mediated neutropenia Neutropenia in lymphoproliferative diseases, hypertension, portal hypertension, autoantibody-mediated neutropenia
G-CSF, GM-CSF	Direct stimulation of committed granulocyte precursors Improved granulocyte function (GM-CSF only)	Unknown	Production failure, i.e., Felty syndrome
Plasmaphoresis	Remove antibodies and circulating immune complexes	Bleeding anemia infection	Autoantibody-mediated neutropenia
Lithium	Enhance granulopoiesis†	Diabetes insipidus Cardiac arrhythmia Convulsion and death	Felty syndrome
Imuran	Immunosuppression	Infections (? malignancy)	Autoantibody, SLE, ? Felty syndrome
ATG, anti-TAC	Eliminate suppressor T cells	Predispose to infections, fever, chills, rigors	Aplastic anemia Suppressor cell-mediated neutropenia

*To be used for limited periods only.
†By direct action on committed granulocytic progenitors (CFU-GM). Increase colony stimulating activity (CSA).

intravenous gammaglobulin is safe and effective for autoantibody-mediated neutropenia. Granulocyte-colony stimulating factor (G-CSF) and granulocyte macrophage colony stimulating factor (GM-CSF) are very promising therapies; the benefits of their use in autoimmune neutropenias, however, remain to be demonstrated. Steroid therapy and splenectomy are the established treatments of immune neutropenia. Both are effective in the appropriate setting but have their drawbacks, particularly in light of their predisposing to infections. This review will also indicate that, although many additional therapies are possible, experience with them is limited. In addition, the use of immunosuppressive therapies shown to be effective in ITP and autoimmune hemolytic anemia may pose grave risks in already neutropenic patients.

AUTOANTIBODY-MEDIATED NEUTROPENIA IN CHILDHOOD

Pure autoantibody-mediated immune neutropenia occurs more commonly in childhood, especially during infancy, than in adulthood. A recent report from one center of 120 consecutive cases in children studied over a 10-year period illustrates that autoimmune neutropenia is probably one of the most common causes of so-called benign neutropenia in infancy and childhood. This type of neutropenia is usually diagnosed before 1 year of age, but serious infections such as sepsis, meningitis, or even pneumonia are uncommon. Many patients are relatively asymptomatic, suffering only from more frequent routine childhood infections. This disease has probably been underdiagnosed in the past because it is usually benign and the total white blood count is often normal, and therefore the differential is omitted. For example, a total white count might be $5{,}000 \times 10^9$ per liter, with only 3 percent polys. The diagnosis is often made because evaluation of a high fever leads to obtaining of a CBC. Once the neutropenia is revealed by the differential analysis of the white blood cells, further work-up usually includes a bone marrow aspiration, which typically reveals normal numbers of the three stem lines, but absence of the most mature myeloid elements.

Because of the *benign* nature of the disease, the majority of these patients require no, or only intermittent, antibiotic treatment for specific infections such as otitis media. Most infants achieve a spontaneous remission by the age of 4 years. Where needed, therapy of the neutropenia was previously attempted with corticosteroids, but this use has been viewed with trepidation. The neutrophil count usually increases in response to 2 mg per kilogram of prednisone, but this increase may be offset by the immunosuppressive action of steroids; in one reported case, fungal sepsis ensued even though the neutrophil count had increased substantially. IVGG has recently been shown to be effective in seven of eight such cases, leading to a prompt increase in the ANC to over 1,500 per microliter. The mechanism of action may be temporary inhibition of reticuloendothelial Fc-receptor function, or decreased antineutrophil antibody synthesis.

Most patients usually require only a single course

of treatment to elevate the neutrophil count temporarily, to resolve a specific infection. We have used a dose-response treatment protocol in these patients, infusing 0.5 to 1.0 g per kilogram per day until the ANC increases to greater than 1,000 per microliter. Our experience suggests that a high proportion of patients with positive direct neutrophil immunofluorescence tests respond acutely to IVGG within 3 days. Deciding whether or not to treat neutropenic patients with IVGG if the direct assay is negative requires further study, but if the patient is symptomatic and has positive indirect immunofluorescense test, IVGG may be worthwhile for diagnostic as well as therapeutic purposes. IVGG does not appear to interfere with neutrophil function (specifically chemotaxis) and has been used in successful resolution of a broad spectrum of clinical infections, including fungal sepsis, recurrent pneumonias, and a chronic leg ulcer. Although IVGG appears to be effective at acutely raising the neutrophil count, anecdotal experience suggests that IVGG may be less effective as a maintenance therapy. Fortunately, few patients need ongoing treatment (repeated infusions), although these may be required with a chronic infection, i.e., an abscess that may require persistent elevation of the neutrophil count to heal, or in certain patients with recurrent severe infections.

Splenectomy has been required in few cases of autoimmune neutropenia, especially because of the tendency toward spontaneous remission. This is particularly important because splenectomy may contribute to immune deficiency in the neutropenic host. Experience with other therapies such as imuran, cyclophosphamide, and vinca alkaloids is limited. These therapies and splenectomy are usually resorted to only in older children and adolescents whose neutropenia is more complicated and who may respond less well to IVGG, develop continued problems with infections requiring ongoing management, and develop other immune cytopenias. Relatively few such cases have been reported, but treatment is uncertain and management is difficult; these patients would likely be candidates for treatment with the new poietins (G-CSF and GM-CSF).

Another setting of immune neutropenia in childhood involves *passive immune neutropenia in the newborn*. This occurs as frequently as 1 in 1,000 to 1 in 2,000 deliveries. The neutropenia in the newborn develops either because of a transplacental transfer of maternal autoantineutrophil antibodies or, more commonly, with alloantibodies directed against the father's neutrophil antigens in a way analogous to erythroblastosis fetalis. The neutropenia may be falsely interpreted as a sign of sepsis. Conversely, sepsis may occur in this setting; in this case neutrophil transfusion would be of little or no benefit, because of the antineutrophil antibodies, unless an antibody specificity is identified so that an appropriately matched transfusion can be used. One well-documented case was treated with intravenous gammaglobulin, suggesting that this form of immune neutropenia would be amenable to this therapy.

Autoimmune neutropenia in adults may be a result of destruction of granulocytes by direct lysis, by complement-binding antibodies, and/or by splenic phagocytosis of opsonized granulocytes. In some series autoantibodies detected on neutrophils are correlated with the presence of Clq-binding immune complexes. Although steroids are usually effective in elevating the neutrophil counts, neutropenia typically recurs when steroids are tapered. There is little experience with plasmapheresis, because it apparently has little effect. IVGG has been used with good response in several adults. Interestingly, the four reported cases have responded to 1 g per kilogram, or less, of IVGG, which is less than the dose required for children with autoimmune neutropenia.

Clinical dilemmas arise when patients with autoantibody-mediated neutropenia also have other manifestations such as lymphadenopathy, splenomegaly, or other autoimmune cytopenias. Patients with multiple autoimmune cytopenias, as exemplified by Evans syndrome, are less responsive to any therapy than patients with only one immune cytopenia. The treatment plan of these more complicated patients should probably start with IVGG if neutropenia is one of the cytopenias; however, these patients may not even respond to splenectomy. For patients with lymphadenopathy and/or splenomegaly, treatment with prednisone may be better and a lasting decrease in adenopathy or splenomegaly may be achieved with a course of steroids. An infectious etiology such as human immunodeficiency virus (HIV), Epstein-Barr virus, or toxoplasmosis should be considered and node biopsy obtained if needed. These patients probably are similar in certain ways to those with Felty syndrome (see below). Even if steroid therapy is not contemplated, patients with lymphadenopathy should have their HIV antibody status determined, because this may alter the approach to therapy (see below). In general, *if continuing therapy is required*, splenectomy should probably be performed. Initial attempts at treatment should include IVGG and steroids, but prolonged administration of immunosuppressive medication is probably a disservice to the neutropenic patient.

Neutropenia associated with immune deficiency appears to be a relatively common cause of what otherwise might be considered idiopathic autoantibody-mediated neutropenia, and indeed these entities are probably part of the same spectrum of disease. In several large series of immunodeficient patients neutropenia, though not documented by antibody studies to be autoimmune, was found in a large number of patients with humoral immunodeficiency, e.g., hypogammaglobulinemia patients. In particular, patients with elevated levels of IgM but subnormal levels of IgG and IgA (so-called hyper-IgM syndrome) have the highest incidence of neutropenia ($\geq$25 percent in one series of the cases). The relationship of the hypogammaglobulinemia to the neutropenia is illustrated by one report describing a threshold level of IgG above which, when the IgG level was maintained by intramuscular gammaglobulin therapy, the neutropenia resolved. Relatively few hypogammaglobulinemia patients have been studied for the presence of neutrophil or other autoantibodies, which is unfortunate because neutropenia has several possible other etiologies such as infections. Autoimmune neutropenia may be inferred to be a relatively common event, however, based on anecdotal cases and on the relatively common occurrence of autoimmune hemolytic anemia and ITP in this same group of patients. Response to prednisone is variable in these patients. Vincristine was used successfully according to one report of five patients. IVGG is clearly the treatment of first choice, not only for the underlying humoral immunodeficiency, but also for reversal of neutropenia. If it is ineffective, then vincristine and eventually splenectomy may be needed. If marked splenomegaly exists, IVGG is unlikely to be effective despite repeated infusion of high doses, and splenectomy should be performed. Careful attention needs to be paid to the risk of postsplenectomy sepsis; both IVGG and antibiotic prophylaxis should probably be given indefinitely. The exact dosage of IVGG to be used remains unknown, but probably should be based on the neutrophil response with at least 3 g per kilogram given within 1 week before the patient is classified as "unresponsive."

Although immune neutropenia in the setting of overt hypogammaglobulinemia is relatively uncommon in relation to the overall number of cases of neutropenia, IgG_2 deficiency and other abnormalities of humoral immunity may be common in so-called pure autoantibody-mediated neutropenia, in both children and adults. Another illustration of "mild" immunodeficiency is elevated levels of IgM in some neutropenic patients with normal IgG and IgA levels. This may represent a form fruste of the hyper-IgM syndrome. The elevated IgM per se is not a specific antineutrophil antibody; more likely it serves as a marker of a pathophysiologic process, presumably related to an aberrant "switch" mechanism whereby the primary IgM humoral response is normally converted to a secondary IgG response. Nonetheless, the number of neutropenic patients with elevated IgM and/or decreased IgG_2 may be considerable. Both types of patients may initially receive IVGG treatment; however, it is not clear that the patient with elevated IgM and normal IgG and IgA will respond to it. Many of these patients are leukopenic adults who are not selectively neutropenic and do not have a marked tendency to develop serious bacterial infection. Another possible approach is plasmapheresis, because IgM is greater than 95 percent intravascular, but these patients usually test negatively for direct antineutrophil antibody; thus, removing the IgM may only treat a symptom. Little experience exists with plasmapheresis or other treatment modalities, although this syndrome is relatively common. The pathophysiology and treatment resemble those of Felty syndrome, which is discussed subsequently.

A recently reported and potentially confusing entity that is likely to occur with increasing frequency is *human immunodeficiency virus–mediated neutropenia*. Autoimmune thrombocytopenia has been well-demonstrated in patients with evidence of exposure to HIV, making autoimmune neutropenia likely in some of these patients. One series described patients who had neutrophil-associated antibodies demonstrated by immunofluorescence. Other nonimmune etiologies of the neutropenia are possible, including leukophagocytosis in the bone marrow. As with ITP in HIV-positive patients, the treatment should probably be IVGG, followed by splenectomy if a tolerable maintenance cannot be achieved with IVGG. When it becomes available antiviral therapy will probably be a useful adjunct. Immunosuppressive therapy should probably be more strictly avoided for the HIV-positive neutropenia patient than for the HIV-positive thrombocytopenia patient. Whether IVGG plays any role in managing such a patient if the neutrophil count is *not* depressed or if the neutropenia is not autoimmune and no response of the neutrophil count to IVGG is seen, remains controversial.

Autoimmune neutropenia may also occur in patients with *lymphoproliferative disease*. It is less common than autoimmune thrombocytopenia or autoimmune hemolytic anemia in this setting, but is rarely seen in chronic lymphatic leukemia, Hodgkin's disease, and nonHodgkin's lymphoma. In the latter case, it may be associated with a predilection to hepatic involvement. Treatment should focus on the underlying disease, but immune cytopenias may occur while patients are in remission; then prednisone, IVGG, and splenectomy are the most important treatments, with others (imuran, cyclophosphamide, cyclosporin) reserved in case of failure.

Neutropenia with the presumed presence of neutrophil antibodies (platelet autoantibodies have been reported after *bone marrow transplantation*) has been seen following bone marrow transplantation. The antibody may be directed to neutrophils of donor origin. Little treatment experience exists. Presumably IVGG would be the first line, as in immunodeficient patients with autoimmune neutropenia.

Another disease entity related to immune neutropenia is *systemic lupus erythematosus (SLE)*. In one report, 53 percent of sera from 57 patients with SLE revealed granulocyte autoantibodies. However, in contrast with other settings in which the possibility of immune neutropenia is not considered sufficiently, in SLE humoral autoimmune neutropenia is probably assumed to occur far more often than it actually does. Several reports of aplastic anemia or other bone marrow problems in lupus are now available, whereas, strikingly, there are *few* documented cases of neutropenia mediated by neutrophil-associated antibodies. Bone marrow hypoplasia/aplasia may play a greater role in neutropenia and other cytopenias in lupus than was previously thought. It is tempting to speculate that part of the pathogenesis of the neutropenia may be related to large granular lymphocytosis and/or the activated interferon-secreting suppressor cell mechanism first described in patients with aplastic anemia by Neil Young—i.e., to a cell-mediated "hostile environment" effect. Unfortunately, too few of these patients have been studied, partly because of the general inaccessibility of neutrophil antibody testing and partly because of the general assumption that adverse events in SLE are autoantibody mediated.

When neutropenia does occur in lupus it is a difficult clinical problem. Intravenous gammaglobulin is unlikely to be helpful, although it is effective for ITP in SLE and should be given a trial, especially if neutrophil-associated or circulating neutrophil-binding antibodies can be demonstrated. Usually high dose steroids are the treatment not only of the neutropenia, but also of the total disease process, with immunosuppressive medication often added to amplify the effect. Although this therapy is effective in many cases, it creates a vulnerability for many opportunistic, especially fungal, infections in a setting where high dose steroids and neutropenia may coexist for weeks. Usually the risk is tolerated because the therapy is needed and the neutropenia is perceived to be short-lived. If the pathogenesis is immediately diagnosed, therapies such as infusion of the anti-TAC monoclonal antibody to cut down interferon production in the marrow or G-CSF/GM-CSF might be useful in severe cases, perhaps combined with a more moderate dose of steroids. Infectious etiology (viral) and treatment of specific infections should also be vigorously pursued. As indicated previously, therapy protocols of cell-mediated immune neutropenia are in their infancy.

Felty syndrome consists of a triad of rheumatoid arthritis (RA), splenomegaly, and leukopenia. The overall incidence of neutropenia in patients with RA is estimated to be 1 percent. Splenomegaly is not an essential feature of Felty syndrome because circulating antibodies have been found in neutropenic patients with RA but without splenomegaly. Anemia, increased susceptibility to infections, and thrombocytopenia have also been found in this syndrome, but to a lesser extent. Bone marrow studies in these patients revealed hyperplasia of lymphoid and monocytoid mononuclear cells, with maturation arrest in the granulocyte series. Consistent with the marrow finding, these patients often fail to show any neutrophil response to infections, corticosteroids, or endotoxin.

The mechanisms of neutropenia in Felty syndrome is obscure and likely to be multifactorial. Different studies have implicated both humoral and cellular mechanisms in the genesis of the neutropenia. T cells and monocytes residing in the spleen have been shown to suppress the colony-forming unit (CFU-C). However, other pathophysiologic mechanisms may contribute to the occurrence of neutropenia, including increased neutrophil-bound IgG activity, maturation arrest of the granulocytic series secondary to humoral inhibitory factor, and lack of myclopoiesis-stimulating factors. Increased circulating immune complexes have been described in as many as 68 percent of patients with RA with neutropenia: these complexes may mediate increased levels of (nonspecific) neutrophil-associated IgG. Splenic sequestration for neutrophils has not been specifically demonstrated, although it seems unlikely in certain patients.

Treatment of neutropenia in Felty syndrome remains uncertain, because effective modalities are lacking and uncertainties surround the pathogenesis. Prednisone therapy is often effective at high dosage for prolonged periods (weeks to months), but relapse of the neutropenia when corticosteroids are discontinued occurs in the overwhelming majority of cases; also, as with SLE, prolonged corticosteroid therapy of neutropenic patients is worrisome. Two studies have suggested that high dose IgG, 2 g per kilogram is unlikely to be beneficial in patients with Felty syndrome, only one in nine patients having even a short-lived response of the neutrophil count. These data support studies indicating that the neutrophil-associated IgG actually represents immune complexes rather than specific antineutrophil antibodies.

Lithium salts in a dose of 900 mg per day for 6 weeks have been used to increase the colony-stimulating activity and blood neutrophil concentration in patients with Felty syndrome, but this effect could not be maintained when therapy was discontinued. Lithium's side effects—including diabetes insipidus, cardiac arrhythmias, convulsion, and death prevent its routine use. Since effectiveness takes weeks, when there is an effect, lithium is not generally accepted as a therapeutic agent in Felty syndrome, although it may be useful in selected patients if the benefits outweigh its side effects.

Splenectomy has been the definitive therapy for reversing the neutropenia in Felty syndrome, although the success rate remains controversial. An initial transient response to splenectomy may be seen as a result of removal of suppressor cells. Neutropenia may recur and has been postulated to be due to activation of suppressor cells in other organs such as the bone marrow. Overall, splenectomy has failed to reverse the leukopenia in one-third of cases in some reports, and relapse rate as high as 30 percent have been reported after initial response. It is therefore recommended that splenectomy be employed only in those patients with clinical evidence of frequent infections, when the ANC is persistently less than 500 and other therapies have been ineffective. Caution in employing this modality is particularly indicated because splenectomy may lower defense against infection. *Haemophilus influenzae* B and pneumococcal vaccines should be given before splenectomy is performed, and antibody response studied. Reduced bone marrow neutrophil mass as well as marrow lymphocytosis before surgery may indicate a poor response to splenectomy.

Other therapeutic approaches to treatment of neutropenia in Felty syndrome (including gold therapy, vincristine, and other cytotoxic chemotherapies) are not well-documented, and currently no good therapy exists for this disease. Future use of growth factors (G-CSF and GM-CSF) is likely to prove particularly useful in these difficult patients.

Another type of neutropenia, described 10 years ago and now recognized to be relatively common, is the syndrome of *T killer cell neutropenia or large granular lymphocytosis* with neutropenia. It may occur with, but usually occurs without, neutrophil antibody. The lymphocytes bear the natural killer phenotype (T8 + leu 11+). This is an interesting syndrome because it appears to be a cellular equivalent of benign monoclonal gammopathy and it is heterogeneous for many parameters. It is apparently not a malignant proliferation of cells, as evidenced by the natural history of these patients. Studies of the T cell receptor have shown both polyclonal and monoclonal rearrangement, as well as germline configuration of the T cell receptor. The pathophysiology of the neutropenia is uncertain because it occurs with and without neutrophil antibodies, and direct suppressive influence of the large granular lymphocytes has not been demonstrated. Fortunately, most of these patients are clinically well. It is not clear what treatment if any should be used; many of these patients have been studied, but few have been treated. IVGG might be considered if neutrophil antibodies are present. If studies suggested a direct effect of the large granular lymphocytes, then high dose steroids, lymphoplasmapheresis, immunosuppresive therapy, or even a monoclonal antibody infusion could be considered. Eventually G-CSF or GM-CSF may become the treatment of choice for neutropenia caused by a maturation defect.

Another category of immune neutropenia is that mediated by *bone marrow suppression.* This has been demonstrated in several cases and, though it may be relatively uncommon, it is probably underdiagnosed. It may be mediated by either antibodies or cytotoxic cells. This problem is difficult to document in vitro, but cell culture systems to assess colony-forming units may be of help. Treatment is likely to be immunosuppressive medicines (steroids, imuran, cyclophosphamide) or antithymocyte globulin, especially if the suppression can be shown to be mediated by T cells.

Hypersplenism is defined as an enlargement of the spleen, with either reduction of a single element or pancytopenia in peripheral blood with at least a normal number of elements in bone marrow. The mechanism of cytopenia in hypersplenism may be multifactorial. One important component is plasma volume expansion, which may be seen as massive splenomegaly and may produce a disproportionate amount of blood, including its cellular elements, in the spleen. The mild pancytopenia usually seen is presumably caused only by this effect of dilution. However, this may be exacerbated by increased destruction or sequestration of blood components in the spleen. Hypersplenism may be primary, in which no etiology can be found, or secondary to different disorders including infectious processes, inflammatory diseases, congestive hypersplenism, storage diseases, malignant diseases, chronic hemolytic disease, and cirrhosis. An epinephrine stimulation test (given intravenously over 15 minutes rather than subcutaneously) may show a dramatic increase in the granulocyte count if neutropenia is caused by hypersplenism rather than another cause in a patient with splenomegaly.

Treatment of hypersplenism is usually related to correction of underlying disorders. In cases of hypersplenism in which the underlying etiology is either unknown or cannot be corrected (especially with associated symptoms, such as abdominal discomfort, pain, or splenic infarction), splenectomy may be indicated. If the hypersplenism is associated with portal hypertension, it often responds to a shunting procedure. Shunting is problematic, however, with the possible recurrence of hypersplenism related to shunt thrombosis. In patients with storage disorders such as Gaucher's disease with cytopenia resulting from massive splenomegaly and plasma volume expansion, splenectomy may not resolve the cytopenia and may worsen the underlying disease. Partial splenectomy, through either surgical or emboli, may be useful in these disorders.

Complications of splenectomy in patients with enlarged spleens are substantial; these include venous thrombosis, infarction of the left lobe of the liver, increased susceptibility to infection, and increased incidence of ischemic heart disease resulting from increased blood viscosity. The very uncommon response to IVGG in this setting would not recommend frequent use of this therapy. Certainly patients who are asymptomatic, with mild to moderate pancytopenia, should be given no therapy.

SUGGESTED READING

Abdou NI, NA Pombejara C, Balentine L, Abdou NL. Suppressor cell-mediated neutropenia in Felty's syndrome. J Clin Invest 1978; 61:738–743.

Bowdler AJ. Splenomegaly and hypersplenism. Clin haematol 1983; 12:467–488.

Bussel J, Lalezari P, Hilgartner M, et al. Reversal of neutropenia with intravenous gammaglobulin in autoimmune neutropenia of infancy. Blood 1983;62:398–400.

Laszlo J, Jones R, Silberman HR, Banks PM. Splenectomy for Felty's syndrome: clinicopathological study, in 27 patients. Arch Intern Med 1978;138:597–602.

Logue GI, Shimm DS. Autoimmune granulocytopenia. Ann Rev Med 1980;31:191–200.

Minchinton RM, Waters AH. Autoimmune thrombocytopenia and neutropenia after bone marrow transplantation. Blood 1985; 66:752.

Murphy MF, Metcalfe P, Waters AH, et al. Immune neutropenia in homosexual men. Lancet 1985;1:217–218.

Pollack S, Cunningham-Rundles C, Smithwick EM, et al. High dose intravenous gammaglobulin for autoimmune neutropenia. N Engl J Med 1982;307:253.

Rothstein G, Clarkson DR, Larsen W, et al. Effect of lithium on neutrophil mass and production. N Engl J Med 1978;298:178–180.

Rustorgi PK, Currie MS, Logue GL. Complement-activating antineutrophil antibody in systemic lupus erythematosus. Am J Med 1985;78:972–976.

Starkebaum G, Singer JW, Arend WP. Humoral and cellular immune mechanisms of neutropenia in patients with Felty's syndrome. Clin Exp Immunol 1980;39:307–314.

Webster ADB, Platts-Mills TAE, Jannossy G, et al. Autoimmune blood dyscrasias in five patients with hypogammaglobulinemia; response of neutropenia to vincristine. J Clin Immunol 1981;1:113.

HEMOPHILIA

ALAN R. GILES, M.D., FRCPC

Generically, the term hemophilia should be applied to all hemostatic disorders resulting from an inherited deficiency of an individual coagulation factor. In common clinical usage, it has become customary to consider only those conditions caused by deficiencies of factor VIII (antihemophilic factor) or factor IX (Christmas factor). The former is by far the most commonly encountered inherited disorder of coagulation and affects approximately one in 10,000 of the male population, whereas the latter is five to ten times less frequent. Factor IX is one of a family of vitamin K-dependent zymogens that, in its activated serine protease form, is responsible for the conversion of a similar zymogen, factor X, to its activated enzymatic product. In contrast, factor VIII is not an enzyme but an essential cofactor for the activation of factor X by activated factor IX. Although they are quite different proteins, deficiency of either results in identical hemostatic consequences. Moreover, both deficiency states are inherited as sex-linked recessive disorders, and thus the clinical phenotype of each is identical. It is essential to appreciate this fact because replacement therapy, which is discussed in detail below, requires a precise diagnosis in order that the correct factor replacement therapy be chosen.

Prior to the middle 1960s, severely affected individuals had an extremely restricted life expectancy because of either the direct or the indirect complications of uncontrolled bleeding into joints, body cavities, and vital organs. In particular, the arthropathy resulting from joint bleeds was responsible for the high morbidity of surviving individuals. The introduction of effective replacement therapy has dramatically changed both the life expectancy and quality of life of these patients. The life expectancy of well-managed hemophiliac patients, is now approaching that of nonhemophilic individuals. However, major problems in their management still remain. These include the acquisition of inhibitors to replacement therapy by some patients, the constant risk of transfusion-transmitted infection, and the significant socioeconomic burden shared by both the patient and the health care system. The following account details the current approach to the management of these conditions. It is likely that the recent enormous increase in knowledge of the molecular biology of these conditions may modify this in the near future. The imminent introduction of replacement therapy using recombinant (genetically engineered) products is an obvious example of this. This and other developments are discussed in this chapter.

GOALS OF HEMOPHILIA THERAPY

The goals of hemophilia therapy are

1. Prevention and treatment of bleeding
2. Management of complications resulting from bleeding
3. Management of the socioeconomic implications of the disorder
4. Comprehensive medical care.

Prevention and Treatment of Bleeding

The cornerstone of modern therapy is the administration of appropriate replacement therapy either to prevent bleeding or to treat bleeding once it occurs. Such therapy must be given expeditiously and according to an appropriate dosage protocol that meets the needs of the prevailing clinical condition of the patient. In emphasizing this, it is extremely important not to neglect appropriate counseling of both the patient and medical attendants, who may not be expert in the management of hemophilia as to appropriate preventive measures that reduce the incidence of bleeding and subsequently the need for replacement therapy. For example, diligent dental prophylaxis reduces the need for surgical procedures. However, many bleeds are spontaneous, resulting from the trauma of everyday living, which cannot easily be avoided. Moreover, it is essential for the individual's social well-being and development that he be encouraged to maintain normal social and physical activities.

The risk of bleeding shows a reasonable correlation with the results of coagulation factor assay. One unit (U) of any coagulation factor is that amount found in 1 ml of plasma taken from a normal individual (100 percent activity). Severely affected hemophiliacs have less than 0.01 U per milliliter (1 percent) factor VIII or factor IX activity and experience major bleeding from birth. Moderately affected individuals have 0.01 to 0.05 U per milliliter (1 to 5 percent) of factors VIII or IX and are less likely to suffer spontaneous bleeding but bleed abnormally when traumatized. Hemophiliacs with over 0.05 U per milliliter (5 percent) factors VIII or IX are only mildly affected and may only require therapy when subjected to significant trauma. Moreover, individuals with 0.18 U per milliliter (18 percent) or more of factors VIII or IX may be totally asymptomatic and may be identified only at the time of major surgical procedures or trauma. Carrier females may have marginal reductions in clotting factor activity, depending on the degree of random inactivation of the normal versus the abnormal gene carried on the X chromosomes. In some cases, extreme lyonization may result in an affected female's having a significant bleeding diathesis. Following major trauma or surgical procedures, some carrier females with marginally depressed factor levels may experience a bleeding tendency.

Blood Products

The nature of the coagulation deficiency state must be precisely identified in order to select the appropriate blood product for replacement. Concentrates of either factor VIII or factor IX are available. Cryoprecipitate was the first available concentrate of factor VIII. In the treatment of classic hemophilia (factor VIII deficiency), this has largely been replaced by medium or high purity lyophilized factor VIII concentrate. However, in the treatment of factor VIII deficiency associated with von Willebrand's disease, cryoprecipitate remains the treatment of choice because it also contains biologically active von Willebrand factor. Generally speaking, the lyophilized concentrates of factor VIII are ineffective in correcting the abnormal bleeding time in von Willebrand's disease, although they apparently contain adequate amounts of von Willebrand factor antigen. It would appear that the multimeric structure is modified during their preparation, and the function of the transfused von Willebrand factor is affected. Because cryoprecipitate is difficult to sterilize by heating procedures (see further on), its use presents a continued risk of transmission of viruses such as human immunodeficiency virus and hepatitis B. Recent reports suggest that the later generation of lyophilized concentrates may preserve von Willebrand factor protein function. Given that these preparations can be effectively sterilized by heating, it is possible that they will become the treatment of choice. Further clinical studies are required, however, before general recommendations can be made. Lyophilized concentrates are preferred because (1) contamination by other plasma proteins is reduced; (2) storage is more convenient (freeze-dried concentrates may be stored in a domestic refrigerator, whereas cryoprecipitate must be stored in a −20°C freezer); (3) replacement volume is minimized even when high doses of factor VIII are given; and (4) as previously discussed, these concentrates appear to be amenable to effective heat sterilization of potentially contaminating viruses.

Factor IX is also available as a freeze-dried concentrate, but the concentrate provided (prothrombin complex concentrate) also contains the other vitamin K–dependent clotting factors, prothrombin (factor II), factor VII, and factor X in equivalent concentrations. However, some of the available products contain little if any factor VII. Highly purified factor IX concentrates have been developed by some agencies, but their approval by the regulatory authorities for general clinical use has not yet been granted.

Administration of Replacement Blood Products

Replacement therapy may be given expectantly (i.e., when bleeding occurs) or prophylactically. Although total prophylaxis (i.e., the maintenance of the clotting factor level within the normal range on an ongoing basis) is theoretically attractive, it is not feasible in practice and undesirable from the standpoints of cost, side effects, and/or risks of treatment. Limited prophylaxis, however, may be useful in certain situations. The modern hemophiliac patient often engages in physical pursuits that were previously untenable prior to the advent of replacement therapy. Given that participation in normal physical activities (with the exception of contact sports) should be encouraged, the judicious use of prophylactic therapy prior to strenuous physical exercise is appropriate. Similarly, elective surgical procedures are managed in this way. Finally, an individual may be particularly at risk of developing recurrent bleeding into a joint or organ, at which time limited prophylaxis (treatment usually administered on alternate days) may halt the progress of this development.

More frequently, therapy is administered expectantly as soon as possible after bleeding occurs and maintained until the danger of rebleeding has passed. The dosage required depends on the severity of the hemophilia and the nature and site of the bleed. Table 1 provides a general outline. It should be emphasized, however, that the intensity of treatment should be based on clinical response. Treatment should be administered as soon as bleeding is suspected. The hemophiliac is often the best judge as to whether or not bleeding is occurring, and it is better to overtreat rather than undertreat. Home administration of clotting factor concentrates significantly improves the efficiency of this approach, since much time can be lost in bringing the patient to the hospital. Clotting factor concentrates may be administered by the patient or a family member who has been appropriately trained. As well as improving efficiency, the direct involvement of the patient and family in medical care often imparts additional social benefits. Such therapy should still be closely supervised to maintain good transfusion techniques, such as the care of venous access and the safe disposal of hypodermic needles.

The dosage given in Table 1 may be calculated according to the body weight of the individual. Approximately twice as much factor IX as factor VIII is required to achieve the same increment in the circulating levels of each. One unit of factor IX per kilogram of body weight elevates the circulating level of factor IX by 1 percent. In contrast, 0.5 U of factor VIII per kilogram of body weight achieves the same increment. Consequently, a 70-kg patient with severe factor VIII deficiency (factor VIII < 1 percent) requires the infusion of 3,500 U of factor VIII to achieve 100 percent activity.

(Calculation: 70 [body weight in kilos] × 0.5 × 100 [increment required] = 3,500 U)

A factor IX–deficient patient of identical body weight requires 7,000 U.

(Calculation: 70 [body weight in kilos] × 1.0 × 100 [increment required] = 7,000 U)

One bag of cryoprecipitate contains 60 to 100 U of factor VIII. Information detailing the formulation is found on the labels of all vials of lyophilized concentrate (factors VIII and IX). As the biologic half-lives of the two coagulation proteins are different (factor VIII — 8 to 12 hours, factor IX — 24 hours), maintenance therapy for factor VIII deficiency requires repeat transfusions every 8 to 12 hours, whereas this can be reduced to 18 to 24 hours in the case of factor IX. When life-threatening bleeding is involved, therapy should be given more frequently.

In planning surgical procedures, it is essential to adopt a team approach. The surgical team must appreciate the restraints imposed on them and give a full account of the precise nature and timing of the procedures to be performed. With the exception of minor procedures, it is advisable to perform a therapeutic trial of concentrate therapy prior to the scheduled surgery. This allows the formulation of an adequate protocol and rules out the possibility of a previously undetected inhibitor. General guidelines to the dosages required are given in Table 1. Therapy should be continued for 7 to 10 days, depending on the nature of the procedure, and further therapy should be administered prior to the removal of sutures or other such supplementary surgical maneuvers.

TABLE 1 Recommended Dosages for Factor Replacement Therapy

Type of Bleed	*Recommended Factor Level (%)*	*Dose of Factor VIII* (U/KG)*	*Dose of Factor IX† (U/kg)*
Mild	30	15	30
Early joint or muscle bleeding			
Epistaxis			
Dental bleeding			
Persistent hematuria‡			
Moderate	50	25	50
Major joint bleeding			
Muscle bleeding			
Gastrointestinal bleeding			
Suspected abdominal bleeding			
Head trauma without neurologic deficit			
Major	100	50	100
Neck, tongue, pharynx bleeding			
Intracranial bleeding			
Surgery			
Compartment syndrome			
Major trauma			

*Subsequent doses of factor VIII are given every 8 to 12 hours.
†Subsequent doses of factor IX are given every 18 to 24 hours.
‡Use of antifibrinolytics contraindicated.

Alternatives to Replacement Therapy

In view of the risks of current replacement therapy, alternative modes of treatment should be considered whenever possible, particularly in individuals with mild to moderate disease. DDAVP (1-deamino-[8-D-arginine], a synthetic vasopressin) includes a moderate increase in factor VIII levels. However, its effect is relatively short-lived. Consequently, it is most useful in procedures such as dental extractions, in which surgical trauma is not prolonged. It can only be used in individuals with mild disease. Similarly, antifibrinolytics such as epsilon-aminocaproic acid and tranexamic acid are useful in similar situations. The latter is better tolerated than the former and is currently preferred. Because DDAVP also enhances fibrinolytic activity, an antifibrinolytic should be given in conjunction with this agent. When such an approach is adopted, it is essential that the medical attendants are familiar with and have available the traditional replacement therapy should this approach not prove efficacious.

Management of Complications of Hemophilia

Arthropathies remain the major complication of this condition. However, modern replacement therapy has significantly reduced this as a major cause of morbidity. Nonetheless, management of pain following this complication is a recurrent problem. Aspirin and aspirin-containing analgesics are contraindicated because of their association with a qualitative platelet function, which exacerbates the underlying bleeding diathesis. Acetaminophen is a satisfactory substitute, but nonsteroidal anti-inflammatory drugs such as ibuprofen may be of more benefit. Surgical maneuvers such as synovectomy or even total joint replacement have been performed with some success, although the long-term outcome remains to be evaluated. The importance of aggressive and expertly supervised physiotherapy should be emphasized. Muscle-wasting resulting from immobilization following joint bleeds is the forerunner of joint instability and eventually leads to permanently damaged joints. Early mobilization and active physiotherapy in association with effective factor replacement therapy are effective in breaking this cycle.

Management of Socioeconomic Implications of the Disorder

Hemophilia presents a significant economic burden to the individual, the family, and the health care system. This relates not only to the cost of therapy but also to the effect of such a disorder on education and employment. It is essential that hemophiliacs and their families receive expert and continuing advice on all such matters.

Advice on genetic counseling and the eugenic options available to hemophilic families is also required.

Traditional laboratory methods allied with classic pedigree analysis permit the diagnosis of the carrier status of approximately 80 to 85 percent of women at risk. Newer methods of DNA analysis have significantly increased diagnostic precision and permit accurate prenatal diagnosis in the very early stages of pregnancy. Access to such diagnostic procedures should be made available to all hemophilic families, together with the necessary counseling required to facilitate their decision making.

Comprehensive Hemophilia Care

The foregoing illustrates the multifaceted problem that hemophilia presents. Modern hemophilia management is facilitated by a team or comprehensive approach. Such programs bring together those specialty areas that may be involved at one time or another in the management of a hemophiliac. The coordination of these activities is the cornerstone of this approach to management. Thus, individuals involved in the medical, physical, and social management act in concert to develop and to optimize the management program. It has been demonstrated that such programs not only dramatically improve the individual's overall management but also significantly decrease the costs of health care delivery in reducing the number of inpatient admissions. Such programs should be established at centers where all the necessary expertise is available.

COMPLICATIONS OF TREATMENT

The complications of treatment relate to the following factors:

1. The development of inhibitors
2. Transfusion-transmitted infectious disorders
3. Allergic reactions
4. Thrombogenicity (prothrombin complex concentrates).

Inhibitor Development

Approximately 10 percent of factor VIII–deficient individuals develop immune-related resistance to replacement therapy. This also occurs in factor IX deficiency, but the incidence is probably less. Hemophiliacs should be tested for the presence of an inhibitor at least every 6 months, although failure of clinical response to replacement therapy may suggest it at any time. The mechanisms responsible for inhibitor development remain unclear, but there appears to be a familial propensity. The intensity and duration of replacement therapy do not appear to be predisposing factors. Once individuals have developed inhibitors, they constitute a significant management problem.

Immunosuppressant therapy alone is of questionable efficacy. Recent studies combining immunosuppressant therapy together with continued factor VIII replacement, intravenous gamma globulin concentrates, and selective immunodepletion have proved beneficial to some patients (see Suggested Reading). Further evaluation is required before this approach can be generally recommended because the facilities required are significant and concern remains regarding the use of immunosuppressant therapy in young individuals. Prothrombin complex concentrates have been demonstrated to bypass factor VIII and factor IX. These concentrates contain zymogens that are active below the factor IX–factor VIII dependent step in the coagulation cascade, i.e., prothrombin, factor VII, and factor X. It is known that the prothrombin complex concentrate fractionation process results in the formation of the activated products of these component clotting factors. Consequently, it was suspected that this activation may explain the bypassing effect observed. Controlled clinical studies have confirmed the potential benefit of such therapy. However, their optimal formulation and use require a clearer definition of the bypassing mechanism involved. This does not show direct correlation with the content of activated clotting factors, as previously supposed. In this regard, there is conflicting evidence concerning the view that the more activated preparations, specifically developed for this indication, are more efficacious than the nonactivated preparations developed specifically for factor IX replacement.

Acute life-threatening bleeds are best managed by the use of heterologous (porcine) factor VIII replacement, since many inhibitor patients have antibodies that do not show crossed species factor VIII specificity. However, the occasional anaphylactic reaction to subsequent infusions suggests that this therapy should be held in reserve for life-threatening bleeding. Alternatively, intensive plasma exchange with human factor VIII replacement can be extremely effective if the appropriate facilities are available. The continued use of human factor VIII replacement is controversial. Although some inhibitor patients develop an anamnestic response, thereby making subsequent therapy impossible, not all patients demonstrate this phenomenon. Such low responders may continue on human factor VIII replacement, although the dosage and frequency of replacement may need adjustment. In some practitioners' experience, even high responders may continue to respond and over time may develop a low responder phenotype. This observation makes the claim of induction of immune tolerance by high-dose factor VIII therapy difficult to interpret. This approach to therapy has the additional disadvantages of an enormous cost and a major increase in the risk of transfusion-transmitted infection (to be discussed). More recently, it appears that effective immunosuppression may be obtained with continued relatively low-dose factor VIII replacement. In some investigators' hands this may prove effective in up to 75 percent of inhibitor patients. However, the heterogeneity of the immune response over time (previously referred to) should still be considered in evaluating the outcome of this approach. Generally speaking, bleeding in most patients with inhibitors should be managed conservatively with techniques such as immobilization, cold compresses, and splinting. Factor VIII therapy may be continued, but each patient must be assessed individually. Those patients who do not respond to factor VIII should receive a clinical trial of prothrombin complex concentrate (75 to 100 U per kilogram of factor IX), as there is no doubt that this approach is successful in some situations. Overall, when a response is observed, it is suboptimal in comparison to the benefits noted following factor concentrate replacement in the noninhibitor patient.

The treatment of this complication is clearly unsatisfactory. It is hoped that research in this area will present better modes of treatment in the near future. At present the use of factor VIIIa is being investigated in clinical studies, and preliminary results using recombinant factor VIIa show promise, although the precise details of dosage protocols require further evaluation. It would appear that the overall dosage required is significantly greater than originally anticipated on the basis of preliminary studies performed with plasma-derived factor VIIa. The use of factor Xa in combination with coagulant active phospholipid is currently undergoing intensive preclinical evaluation in order to establish the limits of efficacy and toxicity prior to clinical study. Studies in hemophilic dogs have demonstrated major promise for this approach as an acutely acting and efficacious factor VIII bypass therapy. Finally, a more detailed understanding of the molecular biology of the deficiency state may allow more accurate predictions regarding those individuals at risk of this difficult complication of hemophilia.

Infectious Disorders

Because of the exposure to many blood donors, the risk of transfusion-transmitted infection is extremely high. All treated hemophiliacs demonstrate evidence of exposure to the hepatitis B virus. Fortunately, few appear to progress to chronic disease. Nonetheless, it is essential that all new hemophiliacs receive vaccination against the hepatitis B virus. The incidence of non-A, non-B hepatitis is also close to 100 percent, although the diagnosis of this condition presents obvious difficulties. The recent demonstration that a significant number of patients with non-A, non-B hepatitis are infected with the newly identified hepatitis C virus raises the possibility that this complication may be significantly reduced with screening of blood donors and the subsequent development of specific immunization procedures.

One of the most devastating problems in the current management of hemophilia relates to exposure to the acquired immunodeficiency syndrome virus (human immunodeficiency virus—HIV). Up to 90 percent of North American hemophiliacs treated prior to 1986 exhibit evidence of exposure to HIV. The precise implications of this remain to be ascertained, but a significant number of hemophiliacs have developed the acquired immunodeficiency syndrome, and many of them have died. Since 1986, all American factor concentrates have been prepared from plasma obtained from HIV seronegative donors, and subsequently the product has been either heat-treated or subjected to solvent detergent processing. Both procedures have been demonstrated to sterilize the final product effectively. Clinical studies of these products have been most encouraging and suggest that the new generation of hemophiliacs will not be at risk for this infection. Similar approaches also show great promise with regard to the transmission of non-A, non-B hepatitis.

Allergic Reactions

Allergic reactions are more commonly seen following the use of cryoprecipitate and may be resolved by switching to freeze-dried concentrates, which contain less contaminant proteins. Most cases respond to antihistamine, but hemophiliacs on home therapy should never be unaccompanied during treatment, and they or their families should have available and be familiar with the use of epinephrine should anaphylaxis occur.

Thrombogenicity of Prothrombin Complex Concentrates

The generation of activated products of the component clotting factors during fractionation has already been referred to with regard to factor VIII–factor IX bypass therapy. This activity may also induce thrombotic complications during their use as regular replacement therapy. It is clear that this side effect also relates to the presence of coagulation-active phospholipids, which may contaminate the source plasma. Recent improvements in fractionation techniques and plasma procurement have significantly reduced the incidence of this complication in the products currently available. However, such complications may still occur when prothrombin complex concentrates are used in high doses, particularly in the presence of liver disease, probably because of reductions in the levels of antithrombin III. As previously discussed, it is hoped that the highly purified factor IX concentrates will be available in the near future and this important complication of the current therapy for factor IX deficiency will be alleviated.

FUTURE DEVELOPMENTS

With the cloning of the genes for both factor VIII and factor IX, new developments in the management of these conditions have resulted and more can be expected in the future. DNA analysis is leading to the more accurate diagnosis of the carrier state in females at risk and to the development of prenatal diagnostic techniques to permit therapeutic termination of affected pregnancies at a very early stage. Cloning techniques and the expression of the gene products have resulted in the availability of recombinant factor VIII equivalent to the plasma product by in vitro and in vivo preclinical evaluation. Clinical studies to date are extremely encouraging and suggest that recombinant factor VIII is completely equivalent to the plasma-derived product. Use of this product should be free of infectious complications, but the problems of inhibitor development will remain. However, with the ever-increasing knowledge of the molecular biology of the proteins involved, the mechanisms of inhibitor development may be clarified, and more appropriate therapy may be developed. Although still in the remote future, gene therapy should no longer be considered an impossible development in the management of these conditions.

SUGGESTED READING

Forbes CD. Clinical aspects of the hemophilias and their treatment. In: Ratnoff OD, Forbes CD, eds. Disorders of hemostasis. New York: Grune & Straton, 1984:177.

Giles AR. By what mechanism could prothrombin complex concentrates promote factor VIII bypassing activity in vivo? Transfus Med Rev 1988; 1:131–137.

Graham JB, Green PP, McGraw RA, Davis LM. Application of molecular genetics to prenatal diagnosis and carrier detection in the hemophilias: Some limitations. Blood 1985; 66:7764–7769.

Lawn RM, Vehar GA. Molecular genetics of hemophilia A. Sci Am 1986; 254:48–65.

Nilsson IM, Berntorp E, Zettervall O. Induction of immune tolerance in patients with hemophilia and antibodies to factor VIII by combined treatment with intravenous IgG, cyclophosphamide, and factor VIII. N Engl J Med 1988; 318:947–950.

Thompson AR. Structure, function and molecular defects of factor IX. Blood 1986; 67:565–572.

White GC II, McMillan CW, Kingdon HS, Shoemaker CB. Use of recombinant antihemophilic factor in the treatment of two patients with classic hemophilia. N Engl J Med 1989; 320:166–170.

VON WILLEBRAND'S DISEASE

ZAVERIO M. RUGGERI, M.D.
THEODORE S. ZIMMERMAN, M.D.

PATHOGENESIS AND CLASSIFICATION

Von Willebrand's disease is a congenital bleeding disorder characterized by a complex hemostatic defect. Abnormal platelet function, expressed by prolonged bleeding time, is a consistent finding and may be accompanied by decreased factor VIII procoagulant activity. The pathogenesis of von Willebrand's disease is based on quantitative and/or qualitative abnormalities of von Willebrand factor, a large multimeric glycoprotein that circulates in plasma complexed with the factor VIII procoagulant protein. These two proteins form the factor VIII-von Willebrand factor complex. When present, the decreased factor VIII procoagulant activity is secondary to the reduced concentration of von Willebrand factor. The von Willebrand factor, but not the factor VIII procoagulant protein, is present in endothelial cells, the subendothelium, platelets, and megakaryocytes, as well as plasma.

Different forms of von Willebrand's disease can be identified by their patterns of genetic transmission as well as von Willebrand factor abnormalities in plasma and the cellular compartment. The distinction of various von Willebrand's disease subtypes is important for correct therapy. These include the following.

Autosomal Dominant Inheritance

Type I. These patients may represent over 70 percent of all cases. Concentrations of factor VIII procoagulant and von Willebrand factor in plasma are decreased, usually to the same relative degree. Concentration of von Willebrand factor in the cellular compartment is normal in the majority of patients, although cases have been reported with low platelet content of the protein. All sizes of von Willebrand factor multimers are present, though there may be a relative decrease in the largest multimers and the structure of individual multimers may be altered. The characteristic hemostatic and laboratory abnormalities result from reduced plasma concentrations of the factor VIII-von Willebrand factor complex.

Type II. Concentrations of factor VIII procoagulant activity and von Willebrand factor may be decreased or normal in plasma. Von Willebrand factor concentration is usually normal in the cellular compartment. Plasma lacks large multimeric forms of von Willebrand factor. Several type II variants have been described based on altered structure and function of von Willebrand factor. With the exception of type IIB variants, ristocetin-induced platelet-von Willebrand factor interaction is decreased.

In type IIB, there is heightened ristocetin induced platelet-von Willebrand factor interaction resulting from an increased affinity of the abnormal von Willebrand factor for the platelet glycoprotein Ib receptor. In some families, this heightened interaction results in chronic thrombocytopenia and the presence of platelet aggregates in the circulation.

Platelet type or so-called pseudo von Willebrand's disease is similar in many respects to type IIB von Willebrand's disease. However, the defect lies in the platelet receptor for von Willebrand factor which has an increased affinity for the protein.

Autosomal Recessive Inheritance

Type III. The patients are homozygous or double heterozygous for abnormal gene(s) inherited from both parents who are usually clinically normal. Factor VIII procoagulant activity is markedly decreased. Von Willebrand factor is undetectable or present in trace amounts both in plasma and in the cellular compartment. These patients are clinically the most severely affected. A subset of patients with complete homozygous deletion of the von Willebrand factor gene is prone to develop antibodies to von Willebrand factor after repeated infusions of concentrates containing the protein.

GENERAL PRINCIPLES OF THERAPY

The aim of therapy in von Willebrand's disease is to correct the prolonged bleeding time and, if present, the abnormality of blood coagulation. To achieve this, both von Willebrand factor and factor VIII procoagulant activity must be raised to normal levels in plasma. A normal concentration of a *functionally normal* von Willebrand factor must be achieved in patients with qualitative abnormalities of the protein.

Most patients with the more common autosomal dominant form of von Willebrand's disease have a relatively mild bleeding tendency. In children, mucosal bleeding, particularly epistaxis and gingival bleeding, are common symptoms. Excessive blood loss following dental extraction, tonsillectomy, or other common surgical procedures is also frequent, as are cutaneous bleeding and easy bruising. Gastrointestinal bleeding is not infrequent and can be without identifiable cause. In females, menorrhagia is not uncommon, particularly after the first menses and in adolescent girls in general. Excess postpartum bleeding can also occur. However, spontaneous joint and muscular bleeding are exceptional.

Bleeding symptoms may be present in patients with normal plasma levels of factor VIII procoagulant activity. Therefore, it is not surprising that effective therapy requires correction of the quantitative and/or qualitative von Willebrand factor defect. If this is not achieved, poor control of bleeding will be observed even if concentrations of factor VIII procoagulant activity are raised to normal or above.

The clinical picture of the recessive form of von Willebrand's disease is more severe. Mucosal and cutaneous bleeding, as well as hemorrhages from the female genital tract, occur more frequently and are of greater severity. Excessive bleeding after dental extractions or surgery can only be controlled by replacement therapy. Hemarthroses and muscular hematomata are not uncommon, and permanent disability may ensue in some cases. In these patients, correction of both the von Willebrand factor and factor VIII procoagulant defect is mandatory. In nonmucosal bleeding, particularly in cases of joint or muscle hemorrhage, raising the factor VIII procoagulant levels may be sufficient for effective hemostasis even when the bleeding time is not normalized. This is fortunate because individuals with homozygous von Willebrand factor gene deletion may develop antibodies to von Willebrand factor which may render von Willebrand factor replacement therapy ineffective.

There are two main approaches to the therapy of von Willebrand's disease. One is replacement therapy, i.e., the infusion of exogenous factor VIII-von Willebrand factor derived from normal plasma. The second is to induce release of endogenous factor VIII-von Willebrand factor from tissue stores using 1-Deamino-[8-D-Arginine]Vasopressin (DDAVP). Replacement therapy is the only possibility in patients with severe (type III) von Willebrand's disease who have markedly reduced levels of the factor VIII-von Willebrand factor related activities in both plasma and tissue stores. Infusion of DDAVP may release cellular factor VIII-von Willebrand factor into the circulation and increase its concentration to adequate levels in patients with the dominant form of von Willebrand's disease and who have normal tissue stores of von Willebrand factor. Occasional patients with type I and a larger percentage of type II variants do not respond to this drug.

DDAVP is contraindicated in both type IIB and platelet type (pseudo) von Willebrand's disease because raising the endogenous von Willebrand factor in either of these disorders results in thrombocytopenia.

REPLACEMENT THERAPY AND BLOOD DERIVATIVES

Replacement therapy is performed by infusing plasma fractions enriched in the factor VIII-von Willebrand factor complex. Infusion of blood derivatives in patients with von Willebrand's disease promotes a delayed increase in factor VIII procoagulant activity that is disproportionate to the amount administered. After the peak reached at the end of the infusion, factor VIII procoagulant activity continues to rise for 12 to 24 hours. On the contrary, von Willebrand factor starts to decrease immediately after the end of the infusion. Therefore, a discrepancy between factor VIII procoagulant activity and von Willebrand factor is found between 12 to 48 hours after treatment. Correction of the bleeding time defect is even shorter than that of the von Willebrand factor plasma levels. The delayed rise of factor VIII procoagulant activity is characteristically observed in all forms of von Willebrand's disease, with the exception of the recessive form in patients who have developed an inhibitor antibody to factor VIII-von Willebrand factor (see below).

Of the available sources of factor VIII-von Willebrand factor, only single-donor cryoprecipitate appears to correct both von Willebrand factor (bleeding time) and factor VIII procoagulant activity. Commercial concentrates of factor VIII-von Willebrand factor prepared from large pools of plasma are effective in raising the factor VIII procoagulant levels, but usually fail to correct the bleeding time, even when they bring the ristocetin cofactor activity up to normal levels. Single-donor cryoprecipitate contains the larger von Willebrand factor multimers that are necessary for shortening bleeding time. Most commercial concentrates of factor VIII-von Willebrand factor have lacked these larger multimers. Correction of both the bleeding time and procoagulant activity are important to achieve normal hemostasis in von Willebrand patients. Correction of the former is particularly important in the case of mucosal bleeding or whenever platelet adhesion to the subendothelium plays a major role in stopping hemorrhage. In most surgical procedures, when primary hemostasis can be bypassed by surgical hemostasis, correcting the factor VIII procoagulant abnormality becomes most important.

In severe bleeding episodes, a dose of cryoprecipitate between 30 and 50 U per kilogram is recommended. This dosage should raise factor VIII procoagulant activity and correct the bleeding time if the material contains the larger von Willebrand factor multimers. This effect on bleeding time, however, is transient and lasts less than 12 hours, probably because the larger forms of von Willebrand factor are rapidly cleared from the circulation. Therefore, cryoprecipitate should be administered twice a day if hemostasis must be kept normal at all times.

Replacement therapy with human blood derivatives, particularly those obtained from large plasma pools, carries a relatively high risk of transmitting viral hepatitis. This is particularly true in patients who have had no or limited exposure to factor VIII-von Willebrand factor concentrates. Single-donor cryoprecipitate is preferred for this reason as well as for its ability to correct the bleeding time and factor VIII-procoagulant activity levels. However, there is a small risk of transmitting the human immunodeficiency virus with cryoprecipitate. Although all donors are screened for antibodies to the virus, single-donor cryoprecipitate is not heat treated.

THE USE OF DDAVP

DDAVP (0.3 μg per kilogram) is the treatment of choice because of the virtual absence of serious side effects. However, it is not equally efficacious in all forms of the disorder. It is not effective in the severe recessive form (type III), in which tissue stores of von Willebrand factor are markedly reduced or absent. On the other hand, most patients with type I von Willebrand's disease will have a complete correction of their hemostatic abnormality lasting for 4 to 6 hours provided that von Willebrand factor concentration in plasma reaches normal levels. In type II disease, the bleeding time may not be corrected even though von Willebrand factor levels are increased to well within normal ranges. This ineffectiveness is due to the fact that the multimeric structure of plasma von Willebrand factor will not be normalized in these patients. However, factor VIII procoagulant levels will be restored to normal, and this may be sufficient for some surgical procedures in which primary hemostasis can be achieved by suturing or cautery. Where this is not possible (as in tooth extraction, gastrointestinal bleeding, or childbirth), normalization of factor VIII procoagulant activity without correction of the bleeding time will usually not secure hemostasis. Cryoprecipitate should be used in type II von Willebrand's disease whenever primary hemostasis must be assured. It also should be used in type I patients who do not obtain an adequate response to DDAVP.

Because DDAVP causes thrombocytopenia in IIB and platelet type (pseudo) von Willebrand's disease, its use should not be attempted in these disorders. Cryoprecipitate is usually effective in type IIB. Cryoprecipitate should be used sparingly in platelet type von Willebrand's disease since large amounts can cause thrombocytopenia.

PREGNANCY AND CHILDBIRTH

During pregnancy, factor VIII-von Willebrand factor levels tend to rise. In many individuals, particularly those with type I von Willebrand's disease, this will be sufficient to restore hemostasis to normal. However, complete correction will not occur in patients with severe von Willebrand's disease (type III) or those producing abnormal von Willebrand factor (type II). It is therefore recommended that the *bleeding time* be followed during pregnancy and, if it has not been corrected, that replacement therapy be given at the time of delivery.

INHIBITOR ANTIBODY DEVELOPMENT AFTER REPLACEMENT THERAPY

In a subset of patients with severe (type III) von Willebrand's disease, replacement therapy will induce the appearance of antibodies directed toward the factor VIII-von Willebrand factor complex. The individuals so affected have a homozygous deletion of the von Willebrand factor gene. These inhibitors may complicate the treatment of bleeding episodes, and correcting the abnormal hemostasis may be impossible when the inhibitor titer is too high. Since antibodies in these cases are specifically directed against von Willebrand factor, inactivation of factor VIII procoagulant activity probably occurs as a result of steric hindrance. Correcting the bleeding time abnormality is therefore more difficult than correcting the coagulation abnormality. This contrasts with the inhibitors seen in hemophilia A, which are directed at the factor VIII procoagulant protein and do not characteristically affect the bleeding time.

From the clinical point of view, management of soft tissue or joint hemorrhages in the presence of von Willebrand factor inhibitors may be satisfactory if plasma factor VIII procoagulant activity is raised. On the other hand, the inability of replacement therapy to shorten the bleeding time is associated with poor control of mucosal bleeding. Reactions have been described in patients with these inhibitors who are infused with factor VIII-von Willebrand factor concentrates. Most of these reactions are probably due to the precipitating nature of the antibodies, with formation of circulating antigen-antibody complexes. Infusion of factor VIII-von Willebrand factor concentrates into these patients will inevitably cause an amnestic rise of the inhibitor titer. Avoiding replacement therapy, on the contrary, may lead to disappearance of the antibody. To choose the correct dosage, antibody titers should be measured before replacement therapy is administered. Plasma factor VIII procoagulant activity and ristocetin cofactor activity should be tested in vitro to evaluate in vivo recovery of infused factor VIII-von Willebrand factor and to determine the successive dosage of replacement therapy often required. Post-transfusional antibody titers should also be monitored at periodic intervals.

ACQUIRED VON WILLEBRAND'S DISEASE

A bleeding diathesis similar to inherited von Willebrand's disease is occasionally seen on an acquired basis. This syndrome has been reported in association with lupus erythematosus, monoclonal gammopathy, hypernephroma, lymphoproliferative disorders, and angiodysplastic lesions. Antibodies to von Willebrand factor have been detected in a minority of these cases. However, von Willebrand factor is usually decreased in plasma, often to an impressive degree. The principles of replacement therapy outlined above apply to these patients. When antibodies have been detected, they should be monitored before and after replacement therapy.

SUGGESTED READING

Ruggeri ZM. Classification of von Willebrand disease. In: Verstraete M, Vermylen J, Lijnen R, Arnout J, eds. Thrombosis and haemostasis. Leuven, Belgium: Leuven University Press, 1987:419.

Ruggeri ZM, Zimmerman TS. Platelets and von Willebrand disease. In: Schick PK, Stormorken H, eds. Semin Hematol. New York: Grune & Stratton, 1985:203.

Zimmerman TS, Ruggeri ZM, Fulcher CA. Factor VIII/von Willebrand factor. Prog Hematol 1983; 14:279–309.

VITAMIN K-DEPENDENT COAGULATION FACTOR DEFICIENCY

MAUREEN ANDREW, M.D.

The importance of vitamin K in blood coagulation was serendipitously discovered in 1929 when bleeding was observed in chickens fed a fat free diet. The bleeding could be prevented by a factor in seeds and cereals, which in 1935 was identified as a fat soluble vitamin, termed K. Over the past 50 years, we have learned that vitamin K is required for the production of active forms for clotting factors II (prothrombin), VII (proconvertin), IX (Christmas factor), and X (Stuart-Prower factor), the coagulation inhibitors protein C and S, and two additional proteins that may not participate in hemostasis, protein Z and protein M. The characteristic chemical feature of the vitamin K-dependent proteins is a unique amino acid residue, gamma-carboxyglutamic acid. Vitamin K is responsible for the post-translational carboxylation of des-γ-carboxyglutamic acid to gamma-carboxyglutamic acid. The gamma-carboxyglutamic acid serves as a calcium binding site on the vitamin K-dependent proteins, allowing these proteins to form so-called calcium bridges with acidic phospholipids. This property is essential for the function of the vitamin K-dependent proteins in the coagulation mechanism. Deficiencies of the vitamin K-dependent coagulation proteins can be congenital (rare) or acquired (common). Deficiencies of factors II, VII, IX, and/or X are associated with bleeding whereas deficiencies of protein C or protein S lead to thrombosis. This chapter focuses on the treatment of the hemorrhagic complications of vitamin K deficiency. The general approach to the treatment of patients with an inherited predisposition to thrombosis (as occurs for proteins C and S) is discussed in a separate chapter.

ACQUIRED DEFICIENCY STATES

Acquired deficiencies for the vitamin K-dependent factors are either secondary to: (1) a lack of vitamin K; (2) inhibition of vitamin K; or (3) as part of other coagulopathies such as liver disease or a consumptive coagulopathy. A vitamin K deficient state results in the inhibition of the vitamin K-dependent carboxylation reactions. The latter results in the production and circulation of noncarboxylated proteins (PIVKA: protein induced by vitamin K absence [or antagonism]) which are functionally defective because they cannot bind calcium. The lack of functional activity for factors II, VII, IX, and X leads to a bleeding disorder which is responsive to treatment with vitamin K. Other acquired deficiencies of the vitamin K-dependent factors lead to a decrease in both the circulating protein as well as activity of the vitamin K-dependent factors.

SOURCES OF VITAMIN K

Vitamin K is a generic term for a group of fat soluble naphthoquinone derivatives. Vitamin K_1 (phylloquinone) is restricted to plants, and vitamin K_2 refers to a family of compounds with similar structures (the menaquinones) that are produced by bacteria in the gastrointestinal tract as well as being present in a variety of natural materials. Vitamins K_1 and K_2 as well as other vitamin K derivatives (e.g., vitamin K_3 or menadione) can be prepared synthetically and used therapeutically. The K vitamins, with the exception of the synthetic water soluble forms (e.g., vitamin K_3) are absorbed from the gastrointestinal tract only in the presence of adequate quantities of bile salts and pancreatic lipase. The daily requirements for vitamin K are estimated at approximately 0.5 to 1.5 μg per kilogram body weight per day for an adult and 1 to 5 μg per kilogram body weight for the newborn infant. In general, green leafy vegetables are high in vitamin K, fruits and cereals are low, and meats and dairy products are intermediate. A normal mixed diet contains 300 to 500 μg of vitamin K per day, an amount more than adequate to supply the dietary requirement of vitamin K.

VITAMIN K DEFICIENCY

Primary vitamin K deficiency is uncommon in healthy persons. This is due to a relatively low requirement for vitamin K, the widespread distribution of vitamin K_1 in plant and animal tissues, and the microbiologic flora of the normal gut, which synthesizes vitamin K_2 in amounts that can supply a large part of the requirement for vitamin K. In contrast, vitamin K deficiency is one of the most common coagulation abnormalities in patients admitted to hospital. Because the intestinal bacteria can produce vitamin K_2, it is extremely rare for an individual fed a diet low in vitamin K to become vitamin K-deficient. Similarly, even if the production of vitamin K_2 by the intestinal bacteria is reduced by broad spectrum antibiotics, a vitamin K deficiency is rare if the individual is maintained on a normal diet. However, the combination of inadequate dietary vitamin K in conjunction with the administration of broad spectrum antibiotics results in a severe vitamin K deficiency.

Certain groups of patients are at high risk for vitamin K deficiency. These groups include breast-fed newborn infants, chronically ill patients with an inadequate dietary intake of vitamin K, patients with disorders that interfere with the absorption of vitamin K (diarrhea, cystic fibrosis, biliary atresia, hepatitis, celiac disease), and patients with poor nutrition who are receiving broad spectrum antibiotics. Bleeding from vitamin K deficiency can present as cutaneous bleeding or gastrointestinal bleeding. Bleeding into the central nervous system is a potentially life-threatening complication that occurs as a manifestation of vitamin K deficiency, particularly in the neonate.

LABORATORY DETERMINATION OF VITAMIN K DEFICIENCY

Screening tests reflecting the decrease in the vitamin K-dependent procoagulants, such as the prothrombin time, activated partial thromboplastin time, and thrombotest are abnormal in vitamin K deficiency. Because other acquired or congenital coagulopathies can give similar screening test abnormalities, confirmatory tests for vitamin K deficiency are often needed. The simplest approach to confirm the diagnosis is to measure the functional amount of the vitamin K-dependent coagulation factors (II, VII, IX, and X). These results are low whereas the levels of the other coagulation factors are normal. The measurement of multiple coagulation factors is of limited usefulness when there is a concomitant coagulopathy such as liver disease. In addition, the newborn infant who is likely to develop vitamin K deficiency has physiologically low levels for the vitamin K dependent factors unrelated to vitamin K deficiency. Because of these limitations, more specific tests for a vitamin K deficiency have been developed. Most of these tests measure the noncarboxylated forms (PIVKAS) of the K-dependent factors that circulate in the plasma of the vitamin K-deficient patient. Our laboratory uses a snake venom from Echis carinatus, which cleaves both carboxylated and noncarboxylated prothrombin to thrombin. The use of Echis carinatus in an assay provides a rapid measurement of the total amount of prothrombin (Echis II) present. This value is then compared to the amount of carboxylated prothrombin (II) as measured in a conventional calcium phospholipid-dependent system. A ratio of II to Echis II of less than 0.80 indicates vitamin K deficiency.

THERAPY

Bleeding can occur as a result of isolated or multiple deficiencies of the vitamin K clotting factors. The former usually occur as a result of a congenital deficiency and are very rare. The latter, an acquired deficiency state, usually results from vitamin K deficiency or a general impairment of hepatic synthesis. The precise deficiency should be defined using the patient's history and appropriate coagulation tests. The specific type and route of therapy is dictated by the specific coagulopathy and by the urgency of the clinical situation. The risks and benefits of each form of therapy should be carefully considered for each patient. The following sections focus on the treatment of vitamin K deficiency.

The route for the administration of vitamin K determines the side reactions and the rapidity of response. Severe anaphylactoid reactions, with hypotension which can be fatal, have complicated intravenous vitamin K even when the solution is diluted and infused slowly. Therefore, intravenous administration of vitamin K should be restricted to those situations where other routes are not feasible and where the risk is justified. If the urgency of the clinical situation dictates the use of vitamin K intravenously, it should be infused no faster than 1 mg per minute. Vitamin K should never be given intramuscularly as a treatment for vitamin K deficiency. Intramuscular vitamin K can result in pain, swelling, and hematoma formation at the site. The preferred systemic route is subcutaneous because it is a safe and effective technique. If vitamin K is given orally, one must be sure that the patient is capable of absorbing it. In addition, oral vitamin K produces a slower correction of the prothrombin time compared with parenterally administered vitamin K. Approximately 50 percent of vitamin K given parenterally will be in the liver within 1 hour, and the coagulation abnormality corrects within 2 to 6 hours. In contrast, if the same dose is given orally, approximately 20 percent of the amount will be located in the liver within 2 hours, and the prothrombin is not corrected for 6 to 8 hours.

The vitamin K preparations available for clinical use are most commonly synthetic derivatives of vitamin K_1 and K_2 as well as the synthetic water soluble forms (e.g., vitamin K_3). The choice of a preparation is determined by the clinical situation. For example, large amounts of the water soluble, synthetic analogue vitamin K_3 should not be administered during pregnancy nor to the newborn because it can result in hemolytic anemia, jaundice, and resultant kernicterus in the newborn. We use vitamin K_3 for oral administration to nonpregnant adults and vitamin K_1 for systemic administration to all other patients.

Prevention of Vitamin K Deficiency

Prophylactic vitamin K (e.g., vitamin K_3 at a dose of 5 mg orally each day) should be given to patients at risk for vitamin K deficiency. The risk is highest for patients with inadequate nutrition who are receiving broad spectrum antibiotics. The risk is lower for patients receiving total parenteral nutrition and for chronically ill patients with inadequate nutrition. Oral administration of vitamin K_1 in the third trimester (5 mg daily) to pregnant women receiving oral anticonvulsant therapy may be helpful in preventing overt vitamin K deficiency in their infants at birth.

The American Academy of Pediatrics recommends that all newborn infants receive vitamin K at the time of birth. Despite the lack of a clinical trial confirming the necessity of vitamin K for all newborns, physicians should administer prophylactic vitamin K to all neonates immediately after birth since the adverse effects are minimal. This should be in the form of vitamin K_1 or K_2, but not a water soluble form such as Vitamin K_3.

A single dose of 0.5 to 1.0 mg, intramuscularly, is recommended. It is possible that effective prophylaxis can be achieved by orally administered vitamin K_1 or K_2. However, it may not be effective due to reduced absorption and regurgitation. The vitamin K needed during the first few months of life comes from breast milk or formula and may be important for prevention of a delayed form of vitamin K deficiency. The American Academy of Pediatrics recommends that milk substitute formulas be supplemented to supply at least 100 μg per liter of vitamin K. The average amount of vitamin K in 14 commercially available formulas is 830 μg per liter, which is considerably greater than breast milk (1 to 2 μg per liter) or cow's milk (15 to 17 μg per liter).

Treatment of Vitamin K Deficiency

Asymptomatic Patients

The treatment of vitamin K deficiency depends upon the clinical status of the patient and the cause of the deficiency. Asymptomatic patients with mildly abnormal coagulation results that are presumed secondary to vitamin K deficiency should be given vitamin K subcutaneously (10 mg). This approach is both therapeutic and diagnostic. The administration of vitamin K results in a correction of the coagulation abnormality within 2 to 6 hours.

Mild Bleeding

A patient bleeding because of vitamin K deficiency should receive 10 to 25 mg of vitamin K subcutaneously (or, if extremely urgent, intravenously). In addition, depending upon the severity of the bleeding, plasma (stored or fresh frozen) can also be given. Administering 10 to 20 ml per kilogram of fresh frozen plasma or stored plasma results in a boost of the vitamin K-dependent factors by approximately 0.1 to 0.2 units for each factor. Fresh frozen plasma is particularly useful when the precise nature of the coagulation factor deficiency is unknown, as all factors are present at approximately 1.0 unit per milliliter. Stored plasma, which has not been immediately frozen, has low levels for the labile factors V and VII, but contains normal amounts of the K-dependent clotting factor. Crossmatching is not required for the administration of plasma, but the plasma should be AB0 compatible with the recipient. The amount of plasma needed to correct totally a severe vitamin K deficiency is so large that it may result in volume overload.

Life-Threatening Bleeding

Any patient with a life-threatening hemorrhage or a hemorrhage into the central nervous system should receive factor IX concentrate (prothrombin complex concentrates) at a minimum dose of 50 units per kilogram in addition to systemic vitamin K (25 mg). Factor IX concentrates are commercially available and are provided in a lyophylized freeze-dried form. They contain relatively uniform amounts of factors II, IX, and X with VII being variable. The use of factor IX concentrates entails a number of potential risks to the patient including the transmission of hepatitis B and nonA-nonB. Patients should also receive hepatitis B immunoglobulin intramuscularly and a hepatitis vaccination as soon as the coagulopathy is corrected and within 24 hours of receiving the factor IX concentrate. Rarely, factor IX concentrates have been reported to precipitate disseminated intravascular coagulation, especially in those patients with liver disease.

Vitamin K deficiency can complicate other coagulopathies such as disseminated intravascular coagulation (particularly if there is hypovolemia or an intracranial hemorrhage as well) or liver disease. If there is any doubt about the diagnosis, the patient should receive vitamin K in conjunction with other supportive care.

Bleeding Due to Oral Anticoagulant Therapy

Patients with bleeding due to excessive anticoagulant therapy pose a particular problem. The oral anticoagulants are competitive antagonists of vitamin K and over correction with vitamin K makes it difficult to resume oral anticoagulant therapy. Excessive anticoagulation without bleeding can be managed by withholding the anticoagulant and monitoring the prothrombin time over time. However, bleeding requires a more aggressive approach. For patients with only moderately prolonged prothrombin time, with minor bleeding, and who need continued anticoagulant therapy, we give low doses of vitamin K (1 to 2 mg orally per day). The rationale for choosing the lowest effective dose is to avoid the problem of refractoriness to further anticoagulant therapy. Larger doses of vitamin K (10 to 20 mg subcutaneously) are recommended for patients with significant bleeding and for patients not needing further anticoagulant therapy. When vitamin K is used for this indication, it should be remembered that the half-life of vitamin K is shorter than that of oral anticoagulants and the prothrombin time often lengthens again after 24 hours if further vitamin K supplementation is not given. Severe, potentially life-threatening, bleeding requires large doses of parenteral vitamin K and treatment with prothrombin complex.

CONGENITAL DEFICIENCY STATES

Congenital deficiencies of the vitamin K-dependent clotting factors are rare and are documented by specific factor assay measurement. The management of the most common, factor IX deficiency (Christmas disease or hemophilia B), is included in another chapter. In general, prothrombin complex concentrates are the most convenient and effective treatment available for factor IX deficiency. Deficiencies of factors II, VII, and X can be treated with either plasma or factor IX concentrates, depending upon the clinical situation.

SUGGESTED READING

Brace L. The pharmacology and therapeutics of vitamin K. Am J Med Technology 1983; 49:457–463.

Prentice CRM. Acquired coagulation disorders. In: Ruggeri ZM, ed. Clinics in haematology. Toronto: WB Saunders, 1985:411.

Shapiro AD, Jacobson LJ, Armon ME, Manco-Johnson MJ, Hulac P, Lane PA, Hathaway WE. Vitamin K deficiency in the newborn infant: prevalence and perinatal risk factors. J Pediatr 1986; 109:675–680.

DISSEMINATED INTRAVASCULAR COAGULATION

JEFFREY I. WEITZ, M.D., FRCPC, F.A.C.P.

Disseminated intravascular coagulation (DIC) is not a single disease entity, but rather is a clinicopathologic syndrome associated with a wide variety of primary disorders (Table 1). The initiating event in intravascular coagulation is local or systemic activation of the coagulation mechanism. In each of the clinical disorders associated with intravascular coagulation, a biologically plausible triggering mechanism has been identified. Activation of the coagulation system leads to thrombin formation. Because of its multiple actions, thrombin causes consumption of platelets and clotting factors and converts fibrinogen to fibrin. The biologic consequences of these events reflect the dynamic balance between clot deposition and fibrin dissolution. The resulting clinical manifestation may be hemorrhage (when depletion of platelets, coagulation factors, and the anticoagulant effects of fibrin degradation products predominate), ischemic tissue damage due to vascular

TABLE 1 Etiology of Intravascular Coagulation

Infection
Hypotension
Malignancy
Obstetrical conditions
Abruptio placentae
Amniotic fluid embolism
Retained dead fetus
Other
Immunologic (incompatible blood transfusion, allograft rejection, immune complex disease)
Metabolic (diabetic ketoacidosis)
Injuries (burns, envenomation)
Vascular abnormalities (cavernous hemangiomas, dissecting aneurysm)

occlusion by fibrin and/or platelet thrombi, or a combination of hemorrhage and thrombosis.

INITIATION OF COAGULATION

The two major mechanisms through which the various diseases associated with intravascular coagulation can activate the coagulation pathway are: (a) endothelial cell injury, and (b) the release of procoagulant material into the circulation.

Endothelial Cell Injury

Endothelial cell injury may be a systemic process or may be localized to a specific anatomical site. Systemic endothelial cell injury may occur with infectious processes, and in many cases, this is the result of endotoxemia. In vitro studies indicate that endotoxin has the potential to perturb the delicate balance between the procoagulant and the anticoagulant activities of endothelial cells. Further, experimental endotoxemia in rabbits results in endothelial sloughing, thereby allowing interaction of the exposed basement membrane with the contact factors of coagulation. Other potential causes of systemic damage to the vascular endothelium include immunologic injury, burns, and acidosis.

Localized vascular abnormalities associated with decreased blood flow may also activate the coagulation system. Examples of this are disseminated intravascular coagulation secondary to giant cavernous hemangiomas (Kasabach-Merritt syndrome) or dissecting aortic aneurysms.

Release of Procoagulant Material

Tissue injury may trigger intravascular coagulation through the release of tissue factor into the circulation. Brain, lung, and placenta are especially rich in this membrane-bound apoprotein, thus explaining the occurrence of intravascular coagulation with head injury or in association with various obstetrical conditions. Blood vessel walls, endothelial cells, and monocytes also contain tissue factor activity that may be increased by various stimuli. Finally, in pathologic states such as acute promyelocytic leukemia, the malignant cells contain tissue thromboplastin.

Procoagulants other than tissue factor may also activate the coagulation system. Purified mucin isolated from adenocarcinomas can directly activate factor X as can a cysteine proteinase isolated from tumor cells. The activated clotting factors present in commercial concentrates of factors II, VII, IX, and X (prothrombin complex concentrates) may produce diffuse intravascular coagulation, especially when these concentrates are given to patients with hepatic disease, since the impaired liver is unable to clear the activated clotting factors. Finally, certain snake venoms contain enzymes that activate prothrombin, convert fibrinogen to fibrin, or activate platelets and hence can trigger intravascular coagulation.

PATHOGENESIS OF DISSEMINATED INTRAVASCULAR COAGULATION

There is increasing evidence that hemostasis is a dynamic process in which the platelets, the coagulation mechanism, and the procoagulant activity of endothelial cells that favor clot formation are balanced by the anticoagulant properties of endothelial cells, circulating inhibitors of thrombin, and the plasma and cellular fibrinolytic enzyme systems. If the stimulus activating the coagulation system results in fibrin formation in excess of that which can be handled by the compensatory fibrinolytic system, intravascular fibrin thrombi accumulate, and the pathologic syndrome of disseminated intravascular coagulation develops (Fig. 1).

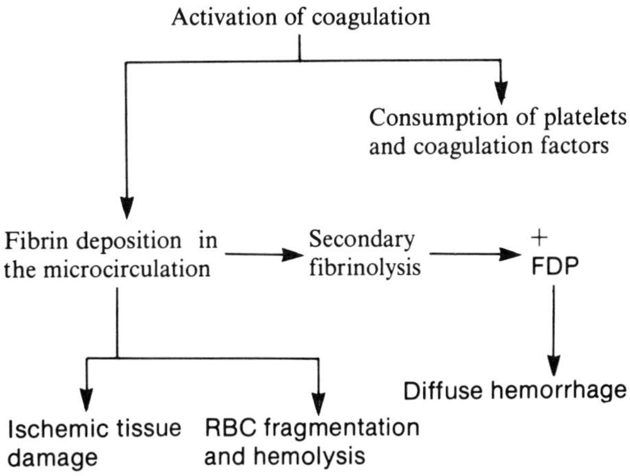

Figure 1 The pathophysiology of disseminated intravascular coagulation. Illustrated are the interactions between the coagulation and fibrinolytic pathways that result in the clinical manifestations of the syndrome.

ROLE OF THROMBIN

All of the clinical, biochemical and pathologic manifestations of disseminated intravascular coagulation can be directly or indirectly explained by the formation of thrombin. Thrombin and other activated coagulation factors are normally inhibited by interacting with antithrombin III. In disseminated intravascular coagulation, antithrombin III is consumed as it complexes with thrombin and other serine proteinases. With depletion of antithrombin III, unopposed thrombin is then free to interact with platelets, fibrinogen, and various coagulation factors (Fig. 2). Thrombin binds to platelets causing platelet release and aggregation. Removal of platelet aggregates by the reticuloendothelial system and the deposition of platelet thrombi in the microvasculature results in thrombocytopenia. Thrombin mediated conversion of fibrinogen to fibrin leads to a decrease in the plasma fibrinogen concentration. Further, contact of fibrin with the endothelium results in the release of tissue plasminogen activator (tPA) from the endothelial cells. The tPA binds to the fibrin and activates plasminogen to plasmin. Plasminogen is incorporated into fibrin as it polymerizes through attachment via its lysine binding sites. The bound plasmin generated in situ is protected from inhibition by circulating alpha-2-antiplasmin and degrades the fibrin, thereby producing fibrin degradation products (FDP) and D-dimer (a product of plasmin-mediated lysis of cross-linked fibrin). Liberated plasmin is rapidly inhibited by alpha-2-antiplasmin, thus leading to a decrease in plasma alpha-2-antiplasmin, and an increase in the concentration of plasmin-alpha-2-antiplasmin complexes. With depletion of alpha-2-antiplasmin, unopposed plasmin can degrade fibrinogen and other clotting factors, thereby contributing to the hemorrhagic state.

Thrombin also acts on factors V, VIII, and XIII. Initially, limited thrombin mediated proteolysis of the zymogens results in their activation, and the increase in activated factors VIII and V may shorten plasma clotting times. With further thrombin attack, however, these coagulation factors are degraded into inactive fragments and their plasma concentration decreases. This leads to a prolongation of the plasma clotting times and impairment of hemostasis.

THROMBOTIC MANIFESTATIONS

The thrombotic manifestations of DIC are the result of fibrin and/or platelet desposition in the microvasculature. Circulatory occlusion produces organ hypoperfusion, which can lead to ischemic tissue necrosis. Because this process is disseminated, all organs are susceptible. Most obvious upon physical examination is skin involvement, which manifests as hemorrhagic necrosis of the digits, nose, and genitalia as a result of occlusion of terminal arterioles or as more diffuse skin infarction (purpura fulminans). The deposition of microthrombi in the renal vasculature may cause hematuria and oliguria, while involvement of cerebral vessels results in nonfocal cerebral dysfunction, which may manifest as an altered level of consciousness or as generalized seizures. Less frequently, especially in those with compromised cardiopulmonary reserve, progressive hypoxemia or respiratory distress syndrome may develop as a result of occlusion of pulmonary vessels.

MICROANGIOPATHIC HEMOLYTIC ANEMIA

Incomplete occlusion of small vessels by microthrombi may retard blood flow, and red cells may be damaged as they traverse the fibrin strands. This leads to microangiopathic hemolytic anemia with reticulocytosis, hemoglobinemia, hemoglobulinuria, and characteristic morphologic abnormalities with the appearance of red cell fragments (schistocytes) and helmet cells.

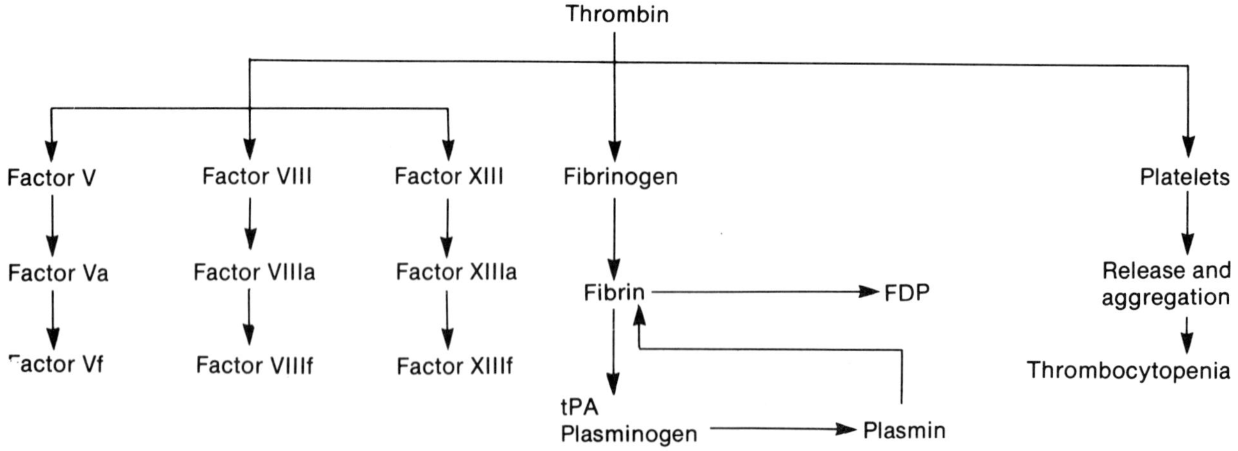

Figure 2 The pivotal role of thrombin in the pathogenesis of the biochemical abnormalities associated with disseminated intravascular coagulation. See text for details.

HEMORRHAGIC COMPLICATIONS

The hemorrhagic complications of disseminated intravascular coagulation are multifactorial in origin. Formation of microthrombi depletes the supply of platelets and coagulation factors, thereby resulting in marked thrombocytopenia and a decrease in fibrinogen, prothrombin, and factors V, VIII, and XIII. In addition to consumption of platelets and clotting factors, secondary activation of the fibrinolytic system and lysis of intravascular thrombi lead to the formation of fibrin degradation products. These fibrin derivatives have anticoagulant properties and they retard fibrin polymerization (which is reflected by a prolongation of the thrombin clotting time) and impair platelet function by interfering with platelet-to-platelet interaction.

LABORATORY MANIFESTATIONS

The laboratory diagnosis of disseminated intravascular coagulation is made by a decreased platelet count and fibrinogen concentration, a prolonged prothrombin time, and increased levels of FDP and/or D-dimer in the presence of clinical evidence of hemorrhage or thrombosis.

Thrombocytopenia, as a result of peripheral platelet destruction, is a cardinal feature of intravascular coagulation. In over 50 percent of cases, the platelet count is less than 50,000 per microliter. The decreased fibrinogen concentration results from a combination of thrombin induced clotting and plasmin induced fibrinogenolysis. Prolongation of the prothrombin time reflects the decrease in factor V and, to a lesser extent, decreases in prothrombin and fibrinogen. The hallmark of intravascular coagulation, however, is the presence of increased levels of FDP and/or D-dimer. Like a decrease in antithrombin III levels, this finding is not specific for intravascular coagulation. Increased levels of FDP (or D-dimer) and low antithrombin III values may be found in patients with hepatic disease.

The presence of schistocytes, as a reflection of microangiopathic hemolytic anemia, provides useful confirmatory evidence for the diagnosis of disseminated intravascular coagulation. However, fragmented red cells are seen only in about one-quarter of the cases of intravascular coagulation, and hence their absence does not exclude the diagnosis.

THERAPY

When faced with the patient with disseminated intravascular coagulation, it is useful to consider: (a) the tempo of the illness, (b) the predominant clinical manifestations (i.e., hemorrhage and/or thrombosis), and (c) the pathologic mechanism responsible for triggering the process.

Tempo of the Illness

The intensity and duration of activation of the coagulation system—the tempo of the process—have a profound influence on the clinical picture. Accordingly, it is important to determine whether the clinical presentation is severe enough to warrant specific therapy and whether the triggering event is self-limited in nature or is ongoing and unlikely to respond to treatment for some time.

In those individuals with biochemical evidence of consumption only, no specific therapy is required other than that indicated for the treatment of the underlying disease. In contrast, specific therapy is necessary if the patient presents with hemorrhagic or thrombotic manifestations, if the underlying disorder is unlikely to respond promptly to treatment (e.g., a malignant process), or if the consumptive process is likely to gain momentum as the disease progresses (e.g., following induction chemotherapy for acute promyelocytic leukemia).

Clinical Manifestations

The clinical picture may be characterized by thrombosis and/or hemorrhage, depending on whether thrombin or plasmin action predominates. Accordingly, antithrombotic therapy should be considered for patients with evidence of tissue hypoperfusion as a result of fibrin deposition in the microvasculature. Patients with hemorrhage as the major manifestation should receive fresh frozen plasma and cryoprecipitate to replace the depleted coagulation factors and platelet concentrates to correct thrombocytopenia. If bleeding perisists despite vigorous replacement, the addition of antithrombotic therapy should be considered.

Pathologic Mechanism

Consideration must be given to the pathologic mechanism triggering the process. This involves assessment of both the location at which activation of the coagulation system is occurring and the trigger for the process. Such evaluation provides insight into the treatment and the prognosis.

ACUTE DISSEMINATED INTRAVASCULAR COAGULATION

The most important aspects of therapy are those directed at treatment of the underlying disorder and general support measures aimed at maintaining blood pressure and tissue oxygenation. The need for further therapy depends on the patient's response to these measures. Thus, if the underlying disorder can be readily treated (e.g., antibiotic administration for sepsis) and the medical condition can be rapidly stabilized, no specific therapy for intravascular coagulation is necessary. In contrast, severe or progressive tissue hypoperfusion as a result of microvascular thrombosis indicates the need for antithrombotic therapy with heparin, while significant bleeding requires aggressive replacement therapy with platelets and clotting factors.

Heparin is given to inhibit the formation of microthrombi. The optimal dose of heparin is uncertain, but it is reasonable to give 1,000 units per hour by continuous intravenous infusion and to titrate the dose according to the clinical response. Once heparin therapy has been initiated, the hemorrhagic manifestations should be treated by vigorous replacement with platelets and clotting factors. Each unit of platelet concentrate can be expected to increase the platelet count by 5,000 to 10,000 per microliter, and a platelet count over 50,000 per microliter is a reasonable target. Fresh frozen plasma provides all the necessary clotting factors (including antithrombin III), while cryoprecipitate is an excellent source of fibrinogen. Clotting factor replacement can be monitored by following the fibrinogen concentration. A fibrinogen level of 1 g per liter is more than adequate to effect normal hemostasis. Any increase in the platelet count and fibrinogen concentration following replacement therapy indicates that the consumptive process is coming under control. Clinically, this is reflected by a decrease in the bleeding.

Vigorous replacement therapy is indicated for patients presenting with severe hemorrhage as a result of intravascular coagulation. Failure to control the bleeding and to raise the platelet count or fibrinogen concentration in these patients indicates ongoing consumption. Accordingly, antithrombotic therapy with heparin should be initiated to block fibrin formation, and vigorous transfusion of platelets and clotting factors should be continued.

Fibrinolytic inhibitors have a limited role in the treatment of patients with intravascular coagulation. The rationale for using these agents is to decrease the concentration of fibrin degradation products and to stabilize the hemostatic plugs. However, by blocking compensatory fibrinolysis, these compounds may potentiate microvascular thrombosis. Accordingly, fibrinolytic inhibitors should be reserved for the rare patient who has evidence of systemic fibrin(ogen)olysis and continues to have life-threatening bleeding despite heparin and vigorous replacement therapy.

CHRONIC DISSEMINATED INTRAVASCULAR COAGULATION

In contrast to acutely ill patients with severe intravascular coagulation, some patients present with subclinical disease manifested only by laboratory abnormalities. Most of these patients have long-standing illnesses such as malignancy or autoimmune diseases. While easy bruising or hemorrhage may occur, a significant number of patients with underlying malignant disease present with venous thrombosis. Signs of microvascular thrombosis, however, are unusual. Another feature unique to this patient group is nonbacterial thrombotic endocarditis with systemic emboli or infarction.

Patients with only laboratory abnormalities require treatment of the underlying disorder and follow-up studies. Those presenting with venous thrombosis or overt skin infarction are treated with heparin. The coumarin derivatives may be less effective at controlling the consumptive process in this patient group, so that long-term treatment with subcutaneous heparin may be necessary. When bleeding manifestations predominate, replacement therapy should be given and heparin added if the hemorrhage continues. The prognosis in these patients depends on the underlying disease, and all efforts must be directed at its control.

SUGGESTED READING

Bick RL. Disseminated intravascular coagulation and related syndromes: etiology, pathophysiology, diagnosis and management. Am J Hematol 1978; 5:2656.

Colman RW, Robboy SJ, Minna JD. Disseminated intravascular coagulation (DIC): an approach. Am J Med 1972; 52:679.

Marder VJ. Consumptive thrombohemorrhagic disorders. In: Williams WJ, Beutler E, Erslev AJ, Lichtman MA, eds. Hematology. New York: McGraw-Hill, 1983.

DEFICIENCY OF NATURALLY OCCURRING ANTICOAGULANTS: ANTITHROMBIN III, PROTEIN C, AND PROTEIN S

PHILIP C. COMP, M.D., Ph. D.

Protein C, protein S, and antithrombin III are plasma proteins that regulate the formation of blood clots in the body. This protective, regulatory effect involves inhibition of the clotting cascade at several levels. The enzymatically active form of protein C, termed activated protein C, inhibits clotting at the levels of factors V and VIII in the cascade. Protein S is a necessary cofactor for the anticoagulant activity of activated protein C. Both protein C and protein S are vitamin K dependent plasma proteins and are structurally similar to the vitamin K dependent clotting factors, such as factors X, IX, VII, and prothrombin. In addition to inhibiting the clotting cascade, activated protein C promotes fibrinolysis, partly by inactivating an inhibitor of tissue plasminogen activator.

Antithrombin III inhibits coagulation by permanently inactivating various active clotting factors, such as the active form of factor X (factor Xa). The rate at which antithrombin III (AT III) inhibits these clotting factors is greatly enhanced by heparin. In the body, heparin is not normally found in the circulation. However, heparan sulfate (a compound closely related to heparin) occurs on the surface of the endothelial cells that line the vascular bed and greatly enhances the rate at which AT III inhibits the active clotting factors in vivo.

LABORATORY DIAGNOSIS OF DEFICIENCY STATES

Measurement of AT III plasma levels is straightforward and can be performed in most large hospital laboratories and by a number of reference laboratories. Detection of functional AT III activity is preferable since some deficient individuals have normal antigenic levels of AT III but have significantly reduced functional activity. Warfarin therapy raises AT III levels as much as 15 to 25 percent in some individuals, and thus an AT III deficient individual receiving warfarin might appear normal. Intravenous heparin therapy lowers the levels of detectable AT III.

Protein C is presently measured by immunologic methods, but functional assays involving the use of snake venom proteins may soon become widely available. Protein S is presently measured by immunologic techniques. Protein S is found in two forms in plasma, and methods that detect the free, functionally active, form of protein S may be particularly useful. The levels of both protein C and protein S are significantly reduced by warfarin therapy, and diagnosis of deficient individuals receiving warfarin involves the comparison of the levels of protein C and protein S to the levels of other vitamin K dependent plasma proteins, such as prothrombin. For this comparative approach to have any validity, the patient must receive stabilized warfarin therapy for at least 2 weeks. During pregnancy, the levels of protein S fall markedly, probably due to hormonal effects. This makes the diagnosis of protein S deficiency during pregnancy difficult. This decrease in protein S can persist several weeks after delivery. Oral contraceptives also lower protein S levels to a significant degree, but the detection of congenital protein S deficiency in women taking oral contraceptives should still be feasible.

Since both heparin and warfarin affect the measurement of these natural anticoagulants, the ideal time to test the patient for possible deficiency is before anticoagulant therapy is initiated. Alternatively, parents of the affected individual may be studied, as may siblings or children who have a history of thromboembolic complications but who are not anticoagulated.

CLINICAL PRESENTATION

Thromboembolic Disease

Patients deficient in either protein C, protein S or antithrombin III are at risk of recurrent thrombophlebitis and pulmonary emboli. Additionally, protein C deficient individuals are at risk of two other thrombotic complications, warfarin induced skin necrosis and purpura fulminans neonatalis. (Table 1)

The median age of onset of thromboembolic disease is approximately 27 years in individuals with heterozygous deficiency of either protein C, protein S or antithrombin III. Patients may present with venous thrombosis as early as 14 years of age and a strong family history is often present. Protein S deficient men often present at an earlier age with their first episode of thrombosis than do protein S deficient women. A protein S deficient son frequently develops deep vein thrombosis before his mother develops similar problems.

While the major thrombotic events reported in protein C, protein S, and AT III deficiencies are throm-

TABLE 1

Deficiency	*Associated Thrombotic Complications*
Protein C	Venous thromboembolism
	Purpura fulminans neonatalis
	Warfarin induced skin necrosis
Protein S	Venous thromboembolism
AT III	Venous thromboembolism

bophlebitis and pulmonary emboli, arterial thrombosis has been reported in each of these conditions. This should be kept in mind when evaluating patients with unexplained arterial clot formation.

Purpura Fulminans Neonatalis

A disastrous thrombotic complication of homozygous protein C deficiency, termed purpura fulminans neonatalis, occurs in affected newborn babies. The infants develop necrotic areas of skin which are histologically characterized by thrombosis of the small vessels in the dermis and underlying tissue. The affected areas of skin are not viable, and if the infant survives this frequently fatal syndrome, extensive scarring occurs. Diagnosis of homozygous protein C deficiency is not particularly easy since normal newborns have only 20 to 30 percent of adult levels and these affected infants frequently have been treated with a variety of plasma products and heparin or warfarin. Measurement of protein C levels in the parents is often the best way to diagnose presumptive homozygous deficiency in the infant. This condition has not been reported in protein S or antithrombin III deficient kindreds.

Warfarin Induced Skin Necrosis

Warfarin induced skin necrosis may occur when warfarin therapy is initiated in heterozygous protein C deficient individuals. Skin necrosis due to clots in the small vessels of the skin occurs, usually on the second or third day of warfarin treatment. The breasts and flanks are frequently affected. Protein C is vitamin K dependent and has a short half-life compared with most of the vitamin K dependent clotting factors. Warfarin causes a substantial and rapid disappearance of protein C activity in the plasma before adequate anticoagulation is achieved. While normal individuals are not significantly affected by this early drop in protein C, heterozygous protein C deficient individuals experience profound decreases in protein C and thus are prone to skin necrosis. Not all protein C deficient individuals develop skin necrosis when warfarin therapy is initiated. Concomitant intravenous heparin may offer protection. Determination of protein C status is prudent before initiating warfarin therapy in an individual with a personal or family history that is compatible with protein C deficiency. Skin necrosis has not been reported in protein S or antithrombin III deficiency.

TREATMENT

Treatment of deep vein thrombosis or pulmonary emboli in patients deficient in protein C, protein S, or antithrombin III requires heparin and the judicious use of warfarin. Objective diagnosis of either deep vein thrombosis or pulmonary emboli is essential. Many of these patients have had recurrent episodes of lower extremity thrombosis and may have postphlebitic damage to the leg veins with accompanying swelling and tenderness, but no active thrombus formation. Bilateral contrast venography with the legs in a dependent position to ensure adequate filling of the calf veins is recommended. As noninvasive alternatives to venography, I^{125} fibrinogen scanning is useful for detecting active clotting in the lower leg, and impedance plethysmography may be used to detect clots in proximal leg veins. Pulmonary angiography should strongly be considered to diagnose pulmonary emboli. In treating patients known to have congenital deficiencies predisposing them to thrombosis, care must be taken not to overdiagnose thromboembolic disease, since in some instances making such a diagnosis may commit the patient to long-term oral anticoagulation. Also, in protein C deficient individuals, this diagnosis may subject the patient to the risk of warfarin induced skin necrosis.

Conventional treatment of individuals who develop thrombosis is initiated with a bolus of intravenous heparin (5,000 to 10,000 units) followed by a continuous infusion of heparin sufficient to keep the activated partial thromboplastin time (aPTT) at 2.0 to 2.5 times the mean of the normal range for the particular aPTT reagent the laboratory is using. Individuals with mild-to-moderate antithrombin III deficiency can often receive successful anticoagulation with heparin, although relatively larger dosages (frequently as high as 2,000 units per hour for a 70 kilogram individual) are required. Heat-treated antithrombin III concentrates are becoming available in North America, and simultaneous infusion of heparin and antithrombin III should be considered in severely antithrombin III deficient individuals who do not respond to the higher dosages of heparin alone. Congenitally deficient individuals may be treated with fibrinolytic therapy, followed by intravenous heparin and warfarin. Also, the use of either streptokinase or, when available, tissue plasminogen activator should be considered very early in the course of therapy.

Warfarin administration should be initiated at approximately the fifth day of heparin therapy, and the heparin should be continued at therapeutic levels until adequate prolongation of the prothrombin time is achieved. An initial warfarin dose of 10 mg is suggested. Once a prothrombin time of 1.5 to 1.8 times the mean normal control range time is achieved, heparin may be discontinued. Oral anticoagulant status should be monitored daily until the patient leaves the hospital. The prothrombin time should then be checked twice a week after discharge for 2 weeks, once a week for a month, and then at least monthly thereafter. Any change in warfarin dosage requires close monitoring until the new level of anticoagulation is achieved.

Warfarin induced skin necrosis poses a threat to protein C deficient patients. Many protein C deficient patients have, however, achieved successful anticoagulation with warfarin and have remained without recurrent thromboembolic disease while receiving the anticoagulant. Unfortunately, the optimal method of initiating warfarin therapy in known protein C deficient patients has not been established. Isolated case reports suggest that the use of very low initial doses of warfarin may be successful; the simultaneous administration of plasma to provide an adequate source of protein C has been employed. Simultaneous heparin administration may, in fact, provide adequate systemic anticoagulation to prevent warfarin induced skin necrosis; this may explain the relative infrequency of skin necrosis. Actual evidence that this is the case is, however, wanting.

Warfarin induced skin necrosis is frequently associated with other medical conditions in addition to venous thromboembolic disease. These include infection, extensive trauma, the postoperative period, and inflammation. Particular caution in initiation of warfarin treatment in such individuals is advised. Similarly, although the simultaneous initiation of heparin and warfarin therapy has been suggested as a means of shortening the hospitalization of patients with venous thrombosis, an initial treatment period with heparin before starting warfarin may reduce inflammatory changes resulting from the intravascular clotting itself and may thus reduce the risk of necrotic complications.

To initiate the warfarin treatment of a known protein C deficient individual, the use of full dose intravenous heparin and small initial warfarin doses is one course of action presently available. Starting warfarin in protein C deficient individuals without heparin coverage is not advisable. Protein C, free from viral contamination and produced by genetic engineering technology, should be available by the end of the decade. Intravenous administration of this protein C during the initiation of warfarin treatment should significantly reduce the risk of skin necrosis.

Once it has occurred, warfarin induced skin necrosis is difficult to treat successfully. The administration of vitamin K and fresh frozen plasma is advisable. Extensive debridement and surgical repair of the necrotic area is often necessary. Long-term heparin administration (with the recognized risk of osteoporosis) is a practical alternative to further attempts at oral anticoagulation.

The treatment of purpura fulminans neonatalis centers on the administration of plasma, which is a source of protein C. Heparin and warfarin have not proven particularly helpful in preventing further appearances of necrotic skin. The major limitation of plasma administration is the short half-life of protein C, which necessitates the infusion of plasma on an every-other-day basis.

OTHER CAUSES OF RECURRENT THROMBOSIS

Congenital deficiency of plasminogen can cause recurrent venous thrombosis, as can inherited fibrinogen abnormalities. Both these abnormalities may be easily detected. Specific assays for plasminogen are readily available, and abnormal forms of fibrinogen in the plasma are frequently associated with a prolonged thrombin clotting time. An acquired abnormality associated with thromboembolism is the nonspecific anticoagulant (also called the lupus anticoagulant). This is an antibody in the plasma which has as its hallmark a prolonged activated partial thromboplastin time when the patient is receiving no anticoagulants.

FUTURE AREAS OF INTEREST

Antithrombin III and protein C prepared by genetic engineering will be useful in treating congenitally deficient patients. However, activated protein C may have a number of interesting clinical uses. The anticoagulant properties of this enzyme do not require the presence of heparin, and this suggests that it may be useful in the anticoagulation of patients with heparin induced thrombocytopenia and in the anticoagulation of severely antithrombin III deficient individuals. Furthermore, activated protein C inactivates an inhibitor of tissue plasminogen activator, and the combination of activated protein C and tissue plasminogen activator may prove useful in the treatment of acute myocardial infarction. The activated protein C should protect the plasminogen activator from inhibition and simultaneously prevent further clot formation in the involved coronary artery.

SUGGESTED READING

Clouse LH, Comp PC. The regulation of hemostasis: the protein C system. N Engl J Med 1986; 314:1298–1304.

Comp PC. Hereditary disorders predisposing to thrombosis. Prog Hemost Thromb 1986; 8:71–102.

Esmon CT. Protein C: biochemistry, physiology, and clinical implications. Blood 1983; 62:1155–1158.

IMMUNE THROMBOCYTOPENIA

RICHARD H. ASTER, M.D.

ACUTE ITP

Acute idiopathic thrombocytopenic purpura (ITP) is a relatively common childhood disorder characterized by a sudden reduction in platelet levels and hemorrhagic manifestations. About one-half of the cases are preceded by an upper respiratory infection or, less commonly, by specific viral infections such as measles or chicken pox. Platelet destruction in acute ITP is thought to be mediated by autoantibodies or immune complexes somehow triggered by exposure to viral antigens, but its exact pathogenesis is not understood. Serologic tests capable of diagnosing acute ITP with precision are not yet available. Accordingly, the diagnosis is made on the basis of clinical and nonspecific laboratory findings and exclusion of other causes of thrombocytopenia.

Therapeutic Approach

Passive Management

Acute ITP is usually self-limited and untreated cases recover spontaneously, often within a week or two, occasionally after 4 to 6 months. Watchful waiting while avoiding trauma is an acceptable form of therapy, especially in mild cases.

Corticosteroids

Carefully conducted clinical trials provide evidence that platelet levels increase more rapidly in children given corticosteroids than in untreated children. Other trials fail to demonstrate this distinction. Considering the relatively minor side effects associated with corticosteroid administration for a few weeks in children, it is reasonable to prescribe prednisone, 2 mg per kilogram daily, for a maximum of 2 or 3 weeks, to symptomatic patients pending resolution of this controversy. Higher doses of prednisone or intravenous prednisolone are recommended for children with profoundly reduced platelet counts (less than 5,000 per microliter) and severe hemorrhagic symptoms. After a few days of treatment, bleeding symptoms often diminish in severity, reflected by clearing of purpuric lesions in the skin and buccal mucosa. At this point, the dose of prednisone can be reduced to 0.5 to 1 mg per kilogram even if the platelet count has not yet risen. Children receiving corticosteroids are subject to the same side effects as adults, i.e., fluid retention, cushingoid changes, psychiatric abnormalities, and increased susceptibility to infection, and they should be followed closely. The medication can be tapered and then discontinued as soon as the platelet count exceeds 50,000 per microliter.

Intravenous Gamma Globulin

Intravenous gamma globulin provides a therapeutic alternative to corticosteroids in patients with severe hemorrhagic symptoms. The dose currently recommended is 0.4 g per kilogram body weight daily for 5 days. About 80 percent of children so treated experience significant elevations in platelet counts, often to normal levels. In approximately half of these cases, the elevation is sustained. In the others, thrombocytopenia recurs, but may respond again to intravenous gamma globulin infusion. Intravenous gamma globulin is thought to impair the ability of macrophages to clear immunoglobulin-coated platelets, but other mechanisms of action are also possible. At the recommended doses, the side effects of intravenous gamma globulin are minor, consisting mainly of fever and headache. There is no evidence that any one of the various commercial preparations available is superior to the others.

Management of Intracranial Hemorrhage

Less than 1 percent of children with acute ITP present with intracranial hemorrhage or develop this complication soon after diagnosis. Such cases require aggressive treatment with high dose corticosteroids, intravenous gamma globulin, and platelet transfusions. Surgical evacuation of subdural or epidural hematoma is sometimes required. It is reasonable to perform a splenectomy in patients capable of tolerating surgery, although the effectiveness of this procedure is not fully established. Exchange transfusion has been employed in a few cases.

Platelet Transfusions

Transfused platelets are rapidly destroyed in children with acute ITP and, except in patients with intracranial hemorrhage, or other severe bleeding symptoms, are contraindicated because of potential infectious complications.

Refractory Cases

Children who remain thrombocytopenic after 4 to 6 months of observation rarely recover spontaneously thereafter. Such patients generally have a different form of autoimmune thrombocytopenia—chronic ITP. Splenectomy is the mainstay of treatment for this disorder (see below). Repeated courses of IV gamma globulin are sometimes effective in symptomatic children. Removal of the spleen in young children results in increased susceptibility to postsplenectomy sepsis. Children undergoing splenectomy should be immunized with pneumococcal and *Haemophilus influenzae* vaccine, and their parents should be cautioned to seek medical consultation at the first sign of infection. If splenectomy must be performed in a child less than 5 to 6 years of age, consideration should be given to prophylactic antibiotic therapy.

CHRONIC IDIOPATHIC (AUTOIMMUNE) THROMBOCYTOPENIC PURPURA

Chronic ITP is generally more insidious in onset than acute ITP of childhood, although the degree of thrombocytopenia and severity of bleeding symptoms vary widely from patient to patient. Women are affected about four times as often as men. The disorder appears to be a true autoimmune condition in which certain glycoproteins on the surface of platelets are the target autoantigens. The underlying cause of chronic ITP is almost certainly a failure of immunoregulation, but the exact basis for this abnormality is unknown. Chronic ITP usually occurs in isolation, but develops in association with a number of other conditions, including Hodgkin's and nonHodgkin's lymphoma, systemic lupus erythematosus, and hyperthyroidism. The diagnosis is made on the basis of clinical and nonspecific laboratory findings that exclude other causes of thrombocytopenia. Serologic methods for detecting and characterizing platelet reactive autoantibodies are becoming more precise, and specific serologic diagnosis may soon be possible.

Therapeutic Approach

Passive Management

Occasional patients with mild thrombocytopenia and minimal hemorrhagic symptoms can be followed without specific therapy, sometimes for many months or even years.

Corticosteroids

Corticosteroids are the primary therapy for patients with more severe thrombocytopenia as well as purpuric lesions. A distinction is often made between patients with wet purpura and those with dry purpura. In the former group, hemorrhagic bullae and generalized oozing from mucosal surfaces is seen, and the risk of intracranial hemorrhage appears to be greater. Such patients should be hospitalized for their initial treatment. The conventional initial dose of prednisone is 1 mg per kilogram per day. Doses two or three times higher are indicated in patients with extensive wet purpura and profound thrombocytopenia (platelets less than 5,000 per microliter). In many patients, there is clearing of purpura before the platelet count rises.

The exact mechanism of corticosteroid action is not known, but they are thought to act by inhibiting the capacity of macrophages to remove antibody-coated platelets from the circulation and, perhaps, by suppressing autoantibody production. Most patients respond with a rise in platelet count within 1 or 2 weeks of the time treatment is initiated. As soon as purpura clears and the platelet count exceeds 100,000 per microliter, the medication can be tapered gradually. A reasonable schedule is to reduce the dose of prednisone by 10 mg per week initially and 5 mg per week after the dose reaches 0.5 mg per kilogram. Platelet counts should be determined weekly and the regimen modified if thrombocytopenia recurs. All patients receiving long-term corticosteroids should be observed for side effects, which include fluid retention, cushingoid features, hypertension, aggravation of diabetes, gastric complications, and psychosis.

Splenectomy

In nearly all patients with chronic ITP, thrombocytopenia recurs as the dosage of corticosteroids is reduced. Some patients can be managed for long periods of time on doses of prednisone sufficiently low to minimize side effects. Others require splenectomy if there is no contraindication to surgery. The benefit of splenectomy derives from removing the major site in which antibody-coated platelets are destroyed and removing a major site of autoantibody production. About 75 percent of patients achieve a permanent remission after surgery. The response rate is higher in younger patients than in persons older than 50 years. Patients who fail to achieve a complete remission can often be managed on low doses of prednisone.

Recurrent Thrombocytopenia

Thrombocytopenia sometimes recurs many years after a splenectomy-induced remission. In most cases, this is a consequence of increased autoantibody production and destruction of platelets in extrasplenic sites. In a minority of cases, the recurrence results from hypertrophy of an accessory spleen, which can be detected by spleen scan. Surgical removal of the accessory splenic tissue is often curative.

Refractoriness to Prednisone and Splenectomy

A number of second line therapies are available for patients who fail to respond initially even to high dose prednisone or in whom splenectomy is ineffective.

Intravenous Gamma Globulin

More than half of patients with chronic ITP achieve an increase in platelet levels following administration of intravenous gamma globulin, 0.4 g per kilogram body weight daily for 5 days. Intravenous gamma globulin appears to act by impairing the ability of macrophages to clear antibody-coated platelets from the circulation, but other mechanisms are also possible. Several commercial preparations of intravenous gamma globulin are available; none has been shown to be clearly superior to the others. The duration of the response to gamma globulin is variable. Some patients have only a modest elevation in platelets for a few days. In others, the platelet count is normalized for several weeks, and sometimes for months. In the majority of cases, thrombocytopenia recurs, but occasional patients develop a sustained remission for reasons not currently understood. Side effects of intravenous gamma globulin are limited to headache and occasional fever, but the current treatment is expensive and should be reserved for patients who fail to respond to prednisone and splenectomy.

Immunosuppression

Several immunosuppressive regimens have been used to treat patients who fail to respond to standard therapy or who are not candidates for splenectomy. The highest response rate appears to have been achieved with vincristine, 1 to 2 mg intravenously every 7 days for 3 to 4 weeks. Some patients achieve a sustained remission, but thrombocytopenia recurs within weeks or months in most. Patients receiving repeated doses of vincristine should be monitored for the development of peripheral neuropathy. It has been suggested that vincristine is more effective if infused slowly over a 6-hour period than when it is given as a bolus injection.

Cyclophosphamide in doses ranging from 50 to 200 mg per day orally with prednisone produces at least a transient elevation in platelet levels after 3 to 8 weeks of treatment in about one-third of cases. A minority of responders develop permanent, unmaintained remissions. Patients receiving cyclophosphamide should take large amounts of fluid daily to prevent cystitis and should have blood counts performed at least weekly. Azathioprine in doses of 100 to 300 mg per day with prednisone leads to platelet elevations in about 25 percent of cases, sometimes after 6 to 9 months of treatment. Side effects of this regimen are minimal, but blood counts should be monitored periodically.

Colchicine

Colchicine, in doses ranging from 0.6 to 1.2 mg four times daily, has been reported to raise platelet levels in some refractory patients. Its mechanism of action is unknown, but inhibition of macrophage function has been suggested. Gastrointestinal side effects may limit therapy in individual patients. Up to 4 to 6 weeks may be required for a therapeutic effect.

Danazol

Danazol is a nonvirilizing, modified androgen found empirically to raise platelet levels in some patients with refractory ITP when given with prednisone. In some series, about one-half of treated patients have achieved significant benefit.

Platelet Transfusions

Platelets transfused to patients with chronic ITP are usually destroyed rapidly and produce little therapeutic benefit. Their use should be limited to patients with severe, life-threatening bleeding, in whom they may be of transient benefit. It may be necessary to give platelet concentrates every few hours to maintain a hemostatic effect in such cases. Platelets can be given preoperatively to patients undergoing splenectomy, but surgery is often tolerated without transfusion. A more sustained elevation in platelet count is achieved if platelets are given after the splenic pedicle is clamped. Alternatively, the transfusion can be given after a single dose of intravenous gamma globulin, 0.4 g per kilogram.

Plasma Exchange

Machine-assisted, therapeutic plasma exchange has been advocated for patients with life-threatening bleeding in an attempt to lower circulating levels of autoantibody. This approach is worthy of trial in critically ill patients, but often is without beneficial effect.

ITP in Pregnancy

Special therapeutic considerations apply in pregnant women with ITP because of the potential effects of treatment on the fetus and the risk of neonatal thrombocytopenia resulting from transplacental passage of autoantibody. Most women can be managed during pregnancy with modest doses of prednisone. In rare instances, splenectomy has been performed successfully in the second or third trimester. Intravenous gamma globulin can also be utilized and is not known to be harmful to the fetus. In general, the severity of thrombocytopenia in the newborn is proportional to the severity of the disease in the mother, but there are many exceptions. Infants with severe thrombocytopenia have been born to women previously splenectomized and who have normal platelet counts. Currently, it is not possible to predict by serologic testing whether an infant will be born thrombocytopenic. There is some evidence that administration of prednisone, 0.5 to 1.0 mg per kilogram, to the mother during the last 2 or 3 weeks of pregnancy reduces the severity of thrombocytopenia in the newborn. Opinions differ as to whether cesarean section should be performed to reduce the chance of intracranial hemorrhage in the infant. When labor is routine, even thrombocytopenic infants generally do well with vaginal delivery. Sometimes, a scalp vein platelet count is performed shortly after rupture of the membranes, and vaginal delivery proceeds if the infant's platelet count is greater than 50,000 per microliter. In infants with lower counts, cesarean section is performed. Probably, a platelet count done on fetal blood obtained by percutaneous sampling of the umbilical vein provides a better index of fetal platelet levels. In affected infants, thrombocytopenia sometimes persists for several months and can usually be managed with prednisone, 1 to 2 mg per kilogram per day. Intravenous gamma globulin, 0.4 g per kilogram per day for 5 days, can also be utilized. With further experience, this may become the treatment of choice. Exchange transfusion is indicated only in severely affected infants who fail to respond to these therapies.

THROMBOTIC THROMBOCYTOPENIC PURPURA

JOHN J. BYRNES, M.D.

Thrombotic thrombocytopenic purpura (TTP) is a relatively rare syndrome that occurs predominantly in young, otherwise healthy, women and much less frequently in men. Without effective treatment, TTP quickly becomes fatal consequent to anemia, hemorrhage, and multiple organ dysfunction. Owing to enhanced agglutination, platelets form microthrombi that deposit in arterioles and capillaries. Exactly what causes the platelets to agglutinate is poorly understood; it appears that von Willebrand factor participates in the process. Several other abnormalities of plasma factors have been described, but the pathogenetic significance of each is not clear. Endothelial injury, recanalization of the thrombi, endothelial cell proliferation, and microaneurysm formation ensue. The consumption of platelets results in thrombocytopenia, and the thrombi in the microcirculation cause shearing of red blood cells, giving the characteristic microangiopathic hemolytic anemia (MAHA). Disturbance in the perfusion of the brain's microcirculation is most readily manifest as clinical findings, and the unpredictable distribution of lesions leads to a diversity of neurologic manifestations. Microthrombi in other organs are less readily evident. Impaired perfusion of the kidneys generally results in renal impairment, though often not severe. Other organs, although suffering impaired perfusion and microinfarctions, may not demonstrate clinical or laboratory abnormalities early in the disease. The triad of consumptive thrombocytopenia, fragmentation hemolysis and waxing and waning, and bizarre neurologic abnormalities was first considered indicative of TTP. Subsequently, the high incidences of renal impairment and fever were noted, and the pentad of findings was popularized. However, depending upon the distribution and severity of organ involvement, the patient with TTP may be virtually asymptomatic or suffering from failure of virtually every organ system.

The outlook for patients with TTP was extremely poor until the beneficial effect of whole blood or plasma infusion was recognized. It has subsequently become apparent that a plasma factor, which is still poorly characterized, can neutralize the abnormal platelet agglutination. Satisfactory clinical response to plasma therapy occurs in approximately 70 percent of patients. Eventually, the tendency to thrombus formation passes, and the plasma requirement abates. However, relapses or recurrent illness can occur.

NECESSARY EXCLUSIONS PRIOR TO THERAPY

Evidence of the consumption of platelets and the presence of schistocytes in the blood smear are essential to diagnosing TTP. A number of alternative disorders may resemble TTP in these and other features and must be excluded before implementing the following therapeutic recommendations. Disseminated intravascular coagulation often has to be considered. However, the clinical setting is generally not appropriate, and the fibrinogen level typically is normal in TTP; there is usually little or no evidence of fibrinogen consumption, fibrin deposition or fibrinolysis. Hemolytic uremic syndrome (HUS) resembles TTP in many features. Differences in the pathogenesis of TTP and HUS are poorly understood. The kidney is the organ primarily involved by microthrombi, and renal impairment is severe in HUS. Acute renal failure shortly after an episode of gastroenteritis, especially in a child, is typical of HUS. The HELLP syndrome (hemolysis, elevated liver enzymes, low platelets) of pregnancy is probably a variant of eclampsia. It is characterized by hemolysis with schistocytes, elevated liver enzymes, and low platelets. During the peripartum period, either HUS, the HELLP syndrome, or overt eclampsia may mimic TTP. Furthermore, there is an association of TTP with pregnancy that engenders more possibility for confusion. Severe vasculitis can resemble TTP; systemic lupus erythematosus, especially with cerebritis, can resemble TTP in many clinical features. Malignant hypertension can cause platelet consumption and fragmentation hemolysis, often with associated neurologic disturbance. In this instance, the pathogenesis of the process is readily evident; control of the blood pressure alleviates the consumption of platelets and red cell fragmentation. These alternative causes of consumptive thrombocytopenia and microangiopathic hemolytic anemia (MAHA) may be difficult to distinguish from TTP, and in some circumstances, a trial of TTP therapy may be warranted. However, the relative hazards of plasma therapy must be considered.

In order to more firmly establish the diagnosis of TTP, the question of a tissue biopsy often arises. Characteristic microvascular lesions of TTP have been found in skin, gingiva, and bone marrow biopsies. One does not routinely obtain a tissue biopsy. TTP is a clinical syndrome that must be treated promptly. Biopsies in TTP, even in fulminant disease, have a substantial percentage of false negatives. Thus, the biopsy result, whether positive or negative for TTP, does not change the case management. Moreover, awaiting the biopsy result often causes temporizing when aggressive therapy should be instituted without delay.

A confirmatory test for TTP would be helpful, especially when alternative explanations cloud the diagnosis. Various plasma abnormalities have been described in TTP and some have been proposed as a diagnostic test. When suspended in untreated TTP plasma, normal platelets will often spontaneously agglutinate.

Such testing is not generally available, and there are a number of possible pitfalls that need to be worked out before its clinical usefulness is established.

BASELINE ASSESSMENT OF THE PATIENT

As treatment is being arranged, it is important to fully assess the status of the patient clinically with laboratory measurements so that response to therapy can be evaluated and adjustments made accordingly. Generally, there is neurologic impairment which may range from subtle subjective manifestations to deep coma. It is necessary to have a precise inventory of symptoms and signs for ongoing reference. The reversibility of neurologic manifestations is remarkable. This probably is due to the microcirculatory level of thrombosis, which results in reversible dysfunction and some microinfarctions, but not gross infarction of the areas of impaired perfusion. Laboratory parameters that are especially important to follow are the platelet count, hematocrit, and the serum lactic dehydrogenase (LDH). The serum LDH reflects the combined hemolysis and other tissue injury, and as such, is an excellent guide to the patency of the microcirculation and is the best overall indicator of disease activity. These values should be obtained prior to treatment as well as daily during the acute phase of management.

The cardiovascular and renal status must be evaluated for the ability to handle the plasma volume challenge that ensues. This generally means the infusion of the equivalent of one plasma volume per 24 hours. Often, there is renal impairment, although it is generally not severe. Most patients with TTP are able to tolerate plasma infusion of this magnitude with an occasional pharmacologic stimulation of diuresis, if a positive fluid balance is developing. If the cardiac or renal function does not permit vigorous plasma infusion, then arrangements for plasmapheresis must be promptly made. Treatment is preferably carried out in an intensive care setting as the central nervous, cardiac, pulmonary, and renal systems may be subject to dysfunction. Strict attention to fluid balance is necessary including daily patient weighing; central hemodynamic pressure measurements are often required for optimal management.

THERAPEUTIC STRATEGY AND RECOMMENDATIONS

Typically, TTP occurs in an otherwise healthy young adult. A number of prodromal conditions and associations with other disorders have been reported, but the relation to the onset and the propagation of the syndrome is generally not clear. After a variable period (weeks to months), this disturbance of platelet equilibrium passes. If the patient has survived the ordeal, the syndrome disappears, often leaving minimal or no residual impairment. Consequently, therapeutic strategy consists of two aspects. First, there is the need to neutralize the factor causing platelet agglutination during this period. Second, measures to terminate or shorten the duration of the underlying abnormality need to be considered, especially if the disorder is becoming protracted. The most effective measure to suppress the abnormal platelet agglutination is plasma infusion, and this is the cornerstone of TTP treatment. Some patients have a reversal of the syndrome with the infusion of only a few units of plasma; most require much more. The daily dose of plasma and the duration of the requirement are extremely and separately variable. The amount of plasma necessary to control the disorder and the duration must be empirically determined for each patient. The nature of the factor in plasma that neutralizes platelet thrombus formation in TTP is unknown. The supernatant of cryoprecipitate is effective, as is outdated plasma. Thus, the factor is relatively stable. As a starting point, I recommend plasma infusion equivalent to one normal plasma volume daily (40 ml per kilogram per day) until the clinical status has stabilized. This means the central nervous system and other organ dysfunction has reversed, the platelet count is rising, the LDH is near normal, and hemolysis is minimal. As the patient improves, the rate of plasma infusion can be gradually tapered. When the indices of platelet consumption and microcirculatory perfusion have returned to normal, plasma infusion is discontinued. Plasma therapy must be resumed if the platelet count falls substantially or there is an increase in LDH, MAHA, or organ dysfunction.

If the cardiac or renal status does not permit vigorous plasma infusion or if the patient is not responding to the infusion of one plasma volume daily, plasmapheresis is recommended. Effectiveness of plasma infusion often is evident within 48 hours. Plasmapheresis should be calculated to provide at least one plasma volume exchange. The replacement fluid is plasma. Plasmapheresis is continued daily until the clinical status has stabilized. Occasionally, larger volume exchanges are necessary. Between plasmaphereses, plasma infusion is continued at whatever rate the patient can tolerate.

Some advocate immediate plasmapheresis if the patient presents with severe neurologic impairment. Partial removal of the platelet agglutinating factor in addition to its neutralization by plasma infusion may be therapeutically useful. A comparative trial of plasma infusion versus plasmapheresis is underway in Canada. As plasma infusion is more readily available and less costly, this is an important issue to settle. If plasmapheresis is planned, plasma infusion should be instituted while arrangements for plasmapheresis are being made; plasma should be the replacement fluid, and plasma infusions can be given between episodes of plasmapheresis. After a satisfactory clinical response is obtained and plasmapheresis is discontinued, plasma infusion is resumed at a rate the patient can tolerate and then slowly tapered. If the patient starts to relapse, plasma infusion should be increased as tolerated. If this does not control the relapse, then plasmapheresis should be resumed. Plasmapheresis without plasma infusion between sessions, gradually discontinued thereafter, can result in a stormy course of brief remissions and relapses.

Antiplatelet agents have been used to impair platelet thrombus formation. This has usually included the administration of aspirin and dipyridamole. In general, I do not recommend their use, especially if the patient is severely thrombocytopenic. Their effectiveness in TTP is marginal and they handicap the platelets' ability to prevent hemorrhage. Anticoagulants likewise have no role. Clinical experience suggests that patients with TTP are more likely to suffer bleeding complications if antiplatelet agents are used. Plasma infusion, in contrast, does not handicap normal hemostasis and more effectively addresses the abnormally enhanced platelet agglutination.

Corticosteroids are often used. Although not proven, they have an apparently beneficial effect, especially when used in conjunction with other effective modalities. Because of this potentially ancillary benefit, I generally give prednisone 1 to 2 mg per kilogram per day or equivalent. This is gradually eliminated when the patient is in remission and does not require further plasma therapy.

The requirement for plasma therapy has extended for many months in some patients. Various therapeutic modalities have been employed in attempting to terminate this requirement. There are a number of reports of the disorder abating after the administration of agents such as vincristine, cyclophosphamide, or azathioprine. There are also reports of protracted plasma dependency resolving after splenectomy. It is necessary to be cautious in accepting a therapeutic role for these measures as many similar, but unsuccessful, attempts do not get reported, and generally the disorder remits spontaneously. Thus, the cessation of TTP may be erroneously credited to the last measure applied. Nevertheless, if the course is becoming protracted, I recommend the administration of vincristine in standard dosage, 1.4 mg per square meter, not to exceed 2 mg, be given intravenously. This can be repeated weekly with the usual precautions in its use. Cyclophosphamide or azathioprine may also bear consideration. Splenectomy has several advocates, although a rationale for its possible effectiveness is not clear. I would consider splenectomy in a patient who responds poorly to continued plasma therapy and in whom several attempts to terminate the process with less drastic measures such as vincristine administration have failed.

Those unfamiliar with the basic pathogenetic process in TTP may be tempted to give platelet transfusions to a severely thrombocytopenic patient, especially if surgery is being contemplated. There are numerous cases reported in the literature where platelet transfusions caused neither adverse effects nor benefits. However, several instances of severe deterioration and death immediately following platelet transfusion have been recorded. In one clear example, platelet transfusions were immediately followed by abrupt neurologic deterioration and death. Fresh, fluffy platelet aggregates were found throughout the cerebral microcirculation, thereby attesting to the hazard of this inappropriate measure. I believe platelet transfusions in TTP are extremely hazardous and of unlikely benefit.

Consequent to the effectiveness of plasma therapy, a few patients are now surviving who have extremely protracted courses of plasma requirement. The plasma requirements in these patients are usually not great, several units a month. One such patient has had chronic TTP for more than 8 years. Several lessons are learned from these patients, which can be extrapolated to more typical acute patients. Infections, such as bacterial or viral illness, or pregnancy can cause a relapse or a several fold increase in the plasma requirement, which then reverts after resolution. When TTP presents during pregnancy, the microvascular thrombotic process involves the placenta, and this often results in the death of the fetus. Occasionally, if the fetus is not dead and the patient responds to therapy, the pregnancy can be continued with successful outcome. Delivery of the fetus does not necessarily terminate the TTP syndrome. However, in all patients with TTP, a search for underlying inflammatory process or associated illness should be undertaken, as addressing such problems may help alleviate the disorder. Furthermore, some patients who go into a complete remission for months or years have a recurrence of TTP precipitated at the time of another illness. Therefore, any patient who recovers from TTP should be monitored for recurrent TTP, especially during subsequent illness.

There are reports of TTP occurring secondary to chemotherapy and other stressful events. Several patients have apparently benefited from plasma therapy. Consequently, the same therapeutic recommendations hold. However, as several reported cases of thrombotic microangiopathy were associated with chemotherapy regimens containing vinca alkaloids, their use in TTP occurring in this setting is not advisable.

As for future treatment, if the beneficial plasma component is identified and a concentrate obtained, and as the therapeutic efficacy of ancillary measures and splenectomy become better understood, then less empiric recommendations for the management of TTP will be possible.

SUGGESTED READING

Bukowski RM. Thrombotic thrombocytopenic purpura: a review. Prog Hemost Thromb 1982; 6:287–337.

Byrnes JJ, Moake JL. Thrombotic thrombocytopenic purpura and the haemolytic uraemic syndrome: evolving concepts in pathogenesis and therapy. Clin Haematol 1986; 15:413–442.

IMMEDIATE AND DELAYED ADVERSE REACTIONS TO TRANSFUSIONS

J. A. McBRIDE, M.D., F.R.C.P.(Edin), FRCPC, F.R.C.P.
PAMELA O'HOSKI, A.R.T.

Blood transfusion in the 1990s is a relatively safe procedure. Nevertheless, in a small number of patients who receive transfusion, complications do occur. Although these complications are generally not serious, they are uncomfortable for the patient. In rare cases, these reactions can be serious and have a morbidity of their own and may even lead to the death of the patient. Serious life-threatening reactions to transfusion are discussed first and less serious but more common reactions later.

LIFE-THREATENING TRANSFUSION REACTIONS

Immediate Immune Hemolysis

Red cell lysis occurs when potent antibodies that are invariably present in the patient's serum react with transfused red cells. Severe hemolysis may be seen after as little as 50 to 100 ml of incompatible red cells have been transfused. For this reason, it is wise to run the first portion of blood into a patient slowly. The patient should be closely monitored during this time. Hemolysis is usually immediate and occurs both intravascularly and extravascularly. The patient frequently complains of pain at the site of injection of the blood, severe crushing chest pain, and pain in the lumbar region that occasionally radiates into the limbs. Fever and chills are common. Tachycardia occurs, and severe shock with hypotension and circulatory failure may develop. Occasionally, the patient develops a hemorrhagic state.

Patients who receive incompatible transfusion while under general anesthesia may not show any of these signs, and indeed, a generalized bleeding tendency may be the first and only sign of a transfusion reaction.

Management

1. Stop the transfusion but maintain an intravenous access with normal saline.
2. Recheck the identity of the blood and the identity of the patient.
3. Obtain post-transfusion recipient blood samples from the arm opposite the site of transfusion. Both a serum and an ethylenediaminetetraacetic acid (EDTA) sample are required.
4. Ensure the return of the appropriate samples and the suspect blood unit, together with its giving set and filter, to the Blood Bank.
5. Collect the first sample of urine passed by the patient after the incident.
6. Maintain an accurate record of fluid intake and urinary output.

When a major transfusion reaction is suspected, the Blood Bank must be informed immediately. A major ABO-incompatible transfusion reaction is almost always the result of a clerical error or the misidentification of a patient or a unit of blood for transfusion. Under these circumstances, there is always the possibility of a second error, and every attempt should be made to detect this error and prevent a second transfusion reaction in another patient.

Treatment

After the immediate acute phase of hemolysis, the patient usually develops hemoglobinuria that may be transient, and jaundice is seen in about 6 to 12 hours. The jaundice is usually mild but may persist for several days. Treatment of this phase of a transfusion reaction is the same as the treatment for shock. The patient's blood volume and urinary output must be maintained, and this can be done by the administration of normal saline. Diuresis can be encouraged by the use of a thiazide diuretic. The aim is to maintain a urinary output of about 100 ml per hour. Mannitol-induced diuresis has been described in much of the older transfusion literature, but there is little experimental evidence to support its use. Vasopressive drugs that restrict blood flow through the kidneys should not be used. If the patient develops a generalized hemorrhagic tendency, treatment consists of replacement of the coagulation factors by cryoprecipitate or fresh frozen plasma. Thrombocytopenia can be corrected by the use of platelet concentrates. In the event that a patient requires further transfusion of red cells, he or she should be transfused with group O cells and if necessary given group AB plasma. Oliguria and rising creatinine and urea levels are the first signs of

TABLE 1 Laboratory Tests Performed at Time of Suspected Hemolytic Transfusion Reaction

1. Find the pretransfusion sample and compare the patient identification data with the post-transfusion sample.
2. Spin and check blood for visual evidence of hemolysis (pretransfusion sample acts as a control).
3. Repeat the ABO group, the Rhesus type, and perform a direct antiglobulin test on pre- and post-transfusion samples side by side.
4. Repeat the cross-match and antibody screen on both samples.
5. In the event that all of these investigations prove negative, consider retesting the donor bag for ABO, Rhesus type, and perform an antibody screen on the plasma.

renal failure, and the clinical picture soon becomes that of acute tubular necrosis. The mortality from acute hemolytic transfusion reaction is estimated to be between 10 and 25 percent.

Infected Blood Product

The transfusion of a blood product contaminated by live bacteria or bacterial toxin fortunately is extremely uncommon. Small amounts of infected blood products, for example, the volume of a platelet transfusion, can result in immediate and severe shock with peripheral circulatory failure and the rapid death of the patient. The organisms responsible are usually gram-negative and may be organisms that in other circumstances are not usually regarded as pathogenic, such as *Serratia marcescens.* Most bacteria do not grow in the cold, but recently bacteremia caused by *Yersinia enterocolitica* has been described in four patients who had received a transfusion of packed red cells that had been stored at 4°C for up to 42 days. The modern tendency to store platelets at room temperature at least increases the possibility for bacterial growth. The diagnosis is suggested by the clinical picture of shock, peripheral failure, high fevers and rigors, hypotension, tachycardia, and frequently vomiting. As in all transfusion reactions, the patient may complain of pain in the arm or in the general area of the vein in which the blood product is being infused. Treatment, which is frequently unsuccessful, consists of aggressive measures to combat shock—the use of plasma volume expanders, steroids, pressor agents, and broad-spectrum antibiotics. It is important that when this complication is suspected, blood samples be taken from the patient for cultures. The blood product bag and any closed segments on the bag should be returned to the Blood Bank for microbiologic culture. It is necessary to inform the supplier of this blood product immediately, because other blood products derived from the same donor unit may be similarly contaminated.

Some plasma products that are thawed in a water bath may become contaminated either through microscopic flaws in the plastic of the bag or by droplet infection at the time of entry for infusion. It is also important when these plasma products are thawed that the temperature during thawing be strictly controlled. The transfusion of overheated blood products that contain coagulated proteins may activate complement, which can produce a pulmonary hypersensitivity transfusion reaction.

Anaphylactic Reactions to Blood

Approximately 1 in 500 of the population is totally deficient in IgA protein. Such patients recognize all subgroups of IgA as foreign, and can, when stimulated, produce complement binding IgG class-specific antibodies. When patients who are IgA deficient have become sensitized, either by previous transfusion or by pregnancy, they can have an anaphylactic reaction to plasma products. Traditionally, the transfusion reaction has been fast and starts almost immediately on beginning the transfusion. Plasma or a plasma product is the usual culprit. Red cell concentrates do contain enough plasma to provoke anaphylaxis. Gamma globulin or Rhesus immunoglobulin, if given intravenously, can also provoke this severe reaction. If a patient has had such a reaction in the past and requires further transfusion, IgA can be removed either by washing donor red cells or by the use of frozen red cells that are washed during processing. If IgA-deficient donors of the appropriate group are available, plasma from such donors may be used with considerable safety. Perhaps the best method for avoiding such a serious side effect, if there is time, is the use of autologous blood for transfusion.

LESS SERIOUS TRANSFUSION REACTIONS

Delayed Hemolytic Transfusion Reactions

Delayed hemolytic transfusion reaction is much milder than the direct reaction described above and occurs from 2 to 14 days after the administration of blood that appears to be cross-match compatible. Following transfusion, the patient is immunized either by an antigen present on the transfused cells to which he or she has never been exposed, or there is a secondary immune response with the renewed production of a previously stimulated antibody. Symptoms are usually mild, the only manifestation of a delayed transfusion reaction may be unexpected failure to maintain the patient's hemoglobin value after transfusion or the development of mild jaundice. There is no real treatment. The major challenge to the physician is the prevention of further delayed transfusion reactions if the patient requires repeated blood transfusions. Prevention depends on the use of accurate records kept by the Blood Bank, in the physician's office, or by the patient. The knowledge that an antibody had at one time been detected in the patient's serum allows the infusion of red cells negative for that particular antigen in the future if transfusion is required. About 15 to 20 percent of patients are good antibody formers and tend to produce multiple antibodies following transfusion. Patients who develop multiple antibodies and still require transfusion are a difficult ongoing clinical problem. The Blood Bank should be informed as far in advance of an intended transfusion as possible in order to allow for extensive search either by computer or by manual screening for suitable antigen-negative, cross-matched compatible red cells. If widespread screening is unsuccessful, suitable blood might be found among the patient's immediate blood relatives. If the patient's clinical condition improves to the point that transfusion is no longer required, he or she should be encouraged to donate red cells to be frozen in the Rare Donor Bank. If the patient requires elective surgery, autologous transfusion should be considered.

Febrile Reactions Following Transfusion of Blood Product

Febrile reactions are common in patients receiving multiple transfusions. In general terms, the frequency and severity of febrile reactions become greater as the number of transfusions increases. This type of reaction is probably attributable to the development in the patient's plasma of antibodies directed against human leukocyte antigens (HLA) carried on leukocytes. These antibodies react in turn with leukocytes in the transfused blood. Fever occurs toward the end of the transfusion. It is necessary to stop the transfusion and initiate a transfusion reaction investigation. Characteristically, the patient's temperature falls once the transfusion has stopped. The reason for stopping the transfusion is that an initial febrile reaction may conceal a more serious transfusion reaction. In patients who are in a chronic transfusion program and experience febrile reactions, it is often advisable to transfuse leukocyte-poor blood. This may be accomplished by the use of a filter or by the simpler and less expensive technique of centrifugation of blood and the removal of the identifiable buffy coat.

Allergic Reactions

Allergic reactions to blood products are relatively common. They usually consist of hives or a wheal and flare reaction. This may occur at any time during the course of the transfusion. It is not usually necessary to stop the transfusion when the allergic reaction is mild, but the person performing the transfusion must be aware that the earliest sign of an anti-IgA potentially anaphylactic reaction is the appearance of a red rash on the skin. Edema of the face and the larynx is uncommon, but laryngeal edema is an important potential complication of any allergic reaction. The transfusion should be slowed, and an antihistamine drug such as diphenhydramine (Benadryl) given. Alternatively, the patient may be given hydrocortisone intravenously. This usually brings the reaction under control, the patient becomes much more comfortable, and the transfusion can continue. Premedication with these same drugs should precede future transfusions.

Noncardiogenic Pulmonary Edema Syndrome

This increasingly recognized complication is an example of transfusion-associated adult respiratory distress syndrome. This syndrome is also known as transfusion-related acute lung injury. The patient usually develops chills and fever within a relatively short time after transfusion starts. The temperature may be persistently raised for up to about 48 hours, and changes of so-called allergic pneumonitis appear on x-ray films within a few hours after the transfusion. Clinical examination of the chest may be negative or may reveal diffuse, fine, basal crepitations. This syndrome is probably caused by an HLA antibody present in the donor plasma. Even when traditional packed cells are used, the packed cell preparation contains up to 80 ml of plasma, which is sufficient to produce this syndrome. The syndrome is usually self-limiting, and all the changes generally clear within 72 hours. Treatment should be expectant, with strict control of transfusion requirements and fluid balance and the vigorous use of diuretics. Steroids may be helpful if the dyspnea and cyanosis are persistent or severe. In the most severe cases, treatment with a respirator may be necessary. Multiparous women have been identified as the donors of the blood that produces these reactions. Implicated donors should be removed from the donor registry.

Pulmonary overload can also occur when patients who are chronically anemic are transfused too rapidly and are given too much volume. The first step is to recognize that the patient has an expanded blood volume and has pulmonary edema. Treatment entails the production of a forced diuresis and strict control of fluid balance. Patients who have an expanded blood volume should be transfused very slowly with well-packed red cells.

Delayed Post-Transfusion Purpura

Delayed post-transfusion purpura is a rare syndrome that occurs in multiparous women 5 to 7 days after a blood transfusion. Characteristically, the patient develops a profound thrombocytopenia that may persist for 4 to 6 weeks. Patients generally respond to plasma exchange and may respond to administration of intravenous gamma globulin. The syndrome is caused by the existence of an alloantibody in the serum of a recipient previously immunized to a platelet antigen (usually anti-Pl^{a1}). If patients who develop this syndrome require future transfusion, it may be prudent to consider the use of washed red cells to remove contaminating platelets.

Graft Versus Host Reaction

This has been described in patients with compromised immune systems following transfusion of blood products that contained immunologically competent lymphocytes. Groups at risk include neonates, patients with congenital immune deficiencies, recipients of both allogeneic and autologous marrow transplants, patients recovering from intensive chemotherapy, and patients with acquired immunodeficiency syndrome. Irradiation of blood and blood products using 1,500 to 5,000 cGy destroys the ability of lymphocytes to produce this syndrome.

Recently, the American Association of Blood Banks has recommended that blood from closely related, directed donors should be irradiated to 1,500 cGy.

Citrate Toxicity

Patients may develop citrate toxicity as a result of ultramassive transfusions of blood or plasma during prolonged surgical procedures or following trauma.

The monitoring of ionized calcium seems to be the optimal way to manage this complication. Replacement of ionized calcium can be accomplished by the administration of calcium chloride or calcium gluconate.

Mild tetany is not uncommon during rapid plasma exchange, as for example during therapeutic plasmapheresis. Management is to slow the infusion rate. Calcium replacement is seldom necessary in these circumstances.

Red Herrings

Occasionally the transfusionist is asked to see a patient who appears to be having a transfusion reaction. This is particularly prone to occur when an underlying event takes place at the same time that the patient is receiving a transfusion for another reason.

1. Such reactions are seen in patients with glucose-6-phosphate dehydrogenase deficiency who have been exposed to an oxidant drug at the same time as they are receiving red blood cells for another reason. In this case it is the patient's own cells that are being lysed, not the transfused cells.
2. After transurethral resection of the prostate, bladder lavage is occasionally carried out with sterile, distilled water. Some of the perfusate finds its way into the venous system and may cause significant intravascular hemolysis.
3. *Clostridium welchii* septicemia, for example following gallbladder surgery, can produce fulminant intravascular hemolysis that may be mistaken for a transfusion reaction if the patient has received a transfusion in the course of the surgery.
4. Almost any cause of intravascular hemolysis, however rare (e.g., paroxysmal nocturnal hemoglobinuria), may superficially appear to be a transfusion reaction when, in fact, the patient's own cells are being lysed.
5. Blood that has been handled poorly, e.g., damaged in an inappropriate condition of storage, may lyse rapidly when transfused into a patient. This produces hemoglobinemia and hemoglobinuria, which may resemble a transfusion reaction.
6. The use of intravenous dimethylsulfoxide has been associated with a reaction that mimics a severe direct transfusion reaction.

TRANSMISSION OF DISEASE

Any blood transfusion carries with it a risk, although a small one, of transmitting disease. Two diseases, syphilis and hepatitis B, are routinely tested for. The transmission of syphilis and hepatitis B by blood transfusion is now a rarity. However, transmission of non-A, non-B hepatitis continues unabated. The causative virus has recently been identified, and the disease is now called hepatitis C. A commercial screening test has been developed, and routine screening of donor blood will begin in the near future. It may still be necessary to continue the already existing surrogate testing to identify donors who have other forms of viral hepatitis.

Malaria and infectious mononucleosis can be transmitted by blood transfusion. Recently, cases of Chagas' disease (caused by *Trypanosoma cruzi*) have been described following transfusion of blood from South American donors. The culture of *Borrelia burgdorferi*, the causative agent of Lyme disease, from the peripheral blood of seven patients, implies that this disease can be transmitted by blood products.

Cytomegalovirus is thought to persist in lymphocytes, and the removal of white blood cells by a micropore filter shows promise as an alternative to the provision of cytomegalovirus-negative donors for patients at risk (e.g., neonates, marrow transplant recipients).

Much has been said about the transmission of the human immunodeficiency virus and its relationship to transfusion. It is now quite clear that in donors who have been exposed to this virus, antibodies can be tested for, and confirmation of the exposure by the use of a Western blot technique should eliminate the majority of potentially infected donors. Other retroviruses, such as human T-cell leukemia virus type 1 (HTLV-1), can also be transmitted by transfusion. The antibody to this virus will soon be routinely tested for by transfusion services. The donor who has recently been exposed to either virus and who has not yet formed antibodies will continue to be a hazard.

SUGGESTED READING

Cohen ND, Munoz A, Reitz BA, et al. Transmission of retroviruses by transfusion of screened blood in patients undergoing cardiac surgery. N Engl J Med 1989; 320:1172–1176.

deGraan-Hentzen YCE, Gratama JW, Mudde GC, et al. Prevention of primary cytomegalovirus infection in patients with hematologic malignancies by intensive white cell depletion of blood products. Transfusion 1989; 29:757–760.

Dzik WH, Kirkley SA. Citrate toxicity during massive blood transfusion. Transfusion Med Rev 1988; 2:76–94.

Grant IH, Gold JWM, Wittner M, et al. Transfusion-associated acute Chagas' disease acquired in the United States. Ann Intern Med 1989; 111:849–851.

Issitt PD. Transfusion reactions. In: Issitt PD, ed. Applied blood group serology. 3rd ed. Miami: Montgomery Scientific, 1985:498.

Laschinger CA, Naylor DG. Anti-IgA antibodies and transfusion reactions in Canada. Can Med Assoc J 1983; 1281:381–382.
Leitman SF, Holland PV. Irradiation of blood products. Transfusion 1985; 25:293.
Levy GJ, Shabot MM, Hart ME, et al. Transfusion-associated noncardiogenic pulmonary edema. Transfusion 1986; 26:278–281.
Nickerson P, Orr P, Schroeder ML. Transfusion-associated *Trypanosoma cruzi* infection in a non-endemic area. Ann Intern Med 1989; 111:851–853.
Popovsky MA. Immune mediated transfusion reactions. In: Nance SF, ed. Immune destruction of red blood cells. Arlington, VA: American Association of Blood Banks, 1989.
Yersinia enterocolitica bacteremia and endotoxin shock associated with red blood cell transfusion—United States, 1987–1988. MMWR 1988; 37:577–578.
Zuck TF, Sherwood WC, Bove JR. A review of recent events related to surrogate testing of blood to prevent non-A, non-B posttransfusion hepatitis. Transfusion 1987; 27:203–206.

NEOPLASTIC DISORDERS

HODGKIN'S DISEASE

GIANNI BONADONNA, M.D.

Over the past 2 decades, treatment of Hodgkin's disease has evolved considerably through innovations in the management of various stages. The impact of various treatments on the 5-, 10-, and 15-year results is now being balanced against delayed morbidity, such as organ damage and second malignancies, produced by the intensity of therapy or the prolonged delivery of given drugs.

Clinicians should be aware that certain procedures or indications that were routine in the past decade (e.g., staging laparotomy, primary radiotherapy for all subsets of patients with nodal disease) should now find more flexible applications in the light of new prognostic factors. Past and present experience confirms that the complexity of clinical evaluation and the modern, sophisticated treatment modalities demand considerable technical resources and qualified personnel. Practicing physicians should therefore carefully and honestly evaluate whether their own experience and the facilities available to them are adequate. If not, patient referral to specialized centers remains a wise professional response.

PROPER STAGING

Proper staging is still important for selecting patients suitable for curative radiotherapy and those who are candidates for a systemic treatment program with or without irradiation.

Table 1 outlines the procedures necessary to carry out correct clinical (CS) and pathologic (PS) staging. In particular, staging laparotomy should be performed only if management decisions depend on the histologic identification of occult abdominal disease and in particular a positive spleen. Thus, laparotomy remains, at present, a necessary procedure in CS IA and IIA without bulky mediastinal adenopathy as the 10-year relapse-free survival of PS IA and IIA treated with subtotal nodal radiotherapy alone is 70 to 85 percent. To histologically document hepatic involvement by Hodgkin's disease today, we can recommend either laparoscopy with multiple biopsies or needle biopsy of suspicious lesion(s) on liver computed axial tomography (CT) scanning. Splenectomy is contraindicated in a child younger than 5 years because of increased risk of fulminant septicemia. As for procedures required under certain circumstances, we recommend the following. CT and magnetic resonance imaging (MRI) are not superior to lymphography for the radiologic diagnosis of retroperitoneal adenopathy below L2; they can be useful to visualize mesenteric nodes whose infiltration by Hodgkin's disease in CS IA and IIA is less than 4 percent. CT scanning and MRI are not routinely recommended to diagnose thoracic lymphoma, but are important in designing the radiation therapy field. Ultrasonography is often useful to diagnose intra-abdominal masses. Gallium whole body scan can be helpful in assessing the site(s) of recurrence, especially in the mediastinum when all the above procedures are either negative or not conclusive. Most of the above mentioned studies should be repeated once the initial treatment is completed to assess the status of complete remission properly or restaging in the presence of a single recurrence.

TABLE 1 Essential Procedures for Proper Staging Besides History and Physical Examination

Chest roentgenogram with mass/thoracic ratio (measurement of the largest transverse diameter of mediastinal mass and the transverse diameter of the thorax at the level T5-T6 on a standing posteroanterior film).
Bipedal lymphography.
Laboratory tests: complete blood count, erythrosedimentation rate, liver function tests, serum uric acid and copper.
Core needle biopsy from posterior iliac crest. Biopsy should be bilateral, especially in the presence of CS III and in patients with systemic symptoms.
Staging laparotomy with splenectomy and multiple biopsies of hepatic and abdominal lymph nodes in CS I-II if therapeutic decision depends on the identification of occult abdominal involvement.
Needle or surgical biopsy of any suspicious extranodal (e.g., osseous, pulmonary, cutaneous) lesion(s).
Cytologic examination of any effusion.

PROGNOSTIC FACTORS

The results of clinical trials performed during the last decade have allowed us to reconsider the various prognostic variables. The major unfavorable prognostic factor is tumor mass (e.g., bulky mediastinal lymphoma, multiple extranodal involvement, five or more splenic nodules). The biologic implications of large tumor volume have been extensively studied: the greater the tumor cell population, the more likely it is to contain significant numbers of various classes of drug resistant cells. Modern clinical research should improve the correct assessment and even quantitation of tumor volume. Disease progression while on chemotherapy or short-term complete remission despite intensive multiple drug regimens indicates poor prognosis because of primary cell resistance. In general, prognosis is inversely related to age, since children and young adults fare better than older people. In particular, patients older than 60 years often present with advanced disease and other medical problems that cause difficulties in the proper staging and treatment of their disease. Recent observations have confirmed that lymphocyte depleted Hodgkin's disease is a rare but very aggressive form of lymphoma whose prognosis is still unfavorable because of widespread nodal and extranodal involvement. The presence of B symptoms carries, in general, unfavorable prognostic significance, epecially in patients with more advanced disease. Patients with stage IIB disease appear to have an adverse prognosis when they manifest all three systemic symptoms; this finding is often associated with bulky mediastinal disease. Males almost always have a less favorable prognosis compared with that of females.

PRINCIPLES OF TREATMENT

In patients with limited disease after adequate staging (PS I-IIA), the aim of current therapy is to provide a high cure rate within a short period of time and through limited morbidity. In patients with advanced Hodgkin's disease (stage IIIB-IV), the aim of therapy is to achieve durable complete remission, in most cases through effective full dose polydrug regimens at the expense of acceptable morbidity. Since a fraction of patients with advanced lymphoma are not cured by drugs, most probably due to primary tumor cell resistance, more attention should be given to the potential of alternating treatments, that is, alternating non-cross resistant drug regimens and alternating chemotherapy with radiotherapy to the site(s) of initial bulky disease. For the management of the intermediate stages (IIB-IIIA), more than one treatment option is available, and in the selection of optimal therapy, physicians should take into consideration some of the known prognostic variables such as disease extent (bulky adenopathy, stage III_1 versus III_2) and systemic symptoms.

Patients resistant to primary drug therapy pose problems since current salvage treatments (second and third line chemotherapy as well as high dose chemotherapy with autologous bone marrow transplantation) appear to induce durable complete response in only a limited number of selected patients.

GUIDELINES TO PRIMARY TREATMENT

Stage IA-IIa With No Bulky Adenopathy

Following staging laparotomy, patients with supradiaphragmatic disease and no bulky mediastinum are treated with subtotal nodal irradiation delivered with high energy equipment at conventional tumoricidal doses (involved areas—40 to 44 Gy, uninvolved areas—35 Gy). In rare cases (4 to 5 percent) with subdiaphragmatic nonbulky Hodgkin's disease, radiotherapy is administered through an inverted Y field including the splenic pedicle in stage I, and through total nodal irradiation (including the mediastinum) in stage II, respectively. With this strategy, the 10-year relapse-free survival (RFS) ranges from 70 to 85 percent; total survival following salvage chemotherapy in relapsing patients ranges from 80 to 95 percent. Late relapses, (i.e., 3 years or more after completion of radiotherapy) are 10 to 13 percent, and they occur more often in patients with stage I disease and a nodular sclerosis histology. In patients not subjected to staging laparotomy, subtotal or total nodal irradiation including a splenic port, RFS may be inferior, but total survival remains similar because, in both situations, the ability to salvage patients with combination chemotherapy after they relapse from radiotherapy is excellent.

Stage IB-IIB With No Bulky Adenopathy

In patients treated as those with the same stage and no systemic symptoms, the 10-year freedom relapse is comparatively lower, but most cases can be salvaged with optimal chemotherapy. However, in a small subset of stage IIB patients presenting with all three systemic symptoms, prognosis is extremely poor since the 5-year freedom from relapse rate is only about 40 percent. In this subset, staging laparotomy is superfluous, and combined modality therapy is recommended. In all other patients with nonbulky, true (i.e., after laparotomy) stage IB-IIB disease with a solitary systemic symptom, subtotal or total nodal radiotherapy appears the treatment of choice and can yield a 10-year RFS of 80 percent or over.

Stage II (A and B) With Bulky Adenopathy and Limited Extranodal Extension

With few exceptions, the majority of oncologists agree that this stage group should now be managed with combined modality therapy. In general, patients present with multiple supradiaphragmatic nodal groups involved and may have extension of tumor into the lung, pericardium, or chest wall. Staging includes only lymphography and two needle bone marrow biopsies. Because effective combination chemotherapy is able to induce prompt tumor shrinkage of compressive symptoms from mediastinal-hilar adenopathy, medical treatment should precede irradiation; radiotherapy can be delivered at conventional tumoricidal doses as mantle or subtotal nodal irradiation including spleen once three to four cycles of the selected combination are completed (i.e., MOPP or one of its variants, ABVD, MOPP alternated with ABVD, see Table 2). Utilizing this strategy, most patients begin the radiation program in complete or almost complete clinical remission, thus avoiding the pulmonary sequelae following primary irradiation of huge mediastinal-hilar adenopathy. With a combined modality approach, both 5- and 10-year RFS and survival rates are over 75 percent.

Stage IIIA

There is still debate as how to treat this patient subset properly, which includes various prognostic groups depending on the extent and the bulkiness of disease. If, through careful surgical staging, patients with CS I or CS II show histologic involvement limited to the lymphatic structures in the upper abdomen that accompany the celiac-axis group of arteries (substage III_1), subtotal or total nodal irradiation can represent the treatment of choice for patients with no bulky adenopathy and minimal splenic involvement (less than 5 positive nodules). In fact, the overall survival results, inclusive of salvage chemotherapy for relapsing patients are comparable with those reported with PS IIA.

The controversy arises when there is involvement of low para-aortic nodes and iliac nodes (substage III_2). Based on the results of numerous trials utilizing systemic drug therapy, when the lymphographic patterns appear typical for retroperitoneal node involvement, most clinicians avoid staging laparotomy and utilize combination chemotherapy with or without radiotherapy. A common approach involves total nodal irradiation followed by chemotherapy (usually six cycles of MOPP), but this form of treatment carries a high risk of acute leukemia even if irradiation is limited to involved fields. A more recent approach consists first in the delivery of three to four cycles of combination chemotherapy to be followed by total nodal irradiation with 30 to 35 Gy if the patient achieves complete or almost complete remission after drug therapy. This approach is particularly useful in patients with extensive Hodgkin's disease and in the presence of bulky mediastinum or para-aortic nodes. In the experience of the Milan Cancer Institute, ABVD plus radiotherapy yielded superior 7-year results (94 percent) when randomly compared to MOPP plus radiotherapy (67 percent) and was devoid of leukemogenesis, irreversible gonadal dysfunction, and cardiac toxicity. In light of modern concepts about drug resistant tumor cells, it appears highly questionable whether further chemotherapy, utilizing the same drug regimen, after completion of the irradiation program is strategically important to influence the duration of complete remission. On the contrary, chemotherapy after extensive irradiation must often be delivered through low dose regimens because of prolonged myelosuppression and may increase the incidence of treatment related sequelae. To make combined treatment even more tolerable as far as myelosuppression is concerned, one may utilize the so-called ping-pong strategy devised at Stanford University, that is the delivery of two cycles of combination chemotherapy alternating with the irradiation of two lymph node regions, starting with central nodal areas. Regardless of the treatment sequence utilized, the frequence of durable complete remission appears invariably superior following combined modality therapy (over 80 percent) compared to total nodal irradiation alone (less than 50 percent). Thus, combined modality appears to be the most effective means to maximize, through the first treatment approach, the chances of cure of stage IIIA disease when low retroperitoneal nodes are positive as well as when extensive splenic involvement (5 or more positive nodules) and/or bulky adenopathy are present.

Over the past 15 years, there have been several attempts to treat stage IIIA disease with combination chemotherapy alone, usually MOPP. With the exception of the results achieved at the National Cancer Institute, both incidence and duration of complete remission following MOPP alone are, in general, inferior compared with combined modality therapy, and the majority of relapses occur in the original sites of disease. Recent data from a randomized trial on stage IIIA disease by the Southwest Oncology Group yielded at 8 years no significant difference in the incidence of complete remission, relapse-free and total survival rates between chemotherapy alone (10 courses of MOPP plus low dose bleomycin) or three cycles of the same drug therapy followed by total nodal irradiation. The above mentioned data, however, do not provide comparative details concerning differences related to disease extent (e.g., substage III_1 versus III_2, less than three versus three or more involved lymph node sites) and bulky lymphoma. At present, there are no long-term results following alternating chemotherapy (e.g., MOPP-ABVD) with or without radiotherapy to initial sites of bulky lymphoma.

Stage IIIB

It remains unresolved at present whether the optimal management of this stage group is combined modality therapy, as above described for stage III_2A, or intensive combination chemotherapy with or without irradiation to the lymphoid regions presenting with bulky disease. The results from the Milan Cancer Institute utilizing ABVD for three cycles followed by subtotal or total nodal irradiation appear excellent: complete remission in 92 percent of cases and 85 percent RFS at 7 years (no bulky lymphoma 96 percent, bulky lymphoma 81 percent). These findings appear superior to those reported after a single drug combination (e.g., MOPP) alone and comparable, though devoid of acute leukemia and sterility, to the results achieved with combined modality therapy utilizing MOPP or similar regimens.

Stage IV (A and B)

This stage group is best managed with intensive, full dose combination chemotherapy. However, it may be possible that irradiation limited to the site(s) of initial bulky disease can further optimize the long-term RFS.

MOPP is still the most widely used drug combination in clinical practice. However, in recent years, the administration of MOPP has been alternated monthly with ABVD (MOPP-ABVD) in the attempt to overcome the problem of primary drug resistance. The largest experience has been achieved so far by investigators of the Milan Cancer Institute; they have shown that in stage IV, there was a superiority of alternating chemotherapy compared to MOPP alone in terms of complete remission (89 percent versus 74 percent), freedom from progression (65 percent versus 36 percent), 8-year relapse-free (73 percent versus 45 percent), and total survival (84 percent versus 64 percent). In particular, the superiority of alternating chemotherapy was evident in the subsets known to be prognostically unfavorable or less affected by MOPP chemotherapy (i.e., age over 40 years, systemic symptoms, nodular sclerosis, and bulky lymphoma).

The alternating treatment is simple to administer (Table 2). MOPP is administered at the classic dose schedule, both when used alone or when alternated with ABVD. Prednisone is administered on cycles 1, 4, 7, and 10. The ABVD regimen is started on day 29 from the initiation of the previous MOPP cycle. All four drugs are given simultaneously as rapid intravenous injections on day 1 and 15 of each cycle. After each ABVD treatment, patients are given no other therapy for an additional 14 days. On day 29 from the initiation of ABVD, the next cycle of MOPP is started. Thus each treatment cycle of both drug regimens takes approximately 1 month. MOPP-ABVD should be administered until complete clinical remission is achieved (median five cycles) followed, after bone marrow and liver biopsies if these organs were known to be involved prior to therapy, by two consolidation cycles (MOPP and ABVD). It is important to administer full dose chemotherapy of both regimens unless peripheral leukocytes are below 3,500 per millimeter cubed and/or platelets below 100,000 per millimeter cubed, respectively, on the planned day of drug administration. In this case, physicians can decide whether to delay therapy for a few days or give chemotherapy, thereby reducing temporarily by 50 percent the dose of mechlorethamine, procarbazine, Adriamycin, and vinblastine. About 40 percent of patients manifest a leukocyte fall to less than 2,500 per millimeter cubed; a platelet fall to under 75,000 per millimeter cubed can be observed only in 15 percent of cases. Complete or almost complete alopecia occurs in only 17 to 20 percent of patients, and severe peripheral neuropathy in 7 percent, respectively. Vomiting is more frequent and severe after ABVD compared to MOPP. The results of MOPP-ABVD are confirmed, so far, by some European and American groups. In particular, a high, durable, complete remission rate was reported by Canadian investigators who have deleted dacarbazine from ABVD to decrease the incidence and the degree of vomiting.

TABLE 2 MOPP and ABVD Regimens

Combination	*Dose (mg/m²)*	*Days of Treatment*	*Frequency*
MOPP			
Mechlorethamine	6 IV	1 and 8	q 28 days
Vincristine	1.4 IV	1 and 8	
Procarbazine	100 PO	1 to 14	
Prednisone*	40 PO	1 to 14	
ABVD			
Adriamycin	25 IV	1 and 15	q 28 days
Bleomycin	10 IV	1 and 15	
Vinblastine	6 IV	1 and 15	
Dacarbazine	375 IV	1 and 15	

* On cycle 1, 4, 7.

SALVAGE THERAPY

Relapse from Primary Radiotherapy

After proper restaging, further irradiation can be delivered, if technically feasible, to patients with marginal or true recurrence followed by combination chemotherapy. Recent results from the Milan Cancer Institute suggest that Adriamycin containing regimens (ABVD, MOPP-ABVD) can yield superior results compared to MOPP (complete remission 90 percent versus 75 percent, 7-year RFS 80 percent versus 55 percent, survival 80 percent versus 45 percent). Whenever possible, as in stage IV disease, chemotherapy should be administered for a minimum of six cycles or to complete tumor remission plus two consolidation cycles.

Relapse from MOPP

If the duration of first complete remission is longer than 12 months, retreatment with MOPP remains the standard approach; it can yield a second complete remission in about 80 percent of patients, and in 75 to 85 percent of cases remission is durable. The same strategy is recommended in patients relapsing from other polydrug regimens. Patients relapsing from MOPP but in whom duration of first complete remission is less than 12 months as well as patients who do not achieve complete remission or show progressive disease during primary chemotherapy require treatment with non-cross resistant regimens. The most widely used salvage chemotherapy in MOPP resistant patients is ABVD. Treatment should be given at full dose to complete remission plus two consolidation cycles. The complete response rate is about 50 percent, and the likelihood of attaining complete remission is higher or lower in relation to A or B symptoms as well as to the anatomic extent of disease. Approximately 20 percent of all MOPP resistant patients remain disease-free at 5 years or more. Comparable results are being obtained with other Adriamycin containing regimens if treatment is promptly instituted at the time of recurrent or progressive lymphoma. There is early evidence that MOPP resistant patients can experience superior results with the cyclical delivery of non-cross resistant regimens such as ABVD and CEP (CCNU, etoposide, and prednimustine) (complete remission 60 percent, 2-year survival in excess of 50 percent).

Relapse from MOPP-ABVD

Patients should be retreated with the same alternating sequence if duration of first complete remission is longer than 12 months. Physicians should avoid risk of cumulative doses of Adriamycin (over 550 mg per meter squared) and of bleomycin (over 200 mg per meter squared). In patients with shorter duration of complete remission, CEP is recommended for a minimum of six cycles. The dose schedule is as follows: CCNU—80 mg/per meter squared orally, on day 1, etoposide 100 mg/per meter squared orally or intravenously from day 1 through 5, prednimustine 60 mg per meter squared orally from day 1 through 5. All drugs are recycled on day 28. Prednimustine can be replaced by an equivalent dose of chlorambucil and prednisone. Complete remission can be achieved in about 40 percent and the 5-year survival is 20 percent.

Salvage with ABMT

In recent years, high dose chemotherapy with autologous bone marrow transplantation (ABMT) has been applied to patients with advanced Hodgkin's disease in relapse or refractory to first or second line chemotherapy. One of the different drug regimens tested so far consists of cyclophosphamide 5 g per meter squared, BCNU 600 mg per meter squared, and etoposide 400 mg per meter squared with total body irradiation. If patients are properly selected (i.e., with age less than 50 years, with no prior radiotherapy, and in first relapse from primary chemotherapy), complete remission can be achieved in more than two-thirds of cases. In this type of patient, the actual RFS rate remains to be determined, but is expected to be in excess of 50 percent at 3 years. Because of severe myelosuppression for about 2 weeks and the persisting uncertainty about patients who may benefit from high dose chemotherapy with ABMT, this form of intensive treatment should be administered at present in specialized centers.

CHEMOTHERAPY IN EARLY STAGES

There is no standard role of chemotherapy in the management of stage I-II of Hodgkin's disease. However, chemotherapy may be indicated under certain circumstances, as summarized in Table 3. Full dose or wide field irradiation in children and adolescents would result in unacceptable bone and muscle growth abnormalities. Pediatric patients are now being treated with combination chemotherapy combined with involved field, low dose radiotherapy, and regardless of stage, 90 percent or more are alive at 10 years. As previously mentioned, another group of patients is those with bulky mediastinal adenopathy extending to the surrounding organs or all three B symptoms. If staging laparotomy is unavailable or considered unacceptable because of the patient's age, medical condition, or the therapeutic philosophy, chemotherapy should be given. If well-tolerated chemotherapy regimens were available, which after adequate long-term experience were associated with low or no leukemia or other neoplasm risk and low or no sterility risk, then chemotherapy would be the preferred treatment. The ABVD combination may represent an effective drug regimen devoid of chronic organ damage. The major disadvantages remain severe nausea and vomiting in at least half of patients. However, at present, it remains to be demonstrated whether a milder chemotherapy will be safer, more tolerable, and as effective as ABVD.

TREATMENT RELATED MORBIDITY

The most serious consequence of curative therapy for Hodgkin's disease is the emergence of second malignancies. Most common among these are acute, nonlymphocytic leukemia, myelodysplastic syndromes including preleukemia, and diffuse aggressive lymphomas. In patients treated with MOPP or one of its variants, i.e., treatment including alkylating agents, procarbazine, or nitrosourea derivatives (BCNU, CCNU), the risk of leukemia within 10 years is 3 to 4 percent. This risk seems to be increased when patients are older than 40 years at the time of systemic treatment and when combined treatment modality is utilized, especially if salvage MOPP is given after radiation failure (over 15 percent). The overall risk of nonHodgkin's lymphomas is about 2

TABLE 3 Indications for Primary Chemotherapy in the Management of Early Stage Hodgkin's Disease

If irradiation cannot or should not be given in full tumoricidal doses, or to appropriate (usually subtotal nodal) fields.
If diagnostic or staging information is inadequate by plan or circumstances.
If appropriate staging and irradiation would result in less than half of the patients enjoying prolonged recurrence-free survival.
If the acute toxicity and long-term complications of chemotherapy can be reduced significantly.

percent. The risk of developing a secondary solid tumor is continuing to increase beyond 10 years (a finding not seen with leukemia), and the risk is highest in older patients; approximately two-thirds of the tumors have occurred so far in the radiation therapy field. Since the selection of agents may be important (ABVD does not appear to be as toxic as MOPP in terms of the development of secondary leukemias), the accrual of more data from patients who receive alternate drug regimens is essential in assessing the relative carcinogenicity of the treatment modalities.

Gonadal dysfunction represents another important iatrogenic toxicity that considerably affects the quality of life in patients with Hodgkin's disease. A few cycles of MOPP or MOPP-like combinations induce azoospermia in 90 to 100 percent of patients, and this finding is associated with germinal hyperplasia and increased FSH levels, with normal levels of LH and testosterone. In addition, only 10 to 20 percent of patients eventually show recovery of spermatogenesis after long periods of time, even up to 10 years. About half of women become amenorrheic, and premature ovarian failure appears dependent upon age (over 30 years: 75 to 85 percent; under 30 years: about 20 percent). This is most probably related to the total dose of drugs, and is a progressive rather than an all-or-none phenomenon. The Milan Cancer Institute has reported that the administration of ABVD chemotherapy produces only a limited and transient germ cell toxicity in males and no drug induced amenorrhea. Thus, to circumvent chemotherapy induced sterility, the use of drug regimens not containing alkylating agents, procarbazine, or nitrosourea derivatives is highly recommended. An alternative for males undergoing MOPP or MOPP-ABVD combinations is represented by sperm storage prior to chemotherapy; however, both physicians and patients should be aware that about one-third of male patients with Hodgkin's disease have low sperm count or sperm motility before starting cytotoxic treatment. The usefulness of the administration of analogues of gonadotropin releasing hormone in males or oral contraceptives in premenopausal women remains to be fully confirmed. Libido tends to decrease after both the diagnosis of Hodgkin's disease and treatment with combination chemotherapy. There is no evidence of teratogenicity in patients treated for Hodgkin's disease.

Pericarditis, both acute and chronic, is the most common symptomatic cardiovascular complication of mediastinal irradiation. The incidence of pericarditis is related to the dose, dose rate, and volume irradiated. Clinically evident pericarditis occurs in about 15 percent following anteroposterior fields from a linear accelerator to a mean mediastinal dose of 44 Gy. Pericardial effusions develop in 25 percent to 30 percent of patients within 2 years of radiation. Surgical stripping of the pericardium remains the only definitive therapy for chronic constrictive pericarditis. Radiation induced myocardial fibrosis at the subclinical level occurs in over 50 percent of irradiated patients. Chronic cardiomyopathy may occur after anthracycline administration only if the cumulative dose of Adriamycin exceeds 400 to 450 mg per meter squared. At the Milan Cancer Institute, cardiac evaluation of patients treated with ABVD plus irradiation failed to detect any clinical and laboratory abnormalities up to 8 years from starting ABVD chemotherapy (maximum cumulative dose of Adriamycin: 300 mg per meter squared).

Acute radiation pneumonitis and chronic restrictive fibrosis are the most important pulmonary complications of mantle irradiation. Both are related to the total dose, dose rate, and volume of lung tissue irradiated. The overall incidence is about 20 percent. Patients with relapsed Hodgkin's disease who receive total body irradiation in preparation for bone marrow transplantation are also at risk for developing pneumonitis. The drugs with greatest potential for pulmonary toxicity are bleomycin and BCNU. In patients treated with ABVD plus radiotherapy, overt bleomycin related lung toxicity is uncommon, and no pulmonary damage was seen in patients given MOPP-ABVD.

SUGGESTED READING

Bonadonna G, Valagussa P, Santoro A. Alternating non-cross resistant combination chemotherapy or MOPP in stage IV Hodgkin's disease. Ann Intern Med 1986; 104:739–746.

Bookman MA, Longo DL, Concomitant illness in patients treated for Hodgkin's disease. Cancer Treat Rev 1986; 13:77–111.

Crnkovich MJ, Hoppe RT, Rosenberg SA. Stage IIB Hodgkin's disease: the Stanford experience. J Clin Oncol 1986; 4:1295–1306.

Santoro A, Bonadonna G, Valagussa P, et al. Long-term results of combined chemotherapy-radiotherapy approach in Hodgkin's disease: superiority of ABVD plus radiotherapy versus MOPP plus radiotherapy. J Clin Oncol 1987; 5:27–37.

Valagussa P, Santoro A, Fossati-Bellani F, et al. Second acute leukemia and other malignancies following treatment for Hodgkin's disease. J Clin Oncol 1986; 4:830–837.

FAVORABLE NONHODGKIN'S LYMPHOMA

MARTIN M. OKEN, M.D.

In the United States, nearly 25,000 people will be diagnosed with nonHodgkin's lymphoma during 1987. This represents an incidence roughly three times that of Hodgkin's disease. The nonHodgkin's lymphomas are a heterogeneous group of neoplasms that vary greatly in their clinical behavior. While some pursue an indolent course for many years, others are highly aggressive tumors leading rapidly to disability and death if not promptly controlled by effective therapy. Histologic classifications of the nonHodgkin's lymphomas are generally complex and hardly without controversy. However, some have succeeded in defining clinically and prognostically relevant subgroups. The Rappaport classification and the Working Formulation of non-Hodgkin's lymphomas are two particularly helpful systems that are currently in wide use (Table 1). The favorable histology lymphomas are those defined as low grade by the Working Formulation. These include small lymphocytic (SL), follicular small cleaved cell (FSC), and follicular mixed small cleaved and large cell (FM) lymphomas corresponding to the Rappaport classification equivalents—diffuse lymphocytic well differentiated (DLWD), nodular lymphocytic poorly differentiated (NLPD), and nodular mixed lymphocytic and histiocytic (NM), respectively. But are the low grade lymphomas truly favorable histologies? Although they tend to grow more slowly than the intermediate or high grade lymphomas, low grade lymphomas are usually widely disseminated at diagnosis; show a persistent tendency to relapse with few, if any, chemotherapeutic cures; and frequently transform late in their course to a more high grade histology. These problems should be kept in mind when considering the currently available treatment approaches and their limitations.

CLINICAL MANIFESTATIONS

The early history of low grade nonHodgkin's lymphoma is characteristically one of painless lymph node enlargement in an otherwise asymptomatic patient. It is common for multiple lymph node groups to be involved and for the bone marrow to be involved at diagnosis. Abdominal and inguinal adenopathy are often prominent, but mediastinal and hilar lymphadenopathy are seldom apparent until late in the disease course. DLWD is not distinguishable from the extramedullary manifestations of chronic lymphocytic leukemia, and a leukemic course may supervene.

Low grade nonHodgkin's lymphomas are usually indolent or slowly progressive at first. Spontaneous regressions are common, occurring in as many as 30 percent of patients with NLPD and in nearly 15 percent of patients with other low grade lymphomas. Occasionally, spontaneous regressions are complete and may persist for months to years. Despite its characteristic slow start, the disease eventually becomes progressive in most patients and leads to clinical deterioration and death. Many manifestations of advanced low grade lymphomas relate directly or indirectly to tumor bulk. Weight loss and pancytopenia are common severe problems late in the disease course. The pancytopenia may be caused by hypersplenism, bone marrow infiltration with lymphoma, the effects of chemotherapy, or a combination of these factors. Occasionally, autoimmune cytopenias are present, particularly in patients with DLWD.

CLINICAL EVALUATION AND STAGING

Initial clinical evaluation and staging procedures have four principal purposes in patients with nonHodgkin's lymphoma.

1. It is essential that the precise histologic diagnosis be confirmed. The need for adequate biopsy material is emphasized. This also permits immunophenotyping to identify B or T cell lineage, immunoglobulin or T cell receptor gene rearrangement studies, and cytogenetic studies where applicable. Most DLWD and all NLPD and NM are B cell lymphomas. At least 85 percent of NLPD and NM tumors have cytogenetic abnormalities that include t(14;18), and a sizable minority of DLWD tumors have trisomy 12 or del(11q).

TABLE 1 The Working Formulation of NonHodgkin's Lymphoma and the Comparative Rappaport Designation

Working Formulation	*Rappaport Classification*
Low Grade	
Small lymphocytic (SL)	Diffuse, lymphocytic, well differentiated (DLWD)
Follicular, predominantly small cleaved cell (FSC)	Nodular, lymphocytic, poorly differentiated (NLPD)
Follicular, mixed, small cleaved, and large cell (FM)	Nodular, mixed, lymphocytic, and histiocytic (NM)
Intermediate Grade	
Follicular, predominantly large cell (FL)	Nodular histiocytic (NH)
Diffuse, small cleaved cell (DSC)	Diffuse, lymphocytic, poorly differentiated (DLPD)
Diffuse, mixed, small cleaved, and large cell (DM)	Diffuse, mixed, lymphocytic, and histiocytic (DM)
Diffuse, large cell (DL)	Diffuse, histiocytic (DH)
High Grade	
Large cell, immunoblastic	Diffuse histiocytic (DH)
Lymphoblastic	Lymphoblastic
Small noncleaved cell (SNC)	Diffuse, undifferentiated, Burkitt and nonBurkitt (DU)

2. The primary role of initial staging evaluation is to determine the optimal treatment strategy. Is the patient curable with radiation therapy? Should treatment be deferred initially? Is active systemic therapy required initially?
3. One must determine whether the patient is threatened by imminent serious complications from the lymphoma such as urinary tract obstruction or bone marrow failure.
4. Finally, it is important to evaluate the patient's overall medical condition to detect the presence of any complicating underlying medical disorders that may impact on the treatment options.

The Ann Arbor staging system, developed for use in staging Hodgkin's disease, is also utilized for adult patients with nonHodgkin's lymphomas. In this system, stage I disease denotes involvement of a single lymph node region. Stage II disease requires involvement of two or more lymph node regions on the same side of the diaphragm. Stage III disease represents involvement of lymph node regions on both sides of the diaphragm with or without splenic involvement. Patients with diffuse or disseminated involvement of one or more extra lymphatic organs or tissues with or without splenic involvement are considered to have stage IV lymphoma. The Ann Arbor staging system is based on the tendency of Hodgkin's disease to spread initially to contiguous lymph node groups. This, however, is not the clinical pattern generally observed in the low grade nonHodgkin's lymphomas. Disease limited to stage I or II distribution accounts for less than 10 percent of properly staged patients. Most patients with DLWD and NLPD present with bone marrow involvement. In contrast to Hodgkin's disease and the higher grade nonHodgkin's lymphomas, advanced Ann Arbor stage does not convey an ominous short-term prognosis to patients with low grade nonHodgkin's lymphomas. It does, however, suggest that the disease is less amenable to curative treatment and will most likely be fatal.

Evaluation should include a careful history with particular attention to possible systemic manifestations of the lymphoma. The B symptoms include fever, sweats, or weight loss greater than 10 percent of body weight. A history of asymptomatic localized or generalized lymphadenopathy, which may wax and wane, should be sought. Physical examination should emphasize evaluation of all lymph node regions including epitrochlear nodes and Waldeyer's ring as well as measurement of the liver and spleen. Laboratory studies to be included in all staging evaluations are a complete blood count with careful evaluation of the peripheral blood smear, blood tests to evaluate liver and renal function, serum uric acid determination, and chest x-ray examination. Bilateral bone marrow biopsies are essential in patients whose clinical stage remains I or II at this phase of the work-up. Patients who still appear to have limited disease should be evaluated with bilateral lower extremity lymphangiography and abdominal computed tomography (CT) scan. The latter is particularly valuable for diagnosing mesenteric node, splenic hilar node, and porta hepatis lymph node involvement. The CT scan is useful even in patients already known to have stage III or IV disease since it frequently provides the baseline documentation of extent of disease that can help gauge completeness of response. Once stage III or IV disease has been documented, further invasive staging procedures are generally unnecessary. Staging laparotomy with splenectomy and open liver biopsy is limited to highly selected patients in whom aggressive curative radiation therapy is considered.

TREATMENT

Principles Guiding the Development of a Treatment Plan In Low Grade NonHodgkin's Lymphoma

It is important to differentiate between what is known about the management of low grade nonHodgkin's lymphoma and what is hypothesized. The latter may be useful in helping to formulate new treatment approaches for study, but the former represents the proper base on which to construct treatment plans for patients not entered into experimental protocols. The following principles are clearly supported by data available in 1989.

1. Stage I and stage II disease is infrequent, but when carefully documented, it is curable with radiation therapy.
2. In stage III and IV low grade nonHodgkin's lymphoma, indolent disease often associated with spontaneous regression may permit delay of treatment for years, apparently without jeopardizing the patient's well-being or long-term prognosis.
3. Moderately intensive combination chemotherapy does not produce better long-term disease control or survival than conservative regimens based on single alkylating agents with or without prednisone. The possible exception to this rule is nodular mixed lymphoma, but the results here are controversial.
4. Clinical trials comparing aggressive newer regimens are in progress, but no conclusive results are yet available. So far, no treatment for stage III-IV low grade lymphoma has proved superior to conservative treatment, which must be considered the current standard.
5. Of the biologic response modifiers, only alpha interferon has been extensively tested to date. It is active and can readily be combined with chemotherapy. Numerous studies are in progress, but until they are completed, a role for interferon is not yet defined.
6. New agents have been introduced into this field slowly, but could have more impact on salvage therapy if they are more aggressively tested.
7. Histologic transformation to higher grade lymphoma is the rule and frequently dominates the late clinical course.

Treatment of Stage I-II Disease

It is important to identify the 5 to 10 percent of patients with low grade nonHodgkin's lymphoma who have stage I or II disease. Approximately 80 percent of these patients can be cured with moderate dose regional radiotherapy. The treatment usually involves 3,000 to 4,000 rads of involved field radiation delivered over a 4-week period. While total lymphoid irradiation has been used in some reported series, its advantage over involved field or extended field treatment is yet to be demonstrated. Patients relapsing after regional radiation therapy may still have long periods of disease control with systemic chemotherapy.

Although some centers combine systemic chemotherapy with curative radiation therapy for stage I and II disease, there has been no clear demonstration that this improves either the cure rate or survival duration. In view of the toxicity risk and possible increased risk of treatment induced leukemia, this combined modality approach cannot be recommended over radiation therapy alone. Because of the distinct possibility of cure, no serious consideration should be given to deferring therapy unless the patient is clearly demonstrated to have stage III or IV disease.

Treatment of Stage III and IV Low Grade Lymphoma

Systemic chemotherapy is the standard treatment for stage III and IV low grade nonHodgkin's lymphoma. The issue of when to start treatment is not completely resolved. However, it is reasonable to defer initial therapy for indolent stage III and IV disease, particularly with NLPD or DLWD histologies, until the development of systemic symptoms, disease progression, or threat of complications. Specific treatment indications include rapid growth or large bulk of disease, anemia, neutropenia, thrombocytopenia, or threatening extranodal disease such as orbital, pulmonary, or progressive hepatic involvement, urethral obstruction, pleural effusion, or ascites. A group of 83 patients studied at Stanford University had treatment deferred for an average of 3 years. This initial approach is appropriate in 50 to 60 percent of newly disgnosed patients with stage III-IV disease.

When chemotherapy is instituted, the mainstays are the alkylating agents cyclophosphamide and chlorambucil given singly or with a corticosteroid, generally prednisone. Each of the regimens outlined in Table 2, yield objective responses—complete response (CR) or partial remission (PR)—in over 90 percent of patients with CR in 50 to 80 percent. Several randomized prospective clinical trials have compared single alkylating agent therapy (with or without prednisone) to moderately intensive combinations such as CVP, C-MOPP, BCNU plus CVP, or Adriamycin plus bleomycin plus CVP. These have consistently shown no difference in CR rate, CR duration (median 2 years), or survival (median 6 to 10 years). For this reason, single agent therapy or the CP regimen is satisfactory treatment unless more rapid tumor lysis is needed. In that case, CVP, C-MOPP, or COPA might be preferable. Durable, long-term remissions have been claimed in over 50 percent of one series of DM patients treated with the C-MOPP regimen. However, late relapses have emerged, and a large Eastern Cooperative Oncology Group ECOG study failed to substantiate the favorable response duration in most patients. Nevertheless, C-MOPP or COPA represent reasonable treatment options in NM because rapid tumor reduction is generally desirable with this more aggressive histology.

Regardless of the regimen, initial chemotherapy should be accompanied by allopurinol therapy to pre-

TABLE 2 Chemotherapy Regimens for Low Grade Lymphomas

Regimen	*Drug*	*Dose, Mode of Administration*	*Schedule*	*Cycle Duration*
Single, daily, oral alkylating agent	Cyclophosphamide or	100 mg/m^2 PO	daily	—
	chlorambucil	4–6 mg/m^2 PO	daily	—
High dose, intermittent oral therapy	Chlorambucil,	30 mg/m^2 PO	d 1	2 weeks
	prednisone	80 mg/m^2 PO	d 1–5	
CP	Cyclophosphamide,	600 mg/m^2 IV	d 1,8	4 weeks
	prednisone	100 mg/m^2 PO	d 1–5	
CVP	Cyclophosphamide,	400 mg/m^2 PO	d 1–5	
	vincristine,	1.4 mg/m^2 IV (max. 2 mg)	d 1	3 weeks
	prednisone	100 mg/m^2 PO	d 1–5	
C-MOPP	Cyclophosphamide,	650 mg/m^2 IV	d 1,8	
	vincristine,	1.4 mg/m^2 IV (max. 2 mg)	d 1,8	4 weeks
	procarbazine,	100 mg/m^2 PO	d 1–10	
	prednisone	40 mg/m^2 PO	d 1–14	
COPA	Cyclophosphamide,	600 mg/m^2 IV	d 1	
	Adriamycin,	50 mg/m^2 IV	d 1	3 weeks
	vincristine,	1.4 mg/m^2 IV (max. 2 mg)	d 1	
	prednisone	100 mg/m^2 PO	d 1–5	

vent hyperuricemia until the tumor mass is reduced. The chemotherapy regimen should be continued until 2 months after maximum tumor reduction is achieved before being discontinued. This may take up to 24 to 30 months for some patients, but generally results in a 2 to 3-year period during which no treatment is required. Remissions can usually be reinduced 2 or 3 times utilizing the initial regimen.

It should be emphasized that the standard treatment approaches for stage III-IV disease as outlined above are palliative and after initial success are unfortunately followed by a continuing pattern of relapse and eventual development of refractory disease. There is a strong tendency for the low grade lymphomas to progress histologically from nodular to diffuse and from small lymphocytic to large cell. Rebiopsy should be performed in patients with refractory disease or in patients in whom the disease has changed its rate of progression in order to rule out such histologic transformation.

Clearly, the trials reported to date showing single agent therapy to be as effective as combination chemotherapy have evaluated regimens of only intermediate intensity. Studies evaluating truly intensive regimens such as ProMACE-MOPP (see chapter on unfavorable lymphoma) combined with total lymphoid irradiation are in progress. Monoclonal antibody therapy, biologic response modifiers such as interferon, and new chemotherapeutic agents including pentostatin, mitoxantrone, and others are also under evaluation. These approaches to the treatment of low grade lymphomas are experimental and should not be used except in the context of formal clinical trials.

SUGGESTED READING

Acker B, Hoppe RT, Colby TV, et al. Histologic conversion in the non-Hodgkin's lymphomas. J Clin Oncol 1983; 1:11–16.

Chabner BA, Johnson RE, Young RC, et al. Sequential nonsurgical staging of non-Hodgkin's lymphomas. Ann Intern Med 1976; 85:149–154.

Cheson BD, Wittes RE, Friedman MA. Low-grade non-Hodgkin's lymphomas revisited. Cancer Treat Rep 1986; 70:1051–1054.

Garvin AJ, Simon RM, Osborne K, et al. An autopsy study of histologic progression in non-Hodgkin's lymphomas. Cancer 1983; 52:393–398.

Gomez GA, Barcos M, Krishnamsetty RM, et al. Treatment of early-stages I and II—nodular poorly differentiated lymphocytic lymphoma. Am J Clin Oncol (CCT) 1986; 9:40–44.

Horning SJ, Rosenberg SA. The natural history of initially untreated low-grade non-Hodgkin's lymphomas. N Engl J Med 1984; 311:1471–1475.

Jones SE. Follicular lymphoma—do no harm. Cancer Treat Rep 1986; 70:1055–1058.

Rosenberg SA. The low-grade non-Hodgkin's lymphomas: Challenges and opportunities. J Clin Oncol 1985; 3:299–310.

The Non-Hodgkin's Lymphoma Pathologic Classification Project National Cancer Institute sponsored study of classifications of non-Hodgkin's lymphomas. Cancer 1982; 49:2112–2135.

UNFAVORABLE NONHODGKIN'S LYMPHOMA

ELLEN R. GAYNOR, M.D.
RICHARD I. FISHER, M.D.

The nonHodgkin's lymphomas (NHL) are a diverse group of diseases both in their natural history and in their responses to therapy. These diseases are related to one another in that all are the result of the malignant transformation of lymphocytes at a particular stage of normal lymphocyte transformation. Over the years, a variety of classification schemes have been proposed; such variety has resulted, at times, in undue confusion. The two most commonly used classification systems in the American literature are the Rappaport system and the Working Formulation Nomenclature (Table 1). From a clinical standpoint, the lymphomas may be conveniently grouped into those that are favorable and those that are unfavorable (see Table 1). These groupings stem from observation of the natural history of these diseases. Favorable lymphomas are generally indolent in their behavior, while unfavorable lymphomas follow a more aggressive clinical course. Paradoxically, lymphomas that are favorable are, in fact, usually not curable, while those in the unfavorable category are frequently curable with aggressive combination chemotherapy. The remainder of this chapter focuses on the approach to treatment of the unfavorable lymphomas.

BURKITT'S AND LYMPHOBLASTIC LYMPHOMA

Lymphomas of the small noncleaved cell (Burkitt's type) are endemic in certain parts of Africa. The disease in these areas appears to be etiologically related to the Epstein-Barr virus. The disease is also seen in this country, although it is rare and its relationship to prior exposure to the Epstein-Barr virus is not as clear. It is primarily seen in the pediatric age group, is frequently associated with bulky disease involving the jaw or abdomen, and often involves the bone marrow and meninges. While it is very aggressive in its clinical behavior, it is also exquisitely sensitive to chemotherapy.

TABLE 1 Classification Systems for NonHodgkin's Lymphoma

Rappaport Classification	*Working Formulation*	*Favorable/ Unfavorable*
Low grade malignancy		
Lymphocytic, well differentiated	Malignant lymphoma, small lymphocytic	Favorable
Nodular lymphocytic, poorly differentiated	Malignant lymphoma, follicular; predominantly small cleaved cell	Favorable
Nodular mixed, lymphocytic and histiocytic	Malignant lymphoma, follicular mixed, small cleaved and large cell	Favorable
Intermediate grade malignancy		
Nodular histiocytic	Malignant lymphoma, follicular, predominantly large cell	Unfavorable
Diffuse lymphocytic, poorly differentiated	Malignant lymphoma, diffuse small cleaved cell	Unfavorable
Diffuse mixed, lymphocytic and histiocytic	Malignant lymphoma, diffuse mixed, small and large cell	Unfavorable
Diffuse histiocytic	Malignant lymphoma, diffuse large cell	Unfavorable
High grade malignancy		
Diffuse histiocytic	Malignant lymphoma, large cell, immunoblastic	Unfavorable
Lymphoblastic	Malignant lymphoma, lymphoblastic	Unfavorable
Diffuse undifferentiated (Burkitt's and non-Burkitt's types)	Malignant lymphoma, small noncleaved cell	Unfavorable

Lymphoblastic lymphoma (LBL) is also an aggressive lymphoma that is usually of T cell origin. The disease is, in many ways, similar to acute lymphoblastic leukemia, and in some instances the distinction between these two diseases is not clear. Like Burkitt's lymphoma, LBL is seen primarily in the pediatric age group, although it is encountered in the adult population. Typically, the disease presents as a mediastinal mass in association with peripheral adenopathy. Bone marrow and central nervous system (CNS) involvement are frequently encountered in this disease.

Because of the systemic nature of both Burkitt's and lymphoblastic lymphoma, and because of the extremely rapid growth rate of these lymphomas, intensive chemotherapy with attention to CNS prophylaxis is standard therapy. For lymphoblastic lymphoma, it is not clear whether the disease is best treated as a very aggressive lymphoma or if it should be treated like acute lymphoblastic leukemia. It is clear, however, that the regimens used for diffuse large cell lymphoma are not adequate therapy for this disease. However, the detailed management of these relatively rare lymphomas is beyond the scope of this discussion. The reader is referred to recent publications for details of management.

DIFFUSE LARGE CELL LYMPHOMA

Of the other unfavorable lymphomas, those most commonly encountered in clinical practice are the various types of large cell lymphoma. While there are morphologic and clinical differences among the large cell lymphomas, in general their management is the same, and they are grouped together in clinical trials. The management of the large cell lymphomas provides the basis for decisions regarding the management of the other unfavorable lymphomas (with the exception of Burkitt's and lymphoblastic lymphomas as discussed above). The remainder of this chapter focuses on the staging and principles of chemotherapeutic approaches to the large cell lymphomas.

Staging

Because of the curative potential of large cell lymphomas and because the only significant chance for cure depends upon the choice of appropriate initial therapy, it is essential to determine the extent of disease at the time of diagnosis. This involves rigorous staging procedures including, as a minimum, chest x-ray, computed tomography (CT) scan, lymphangiogram, and biopsy of the bone marrow and other organs as indicated. Staging laparotomy, as performed routinely in the staging of Hodgkin's disease, is utilized rarely in the staging of NHL. The Ann Arbor Staging System (Table 2) is generally applied to the staging of NHL, although it is clear that this system (which was originally proposed for the staging of Hodgkin's disease) has some shortcomings when applied to the nonHodgkin's lymphomas. Initial patient characteristics that have prognostic significance

TABLE 2 The Ann Arbor Staging Classification

Stage I
: Involvement of a single lymph node region or of a single extranodal organ or site (I_E).

Stage II
: Involvement of two or more lymph node regions on the same side of the diaphragm, or localized involvement of an extranodal site or organ (II_E) and of one or more lymph node regions on the same side of the diaphragm.

Stage III
: Involvement of lymph node regions on both sides of the diaphragm, which may also be accompanied by localized involvement of an extranodal organ or site (III_E) or spleen (III_S) or both (III_{SE}).

Stage IV
: Diffuse or disseminated involvement of one or more distant extranodal organs with or without associated lymph node involvement.

Fever >38°C, night sweats, and/or weight loss >10% of body weight in the 6 months preceding admission are defined as systemic symptoms, and denoted by the suffix B. Asymptomatic patients are denoted by the suffix A.

in large cell lymphoma are the presence or absence of constitutional symptoms, stage IV disease, gastrointestinal tract involvement, bone marrow involvement, bulky disease (which is defined as a tumor mass greater than 10 cm in diameter in a single location), age, and serum lactic dehydrogenase (LDH).

Chemotherapeutic Approaches

The treatment of large cell lymphoma has evolved considerably over the past 20 years (Table 3). When single agent chemotherapy was used, 5 percent of patients achieved a complete remission (CR), and the median survival of patients was 9 months. In 1975, investigators at the National Cancer Institute reported on the C-MOPP regimen. Forty-one percent of treated patients achieved a complete remission, while 37 percent of treated patients achieved long-term remission, which is probably equivalent to cure in this disease. Successful use of combination chemotherapy obviously represents a significant advance as compared with results achieved with single agent therapy.

The introduction of the drug Adriamycin represents a major advance in cancer chemotherapeutics, and the CHOP regimen was one of the first programs to incorporate this drug. This combination has been used extensively in the treatment of large cell lymphoma. Follow-up data of up to 12 years is now available from the Southwest Oncology Group for 418 patients treated in three consecutive studies employing the CHOP regimen. The CR rate is 53 percent, with 30 percent of all treated patients achieving a sustained complete remission. While the initial CR rates are higher with CHOP than with C-MOPP, the percentage of cures is similar when considering the entire group of treated patients. Several points are worth noting, however. First, the CHOP trials were cooperative group studies as opposed to single institution studies. In general, results from single institution studies are better than those from cooperative group trials. Second, in an analysis of the CHOP studies, age was a significant determinant of survival since 45 percent of all patients who were less than 55 years old at the time of treatment were cured with this chemotherapy. Older patients tended to be treated less aggressively with frequent dosage reductions. However, even the older patients who received full doses had a worse prognosis. These facts must be taken into consideration when comparing the CHOP regimen with the more recently reported regimens.

In an attempt to improve on the results achieved with CHOP and in an attempt to address the problem of tumor growth during periods of myelosuppression, several chemotherapy regimens were designed that incorporated the use of nonmyelotoxic drugs at times during the chemotherapy cycle when the patient's bone marrow was maximally suppressed. The M-BACOD regimen incorporates high dose methotrexate with leucovorin rescue at the midpoint of the treatment cycle to prevent tumor growth, which has been seen occasionally with regimens given on a 21 to 28 day cycle. Results are encouraging, with a reported complete response rate of 77 percent and long-term remissions being achieved in 57 percent of patients.

To decrease toxicity and to allow greater usage of this type of approach, the m-BACOD regimen was designed. This regimen uses a much lower dose of methotrexate and can be given on an outpatient basis. With a shorter period of follow-up as compared with the M-BACOD study, results are encouraging, with a 75 percent complete response rate, and with 58 percent of patients remaining in complete remission.

While several regimens address the problem of midcycle tumor growth, other investigators have devised regimens that employ the simultaneous use of two non-cross resistant drug combinations. Such an approach is rational since it appears that a major cause of chemotherapy failure is the presence of, and subsequent selection of, clones of cells that are resistant to therapy. By using alternating non-cross resistant regimens, one hopes to eradicate tumor cells that are resistant to one but not both drug combinations. An example of such an approach is the ProMACE–MOPP regimen. As initially devised, ProMACE was given either until a complete remission had been achieved or until the rate of the tumor response had plateaued. Patients were then treated with an equal number of cycles of MOPP and finally were given additional late intensification cycles of ProMACE. Seventy-three percent of patients so treated achieved a complete remission, with 60 percent of all treated patients experiencing long-term disease-free survival. Subsequent modifications of the ProMACE–MOPP regimen are the ProMACE–CytaBOM and ProMACE d1–MOPP d8 regimens. These modifications of the original regimen have the theoretical advantage of overcoming resistant clones of cells by introducing two non-cross resistant regimens into the initial treatment cycle.

One of the most recently reported chemotherapy approaches to large cell lymphoma is the MACOP-B regimen. This regimen differs from the others in that it involves weekly treatments of myelotoxic drugs alternating with nonmyelotoxic agents. The total duration of treatment is 12 weeks, which is considerably shorter than any previously reported treatment program. Excellent results have been achieved, with 84 percent of patients entering complete remission and 75 percent of all patients achieving long-term remissions.

Specific Therapeutic Approaches

With so many effective regimens from which to choose, it might appear that large cell lymphoma is a relatively easy disease to treat; however, this is not the case. Two questions arise when confronted with a given patient: (1) should all patients be treated in exactly the same way regardless of the initial extent of disease, and (2) what is the most appropriate chemotherapy regimen

TABLE 3 Chemotherapeutic Regimens

Regimen	*Dose and Route*	*Day*	*Frequency*	*Reference*
C-MOPP				
C = cyclophosphamide	650 mg/m² IV	1,8	Repeat every 28 days	5
O = Oncovin	1.4 mg/m² IV	1,8		
P = procarbazine	100 mg/m² PO	1–14		
P = prednisone	40 mg/m² PO	1–14		
COMLA				
C = cyclophosphamide	1,500 mg/m² IV	1	Repeat every 91 days	10
O = Oncovin	1.4 mg/m² IV (max 2.0 mg)	1,8,15		
M = methotrexate	120 mg/m² IV	22,29,36,43,50,57,64,71		
L = leucovorin	25 mg/m² PO × 4	24 hours after methotrexate		
A = cytarabine	300 mg/m²	Same as methotrexate		
CHOP				
C = cyclophosphamide	750 mg/m² IV	1	Repeat every 21 days	2
H = Adriamycin	50 mg/m² IV	1		
O = Oncovin	1.4 mg/m² IV (max 2.0 mg)	1		
P = prednisone	100 mg PO	1–5		
M-BACOD				
M = methotrexate*	3,000 mg/m² IV	1	Repeat every 21 days	15
B = bleomycin	4 mg/m² IV	1		
A = Adriamycin	45 mg/m² IV	1		
C = cyclophosphamide	600 mg/m² IV	1		
O = Oncovin	1 mg/m² IV	1		
D = Decadron	6 mg/m² PO	1–5		
m-BACOD				
m = methotrexate*	200 mg/m² IV	8,15	Repeat every 21 days	16
B = bleomycin	4 mg/m² IV	1		
A = Adriamycin	45 mg/m² IV	1		
C = cyclophosphamide	600 mg/m² IV	1		
O = Oncovin	1.4 mg/m² IV	1		
D = Decadron	6 mg/m² PO	1–5		
ProMACE-MOPP				
Pro = prednisone	60 mg/m² PO	1–14	Repeat every 28 days	7
M = methotrexate*	1,500 mg/m² IV	15		
A = Adriamycin	25 mg/m² IV	1,8		
C = cyclophosphamide	650 mg/m² IV	1,8		
E = etoposide	120 mg/m² IV	1,8		
Followed by MOPP after maximal response				
M = mechlorethamine	6 mg/m² IV	1,8	Repeat every 28 days	
O = Oncovin	1.4 mg/m² IV	1,8		
P = Procarbazine	100 mg/m² PO	1–14		
P = prednisone	40 mg/m² PO	1–14		
ProMACE-CytaBOM				
Pro = prednisone	60 mg/m² PO	1–14	Repeat every 21 days	8
A = Adriamycin	25 mg/m² IV	1		
C = cyclophosphamide	650 mg/m² IV	1		
E = etoposide	120 mg/m² IV	1		
Cyta = cytarabine	300 mg/m² IV	8		
B = bleomycin	5 mg/m² IV	8		
O = Oncovin	1.4 mg/m² IV	8		
M = methotrexate*	120 mg/m² IV	8		
MACOP-B				
M = methotrexate*	400 mg/m² IV	8,36,64		11
A = Adriamycin	50 mg/m² IV	1,15,29,43,57,71		
C = cyclophosphamide	350 mg/m² IV	1,15,29,43,57,71		
O = Oncovin	1.4 mg/m² IV (max 2.0 mg)	8,22,36,50,64,78		
P = Prednisone	75 mg/m² PO	1–84		
B = bleomycin	10 mg/m² IV	22,50,78		

* Leucovorin rescue is given 24 hours after each methotrexate dose.

to use? The answers to these questions are discussed in the next two sections.

Early Stage Disease (Stage I and Stage II [Nonbulky])

With regard to stage, most investigators agree that patients with stage I and stage II (nonbulky) disease should be approached differently than patients with stage II (bulky), stage III, and stage IV disease. There are a few patients who, after meticulous pathologic staging (including a formal staging laparotomy), have pathologic stage I disease. These patients may be cured by radiation therapy alone. In general, this extensive pathologic staging is not, and should not be, undertaken except in institutions where there is the necessary experience in the performance of staging laparotomy. Most investigators advise the use of systemic chemotherapy for patients with early stage disease since, in the majority of cases, large cell lymphoma is a systemic disease at diagnosis. Excellent results have been reported with the use of CHOP chemotherapy in patients with stage I and stage II (nonbulky) disease. An issue that is not resolved at present is whether there is any benefit to radiation therapy in addition to chemotherapy. This question is currently being addressed by cooperative group studies.

Advanced Stage Disease (Stage II [Bulky] Stage III and IV)

For patients with stage II (bulky), stage III and stage IV disease, it is clear that an aggressive chemotherapy approach is mandatory if the patient is to be cured. While it appears that regimens developed subsequent to CHOP give significantly better results, it is important to recognize that each of these regimens is reported by a single institution, and it is invalid to compare these newer regimens with the CHOP regimen in a retrospective manner. Interestingly, the Southwest Oncology Group (SWOG) recently completed a series of phase II studies in which the m-BACOD, ProMACE–CytaBOM, and MACOP-B regimens were tested in a cooperative group setting. These pilot studies demonstrate that such aggressive regimens can be safely used in a cooperative group setting. The complete response rates of 58 to 65 percent that were observed were, as expected, lower than those reported in the single institution studies. Also of interest is the fact that these response rates are not markedly different from the complete response rates seen with the CHOP regimen in cooperative group studies. The increased toxicity and expense of the newer regimens are acceptable if, in fact, response rate and cure rate are improved. However, if there is no difference as compared with the CHOP regimen, such increased risk to the patient is not warranted.

Currently, a randomized trial is being conducted that compares the four regimens: CHOP, m-BACOD, ProMACE–CytaBOM, and MACOP-B. Obviously, the results of this study will have a major impact on the future treatment of large cell lymphoma. Ideally, every eligible patient should be encouraged to participate in this study in order to complete it in a timely fashion.

Until this study is completed, however, there is no correct answer regarding the most appropriate regimen to use in the treatment of nonprotocol patients with advanced stage large cell lymphoma. We believe that the choice of regimen should be dictated by which regimen the treating physician is most familiar with and by the sophistication of the support facilities available to the treating physician. The more aggressive regimens can put the patient at risk for life-threatening toxicity. Such treatment should be undertaken only in situations where the patient can be supported through the complications of therapy. Because we are familiar with the ProMACE-based regimens and because we believe these are effective, we would use one of them in treating a patient who is not participating in a research protocol. For the patient who is not able to tolerate the drug Adriamycin, we believe that the COMLA or C-MOPP regimen is a reasonable alternative.

SALVAGE THERAPY

Patients not achieving complete remission with initial therapy present difficult management problems. While an occasional patient achieves a complete remission with another conventional regimen, the majority of patients cannot be rendered disease-free. At present, there are no outstanding salvage regimens for patients who fail to achieve complete remission with initial therapy. The drugs cis-platinum, amsacrine, etoposide, and ifosfamide, used either alone or in combination, have yielded response in some patients whose initial therapy failed. Duration of remission has, unfortunately, been short in most cases. High dose chemotherapy in conjunction with autologous bone marrow transplant is an alternative salvage approach. While there have been some encouraging results, this approach remains experimental at this time.

Because salvage therapy is frequently unsuccessful in this disease and because the patient's only chance of cure rests with the initial therapy, we recommend that the physician choose therapy wisely, treat aggressively, and modify drug dosages only as specified for each regimen. To do otherwise may unnecessarily deny the patient the possibility of cure.

SUGGESTED READING

Armitage JO, Fyfe MAE, Lewis J. Long term remission durability and functional status of patients treated for diffuse histiocytic lymphoma with the CHOP regimen. J Clin Oncol 1984; 2:898–902.

DeVita VT, Canellos GP, Chabner B, et al. Advanced diffuse histiocytic lymphoma, a potentially curable disease: results with combination chemotherapy. Lancet 1975; 1:248–250.

Fisher RI, DeVita VT, Hubbard SM, et al. Diffuse aggressive lymphomas: increased survival after alternating flexible sequences of ProMACE and MOPP chemotherapy. Ann Intern Med 1983; 98:304–309.

Fisher RI, DeVita VT, Hubbard SM, et al. Randomized trial of

ProMACE-MOPP vs ProMACE–CytaBOM in previously untreated, advanced stage diffuse aggressive lymphoma [abstract]. Proc Am Soc Clin Oncol 1983; 3:c–945.

Fisher RI, Miller TP, Dana BW, et al. Southwest Oncology Group clinical trials for intermediate and high grade non-Hodgkin's lymphomas, in press.

Gaynor ER, Ultmann JE, Golomb HM, Sweet DL. Treatment of diffuse histiocytic lymphoma with COMLA: a 10-year experience in a single institution. J Clin Oncol 1985; 3:1596–1604.

Klimo P, Connors JM. MACOP-B chemotherapy for the treatment of advanced diffuse large cell lymphoma. Ann Intern Med 1985; 102:596–602.

Miller T, Jones SE. Initial chemotherapy for clinically localized lymphomas of unfavorable histology. Blood 1983; 62:413–418.

Skarin AT, Canellos GP, Rosenthal DS, et al. Improved prognosis of diffuse histiocytic and undifferentiated lymphoma by use of high dose methotrexate alternating with standard agents (M-BACOD). J Clin Oncol 1983; 1:91–97.

Skarin AT, Canellos GP, Rosenthal DS, et al. Moderate dose methotrexate (m) combined with bleomycin (B), Adriamycin (A), cyclophosphamide (C), Oncovin (O) and dexamethasone (D), m-BACOD, in advanced diffuse histiocytic lymphoma. Proceedings of the second international conference of malignant lymphoma. Lugano, Switzerland, Boston: Martinus Nijhoff, 1984:59.

T-CELL LYMPHOMA

WALTER J. URBA, M.D., Ph.D.
DAN L. LONGO, M.D.

Mycosis fungoides and the Sézary syndrome are parts of a spectrum of malignant nonHodgkin's lymphomas called the cutaneous T-cell lymphomas (CTCL). They are relatively uncommon, with approximately 400 new cases occurring in the United States each year. The disease can be extremely difficult to diagnose, and it is not uncommon for patients to have undergone multiple skin biopsies and to have received various topical treatments prior to the definitive diagnosis. These disorders are of a chronic nature, and prolonged survival measured in years is the rule rather than the exception. The malignant cells are mature CD4+ lymphocytes. Although some tumors retain the functional characteristics of helper T cells on assay in vitro, most are nonfunctional, and patients rarely develop signs or symptoms related to an excess of T-helper cell function. The disease is characterized by initial involvement of the skin with subsequent spread to peripheral blood, lymph nodes, and other organs.

A staging system for mycosis fungoides has been devised that takes into account the type of skin disease, the presence of histologic and clinical lymph node involvement, and the presence of visceral disease. This staging system can be used to divide patients into three prognostic categories at diagnosis irrespective of subsequent treatment. A very favorable group, with plaque skin disease and no evidence of lymph node or visceral involvement, has a median survival in excess of 8 years. An intermediate group, with cutaneous tumors or more advanced lymph node involvement, has a median survival of 5 years. Finally, the unfavorable group has a median survival of 24 months. These last patients are distinguished by lymph node replacement or effacement by frank lymphoma, or visceral organ involvement.

Since the prognosis of individual patients is highly dependent on the presence or absence of extracutaneous disease, proper staging is extremely important. Following history and physical examination, routine laboratory studies with careful examination of blood smear, chest x-ray film, lymphangiogram, bone marrow aspirate and biopsy, lymph node biopsy, and liver biopsy, disseminated disease is found in approximately 51 percent of patients at presentation. However, when specialized techniques such as cytogenetics or DNA analysis by Southern blotting test to look for clonal rearrangements of the T-cell antigen receptor are used, the incidence of extracutaneous disease at presentation approaches 90 percent. This has major implications for the therapy of patients with CTCL.

Initial therapy is usually directed at the skin. This may include the daily application of topical nitrogen mustard, chronic treatment with psoralen plus ultraviolet light irradiation (PUVA), or total body electron beam radiation therapy (EBRT). These treatments are effective in temporarily controlling skin disease in the majority of patients but are of long-term benefit to only a minority of patients (i.e., probably those 10 percent with truly cutaneous disease). The median duration of response for these therapies is 1 to 2 years, and 10 to 20 percent of patients remain disease-free at 3 years. Long-term disease-free survival is found exclusively in patients with early plaque disease. Remissions induced by topical mustard and PUVA probably require continued maintenance therapy. Unmaintained long-term, disease-free remissions have been observed primarily with EBRT. Preliminary data obtained after prolonged follow-up of patients receiving PUVA suggest that certain patients may remain disease-free for more than 5 years following discontinuation of therapy. These observations indicate that a minority of patients with cutaneous disease may be cured of this malignant neoplasm. Unfortunately, the majority of patients present with extracutaneous disease, for which current therapy is only palliative. This chapter discusses our approach to these two groups of patients and mentions some of the newer therapies for CTCL.

TREATMENT

The only compelling evidence of long-term disease-free survival in patients with mycosis fungoides is following the use of EBRT. We favor EBRT for the small number of potentially curable patients whose disease is limited to the skin (Fig. 1). There is no evidence to suggest that adding total body irradiation or other topical or systemic therapy improves long-term disease-free survival.

Patients with extracutaneous disease are not curable with current therapies. A recent randomized trial found that early aggressive therapy with EBRT and combination chemotherapy does not improve the survival of patients with mycosis fungoides as compared with conservative treatment consisting of the sequential application of topical therapies. If at all possible, patients with extracutaneous disease should be entered in ongoing clinical trials that attempt to improve current therapy. Outside the study setting, in patients without visceral (liver, bone marrow) disease, we prefer the stepwise use of multiple topical modalities without systemic therapy, as described in Figure 2. In patients with visceral involvement, we advocate the use of systemic chemotherapy in addition to the topical modalities.

ELECTRON BEAM IRRADIATION

Electrons have a limited range of penetration, and therefore their radiobiologic effect is limited to the superficial tissues. This provides a means for irradiating the entire body surface area while sparing the deeper tissues. It also spares the mucous membranes, bone marrow, gastrointestinal tract, and other vital organs. The radiation delivery system is complex and employs a linear accelerator that generates a beam that is spread over the entire skin surface by passing it through an aluminum scattering foil. This is technically demanding and requires great attention to detail with regard to the positioning of the patient and the beam. The generally recommended technique consists of treating the patient using anterior, posterior, and four oblique fields arranged in 60-degree increments about the vertical axis during each treatment cycle. A complex six-field cycle requires 2 consecutive treatment days, and two treatment cycles can be delivered per week. Because of the complexity and time required to deliver this therapy properly, it is only available at a limited number of centers. The tolerance of individual patients to the beam is variable, but doses of 200 rad per cycle and total doses of 3,000 to 3,600 rad in 8 to 9 weeks are tolerated well by most patients. The total dose of irradiation is important

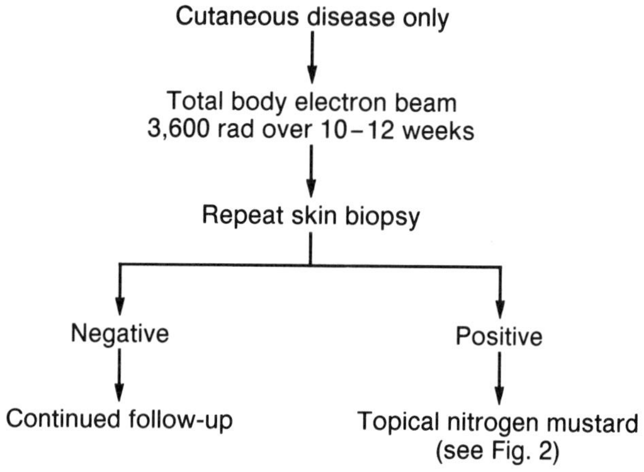

Figure 1 Management of patients who have only cutaneous disease after complete staging.

since patients treated with more than 3,000 rad have a higher complete remission rate and longer disease-free survival than those treated with lower doses. It is not known whether the technique and dose fractionation schedule are equally important. Areas not directly exposed to electrons (such as the soles, perineum, and scalp) need to be treated separately. All of this can take 10 to 12 weeks to complete and is very expensive.

The best results occur in patients with limited plaques and minimal tumor burden. Good results can be achieved in the generalized plaque phase provided that lymphadenopathy is not present. Patients with tumors or generalized erythroderma rarely benefit from total body EBRT therapy.

The patient's eyes must be shielded during therapy to prevent cataracts, and if the eyelids are involved, special lead contact lenses must be employed to protect the eyes. Nearly all patients experience excessive dryness of the skin with various degrees of scalding during treatment. Therapeutically induced epilation, anonychosis, and anhidrosis are short-term effects from which most patients recover within 4 to 6 months. Chronic toxicities may include skin atrophy, hyperpigmentation, and telangiectasia. Using this technique, a majority of patients have complete clearing of their skin lesions. The Stanford group has reported an 84 percent complete remission rate with a median duration of 16 months. Only those patients with disease limited to the skin experience long-term control and possible cure of their disease, whereas the remainder experience recurrent skin or extracutaneous disease.

Orthovoltage radiation therapy can be used at low doses for palliative therapy. Small field or spot treatment in moderate dose fractions (300 to 500 rad) to relatively low total doses (800 to 1,500 rad) can be used successfully to treat plaques and tumors in patients with recurrent disease that does not respond to other forms of therapy.

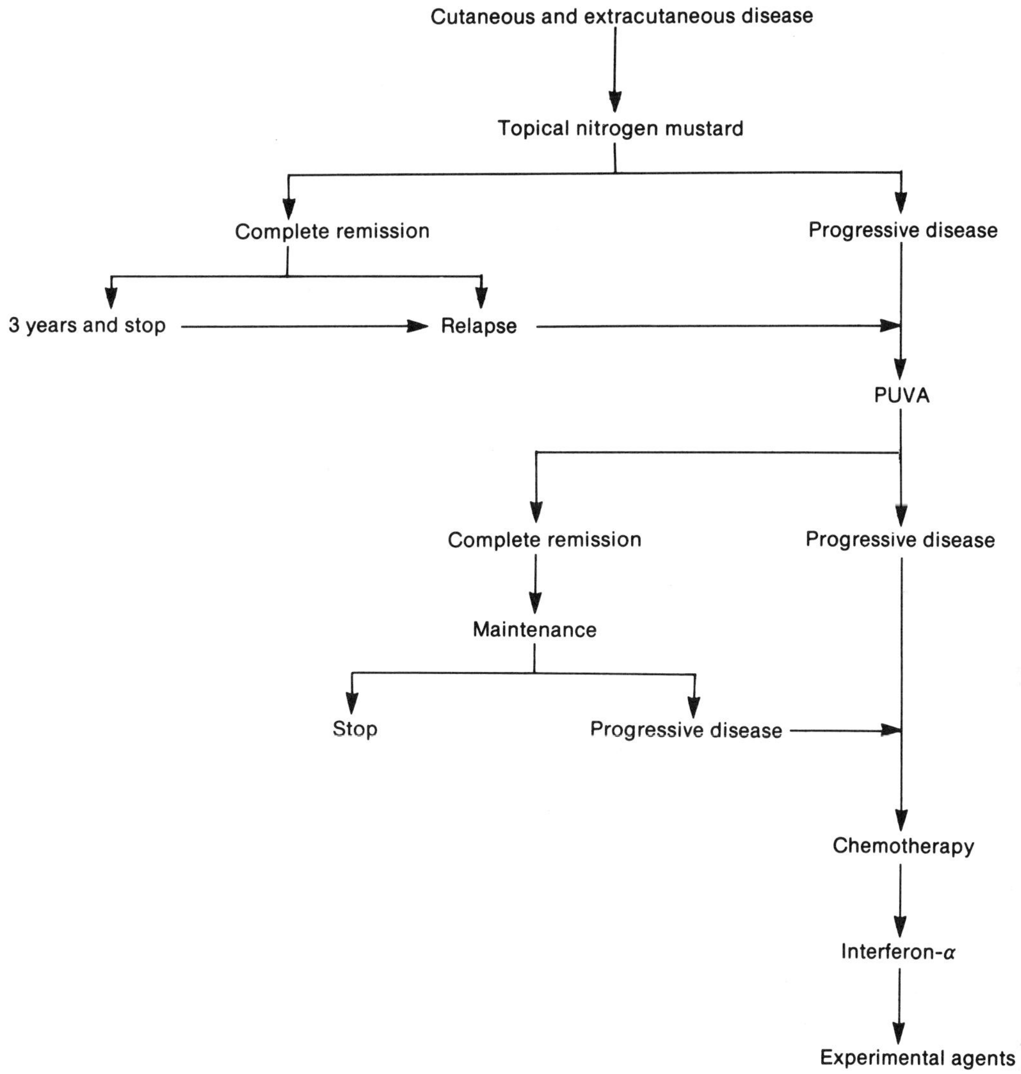

Figure 2 Algorithm for the management of patients found to have extracutaneous disease after complete staging.

TOPICAL CHEMOTHERAPY

Mechlorethamine remains the most commonly used agent for topical therapy. It is particularly useful for patients with early cutaneous stage disease or to supplement other therapeutic approaches to nodal or visceral disease. Complete remissions (CR) have been observed in up to 64 percent of patients. However, relapses occur over time, and only 10 to 15 percent of patients are disease-free at 3 years. Although topical mechlorethamine has excellent palliative potential, it is rarely curative. Its major advantages are that it is relatively nontoxic, inexpensive, and readily available to all patients.

Ten milligrams of mechlorethamine is added to 50 ml of tap water and painted with a brush over the entire body once per day. Lesser amounts are generally applied to the axillary, inguinal, and inframammary regions because of the propensity for irritation. Since secondary neoplasms have occurred in the genital area following topical mechlorethamine, we treat these areas only in the presence of detectable disease. Patients are asked to apply mechlorethamine immediately after bathing because surface oils and greases can interfere with absorption. Therapy is continued daily for 6 to 12 months in responding patients, at which time the frequency of application is decreased to every other day for an additional 1 to 2 years. For those with a complete response, we discontinue therapy at 3 years.

Up to 70 percent of patients treated in this fashion develop an allergic contact dermatitis. In some, treatment can be continued, but in many patients the reaction is so severe that treatment must be stopped and, at times, topical steroids are needed to control the toxic reaction. In these patients, we sometimes try to reinstitute topical therapy using dilute concentrations of mechlorethamine. Diluting 10 mg of mechlorethamine in a bathtub of water may be an effective first step, with the dose being increased by diluting 10 mg in a sink of water prior to administering the agent at full strength again. If these measures fail, we have found that mixing the mechlorethamine in a petrolatum base according to the method of Price and colleagues is quite useful. Using this method, many patients with serious allergic reactions to topical mechlorethamine are able to continue therapy. Although the amount of mechlorethamine applied to the entire skin surface is only 1.5 mg in the ointment-based regimen versus 5 mg in the aqueous solution, early results suggest that the methods are equally efficacious. Patient acceptance of this latter method is excellent, and many prefer this to the daily preparation and application of the aqueous formulation. We find these approaches more beneficial than attempts to desensitize patients via the intravenous injection of mechlorethamine. An increase in the incidence of squamous cell and basal cell carcinoma of the skin has been reported in these patients, however.

In patients who cannot tolerate mechlorethamine, we have rarely employed topical carmustine (BCNU). When 40 to 60 mg of BCNU in alcohol is administered on a daily basis for short courses, good responses in skin lesions have been observed. Some degree of dermatitis is seen in all patients, and it can be severe. More important, bone marrow depression and abnormalities in kidney function have been observed following the topical use of BCNU. These hazardous effects may be lessened without decreasing efficacy by using alternate-day therapy.

PHOTOCHEMOTHERAPY

The combination of 8-methoxypsoralen and long-wave ultraviolet (UV) light has been shown to be effective for CTCL. The methoxypsoralen is given orally at 0.6 mg per kilogram 2 hours prior to treatment of the entire skin surface with UV light in a continuous spectrum of 320 to 380 nm. The psoralen binds covalently to DNA and appears to inhibit DNA synthesis and mitosis in the T lymphocytes in the cutaneous infiltrate. The initial exposure times of patients to long-wave UV light need to be based on the degree of pigmentation before therapy, the patient's ability to tan, and the type of phototherapy units to be used. Patients with a history of sun sensitivity should have shorter initial exposure. Exposure times can be increased with each treatment depending upon patient response, evidence of erythema, and type of photounit used. The initial UV radiation dose is usually between 1.5 and 3 J per centimeter. Exposure times may be increased at each treatment by approximately 0.5 J per centimeter, depending on the presence of erythema. All patients must wear UV radiation-blocking goggles during therapy and UV radiation-blocking sunglasses before and after PUVA.

PUVA is usually given three times a week to start, and then a maintenance schedule is arranged when lesions have completely cleared. The UV radiation exposure (joule per centimeter) during maintenance is usually the same as the last doses used during the clearing phase. Maintenance is usually initiated at a rate of once per week and is decreased as tolerated to as little as once per month. Patients are encouraged to continue therapy because relapse rates are high. Most patients with eczematous or plaque stage lesions respond to PUVA with disease clearing, whereas those with tumors often require additional x-ray therapy. Patients with generalized erythema do not respond well to PUVA. It was previously thought the PUVA was strictly palliative, but a recent study found that five of nine patients with stage IA and 10 of 26 patients with stage IB disease were continuously free of disease 79 months after discontinuation of therapy. This suggests that long-term control can be achieved without chronic maintenance therapy. Acute toxicities of PUVA consist of mild nausea and dry skin with generalized pruritus and erythema. Long-term toxicity is not well defined, but there has been a report of an increased incidence of skin cancer in patients treated with PUVA. The major advantages of PUVA are its relative lack of toxicity, apparent effectiveness, and lack of cross-resistance with other treatment modalities.

Extracorporeal photochemotherapy has also been used to treat CTCL. After oral administration of methoxsalen, a lymphocyte-enriched blood fraction obtained at leukapheresis is exposed to UV light in the laboratory and then returned to the patient. In a recent study, this resulted in responses in 27 of 37 patients with otherwise resistant disease. The responding group included patients with lymph node involvement and exfoliative erythroderma. Although the mechanism is unknown, the generalized improvement in cutaneous and extracutaneous disease suggests that the infused damaged cells may elicit an antitumor immune response to the abnormal T cells. This preliminary study suggests that extracorporeal phototherapy may benefit patients with advanced CTCL that is refractory to other forms of treatment.

SYSTEMIC THERAPY

Single-agent chemotherapy for CTCL can result in response rates as high as 60 to 70 percent; these rates are similar to those reported for other indolent nonHodgkin's lymphomas. The alkylating agents cyclophosphamide and chlorambucil have been used successfully, as have the antitumor antibiotics doxorubicin and bleomycin. Experience with mitotic inhibitors such as vinblastine and VP-16 indicates that they also have significant activity. Our preference is single-agent methotrexate, which can be given daily by the oral route or can be given weekly by intramuscular or intravenous injection. We find no benefit to the use of higher dose methotrexate, which adds the extra complexity of requiring calcium leucovorin rescue. We use methotrexate for patients with visceral disease at presentation but who do not have rapidly progressive disease. We also use methotrexate in patients who develop visceral disease during other forms of therapy.

Combination chemotherapy has increased the response rate and number of complete remissions, but the median duration of these remissions is rarely greater than 1 year, with most patients eventually dying from their disease. To date, no form of chemotherapy, single agent or combination, has resulted in the cure of a significant number of patients.

In patients with rapidly progressing disease or in those no longer responding to methotrexate, we employ combination chemotherapy. A number of regimens useful in the treatment of nonHodgkin's lymphomas are associated with good response rates (Table 1). Any one of these regimens is suitable, and although they have not been tested in patients with CTCL, many of the newer lymphoma regimens are likely to be at least as effective as those listed in Table 1.

Since no single modality has been associated with long-term, disease-free survival in patients with extracutaneous disease, the recent trend has been toward combined modality therapy. This is generally reserved for patients in clinical trials or those in whom single modalities no longer control symptoms. Stanford is currently conducting a randomized study of whole body EBRT alone versus EBRT with adjuvant topical mechlorethamine. There is a trend toward increased disease-free survival in patients receiving adjuvant mechlorethamine, but this approach can only be expected to benefit patients without extracutaneous disease. Topical mechlorethamine has been combined with chemotherapy in at least one study, and its major finding is increased toxicity without a definite improvement in long-term, disease-free survival. A handful of studies have examined the combination of EBRT and systemic chemotherapy. The results are difficult to interpret because the trials were nonrandomized and included patients with various stages of disease and used different chemotherapy regimens. In general, overall response rates approach 100 percent with CR rates of 60 percent or better and median response durations of longer than 1 year. Unfortunately, responders continue to relapse with time. The combined modality therapies are reasonably well tolerated, with acceptable toxicities even when both modalities are administered simultaneously. The cutaneous toxicity from electron beam irradiation that is a component of combined modality treatment may be somewhat exaggerated over that seen when EBRT is used alone, particularly in patients with erythroderma. Although the toxicity of combined modality treatment may be acceptable or tolerable, the cutaneous reactions, myelosuppression, and other drug-related effects are significant. Also, there is always the concern about as yet undefined late toxicities. Is it reasonable to administer this aggressive therapy to patients who have not yet been shown to have curable disease? To answer this question, National Cancer Institute investigators randomized patients to groups of (1) conservative therapy with sequential use of topical mechlorethamine (with oral methotrexate for visceral disease), PUVA, local EBRT as needed, with combination chemotherapy for progressive disease, or (2) aggressive combined modality therapy with simultaneous total skin EBRT and 8 or 16 cycles of CAPO (cyclophosphamide, doxorubicin, etoposide, and vincristine). More than 100 patients were studied, and although patients who received combined therapy had a significantly higher CR rate, there was no significant improvement in disease-free or overall survival. Combined modality therapy resulted in significantly more toxicity. Therefore, routine application of aggressive combined modality treatment cannot be recommended as initial therapy for all patients with mycosis fungoides. We consider this approach for patients with widespread disease in whom a prompt response is necessary to protect them from the undesirable effects of uncontrolled mycosis fungoides.

TABLE 1 Combination Chemotherapy in CTCL

Regimen	*Response Rate (%) (CR + PR)*	*Duration Response (Months)*
CVP	89	16
CVP-B	92	11.5
CHOP/HOP	100	5
COMP	100	11

CR = complete remission;
PR = partial remission;
CVP = cyclophosphamide, vincristine, prednisone;
CVP-B = cyclophosphamide, vincristine, prednisone, bleomycin;
CHOP = cyclophosphamide, doxorubicin, vincristine, prednisone;
HOP = doxorubicin, vincristine, prednisone;
COMP = cyclophosphamide, vincristine, methotrexate, prednisone.

INTERFERON

Interferon alpha (IFN-α) has been demonstrated to be an effective single agent against CTCL. In the National Cancer Institute study, nine of 20 (45 percent) heavily pretreated patients responded to maximally tolerated doses of IFN-α. Responses were usually seen within 3 months of therapy and continued for many months. Complete responses were seen in

15 percent of patients and have lasted up to 42 months, or continuous IFN-α therapy. Responses were seen in both cutaneous and extracutaneous sites. Extremely high doses (50×10^6 units per square meter daily for 4 weeks) were required, and all except one patient required a 50 percent dose reduction. The major dose-limiting toxicity was a flu-like syndrome consisting of malaise, fatigue, anorexia, and mental confusion. Fever with myalgias and arthralgias was also noted. The flu-like syndrome and fever could be partially blocked by pretreatment with acetaminophen and were rarely a chronic problem, since most patients developed tolerance. The fatigue and anorexia, however, were troublesome and usually only responded to a reduction in the dose of IFN. Patients with severe cardiac disease and those in whom a high temperature could be life-threatening should not receive IFN at high doses. Renal and hepatic functions should be monitored closely, as should blood counts, since myelosuppression has been observed.

The optimal dose and schedule for administration of IFN-α are not known. Other investigators have reported similarly high response rates with high-dose IFN-α, but responses also have been noted in patients receiving much lower doses (3×10^6 units per day). A randomized study of high versus low doses of IFN-α was stopped prematurely because of low accrual; 11 of 14 patients receiving high doses of IFN-α responded, whereas three of eight patients responded during low-dose therapy. For patients no longer responsive to other modalities, we recommend daily intramuscular therapy at 50×10^6 units per square meter of body surface area until toxicity develops, when the dose can be reduced by 50 percent. If toxicity persists, we generally decrease the dose to 10 percent of the initial dose. If this is not effective, we discontinue IFN-α. Some patients progressing on low-dose IFN respond to increases in IFN dose. Some patients have achieved long-term disease control on low maintenance doses of IFN. Treatment for up to 1 year has been required to achieve maximal responses in some cases.

SEROTHERAPY

Horse antithymocyte globulin has induced a clinical response in three of four patients following repeated injections. The responses were all partial and short-lived. Passive serotherapy with mouse monoclonal antibodies has also resulted in responses in patients with CTCL. The monoclonal antibody used (T101) recognizes a normal human T-cell differentiation antigen (CD5) that is expressed to a greater degree on CTCL tumor cells (four- to ten-fold). ^{111}In or ^{131}I-labeled T101 has been used to image successfully and specifically lymph node groups containing malignant cells following either intravenous or intralymphatic administration. Therapy with unlabeled antibody has produced dramatic but very transient clinical responses in skin, lymph nodes, and blood. Responses have also been seen with therapeutic doses of ^{131}I-T101 conjugates, but such studies are not yet definitive.

Problems with this approach are applicable for all serotherapy and include heterogeneous expression of the target antigen, modulation of the target antigen, and formation of human antimouse antibodies. New approaches employing these antibodies conjugated with therapeutic quantities of radioactive moieties or toxins have theoretical appeal and are in early clinical testing. Passive serotherapy directed at antigens more restricted to CTCL cells, such as BE-2, may also be interesting to evaluate as therapy for CTCL.

ENZYMATIC INHIBITORS

2′-Deoxycoformycin (2′-dCF) is a potent inhibitor of the enzyme adenosine deaminase that is found in high concentrations in lymphocytes. 2′-dCF has recently been shown to be active at low doses in various lymphoid malignancies, particularly hairy cell leukemia. Investigators using relatively high doses of 2′-dCF have demonstrated its activity in CTCL. Lower and safer doses have not been evaluated in patients with CTCL. However, for patients with progressive disease resistant to other therapies, we recommend a trial of 2′-dCF at 4 mg per square meter intravenously once a week or every other week. Care must be taken to ensure adequate hydration to prevent renal damage. Serum creatinine levels and 24-hour urine samples to check for creatinine clearance should be measured prior to each dose. Myelosuppression, particularly anemia and granulocytopenia, occur (although our experience has been primarily in patients with hairy cell leukemia who already have poor bone marrow function). Significant nausea and vomiting have been noted and require close attention to antiemetic therapy.

OTHER AGENTS

CTCL patients have been treated with cis-retinoic acid. Partial and complete responses have been documented in heavily pretreated patients at a daily oral dose of 100 mg per square meter. Toxicity is primarily cutaneous, and in one patient, therapy was discontinued because of excessive dryness and scaling. The mechanism of action of the vitamin A analogues is poorly understood.

There have been anecdotal reports of complete clearing of extensive ulcerated tumors in patients with CTCL during intravenous administration of acyclovir. The mechanism is not known, but this agent is currently under study.

There also have been anecdotal reports of responses following treatment with either cyclosporine or cimetidine. Leukapheresis has also been applied with some benefit in the treatment of CTCL.

SUGGESTED READING

Bunn PA Jr, Huberman MS, Whang-Peng J, et al. Prospective staging evaluation of patients with cutaneous T cell lymphomas. Demonstration of a high frequency of extracutaneous dissemination. Ann Intern Med 1980; 93:223–230.
Edelson R, Berger C, Gasparro F, et al. Treatment of cutaneous T cell lymphoma by extracorporeal photochemotherapy. Preliminary results. N Engl J Med 1987; 316:297–303.
Hoppe RT, Cox RS, Fuks Z, et al. Electron beam therapy for mycosis fungoides: The Stanford University experience. Cancer Treat Rep 1979; 63:691–700.
Kaye FJ, Bunn PA, Steinberg SM, et al. A randomized trial comparing combination electron-beam radiation and chemotherapy with topical therapy in the initial treatment of mycosis fungoides. N Engl J Med 1989; 321:1784.
Price NM, Deneau DG, Hoppe RT. The treatment of mycosis fungoides with ointment-based mechlorethamine. Arch Dermatol 1982; 118:234–237.
Vonderheid EC, Tan ET, Kantor AF, et al. Long-term efficacy, curative potential, and carcinogenicity of topical mechlorethamine chemotherapy in cutaneous T cell lymphoma. J Am Acad Dermatol 1989; 20:416.
Vonderheid EC, Van Scott EJ, Wallner PE, Johnson WC. A 10-year experience with topical mechlorethamine for mycosis fungoides: Comparison with patients treated by total-skin electron beam radiation therapy. Cancer Treat Rep 1979; 63:681–689.
Winkler CF, Bunn PA Jr. Cutaneous T cell lymphoma: A review. CRC Crit Rev Oncol/Hematol 1985; 1:49.

MALIGNANT MELANOMA

EDWARD T. CREAGAN, M.D., F.A.C.P.

Malignant melanoma comprises approximately 2 percent of newly diagnosed cancer cases in the United States and accounts for 1 percent of cancer deaths. However, the frequency of malignant melanoma has increased disturbingly over the past several decades. There were an estimated 5,600 deaths from this neoplasm in 1986, and melanoma is now reportedly twice as common as Hodgkin's disease. In some studies, the rate of increase in malignant melanoma is exceeded only by that of non-small cell bronchogenic carcinoma. By the year 2000, it is estimated that one individual out of 150 will develop a malignant melanoma. Therefore, the clinician should be familiar with general therapeutic recommendations in melanoma management.

MICROSTAGING

A dominant prognostic variable of malignant melanoma is the vertical penetration of the primary lesion (Fig. 1). A level I lesion is confined to the epidermis and has negligible metastatic potential, whereas a level V lesion involves the subcutaneous fat and has a grave prognosis. Since the determination of levels of invasion may be arbitrary, the specific thickness of the melanoma, measured with an ocular micrometer from the stratum corneum to the deepest penetration of the tumor, is a more reliable predictor of metastatic disease (Table 1)

SURGERY

Primary Excision

Microstaging data provide a rational strategy for localized (stage I) malignant melanoma. However, the optimum extent of resection of the primary lesion is unclear. Among patients with lesions less than 1.0 mm thick in one series, approximately two-thirds had resected margins of 2 cm or less and only 8 percent recurred locally. The survival of patients with lesions less than 2.0 mm thick was not influenced by the margin of excision. Moreover, there was no survival advantage for lesions 2 mm thick or greater by increasing the margin of resection to over 3 cm. On the other hand, survival was substantially decreased if deeper lesions were excised with margins less than 2.0 cm. As a general guideline, lesions 1.69 mm or less can be adequately excised with margins of 1 to 2 cm, while thicker lesions should be excised with a 3 cm margin.

Node Excision

The efficacy of elective node dissection (END) for patients without palpable adenopathy remains unsettled. The World Health Organization (WHO) has prospectively assessed the role of END, and current analysis with 7 to 13 years of follow-up demonstrates no overall survival advantage from END. The study has been criticized since it only included distal extremity lesions, had a female predominance, and not all patients were stratified by tumor thickness. In a Mayo Clinic randomized trial, END did not meaningfully influence survival or interval to metastasis. This study has also been criticized since most patients did not have nodel involvement and most had lesions that were 1.50 mm or less in thickness. This more favorable cohort of patients may not be appropriate to demonstrate the benefit from END.

These two prospective studies showing no obvious benefit from END contrast with retrospective analyses. In one such study, among 122 patients with extremity malignant melanoma, there was a statistically significant survival advantage from END, but the benefit was most evident for lesions between 1.50 to 3.99 mm thick.

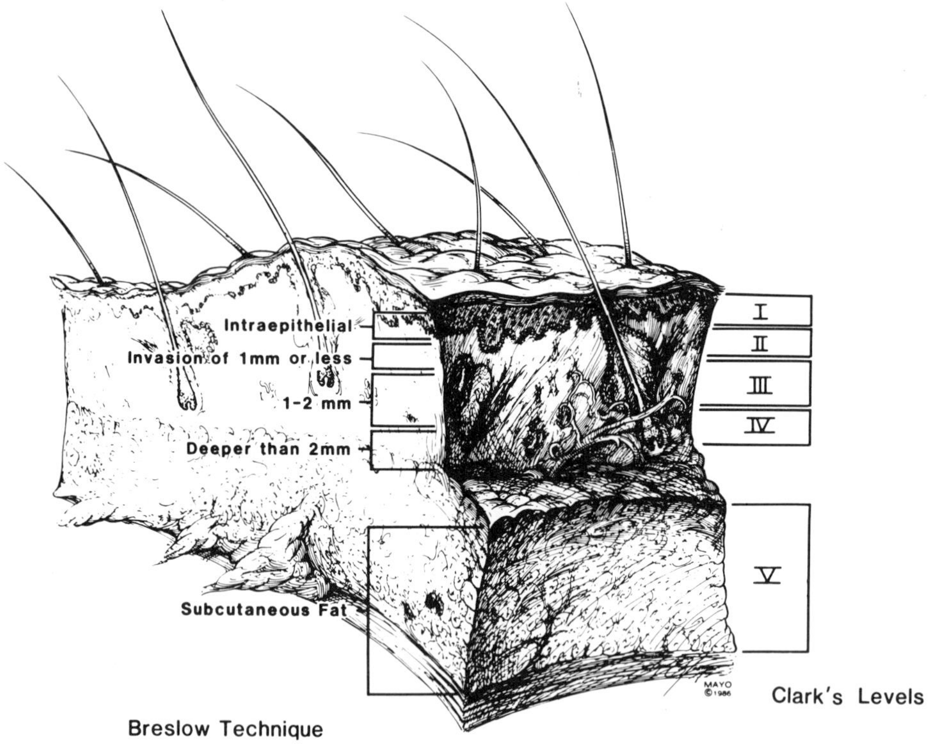

Figure 1 Penetration of malignant melanoma.

The apparent advantage from END emerged between the years 5 and 8 postoperatively. Nevertheless, a 1985 retrospective study could not confirm any benefit from END for these intermediate thickness lesions. Additionally, in this study, END offered no statistically significant advantage for lesions less than 0.76 mm or over 4.0 mm in thickness.

There are no data from prospective trials to address the benefit of elective node dissection for patients with intermediate thickness lesions (1.5 to 3.9 mm). However, it appears from extrapolated experience that the survival benefit may be approximately 5 to 10 percent (Fig. 2). A recommendation for elective node dissection must weigh the limited survival advantage against the patient's age, fitness, and the existence of concomitant medical conditions that could enhance the morbidity of surgery. There may be a subgroup of patients who benefit from END, but the procedure has not yet withstood the scrutiny of a randomized clinical trial and should not yet be regarded as standard treatment.

TABLE 1 Tumor Thickness and 8-year Survival Rates for Stage I Malignant Melanoma

Thickness Range (mm)	*Number of Patients*	Percent Survival
<0.85	190	99
0.85–1.69	178	93
1.70–3.64	151	69
≥3.65	79	38

There is less controversy concerning the surgical management of patients with lesions greater than 1.69 mm thick in the head and neck area and patients with clinically involved regional nodes regardless of primary site. A lymphadenectomy is the generally accepted procedure in these clinical circumstances.

Surgical Management of Distant Metastatic Disease

It is most unusual that a patient with a prior malignant melanoma would have an isolated focus of metas-

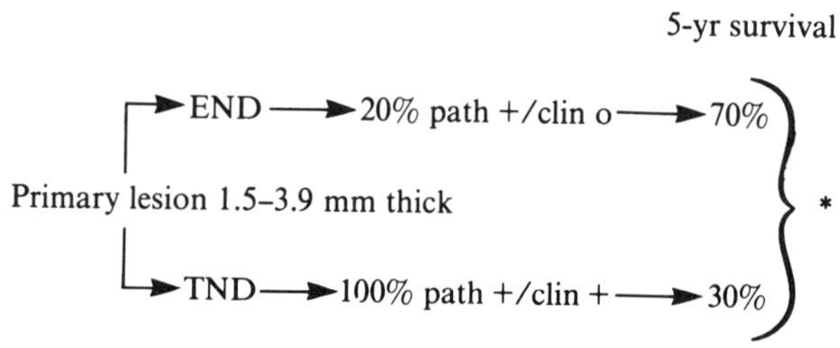

40% benefit applies to the 20% of patients with pathologically involved nodes; therefore, approximately 5–10% possible survival advantage.

Figure 2 Theoretical statistical model of possible benefit from elective node dissection (END) versus therapeutic node dissection (TND) for clinically palpable nodes.

tatic disease. It is incumbent upon the clinician to detect clinically occult metastases prior to considering surgical resection. Yet, if a patient is generally fit and has a disease-free interval of greater than 1 year, surgical resection might be considered, particularly for a pulmonary nodule, soft tissue, or extraregional nodal disease. Even if two metastases are located within the same lobe of the lung, a thoracic surgical opinion would certainly seem indicated. On the other hand, technical considerations may preclude an adequate surgical excision of a single hepatic metastasis. This caveat would also apply to central nervous system lesions if the surgical removal might be fraught with a substantial neurologic deficit. A note of caution: an incomplete resection of metastatic disease often causes grave complications and prolonged hospitalization. The proposed surgery should offer the patient a considerable certainty of complete resection or should not be considered.

The Unknown Primary Malignant Melanoma

An uncommon presentation of malignant melanoma is nodal involvement without an obvious primary site. This situation usually reflects metastasis from a regressed or undetected primary lesion. In cases with ambiguous histology, the detection of S-100 protein within the cells presumes malignant melanoma. A regional lymphadenectomy is recommended in such a case. Although distant metastases eventually occur in most patients, a lymphadenectomy rather than a node biopsy increases the interval between local treatment and both local recurrence and disseminated disease. Prior to surgery, the patient should undergo a thorough physical examination with particular attention to the scalp, genitalia, and mucosal surfaces. A chest x-ray and hematological and chemical parameters, including liver function tests, are advisable. The indiscriminate use of computed tomographic, magnetic resonance, and radionuclide imaging is typically unrewarding in the absence of clinical, chemical, or roentgenographic indications of disseminated disease.

SYSTEMIC THERAPIES

Systemic treatment for disseminated malignant melanoma should include an awareness of the anticipated natural history of the neoplasm. As noted in Table 2, there are a number of well-recognized features, both favorable and unfavorable, of advanced disease. In general, the more favorable characteristics include female sex and ambulatory status. Soft tissue involvement, particularly at a single site, and a disease-free interval of greater than 6 months may portend a more optimistic prognosis. Prior chemotherapy usually indicates a dismal response to subsequent treatment. The long-term prognosis may be relatively promising for patients who have had fully resected metastatic disease, especially from an isolated lesion. Residual disease following surgical excision is an ominous prognostic event.

The decision to commence a chemotherapy trial must clearly include an awareness of the factors listed in Table 3. A clinically fragile patient with indolent soft tissue disease, little psychosocial or familial support, and only a rudimentary grasp of the realistic limitations of treatment would hardly be an ideal candidate. It is the

TABLE 2 Prognostic Factors in Disseminated Malignant Melanoma

Patient	Favorable	Unfavorable
Sex	Female	Male
Performance score	Ambulatory	Non-ambulatory
Treatment	**Favorable**	**Unfavorable**
Prior chemo Rx	None	Any
Resectable metastases	Complete	Incomplete
Metastases	**Favorable**	**Unfavorable**
Site	Soft Tissue	Viscera (Lung, Liver, CNS)
Number	One	One
Disease-free interval	6 months	6 months

TABLE 3 Ideal Criteria for Chemotherapeutic Recommendations

Patient

- Biologically fit despite chronological age.
- No substantial concurrent medical illnesses.
- Psychosocial support; adequate follow-up; reliability.
- Full understanding of risks, benefits, palliation (not cure), and options of symptomatic treatment.

Disease

- Clinically aggressive, typically with symptomatic visceral involvement.
- Histologically documented.
- Measurable or objectively assessible disease.

responsibility of the primary physician to discuss carefully with the patient and significant caregivers the anticipated toxicities of treatment, palliative rather than curative intent, and the practical limitations of therapy. Patients and families should also be aware of alternative symptomatic and supportive management in lieu of chemotherapy.

Imidazole carboxamide (DTIC) is one of the more intensively studied single agents in malignant melanoma. A typical schedule involves 5 days of intravenous treatment each 3 weeks. A randomized clinical trial involving 415 patients notes a response rate of only 14 percent compared with an alternative multiagent regimen. Increasingly complex regimens using DTIC have yet to show any meaningful advantage compared with DTIC alone and may have enhanced toxicities.

Nitrosoureas are another class of agents that can be used against disseminated malignant melanoma. Comparative trials have not been undertaken; however, the various nitrosoureas (BCNU, CCNU, or Methyl-CCNU) seem to be therapeutically equivalent. Overall objective response rates have occured in approximately 15 percent of patients. These agents offer some logistical advantage over DTIC in that BCNU is given intravenously each 6 weeks and CCNU is an orally administered agent. There is no convincing evidence that polychemotherapy with a nitrosourea offers a dramatic advantage compared with single agent regimens. Likewise, combinations of a nitrosourea with DTIC have not been more efficacious that treatment with each agent singly.

In light of the low response rates from commercially available cytotoxic agents, every reasonable effort should be made to enroll the patient in a prospective clinical trial that assesses the impact of strategies in melanoma management.

Biological Response Modifiers (BRM)

Interferons have been intensively investigated as therapy for disseminated malignant melanoma (DMM). The objective response rate is approximately 15 percent with rates of disease progression and survival generally similar to those of chemotherapy regimens. Most regressions occur in soft tissue sites and less frequently influence visceral metastases. The major complications include fatigue, fever, and a flu-like illness; gastrointestinal and myelosuppressive sequelae are usually not significant. Interferons as single agents have only limited usefulness against DMM. Combination programs with chemotherapy, different interferon species, and other BRMs such as tumor necrosis factor and interleukin hold promise and are now being investigated.

Immunotherapy

A number of trials have assessed the impact of *bacillus Calmette-Guerin* (BCG) and other immunostimulants with or without chemotherapy for patients having fully resected high risk lesions, that is, thick lesions or nodal involvement. Overall, results have been conflicting, inconsistent, and have not provided reproducible therapeutic benefit. Based on currently available data, routine adjuvant or prophylactic systemic therapy cannot be recommended.

Endocrine Implications

Limited objective regressions of DMM have occasionally followed additive and ablative hormonal therapies. Tamoxifen has been among the more actively evaluated agents in the advanced disease setting. Cimetidine has also been evaluated by investigational trials. With a few notable exceptions, these agents have shown no predictably meaningful activity against malignant melanoma.

REGIONAL MODALITIES

Radiation Therapy

An increasing number of clinical studies indicate that malignant melanoma is not necessarily a radioresistant neoplasm. Most earlier programs typically utilized individual doses of 200 cGy and total doses of 5,000 to 6,000 cGy. There is some evidence that the dose per fraction and not the total cumulative dose of treatment is the more important factor in the radiosensitivity of malignant melanoma. Four hundred cGy fractions typically adminstered twice or thrice weekly can offer palliation, particularly for painful osseous lesions, with manageable short-term sequelae. At doses over 400 cGy, the complete response rate is significantly improved compared with lower doses. There seems to be no real advantage from doses above this threshold. It is unlikely that palliative radiation therapy influences survival from disseminated disease. However, effective local control of locally recurrent malignant melanoma may enhance patients' survival as compared with those in whom local control is not achieved. Experimental evidence demonstrates that hyperthermia augments the radiation sensitivity of malignant melanoma. The concomitant use of these modalities is generally investigational and cannot yet be considered routine clinical management.

The onset of intracerebral metastases from malignant melanoma is common. Most patients who receive traditional radiation therapy for this problem (that is, approximately 5,000 cGy) have a median survival of approximately 3 to 4 months. The use of high fraction programs with corticosteroids can often ameliorate neurologic symptoms, but it is unclear if this approach enhances overall survival.

Intra-arterial (IA) Therapy

Currently, there are no published, large randomized trials studying IA therapy for patients with fully resected primary melanoma (stage I). Therefore, the technique cannot be endorsed as routine clinical practice. On the other hand, some patients with regionally recurrent disease may derive substantial palliation from either normothermic or hyperthermic perfusion with IA chemotherapy. When used by experienced personnel, complications of this technique are sufficiently low to consider its usefulness in selected circumstances, especially if amputation is being considered as an alternative and other regional modalities are not advisable. However, the majority of patients who develop locally recurrent melanoma succumb from disseminated disease within a year of recurrence. Therefore, it is not apparent from a diverse spectrum of retrospective and uncontrolled studies that regional therapies influence survival.

SURVEILLANCE

All malignant melanomas can potentially metastasize regardless of thickness. For patients with primary lesions less than 0.85 mm, the prognosis is sufficiently favorable to advise a history and physical examination, chest x-ray, routine hematologic and chemical indices including liver function parameters every 3 months for 1 year, then each 6 months during the second and third years, and then yearly thereafter. For individuals with lesions 0.85 to 1.69 mm thick, the aforementioned procedures should be repeated at 3-month intervals during the first 2 years, then each 6 months indefinitely. In light of the more serious prognosis from lesions greater than 1.69 mm thick and those with nodal involvement who are not participating in investigational programs, surveillance is advisable at 3-month intervals for 3 years and at 6-month intervals indefinitely. Sophisticated imaging techniques are usually not warranted on a routine basis, but can be targeted to the specific area of suspected metastatic disease.

The clinician should alert the patient and family to the anticipated signs and symptoms of locally recurrent as well as disseminated disease. It is also important for the clinician to emphasize that the patient is at an increased risk of developing a second primary melanoma and this is another reason for ongoing surveillance. Both the patient and first-degree relatives should be advised to avoid solar damage and to use a No. 15 sunscreen during peak hours of sun exposure.

SUGGESTED READING

Aitken DR, Clausen K, Klein JP, James AG. The extent of primary melanoma excision: a re-evaluation—How wide is wide? Ann Surg 1983; 198(5):634–641.

Amer MH, Al-Sarraf M, Vaitkevicius VK. Clinical presentation, natural history and prognostic factors in advanced malignant melanoma. Surg Gynecol Obstet 1979; 149:687–692.

Balch CM, Milton GW, eds. Cutaneous melanoma: clinical management and treatment results worldwide. Philadelphia: J B Lippincott, 1985.

Balch CM, Soong S, Murad TM, Smith JW, et al. A multifactorial analysis of melanoma. IV. Prognostic factors in 200 melanoma patients with distant metastases (stage III). J Clin Oncol 1983; 1(2):126–134.

Creagan ET. Malignant melanoma. Compr Ther 1981; 7:36–44.

Creagan ET, Ahmann DL, Frytak S, et al. Phase II trials of recombinant leukocyte A interferon in disseminated malignant melanoma: results in 96 patients. Cancer Treat Rep 1986; 70(5):619–624.

Cumberlin R, De Moss E, Lassus M, Friedman M. Isolation perfusion for malignant melanoma of the extremity: a review. J Clin Oncol 1985; 3:1022–1031.

Day CL Jr, Mihm MC Jr, Lew RA, Kopf AW, et al. Cutaneous malignant melanoma: prognostic guidelines for physicians and patients. CA 1982; 32(2):113–122.

Elder DE, Guerry D IV, VanHorn M, et al. The role of lymph node dissection for clinical stage I malignant melanoma of intermediate thickness (1.51–3.99 mm). Cancer 1985; 56:413–418.

Greene MH, Clark WH Jr, Tucker MA, et al. High risk of malignant melanoma in melanoma-prone families with dysplastic nevi. Ann Intern Med 1985; 102:458–465.

Legha SS. Interferons in the treatment of malignant melanoma: a review of recent trials. Cancer 1986; 57:1675–1677.

Luikart SD, Kennealey GT, Kirkwood JM. Randomized phase III trial of vinblastine, bleomycin, and cis-dichlorodiammine-platinum versus dacarbazine in malignant melanoma. J Clin Oncol 1984; 2(3):164–168.

Overett TK, Shiu MH. Surgical treatment of distant metastatic melanoma. Indications and results. Cancer 1985; 56:1222–1230.

Overgaard J. The role of radiotherapy in recurrent and metastatic malignant melanoma: a clinical radiobiological study. Int J Radiat Oncol Biol Phys 1986; 12:867–872.

BRAIN TUMORS

JOHN D. EARLE, M.D.

The treatment of brain tumors is in a state of flux. New technology, better utilization of existing technology, and better understanding of the biology of these tumors have led to new approaches that have created an atmosphere of excitement among those who manage patients with brain tumors. This chapter presents selected highlights of the treatment of primary intracranial tumors of adults, with emphasis on those methods expected to provide the most hope for improved treatment in the future.

Computed tomography (CT) is commonly available, and magnetic resonance imaging (MRI) is becoming available in most tertiary health care centers. CT has virtually eliminated pneumoencephalography, ventriculography, and arteriography for providing information about tumor location, although arteriography is still useful in revealing the relationships of such tumors to larger vessels. Stereotactic procedures rely on this information to guide approaches to these tumors.

High-energy, isocentric, linear accelerators are available to most radiation oncologists. These machines produce deeply penetrating, skin-sparing beams that can be directed at tumors along various paths. The use of wedge filters and tissue compensators facilitates complex treatment plans, thereby resulting in isodose envelopes that adequately encompass irregularly shaped tumors, but minimize the dose to surrounding normal structures. Nowhere is this more critical than with brain tumors.

Commonly available treatment planning computers allow the radiation oncologist to explore and to evaluate multiple competing options rapidly, so that the optimal treatment plan can be selected. More sophisticated treatment planning computers now being designed will generate three-dimensional, optimized treatment plans, thereby allowing even more flexibility than is currently available.

Brain tumors have been studied in prospective clinical trials by a number of cooperative groups. As these studies have matured, data from them have become available to guide treatment and to suggest new avenues for investigation. New trials in areas previously unstudied are being proposed.

More refined analyses have led to a better understanding of brain tolerance to radiation. As radiation oncologists have gained experience with hyperfractionation, accelerated fractionation, and other nonstandard treatment schedules, these have been introduced for the treatment of some brain tumors.

All of these factors are changing the management of patients with brain tumors. Prospective trials are needed to establish the roles of the advances in the treatment of these patients. Several have been mounted to address fractionation schedules, combined radiation and chemotherapy, and use of neutrons with photons. A number of pilot studies are accruing patients to explore new applications of these ideas as well as to explore radiation sensitizers and manipulations of dose level. In selected patients with low-grade astrocytomas, the use of no treatment has been proposed.

PATHOLOGY

Table 1 lists the pathologic entities reviewed here. Standard texts should be consulted for complete listings or for incidence data. The gliomas are the most frequently treated tumors; thus, they raise many of the management problems of the less frequent tumors.

TABLE 1 Pathologic Entities Reviewed

Astrocytoma	Ependymoma
Oligodendroglioma	Meningioma
Glioblastoma multiforme	Pituitary adenoma
Medulloblastoma	Craniopharyngioma
Lymphoma	Pinealoma

The most common of the gliomas are the astrocytomas. Grading has become an issue in managing these patients. There are a number of competing systems of nomenclature. We have used a basic four-grade system with a major break in prognosis between Grades II and III. Grade IV is frequently referred to as glioblastoma multiforme. Caution should be used in reviewing the literature, however, because three-grade systems have been used, and even the four-grade systems may assign different groups of tumors to the same grade or may assign the same group of tumors to different grades. The lack of a completely satisfactory grading scheme has not only impeded review of results, but also has frustrated choices of therapy.

Classification schemes, such as the scheme of Daumas-Duport et al., are proving useful in selecting therapy. Their classification recognizes the distribution of tumor cells within the substance of the central nervous system tissue in which the tumor occurs. Class I designates solid tumors that displace the parenchyma; class III tumors diffusely infiltrate the brain substance they occupy. Class II tumors have a solid central portion, but have infiltrating, isolated tumor cells at the periphery. The implications for treatment are considerable: class I tumors might best be approached with localized treatments—e.g., resection or brachytherapy; class III tumors should be managed with less localized approaches—e.g., external beam irradiation.

Oligodendrogliomas usually occur in lower grades and carry a better prognosis, even when they appear with elements of astrocytoma—a not uncommon occurrence. They frequently are calcified and, in many instances, have been present for long periods of time. The gliomas rarely seed the meninges. When this seeding occurs, high-grade astrocytoma is responsible.

Adult medulloblastoma is being seen more frequently. The extent of resection and invasion of the meninges or into the ventricle are important in predicting the spread of this tumor through the cerebrospinal fluid.

Primary central nervous system lymphoma is another brain tumor being seen with increasing frequency, not only in the immunocompromised host (such as the post-transplantation patient or the patient with acquired immunodeficiency syndrome [AIDS]), but also in those with no known predisposing factor. Once again, newer immunohistochemical techniques have been of great assistance to the pathologist in identifying these tumors. Of paramount importance is accurate staging to detect disease outside the central nervous system in patients for whom central nervous system involvement is not primary but is part of their systemic involvement.

Grade is the most important characteristic of the ependymomas. Only the most malignant or those that have demonstrably spread to the cerebrospinal fluid require treatment of the neuraxis, as for medulloblastoma.

Meningioma is usually a benign tumor, but it can

have malignant characteristics and may recur if not completely removed. In either case, postoperative irradiation decreases recurrence rates and improves survival.

Pituitary adenomas provide the best example of the impact of new tools in neuropathology. With expanding capacity to characterize these tumors immunochemically, the standard histologic classifications of only a decade ago no longer apply. Our understanding of the mixed nature of many of these tumors has simplified treatment recommendations. The pathologist can assist in treatment decisions, not only by identifying completeness of removal (of particular importance in transsphenoidal approaches), but also by carefully observing for invasive characteristics in the submitted meninges. Use of CT and serum markers is allowing identification of microadenomas that need no treatment other than transsphenoidal resection.

Craniopharyngiomas are malignant and require irradiation after excision. They are of particular historic interest because they were the first tumors in the cranial cavity to be approached with the precision, high-dose radiotherapy techniques being applied to the rest of the brain tumors, modified appropriately for location, radiosensitivity, and other factors discussed below.

Pinealomas fall into two groups with regard to radiation approaches. The germinomas are quite sensitive and may need treatment of the neuraxis if spread to the cerebrospinal fluid is documented, whereas the pinealoblastoma, pinealocytoma, teratoma, and glioma are generally localized and more resistant to irradiation.

SURGERY

There is an advantage to removal that is as complete as possible for all of these tumors with the exception of lymphomas and pineal germinomas. For the remainder of the tumors, radiation therapy after resection further decreases the number of viable cells, thereby maximally delaying regrowth to symptomatic size or effecting cure. This removal provides the pathologist with the greatest amount of tissue for making an accurate diagnosis and reporting information upon which to base treatment and an estimation of prognosis. Tumor removal seems most important for high-grade astrocytomas, meningiomas, pituitary adenomas that are large or cystic, craniopharyngiomas, and medulloblastomas.

The newer stereotactic biopsy procedures are making the treatment of undiagnosed brain tumors virtually a thing of the past. Stereotactic removal may be accomplished in cases in which the usual neurosurgical procedure would be impossible. Also, these stereotactic procedures are allowing implantation of radioactive sources into tumors, a treatment method yet to be fully evaluated with regard to its relationship to the standard procedures.

RADIATION THERAPY

The new imaging procedures have revolutionized the determination of the volume to be treated and its relationship to surrounding normal tissues. The use of simple lateral opposed fields for the treatment of these patients should be gone forever. Use of multiple, shaped, intersecting fields is mandatory in order to apply the high doses referred to here. Overdosing of 15 to 20 percent commonly will be the result of the older treatment methods. This must be kept in mind when reviewing the literature to determine normal tissue tolerance.

For class II and III low-grade gliomas and for high-grade gliomas, some data support using CT enhancing volume plus the zone referred to as edema, allowing a 2 cm margin as the tumor volume. However, MRI frequently reveals that areas of abnormality are wider than seen on CT, and stereotactic biopsy procedures only now are accumulating information on the precise anatomic meaning of the abnormalities shown by these imaging procedures. For pituitary adenomas, craniopharyngiomas, nongerminoma pinealomas, meningiomas, and booster doses for medulloblastomas, radiologically abnormal volumes with a 1-cm margin are adequate.

The entire neuraxis must be treated in patients with medulloblastoma, high-grade ependymomas, and tumors that have seeded the cerebrospinal fluid. The cranium is usually treated with lateral opposed fields carefully matched at vertebrae C-2 through C-6 to a posterior spinal field or matched fields if a single field is not long enough. Care must be taken with the junctions, and the usual practice is to move the gaps several times during the course of treatment.

In the 1970s, several investigators pointed out that the usual treatment of 5,000 cGy through large, if not whole, brain fields might not be the best treatment for high-grade gliomas. The Brain Tumor Study Group (BTSG) reviewed several sequential trials and found that median survival was improved as the dose of radiation was increased from that level to 5,500 and 6,000 cGy. In the early 1980s, better understanding of tolerance and of the impact of fraction size led to our adoption of 6,480 cGy in 180-cGy fractions as reasonable, aggressive treatment for high-grade gliomas. With careful limitation of the treated volume, as previously emphasized, doses approaching these levels could be applied to the more resistant of the brain tumors: low-grade gliomas, meningiomas, craniopharyngiomas, and nongerminoma pinealomas.

It became clear that the higher doses needed to control pituitary adenomas, 5,000 to 6,000 cGy, could be given safely. Key to this increase in total dose was not only the volume consideration but also the necessity of keeping the fraction size below 200 cGy. Fractions of 180 cGy per day appear to give a better therapeutic ratio than do larger fraction sizes.

Necrosis usually is associated with use of uncompensated fields, so that significant portions of brain are treated to large fraction sizes. A smooth sigmoid curve appears to describe the relationship between radiation dose (taking fractionation into account) and the probability of radiation necrosis. Care must be taken with the definition of this effect because radiation changes will be observed whenever central nervous system tissue is examined histologically after being exposed to doses of 5,000 cGy or larger.

EXPERIMENTAL TREATMENTS

The search for effective chemotherapy continues to be both a search for effective single agents and trials of multiple agents. The nitrosoureas are the most dependable agents. Procarbazine, bischloronitrosourea (BCNU), and vinblastine are reasonably active and are used by some as adjuvant treatment for high-grade tumors in combination with irradiation. The 8-in-1 vincristine, methylprednisolone, lomustine (CCNU), procarbazine, hydroxyurea, cisplatin, cytosine arabinoside, and imidazole carboxamide regimen has been active and is being investigated by several institutions for recurrent gliomas.

The initial enthusiasm for use of neutrons has been severely curtailed by the sensitivity of neural tissues to neutrons. Necrosis has been found at doses apparently leading to complete ablation of high-grade astrocytomas. Trials of various mixtures of photons and neutron beams continue.

Heavy charged particles, such as protons and alpha particles, are of interest for small, well localized tumors such as pituitary adenomas. These are available in a small number of institutions. The accelerators used must be scheduled in advance because they are used for other purposes such as physics experiments.

Precisely collimated linear accelerator beams applied with multiple stationary or a number of arcs (moving field) or multiple cobalt-60 gamma ray sources (Gamma Knife) are used with carefully planned positioning of the skull in a head frame to treat small (<5-cm diameter) volumes. These take advantage of stereotactic technology (see above). The precise role of this technical application of single high doses (1,500 to 2,500 cGy) remains to be elucidated.

Although brachytherapy has been used in isolated centers, primarily in Europe, for many years, the availability of CT, digital angiography, treatment planning computers, and safer isotopes have made it available in several centers in the United States. Approaches vary widely from large multiple row arrays to arrays with relatively few seeds in three to five rows. Similarly, the role of the implant varies from being the major portion or all of the treatment to being a booster. The facts described in the Daumas-Duport et al. classification noted above are being addressed by relatively few centers yet. Colloidal isotope preparations such as chromic [^{32}P]phosphate are being used for booster treatment of the wall of malignant cysts when the fluid reaccumulation in the cyst is symptomatic. The role of brachytherapy in the management of brain tumors is being developed in pilot studies, most of which are in single institutions. It is unlikely that multi-institutional trials will be mounted in the near future. The goal of our own pilot studies is to treat low-grade gliomas with relatively small implants designed as booster treatment and is mostly confined to tumors that are biopsied stereotactically and demonstrated to be Daumas-Duport et al, class I.

The Radiation Therapy Oncology Group (RTOG) is exploring the tolerance to treatments of 120 cGy twice each day. With 240 cGy each day, patients complete treatment more rapidly, and there may be an increased therapeutic ratio because of the small fraction size and the greater daily dose to the tumor. Some of the glioblastoma multiforme tumors are among the most rapidly growing in man.

The BTSG has established the treatment of high-grade astrocytomas with irradiation and bischloronitrosourea as standard for many centers. The advantage over irradiation alone was observed only after subset analysis of patients judged to have been treated adequately and with certain histologic characteristics and in certain age groups. Thus, it appears that the combination of irradiation with any chemotherapeutic agent(s) should be considered as experimental. Thus far, the hypoxic cell-sensitizing agents have not proven advantageous, but the optimal drugs are only now coming into clinical trials. The pyrimidine nucleic acid analogues are an attractive group of agents being re-examined after having been suspended because of the difficulty of prolonged intracarotid artery infusions in previous tests. More effective combinations of drugs, such as in the 8-in-1 regimen (see above), remain to be investigated.

The advances of recent years have given us new tools for the treatment of brain tumors. There is every likelihood that, with time, these will be used effectively to improve survival for these patients. More experience is needed with some of these methods to determine the optimal way to use them. Combinations of effective methods will likely be necessary in order to maximize survival. Design, accrual, and maturation before analysis of prospective trials will require a decade or more before the full impact of these advances can be assessed accurately.

SUGGESTED READING

Daumas-Duport C, Monsaingeon V, N'Guyen JP, et al. Some correlations between histological and CT aspects of cerebral gliomas contributing to the choice of significant trajectories for stereotactic biopsies. Acta Neurochir [Suppl] (Wien) 1984; 33:185–194.

Kelly PJ, Earnest F IV, Kall BA, et al. Surgical options for patients with deep-seated brain tumors: computer-assisted stereotactic biopsy. Mayo Clin Proc 1985; 60:223–229.

Pezner RD, Archambeau JO. Brain tolerance unit: a method to estimate risk of radiation brain injury for various dose schedules. Int J Radiat Oncol Biol Phys 1980; 7:397–402.

Sheline GE. Radiotherapy of adult primary cerebral neoplasms. In: Oncology of the nervous system. Walker MD, ed. Boston: Martinus Nijhoff, 1983: 223.

Walker MD, Strike TA, Sheline GE. An analysis of dose-effect relationship in the radiotherapy of malignant gliomas. Int J Radiat Oncol Biol Phys 1971; 5:1725–1731.

HEAD AND NECK CANCER

ROLAND T. SKEEL, M.D.
BARRY H. KAPLAN, M.D., Ph.D.

Cancers of the head and neck, excluding skin cancer, represent 4 to 5 percent of all new cancer cases in the United States. In 1989, approximately 43,000 new cases were diagnosed, and 12,400 patients died. This chapter deals primarily with squamous cell cancer of the head and neck, which is by far the most common cancer in this anatomic region. Carcinomas of the salivary glands are mentioned briefly, but thyroid carcinomas, melanomas, lymphomas, and sarcomas are excluded from this discussion.

Squamous cell cancers may originate in the nasal sinuses (4 percent), nasopharynx (1 percent), oral cavity (55 percent), oropharynx (10 percent), larynx (25 percent), and hypopharynx (5 percent). The disease occurs predominantly in men (the male-to-female ratio is greater than 3 to 1) over the age of 40, who usually have a history of smoking and often alcohol use. The combination of the disfigurement and functional impairment associated with these cancers and the socioeconomic problems commonly found in this patient population have led to significant difficulties in evaluating therapy.

Over the past several years, there has been greater research emphasis on a multidisciplinary approach to the treatment of all but the earliest cases. The potential benefits of this approach have carried over into clinical practice, and the involvement of surgeons, radiotherapists, and medical oncologists in the initial evaluation and treatment has now become the standard in many institutions. Other medical specialists and support services are also often needed, including dentists, plastic surgeons, dietitians, and speech pathologists.

STAGING

Since treatment decisions and outcome are highly dependent on the extent of the primary tumor, the local spread, and the presence of metastases, accurate staging is an essential part of the pretreatment assessment. Work-up includes at least panendoscopy with multiple biopsies and a chest roentgenogram. A bone scan is useful both to evaluate local invasion and to look for metastases, and a computed tomographic scan or magnetic resonance imaging of the head and neck area may help to define tumor extent. An esophagogram can also be helpful in selected patients.

The American Joint Committee on Cancer has devised a site-specific staging system for each of the primary head and neck tumor regions and the several subregions. As with other tumors, the tumor (T) stage is dependent on size and extension; the node (N) stage is based on the presence, number, size, and bilaterality of regional nodes; and the metastases (M) stage indicates the presence or absence of distant metastases. Stage groupings for all sites are determined by the composite of tumor, node, and metastatic involvement shown in Table 1.

The prognosis of a particular lesion depends on the site as well as the stage. An early lesion of the piriform sinus or base of the tongue carries a much higher risk of relapse than a comparably staged lesion of the larynx. Similarly, even extensive nodal involvement in cancer of the nasopharynx can often be cleared with radiotherapy alone. There is no substitute for an experienced multidisciplinary team for evaluating these patients.

TREATMENT SELECTION

In general, stage I and stage II cancers of the head and neck are treated with surgery and/or radiotherapy, with cure rates in most sites higher than 50 percent with either modality alone. The choice of treatment is based on site and extent of disease, general physical health status (age, performance status, and nutritional condition), expected morbidity from alternative treatments, rehabilitation potential, and available expertise. Quality of life considerations must be taken into account, and the perspective of the patient weighed together with that of the health care professionals. Even within these early stages, there are patients who are good candidates for chemotherapy as part of their treatment. For example, patients with poor nutritional status at the time of diagnosis or those who have other medical contraindications to immediate surgery may profit from 6 to 9 weeks of effective chemotherapy to allow for hyperalimentation and other supportive measures. Patients with stage I and stage II cancer of the piriform sinus have a high relapse rate such that attempts to add chemotherapy to other modalities seem justified. In the future, it may well be that patients with early-stage cancer with significant relapse rates will benefit the most from adding chemotherapy to their management, but these patients are not commonly treated with chemotherapy at present.

TABLE 1 Stage Grouping for Carcinomas of the Head and Neck

Stage I	T1, N0, M0
Stage II	T2, N0, M0
Stage II	T2, N0, M0
Stage III	T3, N0, M0
	T1, T2, T3; N1, M0
Stage IV	T4, N0 or N1, M0
	Any T, N2 or N3, M0
	Any T, any N, M1

Patients with stage III and stage IV disease without distant metastases are now usually treated with various combinations of surgery, radiotherapy, and chemotherapy. The value of chemotherapy in this group of patients is discussed here. Patients with metastases below the clavicle or recurrent disease following treatment with either radiation or surgery, or radiation and surgery are candidates for palliative chemotherapy.

Because of the evolving nature of the treatments for head and neck cancers, particularly those classified as stage III and stage IV disease, investigational protocols should be considered. If patients are eligible for locally available studies, they usually provide treatment programs that are at least as effective as "standard" treatment and often offer the possibility of significantly more effective therapy than might otherwise be used.

CHEMOTHERAPY FOR RECURRENT OR METASTATIC DISEASE

Patient Selection

Before recommending chemotherapy, the oncologist must be sure it is indicated. Two errors commonly occur. One mistake is to assume that a mass or swelling represents recurrent cancer. Changes, especially edema induced by radiotherapy, stitch granulomas, and intercurrent infections causing lymphadenopathy, can mislead the treating physician. Biopsies or needle aspiration confirming the malignant nature of a suspicious mass should be carried out whenever possible. The other error is to assume that a new mass is recurrent disease rather than a second, potentially curable primary tumor. These patients, especially if they continue to smoke, develop second primaries in the epithelium at risk (head and neck, lung, esophagus) at the rate of 5 percent per year. For example, a single coin lesion in the lung should be assumed to be a second, curable primary and should be resected.

Renal, cardiac, pulmonary, and bone marrow functions are evaluated prior to therapy in order to guide the choice of drugs. Poor renal function with creatinine level over 3.0 mg per deciliter does not preclude the use of cisplatin in moderate doses (e.g., 50 mg per square meter of body surface area) as long as the patient can excrete a water load promptly. On the other hand, such a fluid load in a patient with congestive heart failure may put the patient at risk. By far the most dangerous drug used in these patients is methotrexate. Patients receiving this medication must be well hydrated, have creatinine levels less than 1.5 mg per deciliter, and have no third-space fluid accumulations such as ascites, pleural effusions, or significant edema. The presence of severe emphysema, common in heavy smokers, should lead physicians to avoid bleomycin. Dosages must be reduced and patients must be carefully monitored for bone marrow suppression if the initial white blood cell count is less than 4,000 per microliter or if the platelet count is less than 100,000 per microliter. Even cisplatin can cause significant myelosuppression in patients with compromised marrow function.

Active Single Agents

Chemotherapeutic agents of established activity in squamous cancer of the head and neck include methotrexate, cisplatin, bleomycin, 5-fluorouracil (5-FU), the vinca alkaloids, and mitomycin. Weekly methotrexate, at doses of 40 to 60 mg per square meter, has long been considered standard therapy, with response rates of 20 to 40 percent. There is no good evidence that higher doses of methotrexate with leucovorin rescue are better; in a controlled study by the Eastern Cooperative Oncology Group (ECOG), methotrexate at 240 mg per square meter with rescue yielded a shorter response duration than standard methotrexate. High-dose methotrexate is also extremely dangerous in this debilitated patient population.

The response rate to treatment with cisplatin as a single agent is comparable to the rate obtained with methotrexate. High-dose cisplatin is no more effective than standard doses (50 mg per square meter). 5-Fluorouracil appears to be more active when given as a continuous infusion over several days rather than as an intravenous bolus.

Combination Chemotherapy

The only combination of chemotherapeutic agents that has been shown in a prospective, randomized trial to have a higher overall and complete remission rate than methotrexate alone is a regimen using methotrexate, bleomycin, and cisplatin (MBD). In a study involving 163 patients, MBD produced responses in 48 percent compared with 35 percent for methotrexate alone, with 16 percent complete remissions for MBD versus 8 percent for methotrexate alone. The difference is significant ($p = 0.04$) using a one-sided binary regression test. Ambulatory patients, those without fixed neck nodes, and those without distant metastases responded more often.

Unfortunately, median time to disease progression in this study among responders was only 5.8 months for MBD and 5 months for methotrexate. Median survival was identical at 5.6 months in each group. Poor performance status, distant metastases, a history of heavy smoking, and adjacent organ invasion by the primary tumor were associated with shorter survival, as were weight loss, the presence of tumor in the neck, and heavy alcohol consumption.

Either regimen can be given to patients safely in the office or clinic, although MBD requires a 2-hour intravenous hydration every 3 weeks. The toxicity of both is comparable except for the nausea and vomiting associated with cisplatin administration. Lethal toxicity occurs in only about 3 percent of patients with either regimen and is usually associated with methotrexate-induced leukopenia and mucositis. Thus, since MBD more frequently provides effective palliative therapy, it is the treatment of choice, except for those patients whose medical condition precludes the use of cisplatin or those who cannot tolerate the increased nausea and vomiting. Symptomatic care may be most appropriate for patients who do not wish to undergo any treatment toxicities when the duration of benefit is likely to be brief.

Another regimen that is now being tested in a prospective, randomized trial is in common use in this country. The regimen was developed by Dr. Muhyi Al-Sarraf at Wayne State University and uses a combination of an intravenous bolus of 100 mg cisplatin per square meter and 4- or 5-day infusions of 5-FU at 1,000 mg per square meter per day (DF). The initial report indicated a 27 percent complete remission rate and 70 percent overall response rate for DF, and an ECOG pilot study achieved the same results. Median survival in these studies is 6 to 7 months. Toxicity with this treatment can be severe, especially in obese or cachectic patients or in patients over 65 years of age. The 5-FU dose should be reduced for these patients. The DF protocol requires extensive hospitalization for many of the patients, although some may be able to be treated as outpatients using portable continuous infusion pumps. The determination of whether DF or MBD provides the better palliative therapy or which one if either provides a longer survival than methotrexate must await mature results of randomized clinical trials. The three regimens for the treatment of head and neck cancer (already discussed) are presented in Table 2.

With either of the cisplatin-based regimens, one of a number of intensive regimens to alleviate nausea and vomiting should be begun.

TABLE 2 Regimens for Advanced Squamous Cell Carcinoma of the Head and Neck

Methotrexate

Methotrexate, 40 mg/m² IV bolus day 1. If no toxicity, escalate to 60 mg/m² IV bolus day 8 and continue weekly

MBD

Methotrexate, 40 mg/m² IM days 1 and 15
Bleomycin, 10 U IM days 1, 8, and 15
Cisplatin, 50 mg/m² IV day 4 with induced diuresis*

Repeat cycle every 21 days

DF

Cisplatin, 100 mg/m² IV day 1 with induced diuresis†
5-FU, 1,000 mg/m² in 2,000 ml 5% dextrose in half-normal saline to run over 24 hours daily × 4 or 5 days

Repeat cycie every 21 days

*Cisplatin is given 30 minutes after starting a 2-hour IV infusion of 2 L of 5% dextrose in half-normal saline with 10 mEq of KC1/L. Furosemide, 40 mg, is given intravenously at the start of the infusion, and mannitol, 12.5 g, is given intravenously just before administration of cisplatin. Patient must void at least 200 ml of urine in the first 30 minutes of the infusion, or cisplatin should be withheld and more intensive diuretic therapy administered until that rate of urine output is achieved.

†Oral hydration is begun the evening before treatment. On the morning of treatment an IV infusion of 5% dextrose in half-normal saline with 20 mEq of KC1/L is begun at a rate of 200 ml/hr. Furosemide, 40 mg, and mannitol, 12.5 g, are given intravenously after the first liter. The patient should be voiding freely. Immediately thereafter, cisplatin 100 mg/m², is added to a calibrated solution set and given over a 30-minute period and the second liter of fluid is continued.

CHEMOTHERAPY AS PART OF INITIAL MANAGEMENT

Resectable Cases

An enormous amount of excitement has been generated over the past several years because it has become apparent that patients who have not received prior radiotherapy have a very high response rate to chemotherapy. For example, two cycles of MBD given to previously untreated patients yielded a response rate of 80 percent. Even more interesting is a report of a response rate of 93 percent with 54 percent complete remissions, many documented at surgery, for patients treated with three cycles of DF using a 5-day infusion of 5-FU with cisplatin.

There is no evidence that prior chemotherapy interferes with subsequent surgery and/or radiotherapy; indeed, many surgeons welcome the improved nutritional state and medical condition that several weeks of effective chemotherapy provide. The impression is that these patients become better surgical candidates with improved rates of healing. However, it is true that about 25 percent of these patients refuse surgery following chemotherapy so that it is probably unwise to subject patients with a high surgical cure rate to preoperative chemotherapy, except in highly selected cases.

The hypothesis that these high response rates to chemotherapy translate into improved survival for these patients remains to be proved. One large controlled trial carried out thus far failed to show any benefit from the administration of one course of chemotherapy with bleomycin and cisplatin prior to surgery and radiotherapy.

Several large randomized trials are now ongoing that utilize various combinations and sequences of cisplatin-based chemotherapy combined with surgery, radiotherapy, or both. Given the high response rate of untreated patients to these chemotherapy programs and the radiosensitizing potential of cisplatin, there is cautious optimism that improvements in survival will be seen in the patients treated with multimodal protocol arms including such chemotherapy.

Since the indications for combination chemotherapy in association with surgery or radiotherapy have not yet been clarified, selection of patients not on investigational protocols for multimodality therapy is made on a case by case basis. Most frequently, patients who require a period of hyperalimentation or other medical management receive several cycles of chemotherapy prior to definitive local therapy. Patients with a high probability of relapse and patients with bulky disease are also logical candidates for combined modality approaches.

If preoperative chemotherapy is selected, it is critical that the lesions be mapped accurately endoscopically and tattooed or marked. Once the patient is given chemotherapy, it may be impossible to identify the original borders of the tumor. It is quite common to find small nests of viable tumor cells extending near the original margin of the tumor, even in patients who appear to have achieved a complete remission. For this reason, neither the surgical nor the radiotherapy treatment plan should be changed because the patient received chemotherapy irrespective of response.

Unresectable Cases

In general, patients with unresectable tumors have been identified as inoperable at the time of the initial staging of their disease. Although preoperative treatment with chemotherapy can make these patients' disease appear to become resectable, the results of surgery in controlling the disease are so poor that combined treatment with radiotherapy and chemotherapy is preferred to surgical intervention. Again, there are as yet no data that establish that combined modality therapy with chemotherapy improves survival in these patients. Two methods are commonly used to combine chemotherapy and radiotherapy for this group of patients. One method is similar to the treatment for resectable patients: two or three cycles of MBD or DF are administered prior to starting radiotherapy. The disadvantages of this approach include potentially prolonged hospitalization prior to definitive therapy and patient refusal of definitive therapy. The second method for combining chemotherapy and radiotherapy is to give both treatments simultaneously, so that chemotherapy serves as a radiosensitizer for radiation therapy.

Experimental laboratory data have shown that cisplatin enhances the effectiveness of radiotherapy. Patients with unresectable stage III and stage IV disease can be given 20 mg of cisplatin per square meter weekly concomitantly with intensive radiotherapy at 180 to 200 cGy per day, 5 days per week, to 6,800 to 7,600 cGy. At this dose, about 70 percent of patients achieve a complete or partial response, with the median survival being about 1 year. A current ECOG study comparing this regimen to radiotherapy alone will determine whether and to what degree the combined modality therapy is better. The toxicity of the combined treatment program can be expected to be greater than with radiotherapy alone, with over half of the patients having some vomiting and moderate to severe mucositis and 30 percent having moderate to severe hematologic toxicity.

Cisplatin is administered once a week on Tuesday, Wednesday, or Thursday immediately after radiotherapy during the entire radiotherapy course. Twenty-four hours before the drug administration, a white blood cell count, a platelet count, and a serum creatinine determination are obtained; treatment is withheld for a white blood cell count of less than 2,500 per microliter, a platelet count of less than 40,000 per microliter, or a creatinine level greater than 1.5 mg per deciliter. A fluid intake of 2 to 3 L is necessary for the 24-hour period prior to administration of cisplatin. Patients receive cisplatin within 2 hours following radiotherapy and should have urine output of at least 200 ml in the hour before cisplatin administration. Thirty minutes prior to cisplatin administration and infusion, 1 L of 5 percent dextrose in half-normal saline is started to run over a 2-hour period, followed by a second liter also containing 10 mEq of potassium chloride to run over a 4-hour period. If the patient fails to void 200 ml of urine in the hour prior to cisplatin administration, mannitol, 12.5 g, is given in an intravenous push immediately before cisplatin. The cisplatin is given by slow intravenous push. Urine output is monitored for the next 3 hours, and furosemide, 20 mg by intravenous push, is given if the output falls below 200 ml per hour.

CANCER OF THE SALIVARY GLAND

Only a modest number of reports deal with the chemotherapy of these tumors. Reports of responses of cancers of the salivary gland to doxorubicin (Adriamycin) and cisplatin-containing regimens are in the literature. Much more information about the response of salivary gland tumors to chemotherapy is needed before any firm conclusions can be developed or recommendations made.

SUGGESTED READING

Al-Sarraf M, Pajak TF, Marcial VA, et al. Concurrent radiotherapy and chemotherapy with cisplatin in inoperable squamous cell carcinoma of the head and neck. An RTOG Study. Cancer 1987; 59:259–265.

American Joint Committee on Cancer. Staging cancer at head and neck sites. In: Manual for staging of cancer. Philadelphia: JB Lippincott, 1983:25.

Decker DA, Drelichman A, Jacobs J, et al. Adjuvant chemotherapy with cis-diamminedichloroplatinum II and 120-hour infusion 5-fluorouracil in stage III and IV squamous cell carcinoma of the head and neck. Cancer 1983; 51:1353–1355.

Jacobs C. Adjuvant chemotherapy for head and neck cancer. J Clin Oncol 1989; 7:823–825.

Taylor SG IV. Why has so much chemotherapy done so little in head and neck cancer? [editorial]. J Clin Oncol 1987; 5:1–3.

Vogl SE, Schoenfeld DA, Kaplan BN, et al. A randomized prospective comparison of methotrexate with a combination of methotrexate, bleomycin and cisplatin in head and neck cancer. Cancer 1985; 56:432–442.

THYROID CANCER

IAN D. HAY, B.Sc. (Hons), M.B., Ch.B., Ph.D., F.A.C.P., F.R.C.P. (EDIN, GLASG, & LOND)

Although nodular thyroid disease continues to be common, even in such nonendemic areas as North America, thyroid cancer is rare and accounts for less than 1 percent of all malignant neoplasms. The American Cancer Society estimates that in the United States during 1990, 12,100 new cases will be diagnosed and 1,025 deaths will occur from thyroid cancer. Recent estimates of the incidence of thyroid carcinoma in a southeastern Minnesota community suggest an overall annual incidence rate of approximately 5 per 100,000 population, with papillary tumors accounting for most of the diagnosed cases, with an annual rate of approximately 4 per 100,000.

In most patients with primary thyroid cancer, the tumors are of epithelial origin, being derived from either the follicular or parafollicular cells. A variety of tumors of mesenchymal origin are found but are extremely rare. Malignant nonepithelial thyroid tumors include fibrosarcoma, malignant hemangioepithelioma, and more commonly, lymphomas of various types (spindle cell, giant cell, small cell). The non-Hodgkin's lymphomas seen in the thyroid often arise from glands that show evidence of chronic lymphocytic thyroiditis (Hashimoto's disease). They are treated according to the principles for favorable nonHodgkin's lymphoma outlined elsewhere in this volume.

Most thyroid cancers are well differentiated, and in North America papillary carcinoma (including so-called mixed papillary and follicular carcinoma) accounts for 52 to 81 percent of all cases. Recent studies at the Mayo Clinic suggest that, at present, 84 to 90 percent of thyroid carcinomas are well differentiated, about 7 to 10 percent are less well differentiated, and approximately 2 to 6 percent are undifferentiated (anaplastic). Table 1 illustrates the distribution of the various types of thyroid carcinoma diagnosed during 1935 to 1985, either in the Mayo Medical Center or the surrounding district of Olmsted County.

THERAPY OF DIFFERENTIATED THYROID CANCER

As yet, there is no unified opinion regarding the optimal therapeutic program for patients with differentiated thyroid carcinoma. Although surgical excision of the primary tumor is generally agreed to be the most effective initial treatment, the extent of surgical resection that is necessary to control the disease continues to be debated, and controversy exists concerning not only the amount of thyroid tissue to be resected but also the indication for and the extent of cervical node dissection. Because thyroid hormone treatment is thought to decrease the rates of both mortality and tumor recurrence, the use of postoperative thyroxine has been almost universal. However, the routine use of therapeutic radioiodine to ablate postoperative thyroid remnant tissue continues to arouse controversy. The present state of the art was recently assessed by Mazzaferri, who observed that "initial treatment generally consists of surgery, often followed by ^{131}I therapy, and invariably includes thyroid hormone." External irradiation does have a role to play in the management of recurrent or metastatic disease. However, cytotoxic chemotherapeutic agents have rarely been systematically investigated for the treatment of differentiated thyroid cancer.

PREFERRED APPROACH

Papillary Thyroid Carcinoma

Initial Surgery. Of 1,500 consecutive patients with papillary cancer operated on at the Mayo Clinic during 1945 through 1985, most (67 percent) underwent either bilateral subtotal resection or ipsilateral total and contralateral subtotal lobectomies (so-called near-total thyroidectomy). Total thyroidectomy was performed in only 19 percent of cases, in particular those in which both lobes were grossly involved or in which distant metastases were known to be present. In surgical series like these, there typically has been a more than 5 percent risk of permanent hypocalcemia, and a 1 to 2 percent incidence of permanent unilateral vocal cord paralysis not caused by malignant involvement of the recurrent laryngeal nerve. Most patients having permanent postoperative hypocalcemia had undergone total thyroidectomy, were younger than

TABLE 1 Percent Distribution of Histologic Types of Thyroid Carcinoma Diagnosed in a Community or at a Major Referral Center

Histologic Type	*Olmsted County 1935–1984**	*Mayo Medical Center 1946–1970†*	*Mayo Medical Center 1980–1985‡*
Well differentiated			
Papillary	81	77	80
Follicular	8	7	10
Less well differentiated			
Hürthle cell	5	4	4
Medullary	2	6	4
Undifferentiated			
Anaplastic	4	6	2

*Histologic diagnoses.
†Surgcal cases.
‡Cytologic diagnoses.

20 years, or had tumors 4 cm in diameter or larger. In the past decade, technical modification of the total thyroidectomy procedure and the advent of successful parathyroid autotransplantation have permitted a reduction of the hypoparathyroid rate to the 2 to 3 percent range. No data are available at the Mayo Clinic to show improved survival for papillary cancer with the performance of a total thyroidectomy. However, there is evidence that local tumor recurrence is significantly more frequent after unilateral lobectomy than after bilateral lobar resection, possibly a reflection of the multicentric nature of the primary disease.

Extent of Node Removal. For the treatment of papillary cancer at the Mayo Clinic, surgeons routinely remove all suspicious lymph nodes ipsilateral to the lesion from the paratracheal region and the tracheoesophageal groove down into the anterosuperior mediastinum. If clinical examination or gross examination at thyroidectomy indicates that lymph nodes in the lateral neck are involved, a modified neck dissection is generally performed. In neither the recent Mayo series nor the series of patients reported by Mazzaferri was the extent of node dissection shown to influence either tumor recurrence or the overall survival rate.

Radioiodine Ablation of Remnant. Once the primary tumor has been excised and the clinically suspicious nodes have been removed, the decision must be made as to whether to complete the thyroidectomy by the administration of radioactive iodine to ablate the functioning remnants of presumed normal thyroid tissue. Although evidence from the literature that remnant ablation influences the morbidity and mortality of patients having near-total thyroidectomy for papillary cancer is fragmentary and inconclusive, the practice has gained popularity since the 1977 publication by Mazzaferri and coworkers. In some institutions, ^{131}I is routinely administered postoperatively to all patients with papillary cancer, whereas in others it is restricted to patients with tumors of 1 cm in diameter or larger. Since the majority (possibly about 85 percent) of patients undergoing surgical treatment of papillary cancer are at minimal risk of cancer death (e.g., 1 to 2 percent at 30 years), it is probably more logical to restrict the use of ablative ^{131}I doses to those patients who are at high risk of mortality. Such patients are those over 40 years old at presentation, those having tumors over 4 cm in diameter, or those with nondiploid DNA or higher histologic grade tumors and especially those showing extrathyroidal invasion at neck exploration or evidence of distant metastases.

In those patients selected for ablation, it is our practice to administer, on an outpatient basis, a 29.9-mCi dose of ^{131}I. Typically, such ablation is performed at least 6 weeks after the operation and under optimal conditions of thyroid hormone withdrawal. Our practice is to commence patients on triiodothyronine (Cytomel), 25 μg two or three times daily for 4 weeks, discontinuing the medication 2 weeks prior to performing the neck scan with a 1-mCi ^{131}I diagnostic dose. Although other centers that hospitalize their patients for a 75- to 100-mCi ^{131}I ablative dose may disapprove of lower doses, we have found that a dose of 29.9 mCi reduces visible radioiodine uptake to zero or nearly zero in more than 80 percent of patients after a single outpatient treatment.

^{131}I Treatment of Distant Metastases. Most patients with papillary cancer and functioning distant metastases have a demonstrably abnormal whole body ^{131}I scan only when all functioning thyroid tissue in the neck has been totally ablated. Three days after ablative ^{131}I has been administered, we restart our patients on L-thyroxine, 0.2 mg daily for at least 6 weeks, and then ensure that the serum thyrotropin level measured in a sensitive immunometric assay is adequately suppressed at less than 0.1 mIU per liter. Thereafter we switch to triiodothyronine, 25 μg twice or three times per day for an additional 4 weeks, and then discontinue (as before) this medication 2 weeks prior to performing a whole body scan with a 3-mCi ^{131}I diagnostic dose. Patients with significant ^{131}I retention in metastatic deposits are routinely treated with standard doses of 150 to 200 mCi of ^{131}I in a lead-lined hospital room. Such doses do not induce radiation sickness and ordinarily do not produce damage to any bodily structures, including the lungs.

Treatment should be continued with ^{131}I until all residual uptake is ablated but should be discontinued if any adverse effects of ^{131}I are detected, e.g., persistent bone marrow depression or pulmonary fibrosis. Re-treatment doses are typically given at least 3 months apart to allow for proper assessment of induced tumor regression. Some physicians re-treat their patients only at yearly intervals because of their concern that more frequent treatment is associated with an increased frequency of leukemia, an occurrence that is possibly related to a failure to allow maximal bone marrow recovery.

Post-treatment Follow-up. If scanning shows that the patient is free of disease 1 year after successful therapy of metastatic lesions with ^{131}I, the whole body ^{131}I scan should probably be repeated after another 2 years. Thereafter, if results of scanning continue to be normal, it should be repeated at 3-year and then 5-year intervals. It has recently been suggested that whole body thallium scanning may be more sensitive in detecting metastatic thyroid cancer and might be a useful addition to follow-up schemes for papillary cancer. Thallium scanning has the advantage of not requiring the patient to discontinue suppressive thyroid hormone treatment. However, thallium scanning may sometimes accurately demonstrate subclinical metastatic lesions that cannot be treated with ^{131}I and may not be amenable to surgical intervention. In the search for persistent or recurrent tumor tissue in the neck, high-resolution sonography has proved to be particularly useful and has frequently allowed needle aspiration biopsy of clinically nonpalpable tumor masses. High-resolution computed tomography and magnetic resonance imaging may be used to evaluate disease in the lower neck and mediastinum and a computed tomographic study with contrast administration has become the radiologic procedure of choice for detection of micronodular pulmonary metastases.

If facilities for estimating the concentration of serum thyroglobulin (Tg) are available, this biologic tumor marker should be measured initially at the time of ablative therapy and repeated at least 2 months after complete ablation and probably at yearly intervals thereafter. If the concentration is more than 50 ng per milliliter, while the patient is on suppressive treatment, metastatic deposits are very likely to be present. If the concentration is less than 5 ng per milliliter, results of the whole body scan are almost invariably normal, and this procedure may not be required. Tg assays can be used during suppressive thyroxine therapy, perhaps at 6- to 12-month intervals, to detect the development of a large tumor burden. If the result is above an arbitrary cutoff of 10 ng per milliliter, it can be followed by a ^{131}I whole body scan to localize the disease and to evaluate the possibility of ^{131}I therapy. At intervals of 3 to 5 years, the ^{131}I scan can be done even when the Tg assay is negative in order to detect cases in which the scan is a more sensitive indicator. In patients in whom the Tg level is quite high (e.g., over 50 ng per milliliter) but the ^{131}I scan is negative, closer follow-up with nonisotopic imaging techniques is warranted. Some European authorities have treated such patients with an empirical 100-mCi ^{131}I therapy dose for presumed pulmonary micrometastases. However, in most North American centers, therapy is generally withheld until a treatable lesion is discovered.

External Irradiation Therapy. Although some have found that external irradiation in moderate doses may eradicate microscopic residual disease in patients with grossly complete excision of their tumors, others have found that the routine use of external irradiation has an adverse effect on outcome. Most authors agree that external radiotherapy is indicated for those patients with tumors that concentrate ^{131}I poorly (below 0.03 percent dose per gram of tumor) and also in those patients with osseous metastases who require rapid relief of pain.

Cytotoxic Chemotherapy. Of the currently available chemotherapeutic agents, data are most extensive on doxorubicin (Adriamycin), which seems to be effective in about 30 to 40 percent of patients with differentiated thyroid cancer. Until adequate trials have been completed for most of the standard alkylating agents and antimetabolites, however, the consideration of embarking on a combination chemotherapeutic approach would be premature. In general, as has been recently reported, chemotherapy in patients with papillary carcinoma should be considered only as a last resort.

Follicular Thyroid Carcinoma

Initial Treatment. In contrast to the considerably variable opinions regarding the optimal therapy of papillary carcinoma, most authorities now agree that the majority of follicular thyroid carcinomas should be treated initially with total or near-total thyroidectomy, followed by total ablation of all remaining tissue that concentrates ^{131}I. At the Mayo Clinic, most follicular carcinomas are treated by total lobectomy on the side of the lesion and subtotal lobectomy on the opposite side to obtain a wider margin around the lesion. Because spread to the lymph nodes is so rare, a modified or radical neck dissection is performed in less than 5 percent of cases.

The amount of radioiodine taken up by follicular carcinoma is thought to be dependent on the proportion of well-differentiated follicular structures present in the tumor, and therefore tumors composed predominantly of Hürthle cells rarely take up significant ^{131}I doses. Concentration of ^{131}I is improved if there is no competition from normal thyroid tissue. Consequently, when distant metastases are known or suspected, a total thyroidectomy is almost routinely recommended. When considered as an isolated variable, however, the extent of the initial thyroid operation has not been shown to affect the rate of later tumor recurrence, the rates being similar with either total or subtotal thyroidectomy.

Postoperative Therapy and Follow-up. In our practice, 6 weeks after total or near-total thyroidectomy, patients with follicular cancer regularly undergo whole body ^{131}I scanning to assess whether substantial uptake is demonstrable either in the thyroid bed or in distant functioning metastatic deposits. As noted in the section on papillary cancer, patients at the Mayo Clinic with postsurgical cervical remnants are treated with 29.9 mCi of ^{131}I, and patients with significant retention in metastatic deposits receive a therapeutic ^{131}I dose of 150 to 200 mCi. Thereafter, the frequency of ^{131}I re-treatments, the requirement for thyroid hormone suppression, the mode of follow-up with whole body imaging, the measurement of serum Tg, and the limited role of external irradiation and chemotherapy are as described in the preceding section on papillary cancer.

Outcome in Thyroid Cancer of Follicular Cell Origin

In a recently concluded study of 1,500 patients with papillary cancer treated at the Mayo Clinic during 1945 through 1985, 5 percent of the patients to date have died as a result of papillary cancer. In this group of conservatively treated patients, 19 percent of whom underwent total thyroidectomy and only 15 percent of whom had ^{131}I remnant ablation within 6 postoperative months, the overall mortality observed at 20 years was only 1.5 percent above that expected. Increasing age or the presence of distant metastases seems to have an adverse influence on the survival of patients with either papillary or follicular cancer. The prognosis for patients with follicular thyroid cancer also varies considerably according to the degree of vascular invasion: patients with moderately or markedly invasive tumors have a greatly increased rate of tumor recurrence and cancer mortality. It is generally accepted that patients who have follicular carcinoma (including the Hürthle cell variant, which does not usually respond to ^{131}I treatment) have a higher cumulative mortality rate than patients with papillary or mixed tumors. After 10 years, patients with pure follicular carcinoma have a cumulative cause-specific mortality rate of about 17 percent, and by 25 years, the rate is nearly 27 percent, in contrast to a comparable 6 percent figure for papillary cancer.

Medullary Thyroid Carcinoma

Initial Treatment. This unusual thyroid cancer is derived from the parafollicular or C cells, typically secretes the hormone calcitonin, is frequently familial, and constitutes an essential component of the multiple endocrine neoplasia (MEN) type 2 syndromes. The only effective treatment is surgery. The incidence of multifocal or bilateral disease is around 90 percent in familial cases and is at least 20 percent in patients presumed to have the sporadic disease. Total thyroidectomy is the procedure of choice in initial treatment. Because of a high incidence of metastatic lymphadenopathy, lymph nodes from the central zone of the neck (anterosuperior mediastinum to the thyroid isthmus) should be prophylactically dissected and the lateral compartments of the neck should undergo at least node picking. Once lymph node metastases are present, surgical cure is rare. When the viability of normal parathyroid glands is in question, autotransplantation should be considered.

In the MEN type 2 syndrome, patients with medullary thyroid cancer may also have pheochromocytomas and, more commonly, hyperparathyroidism. Before a neck exploration procedure is considered, the patients should be screened for pheochromocytoma, and if this tumor is present, it should be treated as a first priority. Bilateral total adrenalectomy may be necessary in familial disease, with excision of any extra-adrenal paraganglioma. At the time of neck exploration, the parathyroid glands should be explored, and only those glands that are grossly enlarged should be removed. If diffuse hyperplasia is present, a three-quarter parathyroidectomy or total parathyroidectomy and heterotopic transplantation are proven satisfactory procedures.

Postoperative Therapy and Follow-up. Serum calcitonin levels generally fall soon after successful thyroidectomy but may not reach a nadir for weeks or months. Elevated serum calcitonin levels may persist in the absence of detectable residual tumor, and without evident recurrence or metastases may persist over several years' observation. The serum level of carcinoembryonic antigen has been considered by some to be a more accurate predictor of tumor recurrence during postoperative follow-up. Rising levels of serum calcitonin and carcinoembryonic antigen should raise the question of metastatic or locally recurrent disease, and localizing studies may then be indicated. In the absence of inoperable metastases in the liver, bones, or lung, as detected by magnetic resonance or computed tomographic scanning or by radionuclide (thallium or diphosphonate) imaging, a search should be made for potentially reoperable tumor in the neck or mediastinum, possibly by a combination of high-resolution sonography and computed tomographic or magnetic resonance scanning. Reoperation for cervical metastatic disease is rarely curative, however, and patients may survive for more than 20 years with known metastatic cervical lymph nodes. Overall, the prognosis for patients with medullary cancer is considered to be somewhat worse than that for those with follicular cancer but much better than that seen in undifferentiated cancer.

Rapidly rising serum calcitonin and carcinoembryonic antigen levels or clinical evidence of advancing disease may be an indication for considering chemotherapy. Occasional cases have responded transiently to doxorubicin, but adverse affects have been considerable. Preliminary experience with VP-16 (etoposide) suggests that this agent may confer some benefit with very little morbidity, as may DTIC (dacarbazine). Radiation therapy has little overall effect on recurrent medullary cancer but may provide at least brief palliation when used for spinal metastases. In patients incapacitated by diarrhea, embolization of hepatic metastases may provide palliation when lesser measures have not been helpful.

Anaplastic Thyroid Carcinoma

Initial Treatment. This disease of the elderly represents one of the most lethal human solid tumors. Typically, patients present with a history of recent, rapid thyroid enlargement. Often the tumor may be inoperable at presentation but, when resectable, thyroid lobectomy with wide margins of adjacent soft tissue on the side of the tumor would seem to constitute a safe, appropriately aggressive surgical approach. Tracheostomy may sometimes be necessary to alleviate airway obstruction either on presentation or after the postoperative external irradiation therapy, which tends to be standard practice after an initial surgical procedure.

Alternative Therapy and Prognosis. Because of the strong possibility of recurrence and relapse, surgical therapy is typically followed by external irradiation and/or chemotherapy, even if complete resection of the tumor is confirmed surgically and pathologically. A 6-week treatment composed of doxorubicin and hyperfractionated radiation therapy was described in 11 patients from Memorial Sloan-Kettering, seven of whom showed an initial complete tumor response, but after 6 months only one patient survived. A recent Eastern Cooperative Oncology Group study observed a 33 percent (complete and partial) response after combined doxorubicin and cisplatin, as compared with only 5 percent after doxorubicin alone. Unfortunately, a prolonged response of approximately 3 years was obtained in only two of the 18 patients treated with a combination of drugs. In Sweden, hyperfractionated radiation therapy is currently being employed as a primary treatment, and patients whose tumors were initially inoperable are subsequently undergoing partial exploration procedures and in some cases having significant amounts of tumor resected. Unfortunately, most patients treated in this manner succumb to their disease, although less often by a local, obstructive mechanism.

In a 1971 Mayo Clinic study, all but one of 160 patients with anaplastic cancer died of their disease, usually within 6 to 8 months of diagnosis. In a more recent review of 82 patients having primary surgical treatment at the Mayo Clinic, the 5-year survival rate was only 3.6 percent, and patients had a median survival of 4 months after initial treatment. There is obviously a clear need for improved therapy in this most lethal of thyroid cancers.

SUGGESTED READING

Cady B, Rossi R. An expanded view of risk-group definition in differentiated thyroid carcinoma. Surgery 1988; 104:947–951.

Hay ID, Grant CS, Taylor WF, et al. Ipsilateral lobectomy versus bilateral lobar resection in papillary thyroid carcinoma. Surgery 1987; 102:1088–1094.

Simpson WJ, McKinney SE, Carruthers JJ, et al. Papillary and follicular thyroid cancer: Impact of treatment in 1,578 patients. Int J Radiat Oncol Biol Phys 1988; 14:1063–1072.

Snyder J, Gorman C, Scanlon P. Thyroid remnant ablation: Questionable pursuit of an ill-defined goal. J Nucl Med 1983; 24:659–663.

LUNG CANCER

JAMES R. JETT, M.D.
ROBERT S. FONTANA, M.D.

In the early 1900s, lung cancer was considered uncommon. Now we are experiencing an epidemic of the disease in the United States. In 1988 more than 150,000 Americans acquired lung cancer, and nearly 140,000 died of it. Approximately 85 percent of lung cancer deaths in this country are attributable to tobacco smoking, and lung cancer now is the most common cause of death from cancer among both men and women. The rate of cigarette smoking is gradually decreasing in the United States, and for the first time there is the suggestion of the occurrence of a plateau or even a slight decline in the incidence of lung cancer among white males. This decrease in incidence has not been observed among white females or among blacks. If we achieve the goal of a smoke-free society by the year 2000, we also should experience a substantial reduction in the incidence of this dreaded disease.

DIAGNOSIS

The only proven methods of detecting preclinical lung cancer are the chest roentgenogram and the sputum cytologic examination. Screening of asymptomatic persons at high risk for lung cancer utilizing periodic chest films and sputum cytology tests has not been shown to decrease lung cancer mortality, and therefore mass screening is not recommended.

A chest roentgenogram is likely to be the first significantly abnormal test among patients with symptomatic lung cancer. The flexible fiberoptic bronchoscope is the most common method of obtaining a histologic diagnosis. Tumors that are inaccessible bronchoscopically are often approachable by transthoracic needle aspiration.

Unfortunately, the majority of lung cancer patients present with evidence of metastatic disease. In these patients the diagnosis is frequently established by fine needle aspiration of the tumor or by open lung biopsy. For a detailed discussion of these and other diagnostic procedures, the reader is referred to *Seminars in Respiratory Medicine* 1982; 3:165.

One technique that has received considerable attention at the Mayo Clinic is the use of hematoporphyrin derivative for endoscopic photodetection and demarcation of radiographically occult lung cancers, especially those that are small and difficult to delineate with a standard white lighting system. Others have applied hematoporphyrin phototherapy to larger cancers that obstruct major bronchi, but we prefer the neodymium: yttrium-aluminum-garnet (Nd:YAG) laser in such cases.

STAGING OF LUNG CANCER

There are four major cell types of lung cancer: squamous cell, adenocarcinoma, large cell, and small cell. These four cell types, commonly designated bronchogenic carcinoma, account for almost 90 percent of all lung cancers. However, for therapeutic purposes, lung cancer is generally divided into small cell and non-small cell types.

A new international system for assessing (or staging) the anatomic extent of lung cancers has been adopted by the American Joint Committee on Cancer and by the International Union Against Cancer. Staging is based on the letters T (tumor), N (lymph nodes), and M (metastases), with appropriate suffixes that describe the extent of the cancer (Table 1).

For an in-depth discussion of the new staging system, consult the article by C. F. Mountain. Briefly, lung cancer has been divided into four stages (Table 2). Stage 0 is uncommon and refers specifically to carcinoma in situ. Stage I, stage II, and some stage IIIa lung cancers are considered to be resectable. Stage IIIb and stage IV cancers are not amenable to surgical treatment. The 5-year survival rates for patients with stage I and II cancers are approximately 50 to 60 percent and 30 to 40 percent, respectively. The 5-year survival rates of patients with stage IIIa, IIIb, and IV lung cancers are less than 20 percent. The new staging system offers a uniform basis for communication among scientists from different countries.

TABLE 1 International System for Staging of Lung Cancer—TNM Classification

Primary tumor (T)	
T0	No evidence of primary tumor
TX	Cancer cell in bronchopulmonary secretions; no tumor seen on chest film or at bronchoscopy
TIS	Carcinoma in situ
T1	Tumor ≤3 cm in greatest dimension, surrounded by lung tissue, no bronchoscopic evidence of tumor proximal to lobar bronchus
T2	Tumor >3 cm in diameter, or a tumor of any size that involves visceral pleura, or associated with atelectasis extending to hilum (but not involving entire lung); must be ≥2 cm from carina
T3	Tumor involves chest wall, diaphragm, mediastinal pleura or pericardium; or is ≤2 cm from carina (but does not involve it)
T4	Tumor involves carina or trachea, or invades mediastinum, heart, great vessels, esophagus, or vertebrae; or malignant pleural effusion
Nodal involvement (N)	
N0	No demonstrable lymph node involvement
N1	Ipsilateral peribronchial or hilar nodes involved (includes direct extension)
N2	Metastasis to ipsilateral mediastinal nodes or to subcarinal nodes
N3	Metastasis to contralateral mediastinal or hilar nodes or to scalene or supraclavicular nodes
Distant metastasis (M)	
M0	No (known) distant metastasis
M1	Distant metastasis present-specify site(s)

Modified from Mountain CF. A new international staging system for lung cancer. Chest 1986; 89(Suppl):225-233.

TABLE 2 TNM Subsets for Staging of Lung Cancer

Stage	*TNM Subsets*
0	TIS (in situ)
I	T1 N0 M0 T2 N0 M0
II	T1 N1 M0 T2 N1 M0
IIIa	T3 N0 M0 T3 N1 M0 T1-3 N2 M0
IIIb	AnyT N3 M0 T4-AnyN M0
IV	AnyT AnyN M1

Modified from Mountain CF. A new international staging system for lung cancer. Chest 1986; 89(Suppl):225-233.

MANAGEMENT

Surgery

The treatment of choice for early-stage non-small cell lung cancer is surgical resection. Small cell lung cancer is not generally considered to be a surgical disease and is reviewed separately. All stages 0, I, and II and some stage IIIa non-small cell cancers are best treated surgically. The role of surgery in the T1-3 N2 M0 subset of stage IIIa is controversial. We believe that a few highly selected patients with N2 disease of the squamous cell type should be considered for surgery. In patients with N2 disease documented by mediastinoscopy, the 5-year survival rate is less than 10 percent, and we believe that these patients are not good candidates for resection.

In a recent review of operative mortality, the Lung Cancer Study Group evaluated the 30-day surgical mortality rate encountered in the cooperating group of major institutions. More than 2,000 cases of resected lung cancer were analyzed. The mortality rate was 6.2 percent for pneumonectomies and 2.9 percent for lobectomies. Among patients younger than 60 years of age, the surgical mortality rate was 1.4 percent, whereas in those 60 to 69 years of age, the mortality rate was 4.1 percent. Of 453 patients who were 70 years of age or older, the operative mortality was 7.1 percent. Although others have also reported an operative mortality rate of less than 10 percent in patients over 70 years old, serious medical problems were definitely more common in this group. Thus it appears that, in centers where many pulmonary resections are performed each year, surgery for lung cancer is associated with an acceptable operative risk and age is not an absolute contraindication to thoracotomy. However, careful attention must be paid to potential complicating medical problems as well as to the anticipated quality of life following surgery.

Therapy for Locally Unresectable Non-Small Cell Lung Cancer

Patients with unresectable stage III non-small cell lung cancer that has not spread beyond one hemithorax, the mediastinum, and the ipsilateral supraclavicular nodes are usually treated with radiation therapy. The median survival in this group of patients is 10 to 12 months. Approximately 5 to 10 percent survive 5 years. In a randomized multi-institutional trial, the Radiation Therapy Oncology Group demonstrated that increasing the dose of radiation from 4,000 cGy to 6,000 cGy improved the 2-year survival from 10 to 19 percent and decreased the frequency of local recurrence from 51 to 35 percent.

The majority of patients treated with radiation therapy die of metastatic disease. Accordingly, a number of investigators have advocated the addition of systemic treatment (chemotherapy) to radiotherapy in the treatment of locally unresectable non-small cell lung cancer. Results of uncontrolled studies involving relatively small groups of patients have suggested that the combination of chemotherapy and radiation therapy is superior to radiation alone. A preliminary report by the Cancer and Leukemia Group B observed superior survival in a group of patients treated with vinblastine and cisplatin plus thoracic radiotherapy versus those undergoing treatment with identical thoracic radiotherapy alone. The final report of this study is pending and, if still positive, will need to be confirmed by future studies.

Currently, opinion is divided regarding the proper management of locally unresectable non-small cell lung cancer. Radiation alone or in combination with systemic chemotherapy would be considered appropriate for this stage of disease, and there is no single, optimal program of chemotherapy. Further randomized controlled trials are needed to evaluate the potential benefit of new systemic therapeutic regimens.

Following standard thoracic radiation, approximately 50 percent of patients will have relapses in the chest within the previous radiation portal. Accordingly, investigators are evaluating the role of twice a day radiotherapy (hyperfractionation) for control of local disease. A preliminary report by the Radiation Therapy Oncology Group has suggested the merit of this approach. At present, phase III trials are under way comparing standard fractionated radiotherapy with hyperfractionation. At this time, hyperfractionation thoracic radiotherapy should only be used in a protocol setting until the risks and benefits have been clearly defined.

Therapy for Metastatic Non-Small Cell Lung Cancer

About half of all patients with non-small cell lung cancer have evidence of distant metastases at the time of diagnosis, that is, they have stage IV disease. Previous reports have suggested that a variety of individual chemotherapeutic agents, as well as combinations of these agents, are active against this stage of lung cancer. Rates of response to treatment have ranged from 10 to 50 percent. However, once again, randomized controlled clinical trials have failed to demonstrate the superiority of any individual drug or combination of drugs.

Approximately 15 to 30 percent of patients with metastatic non-small cell lung cancer exhibit some response to chemotherapy, but less than 5 percent show evidence of a complete response or complete remission. Factors that appear to have the greatest influence on patient survival are the initial clinical status (performance score), the extent of metastasis at the time of treatment, the initial response to chemotherapy, and the amount of weight lost prior to treatment.

Some have questioned the value of any form of treatment for non-small cell lung cancer. In fact, several randomized trials have been conducted in which no treatment has been compared with chemotherapy. The most recent of these trials studied supportive care versus treatment with combinations of cyclophosphamide, doxorubicin, and cisplatin or vindesine and cisplatin. Median survival rates were 17 weeks for the group given no chemotherapy, 23 weeks for the group treated with cyclophosphamide, doxorubicin, and cisplatin, and 31 weeks for the group receiving vindesine and cisplatin. The difference in survival following chemotherapy was statistically significant.

At present, there is no standard chemotherapeutic program for patients with stage IV non-small cell lung cancer. Because of this, it is our opinion that all such patients should be offered treatment in a clinical trial (protocol) setting. The reasons for this opinion are as follows: (1) treatment may provide psychological benefit to some patients, (2) patients who respond to treatment may experience amelioration of symptoms, (3) responders tend to survive longer than nonresponders, (4) treatment in a protocol setting provides information that may benefit the patient and society, and (5) failure to treat in a protocol setting hinders advancement of knowledge.

As previously noted, lasers have recently been employed as palliative therapy for lung cancers that have obstructed major air passages. The instrument of choice for treatment of such tumors at the Mayo

Clinic has been the Nd:YAG laser, which provides excellent palliation with some risk. The YAG laser should be reserved for those cases in which all of the more conventional therapies have failed. One exception may be the patient who presents with evidence of marked tracheal obstruction and severely compromised respiration. In this situation, laser treatment may relieve the obstruction enough to make more definitive therapy possible.

In recent years we have also used local endobronchial radiation (brachytherapy), often in combination with YAG laser therapy, for management of unresectable tumors of the trachea and the major bronchi. Brachytherapy tends to induce a more prolonged palliation of endobronchial disease and may decrease the frequency with which repeated laser treatments are required.

Therapy for Small Cell Lung Cancer

Small cell lung cancer accounts for 20 to 25 percent of all bronchogenic carcinomas. It differs from non-small cell lung cancer in rapidity of growth and dissemination, hormonal secretions, and response to therapy. In the majority of patients, small cell lung cancer is disseminated at the time of initial diagnosis. This fact has been documented by the extremely low 5-year survival rates for patients with small cell lung cancer following surgery or thoracic radiotherapy alone.

Small cell lung cancers have features of amine precursor uptake and decarboxylation cells and exhibit neurosecretory granules when examined by electron microscopy. Secretion of dopa decarboxylase, neuron-specific enolase, bombesin, and hormones such as antidiuretic hormone, adrenocorticotropic hormone, and calcitonin has been documented repeatedly. Studies in the early 1970s showed significant responses of these tumors to treatment with combination chemotherapy and radiation therapy. Median survival increased dramatically with combined modality treatment. Unfortunately, the 5-year survival rate remains less than 10 percent.

Although small cell lung cancer may be staged according to the TNM system, it is more commonly classified as either "limited" or "extensive." Small cell lung cancer that is confined to a single hemithorax, the mediastinum, and the ipsilateral supraclavicular nodes is referred to as limited disease (LD), whereas small cell lung cancer that spreads beyond these boundaries is regarded as extensive disease (ED).

The response rate of LD to treatment consisting of combination chemotherapy plus radiation therapy to the primary lung tumor is 70 to 90 percent. Total resolution of clinically detectable disease, or complete response, is achieved in 40 to 60 percent of all cases. The median survival of patients with LD is 12 to 18 months, with a 2-year survival rate of 20 to 30 percent. Five-year survival rates of approximately 10 percent have been reported.

For ED, the overall response to treatment (usually combination chemotherapy) is 60 to 80 percent, with a complete response rate of 20 to 30 percent. The median survival of all patients with ED is 8 to 10 months, and the 2-year survival rate is 5 to 10 percent. Very few patients (1 to 2 percent) survive 5 years.

Major advances in the treatment of small cell lung cancer have reached a plateau since the late 1970s. Since the mid-1970s, the standard treatment regimen for small cell lung cancer has been combination chemotherapy, consisting of cyclophosphamide, doxorubicin, and vincristine (CAV), with or without thoracic radiation. More recently, a combination of etoposide (VP-16) and cisplatin (EP) has proved effective either as initial therapy or if relapse occurs after treatment with CAV.

Recent reports from the Clinical Trials Group of the National Cancer Institute of Canada have described favorable results of a program that alternates CAV and EP every 3 to 4 weeks for a total of six cycles. Those patients in whom complete response is achieved are followed for signs of relapse. Those who have evidence of residual disease after six cycles of treatment receive additional chemotherapy, as tolerated.

The addition of thoracic radiation therapy to chemotherapy has improved the survival of patients with LD. In contrast, thoracic radiation rarely benefits patients with ED, with the possible exception of those who achieve a complete regression of all extrathoracic disease following chemotherapy alone.

Three exciting preliminary reports have appeared in the literature using the combination of hyperfractionated thoracic radiotherapy (twice a day) and systemic chemotherapy with EP. In each of these communications, the two-year survival for LD small cell lung cancer is approximately 60 percent. If these results can be confirmed in phase III trials, this would represent a major advance in our treatment of LD small cell lung cancer. These phase III trials, with survival as the major end point, are in progress.

Radiation therapy for intracranial metastases from small cell lung cancer is effective in 70 to 90 percent of cases. Prophylactic cranial irradiation has been a standard practice since the mid-1970s and has been shown to decrease the frequency of metastasis to the brain. However, it has never been shown to prolong survival. More recently, neuropsychiatric sequelae, including abulia, ataxia, and dementia, have been reported in long-term survivors of small cell lung cancer who have received prophylactic cranial irradiation. The combination of prophylactic cranial irradiation and nitrosourea chemotherapy may be especially toxic to the central nervous system. At present, prophylactic cranial irradiation probably should be reserved for those patients who achieve a complete response to systemic chemotherapy. Ongoing studies are evaluating the efficacy and toxicity of small cumulative doses and fractionations of prophylactic cranial irradiation.

Surgery as the sole treatment of small cell lung cancer was abandoned years ago because it proved ineffective. Now the potential role of surgery in selected cases of limited small cell lung cancer is being reassessed. At this time, no prospective randomized trials have been reported that demonstrate significant prolongation of the survival of patients with small cell lung cancer who have undergone resection of their thoracic tumors in addition to treatment with combination chemotherapy and radiation therapy. Patients undergoing resection of an indeterminate pulmonary lesion who are found to have small cell lung cancer should receive adjuvant chemotherapy and radiation therapy, even if there is no clinical evidence of residual tumor, because of the high frequency of relapse.

SUGGESTED READING

Brutinel WM, Cortese DA, McDougall JC, et al. A two-year experience with neodymium-YAG laser in endobronchial obstruction. Chest 1987; 91:159–165.

Fontana RS, Sanderson DR, Woolner LB, et al. Lung cancer screening: The Mayo program. J Occup Med 1986; 28:746–750.

Ginsberg RJ, Hill LD, Eagan RT, et al. Modern thirty-day operative mortality for surgical resections in lung cancer. J Thorac Cardiovasc Surg 1983; 86:654–658.

Mountain CF. A new international staging system for lung cancer. Chest 1986; 89(Suppl):225–233.

Perez CA, Stanley K, Grundy G, et al. Impact of irradiation technique and tumor extent in tumor control and survival of patients with unresectable non-oat cell carcinoma of the lung. Cancer 1982; 50:1091–1099.

Rapp E, Pater JL, Willan A, et al. Chemotherapy can prolong survival in patients with advanced non small cell lung cancer. J Clin Oncol 1988; 6:633–641.

Ruckdeschel JC, Finkelstein DM, Ettinger DS, et al. A randomized trial of the four most active regimens for metastatic non–small-cell lung cancer. J Clin Oncol 1986; 4:14–22.

Silverberg E, Lubera JA. Cancer statistics, 1988. CA 1988; 38:5–22.

SURGERY FOR BREAST CANCER

UMBERTO VERONESI, M.D.

The new developments in science, the new concepts about the biology of breast cancer, and the changes in the characteristics of breast cancer patients have led in the last 20 years to a substantial change of approach in the treatment of primary breast cancer. The classic Halsted mastectomy, which for nearly a century has been the standard surgery for breast cancer of any type, has been gradually replaced by a variety of operations. Some of these are simply modifications of the Halsted mastectomy, but others are totally new operations and are often associated with radiotherapy. The embarrassing result of this development is that the surgeon today faces a great variety of options and choices without any clear and agreed-on definition of the various indications (Table 1). It is difficult to find two institutions, or even two surgeons in the same institution, that use the same treatment for breast cancer.

TERMINOLOGY

One important achievement would be the agreement on terminology: for instance, one often reads of comparisons between "radical and conservative surgery" for breast cancer, implying that conservative surgery is by definition not radical. I believe this is a poor way to define treatments because the term radical does not refer simply to the extent of the treatment—extensive operations may not be radical (i.e., local or distant recurrences may appear some time after treatment), and limited operations may be totally radical (i.e., local and general control may be complete and definitive). Therefore, I think that the term *radical* should be avoided in favor of others that describe the anatomic extent of the operation, such as total mastectomy, total mastectomy and axillary dissection, quadrantectomy, and so on.

Another source of confusion is the terminology related to conservative surgical procedures. *Partial mastectomy* and *segmental mastectomy* do not appear reasonable, because the term *mastectomy* by definition indicates the total removal of the breast. Wedge resection and tylectomy do not describe the extent of the excision, and lumpectomy and tumorectomy are equally vague. I think three terms would be sufficient to cover the various types of conservative surgery: (1) quadrantectomy—an operation that removes a quadrant of the breast en bloc with the overlying skin and underlying fascia of the major pectoralis muscle, (2) large breast resection—an extensive removal of mammary tissue around the primary tumor (without skin and deep fascia), with a margin of at least 2 cm of normal tissue, and

TABLE 1 Options for Local-Regional Treatment*

Breast	*Axillary Nodes*	*Internal Mammary Nodes*
Mastectomy	total dissection	total dissection
Quadrantectomy	partial dissection	biopsy
Resection	radiotherapy	radiotherapy
Tumorectomy	no treatment*	no treatment*
Radiotherapy		

* In clinically negative patients.

(3) limited breast resection—the removal of the tumor with a margin of normal tissue of less than 2 cm.

ABLATIVE SURGERY

Halsted mastectomy (en bloc removal of the entire breast with its overlying skin, both pectoralis muscles, and the whole content of the axillary fossa) has represented the treatment of choice for any type of breast cancer for almost a century, without substantial criticism, because it fulfilled the needs resulting from the two major dogmas of local–regional spread of breast cancer. The first dogma was that, since the lymphatics of the breast are richly anastomosed, a cancer cell that escapes from the primary tumor rapidly reaches any point in the mammary gland. The second was that the mechanism of axillary invasion is that of lymphatic permeation, whereby the cancer cells fill the lymphatic trunks through a process of continuous intralymphatic proliferation. Although recent studies have shown that neither dogma is defendable—since cancer cells are generally found in close connection with the primary tumor and the mechanism of axillary metastasis is embolic, the intermediate lymphatic vessels being ordinarily free of cancer cells—a number of surgeons still prefer this mutilating operation on the grounds of an unproven safety.

However, many modifications have been introduced in the last 30 years, some directed to the dissection of additional lymph node groups (such as the internal mammary and the supraclavicular). In the 1960s, the dissection of internal mammary nodes appeared a logical step; later it was shown that 25 percent of the cases treated with the classic Halsted mastectomy have metastases in the internal mammary nodes. The Halsted mastectomy therefore appeared to be not radical in one out of four cases, and it was considered reasonable to add the dissection of the internal mammary nodes in the hope of improving long-term results. However, clinical trials carried out in many centers failed to show any advantage in this extended mastectomy over the classic Halsted operation, and today the extended and super-radical operations have only historical importance.

The failure of extended aggressive surgery to improve survival, the emerging concepts on the biology of breast cancer, the awareness that the major problem in breast cancer is the control of distant metastases have induced many surgeons to reduce the extent of the tissue removed. Patey reported his results of a modified mastectomy that spared the major pectoralis muscle. He adopted his new procedure in 1936, and the long-term follow-up of his cases showed improved cosmetic and functional results without any apparent increase in local and distant recurrences. The new procedure, although considered unorthodox and therefore not accepted by most cancer surgeons for many years, slowly gained popularity and today is the most commonly used surgical procedure in breast cancer in many countries.

One of the more ambitious goals, long pursued by surgeons, to remove the psychologic distress caused by mastectomy, has been the surgical reconstruction of the breast. However, as long as the treatment of choice was Halsted mastectomy, the practical possibilities were limited, and the cosmetic results were poor. In recent years, two important developments have made reconstructive breast surgery easier and more widely accepted. The first was the gradual substitution of Halsted mastectomy with less mutilating procedures, which spare the pectoralis muscles and leave an anatomic condition more suitable for reconstruction. The second development was the widespread introduction in plastic surgery of myocutaneous flaps, a technique that makes available to the anterior chest region an abundant, well-oxygenated tissue that, properly reshaped and, where necessary, integrated with a prosthesis, creates an excellent new breast.

There are various alternative possibilities, depending on the extent of ablative surgery and the size of the contralateral breast. In women who have had a modified mastectomy and have a remaining small breast, reconstruction can be simply carried out by inserting a silicone prosthesis. The prosthesis can be placed in a pocket created in the mastectomy site, and the size can be similar to that of the remaining breast. An areolar nipple complex can be made at a later time. If the patient has a large opposite breast, reconstruction at the site of the mastectomy and the reduction of the contralateral breast can be performed in the same operative session.

In patients who have had an extensive mastectomy, the surgeon can make use of a myocutaneous flap, generally taken from the latissimus dorsi muscle. The flap provides a large volume, and the size of superimposed skin padding can be designed as needed.

A number of centers have attempted reconstruction by means of microvascular methods. Large areas of skin and subcutaneous fat can be taken from the buttocks to the chest area and the vessels anastomosed to axillary vessels. Although the results are encouraging, further studies are needed in this field.

The reconstruction can be performed as soon as the skin over the chest wall becomes freely movable, i.e., from 4 to 6 months after mastectomy, but there is an increasing trend to perform the reconstruction immediately, at the same time of the mastectomy. The psychological advantages of this procedure are considerable and we are pushing strongly in this direction.

CONSERVATIVE TREATMENTS

The recent and increasing interest in conservative surgery is mainly the result of modification of the patient population observed in the last 15 years. The introduction of mammography and of intensive education programs has led to a spectacular increase in the number of breast carcinomas of limited dimensions, and in many institutions more than 40 percent of the patients with operable tumors have a carcinoma less than 2 cm in pathologic diameter. Nonpalpable carcinomas of less than 0.5 cm are also more common today, as are noninfiltrating lobular and ductal carcinomas.

In addition, women today are more aware of medical and surgical treatments and an increasing number of women with breast cancer are demanding to participate in the therapeutic decisions, after having been informed of the different approaches and the respective risk for each type of treatment. Finally, it has been stressed that the chance of breast conservation for patients with a limited breast tumor would be an impressive tool for publicizing breast self-examination and participation in screening programs. It is reasonable to think that women would develop an attitude of cooperation with the medical profession if they knew the reward would be preservation of the breast for their alertness instead of a scarring mutilation.

Evaluation of the efficacy of limited surgery of the primary carcinoma alone (extensive breast resection, quadrantectomy) is difficult because it is almost always immediately followed by radiotherapy. The only extensive clinical trial applying limited surgical excision of the tumor without radiotherapy is that conducted by the National Surgical Adjuvant Breast Program (NSABP) in the United States. The trial was initiated in 1976, and preliminary results published recently showed that limited surgical excision without additional radiotherapy exposes the patients to an increased risk of local recurrences.

Many trials have evaluated the efficacy of limited surgery combined with radiotherapy. Probably the trial that has produced the most meaningful results is the Milan trial. It started in 1973, and the accrual of patients was terminated at the beginning of 1980. Altogether, 701 patients entered the trial; 349 were randomly allocated to Halsted mastectomy and 352 to the conservative procedure. Conservative treatment consisted of a breast quadrantectomy, axillary dissection, and radiotherapy on the ipsilateral breast tissue. Up to the end of 1975, patients were further randomized to postoperative radiotherapy on supraclavicular and internal mammary nodes, or no further treatment. Since 1976, in both groups adjuvant chemotherapy with cyclophosphamide, methotrexate, and fluorouracil (CMF) was administered for 1 year when positive lymph nodes were found at the axilla. The accrual was limited to T_1N_0 patients (less than 2 cm at pathologic examination and no palpable axillary nodes).

The quadrantectomy, axillary dissection, and radiotherapy (QUART) procedure consists of the surgical removal of an entire quadrant of the breast with the overlying pectoralis fascia, so that the primary tumor is removed with a very large portion of normal tissue in the three dimensions. The axillary dissection may be performed in continuity when the primary cancer lies in the upper-outer quadrant, or in discontinuity, with a separate incision in all other cases. Radiotherapy on the ipsilateral breast is delivered at the dose of 50 Gy through two opposing tangential fields with high-energy photons, and with a conedown of an additional 10 Gy to the scar with orthovoltage radiotherapy. The updated results show that relapse-free survival and overall survival are not different in the two groups of patients (Fig. 1). There have been seven local recurrences in the Halsted group and eight in the QUART group. Moreover, eight patients in the QUART group developed a second primary tumor in the ipsilateral breast. The results allow us to conclude that mastectomy involves unnecessary mutilation in patients with carcinoma of the breast less than 2 cm in diameter.

A second trial is in progress at the Milan Cancer Institute, comparing two different conservative techniques, the QUART, already described, and the TART (tumorectomy, axillary dissection, radiotherapy), which consists of a limited breast resection plus total axillary dissection and a vigorous radiotherapy, with 45 Gy administered by an external high-energy source and a boost of some 15 Gy through an interstitial implant of Ir^{192} wires. The trial is now completed as 600 patients have already entered the randomized study, and the results will be available in 2 to 3 years.

THE CHOICE OF TREATMENT

At present, it appears reasonable to affirm the following facts: (1) Extended surgical treatments, including the dissection of internal mammary and supraclavicular nodes, have not improved the prognosis and no longer have a role in breast cancer surgery. The same conclusion is applicable to regional radiotherapy. (2) Halsted mastectomy is indicated in special cases, such as very large cancers, deeply situated, with massive axillary metastases, or locally advanced carcinomas after aggressive chemotherapy as a rescue operation. (3) Total mastectomy with axillary dissection appears to be adequate treatment for tumors of medium size (more than 2 to 3 cm in diameter) with or without palpable axillary nodes. (4) Quadrantectomy, axillary dissection, and radiotherapy on the ipsilateral breast is a safe procedure for patients with a small breast cancer (less than 2 to 3 cm in pathologic diameter), with or without palpable axillary nodes. (5) Other more limited conservative procedures are still under evaluation. In Table 2 a series of indications for radiosurgical treatment of breast cancer is shown.

TABLE 2 The Choice of Radio-Surgical Treatment for Breast Cancer*

T^1, $T^2 < 2.5$ cm, $N^0{}_{,1}$	quadrantectomy, axillary dissection, radiotherapy
$T^2 > 2.5$ cm, $T^3N^0{}_{,1,2}$	total mastectomy, axillary dissection ± immediate reconstruction
$T^4N^0{}_{,1,2}$	radiotherapy + Halsted mastectomy or total mastectomy, axillary dissection
T^4 inflammatory	radiotherapy

* The choice of adjuvant treatment (endocrine and/or chemotherapy as well as primary chemotherapy is made according to (1) the local–regional extent of the disease, (2) the prognostic factors, (3) the menopausal status, (4) the indicators of response.

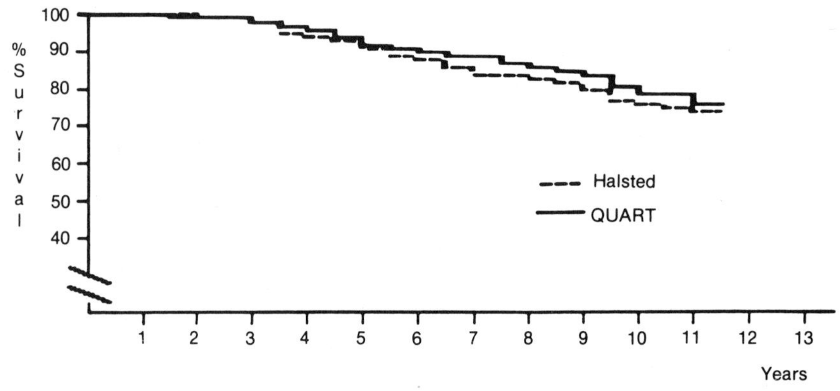

Figure 1 Survival: Halsted vs QUART.

In situ lobular carcinoma and noninfiltrating intraductal carcinoma of the breast are two much discussed pathologic entities in terms of the extent of treatment. The feeling is widespread that conservative procedures should be adopted in both cases, whenever possible. For lobular carcinoma in situ, an occasional finding by the pathologist, a careful follow-up of the patient is considered sufficient. In fact, those patients must be considered at high risk of developing a breast cancer, which, however, appears with equal probability in either breast.

For intraductal noninfiltrating carcinomas, the decision can be made according to the size of the dominant tumor mass. If the tumor mass is less than 2 to 3 cm in diameter, a simple quadrantectomy can be performed; if it is larger or the tumor is multifocal, a total mastectomy is advisable. In both cases, because axillary metastases almost never occur, axillary dissection can be avoided.

Although conservative treatment is now cautiously entering common surgical practice for selected breast cancers, there are a number of unsolved questions about the conservative approach: Will it be possible to expand the indications of quadrantectomy to tumors larger than 2 to 3 cm in diameter? Is simultaneous axillary dissection needed in clinically node-negative patients, or can it be deferred until the appearance of clinically involved lymph nodes? Is postoperative radiotherapy on the remaining breast tissue necessary? Can the surgical procedure of quadrantectomy be replaced by radiotherapy, such as interstitial implantation with radioactive preparations after a simple debulking procedure? These questions remain the object of a number of new clinical trials, which in the next decade will produce more conclusions on the appropriate treatment of breast cancer.

SUGGESTED READING

Fisher B, Bauer M, Margolese R, et al. Five-year results of a randomized clinical trial comparing total mastectomy and segmental mastectomy with or without radiation in the treatment of breast cancer. N Engl J Med 1985; 312:665–673.

Fisher B, Redmond C, Edwin R, et al. Ten-year results of a randomized clinical trial comparing radical mastectomy and total mastectomy with or without radiation. N Engl J Med 1985; 312:674–681.

Harris JR, Hellman S, Silen W. Conservative management of breast cancer. New surgical and radiotherapeutic techniques. Philadelphia: JB Lippincott, 1983.

Strömbeck JO, Rosato FE. Surgery of the breast. Diagnosis and treatment of breast disease. Stuttgart: Thieme Verlag, 1986.

Veronesi U, Rilke F, Luini A, et al. Distribution of axillary node metastases by level of invasion. Cancer 1987; 59:682–687.

Veronesi U, Saccozzi R, Del Vecchio M, et al. Comparing radical mastectomy with quadrantectomy, axillary dissection, and radiotherapy in patients with small cancers of the breast. N Engl J Med 1981; 305:6–11.

ENDOCRINE THERAPY FOR BREAST CANCER

B. J. KENNEDY, M.D.

Hormonal therapies provide an effective means of controlling advanced breast cancer in women (Table 1). The appropriate successful selection of the various modalities can produce tumor regression, rehabilitation of the patient, and prolonged survival. Moreover, because of their effectiveness in management of advanced breast cancer, employment of hormonal therapies as adjuvant therapy has occurred.

BIOLOGIC FACTORS

The response of breast cancer to various hormonal therapies is dependent on specific biologic features of the disease and the patient. A most significant advance in endocrine therapy was the introduction of the estrogen receptor in the 1970s and subsequently the progesterone receptor. The commonly used assay is the dextrancharcoal method expressed in femtomoles per milligram of cytosol protein. Values of less than 3 are negative, values from 3 to 9 are borderline, and values over 10 are positive. The low instance of estrogen receptors in premenopausal women (29 percent) is attributed to the high endogenous estrogens that occupy the receptor sites. These receptor sites were previously thought to be in the cytoplasm but are now recognized to be in the nucleus of the cancer cell. The incidence of receptor positivity is higher in postmenopausal women (60 percent). The progesterone receptor was found to be elevated in tumors with extremely high estrogen receptors (Table 2). Tumors with progesterone receptors but no estrogen receptor are rare.

The physician must be cognizant of the pitfalls of the receptor assays. Improper handling of the tissue at the time of biopsy, lack of cancer cells in the assayed specimen, or other laboratory problems may result in a false-negative receptor report. False-positive results are less likely.

The recent introduction of the monoclonal antibody receptor assay provides additional aid in treatment selection. The procedure can be performed on small specimens (needle biopsies of liver, lung, or bone metastases but not effusions). Furthermore, the percentage of receptor-positive cells can be measured, thus expressing the degree of receptor heterogeneity of the tumor. This assay is not interfered with by the administration of estrogenic hormones or tamoxifen.

All patients are entitled to receptor assays at the time of biopsy. Assays should also be performed on biopsies of recurrent cancer, since the clone of cells in the recurrences may differ from the primary tumor. Knowledge of the receptor status provides a means of selecting the indicated hormonal therapy.

The duration of the history of the disease from mastectomy to recurrence and the duration of the metastatic disease correlate with response to endocrine therapy. A long history of slow dissemination correlates with positive receptors and favorable responses to endocrine therapy. The chronologic and menopausal ages of the patient are important because older women have a higher incidence of receptor-positive tumors and thus a higher response rate to hormonal therapy. The presence of positive receptors implies slow-growing disease. The site of metastatic disease affects the response. Soft-tissue lesions are more responsive to hormonal therapy than osseous metastases; visceral metastases are even less responsive than osseous metastases.

TABLE 1 Treatment Eras of Advanced Breast Cancer

Years	*Treatment*
1940	Endocrine therapies
1960	Single-agent chemotherapy
1970	Combination chemotherapy
1975	Receptors
	Estrogen antagonists
1980	Hormones + chemotherapy

SUCCESSIVE ENDOCRINE THERAPIES

The many hormonal factors involved in breast cancer growth are reflected in the therapeutic regulatory concepts of ablative or administered hormonal therapies. Clinical investigations have developed patterns for successive use of the hormonal therapies, depending on the biologic factors of the tumor and the observed responses to each therapy. The introduction of chemical therapies, especially combination chemotherapies with regression rates exceeding 65 percent, distracted physicians from employing hormonal therapies. With the realization that despite these high

TABLE 2 Probability of Response to Endocrine Therapy According to Estrogen and Progesterone Receptors

Receptor	*% Response to Endocrine Therapy*
ER+PR+	80
ER+PR−	35
ER−PR+	Rare tumor
ER−PR−	>5

rates the cancer was not being cured, these hormonal therapies have gained attention.

ABLATIVE HORMONAL THERAPIES

The growth of specific breast cancers depends on hormonal factors. This dependence has been demonstrated by the stimulation of growth by low doses of estrogenic hormone or regression of tumor upon withdrawal of this hormone.

Ovariectomy

In 1889, Schinzinger first proposed castration as a treatment for breast cancer. Beatson performed the first oophorectomy in 1895. In 1897, Boyd noted differing tumor responses. By 1905, Lett reported improvement in 41 percent of 75 patients under 50 years of age. Although both radiation and surgical castration produced similar results, oophorectomy is preferred because of its faster effect and assurance of total ovarian ablation.

Today, for premenopausal patients with metastatic breast cancer, bilateral salpingo-ovariectomy is still the initial endocrine treatment of choice. In patients who are unselected on the basis of estrogen receptor measurements, objective remission occurs in approximately 40 percent. The median period of remission is 9 to 12 months. The selection of patients for ovariectomy is now limited to those who have a known estrogen receptor–positive tumor. The response rate is almost double that of the rate of unselected patients. In patients with osseous metastases, a history of increased premenstrual pain is another indication of a potential responder. Castration alone is not recommended as an adjuvant therapy at the time of mastectomy.

Adrenalectomy

The beneficial effects of bilateral adrenalectomy in metastatic breast cancer have been unequivocally demonstrated. Overall, approximately 32 percent of patients treated have had an objective response to adrenalectomy. In patients responding to a prior ovariectomy, the response rates have ranged from 41 to 60 percent. Taking account of the estrogen receptor content of the tumor, for those with estrogen receptor–positive tumors, the response rate to adrenalectomy has ranged from 48 to 71 percent.

The selection of bilateral adrenalectomy as treatment of metastatic breast cancer can be aided by consideration of the prognostic factors. Factors unfavorable for adrenalectomy are as follows:

1. Site of metastases: hepatic, central nervous system, or pulmonary lymphatic spread.
2. Age under 45 years.
3. A short, disease-free interval of less than 24 months.
4. No response to prior endocrine therapy.
5. Estrogen receptor–poor tumors.

In contrast, the favorable factors for adrenalectomy are as follows:

1. Soft-tissue and osseous metastases.
2. Age over 45 years.
3. Disease-free interval of longer than 24 months.
4. Objective response to prior endocrine therapy.
5. Estrogen receptor–rich tumors.

It is apparent that if a response to oophorectomy occurred and the estrogen receptors were extremely high, more than 80 percent of these patients will respond to bilateral adrenalectomy.

Hypophysectomy

The role of hypophysectomy in advanced breast cancer is comparable to that of adrenalectomy. The major effect of hypophysectomy is the loss of adrenal function, although aldosterone production is not abolished.

The overall response rate to hypophysectomy is about 36 percent. For premenopausal patients responding to castration or postmenopausal patients responding to administered hormonal therapy, the response rates to hypophysectomy have been 55 percent in premenopausal patients and 70 percent in postmenopausal patients. This is because of the higher number of estrogen receptor–positive patients among postmenopausal women. Considering the estrogen receptor contents, the overall response rate in estrogen receptor–rich tumors was 64 percent. In postmenopausal women demonstrating a response to primary endocrine therapy and in whom the tumor is estrogen receptor–positive, response rates of greater than 80 percent occur.

A comparison of adrenalectomy and hypophysectomy showed similar response rates. Higher response rates occur in receptor–rich tumors and in patients who had responded to prior hormonal therapies. Although these ablative procedures occasionally can result in long-term responses, the use of other therapies has resulted in a marked decrease in treatment with these ablative procedures.

ADMINISTERED HORMONES

Aminoglutethimide

Aminoglutethimide has produced clinical improvement in metastatic breast cancer in postmenopausal women. Its introduction resulted in the term *medical adrenalectomy* because its effectiveness was comparable to that of adrenalectomy. Aminoglutethimide blocks estrogen synthesis by inhibiting conversion of cholesterol to pregnenolone, a major precursor of cortisol and androstenedione, the latter peripherally converted to estrone through the enzyme aromatase. The rate of response to aminoglutethimide increases if the patient had previously responded to some other form of endocrine therapy, and an even greater response rate occurs if the tumor was estrogen receptor positive. Most studies with this agent have compared its response rate (37 percent) with that of adrenalectomy and not that of hypophysectomy. Its effect could be projected to be comparable to that of hypophysectomy.

The usual dosage of aminoglutethimide is 250 mg, four times daily by mouth, plus 40 mg of hydrocortisone daily. The best selection of patients for use of this agent are those with estrogen receptor-rich tumors that respond to an initial endocrine therapy.

Adrenocorticosteroids

Before the introduction of aminoglutethimide, adrenocorticosteroids were employed in patients who were not candidates for adrenalectomy or hypophysectomy. Massive doses of oral cortisone, 300 mg a day or its equivalent, did produce objective responses in 47 percent of patients with estrogen receptor-rich tumors. However, the duration of tumor regression was shorter, and long-term use was complicated by systemic reactions.

Nevertheless, adrenocorticosteroids are helpful in aiding patients subjectively. The use of dexamethasone reduces peritumor edema in central nervous system reactions. The reduction of peritumor edema or lymphocytic infiltration about tumors results in improvement in patients with extensive lung metastases or hepatic metastases with jaundice. The adrenal corticosteroids are of greatest value as nonspecific palliative agents.

Estrogens

In women who are 4 or more years postmenopausal, the administration of estrogenic hormones in pharmacologic doses can be regarded as a primary endocrine therapy for metastatic or inoperable breast cancer. Before the era of estrogen receptors, the objective remission rate was approximately 35 percent. With selection of estrogen-rich tumors, the response rate almost doubles that figure. Remissions last several months to many years, and in the rare patient cure is regarded to have occurred.

The site of the metastatic lesions is of paramount importance. Before the employment of receptors, the objective remission rate was 55 percent for primary lesions, 40 percent for pulmonary metastases, and 22 percent for osseous metastases. The measurement of receptors added significantly to the response rate, but the difference in response by site prevails.

Castration results in improvement of breast cancer in premenopausal women, but in postmenopausal women estrogenic hormone is beneficial. It is evident that a dual, dose-related mechanism is involved. Massive doses of estrogenic hormone in premenopausal women produce tumor regression without evidence of aggravation of the disease, whereas low physiologic doses may stimulate the disease. A mechanism of this action may be a result of suppression of the pituitary gland and/or a direct effect on the stroma of the tissue or cancer cell.

The most commonly utilized estrogenic hormone is diethylstilbestrol, given 5 mg three times a day, using a nonenteric-coated tablet. Approximately 90 percent of the patients begin to improve by the end of 8 weeks, but complete regression may take several months.

Comparative studies of the use of diethylstilbestrol versus the estrogen antagonist, tamoxifen, have been carried out. The response rates are the same. Tamoxifen has fewer side effects; hence it is being used more often. However, no adequate randomized, cross-over study has been done to assess the qualitative differences between these two therapies. It has been found that in patients who respond to tamoxifen, their tumor recurrences may respond to estrogens.

Androgens

The effectiveness of the androgenic hormone depends on the site of the lesion and the age of the patient. Although it is effective in metastatic breast cancer in premenopausal women, androgens are not warranted for primary endocrine therapy in that age group in view of the superior results with castration. In patients who have responded to castration, androgenic hormone is contraindicated because the metabolic breakdown products include estrogenic hormones that might stimulate the tumor.

In postmenopausal women, the androgenic hormone is efficacious in patients with osseous metastases. At this site, the results are similar to those obtained with the estrogenic hormone but less effective in soft-tissue or pulmonary lesions.

The androgenic hormones have been used more extensively because of their subjective and metabolic effects. The anabolic effect may produce prolonged survival of patients, even though no tumor regression occurs. Androgens stimulate erythropoiesis and improve existing anemia secondary to the disease.

The most commonly employed androgen is the oral agent fluoxymesterone, 10 mg given twice a day. Long-acting parenteral agents are not recommended. Careful monitoring of serum calcium levels should be done in those with osseous metastases because of the induced hypercalcemia that may occur at the onset of therapy.

Progestins

The use of massive doses of progestins has produced regressions in 20 to 30 percent of patients. Again, treatment of receptor-rich tumors doubles this response rate. Earlier studies suggested that duration of remission is less than with estrogens. Nevertheless, it is a helpful agent, especially in elderly women who are prone to develop fluid retention with estrogens or androgens.

Medroxyprogesterone acetate, 200 mg given orally every day, or its equivalent is associated with minimal side effects.

Estrogen Antagonist, Tamoxifen

Inhibition of estrogen action at the target tissue level with the estrogen antagonist, tamoxifen, has proved highly successful in the treatment of hormone-responsive breast cancer. In randomized clinical trials of postmenopausal patients, tamoxifen was as effective as high-dose estrogens, androgens, progestins, or aminoglutethimide. However, because of its lack of significant toxicity, tamoxifen is used as the first endocrine treatment of hormone-responsive postmenopausal breast cancer. The dosage is 10 mg given twice a day.

In premenopausal patients, tamoxifen cannot be considered a substitute for ovariectomy because it does not suppress menses and because response to castration does occur after progression during estrogen antagonist therapy. Further, the evidence suggests that combining tamoxifen with other endocrine therapies or chemotherapy offers no advantage.

Sequential endocrine therapy is highly effective in women with hormone-responsive breast cancer, and it can significantly prolong survival. When tamoxifen is employed initially, following relapse, proven effective sequential therapy consists of aminoglutethimide, androgens, and progestational agents. In a randomized study of tamoxifen versus hypophysectomy, use of the latter initially was more effective overall. With replacement of the ablative procedure by amnioglutethimide, this may be the choice for a second hormonal therapy. Which sequence of agents is most effective has yet to be established.

Multiple Endocrine Therapies

The successive employment of multiple endocrine therapies has been emphasized as a means of long-term control of breast cancer before cytotoxic chemotherapy is used. In a study in which patients received two or more endocrine treatments, as the number of successive endocrine therapies increased, the response rate decreased. In that study, the survival of this group of patients was over 7 years from the onset of endocrine therapy (Table 3). With successive endocrine therapies, the duration of response also decreased.

TABLE 3 Response Rates in 69 Patients Receiving Two or More Endocrine Therapies

No. of Therapies	*Response Rate (%)*
1	65
2	43
3	30
4	16
5	0

COMBINED ENDOCRINE THERAPY AND CHEMOTHERAPY

The combined use of chemotherapy and endocrine therapy has been advocated ever since these modalities demonstrated benefit in the treatment of breast cancer. The pharmacologic modes of action are different, and development of cross-resistance seems unlikely. Numerous trials comparing concurrent chemoendocrine therapy with successive uses of endocrine therapy and chemotherapy have shown an occasionally higher initial response rate with the combined treatments but no overall improvement in survival. The lack of benefit may be a result of the failure to take into account the estrogen receptor information.

Combinations of oophorectomy and chemotherapy showed a higher initial response rate, but this was not superior to that of oophorectomy alone followed by chemotherapy upon failure. In studying a subset of postmenopausal patients with estrogen receptor–positive tumors, an overall survival advantage was noted with concurrent use of diethylstilbestrol, 5-fluorouracil, and cyclophosphamide over the use of the hormone alone followed later by the same chemotherapy when the disease progressed. This emphasizes the increasing awareness that subsets of breast cancer must be considered in selecting therapies. Another study using tamoxifen in the chemoendocrine therapy showed no benefit. Hence, even which agents are compared is important.

Continuing studies of chemoendocrine therapy are being pursued. Since hormonal therapies require estrogen receptor–positive tumors, the maximal benefit from chemoendocrine therapy is apparent if the patients with estrogen receptor–positive tumors are selected for study. The inclusion of estrogen receptor–negative tumors masks any beneficial effects of the combination chemotherapy. There is continuing evidence that some interactions between cytotoxic and hormonal agents are inhibitory. These need to be avoided.

ADJUVANT ENDOCRINE THERAPY

The use of adjuvant endocrine therapies began with ovariectomy as a "prophylactic" castration to prevent the recurrence of the disease in premenopausal women. Most studies were done before estrogen receptors were measured. Although ovariectomy at the time of initial mastectomy delayed the onset of recurrence of the disease, the overall survival rate was not different from that of patients in whom ovariectomy was employed at the time of recurrence. It seems apparent that the ovariectomy procedure had an inhibitory effect on cancer cells, regardless of when the procedure was performed. Understanding of the importance of the receptors has resurrected interest in the role of ovariectomy as an adjuvant therapy. Attempts to conduct this in combination with chemotherapy have not been successful; in fact, the combination of ovariectomy and chemotherapy may be detrimental.

Success of adjuvant therapy depends on the delay of onset of recurrence and on increasing the total survival rate over that of patients in whom no adjuvant therapy is employed but appropriate anticancer therapy is employed using agents similar to those in the adjuvant setting if cancer recurs.

Adjuvant chemotherapy and hormonal therapy are effective treatments for breast cancer patients. Because of information that demonstrates prolonged survival, the following statements can be made:

1. For premenopausal women with positive nodes, regardless of hormone receptor status, treatment with combination chemotherapy has become a standard of care using cyclophosphamide (cytoxan), methotrexate, and 5-fluorouracil (CMF) or CAF (A = Adriamycin or doxorubicin).
2. For premenopausal women with positive nodes and estrogen receptor–positive cancer, the adjuvant chemotherapy could be followed by tamoxifen therapy.
3. For postmenopausal women with positive nodes and positive hormone receptor levels, tamoxifen is the treatment of choice.
4. For postmenopausal women with positive nodes and negative hormone receptor levels, chemotherapy may be considered, especially with the patient as a participant in controlled clinical trials.
5. There has been much controversy regarding the treatment of node-negative patients. Part of the confusion is that data combined stage I and stage II breast cancer patients. Since lesions larger than 2 cm in diameter belong to the stage II category, it would be reasonable to follow the same therapeutic recommendations as defined above in node-positive patients.
6. In lesions smaller than 1 cm, the cure rate from surgery or surgery plus radiotherapy is very high. Since the clinical data to date describe only a prolonged disease-free interval and no benefit in survival, adjuvant therapy in these patients is not a standard procedure.
7. For patients with lesions that are 1 to 2 cm, entering into clinical trials is encouraged, since the initial data only demonstrated prolonged disease-free intervals but no survival times. The results of the earlier studies are incomplete with respect to survival.

TABLE 4 Sequence of Therapies in Advanced Breast Cancer

Phase	*Premenopausal*	*Postmenopausal*
I	Castration	Tamoxifen Progestogens Estrogens
II	a. Adrenalectomy or hypophysectomy or glucocorticoids or aminoglutethimide b. Androgens	
III	Chemotherapy	Chemotherapy

Endocrine therapies have an established role in the management of breast cancer. New concepts about their use as adjuvant treatments are being defined, although their role has not been clearly established. The sequence for endocrine therapies in advanced breast cancer can be established for those patients with receptor-positive tumors (Table 4). Careful study of the receptor status at all stages of the breast cancer, the menopausal age, and the site of metastases plays a significant role in the specific selection of endocrine therapies. They should be carefully considered before combination chemotherapies are used.

SUGGESTED READING

Henderson IC. Adjuvant chemotherapy and endocrine therapy in patients with operable breast cancer. Update 1987; 1:1–14.

Kennedy BJ. Current status of adjuvant endocrine therapy for resectable breast cancer. Semin Oncol 1974; 1:119–130.

Kennedy BJ, ed. Breast cancer. Current Clinical Oncology series. New York: Alan R. Liss, 1990.

Kiang DT, Gay J, Goldman A, Kennedy BJ. A randomized trial of chemotherapy and hormonal therapy in advanced breast cancer. N Engl J Med 1985; 313:1241–1246.

Manni A. Tamoxifen therapy of metastatic breast cancer. Lab Clin Med 1987; 109:290–299.
Pritchard KI. Current status of adjuvant endocrine therapy for resectable breast cancer. Semin Oncol 1982; 14:23–33.
Rausch D, Kiang DT. Interaction between endocrine and cytotoxic therapy. In: Stoll BA, ed. Contemporary endocrine therapy in cancer. Basel, Switzerland: S Karger, 1988.
Santen RJ, Boucher AE, Sautner SJ, et al. Inhibition of aromatase as treatment of breast carcinoma in postmenopausal women. Lab Clin Med 1987; 109:278–289.

CHEMOTHERAPY FOR BREAST CANCER

MARTIN D. ABELOFF, M.D.

Breast cancer is one of the most responsive solid tumors to cytotoxic chemotherapy. In the adjuvant setting, combination chemotherapy can provide the opportunity for cure to perhaps 20 percent of patients who would otherwise eventually develop metastatic disease and succumb to breast cancer. Combination chemotherapy can result in significant resolution of tumor masses in 50 to 60 percent of patients with already established metastatic disease, thereby bringing about palliation of symptoms and prolonging life in a small percentage of patients. Before discussing chemotherapy as adjuvant treatment and as therapy for locally advanced and widespread metastatic disease, some general concepts of cytotoxic chemotherapy for breast cancer are reviewed.

GENERAL CONCEPTS

A considerable number of single agents can achieve a 15 to 20 percent objective response rate in patients with measurable metastatic breast cancer. As noted in Table 1, this list of active agents includes representatives from the major categories of cytotoxic drugs. The different spectra of toxicities and the additive (or perhaps synergistic) therapeutic effects allow these drugs to be used most effectively in combination regimens. The most commonly used combinations are outlined in Table 2. Recent studies have indicated that cisplatinum and etoposide may also be an effective combination in breast cancer. Only rarely is single-agent chemotherapy employed in the management of breast cancer.

Clinical data strongly suggests that the response of breast cancer to combination chemotherapy is closely correlated to the dose intensity of treatment, i.e., the amount of drugs delivered per unit of time. It is essential that the effective regimens (see Table 2) be administered at the full dosage of chemotherapy. If hematologic or other toxicities preclude the delivery of the full dosage of chemotherapy, it is common practice to delay therapy for a brief period rather than reduce the doses.

The delivery of the planned doses of chemotherapy has been facilitated by significant improvement in our ability to prevent or ameloriate adverse effects. This is particularly evident in the improved management of nausea and vomiting with antiemetics such as corticosteroids, metoclopramide, and phenothiazines. In fact, anticipatory nausea and vomiting (which occurs before chemotherapy is administered) have also significantly decreased in frequency, probably as a result of more effective antiemetics.

TABLE 1 Active Drugs in Breast Cancer and Major Toxicities

Agents	*Patterns of Toxicity*								
	Cardiac	*Gastro-intestinal*	*Hair Loss*	*Hematologic*	*Neurologic*	*Pulmonary*	*Renal*	*Repro-ductive*	*Tissue Injury Due to Extravasation*
Alkylating agents									
Cytoxan		X	X	X				X	
Alkeran		X		X				X	
Thiotepa		X		X				X	
Mitomycin		X		X		X	X	X	X
Anthracycline									
Adriamycin	X	X	X	X					X
Vinca alkaloids									
Vincristine			X		X				X
Vinblastine			X	X	X				X
Antimetabolites									
Methotrexate		X		X			X	X	
5-Fluorouracil		X		X	X				

TABLE 2 Combination Chemotherapy Regimens

	Agents	Dose		
First Line				
CMF	cyclophosphamide	100 mg/M^2 PO days 1–14		600 mg/M^2 IV day 1
	methotrexate	40 mg/M^2 IV days 1 + 8	or	40 mg/M^2 IV day 1
	5-fluorouracil	600 mg/M^2 IV days 1 + 8		600 mg/M^2 IV day 1
		Repeat every 4 weeks		Repeat every 3 weeks
CAF	cyclophosphamide	100 mg/M^2 PO days 1–14		500 mg/M^2 IV day 1
	Adriamycin	30 mg/M^2 IV days 1 + 8	or	50 mg/M^2 IV day 1
	5-fluorouracil	500 mg/M^2 IV days 1 + 8		500 mg/M^2 IV day 1
		Repeat every 4 weeks		Repeat every 3 weeks
CMFVP "Cooper" continuous	cyclophosphamide	80 mg/M^2 PO daily		
	methotrexate	40 mg/M^2 IV weekly		
	5-fluorouracil	500 mg/M^2 IV weekly		
	vincristine	1.0 mg/M^2 IV weekly (maximum dose 2.0 mg per injection)		
	prednisone	30 mg/M^2 PO daily for 21 days, then taper to 0 over 7 days		
		Continue for 12 weeks; after a 2-week break, maintenance therapy		
CMFVP continuous "SWOG"	cyclophosphamide	60 mg/M^2 PO daily		
	methotrexate	15 mg/M^2 IV weekly		
	5-fluorouracil	300 mg/M^2 IV weekly		
	vincristine	0.625 mg/M^2 IV weekly for 10 weeks, then discontinue		
	prednisone	30 mg/M^2 PO days 1–14		
		20 mg/M^2 PO days 15–28		
		10 mg/M^2 daily days 29–42 then discontinue		
Second Line				
AV	Adriamycin	60 mg/M^2 IV day 1		
	vincristine	1.2 mg/M^2 IV day 1 (maximum dose 2 mg/injection)		
TAV	thiotepa	12 mg/M^2 IV day 1		
	Adriamycin	45 mg/M^2 IV day 1		
	vinblastine	4.5 mg/M^2 IV day 1		
		Repeat every 3 weeks		
MV	mitomycin	20 mg/M^2 IV day 1		
	vinblastine	0.15 mg/kg IV day 1 and day 21		
		Repeat every 6–8 weeks		

ADJUVANT THERAPY

Considerable progress has been made in the last decade in the adjuvant therapy of breast cancer. Based on considerable data from large phase III clinical trials and an overview analysis of available published and unpublished data, the Consensus Development Panel in December 1985 recommended combination chemotherapy as standard therapy for premenopausal patients with histologically positive axillary lymph nodes, regardless of hormonal receptor status. For postmenopausal patients with positive axillary lymph nodes and positive estrogen receptors, the panel recommended use of the antiestrogen tamoxifen as standard care.

Considerable controversy still remains regarding the role of adjuvant chemotherapy for postmenopausal patients with stage II estrogen receptor negative disease. Although the Consensus Development Panel did not recommend cytotoxic chemotherapy as standard practice for these patients, there is enough evidence for a therapeutic effect of adjuvant chemotherapy in postmenopausal patients that such treatment should at least be offered as an option to this group of patients. As was stated repeatedly in the Consensus Development Conference summary, adjuvant chemotherapy should be delivered whenever possible as part of a controlled clinical trial.

There is increasing evidence that adjuvant chemotherapy and antiestrogen therapy are also effective for patients with stage I disease (i.e., node negative) who are at greatest risk for recurrence. Clinical trials are underway to identify the optimal treatment regimens and to assess relative roles of chemotherapy and endocrine therapy.

One of the most significant developments in the management of breast cancer has been the refined ability to select patients most likely to develop recurrent or metastatic disease, and perhaps most likely to benefit from adjuvant therapy. Prognostic factors that indicate a high risk of recurrence include (1) histologically positive axillary nodes with the worst outlook for patients with 10 or more involved nodes, (2) large primary tumor, i.e., pathologic size greater than 3 cm, (3) undifferentiated cancer, as manifested by high nuclear grade, (4) high proliferative capacity, as indicated by a large proportion of cells in S phase and marked aneuploidy or high thymidine labeling index, and (5) negative estrogen and progesterone receptors. A number of biologic parameters are being assessed as prognostic factors including oncogene amplification and expression, growth factor receptors, and protein markers such as cathepsin.

The optimal adjuvant therapeutic regimen has not been established, but certainly the greatest experience has been gained with the CMF, CMFVP, and CAF regimens (see Table 2). Adriamycin-containing regimens have not yet been clearly demonstrated to be better than other adjuvant combinations, but it is reasonable in the non-protocol setting to treat more aggressive disease with the chemotherapy that is most effective in metastatic disease (i.e., Adriamycin-based chemotherapy). Likewise, the optimal duration of therapy is not known, but the evidence suggests that continuing therapy beyond 6 months or (six cycles) of CMF or CAF and 1 year of CMFVP may not give any added benefit. The importance of dose intensity has been further supported by some randomized studies in which therapies of longer duration appear less efficacious than shorter-duration regimens, perhaps because of dose attenuations in the lengthier treatments.

Concepts currently receiving considerable attention in prospective trials of adjuvant therapy include preoperative or perioperative chemotherapy; and increasing dose intensity with weekly multiagent therapy, high dose methotrexate with leukovorin rescue, or 5-fluorouracil infusions. The concept of synchronizing DNA synthesis with endocrine therapy (recruitment) to increase the susceptibility of breast cancer to cytotoxic chemotherapy is being examined in randomized trials. Currently there is no clear-cut evidence that combined chemohormonotherapy is better than either modality alone, but this is still under investigation.

The spectrum of toxicities of chemotherapy (see Table 1) in the adjuvant setting is similar to that in patients with metastatic disease. However, Adriamycin cardiotoxicity is rarely a problem because the total dose of drug (550 mg per square meter) that results in cardiac damage is generally not reached with the shorter-duration (6 months of chemotherapy) adjuvant regimens. The reproductive and endocrine effects of cytotoxic drugs are of particular concern to the patients receiving adjuvant therapy. There is a significant incidence of drug-induced amenorrhea in premenopausal patients, particularly in those over 40 years of age at the time of adjuvant therapy. Menopausal symptoms (hot flashes, vaginal dryness) and questions regarding osteoporosis are frequent concerns of those patients. Estrogen replacement therapy (oral or topical) cannot be recommended in these women; menopausal symptoms are treated symptomatically and supplemental calcium plus exercise is advised as prophylaxis for osteoporosis.

THERAPY FOR LOCALLY ADVANCED DISEASE

The challenge of the management of locally advanced breast cancer is to offer therapy that prevents devastating local complications yet offers the chance of long-term survival by eradicating micrometastases. Patients with technically resectable disease (stage IIIa) should undergo surgical removal of the primary tumor followed by radiation therapy and combination chemotherapy. For patients with technically unresectable disease and/or inflammatory breast cancer (stage IIIb), neoadjuvant or preoperative chemotherapy appears to be the treatment of choice. If the tumor responds adequately to systemic chemotherapy, surgery and/or radiation therapy can then be employed. The optimal integration of chemotherapy, surgery, and radiotherapy has yet to be established, but there is ample evidence that combination chemotherapy can be given, with relatively modest dose modifications, concomitantly with external beam radiation therapy. This type of combined modality therapy, however, requires the attention of experienced medical, radiation, and surgical oncologists.

METASTATIC DISEASE

Although systemic chemotherapy can result in substantial increase in disease-free survival and/or cure for patients with stage I, II, or III breast cancer, such cytotoxic therapy virtually never results in cure in patients with widespread metastases. In addition, some degree of adverse effects (physical, psychological, economic) is probable with combination chemotherapy in patients with advanced disease. Therefore, the decision whether or not to initiate combination chemotherapy for metastatic disease requires an in-depth understanding of the natural history of breast cancer, response data to specific chemotherapy regimens, and appreciation of the toxicity of the available regimen.

Factors that indicate combination chemotherapy should be seriously considered for patients with metastatic disease include (1) estrogen and progesterone receptor negativity, (2) failure to respond to prior endocrine therapy, (3) short disease-free interval of less than 2 years from the time of primary therapy, (4) rapidly progressive metastatic disease, and (5) visceral involvement, particularly hepatic involvement, lymphangitic pulmonary disease, or multiple symptomatic pulmonary nodules. For example, systemic chemotherapy would certainly be the treatment of choice for a young patient with widespread visceral metastases with a short disease-free interval and a receptor negative tumor. An elderly patient with a hormone receptor positive chest wall recurrence after a long disease-free interval would generally not be considered for chemotherapy at that juncture, but would be a more appropriate candidate for local therapy (surgery and/or radiation therapy) in conjunction with endocrine treatment. There are obviously many shades of grey between these two rather extreme examples. Because systemic therapy does not cure metastatic disease, but can provide significant palliation of symptoms and sometimes prolongation of survival, the decision to initiate such therapy requires careful evaluation with the patient and family of the risk/benefit ratio.

Patients who have received chemotherapy, and subsequently relapsed after a disease-free interval of greater than 1 year from the completion of therapy, may respond well to either the same chemotherapeutic regimen or an alternative combination. However, patients who progress during their first-line chemotherapy for metastatic disease or relapse shortly after an initial response generally do not do well. The use of alternative combinations as salvage therapy for patients who failed first-line chemotherapy for metastatic disease must be considered in the context of the patient's general medical status. The response rates of salvage regimens are generally much worse for patients who have received multiple regimens, have poor performance status, have impaired bone marrow function, and have extensive and rapidly progressive visceral disease.

Patients who have not received an Adriamycin-containing regimen as first-line chemotherapy for their metastatic disease generally receive an Adriamycin plus vincristine combination or thiotepa-Adriamycin-Velban (TAV) as their salvage regimen. Patients who have previously received CMF or CMFVP and an Adriamycin-containing regimen have been shown to respond to a mitomycin-Velban combination. However, the toxicities of mitomycin must be seriously considered. Mitomycin can cause prolonged cytopenias, particularly thrombocytopenia, can result in severe tissue necrosis even if slight infiltration occurs, and has been associated with a hemolytic uremic syndrome with hematologic and renal sequelae.

For the patient who is not a good candidate for second- or third-line chemotherapy for metastatic breast cancer, palliation can be achieved by (1) local radiation therapy to painful bony lesions, soft tissue masses, or lesions causing nerve compression, (2) chest tube drainage with installation of sclerosing agents to relieve symptoms secondary to malignant pleural effusion, or (3) judicious use of narcotics and anti-inflammatory agents to relieve pain. There is also a variety of pharmacologic methods of treating hypercalcemia, including mithramycin, calcitonin, diphosphonates, and corticosteroids.

SUGGESTED READING

Bonadonna G. Karnofsky Memorial Lecture: conceptual and practical advances in the management of breast cancer. J Clin Oncol 1989; 7:1380–1397.

Consensus Conference. Adjuvant chemotherapy for breast cancer. JAMA 1985; 254:3461.

Hyrniuk W, Bush H. The importance of dose intensity in chemotherapy of metastatic breast cancer. J Clin Oncol 1984; 2:1281–1288.

Proceedings of NIH Consensus Development Conference on Adjuvant Chemotherapy and Endocrine Therapy for Breast Cancer. NCI Monograph No 1, 1986.

Rouesse J, Friedman S, Sarragin D, et al. Primary chemotherapy in the treatment of inflammatory breast carcinoma: a study of 230 cases from the Institut Gustave-Roussy. J Clin Oncol 1986; 4:1765–1771.

RADIATION THERAPY FOR BREAST CANCER

RICHARD A. STEEVES, M.D., Ph. D.

Radiation therapy is very effective in the treatment of breast cancer. In this chapter, I will focus on its use with curative intent, such as after mastectomy or after surgical removal of the primary tumor alone and with breast conservation. The indications for adjuvant radiation therapy after modified radical mastectomy are not well defined. Many different factors have to be weighed against one another, such as the size, location, and grade of the primary tumor; the number of metastatic axillary nodes removed; whether or not there is extranodal extension of tumor; as well as the age and general health of the patient. While controversy surrounds the question of whether radiation therapy increases the duration of life, there is general agreement that, when grave signs suggest a high likelihood of recurrence, radiation can reduce the risk of recurrence, and may thereby improve the quality of life.

In contrast, when the breast has been conserved, there is little or no argument that it should be irradiated within 2 or 3 weeks of excision of an infiltrating ductal adenocarcinoma. Some might argue that lobular carcinomas in situ or intraductal carcinomas do not need irradiation post excision, but even with these early neoplasms, recurrence rates are so high (20 to 30 percent within 10 years) that radiation is usually recommended for all but the very elderly patient.

The only absolute contraindications against breast irradiation are conditions affecting DNA repair, such as xeroderma pigmentosum. However, there are a number of situations in which prudence should dictate a delay. Perhaps the most common of these is the premenopausal, node-positive patient who is willing to accept adjuvant cytotoxic chemotherapy. In my opinion, such patients should receive systemic therapy as soon as possible after surgery while the theoretical tumor burden is low. These patients should be referred back for radiation as soon as the chemotherapy has been delivered. A much rarer problem is delayed healing at the tumorectomy site or diffuse mastitis following surgery. The radiation oncologist should not be rushed into treating these patients, in spite of the threat of tumor cell growth, and mastectomy may need to be considered if surgical complications cause delayed healing. Multicentric carcinomas or Paget's disease may also require that a mastectomy be performed if all primary malignancies cannot be located and excised.

Finally, we have to appreciate that the size and location of the primary breast cancer does influence the therapeutic options. When is a tumor too big for treatment by tumorectomy plus radiation? The answer ultimately depends on the size of the breast in which the cancer arose. Most surgeons find that tumors occupying more than a quarter of the breast cannot be excised without leaving such a distorted breast that mastectomy would have been cosmetically preferable. Location also plays a role, in that lower inner quadrant tumorectomies often give rise to the poorest cosmetic results.

ANALYSIS OF STAGE, HISTOLOGY, AND SURGICAL MARGINS

The staging is primarily surgical, because clinical judgments of both tumor size and axillary metastases are known to be unreliable. Much emphasis, therefore, is placed on detailed communication with the pathologist regarding the size of the primary tumor, the proximity of the margins, and the extent of involvement of the axillary nodes. Since other factors such as the degree of anaplasia or infiltration by lymphocytes are also of prognostic significance, it is ideal to personally review the slides with the pathologist. This is not meant to lessen the value of a thorough physical examination, for a supraclavicular metastasis that is either not clinically palpable or not detected preoperatively drastically alters the prognosis as well as the treatment plan. Careful assessment is needed of the rate of healing of the surgical scar, the volume of induration or hematoma in the remainder of the affected breast, any arm swelling, as well as a comparison with the opposite breast. A review of the preoperative mammogram, chest x-ray, liver function tests, and bone scan usually completes the staging analysis.

Occasionally, a breast cancer patient is referred for a second opinion after a limited excisional biopsy only, without surgical assessment of her axilla. If she elects to conserve her breast, she should be advised of possible reexcision of the tumor bed around the biopsy site, especially if the margins were not assessed or were not adequate (minimum of 1 cm of normal breast tissue). She should also be informed about the importance of either an axillary dissection or an axillary sampling. There is considerable controversy over which of the two axillary procedures is better. Because axillary metastases are known to skip the lower (level 1) nodes 25 percent of the time, I prefer an axillary dissection that includes not only level 1 but also level 2 nodes (i.e., those behind the pectoralis minor insertion). Only with this procedure can a node-negative axilla and the supraclavicular region be shielded with confidence. Thus, it is not only a better staging procedure, but it offers the potential of sparing a considerable volume of normal tissue from unnecessary radiation.

Another area that is often left unirradiated in axillary node-negative women is the internal mammary node region. However, if such women have central or medial lesions, they still have a 10 percent chance of harboring internal mammary node metastases. Surgical assessment of these nodes is difficult and occasionally hazardous, but radiologic assessment via lymphoscintigraphy is rapidly becoming a simple and routine procedure. Based on the uptake of colloidal ^{99}Te after injection into the rectus abdominis muscle, lymphoscintigraphy provides not only a prognostic assessment equivalent to that of axillary dissection, but also provides the anatomic localization of these nodes to aid in the design of radiation portals that will encompass them. A summary of our treatment policy at the University of Wisconsin is given in Table 1.

SETTING UP TREATMENT FIELDS

Once the work-up outlined above has been completed, the tissue volumes to be treated can be defined as shown in Figure 1. The use of a CT scanner for this purpose is very helpful for improving the precision of dose delivery and for reducing the chance of a so-called geographic miss. This is especially true for the internal mammary nodes, which can be treated by any of four different techniques, depending on whether photons or electrons are used and on whether a direct appositional or an obliquely angled beam is used. Each technique has its advantages and disadvantages. For example, the once popular appositional photon field is used less often now, especially for cancers of the left breast, because of the possibility of cardiac damage in women who may also receive Adriamycin. Better definition of these nodes by lymphoscintigraphy and CT scanning fre-

TABLE 1 Selection of Treatment Areas Based on Clinical Variables*

Location of Primary Tumor (Quadrant)	*Axillary Node Status (Microscopic Evaluation)*	*IMN Status (Lymphoscintigraphy)*	*Treatment Areas*
Outer	−	Often not done	Breast only
Central or inner	−	Normal	Breast + IMN
Central or inner	−	Abnormal	Breast + IMN + SCN
Outer	+	Normal	Breast + SCN + upper axilla
Central or inner	+	Normal }	Breast + IMN + SCN + upper axilla
Any location	+	Abnormal }	

* Abbreviations: IMN = internal mammary nodes
SCN = supraventricular nodes

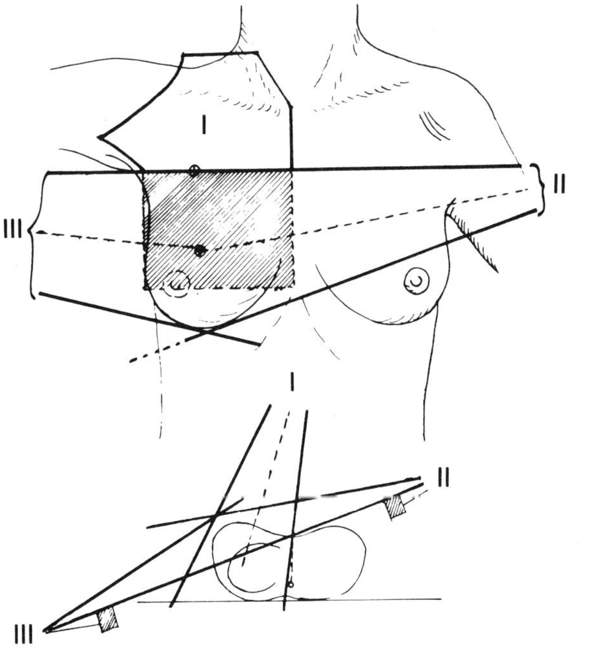

Figure 1 Breast and lymph node regions irradiated in a 3-field treatment geometry are illustrated in coronal and cross sectional projections. Half-beam blocks are shown as shaded areas. I = supraclavicular field; II = medial tangential field to the right breast; III = lateral tangential field to the right breast.

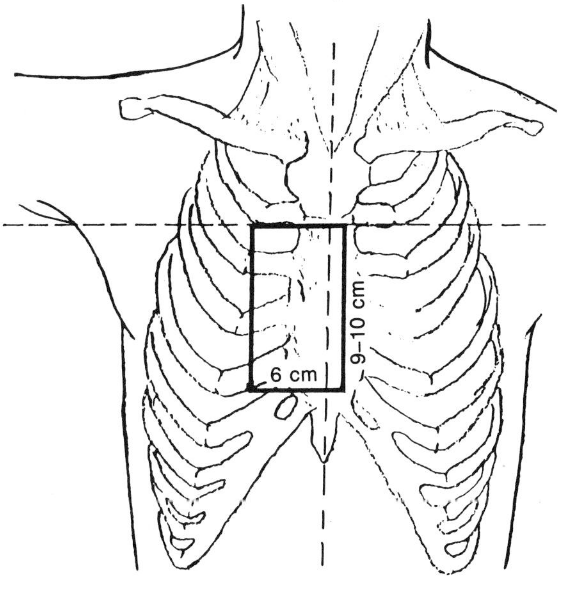

Figure 2 Appositional field used to treat the internal mammary nodes, as related to the sternum and anterior rib cage. The medial border usually extends 1 cm across the midline, and the superior border matches the inferior border of the supraclavicular field, usually near the angle of Louis. The field size is generally 6 by 9 to 10 cm, but this may be modified, as indicated by the results of internal mammary lymphoscintigraphy.

quently allows their inclusion with greater confidence in the tangential beams to the breast and chest wall. This causes less damage to the myocardium and esophagus and less chance of recurrence or rib fracture from underdosing or overdosing, respectively, tissues along the match line between the internal mammary and medial tangential fields.

If the internal mammary nodes are to be treated but not encompassed in the tangential beams, then an appositional field is usually chosen, with borders as shown in Figure 2. These borders may need to be modified after reviewing the lymphoscintigram. I prefer to treat this region with a mixed beam that is composed of 40 percent 1 to 4 MV photons and 60 percent 12 MeV electrons to reduce damage to the myocardium and esophagus (that would result from 100 percent photons) without causing the intense dermatitis and subsequent telangiectasia in the skin (that would result from 100 percent electrons).

The CT scanner is helpful in setting up the tangential fields. Barium filled catheters may be taped to the skin along the anticipated beam margins and adjusted as necessary on the computer display. For example, a treatment beam along the line shown in Figure 3 would spare most of the right lung, but would also miss most of the internal mammary nodes. This type of analysis also aids in calculating any tissue inhomogeneity corrections needed and in planning the design of wedge compensators. To eliminate beam divergence into the lung, half-beam blocking is often used. A half-beam block tailored to the patient's rib cage outline with cerrobend shields more lung than the typical linear block. In addition, it is preferable to angle the longitudinal axis of the treatment couch so that the superior border of each tangential beam does not diverge into the supraclavicular field (see Fig. 1). This improves the cosmetic result and reduces the chance of a rib fracture.

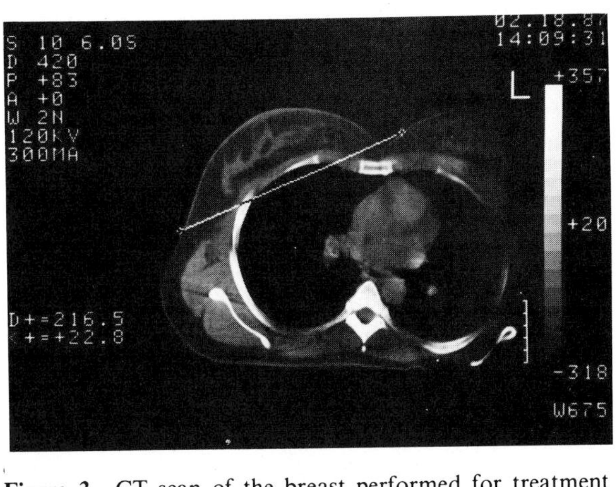

Figure 3 CT scan of the breast performed for treatment planning. Note the barium filled catheters taped over the preliminary skin markings left of the anterior midline and in the axilla.

The most superior lymph nodes in the internal mammary, supraclavicular, and axillary regions are readily encompassed in a single anterior field, the lower half of which is blocked to avoid divergence into the tangential fields as shown in Figure 1. If the medial border of this field is near the patient's midline. lateral angulation of the beam by 15 degrees usually prevents significant radiation of the esophagus and spinal cord. If the surgeon has dissected the axilla enough to remove nodes from level 2 and has left clips at the limit of the dissection, it is wise to shield the axilla distal to the uppermost clips. However, the dose to the upper axilla lags behind the dose to the superficial supraclavicular tissues unless a posterior axillary field is used to give a consistent dose to all areas at risk.

The doses generally used to treat these regions are 50 Gy in 25 fractions over a period of 5 weeks, although slightly lower doses (46 to 48 Gy) in 1.8 Gy fractions are often used if the patient has recently completed cytotoxic chemotherapy. The energy of the photon beam can range from 1 to 6 MV. Cobalt γ-rays have become less popular recently because they are less skin sparing than higher energy x-ray beams. However, the much sharper penumbra associated with x-rays can lead to greater variations in dose along the match lines unless great care is taken with each treatment set-up. Bolusing the skin is not usually needed with cobalt, but may be indicated more often with higher energy x-rays, especially if there has been invasion of the dermal lymphatic vessels. Treatment of all fields each day is essential for good cosmetic results.

TECHNIQUES FOR BOOSTING THE TUMOR BED

If the margins of resection were negative, the bed from which the tumor was excised is usually boosted to 60 Gy. Deep lesion sites are best treated with photon therapy through coned tangential portals, whereas superficial lesion sites can be encompassed with a minimum volume of normal tissue through the use of shaped electron fields. However, if there is any question about the absence of carcinoma cells within a centimeter of the resected margin, then doses of 70 to 75 Gy are preferred. Boost doses of this magnitude cannot be given by external beam with satisfactory cosmetic results, so the dose is delivered with a 2- or 3-plane intersitital implant that is after-loaded with iridium 192. The dose rate is usually 0.4 to 0.5 Gy per hour so that the entire boost dose can be given over a 2- to 3-day period. If care is taken to place the most superficial iridium seeds at least 1 cm deep from the skin, a good cosmetic result is still feasible.

FOLLOW-UP EVALUATION

Critical for effective follow-up by both physical examination and mammography is the use of a baseline examination to document the effects of treatment, such as a defect in the breast tissue from surgery or localized induration around the tumor bed from surgical and radiation scarring. A subsequent change in the physical findings is most important. Certain changes, such as focal areas of fat necrosis within the electron boost portal or fibrosis along a radiation field matchline, can be followed carefully without resorting to a biopsy in an area that may be slow to heal. A small percentage of patients may suddenly develop an inflammatory episode 6 months or so after radiation therapy. Such patients may notice warmth, tenderness, and limited motion in the treated area, particularly in the pectoral muscles. Not to be confused with recurrence or infection, these symptoms generally last for a few weeks and appear to be improved by conservative measures such as aspirin and gentle stretching exercises.

Other complications, such as radiation pneumonitis, pericarditis, or brachial neuropathy, are rare in our experience and are reported among published reports in 0.5 to 2.0 percent of patients. Precise technique and careful attention to detail is required to maintain a low risk of such complications.

The question of radiation carcinogenesis is a complex issue because its incidence must be compared with the natural incidence, not with zero incidence, and the latent period for radiation-induced cancer is long. In addition, there has been inadequate follow-up of a sufficient number of early breast cancer patients following radiation therapy. With regard to the risk of tumor induction in the contralateral breast, it must be remembered that patients with breast cancer are already at increased risk of developing contralateral disease: this is estimated to be 0.5 to 1 percent per year over 20 to 30 years. It is worth noting that among a large number of women irradiated postmastectomy at the Ontario Cancer Foundation in London, the incidence of nonsynchronous cancer in the contralateral breast was the same: 1 percent per year for 20 years of follow-up.

Finally, the cosmetic results are important to record during follow-up, but, unfortunately, there are no uniformly accepted criteria by which to do so. At the University of Wisconsin, we have used the criteria shown in Table 2 to develop more consistent scoring among examiners. We now have 45 patients followed for a minimum of 5 years; our results appear to be similar to those of several others who give no more than 50 Gy to the entire breast, i.e., 80 to 90 percent are judged to have good to excellent results. In general, patients are less critical than their oncologists since, from the patient's perspective, the most important thing is that her breast is retained.

COMBINATION OF BREAST IRRADIATION AND CHEMOTHERAPY

Recent studies from several cancer centers show that the benefits of adjuvant chemotherapy can be applied to conservative surgery and radiation as well as to mastectomy. Opinions still differ, however, regarding the preferred sequence for these two modalities. If the

TABLE 2 Criteria for Scoring Cosmetic Results

A Effects of surgery	
0 Scar unapparent	
1 Scar apparent	
2 Major tissue loss	
B Effects of radiation	
0 None 1 Slight 2 Moderate 3 Severe	skin changes (diffuse or along matchlines) fibrosis (diffuse or focal) retraction of the breast
C Photographic assessment	
1 Excellent—hard to distinguish treated from untreated breast	
2 Good—treated breast slightly different from untreated breast	
3 Fair—treated breast clearly different from untreated breast	
4 Poor—treated breast seriously distorted	

Added scores from all three categories above range from 1 (excellent) to 4 (good) to 9 (worst case).

radiation is administered first, the blood counts may drop more severely during chemotherapy, and the doses as well as the effectiveness of the latter could be compromised. If the chemotherapy and radiotherapy are given concomitantly, there is often a more brisk, acute skin reaction within the irradiated areas and some compromise in the overall cosmetic result. At the University of Wisconsin, we prefer to give all of the chemotherapy first, followed by radiotherapy. While the delayed radiation could theoretically lead to an increased risk of tumor recurrence, we have not seen evidence to support this so far. Severe skin reactions and poor cosmetic results have generally been avoided by treating the whole breast only to 46 Gy, as discussed earlier. Special attention is given to planning the internal mammary node field, especially in women with left sided breast cancers who have received Adriamycin.

GENERAL REMARKS

It is all very well to be able to offer equivalent therapy that preserves most of the breast, but we cannot be complacent about marginal improvements in the survival of breast cancer patients, about continuing difficulties in accurate staging of patients, or about the need for optimal integration of multimodal forms of therapy.

We must also remember that breast cancer has a strong tendency to be multicentric. Gross tumor excision alone, as applied at the University of Toronto, resulted in a 25 percent recurrence rate even in patients with favorable lesions; thus it is important to irradiate the entire breast. Identification of patients with the highest likelihood of local failure is also important. Patients whose tumors have a high proliferative capacity (as measured by nuclear grade and mitotic index) and who have extensive intraductal disease, either within or adjacent to the tumor, deserve special treatment such as an ^{192}Ir interstitial implant after whole breast irradiation.

Although recurrences in the internal mammary nodes are relatively rare, they have a much worse prognosis than recurrences in the preserved breast. As more experience is gained from the use of lymphoscintigraphy in all patients with central or medial lesions, the scans will have more accurate interpretations and will be of better prognostic value. Future use of radiolabelled monoclonal antibodies may also help to evaluate nodes in this region. Routine use of CT scans for treatment planning will ensure that these nodes are encompassed with as much shielding as possible of normal tissues.

From the foregoing remarks, it is clear that all of the questions are not yet answered regarding the long-term effects of radiation used in conjunction with breast conserving surgery. However, it can be safely stated that this approach is no longer experimental, and that women with early breast cancers should be made aware of this.

SUGGESTED READING

Harris JR, Hellman S, Silen W, eds. Conservative management of breast cancer. Philadelphia: JB Lippincott, 1983.

Hellman S, Harris JR. The appropriate breast cancer paradigm. Cancer Res 1987; 47:339–342.

Shank B, Hellman S. Preservative surgery and radiation therapy in the treatment of early breast cancer. In: Nori D, Hilaris B, eds. Radiation therapy of gynecological cancer. New York: Alan R Liss, 1987:251.

Steeves RA, Phromratanaponse P, Wolberg WH, Tormey DC. Cosmesis and local control after irradiation in women treated conservatively for breast cancer. Arch Surg 1990 (in press).

ESOPHAGEAL CARCINOMA

H. GUNTER SEYDEL, M.D., M.S., F.A.C.R.

In 1986, carcinoma of the esophagus afflicted approximately 9,300 new patients in the United States with 8,800 deaths estimated. The predominant tumor type is squamous cell carcinoma; however, adenocarcinomas frequently occur. From 1982 to 1985 at Henry Ford Hospital Department of Therapeutic Radiology, 57 patients with squamous cell carcinoma and nine patients with adenocarcinoma involving the esophagus or gastroesophageal junction were treated with a curative intent. These patients are usually in their fifth or sixth decade, male, smokers, and consumers of alcohol. The presenting symptoms are dysphagia, weight loss, and odynophagia in 90 percent of the patients, with hemoptysis, melena, cough, and dysphagia, as well as other symptoms, occurring in the remaining 10 percent.

DIAGNOSIS

The most widely accepted staging system for carcinoma of the esophagus is that of the American Joint Committee on Cancer: the tumor/nodal involvement/metastasis (TNM) staging system (Table 1). In patients without symptoms or signs of disease other than those related directly to the intrathoracic lesion, minimum examination should include a history and physical examination, electrocardiogram, pulmonary function and biochemical tests as well as hemogram and urinalysis. Tumor-specific tests include an esophagram, chest x-ray, computed tomography of the chest and upper abdomen, as well as triple endoscopy of the larynx, bronchi, and esophagus. Bone scan and liver function tests, most of which are usually included in the biochemical tests, exclude gross metastatic disease. The diagnosis is most frequently established on endoscopy with brushing being positive in 90 percent of cases and a biopsy in at least 70 percent.

TABLE 1 TNM Classification*

Primary Tumor (T)	
TX	Minimum requirements to assess the primary tumor cannot be met.
TO	No evidence of primary tumor.
	Tis carcinoma in situ.
T1	A tumor that involves 5 cm or less of esophageal length, produces no obstruction†, has no circumferential involvement, and no extraesophageal spread‡.
T2	A tumor that involves more than 5 cm of esophageal length without extraesophageal spread‡, or a tumor of any size that produces obstruction or that involves the entire circumference but without extraesophageal spread.
T3	Any tumor with evidence of extraesophageal spread.
Nodal Involvement (N)§	
NX	Minimum requirements to assess the regional nodes cannot be met
NO	No clinically palpable nodes
N1	Movable, unilateral, palpable nodes
N2	Movable, bilateral, palpable nodes
N3	Fixed Nodes
Distant Metastasis (M)	
MX	Minimum requirements to assess the presence of distant metastasis cannot be met.
MO	No evidence of distant metastasis†.
M1	Distant metastasis present.
Stage Grouping	
Stage I	T1, NO, MO
Stage II	T2, NO, MO
Stage III	T3, NO, MO
	Any T, NO, MO
Stage IV	Any T, any N, M1

* Reprinted with permission of JB Lippincott Co., Philadelphia.

† Roentgenographic evidence of significant impediment to the passage of liquid, contrast material past the tumor or endoscopic evidence of esophageal obstruction.

‡ Extension of cancer outside the esophagus is seen by clinical, roentgenographic, or endoscopic evidence of any of the following:

- recurrent laryngeal, phrenic, or sympathetic nerve involvement;
- fistula formation;
- involvement of the tracheal or bronchial tree;
- vena cava or azygos vein obstruction;
- malignant effusion: mediastinal widening itself is not evidence of extraesophageal spread.

§ In the cervical esophagus, any lymph node involvement other than that of cervical or supraclavicular lymph nodes is considered distant metastasis. For the thoracic esophagus, any cervical, supraclavicular, scalene, or abdominal lymph nodes are considered distant metastasis sites.

Synchronous or metachronous tumors occur in 5 to 12 percent of patients. Approximately half of these tumors are head and neck cancers, with the majority of the remaining cancers occurring in the lung. Of the multiple tumors, 25 percent are synchronous and 68 percent occur within 2 years of treatment of the initial esophageal tumor.

In patients with squamous cell carcinoma of the thoracic esophagus (SCCTE) where the primary lesion is less than 5 cm in diameter, 40 percent have localized disease, 25 percent show locally advanced tumor, and 35 percent have distant metastases. For patients with larger lesions, distant metastases are more frequent at presentation. Distant metastases occur in the subdiaphragmatic lymph nodes, liver and other abdominal organs, lungs, supraclavicular nodes, as well as many other sites.

METHODS OF TREATMENT

Treatment by surgery, involving esophagectomy with an esophagopharyngoscopy or gastropharyngostomy or interposition of the large bowel to maintain continuity of the gastrointestinal tract, has a mortality rate of 5 to 30 percent, while the 5-year survival rate of 4 to 30 percent reflects patients' selection in various series.

Radiation therapy with curative doses of no less than 50 Gy following selection criteria of individual investigators produces 5-year survival rates of 3 to 23 percent. The main complication is tracheoesophageal fistula, which may occur in 5 to 18 percent of patients.

Multidrug chemotherapy including 5-fluorouracil, mitomycin C, bleomycin, cis-platinum, and other drugs has response rates (including complete and partial response) of 25 to 50 percent with few, if any, 5-year survivors. This dismal outcome of unimodality therapy has led to the combination of treatment modalities.

Preoperative radiation therapy using 24 Gy in 3 days to 60 Gy in 8 weeks leads to resection of 30 to 67 percent of the patients thus treated, and depends on selection of patients in the individual series. The 5-year survival rate is 4 to 38 percent. No randomized studies have demonstrated the advantage of this over surgery alone or over radiation therapy alone. Postoperative radiation therapy is usually given to high risk patients with locally advanced disease, microscopically or macroscopically unresected tumor, or where lymph node metastases have been confirmed pathologically. The literature reports less than ten 5-year survivors.

Preoperative or postoperative chemotherapy using drugs similar to those previously mentioned has been employed. The most favorable results occur with cis-platinum and bleomycin, with eight out of 21 1-year survivors described in conjunction with surgery. The long-term value of this method of treatment remains to be proven.

Institutional and cooperative clinical trials (including the Radiation Therapy Oncology Group and the Southwest Oncology Group) for patients with localized SCCTE involving a combination of radiation therapy, surgery, and chemotherapy have shown a mean survival of 13 months and 2-year survival rates of up to 28 percent. Complete tumor eradication in the surgical specimen was found in 17 to 29 percent of the patients. Local failure, therefore, remains a major obstacle. Treatment of localized SCCTE currently being used at Henry Ford Hospital combines surgery, chemotherapy, and radiation therapy.

The work-up of patients includes the aforementioned studies as well as the examination of the remaining gastrointestinal tract by endoscopy or radiographic studies to exclude second primary lesions. If localizing symptoms such as rectal bleeding are present, a more extensive work-up for the second primary lesion must be carried out.

Treatment includes preoperative radiation therapy, cis-platinum, and 5-fluorouracil starting on day one. Radiation therapy is given for 5 days per week for 3 weeks at 2 Gy per day for a total of 30 Gy for the lesion in the esophagram and adjacent mediastinum with the margins 5 cm above and below the lesion as defined by barium swallow. The width of the portal is 7 to 8 cm. The radiation therapy is given with parallel opposed anterior and posterior fields. Both fields are treated on each day of treatment. Radiation therapy is stopped when granulocyte counts are less than 1,000 per millimeter cubed and platelet counts are less than 50,000 per millimeter cubed.

Cis-platinum is given at 75 mg per meter squared as an intravenous bolus on days one and 29, with 2,000 cc of fluid over 24 hours prior to administration of the drug. Mannitol (12.5 g in 1,000 cc 5 percent dextrose in half-normal saline) is given prior to injection and 5-fluorouracil is started on day one for 1,000 mg per meter squared per day continuous infusion (days 1 to 4 and days 29 to 32).

Four to 6 weeks following completion of this treatment, patients are evaluated for surgery; candidates undergo an esophagectomy with a gastropharyngostomy or gastroesophagostomy. Occasionally, colonic interpositions are performed. Where the tumor permeates the esophageal wall or where lymph node metastases or other metastases are identified, additional radiation therapy is given to the site of anastomosis and the initial tumor bearing volume for 2,000 Gy in 2 weeks, avoiding the spinal cord. This regimen is started about 4 weeks after surgery or when healing is completed. Those patients who are inoperable or elect not to undergo esophagectomy receive doses of 26 to 30 Gy to the initial volume as in the first series of treatments using lateral or oblique fields and avoiding the spinal cord as well as concomitant chemotherapy.

Patients are examined several times each month for 3 months, then every 3 months for approximately 2 years, and less frequently thereafter. The examination includes barium swallow, hemograms, and other tests, including esophagoscopy, as indicated by the patient's condition.

TREATMENT RESULTS

Among the Henry Ford Hospital patients, preoperative radiation therapy and chemotherapy as described above with subsequent esophagectomy have produced a median survival of 13 months and a 2-year survival rate of 38 percent in 15 patients. Of the 25 patients treated by radiation therapy and chemotherapy without surgery, the median survival was 12 months and the 2-year survival rate was 37 percent. For the 17 patients treated by radiation therapy alone (40 to 65 Gy) before development of this protocol, the median survival was 5 months and the 2-year survival rate was 0 percent.

Dose reductions (25 percent of 5-fluorouracil) were prescribed for stomatitis, and 5-flourouracil was stopped for granulocyte counts below 1,000 per millimeter cubed or platelets less than 50,000 per millimeter cubed. Dose reduction for cis-platinum were 25 percent and 50 percent for WBC nadirs 1,000 to 2,999 per millimeter cubed and less than 1,000 per millimeter cubed respectively, and platelet nadirs between 50,000 and 74,999 per millimeter cubed or less than 50,000 per millimeter cubed.

A multivariate analysis reveals that significant predictors for increased survival are treatment strategy ($p = 0.0003$), increased radiation dose ($p = 0.0005$), and tumor extent as defined by T staging ($p = 0.005$). There are no significant differences among the two multimodality treatment strategies according to the Mantle Cox univariate analysis.

Local tumor control was improved in those patients treated by the multimodality approach as compared with those treated by radiation therapy alone. Among 15 patients undergoing surgery, four had no tumor present in the specimen, and three of these four are alive and without evidence of disease 36 months after surgery. Among the ten 2-year survivors treated by radiation therapy and chemotherapy, all have had clinical and radiographic control of their intrathoracic tumor. An additional three patients with local control of SCCTE had distant metastases during the first 2 years of follow-up. All patients with either gross or microscopic residual tumor in the resected specimen eventually died. Toxicity was due to three tracheoesophageal fistulas in patients treated by radiation therapy alone, one of whom died from acute hemorrhage from the esophagus.

In the patients treated by radiation therapy and chemotherapy, one death was due to sepsis from a severe leukopenia and three deaths were attributed to surgery. Significant nonfatal morbidity included two severe esophageal strictures (both in the multimodality treatment groups) and one case of presumed radiation pericarditis in the radiation therapy alone group. Among the surgical patients, one required a "second look" operation because of an anastomotic leak.

Our data confirms the experience of others. Following combined modality treatment, approximately one-forth of the resected specimens were free of tumor upon esophagectomy. The only treatment-related factor that correlates with long-term survival is complete response with no cancer in the specimen or complete absence of tumor on clinical examination, including the various radiographic studies, in patients who did not undergo surgery. Similar results were obtained in eight patients with adenocarcinoma of the esophagus; however, this limited number of patients precludes definite conclusions. The contribution of surgery to long-term survival remains undetermined in our patient data, as the results in those patients treated by radiation therapy and multidrug chemotherapy are equivalent even when esophagectomy is avoided.

SUGGESTED READING

Coia L, Engstrom P, et al. A pilot study of combined radiotherapy and chemotherapy for esophageal cancer. Am J Clin Oncol 1984; 7:653–659.

Hancock SL, Glatstein E. Radiation therapy of esophageal carcinoma. Semin Oncol 1984; 2(2):144–158.

Kelsen D, Bains M, et al. Combined modality therapy of esophageal cancer. Semin Oncol 1984; 2(2):169–177.

Leichman L, Steiger Z, et al. Preoperative chemotherapy and radiation therapy for patients with cancer of the esophagus — a potentially curative approach. J Clin Oncol 1984; 2:75–79.

Leichman L, Steiger Z, et al. Combined preoperative chemotherapy and radiation therapy for cancer of the esophagus: The Wayne State University, Southwest Oncology Group, and Radiation Therapy Oncology Group Experience. Semin Oncol 1984; 2:178–185. Skinner D. Surgical treatment for esophageal cancer. Semin Oncol 1984; 2:136–143.

Seydel H, Leichmann L, et al. Preoperative radiation and chemotherapy for localized squamous cell carcinoma of the esophagus: A RTOG study. Int J Radiat Oncol Biol Phys 1988; 14:33–35.

Seitz J, Padaut-Cesana J, et al. Cancers nonoperables de l'esophage: Resultats preliminaries d'une chimiotherapie (5-fluorouracile-cisplatinum) avec radiotherapie concomitante. Gastroenterol Clin Biol (France) 1988; 12:736–742.

GASTRIC CANCER

JOHN S. MACDONALD, M.D.

The appropriate treatment approach to adenocarcinoma of the stomach depends upon the extent of the malignancy. In patients with truly localized carcinoma, regional treatment such as surgical resection or surgery plus radiation therapy may be used. In patients with more widespread cancer, either grossly or microscopically disseminated, systemic therapy (usually chemotherapy) must be considered. This chapter discusses an approach to the treatment of patients with gastric cancer based upon the extent of disease that is defined by careful staging.

The diagnosis of gastric cancer depends upon the physician suspecting the presence of this disease in appropriate patients. Individuals in their fifties or older who have a history of dyspepsia, weight loss, iron deficiency anemia, and early satiety are likely to have stomach cancer. Diagnosis requires endoscopic evaluation of the stomach with multiple biopsies of suspicious lesions, masses, or ulcers. Occasionally, no mucosal lesions will be noted in patients with infiltrating submucosal stomach cancer, frequently of the linitis plastica type. In these patients, endoscopic biopsy may be negative and diagnosis requires surgery. Patients with proven or suspected gastric cancer should be considered candidates for gastric resection unless there are compelling reasons (medical contraindications or widespread metastases) that mandate inoperability.

Conceptually, gastric cancer staging may be thought of as answering the following questions: 1) Is the tumor truly localized? 2) Is the tumor locally advanced or locally recurrent (in the gastric bed)? and 3) Is there grossly or microscopically disseminated cancer? In the United States, where stomach cancer is diagnosed relatively late in its course, truly localized cancer is uncommon. Some series show as few as 11 percent of patients have disease confined to the stomach only. Another 11 percent have local nodal disease as the only evidence of extension beyond the stomach. Regional extension of gastric cancer may occur with direct involvement of the lesser and greater omentum, or extension to the liver and diaphragm, the biliary tree, the transverse colon, or the spleen. Extension to the spleen is relatively uncommon, with less than 10 percent of patients exhibiting this finding.

As with many visceral malignancies, nodal metastases are common in gastric cancer patients. Positive regional nodes occur in at least 50 percent of patients, and there are several areas of distant lymphatic dissemination that one should be aware of since detection of these metastatic sites is important in determining appropriate therapy. Virchow's node, commonly in the left supraclavicular area, is an important point of dissemination for a variety of intra-abdominal malignancies, including gastric cancer. The left axillary nodes will occasionally be involved in patients with gastric cancer. The etiology of lymphatic cancer dissemination to this area is unknown. Umbilical (Sister Joseph) nodules also may be seen in patients with gastric carcinoma. Whether this finding represents true lymphatic dissemination of the tumor or results from peritoneal dissemination is not entirely clear. Finding tumors in any of the distant sites of nodal metastases means the patient is incurable, but not necessarily unresectable.

Two other forms of tumor dissemination other than nodal metastases are important in gastric carcinoma. The first is hematogenous spread. These metastases commonly occur in the liver, with the next most common site being the lungs. Adrenal metastases may also occur. Bone and brain metastases are distinctly uncommon in patients with stomach cancer. The second mechanism of metastasis is peritoneal dissemination. In women, the occurrence of ovarian metastases is relatively common (the Krukenberg tumor). A Krukenberg tumor should be suspected when one palpates an ovary in a postmenopausal woman in whom gastric carcinoma is suspected. Normally, the ovary cannot be palpated in postmenopausal women. When it can, it is definitely enlarged and may represent metastatic disease from stomach, large bowel, or breast carcinoma, or it may indicate primary ovarian pathology. A second site of peritoneal dissemination is Blumer's rectal shelf. Tumors here result from drop metastases in the peritoneal space, and may be palpated on rectal exam as a very indurated prerectal mass. Finally, local peritoneal dissemination occurs and is noted intraoperatively by the presence of nodules in the area of the primary gastric cancer. More diffuse intra-abdominal dissemination may be noted in stomach carcinoma patients, with tumors studding the peritoneal surfaces similar to the pattern seen in patients with ovarian cancer.

TREATMENT

As noted earlier, staging affects the therapeutic approaches that may be used for patients with cancer. The first treatment option involves local therapy for localized, resectable gastric cancer. This generally represents surgical resection. The second option is extended local therapy, which may represent surgery plus the use of irradiation for patients with incompletely resectable disease or patients with locally recurrent disease. The third is systemic therapy for patients with metastatic cancer. Patients with disseminated cancer may present with gross metastases or have a high probability of microscopic metastases. In the latter case, adjuvant therapy is considered. The approach to metastatic cancer, gross or microscopic, is generally chemotherapy. A fourth approach to treatment, regional therapy, is investigational at present. Two forms of regional therapy that are of interest in gastric cancer are hepatic artery infusion and intraperitoneal chemotherapy.

All stomach cancer patients should be considered operable and potentially resectable with curative intent until proven otherwise. Patients with fully localized gastric carcinoma are excellent candidates for surgical resection, and approximately 50 to 60 percent of these patients will be cured. The procedure most useful for gastric cancer is the radical subtotal gastrectomy. This procedure is used in patients with lesions in the body and antrum of the stomach. Generally, 70 to 80 percent of the stomach is resected. In patients with cardioesophageal junction lesions, a proximal subtotal gastrectomy may be performed, and in patients with diffuse involvement of the stomach who have no obvious evidence of metastatic disease, a total gastrectomy with the construction of a gastric reservoir pouch may be the only option available. In patients with known metastatic or unresectable locally advanced disease, palliative resection of the stomach tumor should still be considered. Leaving the primary tumor in place results in a high likelihood of bleeding and/or obstruction, and a subtotal gastrectomy is an appropriate option to consider in such patients. Palliative total gastrectomy should not be performed since the palliative results of total gastrectomy with gastric pouch reconstruction are poor in patients with known disseminated disease. Also, patients with a large gastric tumor that requires total gastric resection likely have poor prognosis and will not achieve significant palliation from the procedure.

Long-term survival after gastric resection depends upon the degree of local tumor extension in the resected specimen. Table 1 demonstrates the approximate 5-year survivals according to the degree of pathologic involvement after gastric resection. It should be emphasized that gastric resection, even in patients who are not curable by operation, represents cytoreductive surgery that increases the probability of effective palliation and prolonged survival from combined modality approaches such as the combination of postoperative radiation and chemotherapy.

Locally Advanced Gastric Cancer

There have been significant advances in the treatment of patients with locally recurrent or residual gastric cancer. These advances involve combined modality therapeutic approaches. Although megavoltage radiation alone to an unresectable or recurrent gastric carcinoma does not prolong survival, subgroups of patients

TABLE 1 Initial Pathology and Survival in Gastric Cancer

Extent of Disease	*% 5-Year Survival*
Regional lymph nodes (−)	
Mucosa only	85
Mucosa and gastric wall	52
Through gastric wall	47
Lymph nodes (+)	
Regional only	17
Distant nodes	5

(Adapted from Kennedy BJ. Cancer 26:971)

who receive radiation with concomitant 5-fluorouracil do receive prolonged periods of survival. In 1982, the Gastrointestinal Tumor Study Group demonstrated that 5-fluorouracil plus methyl-CCNU in combination with 5,000 rads of split course radiation resulted in approximately 20 percent of the patients attaining greater than 3-year disease-free survival. This study is important because it indicates that long-term survival is possible in patients with locally unresectable or recurrent gastric carcinoma. This study also demonstrates that the survival advantage is confined to patients in whom the primary tumor is resected. Patients with large, unresectable lesions do not benefit from combined modality therapy. Thus, this evidence also supports the desirability of performing cytoreductive surgery whenever possible in patients with gastric carcinoma. It is important to remember that programs of aggressive surgery and combined radiation plus chemotherapy are toxic. In managing patients who are receiving modern combined modality therapy, intensive nutritional support, including intravenous hyperalimentation, may be necessary. It also should be emphasized that methyl-CCNU may produce leukemia as a late complication of therapy and, therefore, should not be considered a drug of first choice for combined modality programs.

Intraoperative radiation therapy is of investigational interest in the therapy of locally advanced gastric cancer. Workers from Japan pioneered this approach and are currently involved in studies to evaluate intraoperative radiation therapy. This approach has obvious attraction since it allows the radiosensitive organs, such as the small bowel, to be removed from the treatment field, thereby permitting one to position the beam precisely to radiate locally unresectable or residual gastric cancer disease. Whether this approach will be of significant value to patients in the United States with stomach carcinoma is not clear at present.

Advanced Gastric Cancer

Treating patients with advanced gastric carcinoma currently entails the use of chemotherapy. The chemotherapy of stomach cancer is of interest because there are some indications that combination chemotherapy is superior to single agent therapy. Table 2 demonstrates results of a variety of combination chemotherapy regimens used in patients with advanced measurable stomach cancer. As one can see, response rates as high as 50 percent have been reported. The FAM regimen (5-fluorouracil, Adriamycin, and mitomycin C) has been widely used and a summary of the results of FAM, as reported by 12 separate studies, is shown in the table. However, it is important to note that, with over 450 patients treated, the true response rate for this regimen is approximately 34 percent. When all patients treated are evaluated, the median survival is approximately 6 to 7 months. It is not surprising that median survivals are not improved by a regimen that induces a response in less than 50 percent of patients. If one examines survival in responding versus nonresponding patients, one finds that the median survival in patients responding to FAM

TABLE 2 Drug Combinations in Gastric Cancer Therapy

Drug Combination	*# Responses/ # Patients*	*Percent Response*	*Median Duration of Survival (Months)*
5-FU + BCNU	14/34	41	7.7
	5/28	18	3.0
TOTAL	19/62	30	
5-FU + methyl-CCNU	12/30	40	4.7
	12/49	24	4.0
	6/44	14	3.0
	6/29	21	4.5
	5/54	9	4.5
	1/18	6	5.5
TOTAL	42/224	19	
5-FU + mitomycin C	17/53	32	4.5
	6/43	14	6.0
TOTAL	23/96	24	
5-FU + Adriamycin	3/11	27	7.0
Adriamycin + mitomycin C	13/45	29	3.5
Triazinate + mitomycin C	8/28	29	5.0
FAM (5-FU, Adriamycin, mitomycin C)	6/11	55	16.5*
	26/62	42	12.5*
	7/33	21	5.5
	20/45	44	11.5*
	29/84	35	—
	4/22	18	6.2
	25/83	30	5.8
	5/13	38	7.0
	6/27	22	5.5
	20/49	40	6.8
	3/12	25	6.8
	3/18	17	6.0
TOTAL	154/459	34	
EAP (etoposide + Adriamycin + cisplatin)	43/67	64	8
FAMe (5-FU, Adriamycin, methyl-CCNU)	7/15	47	5.6
	3/10	30	8.0
	4/16	25	6.5
	11/39	29	6.0
TOTAL	25/80	31	
5-FU + cytosine arabinoside + mitomycin C	15/27	55	—
	6/16	38	—
	3/18	17	2.5
TOTAL	24/61	39	
FAP (5-FU + Adriamycin + cis-platinum)	10/35	29	7.0
	8/16	50	10.5
	9/17	53	10.0
TOTAL	27/68	40	
FAMtx (5-FU + Adriamycin + methotrexate)	22/62	35	6.0
	59/100	59	9.0
TOTAL	81/162	50	
5-FU + Adriamycin + BCNU	18/35	52	—
FAM + methyl-CCNU	2.18	11	6.2
	12/35	34	6.5
TOTAL	14/53	26	
FAM + triazinate	4/18	22	—

*Survival duration in responders only, not all patients.

is approximately 12 months versus 4 months for patients who do not respond. However, one may not draw the conclusion that response causes prolonged survival, since it may be just as likely that patients who respond to chemotherapy have intrinsically longer survival than patients who do not respond. A striking and disappointing finding with FAM is that only 2 percent of patients develop a complete regression of metastatic disease. It is clear from experience with leukemias, lymphomas, testicular cancer, non-small cell carcinoma of the lung, and ovarian cancer that the most important precondition for long-term disease-free survival is the complete, pathologically proved disappearance of cancer. Chemotherapy regimens that do not produce complete remission do not produce prolongation of survival. Therefore, it must be assumed that FAM, as currently given, represents an effective palliative regimen, but does not provide long-term disease-free survival in many patients with advanced gastric cancer.

Other regimens noted in Table 2 appear capable of producing some percentage of complete regression. The 5-FU, methotrexate, Adriamycin regimen reported by Klein and colleagues, which depends upon a biochemical modulation, produced a response rate of 59 percent with 12 percent complete regressions. This study will need confirmation. A 5-FU, Adriamycin, platinum regimen reported by investigators at the Mayo Clinic also notes a relatively high order of complete regressions. This is significant, although it should be emphasized that other studies from the Gastrointestinal Tumor Study Group and Georgetown University show that 5-FU, Adriamycin, platinum produced response rates inferior to FAM.

Recently there has been much interest in the EAP (etoposide, Adriamycin, platinol) regimen originally described in Germany. This program is reported to produce a 64 percent overall response rate, which includes 21 percent complete responses. These promising preliminary data require confirmation.

The toxicities associated with chemotherapy in gastric cancer are similar to those resulting from the use of cytotoxic drug therapy in any malignancy. Myelosuppression is the most common toxicity, with mucositis also being associated with many of the commonly used drugs (doxorubicin, mitomycin C, 5-fluorouracil and methotrexate). Cis-platinum is nephrotoxic, thereby requiring pretherapy evaluations of renal function and adequate hydration. An unusual complication, the adult hemolytic uremic syndrome, has been seen in patients with stomach cancer who have had an excellent response to chemotherapy. Whether this finding is secondary to the disease or the treatment (chemotherapy) is not entirely clear.

In summary, the use of chemotherapy in stomach cancer for advanced disease is still investigational. No regimen has such well-documented efficacy that it may be recommended as standard. Combination regimens do appear to produce a higher order of partial response than single agents. The North Central Cancer Therapy Group performed a phase III testing of 5-FU, 5-FU plus Adriamycin, and FAM. The response rates were 18 percent, 27 percent, and 35 percent, respectively, thereby demonstrating that combination chemotherapy is superior in regard to response. However, the increase in response rate does not translate into improved survival. Since survival is not improved with current therapy, all patients with advanced gastric cancer should be considered candidates for inclusion in clinical trials.

Other patients who may be candidates for systemic therapy are those with a high risk of recurrence after primary gastric cancer surgery. As noted in Table 1, these patients have nodal involvement or serosal involvement of the tumor at the time of their original gastric resection and therefore have a poor probability of remaining disease-free after surgery only. Such patients are candidates for adjunctive therapy. The value of adjuvant chemotherapy for gastric cancer (Table 3) is still undefined. Single agent chemotherapy in the United States has shown no benefit for patients with resected stomach cancer. Combination chemotherapy, in general, has been disappointing. Three studies utilizing 5-FU and methyl-CCNU have been published. Studies by the Eastern Cooperative Oncology Group and the Veterans' Administration Surgical Oncology Group have demonstrated no survival benefit from adjuvant chemotherapy. On the other hand, one study performed by the Gastrointestinal Tumor Study Group did demonstrate a significant benefit for patients treated with 5-FU and methyl-CCNU. The reason for this discrepancy is not clear. The Southwest Oncology Group and the Middle Atlantic Oncology Program performed studies in which FAM chemotherapy was tested in a prospective randomized fashion versus surgery only. The data from these studies are too immature to tell whether or not FAM will be an effective adjuvant therapy.

One investigational approach to adjuvant therapy is the use of intra-abdominal chemotherapy. Conceptually, this approach may be effective in sterilizing intra-abdominal micrometastatic disease. Intraperitoneal chemotherapy entails the placement of a peritoneal catheter and perfusion of the peritoneal space with a drug-containing solution. This approach has the pharmacologic and pharmacokinetic advantage of produc-

TABLE 3 Adjuvant Therapy of Gastric Cancer

Treatment	*(Study Group)*	*Patients Randomized*	*Survival Benefit*
5-FU + methyl-CCNU	(VASOG)	134	NS
5-FU + methyl-CCNU	(ECOG)	160	NS
5-FU + methyl-CCNU	(GITSG)	142	P<0.03
5-FU + doxorubicin	(NCCTG)		ongoing
FAM	(SWOG)	148	ongoing
FAM	(MAOP)	295	ongoing

5-FU = 5-fluorouracil; FAM = 5-FU + doxorubicin + mitomycin; VASOG = Veterans Administration Surgical Oncology Group; ECOG = Eastern Cooperative Oncology Group; GITSG = Gastrointestinal Tumor Study Group; MAOP = Middle Atlantic Oncology Group; SWOG = Southwest Oncology Group; NCCTG = North Central Cancer Therapy Group; NS = not significant.

ing high concentrations of drug in the peritoneal space. Theoretically, the concentration X time (CXT) product to which the residual tumor may be exposed is large and results in increased cytotoxicity. Only carefully designed clinical trials will define the value of intra-abdominal chemotherapy. Another approach worth evaluating is the use of regional chemotherapy for microscopic disease metastatic to the liver. Evaluation of this technique in gastric cancer using either portal vein or hepatic arterial infusion will require controlled randomized trials.

FUTURE IMPROVEMENTS

It is clear that the management of gastric carcinoma needs improving in many areas. Stomach cancer is diagnosed relatively late in the United States, thereby resulting in a poor prognosis from surgical resection. It is not economically feasible to perform population based mass screening for early detection as is done in Japan. Thus, future improvement in stomach cancer survival in the United States will result from improvements in treatment. The use of innovative combined modality therapy, intraoperative irradiation, or intra-abdominal chemotherapy may improve long-term survival after surgery, but these techniques must be tested in controlled clinical trials to define their roles.

The systemic chemotherapy of advanced gastric cancer can be thought of as a halfway technology. Until a major increase in complete response is obtained, no significant improvement in survival will be seen. In the future, approaches such as biochemical modulations and/or biologic response modifiers may have a significant role in the therapy of disseminated gastric cancer. Improvement in the adjuvant therapy of resected gastric cancer patients will depend upon the identification and application of treatment programs defined as active in patients with advanced stomach cancer.

SUGGESTED READING

Abe M, Takahashi M. Intraoperative radiotherapy: the Japanese experience. Int J Radiat Oncol Biol Phys 1981; 5:862–868.

Howell SB, Pfeifle L, Wung WE, et al. Intraperitoneal cisplatin with systemic thiosulfate protection. Ann Intern Med 1982; 97:845.

Kemeny N, Daly J, Oderman P, et al. Hepatic artery pump infusion: toxicity and results in patients with metastatic colorectal carcinoma. J Clin Oncol 1984; 2:595.

Macdonald JS, Schein PS, Woolley PV, et al. 5-fluorouracil doxorubicin, and mitomycin (FAM) combination chemotherapy for advanced gastric cancer. Ann Intern Med 1980; 93:533.

Macdonald JS, Steele G Jr, Gunderson LL. Cancer of the stomach. In: DeVita VT, Hellman S, Rosenberg SA, eds. Cancer: principles and practice of oncology. Philadelphia: JB Lippincott, 1989:765.

Preusser P, Wilke H, Achterrath W, et al. Phase II study with the combination of etoposide, doxorubicin and cisplatin in advanced measurable gastric cancer. J Clin Oncol 1989; 7:1310.

Schein PS, Stablein DM, Bruckner HW, et al. A comparison of combination chemotherapy and combined modality therapy for locally advanced gastric carcinoma. Cancer 1982; 49:1771.

PANCREATIC CANCER

HAROLD O. DOUGLASS Jr., M.D., F.A.C.S.

This year, nearly 27,000 men and women in the United States will be informed that they have cancer of the pancreas. For virtually all of these unfortunate individuals, this is a sentence of death. For most, the death knell will come within 1 year.

While nearly 60 percent of patients have disseminated tumor (at least liver metastases or ascites and peritoneal implants) at the time of diagnosis, the remainder still have localized disease in the pancreas and adjacent lymphatics. Of this latter group, slightly fewer than half have technically resectable cancers. As an unfortunate result of the nihilism that pervades the treatment of pancreatic cancer, resections are attempted in only a small proportion of those with localized cancer. Yet, with current combined modality, postsurgical adjuvant therapy, nearly 20 percent of those resected can be expected to live 5 years or more.

DIAGNOSIS

A significant part of our failure to successfully control pancreatic cancer results from not recognizing the symptom complexes often associated with the disease; this is combined with a lack of perserverence in the establishment of a definite diagnosis. Four common symptom complexes are typical of pancreatic cancer:

1. The development of mature onset diabetes in a patient whose family history is devoid of other diabetic (one-third of patients with pancreatic cancer are diabetics).
2. Unexplained weight loss, or a patient who diets unsuccessfully and then, without good reason, loses weight with remarkable ease.
3. Newly developed gallbladder symptoms, particularly in male patients over 50 years of age.
4. Symptoms of peptic ulceration sufficient to mandate a study (radiologic contrast or endoscopic) that fails to absolutely confirm the diagnosis.

Among physical signs, it is the expected but missing findings that can lead to the correct diagnosis:

1. In obstructive jaundice, it should be remembered

that biliary stones rarely totally obstruct the biliary tree. Rapidly increasing jaundice (more that 3 mg per deciliter per day), or relatively deep jaundice (probably more than 12 mg and certainly more than 16 mg per deciliter) suggests complete and total obstruction.

2. A deeply jaundiced patient who is not clinically sick, as would be expected in hepatitis.
3. Symptoms of pancreatitis, but expected pain and fever are absent.

Whereas the imaging studies designed to establish the diagnosis of pancreatic cancer were once limited to barium meal examination and angiography, currently ultrasonography, computerized tomography, and magnetic resonance imaging are extensively utilized, with endoscopic retrograde cholangiopancreatography (ERCP) providing diagnostic confirmation (and, ever more frequently, biliary decompression) in selected cases (Table 1). Unfortunately, the limited resolution of most imaging techniques precludes finding the curable lesions. Our experience confirms that ERCP is a more accurate means of identifying smaller lesions, but tumors no bigger than 600 microns in diameter may already have spread to lymph nodes or to the liver.

While the past two decades have witnessed this revolution in the diagnosis of pancreatic cancer as a result of advances in fiberoptic endoscopy and diagnostic imaging, occasional patients are still explored without obtaining a tissue diagnosis. The fear of pancreatic biopsy is complemented by a defeatist attitude with regard to therapeutic intervention.

Histologic confirmation must still be considered critical. Of a series of 100 patients referred without histologic confirmation, 22 had no cancer (Table 2). These patients came from renowned university centers as well as from rural hospitals. We feel secure, now, in this statement, since all have now survived 5 years or more and have shown no evidence of cancer. The story does not end here! Of the remaining 78 patients, 18 had some other kind of cancer, including one lymphoma. From that group of 18, nearly half were eventually cured of their cancers.

No wonder, then, that those patients with signs and symptoms of pancreatic cancer who refer themselves to our GI Service at Roswell Park Memorial Institute for diagnostic studies are vigorously evaluated. For the nonjaundiced patient, this evaluation centers around

TABLE 1 Sensitivity of Four Imaging Techniques to Detect Pancreatic Cancer

Series	*Ultrasound*	*CT Scan*	*ERCP*	*Angiography*
Moosa				
(resectable)	90	60	88	*74*
(not resectable)	84	84	90	*80*
Go	74	79	95	*69*

TABLE 2 Final Histologic Diagnoses of 100 Patients Referred for Treatment of Pancreatic Cancer After Laparotomy but with no Histologic Diagnosis (Roswell Park Memorial Institute)

Histologic Diagnosis	*Number of Cases*
Malignant	
Adenocarcinoma pancreas	60
Periampullary cancer	13
Metastatic cancer	3
Sarcoma	1
Gastric cancer	1
Benign	
Liver cirrhosis	8
Benign biliary	8
Pancreatitis	4
Vascular	2

185

computerized tomography (CT) and gastroduodenoscopy followed by ERCP. Needle aspiration biopsy based on CT, ERCP, or and ultrasonically defined mass often confirms the primary site when surgical exploration otherwise seems indicated only for histologic confirmation of a clinical diagnosis, saving the patient a now unnecessary laparotomy.

The ultrasound examination plays a greater role in the jaundiced patient, since it demonstrates whether biliary ducts are dilated and provides evidence with regard to liver metastases. If, for some reason, operative decompression is not imminent (e.g., there are peritoneal metastases with ascites, or nutritional or cardiopulmonary status must be improved), endoscopic or percutaneous drainage of the biliary tree is performed.

PRETREATMENT CONSIDERATIONS

The frequently accompanying nutritional deprivation of pancreatic cancer can alter a patient's performance status, cardiac output, respiratory mechanics, hepatic function, and enterocyte competence. When jaundice is prolonged or severe, evidence of deteriorating renal function can be reflected in abnormalities of urea and creatinine excretion. The result is a decreased tolerance to therapeutic interventions of all types. In a series of patients treated by pancreatoduodenectomy more than a decade ago, the most significant prognostically adverse finding for in-hospital mortality was an elevation of the blood urea nitrogen (BUN) at time of admission (Table 3).

The initiation of nutritional repletion does not need to await the final confirmation of a diagnosis. Indeed, during the period of the work-up, the patient may become further depleted unless precautions are undertaken to increase protein and caloric intake. While there are elaborate techniques to assess nitrogen balance and energy expenditure, bedside evaluation including a history of weight loss, estimates of caloric (not fluid) intake, and examination for skeletal muscle weakness

TABLE 3 Predictive Factors for Postoperative Mortality for Patients with Obstructive Jaundice due to Cancer (author's data: 1966–1970)

	Mortality Rate for Operation		
	Resection	*All Patients*	*Bypass*
Age			
≥70	14%		20%
<70	19%		34%
Bilirubin			
>16 mg%	24%		22%
≤16 mg%	6%		67%
Duration of jaundice			
≥3 wks		23%	
≤2 wks		0	
Blood urea nitrogen			
>20 mg%		50%	
≤20 mg%		10%	
Serum amylase			
≥150 IU		50%	
<150 IU		10%	
Occult blood in stool negative		20%	
Occult blood in stool positive		20%	

and atrophy (particularly in the extensor groups) combined with a serum albumin level can document the need to institute nutritional support, preferably by the enteral route. Nutritional deprivation is demonstrated by low spike size on the electrocardiogram, weak cough, and poor healing.

That thin critical line of defense of the body against endotoxemia and gram-negative sepsis from the content of the gut, the bowel mucosa, is better nourished by the enteral rather than the parenteral route. The same is essentially true of the liver. A rising BUN rarely accompanies enteral nutrition, but when it accompanies parenteral nutrition, it often indicates a mining of the body's protein resources for amino acids essential to hepatic function (most commonly leucine), thereby discarding less well-utilized amino acids and adding them to the waste heap of the body by their conversion to urea.

EVALUATION FOR SURGERY

Invasive radiology has reduced to two, the absolute indications for surgical intervention for newly diagnosed pancreatic cancer patients, and has left three other relative indications. Absolute indications include potentially curative resection of the pancreas, and the relief of gastric outlet obstruction that is unresponsive to metaclopramide.

Relative indications include biliary drainage when percutaneous or endoscopic stents cannot be passed beyond the cancer, histologic confirmation when percutaneous needle aspiration of the pancreas or biopsy of metastatic sites fail to establish a diagnosis, and accurate staging of localized unresectable cancer in patients in whom a combined radiation-chemotherapy program is planned.

Limitation of the indications for surgical intervention to these few permits a more expeditious patient evaluation. Perhaps the single most valuable study is computerized tomography (CT). Although fat planes tend to fade because of weight loss, a factor that somewhat reduces the value of CT scans generally, the use of intravenous and particularly oral contrast media permits evaluation of a number of critical points that can determine resectability:

1. Diameter of the head of the pancreas;
2. Separation of the superior mesenteric artery from the tumor or mass;
3. Absence of adenopathy at the origin of the superior mesenteric artery;
4. Separation of the vena cava from the mass, and lack of significant compression of this vessel;
5. Absence of adenopathy along the aorta and at the celiac axis;
6. Probable absence of liver metastases;
7. By changing to a lateral position to observe a change in position and shape of the pancreas, a lack of invasion into the retroperitoneum;
8. Occasionally, a dilated pancreatic duct;
9. Distension of the splenic vein with splenomegaly, suggesting obstruction of the vessel and localized portal hypertension;
10. Dilated intrahepatic ducts;
11. Occasionally, identification of cancers that arise in the uncinate process of the pancreas (which may be resectable, but to date are not curable).

The ERCP is still the single most useful test to delineate the site of the cancer within the pancreas. Not only is the ERCP the most accurate diagnostic study, the pancreatogram has, on occasion, been useful in guiding fine needle aspiration to the cancer when computerized tomography or ultrasound could not localize a small tumor, thereby enhancing the frequency of positive cytology reports.

When resection of the pancreas is a consideration, celiac and superior mesenteric angiography can provide useful guidelines for the surgeon. Arterial abnormalities suggesting compression, obstruction or neovascularity are virtually diagnostic of nonresectability or incurability. Venous phase films are obtained between 9 and 15 seconds after injection. Veins not well visualized by 13 seconds are often obstructed, with collaterals appearing on images taken 13 to 15 seconds after dye injection.

The upper gastrointestinal series should include a follow-up view of the stomach at 2 hours. Residual barium in the stomach at that time identifies patients with impaired gastric emptying and who are in need of gastrojejunostomy.

If the tumor is in the body or tail of the pancreas, close inspection of the common bile duct can avert the necessity for a second operative procedure, since a dilated duct portends imminent biliary obstruction.

OPERATIVE FINDINGS

The critical step in the pancreatoduodenectomy has long been considered the separation of the neck of the pancreas from the anterior surface of the superior mesenteric vein. Within the past few years, we and others have found that adherence in this plane does not necessarily require that the operation be aborted. Rather, the neck and a portion of the body of the pancreas can be resected in continuity with a venous segment, the superior mesenteric vein then being reapproximated to the junction of the portal and splenic veins. With the pancreas removed, these structures come together easily: no graft has been necessary in our experience. The maximal safe occlusion time for the superior mesenteric vein is about 40 minutes, but biochemical abnormalities in liver function may be apparent after even shorter intervals of clamping. Although not generally suggested, we administer a small dose of heparin (5,000 units or less) before cross clamping the veins.

The presence of enlarged peripancreatic lymph nodes, even when they contain metastatic cancer, should not dissuade the surgeon from performing a resection, since these nodes will be resected en bloc with the pancreas. A minimal resection for carcinoma in the head of the pancreas includes the bile duct to the level of the midhepatic duct; the gallbladder and lymph nodes in Calot's triangle; the lymphatics around the bile duct and hepatic artery; the lesser omentum and its lymph nodes; the gastric antrum, duodenum and proximal jejunum; the right half of the omentum and the head, neck, and uncinate process of the pancreas with the lymphatics and lymph nodes anterior and lateral to the origin of the superior mesenteric artery at the aorta. If there is any question of tumor in the neck of the pancreas, the resection is extended to the left of the superior mesenteric vein into the body of the pancreas. Total pancreatectomy should include the spleen and the lymph nodes along the splenic artery and around the tail of the pancreas. When indicated, the mesocolon or transverse or right colon can be included in the en bloc resection.

Following partial pancreatectomy, reconstruction of the pancreas by end-to-side anastomosis with three or four sutures between the duct and the ileal mucosa over a silastic stent has reduced the incidence of pancreatic fistula to near zero. Our service is split as to whether a vagotomy should regularly be performed at the time of pancreatectomy.

Far more ominous than cancer in peripancreatic lymph nodes are the findings of cancer invading the peritoneal surface overlying the pancreas, cancer arising in the uncinate process of the pancreas, or metastatic cancer in lymph nodes around the origin of the superior mesenteric artery. When the lymph nodes at the celiac axis are involved, the tumor has progressed beyond the potential for surgical cure.

While carcinoma arising in the body and tail of the pancreas can be resected on rare occasions, cures are so uncommon as to be reportable.

Technically unresectable cancers in patients with no liver, peritoneal, or other distant metastases should be outlined with radiopaque clips to identify the tumor mass for purposes of postoperative radiotherapy. For tumors involving the head of the pancreas, biliary drainage should be performed. We prefer hepaticojejunostomy using either an interrupted jejunal loop with an enteroenterostomy or a Roux-en-Y limb, dividing the hepatic duct to anastomose it end-to-side to the bowel. Duct division should also include ligation and division of the lymphatics extending from the pancreas toward the hilum of the liver. Survival of patients treated in this manner is generally longer (although not significantly so) than for patients in whom a cholecystojejunostomy is performed.

In the presence of extensive and metastatic disease, a cholecystojejunostomy is acceptable provided that the cystic duct is proven to be patent and does not extend down along the common duct (or share a common wall with the common duct), the cystic and common duct then joining within a centimeter of the cancer or the pancreas. This anomaly is remarkably frequent in patients with pancreatic cancer. Some surgeons prefer cholecystogastrostomy, provided that the stomach wall has not been invaded by the cancer. This does not require the construction of a jejunal loop or limb, but often requires mobilization of at least a portion of the gallbladder from its bed, thus risking interruption of venous drainage and infarction.

The question of whether a gastrointestinal bypass should be performed at the time of biliary drainage continues to be debated. The second bypass does not significantly contribute to the overall operative morbidity or mortality. In the absence of obstruction, the stomach still empties via the pylorus, although small bowel content may regurgitate into the stomach through the anastomosis. While as many as 27 percent of patients treated by biliary anastomosis alone will, if they live long enough, need a gatrointestinal bypass, the majority will not. Further, patients' lives are little prolonged by the second procedure.

An exception to this is the second bypass that is needed within 1 to 2 months after the biliary decompression. In these patients, the gastric drainage was most probably indicated at the time of first exploration. The preoperative identification of this group of patients is a problem. Patients who present with epigastric feelings of fullness, nausea, or vomiting are likely candidates for gastroenterostomy. Residual barium in the stomach in any but the most minimal amount also identifies potential candidates for gastroenterostomy. Although these symptoms and radiographic findings may be ameliorated after administration of metaclopramide, a response to pharmacologic stimulation should not deter the surgeon from a decision to bypass. Metaclopramide is of value only in avoiding an operative procedure in a patient in whom metastatic disease has been documented and a percutaneously or endoscopically placed biliary stent has successfully decompressed the biliary tree.

The reverse problem can occur during an exploration for carcinomas of the body and tail of the pancreas. For these patients, the necessity for gastric drainage may have been the indication for surgery, but obstructive jaundice may develop in the early postoperative period. Most commonly, this appearance of jaundice does not reflect rapid growth of the cancer. Rather, it results from an impending obstruction overlooked at the time of laparotomy. Part of the surgical exploration in these patients should include examination for a distended gallbladder and a dilated common bile duct. This latter requires the opening of the peritoneum over the bile duct so that the duct can be closely inspected. Mere palpation or estimation through an intact peritoneal covering is insufficient. In the absence of gross liver metastases, preoperative elevation of the serum alkaline phosphatase or identification of dilated bile ducts on ultrasonographic examination of the liver should also steer the surgeon toward a close inspection of the biliary tree. If the bile duct is 1 cm in diameter or more, internal biliary drainage is indicated.

The most ominous findings encountered at time of laparotomy are peritoneal metastases, particularly if accompanied by even a small amount of ascitic fluid. These often minute, hard, whitish granules or plaques are often difficult to distinguish from granulomata or fat necrosis, and may be the cause of fairly dense adhesions. Although occasionally found over the dome of the liver and on the undersurface of the diaphragm, they are more commonly found deep in the pelvis, near the base of the small bowel mesentery, on the small bowel, and occasionally in the omentum. As the disease progresses, these lesions frequently lead to dense adhesions and small bowel obstruction, a situation in which operative intervention is often unrewarding. Patients with peritoneal metastases may be considered candidates for intraperitoneal chemotherapy.

When abdominal or back pain has led to diagnostic studies and laparotomy, patients should be considered for chemical splanchnicectomy as a part of the operative procedure. Both sides of the celiac axis and aorta should be injected, although the accuracy of injection is impaired when massive lymphadenopathy and metastatic tumor extends along the aorta and surrounds the celiac axis. Depending on the surgeon's preference, 6 percent phenol, 95 percent alcohol, or 50 percent alcohol may be used. The lower strength alcohol, diluted in sterile water, offers as an advantage a volume of up to 25 ml which may be injected on each side. In contrast, the total volume of 95 percent alcohol or 6 percent phenol should not exceed 6 to 8 ml.

In selected patients, pain is due to pancreatic secretion against the obstruction of the cancer. When a dilated pancreatic duct is identified, retrograde drainage by a Peustow procedure can provide dramatic pain relief.

Histologic confirmation of pancreatic cancer is essential. Metastatic tumors within or invading the pancreas can appear as primary disease clinically, by imaging techniques, and in the operating room. While the most common origin of metastases in this site are tumors of the lung, stomach and breast, melanoma, lymphoma and genitourinary tumors have also presented in this fashion. In the presence of extensive metastases, biopsy from the liver or a regional lymph node may be sufficient, particularly since the pathologist may suggest the true nature of those cancers that are treatable.

Fear of hemorrhage, pancreatic juice leakage, and pancreatitis has led many surgeons to feel that the pancreas is an organ not to be biopsied. The problem is compounded, in the case of small and potentially resectable cancers, by the surrounding obstructive pancreatitis caused by the presence of these tumors, which usually arise from ductal tissue. This can make the establishment of the exact location of the cancer within the pancreas difficult.

Large cancers that extend beyond the gland are easily biopsied by shaving off a superficial sliver of tumor. Smaller cancers are best diagnosed by fine needle aspiration biopsy and prompt cytologic examination of the aspirate with the patient still in the operating theater. When facilities or expertise for this are unavailable, needle biopsy by the Tru-Cut technique can often provide adequate tissue. Rather than approach the kocherized gland anteriorly, transduodenal biopsy allows any pancreatic fluid to drain into the duodenum (the needle hole in the opposite duodenal wall is closed with a pursestring or Halsted suture). Up to three biopsy attempts can usually be performed safely by this technique and should provide confirmatory tissue in the majority of cases. Alternatively, the needle can be inserted through the opened bile duct, since it is compression from tumor adjacent to the duct that has caused bile duct occlusion.

Should a significant blood vessel within the pancreas be caught in the biopsy, prompt swelling of the head of the pancreas signifies hemorrhage within the gland. Ligation of the pancreatoduodenal artery just above the superior border of the pancreas promptly stops the bleeding.

POSTOPERATIVE CARE

Following pancreatic resection, it has been our policy not to stimulate the pancreas for up to 10 days to allow healing of the pancreatojejunostomy. Nutrition is maintained intravenously during the first 2 or 3 days, while gradually switching over to an elemental diet fed through a needle catheter jejunostomy. These feedings are maintained once the patient resumes an oral diet by supplementation at night until the patient's caloric intake allows weight to be maintained. The catheter is left in place during radiation therapy in case alimentation becomes insufficient to maintain weight and strength.

Catheter jejunostomies are also inserted when bypasses are constructed and there are no peritoneal or liver metastases, since definitive postoperative therapy will include radiation and chemotherapy. Maintenance of nutritional status has been a key factor in our ability to carry patients through aggressive combined modality therapy, to maintain treatment intensity, and to avoid delays in the treatment schedule.

Patients with pancreatic resection virtually all require enzymatic support to digest the fats in their food. Enzymatic supplements should be selected entirely according to their effective lipase content since the pancreas is the only source of this essential digestive material.

Generally, in patients with pancreatic cancer, the stomach is hypochlorhydric. However, a few patients may have normal acid secretion. Since lipase is rapidly degraded in the presence of a low pH, its efficacy may be enhanced by the addition of H_2 blocking agents.

MULTIMODALITY THERAPY FOLLOWING RESECTION AND FOR LOCALLY INCURABLE DISEASE

Following potentially curative resection of pancreatic cancer, most reports of the last decade often provided little more than anecdotal notations of one or two patients who were long-term survivors. Five-year cure rates were rarely in excess of 5 percent. On the other hand, mortality related to the operation claimed nearly one of every five patients. More recently, operative mortality has been reduced by more than two-thirds, while long-term survival rates have reached as high as 10 to 12 percent in small, single institution series. Nevertheless, it is probably that the mortality and survival statistics in unreported patient series are less optimal.

In 1973, the Gastrointestinal Tumor Study Group (GITSG) was formed to test programs that might improve postsurgical survival. Two leads had already been developed over the course of years. Childs and Moertel at the Mayo Clinic had noted that, in a randomized, doubly blinded trial, patients with locally unresectable pancreatic cancer treated with radiation and 5-fluorouracil survived significantly longer than those whose radiation therapy was accompanied by a placebo. About the same time, Haslam and Cavanaugh reported prolongation of survival when somewhat higher radiation doses were administered.

The GITSG therefore set out to test whether postoperative, combined modality treatment with radiation plus 5-fluorouracil would enhance survival of patients with pancreatic cancer through the format of a randomized, controlled multi-institutional trial. Treated patients were to receive 40 Gy of radiation therapy in a split course through anterior and posterior portals not larger than 400 cm^2 in size. Each course of radiation therapy was to be accompanied by 500 mg per square meter of body surface area of 5-fluorouracil on each of the first 3 days of treatment. Following recovery from radiation therapy, 5-fluorouracil would be given once weekly in the same dose, for a total postoperative period of 2 years.

Initial accrual goals were ambitious, but the rate of patient entry was painfully slow. Many surgeons doubted that patients could tolerate this rigorous therapy following pancreatic resection. By 1980, only 43 eligible patients had been entered, but 2- and 5-year survival information was already available for a considerable proportion of the group. Even in this small group of patients, survival curves were significantly divergent (Table 4). Further, the survival pattern of the untreated controls closely approximated that of a composite group of historic controls.

Although the survival of the treated group of patients was statistically and clinically significantly improved, the GITSG, concerned with the small sample size, elected to stop randomization and enroll a second group of patients for descriptive purposes. These patients were to be treated according to the guidelines of the original protocol. The only adjustment made was for improved radiotherapy technique by allowing patients to be treated by three fields. Thirty patients were accrued in just over 2 years. The survival pattern of this second group of patients virtually overlapped that of the randomized treatment group. Intense review of the pathology, surgery, population characteristics, and treatment programs for all patients entered into both phases of the study permitted the GITSG its conclusion, now based on 51 treated patients. Multimodality, postsurgical adjuvant therapy had enhanced survival of patients following potentially curative pancreatic resection.

The GITSG also tested treatments for patients with locally unresectable pancreatic cancer in whom no distant metastases were present. In the first study, the treatment that had been proposed for the surgical adjuvant trial was tested against a higher dose of radiation therapy (60 Gy) given as a double split course, with or without 5-fluorouracil. The result, apparent within 3 years, confirmed the original Mayo Clinic study: survival of patients who received 5-fluorouracil with their radiotherapy (and subsequent to it, until relapse) was

TABLE 4 Results of Controlled Trial of Postoperative Treatment with 40 Gy and 5-fluorouracil Following Pancreatic Resection

	Controls	*Adjuvant Treatment*
Median disease-free survival	9 months	16 months
Overall survival		
1 year	41%	65%
2 years	14%	38%
3 years	11%	24%
Incidence of liver metastases	50%	32%

TABLE 5 Results of Treatment of Patients with Locally Unresectable Pancreatic Cancer with Radiation Therapy ± 5-fluorouracil

	First Study		*Second Study*	
	Weeks to Progression	*Survival (Weeks)*	*Weeks to Progression*	*Survival (Weeks)*
6,000 Gy	13	23		
6,000 Gy + 5FU	33	40	34	49
4,000 Gy + 5FU	30	42	23	37

significantly superior (36 to 49 weeks) to that of patients treated with radiotherapy alone (23 weeks), but little advantage was documented for the higher dose radiotherapy (Table 5).

Since 5-fluorouracil seemed to potentiate the effects of radiation therapy, it was thought that perhaps a stronger radiosensitizer (Adriamycin) would further enhance survival, but this was not the case. Survival was equivalent. Only toxicity had been enhanced in this randomized study.

If the radiation sensitizer could not improve survival, perhaps hyperfractionation could increase the radioequivalence of the therapy, thus enhancing local tumor control. The results of this phase II trial suggested that there was nothing to be gained by expansion of the concept to phase III.

One question remained: was combined modality therapy better than chemotherapy alone? The Eastern Cooperative Oncology Group had previously attempted to tackle this question, but closed its study because of inadequate patient accrual. The results of the treatment of the few patients entered, however, suggest no advantage of combined modality treatment over treatment with 5-fluorouracil alone. Could the first GITSG trial have suggested that patient survival was due to the 5-fluorouracil alone? Was it possible that radiation therapy might even have been detrimental?

The decade had seen changes in both radiation therapy techniques and in chemotherapy programs. It was thought that perhaps a definitive answer could be found with improved radiation therapy planning, higher radioequivalent dosage, and the addition of a three-drug chemotherapy program in the maintenance phase of the study. A straight course of radiation therapy, 52.4 Gy, accompanied by 5-fluorouracil during the first 3 and last 3 days of the course. After recovery, patients received 8-week cycles of a three-drug combination of streptozocin, mitomycin C, and 5-fluorouracil, a combination that somewhat prolonged survival of patients with advanced pancreatic cancer as compared with the results of 17 other treatment programs evaluated by the GITSG. Patients randomized to the chemotherapy alone arm of this trial were given this same three-drug combination.

This final GITSG trial in locally advanced, nonmetastatic pancreatic cancer confirmed the Group's impression that combined modality therapy provides better quality and longer duration of palliation than either radiotherapy or chemotherapy alone.

CHEMOTHERAPY

Until the advent of computerized tomography, response was usually difficult or impossible to assess in patients with pancreatic cancer. Response evaluation was possible only for patients with large masses palpable through the abdominal wall, hepatomegaly with the liver extending 5 cm or more below the costal margin, or rare discrete tumor nodules in the lungs. All of these findings were associated with far advanced disease and shortened life expectancy (6 to 10 weeks). On occasion, supraclavicular lymph nodes provided a measurable lesion in a patient who might be expected to live longer than 3 months.

Ultrasonography, computerized tomography, and nuclear resonance imaging have permitted more accurate assessment of earlier lesions in the peripancreatic region and of metastases in the liver and in retroperitoneal lymph nodes. Although at times it can be difficult to delineate the head of the pancreas from adjacent first and third portions of the duodenum, studies by the GITSG have shown that survival is prolonged in patients in whom a shrinkage of a mass in this region can be demonstrated.

Unfortunately, the technologic advances that have made possible the assessment of results have not been accompanied by the identification of increasingly effective drugs or by the development of improved drug combinations. When given the critical test of a multi-institutional trial, no single agent has yielded a response rate of more than 20 percent, and no drug combination has provided a clinically important improvement in overall survival. The survival curves for all agents and combinations tested (including 5-fluorouracil, Adriamycin, and mitomycin C) virtually overlap each other, with a single exception. The streptozocin, 5-fluorouracil, mitomycin C (SMF) combination has provided patients with an overall survival that, while statistically significantly superior, is of little clinical importance. For standard therapy, 5-fluorouracil or SMF must be considered, but there is little evidence that these are superior to no antineoplastic treatment when toxicity considerations are added to the equation. Certainly, previously untreated patients with pancreatic cancer can ethically be considered as candidates for new drug programs.

The situation is not totally bleak, however. There are faint suggestions that biologic response modifiers may be of some value in the management of these patients. Even more encouraging are the anecdotal reports of the potential for pharmacologic modulation of pyrimidine metabolism. More than one center has noted prolonged survival and enhanced quality of life for patients treated by 5-

fluorouracil and leukovorin, but the ideal dose of leukovorin has yet to be determined in any gastrointestinal malignancy, even though statistical techniques for doing so (response surface methodology) are now available.

Because of the rather diffuse spread of malignant cells and fairly widespread development of metastases, regional chemotherapy programs have generally failed to impact on this disease. Once again, the absence of truly effective agents plays a role in this failure. Because transperitoneal, venous, and lymphatic routes allow the development of the common sites of metastases, the peritoneal, liver, and lymph node metastases (all of which are at least theoretically accessible to intraperitoneal drug delivery), a critical trial of peritoneal chemotherapy utilizing both water soluble (for peritoneal and portal distribution) and particulate or lipid soluble (for lymphatic incorporation) forms of the chemotherapeutic agents is needed.

TUMOR MARKERS AND MONOCLONAL ANTIBODIES

To date, there has been no tumor marker that would be of value for the identification of pancreatic cancer. The problem is the false positive rate for proposed diagnostic agents. With the annual incidence of pancreatic cancer affecting only 0.01 percent of the population, the value of any test with a false positive rate of more than 1 percent must be considered, at best, very limited. The most successful assays from this standpoint were those involving leukocyte adherence inhibition, but antigen stability problems, the inherent labor intensive technique, and the need for viable leukocytes designate this test as impractical.

Carcinoembryonic antigen, CA 19–9, and other pancreatic tumor associated antigens fail to meet the restrictive criteria necessary for tumor markers to be of aid in diagnosis in pancreatic cancer, and are of only little more value in following the course of the patient's disease. CEA and CA 19–9 are of value when a large tumor or significant liver metastases are present, by which time physical examination alone is almost equally useful. Neuron specific enolase and pancreatic elastase may be of greater value, but critically testing their potential as markers has been limited by the paucity of treatment approaches that will even temporarily alter the progression of advanced disease.

Kaproski's antigen has been applied to a very limited number of patients with pancreatic cancer, at least one of whom had a significant reduction in tumor mass and prolongation of survival. Limited tissue availability and the difficulty in evaluating results have limited the number of trials of immunotherapy. A suggestion that interferons may retard the progression of this disease has not been confirmed in a cooperative or controlled setting.

PAIN, NUTRITION, AND SUPPORTIVE CARE

The potential survival impact of optimal supportive care has probably not been realized in patients with pancreatic cancer. While many of these patients die of progression of cancer with liver metastasis and hepatorenal failure, or the complications of chronic intestinal obstruction due to peritoneal metastases, a significant number die of the complications of malnutrition or of incompletely or unrelieved biliary obstruction with cholangitis, liver abscesses, and endotoxemia.

The most significant problem is that of pain. The multiplicity of the etiologic factors that cause pain in patients with pancreatic cancer have prevented the development of a universal solution resulting from a simplistic approach to its management. A tendency toward increased anxiety and depression in patients with pancreatic diseases, and particularly in those with pancreatic cancer, combined with chronicity of pain and frequent failure to respond to usual analgesic management have made these patients even more refractory to treatment. In addition, patients who have severe pain and those who are depressed do not eat. The result is a compounding of the catabolic state, even when the gastrointestinal tract is intact.

There are at least six distinct pain patterns, three of which arise from the pancreas and are due to the primary tumor, while the rest are due to invasion or metastases. However, patients with pancreatic cancer present with mixtures of these pain syndromes, yet it is probable that each syndrome requires individualized management to provide optimal pain control. The potential for various psychotropic agents must also be evaluated in these patients.

The recognizable discrete patterns of pain in pancreatic cancer can be described as follows:

1. Tumor mass, with invasion of perineural lymphatics. Pain is predominantly epigastric or left subcostal and tends to be more or less continuous, but worse at night.
2. Pancreatic ductal obstruction, but with a nonmalignant obstructed pancreas distal. The histologic picture is that of pancreatitis, which is the result of inflammation as the pancreas attempts to secrete against obstruction. The pancreatic duct is often dilated, pseudocysts may develop. The pain is aggravated by meals, alcohol, and anxiety, and tends to be localized in the epigastrium, radiating to left flank or to the left side of the back. This pain is frequently associated with nausea. The patient may describe the pain in the left upper abdomen as going straight through from front to back.
3. Retroperitoneal invasion with severe back pain, worse at night. The patient has a favorite, often contorted, position in which he or she sits or lies. This position reduces tension or pressure on the retroperitoneum, thereby giving a small but notable amount of pain relief. The position varies from patient to patient, but is often left side down, resembling a fetal configuration. Nausea is not a part of this syndrome.
4. Biliary obstruction, involving either the entire biliary

tree or small intrahepatic segments as a result of metastases. This pain is usually in the right upper quadrant and is associated with anorexia, nausea, and vomiting. The pain may vary, but tends to be worse after eating. Pain may be referred to substernal or scapular region.

5. Liver metastases, with stretching or invasion of Glisson's capsule. This may be described as a vague, dull ache in the right upper abdomen and is associated with a feeling of fullness. Mixed with this may be a sharper pain radiating to the scapula, shoulder, or anterior mediastinum and which is associated with coughing, deep breathing, or attempts at exercise, as the parietal peritoneum is irritated by tumor nodules or adhesions.
6. Intestinal dysfunction with crampy pain of intestinal obstruction due to peritoneal metastases and their adhesions. This pain may present over the entire abdomen or may be localized to any portion and is aggravated by food and by prolonged use of narcotics. Nausea is followed by vomiting as the syndrome progresses. This pain almost always overlies a second discrete pain, which may be present independently, and is related to lymphadenopathy in the base of the small bowel mesentery and around the origin of the superior mesenteric artery. This pain becomes more pronounced as the nodes around the superior mesenteric artery coalesce into a single mass. It begins as a dull ache over the fourth and fifth lumbar vertebrae and occasionally extends both upward and down over the upper sacrum. On occasion, the pain can radiate towards one hip or the other (although towards the left seems more frequent). Beginning as a discomfort, the pain can slowly progress to the intensity of a leaking aortic aneurysm.

While the use of narcotics is the traditional approach to management of cancer pain, some narcotics (particularly codeine compounds) can aggravate the patient's discomfort. Some relief may be provided transiently, but then pain progress as one syndrome is exchanged for another. In other circumstances, aspirin and nonsteroidal anti-inflammatory drugs can significantly potentiate pain relief. When the pain or a major component is due to pancreatic ductal obstruction, 600 mg of aspirin can give more relief than almost anesthetic doses of narcotics. Pain of the pancreatic mass may be relieved by celiac axis blockade with alcohol or phenol in the majority of patients. However, the duration of pain relief from celiac axis blockade can vary from as little as a week to as much as 4 months or more. The presence of other pain syndromes may well explain why relief is fleeting in a number of patients.

It is critical that other approaches to pain relief be examined. As an example, two of our patients who were candidates for celiac axis blocks were taught self-hypnosis with remarkable improvement in pain control and well-being. Finally, one must not overlook the potential for locally applied heat to provide pain relief, particularly at night. Sleep at night can be a precious and scarce commodity for patients with pancreatic cancer. In many cases relief of pain will improve appetite. However, patients with pancreatic cancer, even those without pain, are not spared from the anorexia of cancer. They must be taught the importance of eating, the foods they will most likely tolerate, and how to avoid the odors which are, to them, nauseating. Commercial enteric supplements are of some help, but for many, continuous feedings through a jejunostomy tube can be critical in the battle to maintain weight, strength, and performance status. When possible, these should be given as 10 to 14-hour overnight feedings to free the patient during the day. Nutrition by the enteral route provides critical preferential support for the intestinal mucosa and liver, the defenders of the host from gram-negative sepsis and endotoxemia arising from the gut content.

On rare occasion, the intestinal tract functions poorly or not at all, but the patient with good performance status and otherwise controlled symptoms wishes to keep functioning independently. In this case, total parenteral nutrition can be a suboptimal alternative. In our experience, occasional nutritionally supported patients with otherwise controlled symptoms and no biliary sepsis have survived for as long as 14 months without antineoplastic therapy.

Secondary biliary obstruction can become a serious problem in patients in whom a previously functioning cholecystoenteric bypass ceases to function as progressive tumor obstructs the cystic duct. Whereas formerly we reexplored many patients who were referred for secondary obstruction, we now utilize percutaneous drainage and reassess the tumor load. Only if the catheter cannot be passed beyond the obstruction into the bowel, the tumor has not widely metastasized, and the amount of fluid and electrolyte lost by external drainage threatens patient survival do we offer reexploration (and its attendant risks) to the patient. Survival after reexploration is often brief (10 to 12 weeks).

Liver abscesses, when they occur, are now percutaneously drained with the aid of ultrasonography, usually resulting in control of fever and sepsis. Since the most common cause of the abscesses is obstruction of undrained bile ducts by metastatic disease, survival in this group of patients is only minimally prolonged. However, even this short palliative period is usually of better quality.

For a period of time, ascites may be controlled by administration of high doses of spirinolactone and hydrochlorothiazide, but this requires close monitoring of renal function. Because of high protein content and large numbers of malignant cells, peritineovenous shunts are rarely of value. Our greatest success for the treatment of symptomatic ascites after the failure of diuretics has resulted from treatment with intraperitoneal mitomycin C in large volumes (2 liters) of saline, repeated at 6-week intervals as needed. Since the drug is absorbed from the peritoneal surface, hematologic monitoring is required, as would be the case if the drug were administered intravenously.

AMPULLARY AND PERIAMPULLARY CANCERS

The prognosis of patients with adenocarcinoma of the distal common bile duct, periampullary duodenum, and ampulla of Vater differs considerably from that of patients with pancreatic adenocarcinoma arising only millimeters away. A far greater proportion of patients with periampullary cancers have resectable disease, largely because the location of these tumors causes symptoms of jaundice (sometimes intermittent) and anemia or gastrointestinal bleeding at an earlier stage.

Resection by pancreatoduodenectomy can cure 20 to 45 percent of these patients. However, lymph node metastases do alter their prognosis, and have encouraged us to offer those subset of patients who have nodal metastases a brief course of radiation therapy potentiated by 5-fluorouracil, but no long-term chemotherapy. This has been well tolerated and appears to have improved survival.

Ampullary carcinomas offer a special situation. Papillary tumors have been treated by local resection in poor risk candidates, with a 15 percent long-term cure potential, but we prefer the standard pancreatoduodenectomy, with a potential for cure that is at least twice as high. Patients with ulcerating ampullary cancers have a much worse prognosis. When an ampullary cancer invades into the head of the pancreas, the prognosis is the same as that of pancreatic cancer.

THOUGHTS FOR THE FUTURE

The results of combined modality therapy, either as adjuvant to surgery or as definitive therapy for patients with localized disease, have indicated that a first step has been accomplished in the management of pancreatic cancer. But further intensification of radiation therapy and chemotherapy offer little potential benefit until better chemotherapeutic agents become available or newer approaches show potential value.

Among agents in need of study and development are the biologic response modifiers and growth factor inhibitors. There is already evidence that growth factor inhibitors such as somatostatin analogues have proven their value in at least symptomatic control of islet cell tumors and may have been associated with a few tumor regressions. The results of further trials with interferons could certainly be no worse than those of the multitude of phase II trials of the past decade.

Radiation therapy, whether using particles or x-rays, has probably reached the point of maximum benefit. However, there are possibilities of activity of other forms of radiation, particularly if the target organ can be sensitized. One such example would be photodynamic therapy, a modality that has been utilized to treat tumors elsewhere in the body on more than 3,000 patients worldwide.

It is time for carefully planned innovation in the development of new approaches to this disease.

SUGGESTED READING

Barkin JS, Lindblad AS, Bruckner HW. The evaluation of CT and sonographic pancreatic measurements in determining tumor response. Proc Amer Soc Clin Oncol 1986; 5:22(85)

Childs DS Jr, Moertel CG, Holbrook MA, et al. Treatment of malignant neoplasms of the gastrointestinal tract with a combination of 5-fluorouracil and radiation. A randomized double-blind study. Radiology 1965; 84:843–848.

Dickey JE, Haaga JR, Stellato TA, et al. Evaluation of computed tomography guided percutaneous biopsy of the pancreas. Surg Gynecol Obstet 1986; 163:497–503.

Douglass HO Jr. Carcinoma of the head of the pancreas and periampullary region. In: Nyhus L, ed. Surgery Annual 1974. New York: Appleton-Century-Croft, 1974:161.

Flanigan DP, Kraft RO. Continuing experience with palliative chemical splanchnicectomy. Arch Surg 1978; 113:509–511.

Gastrointestinal Tumor Study Group. Further evidence of effective adjuvant combined radiation and chemotherapy following curative resection of pancreatic cancer. Cancer 1987; 59:2006–2010.

Go VLW, Taylor WF, DiMagno EP. Efforts at early diagnosis of pancreatic cancer: The Mayo Clinic experience. Cancer 1981; 47:1698–1703.

Haslam JB, Cavanaugh PJ, Stroup SL. Radiation therapy in the treatment of irresectable adenocarcinoma of the pancreas. Cancer 1973; 32:1341–1345.

Moertel CG, Frytak S, Hahn RG, et al. Therapy of locally unresectable pancreatic carcinoma: A randomized comparison of high dose (6,000 rads) radiation alone, moderate dose radiation (4,000 rads + 5-fluorouracil) and high dose radiation + 5-fluorouracil. The Gastrointestinal Tumor Study Group. Cancer 1981; 48:1705–1710.

Sarr MG, Cameron JL. Surgical palliation of unresectable carcinoma of the pancreas. World J Surg 1984; 8:906–918.

Sears HF, Herlyn D, Steplewski Z, Kaprowski H. Effects of monoclonal antibody immunotherapy on patients with gastrointestinal adenocarcinoma. J Biol Response Med 1984; 3:138–150.

COLORECTAL CANCER

HERBERT C. HOOVER Jr., M.D.

Colorectal carcinoma remains just second to lung carcinoma as the most common malignancy affecting both males and females in the United States. There are approximately 145,000 new cases with nearly 65,000 deaths each year. The cause of colonic or rectal cancers remains unknown but dietary factors most likely play a role. A number of conditions tend to predispose to malignancies in the large bowel. Among these are chronic ulcerative colitis and familial polyposis. Patients with familial polyposis carry a nearly 100 percent risk of developing carcinoma if total colectomy is not performed.

DIAGNOSIS

Screening for colorectal cancer is important because of the frequency of the disease and its curability if detected at an early stage. Commonly utilized screening tests include digital rectal examination, stool test for occult blood, air contrast barium enema, rigid or flexible sigmoidoscopy, colonoscopy, and carcinoembryonic antigen (CEA) test. Unfortunately, cancers do not always bleed continuously, so occult blood tests are not totally effective in detecting even large cancers. Full colonoscopy is the best screening test, because early lesions are more likely to be detected by direct visualization and biopsy. Shinya and others have shown convincingly that colons kept free of polyps are also kept free of cancer, lending strong support to the polyp-to-cancer transition theory. All patients with unexplained large bowel symptoms, guaiac-positive stools, or gross rectal bleeding should be evaluated by a full colonoscopic examination. If symptoms of colonic disease persist after a negative colonoscopy, an air contrast barium enema should be performed. Being a large and tortuous organ, both radiologic and endoscopic diagnostic procedures can miss significant lesions. Therefore, the two are complementary rather than competitive in their diagnostic potential.

Unfortunately, many large bowel cancers encountered clinically have not been previously sought by screening tests. Consequently, patients present with symptoms representing bowel dysfunction that occurs relatively late in the natural history of this disease. Blood streaking on the stool is the most frequent complaint of patients with rectal cancer, whereas patients with colonic cancer more often complain of pain. Pain in left colon cancer is often colicky, whereas the pain in right colon cancer is usually late and ill defined. The differences occur because of the disparities in the caliber of the colon lumen and differences in the character of the stool, solid or liquid.

Patients found to have colonic and rectal cancers should undergo other diagnostic tests before surgery. Urinalysis can indicate colovesicle fistulas. It is important to obtain a CEA level both preoperatively and at approximately 1 month postoperatively. If an elevated preoperative level fails to return to normal, persistent disease is indicated. CEA levels that are elevated well above normal can make one suspicious of liver metastases. A chest x-ray examination should always be performed to look for lung metastases. Although not uniformly done preoperatively, computed tomographic (CT) scans of the abdomen provide very useful information. As many as 30 percent of patients may have occult hepatic metastases that are not palpable at laparotomy and are shown only by CT scanning. Magnetic resonance imaging (MRI) scanning is proving to be even more effective in detecting small metastases, but is not available in all hospitals. A CT scan also provides useful information relative to retroperitoneal lymph node enlargement, shows the position of both ureters, and indicates any possibility of obstruction as well as the functional status of both kidneys. It can also diagnose extramural spread of rectal cancer and may indicate involvement of adjacent organs, especially the urinary bladder. If a CT scan has not been obtained, intravenous pyelography (IVP) can be useful, especially in patients with large right colon cancers or advanced rectosigmoid lesions where ureteral or bladder involvement is not uncommon. Bone scans or lung CT scans do not usually provide sufficient clinical information to warrant their expense in asymptomatic patients.

TREATMENT: GENERAL CONSIDERATIONS

Since surgical resection is the only effective treatment for most carcinomas of the colon and for all but early rectal carcinomas, the surgeon's goal in treating localized colonic or rectal tumors must be to control the primary tumor and do everything possible to prevent recurrence. Approximately 70 percent of patients present with "totally resectable" primary tumors, but nearly one-half of these patients eventually die of recurrent or metastatic disease. Obviously, microscopic deposits are left behind or are potentially spread at the time of the operation. Thirty to 50 percent of recurrences are local or regional, and therefore potentially avoidable or treatable.

There are a number of predictors of an increased failure rate in colorectal cancer. Clinical factors include symptomatic lesions, youth, elevated CEA, obstruction, perforation, adjacent organ involvement, ulcerated primary tumor, location in the rectum, fixed tumor in the rectum, and circumferential bowel involvement. Pathologic predictors of failure include poorly differentiated histology; deep penetration of the bowel wall; infiltrating deep margins; mucinous, signet ring, or scirrhous adenocarcinomas; lymphatic and lymph node involvement; and venous and perineural invasion. Although all the above factors are beyond the surgeon's control, there is some evidence that surgeons can alter the recurrence or metastatic rate. Modes of spread, whether by direct continuity to surrounding organs, through the peritoneal cavity, through the lymphatic or hematogenous channels, or by direct implantation, are theoretically influenced by surgical techniques.

Commonly accepted techniques that can possibly lower the iatrogenic spread of colorectal cancers include minimal manipulation of tumor, wide resection of bowel and mesentery, and en bloc resection of adjacent organs. Other techniques of possible importance include isolation of the involved bowel segment with tapes; early high ligation of colonic vessels; mechanical measures, such as covering the tumor with gauze or irrigating the bowel lumen with cytotoxic agents; and pelvic lymphadenectomy for advanced rectal cancer. The issue of high or low ligation of the inferior mesenteric artery (IMA) for patients with rectal or sigmoid carcinoma remains controversial, but most recent reports suggest no significant difference in the recurrence or survival rates among patients having ligation of the IMA flush with the aorta, and those in whom the ligation and resection go up just to the left colic branch. Certainly, the more extended operations lead to increased morbidity and cannot be recommended until studies show a more clear benefit in terms of survival. I isolate the involved bowel and perform an early ligation of colonic vessels whenever possible, but do not perform colonic irrigations or radical pelvic lymphadenectomy on a routine basis.

Surgical treatment is designed to remove the primary tumor with generous lateral margins, as well as all regional lymph nodes and lymphatic channels that can be safely extirpated. Because of the segmental nature of spread from colorectal cancers, the margin of normal bowel distal to the tumor need not be extensive. This is especially true in rectal cancer. Several recent studies show that even 2 cm is sufficient for rectal cancers, but 3 to 5 cm should be obtained whenever possible. Longitudinal spread, more than 1 cm beyond the tumor mass, occurs only in patients with retrograde lymphatic obstruction. Prognosis is poor in such patients no matter what procedure is performed. It is important to maximize the lateral margins of resection in potentially curable patients. If a colonic or rectal tumor is adherent to other organs, an en bloc resection is critically important. Peeling tumors away from organs leads to a high rate of local recurrence. En bloc resection adds very little morbidity in the usual situation, and leads to salvage rates nearly comparable with those patients in whom there is no extension to other organs. Rectal tumors most frequently adhere to the vagina, bladder, prostate, or uterus. Sigmoid tumors adhere to ovaries, pelvic side walls, and the bladder. Cecal tumors tend to adhere to the abdominal wall or to small bowel.

PREPARATION FOR RESECTION

In recent years, we have abandoned the clear liquid diet and 3-day bowel preparation in favor of 4 liters of Golytely on the evening before operation. Patients are admitted the afternoon before the operation and started on a clear liquid diet on the day of admission. Oral neomycin and erythromycin base, 1 g each, are given in three doses the afternoon and evening before resection. This provides an excellent bowel preparation without the economic and nutritional consequences of the three day bowel preparation. Cefazolin sodium (Ancef), 500 mg intramuscularly is given on call to the operating room, and two additional doses are given postoperatively.

Since recent data consistently show an increased rate of infectious complications and a diminished survival rate in patients who are transfused at any time during the management of colorectal cancer, we avoid transfusions in these patients whenever possible. This often means that even elderly patients are treated and discharged with hematocrit levels as low as the mid-20s.

TREATMENT: SPECIFIC RECOMMENDATIONS

The extent of resection for colon or rectal cancers varies with the site of the primary tumor based upon the arterial and venous supply of the colon. Anastomoses in any of the resections for lesions above the peritoneal reflection can be performed with either a one- or two-layer handsewn technique or with staplers. Obstructing lesions in the right colon are commonly treated with a one-stage resection, whereas lesions in the more distal colon or rectum are more often treated with a preliminary diverting colostomy followed in several days by a primary resection.

The surgical management of middle and low rectal cancers has changed dramatically in the past 10 to 15 years, with a clear trend toward sphincter-saving procedures. This subject is discussed elsewhere. Generally, patients with tumors 5 cm or greater above the anus can be spared a colostomy, whereas most individuals with tumors palpable within 5 cm of the anal verge are best treated with abdominoperineal resection unless the tumors are small enough for a local resection. Some of these small tumors can also be treated effectively with primary radiation therapy by the Papillion technique. Fulguration is another treatment option, but local excision or radiation is generally preferred. Several recent studies have shown that local excision of small rectal tumors can yield excellent long-term cure rates. Local excision has the advantage of histopathologic examination of the resected specimen, which is not the case with fulguration or radiation. If the locally excised tumor proves to be more deeply invasive than suspected, the patient should undergo a more radical resection if there are no medical contraindications. In all but the most favorable lesions, irradiation should be strongly considered. I reserve local resection for low rectal lesions that are less than 3 cm, polypoid, mobile, and well differentiated histologically and do not penetrate through the full thickness of the rectal wall. Age or general state of health need not influence one's decision when such restrictive criteria are used. Obviously, in patients who are not considered candidates for general anesthesia, more advanced lesions can be managed by local resection and radiation therapy. The use of a resectoscope for the transanal resection of rectal cancers, similar to the transurethral resection of prostatic or bladder neoplasms, has recently been championed, but will require further investigation and follow-up before it can be widely recommended. Recent advances in transrectal ultrasonography allow more accurate preoperative assessment of the depth of penetration of rectal cancers.

Approximately 20 percent of patients with colorectal cancer present with clinically obvious metastatic disease, most commonly to the liver or lungs. Unless the metastatic disease is extensive and the expected survival is short, a palliative resection of the primary tumor is usually indicated to prevent or treat obstruction, bleeding, perforation, and other complications.

MANAGEMENT OF RECURRENT COLONIC OR RECTAL CANCER

Follow-up Schedule to Detect Recurrent or Metastatic Colorectal Cancer

Some of the more difficult decisions in the management of patients with colorectal cancer concern those with recurrent or metastatic disease. Since several modern series report encouraging results in the management of these patients, detection of such disease becomes increasingly important. Approximately 80 percent of these recurrences appear within the first 2 years, and so I recommend follow-up examinations every 3 months for 2 years, every 4 months during the third year, and at 6-month intervals until 5 years, at which time a yearly follow-up is sufficient. At each follow-up examination, a careful history should be taken and a thorough physical examination, including a stool guaiac test, performed. CEA determinations are also important at each visit. Colonoscopic examinations should be repeated at 6 to 12 months, then yearly for 2 or 3 years, and repeated every 2 to 3 years if no polyps or recurrences are found. A chest radiograph should be obtained at 6-month intervals for the first 2 years and yearly thereafter.

Surgical Options for Recurrent or Metastatic Disease

Recurrence in colorectal cancer is not always the dismal situation that many physicians envision. There are several biologic and anatomic characteristics related to colorectal cancer that favor the prospect of surgical control of recurrent disease: recurrent colorectal cancers are usually slow growing, the lymphatic extension is usually palpable, and the soft tissues surrounding the recurrence can generally be removed.

Prognostic Factors

Factors in recurrent colorectal cancer that tend to be more favorable are anastomotic recurrences; stage B2 or B3 (through the bowel wall or invading an adjacent organ but with negative nodes) original primary tumors; or implantation recurrences in the colostomy site, perineal scar, or abdominal wound or in a drain site. Recurrences in the pericolic fat, pelvic recurrences after abdominoperineal resection, or recurrences less than 6 months from the time of the primary resection all tend to be unfavorable for surgical salvage.

Reexploration

An aggressive approach toward patients with recurrent colorectal cancer is appropriate unless an unfavorable outcome is certain. We should think in terms of a cure by a radical procedure in selected patients, or a palliation of symptoms whenever possible. Reexploration in patients with a previously resected colonic or rectal cancer is indicated in any patients with a rising CEA and a negative work-up, including a chest x-ray film, abdominal and pelvic CT scan, and a colonoscopy; isolated pulmonary or hepatic metastases or local recurrences; or patients with unresectable tumors in whom obstruction or bleeding can be palliated. One can expect approximately 25 percent of recurrent colorectal cancers to be resectable with curative intent. Several studies have documented that resection of recurrent colorectal cancers with negative margins significantly increases both survival and the quality of life. However, tumor resections with gross disease left behind (debulking procedures) are rarely, if ever, indicated except to control unremitting symptoms such as bleeding or obstruction. Anastomotic recurrences account for 25 percent of all recurrences in colorectal cancer. Most of these present with bleeding or pain, and 50 to 60 percent can be totally resected in the expectation of almost a 50 percent 5 -year survival if all margins are microscopically clear. This is one area in which close follow-up with stool guaiacs can pay big dividends in salvage.

There is increasing enthusiasm for the role of total pelvic exenteration either for advanced primary tumors of the rectum with involvement of the base of the bladder, or for patients with recurrent rectal cancer involving the bladder. The operative mortality rate is low in experienced hands, and cure rates of 20 to 30 percent are being reported.

Distant Metastases

Metastases from colonic or rectal cancers most commonly involve the liver or lungs. Pulmonary metastases from colonic cancer are rare in the absence of liver metastases, but are more likely from rectal cancers. One should usually consider a preliminary laparotomy to evaluate the liver before embarking on a pulmonary resection for metastases from a colorectal cancer. A 5-year cure rate of 10 to 15 percent can be expected from aggressive approaches if the liver is free of metastases. The role of hepatic resection in isolated liver metastases is evolving. It is evident that total resection of single or even multiple metastases can provide a long-term cure. With single metastases, a cure rate of 30 percent may be anticipated; this drops off quickly as the number of lesions increases. There is no evidence that extended resections provide any more success than wedge resections if the tumor can be totally removed with microscopically negative margins. Recent studies support the use of intra-arterial chemotherapy in patients with unresectable hepatic metastases who have no apparent disease outside the liver. My enthusiasm for that technique is growing.

COMPLICATIONS AFTER COLORECTAL CANCER RESECTIONS

Major complications should be relatively unusual in patients who undergo elective resections of primary colonic or rectal cancers. Wound infections occur in spite of meticulous bowel preparations and systemic antibiotics, but the incidence should be low. Intra-abdominal abscesses are usually secondary to anastomotic leaks. Delayed hemorrhage secondary to inadequately ligated major vessels should be a rare occurrence. Strictures of circular stapled anastomoses are not uncommon, especially when postoperative irradiation is given. These usually occur close to the anus, making dilatation under intravenous sedation relatively straightforward. Rectal resections are frequently associated with urinary and sexual problems. The voiding difficulty is usually transient, but an adequate lymphatic resection for rectal cancer in males generally causes a permanent loss of potency. This possibility should be discussed in advance with all male patients. In patients with colostomies, devascularization with stenosis, retraction, and peristomal hernias are occasionally seen.

Complications are seen more commonly after resections or palliative procedures in patients with recurrent or metastatic colorectal cancer. Many of these patients have been heavily irradiated or have received chemotherapy, both of which can adversely affect anastomotic and wound healing, hemostasis, and resistance to infection.

RESULTS

Survival from colorectal cancer relates closely to the stage of disease at the time of diagnosis. Approximately 20 percent of patients have lesions that have neither extended through the bowel wall nor spread to lymph nodes. Most of these individuals are cured by resection alone. Another 30 percent present with clinically obvious metastatic disease; few of these are cured. This leaves 50 percent of patients who present with localized tumors that have grown through the entire thickness of the bowel wall or have spred to regional lymph nodes. Thirty to 60 percent of these patients can be cured by surgical resection alone. Adjuvant chemotherapy has shown no benefit in most studies and marginal benefits in a few recent ones. Pelvic irradiation definitely diminishes the pelvic recurrence rate in rectal cancers and probably improves overall survival rates. Survival benefits from the resection of recurrent or metastatic colorectal cancer are often difficult to evaluate, but the improved quality of life is often a definite advantage.

HOPES FOR THE FUTURE

Intraoperative radiation therapy is showing encouraging results in advanced carcinoma of the rectum, but is still a research procedure that is not widely available. My own studies using an autologous tumor cell-BCG vaccine (active specific immunotherapy) show some promise for this approach to immune induction in the adjuvant setting. Results of an ongoing national cooperative trial should clarify its potential. Human monoclonal antibodies have the potential for earlier diagnosis of metastases and can possibly deliver radionuclides, chemotherapy, or cell toxins to tumors in doses that could be therapeutic, with less damage to normal tissue than is the case with conventional delivery.

Remarkable advances in the understanding of the molecular biology of all types of cancer give us renewed hope for radically different and improved forms of therapy in the future.

SUGGESTED READING

Herfarth C, Schlag P, Hohenberger P. Surgical strategies in locoregional recurrences of gastrointestinal cancer. World J Surg 1987; 11:504–510.

Hoover HC, Surdyke MG, Dangel RB, et al. Prospectively randomized trial of adjuvant active-specific immunotherapy for human colorectal cancer. Cancer 1985; 55:236–243.

Lopex MJ, Kraybill WG, Downey RS, et al. Exenterative surgery for locally advanced rectosigmoid cancer. Is it worthwhile? Surgery 1987; 102:644–651.

Pezim ME, Nicholls RJ, Chir M. Survival after high or low ligation of inferior mesenteric artery during curative surgery for rectal cancer. Ann Surg 1984; 200:729–733.

Vassilopoulos PP, Yoon JM, Ledesma EJ, Mittelman A. Treatment of recurrence of adenocarcinoma of the colon and rectum at the anastomotic site. Surg Gynecol Obstet 1984; 152:777–780.

OVARIAN CANCER

RICHARD V. SMALLEY, M.D.

Ovarian cancer is the fourth most common fatal form of cancer in women. There are approximately 17,000 new cases each year in the United States, and over 11,000 women in the United States die annually of this disease. The majority of malignant ovarian tumors are epithelial in origin, with serous cystadenocarcinoma accounting for 42 percent, undifferentiated carcinoma accounting for 17 percent, endometrioid carcinoma accounting for 15 percent, and mucinous cystadenocarcinoma accounting for 12 percent. The remainder is equally split between miscellaneous tumors and sex cord, stromal, or germ cell tumors. Ovarian tumors commonly present as a large pelvic mass, and usual symptoms are pain, abdominal distension, and vaginal bleeding. The tumors generally remain confined to the peritoneal cavity, but may metastasize by lymphatics through the diaphragm into the thoracic cavity and beyond late in their course.

STAGING

The International Federation of Gynecology and Obstetrics (FIGO) staging system for primary carcinoma of the ovary is the generally accepted system and is detailed along with 5-year survival figures by stage in Table 1. Accurate and detailed staging is

TABLE 1 FIGO Staging for Ovarian Cancer

	5-yr Survival
Stage I Limited to ovaries	66%
One ovary involved	70%
Both ovaries involved	64%
With ascites or positive peritoneal washings	50%
Stage II Limited to ovaries plus pelvic extension	45%
Extension to uterus and tubes	52%
Extension to other pelvic tissues	42%
With ascites or positive peritoneal washings	42%
Stage III Intraperitoneal but beyond pelvis, including retroperitoneal nodes and/or small bowel and/or omentum	13%
Stage IV Distant metastases outside the peritoneal cavity but including liver metastases	4%

mandatory in order to determine both prognosis and treatment. In addition to history, physical, and bimanual pelvic exam, procedures to be used in the staging of patients are ultrasound and CT scan of the abdomen and pelvis and surgical exploration. The single most important staging procedure (unless a classification of stage III or IV is obvious) is a thorough and extensive surgical exploration of the abdomen and pelvis including multiple biopsies from the left and right inferior side of the diaphragm, a generous omental biopsy, a biopsy of retroperitoneal nodes in the area where the ovarian vessels attach to the aorta, and a biopsy of palpable pelvic or periaortic nodes. Samples of ascites fluid should be obtained or, if no ascites exist, washings from the four quadrants of the abdomen and pelvis should be performed. Since the prognosis correlates with the information obtained from this initial exploration and the future course is influenced by the ability to remove as much grossly visible tumor as possible, it is extremely important that a surgeon experienced in the evaluation and treatment of ovarian tumors perform these procedures. A midline incision in the upper abdomen is needed for adequate exploration and treatment, and the possibility or likelihood of this being performed should be discussed with the patient prior to general anesthesia. During surgery, the primary tumor should be carefully checked for rupture or other breaks in the capsule and, if intact, should be protected from rupture since the 5-year survival is adversely affected by capsular penetration or rupture.

PROGNOSTIC FACTORS

The stage (as discussed above), the histology, the grade of differentiation, and perhaps most importantly, the size of residual tumor following surgery are the factors correlating best with prognosis and dictating subsequent treatment. Serous cystadenocarcinomas and undifferentiated carcinomas are frequently bilateral and tend to be more aggressive than either mucinous or endometrioid carcinomas. While the grade of differentiation is difficult to reproduce amongst pathologists, an estimate of differentiation by an experienced pathologist is helpful and important. Well differentiated (grade 1) tumors have a more benign course than do the less well differentiated (grades 2–3) tumors. Finally, the size of residual tumor following surgery is most important in that the possibility of cure (or at least the likelihood of prolonged disease-free survival for stage III patients) is limited to patients in whom the largest residual tumor is less than 2 cm in diameter.

TREATMENT

Standard treatment for ovarian carcinoma is bilateral salpingo-oophorectomy plus total abdominal hysterectomy (BSO/TAH). This should be adequate treatment for patients with unilateral or bilateral ovarian lesions that are well differentiated and in whom exploration and peritoneal washings are negative and the tumor capsule is intact. The only exception is the patient who strongly desires to have children. In such a patient, a unilateral salpingo-oophorectomy may be performed with a reasonable expectation of cure (75 to 80 percent) provided the tumor is not a grade 2 or 3 serous cystadenocarcinoma. Under any other circumstance, minimal surgery should include BSO/TAH and a surgical attempt at debulking, followed by either abdominal irradiation or systemic chemotherapy. Patients with histologic borderline tumors are discussed below.

Postoperative Treatment

Patients with serous cystadenocarcinoma of grade 2 or 3 differentiation, those with an undifferentiated histology, or those with mucinous or endometrioid carcinoma stage IB or greater warrant aggressive postoperative therapy since the likelihood of cure with surgery alone is less than 50 percent. Although both whole abdominal radiation therapy and systemic chemotherapy provide additional therapeutic benefit, they tend to be mutually exclusive because of cumulative bone marrow toxicity. The choice between the two depends upon the physician's bias and experience as well as the availability of support facilities.

Whole Abdominal Radiation Therapy

In order to be maximally effective, radiation therapy has to be delivered to the whole abdominal cavity in doses of 4,500 to 6,000 rads over 4 to 6 weeks. The most common side effect observed is enteritis. Diarrhea, nausea, vomiting, and weight loss may occur in 75 percent of patients. In most patients, symptoms subside within a few weeks after completion of treatment, but in a quarter to a third, GI distress may persist for months or years. Bowel stenosis and GI bleeding may subsequently develop and require additional surgical intervention. Myelosuppression occurs, and although counts generally return to normal shortly after completion of treatment, the affected bone marrow is never the same and these patients are unable to subsequently tolerate substantial doses of chemotherapy.

The use of radioisotopes, including AU 198 or P32, has been advocated by some. Each of these isotopes emits beta irradiation, the range of which is only 3 to 5 mm. They are therefore effective only with tumors less than 5 mm in diameter. Due to adhesions or loculation, poor distribution following administration may occur; additionally, the possibility of subsequent small bowel obstruction is high. Because of these complications and difficulties, isotope therapy is not frequently used.

Systemic Chemotherapy

A number of cytotoxic agents are active when administered systemically to patients with advanced ovarian carcinoma (Table 2). Several drugs administered together in combination can frequently induce a complete response (CR) and a prolonged disease-free interval. Single agent chemotherapy should be considered in all patients who, by virture of age, amount of bulky disease, or general medical condition, are candidates for palliation rather than curative treatment.

Single Agent Cytotoxic Therapy

Melphalan is as effective as any, is arguably the best tolerated single agent, and is certainly the most frequently used. It is available as a 2 mg tablet and is administered at a dose of 0.2 mg per kilogram daily for 5 days, with each 5-day course repeated every 6 weeks. GI disturbance including nausea, vomiting, diarrhea, and oral ulceration may occur, but such symptoms are infrequent. The most common side effect is bone marrow suppression and some degree of neutropenia (less than 1,500 per millimeter cubed) should be obtained with each cycle. A blood count including hemoglobin, white blood cell count, and differential and platelet count should be performed weekly during the first 2 or 3 cycles until the time (generally 3 to 4 weeks) and degree of nadir for each patient have been established. Subsequent cycles should be delayed until the neutrophil and/or platelet counts have returned to near baseline levels. The dose for subsequent cycles should be decreased by 25 percent if the neutrophil count nadir falls below 500 per millimeter cubed or the platelet count nadir falls below 50,000 per millimeter cubed. An evaluation of tumor status should be performed periodically (every four cycles) by pelvic exam and CT examination of the abdomen and pelvis. Treatment is continued for eight to ten cycles, provided there is stability or regression in the tumor at therapeutic evaluation. Should the tumor progress (i.e., show an increase in size while on treatment), melphalan should be discontinued and another treatment selected.

TABLE 2 Active Cytotoxic Agents in Ovarian Carcinoma

Drug	*Response Rate*
Melphalan	33%
5-Fluorouracil	29%
Methotrexate	18%
Doxorubicin	33%
Mitomycin	16%
Hexamethylmelamine	24%
Cis-platinum	32%
Carboplatin	50%

Combination Cytotoxic Chemotherapy

Combination cytotoxic chemotherapy has a substantially greater degree of antitumor effect and induces a longer duration of response and disease-free interval than single agent cytotoxic chemotherapy. Additionally, although no overall improvement in survival can be demonstrated for the majority of patients receiving combination cytotoxic chemotherapy as compared to single agent treatment, cures can be induced in a small percentage of patients with minimal residual disease (tumors less than 10 to 15 mm) with aggressive chemotherapy following surgery.

A variety of combinations have been utilized, some of which are listed in Table 3. Most investigators concur that cis-platinum is the single most influential drug in these combinations. The most frequently used combination has been cyclophosphamide, hexamethylmelamine, Adriamycin, and cis-platinum (CHAD). However, there is little evidence that the use of hexamethylmelamine adds significantly to this combination. Thus, my preference and recommendation is to utilize a combination of cyclophosphamide, 750 mg per meter squared; Adriamycin, 50 mg per meter squared; and cis-platinum, 50 mg per meter squared administered concurrently and

TABLE 3 Combination Cytotoxic Chemotherapy Regimens

	CA q 3-wk	*CAP q 3-wk*	*CHAD q 4-wk*	*HEXA-CAF q 4-wk*	*CHEX-UP q 4-wk*
Cytoxan	500	750	600 D1	150 PO D1–14	150 PO D1–14
Adriamycin	50	50	25 D1		
Cis-platinum		50	50 D1		30 IV, D1, 8
Hexamethyl-melamine			150 PO D8–22	150 PO D1–14	150 PO D1–14
Methotrexate				40 IV D1, 8	
5-Fluorour-acil				600 IV D1, 8	600 IV D1, 8

All doses are mg/m²

intravenously every 3 weeks. Because Adriamycin is excreted by the biliary system, a dose reduction of 50 percent is required with a bilirubin of one to three times normal, and a bilirubin above three times normal negates the use of Adriamycin. Although this is a relatively low dose of cis-platinum, adequate hydration should be provided to prevent the renal toxicity that can be associated with platinum therapy. Nausea and vomiting are the most troublesome side effects, but these may be blunted by a variety of antiemetics, including a combination of Haldol and lorazepam. Neutropenia occurs with a nadir 10 to 14 days following administration, and a blood count including hemoglobin, white blood cell count, differential and platelet count should be obtained 7 and 14 days following treatment. A dose reduction of 25 percent should be employed in subsequent cycles for neutropenia below 500 per millimeter cubed. Thrombocytopenia is less likely to occur, but dose adjustments should be made accordingly if it is noted. Treatment is continued aggressively for six to eight cycles, or approximately 4 to 6 months, with an evaluation for tumor response performed at the time of the fourth and eighth cycle. If tumor progression is documented following four cycles, treatment should be discontinued. However, with tumor stability or response, treatment is continued through two cycles beyond maximum improvement and the situation should then be re-evaluated. Treatment is warranted until either a plateau in tumor shrinkage or a CR is achieved. If a complete response has been achieved by the end of eight cycles, treatment can be discontinued. Therapeutic efficacy may be evaluated by physical and radiologic examinations including CT scan of the abdomen. In addition, use of tumor markers as discussed below may be utilized. Second look surgery can then be utilized in the event of a clinical CR.

Second Look Surgery

Second look surgery following completion of aggressive chemotherapy serves two functions. Fifty percent of patients who, by physical examination and CT evaluation, have obtained a clinical CR with cytotoxic chemotherapy have residual tumor at second look examination. CA125, a tumor associated antigen shed by ovarian cancer cells, is a useful marker in such patients. A serum level of 60 units or above indicates residual tumor despite a negative physical and radiologic evaluation and circumvents the need for second look surgery. Patients with serum levels of circulating antigen below 60 warrant second look surgery. If tumor is demonstrable at this second staging procedure, which should again include multiple biopsies, palliative treatment is warranted. Should the patient have no demonstrable tumor at second look surgery, the standard recommendation would be no additional therapy. The likelihood of a 5-year disease-free survival (DFI) in this circumstance is about 50 percent, but even with prolonged DFI, there is a high likelihood of eventual relapse. It is my recommendation that all patients undergo additional therapy in the form of investigational treatment.

Investigational Treatment

Intraperitoneal (IP) Therapy

Intraperitoneal Cytotoxic Chemotherapy. Cytotoxic agents are reasonably well tolerated when administered intraperitonealy. The advantage over systemic administration is increased concentration and greater drug exposure. The intraperitoneal use of a number of cytotoxic agents is under active investigation.

Intraperitoneal Biologic Therapy. A number of murine studies suggest that the intraperitoneal injection of biologics results in the stimulation of a variety of effector cells. Interferons are the biologic prototype under current evaluation. The systemic administration of alpha interferon has been associated with a modest degree of antitumor effect in patients with ovarian cancer. Clonogenic assay studies suggest, however, that in order to obtain an antiproliferative effect, the concentration of interferon needed is higher than might be obtained with systemic use. Intraperitoneal administration of interferon has the potential of meeting these concentration requirements in addition to stimulating effector cell activity. Alpha interferon has been administered IP to a small number of patients with minimal residual disease (largest tumor less than 5mm) and has induced responses in some. The use of other biologicals, such as gamma interferon and tumor necrosis factor in combination, is an attractive combination that is capable of stimulating both polymorphonuclear leukocytes and macrophages. Such trials are being organized.

Borderline Tumors

A unique histologic category, the so-called borderline tumors are carcinomas of low metastatic potential. They are characterized pathologically as neoplastic (increased mitotic activity and nuclear abnormalities), but do not demonstrate histologic invasion of the supporting stroma. Metastases occur late, if at all, and the 5-year survival exceeds 80 percent with a 10-year survival in excess of 75 percent. Approximately 25 percent of serous cystadenocarcinomas and 50 percent of mucinous carcinomas are borderline or noninvasive. In patients with borderline tumors, BSO/TAH is generally adequate therapy, certainly in patients with stage I or stage II disease. In the rare patient presenting with stage III or IV disease, generally surgical removal of grossly visible tumor is also adequate therapy. No treatment other than surgery is warranted.

Second Line Therapy

Relapse following primary combined therapy carries an extremely poor prognosis and implies drug resistant disease. Single agent therapy (i.e., 5-FU or high dose Megace) may be tried, but the likelihood of clinical benefit is less than 10 percent. In this circumstance, one should seek ongoing investigations of untried cytotoxic or biologic agents (phase II trials). Recommendations for individual patients in this situation depend on the general clinical status and age of the patient, the availability of investigational studies, and the desires of the patient.

Overall, treatment for patients with ovarian carcinoma is effective but remains palliative. The challenge is to make it curative.

SUGGESTED READING

Bast RC Jr., Klug TL, ST. John E, et al. Radioimmunoassay using a monoclonal antibody to monitor the course of epithelial ovarian cancer. NEJM 1983; 309:883–887.

Berek JS, Hacker NF, Lagasse LD, et al. Survival of patients following secondary cytoreductive surgery in ovarian cancer. Obstet Gynecol 1983; 61:189–193.

Berek JS, Hacker NF, Lagasse LD, et al. Second-look laparotomy in stage III epithelial ovarian cancer: clinical variables associated with disease status. Obstet Gynecol 1984; 64:207–212.

Berek JS, Hacker NF, Lichtenstein A, et al. Intraperitoneal recombinant a-interferon for "salvage" immunotherapy in stage III epithelial ovarian cancer: a Gynecologic Oncology Group study. Cancer Res 1985; 45:4447–4453.

Dembro AJ. Abdominopelvic radiotherapy in ovarian cancer. A 10 year experience. Cancer 1985; 55:2285–2290.

Greco FA, Julian CG, Richardson RL, et al. Advanced ovarian cancer: brief intensive combination chemotherapy and second look operation. Obstet Gynecol 1981; 58:199–205.

Omura G, Blessing JA, Ehrlich CE, et al. Randomized trial of cyclophosphamide and doxorubicin with or without cisplatin in advanced ovarian carcinoma. Cancer 1986; 57:1725–1730.

Ozols R. The case for combination chemotherapy in the treatment of advanced ovarian cancer. J Clin Oncol 1985; 3:1445–1447.

Redman JR, Petroni GR, Saigo PE, et al. Prognostic factors in advanced ovarian carcinoma. J Clin Oncol 1986; 4:515–523.

Richardson GS, Sculli RE, Nikrui N, Nelson JH Jr. Common epithelial cancer of the ovary. N Engl J Med 1985; 312:415, 312:474.

Young RC, Knapp RC, Fruks Z, DiSaia PJ. Cancer of the ovary. In: DeVita VT, Hellman S, Rosenberg SA, eds. Cancer principles and practice of oncology. 2nd ed. Philadelphia: JB Lippincott, 1986: 83.

UTERINE AND ENDOMETRIAL CARCINOMA

GEORGE D. MALKASIAN Jr., M.D.

Over the years, the American Cancer Society has predicted the number of new cases of endometrial cancer expected in any one year and the number of anticipated deaths from that cancer in that particular year. In 1977, the number of anticipated new cases was 27,000, with new cases rising to 39,000 in 1983 and 1984 but declining to 37,000 in 1985, 35,000 in 1987, and 34,000 in 1989. The number of anticipated deaths from the disease peaked at 3,400 in 1983 and declined to 2,900 in 1987. Three thousand deaths were anticipated in 1989. In 1989, endometrial cancer accounted for about 47 percent of all new primary genital cancers and about 12 percent of all deaths from cancers originating in these organs. In 1985, data showed that the probability of a female's developing endometrial cancer was 3.3 percent if she was born in 1975 and 2.4 percent if she was born in 1985.

RISK FACTORS

Hormones

An analysis of women who had used combination oral contraceptives at some time in their lives showed a relative risk of occurrence of endometrial carcinoma of 0.5 percent when compared with women who had never used oral contraceptives. This protective effect took place when combination oral contraceptives had been used for a minimum of 12 months, and it persisted for at least 10 years after the cessation of their use. The relative risk decreased most significantly in nulliparous users (to 0.4 percent when compared with nulliparous never users). On this basis alone, the authors of the study predicted a drop of about 2,000 cases per year in the population at risk.

A case control study of the relationship between exogenous estrogens and endometrial carcinoma identified a 2.3 percent risk when any estrogen had been used for longer than 6 months. In this study, the risk of conjugated estrogens used for any duration was 2.0 percent; when estrogens were used for 6 or more months, this rose to 4.9 percent; when used for 1 year or more, it was 5.3 percent; when used for 2 years or more, it was 8.3 percent; and when used for more than 3 years, it was 7.9 percent. This study also demonstrated that, whereas doses of 0.625 mg per day for 6 months or more were associated with a risk of 1.4 percent, doses of 1.25 mg per day for 6 months or more promoted an increase to 7.2 percent. The risk for 6 or more months of uninterrupted estrogen use is 7.9 percent.

Studies relating the use of sequential contraceptives to endometrial carcinoma are consistent. These all suggest that the 16 days of unopposed estrogen followed by 5 days of a weak progestin do not allow the estrogen effect to be counteracted by the progestin.

Studies of higher dose progestin for longer periods show the incidence of endometrial cancer to be 390:100,000 in estrogen users alone and 49:100,000 among estrogen-progestin users. These figures are compared with 245:100,000 in nonhormone users in the population at large. This same study reports the occurrence of carcinoma among estrogen-progestin users when the progestin had been used for 6 to 10 days, but no cases of carcinoma had been identified in women who had used a progestin for 14 days per cycle. The associations between endometrial carcinoma and feminizing ovarian tumors and between endometrial carcinoma and polycystic ovarian syndrome are both statistically much greater than chance. This increased risk emphasizes the need to sample the endometrium whenever either of these ovarian situations is encountered.

Other Risk Factors

Endometrial cancer occurs significantly more often in patients who are obese or nulliparous. When obesity is defined as 30 percent or more above the upper limit of ideal weight for height and frame, the relative risk of endometrial cancer is 3.5 percent. The relative risk for nulliparous patients is 1.8 percent. The attributable risk or etiologic fraction (the percentage of the total cases that would not have occurred if the factors under consideration had been absent) is calculated at 9.0 percent for long-term use of estrogens but 25.0 percent for obesity and 19.0 percent for nulliparity. This study shows the risk factors of obesity, nulliparity, and unopposed exogenous estrogen exposure to be additive.

Gallbladder disease, hypertension, and diabetes are frequently listed among the risk factors associated with endometrial carcinoma. Mayo Clinic studies demonstrate these conditions to reflect the referral base group under study more commonly. The incidence of these factors in local county patients reflects the occurrence of these diseases in the county population at large. For example, when diabetes was evaluated, the expected and/or observed numbers were 4.3 and 3, respectively, for the local county, 4.0 and 7 for Southeastern Minnesota, 5.3 and 14 for a 100-mile radius referral, 15.7 and 28 for a 500-mile referral, and 22.8 and 45 when referred from beyond that distance.

Pelvic radiation is a risk factor in patients with mesodermal mixed sarcomas of the uterus. Approximately 20 percent of the patients with this histologic subtype have received such treatment.

PATHOLOGY

Reviews of pathology material from uterine cancer registries have identified three subtypes of endometrial carcinoma with very favorable prognoses. These are adenoacanthoma, adenocarcinoma with no defined specific features, and secretory carcinoma. All of these have 5-year survivals for stage I of 87.5 percent, 79.8 percent, and 86.6 percent, respectively. Patients with secretory carcinoma have a 13.6 percent fatal recurrence rate after 5 years. The three subtypes with a significantly less favorable prognosis were papillary carcinoma, mixed adenosquamous carcinoma, and clear cell type. These latter three subtypes together constitute approximately 17 percent of all endometrial carcinomas. The 5-year survivals in stage I patients with these subtypes are 69.7 percent, 53.1 percent, and 44.2 percent, respectively.

A number of authors subdivide the papillary adenocarcinomas into two clinicopathologic types —well differentiated and papillary serous adenocarcinoma. The reported 5-year survivals for these two subtypes are strikingly different (100 percent and 24 percent, respectively).

Mesodermal mixed tumors of the uterus constitute a group of mesodermal mixed sarcomas and carcinosarcomas. When evaluated as separate entities, the 5-year survival rates are similar at approximately 50 percent. If the lesions are grade 1 or 2 and confined to the myometrium, 5-year survival is reported at 60 percent. Higher grade lesions or those with increased depth of penetration have a decreased 5-year survival of 25 percent.

STAGING

In 1971, the Cancer Committee of the International Federation of Gynecology and Obstetrics (FIGO) published a staging categorization for endometrial carcinoma based on clinical evaluation and description (Table 1). Although this FIGO scheme has some clinical usefulness, by today's standards it has some definite deficiencies. For example, in this FIGO classification, the depth of invasion of the myometrium is not defined, and the amount of tumor is not quantitated. Peritoneal cytologic and nodal evaluation (both important staging characteristics) are not properly integrated in this classification. The definitive staging procedures should include (1) sampling of the peritoneal fluid present on entering the peritoneal cavity; (2) assessment of the extent of neoplastic spread; (3) sampling of the pelvic and/or para-aortic nodes; (4) evaluation of the myometrial penetration, i.e., inner, middle, or outer one-third; and (5)

TABLE 1 Staging of Carcinoma of the Corpus Uteri—Federation of Gynecology and Obstetrics Cancer Committee, January 1971

Stage 0 Carcinoma in situ
Stage I Carcinoma confined to the corpus
Stage IA—length of uterine cavity is 8 cm or less
Stage IB—length of uterine cavity is greater than 8 cm
All stage I cases to be graded as follows:
G1—highly differentiated adenomatous carcinomas
G2—differentiated adenomatous carcinomas with partly solid areas
G3—predominantly solid or entirely undifferentiated carcinoma
Stage II Carcinoma involves corpus and cervix
Stage III Carcinoma extends outside the uterus but not outside the true pelvis
Stage IV Carcinoma extends outside the true pelvis or obviously involves mucosa of the bladder or rectum. (Bulbous edema as such does not itself constitute stage IV disease)

description of the cellular subtype and grade. This type of staging is addressed when employing surgery as the first-line treatment approach and then with information from steps 1 through 5 in planning the adjuvant therapy. A common error in clinical versus surgical staging became apparent when 52 patients with surgical stage II disease were evaluated. Of this group, only 24 had been clinically staged correctly. The remainder had been designated as having stage I disease. Further, 23 patients clinically diagnosed with stage II disease were found, in fact, to have stage I disease when the specimen was pathologically evaluated. Table 2 demonstrates the influence of grade of tumor and its correlation with penetration of the myometrium in the most recent Mayo Clinic series of stage I patients. It is evident that the separation of patients into stages IA and IB is an artificial one. A staging categorization for endometrial carcinoma addressing these problems is currently being developed.

A study of the relationship of pathologic grade and myometrial penetration with the frequency of involvement of pelvic and aortic nodes was done by the Gynecological Oncology Group. This study provided the data derived from the FIGO clinical staging and the use of surgical staging. Overall, there was a 23 to 25 percent occurrence of pelvic nodal metastasis with grade 3 tumors and superficial myometrial invasion. Further, about 45 percent of these had aortic nodal involvement. Patients with grade 1 disease and deep invasion had positive pelvic nodes 25 percent of the time, although no aortic nodal involvement was reported. Grade 3 tumors with deep myometrial invasion showed 42 to 43 percent pelvic node involvement and 30 to 35 percent aortic nodal involvement. When the tumor was confined to the endometrium, there was minimal nodal involvement (0 to 1.7 percent) for all practical purposes. When adenocarcinomas, adenoacanthomas, and adenosquamous carcinomas were compared for grade and depth of penetration, they behaved in a similar fashion. Finally the data show that if the sampled pelvic nodes are negative, the number of positive aortic nodes is very small. A little over half of the positive nodes reported were palpable.

An estimated 15 percent of stage I carcinomas have positive peritoneal cytologic findings. The recurrence rate in patients with positive cytology is nearly fourfold greater than in that of patients with negative results. The presence of positive cytology in this group of patients, therefore, is of major concern and justifies more aggressive adjuvant therapy considerations.

Table 3 shows the relationship of survival to stage in the two Mayo Clinic series where the primary approach was extended extrafacial abdominal hysterectomy staying medial to the ureters. In connection with this, bilateral salpingo-oophorectomy was done and palpable nodes were sampled. Two things were evident in this table: (1) the FIGO categories of IA and IB are not of practical use, and (2) the survival did not improve over the two 10-year intervals.

Table 4 correlates the grade and depth of penetration with 5-year survival in stage I patients in the later

TABLE 2 Myometrial Invasion

Stage and Grade	*Depth of Invasion (%)* Inner Third	Middle Third	Outer Third
IA			
G1	89.5	5.8	4.7
G2	69.1	20.4	10.5
G3	60.0	17.1	22.9
IB			
G1	87.1	8.2	4.7
G2	61.1	16.7	22.2
G3	52.0	16.0	32.0
Total	76.8	12.7	10.5

TABLE 3 Survival Rates According to Stage and Grade—Mayo Clinic Study

	Series 1 1953–1962		*Series 2 1963–1972*	
Stage	*No. Patients*	*5-Year Survival %*	*No. Patients*	*5-Year Survival %*
IA	324	83.0	400	92.0
G1	209	88	197	92.7
G2	92	76.1	168	86.5
G3	23	65.2	35	68.2
IB	85	78.9	177	81.3
G1	40	97.5	90	89.6
G2	29	75.9	60	76.4
G3	16	37.5	27	62.9
II	24	75.0	23	69.2
III	44	59.1	—	—
IV	46	13.0	—	—
Total	523	73.8	600	—

TABLE 4 Myometrial Invasion and 5-Year Survival

Stage and Grade	Depth of Invasion (%)		
	Inner Third	*Middle Third*	*Outer Third*
IA			
G1	93.7	83.3	92.3
G2	89.0	71.9	82.4
G3	76.3	60.0	56.3
IB			
G1	93.7	83.3	92.3
G2	87.9	67.0	57.0
G3	76.3	60.0	56.3

Mayo series. It is again evident that both the grade and depth of cellular penetration are the important prognostic factors rather than the subcategories of stage I and other disease characteristics.

Evaluation of patients with surgical stage II disease shows two factors to be of importance in survival: (1) grade of disease, and (2) the extent of involvement of the endometrial cavity. The 5-year survival is 100 percent for those with grade 1 lesions, 75 percent for those with grade 2 lesions, and 50 percent for those with grade 3 lesions. When less than 50 percent of the endometrial cavity is involved, the 5-year survival is 100 percent and falls to 54 percent if a larger amount of the cavity is involved.

THERAPEUTIC APPROACH

The primary approach to all stage I lesions is wide extrafacial hysterectomy with surgical development and removal of a generous vaginal cuff, bilateral salpingo-oophorectomy, pelvic node sampling, and peritoneal cytologic examination done on fluid removed when the abdomen is first opened. Estrogen and progesterone receptor studies should be performed. Depending on the pathologic grade of the tumor, depth of cellular invasion, the presence of positive cytology and/or positive pelvic and/or aortic nodes, additional treatment considerations should be provided as follows: patients who have stages IA and IB grade 1 lesions, regardless of the depth of penetration, should have no further treatment unless (1) the cytologic findings are positive, in which case, chromic phosphate (^{32}P) is used when possible; or (2) the nodes are positive, in which case, appropriate pelvic and aortic areas are irradiated.

Patients with stages IA and IB grade 2 lesions with penetration beyond the inner one-third of the myometrium and/or positive nodes should receive pelvic irradiation approximating 5,000 cGy with appropriate nodal boosts. These patients who are node-negative but whose cytologic findings are positive should be considered for intraperitoneal radioactive phosphate (^{32}P).

Patients with stages IA and IB grade 3 lesions of any depth of invasion or whose lesions are of papillary, adenosquamous, or clear cell type with or without positive nodes should be considered for whole abdominopelvic irradiation, as described by Martinez.

Patients with stage II lesions should be treated by Wertheim hysterectomy with bilateral salpingo-oophorectomy and bilateral pelvic node resection. Surgical sampling and pathologic review of para-aortic nodes should be done if pelvic nodes are metastatically involved. No further treatment is recommended if the lymph nodes are negative on pathologic review. If metastatic nodal disease is present, pelvic radiation with appropriate nodal radiation should be provided. If there are positive cytologic findings and positive nodes are present, whole abdominopelvic radiation is administered in accordance with the Martinez technique.

The question of estrogen replacement is frequently discussed following surgery for carcinoma of the endometrium, particularly in the premenopausal and perimenopausal patient. Today, replacement therapy is generally contraindicated. A retrospective evaluation was done of 47 patients receiving estrogen. Thirty-seven used it vaginally, 7 received it orally, and 6 used estrogen both orally and vaginally for at least 3 months, starting at a median of 15 months after surgery. They reported no increased incidence of recurrence. Despite the absence of a prospective randomized trial to demonstrate the safety of estrogen replacement therapy, a recent survey of gynecologic oncologists showed them to be using such therapy in these patients. This led to the following statement's being issued by the American College of Obstetricians and Gynecologists:

There are no definitive data to support specific recommendations regarding the use of estrogen in women previously treated for endometrial carcinoma. However, responses from a survey of members of the Society of Gynecologic Oncologists indicate that 83% of the respondents approved using estrogen replacement therapy in patients with stage I, grade 1 endometrial cancer; 56% favored using estrogen in cases of stage I, grade II cancer; and 39% would use estrogen in cases of stage I, grade III cancer. The Committee on Gynecologic Practice has concluded that in women with a history of endometrial carcinoma, estrogens could be used for the same indications as for any other women, except that the selection of appropriate candidates should be based on prognostic indicators and the risk the patient is willing to assume. If the patient is free of tumor, estrogen replacement therapy cannot result in recurrence. If an estrogen-dependent neoplasm is harbored somewhere in her body, it will eventually recur; however, estrogen replacement may result in an earlier recurrence. Prognostic predictors (depth of invasion, degree of differentiation, and cell type) will assist the physician in describing the risks of persistent tumor to the patient.

In the absence of estrogen replacement therapy:

1. A well-differentiated neoplasm of endometroid cell type with superficial invasion would render a risk of persistent disease of approximately 5%.
2. A moderately differentiated neoplasm of endometroid cell type with up to one-half myometrial invasion would render a 10–15% risk of persistent disease. The risk would increase to 20–30% for adenosquamous cell type and to approximately 50% for serious papillary tumors.
3. A poorly differentiated neoplasm, regardless of cell type, with invasion of over one-half of the myometrium, would render a 40–50% risk of persistent disease.

Because the metabolic changes of estrogen deficiency are significant, the woman should be given complete information, including counseling about alternative therapies, to enable her to make an informed decision. For some women the sense of well-being afforded by amelioration of menopausal symptoms or the need to treat atrophic vaginitis or osteoporosis may outweigh the risk of stimulating tumor growth.

The need for progestational agents in addition to estrogen is unknown at present.

If only control of vasomotor symptoms is sought, this can be done quite nicely with a progestogen.

Radioactive chromic phosphate (^{32}P) has been shown to be effective in patients with microscopic metastatic residual endometrial carcinoma of the peritoneal cavity. Of patients so treated, 10 of the 15 survived for more than 5 years tumor-free. A joint study addressing this aspect of treatment reports that 10 of 26 patients with positive peritoneal cytologic findings and no other abdominal disease had recurrent disease when no treatment was used beyond the primary surgery. When a similar group of 23 patients with positive peritoneal cytology was studied with intra-abdominal ^{32}P, only three recurrences were observed. A study of 567 surgically treated stage I patients showed that 7 percent of the patients with negative peritoneal cytology and 32 percent of those with positive peritoneal cytology developed recurrences. This is highly significant.

In stage I disease, an evaluation of adjuvant progesterone in the form of 6 methyl-17 hydroxyprogesterone, 1,000 mg, was given within 24 hours of surgery and followed by 500 mg per week for 14 weeks. A randomized, control, placebo-treated group of patients with stage I disease was followed for the same period. Over 5 years, the recurrence rate was identical in the two groups. These patients did not have estrogen and/or progesterone receptor studies done, and such information in a subsequent study would be important. CA 125 levels were studied in 15 patients with recurrent carcinoma of the endometrium. Of these, six had levels over 35 U per milliliter. In those patients with positive levels at the time of recurrence, the test appears to be a means of following response to treatment.

In recent flow cytometric DNA analyses of stage I endometrial carcinoma, the overall 5-year progression-free survival for patients with grade 1 and 2 lesions was 90 percent. Stratification by DNA diploid and DNA nondiploid patterns revealed progression-free survivals of 94 and 64 percent, respectively. Patients with positive peritoneal cytologic findings and a diploid pattern had no relapses, whereas patients with positive peritoneal cytologic findings and a nondiploid pattern had recurrences of their tumors.

When the site of recurrent disease was evaluated in patients with stage I lesions, 2 of 8 with grade 1 lesions, 19 of 27 with grade 2 lesions, and 6 of 17 with grade 3 lesions had recurrences in the abdomen and/or pelvis, where irradiation could have been a useful adjuvant treatment. The remaining lesions recurred outside the abdomen or pelvis, either singly or as multiple sites of recurrence. These findings point out the need for adjuvant therapy in high risk cases, i.e., patients with grade 3 lesions of any pathologic type or adenosquamous, papillary, or clear cell histologic lesions.

When recurrent disease is isolated and amenable to surgery, this is our primary salvage procedure. If surgery is not feasible, radiation therapy is the next choice. Our experience has also demonstrated that radiation therapy has been particularly useful in controlling pain from metastatic disease to bone.

Progesterone treatment for recurrence or advanced primary disease attained popularity in the early 1960s. The most recent evaluation of this form of therapy in our institution shows that these agents have induced an 11.2 percent response in 155 patients so treated. The response rates were 40 percent for Broder's grade 1 tumors, 17.5 percent for Broder's grade 2 tumors, and 2.4 percent for Broder's grade 3 lesions. No Broder's grade 4 tumors responded to progesterone. The survivals from the onset of hormone treatment were 40 percent at 1 year, 19 percent at 2 years, and 8 percent at 5 years. The data show that survival was dependent on the differentiation of the tumor, the tumor volume, and the interval from the time of initial treatment to the onset of progesterone therapy. The progestogens used were 17 hydroxyprogesterone caproate, 6,17 dimethyl-6-dehydroprogesterone, and 6-methyl,6-dehydroprogesterone acetate. None of these produced results better or worse than the others.

In a number of patients who failed to respond to progesterones, an alternative hormonal treatment has been evaluated. Of 46 patients who received tamoxifen, 20 mg per day, 22 failed to respond to progestogens. None of these patients responded to the tamoxifen. There were five responses to tamoxifen among the 24 patients who had not previously been treated with a progestogen.

The soft agar colony formation assay for in vitro testing of sensitivity to gynecologic malignancies was evaluated in 47 patients with carcinoma of the endometrium. Of these, 13 showed positive assay, and 149 drugs were evaluated, with 20 sampled drugs showing sensitivity. The drugs indicating sensitivity in vitro did not behave in a similar fashion in vivo.

Cytotoxic agents used to date have had minimal antitumor activity and have not been particularly useful. The combined programs such as cyclophosphamide, doxorubicin, and cisplatin have reported 10 to 30 percent objective response rates for 1 to 3 months with no significant improvement in survival. One study reported a 40 percent objective response rate to high-dose carboplatin for 1 month. Partial disease regressions have been seen in 28 percent of patients treated with moderate doses of carboplatin for a median of 128 days. Further active antitumor agents are needed for these malignancies, and new trials of any promising agents should be encouraged.

FOLLOW-UP

Follow-up evaluations are scheduled every 3 to 4 months during the first year after primary therapy, every 6 months for the next 2 years, and yearly thereafter. During these follow-up examinations, in addition to screening for recurrent endometrial carcinoma, it is necessary to keep in mind the fact that the relative risk of subsequent breast cancer is 1.3 percent in this population. The increase was noted in patients who had the risk factors common to breast cancer, that is, nulliparity and obesity. Alternatively, the nonobese parous patient with endometrial carcinoma did not seem to be at risk for breast cancer. A temporal relationship exists for those at risk in that the increased incidence occurred 5 or more years after their treatment for endometrial cancer. A borderline increased risk for colon cancer also seems to be present for these patients. However, this is greatest in the first 5 years after therapy. On this basis, periodic mammograms and hemoquant screening of these patients is appropriate. An unusual occurrence of primary carcinoma of the lung was found 10 or more years after treatment for endometrial carcinoma, thereby pointing out the necessity of biopsying all lung lesions occurring late after primary therapy of endometrial cancer before treating them as recurrences.

Current Studies

The areas of interest under prospective study at present are (1) the prospective evaluation of treatment modalities for patients with other poor histologic and anatomic prognostic factors, (2) the evaluation of treatment modalities for patients with stage I, grade 3 disease, (3) the chemotherapeutic manipulation of advanced primary or recurrent disease, (4) the prospective evaluation of estrogen replacement therapy in patients at low risk of recurrence, (5) the value of receptor studies, and (6) further flow cytometric studies incorporating the information with postsurgery treatment protocols.

SUGGESTED READING

Britton LC, Wilson TO, Gaffey TA, et al. Flow cytometric DNA analysis of stage I endometrial carcinoma. Gynecol Oncol 1989; 34:317–322.

Christopherson WM, Alberhasky RC, Connelly PJ. Carcinoma of the endometrium. II. Papillary adenocarcinoma: a clinical pathological study of 46 cases. Am J Clin Pathol 1982; 77:534–540.

Christopherson WM, Connelly PJ, Alberhasky RC. Carcinoma of the endometrium. V. An analysis of prognosticators in patients with favorable subtypes and stage I disease. Cancer 1983; 51:1705–1709.

Creasman WT, Disaia PJ, Blessing J, et al. Prognostic significance of peritoneal cytology in patients with endometrial cancer and preliminary data concerning therapy with intraperitoneal radiopharmaceuticals. Am J Obstet Gynecol 1981; 141:921–927.

Fountain KS, Malkasian GD Jr. Radioactive colloidal gold in the treatment of endometrial cancer: Mayo Clinic experience 1951–1976. Cancer 1981; 47:2430–2432.

Gambrell RD Jr. Prevention of endometrial cancer with progestogens. Maturitas 1986; 8:159–168.

Malkasian GD Jr, Decker DG. Adjuvant progesterone therapy for stage I endometrial carcinoma. Int J Gynaecol Obstet 1978; 16: 48–49.

Malkasian GD Jr, Annegers JF, Fountain KS. Carcinoma of the endometrium: stage I. Am J Obstet Gynecol 1980; 136:872–888.

Malkasian GD Jr. Management of uterine and other gynecologic sarcomas. In: Williams CJ, Whitehouse JMA, eds. Cancer of the female reproductive system. Chichester, England: John Wiley & Sons, 1985:273.

Malkasian GD Jr, Podratz KC, Stanhope CR, et al. CA 125 in gynecologic practice. Am J Obstet Gynecol 1986; 155:515–518.

McDonald TW, Annegers JF, O'Fallon WM, et al. Exogenous estrogen and endometrial carcinoma: case-control and incidence study. Am J Obstet Gynecol 1977; 127:572–580.

Martinez A, Schray MF, Howes AE, Bagshaw MA. Postoperative radiation therapy in epithelial ovarian cancer: the curative role based on 24 year experience. J Clin Oncol 1985; 3:901–911.

Podratz KC, O'Brien PC, Malkasian GD Jr, et al. Effects of progestational agents in treatment of endometrial carcinoma. Obstet Gynecol 1985; 66:106–110.

Turner DA, Gershencon DM, Atkinson N, et al: The prognostic significance of peritoneal cytology for stage I endometrial cancer. Obstet Gynecol 1989; 74:775–780.

Wallin TE, Malkasian GD Jr, Gaffey TA, et al. Stage II cancer of the endometrium: a pathologic and clinical study. Gynecol Oncol 1984; 18:1–17.

RENAL AND UROEPITHELIAL CANCER

BRUCE A. LOWE, M.D.
JAMES A. NEIDHART, M.D.

RENAL CANCER

Renal cancers are the third most commonly diagnosed tumors of the urinary tract in the adult population of the United States. In 1986, there were over 16,000 newly documented cases, and nearly 8,000 Americans died of this malignancy. Adenocarcinomas (which are also called hypernephromas), clear cell carcinomas, and renal cell carcinomas comprise nearly 85 percent of these tumors. Peak incidence occurs in the fifth through sixth decades, but tumors can occur at any age. Occurrence in the pediatric population is rare. There appears to be a male to female predominance of 3:1.

Some understanding of the natural history of renal cancer is essential for therapeutic decisions. Primary renal lesions usually produce few early symptoms, and one-fourth of patients present with advanced stages of disease. Progression is by direct extension, regional lymphatics, or hematogenously. At presentation, the most common metastatic sites are the regional nodes, lungs, bone, and skin. The liver, brain, adrenal, and contralateral kidney are often involved as the disease progresses.

There is wide variation in the clinical presentations of renal cancers and in their rate of progression. The classic triad of hematuria, pain, and palpable flank mass is infrequent, but at least one of these findings can be found in 40 percent of patients. More common are nonspecific symptoms such as weight loss, fever, night sweats, fatigue, and malaise. Laboratory findings of anemia of chronic illness with low serum iron, low iron binding capacity, and normal to high ferritin is ubiquitous. Hypercalcemia reflects aggressive disease and poor prognosis. This constellation of symptoms and findings identifies patients who probably will have rapidly progressive and fatal disease within 6 to 12 months. Approximately 20 percent of patients have slowly progressive disease and will remain relatively asymptomatic for several years. Documentation of rate of disease progression by tumor measurements (exams, x-ray) over time is helpful in recommending therapy.

Much is made of tumor related overproduction of renin, erythropoietin, and parathormone. In fact, the former two problems are unusual and rarely clinically important. Hypercalcemia is usually associated with metastasis to bone and only occasionally responds to indomethacin, although the agent is worth trying. Renin, erythropoietin, and urine polyamine levels have been proposed as tumor markers in renal cancer, although their value as markers is unproven at present. Abnormal liver functions can be present in the absence of liver metastasis and prothrombin time. The etiology is unclear, but a humoral factor has been postulated as the cause.

The excretory urogram with tomography remains the most common and valuable initial diagnostic tool for patients suspected of having renal cancer. Once a renal mass is identified, computerized tomography (CT) is rapidly replacing the traditional contrasted vascular studies as the diagnostic test of choice. Extent of the tumor, extension to adjacent structures, nodal status, and hepatic involvement are readily assessed with CT scans. Currently available machines provide good visualization of the renal vein and vena cava, thereby allowing evaluation of potential tumor thrombi invading the renal vein or vena cava. Ultrasonography in experienced hands can produce studies of comparable worth, especially in children. Magnetic resonance imaging may prove to be an alternative to CT, although more experience with this technique is needed.

Patients should also receive a complete blood count, serum liver function studies, chest x-ray, and CT scan of the abdomen. Radioisotopic bone scan is appropriate for patients with pain or discomfort that is possibly due to bone lesions. Brain scans are not necessary unless clinical symptoms or routine neurologic evaluation suggest a brain metastasis. Radiation is reasonably good therapy for central nervous system (CNS) metastases, although responses are usually partial and transient.

Management of Localized Renal Tumors

Surgical removal of localized tumor is still the primary treatment for renal cancer unless systemic disease or a clinical condition prohibits the operative approach. An extrafascial approach with early control of the vascular supply and removal of the entire kidney en bloc with the contents of Gerota's fascia is the procedure of choice. Gerota's fascia is an excellent barrier to local tumor extension and is only rarely involved. Perinephritic fat extension occurs in approximately 30 percent of patients. Usually, the ipsilateral adrenal is included within the dissection, but recent reports suggest the adrenal can be retained in smaller tumors without reducing the survival rate. For smaller lesions or lower pole tumors, an abdominal approach is adequate. Larger lesions or upper pole tumors require a more extensive exposure, and a thoracoabdominal incision of the pleural and abdominal cavities is usually required. Complete excision of a localized lesion provides a greater than 70 percent chance of 5-year survival.

Neither preoperative nor postoperative radiotherapy have shown definite therapeutic benefit in terms of survival or local recurrence in several randomized trials. Local recurrence is not a common cause of failure in these patients, but can cause considerable flank and back discomfort as the tumor invades the renal bed. Local recurrence can be successfully palliated by regional radiotherapy and/or infarction of the tumor mass. Adjunctive chemotherapy or immunotherapy is not used except in investigational protocols mainly because of a lack of effective agents.

Direct invasion of the renal vein by the tumor can produce large thrombi, occasionally extending into the vena cava and proximally to the right atrium. In the absence of additional metastatic lesions, complete removal of the primary tumor and the caval thrombus can provide long-term survival nearly equal to that of patients with localized tumors. Removal of intracardiac thrombi requries placing the patient on cardiopulmonary bypass and can provide long-term survival in selected patients.

Angioinfarction

Renal cell carcinomas can be large and vascular at the time of diagnosis, thereby making excision difficult and hazardous. Preoperative precutaneous angioinfarction is used in investigational settings to reduce operative complications or occasionally as definitive initial therapy. A variety of materials have been used including steel coils, microspheres, absorbable gelatin sponges, autologous muscle or blood clot, inflatable balloons, and ethanol. Routine angioinfarction in the treatment of primary renal tumors is not indicated. Angioinfarction may also be of value for palliation of local disease that is refractory to radiation therapy, but having defined vascular supply. An investigational protocol should be used in these settings and often offers the patient the best alternative for relief.

Management of Bilateral Renal Tumors or Tumors in a Solitary Kidney

Approximately 2 to 4 percent of patients with renal carcinomas present with either synchronous or asynchronous bilateral disease. Physicians are understandably reluctant to electively make a patient anephric. Partial nephrectomy or bilateral partial nephrectomies in the presence of a small lesion in a solitary kidney or bilateral lesions produce long-term survival similar to that of resectable unilateral disease. Simple enucleation, however, is associated with a high incidence of local recurrence. Dialysis or renal transplantation has provided long-term survival, but should be considered only in those patients with tumors too extensive to remove with simpler methods and who have a good prognosis. The decision to remove both kidneys should be made only after thoughtful multidisciplinary consultation and well-informed patient consent.

Management of Advanced Disease

Spontaneous remission of systemic metastases has been reported infrequently in patients with renal cell carcinoma with and without surgical excision of the primary lesion. This occurs in less than 1 percent of patients and is not justification for removal of a primary lesion in the presence of systemic disease. Nephrectomy in the face of disseminated disease can be performed for the palliation or prevention of symptoms related to the presence of a retroperitoneal tumor.

Patients with a solitary metastasis may derive long-term benefit from surgical removal of the primary and concurrent or subsequent metastasis. Patients considered for such surgery should have slow growing tumors as evidenced by long (over 1 year) intervals from diagnosis to recurrence or repeated tumor measurements showing doubling times of 4 to 6 months. A 5-year survival of about 35 percent has been shown for these patients.

Hormonal Therapy

The use of progestational agents, androgens, and antiestrogens in disseminated renal carcinoma is based upon the observation that these agents will inhibit growth of diethylstilbestrol-induced renal tumors in the Syrian hamster and also on clinical trials carried out by Bloom in the 1960s. Regression of the tumor was seen in approximately 20 percent of patients in these studies. A much lower response rate has subsequently been reported in carefully controlled prospective studies using modern response criteria and diagnostic tools. No survival benefit has been demonstrated with any hormonal therapy. Side effects are generally minimal, but phlebitis and fluid retention do occur, and the benefit-to-risk ratio is marginal. Hormonal therapy should be used only for palliation in patients not desiring or able to enter investigative programs. If some relief of symptoms is not achieved within 3 to 4 months, treatment should be stopped.

Renal tumors remain insensitive to standard chemotherapeutic agents. The most effective single agent identified to date is vinblastine, which has an overall response rate of about 25 percent. While other agents have reportedly produced regression of tumors, combinations of cytotoxic drugs have shown no convincing benefit. No survival benefit has been demonstrated for any chemotherapy regimen. Toxicity of these regimens is often high. Standard anticancer drugs should be used for possible palliation only in select symptomatic patients. If relief is not obtained within several months, treatment should be stopped. Patients who realize that only a new approach can offer possibilities of survival benefit should be considered for and offered formal investigational programs. Most cancer centers now offer protocols exploring new chemotherapeutic agents, imaginative and substantial deviations from standard doses, or new schedules or combinations of available agents.

Spontaneous remissions of renal cancer have been attributed to immunologic rejection and have led many investigators to attempt immunotherapy of these tumors. A number of immunotherapeutic modalities have been employed in the treatment of these patients, including nonspecific immunostimulation with bacille Calmette-Guerin (BCG) or *Corynebacterium parvum.* Adoptive specific immunotherapy has been attempted using transfer factor, xenogeneic immune-ribonucleic acid, or plasma from family members previously cured of renal carcinoma. Anecdotal cases of response have been reported, but no convincing benefit has been documented and most of these treatments have been discarded. Active specific immunotherapy has also been tried using soluble preparations of lysed or irradiated autologous tumor cells polymerized to small particles or admixed with nonspecific immune adjuvants such as skin test antigens or BCG. While a low level (20 percent) response rate has been reported, none of these therapies have proven merit, although experimental approaches continue. A number of natural and recombinant interferons have been used extensively in investigational therapy of disseminated renal carcinoma. A low level response without proven survival benefit seems to exist, but these agents remain investigational. Newer interferons and combinations with chemotherapeutic agents or other biologic response modifiers are currently being explored in a number of clinical trials.

The biologic agent receiving the most recent fanfare is a growth factor called interleukin 2 (IL2). This agent has stimulated great interest and some controversy. Incubation of IL2 with patient's lymphocytes to generate activated killer cells and reinfusion of these cells into the patient has been tried in an effort to increase the putative antitumor effectiveness of IL2. More recently, tumor infiltrating lymphocytes have been incubated with IL2 and infused into the patient. The toxicity of IL2 at doses presently used has been significant and is a major factor that limits treatments. Trials are continuing in the United States.

Another recent innovation is the use of anticoagulants such as Coumadin as therapy for advanced renal cancer. Again, preliminary results are encouraging, but the treatment remains only one of several investigative approaches.

For the patient with localized adenocarcinoma of the kidney, surgical excision remains the mainstay of treatment and may be curative. For those patients with advanced disease, the currently available modalities of therapy can only offer a response rate of around 20 percent and no proven ability to prolong survival. Usually, these patients manifest a steady progression of the tumor with rapid deterioration and death within a year after diagnosis. Approximately 20 percent of patients have a slower tumor progression and do well for years, even without therapy. The rare patient has spontaneous regression of the tumor. Careful clinical trials employing new modalities of therapy should be supported vigorously in the hope of identifying an effective treatment. These trials usually offer the patient the best and only hope for long-term benefit. Patients who wish to pursue therapy with intent of prolonging survival should be offered a well-informed choice of investigative programs. Enthusiastic results of investigative regimens should be interpreted cautiously and followed with carefully designed trials to document benefits. Adenocarcinoma of the kidney has a variable clinical course, and some patients do well with no therapy.

RARE MALIGNANT TUMORS OF THE KIDNEY

Sarcomas rarely occur in the kidney and are thought to arise from the renal capsule, renal vessels, or perinephric fat. In general, the presentation is similar to that of renal cell carcinomas and diagnosis is often delayed. Surgical excision followed by local radiation and chemotherapy has been utilized in the treatment of these tumors. Local recurrence is frequent, and the disease can be palliated by repeated resections of recurrent tumor. The prognosis is generally poor.

Wilms' Tumors

These are generally neoplasms of childhood, but have been reported in the adult population. Histologically, these tumors represent the embryonic nephroblast, and the closer the reproduction of mature elements the more favorable the prognosis. Unlike renal cell carcinoma, these tumors are highly sensitive to radiation and chemotherapy. Treatment consists of surgical excision or debulking followed by radiation and chemotherapy. Survival for those patients with a favorable histology is excellent, even for advanced disease. These patients should receive potentially curative treatment through a national study group if at all possible.

CANCER OF THE UROTHELIUM

Transitional cell carcinoma of the urothelium is the second most common genitourinary malignancy and has an incidence of 1 per 5,000 population with a male predominance. Over 45,000 new cases will present in 1987, resulting in 10,000 deaths. The majority of patients present with localized disease and, properly treated, can expect a 65 to 70 percent 5-year survival. With development of effective chemotherapy, even patients with advanced disease have a 30 to 40 percent 5-year survival. Transitional cell carcinomas are extremely uncommon in children.

Hematuria is the most common complaint at presentation and occasionally produces significant hemorrhage. Bleeding can be intermittent, episodic, and minimal. The demonstration of hematuria on the routine urinalysis is often the only sign of urothelial neoplasms. The presence of more than 2 to 3 red cells per high power field on the urinalysis without explanation should indicate cancer until proven otherwise. Symptoms of voiding dysfunction may predominate in those patients with diffuse carcinoma in situ or papillary lesions of the trigone or bladder neck. Chronic complaints of dysuria, frequency, urgency, and urge incontinence in the absence of infection may indicate a transitional cell tumor of the bladder and should be explored. Patients with advanced disease may present with symptoms due to the invasion of adjacent organs or distant metastasis.

The diagnostic work-up for suspected uroepithelial malignancy should include an excretory urogram, although a normal study does not rule out the presence of cancer. Ultrasonography can be of significant value since the fluid filled bladder enhances visualization of the bladder wall and perivesicle space. Computerized tomography provides a gross assessment of local extension through the bladder wall and involvement of the pelvic lymph nodes which are the most common sites of regional spread. Bipedal lymphangiography offers limited additional information and is rarely necessary. A chest x-ray, thorough history, and physical complete the necessary staging exam. Patients with pain suggestive of bone lesions should receive a bone scan.

Urinary cytology, although not useful as a screening test, can be a sensitive indicator of urothelial malignancy in high grade tumors and in high risk groups. Flow cytometric analysis of the DNA content of epithelial cells obtained by bladder washings correlates with malignant degeneration. Its use as a screening and surveillance test is currently investigational. Endoscopic evaluation of the bladder with biopsies for staging and a pathologic diagnosis is the most sensitive diagnostic test available and should be employed whenever there is suspicion of a bladder tumor. Biopsies can be subject to processing errors and false negative results. Suspicion of in situ cancer with a negative biopsy requires a repeat sampling. These procedures can easily be performed in an ambulatory setting under local or general anesthesia. Flexible endoscopy is increasingly utilized in an effort to improve patient comfort and reduce cost.

Management of Superficial Cancer

In Situ Cancer

The capacity of in situ tumors to metastasize early makes aggressive treatment of these patients mandatory. Effective topical chemotherapy has replaced radical cystectomy or radiotherapy as the treatment of choice. The optimal treatment remains undefined, and a variety of agents are available. Thiotepa has been used for over 20 years as a therapeutic and prophylactic agent after endoscopic resection of small papillary tumors. The standard dosage is 30 mg in 30 ml of sterile water placed into the bladder via a urethral catheter and retained for 1 to 2 hours while the patient rotates to allow coating of the entire bladder surface. It is given weekly for 4 to 6 weeks with a 4 to 6 week waiting period before reevaluation is performed endoscopically. Dose related myelosuppression is the major side effect and must be carefully monitored. Ureteral strictures may be produced. Doxorubicin appears to have an effectiveness equivalent to thiotepa. Dosage ranges from 40 to 80 mg given in 50 ml of sterile water and retained for 1 hour. Absorption appears to be minimal and toxicity is mild. Direct irritation of the bladder causes irritable voiding symptoms in 30 to 50 percent of patients, occasionally to an intolerable degree. Topical mitomycin C is given at a dose of 20 to 40 mg in 40 ml of sterile water. Toxicity is minimal, but cost is high and there is no proven advantage over carefully administered thiotepa. Bacille Calmette-Guerin appears to be equal if not superior to the other agents described, but currently remains investigational and optimal treatment regimens have not been defined. Toxicities are generally mild and include fever, irritative voiding symptoms, and visceral granulomatous reactions. Other biologic response modifiers such as interferons and IL2 are currently being evaluated as topical therapy for bladder cancer. Unsuccessful eradication of an intraepithelial tumor with topical therapy requires more aggressive treatment, and careful followup evaluation is essential.

Phototherapy with a photosensitizing agent such as hematoporphyrin derivative (HPD) and administered laser energy has been used investigationally in the treatment of in situ cancer. HPD is selectively retained by malignant tissues, but is cleared by normal tissues within 24 to 48 hours, theoretically leading to selective destruction of the intraepithelial tumor. Cells with retained HPD exposed to laser light generate superoxide radicals, thereby causing irreversible oxidation of cellular components and cell death. Patients are susceptible to severe skin burns resulting from HPD retained in skin exposed to sunlight.

Superficial Papillary Tumors

Transurethral resection with cold cup biopsies, electroexcision, or laser is the first step in the treatment of superficial papillary transitional cell cancers and is adequate treatment for noninvasive tumors. Although electroexcision is the accepted method of treatment for superficial tumors, the recurrence rate is high (50 to 70 percent) perhaps due to bladder wall implantation of disaggregated tumor cells. Laser treatment offers the theoretical but unproven advantage of destroying tumor cell viability before manipulation and produces less injury to surrounding tissue. The neodymium YAG laser, which emits in the near infrared region, 1,060 nm, is most frequently used. Intravesicle chemotherapy is currently being investigated as an adjunct to surgery.

Management of Invasive Transitional Cell Cancer

Invasion of the bladder muscle requires radical cystectomy with removal of the bladder and adjacent sexual structures followed by urinary diversion. Although patients with tumors confined to the bladder can expect a 5-year survival of nearly 70 percent, the significant impact on sexual function and self image has led to a search for more palatable alternatives. Radiation therapy at doses of 6,000 to 7,000 rads followed by a restaging transurethral biopsy has been reported to salvage the bladder in 40 percent of patients. The remaining 60 percent require radical cystectomy for management of residual tumor. However, significant long-term complications occur, and many patients become bladder cripples with debilitating voiding symptoms. This approach remains investigational.

Preoperative radiation therapy (4,000 to 5,000 rads) has been used to sterilize micrometastasis and to downstage tumors prior to surgery. Complications with full course radiation led to a splitting of the treatment course with sandwiching 2,500 rads preoperatively with another 2,500 to 4,000 rads after surgery. Complications are diminished, but a paucity of well-controlled trials showing a survival advantage has caused many urologists to question the value of radiotherapy except in patients unable to tolerate a major surgical procedure. The value of the YAG laser, BCG therapy, radiation alone, and other intravesicle therapies in treatment of invasive cancer remains unclear, and these treatments remain investigational.

The use of segmental or partial cystectomy is controversial and little used in the United States. Current techniques preserving sexual function and providing continent diversions are making radical surgery more acceptable to many patients.

Management of Advanced Transitional Cell Cancer

The use of systemic chemotherapy in advanced or metastatic uroepithelial cancer is increasing. Several single agents and combinations have been found to produce regression of tumors, although survival advantage has not been proven. Cis-platinum, doxorubicin, vinblastine, methotrexate, cyclophosphamide, and several newer agents have some antitumor activity. Optimum regimens and definite benefits have not been proven, and patients should be considered for investigational programs when possible. Otherwise, treatment should be considered palliative and continued only as long as subjective benefit to the patient is demonstrated.

Treatment of Upper Tract Urothelial Tumors

Transitional cell tumors of the upper tracts have been historically treated by complete nephroureterectomy. Small, low grade, noninvasive ureteral lesions can be removed by segmental ureterectomy alone by percutaneous renal surgery or the ureteroscope. Survival for patients with adequately resected localized cancer is excellent. Successful use of the laser in upper tract tumors has been reported recently in a few patients. Because of the silent nature of upper tract tumors, many patients present with advanced disease, and survival in this case is poor.

Other Tumors of the Urothelium

Squamous cell cancer appears to arise within the urothelium as a response to chronic inflammation, including bilharzial infections. These tumors tend to be aggressive with rapid growth, and are relatively radioresistant and insensitive to chemotherapeutic agents. Surgical excision with wide margins appears to offer the best chance of survival.

Adenocarcinoma of the urothelium is relatively uncommon and is felt to arise from urachal elements or from metaplastic changes within the transitional epithelium. These lesions tend to be resistant to radiation and chemotherapy. Surgical excision appears to be the only treatment.

Sarcomas are rarely reported in the bladder. Overall prognosis is poor despite surgery and radiation therapy. Childhood rhabdomyosarcoma is treatable with radiotherapy, chemotherapy, and local excision, with retention of a normally functional bladder. Long-term survival and cure is frequent.

SUGGESTED READING

Renal Carcinoma

deKernion JB. Treatment of advanced renal cell carcinoma—traditional methods and innovative approaches. J Urol 1983; 130:2–7.

deKernion JB. Renal tumors. In: Walsh P, Gittes R, Perlmetter A, Stamey T, eds. Campbell's urology. Philadelpha: WB Saunders, 1986: 1294.

Javadpour N. Natural history diagnosis and staging of renal cancer. In: Javadpour N, ed. Principles and management of urologic cancer. Baltimore: Williams & Wilkins, 1983: 481.

Montie JE. Management of stages I, II, and III renal adenocarcinoma. In: Javadpour N, ed. Principles and management of urologic cancer. Baltimore: Williams & Wilkins, 1983: 492.

Neidhart JA. Interferon therapy for the treatment of renal cancer. Cancer 1986; 57:1696-1699.

Bladder Cancer

Droller MJ. Transitional cell cancer: upper tracts and bladder. In: Walsh P, Gittes R, Perlmetter A, Stamey T, eds. Campbell's urology. Philadelphia: WB Saunders , 1986: 1343.

Droller MJ. The controversial role of radiation therapy as adjunctive treatment of bladder cancer. J Urol 1983; 129:897–903.

Klimberg IW, Wajsman Z. Treatment for muscle invasive carcinoma of the bladder. J Urol 1986; 136:1169–1175.

Sternberg CN, et al. Preliminary results of M-VAC (methotrexate, vinblastine, doxorubicin, and cisplatin) for transitional cell carcinoma of the urothelium. J Urol 1985; 133:403–407.

Torti FM, Lum BL. The biology and treatment of superficial bladder cancer. J Clin Oncol 1984; 2:505–531.

BLADDER CANCER

RICHARD K. LO, M.D.
FRANK M. TORTI, M.D., M.P.H.

Urothelial transitional cell carcinoma (TCC) presents in four forms: (1) superficial, low-grade tumors, (2) superficial, high-grade neoplasms, and carcinoma in situ (CIS), (3) muscle-infiltrative tumors, and (4) metastatic tumors. Each has profound ramifications for the clinical course and eventual outcome.

TREATMENT OF LOW-GRADE SUPERFICIAL BLADDER CANCER

Endoscopic Treatment

When the presence of bladder cancer is suspected in the course of an investigation for hematuria, a thorough endoscopic examination of the bladder is mandatory. The number, size, appearance, and location of these tumors should be noted on a bladder diagram. This "map" offers a document for subsequent reference when investigating for recurrences, or more appropriately, new occurrences. The tumor is resected transurethrally; the deeper portion of the tumor should be sent as a separate specimen to delineate the depth of invasion. The mucosa adjacent to the tumor, as well as other, more remote, random (preselected) sites, are biopsied using the cold-cup biopsy forceps to minimize cautery artifact. Other suspicious areas are also biopsied to exclude intraepithelial tumor in apparently normal areas. Bimanual examination under adequate relaxation is performed, before and after the resection, noting the presence of any induration or masses. Cytologic examination of a bladder wash specimen, obtained by barbotage, is useful in recognizing the presence of high-grade tumors and/or CIS. In general, because of the decreased intracellular cohesiveness, exfoliation of surface epithelial cells is more common in high-grade tumors than in well-differentiated ones.

When a histologic diagnosis of transitional cell carcinoma is made, and the depth of invasion determined, the patient is stratified into a treatment category. Approximately two-thirds of patients have papillary, superficial tumors, usually of low-grade, which have not penetrated the muscularis propia at presentation. The distinction is made between non-muscle-invading and muscle-invading tumors, for management strategies.

For low-grade, noninvasive papillary tumors, transurethral resection (TUR) offers a definitive, effective, albeit temporary, management. The patient should then be placed on a close surveillance protocol, with cystoscopy and urine cytology performed every 3 months for the first year, extending the intervals to 4 months for the second year, 6 months for the third year, and yearly thereafter. Although most follow-up cystoscopies are performed as an office procedure under local anesthesia, it is mandatory that the entire bladder mucosa be visualized completely. Special attention should be directed to the areas of increased risk for recurrence—sites of previous tumors or severe dysplasia and the dome. The risk of tumor recurrence in superficial tumors after definitive transurethral resection has been reported to range from 50 to 75 percent.

Intravesical Treatment

At the Stanford University Medical Center, we recommend TUR alone for first presentations of low-grade papillary tumors. However, patients developing a second low-grade tumor are offered adjuvant chemotherapy, as are those with multiple (three or more) tumors at presentation. These intravesical chemotherapeutic agents are introduced through a urethral catheter and retained for a total contact time of 2 hours. The choices of intravesical chemotherapeutic agents, with their advantages and disadvantages are listed in the following paragraphs.

Intravesical *thiotepa* is administered at dosages of 30 to 60 mg per treatment, using a 1-mg-per-cubic-centimeter concentration solution in sterile water. The treatment schedule consists of weekly treatments for 6 weeks, followed by monthly maintainance therapy. Cystoscopic evaluation is conducted about 6 months after the first treatment. Complete response in the *treatment* of bladder tumors varies from 30 to 40 percent, with partial responders accounting for an additional 10 percent. Thiotepa can be instilled almost immediately after transurethral resection, it offers the theoretical advantage of killing tumor cells before they have a chance to implant on "injured" mucosa. Given as a *prophylactic* regimen, the rate of recurrence is 20 percent less than controls. The major side effect of thiotepa is myelosuppression, especially immediately after a deep resection. The patient should have a leukocyte and platelet count before the drug is administered, and the treatment should be withheld if the white blood count (WBC) is less than 4000 per cubic millimeter or the platelet count is less than 100,000 per cubic millimeter.

Mitomycin C (MMC), an antitumor antibiotic, is increasingly being used as a primary intravesical chemotherapy agent, rather than as a second-line drug after thiotepa failure. The results of MMC administration for existing bladder tumors are comparable to those with thiotepa, with approximately 45 percent complete response and 25 percent partial response rates. As a prophylaxis, using only one-third of the usual 60-mg dose, twice a month for 12 months and then every month for another year, the recurrence rate can be reduced to 11 percent. The major drawbacks are the relatively high cost, the chemical cystitis with occasionally bladder capacity reduction, and a dermatitis-type rash on the genitalia.

Doxorubicin has been used in both papillary tumors and carcinoma in situ, in treatment as well as in adjuvant settings. In general, there is approximately a 70 percent response rate, complete responders plus partial responders (CR + PR). Given intravesically, doxorubicin is not absorbed systemically. The major side effect is chemical cystitis, especially when it is diluted in water. No cardiotoxicity has been reported after intravesical use.

Bacille Calmette-Guerin (*BCG*) is the first agent used as a nonspecific immunomodulating intravesical agent. Used intravesically, with or without concomitant oral or intradermal administration, BCG showed potent antitumor activity with a reduced tumor recurrence rate (22 versus 46 percent in controls). BCG is also particularly active in flat carcinoma in situ, with an approximately 80 percent response rate, measured by negative urine cytology and cystoscopic findings. Whether this activity is secondary to recruitment of immune defense mechanism or to sloughing of surface mucosa after an intense inflammatory reaction has not been resolved. Vesical irritability and flu-like symptoms are the usual side effects.

Interferons, according to recent reports, using both natural and recombinant interferon preparations, may have a role in limited numbers of patients in the treatment, and perhaps the prevention of recurrences, of superficial bladder cancers. Interferons injected into papillary tumors have shown regression in some cases. The use of poly-I:C, a stimulator of interferon production, has been associated with survival advantage in patients with papillary tumors. In one recent published abstract, recombinant alpha-2b interferon has shown activity against carcinoma in situ and papillary tumors. The eventual role of the interferons, and their relative utility against other intravesical agents, must await careful randomized comparisons.

Others

Laser therapy and photodynamic therapy using hematoporphyrin derivative dessicate targeted tumor cells with their respective energies. They offer the advantage of tumor eradication under guidance, without the need for anesthesia, as in the case of transurethral resection. For the patients predisposed to forming recurrent low-grade, low-stage tumors, laser therapy is simple, effective, with minimal risks, and can be administered in an outpatient setting, under local anesthesia. External beam irradiation has not been shown to be effective in papillary-type superficial bladder cancer. In selected cases of rapidly recurring tumors not amenable to transurethral resection and intravesical chemotherapy, radical cystectomy may be indicated as the definitive treatment.

TREATMENT OF HIGH-GRADE SESSILE TUMORS AND CARCINOMA IN SITU

Carcinoma in situ and sessile tumors have a different biologic behavior than the low-grade papillary tumors. Large, grade 3 to 4 tumors that invade the submucosa have a high propensity for a more progressive biologic behavior, measured both by superficial recurrence and by invasion into the bladder muscle wall. Similarly, diffuse carcinoma in situ has a great potential for muscle invasion. Up to 80 percent of patients with such lesions have been reported to develop invasive bladder cancer within 4 years of diagnosis. Thus, both high-grade sessile tumors and CIS pose a different set of clinical dilemmas from those that tend to recur superficially.

Patients with these tumors tend to present with frequency, dysuria, and only occasional hematuria: a constellation of symptoms similar to that of urinary tract infections. The symptoms are often less threatening to the patient than hematuria, the common presentation of low-grade papillary tumors. The prognosis of, and therefore treatment recommendations for, patients with carcinoma in situ depends on the clinical context in which it is observed. Carcinoma in situ, which presents as a focus of carcinoma in situ immediately adjacent to a visible papillary tumor without other areas of involvement, correlates with progression to invasive bladder cancer. We have termed this presentation type I. It was shown by Althuasen that, of 41 patients with low-grade, low-stage papillary carcinoma, only three developed invasive cancer, whereas nine, or 36 percent, of 25 patients with just atypia in the surrounding urothelium, and 83 percent of patients with frank CIS, developed invasive bladder cancer. Nonetheless, careful, complete resection and adjuvant intravesical treatment is our current approach to type I CIS.

In type II CIS, the in situ carcinoma is present in areas distant from a papillary tumor. This occurs frequently in abnormal areas identified by cytoscopy, but can also be found in cystoscopically normal areas; sampling areas distant from the papillary tumor is mandatory. The appearance of a diffuse carcinoma in situ distant from the papillary tumor indicates the need for more intensive treatment—either more radical surgery or aggressive chemotherapy in appropriate cases. Type III CIS is associated with a total involvement with the urothelium by tumor. Papillary tumors may or may not be present. Patients often have symptoms of bladder irritability, which actually may indicate a very poor prognosis. This clinical syndrome is associated with the 50 to 80 percent incidence of infiltrating cancer. Although cystectomy is the conventional treatment, intravesical chemotherapy has been used with some success to eradicate tumors and preserve the bladder, perhaps temporarily.

It is important, however, to recognize that, although many intravesical chemotherapies are used for high-grade, sessile cancers and carcinoma in situ, the long-term efficacy for most of these treatments is unclear, particularly for the situation of diffuse carcinoma in situ. Furthermore, cystectomy is a therapeutic option with a high probability of cure. We do not present to patients options of less aggressive treatment (with uncertain prognosis), without pointing out the investigational nature of these treatments. When intravesical chemotherapy is used for these more aggressive tumors, the aim must be to alter the biology of the disease substantially, over not only the short period of acute administration but years, since the patient remains at risk of developing invasive or metastatic cancer.

TREATMENT OF INVASIVE BLADDER TUMORS

Approximately one-quarter of patients at initial diagnosis have tumors penetrating into the muscularis. In addition, 15 to 20 percent of those with superficial disease progress to more advanced stages. Muscle invasion usually implies an ominous course. Approximately 10 percent of P1 tumors develop metastatic disease. For those with deeper bladder wall penetration, metastatic spread is found in at least 40 percent. Aggressive therapy is therefore indicated to eradicate local disease and to prevent further tumor dissemination.

Primary Bladder Irradiation

External beam radiotherapy, with cobalt sources using rotational fields, or the more high-energy, linear accelerator–generated photons, with opposing ports, has been used in the treatment of invasive bladder tumors. This method has been advocated for those patients who refuse, or are not considered good surgical risks for, cystectomy. The dismal survival results, however, preclude its use except in patients with high risk of surgical mortality. Five-year survivals range from 13 to 35 percent for patients given 6,000 to 7,000 rad over 30 to 40 fractions. Locoregional failure of up to 68 percent would dictate the need for additional therapy, usually by salvage cystectomy, with the attendant risks plus technical difficulties from fibrosis and potential complications of a heavily irradiated ileal conduit. Interstitial radiotherapy, with or without additional external beam irradiation, has been used in Europe with similar survival rates. The complication rate after external beam radiotherapy is also considerable. Although the early diarrhea and dysuria may be transient, 15 percent of patients suffer permanent bladder and rectal injury, with resultant irritable urinary and rectal symptoms of frequency and possibly incontinence. In rare instances, intractable hematuria from radiation cystitis requires a salvage cystectomy to control the hemorrhage.

Segmental Resection

Segmental resection of a solitary, low-grade lesion is occasionally indicated. Preservation of normal micturition function is an obvious advantage to these patients. Local bladder recurrence (30 percent in low-grade and 80 to 100 percent in high-grade tumors) and the risk of wound implant have been the major drawbacks in the application of this procedure. To maximize the benefit and safety in these patients, strict adherence to selection criteria should be observed. These include a solitary lesion of less than 4 or 5 cm, with no adjacent or distant mucosal dysplasia, no antecedent history of other bladder tumors, and a location preferably in the dome or posterior wall, and with surgical margins of at least 2 cm, without the need to reimplant the ureters. Preoperative radiotherapy, usually 5,000 rad over 25 fractions, should be given to minimize wound implant and to sterilize nodal disease.

Radical Cystectomy

Radical cystectomy remains the mainstay in the management of invasive bladder carcinoma. Improvements in surgical techniques, advances in preoperative evaluation and postoperative care, and selection of patients all contribute to a 5-year survival rate of approximately 50 percent. This is reflected by the reduction of the perioperative mortality rate from 14 percent to 1 or 2 percent. Despite improved radiologic staging methods, unrecognized regional extension and micrometastases contribute substantially to eventual tumor recurrence. Integrated therapy using either a high-dose, short-course method (1,600 to 2,000 rad over 5 fractions) or the more protracted 4,000 to 5,000 rad in 200-rad fractions, combined with extirpative surgery is probably the standard of practice in most parts of the country. Preoperative radiotherapy theoretically minimizes the viability of tumor cells and sterilizes nodal micrometastasis, therefore improving survival over that with cystectomy alone. Improved survival is apparently restricted to those patients who are "downstaged" by the radiation therapy: that is, the pathologic stage (pT stage) is lower than the clinical stage (T stage). Inaccuracies in clinical staging, however, despite advances in radiological imaging techniques, approaches 50 percent, both in over- and understaging. Five-year survivals reached 80 percent for patients with no evidence of tumor in the cystectomy specimen (pTo), contrasted to 30 percent in those with no downstaging (pT = T). Additional factors that improve the probability of downstaging include the total dosage given, and the interval from radiation to cystectomy. Improvements in survival, therefore, can be restricted only to those in which residual tumor is not found in the cystectomy specimen.

Recent data suggest, however, that cystectomy alone can achieve the same survival results as the integrated approach. Radiation therapy has not been shown to reduce the incidence of metastatic disease, the main cause of treatment failure. Furthermore, the rate of pelvic recurrence and incidence of nodal disease have not differed from those of some other contemporary surgery-alone series, negating some of the theoretical arguments for intergrated therapy. Superior survival results from downstaging may reflect only the natural biological behavior of the tumor itself, which may or may not be modified by the radiation therapy. The controversy continues because of the paucity of adequately controlled, randomized studies.

Bilateral pelvic lymphadenectomy is an integral part of the treatment of invasive bladder cancer. Preoperative radiation with 2,000 rad, which delivers approximately 60 percent of the tumorcidal dosage, (compared with the more protracted therapeutic conventional 5,000 or 6,000 rad course), is not sufficient to sterilize metastases in lymph nodes. In addition to being a staging procedure, a meticulous lymph node dissection has been reported to yield a 5-year survival rate of 34 percent in those with nodal involvement. It also provides accurate staging data, with which patients with nodal discasc can be considered for adjuvant chemotherapy because of the poor prognosis.

Urinary drainage after radical cystectomy is usually achieved by means of an intestinal conduit. The Bricker-type uretero-ileal-cutaneous conduit has enjoyed vast popularity in the last 3 decades, with other variations using different portions of the small (jejunum) and large (sigmoid, cecum) bowel. This change in body image and the nuisance in the care of the stoma appliance has been an impediment to patient acceptance of radical cystectomy. Modern drainage procedures, however, should make this argument obsolete. The continent Koch ileostomy reservoir offers the patient the convenience of self-catheterization a few times a day with reservoir capacities of more than 1 liter. Other similar reservoirs and continent bladder substitutions (the Camey procedure, the hemi-Koch technique, the Mainz pouch and "Le bag") have made cystectomy and drainage more palatable. Unfortunately, because of the en bloc removal of the female urethra, together with the bladder, bladder substitution procedures are not applicable in female patients. Furthermore, applying a technique similar to the nerve-sparing type of radical prostatectomy, a radical cystectomy can be performed without interrupting the pelvic plexus of nerves supplying the corpora cavernosa, enhancing the chance of postoperative potency.

TREATMENT OF METASTATIC TRANSITIONAL CELL CARCINOMA

The 5-year survival figure of 50 percent after radical cystectomy for tumors that are apparently localized highlights the inadequacies of definitive therapy in the local treatment of bladder cancer. These statistics can be improved by improvement of diagnostic techniques to identify micrometastasis and treat these patients earlier with chemotherapy, and by development of more effective chemotherapeutic regimens.

A combination chemotherapy regimen, using many of the active chemotherapeutic agents in transitional cell carcinoma (CMV: cis-platinum, methotrexate, and vinblastine), was developed recently at Stanford. A 56 percent objective response rate was achieved (complete plus partial responders), with 28 percent complete responders and some patients now disease-free at 4 and 5 years past treatment. In this schedule, the toxicity was acceptable. The complete response rate of the bladder tumor itself is over 50 percent. Discordant relapses in the central nervous system (CNS) are seen with complete

TABLE 1 CMV Chemotherapy for Transitional Cell Carcinoma

CMV	*D1 (mg/m²)*	*D2 (mg/m²)*	*D8 (mg/m²)*	*Cycle*
Methotrexate	30		30	
Vinblastine	4		4	21 days
Cis-platinum		100		

TABLE 2 Dose Reduction for CMV Chemotherapy: Hematologic Toxicity*

	Percentage of Initial Calculated Dose of Methotrexate and Vinblastine (To be used to adjust for hematologic status for each cycle) for Following No. of Platelets			
WBC	≥150,000	100,000–149,000	75,000–99,000	<75,000
≥35,000	100	100	50†	0†
3,000–3,499	100	100	50†	0†
2,500–2,999	50†	50†	0†	0†
<2,500	0†	0†	0†	0†

* (1) If WBC ≤1,000 (and/or polys ≤500) or if platelets are ≤50,000 during the the previous cycle but counts have returned to the dosing levels, administer only 80 percent of the dose delivered in the last cycle. (2) If WBC ≥3,000 and platelets are ≥100,000, treat on the schedule at the dose specified in the table.
† If the dose at day 1 of the subsequent cycle (day 21) falls into the 0 to 50 percent range, delay the initiation of cycles up to 1 week (day 28). If counts are still in the 50 percent range at week 4 (day 28), treat at the 50 percent dose.

TABLE 3 Dose Reduction for CMV Chemotherapy: Renal Toxicity

A. Methotrexate

Do not give methotrexate on day 8 if any of the following occur (vinblastine can still be given):

1. Creatinine clearance falls by greater than 30 cc/min from the day 1 value.
2. The absolute day 8 value is less than 45 cc/min.
3. Serum creatinine is 2.0 mg% on day 8, regardless of creatinine clearance.
4. Rescue MTX if stomatitis or platelets <75,000.

B. Cis-platinum (to be used to adjust for renal status for each cycle)

Creatinine Clearance (cc/min)	*% Calculated Cis-platinum Dose*
>60	100
45–60	50
<45	0

response at other sites, suggesting the possible need for CNS prophylaxis.

With efficacy of these combination chemotherapeutic regimens, adjuvant therapy studies have been initiated in an attempt to improve the long-term outlook for the patients with invasive disease who are at high risk for recurrence (undownstaged, high-grade, or regional nodal involvement).

SUGGESTED READING

Althuasen AF, Prout GR, Daly JJ. Non-invasive papillary carcinoma of the bladder associated with carcinoma in situ. J Urol 1976; 116:575–580.

Droller MJ. Transitional cell cancer—upper tracts and bladder. In: Walsh PC, Gittes RF, Perlmutter AD, Stamey TA, eds. Campbell's urology, 5th ed. Philadelphia: WB Saunders, 1986; 1343.

Harker WG, Meyers FJ, Freiha FS, et al. Cisplatin, methotrexate and vinblastine (CMV): an effective chemotherapy regimen for metastatic transitional cell carcinoma of the urinary tract. A Northern California Oncology Group Study. J Clin Oncol 1985; 3:1463–1470.

Meyers FJ, Palmer JM, Freiha FS, et al. The fate of the bladder in patients with metastatic bladder cancer treated with cisplatin, methotrexate and vinblastine. A Northern California Oncology Group Study. J Urol 1985; 134:1118–1121.

Torti FM, Lum BL. The biology and treatment of superficial bladder cancer. J Clin Oncol 1984; 2:505–531.

Torti FM, Lum BL. Superficial carcinoma of the bladder: natural history and the role of interferons. Semin Oncol 1986; 13(Suppl 2):57–60.

Torti FM, Lum BL. Aston D, et al. Superficial bladder cancer: the primacy of grade in the development of invasive disease. J Clin Oncol 1987; 5:125–130.

PROSTATIC CANCER

ALEX Y. C. CHANG, M.D., F.A.C.P.

Carcinoma of the prostate is the second most common cancer and the third leading cause of cancer deaths in American men. Frequently, patients present with symptoms and signs of obstructive uropathy such as frequency, dysuria, dripping, and difficulty in urination. The enlarged prostate gland is readily demonstrable by digital rectal examination. However, in the majority of the patients, obstructive uropathy is due to benign prostate hypertrophy. About 25 percent of patients with prostate carcinoma are diagnosed under the impression of benign prostate hypertrophy without palpable nodule (clinical stage A, Table 1). In patients with advanced disease, bone pain and nodular mass in the prostate gland are common. Occasionally, patients may present with deep vein thrombophlebitis or symptoms and signs of spinal cord compression with no or minimal urinary complaints. In these instances, careful digital rectal examination and checking of serum acid phosphatase may reveal additional clues of the presence of prostate carcinoma. The prognosis for patients with prostate carcinoma depends on the following factors: stage of the disease; histologic grade and size of the tumor within each stage; age and performance status of the patient; response to therapy; and presence or absence of dire complications such as renal failure, spinal cord compression, and pulmonary emboli following deep vein thrombophlebitis. The therapeutic approach should take all of these factors into consideration.

STAGING OF PATIENTS

After the diagnosis of prostate cancer is documented pathologically, which can be accomplished by transperineal or transrectal needle core biopsy or transrectal aspiration biopsy, appropriate staging of the disease should be done to assess the tumor burden, prognosis, and treatment. A work-up should include the following:

1. Digital examination of the rectum to determine local disease extension;
2. Radioisotope bone scanning and x-ray study of suspicious or symptomatic bony areas;
3. Prostatic or total serum acid phosphatase or prostate-specific antigen;
4. Determination of other serum enzymes, alkaline phosphatase, lactic dehydrogenase, serum aspartate aminotransferase, and bilirubin;

TABLE 1 Staging Classification by American Urologic System

Stage A	Incidental, clinically latent adenocarcinoma
A_1	Focal locus of adenocarcinoma in TURP* specimen
A_2	Diffuse and multifocal involvement
Stage B	Palpable tumor confined within the capsule of the prostate gland
B_1	Nodule involves a single lobe and is $\leq$ 1.5 cm in diameter
B_2	Nodule involves more than a lobe and is $>$1.5 cm
Stage C	Tumor invades neighboring tissue through direct extracapsular extension
Stage D	Tumor with metastases
D_1	Metastases confined to the pelvic lymph nodes
D_2	Metastases beyond the pelvis

*Transurethral resection of the prostate.

5. Evaluation of renal function and intravenous pyelogram if renal function allows;
6. Evaluation of retroperitoneal space and pelvis by ultrasonogaphy, computed tomography (CT) scanning, or magnetic resonance imaging (MRI);
7. Baseline complete blood count.

Rectal examination is the fundamental test in the screening and diagnosis of prostate carcinoma as well as evaluation of local disease. An objective (not necessarily better) assessment of the pelvic lymph nodes and retroperitoneum can be obtained by any of the following tests: ultrasonography, CT scan, or MRI. It is unclear which test is most useful at the present time. None of these tests is specific or sensitive enough to abandon the practice of pelvic lymphadenectomy. Most treatment centers advocate this surgical practice as part of the staging procedure for medically suitable patients with early disease. Bilateral lymphangiography coupled with needle aspiration biopsy of the suspicious area has been suggested by some investigators, but it has not gained popularity. Blood for prostate or total acid phosphatase determinations should be drawn twice, beginning 24 hours after rectal examination because of its diurnal variation and spurious elevation by prostate massaging. Acid phosphatase concentration is not useful for screening for prostate carcinoma, but it can aid in the assessment of prognosis and tumor response. A normal value does not rule out the presence of stage C or D disease, since 30 to 40 percent of these patients have normal levels. On the other hand, 10 percent and 40 percent of patients with stages A and B disease have increased acid phosphatase. Abnormal acid phosphatase is a poor prognostic sign in patients with stage B or C disease. Recently, prostate-specific antigen has been shown to be more discriminatory in diagnosis of prostatic carcinoma determination than prostate acid phosphatases. It's use will be increased in the future.

THERAPEUTIC APPROACH

Stage A. Patients with stage A_1 (incidental and focal adenocarcinoma) require no further therapy in most instances except the transurethral resection of the prostate gland (TURP) for obstructive uropathy. However, stage A_2 patients need more aggressive treatment, since they have a worse prognosis than patients with stage B_1 disease. Radical prostatectomy with pelvic lymphadenectomy is the preferred treatment for young, healthy patients. The other alternative is radical pelvic radiation, either by external beam or interstitial implantation of ^{125}I. Radical surgery and radiation produce comparable therapeutic results at 10 years after treatment. At 15 years, patients with radical surgery can enjoy a life expectancy similar to that of the general population. The data of radiation therapy at 15 years are not yet assessed. A comparison between the side effects of radical surgery and radiation is also under way. Radical prostatectomy has a mortality rate of 0 to 5 percent and used to carry a high rate of impotence (up to 90 percent). However, recent advances in surgical technique to avoid severance of the sacral parasympathetic nerve and limited dissection of lymph nodes have reduced the incidence of impotence to 20 percent. This is probably lower than that from radical pelvic radiation. Other complications from radical surgery consist of incontinence, urethral stricture (both can be avoided in experienced hands), and complications associated with major pelvic surgery. Hence, for young and healthy patients, radical surgery with nerve sparing is my preferred treatment. Complications from pelvic radiation include lymphedema of the perineal area and lower extremities, urinary frequency and incontinence, urethral stricture, dysuria, radiation enteritis, and proctitis in addition to impotence.

Stage B. The choices of treatment are the same as those for stage A_2 patients: either radical prostatectomy or pelvic radiation.

Stage C. Pelvic radiation is the treatment of choice for stage C patients. Systemic hormonal therapy may improve the survival of these patients, and this requires further investigation, particularly in view of the development of less toxic medicines such as leuprolide and flutamide. Pelvic radiation may be of additional value in local disease control in patients initially treated with surgery.

Stage D. Postoperative pelvic radiation for patients with unsuspected stage D_1 disease has not been shown to have longer disease-free intervals to those of observation. Recently, bilateral orchiectomy following radical prostatectomy has been suggested as an effective alternative treatment. There is little chance to cure patients with stage D_2 disease; therefore the purpose of treatment should be palliation. Hence, asymptomatic patients should only be observed carefully, except in the case of impending complications such as pathologic fracture, spinal cord compression, renal failure, or bilateral hydronephrosis. The Veterans Administration Cooperative Urological Research Group (VACURG) studies demonstrate that early treatment of asymptomatic patients with diethylstilbestrol (DES) or orchiectomy does not prolong survival in patients with stage D disease because of the increased cardiovascular and thromboembolic mortality caused by DES in the first year of therapy, although the number of cancer deaths was reduced.

For symptomatic patients, local therapy with TURP to relieve bladder outlet obstruction and systemic treatment are often required. The first line of systemic therapy has almost always been endocrine manipulation since the report of Huggins and coworkers, who showed that growth of the prostate carcinoma is dependent on androgen. Therefore, androgen ablation is the principle of the treatment. It is also

TABLE 2 Primary Endocrine Treatment of Stage D_2 Prostate Carcinoma

Additive Hormones	*Dose*	*Route*	*Common Side Effects*	*Comment*
DES	1 mg tid	PO	Impotence, gynecomastia, cardiovascular,* thromboembolic†	
Megestrol acetate	40 mg tid	PO	Impotence, thromboembolic, gynecomastia	Fewer side effects than DES; also may be less effective
Goserelin (Zoladex)	3.6 mg	SC	Hot flushes, impotence	
Leuprolide acetate	1 mg/day or 7.5 mg/mo	SC	Hot flushes, impotence, bone pain	
Flutamide	250 mg tid	PO	Gynecomastia, diarrhea, rare hepatic side effects	
Estramustine	4–5 mg/kg tid	PO	Similar to DES	Myelosuppression is rare
Cyproterone acetate	300 mg qd	PO	Nausea and vomiting, edema	Investigational drug in US
Ablative procedure				
Bilateral orchiectomy	—	—	Impotence, psychological trauma	

*Incuding edema, congestive heart failure, myocardial infarction, and cardiac arrest.
†Including deep vein thrombophlebitis, pulmonary emboli, and cerebrovascular accident.

apparent that it is difficult to suppress serum androgen completely and permanently with exogenous estrogen and that prostatic cancer cells eventually develop resistance to androgen ablation after initial response. Table 2 lists most of the treatment options of endocrine manipulation. Estrogen inhibits the secretion of luteinizing hormone from the pituitary gland and hence the production of androgen from the testis. A castration level of testosterone can be maintained in about 90 percent of patients with 3 mg a day (1 mg three times per day) of DES. However 1 mg per day only reduces serum testosterone to castration level in 60 percent of patients. Five milligrams of DES a day has significantly higher cardiovascular and thromboembolic complications than 1 mg of DES, which has the equivalent clinical effectiveness of 5 mg of DES. It is important to realize that there is no randomized study to compare 1 mg versus 3 mg of DES in patients with stage D prostate carcinoma. The incidence of cardiovascular and thromboembolic effects ranges from 5 to 10 percent in patients taking 3 mg of DES. It is not negligible, but it is tolerable in a majority of patients. Leuprolide is a luteinizing hormone releasing hormone (LH-RH) agonist and offers therapy for patients with stage D disease that is equal to 3 mg of DES. It lowers serum testosterone to castration level about 3 weeks after an earlier rise. Its advantage over DES lies in the reduction of cardiovascular and thromboembolic effects. The disadvantages are that leuprolide is given by daily subcutaneous injection and it costs at least 10 times more than DES. LH-RH agonist of long-acting derivation (such as depo-leuprolide or Zoladex) or by nasal spray obviates the inconvenience of leuprolide and has been approved for commercial use. Occasionally, leuprolide causes bone pains in the first few weeks of therapy before it actually relieves the bone pain or other symptoms. This paradoxical action is believed to be due to the initial increase of luteinizing hormone by leuprolide before complete suppression. In patients with suspicious or documented spinal cord compression, the use of leuprolide should be avoided. Therefore, leuprolide is most suitable in patients with severe cardiac decompensation or in those who have experienced deep vein thrombophlebitis and/or pulmonary emboli.

Other first-line additive hormones include megestrol acetate (a progestational agent) or estramustine (a combined estrogen and nitrogen mustard). Megestrol acetate offers a theoretical advantage over DES because progestational agents can compete with androgen at the receptor level and can inhibit the 5α-reductase that converts testosterone into its active molecule, dihydrotestosterone, in addition to the suppression of luteinizing hormone secretion. But the clinical result with megestrol is not better than that with DES. In fact, it may be inferior. Estramustine may have a slightly better effect than DES, but it is an expensive medication. It is interesting to note that its side effects are almost identical to those of DES without increase in myelosuppression or gastrointestinal toxicities. Flutamide is a pure antiandrogen at the receptor level. Another antiandrogen is cyproterone acetate. Ketoconazole has also been tested for its ability to inhibit androgen synthesis. Preliminary reports on flutamide and cyproterone acetate show that they have therapeutic results similar to those of DES, although with fewer side effects. Large randomized studies comparing DES with flutamide are in progress in the United States.

The potential use of an antiandrogen is in the combination with leuprolide for total androgen ablation. Labrie and colleagues have shown that flutamide plus leuprolide may be superior to historical treatment in terms of remission rate and overall survival. Crawford and coworkers have reported that flutamide and leuprolide resulted in longer progression-free survival and median survival (35.6 versus 28.3 months; $p = 0.035$) than leuprolide alone in a randomized controlled study. Bilateral orchiectomy also gives results comparable to those of DES. Most urologists favor this procedure and view orchiectomy as the first treatment of choice, either alone or with flutamide. The reasons patients may refuse orchiectomy are usually emotional and psychological blocks. Bilateral orchiectomy is best indicated for patients who have poor compliance records with oral medication.

Close to 80 percent of patients treated with first-line hormonal manipulation benefit from their therapy, with relief of bone pain, improvement of performance status and anemia, and lessened requirement of analgesics. Objective tumor response usually occurs in 30 to 40 percent of patients who have measurable diseases. The median duration of response is about 12 to 15 months. The median survival for hormonally unresponsive patients is 10 to 12 months, and for responsive patients it is 20 to 24 months. Secondary hormone therapy for those patients who fail or relapse from the first line hormone is ineffective most of the time. Aminoglutethimide and glucocorticoid, megestrol acetate, estramustine, or bilateral orchiectomy has been reported to produce clinical subjective improvement in up to one-third of patients but rarely results in an objective response. Chemotherapy with single or multiple agents is usually used after failure of hormone therapy. There is no proven benefit for chemotherapy in first-line treatment, either alone or in combination with a hormone. Combination chemotherapy has not been conclusively proved as superior to single-agent chemotherapy. The poor results from chemotherapy are due to the fact that this group of patients has decreased or debilitated cardiac, renal, and bone marrow functions, which render them prone to side effects from chemotherapy with reduced tolerance. Also, most stage D prostate cancers are resistant to any given chemotherapy. Cyclophosphamide, 5-fluorouracil, doxorubicin, cisplatin, dacarbazine, and lomustine are frequently used and can produce up to 20 percent objective response rate and an additional 20 percent disease stabilization. The response duration is usually only a few months, and survival is not prolonged. Therefore, chemotherapy should be individualized by taking into consideration each patient's general condition and, in particular, his or her cardiac, renal, and bone marrow function. The median survival of patients receiving chemotherapy is 6 months.

ASSESSMENT OF TREATMENT

The most difficult part of performing clinical studies of prostate carcinoma is evaluating the response in stage D patients. Different response criteria have been employed because 80 percent of patients have only bone metastases without any measurable or evaluable nonosseous disease sites. Their diseases can only be evaluated by bone scan and bone x-ray film, and both are subject to interpretation bias and insensitivity. Bone x-ray study is less sensitive than bone scan. To evaluate any patient receiving treatment for prostate carcinoma, four different assessments have to be made: (1) objective measurable or evaluable nonosseous diseases such as palpable lymph nodes, pulmonary nodules, or hepatomegaly; (2) bone scan and x-ray film for bone diseases; (3) clinical status of the patients, which includes performance status, bone pain assessed by the requirement for analgesics, weight, and hemoglobin levels; and (4) serum acid phosphatase or prostatic-specific antigen level. Concordance in these four areas of assessment may not happen all the time; hence prioritization is necessary. In my opinion, the priority should be assigned according to the following sequences: objective measurable or evaluable nonosseous disease response followed by patient's clinical status response and bone scan response. Because of the large margin of error, changes in acid phosphatase should not be the only criterion used to determine treatment results.

These have been the principles in the development of the response criteria for the Eastern Cooperative Oncology Group studies of the prostate carcinoma. However, the most commonly used response criteria are those of the National Prostate Cooperative Projects, which define the partial response as normalization of acid phosphatase level, improvement of bone scan with greater than 50 percent reduction of increased uptake, greater than 50 percent reduction in measurable lesions (if present), and no new tumors or symptomatic deterioration for 12 weeks. At the same time, this group has claimed that stable disease is favorable to patients, and it includes those patients in the responsive portions of any given treatment.

SUGGESTED READING

Blackard CE. The Veterans Administration Cooperative Urological Research Group of carcinoma of the prostate: A review. Cancer Chemother Rep 1975; 59:225–227.

Crawford ED, Eisenberg MA, McLeod DG, et al. A controlled trial of leuprolide with and without flutamide in prostatic carcinoma. N Engl J Med 1989; 321:419–424.

Eggleston JC, Walsh PC. Radical prostatectomy with preservation of sexual function: Pathological findings in the first 100 cases. J Urol 1985; 134:1146–1148.

Eisenberger MA, O'Dwyer PJ, Friedman MA. Gonadotropin hormone-releasing hormone analogues: A new therapeutic approach for the prostate carcinoma. J Clin Oncol 1986; 4:414–424.

Gittes RF. Serum acid phosphatase and screening for carcinoma of the prostate. N Engl J Med 1983; 309:852–853.

Guinan P, Bush I, Ray V, et al. The accuracy of the rectal examination in the diagnosis of prostate carcinoma. N Engl J Med 1980; 303:499–503.

Labrie F, Dupont A, Belanger A. Complete androgen blockade for

the treatment of prostate cancer. In: De Vita VT, Hellman S, Rosenberg S, eds. Important advances in oncology. Philadelphia: JB Lippincott, 1985:193.
Paulson DF, Uro-oncology Research Group. Radical surgery vs radiotherapy for adenocarcinoma of the prostate. J Urol 1982; 128:502–508.
Pavon-Macaluso M, de Voogt HJ, Viggiano G, et al. Comparison of diethylstilbestrol, cyproterone acetate and medroxyprogesterone acetate in the treatment of prostatic cancer: Final analysis of a randomized phase III trial of the European Organization for Research on Treatment of Urological Cancer. J Urol 1986; 136:624–631.
Peeling WB. Phase III studies to compare goserelin (Zoladex) with orchiectomy and with diethylstilbestrol in treatment of prostatic carcinoma. Urology (Suppl) 1989; 33:45–52.
Perez CA. Carcinoma of the prostate, a vexing biological and clinical enigma. Int J Radiat Oncol Biol Phys 1983; 9:1427–1438.
Stamey TA, Kabalin JN. Prostate specific antigen in the diagnosis and treatment of adenocarcinoma of the prostate. I. Untreated patients. J Urol 1989; 141:1070–1075.
Zincke H, Utz DC, Taylor WF. Bilateral pelvic lymphadenectomy and radical prostatectomy for clinical stage C prostate cancer: Role of adjuvant treatment for residual cancer and in disease progression. J Urol 1986; 135:1199–1205.

TESTICULAR CANCER

DONALD L. TRUMP, M.D., F.A.C.P.

It has been known for many years that germ cell neoplasms of the testis are highly curable. In the 1950s researchers demonstrated that removal of the primary testicular tumor and either retroperitoneal node dissection (nonseminomas) or radiation therapy (seminomas) could cure 50 to 75 percent of patients in whom regional lymph node involvement was not found. Even patients with disseminated metastases were cured on rare occasions with radiation therapy to multiple sites (seminoma) or with single agent chemotherapy (actinomycin D, mithramycin). One of the first reports of the use of combination chemotherapy in adult malignancy was that of Li and co-workers at Memorial Hospital in New York. In 1961, they reported the effect of actinomycin D, chlorambucil, and methotrexate treatment in advanced testicular cancer. Thirty-eight percent of their patients experienced complete regression of all metastatic disease, and 8 percent were free of disease for more than 1 year. The development of cis-platinum based combination chemotherapy regimens now makes it possible to cure most patients with disseminated testicular cancer and offers options for the management of more limited disease, which should enable all patients with stage I and limited stage II disease to be cured.

The two most important parameters to consider in planning therapy for testicular cancer are the histology of the tumor and the stage of disease. Almost all primary tumors of the testis arise from the germ cells which ordinarily, are precursors of the spermatogonia. Tumors derived from these totipotent cells may contain elements differentiating along endodermal, mesodermal, ectodermal, or extraembryonic lines. The array of recognizable tissues contained within a germ cell tumor (GCT) may be quite striking—cartilage, smooth muscle, respiratory or squamous epithelium, or nerve tissues. The two major histologic classes of GCT are pure seminomas and nonseminomas. Germ cell tumors containing any element of nonseminomatous differentiation should be treated as nonseminomatous germ cell tumors (NSGCT).

The histologic diagnosis of GCT is almost always made by examination of an entire testis removed by an inguinal orchiectomy. While it has been frequently emphasized, it merits repeating that there is no role for percutaneous needle aspiration or trans-scrotal orchiectomy in the diagnosis of a testicular mass. Occasionally, a histologic diagnosis of GCT is made by biopsy of extratesticular tissue—usually a supraclavicular lymph node or retroperitoneal mass. Careful clinical examination of the testes, including the use of testicular ultrasonographic examination, usually discloses an unappreciated testicular mass. Even if a testicular mass is not discernible, patients with apparent GCT arising in an extragonadal site should be managed as though they have the usual type of GCT. The rationale for this approach is that primary extragonadal germ cell neoplasms do occur, are usually found in the retroperitoneum or anterior mediastinum, and are highly curable even when widely disseminated.

The clinical staging of patients with testicular GCT is based on careful history and physical examination, chest radiographs, and contrast enhanced abdominal computerized tomographic (CT) scans. If chest x-rays are normal, then chest CT scans are recommended. In view of the accuracy of these procedures, the role of lymphangiography (LAg) is uncertain, and intravenous pyelography as a staging procedure is probably unnecessary. LAg may be useful in planning retroperitoneal lymph node dissection (RPLND) and is often helpful in determining radiation therapy treatment portals, but as a staging procedure, LAg is probably not required.

Measurement of the serum content of the beta subunit of human chorionic gonadotropin (βhCG) and alpha fetoprotein (AFP) is crucial to the accurate histologic classification, staging, and post-treatment monitoring of patients with GCT. Whenever possible, a serum sample should be obtained before orchiectomy. When a diagnosis of GCT is confirmed, the specimen should be analyzed for βhCG and AFP. Both NSGCT and seminomas may produce βhCG: increased βhCG is seen in 40 to 50 percent of advanced NSGCT and in 10 percent of seminomas. No example of a pure seminoma leading to increased serum levels of AFP has been described. Consequently, patients with increased serum AFP and a biopsy revealing only seminoma should be managed as though they have NSGCT.

The most widely employed clinical staging system of GCT is outlined in Table 1. The therapy for GCT is determined by the clinical stage of disease as determined by the procedures noted above.

CLINICAL STAGE I NSGCT

The standard treatment for patients with stage I NSGCT is a retroperitoneal lymph node dissection (RPLND). Thirty percent of patients with clinical stage I disease have microscopic involvement of retroperitoneal nodes—usually at the renal hilum ipsilateral to the primary testis tumor. Sixty to 70 percent of patients with microscopic nodal involvement are cured with RPLND. Even in patients with clinically recognized but resectable retroperitoneal nodal involvement (stage IIB), 40 to 50 percent are cured by resection of involved nodes. Eighty to 90 percent of patients whose retroperitoneal nodes are shown to be histologically free of GCT are cured. It is rare for tumors treated by RPLND to recur in the abdomen: most relapses occur in the mediastinal or supraclavicular nodes or lung parenchyma. While RPLND is not without morbidity, 80 to 90 percent of stage I and 40 to 50 percent of stage II patients are cured after RPLND. The major chronic morbidity of RPLND is infertility due to ejaculatory incompetence. In stage I patients without evidence of retroperitoneal node involvement at surgery, a modified unilateral RPLND may be done with excellent probability of preserving the ability to ejaculate and no compromise in therapeutic efficacy. Patients with ejaculatory failure after RPLND may have fertility restored through pharmacologic means. Ephedrine or imipramine can restore ejaculation in 50 percent of such patients.

The immediate morbidity and potential for infertility following RPLND have led several groups to evaluate a cautious approach to stage I NSGCT. Workers at Memorial Sloan-Kettering Institute in New York City and the Royal Marsden Hospital in Great Britain have carefully followed patients after orchiectomy without treatment to retroperitoneal nodes. This follow-up requires monthly chest x-ray examinations and markers as well as abdominal CT scans every 3 months. Patients followed in this manner do very well. Sixty to 80 percent do not develop recurrent disease. Those who relapse develop tumors either in the lungs or retroperitoneal nodes, and almost all are curable with chemotherapy and surgery. A recent study from the Royal Marsden reported that 125 of 126 patients were cured with this approach. The study showed that patients with lymphatic invasion of the orchiectomy specimen or embryonal carcinoma had substantially higher relapse rates (40 percent) and were deemed unsuitable for a so-called wait and see approach.

The critical elements in the decision to observe stage I patients are the patient's ability to adhere to a meticulous follow-up and the ability of a multidisciplinary team to carry out such a plan. Not only is an experienced clinician required to coordinate careful follow-up and to communicate the absolute necessity of this plan to the patient, but a radiologist equally experienced in the subtleties of CT evaluation of the retroperitoneum and a reliable laboratory for the measurement of AFP and βhCG are necessary. The single most important variable in the prognosis of recurrent GCT is the extent of the tumor. With meticulous follow-up, recurrences may be detected early and at a highly curable stage. Failure of the patient or the team of physicians to adhere to the follow-up regimen compromises the patient's survival. While either RPLND or careful observation is a defensible therapy option for CSI patients, I favor RPLND. It must be remembered, however, that virtually all such patients should be cured of GCT—even if relapse occurs. Therefore, care should be taken to avoid any treatment or follow-up plan that may compromise the ultimate goal.

TABLE 1 Clinical Staging System for Testicular GCT

Stage I	
Disease limited to the testis	
Stage II	
Retroperitoneal nodes shown to contain GCT	
	≤2 cm
	2–5 cm
	>5 cm
Stage III	
Metastases beyond retroperitoneal nodes	

CLINICAL STAGE II NSGCT

Patients with microscopic retroperitoneal lymph node involvement or nonbulky nodes (IIB) are cured in 40 to 60 percent of cases by RPLND. While primary cytotoxic chemotherapy followed by surgery as needed would also cure these patients, the morbidity and potential mortality of 3 to 4 months of cis-platinum based combination therapy are certainly competitive with RPLND.

Patients with lymph node involvement and who have undergone RPLND present an interesting problem for the oncologist. A randomized intergroup trial demonstrates that virtually all (over 95 percent) resected stage II patients can be cured if they receive 2 months of postoperative chemotherapy with a platinum based regimen. However, this study also demonstrates that patients randomized to careful follow-up with chemotherapy administered at the first indication of recurrence also can all be cured. Chemotherapy for recurrent disease consisted of 4 months of treatment. However, 30 to 40 percent of patients never relapse after RPLND. A policy of routine adjuvant chemotherapy would expose these individuals to unnecessary chemotherapy. In view of these data, it is not appropriate to recommend routine adjuvant chemotherapy for patients with stage IIA or IIB NSGCT following RPLND. Patients in whom careful follow-up with monthly chest x-ray exam and markers is not possible can be cured with adjunctive chemotherapy. Patients at higher risk of recurrence (with more than six nodes or nodes over 4–5 cm, with embryonal histology or lymphatic invasion) could be considered for postoperative adjuvant chemotherapy. However, it is not clear that adjuvant chemotherapy in any subgroup improves survival if careful follow-up is possible.

Patients with stage IIC NSGCT disease can be optimally managed by a combined modality approach. Combination chemotherapy (cis-platinum, etoposide, and bleomycin) for 4 to 6 months should form the initial phase of therapy. Thirty to 40 percent of patients with stage IIC disease are rendered free of all radiographic and serologic (AFP and βhCG) evidence of disease with this therapy. Patients with stable, residual radiographic abnormalities and normal serum AFP and βhCG after four to six cycles of therapy should undergo excision of all residual abnormalities whenever possible. In approximately 60 percent of such patients, only fibrosis or necrotic material is found at surgery. Such patients have an excellent prognosis; their relapse rate at 2 years is only 10 to 20 percent. Thirty percent of resected patients have mature teratoma in the resected specimens. These patients have a relapse rate approximately the same as those with resected fibrosis and necrosis. The natural history of unresected mature teratoma is unclear. Patients in whom mature teratoma is not or cannot be completely resected may develop enlarging mature teratoma or recurrent GCT. Consequently, it is not wise to leave mature teratoma unresected. Ten percent of patients who undergo resection of residual radiographic abnormalities have residual GCT, and these individuals have a poorer prognosis. Most investigators recommend 2 additional months of chemotherapy in this situation. The long-term prognosis is still guarded, with recurrence rates approaching 50 percent.

STAGE IIC, III DISEASE

Cure rates for disseminated GCT are 70 to 80 percent. Important progress has been made in the last 5 years in more precisely defining the cure rates of the different subsets of stage III GCT. Einhorn and colleagues have retrospectively and prospectively evaluated the classification system outlined in Table 2. This system differs from others (most notably the Samuels–M.D. Anderson system) in that it more clearly defines patients with a poor prognosis. The Samuels system classifies as poor risk patients those whom the Indiana group has shown to be curable in 80 percent of instances—bulky abdominal disease only. Bosl and co-workers at Memorial have developed a system similar to the Indiana system, which also accurately classifies patients with GCT. Bosl's system utilizes the serum βhCG, AFP, and LDH content, which may add somewhat to the prognostic accuracy.

TABLE 2 Indiana Classification of Extent of Disease

Minimal
Elevated βhCG and/or αFP only
Cervical nodes (± nonpalpable retroperitoneal nodes)
Unresectable, but nonpalpable, retroperitoneal disease
Minimal pulmonary metastases—less than five per lung field and the largest <2 cm (± nonpalpable abdominal disease)
Moderate
Palpable abdominal mass as only anatomical disease
Moderate pulmonary metastases—five to ten pulmonary metastases per lung field and the largest <3 cm or a mediastinal mass <50% of the intrathoracic diameter or a solitary pulmonary metastasis any size >2 cm (± nonpalpable abdominal disease)
Advanced
Advanced pulmonary metastases—mediastinal mass >50% of the intrathoracic diameter or greater than ten pulmonary metastases per lung field or multiple pulmonary metastases >3 cm (± nonpalpable abdominal disease)
Palpable abdominal mass plus pulmonary metastases
8.1—minimal pulmonary
8.2—moderate pulmonary
8.3—advanced pulmonary
Hepatic, osseous, or CNS metastases

The success of platinum based chemotherapy is such that efforts are now being exerted to reduce the toxicity of therapy for patients with highly curable disease (Indiana staged good and moderate risk patients) and to improve the efficacy of therapy for poor risk patients.

GOOD-MODERATE RISK DISEASE

Cis-platinum based chemotherapy is the mainstay of treatment for GCT. It is now clear that VP-16 (etoposide) can replace vinblastine in the cis-platinum Velban, bleomycin (PVB) regimen. The Southeastern Cancer Study Group (SEG) study comparing PVB with bleomycin, VP-16, cis-platinum (BEP) clearly shows less toxicity with BEP (less severe myalgias, abdominal pain, and constipation). There is also indication that survival is superior with BEP therapy. Four cycles of therapy are almost always adequate to induce complete remission or stable radiographic abnormalities with normal AFP and βhCG. As noted above, surgical resection of stable residual radiographic changes is strongly recommended. BEP must be administered properly, however (Table 3). Treatment cycles should be repeated every 3 weeks, and dose modifications for mild–moderate toxicity are not indicated. Ten to 15 percent of patients receiving BEP as outlined experience white blood cell counts of less than 1,000 cumm; platelet counts of under 20,000 cumm are uncommon, although counts of 50 to 75,000 are often seen. With careful hydration, serious renal impairment

TABLE 3 BEP Combination Chemotherapy

Day 1–5	Etoposide 100 mg/m^2 IV
Day 1–5	Cis-platinum 20 mg/m^2 IV
Day 1,8,15	Bleomycin 10U IV or IM
Cycles repeated q21d	

is uncommon; magnesium wasting due to renal tubular injury is frequent. Raynaud's phenomenon occurs in 20 to 30 percent of patients who receive PVB or BEP. Further efforts to reduce the toxicity of BEP therapy are being evaluated in the good risk patients. The SEG has shown that three cycles of BEP are equivalent to four cycles of BEP. The Eastern Cooperative Oncology Group (ECOG) is now comparing BEP to EP (three cycles each) in good and moderate risk patients. This study follows the suggestion of Australian investigators that bleomycin may be deleted from the BEP regimen. Bosl has shown that VP16 plus cis-platinum is equivalent to the VAB6 regimen in advanced seminoma. These data all suggest that further reduction in treatment intensity may be achieved. At this time, three cycles of BEP is the standard therapy in good and moderate prognosis GCT.

POOR RISK DISEASE

It is an interesting phenomenon that an epithelial neoplasm, when widely disseminated, is curable in 30 to 40 percent of cases and is called a poor risk. In fact, such results are remarkable and represent one of the major achievements in oncology in the last 20 years. Nonetheless, therapy for poor risk GCT needs to be improved. Intensive therapy with BEP for four to six cycles followed by resection of residual masses (if markers are normal) is the standard of therapy for poor risk disease. However, only 50 percent of poor risk patients achieve a complete remission. Ozols and colleagues at the NCI have attempted to capitalize on the apparent steep dose response curve for cis-platinum by using twice the standard dose of this drug. In addition, they have combined VP16 with PVB—their regimen PVBV consists of cis-platinum (40 mg per meter squared in hypertonic saline daily for 5 days), VP16 (100 mg per meter squared daily for 5 days), bleomycin (30 U intramuscularly per week), and vinblastine (6 mg per meter squared daily for 2 days). While the neurologic and bone marrow toxicity of this regimen is great, it does have a high response rate. It does appear to be superior to PVB, although it is not clear that this superiority can justify its routine use in poor risk patients. The SEG has completed a study in poor risk patients comparing standard BEP to BEP with high dose platinum, 40 mg per meter squared. Preliminary analysis of this trial fails to reveal striking advantages for the higher dose platinum regimen. In view of the activity of VP-16–isophosphamide–cis-platinum in recurrent or refractory GCT, the Eastern Cooperative Oncology Group is conducting a trial of this regimen (VIP) versus BEP in poor risk patients. At the moment, optimal therapy for poor risk disease is uncertain. BEP is standard therapy and does achieve appreciable cures; however, most investigators agree that the results of BEP need to be improved upon in this subgroup of patients.

SALVAGE THERAPY

Ten to 40 percent of patients treated initially for advanced (stage IIC or stage III) disease fail to achieve complete remission (CR); an additional 10 to 20 percent of those who achieve a complete remission develop recurrent disease, almost always within 2 years of initial systemic therapy. Such patients have a poor prognosis. VP-16–cis-platinum or VIP in PVB failures or isophosphamide–cis-platinum in BEP failures induces complete remission in 20 to 30 percent of patients. Many of these patients are cured. It is not clear, however, that patients refractory or failing intensively administered initial therapy with PVB or BEP can be salvaged with this frequency. Our own experience in this regard is disappointing. Certainly, patients failing to achieve a CR with initial chemotherapy and surgery have a grim prognosis. While VIP, PVBV or very high dose cis-platinum plus VP16 have activity in such patients, cures are infrequent. There is absolutely no place for less than maximally intensive initial therapy with the hope of salvage therapy if CR is not obtained. Salvage of such patients is not easily or reliably accomplished. New approaches such as very high dose chemotherapy with autologous bone marrow support and development of new drugs are needed.

SPECIAL ISSUES

The Other Testicle

The cure rates for promptly diagnosed and appropriately managed testicular GCT are such that consideration of the long-term consequences of curative therapy are an increasingly important issue. One long-term consequence of cure is the development of contralateral, second primary tumor. In most large series, there is a 3 to 5 percent incidence of new primary tumors in patients cured of the initial tumor. For patients 2 years, without evidence of disease after CR is obtained in limited or extensive disease, the risk of a new primary tumor in the other testis equals or exceeds the risk of relapse. We carefully instruct young men cured of their first testis cancer in the use of testicular self-examination.

Fertility and Sexual Function

Many trials have shown that 50 percent of testis cancer patients—regardless of stage of disease—are azospermic or oligospermic at the time of diagnosis. Contralateral testis biopsies in such patients reveal germinal epithelial atrophy, peritubular fibrosis, and occasionally, intratubular carcinoma in situ. The major changes in fertility induced by therapy are ejaculatory incompetence associated with standard RPLND and germinal epithelial damage caused by chemotherapy. Modified RPLND preserves ejaculation in most patients and is appropriate for clinical stage I patients. Ephedrine or amitriptyline restores ejaculation in perhaps 40 percent of individuals who have ejaculatory failure after RPLND. Transient azospermia is induced by PVB in all patients. In 50 percent of patients, however, at least a modest return of spermatogenesis (sperm counts over 20×10^6) occurs 2 or more years following therapy. It is not clear whether these are the same patients who have adequate spermatogenesis prior to therapy or whether therapy causes permanent destruction of germinal epithelium in some and allows return of spermatogenesis in others. Sexual and psychologic function is largely intact in patients cured of testis cancer. Some reports have noted sexual dysfunction associated with RPLND; however, most data indicate that patients cured of testis cancer can anticipate essentially normal sexual and psychologic function.

Extragonadal GCT (EGCT)

Debate continues regarding the genesis of tumors that clinically appear to be EGCT. Two schools of thought exist. The first holds that the tumors (which almost always present as retroperitoneal or anterior mediastinal disease) really are occult or regressed primary testis cancers. The second view is that these tumors are truly primary in extragonadal sites and arise from primordial germ cells misdirected during embryonic migration. The occurrence of EGCT in the pineal region strongly supports this latter hypothesis. Regardless of the pathogenesis of EGCT, it should be managed according to the same principles that guide treatment of testicular primary tumors. Careful clinical and ultrasonographic examination of both testicles is mandatory. Both testicles should be carefully followed after therapy. While some data suggest that EGCT has a poor prognosis, this seems to be related to the stage or extent of disease at diagnosis rather than an intrinsically resistant or more virulent character of this tumor. Intensive therapy should be pursued in NSGCT arising in extragonadal sites, and cure rates in excess of 50 percent should be expected.

Seminoma

Seminomas are extremely radiosensitive and have a relatively indolent and predictable course of metastatic spread. Most patients with seminoma have stage I or low volume stage II disease at diagnosis. Such patients are cured 90 to 100 percent of the time with rather modest doses (30 to 35 Gy) of radiation administered to the retroperitoneum. The necessity for mediastinal radiation in low volume stage II patients is unclear. Patients with extranodal metastases from seminoma may be cured with cis-platinum based therapy. As in patients with NSGCT, the prognosis in such patients is related to the extent of the disseminated disease. Cis-platinum based combination chemotherapy is clearly the treatment of choice for these patients. Management of patients with bulky (stage IIC) retroperitoneal seminoma is controversial. Radiation therapy cures 40 to 60 percent of such patients, and those not cured with radiation can usually be cured with salvage chemotherapy. However, chemotherapy with radiation or resection of residual radiographic abnormalities cures at least 70 to 80 percent of patients. Patients who have received retroperitoneal radiation, and especially those who have received retroperitoneal and mediastinal radiation, have more difficulty receiving full dose chemotherapy. Whether primary radiation with chemotherapy salvage or whether primary chemotherapy is the optimal treatment plan is not clear. A randomized, intergroup trial evaluating these two treatment plans is currently underway.

SUGGESTED READING

Birch R, Williams S, Cone A, et al. Prognostic factors for favorable outcome in disseminated germ cell tumors. J Clin Oncol 1986; 4:400–407.

Bosl GJ, Geller NL, Cirrincione C, et al. Multivariate analysis of prognostic variables in patients with metastatic testicular cancer. Cancer Res 1983; 43:3403–3407.

Bosl GJ, Yagoda A, Golbey RB, et al. Role of etoposide-based chemotherapy in the treatment of patients with refractory or relapsing germ cell tumor. Am J Med 1985; 78:423–428.

Garnick MB, Richie JP. Toward more rational management for stage I testis cancer: watch out for "watch and wait"! J Clin Oncol 1986; 4:1021–1023.

Hoskin P, Dilly S, Easton D, et al. Prognostic factors in stage I nonseminomatous germ cell testicular tumors managed by orchiectomy and surveillance: implications for adjuvant chemotherapy. J Clin Oncol 1986; 4:1031–1036.

Israel A, Bosl GJ, Golbey RB, et al. The results of chemotherapy for extragonadal germ cell tumors in the cisplatin era: the Memorial Sloan-Kettering Cancer Center experience (1975 to 1982). J Clin Oncol 1985; 3:1073–1078.

Ozols RF, Deisseroth AB, Javadpour N, et al. Treatment of poor prognosis nonseminomatous testicular cancer with a high-dose platinum combination chemotherapy regimen. Cancer 1983; 51:1803–3807.

EPIDURAL SPINAL CORD COMPRESSION AND CARCINOMATOUS MENINGITIS

MARK R. GILBERT, M.D.

EPIDURAL SPINAL CORD COMPRESSION

Epidural spinal cord compression (ESCC) occurs in approximately 5 percent of patients with systemic malignancy, making it the second most common neurologic complication. The term ESCC implies that there is spread of cancer into the epidural space, causing deformation of the spinal cord or the cauda equina. Compression of the spinal cord and the resultant neurologic dysfunction, however, often occur weeks to months after the onset of the initial symptoms of metastatic spread to the epidural space. The initial symptom in 95 percent of patients is pain, either localized or occurring in a radicular pattern. Moreover, patients generally have *no* neurologic dysfunction with the onset of pain. Despite the early presence of pain in most patients with epidural metastases, three-quarters of these patients have significant neurologic dysfunction *at the time of diagnosis*. The most common neurologic findings in patients with ESCC are weakness in the extremities, sensory loss (often with a dermatomal sensory level), and ataxia. Urinary and fecal incontinence are also frequent complaints at the time of diagnosis.

The most common types of primary malignancy that cause epidural metastases are breast cancer, lung cancer, prostate cancer, sarcomas, melanoma, and gastrointestinal cancers, primarily that of the colon. Virtually all types of metastatic cancer have been reported to cause ESCC. The relative frequency of a specific tumor type resulting in ESCC may be related to three factors: (1) the overall incidence of the tumor, (2) the propensity of the tumor to spread to bone (i.e., vertebrae), and (3) the overall duration of survival for patients with the malignancy. ESCC is often a late complication not commonly seen in patients with malignancies associated with a short expected survival, such as those who have pancreatic cancer.

There are two routes by which the tumor infiltrates into the epidural space. The more common route is taken by direct extension of a metastatic lesion from the vertebral bones through the cortical margin of bone that surrounds the spinal canal and into the epidural space. In taking the second route, the tumor spreads into the epidural space through the intervertebral foramina. This occurs most commonly with tumors in the retroperitoneal region or tumors that have metastasized to the periaortic lymph nodes. Once the tumor has reached the epidural space, the fatty tissue and blood vessels in this region provide little barrier to rostral and caudal extension of the tumor. The tumor can extend several vertebral levels from the initial region of tumor infiltration.

Diagnosis

Patients with cancer, back pain, and neurologic dysfunction warrant an emergency evaluation (Fig 1). Plain spine radiographs are useful for directing computed tomographic (CT) myelography. I recommend an x-ray survey of the entire spine so that symptomatic but abnormal regions can be evaluated during CT myelography.

Patients with cancer and back pain who have a *normal* neurologic examination require an x-ray study of the symptomatic area. The finding of a lytic or blastic lesion in the vertebral bones indicates that there is a high likelihood (60 to 80 percent) of tumor being present in the epidural space. X-ray films of the remainder of the spine should then be obtained and the patient should undergo CT myelography to examine the regions with bone changes. Patients with normal spinal radiographs are more difficult to evaluate. If the patient's pain is radicular or if the tumor is retroperitoneal or is a lymphoma (both such tumors being likely to have spread into the epidural space through the intervertebral foramina), I proceed with CT scanning of the symptomatic region of the spine. The CT scan is obtained to look for a paraspinous mass or evidence of vertebral bone metastases eroding through the cortical margin of bone surrounding the spinal canal. If the CT scan is positive, the patient should undergo myelography. If it is negative, the patient is observed.

Combined with CT scanning, myelography using water-soluble agents (metrizamide, iohexol) provides excellent detail of the epidural space with a very low incidence of side effects. The finding of ESCC mandates the delineation of the full extent of the tumor because rostral or caudal extension of tumor greater than five vertebral levels commonly occurs. Complete block often necessitates a second installation of the contrast agent from the other side of the block to determine the extent of the lesion. Cerebrospinal fluid (CSF) should be cytologically evaluated at the time of myelography because carcinomatous meningitis can occur concurrently with ESCC or present with similar symptoms.

The role of magnetic resonance image (MRI) scanning, with or without magnetic "contrast" agents (i.e., gadolinium), in the diagnostic evaluation of ESCC is controversial. A direct comparison of MRI and CT myelography has not been made. Nevertheless, I have had several cases in which

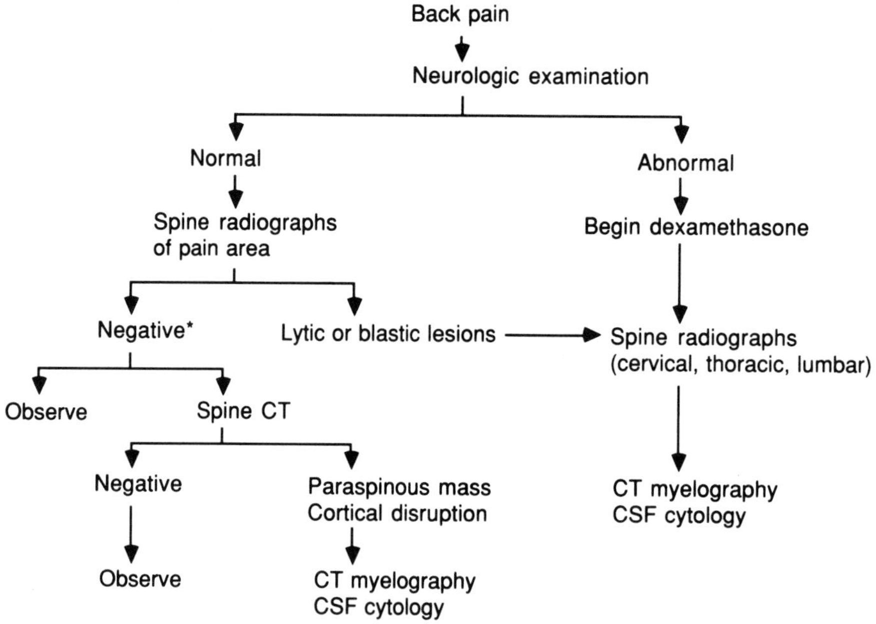

Figure 1 Evaluation of epidural spinal cord compression. *See text.

large epidural deposits of tumor that were found by CT myelography were not demonstrated by MRI scans. In addition, it is unclear whether MRI is able to detect small deposits of tumor in the epidural space at the extending edge of the tumor; if it is not, this limits its usefulness in determining the full extent of disease.

Other diagnoses to consider are carcinomatous meningitis, intramedullary metastases, epidural abscess or hematoma, fungal or tuberculous meningitis, and radiation myelopathy. Rarely, a patient with a parasagittal brain metastasis may present with bilateral (usually asymmetric) lower extremity weakness. Similar findings occur in cases of sagittal sinus thrombosis. Paraneoplastic myelopathy remains a diagnosis of exclusion, as there is no diagnostic test for this condition at present.

Treatment

Corticosteroids

Corticosteroids are highly useful in decreasing edema in the peritumoral region. Prompt institution of steroid therapy for patients with ESCC may prevent vascular compromise of the cord and irreversible dysfunction, thereby allowing time for more definitive treatment of the tumor. In patients presenting with neurologic dysfunction, I recommend high-dose dexamethasone, beginning with a 100-mg bolus, and thereafter 96 mg per day for 3 days. The steroid dose is then tapered off over the next 2 to 3 weeks. In patients with back pain, a normal neurologic examination, and abnormal x-ray studies, I recommend dexamethasone at a dose of 4 mg every 6 hours. This often provides prompt pain relief while diagnostic evaluation is underway.

Surgery

Several studies have shown that a posterior surgical decompression (laminectomy) combined with radiation therapy offers no advantage in outcome or duration of response when compared with radiation treatment alone. There are, however, several indications for surgical intervention:

1. ESCC without a known malignancy. These patients may require a tissue diagnosis before treatment can be initiated. In this case, a needle biopsy may be sufficient.
2. Vertebral instability, particularly of the cervical spine. This may necessitate a debulking and stabilizing procedure.
3. Progression of symptoms during radiation treatment. This may necessitate a surgical decompression to permit completion of the radiation therapy.
4. Recurrence of epidural tumor in a previously irradiated region. This may necessitate surgical decompression to alleviate pain and allow sufficient time for chemotherapy to reduce tumor volume.
5. The possibility of an epidural abscess. This warrants a biopsy procedure.

The most promising surgical technique for treating ESCC is an anterior or anterolateral resection.

Most tumors arise from the vertebral body; therefore the most effective debulking procedure would involve resection of the vertebral body and replacement of the bone with a methacrylate prosthesis. Several studies using this technique have yielded promising results, showing that it provides good symptomatic relief and, in some cases, reversal of dense neurologic dysfunction. The procedure is complex, however, and in patients with widely metastatic disease it is associated with high morbidity and mortality rates. I therefore reserve this technique for patients with limited vertebral involvement who also have a long life expectancy.

Radiation Therapy

Radiation therapy is the primary treatment for patients with ESCC. Radiation ports are carefully defined to prevent recurrence of tumor at the edge of a previous treatment field. Local recurrence would preclude treatment of the new lesion because of overlap of the radiation exposure to the previously treated area of the spinal cord. To prevent this problem, I insist on full delineation of the extent of tumor in the epidural space by myelography and often request a second injection of contrast agent if there is a complete block. Evaluation of other regions of the spine that show abnormalities on x-ray films but are asymptomatic may uncover small epidural deposits of tumor that may benefit from early treatment and assist in planning the radiation treatment port(s).

Chemotherapy

The role of chemotherapy in the treatment of epidural spinal cord compression is limited for most solid tumors, but I have used chemotherapy effectively in patients who have undergone previous irradiation and cannot receive more radiation therapy to that area of the spinal cord. I have had some dramatic success with chemotherapy-sensitive tumors, such as lymphomas, where improvement in neurologic function was noted within days of beginning treatment. For other tumors that are less sensitive to chemotherapy, I recommend a surgical decompression, if cord compression exists, in order to allow time for chemotherapy-induced tumor reduction to occur.

Outcome

The outcome of treatment is directly related to the patient's functional status at the time of diagnosis. Generally, patients who are ambulatory at the time of diagnosis will remain so after treatment. Paraplegic patients rarely regain neurologic function after surgical resection and postsurgical radiation treatment. The key to successful management of epidural tumors, therefore, is early diagnosis. Patients with malignancy who develop back pain warrant an evaluation as outlined in Figure 1. It is through the prompt recognition and treatment of epidural metastases that we can alleviate the associated pain and prevent neurologic dysfunction.

CARCINOMATOUS MENINGITIS

Carcinomatous meningitis is defined as the presence of free-floating tumor cells in the CSF. These cells can cause neurologic dysfunction by local infiltration of nerve roots and brain parenchyma, by obstructing the normal flow of the CSF, and by irritating the surface of the cortex, causing seizures. The evaluation and management of carcinomatous meningitis are appropriate for lymphomatous and leukemic meningitis. Management of the spread of primary brain tumors into the spinal fluid, such as in medulloblastoma and glioblastoma multiforme, requires special consideration and is beyond the scope of this discussion.

The most common manifestation of carcinomatous meningitis is an alteration in cognitive function. This symptom may be related to diffuse infiltration of the brain surface by tumor or to increased intracranial pressure. Patients with carcinomatous meningitis frequently complain of headache, which is also often related to increased intracranial pressure. An increase in intracranial pressure is caused by either communicating or noncommunicating hydrocephalus or a combination of both. Communicating hydrocephalus results from tumor cells infiltrating the arachnoid granulations and preventing CSF resorption. Noncommunicating hydrocephalus results from a collection of tumor cells, usually in the cerebral aqueduct, preventing the outflow of CSF.

Patients with carcinomatous meningitis may also present with isolated cranial nerve or spinal radicular findings. Often, nerve dysfunction may be evident at several levels, indicating the diffuse nature of this process. Symptoms of cranial nerve involvement may include blindness (infiltration of the optic nerve or chiasm), diplopia (usually involvement of cranial nerve III or VI), peripheral facial palsy, and less commonly, facial numbness and hearing loss. Spinal cord involvement tends to show predominantly lumbosacral signs and symptoms because tumor cells have a propensity to collect in the thecal sac. This collection may be caused by gravity-related settling of the tumor cells. Patients may also present with low back pain that often has a radicular component similar to sciatica. Lower extremity weakness, dermatomal pattern sensory loss, incontinence, and selected loss of deep tendon reflexes are common.

Seizures, relatively rare occurrences, may be either focal or generalized. Seizures are believed to be caused by meningeal irritation or infiltration of cortical parenchyma by tumor.

Carcinomatous meningitis is primarily caused by adenocarcinomas, most commonly those of the breast, lung, and melanoma. Leukemic meningitis is common in patients with acute leukemia, particularly those with acute lymphocytic leukemia. Lymphomatous meningitis occurs with nonHodgkin's lymphomas, with a few reported cases occurring with Hodgkin's lymphoma. Lymphoma cells in the CSF are a common finding in primary CNS lymphoma.

Diagnosis

The definitive diagnostic test for carcinomatous meningitis is the demonstration of malignant cells in the CSF. This may require repeated lumbar puncture. The diagnostic yield of a single cytologic analysis of CSF has been reported to be 50 percent. Three CSF analyses increase the sensitivity cytologic examination to approximately 85 percent. Five CSF samples increase the yield of cytology to 95 percent. The spinal fluid, however, is abnormal in almost all patients. Most commonly, the CSF total protein is elevated (80 percent). Other abnormal findings include a pleocytosis (predominantly mononuclear), elevated opening pressure, and a low glucose concentration.

Radiologic studies are often helpful in supporting a diagnosis of carcinomatous meningitis. MRI scanning, particularly with gadolinium administration, may show enhancing deposits along the walls of the ventricles or the cortical sulci. Similar cortical enhancement is sometimes noted on contrast CT scans. Additionally, communicating and noncommunicating hydrocephalus may often be seen with either MRI or CT scanning. CT myelography of the cauda equina region often detects nodular tumor deposits on the nerve roots.

Infectious meningitis, usually a subacute infection such as tuberculosis or a fungal process, may present with findings similar to those of carcinomatous meningitis. Brain metastases, bland or hemorrhagic infarct, or cerebral abscess may present with signs and symptoms of increased intracranial pressure, altered mental status, and headache, which are similar to the common clinical features of carcinomatous meningitis. Other processes that can cause isolated spinal symptoms include ESCC, brachial or lumbar plexopathy, intramedullary metastases, and radiation myelopathy.

Treatment

Radiation Therapy

Radiation therapy was the original means of treating carcinomatous meningitis. Cranial-spinal irradiation, encompassing the entire neuraxis, is necessary if radiation therapy is the only treatment used. However, irradiation of the vertebrae, which provide much of the bone marrow in adults, is associated with significant myelosuppression. Myelosuppression severely limits any future chemotherapeutic treatment and is often severe enough to make the patient dependent on transfusions of blood products. Radiation treatment to the brain is also associated with a chronic neurotoxic syndrome known as leukoencephalopathy. This syndrome usually occurs months to years after treatment and is characterized by a slowly progressive change in personality, leading to changes in cognitive function and often ultimately leading to coma or death. Patients who receive intrathecal chemotherapy after brain irradiation are at a particularly high risk for developing leukoencephalopathy.

As indicated in the following sections of this chapter, I use radiation therapy only for control of local symptoms or to alleviate ventricular outflow obstruction if noncommunicating hydrocephalus exists. This approach usually provides some reversal of local neurologic dysfunction, particularly if cranial nerve palsies are prominent findings. Relief of ventricular outflow obstruction is critical for safe installation of chemotherapy into the lateral ventricles through a reservoir.

Chemotherapy

Intrathecal administration of chemotherapeutic agents is the predominant treatment modality for carcinomatous meningitis. Chemotherapeutic agents administered systemically do not cross the blood-brain barrier in sufficient amounts to achieve tumoricidal levels in the CSF. Chemotherapy can be instilled into either the lumbar thecal space or into the lateral ventricles through a subcutaneous reservoir (i.e., Ommaya reservoir). Lumbar injections can be done with standard lumbar punctures, although studies using radiotracer have shown that 10 to 15 percent of these injections end up in the epidural space or in the subcutaneous fat. Moreover, repeated injections can lead to local scar formation, making subsequent punctures difficult and uncomfortable. Placement of the ventricular reservoir system requires a neurosurgical procedure, but once the ventricular reservoir system is in place, it provides a well-tolerated method of instilling drug into the CSF. I use the reservoir also to obtain an ^{111}Indium DTPA ventriculogram before injecting the drug to ensure that ventricular outflow is not obstructed. Outflow obstruction causes pooling of drug in the lateral ventricles, which can result in a rapidly progressive, often fatal degeneration of brain parenchyma. Patients with outflow obstruction undergo local radiation treatment; clearance of the obstruction is then confirmed with a repeat ventriculogram.

It is unclear whether an advantage exists for either lumbar or ventricular injections. Some recent data from studies of drug delivery in animal models indicate that combined lumbar and ventricular administration of drug is best for achieving adequate concentrations of drug throughout the neuraxis. Ventricular injections provide high concentration of drug in the CSF surrounding the brain, but the levels are significantly lower in the spinal cord region. The reverse, however, is true with lumbar injections. For this reason, I favor a combination of both lumbar and ventricular injections.

Methotrexate is the most commonly used drug for intrathecal injections. It has tumoricidal activity against most solid tumors, leukemias, and lymphomas. Cytosine arabinoside (ara-C) is useful only for leukemias and lymphomas. Thiophosphoramide (Thiotepa) can also be administered intrathecally. This alkylating agent is useful for solid tumors, particularly for breast and lung cancers. I usually administer intrathecal drugs two times per week for 8 to 12 weeks or until the tumor is cleared from the CSF. I continue a maintenance regimen of biweekly injections for 1 year or until there is evidence of progressive disease. The standard dose of methotrexate for adults is 12 mg per injection; ara-C is administered in a dose of 50 mg per injection; and Thiotepa is given in doses of 10 mg.

As described above, intrathecal chemotherapy is associated with a high incidence of leukoencephalopathy. Prior cranial radiation therapy significantly increases the incidence of developing leukoencephalopathy. In my experience, almost all patients who receive both radiation and intrathecal chemotherapy develop leukoencephalopathy within 1 year of completing treatment.

Outcome

Carcinomatous meningitis carries a grave prognosis. The duration of survival is related to the type of primary malignancy and to the extent of neurologic dysfunction at the time of diagnosis. For all tumor types, if the patient is not treated, survival is generally a few weeks. Patients with melanoma have the worst prognosis; despite radiation and chemotherapy, low treatment response rates (20 percent) and short median survival times (3.6 months) have been reported. Patients with carcinomatous meningitis from lung cancer fare only slightly better than patients with melanoma; the treatment response rate is 20 percent and the median survival is 4 months. Patients with breast cancer have the best prognosis, but even in those who are treated, the median survival is only 7.2 months. There are, however, several reports of patients with breast cancer surviving more than 2 years after the diagnosis of carcinomatous meningitis. Unfortunately, most of these patients develop severe neurologic dysfunction from leukoencephalopathy caused by chemotherapy and radiotherapy.

SUGGESTED READING

Findlay GFG. Adverse effects of the management of malignant spinal cord compression. J Neurol Neurosurg Psych 1984; 47:761–768.

Grossman SA, Chen CDP, Thompson G, et al. Cerebrospinal fluid abnormalities in patients with neoplastic meningitis: an evaluation using ^{111}Indium-DTPA ventriculography. Am J Med 1982; 73:641–645.

Harrington KD. Anterior cord decompression and spinal stabilization for patients with metastatic lesions of the spine. J Neurosurg 1984; 61:107–117.

Rodichok LD, Harper GR, Ruckdeschel JC, et al. Early diagnosis of spinal epidural metastases. Am J Med 1987; 70:1181–1187.

Wasserstrom WR, Glass JP, Posner JP. Diagnosis and treatment of leptomeningeal metastases from solid tumors: experience with 90 patients. Cancer 1982; 49:759–772.

Weissman DA, Gilbert MR, Wong H, Grossman SA. The use of computed tomography of the spine to identify patients at high risk for epidural metastases. J Clin Oncol 1985; 3:1541–1544.

HYPERTENSION AND RENAL DISEASE

HYPONATREMIA

JOHN F. WADE III, M.D.
ROBERT J. ANDERSON, M.D.

Hyponatremia is a common electrolyte disorder with a prevalence of 2 to 3 percent in hospitalized patients. Central to the understanding of hyponatremia and its therapy is the concept that the plasma sodium concentration reflects the ratio between the amount of sodium and the amount of water in the body. Hyponatremia results from an excess of water relative to sodium. Such an excess of water occurs from continued water intake (oral or intravenous) in the presence of impaired renal water elimination. Decreased renal water excretion is usually caused by the action of antidiuretic hormone causing the kidney to retain water. Occasionally, decreased renal water elimination is caused by renal failure. The rational treatment of hyponatremia depends on whether it is symptomatic or not, whether it is acute or chronic, and on the underlying cause (Table 1).

SYMPTOMATIC HYPONATREMIA

Since body water is in osmotic equilibrium, positive water balance dilutes plasma, decreasing the sodium concentration and osmolality. This leads to a shift of water from extracellular (low osmolality) to intracellular (normal osmolality) spaces. The subsequent cell swelling can produce central nervous system dysfunction since the brain is encased within a rigid skull. The severity of brain edema and dysfunction depends on the rate and magnitude of the decrease in plasma sodium concentration. Acute marked hyponatremia leads to cerebral edema with progressive anorexia, nausea, vomiting, lethargy, headaches, confusion, seizures, and ultimately transtentorial herniation with cardiopulmonary arrest and death. With a more gradual decline in the plasma sodium concentration, brain cells can extrude osmotically active particles such as sodium and potassium. This decreases cell osmolality and water uptake and mitigates cerebral swelling and dysfunction. The clinical corollary is that acute hyponatremia is often symptomatic while chronic hyponatremia is usually well tolerated.

Acute symptomatic hyponatremia should be considered a medical emergency. Although most symptomatic hyponatremic patients have a plasma sodium concentration of less than 120 mEq per liter, life-threatening hyponatremia can occur with higher concentrations of plasma sodium. The optimal management of acute, symptomatic hyponatremia is currently under debate. Untreated symptomatic hyponatremia can lead to seizures and death. Alternatively, an "osmotic demyelination syndrome" with pontine and extrapontine myelinolysis resulting in pseudobulbar palsy, quadriplegia, a "locked-in" state, and other neurologic deficits has occurred after therapy. Risk factors for the development of neurologic sequelae following treatment of symptomatic hyponatre-

TABLE 1 Causes and Treatment of Hyponatremia

Cause	*Treatment*
Erroneous and factitious hyponatremia and pseudohyponatremia	No specific therapy needed
Normovolemic hyponatremia (SIADH)	Treat underlying disorder Water restriction Hypertonic saline with or without a loop diuretic Loop diuretics with sodium chloride supplementation Demeclocycline Induce urea diuresis
Primary polydipsia	Water restriction
Hypovolemic hyponatremia	Isontonic saline Rarely, hypertonic saline
Hypervolemic (edematous) hyponatremia	Treat underlying disease Salt and water restriction Loop diuretics Converting enzyme inhibitors for heart failure Rarely, dialysis

mia include chronic hyponatremia (>48 hours), overcorrection, a large magnitude of correction (> 15 to 25 mEq per liter), rapid correction (> 1 to 2 mEq per liter per hour), severe underlying disease such as malnutrition, malignancy, or alcoholism and an associated hypoxic event.

One approach to the management of acute, symptomatic hyponatremia is to administer hypertonic sodium chloride (3 percent or, rarely, 5 percent) at approximately 100 ml per hour until seizures and other symptoms resolve. The endpoint of therapy is either cessation of major symptoms or a 10 to 15 percent increase in plasma sodium concentration. Acutely, 3 percent saline increases the plasma sodium concentration because the concentration of the sodium (513 mEq per liter) exceeds that of the plasma. To produce a sustained, significant increase in the plasma sodium concentration, removal of excess free water from the body is necessary. The administration of hypertonic saline results in negative water balance as long as the osmolality of the administered fluid exceeds that of the urine. In patients with a fixed high urine osmolality, 3 percent sodium chloride (osmolality of 1,026 mOsm per kilogram of H_2O) may result in only a slow correction of hyponatremia. In symptomatic hyponatremic patients with a high urine osmolality, administration of a loop diuretic (i.e., 0.5 to 1 mg per kilogram of furosemide) usually results in a large diuresis of isotonic urine. Repletion of urinary electrolytes lost after the administration of furosemide with a small volume of 3 percent sodium chloride functionally results in the rapid removal of a large amount of free water and in an increase in the plasma sodium concentration. In the treatment of symptomatic hyponatremia of unknown or chronic duration, a reasonable plan is to administer 3 percent sodium chloride (with or without a loop diuretic) to increase the plasma sodium concentration by about 10 percent. In the acute treatment of symptomatic hyponatremia, frequent monitoring of the plasma sodium concentration during therapy (i.e., every 2 to 3 hours) is necessary to ensure a rate of correction of less than 1.5 to 2 mEq per liter per hour and a total magnitude of acute correction of less than 15 mEq per liter over 24 to 48 hours. After the discontinuation of 3 percent sodium chloride, water restriction alone should be undertaken to bring about a slower normalization of plasma sodium.

ASYMPTOMATIC HYPONATREMIA

The majority of patients with hyponatremia are asymptomatic. In such asymptomatic patients, the risks of emergent therapy outweigh any potential benefits. The appropriate treatment of asymptomatic hyponatremia depends on the underlying cause of the disorder (see Table 1).

Erroneous and Factitious Hyponatremia

In approximately 20 percent of patients with hyponatremia, the low plasma sodium concentration can be attributed to laboratory error, blood drawing error (i.e., from a vein proximal to an intravenous infusion of hypotonic fluid), or the presence of high blood concentrations of an osmotically active particle, which is usually glucose but may on rare occasions be mannitol or glycine. Rarely, marked hyperlipidemia or hyperproteinemia can artifactually lower the plasma sodium concentration. In the case of hyperglycemia, the osmotic effect of glucose results in a shift of water from the intracellular space to the extracellular space, thereby diluting plasma and producing hyponatremia. In the settings discussed above, hyponatremia occurs without hypotonicity and therefore requires no specific therapy.

Syndrome of Inappropriate Secretion of Antidiuretic Hormone

Once erroneous and factitious hyponatremia have been excluded, it is useful to categorize patients on the basis of the clinical assessment of their extracellular fluid volume status. Most hyponatremic patients (30 to 40 percent) appear to be euvolemic and meet the criteria for the diagnosis of syndrome of inappropriate secretion of antidiuretic hormone (SIADH). Common clinical settings of SIADH include the postoperative state, the presence of intrathoracic and intracranial disease, selected hormone deficiency states (glucocorticoid and thyroid), psychosis, and cancer, and the use of selected medications such as chlorpropamide. In these disorders, the combination of nonosmotic secretion of antidiuretic hormone plus continued water intake leads to positive water balance and hyponatremia.

The treatment of SIADH varies with the severity of the hyponatremia and the magnitude of the increase in urine osmolality. In all cases, recognition and treatment of the underlying disease is important. Asymptomatic patients with mild to moderate hyponatremia may respond to water restriction sufficient to achieve negative water balance. To achieve negative water balance, the sum of the amount of water intake and of water produced by metabolism must be less than that lost through perspiration, breathing, and urination. Negative water balance with an improvement in the hyponatremic patient's condition can usually be accomplished in patients with urine osmolalities of approximately 300 mOsm per kilogram of H_2O. Successful therapy with water restriction thus requires good patient compliance and a relatively low urine osmolality.

For patients with chronic SIADH in whom urine osmolality is higher and compliance is poor, additional therapy directed toward decreasing urinary osmolality, which increases renal water excretion, is often needed. This therapy may consist of a loop diuretic such as furosemide or bumetanide combined with sodium chloride supplementation (intravenous or oral) to prevent hypovolemia. A second line of therapy used to decrease urine osmolality and increase renal water excretion is the administration of a drug that inhibits the ability of antidiuretic hormone to increase renal collecting tubular water reabsorption. Two such agents are demeclocycline (300 to 600 mg twice daily) and lithium. Because of the potential significant toxicity associated with lithium, demeclocycline is usually preferred, except in children, where this tetracycline can interfere with bone growth. The onset of action of demeclocycline is slow, and it may take several days for an effect to be seen. A final form of therapy for chronic SIADH, infrequently used in the United States, is to decrease urine osmolality by inducing a solute (urea) diuresis by administration of 30 to 60 g of oral urea per day. Oral urea is unpalatable and, in our experience, not a practical therapeutic agent.

Occasionally, the clinician encounters a patient with SIADH and moderate to severe hyponatremia in whom it is difficult to determine if any of the symptoms can be attributed to hyponatremia. In such a case, a modest increase of plasma sodium concentration (5 to 10 percent) may be advisable. In this setting, it is tempting to consider normal (0.9 percent) saline therapy. Normal saline (total osmolality of 308 mOsm per kilogram of H_2O; 154 mEq of sodium and 154 mEq chloride) has a higher sodium concentration than plasma and would produce an initial small increase in plasma sodium concentration. If, however, the patient has a fixed high urine osmolality (for example, 616 mOsm per kilogram of H_2O), then worsening of hyponatremia may ultimately occur after administration of normal saline. With a urine osmolality of 616 mOsm per kilogram of H_2O, the 308 mOsm of sodium chloride in the 1 L of normal saline would be excreted in 0.5 L of urine, leaving approximately 0.5 L of free water retained in the body and subsequently causing a slight decrease in the plasma sodium concentration. Thus the key to success in raising a low plasma sodium concentration in disorders associated with high urinary osmolality is either to give the patient a solute (hypertonic saline or urea) with a greater osmolality than the urine or to decrease urinary osmolality (via demeclocycline or loop diuretics). Either approach favors renal free water excretion. When used together, hypertonic saline and furosemide allow for rapid increments in the plasma sodium concentration.

Thiazide diuretics are a relatively common cause of hyponatremia, particularly in frail, elderly women. The pathogenesis of hyponatremia in these patients, who usually appear to be euvolemic, is multifactorial. Thiazides may induce mild volume depletion with enhanced antidiuretic hormone secretion, which results in retention of ingested water. Also, thiazide diuretics exert a renal tubular effect that impairs kidney water elimination. Profound potassium depletion usually accompanies thiazide diuretic–associated hyponatremia. Cessation of the diuretic agent, restoration of any volume deficits through the administration of normal saline, and aggressive potassium repletion constitute the cornerstone of therapy. Repletion of potassium often increases the plasma sodium concentration, presumably because potassium enters cells in exchange for sodium, which is extruded into extracellular fluid.

Normal individuals are capable of excreting large volumes of administered free water. Occasionally, patients with profound psychogenic polydipsia present with euvolemic hyponatremia. In these patients, the rapid ingestion of large volumes of water temporarily exceeds renal excretory capacity. In contrast to patients with SIADH, these patients usually have hypotonic urine (osmolality less than plasma) since the antidiuretic hormone secretion is suppressed. These patients usually need no therapy other than water restriction, as the excess water ingested is rapidly excreted in the urine.

True Volume Depletion

Extracellular fluid volume depletion resulting from gastrointestinal losses (caused by vomiting, diarrhea, blood loss), renal losses (caused by diuretics), skin losses (caused by burns), and other losses or sequestration (caused by pancreatitis, muscle crush injury) is a common clinical setting of hyponatremia. In such cases, the volume depletion leads to antidiuretic hormone release and decreased renal function, which combine to impair renal water excretion. When such patients orally ingest free water or are given hypotonic fluids intravenously, the water is retained, thereby lowering the plasma sodium concentration. Significant weight loss, orthostatic hypotension and tachycardia, decreased skin turgor, dry mucous membranes, and low jugular venous pressure strongly suggest hypovolemia. Often it is difficult to assess extracellular fluid volume status accurately from clinical parameters alone. In circumstances in which volume status remains unclear after clinical evaluation, a spot urinary sodium concentration may be helpful. A urinary sodium concentration of less than 30 to 40 mEq per liter suggests hypovolemia with diminished renal perfusion.

In hyponatremic, volume-depleted patients, the restoration of effective circulating blood volume with appropriate therapy, usually the administration of normal saline, normalizes the plasma sodium concentration. The rate at which the plasma sodium concentration is normalized tends to be slow initially. However, once euvolemia is restored, antidiuretic hormone secretion diminishes and renal function improves, resulting in a water diuresis and a later rapid return of plasma sodium to normal. If hypovolemic patients are symptomatic from hyponatremia, initial administration of 3 percent sodium chloride may rarely be indicated, following the guidelines discussed previously.

EDEMATOUS STATES

Hyponatremia occurring in the presence of an edematous disorder (heart failure, cirrhosis, nephrosis) accounts for approximately 30 percent of all cases of hyponatremia. In these settings, a diminished "effective circulating blood volume" leads to decreased renal perfusion with avid renal salt and water retention. If excess free water is ingested or given intravenously, hyponatremia in the context of an increase in both total body water and salt occurs. Thus in hyponatremic edematous disorders, both salt and water restriction are often indicated. Additional therapy in the hyponatremic edematous states should be directed first against the primary disease state. In patients with heart failure, reduction of preload (venodilation, loop diuretics), and afterload (vasodilators and angiotension-converting enzyme inhibitors) and improvement in myocardial contractility (digitalis) may improve effective circulating blood volume sufficiently to suppress antidiuretic hormone secretion and improve renal perfusion, thereby increasing renal water excretion. In patients with congestive heart failure, loop diuretics and converting enzyme inhibitors appear synergistic with regard to enhancing renal water elimination. Converting enzyme inhibitors potentially improve cardiac output and renal perfusion, which enhance renal hemodynamic parameters and thereby increase renal water excretion. Converting enzyme inhibitors also directly inhibit the ability of antidiuretic hormone to increase collecting tubular water reabsorption.

Increasing the effective circulating blood volume is more difficult in patients with severe hepatic cirrhosis and nephrotic syndrome. Loop diuretics may be beneficial in both conditions. In advanced hepatic cirrhosis, effective arterial blood volume can be restored with a peritoneovenous shunt, although this procedure is usually reserved for patients with severe, refractory ascites or the hepatorenal syndrome. Therapy directed at the primary glomerular pathology may result in amelioration of the nephrotic syndrome. Intravenously administered albumin may temporarily improve renal perfusion and enhance renal water excretion in patients with severe nephrosis. Demeclocycline has also been used in the treatment of chronic hyponatremia of the edematous disorders. Although demeclocycline is efficacious, the drug may accumulate in the body in the presence of liver disease and passive hepatic congestion and lead to severe vomiting and nephrotoxicity. Thus this agent should be used with extreme caution in the setting of cardiac and liver disease.

Hyponatremia associated with edematous states is rarely symptomatic. If it is symptomatic, administration of a loop diuretic with replacement of urinary electrolyte losses through hypertonic saline and peritoneal dialysis and hemodialysis are the preferred modes of therapy.

SUGGESTED READING

Anderson RJ, Chung HM, Luge R, Schrier RW. Hyponatremia: a prospective analysis of its epidemiology and pathogenetic role of vasopressin. Ann Intern Med 1985; 102:164–168.

Arieff AI. Hyponatremia, convulsions, respiratory arrest, and permanent brain damage after elective surgery in healthy women. New Engl J Med 1986; 314:1529–1535.

Sterns RH. The treatment of hyponatremia. Unsafe at any speed? Am Kidney Fund Letter 1989; 6:1–10.

Sterns RH, Riggs JE, Schockett SS. Osmotic demyelination syndrome following correction of hyponatremia. New Engl J Med 1986; 314:1535–1542.

HYPERNATREMIA

PAUL M. PALEVSKY, M.D.
IRWIN SINGER, M.D.

Hypernatremia is a common clinical problem, with a prevalence in hospitalized patients of 0.5 to 2 percent. The maintenance of the serum sodium concentration within the normal range of 135 to 145 mEq per liter depends on homeostatic mechanisms that balance water intake and excretion. Hypernatremia is usually the result of impaired water intake in the setting of increased renal or extrarenal water losses (in excess of electrolyte losses, if any).

In the adult population, hypernatremia is most prevalent among the elderly, who are frequently less able to resist dehydration. Several defenses are impaired with aging: body water content, as a percentage of body weight, decreases; maximal urinary concentrating capacity diminishes; and thirst perception declines.

In adults, hypernatremia occurs primarily in the setting of systemic illness, confounding the ability to attribute symptoms precisely and to attribute morbidity and mortality to the hypertonic stress. Although hypernatremia can serve as a marker for the severity of underlying illness, there is little doubt that substantial morbidity and mortality are directly attributable to the hypernatremic state itself. Mortality rates ranging from 40 percent to greater than 70 percent have been reported, depending on the magnitude and duration of the hypernatremia. Survivors of hypernatremia often exhibit significant decreases in functional capacity and the ability to care for themselves.

Hypernatremia can produce clinically important central nervous system (CNS) dysfunction: confusion, lethargy, weakness, and seizures may be presenting symptoms. In acute hypernatremia, the rise in extracellular fluid osmolality results in intracellular dehydration as water redistributes across cell membranes to maintain osmotic equilibrium. Cellular dehydration results in a loss of brain volume, increases the mechanical traction on intracranial vessels, and can result in intracranial bleeding.

The cerebral response to hypernatremia and other hypertonic states is a function of the rapidity of onset and duration of hypertonicity. In animal studies, acute hypernatremia from hypertonic saline infusion produces a rapid decrease in brain water content and an increase in intracellular electrolyte concentration. Intracellular osmolality increases as a result of cellular water loss and electrolyte accumulation. In chronic hypernatremia the increase in intracellular osmolality is the same; however, the relative contributions of intracellular water loss and solute accumulation differ. Brain water content is relatively preserved in chronic hypernatremia; intracellular osmolality increases primarily as the result of the accumulation of "idiogenic osmoles." These poorly characterized solutes, probably consisting of organic metabolites such as polyols, polyamines, and amino acids, accumulate after several hours of hypertonic stress as part of an adaptive mechanism that conserves intracellular brain volume. Although the accumulation of intracellular "idiogenic osmoles" minimizes cerebral shrinkage and the risk of intracranial bleeding, the production of "idiogenic osmoles" increases the risk of developing cerebral edema during rehydration.

CAUSES

In the majority of patients, hypernatremia develops as a result of the combination of inadequate water intake and increased electrolyte-free water loss. Occasional patients develop hypernatremia as the result of hypertonic sodium intake in the absence of concomitant water intake. The common denominator of all forms of hypernatremia is an inadequate ingestion or administration of water to maintain a normal serum tonicity.

Although impaired water intake and hypernatremia may result from primary hypodipsia, adult hypernatremia is usually secondary to an intercurrent illness or alteration in mental status that has diminished thirst or restricted water intake. The importance of thirst in the regulation of plasma tonicity is exemplified by patients with diabetes insipidus. Despite massive polyuria, patients with diabetes insipidus maintain a serum sodium concentration in the normal range as long as they have adequate thirst perception and unrestricted access to water. In the setting of intercurrent illness or depressed sensorium, their ability to maintain sufficient water intake is diminished, and hypernatremia rapidly develops. Elderly patients with febrile or diarrheal illness, patients with neurologic disease (e.g., stroke or chronic dementia), and patients with acute obtundation or delirium are particularly vulnerable to the development of hypernatremia.

Hypernatremia can be divided into four categories on the basis of total body sodium and water content (Table 1). Pure water deficits, with little change in total body sodium, may develop in patients with increased insensible water losses (e.g., water losses secondary to fever, increased ambient temperature, mechanical ventilation without humidification, or hyperventilation), and in patients with hypothalamic or nephrogenic diabetes insipidus. Hypotonic fluid losses from the gastrointestinal tract, skin, or kidneys, may produce hypovolemia and hypernatremia. Large volumes of hypotonic gastrointestinal secretions can be lost during prolonged vomiting or nasogastric suction, through enterocutaneous fistulae, and in cases of severe diarrhea. Hypotonic polyuria may be produced by diuretic administration, osmotic diuresis caused by the excretion of glucose, mannitol, or urea, or nonoliguric acute renal failure, any of which may result in hypernatremia and volume depletion. Hypertonic sodium gain produces hypervolemic hypernatremia; it is usually iatrogenic, developing from the intravenous administration of hypertonic sodium bicarbonate or sodium chloride solutions. Pure sodium gain from voluntary or iatrogenic oral salt ingestion may also produce hypernatremia and sodium overload. Hypernatremia secondary to dialysis against hypertonic or high-sodium baths has also been described.

DIAGNOSIS

The diagnosis of hypernatremia is made through laboratory testing. Symptoms and physical signs are nonspecific and may be obscured by underlying medical illnesses. Thirst, the hallmark of dehydration, may not be verbalized or perceived as the result of depressed mental status. Classic physical signs of de-

TABLE 1 Causes of Hypernatremia

Pathophysiologic Conditions	*Total Body Sodium*	*Total Body Water*	*Typical Etiologies*
Pure water loss	Near normal	↓	Diabetes insipidus Nephrogenic Hypothalamic Increased insensible losses Fever Mechanical ventilation Hyperventilation
Hypotonic water loss	↓	↓↓	Gastrointestinal losses Vomiting Nasogastric drainage Enterocutaneous fistulae Diarrhea Renal losses Diuretic administration Osmotic diuresis Postobstructive diuresis Nonoliguric ATN
Pure sodium gain	↑	Near normal	Salt ingestion
Hypertonic sodium gain	↑↑	↑	Intravenous hypertonic saline Intravenous sodium bicarbonate

hydration, such as poor skin turgor and sunken eyes, are unreliable in the elderly patients most susceptible to the development of hypernatremia.

Clinical hypernatremia is primarily manifest as central nervous system dysfunction. Although a depressed sensorium may precede hypernatremia, hypernatremia may produce CNS depression, which may range from lethargy to coma, in previously alert patients. Myoclonic twitching and generalized seizures may also develop; seizures are uncommon in patients with chronic hypernatremia, but have been described in as many as 40 percent of patients after the initiation of therapy.

CALCULATION OF WATER DEFICITS

A hypernatremic patient's water deficit may be estimated from his or her serum sodium concentration and body weight. Assuming that total body sodium has remained unchanged and that the hypernatremia is entirely the result of water loss, one may estimate the water deficit through the following equation:

$$\text{Water Deficit} = (\text{Total Body Water}) \times \frac{\text{Serum } [Na^+] - 140}{140}$$

The total body water is usually assumed to be 60 percent of body weight.

Although this formula provides a useful first approximation of the water deficit and can be used to guide initial therapy, several important caveats must be recognized.

First, the assumption that total body water is a fixed percentage of body weight is incorrect; total body water is a function of the patient's age, gender, and percentage of body fat. As a general rule, the total body water is a smaller percentage of body weight in women than in men and declines with age. Thus, while a 25-year-old man may have a water content that is 60 percent of his body weight, body water may comprise only 55 percent of body weight in a 25-year-old woman. At 75 years of age, in men, body water may decrease to 50 percent of body weight, and in women, it may decrease to 45 percent of body weight.

Second, the above-mentioned calculation assumes that changes in serum sodium concentration reflect changes in plasma tonicity. This assumption is correct only if there is no elevation in other osmotically active solutes, such as glucose or mannitol. Because these solutes shift water from the intracellular to the extracellular compartments, an elevation in their concentration dilutes other solutes and decreases the serum sodium concentration. In this circumstance, the calculation of the water deficit must be based directly on the change in plasma osmolality, and not just on the serum sodium concentration.

Finally, the above-mentioned formula assumes that total body sodium and other electrolytes have remained constant. In the setting of depletion or overload of sodium or other electrolytes, the calculation must be corrected by the volume of isotonic sodium (or electrolyte) lost or gained.

THERAPY

The treatment of hypernatremia is water repletion. There are a paucity of data regarding the rapidity with which water deficits should be corrected. Although hypernatremia is potentially lethal, overly rapid water repletion may result in the development of cerebral edema or seizures. Because mortality rates may increase with increasing rates of water repletion, therapy should be instituted promptly, but it should also be sufficiently gradual so as to prevent rapid transcellular fluid shifts.

In hypernatremic patients with hypovolemia and evidence of circulatory compromise, the initial therapy is volume replacement. Isotonic saline or colloid should be administered promptly to correct hypotension and restore plasma volume. Severe acidosis ($pH<7.15$) should also be treated; moderate acidosis, which does not compromise myocardial contractility, does not require rapid bicarbonate supplementation. Undiluted solutions of sodium bicarbonate are hypertonic (a standard 50-ml ampule of 7.5 percent $NaHCO_3$ has a sodium concentration of 892 mEq per liter) and can increase hypernatremia. If bicarbonate must be administered, it can be diluted to isotonicity (e.g., 100 ml of 7.5 percent $NaHCO_3$ added to 1,000 ml of 0.45 percent saline) before infusion.

Once adequate volume replacement has been achieved, the water deficit should be estimated and replacement initiated. Water repletion should be gradual; no more than half of the calculated deficit should be replaced over the first 12 to 24 hours, with the remainder of the deficit corrected during the ensuing 48 to 72 hours. The rate of correction of the serum sodium concentration should not exceed 2 mEq per liter per hour. Throughout the course of therapy, neurologic status should be monitored closely; an abrupt deterioration after initial improvement in mental status may suggest the development of cerebral edema from overly rapid rehydration.

No individual fluid regimen is of documented superiority in the treatment of hypernatremia. Enteral water repletion, administered either orally or by gavage, may be sufficient but is frequently limited by the magnitude of the water deficit or by the patient's underlying medical condition. Intravenous repletion should consist of 5 percent glucose in water or another solution with a low electrolyte content; pure water should not be infused intravenously, as it can cause intravascular hemolysis.

In addition to the repletion of the water deficit, all ongoing fluid and electrolyte losses must be continuously replaced. Plasma electrolytes must be monitored frequently, at a minimum of 6-hour intervals, throughout the course of therapy. Replacement fluid solution should be modified on the basis of response to the prescribed therapy. Insensible water losses may be estimated to be 0.6 ml per kilogram per hour in an afebrile patient, and increase by 20 percent for each 1 °C rise in body temperature. Urinary, gastrointestinal, and other fluid losses must be quantitated and their electrolyte content determined. The replacement fluid prescription should be based on these measured and estimated losses so as to achieve and maintain euvolemia.

The reduction of ongoing fluid losses is also of paramount importance. Fever should be reduced by cooling and through the use of antipyretics to minimize insensible water losses. Ongoing osmotic diuresis should be reduced by controlling hyperglycemia and reducing urea synthesis (by treating catabolic states and avoiding protein loads). Osmotic diarrhea from hypertonic enteral nutritional supplements can be reduced by altering the nutritional prescription or with the use of antidiarrheal agents. The polyuria of hypothalamic diabetes insipidus can be minimized by vasopressin administration. Aqueous vasopressin is used for diagnostic testing, and occasionally for acute therapy; dDAVP, a synthetic analogue of vasopressin, may be administered subcutaneously or intravenously (1 to 2 μg twice daily) during acute illness, or intranasally (10 to 20 μg twice daily) as chronic therapy.

For patients in whom hypernatremia results from the administration of hypertonic saline or bicarbonate or from salt ingestion, treatment requires both water administration and diuresis. Loop-acting diuretics should be used to reduce volume overload. If renal failure prohibits the establishment of diuresis, dialysis may be required.

Since many patients develop hypernatremia as an iatrogenic complication, greater emphasis must be placed on prevention. In patients at high risk for the development of hypernatremia, particularly the elderly and patients with increased fluid losses, fever, or obtundation, more frequent monitoring of the serum sodium concentration is required. Therapy should be initiated early, with prompt treatment of mild hypernatremia, so as to prevent the development of life-threatening water deficits.

SUGGESTED READING

Alvis R, Geheb M, Cox M. Hypo- and hyperosmolar states: diagnostic approaches. In: Arieff AI, DeFronzo RA, eds. Fluid electrolyte and acid-base disorders. New York: Churchill Livingstone, 1985:185.

Cox M, Geheb M, Singer I. Disorders of thirst and renal water excretion. In: Arieff AI, DeFronzo RA, eds. Fluid electrolyte and acid-base disorders. New York: Churchill Livingstone, 1985:119.

Robertson GL. Abnormalities of thirst regulation. Kidney Int 1984; 25:460–469.

Snyder NA, Feigal DW, Arieff AI. Hypernatremia in elderly patients: a heterogeneous, morbid, and iatrogenic unity. Ann Intern Med 1987; 107:309–319.

HYPOKALEMIA

SANDRA M. DONNELLY, M.D.C.M., B.Sc., M.Sc.
EUAN J. F. CARLISLE, M.B., M.D.
KAMEL S. KAMEL, M.D.
MITCHELL L. HALPERIN, M.D.

Hypokalemia is an important electrolyte disorder because it can lead to life-threatening cardiac arrhythmias. It is important to establish the diagnosis as well as to evaluate the clinical setting in which hypokalemia occurred in order to determine the urgency and the form of potassium replacement therapy.

DEFINITION

Although hypokalemia is conventionally defined as a concentration of potassium in the plasma less than 3.5 mmol* per liter, this definition is arbitrary. A concentration of potassium in the plasma of less than 3.8 mmol per liter is uncommon in normal individuals, and values between 3.5 and 3.8 mmol per liter probably represent a degree of hypokalemia. Of greater importance, in a patient with underlying cardiac disease or in a patient taking digitalis, even a level of potassium in the plasma that is within the range of 3.5 to 3.8 mmol per liter may put the patient at some risk of developing a cardiac arrhythmia.

CAUSES

A list of the causes of hypokalemia is provided in Table 1. In broad terms, hypokalemia may be caused by the following.

Decreased Intake of Potassium

By itself, decreased intake of potassium is a rare cause of hypokalemia. Nevertheless, it can lead to a greater degree of hypokalemia and potassium depletion if other causes of potassium loss are already present.

Shift of Potassium From the Extracellular Fluid to the Intracellular Fluid

When transient, hypokalemia caused by a shift of potassium is usually the result of a surge of catecholamines, such as that which occurs in patients with acute stressful conditions such as myocardial infarction, head injury, or delirium tremens. A longer-lasting hypokalemia caused by potassium shift may result from potassium uptake during anabolism, as occurs during refeeding in cachectic patients or in the treatment of pernicious anemia.

Hypokalemia caused by a shift of potassium can also predispose to cardiac arrhythmias and should not be ignored. In this situation, a smaller quantity of potassium is generally required to treat a severe degree of hypokalemia.

Loss of Potassium From the Gastrointestinal Tract

There are three situations in which the gastrointestinal (GI) tract has a clinical impact on hypokalemia. First, loss of an important amount of potassium can occur from the GI tract in patients with diarrhea of small bowel origin or with a villous adenoman. The volume of diarrhea fluid may exceed 20 L per day, and the concentration of potassium in the feces can be as great as 45 to 50 mmol per liter; the usual concentration of potassium in the fecal contents is 10 mmol per liter in a volume of 0.5 L. Second, the hypokalemia of vomiting is not caused by loss of potassium in gastric fluids; rather, the decrease in the concentration of potassium in the plasma is due to renal potassium wasting (see below) and alkalemia inducing a shift of potassium into cells. Finally, in patients with an ileus, potassium cannot be given orally.

Renal Potassium Wasting

The major causes of a high rate of excretion of potassium are a high urine flow rate and a stimulated rate of secretion of potassium in the distal nephron. Clinically, aldosterone and the presence of bicarbon-

TABLE 1 Causes of Hypokalemia

Decreased intake of potassium
Shift of potassium into cells
Hormones
Insulin: treatment of ketoacidosis
Catecholamines (stress-related transient hypokalemia), $beta_2$ agonists
Gain of anions in the intracellular fluid (treatment of ketoacidosis or pernicious anemia, refeeding after cachexia)
Metabolic alkalosis
Others (e.g., anesthesia, hypokalemic periodic paralysis)
Intestinal loss of potassium
Diarrhea, ileus
Excessive loss of potassium in the urine
High urine flow (diuretics, pharmacologic or osmotic)
Stimulation of the potassium secretory process
Increased mineralocorticoid activity (see Table 2)
Increased delivery of nonabsorbable anions such as bicarbonate (caused by vomiting, treatment of saline-responsive metabolic alkalosis, or the use of acetazolamide), beta-hydroxybutyrate, D-lactate, organic anions, anions from drugs in the presence of mineralocorticoids

*mmol = mEq.

ate in the urine are the two most important modulators of the secretion of potassium, independent of the rate of urine flow.

In the presence of hypokalemia, the expected renal response is to conserve potassium maximally; this means that the rate of excretion of potassium should be less than 20 mmol per day. Excretion of potassium is determined by two factors: its concentration in the urine and the rate of urine flow.

$$K_{excretion} = [K]_{urine} \times \text{urine flow}$$

Hence, assessment of the renal handling of potassium requires a separate analysis of these two components. Although it is easy to obtain an assessment of the urine flow rate, the concentration of potassium in the urine does not provide the clinician with an adequate assessment of the activity of the secretory process for potassium. Since the concentration of potassium in the urine is the potassium : water ratio, it is influenced to a major degree by the amount of water abstraction in the renal medulla.

We use the transtubular potassium concentration gradient (TTKG) to assess the activity of the potassium secretory process in the cortical distal nephron. Using a "spot" urine, the TTKG can be calculated through the following formula:

$$TTKG = \{[K]_{urine}/(\text{urine/plasma})_{osm}\}/[K]_{plasma}$$

In the first step of the calculation, an estimate of the concentration of potassium achieved in the cortical distal nephron is obtained by adjusting the value of the concentration of potassium in the urine for the abstraction of water in the renal medulla. Thereafter, to assess the potassium secretory process, this value is divided by the concentration of potassium in the plasma.

Calculating the TTKG can help the clinician sort out the pathophysiology of hypokalemia. A TTKG of less than 2 reflects a normal renal response to hypokalemia and implicates a low intake of potassium, a shift of potassium into the intracellular fluid, or an intestinal loss of potassium as the underlying etiology. However, one must be aware of two caveats: (1) renal loss of potassium may have occurred before the evaluation (e.g., remote use of diuretics or remote vomiting) and (2) a low TTKG can be found in the face of a high rate of excretion of potassium in extremes of polyuria.

By contrast, a higher value for the TTKG points to an enhanced rate of secretion of potassium in the cortical distal nephron. A primary or secondary increase in mineralocorticoid activity may be playing an important role and this can be confirmed, if required, by measuring the levels of aldosterone and renin in the plasma (Table 2).

Another important factor that modulates the secretion of potassium is the presence of nonreabsorbable anions in the urine. Again, using a "spot" urine, the clinician can detect the presence of unusual anions by finding a concentration of sodium plus potassium that exceeds that of chloride by more than 40 mmol per liter. Bicarbonaturia can be confirmed by finding an alkaline pH of the urine. Other anions to be considered are beta-hydroxybutyrate, drugs such as acetosalicylate, or organic anions excreted in unusually large quantities. Hence, using information readily available on the initial evaluation, the cause of hypokalemia should be relatively obvious.

When both a high mineralocorticoid level and a high concentration of bicarbonate are present simultaneously, as in patients with vomiting, the rate of excretion of potassium can be very high, leading to rapidly progressive and severe hypokalemia.

TABLE 2 Causes of Hypermineralocorticoid States

Increased renin and increased aldosterone levels
Renal salt wasting states, including diuretic therapy and Bartter's syndrome
Malignant hypertension
Renal artery stenosis
Renin-secreting tumor
Decreased renin and increased aldosterone levels
Adrenal adenoma
Adrenal hyperplasia
Mg^{++} deficiency
Decreased renin and decreased aldosterone levels
Liddles's syndrome
Licorice ingestion
Agents with mineralocorticoid-like activity (possibly amphotericin B)
Cushing's syndrome

THERAPY

While making an initial assessment of the cause of hypokalemia, the clinician should first consider if the hypokalemia requires therapy urgently. We shall approach the therapy of hypokalemia by first discussing those situations in which treatment is urgent.

Clinical Circumstances in Which Hypokalemia Is a Medical Emergency

Hypokalemia may be life-threatening in three ways. It may induce serious cardiac arrhythmias, including ventricular fibrillation. It may lead to extreme muscular weakness, and if the respiratory muscles are involved, respiratory failure may result. Lastly, it may precipitate hepatic encephalopathy in patients with liver failure. The replacement of potassium must be vigorous if any of these complications are present or likely to occur. Further, even in the absence of these detectable abnormalities, we consider a patient with a concentration of potassium in the plasma of less than 2 mmol per liter as one who needs therapy urgently.

Cardiac Arrhythmias

Few would disagree that hypokalemia, even if it is mild, should be treated aggressively in the setting of cardiac arrhythmias or acute myocardial ischemia. Several studies have shown that during acute myocardial infarction, the incidence of ventricular fibrillation is increased as much as threefold if hypokalemia is present. It has been suggested that hypokalemia may simply be a marker of some other more important factor such as the circulating catecholamine level or the size of the area of myocardial ischemia. Laboratory studies, however, have shown that in animals undergoing coronary artery ligation, the ventricular fibrillation threshold is 25 percent lower when hypokalemia (induced by hemodialysis) is present. Hypokalemia has been observed in 49 percent of patients resuscitated from out-of-hospital ventricular fibrillation. The prognostic significance of this has not been assessed, but it would seem important to correct the hypokalemia rapidly. After a drug overdose, arrhythmias may be induced or exacerbated by hypokalemia resulting from attempts at forced alkaline diuresis.

Muscular Weakness

Biochemical evidence of muscle damage, severe muscular weakness, and rhabdomyolysis may be seen in patients with severe hypokalemia. Weakness may be life-threatening if the respiratory muscles are involved, especially when respiratory acidosis is already present (e.g., in patients with coma, aspiration, or underlying pulmonary disease). This weakness might not be such that it compromises basal functions, but it could be important if a high ventilation rate is required (e.g., in the therapy of severe metabolic acidosis with bicarbonate as may occur in a patient with type 1 renal tubular acidosis associated with enhanced potassium wasting, in some patients who abuse laxatives, or in those who have severe diarrhea). In addition to the carbon dioxide load, treatment of the acidosis may lead to a shift of potassium from the extracellular fluid to the intracellular fluid, worsening the degree of hypokalemia. In such a case, a strong argument can be made for highly aggressive administration of potassium.

Hepatic Encephalopathy

In patients with hepatic cirrhosis, potassium depletion may occur as a result of several mechanisms (e.g., poor intake of potassium, vomiting, diarrhea, secondary hyperaldosteronism, diuretic therapy). Hypokalemia is a potent stimulus for ammoniagenesis, which may precipitate hepatic encephalopathy in those already at risk. Prevention of hypokalemia is therefore important, but it should be noted that these patients are also at an increased risk for acute renal failure. If renal function declines, overenthusiastic treatment with potassium supplements and potassium-sparing diuretics may cause life-threatening hyperkalemia. Regular monitoring of plasma electrolytes and renal function is therefore of particular importance in these patients. In a report on 4,921 patients receiving potassium supplements, seven deaths were attributed, at least in part, to hyperkalemia; three of these patients had liver cirrhosis.

Therapy

After it has been established that one is dealing with an acute medical emergency, two questions arise with respect to therapy.

By What Route Should Potassium Be Administered? It is obvious that potassium should be administered as fast as is safe. The intravenous route is the only one we need consider. The aim of this aggressive therapy should be to minimize the risk of complications from hypokalemia, rather than to increase the concentration of potassium in the plasma to a level within the normal range. Based on the information on hand, we stress that one can treat the patient for a short interval only and that frequent reassessment is mandatory. Indeed, no further recommendation for the dose of potassium can be made without a reappraisal of the concentration of potassium in the plasma.

For emergency treatment of hypokalemia, we recommend the following approach with a central line in place:

1. Estimate the extracellular fluid volume and multiply it by the desired increment in the concentration of potassium in the plasma to provide the initial amount of potassium to be infused. Thus if the extracellular fluid volume is 15 L and the concentration of potassium in the plasma is to be increased by 2 mmol per liter, then 30 mmol can be infused during the first 30 minutes, with the infusion administered at a faster rate during the first several minutes (2 mmol per minute). Even if there is absolutely no shift of potassium into the intracellular fluid during this time, the concentration of potassium in the plasma will not increase to dangerous levels, and even with a reduced cardiac output (e.g., 2 L of plasma per minute), the local concentration of potassium in intraventricular blood should not increase by more than 1 mmol per liter above that of the rest of plasma. Measurement of the concentration of potassium in the plasma must be repeated after 30 minutes.
2. The rate of infusion of potassium over the next hour may be determined from the resulting increase in the concentration of potassium in the plasma. If the concentration of potassium in the plasma has not changed much, then a

large amount of potassium has moved intracellularly and these relatively high rates of infusion of potassium may be continued. If the concentration of potassium in the plasma increases substantially after this infusion, the rate should be reduced accordingly. Again, vigilant follow-up is required.

Concentrations of potassium of as much as 200 mmol per liter may be infused centrally, although lower concentrations (60 mmol per liter) have been recommended if the entry port is within the heart itself (i.e., a Swan-Ganz catheter). It should be noted that if 2 mmol per minute is to be infused initially, this would require 10 ml of a potassium chloride solution of 200 mmol per liter or 33 ml of a solution of 60 mmol per liter per minute. The higher concentration of potassium chloride is advantageous in situations in which the large volumes of infusion may not be well tolerated. These rapid rates of infusion of potassium chloride should take place only in an intensive care setting, and electrocardiographic monitoring is mandatory. The key to safe management lies in frequent monitoring (every 30 to 60 minutes initially) of the concentration of potassium in the plasma.

What Preparation of Potassium Should Be Administered? While on the surface it would seem to be advantageous to administer potassium bicarbonate to patients with severe metabolic acidosis, and potassium chloride to all other patients with serious hypokalemia, it is not necessary to make this differentiation in practice. In the former case, the rate of production of carbon dioxide might be so high that it would be more dangerous to use the potassium bicarbonate preparation initially. Thus we would recommend that potassium replacement begin with the administration of potassium chloride.

Clinical Circumstances in Which Hypokalemia Is Not a Medical Emergency

If it is established that the hypokalemia requires treatment but the clinical situation does *not* constitute an emergency, a new set of questions arises. Only issues that are relevant to the administration of potassium are considered here, and aspects of treatment in special circumstances are considered in a later section of this chapter.

Therapy

By What Route Should Potassium Be Administered? Potassium may be administered either orally or intravenously. The choice of which route to use depends on several factors, including the degree of urgency, the level of consciousness, and the reliability of gut absorption. When paralytic ileus is present (e.g., in severe hypokalemia and during the postoperative period), potassium must be given intravenously.

Oral Therapy. In most patients, replacement of potassium is given orally. Potassium supplementation may be provided by the dietary intake of foods rich in potassium or by potassium formulations.

The dietary intake of foods rich in potassium may be recommended as prophylaxis against hypokalemia. Such foods include meat, fish, fruit, and vegetables. The disadvantage of this form of supplementation is the quantity of food required and the resulting increase in caloric intake. Measures of "high-potassium" foods containing 50 mmol of potassium include 1.5 lb of meat, four baked potatoes, six carrots, six cups of milk, five bananas, or two cantaloupes. An alternative approach is to use salt substitutes (50 to 60 mmol of potassium per teaspoon). Rather than allowing free intake, one should prescribe the amount required for daily use.

Preparations of potassium may be in solid or liquid form (Table 3). The liquid is poorly tolerated, and the vast majority of patients prefer supplements in the solid form. Most tablets are "slow-release," either microencapsulated or in a wax matrix. Serious gastrointestinal side effects, such as hemorrhage, ulceration, and perforation, are infrequent, but patients with impaired gastrointestinal motility (e.g., the elderly and those with scleroderma or esophageal disease) are at increased risk.

Potassium supplementation is usually given as the chloride salt, although other preparations are available (e.g., phosphate, citrate, bicarbonate). In patients in whom there is a tendency towards alkalosis (i.e, in patients treated with diuretics or in those with hyperaldosteronism), it is essential to use the chloride salt, as chloride depletion will aggravate the alkalosis and prevent the development of a positive balance for potassium. In the acidotic patient, however, it may be preferable to use potassium bicarbonate or salts that generate bicarbonate, such as potassium acetate or potassium citrate. If a phosphate deficit is present or anticipated (e.g., in diabetic ketoacidosis or rapid anabolism), potassium phosphate may be given, although care must be taken not to administer the phosphate too rapidly ($<$ 50 mmol of phosphate per 8 hours by mouth).

Intravenous Therapy. If there is a contraindication to using the oral route or if potassium is needed more quickly, potassium may be infused peripherally at a concentration of no more than 40 mmol per liter (higher concentrations may cause thrombophlebitis in small veins). As a rule, the rate of administration of potassium should not exceed 60 mmol per hour. Thus care must be taken when administering large volumes of intravenous fluid ($\geq$ 1.5 L per hour), as might occur in the initial treatment of patients with severe extracellular fluid volume depletion and hypokalemia. Thorough mixing of the added potassium and the intravenous fluid is essential, as pooling of the potassium has occasionally occurred, leading to infusion of

TABLE 3 Type and Content of Potassium in Available Formulations

Type of Formula	*Chloride*	*Bicarbonate*	*Citrate (C) Gluconate (G) Acetate (A)**	*Phosphate*
Liquid	10 to 40 mmol/15 ml		20 mmol/15 ml (G)	7 mmol/15 ml
Packets, tablets for solution	15 to 25 mmol/packet	6.5 to 25 mmol/tablet	20 mmol/15 ml (G) 25 mmol/tablet (C)	3.7 to 14 mmol/tablet
Extended release tablets	6.7 to 20 mmol/tablet			
Extended release capsules	8 to 10 mmol/capsule			
Intravenous additives†	1.5 to 3 mmol/ml		2.4 mmol/ml (A)	4.4 mmol/ml

*Some potassium preparations have varying proportions of alkaline salts and chloride available. These are rarely, if ever, necessary.
†A variety of premixed intravenous fluid solutions containing added potassium are also available.
Results are expressed as millimoles of potassium.

a much higher concentration of potassium than that anticipated.

How Much Potassium Should Be Administered? To answer this question, it is important to know the degree of depletion of potassium and how the potassium was lost, and to have an estimate of the ongoing loss of potassium in the urine.

Degree of Depletion of Potassium. In general, a wide range of deficits of potassium are associated with a given degree of hypokalemia. A concentration of potassium in the plasma of 3 mmol per liter may result from a total body potassium deficit of 100 to 400 mmol, while a concentration of potassium in the plasma of 2 mmol per liter may mean that up to 800 mmol of potassium have been lost. However, factors may be present in an individual patient that cause a shift of potassium from the extracellular fluid to the intracellular fluid, making the degree of hypokalemia more significant relative to the overall deficit of potassium (see Table 1). Hence caution and careful follow-up are mandatory for formulating the plan of treatment.

Type of Potassium Loss. Potassium may be lost in the urine, primarily along with chloride, in patients who have been treated with diuretics. In this case, since the bulk of the potassium was derived from the intracellular fluid (and chloride from the extracellular fluid and/or the diet), there must have been a major shift of cations across the cell membrane (predominantly sodium). The implication for therapy in this situation is that replacement with potassium chloride will permit the sodium to leave the intracellular fluid and be excreted as sodium chloride in the urine, provided that there is not a renal problem that limits the excretion of this "sodium chloride" load.

In a patient with poorly controlled diabetes mellitus or suffering from a catabolic state, the loss of potassium is accompanied by a parallel loss of phosphate. The implication for therapy in this situation is that replacement of phosphate must accompany the replacement of potassium, otherwise hypokalemia may develop. Further, if potassium chloride or potassium bicarbonate is the only form of potassium replacement, the intracellular deficit of potassium will not bc replaced, as there is still an intracellular phosphate deficit. In this case, correction of the potassium deficit must await the replacement of phosphate and other necessary intracellular constituents, such as magnesium and amino acids.

Ongoing Loss of Potassium. More than the anticipated deficit of potassium must be given to a patient with hypokalemia and significant ongoing or anticipated loss of potassium in the urine. For example, if a patient has bicarbonaturia and a high level of aldosterone in the plasma, the concentration of potassium in the urine may be very high. This may occur in a patient who has metabolic alkalosis and hypokalemia and who is being treated with sodium chloride. Even if alkalemia is not present, a wide anion gap in the plasma may have a similar implication in this setting, because anions, such as lactate or beta-hydroxybutyrate, are converted to bicarbonate upon metabolism (once blood flow and insulin become normal). If the concentration of bicarbonate in the plasma increases sufficiently, bicarbonaturia might then result. (This is considered in more detail later in this chapter.)

The second factor to consider is the volume of filtrate delivered to the cortical collecting duct. If a large increase in this delivery is anticipated (e.g., after the administration of a diuretic), much more potassium will need to be administered to place the patient in a positive balance for potassium. It may be worthwhile to diminish this high rate of excretion of potassium by blocking the action of aldosterone through the use of aldosterone antagonists, by inhibiting the secretion of potassium through the use of potassium-sparing diuretics, and by lessening the rate of flow of urine through avoidance of diuretics and lowering the load of sodium.

What Are the Risks of Therapy?

Acute Therapy. During hypokalemia of nonrenal origin, the distal nephron becomes "hyporesponsive" to the kaliuretic actions of aldosterone. This resistance may persist even while the deficit of potassium is corrected acutely; thus if the rate of administration of potassium is not reduced as normokalemia approaches, an inadequate rate of excretion of potassium may lead to hyperkalemia. This again underlines the importance of frequent monitoring of the concentration of potassium in the plasma during the treatment of hypokalemia.

An additional potential danger of the administration of potassium is the presence of intestinal ileus, as large quantities of bicarbonate and potassium may have been sequestered in the intestine, compounding the degree of hypokalemia and metabolic acidosis. During therapy, if this potassium is absorbed rapidly, hyperkalemia might ensue. Alternatively, if bicarbonate is absorbed quickly, a rapid decrease in the concentration of potassium may be anticipated owing to a shift of potassium into cells and perhaps to enhanced kaliuresis.

Chronic Therapy. Hyperkalemia has been observed in 3.6 percent of patients taking potassium supplements. The risk is highest in patients with renal failure, in the elderly, and in diabetics. The simultaneous use of nonsteroidal antiinflammatory agents or beta-blocking drugs may also predispose to hyperkalemia. The concurrent use of potassium-sparing diuretics and potassium supplements is potentially very dangerous and should be considered only under the most unusual circumstances.

SPECIAL CONSIDERATIONS FOR THERAPY

In this section, we arbitrarily divide the special considerations into the following categories

1. States with excessive ongoing loss of potassium in the urine.
2. States in which a shift of potassium into the intracellular fluid can be anticipated.
3. Diuretic-induced hypokalemia, as its prophylaxis has broad clinical application.
4. Adjuncts to therapy.

States with Excessive Ongoing Loss of Potassium in the Urine

In addition to the conditions discussed below, hypokalemia with excessive ongoing renal loss of potassium occurs in primary hyperaldosteronism, amphotericin B administration, and Bartter's syndrome. The underlying mechanisms for potassium loss may be quite different in these three conditions, and the results of pharmacologic therapy are variable. It is often possible to correct hypokalemia caused by primary hyperaldosteronism and amphotericin B administration; in Bartter's syndrome, however, renal potassium loss is usually severe, and it is often not possible to correct the deficit.

Primary Hyperaldosteronism

In patients with primary hyperaldosteronism caused by an adrenal adenoma, the definitive therapy is the resection of adrenal tissue. Potassium replacement, however, is required preoperatively in these patients and in those for whom surgery is not recommended. The aim of therapy is to increase the concentration of potassium in the plasma to greater than 3.5 mmol per liter. Since the ongoing loss of potassium exceeds the normal intake of potassium, both potassium supplements (100 mmol per day) and potassium-sparing diuretics are needed when more severe hypokalemia is present. Large doses of spironolactone (200 to 400 mg per day) or amiloride (5 to 20 mg per day) are not unusual. Since hyperaldosteronism leads to a high concentration of potassium in the urine, it is mandatory that agents that increase the volume of urine not be given to these patients (i.e., diuretics for the treatment of hypertension). Further, a high-salt diet could also lead to an excessive loss of potassium in the urine for the same reason. By contrast, marked restriction of sodium in the diet could reduce the excretion of potassium and, in association with potassium supplements and potassium-sparing diuretics, even lead to hyperkalemia; restriction of sodium intake to 100 to 150 mmol per day is appropriate. Finally, as this condition may result in magnesium deficits and as hypomagnesemia perpetuates an augmented rate of excretion of potassium, deficits of magnesium must also be replaced.

Amphotericin B Administration

Amphotericin B is an antifungal drug commonly used in the treatment of systemic fungal infection. It has many side effects, including the propensity to induce a substantial renal loss of potassium, that may result in hypokalemia. The mechanism is said to be an increased permeability of the luminal membrane to cations (Na^+, K^+, and H^+), thereby simulating some of the actions of aldosterone. Limitation of renal loss of potassium by the addition of amiloride has been tried with varying success. In our experience, these agents have been disappointing, and the only alternative has been to give large supplements of potassium and to avoid a large delivery of sodium and volume to the cortical collecting duct while amphotericin B is acting. Also, if it is anticipated that a large loss of potassium is imminent, supplementation of the intake of potassium at the initiation of therapy might lessen the degree of the resulting hypokalemia.

Bartter's Syndrome

Bartter's syndrome presents a challenging problem of excessive loss of potassium in the urine during hypokalemia. Despite often profound degrees of hypokalemia, renal wasting of potassium can amount to approximately 200 to 300 mmol per day. The consequences of prolonged severe depletion of potassium may include nephropathy in the adult or growth retardation in children. The precise etiology and pathophysiologic mediators of this syndrome are not known, and hence therapy is directed at optimizing the concentration of potassium in the plasma. A concomitant deficit of magnesium may be associated with Bartter's syndrome and, if present, minimizes the effectiveness of therapy of hypokalemia. Therefore, monitoring of the magnesium status of the patient is also required.

The hyperreninemia and hyperaldosteronism that accompany this entity make the aggressive use of dietary supplements of potassium and potassium-sparing diuretics a rational therapy. If these efforts fail to raise the concentration of potassium in the plasma to 3.5 mmol per liter, a trial of prostaglandin synthesis inhibitors may be warranted. Indomethacin (100 to 200 mg per day) is generally used. These drugs, however, have serious gastrointestinal side effects in many patients.

The use of angiotensin-converting enzyme inhibitors has been tried in several patients with variable results. Few side effects are reported, and thus these agents probably warrant a trial in patients who do not achieve the target concentration of potassium in the plasma with the above-mentioned therapeutic measures.

States in Which a Shift of Potassium into the Intracellular Fluid Can Be Anticipated

Diabetic Ketoacidosis

Diabetic ketoacidosis (DKA) is associated with a large deficit of potassium in the intracellular fluid, but not usually in the extracellular fluid; hence hypokalemia is not likely to be present before therapy. The administration of insulin causes an acute shift of potassium into cells; anabolism and the intake of phosphate result in a further shift of potassium into cells. Expansion of the extracellular fluid volume, with a rise in the rate of flow of the urine, is accompanied by the potential to augment the loss of potassium in the urine (aldosterone levels have not yet decreased to very low levels). To prevent a great decrease in the concentration of potassium in the plasma after the initiation of therapy, we recommend that potassium chloride be given intravenously once the concentration of potassium in the plasma decreases to less than 4.5 mmol per liter; we give potassium chloride initially at a rate of 20 mmol per hour, provided that the rate of flow of the urine is at least 1 ml per minute and the concentration of potassium in that urine is at least 20 mmol per liter. This rate of infusion is increased or reduced depending on changes in the concentration of potassium in the plasma. When replacing potassium, it is important to note that a defect in renal potassium secretion has been observed in patients with DKA. Careful follow-up and frequent monitoring of the concentration of potassium in the plasma is therefore mandatory, as changes in its concentration are not easy to predict with any degree of confidence.

Hypokalemia in the Alcoholic

This problem is even more delicate than DKA. The additional issues are the enhanced rate of loss of potassium in the urine because of the profound vomiting associated with alcoholism; an enhanced degree of shift of potassium into cells caused by possible alkalemia or alcohol withdrawal; and the possible presence of ileus (e.g., if pancreatitis is also present). Hence these patients may have overt hypokalemia on admission owing to the exaggerated loss of potassium in the urine, and the oral route for the administration of potassium might not be available.

There is one bright side to the story. Despite the ketoacidosis, it is almost always unnecessary to administer insulin, as life-threatening acidemia is generally not present; thus insulin-mediated potassium shifts can be avoided initially. We recommend that thiamine be given at the outset, and that 40 mmol of potassium be given hourly during the first few hours, provided that the concentration of potassium in the plasma is less than 4 mmol per liter. Perhaps several hundred millimoles of potassium will need to be given. Finally, these patients have a large deficit of phosphate, as well; full replacement of the deficit of potassium must await the replacement of phosphate. The replacement of the deficits of potassium and phosphate should take place over several days and should be administered orally in almost all cases.

Since a significant bicarbonate diuresis can be anticipated (either from a high concentration of bicarbonate per se or from the metabolism of organic anions to bicarbonate), it might be reasonable to add a potassium-sparing diuretic (10 mg amiloride, administered once only) to the initial treatment regimen. Because care must be taken to avoid a large input of potassium while this drug is acting, we are reluctant to use it if ileus is present and the degree of hypokalemia is not very severe.

Severe Metabolic Alkalosis and Hypokalemia

In patients with severe metabolic alkalosis associated with vomiting and extracellular fluid volume contraction, the deficit of potassium may indeed be substantial. In addition, in these patients there is a shift of potassium into cells, which leads to a greater degree of hypokalemia.

One should consider the expected course of events that may occur as therapy is instituted to restore the extracellular fluid volume. As flow to the distal nephron increases in the presence of sustained mineralocorticoid action, the secretion of potassium is augmented and results in further loss of potassium. If the increased flow to the cortical collecting duct contains bicarbonate, wasting of potassium will be even greater. In this situation, aggressive replacement of potassium (potassium chloride, 40 mmol per liter of intravenous saline) should be instituted in anticipation of this effect. The use of amiloride (10 mg, administered once only) to blunt the kaliuresis can play an important role in minimizing this loss of potassium in the urine. We use amiloride if the concentration of potassium in the urine is greater than 50 mmol per liter and the flow rate is higher than 2 ml per minute.

Severe Hyponatremia and Hypokalemia

In a patient who has severe hyponatremia in addition to hypokalemia, one must take care to avoid the danger of too rapid an increase in the concentration of sodium in the plasma when correcting hypokalemia by administering potassium chloride. Administered potassium generally moves intracellularly, causing sodium to move out of the cells and thus increasing the concentration of sodium in the plasma more rapidly than would otherwise take place.

In such a patient, the rate at which the concentration of sodium in the plasma increases should not exceed 0.5 mmol per liter per hour. Thus if such a patient has a total body water of 50 L, a maximum of 25 mmol of sodium plus potassium could be administered during the 1st hour. Note that if 20 mmol of potassium chloride is given during that hour, there is little room to give sodium. In this situation, therefore, we recommend that therapy be initiated with 20 mmol of potassium chloride in as little water as possible and that the electrolyte changes be followed frequently; ongoing losses of sodium and potassium must also be monitored.

Diuretic-Induced Hypokalemia

Diuretic-induced hypokalemia results primarily from the augmented rate of flow of urine together with a high aldosterone level (the result of extracellular fluid volume contraction). The deficit of potassium resulting from diuretic therapy is rarely greater than 120 mmol, and the decrease in the concentration of potassium in the plasma is rarely greater than 0.5 mmol per liter. These effects are established within 1 week of therapy. If more severe hypokalemia develops, other causes of wasting of potassium should be sought.

Although the indications for treatment of hypokalemia are debated, we believe that such indications include the presence of overt cardiac disease, digitalis therapy, and left ventricular hypertrophy. Furthermore, if glucose intolerance or vague symptoms of depletion of potassium develop, a trial of potassium replacement is warranted. In these settings, potassium should be given as the chloride salt.

There are several ways to prevent diuretic-induced hypokalemia. First, the total body deficit for potassium can be minimized by restricting the intake of sodium to approximately 100 mmol per day before the initiation of diuretic therapy. Second, the intake of potassium can be augmented by dietary manipulation or by the use of potassium supplements. Third, potassium-sparing diuretics can be used in conjunction with thiazides. Finally, if one appreciates that excretion of potassium occurs primarily during the first part of the day or when the diuretic is acting, the effectiveness of potassium supplements can be maximized by using them only later in the afternoon when the diurnal excretion of potassium is less and when the action of the diuretic is waning.

Adjuncts to Therapy

Renal loss of potassium can be reduced by the use of potassium-sparing agents; these are most commonly used as prophylaxis against diuretic-induced hypokalemia.

Spironolactone

Spironolactone acts as a competitive inhibitor of aldosterone. Its onset of action is slow, requiring 2 to 3 days to reach its peak effect. Side effects including gynecomastia, gastrointestinal symptoms, impotence, loss of libido, and menstrual irregularities are not infrequent. The usual dose is 25 to 100 mg per day, but up to 400 mg per day may be required with hyperaldosteronism.

Triamterene and Amiloride

Triamterene and amiloride act directly on the distal nephron to reduce the excretion of potassium. In stable patients, these agents are commonly given with thiazide diuretics in combined preparations (e.g., Dyazide, Moduretic). The dose of triamterene is 50 to 300 mg per day; side effects include gastrointestinal symptoms, nephrolithiasis, and megaloblastosis. Amiloride is given in a dose of 5 to 20 mg per day. It is generally well tolerated and has few side effects.

Angiotensin-Converting Enzyme Inhibitors

Angiotensin-converting enzyme inhibitors block the conversion of angiotensin I to angiotensin II, reducing aldosterone secretion and thus reducing renal potassium loss. While not specifically used for the prophylaxis of hypokalemia, they play an important role in the treatment of hypertension and heart failure and may help to prevent hypokalemia in patients who are taking thiazide or loop diuretics for these conditions. The currently available formulations are captopril, enalapril maleate, and lisinopril; the differences among them are small, although the latter two have the advantage of once-a-day administration. The serious side effects initially reported (proteinuria, agranulocytosis) are now less common as lower doses are used; acute renal failure is occasionally seen under certain circumstances (e.g., in patients with bilateral renal artery stenosis or heart failure and in the elderly).

SUGGESTED READING

Brown RS. Extrarenal potassium homeostasis. Kidney Int 1986; 30:116–127.

Ethier JH, Kamel KS, Magner PO, et al. Evaluation of the renal response to hypokalemia and hyperkalemia. Am J Kidney Dis 1990; 15:309–315.

Tannen RL. Diuretic-induced hypokalemia. Kidney Int 1985; 28:988–1000.

Wright FS. Renal potassium handling. Semin Nephrol 1987; 7:174–184.

HYPERKALEMIA

IRA KURTZ, M.D., FRCPC
LEON G. FINE, M.B., Ch.B., M.D.

POTASSIUM DISTRIBUTION

In a normal 70-kg adult there are approximately 3,500 mEq of potassium or approximately 50 mEq per kilogram of body weight. Most of the total body potassium is located intracellularly, with only 65 mEq being distributed in the extracellular fluid compartment. The intracellular concentration of potassium is about 150 mEq per liter, while in the extracellular fluid it is only 3.5 to 5 mEq per liter (the normal range depends on whether serum or plasma is measured). In addition to the extracellular–intracellular compartmentalization of potassium, there is a dynamic turnover of potassium owing to the intake and output of potassium from the extracellular compartment. In a normal adult ingesting approximately 100 mEq of potassium daily, 10 mEq are lost in the stool while 90 mEq are absorbed by the gastrointestinal tract and enter the extracellular compartment. The kidney is responsible for maintaining the constancy of total body potassium by excreting the 90 mEq of potassium which enter the extracellular compartment daily. The plasma potassium concentration is held constant by both renal and extrarenal mechanisms.

Hyperkalemia is caused by either a shift of potassium from the intracellular to the extracellular compartment or a decrease in the renal excretion of potassium. The most common causes of hyperkalemia are listed in Table 1.

PSEUDOHYPERKALEMIA

When whole blood clots, potassium is released from red blood cells, white blood cells, and platelets. The normal plasma potassium level is therefore less than the normal serum level. Abnormal red cell membrane fragility, or an increase in white blood cell number or platelet number can all lead to excess release of potassium when blood clots. This effect is not seen if plasma potassium is measured concurrently. Therefore, if a large discrepancy exists between the serum and plasma levels (greater than

TABLE 1 Etiology of Hyperkalemia

Pseudohyperkalemia
In vitro: Hemolysis, thrombocytosis, leukocytosis
In vivo: Tourniquet + fast exercise
Redistribution
Acute acidemia
Hemolysis
Rhabdomyolysis
Catabolic state
Insulinopenia
Hyperglycemia
Hyperosmolarity
Hypoaldosteronism
Exercise
Beta-adrenergic blockade
Periodic paralysis
Digitalis
Succinylcholine
Arginine hydrochloride
Impaired renal potassium excretion
Renal failure: acute, chronic
Impaired distal tubular flow rate
Hypoaldosteronism, pseudohypoaldosteronism–types I and II
Potassium secretory defect
Spironolactone, triamterene, amiloride, digitalis
Increased intake

0.3 mEq per liter), pseudohyperkalemia should be suspected.

REDISTRIBUTION OF POTASSIUM BETWEEN INTRACELLULAR AND EXTRACELLULAR COMPARTMENTS

Acid-Base Status

An acute lowering of luminal pH in the cortical collecting tubule causes an inhibition of potassium secretion. On the other hand, chronic acidemia causes an inhibition of proximal salt and water reabsorption, thereby increasing the distal delivery of sodium and water, which increases distal potassium secretion. Therefore, acute and chronic acidemia appear to have opposing effects on renal potassium secretion. In addition, acidemia causes potassium to shift from the intracellular to extracellular space. Until recently, it has been accepted as clinical dogma that the potassium concentration changes by 0.5 to 0.6 mEq per liter for every 0.1 unit change in the opposite direction of blood pH. More recent data have suggested that the relationship between blood pH and plasma potassium is not straightforward and depends on a number of factors, such as (1) mineral versus organic acidosis, (2) respiratory versus metabolic acidosis, (3) bicarbonate concentration, and (4) duration of acid-base disturbance.

Mineral versus Organic Acidosis

Results of administration of hydrochloric acid to humans, and studies using in vitro preparations suggest that hydrochloric acid causes a greater increase in plasma potassium concentration than lactic acid or beta-hydroxybutyric acid. Since the cell membrane is less permeable to chloride than the above mentioned organic acid anions, in order to maintain electroneutrality, potassium leaves the cell as protons enter. This occurs to a lesser extent during lactic or ketoacidosis, in which the accompanying organic anions enter the cell along with a proton. The situation is further complicated by the associated abnormalities found in patients with ketoacidosis, such as osmotic diuresis, volume depletion, secondary hyperaldosteronism, insulin lack, decreased dietary intake, and renal insufficiency, all of which can independently alter the plasma potassium level by renal or extrarenal mechanisms.

Respiratory versus Metabolic Acidosis

Respiratory acidosis causes little increase in the plasma potassium concentration compared with similar degrees of metabolic acidosis. The reason for this finding is unclear.

Bicarbonate Concentration

It has been reported that when mineral acid is infused to lower the bicarbonate concentration, and blood pH is maintained constant by lowering the blood P_{CO_2}, the plasma potassium level rises. The results of these studies suggest that changes in the bicarbonate concentration per se affect the plasma potassium concentration. However, these findings have not been confirmed by all investigators.

Duration of Acid-Base Disturbance

As the duration of metabolic acidosis increases, the intracellular buffering capacity rises. As more protons move into cells to maintain blood pH, more potassium tends to leave the intracellular compartment, with the result that hyperkalemia is more severe during chronic acidemia.

Increased K^+ Influx into the Extracellular Fluid Compartment

K^+ may enter the extracellular fluid compartment from intracellular sources, i.e., rhabdomyolysis, gastrointestinal hemorrhage, and catabolic states, or from exogenous sources, such as diet or medications. It is unusual for the plasma potassium to be chronically elevated in these situations unless there is an associated decrease in the renal excretion of potassium or decreased cellular uptake of the potassium load. Normally, renal and extrarenal homeostatic mechanisms prevent the rise in plasma potassium from occurring.

There are certain circumstances under which the rise in plasma potassium is exaggerated:

Hormonal

Insulin lack, aldosterone deficiency and beta-adrenergic blockade all result in decreased potassium tolerance. All three hormonal systems appear to mediate cellular potassium uptake. Marked, sustained hyperkalemia will be present only if renal excretory mechanisms are concomitantly impaired.

Hyperkalemic Periodic Paralysis

Patients with this autosomal dominant disorder present with intermittent attacks of acute paralysis and hyperkalemia. Exercise, potassium loads, and cold can precipitate the attack. The cause of the disorder is unknown, but it appears to result from an abnormal distribution of intracellular and extracellular potassium. Recurrences are prevented prophylactically with a high carbohydrate diet, salbutamol, thiazides, and acetazolamide.

Tissue Breakdown

Release of intracellular potassium occurs in patients with tumor lysis, burns, and crush injuries. Normally the kidney would be able to excrete the increased potassium load. However, as renal failure is frequently present, marked hyperkalemia may result.

IMPAIRED RENAL POTASSIUM EXCRETION

Delivery of Fluid to the Distal Nephron

Recent microperfusion studies of the rat distal tubule have demonstrated that tubular flow rate independent of the luminal Na^+ concentration can alter distal potassium secretion. Patients with disorders causing a decrease in distal flow, such as congestive heart failure or volume depletion, can become hyperkalemic because of a decrease in distal potassium secretion in addition to decreased filtration of potassium by the glomerulus. A urinary sodium concentration of less than 20 mEq per liter and a decreased ability to excrete free water are seen clinically in these patients.

Renal Insufficiency

Patients with chronic renal failure are not hyperkalemic unless the glomerular filtration rate is less than 15 ml per minute. As nephrons are lost, there is a homeostatic increase in potassium excreted by the remaining nephrons. However, acute renal failure is commonly associated with hyperkalemia for several reasons: (1) a decreased glomerular filtration rate, (2) decreased distal flow rate, (3) direct damage to the distal tubule in acute tubular necrosis, (4) the rapidity of the renal failure, which frequently precludes homeostatic mechanisms from developing, and (5) the increased release of potassium into the extracellular fluid which frequently occurs when patients with acute renal failure are catabolic.

Aldosterone Deficiency

Aldosterone stimulates potassium secretion by the cortical collecting tubule and enhances potassium uptake into cells. In the presence of a normal volume status, aldosterone deficiency results in only mild hyperkalemia, since adequate distal tubular flow maintains distal nephron potassium secretion and potassium balance.

Adrenal Enzymatic Defects

The most common enzyme defect in the aldosterone synthetic pathway is 21-hydroxylase deficiency. Patients with this disorder present in childhood with hyperkalemia, salt wasting, failure to thrive, and virilization. Both glucocorticoid and mineralocorticoid synthetic pathways are impaired.

Defects in the final two enzymatic steps in aldosterone biosynthesis have recently been described. In these disorders glucocorticoid synthesis is unimpaired.

Hyporeninemic Hypoaldosteronism

Hyporeninemia is the most common cause of hypoaldosteronism. Although the cause and pathogenesis of the syndrome are quite varied and beyond the scope of this discussion, the clinical presentation is typical. The mean age of most patients is 65 years. Patients are usually asymptomatic at presentation. Half of them have a hyperchloremic metabolic acidosis. Salt wasting is rarely present. Most patients have renal insufficiency, which is caused most commonly by diabetic glomerulosclerosis. The syndrome has also been described in patients with sickle cell disease and obstructive uropathy. Hypertension is found in more than 50 percent of the patients.

The cause of the hypoaldosteronism in these patients is probably multifactorial. All patients have a subnormal increase in plasma aldosterone concentration following volume depletion. Whether this is attributable to a primary defect in adrenal aldosterone synthesis or secretion, or is secondary to adrenal atrophy as a result of prolonged hyporeninemia, is unclear. Interestingly, hyporeninemia is present in most, but not all patients (18 to 21 percent) with this syndrome. Hyporeninemia has been attributed to decreased conversion of big renin to renin, decreased circulating catecholamine levels or autonomic neuropathy, decreased prostaglandin levels, extracellular fluid expansion, and glomerular hyperfiltration.

Potassium Secretory Defect

Some patients with hyperkalemia have normal or elevated renin and aldosterone levels and fail to respond to mineralocorticoid therapy. These patients do not develop a normal kaluresis in response to sodium sulfate, furosemide, or potassium chloride. In addition, some patients appear to have hypoaldosteronism. Clinical examples of this disorder are sickle cell trait and disease, systemic lupus erythematosus, obstructive uropathy, and renal transplantation.

Pseudohypoaldosteronism Types I and II

Pseudohypoaldosteronism type I is characterized by volume depletion, hyperkalemia, salt wasting, hyperchloremic metabolic acidosis, and failure to thrive. Most patients present in infancy. Plasma and aldosterone levels are elevated, and treatment with mineralocorticoids is not effective. The syndrome appears to diminish spontaneously in severity at about 2 years of age. In adults the syndrome is usually associated with tubulointerstitial disease.

Type II pseudohypoaldosteronism is characterized by hyperkalemia, hypertension, hyperchloremic metabolic acidosis, hypoaldosteronism, and hyporeninemia. Mineralocorticoid treatment fails to increase urinary potassium excretion normally, yet increased renal sodium reabsorption is observed in response to mineralocorticoids. Because potassium excretion increases normally in response to intravenous potassium sulfate infusions and not potassium chloride, it has been proposed that the primary defect in this disorder is enhanced electrogenic chloride reabsorption in the distal nephron. This results in a decrease in the lumen negativity which impairs potassium and proton secretion. The enhanced reabsorption of sodium and chloride results in hypertension, hyporeninemia, and hypoaldosteronism.

DRUGS THAT CAUSE HYPERKALEMIA

Captopril

An angiotensin converting enzyme inhibitor, captopril causes a rise in serum potassium level which varies inversely with the glomerular filtration rate and is most severe in those patients with markedly impaired renal function. The mechanism is likely attributable to decreased aldosterone synthesis resulting in a decreased fractional excretion of potassium.

Beta-Blockers

The beta$_2$-receptor has been shown to mediate potassium uptake into cells. Propranolol has a direct effect, blocking the influx of potassium into muscles, and also inhibits renin secretion. This results in a moderate sustained increase in the plasma potassium concentration when the drug is ingested chronically. Hyperkalemia is observed most commonly in diabetics and patients with renal insufficiency and is reversible upon discontinuation of the drug.

Prostaglandin Inhibitors

Indomethacin and other nonsteroidal anti-inflammatory agents have been reported to cause hyporeninemic hypoaldosteronism and hyperkalemia. The hyporeninemia has been attributed to decreased prostaglandin production, since prostaglandin E_2, I_2, and D_2 are stimulants of renin secretion. In a recent study of a patient with Bartter's syndrome, mepacrine (a phospholipase inhibitor) was shown to inhibit prostaglandin excretion without decreasing the plasma renin concentration. It is therefore possible that nonsteroidal anti-inflammatory agents directly inhibit renin release by a non-prostaglandin-dependent mechanism.

Heparin

Chronic heparin therapy has been reported to be associated with hyperkalemia. The hyperkalemia is attributable to a direct impairment of adrenal aldosterone synthesis and, as might be expected, these patients are hyperreninemic.

Spironolactone, Triamterene, and Amiloride

Administration of these diuretics inhibits potassium secretion by the cortical collecting tubule. These drugs should be used cautiously in those patients with diabetic or renal insufficiency.

Digitalis

Digitalis overdose results in an inhibition of sodium-potassium-adenosine triphosphatase activity which prevents cells from actively accumulating potassium, which results in a rise in plasma potassium level.

Succinylcholine

By depolarizing cells, succinylcholine causes a passive leak of potassium from the intracellular to the extracellular compartment. Hyperkalemia may result.

Arginine Hydrochloride

This drug has been reported to cause an efflux of potassium into the extracellular compartment resulting in hyperkalemia.

TREATMENT

General Considerations

In approaching the treatment of hyperkalemia, the clinician must ascertain whether the patient is symptomatic and whether the disorder is acute or chronic. Hyperkalemia should be treated aggressively if there are associated neuromuscular and cardiac abnormalities. The neuromuscular abnormalities include paresthesias and weakness of the extremities, which, in severe cases, may result in symmetric flaccid analysis. Sensory abnormalities are usually mild in comparison to the muscular findings. Cardiac toxicity is the primary reason for treating hyperkalemia. Electrocardiogram abnormalities include an increase in the amplitude of T waves, lengthening of the PR interval, and widening of the QRS complex. Severe hyperkalemia (serum concentrations greater than 8 mEq per liter) results in disappearance of P waves and a sine wave pattern resembling slow ventricular tachycardia. Any disturbance in conduction may be present, including atrioventricular (AV) nodal and fascicular conduction blocks. In patients with chronic hyperkalemia these electrocardiographic abnormalities may be absent. In addition, milder degrees of hyperkalemia may be associated with cardiac toxicity if hyponatremia, hypocalcemia, or acidemia coexists. Treatment is generally indicated in the absence of electrocardiogram abnormalities if the potassium concentration has risen above 6 mEq per liter. Patients with preexisting AV conduction abnormalities may develop Stokes-Adams episodes and complete AV block with only modest hyperkalemia.

Treatment of Acute Hyperkalemia

Treatment of an acute elevation in the plasma potassium concentration involves the following principles: (1) Oppose the effects of hyperkalemia on the cell membrane to minimize cardiac and neuromuscular toxicity; (2) increase the transport of potassium from the extracellular to the intracellular compartment; (3) increase the excretion of potassium; and (4) treat the cause of the hyperkalemia. These principles are summarized in Table 2.

Membrane Antagonism

Calcium increases the threshold potential required to excite the plasma membrane of the cardiac cell. Since

TABLE 2 Treatment of Acute Hyperkalemia

	Dose
Membrane antagonism	
Calcium gluconate (10%)	10–20 ml IV
Sodium bicarbonate	50–100 mEq IV
Sodium chloride	50–100 mEq IV
Redistribution	
Insulin/glucose	20 units regular insulin plus 50 g glucose IV over 1 hour
Sodium bicarbonate	50–100 mEq IV
Increase excretion	
Furosemide	40–80 mg IV
Kayexalate	25–50 g per rectum with sorbitol, or PO
Sodium bicarbonate	50–100 mEq IV
Hemodialysis	
Peritoneal dialysis	

hyperkalemia depolarizes the cardiac cell's resting membrane potential, bringing it closer to the potential required for excitation, calcium, by increasing the difference between the resting and excitation potential, reduces the adverse effect of hyperkalemia. Calcium also reverses the decrease in conduction velocity induced by hyperkalemia by increasing the number of sodium channels in the cell membrane. Calcium is given intravenously as a bolus of 10 to 20 ml of a 10 percent solution of calcium gluconate. The dose may be repeated if no immediate effect is seen. Electrocardiographic monitoring is desirable. If the patient is also being treated with digitalis, hypercalcemia may result in digitalis toxicity, so it is preferable to give the calcium gluconate as a slow infusion over 30 minutes to prevent an acute elevation of the serum calcium concentration.

Hyponatremia may aggravate the cardiac toxicity induced by hyperkalemia, as mentioned previously. The treatment consists of administering hypertonic saline (50 to 100 mEq of sodium chloride) which may reverse the adverse effects of hyperkalemia on the cardiac cell.

Redistribution of Potassium

Insulin-Glucose. Insulin directly stimulates the uptake of potassium into cells, predominantly muscle, by depolarizing the membrane potential. Glucose is given to prevent hypoglycemia during insulin therapy. Ten to 20 units of regular insulin are added to 0.5 liters of 10 percent glucose solution and infused over 1 hour. The treatment is repeated as required. The K^+ concentration should fall 0.5 to 1.2 mEq per liter in 1 to 2 hours.

Sodium Bicarbonate. Sodium bicarbonate reduces hyperkalemia by shifting potassium into cells and by increasing renal potassium excretion. The standard dose is 50 mEq given intravenously over 10 minutes. This dose can be repeated as long as the patient can tolerate the increased sodium intake. Patients with hypocalcemia may be at increased risk of seizures and tetany as the blood pH is increased.

Increased Excretion of Potassium

Diuretics. Although not useful in an acute situation, a diuretic such as furosemide is effective in markedly enhancing the renal excretion of potassium. The usual dose is 40 to 80 mg intravenously. In the presence of renal failure, these agents are less potent.

Resins. Ion-exchange resins such as Kayexalate (Na^+ polystyrene sulfonate) bind potassium in the gastrointestinal tract in exchange for sodium. Each gram of resin binds 1 mEq of potassium in exchange for 2 to 3 mEq of Na^+. The resin may be given orally (25 to 50 g) or as a retention enema (50 g in 200 ml of 10 percent dextrose in water per rectum). Sorbitol is given to prevent the major side effect of constipation. The serum potassium level falls 0.5 to 1 mEq per liter after a 50-g dose within 1 to 2 hours. Since a sodium load is administered during this form of therapy, clinicians should be cautious in prescribing the drug for patients who cannot tolerate volume overload.

Dialysis. Potassium can be removed effectively from the body using either hemodialysis or peritoneal dialysis. The major difference between the two modes of therapy is the rapidity of potassium removal. Hemodialysis is preferred if an acute decrease in the serum potassium concentration is required. The major drawback is the time needed to set up the hemodialysis equipment and the need to have access to the circulation. Using this method, approximately 40 mEq of potassium can be removed during the first hour as opposed to approximately 5 mEq with peritoneal dialysis.

Treatment of Chronic Hyperkalemia

Chronic moderate hyperkalemia (plasma potassium concentration equal to 6 or 7 mEq per liter) is better tolerated by patients than acute hyperkalemia of a similar magnitude. For example, patients with chronic renal failure tolerate very high plasma potassium levels. In treating chronic hyperkalemia, one should be aware that many of these patients have associated diseases such as diabetes mellitus, renal failure, congestive heart failure, hypertension, and cardiovascular disease. One must be wary of the possible detrimental side effects the therapy may have on associated medical disorders.

Diet

In chronic renal failure, the plasma potassium concentration is proportional to the dietary potassium intake. Although this has not been demonstrated in all causes of chronic hyperkalemia, it is also beneficial to reduce the dietary intake in these disorders. The total daily potassium intake should be reduced to less than 60 mEq per day. Since the dietary potassium is normally exchanged for increased sodium, as in patients receiving ion exchange resins, one must be cautious when treating patients who cannot tolerate a volume load. In addition, there is a growing amount of clinical data which indicates that increasing the dietary intake of potassium may be beneficial in lowering the blood pressure in patients with hypertension. The exact mechanism involved in this blood pressure lowering effect is unknown. Whether patients with hyperkalemia and hypertension will experience an increase in their blood pressure during a decrease in dietary potassium intake is also unknown. Dietary salt substitutes containing potassium must be avoided.

Drugs

Drugs that cause an increase in the plasma potassium concentration should be avoided. These drugs include prostaglandin inhibitors, heparin, beta-blockers, angiotensin converting enzyme inhibitors, amiloride, triamterene, and spironolactone. In addition, diabetics who lack the compensatory response of an increase in insulin and aldosterone secretion during glucose infusions are susceptible to life-threatening hyperkalemia.

Acid-Base Balance

Acidemia will often result in an increased plasma potassium concentration. Bicarbonate will ameliorate the hyperkalemia both by raising the plasma pH and by directly shifting potassium intracellularly. Bicarbonate will also cause a potassium diuresis. The low plasma bicarbonate concentration can be corrected by assuming a distribution space of 40 percent of total body weight. As mentioned previously, patients with heart failure may not be able to tolerate the excess volume load associated with this form of therapy, and therefore a diuretic should be given concomitantly.

Prevention of Volume Depletion

Since potassium secretion in the distal tubule is decreased when the luminal Na^+ concentration falls and when luminal flow decreases, the volume status of the patient with chronic hyperkalemia should be adequately maintained.

HYPERCALCEMIA AND HYPOCALCEMIA

RENEE E. GARRICK, M.D.
STANLEY GOLDFARB, M.D.

An understanding of the plasma forms of calcium is a critical first step in assessing the clinical significance of serum calcium values. Calcium exists in serum in three forms: *a non diffusible protein* (primary albumin) bound fraction, constituting approximately 40 percent of the total; *a diffusible nonionized fraction* chelated with bicarbonate, citrate, and phosphate, constituting about 10 percent of the total; and a *free, ionized fraction.* Although the ionized fraction represents the physiologically active moiety, most laboratories measure only total calcium. Thus, it is important to recognize that the ionized fraction may vary independently of total calcium. For example, since 85 to 90 percent of the non diffusible calcium is bound by albumin and only 10 to 15 percent is bound by globulin, hypoalbuminemia will reduce the bound fraction and the total calcium measurement, but will not change the ionized fraction. Therefore, the patient will not exhibit signs or symptoms of hypocalcemia. Conversely, acid-base changes may affect the ionized fraction without changing the total calcium measurement. An alkaline pH will increase the binding of calcium to protein, lowering the ionized fraction, while total calcium is unchanged. Finally, certain forms of hyperglobulinemia may increase total calcium without affecting ionized calcium.

FACTORS REGULATING SERUM CALCIUM

Three systems participate in the regulation of serum calcium: *intestine, bone,* and *kidney.* Dietary calcium is absorbed in the proximal small bowel primarily under the influence of vitamin D and its metabolites; it is deposited into and released from bone under the influence of parathyroid hormone (PTH), vitamin D, and phosphorus; and it is excreted by the kidney. The renal excretion of calcium is regulated by both the filtered load of calcium (glomerular filtration rate × diffusible calcium) and PTH. High levels of PTH increase the reabsorption of filtered calcium in the distal nephron segments. Most clinical disorders of serum concentration can be traced to abnormalities in either intestinal absorption or bone resorption, with the kidney playing a secondary role.

HYPERCALCEMIA

With the advent of the autoanalyzer, the detection of hypercalcemia has become increasingly common. Table 1 lists the major causes of hypercalcemia together with some comments on the associated mechanisms. The most common causes of hypercalcemia are malignancy and hyperparathyroidism. Granulomatous disorders, as a group, are the third most common cause of hypercalcemia.

TABLE 1 Causes of Hypercalcemia

Hyperparathyroidism
Adenoma
Hyperplasia—familial, multiple endocrine neoplasia syndrome
Malignancy associated
Metastatic resorption of bone
Osteoclast activating factors
PTH-like substances (humoral hypercalcemia of malignancy)
$1,25(OH)_2D$ production by tumor
Prostaglandin-mediated bone resorption
Granulomatous disorders
Tuberculosis, sarcoidosis, histoplasmosis, coccidioidomycosis
Drugs
Hormonal therapy of breast cancer
Lithium
Thiazides
Vitamin D and A intoxication
Isoretinoic acid
Systemic disease
Paget's
Addison's
Thyrotoxicosis
Immobilization
Postrenal transplant; polyuric phase of acute renal failure
Familial hypocalciuric hypercalcemia
Breast implants

Signs and Symptoms

Since hypercalcemia frequently occurs in association with other disorders, many of the signs and symptoms present may reflect the primary disorder, rather than the hypercalcemia per se. The major symptoms directly attributable to hypercalcemia are given in Table 2. These findings are independent of the cause of hypercalcemia, and their severity is influenced by the degree of hypercalcemia and perhaps by the rate at which the calcium level rises. Although many patients with mild hypercalcemia (11 to 12 mg per deciliter) are either asymptomatic or complain of only malaise, patients with severe, acute hypercalcemia (usually 15 mg per deciliter or higher) may present with potentially life-threatening nervous system, cardiac, and renal dysfunction. Within this spectrum, symptomatic hypercalcemia is usually characterized by complaints of anorexia, constipation, polyuria, polydipsia, mild confusion and memory lapses. Hypercalcemia may be associated with hypertension, which is most frequently seen with the hypercalcemia of parathyroid, granulomatous, and malignant disease.

TABLE 2 Signs and Symptoms of Hypercalcemia

Gastrointestinal
Anorexia, nausea, vomiting, constipation, pancreatitis
Central nervous system
Confusion, memory loss, stupor, coma
Cardiovascular
ECG changes, hypertension, arrhythmias
Renal
Polyuria, polydipsia, acute and chronic renal insufficiency, nephrolithiasis, nephrocalcinosis
Systemic
Hyperchloremic acidosis, metastatic calcification

With the exception of the electrocardiogram (ECG) and urinalysis, the laboratory findings of hypercalcemia are fairly nonspecific. The ECG changes include shortening of the QT interval and ST-T segment coving. As hypercalcemia progresses, T wave widening and ventricular arrhythmias as well as heart block may occur. Hypercalcemia potentiates the effects of digitalis and may induce digitalis-associated arrhythmias.

The most consistent renal defect in hypercalcemia is a reduction in urinary concentrating ability. This occurs with relatively mild (11 to 12 mg per deciliter) hypercalcemia, and although the defect is typically not severe (urine osmolality is usually isotonic or greater), in some cases the urine may be frankly hypotonic and significant polyuria may ensue. The loss of urinary concentrating ability, coupled with hypercalcemia-induced nausea, vomiting, and anorexia, may lead to significant extracellular volume depletion. Extracellular volume depletion will in turn lead to enhanced proximal tubular sodium and calcium reabsorption and may thereby further exacerbate the hypercalcemia. More marked elevations in serum calcium (>13 mg per deciliter) affect both renal blood flow and glomerular permeability and may lead to acute renal insufficiency. This reduction in glomerular filtration rate and the concomitant impairment in renal calcium excretion, may be important contributory factors in the genesis of the severe hypercalcemia of certain malignancies—most notably multiple myeloma. With the exceptions of lithium- and thiazide-induced hypercalcemia and familial hypocalciuric hypercalcemia, hypercalciuria is present. Long-standing hypercalcemia, such as that seen with hyperparathyroidism and granulomatous disease, may cause nephrolithiasis and/or nephrocalcinosis, and chronic renal insufficiency may ensue.

Therapeutic Modalities

The basic pharmacologic approaches available for the management of hypercalcemia, together with their possible side effects, are outlined in Table 3. Each of these treatments has certain limitations and some are more likely to be beneficial in certain settings.

Saline and Loop Diuretics

Most patients with severe, symptomatic hypercalcemia are depleted of extracellular fluid volume. This loss of both the water and sodium results from the renal tubular effects of hypercalcemia. Also, mental obtundation may limit intake of sodium and water. Infusion of isotonic saline solution by expanding the plasma volume with non-calcium-containing solutions will acutely lower the serum calcium level by dilution. Moreover, increasing urinary calcium excretion is an effective and relatively safe method

TABLE 3 Therapeutic Modalities for Hypercalcemia

Therapeutic Modalities	*Potential Side Effects*
Increased renal excretion	
Saline	Extracellular volume expansion
Loop diuretics	Hypokalemia, hypomagnesemia, volume depletion
Decreased gastrointestinal absorption	
Glucocorticoids (may inhibit vitamin D metabolism)	Hyperglycemia, immunosuppression
Oral phosphates*	Diarrhea, ? worsening of hyperparathyroid bone disease, extravascular calcification
Decreased bone resorption	
Oral phosphates*	
Calcitonin	Resistance frequently develops
Mithramycin	Renal, hepatic, and bone marrow toxicity
Diphosphonates	Osteomalacia (long-term use)
Prostaglandin inhibitors	Gastrointestinal bleeding, renal toxicity, salt retention
Chelation of ionized calcium	
Intravenous phosphates*	Widespread metastatic calcification
EDTA+	Renal toxicity
Removal of calcium	
Dialysis—dialysis plus EDTA	Useful in acute renal failure and chronic renal failure; transient effect

* Also increases calcium movement into bone
\+ Chelation will lower ionized calcium immediately and chelated calcium will be cleared by renal excretion.

of further lowering the serum calcium level. A brisk saline diuresis alone will substantially increase urinary calcium excretion by minimizing tubular calcium reabsorption at those sites where sodium and calcium transport are linked. Although the addition of a loop diuretic such as furosemide can further potentiate calciuria by inhibiting sodium and calcium reabsorption at sites distal to the proximal tubule, the major aim of furosemide therapy is to maintain the saline diuresis and to reduce the risk of saline-induced extracellular volume overload and congestive failure. Thus, when the diuretic is used, it should *not* be administered until after a saline diuresis has been established, and great care must be taken to avoid diuretic-induced extracellar volume depletion because this will serve to increase proximal tubular sodium and calcium reabsorption and thereby aggravate the hypercalcemia. The approach we prefer is as follows:

1. Begin with 1 to 2 L of isotonic saline over 1 hour to produce the initial volume expansion.
2. Administer furosemide, 20 to 40 mg IV and repeat every 4 to 5 hours.
3. Measure urine volume every hour and urine potassium and sodium concentration every 4 to 6 hours.
4. Replace urine volume with saline and added potassium chloride (20 to 40 mEq of potassium chloride per liter is usually adequate).
5. Measure serum electrolytes and calcium every 4 hours.

A urine volume of 250 to 300 ml per hour is the minimum amount required for adequate calciuria, and effective treatment of severe hypercalcemia ($\geq$15 mg per deciliter) may require urine volumes of 400 to 500 ml per hour. Clearly, close monitoring of urinary sodium and potassium losses and serum electrolytes is imperative. Since optimal management requires infusions of large amounts of saline, central venous pressure determinations should be used as a guide for fluid administration. Elderly patients, patients with cardiovascular disorders, and patients with severe hypercalcemia ($>$15 mg per deciliter) are best managed in an intensive care unit with central venous pressure or, where appropriate, Swan-Ganz monitoring. Although saline diuresis is effective therapy for most cases of hypercalcemia, the presence of severe renal insufficiency or congestive heart failure will preclude its use. Further, since serum calcium concentration usually falls relatively slowly with this treatment (2 to 3 mg per deciliter per 24 to 36 hours), when severe, symptomatic hypercalcemia is present, modalities capable of inducing a more rapid decline in calcium level must also be employed.

Glucocorticoids

These agents reduce serum calcium concentration by limiting gastrointestinal absorption either directly or via a reduction in $1,25(OH)_2D$ levels. They are very effective agents for the treatment of hypercalcemia due to *vitamin D intoxication, sarcoidosis,* and perhaps *other granulomatous disorders.* In the case of vitamin D intoxication, glucocorticoids limit the production of the active vitamin D metabolite, $1,25(OH)_2D$, and reduce both gut absorption and bone resorption. In sarcoidosis, glucocorticoids reduce the production of $1,25(OH)_2D$ by the granulomatous tissue and also impair its actions at the level of the gut and the bone. In both vitamin D intoxication and sarcoidosis, very small doses of glucocorticoids may be effective (10 to 15 mg of prednisone or prednisone equivalent per day) and the onset of action is usually between 3 and 5 days. Glucocorticoids may also effectively control the hypercalcemia of certain malignancies—most notably *multiple myeloma, breast cancer,* and *lymphoproliferative disorders*. In these settings, glucocorticoids presumably act through a direct tumorlytic effect and by limiting the production of bone resorbing factors such as osteoclast activating factor. Additionally, certain lymphoproliferative disorders (T cell lymphomas) may produce $1,25\ (OH)_2D$, and in these conditions glucocorticoids may also reduce serum calcium concentration via an inhibitory effect on the production and action of $1,25\ (OH)_2D$. When used for malignancy-associated hypercalcemia, doses of 60 mg per day of prednisone or prednisone equivalent are usually required. In this setting, glucocorticoid therapy has the disadvantage of being relatively slow acting: Serum calcium concentration usually falls 5 to 10 days after the start of therapy. In addition, glucocorticoids may (1) lead to increased risk of infection; (2) worsen the catabolic effects of malignancy, chemotherapy, and poor nutrition; and (3) exacerbate skeletal demineralization through a direct effect. Glucocorticoids are generally ineffective in parathyroid-mediated hypercalcemia or in the management of solid-tumor–associated hypercalcemia due to the presence of PTH-like substances (humoral hypercalcemia of malignancy).

Oral Phosphates

In hypercalcemic patients with normal or reduced serum phosphate levels, oral phosphate supplementation is a very reliable, relatively safe treatment. The anticalcemic effects of phosphate are expressed primarily at the level of the bone where there is reduced calcium resorption and enhanced calcium uptake. Phosphates are usually given as 1.5 to 3.0 g of elemental phosphorus per day in divided doses. Neutra-Phos (250 mg phosphorus per capsule) and other phospho-soda preparations are safe, inexpensive preparations. Serum calcium concentration usually declines with 48 hours. Oral phosphate should never be used if renal insufficiency or hyperphosphatemia is present, since the attendant increment in the calcium-phosphate product will greatly increase the risk of extravascular calcification. Serum calcium, phosphorus, and creatinine levels should be closely followed in the hospital until a therapeutic response is seen and the absence of hyperphosphatemia assured. Diarrhea frequently occurs with large doses of oral phosphate and is a major reason for patient noncompliance.

Calcitonin

This agent inhibits osteoclastic bone resorption. Calcitonin acts rapidly (hours) and has a low incidence of toxicity (rash, flushing, rare allergic reactions). These characteristics would suggest that calcitonin is an ideal drug for the treatment of severe hypercalcemia, or the long-term management of malignancy-associated hypercalcemia. Unfortunately, about 20 percent of patients do not respond to calcitonin and the majority of patients who do initially respond become resistant to its effects after several days of therapy. In some patients, concurrent glucocorticoid therapy (30 to 60 mg per day of prednisone) may prevent the development of resistance, but this effect is generally not long lasting. Despite these drawbacks, its safety and rapid onset of action make calcitonin an attractive agent for treatment of hypercalcemia. Although allergic reactions are rare, prior to therapy a 1.0 unit intradermal skin test should be performed. If the skin test is negative then the recommended initial dose of salmon calcitonin is 4 units per kilogram subcutaneously every 12 to 24 hours. The need for dosage increments is guided by the serum calcium level; the maximum recommended dose is 8 units per kilogram every 6 hours.

Mithramycin

Inferential data suggest that this antitumor agent reduces serum calcium levels by inhibiting osteoclastic bone resorption. The usual hypocalcemic dose is 25 μg per kilogram of body weight, although occasionally smaller doses may suffice (10 to 15 μg per kilogram). Its onset of action is less rapid than that of calcitonin; serum calcium usually begins to fall 10 to 20 hours after administration. If an adequate response is not initially obtained, the dose can be repeated daily for 3 to 4 days. The hypocalcemic effect typically lasts from 2 to 6 days. These dosage regimens are only 10 percent of those used to treat malignancy and they are relatively safe and effective even in the presence of renal insufficiency. When several repeated doses are required, however, renal, hepatic, and platelet dysfunction and bone marrow toxicity (thrombocytopenia) may develop. Although weekly administration of mithramycin has been successfully used in the long-term management of malignancy-associated hypercalcemia, the risk of toxicity necessitates close monitoring of renal, hepatic, and platelet function.

Diphosphonates

Normally, the pyrophosphate (P-O-P) bonds of the bone calcium-phosphate crystal hydroxyapatite are cleaved by local pyrophosphatases. The diphosphonates, which contain a pyrophosphatase-resistant P-C-P bond, prevent bone dissolution in part by chemiabsorption to bone calcium-phosphate surfaces and in part by a cellular action on osteoclasts. Additionally, some diphosphonates interfere with bone formation and thus may lead to osteomalacia. Experimental trials have been conducted with three diphosphonate compounds: ethane-hydroxy-diphosphonate (EHDP), dichloromethylene diphosphonate (Cl_2MDP), and amino-hydroxy-propylidine-diphosphonate (APD).

Both EHDP and Cl_2MDP, administered intravenously, have been shown to be effective in the treatment of malignancy-associated hypercalcemia. Cl_2MDP act slightly more rapidly than EHDP, and a reduction in calcium concentration usually occurs within 24 hours, with a maximum effect observed by 5 days. Neither of these compounds is available for parenteral use in the United States.

Oral EHDP has met with only minimal success as a treatment for malignancy-associated hypercalcemia, and in the United States it is currently approved for use only in Paget's disease and heterotopic calcification (myositis ossificans). Since EHDP interferes with bone formation as well as bone resorption, long-term use may be complicated by osteomalacia. In addition, hyperphosphatemia may occur during the initial phases of EHDP therapy. Oral Cl_2MDP effectively reduces serum calcium concentrations, but oral Cl_2MDP is not available in the United States because of purported side effects (possible hematologic malignancies).

Oral APD has also been successfully used to treat the hypercalcemia of malignancy and hyperparathyroidism. A significant fall in calcium level usually occurs within 72 hours of treatment, but in some cases an adequate response may take longer. Unlike EHDP, therapy with APD is not associated with the development of osteomalacia. Although APD appears to be a promising agent for the treatment of hypercalcemia, it is not yet approved for use in the United States.

Prostaglandin Inhibition

Several early reports suggested that inhibitors of prostaglandin synthesis (NSAIDs) could effectively control malignancy-associated hypercalcemia, presumably by blocking prostaglandin-mediated bone resorption. Along these lines, in vitro studies demonstrated that under certain conditions, the bone resorbing activity of cultured human breast cancer cells could be inhibited by the addition of indomethacin to the cell cultures. However, in recent clinical trials, the systemic administration of indomethacin and related agents only rarely resulted in successful control of the serum calcium. Since the vasodilatory prostaglandins may help to counterbalance the vasoconstrictive effects of hypercalcemia, NSAIDs could theoretically worsen renal function. Given these considerations, prostaglandin inhibitors are not recommended for the routine treatment of hypercalcemia.

Intravenous Phosphate

Infusion of 0.70 mmol per kilogram of phosphate over 10 to 12 hours will rapidly lower the ionized calcium by chelation. The dose-dependent fall in serum calcium occurs almost immediately, and it is one of the most potent therapies available. Although a large portion of the calcium-lowering effect may be due to inhibition of bone resorption, the effect also depends on the deposition of complexed calcium and phosphate in bone and extraskeletal sites. Thus deposits may form in the kidney or the heart, and hypotension, acute renal failure, cardiac arrest, and sudden death have been reported. For these reasons, intravenous phosphate is very rarely indicated for the treatment of hypercalcemia, and it should never be used if renal insufficiency is present.

Sodium-EDTA

Sodium disodium-ethylene diamine tetraacetate (sodium-EDTA) can immediately lower ionized calcium by chelation with the serum ionized fraction. Although the total serum calcium level will not fall until after the chelated calcium has been excreted by the kidney, the immediate reduction of the physiologically active ionized fraction provides protection against the toxicities of hypercalcemia. Reports of severe nephrotoxicity have limited its use, but many of those cases involved higher doses than those currently recommended. However, in view of its potential toxicity, we recommend that its use be restricted to the treatment of severe life-threatening hypercalcemia (arrhythmias, seizures, obtundation) where immediate reduction of ionized calcium is critical. The recommended dose is 15 to 50 mg IV over 4 hours. In patients with renal isufficiency and life-threatening hypercalcemia, sodium-EDTA administration can be used in conjunction with dialysis.

Dialysis

Hemodialysis against a low or calcium-free bath can effectively remove calcium and lower the serum calcium level. This treatment is useful if the hypercalcemia is accompanied by oliguria, or if the patient is unable to tolerate saline infusions. The fall in serum calcium concentration is only transient, however, and this therapy usually only serves as a stopgap measure until other agents can begin to exert their effect.

Therapeutic Approach

The first step in the management of hypercalcemia is to determine whether the total serum calcium measurement accurately reflects the ionized calcium level. In view of the calcium-binding properties of serum proteins (as discussed), the serum albumin concentration must always be considered when interpreting the total calcium value. A useful clinical rule of thumb is that the total serum calcium level is decreased by 0.8 mg per deciliter for every 1 g per deciliter decrement in the serum albumin level. Thus, if the serum calcium level is 11.0 mg per deciliter and the albumin is 1 g per deciliter, the corrected serum calcium level would be 13.4 mg per deciliter, and the symptoms consistent with moderate hypercalcemia would be expected. Conversely, an increase in serum albumin concentration, secondary to hemoconcentration, can result in hypercalcemia due to an increase in calcium binding, but the ionized fraction will be normal and the patient will be asymptomatic. Abnormalities of serum globulins are less common; however, as previously noted, in certain cases of multiple myeloma, calcium binding by the paraprotein can result in marked hypercalcemia without an increase in ionized calcium. Proper interpretation of the laboratory values together with careful history and physical examination will help to avoid unnecessary therapeutic maneuvers.

Acute Hypercalcemia

The initial treatment of acute hypercalcemia is guided by the clinical manifestations and the severity of the hypercalcemia. Rarely, a patient with severe hypercalcemia (>15 mg per deciliter) presents with acute oliguric renal failure along with neurologic and cardiovascular complications (hypercalcemic crisis). This constitutes a medical emergency and immediate reduction of the ionized calcium may be lifesaving. An acute saline infusion is the first treatment to use. If potentially fatal cardiac arrhythmias or shock are present, sodium-EDTA infusion and/or short-term hemodialysis should be instituted. Since hemodialysis reduces calcium only transiently, agents such as mithramycin or calcitonin, which work independently of renal function, must also be employed.

A more common presentation is that of moderate to severe hypercalcemia (13 to 15 mg per deciliter) without associated life-threatening neurologic or cardiovascular complications, and here the therapy must be individualized. If the calcium is in the range of 15 mg per deciliter or higher, our initial approach is calcitonin in combination with saline and furosemide. The selection of calcitonin stems from the fact that, although it is less uniformly effective than mithramycin, it has a faster onset of action and fewer side effects. If the serum calcium level does not fall after 8 to 12 hours of treatment, mithramycin can be added.

In symptomatic patients with mild to moderate hypercalcemia, therapy with saline alone or saline and furosemide will usually suffice. If the serum calcium level remains above 12 mg per deciliter after 12 to 24 hours of brisk saline-furosemide diuresis or if a continuous saline infusion is required to maintain the calcium level at less than 12 mg per deciliter, then additional therapy is usually warranted. This is especially true if the glomerular filtration rate fails to normalize after volume expansion, since not only does renal insufficiency blunt the calciuric response to saline and furosemide, but also hypercalcemia per se can worsen renal function. In this setting the choice of therapeutic agents remains somewhat controversial; however, for the reasons enumerated above, we prefer to try first calcitonin and then mithramycin if calcitonin fails. Other potentially useful agents include oral phosphates, which can safely be employed if the serum phosphate concentration is normal or low and if renal and gastrointestinal functions are intact, and glucocorticoids, which may be effective if the underlying cause of the hypercalcemia is myeloma, lymphoma, or breast cancer.

Chronic Hypercalcemia

Therapy for chronic mild hypercalcemia depends to a certain extent on the cause of the hypercalcemia. In the case of malignancy-associated hypercalcemia, specific treatment directed at the underlying tumor is crucial. Glucocorticoid therapy may be useful for the chronic hypercalcemia associated with sarcoidosis, myeloma, lymphoma, and breast cancer. In the setting of glucocorticoid-unresponsive malignancy, oral phosphates may provide effective control. However, if the serum phosphate level is elevated or if the patient is unable to tolerate the associated gastrointestinal discomfort, then mithramycin at 5 to 7 day intervals is a reasonable alternative. this agent may be effective at reduced doses (10 to 15 μg per kilogram) in this setting. If the use of phosphorus or mithramycin is contraindicated, therapy with calcitonin together with glucocorticoids may be attempted. If effective oral diphosphonates become available, this would be an ideal setting for their use.

Surgery is the most appropriate management for symptomatic chronic hypercalcemia of hyperparathyroidism. Medical management is indicated only in patients in whom surgery has repeatedly failed or is contraindicated. When medical management is necessary, oral phosphates can be used to control the serum calcium level, but these may potentially worsen the bone disease, since at least in some patients the reduction in serum calcium concentration will be accompanied by an increase in PTH release. In postmenopausal women, estrogen therapy may be useful in about 50 percent of cases for management of the hypercalcemia of primary hyperparathyroidism. The management of hyperparathyroidism accompanied by mild asymptomatic hypercalcemia detected on routine screening studies remains a difficult issue. We believe that unless adequate follow-up can be ensured, the risk of bone disease, renal stones, and kidney damage usually justifies surgical intervention.

Special Considerations

Mild asymptomatic hypercalcemia is present in familial hypocalciuric hypercalcemia. Associated findings include hypermagnesemia, low fractional excretion of calcium (<1 percent), and hypercalcemia in family members. Although the serum PTH level may be slightly elevated, parathyroidectomy is of no value and this diagnosis must be excluded prior to parathyroid exploration, particularly if the hypercalcemia is asymptomatic.

The hypercalcemia of hyperthyroidism frequently responds to propranolol. This can be administered intravenously (5 to 10 mg per hour), if acute reduction in calcium is necessary. When propranolol is given orally (80 to 100 mg per hour), the serum calcium level usually declines within five to seven days, during which time specific therapy directed at restoration of a euthyroid state should be initiated. Thiazide-induced hypercalcemia can be effectively treated by discontinuation of the drugs and treatment with saline and furosemide. These patients should be evaluated for possible parathyroid abnormalities and should be questioned regarding their use of over-the-counter vitamin D supplements or calcium supplements.

The mild-alkali syndrome, characterized by hypocalciuria, hypercalcemia, hyperphosphatemia, renal insufficiency, and alkalosis, was more common when large amounts of calcium carbonate and milk were prescribed for the treatment of duodenal ulcer disease. The increased calcium intake alone cannot account for the hypercalcemia; since alkalosis reduces urinary calcium excretion, it is likely that this combination of events is responsible for the maintenance of the elevated calcium. The serum calcium can usually be reduced by discontinuation of both the calcium and the alkali. If these measures fail, other causes of hypercalcemia, including hyperparathyroidism, should be considered.

HYPOCALCEMIA

Etiologic Agents

As discussed earlier, most laboratories measure only total serum calcium concentration, which is the sum of the free-ionized moiety, the complexed calcium, and the protein-bound calcium. Approximately 40 percent of the total calcium is bound by albumin and globulin. Hypoalbuminemia lowers the total serum calcium level by reducing the fraction that is bound to protein. The physiologically relevant ionized fraction is not affected by this reduction, and therefore the patient is asymptomatic. When direct measurement of the ionized fraction is not available, the effect of albumin on the serum calcium level can be approximated by assuming that for every 1-g decrement in the serum albumin, the serum calcium level will fall by 0.8 mg per deciliter.

The etiologic factors in reduced ionized calcium are given in Table 4. Since PTH serves to regulate $1,25(OH)_2D$ synthesis, and since $1,25(OH)_2D$ is necessary for the action of PTH at the level of the bone, abnormalities in one system may not be compensated for by the other. Most cases of hypocalcemia can be linked to abnormalities in the production, metabolism, or response to vitamin D and/or PTH. The removal of calcium from the serum and deposition in extravascular sites can also produce hypocalcemia.

Disorders of Vitamin D

Vitamin D deficiency may occur in a variety of ways. An understanding of the normal metabolic pathways of vitamin D allows one to better predict how a given clinical disorder might disrupt vitamin D synthesis and thereby lead to hypocalcemia. Following absorption from the duodenum and jejunum as a fat-soluble vitamin (D_2, D_3), or dermal synthesis under the influence of ultraviolet radiation (D_3), vitamin D_2 and D_3 are hydroxylated to 25(OH)D. 25(OH)D rapidly leaves the liver and a portion of this intermediate compound is further metabolized by the kidney to form $1,25(OH)_2D$—the most active D metabolite. 25(OH)D also participates in an enterohepatic circulation, and after biliary secretion approximately 80 percent of 25(OH)D or its conjugate forms are reabsorbed by the liver. The blood level of 25(OH)D is not directly influenced by primary changes in parathyroid function, calcium balance, or phosphate balance. The synthesis of $1,25(OH)_2D$ is dependent upon adequate renal function and is stimulated by PTH, hypophosphatemia, and hypocalcemia.

Dietary vitamin D deficiency is very uncommon in the Untied States because milk and other food products are fortified with vitamin D_2. Gastrointestinal disease, primarily gastric surgery, is now the predominant cause of vitamin D deficiency in the United States. Partial gastrectomy, small bowel disease, steatorrhea, malabsorption, and intestinal resection are all associated with impaired vitamin D absorption or enhanced fecal loss of 25(OH)D due to impaired enterohepatic circulation. Hepatobiliary dysfunction may lead to reduced production or enhanced metabolism of 25(OH)D. Drugs that alter hepatic metabolism, such as phenobarbital and phenytoin, may induce vitamin D deficiency via increased metabolism of 25(OH)D and impairment of vitamin D-dependent calcium absorption. Primary biliary cirrhosis is the hepatic disease most frequently associated with vitamin D defi-

TABLE 4 Causes of Hypocalcemia

Disturbances in parathyroid function
Hypoparathyroidism—surgical, infiltrative, idiopathic
Pseudohypoparathyroidism
Pseudoidiopathic hypoparathyroidism
Disturbances in vitamin D
Decreased intake—nutritional deficiency
Decreased absorption—gastrointestinal disorders
Decreased production of 25(OH)D—hepatic disorders
Increased metabolism of 25(OH)D—anticonvulsants, alcohol
Accelerated loss of 25(OH)D—impaired enterohepatic circulation, nephrotic syndrome
Decreased production of $1,25(OH)_2D$
Renal disorders, hyperphosphatemia, hereditary vitamin D-dependent rickets
Resistance to $1,25(OH)_2D$ end-organ effects
Removal of calcium
Hyperphosphatemia
Osteoblastic metastases
Hungry bones
Acute pancreatitis

ciency. The deficiency of 25(OH)D may stem from either diminished production or reduced enterohepatic reabsorption. Losses of vitamin D can also occur via the kidney. The nephrotic syndrome can result in the loss of vitamin D binding protein together with 25(OH)D. In each of these disorders, the serum levels of 25(OH)D are low. The levels of $1,25(OH)_2D$ may be normal or low depending on the presence or absence of hypocalemia-induced secondary hyperparathyroidism.

Hyperphosphatemia per se suppresses $1,25(OH)_2D$ synthesis. Defective $1,25(OH)_2D$ production can occur in association with renal parenchymal disease or as a hereditary defect of 1-hydroxylase activity (vitamin D-dependent rickets). Recently a vitamin D deficiency-like syndrome has been reported in association with elevated $1,25(OH)_2D$ levels, and these patients appear to have end-organ resistance to vitamin D metabolites.

Disorders of the Parathyroid System

Hypocalcemia can arise from either reduced production of PTH (hypoparathyroidism) or end-organ resistance to PTH (pseudohypoparathyroidism). Hypoparathyroidism commonly occurs following thryoid, parathyroid or radical neck surgery. Other causes include infiltrative disorders (amyloidosis, hemochromatosis, malignancy) and idiopathic hypoparathyroidism. The latter disease is often associated with idiopathic adrenal insufficiency, pernicious anemia, hypothyroidism, and diabetes mellitus.

Most patients with pseudohypoparathyroidism have a characteristic short stature, mental retardation, and shortening of the third and fourth metacarpals. Although usually both the kidney and bone demonstrate resistance to the effects of PTH, resistance may rarely exist only at one end organ. Pseudoidiopathic hypoparathyroidism is associated with high PTH levels and a normal renal response to exogenous PTH infusion. Thus, this disorder appears to be due to the secretion of a defective species of PTH. A similar defect may be present in some patients with pseudohypoparathyroidism.

Hypomagnesemia and Hypermagnesemia

With hypomagnesemia of any cause (serum magnesium <1 mg per deciliter), hypocalcemia can occur due to reduced PTH secretion and/or to inhibition of the skeletal effects of PTH. Brisk saline diuresis, loop diuretics, aminoglycosides, and cis-platinum therapy may all increase magnesium excretion. Alcoholism, small bowel disease, and diarrhea are common causes of impaired magnesium absorption.

Increases in serum magnesium (>5.5 mg per deciliter) may suppress PTH release and reduce renal calcium reabsorption and lead to hypocalcemia. Hypermagnesemia frequently occurs during the acute management of eclampsia and during the inadvertent use of magnesium-containing cathartics in patients with renal insufficiency.

Hyperphosphatemia, Pancreatitis, Osteoblastic Metastases and "Hungry Bones"

The removal of calcium from the circulation and its deposition elsewhere can produce severe, acute hypocalcemia. Acute hyperphosphatemia from any cause (infusion, ingestion, use of phosphate enemas and laxatives) can lead to hypocalcemia by chelation with ionized calcium. Severe hyperphosphatemia may be seen with rhabdomyolysis and often accompanies the cytotoxic treatment of lymphoma and leukemia. Hyperkalemia, hyperuricemia, and renal failure may occur in these settings. Chronic hyperphosphatemia can lead to hypocalcemia by reducing $1,25(OH)_2D$ synthesis and enhancing extravascular deposition. The precipitation of calcium soaps appears to be the major mechanism responsible for the hypocalcemia associated with acute pancreatitis. Additionally, pancreatitis may lead to suppression of PTH release.

The osteoblastic metastases which occasionally accompany carcinoma of the breast, prostate, and lung lead to enhanced deposition of calcium into bone. Enhanced bone formation may also occur following the surgical treatment of hyperparathyroidism. When bone formation is greatly stimulated, the skeletal deposition of calcium, phosphate, and magnesium may result in marked reductions in the serum levels of these minerals. This "hungry bone" syndrome is most likely to occur when radiographic evidence of significant osteitis fibrosa and an elevated alkaline phosphatase level are present preoperatively. It is frequently seen following parathyroidectomy in patients with chronic renal failure and secondary hyperparathyroidism.

Signs and Symptoms

The manifestations of hypocalcemia range from a vague feeling of ill health to life-threatening neuromuscular and cardiovascular dysfunction. The development of symptomatic hypocalcemia probably relates to the rate at which the ionized calcium level falls. A relatively small, acute drop in ionized calcium may produce symptoms, whereas moderate chronic hypocalcemia is often asymptomatic.

The symptoms of hypocalcemia are given in Table 5. The hallmark of hypocalcemia is tetany with markedly enhanced neuromuscular irritability. Latent tetany may be

TABLE 5 Signs and Symptoms of Hypocalcemia

Neuromuscular
Paresthesias, tetany, muscle cramps, seizures, anxiety, depression, dementia, movement disorders, proximal myopathy
Cardiovascular
ECG changes, hypotension, congestive heart failure, arrhythmias
Ectodermal
Brittle, dry hair, alopecia, dry skin, cataracts, delayed dentition

detected in otherwise asymptomatic patients by tapping over the facial nerve to produce a facial twitch (Chvostek's sign) or by inflating a blood pressure cuff over systolic pressure for 3 minutes to produce carpal spasms (Trousseu's sign). Clinically, tetany usually begins with circumoral and facial paresthesias. Motor manifestations include stiffness, muscle cramps, and the characteristic spontaneous carpopedal spasms. Other less common complications of severe hypocalcemia include laryngeal stridor with ventilatory failure, frank seizures, hypotension and congestive heart failure due to decreased myocardial contractility, and ventricular arrhythmias. Resistance to digitalis may occur with hypocalcemia. The electrocardiogram reveals a characteristic lengthening of Q-T interval, which is best detected by measuring the QT intervals, since the ST segment is lengthened but the T-wave is not affected.

More chronic manifestations of hypocalcemia include mental retardation in children and psychosis and dementia in adults. In children, delayed or defective dentition and extrapyramidal movement disorders may be present. Anterior and posterior subcapsular cataracts, dermatitits, and patchy alopecia may occur. Although skeletal abnormalities (osteomalacia, osteopenia) are often present, their pathogenesis appears to be more closely linked to deficiencies of vitamin D and phosphate rather than to hypocalcemia per se. Similarly, the occurrence of proximal myopathy is most closely related to the presence of secondary hyperparathyroidism, phosphate depletion, or vitamin D deficiency.

Therapeutic Modalities

The preparations of calcium and vitamin D commonly available are given in Table 6. The calcium preparations vary greatly in their elemental calcium content and this must be taken into consideration when prescribing them. Similar care must be taken when recommending over-the-counter calcium preparations, since some of these compounds contain both calcium and vitamin D. We generally prefer to use calcium carbonate, as it is relatively well tolerated and inexpensive. Numerous vitamin D preparations are available and, as will be discussed, some are more likely to be effective in selected situations. Dihydrotachysterol (DHT), $1,25(OH)_2D$ (calcitriol), and 1α-hydroxycholecalciferol (1α-OH-D_3, available in Europe) do not require renal metabolism to be effective.

Therapeutic Approach

Acute Hypocalcemia

Acute hypocalcemia accompanied by tetany or cardiovascular or respiratory complications demands emergent therapy. Findings of latent tetany alone do not indicate the need for emergency therapy. However, if these are accompanied by early signs of tetany (circumoral paresthesia) or other symptoms, then therapy is warranted. The treatment of acute hypocalcemia of any cause begins with intravenous infusion of 200 to 300 mg of elemental calcium. We prefer to use calcium gluconate since it is less irritating than calcium chloride. Each 10-ml ampule of 10 percent calcium gluconate provides 93 mg of elemental calcium and 2 to 3 ampules can be infused over 10 to 15 minutes. If the symptoms are severe or fail to resolve after the initial therapy, calcium can be administered by continuous intravenous infusion. Fifteen milligrams per kilogram of body weight of elemental calcium (as calcium gluconate) can be administered in D5W every 6 hours. If magnesium depletion is possibly present, blood should be drawn for a magnesium determination, and if renal function is intact, magnesium sulfate should be administered. Several magnesium preparations of varying strengths are available and care must be taken to ensure that the dose of elemental magnesium is appropriate. Each 10-ml ampule of 10 percent magnesium sulfate contains 97 mg of elemental magnesium and one to two ampules can be administered intravenously over a 60-minute period. Every effort should be made to obtain the serum magnesium value as quickly as possible. Until the serum magnesium is available, if magnesium depletion is strongly suspected, intramuscular injections of 2 to 3 ml of a 50 percent magnesium sulfate solution can be given every 4 to 6 hours (2 ml of a 50 percent magnesium sulfate solution

TABLE 6 Therapeutic Modalities for Treatment of Hypocalcemia

Calcium Preparations	*Percent Elemental Calcium*
Calcium carbonate	40
Calcium chloride	36
Calcium lactate	12
Calcium gluconate	8

Vitamin D Preparations	*Daily Antirachitic Dose (μg)**	*Daily Dose in Hypoparathyroidism (μg)**	*Time Required to Achieve Effect (wk)*
Vitamin D_2 (ergocalciferol)	2–10	700–8000	4–8
25(OH)D (calcifediol)	1–5	20–100	2–4
Dihydrotachysterol (DHT)	100–500	250–1000	1–2
$(OH)_2D1,25$ (calcitriol)	.25–.75	.25–2.0	½–1

* These are average doses, individual requirements vary. During dosage titration period serum calcium level should be measured 1 or 2 times per week.

contains 97 mg of magnesium). Once significant magnesium depletion is documented, its cause should be evaluated and oral magnesium (as MgO) or intramuscular magnesium should be continued until the serum value returns to normal. Empiric magnesium therapy is absolutely contraindicated in the presence of renal insufficiency.

Acute Hypocalcemia: Specific Clinical Settings

Postsurgical. Transient hypocalcemia frequently occurs after surgery on the parathyroid glands or adjacent structures. If acute symptomatic hypocalcemia occurs, it should be managed as outlined above. More commonly, subacute hypocalcemia is present and this is best managed with slow, continuous intravenous calcium infusion followed by oral calcium supplementation when oral intake is resumed. Postsurgical hypoparathyroidism often persists for 10 to 14 days, and during this interval we recommend continued oral calcium supplements along with a modest restriction in phosphate intake. If the hypocalcemia or hyperphosphatemia persists beyound 14 days, it is likely that the hypoparathyroidism will be permanent and chronic therapy should be instituted. Close follow-up is important, since even patients with protracted postsurgical hypoparathyroidism may recover and become hypercalcemic on therapy.

Subtotal parathyroidectomy for marked secondary hyperparathyroidism is often complicated by the hungry bone syndrome. If preoperative evaluation reveals evidence of significant PTH-related skeletal disease, the patient is more likely to develop this syndrome, and in this setting it is often helpful to increase the serum calcium level to 11 to 12 mg per deciliter a few days before surgery by calcitriol supplementation (.25 to .5 μg per day). Both calcium and calcitriol should be continued postoperatively and the serum calcium, phosphate, and magnesium levels must be closely monitored. Initially, adequate maintenance of serum calcium may require 1.0 to 2.0 μg per day of calcitriol and 3 to 4 g of oral calcium daily, along with phosphate and magnesium. In very severe cases intravenous calcium may be necessary. As bone healing occurs the calcium requirement falls and the therapeutic regimen must be appropriately adjusted. Since serum alkaline phosphatase levels decline as bone healing occurs, to avoid hypercalcemia the calcium and calcitriol dosages should be reduced as soon as these levels begin to fall.

Hypocalcemia with Acute Hyperphosphatemia. As indicated above, hyperphosphatemia from any cause can lead to hypocalcemia. Usually, the hypocalcemia is associated with only mild symptoms, and in view of the concomitant hyperphosphatemia, calcium therapy should be avoided. Therapy should be aimed at reducing the serum phosphate concentration and at correcting the underlying cause of the hyperphosphatemia.

Chronic Hypocalcemia

Hypoparathyroidism and Hypocalcemia. In hypoparathyroidism the initial therapy is to provide calcium in the range of 2 to 4 g of elemental calcium per day. In patients with mild hypoparathyroidism calcium alone may be sufficient. However, in most cases therapy with vitamin D is also required. As indicated in Table 6, large doses of either vitamin D_2 or calcifediol can be used effectively. The need for these pharmacologic doses reflects the loss of the stimulating effect of PTH on renal $1,25(OH)_2D$ production. Alternatively, one may use smaller doses of either DHT or calcitriol. We prefer to use these compounds and usually begin therapy with calcitriol. The advantage of calcitriol is that it will quickly improve the hypocalcemia, and if the patient become hypercalcemic with therapy, it will resolve quickly upon discontinuation of the drug. The disadvantages are its expense and the fact that it bypasses the renal hydroxylation feedback mechanism that normally serves to regulate the synthesis of $1,25(OH)_2D$ from 25(OH)D. We believe that usually these disadvantages are outweighted by calcitriol's ability to reliably achieve calcemic control without risking the "overshoot" hypercalcemia that frequently occurs with D_2 and calcifediol therapy, or prolonged periods of hypercalcemia that occur with these agents and DHT. The goal of therapy is to maintain the serum calcium level between 8 and 9.5 mg per deciliter. Values within this range protect against the untoward effects of hypocalcemia, but avoid the occurrence of marked hypercalciuria. The hypercalciuria is due to the loss of the renal action of PTH. In all cases of hypoparathyroidism therapy must be individualized. Some patients may require only calcium or calcitriol, whereas others will require both modalities to maintain the serum calcium concentration in an acceptable range. Additionally, there is always a risk of unexpected hypercalcemia, especially in patients receiving both vitamin D and calcium, and thus routine monitoring of the serum calcium level is mandatory.

Finally, in patients with mild hypoparathyroidism receiving only calcium supplements, the addition of thiazide diuretics may maintain the serum calcium level between 9 and 10 mg per deciliter while simultaneously reducing the hypercalciuria. Unless very close follow-up can be ensured, we do not recommend the use of thiazides in conjunction with vitamin D therapy because potentiation of hypercalcemia may occur unpredictably.

Patients with pseudohypoparathyroidism are best managed with calcitriol. In this disorder the depressed levels of $1,25(OH)_2D$ are due, at least in part, to renal unresponsiveness to PTH. Thus, small doses of this preparation will usually suffice.

Chronic Hypocalcemia: Vitamin D Deficiency States. Optimal management of hypocalcemia due to vitamin D deficiency is partly dependent upon the underlying cause of the disorder. The rare patient with nutritional deficiency can be managed with small, physiologic doses of vitamin D_2 (2 to 10 μg daily). Disorders associated with malabsorption can be managed with pharmacologic amounts of vitamin D_2 (100 to 300 μg or more daily). In the presence of malabsorption concurrent magnesium depletion should always be considered. If the vitamin D deficiency is secondary to intestinal resection or impaired enterohepatic circulation, calcifediol therapy (50 to 100 μg daily) may be adequate. In all cases of gastrointestinal dysfunction, adequate calcium intake must be maintained. This can usually be achieved by dietary calcium supplementation to ensure daily intake of 2 to 3 g of elemental calcium. Finally, since certain gastrointestinal disorders, such as Crohn's disease, display less marked resistance to vitamin D, it is critical that the optimal regimen be found for each patient, and in some cases, such as celiac sprue, appropriate treatment of the underlying disorder may obviate the need for exogenous supplementation.

Primary biliary cirrhosis can be adequately managed with calcium (1 to 2 g per day) and either vitamin D_2 or calcifediol. Although larger doses of vitamin D_2 are required, it is less expensive that calcifediol. Altered vitamin D metabolism secondary to anticonvulsants can be treated with vitamin D_2 (250 μg daily) and prevented by doses of 125 to 375 μg weekly. Alternatively, physiologic doses of 25(OH)D can be used. These patients usually do not require calcium supplementation. Similarly, if true (ionized) hypocalcemia is present in association with the nephrotic syndrome and vitamin D deficiency, it can be managed with either vitamin D_2 or 25(OH)D.

In general, states of vitamin D deficiency in which 1-hydroxylation is intact should not be treated with compounds such as DHT and calcitriol. These compounds bypass the renal site of feedback control of $1,25(OH)_2D_3$ synthesis and carry a greater risk of inducing hypercalcemia. Periodic measurement of 25(OH)D levels is useful in assessing adequacy of therapy, and since alterations in a variety of factors, such as endogenous estrogens, renal functions, and dietary calcium intake, may occur over time, all patients receiving long-term calcium and vitamin D supplementation must have their serum values routinely monitored.

Chronic Hypocalcemia-Renal Disorders. Vitamin D-dependent rickets, due to defective renal hydroxylation of 25(OH)D, is best managed with small physiologic doses of calcitriol. As long as dietary calcium intake is adequate (1 to 2 g daily), additional calcium supplementation is usually not required. The hypocalcemia of acute renal failure is usually asymptomatic or associated with only minimal symptoms and the initial therapy should be directed at correcting the serum phosphate level by administration of phosphate binding antacids. During the recovery phase of acute renal failure, especially in the setting of rhabdomyolysis and hyperphosphatemia, hypocalcemia can quickly resolve and frank hypercalcemia may occur. One must anticipate this possibility so that the needed adjustments in the therapeutic regimen can be made. The hypocalcemia of chronic renal insufficiency and end-stage renal disease is usually asymptomatic, and therapy is aimed at preventing or treating the associated secondary hyperparathyroidism and bone disease. Since both hyperphosphatemia and $1,25(OH)_2D$ deficiency contribute to the hypocalcemia, a two-pronged therapeutic approach is useful. The first step is the reduction of hyperphosphatemia with dietary phosphate restriction and phosphate-binding antacids. In early renal insufficiency this alone may be adequate. As renal parenchymal mass decreases, therapy with calcium and then with vitamin D is usually required. An elemental calcium intake of 1 to 2 g per day and vitamin D, as either DHT or calcitriol (.25 to 1.5 μg daily), are useful, since these compounds do not require renal hydroxylation to be effective. The goal of therapy is to maintain the serum calcium level between 10 and 10.5 mg per deciliter and the serum phosphate level between 4 and 5 mg per deciliter. Calcium therapy should not be instituted if hyperphosphatemia is present, and patients receiving such treatment must have their blood levels of calcium and phosphate routinely monitored.

HYPOPHOSPHATEMIA AND PHOSPHATE DEPLETION

GEORGE C. YU, M.D.
DAVID B. N. LEE, M.D.

Phosphorus is an essential element for all human tissues and is the major intracellular anion. It exists in both organic and inorganic forms. Organic phosphorus comprises the phospholipids, nucleic acids, and phosphoproteins that are needed for cellular integrity and metabolism. Intracellular inorganic phosphorus provides substrate for the synthesis of a large number of life-sustaining phosphorus compounds, including adenosine triphosphate (ATP). Serum phosphorus is mostly in inorganic forms consisting of orthophosphate ions. In an adult the normal serum phosphorus concentration ranges from 3.0 to 4.5 mg per deciliter. The human body contains about 600 to 700 g of phosphorus, of which 80 to 85 percent is found in bone, 10 to 15 percent in soft tissue, and only about 1 percent in the extracellular fluid (ECF).

Average dietary phosphorus intake varies from 800 to 1,200 mg per day. The percentage of dietary phosphorus absorbed by the intestine remains remarkably constant at 60 to 65 percent over a wide range of phosphorus intake (4 to 30 mg per kilogram per day). Thus, the dietary intake of phosphorus is an important determinant of the amount of phosphorus absorbed. In addition, phosphate absorption is regulated by vitamin D, mainly through the action of its active metabolite 1,25-dihydroxyvitamin D ($1,25\ (OH)_2D$). Phosphorus is present in most food, especially red meat, dairy products, fish, poultry, and the legumes. The phosphorus, absorbed as phosphate ions from the intestinal lumen into ECF, is handled by two general processes: an intracellular-extracellular phosphate shift mechanism and the renal phosphate excretory mechanism. The absorbed phosphate is first "buffered" by shifting into the soft tissue cells (and probably also the skeleton). Any excess phosphate is ultimately excreted by the kidneys. Shifts of phosphate between extracellular and intracellular compartments cause acute changes in serum phosphorus levels without changes in total phosphorus balance. Renal phosphate excretion is determined by the difference between phosphate filtered at the glomerulus and phosphate absorbed by the tubule. Normally, about 85 percent of the filtered phosphate is reabsorbed by the tubule, and the remaining 15 percent is excreted in the urine. The maximal tubular phosphate reabsorptive capacity (TmP) plays a major role in the maintenance of long-term, steady-state serum phosphorus concentration, i.e., the higher the TmP the higher the serum phosphorus concentration. The total body phosphorus balance is maintained by urinary excretion of the excess phosphate absorbed by the intestine. In an individual who is in phosphorus balance, urinary phosphate would equal the phosphate absorbed. Factors that may influence renal phosphate reabsorption are listed in Table 1.

It is important to distinguish the terms hypophosphatemia, phosphorus deprivation, and phosphorus depletion. *Hypophosphatemia* simply means a serum phosphorus concentration below the range found in the normal population. Sustained hypophosphatemia encountered in clinical practice generally represents conditions with abnormal reduction in TmP, rather than phosphorus deprivation or depletion. Reduction in TmP can be caused by excessive parathyroid hormone secretion or by intrinsic tubular transport defects. *Phosphorus deprivation* is generally used to mean selective omission of phosphorus from the diet, sometimes accompanied by the administration of intestinal phosphate binders. This should be distinguished from complete starvation, which implies total caloric deprivation. Starvation leads to a catabolic state with loss of water, nitrogen, potassium, phosphorus, and magnesium in the same proportion as in the tissues. The phosphorus content of the remaining tissue would therefore be normal for the reduced body mass. Thus, hypophosphatemia is not a feature of starvation per se. *Phosphorus depletion* indicates a state in which actual reduction in the body phosphorus store occurs. The distinction between phosphorus deprivation and phosphorus depletion is important because many biochemical changes attributed to phosphorus depletion in fact develop within hours of phosphorus removal from the diet, i.e., long before appreciable net phosphorus loss from the body can occur.

Hypophosphatemia associated with ample phosphate in the urine suggests an abnormally low TmP as the cause of the reduction in serum phosphorus concentration. In such conditions, total body phosphorus balance may still be maintained, and phosphorus depletion may not develop. The laboratory hallmark of phosphorus deprivation and phosphorus depletion is hypophosphatemia associated with the virtual absence of phosphate in the urine. The reappearance of phosphate in the urine indicates phosphate repletion through either exogenous phosphate administration or endogenous release of phosphate into ECF. The latter condition may be brought about by catabolic states such as starvation or the administration of large doses of glucocorticoids.

TABLE 1 Factors Influencing Renal Handling of Phosphates

Decreased Renal Phosphate Absorption
Hormonal
Parathyroid hormone
Glucocorticoids
Sex hormones
Calcitonin
Thyroid hormone
Metabolic
High dietary phosphate intake
Metabolic acidosis
Alcoholism
Urinary alkalinization
Diuresis
Diuretics
Osmotic load
Extracellular fluid volume expansion
Increased Renal Phosphate Absorption
Hormonal
Insulin
Vitamin D metabolites
Growth hormone
Metabolic
Dietary phosphate restriction
Hypercalcemia
Hypermagnesemia

CAUSES OF HYPOPHOSPHATEMIA AND PHOSPHORUS DEPLETION

Hypophosphatemia may result from three general mechanisms. They are increased phosphate shift into cells and bone, decreased intestinal phosphate absorption or increased intestinal loss of phosphate, and inappropriate urinary phosphate loss through reduction in renal phosphate reabsorptive capacity. Chronic, stable hypophosphatemia of moderate severity (serum phosphorus level 1.5–2.5 mg per deciliter) is generally caused by a reduction in the maximal renal phosphate absorptive capacity and does not manifest characteristics of the phosphorus depletion syndrome. Severe hypophosphatemia (serum phosphorus level < 1.5 mg per deciliter), on the other hand, is often associated with phosphorus deprivation or depletion and may be accompanied by clinical manifestations of the phosphorus depletion syndrome. It is obvious, however, that hypophosphatemia does not always indicate phosphorus depletion. Table 2 summarizes the hypophosphatemic disorders encountered in clinical practice.

TABLE 2 Conditions Associated with Hypophosphatemia

Conditions	*Altered Phosphate Metabolism:* *Increased Transcellular Shift*	*Decreased Intestinal Absorption*	*Reduced Renal Reabsorption*
Carbohydrate load	+		
Nutritional recovery syndrome and hyperalimentation*	+		
Respiratory alkalosis	+		
Rapid cell growth*	+		
"Hungry bone syndrome"	+		
Selective dietary phosphorus deprivation*		+	
Administration of phosphate binding antacids*		+	
Vomiting		+	
Prolonged nasogastric suction		+	
Severe malabsorption disorders		+	
Hyperparathyroidism			+
Primary renal tubular disorders			+
Secondary renal tubular disorders			+
Acidosis	+		
Severe burns*	+		
Gout	+		
Sodium lactate administration	+		
Abnormal vitamin D metabolic states		+	+
Oncogenic hypophosphatemia		+	+
Hemodialysis*		+	+
Diabetic ketoacidosis*	+	+	+
Alcoholism*	+	+	+
Postrenal transplantation	+	+	+

* Conditions that may cause severe hypophosphatemia and phosphorus depletion.

Hypophosphatemia Associated with Increased Phosphate Shift into Cells and Bone

The most common cause of acute hypophosphatemia in hospitals is the intravenous administration of carbohydrate, usually glucose. The reduction in serum phosphorus concentration is usually modest and transient. Fructose administration, on the other hand, may lead to more prolonged and pronounced decrease in serum phosphorus. This is due to the intracellular trapping of phosphate as fructose-1-phosphate. The lack of negative feedback by the end-product fructose-1-phosphate on the enzyme fructokinase allows for the continual cellular uptake of phosphate. Severe hypophosphatemia may develop especially in those with congenital fructose intolerance.

The nutritional recovery syndrome was first observed during rapid refeeding of severely malnourished prisoners of war. The modern equivalent of this syndrome can be seen in intravenous feeding of patients with severe debilitation or anorexia nervosa, especially if the hyperalimentation solutions are deficient in phosphates. The anabolic state from refeeding promotes an intracellular shift of phosphate and may lead to severe hypophosphatemia, frequently associated with hypokalemia and hypomagnesemia.

Respiratory alkalosis is a common cause of moderate to severe hypophosphatemia. Hyperventilation leads to a reduction of intracellular carbon dioxide and an increase of intracellular pH, which activates phosphofructokinase. This results in accelerated glycolysis, and the enhanced glucose phosphorylation promotes transcellular phosphate influx. Salicylate overdose and gram-negative sepsis are thought to cause hypophosphatemia through respiratory alkalosis. In addition, the massive release of catecholamines with sepsis also promotes cellular uptake of phosphate.

Rapid tumor growth may cause hypophosphatemia by increasing phosphate demand for cell proliferation and growth. An interesting case of recurrent, severe hypophosphatemia has been reported in a patient with T cell lymphoblastic leukemia accompanied by an increase in tumor burden followed by hyperphosphatemia after chemotherapy. The underlying mechanism of hypophosphatemia was thought to be the rapid tumor growth and the high intracellular phosphate content of a lymphoblast compared with a mature lymphocyte.

The "hungry bone syndrome" is a rare disorder in which hypophosphatemia develops as a result of therapy leading to rapid new bone formation in a severely demineralized skeleton. This may follow subtotal parathyroidectomy in a patient with primary or secondary hyperparathyroidism.

Hypophosphatemia Associated with Decreased Absorption or Increased Loss of Phosphate in the Intestine

Because of the universal presence of phosphate in food, selective dietary phosphorus deficiency is generally achieved only under experimental conditions. Certain aluminum- and magnesium-containing antacids avidly bind to intestinal phosphate and render it nonabsorbable. When this condition is superimposed on poor oral intake, vomiting, or prolonged nasogastric suction severe hypophosphatemia may result. Malabsorptive disorders, per se, rarely cause significant net phosphate loss.

Hypophosphatemia Associated with Reduced Maximal Renal Phosphate Reabsorptive Capacity

Hyperparathyroidism is a common cause of moderate hypophosphatemia. Parathyroid hormone reduces renal phosphate reabsorptive capacity and leads to a low serum phosphorus concentration. Primary renal tubular disorders associated with hypophosphatemia include renal tubular acidosis and the Fanconi syndrome. The conditions that lead to secondary renal tubular dysfunction and renal phosphate wasting are listed in Table 1.

Hypophosphatemia Associated with Both Increased Intracellular Phosphate Shift and Decreased Renal Phosphate Reabsorptive Capacity

Acidosis induces decomposition of intracellular organic compounds with release of inorganic phosphate, which is subsequently excreted in the urine. Hypophosphatemia generally develops during the treatment of acidosis from resynthesis of organic compounds and intracellular shift of inorganic phosphate.

Severe burn injury may also induce hypophosphatemia. The lowest serum phosphorus level is commonly seen on the fifth day. Hypophosphatemia may last from 2 to 10 days. Possible mechanisms include respiratory alkalosis, gram-negative sepsis, and pain as well as rapid tissue build-up. These patients also have an inappropriate phosphaturia in the face of severe hypophosphatemia, thus suggesting a defect in renal tubular phosphate reabsorption.

The hypophosphatemia of untreated gout has been attributed to respiratory alkalosis produced by pain-induced hyperventilation and a reduction in renal phosphate reabsorption secondary to tubular damage.

Sodium lactate infusion promotes phosphaturia through volume expansion. The lactate also increases hepatic glucose production and consequent intracellular phosphate shift.

Hypophosphatemia Associated with Reduced Renal Phosphate Reabsorptive Capacity and Decreased Intestinal Absorption of Phosphate

Hypophosphatemia, renal phosphaturia, and impaired intestinal absorption of calcium and phosphate are common features of vitamin D-deficient, -dependent, and -resistant rickets or osteomalacia.

Oncogenic hypophosphatemia is an interesting entity associated with mesenchymal tumors. The underlying mechanism is unclear but may be related to an increased sensitivity to the phosphaturic effect of parathyroid hormone, a reduced level of $1{,}25(OH)_2D$ or the production of an unknown phosphaturic agent.

Severe hypophosphatemia has been described in dialysis patients and attributed to a combination of phosphate loss through dialysis and intensive use of phosphate-binding antacids.

Hypophosphatemia Associated with Increased Intracellular Phosphate Shift and Reduction in Both Renal Phosphate Reabsorptive Capacity and Intestinal Absorption of Phosphate

In clinical practice, severe hypophosphatemia is often encountered in patients recovering from diabetic ketoacidosis and alcohol withdrawal. Patients with diabetic ketoacidosis often have decreased phosphate intake from anorexia, nausea, and vomiting prior to hospitalization. Concomitant metabolic acidosis enhances breakdown of intracellular organic phosphates, and the catabolic effects of insulin deficiency promote a phosphate shift into the ECF, thereby leading to increased phosphaturia. Glycosuria and ketonuria induce further renal phosphate loss. Before treatment, despite normal or even increased serum phosphorus concentrations, these patients have a total body phosphorus deficit. During treatment, insulin administration promotes glycolysis and oxidative phosphorylation with a rapid shift of phosphates into the cells. In addition, vigorous fluid replacement may enhance renal phosphate excretion. Usually, 6 to 12 hours following the initiation of therapy for diabetic ketoacidosis, the serum phosphorus level may fall precipitously.

Another clinical setting in which severe hypophosphatemia often arises is in the hospitalized patient with chronic alcoholism. The patient may have decreased phosphate intake from poor diet or vomiting. Steatorrhea and malabsorption due to chronic pancreatitis and alcoholic cirrhosis may lead to vitamin D deficiency and resultant secondary hyperparathyroidism. Both entities lead to increased renal and intestinal loss of phosphates. In addition, concomitant alcoholic ketosis, hypokalemia, and hypomagnesemia may promote further renal phosphate clearance. During hospitalization, nutritional repletion with intravenous glucose solution leads to increased cellular phosphate uptake. This transcellular phosphate shift is further enhanced by respiratory alkalosis from alcohol withdrawal, hepatic encephalopathy, or concomitant sepsis. The use of phosphate-binding antacids for gastrointestinal bleeding or lactulose further aggravates hypophosphatemia. Typically, severe hypophosphatemia can develop 24 to 72 hours following hospital admission.

Hypophosphatemia may be seen in one-third of renal transplant recipients. Reduced renal phosphate reabsorptive capacity is an important contributing factor. The possible mechanisms for renal phosphate wasting include persistent hyperparathyroidism, subnormal graft function, corticosteroid and diuretic therapy, and chronic volume expansion. The use of phosphate-binding antacids for peptic ulcer prophylaxis leads to decreased intestinal absorption of phosphate. In addition, the resolution of hyperparathyroidism coupled with an increase in circulating 1,25 $(OH)_2D$ may promote healing of renal osteodystrophy with rapid cellular influx of calcium and phosphorus. In some chronically malnourished uremic patients, a post-transplant anabolic state may promote a further intracellular shift of phosphate for cell synthesis.

CLINICAL CONSEQUENCES OF SEVERE HYPOPHOSPHATEMIA AND PHOSPHORUS DEPLETION

Multiple organ dysfunction may occur as a result of severe hypophosphatemia and phosphorus depletion. These disturbances from hypophosphatemia invariably occur in patients with chronic debilitation, often in the setting of pre-existing cellular injury. Acute hypophosphatemia in experimental animals resulting from transcellular phosphate shift is not associated with manifestations of the phosphorus depletion syndrome.

The clinical sequelae of severe hypophosphatemia and phosphorus depletion are the results of three critical biochemical disturbances. First, the level of 2,3-diphosphoglycerate (2,3-DPG) in the erythrocyte is decreased, leading to increased oxygen affinity of the hemoglobin and resultant tissue hypoxia. Second, there is a decrease in the intracellular concentration of ATP, the energy source needed for cell functions. Third, inorganic phosphate is a crucial cofactor in the glyceraldehydephosphate-dehydrogenase step of the Embden-Meyerhof pathway, and a deficiency of intracellular inorganic phosphate may impair glycolysis.

The critical determinants of cellular injury appear to be the level of inorganic phosphate and adenine nucleotide in the cytosol. When cytosolic ATP decreases below a critical level, cellular dysfunction or necrosis may ensue. The cytosolic inorganic phosphate is essential for the formation of ATP from ADP. In addition, intracellular inorganic phosphate has an important role in determining the cellular pool of adenine nucleotides. Normally, ATP, ADP, and adenosine monophosphate (AMP) are related by the following reaction:

$$2\ ADP \gtrless AMP + ATP$$

A major degradation pathway for AMP is the irreversible deamination to inosine monophosphate (IMP) through the action of AMP-deaminase. This enzyme is inhibited by a normal intracellular phosphate concentration. Therefore, a significant reduction in intracellular inorganic phosphate may result in AMP degradation and a decrease of the total adenine nucleotide pool. In addition, a drop in ATP concentration enhances the action of 5 ′ nucleotidase, which further reduces the amount of nucleotides. Any demand in energy production may place the cell in danger of disintegration from a further decrease in intracellular ATP concentration. The various systemic dysfunctions in severe hypophosphatemia and phosphate depletion are listed in Table 3.

TABLE 3 Clinical Manifestations of Severe Hypophosphatemia and Phosphorus Depletion

Cardiac
Reversible cardiomyopathy
Depressed vascular response to vasopressors
Respiratory
Acute respiratory failure
Hyper- or hypoventilation
Neurologic
Paresthesia
Confusion
Seizures
Coma
Intention tremor
Ataxia
Guillain-Barré-like syndrome
Muscular
Generalized weakness
Proximal myopathy
Rhabdomyolysis
Hematologic
Reduced red cell 2,3-DPG
Hemolytic anemia
Impaired leukocytic chemotaxis, phagocytosis, and bacterial killing
Platelet dysfunction
Skeletal
Osteomalacia with bone pain and pseudofractures
Nonosteomalacic bone disease
Renal
Hypophosphaturia
Hypercalciuria
Hypermagnesuria
Hyperchloremic metabolic acidosis
Endocrine
Functional hypoparathyroidism
Glucose intolerance

Experimental evidence points to a significant impairment of the cardiovascular system in severe hypophosphatemia. An increased cardiac index was found in critically ill hypophosphatemic patients given phosphorus replacement. Cardiac arrhythmia can occur in acute hypophosphatemia. Reversible congestive heart failure has been found in patients taking large amounts of phosphate-binders. Decreased vascular reactivity to angiotensin II and norepinephrine has been shown in phosphorus-depleted animals.

Acute respiratory failure from respiratory muscle weakness is a serious complication of severe hypophosphatemia. Reversible hypophosphatemia-induced diaphragmatic weakness and pulmonary insufficiency has been demonstrated. Hypophosphatemia may induce hyperventilation, possibly the result of poor tissue oxygenation from decreased erythrocyte 2,3-DPG levels. Hyperventilation leads to respiratory alkalosis and further lowering of the serum phosphorus. The vicious cycle may finally induce hypoventilation due to respiratory muscle fatigue.

Various neurologic manifestations may follow phosphorus depletion. Severe hypophosphatemia can result in a metabolic encephalopathy with paresthesia, tremor, ataxia, weakness, irritability, confusion, seizure, and eventually coma. This has been shown in patients receiving phosphate-deficient hyperalimentation and could be prevented with adequate phosphate supplementation.

Muscle biopsy of hypophosphatemic alcoholics has revealed a decrease in cellular phosphorus and an increase in intracellular sodium, chloride, and water. This may account for the generalized weakness or proximal myopathy seen in some hypophosphatemic patients. Severe hypophosphatemia may induce rhabdomyolysis with elevations of serum creatine phosphokinase levels. This is usually asymptomatic or clinically mild. Occasionally, profound weakness, muscle pain, and acute myoglobinuric renal failure may develop.

A fall in serum phosphorus level leads to a decrease in intracellular inorganic phosphate in the erythrocyte. This in turn leads to impaired glycolysis with a fall in intracellular ATP. The elasticity of the red cell membrane is maintained by a microfilament system dependent on ATP for energy sources. Therefore, insufficient ATP causes erythrocyte rigidity and may lead to fragmentation in the microcirculation. Hemolytic anemia may occur when serum phosphorus concentration falls below 0.5 mg per deciliter. Another important biochemical consequence of hypophosphatemia in erythrocytes is the drop in 2,3-DPG, which leads to a leftward shift in the hemoglobin-oxygen dissociation curve. The increased oxygen binding by the red cell results in decreased peripheral oxygen delivery and tissue hypoxia.

Experimental studies have shown defects of chemotaxis, phagocytosis, and bacterial killing in leukocytes of hypophosphatemic animals. This may be related to impaired microtubular actions from low cellular ATP and abnormal membrane synthesis.

Thrombocytopenia, decreased platelet survival, and impaired clot retraction have been demonstrated in experimental hypophosphatemic animals. These may be due to a reduction of platelet ATP content. However, similar clinical findings have not been observed in humans.

Osteomalacia and pathologic fractures have been described in antacid-induced phosphate depletion. A recent study reported ten male patients with chronic hypophosphatemia due to renal phosphate wasting and with bone disease other than osteomalacia. These patients have decreased parathyroid hormone, osteopenia, normal osteoid volume, and calcification front. A possible X-linked transmission was proposed.

Phosphorus depletion leads to hypophosphaturia, hypercalciuria, and hypermagnesuria. Measurements of these urinary electrolytes have been proposed as diagnostic criteria for a true phosphorus deficient state.

Metabolic acidosis may also result from severe hypophosphatemia via three mechanisms. First, a decrease in titratable acid excretion follows hypophosphaturia. Second, a fall in renal ammonia excretion secondary to hypophosphatemia leads to decreased acid clearance. Third, reduced renal tubular bicarbonate reabsorption occurs and leads to a hyperchloremic metabolic acidosis. Clinically the degree of acidosis is usually mild as a result of skeletal buffering from mobilization of both phosphorus and bicarbonate. However, severe metabolic acidosis has been observed in hypophosphatemic malnourished children receiving hyperalimentation. This may be related to defective mobilization of skeletal buffers.

Hypophosphatemia has been shown to cause glucose intolerance, probably due to insulin resistance. A state of functional hypoparathyroidism exists in severe hypophosphatemia and phosphorus depletion.

DIAGNOSTIC APPROACH

As with most disorders, appropriate therapy rests upon accurate diagnosis. Generally, the cause of hypophosphatemia is apparent from the history or clinical setting in which it occurs. Measurement of urinary phosphorus level is helpful in difficult cases. A fractional phosphate excretion of under 10 percent or 24-hour phosphorus output of less than 100 mg should direct attention to causes other than renal phosphate wasting. Such patients may have transcellular phosphate shift, increased nonrenal loss, or decreased phosphate intake or absorption. Transcellular phosphate shift is the most common cause of hypophosphatemia in the hospitalized patient.

Renal phosphate wasting is suggested by a urinary fractional phosphate excretion of greater than 20 percent or a 24-hour phosphorus output of more than 100 mg in the face of hypophosphatemia. An associated increase in urinary glucose, amino acid, bicarbonate, and uric acid points to Fanconi's syndrome as the underlying disease. Measurement of serum calcium and parathyroid hormone levels distinguishes hyperparathyroidism from the other causes of renal phosphate leak.

TREATMENT

At normal body pH (7.40), serum phosphorus exists in two forms, $H_2PO_4^-$ and $HPO_4^=$. Their relationship can be expressed by the following chemical reaction:

$$H_2PO_4^- \rightleftharpoons H^+ + HPO_4^=$$

The relative proportion of these ions in the serum can be calculated from the Henderson-Hasselbalch equation:

$$pH = pK + \log [HPO_4^=]/[H_2PO_4^-]$$

Since normal serum pH is 7.40 and the physiologic pK is 6.80, we have:

$$7.40 = 6.80 + \log [HPO_4^=]/[H_2PO_4^-]$$

or

$$0.60 = \log [HPO_4^=]/[H_2PO_4^-]$$

Antilog 0.60 = 4, therefore:

$$[HPO_4{}^{=}]/[H_2PO_4{}^{-}] = 4$$

or

$$[HPO_4{}^{=}] = 4\ [H_2PO_4{}^{-}]$$

Since the orthophosphate ions are expressed in molar concentration in the Henderson-Hasselbalch equation, the *molar* ratio of $HPO_4{}^{=}$ to $H_2PO_4{}^{-}$ is 4:1 under normal serum pH. A solution containing the two orthophosphate ions in this ratio has a pH of 7.40 and is commonly called a "neutral phosphate" solution.

It follows that in normal serum, every 5 mmol of serum phosphate contains 4 mmol of divalent phosphate and 1 mmol of monovalent phosphate, giving a total of nine negative charges per five phosphate ions, or a valence of 9/5 = 1.8. Therefore, the interconversion of serum phosphate from millimoles to milliequivalents at normal serum pH is: 1 mmol = 1.8 mEq.

It is also apparent that changes in pH affect the ratio of the phosphate ions and thus alter the concentration of the solution expressed in milliequivalents per liter. To avoid confusion, all therapeutic phosphate preparations should be expressed in millimoles per liter and elemental phosphorus in milligrams per deciliter, since these concentrations are independent of pH. Each millimole per liter of phosphate contains 3.1 mg per deciliter of elemental phosphorus. For example, the concentration of elemental phosphorus in 40 mmol per liter of K_2HPO_4 can be calculated as follows: atomic weight of P = 31; 40 mmol per liter K_2HPO_4 contains 40 mmol per liter P, therefore it has 40 × 3.1 mg per deciliter = 124 mg per deciliter P.

MODES OF THERAPY

Asymptomatic moderate hypophosphatemia usually requires attention only to the underlying etiologic agent. For hyperalimentation solutions, the addition of 15 mmol per liter of phosphate normally prevents hypophosphatemia. The judicious use of phosphate-binding antacids in patients with peptic ulcer disease or chronic renal failure avoids hypophosphatemia. For patients with respiratory alkalosis, treatment of the underlying disorder (sepsis, acute gout, or metabolic encephalopathy) reverses the hypophosphatemia.

Treatment of hypophosphatemia in patients with diabetic ketoacidosis remains controversial. Despite normal or elevated levels of serum phosphorus before treatment, these patients become hypophosphatemic and hypophosphaturic when given fluids and insulin. Clinical manifestations of severe hypophosphatemia usually do not develop however, and serum phosphorus normalizes with resumption of oral intake. In addition, several studies have failed to show improvement in insulin requirement, degree of acidosis, glucose metabolism, and red cell abnormalities with phosphate supplementation. Nonetheless, the small proportion of patients who present with hypophosphatemia *prior* to treatment require close monitoring. They have significant phosphorus depletion and are likely to develop severe hypophosphatemia during treatment for diabetic ketoacidosis. These patients may benefit from phosphate administration.

Chronic alcoholics, on the other hand, frequently have phosphorus depletion at the time of hospitalization. Frequent monitoring of their serum phosphorus levels is indicated. Oral phosphate supplementation may be given when an evolving trend toward hypophosphatemia becomes clear, so that a full-blown phosphorus depletion syndrome may be aborted.

For patients with severe hypophosphatemia associated with clinical manifestations of phosphorus depletion, therapy should be instituted without delay. As a general rule, oral therapy is preferred unless the patient cannot tolerate oral feeding or has continual seizures or coma.

TABLE 4 Commonly Available Phosphate Preparations

Preparations	*Phosphorus (1g)*	*Na (mEq)**	*K(mEq)**
Oral			
Skim milk	1,000 ml	28	39
Neutra-Phos	300 ml or 4 caps	28	28
Neutra-Phos-K	300 ml or 4 caps	0	57
Fleet Phospho Soda	6.2 ml	57	0
K-Phos neutral tabs	4 tabs	50	5
K-Phos tabs	7 tabs	0	26
Parenteral			
Hyper-Phos-K	15 ml	0	50
In-Phos	40 ml	65	8
Sodium phosphate	11 ml	45	0
Potassium phosphate	11 ml	0	45

Adapted from Lee DBN, et al. Disorders of phosphorus metabolism. In: Bronner F, Coburn J, eds. Disorders of mineral metabolism. Vol III. New York: Academic Press, 1981.
* In 1 g of phosphorus.

Skim milk has about 1 g per liter of both phosphorus and calcium. It is a safe and desirable form of phosphorus supplementation. If the patient cannot tolerate lactose or substantial fluid intake, a commercial phosphate preparation may be used. A total daily amount of 2 to 3 g of elemental phosphorus may be given in two to four divided doses. Mild diarrhea is a frequent side effect. Various commonly available phosphate preparations are listed in Table 4.

In the patient requiring parenteral phosphate, caution must be exercised to prevent hyperphosphatemia. The volume of distribution of the administered phosphate varies widely among individuals and is affected by the serum pH, glucose, and insulin availability. In addition, phosphorus-depleted patients are extremely hypophosphaturic and may remain so for some time despite correction of their hypophosphatemia. Consequently, they are vulnerable to developing hyperphosphatemia when a large quantity of phosphate is given parenterally over a short period of time. We recommend that no more than 1 g of elemental phosphorus be given by steady infusion over 24 hours. In patients with renal failure or oliguria, potassium phosphate preparations should be avoided. An initial phosphate dose of 0.08 mmol per kilogram of body weight (2.5 mg per kilogram of body weight) may be given over 6 hours. The dose may be increased to 0.16 mmol per kilogram (5.0 mg per kilogram) if the patient has serious life-threatening clinical manifestations. Thereafter, serum phosphorus, calcium, potassium, and magnesium should be determined and the rate of phosphate infusion adjusted accordingly. Parenteral phosphate infusion should be discontinued when the serum phosphorus level is higher than 2 mg per deciliter or the serum calcium level is less than 8 mg per deciliter.

The hazards of parenteral phosphate therapy include hyperphosphatemia, hypocalcemia, hypomagnesemia, metastatic calcification, hypotension, and renal failure. Diuresis may accompany phosphate administration and lead to dehydration, hypokalemia, and hypernatremia. Patients with renal failure receiving parenteral phosphate therapy are especially susceptible to serious complications.

HYPOMAGNESEMIA AND HYPERMAGNESEMIA

NACHMAN BRAUTBAR, M.D.

BODY MAGNESIUM

Distribution

Body magnesium is distributed in three major compartments—in (1) extracellular fluid, 1.3 percent; in (2) intracellular fluid, 13 percent; and in (3) bone, 67 percent. Thus, magnesium is mainly located in areas that are poorly accessible to study, i.e., the intracellular and the bony compartments. Unfortunately, most of the available data on magnesium metabolism are derived from measurements of the blood concentration of magnesium. The limitations of such information is obvious.

Balance

The role of magnesium has recently been reviewed by Flink et al and by Seelig et al who concluded that at least 6 mg per kilogram per day is required to maintain magnesium *balance.* The Food and Nutrition Board of the National Academy of Sciences recommend an intake of 300 to 350 mg per day for adults or approximately 5 mg per kilogram per day. The requirement for magnesium may increase in pregnant women or in adolescents. Table 1 shows magnesium requirements for various age groups.

The magnesium content of food as calculated from tables of food consumption and from chemical analysis shows that, in a mixed general American diet, the intake of magnesium is closely correlated with the number of calories consumed. This is true as long as the calories are not consumed in the form of alcohol or sugar, since both have little or no mineral content and can also cause renal wasting of magnesium. Magnesium is found in great concentration in nuts, green vegetables, soybeans, chocolate, and whole cereal grains. In some countries, the drinking water contains some magnesium that depends on the hardness of the water.

TABLE 1 Daily Requirements for Magnesium

	Age in years	*Daily Need in mg (mEq)*
Infants	0.5–0.5	50 (4.2)
	0.5–1.0	70 (5.8)
Children	1–3	150 (12.5)
	4–6	200 (16.6)
	7–10	250 (20.8)
Males	11–14	350 (29.2)
	15–18	400 (33.3)
	>19	350 (29.2)
Females	11–14	300 (25.0)
	>15	300 (25.0)
	Pregnancy	450 (37.5)
	Lactation	450 (37.5)

HYPOMAGNESEMIA AND MAGNESIUM DEPLETION

Definitions

Hypomagnesemia can develop without concomitant magnesium losses, and cellular magnesium depletion can occur in the presence of normomagnesemia. However, low plasma magnesium levels may not always indicate magnesium depletion. Since magnesium is primarily an intracellular cation, in clinical reports and experimental studies that only measure serum magnesium, it is sometimes extremely difficult to judge precisely the status of body magnesium content and with all its limitations, the serum magnesium level remains the prime clinical diagnostic tool. If patients are found to be hypomagnesemic, it is safe to assume that, in most cases, the hypomagnesemia is asociated with some degree of magnesium depletion. Special care and a high index of suspicion should be utilized in those patients who may be magnesium depleted, but whose serum magnesium is normal or only very slightly reduced. In these special cases, the clinician may look for other laboratory and clinical findings associated with magnesium depletion.

To aid in the diagnosis of *magnesium depletion*, several investigative tools are available. The magnesium retention test has been used in the study of magnesium depletion and in the evaluation of magnesium balance. The test is relatively easy to perform and requires the intravenous loading of magnesium and the collection of urine. In a normal subject, 75 to 80 percent of an administered load is excreted in the urine within 24 hours. In a magnesium deficient individual, less than 75 percent of the administered magnesium is excreted in this period of time, provided no tubular defect in magnesium reabsorption is present. Retention of less than 20 percent indicates that magnesium depletion is unlikely.

Prevalence of Magnesium Depletion in Men

The prevalence of hypomagnesemia (serum magnesium < 1.53 mEq per liter) among 5,100 ambulatory and hospitalized patients is approximately 10.2 percent. However, caution should be exercised in the interpretation of these data regarding the presence and/or the severity of magnesium depletion since these studies did not evaluate other definitive parameters of magnesium depletion. However, it is safe to conclude that hypomagnesemia and possibly magnesium depletion are common in the clinical practice of medicine.

Causes of Hypomagnesemia and Magnesium Depletion

The causes and disease entities where magnesium depletion and hypomagnesemia are common are shown in Table 2.

Redistribution of Magnesium in Hypomagnesemia Without Net Magnesium Losses

Hypomagnesemia without a net total body magnesium loss occurs from maldistribution of magnesium from the blood to the intracellular, bone, and soft tissue com-

TABLE 2 Causes of Hypomagnesemia and Magnesium Depletion

Decreased Intake	Excessive Urinary Losses
Protein-calorie malnutrition	Diuretic therapy (especially "loop" agents)
Starvation	Diuretic phase of acute renal failure
Prolonged intravenous therapy	Chronic alcoholism
Decreased Intestinal Absorption	Primary aldosteronism
Malabsorption syndromes, including nontropical sprue	Hypercalcemic states: malignancy, hyperparathyroidism, and vitamin D excess
Massive surgical resection of the small intestine	Renal tubular acidosis
Neonatal hypomagnesemia with selective malabsorption of magnesium	Diabetes, especially during and following treatment of acidosis
Excessive Losses of Body Fluids	Hyperthyroidism
Prolonged nasogastric suction	Idiopathic renal magnesium wasting
Excessive use of purgatives	Chronic renal failure with renal magnesium wasting
Intestinal and biliary fistulas	Gentamicin toxicity
Severe diarrhea as in ulcerative colitis and infantile gastroenteritis	Tobramycin nephrotoxicity
Rarely, prolonged lactation	Cisplatinum nephrotoxicity
	Miscellaneous
	Idiopathic hypomagnesemia
	Acute pancreatitis
	Porphyria with inappropriate secretion of antidiuretic hormone
	Multiple transfusions or exchange transfusions with citrated blood
	Bartter's Syndrome

partments. Refeeding after starvation is associated with hypomagnesemia without magnesium losses from the body. This hypomagnesemia is attributable to increased trapping of the cation in newly formed tissue. The same mechanism is responsible for the development of hypomagnesemia in patients maintained with intravenous feedings containing glucose, amino acids, and inadequate amounts of magnesium. Potts and Roberts found that hypomagnesemia commonly develops following parathyroidectomy from hyperparathyroidism. This reduction in serum levels was attributed to the fall in circulating parathyroid hormone (PTH) levels and the restoration of normal cellular function. The hypomagnesemia complicating *acute pancreatitis* is most likely due to deposition of magnesium in injured tissues.

Hypomagnesemia Due to Reduced Dietary Intake Without Losses of Magnesium

Reduced oral intake of magnesium in adults has been associated with hypomagnesemia and evidence of magnesium depletion. During long-term dietary magnesium restriction (> 6 weeks), signs of hypomagnesemia such as Trousseau sign, abnormal skeletal muscle electromyograms, and spasticity may develop. Both plasma and red blood cell magnesium levels and urinary magnesium excretion became significantly reduced by 7 days of dietary magnesium restriction. All these clinical findings can be reversed after the administration of magnesium salts. Thus, hypomagnesemia and magnesium depletion can develop when magnesium intake is severely reduced despite the absence of excessive losses of magnesium from the body. Magnesium depletion in these patients is caused by the constant cellular need for magnesium by the turnover of tissue. Relatively reduced magnesium intake in settings in which magnesium requirements are increased (pregnancy and infancy) could also result in magnesium depletion. The formation of new tissue in pregnancy requires that dietary magnesium be higher compared to that of nonpregnant women of the same age.

Protein calorie malnutrition is commonly associated with magnesium depletion. Reduced urinary magnesium excretion, negative magnesium balance, and reduced red blood cell magnesium content have been described. The mechanism is related to both reduced intake and reduced intestinal absorption of magnesium

Hypomagnesemia With Net Loss of Total Body Magnesium

Gastrointestinal Losses. Increased intestinal loss is a common cause of magnesium depletion and hypomagnesemia, especially in disease entities that produce *steatorrhea,* such as nontropical sprue, short-bowel syndrome, and malabsorption secondary to inflammation of the intestinal wall or pancreatic insufficiency.

Biliary fistulas and *prolonged nasogastric suction* with the administration of *magnesium-free parental fluids* are commonly associated with hypomagnesemia and magnesium depletion. Acute pancreatitis is frequently associated with hypocalcemia and hypomagnesemia. The mechanism is not clear, but is at least partially attributable to the deposition of magnesium within the fatty soaps of injured tissues in and around the pancreas.

Renal Losses. Magnesium depletion, hypomagnesemia, and negative magnesium balance can result from impaired renal reabsorption of the cation. The various disease entities associated with renal magnesium wasting are shown in Table 3.

Several drugs that cause renal wasting have been described. "Loop" diuretics (e.g., furosemide), may be associated with severe hypomagnesemia. This is associated with a marked reduction in muscle potassium content which is not improved by potassium supplementation, but which was reversed after intravenous magnesium administration. Thus, hypomagnesemia is common in patients receiving potent diuretics, and muscle potassium depletion may be a serious complication of this magnesium depletion.

Cisplatinum administration is associated with a nephropathy and with hypomagnesemia secondary to increased urinary excretion of magnesium. The pathogenetic factor responsible for the magnesium wasting is not clear. The possible mechanisms to be considered include (1) the direct effect of cisplatinum on the renal absorption of magnesium and (2) the interstitial nephritis secondary to cisplatinum with damage to the loop of Henle and, in turn, reduced magnesium absorption.

Aminoglycosides may be associated with nephrotoxicity and urinary magnesium wasting. Although the precise mechanism underlying the magnesuria is not known, some indirect information is available. The nephrotoxic effect of aminoglycosides is exerted mainly on the proximal tubule. It is possible that inhibition of proximal magnesium transport leads to increased magnesium delivery to the loop of Henle, thereby exceeding the loop's reabsorptive capacity and thus resulting in magnesuria. A possible direct effect on the loop of Henle cannot be ruled out.

Phosphate depletion is commonly associated with hypomagnesemia and renal magnesium wasting. The magnesuria is correlated with the degree of the hypophosphatemia and the administration of phosphate.

TABLE 3 Conditions Associated with Renal Wasting of Magnesium

Primary renal magnesium wasting
Loop diuretics
Diabetic ketoacidosis (osmotic diuresis)
Bartter's syndrome
Hyperaldosteronism
Syndrome of inappropriate ADH secretion
Alcoholism
Hypercalciuria or salt-wasting states
Amphotericin toxicity
Aminoglycosides (gentamicin)
Cisplatin

Prevention and Therapy of Magnesium Depletion and Hypomagnesemia

Basic Concepts That Determine the Relationship Between Millimoles, Milligrams, and Milliequivalents

Magnesium has an atomic weight of 24.312 and an atomic number of 12; it carries the valency of 2. Millimoles (mmol) are weight (in mg) divided by the atomic weight, and milliequivalents are mmol times valence. For example, let us take the most commonly used salt of magnesium, $MgSO_4$. The atomic weights of this compound are as follows: Mg, 24; S, 32; and O_4, 64. Therefore, 1 g mol of $MgSO_4$ is 120. That means that for each mol of $MgSO_4$ given to the patient, we deliver 24:120 × 100% of elemental magnesium, which means 20 percent of this weight is elemental magnesium. Therefore, 2 ml of 50 percent of a $MgSO_4$ ampule delivers about 4 mmol or 8 mEq per milliliter of Mg.

Prevention. In this category, we can include the following groups of patients: (a) patients on total parenteral nutrition, (b) patients with chronic diarrheal conditions who waste magnesium, (c) patients with renal wasting of magnesium, and (d) lactating females and growing youngsters. In this group of patients, both oral and intravenous supplementation can be used. In groups (a) to (c), the most appropriate route is the parenteral route, which can be either intramuscular or intravenous. In these patients, 15 to 25 mmol of magnesium should be considered as adequate to prevent depletion. In groups (c) to (d), oral intake is advised. Several preparations are available. Magnesium gluconate tablets, 500 mg, deliver 1.2 mmol of magnesium per tablet. In each 15 g of magnesium sulfate powder there are 12.5 mmol of magnesium. Four hundred mg tablets of $Mg(OH)_2$ deliver 7 mmol. Our own experience has shown that patients readily tolerate magnesium gluconate administered orally. Although $MgSO_4$ powder delivers more magnesium, the side effects of diarrhea and abnormal cramps are disturbing. In all cases, the physician must make sure that renal function is normal. In some patients who require total parenteral nutrition (TPN), intravenously delivered $MgSO_4$ can be used even in the case of renal failure. This procedure needs the monitoring of daily magnesium blood levels. The intravenous dose should not exceed 4 mmol per day.

Treatment

In patients whose clinical and chemical evidence indicate magnesium depletion, such as in the alcoholic patient or in the diabetic with ketoacidosis, administration of intravenous magnesium is indicated. The dose should be considered in relation to renal function. If renal function is normal, the administration of $MgSO_4$, intramuscularly or intravenously, at doses of 16 to 20 mmol per day for several days is recommended. Daily determination of serum magnesium levels should be undertaken.

Maintenance. In patients who have already established a clinical condition that leaves them prone to develop Mg depletion, a daily maintenance oral or intravenous dose should be determined. Again, renal functional assessment is an integral part of the management of these patients.

Emergency Administration. In the patient who develops severe hypomagnesemia and hypocalcemia and who exhibits one or more of the complications of magnesium depletion, administration of high intravenous doses of magnesium supplements are imperative. In these cases, 4 ml of 50 percent $MgSO_4$ diluted in 500 ml of 5 percent glucose and water should be given over a period of 10 to 15 minutes followed by continuous intravenous administration of $MgSO_4$ at a daily dose of 20 mmol per day. To prevent magnesium toxicity and death, renal function measurement is important in any of these cases.

HYPERMAGNESEMIA AND MAGNESIUM TOXICITY

Since large loads of magnesium can easily be eliminated in the urine when renal function is normal, it is unusual to encounter hypermagnesemia unless renal function is impaired. Table 4 lists the various clinical conditions in which hypermagnesemia has been noted. As the glomerular filtration rate declines, absolute magnesium excretion falls, and this may result in hypermagnesemia. As long as the patient remains on a normal diet, the serum levels of magnesium stabilize at around 2.5 mEq per liter. However, when patients with chronic renal failure are treated with magnesium containing antacids, the plasma level can reach 14 to 16 mEq per liter, thus providing symptoms of toxicity.

Many geriatric patients risk the development of magnesium toxicity owing to (1) reduced renal function with age, (2) increased consumption of antacids containing magnesium, and (3) increased intake of vitamins containing mineral salts as magnesium. The sources of magnesium can be classified as magnesium-containing antacids, magnesium-containing laxatives, and urologic lubrication solutions containing magnesium.

Signs and Symptoms

The signs and symptoms of hypermagnesemia are the result of the pharmacologic effects of this ion on the ner-

TABLE 4 Conditions Associated with Hypermagnesemia

Acute renal failure
Chronic renal failure
Infants of mothers treated with Mg for eclampsia
Adrenal insufficiency
Administration of pharmacologic doses of Mg and use of oral purgatives or rectal enemas containing Mg, especially in patients with impaired renal function

vous and the cardiovascular systems. Deep tendon reflexes are usually lost when blood magnesium concentration exceeds 6 mEq per liter. Respiratory paralysis, narcosis, hypotension, and abnormal cardiac conduction may occur as blood levels of magnesium approach 10 mEq per liter.

The diagnosis of magnesium toxicity in the elderly patient is of great importance since they are the ones to utilize much of the magnesium-containing medications, and also they commonly have reduction in renal function, at least 50 percent of glomerular filtration rate (GFR). Several reports have suggested a relationship between the blood levels of magnesium and the symptoms. However, there seems to be a great deal of variability from one individual to another; some report drowsiness and altered levels of consciousness at levels of 5 mEq per liter whereas, at the same levels, others report normal mental responses with these blood magnesium levels. The most common clinical signs and symptoms described in patients whose blood magnesium rose to 4 mEq per liter were drowsiness, lethargy, and diaphoresis.

Treatment

Discontinuation of magnesium ingestion or administration and the intravenous injection of calcium compounds are the initial steps in the treatment of symptomatic hypermagnesemia. The administration of 100 to 200 mg of calcium may be adequate to reverse the manifestations of hypermagnesemia, but greater amounts may be required. Peritoneal or hemodialysis may be needed to lower the concentration of blood magnesium in patients with severe hypermagnesemia.

RESPIRATORY ACIDOSIS

KARLMAN WASSERMAN, M.D., Ph.D.
RICHARD CASABURI, M.D., Ph.D.
DARRYL Y. SUE, M.D.

Respiratory acidosis is the acid-base state in which the arterial carbon dioxide (CO_2) pressure ($PaCO_2$) is elevated above its normal value (38 to 42 mm Hg at sea level, but less at higher altitudes). The increase in dissolved CO_2 causes a shift in the bicarbonate buffer system so that more carbonic acid is formed, which then dissociates in the body fluid to increase the hydrogen ion (H^+) concentration (and thus decreases the pH). This acidosis is referred to as respiratory acidosis because the mechanism for regulation of $PaCO_2$ is ventilation of the blood perfusing the lungs. Respiratory acidosis occurs when alveolar ventilation decreases relative to metabolic CO_2 production. Clinically, respiratory acidosis is observed in many conditions and may develop rapidly (as acute acidosis) or gradually (as chronic acidosis).

ACUTE RESPIRATORY ACIDOSIS

Acute respiratory acidosis occurs because of an abrupt decrease in alveolar ventilation (the proportion of ventilation that is effective in producing pulmonary gas exchange) relative to the CO_2 produced by metabolic processes. Because of the rapidity with which the $PaCO_2$ increases, there is not sufficient time for compensatory mechanisms (principally renal bicarbonate generation) to respond to prevent a decrease in pH. The primary mechanisms for acute respiratory acidosis are (1) failure of the ventilatory control mechanism to sense the CO_2 stimulus adequately and thereby regulate it; (2) a defect in the respiratory pump resulting from failure of respiratory muscle function; and (3) increased work of breathing and inefficiency in gas exchange resulting from pulmonary pathologic factors.

CHRONIC RESPIRATORY ACIDOSIS

Chronic respiratory acidosis is the state in which the $PaCO_2$ has elevated gradually, allowing sufficient time for a compensatory increase in bicarbonate to occur, with the result being that the arterial pH is usually in the normal range (7.38 to 7.42). In this state, the kidneys have had sufficient time to generate bicarbonate, and metabolic compensation for the respiratory acidosis is usually complete. Respiratory acidosis appears to be the one simple acid-base disturbance that can be completely compensated. Although some authorities maintain that in chronic respiratory acidosis, the pH is low and the degree of acidemia is greater for greater degrees of CO_2 retention, this conclusion is generally based on data collected from experiments with animals. In most mammals, the respiratory system is used to control body heat as well as pH, whereas in humans, it is used primarily to control pH and is not needed for heat elimination. This might account for the more precise pH regulation observed in humans in contrast to that of animals with fur coats.

MECHANISM OF CO_2 REGULATION

CO_2 regulation is accomplished by chemoreceptors that control ventilation. In humans, these receptors include the chemoreceptors in the medulla in close relation to the floor of the fourth ventricle that respond to pH changes of both cerebrospinal fluid and blood, and the carotid bodies that are perfused by a branch of the internal carotid artery near the bifurcation of the common carotid artery. The operative stimulus to the chemoreceptive cells appears to be the H^+ generated by CO_2 and not CO_2 itself. Thus the chemoreceptor stimulation that occurs in association with the high $PaCO_2$ of chronic compensated respiratory acidosis is not substantially different than that which occurs when the $PaCO_2$ and acid-base status are normal. In situations in which the bicarbonate level is low, such as chronic metabolic acidosis, the CO_2 is sensitively regulated because any change in $PaCO_2$ produces a greater H^+ change than occurs when the bicarbonate level is high. Because of the location of the respiratory chemoreceptors, it is the arterial and cerebrospinal fluid pH values that appear to be the set point around which the ventilatory control mechanisms operate.

PATHOPHYSIOLOGY

Mechanisms causing respiratory acidosis include the following: (1) central respiratory depressants (drugs, central nervous system infection, brain injury); (2) idiopathic loss of respiratory drive (primary alveolar hypoventilation); (3) impaired chemoreceptor function; (4) muscle or motor end-plate dysfunction; (5) chest wall deformity or extreme obesity; and (6) mechanical limitation to pulmonary ventilation or gas exchange. If the pathophysiology is of central origin, breathing appears to be slow and shallow and, if acute, the patient may lapse into coma. If the cause is acute failure of the respiratory pump (respiratory muscle failure) or air flow obstruction, the patient becomes tachypneic and complains of breathlessness.

The most common cause of respiratory acidosis is air flow obstruction such as that associated with one of the obstructive lung diseases (bronchial asthma, bronchitis, emphysema). Chronic respiratory acidosis is commonly associated with obstructive lung disease. It is difficult for patients with these diseases to maintain $PaCO_2$ in the normal range because of the combination of high respiratory work, inefficiency of gas exchange associated with intrapulmonary mismatching of ventilation and perfusion, and lung hyperinflation putting the diaphragm at a mechanical disadvantage. Many of these patients therefore ventilate inadequately, allowing their $PaCO_2$ to increase. Because this generally occurs gradually, the renal generation of bicarbonate is usually sufficient to maintain the arterial pH near the normal range.

Chronic respiratory acidosis also occurs in patients with chest wall deformities such as kyphoscoliosis. Similarly, the morbidly obese patient may retain CO_2 (obesity-hypoventilation or the pickwickian syndrome).

Central respiratory depression secondary to ingestion or injection of drugs that have respiratory depressant properties is another common cause of CO_2 retention. Central respiratory depression can usually be distinguished from the mechanical causes of respiratory acidosis by observation of the patient's pattern and rate of breathing. Respiratory depression is associated with bradypnea and mechanical limitation to breathing is associated with tachypnea.

SYMPTOMS AND SIGNS

Virtually all of the symptoms of respiratory acidosis are secondary to the consequent acidemia. The symptoms and signs of acute respiratory acidosis without associated hypoxia are (1) tachypnea, (2) dyspnea on exertion, (3) asterixis, (4) obtundation, (5) coma, (6) headache, (7) papilledema, (8) heart failure, (9) hypertension, and (10) arrhythmia. Other manifestations may occur if hypercapnia is accompanied by hypoxia; compensated respiratory acidosis in which the pH is normal generally does not cause symptoms. Tachypnea and dyspnea are secondary to the acute decrease in arterial and cerebrospinal fluid pH. The cause of the twitching of muscles held in sustained contraction, best marked by the inability to hold the wrists in extension (asterixis), is uncertain but seems to be related to the effect of pH on the transmembrane potential of the peripheral nerves. Headaches and the papilledema may occur secondary to cerebral vasodilation caused by the low pH. Obtundation and coma may also be precipitated by the acute central nervous system acidosis. Heart failure and arrhythmia may result from the direct effects of acidemia on Ca^{++} and K^+ flux in the myocardium as well as from the increased pulmonary and peripheral vascular resistance that accompanies systemic acidosis.

A variety of central nervous system signs can be precipitated by pH disturbances that result from acute changes in $PaCO_2$. When the pH decreases to less than 7.35, asterixis is commonly noted. When the pH decreases to less than 7.30, asterixis tends to disappear but obtundation supervenes. The patient becomes semicomatose and eventually lapses into coma. Generally these effects can be quickly reversed by ventilating the patient and returning the pH to normal.

Neurologic effects can also be induced by an acute decrease in $PaCO_2$ in patients with chronic respiratory acidosis by the creation of alkalemia. When the pH is greater than 7.55, seizures are common, and they are almost inevitable when the pH is increased to more than 7.60. This is especially likely to occur if the blood bicarbonate level is elevated, because a small decrease in $PaCO_2$ results in a greater alkaline swing than that which occurs when the bicarbonate level is normal.

TREATMENT

Because respiratory acidosis always results from insufficient ventilation of the blood perfusing the lungs (alveolar ventilation), treatment is directed at increasing the alveolar ventilation. The method of choice depends on the mechanism of disease and the urgency of treatment.

Acute Respiratory Acidosis

The elevation of $PaCO_2$ that occurs with severe acute respiratory acidosis generally necessitates immediate treatment because of the effects of central nervous system acidosis on the central nervous system (e.g., lethargy, coma) and the hypoxemia that usually accompanies this elevation. Treatment is directed at restoring a sufficient amount of alveolar ventilation by reversing the condition that led to the hypoventilation and/or by providing artificial ventilation to the patient.

Patients with central depression of ventilation may have central nervous system injury or disease or may have taken sedatives or narcotics. These patients may need to receive mechanical ventilation until the central nervous system damage is reversed or the effects of depressant drugs have disappeared. In both cases, maintenance of an effective airway is important. For patients known to have or suspected of having opiate depression of respiration, the specific antagonist naloxone is useful, and other specific pharmacologic antagonists may be available in the future. For depression of respiration caused by the use of other drugs, such as long-acting sedative-hypnotics, supportive care including mechanical ventilation seems to be the most appropriate treatment. Efforts to enhance elimination of such drugs by hemodialysis or other means are not usually beneficial, and nonspecific respiratory stimulants are of little value. Patients in whom central depression of ventilation is the cause of respiratory acidosis may initially have normal lung function, but complications of altered mental status and supportive care may lead to secondary pulmonary problems such as atelectasis and aspiration pneumonia.

Some neuromuscular and chest wall abnormalities that lead to acute respiratory acidosis can be effectively treated, while others are benefited only by supportive care. Patients with neuromuscular diseases such as myasthenia gravis, Guillain-Barré syndrome, and muscular dystrophy generally do not develop respiratory acidosis until the vital capacity reaches less than 40 percent of the predicted value or less than approximately 1,200 ml in the typical adult patient. Some investigators believe that, in this setting, the measurement of maximal inspiratory and expiratory pressure generated at the mouth has particular predictive value for the development of respiratory acidosis. These patients should be monitored with frequent vital capacity measurements as well as by neurologic assessment. Treatment should be individualized on the basis of the type of neuromuscular problem. It should also be noted that because patients with respiratory muscle weakness have particularly ineffective coughing and breathe at low lung volume, they are prone to lung infection and atelectasis that further decrease the respiratory ability to ventilate and oxygenate the blood.

The largest group of patients with acute respiratory acidosis are those with chronic obstructive lung disease who have acute decompensation. These patients, some of whom have chronic respiratory acidosis as well, may have mechanical and ventilatory control abnormalities that need to be identified and corrected. First, because the primary problem is airway obstruction, bronchodilators are useful (theophylline, aerosolized and oral beta-adrenergic agonists, and, in some cases, anticholinergic agents such as ipratropium bromide). Corticosteroids are often given to those patients whose obstruction is partially due to asthma, but these should be used judiciously. Airway secretions are an important component of obstruction. Suctioning, coughing, mucolytic agents, and mechanical mobilization of secretions may be of value. Antibiotics that work against usual airway pathogens such as *Haemophilus influenzae* and *Streptococcus pneumoniae* are generally regarded as effective. Second, it is now recognized that respiratory muscle fatigue is an important aspect of acute respiratory failure in these patients. This should be treated by correction of electrolyte abnormalities such as hypokalemia and hypophosphatemia or by "resting" the respiratory muscles through the use of mechanical ventilation. Improvement of respiratory muscle function after the administration of theophylline or dopamine has been reported; these drugs may cause the respiratory acidosis to lessen while the underlying mechanical derangement is corrected. Third, because central respiratory depression is often a factor in acute decompensation, the use of sedatives and narcotics should be avoided. Fourth, although it is often anticipated that oxygen administration will worsen acute respiratory acidosis in patients with chronic obstructive lung disease by suppressing the output of the carotid bodies, its benefit in improving central nervous system oxygenation and in relieving pulmonary artery hypertension generally outweighs its adverse effects. Oxygen should be given at a low concentration (24 to 30 percent), and the consequent acid-base status should be carefully monitored. Finally, endotracheal intubation and mechanical ventilation should be considered for those patients who cannot be managed otherwise.

It is important to remember that patients with chronic lung diseases other than chronic bronchitis and emphysema can also have acute respiratory acidosis. These conditions include severe asthma, restrictive lung disease (especially disease caused by chest wall deformity), and adult respiratory distress syndrome. Although the management of acute respiratory acidosis is generally similar in each of these disorders, specific treatment of the underlying problem may be different.

After the patient with acute respiratory acidosis begins receiving mechanical ventilation, adjustments are made to give the appropriate $PaCO_2$ value. This is generally the $PaCO_2$ that results in an acceptable pH value (7.35 to 7.42). This $PaCO_2$ may not necessarily be within the normal range if the plasma bicarbonate value is high (in cases of chronic respiratory acidosis or metabolic alkalosis) or low (in cases of chronic respiratory alkalosis or metabolic acidosis). $PaCO_2$ and alveolar ventilation are inversely related, but the volume of air per minute provided to the patient, the minute ventilation ($\dot{V}E$), is related to alveolar ventilation as the sum of alveolar ventilation plus dead space ventilation.

The adult patient with normal lungs usually has a $\dot{V}E$ of 7 L per minute and a dead space ventilation of approximately 2.3 L per minute. For the production of CO_2 at rest, this ventilation is sufficient to maintain a $PaCO_2$ at 40 mm Hg. In patients with abnormal lungs, the dead space ventilation is increased, so that the $\dot{V}E$ must increase to maintain a normal $PaCO_2$. Furthermore, if the metabolic rate increases as a result of fever, infection, or physical activity, the $\dot{V}E$ must also increase proportionally to maintain a normal $PaCO_2$. Thus the relationship of $\dot{V}E$ to $PaCO_2$ and the amount of $\dot{V}E$ ordered for the patient undergoing mechanical ventilatory support may vary considerably.

The required ventilation for a desired $PaCO_2$ for given values of the ratio of dead space volume to tidal volume (VD/VT) (or, equivalently, the ratio of dead space ventilation to $\dot{V}E$) is shown in Figure 1. This nomogram assumes a constant CO_2 production of 200 ml per minute. The VD/VT ratio can be determined at the intersection of the $PaCO_2$ value (measured by arterial blood gas analysis) and the $\dot{V}E$ (measured by the mechanical ventilator). Alternatively, from a given $PaCO_2$ and $\dot{V}E$ and an assumed constant VD/VT ratio, the necessary $\dot{V}E$ for any desired PCO_2 value can be determined.

A special problem of acute respiratory acidosis may occur during weaning from mechanical ventilation if the patient cannot provide sufficient spontaneous ventilation to maintain arterial pH and PCO_2 as mechanical ventilation is withdrawn. This may be caused by insufficient resolution of the underlying lung disease, the increased load imposed on the patient by the endotracheal tube or ventilator circuit, respiratory muscle fatigue, electrolyte abnormalities, malnutrition, infection, or patient anxiety. Correction of these contributing factors is necessary for successful withdrawal of mechanical ventilation.

Chronic Respiratory Acidosis

Patients with chronic respiratory acidosis have an increased serum bicarbonate concentration that results in a nearly normal pH. Thus the elevated $PaCO_2$ itself does not require treatment. However, the increased CO_2 in the alveolar gas displaces the oxygen resulting in chronic hypoxemia. Because patients with chronic respiratory acidosis almost always have parenchymal lung disease (except those with chest wall deformities such as kyphoscoliosis), the resultant hypoxemia may be severe. The treatment is directed at increasing the PaO_2 directly and/or by indirectly raising the PaO_2 by reducing the $PaCO_2$.

Oxygen

Long-term studies have shown that supplemental oxygen has a beneficial effect in patients with chronic obstructive lung disease. The goal is reduction of pulmonary hypertension that leads to right ventricular failure and its complications. Although there is concern that inhibition of hypoxic drive with the administration of oxygen may cause respiratory acidosis to worsen, it seems that stable patients with chronic respiratory acidosis tolerate oxygen safely. Oxygen is usually administered at low concentrations sufficient to increase the PaO_2 to approximately 60 mm Hg or to increase the oxyhemoglobin saturation to more than 90 percent. In patients with sleep-disordered breathing syndromes, nocturnal hypoxemia associated with apnea may sometimes be treated with oxygen. In some patients, however, the periods of apnea may be prolonged with oxygen administration. It is therefore appropriate to monitor the effect of oxygen in such patients with appropriate studies.

Long-term Mechanical Ventilation

Long-term mechanical ventilation, either nocturnal or continuous, may be helpful in selected patients. Patients with mild-to-moderate respiratory muscle weakness in particular may require supplemental ventilation from negative-pressure or positive-pressure ventilation during sleeping hours, although they have sufficient muscle strength during the day to support ventilation. Other patients may require longer periods of ventilatory assistance. Patients and their families may require considerable training and orientation to use the mechanical ventilator at home.

Nasal Continuous Positive Airway Pressure

Patients with significant obstruction of the upper airway during sleep (obstructive sleep apnea syn-

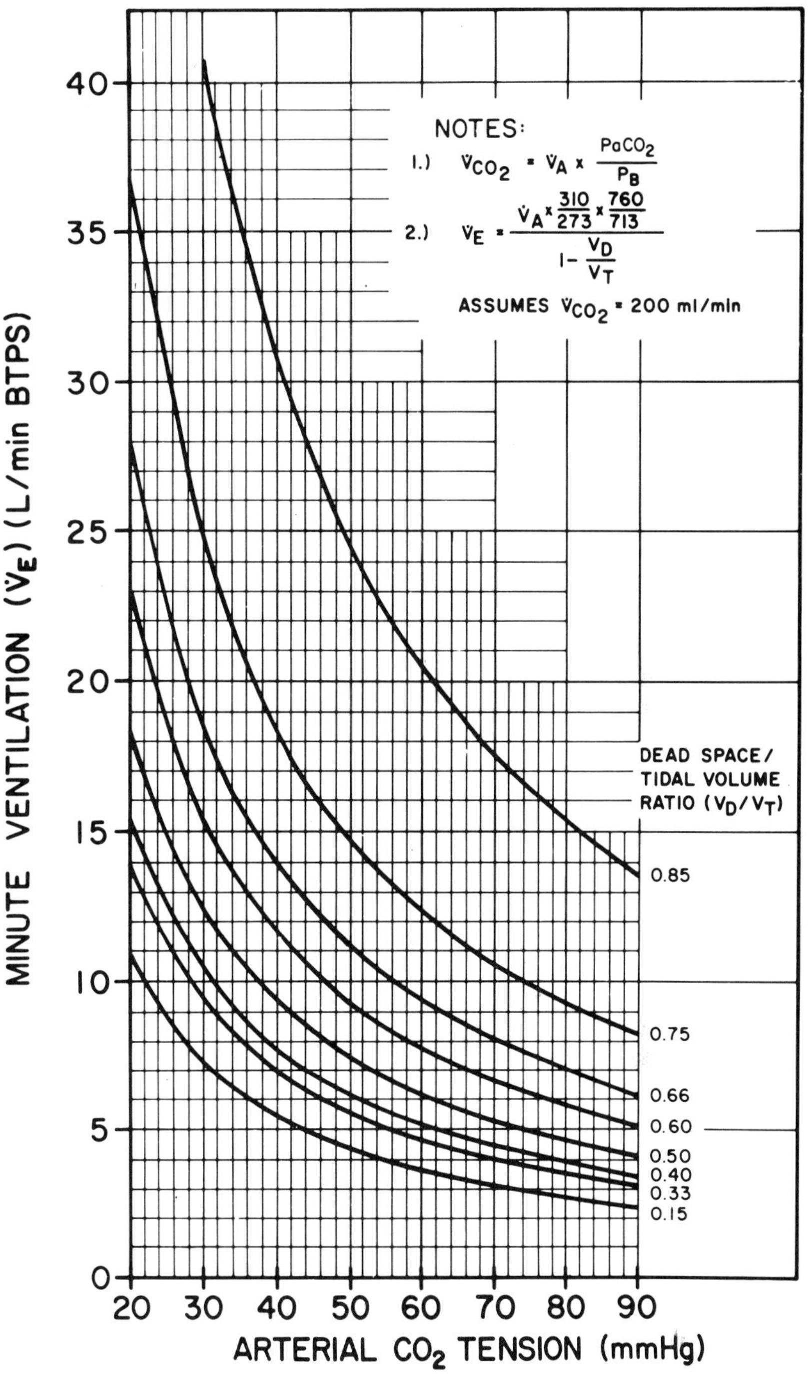

Figure 1 The $\dot{V}E$ is selected according to the desired $PaCO_2$. These curves have been drawn for an average adult with a CO_2 production ($\dot{V}CO_2$) of 200 ml per minute (STPD). However, this nomogram yields good results even when the $\dot{V}CO_2$ is not 200 ml per minute, since a $\dot{V}CO_2$ differing mildly from this value is compensated for by a false estimate of VD/VT, thereby providing a relatively valid $\dot{V}E$. When the $\dot{V}CO_2$ is known to differ from 200 ml per minute, the true VD/VT value can be estimated by multiplying the measured $\dot{V}E$ value by the measured $\dot{V}CO_2$ divided by 200 before determining the intersection of the $\dot{V}E$ and $PaCO_2$ lines.

drome) may be helped by the application of nasal continuous positive airway pressure (nasal CPAP). Positive pressure applied over the nose during sleep may reduce the periods of obstructive apnea and decrease the duration of hypoxemia. Patients considered for nasal CPAP should be studied during sleep for the presence of obstructive sleep apnea, and testing of the benefit of nasal CPAP should be performed. Supplemental oxygen administration is sometimes combined with nasal CPAP. Surgical approaches to obstructive sleep apnea include uvulopalatoplasty and tracheostomy; patients should be carefully selected for these procedures. Finally, in some obese patients with obstructive sleep apnea, reduction of weight by the use of severely restricted diets or by surgical procedures may be indicated.

Improving Respiratory Muscle Function

There is some evidence that the strength and endurance of the inspiratory muscles improves after specific training of these muscles. Some investigators have found that training of the inspiratory muscles achieved by inhalation through a device with a small orifice improves exercise tolerance in patients with chronic obstructive lung disease. The role of respiratory muscle training in the prevention or management of chronic respiratory acidosis is unclear. Similarly, it has been suggested that theophylline and dopamine have a beneficial effect on the strength and endurance of the diaphragm but, again, the precise effect of these drugs on respiratory acidosis is not known.

Drug Therapy

Doxapram Hydrochloride. Doxapram hydrochloride is a reliable respiratory stimulant with a wide range of doses that may be used safely (toxicity is usually manifested by hypertension and seizures). It stimulates both central and peripheral chemoreceptors. At present, in the United States it is available only as an intravenous preparation, so it may be used for short-term therapy only. It has been found useful in the treatment of primary alveolar hypoventilation syndrome. It may also be used in treating hypoventilation secondary to chronic lung diseases, but, as with the use of other respiratory stimulants, dyspnea may be exacerbated. The drug may be administered by constant intravenous infusion, with 3 to 6 mg per minute being an effective dose.

Progesterone. This hormone has been found effective in the treatment of some patients with chronic CO_2 retention secondary to obesity-hypoventilation syndrome. Progesterone seems to act as a central respiratory stimulant, but it does not appear to be an especially potent stimulant. Oral forms are available, and chronic therapy has been accomplished. Medroxyprogesterone in a dose of 20 mg three times per day has been used with success. Potential side effects are thromboembolism and impotence in the male.

Almitrine. Almitrine is a respiratory stimulant currently unavailable in the United States. It has been studied in patients with chronic obstructive pulmonary disease and has been found capable of reducing $PaCO_2$ and increasing PaO_2 when administered chronically by the oral route. Respiratory stimulation takes place by sensitization of the carotid chemoreceptors. A seemingly independent effect is enhancement of hypoxic pulmonary vasoconstriction, which may serve to improve oxygenation by reducing ventilation-perfusion inequality.

Acetazolamide. This drug is not actually a respiratory stimulant, but may be used to "decompensate" a compensated respiratory acidosis. Acting as a carbonic anhydrase inhibitor, it facilitates a bicarbonate diuresis, leading to a mild hyperchloremic metabolic acidosis. The relative acidosis stimulates ventilation to reduce $PaCO_2$. This approach, while useful, is not without hazard; if the patient is unable to increase ventilation in response to the induced acidemia, dyspnea and the consequences of metabolic acidosis will ensue. The drug may be administered orally or intravenously in a single dose of 250 to 500 mg. Subsequent doses depend on the arterial blood gas and pH response.

Aminophylline. This agent, given in usual doses, is a mild respiratory stimulant that acts on the central nervous system. It may be especially useful when hypoventilation is associated with Cheyne-Stokes breathing.

Methylphenidate Hydrochloride and Caffeine. Methylphenidate hydrochloride (Ritalin) and caffeine have been used as respiratory stimulants, apparently functioning to increase the general level of arousal. They are useful in some narcoleptic patients.

SUGGESTED READING

Aldrich TK. Respiratory muscle fatigue. Clin Chest Med 1988; 9:225–236.

Altose MD, Hudgel DW. The pharmacology of respiratory depressants and stimulants. Clin Chest Med 1986; 7:481–494.

Johanson WG, Peters JI. Respiratory failure: pathophysiology and treatment. In: Murray JF, Nadel JA, eds. Textbook of respiratory medicine. Philadelphia: WB Saunders, 1988:2017.

Weinberger SE, Schwartzstein RM, Weiss JW. Hypercapnia. New Engl J Med 1989; 321:1223–1231.

RESPIRATORY ALKALOSIS

RICHARD M. EFFROS, M.D.

Respiratory alkalosis occurs when the rate of alveolar ventilation exceeds that needed to keep arterial carbon dioxide partial pressure ($PaCO_2$) below 38 mm Hg and consequently results in an alkalosis. Implicit in this definition is the assumption that alveolar ventilation is increased relative to the rate at which carbon dioxide (CO_2) is produced. Furthermore, it is assumed that the alveolar hyperventilation is not secondary to an underlying metabolic acidosis. It must be emphasized that it is the alveolar ventilation rather than the total ventilation that must increase under these circumstances; ventilation of dead space within the lungs does not contribute to the loss of CO_2. The relationship between arterial carbon dioxide pressure ($PaCO_2$), alveolar ventilation ($\dot{V}_A$), and CO_2 production ($\dot{V}co_2$) can be readily understood in terms of the following alveolar ventilation equation:

$$PaCO_2 = \frac{\dot{V}co_2 P_B}{\dot{V}_A}$$

where P_B is the atmospheric pressure. Not uncommonly, dead space and total ventilation is increased in patients with severe lung disease, but V_A is actually reduced and hypercapnia is consequently observed. Diagnosis of respiratory alkalosis must depend on measurements of Pco_2 and pH. Hyperventilation can be quite subtle and is frequently overlooked by clinicians. Furthermore, it is difficult to distinguish between total and alveolar hyperventilation and between primary and secondary disorders without arterial blood data.

After the onset of acute respiratory alkalosis, the level of plasma bicarbonate decreases rapidly by approximately 4 mEq per liter, from 24 to 20 mEq per liter, when the $PaCO_2$ is decreased from 40 to 20 mm Hg. This change in bicarbonate is related in large part to tissue and blood buffering, and to a lesser extent, to lactate accumulation. Under these circumstances, actual pH is 7.6 rather than 7.7, the pH which would have been observed had the level of bicarbonate not decreased. Over the next few days, renal excretion of bicarbonate may result in an additional decrease in bicarbonate to 15 mEq per liter, with a further improvement of arterial pH to 7.49.

CAUSES RELATED TO HYPOXIA

High Altitude Exposure

Hypoxia is an inevitable consequence of residence at high altitudes (Table 1). The response of the peripheral chemoreceptors to acute hypoxia is stimulation of the respiratory center, causing the Pco_2 to decrease rapidly. Increased ventilation is helpful because it tends to increase the partial pressure of oxygen (Po_2). Over the next few days, the kidneys respond to the respiratory alkalosis by increasing bicarbonate excretion. This causes the arterial pH to return toward normal and reduces the restraint on ventilation exerted by alkalosis. Ventilation consequently increases further, and there are additional decreases in the Pco_2 and increases in the Po_2 during this period of compensation. In some individuals, the hyperventilatory response to hypoxia appears to be less than optimum, and these patients may complain of dyspnea, malaise, headaches, insomnia, anorexia, nausea, and vomiting after a day or two of residing at high altitudes. These symptoms are referred to as "acute mountain sickness" and are probably related to hypoxia rather than hypocapnia. They can be avoided if a metabolic acidosis with secondary hyperventilation is induced through administration of acetazolamide before ascent into high altitudes. It should be noted that long-term residents of high altitudes seem to lose their sensitivity to hypoxia and typically have less severe hypocapnia and are less hypoxic than visitors. In a small number of natives, decompensation eventually develops with severe hypoxemia, polycythemia, and cor pulmonale. At altitudes over 8,000 feet, acute pulmonary edema, retinal hemorrhage, and cerebral edema may occur. The onset of these events is unpredictable, and pulmonary edema is more commonly seen in healthy young people. It may recur in these individuals and has not been linked to respiratory alkalosis.

TABLE 1 Causes of Respiratory Alkalosis

Hypoxia
High altitudes
Lung disease
Pneumonia
Pulmonary vascular disease
Pulmonary restrictive disease
Pulmonary obstruction (early)
Anemia
Hypotension
Central nervous system
Anxiety
Central nervous system injuries
Cerebrovascular disorders
Tumors
Infections
Other causes
Drugs
Salicylates
Xanthines
Catecholamines
Nicotine
Progestational agents
Gram-negative sepsis
Liver failure
Mechanical ventilation
Treatment of metabolic acidosis

Lung Disease

Hypoxia can occur with a wide variety of pulmonary diseases and stimulates ventilation. In restrictive disease associated with decreased lung or chest wall compliance, patients characteristically remain hypocapnic until late stages, when $\dot{V}_A$ becomes compromised. Hypocapnia may also be seen in association with asthma and relatively mild obstructive lung disease, but CO_2 retention eventually occurs as obstruction worsens. Pulmonary vascular and embolic disease are usually associated with respiratory alkalosis. Pneumonias also tend to stimulate ventilation, and hyperventilation may be observed in as many as 10 percent of patients with pulmonary edema. It should be emphasized that the degree of hyperventilation found in patients with these pulmonary disorders is often out of proportion to the amount of hypoxia seen and seems to be related in part to the stimulation of pulmonary parenchymal receptors that respond to stretch or deformation. Thus even if administration of oxygen in these individuals corrects the arterial Po_2, it may fail to eliminate the respiratory alkalosis. Chronic hyperventilation is frequently observed in the presence of intrapulmonary or intracardiac shunting of venous blood into the systemic arteries.

Anemia and Hypotension

If sufficiently severe, either anemia or hypotension may result in tissue hypoxia and hyperventilation. The tendency for anemia to stimulate ventilation is particularly pronounced if an acute loss of blood has occurred.

CAUSES RELATED TO THE CENTRAL NERVOUS SYSTEM

Anxiety

Anxiety is probably the most common cause of respiratory alkalosis. This may be a transient problem related to acute stress, or it may recur in individuals who chronically hyperventilate. Episodes of hyperventilation may be initiated by anxiety, anger, or grief, and patients experiencing these emotions are particularly likely to be symptomatic.

Central Nervous System Injury

Any injury involving the brainstem may result in hyperventilation; this sign generally indicates a poor prognosis. Cerebrovascular disorders, tumors, and infections may be responsible for moderate or severe hyperventilation, and CO_2 tensions may decrease dramatically. Respiration may become extremely regular, having an increased rate and depth of ventilation, and the patient is usually (although not always) unconscious. Alternatively, patients with central nervous system disease may manifest Cheyne-Stokes respiration with episodes of hyperventilation interrupted by apneic spells. The level of the $PaCO_2$ is then dependent on the stage of respiration during which blood is sampled; it is characteristically lower during the apneic phase. This pattern of ventilation is also seen in patients with severe congestive heart failure in whom prolonged circulation times may contribute to this cyclic ventilatory abnormality.

Drug Toxicity

High doses of salicylates stimulate medullary chemoreceptors and cause hyperventilation. The Pco_2 may decrease to 30 mm Hg if the patient is taking a dose of 4 g of aspirin per day and to 10 mm Hg if the dose is 12 g per day. This hyperventilation occurs independent of the metabolic acidosis that follows and persists even if metabolic acidosis is corrected. The metabolic acidosis is in turn related to the uncoupling of oxidative phosphorylation and may be accompanied initially by hyperglycemia, and later by hypoglycemia with ketosis and lactic acidosis. Acutely, patients experience nausea, agitation, confusion, seizures, and coma. Tinnitus is common with chronic salicylate ingestion. Young children are more likely to present at the hospital with metabolic acidosis.

Respiratory alkalosis may also be related to the use of theophyllines, catecholamines, progestational compounds, and nicotine.

OTHER CAUSES

Hyperventilation is observed in more than 50 percent of patients with gram-negative sepsis and may precede other manifestations such as fever, hypotension, and metabolic acidosis. Gram-positive sepsis may also cause hyperventilation in some patients.

Not uncommonly, respiratory alkalosis is observed after correction of metabolic acidosis. The delay in slowing of ventilation is presumably related to persistence of acidosis in the cerebrospinal fluid, and care must be taken to avoid correcting the metabolic acidosis too rapidly with bicarbonate infusions. Another common iatrogenic problem is encountered in patients with chronic CO_2 retention who are placed on ventilators. If mechanical ventilation is overly vigorous, the underlying compensatory metabolic alkalosis will become evident, and if this is sufficiently severe, it may result in seizures and death, even when the Pco_2 level remains above normal.

Virtually any kind of severe liver disease with hepatic failure can be associated with moderate or severe respiratory alkalosis, and levels of arterial Pco_2 of less than 25 mm Hg carry a grave prognosis.

By the end of the first trimester of pregnancy, the $PaCO_2$ decreases by approximately 12 mm Hg and stays close to this level throughout the remainder of the pregnancy. During childbirth, the $PaCO_2$ decreases even further and may cause a typical hyperventilation syndrome. It is generally believed that this response to pregnancy is related to the level of progesterone, and ventilation returns to normal as this level declines with the termination of pregnancy. Mild hyperventilation is also common during the progestational stage of the menstrual cycle.

Fever, hypotension, delirium tremens, hyperthyroidism, heat stroke, and heat exhaustion have all been reported to cause hyperventilation.

SYMPTOMS AND SIGNS

Patients with respiratory alkalosis are usually unaware of the fact that they are hyperventilating. They may complain of difficulty breathing and hyperventilation may actually induce bronchospasm. Other common complaints are a sense of imminent doom and substernal or epigastric discomfort, which can resemble that of angina or pulmonary embolism. These symptoms may be particularly confusing because respiratory alkalosis can also result in depressions of the ST segments of the electrocardiogram that resemble those of myocardial ischemia. It has been suggested that respiratory alkalosis may aggravate myocardial ischemia in patients with either arteriosclerotic coronary artery disease or Prinzmetal's angina by increasing the affinity of hemoglobin for oxygen or by promoting coronary artery constriction. In the presence of coronary artery disease, hypocapnia can promote both atrial and ventricular arrhythmias that may respond to correction of the arterial Pco_2.

Chest discomfort may also be related to mitral valve prolapse, which appears to be enhanced by hyperventilation. When related to anxiety, hyperventilation is often accompanied by aerophagia, with a sensation of bloating and cramping, and the patient may complain of palpitations. Lightheadedness and confusion may be encountered when the PCO_2 level acutely decreases to less than 25 mm Hg. Paresthesias are common. They are usually, but not always, bilateral and are characterized by numbness about the mouth and extremities. If hyperventilation is sufficiently severe, carpopedal spasm, syncope, or seizures may follow. The neuromuscular complications of respiratory alkalosis appear to be related to a decrease in ionized calcium in the serum and perhaps to the alkalosis itself.

Symptoms and signs of acute respiratory alkalosis are summarized in Table 2. This disorder is responsible for many of the symptoms associated with "neurocirculatory asthenia" and "panic disorders."

TABLE 2 Symptoms and Signs of Acute Respiratory Alkalosis

Dyspnea
Substernal and epigastric discomfort
Anxiety
Confusion
Diaphoresis
Aerophagia
Paresthesias
Carpopedal spasm
Dizziness
Syncope
Seizures
Arrhythmias in patients with coronary artery disease

THERAPY

Treatment of respiratory alkalosis is frequently more perplexing than is its detection. Generally treatment is not needed unless the arterial pH exceeds 7.5, and therapy is seldom indicated in cases of chronic respiratory alkalosis. In patients with primary hyperventilation secondary to anxiety, rebreathing into a relatively noncompliant paper bag about the size of a lunch bag quickly increases the $PaCO_2$ and reverses symptomatology. Rebreathing must continue as long as the patient continues to hyperventilate. Reassurance and other modes of relieving anxiety may be needed. Beta-adrenergic blockade has recently been reported to be helpful, presumably because it reduces adrenergic stimulation of ventilation. Tricyclic antidepressants may be useful in mitigating symptoms associated with panic attacks.

$PaCO_2$ tensions can be increased by raising inspired CO_2 tensions or, if the patient is mechanically ventilated, by increasing the dead space of the ventilator. These maneuvers stimulate respiration and may promote fatigue. Furthermore, attempts to increase the $PaCO_2$ in patients with respiratory alkalosis associated with serious illness are seldom helpful, although they may reverse arrhythmias in patients with coronary artery disease. In patients with brain injury, increasing the $PaCO_2$ may cause more damage by increasing cerebral perfusion and intracerebral pressure.

Relief of hypoxia by administration of oxygen (or by return to normal altitudes) can reverse respiratory alkalosis secondary to hypoxemia.

Salicylate poisoning can be treated by urinary alkalinization and diuresis, and these measures can increase salicylate excretion by an order of magnitude. Alkaline fluids that contain both potassium and glucose are generally administered, but care must be taken that the patient does not become overhydrated, since some patients with salicylate poisoning seem predisposed to pulmonary edema. Furthermore, administration of alkaline solutions is contraindicated in patients with severe respiratory alkalosis. Either hemodialysis or hemoperfusion is indicated when blood levels of salicylate are very high or when severe neurologic signs or cardiovascular complications appear. In addition, it may be possible to remove tablets from the stomach by gastric lavage, and the absorption of residual medication from the gut can be enhanced by administering activated charcoal with sorbitol.

SUGGESTED READING

Ferguson A, Addington W, Gaensler E. Dyspnea and bronchospasm from inappropriate postexercise hyperventilation. Ann Intern Med 1969; 71:1063–1072.

Leibowitz MR. Imipramine in the treatment of panic disorder and its complications. Psychiatr Clin North Am 1985; 8:37–47.

McHenry PL, Cogan OJ, Elliott WC, Knoebel SB. False-positive ECG response to exercise secondary to hyperventilation: cineangiographic correlation. Am Heart J 1970; 79:683–687.

Okel BB, Hurst JW. Prolonged hyperventilation in man: associated electrolyte changes and subjective symptoms. Arch Intern Med 1961; 108:757–762.

Rice RL. Symptom patterns of the hyperventilation syndrome. Am J Med 1950; 8:691–700.

Saltzman HA, Heyman A, Sieber HO. Correlation of clinical and physiologic manifestations of hyperventilation. N Engl J Med 1963; 268:1431–1436.

Tavel ME. Hyperventilation syndrome with unilateral somatic symptoms. JAMA 1964; 187:301–303.

Tavel ME. Hyperventilation syndrome: hiding behind pseudonyms? Chest 1990; 97:1285–1287.

METABOLIC ACIDOSIS

JAIME URIBARRI, M.D.
HUGH J. CARROLL, M.D.

Normal metabolic processes generate daily approximately 1 mEq of hydrogen ion per kilogram of body weight, leading to the daily consumption of the same amount of buffer, which for practical purposes can be designated as bicarbonate. Reversal of this physiologic tendency toward metabolic acidosis is normally accomplished by two renal mechanisms: (1) complete renal tubular reabsorption of all filtered bicarbonate and (2) generation of new bicarbonate by a mechanism that excretes acid in the urine.

Metabolic acidosis is caused by a diminution in body bicarbonate content. The mechanisms of this process include loss of bicarbonate in stool or urine, failure of the kidney to generate new bicarbonate appropriately, generation of acid by metabolic processes (e.g., ketoacids and lactic acid), and ingestion of acids or their precursors (e.g., methanol, ethylene glycol).

COMPENSATORY MECHANISMS

All of the four primary acid-base disorders are tempered by compensatory alterations in the parameters not primarily involved. In the case of metabolic acidosis, the acidemia caused by the decrease in serum bicarbonate stimulates central and peripheral chemoreceptors, and hyperventilation ensues. This compensatory decline in carbon dioxide partial pressure (Pco_2) raises the blood pH toward (although not to) the normal level. A useful approximation of appropriate respiratory compensation for metabolic acidosis is given by the following formula:

$$\Delta Pco_2 = (\Delta HCO_3 \times 1.2) \pm 2$$

Respiratory compensation usually reaches its appropriate level within 12 to 24 hours. If Pco_2 is inappropriately high, two causes should be considered: (1) acidosis of short duration or (2) a complicating primary respiratory acidosis. If Pco_2 is inappropriately low, respiratory alkalosis is also present and its cause must be sought.

Renal compensation for metabolic acidosis relies upon an increase in ammonia excretion and may require more than 24 hours to be fully established.

Although it is not truly a compensatory mechanism, metabolic alkalosis complicating metabolic acidosis ameliorates the acidosis or restores the pH to normal. If the alkalosis is more severe than the acidosis, the pH rises to levels higher than normal.

THE ANION GAP

The concentration of serum cations must equal the concentration of serum anions. For purposes of defining the anion gap, we designate sodium, chloride, and bicarbonate as the "measured ions." Albumin, sulfate, phosphate, and organic anions (a total of 23 mEq per liter) are the "unmeasured anions," and potassium, calcium, and magnesium (a total of 10 mEq per liter) are the "unmeasured cations." Although the anion gap is estimated as Na- (Cl + HCO_3), it is actually determined by the difference between unmeasured cations and unmeasured anions. Thus, in ketoacidosis, an accumulation of 12 mEq per liter of organic acid increases the level of unmeasured anions from 23 to 35 mEq per liter, and thus the anion gap is 35 − 11 = 24 mEq per liter. In renal tubular acidosis (RTA), the normal anion gap reflects the normal concentrations of unmeasured ions.

CLASSIFICATION OF METABOLIC ACIDOSIS ACCORDING TO THE ANION GAP

The anion gap (normally 12 ± 4 mEq per liter) serves as a useful point of departure for classifying metabolic acidosis (Table 1). However, proper interpretation of the anion gap for the differential diagnosis of metabolic acidosis requires the recognition of conditions that may alter the anion gap independently of acid-base disorders. For example, hyperglobulinemia, as in multiple myeloma, may reduce serum sodium without reducing chloride or bicarbonate and to the same extent reduces the anion gap. Similarly, in hypoalbuminemic states, chloride replaces the anions normally contributed by albumin, and the resulting hyperchloremia decreases the anion gap. Thus, a cirrhotic patient with hypoalbuminemia and hyperchloremia who has suffered rupture of esophageal varices and shock might develop lactic acidosis and manifest a normal anion gap because the accumulation of lactate in his blood has simply raised an initially low anion gap into the normal range.

The causes of acidosis with increased anion gap are usually apparent from the clinical presentation and, except for uremic acidosis, which is readily identified by assessment of renal function, these disorders tend to develop very rapidly. Ketoacidosis is diagnosed by a positive serum ketone test (Acetest). Lactic acidosis is usually suggested by tissue underperfusion, ethanol intoxication, or severe liver disease and is confirmed by a high serum lactate level and, in a patient with short bowel syndrome and neurologic abnormalities, by D-lactic acidosis. Acidosis resulting from ingestion of toxins may be suspected on the basis of the history and is confirmed by measurement of the concentration of toxins in the blood; a serum osmolar gap in excess of 10 mOsm per liter in an appropriate clinical setting supports the diagnosis of ethylene glycol or methanol poisoning. The serum osmolar gap is estimated as the difference between the measured osmolality and that estimated from the following formula:

$$\text{serum osmolality} = \text{serum sodium} \times 2 + \text{BUN}/2.8 + \text{glucose}/18$$

Clinically, the most common cause of an increased osmolar gap is ethanol intoxication, which can cause lactic acidosis and ketoacidosis.

In those cases in which bicarbonate is not replaced by an "unmeasured" anion, the chloride is elevated and hyperchloremic acidosis results. Serum chloride must always be interpreted in relation to serum sodium; with states of dehydration, water retention, or salt loss, serum chloride varies with serum sodium. Thus a dehydrated patient with lactic acidosis may present with hyperchloremia, while a patient with fecal loss of bicarbonate may have a hyperchloremic acidosis despite a serum chloride level that is absolutely low. A common error is to mistake compensated respiratory alkalosis (low bicarbonate and high chloride) for hyperchloremic acidosis; the problem is quickly resolved by measurement of blood pH.

The cause of hyperchloremic acidosis is usually apparent from the history and clinical findings. When the cause is not clear, measurement of net acid excretion (titratable acidity + ammonia − bicarbonate) distinguishes renal acidosis (low or normal net acid excretion) from extrarenal acidosis (increased net acid excretion). It has been suggested that the urinary anion gap (urinary sodium + potassium − urinary chloride) is a rough but useful estimate of ammonia excretion. If the urinary anion gap is negative, the ammonia excretion will be greater than normal and the acidosis is extrarenal. A positive urinary anion gap, on the other hand, will indicate low ammonia excretion and suggest acidosis of renal origin. These calculations are useful only when the urine has an acid pH and is not infected. The glomerular filtration rate (GFR) may be frankly below normal in the presence of hyperchloremia, in which case the diagnosis of early uremic acidosis may be made; if the GFR is normal or only minimally impaired, RTA is present.

TABLE 1 Classification of Metabolic Acidosis According to the Anion Gap

Increased anion gap (normochloremic acidosis):
Ketoacidosis
Beta-hydroxybutyric acidosis
Lactic acidosis
D-lactic acidosis
Uremic acidosis
Salicylate, methanol, ethylene glycol, and paraldehyde intoxications
Normal anion gap (hyperchloremic acidosis):
Renal tubular acidosis
Early uremic acidosis
Intestinal loss of bicarbonate
Urinary diversion procedures
Acidosis caused by chloride-containing acids (e.g., hydrochloric acid, ammonium chloride, arginine hydrochloride, lysine hydrochloride)
Acidosis caused by the use of anion-exchange resins (e.g., cholestyramine)
Ketoacidosis during recovery phase
Dilutional acidosis
Acidosis following respiratory alkalosis
Acidosis caused by a shift of H^+ from the cell
Acidosis caused by the use of acetazolamide
Organic acidosis with narrow normal anion gap

TREATMENT

Attempts should always be made to reverse the underlying disorder. If conditions cannot be re-established in which the patient can maintain his own bicarbonate balance, the patient must be provided in the long-term with bicarbonate or with a bicarbonate precursor such as citrate; in the patient with renal tubular acidosis or uremia who presents with severe acidosis, bicarbonate is a required part of the immediate therapy. The patient with diabetic ketoacidosis, however, usually has two major sources of endogenous bicarbonate: (1) the ketone anions, which produce bicarbonate on their metabolism, and (2) the bicarbonate-generating capacity of the renal tubules. In the great majority of diabetics, these two sources suffice and exogenous bicarbonate is unnecessary, but in some instances of diabetic ketoacidosis or in other varieties of acidosis in which the patient has the capability ultimately to reverse the acidosis, severe acidemia must be directly dealt with and bicarbonate must be given.

The relationship between bicarbonate dosage and the increase in serum bicarbonate is curvilinear; the lower the level of serum bicarbonate, the less is its increase for a given quantity of alkali. As a useful approximation, it may be calculated that 2 mEq of bicarbonate per kilogram of body weight will raise serum bicarbonate by 4 mEq per liter in mild acidosis but only 2 mEq per liter in severe acidosis. The amount actually required to produce a given effect in a given individual is hard to calculate for several reasons—for example, in lactic acidosis, bicarbonate therapy may stimulate the glycolytic pathway to produce more lactic acid, and in diabetic ketoacidosis (DKA), the metabolism of ketones may produce additional alkali. An acceptable approach is to give one or two ampules of bicarbonate (44 to 88 mEq) initially with repetition of the same dosage as indicated by the results of repeated blood gas measurement.

The precise conditions under which bicarbonate should be given is to some extent a matter of individual experience, but most physicians consider administration of bicarbonate when the pH falls below 7.1. A particular hazard of acidosis is cardiovascular collapse due to arteriolar dilation and decreased myocardial contractility. In general, older patients and patients with diminished myocardial reserve tolerate acidosis very poorly, and therefore bicarbonate therapy should probably begin at a pH of 7.2.

The following reasons have been given for avoiding rapid correction of severe acidosis:

1. "Overshoot alkalosis" caused by the summation of exogenous bicarbonate and that which results from the metabolism of organic anions.
2. Elevation of pH at such a rapid rate that low levels of red blood cell 2,3-diphosphoglycerate cannot increase rapidly enough to avoid tissue hypoxia.
3. Alkalosis caused by persistent hyperventilation in the presence of bicarbonate administration.
4. Paradoxical central nervous system (CNS) acidosis caused by the fact that carbon dioxide can enter the CNS more rapidly than bicarbonate.

It must be pointed out, however, that these arguments have been overemphasized and should not cause the physician to deny the patients the beneficial effect of at least modest amounts of bicarbonate when acidosis is severe. The administration of bicarbonate for specific indications is discussed later in this chapter.

Metabolic Acidosis in Specific Clinical States

Diabetic Ketoacidosis

In the average patient with DKA, the anion gap approximately equals the decrement in serum bicarbonate concentration and the test for ketones in serum and urine is strongly positive. However, neither of these two conditions is mandatory. In some patients, the anion gap exceeds the decrement in bicarbonate because ketone excretion has not been excessive and the retained ketones accumulate preferentially in the extracellular space, whereas in other patients, excretion of large amounts of ketones makes the anion gap somewhat smaller and the serum chloride somewhat higher. The occurrence of frank hyperchloremia, however, is unusual unless the serum sodium is also elevated. The patient may have DKA with a weakly positive or, rarely, a negative Acetest reaction if most or all of the ketoacid is in the reduced form as beta-hydroxybutyric acid. The conditions under which this event occurs are those in which tissue oxygenation is markedly reduced (e.g., septic shock), and in this event, serum lactate is usually higher than the 3 to 4 mEq per liter usually found in DKA.

When the diagnosis of DKA has been confirmed, a flow sheet is prepared in which the patient's clinical and chemical indices and fluid balance are carefully recorded.

Insulin. The patient should receive regular insulin as an intravenous bolus of 10 to 20 U, followed by either an intravenous infusion at a rate of 0.1 U per kilogram per hour or intramuscular injections of 10 U per hour. Insulin administration is continued at this rate until the serum ketone reaction becomes negative. If the blood glucose decreases to less than 300 mg per deciliter before the disappearance of serum ketones, glucose-containing solutions should be substituted and insulin administration continued at the same rate.

Fluids. Water and salt replacement is needed in all patients. Theoretically, the patient should receive hypotonic saline because he has lost water in excess of salt, but the fear of cerebral edema has popularized the practice of starting fluid replacement therapy with 1 L of normal saline and thereafter alternating normal saline with half-normal saline. The actual rate of infusion is determined by the needs of the individual, but the state of dehydration (4 to 5 L of water in adults) is such that 1 L is commonly administered with the first hour; most patients require 4 to 6 L during the first 24 hours. Many pediatric textbooks advise the administration of large amounts of hypotonic solution, but the ubiquity of cerebral edema in DKA and the propensity of children to die of or be disabled as a result of cerebral herniation suggest that avoidance of plasma hypotonicity in children is a prudent measure, and that small volumes of more concentrated salt solutions should be used in children than is currently the practice.

Potassium. Although potassium depletion is a universal phenomenon in DKA, the serum potassium level may range from low to high; usually it is slightly elevated. The effects of several events—e.g., insulin administration, an increase in blood pH, glycogen synthesis—combine to cause a decline in serum potassium, sometimes precipitously, and care must be taken to avoid hypokalemia. If at the start of therapy serum potassium is less than 5 mEq per liter and urine output is normal, potassium administration can be started at a rate of 10 mEq per hour and thereafter modified according to the results of repeated serum potassium levels. Although it is appropriate to be cautious with regard to the rate of potassium administration, no upper limit (e.g., 20 to 30 mEq per hour) can be arbitrarily assigned. If, for example, a patient has life-threatening acidosis and must receive bicarbonate, while the serum potassium is already very low, the intracellular shift of potassium may cause lethal hypokalemia unless potassium is administered at a rate much more rapid than those cited.

Bicarbonate. Treatment with insulin not only stops excessive gluconeogenesis and restores normal glucose metabolism, it also stops mobilization of fatty acids, the precursors of ketoacids, and the blood pH increases as glucose decreases. The blood pH increases primarily because the ketone anions, acetoacetate, and beta-hydroxybutyrate are converted to bicarbonate, but renal generation of bicarbonate also makes a contribution. As noted earlier, insulin alone is usually sufficient to improve serum bicarbonate, and administration of bicarbonate is therefore not necessary. In many patients, when the anion gap returns to normal levels (indicating metabolism of all bicarbonate precursors), only a modest increase in serum bicarbonate occurs, and at this point, the chemical pattern of the blood is that of hyperchloremic (normal-anion gap) acidosis. This chemical pattern obtains because a significant portion of the ketone anions are excreted in the urine before the patient's admission to the hospital. Despite this failure of serum bicarbonate to increase promptly to normal levels, blood pH is usually satisfactory because hyperventilation persists for many hours and, eventually, renal generation of bicarbonate normalizes the serum bicarbonate level. Although routine administration of bicarbonate to patients with DKA is not necessary, small amounts should be given to patients with severe acidosis. For example, as was discussed earlier in this chapter, bicarbonate should be given to older patients with poor myocardial reserve when the arterial pH is less than 7.2, and to younger patients when the pH decreases to less than 7.1.

Phosphate. The routine administration of phosphate is probably unnecessary in most patients with DKA, but the serum level should be followed and phosphate supplement should be given if the serum level decreases to less than 2 mg per deciliter. Phosphate can be given as the potassium salt, and the total intravenous dose should not exceed 1 g of phosphorus per day. Excessively rapid administration of phosphate can lead to hypocalcemia.

Indices of Successful Treatment. The endpoint in the treatment of DKA should be the disappearance of ketone anions from the patient's serum. This is best indicated by a negative Acetest reaction and usually coincides with the disappearance of the excess anion gap. Early in the treatment period, despite a decrease in the total ketone concentration, the Acetest reaction may suggest that ketonemia is worsening. This is because the test measures acetoacetate and acetone and not beta-hydroxybutyrate, and with the improvement of the oxidation status of tissues, the ratio of acetoacetate to beta-hydroxybutyrate increases. Normalization of the anion gap is usually a less reliable marker for the disappearance of ketonemia because substantial laboratory errors are often associated with its measurement. Delayed excretion of acetone by lungs and kidneys may sometimes explain a normal anion gap and a positive serum Acetest, since acetone is not a charged moiety.

Alcoholic Ketoacidosis

Alcoholic ketoacidosis typically occurs in chronic alcoholics after a binge during which they have eaten poorly and vomited severely. The possible mechanisms of this acidosis include insulin deficiency caused by hypoglycemia induced by fasting, and an increase in lipolysis. The latter mechanism may be caused by vomiting, which causes an increased secretion of glucocorticoids and catecholamines, and by the ketogenic effect of alcohol or alcohol withdrawal. The Acetest reaction may be only weakly positive in those instances in which most of the ketone anions are in the form of beta-hydroxybutyrate rather than acetoacetate. A modest degree of lactic acidosis may accompany alcoholic ketoacidosis.

The administration of glucose without bicarbonate or insulin terminates alcoholic ketoacidosis easily. An initial dose of 150 ml per hour of any solution containing 5 percent dextrose is reasonable. As in the case of diabetic ketoacidosis, serum levels of potassium and phosphate tend to decrease during treatment, and these ions should be provided according to need. Hyperglycemia is frequently observed during recovery and may reflect the transient inability of the liver to handle a glucose load.

Lactic Acidosis

Lactic acid, the product of glycolysis, is produced by most tissues and carried to the liver and kidney to be oxidized and converted back to glucose. When oxidative processes are interfered with (e.g., with severe liver disease), particularly when the blood supply and therefore the oxygen supply to the liver is reduced, the excess lactic acid titrates the body buffers and metabolic acidosis results. Tissue hypoxia is by far the most common cause of lactic acidosis. Other causes of this disorder are listed in Table 2. Excessive intake of alcohol can induce severe lactic acidosis because the oxidation of alcohol interferes with the mechanism that ordinarily oxidizes lactate to pyruvate. When the alcohol has been metabolized, the lactic acidosis quickly resolves and, curiously, does not recur when the patient drinks again.

Some aspects of the treatment of lactic acidosis are disputed, but the consensus is that the underlying abnormality must be reversed. Lactic acidosis is a metabolic emergency and should be treated in an intensive care unit with appropriate monitoring of metabolic and hemodynamic parameters. Volume replacement is commonly necessary, but care must be taken to prevent fluid overload.

Although bicarbonate does not improve the underlying disorder, it does protect against the harmful effects of extreme acidemia and should be administered when the arterial pH is less than 7.15. A few clinical reports and experimental studies suggest that bicarbonate therapy for the treatment of lactic acidosis may have some detrimental effects (e.g., negative cardiovascular response, reduction of lactate extraction by the liver, and direct stimulation of lactate production), but no significant adverse effects have been clearly documented in humans. Sufficient bicarbonate should be administered to increase the pH to at least 7.2. Because of the potential for volume overload when bicarbonate is being administered, furosemide may be needed, and if the patient has renal failure, dialysis may be indicated. Recovery from lactic acidosis is commonly characterized by "overshoot alkalosis" as the large amounts of lactate are converted to bicarbonate while hyperventilation persists. Dichloroacetate, an experimental drug that enhances the oxidation of lactate, has shown some initial encouraging results, but larger clinical trials are needed.

Chronic lactic acidosis may occur in patients with cancer, and in general it is not advisable to treat this disorder with bicarbonate. The bicarbonate increases glycolysis and more lactate is formed and excreted in the urine. To provide substrate for this process, protein is broken down and converted to glucose. Hence, in the end, such treatment of this form of lactic acidosis may markedly accelerate cachexia.

TABLE 2 Causes of Lactic Acidosis

Type A (caused by tissue hypoxia)
Circulatory shock
Severe anemia
Cardiopulmonary arrest
Type B
Drugs and Toxins
Biguanides, alcohol, fructose, sorbitol, xylitol, methanol, epinephrine, ethylene, glycol, streptozotocin, papaverine, isonazid, salicylates
Idiopathic
Diabetes, neoplastic diseases, liver disease, renal failure
Congenital enzymatic defect
Glucose-6-phosphatase deficiency, fructose-1, 6-diphosphatase deficiency, pyruvate carboxylase deficiency, pyruvate dehydrogenase deficiency

D-Lactic Acidosis

The lactic acid produced by humans is the L-isomer. In patients with the short bowel syndrome D-lactic acid is produced by the action of colonic bacteria on unabsorbed dietary carbohydrates.

The critical elements in the diagnosis of D-lactic acidosis include (1) rapid development of a high anion gap acidosis; (2) laboratory reports of normal serum lactate levels; (3) a negative Acetest reaction; and (4) the appearance of characteristic neurologic findings (e.g., confusion, disorientation, slurred speech, staggering gait, nystagmus, and delirium). The diagnosis is confirmed by measurement of the serum and urinary D-lactate levels, a procedure identical to the measurement of L-lactate, except for the substitution of D-lactate dehydrogenase (LDH) for L-LDH in the reaction mixture. The development of D-lactic acidosis seems to be caused by a defect in the utilization of as well as by the overproduction of D-lactic acid, since ordinarily humans metabolize D-lactate quite effectively.

For the acute attack, therapy may include administration of intravenous fluids and bicarbonate but relies most on the elimination of the offending colonic bacteria by the administration of oral antibiotics. Subsequent management may include recolonization of the large intestine with Julia flora, a population of bacteria that do not produce D-LDH, and a low-carbohydrate diet.

Salicylate Intoxication

Although salicylate intoxication is generally included in the differential diagnosis of high anion gap metabolic acidosis, the earliest abnormality and the one most commonly found in patients admitted with salicylate intoxication is respiratory alkalosis, which is attributable to the direct effects of salicylate on the respiratory center. When acidosis does occur, it results in part from the compensatory loss of bicarbonate during the phase of hyperventilation and also from interference with metabolic pathways that lead to the accumulation of organic anions (lactate + ketones). The salicylate ion itself may make a small contribution to the anion gap. The toxicity of salicylate depends on its intracellular concentration, and its rate of cellular penetration depends on the concentration of unionized salicylic acid. Thus, acidemia increases the toxicity of salicylate by increasing the rate of its cellular penetration.

The treatment of salicylate intoxication relies primarily on promoting salicylate excretion by alkalinization of urine with administration of bicarbonate. An alkaline blood pH reduces the cell uptake of salicylate, but the blood pH should be monitored hourly, and if it is found to exceed 7.55, acetazolamide should be given to increase bicarbonate excretion. In patients with severe toxicity and worsening neurologic symptoms, hemodialysis should be performed.

Toxic Organic Acidosis Caused by Ethylene Glycol and Methanol

Methanol and ethylene glycol (the latter usually in the form of antifreeze) are sometimes ingested as substitutes for alcohol. Although neither is toxic, both are broken down into toxic organic compounds, most of which are strong acids. Therefore, although patients present with certain individual clinical characteristics, two common features are seen: severe anion gap acidosis and an increased osmolar gap, the latter representing that portion of the ingested substance that has not yet been converted to organic acid. Although fairly typical symptoms may point to the correct diagnosis, confirmation can be rapidly obtained by identification of toxic compounds in the serum. Some hospital laboratories and many commercial laboratories are equipped with constantly available chromatographic apparatus for this type of diagnosis.

Ethylene Glycol Intoxication. Ethylene glycol is metabolized to a series of compounds including glycolic, glyoxalic, and oxalic acids. During the early stages of ethylene glycol intoxication, one finds in addition to profound metabolic acidosis a CNS dysfunction characterized by ataxia, confusion, coma, and seizures. Patients may then develop cardiopulmonary failure and later acute tubular necrosis. The anion that accumulates is predominantly glycolate, but lactate may also accumulate because of the increased production of NADH. In this clinical setting, the appearance of large amounts of urinary oxalate crystals favors the diagnosis of ethylene glycol poisoning.

Therapy is based on the administration of ethanol to prevent ethylene glycol metabolism while simultaneously correcting the severe acidosis and removing ethylene glycol. Unlike ketone anions and lactate, glycolate is not a bicarbonate precursor, and bicarbonate must be administered to treat the acidosis. The loading dose of ethanol is 0.6 g per kilogram of body weight given either intravenously or orally, and the maintenance dose is 0.15 g per kilogram per hour in chronic alcoholics and 0.07 g per kilogram per hour in nonalcoholics. Hemodialysis removes ethylene glycol and glycolate efficiently and should be used in severely intoxicated patients. The ethanol dosage should be increased by 50 percent when hemodialysis is used. Recently, a specific inhibitor of alcohol dehydrogenase—4,methylpyrazole—has been used to treat ethylene glycol poisoning.

Methanol Intoxication. Metabolic acidosis in methanol intoxication results from the metabolism of methanol to formic acid. A prominent complication is optic neuritis, which can cause blurred vision and may progress to blindness. Funduscopic examination may reveal retinal edema and inflammation of the optic disc. As in the case of ethylene glycol poisoning, excessive production of NADH during the metabolism of methanol leads to an excessive production of lactic acid. A diagnostic clue to severe methanol intoxication can be missed if measurement of the osmolar gap is delayed; because methanol is continuously metabolized, the serum osmolar gap may have returned to normal. However, measurement of serum formate concentration provides confirmation of the diagnosis in the latter case. The treatment of methanol intoxication is the same as that of ethylene glycol poisoning.

Chronic Renal Failure

Advanced renal disease of any cause tends to be associated with some degree of acidosis by the time the GFR decreases to less than 20 ml per minute. The predominant mechanism of the acidosis is diminished ammonia production. The acidosis of advanced renal failure is associated with retention of anions such as sulfate and phosphate, with an elevation in the anion gap. However, with milder degrees of renal insufficiency, the acidosis may be hyperchloremic before significant retention of anions occurs. Predominantly tubulointerstitial renal disease may present with defective excretion of ammonia earlier, and hyperchloremic acidosis that is out of proportion to the decline in the GFR may be found.

In renal disease, the rate of acid production is unchanged and the alkali requirement for neutralizing the daily acid production does not usually greatly exceed 1 mEq per kilogram of body weight per day. For patients who tolerate oral bicarbonate pills poorly, Shohl's solution (sodium citrate with some citric acid for flavoring) may be used. One milliliter of Shohl's solution provides 1 mEq of bicarbonate. The serum bicarbonate level should be kept close to the normal range in order to limit progressive bone disease. In children, the goal should be to maintain a normal serum bicarbonate concentration.

Gastrointestinal Loss of Bicarbonate

Fecal, pancreatic, or biliary loss of bicarbonate causes hyperchloremic metabolic acidosis and hypokalemia. The amount of bicarbonate lost depends on the type of diarrhea. For example, in malabsorption syndrome, some of the organic acids produced by bacteria are titrated by bicarbonate and excreted in the stools as the salts of the organic anions. The alkali loss in the stools can be approximated by measuring the stool anion gap (Na + K − Cl). Alkali, fluid, and potassium are replaced according to the patient's specific needs.

Urinary Diversion Procedures

The association of hyperchloremic metabolic acidosis with urinary diversion procedures is well known. In the past, when ureterosigmoidostomy was the procedure of choice, the incidence of acidosis was nearly 80 percent. Later, with the use of other diversion procedures such as the ileal conduits, the incidence of metabolic acidosis diminished markedly. The mechanism of acidosis seems to be excessive urinary loss of bicarbonate secondary to active chloride absorption in exchange for bicarbonate, which normally takes place in the terminal ileum and ascending colon. Close follow-up of serum bicarbonate is required during the period after surgery to determine whether and how much alkali therapy is needed. Progressive renal insufficiency is common and is caused by obstruction due to ureteral stenosis, stones, and recurrent malignancy. Patients may become salt- and volume-depleted, a condition that markedly worsens the metabolic acidosis and often necessitates hospital admission for water and electrolyte replacement as well as for treatment of acidosis.

Renal Tubular Acidosis

RTA comprises a set of disorders characterized by hyperchloremia associated with hypokalemia of varying severity. In proximal RTA, a low threshold for bicarbonate excretion prevents the maintenance of normal serum bicarbonate, while in distal RTA, the crucial dysfunction is an inability to maintain high concentrations of hydrogen ion in the urine. The diagnosis of distal RTA can be made outright in a patient with hyperchloremic acidosis, frank acidemia, and inappropriately "alkaline" urine (pH > 5.5). In proximal RTA, the urine pH may become fairly acidic and may overlap with the range found with distal RTA. Hence, an acid load is sometimes needed to distinguish proximal from distal RTA. If a documented decrease in plasma bicarbonate of 3 to 5 mEq per liter is not accompanied by a decline in urine pH to less than 5.5, the diagnosis of distal RTA is confirmed. The administration of furosemide can be substituted for an acid load, since furosemide promotes hydrogen ion secretion by increasing the distal delivery of sodium.

Proximal Renal Tubular Acidosis. Defective reabsorption of bicarbonate by the proximal nephron may occur as an isolated event in children, but most commonly it occurs as part of a generalized proximal tubular dysfunction (Fanconi's syndrome). Carbonic anhydrase inhibitors produce the same alteration in acid-base metabolism as proximal RTA.

For acidosis to be corrected, large amounts of bicarbonate must be administered because the low tubular threshold causes the bicarbonate to be wasted. As the excess bicarbonate passes through the collecting tubule, excessive secretion of potassium occurs, and hypokalemia is a common consequence of bicarbonate therapy in the treatment of proximal RTA. Despite this difficulty, even mild acidosis should be treated in children because acidosis severely impairs growth. Volume depletion with thiazide diuretics and a low-salt diet may increase the renal bicarbonate threshold and reduce bicarbonate requirements. Alkali is usually given as sodium bicarbonate or as Shohl's solution with potassium supplements. As an alternative, part of the alkali replacement can be given as oral potassium citrate.

Distal Renal Tubular Acidosis. Acidosis is more severe in distal RTA than in proximal RTA, and the severe chronic acidosis leads to potassium wastage. Hence patients commonly present with weakness caused by profound hypokalemia. Nephrolithiasis, nephrocalcinosis, and pyelonephritis frequently complicate distal RTA and may led to progressive renal insufficiency. The daily dosage of alkali required to correct acidosis is determined by trial; since varying but modest amounts of bicarbonate may be excreted in the urine, the dosage is generally in the range of 1 to 3 mEq per kilogram per day. Although potassium supplementation is necessary for patients with acidosis and hypokalemia, it is not regularly required if the alkali supplements are keeping the blood pH within the normal range. In the acute phase of therapy, when acidosis and hypokalemia are severe, therapy should always be directed first at correction of the serum potassium in order to avoid acutely worsening hypokalemia with respiratory paralysis and potentially lethal cardiac arrhythmias.

Hyperkalemic Hyperchloremic Acidosis (Type IV RTA)

In a variety of clinical circumstances in which the common pathophysiologic feature is a lack of aldosterone or that the collecting tubules apparently fail to respond to aldosterone, hyperchloremic acidosis presents with sustained elevation in serum potassium.

A noteworthy feature of the hyperkalemic state is that the electrocardiogram is usually unaffected. The most common cause of sustained hyperkalemia is the syndrome of hyporeninemic hypoaldosteronism (SHH). In this disorder, renin, and consequently aldosterone, are suppressed by volume expansion caused by a primary but unexplained exaggeration in renal salt reabsorption. About half of the patients with this disorder are diabetics, two-thirds have elevated blood pressure, and most have mild-to-moderate renal insufficiency. Interstitial nephropathy, acute glomerulonephritis, and urinary tract obstruction are other common causes of sustained hyperkalemia. The principal cause of the acidosis is suppression of ammonia production due to an excess of body potassium, but the lack of aldosterone, in addition to limiting potassium secretion, also limits hydrogen ion secretion. A liberal salt intake combined with the use of diuretics can diminish the excess total body salt and water and enhance the excretion of potassium, while permitting at least partial return of plasma renin and aldosterone. With this regimen, blood pressure may also decrease. Part of the sodium may be given as bicarbonate or citrate in addition to chloride. Relief of hyperkalemia may ameliorate acidosis. If the suggested program is inadequate, mineralocorticoid replacement can be added (e.g., fluorohydrocortisone 0.1 mg per mouth daily), although mineralocorticoid replacement alone is not appropriate therapy. In many patients, the hyperkalemia is mild and well tolerated. Such individuals may not require therapy. Nevertheless, in these patients, care must be taken to avoid clinical conditions and drugs that may provoke hyperkalemia by reducing distal sodium delivery, reducing aldosterone, or hampering potassium secretion—for example, volume depletion, nonsteroidal anti-inflammatory agents, angiotensin-converting enzyme inhibitors, beta-blockers, heparin, and potassium-sparing diuretics. The underlying cause of type IV RTA should always be sought and, if possible, treated. For example, in patients with obstructive uropathy, relief of obstruction could reverse the defect. Chronic administration of ion-exchange resins (e.g. Kayexalate) is often unsatisfactory because of severe constipation or undesired sodium retention.

Pseudohypoaldosteronism. Pseudohypoaldosteronism type I is a congenital and often transient disorder of infants in which the renal facet of a generalized unresponsiveness to aldosterone is reflected in salt loss, dehydration, hyperkalemia, and hyperchloremic acidosis. A similar disorder may present after infancy as a consequence of chronic renal insufficiency, most often because of tubulointerstitial disease, and is generally described as salt-losing nephropathy. In these disorders, the available evidence shows elevated plasma renin and aldosterone. Treatment consists primarily of supplementation with salt and alkali, sometimes accompanied by thiazide diuretics.

Pseudohypoaldosteronism type II, which is probably identical to Gordon's syndrome, is a variant of hyporeninemic hypoaldosteronism and is treated similarly. In this disorder, primary salt retention is believed to be caused by the inappropriate reabsorption of chloride in the collecting tubule; failure to establish a negative charge in the lumen limits the secretion of both potassium and hydrogen. As in all disorders in which potassium retention leads to hyperkalemia, suppression of ammonia production worsens the acidosis.

SUGGESTED READING

Batlle DC, Hizon M, et al. The use of the urinary anion gap in the diagnosis of hyperchloremic metabolic acidosis. N Engl J Med 1988; 318:594.

Halperin ML, Hammeke M, et al. Metabolic acidosis in the alcoholic: a pathophysiologic approach. Metabolism 1983; 32:308.

Jacobson D, Bredsen JE, Eidel I, Ostborg J. Anion and osmolal gaps in the diagnosis of methanol and ethylene glycol poisoning. Acta Med Scand 1982; 212:17.

Oh MS, Carroll HJ. The anion gap. N Engl J Med 1979; 197:814.

Oh MS, Carroll HJ, Uribarri J. Mechanism of normochloremic and hyperchloremic acidosis in diabetic ketoacidosis. Nephron 1990; 54:1.

Oh, MS, Uribarri J, Carroll HJ. Electrolyte case vignette: a case of unusual organic acidosis. Am J Kidney Dis 1988; 11:80.

Rocher LL, Tannen RL. The clinical spectrum of renal tubular acidosis. Ann Rev Med 1986; 37:319.

METABOLIC ALKALOSIS

ROBERT G. LUKE, M.B., Ch.B
JOHN H. GALLA, M.D.

DIAGNOSIS

Metabolic alkalosis is the most common acid-base disorder in hospitalized patients. Alkalemia is the elevation of arterial blood pH above normal; alkalosis is defined as a tendency toward elevation of arterial blood pH. This difference is important diagnostically because in mixed disturbances, alkalosis may conceal a primary metabolic or respiratory acidosis. Metabolic alkalosis occurs when an acid-base disturbance tends to increase primarily the plasma bicarbonate concentration; the usual associated increment in arterial carbon dioxide concentration ($PaCO_2$) is a secondary and compensatory phenomenon and never fully corrects arterial pH to normal in the absence of an associated primary respiratory acidosis. Patients with hypochloremia and hyperbicarbonatemia may have either respiratory acidosis or metabolic alkalosis; the anion gap tends to be elevated in metabolic alkalosis but not in respiratory acidosis unless there is associated lactic acidosis caused by severe hypoxia. Clearly the determination of arterial pH and $PaCO_2$ is essential before the treatment of hypochloremic hyperbicarbonatemia is instituted in order to determine an accurate acid-base diagnosis. On the average, respiratory compensation for chronic metabolic alkalosis is $PaCO_2$ increase of 0.6 mm Hg for each milliequivalent increase in the plasma bicarbonate concentration above normal. In extreme metabolic alkalosis, the $PaCO_2$ may reach 60 mm Hg or more. It is especially important to recognize that the latter situation is not a primary respiratory disorder, since treatment aimed primarily at reducing $PaCO_2$ produces a life-threatening increase in arterial pH. In primary metabolic alkalosis, specific acid-base therapy is generally indicated when the plasma bicarbonate concentration is greater than 33 mEq per liter or the arterial pH is greater than 7.50.

The clinical manifestations of metabolic alkalosis per se are difficult to separate from those of the commonly associated pathophysiologic states such as volume or potassium depletion. However, neuromuscular irritability, cardiovascular instability and arrhythmias, and mental confusion are common when alkalosis is severe. The potential adverse effects of compensatory hypoventilation on other pulmonary functions or on the development of infections of the respiratory tract in the seriously ill patient or the immunocompromised host may be significant. Metabolic alkalosis is clearly not an innocuous condition; in one large series, for patients with an arterial pH of 7.65 or greater the mortality rate was 80 percent. Again, associated conditions may be important, but treatment of the metabolic alkalosis per se in such circumstances is a medical emergency and requires a rapid assessment of the relevant causative mechanisms in order to prescribe corrective therapy, as discussed below.

Metabolic alkalosis can be divided into two phases: generation (loss of hydrogen ion from or gain of bicarbonate by the body) and maintenance. In the absence of the conditions outlined in Table 1, it is difficult to exceed the capacity of the normal kidney to excrete administered bicarbonate or its metabolic precursors such as citrate or carbonate. Iatrogenic acute metabolic alkalosis related to oral or intravenous sodium bicarbonate administration is thus usually transient in the presence of a normal kidney. Especially when sodium bicarbonate has been given intravenously, transient metabolic alkalosis may also occur as the accumulated organic anions of diabetic ketoacidosis or lactic acidosis are metabolized to bicarbonate secondary to insulin administration and/or volume repletion. Since base loading alone rarely produces a sustained elevation of plasma bicarbonate concentration by more than 2 to 3 mEq per liter in the absence of bicarbonate-retaining mechanisms, the focus of this chapter is on the treatment of chronic metabolic alkalosis in which one of the sustaining causes is virtually always evident. On occasion, the pathogenesis of the generation phase of metabolic alkalosis is obscure and cannot be established by the time the physician is faced with the clinical problem. This, however, need not deter effective therapy. The paramount question to be answered by the physician prior to initiation of appropriately designed therapy is: Why is this patient's kidney not excreting the retained extracellular bicarbonate?

THERAPEUTIC OPTIONS

The mechanisms listed in the first column of Table 1 are almost always responsible for the inability of the kidney to excrete the retained extracellular bicarbonate. In many patients, multiple mechanisms may contribute and interact. In most, the major mechanism relates to either chloride depletion or mineralocorticoid excess potassium depletion. Associated potassium depletion is also common with chloride metabolic alkalosis, but in general the alkalosis *can* be corrected in such patients without concomitant restoration of potassium balance; for the second group, by contrast, repletion of potassium is necessary for correction of metabolic alkalosis. There are, however, cogent clinical reasons to also correct the associated potassium depletion during treatment of metabolic alkalosis even when it is primarily due to chloride depletion. Not included in Table 1 is the recent observation that hypoproteinemia may also be

TABLE 1 Causes and Treatment of Maintained Elevation of Plasma Bicarbonate on Chronic Metabolic Alkalosis

Mechanism	*Causes of Maintained Elevation of HCO_3*	*Therapeutic Options*
Chloride depletion (chronic vomiting)*	Chloride depletion	Replace chloride as NaCl, KCl, or HCl
	Continuing H^+ loss	Cimetidine
	Ineffective CBV	Improve cardiac output; acetazolamide
	Moderately depressed GFR	NaCl; restore ECF or cardiac output
	Severely depressed GFR (at least temporarily irreversible)	HCl; dialysis against high chloride dialysate
Potassium depletion—mineralocorticoid excess (Bartter's syndrome)	Potassium depletion (depresses GFR and increases tubule reabsorption of bicarbonate)	Discontinue diuretic; KCl; amiloride, triamterene or spironolactone; indomethacin; magnesium repletion
With hypertension (primary aldosteronism)	Excess mineralo- and/or glucocorticoid activity	Low-NaCl diet—remove adenoma Spironolactone (primary aldosteronism); Treat hypertension—KCl Spironolactone (secondary aldosteronism); Pituitary surgery or irradiation Remove ACTH-producing tumor or adrenal tumor—metyrapone or aminoglutethimide (Cushing's syndrome)
Base loading (multiple blood transfusions)	Administration of $NaHCO_3$ or its precursors (e.g., citrate) *plus* bicarbonate-maintaining cause	Stop base; correct underlying cause (above)
With hypercalcemia and hypoparathyroidism (milk-alkali syndrome)	Depression of GFR and enhanced tubular reabsorption of bicarbonate	Stop high intake of base and calcium; replete chloride and ECF volume deficit

*Example of clinical cause.
CBV = circulating blood volume.

associated with mild alkalosis, which resolves with the restoration of the serum protein concentration to normal.

In most patients, the history and physical examination will be strongly suggestive of the mechanisms responsible for the maintenance of the elevated plasma bicarbonate concentration. If the cause is not obvious, determination of urinary chloride and potassium concentrations may be helpful. Patients with chloride depletion metabolic alkalosis have a urinary chloride concentration less than 10 mEq per liter except when renal chloride wasting is the cause of chloride depletion, as for example within the period of therapeutic efficacy of administered diuretics or in severe chronic potassium depletion (plasma potassium < 2.4 mEq per liter); in the latter instance, chloride will not be retained until repletion of potassium is initiated. Unless these rather unusual circumstances of renal chloride wasting are present or the patient is ingesting diuretics surreptitiously, a urinary chloride concentration greater than 20 mEq per liter usually suggests that therapy other than chloride repletion is necessary.

Metabolic alkalosis is often also associated with increased urinary potassium excretion, and a urinary potassium concentration of greater than 30 mEq per liter despite hypokalemia would be anticipated unless potassium depletion is profound (i.e., a deficit greater than 500 mEq in an adult man of average weight). In such circumstances, the urinary potassium concentration may be less than 20 to 30 mEq per liter and yet potassium depletion may be a major contributory cause of the metabolic alkalosis. Primary potassium losses from the bowel, as that which occurs with laxative abuse or villous adenoma of the colon, are also associated with low urinary potassium concentrations.

A urinary sodium concentration of greater than 20 to 30 mEq per liter is unusual in chloride depletion alkalosis, especially when urinary pH is acidic (less than 5.5) as is customary when the kidney is conserving bicarbonate. In acute-on-chronic vomiting, as the plasma bicarbonate concentration is further elevated above its chronic stable high plasma level, transient renal wasting of sodium bicarbonate may occur. This clinical state is sometimes termed disequilibrium metabolic alkalosis. In such patients, urinary sodium concentration may be greater than 20 mEq per liter —even in the presence of overt clinical volume depletion—but the urine is quite alkaline (i.e., the pH is greater than 6.5 and contains significant amounts of bicarbonate, and the urine chloride concentration is less than 15 mEq per liter).

If the kidney function is severely depressed and the glomerular filtration rate (GFR) cannot be improved by increasing cardiac output or improving effective circulating blood volume, some form of dialysis using a dialysate with a chloride concentration significantly above that in the patient's plasma may be necessary (see Table 1).

Patients who have alkalosis caused by mineralocorticoid excess potassium depletion can be subdivided into those with a normal or low blood pressure and plasma volume and those with extracellular fluid (ECF) volume expansion and high blood pressure (see Table 1). In the former case, mineralocorticoid excess is associated with renal wasting of sodium chloride and hence an inability to develop hypertension. In the latter case, an intact kidney responds to mineralocorticoid excess with both sodium chloride retention and potassium loss.

A particularly vexing therapeutic problem is posed by those patients who can best be described as belonging to the group representing the differential diagnosis of Bartter's syndrome (Table 2). Bartter's syndrome is thus important beyond its frequency of occurrence because it illustrates the pathophysiology and treatment of the several much more common conditions listed in Table 1. It further illustrates how several mechanisms may interact with one another to maintain an elevated plasma bicarbonate concentration. The syndrome is characterized by normotension; a tendency to renal sodium, chloride, and potassium wasting; and marked stimulation of the renin-aldosterone system and of renal prostaglandin (Pg) production. Some cases are familial and develop in childhood, although the syndrome may also be diagnosed for the first time in adult life. One plausible explanation for the syndrome is a defect in sodium chloride reabsorption in the thick ascending limb of the loop of Henle with increased delivery of sodium and fluid to the more distal potassium secretory sites. Potassium loss is accelerated by both macula densa and baroreceptor stimuli for renin release and the resultant hyperaldosteronism. Potassium depletion stimulates renal synthesis of PgE_2, which in turn further impairs sodium chloride reabsorption in the thick ascending limb and sets up a vicious circle. Diuretic abuse, which may be continually denied by the patient (usually female), mimics the syndrome by impairing sodium chloride transport in the thick ascending limb of the loop of Henle (furosemide) or in the cortical diluting segment (thiazides). Urinary chloride concentration is high in diuretic abuse only during the therapeutic duration of action of the drug. Bulimia may also mimic the syndrome, but the urinary chloride concentration in patients with bulimia is usually low during the metabolic alkalosis. Once the diagnosis is made, the need for therapy is obvious in the case of diuretic abuse or bulimia; expert psychiatric help is usually needed.

SPECIFIC THERAPY

For full correction of metabolic alkalosis, the chloride deficit must be replaced, usually intravenously. Judicious selection of the accompanying cation—sodium, potassium, or hydrogen ion—depends on careful assessment of (1) ECF volume status and the presence or absence of cardiac failure, (2) the presence and degree of associated potassium depletion, and (3) the degree of impairment and reversibility of the depression of the GFR. If the kidney is capable of excreting sodium and/or potassium, it will excrete bicarbonate with those cations and thus rapidly correct the metabolic alkalosis as chloride is made available. When renal function is too severely depressed by acute or chronic intrinsic renal disease, however, or when there is intractable congestive cardiac failure, especially with hyperkalemia, administration of chloride with sodium or potassium may not be feasible. Two therapeutic strategies may be taken in such situations: infusion of chloride as hydrochloric acid (HCl), or providing chloride by dialysis across the peritoneal or hemodialysis membrane so that potassium status, sodium status, and plasma volume can be contemporaneously corrected. An additional indication for HCl is when speed of correction is essential and if there is doubt about the capacity of the kidney to excrete bicarbonate rapidly enough (Table 3).

Administration of isotonic sodium chloride is the preferred therapy if, as is most commonly the case, there is associated ECF volume depletion. This simultaneously corrects the chloride deficit, the ECF volume deficit, and the associated depression in GFR. Even though repletion of potassium is not essential for the correction of the alkalosis, potassium administration is usually indicated because some degree of

TABLE 2 Differential Diagnosis of Bartter's Syndrome

Diagnosis	*Comment*
Diuretic abuse	Low urine chloride when not ingesting diuretics
Bulimia	Low urine chloride; disequilibrium metabolic alkalosis may occur (see text)
Laxative abuse	Metabolic alkalosis usually not severe
Magnesium depletion	May complicate diuretic abuse or Bartter's syndrome
Bartter's syndrome	High urinary chloride

TABLE 3 Indications for Hydrochloric Acid Administration

Arterial pH > 7.55 and NaCl or KCl administration is contraindicated

Need for immediate amelioration of metabolic alkalosis because of:
- Hepatic encephalopathy
- Cardiac arrhythmia
- Digitalis intoxication
- Central nervous system effect of high arterial pH
- Arterial pH > 7.6 when initial renal response to NaCl or KCl or acetazolamide is likely to be sluggish or is in doubt

potassium depletion is usually present and because kaliuresis may occur as plasma volume, GFR, and urinary flow rate are restored to normal. Potassium can be provided conveniently by adding KCl to isotonic saline in a concentration of 10 to 20 mEq per liter. In most patients with overt signs of volume contraction, such as hypotension (including postural hypotension), tachycardia, and diminished skin turgor, administration of 3 to 5 L of 0.15 M NaCl is necessary to correct volume deficits and metabolic alkalosis. The physician must also include replacement of ongoing losses in the fluid and electrolyte replacement schedule. As the chloride deficit is corrected, a brisk alkaline diuresis should occur with a fall in plasma bicarbonate concentration. This alkaline diuresis may increase urinary potassium losses and reinforces the point of concurrently replacing potassium to avoid the effects of hypokalemia.

When the ECF volume is assessed to be normal, total body chloride deficit in milliequivalents can be estimated by the formula: body weight $\times$ 0.2 $\times$ the desired increment in the plasma chloride concentration. If there is associated hypokalemia, as is customary, the deficit can be repleted conveniently by either oral or intravenous KCl.

Some recent animal studies in our laboratories suggest that chloride depletion, independent of volume depletion, may contribute not only to maintenance of chronic metabolic alkalosis, but also to a reduction in the GFR and to stimulation of the renin-aldosterone system. This may explain the occasional patients we have seen with hypochloremic metabolic alkalosis, hypertension in the recumbent position, and a significant elevation of serum creatinine but without overt sodium or volume depletion. In such patients—although not as yet under study conditions of metabolic balance—administration of KCl alone has been associated with restoration of a normal serum creatinine level, amelioration of hypertension, and correction of both potassium deficits and alkalosis: even when quite severe, potassium depletion by itself is associated with only a slight-to-moderate depression of the GFR. Our studies suggest that chloride depletion leads to depression of the GFR in part via activated tubuloglomerular feedback and to stimulation of renin release from the kidney by a macula densa mechanism.

In the clinical setting of ECF volume overload and/or congestive cardiac failure in association with chloride depletion and metabolic alkalosis, administration of NaCl is clearly inadvisable. As in euvolemic patients, hypokalemia may facilitate repletion of chloride as KCl, but KCl may also be contraindicated either because of concurrent hyperkalemia or concern about the ability to deal with the potassium load in the presence of renal failure. If renal function is still reasonable in this situation (serum creatinine < 4 mg per deciliter), the use of acetazolamide in a dosage of 250 mg two or three times daily can be considered. Such an approach could be used for a patient with an acute exacerbation of chronic lung disease and cor pulmonale who develops metabolic alkalosis after therapeutic reduction in $PaCO_2$ in the presence of hyperkalemia. Occasionally, the judicious intermingling of acetazolamide with a loop diuretic in these patients with cor pulmonale will dampen the magnitude of the chloride depletion. If acetazolamide is used in a patient without hyperkalemia, KCl should be concurrently administered because the risk of development of hypokalemia during the ensuing alkaline diuresis is high. Administration of acetazolamide should be stopped when the plasma bicarbonate concentration approaches baseline levels for that patient, and plasma electrolyte composition should be followed daily during its administration.

When the kidney is incapable of responding to chloride repletion or when dialysis is necessary for the control of renal failure, exchange of bicarbonate for chloride across the semipermeable membrane used during hemodialysis or peritoneal dialysis is an effective mechanism for correcting metabolic alkalosis. Current routine dialysate solutions for both peritoneal dialysis (including continuous ambulatory peritoneal dialysis) and hemodialysis contain concentrations of bicarbonate or its metabolic precursors, such as acetate, equivalent to 35 mEq per liter and therefore must be modified in circumstances of metabolic alkalosis. In an emergency, peritoneal dialysis can be performed against solutions of 0.15 M NaCl with appropriate maintenance of plasma potassium, calcium, and magnesium concentration by intravenous infusion. Most large hospital pharmacies, however, can prepare appropriate special dialysate solutions for both hemodialysis and peritoneal dialysis in these circumstances.

The indications for the use of intravenous HCl administration are given in Table 3. Again, most hospital pharmacies are capable of making up sterile HCl as 100 mEq per liter (i.e., a 0.1-M solution), The amount of HCl (in milliequivalents) needed to correct alkalosis is calculated by the formula: 0.4 $\times$ body weight (kg) $\times$ desired decrement in plasma bicarbonate concentration (mEq per liter). Since the goal of such therapy is to get the patient out of the danger zone in terms of acid-base balance, it is usually prudent to plan initially to restore the plasma bicarbonate concentration halfway toward normal. The HCl must be given through a catheter placed in the vena cava or a large vein draining into it, and placement of the catheter must be confirmed radiographically, since extravasation of HCl can lead to sloughing of the mediastinal tissues. The rate of infusion should not exceed 0.2 mEq per kilogram of body weight per hour. The patient is best managed in an intensive care unit with frequent measurement of arterial blood gases and electrolytes. The above formula does not allow for ongoing loss of hydrogen ion or gain of base by the ECF. An alternative to HCl is ammonium chloride, which may be administered via a peripheral vein. The rate of infusion should not provide more than 300 mEq NH_4^+ per 24 hours, and NH_4Cl should be avoided in the presence of renal or hepatic insufficiency. We use HCl only when indicated (see Table 3) but prefer it to NH_4Cl in such circumstances. NH_4Cl is certainly contraindicated in patients with liver or renal failure. The HCl salts of the cationic amino acids lysine or arginine should probably not be used because of the association with dangerous hyperkalemia. Again, we prefer HCl.

Additional therapeutic approaches are necessary in the following clinical situations associated with chloride depletion metabolic alkalosis. In the presence of pernicious vomiting or the surgical requirement for continual removal of gastric secretions, metabolic alkalosis will continue to be generated and replacement of pre-existing deficits may be complicated by these ongoing losses. In these circumstances, the administration of an H_2 receptor blocker, such as cimetidine or ranitidine, will blunt acid production of the stomach and decrease gastric HCl losses. Fairly high doses of cimetidine may be required—e.g., as much as 200 to 600 mg of intravenous cimetidine every 4 hours; omeprazole, an inhibitor of H^+K^+ ATPase, is now available for this purpose and may be more efficacious. Because serious side effects such as acute confusion can complicate these dose levels, it is reasonable to check the pH of the gastric aspirate to determine the lowest effective dose. Even in the presence of achlorhydria, however, gastric secretions contain significant amounts of sodium, potassium, and chloride.

Although diarrhea is normally associated with metabolic acidosis, in two circumstances metabolic alkalosis can occur in association with increased fecal loss of fluid. About 10 to 15 percent of villous adenomas are associated with alkalosis; these require surgical removal after correction of the sodium chloride, potassium, and volume deficits. The second condition is the rare familial disease of chloridorrhea in which massive amounts of chloride, potassium, and fluid are secreted into the ileum because of a transport defect. This condition has been responsive only to continued repletion of these losses by supplementation of the dietary intake.

POTASSIUM DEPLETION-MINERALOCORTICOID EXCESS

In humans, severe potassium depletion is associated with a mild-to-moderate metabolic alkalosis unless there is complicating chloride depletion or mineralocorticoid excess, in which circumstance severe metabolic alkalosis may occur. In the presence of normotension, the cause of the metabolic alkalosis can usually be determined by the differential diagnosis. Administration of thiazide or loop diuretics should be discontinued. Oral HCl given in the liquid form diluted with fruit juice or in the slow-release form can be given in doses of up to 40 to 60 mEq four or five times per day. If serious effects of potassium depletion and/or metabolic alkalosis are present, such as cardiac arrhythmias or muscle paralysis, intravenous HCl may be given at rates as high as 40 mEq per hour in concentrations not to exceed 60 mEq per liter. These are high rates and should be employed only if life-threatening hypokalemia and/or metabolic alkalosis is present; the patient should be monitored by electrocardiogram and frequent determinations of plasma potassium concentration (Table 4). It is critical that the solution used to administer potassium or the solution given immediately before the administration of potassium (for example, in the emergency room) not contain glucose, since this will stimulate insulin secretion and cause hypokalemia to worsen. Once potassium repletion is clearly under way, the presence of glucose in the infusion may facilitate cellular potassium repletion, but hypokalemic nephropathy may impair free water excretion and plasma sodium concentration should also be monitored if a free water load is being administered.

Because Bartter's syndrome probably comprises several disorders with different pathophysiologies, the degree to which other solute deficiencies, such as sodium, chloride, magnesium, or calcium deficiencies, occur in or contribute to the disorder varies. Nevertheless, the principal goal of therapy is to prevent the loss of excessive potassium in the urine. Angiotensin-converting enzyme inhibitors—in particular, enalapril in doses of 20 to 40 mg per day—have been shown to correct hypokalemia, hypomagnesemia, and alkalosis; caution is necessary during the first few days of treatment because of possible hypotension. Potassium-sparing diuretics (amiloride, 5 or 10 mg daily; triamterene, 100 mg twice daily; or spironolactone, 25 to 50 mg four times daily) are effective for this purpose, but dietary potassium supplementation is often also needed. Spironolactone may produce tender gynecomastia in men. Renal production of PgE_2 is increased and may contribute to sodium, chloride, and potassium wasting; Pg synthetase inhibitors such

TABLE 4 Estimation of Potassium Deficit

*Corrected Plasma Potassium Concentration (mEq/L)**	*Approximate Total Body Potassium Deficit*	
	%	*Total (mEq)†*
3–3.5	5	100–200
2.5–3.0	5–10	200–400
2–2.5	10–15	300–600
<2.0	15–20+	500–800+

*Increase plasma K by 0.6 mEq per 0.1 increment in arterial pH.
†For 70-kg man.

as indomethacin or ibuprofen may blunt, but usually do not completely correct, the hypokalemic alkalosis. Because magnesium depletion may increase urinary potassium wasting, an attempt should be made to correct hypomagnesemia and replete magnesium stores. The degree to which the correction of magnesium depletion blunts the alkalosis is uncertain, however, and magnesium salts usually produce an unacceptable degree of gastrointestinal irritation that may compound the patient's problems. Oral magnesium oxide can be given in doses of 250 to 500 mg four times daily (12.5 to 25 mEq Mg). If severe hypomagnesemia is contributing to seizures or tetany, 4 ml of a 50 percent solution of magnesium sulfate (16 mEq Mg) can be given in 100 ml of 5 percent glucose over 10 to 20 minutes.

In the group of alkaloses characterized by an excess of mineralocorticoid, therapy is directed at either removal of the source or blockade of the mineralocorticoid. Hypertension, often severe, may complicate many of these disorders (specific therapy for this is discussed elsewhere in this text). Since mineralocorticoids directly and indirectly stimulate potassium and hydrogen ion secretion (equivalent to bicarbonate reabsorption) in the distal convoluted tubule and collecting duct (in part in exchange for sodium), the administration of potassium-sparing diuretics will effectively reverse the adverse effects of mineralocorticoid excess on sodium, potassium, and bicarbonate.

The stimulation of net sodium reabsorption and potassium secretion by the effect of excess mineralocorticoid on the kidney may also be ameliorated by adjustments to diet. If hypokalemia and potassium depletion develop, as is common, bicarbonate reabsorption in the proximal tubule of the kidney is stimulated and alkalosis is further intensified. By contrast, the stimulated sodium reabsorption produces volume expansion which tends to diminish fluid and HCO_3 reabsorption in the proximal tubule; however, as noted, distal bicarbonate reabsorption is stimulated by the mineralocorticoid. Thus the restriction of sodium and the addition of potassium to the diet should aid in the control of the alkalosis as well as the hypertension that often accompanies these disorders.

Many primary disorders of mineralocorticoid excess are definitively treated by tumor ablation. Adrenocorticotropic hormone-secreting pituitary tumors may be removed by transsphenoidal resection or ablated by irradiation. With adrenal tumors, adrenalectomy—either unilateral or bilateral as appropriate—is curative. In the ectopic adrenocorticotropic hormone syndrome, the ideal treatment of the secreting tumor can rarely be accomplished. In this instance and in metastatic adrenal tumors, metyrapone, which inhibits the final step in cortisol synthesis, and aminoglutethimide, which inhibits the initial step in steroid biosynthesis, will blunt the myriad manifestations of excess cortisol. In 11 beta-hydroxysteroid dehydrogenase deficiency, dexamethasone has been shown to correct the hypokalemic alkalosis. In those disorders in which curative surgery cannot be carried out, mitotane (p,p-DDD), which produces selective destruction of the zona fasciculata and reticularis and leaves aldosterone production intact, has also been used to control effectively many of the manifestations of the disease. To the extent that severe fluid and electrolyte disturbances are due to aldosterone production, this drug may not suffice. Thus, metyrapone or aminoglutethimide may be better choices when hypokalemic alkalosis is present. Cisplatin has also recently been used in the treatment of adrenal malignancies; however, a detailed discussion of the use of such drugs is beyond the scope of this review.

Among the alkaloses associated with excess exogenous base administration, the milk-alkali syndrome, characterized by metabolic alkalosis, hypercalcemia, and renal insufficiency, is now infrequently seen. Cessation of alkali ingestion and the calcium sources (often milk and calcium carbonate) and chloride and volume repletion for the commonly associated vomiting will usually lead to the prompt resolution of all abnormalities. Occasional occult sources of base loading are citrate in blood transfusions or release of base by metastases in bone.

MIXED ACID-BASE DISTURBANCES

SANDRA SABATINI, M.D., Ph.D.
NEIL A. KURTZMAN, M.D.

Mixed acid-base disturbances are defined as the coexistence of two or more simple acid-base abnormalities. The diagnosis and treatment of acid-base disorders often stress the physician needlessly. While these disorders pose some of the most challenging problems encountered in clinical medicine, the proper diagnosis should not be difficult given the state of our knowledge of acid-base physiology today. Given the many pathophysiologic processes that can alter plasma bicarbonate and arterial CO_2 tension, it is evident that the presence of one acid-base abnormality does not preclude the development of additional disturbances that have independent effects on acid-base equilibrium. Indeed, the complicated medical problems that breed one acid-base abnormality are just as likely to spawn another.

Among hospitalized patients, mixed acid-base disorders in which two components can be identified occur quite frequently. On rare occasions, three acid-base disturbances may be identified. Because the individual components of mixed acid-base disorders may be additive or counteracting as regards plasma pH, the resultant change in blood hydrogen concentration may be deceptively slight or alarmingly severe.

Table 1 summarizes the simple acid-base disturbances, indicating the primary event as well as the compensatory change (secondary event) which one expects in order to keep blood pH as close to 7.4 as possible. For example, in metabolic acidosis the maximum fall in arterial Pco_2 tension is approximately 1 to 1.5 mm Hg per milliequivalent (mEq) decrement in the plasma bicarbonate concentration. This requires that the patient have normal lungs, normal kidneys, and no underlying disease, and even then the arterial Pco_2 will rarely fall below 20 mm Hg. In such a circumstance one would expect that at an arterial pH of 7.3 the primary fall in plasma bicarbonate would be equal to 12 mEq per liter and the maximum decrement in arterial CO_2 tension in an attempt to compensate would be 25 mm Hg.

Compensation in the simple acid-base disorders is almost never complete except in chronic respiratory alkalosis. Thus, the finding of a normal plasma pH in a patient with an acid-base disorder other than chronic respiratory alkalosis immediately suggests the presence of a mixed acid-base disturbance.

The correct diagnosis of acid-base disorders can be made from a good history plus the proper interpretation of simple laboratory tests. These laboratory tests include serum electrolytes, the anion gap, arterial blood gases and pH, and occasionally urine electrolytes. The integration of these variables will assess the presence and degree of respiratory or metabolic compensation, and will thus determine whether uncomplicated or mixed acid-base disorders are present. Remember, the simple acid-base disorders may mimic mixed abnormalities if the former are acute in origin or are overcompensated. These "copy cats" are usually metabolic, as the time for full changes by the kidney requires 24 to 48 hours; changes in ventilation may occur in the space of a few breaths.

The most useful piece of information in unraveling the diagnosis of an acid-base disorder is the medical history. The presence of known underlying diseases should heighten the clinical suspicion that a specific acid-base

TABLE 1 Primary and Secondary Changes in Arterial pH, Pco_2 Tension, and Plasma HCO_3 in the Common Acid–Base Disorders

Acid–Base Disorder	*Blood pH*	*Primary Change*	*Secondary Compensation*	*Note*
Metabolic acidosis	↓	↓HCO_3	↓Pco_2 1–1.5 mm Hg/mEq ↓HCO_3	Pco_2 rarely lower than 20 mm Hg
Metabolic alkalosis	↑	↑HCO_3	↑Pco_2 0.2–0.9 mm Hg/mEq ↑HCO_3	Steady state H^+ excretion approximately equal to premorbid state
Acute respiratory acidosis	↓	↑Pco_2	↑HCO_3 (slight) 1 mEq/10 mm Hg↑	HCO_3 should be approximately equal to 24–29 mEq/L
Acute respiratory alkalosis	↑	↓Pco_2	↓HCO_3 2 mEq/10 mm Hg↓	Immediate cell buffering with hemoglobin, phosphate, proteins
Chronic respiratory acidosis	↓	↑↑Pco_2	↑↑HCO_3 5 mEq/10 mm Hg↑	↑Net acid excretion, ↑proximal HCO_3 reabsorption ($HCO_3 \leq 40$ mEq/L)
Chronic respiratory alkalosis	↑,NL	↓Pco_2	↓HCO_3 5 mEq/10 mm Hg↓	Begins in 2 hours with ↑ renal H^+ excretion (complete in 2–3 days); blood pH may be NL; hyperchloremia; profound hypophosphatemia

$pH = pKa + \log\frac{HCO_3}{(0.03)(Pco_2)}$; pKa = 6.1; 0.03 = solubility coefficient of dissolved CO_2; NL = normal disorder will be found (Table 2). In cardiopulmonary arrest, for example, both respiratory acidosis and metabolic acidosis are characteristically observed; in septic shock, mixed respiratory alkalosis and metabolic acidosis is common (lactic acidemia); in chronic obstructive pulmonary disease, respiratory alkalosis or respiratory acidosis may coexist with metabolic alkalosis, the metabolic alkalosis commonly being the consequence of diuretics or vomiting. Diarrhea is the most common cause of an acid-base abnormality—metabolic acidosis. A history of diarrhea superimposed on a patient with chronic lung disease (respiratory acidosis or respiratory alkalosis), hepatic decompensation (respiratory alkalosis), or vomiting (metabolic alkalosis) will cause a wide variation in the change of arterial pH. In the patient with severe diarrhea and respiratory acidosis, a marked decrease in arterial pH occurs; diarrhea and respiratory alkalosis will cause a slight increase in arterial pH, and diarrhea and gastric alkalosis will cause no change in arterial pH. Primary respiratory alkalosis should always be expected in the pregnant female and in patients with chronic liver disease. Chronic hypocapnia causes a low plasma bicarbonate concentration. Indeed, the finding of a normal plasma bicarbonate concentration in a patient with hepatic decompensation should immediately bring to mind the diagnosis of a mixed acid-base disorder—the cause of which should be carefully sought. The importance of the history cannot be overemphasized; it is always obtainable when one remembers that yesterday's laboratory data become today's medical history.

TABLE 2 Common Causes of Acid-Base Disorders

Metabolic acidosis
Chloride (normal anion gap) (hyperchloremia)
Gastrointestinal loss of HCO_3 (e.g., diarrhea)
Renal loss of HCO_3 (e.g., renal tubular acidosis)
Hyperalimentation, NH_4Cl ingestion
Hypoaldosteronism
Anion gap (normal plasma chloride concentration)
Ketoacidosis, lactic acidosis
Renal failure
Ingestion (salicylates, ethylene glycol, methanol, paraldehyde)
Metabolic alkalosis (normal or low plasma chloride concentration)
Vomiting or nasogastric suction
Mineralocorticoid excess
Diuretics
Respiratory Acidosis (normal or low plasma chloride concentration)
Pulmonary edema
Acute exacerbation of underlying lung disease
Severe asthma
Pneumonia
Drug overdose
O_2 administration to a patient with chronic hypercapnia
Sleep apnea syndrome
Chronic obstructive pulmonary disease (COPD)*
Pickwickian syndrome
Respiratory alkalosis (hyperchloremia)
Hypoxemia (pulmonary embolus, congestive heart failure, high altitude, anemia)
Pulmonary disease (interstitial fibrosis, pneumonia, COPD)*
Stimulation of respiratory center (psychogenic, liver failure, salicylates, pregnancy, progesterone, cerebrovascular accident/infection, pontine tumors)
Mechanical ventilation

* COPD is more commonly associated with respiratory alkalosis and is secondary to the central hypoxic drive.

RELIABILITY OF BLOOD GAS MEASUREMENTS

As mixed acid-base disorders are more likely to be disguised and are probably more common in hospitalized patients than are simple acid-base disorders, it is critical for the physician to determine the validity of blood gas measurements. At the time the arterial blood gases are drawn, virtually every patient will have a venous bicarbonate concentration measured simultaneously. Venous total CO_2 and the calculated bicarbonate concentration from the arterial blood gas should differ by no more than 1 to 2 mEq per liter. Plasma bicarbonate concentration can easily be calculated from the Henderson-Hasselbalch equation:

Eq. A

$$\text{pH} = \text{pKa} + \log\frac{[HCO_3]\ \text{(mmol per liter)}}{0.03 \times P_{CO_2}\ \text{(mm Hg)}}$$

where: $pK_a = 6.1$, the dissociation constant for the HCO_3/H_2CO_3 buffer system; and 0.03 = the solubility coefficient of dissolved CO_2 in whole blood at 37 °C. An alternative is:

Eq. B

$$[H^+]\left(\begin{matrix}\text{nmol per liter}\\ \text{or nanoEq)}\end{matrix}\right) = \frac{24 \times P_{CO_2}\ \text{(mm Hg)}}{[HCO_3]\ \text{(mmol per liter)}}$$

If the normal P_{CO_2} is 40 mm Hg and HCO_3^- concentration is 24 mEq per liter, then the normal H^+ concentration is 40 nanoEq per liter. Thus, to use Equation B, one must convert measured pH to H^+ concentration. A simple rule of thumb is as follows:

1. For every 0.1 *increase* in pH, multiply the H^+ concentration by 0.8 (e.g., pH = 7.5, then $H^+ = 40 \times 0.8 = 32$ nanoEq per liter).
2. For every 0.1 *decrease* in pH, multiply the H^+ concentration by 1.25 (e.g., pH = 7.2, then $H^+ = 40 \times 1.25 \times 1.25 = 63$ nanoEq per liter).

In essence, this equation can be reduced to a proportional relationship so that the blood pH is directly related to the ratio between the *metabolic* component of acid base (i.e., the blood bicarbonate concentration) and the *respiratory* component (i.e., the arterial CO_2 tension):

Eq. C

$$\text{pH} \propto \frac{\text{Metabolic Component}}{\text{Respiratory Component}}$$

THE PLASMA CHLORIDE CONCENTRATION

Essential to the dissection of acid-base disorders is an initial assessment of the plasma chloride concentration (normally 100 mEq per liter). The plasma chloride changes for only two reasons: a change in hydration, or a change in acid-base status. It is easy to distinguish between these by examining the plasma sodium concentration (normally 140 mEq per liter). The normal ratio of the plasma sodium to plasma chloride concentration = 140 mEq per liter over 100 mEq per liter = 1.4. If the plasma chloride concentration increases parallel and proportional to the rise in plasma sodium concentration, then a change in the state of hydration has occurred, i.e., dehydration. Dehydration should be suspected in the elderly, particularly in hot weather, or in the comatose patient who is unable to express a feeling of thirst. Hyperchloremia occurs in this instance if there is inadequate water replacement secondary to inadequate intake or large obligatory losses of free water by the skin and lungs. Dehydration can also be caused by vomiting or diarrhea, and these disorders in turn are virtually always associated with an acid-base disturbance. On the other hand, if the plasma chloride concentration falls in proportion to a decrease in plasma sodium concentration, then cellular overhydration is present. Overhydration commonly occurs from the injudicious administration of hypotonic fluids to hospitalized patients with impaired urinary diluting capacity either secondary to an inadequate circulation (heart failure) or to intrinsic renal disease.

If the plasma chloride concentration changes out of proportion to the serum sodium concentration and the ratio is not 1.4, then an acid-base disturbance is present. Of the four simple acid-base disorders, two are always associated with hyperchloremia and two are associated with a normal (or low) plasma chloride concentration (see Table 2). Hyperchloremia occurs in metabolic acidosis (nonanion gap) and compensated respiratory alkalosis. The simple disorders should be easily recognizable by the fact that the former will be associated with acidemia and the latter with either alkalemia or a near normal arterial pH. Both will be associated with a low arterial P_{CO_2}. A low plasma chloride concentration occurs in metabolic alkalosis and compensated respiratory acidosis. While both of these will be associated with an increase in P_{CO_2} tension, the arterial pH will never be normal. Metabolic alkalosis will have an increase in arterial pH, whereas respiratory acidosis, regardless of the degree of compensation, will be associated with an acid blood pH. In addition to Table 2, the common causes of the simple acid-base disturbances are found in the chapters *Metabolic Acidosis, Metabolic Alkalosis, Respiratory Acidosis,* and *Respiratory Alkalosis*.

ANION GAP

Assessment of acid-base abnormalities includes calculation and interpretation of the anion gap and is equal to:

$$AG = \text{plasma Na} + K - (\text{plasma Cl} + HCO_3)$$
$$AG = 12 - 16 \text{ mEq per liter}$$

The anion gap is simply a measure of the unmeasured anions or cations present in blood. The anion gap changes as the arterial pH changes, primarily as a result of the normally negative charges on the anionic protein, albumin. Other less important anions are phosphate and sulfate. When the body makes excess endogenous anions (acetoacetatic acid, lactic acid, beta-OH-butyric acid) the anion gap increases, and is exactly equal to the decrement in plasma bicarbonate concentration—anion gap acidosis (see Table 2). Plasma chloride concentration stays normal because the addition of acid is neutralized to a certain extent by the bicarbonate buffer system. If acidosis is present, but the anion gap is normal (12 to 16 mEq per liter), bicarbonate has been lost from the body, usually by the gastrointestinal tract or by the kidney. The loss of bicarbonate results in an acidosis with hyperchloremia, therefore the anion gap is normal. The anion gap increases in metabolic alkalosis as a combination of the increase in blood pH and lactate production. This may be masked, however, when one remembers that approximately one-third of hospitalized patients with metabolic alkalosis will also have an associated respiratory acidosis or respiratory alkalosis. If a mixed disorder is present, such as diabetic ketoacidosis (anion gap acidosis) and vomiting (metabolic alkalosis), the change in the gap will be much greater than the decrement of the plasma bicarbonate concentration. In this mixed abnormality both acid-base disorders will increase the anion gap; the acidosis will tend to decrease the plasma bicarbonate concentration while the alkalosis will tend to increase the bicarbonate concentration.

The anion gap is also of value to assess the unmeasured cations, such as calcium, magnesium, and certain cationic proteins. Hypercalcemia is associated with a decrease in the anion gap, as is the presence of the cationic myeloma protein.

Many nomograms have been developed to aid the clinician in the diagnosis of acid-base disorders. In general, these are of no value in mixed acid-base disorders. At pH 7.4 the normal hydrogen ion concentration of the blood is 40 nmol per liter; thus, the finding of a normal pH in the presence of an abnormal P_{CO_2} and plasma bicarbonate concentration virtually defines a mixed metabolic-respiratory disorder (P_{CO_2} tension and plasma bicarbonate concentration change in the *same* direction). Plasma pH is most affected when the P_{CO_2} and plasma bicarbonate change in the opposite direction. Remember, pH is proportional to plasma HCO_3 concentration divided by the arterial P_{CO_2} tension.

CLINICAL EXAMPLES

Case One

A 38-year-old man with adult-onset insulin-dependent diabetes mellitus developed anorexia, nausea, and intermittent chest pain. After three days he became lightheaded, developed intractable chest pain, and was admitted to the hospital. Blood pressure on admission was 70/50 mm Hg, heart rate 120 per minute, respirations 28 per minute. He was diaphoretic and the electrocardiogram revealed anteroseptal myocardial infarction, age undetermined.

He was noted to have the following blood gases and electrolytes: pH 7.41; Pco_2 14 mm Hg; Po_2 50 mm Hg; Na 128 mEq per liter; K 5.9 mEq per liter; Cl 92 mEq per liter; HCO_3 8 mEq per liter; glucose 522 mg per deciliter; creatinine 1.8 mg per deciliter; blood urea nitrogen 40 mg per deciliter.

The finding of a normal arterial pH in an obviously ill patient with hypotension suggests immediately that at least two acid-base abnormalities are present, and that they are counterbalancing as regards arterial pH. The presence of metabolic acidosis was established by a plasma venous bicarbonate concentration of 8 mEq per liter. The degree of hyperventilation exceeds that which would be anticipated purely as a result of this decrement in bicarbonate (Pco_2 14 mm Hg). The ratio of plasma sodium to plasma chloride concentration was normal (1.4), suggesting that cell hydration was normal, but the noted acidosis however, was normochloremic (i.e., anion gap). The calculated anion gap was increased to 34 mEq per liter (plasma Na + K − [plasma Cl + HCO_3]). The normal anion gap varies between 12 and 16 mEq per liter and represents the anions normally present in blood which are not measured routinely (phosphate, sulfate, organic acids). Metabolic acidosis secondary to a gain of any acid other than hydrochloric acid will be associated with an increased anion gap. The likely gained acids in this patient are a combination of lactic acid and keto acid overproduction. While the acidosis of chronic renal failure is an anion gap metabolic acidosis, this possibility is excluded because renal function is only mildly impaired (serum creatinine concentration 1.8 mg per deciliter). Unless it is determined that exogenous acid was given, the most reasonable possibilities include endogenous production of keto acids in a diabetic or lactic acid secondary to circulatory shock. The longstanding diabetes mellitus suggests that diabetic ketoacidosis is present, but blood ketone measurement was found to be 2+, consequently the ketonemia is only moderate. The presence of profound hypotension makes lactic acidosis a more likely possibility, and further documentation could be achieved by measuring lactate plasma pyruvate ratio, normal being 1 mEq per liter over 0.1 mEq per liter.

Case Two

A 30-year-old woman was brought to the clinic because of weakness and malaise of three months' duration. Physical examination revealed muscle tenderness in the upper arms and thighs, and decreased deep tendon reflexes. Routine laboratory values were: Na 140 mEq per liter; K 1.8 mEq per liter; Cl 118 mEq per liter; HCO_3 12 mEq per liter; pH was 6.90; Pco_2 60 mm Hg; Po_2 52 mm Hg; urine pH was 6.92; chest roentgenogram normal; routine abdominal x-ray film revealed nephrocalcinosis.

This patient had hyperchloremic metabolic acidosis with a normal anion gap of 12 mEq per liter. Were this the sole acid-base abnormality, the arterial Pco_2 should have been 20 mm Hg, yet this patient had a Pco_2 of 60 mm Hg. The profound decrease in arterial pH (6.9) demonstrates the degree of acidemia which may develop when respiratory acidosis and metabolic acidosis occur simultaneously. The finding of nephrocalcinosis on an abdominal roentgenogram in a patient with metabolic acidosis and high urine pH strongly suggests the presence of distal renal tubular acidosis, an anion gap metabolic acidosis. Hypokalemia per se is not a classic feature of all patients with distal renal tubular acidoses, as many now have been reported with hyperkalemia. Hypokalemia in this patient caused a complicating factor to occur, evidenced by marked weakness, malaise, and a second acid-base disorder, namely, respiratory acidosis. Profound potassium depletion may cause paralysis of the respiratory muscles and thus prevent the normal compensatory changes that would be expected to accompany uncomplicated metabolic acidosis, i.e., a decrease in arterial Pco_2. Shortly after potassium replacement was initiated, Kussmaul respirations began, the Pco_2 fell, and plasma pH began to rise. The patient, in the face of profound acidemia, was able to lower her arterial Pco_2 tension. The calculated pH was now in the range of approximately 7.2.

Since renal tubular acidosis of the distal type is attributable to renal retention of acid, appropriate therapy is sodium bicarbonate. Proximal renal tubular acidosis, on the other hand, is attributable to massive bicarbonate loss from the proximal tubule along with the loss of glucose and amino acids. This form of hypokalemic hyperchloremic renal tubular acidosis may be quite refractory to bicarbonate therapy, and the addition of a mild diuretic may be of value. The diuretic, usually a thiazide, causes some volume contraction, and increase proximal bicarbonate reabsorption.

Case Three

A 60-year-old man with a history of chronic obstructive pulmonary disease presented with a seven-day history of cough and dyspnea. Chest roentgenogram revealed a left lower lobe infiltrate and the following laboratory values: pH 7.33; Pco_2 75 mm Hg; Po_2 44 mm Hg; Na 140 mEq per liter; K 4 mEq per liter; Cl 94 mEq per liter; bicarbonate 39 mEq per liter; U_{Na} 7 mEq per liter. From the outpatient clinic records he was known to have hypertension, a modest systemic acidemia, and an arterial Pco_2 greater than 50 mm Hg. Because of impending respiratory failure, he was placed on a ventilator, and the Pco_2 was rapidly brought to 40 mm Hg. While his cyanosis improved markedly, his mental status quickly deteriorated and he became somewhat combative. Since the plasma bicarbonate concentration remained 39 mEq per liter after the ventilator Pco_2 was decreased to 40 mm Hg, the calculated pH from the Henderson-Hasselbalch equation was 7.66! This is an example of a patient with overcompensated respiratory acidosis.

Because of the past history of hypertension, the patient was given thiazide diuretics, and the following morning he became extremely disoriented; his laboratory values were P_{CO_2} 40 mm Hg, bicarbonate 38 mEq per liter, and an arterial pH of 7.66. At this point the patient had developed "posthypercapnic metabolic alkalosis."

Chronic hypercapnia enhances the renal excretion of acid and chloride. At the same time, however, it stimulates bicarbonate reabsorption by the proximal tubule. Renal compensation does not occur immediately, but rather is a gradual process occurring over several days. Following the return of the P_{CO_2} to normal, renal retention of chloride occurs in parallel with an increase in bicarbonate excretion. A rapid decrease of arterial P_{CO_2}, as can be caused by a ventilator, causes an immediate rise in arterial pH. The plasma bicarbonate concentration will remain close to that which was observed prior to use of the ventilator (e.g., approximately 39 mEq per liter), as the renal adjustment takes approximately 24 hours to occur. This alkalemia is the consequence of overcompensated respiratory acidosis.

If patients with hypercapnia are placed on a low-salt diet or are treated with diuretics as was this patient, proximal bicarbonate reabsorption will be enhanced as a consequence of volume contraction. Excretion of excess bicarbonate will not occur, and the patients are likely to develop "post-hypercapnic metabolic alkalosis." Correction of this type of metabolic alkalosis can be accomplished by salt administration. This syndrome may also occur if effective arterial volume is contracted for any reason, such as congestive heart failure. In this instance, successful treatment of the heart failure is required to correct the alkalosis, and salt administration is contraindicated.

Acetazolamide (250 to 1,000 mg daily), a carbonic anhydrase inhibitor, may be given on an acute basis to enhance the renal excretion of bicarbonate. This mild diuretic acts in the proximal tubule to prevent bicarbonate reabsorption.

Case Four

A 48-year-old man was admitted to the hospital because of protracted vomiting of 5 days' duration. On physical examination his blood pressure was 80/60 lying and in the upright position fell to 70/0. Routine laboratory values were: Na 127 mEq per liter; K 6.7 mEq per liter; Cl 80 mEq per liter; pH 7.30; P_{CO_2} 19 mm Hg; HCO_3 9 mEq per liter; creatinine 7.2 mg per deciliter; U_{Na} 30 mEq per liter; U_{Cl} 4 mEq per liter. He was mildly icteric.

The anion gap in this patient was 45 mEq per liter and the plasma chloride concentration was low in relationship to a plasma sodium concentration of 127 mEq per liter (calculated chloride should be 90 mEq per liter). The finding of an increased anion gap and a decreased plasma chloride concentration should immediately suggest at least two acid-base disorders. Upon examination of the arterial pH, one sees a mild acidemia in the face of a low plasma bicarbonate concentration and a low P_{CO_2}. Thus relative normalization of the arterial pH suggests two offsetting acid-base disorders. Based on the history of vomiting and the low plasma chloride concentration, metabolic alkalosis is probably one of the disorders. Analysis of the plasma bicarbonate concentration and the arterial P_{CO_2} and pH suggest metabolic acidosis. The metabolic acidosis could indicate a patient with chronic renal failure, a finding further suggested by substantial quantities of sodium in the urine. Analysis of the urine chloride, however, which was vanishingly low, tells you that this is not a patient with chronic renal failure, because approximately equivalent amounts of sodium and chloride should have been present in the urine. In this setting, the urine chloride level is an index of the state of effective arterial volume and is characteristic in patients with vomiting. The anion excreted with the sodium in this instance was bicarbonate. Analysis of the urine revealed a pH of 6.8. Subsequent hydration with intravenous sodium chloride resulted in a rise in urinary chloride excretion; a fall in plasma creatinine concentration to 0.8 mg per deciliter; and arterial pH of 7.47, P_{CO_2} 33 mm Hg, and HCO_3 17 mEq per liter. Abnormal liver function tests were obtained. Reanalysis of this patient revealed that he had three and not two primary acid-base disorders: metabolic alkalosis secondary to vomiting, metabolic acidosis secondary to hypotension and poor tissue perfusion, and a respiratory alkalosis that is of central origin in patients with chronic liver disease.

Case Five

An obtunded 68-year-old woman was brought to the emergency room; her laboratory values were: pH 7.15; P_{CO_2} 15 mm Hg; P_{O_2} 70 mm Hg; Na 168 mEq per liter; K 3.8 mEq per liter; Cl 122 mEq per liter; HCO_3 5 mEq per liter.

The intern in the emergency room made a presumptive diagnosis of hyperchloremic metabolic acidosis. Careful analysis of the plasma electrolytes, however, revealed that the plasma sodium concentration was 168 mEq per liter and that the plasma chloride concentration had risen in direct proportion (i.e., by 20 percent) to the plasma sodium concentration. Thus, it was obvious that this was a markedly dehydrated patient as well as one with metabolic acidosis of the anion gap type (45 mEq per liter). Subsequently, blood lactate levels were found to be markedly elevated and the lactate to pyruvate ratio, normally 10:1, was increased. The cause of the profound lactic acidosis in this patient was tissue hypoxia secondary to marked dehydration, volume contraction, and pulmonary disease. Of particular note is the finding that the P_{O_2} was only 67 mm Hg when the P_{CO_2} was 15 mm Hg. While this case does not represent a mixed acid-base disorder, it does demonstrate the importance of interpreting the plasma chloride concentration pari passu with the arterial blood gases.

Case Six

A 64-year-old diabetic woman presented to the clinic with a five-day history of diarrhea. Known medications included insulin, a diuretic, phosphate binders, and oral calcium supplement. Laboratory data were: Na 140 mEq per liter; K 5 mEq per liter; Cl 125 mEq per liter; pH 7.24; Pco_2 26 mm Hg; HCO_3 10 mEq per liter; creatinine 5 mg per deciliter; glucose 200 mg per deciliter.

Note that the plasma sodium concentration was normal, the chloride and the creatinine levels were elevated, and that metabolic acidosis was present. The calculated anion gap was 10 mEq per liter ($Na + K - [Cl + CO_2]$). Were the metabolic acidosis solely the result of chronic renal failure, inferred from the patient's known medications and confirmed by the creatinine concentration of 5 mg per deciliter, an anion gap acidosis should be present (i.e., normal plasma chloride concentration). Since hyperchloremia was present, however, the patient must have another acid-base abnormality, either respiratory alkalosis or nonanion gap acidosis. With the history of diarrhea and the laboratory data, the correct diagnosis is nonanion gap metabolic acidosis, superimposed on the anion gap acidosis of renal failure. The key clue is the finding of hyperchloremia in a patient with renal failure.

THERAPY

Once the etiologic agents of the acid-base disorders are identified, the treatment is simple. A few points are worth remembering:

First, most forms of metabolic alkalosis do not require immediate correction unless the alkalemia is severe (pH >7.55) or has occurred acutely. Attention to the state of volume (NaCl) and its replacement often causes enough bicarbonaturia that acid-base balance returns to normal. Acetazolamide (250 to 1,000 mg daily for 24 to 48 hours) will enhance bicarbonate excretion enough to decrease systemic pH toward normal. Rarely, NH_4Cl, $CaCl_2$, arginine, or lysine may be necessary. Dilute infusion of HCl is a safe measure when used by those with experience. HCl (100 to 200 mmol) is given in a large vein up to a concentration of 200 to 300 mmol over a 24-hour period. The deficit is calculated according to the extracellular space (approximately 20 percent of body weight), and a portion of the deficit is given with careful monitoring of pH and Pco_2 approximately every 3 to 4 hours.

Second, acidemia requires treatment if the pH is less than 7.20. Bicarbonate is the treatment of choice if parenteral therapy is being given. Sodium lactate offers no advantage and requires conversion to bicarbonate before its potential as a base is recognized. Severe liver disease or hypotension with poor tissue perfusion further impairs the usefulness of lactate as an alkalinizing agent. Bicarbonate (or acetate) dialysis may be considered if the acidemia is severe or is worsening despite parenteral bicarbonate therapy. Using this technique, control of the patient's volume status may be easily managed. This is of particular importance in patients with severe cardiovascular disease. Oral alkali therapy may be given in the form of bicarbonate, citrate, (Shohl's solution), or gluconate, the latter two requiring conversion to base in vivo.

Third, ion shifts tend to occur simultaneously with the acid-base disorders. Hyperkalemia generally accompanies metabolic acidosis and is attributable to a shift of potassium from the intracellular space to the extracellular fluid. Patients with protracted diarrhea, renal tubular acidosis, and diabetic ketoacidosis will generally be potassium depleted despite hyperkalemia and require oral or parenteral replacement. If parenteral therapy is chosen, potassium should not be given at a rate greater than 60 mEq per hour and should not begin until urine output is ascertained. The plasma potassium concentration should be monitored carefully. Hypokalemia accompanies metabolic alkalosis and may be profound during protracted vomiting secondary to large urinary losses of potassium. Potassium supplementation may be necessary in this instance. In syndromes associated with mineralocorticoid excess, spironolactone (300 to 600 mg daily) may be of value.

Profound hypophosphatemia may also occur during the treatment of ketoacidosis. This is attributable to a shift of phosphate from the extracellular fluid to the cell interior, a phenomenon similar to that seen with potassium. Hypophosphatemia may cause myocardial dysfunction, rhabdomyolysis, leukocyte dysfunction, and decreased 2-3 diphosphoglycerate. Milk is an excellent source of phosphate (33 mmol per liter), as is Fleet Phospho-Soda (15 to 30 ml 4 times daily). If parenteral phosphate is required, sodium or potassium phosphate may be given. These preparations contain 3 mmol per milliliter of phosphate, and in most instances up to 20 mmol every 8 hours may be safely given. While hypocalcemia and metastatic calcification are the major risks of parenteral phosphate therapy, they are easily avoided if the rate of infusion is slow and plasma calcium and phosphate concentrations are monitored carefully.

A reduction in ionized fraction of total serum calcium tends to occur in alkalosis, the most dramatic instances being seen in patients with respiratory alkalosis. This is the result of increased binding of calcium to the anionic protein, albumin, and generally does not require treatment other than to correct the underlying acid-base disorder. In acidotic states plasma ionized calcium may be slightly increased; however, large quantities of calcium (and magnesium) may be lost in the urine. Some of these conditions may require supplementation (diabetic ketoacidosis, for example) and some may not (renal tubular acidosis).

ACUTE INTERSTITIAL NEPHRITIS

PETER S. HEEGER, M.D.
ERIC G. NEILSON, M.D.

Acute tubulointerstitial nephritis, often referred to as simply "acute interstitial nephritis," accounts for nearly 15 percent of cases of acute renal failure. Individuals with acute interstitial nephritis typically experience a sudden decrease in renal function, with the hallmarks of acute interstitial injury on renal biopsy manifested by mononuclear cell infiltrates (lymphocytes and plasma cells), occasional eosinophils, tubular destruction, and relatively normal glomeruli. It is also important that as many as 25 percent of patients with chronic renal failure have sustained injury from the concealed, long-term sequelae of what probably began as acute interstitial inflammation. In such patients, biopsy reveals progressive pathologic injury involving interstitial fibrosis, tubular atrophy, and tubular drop-out with or without senescent glomerular tufts. Largely because of the work done in experimental systems, there is now a growing knowlege of the pathophysiologic mechanisms involved in the production of interstitial injury. Applying this insight to human renal disease has resulted in a reasoned clinical method for evaluating patients suspected of having acute interstitial nephritis, and in a firmer groundwork for the discussion of therapeutic options. The approach we use emphasizes the diagnosis, the removal of potentially causative agents, and attempting to treat the destructive lesion with chemotherapy when necessary.

ETIOLOGY

A wide variety of etiologic factors have been implicated in the development of acute interstitial nephritis. Most prominent among them is exposure to a multitude of drugs. Frequent offending agents include penicillinlike compounds, the cephalosporins, rifampin, sulfonamides, phenytoin, allopurinol, furosemide, alpha-interferon, and nonsteroidal anti-inflammatory drugs. A number of systemic infections such as diphtheria, scarlet fever, subacute bacterial endocarditis, human immunodeficiency virus, and Epstein-Barr virus infection are also associated with interstitial nephritis. Diphtheria and scarlet fever, however, are more commonly seen as etiologic factors in the pediatric age group. Finally, acute interstitial nephritis may be a manifestation of a local or systemic autoimmune phenomenon like sarcoidosis, Sjögren's syndrome, systemic lupus erythematosus, antitubular basement membrane disease, or the tubulointerstitial nephritis-uveitis (TINU) syndrome. Occasionally the presentation of interstitial nephritis is simply idiopathic.

CLINICAL PRESENTATION

The diagnosis of interstitial nephritis is relatively straightforward in the classic setting in which a rapidly rising serum creatinine level (0.3 to 0.5 mg per deciliter per day), accompanied by fever, rash, and eosinophilia, occurs 10 to 15 days after treatment with a pharmaceutical agent is started. Unfortunately, this presentation of a hypersensitivity reaction is the exception, not the rule. Skin rash occurs in less than 50 percent of patients, fever in approximately 75 percent, eosinophilia in about 80 percent, and the triad is found in less than 30 percent. Normal-sized or enlarged kidneys as detected by ultrasonography or radiographic methods are the rule. The physician must therefore first systematically exclude prerenal and obstructive causes of acute renal failure from the differential diagnosis and then proceed to distinguish interstitial nephritis from acute tubular necrosis, glomerulonephritis, or vasculitis. A careful urinalysis is usually helpful in this regard. In interstitial nephritis, the urinalysis reveals mild-to-moderate proteinuria (although the nephrotic syndrome has been reported, especially with use of alpha-interferon and nonsteroidal anti-inflammatory drugs), and microscopic hematuria may be present. Sterile pyuria and/or white blood cell casts are usually encountered, but red blood cell casts are so rare that their presence should suggest the alternative diagnosis of glomerular injury. Eosinophiluria supports the diagnosis of interstitial nephritis, although, again, this finding is not entirely sensitive or specific and must be considered in the context of the clinical setting. Eosinophils in the urine can best be demonstrated by Hansel's stain, where in one study the sensitivity of interstitial nephritis was 100 percent, compared with 18 percent for Wright's stain. False-positive reactions (e.g., from prostatitis) decrease the specificity and the positive predictive value of this finding.

In many situations, the precise diagnosis may not be certain from the clinical data alone, and a renal biopsy is usually warranted to clarify the form of injury. If the patient has acute interstitial nephritis, this diagnosis must be made as quickly as possible. Minimizing the time that elapses from the onset of renal injury to the institution of appropriate therapy allows the greatest possibility for return of normal renal function. In experimental interstitial nephritis, substantial interstitial fibrosis can develop in as little as 10 days. The biopsy is therefore usually needed to offer additional information on the extent and character of the lesion as well as on the prognosis and therapeutic modalities that will be necessary. We recommend routine biopsies in all cases of suspected interstitial nephritis, provided that the patient is medically stable enough to tolerate a biopsy and if his general condition is such that he is capable of tolerating immunosuppressive therapy. Although a "classic" presentation may be managed without a biopsy, additional information regarding the extent of fibrosis and the amount of mononuclear cell infiltration, both of which tend to correlate inversely with the reversibility of injury, can provide further perspective on the aggressiveness with which one should pursue therapy. Thus, for example, a patient with advanced renal insufficiency and marked interstitial fibrosis may be more appropriately diagnosed as having irreversible interstitial injury and may therefore be treated conservatively and spared the potential complications of immunosuppressive therapy. The approach to the diagnosis of acute interstitial nephritis is outlined in Figure 1.

MECHANISMS OF DISEASE

A general understanding of the underlying pathophysiologic processes leading to interstitial injury is helpful in the selection of appropriate therapy. We believe that virtually all forms of human interstitial nephritis have an immunologic basis, and several reports in the clinical literature are consistent with this view. Most of the detailed information, however, comes from studies in experimental animals.

Rodent models of interstitial nephritis implicate both humoral and/or cellular arms of the immune system in the expression of the disease. In one form of experimental interstitial nephritis—antitubular basement membrane disease—antibodies and T lymphocytes are directed against an antigen attached to the tubular basement membrane. In other circumstances, some animals with a genetic predisposition to interstitial nephritis lose their protective immunologic tolerance to self-antigens and subsequently develop an immune response against themselves. In other situations, molecular mimicry from infectious agents, and drugs acting as a hapten-bridge with the tubulointerstitium, can target an immune response towards previously unrecognized (or unexposed) self-antigens. Other drugs can damage interstitial structures through toxic mechanisms and thereby produce novel antigens that are immunogenic. Obviously, avoidance or removal of exogenous factors that

Figure 1 Approach to the diagnosis of acute interstitial nephritis.

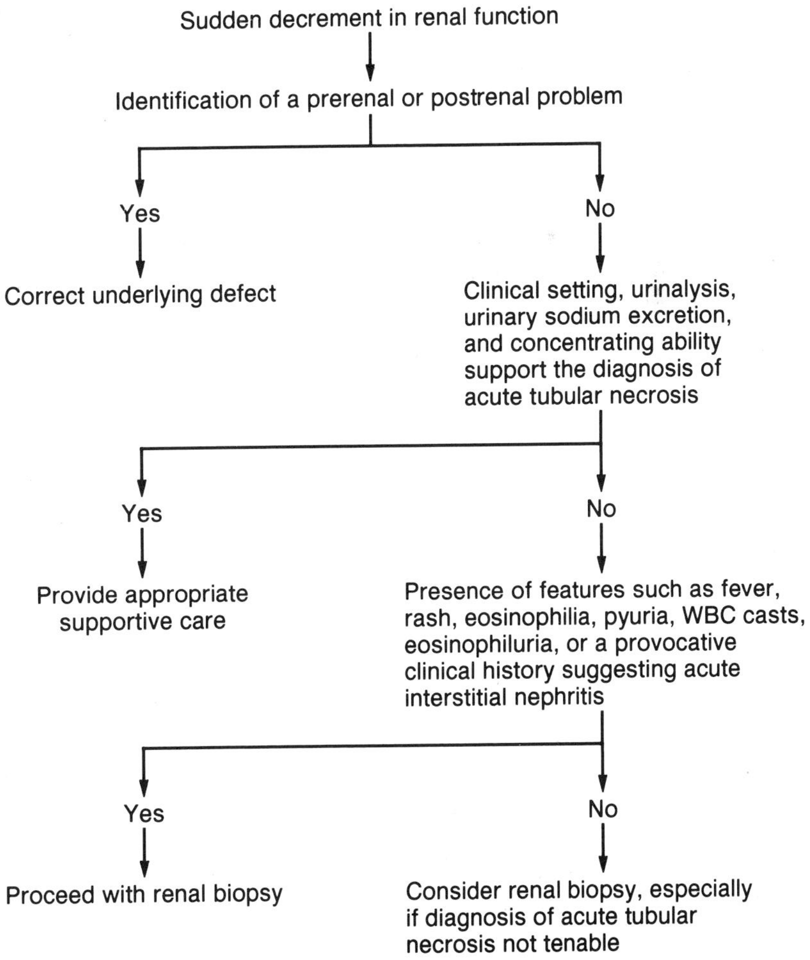

mimic or lead to antigen expression is the first step in the treatment of interstitial nephritis.

Once the target nephritogenic antigen is recognized by the immune system, several immunoregulatory factors can modulate the severity of disease. Although a detailed discussion of these factors is beyond the scope of this chapter, suppressor T-cell networks, anti-idiotypic networks, and the regulation of major histocompatibility complex (MHC) molecule expression can be considered among these variables. Therapies that make use of these endogenous control mechanisms are at the forefront of immunologic research; these are mentioned at the end of this chapter.

Actual damage to the kidney can be mediated by several effector mechanisms. Primary immune deposits are uncommon but can produce inflammation and injury through complement activation and the chemotaxis of other effector cells. The humoral response may preferentially produce IgE antibodies which then bind to eosinophils, basophils, and mast cells, leading to a coordinated hypersensitivity response. These cells release proteases, leukotrienes, superoxides, and peroxides that directly and indirectly cause tissue injury. Complement activation through the alternative pathway may play an additional role in some situations.

The hallmark of active interstitial nephritis is the presence of mononuclear cells, particularly T lymphocytes. Experimental work has revealed that populations of helper T cells can induce a second population of effector cells. These effector T cells cause injury through several discrete mechanisms including (1) delayed-type hypersensitivity with the release of inflammatory lymphokines, (2) cell-mediated cytotoxicity through protease release, and (3) the production of lymphokines that modulate the biosynthesis of extracellular matrix in epithelial cells and fibroblasts. The importance of this last mechanism cannot be overemphasized. It has become clear that the degree of fibrosis found on histologic examination of renal tissue is the best correlate of clinical renal function and that more extensive fibrosis implies a worse prognosis for recovery. The majority of therapeutic interventions probably modify some element of the effector response, although the exact mechanisms are not clear.

TREATMENT

Once the diagnosis of acute interstitial nephritis has been firmly established, the first and most obvious intervention is to identify and discontinue the use of any potential offending drugs or to treat any underlying systemic infection. In some cases, this may constitute definitive therapy. Renal function, as assessed by daily blood urea nitrogen (BUN) and/or creatinine measurements, should improve within several days of removal of potential inciting immunogenic stimuli.

For those patients whose condition does not improve or in whom the disease process appears to be idiopathic, treatment with corticosteroids should be instituted as adjunctive therapy. One should realize, however, that there are only marginal published clinical data to support its widespread use. One often quoted report of 14 patients with methicillin-induced interstitial nephritis suggests that treatment with corticosteroids leads to a faster (9 days vs. 54 days) and fuller recovery of renal function (a lower final creatinine level), but this is a retrospective, nonrandomized, nonblinded study. Although numerous other similar reports and anecdotes pervade the clinical literature, no properly designed study has yet been published. Nevertheless, many physicians have treated patients with acute interstitial nephritis whose conditions have improved temporally (and probably causally) with the initiation of steroid therapy. We therefore recommend beginning steroid treatment in a patient with biopsy-proven interstitial nephritis that does not demonstrate significant fibrosis and that has not immediately responded to withdrawal of potential inciting factors. Since the likelihood of recovery of renal function decreases when azotemia persists for more than 1 to 2 weeks, therapy should be initiated early. Prednisone in a dose of 1 mg per kilogram per day (or in the patient incapable of oral intake, an equivalent dose of intravenous prednisolone) is recommended, and this treatment should be maintained for approximately 4 to 6 weeks. If the patient does not show some signs of improvement within the first 1 to 2 weeks of therapy, a second drug (e.g., cyclophosphamide) should be added, and if no progress is realized after 5 to 6 weeks, plans should be made to stop the chemotherapy completely. We believe that the risk/benefit ratio of a well-defined course of steroid therapy is favorable. We are unaware of any cases of acute interstitial nephritis in which the maintenance of improved renal function has been dependent on steroids, except in the setting of acute interstitial nephritis from sarcoidosis. It should be noted, however, that steroids themselves improve the glomerular filtration rate by 10 to 25 percent independent of any specific effect they may have on the destructive tubulointerstitial lesion. The mechanism for this is not fully known, but it seems to be related to volume expansion. As a result of this nonspecific effect, one may anticipate aggravated heart failure or pre-existing hypertension. Also, because steroid treatment results in accelerated protein catabolism, the patient with renal failure is at higher risk for developing hyperkalemia, hyperphosphatemia, and hyperuricemia out of proportion to the degree of renal compromise. The diabetic patient will additionally develop a worsening of serum glucose that may require a change in insulin therapy.

The mechanism whereby corticosteroids exert a beneficial influence in the treatment of acute interstitial nephritis can only be inferred from their known effects on other immunologic processes. A specific assessment of their action has not been made in either human or experimental interstitial nephritis. Corticosteroids are known to impair cell-mediated immunity and have been shown to abrogate delayed-type hypersensitivity responses in humans. Numerous investigators have noted that pharmacologic doses of steroids inhibit production of interleukin 1, interleukin 2, and gamma interferon by macrophages and T cells, and may impair T-cell responsiveness to these and other lymphokines. There is some evidence that steroids suppress antibody production. In addition, steroids stabilize lysosomal membranes, and thereby suppress the release of proteolytic enzymes. It is therefore reasonable to speculate that the beneficial effects of corticosteroids in interstitial nephritis interrupt the effector phase of the immune response through one or more of the above mechanisms.

In a small number of patients with acute interstitial nephritis who do not respond to steroid therapy alone, a more aggressive intervention may be required to produce a remission. In the occasional patient who has little to no fibrosis on renal biopsy and who has not responded to the removal of inciting factors and to 1 to 2 weeks of daily prednisone treatment, cytotoxic treatment may be offered as adjunctive therapy. Under these conditions, it would be reasonable to begin cyclophosphamide at a dosage of 2 mg per kilogram per day in addition to the steroids. If no response is noted within 5 to 6 weeks, the cyclophosphamide should be discontinued and the steroids tapered over several weeks. On the other hand, if an improvement in renal function coincides with the initiation of cyclophosphamide therapy, then, based on anecdotal experience, treatmment should be continued for 1 year. As always, with cyclophosphamide, the white blood cell count must be monitored closely and the drug discontinued or decreased in dosage if the total white blood cell count decreases to less than 3,500 per cubic millimeter (2,000 neutrophils). We do not believe that cyclophosphamide poses a serious oncogenic threat within this time frame, and there is only a small chance of its limiting fertility. Given that fertility is likely to be decreased with chronic renal failure, we tend to accept these risks with consultation and guidance from the patient. While there is no controlled clinical data to support the use of cyclophosphamide, there are anecdotal reports in which a response was noted in several patients. In addition, cyclophosphamide is extremely effective in preventing irreversible damage in experimental interstitial nephritis, provided that it is given early at an appropriate dosage. Unfortunately, because of the limited numbers of patients, it is not likely that cytotoxic therapy will be systematically evaluated in controlled trials. The possible beneficial effect of cyclophosphamide seems to be mediated through the functional inhibition of T cells, in that cyclophosphamide has been demonstrated to abrogate the delayed-type hypersensitivity response in the experimental animals. Within the context of the experimental design, cyclophosphamide did not affect the humoral response.

Finally, one of the most important features of immunosuppressive management is knowing when to stop treatment. With all of the interventions mentioned above, it takes time for the maximum effect to be achieved. Within several weeks, however, one should be able to make a rational decision to provide no further treatment. Protracted treatment in patients with renal failure can lead to metabolic and infectious complications that occasionally prove fatal. The positive renal transplant experience and the consistent improvement in dialytic techniques have demonstrated that patient survival and well-being must always take precedence over attempts to treat hopeless renal failure. It is clearly preferable, at some point, to accept the irreversibility of progressive renal insufficiency and plan for chronic dialysis and/or renal transplantation rather than prolong treatment with powerful immunosuppressive agents. Figure 2 summarizes our approach to limiting tubulointerstitial destruction.

Experimental Therapy

Data from experimental animal studies support the use of cyclosporin A in the therapy of acute interstitial nephritis. This drug has been shown to be an effective prophylactic and therapeutic agent probably by a direct inhibition of T-cell activation. With a small but growing experience with this therapy in the treatment of autoimmune diseases in humans, we can anticipate the occasional use of this drug in the treatment of interstitial nephritis. Nevertheless, since its long-term administration in some transplant settings has raised questions about its ability to induce fibrogenesis, there will be some gegenhalt in getting a large experience with its various effects. We believe further evaluation of the beneficial effects of cyclosporin is warranted, since it is likely that the drug will be used for only a limited time in any given patient.

The use of plasmapheresis may also be considered in those rare patients who, in addition to meeting the criteria for cyclophosphamide therapy, have antitubular basement membrane antibodies demonstrable by renal immunofluorescence. The rationale for this is parallel to the rationale for treating antiglomerular basement membrane disease with plasmapheresis, cyclophosphamide, and steroids—namely, that antitubular basement membrane antibodies are playing a critical role in the disease process and that their removal disturbs an immune effector mechanism that contributes to renal injury. Normally we would use 3- to 4-liter exchanges every day for 5 days, and every other day for a second week. Anecdotal reports on its limited use have been mixed.

One of the forefronts of immunologic research is the use of antigen-specific therapy in the treatment of

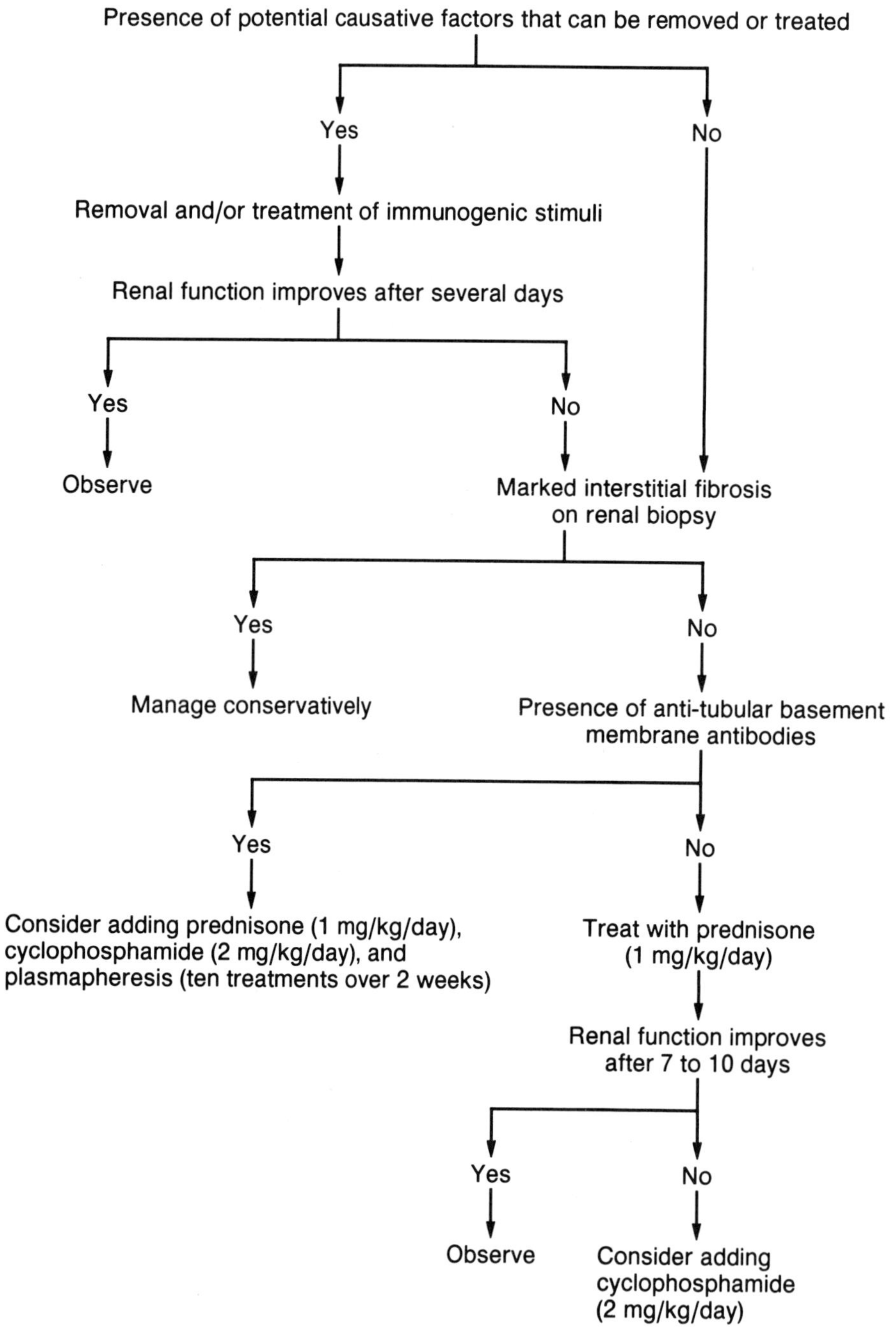

Figure 2 Treatment of acute interstitial nephritis.

immune-mediated diseases. Studies in experimental intersitial nephritis have shown that the induction of a specific suppressor T-cell response prevents the induction of disease. Additionally, anti-idiotypic antibodies (antibodies directed towards unique gene products of the T-cell receptor variable region that are in or near the antigen-binding site) have been demonstrated to decrease the severity of interstitial injury, even after the disease is well established. Although there are many practical obstacles to overcome before such therapy can be used in humans, these novel approaches hold considerable promise for the future.

Supportive Therapy

While a variety of specific renal tubular disorders, electrolyte abnormalities, and acid-base disturbances attend the development of chronic interstitial nephritis, the complications of acute interstitial nephritis are, in essence, the general complications of acute renal failure. Thus the supportive therapy of acute interstitial nephritis may involve the treatment of volume overload, hyponatremia, hyperkalemia, hypocalcemia, hyperphosphatemia, and acidosis. (These aspects of patient care are discussed in standard textbooks of nephrology and therefore will not receive further attention here.) Some recent evidence also suggests the potential efficacy of dietary protein restriction in slowing the progression of some forms of chronic renal insufficiency. Interestingly, the cellular lesions of experimental interstitial nephritis can be largely attenuated by dietary protein restriction, probably through a nonspecific inhibition of T-cell function. Bearing in mind that this finding has not been formally investigated in humans, one may consider decreasing protein intake to approximately 0.5 to 0.6 g per kilogram per day in those patients left with chronic renal insufficiency after an episode of acute tubulointerstitial nephropathy. However, considering the overall catabolic and relatively malnourished state of most hospitalized patients with acute renal failure, protein restriction during the acute phase is probably best delayed until ambulatory health is fully established and the patient may be treated on an outpatient basis.

SUGGESTED READING

Galpin JE, Shinberger JH, Stanley TM, et al. Acute interstitial nephritis due to methicillin. Am J Med 1978; 65:756–765.

Laberke HG, Bohle A. Acute interstitial nephritis: correlations between clinical and morphological findings. Clin Nephrol 1980; 14:263–273.

Neilson EG. Pathogenesis and therapy of interstitial nephritis. Kidney Int 1989; 35:1257–1270.

Nolan CH, Angel M, Kelleher SP. Eosinophiluria: a new method of detection and definition of the clinical spectrum. New Engl J Med 1986; 315:1516–1519.

Tsokos GC. Immunomodulatory treatment in patients with rheumatic diseases: mechanisms of action. Semin Arthritis Rheum 1978; 17:24–38.

POSTSTREPTOCOCCAL GLOMERULONEPHRITIS

FRANK G. BOINEAU, M.D.
JOHN E. LEWY, M.D.

In its typical form poststreptococcal glomerulonephritis has various manifestations, including edema, hematuria, oliguria, proteinuria, reduced glomerular filtration rate, and hypertension. Many patients do not have all of the typical features, and the symptoms and signs may be very mild. This is especially true in family contacts, in whom this disease often goes unrecognized unless the family member is examined and laboratory evidence of the disease is sought.

CLINICAL FEATURES

Epidemiology

Acute poststreptococcal glomerulonephritis (APSGN) is extremely rare before the age of 2 years. Thereafter it may occur at any age, but is most common in school-aged children. In many studies, the mean age of onset of the sporadic form of APSGN is approximately 7 years. The male to female ratio is 2:1.

Preceding Infection

APSGN has long been known to follow certain types of group A beta-hemolytic streptococcal infections of either the throat and upper respiratory tract or skin. Upper respiratory infections are associated with most cases of APSGN in the northern United States, whereas skin infections are frequently associated with cases in the South. The latent interval is usually 8 to 14 days after an upper respiratory infection, while the latent interval after skin infection is usually longer (21 to 28 days). Direct culture of streptococcal organisms from the pharynx or skin is not common, but serologic evidence of a preceding group A beta-hemolytic streptococcal infection is usually present. After an upper respiratory tract infection, the antistreptolysin O (ASO) antibody titer is elevated in about 90 percent of the patients with APSGN. After skin infections, the ASO titer is elevated in only about half of the patients, but Streptozyme (Wampole Laboratories), antihyaluronidase, or antideoxyribonuclease B antibody titers are usually elevated. If titers of antibodies to these streptococcal antigens are not elevated when APSGN is recognized, serial quantitation of the titers usually reveals a significant rise over 1 to 3 weeks after onset of the clinical illness.

Clinical Manifestations at Onset

Typically the child or adult with APSGN has a history of gross hematuria and edema. He may also have oliguria or anuria, and gastrointestinal, pulmonary, and/or central nervous system manifestations. Because neither gross hematuria nor edema may be present in an individual patient, and the predominant symptoms may be related to the gastrointestinal, central nervous system, or pulmonary system, APSGN must be considered when these symptoms are present, and the urine carefully examined. The presence of microscopic hematuria or proteinuria or both, should alert the physician to pursue the diagnosis of APSGN.

The presenting signs in patients with APSGN mirror the symptoms recorded above. Elevation in blood pressure above 140/90 is present in from 30 to 80 percent of patients. Other evidence of an expanded extracellular fluid volume is often noted. Skin infection may also be present.

Laboratory Data at Onset

Laboratory data at the time APSGN is diagnosed reflect the reduced glomerular filtration rate, serologic evidence of a preceding streptococcal infection, and consumption of complement. It is well to remember that the degree of hematuria and proteinuria may be very mild and that nephrotic range proteinuria is uncommon. Thus the diagnosis of APSGN must be considered in patients with mild degrees of hematuria and proteinuria.

PREFERRED APPROACH TO MANAGEMENT AND DRUG THERAPY

Hospitalization

Many patients with APSGN can be treated at home. The principal considerations are the severity of the clinical abnormalities and the family's and physician's ability to provide close observation and care at home. Patients with moderate to severe reduction in renal function (creatinine clearance less than 50 ml per minute per 1.73 m^2 or blood urea nitrogen greater than 50 mg per deciliter) and those with oliguria or anemia; any symptoms of hypertensive encephalopathy, including lethargy, vomiting, or ophthalmologic changes; and significant edema or pulmonary congestion should be hospitalized. If hypertension is absent or mild and responds promptly to antihypertensive measures, including bed rest and medication, hospitalization can often be avoided.

Bed rest is an extremely controversial therapeutic modality. It was once considered appropriate to maintain bed rest until all signs of nephritis were past. However, it appears that ambulation has not been associated with worsening of any variables of renal function once gross hematuria, edema, hypertension, and azotemia have resolved. Children will not comply with a regimen of complete bed rest even if the physician or parents desire it. The conflict that arises in attempting to impose complete bed rest on an unwilling child is probably not worth its questionable advantages. A reasonable guide is that patients who have gross hematuria, hypertension, edema, evidence of circulatory congestion, or moderate to severe depression of renal function be kept on bed rest as much as possible.

Nutritional Management

Alterations in diet depend on the severity of the edema, renal failure, and hypertension. If the blood urea nitrogen concentration is less than 75 mg per deciliter, dietary protein need not be restricted. If the blood urea nitrogen concentration is above this level, intake should be restricted to 0.5 g per kilogram of body weight per day of proteins of high biologic value until renal function improves and the blood urea nitrogen concentration spontaneously decreases to below 75 mg per deciliter. Calorie intake should be maintained as near to normal as possible to reduce catabolism. In patients with hypertension or edema, sodium intake should be restricted to 1 to 2 g each day. More severe degrees of sodium restriction are usually not required and lead to poor caloric intake. Fluid balance should be carefully monitored, and fluid should be restricted in the presence of severe edema, oliguria, or anuria. In these patients, fluid intake should not exceed the sum of urine output and insensible water loss minus planned weight loss. Measurement of body weight daily, or more often if needed, is an effective way to determine whether fluid intake is appropriate. Fluid and sodium restriction with a decrease in extracellular volume will assist in the management of hypertension. Once edema has resolved, fluid intake should be restricted to insensible water loss plus measured fluid output as long as oliguria persists.

Treatment of Hypertension

Hypertension may be mild or severe. There is considerable disagreement regarding levels of blood pressure in APSGN which require therapeutic intervention. Hypertension often resolves with bed rest alone. If the diastolic blood pressure is below 100 mm Hg and falls further with the patient on bed rest, sodium restriction and continued bed rest are sufficient. If the blood pressure does not decline in 2 to 4 hours, or symptoms of encephalopathy develop (headache, nausea, vomiting, seizures), treatment should be instituted promptly. Hydralazine, 0.15 mg per kilogram up to 10 mg, given intramuscularly, is usually quite effective in reducing the blood pressure in this disease. The dose may be repeated in 4 to 6 hours if needed. If hypertension responds to the above measures only transiently, hydralazine may be given orally (0.7 mg per kilogram of body weight per day) in four divided doses. Hydralazine can gradually be increased, if needed, to a maximum of 200 mg per day orally. An effective dose should be continued until the blood pressure has been normal for 24 to 48 hours, and then the drug may be tapered and discontinued if the blood pressure remains normal. Sustained hypertension is infrequent, but may require sustained hydralazine therapy. Occasionally the blood pressure remains moderately, but persistently elevated, and treatment with oral methyldopa or propranolol is useful. Intravenous nitroprusside or diazoxide has been used successfully to treat severe acute hypertension. Hypertension in APSGN is largely attributable to an expanded

TABLE 1 Common Antihypertensive Drugs Used in Acute Poststreptococcal Glomerulonephritis

Drug	*Initial Dose/Route (mg/kg)*	*Dose Interval (hour)*	*Maximum Dose*	*Common Side Effects*
Direct vasodilators				
Hydralazine	0.1–0.4 IV or IM	4–6	20 mg/dose	Tachycardia, palpitations
Diazoxide	3–10 IV over 30 min	Repeat once in 0.5 hour if needed	10 mg/kg/dose	Dizziness, tachycardia, nausea, rapid fall in BP, hyperglycemia, fluid retention
Nitroprusside	0.5–8 μg/kg/min	Constant infusion		Tachycardia, fluid retention, nausea, dizziness, cyanide poisoning
Hydralazine	0.25 PO	4–6	200 mg/day	Tachycardia, palpitations
Adrenergic inhibiting drugs				
Propranolol	1–2 PO	6–12	10 mg/kg/day	Lethargy, fatigue, bradycardia
Alpha-Methyldopa	2–3 PO	6–8	40–60 mg/kg/day	Lethargy, fatigue, depression
Drugs that reduce plasma volume				
Furosemide	1–4 PO	12–24	8 mg/kg/dose	Hypokalemia, metabolic alkalosis, postural hypotension
Chlorothiazide	5 PO	12	20 mg/kg	Hypokalemia, metabolic alkalosis, postural hypotension

Adapted from Portman RJ, Robson AM. Controversies in pediatric hypertension. In: Tune BM, Mendoza SA, eds. Pediatric nephrology. New York: Churchill Livingstone. 1984:282.

extracellular fluid volume. Renin levels at the onset of the disease are characteristically normal or suppressed. Common antihypertensive drugs used in APSGN are listed in Table 1. Diuretics can be important in lowering the blood pressure. Furosemide, 2 mg per kilogram orally or 1 mg per kilogram intravenously, is often effective in producing a diuresis and lowering of the extracellular fluid volume. An improvement in encephalopathy has been seen in patients treated with intravenous furosemide even when only minimal or no changes in blood pressure have occurred. These observations imply that edema of the central nervous system plays an important role in hypertensive encephalopathy in APSGN.

Treatment of Edema

If there is fluid overload, diuretics are indicated to reduce edema, to test renal responsiveness, and as an adjunct in the treatment of hypertension. Persistent edema can be treated with oral furosemide, 2 mg per kilogram once or twice daily. Hydrochlorothiazide, 2 mg per kilogram per day, is effective when renal function is normal or nearly normal, but not when there is marked depression of the glomerular filtration rate. Pulmonary congestion in APSGN usually reflects fluid overload and not myocardial failure. It is therefore *not* responsive to administration of digitalis. Vascular congestion can usually be treated effectively with fluid and sodium restriction and the use of diuretics as outlined above.

Antibiotics

Cultures of the throat and skin lesions if present should be obtained in all patients with suspected APSGN and all immediate family members. Those with positive cultures should be treated with appropriate antibiotics. In patients with suspected APSGN, even if beta-hemolytic streptococcus is not cultured, it is probably safest to treat with a ten-day course of penicillin (or erythromycin in penicillin-sensitive patients) Additional antibiotics are not used unless infectious complications are present. Prophylactic antibiotics are not indicated in this disease, since recurrences of APSGN are very rare.

Subclinical Cases

Subclinical asymptomatic cases of APSGN have been reported by several investigators. When first-degree relatives of an index case were studied, the ratio of subclinical to clinical disease was 4 and there was documented evidence of APSGN occurring in about 33 percent of household patient contacts. Thus it seems prudent to recommend evaluation of household family members (throat or skin culture, physical examination, and urinalysis) when an index case of APSGN is identified. If symptoms of acute nephritis develop in family members, serologic and renal function tests should be performed. Serial evaluation of family members is not indicated. The prophylactic treatment of household members with antibiotics is controversial and currently, unless skin or throat cultures are positive, prophylactic treatment is not indicated.

Renal Biopsy

In a typical case of APSGN, a renal biopsy is not required to diagnose the disease. There are however, times when a renal biopsy should be considered, either because of atypical presentation or because resolution does not follow the expected course. The reasons for considering a renal biopsy are listed in Table 2. None of these is an absolute indication, but should alert the physician that APSGN may not be present and a renal biopsy should be considered for diagnostic reasons. If a renal biopsy is considered, it should be done early, since pathologic changes such as generalized proliferation tend to become focal, and subepithelial deposits of immunoglobulin G (IgG) and complement tend to resolve after the first few weeks of the illness, making the diagnosis of APSGN more difficult. It should be emphasized that there are no pathognomonic features of APSGN and the renal biopsy must be interpreted in conjunction with the clinical findings.

Immunosuppressive Therapy

Corticosteroids and other immunosuppressive drugs are not indicated in the treatment of acute poststreptococcal glomerulonephritis. Mild or moderate cases have an excellent prognosis with supportive therapy, particularly in children. Even in cases of severe APSGN, supportive therapy alone frequently results in complete recovery of renal function. Recent studies, that have compared supportive care with immunosuppressive plus anticoagulant therapy in a nonrandomized fashion in crescentic glomerulonephritis of poststreptococcal origin in adults, suggest that the renal outcome is equally good in the two groups. Thus the known risks of immunosuppressive medications are not justified in APSGN even when there are diffuse crescents on the biopsy specimen.

COURSE AND PROGNOSIS

Resolution of the Acute Phase

The overt manifestations of APSGN, which include gross hematuria, edema, reduced urine output, hypertension, and central nervous system symptoms, usually resolve in the first 1 to 2 weeks of the illness in most patients. Diuresis with loss of edema is usually complete by the end of the second week or sooner. Even those with severe renal failure will begin to show an improvement in the glomerular filtration rate in the first 2 to 3 weeks after the clinical onset of the disease. Hypertension disappears in many patients once they begin bed rest or after a short course of antihypertensive treatment. An improvement in the glomerular filtration rate and renal blood flow results in diuresis with loss of edema and return of plasma volume to normal. This is one of the factors leading to a decrease in blood pressure. The total hemolytic or third component of complement (C3) usually returns to normal within 6 weeks after the clinical onset of APSGN. Failure of complement to return to normal suggests that the patient may have membranoproliferative glomerulonephritis instead of APSGN. Microscopic hematuria will persist after gross hematuria disappears, but it too will gradually resolve. Complete disappearance of hematuria may take several months to several years. Occasionally, intermittent or orthostatic proteinuria is noted. Some studies of sporadic APSGN in adults have documented persistence of abnormal proteinuria for 2 years or more. Such persistent proteinuria, especially if associated with hypertension and a reduced glomerular filtration rate, may be a manifestation of a chronic form of glomerulonephritis. If the nephrotic syndrome is present at onset, it tends to be very transient and disappears in the early phase of the illness.

TABLE 2 Relative Indications for Renal Biopsy in Suspected Acute Poststreptococcal Glomerulonephritis

At onset of illness
Absence of reduced serum complement
Anuria
Nephrotic syndrome
Prior history of renal disease
Retarded linear growth in children
Family history of nephritis
During period of expected resolution
Persistence of oliguria beyond 3 weeks
Low C3 or total hemolytic complement beyond 6 weeks
Gross hematuria beyond 3 weeks
Persistence of hypertension

Long-Term Prognosis

The long-term prognosis of APSGN is controversial and depends on the age of the patient at the onset of illness, the severity of the acute disease, and epidemiologic considerations. The prognosis of epidemic APSGN in children seems very favorable, even in those with severe acute disease. Severe oliguria and the presence of diffuse crescents on biopsy suggest a more guarded prognosis.

The long-term prognosis of the sporadic form of APSGN is less favorable in adults than in children. Severe initial disease with a creatinine clearance below 40 ml per minute per 1.73 m^2, persistent heavy proteinuria (above 2 g a day), and older age at the time of onset contribute to a guarded prognosis.

Serial renal biopsies in adult patients with APSGN have demonstrated chronic findings such as glomerulosclerosis, varying degrees of interstitial fibrosis, and arterial changes in one-third to one-half of some series. Whether these changes represent progression of disease or simply healing of the acute process and static pathologic changes is unknown. The incidence of progression to end-stage renal disease is much less than that of the chronic changes found on histopathologic examination of tissue. A review of recent literature with medium- to long-range follow-up of adults reveals that chronic renal failure develops in 3 percent of the cases of sporadic, symptomatic APSGN. Follow-up studies of longer duration will better answer the question of long-term functional outcome in APSGN.

LUPUS NEPHRITIS

HOWARD A. AUSTIN III, M.D.
JAMES E. BALOW, M.D.

The prognosis of lupus nephritis has dramatically improved over the past few decades. There is broad acceptance (if not stringent proof) of the fact that corticosteroids and immunosuppressive drugs have contributed to this. However, the lack of a consensus regarding indications for, as well as the type and duration of, therapy continues to perplex the clinician dealing with lupus nephritis. Solace comes, however, with the realization that many types of therapy are effective, and that recent research efforts have focused on the development of regimens with reduced rates of iatrogenic complications. Until definitive proof of superior efficacy of particular forms of treatment becomes available, one of the major tasks of the clinician is to become familiar with the intricacies of each drug therapy so that risks can be minimized and realistically communicated to the patient with lupus nephritis.

SPECTRUM OF RENAL DISEASE

In practice, renal biopsy is most rewarding if the patient has clinical evidence of kidney involvement: abnormal sediment, proteinuria, and/or azotemia. Prognostic information gained from careful assessment of the types of histologic changes can be particularly helpful in patients presenting with urinary abnormalities, but whose lupus is of uncertain duration. The World Health Organization (WHO) classification system has helped to standardize the definitions of the major types of lupus nephritis (Table 1). Also shown in the table are other classes that are more rare, but may predominate. Varying grades of active and chronic irreversible lesions further characterize the spectrum of histologic changes. Controversy centers around the weak prognostic value of the conventional WHO classification system. Moreover, transitions among classes are observed. Specification of the severity, extent of activity, and chronicity has been found to increase the prognostic information derived from the renal biopsy.

INDICATIONS FOR THERAPY

The decision to initiate therapy is generally based on several clinical, laboratory, and pathologic measures. Unfavorably changing factors, such as urinary sediment, proteinuria, renal function, and lupus serologic tests, are considered signs of activity, but there is much debate about the merits of making therapeutic decisions on these clinical features alone. It is best to consider that pathologic features supplement rather than replace clinical measures. Pathologic data are especially helpful when the previous course of disease is uncertain and when sequential clinical observations (for example, rate of change in renal function) are lacking. Responses to therapy depend on the presence of potentially reversible renal disease. Thus, chronic, irreversible, or fixed anatomic and functional changes should be carefully delineated prior to judging the need for and potential response to immunosuppressive therapy. Chronic histologic changes are likely to be associated with loss of kidney functional reserve and the ability to compensate for ongoing renal injury. Patients with these background lesions are at substantial risk of progressive azotemia with continued activity of lupus nephritis. Although the course of patients with both active and chronic lesions may be favorably affected by immunosuppressive therapy, patients with exclusively chronic disease should be spared the risks of these treatments.

As shown in Table 2, clinical and pathologic indications for therapy in lupus nephritis have been delineated according to their relative strengths. Major indications generally prompt rather aggressive therapeutic intervention. Intermediate indications considered individually may warrant moderate therapy; occasionally, more intensive therapy is employed if two or more features characterize the clinical picture.

Major Indications for Aggressive Induction Therapy

Aggressive therapy is indicated for the following problems: (1) rapidly progressive glomerulonephritis; (2) nephritic sediment of recent onset with concomitant azotemia; (3) substantial fibrinoid necrosis; or (4) cellular crescents on renal biopsy. Historically, these findings have prompted the use of high-dose corticosteroids; this approach is still widely practiced and is frequently effective (Table 3). Prednisone (1 mg per kilogram per day) is initiated in single daily doses. Controversy arises in regard to duration of therapy. Though divided doses and prolonged corticosteroid therapy (more than 8 to 12 weeks) are undoubtedly effective in achieving immuno-

TABLE 1 Major Classes of Lupus Nephritis

World Health Organization classification
Normal/minimal disease
Mesangial disease
Focal proliferative GN
Diffuse proliferative GN
Membranous GN
Other classes
Membranoproliferative GN*
Crescentic GN*
Mixed membranous and proliferative GN
Sclerosing disease
Interstitial nephritis

* GN = glomerulonephritis
Generally considered subsets of diffuse proliferative GN

TABLE 2 Indications for Therapy in Lupus Nephritis

Clinical	*Pathologic*
Major indications	
Rapidly progressive GN*	Diffuse proliferative GN
Nephritic urinary sediment of recent onset with azotemia	Fibrinoid necrosis †
	Cellular crescents†
Worsening nephritic sediment	Hyaline thrombi and extensive subendothelial deposits‡
Intermediate indications	
Nephritic sediment	Focal proliferative GN
Slowly progressive azotemia	Scattered subendothelial deposits
Worsening proteinuria§	
Worsening anti-DNA titers	Mesangial nephritis
Worsening serum complement	Membranous GN
	Subepithelial deposits#
	Interstitial nephritis**
Weak/poor indications	
Fixed azotemia	Glomerular sclerosis††
Fixed proteinuria	Fibrous crescents††
Fixed abnormal anti-DNA	Tubular atrophy††
Fixed abnormal complement	Interstitial fibrosis††
	Intramembranous deposits††

* GN = Glomerulonephritis
Defined as combinations of endocapillary proliferation, necrosis, sclerosis, and capillary loop thickening in more than 50% of glomeruli.
† Present in ≥25% of glomeruli.
‡ Indicating heavy immune complex deposition.
§ Especially movement from low grade to nephrotic range proteinuria.
\# May be present predominantly in membranous but also in treated or chronic stages of proliferative nephritis.
** Mononuclear infiltrate composed of lymphocytes, macrophages, and plasma cells.
†† Weak indicators if these lesions predominate or are unaccompanied by other active lesions.

TABLE 3 Therapeutic Options in Lupus Nephritis

Aggressive induction therapy for major indications

1. High-dose prednisone: 1.0 mg/kg per day for 4 to 6 weeks. Taper to alternate-day by 8 weeks. If inadequate response, excessive dose dependency, or flare with tapering, consider adding cytotoxic agents. Maintenance goal ≤0.3 mg/kg every other day.*
2. Pulse methylprednisolone: 1.0 g/m² daily for 3 doses. Repeat single (1.0 g/m²) doses may be given monthly up to 6 months if active nephritis persists. Pulse therapy is accompanied by prednisone, 0.5 mg/kg per day for 4 weeks with tapering to alternate day by 8 weeks.†
3. Experimental: (a) Pulse cyclophosphamide—single doses of 0.5–1.0 g/m² monthly for up to 6 months; oral prednisone, 0.5 mg/kg per day for 4 weeks with tapering to alternate day by 8 weeks; (b) Plasma exchange—daily or alternate-day 4-L exchanges plus prednisone and cyclophosphamide.

Alternative induction and maintenance therapy

1. Moderate-dose prednisone: 0.5 mg/kg per day or 1.0 mg/kg alternate days for 4 to 6 weeks. Taper to minimal dose of alternate-day prednisone to control active disease.
2. Azathioprine: 2 mg/kg per day for 6 month intervals. ‡§
3. Cyclophosphamide: 2 mg/kg per day for 6 month intervals.†#
4. Low-dose cyclophosphamide plus azathioprine: 1 mg/kg per day of each drug for 6 month intervals.‡#
5. Pulse cyclophosphamide: 0.5–1.0 g/m² IV every 3 months.‡**

* Considerably higher and/or longer doses of prednisone are advocated by some, but with considerable escalation of side effects and obscure evidence of advantage.
† Experience with use of pulse therapy for maintenance is limited.
‡ Options 2, 3, 4, and 5 used together with moderate-dose prednisone. All are continued if nephritis is persistently active or repeated if relapses occur.
§ Monitor white blood cell counts, liver function tests.
\# Taper dose of cyclophosphamide to keep total neutrophils ≥2,000/mm³. Encourage oral hydration and frequent voiding.
** Initiate pulse cyclophosphamide at 0.75 g/m² (or 0.5 g/m² if glomerular filtration rate ≤ 30 ml/min) given over 30 min. Modify subsequent doses so that white blood cell count falls but that nadir at 10 to 14 days does not go below 2,000/mm³ total. Administer 3 L of intravenous fluids in the 24-hour period after pulse cyclophosphamide and encourage frequent bladder emptying.

suppression, the physician should carefully balance this against the potential for iatrogenic problems. Thus, we make a strong effort to taper to alternate-day prednisone within 8 weeks of starting therapy. Consideration of alternative approaches to induction therapy is appropriate under the following circumstances: (1) unwillingness of the patient to accept the potential side effects of high-dose oral corticosteroids (such as cosmetic changes or fear of degenerative bone disease); (2) failure to tolerate corticosteroids (for example, major infection, severe diabetes, uncontrolled hypertension, gastrointestinal bleeding, psychosis); (3) inadequate response to corticosteroid therapy; or (4) clinical and/or histologic features of severe lupus nephritis suggesting increased risk of renal functional deterioration.

Pulse methylprednisolone (1 g per square meter) given intravenously daily for 3 days is a popular alternative form of aggressive induction therapy (see Table 3). Based on our own studies of this mode of treatment, maintenance doses of single pulses of methylprednisolone (1 g per square meter) can be given monthly for up to 6 months. In addition, moderate-dose prednisone (0.5 mg per kilogram per day) is given for 4 weeks, followed by tapering to alternate days by 8 weeks. There have been no formal comparative trials of pulse versus conventional high-dose corticosteroids in lupus nephritis. The current widespread use of pulse methylprednisolone is primarily based on the consensus that it is at least as effective as oral prednisone but has fewer side effects. Attitudes about this form of therapy are highly polarized, however. Most enthusiasts have used pulse therapy in early, active disease and most nihilists have used it in desperation for advanced chronic diseases when other treatment has failed. When considering pulse methylprednisolone as an alternative, it is crucial to remember that megadose therapy will be no more or less effective than any other choice unless potentially reversible renal pathologic factors are present.

Experimental treatments may be considered in patients with major forms of lupus nephritis, but should be administered under the guidelines of approved protocols from research centers. Plasma exchange is not strongly believed to be more effective or safer than conventional immunosuppressive drug therapy in lupus nephritis, but final results of controlled trials are pending. Also listed in Table 3 is experimental pulse cyclophosphamide therapy for severe lupus nephritis. In this National Institutes of Health (NIH) protocol, intravenous cyclophosphamide can be given in doses ranging between 0.5 to 1.0 g per square meter monthly for 6 months as induction therapy. Patients participating in this study may be randomized to receive an additional 2 years of pulse cyclophosphamide every 3 months as maintenance therapy. These regimens are well tolerated, but their efficacy relative to pulse methylprednisolone is currently under investigation. In a previous study, favorable renal outcomes were observed in patients randomized to receive pulse cyclophosphamide every 3 months as induction and maintenance therapy for an average of 4 years. The optimal duration of cytotoxic drug therapy for lupus nephritis remains to be clarified.

Alternative Induction and Maintenance Treatments

The remaining major indications for treatment listed in Table 2 are more controversial: (1) worsening nephritic urinary sediment; (2) diffuse proliferative glomerulonephritis; and (3) hyaline thrombi with extensive subendothelial immune complex deposits on renal biopsy. Considered individually, none of these items necessarily warrants aggressive or experimental therapy. This is especially evident when the diagnosis of diffuse proliferative glomerulonephritis is ascertained. Additional descriptions of the type and extent of active lesions or evidence of renal functional impairment are helpful to define the severity of this type of lupus nephritis, and thereby modify the strength of the indications for therapy. Generally, these features of lupus nephritis are treated with high-dose prednisone or with moderate-dose prednisone plus one of the following cytotoxic regimens: (1) oral cyclophosphamide, (2) oral azathioprine, (3) low-dose combined cyclophosphamide and azathioprine, or (4) intravenous pulse cyclophosphamide (see Table 3). The decision on which cytotoxic agent(s) to employ and when is difficult in lupus nephritis and cannot be based on a wide consensus regarding the superiority of any one of these choices. Thus, at the present time the decision to use cytotoxic drugs rests on recent evidence of their efficacy in therapeutic trials and on the desire to avoid the long-term side effects of high doses of corticosteroids. As opposed to the typically insidious side effects of corticosteroids, the majority of side effects of even the conventional orally administered cytotoxic drugs can be minimized by careful monitoring of white blood cell counts. Increased risk of viral infection, particularly herpes zoster, does not appear to be avoidable by available monitoring techniques, but concern for more ominous complications, such as malignancy, has almost certainly been overstated. We are currently enthusiastic about the ability of intermittent pulses of intravenous cyclophosphamide to reduce the risks of chronic bone marrow depression, gonadal toxicity, and bladder complications of conventional oral cyclophosphamide. To date, malignancy has not occurred in any patient treated with intermittent cyclophosphamide after median follow-up approaching 1 decade. Although the administration of intravenous cyclophosphamide is cumbersome, relatively costly, and frequently associated with several hours of susceptibility to nausea and vomiting, we feel that the intermittent pulse regimen reduces the risks of major complications compared with treatments that involve daily exposure to a potentially toxic agent. Thus, in our current practice, we rarely treat patients who have lupus nephritis with daily oral cyclophosphamide.

It is likely that each patient will assign a different weight to the various risk factors involving corticosteroids and cytotoxic drugs. These considerations should be balanced against the personal bias of the physician as to what constitutes the most unacceptable side effects of treatment (assuming that several forms of therapy each have some efficacy). In practice, the physician should repeatedly taper corticosteroids to identify the minimum dose required for control of disease activity. As a general rule, serious consideration should be given to the addition of cytotoxic drugs if the patient cannot be successfully switched to alternate-day prednisone within 8 weeks of initiation to daily corticosteroids because of flares of nephritis. Cytotoxic drugs should also be considered if unsatisfactory therapeutic responses to corticosteroids are observed, or excessive maintenance doses are required to achieve a complete remission of signs of active nephritis (see Table 3).

Regarding the specific choice of cytotoxic therapy, azathioprine is rarely used because it has produced the least favorable results as assessed by improvement in urinary sediment or preservation of renal function. More promising results (based on the same measures of outcome) have been observed with regimens containing cyclophosphamide, particularly the combination of low-dose cyclophosphamide and azathioprine or intermittent pulse cyclophosphamide (see Table 3). Hopefully, a proper perspective on the regimen of cyclophosphamide with the highest therapeutic index will be forthcoming with additional periods of follow-up in clinical trials. There is no convincing evidence that other alkylating agents, such as chlorambucil or nitrogen mustard, are either more efficacious or less toxic than cyclophosphamide, but only meager data have been presented.

Intermediate Indications for Therapy

The factors listed as intermediate indications in Table 2 may identify active nephritis and are considered to warrant limited therapeutic intervention in most cases, but the presence of multiple adverse features may prompt more aggressive therapy. Unfortunately, one cannot easily ascertain whether these individual clinical and pathologic features (especially mesangial and focal proliferative glomerulonephritis) indicate intrinsically mild forms or rather early forms of lupus nephritis. Therefore, essentially all of the listed clinical and pathologic features should prompt careful monitoring for evidence of subsequent transitions and disease progression. Therapy is usually initiated with short courses of high- or moderate-dose prednisone with rapid tapering to alternate-day therapy within 8 weeks (see Table 3). If disease remits and remains quiescent, no further treatment is required aside from the smallest dose of prednisone needed to control extrarenal lupus symptoms. On the other hand, reappearance of the intermediate indications or emergence of any of the major indications for therapy may prompt retreatment with prednisone, and the addition of pulse therapy, and/or of the maintenance forms of cytotoxic drug therapy. Some authors feel that membranous lupus nephritis does not warrant specific treatment unless symptomatic nephrotic syndrome is present. It has been our practice to include such patients in protocols involving moderate-dose prednisone and cytotoxic drug therapy. The low rate of renal failure in patients with pure membranous lupus nephritis underscores the need for a generally conservative approach to treatment. However, mixed membranous and proliferative lesions as well as transformations from membranous to more aggressive forms of nephritis do occur and should prompt intensification of therapy. Interstitial nephritis is usually a component of, and parallels the severity of, lupus glomerulonephritis. Interstitial nephritis is rarely the predominant lesion. However, interstitial infiltrates of mononuclear cells are a sign of active nephritis and should be considered in the therapeutic decision.

Weak and Poor Indications for Therapy

Clinicians are frequently faced with patients exhibiting chronic, indolent abnormalities of urinary sediment, renal function, and lupus serologic tests. It may be difficult in many patients to distinguish ongoing smoldering nephritis from the prolonged effects of previous nephron injury. As indicated in Table 2, fixed azotemia or proteinuria, as well as fixed abnormalities of anti-DNA antibodies or serum complement, are usually weak signs of disease activity. Verification by repeat renal biopsy of the activity of lupus nephritis can often be extremely helpful when therapeutic decisions are necessary. Predominant glomerular sclerosis, fibrous crescents, tubular atrophy, interstitial fibrosis, or intramembranous deposits suggest irreversible disease and indicate that continued therapeutic trials are unwarranted. The temptation toward "one last effort" to treat the patient who appears to be slowly progressing to end-stage renal failure should be resisted unless clear signs of active glomerular disease are present. Recent evidence suggests that nonimmunologic factors can be responsible for progressive renal insufficiency, which can be mistakenly interpreted as a sign of active lupus nephritis.

ASSESSMENT OF THERAPEUTIC RESPONSE

Prevention of end-stage renal failure has been the major objective of treatment of lupus nephritis. However, experience at our own and many other centers indicates that the risk of renal failure is approximately 25 to 35 percent after ten years of treatment, even in patients with diffuse proliferative lupus nephritis. This low rate of renal failure in patients with lupus nephritis has weakened our ability to judge the absolute merits of different forms of immunosuppressive therapy by strong renal functional criteria. The question of what constitutes valid measures of outcome by which to judge treatment in lupus nephritis remains controversial. Some clinicians prefer conventional corticosteroid therapy because of the controversial evidence that cytotoxic drugs are more efficacious or are associated with enhanced survival. Others have become strongly disenchanted with corticosteroids because of the relatively high rate of patient dissatisfaction and the impressive array of side effects. Unfortunately, the real risks of cytotoxic drugs in lupus nephritis have not been fully characterized and a concern for late malignancy continues to dominate decision-making. Admittedly, a complete and proper perspective on this issue is lacking.

Our own approach emphasizes the need to minimize corticosteroid exposure even when these agents are effective in controlling clinical and pathologic manifestations of disease activity. Data demonstrating that cytotoxic drugs reduce the likelihood of progressive renal scarring and functional deterioration compared with "conventional" oral corticosteroid therapy alone have provided substantial support for their use for many of the indications outlined above. Nonetheless, decisions regarding initiation of cytotoxic drugs are difficult and involve a complex interaction of factors, including clinical and histologic features on presentation, completeness of response to corticosteroids, and concerns regarding toxicities of both corticosteroids and cytotoxic drugs.

GOODPASTURE'S SYNDROME

ANDREW J. REES, M.B., M.Sc.

The term Goodpasture's syndrome was originally applied to all patients who had necrotising glomerulonephritis and pulmonary hemorrhage. Nowadays it is used most frequently to describe only those patients in whom the syndrome is caused by autoantibodies to the glomerular basement membrane (anti-GBM). These autoantibodies have highly restricted specificity and probably react exclusively with determinants in the glomerular non-collagenous-1 domain of type IV collagen. Nevertheless it is important to remember that anti-GBM antibodies are the cause of disease in less than half the patients who present with pulmonary hemorrhage and nephritis; other causes include various types of systemic vasculitis, systemic lupus erythematosus, and occasionally cryoglobulinemia. These disorders differ substantially in their response to therapy. This chapter deals exclusively with the management of anti-GBM antibody-mediated disease, except to contrast differences in clinical presentation.

Two aspects of antibody-mediated Goodpasture's syndrome have ensured that its importance far exceeds its prevalence, and both have obvious consequences for therapy. First, anti-GBM disease is almost always severe and frequently life threatening and may evolve with great rapidity accompanied by complete loss of renal function within 24 hours. Up to 4 litres of blood may be lost into the lungs within a similar time. Thus the urgency of treatment should be as required for a potential medical emergency. Second, anti-GBM disease is the first type of glomerulonephritis in which the pathogenesis—autoimmunity to the GBM—is known and can be quantified by serum assay for anti-GBM antibodies. This means that it is possible to diagnose the disease noninvasively, design rational therapies to remove anti-GBM antibodies, and monitor the effectiveness of these treatments. It has also been possible to study the relation between circulating anti-GBM antibodies and the injury they cause and to show the importance of secondary factors such as intercurrent infection and cigarette smoke on the course of the disease. Thus, a better understanding of the pathogenesis has broadened the approach to management; this broader approach will be emphasized here.

CLINICAL ASPECTS

Anti-GBM disease affects people of both sexes and of all ages. Most commonly it presents during the third decade, but there is a second peak in incidence—patients over 60 years of age. Originally it was suggested that most patients were male, but this greatly exaggerates the sex difference; most current series of anti-GBM disease describe sex ratios of less than two to one. Some authors have found elderly female patients to be less severely affected than other groups, but this has not been our experience.

It is unclear what initiates anti-GBM antibody synthesis. Despite repeated claims and a few suggestions reported in anecdotes, there is no convincing evidence to generally link anti-GBM disease with exposure to hydrocarbon fumes. Equally unconvincing is the evidence that specific viral infections cause anti-GBM disease. An association with Hodgkin's disease (or its treatment) has also been noted. There is, however, strong evidence of inherited predisposition to anti-GBM disease. The frequency of the class II major histocompatability antigen (HLA-DR2) is greatly increased, and there is also an association with immunoglobulin (Gm) allotypes. Inheritance also apears to influence the severity of anti-GBM nephritis and the intensity of the autoantibody response.

Patients with anti-GBM antibodies usually present with glomerulonephritis, which is associated with hemoptysis or a past history of hemoptysis in a half to three-quarters of patients. Only rarely do patients with anti-GBM antibody-mediated nephritis have the signs or symptoms suggestive of generalized disease—rashes, arthralgia, myalgia, or fever—that are so characteristic of other types of rapidly progressive nephritis. Typically, the glomerulonephritis is severe and in untreated patients progresses to renal failure in weeks or months. Sometimes, especially in the presence of intercurrent infection, progression is much more rapid accompanied by destruction of all renal function in hours or days. Presently it is impossible to tell whether an individual who presents with comparatively little renal injury is at risk from sudden deterioration or whether they come from the subgroup of patients with truly indolent disease. Evidence from renal biopsies, including those from patients who have already developed renal failure, suggest an explosive final event in that the crescents all appear to be at a similar stage of their evolution. This is in contrast to the appearances of renal biopsies from patients with other causes of rapidly progressive nephritis in whom crescents are found in all phases of evolution from cellular to fibrous and often coexist with sclerosed glomeruli, which imply past episodes of disease.

The severity of pulmonary hemorrhage is more variable still, with none apparent in 25 to 50 percent of patients. In the remainder, pulmonary hemorrhage usually precedes evidence of nephritis, is episodic, and varies in severity from mild hemoptysis to severe respiratory failure. The presence and severity of pulmonary hemorrhage is not influenced by differences in the specificity of anti-GBM antibodies, which appears to be the same irrespective of clinical presentation; rather, it depends on external factors. The most important of these in our experience is exposure to cigarette smoke as almost all current cigarette smokers have pulmonary hemorrhage, whereas, it is rare in nonsmokers. Smoke may also precipitate acute pulmonary hemorrhage, as may intercurrent infection and fluid overload. Experimentally high concentrations of inspired oxygen have the same effect. Avoidance of circumstances known to aggravate injury caused by anti-GBM antibodies is as crucial to effective management of antibody-mediated nephritis as are attempts to control antibody levels and to suppress inflammation.

The effectiveness of therapy in anti-GBM disease is greatly influenced by the speed of diagnosis because of the rapidity with which the disease can progress. Anti-GBM disease can often be suspected clinically, even in the absence of pulmonary hemorrhage, because of the combination of nephritis, evidenced by the urinalysis and microscopy, and deteriorating renal function, which are not accompanied by the signs of generalized illness typical of other types of rapidly progressive glomerulonephritis. Glomerulonephritis is confirmed by renal biopsy and pulmonary hemorrhage is confirmed by the presence of anemia, hemoptysis, alveolar shadows on chest film, an *increased* diffusing capacity for carbon monoxide (kCO) after correction for lung volumes, and the patient's hemoglobin concentration. The specific diagnosis is confirmed by demonstrating anti-GBM antibodies either in the serum by radioimmunoassay (an alternative test using indirect immunofluorescence is not sensitive enough) or in kidney tissue by immunohistochemical demonstration of linear deposition of immunoglobulin along the GBM. Linear staining of the alveolar basement membrane is variable, and its absence on biopsy specimens cannot be used to exclude anti-GBM disease. Both serum and tissue diagnosis are equally effective, but the radioimmunoassay has the advantage that serial measurements can be used to follow the patient's response to treatment and to ensure the suppression of anti-GBM antibodies before renal transplantation is undertaken. Lastly, our view is that the diagnosis of anti-GBM antibody-mediated nephritis is a medical emergency, which should be confirmed or refuted within the first few hours after patient presentation.

APPROACHES TO TREATMENT

The immediate aim of treatment in anti-GBM disease is to control pulmonary hemorrhage and glomerular inflammation as swiftly as possible, thereby providing the best chance of healing and repair. Simultaneously, it may be necessary to treat infection and to support renal and pulmonary function. The longer-term objective is to suppress anti-GBM antibody synthesis permanently. Before discussing our preferred regimen, it is important to recognize the grim prognosis for untreated patients. In their 1973 survey, Wilson and Dixon reported that 25 of their 53 patients died and only seven retained useful renal function. Even now, with the general availability of dialysis and with better diagnosis of less severely affected cases, less than 15 percent of untreated patients reported in the literature in all reported series of more than five patients who presented with raised plasma creatinines, have retained useful renal function.

Immunosuppressive drugs by themselves appear to have little influence on the course of anti-GBM antibody-mediated nephritis whether prescribed singly or in combination; this observation is in contrast with their effectiveness in treating other types of rapidly progressive nephritis. It is possible that pulmonary hemorrhage is controlled by drugs more easily than is nephritis as intravenous boluses of methylprednisolone have been reported to be effective. However, this has not been our experience.

In the past, bilateral nephrectomy was advocated for treating severe pulmonary hemorrhage in patients with anti-GBM, antibody mediated disease. The original rationale for bilateral nephrectomy was that removal of the GBM would minimize the stimulus to further anti-GBM synthesis. However, not surprisingly, since the autoantigen is found in lungs as well as kidneys, nephrectomy has no effect on anti-GBM antibody titres and with hindsight, the case reports that originally suggested benefit are unconvincing. This approach is strongly contradicted and should be abandoned as ineffective and potentially dangerous.

Against this background, it was argued that effective treatment should include measures to rapidly reduce the concentration of anti-GBM antibodies, as well as measures to limit their synthesis and to suppress inflammation. Thus a treatment regimen was developed that combined repeated large volume plasma exchange with cytotoxic drugs and steroids. It would be ideal to assess the effectiveness of this treatment regimen with a prospective controlled trial, but unfortunately this cannot be done because of the rarity of anti-GBM disease, the rapidity with which it progresses, and the inherited influences on its severity. Consequently, the usefulness of therapy has had to be judged by its ability to control anti-GBM antibody titres, to suppress disease activity, and by the frequency and severity of the complications.

MANAGEMENT

Specific Therapy

Our standard regimen for treating Goodpasture's syndrome is outlined in Table 1. It consists of daily whole volume (4 L for adults) plasma exchanges for albumin, combined with prednisolone 60 mg daily, cyclophosphamide (3 mg per kilogram scaled down to the nearest 50 mg), and azathioprine 1 mg per kilogram. The regimen is modified in patients over the age of 55 years who receive cyclophosphamide 2 mg per kilogram scaled down to the nearest 50 mg and no azathioprine. Plasma exchanges are performed for 14 days or longer until clinical evidence of continuing injury has subsided. Plasma exchanges are restarted if disease activity recurs or if the anti-GBM antibody titre increases rapidly after the first course of exchanges has been completed, albeit both circumstances are rare. Five plasma exchanges are routine when a second course is required. Cyclophosphamide and azathioprine are discontinued after 8 weeks, provided that anti-GBM antibody titres are no longer detectable. The prednisolone dose is also rapidly reduced. Patients receive 60 mg of prednisolone daily for 1 week, and then, the dose is reduced at weekly intervals to 45 mg daily, 30 mg daily and then 20 mg daily. Thereafter the dose of prednisolone is reduced by decrements of 5 mg weekly until it is stopped after 8 weeks.

Plasma Exchange

The development of automatic techniques for plasma separation by centrifugation or filtration opened the way

TABLE 1 Plasma Exchange Regimen

Plasma exchange	Daily 4 L exchanges for albumin for 2 weeks
Steroids	Prednisolone, 60 mg daily for 7 days, thereafter 45, 30, 20, 15, 10, and 5 mg for 1 week each
Cytotoxic drugs	Cyclophosphamide 3 mg/kg (down to nearest 50 mg) Azathioprine 1 mg/kg (down to nearest 50 mg) Each given concurrently for 8 weeks

for therapeutic plasma exchange. This is a technique in which whole blood is removed from a patient and separated into its plasma and cellular constituents before the cells are reinfused with fresh albumin instead of the patient's plasma, which is discarded. A single 4 L plasma exchange removes approximately 90 percent of an intravascular marker, such as Evans Blue, injected intravenously at the start of plasma exchange, and 45 percent of IgG and is a highly effective way to remove circulating autoantibodies. Unfortunately, anti-GBM antibodies are rapidly resynthesized and repeated exchanges as well as the concurrent administration of immunosuppressive drugs are needed to reliably reduce their concentration in most patients.

Venovenous circuits can be used for plasma exchange, but the repeated exchanges needed to treat anti-GBM disease demand more effective vascular access. Arteriovenous shunts and central vein catheters are both suitable, but I prefer the latter as they are less liable to become infected. All types of cell separators are equally effective at removing IgG, and so, the choice between centrifugation and filtration is a personal one depending on the facilities available. Albumin solutions should be used as the plasma substitute and should have potassium and calcium added in sufficient amount to bring their concentrations into the physiologic range. Plasma exchange removes coagulation factors as well as immunoglobulins; these factors are returned as two units of fresh frozen plasma at the end of exchange in all patients who are at risk of bleeding, including those with fresh pulmonary hemorrhage or those who have had recent renal biopsies. The anticoagulation needed to prevent clotting in the extracorporeal circuit also poses a potential danger for these patients, but only a slight one as most of the anticoagulant is discarded with the patients plasma rather than being returned to the patient.

Plasma exchange shares the complications of all extracorporeal circuits, such as infection of vascular access sites and embolism. In addition, there is a tendency to fluid overload in patients with renal failure because the sodium concentration of most plasma substitutes is greater than that of plasma. Thus, each whole volume exchange is often associated with a sodium load of 100 to 150 mmoles. Fluid overload should be anticipated by daily measurement of body weight, and excess fluid should be removed by appropriate use of diuretics or dialysis. Acute hypervolemia associated with severe hypertension can be a problem, especially in children, because of rapid redistribution of fluid, which is caused by the sudden increase of plasma albumin concentration to normal levels in previously hypoalbuminemic patients. Finally, repeated plasma exchange can cause thrombocytopenia because of platelet destruction in the circuit. Table 2 outlines practical considerations to minimize complications.

TABLE 2 Practical Considerations to Minimize the Dangers of Plasma Exchange

Proper extracorporeal technique to prevent air embolism
Accurate volume replacement to maintain blood volume
Sterile technique to minimize the risk of infection
Use of albumin solutions not contaminated with vasoactive substances
Addition of potassium chloride (1.4 mmol) and calcium gluconate (0.45 mmol) to each 400 ml unit of albumin to prevent acute electrolyte disturbances
Diluting replacement albumin solutions given to hypoalbuminemic patients because of the risk of acute hypervolemia
Prevention of chronic fluid overload caused by sodium loading imposed by exchanges

Cytotoxic Drugs

Anti-GBM antibody titres rapidly return to preexchange values without the concomitant use of cytotoxic drugs. The main drug used is cyclophosphamide, which is an alkylating agent that is rapidly converted by hepatic microsomes to a series of active metabolites. These metabolites are incorporated into host DNA at all stages of the cell cycle, but cells are only killed during division. In man, cyclophosphamide, in daily doses over 2 mg per kilogram, suppresses primary antibody responses and, when used with plasma exchange, has been found to significantly shorten the duration of anti-GBM antibody synthesis in Goodpasture's syndrome. The principal early complication of cyclophosphamide is bone marrow suppression, which may occur at any stage and should be anticipated by daily measurement of the leucocyte count and prevented by appropriate reduction of the dosage. Later complications include hemorrhagic cystitis caused by excretion of toxic metabolites, infertility—especially in males, and a small but perceptible risk of malignancy. In the doses advocated here, short-term and long-term risks are minimal.

I use a small dose of azathioprine in conjunction with cyclophosphamide, but it is very difficult to quantify its effectiveness. Azathioprine is a purine analogue that is only incorporated during DNA synthesis, i.e., during cell division. In high doses, it is immunosuppressive, but in the dosage given here (1 mg per kilogram), azathioprine probably acts as an anti-inflammatory drug that is thought to be particularly effective at depressing monocyte-induced injury. In the dosage used here, it adds to the bone marrow suppression caused by cyclophosphamide and can occasionally cause an idiosyncratic reaction characterized by fever and diarrhea. The mechanism of this reaction is not clear.

Prednisolone

Corticosteroids are the most powerful anti-inflammatory drugs available, and they also have some immunosuppressive properties. The pharmacologic aspects of these drugs are discussed extensively in other chapters. In anti-GBM antibody-mediated injury, they are used predominantly for their anti-inflammatory properties and are prescribed in short, intensive courses to control the inflammatory response until anti-GBM antibody synthesis has been suppressed. There is no rationale for continuing their use beyond this point.

Patients with Goodpasture's syndrome may require supportive treatment for renal or respiratory failure, as well as for anemia.

Renal Failure

Patients with Goodpasture's syndrome may progress to end-stage renal failure within 24 hours and so need to have their renal function assessed daily in the early stages of their disease. Dialysis may be needed either because of azotemia or fluid retention (exacerbated by plasma exchange or blood transfusion), which can cause new life-threatening pulmonary hemorrhage. The choice between hemodialysis and peritoneal dialysis is controversial. Hemodialysis imposes the practical risks of further heparinization as well as adding to the duration of "machine treatment." It also carries the theoretical risk that complement activation by dialysis membranes may aggravate injury, either by priming neutrophils and activating monocytes or by sequestration of neutrophils in pulmonary capillaries adjacent to the site of antibody binding. Peritoneal dialysis has neither of these problems, but does carry the risk of infection. My own preference is to use peritoneal dialysis whenever possible.

Respiratory Failure

The treatment of respiratory failure in patients with anti-GBM disease is also controversial; although a hypoxemia may need to be corrected by oxygen therapy, there are sound experimental reasons for being anxious about such therapy. Oxygen toxicity exacerbates anti-GBM antibody-mediated pulmonary injury in rats and rabbits, at least in part, by increasing alveolar-capillary-endothelial cell permeability and thus the accessibility of the GBM to circulating antibody. It is impossible to test whether high concentrations of inspired oxygen have similar effects in patients with Goodpasture's syndrome. Nevertheless, it seems prudent to limit the inspired oxygen concentration to the absolute minimum necessary to maintain safe levels of arterial oxygen concentration. Continuous positive airway pressure should be used as required.

Anemia

Some patients with Goodpasture's syndrome are anemic and may present with a hemoglobin concentration of less than 5 g per deciliter. Care must be taken to avoid hypervolemia, which exacerbates pulmonary hemorrhage, when blood transfusions are being given.

Infection

Intercurrent infection is the most powerful cause of relapse with anti-GBM disease and appears to produce the effect by enhancing the potency of inflammatory mediators rather than by changing anti-GBM antibody synthesis. Meticulous care must be taken to prevent infection during the course of treatment, especially as the risks substantially increase by the presence of indwelling catheters (intravenous, peritoneal, or urinary) and by the use of high doses of steroids.

Other Nonspecific Measures

Cigarette smoking has been identified as an important cause of pulmonary hemorrhage in patients with Goodpasture's syndrome, and resumption of smoking can precipitate relapse. These data provide exceptionally powerful reasons for stopping patients with this disease from smoking. Goodpasture's syndrome has frequently been associated with exposure to hydrocarbon fumes. Whether or not the nature of this association and its effects are analogous to those of cigarette smoke, it again seems prudent to limit such exposure as much as possible.

RESULTS OF THERAPY

We have used plasma exchange to treat antibody-mediated Goodpasture's syndrome for the past 10 years and during this time have treated 49 patients. Since 1980, we have also performed serial assays of anti-GBM antibodies and advised on the management of a further 71 patients treated in other units throughout the United Kingdom.

Control of Anti-GBM Antibody Titre

Anti-GBM antibody titres fell immediately after starting therapy in all patients treated with the combination plasma exchange and immunosuppressive drugs, and there has been little tendency for anti-GBM antibody titres to increase once the concentrations have been reduced to background values. Long-term, possibly permanent, disappearance of anti-GBM antibodies was achieved within 8 weeks in 29 of 30 patients who received a full course of the plasma-exchange regimen. A full course was defined as at least 12 plasma exchanges and 8 weeks of treatment with cyclophosphamide. In contrast, anti-GBM antibodies persisted for much longer in patients who did not receive complete tretment, and only three of 33 patients cleared of antibodies by 8 weeks; the autoantibodies persisted for more than a year in 12 of these patients. Thus it appears that cyclophosphamide and plasma exchange act synergistically to promote long-term control of anti-GBM antibody synthesis.

Renal Function

Nephrons that have been destroyed cannot regenerate, and so it comes as no surprise that the degree of improvement of renal function depends on the severity of injury at the time treatment is started. The plasma exchange regimen has been used on 58 dialysis-dependent patients with anti-GBM disease under our direct or indirect supervision, and none regained useful renal function despite control of autoantibody titres. Similarly, the results in patients whose serum creatinines exceed 600 μ moles per L (6.8 mg per deciliter) at the start of treatment have not been encouraging, with improvement in only one of 12 such patients. By contrast, renal function improved in 13 of 15 patients with plasma creatinines that were rapidly increasing, but were less than 600 μmoles per L (6.8 mg per deciliter), who were treated by us and in 2 of 5 patients monitored by us, but treated elsewhere in the United Kingdom. Improvement in these patients was evident as soon as the plasma exchange regimen was started, which argues strongly that it was a direct result of treatment. Seven patients with biopsy-proved nephritis, whose serum creatinines were within the normal range, were also treated and showed improvement when assessed, by changes of serum creatinine to within normal range or by improvement of the urine sediment. Thus the plasma exchange regimen is effective treatment for nephritis in Goodpasture's syndrome provided that it is introduced before the kidneys have been severely damaged. In a few patients, late deterioration of renal function because of progressive fibrosis has occurred without recurrence of detectable anti-GBM antibody synthesis. These patients have not been treated by reintroduction of plasma exchange or drug therapy, but have received nonspecific treatment until dialysis or transplantation was performed.

Mortality

The overall mortality at 8 weeks in patients treated at Hammersmith was 16 percent (eight of 49 patients). In three of these, mortality was unrelated to the regimen—unsuitability for long-term dialysis in two and a myocardial infarction in the third—and in the remaining five, pulmonary hemorrhage was the cause of death. All the patients who had uncontrollable pulmonary hemorrhage had concomitant infections.

Pulmonary Hemorrhage

Pulmonary hemorrhage in anti-GBM antibody-mediated disease has a much greater tendency to be episodic than nephritis, and the lungs have a much greater capacity to recover. In all, 56 patients had evidence of pulmonary hemorrhage when treatment was started, and it improved in 51. All the remaining patients died of respiratory failure. Relapses of pulmonary hemorrhage that occurred were related to infection, fluid overload, or in one patient, resumption of cigarette smoking. None of the patients who recovered has developed pulmonary fibrosis of sufficient severity to be visible radiologically. Possibly, this is because pulmonary blood is very focal and thus even widespread pulmonary hemorrhage can be disseminated from a small lesion.

MONITORING THE EFFECTS OF THERAPY

The effects of treatment should be monitored meticulously by repeated assessments of disease activity, fluid balance, and possible complications (Table 3). Routine investigations include daily measures of body weight, urine microscopy, serum creatinine, and full blood count. Chest radiographs and kCO are assessed three times weekly when clinically indicated. Cultures of urine, sputum, and vascular access sites are taken three times weekly, but antibiotics are given only when clinically indicated. Whenever possible, it is helpful to monitor anti-

TABLE 3 Routine Monitoring of Patients with Goodpasture's Syndrome

System	*Investigation*	*Frequency*
General	Weight	Daily
	Routine clinical examination	At least daily
	Blood pressure	4 hourly
Hematologic	Hemoglobin White cell count Platelets	Daily
Renal	Urine sediment Serum creatinine	Daily
Pulmonary	Chest radiography kCo	3 times weekly
Immunologic	Bacteriologic cultures of urine, throat, vascular access site	3 times weekly
	Anti-GBM antibody titres	Daily for 2 weeks; thereafter 3 times weekly until undetectable, then monthly

GBM antibody titres frequently. We measure anti-GBM antibody titres daily for the first 2 weeks and then three times weekly, but this is not essential. However, it is important to measure antibody titres initially to confirm the diagnosis, secondly at the end of therapy to assess the need for continuous immunosuppression, thirdly before transplantation in patients who develop end-stage renal failure, and fourthly in all patients with deteriorating renal function so as to distinguish active disease from progressive scarring.

PATIENT SELECTION

The plasma exchange regimen described here is arduous and exposes the patient to discomfort as well as some risk. It should not be used indiscriminately, but should be reserved for those patients who are likely to benefit. Presently, we offer plasma exchange to all patients with active pulmonary hemorrhage and all those with nephritis and declining renal function. We also treat the majority of patients with nephritis and creatinines within the normal range, but who have clinical or morphologic evidence of active nephritis. Patients who are anuric, but do not have pulmonary hemorrhage, are not treated, except occasionally to limit the duration of anti-GBM antibody synthesis and allow earlier renal transplantation.

Although this plasma exchange appears to be the first consistently effective treatment for anti-GBM disease, it is clearly unsatisfactory, being cumbersome and lacking specificity. Presently, understanding of autoimmunity and the control of autoantibody responses are advancing rapidly and hopefully will result in the development of more specific ways to suppress anti-GBM antibody synthesis. It is also depressing that so many patients present after their kidneys have been destroyed, and this clearly indicates the need for earlier diagnosis.

IDIOPATHIC RAPIDLY PROGRESSIVE GLOMERULONEPHRITIS

PETER I. LOBO, M.D.
W. KLINE BOLTON, M.D.

A diagnosis of rapidly progressive glomerulonephritis (RPGN) is conventionally made in patients presenting with a rapid loss of renal function associated with glomerulonephritis, usually with extensive glomerular crescent formation, on renal biopsy. Deterioration in renal function is considered "rapid" if there is a doubling of serum creatinine or a halving of the creatinine clearance within 3 months or less. Immunopathogenetically, RPGN is divided into three main categories:

1. Immune-complex–induced RPGN, comprising 30 to 40 percent of cases with RPGN. It is frequently associated with postinfectious processes (e.g., poststreptococcal nephritis) or a form of systemic immune complex disease (e.g., lupus nephritis, vasculitis, and cryoglobulinemia). Characteristically, this category is associated with granular immune deposits.
2. Anti-glomerular basement membrane (GBM) antibody–induced RPGN, comprising 20 to 30 percent of cases of RPGN.
3. RPGN without glomerular immune deposits (no immune deposits [NID], or "pauci-immune" deposits), comprising approximately 30 to 40 percent of patients with RPGN.

The term "idiopathic" RPGN applies to those types of glomerulonephritis of unknown etiology, regardless of whether crescents are present or not. It includes all three categories described above since its etiologies, except as delineated by specific diseases, are unknown, regardless of the fluorescence or ultrastructural appearance. RPGN associated with immune deposits, as immune complexes or anti-GBM disease, is addressed in other chapters of this text. Therefore this chapter addresses only the NID or "pauci-immune" deposit subtype of idiopathic RPGN associated with crescents.

Most patients with NID-RPGN have a primary renal disease of uncertain etiology and pathogenesis. Some patients with this subtype of RPGN have a form of vasculitis (e.g., polyarteritis nodosa) with inflammation confined to the glomerular capillaries. The presence of antineutrophil cytoplasmic antibodies (ANCA, a marker of vasculitic disease) in some of these patients supports this concept. The therapeutic approaches to each of these categories may differ. This chapter deals with the therapy of the NID subtype of idiopathic RPGN.

DIAGNOSIS

Few true emergencies exist in the area of nephrology. One of these, however, is RPGN, especially the crescentic variety. It is critical to make the correct diagnosis to avoid needless and inappropriate therapy for other disease processes, and yet to make the diagnosis that directs therapy at the specific type of RPGN. We routinely perform an emergent renal biopsy in any patient with the de novo clinical presentation of RPGN if no obvious precipitating cause is found (e.g., vasomotor nephropathy, trauma, acute interstitial nephritis with eosinophils in the urine, and an allergic exposure). We perform a biopsy in patients with nosocomial acute renal failure with atypical manifestations such as red blood cell casts, heavy hematuria, and/or proteinuria in the absence of overt causes; with oliguria or anuria in the absence of pressors or obvious causes of severe acute tubular necrosis; and with systemic diseases that have a clinical presentation consistent with the diagnosis of RPGN. Biopsies are also performed in patients with known pre-existing disease who have a sudden change in renal function consistent with RPGN. In our geographic region, one-third of all patients who undergo biopsy are found to have glomerulonephritis. Twenty percent of these have crescents (7 percent of the total number of biopsies). Approximately 12 percent of patients with glomerulonephritis (4 percent of total biopsies) have the clinical course of RPGN. A diagnosis of idiopathic NID-RPGN is made when the biopsy shows greater than or equal to 20 percent cellular crescents in the glomeruli and if immunofluorescence fails to detect anti-GBM antibody or significant immune complex deposits. The idiopathic nature of RPGN is also verified by the absence of antistreptococcal, antinuclear, anti-GBM, and hepatitis B surface antigen antibodies and cryoglobulins. The presence of ANCA does not exclude the diagnosis of idiopathic RPGN, but it becomes necessary to exclude the possibility of systemic necrotizing vasculitis, including Wegener's granulomatosis and polyarteritis.

PROGNOSIS

The prognosis of idiopathic RPGN in general has been poor. Precise figures are difficult to obtain from the existing literature, as most series consist of patients with several types of RPGN. Additionally, follow-up is usually of short duration, and the patients have received variable forms of therapy. However, available data would indicate that 75 percent of such patients become dialysis dependent (or die) within months if they are untreated or treated only with oral steroids and/or immunosuppressive agents.

Recent advances in the therapy of idiopathic RPGN are related to the introduction of intravenous bolus injections of methylprednisolone and plasma exchange. In this chapter, we emphasize our experience with intravenous bolus injections of methylprednisolone (pulse therapy).

TREATMENT REGIMEN

We have used the following regimen at our institution over the past several decades. With pulse methylprednisolone therapy, methylprednisolone is administered intravenously in doses of 30 mg per kilogram of body weight given over a 20-minute period with monitoring of blood pressure. The methylprednisolone is given over a period not greater than 20 minutes and not less than 15 minutes. It is ascertained that patients are volume replete and have not received diuretics within the past 3 hours, and they should not receive any diuretics for 24 hours after therapy. The methylprednisolone should be administered as soon as the patient is stabilized and volume repleted. The maximum dose administered at any single time must not exceed 3 g. This dose of methylprednisolone is repeated every other day for a total of three doses. Forty-eight hours after the last dose of methylprednisolone is administered, treatment with oral alternate-day prednisone is instituted, as detailed in Table 1.

We have a few patients treated with cyclophosphamide or dipyridamole. For such patients, we administer approximately 100 mg per day of cyclophosphamide and 200 mg per day dipyridamole in divided doses. The dose of oral prednisone is adjusted for any patient 60 years of age or older; such patients receive 75 percent of the dose recommended in Table 1. The regimen is accelerated to the next steroid dose (Table 1) if the patient develops and maintains normal renal function for 1 month. Thus the shortest duration of treatment in responding patients is approximately 1 year, and the longest duration is approximately 5 years. Reactivation of disease, documented clinically and with repeat biopsy, is treated as de novo RPGN according to protocol; treatment is repeated as often as three times if the response has previously been good.

Patients we have excluded from treatment with pulse methylprednisolone therapy include those with an unexplained acute febrile illness, overt psychosis, active peptic ulcer, terminal irreversible illness, and

TABLE 1 Protocol for Administering Oral Prednisone Therapy

*Alternate-Day Dose of Prednisone**	*Duration of Theapy (mos.)*
2.00 mg/kg	0.5
1.75 mg/kg	1.0
1.50 mg/kg	3.0
1.25 mg/kg	6.0
1.00 mg/kg	6.0
0.75 mg/kg	6.0
0.50 mg/kg	6.0
0.25 mg/kg	6.0
0.125 mg/kg	12.0
0.0625 mg/kg	12.0

*75 percent of dose for patients 60 years of age or older.

those who have undergone major surgery within the past 2 weeks. We do not permit the use of any steroidal medications, aspirin, phenylbutazone, or other steroid-type drugs while patients are taking methylprednisolone and prednisone.

CRITERIA FOR RESPONSE

Patients are considered to be treated adequately if they survive for 6 weeks or longer, since more than 90 percent of patients respond within the first 6 weeks. Patients' conditions are considered to be stable or improved if the serum creatinine level remains stable or is decreased by 30 percent or more or if the patients were receiving dialytic support and are able to discontinue it.

Table 2 provides the results of treatment with pulse therapy with methylprednisolone in our patients with idiopathic RPGN. Data presented pertain to the average percentage of crescents, whether or not patients were improved, and whether they were receiving dialysis and were able to discontinue it. Twenty-one patients had the histologic diagnosis of idiopathic NID-RPGN. Sixteen of the 21 patients (76 percent) who received pulse therapy showed an improvement. Ten of 15 patients who received pulse therapy and were receiving dialysis were able to discontinue dialysis. An analysis of response relative to the extent of glomerular involvement with crescents showed that 75 percent of patients with 60 percent or more crescents improved with pulse therapy and that 64 percent of patients who received dialysis with 60 percent or more of the glomeruli involved with crescents were able to discontinue dialysis. Ninety percent of patients who were oliguric showed improvement with pulse therapy.

We have also evaluated the effect that associated glomerulosclerotic lesions have on the response to pulse therapy in these patients. Of patients with less than 33 percent glomerular obsolescence, 92 percent demonstrated initial improvement and 85 percent continued to show long-term improvement. The response in those patients exhibiting a glomerular obsolescence of more than 33 percent was not as promising. Seventy-one percent of these patients had initial improvement, with only 36 percent maintaining improvement over the long-term. More importantly, a short duration of disease before the institution of therapy was significantly associated with less chronicity and better response to therapy. This again emphasizes the importance of early biopsy with this disease.

TABLE 2 Results of Pulse Methylprednisolone Therapy in the Treatment of Idiopathic NID-RPGN

Total number of patients	21
Mean age	59
Percentage of crescents	69
Percentage of patients whose condition improved	76
Number of patients requiring dialysis	15
Number of patients in whom dialysis was discontinued	10

COMPLICATIONS

Our treatment regimen has been associated with no major complications. There have been complaints of a metallic taste in the mouth, muscle weakness, "seeing bright lights" and other psychotropic effects, nausea, arthralgia, and discomfort at the site of infusion. Arrhythmia was noted in one patient with a previous cardiac abnormality. No patient has had decreased blood pressure. In patients observed over a long period, we have noted cataracts, cushingoid facies, acne, hirsutism, and occasionally, glaucoma. Our experience over the past two decades indicates that a significant steroid-associated side effect such as myocardial infarct, pulmonary embolus, or stroke may be expected once in each 12 patient years of therapy.

OTHER TYPES OF THERAPY

A comparison of pulse therapy with methylprednisolone with the other types of therapy for RPGN is difficult to make because of the general lack of discrimination in including patients with different diagnoses in the category of RPGN. Nevertheless, several other general types of treatment have been used successfully. *Conventional therapy* consists of all types of therapy other than pulse therapy, quadruple therapy, and plasma exchange. *Quadruple therapy* consists of prednisone, dipyridamole, cyclophosphamide or azathioprine, and anticoagulation. Regimens of *pulse therapy* other than our own include those consisting variously of 1 g daily administered for up to 11 days or given on an alternate-day schedule or on other schedules. The results of these latter regimens have not necessarily been comparable to our experience. *Plasma exchange therapy* is given in combination with immunosuppressive agents (i.e., prednisone, cyclophosphamide, and azathioprine).

Approximately 25 percent of patients show improvement with a variety of types of therapy (e.g., prednisone alone or combined with azathioprine). This contrasts markedly with the results of quadruple therapy, pulse therapy, and plasma exchange treatment, all of which result in a response in approximately 75 to 80 percent of patients.

We prefer to treat idiopathic RPGN with pulse therapy for several reasons. Quadruple therapy, while apparently effective in non-anti-GBM disease, does require the use of anticoagulants and cytotoxic drugs; and the potential for infection and other complications may therefore be higher. The patient who eventually experiences a relapse, progresses to chronic renal failure, or requires transplantation may already have received enough cytotoxic therapy to increase his or her susceptibility to malignant disease after the institution of immunosuppressive therapy during the transplant period. In addition, a significant number of patients—perhaps half—treated with quadruple therapy eventually progress slowly to chronic renal failure. In our experience, fewer patients treated with pulse therapy alone gradually progress to renal failure. Since the rate of response to pulse therapy in patients with oligoanuria and high degrees of crescent formation is comparable with or better than the rate of response to quadruple therapy and because progression of fibrosis to end-stage disease appears to be less (and the side effects are less), we believe that pulse therapy is indicated over quadruple therapy.

Plasma exchange in combination with prednisone, azathioprine, and cyclophosphamide has been used for a wide variety of types of glomerulonephritis. The complication rate during the initial period of exchange may be higher than that of pulse therapy. Once again, this type of therapy may possibly be associated with the later higher risks of malignant disease because cyclophosphamide is given as part of the regimen. It is also possible that some protective factors that are circulating may be removed as well as harmful factors; we have seen several patients with glomerulonephritis whose conditions actually appeared to deteriorate with the initiation of plasma exchange. In addition, plasma exchange is much more expensive and is inconvenient for the patient. Since the results of therapy with plasma exchange appear to be comparable to those of pulse therapy for idiopathic RPGN, we continue to prefer pulse therapy.

Steroid pulse therapy in idiopathic NID-RPGN has generally not included the use of concomitant cytotoxic agents. Currently there is increasing evidence to implicate a vasculitic process with some patients having idiopathic RPGN. It would therefore seem reasonable to add cyclophosphamide to pulse therapy in those patients with circulating ANCA, as this subgroup may represent a forme fruste of vasculitis. After all, long-term therapy with cyclophosphamide appears to be beneficial for polyarteritis nodosa and Wegener's granulomatosis.

It remains to be determined whether newer approaches (e.g., the use of cyclosporine and normal pooled human gamma globulin) will also be effective for idiopathic RPGN. The latter approach has been used with some success in the therapy of Kawasaki disease and ANCA-positive systemic necrotizing vasculitis.

MECHANISM OF DRUG ACTION

The exact mechanism by which pulse therapy with methylprednisolone followed by an alternate-day regimen of prednisone achieves its beneficial effects is not known. The rationale for using pulse therapy was derived from the similarities between crescentic glomerulonephritis and the interstitial reaction that occurs with transplant rejection. Prednisone and large doses of methylprednisolone are known to impair lymphocyte function and to have a dramatic effect on macrophages and monocytes, with depletion of their numbers and impairment of their ability to phagocytose and present antigens. Fibroblast formation is impaired, and lysosomal membranes are stabilized. Arachidonic acid metabolites may also be decreased. It has been our experience that the use of larger doses of methylprednisolone given over 20 minutes is associated with a slightly better response rate than methylprednisolone given in smaller doses over a longer period of time. However, no specific studies on this have been performed.

SUGGESTED READING

Bolton WK. The role of high-dose steroids in nephritic syndromes: the case for aggressive use. In: Narins RG, ed. Controversies in nephrology and hypertension. New York: Churchill Livingstone, 1984: 421.

Bolton WK, Sturgill BC. Methylprednisolone therapy for acute crescentic rapidly progressive glomerulonephritis. Am J Nephrol 1989; 9:368–375.

Couser WG. Rapidly progressive glomerulonephritis: classification, pathogenetic mechanisms, and therapy. Am J Kidney Dis 1988; 11:449–464.

Jacquot C, Baran D, Vendeville B, et al. Update on immunosuppressive therapy in human and experimental glomerulonephritis. Adv Nephrol 1988; 17:77–99.

HEMOLYTIC-UREMIC SYNDROME

BRIAN T. STEELE, M.D., FRCPC

Outside of the neonatal period, hemolytic-uremic syndrome (HUS) is rivaled only by acute poststreptococcal glomerulonephritis as a common cause of acute renal failure in children. Indeed in the age group where it is most commonly seen (1 to 4 years), it is by far the most common cause of acute renal failure. Since its original description more than 30 years ago, it has become clear that there are many different causes for the syndrome of microangiopathic anemia, thrombocytopenia, and acute renal failure. In considering the treatment of HUS, an analogy could be made with nephrotic syndrome where common principles of therapy often apply, but where specific therapies are also considered. Just as the close hematologic and pathologic relationships between HUS and thrombotic thrombocytopenic purpura do not imply similar treatment or prognosis, so might HUS in a young child differ from the same syndrome postpartum or postchemotherapy. Most patients recover from HUS despite both a poor understanding of etiology and a lack of specific therapy. Many discussions on this syndrome have focused on concepts of pathogenesis with possible therapy, while acknowledging that the improved mortality and morbidity over the last 10 years is a reflection of good supportive care. Some details of this supportive care will be emphasized first.

ASSESSMENT OF FLUID BALANCE

A clinical assessment for dehydration or fluid overload is important, and the degree of fluid imbalance is often determined by the timing of the diagnosis. Typically, the child has been unwell for several days with a gastrointestinal upset, predominantly blood-stained diarrhea. At the time of diagnosis, some may have a marked deficit of extracellular fluid, while others may be hypertensive and edematous from over-generous fluid replacement in the presence of insidious or unrecognized renal failure. Thus, some patients will require volume expansion to encourage urine flow, while others will require severe fluid restriction until a diuresis occurs with recovery. When the patient's hydration is normal, the desired maintenance fluid should be given as a replacement of insensible losses (approximately 400 ml per m^2 per day) plus urine plus gastrointestinal losses. Intravenous and not oral fluids are initially required until the patient's nausea has disappeared and the abdomen is soft.

Maintaining urine flow is fundamental to the management of acute renal failure since nonoliguric renal failure is easier to manage than established anuric renal failure. If oliguria or anuria is present, a single dose of furosemide (3 mg per kilogram over 30 minutes) is safe and often worthwhile.

Hypertension at the time of diagnosis usually reflects fluid overload and is likely to improve after diuresis or fluid restriction. Headaches or visual symptoms can be expected in young children with a diastolic blood pressure greater than 90 mm Hg, and urgent therapy is then necessary. Intravenous hydralazine, perhaps with a beta-blocker such as labetalol, is usually effective and safer than more potent agents such as intravenous diazoxide or sublingual nifedipine.

ELECTROLYTE DISORDERS

Hyperkalemia is the most serious biochemical disturbance with life-threatening arrhythmias likely if the serum potassium is greater than 7.0 mmol per liter. Despite the concomitant hemolysis, hyperkalemia does not seem to be more severe in HUS than other causes of acute renal failure. If a metabolic acidosis is present, the serum potassium will fall with sodium bicarbonate treatment. With continued severe hyperkalemia, other drugs such as calcium gluconate 10 percent or hypertonic glucose are likely to produce only a temporary improvement which allows time for dialysis to be instituted. With good nursing skills, Kayexalate, a sodium polystyrene sulfonate resin may be used rectally, but is rarely tolerated by mouth.

Hyponatremia is common and most often is a reflection of water overload rather than salt depletion from gastrointestinal losses and dehydration. The importance of hyponatremia as an explanation for seizures and other central nervous system abnormalities in HUS has probably been overstated, and intracerebral thrombotic lesions may be a more likely explanation. A serum sodium less than 120 mmol per liter is difficult to ignore, and although a small infusion of hypertonic saline may add to the problems of fluid overload, it is justified if the patient is symptomatic.

HEMATOLOGIC ABNORMALITIES

The severity of microangiopathic hemolytic anemia in HUS is variable and does not correlate well with the severity of renal failure or thrombocytopenia. A rapid hemolysis will be tolerated less well, but most children remain relatively asymptomatic with a hemoglobin greater than 70 g per liter. A transfusion of packed red cells is advisable below this level and should be given cautiously (a maximum of 10 ml per kilogram) if the patient is edematous, hypertensive, or anuric. Platelet transfusions are rarely required in HUS and theoretically could accentuate the thrombotic injury to the kidney or brain. Platelet counts below 100×10^9 per liter are invariably seen, but levels below 15×10^9 per liter are rare. Unlike disseminated intravascular coagulation, clinical bleeding is uncommon despite thrombocytopenia and azotemia. It is advisable, however, to have platelets available with any surgical or dialysis procedure.

A leukocytosis is commonly seen at the time of presentation and in itself does not imply bacterial sepsis and the need for systemic antibiotics.

EXTRARENAL MANIFESTATIONS

Widespread extrarenal thrombotic lesions have been reported in patients who died early in the course of the disease. With the exception of the central nervous system and colon, extrarenal manifestations of HUS are clinically uncommon. Subtle signs within the central nervous system such as lethargy, disorientation, or aphasia may be difficult to interpret in a young child with renal failure. Seizures and coma may follow, and computerized tomography is a worthwhile investigation since small basal ganglia infarcts are virtually pathognomonic of HUS. Early treatment with anticonvulsants, fluid restriction to minimize cerebral edema, and close monitoring of the airway and gas exchange is desirable in those patients with proven or suspicious central nervous system involvement.

Bloody diarrhea and abdominal tenderness are usually transient but can be troublesome in some patients. Characteristic radiologic abnormalities can be seen in the transverse colon, but neither a barium enema nor sigmoidoscopy are likely to help in patient management. Gangrene of the bowel and perforation requiring surgery are rare complications.

INDICATIONS FOR DIALYSIS

There are two relatively clear indications for dialysis:

1. Hyperkalemia with arrhythmias or rising potassium levels (greater than 7.0 mmol per liter), despite treatment, and
2. Fluid overload in an oliguric patient, producing either pulmonary edema or uncontrolled hypertension.

A less clearly defined indication for dialysis is the patient with prolonged anuria but neither of the above two indications. Such a patient is likely to be severely catabolic and increasingly uremic. Early dialysis will prevent uremic complications such as gastrointestinal bleeding, and fluid removal allows good nutritional support. It can be difficult to decide on the timing of such dialysis since many patients are anuric for less than 1 week. Peritoneal dialysis is usually the preferred choice, although some centers have a bias towards hemodialysis. The latter requires vascular access and maintenance of this access between dialysis treatments. The main contraindication to peritoneal dialysis is the patient with major abdominal signs from severe colitis.

SPECIFIC THERAPY

There is little evidence that patients with HUS have benefitted from any specific therapy. Enthusiasm for therapy based on new concepts on the pathogenesis of HUS has usually been followed by disappointing trial results or case reports of failed treatment. A major difficulty in proving the effectiveness of any new therapy is the high recovery rate with supportive care alone. It has been calculated that more than 300 children with HUS would be required for any treatment trial that would give statistical credibility. Large pediatric centers rarely see more than 15 patients in 1 year. Specific therapy that has been advocated includes the following:

Heparin. This was advocated for many years but did not seem to hasten recovery. Moreover, there have been reports of fatal hemorrhage from heparin therapy and its use can no longer be justified.

Antiplatelet Agents. Aspirin and dipyridamole are not easy to take orally in the acute stage of the disease. Ths most desirable dose of each drug may still be controversial, but previous regimens have not shown any improvement in outcome.

Fibrinolytic Therapy. Streptokinase, urokinase, and defibrodide have all been used in small numbers of patients. The reported success has not differed from the expected course of the disease, even in patients where the infusion was made directly into the renal arteries. Spontaneous hemorrhage into infarcted areas within the brain is rare but has occurred in patients untreated with heparin, antiplatelet, or antifibrinolytic agents. Thus, all of these drugs pose some risk to the patient and are without a proven benefit.

Plasma Infusion or Exchange. Plasma has been advocated following the observation of a deficient plasma factor that normally stimulates vascular prostacyclin. Treatment failures have been described and large controlled trials have not been done. Repeated plasma infusions to an anuric child are likely to complicate fluid overload, and plasma exchange requires large vessel access and again poses the potential for increased morbidity and mortality.

Vitamin E. Low plasma vitamin E levels are sometimes found with HUS. Consequently, these patients may have a reduced antioxidant potential, favoring the selective destruction of prostacyclin synthetase. One uncontrolled study of 16 children has claimed good results, but more convincing evidence of efficacy is still required.

Prostacyclin. A constant infusion of prostacyclin might theoretically bypass the need for plasma or vitamin E. Large trials have not been done, but again reports of treatment failure suggest that recovery depends on factors other than normal prostacyclin levels.

ATYPICAL CASES OF HUS

There have been many attempts to classify types of subgroups of HUS. It is generally agreed that the epi-

TABLE 1 Prognosis of HUS

Excellent Prognosis	*Guarded Prognosis*	*Poor Prognosis*
Age 1–4 yr	Older children	Absent prodrome
Clustering of cases	Adult	Recurrent episodes
Bloody diarrhea prodrome	Atypical prodrome	Family history Low C_3
?Verotoxin in stools		

demic form occurring in young children is almost always associated with a good prognosis. These patients usually have a bloody diarrhea prodrome, and recent work suggests that this prodrome is associated with a verotoxin-producing *E. coli*. Not all of these patients present during epidemics, and a sporadic presentation with the same prodrome will also have a good prognosis. Table 1 indicates which patients are likely to have a guarded or poor prognosis. Despite such divisions, a predictable outcome is not always possible so that, for example, older patients with an atypical prodrome can also recover completely. Most large series of HUS include atypical cases who have done poorly. However, the total number of such cases is small and the real significance of each atypical presentation has not been determined. As an example, HUS is rarely associated with chicken pox and such reported cases have not recovered from acute renal failure. This apparent bad risk factor would be less significant if there were unreported cases following chicken pox who did recover. Some atypical cases of HUS are indistinguishable from thrombotic thrombocytopenic purpura and, as a confusing example, both syndromes have been described after mitomycin therapy. HUS registries have been set up, and it is hoped that controlled, multicentered trials with specific therapy can be done on selected atypical patients. Until this happens, atypical patients with a poor prognosis are likely to receive overtreatment rather than undertreatment, i.e., a combination of plasma exchange, vitamin E, or prostacyclin.

MANAGEMENT AFTER THE ACUTE STAGE

After renal function improves, an uncomplicated course can be anticipated with complete renal recovery in most cases. It is important to avoid further renal insults, particularly fluid depletion in a patient with a renal concentrating defect. Incomplete recovery can present in later years with severe hypertension or chronic renal failure. Persistence of proteinuria, hypertension, azotemia, or polyuria with polydipsia after the initial period of hospitalization is an important observation and requires further investigation and, in some cases, renal histology.

A rebound thrombocytosis is common during recovery and does not seem to affect the prognosis, even with platelet counts greater than $1{,}000 \times 10^9$ per liter. A stable hemoglobin, less than 90 g per liter in the recovery phase is often best treated with a blood transfusion. This provides faster rehabilitation, particularly in the patient who has had a prolonged period of catabolism.

SUGGESTED READING

Derereyn G, Proesmans W, Machin SJ, Lemmen SF, Vermylen J. Abnormal prostacyclin metabolism in the hemolytic uremic syndrome: equivocal effects of prostacyclin infusion. Clin Nephrol 1982; 18:43–49.

Fong TSC, de Chadarevian JP, Kaplan BS. Haemolytic uraemic syndrome: current concepts and management. Pediatr Clin North Am 1982; 29:35–56.

Kaplan BS, Drummond KN. The hemolytic uremic syndrome is a syndrome. N Engl J Med 1978; 298:964–966.

Karmali AM, Steele BT, Petric M, Lim C. Sporadic cases of haemolytic uraemic syndrome associated with faecal cytotoxin and cytotoxin-producing escherichia coli in stools. Lancet 1983; 1:619–620.

Powell HR, McCredie DA, Taylor CM, Burke JR, Walker RG. Vitamin E treatment of haemolytic uraemic syndrome. Arch Dis Child 1984; 59:401–404.

Remuzzi G, Marchesi D, Mecca G. Haemolytic uraemic syndrome: deficiency of plasma factor(s) regulating prostacyclin activity? Lancet 1978; 2:871–872.

Steele BT, Murphy N, Chuang SH, McGreal D, Arbus G. Recovery from prolonged coma in hemolytic uremic syndrome. J Pediatr 1983; 102:402–404.

Trompeter RS, Schwartz R, Chantler C, Dillon MJ, Hancock GB, Kay R, Barratt TM. Haemolytic uraemic syndrome: an analysis of prognostic features. Arch Dis Child 1983; 58:101–105.

IgA NEPHROPATHY (BERGER'S DISEASE)

BRUCE A. JULIAN, M.D.
A. WARMOLD L. VAN DEN WALL BAKE, M.D., Ph.D.

IgA nephropathy has become recognized in many countries as the most common form of primary glomerulonephritis in the 22 years after its description by Berger and Hinglais. Originally entitled *les dépôts inter-capillaires d'IgA-d'IgG,* this entity has also been labelled *mesangial IgA disease, IgA-IgG nephropathy,* and *IgA mesangial glomerulonephritis.* Because of the enthusiasm of its champion and the evolving controversies about the pathogenesis of this disorder, the eponym *Berger's disease* has gained increasing favor. The hallmark feature of this kidney disease is the dominant presence of IgA in the mesangium on immunofluorescence examination of the glomeruli. Light microscopy shows variable degrees of mesangial expansion and hypercellularity. Indistinguishable immunohistologic patterns may be found in the kidney biopsy specimens of patients with nephritis caused by Henoch-Schönlein purpura. Furthermore, similar pathologic findings have been described in patients with a wide spectrum of diseases, including dermatitis herpetiformis, psoriasis, ankylosing spondylitis, celiac disease, regional enteritis, ulcerative colitis, carcinomas (especially of the colon, oral pharynx, and lung), IgA monoclonal gammopathy, alcoholic cirrhosis, chronic hepatitis, and mycosis fungoides. IgA nephropathy in patients with these latter conditions is often referred to as secondary, IgA nephropathy. Secondary IgA nephropathy is in contrast to primary IgA nephropathy, which is seen in patients with the idiopathic form (Berger's disease) or Henoch-Schönlein purpura, considered by some investigators to be the "systemic form" of this process. The discussion in this chapter is devoted to Berger's disease.

DIAGNOSTIC FEATURES

Immunohistologic Features

The diagnosis of IgA nephropathy requires an immunofluorescence examination of kidney tissue. Mesangial deposits of IgA are found in all glomeruli, even in those with a normal histologic appearance or minimal changes. Occasionally the IgA deposits may extend to the peripheral capillary loops. IgG and/or IgM are detected less often. C3 (the third component of complement) is usually found in a similar mesangial distribution. Other components of the alternative complement pathway, including properdin and Factor H (β1H), as well as the membrane attack complex (C5b–9) are often detected. The absence or minimal intensity of the staining for C1q is a useful criterion to separate IgA nephropathy from lupus nephritis if IgG is present. When light chain-specific antibodies are used, the intensity of immunofluorescence staining for lambda often exceeds that for the kappa isotype. Light microscopy usually shows mild mesangial proliferation and matrix expansion, although the pattern may vary within a biopsy specimen and be segmental (only a portion of a glomerulus affected) or focal (not all glomeruli affected). Segmental sclerosing lesions and cellular crescents are less common. Electron-dense deposits in the mesangial and paramesangial areas are usually easily found on electron microscopy. Small deposits may be located infrequently in the subendothelial or subepithelial areas.

Clinical Features

IgA nephropathy usually presents clinically as one of two syndromes. The most characteristic syndrome is an episode of *macroscopic hematuria* concurrent with an infection of the upper respiratory tract or with gastroenteritis. In contrast to the 10- to 14-day delay for the onset of macroscopic hematuria in patients with poststreptococcal glomerulonephritis, the urinary blood in patients with IgA nephropathy appears 1 to 2 days after the onset of symptoms and is rarely accompanied by hypertension or edema. Some patients, especially children, experience loin pain. The episode generally lasts only a few days but may recur with a similar illness months or years later. Strenuous exercise or a nonspecific febrile illness also occasionally induces macroscopic hematuria. Examination of the urinary sediment by phase contrast microscopy reveals deformed red blood cells indicating glomerular bleeding rather than bleeding from a site in the urinary tract. Macroscopic hematuria is more common in children and adolescents than in adults, and its frequency decreases with increasing age. The second manner by which IgA nephropathy often presents is asymptomatic *microscopic hematuria* accompanied by variable degrees of proteinuria. This syndrome is usually discovered on routine urinalysis testing performed during insurance, employment, or check-up examinations. Less common presentations include nephrotic syndrome, chronic renal insufficiency, and malignant hypertension. In a few patients, the first evidence of renal dysfunction is macroscopic hematuria with acute renal insufficiency; renal biopsies in these individuals may show large cellular crescents in many of the glomeruli or tubular necrosis accompanied by red blood cell casts.

IgA nephropathy is diagnosed most frequently in the second and third decades of life. The likelihood of documenting the disease depends greatly on the threshold for performing the requisite renal biopsy. In several geographic regions with an apparently low incidence of IgA nephropathy, subsequent screening programs with follow-up evaluation substantially increased the incidence of known disease. In some regions, genetic factors probably influence the prevalence of IgA nephropathy. The disease is two to three times more common in males than in females and is distinctly rare in some ethnic groups, especially blacks. Families with multiple members with IgA nephropathy have been described, including some with members affected by Henoch-Schönlein purpura. Furthermore, several studies have shown abnormalities of the IgA immune system affecting both patients with biopsy-confirmed disease and unbiopsied first-degree relatives with hematuria. Nonetheless, no human leukocyte antigen (HLA), restriction fragment length polymorphism, or other genetic marker has been clearly linked with IgA nephropathy in family studies. In our experience, familial IgA nephropathy is clinically indistinguishable from the sporadic form (individuals without a relative known to be affected by the disease).

Prognosis

Shortly after its description in 1968, IgA nephropathy was assumed to follow an uneventful course and was frequently referred to as "benign recurrent hematuria." However, over the intervening years, an indolent progressive loss of renal function has been observed in a large proportion of patients. As many as 20 to 30 percent of patients reach end-stage renal failure after 20 years of known disease. The clinical markers for an unfavorable long-term prognosis include proteinuria greater than 2 g per day, older age at diagnosis (perhaps indicating a longer duration of disease), hypertension, and male gender. Of these, the magnitude of proteinuria has the greatest predictive power. Serum IgA concentrations have been reported to be increased in as many as 50 percent of patients, but the finding is not unique to patients with IgA nephropathy. Moreover, the levels have not correlated with the subsequent clinical course. In our longitudinal studies, we found that all six patients with a deficiency of the C4A complement protein progressed to chronic renal insufficiency compared with only 47 percent of the patients without C4A deficiency, despite similar ages at apparent clinical onset and duration of observation. The prognosis of IgA nephropathy sometimes differs between ethnic groups, perhaps reflecting the varied methods of ascertainment of patients and differences in the threshold for performing renal biopsies. Although IgA nephropathy is uncommon among blacks, the clinical course in this racial group appears to be worse than in whites. Whether this less favorable outcome arises from a higher prevalence of hypertension due to causes independent of IgA nephropathy remains unclear. From the histologic perspective, the features frequently associated with progression to renal insufficiency include segmental glomerular sclerosis, interstitial fibrosis, and extension of the IgA immune deposits to the peripheral capillary walls as observed by immunofluorescence staining or by electron microscopy.

Some patients spontaneously enter a prolonged quiescent phase and maintain normal renal function. In our experience, the urinalysis becomes normal for years in about 20 percent of patients. Nevertheless, some of these patients remain hypertensive. Repeat renal biopsies performed during clinical remission generally show persistent immunohistologic findings diagnostic of IgA nephropathy. In fact, resolution of the immune deposits has been described only rarely during clinical remission; one patient was treated with glucocorticoids.

Pregnancy and IgA Nephropathy

Because IgA nephropathy commonly affects young adults, the safety of pregnancy in women with the disease is frequently of concern. Surprisingly, relatively few studies have addressed this issue. Case reports have described irreversible decline of renal function associated with worse hypertension in gravid women with IgA nephropathy. Hypertension may first appear during pregnancy and often foreshadows recurrence of hypertension during subsequent gestations and permanent hypertension. Pre-existing renal insufficiency with a serum creatinine concentration of more than 2 mg per deciliter has been associated with increased fetal loss and growth retardation as well as loss of maternal renal function. Although patients with familial IgA nephropathy comprise a small minority of the total patient population, prospective parents may ask their physician for genetic counseling prior to pregnancy. At present, neither the genetic basis nor the mode of inheritance has been elucidated for familial IgA nephropathy.

PATHOGENESIS

Despite intensive efforts by many investigators in centers throughout the world, the pathogenesis of IgA nephropathy has been, at best, only partially uncovered. As in many diseases, it is probable that a truly effective and safe therapy will be developed only after our insight into the pathogenesis has become more complete. We will briefly review some of the generally accepted concepts and focus on areas of controversy.

Circulating IgA-Containing Immune Complexes

The mesangial deposits of IgA, often accompanied by other immunoglobulin isotypes and complement, arise from the circulation rather than are synthesized locally in the kidney. This is most clearly shown by the transplant experience whereby mesangial deposits of IgA recur in the allograft of many patients after several years. Conversely, it has been documented that the immune deposits in a kidney with mesangial IgA deposits inadvertently transplanted into a recipient suffering from another type of renal disease disappeared within several months. Other features illustrating the systemic nature of IgA nephropathy include the vascular deposits of IgA in muscle and skin of some patients and the abnormalities of the circulating IgA reported in many patients. The prevalence of IgA deposits in the skin is controversial, and the predictive value of a skin biopsy is too low to render it a suitable diagnostic alternative to a kidney biopsy.

The appearance of the mesangial IgA by immunofluorescence and electron microscopy strongly suggests an immune complex pathogenesis. It is not clear, however, whether the mesangial immune complexes are deposited as such from the circulation or, alternatively, are formed in the mesangium through an *in situ* mechanism. Using a variety of techniques, many investigators have found immune complexes in the circulation that contain IgA, complement, and frequently, other immunoglobulin isotypes. However, in recent studies, the prevalence of such complexes was lower (25 to 50 percent of patients) than in earlier reports. Despite occasional descriptions of microbial or alimentary antigens in the mesangial deposits, in most patients, the identity of the antigens inciting formation of the complexes remains unknown.

IgA Subclass

Of the two subclasses of IgA in man, only the IgA1 subclass appears to be involved in this disease. There is general agreement that the mesangial IgA is exclusively IgA1 in most patients. The IgA in the circulating immune complexes is also restricted to IgA1, and the increased serum concentration of total IgA detectable in 50 percent of patients is caused by an increased concentration of this subclass. The percentage of the total IgA produced by lymphocytes from the peripheral blood, bone marrow, and tonsils that is IgA1 is greater than that in normal controls. Recent studies have shown that patients manifest an immune hyper-responsiveness to influenza vaccination, also limited to the subclass IgA1.

IgA Molecular Form

IgA occurs in two molecular forms in man: the monomeric form that predominates in the circulation and the polymeric form that is found mainly in mucosal secretions. The pathogenetic role of the polymeric forms of IgA in IgA nephropathy is highly controversial. Much recent work has shown no increase in the proportion of the polymeric forms in the serum total IgA, the IgA produced in response to vaccination, the IgA in immune complexes, or the IgA produced by lymphocytes from the blood or bone marrow. Nonetheless, two studies suggested that polymeric IgA, which may be phlogistically more active than monomeric IgA, may comprise a pathogenetically significant fraction of the mesangial IgA. Unfortunately, the deposited IgA is technically difficult to isolate and characterize.

Metabolism of IgA1 and Circulating IgA1-Containing Immune Complexes

The amount of circulating IgA1 and IgA1-containing immune complexes may increase theoretically through either of two mechanisms: decreased catabolism or increased synthesis. Until recently, the study of the catabolism of IgA-containing immune complexes has been approached by only a very indirect method, using IgG- or complement-coated red blood cells to gauge the function of the mononuclear phagocytic system. In these analyses, a prolonged elimination half-life has been found, but its relevance to the disposal of IgA-containing immune complexes is unclear. The rate of removal of altered red blood cells measures predominantly splenic function, and the observed abnormalities may be secondary rather than primary. Two recent studies using aggregated human IgA have, unfortunately, yielded conflicting results; the role of a postulated disturbed clearance of IgA-containing immune complexes therefore remains uncertain.

Compared with the findings in the catabolism studies, the data supporting an increased synthesis of IgA1 as a mechanism leading to increased circulating levels of IgA are much more solid. Numerous experiments using peripheral blood lymphocytes have shown both increased and normal synthetic rates for IgA. The basis for an increased synthetic rate has been postulated to be an increased function of helper T cells or a decreased function of the suppressor T cell subset. The relative contribution of the IgA1 subclass to the total IgA produced by blood mononuclear cells was increased. In interpreting these results, we should remember that peripheral blood cells comprise a negligible *in vivo* source of plasma immunoglobulin and are cells in transit from one lymphoid organ to another. Although IgA1 is produced in both compartments (systemic and mucosal) of the IgA immune system, there has been considerable debate about which compartment predominates as the origin of the mesangial IgA. An increased production of IgA1 has been shown for the bone marrow and the tonsils of patients with IgA nephropathy. We tend to view the bone marrow rather than the mucosal compartment as the origin of the mesangial IgA1. In healthy humans, the bone marrow is the predominant source of plasma IgA, and the contribution from the mucosal surfaces is very small. Mucosal infections certainly play an important clinical role in IgA nephropathy, however, as illustrated by their frequent association with episodes of macroscopic hematuria. Perhaps such infections, usually those in the upper respiratory tract, lead not only to a local immune response, but also to a circulating antibody response through increased synthesis of IgA in the bone marrow. Indeed, evidence for such a sequence of events has been observed in experimental animals. The IgA1 hyper-responsiveness would produce elevated plasma levels of IgA1 and IgA1-containing immune complexes after many everyday infections. Possibly an increased permeability of the mucosae permits antigens greater access to the circulation, thereby contributing to the formation of immune complexes. However, evidence for such an increased permeability is not firm. Moreover, although the barrier function of the mucosa is often compromised in inflammatory bowel disease, this group of diseases is only rarely complicated by secondary IgA nephropathy.

Other Pathogenetic Considerations

The immune hyper-responsiveness described above is probably not the sole pathogenetic factor in IgA nephropathy. Other disease states also characterized by increased plasma levels of IgA1 or IgA1-containing immune complexes (such as IgA myeloma and acquired immunodeficiency syndrome) generally do not manifest mesangial deposits of IgA1. Another, yet unidentified, factor must determine whether or not the elevated plasma level of IgA1 will lead to mesangial deposition, which causes inflammatory damage. In our opinion, the identification of this factor (or factors) will greatly improve our understanding of this disease. Theoretically, the factor may entail a biochemical characteristic of the IgA1 unrelated to its antigen specificity or, conversely, it may involve the capacity of the IgA1 to bind antigen. Examples of the first category include charge, size, and glycosylation of the IgA1 molecule. With respect to antigenic specificity, autoantigens (whether native to the glomerulus or not) or exogenous antigens may play a role. In recent years, several studies have described immunoglobulin binding to glomerular structures. One such interaction encompasses the binding of IgA-fibronectin aggregates to collagen; another encompasses the binding of autoantibodies of the IgG isotype to glomerular antigens. Investigators from Japan have observed that glomerular eluates from patients with IgA nephropathy frequently recombine with autologous glomeruli but less frequently with glomeruli from other patients or controls.

Mesangial Cell Physiology

Recent data pertaining to mesangial cell physiology may have important implications for the pathogenesis of IgA nephropathy. The emergence of mesangial cell culture techniques has greatly advanced our understanding of the physiology of these cells. The results have changed our previous perception of the mesangial cells as merely "innocent bystanders" in this disease to one in which they are seen as actively participating in the disease. Mesangial cells possibly express surface receptors for IgA and thereby may play an active role in the accumulation of the mesangial immune deposits. Furthermore, the mesangium appears capable of synthesizing a large array of inflammatory mediators and expressing receptors for such mediators. Consequently, mesangial cells may mediate the inflammation and sclerosis which characterize the glomerular damage in more advanced disease. Overall, considerable uncertainty persists regarding the inflammatory mechanisms damaging the glomerulus after the IgA has been deposited in the mesangium. Complement almost certainly plays an important role, as illustrated by the nearly universal finding of mesangial deposits of C3, components of the alternative pathway, and the membrane attack complex. Whether IgA alone is capable of activating the alternative pathway, or whether another co-deposited isotype or perhaps a certain biochemical property of the antigen is necessary remains hotly debated. The wide spectrum of clinical and histologic expression of IgA nephropathy, ranging from almost normal histology to crescentic glomerulonephritis, suggests that various inflammatory mechanisms may be activated, depending on the patient and the phase of the disease.

Thus many aspects of the pathogenesis of IgA nephropathy unfortunately remain unclear, despite considerable research devoted to the issue. Some of the controversy has arisen because cross-sectional studies frequently have not considered the clinical phase of the patients. We expect that longitudinal studies and basic research regarding mesangial cell physiology and immune regulation will provide sorely needed insight into the pathogenesis of IgA nephropathy.

TREATMENT

Despite the intensive efforts of many centers around the world to uncover the pathogenesis of IgA nephropathy, no consensus has emerged to permit a unified disease-specific approach to treatment, either for the short-term or long-term. Many of the claims of improved proteinuria or stabilization of renal function resulting from treatment have arisen from anecdotal observations or after retrospective review. Unfortunately, only a few controlled treatment trials, generally with few patients, have been conducted to date (Table 1).

Acute Clinical Presentation

Acute renal dysfunction sometimes complicates an episode of macroscopic hematuria. As noted above, renal biopsy specimens occasionally show nu-

TABLE 1 Results of Controlled Trials in the Treatment of Chronic IgA Nephropathy

Treatment Regimen (treatment interval; country)	*Results*
Aspirin + dipyridamole (3 yrs; Hong Kong)	No benefit
Azathioprine + acenocoumarol; or indomethacin (various intervals; Bulgaria)	No benefit
Cyclophosphamide + dipyridamole + warfarin (3 yrs; Singapore)	Creatinine clearance stabilized; proteinuria decreased
Cyclosporine (4 mos; Hong Kong)	Creatinine clearance and proteinuria decreased
Eicosapentaenoic acid (1 yr; Japan)	Slowed decline of creatinine clearance
Eicosapentaenoic acid (2 yrs; Australia)	No benefit
Phenytoin (2 yrs; Australia)	No benefit
Phenytoin (1 yr; Spain)	Hematuria decreased
Prednisolone or prednisone, daily (4 mos; Hong Kong)	Proteinuria decreased in patients with mild glomerular pathology; creatinine clearance unchanged after 3 yrs
Tetracycline, daily (1 yr; Australia)	Hematuria decreased

merous glomerular crescents consistent with the histologic diagnosis of immune complex–positive crescentic glomerulonephritis. Some patients in this setting have been treated with plasmapheresis and/or glucocorticoids and/or cytotoxic agents and/or anticoagulants. Anecdotal reports of early treatment-associated improvement in renal function often described progressive renal insufficiency after longer observation. Alternatively, some authors have reported spontaneous resolution of renal dysfunction in this setting. For patients with macroscopic hematuria and tubular necrosis with large casts of red blood cells in the biopsy specimen, supportive therapy entailing control of blood pressure and dialysis as necessary will suffice, and the renal function often returns to the previous baseline.

Chronic Disease

General

Because of the frequently indolent clinical course and the variable histologic findings of IgA nephropathy, assessment of the results of medical intervention requires prolonged monitoring of many patients. Hypertension often reflects progressive renal damage and, in turn, undoubtedly accelerates the rate of deterioration of renal function. Its control remains the cornerstone of long-term therapy. Whether angiotensin-converting enzyme inhibitors with the postulated better control of intraglomerular capillary hypertension offer an advantage over other classes of agents in the setting of equal control of systemic blood pressure remains unclear. Moderate salt restriction may improve the effects of the pharmacotherapeutic regimen and should be routinely prescribed. The restriction of dietary protein intake to about 0.9 g per kilogram per day has been proposed to slow the progressive course of renal failure in a wide variety of renal diseases. A multicenter trial to test this mode of treatment is currently underway in the United States. Additionally, investigators in Italy have suggested that a gluten-free diet selectively benefits patients with IgA nephropathy. Their studies showed lower levels of circulating IgA-containing immune complexes and lesser microscopic hematuria after patients switched to the special diet. However, the long-term efficacy of this approach has not been tested.

Infection/IgA Synthesis

Because macroscopic hematuria frequently coincides with an upper respiratory tract infection, eradication of septic foci in the oropharynx has been advocated in several centers. In a controlled trial, treatment with daily tetracycline over a 12-month interval reduced the magnitude of hematuria. However, the possible benefit for renal function over the longer term has not yet been assessed. In another center, tonsillectomy to remove the site of recurrent infection was proposed to improve the course of IgA nephropathy. Patients undergoing the procedure experienced fewer bouts of macroscopic hematuria, and the magnitude of microscopic hematuria and proteinuria decreased compared with the values before surgery. In addition, 2 years later the percentage of circulating lymphocytes producing polymeric IgA had significantly decreased. Nonetheless, this mode of therapy has not yet undergone rigorous testing. The finding that approximately half of the patients with IgA nephropathy have increased serum IgA concentrations predictably led to efforts to lower the IgA blood levels. Phenytoin decreases the serum IgA concentration and has been tested in two prospective controlled trials. However, the only clinical improvement with dosage regimens that achieved therapeutic anticonvulsant blood concentrations was a decreased magnitude of hematuria in one study; no histologic manifestation of disease activity improved during this interval.

Immunosuppression

In the absence of a disease-specific therapy derived from studies of the pathogenesis of IgA nephropathy, several investigators have pursued treatment plans using agents with broad immunosuppressive effects. Most of the attention has been focused on glucocorticoids, either alone or combined with azathioprine. A controlled trial of daily glucocorticoid therapy for 4 months in nephrotic adults with IgA nephropathy in Hong Kong was shown to have no beneficial effect on creatinine clearance after 3 years. However, the magnitude of proteinuria markedly decreased, sometimes to within the normal range, in a subset of patients with mild glomerular pathologic changes. A few patients displayed a steroid-dependent pattern in the subsequent clinical course. This response is reminiscent of the pattern for patients with minimal change glomerulonephritis (see below).

Several retrospective studies have suggested that glucocorticoid therapy is of benefit in patients with IgA nephropathy. In a nonrandomized study in the United States, six children with histologic features associated with progressive disease were treated with prednisone on an alternate-day basis for a mean period of 36 months. At the end of a mean observation period of 54 months, all had preserved normal renal function and a normal urinalysis. Four patients underwent repeat renal biopsy. All showed mesangial IgA deposits of an intensity similar to that of the earlier biopsies. The clinical course of these treated patients was compared with that of 15 untreated controls with similar pathologic and clinical findings chosen retrospectively. Four of the controls progressed to chronic renal insufficiency over a mean observation period of 96 months; each had persistently abnormal urinalyses. Only one of the 15 had a normal urinalysis at the last follow-up examination, and four had proteinuria greater than 1 g per day. The authors postulated that alternate-day prednisone therapy was beneficial and merits testing in a prospective controlled trial. A retrospective study from Japan included 29 patients with proteinuria greater than 2 g per day who had been treated with 40 mg prednisolone per day. The dosage was slowly tapered, and all patients received prednisolone for at least 1 year. In review, the outcome was predictable based on the creatinine clearance at the start of therapy. Each patient who preserved renal function had a creatinine clearance greater than 70 ml per minute before treatment. Patients with a lower creatinine clearance developed progressive renal insufficiency. This study also analyzed the effect of the same prednisolone schedule on the renal function of patients with moderate proteinuria. Thirty-four patients with proteinuria ranging from 1 to 2 g per day were assigned to two groups. Eleven patients received prednisolone; 23 received only nonsteroidal anti-inflammatory drugs and/or antiplatelet drugs. The mean values for serum creatinine concentration and proteinuria and the prevalence of hypertension did not differ between the two groups before treatment. All patients receiving prednisolone maintained normal renal function during the mean 92-month follow-up period. By contrast, 14 in the other group developed chronic renal insufficiency (eight progressed to end-stage renal failure) after a mean follow-up of 72 months. The authors suggested that prednisolone therapy may stabilize the clinical course of IgA nephropathy if started during the early stages of disease. In an uncontrolled study in the United States, azathioprine was combined with prednisone for the treatment of 10 children with decreased renal function, proteinuria greater than 1 g per day, and hypertension. Prednisone in a dosage of 60 mg per m^2 per day (initially administered in divided doses) was tapered to 60 mg per m^2 every other day to complete 1 year of therapy. Each child also received 2 to 3 mg azathioprine per kilogram per day. The mean serum creatinine concentration did not change after 2.6 years of observation. The mean proteinuria decreased from 4.1 g per day to 2.4 g per day; the magnitude of microscopic hematuria and the frequency of macroscopic hematuria also decreased. The authors suggested that a controlled trial should be done to test this treatment regimen. Each patient developed some cushingoid features. Eight had a significant increase in blood pressure; one patient developed osteonecrosis of the femoral heads.

Treatment with glucocorticoids certainly benefits a minority of patients with nephrotic-range proteinuria in whom the renal biopsy specimens show minimal cellular proliferation or expansion of the matrix and fusion of the epithelial foot processes on electron microscopy. Although some investigators propose that this clinical circumstance represents the coincidental occurrence of minimal change glomerulonephritis and IgA nephropathy, we believe that these patients comprise a subset of patients with IgA nephropathy. Most of the adults reported with this syndrome have been of oriental ancestry. As in minimal change glomerulonephritis, the proteinuria is quite selective, and thus small proteins such as albumin comprise a large fraction of the total amount of protein excreted. Treatment with glucocorticoids clears the nephrotic syndrome, although the signs and symptoms may recur after treatment has been discontinued. Of interest in a recent report, the mesangial deposits of IgA resolved in one patient with glucocorticoid-responsive nephrotic syndrome on renal biopsy during a clinical remission. Selective proteinuria in IgA nephropathy may be more common than previously considered. A center in Singapore characterized the proteinuria of 98 patients with IgA nephropathy and found a selective pattern in 46 percent of the patients. Patients with nonselective proteinuria more often progressed to chronic renal insufficiency over the 4 years of observation, although at the start of the study, the mean serum creatinine concentration in these patients did not differ from that in the group with selective proteinuria. The degree of selectivity of the proteinuria is usually not examined for a large series of patients entering treatment protocols but should be included as part of the analysis in future trials.

Eicosapentaenoic Acid

Eicosapentaenoic acid, an omega-3 fatty acid in fish oil that has been reported to slow the deterioration of renal function in several experimental models of renal disease, has been tested recently for efficacy in the treatment of IgA nephropathy. Fatty acids are the precursors of vasoactive eicosanoids. Presumably because of the substitution of omega-3 fatty acids for arachidonic acid (the usual omega-6 substrate), the resulting cyclooxygenase metabolites have lesser platelet aggregative and vasoconstrictive properties. Furthermore, eicosapentaenoic acid has immunosuppressive actions that may benefit glomerular disease. In a small prospective controlled trial in Japan, fish oil supplements taken for 1 year significantly slowed the rate of deterioration of renal function compared with untreated controls. However, in a later 2-year prospective trial in Australia, no benefit for creatinine clearance was apparent in either patients with normal or increased serum creatinine concentrations at the start of therapy. The proteinuria decreased significantly not only in the treated subjects, but also in the group receiving no treatment. The treatment was well tolerated; no clinical bleeding or decreased platelet function was observed. An uncontrolled pilot study in the United States with 11 patients showed that proteinuria decreased and glomerular filtration rates increased during a 1-year treatment with omega-3 polyunsaturated fatty acids. A randomized study is currently in progress.

Other Drugs

Other immunosuppressive or anti-inflammatory agents alone or in combination have been sporadically evaluated in IgA nephropathy. A possible therapeutic role for cyclosporine was postulated after an anecdotal case report, but a 12-week controlled trial with this drug failed to show any benefit. The decrease in proteinuria accompanied a treatment-associated decrease in the creatinine clearance. Small groups of patients in Bulgaria treated with azathioprine combined with acenocoumarol or with indomethacin alone for periods up to several years showed no discernible improvement compared with untreated subjects. A controlled study using antiplatelet therapy with aspirin and dipyridamole found no benefit in the clinical course of IgA nephropathy. Danazol (a heterocyclic steroid that increases the serum complement levels of patients with hereditary angioneurotic edema) increased the ability of patients' sera to remove intraglomerular immune deposits in kidney biopsy specimens. In an uncontrolled trial with seven patients, treatment for 4 to 10 months coincided with decreased proteinuria and the serum creatinine concentrations did not change. Serum concentrations of complement proteins also did not change. A combination of low-dose cyclophosphamide, dipyridamole, and low-dose warfarin was administered to 27 patients with IgA nephropathy for 3 years in a controlled trial in Singapore. At the end of the 3 years, the renal function remained stable and the proteinuria had significantly decreased. By contrast, in the untreated controls, the creatinine clearance significantly decreased and the magnitude of proteinuria was unchanged.

Transplantation

For patients reaching end-stage renal failure, transplantation affords an excellent therapeutic option. Recurrent disease, as defined by the appearance of the characteristic immunohistologic features, has been documented in about 50 percent of patients by 2 years post-transplant. In one study, IgA nephropathy recurred only in patients with persistently increased levels of IgA-containing immune complexes in the circulation post-transplant. However, the loss of the allograft from recurrent disease has only rarely been reported. The milder clinical course has been attributed by some authors to the immunosuppressive therapy beginning at the first exposure of the allograft to the milieu in the recipient. Kidneys from living-related donors do not appear to be at greater risk than cadaveric allografts for recurrent disease, and we continue to use family members as donors after the customary evaluation.

SUGGESTED READING

Clarkson AR, ed. IgA nephropathy. Boston: Martinus Nijhoff Publishing, 1987.

D'Amico G, Imbasciati E, Barbiano di Belgioioso G, et al. Idiopathic IgA mesangial nephropathy: clinical and histological study of 374 patients. Medicine 1985; 64:49–60.

Feehally J. Immune mechanisms in glomerular IgA deposition. Nephrol Dial Transplant 1988; 3:361–378.

Julian BA, ed. Proceedings from the national symposium on IgA nephropathy. Am J Kidney Dis 1988; 12:337–453.

SCHÖNLEIN-HENOCH PURPURA

GEORGE B. HAYCOCK, M.B., B.Chir.
J. STEWART CAMERON, M.D.

Schönlein-Henoch (anaphylactoid) purpura is a fairly common disorder of childhood, much less frequently seen in adults, characterized by a distinctive rash, colicky abdominal pain, arthropathy, and glomerulonephritis. It usually follows a respiratory infection; in a few cases, withdrawal of a specific food such as milk protein brings prompt relief, with relapse upon dietary challenge. These epidemiologic features, together with the finding of increased serum immunoglobulin A (IgA) concentration in about half the cases and the presence of deposits of IgA and the 3rd component of complement (C3) in skin and renal biopsy material, suggest an immunologic basis for the syndrome, but little is known of the mechanisms involved. The disease is most common in winter and early spring, affects boys more often than girls, and has its highest incidence between 2 and 12 years of age. The great majority of cases are benign and self-limiting, and do not require hospital attention; most published accounts of the syndrome, being based on hospital cases, are heavily biased by patient selection toward the ''bad'' end of the spectrum. Exceptional patients (usually older children or rarely adults) run a chronic, relapsing course over many months or years; it is not known what causes these patients to behave differently from the majority, in whom the illness resolves completely within three months.

SIGNS AND SYMPTOMS

Rash. The rash affects the extensor surfaces of the limbs, especially the legs, and the buttocks. It is often particularly dense over the ankles. It begins as a pinkish, papular eruption resembling urticaria, but rapidly becoming obviously purpuric so that the mature rash is maculopapular in nature, with petechiae both within and between the raised lesions. Ecchymoses and even hemorrhagic bullae are occasionally seen. The lesions may be precipitated or localized by trauma. Involvement of the face and scalp is virtually confined to young patients (<2 years of age).

Arthropathy The arthropathy principally affects the large limb joints, especially knees, ankles, and wrists. Pain may be severe but joint swelling is generally slight or absent. When present, it is usually attributable to periarticular edema rather than to an intra-articular effusion. The swelling often extends diffusely over the dorsum of the carpus or tarsus without being anatomically related to any single joint.

Abdominal Pain. Abdominal pain occurs in most cases and may be the presenting symptom. It varies from mild colic to severe pain with peritoneal signs, mimicking an acute abdominal emergency. Hematemesis and melena may occur. The symptoms arise from hemorrhagic vasculitis of the intestine. Intussusception is an infrequent but serious complication. *Protein-losing enteropathy* is occasionally seen, resulting in hypoproteinemic edema even in patients without proteinuria, an important diagnostic consideration. However, edema may on occasion be seen in children with a normal serum albumin concentration; the reasons for this are not known.

Renal Involvement. Renal involvement occurs in 30 to 70 percent of patients seen in the hospital. The clinical features are those of a glomerulonephritis, ranging from minimal urinary abnormalities with no measurable alteration in renal function, through an acute nephritic syndrome with hypertension and circulatory congestion, to rapidly progressive glomerulonephritis with deterioration to end-stage renal failure in weeks or months. The nephrotic syndrome may occur, but must be carefully distinguished from protein-losing enteropathy and incidental edema.

Histologically, the appearance in involved skin are those of a leukocytoclastic vasculitis with deposition of IgA, C3, properdin, late-acting complement components (C5 through C9) and fibrin in dermal capillaries. The typical renal finding is focal and segmental lesions, often superimposed on a mesangial proliferative glomerulonephritis, with mesangial deposition of the same immune components as are seen in affected skin, IgA predominating. In severe cases, the focal, segmental lesions are so widespread that they coalesce, but they do not have the uniform homogeneity of a truly diffuse, proliferative glomerulonephritis. The lesion cannot be distinguished on histologic grounds from that of idiopathic IgA nephropathy (Berger's disease). Minor segmental extracapillary crescent formation is common, but severe, extensive, diffuse crescent formation occurs in the most severely affected patients and has the same significance as in other types of proliferative glomerulonephritis: if a majority of glomeruli are involved, prognosis for renal function is poor. However, Schönlein-Henoch purpura is a rare cause of end-stage renal failure: of 200 children aged less than 15 years treated for end-stage renal failure at Guy's Hospital up to the end of 1985, the cause was Schönlein-Henoch purpura in only eight.

MANAGEMENT

Most patients with Schönlein-Henoch purpura need no treatment, except perhaps mild analgesia for joint pain. However, abdominal pain may be severe enough to justify the use of opiate analgesics. Oral glucocorticoid therapy is claimed to be dramatically helpful in patients with severe abdominal symptoms, although this opinion is based on uncontrolled, anecdotal reports; a short trial of prednisone or prednisolone in a dosage of 1 to 2 mg per kilogram of body weight per day is worth attempting if analgesics alone are ineffective in controlling pain without excessively sedating the patient. Gastrointestinal bleed-

TABLE 1 Clinical and Biopsy Findings and Details of Treatment of 5 Children with Severe Schönlein-Henoch Purpura and Glomerulonephritis

Patient No.	*Age/Sex*	*Crescents (%)*	*Nephrotic Syndrome*	*Pretreatment GFR (ml/min/1.73 m)*	*Post-treatment GFR (ml/min/1.73 m)**	*Follow-up (months)*	*Methylprednisolone*	*Plasma Xch*	*Aza or Cyclo*
1	8/M	0	+	33	117	38	+	−	−
2	12/M	61	+	22	76	31	+	+	Cyclo
3	5/M	17	−	17	90	18	+	−	Aza
4	13/F	21	+	40	137	34	+	−	Aza
5†	6/M	100	+	0	35	1½	+	+	Cyclo

* These values are those obtained at latest follow-up, i.e., at the end of the follow-up period indicated in the table.
† This patient was still under treatment at the time of writing. He had required hemodialysis for 3 weeks and was anuric for most of that time.
GFR=glomerular filtration rate; Xch=exchange; Aza=azathioprine; Cyclo=cyclophosphamide.

ing may occasionally require blood transfusion. The possibility of intussusception should always be borne in mind in a patient with severe abdominal pain and lower gastrointestinal bleeding. Such patients should be managed in close consultation with a surgeon well acquainted with the disease and its abdominal manifestations. Investigation by abdominal ultrasonography and contrast enema may be necessary in some cases; laparotomy should not be performed without verification of the presence of an intussusception by such techniques, since patients operated on unnecessarily do not do well.

Most patients with Schönlein-Henoch purpura and glomerulonephritis recover completely without specific treatment. *Rational management depends on identification of those who are at particular risk for the development of progressive disease.* These include those who, either at presentation or during the subsequent course of the illness, show evidence of reduced renal function (elevated plasma creatinine concentration) or the nephrotic syndrome. Plasma creatinine and albumin concentrations should therefore be monitored once or twice weekly during the active phase of the disease and subsequently, while hematuria and proteinuria persist, at lengthening intervals. If one or both of these is found to be abnormal, renal biopsy should be performed. Patients should be selected for treatment if (1) renal function shows progressive deterioration, irrespective of the biopsy findings, or (2) the biopsy reveals extracapillary glomerulonephritis with extensive crescent formation. Patients in these two categories have universally been found to have a poor prognosis without treatment, most progressing to end-stage renal failure within months or, at most, a year or 2.

Drugs that have been used in the treatment of severe Schönlein-Henoch nephritis include oral and parenteral corticosteroids, azathioprine, alkylating agents such as cyclophosphamide, anticoagulants, and antiplatelet agents in various combinations. In the absence of controlled studies, results are hard to interpret, but have generally been disappointing. Patients with a severe nephrotic syndrome, but normal renal function, and without severe crescent formation, are best left untreated.

In our hands, a combined regimen based on high-dose parenteral steroids, plasma exchange, and azathioprine or cyclophosphamide has been more successful in the severest cases and we continue to use it. Treatment is initiated with intravenous methylprednisolone, 600 mg per square meter of body surface area, six doses being given on alternate days, followed by oral prednisolone, 60 mg per square meter on alternate days. If no improvement has occurred after the first three doses, plasma exchange is begun. Each exchange is of twice the patient's plasma volume (estimated as 50 ml per kilogram of nonedematous body weight), and the procedure is repeated ten times over a 2-week period and six times over the subsequent 2 weeks. If no improvement has been seen by the end of the first week of plasma exchange, then oral cyclophosphamide or azathioprine, 2 to 3 mg per kilogram of body weight per day, is added and is continued for 8 weeks. Prednisolone is continued at the full dosage until renal function has normalized or ceased to improve, and then slowly reduced over several months while renal function is serially measured.

In the last 6 years, since this policy was introduced, 16 children have met our criteria for renal biopsy, of whom five were considered to warrant treatment according to the protocol described above. The other 11 all recovered completely without specific therapy. The salient clinical and histologic features of the five treated patients are summarized in Table 1.

The rather rare adult patients with Schönlein-Henoch purpura do not seem to differ from their younger counterparts in any respect, although it has been alleged that their general prognosis is poorer; this probably results from greater selection of patients for hospital investigation. Many middle-aged patients given a diagnosis of Schönlein-Henoch purpura are in fact suffering from other forms of vasculitis, such as the microscopic form of polyarteritis or Wegener's granulomatosis, and the diagnosis must not be accepted without evidence of renal and/or cutaneous vascular deposition of IgA.

An unknown number of children affected with Schönlein-Henoch purpura develop hypertension 5 to 15 years later; thus an annual check of blood pressure is worthwhile for a decade or 2 following a severe attack of the disease.

MINIMAL-CHANGE DISEASE IN IDIOPATHIC NEPHROTIC SYNDROME

AMIR TEJANI, M.D.

Nephrotic syndrome is a clinical entity defined by proteinuria, edema, and hypoalbuminemia. In children, the proteinuria is greater than 40 mg per m^2 per hour, and in adults, greater than 3 g per 24 hours. The serum albumin is less than 2.5 g per deciliter, and in more than 50 percent of children it can be as low as 1 to 1.5 g per deciliter. The edema of nephrotic syndrome is generalized, unlike that of glomerulonephritis, which is mostly seen as puffiness around the lower eyelids. In children, the presentation is frequently explosive, with the edema involving the face, abdomen, and scrotum, as well as the limbs. Hypercholesterolemia and hyperlipidemia, although considered unnecessary in defining the nephrotic syndrome, are almost always present.

This entity can be seen in a variety of clinical settings. Nephrotic syndrome can occur secondary to lupus nephritis, diabetic nephropathy, sickle cell disease, human immunodeficiency virus (HIV)-associated nephropathy, and a host of other diseases. When it occurs as a primary condition, is not associated with any other systemic disorder, and the morphology is characterized by spreading and fusion of the epithelial cell foot processes over an unaltered glomerular basement membrane, the entity is called minimal change disease. This chapter deals with minimal-change nephrotic syndrome (MCNS), with emphasis on its diagnosis and therapy.

The pathogenesis of MCNS is unknown. There is a paucity of immunologic involvement, and studies have shown circulating or in situ immune complex deposition to be mostly noncontributory. This scarcity of immunologic involvement suggests that capillary permeability in patients with MCNS may be altered by nonimmunologic stimuli. A variety of lymphokines and cytokines have been identified in patients with MCNS, suggesting altered T cell function. The role of T cell as an effector, suppressor, or mediator of altered glomerular permeability has not been established, but current postulate is that T cell–induced cytokines and lymphokines alter the glomerular permeability leading to the proteinuria. Based on this premise, newer drugs have been used in refractory MCNS with salutary results.

CLINICAL EVALUATION AND DIAGNOSIS

Edema is often the first symptom noted, frequently shortly after a nonspecific upper respiratory infection. Progression to a fully manifested nephrotic syndrome with heavy proteinuria and anasarca is more the norm in MCNS than in other forms of primary nephrotic syndrome and is particularly common in children.

In order to distinguish MCNS from other disorders that can mimic the clinical presentation such as membranous nephropathy and membranoproliferative glomerulonephritis, it is helpful to give careful attention to urinary sediment, the presence or absence of hypertension, and renal function. Gross hematuria is rare in all age groups, and its presence should cause one to question seriously the diagnosis of MCNS. However, persistent microscopic hematuria may be seen in almost 25 percent of all MCNS patients. Hypertension is seen in only a minority of pediatric MCNS patients at presentation (5 to 7 percent), but may be seen more frequently in adult patients. Decreased renal function as determined by a rise in serum creatinine at presentation is also not seen in more than 5 percent of patients. However, nitrogen retention manifested as a rise in blood urea nitrogen (BUN) may be seen frequently in both adults and children. Patients whose nephrotic syndrome is caused by postinfectious glomerulonephritis or membranoproliferative glomerulonephritis have a decrease in the third component of complement, whereas the C3 level is normal in patients with MCNS.

The most useful predictor of whether the patient with nephrotic syndrome has MCNS is the patient's age at the onset of the disease. The proportion with minimal change decreases from 96 percent at age 1 to 4 years to less than 50 percent at 10 years of age. Eighty percent of children with MCNS are younger than 6 years of age at the time of diagnosis, with two-thirds presenting between the ages of 1 and 5 years and only 5 percent presenting during the second decade. Because of the heavy preponderance of MCNS in children younger than 6 years of age, it is our policy not to perform a renal biopsy in patients who present with the nephrotic syndrome at an age younger than 6 years at onset, but to administer a course of steroid therapy. A helpful guide for response to steroid therapy can be obtained by using the selectivity protein index. Differential protein clearances using the ratio of IgG to transferrin clearance show that when the selectivity protein index is less than 10 percent, eighty-five percent of patients respond to steroid therapy.

THERAPY

Symptomatic Therapy

Symptomatic therapy includes dietary manipulation, the use of diuretics, and in selected cases, the addition of parenteral albumin. For most patients with MCNS that is treated with corticosteroid therapy, none of these approaches may be necessary. Modest restriction in sodium intake is recommended in adults, but is difficult to enforce in children. If edema is gross and of particular concern, an oral diuretic like hydrochlorothiazide, in a dose of 2 mg per kilogram per day for children or 25 mg orally twice per day for adults, may be used. Frequently, however, a stronger diuretic such as furosemide may be necessary. In children, furosemide is administered orally in a dose of 2 to 4 mg per kilogram or intravenously in a dose of 1 mg per kilogram. For adults, equivalent doses are 20 mg orally or intravenously. Two doses of furosemide per day is usually adequate. Because of the risk of further volume depletion in a patient who already has intravascular contraction, the use of diuretics in a nephrotic patient should be closely monitored. Serum electrolytes, urine output, and body weight must be monitored on a daily basis. Additional concerns are those of hypokalemia, hyponatremia, and alkalosis.

In patients whose edema is immobilizing or in whom there is pulmonary compromise caused by the edema, intravenous albumin followed by furosemide may be necessary. Albumin is administered in a dose of 0.25 to 1 gm per kilogram (25 percent salt-poor albumin) followed by intravenous furosemide in a dose of 0.5 to 2 mg per kilogram of body weight. In most patients with MCNS, this therapy leads to prompt diuresis, with the only exceptions being patients with intrarenal edema caused by the overall nephrotic state. Therapy designed to improve the oncotic pressure in the vascular compartment, however, is nonspecific, and reaccumulation of edema fluid due to the persistent proteinuria requires specific therapy.

Corticosteroid Therapy

For all patients with MCNS, whether the disease is biopsy proven or clinically diagnosed, an 8-week course of corticosteroids is recommended. For children, prednisone is administered in a dose of 60 mg per square meter of the body surface area (maximum dosage of 80 mg per day). This can be given in a single dose or divided into two or three doses. After 4 weeks, the dose is reduced to 40 mg per square meter^2 per day given every other day. Therapy is abruptly discontinued at the end of 8 weeks. For adults, equivalent doses are 1 mg per kilogram daily for the first 4 weeks, after which it is reduced to 0.75 mg per kilogram every other day for the next 4 weeks. More prolonged therapy (up to 20 weeks) may be required in adults older than 40 years of age.

Response to Steroid Therapy

The natural history of MCNS suggests that in 85 percent of steroid-responsive patients, proteinuria will resolve within 4 weeks, and in 90 percent, within 8 weeks. More prolonged therapy may be required in adults. However, prolonged remission or cure after a course of steroid therapy is seen in only 6 to 10 percent of children and in 10 to 12 percent of adult patients. In general, a subsequent relapse is the usual course, and most patients have more than one recurrence of proteinuria. Patients who have no relapse during the first 6 months after their initial response to steroids are likely to have none or only a few relapses over the subsequent 18 months. However, approximately 50 percent of patients have multiple relapses at frequent intervals and require prolonged courses of prednisone. For a relapse in a child, prednisone is again administered in a dose of 60 mg per square meter of the body surface area until the patient is free of proteinuria for 1 week, and the dose is then reduced to 40 mg per m^2 every other day to be given for a total of 8 weeks. For an adult, a similar course using a dose of 1 mg per kilogram per day is employed. Subsequent relapses are also treated in the same manner. The use of intermittent steroid therapy may prevent relapses but will not alter the natural history of the disease. When prednisone is used for more prolonged periods than those recommended here, corticosteroid toxicity becomes a major concern. Steroid toxicity in children leads to arrest of linear growth in addition to aseptic necrosis of the femoral heads, gastrointestinal hemorrhage, and osteoporotic bone damage. In adults, the more common signs of steroid toxicity are myopathy, hypertension, and steroid-induced psychosis. When steroid toxicity is unacceptable or steroid resistance develops, cytotoxic drugs may be considered. It is necessary to have a renal biopsy before the institution of cytotoxic therapy to confirm the diagnosis of MCNS and also to ascertain whether the morphologic lesion will respond to cytotoxic therapy.

Cytotoxic Therapy

Cyclophosphamide has been used extensively in children for a relapse in MCNS. The dose of cyclophosphamide is 2.5 to 3 mg per kilogram given for a period of 8 weeks. This therapy produces a prolonged remission in almost 80 percent of children with MCNS. When cyclophosphamide is used in the dose recommended, its serious side effects, such as hemorrhagic cystitis, alopecia, and leukopenia, are rarely seen. When this agent is used for the duration recommended, the risk of azoospermia in men and gonadal dysfunction in the female is also low. Cumulative doses in excess of 300 mg per kilogram in men and 500 mg per kilogram in women are associated with a high incidence of gonadal toxicity. Thus a dose of 3 mg per kilogram per day for 8 weeks will give a cumulative dose of 180 mg per kilogram, which is well under the toxic range. Dosing for adults is not well-established since there is not a large enough body of experience with cyclophosphamide in adults with MCNS. Second and subsequent courses of cyclophosphamide can be given in children; however, there should be an interval of at least 6 months between two courses to avoid cumulative damage to the gonads. Caution must also be exercised when one is using more than two courses in any given patient, since the risk for the development of neoplasm and chromosomal injury is not known.

Chlorambucil for the treatment of MCNS has not been used as extensively in the United States as in Europe. For children, the dose should be 0.1 mg per kilogram of body weight per day, and this should be increased to 0.2 mg per kilogram per day after 1 week. The drug is given for 8 to 12 weeks. Dosing and schedule for adults is again not available, since experience with this drug in adult patients is limited. Chlorambucil is as effective as cyclophosphamide in inducing a sustained remission in patients with MCNS. The toxicity of chlorambucil is similar to that of cyclophosphamide, but in addition to its gonadal toxicity, it also tends to produce focal seizures, and hence its use for second or subsequent courses is frowned upon by most pediatric nephrologists.

Newer Modalities

The understanding that proteinuria is injurious to the kidney has recently led to a search for other agents that may ameliorate if not remit the proteinuria. With the current concept that T-cell alterations are mediating the glomerular injury in MCNS, *levamisole*, a T-cell stimulant, has been tried and found to be effective in half of the approximately 30 patients who have received the drug over a 3-month period. Currently *cyclosporine*, a specific modulator of T-cell function, has supplemented levamisole, and there has been a small but substantial experience in the use of cyclosporine in MCNS in both adults and children. At 132 centers worldwide, the drug has now been administered to more than 200 adults and children with MCNS, all of whom had been having frequent relapses and were steroid dependent. A complete remission has been obtained in more than 80 percent of the patients.

The drug is started in a dose of 6 to 7 mg per kilogram daily, either in a single dose or in two divided doses. The dose is then titrated to maintain a whole blood trough level of 100 to 200 ng per milliliter using a high-pressure liquid chromatography method. Staying within this range reduces the potential for nephrotoxicity which is an integral part of cyclosporine therapy. If the administration of the drug is limited to an 8-week period, no marked rise in serum creatinine occurs, and the nephrotoxicity (if any is present) is reversible.

Unfortunately, when cyclosporine is discontinued abruptly after 8 weeks of therapy, a majority of patients experience a relapse within 3 to 6 months. More recently, the drug has been given in 6-mg doses for up to 6 months and is then gradually tapered over the next 6 months. When the drug is used in this manner, a more sustained remission can be obtained, but the potential risk of nephrotoxicity is enhanced. Since serial measurements of serum creatinine do not reflect the histologic damage caused by cyclosporine, renal biopsies are necessary when the drug is used for 6 months or more. Also the drug is currently not approved for nontransplant usage. The role of cyclosporine in the treatment for MCNS is unsettled, but it appears to be useful primarily in steroid-dependent patients who exhibit signs of steroid toxicity.

COMPLICATIONS

Clinicians need to be aware of two major complications: the development of peritonitis and vascular thrombosis. The peritonitis associated with MCNS is always seen during relapse and in the presence of ascites. The causal organism most often is *Streptococcus pneumoniae*, and many centers attempt to prevent this by the use of pneumococcal vaccine. In patients with MCNS where the predominant protein lost in the urine is albumin, vaccination is safe and effective, and long-lasting immunity against most serotypes of *Pneumococcus* is achieved. Hence prophylactic antibiotic chemotherapy with penicillin or Bactrim may be advisable in patients with a morphologic lesion other than MCNS but is unnecessary in MCNS. In patients whose histologic lesion is IgM nephropathy or focal segmental sclerosis, significant losses of gamma globulins render vaccination noneffective.

The hypercoagulability associated with the nephrotic syndrome is not well understood but is believed to be a consequence of increased synthesis of clotting factors, urinary loss of plasminogen, and platelet dysfunction. Although renal vein thrombosis is more frequently seen in adults, it does tend to occur in children with heavy proteinuria. No firm guidelines have been established for the management of thrombosis in patients with nephrotic syndrome, but systemic anticoagulation is often required and should be considered.

SUGGESTED READING

Grupe WE. Minimal change disease. Semin Nephrol 1982; 2:241–252.

Tejani A. Relapsing nephrotic syndrome. Nephron 1987; 45:81–85.

Tejani A, Butt K, Trachtman H, et al. Cyclosporine-induced remission of childhood nephrotic syndrome. Kidney Intern 1988; 33:729–734.

MEMBRANOUS NEPHROPATHY

CECIL H. COGGINS, M.D.

Membranous nephropathy (which is also called idiopathic membranous, epimembranous, or extramembranous nephropathy, glomerulonephropathy, or glomerulonephritis) is the most common biopsy diagnosis in adult patients with nephrotic syndrome, accounting for about 25 to 35 percent of cases. Its clinical presentation is proteinuria, with or without the full-blown nephrotic syndrome. There are no clinical or laboratory features specific for the disease, so its identification depends on the performance of a renal biopsy.

In mild cases the biopsy findings on light microscopic examination may appear quite normal and be indistinguishable from minimal change nephropathy. More commonly, however, hematoxylin and eosin and periodic acid-Schiff stains show a diffuse and global change consisting of uniform thickening of the glomerular capillary walls. Silver stains and immunofluorescence and electron microscopic studies demonstrate the abnormalities in greater detail. Electron-dense deposits of varying sizes and shapes are present on the subepithelial surface of the capillary basement membrane. These appear to correspond to finely granular deposits containing IgG and C3 (and sometimes IgA and IgM) which are seen with fluorescence microscopy. As the deposits thicken, the normal basement membrane material appears to grow out between them. This membrane material stained with silver gives the "spiked" appearance characteristic of the disease.

Most patients with this biopsy picture have idiopathic disease, but 20 to 30 percent of cases in most series are associated with and presumably caused by systemic disease. Systemic lupus erythematosus is the most common association, but tumors, drugs, toxins, sickle cell disease, and particularly infections, including hepatitis and parasitic diseases, are also seen. In some cases cure of the associated disease leads to a remission of the membranous nephropathy; in others the renal disease persists. Membranous nephropathy occurs in patients of all ages, though its peak incidence is between ages 35 and 55. In childhood it is much less common than minimal change nephrosis and tends to occur in older children in an age distribution continuous with young adults. There is a male predominance of approximately 2:1. Perhaps as many as 30 to 50 percent of patients with membranous histologic findings have asymptomatic (less than nephrotic) proteinuria.

The cause of membranous nephropathy and the pathogenesis of its accompanying proteinuria are not well understood. Evidence from experimental models suggests that the basement membrane deposits may be the result of in situ formation of immune complexes, the result of a reaction between circulating antibodies with antigens (either endogenous or exogenous) lodged in the glomerular capillary wall.

The course of the disease is variable. After 10 years of observation perhaps a third of patients will be in renal failure, a third will have persisting proteinuria with preserved renal function, and a third will be apparently cured. Patients who have less than 2 g of proteinuria at some time during their disease course, female patients, and children appear to have relatively good prognoses.

MANAGEMENT OF MEMBRANOUS NEPHROPATHY

Evaluation

When a biopsy specimen in a patient with proteinuria demonstrates membranous nephropathy the physician should be alert for the possible presence of associated diseases (Table 1). A careful history and physical examination will identify many of these diseases. Laboratory investigations, including antinuclear antibodies, anti-DNA antibodies, complement, antithyroid antibodies, hepatitis B antigens and antibodies, serologic tests for syphilis, hematocrit, and blood glucose, may be useful. The importance of a search for malignancy in a patient presenting with membranous nephropathy is difficult to assess. Although some series have found neoplasms in about 10

TABLE 1 Diseases Associated with Membranous Nephropathy

Immunologic abnormalities:
Systemic lupus erythematosus*
Rheumatoid arthritis, Sjögren's syndrome, Hashimoto's thyroiditis, dermatitis herpetiformis, myasthenia gravis, Guillain-Barré syndrome, Weber-Christian panniculitis, dermatomyositis
Infections:
Hepatitis B, especially in childhood*
Quartan malaria, schistosomiasis, leprosy, congenital and acquired syphilis, hydatid disease, filariasis, and scabies may be significant causes in areas where they are prevalent
Neoplasms:
Cancers of the lung,* breast,* colon, stomach, kidney, esophagus, carotid body, and melanoma
Lymphoma (more frequent association with minimal change lesion in Hodgkin's disease) and leukemia
Drugs and toxins:
Gold therapy for rheumatoid arthritis*
Penicillamine*
Captopril* and enalapril
Nonsteroidal prostaglandin antagonists*
Mercury (in skin-lightening cosmetics), other heavy metals, tri- or paramethadione, volatile hydrocarbon solvents
Other conditions:
Diabetes mellitus, sarcoidosis, sickle cell disease

* Signifies relatively frequent causes.

percent of patients with membranous nephropathy, it is not clear how many of these tumors were unknown at the time of the renal biopsy. It would seem likely that approximately 5 percent of adult patients with membranous nephropathy might have an underlying malignancy that was not obvious at the time of biopsy, and that some of this 5 percent would have untreatable disease. This likelihood might be expected to vary with the patient's age, and should be interpreted in relation to the age incidence of malignancies in a population without nephrotic syndrome.

Treatment

General

Patients with membranous nephropathy will of course benefit from salt restriction, adequate dietary protein, and appropriate use of diuretics, as do patients with nephrotic syndrome from other causes. Some patients appear to achieve symptomatic benefit as well from the combination of nonsteroidal agents such as indomethacin or meclofenamate with diuretics. This may, however, reduce the glomerular filtration rate.

Associated Disease

When an underlying cause or associated disease is present, every effort should be made toward its successful treatment. With the removal of an underlying cause the membranous nephropathy will often, but not always, remit.

Asymptomatic Proteinuria

Although there is evidence that proteinuria in the 1 to 2 g per deciliter range will remit with prolonged low-dose steroid therapy, there is also evidence that the prognosis for such patients is good without treatment. There would seem little urgency in treating such patients and no evidence that the disease is more harmful than the treatment.

Nephrotic Syndrome with Normal Glomerular Filtration Rate

Corticosteroids. In a large collaborative trial in the United States, prednisone therapy was randomly and prospectively compared with placebo. The patients were adults with idiopathic membranous nephropathy and nephrotic syndrome. The treatment consisted of oral alternate-day prednisone in an average dose of 125 mg every other day for a period of two months with tapering over an additional 4 to 8 weeks. Treated patients had more frequent remissions of proteinuria, but the occurrence of relapses led to few long-term differences between the groups. Of greater importance was that fewer of the treated patients progressed toward renal failure during the period of observation. The steroid therapy was well tolerated with very few side effects. In some series, untreated patients have done almost as well as the treated ones in this controlled trial, while in others untreated patients have done badly. Clearly there is wide variability in the course of untreated patients with this disease. Recognized prognostic indices such as sex, age, and quantity of proteinuria account for only some of the differences. If it were possible to identify which patients would specifically benefit from steroids, then therapeutic decisions would be easy. Unfortunately this has not been possible. A number of uncontrolled observations have also suggested that corticosteroid therapy is helpful in this disease, while others failed to demonstrate benefit.

Immunosuppressive Therapy. In an Italian trial six months of alternating steroids and chlorambucil was compared with no therapy in a randomized prospective design. The initial month began with three 1-g pulses of intravenous methylprednisolone followed by daily oral methylprednisolone (0.4 mg per kilogram per day) or prednisone (0.5 mg per kilogram per day). At the end of the first month the steroid was stopped and chlorambucil (0.2 mg per kilogram per day orally) was given for a month. This two-month cycle was repeated three times for a total duration of six months of therapy. At the end of three years' follow-up, 23 of 32 of the treated patients (72 percent) were in complete or partial remission compared with 9 of 30 controls (30 percent), and there was a small but statistically significant elevation of serum creatinine in the controls as compared with the treated group. Short-term complications of this vigorous therapy were said to be few. A longer follow-up will be necessary before it is clear that the benefits of such treatment outweigh the risks. Other studies have suggested benefit from cyclophosphamide combined with prednisone or anticoagulants.

Nephrotic Syndrome with Renal Insufficiency

There is little evidence to suggest that the treatments described above will restore renal function once the serum creatinine concentration has risen to the range of 3 or 4 mg per deciliter, and it is probably safer to proceed in these patients with conservative measures for the management of chronic renal failure, including tight control of hypertension and reduction of dietary protein intake. These approaches are described in the chapters on nutritional and dialytic management of renal failure.

In light of the above information, it is my practice to treat patients with membranous nephropathy and nephrotic proteinuria with a two-month course of alternate-day steroids, as described above. In asymptomatic patients with only 1 or 2 g per deciliter of proteinuria, I am content to follow blood pressure, urine protein, and serum creatinine concentrations at intervals of a few months. In patients who remain severely symptomatic or who demonstrate rising serum creatinine levels for 2 to 3 months following steroid treatment I consider the use of cyclophosphamide, 2 mg per kilogram (if tolerated) combined with 60 mg of prednisone every other day, or a 6-month course as described in the Italian study above, though I am unconvinced so far that the long-term benefits outweigh the risks. The use of a program of intense diuresis combined with indomethacin or meclofenamate has been suggested, but the combination is a powerful one for reducing the glomerular filtration rate—sometimes profoundly—and in my hands has not produced dramatic reductions in urinary protein.

Complications of Membranous Nephropathy

General

Hypovolemia resulting from hypoproteinemia combined with overvigorous diuretic therapy may impair renal function in membranous nephropathy as it may in other forms of nephrotic syndrome. Allergic interstitial nephritis may result from the use of diuretics, antibiotics, or other drugs and be superimposed on the underlying membranous nephropathy. It is discussed further in the chapter *Acute Interstitial Nephritis* and should be considered particularly in patients in whom there is a sudden increase in the rate of decline of renal function.

Renal Vein Thrombosis

One complication that seems to appear quite frequently in patients with membranous nephropathy is renal vein thrombosis. This complication (so common that it was formerly thought to be a major *cause* of membranous nephropathy) has been reported in up to 50 percent of patients in some series, but probably averages something like 10 to 15 percent. When this complication leads to thromboembolism it should be treated with heparin followed by long-term warfarin. Treatment usually leads to the disappearance of clot on subsequent angiographic studies and to a protection against further embolism. It is not clear when to discontinue the treatment; the tendency to thrombosis probably remains as long as the nephrotic syndrome does.

When renal vein thrombosis is present without any evidence of acute or chronic embolization, it is not clear that serious reduction in renal function or increase in proteinuria results. In patients who show no evidence of embolization then, it may not be necessary to perform routine renal vein angiograms.

Rapidly Progressive Glomerulonephritis

A clinical picture of rapidly progressive glomerulonephritis with the biopsy finding of crescentic glomerulonephritis superimposed on membranous nephropathy is occasionally seen. Antibodies directed against glomerular basement membrane antigens may or may not be present. There is no evidence to recommend any different management from that indicated in the classic form of rapidly progressive glomerulonephritis as discussed in the chapter *Idiopathic Rapidly Progressive Glomerulonephritis.*

Transplantation

In patients in whom membranous nephropathy has progressed to end-stage renal failure, transplantation is often performed. Although the membranous lesion may occasionally recur in the transplanted kidney, it frequently does not impair its function.

FOCAL SEGMENTAL GLOMERULOSCLEROSIS

ALAIN MEYRIER, M.D.

Often referred to as a disease, focal segmental glomerulosclerosis (FSGS) is actually a lesion. Not every lesion of focal sclerosis should be called FSGS; fibrotic scars following injury to the glomerulus may be the consequence of extremely different diseases, such as IgA nephropathy, Henoch-Schönlein purpura, and lupus nephritis. Also, FSGS may be discovered in a wide spectrum of clinical settings, and there is no convincing evidence that these various conditions share a common pathophysiologic pathway.

Schematically, FSGS can be discovered by histology in three types of patients. First is the patient with nephrotic syndrome (NS), which often differs from lipoid nephrosis (or minimal change disease [MCD]) only by nuances. Whether NS accompanied by lesions of FSGS is or is not the same disease as MCD is so far not settled. Some nephrologists (and especially pediatricians) consider MCD and FSGS to be simply two facets of the same immunologic disease and believe that the only point of importance is their sensitivity or resistance to steroid treatment. Others (including myself) believe that FSGS, a condition that differs from MCD by its glomerular lesions, poor sensitivity to treatment, risk of developing into end-stage renal disease (ESRD), and which may relapse almost instantly after renal transplantation, is also caused by a different mechanism. Second is the patient with non-nephrotic proteinuria and an indolent course toward slowly progressive chronic renal failure, often accompanied by hypertension. Patients of the third type may have any one of various conditions that induce glomerular hyperfiltration and/or hypertension. The interested reader will find an excellent review on this topic by Rennke and Klein (see the Suggested Reading list at the end of this chapter).

This chapter concentrates mainly on the treatment of patients with FSGS accompanied by NS and is more sketchy with regard to the management of the two other varieties of FSGS, where management is based on measures that apply to the majority of chronic glomerular diseases.

CLINICAL PRESENTATION

FSGS With Nephrotic Syndrome

Most patients with nephrotic FSGS present with edema. However, its onset can be more progressive in NS than in MCD. In MCD, the disease onset is often explosive: a patient may wake up one morning with puffy eyes and swollen hands and within a few hours after arising observe that his ankles are also swollen. By contrast, despite the fact that a similar amount of protein is excreted in 24-hour urine and equivalent hypoalbuminemia, the patient with FSGS may have slow appearance of edema, which makes the dating of disease onset imprecise. Thus in some patients, the glomerulopathy is discovered only when proteinuria is found during some form of systematic investigation, such as military induction or a spot dipstick check at the workplace.

FSGS Without Nephrotic Syndrome

The presenting features of FSGS without nephrotic syndrome are proteinuria or hypertension and sometimes renal insufficiency. This set of abnormalities is simply indicative of chronic glomerulonephritis. For reasons that might pertain to pathophysiology, many adult patients with this condition that have come to our attention have had an atheromatous background (in the broad sense), with hypertension that has often preceded the probable onset of the glomerulopathy.

These patients do not respond to corticosteroid therapy. The spontaneous course of this disease is characterized by a slow progression to chronic renal failure. However, an analysis of my last 28 patients showed that the progression was slow and that the average interval from the time of discovery of proteinuria to the time of renal failure was 7.75 years.

Hyperfiltration FSGS

This variety of FSGS may complicate a vast array of conditions accompanied by glomerular hyperfiltration. As in non-nephrotic FSGS, management should include the general, nonspecific measures analyzed in Table 1.

TABLE 1 General Measures in the Management of FSGS

1. Restrict sodium intake when indicated by extracellular fluid inflation.
2. Add furosemide in case of resistance to sodium restriction.
3. Restrict daily protein intake to 0.7 g/kg.
4. Recommend a low-cholesterol diet. Adding HMG CoA reductase inhibitors has proved beneficial in animal experiments but its effect in the human disease remains to be evaluated.
5. Treat hypertension with diuretics, and if necessary, add converting-enzyme inhibitors; if additional blood pressure control is needed, add calcium-blocking agents.

DIAGNOSTIC WORK-UP

The presence of abundant proteinuria should lead to the usual diagnostic work-up appropriate to any glomerular disease accompanied by NS.

Step 1: Assess the Presence of Nephrotic Syndrome

Proteinuria in excess of 4 g per 24 hours in an adult or 50 mg per kilogram per day in a child and serum albumin values less than 3 g per deciliter are sufficient to define NS. High serum cholesterol levels are also often found, although hyperlipidemia is not mandatory for the diagnosis of NS.

Step 2: Seek Indices of Glomerular Lesions

In contrast to MCD, when NS is accompanied by lesions of FSGS, proteinuria is generally nonselective and occasionally patients present with microscopic hematuria. Cellulose acetate electrophoresis of concentrated urinary proteins affords valuable indications; for example, a single large spot of albumin with only a trace in the beta globulin region is indicative of selective proteinuria and usually corresponds to MCD. Conversely, an aspect of "diluted serum" with the presence of all protein fractions including globulins is usually found when NS is accompanied by FSGS. Microscopic hematuria can be detected by dipstick examination or, when minimal, can be assessed by a spot sample of urine collected in the morning and examined under the microscope. Both abnormalities (nonselective proteinuria and microscopic hematuria) are good indications for the possibility of the ominous lesion of FSGS. The finding of increased leukocyte counts in the morning urine sample in the absence of urinary infection can be indicative of renal interstitial lesions, which can also be a feature of FSGS, as discussed below.

Step 3: Measure Renal Function

The simplest means of determining renal function is to check the serum creatinine level. However, the glomerular filtration rate (GFR) must be more precisely measured by calculating creatinine clearance on 24-hour urine. In some cases in which NS is severe, especially when the patient has been treated with diuretics, serum creatinine levels may be increased because of functional, reversible renal insufficiency only. In other cases, even a slight reduction in the GFR is indicative of severe glomerular lesions, as the decrement in renal function does not appear until at least 30 percent of the nephrons have been lost.

Step 4: Perform Renal Biopsy

This step is mandatory in the treatment of the adult with NS. Nephrologists caring for children are less prone to undertake renal biopsy early, for two reasons. The first reason is that renal biopsy is performed less routinely in this age group than in adults; the second reason is that in childhood, response to corticosteroid therapy is usually considered more important than determining whether the patient has the MCD or FSGS variety of nephrosis. Pediatricians therefore often skip Step 4 and seek tissue diagnosis only in the event of resistance to an appropriate course of corticosteroid treatment.

The biopsy should be referred to a pathologist familiar with renal diseases. Two samples must be taken, one for light microscopy and the other for immunofluorescence. A small portion of the latter should be fixed separately in glutaraldehyde and prepared for electron microscopy, when feasible. The number of glomeruli in the light microscopy sample is important. It has been known since 1957 not only that the lesions of FSGS are focal and segmental—that is, affecting some glomeruli while sparing others—but also that they begin and predominate in the juxtamedullary glomeruli, which are located in the deeper regions of the cortex. Therefore when the biopsy contains fewer than ten glomeruli and when the renal fragment is superficial, lesions of FSGS can escape detection and a false diagnosis of MCD can be made. This occurs frequently, especially in patients with NS of recent onset. This limitation with regard to tissue diagnosis may be the simplest explanation for resistance to steroid treatment. This is why the clinician should keep in touch with the pathologist. In a patient initially considered to exhibit only MCD, resistance to treatment requires a new deliberation on the biopsy material. Clues that the glomerulopathy is in fact FSGS include (1) the presence of focal IgM and C3 deposits by immunofluorescence; (2) tubular and interstitial lesions in the absence of any alternative explanation (such as the use of nonsteroidal anti-inflammatory drugs); and (3) incipient lesions of FSGS on the sample studied by electron microscopy. The lesion of FSGS begins with alterations in podocytes, followed by hyaline deposits in the nearby mesangium and by adhesion of capillary loops to Bowman's capsule.

Step 5: Start Treatment

The response to steroid treatment can be used both as an additional mode of classification of idiopathic nephrosis (as steroid-sensitive, steroid-dependent, or steroid-resistant) and as the best means of predicting the risk of development of renal failure. This is illustrated in Table 2, which depicts the differing rate of development to ESRD in patients with FSGS who have responded to treatment, as compared with those who have exhibited resistance to treatment.

MANAGEMENT

General Measures

Controlling Edema

Diet. A patient with FSGS and NS usually presents with edema, and the first measure of treatment is to recommend low sodium intake. An interview with a dietician is helpful, especially for the parents of a nephrotic child. High protein intake used to be recommended in order to compensate for the protein loss in the urine. It has recently been shown that a high-protein diet in fact increases the urinary protein output and possibly aggravates the rate of development of the lesions of FSGS. Therefore instead of advising forced protein intake, the dietician should recommend moderate protein restriction in the order of 0.7 g protein per kilogram per day.

Diuretics. For a long time it was believed that nephrotic edema was explained by hypovolemia, stimulating tubular reabsorption of sodium, and that hypovolemia was itself caused by hypoalbuminemia and low-protein oncotic pressure eliciting a shift of fluid into the interstitial space. Extreme care was therefore usually recommended with regard to the use of diuretics in order to avoid further hypovolemia and the attendant hazards of orthostatic hypotension and functional renal insufficiency. It is now known that most nephrotic patients have normal or increased blood volume and that sodium retention is not provoked by a humoral factor but proceeds from an intrarenal disorder. This is probably especially true of

TABLE 2 Risk of Developing ESRD in FSGS According to Response to Treatment

Source	*Mean Follow-up*	*Patients with ESRD at End of Follow-Up*
Seven papers published between 1973 & 1987	5.3 ± 2.4 yrs (in 227 patients)	Responders: 5/75 (6.66%) Nonresponders: 86/152 (56.6%)

patients with FSGS as opposed to those with MCD. The use of diuretics is therefore by no means contraindicated in patients with this condition. Furosemide is well adapted to the treatment of nephrotic edema. The initial dosage is one 40-mg tablet per day for adults and 1 to 3 mg per kilogram per day for children. The effect of furosemide is rather unpredictable. If it is efficacious, the patient (or, in the case of the child, the parents) must be instructed to monitor and record body weight daily on arising in the morning, always using the same scale. The efficacy of the drug is judged by progressive loss of weight paralleled by diminution of edema. Treatment should be tapered or stopped before ankle edema has totally disappeared, in order to avoid dehydration and blood volume contraction. A trace of ankle edema in the evening reflects a "safety margin."

In nephrosis in general and in FSGS in particular, resistance to diuretic treatment occurs frequently and calls for an increase in the dosage. However, what appears to be resistance to the diuretics may be due to noncompliance to the diet. Such noncompliance can be easily detected by sodium output assessment in 24-hour urine; an adult patient with persistent edema, stable body weight, and daily sodium excretion of more than 80 mEq per day is not resistant to diuretics but simply ingests more than 5 g of sodium chloride per day. Such patients should again be referred to the dietician.

Serum potassium levels should be monitored at regular intervals. Low potassium and increasing bicarbonate levels call for potassium supplements and, if necessary, intermittent addition of potassium-sparing agents such as spironolactone or amiloride. In some cases, despite limitation of sodium intake and high doses of furosemide and spironolactone, the patient continues to exhibit massive edema and anasarca. For these patients, a temporary effect of diuretics can be obtained by intravenous administration of salt-poor albumin (1 g per kilogram of body weight) immediately followed by intravenous injection of furosemide (1 mg per kilogram of body weight). The albumin infused is promptly excreted in the urine, reflected by a brisk spike of albuminuria on the following day. This procedure can achieve negative sodium balance and the loss of a few pounds of edema. However, it is not reasonable to multiply albumin infusion, as its effect is short and salt-free albumin is expensive.

Nephrotic FSGS can lead to chronic renal failure. This is the case in two-thirds of patients resistant to steroids and immunosuppressive agents, in whom glomeruli undergo progressive destruction. Chronic glomerulonephritis progressively develops. Glomerular destruction often diminishes the basement membrane surface area available for protein leakage, and the diminution of albuminuria can be accompanied by a progressive increase in serum albumin levels. This by no means reflects an improvement in the patient's condition, but only the transition to ESRD. In this case, control of edema requires that one increase the furosemide dosage, guided by this rule of thumb: daily dosage in milligrams = 4,000 divided by creatinine clearance in milliliters per minute.

Treatment of Hypertension

In cases of hypertension, antihypertensive therapy is mandatory, both to protect the patient from the left ventricular and the atheromatous consequences of high blood pressure and to slow the progression of the renal disease. Currently, angiotensin-converting enzyme inhibitors and calcium channel blockers are the best agents for controlling hypertension in patients with FSGS and chronic glomerulonephritis.

Limiting the Risk of Thrombosis

Nephrotic patients are definitely at risk for thromboembolic accidents due to a sum of factors leading to hypercoagulability. Some nephrologists believe that the patients should be systematically treated with oral anticoagulants. In fact, such treatment is probably excessive, and the hazards of anti–vitamin K therapy counterbalance its potential advantages. However, the patient should at least be systematically treated with platelet antiaggregants. Daily administration of 100 mg of aspirin, a dosage that inhibits thromboxane but not prostacyclin production, is safe and should be recommended. In the event of episodes entailing additional risk of thrombosis (e.g., trauma, infection, surgery), the nephrotic patient should be temporarily treated with heparin.

Prevention and Treatment of Infection

Before antibiotics came into use, patients with nephrosis usually died of infection. Susceptibility to bacterial infection remains a significant problem. Skin erosions linked to severe edema can open the way to streptococcal or staphylococcal lymphangitis. It should be detected and treated early. Another type of infection to which patients with nephrosis are prone is pneumococcal sepsis. Vaccination against such organisms should be considered before one embarks on the use of a high-dose steroid regimen or immunosuppressive treatment.

Specific Measures

In this context, "specific measures" refers to the use of drugs directed toward suppression or diminution of proteinuria. These drugs are steroids, alkylating agents, azathioprine, and a newcomer, cyclosporin A (CsA). However, one should remember that the pathophysiology of FSGS is unknown, and that its possible immunologic nature is only suspected. Therefore when the use of corticosteroids or CsA reduces proteinuria in a patient with FSGS, this does not necessarily mean that the regimen has only had a "specific" effect on the immune system. Such an effect could also be due to a local, nonspecific action on glomerular permeability to proteins.

Corticosteroids

Corticosteroids remain the mainstay of treatment in nephrotic FSGS. However, the corticosensitivity of FSGS is distinctly less than that of MCD. Table 3 summarizes the data of 21 papers published between 1961 and 1986. Complete remission is rare in FSGS. Of note is the relative frequency of partial remission, a situation characterized by the diminution of proteinuria, which in turn induces an increase in serum albumin levels and clinical improvement. Although usually considered "favorable," partial remission is generally maintained by continuous steroid treatment. In such a case, when the threshold of sensitivity to steroids is high, the patient develops long-term steroid toxicity.

As stressed by the Toronto group, corticosteroid treatment should always be attempted in patients with nephrotic FSGS. Response to treatment, although inconstant, usually dictates a favorable long-term prognosis. On the other hand, if the patient is resistant to treatment with steroids, high-dose treatment should not be maintained for an unreasonable period of time.

The steroids that should be used are oral prednisolone or prednisolone. For adults, our schedule (based on personal experience and on data from the literature) consists of the following steps:

1. An initial dose of 2 mg per kilogram of prednisone every other day (alternate-day schedule) is given in a single dose taken at 8 AM.
2. Twenty-four-hour protein excretion is monitored at weekly intervals and serum albumin levels every other week.
3. In case of remission, dosage is maintained for 3 months and tapering is begun, stepwise and progressively, with each step being maintained for 2 weeks. Such slow tapering is intended to prevent a rebound phenomenon with exacerbation of proteinuria, which is often wrongly interpreted as corticodependency. Suppression of corticosteroid therapy should be reached at 1 year. Reappearance or exacerbation of proteinuria at a certain corticosteroid dosage reflects corticodependency. This is a matter of concern when the dose is more than 40 mg administered every other day—that is, 20 mg per day—as this finally leads to long-term steroid side effects. When this is the case, some form of immunosuppressive treatment should be considered, but this decision depends largely on the patient's status and on the risk/benefit ratio.
4. Corticoresistance is defined by the persistence of NS despite adequate corticosteroid treatment. Steroid resistance is more than probable when proteinuria and serum albumin levels are unchanged after 4 months of treatment at an adequate dosage. In these patients, continuing steroid treatment is of no avail and usually leads to complications. Before deciding that a patient is corticoresistant, one should end the protocol by three pulses of 1 g of methylprednisolone at 1- to 2-day intervals. In my experience, when steroid treatment is ineffective, it does not need to be stopped progressively, and we do not believe that adrenal atrophy is a problem in patients so treated.

TABLE 3 Overall Results of Corticosteroid Treatment in Idiopathic Nephrotic Syndrome*

Disease	*No. of Patients*	*Complete Remission*	*Partial Remission*	*Failure*
MCD	302	244 (81%)	26 (8.5%)	32 (10.5%)
FSGS	153	39 (25.4%)	19 (12.7%)	95 (61.9%)

*Based on the data of 21 reports published between 1961 and 1986.

Nephrologists have agreed that a shorter treatment schedule should be used for children. Treatment begins with a prednisone dosage of 60 mg per m^2 per day for 1 month, after which time alternate-day steroid therapy is provided for 4 to 5 months in steroid-responsive cases. If proteinuria persists, three pulses of methylprednisolone, 1,000 mg per 1.73 m^2, are administered 48 hours apart. Absence of response defines resistance, and steroid treatment should be abandoned.

The response of nephrotic FSGS to treatment is rarely all-or-nothing. One frequent response is corticodependency. Other patients exhibit repeated relapses necessitating successive courses of corticosteroid treatment. Steroid resistance, steroid dependency, or a multirelapsing course should lead one to consider immunosuppressive treatment.

Alkylating Agents

Alkylating agents denature cell DNA, especially in the immune system, and are therefore alternatively termed "cytotoxic agents."

Mechlorethamine. This was the first alkylating agent used in the treatment of NS. This compound must be injected by a strict intravenous route. In my experience, it is poorly tolerated and its efficacy is not superior to that of oral cyclophosphamide or chlorambucil. Some pediatricians have claimed that intravenous mechlorethamine obtained remission where cyclophosphamide or chlorambucil had failed, but such encouraging data have not been confirmed by many others, including my personal experience.

Cyclophosphamide. Cyclophosphamide can be administered intravenously in a single injection of 700 mg per m^2, which is repeated at monthly intervals over 3 months. Leukopenia appears within 10 days and regresses spontaneously. Once degraded, part of the molecule of cyclophosphamide (acrolein) is excreted in the urine and is aggressive to the bladder mucosa. Forced diuresis is recommended, although this is often impossible to achieve as nephrotic patients are generally oliguric.

Oral cyclophosphamide should be given at a much lower dose than that recommended in the past. A dose of 2 to 3 mg per kilogram per day administered for 3 months entails limited short-term risk of toxicity and low long-term risk of sterility in the male.

Chlorambucil. This is an alternative oral alkylating agent. The usual dosage is 0.2 mg per kilogram per day. The cumulative dosage should not exceed 1,000 mg. There are no convincing data showing its superiority to cyclophosphamide, and its long-term oncogenic potential has been stressed in several publications.

The overall results of cytotoxic treatment in nephrosis in general and in FSGS in particular are shown in Table 4, which summarizes data published between 1966 and 1986. These data are only superficially clear-cut. First, the indications for the use of alkylating agents were not only steroid-resistance, but also steroid-dependence and multirelapsing cases in which the results of the cytotoxic regimen are much more favorable. Second, cases considered to be "successful" include those in which complete stable remission or partial remission was achieved, corticodependent cases in which there was a possibility of diminishing the level of corticosensitivity, and cases with spacing of relapses.

Despite these restrictions, it is certain that alkylating agents can improve the condition of some patients—especially children—who have corticoresistance or corticodependency and steroid toxicity. An appropriate treatment schedule consists of the following steps:

1. Treatment is indicated only in patients who are truly corticosteroid resistant, dependent on high doses of steroids, or have a relapsing course with more than three relapses per year.
2. Young male patients (or the parents of a nephrotic boy) should be advised that alkylating agents, even when administered at low dosage and for a limited period of time, entail some risk of long-term sterility.
3. Such agents should not be prescribed alone, but should be administered in combination with low-dose prednisone (0.2 mg per kilogram per day).
4. One should accept the failure of treatment and discontinue the cytotoxic drugs before complications occur. The success rate of alkylating agents in FSGS is approximately 25 percent. Therefore patients with resistance to steroids and to a 4-month course of alkylating agents should not be treated obstinately with a higher dosage and/or for longer periods of time, as this only leads to increased drug toxicity, short-term risk of opportunistic infections, and long-term risk of malignancy.

TABLE 4 Overall Results of Immunosuppressive Treatment (CsA Excluded) in Idiopathic Nephrotic Syndrome*

Disease	*No. of Patients*	*Complete Remission*	*Partial Remission*	*Failure*
MCD	152	114 (75%)	11 (7%)	27 (18%)
FSGS	63	11 (16%)	13 (20%)	39 (64%)

*Based on data published between 1966 and 1986.

Azathioprine

The antimetabolite azathioprine had the reputation of being mostly inefficient in the treatment of nephrosis with or without the lesion of FSGS. A study was published in 1986 by Cade et al on cases of nephrosis, including some with FSGS. They observed progressive reduction of proteinuria, leading to complete remission within 18 months. It is thus possible that the efficacy of azathioprine in nephrosis has been underestimated because of insufficient duration of treatment. Azathioprine has been used in the field of organ transplantation for three decades, and its use can be considered easier and safer than that of alkylating agents. The initial dosage is 3 mg per kilogram per day, but in most cases it must be reduced to 2 mg per kilogram per day due to leukopenia and/or thrombocytopenia. Monitoring should include regular blood counts and liver tests, since azathioprine toxicity, when present, is essentially hematologic and, in some instances, hepatic.

Cyclosporin A

CsA is an immunosuppressive agent which, at least in the United States, has so far been used almost exclusively in organ transplantation. Its side effects are numerous (Table 5). Since 1985, an increasing body of evidence has shown that CsA may be effective in the treatment of NS. My personal experience as Coordinator of two studies made by the French Society of Nephrology is based on 94 cases with all forms of nephrosis. CsA treatment yields the best results in patients with MCD with corticodependency, having a success rate of approximately 80 percent. Stable remissions are achieved with relatively low doses and

TABLE 5 Side Effects of Cyclosporin A Treatment

Minor	
	Gastrointestinal disturbances, tremor, hirsutism, distal paresthesias
	Gum hyperplasia
	Reversible renal insufficiency (functional, due to renal vasoconstriction)
	Controllable hypertension
	Hypomagnesemia, hyperkalemia
	Increase in liver enzymes
Major	
	Severe, uncontrollable hypertension (rare)
	Chronic renal insufficiency, with definitive tubulointerstitial and vascular lesions (in case of long-term overdosage)
	Lymphoma (exceptional)

allow drastic dose reduction or even suppression of steroids, thereby reversing features of steroid toxicity. In a patient with steroid-resistant NS and lesions of FSGS, response to CsA is much less satisfactory. However, in 20 percent of patients with NS that was totally resistant to steroids and alkylating agents, CsA achieved at least partial remission with definite improvement in the clinical status (i.e., suppression of edema and reasonable stability of renal function).

When CsA treatment is considered in a patient with FSGS, I recommend the following inclusion/exclusion criteria. First, treatment should be restricted to patients whose social and intellectual background is adapted to meticulous compliance to dosage and stringent clinical and biological follow-up. Second, patients with the following features should be excluded: serum creatinine in excess of 1.5 mg per deciliter; uncontrolled hypertension; and tubulointerstitial lesions and/or vascular lesions on pre-CsA renal biopsy.

CsA can be efficacious alone, but it is presumed to be more active when coprescribed with a small dose of prednisone (10 to 15 mg per day). Initial CsA dosage should not exceed 5 mg per kilogram per day given in two doses 12 hours apart—that is, 2.5 mg per kilogram at 8 AM and 8 PM. Whole blood CsA levels should be measured by radioimmunoassay, and trough levels 12 hours postdose should not exceed 500 ng per milliliter with the polyclonal antibody or 200 ng per milliliter with the specific monoclonal antibody. This monitoring should be performed weekly during the first weeks of treatment until stable levels are attained. Such levels necessitate dose titration, and the final dosage, which varies among patients, is usually approximately 3 to 7 mg per kilogram per day. Serum creatinine levels should be monitored at the same weekly intervals. An increase in serum creatinine in excess of 30 percent over baseline on two consecutive assessments should lead to a 25 percent CsA dose reduction. When no diminution of serum creatinine is obtained despite two further dose reductions, the CsA regimen should be abandoned. Heeding these precautions, we have observed only one case of definite renal toxicity in the last 26 patients with nephrosis who have received this treatment.

When nephrotic FSGS responds to CsA, proteinuria usually starts diminishing after several weeks. Remission is obtained slowly and is often only partial. Nevertheless, even when albuminuria persists in the order of 2 to 3 g per 24 hours, serum albumin levels increase and edema regresses. Complete remission can also be observed. Such remission is usually "cyclosporine-dependent," and each attempt to taper dosage to a stop is followed by a recurrence of NS.

Given that most patients are "CsA dependent" and knowing that when CsA is nephrotoxic, tubulointerstitial and vascular lesions precede the diminution of the GFR, we recommend that one should decide to continue CsA therapy for more than 1 year only when a repeat renal biopsy shows absence of significant lesions attributable to this drug. Interestingly, it has been ascertained by repeat renal biopsies that in some cases in which CsA had achieved remission of NS, the glomerular lesions of FSGS continued to develop. This explained the progressive reduction of renal function, which therefore was not attributable only to the toxicity of CsA. However, this also means that CsA had no obvious effect on the unknown process that leads to glomerular injury.

Considering the present state of experience with CsA, this drug should certainly not be indiscriminately prescribed for every patient with corticosteroid-resistant nephrotic FSGS, but neither should it be adamantly rejected on the basis of its renal toxicity. It is simply not yet a routine treatment, and still needs continuing evaluation in controlled studies.

RENAL TRANSPLANTATION

As discussed earlier in this chapter, a patient with nephrotic FSGS who has resisted treatment(s) has a 60 percent chance of developing ESRD and of requiring dialysis. Renal transplantation may be considered in some of these cases. Recurrence of FSGS in the renal transplant is possible, a risk that seems greater when the kidney has been donated by a relative than when harvested from a cadaver. This indicates that living-related donor transplantation should be reluctantly considered in patients with FSGS.

The recurrence rate of FSGS with a cadaver transplant is not as great as previously thought. Of 1,080 transplantations performed in three Paris transplant centers, 51 recipients suffered from FSGS. In thirty-five of these patients, there was no recurrence. In the sixteen remaining cases, proteinuria recurred soon after transplantation. Of these, five patients exhibited only persistent proteinuria, whereas in eleven, repeat renal biopsy showed recurrence of the lesion of FSGS on the transplant. However, of these eleven patients, seven had renal function that remained stable, and in only four it deteriorated to loss of the graft. Two underwent retransplantation, and both lost their second graft because of FSGS. These data show that the risk of recurrence of FSGS in a renal transplant is reasonably small. Therefore, I do not consider that FSGS is a contraindication to renal transplantation with a cadaver kidney.

SUGGESTED READING

Cade R, Mars D, Privette M, et al. Effect of long-term azathioprine administration in adults with minimal-change glomerulonephritis and nephrotic syndrome resistant to corticosteroids. Arch Intern Med 1986; 146:737–741.

Meyrier A, Simon P. Treatment of corticoresistant idiopathic nephrotic syndrome in the adult. In: Grünfeld JP, ed. Advances in nephrology. Chicago: Year Book Medical Publishers, 1988:127.

Niaudet P, Habib R, Gagnadoux MF, et al. Treatment of severe childhood nephrosis. In: Grünfeld JP, ed. Advances in Nephrology. Chicago: Year Book Medical Publishers, 1988:151.

Rennke HG, Klein PS. Pathogenesis and significance of nonprimary focal and segmental glomerulosclerosis. Am J Kidney Dis 1989; 13:443–456.

Schena P, Cameron JS. Treatment of proteinuric idiopathic glomerulonephritides in adults: a retrospective study. Am J Med 1989; 85:315–326.

Tejani A, Butt K, Trachtman H, et al. Cyclosporine A induced remission of relapsing nephrotic syndrome in children. Kidney Int 1988; 33:729–734.

MEMBRANOPROLIFERATIVE GLOMERULONEPHRITIS

DANIEL C. CATTRAN, M.D.

Membranoproliferative glomerulonephritis (MPGN) is a chronic nephritis that has had a number of different labels over the past 20 years, including lobular glomerulonephritis, mesangiocapillary glomerulonephritis, and chronic hypocomplementemic glomerulonephritis.

The prevalence of the disease is decreasing worldwide. During the 1970s, it represented approximately 10 percent of the annual total in several renal biopsy surveys, including our own, but during the last 5 years, its incidence has dropped in many reviews to less than 5 percent. It remains an important type of glomerulonephritis, however, since more than 50 percent of the patients eventually progress to end-stage renal failure. The list of secondary causes has increased, and although it is dominated by systemic diseases such as mixed essential cryoglobulinemia and systemic lupus erythematosus, other causes (e.g., malignancies including lymphoma, carcinomas, and infections such as subacute bacterial endocarditis and acquired immunodeficiency syndrome) have also been recognized as etiologic agents.

The lobular pattern observed on light microscopy represents an accentuation of the segmental nature of the glomerulus and is caused by proliferation of the mesangial cells and their associated matrix. The mesangial expansion extends out and around the capillary loops, and the subsequent laying down of new basement membrane on the surface of this matrix produces the double-layered appearance to the glomerular basement membrane and the classic "tram tracking" noted on periodic acid-Schiff (PAS) staining. The two major variants of MPGN are distinguished by their appearance on electron microscopy. Type I has subendothelial deposits and type II has a ribbonlike continuous "deposit" of electron-dense material within the basement membrane. A less common type III has features of type I combined with subepithelial deposits.

There does appear to be a genetic marker or link of the disorder to a particular major histocompatibility complex—i.e., the extended haplotype HLA B8, DR3, SCO1, GLO2, with a relative risk score of 15 to 1. The actual pathogenesis of the disorder, however, remains obscure. Discovery of the unique autoantibody C3 Nephritic Factor (C3NeF) was initially believed to be a major link to disease pathogenesis, but its importance has been reduced by the finding of the antibody in patients without significant renal disease, in patients with no functioning renal mass, in patients who had undergone bilateral nephrectomy, and even in patients with secondary forms of the disorder. The role of cell-mediated immunity also remains poorly defined, and although there is some in vitro evidence to support T cell malfunction, in vivo these cells appear to perform normally.

It has been recognized for the past decade that platelet survival is significantly reduced in patients with active MPGN. Although this abnormality may not be of primary pathogenetic importance, it has been the rationale for several different treatment protocols.

Eighty percent of patients with MPGN have the type I variant, 10 to 20 percent have type II, and less than 5 percent type III. The mode of presentation of MPGN is extremely variable and includes the acute nephritic syndrome (10 to 20 percent of patients), asymptomatic proteinuria (20 to 30 percent), and the nephrotic syndrome (10 to 20 percent). Other findings at onset include gross hematuria in 5 to 10 percent of patients, hypertension in as many as 20 percent, and asymptomatic but significant elevations of serum creatinine values in a further 10 to 20 percent.

Type I MPGN can be seen in patients of any age, although it is most common in patients between the ages of 5 and 40 years. Type II, on the other hand, is almost always seen in patients 3 to 20 years of age. The third component of complement (C3) may be depressed in type I but is very commonly depressed in type II and can be extremely low. A C3 level of less than 10 percent of normal in a patient with no evidence of systemic disease is almost pathognomonic for idiopathic type II MPGN. In many cases of type II and some type I MPGN, the autoantibody C3NeF is present and is the likely cause of this hypocomplementemia. The precise relationship between the complement abnormalities and immunopathogenesis is poorly defined, but the important clinical point is the lack of correlation between the level of the complement components and disease activity. Sex distribution is the same for all types of MPGN, and although whites are the race most commonly affected, the disease has been reported in both blacks and Asians. Table 1 outlines the common clinical, laboratory, and pathologic features of types I and II MPGN. Type II MPGN is the one associated with partial lipodystrophy (in 5 percent of patients), but otherwise it and type III MPGN, by mode of presentation and survival, are indistinguishable from type I MPGN. The natural history of patients with MPGN has been difficult to determine because many have received drug treatment either because they had an acute, catastrophic presentation or because the physician believed that the process was going to be progressive and wanted to "do something." Most series of untreated patients have indicated that the overall 50 percent actuarial renal survival in types I, II, and III MPGN is reached between the 8th and 12th year after presentation.

MANAGEMENT

Prognosis

There is no proven definitive treatment for MPGN. A major problem in interpreting therapeutic efficacy is the fluctuations that occur in the natural history of many MPGN patients. This variability includes periods of acute deterioration and rapid spontaneous improvement in both the glomerular filtration rate and proteinuria in as many as one-third of patients. However, there are certain clinical features associated with a poor prognosis, including a persistent nephrotic range proteinuria lasting for more than 6 months and/or a progressive decline in creatinine clearance over a similar time frame. Unfavorable histologic features include significant glomerulosclerosis and crescent formation. By contrast, isolated focal and segmental MPGN lesions rather than diffuse involvement carries with it a much more benign prognosis.

Features of no prognostic importance include a nephritic presentation, the initial creatinine and proteinuria values, the age of onset, gender, and the complement profile.

Anticoagulants

The following comments with regard to drug therapy are limited to type I MPGN since there have

TABLE 1 Pathologic Variates and Their Clinical Features

Clinical	*Type I*	*Type II*
Mean age	18 yrs	12 yrs
Age range	5–60 yrs	3–35 yrs
Sex (M/F)	1/1	1/1
Blood pressure	N/↑	N/↑
Urinalysis	Active	Active
24-hour protein	0.1–>5 g	0.1–>5 g
Creatinine clearance	N/↓	N/↓
C3	N/↓	↓↓
Renal survival*		
5 yrs	85%	85%
10 yrs	60%	60%
Pathology		
Light microscopy	Mesangial cell proliferation and increased mesangial matrix, classic double contouring of basement membrane	Mesangial cell proliferation, apparent basement membrane thickening that tends to be segmental
Immunofluorescence	Peripheral C3, ± IgG ± mesangial deposits	C3-interrupted peripheral deposits ± "mesangial rings"
Electron microscopy	Subendothelial ± paramesangial deposits with mesangial matrix interposition and basement membrane splitting	Intramembranous diffuse dense "deposits" in the capillary loops ± mesangium and rarely Bowman's capsule and proximal tubule membrane

*From presentation.

been no series large enough to permit valid conclusions to be drawn relative to type II or type III. The most intriguing therapeutic trial was the use of a combination of aspirin (975 mg per day) and dipyridamole (325 mg per day). The study was a well-designed, randomized, 1-year trial. The rate of change in renal function was measured not only by the standard creatinine clearance but also by the more precise radioisotope iothalamate method. An additional interesting feature of this study was the monitoring of the patient's platelet survival times. At follow-up there was both better preservation of the glomerular filtration rate and better platelet survival in the drug-treated group compared with the control group. There was no improvement in the urine sediment activity, the complement profile, or the severity of proteinuria. The majority of the treated patients continued to receive the medication, and after an average of 4 years of follow-up, they had a lower percentage of end-stage renal failure than the control group. This drug combination can produce problems, especially in the more advanced renal failure patients, and three of the treated patients (15 percent) had to discontinue the medication because of bleeding complications.

Another trial used a regimen of warfarin combined with dipyridamole and was also shown to have a beneficial effect. These results were much less convincing considering the sample size and complication rate; the trial was designed to be a randomized, crossover prospective study of 22 patients, but because of problems, only 13 completed the study. Significant side effects included one death due to a cerebrovascular accident, two significant hemorrhagic episodes (in two patients), and a duodenal ulcer (in one patient). I do not use or recommend this regimen.

The introduction of anticoagulant therapy and antiplatelet agents was based on the observation that platelet survival time is reduced in patients with MPGN. These drugs may reduce platelet-derived growth factor release, decrease smooth muscle cell proliferation, and reduce chemotaxis of monocytes and neutrophils to the area, thereby helping to limit the severity of injury. The aspirin and dipyridamole may also act via inhibition of intrarenal prostaglandin synthesis and/or through a change in the balance between platelet thromboxane production and endothelial cell prostacyclin release.

Anticoagulant Plus Cytotoxic Agents

An uncontrolled study done in the early 1970s combined a cytotoxic agent with an oral anticoagulant and dipyridamole and showed this therapy to produce a dramatic improvement in MPGN. A more rigorous, prospective study done by our group using a similar therapy showed it to be of no benefit in the treatment of MPGN, and I therefore believe that this approach should no longer be considered for these patients.

Corticosteroids

An alternate therapeutic approach has been prednisone therapy. Studies of this therapy have been confined to children, and although the studies have been performed over the long-term, they have been uncontrolled. The authors' latest results indicate that steroid treatment for patients with type I MPGN results in a significant improvement in both renal survival and severity of proteinuria. It is interesting to note that this beneficial effect was demonstrated only after 3 years of treatment and only if the prednisone was initiated within 12 months of presentation. The dose is substantial; alternate-day prednisone is begun at 2 to 2.5 mg per kilogram and is reduced to 1.5 to 2.5 mg per kilogram after 1 year, to 1 to 1.5 mg per kilogram after 2 years, and to 0.8 to 1.5 mg per kilogram after 3 years. These patients are still receiving significant prednisone in a dose between 0.2 and 1 mg per kilogram at 4 years. The International Study of Kidney Disease in Children (ISKDC) carried out a prospective randomized trial to test this regimen. In MPGN patients with a glomerular filtration rate of greater than 40 ml per minute and significant proteinuria, they compared the effects of prednisone, 40 mg per m^2 given on alternate days, with those of placebo. Patients excluded from the study were those with any evidence of systemic disease and those previously treated with steroids or immunosuppressive drugs. There were 37 patients entered into the study, 23 of whom received treatment and 14 of whom received placebo. There was better preservation of creatinine clearance in the prednisone group; however, survival rates at Years 2 through 5 were not different, and significant side effects did occur in the treated patients. These included seizures (in 8 percent of patients), severe hypertension (in 4 percent), growth retardation (in 4 percent), osteoporosis (in 4 percent), glycosuria (in 4 percent), and cushingoid features and obesity (in 8 percent). Taking into account the risks of therapy, they concluded that the marginal improvement in preservation of the glomerular filtration rate did not outweigh the risks.

Other Therapeutic Approaches

Other treatment routines have been advocated. These have included the long-term use of nonsteroidal anti-inflammatory drugs (NSAIDs) and more recently, the immunosuppressive agent cyclosporine. The former is associated with a significant reduction in the glomerular filtration rate, although uncontrolled trials have shown some evidence to suggest that the improvement in proteinuria is disproportionate to the reduction in the glomerular filtration rate. This reduction in the glomerular filtration rate may be acceptable, especially if the patient is rescued from severe hypoalbuminemia and the associated debilitating edema. Cyclosporine may act through its suppression of T-cell activity or have an effect similar to that of the NSAIDs, with the improvement in proteinuria being related to an overall reduction in the glomerular filtration rate. This drug does have other significant side effects and its use must be considered experimental.

My own approach to this disorder is conservative. We are now very familiar with the patients (as many as one-third of those with the disease) who spontaneously improve after an acute nephritic syndrome presentation. If severe proteinuria (>4 g per day) or persistent and increasing creatinine (>1.5 mg per deciliter but less than 4 mg per deciliter) persists for more than 6 months, I initiate therapy using a low dose of aspirin (325 mg per day) combined with dipyridamole (225 mg per day). If the glomerular filtration rate stabilizes and proteinuria does not worsen over 6 months and if the patient is tolerating the medication without problems, I have the patient continue with this regimen indefinitely. If, however, during this period, the patient's condition deteriorates but the glomerular filtration rate is still greater than 50 percent of normal, I may try alternate-day prednisone or other experimental therapy, although only after the risk-to-benefit ratio has been carefully considered. On the other hand, if the initial biopsy shows only focal segmental lesions and the proteinuria remains at less than 3 g per day (<40 mg per kilogram) with good preservation of serum albumin and a serum creatinine of less than 1.5 mg per deciliter, I limit my treatment to symptomatic therapy—i.e., diuretics for edema, antihypertensive drugs (I use the angiotensin-converting enzyme inhibitors) for blood pressure control, and a modest restriction in dietary protein intake.

SPECIAL ASPECTS OF MPGN

As many as 100 percent of patients with type II MPGN have a recurrence in the renal allograft. Despite the presence of the dense "deposits," however, transplant survival seems to be unaffected and is equal to that of other primary types of glomerulonephritis. By contrast, although the recurrence of type I lesions occurs much less frequently (in 20 to 30 percent of patients), long-term preservation of the graft may be adversely affected. If patients with type I MPGN have had a rapid deterioration in native kidney function, a similar pattern is more likely to occur in their transplant allograft. Despite this problem, I still recommend transplantation for all patients with end-stage MPGN renal disease.

SUGGESTED READING

Cattran DC, Cardella CJ, Roscoe JM, et al. Results of a controlled drug trial in membranoproliferative glomerulonephritis. Kidney Int 1985; 27:436–441.

Donadio JV, Anderson CF, Mitchell JC, et al. Membranoproliferative glomerulonephritis: A prospective clinical trial of platelet-inhibitor therapy. N Engl J Med 1984; 310:1421–1426.

Donadio JV, Offord KP. Reassessment of treatment results in membranoproliferative glomerulonephritis, with emphasis on life-table analysis. Am J Kidney Dis 1989; 14:445–451.

McEnery PT, McAdams AJ, West CD. The effect of prednisone in a high-dose, alternate-day regimen on the natural history of idiopathic membranoproliferative glomerulonephritis. Medicine 1986; 64:401–424.

Watson AR, Poucell S, Thorner P, et al. Membranoproliferative glomerulonephritis type I in children: Correlation of clinical features with pathologic subtypes. Am J Kidney Dis 1984; 9:141–146.

MESANGIAL PROLIFERATIVE GLOMERULONEPHRITIS

ARTHUR H. COHEN, M.D.
SHARON G. ADLER, M.D.

Glomerular lesions with mesangial IgM deposits (in this chapter to be synonymous with mesangial proliferative or injury glomerulonephritis or "IgM nephropathy") represent a somewhat controversial glomerulopathy. Since the initial emphasis of this immunopathologic "entity" in the mid-1970s, reports have both attested to, and disagreed with, the concept of it as a distinct pathologic or clincopathologic process.

The precise categorization of this "lesion" is difficult. One prevailing view is that in patients with nephrotic syndrome, glomerulonephritis with mesangial IgM deposits is part of a spectrum of injury with a common pathogenesis that includes minimal change disease at the benign end and focal and segmental glomerulosclerosis at the more malignant end. The mesangial "injury" lesion, because of clinical and pathological similarities to each of the others, is in an intermediate position. In support of this concept is the occasional finding of transitions between these three lesions in patients who undergo serial biopsies. A polar view is that it is a distinct entity unto itself. An intermediate consideration is that, regardless of the categorization, the presence of mesangial IgM deposits in glomeruli in a patient with nephrotic syndrome might be a marker for a poor response to corticosteroids and/or progression to renal failure, despite the relatively normal appearance of glomeruli.

This ''lesion'' is defined by its immunopathologic features: IgM (and often C3) granular deposits in all mesangial regions of all glomeruli. The light microscopic appearance may vary, ranging from normal glomeruli (''mesangial injury'') to those with moderate degrees of mesangial hypercellularity. In general, all glomeruli in a biopsy are reasonably similar to one another. Capillary lumina are patent, and capillary walls and basement membranes are thin and single-contoured. Unless complicated, there are no segments of sclerosis. Ultrastructurally, there are small electron dense deposits in mesangial regions in approximately 50 percent of the cases. When heavy proteinuria is present, the foot processes of visceral epithelial cells are completely effaced. The morphologic features of mesangial proliferative glomerulonephritis may also be associated with diffuse mesangial IgA deposites (Berger's disease), isolated C3 deposits, predominant 1gG deposits, or no Ig or complement deposits. Thus ''IgM nephropathy'' is but one portion of a heterogenous group of disorders having mesangial proliferation or hypercellularity in common.

There are four common presentations of this form of glomerular injury: asymptomatic proteinuria, heavy proteinuria often in the nephrotic range, isolated microscopic hematuria, or heavy proteinuria with hematuria. Mild hypertension is present in up to one-third of the patients. Laboratory studies are not diagnostically helpful. Serum albumin is low and hyperlipidemia is present in association with the nephrotic syndrome. Mild to moderate azotemia may be present in 25 to 50 percent of patients at the time of diagnosis. Serum complement and immunoglobulin levels are usually normal. Antibodies to nuclear or streptococcal antigens are absent. Genetic determinants have not been identified.

The clinical course is variable and, for the most part, depends upon the initial manifestation. Patients with isolated hematuria usually maintain normal renal function for a considerable period of time, although microscopic hematuria persists, occasionally punctuated by bouts of gross hematuria. Apparently, those with low-grade proteinuria also have a good long-term prognosis. On the other hand, patients with heavy proteinuria may progress to renal insufficiency. This usually occurs within several years of the onset and is heralded by increasing proteinuria and hypertension. It is invariably in patients who are, or have been, steroid-dependent, or, more commonly steroid-resistant and who have persistent heavy proteinuria, often with hematuria. In most instances, repeat renal biopsy discloses either the same lesion or segmental glomerulosclerosis and variable presence of mesangial IgM deposits.

The approach to therapy has not been well defined. The most common indication for treatment is the nephrotic syndrome. The effects of therapy on isolated microhematuria, non-nephrotic range proteinuria, and progressive azotemia are less well appreciated. Reports from the United Kingdom in the early 1970s suggested that the prevalence of steroid-responsiveness in patients with primary mesangial proliferative glomerulonephritis was low. As a result, few patients were subsequently treated. More recently, however, many investigators have approached therapy in a manner similar to that given patients with minimal change disease. Utilizing high dose oral prednisone (i.e., 60 mg per day or 120 mg every other day in adults or equivalent in children), the nephrotic syndrome has been reported to respond in up to 65 percent of patients, although frequent relapses, steroid dependence, and partial remissions are common. Nephrotic patients with prominent hematuria are less likely to respond to steroids than those without hematuria.

The use of cytotoxic agents is more controversial than corticosteroids. However, in a few cases, agents such as chlorambucil or cyclophosphamide have been utilized for their steroid-sparing effects in patients with frequently relapsing or steroid-dependent nephrotic syndrome. An occasional report has suggested that cytotoxic agents may be useful in inducing remission in small numbers of steroid-unresponsive patients. Cyclosporine has now been utilized in patients with minimal change disease and focal and segmental glomerulosclerosis who are either steroid-resistant, steroid-dependent, or frequent relapsers. The usefulness of this agent in mesangial proliferative glomerulonephritis remains to be determined. Similarly, the efficacy of nonsteroidal agents, angiotensin coverting enzyme inhibitors, and low-protein diets in inducing remission or amelioration of nephrotic syndrome has not been specifically studied.

In summary, mesangial proliferative glomerulonephritis with IgM deposits is an uncommon form of renal disease. Its pathogenesis is poorly understood, but some now believe that it may be an intermediate form in a spectrum of disorders including minimal change disease and focal and segmental glomerulosclerosis. The prognosis also appears to be intermediate, with end-stage renal disease developing in a substantial, but not a precisely quantitiated number of patients over the course of many years. Patients most often present with nephrotic syndrome, but less common manifestations include non-nephrotic range proteinuria and macroscopic or microscopic hematuria. Steroid responsiveness occurs in 25 to 65 percent of patients. In a small number of patients, cytotoxic agents may be useful adjuncts in treating steroid-unresponsive, steroid-dependent, or frequently relapsing nephrotic syndrome. A prospective randomized controlled trial, although difficult to achieve for this group, would be useful to define better the natural history and responsiveness to therapy of this from glomerular injury.

HYPERTENSIVE EMERGENCIES AND URGENCIES

STANLEY S. FRANKLIN, M.D.

Over the past 30 years, with the development and increasing use of effective antihypertensive agents in the therapy of hypertension, there has been an associated steady decline in the incidence of accelerated and malignant hypertension. Therefore, high blood pressure rarely constitutes a medical emergency; this is despite the large number of patients with chronic hypertension. Indeed, the hypertensive crisis probably occurs in less than 1 percent of the hypertensive population. In the majority of these cases, the hypertensive emergency represents a failure of early diagnosis or inadequate drug therapy.

Not all patients who present with severe hypertension have true hypertensive emergencies. In their 1984 report, The Joint National Committee on Detection, Evaluation, and Treatment of High Blood Pressure proposed an operational classification of hypertensive emergencies and urgencies. On the one hand, *emergencies* were defined as situations in which greatly elevated blood pressure must be lowered within 1 hour to reduce actual patient risk and on the other, *urgencies* were defined as situations in which severe elevations in blood pressure were not causing immediate end organ damage but which should be controlled within 24 hours in order to reduce potential patient risk.

A physician's first task is to diagnose accurately if a patient's severe hypertension represents (1) a true hypertensive emergency, (2) urgent hypertension, or (3) labile hypertension without evidence of an immediate threat to the vasculature or vital organs. If a true hypertensive emergency exists, the physician must choose the proper antihypertensive agent, or agents, and make a decision with regard to how rapidly and to what extent blood pressure should be lowered. The question of the desirability of a rapid lowering of blood pressure must necessarily take into account the risk of excessive delay in lowering the pressure versus the risk of neurologic or cardiac damage brought about by excessive reduction.

DIFFERENTIAL DIAGNOSIS OF A POTENTIAL HYPERTENSIVE CRISIS

A true hypertensive emergency is a life-threatening condition that requires the immediate lowering of blood pressure; both idiopathic and secondary hypertension can lead to a hypertensive emergency. The diagnosis is not based on any specific level of blood pressure, but rather on numerous factors that include the rapidity in rise of blood pressure, the duration of the hypertension, and the clinical determination of the immediate direct threat to the patient. For example, a young woman with eclampsia could develop a hypertensive emergency with a blood pressure of only 170/110 mm Hg, whereas a patient with longstanding hypertension may not be in a crisis situation with a blood pressure of 250/150 mm Hg.

Conditions that can be classified as a true hypertensive emergencies are shown in Table 1. Hypertensive encephalopathy represents an emergency characterized by markedly elevated blood pressure with symptoms and signs of increased intracranial pressure or cerebral edema. Frequent symptoms are severe headache, altered mental status (e.g., irritability, lethargy, or confusion), nausea or vomiting, seizures, or focal neurologic signs. The hypertensive crises of toxemia of pregnancy, pheochromocytoma, or of drug-induced catecholamine excess syndromes frequently are associated with an extremely rapid rise in blood pressure to crisis level, which can cause an acute intracranial bleed, even in the absence of hypertensive encephalopathy. In contrast, malignant hypertension, which can be defined as severe hypertension with hemorrhages, exudates, and papilledema of the optic fundi, may not represent a true hypertensive emergency unless it is also associated with encephalopathy. Other life-threatening presentations that demand immediate lowering of malignant hypertension are decreasing visual acuity, the onset of acute renal failure, mesenteric insufficiency, acute gastrointestinal hemorrhage, or acute pancreatitis.

Moderate to severe elevations in blood pressure, without features of accelerated malignant hypertension, may constitute a true hypertensive emergency when complicated by refractory pulmonary edema, crescendo angina or recent myocardial infarction, dissecting or leaking aneurysms, intracranial hemorrhage, or postoperative bleeding at vascular suture lines.

In contrast to the true hypertensive emergency, Table 2 lists urgent hypertension, which requires a slower reduction in blood pressure. A review of the clinical manifestations and of the differential diagnostic features of each of the entities listed in Tables 1 and 2 is clearly beyond the scope of this presentation. However, accurate clinical diagnosis represents the keystone to successful therapeutic management of these high-risk patients.

TABLE 1 Hypertensive Emergencies

Hypertensive encephalopathy
Eclampsia
Pheochromocytoma crisis
Drug-induced catecholamine excess syndromes
Accelerated malignant hypertension with decreasing vision, acute renal failure, mesenteric insufficiency, acute GI hemorrhage, or acute pancreatitis
Intracranial or subarachnoid hemorrhage
Dissecting aneurysm or leaking abdominal aortic aneurysm
Refractory crescendo angina or myocardial infarction
Refractory pulmonary edema
Postoperative bleeding at vascular suture lines

TABLE 2 Hypertensive Urgencies

Accelerated and malignant hypertension (uncomplicated)
Hypertension associated with coronary disease
Hypertension associated with incipient congestive heart failure
Severe hypertension in a kidney transplant patient
Moderate to severe elevations in blood pressure (≥ 120 mm Hg diastolic) with minimal end-organ damage and no impending complications

POTENTIAL DANGERS OF RAPID LOWERING OF BLOOD PRESSURE

Whenever arterial blood pressure rises too high or falls too low, the cerebral arteries constrict or dilate as required to ensure a constant cerebral blood flow. This phenomenon, referred to as autoregulation, occurs primarily in the small resistance arterioles of the cerebral arteries. In normotensive subjects, cerebral blood flow is autoregulated down to a mean blood pressure of 60 mm Hg. As the blood pressure decreases below this critical level, no further dilation of the vascular bed of the brain can compensate for the decreased perfusion pressure and, thus, cerebral blood flow decreases. Early symptoms of hypoxia follow such as lightheadedness, confusion, and dimming of vision. If mean blood pressure decreases below 35 to 40 mm Hg, somnolence and loss of consciousness ensue. On the other hand, if blood pressure exceeds the upper limit of autoregulation (150 to 200 mm Hg of mean blood pressure), cerebral blood flow increases and hypertensive encephalopathy may develop. In chronically hypertensive patients, there is a shift of the autoregulatory cerebral blood flow curve to the right; this implies that a chronically hypertensive patient has a greater resistance to autoregulatory breakthrough of cerebral blood flow than his normotensive counterpart. Thus, these chronically hypertensive patients reach the lower limit of autoregulation and subsequently suffer a decrease in cerebral blood flow at a mean arteriolar pressure easily tolerated by normotensive patients. This is not an argument to be used against the treatment of severe hypertension, but it does illustrate the necessity for careful, gradual, and not excessive reduction in blood pressure, which can prevent ischemia to the vital organs of the body. Over a period of months, with successful treatment of hypertension, there appears to be a readaptation of cerebral blood flow autoregulation to a more normal curve.

Hypertensive encephalopathy is best explained as a severe hypertensive state in which there is a decompensation of the normal cerebral autoregulation of blood flow that results in breakthrough hyperperfusion, damage to the blood brain barrier with the subsequent development of increased permeability, petechial hemorrhage, infarction, and necrosis. Cerebral edema is not a necessary or obligatory component of hypertensive encephalopathy. The autoregulation of cerebral blood flow may be lost in the presence of cerebral ischemia or edema as well as from local tissue acidosis that results from an acute intracerebral hemorrhage or thrombosis. In the presence of a completed cerebral thrombosis, minimal reduction in systemic arterial blood pressure may lead to further ischemia to the compromised area of the brain, which may cause an enlargement of the original infarct with worsening of neurologic symptoms. Deterioration in cerebral blood flow during reduction in systemic blood pressure may result in part from a steal syndrome, in which the normal surrounding areas of the brain maintain normal cerebral blood flow at the expense of the injured area. Disturbed autoregulation of cerebral blood flow has recently been observed in patients with accelerated malignant hypertension who develop acute neurologic signs and symptoms in association with rapid and excessive lowering of blood pressure.

From the preceding discussion, it is obvious that blood pressure ought not be reduced to values below the autoregulatory range for cerebral or myocardial blood flow. Numerous studies have shown that critical blood flow is maintained in the normal range if hypertensive pressures are not reduced to mean values below 120 mm Hg. Therefore, an initial blood pressure reduction to a mean value of 130 to 120 mm Hg, which translates into a blood pressure of 170/110 to 160/100, respectively, would appear to be a safe level for initial blood pressure reduction. However, there may be the rare patient who develops deteriorating neurologic symptoms at this level, especially if there is an unrecognized completed stroke in association with accelerated malignant hypertension. The prevention of both neurologic and myocardial damage in these high-risk hypertensive emergency situations would argue strongly for the selection of an antihypertensive agent with both a short onset and a brief duration of action; thus, if disturbing cerebral or myocardial symptoms develop with the lowering of blood pressure, the infusion of medication could be discontinued in order to allow for a rapid return of blood pressures towards previous baseline levels and, hopefully, prevention of irreversible tissue damage.

CLINICAL STRATEGIES IN REGARD TO DIAGNOSIS AND THERAPY

During the initial evaluation of the severely hypertensive patient, an effort should be made to triage the patient into one of several categories: a *pseudohypertensive crisis* patient, i.e., one with labile hypertension without evidence of an immediate threat to the vasculature or vital organs, can be treated with sedation and reassurance and sent home; a *true hypertensive emergency* state that frequently requires parenteral therapy and intensive care unit observation; and finally, the *intermediate state of urgent hypertension* which, depending on the circumstances, can be treated with rapidly acting oral antihypertensive agents either inside or outside the hospital.

A brief but concise history and physical examination are necessary to establish an accurate etiologic diagnosis and to determine the status of the cerebral, cardiac, and renal function (Table 3). This has an important clinical bearing on the safety of subsequent reduction of blood

TABLE 3 Check List of Useful Information for the Assessment of Hypertensive Urgencies and Emergencies

Date of onset of hypertension and when it become severe or accelerated.
Recent and past antihypertensive drug history
Status of circulatory blood volume and possible presence of congestive heart failure
Optic fundi evidence of hemorrhages, exudates, and/or papilledema
Clinical picture compatible with hypertensive encephalopathy
Neurologic findings compatible with an evolving or completed stroke
History or ECG evidence of coronary artery disease
Proteinuria, active urinary sediment and/or elevated serum creatinine suggestive of acute or chronic hypertensive renal disease
History compatible with a high catecholamine state
Clinical and laboratory evidence of a potential high renin-angiotensin state

Table 4 Drugs Recommended for Hypertensive Emergencies and Urgencies

Hypertensive emergencies treated with parenteral drug therapy
Sodium nitroprusside
Diazoxide
Trimethaphan camsylate
Nitroglycerin
Hydralazine
Phentolamine
Hypertensive urgencies treated with oral antihypertensive agents
Clonidine
Nifedipine
Labetalol
Minoxidil
Angiotensin-coverting enzyme inhibitors (captopril, enalapril)

pressure values. Of special note is the onset of hypertension and knowledge about past and more recent use of antihypertensive drug therapy. The majority of patients have chronic hypertension, and although it may be severe, they do not necessarily have resistant hypertension. Clinical assessment, often accompanied by screening laboratory tests, electrocardiograms, and chest films are of paramount importance in answering the following questions: How rapidly should the blood pressure be lowered?; What is the first end point in blood pressure reduction?; What agent or agents should be used?; What should be the route of administration?; and finally is there a need for intensive care unit monitoring?

STRATEGY FOR PROPER DRUG SELECTION

The ideal medication for *hypertensive emergencies* should have a rapid onset and a brief duration of action, be easy to administer and monitor and not adversely to affect critical organs such as the brain, heart, or kidneys, and have few side effects. Such an ideal drug is not available. Drugs recommended for use in hypertensive emergencies and urgencies are shown in Table 4.

Sodium Nitroprusside

Sodium nitroprusside is predictably the most effective drug used in the treatment of hypertensive emergencies. The mechanism of action is that of direct peripheral vasodilatation with a balanced effect on both capacitance and resistance blood vessels. When administered by intravenous infusion, the antihypertensive effect of nitroprusside is apparent within seconds and is highly dose-dependent. After discontinuation of therapy, blood pressure rises rapidly to previous levels within 1 to 5 minutes. In many centers, nitroprusside has become the drug of choice for maintaining hypotension during surgery because of its ease of administration and its sparing of sympathetic reflexes. Serious toxicity and death from cyanide accumulation have rarely occurred, and then only with a total dose that exceeds 300 mg per hour. Safe maximum doses recommended for short-term use have ranged from 0.5 to 1.5 mg per kilogram per hour. Since nitroprusside reduces both venous return and afterload, it can be used safely and effectively in the presence of cardiac failure. It may be used in cases of dissecting aneurysm, but should be combined with intravenous propranolol in order to reduce effectively the myocardiac contractility. In patients who have become refractory to phentolamine, it may even be the drug of choice in the treatment of pheochromocytoma.

The suggested protocol for nitroprusside use that follows appears efficacious. Sodium nitroprusside is supplied as a 50 mg lyophilized powder, which can be dissolved in 500 ml of 5 percent dextrose in water, thereby yielding a final concentration of 100 μg per ml. Infusions are started at a rate of approximately 0.5 μg per kilogram of body weight per minute by means of infusion pump (IVAC, Holter, or Harvard). There are three phases to nitroprusside administration as follows:

1. Initial titration phase. In this phase, infusion rates are doubled every 3 to 5 minutes until blood pressure falls. When this occurs, the infusion can be turned off until the blood pressure begins to turn upward once again.
2. Stabilization phase. In this phase, the nitroprusside infusion is restarted at rates half way between the last two values of the titration phase. If there is a fluctuation in blood pressure, the rate is adjusted until the pressure is stabilized.
3. Discontinuation phase. At this point, oral antihypertensive agents are used concurrently with the nitroprusside. The nitroprusside infusion can be discontinued at 4 to 6 hour intervals to determine new baseline blood pressures and to assess the need for continuation of parenteral therapy.

The use of nitroprusside requires careful monitoring of the patient in an intensive care unit and the use of an arterial line to monitor blood pressure accurately. Experienced nursing care for assessment of blood pressure and cardiac and neurologic status is necessary to ensure safe management.

Nitroprusside crosses the placenta, and its metabolites may accumulate in the fetus; therefore, in eclampsia it is not the drug of choice.

Diazoxide

Diazoxide is a benzothiadiazine derivative that is closely related chemically to thiazide diuretics. Diazoxide exerts its hypotensive effect by reducing arteriolar vascular resistance through direct relaxation of arteriolar smooth muscle. It has little effect on capacitance vessels and no direct effect on the heart or autonomic reflexes. Consequently, when the drug decreases arterial pressure, baroreceptor reflexes are activated, thereby leading to an increase in heart rate, myocardial contractility, stroke volume, and cardiac output. In addition to increased sympathetic reflex activity, diazoxide has several other recognized disadvantages. With the bolus administration of 300 mg of diazoxide, blood pressure may rapidly decrease to normal or even to subnormal levels. An alternate method of multiple small intravenous injections of 50 to 100 mg of diazoxide at 10 minute intervals would appear to produce a more controlled reduction in blood pressure. However, the duration of action of diazoxide is from 2 to 12 hours or more, thereby preventing rapid return of blood pressure to baseline levels in the presence of any deterioration in neurologic or cardiac function. Therefore, it would appear that diazoxide is not the drug of choice in treating (1) hypertensive encephalopathy, (2) eclampsia, (3) dissecting or leaking aneurysms, (4) refractory hypertension in association with angina or myocardial infarction, and (5) impending or completed strokes that are either hemorrhagic or thrombotic in nature.

Trimethaphan Camsylate

Trimethaphan camsylate is a short-acting ganglionic blocking drug which has long been in use. The advantages of trimethaphan are that it is potent, acts rapidly, and has a hypotensive action that can be reversed rapidly by stopping the infusion and placing the patient in a Trendelenburg position. However, its adverse effects are many and result from its ganglionic blockade action. These include paralytic ileus, urinary retention, and the development of tachyphylaxis. Because of the availability of newer drugs with fewer side effects, trimethaphan is seldom used today. However, it can be used as a substitute when nitroprusside is not available.

Nitroglycerin

Nitroglycerin has recently been released for intravenous administration. In a manner similar to that of sodium nitroprusside, its features are rapid onset and offset of action with the ability to titrate blood pressures by careful control infusion rates. At low infusion rates, venodilatation is the predominant effect, whereas at higher doses arteriolar dilatation also occurs. Thus, nitroglycerin infusions reduce both preload and afterload without appreciable changes in heart rate.

When hypertension has not responded to analgesia and sedation, intravenous nitroglycerin would appear to be the drug of choice in the management of hypertensive patients who present with crescendo angina or myocardial infarctions in evolution. There is evidence that intravenous nitroglycerin may dilate collateral blood vessels and improve perfusion to ischemic areas of the myocardium, whereas sodium nitroprusside may decrease perfusion to ischemic myocardium in patients with severe coronary artery disease. Moreover, cardiac output is improved to a greater extent with nitroglycerin than with nitroprusside when pre-treatment pulmonary capillary wedge pressures are increased.

The method of administration is similar to that recommended for sodium nitroprusside. Since nitroglycerin is rapidly absorbed into plastic from solution, glass containers and special intravenous tubing should be utilized for its administration. Headache, nausea, and vomiting are the most frequent side effects.

Hydralazine

Hydralazine, like diazoxide, reduces arterial blood pressure by direct relaxation of arteriolar smooth muscle without much effect on venous capacitance. Thus, sympathetic overactivity is frequently noted with the same contraindications to its use as were described for diazoxide. Hydralazine is still considered the drug of choice for the treatment of eclampsia. Reflex tachycardia and palpitations may occur, but the risk of myocardial ischemia is minimal in young women with freedom from significant coronary atherosclerosis.

Phentolamine

Phentolamine is a short-acting alpha-adrenergic blocker that is specifically indicated in patients with disorders associated with high circulating levels of catecholamines. This would include (1) pheochromocytoma; (2) hypertensive crisis associated with monoamine oxidase inhibitors; (3) drug overdoses with phencyclidine, cocaine, or LSD; and (4) hypertensive rebound following sudden discontinuation of agents such as clonidine or guanabenz. Intravenous administration of phentolamine is associated with tachycardia and frequently with symptoms of abdominal pain, cramps, nausea, vomiting, and diarrhea. Because of these symptoms and the drug's tendency towards tachyphylaxis, nitroprusside infusions represent an alternative mode of therapy for the described clinical emergencies.

For the urgent hypertensive patient (see Table 2), the administration of antihypertensive therapy by intravenous infusion is most often not necessary. However, several oral agents have been shown to be effective and relatively safe in treating urgent hypertension (see Table 4). Currently, it is difficult to choose between these agents on the basis of efficacy and safety because no randomized comparative studies have yet been published.

Clonidine

Oral clonidine loading has been used successfully in a large percentage of patients with hypertensive urgencies. Clonidine is absorbed rapidly, and its antihypertensive effects are noted within 30 minutes with peak levels being achieved within 2 to 4 hours. An initial dose of 0.2 mg of clonidine is given orally, followed by 0.1 mg hourly for several hours, or until blood pressure has reached the desired level. Because clonidine is a central $alpha_2$-agonist, there is no interference with normal baroreceptor reflex control of blood pressure. The average total dose of clonidine required to control hypertension initially is 0.45 mg, the range being between 0.2 to 0.7 mg. For chronic use, approximately one-half of the total loading dose is given daily in split doses—in the morning and at bedtime. The main contraindication to use is second or third degree heart block or sick sinus syndrome.

Nifedipine

When given either sublingually or orally, nifedipine can promptly reduce blood pressure. There is no evidence for more rapid absorption of oral nifedipine when the soft capsule is chewed and swallowed. The blood pressure lowering effect peaks within 15 to 30 minutes and remains effective for up to 3 to 5 hours.

The hemodynamic effects of nifedipine are variable, but in general, an increase in heart rate and cardiac output are noted, along with a reduction in left ventricular end-diastolic pressure in patients with impaired left ventricular function. In the absence of significant cerebrovascular disease, the acute oral administration of nifedipine has been associated with preservation or improvement of cerebral blood flow; however, in the presence of significant cerebrovascular disease, nifedipine, which penetrates the blood-brain barrier, can dilate the cerebral vessels and lead to an uneven cerebral perfusion attributable to an intracranial "steal" effect. Furthermore, the calcium antagonist effect of nifedipine on the coronary vessels can lead to generalized vasodilatation, but in the presence of significant coronary artery disease, can produce a "steal" effect from a segment of fixed, obstructed coronary artery. This may explain the occasional occurrence of the paradoxical worsening of angina pectoris or the appearance of ischemic ECG changes with or without the associated angina that follows the oral administration of nifedipine.

Oral or sublingual nifedipine would appear to be an effective and safe agent in the control of hypertensive urgencies, with the possible exception of patients with cerebrovascular or coronary disease. Furthermore, a drug such as nifedipine, which dilates cerebral vessels and increases cerebral blood flow, may cause an immediate increase in intracranial pressure; therefore, this agent should be used with extreme caution in patients with malignant hypertension because of its potential for cerebral herniation.

Labetalol

Labetalol is a combination alpha- and beta-adrenergic blocker, which in an oral dose of 200 to 400 mg, results in a gradual decrease in blood pressure that begins within 2 hours. Large, single doses of intravenous labetalol appear to be less effective than diazoxide in controlling blood pressure, but may lead to severe prolonged hypotension. Because labetalol is lipid-soluble and has a considerable first pass hepatic metabolism, the oral dosage range to produce controlled hypotension varies considerably. For this reason, the antihypertensive effect of labetalol is not nearly as predictable as it is with oral clonidine or nifedipine. Also, labetalol is contraindicated in patients with congestive heart failure, asthma, sinus bradycardia, or atrial ventricular block graded in first degree.

Minoxidil

Minoxidil is a potent, oral active vasodilator that works predominantly at the arteriolar level. This drug is usually reserved for patients who are refractory to conventional therapy. The reason for this is that minoxidil is usually given as triple therapy along with a beta-blocker or clonidine and vigorous diuretic therapy. The rationale for this type of triple therapy is to overcome severe reflex sympathetic overactivity and marked sodium and fluid retention. Because of the effectiveness of this regimen, minoxidil will undoubtedly continue to be used in the role of a last-resort antihypertensive agent. Chronic use in women is also made difficult by its tendency to cause hypertrichosis.

Angiotensin-Converting Enzyme Inhibitors

Angiotensin-converting enzyme inhibitors (captopril and enalapril) are frequently effective in acutely lowering blood pressure in hypertensive urgencies, especially when in association with accelerated malignant hypertension and renal insufficiency. The major problem with the use of these agents is that the urgent hypertensive patient is in need of close observation to detect a possible first-dose hypotensive response; this tends to occur frequently in salt-depleted vasoconstricted patients. Significant hyperkalemia may also be a problem when these agents are used in patients with renal insufficiency, and one must also be aware of a precipitous deterioration in renal function when these agents are administered to patients with bilateral renal artery stenosis. Although angiotensin-converting enzyme inhibitors are undoubtedly important antihypertensive agents in severe and resistant hypertension, one must be extremely cautious when they are used in the urgent hypertensive patient.

In summary, therefore, the physician must use clinical judgment in deciding which patient has a true hypertensive emergency and which has a less severe, urgent hypertension that can be lowered more slowly and with oral agents. Thus, accurate diagnosis determines (1) selection of the route of administration, (2) selection of a specific agent, (3) the need for special monitoring, and (4) determination of how rapid the initial blood pressure should be lowered.

In the true hypertensive emergency, blood pressure should be lowered in a controlled manner in order to mediate blood pressure levels below the danger level of hypertensive catastrophe, but above the level of impaired of autoregulatory control of cerebral and myocardial blood flow. This is best achieved by using parenteral drugs that can be given via slow infusion in a controlled manner, by using a drug that has a rapid onset and offset of action, and by using it in a setting where optimal monitoring of myocardial and cerebral function can be achieved—in an intensive care unit with specially trained nurses in attendance. Sodium nitroprusside would appear to be the drug of choice in a variety, but not in all, hypertensive emergency states. In contrast, in the urgent hypertensive state, several oral antihypertensive agents have been shown to be effective and relatively safe; the need for hospitalization depends on individual circumstances.

RENOVASCULAR HYPERTENSION

MORTON H. MAXWELL, M.D.
ABRAHAM U. WAKS, M.D.

Renovascular hypertension (RVH) is defined as high blood pressure caused by occlusive disease of a main renal artery or of a primary branch that is potentially curable by reconstitution of vessel patency. Since renal artery stenosis may be present without causing hypertension, the diagnosis of RVH must be made retrospectively after correction of the occlusive disease. However, a tentative diagnosis may be suspected by certain anatomic findings and functional tests. The incidence of RVH varies widely depending on methods of patient selection. Several studies have shown a prevalence of RVH of 3 to 6 percent in hospital referral populations with the remaining patients mainly having essential hypertension.

TYPES OF LESIONS

Although there are multiple etiologies of RVH, 90 to 95 percent of cases present with two principal lesions: atherosclerosis and fibrous dysplasia. In the national Cooperative Study of Renovascular Hypertension, patients with atherosclerotic lesions constituted 60 percent of cases of renovascular disease; the lesions had a striking predilection for the osteum and proximal one-third of the main renal artery. The left side was more frequently involved than the right, and approximately one-third of patients had bilateral lesions. Fibrous dysplasia was present in 35 percent of patients with renovascular disease mainly involving the middle and distal third of the renal artery, and commonly extending into the primary branches. The right side was more commonly affected than the left. When bilateral disease was present from either major disease entity, one side usually predominated.

PATHOPHYSIOLOGY

The pathophysiology of RVH involves the release of renin from the ischemic kidney. However, RVH may be divided into two-kidney and one-kidney models. In the two-kidney model, the ischmeic (ipsilateral) kidney secretes an excess of renin and retains sodium and water; whereas the opposite (contralateral) intact kidney loses sodium and water. In this model, there is an overall negative sodium balance, a persistence of elevated plasma renin activity, and a continual blood pressure responsiveness to inhibitors of the renin-angiotensin systems. Clinical variants of the two-kidney model are unilateral main or segmental stenosis and a solitary kidney with segmental renal artery stenosis.

In contrast, the one-kidney model secretes renin and conserves sodium—the absence of a contralateral kidney thereby preventing sodium loss and leading to eventual expansion of total body sodium and extracellular fluid volume. Fluid volume expansion suppresses renin; hence, hypertension in the one-kidney model is relatively insensitive to the inhibitors of the renin-angiotensin system. Clinical variants of the one-kidney model are bilateral, high grade, main renal artery stenosis; solitary kidney with main renal artery stenosis; and unilateral main renal artery stenosis with contralateral loss of excretory function secondary to nephrosclerosis or parenchymal renal disease.

CLINICAL CHARACTERISTICS

The natural history of renovascular disease depends on the etiology. In terms of clinical characteristics, two prototypical patterns of RVH are recognized. First, there is the young or middle-aged woman with fibrous dysplasia who has hypertension of brief duration that is moderate to severe in intensity, minimal evidence of target organ damage, and a systolic–diastolic epigastric bruit that lateralizes from the midline to the right upper quadrant. Second there is the elderly male with atherosclerotic renovascular disease who has had mild hypertension for many months that has recently accelerated to severe values and has demonstrated grade III or IV optic fundi, cardiomegaly, and azotemia. An abdominal bruit may or may not be present. More common than either of the two prototypical patterns is RVH that cannot be clearly separated from the clinical picture of essential hypertension.

Fibrous Dysplasia

Diffuse medial fibroplasia accounts for 70 to 80 percent of fibrous dysplasia, is often bilateral, and shows slow progression. Dissection, thrombosis, or rupture are unusual. Studies from the Cleveland and the Mayo Clinic, which utilized serial arteriography, revealed progression in 33 percent of patients during a 3-year follow-up period. No patient progressed to total occlusion during follow-up of up to 11 years. In contrast, patients with localized, intimal, medial, or adventitial hyperplasia often demonstrate rapid progression.

Atherosclerosis

Atherosclerotic lesions are part of a systemic disease that involves different segments of the vascular system. Mortality is higher because of cardiovascular events and target organ disfunction. Renal lesions tend to progress in 44 to 50 percent of the patients, as reflected by impairment of renal function and loss of renal mass. Total occlusion was observed in 16 percent of the patients followed by the Cleveland Clinic.

THERAPY

The therapeutic goals are (1) reversal of hypertension, and (2) restoration of renal blood flow, preservation of renal tissue, and improvement of renal function. Medical therapy with antihypertensive drugs may control the hypertension, but has no effect on the progression of the disease. Therefore, every effort should be made to find patients that can benefit from angioplastic or operative procedures.

The diagnosis of RVH involves careful risk-benefit and cost-benefit analysis when one is evaluating individual patients. The availability of newer antihypertensive drugs that are usually successful in lowering blood pressure in patients with RVH and the development of percutaneous transluminal angioplasty (PTA) as an alternative to operative treatment drastically change the decision matrix.

DIAGNOSTIC STRATEGIES

With regard to the need for aggressive work-up, the hypertensive population can be classified into three subgroups.

Patients in Whom Intervention with Possible Cure or Improvement of Hypertension is Preferable to Long-Term Drug Therapy

This group includes: children; patients with severe or accelerated hypertension; hypertension that is uncontrollable (poor blood pressure response, adverse side effects, lack of compliance) with antihypertensive drug therapy; progressive diminution of kidney function; and progressive hypertension after kidney transplantation. Angiography should be used here as the initial diagnostic procedure and PTA may be attempted during the same procedure. Blood pressure response as well as reductions in plasma renin levels after successful dilation confirm the diagnosis of RVH. Thus, PTA is used as a definitive diagnostic test as well as a therapeutic modality.

Patients Suspected of Having RVH

Patients with inappropriate age of onset, abrupt worsening of hypertension, or systolic–diastolic epigastric bruits should be screened for RVH with digital subtraction intravenous angiography, rapid sequence intravenous urography, or radioisotope studies, which are followed by arteriography only if screening tests are positive.

Patients with Moderate Hypertension Who Are Not Suspected of Having RVH

This group of asymptomatic patients represents the majority of the hypertensive population and are usually treated medically. Patients with marked response to angiotensin–converting enzyme (ACE) inhibitors or patients who do not respond to diuretics are more likely to have renin dependent hypertension, which includes RVH, thereby representing the best group for further diagnostic work-up.

MEDICAL THERAPY

Since the introduction of the oral converting enzyme inhibitor, captopril, which is often used concomitantly with a diuretic, successful control of hypertension has been reported in 85 to 90 percent of renovascular hypertensive patients. Similar results will likely occur with the use of the other ACE inhibitor, enalapril.

The greater effect of captopril is undoubtedly related to the specificity of action on underlying pathophysiological mechanisms of RVH. The acute depressor response to captopril correlates with the pre-treatment plasma renin activity; in contrast, the long-term response correlates poorly with renin levels. Although the vasodilatory action of captopril is not accompanied by significant sodium or volume retention, the addition of a diuretic greatly enhances its activity. Since many patients with RVH are extremely sensitive to the blood pressure lowering effect of captopril, a test dose of 6.25 mg (¼ tablet) should be given initially, followed by a dose of 12.5 mg, then increased to 25 mg 2 times per day or 3 times per day as necessary to obtain an optimal blood pressure response. By maintaining the total daily dose of captopril at no greater than 100 mg daily, serious side effects, such as leukopenia and membranous glomerulopathy, can be largely avoided. Captopril must be used with caution and in substantially lower doses in patients with renal insufficiency.

In patients with high-grade bilateral renal artery stenosis, effective control of blood pressure may contribute to slow progressive reduction in renal function by lowering perfusion pressure. In addition, several reports have described reversible acute renal failure after treatment with converting enzyme inhibitors such as captropril or enalapril in patients with bilateral renal artery stenosis, unilateral stenosis with contralateral renal dysfunction, or a single kidney with renal artery stenosis. Renal failure may occur even when there is no significant reduction in blood pressure from the converting enzyme inhibitor.

The complication of renal failure is best understood by considering the role of angiotensin II in the control of glomerular filtration. Angiotensin II, by preferentially constricting the efferent arteriole, maintains the glomerular filtration rate during hypoperfusion. Converting enzyme inhibitors therefore cause a selective dilation of the efferent arteriole by blocking angiotensin II, with a resulting decrease in renal perfusion and glomerular filtration. The overall incidence of converting enzyme-inhibitor-induced renal failure in the treatment of RVH is not known. Considering that bilateral, hemodynamically significant renal artery stenosis occurs in less than 10 percent of all renovascular patients, the majority of patients with RVH can be given converting enzyme inhibitors without the danger of renal failure.

The question of medical versus operative therapy for RVH continues to be a subject of controversy. The 1973 report of Hunt and Strong from the Mayo Clinic is the most extensive study that compares medical and operative therapy. Two hundred and fourteen patients with RVH were placed on drug therapy. From this initial group, 100 patients were selected for operative therapy after 3 months of unsuccessful medical treatment. Over the 7- to 14- year follow-up period of the atherosclerotic group, 30 percent of operatively treated patients died, as compared to 70 percent of the medically treated group. There was no significant difference in mortality for medical versus operative therapy in patients with fibrous dysplasia. Because the patients in this study were not selected randomly, one must use caution in the interpretation of results. Moreover, with newer, more effective drug therapy, the long-term prognosis of RVH may be improved.

A prospective, randomized study of RVH at Vanderbilt University, which compared medical versus operative therapy, has been ongoing for more than 12 years. Although this study has not been reported in detail, Dean has reported a 41 percent incidence of progression of renal artery stenosis in medically treated patients, demonstrated either by a significant decrease in renal length, and hence functioning renal mass, or by a decrease in creatinine clearance. Of great significance was the presence of continued good blood pressure control with medical therapy in 15 of 17 (88 percent) patients who showed deterioration of renal function. Thus, drug therapy cannot stop the progression of renal artery stenosis, despite good blood pressure control. In as many as 40 percent of cases, progressive renal artery stenosis may eventually impair renal function in the affected kidney.

With the use of currently available antihypertensive medication, good blood pressure control can probably be obtained in 85 to 90 percent of patients with RVH. Medical failures probably represent high-grade stenoses with extremely elevated, autonomous production of renin or severe bilateral renal artery stenosis with superimposed salt and water retention. Because of possible progression of renal artery stenosis, monitoring of kidney function is mandatory in patients receiving medical treatment. This monitoring is vital because blood pressure may continue to be well controlled with medications despite progressive loss of renal function. Moreover, serum creatinine or creatinine clearances may not change in the presence of progressive unilateral renal artery stenosis because of a counterbalancing improvement in renal function in the contralateral kidney without arterial stenosis. Thus, both creatinine clearance and renal size are important signs to follow. Renal size can be assessed by computed tomography, ultrasonography, or intravenous urography. It is important to note that a 10 percent loss in renal length is equivalent to a 30 percent loss in functioning renal mass since the kidney is shaped like an ovoid ellipsoid.

PERCUTANEOUS TRANSLUMINAL ANGIOPLASTY

The development by Gruentzig and associates of catheters fitted with an expansible balloon to dilate vascular obstructive lesions has stimulated interest in the possibility of correcting occlusive renal artery disease and benefitting RVH without the risks of surgery. The efficacy of renal PTA is difficult to determine because most early reports are relatively small in sample size, are largely retrospective and nonrandomized, and consist primarily of short-term (12 months or less) clinical follow-up. In general, success rates appear to be higher in (1) fibrous dysplasia as compared to atherosclerotic disease; (2) vessels with only one or two short stenoses, rather than more extensive disease; and (3) in stenoses located completely within the renal artery, rather than lesions that include the aortic wall or renal artery orifice. Only occasional success has been reported in occluded renal arteries.

The most comprehensive series to date is that of Sos and associates, reported in 1983 (Table 1). In this study, 89 patients with RVH, 51 with atheromatous stenosis, and 31 with fibrous dysplasia were followed for an average of 16 months (range 4 to 40 months) after angioplasty therapy. Angioplasty was technically successful in 87 percent of patients with fibrous dysplasia, but in only 57 percent of those with unilateral atherosclerotic lesions. Technical failure in atherosclerotic lesions resulted from both ostial lesions, which could not be successfully dilated, and total occlusion of the vessels, which rarely allowed passage of a catheter. After successful angioplasty, blood

TABLE 1 Success Rate of Angioplasty in Renovascular Hypertension

Type of Lesion	*Number of Patients*	*Technical Success %*	*Improved Hypertension %*	*Overall Benefitted %*	*Major Complications %*
Fibrous Dysplasia					
Combined lesions	31	87	93	81	6
Atherosclerosis					
Combined lesions	51	37	84	31	8
Unilateral lesions	31	57	82	47	

(By permission of Sos, et al. N Engl J Med 1983; 309:274.)

pressure was reduced to normal or was improved in 93 percent of patients with fibrous dysplasia and in 82 percent of those with unilateral atheromatous disease.

Therefore, the overall benefit rate (percent technically successful multiplied by percent improved) was 81 percent in fibrous dysplastic disease and only 47 percent in unilateral atherosclerotic lesions. Much poorer results were obtained in bilateral atherosclerotic lesions, largely attributable to a high rate of technical failures. In a later report by Sos and associates, angiographic follow-up in 14 patients at 1 year and 13 patients at 2 years showed no evidence of restenosis or deterioration in blood pressure control, thereby suggesting that restenosis is unusual when full technical success has been obtained. In contrast, other investigators have noted a restenosis rate of 10 to 17 percent.

In addition to improved blood pressure control, successful angioplasty may stabilize or improve renal function. In the Sos series, there was a 12 percent increase in kidney size in patients who had technically successful angioplasties. Others have noted improved renal function in approximately 50 percent of azotemic patients after successful angioplasty.

The morbidity and mortality from angioplasty for both atheromatous and fibrous dysplastic disease of the renal arteries appear to be less than that from operative therapy. However, emergency operative repair of renal artery dissections was necessary in 6 percent of patients treated by Sos; this is higher than the usual 1 to 2 percent dissections reported by others and is perhaps explainable by more advanced atheromatous disease and the participation of many angiographers with varying experiences. Also to be considered is that follow-up operative therapy would have been necessary in those patients with technical failures. Other potential complications are massive hematoma, subsegmental infarcts, distal embolization, and acute deterioration in renal function. Most of these latter complications are self-limited and reversible. Randomized clinical trials of angioplasty versus surgery are needed to establish the long-term rate of complications and patency of arteries.

Informed consent of the patient requires explanation of the potential need for emergency operative correction of possible renal artery dissections. Thus the patient should be judged a good operative risk, and a surgical support team should be available prior to undertaking angioplasty therapy. Blood pressure should be monitored for at least 24 hours after the procedure, and if hypotension develops, the patient should be treated with short-term volume or vasopressor support. Because PTA may be done under local anesthesia, patients generally can be discharged from the hospital within several days of their procedure as compared to 1 to 2 weeks of hospitalization after surgery.

OPERATIVE INTERVENTION

In 1974, the National Cooperative Study on Renovascular Hypertension summarized operative results as follows. In 300 patients with atherosclerotic renal artery disease who underwent operative intervention, there were cure, improvement, failure, and mortality rates of 41, 15, 32, and 12 percent, respectively. In contrast, in 179 patients with fibrous dysplasia, there were cure, improvement, failure, and mortality rates of 64, 11, 25, and 3 percent, respectively. The unacceptably high mortality rate in individuals with atherosclerotic lesions reflected a high prevalence of generalized atherosclerosis, angina pectoris, previous myocardial infarctions, left ventricular hypertrophy, and impaired renal function.

When cardiovascular risk factors are considered in order to optimize patient selection, and only patients operated on by experienced personnel in specialized centers are included in the series, overall operative results are more impressive. Tables 2 and 3 summarize the more recent operative results in atherosclerotic and fibrous dysplastic RVH, respectively. Operative mortality has been reduced to 3 percent in patients with underlying atherosclerotic disease and to 1 percent or less in those with fibrous dysplastic RVH. Whereas one-third of atherosclerotic patients are cured by successful reconstructive surgery, as compared to two-thirds with underlying fibrous dysplastic disease, the overall benefit rate (improvement or cure of hypertension) was 85 percent versus 96 percent, thus supporting the efficacy of operative intervention in selected cases, regardless of underlying etiology of the renal artery stenosis or age of the patient.

Frequently omitted from a discussion of the management of RVH is the long-term adverse effects of uncorrected renal artery occlusive disease on renal function.

TABLE 2 Operative Results in Atherosclerotic Renovascular Hypertension

Reference	*Number of Patients*	*Cured No., (%)*	*Improved No., (%)*	*Failures No., (%)*	*Died No., (%)*
Dean et al (1977)	78	28 (36%)	39 (50%)	11 (14%)	1 (1%)
Stanley & Fry (1977)	105	29 (28%)	55 (52%)	18 (18%)	3 (3%)
Lankford (1979)	52	15 (29%)	30 (58%)	4 (8%)	3 (6%)
Novick et al (1981)	100	39 (40%)	50 (51%)	9 (9%)	2 (2%)
Totals	335	111 (33%)	174 (52%)	42 (13%)	9 (3%)

TABLE 3 Operative Results in Fibrous Dysplastic Renovascular Hypertension

Reference	*Number of Patients*	*Cured No., (%)*	*Improved No., (%)*	*Failures No., (%)*	*Died No., (%)*
Korobkin (1976)	19	14 (81%)	1 (5%)	2 (14%)	1 (5%)
Stanley & Fry (1977)	159	101 (63%)	53 (33%)	6 (4%)	0 (0%)
Lankford (1979)	25	14 (56%)	20 (40%)	0 (0%)	1 (4%)
Totals	203	129 (64%)	64 (32%)	8 (4%)	2 (1%)

As discussed earlier, as many as 40 percent of patients with atherosclerotic renal artery stenosis show deterioration of renal function over a period of several years while on medical therapy. Recent studies (Table 4) have shown that 68 percent of patients have a marked improvement in renal function, as well as significant improvement in blood pressure when successful reconstructive surgery was performed. Indeed, the presence of a complete renal artery stenosis may still be compatible with operative improvement in renal function.

The most dependable predictors of improvement in renal function and blood pressure control after operative correction of occluded renal arteries are (1) renal length of 9 cm or greater; (2) arteriographic demonstration of a patent distal vessel, without evidence of severe intrarenal stenosis; (3) demonstration of an early nephrogram phase during arteriography; and (4) demonstration of an abundant collateral circulation, frequently with retrograde flow through the occluded vessel.

Because RVH is frequently a bilateral disease, which is progressive, one should avoid ablative treatment of RVH whenever possible. However, there are occasions when reconstructive surgery has a minimal chance of success, thereby making it necessary for either partial or total nephrectomy to be the operative treatment of choice. Such indications are as follows (1) renal atrophy, with length less than 9 cm; (2) main renal artery occlusion with renal infarction; (3) unilateral parenchymal disease; (4) segmental renal infarction; (5) segmental renal hypoplasia (Ask-Upmark kidney); and (6) noncorrectable renovascular disease such as intrarenal aneurysm or arteriovenous malformation.

Of the many operative procedures used to treat RVH, aortorenal bypass has emerged as the single most preferred operative treatment. In the past, satisfactory results have been obtained by using saphenous veins, although more recently a higher success rate has been reported by means of autogenous arterial grafts. Technical success rates in experienced hands now range between 95 and 97 percent.

Particularly challenging are renovascular lesions that extend into the renal arterial branches. Previously, these patients would have been candidates for nephrectomy. With the advent of microvascular extracorporeal operative techniques, renal revascularization may be the treatment of choice. However, it has been the experience of many surgeons that the main renal artery and its branches frequently can be repaired in situ, particularly when disease-free branches occur outside the renal hilus, by means of aortorenal bypass, which is the preferred technique.

There are occasions when other reconstructive tech-

TABLE 4 Operative Results in Renovascular Hypertensive Patients with Azotemia

Reference	*Number of Patients*	*Cure No., (%)*	*BP Results Improved No., (%)*	*Failure No., (%)*	*Improved Renal Function No., (%)*
Dean (1979)	25	9 (36%)	15 (60%)	1 (4%)	15 (60%)
Libertino (1980)	15	10 (67%)	5 (33%)		13 (87%)
Novick (1983)	51				34 (67%)
Totals	91	19 (47%)	20 (50%)	1 (3%)	91 (68%)

niques are preferable to aortorenal bypass. A splenorenal bypass may be the operation of choice when the stenosis is on the left side and when mobilization and use of the aorta may be hazardous owing to previous aortorenal operations, severe degenerative atherosclerosis, or complete aortic thrombosis. Since a splenorenal bypass involves only a single vascular anastomosis without the need for cross- clamping of the aorta, less operating time is required than for many of the more conventional reconstructive procedures, and thus may be indicated in the poor surgical risk patient. An aortorenal reimplantation procedure may be used to treat renovascular disease caused by a short, fibrous lesion, such as intimal fibroplasia or true fibromuscular hyperplasia, that involves the proximal one-third of the renal artery. This operation is particularly well suited to the anatomical variant of an anomalous high orgin of the renal artery since an adequate amount of disease-free distal renal artery is a prerequisite for successful surgery.

The transfer of a kidney from one site to another in the same patient is termed renal autotransplantation. Autotransplantation has been used in patients with renovascular disease secondary to renal trauma, staghorn renal calculus, extensive ureteral loss, or tumors occurring in a solitary kidney. Other candidates for renal autotransplantation in the operative treatment of RVH are patients with a surgically difficult aorta, in whom relatively disease-free iliac arteries are present and in patients with extensive branch renal artery lesions that cannot be repaired by conventional revascularization techniques in situ. However, whenever possible, conventional in situ renal revascularization techniques should be used for the above indications because these techniques are associated with significantly reduced operative time and postoperative morbidity.

Certain general precautions can be taken to minimize renovascular operative morbidity and mortality. Atherosclerotic lesions of the renal artery are frequently associated with generalized vascular disease. When indicated, prophylactic coronary or carotid bypass surgery should be performed in patients with associated renal artery stenosis; these lesions should be corrected prior to operative repair of renal arteries—otherwise a high incidence of stroke and myocardial infarction occurs during routine renal artery bypass. In the presence of significant impairment in cardiac function, a Swan-Ganz flow catheter should be used to monitor the patient during renovascular surgery. Refractory hypertension should be treated with parenteral sodium nitroprusside infusions before, during, and after operative procedures.

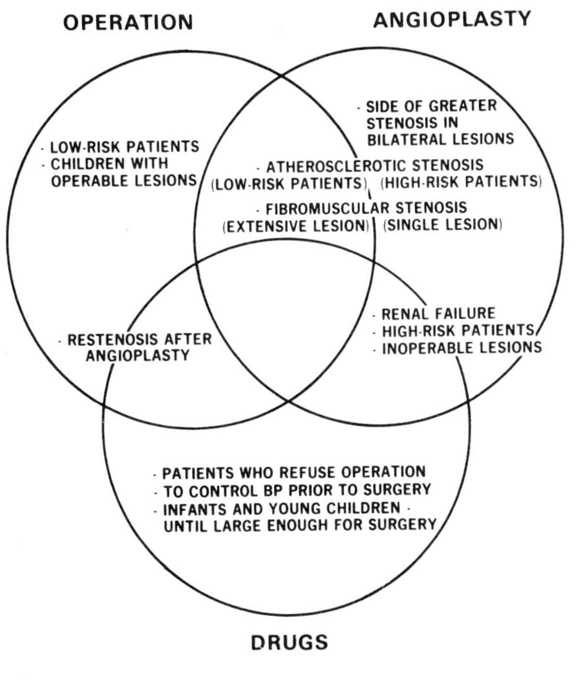

Figure 1 Treatment modalities in patients with renovascular hypertension.

CHOICE OF THERAPY AND CLINICAL MANAGEMENT

Reconstruction of vessel patency by operation or by PTA is preferable to medical therapy for the following reasons:

1. Patient can discontinue antihypertensive drugs, which results in substantial reduction of cost as well as avoidance of side effects.
2. Renal artery lesions, especially atherosclerotic, may worsen and thereby cause an increase in hypertension and reduction of renal function.
3. Operative techniques have been improved.
4. The introduction of transluminal angioplasty helps to avoid complicated and risky operative procedures.

Medical therapy should be favored for the following subgroups:

1. Patients with extensive bilateral and/or segmental lesions that are both inoperable and nondilatable.
2. Infants and young children who are not large enough for surgery.
3. Patients who refuse invasive procedures.
4. High-risk patients with nondilatable lesions.

All other patients, including high–risk patients, should be considered for invasive procedures.

PTA should be attempted as the initial procedure in all patients with RVH, unless technically unfeasible. PTA may be attempted at the time of initial arteriography when stenosis is demonstrated, regardless of its type or degree. If initial dilation by PTA is successful, as judged by the radiologic appearance and confirmed by a decreased pressure gradient, then the short-term blood pressure response offers the most accurate and practical diagnosis of RVH; if the blood pressure falls significantly, the diagnosis of RVH is established, even if the blood pressure should subsequently increase because of restenosis. When PTA is not technically feasible or is initially unsuccessful in dilating a stenotic lesion, the diagnostic confirmation of RVH should be obtained and surgery is recommended unless contraindicated.

Specific indications for surgery are (1) progressive fibrous dysplasia lesions, usually associated with intimal fibroplasia and subadventitial fibroplasia; (2) atherosclerotic-ostial lesions in patients with progressive decrease in renal function despite good response to medical management; and (3) patients whose hypertension or azotemia responds only transiently to successful angioplasty (PTA might be reattempted in such cases prior to operative procedures).

To conclude, the choice of treatment depends on two principal considerations: control of blood pressure and preservation of renal function. The outcome of PTA or surgery depends on (1) accurate diagnosis of renin mediated hypertension, (2) technically successful procedure, and (3) type of renal artery disease (with more favorable results in patients with fibromuscular hyperplasia).

The introduction of PTA has modified the decision matrix (Figure 1) in the management of renal artery stenosis and should be attempted in amost every patient with an arteriographically demonstrable lesion, regardless of its severity. Immediate blood pressure response may then be used as the "ultimate" diagnostic test. The introduction of ACE inhibitors has increased the success rate of medical therapy, and they are also useful in patients with poor blood pressure response to surgery. However, their use involves the risk of renal failure in the patient with high-grade stenosis.

HYPERTENSION IN PREGNANCY

MARSHALL D. LINDHEIMER, M.D.
ADRIAN I. KATZ, M.D.

High blood pressure complicates approximately 10 percent of all gestations; in nulliparas the incidence is almost 20 percent, and 40 to 50 percent of women carrying twins develop hypertension. Furthermore, high blood pressure in pregnancy remains an important cause of fetal loss and maternal morbidity. Nevertheless, hypertension associated with pregnancy remains an understudied area of reproductive medicine beset by considerable controversy. Thus, current textbooks and reviews may advise diametrically opposite approaches to management: the reader of the first edition of this text, for example, will find in it contrasting opinions to those expressed below. Our contribution, a brief survey of hypertension in pregnancy, focuses on preeclampsia as well as on the results of recent drug trials of agents used to treat chronic hypertension in pregnancy.

BLOOD PRESSURE IN NORMAL PREGNANCY

Mean blood pressure decreases early in pregnancy and by midtrimester diastolic levels are often 10 mm Hg less than before conception. Blood pressure then increases gradually, approaching prepregnancy values near term. Cardiac output also changes in pregnancy, increasing by 40 to 60 percent above the nongravid state during the first trimester and remaining relatively constant thereafter. Thus the decrement in pressure during gestation is due to a marked decrease in peripheral vascular resistance.

The physiologic changes described above mean that norms for pregnancy must be lowered: Diastolic levels exceeding 75 mm Hg in the second trimester and 85 mm Hg in the third trimester are abnormal. Perinatal mortality rates increase significantly when mean arterial pressures exceed 90 mm Hg in midtrimester and 95 mm Hg in late pregnancy—all values that would not be of great concern in nonpregnant patients. Another interesting aspect of the cardiovascular alterations in pregnancy is the slow pressure rise that follows the midtrimester nadir, because it demonstrates that increasing vasoconstrictor tone is a feature of late pregnancy in normal women as well as in those who develop preeclampsia (see below).

CLASSIFICATION OF HYPERTENSION IN PREGNANCY

There are many classifications of the hypertensive disorders of gestation, which is a source of confusion to the reader. We recommend the classification suggested by The American College of Obstetricians and Gynecologists, which is both sound and concise. It considers pregnancy-associated hypertension in only four categories: preeclampsia and eclampsia, chronic hypertension (of whatever cause), chronic hypertension with superimposed preeclampsia, and late transient hypertension.

Preeclampsia — Eclampsia

Category 1 accounts for more than 50 percent of the hypertensive disorders complicating gestation. In preeclampsia the high blood pressure is associated with proteinuria, edema, and at times coagulation or liver functon abnormalities or both. This disease occurs primarily in nulliparas, usually after the 20th gestational week, and most frequently near term. Preeclampsia can progress rapidly to a convulsive phase termed eclampsia, a dramatic and life-threatening event. The eclamptic convulsion is usually preceded by a number of premonitory symptoms and signs, including headache, severe epigastric pain, hyperreflexia, and hemoconcentration, but it can also appear suddenly and without warning in a seemingly stable patient, with only minimal blood pressure elevations. This is why attempts to categorize preeclampsia as "mild" or "severe" (in the latter case, increases in diastolic and systolic levels to 110 and 160 mm Hg or higher, heavy proteinuria, and neurologic signs and symptoms) can be misleading. *Therefore, the appearance of de novo third trimester hypertension in a nullipara whether or not other signs are present is sufficient reason to hospitalize her.*

One form of preeclampsia whose clinical appearance may be misleadingly benign affects patients presenting with minimal changes in platelet counts and/or liver function tests and almost no evidence of hypertension. While most preeclamptic women with coagulation abnormalities and/or hepatic involvement have other markers of severe disease, an occasional gravida has only a borderline elevation in blood pressure, little or no proteinuria, a small decrement in platelet count, and minimal elevations of liver enzyme values. Such patients, however, can rapidly progress to a syndrome characterized by hemolysis and marked signs of both liver dysfunction and coagulation changes. The bilirubin level may become elevated; transaminase values often exceed 1,000 to 2,000 IU, circulating platelet counts frequently decrease to below 40,000 per cubic millimeter, and evidence of microangiopathic hemolysis appears on the blood smear. (In the literature this is called the HELLP syndrome, an acronym for Hemolysis, Elevated Liver enzymes, and Low Platelet count.) This uncommon form of preeclampsia is life-threatening and constitutes a medical emergency. Fortunately, most patients survive with supportive care, the abnormalities abating two days to one week after evacuation of the uterus. There have been maternal deaths associated with this syndrome, however, which in some instances were due to a failure to appreciate the severity of the situation at an early stage.

Chronic Hypertension (of Whatever Cause)

Category 2 includes approximately one-third of all cases of high blood pressure in pregnancy, and in most cases the underlying pathologic factor is essential hypertension. In some, however, the hypertension is secondary to such conditions as kidney disease, renal artery stenosis, coarctation of the aorta, pheochromocytoma, primary aldosteronism, and in very rare instances a renin-secreting tumor. These patients, whose hypertension predates the gestation, are more prone to superimposed preeclampsia (the third category, see below), but otherwise pregnancy seems to have little influence on the course of their underlying disease: fetal outcome appears related to the extent of end-organ damage before conception, and to the severity of the preeclamptic complication. In fact, some hypertensive diseases may be ameliorated by gestation: Normalization of blood pressure has been described during pregnancy in a woman with renal artery stenosis; gestation has ameliorated the tendency to lose potassium in some patients with primary aldosteronism; and gestational increases in circulating free cortisol may ameliorate certain uncommon forms of high blood pressure characterized by overproduction of desoxycorticosterone or other mineralocorticoids (categorized in the literature as dexamethasone suppressible hypertension).

There are exceptions to the generally favorable outcome for category 2 patients. Certain women with systemic renal diseases, mainly scleroderma and periarteritis nodosa, do poorly during gestation, and both entities have been associated with maternal deaths. Thus, one should advise against conception or continuing gestation in women with these collagen diseases. Another hypertensive disorder with catastrophic potential is pheochromocytoma. In the past, pheochromocytoma was associated with maternal mortality rates in excess of 40 percent. Most of these deaths were due to fulminating disease at times mistaken for preeclampsia, and the true nature of the tumor remained unsuspected and was found only at autopsy. More recently, a greater percentage of these cases are being diagnosed prenatally, and because the tumor is resected or managed medically through term (using alpha-adrenoceptor inhibiting drugs), a successful outcome for both mother and fetus is achieved. Thus screening for pheochromocytoma is indicated when hypertension has predated conception or was discovered during early pregnancy.

Chronic Hypertension with Superimposed Preeclampsia

Women in category 2 have a high propensity to develop superimposed preeclampsia. (This complication may occur in 20 to 40 percent of women with hypertensive disorders predating conception, and the combination represented by category 3 affects 10 to 15 percent of all women with hypertension in pregnancy.) In our experience hypertensive gravidas with superimposed preeclampsia are most often multiparas whose disease accelerates during the early and middle parts of the third trimester. If their gestation is allowed to continue, they often manifest extremes of hypertension, heavy proteinuria, decreasing renal function, and a susceptibility to hepatic and coagulation-type syndromes, and the fetus often succumbs. In essence, the combination of another hypertensive disorder and superimposed preeclampsia may produce an acute medical emergency, and the women with this condition have the poorest fetal outcome. Furthermore, there is a good probability that this dangerous complication will recur in subsequent pregnancies.

Late or Transient Hypertension

Category 4, which includes a number of women who are otherwise difficult to classify, is characterized by the appearance of hypertension only (*without proteinuria*) late in pregnancy or in the immediate puerperium, and the blood pressure returns to normal by the 10th postpartum day. Among such patients may be nulliparas who may have early preeclampsia but have manifested no other signs of the disease, and it is prudent to manage them as if preeclampsia were present. Another group develops hypertension during two or more pregnancies and again become normotensive soon after delivery (manifesting an entity once erroneously labeled "recurrent toxemia"). The outcome of such pregnancies, however, is usually good compared with the more reserved prognosis in patients with preeclampsia. There is evidence that transient hypertension in such gravidas is a forerunner of essential hypertension later in life, analogous to the situation of women with gestational diabetes who eventually become frank diabetics.

It should be noted that the classification scheme above avoids a number of terms in the current literature that we find misleading. For example, "gestational," "pregnancy-induced," and "pregnancy-associated" hypertension do not differentiate between the more serious preeclampsia and the rather benign transient hypertension of pregnancy. The term "toxemia" is archaic (no one has ever identified a toxin in the blood of such women), and its use in the older literature covers a variety of different forms of hypertension and is thus especially confusing. Another classification "EPH gestosis," which mainly appears in European publications, categorizes patients on the basis of symptomatology such as E for edema, P for proteinuria, and H for hypertension, the individual being defined as mono- or polysymptomatic. We see little value in such a schema, because edema alone occurs in 80 percent of normal gestations, proteinuria may be observed in gravidas with renal disease who have no hypertension, and high blood pressure is a manifestation of all the etiologic entities described above.

Finally, one should be aware of two uncommon conditions: "late postpartum eclampsia" (hypertension and convulsions occurring days to weeks after delivery), the existence of which was once debated, and "postpartum hypertension" (in women who were normotensive during gestation), which is characterized by abnormal increments in blood pressure 2 weeks to 6 months after delivery. The latter, about which little is known, is rather benign, the blood pressure becoming normal within one year of delivery.

DIAGNOSIS, CLINICAL COURSE, AND PATHOPHYSIOLOGY

It can be very difficult to distinguish clinically among preeclampsia, essential or secondary hypertension, renal disease, and combinations of these entities. For example, certain women with undiagnosed hypertension experience the physiologic decrement in mean blood pressure early in gestation and have normal levels when first examined near midpregnancy. Later, when frankly elevated pressures are recorded near term, they are erroneously labeled as preeclamptics. Also, an accelerated phase of essential hypertension (albeit a rare event during gestation), pheochromocytoma, and certain renal diseases (e.g., glomerulonephritis, lupus erythematosus) occurring late in pregnancy may all mimic preeclampsia. Such diagnostic problems are illustrated best in reports of cases in which the cause of hypertension complicating pregnancy has been determined by renal biopsy. These studies reveal that the clinical impression of preeclampsia could be erroneous in more than 15 percent of nulliparas and in 50 percent or more of multiparas, and that unsuspected renal disease was uncovered in 10 to 20 percent of the cases. In one of these reports, in which an academic obstetrician and a nephrologist recorded their impressions prior to biopsy, a correct diagnosis was made on clinical grounds in only 58 percent of the patients. However, renal biopsy is rarely indicated prepartum; in the absence of a morphologic diagnosis, a nullipara developing high blood pressure in late pregnancy and manifesting proteinuria, elevated plasma urate levels, and decrements in platelet counts is the patient in whom the diagnosis of preeclampsia is most secure. Some suggest that the presence of a low circulating antithrombin III level also increases the sensitivity of this diagnosis. In any event, it is always better to *overdiagnose* preeclampsia. The pathophysiology is such that when this disease is neglected, fetal and occasionally maternal prognosis is poor, while early intervention often results in a successful outcome for both mother and child.

Pathophysiology of Preeclampsia

Women with preeclampsia may have a reversal of the normal diurnal blood pressure rhythm (morning peaks and nighttime nadirs), so that the highest levels occur during the night. Thus one may be unaware of dangerous pressure elevations if only daytime values are recorded.

Hypertension in preeclampsia is characteristically labile, reflecting the intense sensitivity of the vasculature to endogenous pressor peptides and catecholamines. Whereas normal pregnant women are extremely resistant to the pressor effects of infused angiotensin, those in whom preeclampsia is destined to develop have increased pressor responsiveness to this peptide weeks before the appearance of clinical manifestations. Similar alterations occur in women with chronic hypertension who develop superimposed preeclampsia. The vasculature of preeclamptics is also quite sensitive to infused norepinephrine and vasopressin. These alterations in vascular sensitivity may be due to decreased prostacyclin levels or increases in vasoconstricting thromboxane concentrations or both, changes which also have been linked to coagulopathies associated with preeclampsia.

Glomerular filtration rate (GFR) decreases in preeclampsia partly due to a characteristic renal lesion that consists mainly of intracapillary cell swelling ("glomerular endotheliosis"). The drop in GFR is approximately 25 percent in mild cases. Because renal hemodynamics increase about 50 percent in normal pregnancy, the GFR in preeclamptic women often remain above prepregnancy values. Levels of serum creatinine and urea nitrogen of 0.9 mg and 15 mg per deciliter respectively, considered normal in nonpregnant subjects, indicate decreased function in gravidas and should concern the clinician. This is because renal function in preeclamptics with plasma creatinine concentrations between 1 and 1.5 mg per deciliter (which are seemingly benign but already represent a 50 percent loss of GFR for pregnancy) has been known to deteriorate suddenly and progress to acute tubular (and rarely cortical) necrosis.

Uric acid clearance is also increased in normal gestation but reduced in preeclampsia. These decrements may occur earlier and be more profound than those in GFR, and uric acid levels above 4.5 mg per deciliter are already suspect in gravidas. The level of hyperuricemia correlates with the extent of the renal lesion in preeclampsia, as well as with fetal outcome.

Salt handling and volume homeostasis are also altered in preeclampsia. The ability to excrete sodium is decreased, but the degree of impairment varies and severe disease can occur in the absence of edema (the so-called dry preeclamptic). It is important to recognize that even when interstitial edema is present, plasma volume is decreased and hemoconcentration occurs. In most instances central venous and pulmonary capillary wedge pressures are low, and when studied prior to any therapeutic intervention cardiac output is decreased compared with normal gestation. Uteroplacental blood flow is also impaired in preeclampsia, this being one reason for the increased incidence of fetal loss and intrauterine growth retardation. The combination of low plasma volume and cardiac output, decreased central venous and pulmonary wedge pressures, and suboptimal uterine blood flow are the major reasons why most experts avoid the use of diuretics in preeclampsia.

MANAGEMENT

Preeclampsia

Women in whom preeclampsia is suspected should be hospitalized, an approach which diminishes the frequency of convulsions (and other consequences of diagnostic error), and enhances fetal survival. Such "prophylactic" hospitalization may appear overly expensive, but it delays termination of the pregnancy and reduces the higher costs incurred by very premature infants in intensive care nurseries. If blood pressure decreases to less than 100 mm Hg diastolic, and renal and hepatic function as well as coagulation indices remain normal over a period of several days, an occasional informed and trustworthy patient may be allowed to return to a quiet home environment, but in this case she should be evaluated twice weekly until delivery.

In general, induction is the therapy of choice near term, whereas attempts can be made to postpone action if pregnancy is at an early stage (mainly before 32 weeks). If a decision is made to temporize, several antihypertensive agents considered safe and effective in pregnancy are available (Tables 1 and 2). However, if severe hypertension (diastolic levels above 105 mm Hg in most women, above 100 mm Hg in teenage gravidas) persists after 24 to 48 hours of treatment, delivery is indicated regardless of the stage of gestation, since the mother is at risk and further delay rarely saves the fetus. Advances in neonatology have been such that most infants weighing 1,500 g or more survive better in a premature nursery than in the womb of a woman with preeclampsia. The appearance of clotting abnormalities, decreasing renal function, and signs of impending convulsions (headache, epigastric pain, and hyperreflexia) are indications for termination of pregnancy. Persistence of hemoconcentration, increasing hyperuricemia, and proteinuria may be signs that the fetus is in jeopardy. Obstetricians have an armamentarium of tests to evaluate fetal well-being, certain patterns of fetal heart rhythm recordings being among the most reliable indication of fetal jeopardy.

Treatment of the Acute Hypertensive Crisis

There is controversy concerning how aggressively acute hypertension near term should be treated. Some authorities believe that reductions in maternal blood pressure tend to decrease uteroplacental perfusion, and caution against large or precipitous decrements in mean arterial pressure, because placental blood flow is already compromised in preeclampsia. Others believe that uteroplacental blood flow autoregulates appropriately and

TABLE 1 Guidelines for Treating Severe Hypertension Near Term or During Labor

The degree to which blood pressure should be decreased is disputed. Levels between 90 and 105 mm Hg diastolic are recommended.

- Hydralazine administered intravenously is the drug of choice. Use low doses (start with 5 mg, then give 5 to 10 mg every 20 to 30 minutes) in order to avoid precipitous decreases. Side effects include tachycardia and headache. Neonatal thrombocytopenia has been reported.
- Diazoxide is recommended for the occasional patient whose hypertension is refractory to hydralazine. Use 30-mg mini-boluses, since maternal vascular collapse and death have been associated with the customary 300-mg dose. Side effects include arrest of labor and neonatal hyperglycemia.
- Experience with parenteral labetalol is growing, and this drug may replace diazoxide as the second-line drug.
- Favorable results have been reported with calcium-channel blockers. However, if magnesium sulfate is being infused, the magnesium ion may potentiate the effect of calcium-channel blockers, resulting in precipitous and severe hypotension.
- Do not use sodium nitroprusside (fetal cyanide poisoning has been reported in animals), or loop diuretics (e.g., furosemide) (see text). However, in the final analysis, maternal well-being will dictate the choice of therapy.

Parenteral magnesium sulfate is the drug of choice for preventing impending eclamptic convulsions. Therapy should continue for 12 (and sometimes 24) hours into the puerperium, since one-third of patients with preeclampsia have convulsions after childbirth.

Reprinted with permission from Lindheimer MD, Katz AI. Hypertension in pregnancy. N Engl J Med 1985; 313:675–680.

TABLE 2 Antihypertensive Drugs for the Treatment of Chronic Hypertension During Pregnancy

α_1-Receptor agonists	Methyldopa is the most extensively used drug of this group; its safety and efficacy have been supported in randomized trials. Follow-up studies of children born to mothers who received methyldopa revealed normal physical and mental development up to 10 years of age.
β-Receptor antagonists	These agents, especially atenolol and metoprolol, have undergone considerable testing and appear to be safe and efficacious if used in late pregnancy. However, intrauterine growth retardation has been noted when the drug is started in early midgestation. Fetal bradycardia has also been reported, and animal data suggest the possibility of a decreased ability of the fetus to tolerate hypoxic stress.
α- and β-Receptor antagonists	Labetalol appears to be as effective as methyldopa. A possible association with retroplacental hemorrhage is under investigation.
Arteriolar vasodilators	Hydralazine is used frequently as adjunctive therapy with methyldopa and β-receptor antagonists. Neonatal thrombocytopenia has been reported. There has been only limited experience with minoxidil, and therefore this agent is not recommended at present. Trials with calcium-channel blockers during pregnancy look promising.
Converting-enzyme inhibitors	Captopril, which causes fetal death in several animal species, has been associated with renal failure in the newborn when administered to humans. Do not use in pregnancy.
Diuretics	Many authorities discourage their use, though some continue these medications if they were prescribed before gestation. The latter view has been endorsed by a National Institutes of Health consensus group.
Miscellaneous	Serotonin antagonists (e.g., ketanserin) are currently under investigation. Do not use ganglion-blocking agents.

Modified with permission from Lindheimer MD, Katz AL. Hypertension in pregnancy. N Engl J Med 1985; 313:675–680.

prefer a more aggressive approach in treating the hypertension. Data from studies in human beings are scarce, but there are documented instances in which precipitous reductions in blood pressure were accompanied by signs of fetal distress, even when diastolic levels remained at or above 80 mm Hg. Thus, when treating acute elevations of blood pressure in late pregnancy or during labor, we recommend an intermediate approach (see Table 1) in which antihypertensive agents are withheld as long as maternal pressure is only mildly elevated. When diastolic pressure is 105 mm Hg or higher, parenteral hydralazine is given cautiously and is successful in most instances. Diazoxide administered in small doses (30 mg boluses) or labetalol (20 mg IV) is restricted to the occasional resistant case. Successes have been recorded when calcium-channel blockers (e.g., oral nifedipine) have been used, and in 1990 this group of drugs was undergoing extensive testing. Despite anecdotal reports of the usefulness of sodium nitroprusside, this agent should be avoided because cyanide poisoning and fetal death have been observed in laboratory animals. In the last analysis, however, the mother's well-being should take precedence even if the therapy necessary to control pressure may potentially harm the fetus.

Magnesium sulfate is the drug of choice in North America for impending convulsions or frank eclampsia, although its use evokes controversy. The mode of action of magnesium sulfate is poorly understood, but as a result of empiric success, it remains the standard by which all others must be assessed.

Magnesium sulfate is administered parenterally either by intramuscular or intravenous injections. In the former regimen, a loading injection of 20 ml of 20 percent magnesium sulfate solution (4 g) is first given intravenously at the rate of 1 g per minute, immediately followed by 20 ml of 50 percent magnesium sulfate solution, half (5 g) of which is injected into each buttock through a 3-inch-long, 20-gauge needle. Every 4 hours thereafter, 10 ml of a 50 percent solution (5 g) is similarly injected intramuscularly into alternate buttocks, after ascertaining that the patellar reflex is present, respirations are not depressed, and urine flow was above 100 ml during the preceding 4 hours.

An intravenous regimen is used at the University of Chicago's Lying-in Hospital. A loading dose of 4 to 6 g of magnesium sulfate in a 10 percent solution is infused over a 10-minute period (it must never be given as a bolus), after which a sustaining solution of 24 g of magnesium sulfate in 1 liter of 5 percent dextrose solution is delivered at a rate of 1 g per hour. Blood levels of magnesium and deep tendon reflexes are monitored, and the infusion rate may be increased to 2 g per hour if the patient remains hyperreflexic or if plasma magnesium levels remain below 5 mg per deciliter. Once levels exceed 9.5 mg per deciliter, however, the drug is more likely to lead to respiratory and cardiac depression. In such instances the infusion should be decreased or temporarily stopped with the aim of maintaining levels between 5 and 9.5 mg per deciliter throughout labor. Following delivery magnesium sulfate treatment is usually continued for 12 to 24 hours, depending on the clinical severity of the preeclampsia. A vial of calcium gluconate should be kept at the bedside as an antidote for the sudden appearance of magnesium toxicity.

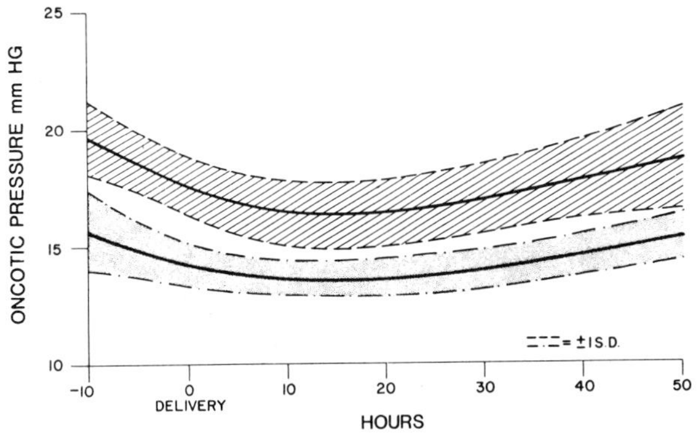

Figure 1 Intrapartum and postpartum plasma colloid oncotic pressure in nine normotensive gravidas (upper curve) and nine severe preeclamptics (lower curve). (From Zinaman M, Rubin J, Lindheimer MD. Serial plasma oncotic pressure levels and echoencephalography during and after delivery in severe preeclampsia. Lancet 1985; 1:1245-1247. Reprinted with permission.)

Volume Expansion

The literature contains claims that volume expansion may reduce blood pressure during preeclampsia and currently there are advocates for the use of such therapy in selected patients. This approach has been prompted by repeated observations that many preeclamptics present with decreased cardiac output, central venous and pulmonary capillary wedge pressures, and occasionally have postpartum vascular collapse. It has also been noted that hemodilution precedes the occasional improvement in hospitalized patients before delivery. In one well-documented study the rapid replenishment of intravascular volume with a commercial stable-protein substitute decreased blood pressure for periods of 24 hours or more in third trimester hypertensives. The authors further demonstrated that the decrement in pressure coincided with an increase in plasma volume. While the results appear impressive, most of the patients under study had only mild disease, and a review of available documentation by other authors who have used volume expansion reveals equivocal or unconvincing results.

Currently we recommend against "volume expansion" in preeclampsia for the following reasons: Myocardial performance may be compromised in severe cases, and volume expansion (especially with saline) may enhance vascular reactivity. Furthermore, the infusion of crystalloids alone decreases oncotic pressure (which is already markedly decreased in preeclampsia) and this can lead to pulmonary and cerebral edema, especially after childbirth when plasma oncotic levels decrease further (Fig. 1) while central volume and pressures tend to rise. Our current recommendations therefore are to minimize crystalloid infusions into preeclamptic women in labor (goal should be <75 ml per hour). Most problems of apparent poor renal perfusion will resolve quickly postpartum, and if fluid therapy does seem necessary, a colloid infusion is preferable and should be given concurrently with hemodynamic monitoring (i.e., a central venous pressure line).

Anticoagulation and Antiplatelet Therapy

Past reports on the use of heparin or aspirin in the management of preeclampsia have been contradictory, the majority showing these drugs to have limited efficacy at best. Also, administration of anticoagulants to patients with frank hypertension and a disease sometimes complicated by cerebral bleeding or subcapsular liver hematomas appears to us too hazardous, especially when other approaches succeed. In one instance, the latter complication occurred insidiously in a gravida under our care who received anticoagulants for thrombophlebitis and had begun to manifest minimal signs of preeclampsia.

It has been recently suggested that a combination of antiplatelet agents can prevent preeclampsia if started early in pregnancy. Some investigators report mounting evidence that low-dose aspirin, which decreases thromboxane but spares prostacyclin production, may prevent preeclampsia. Others, believing that hypertension is related to low dietary calcium, are investigating whether supplemental calcium will prevent preeclampsia.

Special Considerations

Monitoring of central venous or pulmonary capillary wedge pressures may be required in severe or complicated cases, especially during operative procedures. It is our experience, however, that the need for Swan-Ganz catheterization (a procedure that causes a certain morbidity) during preeclampsia is uncommon, and virtually all cases of preeclampsia can be managed using clinical acumen and an occasional central venous catheter. Patients with marked coagulation changes and severe right upper quadrant pain should be considered for ultrasonographic or (postpartum) computed tomographic scanning of the liver which may reveal subcapsular hemorrhages that can rupture and produce an acute emergency.

CHRONIC HYPERTENSION IN THE ABSENCE OF PREECLAMPSIA

There is a great deal of literature documenting the increased risk associated with pregnancy in women with chronic hypertension. Complications include superimposed preeclampsia, accelerated rise of pressure to a malignant phase, placental abruption, acute renal tubular and cortical necrosis, intrauterine growth retardation, and midtrimester fetal death. Such events seem to correlate with the age of the gravida and the duration of her high blood pressure. Thus the majority of these complications occur in women 30 years of age or over, or in those whose preexistent hypertension has caused end organ damage (primarily nephrosclerosis). On the other hand, more than 85 percent of patients with essential hypertension have uncomplicated gestations.

Women with chronic essential hypertension often manifest reductions in blood pressure by midpregnancy which may exceed those observed in normotensive gravidas. In fact, failure of this decrement to occur or increments in blood pressure in early pregnancy or midtrimester portends a reserved prognosis.

Fetal outcome is poorer in hypertensive women with superimposed preeclampsia than in previously normotensive women with this complication, and it is the combination of chronic hypertension and preeclampsia that seems responsible for most cases of cerebral hemorrhage in pregnancy. As was the case for previously normotensive patients, the marked increase in morbid events is due primarily to the specific pathophysiology of preeclampsia. This includes marked increments in pressor responsiveness to infused angiotensin weeks before the appearance of clinical manifestations of superimposed disease such as coagulation changes, liver function abnormalities, or both.

As was the case for women with pure preeclampsia, the gravida with chronic hypertension and superimposed disease must be hospitalized and her hypertension controlled. A substantial number of these patients present between the 25th and 30th gestational weeks and the wish to temporize may be strong. However, the fetal prognosis of chronic hypertensives with early third trimester superimposed preeclampsia is quite poor, and many clinicians consider delaying actions too risky for maternal well-being; thus most terminate the gestation.

There is controversy about whether women with mild blood pressure elevations should be treated during pregnancy, and a National Institutes of Health consensus group has recently recommended withholding treatment until diastolic levels exceed 100 mm Hg.

The use of antihypertensive agents in pregnancy is summarized in Table 2. It is only in the past decade that efforts have been made to determine the efficacy and safety of these drugs in pregnant women. Many of the published studies are limited in scope and often were performed at the request and with the support of pharmaceutical companies. There is a critical need for large, multicenter clinical trials using the combined services of obstetricians, hypertension specialists, epidemiologists, and statisticians. Currently methyldopa, on occasion combined with hydralazine, is the drug most often used in the United States. This medication has been administered to gravidas for several decades and is thus considered "safe" in pregnancy, and it has been demonstrated to be effective in a meticulously performed controlled trial. Several beta-adrenoceptor antagonists, and the combined alpha- and beta-blocking agent labetalol (see Table 2) have also undergone trials and are used more frequently. These drugs have the advantage of being administered but once or twice daily, which facilitates patient compliance. However, beta-blocking agents cross the placenta and cause fetal bradycardia, thus restricting the value of alterations in fetal heart rate in evaluating the course of labor. They may also cause growth retardation. Experimental studies suggest that beta-blocking agents may compromise the ability of the fetus to tolerate hypoxic stress, and one investigator has suggested that labetalol may be associated with retroplacental bleeding. It is for reasons such as these that we continue to use methyldopa as our primary drug in treating chronic hypertension in pregnancy.

Diuretics

There is controversy concerning the use of diuretics during gestation, and currently most obstetricians avoid their use in pregnant women. These drugs were once used "prophylactically" to avoid preeclampsia, but results of a meta-analysis of those trials suggest that diuretic agents have only marginal benefits, although they are apparently harmless.

Saluretic drugs are successful in mobilizing edema fluid, but it is unclear whether such therapy influences favorably the course of pure or superimposed preeclampsia. It remains to be established whether the normal increments in maternal extracellular volume are required for optimal uteroplacental perfusion, but some investigators claim that diuretics limit the "physiological hypervolemia" of pregnancy and are associated with decreased weight of the neonate. As already noted, cardiac output, intravascular volume, and central venous as well as pulmonary capillary wedge pressures are low in many hypertensive gravidas. Thus saluretic agents should not be used as the initial treatment of these patients, because mobilization of the intravascular fluid may conceivably decrease cardiac output further and compromise placental perfusion.

Although we do not recommend the use of diuretics during gestation, there are two exceptions. First, they should be used in gravid women with heart disease, for the same indications as in nonpregnant women. Second, we occasionally prescribe diuretics for women with chronic hypertension refractory to antiadrenergic agents and vasodilators (especially if the refractoriness appears due to excessive sodium retention secondary to the antihypertensive agent's action), in particular when the fetus is immature and termination of the pregnancy is the only alternative.

HYPERTENSION IN THE ELDERLY

GEORGE L. BAKRIS, M.D., F.A.C.P.
EDWARD D. FROHLICH, M.D., F.A.C.C.

Two types of hypertension exist in the elderly population. Those are isolated systolic hypertension, defined by the Joint National Committees Fourth Report (1988) as a systolic pressure greater than 139 mm Hg with a diastolic pressure of less than 90 mm Hg, and diastolic hypertension, defined as a pressure of greater than or equal to 90 mm Hg.

Patients older than 60 years of age with systolic hypertension have a lower cardiac output and left ventricular ejection fraction with a significant increase total peripheral resistance when compared to age-matched controls. In addition, this population has a more contracted intravascular plasma volume compared to controls. Moreover, systolic hypertension is a disease that involves reduced large vessel compliance in conjunction with these preceding factors. Diastolic hypertension in elderly patients has a pathophysiology similar to those younger than age 60. Studies have shown, however, that older populations have an increased total peripheral and renal vascular resistance as well as left ventricular mass. Furthermore, since this population has a greater likelihood of occlusive atherosclerotic disease, unilateral or bilateral renal artery stenosis may elevate de novo hypertension or exacerbate already existing hypertension.

THERAPEUTIC ALTERNATIVES

Numerous studies have shown that lowering arterial pressure below a level of 140/90 mm Hg yields a significant decrease in cardiovascular as well as cerebral morbidity and mortality. When dietary sodium restriction($\leq$2 g per day) alone does not adequately reduce arterial pressure to an acceptable level ($\leq$140/90 mm Hg), addition of various antihypertensive agents will serve to further potentiate these pressure reductions. These agents include diuretics, calcium antagonists, angiotensin converting enzyme (ACE) inhibitors, central alpha-adrenoreceptor agonists (e.g., methyldopa, clonidine), and beta-adrenoreceptor blockers. Any one of these agents is effective for reducing both isolated systolic as well as diastolic hypertension in the elderly. However, with the available therapeutic armamentarium in the 1990s one should consider the coexistence of other pathophysiologic conditions such as peripheral vascular disease, lung disease, heart or kidney disease, as well as a history of previous strokes before prescribing antihypertensive medications for this population.

Diuretics, although effective for lowering arterial pressure in the elderly and relatively inexpensive, may be associated with certain adverse metabolic effects that may mitigate their use in certain patients. These agents should be used with caution for patients with hyperlipidemias, gout, and diabetes mellitus or those prone to cardiac arrhythmias. In addition, various antihypertensive agents have other untoward effects that may limit their tolerance by this population. These include sedation and orthostatic hypotension by the central α-adrenoreceptor agonists and exacerbation of pulmonary or peripheral vascular disease by β-adrenoreceptor antagonists. Both the calcium antagonists and, however, are efficacious in lowering arterial pressure in the elderly without adverse metabolic effects. Therefore, it has now become possible for physicians to tailor antihypertensive therapy for each patient, taking into account their particular set of problems rather than routinely prescribing one medication for all patients.

PREFERRED APPROACH

Medical Treatment

Isolated Systolic and Combined Diastolic Hypertension Without End Organ Dysfunction

Epidemiologic studies have shown that reduction of arterial pressure in the elderly may be achieved with any antihypertensive agent regardless of whether it is isolated systolic or diastolic hypertension. Preliminary data from the Systolic Hypertension in the Elderly Patients Study (SHEPs) have demonstrated that low dose thiazide diuretics (i.e., 12.5 to 25 mg per day) adequately reduces elevated systolic pressures to normal levels. However, the definitive long-term study to assess risks versus benefits of this therapy is still in progress. Nevertheless, the Medical Research Council trial suggested that there is benefit in treating such patients.

Diuretics lower arterial pressure primarily by increasing urinary sodium excretion and reducing extracellular fluid volumes; and this may promote, in elderly patients with poor oral intake of fluids, a volume-contracted state. This could then result in significant prerenal azotemia, orthostatic hypotension, and tachycardia, thereby overshadowing the beneficial effects of the antihypertensive drug. Furthermore, diuretics may provoke certain metabolic effects including: elevation of serum cholesterol, triglycerides, and low density lipoprotein cholesterol; hypokalemia and possible consequent cardiac dysrhythmias; inhibition of insulin release that may increase blood glucose by 10 to 15 percent; and lastly, inhibition of uric acid secretion by the renal tubule thereby increasing serum uric acid levels and precipitating a gouty attack in predisposed individuals.

In general, we employ diuretics in elderly who are either volume-expanded or those who are already receiving other antihypertensive agents in order to enhance their effectiveness. We would also employ diuretics in patients with cardiac or renal insufficiency as well as elderly subjects with hypoalbuminemia associated with massive proteinuria or cirrhosis. The thiazides are prescribed for patients without impaired renal function (i.e., serum creatinine of $\leq$1.6 mg per deciliter) and are started in doses of 12.5 mg per day and can be increased to a maximum of 25 mg daily. In contrast, loop diuretics (i.e., fuorsemide or bumetanide) are more effective in patients with renal insufficiency (i.e., serum creatinine of $\geq$1.7 mg per deciliter) in doses of 40 to 80 mg or 2 to 4 mg, respectively, once or twice daily.

The calcium antagonists are all equally efficacious in reducing both isolated systolic as well as diastolic pressures. Furthermore, they are available in sustained release formulations and can, therefore, be given conveniently in once or twice daily doses. We generally start therapy with sustained released verapamil (120 to 240 mg daily), sustained-release diltiazem (90 mg twice daily) or sustained-release nifedipine (30 mg daily) as single agents. These long-acting preparations are not as frequently associated with significant side effects when compared to conventional dosing. Furthermore, some calcium antagonists decrease myocardial oxygen demand and are more beneficial in states of cardiac and renal functional impairment. The dosage of these medications, as with all medications in the elderly, should be governed by the rule, "start low and go slow." The reasons for this adage are summarized in Table 1. The more prominent side effects of these agents include constipation for verapamil; headache, orthostatic hypotension, and peripheral edema for nifedipine; and nausea or mild peripheral edema with diltiazem. As their doses are increased the side effects may become more prominent.

TABLE 1 Factors Affecting Drug Disposition in Elderly Patients

Age-Related Decreases in Physiologic Parameters	*Pathologic Condition*
Absorption	
Absorptive surface	Diarrhea
Gastrointestinal motility	Malabsorption syndromes
Volume of Distribution	
Cardiac output	Congestive heart failure
Total body water	Dehydration
Lean body mass	Edema or ascites
Serum albumin	Hepatic failure
Metabolism	
Hepatic blood flow	Congestive heart failure
Excretion	
Renal blood flow	Hypovolemia
Glomerular filtration rate	Renal insufficiency
Tubular secretion	Renal insufficiency

Angiotensin converting enzyme inhibitors, like the calcium antagonists, are relatively devoid of metabolic side effects and are effective in reducing arterial pressure in the elderly. Their initial starting doses and side effects are noted in Table 2. In general, these agents have not been employed in initial therapy of elderly hypertensive patients because in our experience and that of others they may not be as effective as the calcium antagonists or diuretics in patients with low renin states. We frequently add a diuretic to potentiate the antihypertensive effects of ACE inhibitors, especially in isolated systolic hypertension. Moreover, they may also be employed as second drugs when a calcium antagonist or another agent fails to control pressure adequately or if adverse effects are experienced.

The β-adrenoreceptor blockers reduce arterial pressure in the elderly, and they are of particular value in those patients with a previous myocardial infarction. Those agents with intrinsic sympathomimetic activity (ISA), e.g. pindolol or acebutalol, however, may not protect against a second myocardial infarction, but may be used in patients in which bradycardia limits the use of non-ISA compounds.

The central α-adrenoreceptor agonists (methyldopa, clonidine) are effective in controlling pressure in both isolated systolic and diastolic hypertension. However, they may be associated with adverse reactions, the most frequent of which are sedation, dry mouth, and sexual dysfunction. We start with doses of 250 mg or 0.1 mg twice daily for methyldopa or clonidine, respectively. We infrequently use the postganglionic neuronal inhibitors (e.g., guanethidine, guanabenz) or the α-adrenoreceptor antagonists (e.g., prazosin or terazosin) in the elderly patient because of its most frequent side effect of postural hypotension.

TABLE 2 A Comparison of Angiotensin Converting Enzyme Inhibitors in the Elderly

	Captopril	*Enalapril*	*Lisinopril*
Dosage (mg)*	6.25–25 bid	5–30 qd	10–40 qd
Elimination	Renal	Renal	Renal
Pro Drug	No	Yes (converted to enalaprilat by liver)	No
Adverse Effects	Cough Angioedema Renal Insufficiency Hyperkalemia Dysgeusia Skin Rashes	Cough Angioedema Renal Insufficiency Hyperkalemia	Cough Angioedema Renal Insufficiency Hyperkalemia

*Dose should be adjusted in patients with renal failure

Arterial Hypertension with Myocardial Dysfunction

Patients with either left ventricular hypertrophy or moderately impaired cardiac function defined as a an ejection fraction of ≤35 percent are at significant risk for a cardiac event. In the absence of poor myocardial contractility in this population, we generally use the calcium antagonist diltiazem since it tends to have less negative inotropic effects. In addition, low doses of a thiazide controls expanded intravascular volume. If these agents fail to adequately control arterial pressure, the ACE inhibitors (i.e., lisinopril or enalapril) 10 or 20 mg daily, respectively, or captopril 12.5 mg twice daily are used. Furthermore, the shorter-acting ACE inhibitor, captopril, does not exacerbate preexisting renal insufficiency in patients with congestive heart failure when compared to longer-acting preparations. Both classes of agents (calcium antagonists and ACE inhibitors) reduce left ventricular mass and may improve myocardial function, particularly in the patient with prior left ventricular decompensation. If neither of these agents fail to control arterial pressure, the calcium antagonist and ACE inhibitor may be used together or a central α-adrenoreceptor agonist may be added. In patients with impaired left ventricular function, we avoid antihypertensive agents that have negative iontropic effects such as β-adrenoreceptor blockers or certain calcium antagonists in favor of an ACE inhibitor, and not infrequently a loop diuretic is added to improve volume status. Remember, in patients with cardiac failure there is a state of secondary aldosteronism; and, if an ACE inhibitor is utilized, one must be careful of inducing hyperkalemia if potassium supplements are also used.

Arterial Hypertension with Renal Dysfunction

Numerous elderly patients have renal dysfunction secondary to long-standing hypertension, diabetes mellitus, or mild congestive heart failure. In these patients, we first assess their volume status. Patients with severe hypoalbuminemia (albumin ≤2.0) generally have intravascular volume contraction unless there is significant associated myocardial dysfunction. These patients require a loop diuretic to improve volume status. In addition, when an ACE inhibitor is used, a reduction of arterial pressure and urinary protein excretion is to be expected. In patients with proteinuria secondary to diabetic nephropathy, who also have type IV renal tubular acidosis or in patients who cannot take ACE inhibitors, a calcium antagonist (e.g., diltiazem, 90 mg twice daily) may be of particular value. We select diltiazem since, in a recent clinical study by Bakris (1990), it was as efficacious as ACE inhibitors for reducing proteinuria in diabetic patients. Recent evidence also suggests that verapamil has similar antiproteinuric effects to ACE inhibitors. In patients who are not hypersensitive to ACE inhibitors or who do not have type IV renal tubular acidosis, we frequently add a calcium antagonist to the ACE inhibitor (or vice versa) if pressure is not adequately controlled. Under this circumstance, we have demonstrated an additive effect on lowering urinary protein excretion as well as improved volume homeostasis. It is important to evaluate every patient with renal functional impairment for the real possibility of bilateral renal artery stenosis so that the adverse effect of further loss of renal function produced by ACE inhibitors. Even after initiation of therapy with this important precaution, we continue to check blood chemistries within 1 week for renal functional deterioration and then periodically to be sure that serum potassium and creatinine have not risen significantly; this is further evidence to suggest bilateral renal artery stenosis.

SUGGESTED READING

Bakris GL, Frohlich ED. Hypertension in the elderly: Rationale for therapy. In: Maldenado M, ed. Hypertension and renal disease in the elderly. Boston: Blackwell Scientific, in press.

Frohlich ED. Hypertension in the elderly. In: Cassel C, Walsh E, Reisenberg D, Sorenson L, eds. Geriatric medicine. New York: Springer Verlag, 1990:141.

Joint National Committee—The 1988 Report of the Joint National Committee on Detection, Evolution and Treatment of High Blood Pressure. Arch Intern Med 1988; 148:1023.
Kannel WB. Blood pressure and the development of cardiovascular disease in the aged. In: Chaird FI, Dall J, Kennedy RD, eds. Cardiology and old age. New York: Plenum Press, 1976:127.
Kawanamoto A, Shimada K, Matsubayashi K, et al. Cardiovascular regulatory functions in the elderly patients with hypertension. Hypertension 1989; 13:401.
Perry HM Jr, McDonald RH, Halley SB, et al. Pilot study (SHEP-PS): Morbidity and mortality experience. J Hypertens 1986; 4(suppl 6):521.
Strassen J, Fagard R, VanHoff R, Amery A. Mortality in various intervention trials in elderly hypertensive patients. A review. Eur Heart J 1988; 9:215.

HYPERTENSION IN CHRONIC RENAL FAILURE, DIALYSIS, AND/OR TRANSPLANTATION

JAMES F. WINCHESTER, M.D., F.R.C.P.(Glas)

Systemic hypertension is the most important factor contributing to the decline in renal function and to the development of cardiovascular disease in patients with chronic renal parenchymal disease, both in the predialysis phase, as well as after initiation of dialysis or after a successful renal allograft. Since the kidney is the central organ controlling blood pressure, by virture of its regulatory control of vascular tone and central blood volume, arterial hypertension is an almost constant feature in chronic renal failure from all causes. In patients who are dehydrated, or have "salt-losing" nephropathy (in some patients with tubulointerstitial renal disease), hypertension may be absent. In most renal diseases, however, as renal function deteriorates, hypertension supervenes, along with failure of regulatory and compensatory machanisms of vasopressor and vasodepressor responses, as well as sodium–fluid control. Additionally, systemic hypertension, by producing renal vascular lesions, contributes to the progression of ischemia of the juxtaglomerular apparatus (which stimulates secretion of renin, to further exacerbate renal ischemia), and eventually to vascular narrowing, glomerular obstruction, and sclerosis.

Evidence indicates that control of hypertension slows the progression of certain renal diseases (diabetes mellitus, chronic glomerulonephritis, and primary hypertensive nephrosclerosis), as well as reduces the complications of hypertension, such as congestive heart failure, stroke, and diabetic retinopathy. Although hypertension complicating renal disease is more difficult to control than in patients without primary renal disease, with the advent of modern therapeutic drugs, adequate control of blood pressure is now easily within the grasp of the physician.

FREQUENCY AND PATHOPHYSIOLOGY OF HYPERTENSION IN RENAL DISEASE, DIALYSIS, OR TRANSPLANTATION

Renal disease is responsible for 5 to 7 percent of all cases of hypertension in the community, while essential hypertension (92 percent) and endocrine factors account for the rest. Even in essential hypertension the kidney may have a pivotal etiologic role, but this is more clearly defined in primary renal disease. Hypertension is present in 80 percent of patients with chronic renal failure initiating dialysis, and in about 70 percent of those with tubulointerstitial renal disease; the incidence is even higher in glomerular and polycystic renal disease, and almost invariable in diabetic nephropathy and nephrosclerosis. Accelerated hypertension with grade III or IV hypertensive retinal changes (today quite erroneously called "malignant hypertension") may occur frequently (10 to 20 percent) in patients with renal hypertension, and is more frequent in patients without primary renal disease, but with renal artery stenosis.

Many factors influence blood pressure control in the patient with renal disease, to produce hypertension. In end-stage renal disease sodium retention (and consequent intravascular volume increase) is more frequently responsible for hypertension (80 percent) than is renin-dependency (20 percent) (Table 1). It has been appreciated that even early in the course of renal disease, alteration of hemodynamics occurs, with cardiac output as well as total peripheral resistance increasing; since these changes are physiologically abnormal, hypertension results in patients who do not increase vascular compliance to compensate.

Recently it has been demonstrated that hormonal factors also may be important in the pathogenesis of hypertension in renal disease, ranging from reduction of vasodilators (kallikrein, prostacyclin) to elevation of vasoconstrictors (angiotensin II, thromboxane), although their precise role (excluding angiotensin II) is not well defined at present. Other factors, such as high total exchangeable sodium and decreased response to catecholamines, calcium, etc., may also be important. The main factors in the pathogenesis of hypertension in patients with renal

TABLE 1 Pathogenetic Factors in Hypertension Complicating Chronic Renal Failure and Dialysis

	CRF	*Dialysis*	
Increased		C	UC
Extracellular fluid	+	+	Normal or low
Plasma volume	+	+	Normal or low
Total Na	+	+	low
Renin, angiotensin II	+	Normal	++
Total peripheral resistance	+	Normal	++
Cardiac output (early in CRF*)	+	Normal	Low
Baroreceptor dysfunction	+	+	+
Catecholamines	+	+	+
Decreased			
Vasodilators	+	+	+
Bradykinin	+	+	+
Prostaglandins	+	+	+
Other			
Vascular abnormalities	?		
Calcium	?		

CRF =chronic renal failure;
UC =uncontrollable, C =controllable hypertension by dialysis.

disease are: diseased native kidneys, allograft rejection (acute or chronic), renal insufficiency, acute ureteral obstruction, recurrence of original disease in transplant, de novo glomerulonephritis, persistence of original hypertension, genetic predisposition to hypertension, volume expansion, antirejection therapy (steroids, cyclosporine), and transplant renal artery stenosis.

In the renal transplant recipient many of the factors operative prior to transplant remain important, but several new factors become operative. The incidence of hypertension following transplantation ranges from 20 to 80 percent, but is usually between 40 and 50 percent. Hypertension arises de novo in 15 percent of patients without pretransplant hypertension, and is relieved (probably by normalized sodium and water balance) in 30 to 40 percent of transplant recipients. Recent reports strongly link the presence of diseased native kidneys to the prevalence and severity of hypertension in transplant recipients, and benefits of native nephrectomy to control of hypertension. The prevalence of hypertension in transplant patients is relatively constant with time after transplant, but is higher in the first 3 months (due partly to the higher steroid dosage used in this early phase) and in cadaveric allograft recipients. Cyclosporine is also associated with hypertension, but the mechanism(s) by which it produces hypertension is unknown, although nephrotoxicity of cyclosporine and its effects on renal prostaglandins have been suggested. It remains to be seen whether the hypertension associated with cyclosporine will persist in the long term.

During rejection, hypertension occurs. Since thromboxane is released during rejection, it is conceivable that the local and systemic effects of thromboxane, coupled with acute sodium and water retention, may produce the rise in blood pressure seen during a rejection crisis. As in primary renal disease, continued hypertension results in reduction of renal function and hypertension in the renal transplant patient, and is also associated with reduced kidney function and graft survival. However, in these hypertensive subjects, initial graft function is poorer than in the nonhypertensive transplant recipient.

PHARMACOLOGIC PRINCIPLES OF ANTIHYPERTENSIVE AGENTS USED IN RENAL DISEASE

Nonpharmacologic methods (apart from sodium restriction) are of no use in the management of hypertension in the patient with chronic renal failure. Modern therapeutic drugs have considerably improved and eased the control of hypertension in this group of patients. However, some drugs may influence changes in renal hemodynamics (Table 2), and therefore renal function, while others may produce immunologic glomerular lesions (captopril), or interstitial nephritis with or without gout (thiazides, furosemide). It is therefore worthwhile for the nephrologist to become familiar with the mode of action and dosage alterations necessary in the face of reduced renal function for certain drugs used in the treatment of hypertension in chronic renal failure (Table 3). Additionally, sudden withdrawal of drugs may be hazardous, as may drug interactions (Table 4). The following section will outline the major pharmacologic agents used in this regard.

Diuretics

Diuretics are the agents most often used in renal disease patients to control hypertension as well as the edema complicating nephrotic syndrome or fluid retention of renal disease, or after renal transplantation. They are inexpensive, efficacious, have manageable side effects, and most importantly have synergistic activity with most of the other antihypertensive agents.

Thiazides (e.g., *hydrochlorothiazide*, 50 to 100 mg per day; *metolazone* 5 mg per day), which act by reducing plasma volume initially, but later by reducing total peripheral vascular resistance, are particularly useful in treating hypertension complicating mild to moderate renal failure. However, whereas hydrochlorothiazide loses its effectiveness at a glomerular filtration rate (GFR) of less than 10 ml per minute, metolazone may retain some diuretic activity. In general, however, thiazides and metolazone lose effect or have less effect at a GFR of less than 30 ml per minute, and loop diuretics (*furosemide, bumetanide, ethacrynic acid*), which are more potent natriuretic agents, may be required.

Potassium-sparing diurectics (*spironolactone, triamterene,* and *amiloride*) may be useful in patients receiving high-dose diuretics or those who have secondary hyperaldosteronism (spironolactone), but great caution should be exercised in the use of these agents, since in the presence of renal failure, hyperkalemia and its attendant dangers may occur. This is particularly likely to occur in patients with a GFR of less than 20 ml per minute, or with

TABLE 2 Antihypertensive Drugs Affecting Renal Function

Class	*Drug*	*Effect on Renal Blood Flow*	*Effect on Glomerular Filtration Rate*
Diuretic	Thiazide	None	None
	Furosemide	Increased	None
Central agent	Methyldopa	Reduced 8%	Reduced 13%
Adrenergic blocker	Guanethidine	Reduced	Reduced
Beta-blocker	Propranolol	Reduced	Reduced
	Nadolol	Increased	None
Vasodilator	Hydralazine	Increased	None
	Nitroprusside	Increased	None
ACE inhibitor	Captopril	Increased	None
	Enalapril		

diabetes mellitus, type IV renal tubular acidosis (hyporeninemic hypoaldosteronism), or catabolic states, in patients taking nonsteroidal anti-inflammatory agents or potassium supplements, and possibly in patients taking angiotensin-converting-enzyme inhibitors or beta-blockers.

Since the diuretics are excreted by the kidney, renal impairment slows their excretion, and consequently side effects are more common in this patient group. Common side effects are hypokalemia, hyperlipidemia (although this has recently been questioned), hyperuricemia, hyperglycemia, hypercalciuria (furosemide), hypercalcemia (thiazides), and ototoxicity (loop diuretics). The major side effect of potassium-sparing diuretics is hyperkalemia. Spironolactone may produce gynecomastia, skin rash, epigastric discomfort, hyperhidrosis, ataxia, and alopecia, while amiloride and triamterene can produce nausea, vomiting, muscle cramps, and dizziness. All three potassium sparers have been associated with reductions in GFR and elevations in blood urea nitrogen in patients with underlying renal disease.

Central Acting Agents

Methyldopa

The pharmacologic activity of methyldopa is poorly understood. It was hypothesized that methyldopa caused

TABLE 3 Antihypertensive Drugs for Which Dosage Reduction is Necessary in Chronic Renal Failure

Class	*Drug*	*Glomerular Filtration Rate* 50	30	< 10
Diuretic	Thiazide	None	Ineffective at GFR < 30	
	Metolazone	None	None	Ineffective
	K sparing	None	Contraindicated	
	Furosemide	None	Increase	Increase
Central agent	Methyldopa	None	Dose q 8–12hr	Dose q 12–24 hr
	Clonidine	Reduced	Reduced	Reduced
	Reserpine	None	None	None
	Guanabenz	None	None	None
Adrenergic blocker	Guanethidine	None	None	None
Beta-blocker	Propranolol	None	None	None
	Atenolol	None	Reduced 50%	Reduced 75%
	Timolol	None	None	Reduced
	Nadolol	None	Reduced50%	Reduced 70%
	Acebutolol	None	Reduced 50%	Reduced 75%
Beta-/alpha-blocker	Labetalol	None	None	None
Vasodilator	Hydralazine	None	None	Reduced
ACE inhibitor	Captopril	Reduced	Reduced	Reduced++
	Enalapril	None	Reduced 50%	Reduced 75%

TABLE 4 Drugs That Have Produced Hypertensive Crisis on Abrupt Withdrawal or Have Activity Blunted or Increased by Other Drugs

Produce Hypertension on Withdrawal	*Action Blunted or Increased by Other Drugs*
Diuretic (usually in combination)	Excess salt intake
Thiazide	Indomethacin
Furosemide	Oral Anticoagulants
Spironolactone	Salicylates
Central agent	
Methyldopa	Tricyclic antidepressants, propranolol
Clonidine	
Adrenergic blocker	
Guanethidine	Monoamine oxidase inhibitors, tricyclic antidepressants, chlorpromazine, amphetamines, and ephedrine (alcohol, alpha-, beta-blockers reserpine)
Bethanidine	
Alpha-/beta- blocker	
Labetalol	(Cimetidine increases bioavailability)
Beta-blocker	
Propranolol	Methyldopa, clonidine
Calcium channel blocker	
Nifedipine	(Beta-blocker occasionally)
Vasodilator	
Sodium nitroprusside	? Salicylates
Hydralazine	? Monoamine oxidase (MAO) inhibitors
ACE inhibitor	
Captopril	Indomethacin ? Salicylates
Enalapril	? Indomethacin
Antiangiotensin	
Saralasin	(Occasionally pressor)

either depletion of intracellular norepinephrine stores or formation of a false neurotransmitter, but it now appears that the most likely site of action is the stimulation of alpha$_2$ receptors in the brain stem vasomotor center by the active metabolite alpha-methylnorepinephrine. The plasma half-life of methyldopa doubles from the normal of 1.8 hours in the presence of renal failure, and dosage adjustment (dose or time of administration) is required. Methyldopa causes a 30 percent fall in peripheral resistance, a 10 percent fall in cardiac output, but also a reduction in renal vascular resistance which maintains renal blood flow and function. Tolerance to methyldopa occurs in 20 to 50 percent of patients owing to its antinatriuretic effects, especially in the presence of renal impairment, necessitating the concomitant use of diuretics.

Common side effects (15 to 50 percent) are sedation and orthostatic hypotension. Less common side effects are sexual dysfunction, depression, Coombs positive test (rarely Coombs positive hemolytic anemia), positive antinuclear antibody, and rarely thrombocytopenia, leukopenia, hepatitis, galactorrhea, and hyperpyrexia. All these side effects require discontinuation of the drug; however, caution should be exercised in discontinuing the drug, since rapid withdrawal has been associated with rebound hypertension (see Table 4). In addition, accelerated hypertension has been reported in a patient taking propranolol, as a result of possible drug interaction. The usual dosage regimen is 250 mg twice daily increasing to a maximum of 1,000 to 2,000 mg per day in divided doses at 12- to 24-hour intervals when renal function is severely impaired.

Clonidine

Clonidine given intravenously produces a brief rise and subsequent fall in blood pressure owing to direct stimulation of peripheral alpha-adrenergic receptors and later to stimulation of presynaptic alpha$_2$-adrenergic receptors in the medulla oblongata of the brain. Long-term reduction in blood pressure is associated with reduced discharge rate of preganglionic adrenergic nerves and bradycardia, because of both a decrease in sympathetic and an increase in vagal tone. Both plasma norepinephrine and plasma renin fall in the long term in patients receiving clonidine.

Elimination half-life is 8.5 hours; this is prolonged markedly in patients with renal failure, requiring dosage adjustment. GFR is usually reduced, but even when filtration is unaltered sodium excretion is also reduced. The most frequent side effects are dry mouth, sedation, and constipation. Impotence may also result and orthostatic hypotension is rare. Sodium and fluid retention occur and diuretic therapy may be required for optimal care.

Sudden withdrawal of clonidine may result in a hypertensive crisis within 8 to 12 hours after the last dose of chronic therapy, associated with a rise in catecholamines in plasma and urine. Treatment involves reinstitution of clonidine or alpha-adrenergic blockade with drugs such as phentolamine, or combined alpha–beta-blockers such as labetalol. Drug interaction occurs with tricyclic antidepressants, and clonidine should probably not be used in patients with depression.

The usual dose is 0.05 to 0.1 mg twice a day, increasing to a maximum of 0.15 to 0.3 mg twice a day orally. In certain patients the transdermal formulation of clonidine (TTS) may be used, with a patch of clonidine being applied to the skin for an entire week. When discontinuation of clonidine is necessary it should be done slowly over a period of a week. The maximum daily dose of 0.8 mg should be given in 2 divided doses and caution should be exercised at doses exceeding 1.0 mg per day.

Guanabenz

Guanabenz is an aminoguanidine which, like clonidine, stimulates alpha$_2$ receptors in the medullary brain stem. The result is reduction in peripheral sympathetic activity, and 20 percent reduction in renal plasma flow and

GFR which is not sustained after 1 week of therapy. Associated with this is a 10 percent increase in plasma volume which is sustained during chronic therapy. Less than 1 percent of the drug is excreted in the urine unchanged and the onset of hypertensive activity begins within 1 hour of a single oral dose.

Most of the work done on this drug has been done in patients with normal kidney function and little is known of its effects in renal insufficiency. It appears, however, that little or no dosage adjustment is necessary in patients with renal insufficiency, since the drug is mainly excreted through hepatic metabolism. Side effects are similar to those of clonidine, with drowsiness, dry mouth, and mild depression; sexual dysfunction and orthostatic hypotension are less common, and catecholamine excess rebound hypertension has also been reported with rapid withdrawal of this drug. Although an increase in plasma volume is reported, guanabenz appears to have less salt and fluid retention than either methyldopa or clonidine. The usual dose is 4 to 32 mg orally at 12-hour intervals.

Neuronal Uptake Inhibitors

Reserpine

Reserpine has been employed successfully for more than 3 decades for mild to moderate hypertension, but its use has decreased because of newer agents which possess more favorable side effect profiles and efficacy. Reserpine selectively inhibits the sympathetic nervous system by depletion of catecholamine stores of norepinephrine both peripherally and centrally. The antihypertensive effect is primarily mediated by peripheral sympathetic blockade, due to inhibition of norepinephrine reuptake at peripheral nerve endings, thereby exposing norepinephrine to monoamine oxidase. At the start of therapy with reserpine, particularly with large doses, there may be transient sympathomimetic responses, but with continued use a gradual reduction in total peripheral resistance and blood pressure often accompanied by bradycardia occurs. This is accompanied initially by a decrease in cardiac output, but this returns to pretreatment values over the long term, while total peripheral resistance remains reduced. Reserpine also has been shown to decrease renal blood flow and GFR, but again, with chronic therapy these variables return to pretreatment levels, although suppression of renin release is maintained.

Oral absorption of reserpine is rapid but incomplete with only 40 percent bioavailability. There is a biphasic distribution profile, and after oral dosing the onset of antihypertensive action may take a few days to weeks despite peak blood levels being observed within 1 to 3 hours. Following parenteral administration, however, the onset of effect is seen within 1 to 3 hours. Reserpine is extensively metabolized in the liver via hydrolysis and demethylation, and excretion of the drug has been shown to be slow in patients with impaired renal function, with an increase in the normal half-life (50 to 100 hours) being observed. This, however, is seen mainly in patients with a GFR less than 10 ml per minute.

The most frequent side effects are sedation, bradycardia, nasal congestion, impotence, and diarrhea. Sedation is due to reduction in norepinephrine, serotonin, and dopamine in the brain, and the patient may also complain of nightmares. Bradycardia is also seen in patients susceptible to congestive heart failure, which may be precipitated in bradycardic patients, especially in those with fluid retention due to reserpine. Particularly serious effects are mental depression, activation of peptic ulcer, and parkinsonism. Depression in particular is variable and may take 2 to 8 months to develop. The depression is treated by discontinuation of the drug, but symptoms may persist for several months thereafter—not surprisingly, since the duration of action of reserpine may be 1 to 6 weeks following discontinuation of oral therapy.

The usual dosage is 0.1 to 1.0 mg daily taken in 2 to 3 divided doses. Caution should be exercised at high doses in patients with renal insufficiency, and the drug is contraindicated in patients with a history of depression. The effects of reserpine are increased with concomitant diuretic administration.

Guanethidine

Guanethidine is used only in the treatment of severe therapy-resistant hypertension. Guanethidine is particularly effective when used with a diuretic, permitting a lower dosage, controlling sodium and fluid retention, and preventing tolerance which is a feature with this drug. Guanethidine depletes norepinephrine stores from neurosecretory granules of postganglionic sympathetic nerve endings. The result is a gradual reduction in blood pressure with bradycardia and decreased pulse pressure. Guanethidine is more effective in decreasing systolic pressure than diastolic, and this is associated with a slight decrease in or unchanged total peripheral resistance. Guanethidine may blunt positional cardiovascular reflexes, which in turn cause problems with postural and postexercise hypotension.

The drug has various effects on renal blood flow and GFR; the overall effects are usually clinically insignificant. Progression to azotemia or oliguria has not been found except in those patients with severely compromised renal function prior to therapy. Guanethidine appears to compromise renal function in the acute phase of therapy, but not with chronic therapy. Therefore, in the presence of compromised renal function, the drug should be used with caution. Guanethidine is associated with sodium and water retention and subsequent increase in plasma volume. An increase in peripheral renin concentrations occurs in those patients with decreased plasma renin prior to drug therapy. Plasma renin activity does not decrease with guanethidine therapy. As mentioned above, tolerance may develop in some patients on long-term therapy.

The major adverse affects of guanethidine are: bradycardia, dizziness, weakness, syncope, sexual dysfunction, nasal congestion, diarrhea, weakness, postural and postexercise hypotension, precipitation of cardiac failure in susceptible patients, edema, increased weight, and dyspnea due to sodium retention. It is therefore recommended that the drug be administered with a diuretic.

Fifty percent is excreted unchanged by the kidney, the rest being metabolized in the liver. Because of the long half-life (5 days), it can be administered once daily. Approximately 15 days are required for steady-state reduction in blood pressure following any dosage adjustment. Its therapeutic effects are antagonized by tricyclic antidepressants and chlorpromazine. The usual dose is 20 to 50 mg once daily, which may be increased to 100 mg if required. It is usually held in reserve for patients resistant to all other antihypertensive agents, and because of its effect on renal function it should be used with caution or not at all in patients with moderate to severe renal insufficiency.

Guanadrel

Guanadrel is similar to guanethidine, but has a shorter duration of action. As with guanethidine, the effect on blood pressure is greater in the standing than in the supine position. Peak plasma concentrations are achieved within 1.5 to 2 hours, and the elimination half-life is 10 hours with 85 percent elimination of the drug (40 percent unchanged) in the urine. Individual response to the drug is variable, but the tolerance and sodium retention induced by this drug are ameliorated by concomitant diuretic therapy. The usual dose is 2.5 mg twice a day to start, rising to 20 to 75 mg per day at 12-hour intervals. The same precautions should be taken as for guanethidine, and the side effect profile is similar.

Alpha-Receptor Blockers

Prazosin

Prazosin exerts its antihypertensive effect by vasodilation effected by direct vascular smooth muscle relaxation as well as alpha-adrenergic receptor blockade, which interferes with peripheral sympathetic function. A functional alpha-adrenoreceptor blockade occurs by virtue of the fact that prazosin blocks the postsynaptic $alpha_1$ receptors, but does not block the presynaptic $alpha_2$-adrenergic receptors. This allows more epinephrine to occupy the $alpha_2$ receptor site via a negative feedback mechanism to inhibit its own release. This may explain the lack of tachycardia, tolerance, and renin release associated with prazosin therapy. In patients with impaired GFR the drug has not been shown to affect renal function adversely nor does it increase plasma renin activity.

The drug is well absorbed but variable and is 90 percent protein bound. It is extensively metabolized in the liver by demethylation and its plasma half-life is 2.5 to 4 hours. Only 6 percent of the oral dose is excreted unchanged in the urine, and in conjunction with the high protein binding demonstrates that there is little need for alteration in drug dosage in patients with renal failure. On the other hand, patients with severely compromised renal function appear to be more sensitive to the effect of prazosin, and although no formal dosage guidelines are available, lower dosages should be used in such patients with careful titration of the dose. Prazosin exhibits a "first dose" hypotensive effect, and patients should be forewarned about this potential orthostatic effect and perhaps advised to take the first dose immediately prior to retiring to bed. The overall side effects of prazosin are: postural hypotension, dizziness, syncope, occasional skin eruptions, dry mouth, diarrhea, nausea, irritability, mental depression and fluid retention.

The usual starting dose of prazosin is 1 mg twice daily. The dosage can be increased up to a maximum of 40 mg in 2 or 3 divided doses daily. Prazosin is usually administered as a second-line drug when beta-blockers or central inhibitors are contraindicated or poorly tolerated.

Other alpha-adrenergic blocking drugs such as *phenoxybenzamine* and *phentolamine* are little used in renal disease patients except in hypertensive crises, during clonidine or guanabenz withdrawal after tyramine ingestion in patients taking monoamine oxidase inhibitors, or in pheochromocytoma.

Mixed Adrenergic Blockers

Labetalol

Labetalol is a unique antihypertensive agent that combines both alpha- and beta-adrenergic receptors blockade in a ratio of 1:7. The beta-blockade is nonselective, while alpha antagonism predominantly affects the postsynaptic alpha receptors. In addition, labetalol possesses mild intrinsic sympathomimetic activity. The renal effects of labetalol have not been extensively evaluated, but several studies have shown no deleterious affects on GFR or renal plasma flow. Since 20 to 40 percent of labetalol is excreted by the kidney, it is likely that in patients with renal insufficiency it may prove necessary to reduce the dosage to avoid hypotension, bradycardia, and other adverse affects. Labetalol as a single therapy is likely to be comparably effective to beta-blocker, or beta-blocker–vasodilator combinations.

Generally labetalol is well tolerated; side effects are usually light-headedness, headache, gastrointestinal symptoms, and tingling in the scalp. Rarely postural hypotension, dyspnea, depression, or sexual dysfunction may be reported, and are likely to be related to the drug's beta-blocker activity. There are few reports of development of antinuclear antibody titers in patients receiving labetalol.

The usual dosage is 300 to 1,200 mg per day orally in 2 divided doses and the drug may also be administered intravenously in 20- to 80-mg boluses given at 10- to 20-minute intervals for a total loading dose of 300 mg. The drug has been shown to be useful as monotherapy in control of hypertension during hypertensive crises including pheochromocytoma and clonidine withdrawal.

Beta-Adrenergic Blockers

There are several beta-blockers now available in the United States for the treatment of mild to severe hypertension. $Beta_1$ receptors appear primarily in the heart and cause tachycardia, enhancement of atrial ventricular conduction, and myocardial contractility with subsequent increase in cardiac output. $Beta_2$ receptors are located primarily on vascular smooth muscle and cause vasodilation, and reduction in peripheral resistance, bronchodilatation, gluconeogenesis, and insulin release. The exact mechanism by which beta-blockade produces a reduction in blood pressure has not been elucidated. A decrease in cardiac output is common to all beta-blockers, but the maximum hypotensive action is not seen until several days or even weeks after starting therapy. A slower, more gradual lowering of peripheral resistance occurs before blood pressure reduction becomes evident, and it is more likely that resetting of the baroreceptors brings about a fall in blood pressure.

Almost all beta-blockers inhibit renin release from the kidney. While there is a tendency for low renin hypertensive patients to respond less well to beta-blockers, and some may exhibit a paradoxical pressor response, in general beta-blocking drugs lower blood pressure in patients with high or low renin hypertension. However, animals made hypertensive with angiotensin II infusion do not respond to *propranolol* or captopril. Reduction in renin fails to explain the slow fall in peripheral resistance and blood pressure, since plasma renin falls immediately after institution of therapy. In addition, pindolol, which has little or no effect on plasma renin activity, is an effective antihypertensive agent. Certain of the beta-blockers which possess intrinsic sympathomimetic activity (*pindolol, acebutolol*) may induce vasodilation by action on vascular smooth muscle mediated through $beta_2$ adrenergic receptor stimulation, which may not be associated with reduction in cardiac output.

The $beta_1$ selective adrenergic blockers are *acebutolol, atenolol,* and *metoprolol*. The nonselective beta-blockers are *propranolol, nadolol, timolol,* and *pindolol*, which act as competitive antagonists of both $beta_1$ and $beta_2$ adrenoreceptors to produce bradycardia, reduce myocardial contractility, and inhibit renin release. In adition, bronchoconstriction may occur in asthmatic patients and reduction in glycolysis, insulin, and gluconeogenesis are observed, as is spontaneous hypoglycemia. Muscle tremor may also be reduced.

Nonselective Beta-Blockers

Propranolol may produce a 10 to 15 percent decline in renal blood flow and GFR, which may be worse in hypertensive patients who do not have a hypotensive response to drug, probably by unmasking the effects on renal alpha-adrenergic vascular receptors. In the case of nadolol and pindolol, renal blood flow and GFR are relatively well preserved even in the face of a decline in cardiac output. The effects of timolol on GFR and renal hemodynamics have been studied very little.

All of the nonselective beta-blockers are well absorbed from the small intestine, but in the case of propranolol, and the $beta_1$ selective drug acebutolol, only 40 percent of the orally administered dose reaches the systemic circulation, by virtue of extensive hepatic first-pass metabolism. Also in the case of propranolol, hepatic metabolites may retain some beta-blocking activity. Propranolol is highly lipid soluble, has a large volume of distribution, and is over 90 percent bound to plasma proteins. Beta-blockers that are eliminated more quickly from the body are highly lipid soluble, and these include propranolol and timolol. Nadolol, on the other hand, is relatively insoluble and is excreted virtually unchanged by the kidneys, with a long plasma half-life of 14 to 17 hours. Pindolol is intermediate, with about 40 percent of the drug being excreted unchanged in the urine. Metoprolol in the presence of renal impairment should be administered at long intervals, for example, 36-hour intervals for moderate reduction in renal function (20 to 50 ml per minute), and 48 to 60-hour intervals for severe renal impairment (< 10 ml per minute); this requires individual titration. Atenolol and acebutolol (the latter of which has the active metabolite diacetolol) should also be reduced in dosage when there is renal impairment (see Table 3).

In general, no dosage modification is necessary for propranolol, timolol, and pindolol in renal failure, although the normal interpatient variation in the bioavailability and metabolism of these substances is greater when renal disease is present. Therefore, each agent should be administered cautiously and in the smallest possible therapeutically effective dose.

Side effects related to beta-blocking activity are sinus bradycardia, atrioventricular conduction delay, congestive heart failure, bronchospasm, peripheral vascular insufficiency, and disturbances in carbohydrate metabolism. Adverse effects probably not related to adrenergic beta-blocker activity include skin rash, keratoconjunctivitis, and positive antinuclear antibody titers. Psychiatric effects seen more commonly with the highly lipid soluble drugs are depression, nightmares, decreased libido, and impotence.

Propranolol should be administered at 12-hour intervals, as should timolol and pindolol. Nadolol can be administered at 24-hour intervals unless, as mentioned above, renal failure is present. The usual dosage of propranolol is 20 to 320 mg daily, timolol, 20 to 80 mg daily; and pindolol, 5 to 40 mg daily.

$Beta_1$ Selective Antagonists

These drugs are commonly referred to as "cardioselective" and reduce heart rate and myocardial contractility as well as reducing renin secretion. *Acebutolol, atenolol,* and *metoprolol* are the drugs available in the United States.

The oral availability of metoprolol is reduced to 40 to 50 percent because of extensive first pass hepatic metabolism, and, as with propranolol, large interpatient variability in dosing requirements is seen. The drug is highly lipid soluble, but only slightly bound to plasma proteins and is cleared from the body primarily by hepatic metabolism to inactive compounds which are excreted in the urine. In renal failure dosage reduction is not necessarily required, although adjustment of dosage may be necessary in patients with renal disease on an individual basis.

Atenolol is excreted virtually intact by the kidneys, its bioavailability is 40 to 50 percent, and because of its dependence on renal excretion, the dose of the drug should be modified when renal insufficiency is present. In moderate insufficiency the dosage should be reduced by 50 percent and when renal failure is severe by 75 percent. Side effects of atenolol and metoprolol are primarily cardiac, including bradycardia, atrioventricular conduction delay, and congestive heart failure. This is especially true when large doses are administered, since the $beta_1$ selectivity is overcome, with resultant blocking of the $beta_2$ receptors which results in bronchospasm, Raynaud's phenomenon, and abnormalities in carbohydrate metabolism. Psychiatric side effects are probably not related to beta-receptor activity, but to lipid solubility. Such side effects are less common with atenolol because of its low lipid solubility. Very few studies have been performed on the renal effects of metoprolol, acebutolol, and atenolol, but the work so far fails to demonstrate any detrimental effects on renal blood flow or GFR. The usual dose of metoprolol is 50 to 200 mg daily divided at 12-hour intervals, of atenolol, 50 to 100 mg daily at 24-hour intervals unless renal failure is severe; of acebutolol, 200 to 400 mg per day.

As with all beta-blockers, these should not be discontinued abruptly, since they may precipitate a hypertensive crisis or result in coronary spasm in patients with angina. This effect may be exacerbated in patients receiving concomitant nifedipine. There are also a few reports of severe hypertension, exacerbation of angina, and congestive heart failure in patients receiving both beta-blockers and nifedipine.

Beta-blockers increase serum triglycerides and decrease high-density lipoprotein concentrations, but do not influence serum low-density lipoprotein concentrations. The least changes occurring in lipids occur with drugs which possess intrinsic sympathomimetic activity.

Vasodilators

The orally effective vasodilators are hydralazine, minoxidil, and nifedipine, while the parenteral agents are diazoxide, nitroprusside, and trimethaphan. Nifedipine will be discussed in the section on calcium channel blockers.

Hydralazine

Hydralazine exerts its antihypertensive action via relaxation of arterial smooth muscle, possibly by binding with calcium or other trace metals necessary for vascular contraction. The main effect is depression of diastolic more than systolic blood pressure, and is associated with little or no orthostatic hypotension. There is an accompanying reflex increase in heart rate, cardiac output, and stroke volume, but this is not observed in elderly patients in whom baroreceptor sluggishness is well recognized. Hydralazine increases GFR, renal tubular function, and urine volume, accompanied by an acute rise in renal blood flow, although this returns to normal with chronic use, as does GFR. Plasma renin activity is also increased. Sodium and fluid retention with resultant increase in plasma and extracellular fluid volume may occur, and tolerance to the effects of the drug may develop with prolonged use. Accordingly, the administration of a diuretic or a beta-blocker may maintain the therapeutic efficacy. Most of the adverse effects associated with hydralazine are due to vasodilation and reflex cardiovascular responses. Patients complain of palpitation, headache, and flushing, and in some patients with angina there may be aggravation of anginal symptoms (this occurs in approximately 7 percent of predisposed patients when the drug is used alone). The angina is caused by increased myocardial oxygen demand and is also associated with ECG changes in patients with underlying atherosclerotic heart disease.

A syndrome similar to sytemic lupus erythematosus is associated with large doses of the drug (more than 400 mg per day), but this is variable, since the syndrome has occurred in patients receiving low doses (75 g per day). Patients with slow acetylation of the drug in the liver are at a greater risk of developing this syndrome than are fast acetylators. Typical symptoms include polyarthralgia, fever, dermatitis, malaise, pleuritic chest pain, antinuclear antibodies, leukopenia, and lupus erythematosus cells. The drug should be discontinued in patients developing this syndrome.

Fifty to 90 percent of hydralazine is rapidly absorbed, with the higher values being achieved in slow acetylators. Peak plasma levels of drug and metabolites occur within 1 to 2 hours. Hypotensive activity occurs within 30 minutes and has a duration of approximately 2 to 4 hours. Accumulation of hydralazine occurs in patients with severely compromised renal function; in these patients hydralazine dosage intervals should be increased to 8 to 16 hours for fast acetylators and 12 to 24 hours for slow acetylators. Although there is no conclusive evidence regarding increased hydralazine toxicity in renal failure, the usual starting dose is 25 mg 3 or 4 times daily, advancing to a maximum of 200 mg per day; this may be exceeded in patients in whom the benefits outweigh the risk of developing the lupus syndrome. The hydralazine is usually given as a third-line drug in combination with diuretics and beta blockers.

Minoxidil

Minoxidil is a piperidino-pyrimidine derivative with unusually potent vasodilating properties. Like diazoxide and hydralazine, it interferes with calcium uptake into cell membranes or vascular smooth muscle, and the vasodilating activity is confined mainly to the arterial resistance bed. As a result there is increased tissue blood flow, a fall in peripheral vascular resistance, and decreased ventricular afterload, but an increase in cardiac preload because of the absence of venodilator effects. There is a consequent increase in left ventricular stroke volume accompanied by adrenergically mediated increases in heart rate so that cardiac output is markedly enhanced.

The most frequent side effects seen with minoxidil are sodium and fluid retention, with marked edema formation occurring rapidly; in some cases it may be quite dramatic. The degree of fluid retention correlates with the total dose of minoxidil and the degree of renal impairment. Fluid retention is not related to altered renal blood flow, nor to renin-mediated hyperaldosteronism (normal levels of aldosterone are observed with chronic therapy). It may be that the drug has a direct effect on the renal tubule, although even in patients who are functionally anephric (dialysis patients) intradialytic weight gain may also be increased. Patients receiving minoxidil require concomitant administration of high ceiling diuretics (furosemide or bumetanide). In addition to weight gain, minoxidil produces tachycardia and palpitation, and in some patients myocardial infarction and angina pectoris have been reported. Electrocardiographic abnormalities, including ST depression and T wave flattening in the lateral chest leads, have been seen in many patients receiving minoxidil. Pericarditis with effusion and occasional tamponade has been described in 3 to 10 percent of patients treated with minoxidil. This is commonly seen in patients with some degree of renal impairment and may be accompanied by other serosal effusions. The frequency of small pericardial effusions is markedly increased in dialysis patients receiving minoxidil. Reversible hypertrichosis occurs in the majority of patients treated with minoxidil for more than six weeks. The hair growth involves the forehead, temples, eyebrows, forearms, and back and is due to growth of lanugo hair. Increased cutaneous blood flow may play a role. The hair growth is reversible within one to two months after discontinuation of minoxidil.

Minoxidil has variably been reported to increase or decrease renal blood flow. Renal vascular resistance either falls or remains stable. The decline in glomerular filtration rate seen in patients with severe or malignant hypertension and azotemia, may be ameliorated by the use of minoxidil. In other patients there seems to be no clear-cut effect of minoxidil on GFR.

Ninety-five percent of minoxidil is absorbed from the gastrointestinal tract and distributed to the arterial vasculature where there is extensive tissue binding. Minoxidil is conjugated with glucuronide and excreted in the urine. Since the glucuronide derivative has a slight antihypertensive action it may be necessary to reduce the dose of the drug in severe renal insufficiency. Minoxidil is generally reserved for cases of refractory hypertension, often in the setting of severe renal insufficiency. The usual starting dose is 2.5 mg twice a day, increasing to the maximum of 40 mg per day, with any increases being at weekly intervals. For acute and chronic therapy it is necessary to administer beta-adrenergic–inhibiting drugs and loop-acting diuretics along with minoxidil.

Diazoxide

Diazoxide is a benzothiadiazine, related chemically to chlorothiazide. It is an important vasodilator, but does not have diuretic activity. The drug is a direct vasodilator, relaxes arterial tone, and reduces peripheral vascular resistance. Competition for calcium receptor sites in vascular smooth muscle and depletion of arterial muscle intracellular calcium or blocking of its release are thought to mediate the vasodilator activity. In addition, an effect on cyclic adenosine monophosphate may also be involved. Oral and parenteral administration of diazoxide decreases urine volume and electrolyte excretion. The mechanism for the antinatriuresis is not clear, but there may be a direct action on the renal tubule or by an intrarenal hemodynamic alteration. Accompanying this antinatriuresis and prompt retention of sodium and water is an increase in plasma renin activity. Although the increase in plasma renin activity is felt to be unrelated to changes in plasma volume, extracellular fluid, or sodium excretion, there is a marked reduction in renal vascular resistance, and total renal blood flow is increased. There are, however, reports of profound hypotension with subsequent worsening of renal function in patients receiving the initial dose of diazoxide. This is uncommon, and in most patients glomerular filtration rate is unchanged.

The major adverse effects are due to the vasodilator properties, with excessive hypotension and reflex tachycardia occurring. Heart rate, stroke volume, and cardiac output increase when arterial pressure falls, and because of increased myocardial oxygen demand, ischemic heart disease or infarction may be exacerbated. When diazoide is given acutely, as many as 50 percent of the patients develop ST and T wave changes. Other common side effects include gastrointestinal discomfort, sodium and water retention, and irritation at the site of infusion, as well as postural hypotension. Diazoxide inhibits insulin release and is associated with significant hyperglycemia. The hyperglycemia is usually transient and rarely requires treatment with insulin or oral hyperglycemic agents, although ketoacidosis and nonketotic hyperglycemic hyperosmolar coma have been reported. Serum half-life of diazoxide is increased as renal function decreases; diazoxide half-life ranges from 20 to 36 hours, and the antihypertensive activity is approximately one-third of its chemical half-life.

Since the drug is very highly protein bound it is given usually in 300-mg boluses, with a redistribution phase of 10 minutes (up to 3 hours is reported in patients with renal failure). The drug can also be given by slow intravenous infusion. In patients with severe renal insufficiency it is suggested to initiate therapy with half the usual dose (150 mg) intravenously, and repeat every 20 minutes as necessary to achieve a satisfactory therapeutic result. At the time of writing diazoxide is used only in the intravenous form for the control of hypertension and hypertensive crisis.

Nitroprusside

Sodium nitroprusside is an effective vasodilator for managing acute hypertensive emergencies, heart failure, and other vasoconstrictive diseases. The agent is given parenterally, is extremely potent, and is considered to be the drug of choice in the management of hypertensive emergencies. The onset of action is within 2 minutes of intravenous infusion and rapidly disappears when the drug infusion is discontinued. Direct peripheral dilation occurs in both arterial and venous systems. Postulated mechanisms for action include adenyl cyclase activation, and inhibition of phosphodiesterase, possibly mediated by oxidation of specific sulfhydryl groups at smooth muscle receptors. Sodium nitroprusside produces renal vasodilation in hypertensive patients, but little alteration in renal blood flow or glomerular filtration rate, although there is evidence of a slight decrease in renal vascular resistance. Renal vein and systemic venous renin concentrations rise.

The major adverse effects of nitroprusside are excessive reduction in blood pressure associated with catecholamine release to promote diaphoresis, anxiety, psychosis, headache, palpitation, dizziness, retrosternal discomfort, and abdominal pain. All these symptoms are abolished by rapid reduction of the rate of infusion. It is therefore important that nitroprusside be used where there are adequate facilities for close or continued monitoring of blood pressure. The prolonged use of nitroprusside is associated with cyanide and thiocyanate accumulation and reaction of nitroprusside with hemoglobin to form methemoglobin and other unstable intermediate radicals. Ten percent of the cyanide produced by infusion of nitroprusside (there are five cyanide groups on the molecules) is found in plasma, while the remaining four cyanide equivalents are converted to thiocyanate in the liver.

Thiocyanate is excreted by the kidneys. Not surprisingly, patients with hepatic or renal dysfunction accumulate excessive quantities of cyanide and thiocyanate. Cyanide blood levels above 50 mg per deciliter have been associated with toxicity. Additionally, tachyphylaxis may be an indication of cyanide accumulation, since it is suggested that cyanide antagonizes directly the effects of nitroprusside on smooth muscle. Other manifestations of cyanide toxicity include metabolic acidosis, dyspnea, headache, vomiting, dizziness, ataxia, loss of consciousness, coma, absent pulse, reflexes, dilated pupils, pink skin color, severe hypertension, and shallow respiration. In patients with renal insufficiency there is greater risk of thiocyanate toxicity with nausea, vomiting, diarrhea, skin erruptions, arthralgia, muscle cramps, irritability, decreased vision, motor aphasia, disequilibrium, psychosis, and depressed thyroid function. A thiocyanate serum concentration above 10 mg per deciliter in an asymptomatic patient should not, by itself, be a contraindication to continuing therapy. In patients receiving nitroprusside for less than 72 hours, blood levels are not helpful, but after this period, cyanide toxicity may be treated in such patients by infusions of sodium thiosulfate or hydroxocobalamin or in severe cases with dialysis.

Although no specific dosing recommendations are available, thiocyanate metabolites accumulate in patients with renal insufficiency and such patients should be monitored closely for signs of thiocyanate toxicity. In addition, patients with hepatic insufficiency may also be at risk. The usual starting dose is 0.5 μg per kilogram per minute titrated against blood pressure response. Since nitroprusside is sensitive to light-induced decomposition, the containers should be protected from the light by wrapping with aluminum foil or other opaque material. Even so, fresh solution should be made up every 6 hours. In the event of cyanide or thiocyanate toxicity, hemodialysis and peritoneal dialysis may be extremely useful methods for removing the poison.

Trimethaphan

Trimethaphan is a rapidly acting parenteral agent with peak activity 5 minutes after injection. It inhibits postsynaptic ganglionic acetylcholine receptor sites and diminishes adrenergic control of resistance and capacitance vessels. As a result, arterial and venous smooth muscle tone is decreased. Subsequently a decrease in venous return and cardiac output occurs as well as a decrease in total peripheral resistance. Trimethaphan may also produce vasodilation by releasing histamine from mast cells. The anticholinergic effects of this drug produce its side effects; urinary retention and constipation may follow prolonged administration, as can paralytic ileus and visual disturbances, including mydriasis and loss of visual accommodation. Marked hypotension is more likely to be a major side effect, and in some cases blood pressure may be difficult to stabilize. Hypotension may last for 10 to 15 minutes after the infusion is stopped and necessitate the administration of intravenous fluids and placing of the patient in the Trendelenburg position. In some patients GFR and renal blood flow may be reduced and renal vascular resistance increased. The drug should be used with caution in patients with renal disease, but there are no guidelines for dosage modification. Trimethaphan is mostly used in patients with disrupted vascular integrity, as may be seen in cerebral hemorrhage or aortic aneurysm.

Calcium Channel Blockers

Nifedipine is the first in the series of recently introduced calcium channel blocking drugs for the treatment of cardiovascular disorders. With this group of drugs electrophysiology studies indicate that calcium movement across the vascular smooth muscle cell is inhibited and the normal excitation contraction process is thereby blocked. Accordingly, vasodilatory effects are observed. Vascular smooth muscle in the coronaries and peripheral vascular tree are affected equally. The hemodynamic effects are decreased in peripheral resistance and mean arterial blood pressure, along with a decrease in left ventricular end-diastolic pressure. Coronary blood flow is increased along with heart rate, cardiac output, and plasma renin activity. Nifedipine is rapidly and completely absorbed from the mouth and gastrointestinal mucosa. Indeed, its onset of action may range from 3 minutes when administered sublingually to 20 minutes by the oral route. It is 90 percent protein bound and is metabolized by oxidation to inactive metabolites excreted by the kidneys. Little is known of the effect of renal impairment on nifedipine kinetics. Side effects include hypotension, headache, flushing, and leg edema. In general, the drug is well tolerated except at high doses, where symptoms common to other vasodilators occur, such as headache, flushing and so on.

Although not yet approved by the United States Food and Drug Administration for the treatment of hypertension, nifedipine and agents in this class (verapamil, diltiazem) are likely to be approved in the near future. The usual starting dose for chronic therapy with nifedipine is 10 mg 3 times a day by mouth, increased to a maximum of 30 mg 3 times a day. In addition, in hypertensive emergencies, rapid reduction of blood pressure may be achieved by sublingual doses of nifedipine (10 mg every 20 to 30 minutes until satisfactory reduction in blood pressure occurs).

Angiotensin-Converting-Enzyme Inhibitors

Captopril

Captopril is an orally active inhibitor of kininase II (angiotensin-converting-enzyme). Thus, a conversion of angiotensin I to angiotensin II, the powerful vasoconstrictor, is blocked. It has been shown that drugs in this class produce a fall in angiotensin II levels, but a rise in plasma renin activity with chronic use. Angiotensin II is a potent vasoconstrictor peripherally and also will induce vasoconstriction of the afferent and efferent glomerular arterioles. Consequently, angiotensin-converting-enzyme (ACE) inhibitors reduce intraglomerular hypertension as well as systemic hypertension. This may have a beneficial role in the reduction of proteinuria, as reported in diabetic patients with captopril, and may eventually be associated with preservation of renal function in patients with diabetes and other renal diseases. Although this has been demonstrated in animals it has not yet been proved in man. Captopril lowers total peripheral resistance without producing changes in heart rate, cardiac output, or pulmonary capillary wedge pressure.

Significant adverse effects from captopril include skin rashes, angioneurotic edema of the face and mucous membranes, stomatitis, eosinophilia, fever, altered taste sensation, leukopenia, and occasionally agranulocytosis. In addition, heavy proteinuria as a result of captopril treatment has been reported. Most of these side effects are felt to be related to the presence of a sulfhydryl group on the molecular structure of captopril, as is seen with other sulfhydryl-containing compounds such as penicillamine. Captopril may be associated with "first dose effect" hypotension, especially in patients who are volume depleted. Most of the side effects of captopril are observed at high dose levels. Acute renal failure may be observed in patients with bilateral renal artery stenosis, because of reduction in renal blood flow or arterial stenosis in a solitary kidney, or renal allograft.

In the fasting state 75 percent of captopril is absorbed from the gastrointestinal tract, but this is reduced by 55 percent if there is food in the stomach. The drug is 30 percent plasma protein bound, while 50 percent is oxidized at the sulfhydryl group and the unmetabolized portion of captopril is excreted unchanged in the urine. Its half-life is markedly increased in patients with moderate to severe renal dysfunction, and dosage reduction is necessary in the presence of significant renal impairment. The maximum effect of the drug is often not achieved in less than 2 weeks with slow and careful titration of the dosage. The drug is usually given along with a diuretic.

Enalapril

Enalapril is a recently introduced non-sulfhydryl–containing ACE inhibitor that produces lowering of angiotensin II and aldosterone levels. Recent results show that in patients with mild to moderate and severe hypertension the drug is extremely effective, particularly in severe hypertension when combined with an oral diuretic. The side effect profile is quite different from that of captopril in that skin rashes, taste disturbance, leukopenia, and proteinuria are markedly reduced or absent. The peak blood levels of enalapril occur 1 hour after oral administration, and this does not depend on whether the stomach is full or empty. Enalapril action is mediated through the formation of enalaprilat—a diacid metabolized in the liver—which is the active drug. The peak antihypertensive action is approximately 4 to 6 hours after oral absorption and there is no first dose effect. The duration of action of enalapril is prolonged, with a half-life for enalaprilat of approximately 12 hours; hence the drug is given in a single daily dosage. The excretion of enalaprilat is markedly impaired as the GFR falls below 30 ml per minute and enalapril dosage should be reduced (see Table 3).

MANAGEMENT OF THE PATIENT WITH HYPERTENSION COMPLICATING CHRONIC RENAL FAILURE

Management of hypertension in patients with renal disease and replacement therapy is shown in Figure 1. It is now clear that adequate control of blood pressure in patients with chronic renal failure may slow the previously inexorable progression to end-stage renal failure in a variety of renal diseases, including glomerulonephritis, diabetes mellitus, and hypertension. The change in the rate of progression has not been determined with any certainty for the individual patient, but most physicians agree that aggressive control of blood pressure is a worthwhile goal, provided that therapeutic approaches do not endanger residual renal function. For this reason it is recommended that a gradual reduction in blood pressure into the normal range for age—to prevent the dramatic falls in GFR and occasional acute renal failure that may accompany treatment with some of the drugs outlined above—be attempted over a period of a few days to weeks. In the case of "accelerated" hypertension the benefits of rapid reduction in blood pressure far outweigh any potential reduction in GFR. Moreover, patients requiring dialysis as a result of "accelerated" hypertension per se or its treatment may recover renal function to the point at which dialysis may not be required (at least for some time).

Salt restriction (1–2 g sodium per day, 34–68 mEq per day) has proved valuable in motivated patients, but in most it is difficult to enforce, and diuretic therapy is a reasonable substitute. As GFR falls below 30 ml per

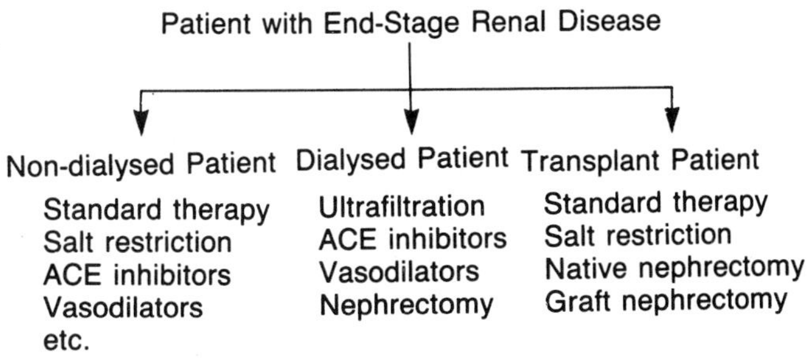

Figure 1 Management of hypertension in renal disease.

minute "loop" diuretics are required, and as GFR approaches 10 to 15 ml per minute high doses of furosemide (> 200 mg per day) may be required for control of blood pressure and edema. In the classic "stepped care" method of treating hypertension one should then choose to introduce one or more of the potent antihypertensives, such as central agents, alpha-blockers, beta-blockers, vasodilators, and ACE inhibitors, adding the drugs in order of potency. With modern drugs that possess more acceptable side effect profiles, however, it is eminently reasonable to go directly to the most potent drugs as a first step. Drugs such as ACE inhibitors (particularly enalapril) may offer specific theoretical and hopefully clinical benefits to the patient with progressive renal disease (inhibition of angiotensin II–mediated efferent glomerular arteriolar vasoconstriction, and subsequent reduction of intraglomerular hypertension), as has been recently demonstrated in diabetic patients in whom quantitative reduction in proteinuria followed captopril treatment of high blood pressure.

Even with the more potent drugs, combination with diuretics (which counteract the sodium-retaining properties of some of the antihypertensives and may prevent tolerance or tachyphylaxis) may be synergistic or at least additive to their effects. With potent vasodilators which produce reflex tachycardia, beta-blockers may be particularly helpful in reducing this disturbing side effect. Minoxidil in particular may require the addition of high-dose diuretic therapy to obviate the often massive edema that accompanies its use. ACE inhibition with captopril is felt to be particularly useful in scleroderma or other vasculitides. In some patients blood pressure is truly refractory to treatment, after noncompliance is ruled out, and high-dose combinations of ACE inhibitors, minoxidil, and beta-blockers may be required before (rarely) considering nephrectomy for the control of hypertension.

MANAGEMENT OF THE DIALYSIS PATIENT WITH HYPERTENSION

Patients initiating hemodialysis are commonly hypertensive (80 percent), and taking medication for its control. Following initiation of dialysis and control of fluid balance by ultrafiltration during hemodialysis or peritoneal dialysis, blood pressure comes under control and reduction in dosage or number of antihypertensive drugs becomes possible in the majority of patients. In approximately 20 percent of patients blood pressure control remains difficult, weight gain between hemodialyses may be high, blood pressure reduction with ultrafiltration may be difficult to achieve without inducing intradialytic hypotension and symptoms of cramping, and potent antihypertensives may be required. Provided that dry "target" weight is sought in dialysis patients, and adjusted as needed, rarely, with modern drug therapy, is nephrectomy necessary for control of hypertension. In the patient with poorly controlled blood pressure, nephrectomy may be considered if transplantation is contemplated.

Patients undergoing continuous ambulatory peritoneal dialysis (CAPD) have more easily controllable hypertension than those undergoing hemodialysis, probably because of easier and smoother control of salt and/or water balance achieved through peritoneal osmotic ultrafiltration. It has been shown in several studies that the numbers of patients receiving no antihypertensive drugs is greater, and the number of drugs per individual patient is less in CAPD patients than in hemodialysis patients. Patients receiving hemodialysis therapy are often on sodium-restricted diets (60 mEq per day), but this is not usually necessary or desirable in CAPD, since hypotension from excessive ultrafiltration is frequently observed.

MANAGEMENT OF HYPERTENSION COMPLICATING TRANSPLANTATION

Careful management of hypertension in the successful transplant recipient is of special concern, since continued hypertension contributes to graft loss and to cardiovascular events following transplantation. As in the dialysis patient, volume deregulation is the most common anomaly responsible for hypertension. accordingly, diuretic therapy may be particularly helpful. Every attempt should be made to reduce steroid dosage to the minimum required for prevention of rejection, and the same approach should probably be taken for reduction in cyclosporine dosage, since cyclosporine administration is associated with hypertension. In the patient with clear-cut acute rejection the dosage of antihypertensive drugs may need to be increased temporarily, until the rejection episode is moderated. In the case of chronic rejection, however, control of blood pressure may not respond to therapy directed at moderating rejection. Similarly, in the patient with transplant renal artery stenosis, failure to control blood pressure along with reduced renal function should stimulate a search for and correction of the renal artery lesion.

The ACE inhibitor captopril should be used with caution in transplantation-associated hypertension because of the potential for inducing neutropenia (this could be particularly hazardous in patients receiving azathioprine). While this may not be true for enalapril, ACE inhibitors in general probably should not be used until renal artery stenosis is excluded, since reduction in function of the single kidney may be induced in the presence of renal artery stenosis.

Removal of native kidneys in transplant recipients with complication hypertension has recently been shown to be a useful measure and is associated with substantial reductions in blood pressure.

URINARY TRACT INFECTION

CALVIN M. KUNIN, M.D.

Treatment of urinary tract infections can be one of the most gratifying experiences in clinical practice. This is because the patient usually has a reasonably specific complaint, definitive diagnosis can readily be made by microscopic examination of the urine and confirmed by culture, and a wide variety of effective antimicrobial agents are available for therapy. As with most infectious diseases, the efficacy of treatment or prophylaxis depends on (1) characteristics of the host, (2) the nature of the invading microorganism, (3) the physician's understanding of the natural history of the disease, and (4) the efficacy of chemotherapy. The overall goal of management is to eradicate the invading organism from the entire system. Almost as important is the necessity to anticipate, prevent, or treat recurrences. At times it is necessary to recognize failure and withhold antimicrobial therapy unless it is essential for the treatment of sepsis.

GENERAL CONSIDERATIONS

The Host

Urinary tract infections are best categorized in relation to host factors. These are conveniently divided into simple or uncomplicated (medical) infections, which occur in a patient with an otherwise normal tract, and complicated (surgical) infections, in which the integrity of the voiding mechanism is impaired or a foreign body is present. In addition, important considerations are the patient's age, sex, and renal function, and the presence of conditions such as diabetes and polycystic disease, which predispose the kidneys to infection. Uncomplicated infections, most often encountered in females, are generally the easiest to treat, whereas those in which a foreign body, such as a catheter or stone, is present in the urinary tract are the most difficult to treat. Because complicated infections tend to be resistant to therapy or to recur soon after treatment, the microorganisms often become resistant to commonly used antimicrobial agents. The ease of management of infections of the urinary tract according to type of patient, clinical characteristics, invading organism, and probability of tissue invasion is outlined in Table 1.

There has been considerable interest in the use of tests to "localize" the site of infection as a means of defining the need for more intensive or prolonged therapy. Theoretically, those infections associated with tissue invasion in some part of the urinary tract (a far more accurate description than "upper" versus "lower" tract infection) should be more difficult to manage and might be expected to indicate a greater potential for renal damage than those with bladder bacteriuria.

This concept may be illusory. Many female patients, for example, with uncomplicated infections (as many as 50 percent) are found by various localizing procedures to have evidence of upper tract infection. Yet their ultimate prognosis remains excellent and urologic studies in similar populations rarely detect significant structural abnormalities. For these reasons localization studies should be considered as research tools. I believe that the clinician will do far better simply to estimate the likelihood of tissue invasion from the clinical guides presented in Table 1. The most that can be concluded at this time is that patients likely to have tissue invasion will respond poorly to single-dose therapy.

The Microbe

Most urinary tract infections are caused by Gram-negative enteric organisms found in the gut. Their common occurence in urinary tract infections is used as one of the arguments to support the concept of the ascending route of infection. Anaerobic fecal flora, although present in 100 to 1,000 times greater abundance in the stool than *Escherichia coli*, rarely produce urinary tract infections. This may be because they do not grow well in urine. Anaerobes should not

TABLE 1 Guidelines to Management of Urinary Tract Infection

Ease of Management	*Type of Patient*	*Clinical Characteristics*	*Organism*	*Probability of Tissue Invasion*	*Therapy*
Excellent	Female, child or adult	Few previous episodes; reliable, with good follow-up available; less than 2 days between onset of symptoms and treatment	Usually *E. coli*, sensitive to most agents	Low	1 dose amoxicillin, sulfonamide, TMP/SMZ,* kanamycin
Good	Female, child or adult	Few previous episodes, follow-up poor	Usually *E. coli*, sensitive to most agents	High or low	3–10 days Prophylaxis for closely spaced recurrences
Fair	Female, child or adult	Many previous episodes, history of early recurrence, diabetes, or postrenal transplant	Variable, tends to have more resistant bacteria, susceptibility tests essential	High	4–6 weeks Prophylaxis for closely spaced recurrences
Fair	Adult male	Recurrent infections, some underlying anatomic abnormality	Variable, susceptibility test needed	High, often prostatic colonization	4–6 weeks Prophylaxis for closely spaced recurrences
Poor	Male or female	Neurogenic bladder, large volume residual urine	Variable, susceptibility test needed	High	Intermittent catheterization (treatment for symptomatic infections only)
Very Poor	Male or female	Continuous drainage required	Variable, susceptibility tests needed	Very high	Indwelling catheter closed drainage (treatment for sepsis only)

*Trimethoprim-sulfamethoxazole

be discounted, however, since polymicrobial infection with these bacteria is now commonly encountered in longstanding renal and perirenal abscesses. The mechanism whereby the bacteria reach the kidney is not clear.

The most common organisms encountered in uncomplicated infections are Enterobacteriaceae. Of these, *E. coli* is seen the most frequently and accounts for roughly 80 percent of infections. The second most common organism in females with uncomplicated infection is *Staphylococcus saprophyticus*, accounting for about 10 to 15 percent of infections. These two very different organisms, one a gram-negative rod encountered in the gut, the other a gram-positive coccus located on the skin surface, imply different mechanisms of infection. The exact reason, however, remains to be clarified.

Microorganisms more commonly encountered in complicated infections are *Klebsiella, Proteus, Enterobacter, Pseudomonas, Providencia, Serratia,* and *Morganella.* These organisms, as well as *Acinetobacter* and *Candida*, are often encountered in patients subjected to instrumentation, particularly those with indwelling catheters. Among the gram-positive bacteria, *Staphylococcus aureus* and Group D streptococci are particularly important. *S. aureus* infections are quite different from those produced by *S. saprophyticus*, in that *S. aureus* tends to be much more invasive. Most infections with this organism result from bacteremia which leads to metastatic abscesses in the kidney.

Occasionally unusual or fastidious bacteria may produce urinary infections. These may at times be difficult to detect. For example, *Haemophilus influenzae* does not grow well in culture media commonly used to detect enteric bacteria and may go undetected unless suspected. For this reason it is critical to perform Gram stains and acid-fast stains on urine from patients who exhibit pyuria in the absence of positive routine bacteriologic cultures.

There has been considerable debate in the literature concerning the role of lactobacilli, anaerobic streptococci and diphtheroids, as a cause of the so-called urethral syndrome. This syndrome is characterized by dysuria with or without accompanying pyuria. It now appears that some of these patients, particularly those with pyuria, may have either "low-count" (less than 100,000 per milliliter) bacteriuria with *E. coli* or are infected with *Chlamydia* or *Mycoplasma.* The significance of this relationship is quite important for therapy.

Natural History

Our understanding of the natural history of urinary tract infections has undergone profound change in recent years. Although urinary tract infections are common in females, they rarely lead to renal damage sufficient to produce end-stage renal failure. The most important problem is management of morbidity, or the symptoms of infection. Most *recurrent* infections in females are the result of reinfection with a new serotype of *E. coli* or a new bacterial species derived from the gut and transferred to the periurethral region, or are the result of local colonization with *S. saprophyticus.*

Most infections in males are acquired as a result of instrumentation but may appear without any discernable predisposing factor. Recurrent infections in males are often caused by silent colonization of the prostate, usually with the same organism as in the previous infection, unless they are instrumented. Renal disease is usually caused by a longstanding combination of obstruction or foreign bodies and infection. As regards the relative importance of risk factors, in general it is better to have a colonized but well-functioning urinary tract than a sterile obstructed system. The major exception is urinary tract infection in the diabetic. These individuals do not appear to acquire infections more often than others, but once these infections have been acquired, they tend to persist and may at times produce severe complications such as renal papillary necrosis, xanthogranulomatous or emphysematous pyelonephritis, and perirenal abscesses.

Chemotherapeutic Agents

A wide variety of drugs are available for the treatment of urinary tract infections. These are listed in Table 2 according to whether they occur in nature (antibiotics) or are synthetic compounds, and with comments concerning their indications. I do not like the term "urinary antiseptics," since it implies some special feature of the action of the drugs. Rather, the most important predictors of efficacy are the concentration achieved in the urine, and the susceptibility of the microorganisms to the agent. The choice of drug depends on these factors as well as on their relative cost, ease of absorption from the gastrointestinal tract, rate of acquisition of resistance, and side effects.

One compound not mentioned in Table 2 is water. A brisk water diuresis accompanied by frequent emptying of the bladder can markedly lower bacterial concentrations in the urine and occasionally clear the tract of bacteria. This probably accounts for the spontaneous clearing of bacteriuria in some females with uncomplicated infections. Antimicrobial therapy, however, is so much more powerful that, for practical purposes, the patient need not be instructed to drink large quantities of water when treated. Furthermore, although there are anecdotal accounts of the value of a female voiding after intercourse, this has not been subjected to clinical trial and is unnecessary when bedtime or postcoital antimicrobial prophylaxis is used.

An issue that has been repeatedly debated is the relative importance of urinary versus renal concentrations of a drug for treatment of infection. It is now clear that virtually all of the commonly used drugs are concentrated to some extent in the tubules and renal interstitium. This depends on how well they are concentrated by the kidney and the extent of back diffusion that occurs. The latter is determined in part by the pKa of the drug and pH of the urine. In general, the best guide to renal concentration is the concentration of the drug in the urine rather than in the blood.

The only exception is with methenamine and its salts (hippurate or mandelate). Methenamine produces its antibacterial effect by the breakdown in acid urine into formaldehyde and ammonia. This occurs primarily in the bladder. Therefore these agents are reserved for prophylaxis and should not be used to attempt to eradicate infection, particularly if tissue invasion is suspected.

Newer Agents

Aztreonam is a novel "monobactam" that is highly resistant to enzymatic hydrolysis by plasmid-mediated beta-lactamases. It is highly active against most strains of Enterobacteriaceae and *Pseudomonas,* but relatively inactive against gram-positive and anaerobic bacteria.

Imipenem is the first of a new class of "carbapenem" antibiotics. It has potent activity against a broad range of gram-positive and gram-negative and anaerobic bacteria. The drug is excreted by the kidneys, where it is hydrolyzed by an enzyme on the brush border of the renal tubular cell. Cilastatin, given simultaneously, inhibits this inactivation. The combination has the advantage over the "third-generation" cephalosporins and aztreonam of being active against enterococci.

Amdinocillin, formerly known as mecillinam, differs from the other beta-lactam antibiotics in binding principally to penicillin-binding protein 2. Other beta-lactams tend to bind more avidly to penicillin-binding proteins 1 and 3. It has a narrow antimicrobial spectrum which includes only gram-negative bacteria but not *Pseudomonas,* indole positive *Proteus,* or anaerobic bacteria. Because of its unique mode of action it may be synergistic with other beta-lactam antibiotics. However, this has to be determined on an individual basis. It may be of value in limited circumstances and should be considered a "specialty agent" to be used only when there is adequate laboratory control.

Clavulanic acid is a weak beta-lactam antibiotic that binds avidly to the family of plasmid-mediated TEM beta-lactamases produced by *E. coli, S. aureus,* and other bacteria. It is available as a combination with amoxicillin for oral use and with ticarcillin for

TABLE 2 Antimicrobial Agents Commonly Used in the Treatment of Urinary Tract Infection

Agent	*Comment*
Oral therapy	
Beta-lactam antibiotics	These agents are all active against the common coliform organisms found in urinary tract infections. Among these, ampicillin is about the least expensive. Amoxicillin has the advantage of less gastrointestinal upset, and carbenicillin indanyl sodium is useful for *Pseudomonas.* The oral cephalosporins are more expensive and no more effective. Amoxicillin/clavulanic acid may be useful for beta-lactamase-producing organisms.
Penicillin G	
Amoxicillin	
Amoxicillin/Clavulanic acid	
Carbenicillin indanyl sodium	
Cephalexin	
Cephradine	
Cefaclor	
Synthetic Compounds	These are synthetic compounds useful in the treatment or prophylaxis of infection. Trimethoprim and nitrofurantoin are most useful in long-term prophylaxis. Sulfonamides are most useful in initial episodes of infection. The other agents are useful back-up drugs. The methenamine salts are used only for prophylaxis. The new quinolones (norfloxacin and ciprofloxacin) are effective agents but expensive. The older quinolones (nalidixic acid, oxalinic acid, and cinoxacin) are often effective.
Sulfonamides	
TMP/SMZ*	
Nitrofurantoin	
Quinolones	
Methenamine	
Mandelate	
Hippurate	
Tetracyclines	These are effective drugs, but they may lead to overgrowth of *Candida,* and resistance may rapidly develop. They are useful in *Chlamydia* infections and prostatitis.
Tetracycline	
Oxytetracycline	
Doxycycline	
Minocycline	
Other Agents	Staphylococcal infections are best treated with nafcillin, oxacillin, cloxacillin, or dicloxacillin. Anaerobic infections may be treated with clindamycin, metronidazole, or chloramphenicol. Flucytosine may be used for *Candida* infections.
Parenteral Therapy	
Beta-lactams	These agents are all equally effective if the organisms are susceptible. Second- and third-generation cephalosporins generally have a broader spectrum of activity against gram-negative bacteria but have variable activity against *Pseudomonas* and are not effective against enterococci.
Ampicillin	
Ampicillin/Sulbactam	
First-, second-, and third-generation cephalosporins	
Carbenicillin	These agents may be preferred over cephalosporins for treatment of urinary infection caused by *Pseudomonas* and enterococci. To avoid aminoglycosides, they may be of particular value in the patient with renal failure.
Ticarcillin	
Piperacillin	
Azlocillin	
Mezlocillin	
Aminoglycosides	Streptomycin is not commonly used because of the rapid development of resistance. Gentamicin and tobramycin are almost equally effective, and gentamicin is less expensive and no more nephrotoxic. Amikacin is preferred for multiresistant bacteria.
Streptomycin	
Gentamicin	
Tobramycin	
Amikacin	
Netilmicin	

*Trimethoprim-sulfamethoxazole

parenteral use. The combination is an effective and rational approach to the problem of resistance; it is more expensive than the parent antibiotics and, because of added expense, should be used only for resistant strains. Ampicillin/sulbactam serves the same purpose and is available for parenteral use.

The older quinolones include nalidixic and oxolinic acid, and cinoxacin. The newer derivatives include norfloxacin, ciprofloxacin, enoxacin, and amifloxicin. These are much more active than the older agents against both gram-negative bacteria, including *Pseudomonas,* and gram-positive bacteria, including staphylococci. They are promising for treatment of systemic as well as urinary tract infections.

Aztreonam, imipenem with cilastatin, and amdinocillin are administered parenterally. Clavulanic acid may be given by the oral or parenteral routes. The new quinolines are absorbed from the gut.

Despite the attractiveness of the new agents for the treatment of urinary tract infections, they tend to be expensive and may not be cost effective when the organism is susceptible to older drugs.

Duration of Therapy

The duration of treatment needed to eradicate infection appears to be closely related to the probability that bacteria have invaded tissue. The less likely this possibility, the shorter the course of therapy may be. Single-dose therapy has been used successfully in selected female populations with uncomplicated infections from *E. coli* who seek medical help shortly after becoming symptomatic. It is much less effective in those who delay treatment. It is not recommended in patients with highly recurrent infections, those whose follow-up might be poor, and patients with diabetes or structural abnormalities. Males should not be treated with single-dose therapy because they may have prostatic involvement which will not respond. The advantages of single-dose therapy, for those in whom it is indicated, are that it is simple, effective, inexpensive, well tolerated, and preferred by patients, and that compliance is assured, there are fewer side effects, and less risk of development of resistant organisms. It can also be used as a test for localization of infection, since failure to eradicate bacteriuria after 2 to 3 days strongly suggests tissue invasion or the presence of a resistant strain. It is doubtful, however, that failure to respond to single-dose chemotherapy can be used to indicate the need for urologic investigation. Finally, single-dose therapy is not recommended for treatment of the urethral syndrome from *Chlamydia* and it has not been adequately tested for efficacy against infections from *S. saprophyticus*.

Intermediate duration of therapy is considered to be somewhere between 3 and 14 days of treatment. Most trials indicate that 10 days of therapy for uncomplicated infection is nearly as effective as 2 weeks of therapy, and several studies indicate that 3 days of therapy is nearly as effective as 10 days of therapy. Unfortunately, there are few comparative studies of 1 day of treatment versus 3 and 10 days of treatment. My own bias is to use a conservative approach, recognizing the heterogeneity of the populations that investigators define for their studies. I prefer the 3- to 10-day method for most patients with uncomplicated infection, using follow-up cultures as a guide to relapse or presence of resistant bacteria.

Long-term therapy of 4 to 6 weeks or longer appears to be useful in individuals with marked tissue invasion, such as diabetics, patients with underlying structural abnormalities, children, and those who demonstrate early relapse after shorter courses.

Prophylactic therapy is highly effective for patients with frequent, closely spaced, recurrent infection. Although it has been shown that postcoital use of antimicrobial agents is effective, I prefer to use a regimen of small doses of an effective agent at bedtime. The preferred agents are trimethoprim, alone or combined with sulfamethoxazole, or nitrofurantoin, but other agents such as methenamine salts or quinolones and related drugs may be used. It must be remembered, however, that regardless of the duration of prophylaxis (at least up to 6 months), recurrent infection in females will occur at about the same rate as after a short course of treatment.

Another form of prophylaxis is the use of antibiotics in infected patients before instrumentation or surgery on the urinary tract. It is now clear that treatment markedly reduces septic complications postoperatively.

TREATMENT AND PROPHYLAXIS OF SPECIFIC CONDITIONS

Asymptomatic Bacteriuria

This is not a clinical entity, but rather a laboratory finding. Patients in very different risk groups may not exhibit symptoms yet have large numbers of bacteria in their urine. For example, prepubertal girls with asymptomatic bacteriuria are at low risk for developing renal disease, whereas elderly individuals with the same findings but who have an indwelling catheter are at high risk for developing pyelonephritis and sepsis.

It is relatively easy to eradicate bacteriuria in young girls yet virtually impossible in patients with a catheter in place. For these reasons, asymptomatic bacteriuria should be considered only as an indicator of the presence of infection and as a guide to the efficacy of therapy.

Urethral Syndrome

This is a clinical entity in which the patient complains of dysuria but is not found to have significant bacteriuria by the usual criterion of 100,000 bacteria per milliliter of urine. About 75 percent of women with the urethral syndrome have pyuria and are infected with either a coliform bacteria present in counts of 10 to 1,000, or with *Chlamydia trachomatis*. The latter infection requires at least 7 days of treatment with tetracycline.

PROSTATIC INFECTION

It is believed that the prostate is often colonized with urinary tract infections and is a source of recurrent infections. Despite elegant attempts to define how various antimicrobial agents enter the prostatic fluid and the attempt to use lipid-soluble drugs (such as trimethoprim, minocycline, and rifampin) for this purpose, response to therapy has been relatively poor. For this reason, I prefer to use long-term bedtime prophylaxis (as described previously) when the patient does not respond to shorter and more intensive courses.

Prostatic colonization must be differentiated from acute bacterial prostatis. The latter is a severe form of acute infection requiring aggressive management, usually with parenteral agents as in the treatment of generalized gram-negative sepsis. Penetration of drugs into the acutely inflamed prostate does not appear to be a problem. These patients are generally treated with an aminoglycoside antibiotic plus additional agents effective against enterococci and gram-negative bacteria.

Acute Pyelonephritis

This syndrome may be encountered in otherwise healthy young women as part of the natural history of uncomplicated infection or may be a serious complication in individuals with complicated infections. In either case, until bacteriologic information is available, it seems reasonable to treat the patients with the parenteral agents most likely to be effective against the invading organism. A useful guide to choosing a drug is the history of agents used in the past by the patient and antimicrobial susceptibility patterns in an individual institution. For example, a young woman not previously treated with antibiotics may respond well to ampicillin or a first- or second-generation cephalosporin, whereas a patient who was treated on multiple occasions may require use of amikacin. I generally prefer to begin with an aminoglycoside antibiotic and ampicillin and change therapy depending on susceptibility tests. Other experts may prefer to begin therapy with a third-generation cephalosporin or extended-spectrum penicillin and then switch to a less expensive agent once the pattern of susceptibility has been determined.

Management of chronic pyelonephritis requires clear definition that an active infection is present. There is no need to treat inactive, noninfected scarred kidneys. The presence of significant bacteriuria is an excellent guide to therapy. I prefer to monitor the urine for bacteria as an indicator of response or need for further treatment. The duration of therapy is then tailored to the patient (see Table 1).

Fungal Infections

Candida and *Torulopsis* infections of the urinary tract may occur in patients receiving catheter drainage and in diabetics who are repeatedly treated with antibiotics. Occasionally fungus balls may obstruct the ureters. These patients may be managed with oral flucytosine, bladder irrigations with amphotericin B, or short courses of systemic amphotericin, in sequence, as needed. Bladder irrigations should not be done routinely for patients with asymptomatic candiduria particularly in patients with indwelling urinary catheters. This may lead to recolonization with multiresistant microorganisms.

CONDITIONS IN WHICH FAILURE MUST BE RECOGNIZED

Patients in whom there is a persistent foreign body, such as a stone or catheter, respond only transiently to chemotherapy. For these patients, the objective is to either remove the foreign body or at least assure good urine flow whenever possible. Treatment should be reserved for episodes of sepsis. No one really knows how long to treat such episodes, since frequently the blood stream will clear spontaneously. In general, however, it seems best to treat the patients as though they had acute pyelonephritis, as described previously.

Bacteriuria in the elderly should probably not be treated aggressively. It has been found in several surveys that 10 percent or more of women older than 65 years of age have asymptomatic bacteriuria but relatively normal renal function. It seems reasonable to reserve treatment for symptomatic episodes.

SUGGESTED READING

Johnson JR, Roberts PL, Stamm WE. *P. fimbriae* and other virulence factors in *Escherichia coli* urosepsis. J Infect Dis 1987; 156:225–229.

Kass EH, Svanborg-Eden C, eds. Host-parasite interactions in urinary tract infections. Chicago: University of Chicago Press, 1989.

Kunin CM. Detection, prevention, and management of urinary tract infections. 4th ed. Philadelphia: Lea and Febiger, 1987.

Sheinfeld J, Schaeffer AJ, Cordon-Cardo C, et al. Association of the Lewis blood-group phenotype with recurrent urinary tract infections in women. New Engl J Med 1989; 320:773–777.

Stamey TA. Recurrent urinary tract infections in female patients: an overview of management and treatment. Rev Infect Dis 1987; 9:S195–S210.

NEPHROLITHIASIS

CHARLES Y. C. PAK, M.D.

Nephrolithiasis is a common disorder affecting 1 to 5 percent of the population, with an annual incidence rate of 0.1 to 0.3 percent in the Western world. It may result in considerable morbidity by causing obstruction, hematuria, or infection.

Although the ultimate symptomatic presentation may be the same, it is clear that nephrolithiasis is heterogeneous with respect to composition and etiologic factors. Renal stones typically contain calcium (calcareous calculi, composed of calcium oxalate and/or calcium phosphate). They are less commonly composed of uric acid, cystine, or struvite (magnesium ammonium phosphate) (noncalcareous calculi). Many patients with stones have been found to suffer from a variety of physiologic or metabolic disturbances, including hypercalciuria, hyperuricosuria, hyperoxaluria, and hypocitraturia. Some of these derangements may be endocrinologic, involving altered metabolism of parathyroid hormone and vitamin D.

The above recognition has led to the refined classification and treatment of nephrolithiasis. Thus, it has been possible to formulate reliable diagnostic criteria on the basis of underlying metabolic derangements in patients with nephrolithiasis. Moreover, treatments could be specifically selected for the ability to "reverse" the particular underlying physiologic disturbances.

This selective approach argues for a thorough diagnostic differentiation of various causes of nephrolithiasis and emphasizes the need for a careful selection of treatment program for each cause of nephrolithiasis. Its feasibility and practicality are considered in detail here.

METABOLIC CLASSIFICATION OF NEPHROLITHIASIS

A simple and logical method of diagnostic differentiation of nephrolithiasis is the categorization on the basis of underlying physiologic abnormalities (Table 1). This classification assumes that these physiologic disturbances are pathogenetically important in stone formation. Although complete validation is lacking, it is generally agreed that excessive renal excretion of calcium, oxalate, uric acid, or cystine may contribute to stone formation by rendering the urinary environment supersaturated with respect to stone-forming salts. Hypocitraturia increases urinary saturation and reduces inhibitor activity against the crystallization of calcium salts. This classification is based on major or principal physiologic abnormalities. It is recognized that several disturbances may coexist in a given disorder. Hypercalciuria is considered to be heterogeneous, comprising six separate entities.

THERAPEUTIC CONSIDERATIONS

Improved elucidation of pathophysiology and formulation of diagnostic criteria for different causes of nephrolithiasis have made feasible the adoption of a selective or an optimum treatment program. Such a program should (1) reverse the underlying physiologic derangements, (2) inhibit new stone formation, (3) overcome nonrenal complications of the disease process, and (4) cause no serious side effects.

The rationale for the selection of a certain treatment program according to its ability to reverse physiologic abnormalities as outlined previously is the assumption that the particular physiologic aberrations identified with the given disorder are etiologically important in the formation of renal stones and that the correction of these dis-

TABLE 1 Classification of Nephrolithiasis

Calcareous Renal Calculi	*Noncalcareous Renal Calculi*
Hypercalciuria	Uric acid stones
Resorptive	Cystine stones
Absorptive	Cystinuria
Primary 1,25-dihydroxyvitamin D_3 excess	
Renal phosphate leak	Infection stones
Combined renal tubular disturbance	Infection with urea-splitting organisms
Hyperuricosuria	
Hyperoxaluria	
Primary	
Secondary	
Hypocitraturia	
No "metabolic" abnormality	

turbances would prevent stone formation. Moreover, it is assumed that such a selective treatment program would be more effective and safe than a "random" treatment. Despite a lack of conclusive experimental verification, these hypotheses appear reasonable and logical.

General Treatment Measures

In patients with calcium stones, moderate oxalate restriction should be imposed by discouraging ingestion of dark greens (such as spinach), rhubarb, brewed tea, and chocolate. Ascorbic acid supplementation should be denied because of potential metabolism of vitamin C to oxalate. A high sodium intake should be discouraged; the avoidance of "salty" foods and using salt shakers should be advised. A moderate dietary calcium restriction is advisable in patients with intestinal hyperabsorption of calcium (by limiting dairy products and dark roughage). In patients with hyperuricosuria and hypocitraturia, there should be an increased intake of fruit juices and an avoidance of excessive animal protein intake. All patients with any form of calculi should be encouraged to drink sufficient fluids to achieve a minimum urine output of 2 L per day.

Selective Treatment Programs

Nephrolithiasis has a high recurrence rate of 50 to 80 percent. The objective of medical treatment is the prevention of further stone formation. Specific treatments should be considered for patients with recurrent nephrolithiasis, especially in those with active disease (for example, stone formation or growth within 3 years of examination). In patients with a single stone episode, selective treatments should also be considered if metabolic derangements (such as hypercalciuria) are disclosed and if patients are in the "high-risk" group in which recurrence is likely (i.e., young adult white men with a family history of stones).

Primary Hyperparathyroidism (Resorptive Hypercalciuria)

Parathyroidectomy is the optimum treatment for nephrolithiasis of primary hyperparathyroidism. Following removal of abnormal parathyroid tissue, the urinary calcium level is restored to normal, commensurate with a decline in serum concentration of calcium and in intestinal calcium absorption. Urinary environment becomes less saturated with respect to calcium oxalate and brushite (calcium phosphate), and its limit of metastability of these calcium salts increases. There is typically a reduced new stone formation rate, unless urinary tract infection is present. Parathyroidectomy is contraindicated in renal hypercalciuria and in absorptive hypercalciuria.

There is no established medical treatment for the nephrolithiasis of primary hyperparathyroidism. Although orthophosphates have been recommended for disease of mild-to-moderate severity, their safety or efficacy has not yet been proven. They should be used only when parathyroid surgery cannot be undertaken. In postmenopausal women with primary hyperparathyroidism, estrogen (e.g., conjugated estrogen 0.625 mg per day for 25 days each month) may control the hyperparathyroid state and might be useful in those in whom parathyroid surgery is contraindicated or refused.

Absorptive Hypercalciuria

The presumed principal defect of absorptive hypercalciuria is the intestinal hyperabsorption of calcium that accounts for hypercalciuria and calcium nephrolithiasis. This condition may be subdivided into two types. In type I, the intestinal absorption and the renal excretion of calcium are increased during a high as well as during a low calcium diet. In type II, a normal urinary calcium concentration may be restored by dietary calcium restriction alone, although hypercalciuria is present on a high calcium diet. The hyperabsorption of calcium is believed to occur independently of renal phosphate leak or 1,25-dihydroxyvitamin D_3 excess.

Absorptive Hypercalciuria Type I. There is currently no treatment program capable of correcting the basic abnormality of absorptive hypercalciuria, although several drugs are available that have been shown to restore normal urinary calcium excretion.

Sodium cellulose phosphate best meets the criteria for optimum therapy. When given orally, this nonabsorbable ion exchange resin binds calcium and inhibits calcium absorption. However, this inhibition is caused by limiting the amount of intraluminal calcium available for absorption and not by correcting the basic disturbance in calcium transport.

The above mode of action accounts for the two potential complications of sodium cellulose phosphate. First, the treatment may cause magnesium depletion by binding dietary magnesium as well. Second, sodium cellulose phosphate may produce secondary hyperoxaluria by binding divalent cations in the intestinal tract, reducing divalent cation-oxalate complexation, and making more oxalate available for absorption. These complications may be overcome by oral magnesium supplementation (1.0 to 1.5 g magnesium gluconate twice daily, separately from sodium cellulose phosphate) and moderate dietary restriction of calcium (by avoidance of dairy products) and oxalate. Under such circumstances, sodium cellulose phosphate at a dosage of 10 to 15 g per day (given with meals) has been shown to lower urinary calcium without significantly altering urinary oxalate or magnesium, to reduce urinary saturation of calcium salts, and to retard new stone formation. This drug therapy is contraindicated in other forms of hypercalciuria because it may overly stimulate parathyroid function or embarrass skeletal status. It should be used with caution in postmenopausal women and growing children, because of potential dangers of exaggerating bone loss or impairing skeletal growth. Thus, the restrictive use of sodium cellulose phosphate in absorptive hypercalciuria type I alone mandates an accurate diagnostic evaluation.

Thiazide exerts the same hypocalciuric action and physicochemical effects in absorptive hypercalciuria as in renal hypercalciuria (see treatment of renal hypercalciuria for action, type, and dosage). Unfortunately, the intestinal hyperabsorption of calcium is not corrected by this treatment in absorptive hypercalciuria, unlike in renal hypercalciuria. Perhaps owing to this reason, some patients with absorptive hypercalciuria type I show an attenuation of hypocalciuric action of thiazide after 2 years of treatment. Moreover, thiazide treatment may cause hypocitraturia (inhibitor deficiency).

Because of the previously mentioned problems with thiazide therapy and difficulties in diagnostic differentiation, the following practical treatment regimen has often been employed. All patients with absorptive hypercalciuria type I may be begun first on a combined therapy with thiazide (e.g., trichlormethiazide, 4 mg per day) and potassium citrate (30 to 60 mEq per day in divided doses in order to prevent hypocitraturia or raise the urinary citrate level). When thiazide is ineffective in controlling hypercalciuria, sodium cellulose phosphate or orthophosphate may be substituted for 6 to 12 months (after which thiazide may again be effective in lowering the urinary calcium level).

Absorptive Hypercalciuria Type II. In type II hypercalciuria no specific drug treatment may be necessary. Normal urinary calcium may be obtained by a moderate dietary calcium restriction. Because urinary output is often low in this condition, a high fluid intake sufficient to produce urinary volume of at least 2 L per day should be encouraged.

Renal Hypercalciuria

Renal hypercalciuria is characterized by a "primary" impairment in the renal tubular reabsorption of calcium, secondary hyperparathyroidism, and compensatory intestinal hyperabsorption of calcium from the parathyroid hormone-dependent stimulation of 1,25-dihydroxyvitamin D_3 synthesis.

Thiazide is ideally indicated for the treatment of renal hypercalciuria. This form of diuretic has been shown to correct the renal leak of calcium by augmenting calcium reabsorption in the distal tubule and by causing extracellular volume depletion and stimulating proximal tubular reabsorption of calcium. The ensuing correction of secondary hyperparathyroidism restores normal serum 1,25-dihydroxyvitamin D_3 levels and intestinal calcium absorption. Physicochemically, the urinary environment becomes less saturated with respect to stone-forming salts (calcium oxalate and brushite) during thiazide treatment, largely because of the reduced calcium excretion. Moreover, urinary inhibitor activity is increased by a heretofore undisclosed mechanism.

These effects are shared by hydrochlorothiazide, 25 to 50 mg twice daily, chlorthalidone, 50 mg per day, or trichlormethiazide, 4 mg per day. Excessive sodium intake must be avoided because it could attenuate the hypocalciuric action of thiazide.

Side effects are mostly due to extracellular volume depletion and hypokalemia. Thiazide treatment should be avoided or stopped in the presence of excessive extrarenal loss of fluids and electrolytes. Renal excretion of citrate, an inhibitor of stone formation, may decline due to potassium loss. Thus, it is our practice to routinely provide potassium citrate (30 to 60 mEq per day in divided doses) whenever thiazide (without potassium-sparing agent) is given.

Concurrent use of triamterene, a potassium-sparing agent, should be undertaken with caution because of reports of triamterene stone formation. Amiloride may potentiate the hypocalciuric action of thiazide or may itself reduce urinary calcium, but it does not alter citrate excretion. In patients with normal citrate excretion, amiloride (5 mg per day) in combination with thiazide (e.g., hydrochlorothiazide, 50 mg per day) without potassium citrate supplementation, may be useful.

Thiazide is contraindicated in primary hyperparathyroidism because of potential aggravation of hypercalcemia.

Primary 1,25-Dihydroxyvitamin D_3 Excess

Primary enhancement of the renal synthesis of 1,25-dihydroxyvitamin D_3 is believed to cause intestinal hyperabsorption of calcium, parathyroid suppression, and hypercalciuria. There is no known agent capable of correcting this disturbance. The same treatment guidelines as with absorptive hypercalciuria type I would be advised.

Renal Phosphate Leak

Previously referred to as absorptive hypercalciuria type III, renal phosphate leak is characterized by the secondary stimulation of 1,25-dihydroxyvitamin D_3 synthesis resulting from impaired renal tubular reabsorption of phosphate and hypophosphatemia.

Oral administration of orthophosphate (neutral or alkaline salt of sodium and/or potassium, 0.5 g phosphorus three or four times per day) has been shown to lower serum concentration of 1,25-dihydroxyvitamin D_3. Although not yet proved, this treatment may restore normal calcium absorption. The treatment reduces urinary calcium, probably by directly altering renal tubular reabsorption of calcium and/or by inhibiting calcium absorption. Urinary phosphorus is markedly increased during therapy, a finding reflecting the absorbability of soluble phosphate. Physicochemically, orthophosphate reduces urinary saturation of calcium oxalate but increases that of brushite. Moreover, the urinary inhibitor activity is increased, owing probably to the stimulated renal excretion of pyrophosphate and citrate.

Minor gastrointestinal disturbances (including abdominal bloating and diarrhea) may develop during treatment. Although controversial, this treatment program has been reported to cause soft tissue calcification and parathyroid stimulation.

Combined Renal Tubular Disturbances

Some patients may have renal calcium leak as well as excessive 1,25-dihydroxyvitamin D_3 production occurring primarily or secondarily from renal phosphate leak. They present with fasting hypercalciuria with normal parathyroid function. Thiazide with potassium citrate (as described for renal hypercalciuria) represents a reasonable initial treatment approach. If persistent hypophosphatemia is present, orthophosphate may be used as well.

Hyperuricosuric Calcium Oxalate Nephrolithiasis

In this condition hyperuricosuria develops, usually from dietary "overindulgence" with purine-rich foods and occasionally from uric acid overproduction. The ensuing hyperuricosuria is believed to cause calcium stone formation from urate-induced calcium oxalate crystallization.

Allopurinol (300 mg per day) is the physiologically meaningful drug of choice in hyperuricosuric calcium oxalate nephrolithiasis, if hyperuricosuria is severe (greater than 800 mg per day) or if hyperuricemia coexists. Physicochemical changes ensuing from restoration of normal urinary uric acid by allopurinol include a reduction in urinary saturation of monosodium urate and a commensurate increase in the urinary limit of metastability of calcium oxalate. Thus, the spontaneous nucleation of calcium oxalate is retarded by treatment, probably via inhibition of monosodium urate–induced stimulation of calcium oxalate crystallization.

Side effects of allopurinol are uncommon in patients with stones, although hepatotoxicity, bone marrow depression, and rash have been reported. The complication of xanthine stone formation is rare.

If hyperuricosuria is mild to moderate (less than 800 mg per day) a moderate dietary purine restriction may be helpful, although usually impractical. If hyperuricosuria and stone formation persists, allopurinol or potassium citrate may be used. The latter drug is preferred if hypocitraturia is also present.

In patients with combined disturbances, allopurinol may be given with other agents (e.g., allopurinol and thiazide for patients with hyperuricosuria and hypercalciuria).

Hyperoxaluria

Primary Hyperoxaluria. Primary hyperoxaluria is caused by an accelerated oxalate synthesis. Magnesium gluconate (4 g per day in divided doses) and large doses of pyridoxine may lower urinary oxalate in some patients. Orthophosphate (0.5 g phosphorus three to four times per day orally) may be useful in controlling stone formation, probably by increasing inhibitor activity.

Secondary Hyperoxaluria. In ileal disease (surgical resection, intestinal bypass, inflammatory disease), urinary oxalate may be high secondary to intestinal hyperabsorption of oxalate (enteric hyperoxaluria). Other factors that may contribute to stone formation include low urine volume, low urinary acidity (predisposing to uric acid lithiasis), hypocitraturia, and hypomagnesiuria. Dietary oxalate restriction should be imposed. A high fluid intake should be encouraged. Magnesium gluconate (0.5 to 1.0 g four times per day orally) may be tolerated without aggravating diarrhea. Potassium citrate (40 to 120 mEq in divided doses) may augment citrate excretion and raise urinary pH. If bone disease is also present, 25-hydroxyvitamin D (50 μg per day) may be given with calcium supplements. Should hypercalciuria ensue, thiazide may be added.

Hypocitraturia

Renal Tubular Acidosis. Distal renal tubular acidosis (complete and incomplete) may be found in some patients with calcium nephrolithiasis. Acidosis may cause hypercalciuria by impairing renal tubular resorption of calcium, at least during the early stages of the disease before a significant renal impairment ensues. Because of high urinary pH, more phosphate is dissociated. Thus the urinary environment may become supersaturated with respect to calcium salts, particularly calcium phosphate. There is a defective renal excretion of citrate; this defect may therefore facilitate the crystallization process in urine.

Potassium citrate (40 to 100 mEq per day in divided doses) may correct the acidosis, reduce urinary calcium, augment urinary citrate, and retard the crystallization of calcium salts. This alkali therapy may also improve calcium balance by lowering urinary calcium and increasing intestinal calcium absorption. It should be used with caution in patients with renal insufficiency (glomerular filtration rate less than 40 ml per minute).

Other Causes. Hypocitraturia is present in approximately 50 percent of patients with calcium nephrolithiasis, even in the absence of renal tubular acidosis. Other causes of hypocitraturia include metabolic acidosis of enteric hyperoxaluria and thiazide-induced potassium depletion. Chronic diarrheal states (other than ileal disease) may also cause hypocitraturia. A strenuous physical exercise and ingestion of a high acid-ash diet (animal protein) may contribute to reduced citrate excretion. In some patients, the cause for the hypocitraturia remains unknown (idiopathic).

Potassium citrate (usually 30 to 60 mEq per day in divided doses) sufficient to restore normal urinary citrate is recommended. In chronic diarrheal states with fast intestinal transit or adhesions, a liquid form of potassium citrate may be preferable. In remaining conditions, the tablet form given with meals may be better tolerated and may provide a more consistent rise in citrate excretion.

Uric Acid Stones

The critical determinant in the formation of uric acid stones is the passage of unusually acid urine (pH 5.5) in which uric acid is stable. Uric acid lithiasis is found in gout, secondary causes of purine overproduction (e.g., myeloproliferative states and malignancy), and chronic diarrheal syndromes.

The oral administration of sodium alkali may increase urinary pH and create an environment in which uric acid is unstable. Although this treatment may inhibit the formation of uric acid stones, it may cause complication of calcium stone formation. In contrast, potassium citrate (30 to 60 mEq per day in divided doses) sufficient to raise urinary pH to a range of 6 to 6.5 may be helpful in the prevention of uric acid lithiasis, without producing a significant risk of calcium stone formation.

Allopurinol may be used to control hyperuricosuria (if present); a dose of 300 mg per day is generally sufficient to restore normal urinary uric acid. Dietary purine restriction is seldom practical. Probenecid is contraindicated because of its uricosuric action.

Patients with uric acid lithiasis may also form calcium stones, as manifestations of gouty diathesis. Potassium citrate is the preferred treatment for the prevention of both uric acid and calcium stones.

Cystine Stones

Stone formation is the result of an excessive renal excretion of cystine and the low solubility of this dicarboxylic acid in the normal pH of urine.

The initial treatment program includes a high fluid intake to promote an adequate urine flow (minimum of 2 L per day) and soluble alkali (e.g., potassium citrate 40 to 80 mEq per day in divided doses) to raise urinary pH to 6.5 to 7, in order to lower cystine concentration and raise cystine solubility. If this program is ineffective, D-penicillamine (1 to 2 g per day in divided doses) may be used. This treatment reduces cystine excretion by forming a more soluble mixed disulfide with cysteine. The dose of D-penicillamine should be adjusted in order to maintain cystine concentration in urine below saturation. Potential side effects include nephrotic syndrome, dermatitis, pancytopenia, and arthralgia. Vitamin B_6 (50 mg per day) should be added to avoid pyridoxine deficiency.

Alpha-mercaptopropionylglycine, an analog of D-penicillamine (soon to be released by the Food and Drug Administration), may also reduce cystine excretion. There is some evidence that it may cause fewer side effects than D-penicillamine.

Infection Stones

Urinary tract infection sometimes accompanies nephrolithiasis. When urea-splitting organisms (*Proteus*, certain species of *Staphylococcus, Pseudomonas, Klebsiella*) are responsible for infection, stones typically contain struvite (magnesium ammonium phosphate) with varying amounts of apatite.

In some patients, struvite stones may have formed *de novo* as a consequence solely of infection. In others, specific metabolic disorders associated with the formation of other types of renal stones could be identified; these derangements include hypercalciuria, hyperuricosuria, hyperoxaluria, and cystinuria. Struvite stone formation in the latter group probably results from a metabolic disorder causing formation of nonstruvite stones and resulting in urinary tract infection with urea-splitting organism, eventually leading to formation of struvite stone.

The physicochemical basis for struvite lithiasis is probably the same whether such a stone forms primarily or secondarily. The initial event is the formation of ammonium in urine on enzymatic degradation of urea by bacterial urease. The ammonia undergoes hydrolysis to form ammonium and hydroxyl ions. The resulting alkalinity of urine stimulates the dissociation of phosphate to form more trivalent phosphate ions and lowers the solubility of struvite. The activity product or the state of saturation of urine with respect to struvite is therefore increased. Stone formation ensues when sufficient oversaturation is reached.

If a longstanding effective control of infection with urea-splitting organisms can be achieved, there is some evidence that new stone formation can be averted or some dissolution of existing stone may occur. Unfortunately, such a control is difficult to obtain with antibiotic therapy. If there is an existing struvite stone, it is difficult to clear the infection completely because the stone often harbors the organisms within its interstices. Even if "sterilization" of urine had been achieved by antibiotic therapy, reinfection could occur by a harbored organism. For these reasons it has been customary to recommend surgical removal of struvite stones.

Prevention of new stone formation requires sterilization of urine with an appropriate antibiotic therapy or prevention of the generation of ammonium and hydroxyl ions with urease inhibitors (e.g., acetohydroxamic acid 250 mg three times per day).

SUGGESTED READING

Pak CYC. Citrate and renal calculi. Min Elect Metab 1987; 13:257–266.
Pak CYC. Kidney stones. In: Foster DW, Wilson JD, eds. Williams textbook of endocrinology. Philadelphia: WB Saunders, 1985:1256.
Pak CYC. Pathogenesis of hypercalciuria. In: Peck WA, ed. Bone and mineral research/4. New York: Elsevier, 1986:303.
Pak CYC, ed. Renal stone disease: pathogenesis, prevention, and treatment. Boston: Martinus Nijhoff, 1987.
Pak CYC, Fuller C, Sakhaee K, Zerwekh JE, Adams BV. Management of cystine nephrolithiasis with alpha-mercaptopropionyl-glycine-(Thiola). J Urol 1986; 136:1003–1008.

OBSTRUCTIVE UROPATHY

SAULO KLAHR, M.D.

In humans, the effects of urinary tract obstruction on renal function are diverse. Not only are there marked reductions in the renal blood flow and glomerular filtration rate, but there are also significant changes in renal tubular function. Partial chronic obstruction of the urinary tract can cause progressive atrophy and destruction of nephrons and ultimately chronic renal insufficiency. Unilateral complete obstruction may be well tolerated for several days; however, if the obstruction persists for more than 1 week, some permanent damage ensues. By the end of 3 weeks of complete obstruction, recoverable function is usually nil. On the other hand, acute complete bilateral obstruction results in renal failure. Because obstruction generally is a remediable cause of kidney failure, early and accurate diagnosis and prompt treatment are vital to the preservation and restoration of renal function.

The clinical manifestations of urinary tract obstructions vary. Bilateral complete obstruction of urine flow is manifested as anuria. Partial obstruction can cause fluctuating urine output, alternating from oliguria to polyuria; urinary tract infection that is usually refractory to treatment; abdominal or flank pain; or unexplained acute or chronic renal failure. Obstruction must always be included in the differential diagnosis of acute renal failure, especially when urine output fluctuates or anuria occurs suddenly (Tables 1 and 2).

GENERAL THERAPEUTIC CONSIDERATIONS

After the diagnosis of urinary tract obstruction has been established, a decision should be made as to whether or not to undertake surgical or instrumental procedures. High-grade or complete bilateral obstruction presenting as acute renal failure requires intervention as soon as possible. In these patients, the site of obstruction frequently determines the approach. If the obstructive lesion is distal to the bladder, passage of a urethral catheter may suffice, although this may require the aid of a urologic surgeon. In some cases, suprapubic cystostomy may be necessary. On the other hand, if the lesion lies proximal to the bladder (upper tract lesion—e.g., a malignant infiltration of the trigone by cervical or prostatic adenocarcinoma), then placement of nephrostomy tubes at the time of ultrasonography or passage of a retrograde ureteral catheter should be undertaken. Tubes should be placed in both obstructed renal calyces, since the potential for recovery of function by either kidney is not easily predicted at the time of the procedure. Such an approach may alleviate the need for dialysis and allows the physician time to determine the specific site and character of the obstructing lesion. Further, the nephrostomy tube may be useful for the local infusion of pharmacologic agents with which to treat infection, malignancy, or calculi. In patients with obstruction complicated by urinary infection and gener-

TABLE 1 Causes of Upper Urinary Tract Obstruction

Urolithiasis	Uterine prolapse
Transitional cell cancer of the pelvis/ureter	Diseases of the gastrointestinal tract
Blood clot	Crohn's disease
Renal papillae	Diverticulitis
Fungus ball	Appendiceal abscess
Ureteral ligation	Pancreatic lesions
Primary obstruction of the ureteropelvic junction; intrinsic (congenital) vs. acquired (vessel crossing postsurgical)	Diseases of the retroperitoneum
Ureteral valve	Retroperitoneal fibrosis
Ureteral polyp	Tuberculosis
Vascular lesions	Sarcoidosis
Abdominal aortic aneurysm	Radiation fibrosis
Iliac artery aneurysm	Retroperitoneal hemorrhage
Retrocaval ureter	Primary retroperitoneal tumors (e.g., lymphomas, sarcomas)
Puerperal ovarian vein thrombophlebitis	Secondary retroperitoneal tumors (e.g., cervix, bladder, colon, prostate)
Fibrosis following vascular reconstructive surgery	Lymphocele
Diseases of the female reproductive tract	Pelvic lipomatosis
Pregnancy	
Mass lesions of the uterus and ovary	
Ovarian remnants	
Gartner's duct cysts	
Tubo-ovarian abscess	
Endometriosis	

TABLE 2 Causes of Lower Urinary Tract Obstruction

Phimosis	Prostatic calculi
Meatal stenosis	Neurogenic bladder
Paraphimosis	Benign prostatic hyperplasia
Urethral stricture	Psychogenic urinary retention
Urethral stone	Bladder calculus
Urethral diverticulum	Bladder cancer
Periurethral abscess	Ureterocele
Posterior urethral valves	Trauma
Anterior urethral valvess	Straddle injury
Urethral surgery	Pelvic fracture
Prostatic abscess	

alized sepsis, appropriate antibiotics and other supportive therapy are indicated.

In patients with low-grade acute obstruction or partial chronic obstruction, surgical intervention may be delayed for a few weeks or even months. However, prompt relief of partial obstruction is indicated when: (1) there are multiple repeated episodes of urinary tract infection; (2) the patient has significant symptoms (flank pain, dysuria, voiding dysfunction); (3) there is urinary retention; and (4) there is evidence of recurrent or progressive renal damage. The presence of postvoid residual urine, urinary extravasation, ureterovesical reflux, or dilatation of the collecting system in the face of sterile urine are not indications for surgical intervention.

MANAGEMENT

Stones are by far the most common cause of ureteral obstruction. The immediate treatment for ureteral stones consists of relief of pain, elimination of obstruction, and control of infection. Relief of pain in acute renal colic is best accomplished by intramuscular injection of adequate doses of a narcotic analgesic. If the stone is less than 5 mm, urologic instrumentation or surgical intervention is not required, since 80 to 90 percent of these ureteral stones will pass spontaneously. Among ureteral stones in the 5- to 7-mm range, however, only 40 to 50 percent will pass, and stones larger than 7 mm will rarely pass spontaneously. High fluid intake to produce urine volumes of at least 1.5 to 2 L daily help pass the stone. The urine must be strained through a gauze sponge to recover the calculi and the stone should be sent for analysis. If a stone completely blocks a ureter and does not move, surgical treatment should commence within a few days. However, if the obstruction is partial, the urine sterile, and the pain manageable, the patient may be observed for weeks or months before surgical therapy is undertaken.

Surgical intervention for renal/ureteral calculi is indicated when there is complete obstruction, unremitting colic, urinary tract infection, and urosepsis, a calculus that is too large to pass (i.e., >7mm) or that has failed to move despite a trial of time (usually months) and increased fluid intake. The surgical therapy for urolithiasis has undergone marked changes during the past 5 years.

Until 1980, the standard approach in treating renal or ureteral calculi *above the pelvic brim* was an open surgical procedure. This was usually accomplished by an anterior abdominal or posterior lumbocostal approach. With these procedures, the usual hospital stay was 4 to 7 days with a convalescence of 2 to 6 weeks.

Because of technologic advances in radiologic imaging modalities and the realization that interventional radiologic techniques may be applied to the urinary tract, a whole new branch of urologic surgery has developed: endourology. Endourology refers to the closed, controlled manipulation of the entire urinary tract. The ability of the interventional radiologist to place a percutaneous nephrostomy and dilate the tract to as large as 12 mm has provided the urologist with a direct conduit to the kidney for the removal of obstructing renal and upper ureteral calculi. The urologist can introduce a variety of rigid or flexible endoscopes through the nephrostomy tract to visualize directly and grasp calculi less than 1.5 cm in diameter. For larger stones, powerful lithotriptor probes have been devised that can use ultrasonic or electrohydraulic energy to disintegrate calculi under direct vision. From its inception in 1976, endourology has garnered rapid acceptance and development in the urologic and radiologic communities. Endourologic methods are currently successful in treating obstructing calculi in 98 percent of patients. In addition, this approach results in a short hospital stay (3 to 4 days) and a convalescence of only 4 to 7 days.

In 1980, another major development in the treatment of symptomatic renal and upper ureteral calculi occurred: extracorporeal shock wave lithotripsy. This technology, developed by Chaussy, Schmiedt, and co-workers in Germany, involves the focusing of extracorporeally electrohydraulically generated fluid-borne shock waves to disintegrate the calculus. The patient is given a general or spinal anesthetic and submerged in a tub of degassed water. A spark plug electrode sits in the bottom of the tub within an ellipsoid container. When fired, the electrode generates a shock wave that bounces off the sides of the ellipsoid container in such a manner that a second focal point is created above the ellipsoid where the shock waves converge. Using dual fluoroscopic control, the patient can be maneuvered until the stone lies completely within the second focal point. The shock waves travel through the water and the patient's body to impact on the stone. Approximately 15,000 lb of pressure per square inch is generated by each shock wave at the second focal point. An average of 2,000 shock waves are given over the 45-minute treatment period. The method is highly effective for calculi in the 7- to 15-mm range; in 90 percent of these patients, the stone is disintegrated and all particulate matter passes within 3 months. In general, these patients experience little morbidity, and the duration of the hospital stay is only 1 to 3 days. In selected patients, the treatment is performed on an outpatient basis, and most patients return to work within 2 to 3 days.

For obstructing calculi *below the pelvic brim,* the best approach remains transurethral. In many cases, these calculi can be removed from the ureter using a variety of stone baskets or loops. This approach is successful in more than 70 percent of patients. When this fails, one can attempt to dilate the ureter and pass a rigid ureterorenoscope to allow for direct endoscopic manipulation of the calculus. Indeed, electrohydraulic and ultrasonic probes have been designed to enable the urologist to destroy larger distal ureteral calculi in situ through the ureterorenoscope. The ureterorenoscope can also be used for upper ureteral calculi; however, because impaction or proximal migration of the stone sometimes occurs, the success rate is only 70 percent. In the distal ureter, the use of either the fluoroscopic or direct endoscopic maneuver has a success rate that exceeds 95 percent. Thus the need for an open surgical approach for the distal ureteral calculus is rare. Finally, for distal ureteral calculi, an approach via a percutaneous nephrostomy or on the extracorporeal shock wave lithotriptor is difficult and should be attempted only when transurethral methods have failed and surgical therapy is not feasible.

Broad-spectrum antibiotics are useful when infections complicate renal calculi. The choice of drugs should be based on the sensitivity studies of the organism isolated from the urine. However, antimicrobial therapy without relief of obstruction is not effective in controlling the infection. Therefore, when primary or secondary obstruction accompanies renal calculi, temporary relief of obstruction should be instituted promptly by insertion of a retrograde ureteral catheter. If the attempted retrograde catheter diversion is unsuccessful, a percutaneous nephrostomy tube can be placed. Whenever possible, relief of obstruction and infection should be achieved before stone manipulation and open surgery.

In summary, a stone less than 5 mm in diameter is likely to be passed without the need for surgical intervention. Even when stone removal appears necessary, in 95 percent of patients this can be achieved with extracorporeal shock wave lithotripsy or via a percutaneous nephrostomy alone, regardless of the size or location of the calculus. Surgical therapy is largely reserved for the few patients in whom the aforementioned measures fail. Earlier intervention is certainly indicated for patients in whom the history, laboratory data, and radiologic studies suggest complete obstruction, for the patient with infected urine, or for the patient with partial obstruction whose stone remains in the same position in the ureter for more than a few months.

Obstruction of the ureter by blood clots, a fungus ball, and papillary tissue can be managed by techniques similar to those employed in the treatment of stones. Significant obstruction attributable to neoplastic, inflammatory, and neurologic diseases must be treated aggressively, since it is unlikely to remit spontaneously. A decision as to whether to divert the urine in patients who have metastatic malignant disease must be made on an individual basis.

Patients with sterile hydronephrosis secondary to advanced pelvic malignancy and a short life expectancy are usually not considered for percutaneous nephrostomy, while those with a reasonable prospect for tumor response to chemotherapy and radiotherapy are strong candidates for the procedure.

The Role of Nephrostomy in the Management of Upper Ureteral Obstruction

Nephrostomy refers to the insertion of a tube through the kidney into the renal pelvis to provide immediate renal urinary drainage. Until the 1950s, all nephrostomy tubes were placed via an open surgical approach. This resulted in significant morbidity and mortality rates, since patients requiring emergency nephrostomy tube placement were often quite debilitated. In 1955, Goodwin reported the first case of a needle-derived nephrostomy tube placed under fluoroscopic guidance. The technique did not gain popularity until the 1970s, when the advent of ultrasonography and improved methods of fluoroscopy made the percutaneous approach more feasible. Currently, almost all nephrostomy tubules are placed percutaneously by an interventional radiologist or urologist. This is usually done with the patient under local anesthesia and takes less than 40 minutes.

The most common indications for placement of a nephrostomy tube are to provide a conduit to the kidney for percutaneous stone removal and to relieve ureteral obstruction secondary to neoplasia; inflammatory disease; or lower tract, extrinsic, or intrinsic obstruction in which the patient's condition does not permit a more definitive surgical procedure. Likewise, unmanageable infection behind an obstructed system is another common indication. It is not unusual to note dramatic clinical improvement within hours of percutaneous drainage in the patient with urosepsis.

The immediate complications of nephrostomy are perirenal hemorrhage and acute obstruction from clot formation. One of the more serious delayed complications is dislodgement of the nephrostomy tube. This is considered an emergency; the tube should be replaced immediately, otherwise the tract will seal off, usually within 24 hours. Another problem occurring after nephrostomy tube removal is the exsanguinating hemorrhage from a renal pseudoaneurysm. This occurs in 0.5 to 1 percent of patients and is best managed by immediate selective embolization of the affected vessel. Long-term complications, such as infection, calculus formation, and pyelonephritis, are significant and may lead to renal failure.

Except in unusual circumstances, long-term urinary diversion by the nephrostomy tube is not recommended. In many patients, however, several years may pass without the development of serious complications from their nephrostomy tubes. Also, in patients with extrinsic obstruction secondary to metastatic carcinoma, the nephrostomy tract can be used to manipulate a catheter into the bladder. A small tube can be placed through the affected flank and kidney with its pigtail end left in the bladder. The external portion of the stent can be clamped, thereby providing unobstructed flow from the affected kidney to the patient's bladder. This eliminates the need for external drainage bags and also facilitates in the changing of the tube. In essence, all nephrostomy tubes or indwelling stents are changed every 3 months to decrease the build-up of concretions and to preclude breakage of ureteral stents within the collecting system.

For chronically obstructed kidneys, a period of percutaneous drainage may permit significant restoration of renal function. With this knowledge and with periodic determination of split renal function studies, treatment can be planned effectively. A lack of significant improvement in function might suggest, for example, that nephrectomy rather than reparative surgery should be undertaken.

Lower Urinary Tract Obstruction

Bladder neck and urethral obstruction should be surgically repaired in ambulatory patients who have recurrent infections, especially when associated with reflux, evidence of renal parenchymal damage, total urinary retention, repeated bleeding, or other severe symptoms. Difficulties with voiding secondary to benign prostatic hyperplasia do not always follow a progressive course. Therefore, a man with minimal symptoms, no infection, and a normal upper urinary tract may be followed safely until he and his physician agree that surgery is desirable. Urethral stricture in men that is secondary to infection or trauma is frequently treated by simple dilation or direct vision internal urethrotomy. In these patients, radiographic and endoscopic follow-up care is essential to rule out recurrence. The incidence of bladder neck and urethral obstruction in women is low and has been overestimated in the past; hence urethral dilation, internal urethrotomy, meatotomy, and revision of the bladder neck are seldom indicated. In some patients, suprapubic cystostomy may be necessary for bladder drainage. This is especially indicated in patients who are unable to void after sustaining injury to the urethra or who have an impassable urethral stricture.

Again, advances in urologic instrumentation have further decreased the indications for open surgery. Almost all suprapubic cystotomies are performed using a percutaneous approach under fluoroscopic guidance. Open cystotomy is rarely performed. In addition, a closed transurethral approach is used to treat the majority of patients with prostatic hyperplasia (≥60 g of tissue), urethral strictures, bladder neck contractures, bladder calculi, and superficial bladder tumors.

When obstructive uropathy is a consequence of neuropathic bladder function, urodynamic studies are essential to establish a treatment regimen. In all cases, the main therapeutic goals are to establish the bladder as a site of urine storage without causing renal parenchymal injury and to provide a mechanism for bladder emptying that is acceptable to the patient. In general, these patients fall into one of two groups: those with bladder atony secondary to lower motor neuron injury and those with unstable bladder function attributable to upper motor neuron disease. In both cases, ureteral reflux and renal parenchymal injury may occur, although it is more common with the hyperactive upper motor neuron bladder. This problem may be potentiated by sphincter-detrusor dyssynergia or by using either external compression (Credé's maneuver) or by increasing abdominal pressure (Valsalva's maneuver) to aid voiding.

Patients with neurogenic bladder function caused by diabetes mellitus are classic examples of lower motor neuron disease. Voiding at regular intervals is one method to aid satisfactory bladder emptying in such patients. Occasionally, these individuals respond to cholinergic medications. Recent reviews on the use of bethanechol chloride (Urecholine), 50 mg orally, have seriously questioned its long-term value. In such patients, overdistention of the bladder impairs emptying, since detrusor contraction is essential to sphincter relaxation. Thus, bladder outlet obstruction may be a major problem. Alpha-adrenergic blockers such as phenoxybenzamine hydrochloride relax urethral sphincter tone but have only limited success because of side effects. Table 3 summarizes the drugs used in the treatment of lower urinary tract dysfunction and their proposed mechanism of action.

Another alternative for men with a flaccid bladder is external sphincterotomy. This transurethral procedure may be successful in relieving outlet obstruction and promoting bladder emptying, but it has the disadvantage of urinary incontinence and requires that the patient wear an external collection device. In men, this problem can be obviated by the use of a penile clamp; however, the clamps often result in significant morbidity owing to urethral erosion and penile edema. In women, the incontinence associated with external sphincterotomy precludes its use. In addition, the implantation of newly developed artificial urinary sphincters has been partially successful. Although these devices are promising, problems

TABLE 3 Drugs Used in the Treatment of Lower Urinary Tract Dysfunction

Drugs that facilitate urine storage
1. By increasing urethral tone
   - Beta-blockers (propranolol hydrochloride)
   - Alpha-adrenergic agonists (imipramine hydrochloride, phenylpropanolamine hydrochloride)
2. By inhibiting bladder (detrusor) contractility
   - Anticholinergic agents (propantheline hydrochloride)
   - Smooth muscle depressants (imipramine hydrochloride, dicyclomine hydrochloride, oxybutynin chloride)
   - Alpha-adrenergic antagonists (prazosin hydrochloride, phenoxybenzamine hydrochloride)

Drugs that facilitate voiding
1. By increasing bladder (detrusor) contractility
   - Cholinergic agents (bethanechol chloride)
2. By decreasing sphincter tone
   - Alpha-adrenergic antagonists (prazosin hydrochloride, phenoxybenzamine hydrochloride, clonidine hydrochloride)
   - Skeletal muscle relaxants (diazepam, dantrolene sodium)

with their longevity have hindered their widespread acceptance.

The most ideal treatment for patients with significant residual urine and recurrent bouts of urosepsis is clean intermittent catheterization (CIC) performed at regular intervals. Ideally catheterization should be performed four to five times per day such that the amount of urine drained from the bladder does not exceed 300 to 400 ml. This technique has met with considerable success in almost all age groups but requires patient acceptance and careful training.

In patients with unstable bladder function attributable to upper motor neuron lesions, the major goal is to improve the storage function of the bladder. Pharmacologic maneuvers include the use of anticholinergic agents such as oxybutynin chloride (Ditropan), 5 mg every 4 to 6 hours. Adjunctive therapy such as CIC is frequently necessary to ensure complete bladder emptying and prevent incontinence.

In all patients with neurogenic bladders, chronic indwelling catheters are to be avoided if possible. In addition to problems of external drainage, bladder stones, urosepsis, and urethral erosion, chronic indwelling catheters are associated with the occurrence of squamous cell carcinoma of the bladder. Patients managed in this fashion for more than 5 years should undergo yearly cystoscopic examinations.

Finally, surgical diversions are indicated for (1) deterioration of renal function despite conservative measures, (2) intractable incontinence, (3) a small contracted bladder, and (4) multiple bladder fistulae. Intermittent bacteriuria is seldom an indication for this treatment, since it is common to all therapeutic approaches to the neurogenic bladder. The ileal conduit is the operation of choice for permanent diversion. Although many individuals do well after this procedure, operative mortality, postoperative intestinal obstruction, and stomal obstruction are complications that make the operation far from ideal. Further, recent studies have indicated that in as many as 80 percent of patients, there will be a progressive decline in renal function. A continent form of ileal diversion has become available: the Koch pouch. With this procedure, an ileal reservoir with a 300- to 500-ml capacity is made. A continent stoma is placed in the right lower quadrant of the abdomen, which the patient must empty by catheterization four times per day. This method of diversion alleviates the need for any external collection devices.

In patients requiring short-term indwelling urethral catheters, good care is necessary to prevent urinary tract infection. Men are instructed to cleanse the glans twice per day with an antimicrobial soap and then to apply an antibiotic ointment. Given specific indications for catheter drainage, proper patient selection, aseptic technique, closed urinary drainage, the judicious use of systemic antimicrobials, and proper catheter care, the indwelling urethral catheter is a satisfactory means of short-term diversion, and in rare instances, of long-term urinary diversion. The principles of closed drainage are that the system never be open, that the urine in the drainage tube never come in contact with the urine in the collecting bag, and that, at all times, the bag be in a dependent position. Cultures can be obtained by clamping the catheter for a few minutes and then using a small needle and syringe to aspirate urine from the lumen of the catheter. I prefer not to break the drainage system for catheter irrigation or for the use of antibiotic irrigating solutions to reduce infection, as has been advocated by some. In patients requiring long-term catheter drainage, intermittent irrigation with an acid citrate solution is useful in reducing encrustation.

In the past, there has been some concern and controversy regarding the possible complications of rapid decompression of a severely distended bladder. It has been advised that the grossly distended bladder be drained slowly over a period of hours rather than all at once. It has also been suggested that rapid emptying of the distended bladder may be followed by hypotension and syncope or hemorrhagic cystitis attributable to sudden decompression of stretched mucosal blood vessels. These concerns appear unjustified, since it has been found that the intravesical pressure in patients with acute urinary retention falls precipitously to near-normal values after the first deciliter of urine is withdrawn, indicating that any sudden decompressive effect on blood vessels would be maximal during the removal of the initial volume of urine.

Fetal Uropathies

Modern real-time ultrasonography equipment and interpretation have presented physicians with a new type of patient: the fetus. One condition, namely obstructive uropathy, appears to be amenable in some cases to treatment in utero. The most common sites of obstruction found during development include the ureteropelvic junction, the ureterovesical junction, and the posterior urethral valves. Antenatal intervention is probably indicated whenever the function of both kidneys is threatened. The amount of amniotic fluid may represent an indirect guide to assess renal function in the fetus. The risk of invasive procedures for the mother, and in particular the fetus, must be weighed against the potential benefits. Additional information is needed in this area of prenatal intervention before firm guidelines can be suggested.

Postobstructive Diuresis

Postobstructive diuresis refers to the marked polyuria that can occur after relief of urinary tract obstruction. This polyuria is usually associated with the excretion of large amounts of sodium,potassium, magnesium, and other solutes. Although self-limited (it may last several days), the losses of salt and water may be of such magnitude as to cause hypokalemia, hyponatremia or hypernatremia, hypomagnesemia and/or marked contraction of the extracellular fluid (ECF) volume, and peripheral vascular collapse. In many patients, however, a brisk diuresis after relief of urinary tract obstruction may be physiologically appropriate rather than caused by an inability of the postobstructed kidney to maintain volume and solute homeostasis. A postobstructive diuresis is appropriate and does not compromise the volume status of the patient when it is caused by excretion of excess salt, water, and urea retained during the period of obstruction. This diuresis is transient and usually subsides within the first day or two after relief of obstruction without causing depletion of the ECF volume. It is often impossible, however, to distinguish such patients from those who have a true defect in tubular reabsorption of salt and water on the basis of urine volume and composition alone. Thus replacement therapy should be guided by clinical and laboratory evidence of the adequacy of the ECF volume and not by the volume of the urine only.

It is well established that postobstructive diuresis may be artificially prolonged by overzealous administration of salt and water after relief of obstruction. Replacement of excreted salt and water maintains a state of expansion of the ECF and hence results in the continuous excretion of the excess salt and water administered. Thus fluid replacement may be justified only when excessive losses of sodium and water occur that are inappropriate for the volume status of the patient and are presumably caused by an intrinsic tubular defect in the reabsorption of sodium and water.

For patients with postobstructive diuresis, the appropriate fluid replacement depends largely on what is excreted. Although intravenous fluid administration may be necessary, urinary losses should be replaced only to the extent necessary to prevent hypovolemia, hypotension, hypokalemia, and/or hypomagnesemia. Excessive fluid administration only prolongs the duration of the postobstructive diuresis. Orthostatic hypotension and tachycardia are perhaps the best indicators of when intravenous fluid administration is needed. To distinguish between inappropriate diuresis and the excretion of fluid retained or excess fluid administration, it may be necessary to decrease the rate of intravenous fluid administration to levels below those of urinary output and observe the patient carefully for signs of volume depletion (hypotension, tachycardia, and stabilization or elevation in the level of blood urea nitrogen, which was previously decreasing). In the case of inappropriate diuresis, appropriate fluid replacement consists of the prompt quantitative replacement of urinary losses of water, sodium, potassium, and magnesium. This is best accomplished by frequent measurements of urine volume and serum and urine electrolytes. With massive diuresis, such measurements may be required every 6 hours. The patient's body weight should be measured daily and occasionally even more often. Fluids administered should be tailored to match the urinary excretion of water and electrolytes.

In most instances, urinary losses of salt and water may be replaced with solutions of 0.45 percent sodium chloride to which sodium bicarbonate and potassium chloride have been added. Replacement of magnesium may be accomplished by adding magnesium sulfate (supplied as 2-ml ampules containing 8 mEq magnesium) to the sodium chloride solution. Sometimes replacement of phosphate losses may be necessary. Either 42 percent sodium phosphate (15-ml ampules containing 45 mmol phosphate and 60 mEq sodium) or 46 percent potassium phosphate (15-ml ampules containing 45 mmol phosphate and 66 mEq potassium) may be added to 5 percent dextrose or 0.45 percent sodium chloride solutions.

SUGGESTED READING

Elder JS, Duckett JW Jr, Snyder HM. Intervention for fetal obstructive uropathy: has it been effective? Lancet 1987; 2:1007–1010.

Smith AD. Endourology update. In Urol Clin North Am 1988; 15:295–554

Wein AJ, Arsdale KN. Non-surgical management of neuropathic voiding dysfunction. Semin Urol 1985; 3:216–237.

CYSTIC DISEASE OF THE KIDNEY

VICENTE E. TORRES, M.D.

A cyst is a gross cavity lined by epithelium or abnormal tissue usually containing fluid or other material. Renal cysts are usually of tubular origin and are lined by tubular epithelium. Many heterogeneous conditions—whether congenital, developmental, or acquired and with or without a genetic cause—that have in common the presence of renal cysts are classified as "renal cystic diseases." There have been many more or less arbitrary provisional classifications of these diseases. In one such classification, based on pathogenetic considerations, they are divided into (1) those caused by defects of metanephric differentia- (cystic dysplasias), (2) those associated with hereditary interstitial nephritis, and (3) those with tubular epithelial hyperplasia without dysplasia, (4) cystic conditions of inflammatory or neoplastic origin, and (5) renal cystic diseases of nontubular origin. Only the most common of these disorders are discussed in this chapter (Table 1).

MULTICYSTIC RENAL DYSPLASIA

Renal cystic dysplasias comprise a spectrum of renal abnormalities resulting from an interference with the normal metanephric differentiation. Multicystic renal dysplasia is a result of an early inhibition of ampullary activity. The ureter is absent or atretic, and the kidneys consist of a grapelike cluster of cysts. When bilateral, multicystic renal dysplasia is incompatible with life. When unilateral or segmental, it can be diagnosed in the newborn or go undetected and be discovered years later as an abdominal mass or an incidental finding.

Treatment

Because these kidneys tend to decrease in size, most authors recommend a nonsurgical approach when the diagnosis of multicystic renal dysplasia can be firmly established by noninvasive techniques. In the newborn, it is essential that this condition be differentiated from hydronephrosis, since the treatment is markedly different. Excretory urography is frequently unsatisfactory because of decreased renal concentrating ability and glomerular filtration in the newborn, resulting in poor visualization of hydronephrotic kidneys, as well as because of the occasional puttering of contrast material in delayed films in multicystic kidneys. Renal scintigraphy has similar limitations. The most useful diagnostic technique is ultrasonography. The criteria to distinguish multicystic renal dysplasia from congenital hydronephrosis include the presence of interfaces between the cysts, nonmedial location of the larger cysts, absence of identifiable renal sinus, and absence of parenchymal tissue. The diagnosis can be confirmed by retrograde pyelography showing an absent or atretic proximal ureter and by angiography revealing an absent or hypoplastic renal artery.

Clear indications for surgical removal of a multicystic dysplastic kidney are pain, increase in size, infection, and hypertension with lateralizing renal vein renin studies. Some authors, however, recommend nephrectomy of all multicystic dysplastic kidneys because of the risk of hypertension or malignant degeneration. Since most patients with unilateral multicystic kidneys diagnosed during infancy or early childhood have been treated surgically, the natural history of this condition is unclear. Considering the large population at risk, very few cases of proven causally related hypertension have been reported. With regard to the risk of malignancy, two Wilms's tumors and four renal cell carcinomas have been reported in unilateral multicystic kidneys. Of interest is that four carcinomas developed in women, three of whom were young (25, 26, and 33 years of age). The early development of renal cell carcinoma in these patients may support the concept that a dysplastic kidney has a significantly increased likelihood of malignant degeneration.

MEDULLARY CYSTIC DISEASE

Medullary cystic disease and nephronophthisis are synonymous terms that denote a heterogeneous group of diseases characterized by small kidneys with interstitial nephritis and cysts in the cortical medullary junction, clinically characterized by an insidious onset, polydipsia and/or polyuria, benign urinary sediment, mild proteinuria, frequent sodium wasting, and relentless progression to renal failure. The pathogenesis of these disorders is not known, but a primary

TABLE 1 Renal Cystic Disease

Multicystic renal dysplasia
Medullary cystic disease
Simple renal cysts
Medullary sponge kidney
Autosomal recessive polycystic kidney disease
Autosomal dominant polycystic kidney disease
Tuberous sclerosis
von Hippel-Lindau disease
Acquired cystic kidney disease
Multilocular cysts
Cystic disease of the renal sinus

tubular basement membrane defect and autoimmune mechanisms have been considered likely. Two main forms are recognized on the basis of inheritance and age at diagnosis, a juvenile recessive form and an adult dominant form. Sporadic presentations may represent recessive cases in families with a small offspring or new dominant mutations. The autosomal recessive form is frequently associated with extrarenal abnormalities such as retinitis pigmentosa (renal-retinal syndrome), skeletal abnormalities (cono-renal syndromes including chondroectodermal dysplasia, asphyxiating thoracic dystrophy, Saldino-Mainzer syndrome, and peripheral dysostosis with medullary cystic disease), congenital hepatic fibrosis, and central nervous system abnormalities (cerebro-oculo-hepato-renal syndrome). A renal disease consistent with medullary cystic disease also occurs in two additional autosomal recessive syndromes, the Laurence-Moon-Bardet-Biedl syndrome (obesity, polydactyly, retinitis pigmentosa, mental retardation, and hypogenitalism) and Alström's syndrome (obesity, diabetes mellitus, retinitis pigmentosa, and nerve deafness).

Treatment

The treatment of medullary cystic disease is supportive. Hypertension is not a prominent manifestation of the disease but, when present, it should be carefully controlled. Volume contraction and prerenal azotemia, unnecessary sodium restriction, and diuretics should be avoided because of the tendency to sodium wasting. Some patients may require sodium chloride supplementation to maintain sodium balance during a phase of their disease. Administration of sodium bicarbonate may be necessary to correct a renal tubular acidosis. Osteomalacia or secondary hyperparathyroidism should be treated if present. In children with failure to thrive, consideration might be given to treatment with growth hormone. Eventually, dialysis and/or renal transplantation are needed. Precautions should be taken to use only unaffected relatives for living-related kidney transplantation. The living-related donors should undergo meticulous diagnostic evaluation and should be at least 10 years older than the affected child or sibling. The patient and his or her family should be provided with genetic counseling based on the mode of inheritance.

SIMPLE RENAL CYSTS

Simple cysts, like most renal cysts of tubuloepithelial origin, are believed to originate from diverticula and localized defects in the tubular wall. The frequency of both tubular diverticula and cysts increases with age. More than 50 percent of people older than 50 years of age have at least one cyst on postmortem examination.

Evaluation and Treatment

Simple cysts most often produce no symptoms and require no specific treatment. Differentiation from more severe conditions, such as renal cell carcinoma and, when multiple, polycystic kidney disease, is therefore essential. Characteristic features on ultrasonography (lack of internal echoes, smooth walls, and enhancement of echoes deep to the lesion) and computed tomography (CT) (density near that of water, thin wall, sharp interface, and no enhancement with contrast material) allow one to distinguish clearly between a benign simple cyst and a renal cell carcinoma in the majority of cases. The presence of a few delicate septa within a cyst is of no clinical significance. When these criteria are not met, percutaneous needle aspiration or, rarely, angiography is necessary. Calcification confined to the cyst wall is not an indication for puncture if all of the CT characteristics for a benign renal cyst are seen. Some findings on ultrasonography or CT, such as a discrete nodule in the wall of the cyst, constitute an indication for surgery regardless of the result of cyst aspiration. Differentiation of multiple simple cysts from mild forms of polycystic kidney disease is difficult and requires a careful family history, search for cysts in other organs, and a careful assessment of clinical correlations.

The incidental discovery of simple renal cysts should not distract one from other more important lesions. They can rarely cause abdominal or flank pain, microscopic or macroscopic hematuria, and renin-dependent hypertension, but other causes of these manifestations should always be sought. For example, simple cysts are often found in the vicinity of a renal cell carcinoma ("sentinel cysts"). Patterns of extrinsic compression and infundibular obstruction caused by cysts on excretory urography are often found to be of no functional significance by furosemide radioactive renal scan.

At present, surgery is indicated only in the rare cases in which there is still doubt regarding the precise diagnosis after using less invasive investigations, in the rare complicated cyst that cannot be adequately treated percutaneously, and in the symptomatic cyst that recurs rapidly after percutaneous drainage. Percutaneous aspiration of a renal cyst is easily accomplished and should be done for diagnostic purposes whenever a cyst might be responsible for pain, obstruction, or hypertension. In some cases, there is no reaccumulation of cyst fluid, and the aspiration is of therapeutic value. Reaccumulation of cyst fluid, however, occurs in 30 to 80 percent of the cases. Several sclerosing agents, including glucose, phenol, bismuth phosphate, iophendylate iodophenylundecanoate (Pantopaque), and ethanol have been used to prevent the reaccumulation of fluid. The best results are obtained with ethanol, but because of the highly sclerosing properties of this substance, introduction of a pigtail catheter into the cyst is required. The technique described by Bean is usually followed; the cyst contents are totally aspirated, and 25 percent of the original cyst volume is replaced with 95 percent ethanol. The patient is then placed in the supine and prone positions and both lateral decubitus positions for 5 minutes to allow adequate contact of the alcohol with all the areas of the cyst wall. The alcohol is then aspirated, and the catheter is removed. It has been shown that after 1 to 3 minutes of contact with the ethanol, the epithelial cells lining the cyst walls become fixed and nonviable, without significant damage to the adjacent normal renal parenchyma. When performed by a radiologist with extensive experience, this procedure is relatively safe, with less than 1 percent of major complications and less than 10 percent of minor complications. The most common major complication is perirenal hemorrhage. The most common minor complication is pain following the procedure, which may persist for several days. Infections of simple renal cysts are very rare, usually occur in female patients, and are caused by *Escherichia coli*. The treatment of infected simple cysts consists of drainage combined with antibiotic therapy. Although surgery used to be required for cyst drainage, percutaneous drainage is equally successful.

MEDULLARY SPONGE KIDNEY

Medullary sponge kidney is a common disorder characterized by tubular dilatation of the collecting ducts and cyst formation strictly confined to the medullary pyramids, especially their inner, papillary portions. It is regarded as a nonhereditary disease, but autosomal dominant inheritance has been suggested in several families. It is usually a benign disorder that may remain asymptomatic for life, but mild tubular function abnormalities, such as a concentration defect, a reduced capacity to acidify the urine after ammonium chloride administration, and a reduced maximal excretion of potassium after potassium chloride loading are common. The diagnosis of medullary sponge kidney is usually established during the course of evaluation of episodes of renal colic, hematuria, or urinary tract infections. Nephrolithiasis is the major complication. Patients with medullary sponge kidney have a higher rate of stone formation than other patients with nephrolithiasis. It is uncertain whether hypercalciuria and hyperparathyroidism are more prevalent in these patients than in other patients with nephrolithiasis. Women with medullary sponge kidney and nephrolithiasis are more likely to have cystoscopic examinations and higher rates of urinary tract infections than other women with nephrolithiasis. There is no evidence that medullary sponge kidney per se that is unrelated to the nephrolithiasis predisposes to urinary tract infection. Hypertension does not occur more frequently in these patients than in the general population. The renal function remains normal except in rare patients with complicated nephrolithiasis and chronic pyelonephritis.

Treatment

Patients with medullary sponge kidney should be informed of the benign nature of this disorder, provided that the nephrolithiasis is controlled. Unnecessary repetitious investigations for hematuria should be avoided. As in other patients with nephrolithiasis, metabolic factors contributing to the formation of stones should be identified and treated. Adequate fluid intake to maintain a 24-hour urine volume of more than 2.5 L in men and 2.0 L in women is essential. Thiazide or orthophosphate may be effective in the patients who continue to form stones. Alkali as potassium citrate may be a more simple alternative to orthophosphate treatment in the patients with medullary sponge kidney and impaired distal acidification with hypocitric aciduria. Because of the blunted kaliuretic response to potassium loading reported to occur in patients with medullary sponge kidney, potassium plasma levels in patients treated with potassium citrate should be rechecked, but hyperkalemia in these patients has not been a problem. As in other patients with nephrolithiasis, urinary tract infections should be aggressively treated, the results of therapy adequately assessed, and chronic suppression or prophylactic therapy instituted if one is unable to eradicate the infection or in patients with frequent recurrences. The treatment of patients with medullary sponge kidney and infected stones with urea-splitting organisms may pose a special problem since complete removal of the stone and adequate acidification of the urine with ammonium chloride may be difficult to achieve in these patients. The roles of surgery and percutaneous or extracorporeal lithotripsy in these patients are not different from those in other patients with nephrolithiasis.

AUTOSOMAL RECESSIVE POLYCYSTIC KIDNEY DISEASE

Autosomal recessive polycystic kidney disease is characterized by various combinations of bilateral renal cystic disease and congenital hepatic fibrosis. The cysts in this disorder result from giantism of the collecting tubules. They are elongated, of similar size, and extend from the medulla to the cortex. Congenital hepatic fibrosis is a developmental abnormality that leads to portal hypertension and is characterized by enlarged and fibrotic portal areas with an apparent proliferation of bile ducts, absence of central bile ducts, hypoplasia of the portal vein branches, and sometimes, prominent fibrosis around the central veins. It can also occur as an isolated finding or in association with renal dysplasia and hereditary tubulointerstitial nephritis. In newborns and infants, the clinical presentation of autosomal recessive polycystic kidney disease is dominated by the manifestations of the renal disease, and in older children and adolescents, by the manifestations of portal hypertension. In older children and adolescents, the cystic dilatation of the collecting tubules may be less pronounced and can be confused with medullary sponge kidney. The differential diagnosis of autosomal recessive and autosomal dominant polycystic kidney diseases in infancy or childhood is usually possible on the basis of the family history and the findings on excretory urography, ultrasonography, and CT. Liver histology is sometimes needed to establish the diagnosis.

Treatment

Autosomal recessive polycystic kidney disease is not always fatal, as was initially believed, and some patients may have a prolonged survival. In fact, the enlarged kidneys may decrease in relative size in patients who survive the neonatal phase of the disease, while the renal function may remain stable for many years or slowly progress to renal failure (Fig. 1). Accurate blood pressure assessment and strict control are essential in these young children. Many require dialysis or renal transplantation at an early age. The surviving patients and those who present during later childhood or adolescence are likely to require treatment for portal hypertension to prevent life-threatening hemorrhages from esophageal varices. The liver function tests are usually normal, although mild elevations of the serum alkaline phosphatase and transaminase can occur. These patients are good candidates for portal systemic shunting procedures, with portocaval shunting being preferred by some. The renal disease may progress to renal failure years after successful shunting. Patients with associated nonobstructive intrahepatic biliary dilatation (Caroli's disease) may have recurrent episodes of cholangitis and may require antimicrobial therapy. Partial hepatectomy can be considered in patients with recurrent episodes of cholangitis and segmental dilatation of the intrahepatic bile ducts.

AUTOSOMAL DOMINANT POLYCYSTIC KIDNEY DISEASE

Autosomal dominant polycystic kidney disease (ADPKD) is an autosomal dominant multisystem disease with high penetrance, mainly affecting the kidney, and with a wide range of ages of clinical presentation and a great variation in severity. The ADPKD gene has been localized proximal to the alpha hemoglobin region in the short arm of chromosome 16, and flanking markers on both sides of the ADPKD gene are now available. The lack of linkage between ADPKD and these markers in a few families indicates that ADPKD is caused by at least two genes, ADPKD1 and ADPKD2 (genetic heterogeneity). Preliminary results of ongoing studies suggest that ADPKD1 accounts for approximately 90 percent of ADPKDs and that ADPKD2 families have a milder expression of the disease.

Presymptomatic Diagnosis

Because of the genetic heterogeneity, a presymptomatic diagnosis of ADPKD by DNA linkage analysis is possible only in families in which linkage to the markers on chromosome 16 can be reasonably established. Otherwise, ultrasonography continues to be the preferred method for presymptomatic diagnosis. The accepted definition of an affected individual in

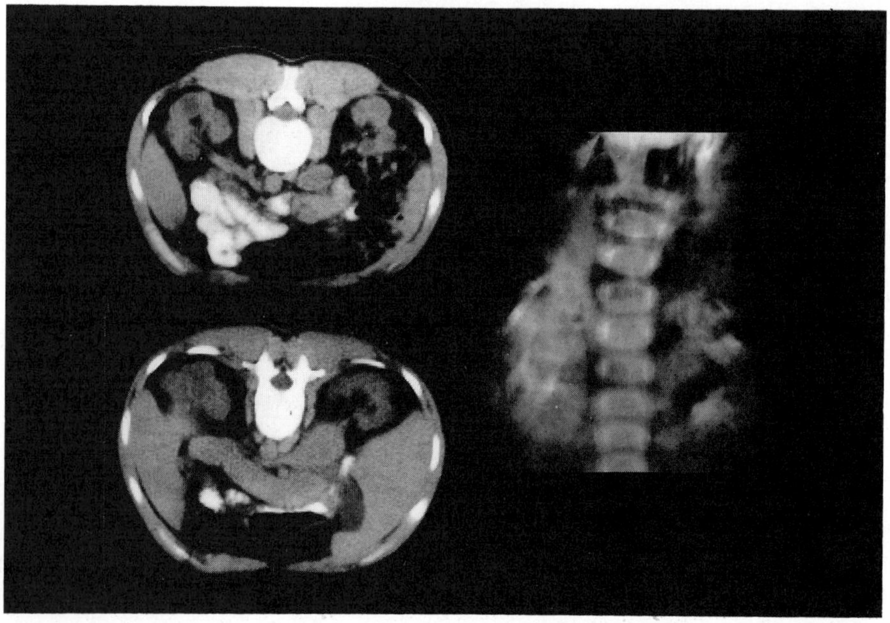

Figure 1 *Left,* Excretory urography in a 12-month-old male with ADPKD showing large kidneys with a characteristic nephrogram of radiating streaks of contrast. *Right,* CT scan of the abdomen 20 years later showing a relative reduction in the size of the kidneys, multiple renal cysts, and a prominent inferior vena cava consistent with previous portocaval shunting.

the presence of a positive family history is at least one cyst in each kidney and at least two cysts in one kidney. Using this definition, the probability that an at-risk subject carries the ADPKD gene after ultrasonography has yielded negative results has been estimated to be 34 percent for patients 15 to 20 years of age, 14 percent for those 20 to 30 years of age, and 5 percent for those older than 30 years of age. This is a conservative estimate, and other studies have suggested that more than 95 percent of ADPKD gene carriers 20 years of age or older can be correctly identified by ultrasonography.

Many individuals at risk, as well as some physicians, question the value of the presymptomatic diagnosis of a disease for which there is no cure. A presymptomatic diagnosis of ADPKD should not be made without adequate genetic counseling, which should include a well-informed discussion of the medical facts, including the diagnosis, pathogenesis and manifestations of the disease, and available management, as well as the inheritable pattern and options for dealing with the inheritable risk. Especially important in this genetic counseling is the avoidance of an unwarranted pessimism, since it has become apparent in recent years that many patients with ADPKD have a normal life expectancy and since solutions for many of the problems encountered by ADPKD patients are now available. Under these conditions, the presymptomatic evaluation of individuals at risk for ADPKD can help avoid the rampages of years of untreated hypertension, preventable complications, unnecessary medical evaluations, and much anxiety. On the negative side, individuals at risk for ADPKD should be informed of the impact that a positive diagnosis of the disease will have on their insurability.

Treatment

Despite major advances in the understanding of the process of cystogenesis and some observations that bear hope that the rate of cyst growth may someday be affected by pharmacologic intervention, the therapy of ADPKD at present is still restricted to the treatment of its symptoms and complications. The main renal manifestations of ADPKD are abdominal or flank pain caused by cyst enlargement, bleeding, nephrolithiasis, or infection; hematuria; hypertension; and renal insufficiency. Whether patients with ADPKD are at increased risk for developing gout, especially during diuretic therapy, is uncertain. Renal cell carcinomas in ADPKD patients are rare and possibly not more frequent than in the general population, although they are more frequently bilateral when they occur. The extrarenal manifestations of ADPKD include hepatic cysts, intracranial aneurysms, cardiac valve abnormalities, dilatation of the aortic root, and rarely, aortic aneurysms. It has been suggested that ADPKD patients have an increased incidence of diverticulosis and diverticulitis, but this association needs further confirmation.

Patients with ADPKD often have a sensation of flank or abdominal fullness or heaviness, but this sensation is not painful and requires no analgesics. In a small subset of patients, the renal enlargement and distortion are accompanied by chronic, severe, disabling flank pain. These patients often become analgesic or narcotic dependent. As is the case in other patients with chronic pain, the evaluation and treatment of these patients are difficult. Other renal causes of the pain, such as an infected renal cyst or undetected uric acid calculi, as well as extrarenal processes, need to be ruled out. A psychologic assessment and an understanding and supportive attitude on the physician's part are essential. Reassurance and changes in lifestyle with avoidance of certain activities may provide some relief. In some cases, a pain clinic evaluation and the use of transcutaneous electric nerve stimulation (TENS), celiac plexus, or sympathetic lumbar blocks may be helpful. In other situations, especially when CT reveals considerable distortion and stretching of the kidney by large cysts and conservative measures have been exhausted, surgical decompression through a lumbotomy or flank incision should be considered. The use of intraoperative ultrasonography to help in the localization of the deeper cysts is helpful. Recent experience indicates that this surgery provides sustained pain relief in approximately 70 percent of these patients without an adverse effect on renal function (Fig. 2). Percutaneous needle aspiration may be of some diagnostic and prognostic value, but it does not provide permanent pain relief. There is little experience with the use of ethanol sclerosis in ADPKD, but because of the large number of cysts, it seems doubtful that it can be safely and effectively accomplished in the majority of patients with chronic, severe pain.

Episodes of hemorrhage in a polycystic kidney are usually confined inside cysts or lead to gross hematuria. They are self-limited and usually can be treated at home with bed rest, hydration, and analgesics such as acetaminophen with codeine. Rarely, the episodes of bleeding are more severe with extensive subcapsular or retroperitoneal hematomas and significant decreases in hematocrit or hemodynamic instability and require hospitalization and investigations with CT or angiography. Urinary tract obstruction by a hemorrhagic cyst or a clot may also require hospitalization and stent placement. In cases of unusually severe or persistent hemorrhage, segmental arterial embolization or surgery needs to be considered. The episodes of bleeding in a polycystic kidney can sometimes be explained by trauma or unusual physical activity or may be triggered by the use of an anticoagulant medication or by uncontrolled hypertension. Often there is no obvious cause. ADPKD patients should be advised against the practice of contact sports and the use of constrictive belts.

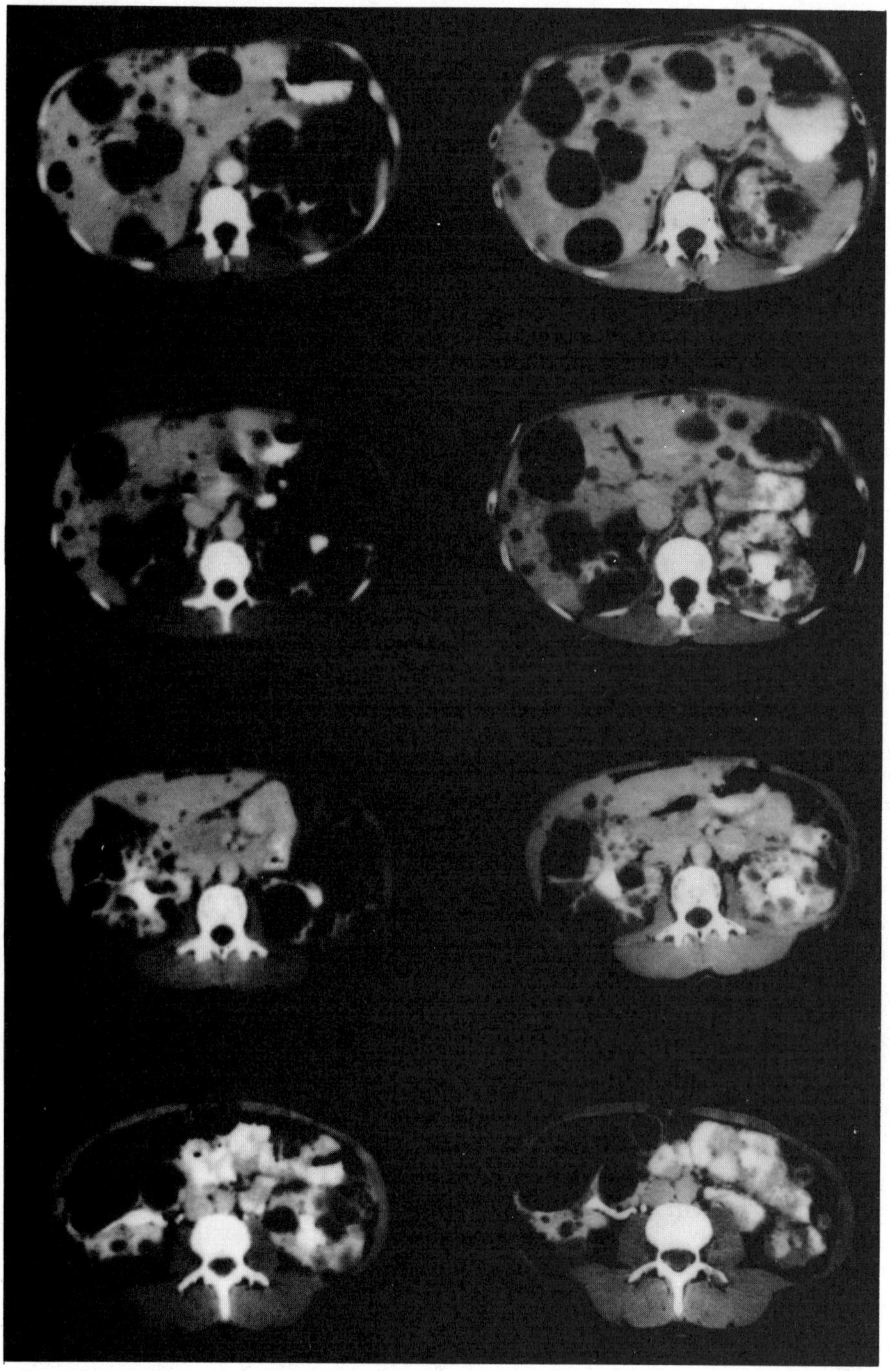

Figure 2 Contrast-enhanced CT scans of the abdomen before (left) and after (right) surgical decompression of a left polycystic kidney.

Early detection and strict treatment of hypertension and correction of other cardiovascular risk factors are most important in ADPKD, since cardiovascular complications constitute the main cause of death for patients with this disease. In addition, several studies have shown that ADPKD patients with hypertension are more likely to have a faster deterioration of renal function than those without. The pathogenesis of hypertension in ADPKD is not completely understood, and therefore the best antihypertensive treatment has not been established. Most studies on the pathogenesis of hypertension in ADPKD are consistent with the hypothesis of an increased intrarenal angiotensin effect, with a reduced renal blood flow, increased filtration fraction, and an abnormal renal handling of sodium leading to an absolute or relative expansion of the extracellular fluid volume and hypertension. Given the central role that the renin angiotensin system is thought to play in this pathogenetic scheme, a converting enzyme inhibitor may be the antihypertensive agent of choice in the presence of normal or near-normal renal function, but this requires further study. It has also been observed that the hypertension in ADPKD becomes less severe with the progression of the renal insufficiency, possibly because of a tendency to sodium wasting. For this reason, diuretics should be administered with caution in these patients to avoid volume contraction and deterioration of renal function. With the currently available antihypertensive medications, the use of diuretics in ADPKD is often unnecessary and contributes to hyperuricemia, hyperlipidemia, hypokalemia, and hyperreninemia, which may have a negative effect on the course of the disease.

It has been assumed that nephrolithiasis, which occurs in 20 percent of ADPKD patients, is caused mostly by the anatomic obstruction of the collecting system by the cysts. In a recent study, the chemical composition of the stones (mainly uric acid and calcium oxalate) and the frequency of hypocitraturia and low urine pH suggest that both metabolic and mechanical factors are responsible for the frequent occurrence of nephrolithiasis in these patients. Identification and treatment of these metabolic factors should be performed as in other stone-forming patients. Both percutaneous lithotripsy and extracorporeal shock wave lithotripsy have been performed in patients with ADPKD, but the experience with these procedures is so limited that no conclusions should be reached on their safety with regard to this disease.

Infection of a renal cyst in ADPKD is usually the result of a retrograde infection from the urinary bladder. Unnecessary urinary tract manipulations should therefore be avoided. When absolutely necessary, antimicrobial prophylaxis should be prescribed. The findings on CT or magnetic resonance imaging are not specific, and the results of nuclear medicine scans, such as gallium and indium-111 leukocyte scans, are not always positive. The failure of conventional antibiotic therapy, despite favorable in vitro sensitivities, may be the best single diagnostic indicator of renal cyst infection. The treatment of infected renal cysts poses a special problem because of the variable penetration of different antibiotics. Most antibiotics enter the proximal, nongradient cyst to some extent. However, only lipid-soluble antibiotics (e.g., ciprofloxacin, trimethoprim, chloramphenicol, and metronidazole) and not other more conventionally used polar lipid-insoluble antibiotics (e.g., aminoglycosides, penicillins, and cephalosporins) enter the distal, gradient cysts well. The initial treatment of an acutely ill patient with a suspected cyst infection should be an appropriate wide-spectrum antibiotic combination, such as ampicillin and aminoglycoside, because adequate treatment of septicemia takes precedence over the treatment of cyst infections. In addition, it is difficult to separate a cyst from a parenchymal infection in ADPKD, and both may occur simultaneously. Patients with no response to the initial therapy after 5 days of treatment should begin receiving a lipid-soluble agent if the in vitro sensitivities are favorable. In refractory cases, the possibility of an anaerobic or hematogeneously disseminated gram-positive infection should be considered.

A decline in renal function eventually occurs in most patients with ADPKD. The relative sparing of the renal parenchyma on ultrasonography or CT at the time of the initial evaluation is helpful in establishing a prognosis. ADPKD patients have a prolonged period of stable renal function followed by a slow decline. Therefore it is unnecessary to recheck the renal function more than once every 1 to 3 years until significant deterioration of renal function has already occurred. With well-known limitations, a reciprocal plot of plasma creatinine against time is useful in the follow-up of patients with depressed renal function and may alert the physician to the possibility of an intercurrent renal disease or complication if a major diversion from the initial slope occurs. The prevention and treatment of renal insufficiency in ADPKD should include the avoidance of nephrotoxic drugs and the chronic use of analgesics; prevention, early detection, and treatment of complications; strict control of hypertension; and a prudent diet with mild protein (0.8 g per kilogram of ideal body weight) and phosphorus restriction when the renal function starts to deteriorate. Preliminary results from a study in progress indicate that surgical decompression of polycystic kidneys in patients with advanced renal insufficiency and a decline in renal function does not have a beneficial effect. Whether earlier intervention might have a long-term beneficial effect is not clear. At present, protection of renal function is not an indication for surgery in patients with ADPKD.

When end-stage renal disease occurs, dialysis and, in the younger patients, renal transplantation are indicated. Patients with ADPKD receiving maintenance hemodialysis do as well as and possibly better than patients with other types of renal disease, probably because they maintain a higher hemoglobin. Bleeding secondary to heparinization during dialysis rarely occurs and can usually be satisfactorily managed by using low or regional heparinization. The evaluation of living-related donors for renal transplantation is not different from that for other diseases, but CT and DNA linkage analysis (in informative families) should be considered in the young patient to rule out the presence of ADPKD. The inclusion of CT of the abdomen, magnetic resonance imaging of the circle of Willis, and an evaluation of the colon is advisable in the pretransplant evaluation of the recipient. Bilateral nephrectomy before transplantation is indicated in patients with a history of infected cysts or, rarely, in patients with massive organ enlargement with kidneys extending into the pelvis. Most ADPKD patients do not need bilateral nephrectomy before transplantation. There has been some concern that these patients might be at an increased risk for developing a renal cell carcinoma in the native kidneys. So far, this has not been a problem, but more information is needed on long-term renal allograft recipients with ADPKD who have not had a bilateral nephrectomy. After renal transplantation, ADPKD patients may have an increased, although small, risk for some morbidity events related to the extrarenal manifestations of the disease. Overall, however, the long-term outcome of renal transplantation in patients with ADPKD is similar to that of patients with other renal diseases with the exclusion of diabetes mellitus.

Hepatic cysts are frequently associated with ADPKD and usually develop later than the renal cysts. Recent studies indicate that the patient's age, the degree of renal impairment, the female gender, and the number of pregnancies the patient has had correlate with the presence and severity of the cystic liver disease. The latter factors suggest that estrogen has an effect on the development of hepatic cysts in ADPKD. This may have some practical implications when one is advising a patient with significant liver cystic involvement on the safety of future pregnancies or the use of oral contraceptives or postmenopausal estrogens. Preliminary observations that the epithelium lining the hepatic cysts is sensitive to hormones that have an effect on the biliary system, such as secretin, suggest that these cysts might also be influenced pharmacologically. For example, it has been shown in one patient that cimetidine reduces the secretion rate of unroofed hepatic cysts, possibly by inhibiting gastric acidity and secretin secretion. Despite the frequency of their occurrence, hepatic cysts rarely become symptomatic or cause laboratory abnormalities. As in the kidney, intracystic hemorrhage causes acute pain and is most often self-limited. Chronic symptoms usually result from liver enlargement and compression of adjacent structures. Sometimes the enlargement is caused by only a few dominant, very large cysts that can be treated by percutaneous drainage and ethanol sclerosis (Fig. 3). Extended cyst fenestration and segmental hepatic resection should be reserved for those rare patients with massive polycystic liver disease who are disabled by marked abdominal distention and physical disability, early satiety and weight loss, and respiratory compromise, or who have obstructive jaundice or portal hypertension caused by extrinsic cyst compression. Segmental hepatic resections are often possible without detriment to the liver function because even patients with massive polycystic liver disease frequently have relative sparing of a few hepatic segments (Fig. 4). Rarely, when there is no relative sparing of any hepatic parenchyma or when there is evidence of hepatic insufficiency (which is exceptionally rare in polycystic liver disease), liver transplantation can be considered. Obviously, these surgical options are associated with significant morbidity and mortality rates and should be considered only for highly symptomatic patients in centers with sufficient expertise with these procedures.

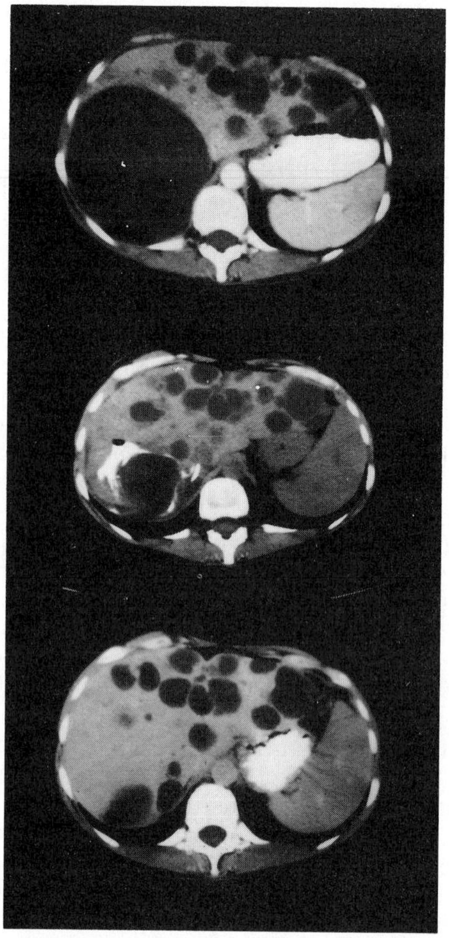

Figure 3 Ethanol sclerosis of a dominant hepatic cyst. *Top*, CT scan showing a large, dominant cyst in the right hepatic lobe. *Middle*, The cyst has been drained and a small amount of contrast material has been injected into the cyst before ethanol sclerosis; a small, adjacent cyst, previously concealed by the dominant cyst, is now seen. *Bottom*, Three months after the ethanol sclerosis, the large dominant cyst is no longer present.

A rare complication of polycystic liver disease is hepatic cyst infection. Usually, this occurs in patients who are immunosuppressed, are receiving maintenance hemodialysis, or who have undergone renal transplantation. Enterobacteriaceae in pure culture are the microorganisms more commonly recovered. The best management is percutaneous drainage combined with antibiotic therapy. Ciprofloxacin is concentrated severalfold in the liver cysts relative to the serum. There is little information on the liver cyst pharmacokinetics of other antibiotics. Surgical drainage or resection and long-term antibiotic suppression may be needed for those patients in whom percutaneous drainage is not possible or successful.

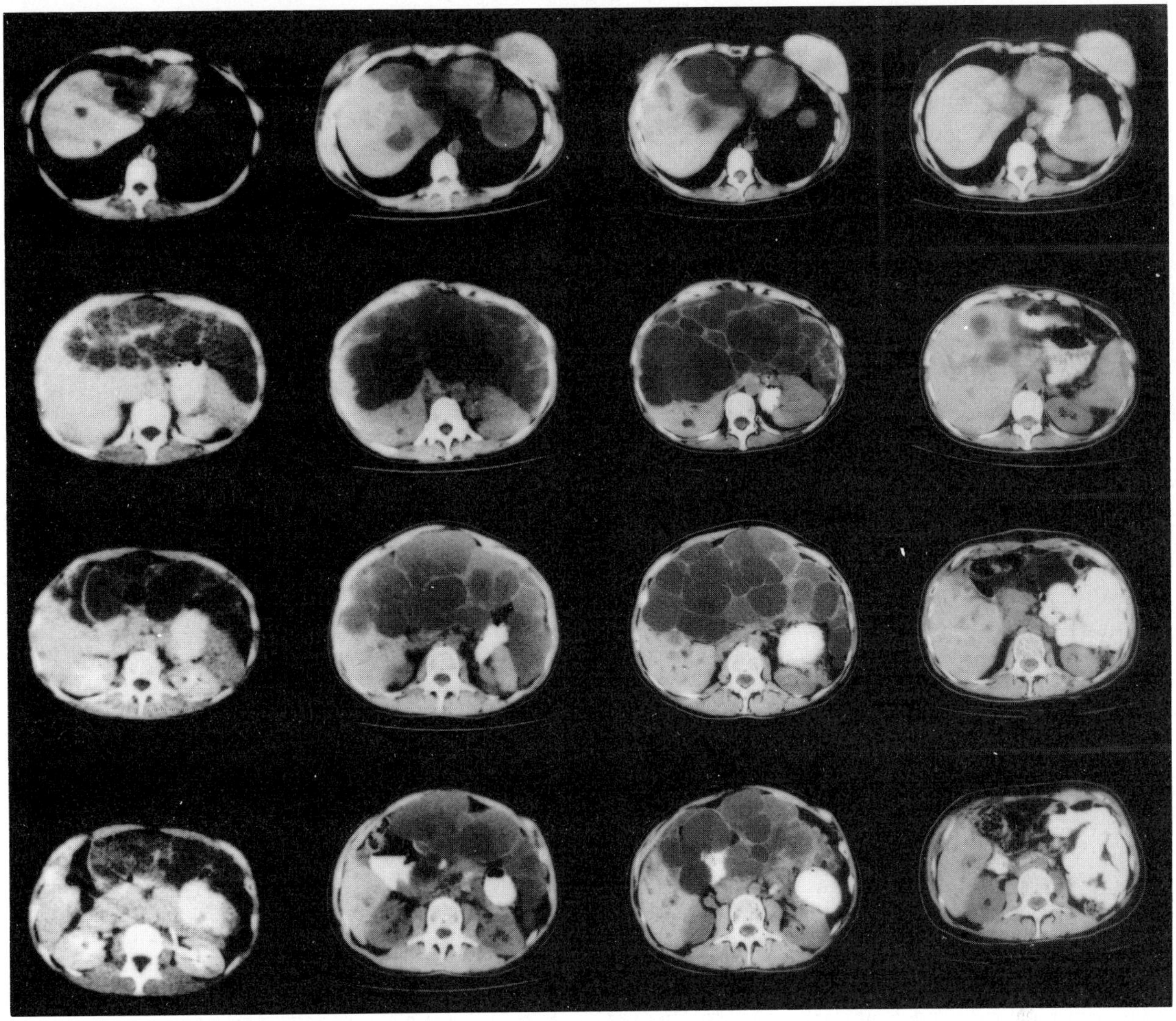

Figure 4 Massive polycystic liver disease. CT scans of the abdomen obtained 10 years before (left), 4 years before (center left), 1 month before (center right), and after (right) a combined hepatic resection fenestration procedure.

The association of intracranial aneurysms and ADPKD is well supported by numerous case reports, autopsy studies, population-based studies, and small prospective angiographic studies. At present, the true prevalence and natural history of these aneurysms in ADPKD are uncertain. Through the use of a decision analysis using the best available information on the prevalence and natural history of intracranial aneurysms in ADPKD, it was concluded that routine cerebral angiography of patients with ADPKD could not be justified. The decision analysis did not take into consideration that the risk of rupture of a previously diagnosed unruptured, asymptomatic intracranial aneurysm is heavily dependent on its size. Aneurysms less than 8 mm in diameter have a low risk of rupture. Current CT and magnetic resonance imaging technologies are well suited to detect aneurysms with a diameter exceeding 8 mm. A prospective study using these technologies at the Mayo Clinic has shown that asymptomatic, large intracranial aneurysms at risk for rupture that are detectable by CT or magnetic resonance imaging are very rare in ADPKD. On the basis of this study, it seems reasonable to restrict these noninvasive, presymptomatic evaluations to patients with a family history of intracranial aneurysms, since they appear to be at an increased risk, as well as to those with vaguely suggestive symptoms, those who will undergo major elective surgery, those in a high-risk occupation, and those who request these evaluations for the purpose of reassurance. The patients with focal neurologic symptoms or sudden onset of severe, localized headaches suggestive of a warning leak should undergo cerebral angiography. Surgery is indicated for symptomatic intracranial aneurysms as well as for asymptomatic aneurysms measuring 10 mm or more in diameter. The management of asymptomatic, unruptured aneurysms 6 to 9 mm in diameter is controversial. Asymptomatic aneurysms less than 6 mm in diameter have a low likelihood of rupture and should be restudied annually. If symptoms develop and/or the aneurysm enlarges, surgery should be considered. The preferred surgical technique involves clipping of the aneurysm at its neck. The overall mortality or severe morbidity rate associated with this procedure for a single unruptured aneurysm is approximately 2 to 7 percent when performed by experienced surgeons using the operating microscope. The risk varies with the location of the aneurysm, its configuration, and the accessibility of its neck to surgical clipping. With multiple aneurysms, the risk is increased for each additional aneurysm. If clipping is successful, it is considered a cure. If clipping of the aneurysm is not possible, other less optimal surgical procedures such as carotid ligation and detachable balloon techniques with or without extracranial to intracranial arterial bypass may be used.

Physicians caring for patients with ADPKD should be aware of the disease's association with cardiovascular abnormalities, especially mitral valve prolapse, aortic insufficiency, and aortic aneurysms, and with colon diverticula. Patients with associated cardiovascular abnormalities should be informed of the importance of strict blood pressure control and endocarditis prophylaxis. Because of the possible increased risk for colonic diverticulosis, these patients should be advised to follow a high-fiber diet and to avoid constipation.

TUBEROUS SCLEROSIS

Tuberous sclerosis is an autosomal dominant disease with high penetrance, an extremely variable expression, and a high rate of spontaneous mutation. It may affect the central nervous system (cortical tubers, subependymal nodules, and giant cell tumors), skin (facial angiofibroma or adenoma sebaceum, fibrous plaques, periungual or subungual fibromas, hypomelanotic macules, and shagreen patches), retina (hamartoma), kidneys (angiomyolipomas and cysts), heart (rhabdomyoma), and lungs. Other organs may also be involved, and cysts can occur in the liver. The association of renal cysts and angiomyolipomas is pathognomonic of tuberous sclerosis. In the absence of a family history or angiomyolipomas, the renal cystic disease can be confused with ADPKD.

Treatment

Renal angiomyolipomas require no treatment except in the event of life-threatening bleeding, which may require arterial embolization or segmental nephrectomy or enucleation. Patients with severe, diffuse bilateral cystic involvement often have hypertension and may develop renal failure, usually in the second or third decade of life. The treatment of hypertension and renal failure in these patients is similar to that in ADPKD. Bilateral nephrectomy performed before renal transplantation is indicated in these patients because of the risk of bleeding caused by the angiomyolipomas and because of a likely increased risk for renal cell carcinoma in tuberous sclerosis.

VON HIPPEL-LINDAU DISEASE

Von Hippel-Lindau disease is an autosomal dominant disorder with high penetrance and variable expression. It affects most frequently the cerebellum, medulla oblongata, spinal cord (hemangioblastomas), retina (angiomatosis), kidney (cysts, hemangiomas, adenomas, and carcinomas), pancreas (cysts and, rarely, tumors), and adrenal gland (pheochromocytoma). The renal cysts are usually multiple and limited in number. Occasionally the kidneys may be diffusely cystic, with characteristics resembling those of ADPKD. Some of the patients described in the literature as having renal cell carcinomas and ADPKD probably had von Hippel-Lindau disease.

Treatment

An effort to spare renal tissue in the treatment of renal cell carcinoma in this disease has been recommended, since bilateral and multiple carcinomas are likely to be present or develop subsequently. Early diagnosis of these lesions is essential and CT of the abdomen performed annually is recommended. The renal cysts usually require no treatment. For those patients who have extensive cystic disease and renal failure that require dialysis, nephrectomy should be performed because of the risk of carcinoma.

ACQUIRED CYSTIC KIDNEY DISEASE

The term "acquired cystic kidney disease" denotes the cystic degeneration of the renal parenchyma in end-stage kidneys that is probably the result of prolonged uremia. It occurs most often in patients receiving maintenance hemodialysis or peritoneal dialysis, but it has also been described as occurring before the initiation of dialysis after prolonged uremia in native as well as in transplanted kidneys with chronic rejection. The number of patients with cysts, as well as the number and size of the cysts, increases with the duration of uremia and dialysis. The frequency of acquired cystic kidney disease depends on the sensitivity of the diagnostic techniques. Contrast-enhanced CT with thin sections has greater resolution than ultrasonography, and both underestimate the number of cysts observed by direct examination of the kidneys. Using sensitive CT techniques, multiple renal cysts are observed in approximately 80 percent of patients who have been receiving hemodialysis for more than 3 years. It is usually a silent process. Symptoms are related to complications, which include intracystic bleeding, gross hematuria, retroperitoneal hemorrhage, cyst infection, and malignant transformation.

Treatment

As in the treatment of ADPKD, the treatment of a cyst hemorrhage is usually conservative, consisting of bed rest and analgesics. Regional heparinization should be used for dialysis. Occasionally, renal artery embolization or nephrectomy is required. Percutaneous drainage in addition to antibiotic therapy is an alternative to surgical drainage or nephrectomy in the treatment of cyst infection in acquired renal cystic disease. It has been estimated that 20 percent of patients with acquired renal cystic disease have tumors, adenomas, or adenocarcinomas. The categorization of these tumors as adenomas or carcinomas is difficult and depends on size and cytologic features. Most tumors less than 3 cm in diameter do not metastasize, but exceptions do occur. It has been estimated that 5 percent of the patients with acquired cystic disease and solid tumors develop metastases. Thus as many as one in 200 patients with acquired renal cystic disease develop metastatic renal cell carcinoma. Whether renal cell carcinomas will become a major medical problem in patients who are maintained on long-term hemodialysis or peritoneal dialysis is uncertain. Until more information becomes available, it seems reasonable to screen these patients after 3 years of dialysis by either ultrasonography or CT and to repeat the study annually or possibly every second year. Small renal tumors measuring less than 3 cm in diameter should be followed at 6-month intervals. Surgical intervention is indicated for large solid tumors or when there is evidence of progressive tumor enlargement. Because of the frequent multicentricity of these tumors and current availability of erythropoietin, bilateral nephrectomy is recommended. Although acquired renal cystic disease can regress after renal transplantation, there have been some reports of patients with acquired renal cystic disease developing a metastatic renal cell carcinoma years after renal transplantation. A recent report has suggested that 2 percent of deaths occurring among patients who have undergone renal transplantation are secondary to metastatic renal cell carcinoma arising from the native kidneys. It therefore seems prudent to recommend that patients with renal failure, especially those who have been receiving dialysis for more than 1 or 2 years, should have an evaluation of the native kidneys by CT or ultrasonography before transplantation. Patients with solid tumors should undergo bilateral nephrectomy before transplantation.

MULTILOCULAR CYST

The multilocular cyst or multilocular cystic nephroma is a well-defined entity consisting of a well-circumscribed, encapsulated renal mass composed of multiple noncommunicating cysts of varying size. The loculi of the cysts are lined with flattened or plump reactive epithelial cells. In some cases, proliferation of these cells has been interpreted as evidence of their neoplastic nature, and occasionally histologic evidence of renal cell adenocarcinoma is found. The biologic course of these tumors is usually benign. Approximately half of the cases occur in children and the other half in adults.

Treatment

The treatment of choice, when technically possible, is partial nephrectomy. At the time of surgery, thorough tissue sampling for histologic studies and frozen sections should be used to rule out the presence of a renal cell carcinoma that would require a total nephrectomy.

CYSTIC DISEASE OF THE RENAL SINUS

The cystic disorders of the renal sinus are benign conditions. The most common cysts in this area are of lymphatic origin and are often multiple and bilateral. Despite considerable distortion of the calices and infundibula, the pressure in these lymphatic cysts is usually low, not causing significant functional obstruction. Ultrasonography and CT have facilitated the differential diagnosis of these cysts from other benign conditions such as renal sinus lipomatosis, as well as from serious diseases such as neoplasms of the renal pelvis and kidney or ADPKD.

Treatment

The therapeutic approach to these cysts should be conservative, since the cystic disease of the renal sinus is a benign condition.

SUGGESTED READING

Elzinga LW, Barry J, Torres VE, Zincke H. Cyst decompression surgery for autosomal dominant polycystic kidney disease (ADPKD): long-term result of renal functional and symptomatic responses. Kidney Int 1990; 37:247.

Elzinga LW, Golper TA, Rashad AL, et al. Ciprofloxacin activity in cyst fluid from polycystic kidneys. Antimicrob Agents Chemother 1988; 32:844–847.

Everson GT, Emmett M, Brown WR, et al. Functional similarities of hepatic cystic and biliary epithelium: studies of fluid constituents and in vivo secretion in response to secretin. Hepatology 1990; 11:557–565.

Gardner KJ, Bernstein J, eds: The cystic kidney. The Netherlands: Kluwer Academic Publishers, 1990.

Grantham JJ, Gardner KD, eds. Problems in diagnosis and management of polycystic kidney disease. Kansas City, MO: PKR Foundation, 1985.

Newman KD, Torres VE, Rakela J, Nagorney DM. Treatment of highly symptomatic polycystic liver disease: preliminary experience with a combined hepatic resection fenestration procedure. Ann Surg 1990; 212:30–37.

Sujansky E, Kreutzer SB, Johnson AM, et al. Attitudes of at-risk and affected individuals regarding presymptomatic testing for autosomal dominant polycystic kidney disease. Am J Med Genet 1990; 35:510–515.

Telenti A, Torres VE, Gross JB Jr, et al. Hepatic cyst infection in autosomal dominant polycystic kidney disease. Mayo Clin Proc 1990; 65:933–942.

RENAL COMPLICATIONS OF CARCINOMA, LEUKEMIA, MALIGNANT LYMPHOMA, AND WALDENSTRÖM'S MACROGLOBULINEMIA

LUIS BAEZ-DIAZ, M.D.
MANUEL MARTINEZ-MALDONADO, M.D.

GLOMERULOPATHIES IN CANCER

Glomerular proteinuria is a well-recognized renal complication in cancer patients. Proteinuria can be massive enough to induce the nephrotic syndrome; it can be seen in patients with carcinomas as well as in those with hematologic neoplasia. In about 10 percent of patients with nephrotic syndrome, an underlying carcinoma can be found. The most common glomerular histopathologic disorder associated with carcinoma is membranous nephropathy. Lung cancer and gastrointestinal tumors are the most common solid tumors associated with nephrotic syndrome. Some patients will achieve long-lasting remission of their proteinuria if given effective curative treatment for their underlying tumor. Most patients, however, have a poor prognosis, with a median survival of 3 to 6 months. Survival in these patients reflects the biology of the tumor rather than the associated renal pathology.

The nephrotic syndrome is not infrequent in patients with hematologic neoplasia. It can be seen with a variety of lymphoproliferative tumors, but it is most common in Hodgkin's disease. In our experience it is most commonly found when Hodgkin's disease is of the mixed cellular type. Renal biopsy has revealed a histopathologic picture of minimal or nil disease in the majority of these patients. Proteinuria or the nephrotic syndrome may appear concomitantly with the diagnosis of lymphoma. There is no relation between the stage of the disease and the nephrotic syndrome (or proteinuria). It may occur with localized as well as with widely disseminated disease. The proteinuria, however, seems to follow the activity of the disease. After curative treatment of Hodgkin's disease with combination chemotherapy or radiation, the proteinuria remits. In rare cases the proteinuria may persist despite remission of the underlying lymphoma.

SECONDARY TUMORS

Metastasis to the kidney is a frequent finding at autopsy in patients with disseminated carcinomatosis. This is particularly striking in cases of lung, breast, and stomach cancer; these tumors also are the most common secondary malignancies associated with renal involvement. Fewer than 5 percent of patients have renal parenchymal destruction severe enough to cause significant renal impairment. The diagnosis of renal metastasis is made ante mortem in less than 20 percent of cases.

Plain abdominal films and intravenous pyelography are good screening tests for the detection and evaluation of renal metastasis and infiltration by malignant neoplasia. Intravenous pyelography and nephrotomography can detect 80 percent of the renal lesions. Ultrasonography is helpful in differentiating between a cystic or a solid mass lesion, but when such a distinction cannot be made, angiography and computed tomography are frequently used to determine the nature of renal masses. When a tissue diagnosis is needed it can be established by aspiration cytology of the renal mass or parenchyma with a 22-gauge needle; percutaneous needle biopsy may be necessary in some cases.

Metastatic involvement limited to the kidney is seen in less than 10 percent of cases; in the great majority of patients other distant metastases are present. As a consequence, prognosis is generally poor. Treatment is usually palliative unless effective systemic therapy is available for the underlying tumor (e.g., small cell lung cancer). In cases of severe pain or life-threatening hematuria secondary to unilateral metastasis, palliative radiation therapy can afford temporary relief. Angiographically directed arterial embolization using blood clots or synthetic material can also stop pain and gross hematuria. The effects of embolization, however, are often transient. The procedure can be repeated on several occasions, but in a number of patients a more definite treatment will be needed. Nephrectomy may be necessary if these procedures fail; unilateral solitary metastasis can be managed by metastasectomy. Both metastasectomy and nephrectomy can prolong life if speed of disease spread is slowed.

Renal infiltration in leukemias or lymphomas can be

a presenting manifestation of the disease, but most commonly it is seen when the disease is advanced and/or relapsing. Treatment is usually in the form of systemic combination chemotherapy, since the kidney is rarely the only site of disease activity. Chemotherapy penetrates well into the renal parenchyma and complete renal tumor regression is seen in the majority of cases. Chemotherapeutic drugs that are metabolized or excreted by the kidneys should be withheld as initial drug therapy. These include methotrexate, bleomycins, and cisplatin. These drugs can subsequently be incorporated as part of the therapeutic regimen when improvement in renal function occurs. Radiation therapy can also be used later to complement the effect of the drug therapy. Kidney radiation is maintained below 2,000 rads to avoid radiation damage to the renal parenchyma. Unfortunately, despite aggressive management, more than 50 percent of patients will have relapse of their disease.

Neoplasia can metastasize to the retroperitoneal nodes and structures and give rise to ureteropelvic obstruction and hydronephrosis. The most common extrapelvic carcinomas producing this syndrome are gastrointestinal tumors and breast cancer. Aggressive management of urinary obstruction in these patients can improve the quality of life.

Urinary diversion is the best palliative approach when obstruction results from tumors that respond poorly to radiation and chemotherapy. This can be accomplished by nephrostomy or ureterostomy, or ureteral catheters can be introduced antegrade via a percutaneous nephrostomy or retrograde by cystoscopy. Complications of these procedures include catheter malfunction secondary to migration, displacement, or occlusion, and bacteriuria associated with cystitis and its symptoms. The catheters can be left in place and changed every 3 to 5 months in those patients with unremitting obstruction.

Aggressive management of lymphoma or leukemia can lead to cure of the disease. Urinary tract obstruction as a result of these diseases usually remits if systemic and local therapy are successful. Our approach to such patients is to relieve the obstruction by placing catheters before the patients begin a regimen of combination chemotherapy. After an initial two to three cycles of drug therapy, the cytotoxic response is magnified with adjuvant radiotherapy. The ureteral catheters can then be removed.

MALIGNANT PARAPROTEINEMIC DISORDERS

Malignant paraproteinemic disorders represent neoplastic transformations of terminal B cells and plasma cells. Their clinical manifestations are dominated by invasion and destruction of tissue by neoplastic cells and/or byproducts. In addition, abnormal immunoglobulins may contribute to the picture.

Renal abnormalities in multiple myeloma are discussed in the chapter *Multiple Myeloma and Related Monoclonal Gammopathies* and need not concern us further.

Bence Jones protein can be detected in 30 percent of patients with Waldenström's macroglobulinemia. Variable degrees of renal insufficiency can be found in 20 percent of cases. Tubular abnormalities and "myeloma kidney"-type lesions are rarely found on renal biopsy specimens. Instead, and in contrast to patients with myeloma, glomerular lesions are more common. These include amyloid deposits, immune-complex glomerulonephritis, and subendothelial deposits of IgM paraprotein. The subendothelial deposits of IgM can be so voluminous as to occlude partially or completely the capillary lumen. In 50 percent of cases a lymphoplasmacytic infiltrate can be found in the renal interstitium, mostly confined to the superficial cortex. This infiltration is a manifestation of the lymphomatous nature of Waldenström's macroglobulinemia, which is usually associated with visceral involvement and lymphadenopathy.

Most patients with macroglobulinemia develop signs and symptoms of hyperviscosity during the course of their disease (Table 1).

Hyperviscosity is more frequent than in other paraprotein disorders as a result of the large amount of circulating immunoglobulin (IgM, 4 to 7 g per deciliter) and the physicochemical characteristics of the protein. Some of these characteristics are large size, abnormal shape, cryoprecipitability (30 percent of cases), and the mostly intravascular localization of the protein.

While patients have individual thresholds, 50 percent of patients will become symptomatic when serum relative viscosity (compared with water, which has a value of 1) reaches values of 4 to 5.

Waldenström's macroglobulinemia can be treated with cytotoxic drugs and prednisone, which reduce the tumor-cell population and decrease production of the macroglobulin. However, the biologic half-life of the protein is long (6 days), and life-threatening complications of hyperviscosity can persist. Therefore, rapid removal of the protein should be accomplished by plasma exchange. Removal of 4 to 5 L of plasma decreases the protein concentration by approximately 80 percent. This is followed by rapid reduction of blood viscosity and immediate subjective relief. Signs and symptoms of hyperviscosity can be controlled for prolonged periods with plasma exchange. We have successfully used plasmapheresis as the only modality

TABLE 1 Clinical Manifestations of Hyperviscosity Syndrome

Neurologic (Bing-Neel Syndrome)
Altered sensorium, headaches, dizzines, vertigo, diplopia, blindness, ataxia, paresthesia, paralysis
Ocular
Venous engorgement, retinal hemorrhages, papilledema
Cardiac
Cardiomegaly, congestive heart failure
Renal
Hematuria, impaired urine concentration, azotemia
Others
Epistaxis, bleeding gums, acrocyanosis, purpura, ear bleeding

of treatment in some patients refractory to cytotoxic drugs. We use a blood cell separator with continuous flow centrifuge for plasma exchange, but other cell separators work as well. Under emergency conditions, if a blood cell separator is not available, therapeutic plasma exchange can be accomplished by phlebotomy into collection bags with a suitable anticoagulant (ACD), and separation of cells from plasma can be followed by reinfusion of cellular elements. If a centrifuge is not available, blood cells can be allowed to settle spontaneously, the plasma decanted, and the cells reinfused.

Complications of this treatment include hemorrhagic diathesis from removal of clotting factors, thrombocytopenia, hypocalcemia from citrate anticoagulation, and even vascular collapse from over-vigorous exchanges. This can be kept to a minimum by allowing only trained personnel to carry out the procedure.

ACUTE TUMOR LYSIS SYNDROME

One of the most dramatic electrolyte and metabolic disturbances seen in cancer patients is the so-called acute tumor lysis syndrome. It is primarily seen in hematologic neoplasias that have a large tumor cell mass, a high growth rate of tumor cells, and exquisite sensitivity to systemic antineoplastic drugs. The most common tumors in which the syndrome is seen are poorly differentiated lymphomas, Burkitt's lymphoma, and acute lymphoblastic leukemias, although the syndrome can occur to a lesser degree in other tumor cell categories (Table 2).

The metabolic and electrolyte disorders can best be explained by the sudden death of chemosensitive tumor cells. This releases amounts of intracellular electrolytes and nucleic acid metabolites, resulting in hyperuricemia, hyperkalemia, hyperphosphatemia, and hypocalcemia. Varying degrees of renal insufficiency are associated with this syndrome. The major causes of renal failure are acute uric acid nephropathy due to intratubular precipitation of uric acid, and acute nephrocalcinosis secondary to marked hyperphosphatemia.

TABLE 2 Neoplasia Most at Risk of Acute Tumor Lysis Syndrome

Burkitt's lymphoma/leukemia syndromes
Poorly differentiated lymphomas
T-cell lymphoblastic lymphomas
Acute lymphoblastic leukemia
Lymphomas/leukemias with high tumor cell mass, (LDH >1,000, massive marrow invasion, bulky abdominal masses)

Because renal clearance is the primary mechanism of excretion of uric acid and phosphates, patients with prior renal insufficiency are more likely to get worse and exhibit dramatic complications. Tumor lysis, with its accompanying metabolic and electrolyte abnormalities, is most marked 24 to 48 hours after the administration of chemotherapeutic agents; it may last 5 to 7 days after drug therapy. It is most severe during the initial treatment and less so in subsequent drug trials. Death can result from hyperkalemia, hypocalcemia, or from renal failure and uremic complications. The best therapy for the tumor lysis syndrome is its prevention by early identification of patients most at risk (see Table 2) and the institution of prophylactic measures prior to antineoplastic drug treatment (Table 3).

NEPHROTOXIC COMPLICATIONS OF ANTICANCER TREATMENT

Radiation Nephritis

Radiation-induced nephritis is seen following radiotherapy for testicular, ovarian, and other abdominal and

TABLE 3 Management of Acute Tumor Lysis Syndrome

Pre-chemotherapy
Correct initial electrolyte and fluid disorder
Correct baseline renal and prerenal azotemia, if possible
Maintain adequate hydration and urine output
Allopurinol 24–48 hr prior to therapy (300/mg/m^2)
Alkalinize urine to pH >7.0 (NaHCO infusion: 7.5% bicarbonate in 5% glucose)
Start oral phosphate binding antacids
Dialysis for established renal failure or unresponsive electrolyte or metabolic abnormalities
Continuous flow leukophoresis might be indicated for patients with a high circulating blast count (WBC >100,000/m^3)
Post-chemotherapy
Dialysis is required for developing renal failure or life-threatening electrolyte disorder
Discontinue urine alkalinization when uric acid homeostatis is achieved (to avoid $CA_3[PO_4]2$ precipitation)
Treat symptomatic hypocalcemia after correction of hyperphosphatemia

pelvic tumors. Its incidence is highest in patients with prior renal disease and in patients receiving radio-potentiating anticancer drugs such as adriamycin, 5-fluorouracil, actinomycin D, bleomycins, and cisplatin. The incidence of nephrotoxicity is proportional to the total dose of radiation delivered to the kidneys. Total doses of 2,000 rads or less are associated with minimal transient toxicity. When doses beyond 2,300 rads are given, irreversible renal damage is to be expected.

Five clinical syndromes are recognized: (1) acute radiation nephritis, (2) chronic radiation nephritis, (3) asymptomatic proteinuria, (4) benign hypertension, and (5) late malignant hypertension.

Acute radiation nephritis is usually seen within a year following radiotherapy to the renal beds, but it can occur as early as 2 to 3 months in young adults and children. The clinical manifestations include anemia, edema, proteinuria, systemic hypertension, and azotemia. Prognosis depends on the severity of malignant hypertension and on the recovery of renal function.

Chronic radiation nephritis can follow acute nephritis but can present de novo 2 to 5 years after radiotherapy. The manifestations are those of chronic renal failure. Asymptomatic proteinuria, and isolated benign or malignant hypertension can develop up to 10 years after treatment. These can persist and eventually lead to cardiac failure and renal insufficiency. There are cases in the literature of severe malignant hypertension after unilateral renal irradiation with curative results after removal of the damaged kidney.

The histopathologic changes induced by radiation nephritis depend on the dose of radiation given and the time when the pathologic specimen is examined. All renal structures are affected. Early changes are seen in the glomerulus and tubules, but with time, interstitial fibrosis and glomerular sclerosis ensue.

Treatment is supportive and special attention should be paid to control of systemic hypertension and uremia. Dialytic therapy might be needed when renal failure is acute and in patients who progress to chronic renal failure. With the newer techniques in radiation delivery, it is expected that renal toxic complications will decrease, although an increase in late complications might occur, since patients so treated are surviving longer.

NEPHROTOXICITY OF ANTICANCER DRUGS

Cisplatin

Cisplatin (cis-diammine dichloride platinum) (Table 4) is the only metal coordination complex in clinical use today. Since its discovery in 1965, it has become a major component in combination chemotherapy for testicular cancer, ovarian tumors, and head and neck cancer. Its mechanism of action lies in the ability to form bifunctional covalent links with DNA, leading to interstrand and intrastrand crosslinking of DNA bases. Adverse reactions to the drug include moderate myelosuppression, ototoxicity, peripheral neurotoxicity, and hypersensitivity reactions. Limitations of its usefulness are the result of its side effects—nausea and vomiting—and its nephrotoxicity. Renal toxicity includes reversible tubular dysfunction, manifested clinically by hypomagnesemia in 50 percent of treated cases and by acute renal failure secondary to tubular necrosis.

Initial clinical trials with this drug in doses of 40 to 100 mg per square meter resulted in an incidence of renal failure of 40 percent of patients. Changes in dose and schedule accompanied by vigorous hydration and diuresis have decreased the incidence of renal failure to less than 5 percent. A commonly used regimen consists of 20 mg per square meter daily for 5 days repeated every 21 days. One liter of normal saline is given before and after each dose for the 5 days. This is accompanied by minimal nephrotoxicity; nausea and vomiting also are less incapacitating. Despite this approach, severe hypomagnesemia frequently develops requiring oral or parenteral magnesium supplementation. Cisplatin should not be used in patients with established renal failure. We have used this 5-day schedule without inducing further renal deterioration in patients with mild elevations of serum creatinine and in some whose creatinine clearance rates were 40 ml per minute or less.

Methotrexate

Methotrexate is an antifolate class of antimetabolite with a wide spectrum of applications in clinical medicine. Because of its cytotoxic and immunosuppressive effects, it is used for the treatment of psoriasis, rheumatic disorders, and other immune-related disorders. Nevertheless, it is used most commonly in the treatment of hematologic neoplasia and solid tumors. In these conditions it is part of curative chemotherapeutic regimens, especially in patients with acute lymphoblastic leukemia and choriocarcinoma. The drug is given intravenously but can be well absorbed orally when doses of 25 mg per square meter or less are given.

Methotrexate's mechanism of action is inhibition of the enzyme dehydrofolate reductase. This inhibition results in the intracellular depletion of folates in the reduced state. Reduced folates, mainly tetrahydrofolates, are one-carbon group donors in enzymatic reactions leading to the synthesis of purine nucleotides and thymidylate. Rescue from the toxic effects of the drug can be accomplished by administering (1) reduced folates in the form of leucovorin (N-5 formyltetrahydrofolate); (2) thymidine, which restores intracellular thymidine triphosphate; and (3) carboxypeptidase-g, an enzyme that hydrolyzes and inactivates methotrexate.

Dose-limiting toxic reactions include bone marrow suppression and mucositis. Ninety percent of the drug is excreted intact in the urine; as a result, systemic toxicity is proportional to the renal clearance of the drug. In doses higher than 100 mg, leucovorin rescue (24 to 36 hours after drug administration) is given to prevent life-threatening reactions. At high doses (1 to 10 g per square

TABLE 4 Nephrotoxicity of Anticancer Drugs

Drug	*Mechanism of Action*	*Renal Excretion*	*Commonly Used Dose and Schedule*	*Nephrotoxicity**	*Renal Abnormalities*	*Management and Recommendations†*
Cisplatin	DNA alkylator	30% in urine at 48 hours	50–100mg/m² every 3–4 weeks 20 mg/m²/day × 5 days every 21 days	4–30%	Transient tubular dysfunction Hypomagnesemia (40%) Acute tubular necrosis	Vigorous hydration (pre- and post-therapy) Mannitol and loop diuretic Modify dose for Cr Cl <60 cc/min
Methotrexate	Antimetabolite	90% intact drug in urine	2.5–5mg PO/day 50 mg/m² IV per week; 1–10 g/m² IV (high dose with rescue)	10%	Direct tubular toxicity Intratubular precipitation	Vigorous hydration, urine alkalinization and leucovorin rescue for high-dose therapy D/C drug for CrCL 50 cc/min
Mitomycin C	Antibiotic, alkylator	10% unchanged drug in urine	10–20 mg/m² IV every 6–8 weeks	10%	Thrombotic glomerular angiopathy	Antiplatelet agents, steroids, immune suppression, and plasma exchange for hemolytic syndrome
Cyclophosphamide	Alkylator	75% in urine (native drug +metabolites)	50–100 mg/m²/day 1–1.5 g/m² IV every 21 days	10%	Transient tubular dysfunction Acute hemorrhagic cystitis Bladder fibrosis and telangiectasia	1–2 L hydration Hemorrhagic cystitis Diuresis and catherization Cystoscopy and cauterization Intravesical formalin
Mithramicin	RNA synthesis inhibition	30% unchanged at 2 hours	20–50 μg/kg IV once or twice per week (for hypercalcemia)	20–40%	Tubular dysfunction Acute tubular necrosis Hemolytic uremia syndrome	Discontinue drug if proteinuria develops Plasma exchange
Streptozotocin	Antibiotic, alkylator	20% unchanged in urine	50 mg/m² IV ×5 days	20–60% dysfunction	Renal tubular dysfunction Fanconi RTA Nephrogenic DI Acute tubular necrosis	Discontinue drug at onset of proteinuria

* Can vary depending on dose, schedule, and duration of treatment.
† See text for further recommendations.

meter) acute renal failure can occur, due to direct tubular damage by the drug or by intratubular precipitation and crystallization. A delay in renal clearance of the drug will then result in severe bone marrow suppression, generalized mucositis, severe skin rash, and death. To avoid this complication of high-dose methotrexate treatments, vigorous hydration and urine alkalinization to enhance drug excretion and its urine solubility have been used with good results. Determination of methotrexate levels by radioassays is of the utmost importance if high doses of methotrexate and leucovorin rescue are to be used. Drug levels greater than 5×10^{-7} M 48 hours after initial drug treatment are indicative of impaired drug excretion and should be followed by increased leucovorin rescue (25 to 100 mg per square meter every 6 hours) and hydration until the drug levels fall to less than 1×10^{-7} M. In cases of acute renal failure, dialysis and hemoperfusion have been tried, but they are usually not effective owing to the large size of the methotrexate molecule and its plasma protein affinity.

Mitomycin C

Mitomycin C is an antitumor antibiotic isolated from *Streptomyces caespitosus*. It functions as a DNA alkylator leading to interstrand crosslinking of DNA bases, resulting in inhibition of DNA synthesis and cell death. Myelosuppression is the main dose-limiting toxic reaction, but renal toxicity can be identified in fewer than 10 percent of cases. In 50 percent of cases of drug-induced renal failure, a microangiopathy manifested by hemolytic anemia, thrombocytopenia, and organ dysfunction is present. The syndrome closely resembles hemolytic-uremic syndrome both clinically and histopathologically. Most patients have an underlying adenocarcinoma, usually of gastrointestinal origin. Circulation immune complexes are frequently detected in the serum of these patients, but their relationship to the pathogenesis of this syndrome is still obscure. Renal pathologic studies reveal thrombotic microangiopathic lesions in the glomerulus and arterioles. Similar lesions are encountered in other affected organs. Prognosis is poor and in patients with acute renal failure mortality is high. Treatment has included high doses of steroids, plasmapheresis, antiplatelet agents, and immunosuppressive drugs, yet improvement is seen in fewer than 40 percent of cases. Ironically, patients who develop this carcinoma-related hemolytic-uremic syndrome are usually patients who have benefited from mitomycin C therapy. (See also the chapter *Hemolytic-Uremic Syndrome.*)

Cyclophosphamide

Cyclophosphamide, the most commonly used alkylating agent, has cytotoxic as well as immunosuppressive effects. Usually administered intravenously, it is well absorbed by the oral route. In addition to its potent carcinogenic and mutagenic effects, it induces myelosuppression, alopecia, nausea, and vomiting.

Following prolonged use or high doses (1 to 2 g per square meter), acute and chronic bladder toxicity results. In addition to acute hemorrhagic cystitis, chronic cystitis, bladder fibrosis, and telangiectasia, an increased incidence of renal and bladder tumors has been found after chronic administration of the drug.

The toxic effects on the bladder appear to be the result of acrolein, a metabolite of the parent compound. Acrolein is excreted in the urine; thus it comes in contact with the urothelium, leading to irritation and ulcerations.

Acute hemorrhagic cystitis occurs in up to 10 percent of patients treated with high doses of cyclophosphamide. Vigorous hydration and diuresis reduce the incidence of this complication. Cyclophosphamide impairs tubular function and potentiates the effect of antidiuretic hormone on the collecting duct. Therefore, care must be taken to avoid severe hyponatremia during hydration.

Life-threatening bleeding can occur as a result of drug-induced cystitis. Most episodes, however, are transient and respond to conservative management and discontinuation of the drug. Patients suffering profuse and unremitting bleeding may require cystoscopy and cauterization of bleeding sites. If these measures fail, bladder irrigation with a 1 to 4 percent formalin solution is effective in more than 90 percent of cases. Evacuation of bladder blood clots and cauterization of bleeding vessels must be carried out. It is also essential to exclude by cystogram the possibility of ureteral reflux, since formalin instillation into the ureters leads to fibrosis. Irrigation is performed with 500 ml of a 1 percent formalin solution for 10 minutes. The solution should not be left in contact with the bladder mucosa for prolonged periods of time. In most instances bleeding will cease after one treatment; if not, irrigation with a 4 percent formalin solution can be attempted.

Mithramycin

Mithramycin is an inhibitor of DNA-directed RNA synthesis with activity against testicular tumors and glioblastomas. Its major use, however, is in the treatment of hypercalcemia, since it reduces the number of bone-resorbing osteoclasts. Doses of 25 to 50 μg per kilogram given for 5 days are nephrotoxic, with elevation of blood urea nitrogen and creatinine concentrations noted in 20 to 40 percent of cases. Proteinuria is reported to occur in up to 80 percent of patients treated with this dose range. Hematuria can be a sign of toxicity, but is usually a manifestation of drug-induced generalized hemorrhagic diathesis with depression of clotting factors and thrombocytopenia. A hemolytic uremic syndrome may ensue. The use of mithramycin is contraindicated in patients with hepatic and kidney dysfunction and in patients with coagulation disorders. Close monitoring of changes in lactic dehydrogenase, blood urea nitrogen, and creatinine concentrations, as well as coagulation variables, is indicated when using this drug.

Streptozotocin

Streptozotocin, an antibiotic, is another DNA alkylating agent. It has recently been approved for clinical use by the United States Food and Drug Administration. It has a limited spectrum of antitumor activity. Its main use is in the treatment of pancreatic islet cell tumors and malignant carcinoid. The nephrotoxicity of streptozotocin has proteinuria as its earliest manifestation. This abnormality heralds the development of severe renal dysfunction and is an indication to discontinue the drug until improvement occurs. Multiple tubular abnormalities, including Fanconi's syndrome, renal tubular acidosis, and nephrogenic diabetes insipidus, have been reported with the use of this drug. Renal failure and acute tubular necrosis are seen in 10 percent of cases. Use of streptozotocin is contraindicated in patients with renal disease. Proteinuria and serum creatinine levels are used to monitor toxicity.

CONSERVATIVE, NONDIALYTIC MANAGEMENT OF ACUTE RENAL FAILURE

JOEL D. KOPPLE, M.D.

Patients with acute renal failure have widely varying abnormalities in metabolic and nutritional status. Some patients show no evidence of negative nitrogen balance and have normal hydration, plasma electrolyte concentrations, and acid–base status. These patients usually have no severe catabolic underlying illnesses and they are not oliguric. The cause of their acute renal failure is typically an isolated, noncatabolic event such as the administration of radiocontrast dye or aminoglycosides. However, most patients have some degree of negative nitrogen balance and have altered fluid, electrolyte, or acid–base status. There is often overhydration, azotemia, hyperkalemia, hyperphosphatemia, hypocalcemia, hyperuricemia, and a metabolic acidosis with a large anion gap.

The net protein degradation in acute renal failure can be massive, with net losses of 150 to 200 g of protein per day or more. Patients are more likely to be catabolic when the acute renal failure is caused by shock, sepsis, or rhabdomyolysis. Enhanced net protein degradation can accelerate the rate of rise in plasma potassium, phosphorus, and nitrogenous metabolites and the fall in blood pH. In nonuremic humans, wasting and malnutrition may impair normal wound healing and immune function and increase morbidity and mortality. It is therefore likely that the profound catabolic status of many patients with acute renal failure increases their risk of delayed wound healing and infection, prolongs convalescence, and increases mortality. In my experience, patients who have acute renal failure caused by shock or sepsis and who are unable to receive adequate nutrition via the gastrointestinal tract have an 80 to 85 percent mortality rate.

A number of studies have evaluated the role of parenteral nutrition in the management of patients with acute renal failure. Patients have usually received mixtures of the nine essential amino acids, with or without nonessential amino acids, and dextrose, fat emulsions, vitamins, and minerals. The average total amino acid intake in these studies has varied from as little as 16 g per day to approximately 70 to 100 g per day. Some investigators have provided rather small quantities of calories while others have tried to match or exceed daily energy expenditure. The results of these studies have been conflicting. Some but not all reports have suggested that total parenteral nutrition (TPN) may decrease the magnitude of negative nitrogen balance and improve the survival of patients. The essential amino acid preparations are reported to decrease serum urea nitrogen (SUN) levels or the urea nitrogen appearance (UNA, net urea generation); not all studies have confirmed these results. There are also conflicting data from animal studies as to whether parenteral nutrition can accelerate the rate of recovery of renal function. The discrepant results from these studies are probably due to the following factors:

1. The clinical course of patients with acute renal failure is so complex and variable that large numbers of patients may need to be studied to show statistically significant improvement with nutritional therapy.
2. Many studies were retrospective or not randomly controlled. This may have led to unintentional biases in the results.
3. The prospective studies of parenteral nutrition in patients with acute renal failure have compared different types of nutritional therapy (e.g., hypertonic glucose with amino acids versus hypertonic glucose without amino acids; essential amino acids versus mixtures of essential and nonessential amino acids). No prospective study has compared the response in patients receiving nutritional therapy with the results in patients receiving no energy or amino acids.
4. It is probable that catabolic patients with acute renal failure may need both good nutrition and metabolic intervention to suppress catabolic processes and promote anabolism. Pharmacologic agents, not yet developed, may be necessary to improve the ability of these patients to utilize nutrients.
5. The optimal nutrient composition of the TPN infusates has not been defined, and the use of suboptimal preparations of nutrients may reduce the clinical benefits of nutritional therapy.

From the available data, it is not possible to recommend a definitive nutritional regimen for patients with acute renal failure. The following therapeutic approach is based upon my analysis of the literature and personal experience.

USE OF THE UREA NITROGEN APPEARANCE

The amount of amino acids to be prescribed for a patient with renal failure can be determined from the patient's UNA. The UNA is a simple, inexpensive, and accurate measure of net protein breakdown (degradation minus synthesis). The usefulness of the UNA is based on the fact that urea is the major nitrogenous product of protein and amino acid metabolism, and that the UNA usually correlates closely with total nitrogen output. UNA is calculated as follows:

$$\text{UNA} = \text{urinary UN} + \text{dialysate UN} + \text{change in body UN}$$

$$\text{Change in body UN} = (\text{SUN}_f - \text{SUN}_i) \times \text{BW}_i \times 0.60 \text{ L per kilogram} + (\text{BW}_f - \text{BW}_i) \times \text{SUN}_f \times 1.0 \text{ L per kilogram}$$

Where UNA and UN are given in grams per day, i and f are the initial and final values for the period of measurement, SUN is serum urea nitrogen (grams per liter), BW is body weight (kilograms), 0.60 is an estimate of the fraction of body weight that is water, and 1.0 is the volume of distribution of urea in the weight gain or loss. Usually, the period of measurement of the UNA and the change in body urea nitrogen is either 24 hours or, in patients undergoing frequent dialysis, the interdialytic interval.

The estimated proportion of body weight which is water may be increased in patients who are edematous or lean and decreased in individuals who are obese or infants. Changes in body weight during the period of measurement of UNA are assumed to be due entirely to changes in body water. In patients undergoing hemodialysis or intermittent peritoneal dialysis, the urea concentration in dialysate is low and difficult to measure accurately; hence, UNA is usually calculated during the interdialytic interval and then extrapolated to 24-hour periods.

In my experience, the relationship between UNA and total nitrogen output in chronically uremic patients not undergoing dialysis is as follows:

$$\text{Total nitrogen output} = 0.97\ \text{UNA} + 1.93$$

where total nitrogen output and UNA are expressed in grams per day. If the individual is in more or less neutral nitrogen balance, the UNA will also correlate closely with nitrogen intake; nitrogen intake may be increased by approximately 0.5 g per day to adjust for unmeasured losses through skin, respiration, and flatus. Pregnancy, large protein losses such as are found in the nephrotic syndrome or with peritoneal dialysis, and acidosis in individuals with sufficient kidney function to excrete large quantities of ammonia may cause the UNA to underestimate total nitrogen intake or output. In general, the UNA will underestimate total nitrogen output by an amount equal to the nitrogen content of the lost protein or ammonia nitrogen.

Sargent and Gotch have developed a technique for assessing UNA in hemodialysis patients which is based on the SUN and body weight at the beginning of two consecutive hemodialyses and at the end of the first dialysis. From these data—the residual renal function, the mass transfer characteristics of the dialyzer, the blood and dialysate flow rates, and the duration of the hemodialysis procedure—the net urea generation can be calculated. Although this technique is useful, it requires a somewhat complicated computer program for calculation, and, in my preliminary experience, it does not appear to offer significant advantages over the method described here.

AMINO ACID AND PROTEIN INTAKE

A typical composition for TPN solutions in adult patients with acute renal failure is shown in Table 1. Two of the most controversial issues regarding the nutritional management of patients with acute renal failure are the quantity of nitrogen and the composition of the amino acid preparations that are administered enterally or parenterally. Some nephrologists infuse only small quantities of the nine essential amino acids, with arginine sometimes added. Others have recommended mixtures of larger amounts of essential and nonessential amino acids.

The use of essential amino acid solutions is reported to reduce the UNA, the SUN, and possibly the serum potassium or phosphorus level; to ameliorate uremic toxicity; and to reduce the need for dialysis treatments. The larger quantities of essential and nonessential amino acids may be more effective at improving nitrogen balance, but the UNA is often much greater, and the need for dialysis treatments may be increased. Some nephrologists have the impression that for the same quantity of nitrogen infused, the essential amino acids may be used more efficiently than mixtures of essential and nonessential amino acids. There is also no clear-cut evidence that TPN with the essential amino acids reduces morbidity or mortality more than does TPN with essential and nonessential amino acids; however, current data do indicate that morbidity and mortality are not greater with essential amino acid solutions.

My method for selecting the quantity and type of amino acids or protein to be given to the patient with acute renal failure is as follows: Patients are prescribed a low dietary or intravenous nitrogen intake if there is a low rate of UNA (i.e., 4 to 5 g of nitrogen per day or less), no evidence of severe protein malnutrition, and the anticipation that the patient will recover renal function within the next 1 to 2 weeks. A severely reduced glomerular filtration rate (GFR) and the desire to avoid dialysis therapy are other factors that suggest the use of a low nitrogen intake. Under these conditions, one may use 0.55 to 0.60 g of protein per kilogram per day of primarily high-quality protein, or lower quantities of protein supplemented with essential amino acids or keto acids (as will be discussed). At least 35 g per kilogram per day of this protein should be of high biologic value. This diet may be particularly well tolerated if the patient has a residual GFR of about 4 to 15 ml per minute. Alternatively, the essential amino acids may be given, since they seem to be utilized more efficiently. In the latter case, one may prescribe a diet providing 0.04 to 0.30 g per kilogram per day of protein of miscellaneous quality (about 3 to 21 g per day) supplemented with 0.20 to 0.30 g per kilogram per day of the nine essential amino acids (approximately 14 to 20 g per day). The lowest quantities of protein are prescribed for the patients who have the most severe renal failure (i.e., GFR less than 3 to 4 ml per minute) and who are not very catabolic. Much of this small quantity of protein is provided in the high-calorie, low-protein foodstuffs that are the source of most of the energy intake. In clinically stable, chronically uremic patients who are not undergoing dialysis therapy and who have a low UNA, these diets should maintain neutral or near neutral nitrogen balance. Where available, ketoacid or hydroxyacid formulations may be substituted for the essential amino acids. This may further increase the efficiency of nitrogen utilization. Patients who are unable to receive oral or enteral nutrition may be given 0.30 to 0.50 g per kilogram (about 21 to 30 g per day) of essential amino acids intravenously, with or without arginine. No more than 40 g per day of the essential amino acids are given. These regimens should minimize the rate of accumulation of nitrogenous metabolites and, unless the patient is severely catabolic, will usually maintain neutral or only mildly negative nitrogen balance. Hence, the need for dialysis therapy may be minimized or avoided.

I prescribe a higher nitrogen intake, up to 1.0 to 1.2 g per kilogram per day of protein or amino acids, for those patients who are more catabolic and have a higher UNA (greater than 5 g of nitrogen per day) or are severely wasted, are undergoing regular dialysis therapy, and either have or are anticipated to have acute renal failure for more than 2 weeks. When protein is administered orally or enterally, at least 50 percent should be of high biologic value. In comparison to small quantities of amino acids, these larger nitrogen intakes may improve nitrogen balance. However, the UNA will almost invariably rise, and the increased azotemia and—in those patients receiving TPN—the large volume of fluid necessary to provide this amount of amino acids may increase the requirements for dialysis. Patients with greater residual renal function, higher fluid tolerance, and a healthy cardiorespiratory system usually are more tolerant of these larger nitrogen and water intakes. With the appropriate use of dialysis or intermittent or continuous arterial-venous hemofiltration, these higher nitrogen intakes are well tolerated by most patients.

When renal failure persists for more than 2 to 3 weeks, patients undergoing regular dialysis treatment are treated, as are maintenance dialysis patients, with about 1.0 to 1.2 g per kilogram per day of protein or amino acids for maintenance intermittent hemodialysis and 1.2 to 1.5 g per kilogram per day for maintenance intermittent or continuous ambulatory peritoneal dialysis. At least 50 percent of the protein should be of high biologic value.

The optimal amino acid composition for enteral or parenteral nutrition in acute renal failure has not been established. As indicated above, there is some evidence that when nitrogen intake is very low, provision of the nine essential amino acids alone (histidine, isoleucine, leucine, lysine, methionine, phenylalanine, threonine, tryptophan, and valine) may be the more efficient treatment and may result in a lower UNA and more positive nitrogen balance for any level of nitrogen intake.

The proportion of each of the essential amino acids traditionally has been designed according to the recommended daily allowances for each of the amino acids as defined by Rose. More recently, some investigators have recommended increasing the proportion of the branched-chain amino acids and reducing the content of some of the other essential amino acids. With higher nitrogen intakes (greater than 5 to 6 g of nitrogen per day) it is important to give both essential and nonessential amino acids. Patients who receive large quantities of amino acids (i.e., greater than 40 g per day) have a nutritional requirement for nonessential amino acids, particularly for the urea cycle amino acids such as arginine. The reason is that a large intake of essential amino acids with no nonessentials can lead to severe alterations in the plasma amino acid pattern and to hyperammonemia.

There is evidence, still not conclusive, that the three branched-chain amino acids (isoleucine, leucine, and valine) may have a specific anabolic effect in acutely ill patients without renal failure. If this effect is also present in acute renal failure, it may justify giving a larger proportion of the nitrogen in the form of branched-chain amino acids. The plasma concentrations of the branched-chain amino acids tend to be decreased in acute renal failure, which may be another reason for giving them in larger proportions. These observations suggest that for the essential and nonessential amino acid mixtures, it may be preferable to give a high ratio of essential to nonessential amino acids (e.g., 3:1 or 4:1). The three branched-chain amino acids may account for 40 to 50 percent of the essential amino acids in this preparation. These formulations of essential and nonessential amino acids are not currently available in the United States. More research is clearly necessary to examine the role of such preparations in patients with acute renal failute. When I administer TPN providing essential and nonessential amino acids I currently use preparations that contain essential to nonessential amino acids for uremic patients, in a ratio of 1:1 to 2:1. Mixtures of these essential and nonessential amino acids may be combined with commercially available essential amino acid solutions to obtain a higher essential: nonessential ratio; however, such preparations are costly and have not been tested in cases of acute renal failure.

ORAL OR ENTERAL VERSUS PARENTERAL NUTRITION

For patients who are able to obtain nutrition by eating or by enteral tube feeding, it is usually preferable to provide nutrition in this way rather than intravenously. Parenteral nutrition can be more hazardous, provides greater fluid loads, and is more costly. However, many patients with acute renal failure are obtunded, severely ill, or debilitated. In these patients, the risk of aspiration of food or enteral feeding preparations is very great, and parenteral nutrition may be safer. The recent development of a technique for the percutaneous insertion of a gastrostomy tube may reduce the risk of enteral feeding in some debilitated or severely ill patients.

There are liquid protein or chemically defined (elemental) preparations for patients who must be nourished by enteral tube or gastrostomy. Since amino acids seem to be utilized more efficiently than protein, I am inclined to use them rather than protein for patients in whom it is important to reduce the UNA and avoid dialysis therapy. As indicated above, experimental data indicate that when patients receive large quantities of amino acids (greater than 40 g per day), they require nonessential as well as essential amino acids. If patients are receiving frequent dialysis therapy or if their GFR is sufficiently great that they do not need dialysis, there may be no advantage to using amino acids instead of high-quality protein.

Patients are given parenteral nutrition when they are unable to receive nutrients safely via the enteral tract. In general, TPN is started as soon as it is determined that the patient has acute renal failure and is unable to receive enteral nutrition. This treatment strategy differs from that recommended for other acutely ill patients in whom TPN usually is begun after it is determined that the patient will not be able to receive enteral nutrition for a defined number of days, usually about 7. This difference in treatment stategy is based upon suggestive evidence that parenteral nutrition may improve survival in patients with acute renal failure, if it is started early. The total quantity of nitrogen and the proportion of individual amino acids to be administered should be determined as described previously and in Table 1.

ENERGY, VITAMINS, AND MINERALS

Since patients with acute renal failure are usually in negative nitrogen balance, I tend to employ large quanti-

TABLE 1 Composition of Total Parenteral Nutrition for Adult Patients with Acute Renal Failure

Intake[a]	*Quantity*
Energy[b]	35–50 kcal/kg/day
70% dextrose (D-glucose) (500 ml)	350 g/L
Essential and nonessential amino acids (4.25–5.0%) [c], *or*	42.5–50 g/L
Essential amino acids (5.0%)[c]	12.5–25 g/L
Electrolytes[d]	
Sodium[e]	40–50 mEq/L
Chloride[e]	25–35 mEq/L
Potassium	≤ 35 mEq/day
Acetate[e]	35–40 mEq/L
Calcium	10 mEq/day
Phosphorus	8 mmol/day
Magnesium	8 mEq/day
Iron	1.0 mg/day
Other trace elements[f]	See text
Vitamins	
Niacin	20 mg/day
Thiamin HCl (B_1)	2 mg/day
Riboflavin (B_2)	2 mg/day
Pantothenic acid	10 mg/day
Pyridoxine HCl (B_6)	10 mg/day
Ascorbic acid (C)	60–100 mg/day
Biotin	200 mg/day
Folic acid[g]	1 mg/day
Vitamin B_{12}[g]	3μg/day
Vitamin A	See text[h]
Vitamin D	See text[i]
Vitamin K[g]	10 mg/week
Vitamin E	10 IU/day[j]

Note: These recommendations should be considered tentative. The composition and volume of the infusate may be modified if patients are volume overloaded, very uremic, or acidotic; if serum electrolyte concentrations are not normal or relatively constant; or if dialysis therapy is not readily available.

[a] The nutrients listed below are added to each 1-L bottle containing crystalline amino acids and 70% dextrose, except for the vitamins and trace elements, which should be added to only one bottle per day. The total volume per bottle will usually be slightly greater than 1 L because of the electrolyte and vitamin additives.

[b] Energy intake (including calories derived from amino acids) is usually maintained at 35–50 kcal/kg/day; add 70% dextrose and lipids to attain this level. The dextrose in parenteral solutions is provided as dextrose monohydrate. The energy thus provided by dextrose monohydrate is approximately 3.4 kcal/g, for amino acids, it is about 3.5 kcal/g. Infuse 25–50 g/day of lipids to prevent essential fatty acid deficiency and to produce more balanced sources of fuel substrates. A 20% lipid emulsion provides the most fat calories per milliliter of water (2.0 kcal/ml). A total of 1.5–2.5 L/day of TPN solutions may be necessary to provide sufficient amino acids and energy. The fluid load necessary to provide this quantity of amino acids, lipids, and dextrose increases the need for dialysis, hemofiltration, ultrafiltration, or CAVH.

[c] Usually, when the UNA is greater than 5 g N/day, 1.0 g/kg/day of essential and nonessential amino acids is given. If the UNA is 4–5 g N/day or less, 0.30 to 0.50 g/kg/day of essential amino acids may be administered. No more than 30–40 g/day of essential amino acids (without nonessential amino acids) are given. See text for a more detailed discussion of the amounts and types of amino acid preparations administered. The prescribed amino acids often may be provided in less than 500 ml of solution, and the volume of 70% dextrose may be increased to bring the volume up to one liter and to provide additional calories.

[d] The amounts of electrolytes intrinsically present in the amino acid solutions should be considered.

[e] Refers to final concentration of electrolytes after any extra 70% dextrose has been added.

[f] Patients receiving TPN for more than 7 to 14 days may need zinc (up to 5 mg/day), copper (up to 0.5 mg/day), and other trace elements (see text).

[g] Given orally or parenterally and not in the TPN solution because of antagonisms.

[h] Vitamin A should be avoided unless TPN is continued for more than several weeks.

[i] Currently, 1,25-dihydroxycholecalciferol is not commercially available for parenteral administration.

[j] May need to be increased with use of lipid emulsions.

ties of calories to minimize net protein breakdown. There is no easy way to estimate the energy requirements for patients with acute renal failure; I therefore empirically administer 35 to 50 kcal per kilogram per day. The higher energy intakes (i.e., 50 kcal per kilogram per day) are used for patients who have a higher UNA, who tend to be severely ill, and who are not very obese. If nitrogen balance, determined by the difference between the patient's nitrogen intake and the nitrogen output calculated from the UNA, is negative, I try to provide an energy intake close to 50 kcal per kilogram per day. Recently, indirect calorimetry has been used to estimate energy expenditure in acutely ill patients with renal failure. In this case, the daily energy requirement is determined by multiplying basal energy expenditure by 1.25. Most researchers believe that there is little nutritional advantage to administering more than 50 kcal per kilogram per day to catabolic patients. Moreover, with high energy intakes, the large quantity of carbon dioxide produced from the infused carbohydrate and fat can cause hypercapnia if pulmonary function is impaired.

Since most patients with acute renal failure do not tolerate large water intakes, glucose is usually administered in a 70 percent solution. The glucose and amino acid solutions are mixed so that the amino acids and energy are provided simultaneously (see Table 1). Patients receiving TPN for more than 5 to 7 days should receive lipid emulsions. Preferably 50 to 100 g per day of lipids should be infused daily, but no less than twice weekly to prevent essential fatty acid deficiency and to balance the energy sources. Ten percent and 20 percent lipid emulsions are available. They are approximately isotonic with plasma and provide 1.1 and 2.0 kcal per milliliter, respectively. By comparison, 70 percent dextrose (the dextrose is provided as D-glucose monohydrate) yields about 2.38 kcal per milliliter and is the parenteral solution that gives the most calories per milliliter. I rely on dextrose as the major source of calories because dextrose is the primary energy source for several tissues and is well utilized by virtually all tissues. Also, 70 percent dextrose is much less expensive per calorie than are lipid emulsions, and hyperglycemia is readily treated with insulin. For these reasons, in acutely uremic patients receiving parenteral nutrition, glucose is used as the major source of calories, and lipids are given daily, but in lesser amounts.

The vitamins and minerals recommended for TPN are shown in Table 1. For patients receiving enteral nutrition, similar quantities of minerals and vitamins can be used. The recommended intake of minerals is tentative and must be adjusted according to the clinical status of the patient. If the serum concentration of an electrolyte is increased, it may be advisable to reduce the quantity infused or not to administer it at the onset of parenteral nutrition. The patient must be monitored closely, however, because the hormonal and metabolic changes that often occur with initiation of TPN may cause the serum electrolytes to fall rapidly. This is particularly likely with serum potassium and phosphorus. On the other hand, a low concentration of a mineral may indicate that there is a need for a greater than usual intake of that element. Again, metabolic changes and the patient's low GFR can lead to a rapid rise in the serum level during repletion.

Trace element requirements in acute renal failure are not defined. At present, I add 1.0 mg per day of iron to TPN solutions. Other trace elements may be given, including zinc, up to 5 mg per day, and copper, up to 0.5 mg per day. When trace elements are given to patients with acute renal failure, blood concentrations must be carefully monitored to ensure that excess levels do not occur.

Vitamin requirements have not been well defined for patients with acute renal failure. Much of the recommended intake is based on information obtained from studies in chronically uremic patients, normal individuals, or nonuremic acutely ill patients. Vitamin A is probably best avoided because in chronic renal failure, serum vitamin A levels are elevated and small doses of vitamin A have been reported to cause toxicity in uremic patients. Also, since most patients with acute renal failure will receive TPN for only a few days or weeks, it is unlikely that a deficiency will occur for this fat-soluble vitamin.

The nutritional requirement for vitamin D in patients with acute renal failure has not been defined. Although vitamin D is fat soluble and vitamin stores should not become depleted during the few days to weeks that most patients with acute renal failure receive TPN, the turnover of its most active analogue, 1,25-dihydroxycholecalciferol, is much faster. This may indicate that there is a need for this analogue in patients with acute renal failure. At the present time, a parenteral preparation of 1,25–dihydroxycholecalciferol is not commercially available. Although vitamin K is fat-soluble, vitamin K deficiency has been reported in some nonuremic patients who were not eating and were receiving antibiotics. Vitamin K supplements are therefore given routinely to patients receiving TPN (see Table 1). Ten mg per day of pyridoxine hydrochloride (8.2 mg per day of pyridoxine) are recommended because studies in patients undergoing maintenance hemodialysis indicate that this quantity may be necessary to prevent or correct vitamin B_6 deficiency. Patients should probably not receive more than 60 to 100 mg per day of ascorbic acid because of the risk of increased serum oxalate concentrations.

It must be recognized that the nutrient intake of patients with acute renal failure must be carefully reevaluated each day and sometimes more frequently. This is particularly important for these patients because they may undergo rapid changes in their clinical and metabolic condition.

PERIPHERAL OR SUPPLEMENTAL PARENTERAL NUTRITION, ANABOLIC HORMONES

Parenteral nutrition through a peripheral vein avoids the problems of inserting a catheter into the inferior vena cava and is safer. There are several limitations to peripheral parenteral nutrition. First, the osmolality of the infusate must be restricted to about 600 mOsm per kilogram H_2O to reduce the risk of thrombophlebitis. Since the osmolality with typical TPN solutions is approximately 1,800 mOsm per kilogram H_2O to reduce tonicity of the infusates it is necessary to use a larger volume of fluid and/or a lower intake of nutrients. Second, the needles or catheters must be changed frequently, usually every 18 to 48 hours to prevent thrombophlebitis. Heparin, 500 units per liter, and cortisol, 5 mg per liter, may reduce the risk of thrombophlebitis and allow the patient to receive somewhat more hypertonic solutions (e.g., about 900 mOsm) and to extend the duration that the catheter can be left in a peripheral vein.

Some patients with acute renal failure are able to ingest or be tube fed only part of their daily nutritional requirements. Peripheral infusions may enable these patients to receive adequate nutrition without resorting to TPN. In the latter cases it is often most practical to infuse 8.5 to 10 percent amino acids or 20 percent lipid emulsions into a peripheral vein and administer as much as possible of other essential nutrients, including carbohydrates, through the enteral tract. The peripheral vascular accesses used for hemodialysis can also be used for parenteral nutrition. However, this technique probably increases the hazard of thrombophlebitis and infection, and it should not be used in patients who will need a hemodialysis access for extended periods.

Parenteral nutrition has been administered with continuous arteriovenous hemofiltration (CAVH) to provide intravenous nutrition and, at the same time, control the water and mineral balance and reduce the accumulation of metabolic products from the infused nutrients or from endogenous substrates. Large amounts of water, minerals, urea, and other metabolites can be removed by CAVH. On the other hand, the quantity of glucose, amino acids and protein lost during CAVH is small, even when patients are receiving parenteral nutrition. Hence, it is often easier to administer adequate amino acids and energy to patients with acute renal failure when they undergo CAVH. CAVH may reduce the frequency with which hemodialysis is needed in patients with acute renal failure.

In patients who have marginally adequate intakes, supplemental amino acids and glucose may be given during hemodialysis treatment. Some nephrologists infuse 20 or 30 g of the nine essential amino acids at the end of dialysis therapy. However, since most patients who need nutritional supplements have decreased intake of energy and total nitrogen, I give 40 to 42 g of essential and nonessential amino acids and 200 g of D-glucose (150 g of D-glucose if dialysate contains glucose). This preparation is infused into the blood leaving the dialyzer at a constant rate throughout the dialysis procedure to minimize disruption of the amino acid and glucose pools which occurs with hemodialysis. Patients who have low serum concentrations of phosphorus or potassium at the start of the dialysis treatment may need supplements of these minerals. With such infusions, plasma amino acids and glucose do not fall during dialysis and over 85 percent of the infused amino acids are retained. The infusion is not stopped until the end of hemodialysis. Also, the patient should eat some carbohydrate 20 to 30 minutes before the end of the infusion. Otherwise, the infusion must be tapered or a peripheral infusion of glucose must be started to prevent reactive hypoglycemia.

Intravenous nutrition that is given only during hemodialysis is probably inadequate for stressed acutely uremic patients because their oral or enteral intake is usually very low, their nutritional needs are high, and the nutritional supplements are given only intermittently, when the patient receives hemodialysis treatment. It is possible that intravenous nutrition during hemodialysis may be of value only for patients who have a daily nutritional intake that is slightly suboptimal.

Insulin and anabolic steroids have been used to reduce the UNA and improve nitrogen balance in acutely ill patients, including those with acute renal failure. Although some studies indicate that these hormones have an anabolic effect, other studies have failed to confirm this. The therapeutic value of these hormones for promoting anabolism in catabolic patients with acute renal failure is not established.

NUTRITIONAL AND NONDIALYTIC MANAGEMENT OF CHRONIC RENAL FAILURE

JOEL D. KOPPLE, M.D.

Nutritional therapy for patients with chronic renal failure has three major goals. These are (1) to retard the rate of progression of renal failure (in the nondialyzed patient), (2) to maintain good nutritional status, and (3) to prevent or improve the uremic syndrome. A reduction in the intake of certain nutrients may retard the progression of renal disease and, in patients with advanced renal failure, reduce uremic toxicity. However, there is much evidence that many patients undergoing maintenance dialysis have wasting and malnutrition. The wasting is usually mild or moderate, but frequently it can be severe. Since in the Western world maintenance dialysis therapy is readily available, it is more advisable to provide a diet for a patient with renal failure that maintains good nutritional status than to prescribe a nutritional therapy that may reduce uremic toxicity at the expense of inducing malnutrition. A proposed recommended intake for adult uremic patients and patients undergoing maintenance hemodialysis or continuous ambulatory peritoneal dialysis (CAPD) is shown in Table 1.

Note: When the recommended nutrient intake is given in terms of kilograms of body weight, this refers to the Metropolitan Life Insurance's desirable body weight, expressed according to the age, height, sex, and frame size of the patient.

Monitoring Nitrogen Intake: Urea Nitrogen Appearance and the Serum Urea Nitrogen to Serum Creatinine Ratio

It is important to ensure that the dietary protein intake in patients with renal failure is neither too low nor too high. Thus, it is of value to estimate accurately a patient's actual nitrogen intake. Since urea is the major

TABLE 1 Recommended Daily Intakes for Nondialyzed Patients with Chronic Renal Failure and Patients Undergoing Maintenance Hemodialysis or Continuous Ambulatory Peritoneal Dialysis

	Chronic Renal Failure[*†]	*Hemodialysis (HD) and Continuous Ambulatory (CAPD) or Cyclic Peritoneal Dialysis (CCPD)*
Protein[‡]	0.55–0.60 g/kg/day (about ≥35 g/kg/day high biological value); maximum intake is 45 g/day Very-low-protein diet (about 0.28 g/kg/day of protein of any biologic value) supplemented with either a ketoacid and amino acid mixture or essential amino acid mixture	HD: 1.0–1.2 g/kg/day; ≥50% high biologic value protein; 1.2 g/kg/day is prescribed unless patient has normal protein status with intakes of 1.0–1.1 g protein/kg/day CAPD: 1.2–1.3 g/kg/day; ≥50% CCPD: High biologic value protein; for malnourished patients, up to 1.5 g/kg/day may be given
Calories[§]	≥35 Kcal/kg/day unless the patient's relative body weight is >120%	
Fat (% of total calorie intake)[**††]	40–55	40–55
Polyunsaturated:saturated fatty acid ration[††]	1.0:1.0	1.0:1.0
Carbohydrate[‡‡]	Rest of nonprotein calories	Rest of nonprotein calories
Total fiber intake[††]	20–25 g/day	20–25 g/day
Minerals		
Sodium	1,000 to 3,000 mg/day[§§]	750 to 1,000 mg/day[§§]
Potassium	40 to 70 mEq/day	40 to 70 mEq/day
Phosphorus	4 to 12 mg/kg/day[***]	8 to 17 mg/kg/day[***]
Calcium	1,400 to 1,600 mg/day[†††]	1,400 to 1,600 mg/day[†††]
Magnesium	200 to 300 mg/day	200 to 300 mg/day
Iron	10 to 18 mg/day[‡‡‡]	10 to 18 mg/day[‡‡‡]
Zinc	15 mg/day	15 mg/day
Water	Up to 3,000 ml/day as tolerated[§§]	Usually 750 to 1,500 ml/day[§§]
Vitamin supplements	Diets to be supplemented with these quantities	
Thiamin	1.5 mg/day	1.5 mg/day
Riboflavin	1.8 mg/day	1.8 mg/day
Pantothenic Acid	5 mg/day	5 mg/day
Niacin	20 mg/day	20 mg/day
Pyridoxine HCI	5 mg/day	10 mg/day
Vitamin B_{12}	3 μg/day	3 μg/day
Folic Acid	1 mg/day	1 mg/day
Vitamin A	None	None
Vitamin D	See text	See text
Vitamin E	15 IU/day	15 IU/day
Vitamin K	None[§§§]	None[§§§]

[*] GFR> 4–5 ml/min and ≤ 70 ml/min/1.73 meters squared.
[†] When recommended intake is expressed per kg body weight, this refers to the patient's desirable weight as determined from the Metropolitan Life Insurance tables.
[‡] The protein intake is increased by 1.0 g/day of high biologic value protein for each g/day of urinary protein loss.
[§] This includes energy intake from dialysate in CAPD and CCPD patients.
[**] Refers to percent of total energy intake (diet plus dialysate).
[††] These dietary recommendations are considered less crucial than the others.
[‡‡] Should be primarily complex carbohydrates, if tolerated by the patient.
[§§] Can be higher in nondialyzed chronic renal failure or maintenance dialysis patients who have greater urinary losses or in CAPD or CCPD patients.
[***] Phosphorus intake should be 4–9 mg/day for patients ingesting a very-low-protein diet supplemented with ketoacids or amino acids; with the 0.55–0.60 g protein/kg/day diet, a phosphorus intake of 8–12 mg/kg/day is more tolerable. Phosphate binders are usually needed as well (see text).
[†††] Dietary intake must be supplemented to provide these levels.
[‡‡‡] ≥10 mg/day for males and nonmenstruating females; ≥18 mg/day for menstruating females.
[§§§] Vitamin K supplements may be needed in those who are not eating and are receiving antibiotics.

nitrogenous product of protein and amino acid metabolism, the urea nitrogen appearance (UNA, net urea generation) usually correlates closely with, and can be used to estimate, total nitrogen output. UNA is calculated as follows:

UNA = urinary urea nitrogen (UN) + dialysate UN + change in body UN

Change in body UN = $(SUN_f - SUN_i) \times BW_i \times$ 0.60 L per kilogram + $(BW_f - BW_i) \times SUN_f \times$ 1.0 L per kilogram

Where UNA and UN are given in grams per day, and final values for the period of measurement, SUN is serum urea nitrogen (g per liter), and BW is body weight (kg). The fraction of body weight that is water is represented by 0.60. Greater or lesser numbers may be used depending on whether the patient is lean, edematous, obese, old, or young. The assumption is made that in a uremic patient any change in BW occurring during a 1 to 3 day interval is attributable to accrual or to loss of water. Therefore, the fraction of weight change that represents gain or loss of water is taken as 1.0.

In our experience, the relationship between UNA and total nitrogen output in chronically uremic patients not undergoing dialysis is as follows:

Total nitrogen output (g per day) = 0.97 UNA (g per day) + 1.93 (g per day).

Since protein contains about 16 percent nitrogen, the relation between UNA and net protein breakdown in these patients can be estimated from the following equation:

Net protein breakdown (g per day)=6.1 UNA (g per day) + 12 (g per day)

If patients are in neutral balance, this same equation can be used to estimate protein intake; about 3.0 g per day of protein may be added to the value to adjust for unmeasured nitrogen losses.

In nondialyzed patients with chronic renal failure, there is a direct correlation between the ratio of the serum urea nitrogen (SUN) to the serum creatinine and the protein intake. This relationship can be used to estimate daily protein intake or, conversely, to select the optimal quantity of protein to be prescribed for a patient. Although this technique is easy to use and fairly accurate, several factors may reduce its usefulness. A urine flow less than 1,500 ml per day may increase the SUN:serum creatinine ratio for a given protein intake because, in contrast to the creatinine clearance, the urea clearance tends to fall progressively as urine flow decreases below this level. The SUN:serum creatinine ratio increases with catabolic stress and with reduced muscle mass, as is found in women, children, and very wasted men. Also, with a change in dietary protein, a period of 2 to 3 weeks may be necessary for the SUN to stabilize and the SUN:serum creatinine ratio to reflect the new protein intake. In clinically stable, chronically uremic men with a protein intake of 20, 40, or 60 g per day, the SUN:serum creatinine ratio should be, on an average, 3.4, 6.0, and 8.6, respectively.

Protein Intake

A number of studies in both rats and humans with renal insufficiency indicate that a diet low in protein and phosphorus may retard the rate of progression of renal failure. This effect has been observed not only in patients with advanced renal failure, but also in those with mild-to-moderate renal failure (serum creatinine values of 2 to 6 mg per deciliter). Although each of the studies carried out in humans suffers from weaknesses in experimental design, almost all reports indicate that in some patients such diets may retard progression of renal failure. The most dramatic effects have been reported with ketoacid- and hydroxyacid-supplemented diets. There are several ketoacid and hydroxyacid formulations currently in use. They usually provide four essential amino acids (histidine, lysine, threonine, and tryptophan) and the ketoacid or hydroxyacid salts of the other five essential amino acids. The ketoacids and hydroxyacids have the same structure as the respective essential amino acids except that the alpha-amino nitrogen is removed and a keto or hydroxy group is substituted.

Chronic Renal Disease with GFR Greater Than 70 ml per Minute per 1.73 Meters Squared

Most studies of the effects of diets low in protein and phosphorus on the rate of progression of renal failure have examined patients with moderately advanced to advanced renal failure (serum creatinine$\geq$5 mg per deciliter). Hence, there is virtually no information concerning the optimal dietary protein (or phosphorus) prescription for patients with chronic renal disease and mild impairment in renal function. Until more information is available, it is recommended that protein (and phosphorus) intake should be restricted for patients with GFR greater than 70 ml per minute per 1.73 meters squared only if there is evidence that renal function is continuing to decline. In this latter case, the patient is treated as indicated in the following paragraph.

Chronic Renal Disease with GFR 5 to 70 ml per Minute per 1.73 Meters Squared

It is the author's policy to discuss with the patient the evidence that low protein, low phosphorus diets may retard progression and to indicate that the data, although not conclusive, are strong enough to justify the patient ingesting a restricted protein and phosphorus diet. If the patient agrees to dietary treatment, the patient is prescribed a diet providing about 0.60 to 0.70 g protein per kilogram per day. At least 0.35 g per kilogram per day of the protein should be of high biologic value (eggs, meat, fish, and milk and its products), because these proteins contain a high proportion of essential amino acids that are present roughly in the proportions required by humans. Hence, these proteins are utilized more efficiently than are proteins of lower quality. On the other hand, low quality proteins, which are prevalent in foods derived from plants (e.g., grains and vegetables), are particularly valuable for increasing the palatability and acceptability of the diet. At least 12 to 16 g per day of low-quality protein seem to be necessary for a palatable diet. An intake of 0.55 to 0.60 g protein per kilogram per day provides about 30 to 35 g per day for women and small men and about 40 g per day for normal sized men. In general, we do not prescribe more than about 45 g per day of protein for any patient with a GFR below 10 ml per minute. In clinically stable patients, the SUN can almost always be maintained below 90 mg per deciliter with these low protein diets until the GFR falls below 4 to 5 ml per minute. This amount of protein should maintain neutral or positive nitrogen balance and should not be excessively burdensome for most patients.

Amino acid- and ketoacid-supplemented diets may also be offered to the patient. Currently, these diets generally provide about 0.28 g protein per kilogram per day (16 to 20 g protein per day) supplemented with about 10 to 20 g of the essential amino acids or mixtures of essential amino acids and ketoacids. Since the amino acid and ketoacid supplements provide sufficient essential amino acids, the protein derived from food does not have to be of high biologic value, thereby increasing the patient's freedom of food selection. In the author's experience, most, but not all, patients seem to prefer the 0.55 to 0.60 g protein per kilogram per day diet over the essential amino acid-supplemented diet. This former diet is less expensive than is the essential amino acid-supplemented diet.

There are several potential advantages to using amino acid or ketoacid formulations. First, with more advanced renal failure (i.e., GFR $<$ 15 to 25 ml per minute per 1.73 meters squared), potentially toxic products of nitrogen metabolism begin to accumulate in increasing quantities. Since the ketoacids and hydroxyacids lack the alpha-amino group, for the same intake of amino acid equivalents less nitrogen is provided and there is less generation of potentially toxic nitrogenous compounds. Second, because the amino acid and ketoacid preparations do not contain phosphorus (or potassium), the content of these elements in the diet can be markedly decreased (see section on recommended phosphorus intake). Third, by modifying the proportions of individual amino acids, ketoacids, or hydroxyacids in the diet, it may be possible to normalize more of the altered plasma and muscle-amino acid concentrations that develop in advanced renal failure—whether this normalization is of value to the patient is not yet established. Finally, as indicated above, these semisynthetic diets may be more effective at retarding the rate of progression of renal failure.

Given the dramatic results described with certain ketoacid formulations, it would seem reasonable that when the GFR decreases to about 25 ml per minute per 1.73 meters squared, patients should be prescribed a diet providing 0.28 g protein per kilogram per day supplemented with a mixture of about 13 to 18 g of ketoacids and amino acids, if the formulation is available. Ketoacid supplements have not yet been approved for clinical use in the United States. Where ketoacids are not available, essential amino acid supplements may be substituted for the ketoacid mixture or patients may be prescribed 0.55 to 0.60 g protein per kilogram per day with at least 0.35 kg per kilogram per day of protein of high biological value. All three of these diets generally maintain neutral or positive nitrogen balance and generate a low UNA. The protein content of each of the diets prescribed for patients with mild-to-severe renal failure should be increased by 1.0 g per day of high biologic value protein for each gram of protein excreted in the urine each day. Whether the ketoacid- or essential amino acid-supplemented very-low-protein diets should be prescribed for patients with a GFR above 25 ml per minute per 1.73 meters squared is not known.

When the GFR falls below 5 ml per minute per 1.73 meters squared, there is no conclusive evidence that patients fare as well with low nitrogen diets as with regular dialysis therapy and higher protein intakes. Since these latter patients may be at high risk for wasting or malnutrition, it is recommended that maintenance dialysis treatment or renal transplantation should be inaugurated at this time. Patients with diabetes mellitus may develop uremic symptoms at a higher GFR; thus, such individuals are often started on maintenance dialysis or undergo renal transplantation when their GFR is between 5 and 10 ml per minute per 1.73 meters squared.

Adherence to low-protein, low-phosphorus diets requires a major change in dietary habits and even in lifestyle. Prior to beginning dietary therapy, the patient and, if possible, close family members or other participants in his or her support network must be informed of the magnitude of this undertaking and must agree to the commitment. Otherwise, there is small likelihood that the patient will adhere successfully to this dietary prescription.

Maintenance Dialysis Therapy

Patients undergoing hemodialysis 3 times per week should receive a minimum of 1.0 and preferably 1.2 g of protein per kilogram per day (Table 1). Patients undergoing CAPD should receive 1.2 to 1.3 g per kilogram per day of protein. In malnourished CAPD patients, up to 1.5 g protein per kilogram per day can be taken. At least half of their dietary protein should be of high biologic value.

Energy Intake

Studies of energy expenditure in nondialyzed chronically uremic patients and patients undergoing maintenance hemodialysis indicate that energy expenditure is normal during resting and sitting, following ingestion of a standard meal, and with graded exercise. Nitrogen balance studies in nondialyzed chronically uremic patients indicate that the amount of energy necessary to ensure neutral or positive nitrogen balance is approximately 35 Kcal per kilogram per day. However, virtually every survey of energy intake in nondialyzed chronically uremic and hemodialysis patients indicates that, on average, it is lower than this level and usually 30 Kcal per kilogram per day or less.

We currently recommend that nondialyzed chronically uremic patients and patients undergoing maintenance hemodialysis or CAPD should receive about 35 Kcal per kilogram per day. Patients who are obese with an edema-free body weight greater than 120 percent of desirable body weight may be treated with lower calorie intakes. There are many commercially available high-calorie foodstuffs that are low in protein, sodium, and potassium. A nephrology dietitian can recommend these foodstuffs as well as other low-protein high-calorie foods that can be prepared easily at home.

Hyperlipidemia

A large proportion of chronically uremic and dialysis patients have type IV hyperlipoproteinemia with elevated serum triglyceride levels and a low serum HDL cholesterol. Since in uremic patients these alterations in serum lipoproteins may contribute to the high incidence of atherosclerosis and cardiovascular disease, attention has been directed toward reducing serum triglycerides and increasing HDL cholesterol. Elevated serum triglyceride levels in uremia appear to be caused primarily by impaired clearance from blood. Also, since diets in renal failure are usually restricted in protein, sodium, potassium, and water, it is often difficult to provide sufficient energy without resorting to a large intake of purified sugars, which can increase triglyceride production. Serum triglycerides may be lowered by feeding a diet in which the carbohydrate content is reduced to supply 35 percent of calories, the fat content is increased to provide 50 to 55 percent of calories, and the polyunsaturated:saturated fatty acid ratio is raised to 1:1.

Although elevated serum triglyceride levels do not appear to be a strong risk factor for arteriosclerotic disease, this dietary treatment should be employed at least for uremic patients with markedly elevated serum triglyceride levels (e.g., greater than 1.5 to 2.0 times the upper limits of normal). L-carnitine, 1.0 g per day orally, may also decrease serum triglyceride concentrations, and patients with this magnitude of hypertriglyceridemia who have low serum carnitine should probably also be given a trial period with this compound. Low serum HDL-cholesterol levels are a strong risk factor for cardiovascular disease. Serum concentrations may increase with daily exercise.

Mineral and Water Intake

Sodium and Water

As renal failure progresses, both the glomerular filtration and fractional reabsorption of sodium fall progressively. Thus, sodium balance is usually well maintained in patients with chronic renal failure when they ingest a normal salt intake. However, there is an impaired ability to handle both a sodium load and to conserve sodium normally during intake of a low-sodium diet. Normally, only about 1 to 3 mEq per day of sodium are excreted in the feces, and in the non-sweating individual, only a few mEq per day of sodium are lost through the skin. If sodium intake exceeds the ability of the kidney to excrete sodium, sodium and water retention, hypertension, edema, and congestive heart failure may develop. Certain conditions predispose to sodium retention and may dictate earlier restriction of sodium or water intake or the use of diuretic agents. These conditions include congestive heart failure and advanced liver disease. When the GFR falls below 4 to 10 ml per minute, the ability to handle even a normal sodium intake may fall. In addition, in renal failure, hypertension may be more easily controlled with sodium restriction and may be accentuated with normal or increased sodium intakes. On the other hand, if sodium intake is not sufficient to replace obligatory renal sodium losses, sodium depletion and contraction of extracellular fluid volume may occur and may lead to reduced renal blood flow and further impairment of GFR. Hence, when evaluating patients with renal failure who do not have evidence of fluid overload or hypertension, they should be given a careful trial of sodium loading to assess whether renal function may be improved.

In general, if sodium balance is well controlled, the patient's thirst adequately controls water balance. However, when the GFR falls below 2 to 5 ml per minute, the water intake often must be controlled independently of sodium to prevent overhydration. In diabetics, hyperglycemia may increase thirst and enhance positive water balance. In patients whose total body water is at the desired level, urine excretion may be a good guide to water intake. Daily water intake should equal the urine output plus approximately 500 ml to adjust for insensible losses.

Most nondialyzed chronically uremic patients maintain sodium and water balance with an intake of 1,000 to 3,000 mg of sodium per day and 600 to 3,000 ml of fluid per day. However, the requirement for sodium and water varies markedly, and each patient must be managed individually. Usually, patients undergoing maintenance hemodialysis or peritoneal dialysis are severely oliguric or anuric. For hemodialysis patients, sodium and total fluid intake generally should be restricted to 1,000 to 1,500 mg per day and 700 to 1,500 ml per day, respectively. Patients undergoing CAPD usually tolerate a greater sodium and water intake because salt and water can be easily removed by using hypertonic dialysate. By maintaining a larger dietary sodium and water intake, the quantity of fluid removed from the CAPD patient and, hence, the daily dialysate volume can be increased. This may be advantageous since with CAPD, the daily clearance of small molecules is directly related to the volume of dialysate outflow. With this in mind, some nephrologists have recommended a larger dietary sodium and water intake for CAPD patients in order to increase the hypertonic dialysate and thus increase dialysate outflow. This treatment may be undesirable for obese or hypertriglyceridemic patients because of the greater need for hypertonic glucose exchanges that increase the glucose load. Also, there is the potential disadvantage that some patients may become habituated to high salt and water intakes; if they are changed to hemodialysis therapy, they may have difficulty curtailing ingestion of sodium and water.

One way to monitor sodium requirements in nondialyzed patients is to follow carefully the body weight, blood pressure, and serum sodium. When sodium intake is inadequate, there is often negative water balance, a decrease in body weight, and a fall in blood pressure. Excessive sodium intake is often associated with positive water balance, a rise in body weight, and an increase in blood pressure. Serum sodium concentrations may rise, fall, or not change depending upon the water balance. On the other hand, a decrease in serum sodium in the presence of an unchanging or falling body weight usually indicates that there is a need for more sodium. The dietary sodium requirement may also be determined by decreasing or raising sodium intake for several days and monitoring body weight, blood pressure, appearance of edema, serum creatinine or clearance, serum sodium, and urinary sodium output. The optimal dietary sodium can be assessed by comparing the effects of the sodium intake on excess water gain or loss, the blood pressure, and the creatinine clearance.

In nondialyzed chronically uremic patients or patients undergoing maintenance dialysis who gain excessive sodium or water despite attempts at dietary restriction, furosemide may be used to increase urinary sodium and water excretion.

Potassium

Most patients who have nonoliguric advanced renal failure or who are undergoing maintenance dialysis can tolerate up to 70 mEq of potassium per day without hyperkalemia. Patients with hyporeninemic hypoaldosteronism, however, may be intolerant to this amount of potassium unless they are given a mineralocorticoid, such as 9-alpha-fluorohydrocortisone. In some patients who are given this mineralocorticoid, sodium retention with hypertension or congestive heart failure may occur. In susceptible patients, this usually can be prevented by administering a diuretic simultaneously with the mineralocorticoid.

Phosphorus

It is important to restrict phosphorus intake to prevent or to minimize hyperparathyroidism and possibly to retard the rate of progression of renal failure (as already discussed). The degree to which dietary phosphorus should be reduced is not well established. Clearly, phosphorus restriction should be employed to keep serum phosphorus within normal levels. However, some nephrologists have questioned whether in order to prevent or to ameliorate hyperparathyroidism, the phosphorus intake should be reduced to maintain a normal renal tubular reabsorption of phosphorus; this would require a very low phosphorus intake. The restriction of phosphorus intake that may be necessary to retard the progression of renal failure is not known. The phosphorus intake can be reduced to 300 to 500 mg per day with the essential amino acid- or ketoacid-supplemented very-low-protein diets. One small clinical trial suggests that a prescribed phosphorus intake of 6.5 mg per kilogram per day will slow progression more than an intake of 12 mg per kilogram per day.

Until more information is available, it seems prudent to use a combination of dietary phosphorus restriction and chemical binders of phosphate to maintain the morning serum phosphorus concentrations well within the normal range. Since there is a rough correlation between the protein and phosphorus content of the diet, it is easier to restrict phosphorus if protein intake is reduced. With a 0.55 to 0.60 g per kilogram per day protein diet, phosphorus intake can be decreased to 10 to 12 mg per kilogram per day and sometimes to as low as 8 mg per kilogram per day. This level of dietary phosphorus restriction usually does not maintain serum phosphorus levels within normal limits in patients with a GFR under about 15 ml per minute, and phosphate binders are therefore also employed.

Formerly, the two most commonly used phosphate binders were aluminum carbonate and aluminum hydroxide. Usually, 2 to 4 capsules are taken 3 to 4 times per day as needed. Greater doses may be used if necessary. Recent evidence that aluminum-induced osteomalacia is causally related to the total lifetime dose of aluminum phosphate binders has made many nephrologists reluctant to use them. However, the hazards of severe uncontrolled hyperparathyroidism would seem to outweigh the potential dangers of aluminum-induced osteomalacia. Thus, if serum phosphorus levels cannot be maintained within normal limits by diet alone, phosphate binders are used.

Several nonaluminum phosphate binders are now being investigated. Calcium carbonate and calcium citrate both appear to bind phosphate effectively. These calcium binders can be given in divided doses with meals and should not be given unless the serum phosphorus level is normal in order to avoid precipitation of calcium phosphate in soft tissues. Thus, hyperphosphatemic patients may be treated with an aluminum binder of phosphate until serum phosphorus falls to normal. At that time, they may be changed to calcium carbonate or calcium citrate. Normally, patients should probably not receive more than about 5.0 g per day of calcium carbonate or 8.3 g per day of calcium citrate (about 2.0 g per day of elemental calcium) in order to prevent excessive accumulation of calcium in soft tissues. Calcium carbonate also may counteract the metabolic acidosis frequently found in patients with renal failure. Calcium citrate may be advantageous for the same reason, since the citrate may be metabolized to generate bicarbonate.

As previously indicated, since the essential amino acid and ketoacid supplements do not contain phosphorus, one advantage to diets providing these formulations with about 0.28 g of protein per kilogram per day is the greater degree to which the phosphorus intake can be reduced, often to as low as 4 to 6 mg per kilogram per day. If future studies confirm that these very low phosphorus intakes are both safe and beneficial for patients with mild, moderate, or severe renal insufficiency, this would provide additional justification for the use of these semisynthetic diets.

Calcium

Patients with chronic renal failure have an increased dietary calcium requirement because there is often both vitamin D deficiency and resistance to the actions of vitamin D. These disorders, which lead to impaired intestinal calcium absorption, are compounded by the low calcium content of diets for uremic patients. A 40 g protein diet, for example, provides only about 300 to 400 mg per day of calcium. Dietary calcium intake is low because many foods that are high in calcium are high in phosphorus (e.g., dairy products) and are therefore restricted for uremic patients.

Chronically uremic patients usually require about 1,200 to 1,600 mg per day of calcium for neutral or positive calcium balance, and the diet, therefore, should be supplemented with elemental calcium. Probably, a good target level for total daily calcium intake (food plus supplemental calcium) is 1,400 to 1,600 mg per day. As indicated, up to 2 g of elemental calcium may be given as calcium salts to bind phosphate. Supplemental calcium therapy should not be initiated unless the serum phosphorus concentration is normal (i.e., 3.5 to 4.5 mg per deciliter) to prevent calcium phosphate deposition in soft tissues. Also, frequent monitoring of serum calcium is important since hypercalcemia may develop, particularly if serum phosphorus should fall to low or low-normal levels. Patients undergoing maintenance hemodialysis or peritoneal dialysis may also require 1.0 g per day of supplemental calcium even though there is net calcium uptake from dialysate.

Calcium comprises 40 percent of calcium carbonate, 24 percent of calcium citrate, 18 percent of calcium lactate, and 9 percent of calcium gluconate. Oral calcium chloride should be avoided in uremic patients because of its acidifying properties. As indicated above, calcium carbonate and calcium citrate have both been shown to be effective intestinal phosphate binders. Several proprietary calcium carbonate or calcium citrate tablets have been given a pleasant flavor and are well accepted.

Magnesium

In chronically uremic patients, there is net absorption from the intestinal tract of about 50 percent of ingested magnesium (net absorption is the difference between dietary intake and fecal excretion). The absorbed magnesium is excreted primarily by the kidney, and in renal failure, hypermagnesemia may occur. However, the restricted diets of uremic patients are low in magnesium (usually about 100 to 300 mg per day for a 40 g protein diet), and their serum magnesium levels are usually normal or only slightly elevated. Clinically significant hypermagnesemia usually occurs only when there are additional sources of magnesium intake such as magnesium-containing antacids and laxatives. The nondialyzed chronically uremic patient requires about 200 mg per day of magnesium to maintain neutral magnesium balance. The optimal dietary magnesium allowance for the dialysis patient has not been defined.

Trace Elements

Increased or decreased tissue levels of many trace elements are often observed in patients with chronic renal failure. Adverse clinical effects have not been identified for most of these disorders. Dietary requirements for trace elements have not been defined for uremic patients. Many trace elements are bound avidly to serum proteins, and when present in dialysate, even in small quantities, they may be taken up in the blood. It is therefore recommended that trace elements be removed routinely from the dialysate prior to use.

Since iron deficiency is common and can cause anemia, chronically uremic and dialysis patients may be given oral iron supplements. Ferrous sulfate, 300 mg 3 times a day after meals, may be used. Patients who do not tolerate this or other oral iron supplements or who have iron deficiency are usually best treated with intramuscular or intravenous iron.

The zinc content of most tissues is normal in renal failure. However, serum and hair zinc may be low, and the red cell zinc is increased. Some reports indicate that dysguesia and impaired sexual function, which occur commonly in renal failure, may be improved by giving patients zinc supplements. There is not yet sufficient evidence that routine zinc supplementation is beneficial; additional studies are clearly indicated. It is probably of value to ensure that patients ingest the recommended dietary allowance for zinc, 15 mg per day.

Increased body burden of aluminum has been implicated in dialysis patients as a cause of a progressive dementia syndrome, osteomalacia, and anemia. Current data suggest that both contamination of dialysate with aluminum and ingestion of aluminum binders of phosphate may contribute to the excess body burden of aluminum. Recent evidence that bone aluminum levels correlate with total lifetime dosage of aluminum binders of phosphate have led many nephrologists to use aluminum binders more sparingly and to rely more upon low phosphorus diets to control serum phosphorus levels. As indicated above, calcium carbonate and calcium citrate have also been used in place of aluminum hydroxide or carbonate to bind phosphate.

Alkali

Metabolic acidosis is common in nondialyzed patients with chronic renal failure because of the impaired ability of the kidney to excrete acidic metabolites and/or the renal losses of bicarbonate. Acidosis can promote bone reabsorption and many symptoms. Ingestion of low-nitrogen diets may prevent or reduce the severity of the acidosis by decreasing the endogenous generation of acidic products of protein metabolism. Alkali supplements are usually effective for preventing or treating acidosis. Calcium carbonate or calcium citrate, may correct mild acidosis and provide needed calcium. In cases of more severe acidosis, sodium bicarbonate or citrate may be administered orally or intravenously. If the nondialyzed uremic patient is not oliguric and is not particularly likely to develop edema, sodium is usually readily excreted when administered as sodium bicarbonate or citrate. Alkali therapy should probably be initiated if the arterial pH is below 7.35 or the serum bicarbonate is less than 20 mEq per liter. Before implementing alkali therapy, it must be ascertained whether the low serum bicarbonate is not a compensatory response to chronic respiratory alkalosis. If acidosis is severe and not controlled by the foregoing measures, hemodialysis or peritoneal dialysis may be employed.

Fiber Intake

A number of studies suggest that dietary fiber intake may lead to a lower incidence of constipation, irritable bowel syndrome, diverticulitis, neoplasia of the colon, and possibly greater glucose tolerance. Since the patient with renal failure also may benefit from fiber intake, we currently prescribe 20 to 25 g per day of total dietary fiber. There are so many more important nutritional restrictions on the dietary intake of the chronically uremic and dialysis patient, however, that we do not insist vigorously that the patients adhere to a high fiber diet.

Vitamins

Unless supplements are given, uremic patients have a tendency to develop deficiency of the water soluble vitamins. Vitamin deficiencies are due to poor intake, altered metabolism (attributable to medicinal intake and, possibly, to uremia per se), or to losses into dialysate. Thus, deficiency of water soluble vitamins tends to occur more frequently in dialysis patients. Vitamin B_{12} deficiency is uncommon in uremia because this vitamin is protein-bound in plasma.

In renal failure, the daily requirements for most vitamins are not well defined. There is evidence that, in addition to vitamin intake from foods, the following daily supplements of vitamins can prevent or correct vitamin deficiency: pyridoxine hydrochloride, 5 mg in nondialyzed patients and 10 mg in hemodialysis or peritoneal dialysis patients; ascorbic acid, 60 mg; folic acid, 1 mg; and the recommended daily allowance for normal individuals for the other water soluble vitamins. High serum oxalate levels have been described in chronically uremic patients given large doses of ascorbic acid; therefore, the recommended supplement for vitamin C has been limited to the recommended dietary allowances for healthy adults. Since serum retinol binding protein and vitamin A are elevated, supplemental vitamin A is not recommended. Additional vitamin E and K are probably not necessary. An exception is the patient who receives antibiotics for extended periods of time and who is not ingesting sufficient quantities of vitamin K; such individuals may need supplements of this vitamin. Treatment with vitamin D analogues is discussed in the chapter on renal osteodystrophy.

Some authors have reported that maintenance hemodialysis patients not receiving vitamin supplements may not develop water soluble vitamin deficiencies. They have recommended that vitamin supplements should not be prescribed routinely to maintenance dialysis patients. However, these patients were generally followed for less than 1 year and it is possible that with longer periods of time, the incidence of vitamin deficiency may increase. Poor nutrient intake is common in chronically uremic patients, and recent reports continue to show that many renal failure patients have evidence of vitamin deficiencies. Since water soluble vitamin supplements are safe, it would seem wise to use them routinely until these issues are more completely resolved.

Methods for Attaining Successful Nutritional Therapy

Successful dietary therapy usually requires that the patient make a major change in his lifestyle. The patient must procure special foods, prepare special recipes, usually must forego or severely limit his intake of many favorite foods, and is often compelled to eat foods that he may not desire. There are demands made on the time, the effort, and the emotional support system of his family or close associates.

In order to ensure successful dietary therapy, patients with renal failure must undergo extensive training concerning the principles of nutritional therapy and the design and preparation of diets. Also, they need continuous encouragement regarding dietary adherence. They must receive repeated retraining regarding their nutritional therapy, and their dietary intake and nutritional status must be closely monitored. Patients who are not monitored carefully usually do not adhere closely to their diets. They may eat too little rather than too much, particularly when undergoing maintenance dialysis therapy.

A team approach to dietary management is often critical. The team should include the physician, dietitian, close family members, the nursing staff, and, when available, psychiatrists or social workers. The diet plans should be designed specifically for each patient and should take into account his or her individual tastes. At each visit, the physician should discuss dietary intake with the patient. The adequacy of energy and protein intake and nutritional status should be frequently assessed. The dietitian is often the best qualified person to perform anthropometric measurements of nutritional status because of her training, interest in nutritional therapy, and access to the patient. The physician must strongly support the efforts of the dietitian. Generally, the spouse or other close relatives or friends should work closely with the patient to provide moral support and to assist with the acquisition and preparation of foods. Nurses, psychiatrists, and social workers can encourage patients and help them work through emotional conflicts that can affect dietary compliance. They are also a valuable source of information concerning the patient's attitude toward dietary therapy, his ability to adhere to the diet, and his actual dietary intake. The important lesson is that if dietary therapy is prescribed to a patient, it requires a major commitment and effort by the patient and the medical staff to attain good results.

The most sensitive, reproducible, and readily available methods for assessing nutritional status in chronically uremic and dialysis patients include the serum albumin and total protein, relative body weight (patient's weight × 100 divided by body weight of a normal person of the same age, height, and sex), patient's weight expressed as a percentage of his weight prior to his illness, triceps and subscapular skinfold thickness, and midarm muscle circumference or cross-sectional area. Serum transferrin may also be helpful; in my experience, values are usually low even in well-nourished patients with chronic renal failure and decrease further when malnutrition is present.

USE OF DRUGS IN RENAL FAILURE

RICHARD J. GLASSOCK, M.D.

The purpose of this section is to provide the reader with a brief overview of the common and frequently confusing problem of administering a variety of therapeutic agents to patients with renal disease, particularly to those in whom the disease has progressed to some degree of renal functional impairment (e.g., decreased glomerular filtration rate). As many drugs are excreted unchanged by the kidney, impairment in overall renal function may alter the pharmacokinetics of the drug so that, with normal dosage, toxic quantities of the compound may accumulate in various body fluids. Alternatively, an attempt to adjust the dosage of chemotherapeutic agents based on an approximation of renal function may lead to inadequate tissue levels and thereby to failure to attain a desired chemotherapeutic effect. It is therefore necessary for all physicians dealing with potent pharmacologic agents to understand and appreciate the perturbations that occur in the absorption, fate, and metabolism of drugs in patients with renal disease, and thus, that they may intelligently and effectively use these agents in the presence of renal disease.

BASIC PRINCIPLES

Absorption of Drugs

Oral Absorption. The oral absorption of a drug is affected by a number of factors including solubility, gastrointestinal transit time, stability of the agent to acid pH, and proteolytic digestion. Absorption of fat-soluble drugs may be interfered with by steatorrhea or concomitant lipid administration. Achlorhydria, deficient salivary excretion, gastritis, and concomitant bowel abnormalities seen in patients with renal disease thus may interfere with the oral absorption of agents. Antacids, provided to patients with renal disease receiving glucocorticoids or in connection with an attempt to deplete phosphate stores, may reduce the bioavailability of certain drugs (e.g., digoxin, iron, salicylates, tetracyclines, and other antimicrobials).

Hepatic metabolism of orally administered agents (first-pass effect) reduces the oral effectiveness of drugs. Agents with important first-pass metabolism are listed in Table 1.

Topical, Buccal, and Sublingual Absorption. Drugs with important hepatic first-pass metabolism or those affected by low pH or tryptic digestion may be effectively administered by these routes. Such drugs include organic nitrates, nifedipine, clonidine and scopolamine. Additional techniques for administering these drugs by topical routes may be developed in the future. Cutaneous absorption through ointments and drug-impregnated adhesive patches may provide slow absorption and stable therapeutic levels.

Rectal Absorption. Drugs that are irritating to the gastric mucosa or cannot be given by mouth because of nausea can frequently be given rectally. Examples include sedatives and antiemetics, and nonsteroidal anti-inflammatory agents.

Parenteral Absorption. The intravenous route is preferred if complete absorption and avoidance of the first-pass effect is desired or if the agent is irritating when injected intramuscularly or subcutaneously. Absorption with intramuscular or subcutaneous injection may be poor in states of circulatory collapse. In addition, some drugs are so insoluble that absorption from intramuscular routes may be very poor. Phenytoin is an example of a drug that is poorly absorbed from intramuscular sites. Certain compounds must be administered intravenously with caution because if high concentrations are achieved rapidly, they may exert adverse effects on cardiac contractility (e.g., methylprednisolone, high concentrations of potassium

TABLE 1 Drugs Having Important Hepatic "First-Pass" Metabolism

Amitriptyline	L-DOPA
Aspirin	Nitroglycerine
Isoproterenol	Paracetamol
Lidocaine	Prazosin
Metoprolol	Proproxyphene
Mepiridine	Propranolol
Morphine	Nifedipine

salts). Irritating or sclerosing agents given intravenously must be administered slowly and with great care.

Inhalation. Topical application of drugs to the bronchial mucosa may be prescribed when concentration of the drug in lung tissue is desirable. However, with repeated use, systemic effects can be anticipated.

DRUG METABOLISM

Drugs are metabolized and/or excreted in a number of ways:

1. Excretion by the kidney unchanged through a process of glomerular filtration and/or tubular secretion (e.g., digoxin and penicillin, respectively).
2. Oxidation and/or conjugation to more polar compounds (e.g., sulfates or glucuronides) in the liver with subsequent excretion by the kidney and/or liver via the bile. Liver metabolism of drugs is carried out in part by a system of mixed function microsomal enzymes, the terminal oxidase enzyme being called cytochrome P-450. Cytochrome P-450 transforms the parent drug into a more polar compound. This enzyme system may be induced by many agents, particularly alcohol, barbiturates, and anticonvulsants. The action of this enzyme system may make drugs more readily excretable by the kidney or the liver, but may also convert them into more toxic metabolites (e.g., paracetamol). It is important to recognize that drugs that influence hepatic blood flow alter the delivery of agents to the important hepatic microsomal metabolizing systems and thus their hepatic conversion and degradation. For example, cimetidine and propranolol, by virtue of their ability to reduce hepatic blood flow, may have important drug interactions in terms of hepatic metabolism.
3. Conversion in the liver, kidney, and peripheral tissues to more active compounds (e.g., prednisone to prednisolone, cholecalciferol to 1,25-cholecalciferol), which can then be excreted by the kidney or further metabolized by the liver or other tissues.

Therefore, in considering the fate of drugs in kidney disease, careful attention must be given to the state of liver function concomitantly as well as to the interaction of compounds that influence hepatic blood flow, cytochrome P-450 oxidase system, and the renal secretory and reabsorption processes.

PHARMACOKINETICS OF DRUGS

The volume of distribution (VD) of a drug after any route of administration depends on a multitude of factors, including its molecular size, charge, and solubility in water and lipid, its conversion to other polar metabolites, and its specific binding to tissue or plasma proteins. The *apparent* VD at equilibrium is calculated:

$$V_D(\text{liters}) = \frac{D}{C_P}$$

where D = dose in milligrams and C_P is the plasma concentration in milligrams per liter.

The apparent VD is an abstract rather than an absolute term and does not specify that all or most of the drug is in a specific fluid compartment (i.e., plasma or total body water). Drugs with high tissue binding properties or those with lipid solubility frequently have apparent VD greater than total body water or even total body weight. Knowledge of the apparent VD is of principal value in determining the loading dose of a given drug required to achieve a desired initial therapeutic, nontoxic level in the plasma. Alternatively, if VD is known and if the plasma level can be measured, the total body content of the drug can be readily calculated. Thus, total body content (TBC) equals VD × CP. It must be emphasized that calculations given for the determination of apparent VD assume that no drug elimination has taken place. Drugs that are rapidly eliminated or extremely slowly equilibrated in various tissue or fluid compartments may not be so simply calculated.

DRUG ELIMINATION

Drug elimination manifests one or the other of two kinds of kinetic pathways. Drugs manifesting first-order kinetics are removed in proportion to the plasma concentration raised to the first power. After administration, such drugs distribute into body compartments (the alpha-phase) and then the plasma concentration falls less rapidly in a log-linear relationship (the beta-phase) with time. If the drug equilibrates with multiple components (water, fat, bone), the plasma disappearance rate may be complex and multiexponential. The half-time of disappearance of the drug demonstrating first-order kinetics and one compartment distribution can be determined when the plot of the logarithm of the CP versus time assumes a straight-line relationship. The time for the CP to fall to one-half of its original concentration equals the half disappearance time or $\tau½$. The $\tau½$ varies widely depending on the site or sites of drug elimination and on the VD. As a general rule, unless metabolism and excretion are not in equilibrium, administration of a given dose of drug at each $\tau½$ leads ultimately to a plateau level with a peak concentration of the drug in the plasma (CP) *twice* the value achieved by the first or loading dose and a trough level *equal* to the value achieved by the first dose. This new steady state is achieved in approximately 5 × $\tau½$. A constant infusion of a drug eliminates both peak and trough levels, but it takes approximately the same amount of time to achieve a steady CP. Drugs with extremely short half-lives (e.g., lidocaine) are most conveniently given by infusion rather than by intermittent boluses once a desired plasma level has been achieved by initial administration of the drug. Infusion rates for constant infusions can be calculated by assuming a desired plasma level (CP) and knowing the VD and the $\tau½$. Since during each $\tau½$ one-half of the total body dose must be replaced, the dose each $\tau½$ equals VD time CP divided by two. Thus the dose each $\tau½$ divided by the $\tau½$ in minutes equals the infusion rate in mg per minute.

Some drugs do not manifest simple first-order kinetics or multicompartmental, multiexponential disappearance curves, but rather the rate of metabolism and elimination is affected by the Cp. In general, these drugs saturate the hepatic metabolizing enzyme systems and include salicylates, ethyl alcohol, methyl alcohol, and phenytoin. Thus, doubling the dose more than doubles the plasma concentration, and if the metabolic capacity is exceeded, toxic levels of the drug rapidly accumulate. The removal rate of the agent is therefore greatly affected by the plasma concentration and a true $\tau^{1/2}$ cannot be determined. The metabolism of these drugs is called zero-order kinetics. The steady state level of drugs of this class must be determined from Michaelis-Menten enzyme kinetics, where Cp (steady state) equals K_m times the dose per unit time, divided by the V_{max} minus the dose per time. K_m equals the Cp when enzymes are one-half saturated and V_{max} is the maximum rate of metabolism of the drug (usually defined by hepatic metabolism).

Because of these considerations, the time to reach a steady state is unpredictable, and depending on the state of hepatic enzyme function, drugs may accumulate to toxic levels or fall to subtherapeutic concentrations. Plasma level monitoring may therefore be required for precise adjustment of dosage. Drug accumulation and/or dissipation may be estimated by administering single extra doses of the agent in question and by measuring the effect on Cp after a few hours or a few days.

Some drugs, most notably salicylates, are handled by both first-order (renal elimination) and zero-order kinetics (hepatic metabolism). Adjustment of dosages may be difficult when both liver disease and renal disease are present.

Drug Clearance Rates

This is a useful concept as it describes the totality of removal of the given drug (but does not give information regarding the removal of unwanted toxic metabolites not measured in a given assay). The clearance of any drug (in liters per minute) is equal to the removal of the drug per unit time in milligrams per minute, divided by the average Cp during the interval in milligrams per liter. Since most drugs manifest first-order kinetics, the clearance concept can be translated into an elimination rate constant (K_e).

$$K_e = \frac{0.693}{\tau^{1/2}}$$

This is where K_e represents the fraction of a given amount of drug which will be eliminated per unit of time.

Plasma clearance of a drug (Cl) in liters per hour may be calculated as follows:

$$Cl = K_e \times V_D$$

The effect of changing Cl and V_D upon $\tau^{1/2}$ can therefore be estimated as follows:

$$\tau^{1/2} = \frac{0.693 \times V_D}{Cl}$$

Thus, $\tau^{1/2}$ is prolonged when Cl decreases or when V_D increases. However, if V_D is increased as a consequence of diminution of binding to tissue proteins then access of the drug to important intracellular metabolic sites might be enhanced leading to an increase in metabolic rate and a shortening of $\tau^{1/2}$.

For drugs that are highly dependent on hepatic blood flow for metabolism, the plasma clearance rate should be *less* than the hepatic blood flow and drug extraction; if not, the drug may escape hepatic metabolism and accumulate in the plasma.

The value of K_e for individual drugs can be used effectively in determining appropriate infusion rates for those drugs manifesting first-order kinetics. The rate of infusion required to maintain a constant amount of drug in the body is equal to the rate of elimination of the drug from the body or $K_e \times C_P \times V_D$.

Table 2 lists the values for K_e for selected agents (in K_e per hour) in subjects with normal renal function (e.g., GFR is >100 ml per minute) and in patients who are essentially anephric from end-stage renal disease (adapted

TABLE 2 Elimination Rate Constant: K_e for Selected Agents (K_e per hour) in Normal Patients and those with End-stage Renal Disease (ESRD)

Drug	*Normal*	*ESRD*
Penicillin G	1.40	0.05
Ampicillin	0.70	0.10
Amoxicillin	0.70	0.10
Cloxacillin, Oxacillin	1.40	0.35
Methicillin	1.40	0.17
Nafcillin	1.20	0.48
Ticarcillin	0.60	0.06
Cephalothin	1.40	0.04
Cephazolin	0.40	0.04
Cephalexin	1.00	0.03
Gentamicin	0.30	0.01
Tobramycin	0.36	0.01
Amikacin	0.40	0.04
Tetracycline	0.08	0.01
Doxycycline	0.03	0.03
Chloramphenicol	0.30	0.20
Clindamycin	0.47	0.10
Erythromycin	0.50	0.14
Trimethoprim	0.60	0.02
Vancomycin	0.12	0.003
Sulfamethoxazole	0.70	0.70
Lidocaine	0.40	0.36
Procainamide	0.22	0.01
Propranolol	0.20	0.16
Quinidine	0.07	0.06
Digitoxin	0.004	0.003
Digoxin	0.017	0.006

* Adapted from Anderson RT, Bennett WM, Gambertoglio J, Schrier R. Fate of drugs in renal failure. In: Brenner B, Rector F, (eds). The Kidney. 2nd ed. Philadelphia: WB Saunders, 1981.

from references given in suggested reading). It should be noted that for some drugs K_e falls dramatically (e.g., Vancomycin, $K_e = 0.12$ in normal and $K_e = 0.003$ in end-stage renal disease), whereas for other drugs the K_e changes little or not at all (e.g., doxycycline, $K_e = 0.03$ in normal and $K_e = 0.03$ in end-stage renal disease).

Determination of Bioavailability

An approximation of the drug absorbed and that which escapes the first-pass effect can be determined by calculating the area under the curve. A plot of the CP versus time, using integral calculus and first-order kinetics (excluding the distribution or alpha-phase by extrapolating back to zero time on the vertical axis from the exponential decay) permits an estimate of the amount of drug absorbed and delivered to the plasma. This amount is proportional to the amount administered after consideration of the VD.

Effects of Protein Binding

Many drugs are bound to albumin or to anionic glycoproteins (Table 3). High affinity binding to plasma proteins results in drugs having a small apparent VD, usually equal to the plasma volume. The bound drug is frequently inactive metabolically and may not enter normal pools of degradation. The drug must be displaced at its site of action for reaction with a receptor of high affinity, or as a consequence of increased dose administration, all binding sites must be saturated so as to permit free and active drug to accumulate. The displacement of protein bound fraction by other drugs not only increases the free active drug, but also increases VD, which may have an effect on metabolic clearance rates (already discussed). Examples of these interactions include aspirin and warfarin or sulfonamides and warfarin. Lowered concentration of tissue binding sites, as a consequence of hypoalbuminemia in nephrotic syndrome, may greatly alter the concentration of free metabolically active drug, even with usual oral doses.

Acetylsalicylic acid (aspirin) is an excellent example of the effect of protein binding of VD. In low doses of acetylsalicylic acid, the VD of aspirin is 0.2 L per kilogram, whereas the high doses VD is approximately 0.6 L per kilogram. These values represent VD for total drug. The VD for (unbound) free acetylsalicylic acid would be about equal in either case. Displacement of bound and inactive drug by other compounds has profound effects on the interpretation of assays which measure only *total* CP. For example, in renal failure, retained acidic compounds may displace phenytoin from albumin, thus increasing the CP of free drug. Whereas a therapeutic CP of phenytoin in a normal subject with a GFR of 100 ml per minute and a serum creatinine of 1.0 mg per deciliter might be 15 mg per liter, the same biologic anticonvulsant effect can be achieved with a *total* CP of 7.5 mg per liter in a patient with advanced renal failure and a serum creatinine of 8 to 10 mg per deciliter. The CP of metabolically active free drug would remain at approximately 1 to 2 mg per liter in both circumstances. For patients undergoing hemodialysis, the free, unbound level of many drugs can be measured conveniently by collecting a plasma ultrafiltrate. Alternatively, salivary levels may be determined. Contrariwise, hyperalbuminemia and increased concentration of acidic-binding proteins may actually reduce the effective active drug level and apparent VD. Whenever one is using *total* CP to monitor the effectiveness of the therapeutic program, one must be cognizant of the effect not only of plasma protein binding, but also of the fact that the assay may either detect ineffective metabolites or fail to detect toxic metabolites having differing pathways of metabolism and excretion. Table 3 lists drugs that bind to albumin or other plasma glycoproteins.

Renal Excretion

Drugs may be excreted by the kidney by glomerular filtration alone, by a combination of glomerular filtration and secretion, and by predominantly tubular secretion. In addition, some drugs may be filtered and subsequently reabsorbed to variable extents. The process of glomerular filtration rate is affected by the molecular size, shape and charge of the compound, as well as protein binding. Uncharged, cationic and anionic molecules $<5{,}000$ daltons molecular weight or less (<17 Å in average molecular radius) is, in general, filtered across the glomerular capillary wall equally as well as water. Molecules bound to plasma proteins have restricted filtration, which depends on the molecule to which they are bound and to the presence or absence of net cationic or anionic charges. Cationic molecules in the vicinity of 10,000 to 40,000 daltons molecular weight are *more* readily filtered, and anionic molecules of similar molecular weight are *less* well filtered than neutral molecules. Both organic bases and organic acids may be secreted and/or reabsorbed by the proximal tubule, and this process manifests saturation kinetics and competitive inhibition. The secretion of some compounds by the proximal tubule may be inhibited by drugs (e.g., probenemid and penicillin). High concentrations of endogenous organic compounds (e.g., lactic acid, acetic acid) may interfere with the secretion of other similar acidic compounds. Some drugs acting on the kidney require initial glomerular filtration and/or tubular secretion so that they may reach their sites of action within the lumen of the distal portions of the nephron (e.g., furosemide and ethacrynic acid).

Assessment of Renal Function Relative to Drug Administration

Since glomerular filtration rate (GFR) is the parameter most readily assessed and seems to be the single most important renal function parameter in determining renal elimination of many drugs, the determination of GFR or an estimate thereof has become the standard reference for determining drug dosages in renal failure. Nonetheless, one should not neglect the fact that tubular function (e.g., secretion, reabsorption, and nonspecific back diffusion) also plays a role in the elimination of drugs in renal failure. Furthermore, urinary pH per se may dramatically

TABLE 3 Selected Pharmacokinetic Properties of Therapeutic Agents in Normal Patients and those with End-Stage Renal Disease (ESRD)†

Drug	*Excreted Unchanged (%)*	*Protein Bound (%)*	*VD (L/kg)*	*Normal C (ml/min/kg)*	*τ½ (hour)*		*Fo ESRD*
					Normal	*ESRD*	
Analgesic and anti-inflammatory agents							
Codeine	5-17	7	3-4	—	3.4	—	?
Morphine	<10	35	1-3.4	—	2.0	—	?
Meperidine	*	65	3.1	—	3.0	—	?
Aspirin	<1	90	0.21	—	2-40*	2-40	1.0
Paracetamol	<1	20	1.0	—	2.0	2.0	1.0
				18-30 oxypurinol		prolonged	
Colchicine	5-20	31	2.1	1.3	19	40	0.07
Indomethacin	15	99	0.78	1.3	6	6	1.0
Probenecid	4-10	83-94	0.13	—	3-17	3-17	?
Phenylbutazone	1-10	90	0.15	—	60	42	1.4
Prednisone	12	50-80	0.4-1.0	—	2.5-3.5	2.5-3.5	1.0
Antihypertensive agents							
Clonidine	50	20	3.2	3.0	7-12	24	—
Diazoxide	20	90	0.18	0.1	15-30	20-53	0.45
Guanethidine	50	0	60.0	5.0	120	245	0.50
Hydralazine	<5	90	1.6	—	2-3	prolonged	0.40
Minoxidil	12	0	3.4	?	3-4	3-4	1.0
Methyldopa	65	<20	0.69	3.3	1.8	3.6	0.40
Captopril	25	30	2.0	13.0	2.0	increased	?
Prazosin	<1	97	0.94	?	3.0	?	?
Reserpine	—	—	78.0	—	46-168	14-60+	0.48
Antimicrobials							
Gentamicin	>95	<0	0.25	1.2	2.0	60	0.03
Amikacin	>95	<0	0.25	1.2	2.0	70	0.03
Tobramycin	>95	<0	0.23	1.2	2.0	60	0.04
Streptomycin	>95	<0	0.26	1.3	2.0	65	0.03
Spectinomycin	75	>0	0.20	1.0	1.6	30	—
Cefaclor	62	25	0.36	5.5	0.7	2.5	0.30
Cefadroxil	90	20	0.30	2.5	1.3	25	0.15
Cephamandole	>95	74	0.19	2.8	1.0	10	0.08
Cefazolin	>90	85	0.14	1.0	2.5	24-50	0.07
Cefonicid	>95	98	0.09	0.3	3.5	17-56	0.07
Ceforamide	80	80	0.15	1.0	2.5	30	—
Ceproxadine	70	—	0.35	4.0	1.0	40	—
Cefsulodin	50	—	0.26	2.0	2.0	10	—
Cephacetrile	>90	30	0.37	3.4	1.0	10-30	—
Cephalexin	95	15	0.33	3.6	1.0	10-20	0.05
Cephalothin	>50	70	0.32	8.2	0.5	18-20	0.20
Cephapirin	50	60	0.22	4.3	0.6	1.7	0.30
Cephadrine	90	14	0.32	5.3	0.7	8-15	0.06
Moxalactam	>80	50	0.28	1.7	2-4	19-30	0.07
Penicillin G	>90	60	0.23	5.3	0.5	6-20	0.01
Ampicillin	90	18	>0.45	2.7	0.8-1.5	20	0.09
			0.30				
Azlocillin	65	28	0.18	2.6	0.8	5	0.17
Carbenicillin	80	50	0.13	15.0	1.0	10-20	0.07
Methicillin	>85	40	0.45	6.1	0.7	4	0.70
Piperacillin	>60	21	0.20	2.6	1.0	3.3	0.30
Ticarcillin	85	65	0.21	1.9	1.2	10-25	0.11
Oxacillin	90	90	0.21	4.7	0.5	1.0	0.50
Cloxacillin	95	95	0.20	—	0.5	0.8	0.75
Dicloxacillin	95	95	0.1-0.2	—	0.7	1.0	0.70
Nafcillin	>85	85	0.28-0.70	—	0.6	1.2	0.41
Amoxicillin	50-70	17	0.66	6.5	0.9-2.3	10-15	0.11
Erythromycin	5-15	80	0.6-0.78	6.0	1-2	3-7	0.40
Clindamycin	15	80	1.2	8.0	2	2.0	0.90
Lincomycin	5-15	70	0.6-1.2	1.2	6	10	0.60
Sulfisoxazole	50	90	0.16	0.3	5-6*	11	0.50
Sulfamethoxazole	0.20	65	0.25-0.36	0.3	9-11	30-60	0.29
Trimethoprim	50	70	2.1	2.2	8-11	24-30	0.50

Table continues

TABLE 3 Continued

Drug	*Excreted Unchanged (%)*	*Protein Bound (%)*	*VD (L/kg)*	*Normal C (ml/min/kg)*	*T½ (hour)*		*Fo ESRD*
					Normal	*ESRD*	
Tetracycline	50	65	1.3–1.6	2.0	6–15	7–75	0.16
Chlortetracycline	50	65	1.2	3.0	6	9	0.67
Minocycline	<10	70	0.4	0.6	12	14	1.0
Doxycycline	20–50	70	0.4	0.6	15–24	25	1.0
Demeclocycline	40–50	75–90	1.8	1.7	12	50	0.24
Rifampin	5–15	60–90	0.93	3.0	2.3	3–5	1.0
Ethambutol	70	25	1.6–2.3	8.6	3.0	8	0.30
PAS	50	60	0.24	4.0	0.7	20	0.04
Cycloserine	50	—	—	—	8–12		—
INH	5% rapid acetylator 25% slow acetylator	0	0.6	7.0	0.7–2.0	4–8	0.75
Chloramphenicol	5–10	50	0.6–1.0	2.5	2–4	3.5–7	0.60
Vancomycin	>90	<10	0.5	0.8	7.0	240	0.03
Nalidixic acid	2–15	93	0.4	2.3	2.0	2.0	1.0
Nitrofurantoin	30–50	60	0.5	19.4	0.3	1.0	0.36
Amphotericin B	3	95	4.0	0.13	360	360	0.60
Flucytosine	85	3			5	70	0.07
Miconazole	0	98	21.0	10.0	24	24	1.0
Metronidazole							
Antineoplastic and immunosuppressive agents							
Adriamycin							
Dactinomycin							
5-Fluoruracil		Metabolism not appreciably altered in renal disease, but data incomplete.					
Melphalan							
Procarbazine							
Vinca alkaloids							
Cyclosporine	?	lipoproteins	3–20	4–70	variable	variable	variable
Streptozotozin	10–20	—	0.5	—	0.25	?	?
Acyclovir	60–90	15	0.53	4.2	2.0	20	0.1
Amantadine	100	0	5.1	4.9	12.0	7–13d	0.01
Vidarabine	40–60	?	?	3.5	2.0		?
Cytarabine	6	?	?	2.0	0.5–3.0	?	?
Bleomycin	60	?	0.35	8.0	0.5–9	20	0.02
Cyclophosphamide	10–15	60	0.45	1.1	4–7.5	10	0.89
Azathioprine	10–30	30	1–4	—	3	3–4	0.9–1.0
Cisplatinum	?	?	?	?	3.2	1.7	1.0
Methotrexate	80	50	0.3–0.8*	0.7	10	64	0.16
Beta-adreneric-blocking agents							
Metoprolol	5–10	12	0.69	10–20	2–5	1.0	—
Propranolol	<5	95	3.9	4.0	4.0	3.2	1–1.2
Nadolol	70	25	1.5	1.0	14–24	45	0.5
Pindolol	37	27	2.1	7.0	3–4	3–4	1.0
Atenolol	75	<5	1.2	1.3	6–9	42	—
Cardiac and anti-arrhythmic agents							
Lidocaine	<3	60	1.5	8.0	2.0	3.0	1.0
Procainamide	50–60	15	2.0	12	2.0	8	0.25
Propranolol	<5	95	3.9	4	4.0	3.2	1.0–1.2
Quinidine	15	80–90	2.0–3.0	4	6	6	1.0
Digitoxin	33	90	0.5–0.7	0.05	145	200	0.73
Digoxin	70–80	25	7.1*	1.8	36–42	80–180	0.36
Bretylium	80	—	—	—	4–17	32	?
Verapamil	?	?	?	?	?	?	?
Diuretic agents							
Spironolactone	<10	98	—	—	16–19	prolonged	?
Triamterene	4	50	3.6	14.0	2.0	10.0	?
Amiloride	52	?	?	?	—	—	?
Metalozone	>90	95	?	?	6.0	increased	—

TABLE 3 Continued

Drug	Excreted Unchanged (%)	Protein Bound (%)	VD (L/kg)	Normal C (ml/min/kg)	τ½ (hour) Normal	τ½ (hour) ESRD	Fo ESRD
Thiazides	>80	95	1.5	—	9–2.5	prolonged	—
Chlorthalidone	50	98	3–13	—	54.0	100	?
Ethacrynic acid	?	95	0.1	—	1–3	prolonged	?
Acetazolamide	—	90	0.3	—	8.0	prolonged	—
Bumetamide	—	—	0.9	—	0.9	prolonged	?
Furosemide	40–95	60	0.12	2.0	0.5	1.4	0.4
Hypoglycemic agents							
Chlorpropamide	47	80	0.2	—	25–42	—	—
Insulin	<1	0	0.2	—	—	—	—
Tolbutamide	<5	95	0.2	—	4–8	3.9	1.0
Sedatives and tranquilizing agents							
Phenobarbital	40	50	0.75	?	60–150	100–150	0.7
Pentobarbital	10	50	0.99	?	22	22	1.0
Phenothiazines	<1	90	7–9	?	11–24	?	?
Haloperidol	<1	90	2.3	?	10–36	?	?
Tricyclics	<5	95	17–27	?	12–56	?	?
Lithium	100	0	0.67	0.35	8–41	640	0.05
Diazepam	?	?	0.74	?	25	90	1.0
Chlordiazepoxide	?	?	0.30	?	10	—	?
Miscellaneous							
Theophylline	50–70	7–10	0.3–0.7	0.65	3–12	—	—
Terbutaline	50–70	?	0.94	3.8	3	?	?
Diphenhydramine	<4	98	3.3	5.2	3.8	—	—
Cimetidine	40–80	13–16	0.45–1.15	3.0	1.4–2.4	3–10	0.37
Heparin	0	>90	0.06	0.5	1.5	1.5	1.0
Warfarin	<1	97	0.11	0.05	33	30	1.1
Allopurinol	30	<5	0.6	2.8	—	2–8	?
Phenytoin	2	90*	0.6	V_{max}= 8.4 mg/kg/d	24	reduced— no change	1.0–1.2 1.2

† Adapted from the references
* Decreased in uremia

affect the renal excretion of drugs even in the absence of changes in GFR. For example, acetylsalicylic acid excretion is enhanced in alkaline urine, and the excretion of quinidine is enhanced in acid urine and the excretion of weak acids is enhanced in acid urine. Urinary pH may also affect the binding of certain drugs to intrarenal membrane sites and determine their accumulation in renal tissue (e.g., gentamicin).

GFR can be measured directly by classic techniques involving the constant infusion of a glomerular filtration marker molecule, such as inulin, and using the classic formula for calculation of renal clearance: GFR (ml per minute) = urine concentration (mg per milliliter) × urine volume (ml per minute), divided by plasma concentration (mg per milliliter). However, the constant infusion method is not practical for the determination of GFR and drug dosage under clinical circumstances and is unsuitable for nonsteady-state conditions.

Measurement of the endogenous clearance of creatinine is a satisfactory substitute, since creatinine is a nearly, but not completely, ideal marker of glomerular filtration rate, at least when renal function is nearly normal. Short-term collection of urine for 4 to 24 hours, measurement of the plasma creatinine at the mid-point, and calculation of creatinine clearance using the above clearance formula can give a reliable estimate of GFR, provided the collections are made during adequate urine flow (at least 1 to 2 ml per minute), no residual urine is present, and steady-state conditions prevail. Unfortunately, creatinine clearance is not a valid measurement of true GFR when renal disease is moderate or severely advanced, or if massive proteinuria is concomitantly present. Under these circumstances, creatinine clearance may, in fact, overestimate the true GFR (as assessed by inulin clearance) by as much as 50 to 400 percent. A better estimate of the true GFR in these circumstances can be obtained by averaging the sum of the creatinine clearance and the urea clearance. Other rapid methods of obtaining a better estimate of true GFR involve the use of injection of radioisotopes, such as ^{51}Cr EDTA or ^{125}I iophthalamate.

When these methods are not available or when time is of the essence, the serum creatinine alone may be used as a rough approximation of GFR in certain situations. Such formulas have been devised from empiric analysis of a comparison of serum creatinine and GFR in large numbers of patients. One such formula is as follows: 140 − age (years)/S_{Cr} (mg per deciliter) = creatinine clearance in ml per minute per 70-kg body weight. For females, the value should be multiplied by 0.85. Estimated creatinine clearance can be corrected to body surface area by the following formulas: body surface area = (weight in kg)$^{0.425}$ × (height in centimeters)$^{0.725}$ × 71.84 divided by 10,000. The corrected creatinine clearance in ml per minute per 1.73 m^2 = the creatinine clearance (uncorrected) × 1.73 divided by the calculated body surface area.

Such nomograms and formulas, used to estimate creatinine clearance and GFR from isolated values of serum creatinine, should be used with extreme caution in individuals who are extremely muscular, who are wasted, who have lost muscle mass from amputation, or who have active muscle necrosis. The nomograms were derived from healthy, ambulatory individuals of normal body habitus and normal conditioning. They may not, in all instances, apply to hospitalized patients, particularly the aged and the infirm. They, of course, *cannot* and *must not* be applied to non-steady-state conditions or in circumstances in which false elevations of the serum creatinine may be encountered. A falsely elevated serum creatinine concentration may be seen in patients with extreme hyperglycemia, in patients with accumulation of ketoacids, and in situations in which colored compounds have accumulated in the plasma, interfering with the colorimetric determination of creatinine. Furthermore, some drugs may accumulate in plasma which cause an elevation in the serum creatinine without a comparable change in creatinine clearance. These drugs include cimetidine and trimethoprim-sulfa. When doubt exists, and toxic compounds are to be used, short-term radioisotopic methods of measurement of GFR, such as chromium EDTA and I^{125} - labeled iophthalamate, may be of great value.

The measurement of GFR under non-steady-state conditions (a rising or falling serum creatinine) may make calculation of drug dosage difficult or impossible. However, an extremely rough estimate of GFR can be obtained by the following formula:

Creatinine clearance

$$[293 - 2y] \times = \frac{\left[1.035 - 0.01685\,(C_{s_1} + C_{s_2})\dfrac{(C_{s_1} - C_{s_2})}{t}\right]}{C_{s_1} + C_{s_2}} f$$

where

- y = patient age in years
- C_{s_1} = first serum creatinine
- C_{s_2} = second serum creatinine
- t = time in days
- f = 1.0 (70-kg males)
  = 0.85 (females) (from Reference 3)

All of these nomograms and estimates are based on the assumption that under steady-state conditions, normal males excrete 20 to 26 mg per kilogram creatinine per day and females excrete 17 to 20 mg per kilogram creatinine per day largely derived from the metabolism of muscle creatinine and to a minor extent from the oral consumption of meat products. Knowledge of these average values, urine volume, and urine concentration of creatinine may give some further evidence as to the validity of timed urine collections. Major deviations from predicted values, in the absence of disorders of muscle bulk and acute muscle disease, may give rise to suspicion of inadequate urinary collections.

Finally, measurements of blood urea nitrogen are unsatisfactory measurements for estimating GFR for the purpose of calculating drug doses, except when used in combination with creatinine clearance in the calculation of markedly reduced GFR, as already mentioned. The blood urea nitrogen is influenced greatly by the state of hydration, protein intake and the overall catabolic state. In fact, substantial increases in blood urea nitrogen may occur in the presence of only trivial declines in glomerular filtration rate, and low blood urea nitrogens may be found in patients with profound reduction in GFR maintained on low protein diets or those with profound concomitant liver disease. Estimation of drug dosage based on blood urea nitrogen in patients with liver disease could lead to disastrous consequences.

Lean Body Mass

The concept of lean body mass is an important determinant of drug dose, especially for drugs that distribute in the water component of the body only. Calculating drug dosage on the basis of total body weight in the very obese overestimates safe limits, as the total body water is only a smaller fraction of total body weight. Unless the drug in question is known to be highly lipophilic, it is wiser to use the lesser of either actual or lean body weight in calculation of drug doses based on weight parameters. Dosages of drugs metabolized predominantly by hepatic metabolism are better based on total body surface area (in m^2) than on total body weight. Drug doses for children should be calculated on the basis of body surface area, rather than on body weight. Unless the drug is known to be highly lipophilic, it is wiser to use the lesser or actual or lean body weight. Lean body weight for males (in kg) can be calculated as 0.73 × the height (in cm) −59.42 and for females lean body weight (in kg) is equal to 0.65 × the height (in cm) − 50.74.

Loading Dosage of Drugs in Renal Diseases

If protein binding, the volume of distribution, and tissue sensitivity to a drug are unaltered in renal failure, a loading dose (LD) equivalent to that for normal subjects may be given.

$$LD = VD \times CP$$

For example, for the administration of gentamicin in a 70-kg man, having a VD equal to 0.25 L per kilogram and a desired CP equal to 6 μg per deciliter (6 mg per liter):

$$\begin{aligned} \text{LD} &= (0.25 \times 70)\ (6\ \mu g \text{ per deciliter}) \\ &= (17.5\ L)\ (6 \text{ mg per liter}) \\ &= 105 \text{ mg} \\ &= 1.5 \text{ mg per kilogram} \end{aligned}$$

A loading dose might be reduced if the individual has an unusual sensitivity to toxic effects, is receiving concomitantly drugs that would influence VD or the drug's toxic effect, or, in the presence of liver disease, if the drug is extensively metabolized by the hepatic microsomal systems.

Modification of Drug Dosage in Renal Failure

The degree of modification of drug dosage required when renal function is impaired depends on the major metabolic fate of the drug (i.e., hepatic metabolism, renal excretion), the disposition and potential toxicity of secondary metabolites, the seriousness of the disease being treated, the seriousness and reversibility of the undesired effects of the drug, the availability of accurate monitoring assays of the plasma drug concentration, the amount of drug excreted unchanged in the urine, protein binding, and displacement from binding sites by organic metabolites retained in uremia.

Three basic modifications may be employed in patients who have renal disease. These are:

1. *Method A.* Extension of the dosage interval, retaining normal doses after appropriate initial loading dose.
2. *Method B.* Reducing maintenance dose, but retaining normal dosing interval after an appropriate initial loading dose.
3. *Method C.* Conversion to continuous infusion, utilizing plasma drug clearance and/or elimination rate constant parameters.

The choice of these alternatives depends on the availability of preparations in parenteral forms, the pharmacologic properties of the agents, and the peculiar advantages and disadvantages of each choice. Prolonging dosage interval while maintaining normal individual doses (method A), of necessity, produces wider swings between peak and trough levels and may expose patients to toxic levels and subtherapeutic levels for periods of time. Reducing individual doses while maintaining the same dose interval (method B) may produce a somewhat smoother plasma concentration time curve, but if errors have been made in estimating true renal function, patients may be exposed to potentially toxic levels of compounds as they accumulate. The choice of constant infusion (method C) is more difficult and time consuming and requires careful monitoring and accurate infusion devices.

Although the choices among these possibilities may be difficult and at times must be made on a highly arbitrary basis, careful attention to the aforementioned underlying pharmacologic principles often averts unnecessary toxicity and yet achieves maximum benefit from the agent. When in doubt, appropriate measurement of plasma levels (taking into account problems of estimating truly effective drug concentration) is required.

In order to simplify the dosing modifications that can be applied to patients with renal disease for the foregoing categories, nomograms have been devised that are based on known pharmacokinetic parameters of drugs in situations of normal renal function and profoundly reduced (anephric) conditions of renal function. In many instances these nomograms are based on an assumption of a plasma clearance fraction (F) of a drug as a linear function of estimated glomerular filtration rate of creatinine clearance. Each drug has a typical, although not invariable, F for each ratio of normal-to-abnormal plasma drug clearance, depending on renal function. The term F applies to the plasma clearance of the drug in patients with normal renal function for their age, sex, and body habitus compared to the plasma clearance of the drug in anuric patients (F = 1 with normal renal function, F = 0 in anephric subjects for drugs solely cleared by the kidney). Using the F value for each drug, as determined from a plot of F and GFR, it is possible to calculate adjustments in drug dosage to be made using either method A or method B (already discussed). Such a nomogram is reproduced in Figure 1. For method A, changing to a new interval, but retaining the same dose, the new interval is equal to the normal interval divided by F from nomogram.

For method B, changing to a new dose, but retaining the same interval, the new dose is equal to the normal dose times F from nomogram. For method C, changing the rate

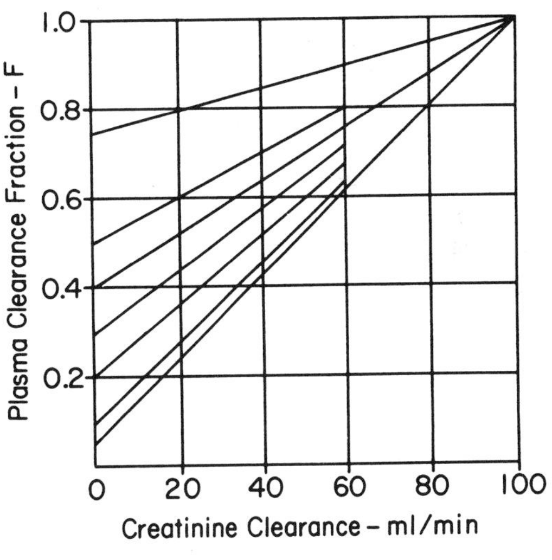

Figure 1 An example of the use of plasma clearance fraction (F) in determining drug dosage in patients with impaired renal function. A line is drawn connecting the F_0 (plasma clearance in anuria) (Table 2) and the normal renal function point at the upper right corner. The point at which this line intersects the patient's creatinine clearance equals the plasma clearance fraction (F). F is the fraction of plasma clearance of a drug relative to plasma clearance with normal renal function. This value is used in calculation of dose or dose interval (see text). (From Cutler R, Krichman KH, Blair A. Drugs in renal failure. In: Massry S, Glassock R, eds. Textbook of nephrology. Baltimore: Williams & Wilkins, 1983:842. Reproduced with permission of author and publisher).

of administration, the new dose per unit time is equal to the normal dose per unit time, times F from nomogram. An example might include the determination of gentamicin dosage in a 50-kg, 70-year-old male with a serum creatinine of 6 mg per deciliter. A normal dose can be assumed as 1.5 mg per kilogram every 8 hours, or 75 mg per dose. The F_O for gentamicin is equal to 0.03 (i.e., only 3 percent of the given dose of gentamicin is eliminated by nonrenal routes in anephric man). GFR may be estimated, from the foregoing reference formula using age and sex, as 8 ml per minute. The value of F by inspection of the nomogram equals 0.07; therefore, using method A, 8 hours divided by 0.07 equals 114 hours or a dose of 1.5 mg per kilogram should be administered approximately every 4.8 days. For method B, 75 mg times 0.07 equals 5.25 mg administered every 8 hours.

Another method of estimating dosage modifications in renal failure does not require reference to the F nomograms and may be useful for drugs with long $\tau½$ in which usual dosing intervals are equal to or less than the normal serum $\tau½$. For method A, the dosing interval in renal failure for drugs without significant extrarenal elimination equals the normal dosing interval times the ratio of the patient's creatinine clearance, divided by a normal creatinine clearance. This method may not be applicable to drugs with significant extrarenal elimination. In this instance, the formula may be modified as follows: For method A, the new dosing interval equals a normal dose interval $\times$ 1/f(K_f − 1) + 1, where f equals the fraction of the drug excreted unchanged by the kidney and K_f equals the ratio of the patient's glomerular filtration rate divided by a normal GFR. Method B, the reduction in dosage size using the same interval, may be most applicable for drugs with very short half-lives in which it is desirable to maintain a relatively constant serum level without resorting to constant infusion. This method may be hazardous if renal function is incorrectly assessed and may expose patients to increased hazards of nephrotoxicity. This may be calculated as follows:

$$\text{Dosing in renal failure} = \frac{\text{normal dose} \times \text{normal creatinine clearance}}{\text{patient's creatinine clearance}}$$

This is where normal clearance is judged by age, sex, and body habitus.

This formula is applicable primarily for drugs that are excreted largely unchanged in the urine. When significant extrarenal routes of metabolism are present, the formula may be modified as follows:

$$\text{Dosing in renal failure} = \text{normal dose} \times f\,(K_f - 1) + 1$$

For many drugs having both renal and hepatic elimination routes, both methods are used, and in critical situations, blood levels may need to be monitored closely, especially for drugs with low therapeutic indices, such as digitalis, lidocaine, gentamicin, theophylline, and methotrexate.

Method C, involving the use of constant infusion of drugs and applying elimination rate constants for calculation of usual dose, the following formula may be used: the dose/unit time in renal failure equals the usual maintenance dose per unit time, times the Ke in end-stage renal failure, divided by the Ke in normal renal function.

If as is frequently the case the patient is not in end-stage renal failure or anephric, the Ke in renal failure may be approximated as follows: Ke (in renal failure, but not anephric) equals Ke (by nonrenal routes), plus alpha times the patient's GFR, where alpha equals the slope of the straight line between Ke and GFR. Examples of these are as follows: Method A—new dose interval equals normal dose interval times Ke in normal renal function divided by estimated Ke in renal failure, but not in anephric man.

As can be seen, using these approximations and taking into account assumptions about nonrenal excretion in linearity between GFR and Ke, one can arrive at approximately similar total doses being administered over a 24-hour period with intervals used varying from normal to many days. These should be viewed as approximations only. The peak values and trough values vary between the chosen methods. For applications of these formulas in nomograms to commonly employed drugs, Table 3 lists a variety of agents according to the percent prone to protein binding, volume of distribution, normal plasma clearance, $\tau½$ in hours in normal and in end-stage renal disease, and F_O for anephric man. It should be recognized that protein binding is influenced by uremia and the concomitant administration of drugs that may displace agents from binding sites and that the volume of distribution may be affected by protein binding and other factors. Several drugs do not manifest first-order, single compartment exponential kinetics and may have multiexponential disappearance curves. Other drugs demonstrate zero-order kinetics, and in these latter instances true $\tau½$s may not be calculated.

Adjustment of Drug Dosage for Patients on Dialysis

For drugs that have negligible removal rates with dialysis (hemodialysis or peritoneal dialysis), no dosage adjustment other than for the level of impaired native renal function is required. However, if the drug can diffuse across the hemodialysis or peritoneal membrane, and if effective plasma or tissue levels are to be maintained, intra- or postdialytic dosage modifications are required. During hemofiltration, if a significant fraction of low-molecular-weight proteins are being removed through the semipermeable membrane, additional dosage adjustments are required for drugs partially bound to such low-molecular-weight proteins. Knowledge of the removal rates of the drug by dialysis is required, and this depends on factors such as the type of dialysis, the surface area of the dialyzer, the membrane parameters, the blood flow, and the dialysate flow.

Drug clearance by the dialyzer (C_D in ml per minute) is equal to Q, the blood flow through the dialyzer, times the arterial drug concentration minus the venous drug concentration divided by the arterial drug concentration. If C_D is known, the amount of drug removed during a given dialysis treatment regimen can be calculated by drug removal (total mg) equals CD in ml per minute times total time of dialysis in minutes times the mid-point arterial drug concentration in mg per milliliter. This calculated amount of drug can be administered at the end of the dialysis and a new dosing schedule calculated. Drugs that are efficiently cleared by dialysis and require adjustments include aminoglycosides, cephalosporins, penicillins, sulfonamides, isoniazid, ethambutol, procainamide, quinidine, azathioprine, cyclophosphamide, methotrexate, lithium, methyldopa, and aminophylline. For details of specific drugs and the recommendations regarding dosage modification in dialysis, as well as in renal failure, the reader is referred to the following list of publications upon which this review is based.

REFERENCES

Cutler R, Krichman K, Blair AD. Pharmacokinetics of drugs and the effects of renal failure. In: Massry S, Glassock R, (eds). Textbook of nephrology. Baltimore: Williams & Wilkins, 1983.

Anderston RT, Bennett WM. Gambertoglio J, Schrier R. Fate of drugs in renal failure. In: Brenner B, Rector F, (eds). The kidney. 2nd ed. Philadelphia: WB Saunders, 1981.

Brater DC, Lancaster, Texas: Improved therapeutics, 1982.

Bennett WM. Use of drugs in renal failure and dialysis. In: Massry S, Glassock R, (eds). Textbook of nephrology. Baltimore: Williams & Wilkins, 1983.

Anderson RT, Schrier R. Clinical use of drugs in patients with kidney and liver disease. Philadelphia: WB Saunders, 1981.

ENDOCRINE AND METABOLIC DISORDERS

HYPOPITUITARISM

PETER O. KOHLER, M.D.
RICHARD M. JORDAN, M.D.

Hypopituitarism may involve the loss of one or more of the six anterior pituitary hormones. The hormone deficiencies may be caused by a lesion involving the pituitary gland itself or one in the hypothalamus, where the anterior pituitary control factors are released. The primary disease processes leading to hypopituitarism will not be discussed in this chapter. After an evaluation into the extent of the hormone deficiency, replacement hormone therapy should be initiated with several goals in mind. The overall aim is to restore normal function, but specific goals depend on the age of the patient, the status with regard to growth, interest in reproduction, and the number of anterior pituitary hormones that are deficient. Treatment of patients with posterior hormone deficiency is discussed elsewhere in this book.

Treatment of the hypopituitarism is performed by administration of either the deficient anterior pituitary hormone such as growth hormone or the target organ hormone that is decreased as a result of inadequate anterior pituitary hormone secretion. Examples of target hormone therapy include direct use of thyroid, adrenal, or gonadal hormones. In the future, use of a hypothalamic-releasing hormone for patients with hypothalamic lesions and adequate pituitary responsiveness will probably increase. Experimentally, gonadotropin-releasing hormone (GnRH) or analogs have been used to induce fertility, and growth hormone-releasing hormone, which stimulates growth hormone release, provides a potential treatment of a hypothalamic lesion causing growth retardation in children. Paradoxically, continuous rather than episodic administration of GnRH can turn off luteinizing hormone (LH) and follicle-stimulating hormone (FSH) secretion and has been used to treat patients with conditions such as precocious puberty or prostate cancer.

PROLACTIN DEFICIENCY

Deficiency of prolactin produces no obvious clinical disorder other than failure of lactation at the time of parturition. Also, human prolactin is available only for experimental use. Therefore, prolactin replacement is not presently part of the treatment for anterior pituitary hormone deficiency.

GROWTH HORMONE DEFICIENCY

Insufficient growth hormone leads to growth retardation and dwarfism with normal body proportions in the child with this deficiency. Growth hormone deficiency may also cause hypoglycemia as well as growth retardation in the child, but hypoglycemia is not a problem in adults with growth hormone deficiency. Treatment of growth hormone deficiency in children is with the human growth hormone, which restores growth and resolves hypoglycemia.

Previously the growth hormone used for treatment of growth retardation was extracted from human pituitary glands. However, concern about Creutzfeldt-Jakob slow virus contamination of the growth hormone preparation caused it to be withdrawn from the market in the United States. Human growth hormone is still used in Europe, where there has been only a single questionable incident of Creutzfeldt-Jakob disease in a patient who received growth hormone many years earlier.

The growth hormone available in the United States is produced with recombinant DNA technology in the bacteria *Escherichia coli*. The two preparations available include a methionyl growth hormone (produced by Genentech and marketed under the trade name Protropin) and a methionyl-free growth hormone (marketed by Eli Lilly under the trade name Somatropin). Previous studies with the human pituitary–derived growth hormone had established a dosage of 0.06 to 0.1 IU per kilogram three times a week, usually given intramuscularly. The new recombinant DNA growth hormone preparations have a potency in the range of 2 to 2.4 IU per milligram, and the usual recommended dose for treatment is now 0.1 mg per kilogram three times a week, usually given subcutaneously. This latter route of administration is often less painful and has been shown to produce a somewhat more prolonged growth hormone elevation in the blood without any increased incidence of antibody generation or allergic reaction.

The hormone should be given at the earliest possible age after growth hormone deficiency is established because older patients respond less well to treatment. Coordination of the growth hormone administration with other hormone treatment is very important to maximize the ultimate height. Other pituitary hormone deficiencies must be identified. Occasionally, growth hormone treatment will unmask hypothyroidism. Therefore, all patients should have thyroid studies performed after initiation of therapy. If present, hypothyroidism should be treated with an oral dose of l-thyroxine (T_4) in the range of 75 to 100 μg per square meter of body surface area. Triiodothyronine (T_3) can also be used but has no advantage over T_4, which is converted to the more potent T_3 in the patient. Adequacy of hormone replacement is ordinarily made by clinical judgment and by measuring the thyroid hormone levels in the blood (Table 1).

Glucocorticoid deficiency should also be treated when present in the growth hormone–deficient patient. However, it is important that this not be treated with excessive doses of glucocorticoids, which could impair the response to growth hormone. For this reason, the glucocorticoid dosage is slightly lower than that which is used to treat glucocorticoid–deficient patients who are not receiving growth hormone. Hydrocortisone is often used because of the shorter duration of action at an oral dose of 10 mg per square meter of body surface area per day; two-thirds of the dose is usually given in the morning and one-third given before the evening meal. If prednisone is used for treatment, it should also be given in a low dose-equivalent amount (Table 2).

Sex hormone replacement in the growth hormone–deficient patient with hypothalamic-pituitary hypogonadotropism should also be done with care to achieve the optimal response to growth hormone. Initiation of treatment with gonadal hormone should be delayed until the patient has begun to achieve a reasonable height, such as 5 feet, 6 inches in boys or 5 feet, 2 inches in girls. Occasionally, some children will not achieve even these modest heights and need to receive gonadal replacement therapy earlier. Initiation of testosterone cypionate (Depo-Testosterone) treatment in boys provides a growth spurt but also leads to maturation and fusion of the epiphyses. Therefore, initial replacement in boys should be low, such as testosterone enanthate or testosterone cypionate at a dose of 50 to 100 mg intramuscularly monthly. This dose is increased later to adult ranges. In girls receiving growth hormone treatment, estrogens are usually withheld (unless there is a problem in social adjustment) until the patient begins to reach a reasonable target height. Then treatment with an estrogen such as conjugated estrogen (Premarin), 0.625 to 1.25 mg per day orally for days 1 through 25 of each month, can be initiated. After several months, medroxyprogesterone (Provera) at a dose of 5 to 10 mg per day can be given orally on days 21 through 25 of each month to induce a secretory endometrium and withdrawal bleeding (see Table 1).

The side effects of growth hormone treatment are minimal. Growth hormone preparations occasionally induce allergic reactions, such as a local pain, erythema, and swelling. Pain at the injection site is more severe with intramuscular than with subcutaneous injections. In addition, antibody formation can occur with all growth hormone preparations. There are rare instances during which response to growth hormone appeared to be blunted in patients with high antibody titers. In an occasional patient, switching from synthetic methionyl growth hormone to human pituitary growth hormone appears to cause resumption of growth. However, in most patients there is little correlation between antibody titers and the rates of growth. Recent preparations of the recombinant DNA–derived

TABLE 1 Anterior Pituitary Hormone Replacement in Hypopituitarism

Drug	*Dosage Schedule*
Adrenal	
Hydrocortisone	20 mg in AM; 10 mg in PM
Cortisone acetate	25 mg in AM; 12.5 mg in PM
Prednisone	5 mg in AM
Fluorohydrocortisone	0.05 to 0.1 mg daily (usually unnecessary)
Thyroid	
l-Thyroxine	0.10 to 0.20 mg daily
Gonadal (men)	
Testosterone enanthate in oil	200 to 300 mg IM every 2 to 3 weeks
Testosterone cypionate	100 to 250 mg IM every 2 to 4 weeks
Gonadal (women)	
Conjugated estrogens	0.625 to 1.25 mg, first 25 days each month
Ethinyl estradiol	0.02 to 0.05 mg, first 25 days each month
Medroxyprogesterone acetate	10 mg/day, on day 20 to 25 each month

Modified from Kohler PO, Jordan RM, eds. Clinical endocrinology. New York: John Wiley & Sons, 1986.

TABLE 2 Glucocorticoid Replacement

	*Anti-Inflammatory Potency**	*Equivalent Potency (mg)*	*Sodium-Retaining Potency*
Short-acting (biologic half-life of less than 12 hours)			
Hydrocortisone	1	20	2+
Cortisone	0.8	25	2+
Intermediate-acting (biologic half-life of 12 to 36 hours)			
Prednisone	3.5	5	1+
Prednisolone	4	5	1+
Methylprednisolone	5	4	0
Triamcinolone	5	4	0
Long-acting (biologic half-life of more than 48 hours)			
Paramethasone	10	2	0
Betamethasone	25	0.60	0
Dexamethasone	30	0.75	0

* The potency of cortisol (hydrocortisone) is arbitrarily set at 1. Modified from Azarnoff DL, ed. Steroid therapy. Philadelphia: WB Saunders, 1975.

growth hormone contain fewer *Escherichia coli* impurities than initial investigative preparations so that reactions to bacterial proteins are rare. Synthetic growth hormone may be less effective in maintaining blood glucose levels than the original pituitary preparations, possibly owing to loss of other contaminating hormones. During growth hormone treatment, careful growth curves should be maintained so that diminution in the growth velocity will be observed and evaluated appropriately.

GONADOTROPIN DEFICIENCY

The treatment of pituitary hypogonadism must be considered with a view to whether sexual maturation or fertility is the goal. When the induction of fertility is desired, treatment with human pituitary gonadotropins and human chorionic gonadotropin (hCG) or GnRH or a feedback inhibiting agent such as clomiphene citrate must be used. Usually, the goal of therapy is the development or preservation of sexual maturation. This goal is ordinarily achieved using replacement with synthetic or natural gonadal steroids. Some clinicians have used hCG to produce a pharmacologic puberty in boys. However, this agent requires several injections per week, is more expensive, and has no advantage over testosterone in most patients.

Boys or men requiring androgen treatment respond best to long-acting injectable testosterone preparations such as testosterone enanthate or testosterone proprionate. The dosage of these agents ranges from 150 to 300 mg by intramuscular injection at intervals of 2 to 3 weeks (see Table 2). Lower doses of steroids are ordinarily given when the patient is receiving growth hormone therapy. Oral androgen preparations are not as potent and the 17-alpha-alkylated steroids may cause cholestatic jaundice and hepatitis. For that reason and because of their greater potency, the parenteral preparations are preferred.

Side effects of testosterone injection are infrequent or transient at these doses. They include acne, increased libido, insomnia, and nightmares. Transient gynecomastia with local tenderness occurs in 50 percent of boys treated with injections. This usually recedes with continuation of treatments. Changes in liver function tests have been reported but are rare.

Girls who need the development of sexual maturation are treated with conjugated estrogens in doses of 0.625 to 2.5 mg daily for days 1 through 25 of each cycle. A dose of 1.25 mg daily appears to be effective in most patients. This is also a dose that preserves bone density as well as developing or maintaining the secondary sexual characteristics. Ethinyl estradiol in doses of 0.02 to 0.05 mg daily also can be used. Estrogen therapy to women should usually be done in a manner that simulates normal menstrual periods. Medroxyprogesterone in a dose of 5 to 10 mg daily on days 20 through 25 will allow withdrawal endometrial bleeding and prevents hyperstimulation of the endometrium by the estrogens. This is thought to protect against the development of endometrial carcinoma from continuous estrogen stimulation in the postmenopausal patient on estrogen treatment.

ACTH DEFICIENCY

In chronic hypopituitarism with adrenocorticotropic hormone (ACTH) deficiency, adrenal steroids are usually replaced with hydrocortisone at doses of 10 to 15 mg per square meter of body surface area per day or equivalent doses of a longer-acting corticosteroid preparation (see Table 1). ACTH itself is not used because of the need for parenteral administration. In most adults, hydrocortisone given in a split dose of 20 mg each morning and 10 mg before the evening meal roughly simulates a physiologic adrenal steroid secretion pattern. Alternatively, prednisone, which is less expensive, may be given in a single dose of 5 to 7.5 mg each morning. Occasionally prednisone is given in a dose of 5 mg in the morning and 2.5 mg in the evening. A total prednisone dose of 7.5 mg is slightly supraphysiologic in some patients. In addition, the biologic effective life of prednisone of about 36 hours makes the split dose regimen for prednisone somewhat questionable. However, this is done in many medical centers with apparent good results. In patients with pituitary hypopituitarism, mineralocorticoid replacement is usually not necessary, since reasonable aldosterone secretion is preserved. Only severe salt restriction may present a problem to the patient with pituitary ACTH deficiency and intact adrenal glands.

The side effects of excess glucocorticoid treatment include the development of cushingoid features with rounding of the face, truncal fat deposition, easy bruising, and lowered resistance to skin and other infections. Decreased bone density and a tendency to develop fractures may occur after excess glucocorticoid hormone treatment. Hypertension and edema may occur with excess salt-retaining steroid preparations. Psychiatric reactions to corticosteroids may occur at pharmacologic doses, although this does not appear to be a problem with physiologic replacement levels. Other less common side efects are cataracts and pseudotumor cerebri, but these are not usually a problem at lower replacement doses.

Patients taking glucocorticoid medications should carry identification indicating that they need additional corticosteroids in the event of an accident or serious illness. A bracelet or necklace may be obtained from the Medic Alert Foundation in Turlock, California. The clinical rule for managing patients with injuries or intercurrent illness is to double the daily corticosteroid dose for moderate illness and to triple it for severe illness, giving it parenterally if necessary. Calculations of maximal adult human cortisol production rates have been in the range of 300 mg per day. Therefore, this equivalent is probably the maximal dose needed since pharmacologic doses do not appear to be necessary unless the patient has cerebral edema.

THYROID–STIMULATING HORMONE DEFICIENCY

Human thyroid-stimulating hormone (TSH) is not available for treatment purposes, and thyrotropin-releasing hormone injections are not practical. However, the treatment of TSH deficiency with thyroid preparation is easily accomplished with the oral administration of thyroxine (T_4) in a dose of 100 to 200 μg per day or 75 to 100 μg per square meter of body surface area per day. In older patients, and particularly those with evidence of ischemic heart disease, replacement therapy should be done gradually with an initial dose of 25 μg per day. This should be increased by 25 μg increments every 2 weeks to a total dose of 100 to 150 μg per day. If the patient begins to develop chest pain during this replacement therapy, the final dose must be lowered so that hypothyroidism is treated without causing angina.

These patients should have electrocardiographic evaluation prior to and during the thyroid hormone replacement. There has been some debate over the relative merits of T_4 or triiodothyronine (T_3) for treatment of hypothyroidism, particularly in elderly patients with potential coronary artery disease. T_4 is converted to T_3 in the patient, giving relatively constant blood levels of both T_4 and T_3. The administration of T_3 with the shorter half-life of less than 1 day in the blood has been stated to have the advantage of being able to be withdrawn rapidly if given in excessive doses. However, T_4, which has a half-life of about 7 days, has the advantage of more constant blood levels and is probably the preferred form of treatment.

Patients who receive thyroid hormone should be watched carefully for possible ACTH deficiency if they are not on ACTH replacement therapy. There are some reports of thyroid replacement therapy precipitating adrenal crisis in patients who have ACTH deficiency and are not receiving cortisol replacement. This presumably occurs because thyroid hormone treatment causes increased cortisol metabolism. Although this seems to be a rare problem, it is still important to search for ACTH deficiency before and during thyroid hormone replacement therapy in a patient with other evidence of hypopituitarism.

Excess thyroid hormone treatment may cause hypermetabolism. There is also now evidence that chronic thyroid hormone overtreatment may produce osteopenia.

ACUTE PITUITARY INSUFFICIENCY

The development of acute pituitary insufficiency such as after trauma or pituitary apoplexy is a medical emergency. The major requirement is for adequate doses of corticosteroids and careful fluid management of the patient. Infusion of 300 mg of soluble hydrocortisone (e.g., Solu-Cortef) over a 24-hour period with saline and adequate monitoring of electrolytes are critical. Initially, a 100-mg intravenous bolus is helpful. The patient must be watched carefully so that circulation is adequately maintained with adequate fluid intake. Glucocorticoids are necessary to excrete a water load and to prevent the patient with hypopituitarism treated only with water or 5 percent dextrose in water from becoming water intoxicated and hyponatremic. ACTH deficiency is more likely to present in this manner than with the vascular collapse found in a patient with adrenal insufficiency and impaired or absent mineralocorticoid function. When a patient has pituitary tumor infarction, much larger doses of synthetic glucocorticoid are given to reduce edema of the infarcted tissue, thus decreasing compression of surrounding tissue. Administration of dexamethasone, 2 mg every 4 hours intravenously, is recommended in this situation. Urine flow must be monitored.

If the patient is also hypothyroid, T_4 should be given,

but the need is usually less urgent since the half-life of T_4 in the blood is 7 days. The replacement therapy ordinarily should consist of a normal daily requirement such as 100 to 150 μg T_4 orally if possible or, if not, 50 to 75 μg intravenously. The elderly patient needs to be monitored for possible problems with angina. When the patient remains comatose and is thought to be unresponsive because of hypothyroidism, larger doses of intravenous T_4 such as 300 to 400 μg may be given. However, the efficacy of larger doses of T_4 in hypopituitary patients is less well established than in myxedema coma from primary hypothyroidism. Acute deficiency of other hormones such as LH and FSH is not an emergency. Levels of gonadal hormones can be corrected when the patient recovers from the acute condition.

SUGGESTED READING

Hoffman CP, Crowley WF. Induction of puberty by long-term pulsatile administration of low dose gonadotropin-releasing hormone. N Engl J Med 1982; 307:1237–1241.

Lam KS, Tse VK, Wang C, Yeung RT, Ma JT, Ho JH. Early effects of cranial irradiation on hypothalamic pituitary function. J Clin Endocrinol Metab 1987; 64:418–424.

Preece MA. The effect of administered corticosteroids on the growth of children. Postgrad Med J 1976; 52:625–630.

Ranke MB, Bierich JR. Treatment of growth hormone deficiency. Clin Endocrinol Metab 1986; 15:495–510.

ANOREXIA NERVOSA AND BULIMIA

ROBERT A. VIGERSKY, M.D., F.A.C.P.

ANOREXIA NERVOSA

Anorexia nervosa has become a widespread, almost epidemic disorder that has been estimated to affect up to 10 percent of teenage girls in Europe and the United States. It is rarely seen in underdeveloped countries. Young men represent about 10 percent of the total number of cases. Because of the large number of affected persons and the protean manifestations of this disorder, many physicians may have primary care and/or consultative encounters with patients with anorexia nervosa. Although the principles of treatment related to endocrinology and metabolism are described in this chapter, the foundations for treatment are based on the ability to make the proper diagnosis. Criteria for the diagnosis of anorexia nervosa that allow for the inclusion of a wider range of patients than may be used in research studies are listed in Table 1. Adherence to these diagnostic criteria should prevent multiple referrals for evaluation of isolated aspects of the disorder and promote earlier treatment.

Anorexia nervosa is a psychiatric disorder with multiple medical and endocrine manifestations. Although treatment of anorexia nervosa should be a multidisciplinary endeavor, the effort should be led by a psychiatrist who has experience in treating such patients. The inter-

TABLE 1 Diagnostic Criteria for Anorexia Nervosa

Standard Criteria	*Modifying Features*
Age at onset before 25	Patients may present at a later age but have had earlier eating behavior abnormalities that had remitted.
Weight loss of at least 25 percent of original body weight	Patients' weight may fluctuate widely particularly in a bulimic phase. Weight may be close to "ideal body weight" at the time of the first visit.
A distorted, implacable attitude toward eating food or weight that overrides hunger, admonitions, reassurances, and threats	This feature may be vigorously denied by the patient and may require evidence from family or friends.
No known medical illness that could account for the weight loss	Patients may have numerous and real symptoms. However, all are correctable with weight gain. The syndrome is rare in patients from low socioeconomic groups.
No other known psychiatric disorder	Patients may be depressed and even suicidal. This does not exclude them from the diagnosis.
At least two of the following: amenorrhea, lanugo hair, bradycardia, periods of overactivity, episodes of bulimia, and vomiting (usually self-induced)	Some patients may have only one of the standard criteria features. Additional features should be diuretic and/or laxative abuse, hypothermia, and hypercarotenemia. Amenorrhea may be primary or secondary. Exercise may often be excessive and surreptitious.

nist, pediatrician, or endocrinologist provide follow-up for the nonpsychiatric manifestations of the disorder. Since anorexia nervosa may have numerous symptoms, knowledge of what to anticipate and the use of appropriate consultation may not only assist in the recovery of the patient but, more importantly, may prevent unnecessary morbidity and mortality. The published mortality rate of up to 10 percent may be an overestimate now that there are more mild cases and the syndrome is recognized earlier, but anorexia nervosa is still a potentially lethal disease if not diagnosed early and treated aggressively.

Endocrine and Metabolic Disorders

Although numerous abnormalities of the endocrine system have been demonstrated, most are corrected with weight gain and require no specific therapy. The well-informed physician recognizes these abnormalities as secondary to the weight loss per se and is not tempted to intervene unnecessarily. However, documentation of these abnormalities may be helpful in following improvement and in educating the patient as to the medical implications of the weight loss.

Thyroid Disorders

Patients with anorexia nervosa have many clinical features of hypothyroidism, including bradycardia, dry skin, constipation, and hypothermia. In fact, one of the more common complaints of patients with anorexia nervosa is that of feeling cold all the time. Routine thyroid function tests show low or low-normal serum thyroxine (T_4) levels. Resin triiodothyronine (T_3) uptake (RT_3U) may be at the upper end of the normal range or frankly high. However, direct measurement of free T_4 by dialysis or calculation of the free thyroxine index ($T_4 \times T_3RU$) is generally normal. Anorexia nervosa patients have profoundly low serum T_3 levels that are directly correlated to the severity of weight loss and result from altered peripheral deiodination of T_4. This constellation of laboratory studies is similar to the low T_3 levels seen in the euthyroid sick syndrome. Patients with anorexia nervosa have an impaired response of thyroid-stimulating hormone (TSH) to thyrotropin-releasing hormone (TRH) with a delay of the peak. Treatment of these patients with thyroid hormones is not indicated except in the rare patient who has true primary or secondary hypothyroidism. Basal serum TSH and the TSH response to TRH are the most helpful diagnostic studies. In addition, the reverse T_3 (3,3′,5-triiodothyronine) value will be low in hypothyroidism, whereas it is normal or elevated in anorexia nervosa. Treatment of true hypothyroidism in a patient with anorexia nervosa does not differ from that in a patient without the disorder. In the recovery phase of anorexia nervosa, T_3 levels may rise and be associated with symptoms suggestive of mild hyperthyroidism.

Pituitary-Gonadal Axis Disorders

Amenorrhea, primary or secondary, is a common presenting complaint in women with anorexia nervosa. About 70 percent of patients cease menstruation prior to or just at the onset of weight loss, suggesting stress-induced effects on the hypothalamic-pituitary-ovarian axis. The degree that exercise plays in the person's weight loss may be a major factor in determining at what weight menses ceases. Most women resume menses with a gain in weight to about 10 percent greater than that at the time of menarche (Table 2). However, about 30 percent of women do not regain normal menstrual function. This, again, may represent stress and/or exercise.

The failure of the hypothalamus to produce normal amounts of gonadotropin-releasing hormone (Gn-RH) to stimulate the pituitary gonadotroph produces severe hypogonadotropic hypogonadism in patients with anorexia nervosa. The administration of Gn-RH acutely and chronically produces normal serum luteinizing hormone and follicle-stimulating hormone responses. Indeed, ovulation and pregnancies have been achieved with the chronic administration of Gn-RH, indicating a normal pituitary gonadotroph and normal ovarian function given the appropriate stimulus. However, pregnancy is contraindicated in patients with anorexia nervosa because of the high risk of intrauterine growth retardation of the fetus. In the 30 percent of anorexia nervosa patients who have recovered their weight but are still amenorrheic, one or two courses of clomiphene citrate (Clomid), 50 to 100 mg per day for 7 days, often stimulates ovulation. This should not be attempted until the patient's weight has been stable for 4 to 6 months and it is certain that she is not maintaining a borderline weight by engaging in vomiting or vigorous exercise.

Although weight gain restores the hypothalamic-pituitary-ovarian axis to normal, it is not clear whether all patients with anorexia nervosa should be treated in the interim with estrogens. The main consideration for this should be the state of bone mineral. Several studies have demonstrated severe osteopenia in women with anorexia nervosa, the etiology of which is undoubtedly a combination of hormonal (hypoestrogenism and perhaps hypercortisolism) and nutritional factors. Of note is that those patients with anorexia nervosa who exercise have higher bone densities than those who do not. Thus, the duration of the weight loss, the role that exercise plays in achieving and maintaining the weight loss, and the actual bone density are all factors in determining whether to treat with estrogen. Therefore, bone densitometry of the lumbar spine and hip by either dual-photon absorptiometry or quantitative computed tomography should be performed in all patients with anorexia nervosa.

In addition to the osteopenia, estrogen treatment should be given to those sexually active women who complain of dyspareunia. Therapy should consist of conjugated estrogens (Premarin, 0.625 mg, days 1 to 25) and the addition of medroxyprogesterone acetate (Provera, 10 mg, days 16 to 25) on a monthly basis. Breast engorgement

TABLE 2 Minimal Weight for Particular Height Necessary for the Onset or Restoration of Menstrual Cycles

Height		Menarche or Primary Amenorrhea			Secondary Amenorrhea		
		Minimal* Weight (10th Percentile)		Average Weight (50th Percentile)	Minimal† Weight (10th Percentile)		Average Weight (50th Percentile)
(inches)	(cm)	(lb)	(kg)	(kg)	(lb)	(kg)	(kg)
53.1	135	66.7	30.3	34.9	74.6	33.9	38.9
53.9	137	68.6	31.2	36.0	76.8	34.9	40.1
54.7	139	70.6	32.1	37.0	79.0	35.9	41.2
55.5	141	72.6	33.0	38.0	81.2	36.9	42.4
56.3	143	74.4	33.8	39.0	83.4	37.9	43.5
57.1	145	76.3	34.7	40.1	85.6	38.9	44.7
57.9	147	78.3	35.6	41.1	87.8	39.9	45.8
58.7	149	80.3	36.5	42.1	90.0	40.9	47.0
59.4	151	82.3	37.4	43.1	92.2	41.9	48.1
60.2	153	84.3	38.3	44.2	94.4	42.9	49.3
61.0	155	86.2	39.2	45.2	96.6	43.9	50.4
61.8	157	88.2	40.1	46.2	98.8	44.9	51.5
62.6	159	90.2	41.0	47.2	101.0	45.9	52.7
63.4	161	92.2	41.9	48.3	103.2	46.9	53.8
64.2	163	93.9	42.7	49.3	105.4	47.9	55.0
65.0	165	95.9	43.6	50.3	107.6	48.9	56.1
65.7	167	97.9	44.5	51.4	109.8	49.9	57.3
66.5	169	99.9	45.4	52.4	112.0	50.9	58.4
67.3	171	101.9	46.3	53.4	114.0	51.8	59.6
68.1	173	103.8	47.2	54.4	116.2	52.8	60.7
68.9	175	105.8	48.1	55.5	118.4	53.8	61.8
69.7	177	107.8	49.0	56.5	120.6	54.8	63.0
70.5	179	109.6	49.8	57.5	122.8	55.8	64.1
71.3	181	111.8	50.8	58.5	125.2	56.9	65.3

* Equivalent to 17 percent fat/body weight.
† Equivalent to 22 percent fat/body weight.
Reprinted with permission from Frisch RE. Food intake, fatness, and reproductive ability. In: Vigersky RA, ed. Anorexia nervosa. New York: Raven Press, 1977.

and fluid retention are common side effects in anorexia nervosa patients given this regimen, however. Calcium supplementation of 1,000 to 1,500 mg of elemental calcium per day is also advisable. Finally, since immobilization induces negative calcium balance, bed rest should not be used as an initial phase of a behavior modification treatment program.

Men with anorexia nervosa also have hypogonadotrophic hypogonadism with symptoms of decreased libido and potency, diminished strength, and decreased shaving frequency. Moreover, osteopenia has been reported in men with other forms of hypogonadotrophic hypogonadism. Like women with the disorder, most anorexic men recover gonadal function with weight gain. Depending on the chronicity of the anorexia nervosa, the bone density values, and the status of the primary therapy, intramuscular testosterone enanthate (Delatestryl, 200 mg every 2 weeks or 300 mg every 3 weeks) should be given. However, adolescents just entering therapy should have androgen therapy withheld to avoid premature sexual stimulation and imagery before these issues can be dealt with psychologically. Although oligospermia has been reported in men with anorexia nervosa, insufficient evidence exists to suggest a causal relationship.

Pituitary-Adrenal Axis Disorders

In the early part of the century, anorexia nervosa patients were often considered adrenally insufficient. It is now known that many patients have adrenocortical hyperfunction, as documented by an increased cortisol production rate and increased levels of urinary "free" cortisol. In addition, there are abnormalities in the diurnal rhythm of serum cortisol in over 50 percent of patients. Studies have documented elevated levels of corticotropin-releasing hormone (CRH) in the cerebrospinal fluid of anorexia nervosa patients and a blunted adrenocorticotropic hormone (ACTH) response to exogenously administered CRH. These abnormalities correct with weight gain. Results of dexamethasone suppression tests are frequently abnormal in anorexia nervosa patients but are most likely related to the concomitant depression rather than a specific abnormality. Despite the abnormally high cortisol secretion, there is no evidence of Cushing's syndrome in patients with anorexia nervosa. The only deleterious effect of the hypercortisolism may be its contribution to the osteopenia. No specific treatment of the adrenal abnormalities is necessary.

Other Hormone Disorders

Serum growth hormone levels are often elevated in patients with anorexia nervosa and may be "inappropriately" stimulated by TRH. Obviously, these patients are not acromegalic, probably because of the low levels of somatomedin C. The elevated growth hormone levels may be an attempt to defend against hypoglycemia and require no specific therapy. Linear growth is maintained in adolescents with anorexia nervosa, and ultimate height attained is close to that predicted prior to the illness.

Serum prolactin levels are normal in patients with anorexia nervosa and respond to TRH in a quantitatively normal way, but there is a delayed peak response.

A few studies have suggested that women with anorexia nervosa have elevations of serum testosterone levels. This is not a constant finding and does not require any specific therapy. The excessive hair growth is usually of the lanugo type and is probably due to the elevated cortisol secretion.

Patients with anorexia nervosa may have partial diabetes insipidus. This is usually asymptomatic and requires no specific therapy if found. However, if diabetes insipidus is found, a hypothalamic disorder (e.g., tumor, sarcoid) should be suspected.

Metabolic Abnormalities

Electrolyte disorders show a variety of patterns depending on the manner in which weight loss is achieved (e.g., vomiting, restricting calories, diuretic and/or laxative abuse). The most serious metabolic abnormality is hypokalemia. This and the often attendant alkalosis are usually seen in patients who have abused diuretics and/or laxatives in order to achieve weight loss or in those who are chronic vomiters. This finding requires hospitalization for prompt intravenous correction of potassium loss. Serum electrolyte values should be monitored daily until they return to normal. An oral potassium supplement should then be used, since the total-body potassium level is still depleted.

Hypophosphatemia may be present prior to the initiation of primary therapy. Even if phosphate levels are initially normal, total-body phosphate stores are usually low. Serum phosphate levels may become precipitously lower during nutritional rehabilitation causing intracellular adenosine triphosphate depletion and cellular hypoxia. Clinically, this may produce respiratory or cardiac failure, seizures, altered mental status, or myoneuropathy. Intravenous or oral phosphate supplements should be administered depending on the severity of the hypophosphatemia and the overall clinical status. Daily measurement of the serum phosphate concentration is advisable during the initiation of nutritional rehabilitation.

Other abnormalities in mineral metabolism that may be seen in anorexia nervosa include low levels of magnesium, zinc, and copper. If hypocalcemia is present, hypomagnesemia may be its cause and replacement therapy prevents tetany and arrhythmias.

Primary Treatment

Patients with anorexia nervosa are often resistant to being entered into any type of treatment program. Reassurances that the patient will not be permitted to become obese and that many somatic complaints will improve with weight gain are often helpful approaches. The initial approach depends on the severity of the weight loss and the method by which it has been achieved. On presentation to the physician, all patients should have a complete physical examination, electrocardiogram, chest roentgenogram, urinalysis, determination of electrolyte levels, and evaluation of renal and hepatic function. If the weight loss is moderate (25 percent or less), the duration is relatively short (4 months or less), and no severe metabolic abnormalities are present, treatment may be initiated on an outpatient basis. The initial aim of therapy whether inpatient or outpatient is nutritional rehabilitation. Patients with anorexia nervosa suffer from the nonspecific symptoms of starvation such as insomnia, depression, and irritability, which are easily reversible with weight gain. Improvement in body image and the overestimation of an object's size also improve with weight gain. On the other hand, programs focusing only on weight gain are doomed to failure. Patients quickly learn to escape from the medical care system by rapidly gaining weight, only to lose it shortly thereafter. Moreover, rapid weight gain may be dangerous in that it may stimulate suicidal thoughts and attempts.

Behavioral therapy, family therapy, and traditional psychotherapy under the supervision of an experienced psychiatrist and a team of health care professionals including dietitians, social workers, and nurses are critical components to the success of treatment.

The help of a dietitian is useful at the outset in providing the patient with a nutritionally balanced meal plan that ultimately will provide an additional 1,000 calories per day to the patient. Since patients with anorexia nervosa have diminished gastric emptying and increased gastric volume following a meal, the calories should be added progressively over 1 to 3 weeks. The use of metoclopramide (Reglan, 10 mg 1 hour prior to meals) may prevent or improve symptoms related to gastric fullness.

The decision to hospitalize a patient with newly diagnosed anorexia nervosa should be based on severe, acute weight loss and/or the presence of severe metabolic changes such as hypokalemia with or without alkalosis (Table 3). Patients with established longstanding anorexia nervosa may be hospitalized for the same reasons or because of the failure of an outpatient treatment program. Suicidal thoughts or preoccupation also mandate hospitalization. Although the specific cause of death is not gener-

TABLE 3 Indications for Hospitalization of Patients With Anorexia Nervosa

Rapid and severe weight loss
a. To less than 25 percent of *ideal* body weight
b. Of more than 25 percent *initial* weight in less than 3 months.
Hypokalemia with or without alkalosis
Azotemia
Hypophosphatemia
Development of lethargy and listlessness
Suicidal thoughts
Lack of family involvement or pathologic family environment
Failure of an outpatient program

ally known in these patients, it is not unlikely that the combination of the severe sinus bradycardia (as low as 28 beats per minute), hypotension, hypokalemia, and hypocalcemia predispose the patient to lethal arrhythmias.

Patients with anorexia nervosa rarely need oral or parenteral hyperalimentation. However, the development of cardiac arrhythmias, particularly in the presence of normokalemia, lethargy in a usually hyperactive patient, or a severe febrile illness is an indication for the initiation of oral hyperalimentation via a nasogastric tube with a nutritionally complete formula such as Sustacal.

Pharmacotherapy

Few double-blind trials of any drugs have been performed in anorexia nervosa. Cyproheptadine (Periactin), 4 to 8 mg four times a day, has limited success in some series. It is a serotonin and histamine antagonist that produces weight gain in animals, children, and geriatric patients. Phenothiazines, tricyclic antidepressants, and monoamine oxidase inhibitors have also been used successfully by some groups. If depression is a major component of the illness, amitriptyline, beginning at 25 mg per day and increasing to 75 to 150 mg per day, seems to be effective.

BULIMIA

Bulimia is diagnosed in patients who have recurrent episodes of binge eating of high-calorie foods in discrete time periods. The binges are usually terminated by self-induced vomiting. Such patients often have multiple fluctuations in weight of 10 pounds or more and feel guilty and depressed after these episodes. It may be present at any weight although often is part of the anorexic syndrome. The incidence of normal-weight bulimia is unknown since the disorder has only recently become evident. However, if one distinguishes between bulimic behavior and clinically significant bulimia, there is a prevalence of 1.3 percent in college women.

The principles of medical treatment of bulimia are similar to that of anorexia nervosa and depend on the weight and metabolic state of the patient. A similar medical evaluation should be given to all normal-weight bulimic patients as to those with anorexia nervosa. Low-weight bulimic patients often have more severe hypokalemia compared with weight-matched anorexia nervosa patients and thus should be aggressively treated with intravenous replacement.

Bulimic patients often have esophagogastritis, which can be effectively treated with histamine antagonists such as cimetidine or ranitidine, and poor gastric emptying, which may respond to metoclopramide.

Few endocrine studies of normal-weight bulimic patients have been done in order to assess whether there are abnormalities specific to this illness. Urinary "free" cortisol levels and the ACTH response to CRH are normal although almost 50 percent of bulimic patients have abnormal results of overnight dexamethasone suppression tests. This seems to be related to the degree of depression present in the patient. Basal thyroid function test results are usually normal. The TSH response to TRH is usually normal but has been reported to be blunted in 30 percent of patients. Finally, basal and clonidine-stimulated growth hormone levels are indistinguishable from normal.

Normal-weight bulimic patients may have oligomenorrhea or amenorrhea, but the incidence of this is much less than in anorexia nervosa. The hormonal characteristics and consequences of the menstrual abnormalities have not been well studied.

From the above, it should be obvious that it is rarely necessary to provide any specific endocrine therapy to bulimic patients.

SUGGESTED READING

Andersen AE. Practical comprehensive treatment of anorexia nervosa and bulimia. Baltimore: Johns Hopkins University Press, 1985.

Ferrari E, Brambilla F, eds. Disorders of eating behavior: a psychoneuroendocrine approach. Oxford, England: Pergamon Press, 1986.

Mitchell JE, Seim HC, Colon E, Pomeroy C. Medical complications and management of bulimia. Ann Intern Med 1987; 107:71–77.

Rigotti NA, Nussbaum SR, Herzog DB, Neer RM. Osteoporosis in women with anorexia nervosa. N Engl J Med 1984; 311:1601–1606.

Vigersky RA, ed. Anorexia nervosa. New York: Raven Press, 1977.

ACROMEGALY

THAD C. HAGEN, M.D.

Acromegaly is a disease with multiple clinical stigmata secondary to growth hormone (GH) hypersecretion. These stigmata are the familiar bony changes including enlargement of the mandible, distal phalanges, and frontal bones, which in concert with generalized soft tissue hyperplasia result in the typical appearance. In addition, visceromegaly results in an increased incidence of obstructive lung disease, dilated cardiomyopathy, and numerous gastrointestinal complaints. Furthermore, degenerative arthritis, hypertrophic osteoarthropathy, and perineural hypertrophy with nerve entrapment are frequent problems requiring therapeutic intervention. Lastly, but importantly, the presence of diabetes mellitus requiring therapy is common.

PATHOGENESIS

An extensive review of the pathogenesis of acromegaly is beyond the scope of this chapter; however, a brief discussion will allow some insight into the interpretation of therapeutic results and possibly the establishment of therapeutic goals.

The hallmark of acromegaly is GH hypersecretion generally from a pituitary tumor or somatotrophic cell hyperplasia. The differentiation of these pathologic features is of considerable interest in understanding the pathogenesis, but is of little importance clinically in developing a therapeutic plan. If the lesion is somatotrophic cell hyperplasia, it is reasonable to conclude that some disorder in the regulation of GH secretion is etiologic and thus removal of pituitary tissue does not correct the primary defect. Ample evidence for this hypothesis exists since many patients continue to have abnormal or so-called paradoxical GH responses after surgical resection of a "tumor" in spite of a significant drop in basal GH levels, frequently into the normal range. Alternatively, if the tissue specimen is a typical adenoma, one might conclude that it arose de novo within the pituitary gland, and resection of the adenoma cures the disease. There are many examples of patients reported in the literature wherein GH secretory dynamics are completely normal postoperatively. These two hypotheses are not mutually exclusive since one could envision a period of somatotrophic cell hyperplasia that progresses to adenoma formation.

An additional pathogenetic mechanism for disordered GH regulation is ectopic hormone production. Clinicians now well recognize that ectopic GH releasing hormone (GHRH) production can occur typically from pancreatic islet cell tumors and carcinoid tumors. In addition, sporadic reports of ectopic GH production have appeared in the literature, including one extensively evaluated patient in which this entity seems clearly established.

THERAPY

The therapeutic goals of the treatment of acromegaly are twofold; first, reduction of GH secretion, which corrects the multiple sequelae including soft tissue hyperplasia, visceromegaly, and diabetes mellitus, and second, reduction in the size of a pituitary tumor and correction of visual impairment and other neurologic symptoms. The therapeutic approaches in my opinion are surgery and radiotherapy that are intended to be definitive, followed by medical approaches that are adjunctive.

Surgery

When a tumor in the anterior pituitary is identified in the acromegalic patient by current state-of-the-art computed tomography or magnetic resonance imaging, the treatment of choice is surgery. Absence of an identifiable tumor precludes this approach because "exploratory" pituitary surgery is inappropriate for this disease. The advent of the transsphenoidal approach to pituitary surgery has significantly increased the role of surgery in pituitary diseases because the morbidity and mortality of the procedure is far less than the transfrontal approach. In patients with small tumors that are completely within the sella turcica, stage I (microadenomas, 10 mm or less), or larger intrasellar tumors with suprasellar extension, stage II, the success rate of surgery as defined by a fall in basal GH to normal is 75 to 90 percent with the highest success rate in stage I tumors. The results can be rather dramatic: GH levels may fall within hours, and soft tissue signs begin to disappear within weeks. In patients with stage III and IV tumors, the results of surgery are more disappointing, and at best only 50 percent of patients note normalization or significant lowering of GH levels. The choice of operative intervention as primary therapy, and the approach, i.e., transsphenoidal or transfrontal, is made by the anatomic characteristics of the tumor. Generally tumors with extensive lateral extension need a transfrontal approach, whereas those extending anteriorly and inferiorly into the sphenoid sinus may be approached transsphenoidally. Tumors with extensive midline suprasellar extension and visual impairment are best treated by surgical decompression and subsequent radiotherapy, rather than primary radiotherapy, which is relatively contraindicated by the presence of optic nerve involvement.

Mortality is unusual with transsphenoidal surgery, generally less than 2 percent, whereas it is higher with the transfrontal approach; however, the latter is reserved for more complicated patients. Morbidity is also unusual with transsphenoidal surgery, being limited mainly to cerebrospinal fluid rhinorrhea and/or meningitis, with rare visual impairment. The transfrontal approach of course adds the possibility of postoperative seizures. In addition, postoperative hypopituitarism is a concern, most commonly in those patients in whom preoperative function was impaired; however, up to 10 to 15 percent of patients develop hypopituitarism secondary to transsphenoidal surgery. In contrast, up to 40 percent of patients with preoperative impairment of pituitary function have been reported to regain function postoperatively.

In those unusual patients with ectopic production of GHRH or GH, the therapeutic approach is surgical resection of the tumor source where feasible.

Radiotherapy

The second line of definitive therapy is conventional radiotherapy with doses between 4,000 and 5,000 rads delivered generally over a 6-week course. Most reported studies indicate that significant reductions in basal GH levels occur in approximately 50 percent of patients in the first posttherapy year and in 75 to 80 percent by the end of the second year. Occasionally a patient does not achieve meaningful results for 3 to 5 years. Unfortunately, much of the data in the literature is oriented to a therapeutic endpoint of basal GH levels less than 10 ng per milliliter. With the advent of transsphenoidal surgery, fewer patients have been treated primarily with radiotherapy in recent years when the more stringent criterion of lower basal GH levels has been applied. The reason for this newer therapeutic goal is discussed next.

Radiotherapy is also used as an adjunct to surgery in patients with large tumors, particularly when longstanding optic nerve involvement exists, wherein surgery is used to reduce the tumor size prior to radiation.

Complications of radiotherapy are predominantly endocrine, with an incidence of panhypopituitarism in the range of 20 percent. Deficiencies of luteinizing hormone and follicle-stimulating hormone alone are more common with a reported incidence of up to 50 to 60 percent. Other complications, including optic nerve injury; hypothalamic injury; and skin, bone, or soft tissue injury are rare with available equipment and dosing schedules.

Medical Therapy

The use of currently available pharmacologic agents is adjunctive for patients who have had an unsuccessful surgical result or are awaiting the effects of radiotherapy. Bromocriptine, a potent dopamine agonist, is the available agent and is well known for its efficacy in prolactin-secreting disorders. Unfortunately, only 30 to 50 percent of acromegalic patients sustain a fall in GH levels adequate to achieve clinical improvement. This fall is obtained with significant side effects of nausea, often recurring after careful titration from a low starting dose of 1.25 to 2.50 mg per day because of the need to use high doses of 20 mg per day or more to achieve an effect. The likelihood of success with this agent can be enhanced by a determination of the acute GH response to bromocriptine, or alternatively, by the use of the agent in patients with a "paradoxical" GH suppression by oral L-dopa. In some patients wherein a biochemical response occurs, it is possible that a reduction in tumor size occurs as is often the case with prolactinomas.

An analog of somatostatin, SMS 201-995, which has a longer half-life than natural somatostatin, may also hold some promise. This agent was recently released as Octreotide, for the treatment of metastatic carcinoid and vasoactive intestinal polypeptide-secreting tumors. The agent has been reported to decrease GH and somatomedin-C in approximately 75 percent of treated patients. A regimen of 100 μg every 8 hours appears to be optimal, and increasing the dose does not enhance effectiveness, whereas less frequent administration does reduce efficacy. This dose is not associated with a suppression of insulin such that diabetes mellitus is worsened and, furthermore, is not followed by rebound GH hypersecretion. Unfortunately, cholelithiasis is a significant side effect, and the need for frequent injection and cost may be a problem. At present, the Food and Drug Administration has not approved Octreotide for the treatment of acromegaly, so this agent is still considered investigational.

MONITORING OF THERAPEUTIC RESULTS

The definitive approach to the treatment of acromegaly is surgical resection of a pituitary tumor where a tumor is clearly demonstrated. In the absence of a tumor, radiotherapy is the primary therapy. In patients with extensive tumors, a combination of surgery and radiotherapy may be employed. Occasionally it is necessary to try medical therapy as an adjunct to definitive approaches where they were unsuccessful or when awaiting a clinical response.

The results of therapy are generally monitored by following basal GH concentrations, in addition to symptoms and physical signs. Optimally, basal GH levels should be less than 5 ng per milliliter. When the levels are higher, and in some patients with basal levels less than 5 ng per milliliter, the disease clearly remains active, albeit improved. One explanation for this continued activity is the continued abnormal GH secretory dynamics, e.g., a rise following meals, which would account for an increased mean GH concentration throughout the day. Measurement of somatomedin-C levels, which are dependent upon the mean level of GH, are often confirmatory of this situation. In general, somatomedin-C levels are useful as an additional mode of biochemical monitoring of acromegaly.

Finally, the numerous conditions that often accompany acromegaly need therapeutic intervention, and an awareness of the increased incidence of neoplasia in acromegalic patients must be borne in mind.

SUGGESTED READING

Baskin DS, Boggan JE, Wilson CB. Transsphenoidal microsurgical removal of growth hormone-secreting pituitary adenomas. A review of 137 cases. J Neurosurg 1982;56:634–641.

Eskildsen PC, Svendsen PA, Vang L, Nerup J. Long-term treatment of acromegaly with bromocryptine. Acta Endocrinol (Copenh) 1978;87:687–700.
Guillemin R, Brazeau P, Bohlen P, Esch F, Ling N, Wehrenberg WB. Growth hormone-releasing factor from a human pancreatic tumor that caused acromegaly. Science 1982;218:585–587.
Ho KY, Weissberger AJ, Marbach P, Lazarus L. Therapeutic efficacy of the somatostatin analog SMS 201-995 (Octreotide) in acromegaly. Ann Intern Med 1990;112:173–181.
Klein I. Acromegaly and cancer. Ann Intern Med 1984;101:706–707.
Lamberts SWJ, Uitterlinden P, Verschoor L, Van Dongen KJ, Del Pozo E. Long-term treatment of acromegaly with the somatostatin analogue. SMS 201–995. N Engl J Med 1985;313:1576–1580.
Melmed S, Brownstein GD, Horvath E, Ezrin C, Kovacs K. Pathophysiology of acromegaly. Endocr Rev 1983;4:271–290.
Melmed S, Ezrin C, Kovacs K, Goodman RS, Frohman LA. Acromegaly due to secretion of growth hormone by an ectopic pancreatic islet-cell tumor. N Engl J Med 1985;312:9–17.

PROLACTINOMA

ASHLEY GROSSMAN, B.A., B.Sc., M.D., M.R.C.P.
MICHAEL BESSER, D.Sc., M.D., F.R.C.P.

Hyperprolactinemia may be defined as the persistent elevation of serum prolactin outside of the normal range. Transient elevations of circulating prolactin may follow many drugs, surgery, exercise, food, and certain types of stress, such that fasting levels from rested supine subjects taken with minimal trauma are necessary to establish the diagnosis. Furthermore, since serum prolactin rises nocturnally, a standardized time of sampling may be important, especially when samples are taken on repeated occasions. There has been some discussion as to the upper limit of the normal range for serum prolactin, and this limit is rendered difficult to establish because standards and other laboratory reagents vary and because the distribution is skewed with a "tail" extending up to 800 to 1,000 mU per liter (40 to 50 ng per milliliter). However, we accept an upper limit of the normal range as 360 mU per liter (18 ng per milliliter); values persistently above this level require further investigation.

CAUSES OF HYPERPROLACTINEMIA

Although hyperprolactinemia may result from a variety of conditions, few of these give rise to any diagnostic confusion (Table 1). In the case of drugs increasing serum prolactin by interfering with the synthesis and release of dopamine (reserpine, methyldopa) or its pituitary action (major tranquilizers, antiemetics), levels of circulating prolactin up to 5,000 mU per liter (250 ng per milliliter) may be achieved. In most instances, a trial of stopping treatment is the only way in which to establish whether or not the high serum prolactin is secondary to the drug therapy. Similarly, in patients with primary hypothyroidism and hyperprolactinemia, a prolonged trial with thyroxine is necessary since there is evidence that the elevated serum prolactin associated with hypothyroidism may take many months to fall to within the normal range, considerably longer than for the fall in thyroid-stimulating hormone (TSH). Patients with

TABLE 1 The Causes of Hyperprolactinemia

Physiologic
Sleep
Coitus
Stress
Psychological (e.g., fear)
Physical (e.g., exercise)
Nipple stimulation
Pregnancy
Suckling
Pathologic
Diseases of the pituitary
Prolactinoma
Combined prolactin/growth hormone–secreting tumors
Empty sella syndrome
Functionless pituitary tumors producing stalk-vessel obstruction
Disease of the hypothalamus
Craniopharyngioma
Sarcoidosis; tuberculoma
Encephalitis
Irradiation
Head trauma
Germinoma ("pinealoma")
Metastatic or primary neoplasm
Histiocytosis X
Rathke's pouch cyst
Surgical stalk section
Irritative lesions of chest wall
Herpes zoster
Chest trauma
Thoracic burns
Drug-induced
Dopamine receptor antagonist
Chlorpromazine
Pimozide
Haloperidol
Metoclopramide
Sulpiride
Domperidone
Estrogens
Reserpine
Methyldopa
Opiates
Miscellaneous
Hypothyroidism
Chronic renal failure

hyperprolactinemia secondary to renal failure show a diminution in dopamine sensitivity at the level of the lactotroph, such that the production rate of prolactin increases in addition to its fall in clearance. Although hyperprolactinemia responds well to treatment with bromocriptine (see next section), researchers have suggested recently that the hyperprolactinemia may be secondary to zinc deficiency and so may respond to dietary supplementation with zinc. Finally, modestly elevated levels of serum prolactin, usually less than 1,000 mU per liter (50 ng per milliliter), are frequently seen in patients with polycystic ovary or Stein-Leventhal syndrome. Some of these patients show a normalization of serum prolactin following conventional therapy aimed at lowering the elevated free androgens characteristic of the syndrome. However, since prolactin itself may increase certain adrenal androgens such as dehydroepiandrosterone-sulfate (DHA-S), direct treatment of the hyperprolactinemia with bromocriptine may also be necessary.

PROLACTINOMAS

In the absence of any obvious cause, hyperprolactinemia is usually assumed to be secondary to a prolactin-secreting microadenoma, a microprolactinoma. These tumors are common, occurring in about 10 percent of an unselected population, but only become manifest if the secretory rate of the tumor is greater than the secretion rate of the normal pituitary. It is becoming increasingly clear that many cases of so-called "functional hyperprolactinemia" are also manifestations of prolactinomas, and it remains dubious if any truly functional syndromes actually exist. We consider that the optimum first-line therapy of patients with microprolactinomas is dopamine agonist therapy, most commonly bromocriptine. The majority of such patients respond to bromocriptine with a fall in serum prolactin to within the normal range and a consequent improvement in symptomatology (usually galactorrhea, menstrual irregularity, infertility and dyspareunia in women, and impotence in men). However, it is essential that the bromocriptine be given according to a precise regimen in order to avoid side effects after the start of treatment. Bromocriptine activates dopamine receptors in the central nervous system (CNS), including the area postrema, as well as on the pituitary lactotrophs, and so bromocriptine may cause side effects such as nausea and vomiting and postural hypotension. These adverse effects diminish due to tachyphylaxis and thus can be frequently abolished, and always minimized, if the drug is increased in dosage gradually and always given in the middle of a bulk meal in order to delay absorption. We find that a dose of 1.25 mg taken in the middle of an evening snack just before retiring is useful for initiation of therapy; in the absence of side effects, this dose is moved forwards to the middle of the evening meal after 3 to 7 days. A second daily dose of 1.25 mg is added after a further 3 to 7 days in the middle of breakfast or lunch, and the dose thereafter gradually increases at intervals until the serum prolactin becomes normal. This normal level of prolactin is usually achieved at a dose of 2.5 mg twice or three times a day. When a therapeutic dose has been obtained, it may be possible to transfer the total daily requirement to a once-daily administration.

Occasionally, patients are unable to tolerate bromocriptine due to persistent side effects despite correct introduction of therapy. These side effects may also include those due to the alpha-adrenergic receptor blocking activity of bromocriptine, such as nasal congestion, as well as central actions such as drowsiness, whereas psychiatric disturbances (including the rare psychosis) may occur on any dopamine agent. Alternative preparations may produce fewer of the side effects in occasional patients, although none is generally available except on a clinical trial basis: lisuride is shorter acting than bromocriptine and is more prone to induce nausea and vomiting; pergolide has the advantage of a long duration of action at conventional doses; and transdihydrolisuride (terguride) may generally be better tolerated. There is some evidence that the ergot, cabergoline, may last for several days after a single dose. Another approach is to administer bromocriptine as a single 50-mg depot injection (Parlodel LAR), which produces a rapid rise in circulating bromocriptine that is maintained for 4 to 6 weeks. Any side effects are then experienced within the first 24 hours, and thereafter the patient may be transferred to a therapeutic dose of oral bromocriptine at 2 to 4 weeks. In our experience, this method has allowed many apparently intolerant patients to be initiated onto oral bromocriptine when other methods have failed. For patients unable or unwilling to take oral medication, this injectable formulation may be repeated at monthly intervals.

Even more infrequently, some patients are found relatively or totally resistant to the effects of oral bromocriptine and are noted to have a clinically insignificant fall in serum prolactin even when high doses (i.e., 20 to 60 mg daily) are given. In order to differentiate this from patient noncompliance, it has been found that serum prolactin measured 24 to 48 hours after a single dose of depot bromocriptine is a reliable guide to the prolactin level likely to be achieved on high-dose oral therapy. Such resistance to bromocriptine in almost all cases generalizes to other dopamine agonist drugs. In such patients, as well as in patients intolerant of all modalities of dopamine agonist therapy, transsphenoidal microadenomectomy may be considered (Fig. 1). In this relatively minor procedure, the pituitary is approached either pernasally or retrolabially, and the adenoma selectively removed while leaving the normal pituitary intact. In experienced hands, this procedure produces an immediate "cure" rate (i.e., a normalization of serum prolactin) of 70 to 90 percent, although the figure falls as the preoperative serum prolactin rises, especially over 4,000 mU per liter (200 ng per milliliter). Complications of the procedure are uncommon, but may be serious: these include damage to local structures, cerebrospinal fluid (CSF) rhinorrhea, and meningitis. Hypopituitarism is also infrequent in the case of microprolactinomas, but transient diabetes insipidus is more commonly seen (about 10 percent) and may some-

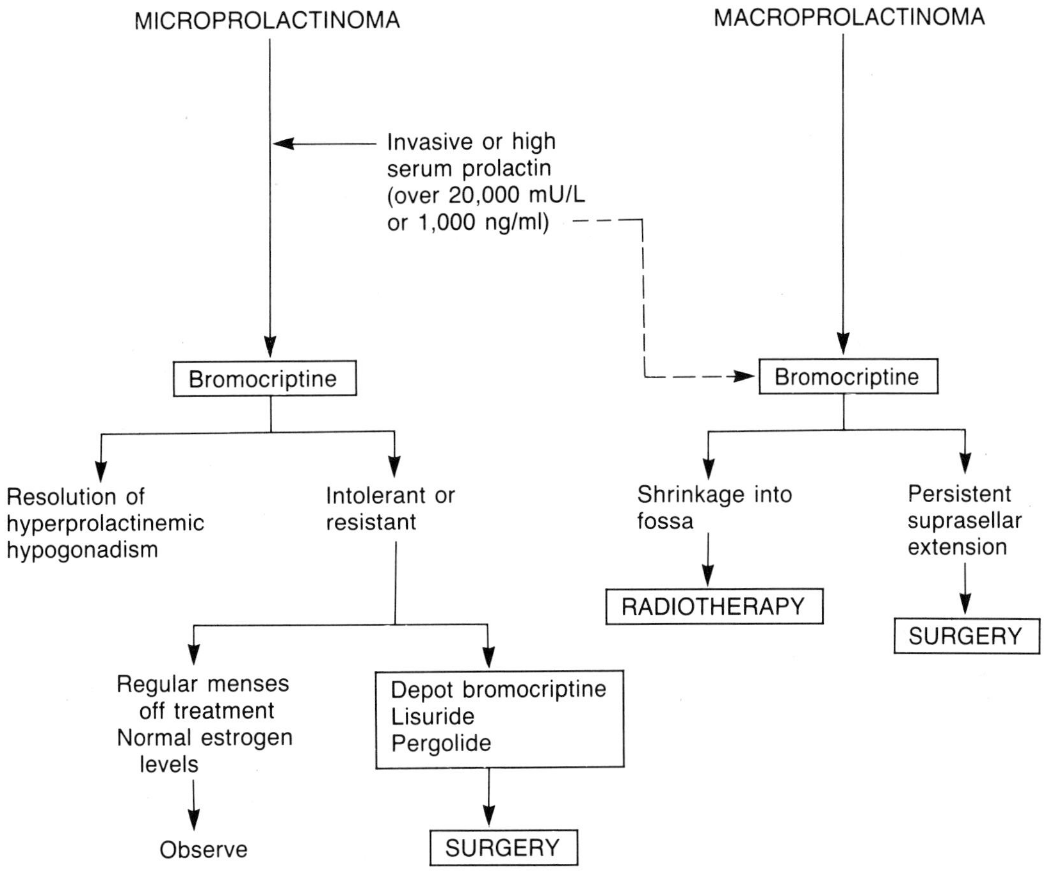

Figure 1 Possible management pathways after CT scanning in a patient with a prolactinoma. Note: All patients, especially following surgery or radiotherapy, require long-term follow-up.

times be permanent. More importantly, recent data have suggested that there is a high rate of recurrence following such surgery, and patients may exhibit 40 to 50 percent recurrent hyperprolactinemia at 5 years postoperation (not all centers agree with these figures). Therefore, our practice is to advise transsphenoidal surgery only when other therapeutic options have failed or are inapplicable.

In patients unresponsive to dopamine agonist therapy, the question arises as to whether hyperprolactinemia always requires treatment. The natural history of the microprolactinoma is generally benign, with few patients showing progressive increases in tumor size or secretion even over many years of follow-up. Also, a minority of patients show a spontaneous normalization of their elevated serum prolactin over time; this normalization appears to be particularly common post partum and when the initial serum prolactin is less than 2,000 mU per liter (100 ng per milliliter). However, an elevated serum prolactin may cause subtle changes in mood, libido, and weight, and we consider that every patient with persistent hyperprolactinemia and oligo- or amenorrhea should have at least a trial of dopamine agonist therapy. Furthermore, it has been clearly shown that the estrogen deficiency secondary to hyperprolactinemia (and androgen deficiency in men) is associated with long-term osteoporosis. In our opinion, an elevated serum prolactin in a female should always be treated unless she has a normal plasma estradiol and she is having menses at least in alternate months. Even then, it would be prudent to assess the patient at 6-month or yearly intervals for any evidence of tumor progression.

Macroprolactinomas

Every patient with hyperprolactinemia should have a good quality plain skull roentgenogram (posteroanterior and lateral) and preferably a high-resolution computed tomography (CT) scan prior to treatment. A macroprolactinoma is defined as a prolactin-secreting pituitary tumor greater than 1 cm in diameter and may extend out of the fossa to invade the cavernous sinuses or suprasellar space to produce characteristic clinical features. In such cases, our first-line treatment is the use of dopamine agonist therapy to normalize the serum prolactin and induce tumor shrinkage, as upwards of 75 percent of such tumors regress in size on such treatment. Local compressive symptoms often improve days or even hours after the initiation of therapy, and marked tumor shrinkage is usually evident within 4 to 6 weeks. Although there is some debate as to whether further shrinkage may be obtained beyond this time, we have observed progressive diminution in size of prolactinomas over many months of treatment. However, when tumor mass has clearly attained a plateau, definitive therapy is required since dopamine agonist therapy alone is rarely curative. There are scattered reports of irreversible tumor necrosis following bromocriptine, but most observers have reported a recrudescence of the hyperprolactinemia and reexpansion of the tumor mass when the bromocriptine is stopped. We would advise external beam radiotherapy delivered as 45 Gy (4,500 rads) from a linear accelerator in daily fractions of less than 2 Gy (200 rads) via three portals: this minimizes medium-term sequelae such as hypopituitarism and avoids long-term sequelae such as radiologic damage to surrounding structures or oncogenesis. However, where there is still evidence of extrasellar tumor extension involvement, despite an adequate trial of dopamine agonist therapy, surgical decompression (transsphenoidal where possible, otherwise transfrontal) is required prior to radiotherapy (see Fig. 1). Surgical treatment alone may occasionally render the patient normoprolactinemic, but there is a high risk of recurrence of macroadenomas that approaches 100 percent by 10 years. Radiotherapy not only reduces this risk to at least below 10 percent, and probably less than 5 percent, but also produces a gradual decline in tumor prolactin secretion such that one may eventually be able to stop bromocriptine altogether after 2 to 10 years. Although radiotherapy always produces growth hormone deficiency within 2 years, this deficiency appears to be of no consequence in adults. Gonadotropin deficiency may develop, but this deficiency is not usually seen for several years. TSH and adrenocorticotropic hormone (ACTH) deficiencies develop only exceptionally within the first 10 years, although there are few long-term data. In addition to prevention of tumor regrowth after mass reduction, radiotherapy also protects against macroprolactinoma enlargement that may otherwise occur during pregnancy.

Some authorities have suggested that long-term dopamine agonist therapy to shrink prolactinomas may increase the fibrous tissue content of these tumors and thus heighten the risk and morbidity of any subsequent operative intervention. We can only repeat that this has not been the general experience, and the decrease in tumor mass seen in the majority of prolactinomas after bromocriptine may obviate the need for operative intervention and increase the accessibility of such tumors still requiring surgical debulking.

Pseudoprolactinomas

In the case of large pituitary tumors, hyperprolactinemia may be secondary either to true tumor secretion or to disturbance of the portal vasculature leading to compression of the stalk and disruption of the delivery of dopamine to the lactotrophs. Such tumors, which may include "functionless" pituitary tumors, craniopharyngiomas, and granulomas, may thus be associated with (but not actively secreting) high levels of prolactin; levels of up to 8,000 mU per liter (400 ng per milliliter) have been recorded with these so-called "pseudoprolactinomas." It is important to realize that although these pseudoprolactinomas rarely shrink significantly with bromocriptine, normalization of an elevated serum prolactin may still give rise to remission of many clinical symptoms. We consider that any large pituitary tumor with an extrasellar extension that is associated with a serum prolactin below 1,000 mU per liter (50 ng per milliliter) is unlikely to be a prolactinoma and should be treated surgically in the first instance. As the serum prolactin progressively increases above 1,000 mU per liter, the probability increases that the tumor is a prolactinoma and may thus shrink with dopamine agonist therapy. We therefore treat all such patients with levels above 1,000 mU per liter initially with bromocriptine, while carefully monitoring the pressure symptoms of the patient, especially the visual pathways, for evidence of a change in tumor size. If, after 4 to 6 weeks, there is unequivocal evidence in favor of a regression in size, we would advise continuation with this treatment and monitoring of further shrinkage. No response by 6 weeks, or a progression in visual loss before that time, demands urgent surgical decompression.

Prolactinoma and Pregnancy

There has been considerable debate as to the risk of a prolactinoma enlarging during pregnancy sufficient to cause a symptomatic disturbance, i.e., severe headache or visual loss. The consensus view would be that pregnancy-related tumor expansion approaches 20 percent in the case of macroprolactinomas and is less (possibly much less) than 5 percent for microprolactinomas. We have suggested that the definitive therapy for macroprolactinomas should be external-beam radiotherapy since this therapy abolishes the risk of pregnancy-related problems. However, there is a risk in the medium-term that this therapy induces hypogonadism, which must be taken into account when arranging the precise timing of any treatment plan. For microprolactinomas, radiotherapy is unnecessary.

We advise patients starting on bromocriptine to use mechanical contraception in order to establish regular ovulatory cycles; when three such cycles have been documented, contraception may be stopped. When a menstrual period is 2 to 3 days overdue, a sensitive test for serum human chorionic gonadotropin (hCG) establishes conception and allows bromocriptine to be stopped. We then monitor the patient during pregnancy for symptoms (e.g., headache) and signs (e.g., field defects) of tumor expansion. In the unlikely event of an expansion being demonstrated, oral bromocriptine can be reinstituted since it shrinks the tumor during pregnancy and may be continued up to, and beyond, delivery. If giving bromocriptine during pregnancy proves essential, the patient may be reassured that there is no evidence of teratogenicity. Nevertheless, we do not recommend that bromocriptine is routinely continued during pregnancy, but is used only when there is a positive indication. In an uncomplicated pregnancy, the question as to whether or not the patient should be advised to breast feed is a difficult one because there is an increased (albeit small) risk of galactocele formation and subsequent mastitis; the physician needs to take the needs and concerns of the mother closely into account in formulating the appropriate advice.

Postpartum pituitary reassessment including a repeat CT scan demonstrates if pregnancy has produced either progression or regression in the prolactinoma, thus altering the requirements for treatment.

In untreated patients with prolactinomas, an estrogen-containing oral contraceptive may induce further tumor growth and should never be used alone. Once patients have a normal serum prolactin on treatment, the oral contraceptive may be carefully used so long as the patient remains on bromocriptine and her serum prolactin is checked regularly.

SUGGESTED READING

Grossman A, Besser GM. Regular review: prolactinomas. Br Med J 1985; 290:182–184.

Molitch ME. Pregnancy and the hyperprolactinemic woman. N Engl J Med 1984; 310:1364–1370.

Randall RV, Laws ER, Abboud CF, Ebersold MJ, Kao PC, Scheithauer BW. Transsphenoidal microsurgical treatment of prolactin-secreting pituitary adenomas, results in 100 patients. Mayo Clin Proc 1983; 58:108–121.

Serri O, Rasio E, Beauregard H, Hardy J, Somma M. Recurrence of hyperprolactinemia after selective transsphenoidal adenomectomy in women with prolactinoma. N Engl J Med 1983; 309:280–283.

Sheline GE, Grossman A, Jones AE, Besser GM. Radiation therapy for prolactinomas. In: Secretory tumors of the pituitary gland. New York: Raven Press, 1984:93.

Vance ML, Evans WS, Thorner MO. Bromocriptine. Ann Int Med 1984; 100:78–91.

DIABETES INSIPIDUS

JOSEPH G. VERBALIS, M.D.
ALAN G. ROBINSON, M.D.

Diabetes insipidus is literally the excretion of a dilute (tasteless) urine. Once an osmotic diuresis is excluded, hypotonic polyuria may be caused by the absence of vasopressin (hypothalamic, or central, diabetes insipidus), lack of renal response to vasopressin (nephrogenic diabetes insipidus), or physiologic suppression of vasopressin in response to ingestion of water (primary polydipsia). We have assumed that appropriate testing to allow accurate differential diagnoses between these three conditions is accomplished prior to beginning therapy. We have also assumed that the etiology for the lack of vasopressin (tumor, trauma, infiltrative disease, or idiopathic) has been diagnosed and treated appropriately.

GOALS

Maintain a Normal Life Style

Most patients with diabetes insipidus have an intact thirst mechanism and are able to drink sufficient water to maintain a relatively normal state of metabolic balance. Since lack of vasopressin per se does not cause progressive morbidity nor secondary complications in other vital systems, in many cases the major manifestation is the inconvenience of thirst and frequent urination. Therefore therapeutic agents should be effective in the prevention of polyuria and nocturia, convenient for the patient's life style, and easy for the patient to administer and monitor. The patient should have sufficient knowledge of the mechanism of the therapy so that he or she can be flexible with dosage and timing depending upon daily activities. Finally, because of the benign course of the disorder, the safety of any therapy must be an overriding consideration. Additionally, even with the use of safe and effective therapy, overtreatment should be avoided because the side effects from this are often more detrimental than from undertreatment.

Control of Potentially Life-Threatening Situations

The benign nature of diabetes insipidus is predicated on the ability of the patient to respond appropriately to an intact thirst center. In any situation in which the patient is either unable to sense thirst or unable to respond by drinking water, the disease is potentially life-threatening. If the patient becomes unconscious (e.g., after an accident), no abnormality may be noted when first seen by a physician because of the persistent effect of therapy. However, as the therapeutic agent reaches its normal duration of pharmacologic effect, polyuria may recur abruptly, and the large volumes of urine may produce severe dehydration and cardiovascular collapse in just a few hours. To avoid this threat, every patient with diabetes insipidus should carry a medical card indicating that diabetes insipidus is present and should wear a Medic-Alert tag indicating the disorder. Diabetes insipidus is rare, and in an emergency the patient may be seen by a physician who is unfamiliar with the disorder, and so the Medic-Alert tag and card should indicate that vasopressin may need to be administered and should also contain the name and telephone number of a physician who is familiar with the disorder, has been involved in the therapy of the patient, and can be contacted.

AVAILABLE AGENTS

Water

Water is listed as an agent to treat diabetes insipidus to emphasize that water alone taken in sufficient quantity corrects any metabolic abnormality secondary to diabetes insipidus. All of the therapies described next are designed to reduce the amount of water intake necessary to a tolerable level. The tolerable level of water intake varies from patient to patient and from day to day in a given patient. The physician (and a knowledgeable patient) should not be disturbed that occasional lapses in pharmacologic treatment require temporary increases in water ingestion. In fact, such lapses are at times beneficial in order to avoid overtreatment and subsequent water intoxication.

Antidiuretic Hormones

L-Arginine Vasopressin

L-Arginine vasopressin is the natural vasopressin of man and all mammals except the pig.

Aqueous vasopressin is a buffered solution of L-arginine vasopressin, which can be given parenterally. It is provided in 1-ml snap-top vials at a concentration of 20 U per milliliter. It is usually given subcutaneously with an onset of action within 1 to 2 hours and duration of effect from 4 to 8 hours. Intravenous bolus administration should be avoided because of an even shorter duration of action and because of potential pressor effects (hypertension, angina).

1-(3-Mercaptopropionic Acid) -8-D-Arginine-Vasopressin (Desmopressin)

Desmopressin is a synthetic analog of L-arginine vasopressin in which the terminal amino group of cystine has been removed and dextro-arginine has been substituted for levo-arginine in position 8. Removal of the terminal amine prolongs the half-life of the drug in plasma, and substitution of D for L-arginine in position 8 reduces the pressor activity. The agent is approximately 2,000 times more specific for prolonged antidiuresis than is natural L-arginine vasopressin. Desmopressin for clinical use is available for administration intranasally, subcutaneously, or intravenously. The intranasal preparation is a buffered aqueous solution containing 100 μg per milliliter. Fifty to 200 μl can be loaded into a soft plastic tube and administered by blowing into the nose. The onset of action is rapid, and the duration of effect is from 6 to 24 hours. Despite this large range of duration of effect between individuals, in a given patient the effect of similarly administered doses is reproducible. Desmopressin is also available in 2-ml vials of 4 μg per milliliter for parenteral injection. When administered parenterally, 5 to 10 percent of the agent produces an effect similar to that produced when administered intranasally.

Lysine Vasopressin

Lysine vasopressin is the naturally occurring vasopressin of the pig. A synthetic form is available in an aqueous buffer of 50 U per milliliter to be used as a nasal spray. The agent comes in a plastic atomizer bottle and can be sprayed directly into each nostril. Absorption of the vasopressin occurs rapidly across the nasal mucosa, but the duration of effect is only 2 to 6 hours.

Orally Administered Pharmacologic Agents

Chlorpropamide

Chlorpropamide (Diabinese) was discovered by serendipity to decrease free water excretion in patients with diabetes insipidus. The major action is to enhance the effect of vasopressin on the renal tubule by increasing the hydroosmotic action of vasopressin. In experimental studies, vasopressin is necessary for chlorpropamide to exert its antidiuretic effect; therefore the drug is most often used in patients with partial diabetes insipidus and some ability to secrete vasopressin. The usual dose is 100 to 500 mg orally per day, and maximum antidiuresis is observed after 4 days of therapy. One must be cautious of the development of hypoglycemia when treating diabetes insipidus, especially in children and in cases of concurrent hypopituitarism.

Carbamazepine

Carbamazepine (Tegretol) has been shown to cause the release of antidiuretic hormone in patients with partial diabetes insipidus. The dosage used is 200 to 600 mg per day. Before prescribing this drug, the physician should be thoroughly familiar with the potential toxicity.

Clofibrate

Clofibrate (Atromid-S) has also been shown to stimulate the release of endogenous arginine vasopressin. Patients with partial diabetes insipidus may respond to 500 mg every 6 hours with a decreased urinary volume. However, because of the possibility of an increased incidence of gallbladder disease and carcinoma in patients taking clofibrate, the agent cannot be recommended for routine treatment of diabetes insipidus.

Thiazide Diuretics

Thiazides are usually thought of as diuretic rather than antidiuretic agents, but they also decrease urine volumes in patients with both hypothalamic and nephrogenic diabetes insipidus. The mechanism is clearly different than that of the other oral agents and is probably secondary to primary natriuresis with subsequent volume contraction, decreased ultrafiltrate, and increased proximal tubular reabsorption of salt and water. Hydrochlorothiazide at a dose of 50 to 100 mg per day is usually sufficient. Potassium replacement should be given as necessary to prevent hypokalemia.

Indomethacin (Indocin)

Prostaglandin E in the renal medulla is thought to inhibit the action of vasopressin. Indomethacin, which decreases the concentration of medullary prostaglandin E, results in an increased responsiveness of the distal tubule to vasopressin and enhances the effect of administered antidiuretic hormones. Although this should not be considered primary therapy for diabetes insipidus, it is important to be aware of this action in those patients for whom the drug is prescribed for other reasons.

CLINICAL SITUATIONS

Acute Postsurgical Diabetes Insipidus

Acute postsurgical diabetes insipidus occurs frequently following surgery in the hypothalamic pituitary area. Often the patient is receiving high doses of glucocorticoids, and hyperglycemia with glycosuria may confuse the initial diagnosis of diabetes insipidus. Once the diagnosis is ascertained, the only pharmacologic therapy is an antidiuretic hormone. However, since many neurosurgeons fear water overload and brain edema after this type of surgery, the patient is sometimes treated with intravenous fluid replacement for a considerable time prior to the use of an antidiuretic hormone. If the patient is awake and able to respond to thirst, one can treat with an antidiuretic hormone and allow the patient's thirst to be the guide for water replacement. If the patient is unable to respond to thirst, either from a decreased level of consciousness or from hypothalamic damage to the thirst center, fluid balance may need to be maintained by intravenously administered fluid. Urine osmolality and serum sodium *must* be checked every several hours during the initial therapy and then at least daily until stabilization or resolution of the diabetes insipidus. One must also be careful with water replacement because excess water during continued administration of vasopressin can create a syndrome of inappropriate antidiuresis and potentially severe hyponatremia.

In some cases, transient postoperative diabetes insipidus is part of a "triphasic" pattern that has been described with stalk section. The initial diabetes insipidus (first phase) is due to axon shock and lack of function of the damaged neurons. This phase lasts from several hours to several days and is followed by an antidiuretic phase (second phase) that is due to the uncontrolled release of vasopressin from the disconnected posterior pituitary or from the remaining severed neurons. Overly aggressive administration of fluids during this second interphase does not suppress the vasopressin and leads to hyponatremia. Antidiuresis lasts 2 to 14 days, at which time the diabetes insipidus (third phase) may return.

Postoperatively, desmopressin for parenteral administration may be given in a dose of 1 to 4 μg subcutaneously or intramuscularly. Prompt reduction in urine output should be experienced, and the duration of effect is 6 to 24 hours. Usually the patient is hypernatremic with a dilute urine when therapy is started. One should follow the urine osmolality and urine volume to be certain the dose was effective and check the serum sodium to insure some improvement of hypernatremia. We allow some return of polyuria prior to administration of subsequent doses of desmopressin (unless the polyuria occurs during the night) because postoperative diabetes insipidus is often transient. If diabetes insipidus persists, the patient is switched to maintenance therapy for chronic disease, as described next.

Acute Traumatic Diabetes Insipidus

Acute traumatic diabetes insipidus can occur after an injury to the head, usually an automobile accident. Diabetes insipidus is more common with injuries to the lateral skull that result in a shearing action on the pituitary stalk and/or cause hemorrhagic ischemia of the hypothalamus and posterior pituitary. After head trauma the diabetes insipidus is recognized by hypotonic polyuria in the face of an increased serum osmolality. Management is similar to postsurgical diabetes insipidus as outlined previously with the exception that the possibility of anterior pituitary insufficiency must be considered and the patient given stress doses of hydrocortisone until anterior pituitary function can be definitively evaluated.

Chronic Complete Diabetes Insipidus

Complete diabetes insipidus describes cases in which there is no vasopressin in the circulation and no ability to concentrate urine with a standard dehydration test. These patients require replacement with some form of antidiuretic hormone. The treatment of choice is desmopressin. First, the patient must be taught to use the rhinyl catheter and to measure an appropriate dose of desmopressin. A solution of saline can be utilized to fill the tubing for practice of administration. Once an appropriately measured dose is in the catheter, the patient can hold it in a U-shape with the two ends in a superior position, allowing the measured dose of hormone to roll to the dependent loop of the tube. The patient then raises the catheter to the mouth and inserts about one-half inch (1.25 cm) into the nostril, being careful to maintain the other end above the nadir of the U. The patient then takes a moderate inspiration and holds his or her breath while placing the other end of the catheter in his or her mouth. Blowing through the catheter with a swift puff as one might imagine doing to blow a ball out of a straw delivers the hormone high into the nose. A physician or assistant trained in the proper use of the rhinyl catheter should train the patient. Inadequate training causes wasted hormone because of dripping out of the end of the catheter, swallowing the hormone, or blowing it into the external nares in a position too low for absorption.

In initiating treatment, having the patient test 50, 100, and 200 μl of the drug is useful. This testing is best done in a controlled environment wherein each voided urine can be measured for volume and osmolality. The next desirable situation would be to measure volume and specific gravity or, as a last resort, volume alone. In fact, measurement of urinary volume can provide a good index of the duration of drug action. The patient is allowed to escape from any previous medication, thereby establishing a baseline polyuria. In patients with complete diabetes insipidus, polyuria returns promptly. Once polyuria of about 4 ml per minute is established, 50 μl of desmopressin is administered. A decrease in urinary volume occurs 1 to 2 hours later. The duration of effect of the dose is 6 to 24 hours, usually around 12 hours. Establishing this duration of action in individual patients is helpful in planning therapy and in assuring the patient (and the physician) that early administration of a second dose of drug (which may be necessary, as described next) does not lead to any adverse effect. If the nasal spray is used, a similar duration of action should be determined.

Having tested three doses of drug, deciding the dose and time of day to administer the drug is necessary. Individualization of this protocol cannot be overemphasized. Occasional patients maintain satisfactory control of urine output with a single dose per day, but most patients require two doses per day. Two small doses per day (e.g., 50 μl) is more cost effective than one large dose (e.g., 200 μl). Since the biologic half-life of desmopressin is about 4 hours, doubling the dose extends the duration only by that amount of time. When a single dose of drug per day is used, many authors suggest that this dose be given at bedtime in order to allow the patient to sleep throughout the night. We find that many patients would rather have the drug administered in the morning in order to allow a full day of work or other activities without interruption for frequent voiding. A single episode of nocturia may be preferable to multiple interruptions of the workday. Where two doses of desmopressin are necessary, the time of administration should again be based upon the activity of the patient for that day. Almost always the first dose should be given in the morning in order to allow an uninterrupted workday. Timing of the second dose should be individualized. If the patient is home for the evening, it is usually best to delay the administration of the second dose until late in the evening in order to allow a full night's sleep. If the patient is going out for the evening and by experience knows that polyuria occurs prior to returning home, it is best to administer the second dose of medication in the late afternoon or early evening in order to allow an evening free of worry about polyuria. If this dose is insufficient to allow an adequate night of sleep, a third dose of medication may be taken on that particular day just prior to bedtime. Three doses of 50 μl taken in this manner are readily accepted by a patient who has already tolerated 200 μl as a single dose during the initiation of therapy.

The obvious danger of a flexible program is the possibility that the patient takes repeated doses of desmopressin to always maintain urine volume at a low output and then becomes volume expanded, natriuretic, and hyponatremic. To avoid this complication, at least once and preferably two to three times a week, the patient should withhold desmopressin until pronounced polyuria recurs with excessive thirst. This procedure guards against hyponatremia occurring from overzealous use of desmopressin and provides ongoing documentation that diabetes insipidus persists. The latter is especially useful in cases of postsurgical or posttraumatic diabetes insipidus where renewed ability to secrete vasopressin may occur within the first year after the initial insult.

The only disadvantage of desmopressin is expense. Because of the expense, some physicians prescribe a combination of an oral agent with administered desmopressin to prolong the action of desmopressin and to decrease the expense. Both chlorpropamide and indomethacin prolong the effect of an administered dose of desmopressin. However, our feeling is that potential complications from agents that are not otherwise indicated make this attempt to decrease the cost of therapy undesirable. It is important to recognize that when any of the oral agents described previously are given for routine medical indications, they may augment the effect of desmopressin and predispose the patient to water retention and hyponatremia. Thus the dose of desmopressin may have to be altered if any such agent is utilized for treatment of another disease.

Chronic Partial Diabetes Insipidus

"Partial" diabetes insipidus refers to patients who have some endogenous secretion of vasopressin, but not a sufficient amount to achieve maximum urinary concentration and to keep the patient asymptomatic regarding polyuria and thirst. Most patients do not become hypernatremic, but do complain of excessive thirst and polyuria. Probably the safest form of therapy for these patients is also desmopressin. The guidelines for initiating and maintaining therapy in partial diabetes insipidus are essentially identical to that described before for the treatment of complete diabetes insipidus with the exception that these patients often tolerate a somewhat less frequent administration of the agent because the intensity of the polyuria and of the thirst is not so severe.

In some of these patients, administration of pharmacologic agents that increase the effectiveness of vasopressin may be preferable. In an occasional patient with the unhappy concurrence of diabetes insipidus and either diabetes mellitus or congestive heart failure, treatment of both diseases with a single agent may be appropriate—chlorpropamide for diabetes mellitus and thiazide diuretics for congestive heart failure. One of these agents is prescribed as necessary to treat the primary disease, e.g., diabetes mellitus or congestive heart failure, and the effect upon the diabetes insipidus is observed. The need for further therapy with an antidiuretic hormone depends upon the response.

If a patient with partial diabetes insipidus is unable to utilize desmopressin because of poor vision or for economic reasons, chlorpropamide is an acceptable alternative. Therapy can be initiated with 100 mg per day and increased every 4 days until appropriate antidiuresis is obtained. Usually little further antidiuresis is obtained by doses above 500 mg per day. When beginning an oral agent, the appropriate index of therapeutic effectiveness is the 24-hour urine volume and the patient's symptomatic response in terms of thirst. In patients with coexistent panhypopituitarism and lack of adrenocorticotropic hormone (ACTH) and growth hormone, the increased potential for hypoglycemia during treatment with chlorpropamide must be recognized, and frequent feedings given and routine blood sugars obtained. In mild cases of partial diabetes insipidus, a trial of thiazide diuretics may be undertaken. Some patients have sufficient reduction of urine output and decrease of thirst on this agent alone, so that they are satisfactorily controlled.

We do not use clofibrate or carbamazepine for the treatment of partial diabetes insipidus. In our opinion, the side effects of each of these agents are too great to justify their use to treat a disease for which other acceptable forms of therapy are available. Furthermore, patients with partial diabetes insipidus who respond to treatment with any oral agents usually respond to either chlorpropamide or thiazides.

Diabetes Insipidus in Pregnancy

A number of cases of adult onset diabetes insipidus have had their onset during pregnancy. The diabetes insipidus has generally not interfered with the progress of parturition and lactation. The agent of choice to treat diabetes insipidus in pregnancy is again desmopressin. This agent has four to 75 times less oxytocic activity than does arginine vasopressin or lysine vasopressin, so that one is able to obtain potent antidiuresis with a minimum uterotonic action.

When diabetes insipidus occurs in pregnancy, it may be especially severe because of the effect of increased serum oxytocinase activity to decrease the effectiveness of endogenously secreted vasopressin. Similarly, in patients with diabetes insipidus who become pregnant, the dose of desmopressin may have to be increased during the pregnancy because of oxytocinase. In women who have the onset of diabetes insipidus during pregnancy, the same protocol for initiation of therapy as in complete diabetes insipidus can be undertaken. These patients may require a three-times-a-day schedule of administered desmopressin. At parturition, the patient is usually alert enough to take intermittent doses of desmopressin intranasally. The only caution is that excessive amounts of fluids should not be administered because this may cause water intoxication and hyponatremia. After parturition, the dosage of desmopressin may have to be adjusted downward because of decreased serum oxytocinase activity.

One should note that desmopressin does not have specific approval for use in pregnancy, but would logically be the appropriate agent where some therapy must be given. Any of the oral agents described before have the potential for teratotoxicity. Lysine vasopressin gives unacceptable levels of control in most normal subjects, which is magnified in pregnant women. Arginine vasopressin has the potential for inducing uterine cramps and must be given by injection. Since desmopressin is similar to the natural hormone, has no known teratogenic effects, and provides adequate control of antidiuresis, it is the best agent to prescribe.

Diabetes Insipidus with Inadequate Thirst

Inadequate thirst constitutes the most difficult management problem of patients with diabetes insipidus. Some patients secrete vasopressin under certain circumstances, but do not respond normally to increases of serum osmolality with either thirst or with secretion of vasopressin. These cases represent a variant of partial diabetes insipidus, and there is the potential for response to oral agents. A trial of chlorpropamide up to 500 mg per day is indicated because in some cases this therapy not only decreases the urine volume, but increases the recognition of thirst as well. If chlorpropamide is ineffective, desmopressin is the agent of choice.

To determine the duration of action of desmopressin, it may be necessary to give a water load either orally or intravenously to bring the sodium level into the normal range and to assure a good urine output. Desmopressin can then be administered, as described previously, with the difference that voided urine is matched volume for volume with administered fluid until the antidiuresis is terminated. At this point, a second dose of desmopressin is administered as in Chronic Complete Diabetes Insipidus. Once the duration of effect of desmopressin is established, the patient must be prescribed a rigid regimen of desmopressin and water intake. The measurement of volumes of fluid to be administered over a given duration of time each day is usually necessary. Even with this careful monitoring of desmopressin and water, regular measurement of serum sodium is necessary because these patients are prone to develop water intoxication with hyponatremia or, alternatively, recurrent dehydration with hypernatremia.

Influence of Diabetes Insipidus on Other Therapeutic Decisions

Routine Surgical Procedures

For most surgical procedures, desmopressin intranasally the morning of the surgery and then careful administration of intravenous fluids during the surgery provide adequate control of fluid balance. For long procedures, serum sodium should be checked during the procedure and in all cases at the end of surgery. If the patient is unable to administer desmopressin intranasally before or after the surgical procedure, parenteral desmopressin is used.

Diabetes Insipidus with Panhypopituitarism

Because the etiology of diabetes insipidus is frequently a sellar or suprasellar tumor, it is commonly accompanied by panhypopituitarism. In these cases, either hypoadrenalism or hypothyroidism causes an inability to excrete a water load. In a patient with diabetes insipidus, there may be no polyuria when hypoadrenalism and/or hypothyroidism is present, and consequently the diagnosis of diabetes insipidus may go unsuspected during initial evaluation. As the patient receives thyroid hormone and (more dramatically) hydrocortisone, a prompt increase in urine output and obvious manifestations of diabetes insipidus occur. At this time, the patient requires evaluation of complete or partial diabetes insipidus and initiation of therapy as outlined in Chronic Complete Diabetes Insipidus and Chronic Partial Diabetes Insipidus.

In patients taking maintenance therapy for diabetes insipidus, hypoadrenalism, and hypothyroidism, maintenance of the treatment of all three conditions is essential. Patients who continue treatment for diabetes insipidus but interrupt the treatment of adrenal or thyroid deficiency are extremely prone to water intoxication and hyponatremia.

Craniopharyngioma

In patients with craniopharyngioma or other suprasellar lesions treated by transfrontal cranial surgery, there is great danger of damaging the neurohypophyseal system and causing permanent diabetes insipidus. This is an almost invariable outcome of attempts at radical, complete removal of a craniopharyngioma. Life-long diabetes insipidus is sufficiently onerous that this possibility provides a continuing stimulus to develop safer modes of therapy for craniopharyngioma, as has been described with stereotaxic implantation of radioisotopes into cystic lesions.

Granulomatous Diseases

Diabetes insipidus in these cases may be partial or complete and may require specific therapy, as described previously. In some cases, there has been remission of the diabetes insipidus with appropriate therapy for the underlying condition, but remission is so rare that to attempt to tailor therapy for the granulomatous disease to specifically try to effect a cure of diabetes insipidus is probably not indicated.

Diabetes Insipidus in Patients with Cardiovascular Disease

A few patients with coronary vascular disease may experience angina pectoris after lysine vasopressin or injected L-arginine vasopressin. This problem has been eliminated by desmopressin because of the markedly reduced pressor activity in the dosage used to produce antidiuresis.

SUGGESTED READING

Czernichow P, Robinson AG, eds. Diabetes insipidus in man. Basel: S. Karger, 1984.

Richardson DW, Robinson AG. Desmopressin. Ann Intern Med 1985; 103:228–239.

Robertson GL. Posterior pituitary. In: Felig P, Baxter JD, Broadus AE, Frohman LA, eds. Endocrinology and metabolism. New York: McGraw-Hill, 1987.

Robinson AG. Disorders of antidiuretic hormone secretion. In: Ney RL, ed. Clinics in endocrinology and metabolism. Vol. 14. London: WB Saunders, 1985:55.

Robinson AG, Verbalis JG. Clinical disorders of the neurohypophysis. In: Smith CW, ed. The peptides, chemistry and biology of neurohypophyseal hormones. New York: Academic Press, 1986:1.

Schrier RW, ed. Vasopressin. New York: Raven Press, 1985.

PRIMARY HYPOTHYROIDISM

LEONA BRENNER-GATI, M.D.

Primary hypothyroidism is a condition in which the thyroid gland is incapable of producing sufficient quantities of thyroid hormone to maintain a state of euthyroidism. The defect is at the level of the thyroid gland. In the United States, primary hypothyroidism is caused most commonly by autoimmune thyroiditis and by thyroid ablative therapy for hyperthyroidism. In adults, exposure to goitrogenic substances such as lithium or iodide is a less common cause of primary hypothyroidism; in the pediatric population, thyroid dysgenesis and inborn errors of thyroid hormone biosynthesis are important etiologic considerations.

The clinical manifestations of hypothyroidism are protean. The goal of therapy is to restore the concentration of thyroid hormones to a level at which biochemical parameters are normalized and symptoms and signs of hypothyroidism are abolished. The clinical spectrum of hypothyroidism is wide; on the one hand, sometimes the presence of primary hypothyroidism is detected by only a single biochemical abnormality that is the hallmark of this disorder, an elevated serum thyroid-stimulating hormone (TSH) concentration. On the other hand, the chronic effects of long-standing severe hypothyroidism manifest themselves as the characteristic clinical picture of myxedema with abnormalities of the skin, cardiorespiratory, reproductive, gastrointestinal, and neuromuscular systems. In almost all patients with primary hypothyroidism, the therapeutic approach is the administration of thyroid hormone. Occasional exceptions include the elimination of goitrogenic substances (e.g., iodide, lithium) when this etiology is apparent or the administration of iodide to the rare patient with an iodide trapping defect or dehalogenase deficiency. Even in these uncommon circumstances, however, it may be easier or more effective to treat with thyroid hormone, particularly if the goitrogenic substance cannot be withdrawn.

PREPARATIONS AVAILABLE

Three types of oral preparations for the treatment of hypothyroidism are available (Table 1). These include (1) pure synthetic preparations of levothyroxine sodium or liothyronine sodium, (2) a synthetic combined formulation of levothyroxine sodium and liothyronine sodium (liotrix), and (3) crude hormone extracts prepared from animal thyroid glands (beef or pork). A consideration of each of these types of preparations readily reveals why the agent of choice for the long-term treatment of primary hypothyroidism is levothyroxine sodium.

Levothyroxine Sodium

Levothyroxine (L-T_4) is approximately 40 percent as active when administered orally as when given by intravenous injection. Formulation of L-T_4 as a sodium salt improves its solubility and absorption, such that absorption ranges from 50 to 80 percent. The variability in absorption is caused by differences in particle size and binders in various formulations; different products are likely to have different bioavailabilities. Absorption is increased in the fasting state. The variable content of L-T_4 in particular preparations has also been a concern. In the early to the mid-1980s, problems created by an increase in the levothyroxine content of a widely used brand of thyroid hormone led to better quality control measures, such as high-pressure liquid chromatography standardization of thyroid hormone content. In fact, recent studies of two commercially available preparations, Synthroid and Levothroid, as to their L-T_4 content (determined by high-pressure liquid chromatography) and their ability to normalize serum TSH levels have revealed no differences between the two products. In addition, the L-T_4 content was found to be as stated by the manufacturer. Yet one particular generic product was found to have only 34 percent as much levothyroxine sodium as stated by the manufacturer. These findings appear to dictate caution in the use of generic levothyroxine sodium products.

The half-life of absorbed thyroxine (T_4) is approximately 7 days in a euthyroid individual. The plasma half-life of T_4 is decreased in hyperthyroidism and prolonged in hypothyroidism. Because of its long half-life, levothyroxine sodium can be taken once a day or even once a week at higher than daily maintenance doses (0.5 to 2.0 mg a week) in situations where compliance or administration is a real problem. Once a steady state level has been attained on a daily maintenance regimen, occasional omission of a dose does not cause any significant alteration in serum levels of thyroid hormones or TSH. One of the major advantages of levothyroxine sodium therapy is the constancy of serum levels because of the large peripheral pool of T_4 that turns over relatively slowly (compared with triiodothyronine [T_3]). Since 80 percent of T_3 in a normal individual is derived from peripheral monodeiodination of T_4, the stable levels of T_4 achieved enable stable levels of T_3 to be attained. Thus the use of levothyroxine sodium allows for easier monitoring of serum T_4 levels and serum T_3 concentrations if desired. In addition to providing a storage pool of T_4 that can compensate for declines in the unbound fraction of T_4 when doses are missed, initiation of therapy with levothyroxine sodium results in a more gradual rise in free thyroid hormone concentration than observed with liothyronine sodium because of the need to saturate a larger number of T_4 protein binding sites. This gradual increase in free thyroid hormone levels could be of importance when initiat-

TABLE 1 Oral Thyroid Hormone Preparations

Preparation	*Generic Name*	*Brand Names*	*Comments*
Synthetic			
Levothyroxine sodium*	Levothyroxine	Levothroid	
		Synthroid	Tartrazine-containing products
Liothyronine sodium	Liothyronine	Cytomel	
Combination of levothyroxine sodium and liothyronine sodium	Liotrix	Euthroid	1 grain = 60 μg T_4 + 15 μg T_3
		Thyrolar	Tartrazine-containing products 1 grain = 50 μg T_4 + 12.5 μg T_3
Crude Hormone			
Desiccated animal thyroid	Desiccated thyroid	Thyroid USP	Bovine or pork thyroid glands
		Thyroid Strong tablets	1 grain = 1½ grain thyroid USP
		S-P-T	Pork thyroid suspended in soybean oil
		Thyrar	Bovine thyroid
Thyroid extract	Thyroglobulin	Proloid	Pork thyroid

*Preferred preparations for the treatment of hypothyroidism (see text).

ing therapy in an elderly patient or in a patient with long-standing hypothyroidism (see next section). When rapid correction of the hypothyroid state is required, such as when treating myxedema coma, a high loading dose of levothyroxine sodium is necessary to saturate the peripheral binding pool (see the chapter entitled *Myxedema Coma*).

Liothyronine Sodium

The sodium salt of liothyronine (L-T_3) is more potent than levothyroxine sodium, such that 25 μg of liothyronine sodium is roughly equivalent to 100 μg of levothyroxine sodium. Liothyronine sodium is almost completely absorbed from the gastrointestinal tract following oral administration. Although T_3 is greater than 99 percent bound to circulating serum proteins, it is less extensively protein bound than T_4 and thus has a shorter serum half-life of 1 to 2 days in an euthyroid individual. Liothyronine sodium has a faster onset but a shorter duration of action compared to levothyroxine sodium and is best administered as two or three daily doses. Even when the daily maintenance dose is administered in several divided doses, significant fluctuation in T_3 levels throughout the day is observed. These peaks and troughs make it difficult to determine the proper maintenance dose based on serum T_3 measurements. In addition, the potential for peak levels of T_3 to reach the supraphysiologic range is a concern when treating elderly patients and those with coronary artery disease. Two instances when administration of liothyronine sodium seems warranted are when a rapid onset of thyroid hormone effect is crucial, as advocated by some endocrinologists in the initial treatment of myxedema coma, or when a rapid decline in thyroid hormone levels is desired, such as prior to radioactive iodine scanning in patients with thyroid cancer.

Mixtures of Levothyroxine Sodium and Liothyronine Sodium

A synthetic preparation of levothyroxine sodium and liothyronine sodium in a 4:1 weight ratio (liotrix) is available for clinical use. Since the majority of T_3 is produced by the peripheral monodeiodination of T_4, there is little rationale for the use of liotrix. When encountering patients maintained on liotrix, the approximate clinical equivalence is 1 grain thyroid equivalent of liotrix equals 100 μg levothyroxine sodium. However, the actual thyroid hormone content in the two commercially available preparations is different. A 1-grain thyroid equivalent tablet of Thyrolar contains 50.0 μg of levothyroxine sodium plus 12.5 μg of liothyronine sodium, whereas a 1-grain thyroid equivalent tablet of Euthroid contains 60 μg of levothyroxine sodium plus 15 μg of liothyronine sodium.

Crude Hormone Preparations

Natural thyroid hormone preparation are derived from animal (beef or pork) thyroid glands and include desiccated thyroid and thyroglobulin. Prior to 1985, the United States Pharmacopeia (USP) required that thyroid and thyroglobulin be standardized only by their iodine content, which is a poor indicator of biologic potency. Current standardization requirements call for specification of levothyroxine and liothyronine content; unfortunately, difficulty with direct measurement of actual hormonal content had been responsible for discrepancies between measured thyroid hormone content and clinical equivalence. Some manufacturers have used bioassay to standardize metabolic potency. However, different batches may be of equal potency by bioassay yet differ in the ratio of levothyroxine to liothyronine. A reasonable assumption is that concentrations of levothyroxine and liothyronine and the ratios of these hormones in commercially available crude thyroid hormone preparations vary among manufacturers and probably among lots as well.

The approximate clinical equivalence of thyroid and thyroglobulin is 1 grain (60 to 65 mg) equals 100 μg of levothyroxine sodium. Of note, one particular thyroid preparation—Thyroid Strong tablets—is 50 percent stronger than ordinary desiccated thyroid, such that 1 grain of Thyroid Strong is equivalent to 1.5 grains of desiccated thyroid. It contains T_4 and T_3 in an approximate ratio of 2.5:1.0 and thus is enriched in T_3 compared with many crude thyroid preparations.

THERAPEUTIC APPROACH

As discussed previously, several factors make levothyroxine sodium the agent of choice for the treatment of hypothyroidism. A major consideration with respect to the therapeutic approach is the dose at which to initiate thyroid hormone replacement. Factors that must be taken into account include the patient's age, duration and degree of hypothyroidism, and the presence of other systemic disorders, in particular, atherosclerotic disease. The usual maintenance dose of levothyroxine sodium in an adult patient is 1.5 to 2.0 μg per kilogram. Recent studies have documented a decrease in thyroid hormone replacement dose with advancing age. Furthermore, patients with long-standing myxedema are exquisitely sensitive to low doses of thyroid hormone, and persons with diagnosed or subclinical cardiac disease can experience cardiac decompensation if thyroid hormone therapy is undertaken too aggressively. For these reasons, a judicious approach to the initiation of thyroid hormone treatment is warranted in the elderly, in persons with long-standing moderate to severe hypothyroidism, and in patients with known or suspected cardiac disease. I believe that all patients 65 years of age or older, those with known cardiac disease, and patients with long-standing significant hypothyroidism who are 50 to 65 years of age should be started on 25 μg of levothyroxine sodium a day (Table 2). (This present discussion excludes the use of levothyroxine sodium in myxedema coma, an endocrine emergency that necessitates the immediate administration of high doses of thyroid hormone, as discussed in the chapter entitled *Myxedema Coma.*) All patients in this group should have a baseline electrocardiogram prior to initiating thyroid hormone treatment. Subsequent incremental increases should be small: 12.5 to 25.0 μg each. Since it takes at least 4 weeks to attain new steady state levels of thyroid hormone and additional time for full tissue effects to be manifested, dosage increases should be made only after 6 to 8 weeks in this group of patients. It is important to recognize that in some patients with cardiac disease, it is impossible to prescribe full replacement doses of thyroid hormone without provoking unacceptable exacerbations of angina, arrhythmias, or heart failure. In patients with severe hypothyroidism who are younger than 50 years of age and thus less likely to have occult coronary artery disease, a starting dose of 50 μg of levothyroxine sodium is reasonable.

Most patients in the 50 to 65 age group with only mild hypothyroidism and no known cardiac disease can also be started safely on 50 μg levothyroxine sodium daily. Younger patients (under 50 years) with no potentially complicating medical problems can receive a starting dose of 100 μg levothyroxine sodium. However, it may be wise to administer a smaller initial dose to a patient who is newly hypothyroid after radioiodine therapy for Graves' disease or other conditions of autonomous thyroid hyperfunction. In these situations, the patient may have some residual autonomous function and may require less than the anticipated thyroid hormone replacement dose. The usual daily maintenance dose of levothyroxine sodium in the nongeriatric population is 100 to 150 μg. Daily maintenance doses of 50 to 150 μg are seen in the elderly.

In the pediatric population, the dosage of thyroid hormone per unit body weight is substantially higher than that in adults. A more aggressive approach to the initiation and continuation of thyroid hormone replacement is employed with children because of the deleterious effects of thyroid hormone deficiency on the maturing nervous system and on growth and development in general. As soon as the diagnosis of hypothyroidism is made, treatment should be initiated and full maintenance doses achieved rapidly. See Table 2 regarding current recommendations for the administration of thyroid hormone to children.

Once thyroid hormone treatment has been started, monitoring of blood tests and assessment of clinical symptoms and signs must be undertaken to determine the proper maintenance dose of levothyroxine sodium. Unfortunately, no reliable tests are readily available to assess tissue levels of thyroid hormone and end-organ responses. Early clinical signs of improving thyroid status include diuresis, decrease in puffiness, and increase in serum sodium levels if hyponatremia was present previously. Subsequently, increases in pulse rate and psychomotor activity are noted, as well as improvements in appetite, lethargy, and constipation. Skin and hair changes are noted after several months of therapy.

However, it is notoriously difficult to determine if a patient is on optimal thyroid hormone therapy based on clinical criteria alone. Optimal thyroid hormone replacement in primary hypothyroidism is generally considered to be the dose that restores serum TSH to the normal range. In recent years, highly sensitive TSH assays have been developed (and are avail-

TABLE 2 Therapy of Hypothyroidism with Levothyroxine Sodium*

Patient	*Initial Dose (μg)*	*Increment of Dose Increases (μg)*	*Frequency of Dose Increases (Weeks)*	*Daily Maintenance Dose (μg)*	*(μg/kg)*
Adults					
Older than 65 years	25	12.5–25.0	6–8	50–150 or	<1.5–2.0
Heart disease	25	12.5–25.0	6–8	50–150 or	<1.5–2.0
Chronic, marked hypothyroidism					
Older than 50 years	25	12.5–25.0	6–8	50–150 or	<1.5–2.0
Younger than 50 years	50	25	4–6	100–150 or	1.5–2.0
Mild hypothyroidism					
50 to 65 years old	50	25	4–6	50–150 or	<1.5–2.0
Younger than 50 years with no complications	100	25	4	100–150 or	1.5–2.0
Children					
0–6 months	25	12.5	2–4	25–50 or	8–10
6–12 months	25	12.5–25.0	2–4	50–75 or	6–8
1–12 years	25–50	12.5–25.0	4–8	75–150 or	2–5†
Over 12 years	50	25	4–8	100–200 or	2–3

*Excluding myxedema coma.
†Average maintenance dose is about 3.5 μg/kg/day.

able for clinical use) that can distinguish a subnormal or suppressed TSH level from a TSH level in the normal range. Use of these sensitive immunoradiometric or enzyme-linked immunoassays now allows for very accurate titration of thyroid hormone doses and avoidance of overreplacement. Since the introduction of a sensitive TSH assay at my institution, many patients have required a reduction in the maintenance dose of thyroid hormone because of the finding of a suppressed TSH level. With the advent of more sensitive TSH assays (and increased T_4 content in current preparations), the daily maintenance dose of levothyroxine sodium appears to be lower than previously thought. The range for the daily maintenance dose of levothyroxine sodium for the adult population was considered to be 100 to 200 μg a day or 2.0 to 2.5 μg per kilogram. Recent studies and experience indicate that a range of 50 to 150 μg a day or less than 1.5 to 2.0 μg per kilogram per day is more appropriate. When a patient on a previously established stable maintenance dose of levothyroxine sodium is discovered to have a suppressed TSH level, a decrease in the dose of 12.5 to 25.0 μg daily is advisable. Since patients with long-term suppression of TSH may require several weeks for recovery of pituitary function, a follow-up TSH value in 4 to 6 weeks would be a good time for reassessment. One can cite many compelling reasons to support the avoidance of long-term overreplacement with thyroid hormone. These include aggravation of cardiac disorders or other diseases such as hypertension or diabetes caused by even small thyroid hormone excess. Another important deleterious consequence of excessive thyroid hormone therapy is increased bone demineralization and an increased propensity for the development of osteoporosis.

Use of the serum TSH value to determine thyroid hormone dose in the adult with primary hypothyroidism is more accurate than relying on the serum T_4 level because of the wide range of normal values for serum T_4. In almost all adult patients with primary hypothyroidism, the patient's own pituitary is the best sensor of appropriate circulating free thyroid hormone concentrations. However, an important exception is the patient with long-standing marked hypothyroidism in whom a lag time of weeks to months between restoration of normal thyroid hormone levels and complete normalization of serum TSH can be observed. One possible explanation for this lag time is the presence of pituitary thyrotrope hyperplasia secondary to chronic myxedema.

Shortly after the initiation of thyroid hormone therapy in a patient with primary hypothyroidism, a decline in serum TSH level should be observed. Incremental increases in serum T_4 level with increasing thyroid hormone doses (as outlined in Table 2) should also be accompanied by further decreases in serum TSH. If the serum TSH has not normalized by the time the serum T_4 is in the mid-normal range in a patient with long-standing hypothyroidism, one is prudent, particularly in the elderly, to delay additional increases in thyroid hormone dosage for 1 to 2 months to determine if the TSH serum level declines further. Similarly, children with congenital hypothyroidism may have a persistent elevation of serum TSH concentration even after serum T_4 levels and growth and development are normalized. For this reason, the attainment of serum T_4 levels in the mid to high normal range is the most important biochemical parameter in congenital hypothyroidism.

Patients on levothyroxine sodium with normal TSH values usually have total and free T_4 levels in the normal to slightly supranormal range. Serum T_3 levels are usually within the normal range. Patients being treated with liothyronine sodium alone have low serum T_4 levels, and biochemical monitoring must rely heavily on serum TSH because of the daily fluctuation in serum T_3 levels described before. In patients treated with crude thyroid hormone preparations or mixtures of levothyroxine sodium and liothyronine sodium, serum thyroid hormone levels are subject to variability based on the content of T_4 and T_3 in particular formulations. Again, serum TSH is of primary importance for biochemical monitoring, with serum T_4 values providing additional helpful information.

MANAGEMENT

Adrenal Insufficiency

It is imperative to consider the possibility of coexisting primary adrenal insufficiency that, when present with primary hypothyroidism, constitutes Schmidt's syndrome. The administration of thyroid hormone to a hypothyroid patient with inadequate adrenal function can precipitate adrenal crisis. In nonemergencies, if there is any doubt as to adrenal status, one should perform a rapid adrenocorticotropic hormone stimulation test prior to starting thyroid hormone treatment. In a hypothyroid emergency (see chapter on *Myxedema Coma*), stress dose steroids are given to guard against the possibility of absolute or relative adrenal insufficiency.

Subclinical Hypothyroidism

The term "subclinical" hypothyroidism refers to the finding of an elevated serum TSH concentration in a clinically euthyroid individual with normal total and free serum thyroid hormone levels. This type of patient has a failing thyroid gland that is usually caused by autoimmune processes or postablative treatment for hyperthyroidism. Considerable controversy exists over whether or not to treat a patient with subclinical hypothyroidism. On the one hand, one could argue that the compensatory increase in serum TSH is maintaining the patient in a metabolically normal status. On the other hand, the fact that the

TSH level remains elevated indicates that the circulating levels of thyroid hormone are inadequate, unless one invokes an altered pituitary set point for thyroid hormone negative feedback inhibition of TSH secretion. Subtle improvements in symptoms potentially attributable to mild hypothyroidism and in cardiac contractility in patients with subclinical hypothyroidism have been reported. Considering that TSH is a goitrogenic substance and that a significant number of patients with subclinical hypothyroidism go on to develop frank hypothyroidism, my bias is to treat these patients with thyroid hormone replacement.

Therapeutic Failures

A therapeutic failure is the inability to normalize biochemical parameters or to alleviate the symptoms or signs of hypothyroidism with routine or even supranormal thyroid hormone replacement doses. The most common cause for this situation is patient noncompliance. Even with repetitive physician reinforcement as to the importance of lifelong necessity of thyroid hormone medication, some patients seem incapable of complying. Supervised administration could be arranged to assess this possibility. Other reasons for treatment failure include poor absorption owing to malabsorption or bioavailability problems related to product formulation. As discussed previously, stated and actual thyroid hormone content of particular preparations may not be in accord; therefore the patient may be ingesting less thyroid hormone than expected. In some circumstances, a change to a brand product of reported reliability may be helpful. If the patient is taking a bile acid–binding resin, thyroid hormone should be taken at least 1 hour before or 4 hours after the resin, since these medications can impair thyroid hormone absorption. Rare cases of rapid hormone degradation can be determined by means of radiotracer studies, if one wishes to pursue that diagnosis. For all practical purposes, the approach to rectifying treatment failures caused by malabsorption, rapid degradation, or bioavailability problems would be to increase the dose of thyroid hormone replacement until adequate levels can be achieved.

A rare condition that ought to be kept in mind when considering thyroid hormone treatment failures is thyroid hormone resistance syndromes. These are a category of conditions within the syndrome of inappropriate TSH secretion. Patients with these syndromes have pituitary and peripheral tissue resistance to thyroid hormones. They require high doses of thyroid hormone and free thyroid hormone concentrations in the supranormal range to ameliorate clinical signs and symptoms of hypothyroidism and to effect a fall in TSH levels. Many patients reported with these syndromes had been misdiagnosed in the past and improperly subjected to thyroid surgery or radioiodine treatment for goiter and presumed hyperthyroidism. If thyroid hormone resistance is suspected, the patient should be referred to an institution with a special interest or experience in diagnosing these syndromes.

Drug Interactions

Initiation of thyroid hormone therapy and restoration of a eumetabolic state may affect therapeutic regimens involving a number of drugs. It addition, certain drugs affect thyroid hormone metabolism and/or pharmacokinetics. Several particular situations in which the patient needs to be monitored closely will be discussed.

Thyroid replacement may potentiate the effects of oral anticoagulants, apparently by increasing the catabolism of vitamin K–dependent clotting factors. Some investigators have suggested that oral anticoagulant dosage be decreased by one-third when therapy with thyroid hormone is begun, with subsequent anticoagulant dose adjustment based on frequent prothrombin time determinations. Thyroid hormone therapy may increase the required dosage of insulin or oral hypoglycemic agents in diabetic patients; conversely, decreasing the daily maintenance dose of thyroid hormone may precipitate hypoglycemic reactions. Diabetics need to be monitored carefully when thyroid hormone therapy is initiated or dose changes are made. Thyroxine increases the adrenergic effect of catecholamines and sympathomimetics. Concomitant use of these agents and thyroid hormone can increase the risk of coronary insufficiency. In addition, the therapeutic effectiveness of digitalis glycosides may be decreased by initiating thyroid hormone replacement, with potential exacerbation of congestive heart failure and arrhythmias. Administration of thyroid hormone in conjunction with imipramine and other tricyclic antidepressants may enhance antidepressant activity and has been associated with cardiac arrhythmias. Estrogens increase thyroxine binding globulin concentration and can cause a decrease in free T_4 levels in a patient with a completely nonfunctioning thyroid gland. Two types of agents that frequently affect thyroid hormone pharmacokinetics and metabolism are bile acid sequesterants (discussed before) and antiseizure medications such as phenytoin which increase the metabolism of thyroid hormones and sometimes necessitate an increase in thyroid hormone maintenance dosage.

Side Effects

Other than the adverse effects of hyperthyroidism associated with overreplacement or acute overdose, thyroid hormones are virtually without known side effects. The only notable exception would be a patient with tartrazine sensitivity who could have an allergic reaction to the dye additive (yellow dye No. 5) in the tablets. Thyroid hormone preparations that contain tartrazine are yellow-colored 100-μg and green-colored 300-μg tablets of Synthroid and the 0.50, 1-, and 3-grain thyroid equivalent tablets of Euthroid. Although the incidence of tartrazine sensitivity is low, it frequently occurs in patients who are sensitive to aspirin.

REASSESSMENT OF THE DIAGNOSIS OF HYPOTHYROIDISM

Frequently, patients are encountered who had been placed on thyroid hormone replacement therapy in the past without adequate documentation of the diagnosis of hypothyroidism. If one is compelled to substantiate the diagnosis, the most straightforward way is to discontinue thyroid hormone treatment. In many instances, "replacement" doses of thyroid hormone have resulted in suppression of pituitary TSH secretion that can persist for many weeks after thyroid hormone is stopped. During this period, symptoms and signs of clinical hypothyroidism may appear in conjunction with falling thyroid hormone levels. By 1 to 2 months, pituitary function has resumed in normal individuals, and thyroid hormone levels begin to rise. In patients with primary hypothyroidism, TSH levels become unequivocally elevated, and the diagnosis of primary thyroid gland dysfunction is verified. Of course, patients with secondary (pituitary) or tertiary (hypothalamic) hypothyroidism do not develop an elevated TSH level. Further investigation of these patients would be necessary (see the chapter entitled *Hypopituitarism*).

SUGGESTED READING

DeGroot LJ, Larsen PR, Refetoff S, Stanbury JB. The thyroid and its diseases. 5th ed. New York: John Wiley & Sons, 1984:546.
Ingbar SI. The thyroid gland. In: Wilson JD, Foster DW, eds. Textbook of endocrinology. 7th ed. Philadelphia: WB Saunders, 1985:682.
Utiger RT. The thyroid: Physiology, hyperthyroidism, hypothyroidism and the painful thyroid. In: Felig P, ed. Endocrinology and metabolism. 2nd ed. New York: McGraw-Hill, 1986:389.
Fish LH, Schwartz HL, Cavanaugh J, et al. Replacement dose, metabolism, and bioavailability of levothyroxine in the treatment of hypothyroidism. N Engl J Med 1987; 316:764–770.
Hennessey JV, Evaul JE, Tseng YC, et al. l-Thyroxine dosage: A reevaluation of therapy with contemporary preparations. Ann Intern Med 1986; 105:11–15.

MYXEDEMA COMA

BASIL RAPOPORT, M.B., Ch.B.

Myxedema coma is a medical emergency with a reported fatality rate as high as 80 percent. As its name suggests, this condition involves a diminished level of consciousness in association with severe hypothyroidism. Fortunately, myxedema coma is encountered only rarely in clinical practice, and only approximately 100 cases have been reported in the literature. This figure must be considered in the light of hypothyroidism being a common clinical condition. That is, few patients with hypothyroidism develop myxedema coma. In recent years, however, with increasing attention being focused on the problem, the diagnosis of myxedema coma is being made more frequently. One possible reason for its apparent rarity is that cases of myxedema coma may remain unrecognized. Thus seriously ill persons dying with a multitude of medical problems, such as respiratory failure and infection, may have unrecognized hypothyroidism that contributes to their demise.

Myxedema coma may present as the end manifestation of chronic, severe primary thyroid failure. In this situation, patients with untreated hypothyroidism, with all the classic signs and symptoms of this condition, slowly lapse into stupor, coma, and then death. A more common presentation, however, is that of myxedema coma precipitated in patients with moderate or unrecognized hypothyroidism by a superimposed acute medical illness, particularly an infection, or following the administration of sedatives or narcotics. Myxedema coma should therefore be considered in all stuporous or comatose patients, particularly when hypothermia is also present and when a reason for the diminished level of consciousness is not clearly evident.

WHEN TO TREAT

Evidence suggests that the early and aggressive therapy of myxedema coma significantly reduces its mortality (Table 1). Indeed, in the absence of irreversible or untreated associated illness, recognized myxedema coma should now rarely be a direct cause of death. Important factors determining the mortality rate in myxedema coma are the duration of coma and the speed with which therapy is instituted. For this reason, and because laboratory confirmation of myxedema may be delayed for hours or even days, therapy should begin when the diagnosis is seriously suspected, even before it has been established with certainty. The rationale for this approach is that the recommended therapeutic regimen is of little risk if the patient

TABLE 1 Treatment of the Acute Phase of Myxedema Coma

Treat on suspicion
Maintain adequate ventilation:
- Perform tracheal intubation or tracheostomy
- Institute mechanical ventilation
- Monitor blood gases

Treat shock with plasma expanders rather than adrenergic agents
Administer T_4, 300–500 μg IV, then 75–100 μg IV daily
Administer hydrocortisone, 50–100 mg IV every 8 hours
Treat hypothermia by passive warming
Provide intravenous fluids:
- Provide free water sparingly
- Provide intravenous glucose if hypoglycemic

Treat precipitating illness
Provide all medications intravenously

ultimately proves to be euthyroid. Euthyroid persons tolerate the short-term administration of a large dose of thyroxine (T_4) very well. In contrast, the delay of therapy can make the difference between survival and death.

MAINTENANCE OF VITAL BODY FUNCTIONS

Respiratory failure is a major cause of death in myxedema coma and may occur for many reasons. Severe myxedema decreases the sensitivity of the brain-stem respiratory centers to hypoxia and hypercarbia. In addition, a frequent precipitating event in myxedema coma is pneumonia or an exacerbation of chronic obstructive pulmonary disease.

Although the development of respiratory failure may be insidious, it may also occur rapidly and need immediate treatment. The airway should first be inspected and, if necessary, cleared. In particular, enlargement of the tongue that may be associated with longstanding hypothyroidism may contribute to upper airway obstruction. If the respiratory failure is acute, artificial ventilation should be initiated immediately, either mouth to mouth or with an Ambu bag and an airway. Forward pressure on the mandible is important because of the possibility of tongue enlargement. At the earliest opportunity the patient should undergo tracheal intubation and mechanical ventilation should be instituted. Arterial blood should be obtained and sent to the laboratory for the analysis of blood gases to ensure that adequate ventilation is being achieved. A tracheostomy should be performed if mechanical ventilation is prolonged.

As in cardiopulmonary arrest from any cause, the patient's electrocardiogram should be monitored during the acute phase and an intravenous line inserted for the administration of medications. Hypotension is particularly ominous and difficult to treat because hypothyroid patients are relatively insensitive to adrenergic agents. Alpha-adrenergic agents should be avoided because patients with profound myxedema already have severe peripheral vasoconstriction. In addition, the combination of adrenergic agents together with large doses of thyroid hormones, particularly triiodothyronine (T_3), has been associated with serious tachyarrhythmias. Because myxedematous patients usually have a diminished plasma volume, it is more important to provide volume in the form of plasma expanders while central venous pressure is being monitored.

The patient should be transferred as soon as possible to an intensive care unit where vital signs are more easily monitored and specialized nursing care is available. With the patient now being adequately ventilated and perfused, a venous blood sample should be drawn and sent to the laboratory for the determination of serum T_4 and free T_4 index (or free T_4 by radioimmunoassay), cortisol, hemoglobin, hematocrit, white blood cell count and differential, serum electrolytes, blood urea nitrogen, creatinine, glucose, creatine phosphokinase (CPK), serum glutamic oxaloacetic transaminase (SGOT), and lactic dehydrogenase (LDH). Some of these tests will be important for later management, while others, such as the white blood cell count and serum sodium level, are for more immediate management. Patients with longstanding myxedema may be anemic for a variety of reasons, and whole blood may be administered if the hematocrit is below 25 to 30 percent.

The above description is for management of myxedema stupor or coma in patients with acute respiratory failure. In other patients, the onset of anoxia and hypercarbia with progressive mental impairment may be slow and insidious, and it may be reversed by other measures without the need for emergency cardiopulmonary resuscitation.

Assisted ventilation may be necessary for a prolonged period of time, as long as 1 or 2 weeks after the institution of thyroxine therapy. I have observed this phenomenon in a patient with unrecognized hypothyroidism who underwent elective surgery and in whom the diagnosis of myxedema coma was made postoperatively when the patient failed to regain consciousness or to resume spontaneous ventilation. The reasons for the prolonged acute respiratory failure are not clear but may include intercostal and diaphragmatic muscle weakness, obesity, atelectasis, and pneumonia.

THYROID HORMONE ADMINISTRATION

Thyroid hormone should be administered as soon as adequate respiration and perfusion have been established. It should be appreciated that there is considerable controversy as to the correct form of thyroid hormone therapy in myxedema coma. Because of the rarity, gravity, and complicated nature of the condition, it is unlikely that controlled clinical trials with different hormone regimens will ever be performed. However, available evidence supports the likelihood that the improvement in the mortality rate in myxedema coma, as reported in more recent series, follows the early use of a large dose of intravenous thyroxine (T_4).

There is obviously a paradox in this form of therapy, in that severe myxedema in the absence of coma is traditionally treated cautiously by administering small doses of thyroid hormone and waiting for the effects to be fully developed before increasing the dose. In the case of myxedema coma, however, the immediate threat to life from the myxedema itself takes precedence over the potential deleterious effects of too-rapid thyroid hormone administration. In other words, the risk of a serious cardiac arrhythmia is the price that must be paid for the more immediate and far greater risk of death from myxedema coma itself.

L-Thyroxine should be administered as an intravenous bolus of 300 to 500 μg, depending on the size of the patient (approximately 7 μg per kilogram with a maximum of 500 μg). The rationale for this dose is that the T_4 pool size is approximately 700 μg in the average euthyroid 70-kg adult. The use of intravenous T_4 rather than T_3 is preferable for a number of reasons. First, an intravenous preparation of T_4, unlike T_3, is commercially available. Second, the disposal rate of T_4 is considerably slower than that of T_3. It is therefore possible to administer T_4 as a single dose rather than as multiple doses throughout the day. Third, in humans extrathyroidal thyroxine is the major source of T_3 production in that T_4 undergoes monodeiodination to T_3 in the peripheral tissues. The relatively stable T_4 pool functions as a depot, so that the peripheral T_3 concentration remains stable. In contrast, when T_3 is administered, serum T_3 levels fluctuate widely and may be associated with a higher incidence of cardiac arrhythmias. Fourth, it is easier to monitor levels of T_4 than T_3 in serum because of the simpler and more widely available assays for T_4.

Not all endocrinologists use T_4. An alternative is to administer T_3 (20 to 40 μg) intravenously at 6-hour intervals during the acute phase of myxedema coma. The rationale for this is that the metabolic effects of T_3 occur more rapidly than do those of T_4. In addition, it is argued, the acute illness that generally coexists with myxedema coma decreases the peripheral conversion of T_4 to T_3, and T_3 therefore bypasses this metabolic block. Despite these theoretic advantages of T_3, however, the most recent reports on therapy for myxedema coma, in which T_4 was used, have indicated survival rates superior to those previously reported when T_3 was administered. Although I prefer the use of T_4, it must be admitted that the most important factor influencing survival is probably the early recognition and treatment of myxedema coma with thyroid hormone in any form, as well as management of the usually serious underlying precipitating condition.

If intravenous thyroxine is not available, or if one chooses to administer intravenous T_3, the preparation may be made by dissolving T_4 or T_3 powder in a few drops of 0.1 N NaOH. The solution is then diluted with sterile normal saline containing 1 percent albumin (to prevent nonspecific binding of the thyroid hormone to the container) and passed through a sterile millipore filter (0.22 μm). Alternatively, crushed tablets may be administered through a nasogastric tube. In this case the dose should be increased by half, that is, 750 μg of T_4, because absorption of T_4 from the gastrointestinal tract is incomplete in euthyroid persons. However, intragastric administration is less reliable than the intravenous route in severe hypothyroidism because of decreased intestinal motility and absorption.

On the second day of treatment, if the serum T_4 level is less than 5 μg per deciliter, and the patient is still stuporous or comatose, a second intravenous dose of 300 to 500 μg of T_4 should be administered. This is particularly important if there is coexistent bacterial infection, such as pneumonia. The rationale for this approach is that bacterial infection may seriously diminish the response to T_4 because polymorphonuclear leukocytes metabolize thyroxine and render the T_4 metabolically inactive.

Further T_4 administration is dictated by the clinical response. If the patient remains stuporous or comatose and is unable to take oral medications, 75 to 100 μg of T_4 should be administered daily intravenously in a single dose. It should be recognized that in severe hypothyroidism the metabolic clearance of T_4 is diminished, and that these doses of intravenous T_4 may temporarily elevate the serum T_4 levels above the normal range. These values will normalize as euthyroidism is attained and the metabolic clearance of T_4 returns to normal. However, this aspect of therapy does not present much difficulty, serum T_4 levels may be monitored and T_4 administration adjusted accordingly.

When the patient is able to take medications by mouth, a physiologic replacement dose of T_4 (100 to approximately 200 μg per day) should be instituted. The requirement for a greater oral than intravenous dose reflects the fact that absorption of ingested thyroxine is not complete.

It is not recommended that serum T_3 levels be monitored, because values may not attain the normal range during the acute phase, especially if the patient has a severe coexisting illness or is also receiving glucocorticoids. Serious nonthyroidal illness as well as glucocorticoids decrease the peripheral conversion of T_4 to T_3. However, the results with T_4 therapy have been satisfactory, even in patients receiving glucocorticoids in whom the T_3 level remains suppressed. Elevated TSH levels associated with primary hypothyroidism usually begin to decrease within 24 hours of initiation of T_4 treatment and subsequently normalize over a period of a few days to a week. It should be recognized, however, that glucocorticoids also suppress TSH secretion and make interpretation of the serum TSH level difficult.

GLUCOCORTICOID ADMINISTRATION

Hydrocortisone should be administered intravenously at stress doses (50 to 100 mg three times a day). Although there has been no clinical study to support this therapy, and neither is it likely that such a study will even be undertaken, this approach is justified because of the increased risk of associated adrenal insufficiency. Thus coexisting primary adrenal insufficiency may occur together with autoimmune primary hypothyroidism (Schmidt's syndrome). In addition, hypothyroidism may be secondary to pituitary insufficiency.

Steroid hormone metabolism is decreased during hypothyroidism. That is, during hypothyroidism, limited adrenal steroid production may be sufficient for a normal response to stress. With the restoration of euthyroidism, however, adrenal steroid use is greatly increased. This, together with the frequently coexisting severe illness, will increase the need for adrenal glucocorticoid production, which may be beyond the capacity of the adrenals if their functional reserve is diminished. This situation increases the risk of acute adrenal insufficiency and shock. It is important to draw a blood sample for analysis of serum cortisol concentration prior to beginning hydrocortisone therapy. If this level is elevated, consistent with the stress of the coexistent acute medical illness, and if there is rapid clinical improvement within a few days (before significant pituitary-adrenal axis suppression is induced), the dose of hydrocortisone may be tapered rapidly and the hormone discontinued. Obviously, if the endogenous serum cortisol level is subnormal during the period of stress, cortisol therapy must be continued and may be tapered to physiologic replacement doses as the illness resolves.

HYPOTHERMIA

Temperatures as low as 75 °F have been recorded in myxedema coma. Severe hypothermia (less than 90 °F) is of serious prognostic significance. Despite the hypothermia, shivering does not occur in this condition. It is important to recognize that monitoring body temperature in patients with myxedema coma is only possible with a thermometer calibrated for lower temperatures. If a routine clinical thermometer is used, the hypothermia may not be appreciated. Despite the hypothermia, active warming with a heating blanket is not recommended. Instead the patient should be passively warmed with an ordinary blanket. Thyroid hormone administration is the most effective way to restore body temperature to normal. A rise in body temperature from subnormal levels should be evident within 24 hours of thyroid hormone therapy. Active warming with a heating blanket is potentially dangerous because patients with myxedema coma typically have a decreased plasma volume and intense peripheral vasoconstriction. Peripheral vasodilatation under these circumstances produces shock.

TREATMENT OF THE PRECIPITATING ILLNESS

Although myxedema coma may occasionally occur because of profound hypothyroidism per se, the condition is more frequently caused by a coexistent acute medical illness. The most common cause is infection, either pneumonia or urinary tract infection. The diagnosis of acute infection may be obscured in myxedema coma because fever and leukocytosis may appear only at a later stage, following the administration of thyroid hormone. It is therefore important to obtain blood cultures as well as a portable chest roentgenogram at an early stage during the management of myxedema coma. Careful examination of the urine is also mandatory. Although recommended by some, I would not suggest the use of empiric broad-spectrum antibiotic therapy unless a source of infection is clearly demonstrated. Other common precipitating causes of myxedema coma include drugs (particularly sedatives and narcotics), gastrointestinal bleeding, myocardial infarction, and chronic obstructive pulmonary disease. If present, these disorders should be treated by the usual means. If the patient does not regain consciousness within 24 hours, the possibility of cerebrovascular accident should be considered, even if localizing neurologic signs were not present at the outset.

Intravenous fluids should be administered carefully. Hyponatremia is frequently present in myxedema coma because of diminished free water clearance in severe hypothyroidism. This may occur because of increased vasopressin activity as well as because of decreased glomerular filtration. It is therefore important to avoid excess intravenous administration of free water. Despite the hyponatremia, total body sodium and water content is increased. The hyponatremia is best treated by correction of the hypothyroidism with thyroxine. Hypertonic saline should only be given if the hyponatremia is profound. Adequate thyroid hormone therapy is associated with a gratifying diuresis and return of the serum sodium level to normal. Hypoglycemia is rarely present but should be considered, especially when hypothermia is present. The treatment is intravenous glucose.

During the acute phase of myxedema coma all drugs, such as digoxin for coexisting congestive heart failure, should be administered intravenously. This is because peripheral vasoconstriction may decrease absorption of medication given by other routes. It must also be appreciated that the clearance of administered drugs is usually impaired during the hypothyroid phase.

The rationale for measuring serum CPK, SGOT, and LDH values at the outset of therapy is that serum levels of these enzymes are commonly elevated in severe hypothyroidism because of their decreased metabolic clearance rate. With thyroid hormone therapy, these enzyme concentrations will gradually return to the normal range. Their use for the diagnosis of myocardial infarction may therefore be unreliable, unless serum values are known prior to the institution of thyroid hormone therapy. Thus elevated serum enzymes do not in themselves support a diagnosis of myocardial infarction. On the other hand, a failure of these enzyme concentrations to decrease as euthyroidism is restored, or an increase above already elevated levels, should raise the suspicion of tissue damage.

As for any comatose patient, careful and specialized nursing is essential. The patient requires frequent turning, and urinary retention and fecal impaction should be recognized and treated appropriately.

PROPHYLAXIS OF MYXEDEMA COMA

One important, and frequently overlooked, feature of myxedema coma in its prevention. With the advent of the use of radioactive iodine for the treatment of hyperthyroidism, there is an increasingly large population of intrinsically hypothyroid patients requiring exogenous thyroxine treatment. It is important to reinforce continually in these patients the need for lifelong thyroxine ingestion and the potential consequences of the discontinuation of this therapy. All too frequently patients discontinue their medications because they "feel so well" on the medication that they do not appreciate the need for this agent.

SUGGESTED READING

Forester CF. Coma in myxedema. Arch Intern Med 1963; 111:100–109.
Holvey DN, Goodner CJ, Nicoloff JT, Dowling TJ. Treatment of myxedema coma with intravenous thyroxine. Arch Intern Med 1964; 113:89–96.
Nicoloff JT. Myxedema coma. Pharmacol Ther 1976; 1:161–169.
Ridgway EC, McCammon JA, Benotti J, et al. Acute metabolic responses in myxedema to large doses of intravenous l-thyroxine. Ann Intern Med 1972; 77:549–555.
Wartofsky L. Myxedema coma. In: Ingbar SH, Braverman LE, eds. Werner's the thyroid. Philadelphia: JB Lippincott, 1987:1227.

HYPERTHYROIDISM IN GRAVES' DISEASE

SIDNEY H. INGBAR, M.D.

This discussion describes the approach I employ in treating the patient who is thyrotoxic as a result of hyperthyroidism in Graves' disease. At the outset, however, it is important to note that not all hyperthyroidism is due to Graves' disease and not all thyrotoxicosis is a reflection of hyperthyroidism. To understand why this is the case requires a definition of terms. Thyrotoxicosis is the clinical and biochemical complex that results from the sustained delivery to the peripheral tissues of excessive quantities of thyroid hormones, wherever their source and whatever the cause. Hyperthyroidism is the term denoting that such hormone excess results specifically from sustained thyroid hyperfunction, leading to increases in both hormone formation and hormone secretion. As can be seen in Table 1, which lists the major causes of thyrotoxicosis and their principal means of treatment, differentiation between the hyperthyroid and nonhyperthyroid varieties of thyrotoxicosis is of major importance because their etiology, pathogenesis, treatment, and prognosis differ so radically.

In the hyperthyroid variety, treatment is principally directed at bringing to an end the excess secretion of hormone. This goal is accomplished mainly with antithyroid agents or the use of radioactive iodine or surgery; iodine and glucocorticoids can be used, in addition, when hyperthyroidism is severe and life-threatening. Additional measures, such as the use of adrenergic blocking agents, sedation, and bed rest, are useful, often very much so, but are merely adjunctive.

In the nonhyperthyroid varieties, thyrotoxicosis variously results from the witting or unwitting ingestion of excess quantities of hormone; synthesis of hormone at some ectopic site, usually a functioning metastatic carcinoma; or more commonly, inflammatory disease that leads to the unregulated leakage of hormone from the gland. As evidenced by low values of the thyroid radioactive iodine uptake, new hormone synthesis is suppressed in all nonhyperthyroid varieties of thyrotoxicosis. In these disorders, therefore, measures intended to decrease hormone synthesis are to no avail. Instead, treatment comprises withdrawal of the exogenous hormone in the case of factitious thyrotoxicosis; destruction or removal of the ectopic site, when that is the source of hormone; or in the case of inflammatory disorders, watchful waiting while the disease runs its course, often together with the palliative measures already mentioned and glucocorticoids when the patient is significantly symptomatic.

GENERAL CONSIDERATIONS

Several aspects of the pathogenesis and natural course of hyperthyroidism in Graves' disease bear importantly on its treatment and will, therefore, be briefly considered. Graves' disease is one of several closely related autoimmune thyroid diseases, the others being Hashimoto's disease and primary myxedema. In these disorders, patients with a genetically determined abnormality of immune regulation become sensitized to, and develop antibodies against, various antigens within their thyroid gland and often other tissues as well. It is generally agreed that thyroid hyperfunction in Graves' disease results from the action of a class of IgG immunoglobulins that are antibodies to the thyrotropin (TSH) receptor. They bind to the TSH receptor, as a consequence of which they inhibit the binding of TSH; like TSH, they activate adenylate cyclase within the plasma membrane of the follicular cell, increase the intracellular cyclic adenosine monophosphate concentration, and thereby initiate a chain of biochemical sequelae that result in thyroid growth and hyperfunction. These pathogenic IgG immunoglobulins can be detected in vitro through their ability to inhibit the binding of TSH to thyroid membranes or their thyroid-stimulating activity, as judged from activation of adenylate cyclase, increased radioiodine accumulation, or hormone release. Hence, they are designated TSH-binding inhibitory IgG (TBII) or thyroid-stimulating IgG (TSI), respectively.

TABLE 1 Disorders Associated with Thyrotoxicosis

Nature of Disorder	*Primary Mode of Therapy*	*Secondary Therapy*
Thyrotoxicosis with hyperthyroidism		
Syndromes of TSH excess		
TSH-producing tumor	Pituitary adenectomy	
Inappropriate TSH secretion	Uncertain*	
Graves' disease	Antithyroid agents	Adrenergic blocking agents
	Radioiodine	Iodine
	Subtotal thyroidectomy	Glucocorticoids
Toxic adenoma	Radioiodine	Adrenergic blocking agents
	Subtotal thyroidectomy	
Toxic multinodular goiter	Radioiodine	Adrenergic blocking agents
Thyrotoxicosis without hyperthyroidism		
Thyrotoxicosis factitia	Withdraw hormone	Adrenergic blocking agents
Ectopic thyroid	Destroy ectopic tissue	
Hormone leakage (thyroiditis)		
Subacute thyroiditis	Analgesics	
	Glucocorticoids	
	Adrenergic blocking agents	
Chronic thyroiditis with transient thyrotoxicosis	Adrenergic blocking agents	

* Optimum treatment is uncertain. Hyperthyroidism can be controlled by the same measures as in Graves' disease, but tends to recur, and the concern is that a pituitary tumor might develop if the thyroid is ablated. Isolated reports suggest that treatment with bromocriptine, T_3, or 3,5,3′-triiodothyroacetic acid (TRIAC) may be effective.

It has recently become evident that in patients with autoimmune thyroid disease, there also exists a class of IgG that binds to the TSH receptor and that therefore has TBII activity, but that does not activate adenylate cyclase. Rather, this class inhibits stimulatory responses to TSH and TSI. "Blocking antibodies" of this type have been implicated in the pathogenesis of some cases of nongoitrous myxedema.

As in other autoimmune disorders, hyperthyroidism in Graves' disease tends to be cyclic, undergoing periods of apparently spontaneous remission and exacerbation of varying duration. Because of associated chronic thyroiditis, patients tend to develop over many years progressive thyroid failure, even if their hyperthyroidism has not been treated by thyroid ablation, as by surgery or radioactive iodine. These aspects of the natural history of the disease have an important bearing on the outcome and therefore the choice of therapy.

Unfortunately, as yet no mode of therapy is directed primarily at the underlying immunologic cause of the disease. The commonly used antithyroid agents, 6-n-propylthiouracil (PTU) and methimazole, or carbimazole in the United Kingdom, act to inhibit both the organic-binding of thyroid iodine and the coupling of iodotyrosines to yield iodothyronines. There is some evidence that they may influence immune processes in vitro and that they may decrease the synthesis of thyroid directed antibodies in vivo, but it is unlikely that they have any effect that persists after their use is discontinued or that they influence the long-term course of the disorder. If this is indeed the case, then whether the patient experiences an immediate exacerbation of thyrotoxicosis when treatment is withdrawn or remains well for months, for years, or forever depends on the natural history of the disease in that particular patient. This seeming lack of a long-term effect of antithyroid agents undoubtedly accounts for the relatively low frequency of long-term or permanent remission that follows the usual course of antithyroid therapy.

Subtotal thyroidectomy and radioactive iodine destroy thyroid tissue, and, if sufficient tissue is destroyed, the disease can no longer manifest itself in hyperthyroidism. Therefore, the effect of such treatment is long-lasting, and, once an euthyroid state is achieved, recurrences of hyperthyroidism are rare. On the other hand, both surgery and radioactive iodine are prone to cause hypothyroidism with disturbing frequency. The cumulative frequency with which hypothyroidism follows ablative therapy increases progressively over the years as chronic thyroiditis erodes the function of a gland that has been partly destroyed.

Thus the relative long-term ineffectiveness of antithyroid therapy and the propensity of surgery and radioactive iodine to induce hypothyroidism pose the therapeutic dilemma in the management of patients with hyperthyroidism in Graves' disease. As a result, and as a recent formal survey of endocrinologists discloses, there is no general agreement concerning the optimum mode of therapy in the patient who presents with an initial episode of hyperthyroidism. In general, the therapeutic decision depends upon a number of factors. Mild disease, the absence of marked thyromegaly, and the fact that the patient is young weigh the decision toward antithyroid therapy, especially if the patient is a woman. Patients with more severe disease and a large, highly vascularized goiter are less likely to experience a long-term remission after a course of antithyroid therapy; in them, ablative therapy is more seriously considered: surgery in young women of childbearing age and radioactive iodine in others. In patients in the fifth decade of age and older, I lean strongly toward the use of radioactive iodine. Superimposed on these considerations is a judgment concerning the likelihood of adequate patient compliance. Anticipated or demonstrated poor patient compliance weighs the decision toward ablative therapy, i.e., surgery or radioactive iodine.

When an initial therapeutic recommendation has been formulated, I discuss with the patient in simple terms the nature of his or her disease, its natural course, and the various advantages and limitations of the several therapeutic options available. In such discussions, the patient has the opportunity to express particular concerns, such as the fear of surgery or radioactive iodine or the desire to "get it over with as quickly as possible." Ultimately, I make a strong therapeutic recommendation, which is almost always accepted, and a therapeutic plan is adopted to which both the physician and the patient are amenable. I find that this approach enhances patient confidence and compliance, minimizes later surprises, and in general fosters a favorable physician-patient relationship for a disease whose care should extend over many years.

ANTITHYROID THERAPY

Partly because of the age- and sex-distribution of patients with Graves' disease that I see and partly because of my personal inclination, I most often initiate treatment with antithyroid agents, usually 100 mg of PTU given thrice daily at 8-hour intervals. The approximately equivalent dose of methimazole is 30 mg daily, but I usually employ PTU because of its effect to inhibit the peripheral conversion of thyroxine (T_4) to triiodothyronine (T_3), hastening the therapeutic benefit that it brings. Patients with more severe disease, or those in whom a more rapid response is desired, are given higher doses, up to 600 mg daily. Improvement is not immediate since PTU and methimazole act by inhibiting hormone synthesis rather than release. As a result, a decrease in hormone secretion and clinical improvement do not occur until significant depletion of intrathyroid stores of hormone has taken place. The duration of this apparent latent period varies with several factors, including the severity of the hyperthyroidism, the hormonal iodine content of the gland, and the dose of antithyroid agent administered. Generally, however, some improvement can be expected in about 2 weeks, with a return to a normal metabolic state in 6 weeks to 2 months. Some patients, especially those with large vascular glands, are resistant to the usual doses of antithyroid agents; in them, larger doses, for example, 1,200 mg daily, may be required.

Clinical improvement is accompanied by a decrease in serum T_4 and T_3 concentrations, but the values do not always correlate well with the clinical state. Thus some patients remain thyrotoxic despite a normal serum T_4 concentration, probably because the serum T_3 concentration remains high. In others, an euthyroid clinical state is apparently sustained by a normal serum T_3 concentration, although the serum T_4 concentration is subnormal. There is accumulating evidence that patients in whom serum T_3 concentrations remain high relative to serum T_4 concentrations during antithyroid therapy are less likely to experience a long-term remission after such therapy is withdrawn.

Once achieved, an euthyroid clinical state can usually be maintained by doses of PTU in the order of 150 to 300 mg daily, and, once a maintenance dose is established, the patient is seen at intervals of 1 and then 2 months. Some patients require only small doses for the maintenance of the euthyroid state; I have the impression that these are patients who are hyperthyroid despite an underlying pronounced chronic thyroiditis, a condition euphemistically referred to as "Hashitoxicosis." An important element in following the patient is to observe the size of the thyroid gland. In about one-third of patients, the thyroid decreases in size. This decrease is probably a reflection of a decreasing level of TSI and is a favorable omen that a long-term remission will follow withdrawal of antithyroid therapy. In some patients, the thyroid gland enlarges instead, often with the appearance of a thrill or bruit. On the one hand, this enlargement may signal overtreatment with resulting hypothyroidism, which may be symptomatic. Symptoms and thyromegaly both respond readily to a decreased dose of antithyroid agent or to the provision of supplemental thyroid hormone. On the other hand, in a small proportion of patients, enlargement of the thyroid gland during antithyroid therapy is a reflection of intensification of the disease that may require an increase in the dose of antithyroid agent.

Adverse reactions to antithyroid agents occur in a small percentage of patients. The most feared is agranulocytosis, an immunologic response that most often occurs after a few weeks of initial exposure to the therapeutic agent, but may occur after a much longer interval. During a second or third course of the agent, it may appear within a few days. Agranulocytosis may be preceded by a period of drug-induced granulopenia, which may be hard to recognize since lymphocytosis and granulopenia occur in some patients with hyperthyroidism before therapy is initiated or may reflect the presence of an intercurrent viral infection.

Dealing with this problem is difficult, but several measures are of assistance. I always obtain baseline total and differential leukocyte counts before therapy begins, when the patient is seen again several weeks later, and when an euthyroid state has been achieved. Little benefit is to be derived from obtaining serial leukocyte counts thereafter since granulopenia and agranulocytosis can appear precipitously within a few days after granulocyte counts have been shown to be normal. However, if a sore throat or fever (or rash) develops, the patient is warned to call and to discontinue taking the antithyroid agent until he or she has been examined. This admonition should be repeated from time to time, and for medicolegal purposes, a note to the effect that this warning has been given should be placed in the patient's record. If granulopenia is found, frequent serial granulocyte counts are obtained, and, if a downward trend is detected, the drug is discontinued. More often, granulopenia remits, and therapy can be continued.

Probably the most common adverse reaction to the antithyroid agents is a rash, which may take many forms. Other toxic reactions include drug fever, cholestatic hepatitis, arthralgias and myalgias, neuritis, loss of taste sensation, thrombocytopenia, loss or altered pigmentation of the hair, and toxic psychoses. Administration of antihistamines may alleviate the rash and allow treatment with the original antithyroid agent to continue. As an alternative, the other antithyroid agent may be substituted. Under these circumstances, I discontinue antithyroid therapy altogether in view of the possibility that occult hypersensitivity reactions may take place since polyarteritis nodosa and lupus-like syndromes as a consequence of antithyroid therapy have been reported. Similarly, I never substitute one antithyroid agent for another in patients who have developed severe granulopenia or agranulocytosis since studies have shown that lymphocytes of patients who have developed agranulocytosis while taking PTU undergo blast transformation when exposed in vitro to methimazole. In sum, in patients with major hypersensitivity reactions to one or both of the classical antithyroid agents, one should resort to alternate modes of treating hyperthyroidism. These include radioiodine or surgery, often while manifestations of thyrotoxicosis are being controlled with a beta-adrenergic antagonist; administration of iodine or iodine-containing agents; use of lithium salts, which have a mild antithyroid effect; or such dramatic and infrequently employed measures as plasmapheresis and resin hemoperfusion in patients who are truly ill.

The most common and difficult decision confronting the physician with respect to patients being treated with PTU or methimazole is when to discontinue treatment, the hope being that an euthyroid state will persist. Unfortunately, there are no truly effective guidelines. As already noted, a decrease in goiter size during treatment is a reasonable indication that activity of the disease has abated and that a remission of reasonable duration may follow withdrawal of treatment; whereas persistence of an elevated serum T_3 concentration despite normalization of the serum T_4 may herald a contrary outcome. Efforts have been made to employ various other laboratory tests as predictors of prognosis. Although statistically related to outcome, thyroid suppression and tests of thyrotropin releasing hormone (TRH) responsiveness are poor indicators of prognosis in the individual patient. Controversy exists as to whether the persistence or absence of high titers of TBII or TSI are forerunners of prompt relapse or prolonged remission, respectively. In view of this uncertainty, the usual duration of a course of antithyroid therapy becomes somewhat arbitrary. The best data available indicate, not surprisingly, that the longer the course of treatment, the more likely a long-term remission will occur after treatment is withdrawn. Generally, I employ a treatment period of 12 to 18 months. Treatment is then withdrawn, and the patient is seen initially at 2 or 3 weeks and then at intervals progressively lengthening to 1 year. Serum T_4 and T_3 concentrations are measured at follow-up visits since an elevation of the serum T_3 may presage the emergence of thyrotoxicosis while the patient still appears euthyroid. Approximately 50 percent of patients treated in this manner experience a long-term remission; in the remainder, hyperthyroidism reemerges within several weeks or recurs at some interval, sometimes many years, thereafter. When this occurs, I most often recommend surgery or radioactive iodine therapy, but many patients prefer to undertake another course of antithyroid treatment, and there is no reason to discourage this approach if the patient is aware that the likelihood of a long-term remission after a second course of treatment is smaller than after the first.

SUBTOTAL THYROIDECTOMY

Subtotal thyroidectomy is an effective means of treating hyperthyroidism in Graves' disease, as many years of experience have demonstrated. It is infrequently followed by recurrence, but more often is followed by hypothyroidism, which sometimes occurs soon after an operation, but also appears in succeeding years. The frequency of postoperative hypothyroidism varies inversely with that of recurrence, depending upon the quantity of thyroid tissue left in situ and probably the degree of associated chronic thyroiditis. In the hands of experienced thyroid surgeons, subtotal thyroidectomy is a safe procedure; both immediate and delayed postoperative complications occur in only a low percentage of patients. By and large, however, this is not the case when the operation is performed by someone who lacks continued operative experience in this area.

Because of the tendency of subtotal thyroidectomy to lead to hypothyroidism, though less often than radioiodine does, and because the frequency of operative complications is greater than that of antithyroid therapy, I rarely recommend subtotal thyroidectomy as the initial therapy in the patient experiencing a first episode of hyperthyroidism in Graves' disease, preferring to rely in general upon antithyroid agents in children and young adults and radioiodine in those who are older. Exceptions include patients with severe hyperthyroidism, usually with large, hypervascular goiters, especially if they are young women or adolescents, in whom I prefer not to use radioactive iodine. In my experience, patients with severe thyrotoxicosis and large goiters are often difficult to bring under control with antithyroid agents and, more importantly, are unlikely to experience a long-term remission after a course of such treatment. Another category of patients in whom I may recommend surgery as the initial mode of therapy comprises those young patients who for personal reasons strongly desire to deal with the disease quickly and definitively and who do not wish to face possible recurrences after one or more courses of antithyroid agents.

Unlike other clinics, in which radioiodine is routinely recommended for the recurrences that follow one or more courses of antithyroid therapy, I often recommend surgery if the patient is a child or young adult and especially if the patient is female. I also recommend surgery in young patients who are noncompliant with a medical regimen.

Unless there are compelling reasons to the contrary, I strongly believe in the importance of rendering the patient euthyroid with medical therapy before subtotal thyroidectomy is performed. Generally, I initiate therapy with antithyroid drugs, though I may use larger doses than usual in order to obtain control more rapidly. After an euthyroid state has been restored, and not before, iodides are added to the regimen, usually in the form of saturated solution of potassium iodide, several drops two or three times daily. Although the value of iodides in bringing about involution of the gland and reducing its vascularity has been questioned, recent direct measurements have shown that the latter effect does take place. Some advocate discontinuing antithyroid therapy and replacing it with iodides once an euthyroid state has been achieved. I believe this approach to be an error since it permits thyroid iodine stores to reaccumulate during the preoperative period. Others, as a matter of convenience, set a target date for surgery on the presumption that an euthyroid state can necessarily be achieved within a defined period, a presumption that is infrequently justified.

Although it would certainly be both convenient and cost effective if one could safely carry out thyroidectomy in a patient whose pre- and intraoperative regimen consisted only of a few days of treatment with adrenergic blocking agents, and although several reports suggest that this approach may be safe and effective, I conservatively resist this approach, recognizing that thyroid storm can develop in patients receiving propranolol and believing that a prompt return of the patient to a normal routine after an operation is more likely to occur if, before operation, the patient has undergone the return toward a normal constitutional state that the full preoperative regimen permits.

RADIOIODINE

Ironically, early concerns about the use of radioactive iodine in the treatment of hyperthyroidism, i.e., leukemogenesis, carcinogenesis, and the induction of genetic damage, have proved to be unfounded, at least in adults, and indications of a low frequency of other late complications have given way to the realization that in a great many patients hypothyroidism either develops soon after iodine-131 therapy or continues to do so for years thereafter. I believe this development to be caused by the destructive effect of the radioiodine (and its possible inhibition of thyroid cell replication) combined with that of the chronic thyroiditis that is almost always associated with hyperthyroidism in Graves' disease. Nonetheless, because radioiodine is capable of curing hyperthyroidism in a way that antithyroid agents do not and because it is essentially devoid of known complications apart from hypothyroidism, it plays a major role in the management of patients with Graves' disease. Opinions vary widely as to the type of patient in whom iodine-131 therapy should be used. Some use it to treat almost all patients, including children. However, children are prone to developing thyroid tumors and other nodular lesions after exposure to thyroid radiation, and the effects of hypothyroidism can be particularly damaging during childhood. Therefore, I and most others never use iodine-131 to treat children with hyperthyroidism. Yet some who never use radioiodine to treat children, use it routinely in almost any adult. Others, believing that long-term genetic effects have not been fully excluded, abjure its use in women who plan to have children. I lean toward the latter approach and resort to surgery in this group when ablative therapy is indicated. An additional consideration that also moves me toward this stance is the recognition that the younger the patient the more time there is for hypothyroidism to develop within the patient's lifespan. Hypothyroidism is also a complication of surgery, of course, but to a lesser degree. In patients who are middle-aged or older or in those whose family is complete, genetic damage is not a consideration, and delayed hypothyroidism is less of a problem. As a consequence, I usually treat patients of this type with iodine-131.

Research on radioiodine therapy has concentrated on means of reducing subsequent hypothyroidism. Smaller than usual doses are less likely to result in hypothyroidism in the short term, but more often fail to control hyperthyroidism; there is no convincing evidence that they decrease the frequency of hypothyroidism in the long term. The latter is true whether or not antithyroid agents or iodides are employed to control hyperthyroidism in the early months after treatment. Similarly, the practice of administering larger doses per unit thyroid weight in patients with larger glands, and smaller doses for smaller glands, has failed to achieve the objective of obtaining both early control of hyperthyroidism and a decreased frequency of delayed hypothyroidism. As a consequence, when I use radioiodine, I and the patient accept the fact that the patient has an approximately 20 percent likelihood of becoming hypothyroid in the first year and about a 50 percent likelihood of doing so by 10 years after treatment. Some physicians purposely administer large doses of radioiodine, accepting that hypothyroidism is almost sure to develop, but desiring to bring the hyperthyroidism definitely to an end. The rationale is that hypothyroidism is usually treated with ease. I would not fault this approach in patients who are likely to be compliant and particularly in the elderly, in whom inadequately treated or recurrent hyperthyroidism may represent a serious threat.

In patients who are to receive iodine-131 therapy, I first determine the 24-hour thyroid iodine-131 uptake and then administer a total therapeutic dose calculated to deliver about 80 μCi or approximately 3×10^6 Bq per gram of estimated thyroid weight. Clinical improvement is usually delayed and progressive. Usually some improvement is evident in a few weeks, but the full early effect of treatment may not be realized for 3, 4, or even 6 months. During this period, propranolol is useful in controlling troubling manifestations of thyrotoxicosis.

Approximately 15 to 20 percent of patients, most commonly those with larger goiters, fail to achieve an euthyroid state within the first 6 months after the usual doses of radioactive iodine. This failure is commonly signaled by a lack of improvement in serum T_4 and T_3 concentrations by several months after treatment. In such patients, a second dose, approximately two-thirds the magnitude of the first, is administered. In a small proportion of patients, perhaps 5 percent, a third dose is required.

Although the likelihood of hypothyroidism is increased, I generally give somewhat larger doses of iodine-131 to elderly patients, particularly those with associated cardiovascular disease, in whom rapid and definitive control of thyrotoxicosis seems especially important. Further, such patients are almost always brought to an euthyroid state with antithyroid agents before radioiodine is administered in order to prevent the release of damaging quantities of hormone if radiation thyroiditis was to occur, as it commonly does approximately 2 weeks after radioiodine is administered. When this regimen is employed, antithyroid therapy is discontinued for 3 days, radioiodine is administered, and the antithyroid agent resumed 2 or 3 days later. Several months later, antithyroid therapy is gradually withdrawn so that the efficacy of the administered iodine-131 can be assessed.

A small proportion of patients become transiently hypothyroid several months after the dose of iodine-131, as is also the case in patients treated surgically. In most instances, this development occurs because, in a manner analogous to the adrenocorticotropic hormone secretory mechanism, the TSH secretory mechanism that has been subjected to prolonged feedback suppression requires some time to recover. This suppression is evidenced by inappropriately subnormal serum TSH concentrations and TRH responses coincident with subnormal serum T_4 and T_3 concentrations. With time, usually weeks but sometimes months, recovery of normal homeostatic control occurs. At that time, serum T_4, T_3, and TSH concentrations normalize if an euthyroid state is to be achieved; whereas serum T_4 concentrations remain low and TSH concentrations become elevated if the patient is destined to become permanently hypothyroid. Thus, if early postablative hypothyroidism is mild, patients can merely be observed over the next several months to see whether symptoms and chemical evidence of hypothyroidism abate. When hypothyroidism is more pronounced, treatment with synthetic T_4 in full replacement doses is initiated. Approximately 1 year later, measures are undertaken to determine if the patient is permanently hypothyroid, and several options are available for doing so. One approach is to discontinue levothyroxine sodium and to observe the patient for 6 weeks. At that time, serum T_4, T_3, and TSH concentrations reflect the true functional capability of the thyroid. An alternate approach can shorten the period of evaluation. Here, levothyroxine sodium is discontinued and a replacement dose of liothyronine sodium (approximately 75 μg daily) is substituted for a period of 4 weeks. At that time, the serum T_4 concentration is measured. Values less than 1.0 μg per deciliter indicate that the patient is truly hypothyroid; values greater than 1.0 μg per deciliter suggest that thyroid function is normal and that liothyronine sodium can be discontinued. Intrinsic euthyroidism can then be verified by demonstrating a normal serum TSH concentration several weeks later. This same procedure can be employed when one sees a patient already receiving replacement therapy for presumed hypothyroidism in whom one wishes to establish a definitive diagnosis.

IODINE

Iodine is an extremely valuable agent in the treatment of hyperthyroidism under the special conditions in which it is indicated. The action of iodine to decrease serum thyroid hormone concentrations and to alleviate thyrotoxicosis is much more rapid than that of the antithyroid agents owing to the fact that iodine acts principally to inhibit the intrathyroid mechanisms that lead to hormone release rather than synthesis. A secondary and undesirable effect of iodine is to increase glandular stores of hormonal iodine, creating a potential reservoir for subsequent excessive hormone release. For this reason, I do not undertake the use of iodine lightly and, except in patients being prepared for surgery, reserve its use for patients in whom rapid amelioration of thyrotoxicosis is critical. In this circumstance, concomitant use of antithyroid agents in large doses is strongly indicated for two reasons. First, patients in whom thyrotoxicosis is sufficiently critical to require treatment with iodine also require a major effort to inhibit ongoing hormone synthesis. Second, when used with iodine, large doses of antithyroid agents substantially decrease the degree of enrichment of thyroid iodine stores that would otherwise ensue. Patients sufficiently ill to receive iodine generally merit both hospitalization and adjunctive agents, such as adrenergic blocking agents and occasionally corticosteroids.

In patients who are not in actual or impending thyroid storm, but who are sufficiently ill to receive iodine, I initiate treatment with PTU in large doses, 600 mg daily or more, several hours before tretment with iodine begins. Saturated solution of potassium iodide is then begun in doses of several drops two or three times daily. The precise quantity of iodine required is admittedly uncertain and may vary from patient to patient; but in my experience, this quantity has been effective in almost all patients. Iodine therapy should not be discontinued too soon or too abruptly since abrupt discontinuation sometimes makes possible accelerated release of hormonal stores that may have become somewhat enriched. For this reason, I continue administering iodine together with large doses of antithyroid agents for several weeks until the effect of the latter to decrease hormone stores is strongly expressed and clinical improvement achieved. Doses of iodine are then tapered over the next several weeks.

ADJUNCTIVE THERAPY

Adrenergic Blocking Agents

The beta-adrenergic blocking agent propranolol plays an important role in managing patients with hyperthyroidism, because of its ability to decrease many of the sympathomimetic manifestations of thyrotoxicosis. In patients with actual or impending thyroid storm, its use may be critical. In less severely ill patients and in the absence of contraindications, such as myocardial failure or bronchial asthma, I often use propranolol to decrease palpitations and lower heart rate and to decrease perspiration and tremor. I use it in particular while awaiting the results of laboratory tests to confirm a diagnosis of hyperthyroidism and while awaiting the therapeutic response to antithyroid agents or radioactive iodine. Doses of 20 to 40 mg four times daily generally suffice; these are reduced and withdrawn altogether as the patient achieves an euthyroid state. As already indicated, I do not favor use of propranolol as the sole pre- and intraoperative therapy in patients undergoing subtotal thyroidectomy. Neither do I recommend chronic use of propranolol in the pregnant woman with hyperthyroidism. Although opinions concerning its safety in pregnancy vary, some indicate that growth retardation, low Apgar scores, and fetal hypoglycemia and bradycardia may attend its use.

Glucocorticoids

High doses of adrenal glucocorticoids play a poorly understood but useful role in the treatment of patients with Graves' disease and severe hyperthyroidism, in whom rapid relief of thyrotoxicosis is critical. One component of the beneficial effect of glucocorticoids stems from their ability to inhibit the peripheral deiodination of T_4 to yield T_3; this effect is not confined to patients with hyperthyroidism, being seen in euthyroid subjects as well. The second effect is more obscure in its origin, has been demonstrated only in patients with Graves' disease, and comprises a reduction in serum T_4 concentration that is evident within 1 or 2 days and is apparently due to inhibition of hormone release. In view of the slow turnover of IgG, this prompt effect is unlikely to reflect an inhibition of TSI synthesis, but doubtless results from an effect of the glucocorticoids on some component of the immune system, possibly lymphocytes that are producing TSI within the thyroid itself. I have employed glucocorticoids infrequently, confining their use to patients sufficiently ill to warrant concomitant treatment with iodides and propranolol. Under these conditions, I have given doses of prednisone or dexamethasone equivalent to 300 mg of hydrocortisone daily.

Ipodate Sodium

This iodinated x-ray contrast agent is one of several that both inhibit the peripheral conversion of T_4 or T_3 and provide large quantities of iodine that act directly on the thyroid to inhibit hormone release. Doses of 1.0 g daily have been shown to produce a prompt decrease in serum T_4 and T_3 concentrations, together with alleviation of thyrotoxicosis. I have no direct experience with use of this agent, but would caution that large doses of antithyroid agents be administered concomitantly and ipodate withdrawn slowly, as in the use of iodine alone.

FOLLOW-UP

From their first visit, patients with Graves' disease should be informed that they will require lifetime, if ultimately infrequent, follow-up. There are many reasons why this is the case. Approximately 50 percent of patients who remain euthyroid after one or more courses of antithyroid therapy develop thyroid failure 20 or more years later. Others, in contrast, develop recurrent hyperthyroidism; the longest interval between remission and later relapse that I have seen has been 28 years. Among patients treated with radioiodine or surgery, continuing surveillance has revealed the development of hypothyroidism in several percent each year. Finally, the passage of years may permit the emergence of other autoimmune diseases with which Graves' disease is associated, such as pernicious anemia, idiopathic adrenal atrophy, or diabetes mellitus. These considerations make reexamination of the patient with Graves' disease at regular intervals mandatory, even though hyperthyroidism no longer appears to be a problem.

SUGGESTED READING

Halnan K. Risks from radioiodine treatment of thyrotoxicosis. Br Med J 1983; 287(2):1821–1822.

Hedley AJ, Bewsher PD, Jones SL, et al. Late onset hypothyroidism after subtotal thyroidectomy for hyperthyroidism: implications for long-term follow up. Br J Surg 1983; 70:740–743.

Romaldini JH, Bromberg N, Werner RS, et al. Comparison of effects of high and low dosage regimens of antithyroid drugs in the management of Graves' hyperthyroidism. J Clin Endocrinol Metab 1983; 57:563–570.

Sugrue DD, Drury MI, McEvoy M, Heffernan SJ, O'Malley E. Long term follow-up of hyperthyroid patients treated by subtotal thyroidectomy. Br J Surg 1983; 70:408–411.

Tamai H, Nakagawa T, Fukino O, et al. Thionamide therapy in Graves disease: relation of relapse rate to duration of therapy. Ann Intern Med 1980; 92:488–490.

Wood LC, Ingbar SH. Hypothyroidism as a late sequela in patients with Grave's disease treated with antithyroid drugs. J Clin Invest 1979; 64:1429.

Wu SY, Shyh TP, Chopra IJ, Solomon DH, Huang HW, Chu PC. Comparison of sodium ipodate (Oragrafin) and propylthiouracil in early treatment of hyperthyroidism. J Clin Endocrinol Metab 1982; 54:630–634.

THYROID STORM

JACOB M. ROBBINS, M.D.

Thyroid storm or thyrotoxic crisis is an extreme state of hyperthyroidism judged severe enough to be life-threatening. Inasmuch as there are no definite criteria on which to base the diagnosis, the decision to begin therapy for this medical emergency is dictated by clinical judgment alone. In almost all cases, thyroid storm develops when a patient with untreated or incompletely controlled hyperthyroidism encounters a stress, such as surgical or accidental trauma, or an intercurrent illness, such as a severe infection. In this setting, it is often difficult to attribute the symptoms and signs to thyrotoxicosis rather than to the associated illness. Since the disease may be rapidly fatal and since mortality from thyroid storm has been greatly reduced by therapeutic regimens such as the one described next, treatment should begin as soon as the diagnosis is seriously entertained.

The manifestations of thyroid storm are usually those of exaggerated thyrotoxicosis, including severe agitation (often of psychotic proportions), extreme tachycardia, gastrointestinal symptoms (notably diarrhea), and fever. Cardiac arrhythmias, congestive heart failure, and jaundice may be present. Apathetic hyperthyroidism, progressing to stupor and coma, may confound the recognition of thyrotoxic crisis, and only the finding of a goiter with elevated serum thyroid hormone levels may lead to the correct conclusion. The laboratory findings in thyroid storm are indistinctive, although the free thyroxine (T_4) concentration may be higher than is usually seen in thyrotoxicosis. Furthermore, the effects of severe illness—decreased thyroxine transport protein levels and interference with the extrathyroidal production of triiodothyronine (T_3)—are factors to be considered in interpreting the hormone levels.

PRINCIPLES OF TREATMENT

Therapeutic intervention should be prompt, vigorous, and multifactorial (Table 1). It should be directed toward inhibition of thyroidal production and release of thyroid hormones; inhibition of monodeiodination of T_4 (a major source of T_3 production in peripheral tissues); interference with the action of thyroid hormone on the cardiovascular and central nervous systems by antiadrenergic therapy; reduction of fever; "support" therapy, including glucocorticoids, fluids and electrolytes, glucose, B vitamins, and sedation if required; treatment of the associated illness (e.g., infection, cardiac failure, diabetic ketoacidosis); and, if these combined therapies fail, extracorporeal removal of thyroid hormone.

Inhibition of Thyroid Hormone Synthesis and Release

Thyroid Hormone Synthesis

Blockade of organification of thyroidal iodine should be instituted immediately by administering a thionamide drug in high dosage. Of the two available agents, 6-n-propylthiouracil (PTU) and methimazole (Tapazole), PTU is preferred because it has the additional effect of inhibiting conversion of T_4 to T_3 in peripheral tissues. The recommended daily dose is 800 to 1,200 mg of PTU or 80 to 120 mg of methimazole, given orally. Because organification blockade must precede the administration of iodide, a large initial dose (800 mg PTU or 80 mg methimazole) may be used, followed by 200 mg PTU or 20 mg methimazole every 4 to 6 hours. Methimazole, which has a longer duration of action, can be given as infrequently as every

TABLE 1 Approaches to the Treatment of Thyroid Storm

Reduction of the circulating thyroid hormone level
Drugs to inhibit thyroid hormone synthesis
Propylthiouracil*
Methimazole
Drugs to inhibit thyroid hormone release
Iodide* (NaI IV or saturated solution of KI orally)†
Lithium carbonate
Extracorporeal removal of thyroid hormone‡
Plasmapheresis*
Exchange transfusion
Peritoneal dialysis
Inhibition of peripheral T_3 formation
Propylthiouracil*
Glucocorticoid*
Propranolol
Iopanoic acid
Blockade of thyroid hormone effects by antiadrenergic drugs
Propranolol*
Atenolol or metoprolol
Reserpine
Guanethidine
"Support" therapy
Glucocorticoid
Fever reduction by physical methods
Fluid and electrolyte replacement
Glucose infusion
Vitamin B complex
Sedation (if required)
Treatment of congestive failure and/or cardiac arrhythmia
Diagnosis and treatment of intercurrent illness§

* The preferred method
† Do not begin until thyroidal iodine organification is blocked
‡ To be used if other treatments fail
§ Almost always present unless trauma was the precipitating event.
Note that thyrotoxicosis may alter the sensitivity to required drug therapy.

8 to 12 hours. If required, crushed tablets are given by nasogastric tube.

Thyroid Hormone Release

Blockade of thyroid hormone release is effected by iodide in high dosage, beginning no sooner than 1 hour after initiating the organification blockage to avoid new hormone synthesis. The daily dose is 750 mg to 1 g, given by continuous intravenous infusion of sodium iodide or orally as potassium iodide solution USP (saturated solution), 300 mg (0.3 ml or 14 drops) every 8 hours. This amount of iodide is probably more than is needed to maximally block hormone release, but the optimum dosage is not known precisely. Lugol's solution (strong iodine solution USP) contains 5 percent iodine plus 10 percent potassium iodide or about 150 mg iodine per milliliter.

Lithium ion is an alternate agent capable of blocking thyroid hormone release, and it can be used before the onset of organification blockade since it is not a substrate for new hormone synthesis as is iodide. There is also evidence that its effect is additive to that of iodide; this additivity has a potential advantage since release is not blocked completely by either lithium or iodide. Although lithium has been used successfully to treat thyroid storm, it has the disadvantage of potentially serious cardiovascular and central nervous system toxicity with a narrow margin of safety between the therapeutic and the toxic levels. It is given orally as lithium carbonate, with a loading dose of 600 mg followed by 300 mg three to five times per day. The serum lithium level must be measured at least once a day and not be permitted to exceed 1.5 mEq per liter. Its effect begins promptly when the blood level reaches 0.6 to 0.8 mEq per liter. Caution is required when it is used in a patient with cardiovascular or renal failure or cardiac arrhythmia.

Peripheral T_3 Formation

Reduction of peripheral T_3 formation can be achieved with PTU, as already mentioned. Reduction is also effected by several other agents, one of which is a glucocorticoid such as hydrocortisone. As with PTU, the use of a glucocorticoid has an additional indication in thyroid storm (to be discussed). Propranolol, used for its beta-adrenergic blockade action, also inhibits 5′-deiodination of T_4, but is less potent than either PTU or cortisol. It seems unnecessary to add still another monodeiodination inhibitor; however, two that have been advocated are iopanoic acid (Telepaque) or sodium ipodate (Oragrafin), in a dose of 1 g daily by mouth. Although these agents also release iodide, it is not known whether the amount would be sufficient to block thyroid hormone release from the gland.

Combined therapy of uncomplicated hyperthyroidism with PTU, 150 mg every 6 hours; saturated potassium iodide, 3 drops every 6 hours; and dexamethasone, 2 mg every 6 hours has been shown to restore a normal serum T_3 level within 24 hours. Radioactive iodine therapy has no role in the immediate therapy of thyroid storm since it may increase thyroid hormone release within days after its administration, and the therapeutic response usually does not begin for several weeks. Radioiodine is ineffective when thionamide or iodide therapy is in progress, but can be administered when lithium alone is used to block secretion since this drug does not affect iodine-131 uptake and retention.

Blockade of Hormone Action

Antiadrenergic drugs (beta-blockers) effectively reduce the cardiovascular and psychomotor manifestations of hyperthyroidism. The drug of choice, because of wide experience and because of its additional action to reduce peripheral T_3 production, is propranolol. It may be given intravenously (2 to 10 mg at a rate of 1 mg per minute) for prompt effect or orally in a dose of 40 to 80 mg every 4 to 6 hours. These are larger doses than are used in treating uncomplicated hyperthyroidism. Intravenous therapy is hazardous and requires continuous monitoring of the electrocardiogram. Central venous pressure can also be monitored. Although propranolol must be used cautiously when congestive failure is present, there is evidence for an overall benefit if the cardiac failure is treated concomitantly. When there is bronchospasm or peripheral vascular disease, the more specific $beta_1$-blockers, such as atenolol or metoprolol, should be used instead of propranolol. Oral doses having equivalent cardiovascular effects are 40 mg propranolol or 50 mg metoprolol twice a day and 25 mg atenolol once a day. There has been little experience with these newer agents in treating thyrotoxicosis, and their effect on the psychomotor manifestations is unknown. However, only propranolol is lipid-soluble and thus readily available to the central nervous system (CNS). It is also the only drug provided for intravenous use.

Reserpine and guanethidine, drugs that deplete tissue catecholamines, are also effective. High doses have been recommended: reserpine intramuscularly, 1 to 3 mg every 4 to 8 hours (after a test dose of 0.25 mg), and guanethidine orally, 1 to 2 mg per kilogram every 4 to 6 hours. Because of serious side effects, these agents are less desirable than propranolol, and the optimum dose should be determined by titration. Both cause hypotension, and reserpine produces CNS depression, which may or may not be tolerable depending on the patient's clinical status. These drugs have a slower onset of action than propranolol, and the effects also take much longer to disappear when therapy is stopped.

"Support" Therapy

Glucocorticoid Therapy. High-dosage glucocorticoids are thought to be beneficial in treating thyrotoxic crisis. In addition to inhibiting peripheral T_3 formation, glucocorticoids may correct a state of relative adrenal insufficiency. This hypothetical diagnosis is based on the known increase in cortisol degradation occurring in hyperthyroidism and on the possibility that this degradation could exceed the increased secretion that also takes place. Other effects of high-dose glucocorticoids, such as reduction in fever and maintenance of blood pressure, may be equally or more important in explaining the apparent benefits of such therapy. The recommended dose of hydrocortisone, 200 to 400 mg per day, can be given intravenously or orally at 6-hour intervals and can be replaced by an equivalent amount of a synthetic corticosteroid (e.g., prednisone, 50 to 100 mg per day, or dexamethasone, 8 to 15 mg per day).

Fever. Control of fever, which may reach a high level, is an important aspect of therapy. Although an antipyretic drug might be used, it is probably wiser to employ a physical method such as a cooling blanket or sponge baths. Salicylates should be avoided since they inhibit binding of thyroid hormone to the serum transport proteins, thereby raising the free hormone level. Salicylates also appear to have a thyromimetic effect peripherally. Pharmacologic blockade of the thermoregulatory center, to reduce the shivering response to cooling, may be accomplished by the use of chlorpromazine and meperidine, 25 to 50 mg IV every 4 to 6 hours. Larger doses up to 100 to 200 mg every 6 hours may be needed in the severely agitated patient.

Nutrition. In addition to the maintenance of fluid and electrolyte balance, attention should be given to the catabolic effects of severe thyrotoxicosis. Intravenous glucose infusion should be supplemented with B-complex vitamins in "therapeutic" doses.

Sedation. For the treatment of CNS excitement, sedation may be indicated. Barbiturates have a potential further benefit in that investigators have shown, in animals, that phenobarbital enhances the degradation of thyroid hormones by the liver and thereby ameliorates the effects of excess hormone.

Treatment of Intercurrent Illness

Since thyrotoxic crisis is often triggered by an intercurrent illness, it is essential to diagnose the associated disease and to treat it appropriately. One must also be aware that the complex nature of the crisis may make the diagnosis difficult and that the medication used to treat the crisis, notably high-dose corticosteroids and antipyretics, may obscure the diagnosis of an infection. In addition, the management of the associated illness may be affected by the hyperthyroid state. Important examples are the increased digitalis dosage required to treat congestive heart failure and to maintain an adequate blood level of the drug, the increased insulin requirement in managing concomitant diabetes mellitus, and the increased anticoagulant potency of dicumarol. Required surgical therapy should be delayed for at least 24 to 48 hours if possible.

Extracorporeal Removal of Thyroid Hormones

The combined therapies outlined previously are successful in most cases of thyroid storm. However, if the thyroid hormone levels do not respond rapidly enough to the drugs and if the hormone effects are not controlled adequately, it is possible to remove the hormones by a dialysis procedure or plasma withdrawal. Several methods have been used with significant success. Hemodialysis utilizing an ion exchange resin or charcoal to retain hormone in the dialystate is effective, but a straightforward alternative approach is to use a method capable of removing the transport proteins to which the hormones are strongly attached. The latter can be accomplished by plasmapheresis, exchange transfusion, or peritoneal dialysis. The quantity of plasma to be removed can be judged from the fact that the exchangeable T_4 space, or serum-equivalent volume, is about 10 L. The serum-equivalent volume for T_3 is about 30 to 40 L. Reduction of serum T_4 to almost normal has been achieved by removing 3 to 4 L of blood, or the plasma equivalent, over 12 to 24 hours. An amount of T_4 roughly equivalent to that in 2 L of plasma can apparently be removed by peritoneal dialysis over a period of about 72 hours. There is also evidence that intracellular thyroid hormone can be depleted during plasma withdrawal. The ideal replacement fluid should contain T_4 binding protein but be low in T_4 and T_3 content. Albumin is, therefore, preferred over whole plasma.

EFFECTIVENESS OF THERAPY

In former years, thyroid storm was a frequent complication of thyroidectomy for hyperthyroidism. It is now a rare occurrence, and, given the imprecise diagnostic criteria, it is difficult to define its prevalence or to evaluate the success of therapeutic procedures. Nevertheless, with the application of the methods described previously, the mortality from thyrotoxic crisis appears to have decreased from about 90 percent to perhaps 10 to 20 percent. The persistence of deaths from this complication calls for vigorous therapy when the diagnosis is suspected.

SUGGESTED READING

Brooks MH, Waldstein SS. Free thyroxine concentrations in thyroid storm. Ann Intern Med 1980; 93:694–697.

Croxson MS, Hall TD, Nicoloff JT. Combination drug therapy for treatment of hyperthyroid Graves' disease. J Clin Endocrinol Metab 1977; 45:623–630.

Nicoloff JT. Thyroid storm and myxedema coma. Med Clin North Am 1985; 69:1005–1017.

Rosenberg IN. Thyroid storm. In: The thyroid. Physiology and treatment of disease. International encyclopedia of pharmacology and therapeutics, section 101. Oxford: Pergamon Press, 1979:301.

Schlienger JL, Faradji A, Demangeat C, et al. Quantitative evaluation of thyroid hormone extraction by continuous plasma exchange in euthyroid subjects. Presse Med 1983; 12:499–502.

THYROIDITIS

MARTIN I. SURKS, M.D.

The diverse group of disorders that produce inflammation of the thyroid result in a variety of clinical syndromes that may include hypothyroidism and hyperthyroidism. Since some of these disorders may be selflimited, management of the abnormal metabolic states may often be different from standard management of hypothyroidism and hyperthyroidism due to other causes. An understanding of the natural history of the different types of thyroiditis is therefore important for appropriate patient management. Several forms of thyroiditis that occur very rarely, such as acute suppurative thyroiditis and Riedel's thyroiditis, are not discussed here; discussions of the management of these disorders are found in standard textbooks.

HASHIMOTO'S THYROIDITIS

Many patients with Hashimoto's thyroiditis present with a syndrome consisting of goiter and hypothyroidism. Therapy with thyroid hormone is employed in these patients both to relieve the hypothyroidism and to decrease the size of the goiter. As in other forms of hypothyroidism, L-thyroxine is the therapeutic agent of choice in these patients, and the mode of administration of the drug is also in accord with that in other hypothyroid disorders. When L-thyroxine is employed for treatment, we recommend the use of the brand name agents, Synthroid or Levothroid, since published reports suggest that the potency of some generic L-thyroxine preparations may be variable. In most patients, therapy with L-thyroxine should relieve both the clinical symptoms and signs of hypothyroidism and also reestablish normal serum concentrations of L-thyroxine (T_4), L-triiodothyronine (T_3), and thyroid-stimulating hormone (TSH). Not only will the decreased serum T_4 and T_3 concentrations of hypothyroid patients with Hashimoto's thyroiditis return to normal with L-thyroxine treatment but the daily variation in serum hormone concentrations will also be small, similar to that in euthyroid patients who do not have thyroid disease. When some other thyroid hormone preparations containing both T_4 and T_3 are employed, a large increase in the serum T_3 concentration may occur after ingestion of the medication, and the relief of hypothyroidism may not be associated with normal serum T_4 and T_3 levels.

The rate of administration and dose of L-thyroxine in Hashimoto's thyroiditis depend on several nonthyroidal factors, such as the patient's age and associated medical conditions. In young patients who are otherwise in good health, the full daily replacement dose can be estimated to be between 0.075 and 0.15 mg and can be administered daily. L-Thyroxine has a slow rate of metabolism in euthyroid persons (half-life of 6 days), which is even slower in patients with hypothyroidism. The rate of equilibration of L-thyroxine that is administered daily will therefore also be quite slow. In fact, 4 to 8 weeks may be required before a new L-thyroxine dose is fully equilibrated in a hypothyroid patient. Because of these factors, patients should be instructed that their symptoms will be relieved slowly. This will avoid disappointment in the slow initial rate of improvement. Patients should also be instructed to return after 2 months of treatment for clinical evaluation and for measurement of serum T_4 and TSH concentrations. Relief of the clinical symptoms and normalization of serum T_4 and TSH levels indicate that the administered dose of L-thyroxine is appropriate for the patient and should be maintained. Therapy is generally lifelong, and the patient should be evaluated by clinical examination and laboratory measurements on an annual basis thereafter. Annual reevaluation should allow the clinician to detect and correct changes in thyroxine requirements (usually small) and to assess patient compliance. The physician should also evaluate the patient for other autoimmune disorders that are associated with Hashimoto's thyroiditis, such as pernicious anemia, rheumatoid arthritis, adrenal insufficiency, and Sjögren's syndrome. When patients are restored to the euthyroid state by the appropriate dose of L-thyroxine, the goiter also decreases in size. However, some thyroid enlargement, possibly depending on the degree of fibrosis in the gland, may remain even after adequate treatment.

If the clinician determines that the patient is not euthyroid, or if serum T_4 and TSH concentration are not normalized by 2 months of treatment with the initial dose of L-thyroxine, the dose should be increased. If, however, the serum T_4 concentration is increased or if the serum TSH concentration is suppressed as determined by a sensitive TSH measurement, the dose of L-thyroxine should be decreased. In either case, the patient should be reevaluated after 1 to 2 months of treatment with the new dose of L-thyroxine and, if laboratory test results are normal, evaluated on an annual basis thereafter.

Although the general principles of patient management are the same, the initial dose and rate of increase of L-thyroxine dosage should be markedly different in patients with Hashimoto's thyroiditis who also have significant cardiovascular disease and in older patients who may have subclinical arteriosclerotic heart disease. Relief of hypothyroidism is associated with an increase in cardiac output, cardiac work, and oxygen consumption. Because of these factors, thyroid hormone treatment has been associated with precipitation of angina pectoris, myocardial infarction, and sudden death in some patients. Thus, in this group of patients, the principles of therapy include initial treatment with a low dose of L-thyroxine, generally 0.025 mg per day, and increasing the dose of L-thyroxine by 0.025 mg per day every 4 to 8 weeks. The very gradual relief of hypothyroidism by this regimen should be associated with a gradual increase in cardiac work and oxygen consumption and thus minimize the possibility of myocardial complications. To avoid disappointment with the very slow rate of improvement of the hypothyroidism, the patient and family should be instructed that it is in the interests of the patient's safety that the hypothyroid syndrome will be relieved over 4 to 8 months rather than in 4 to 8 weeks as in younger persons.

Some patients with Hashimoto's thyroiditis present with thyroid enlargement and with few, if any, symptoms of hypothyroidism. Indeed, Hashimoto's thyroiditis may occur with characteristic goiter and a high titer of antithyroid antibodies but with normal serum T_4, T_3, and TSH concentrations. Treatment of these patients with L-thyroxine is somewhat controversial, since some clinicians believe that treatment with L-thyroxine should be restricted to patients with symptomatic hypothyroidism. Although observation alone in highly motivated, reliable patients may be satisfactory, these optimal circumstances do not occur in many settings. In my view, there are several reasons why all patients with Hashimoto's thyroiditis should be treated with L-thyroxine. First, the disease is generally progressive so that clinically apparent hypothyroidism will likely occur in the patient's lifetime. If a patient with untreated Hashimoto's thyroiditis is lost to follow-up, a slowly developing syndrome of hypothyroidism may remain unrecognized for a long period of time, even years, and seriously disrupt the quality of the patient's life. Second, patients with Hashimoto's thyroiditis without hypothyroidism appear to be at high risk for development of acute iodide-induced hypothyroidism. These patients apparently have the Wolff-Chaikoff phenomenon when exposed to excess inorganic iodide but may fail to adapt to the continued presence of iodide. Hypothyroidism may also develop when patients with Hashimoto's thyroiditis are treated with lithium. Since daily treatment with L-thyroxine is safe, inexpensive, and effective, it should be recommended to all patients with Hashimoto's thyroiditis irrespective of the presence of clinical hypothyroidism.

SUBACUTE THYROIDITIS (VIRAL THYROIDITIS, GRANULOMATOUS THYROIDITIS, DE QUERVAIN'S THYROIDITIS)

Patients with subacute thyroiditis frequently present with pain in the anterior neck and with radiation of the pain to the jaws and ears. Examination reveals tenderness, which occasionally is exquisite, over the affected area of the thyroid gland. Although the disease was originally described as a painful thyroiditis, clinicians should be aware that the degree of pain may be variable. Indeed, in some patients, pain or tenderness on palpation may not occur at all. Management of this syndrome depends on the severity of the pain and the patient's response to various analgesic agents. Analgesics such as acetylsalicylic acid and acetaminophen should be employed for mild to moderate neck discomfort, and these medications may significantly relieve neck pain in some patients. In patients with severe neck pain or in those who fail to obtain sufficient relief from these analgesics, treatment with glucocorticoids in high dosage generally results in a rapid relief of pain. A typical regimen to begin treatment is prednisone, 40 to 60 mg per day in divided doses. The pain is usually completely relieved within 12 to 24 hours. The dose of prednisone is then rapidly decreased to the minimal dose that maintains the patient without distress. Since the duration of viral thyroiditis is often several weeks to several months, prednisone in maintenance doses should be given as long as neck pain recurs when the dosage is decreased.

Patients with subacute thyroiditis with or without pain frequently have symptoms of both hyperthyroidism and hypothyroidism during the course of the disorder. Hyperthyroidism is often observed during the early stages of the disease, mainly in the first 3 months. Since the hypermetabolism results from leakage of thyroglobulin from the inflamed thyroid gland into the circulation rather than from an overproduction of thyroid hormones, the syndrome is clearly self-limited. Once the involved thyroid tissue has discharged all of its stored thyroglobulin, the hypermetabolism will be attenuated. Although self-limited, the hypermetabolism may be associated with a clinical syndrome that warrants treatment in some patients. Because of the nature of the disorder, only symptomatic relief of hypermetabolism can be offered to the patient. This is accomplished through the use of beta-sympathetic antagonists such as propranolol. Doses of 20 mg of propranolol three or four times each day are generally sufficient to relieve the symptoms of hypermetabolism. In the patient on beta-adrenergic blocker therapy, the pattern of change in the serum T_4 level will generally predict the course of the hyperthyroid phase of the disease. Thus, if the serum T_4 level falls into the normal range, clinical euthyroidism quickly follows and the beta-adrenergic blocking agents should be discontinued.

The hyperthyroid phase of subacute thyroiditis may be followed by permanent euthyroidism. However, in some patients the euthyroid state may be preceded by several weeks to several months of hypothyroidism. The hypothyroid phase of the disease probably represents the interval of time between peripheral metabolism of released thyroid hormones and sufficient recovery of the thyroid gland so that it can produce and secrete an adequate amount of thyroid hormone. If it occurs, the hypothyroid phase of the disease may require replacement therapy with thyroid hormones but for only a short period of time (weeks to several months in most cases). Since the disease completely resolves in almost all patients, long-term treatment with L-thyroxine is contraindicated. It is possible that some patients with subacute thyroiditis may have neither neck pain nor hyperthyroidism but may present with symptoms of hypothyroidism. Since these patients require only temporary treatment with L-thyroxine, it is clear that effort should be made to establish the etiology of the hypothyroidism before treatment is initiated.

POSTPARTUM THYROID DYSFUNCTION

Thyroid dysfunction that occurs in the postpartum period has been recognized with increasing frequency in recent years. Two to ten percent of postpartum women may suffer from a syndrome of unknown etiology that has elements that are common to both Hashimoto's thyroiditis and subacute thyroiditis. Characteristics that are related to Hashimoto's thyroiditis include a diffuse, firm enlargement of the thyroid gland, the presence of antithyroid microsomal antibodies in serum, and lymphocytic infiltration of the thyroid gland. Despite these similarities to Hashimoto's thyroiditis, the biphasic clinical course of the disorder is more closely comparable to that of subacute thyroiditis. Patients with this disorder generally present with symptoms and signs of hyperthyroidism during the first 2 to 5 months after childbirth, with spontaneous resolution of the hyperthyroidism and development of hypothyroidism between 6 and 10 months after childbirth. Since the hypothyroidism is also self-limited, patients generally become euthyroid and remain euthyroid until the next childbirth, when the entire syndrome usually recurs. Many patients do not exhibit the entire biphasic clinical course but may develop only hyperthyroidism during the first 6 months of the postpartum period or only hypothyroidism between the sixth and twelfth months after delivery. The occurrence of these metabolic disorders and their relationship to the postpartum period should alert the clinician to the diagnosis of portpartum dysfunction so that life-long therapy is not entertained.

In the hyperthyroid phase of the disorder, the diagnosis can easily be made by determination of thyroidal radioactive iodine uptake, which is decreased. Since the hypermetabolic disorder probably results from unregulated release of thyroglobulin into the circulation rather than overproduction of thyroid hormones, therapy should be symptomatic only. In practice, beta-adrenergic blocking agents such as propranolol are usually used. Doses of 20 mg three or four times each day are generally adequate to alleviate the symptoms of hypermetabolism. Clinicians should measure the serum T_4 level at weekly intervals and when it decreases into the normal range, the beta-adrenergic blockers can generally be discontinued.

The hypothyroid phase of the disorder appears clinically similar to goitrous hypothyroidism of other etiologies. The presence of antithyroid microsomal antibodies in serum and lymphocytes in the thyroid on aspiration biopsy would indicate that the etiology of the disorder is Hashimoto's thyroiditis. However, the relationship of the hypothyroidism to the postpartum period raises the strong probability that the hypothyroidism may be transient, since it is likely the result of postpartum thyroid dysfunction. Thus, if treatment is necessary, the physician should administer L-thyroxine in the doses recommended previously for a limited time only. L-Thyroxine therapy should be discontinued after 3 to 6 months. After L-thyroxine is discontinued, serum T_4 and TSH concentrations will generally be in the normal range and indicate that patients are in the euthyroid state.

SILENT THYROIDITIS

A clinical syndrome that is similar to postpartum thyroid dysfunction may occasionally occur in patients who are not in the postpartum period. The pathology and natural history of this syndrome, silent thyroiditis, are almost identical to those of postpartum thyroid dysfunction. Despite many similarities, it is unclear whether silent thyroiditis and postpartum thyroid dysfunction represent the same disorder. The fact that elevated serum titers of antithyroid microsomal antibodies are less frequently observed in silent thyroiditis than in postpartum thyroid dysfunction suggests that they may be different but related disorders. Since the natural history of silent thyroiditis is the same as that of postpartum thyroid dysfunction, therapy of silent thyroiditis is as described previously for postpartum thyroid dysfunction.

SUGGESTED READING

Amino N, Iwatani Y, Tamaki H, et al. Postpartum autoimmune thyroid syndromes. In: Walfish PG, Wall JR, Volpe R, eds. Autoimmunity and the thyroid. Orlando, FL: Academic Press, 1985:289.

Hall R, Evered DC. Autoimmune thyroid disease; thyroiditis. In: DeGroot LJ, Cahill GF, Odell WD, et al, eds. Endocrinology, Vol 1. New York: Grune & Stratton, 1979:461.

Nikolai TF, Coombs GJ, McKenzie AK. Lymphocytic thyroiditis with spontaneously resolving hyperthyroidism (silent thyroiditis) and subacute thyroiditis—long-term follow-up. Arch Intern Med 1981; 141:1455.

Volpe R. Subacute thyroiditis. Prog Clin Biol Res 1981; 74:115–134.

DIFFUSE AND MULTINODULAR NONTOXIC GOITER

MONTE A. GREER, M.D.

Nontoxic goiter is a common affliction. In the many areas of the world where goiter is endemic, the cause is almost always iodine deficiency. However, in the United States, iodine deficiency has essentially been eradicated. Although thyroid enlargement occurring in nonendemic goiter areas is usually classified as "sporadic," this term is misleading. Sporadic is defined as occurring in isolated single instances. This pattern of occurrence is not precisely the case in sporadic goiter since there is a strong family pattern of thyroid enlargement, regardless of the geographic region within which the patients reside. Fifty percent of patients with goiter in nonedemic areas have one or more close relatives with thyroid hypertrophy or other thyroid diseases.

The etiologic agent of nontoxic goiter in an individual patient is rarely determined definitely. Some cases may represent thyroid neoplasia, chronic thyroiditis, or early Graves' disease without thyrotoxicosis. Probably most represent some inborn error of metabolism too subtle to be diagnosed by currently available techniques. The usual battery of diagnostic tests, including measurement of plasma thyroid hormones, thyroid-stimulating hormone (TSH), thyroid-directed antibodies, fine-needle biopsy, and thyroid radioiodine uptake and/or scan, usually do not lead to a more precise definition of the etiology than can be accomplished by a clinical assessment. This chapter covers treatment primarily for patients in whom a specific pathologic diagnosis has not been made.

Diffuse goiter is caused by some general phenomenon that affects the whole thyroid gland. However, for different regions of the gland to have variable growth characteristics is common. Clones of thyroid follicles with greater growth potential, whether autonomous or in response to hormonal stimulators, form lobes or nodules that stand out from the paranodular tissue. These areas may be hypofunctional or "cold" with respect to the iodine metabolism of the paranodular tissue, but may have a greater growth response to TSH than the rest of the gland.

TREATMENT

Thyroid Hormone

The primary weapon in treating nontoxic goiter is exogenous thyroid hormone. The rationale for its use is based on the principle of negative feedback control of TSH secretion by circulating thyroid hormone. For each patient, there is an individual "set point" for plasma thyroid hormone concentration. The sensor is located in the pituitary thyrotrope, which functions like a thermostat; the thyroid functions like a furnace. When the efficiency of a furnace is impaired, as by a blocked fuel line or a malfunctioning burner, the thermostat sends signals more frequently, and the furnace must work harder to provide an adequate amount of heat. The analogy holds for the pituitary-thyroid relationship.

Impaired production of thyroid hormone, such as that caused by a subtle biosynthetic defect or by inhibitory drugs, allows an adequate production of thyroid hormone only if TSH secretion is increased. This higher concentration of TSH, in addition to increasing the output of thyroid hormone, also causes hypertrophy and hyperplasia of the gland. As soon as the thyroid is stimulated sufficiently to produce enough hormone to reach the set-point concentration in the thyrotrope, TSH secretion is shut off. A lower concentration of TSH is necessary to maintain normal production of thyroid hormone by thyroid cells that have mildly impaired function if a goiter is present since thyroid secretion is proportional to the mass of functional thyroid tissue. The above described relationships clarify why plasma TSH concentration is rarely above normal in euthyroid patients with nontoxic goiter.

The objective of treatment is to reduce the size of the goiter or to alleviate the complaints of the patient by the most innocuous, simple, and inexpensive technique available. Providing thyroid hormone exogenously meets this goal in the majority of patients.

That the underlying etiologic factor in nontoxic goiter is rarely ascertained, makes little practical difference in management. Treatment is basically identical whether the goiter is caused by impaired production of thyroid hormone due to deficient enzymatic machinery in the cell, destruction of tissue due to chronic thyroiditis, or inadequate iodine substrate. Exogenous thyroid hormone reduces TSH secretion and allows regression of the hypertrophied gland to the same degree as would be attained by surgical hypophysectomy.

Although any form of physiologically active thyroid hormone depresses TSH secretion, levothyroxine (T_4) has generally supplanted all other substances. Being a synthetic product, T_4 is readily standardized and of uniform potency among reputable manufacturers. Since T_4 is the major secretory product of the thyroid and undergoes extensive extrathyroidal degradation to triiodothyronine (T_3), essentially normal plasma levels of both T_4 and T_3 can be maintained by the administration of T_4 alone. T_4 has a relatively long half-life in plasma (7 days), and the conversion of T_4 to T_3 (primarily in the liver and kidneys) goes on at a steady rate. Therefore the administration of the required daily quantity of T_4 in a single dose maintains a stable plasma concentration of both T_4 and T_3, similar to the situation that would exist if all thyroid hormone were being secreted directly from the thyroid.

T_3 has a short half-life in plasma (approximately 1 day), and supplying this hormone in a single daily dose causes marked fluctuations in plasma T_3 concentration. Although investigators have not shown that these swings in plasma T_3 concentration are deleterious, there is a potential risk that marked elevations of thyroid hormone concentration above the normal physiologic limits, even for relatively short durations, might increase the damage to an impaired myocardium. T_3 is also more expensive than T_4. Since, in physiologically equivalent doses, it is not more efficacious in suppressing TSH secretion, use of this hormone instead of T_4 is illogical.

Preparations from animal thyroid glands, such as desiccated thyroid or purified thyroglobulin, have proven their effectiveness in a century of use. However, since they come from a pool of animals with an uncertain history, their concentration of thyroid hormone and their ratio of T_4 and T_3 can vary from batch to batch and from manufacturer to manufacturer. Since the cost of desiccated thyroid is only slightly less than that of T_4, T_4 is generally preferred.

A combination of T_4 and T_3 in approximately the ratio found in the human thyroid gland is also commercially available. However, the cost of this material is considerably more than that of T_4 alone, and, since oral ingestion of this combination also causes spikes in plasma T_3 concentration, its employment is not generally favored.

The quantity of thyroxine necessary to suppress plasma TSH secretion completely varies among different individuals, but the average daily requirement is 0.15 mg. The requirement for thyroid hormone is roughly proportional to body size. I have seen nontoxic nodular goiter develop in patients who were receiving 0.1 mg daily of T_4 for inappropriate reasons (for example, the treatment of obesity) in whom the goiter shrank dramatically when the dosage of T_4 was increased to 0.2 or 0.3 mg daily.

Theoretically, the minimum quantity of T_4 required to reduce plasma TSH concentration to subnormal levels should be employed. Most current commercial assays are adequate to distinguish between a subnormal and low normal plasma TSH concentration. I usually begin treatment with a daily dose of 0.1 to 0.2 mg T_4 (depending on body size) in an otherwise healthy individual. If the goiter regresses promptly, the dosage is continued indefinitely.

If no reduction in the size of the goiter is produced within 1 month, plasma TSH is measured. If TSH is still in the normal range, the dose of T_4 is increased by 0.1 mg per day until TSH is suppressed to just below normal. Only rarely do patients require more than 0.3 mg of T_4 daily to suppress TSH secretion adequately. In such patients, the rare conditions of thyroid hormone resistance and TSH-secreting pituitary tumor should be evaluated.

Suppressive therapy with T_4 does not change the underlying problems that caused the goiter in the first place. Therefore, if T_4 is discontinued after the goiter regresses, it recurs in the majority of patients. For this reason, I recommend that T_4 therapy be continued for the patient's lifetime.

The longer the goiter has been present, the more likely that it will develop "nodular" areas rather than presenting as a diffuse, relatively symmetric mass. These nodules are often histologically different from the paranodular tissue and from each other. They presumably represent geographic areas within the thyroid that have developed from aberrant clones. One or more of the nodules may develop autonomy from TSH and undergo little regression with treatment with T_4 in comparison to the paranodular tissue or to the TSH-sensitive nodules. The nodules thus are more readily delineated as the paranodular tissue shrinks under therapy and may suggest actual growth of the autonomous nodules, causing undue alarm that the nodules may be malignant. Careful measurements of the size of the nodules at each patient visit allows a decision about whether the nodules are actually growing in spite of adequate suppressive therapy. If they are objectively enlarging for a period of 2 months under these conditions, surgical removal is advisable because of the risk of malignancy.

In some patients, thyroid enlargement represents a nonthyrotoxic stage of Graves' disease or of multinodular toxic goiter. The differentiation from Graves' disease may be particularly difficult before hyperthyroidism develops or if the patient is in remission from thyrotoxicosis after treatment with antithyroid drugs. A significant goiter may exist, radioiodine uptake may be normally suppressed by T_4 treatment, and the TSH response to thyrotropin releasing hormone may be normal. Treatment with thyroid hormone does not decrease the size of the goiter, and it may result in a supranormal concentration of thyroid hormone through the combination of both exogenous and endogenous contributions if the patient's thyroid function is independent of TSH. Eventually, manifest thyrotoxicosis appears in many of these patients.

Special Considerations

Although elderly patients or those with known coronary insufficiency risk myocardial infarction if their thyroid hormone concentration is raised to a supranormal level, this is not a problem in treating nontoxic goiter since there is a compensatory suppression of endogenous thyroid function equivalent to the dose of T_4 given. Only if the exogenous hormone exceeds that produced by the patient's own gland would any hyperthyroidism be produced. To minimize the possibility of this happening, I begin with 0.1 mg of T_4 daily and measure plasma TSH at the end of 1 month. If there have been no adverse effects of the T_4, the plasma TSH is still in the normal range, and the goiter has not decreased in size, I increase the dose to 0.2 mg or higher. In the majority of elderly patients, 0.1 mg T_4 daily is sufficient to suppress plasma TSH to the subnormal range. Elderly patients have usually had their goiter for many years and are unconcerned about the cosmetic problem. Since the probability that thyroid enlargement decreases significantly with T_4 therapy is inversely proportional to the length of time it has been present, observation rather than therapy may be the wisest course in the aged, unless hypothyroidism is a concern. As long as a normal pituitary-thyroid feedback relation exists and the amount of administered T_4 does not exceed the physiologic equivalent of thyroid secretion, no increased metabolic effect is produced by thyroid hormone therapy. In some elderly patients (and in some younger ones), a recent history of rapid diffuse or nodular goiter development may cause considerable concern that a malignancy has developed. However, if plasma TSH is elevated, the goiter may dramatically shrink or disappear; even what appear to be hard, fibrotic nodules that one would not expect to change at all may disappear.

In a few patients, the goiter is caused by ingestion of drugs (for example, high doses of iodide or drugs like amiodarone with a high iodine content) that inhibit formation of thyroid hormone in susceptible individuals and thus reduce negative feedback on TSH secretion. Removal of the offending agent from the patient's regimen suffices to produce regression of the enlarged gland. When removal is not possible, thyroid hormone can be added, as discussed before.

Surgery

Surgery should be reserved for patients who do not respond adequately to medical management, in whom thyroid malignancy is suspected, or for whom the cosmetic problem is important. If the goiter is due to an underlying biosynthetic defect in hormone formation, extirpation of a major portion of the gland only compounds the problem because it results in removal of the compensatorily increased mass of tissue that allows the patient to produce sufficient thyroid hormone. Although the patient is euthyroid before thyroidectomy, there is a high probability that hypothyroidism will ensue after thyroidectomy. The risk of the surgery is generally justified only if a serious cosmetic problem exists or, in rare instances, if the gland is large enough to cause physical disability by tracheal or esophageal compression. It is important to choose an experienced thyroid surgeon to minimize the risks of hypoparathyroidism and recurrent laryngeal nerve paralysis.

Radioiodine

Although rarely utilized, ^{131}I given in relatively high doses may also cause a significant shrinkage of nontoxic goiters that are refractory to treatment with thyroid hormone. The risk of malignancy or bone marrow depression with this dosage is inconsequential, and it is a much simpler, cheaper, and safer form of therapy than surgery, which can always be employed later if necessary.

SUGGESTED READING

Cassidy CE. Simple goiter and thyroid nodules. Pharmacol Ther 1976; 1:95–99.

Greer MA, Astwood EB. Treatment of simple goiter with thyroid. J Clin Endocrinol Metab 1953; 13:1312–1331.

Homoki J, Garbrecht D, Loos U, Teller WM. Treatment of juvenile euthyroid goiter with thyroxine as compared to treatment with the combination of thyroxine and triiodothyronine. Monatsschr Kinderheilkd 1985; 133:532–536.

Studer H, Peter HJ, Gerber H. Natural heterogeneity of thyroid cells: the basis for understanding function and nodular goiter growth. Endocr Rev 1989; 125–135.

SINGLE THYROID NODULE

MARVIN C. GERSHENGORN, M.D.

The goal in management of a patient with a single (or solitary) thyroid nodule is to decide whether the nodule is likely to harbor a carcinoma so as to recommend operating on all malignant lesions while limiting the number of operations performed on patients with benign disease. A small number of endocrinologists recommend that all nodules be excised, whereas others, also a small group, advise excision only if malignancy is proved. I assume that all single nodules may harbor a carcinoma and utilize a series of diagnostic maneuvers that provide information as to whether there is an increased or decreased likelihood of a nodule's being malignant. In some patients, moreover, the fine-needle aspiration biopsy technique, which I employ in all such patients, provides a definitive, preoperative diagnosis of malignancy. The observation that the detection rates of thyroid carcinoma in surgical series range from 20 to 60 percent, a far greater prevalence of cancer than in the general population (approximately 4 percent of all nodules), attests to the validity of this type of approach.

CLINICAL CONSIDERATIONS

The clinical history of the patient with a single thyroid nodule offers the first insight into the likelihood that a nodule might harbor a carcinoma. A reliable observation that indicates that the nodule is of recent development and/or is growing perceptibly increases the chance of malignant disease. The risk is increased further if either of the aforementioned events has occurred while the patient was taking thyroid hormone replacement or suppression medication. The age of the patient also is important, since the proportion of malignant lesions is higher in patients under age 40; most thyroid nodules are found in patients over age 40. Thus the younger the patient, the more likely it is that a nodule is a carcinoma. The patient's sex is important because nodular thyroid disease occurs in females approximately four times more frequently than in males, but the female-to-male ratio for carcinoma is only about 2:1. Thus a nodule in a male is more likely to be malignant than one in a female. A history of radiation exposure of the head, neck, or anterior chest, especially if the dose received was greater than 100 rad and occurred more than 5 years previously, increases the likelihood of malignancy, since exposure to ionizing radiation has been found to be associated with an increased incidence of nodular thyroid disease in general and an increased proportion of nodules that harbor a carcinoma. (Although physicians had feared that carcinomas found in patients who have been exposed to ionizing radiation might behave aggressively, most tumors in these patients have been papillary carcinomas whose biologic behavior appears to be identical to similar tumors in nonirradiated patients.) The likelihood of malignancy significantly increases if the history includes voice change, stridor, and dyspnea, suggesting vocal cord paresis or paralysis; Horner's syndrome, suggesting cervical sympathetic nerve damage; dysphagia, suggesting impingement on the esophagus; or a superior vena cava syndrome. Last, a family history of thyroid carcinoma suggests that a nodule may be a medullary carcinoma.

The finding on physical examination of a single thyroid nodule is important since, although apparently uninodular glands are commonly shown to contain multiple nodules at surgery, the likelihood of a clinically solitary nodule's being a carcinoma is significantly greater than that of a nodule in a multinodular gland. In contrast to some endocrinologists, I think that a single dominant nodule in a multinodular gland must also be viewed with increased suspicion of harboring a carcinoma. Several characteristics of the nodule are important. Its consistency has limited value, since a firm or hard nodule may be caused by calcification following hemorrhage into a benign lesion, and soft nodules can be malignant. In the absence of calcification, however, a firm, sharply demarcated nodule is more likely to be malignant. Evidence of extension beyond the thyroid capsule or of fixation to surrounding tissues is highly suggestive of malignancy. Rapid growth, especially when the nodule is also tender, is usually caused by hemorrhage into a previously existing nodule. Since most nodules are benign, these lesions are usually benign. However, because malignant lesions may have cystic components and since hemorrhage may occur in any nodule, especially those greater than 2.5 cm in diameter, these findings do not exclude malignancy. Enlargement of the cervical lymph nodes and laryngeal and cervical sympathetic nerve impairment strongly favor malignancy.

LABORATORY EVALUATION

Laboratory evaluation of patients with nodular thyroid disease, especially fine-needle aspiration biopsy and the radioisotopic "thyroid scan," plays the major role in determining the likelihood of malignancy. Measurements of serum thyroid hormone and thyroid-stimulating hormone (thyrotropin, TSH) levels, and antimicrosomal and antithyroglobulin titers are employed to exclude known causes of nodular thyroid disease and to determine the patient's thyroid status. (Serum thyroglobulin determination is not of diagnostic value; it is useful in following patients after initial therapy for thyroid carcinoma.)

Scintillation scanning with radioactive iodine or technetium-99m has been used for many years in the evaluation of the thyroid nodule. Its value is based on the fact that most malignant neoplasms accumulate little or no radioiodine and appear as nonfunctioning ("cold") or hypofunctioning areas on the scintiscan. This appearance is because thyroid cancers are less efficient in their capacity to take up radioiodine than normal thyroid tissue. However, the finding of a cold nodule on the scintiscan indicates only that there is an increased likelihood of malignancy; most cold nodules are benign. Conversely, a clinically palpable nodule that appears to function as well as the surrounding tissue and is not delineated on the scan may, in fact, be hypofunctioning; it is important to note that to be detectable a hypofunctioning nodule must measure at least 0.8 cm, and even then it may be undetectable if situated at the margin of the gland, if surrounded by sufficient normally functioning thyroid tissue, or if radioiodine uptake by the thyroid is low. Such errors are less common when the location of the nodule on physical examination is carefully noted at the time of scintiscanning and when imaging is performed with iodine-123 (or technetium-99m), which allows for high count rates. In some instances, oblique views are useful. Then a nodule may be classified as hypofunctioning when there is unequivocal demonstration of radioiodine within it, but less than in the surrounding tissue. The function of nondelineated but clinically palpable nodules should be classified as indeterminate but evaluated as if they were cold. The finding of a hyperfunctioning ("hot") nodule (toxic adenoma) that suppresses function in the remainder of the gland weighs most heavily against the likelihood of malignancy, since this type of nodule is very rarely, if ever, malignant. Most cases in the literature that purport to document the finding of a malignant hyperfunctioning nodule are clearly instances of incidental "occult" carcinoma in patients with toxic adenoma. In most instances, technetium-99m may be substituted for radioactive iodine for scintiscanning in the evaluation of a thyroid nodule. However, there have been several reports of nodules that appeared functional on technetium scintiscan but were nonfunctional (cold) on radioiodine scan, presumably owing to their ability to trap iodide but not to bind it to proteins.

Even though thyroid scintiscanning is useful as just outlined, some endocrinologists recommend that it need not be employed in these patients if fine-needle aspiration biopsy is planned. This recommendation arises primarily from a cost-effectiveness analysis. However, I continue to use scintiscanning because it provides important information that is particularly useful in managing patients in whom the fine-needle aspiration biopsy does not yield a diagnosis of malignancy and in patients who have hyperfunctioning nodules, some of which may not be associated with frank thyrotoxicosis.

I measure plasma calcitonin concentration in selected patients, for example, those with a family history of thyroid cancer or other tumors that may be components of the multiple endocrine neoplasia syndromes. When plasma calcitonin level is elevated, a diagnosis of medullary carcinoma or its premalignant state, parafollicular cell (or C cell) hyperplasia, may be made with virtual certainty.

Fine-needle aspiration and large-bore needle biopsy have significantly improved the preoperative diagnosis of thyroid nodules. In my experience, the fine-needle aspiration technique, which employs a 22-gauge or smaller needle, is easy to perform, thus allowing for sampling of multiple sites with a suspicious lesion, and is without serious complications. The theoretical complication of the spread of tumor along the needle track has not occurred in several large series. I do not attempt to make a specific diagnosis of the thyroid lesion but try more generally to differentiate malignant from benign conditions. I have adopted a simple classification that grades a cytopathologic specimen on a scale from benign—class 1 or 2—to suspicious—class 3—to malignant—class 4 or 5—which has proved useful (Table 1). In this classification, only class 5 is considered a definitive diagnosis. In my experience, as well as that of others, satisfactory specimens are obtained in over 95 percent of cases and are correctly categorized in approximately 90 percent. A false-negative diagnosis is made in approximately 6 percent of aspiration specimens, and the incidence of false-positive diagnoses is less than 5 percent. For best results, it is important to have the aspiration sample analyzed by a cytopathologist who has gained experience with this type of specimen. If the aspiration specimen demonstrates a malignancy (class 5) or is highly suspicious for malignancy (class 4), surgery is recommended. If the specimen is class 1, 2, or 3, a trial of suppression therapy is usually initiated. The follow-up during suppression therapy and the duration of the trial of suppression are heavily influenced by the cytopathologic results. The fine-needle aspiration technique also is of value in the management of simple cysts because their total evacuation without reaccumulation of fluid obviates the need for surgical excision.

TABLE 1 Thyroid Cytopathologic Classification*

Benign, Class 1. Normal-appearing follicular cells, especially in follicles containing colloid, with or without inflammation.
Benign, Class 2. Follicular cells with mild to moderate atypia or abundant cohesive follicular cells.
Suspicious, Class 3. Occasional follicular cells with moderate to marked atypia or abundant, noncohesive follicular cells.
Malignant, Class 4. Many noncohesive follicular cells with marked to severe atypia.
Malignant, Class 5. Atypical papillary structures with psammoma bodies or pleomorphic cells with amyloid or immunoreactive calcitonin.

*Adapted from Ramacciotti et al. Arch Intern Med 1984; 144:1169

In contrast to the preference for aspiration biopsy, several groups have advocated using large-bore needle biopsy and have reported a high rate of correct diagnoses. False-negative and false-positive diagnoses occur about as often as with the fine-needle technique. However, even in experienced hands, the large-bore needle biopsy procedure can be complicated by hematomas, tracheal puncture, and transient laryngeal nerve palsy. In my opinion, since the fine-needle aspiration biopsy technique appears to be at least as accurate as large-bore needle biopsy and is virtually free of complications, it is the procedure of choice for preoperative diagnosis of solitary thyroid nodules and should be employed routinely.

THERAPEUTIC PLAN

The use of a trial of suppression therapy with thyroid hormone in patients in whom there is no contraindication, such as coronary artery disease or in the elderly, has been advocated. Even in the latter group of patients, careful adjustment of the hormone dose can permit a cautious trial of suppression therapy. The utility of this procedure is based on the observation that thyroid tissue, including adenomas, grows in response to TSH stimulation and involutes when pituitary TSH secretion is inhibited by thyroid hormones and circulating TSH levels decline. Adequate suppression can now be estimated by the measurement of serum TSH using a highly sensitive TSH immunoassay. A nodule that fails to regress or continues to grow with adequate suppression therapy is more likely to be malignant. Some nodules become impalpable with thyroid hormone therapy and almost certainly represent benign lesions. However, many nodules diminish in size but remain clinically palpable, a finding that is not helpful in judging whether they are benign or malignant, since even some thyroid carcinomas can grow in response to TSH.

The following is my approach to the management of a single thyroid nodule (Fig. 1). After the initial history and physical examination, I assess every patient's thyroid status by determining serum concentrations of thyroid hormones and TSH, and an index of the thyroxine-binding proteins. I measure antithyroid antibodies and perform a thyroid scintiscan. The scintiscan is best performed with iodine-123 or technetium-99m. A nodule that appears to function with

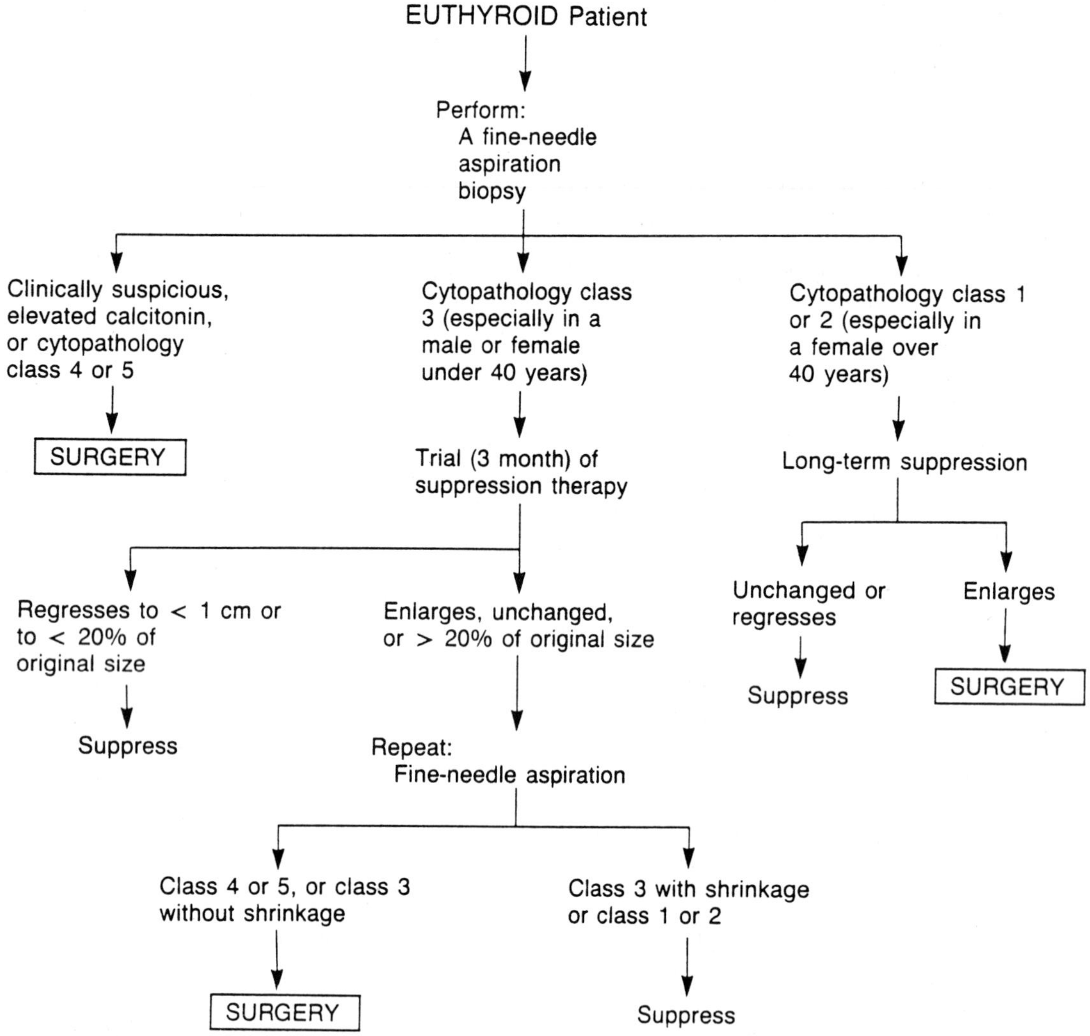

Figure 1 Management of single cold thyroid nodule in a euthyroid patient.

technetium-99m should be retested with iodine-123, except when the surrounding tissue is suppressed. Oblique views are taken if the nodule is not well delineated by frontal scan. Patients with a hot (or hyperfunctioning) nodule that is suppressing the remainder of the thyroid gland have virtually no chance of harboring a malignancy. A nodule that on scintiscan shows substantially more radioactivity within it than in the surrounding normal thyroid is also generally benign. In the patient, who is hyperthyroid, with an apparent solitary hot nodule, I recommend treatment with radioactive iodine to destroy its function and reduce its size. Repeat radioiodine treatment is given at 6-month intervals as required.

In euthyroid patients with an apparently hyperfunctioning nodule, I perform a triiodothyronine (T_3) suppression test by administering 25 μg of T_3 four times a day for 7 to 10 days so as to determine whether the nodule is functioning autonomously or is simply hypertrophic thyroid tissue and can be suppressed with thyroid hormone. If the nodule is hypertrophic, I administer suppression therapy indefinitely. If the nodule is functioning autonomously and the patient is over 40 years of age, I recommend treatment with radioactive iodine to prevent the development of hyperthyroidism. If the patient is under 40 years of age, my recommendation is influenced by the size of the nodule. If the nodule is larger than 2.5 cm, I recommend radioactive iodine treatment while the patient is taking thyroid hormone for suppression of the extranodular tissue, since with time nodules of this size tend to enlarge and then produce hyperthyroidism. If the nodule is smaller than 2.5 cm, I observe the patient for the possible development of hyperthyroidism and for tumor growth. The patient may be treated with thyroid suppression therapy, but take care to avoid hyperthyroidism.

Further work-up for the possibility of malignancy

is performed in glands that contain cold or hypofunctioning nodules or in which a palpable nodule is so situated that the presence or absence of function cannot be confidently decided by scintiscan. I perform fine-needle aspiration biopsy at multiple sites within the nodule(s). Also, I measure plasma calcitonin levels without stimulation in patients with a family history of thyroid cancer and after stimulation if the basal calcitonin level is not elevated in patients with a family history of medullary carcinoma or other components of the multiple endocrine neoplasia syndrome. I recommend surgical excision when there is a cytologic diagnosis of malignancy (class 4 or 5); when the plasma calcitonin level is elevated; or when there is cervical lymph node enlargement, fixation to surrounding tissues, or pressure symptoms.

It is important to note that I do not consider the cytologic diagnosis of benign disease definitive, especially in patients who are under 18 years of age and in those who have a history of high-risk radiation exposure, particularly if it occurred more than 5 years previously. In this group of higher risk patients, I may repeat the fine-needle aspiration biopsy.

The remaining patients—those in cytopathologic classes 1, 2, or 3 without a clinical reason for operation—are given suppression therapy. A trial of suppression therapy lasts only 3 months in patients whose risk of harboring a malignancy is still considered high, that is, if there is a definite cold nodule greater than 1 cm in diameter in a male or in a female under 40 years of age or whose cytopathology was class 3. If such a nodule does not decrease in size, repeat fine-needle aspiration biopsy is performed. If the cytopathologic finding is class 3 and the nodule has not decreased in size or changes to class 4 or 5, surgical excision is recommended. If the cytopathologic result returns as class 1 or 2 or class 3 and the size of the nodule is decreasing progressively, suppression therapy is maintained. In a patient in whom the repeat fine-needle aspiration specimen was class 3 and the size of the nodule stabilizes at 1 cm or larger (or greater than 20 percent of its original dimension in the case of a large nodule), repeat fine-needle aspiration biopsy may be recommended after 1 year.

Long-term suppression therapy is recommended for patients with a cytopathologic classification of 1 or 2, especially if they are females over the age of 40. These patients are followed at regular intervals for evidence of nodule growth. They are continued on suppression therapy indefinitely if the nodule does not grow. If the nodule grows while the patient is taking thyroid hormone, a repeat fine-needle aspiration is performed and surgical excision is recommended unless the specimen is class 1 or 2, or a benign process, such as a hemorrhage, is found. I assume that some tumors that respond to suppression therapy may be differentiated carcinomas; however, it appears safe to continue suppression if the nodule does not increase again in size and there are no findings strongly suggesting malignant behavior. Last, patients whose nodules are less than 1 cm in diameter are placed on long-term suppression therapy. If the nodule remains unchanged or regresses, suppression is continued indefinitely.

It now appears well documented that employing an approach to the management of the single thyroid nodule such as that outlined here, which includes both fine-needle aspiration biopsy and radioisotopic scanning, substantially increases the accuracy of preoperative diagnosis. This approach results in a decrease in the number of excisional biopsies performed for benign disease and in a reduction in the number of carcinomas left in situ.

SUGGESTED READING

Ashcraft MW, Van Herle AJ. Management of thyroid nodules. II. Scanning techniques, thyroid suppressive therapy, and fine needle aspiration. Head Neck Surg 1981; 3:297–322.

Gershengorn MC, McClung MR, Chu EW, et al. Fine-needle aspiration cytology in the preoperative diagnosis of thyroid nodules. Ann Intern Med 1977; 87:265–269.

Gershengorn MC, Robbins J. Thyroid neoplasia. In: Green WL, ed. The thyroid. New York: Elsevier, 1987:293.

McConahey WM, Hay ID, Woolner LB, et al. Papillary thyroid cancer treated at the Mayo Clinic, 1946 through 1970: Initial manifestations, pathologic findings, therapy, and outcome. Mayo Clin Proc 1986; 61:978–996.

Ramacciotti CE, Pretorius HT, Chu EW, et al. Diagnostic accuracy and use of aspiration biopsy in the management of thyroid nodules. Arch Intern Med 1984; 144:1169–1173.

DIABETES MELLITUS

ROBERT G. CAMPBELL, M.D.
DAVID J. BRILLON, M.D.

Diabetes mellitus is a complex heterogeneous disorder of carbohydrate metabolism with multiple etiologic factors. The hyperglycemia associated with this syndrome is the result of either absolute or relative insulin deficiency or insulin resistance or both. Continued progress in the treatment of this disorder accounts for the increasing longevity of the diabetic patient and the increased prevalence of the disease. It is estimated that over 5 percent of the population of the United States has this disorder. It is the fifth leading cause of death in the United States and a leading cause of blindness and kidney disease. Such statistics continue to prevail in spite of the availability of insulin for over 60 years in the treatment of diabetes. These grim statistics highlight the importance of continuing to develop new approaches and to refine the management of the patient with diabetes.

Considerable evidence suggests that there is a close relationship between metabolic control and microvascular complications associated with diabetes. The potential now exists to substantiate this thesis in humans. The recent feasibility of patient self-monitoring of blood glucose levels and the use of glycosylated hemoglobin to assess metabolic control accurately over several weeks provide the methods to achieve close to normal blood glucose levels while avoiding both hyperglycemia and hypoglycemia.

Thus the overall aims of the therapy for both type I insulin-dependent diabetes mellitus (IDDM) and type II non-insulin-dependent diabetes mellitus (NIDDM) should be directed at (1) attaining glycemic control with minimal hypoglycemia, and (2) preventing the microvascular, cardiovascular, and neurologic complications associated with diabetes. To achieve these aims will require a redirection of the classic patient-health care team relationship to involve the patient more directly in day-to-day medical management while allowing sufficient flexibility to maintain a stable quality of life.

DIETARY TREATMENT

Appropriate dietary management is an essential component in the overall therapeutic plan for all patients with diabetes. The dietary program includes determining caloric needs to achieve desired body weight, distribution of daily nutrient intake, and proportions of individual nutrients that make up the daily caloric intake, all directed to ensure proper nutrition.

In a large majority of NIDDM patients who are characteristically overweight at the time of diagnosis, caloric restriction forms the basis of their treatment. In contrast, with IDDM patients weight maintenance is the usual goal, with close attention paid to relationships between timing and nutrient content of a given meal and the time course of insulin administration. To achieve any measure of compliance in the patient following a dietary regimen requires continued reinforcement and education while making allowances for preferred food habits and style of life.

Total Caloric Intake

Basal energy expenditure, which represents approximately 75 percent of total energy requirements, is directly related to percent of lean body mass or skeletal muscle. This amounts to approximately 25 kcal per kilogram body weight per day. Total energy expenditure is largely dependent on degree of physical activity, but generally requirements in a sedentary individual are about 30 kcal per kilogram. Energy expenditure on a per kilogram body weight basis may be slightly lower in obese subjects in that the ratio of lean body mass to absolute body weight is decreased. Establishing a goal for the patient in terms of daily caloric intake is dependent on whether it is necessary to maintain, increase, or decrease body weight to achieve close to a desirable body weight. A host of approaches to weight reduction depend on degree of caloric restriction, rate and amount of weight loss desired, nutrient composition, and psychosocial and behavioral components. These various methods are well described in the chapter on *Obesity*. However, in spite of the availability of this wide variety of approaches for weight reduction, the long-term success for maintaining weight loss is poor. NIDDM patients with significant symptoms related to uncontrolled diabetes may have initial symptomatic benefit associated with weight loss. Such symptomatic relief associated with decreased glucosuria may serve to reinforce the weight loss program. However, improvement in metabolic control occurs well before the patient achieves his or her prescribed weight loss. If the beneficial effects on glycemic control are realized and normoglycemia results, the patient may maintain the motivation not to regain the lost weight. Unfortunately, this rarely occurs. In fact, the greater the degree of obesity, the greater the incidence of regaining the weight lost.

Nutrient Composition of the Diet

For adults consuming a eucaloric diet, the recommended intake of protein is 0.8 g per kilogram of body weight, which contributes about 15 percent of total calories. Recent recommendations advocate liberalizing the amount of carbohydrate up to 55 to 60 percent of total calories as complex carbohydrates, with the remainder of calories as fat, restricted to less than 35 percent of total calories. Rapidly absorbed sugars should be avoided. This degree of fat restriction is not feasible in some patients because of the available food selection and its palatability. With such restriction all components should be proportionally reduced. Because of the high risk of cardiovascular disease associated with diabetes, patients with diabetes should be prescribed a fat-modified diet with saturated fat constituting less than 10 percent, polyunsaturated fat less than 10 percent and the rest as monounsaturated fat. The cholesterol content of the diet should not exceed 300 g per day. Recently attention in the lay press has been given to the incorporation of fish oils (omega-3 fatty acids) into the fat content of diets. Several studies have demonstrated a deleterious effect on glycemic control from the use of these fatty acids in NIDDM subjects. This effect is believed to be secondary to enhanced hepatic glucose production.

A practical goal for fiber intake would be 25 g per 1,000 kcal of food intake. This level of intake may prove to be beneficial, although the level of maximal benefits has not yet been established. Such supplementation may only be effective if the level of carbohydrate exceeds 50 percent of total calories. Careful attention must be paid to insulin schedules in patients consuming high-fiber diets, as variation in nutrient absorption may occur, resulting in hypoglycemia.

Other factors such as the glycemic effect of a given nutrient contribute to postprandial blood glucose levels. Classification of foods by glycemic responsiveness may prove to be a good educational tool for the patient, particularly those who may be on a more intensive insulin regimen. Results of some studies, however, question whether classification of individual foods by glycemic effect remains useful when these foods are included in a mixed meal. Further research is required to determine how this glycemic index of foods can be incorporated into the current exchange system.

The current recommendation for sodium intake is 1,000 mg per 1,000 kcal, not to exceed 2,000 mg a day. Such salt restriction in certain patients with poorly controlled diabetes and autonomic neuropathy may be deleterious because of fluid imbalance and associated hypotension. Therefore it is best to reserve sodium restriction for those patients who have clinical indications such as hypertension, with close attention being paid to those patients with significant hyperglycemia and glucosuria. There is little evidence to suggest use of supplemental vitamins and minerals in the diabetic, except under conditions of very low caloric weight reduction diets.

The contraindications of alcohol in the diabetic patients are no different than those for the general public; however, indiscriminate use of alcohol may mask the symptoms of hypoglycemia. Including alcohol in the diet plan may be individualized to the patients' wishes and appropriate caloric adjustments may be made. It is not appropriate to include alcohol in a weight reduction diet because it is difficult to design a nutritionally sound program around such a regimen.

Use of nutritive (fructose and sorbitol) and nonnutritive (aspartame and saccharin) sweeteners has proved to be a valuable adjunct in the dietary management of the diabetic. The caloric contribution of the nutritive sweeteners can be substantial and they should not be substituted for noncaloric sweeteners in the meal plan. Because of controversy over the possible metabolic effects of long-term use of sweeteners in humans, it is well advised to use a variety of sweeteners so as to distribute any potential risks. At this time, it is generally agreed that the benefits of appropriate use of sweeteners in the management of diabetes outweigh their potential risks.

Distribution and Nutrient Composition of Meals

Basic goals of meal planning should emphasize consistency in meal size and nutrient content and reasonable regularity in their timing but with a sufficient degree of flexibility directed to achieving good compliance. The timing and nutrient content of meals in patients on insulin are chiefly related to time course of action of insulin administered and the patient's activity pattern, with the air of avoiding hypoglycemia. The basic pattern includes three individual meals and two to three snacks with 15 to 20 percent of calories at breakfast, 30 percent each at lunch and dinner, and the remainder as snacks. Calories as carbohydrates are distributed in a similar pattern but may be influenced in part by previous dietary habits. The timing of snacks is adjusted to the insulin schedule selected. One distinct advantage of a multiple insulin dose regimen is that the patient may adjust insulin doses on the basis of meal size, timing of the meal, and its nutrient content. The potential for dietary flexibility may enhance compliance to a greater degree than the more usual fixed meal schedule.

PHYSICAL ACTIVITY AND EXERCISE

Although there is little evidence to suggest that exercise directly affects the treatment of diabetes, the benefits of a daily exercise program are obvious in terms of the overall well-being of the patient. Any amount of exercise will improve cardiovascular fitness and possibly decrease the number of cardiovascular risk factors. There is evidence that a consistent exercise regimen accompanied by appropriate caloric intake will alter body composition by increasing lean body mass, e.g., muscle, at the expense of adipose tissue. This results in enhanced effectiveness of insulin, reducing insulin requirements and improving metabolic control, particularly in the type II diabetic patient. Physical activity itself increases sensitivity to insulin; thus insulin requirements decrease. This concept should be reinforced to the patient, as time and degree of physical activity will acutely alter metabolic control, resulting in either hyperglycemia and ketosis or sometimes precipitous hypoglycemia. Self-monitoring of blood glucose level will prove extremely helpful to the patient in predicting what amount of exercise will alter a given blood glucose level. He or she then can develop a given algorithm for an insulin regimen and nutrient intake based on the amount of physical activity.

ORAL HYPOGLYCEMIC AGENTS

The cornerstone of treatment for the NIDDM patient is diet and exercise. Frequently elimination of simple carbohydrates from the diet may improve metabolic control dramatically prior to any significant weight loss.

In patients who do not respond to diet after a 6- to 8-week trial and continue to maintain fasting blood glucose levels over 150 mg per deciliter, oral agents should be used regardless of age of onset. If the patient continues to have fasting blood glucose levels higher than 200 mg per deciliter after dietary trial and has clinical symptoms related to hyperglycemia, insulin may be required initially until satisfactory control is obtained. This often is the case with younger (under 40 years) nonobese patients.

In patients under 40 years of age, either oral agents or insulin may be indicated, depending on patient acceptance and motivation. New onset diabetics appear to respond better to oral agents than those with longstanding disease. However, about 10 percent of patients fail to respond to oral agents initially, and in another 20 percent the drugs are ineffective after initial treatment of 1 to 2 years. In either case, insulin has to be substituted.

Several kinds of sulfonylureas are available, differing in potency of pancreatic (stimulation of B cell insulin secretion) and extrapancreatic effects and site of metabolism and excretion. As outlined in Table 1, the second-generation sulfonylureas, analogues of the original sulfonylureas, are considerably more potent but not necessarily more effective than the first-generation drugs. The difference in duration of action dictates the frequency with which the drug is usually given. The major complication of the longer acting drugs, primarily chlorpropamide, is hypoglycemia. This drug should be used with caution, if at all, in the elderly patient. This compound also may potentiate antidiuretic hormone action on the kidney, causing water retention and hyponatremia. Chlorpropamide, acetohexamide, and tolazamide should be used cautiously in patients with decreased renal function because of their route of excretion. A disulfiram (Antabuse)-like reaction with alcohol ingestion has been reported with sulfonylureas and particularly chlorpropamide; however, it has not yet been reported in any second-generation group of drugs. Drug interactions, pharmacokinetic and pharmacodynamic, must be considered at all times, particularly in the aged, who commonly are taking two or more medications at any given time. Drug interactions as a result of changes in protein binding are less common with the second-generation sulfonylureas, and therefore these agents may be favored for use when a patient is on medication that could cause displacement from plasma binding sites.

It is generally agreed that all the sulfonylureas are effective, and the choice of a given agent is based on individual patient needs, drug metabolism, and desired dosage schedule. The usual approach is to increase the dosage gradually, depending on the metabolic response. If a given agent fails at maximal doses, another sulfonylurea should be tried. As already mentioned, up to 20 percent of NIDDM patients may have either a primary or a secondary failure of treatment within the first 1 to 2 years, usually related to noncompliance with dietary regimen. However, for unclear reasons a significant number of patients simply do not respond to oral agents and therefore must be placed on insulin.

INSULIN THERAPY

The basic approach to insulin treatment in the diabetic depends largely on the patient's acceptance and motivation and the physician's philosophy of dia-

TABLE 1 Properties of Sulfonylureas Available in the United States

Generic Name	*Dosage Equivalent (mg)*	*Daily Dosage Range (mg)*	*Duration of Action (hr)*
First generation			
Tolbutamide	1,000, given two to three times day	500–3,000	6–12
Acetohexamide	500, given once or twice a day	250–1,500	12–18
Tolazamide	250, given once or twice a day	100–1,000	10–18
Chlorpropamide	250, given once a day	100–750	24–72
Second generation			
Glipizide	7.5, given once a day	2.5–40	18–30
Glyburide	5, given once a day	1.25–20	10–30

TABLE 2 Target Blood Glucose Levels for a Young, Otherwise Healthy Patient with Insulin-Dependent (Type 1) Diabetes

	Ideal (mg/dl)	*Acceptable (mg/dl)*
Pre-meal	70–105	70–130
1 hour after meal	100–160	100–180
2 hours after meal	80–120	80–150
2 AM to 4 AM	70–100	70–120

betic management. Those who believe there is an important relationship between metabolic control and complications will define "acceptable" control more rigidly (Table 2) and design the insulin regimen to closely mimic the normal insulin secretory pattern. Those who do not support this thesis will choose a less intensive insulin treatment program. The intensive method of insulin treatment requires a high degree of commitment of time, motivation, and in-depth understanding of diabetes on the part of both physician and patient. Ideally, the physician should have the services of a dietitian with expertise in diabetes and dedicated to such a program. If such resources and health care team members and patient commitment are lacking, a less intensive insulin program should be considered.

The basic insulin preparations available are outlined in Table 3 and differ in onset of action, time of peak effect, duration of action, source (beef, pork, beef-pork, or human synthetic insulin), and degree of purity. The time and course of action of these preparations, listed in Table 3, may be highly variable, depending on site of injection, presence of insulin antibodies, and individual patient responses, and should serve only as a guide for designing a given insulin regimen.

Total daily insulin requirements of stable IDDM patients, within 20 percent of desired body weight, range from 0.5 to 1.0 U per kilogram body weight per day. Newly diagnosed patients require as little as 0.3 U per kilogram during the early phase of their disease owing to continued endogenous insulin secretion. Insulin requirements of this group of patients may fall significantly during the initial phase of treatment. This so-called honeymoon period may be brief (weeks) or may last as long as 2 to 3 years. Established insulin requirements for IDDM patients approximate 0.6 to 0.9 U per kilogram per day. The insulin requirement gradually increases during pregnancy from 0.6 U per kilogram in the first trimester to 1.0 U per kilogram in the third trimester. Insulin requirements may vary widely during periods of intercurrent illness, change in physical activity, psychosocial-induced stress, and dietary noncompliance.

TABLE 3 Time Course of Action of Various Insulin Preparations

Class	*Type*	*Peak Effect (hr)*	*Duration of Action (hr)*
Rapid	Regular crystalline insulin	2–4	6–8
	Semilente	2–6	10–12
Intermediate	Neutral protamine (NPH)	6–12	18–24
	Lente	6–12	18–24
Long acting	Protamine zinc (PZI)	14–24	36
	Ultralente	18–24	36

Insulin treatment regimens may be classified as follows: conventional, multiple subcutaneous injections, and continuous subcutaneous insulin infusion (CSII). The choice of these treatment programs is dependent on time course of action of insulin used, number of injections a day acceptable to the patient, frequency and method of assessing metabolic control, patient motivation and degree of availability, and commitment of the health care team to interact with the patient. For instance, it is virtually impossible to manage safely and intensively a patient on a multiple-component insulin regimen unless the patient is willing to do home blood glucose monitoring. Therefore, the great majority of IDDM patients are best started on conventional therapy and then considered, depending on resources available and patient motivation, for a more intensive insulin regimen.

Conventional insulin therapy involves the initial use of one or two injections of an intermediate-acting insulin (NPH, Lente) with or without a short-acting preparation (Regular, Semilente) to cover the postprandial-induced hyperglycemia. Newly diagnosed patients may be managed effectively for 2 to 3 years on a single-dose multiple-component regimen. However, when total insulin dose exceeds 50 U per day, middle to late afternoon intermediate-acting insulin-induced hypoglycemia may occur, requiring a split-dose regimen. On the split-dose regimen, approximately two-thirds of the total daily dose is given before breakfast and one-third before dinner. The morning dose is divided as one-third short-acting and two-thirds intermediate-acting, whereas the proportions of short-acting to intermediate-acting in the evening injection are divided equally. If hypoglycemia is suspected during sleep, the intermediate-acting insulin may be given as a separate dose at bedtime so that its peak action is closer to waking hours and its effect is easily monitored. Also, this regimen may be effective in counteracting the progressive early morning rise in blood glucose, the "dawn phenomenon" seen in some IDDM patients. Prior to the advent of home blood glucose monitoring, good metabolic control on the above regimen without hypoglycemia was difficult to achieve when urine glucose determinations were the sole estimate of control. Preprandial adjustments in short-acting insulin dose made on the basis of patient-determined blood glucose concentrations and anticipated nutritional intake make it possible to achieve good to excellent glycemic control on these programs safely.

If the patient accepts the challenge of performing home glucose monitoring and an experienced diabetes team is available to advise the patient, other multiple insulin injection techniques may be considered. Other such methods include the use of preprandial short-acting insulin along with intermediate-acting insulin given at bedtime, one-quarter of the total dose given in each of four injections, or the use of long-acting Ultralente given as 40 to 50 percent of total daily dose, with short-acting insulin given premeal in equal amounts (approximately 20 percent of total dose with each injection). These latter two multiple dose regimens allow a wide range of flexibility to the patient in terms of daily living activities, such as size and timing of meal taking and exercise.

The most effective method to mimic normal insulin secretion is the CSII regimen. This intensive approach involves the use of constant insulin delivery into a subcutaneous abdominal site via a programmable insulin pump. Consistent basal insulinemia may be achieved on a 24-hour basis. The infusion is supplemented with a preprandial insulin bolus given 15 to 30 minutes before meals. Typically, the basal insulin infusion rate averages 0.5 to 1.0 U per hour, with pre-meal bolus size adjusted according to time, nutrient content, and duration, degree, and timing of exercise.

Excellent control can be achieved with CSII; however, use of this method is not without significant risk, e.g., hypoglycemia, pump failure. Therefore it should be reserved for the highly motivated and dedicated patient who has constant access to a trained diabetes health care team.

Insulin therapy in type II diabetes is hardly different from that in patients with IDDM, with the exception that the obese patient is more insulin-resistant, requiring up to and sometimes in excess of 100 U of insulin per day. A single dose of intermediate-acting insulin often is adequate for the majority of patients. Unfortunately, improved metabolic control with either oral agents or more typically with insulin can be accompanied by weight gain. This is caused in part by continued dietary noncompliance in the face of diminished caloric losses secondary to the decreased glycosuria associated with improved control.

HAZARDS OF THERAPY

The major hazard of drug treatment and insulin therapy is hypoglycemia, particularly in those patients in whom efforts are directed to normalize pre- and postprandial blood glucose levels. The common precipitating events include a missed meal, inappropriate or unplanned exercise, unphysiologic insulin replacement, unusual insulin absorption, abnormal glucose counterregulation, and perhaps most important, behavioral and psychosocial stress.

Typically the symptoms of adrenergic nervous system activation such as sweating, nervousness, palpitations, tremors, and hunger may be readily recognizable by the patient; however, nocturnal hypoglycemia is not an uncommon event and may go unnoticed by the patient. The glycemic threshold for activation of the protective glucose counterregulatory events may be quite variable among patients and is subject to change, depending on level of metabolic control. In some instances, patients with normalization of glycemic control may be virtually asymptomatic, with blood glucose levels below 30 mg per deciliter. Unrecognized hypoglycemia may also lead to erratic glycemic control, as the release of counterregulatory hormones results in hyperglycemia and ketosis. As diabetes progresses, subtle deficits of autonomic function can occur, leading to further blunting of the adrenergic-induced warning symptoms and diminished metabolic counterregulation. Such defects will result in unrecognized hypoglycemia and neurologic impairment, e.g., behavioral change, disorientation, and unconsciousness. Thus the major harmful effects of recurrent hypoglycemia to patients are (1) worsening of diabetic control, (2) precipitating injury to themselves or others via accident, and (3) permanent neurologic damage. The use of home glucose monitoring has proved invaluable in allowing documentation of hypoglycemia by the patient so that new therapeutic strategies may be planned to prevent future hypoglycemic events.

MONITORING OF METABOLIC CONTROL

Assessment of day-to-day or short-term metabolic control involves home or self-monitoring of blood glucose and urine testing for glucose and ketones. The current recommendation of the American Diabetes Association is that self-monitoring of blood glucose is preferable to urine testing in any patient requiring insulin because it facilitates both the prevention of hyperglycemia that cannot be detected by urine testing and the prevention of hypoglycemia. With the improved technology that has made the finger-pricking process simple and painless, along with the availability of a variety of blood testing strips and portable battery-operated meters, this technique is now feasible, practical, and acceptable to the large majority of patients. At the minimum, all patients should know how to do self-monitoring of blood glucose, keep testing materials available in order to detect and prevent hypoglycemia, and monitor control during intercurrent illness.

Urine glucose measurement is useful when the renal threshold for glucose is normal. It is determined only on a specimen obtained after emptying the bladder 30 minutes before (double voiding). Under the above conditions, a urine free of glucose indicates the blood glucose level is below 180 mg per deciliter. Routine urine testing before meals and bedtime can provide a record indicative of reasonable symptom-free metabolic control. However, such a rough guide to blood glucose levels is of little help in detecting rapid changes in glycemic control or preventing anticipated hypoglycemia. Measurement of urine glucose level and ketones during intercurrent illness is important even when the patient is doing self-monitoring of blood glucose, as ketosis may go undetected unless tested. Therefore it is good practice to continue to monitor urine glucose concentration and ketones, even when performing home blood glucose testing.

Longer term assessment of metabolic control utilizes measurements of glycosylated hemoglobin A_{1c}. Hemoglobin A_{1c} values are an accurate estimation of the mean level of blood glucose over a period of 4 to 8 weeks and are only minimally affected by acute changes in glycemic control. Periodic measurements should be used to document and confirm that the patient's self-monitoring of blood glucose record is a correct reflection of his or her glycemic control. Well-kept records of home blood glucose values, meal taking, and insulin dosage, in combination with periodic hemoglobin A_{1c} determinations, are the essential components to achieving consistent long-term metabolic control in the diabetic patient.

SUGGESTED READING

American Diabetes Association. Clinical practice recommendations 1989–1990. Diabetes Care 1989; 13:1–59.

American Diabetes Association. The physicians' guide to type II diabetes: Diagnosis and treatment. Alexandria, VA: American Diabetes Association, 1984.

Gerich J. Oral hypoglycemic agents. N Engl J Med 1989; 321:1231–1245.

Olefsky JM, Sherwin RS. Diabetes mellitus: Management and complications. New York: Churchill Livingstone, 1985.

Schade DS, Santiago JV, Skyler JS, et al. Intensive insulin therapy. Princeton, NJ: Excerpta Medica, 1983.

Skyler JS, Skyler DL, Seigler DE, et al. Algorithms for adjustment of insulin dosage by patients who monitor blood glucose. Diabetes Care 1981; 4:311–318.

DIABETIC KETOACIDOSIS

DAVID S. SCHADE, M.D.

Diabetic ketoacidosis (DKA) exists when the blood glucose concentration exceeds 250 mg per deciliter and the blood pH is less than 7.2. It is a life-threatening medical emergency that is treatable in all patients. Prompt diagnosis and initiation of therapy is essential. In the majority of patients, a history of polyuria, polydipsia, and excessive thirst combined with hyperventilation should strongly suggest the diagnosis. However, when a coexistent medical condition exists (such as pneumonia, myocardial infarction, or acute appendicitis) the clinical presentation may be confusing and the physician must maintain a high level of suspicion. Common signs and symptoms of patients presenting in DKA are listed in Table 1.

DKA is usually precipitated by an acute medical condition (often an infection). Therefore, the initial laboratory assessment must include a complete blood cell count; urinalysis; plasma ketone and electrolyte determinations; cultures of the blood, urine, and throat; an electrocardiogram; and a chest roentgenogram. Admission of the patient to an intensive care unit is essential to permit close monitoring of vital signs and mental status and administration of fluids, medications, and insulin.

PREFERRED TREATMENT

Specific treatment of DKA can be divided into six areas: fluid therapy, insulin therapy, potassium administration, bicarbonate administration, other treatments, and recovery. Although all of these areas must be considered simultaneously by the physician who is treating the patient with DKA, they will be discussed separately here. It must be remembered that alterations in one area may have major effects on another.

TABLE 1 Common Presenting Symptoms and Signs in Diabetic Ketoacidosis

Signs and Symptoms	
Abdominal pain	Somnolence
Dehydration	Tachycardia
Hyperventilation	Thirst and polyuria
Hypotension	Warm, dry skin
Hypothermia	Weakness, anorexia
Impaired consciousness or coma	Weight loss
Nausea and vomiting	Visual disturbances

Fluid Therapy

Correction of dehydration is essential to correcting the metabolic derangements in DKA. All patients presenting in DKA are dehydrated, having lost 5 to 10 percent of their usual body weight. The dehydration results from the hyperglycemia-induced diuresis, acidosis-induced hyperventilation, and vomiting. Appropriate guidelines for the fluid management of these patients are provided in Table 2. In most patients, an isotonic saline drip should be started, changing to one-half normal saline when the serum sodium level is greater than 140 mEq per liter and the cardiovascular system has stabilized. Since water is lost in excess of sodium during the development of DKA, "free" water must eventually be provided to correct the metabolic abnormalities. In patients who are hypernatremic or in congestive heart failure when first seen, one-half normal saline should be infused as the initial fluid.

Insulin Therapy

Since all patients in DKA are insulin deficient (either relative or absolute), administration of this hormone is essential to inhibit both glucose and ketone body production. Insulin has major beneficial effects throughout the body that will enhance the correction of the metabolic abnormalities. However, frequent monitoring of the plasma potassium concentration is essential, since insulin augments the movement of this cation into cells. For almost all patients, an intravenous infusion of 0.1 unit per kilogram per hour of regular insulin is adequate (Table 3). Most authorities recommend that the patient be given an initial bolus of 10 units of insulin intravenously at the start of treatment, although published studies have not demonstrated that this approach is necessary. The practical reason to give a bolus dose is that the physician is certain that the patient has received at least some insulin. Although not preferred, intramuscularly administered insulin may also be used when no apparatus is available to regulate the intravenous infusion rate. Appropriate dosages for the intramuscular route are also given in Table 3.

TABLE 2 Fluid Therapy in Diabetic Ketoacidosis

Hour 1—15 ml/kg of isotonic sodium chloride (500 ml/M²/h). If patient is elderly or has heart disease, administer fluid cautiously, e.g., according to central venous pressure.
Hour 2—15 ml/kg. Continue isotonic sodium chloride unless patient is hypernatremic, in congestive heart failure, or is a child. In this case consider one-half normal isotonic sodium chloride.
Hour 3—Reduce fluid rate to 7.5 ml/kg/h. Change fluid to one-half normal isotonic saline.
Hour 4—Adjust fluid rate to meet clinical need. Consider rate of urine output in fluid replacement calculation.
When blood glucose level approaches 300 mg/dl, change fluid to 5% dextrose in one-half normal saline.
Continue fluid therapy including intravenous administration of insulin, if necessary, until patient can ingest food without vomiting. Then change to regular insulin administered subcutaneously every 4 to 6 hours, giving the first subcutaneous dose before discontinuing the intravenous infusion.

Potassium Administration

Adequate administration of potassium in DKA is essential to ensure a successful outcome (Table 4). Four points should be considered when deciding on the dose of potassium to administer:

1. The total-body potassium level is depleted in all patients presenting in DKA.
2. The presenting plasma potassium level may be increased, normal, or low.
3. The plasma potassium concentration will decline during the administration of fluid and insulin.
4. Inappropriate potassium administration (or lack of it) can lead to cardiac arrhythmias and death.

Therefore, frequent monitoring of the potassium concentration (every 2 hours) during the initial 12 hours of treatment is indicated.

DKA is one of the few clinical situations in which large amounts of potassium may need to be given. The principal caveat is that the patient must have at least some urine output (40 ml per hour) before administration of large doses of potassium. The reason for this precaution is that much of the potassium given initially may be excreted in the urine, and severe hyperkalemia can result from the combination of oliguria and potassium administration.

Bicarbonate Administration

The most controversial issue in the management of DKA is the administration of sodium bicarbonate. Classically, bicarbonate has been administered with the rationale of correction of the metabolic acidosis. However, most studies report that the metabolic acidosis is not corrected more quickly and that the patients receiving bicarbonate do not have an improved outcome. The reason that caution is advised in administering bicarbonate is that when the extracellular fluid pH is raised with bicarbonate, the intracellular fluid pH may actually decline. Therefore, bicarbonate administration should be reserved for those patients who have a clinical problem not responsive to standard therapy and that is aggravated by acidosis (e.g., cardiovascular shock or life-threatening cardiac arrhythmias. Giving bicarbonate based only on an arbitrary pH measurement should be discouraged. An appropriate method to give bicarbonate intravenously is to infuse one ampule (50 mEq) of sodium bicarbonate over 10 to 15 minutes and then to assess the patient's clinical response. Most authorities do not recommend continuing to administer bicarbonate once the blood pH has risen above 7.1.

TABLE 3 Insulin Administration in Diabetic Ketoacidosis

Use regular (short-acting, soluble) insulin only
Intravenous route (preferred)
  Give bolus dose of 0.15 U/kg. Administer continuous infusion of 0.1 U/kg/h.
  Before connecting infusion tubing to patient run 30 ml of insulin solution through the tubing to saturate tubing adsorption sites.

Changing the insulin infusion rate
  If no biochemical response is detected by 2 to 4 hours, then double the infusion rate (be sure to check all infusion lines for patency).
  If blood glucose level declines below 300 mg/dl, then half the infusion rate (do not stop the insulin infusion).
  If subcutaneous insulin therapy is begun, then discontinue intravenous infusion 30 minutes later.

Intramuscular route (recommended only if no method is available to regulate intravenous insulin infusion rate)
  In first hour of therapy give 0.5 U/kg. Then administer 0.1 U/kg each hour thereafter until blood glucose level is reduced to 300 mg/dl. Then inject 0.1 U/kg of insulin every 2 hours as necessary to maintain blood glucose concentration at 300 mg/dl.

Phosphate Administration

Although most patients in DKA are phosphate depleted, administration of phosphate is not essential in the treatment of DKA. However, it does have the advantage of administration of potassium without the concurrent administration of chloride, thus reducing the possibility that hyperchloremia may occur during or following DKA therapy. Phosphate administration may also be beneficial on theoretical grounds, i.e., decreasing tissue anoxia. Caution is indicated, however, since excessive phosphate administration has induced hypocalcemia and seizures. Most authorities recommend that phosphate be given as potassium phosphate in the amount of 1 ampule (44 mmol) every 12 hours for the initial 24 hours.

Other Considerations During Initial Therapy

Death that occurs during the therapy for DKA is usually avoidable if the physician considers all aspects of patient management. In comatose patients, an airway must be maintained and a nasogastric tube placed for stomach drainage to prevent aspiration pneumonia. A precipitating cause of DKA must be aggressively pursued and treated. This usually involves the administration of antibiotics since infection is the most common cause of DKA. Cardiac monitoring is recommended in all adult patients, but in the patient suspected of having a myocardial infarction it is essential. Nasal oxygen is recommended as a routine adjunct to therapy. Low doses of subcutaneously administered heparin (5,000 units every 12 hours) are frequently recommended for comatose or elderly patients.

TABLE 4 Potassium Replacement in Diabetic Ketoacidosis

Add potassium to replacement fluid therapy. If concentration of potassium in infusate is 20 to 40 mEq per liter, infuse into central vein if possible.

Replacement of potassium is based on the plasma potassium concentration.
  If the potassium level is
    less than 3 mEq/L, infuse 0.5 mEq/kg/h
    3 to 4 mEq/L, infuse 0.4 mEq/kg/h
    4 to 5 mEq/L, infuse 0.3 mEq/kg/h
    5 to 6 mEq/L, infuse 0.1 to 0.2 mEq/kg/h
    6 mEq/L, withhold potassium until level is below 6.0 mEq/L

Confirm adequate urine output before administering potassium if plasma level is greater than 6.0 mEq per liter.

Initially, the electrocardiogram (lead II) may be used as a guide to plasma potassium concentration.

Recheck plasma potassium level every 2 hours if it is less than 4 mEq per liter or greater than 6 mEq per liter.

Administer potassium as potassium chloride or as potassium phosphate. However, do not exceed 90 mmol of potassium phosphate in 24 hours because of the danger of hypocalcemia.

Recovery

As the patient improves, the question always arises as to when to stop intravenous insulin therapy and change to subcutaneous administration of insulin. This decision requires clinical judgment and depends on the clinical response of the patient and the presence of any concurrent disease. In general, the patient should not be started on subcutaneous insulin therapy until the acidosis has resolved (i.e., pH greater than 7.3 or plasma bicarbonate level above 20 mEq per liter); liquid feedings are tolerated; the usual state of mental functioning has been regained; and no major complications of the diabetic therapy are still present (e.g., cerebral edema, severe hypokalemia).

The conversion of the patient to subcutaneous administration of insulin is not difficult if the physician adheres to the following guidelines. First, and most important, the subcutaneous insulin dose must be given at least 30 minutes before discontinuing the intravenous dose because of the very short half-life of intravenous insulin. Second, only regular insulin should be administered for the first 24 hours after stopping the intravenous therapy to achieve a rapid onset of action and to permit frequent changes in insulin doses. Thus, regular insulin (usually 5 to 15 units) is given every 4 hours for the first 24 hours. Third, the change from intravenous to regular insulin should be made in the morning when a full staff of nurses is available to observe the patient if metabolic decompensation recurs. Finally, the total daily dose of insulin is likely to exceed the patient's usual pre-DKA daily dose because of insulin resistance, which occurs for 2 to 4 weeks following an episode of DKA.

Discharge of the patient from the hospital is recommended as soon as possible after the patient has been stable for 24 hours on subcutaneous insulin therapy and is tolerating solid food. Normalization of the blood glucose concentration should not be expected prior to discharge (and, in fact, is rarely achievable). However, if a precipitating cause has been identified (e.g., pneumonia), it must be under control prior to discharge or the patient will experience recurrent DKA within several days of discharge. In many cases (e.g., myocardial infarction), treatment of the precipitating cause will require a longer hospitalization than treatment of the DKA.

On discharge, the patient should always be instructed to call the physician immediately when he develops an infection or has severe hyperglycemia or ketone bodies in the urine. Aggressive insulin therapy at this time may prevent hospitalization. However, whenever the patient becomes dehydrated, hospitalization is indicated. The more rapidly that this situation is treated with intravenous administration of fluids and insulin the more rapid is the correction of the DKA and the more quickly the patient can be discharged. For an ill patient to wait "until the last minute" to call a physician is not only extremely hazardous but also results in increased morbidity and expense.

SUGGESTED READING

Foster DW, McGarry JD. The metabolic derangements and treatment of diabetic ketoacidosis. N Engl J Med 1983; 309:159–169.

Keller U. Diabetic ketoacidosis: current views of pathogenesis and treatment. Diabetologia 1986; 29:71–77.

Kreisberg RA. Diabetic ketoacidosis: new concepts and trends in pathogenesis and treatment. Ann Intern Med 1978; 88:681–695.

Schade DS, Eaton RP, Alberti KGMM, Johnston DG. Diabetic coma. Albuquerque: University of New Mexico Press, 1981.

Sperling MA. Diabetic ketoacidosis. Pediatr Clin North Am 1984; 31:591–610.

HYPEROSMOLAR NONKETOTIC COMA

JOHN E. GERICH, M.D.

Hyperosmolar nonketotic coma is characterized by severe hyperglycemia (usually greater than 600 mg per deciliter), hyperosmolarity (usually greater than 350 mOsm per liter), and dehydration. In its classic form, hyperosmolar nonketotic coma is distinguished from ketoacidosis by the lack of severe acidosis (plasma bicarbonate usually greater than 18 mEq per liter) and ketosis (plasma ketones usually less than 2+ undiluted Acetest) in the presence of severe hyperglycemia. However, ketoacidosis is also a hyperosmolar condition and hyperosmolar nonketotic coma can be accompanied by some ketosis and some acidosis; with the latter often being due to lactate accumulation.

The typical patient is usually middle-aged or elderly, has no prior history of diabetes mellitus (or only mild non-insulin-dependent diabetes), and has some recent acute illness such as infection, trauma (e.g., burns), myocardial infarction, or cerebrovascular accident. Usually, the acute illness is superimposed on a chronic process for which the patient is being medicated, such as hypertension, congestive heart failure, or arthritis. Diuretic and steroid treatment, which have been implicated in facilitating development of the condition, are common. Nevertheless, in up to 20 percent of cases, patients may be under 40 years of age, have no underlying illness, and present with no precipitating condition other than an apparently insignificant viral syndrome.

PATHOGENESIS AND PRINCIPLES OF TREATMENT

Severe dehydration is always present in hyperosmolar nonketotic coma, and it is generally considered to be the major factor in the pathogenesis of this condition. An acute illness in a person who has a limited capacity to respond to stress with an appropriate increase in insulin secretion occurs in conjunction with an antecedent condition or medication that predisposes to the development of dehydration. The acute stress leads to hyperglycemia, which ordinarily would be mild but the resultant osmotic diuresis, when superimposed on either diuretic therapy, diminished thirst perception, other fluid losses (e.g., vomiting or diarrhea), or impaired renal function, results in progressive dehydration. This dehydration ultimately reduces organ perfusion, which reduces excretion of glucose, permitting development of severe hyperglycemia; limits mobilization of free fatty acids from adipose tissue for ketone body production; produces cerebral dysfunction; and can ultimately lead to circulatory collapse and death. The condition usually develops insidiously over many days, and an appreciable number of cases occur in nursing home residents and hospitalized patients in whom fluid imbalances are produced by poorly monitored diuretic treatment or administration of hypertonic intravenous solutions (e.g., glucose and/or mannitol).

Since severe dehydration appears to be the critical element in both causing this condition and determining its morbidity and mortality, therapy is primarily directed at correcting fluid deficits; secondary considerations involve correcting or preventing associated electrolyte abnormalities (in particular, hypokalemia), diminishing hyperglycemia, and identifying and treating the precipitating acute illness.

PREFERRED TREATMENT

The First Hour

The diagnosis of hyperosmolar nonketotic coma should be considered in all patients who are comatose or semicomatose. As in all such patients, an intravenous line and adequate airway should be established. With insertion of the intravenous line, blood should be drawn for laboratory determination of glucose, electrolytes, blood urea nitrogen (BUN), drug screen, and alcohol level. A sample of blood should be immediately tested for glucose and ketones using commercially available strips to distinguish between hypoglycemia, ketoacidosis, and hyperosmolar nonketotic coma. A careful physical and neurologic examination and electrocardiogram should be performed. At this point, an extremely high blood glucose level with negative or only slight ketonemia would be presumptive evidence for the diagnosis of nonketotic hyperosmolar coma.

While awaiting laboratory confirmation, it is essential to initiate fluid therapy. If the patient is normotensive, one-half normal saline should be infused at a rate of 15 to 30 ml per minute (1 to 2 L over 1 hour); if the patient is hypotensive, normal saline should be used. Reestablishment of an adequate circulating volume is critical in preventing avoidable complications (myocardial infarction, stroke, acute renal failure) and permitting excretion of glucose. It is not essential to start insulin at this time.

By the end of the first hour, laboratory confirmation of the diagnosis should be available and, with fluid therapy initiated, the patient may undergo other emergency diagnostic procedures to identify precipitating or other factors. Patients may be hypernatremic or hyponatremic; the plasma bicarbonate level is usually greater than 18 mEq per liter, the plasma potassium concentration is less than 6 mEq per liter, and the BUN value is elevated. The patient's osmolarity may be calculated using the following formula:

$$\text{mOsm/L} = 2(\text{Na+K}) + \frac{\text{Plasma glucose}}{18} + \frac{\text{BUN}}{2.8}$$

A rough estimate of the patient's fluid deficit may be calculated as well:

$$\text{Deficit (in liters)} = 24\ \text{L}\left(1 - \frac{\text{Patient's osmolarity}}{280\ \text{mOsm/L}}\right)$$

This represents a minimal estimate, since there is both extracellular and intracellular dehydration and this formula takes into consideration only extracellular dehydration. Nevertheless, it provides a reasonable guideline for the administration of fluids during the first 6 to 8 hours of treatment.

Another helpful procedure is to initiate a flow sheet that details the therapeutic steps taken, the laboratory results, and the status of the patient.

Hours 2 Through 8

During the initial 2 hours of therapy, most patients should receive 2 to 4 L of fluid. With renal excretion of glucose established, this hydration alone can reduce an initial blood glucose value of 1,000 mg per deciliter by 200 mg per deciliter. The serum potassium concentration should decrease, and the potential development of hypokalemia, especially in patients being or to be treated with insulin, should be guarded against. Therefore, at 2 hours the plasma glucose and electrolyte values should be rechecked on a stat basis.

At reception of the 2-hour values for plasma glucose and electrolytes, a decision can be made regarding the need for insulin and potassium therapy. If the plasma glucose level has decreased more than 100 mg per deciliter and is less than 700 mg per deciliter and if the serum potassium concentration is above 4.5 mEq per liter, continued rehydration may be the only therapy necessary at this time. Too rapid a fall of plasma glucose levels should be avoided in order to prevent dangerous fluid shifts. With a rapid and marked reduction in extracellular osmolarity, fluid moves intracellularly from the extracellular space; this shift of fluid may lead to cerebral edema, a condition that has an extremely high mortality. In addition, the rapid efflux of fluid intracellularly could cause acute reduction of the plasma volume, hypotension, and vascular collapse. Thus, if the serum sodium value has remained below 135 mEq per liter or if the patient has had a decrease in blood pressure, rehydration should be continued with normal saline rather than one-half normal saline. The rate of fluid administration may proceed at 10 to 20 ml per minute supplemented with oral intake (water) if the patient is alert.

At 2 hours after initiating therapy, insulin therapy should be started if the plasma glucose level has not decreased appreciably and is greater than 700 mg per deciliter. However, it must be remembered that patients with hyperosmolar nonketotic coma are sensitive to insulin, insulin therapy usually necessitates administration of potassium to prevent hypokalemia, and the plasma glucose value should not be decreased to less than 250 mg per deciliter during this period of treatment.

Taking these factors into consideration, if insulin therapy is indicated it can usually be administered safely at a rate of 3 to 6 units per hour in the following manner: add 100 units (1 ml of U-100 human regular insulin) to 1 L of normal or half-normal saline and infuse it at a rate of 30 to 60 ml per hour. It is important that 100 ml of this solution be run through the tubing to coat the walls and prevent subsequent adherence of the insulin to the tubing. For precise regulation of the insulin delivery, it is advisable to use one of the commercially available infusion systems to control the flow rate.

Also, if the initial potassium concentration was normal or low and if there was only prerenal azotemia, it would be appropriate at this point to administer potassium in conjunction with insulin therapy, since the latter reduces serum potassium levels. Potassium chloride should be added to the saline being administered for hydration and given at a rate of 30 to 60 mEq per hour.

It is important to monitor the patient carefully during this period for changes in clinical state and for development of hypoglycemia and hypokalemia. Therefore, 1 hour after starting the insulin and potassium infusions, plasma glucose and electrolyte values should be reassessed and the infusion rates of insulin and potassium should be adjusted accordingly. If the plasma glucose level has not decreased at least 50 mg per deciliter after 1 hour of continued hydration and insulin therapy, this indicates the presence of insulin resistance. The infusion rate of the insulin should be doubled and the response to this maneuver assessed again in 1 hour.

If the plasma glucose level has not decreased by 50 to 100 mg per deciliter at this time (2 hours of insulin therapy), the insulin infusion rate should be doubled again and this process repeated until a satisfactory response is achieved.

Once the plasma glucose level is between 200 and 300 mg per deciliter, glucose-containing solutions (5 percent dextrose in water or saline) may be substituted for the saline being used for rehydration to prevent the fluid shifts described previously and hypoglycemia.

It is important that insulin therapy not be discontinued prematurely or that subcutaneous insulin be started prematurely. The former may result in relapse, and the latter may lead to erratic absorption of insulin.

During this period (2 to 8 hours), measures should be undertaken to evaluate the precipitating and associated conditions of the patient and other supportive procedures instituted if necessary (e.g., oxygen, antibiotics, cardiac drugs).

Hours 8 to 24

By 8 hours, most patients have received 6 to 12 L of fluid and have had their plasma glucose levels reduced to 200 to 300 mg per deciliter. Although plasma sodium and potassium levels should be normal, deficits may remain for these electrolytes, as well as for phosphorus and magnesium. However, further repletion can be made over several days with oral intake. Most patients continue to have carbohydrate intolerance or frank diabetes mellitus. Therefore, it is important when terminating intravenous insulin to consider subsequent antidiabetic therapy. Those patients previously requiring insulin will continue to need insulin. Patients previously treated with oral hypoglycemic agents may require insulin temporarily until acute stress subsides. Ultimately, most patients not previously known to be diabetic and those previously treated with oral hypoglycemic agents may be managed satisfactorily with oral hypoglycemic agents. A few patients (usually those who are very obese) may end up being managed only by restriction of calories.

In the transition period, the subcutaneous insulin therapy that is required may be initiated as follows: in patients who are able to eat, 0.1 to 0.2 unit per kilogram of regular insulin can be given 30 minutes prior to meals and the dose adjusted upward or downward depending on the subsequent pre-meal plasma glucose level. Overnight coverage can be obtained using an intermediate-acting insulin (NPH or Lente) at the evening meal along with (0.1 to 0.2 unit per kilogram) or in lieu of (0.2 to 0.4 unit per kilogram) of the regular insulin for that meal. Later a pre-breakfast dose of intermediate-acting insulin may be used in lieu of a pre-lunch dose of regular insulin.

For patients who are unable to eat, satisfactory glycemic control may be achieved by subcutaneous administration of 0.1 to 0.2 unit per kilogram of regular insulin at 6-hour intervals with preinjection plasma glucose determinations used to evaluate the amount of the next dose. It is important to realize that during this intermediate period, insulin requirements may be increased above what the patient may require 24 to 48 hours later and that near normoglycemia is not a safe or realistic goal. Preprandial and 6-hour plasma glucose concentrations between 100 and 200 mg per deciliter are satisfactory. As insulin requirements decrease and patients resume a normal diet, institution or reinstitution of oral hypoglycemic agents may be considered prior to discharge while the patient is under careful surveillance.

Hyperosmolar nonketotic coma is a medical emergency. If therapy is delayed or inadequate, it carries a mortality rate as high as 80 percent. If treated promptly and adequately, the mortality of this condition is determined by the seriousness of the patient's underlying and precipitating illness. The key element in successful therapy is early and adequate correction of dehydration.

SUGGESTED READING

Arieff AE, Carroll HJ. Nonketotic hyperosmolar coma with hyperglycemia: clinical features, pathophysiology, renal function, acid-base balance, plasma-cerebrospinal fluid equilibria and the effects of therapy in 37 cases. Medicine 1972; 51:73-94.

Feig PU, McCurdy DK. The hypertonic state. N Engl J Med 1977; 297:1444-1454.

Feig PU. Hypernatremia and hypertonic syndromes. Med Clin North Am 1981; 65:271-290.

Gennari FJ. Serum osmolality. N Engl J Med 1984; 310:102-105.

Gerich J, Martin M, Recant L. Clinical and metabolic characteristics of hyperosmolar nonketotic coma. Diabetes 1971; 20:228-238.

Podolsky S. Hyperosmolar nonketotic coma: death can be prevented. Geriatrics 1979; 34:29-42.

DIABETIC RETINOPATHY

LLOYD M. AIELLO, M.D.
JERRY CAVALLERANO, O.D., Ph.D., F.A.A.O.

Diabetic retinopathy, a major complication of diabetes mellitus, is the leading cause of "severe" visual loss to 5/200 levels or less in persons between 20 and 60 years of age in the United States and other technologically advanced nations. Diabetes is also the leading cause of "moderate" visual loss to the 20/200 to 20/400 range.

The national and personal impact of visual loss from diabetes is significant. There are approximately 6 million or more persons in the United States known to have diabetes mellitus and an additional 4 to 6 million who have diabetes mellitus but are not aware of it. Approximately 7 percent of those with diagnosed diabetes mellitus, or 400,000 persons, have macular edema. By the time a person has had diabetes mellitus for 20 years or more, there is a 25 percent chance that diabetic macular edema will be present. Two hundred thousand patients with macular edema only are at risk of moderate visual loss, and another 200,000 patients with macular edema who have associated proliferative diabetic retinopathy are at risk of both moderate visual loss and severe visual loss. An additional 200,000 patients with proliferative diabetic retinopathy with no accompanying macular edema are at risk of severe visual loss.

If the 400,000 patients with diabetic macular edema are not treated with laser photocoagulation, approximately 50 percent will experience a significant loss of vision in one or both eyes within a 5-year period. A significant loss of vision is defined as doubling of the visual angle; that is, a decrease of approximately two or more lines on the standard eye chart that formerly could have been read. Of this group with visual loss, 66,000 would have vision loss from untreated macular edema sufficient to cause legal blindness; that is, best corrected visual acuity of 20/200 or less.

RESULTS OF TREATMENT

In 1976, the Diabetic Retinopathy Study (DRS) conclusively demonstrated that panretinal photocoagulation reduces the risk of severe visual loss from proliferative diabetic retinopathy by at least 50 percent. The Early Treatment Diabetic Retinopathy Study (ETDRS), in December 1985, demonstrated that focal laser photocoagulation reduces the risk of moderate visual loss attributable to macular edema by a factor of 50 percent. Of the 600,000 patients at risk for visual loss, there can be an overall decrease of risk by 50 percent or more if appropriate laser treatment is undertaken in a timely fashion.

The results of the ETDRS are expected to increase by 50 percent the number of diabetic patients who would be considered candidates for some type of laser photocoagulation. The potential is to decrease significant visual loss in approximately 100,000 diabetic patients, saving 33,000 of them from legal blindness. The DRS and ETDRS results, therefore, underscore the need for those with diabetes to have their eyes examined regularly to determine if they have clinically significant diabetic macular edema or high-risk characteristics of diabetic retinopathy.

STANDARD OF EYE CARE

The findings noted previously provide a compelling reason for physicians to refer their diabetic patients for regular eye examinations. Standards of eye care should be established along the guidelines established by the Kentucky Diabetes Foundation and accepted by the American Academy of Ophthalmology as the standard of care.

The eye care in a patient with diabetes mellitus encompasses a partnership among the patient, the primary care physician, the endocrinologist, the optometrist, and the ophthalmologist. The primary care physician and endocrinologist play a fundamental role in the medical management, education, and coordination of the care for a person with diabetes mellitus. Guidelines for the interaction of the health care team should include the following considerations:

1. All patients should be informed that sight-threatening eye disease is a common complication of diabetes mellitus and is often present, even with good vision. Early detection and appropriate treatment of diabetic eye disease significantly reduce the risk of visual loss.
2. Persons with insulin-dependent diabetes mellitus (IDDM) should have an ophthalmic evaluation with photography after 5 years' duration of diabetes and on a yearly basis thereafter. This examination should include (a) a history of visual symptoms, (b) measurement of visual acuity and intraocular pressure, (c) ophthalmoscopic examination through dilated pupils, including stereoscopic evaluation of the macula, and (d) seven standard stereo fundus photographs of the retina. Fundus photography, while perhaps underutilized in the past, is of increasing significance. One study indicates that up to 50 percent of small vessel proliferation may be overlooked in examination even by retinal specialists in patients with dilated fundus examinations.
3. Those with non-insulin-dependent diabetes mellitus (NIDDM) should have an ophthalmic examination on diagnosis of diabetes and at least yearly thereafter.
4. After the initial eye examination, a person with diabetes mellitus should receive an ophthalmic examination on an annual basis. Fluorescein angiography is not necessary except for purposes of clinical research or specifically to determine the presence of "treatable lesions" with clinically significant macular edema.
5. Preferably any diabetic woman contemplating pregnancy should have an ocular examination shortly before the onset of pregnancy. In the event of significant retinopathy, pregnancy may be deferred until the retinopathy is appropriately controlled. If panretinal photocoagulation or other laser therapy is necessary, it is best done before pregnancy. Subsequent pregnancy is often undertaken successfully without significant progression following appropriate laser photocoagulation treatment.
6. Any woman with IDDM who becomes pregnant should have a thorough eye examination early in her first trimester, at the beginning of each trimester, and 2 to 3 months post partum, if there is no significant retinopathy. More frequent examinations are indicated in the presence of significant nonproliferative diabetic retinopathy. If high-risk characteristic proliferative diabetic retinopathy is present, laser photocoagulation should be considered immediately. If neovascularization is evident, whether high-risk characteristics are present or not, and in advanced preproliferative diabetic retinopathy, laser photocoagulation should also be considered. Treatment of macular edema is appropriate during pregnancy when it is clinically significant.
7. Patients with diabetes mellitus should be referred promptly to an ophthalmologist specializing in retinal disease for unexplained visual symptoms, reduced corrected visual acuity, increased intraocular pressures, any retinal abnormalities, and any other pathologic process that threatens vision. It is incumbent on the primary care physician, endocrinologist, and optometrist to consider this point.
8. All patients should be under the care of retinal specialists experienced in the management of diabetic retinopathy for the following conditions:
   a. Preproliferative diabetic retinopathy, which consists of multiple cotton-wool spots, multiple intraretinal microaneurysms and hemorrhages, intraretinal microvascular abnormalities, and venous beading.
   b. Proliferative diabetic retinopathy, characterized by retinal neovascularization, preretinal or vitreous hemorrhage, preretinal or vitreous fibrosis, and traction on the retina with or without traction retinal detachment.
   c. Macular edema, characterized by thickening of the retina and hard lipid exudates.
9. Laser photocoagulation therapy has been proven effective in reducing the risk of severe and moderate visual loss in patients with high-risk proliferative diabetic retinopathy and clinically significant macular edema as previously described. Vitrectomy is effective in restoring certain amounts of vision in patients with recent traction retinal detachments and persistent vitreous hemorrhages. Both laser treatment and vitrectomy should be performed by a retinal specialist (ophthalmologist) experienced in these procedures.
10. Visual function rehabilitation should be performed by appropriately skilled ophthalmologists and optometrists once the retinopathy is in a quiescent stage. Vocational rehabilitation requires the team work of the primary care physician, endocrinologist, other subspecialists, and optometrists skilled in the care of the diabetic patient.

RISK FACTORS

The causes of diabetic retinopathy remain uncertain and unproved; however, there are certain relationships that may be helpful in clinical practice. The most well-established risk factor for diabetic retinopathy is the duration of the diabetes. Diabetic retinopathy develops sooner after the diagnosis of NIDDM than after the diagnosis of IDDM.

In regard to IDDM, retinopathy rarely makes an appearance before a 5-year duration of diabetes, but 60 percent have some form of retinopathy by 10 years of diabetes. Proliferative retinopathy, the most sight-threatening type, is present in 40 to 50 percent of patients with IDDM of 20 years or more. In one study of patients with IDDM followed from the onset of diabetes, a 60 percent cumulative incidence of proliferative diabetic retinopathy was found by 40 years. In summary, in patients with IDDM, background retinopathy commonly develops after 5 years of diabetes and is virtually ubiquitous by 15 to 20 years. Proliferative diabetic retinopathy is uncommon before 10 years, develops during the second decade, and becomes very common after 20 years. Patients with very young onset are relatively immune from developing significant eye disease until after puberty.

Those with NIDDM of older age at onset showed two major differences: (1) retinopathy is present in about 20 percent at onset of diabetes, probably reflecting the uncertain date of onset; and (2) the percent ever developing any retinopathy or proliferative diabetic retinopathy is lower, with 60 to 80 percent developing retinopathy and 10 to 20 percent developing proliferative diabetic retinopathy. Patients who were older at onset of the diabetes who do develop proliferative diabetic retinopathy appear to do so after a shorter duration of diabetes than their younger cohorts.

The presence of joint contractures in young patients poses another risk factor for the development of diabetic retinopathy. Statistics suggest that joint contractures may be associated with significant retinopathy, and these patients should be referred immediately for a complete eye examination.

Pregnancy may also be considered a risk factor for the progression of diabetic retinopathy, and progression of existing retinopathy may be rapid in some women during pregnancy. Preferably, the patient should be examined prior to onset of a planned pregnancy or at least early in the first trimester in an effort to evaluate the possible complications that may occur during pregnancy in the presence of preexisting retinopathy.

Hypertension and renal disease are significant risk factors in the development and progression of diabetic retinopathy. The presence of hypertension or renal disease, particularly proteinuria, should alert the physician to the possibility of the presence or impending onset of proliferative diabetic retinopathy. Approximately 50 percent of patients with proliferative diabetic retinopathy have accompanying renal disease. If renal disease (proteinuria) is not present at the time the retinopathy is diagnosed or within the next 1 or 2 years, it is unlikely to develop; however, in the presence of significant proteinuria, the proliferative diabetic retinopathy may progress rapidly, particularly if there is associated renal retinopathy. Unfortunately, laser treatment is less effective in the presence of renal retinopathy; therefore, even the earliest signs of proteinuria should alert the physician to careful follow-up of potential serious diabetic eye disease and consideration of earlier laser photocoagulation.

Glycemia level is a presumed risk factor for diabetic retinopathy, and most studies have supported the association between lower glycemia and lower prevalence of retinopathy. These studies, however, do not conclusively demonstrate that altering glycemia levels alters the risk of retinopathy or that the associations between glycemia and retinopathy are more than associations between two components of a single syndrome. One randomized clinical trial suggests that attempts at normalization of blood glucose levels may result in worsening of retinopathy early on, with the reduction or reversal of this negative effect within 3 years. Most likely, many other factors impact on retinopathy, the balance of which determines a patient's risk for the development of retinopathy.

There is also a genetic component in determining the risk of proliferative diabetic retinopathy. HLA-associated factors may influence retinopathy, and a particular HLA phenotype, DR4/0, 3/0, and X/X (non 3 or 4) may be associated with a fourfold increase in the risk of proliferative diabetic retinopathy. Among nonmyopic patients, that risk increase is over tenfold, whereas among myopes, the risk differs little from other HLA-DR phenotypes.

Cigarette smoking is not a major risk factor for retinopathy, although its other detrimental effects on health are sufficient to discourage smoking.

Once significant retinopathy develops, local factors within the eye itself relating to the type and severity of retinopathy are the best predictors of long-term visual outcome. The most important of these is neovascularization on the optic disc along with preretinal or vitreous hemorrhage, severe intraretinal hemorrhages and microaneurysms, and venous beading. Additional local risk factors for severe visual loss documented in the DRS were elevated new vessels and fibrous proliferations, extensive retinopathy with hemorrhages and microaneurysms, arterial abnormalities, venous beading and perivenous exudates, and decreased visual acuity. Furthermore, in eyes with active new vessels plus localized traction retinal detachment and/or severe fibrous proliferation, the overall prognosis is worse with or without photocoagulation, although the risk of severe visual loss was reduced by about 50 percent by photocoagulation.

Inappropriate eye examination or referral can also be considered a risk factor for the development of proliferative diabetic retinopathy.

STAGES OF DIABETIC RETINOPATHY AND THEIR TREATMENT

Generally, retinopathy can be divided into two major categories: (1) nonproliferative diabetic retinopathy and (2) proliferative diabetic retinopathy. Background, transitional, and preproliferative retinopathies are all stages of nonproliferative diabetic retinopathy. New vessels either away from or at the nerve head or fibrous proliferation signify proliferative disease. Macular edema can be present at any stage of retinopathy.

Nonproliferative Diabetic Retinopathy

Background Diabetic Retinopathy

Microaneurysms are the earliest clinical manifestations of diabetic retinopathy and appear as small, round, deep intraretinal red dots and somewhat larger as very small hemorrhages (blotches). These lesions appear in some patients after 5 to 7 years of diabetes and in almost all patients with diabetes of 20 years' duration. They tend to come and go over periods of months and years. It is rare for a patient to have shown no evidence of retinopathy after 35 or 40 years of diabetes. This early phase of nonproliferative diabetic retinopathy is best referred to as background diabetic retinopathy, to highlight its almost universal occurrence and its general lack of prognostic significance. Macular edema may be present when these changes occur near the center of the macula and are discussed under the separate entity of macular edema. In general, however, background changes are predominantly intravascular or perivascular and of little significance.

Transitional Diabetic Retinopathy

As the retinal disease progresses, the earliest additional changes such as soft exudates (cotton-wool spots), venous caliber abnormalities (beading or link sausage appearance), arteriolar abnormalities (white threads similar to those seen in hypertension), and intraretinal microvascular abnormalities appearing as irregular tortuous retinal vessels occurring in the early stages would be considered transitional. These changes are no longer merely intravascular or perivascular but are seen clinically away from the major vascular networks. Some of these eyes remain stable over many years and/or only gradually develop further changes. If the changes progress rapidly and the combination of these lesions described previously becomes extensive or becomes associated with intraretinal hemorrhages, then the more extensive phase or preproliferative diabetic retinopathy has occurred. Therefore, transitional retinopathy may progress, regress, or remain remarkably stable over a long period of time and does not necessarily indicate that the more advanced stages of preproliferative diabetic retinopathy or proliferative diabetic retinopathy will develop.

Preproliferative Diabetic Retinopathy

Preproliferative diabetic retinopathy is characterized by more extensive degrees of soft exudates, venous caliber abnormalities, arteriolar abnormalities, and intraretinal microvascular abnormalities with an increase in the extent of hemorrhages and microaneurysms. These patients are at significant risk of the development of proliferative diabetic retinopathy. Patients in the transitional and the preproliferative stages of diabetic retinopathy should be referred immediately to an ophthalmologist for consideration of potential early laser photocoagulation treatment. Associated with preproliferative diabetic retinopathy, in some cases, is optic disc edema, an often asymptomatic condition detected on routine examination. The course of disc edema is usually benign, and it usually resolves spontaneously over a period of several months. Disc edema is sometimes seen in patients with poor control of their diabetes earlier in the course of the disease, perhaps with less than 5 or 10 years' duration of diabetes. On the other hand, those with diabetes of longer duration may develop optic disc edema that goes on to neovascularization of the optic nerve head. In either case, neurologic evaluation is advisable to rule out other causes of disc edema, particularly if it is bilateral.

Laser treatment may be advisable in the presence of *severe* preproliferative diabetic retinopathy. The ETDRS examined the question: When in the course of diabetic retinopathy is it most effective to initiate panretinal photocoagulation to prevent the progression to high-risk proliferative retinopathy and severe visual loss? The ETDRS was initiated in 1979 and enrolled 3,711 patients. The ETDRS research group concluded that scatter laser treatment significantly reduces the risk of severe visual loss. The rates of severe visual loss were low whether scatter treatment was given early or deferred until the development of high-risk proliferative retinopathy. In the ETDRS, patients were followed by a retinal specialist every 4 months. This study further underscores the need for those with diabetes to have their eyes examined regularly and carefully. It is reasonable to consider panretinal photocoagulation in one eye and observe the other eye until high-risk characteristics develop and then immediately institute panretinal photocoagulation in the untreated eye.

Proliferative Diabetic Retinopathy

Proliferation of new blood vessels from the surface of the retina into the vitreous space is the most dangerous stage of diabetic retinopathy. This disease may occur in as many as 60 percent of patients with IDDM by the time they have had diabetes for 40 or more years. Often associated with extensive capillary closure, proliferation may represent an abortive attempt by the eye to revascularize the ischemic retina. The walls of these newly formed blood vessels are lined with endothelial cells only and therefore are likely to rupture and bleed. Since the vitreous may contract frequently in diabetes, these fragile vessels are pulled forward, causing bleeding into the preretinal vitreous space. Cobwebs or floaters may be an early symptom. Large hemorrhages cause a sudden, painless loss of vision. The presence of vitreous or preretinal hemorrhage associated with neovascularization, particularly on the optic nerve head, places the eye at great risk of severe visual loss even if the vision remains good. If the new vessels on the optic nerve head are equal to or greater than one-half disc area in size, even in the absence of a hemorrhage, these vessels on the optic nerve head constitute high-risk characteristics, carrying a 25 to 40 percent risk of severe visual loss over 2 years, and in most cases demand prompt photocoagulation, which reduces the risk by about 60 percent. Lesser degrees of proliferative diabetic retinopathy, including neovascularization less than one-half the disc area and neovascular edema of any size, may be prudently watched, or only one eye may be treated because of the risks associated with photocoagulation. The purposes of panretinal photocoagulation with the argon laser are to halt the progression of retinal neovascularization, decrease the risk of repeat vitreous and preretinal hemorrhage, and prevent traction detachments.

Laser photocoagulation is the accepted standard of care, based on the findings of the DRS. In 1976, the DRS reached the following conclusions:

1. Extensive panretinal photocoagulation reduces the risk of severe visual loss from proliferative diabetic retinopathy by 50 percent. Laser treatment itself, however, causes a persistent decrease in visual acuity of one line on the Snellen Eye Chart in 11 percent of these cases and greater than or equal to two lines in 3 percent.
2. Eyes with DRS high-risk characteristics (neovascularization greater or equal to standard photograph 10A [i.e., new vessels covering ¼ of the disc area] alone or less extensive neovascularization and/or edema greater than one-half the disc area plus vitreous or preretinal hemorrhage) have a 2-year risk of severe visual loss of 25 percent. This benefit outweighs the risk of visual acuity decrease due to photocoagulation. Photocoagulation should usually be carried out as soon as possible in the presence of high-risk characteristics.
3. Eyes with severe nonproliferative retinopathy or proliferative retinopathy without high-risk characteristics have a 2-year risk of severe visual loss of 3 to 7 percent. The risk of visual acuity decrease from panretinal photocoagulation therefore assumes greater relative importance. Photocoagulation of one eye with careful observation of the other eye, if both are at the same stage, may be desirable. Careful follow-up is essential, with photocoagulation recommended if high-risk characteristics develop.

In October 1989, the ETDRS reached the following conclusions:

1. Focal laser treatment is effective for reducing the risk of visual loss from diabetic macular edema.
2. Scatter (panretinal) laser treatment reduces the risk of severe visual loss. Provided that careful follow-up is maintained, it is safe to defer scatter treatment until retinopathy approaches or reaches the high-risk stage. In eyes with mild to moderate nonproliferative retinopathy, the rate of progression to this high-risk stage is very low. ETDRS results do not support early scatter treatment in these eyes. *Careful follow-up is essential.*
3. Aspirin treatment does not alter the progression of diabetic retinopathy. The dosage of aspirin used in the ETDRS (650 mg per day) neither prevented the development of high-risk proliferative retinopathy nor increased the risk of vitreous hemorrhage. Results indicate that there is no ocular reason for those with diabetes to avoid taking aspirin when it is needed for treatment of other problems.

Macular Edema

Although proliferative diabetic retinopathy is responsible for the most severe visual loss, diabetic macular edema is the most common cause of visual acuity reduction among persons with diabetes mellitus. As a complication of diabetic retinopathy, macular edema has become increasingly recognized in the past decade. Diabetic macular edema is not only an important cause of legal blindness, but it is also a major cause of partial visual impairment. These patients may have occupational disabilities that are not reported in any of our blindness statistics.

Diabetic retinopathy may alter the structure of the macula, thereby significantly altering its function in any of the following ways:

1. By macular edema, that is, a collection of intraretinal fluid in the macular portion of the retina with or without lipid exudates and with or without cystoid changes
2. By nonperfusion of parafoveal capillaries with or without intraretinal fluid
3. By traction in the macula by fibrous proliferation causing dragging of the retinal tissue, surface wrinkling, or detachment of the macula
4. By intraretinal or preretinal hemorrhage in the macula
5. By lamellar or full-thickness hole formation
6. By any combination of the above

Items 1 and 2 are discussed in this section, and items 3 and 4 are discussed in the section on vitreous hemorrhage. Usually no treatment is indicated for lamellar or full-thickness hole formation.

The ETDRS, the long-term multicenter randomized clinical trial described previously, was also designed to determine whether photocoagulation is effective in the treatment of diabetic macular edema. The ETDRS has reported its conclusions and results in the *Archives of Ophthalmology*, December 1985, with suggested clinical applications.

Focal argon laser photocoagulation in eyes with clinically significant macular edema reduces the risk of moderate visual loss by about 50 percent, increases the chance of improvement in visual acuity of one line or more on the Snellen Eye Chart, and is not associated with adverse effects on visual field or color vision as measured in the ETDRS. Because the principal benefit of treatment is to prevent further decrease in visual acuity, focal argon laser photocoagulation should be considered even in eyes with normal visual acuity if clinically significant macular edema is present. Although these conclusions are based on eyes with mild-to-moderate nonproliferative diabetic retinopathy (transitional retinopathy) that should not have had past or concurrent scatter photocoagulation, it seems reasonable to extend them to eyes with severe nonproliferative or proliferative diabetic retinopathy associated with clinically significant macular edema as well. The treatment strategy includes determination of clinically significant macular edema, finding treatable lesions on fluorescein angiography, and argon laser photocoagulation to focal and diffuse leaks.

Factors that favor prompt photocoagulation for ETDRS clinically significant diabetic macular edema as well as for DRS high-risk characteristics include hypertension, fluid retention, elevated blood lipid levels, renal failure, anticipated cataract surgery, progressive lens opacities, and reduced visual acuity at the time of examination.

Vitreous Hemorrhage and Traction Retinal Detachment

Photocoagulation has significantly reduced the risk of progressive neovascularization with vitreous hemorrhage and traction detachment. As a result, there has been a considerable decrease in the volume of vitrectomy surgery for diabetic eye disease; however, on occasion, recurrent vitreous hemorrhage or traction detachment of the macula may require vitrectomy surgery. In the Diabetic Retinopathy Vitrectomy Study (DRVS), 616 eyes with recent severe diabetic vitreous hemorrhage reducing visual acuity to 5/200 or less for at least 1 month were randomly assigned to either early vitrectomy or deferral of vitrectomy for 1 year. After a 2-year follow-up, 25 percent of the early vitrectomy group had a visual acuity of 10/20 or better compared with 15 percent in the deferral group. In patients with IDDM who were on the average younger and had more severe proliferative retinopathy, there was a clear-cut advantage for early vitrectomy as reflected in the percentage of eyes recovering visual acuity of 10/20 or better (36 versus 12 percent in the deferral group; $p = 0.0001$). No such advantage was found in the NIDDM group (16 percent in the early group versus 18 percent in the deferral group). Furthermore, among eyes in the deferral group, spontaneous clearing of vitreous hemorrhage occurred more frequently in those with NIDDM and in a mixed group (29.2 and 20.7 percent, respectively) than in the IDDM group (16.4 percent). Deferral may often be the preferred choice for those with NIDDM or in the mixed group, especially in patients who have adequate vision in the fellow eye.

Careful evaluation, follow-up, and selection of cases for intervention are important for success; therefore, it seems important that these patients are treated by those ophthalmic surgeons who have considerable diabetic vitrectomy experience.

REMISSION

The proliferation of fibrous tissue is an early signal for remission of neovascular disease. The hazard of this remission is the proliferation of fibrous tissue with traction on the retina, resulting in traction detachments of the retina. Vitrectomy is indicated in these circumstances; however, the major risk of vitrectomy is neovascular glaucoma, which occurs in 10 to 20 percent of carefully chosen cases. The closure of the filtration angle with the progression of new vessels on the iris into the angle results in an eye that does not respond well to treatment and ultimately becomes blind.

Following this period of fibrous proliferation, most eyes enter into a full-remission phase, known as involutional quiescent diabetic retinopathy. This stage is characterized by thinning of the fibrous tissue with reduction in vascularity of the fibrous tissue, thinning of the retinal arterioles, pallor of the optic nerve head, and residual wispy fibrous proliferation extending into the vitreous without traction. If the central vision has not been destroyed during the active stage of the disease, it may remain quite good, although there is a decrease in the electrophysiologic activity of the retina and central vision gradually becomes dimmer, with few patients retaining 20/20 vision.

VISUAL FUNCTION REHABILITATION

Although diabetic retinopathy is a potentially sight-threatening complication of diabetes that requires timely and appropriate referral and intervention, there are other ocular and visual complications of diabetes that need to be addressed. Diabetes affects all structures of the eye, and patients may need to be counseled concerning these effects in response to reported symptoms or specific questions.

A common question of patients with diabetes is their ability to wear hard or soft contact lenses on either a daily basis or for periods extending up to 2 weeks. There are some definite considerations that need to be made, and cases need to be evaluated individually by appropriate eye examination and contact lens evaluation. Some general principles, however, do pertain in advising the diabetic patient about contact lenses.

There is clinical evidence that the cornea of a person with diabetes does injure more easily, and heal more slowly, than the cornea of a person who does not have diabetes. Furthermore, diminished tear secretion or poor tear quality, resulting from either insulin injections or the diabetic condition itself, as well as from a variety of other factors, may make a contact lens wearer with diabetes less able to support a corneal contact lens, particularly a soft contact lens, or wear a contact lens with comfort. Reduced corneal sensitivity, comparable to the type of peripheral neuropathy that may accompany the diabetic condition, may also result in the overwearing of a contact lens that might otherwise have caused a person to remove an uncomfortable lens. Any of the above complications can result in an increased incidence of corneal abrasion, ulceration, or ocular infection. Moreover, because of the potential for complications with contact lenses, it is advisable for diabetic patients to avoid extended-wear contact lenses under most circumstances.

Ocular symptoms that may concern a diabetic person are numerous and varied, and it is helpful to address these issues, if only to reassure a patient. Perhaps the most common complaint concerns blurring of vision. When blurring occurs in conjunction with laser treatments or diabetic macular edema, it is helpful to educate the patient on the effects of elevated blood glucose levels on visual acuity. A newly acquired distance blur, in conjunction with increased ease of reading for a presbyopic person undergoing treatment or observation for retinopathy, is frequently nothing more than a reflection of elevated blood glucose levels resulting in a myopic shift in refraction.

Laser treatment itself, however, can cause visual changes, either by itself or in conjunction with the retinopathy for which it is applied. A common symptom associated with panretinal photocoagulation is a recognizable change in scotopic vision and decreased ability to adapt to darkness and light. Although these problems cannot be totally eliminated, explaining that laser treatments may selectively damage portions of the retina responsible for scotopic vision in an effort to preserve central vision may be reassuring to many patients. The use of appropriate filtering lenses, particularly amber-shaded lenses that filter out blue light and ultraviolet light, can be effective in providing a subjective improvement in visual function.

Another common complaint, especially in the presence of diabetic maculopathy, is the inability to distinguish colors properly, particularly blue and yellow. These distortions of color perception are the result of damage to color-sensitive cone cells, which are most densely packed in the macula area of the retina. Although there is no treatment for this acquired color vision loss, advising the patient that these changes are a complication of the maculopathy is frequently reassuring. Once again, use of appropriate filtering lenses may result in a subjective improvement for the patient and may even retard or prevent further progression of color vision loss.

Glare, resulting from cataracts, vitreous opacities, vitreous hemorrhage, or laser treatment, is another visually debilitating complication of diabetes. Again, management may involve the use of appropriately selected filtering lenses and patient education.

A challenging problem to manage involves the loss of visual function or visual acuity, even when a patient is undergoing laser photocoagulation. Laser treatment is effective in halting or retarding severe and moderate visual loss from proliferative retinopathy and macular edema. Varying lesser degrees of visual loss, however, can still occur, and a patient with 20/20 vision may believe that his eyes are changed, even though good central vision has been preserved. Moreover, vision may stabilize at a level weaker than 20/20, and a patient may need to be advised that visual changes may result as a consequence of and despite appropriate laser treatment.

When visual acuity is reduced, a patient needs to be referred for proper low vision evaluation. Distance vision may be enhanced by telescopic aids, contact lenses, or other low vision devices. It is reading vision, however, that most patients seem anxious to preserve, and proper low vision management may involve various optical and nonoptical aids or merely the proper use of reading light. Nonoptical aids include large-print books, large-print playing cards and phone dials, or other devices designed to provide ease of viewing. The problem of filling syringes or reading glucometers or blood sugar test strips requiring precise color vision may be overcome with bar type magnifiers to fit on standard syringes or electrical devices that can read test tape colors either verbally or in large-print numerical forms.

The patient may also need encouragement in the use of various "traditional" magnifiers. These magnifiers can be either hand-held or worn as eyeglasses. The hand-held magnifiers provide the advantage of allowing reading material to be held at a standard distance from the eye, but the patient with a shaky hand or reading material requiring two hands to hold may make their use impossible. Spectacle or eyeglass magnifiers provide the advantage of freeing the hands to hold reading material and their use is more in keeping with the type of reading to which a person is accustomed. Their disadvantage, however, is that the stronger a spectacle magnifier becomes, the closer a person must hold the reading matter to the eyes. A 4× magnifier may enable a person to read a telephone directory, but the directory may be only 2 to 4 inches from the eyes. In any case, the more powerful the magnifier, either for distance or for reading, the smaller is the field of vision, and it is advisable that magnifiers be individually prescribed by a low-vision expert who can determine the best combination of magnification and convenience. Closed-circuit televisions provide an expensive alternative to the use of glass magnifiers and certainly should not be prescribed until an ocular situation has stabilized.

The diabetic patient needs to be reassured that only rarely does diabetic retinopathy or maculopathy result in total blindness or the inability to see any light. The decreased risk of visual loss resulting from appropriate laser intervention and the enhancement of vision less than 20/20 by various optical aids provide hope for those with diabetic retinopathy. Education and regular eye examinations are important in preventing and coping with visual loss.

It is obvious that a carefully coordinated medical team is necessary to provide the optimal care for a patient with diabetes mellitus in an effort to decrease the risk of visual loss. The internist, endocrinologist, and family physician must manage the complex medical control of diabetes and try to prevent the progression of the complications of the disease such as hypertension and renal failure. The timely referral of the patient to the ophthalmologist is the second key to the minimization of the risk of complications from diabetic eye disease. The standard of eye care outlined above is of paramount importance. The most important function for the internist in the management of diabetic eye disease is timely referral for a definitive diagnosis and treatment. The patient's physician and optometrist in concert with the ophthalmologist are key members of the team attempting to limit the ravages of diabetic eye disease. Therapy for at least some of these disorders, particularly retinopathy, has improved significantly in the past 20 years. The prognosis for retinopathy may be improved still further pending the results of the currently promising research into factors governing neovascularization.

SUGGESTED READING

Aiello LM, Ferris F. Diabetic macular edema. Ophthalmology Annual. Vol. 3. Norwalk: Appleton-Century-Crofts, 1987:175.

Aiello LM, Rand LI, Weiss JN, Sebestyen J, Wafai MZ, Bradbury M, Briones JC. The eyes and diabetes. In: Marble A, et al, eds. Joslin's diabetes mellitus. 12th ed. Philadelphia: Lea & Febiger, 1985.

Diabetic Retinopathy Study Research Group. Preliminary report on effects of photocoagulation therapy. Am J Ophthalmol 1976; 81:1-14.
Diabetic Retinopathy Study Research Group. Photocoagulation of proliferative diabetic retinopathy. The second report of Diabetic Retinopathy Study findings. Ophthalmology 1978; 85:82-106.
Diabetic Retinopathy Study Research Group. Four risk factors for severe visual loss in diabetic retinopathy: the third report from the Diabetic Retinopathy Study. Arch Ophthalmol 1979; 97:654-655.
Diabetic Retinopathy Vitrectomy Study Research Group. Early vitrectomy for severe hemorrhage in diabetic retinopathy: two-year results of a randomized trial. Diabetic Retinopathy Vitrectomy Study report 2. Arch Ophthalmol 1985; 103:1644-1652.
Diabetic Retinopathy Vitrectomy Study Research Group. Two-year course of visual acuity in severe proliferative diabetic retinopathy with conservative management. Ophthalmology 1985; 92:492-502.
Early Treatment Diabetic Retinopathy Study Research Group. Photocoagulation for diabetic macular edema: Early Treatment Diabetic Retinopathy Study report number one. Arch Ophthalmol 1985; 103:1796-1806.
Early Treatment Diabetic Retinopathy Study Research Group. Treatment techniques and clinical guidelines for photocoagulation of diabetic macular edema: Early Treatment Diabetic Retinopathy Study report number 2. Ophthalmology 1987; 94:761-774.
International Ophthalmology Clinics 1987; 24(4).
Klein R, Klein BE, Moss SE, Davis MD, DeMets DL. The Wisconsin Epidemiologic Study of Diabetic Retinopathy: II. Prevalence and risk of diabetic retinopathy when age at diagnosis is less than 30 years. Arch Ophthalmol 1984; 102:520-526.
Klein R, Klein BE, Moss SE, Davis MD, DeMets DL. The Wisconsin Epidemiologic Study of Diabetic Retinopathy: III. Prevalence and risk of diabetic retinopathy when age at diagnosis is 30 or more years. Arch Ophthalmol 1984; 102:527-532.
Klein R, Klein BE, Moss SE, Davis MD, DeMets DL. The Wisconsin Epidemiologic Study of Diabetic Retinopathy: IV. Diabetic macular edema. Ophthalmology 1984; 91:1464-1474.
Klein R, Klein BE, Moss SE, Davis MD, DeMets DL. The Wisconsin Epidemiologic Study of Diabetic Retinopathy: VI. Retinal photocoagulation. Ophthalmology 1987; 94:747-753.
Rand LI, Krolewski AS, Aiello LM, Warram JH, Baker RS, Maki T. Multiple factors in the prediction of risk of proliferative diabetic retinopathy. N Engl J Med 1985; 313:1433-1438.
Rand LI, Prud'homme GJ, Ederer F, Canner PL, and the Diabetic Retinopathy Study Research Group. Factors influencing the development of visual loss in advanced diabetic retinopathy: Diabetic Retinopathy Study Report Number 10. Invest Ophthalmol 1985; 26:983-991.

DIABETIC NEUROPATHY

AARON VINIK, M.D.

Neuropathy is recognized as a common and often disabling complication in patients with diabetes. Although there are no good studies of the natural history and evolution of the symptom-complex and there are no "gold standards" for the evaluation of the different modalities of sensory, motor, and autonomic nerve function loss that accompany the condition, there are sufficient retrospective data to allow at least a composite picture of the clinical presentations and approaches to management that have emerged. In many instances there have not been appropriate controlled studies of the treatment modalities offered and the suggestions made are those that I have employed or tried with a reasonable degree of success.

On the basis of a large study of 4,400 patients observed for up to 25 years it has been estimated that neuropathy develops in at least 25 percent of subjects whose diabetes is well controlled. If the control is average, then neuropathy emerges in 50 percent; and if the control is poor, some form of neuropathy that is clinically evident occurs in 75 percent of subjects who have had diabetes for 15 to 20 years or more. If, however, one resorts to sophisticated tests of nerve function, then almost 100 percent of subjects have the disorder. The diabetic neuropathies may be broadly divided into somatic and visceral. The major clinical features of the different neuropathies are presented along with the clinical as well as the laboratory approach to diagnosis and the currently recommended form of treatment.

CLINICAL FEATURES

Symmetrical Polyneuropathy

Symmetrical polyneuropathy is the most common and widely recognized form of diabetic neuropathy. The onset is usually insidious, but occasionally it occurs following stress or initiation of therapy for diabetes. The deficit is predominantly sensory with lesser involvement of motor fibers. Signs include depression or loss of ankle jerks and vibratory sensation with calf tenderness and hyperalgesia in some. The neurologic deficit is peripheral, involving the distal sensorimotor nerves in a glove and stocking distribution. The lower extremities are affected most severely. The stocking distribution is not a single line of loss of one modality of sensation, but rather there are multiple glove and stocking levels, one for each modality. In general, the long fibers that are most seriously affected, such as those for position sense and touch, have the highest stocking level and the short pain fibers have the lowest stocking level. If all the levels coincide, then one must be alert to the possibility of a conversion reaction or hysteria. The long and short fibers are affected differentially. The condition starts distally and proceeds proximally. The type of neuropathy varies with the type of nerve fiber involved. Large fibers are associated with loss of position and vibration sense and half of light touch. The symptoms may be minimal, such as walking on cotton wool; floors may feel strange, pages of a book cannot be turned, or coins cannot be discriminated. In contrast, the small fiber neuropathy is associated with loss of pain sensation and loss of the awareness of temperature differences. Motor weakness is not unusual, but a very characteristic feature is the wasting of the small muscles of the hands and feet. This muscle wasting usually occurs in very advanced cases and may resemble that of motor neuron disease, which, however, has no sensory component. Loss of the deep tendon reflexes is a hallmark.

Pain and paresthesias occur with nocturnal exacerbation in the feet more than the hands. Spontaneous episodes of pain may be severely disabling. The pain varies in intensity and in its character. It may be described as burning, lancinating, stabbing, tearing, aching, or like a dog gnawing at the bones. This is often accompanied by paresthesia or episodes of distorted sensation, such as pins and needles or tingling. The lower legs may be exquisitely tender to touch, and any disturbance of the follicles of hair results in excruciating pain, which may preclude carrying on with daily activity that involves repeated contact of the lower limbs with foreign objects, such as sitting at a desk. Pain often occurs at the onset of the disease and is often made worse by initiation of therapy with insulin or sulfonylureas. In this early form of the painful syndrome the condition often remits spontaneously and supportive therapy is all that is required. Unfortunately, there is another variety that tends to start later in the condition, often after many years, and in which the pain persists and becomes debilitating, often leading to habituation to narcotics and analgesics and finally to addiction. This latter variety, although not all that frequent, is resistant to all forms of intervention and can be most trying to the patient and physician.

Neuropathic (Perforating) Ulcer

Loss of protective sensation and repetitive trauma, such as walking, may produce an ulcer. This occurs most frequently over metatarsal heads but also at other areas of increased pressure. Loss of tone in the small muscles of the feet leads to an imbalance between the flexors and extensors and ultimately results in the classic hammer toe. This leads to increased pressure over the ball of the foot corresponding to the heads of the metatarsals. Also, the normal person constantly shifts the area of pressure in the foot while walking or running, whereas the diabetic with neuropathy is unable to do so because of the lack of the sensory input from the soles of the feet. This constant pressure causes calluses with increase in pressure and ultimately ulceration in the high-pressure areas. Infection develops after the skin breaks down. Infection in the milieu of ischemia can eventually lead to gangrene.

Neuropathic Arthropathy (Charcot's Joints)

Neuropathic arthropathy occurs in the presence of impaired sensations of pain and proprioception, intact motor power, and repeated minor trauma, usually occurring in the foot with normal pulses and warmth. The clinical course is painless, nonedematous swelling of the foot, which becomes shorter, wider, everted, and externally rotated with flattening of the arch. The gait becomes abnormal, and clubfoot occurs. It is limited to the ankle and tarsal joints in diabetes. Pathologic roentgenographic features include bone lysis, fragmentation, and eburnation; disarticulation and dissolution of the joints; and bony overgrowth and calcification in and around involved joints. Eventually pressure ulcers, infection, and osteomyelitis develop.

Single and Multiple Mononeuropathies

Focal and multifocal diabetic neuropathies cause neurologic deficits confined to the distribution of a single nerve or multiple single nerves in a mononeuropathy or a mononeuropathy multiplex. The onset is typically acute, often heralded by severe pain, and the differential diagnosis must generally exclude a vascular catastrophe.

Cranial Nerve Lesions

Isolated or multiple palsies primarily occur in the older age group sometimes in the absence of other evidence of neuropathy. The onset is generally abrupt; it is painless in 50 percent, but it may also be extremely painful. The third cranial nerve lesion is most common. It characteristically presents with a sudden onset of a severe headache with ptosis, but in contrast to rupture of an anterior communicating aneurysm, the pupils are usually spared. The sixth nerve is less commonly involved, and the fourth nerve is seldom involved. The seventh nerve is not infrequently affected, resulting in isolated Bell's palsy. All other cranial nerves have been reported to be involved but much less commonly.

Isolated Peripheral Nerve Lesions

Palsies of isolated peripheral nerves involve the ulnar, median, radial, and femoral nerves and the lateral cutaneous nerve of the thigh, which presents as unexplained pain and hyperesthesia in the upper outer quadrant of the thigh and the peroneal nerves. The carpal tunnel syndrome occurs twice as frequently in a diabetic population compared with a normal healthy population and may be related to repeated undetected trauma, metabolic changes, or accumulation of fluid or edema within the confined space of the carpal tunnel. The nerves involved are usually motor, but pure sensory lesions occasionally occur.

Diabetic Amyotrophy

Diabetic amyotrophy may be recognized by the triad of pain, severe muscle atrophy in the limb–girdle distribution, and muscle fasciculation. The onset is usually acute, but it may be subacute and gradually evolve over weeks. Patients also have generalized weight loss and cachexia, and the term used to describe this syndrome is *diabetic cachexia*.

Asymmetrical proximal muscle weakness and wasting of lower extremities involving predominantly the iliopsoas, quadriceps, and adductor muscles occur. Patients often cannot stand unsupported, climb stairs, or rise from the kneeling or sitting position. The differential diagnosis is Cushing's syndrome, thyrotoxicosis, or a neoplasm that produces a proximal myopathy without evidence of nerve lesions and with intact reflexes. Also to be considered are the proximal neuropathies, for example, Gullain-Barré syndrome, in which there is no pain or fasciculation. Diabetic amyotrophy is often accompanied by pain in the thigh muscles and sometimes lumbar or perineal regions. The knee jerks are depressed, but little or no sensory involvement is found. The anterolateral muscle group in the lower leg may also be involved, producing the anterior compartment syndrome. This syndrome occurs primarily in older patients who frequently have only mild diabetes.

Truncal Mononeuropathy (or Radiculopathy)

Truncal mononeuropathy is primarily a sensory neuropathy with root distribution that is almost always unilateral and asymmetrical. The sex distribution is equal; primarily older patients but occasionally those with juvenile insulin-dependent diabetes mellitus (IDDM) of long duration are affected. Truncal mononeuropathy is usually associated with peripheral neuropathy and may resemble diabetic cachexia. Hyperesthesia is often found in the root distribution, and the clinical presentation may be acute abdominal or thoracic crisis. Most commonly the condition needs to be differentiated from herpes zoster infection in the prevesicular phase. Nocturnal exacerbation of pain is troublesome, but there is spontaneous resolution, usually within 3 months of the onset.

Autonomic Neuropathy

Diabetic autonomic neuropathy may involve any system in the body. Its manifestations are protean, and the onset is often insidious. Results of cardiovascular reflex tests indicate the prevalence is 17 to 40 percent. Thirty-one percent of teenagers with IDDM have abnormal test results. The relationship with sensorimotor neuropathy is variable, but in general these disorders coexist. In patients with peripheral neuropathy, 50 percent have asymptomatic autonomic neuropathy. Asymptomatic neuropathy may not alter morbidity and mortality, but once symptoms occur the anticipated mortality is 44 percent within 2½ years. With gastroparesis, 35 percent of patients die within 3 years, usually of aspiration pneumonia. It is therefore vitally important to make this diagnosis early so that appropriate intervention can be instituted. In the section that follows, the clinical presentations of autonomic neuropathy, the diagnostic tests, and the various forms of management currently available are discussed.

Pupillary Abnormalities

Pupillary abnormalities may precede all other evidence of autonomic dysfunction if careful pupillometry testing is carried out. The Argyll Robertson type pupillary responses in which the pupils react slowly to light, if at all, and accommodate normally may be found. However, these pupillary abnormalities do not tend to produce any significant functional deficit unless associated with failure of dark adaptation and difficulty with driving at night.

Orthostatic Hypotension Without Compensatory Tachycardia

Orthostatic hypotension is defined as a fall in the systolic blood pressure of greater than 30 mm Hg within 2 minutes of standing. It is obstensibly due to disease of the autonomic nervous system involving the peripheral nerves with a reduction in the synthesis and release of norepinephrine at postganglionic sympathetic neurons. It is not caused by an insensitivity to norepinephrine since in diabetic patients with autonomic neuropathy there is a tenfold increase in the sensitivity to norepinephrine as occurs in other conditions associated with sympathetic denervation. There may be a cardiac element with decrease in inotrophic and chronotrophic responses of the heart because of cardiopathy involving the autonomic nervous system. Especially prominent may be the provocation of hypotension soon after the administration of insulin and its exacerbation by drugs that accentuate hypotension, such as nitroglycerin, ganglionic blocking drugs, and diuretics.

Vasomotor Instability

Skin Temperature Reversal. Tachycardia of greater than 90 to 100 beats per minute due to autovagotomy and dependent edema due to loss of the tone of the small peripheral blood capillaries occur.

Cardiac Denervation. Autonomic neuropathy has now been reported as involving the cardiovascular system with dysfunctions of both diastolic filling and systolic ejection. This leads to impaired exercise tolerance dysrhythmias and painless myocardial infarction with a risk of sudden death.

Respiratory Dysfunction. Respiratory dysfunction in patients with autonomic neuropathy is the failure of initiation of respiratory drive under conditions of hypoxia. Thus, patients have to rely on CO_2 accumulation, and this constitutes a real danger during induction of anesthesia when oxygen levels are maintained and CO_2 is driven off.

Motor Disturbances of the Gastrointestinal Tract

Esophageal Enteropathy. If sophisticated tests on the upper gastrointestinal tract are performed in patients with diabetes, esophageal enteropathy is extremely common; rarely, however, patients may present with dysphagia, retrosternal discomfort, and heartburn.

Gastroparesis Diabeticorum. The clinical syndrome of gastroparesis diabeticorum comprises anorexia, nausea, vomiting, fullness, and early satiety. Not infrequently, patients complain of vomiting of meals that were ingested some days before hand. Meals such as those containing garlic sausage or seasoning may be tasted on their breath for days after the meal. Physical examination often reveals a hippocratic succussion splash because of the gastroparesis in which initially there is delayed emptying of solids and subsequently of liquids. Poor and irregular absorption of fuels accentuates poor diabetes control. There is also a risk with the ingestion of soluble fibers such as guar and pectin of the development of fiber bezoars. Thus, extreme care must be exercised in prescribing fiber in the diet.

Diabetic Enteropathy. Enteropathy involving the large colon is common, producing constipation in up to two-thirds of patients with long-standing diabetes. The opposite situation tends to be a form of troublesome and explosive diabetic diarrhea that has been called paroxysmal nocturnal diarrhea. The paroxysms occur explosively "out of the blue," and the patients may end up in a pool of liquid feces in embarrassing situations. The enteropathy is usually associated with the loss of perirectal and perianal sensation, and consequently the patients are often not aware of soiling themselves. Sphincteric control and tone is lost, and, thus, feces cannot be retained. The condition often varies from day to day. It does not necessarily occur at night but may occur at any time of the day and fluctuates from season to season.

Genitourinary Tract Disturbances

Neurogenic Vesical Dysfunction. The earliest and most frequent form of neurogenic vesical dysfunction is loss of bladder sensation. The patient is unaware that the bladder is full. Motor function tends to remain intact, and the usual problem is dribbling with overflow continence. One is often surprised when examining such patients to find a bladder at the level of the umbilicus.

Impotence. The most common form of organic sexual dysfunction in male diabetics is erectile impotence. In general, physicians tend to shy away from asking questions related to sexual dysfunction that they feel may lead to a greater degree of dissatisfaction by the patient. Up to 75 percent of male patients who have had diabetes for 15 to 20 years suffer some degree of erectile impotence. In evaluating such patients it is important to exclude psychogenic causes, and the major differentiating feature is that the impotence is gradual in onset, is associated with the loss of nocturnal erections, and is uniform with all partners. Vascular causes can be excluded by a history of buttock claudication and by using Doppler ultrasonography to determine the penile-brachial arterial ratio. If vascular and psychogenic causes are excluded, the clinical examination of perianal sensation includes stroking alongside the anus and watching the anus contract (the anal wink reflex) or applying pressure to the glans penis, which causes a reflex contraction of the anal sphincter. These reflexes and sensation are lost owing to parallel loss of somatic and autonomic sacral segments S2, S3, and S4.

Retrograde Ejaculation. Retrograde ejaculation may be diagnosed by the presence of azoospermia in the ejaculate or the finding of live motile sperm in the urine post coitus. This may be important to diagnose in the relatively young diabetic who desires to procreate, in which case sperm may be recovered from the urine and artificial insemination of the patient's partner carried out.

Sweating Disturbances

A sudomotor dysfunction with distal anhidrosis and bilateral symmetrical loss of the thermoregulatory response may occur. This disorder may be troublesome to patients who do not perspire in their lower limbs and have as a reflex excessive perspiration of the upper body and face. There may also be areas of symmetrical anhidrosis or gustatory sweating.

Unawareness of Hypoglycemia

An important cause of erratic control of diabetes is an unawareness by patients of a severe hypoglycemic reaction due to the lack of secretion of epinephrine in response to the hypoglycemia. These patients also have a reduction in the glucagon response and, thus, the blood glucose levels are unable to return to near-normal levels. However, patients with diabetes who have been intensively treated with either pump therapy or intensive conventional therapy have a similar reduction in epinephrine and glucagon responses to hypoglycemia, which may be difficult to distinguish from autonomic dysfunction. The critical issue here is that one must be careful not to overtreat these cases.

DIAGNOSIS

The diabetic neuropathies represent a diverse group of disabling complications that can be confused with a variety of other conditions. The diagnostic procedures used to identify these neuropathies are listed below:

1. Clinical findings. A thorough clinical examination is performed with special attention to the feet and observation of dryness, shiny skin, cracking of the skin, ulceration, and loss of hair. Many bedside tests allow the diagnosis of autonomic neuropathy to be made, but there are special situations requiring more sophisticated testing.
2. Electrophysiologic studies. These studies are helpful to corroborate the suspicion of diabetic neuropathy, and certain patterns are characteristic but not necessarily diagnostic. Means of evaluation of thermal sensitivity and loss of vibration sense are now available in specialized units but have not been thoroughly studied for sensitivity, specificity, and reproducibility. The following may be noted: demyelinization results initially in slowing of nerve conduction velocities; axonal degeneration initially results in decreased amplitude of action potentials; and denervation of muscle units by axonal loss results in fibrillation potentials and sharp waves in resting muscle.
3. Biopsy. Biopsy may be helpful to exclude other causes such as the familial hypertrophic forms, amyloid, and sarcoid and other granulomas, but again

the pathology is not unique. A microvascular occlusive picture may, however, be pathognomonic of diabetes.

4. Special tests of autonomic cardiovascular function
   a. Resting heart rate greater than 100 beats per minute (normal less than 100 beats per minute)
   b. Beat-to-beat heart rate variation. With the patient at rest and supine, breathing 6 breaths per minute with heart rate monitored by an electrocardiogram (ECG), a difference (maximal-minimal) in heart rate greater than 15 beats per minute is normal.
   c. Valsalva maneuver. The subject blows into the mouthpiece of a manometer to 40 mm Hg for 15 seconds with continuous ECG monitoring before, during, and after. Normally patients develop tachycardia and peripheral vasoconstriction during strain; with an overshoot rise in blood pressure and bradycardia on release. The Valsalva ratio is longest RR interval to shortest RR interval = 1.21.
   d. Heart rate response to standing. The subject stands with continuous ECG monitoring and the RR interval is measured at beats 15 and 30. The 30/15 ratio is normally greater than 1.03. A normal result is tachycardia at beat 15 and bradycardia at beat 30.
   e. Systolic blood pressure response to standing. The response is abnormal if blood pressure falls to less than 30 mm Hg within 2 minutes of standing.
   f. Diastolic blood pressure rise to sustained exercise. A handgrip dynamometer is squeezed to 30 percent of maximum (predetermined in the subject) for 5 minutes. The normal response is a diastolic blood pressure rise of greater than 16 mm Hg.
   g. Examination of the ECG reveals a prolonged QTc interval in patients with cardiac autonomic neuropathy.
   h. Pain with compression of the testis is normal and is lost with autonomic neuropathy.
5. Special tests of bladder function. In suspected cases of a vesical dysfunction there may be a need to do special tests, including cystometry, sphincter electromyography, uroflometry, urethral pressure profile, and an electrophysiologic test of bladder innervation.
6. Special tests of penile function. A variety of tests have been developed to quantitate erectile impotence. These are, in essence, designed to exclude psychogenic from organic and vascular from neuropathic disorders and include Doppler ultrasound measurement of brachial arterial and penile systolic blood pressure; penile tumescence measurement by strain gauge; and bulbocavernosus reflex response latency.
7. Insulin hypoglycemia test of pancreatic polypeptide and catecholamine responses
8. Supine and erect catecholamines
   a. Hyperadrenergic responses
      (1) End organ resistance
         (a) Defect in postsynaptic alpha-1-, alpha-2-, or beta-adrenoreceptors
         (b) Defect in response distal to receptor in mediation of vasoconstriction
      (2) Abnormal number or function of alpha-2-adrenoreceptor with resultant decrease in feedback inhibition of norepinephrine release
   b. Hypoadrenergic responses
      (1) Denervation of sympathetic nerve to periphery with resultant decrease in norepinephrine storage
      (2) Defect in release of adequately stored norepinephrine
         (a) Mechanical abnormality of release
         (b) Abnormal number and function of alpha-2-adrenoreceptors
9. Pressure–motility studies of intestinal function
10. Solid-phase, radiolabeled gastric emptying studies. A positive test is retention of more than half of the radioactivity in the stomach for longer than 100 minutes.

MANAGEMENT

Management may be divided into symptomatic, palliative, and supportive measures, and in certain instances specific therapy.

General Measures

Control of the diabetes may be important. Although there are retrospective studies that suggest that diabetic neuropathy increases in prevalence in direct proportion to the degree of paucity of control, of all the complications of diabetes, including retinopathy and nephropathy, this particular complication is one that indeed has been shown to improve with better diabetes control. On occasion, patients who have tremendous pain with peripheral neuropathy may benefit from a period of intravenous insulin administration irrespective of the degree of improvement in glycemic control or hemoglobin A1.

General nutrition is also important. A variety of factors have been implicated in the pathogenesis of neuropathy, including vitamin B_{12} deficiency, vitamin A deficiency, vitamin pyridoxine (B_6) deficiency, and a host of macronutrient and micronutrient deficiencies. There are studies that suggest that correction of these deficiencies may be of benefit, but these studies have not been controlled, and the present recommendation would be to maintain adequate and healthy nutrition without truly supportive evidence for any specific macronutrient and micronutrient as a therapeutic bomb.

Trials of "Specific" Therapy

Aldose Reductase Inhibitors

The trials of aldose reductase inhibitors are still very much in the research arena, and although there are some promising reports on improvement in symptoms and some of the objective measures of neuropathy, the degree of benefit obtained has not been by any means outstanding. It is too early to evaluate the place of aldose reductase inhibitors in the management of diabetic neuropathy.

Myoinositol

Myoinositol deficiency has been reported in animal models and intolerance to myoinositol in diabetes occurs in humans. There are no good studies suggesting that myoinositol supplements of the normal diet will improve neuropathy, although this may occur in animal models. However, in desperate situations patients who have a normal intake of myoinositol of around 800 mg per day may have this increased to 1,600 mg per day. This is easily obtainable by purchasing brewer's yeast from a pharmacy. It comes in 400-mg and 800-mg tablets.

Pain Control

Pain control may represent one of the most trying problem areas for both physician and patient. All patients are depressed, and the depression does not appear to be a function of the extent or severity of the neuropathy but rather a sense of uselessness, "weakness" not due to a muscle deficit, and a notion that the situation is hopeless. Admitting these patients to various drug trials has yielded improvement in about 50 percent of subjects simply on admission or with the administration of placebo. This appears to be a trial effect and occurs often before institution of drug therapy. It is therefore compelling that physicians need to treat these patients with compassion, sympathy, and understanding and help provide a sense of hope. Simple maneuvers, such as wearing body stockings to decrease movement of hair follicles, can be helpful.

Analgesics

Drugs that have been tried include various analgesics, and care must be exercised in their use because of any habit-forming potential.

Phenytoin

Phenytoin (Dilantin), long advocated in the treatment of pain, tends to cause toxicity with macrocytic anemia, hypertrophic gums, and ataxia before a therapeutic effect is observed.

Carbamazepine

Carbamazepine is useful in the management of epilepsy in children. It has been of some benefit in certain patients and in general results in toxicity without a truly beneficial effect.

Clonidine

Clonidine has been successful in the management of patients who have been withdrawn from alcohol and other drugs and seems to work reasonably well in many causalgic situations. Initially, a small dose of 75 μg is given at night to avoid hypotension and sleepiness, and then the dose is increased gradually until a desired effect is achieved. About one-third of the patients respond.

Amitriptyline

The dose of amitriptyline is 50 to 150 mg orally at bedtime plus fluphenazine, 1 to 2 mg orally. As mentioned earlier, many of these patients are depressed and a trial of imipramine alone or amitriptyline given together with fluphenazine may be of benefit.

Mexiletine

Mexiletine (a structural analogue of lidocaine) has recently been reported to relieve pain, dysesthesia, and paresthesia in patients with painful diabetic neuropathy, without changes in tendon reflexes, vibration thresholds, or blood pressure response to standing or beat-to-beat variation in heart rate. Side effects include nausea, hiccup, and tremor but do not usually necessitate drug withdrawal. Doses should begin with 150 mg the first week, 300 mg the second week, and increase to 10 mg per kilogram per day thereafter.

Capsaicin

It has been noted that capsaicin, an extract of red peppers, is capable in certain animal models of depleting the neuropeptide substance P and thus ostensibly blocking pain neurotransmission. In humans, topical application has provided relief of pain in herpes zoster neuralgia and neuralgia from other causes. Current research on topical application in diabetic neuropathy favors a similar action. The compound may be purchased over the counter as Zostrix (0.025 percent capsaicin) and will be marketed for neuropathic pain as Axsain TM (0.075 percent capsaicin). It does, however, produce significant burning upon application, especially to tender areas, and repeated application is necessary to provide relief.

Pentoxifylline

Current theories of the pathogenesis of neuropathy include the suggestion that there may be a microvascular component with reduction in blood flow via the vasa nervorum. For this reason it seems that in patients who appear to have a vascular element to this painful syndrome, the rheologic agent pentoxifylline (Trental) may be helpful. The drug is a methyl-xanthine derivative and decreases blood viscosity, thereby permitting enhanced oxygenation of tissues.

The usual dose is 400 mg three times per day and should be given for at least 8 weeks before conclusions as to its efficacy are reached. Side effects are uncommon, but as with other xanthine derivatives, arrhythmias, orthostasis, and angina need to be watched for.

Transcutaneous Electrical Nerve Stimulation

Transcutaneous electrical nerve stimulation needs to be tried if only because it is probably one of the most benign approaches to management. What generally happens is that the patient tries it once or twice without moving the electrode patches around sufficiently to identify sensitive areas and gives up. If one is persistent and moves the electrodes to multiple areas, often not in the distribution of the nerves involved, then salutary results may be obtained.

Neuropathic Ulcers

Neuropathic ulcers constitute the greatest hazard to loss of limbs in patients with diabetes. Meticulous foot care includes drying between the toes after bathing, applying drying powder and softening creams such as lanolin, and daily inspection of the feet. In addition, proper nail trimming is essential to the prevention of foot ulcers.

If one finds marked loss of sensation with the development of ulcers in the pressure areas, then the purchase of a shoe one size larger than regular with an insert of Plastozet or Alzet that molds to the foot and distributes the pressure can result in healing of ulcers within several months.

Ulcer care requires debridement of necrotic tissue, repeated sterile dressings, and removal from further pressure with supportive devices or even bed rest or a plaster cast. Infection must be aggressively treated with appropriate antibiotics, often for at least 3 weeks, and the underlying osteomyelitis excluded by roentgenography. Inadequate care of ulcers probably constitutes the single greatest cause of mismanagement of patients with diabetes, often resulting in medicolegal proceedings.

Charcot Joints

Once the joint has undergone complete destruction there is total loss of joint pain and perception, and the only means of treatment is with orthotic devices.

Mononeuropathies

Physiotherapy is important to prevent contractures, and the joints should be protected until spontaneous recovery occurs.

Postural Hypotension

The management of postural hypotension in the patient with diabetic autonomic neuropathy can be complex. One has to tread a narrow path between elevating the blood pressure in the standing position and ensuring that supine hypertension does not occur. The situation is further complicated by the complex nature of the pathogenesis of the neuropathy.

Supportive Garments

The first step in treating postural hypotension should always be to attempt to increase venous return from the periphery with supportive elements such as total-body stockings. These stockings should be applied while the patient is lying in bed and should not be taken off until the patient returns to the supine position. Some people of course find them uncomfortable and do not like to wear them during the summer.

Drug Therapy

The treatment with 9-alpha-flurohydrocortisone (0.5 mg per day) and supplementary salt (2 to 6 g) may relieve symptoms of postural hypotension although there is the inherent danger of the development of edema, congestive heart failure, and supine hypertension. In fact, one does not see relief of the symptoms until edema occurs. In the event that these measures fail, if the alpha- and beta-adrenergic receptor status is known one can make a reasonable guess as to which drug the patient is likely to respond. If there is dopamine excess, metoclopramide (Reglan) 10 mg three times a day, may be useful. If there is an alpha-adrenergic receptor excess, then the alpha-antagonist yohimbine (10 mg three times a day) is helpful. In the event that beta-adrenergic receptors are increased in number as occurs in a small portion of cases, propranolol (Inderal), 10 mg four times a day or more may be of value. If however, there is an alpha-adrenergic receptor deficiency, then the use of clonidine may paradoxically raise blood pressure rather than decrease it. One needs, of course, to start with a small dose and then increase the dose up to as much as 400 μg per day. In the event that all of these measures fail, then the direct alpha-adrenergic agonist midodrine (Gutron), 2.5 to 40 mg every 6 hours, or dihydroergotamine, 2.5 to 40 μg every 6 hours with 15 mg of caffeine, may be of value.

Gastropathy

The initial management of gastropathy should include multiple small feedings with a reduction in the fat content, which tends to delay gastric emptying. If this is not helpful, metoclopramide given 10 mg orally up to four times per day may be of value. However, if there is marked gastroparesis with a large gastric residual volume filled with fluid, then the drug is poorly absorbed and one needs to begin therapy with intravenous administration of nutrients and drugs and gastric suction until it has been shown that the stomach is beginning to empty and only then to switch to oral treatment. Other agents such as cholinergic agonists (bethanechol chloride 10 mg orally four times a day) and cholinesterase inhibitors (pyridostigmine bromide, 180 mg orally three times a day) may produce marked drying of secretions in the mouth, blurring of vision, and colic without enhancing gastric emptying. An investigational drug, domperidone, 10 to 40 mg every 6 hours, has proved to be useful in some people but probably is of no greater value than metoclopramide.* In the event that all else fails a jejunostomy tube is placed transabdominally and feeding is provided by this route into an area of bowel that has normal function. Nutrients are given over the nighttime period freeing the patient for daily activities during the day. This simplifies matters and allows one to tailor the insulin requirements to the nocturnal feeding.

Enteropathy

Diabetic enteropathy can be the most trying and difficult of all diabetic complications to treat. The following measures may be useful:

1. Antibiotics. A broad-spectrum antibiotic is usually the treatment of choice. Tetracycline or trimethaprim-sulfamethoxazole may be used, but metronidazole (Flagyl), in a dose of 750 mg three times a day, seems to be the most effective.
2. Cholestyramine. The dose is 4 g mixed in fluid given orally three times a day. There is often retention of bile, which may be highly irritating to the gut; binding of bile salts may be of considerable help.
3. Diphenoxylate hydrochloride plus atropine. The use of diphenoxylate is a last resort measure, and one should be very careful since toxic megacolon can occur. I recommend Lomotil, 2 mg orally with each diarrheic stool.
4. Gluten-free diet
5. Pancreatic exocrine insufficiency. Many patients have evidence of pancreatic exocrine insufficiency, and replacement of the exocrine secretions with 1 to 3 tablets of Viokase with each meal may be helpful.
6. Withdrawal from narcotics
7. Clonidine may prove useful in the management of some of these patients, but only a small trial in a few patients has determined its efficacy. In resistant cases I have used a combination of a somatostatin analogue together with lithium and been able to treat successfully cases refractory to all other forms of intervention.

Cystopathy

Probably the first step in the management of patients who are unable to detect a full bladder is to educate the patient to do repeated palpations of their lower abdomen to determine whether the bladder is full. They will often be able to initiate micturition simply by applying pressure to the bladder, otherwise known as Credé's maneuver. When this fails, one may consider the use of parasympathomimetics such as bethanechol chloride (10 mg orally four times a day), but in general this produces colic without allowing adequate bladder emptying. The most useful and simple approach seems to be repeated bladder self-catheterizations, and it is surprising how few infections occur. In male patients bladder neck surgery can be done to relieve the spasm of the internal sphincter. Continence is preserved because of the somatic supply of the external sphincter.

Erectile Failure

As mentioned earlier, erectile failure is probably one of the most significant, to the patient at least, presentations of autonomic dysfunction and results in a great degree of sexual dissatisfaction. Counseling and management of behavioral problems is cardinal to the care of these patients. Today a number of treatment modalities are available, including inflatable devices that have been used with some degree of success. These devices operate on the principle of obstruction of venous outflow aided by negative pressure to increase inflow. The alpha-adrenergic antagonist yohimbine, 10 mg three times a day, may help in about one-third of cases. Lastly, the direct intrapenile injection of regitine and papaverine has met with some success. However, this regimen invariably results in a small proportion of patients who develop infections, priapism, and ultimately fibrosis. It does, however, provide the patient with relief of a symptom for a period of time of months to years. If nothing is effective, the use of rigid and semirigid protheses can be discussed with the patient and his partner. (see chapter on *Organic Impotence*).

Gustatory Sweating

Gustatory sweating and sudomotor disturbance appear to respond to some degree to propantheline hydrobromide and to scopalamine patches.

Hypoglycemic Unresponsiveness–Brittle Diabetes

If the notion or belief is that autonomic neuropathy may reverse with intensive therapy, then normalization of blood glucose levels and glycosylated hemoglobin levels is the objective. However, there is considerable risk to these patients who are not aware of hypoglycemia since they lack the counterregulatory response to mount a means of combating their fall in blood glucose concentration. Thus, if pump therapy is to be used, one should elect to use long-acting insulins with very small boluses. In general, one should not aim for normal glycosylated hemoglobin values and normal blood glucose levels when this complication supervenes.

SUGGESTED READING

Asbury AK. Focal and multifocal neuropathies of diabetes. In: Dyck PJ, et al, eds. Diabetic neuropathy. Philadelphia: WB Saunders, 1987.

*Another agent currently being investigated is the cholinergic agonist cisapride. In ongoing studies 10 mg three times per day, increasing to 20 mg three times per day, has proved helpful to some patients, and headaches appear, so far, to be the only untoward effect.

Bradley WE. Aspects of diabetic autonomic neuropathy (workshop with fifteen articles). Ann Intern Med 1980; 92:289–342.
Dyck PJ, Karnes J, O'Brien PC. Diagnosis and classification of diabetic neuropathy and association with other complications. In: Dyck PJ, et al, eds. Diabetic neuropathy. Philadelphia: WB Saunders, 1987.
Ewing DJ, Martyn CN, Young RJ, et al. The value of cardiovascular autonomic function tests: 10 years experience in diabetes. Diabetes Care 1985; 8:491–498.
Jacober SJ, Vinik AI, Narayan A, Strodel WE, et al. Jejunostomy feeding in the management of gastroparesis diabeticorum. Diabetes Care 1985; 9:217–219.
Kahn JK, Zola B, Juni JE, et al. Radionuclide assessment of left ventricular diastolic filling in diabetes mellitus. J Am Coll Cardiol 1985; 7:1303–1309.
Kahn JK, Zola B, Juni JE, et al. Decreased exercise heart rate in diabetic subjects with cardiac autonomic neuropathy. Diabetes Care 1986; 9:389–394.
Levitt NS, Vinik AI, Sive AA, et al. The effect of dietary fiber on glucose and hormone responses to a mixed meal in normal subjects and in diabetic subjects with and without autonomic neuropathy. Diabetes Care 1980; 4:515–519.
Pellegrini CA, Broderick WC, Van Dyke D, et al. Diagnosis and treatment of gastric emptying disorders: clinical usefulness of radionuclide measurements of gastric emptying. Am J Surg 1983; 145:143–151.
Sobotka PA, Liss HP, Vinik AI. Impaired hypoxic ventilatory drives in diabetics with autonomic neuropathy. J Clin Endocrinol Metab 1986; 62:658–663.
Vinik AI, et al. Diabetic neuropathy. S Afr J Hosp Med 1978; 196–203.
Young RJ, Clarke BF. Pain relief in diabetic neuropathy: the effectiveness of imipramine and related drugs. Diabetic Med 1985; 2:363–366.
Zola B, Kahn JK, Juni JE, et al. Abnormal cardiac function in diabetics with autonomic neuropathy in the absence of ischemic heart disease. J Clin Endocrinol Metab 1986; 63:208–214.

INSULIN ALLERGY AND INSULIN RESISTANCE

ALAN R. SHULDINER, M.D.
JESSE ROTH, M.D.

Insulin provides lifesaving therapy for patients with type I (insulin-dependent) diabetes mellitus and may play an important role in the treatment of many patients with type II (non–insulin-dependent) diabetes. Shortly after the introduction of insulin therapy in the early 1920s, adverse reactions were recognized, some of which have an immunologic basis. The host's immune response may involve both humoral and cellular components of the immune system, and the patient may manifest resistance to insulin as a result of circulating antibodies against insulin or local or systemic allergic reactions. Before the widespread use of highly purified insulin, it had been estimated that as many as 15 to 55 percent of patients receiving insulin for the first time manifested localized allergic reactions. Today, the incidence of local insulin allergy appears to be much less, since highly purified insulins are significantly less allergenic. Clinically significant systemic insulin allergy or insulin resistance caused by circulating anti-insulin antibodies is even rarer and occurs in only about 0.1 percent of patients receiving insulin.

Insulin allergy usually occurs within weeks to months of initiating therapy. Some insulin-allergic patients give a history of interrupted use of insulin. Interestingly, up to one-third of patients who have an allergy to insulin also report an allergy to penicillin. There has been no clear association between insulin allergy and atopic diseases such as allergic rhinitis or asthma. Although exposure to insulin or accompanying antigens is necessary, it appears that the tendency to develop an immune response to insulin may be genetically determined. For example, patients with histocompatibility antigens HLA-B7, HLA-DR2, and HLA-DR3 appear to have a greater likelihood of developing insulin allergy than those who do not bear these antigens.

Type I diabetes is characterized by autoimmune-mediated destruction of the beta cells of the endocrine pancreas, and anti-insulin and anti-islet cell antibodies can often be detected before the clinical manifestations of diabetes become apparent. A detailed review of these immunologic mechanisms is beyond the scope of this chapter.

Insulin

Insulin is a two-chain polypeptide of molecular weight of approximately 5,700 daltons, derived from the single-chain peptide precursor proinsulin. Insulins have been isolated from over 40 vertebrate species from mammals to cyclostome fish and their amino acid sequences determined. Not surprisingly, the amino acid sequence of the insulin molecule is well conserved throughout this period of evolution. However, there are two regions in which major interspecies variations occur: (1) amino acids 8, 9, and 10 of the A-chain, and (2) residue 30 of the B-chain (Table 1). Interestingly, the C-peptide region which is excised when proinsulin is converted to insulin, is much less well conserved evolutionarily.

Until recently, commercially available insulins were prepared by extraction from beef and pork pancreases. Beef insulin differs from human insulin by three amino acids, whereas pork insulin differs from human insulin by only one amino acid (see Table 1). Although these closely related insulins have equal biopotency, it has been generally noted that the

TABLE 1 Differences in Amino Acids of Some Mammalian Insulins

	A-Chain			B-Chain
Species	*A-8*	*A-9*	*A-10*	*B-30*
Human	Thr	Ser	Ile	Thr
Pork	Thr	Ser	Ile	Ala
Beef	Ala	Ser	Val	Ala

greater the difference in primary structure from human insulin, the greater the antigenicity in humans. Thus, human insulin tends to be less antigenic than pork insulin, which tends to be less antigenic than beef insulin.

Species variations within the insulin molecule are not the only determinants of antigenicity, however, since human insulin (derived from recombinant DNA technology or by chemical modification of pork insulin) also appears to be antigenic in humans. It has been shown, for example, that dimeric and other aggregated forms of insulin are more antigenic than monomeric insulin. The subcutaneous route and use of depot forms may render insulin antigenic despite structural identity to endogenously produced insulin.

Peptide Impurities

Commercial insulin preparations in the United States before the early 1970s (USP insulin) contained approximately 8 percent protein impurities. These protein impurities included (1) higher molecular weight species, such as proinsulin, proinsulin derivatives, and multimeric insulins; (2) chemically modified insulins, such as esterified insulins, desamido insulins, or insulins in which the secondary or tertiary structure has been disrupted; and (3) proteins of lower molecular weight, such as glucagon, pancreatic polypeptide, vasoactive intestinal peptide, somatostatin, and possibly other peptides of pancreatic origin (Table 2).

In 1974, more extensive purification of commercial insulins in the United States excluded both high and low molecular weight impurities in preparations designated "single peak" insulins. These preparations were 98 percent pure and were clearly less antigenic than previously available preparations. By 1980, commercial insulin preparations were further purified by chromatography on modified celluloses to yield "single component" or "monocomponent" insulins. Monocomponent insulins are more than 99 percent pure and contain less than 10 ppm proinsulin. As might be expected, monocomponent insulins are even less antigenic than single-peak preparations.

In 1983, human insulin became commercially available from two different sources. Human insulin (Eli Lilly & Co) is produced by recombinant DNA

TABLE 2 Potential Antigens in Commercially Available Insulins

Antigen	*Preparation*
Insulin	All (beef>pork>human)
Peptide impurities	
Proinsulin	USP and single peak
Multimeric insulins	All
Modified insulins	USP and single peak
Glucagon	USP and single peak
Pancreatic polypeptide	USP and single peak
Somatostatin	USP and single peak
Microbial contaminants	Recombinant DNA human
Pharmacologic additives	
Zinc	All
Protamine	NPH; PZI*
Preservatives	All
Buffers	All

*NPH = neutral protamine Hagedorn insulin; PZI = protamine zinc insulin.

technology in which bacteria are genetically engineered to produce the human form of either insulin A-chain or B-chain. Once isolated, the A- and B-chains are chemically joined to yield intact human insulin. Alternatively, semisynthetic human insulin (Squibb-Novo) is derived from pork insulin by replacing alanine at the B-30 position with threonine, correcting the only difference between the two. Potential impurities in recombinant DNA human insulin are microbial products, whereas potential impurities from semisynthetic sources include pork insulin or insulin in which the carboxyl terminal amino acid is absent.

Pharmaceutical Additives

Pharmaceutical additives may also be antigenic. Virtually all commercially available insulin preparations contain small quantities of zinc to promote crystallization during the purification process. Neutral protamine Hagedorn insulin and protamine zinc insulin contain the positively charged polyanion protamine. Protamine may be antigenic by itself or may enhance an allergic response to insulin (the so-called schlepper phenomenon). Lente insulins lack protamine but contain a higher concentration of zinc and an acetate rather than a phosphate buffer. Finally, minute quantities in commercial preservatives present in insulins could be antigenic; the nature and concentrations of preservatives may vary among commercial preparations.

In summary, the greater the similarity in primary structure to human insulin, the less antigenic the insulin tends to be, but allergy associated with the injection of insulin may not specifically involve insulin as the offending antigen. Potential antigens present in commercially available insulins are listed in Table 2. In general, purer preparations tend to be less antigenic than cruder preparations, and regular insulin tends to be less antigenic than sustained-action preparations. However, among regular insulins of similar purity from different commercial sources, one cannot predict which preparation will be less antigenic for a particular patient. Similarly, among commercially available intermediate and long-acting insulins, one cannot predict which will be least antigenic. These points are important when considering insulin therapy for patients with diabetes and when considering treatment options for patients with insulin allergy.

The Immune Response

Both cellularly and humorally mediated immunologic responses may be elicited from the host by insulin. The triggering of each of these immunologic mechanisms may determine the character as well as the severity of the allergic response.

The Gell and Coombs classification neatly characterizes the immunologic mechanisms that cause insulin allergy (Table 3). Type I reactions are IgE-mediated; the antigen cross-links IgE on the surface of mast cells, causing release of mediators such as histamine and lymphokines, resulting in an immediate local reaction. When this reaction is severe, a systemic anaphylactic reaction may ensue. Type II reactions have not been recorded with insulin. Type III immune reactions involve the formation of antigen-antibody complexes that result in complement fixation, leukocyte attraction, and an inflammatory response. These reactions may manifest themselves as local Arthus-like reactions or as systemic serum sickness–like reactions. Alternatively, when an anti-insulin antibody of high capacity is present, insulin resistance may result. Virtually all classes of antibody molecules have been identified in patients with this form of insulin resistance. Finally, type IV reactions are cell-mediated and are characterized by local delayed hypersensitivity.

TABLE 3 Gell and Coombs Classification of Immunologic Reactions to Insulin

Class	*Mechanism*	*Clinical Manifestations*
Type I	IgE→mast cell degranulation	Local immediate anaphylaxis
Type II	Cytotoxic	None described
Type III	IgG→complement fixation	Local Arthus reaction Serum sickness Insulin resistance
Type IV	Lymphocyte-mediated	Local delayed hypersensitivity

Adapted from Grammer L. Insulin allergy. Clin Rev Allergy 1986; 4:189–200.

Local Insulin Allergy: Diagnosis and Treatment

Local insulin allergy occurs most commonly within the first few weeks or months of beginning insulin therapy. Complaints include erythema, swelling, and itching or burning as well as induration or wheal formation from 1 to 5 cm in diameter at the site of injection. Local allergy may occur immediately after injection and subside rapidly when a type I immunologic mechanism is involved, or its appearance might be delayed for several hours after injection and persist for as many as 24 to 48 hours when a type III or type IV mechanism is involved. Occasionally, patients show a biphasic allergic response, implying that more than one mechanism may be responsible.

Prior to making the diagnosis of local insulin allergy, the injection technique should be carefully scrutinized since nonsterile techniques or excessive trauma can cause an inflammatory response that can mimic cutaneous allergy. Treatment of local insulin allergy that is mild or even moderate may consist simply of reassurance, since an overwhelming majority of local allergic reactions are self-limited and cease to occur within 1 to 3 months.

For severe or intolerable local reactions, skin testing with the individual components of the insulin preparation often helps to identify the offending antigen; a less antigenic preparation may then be substituted. Individual components are available on request from Eli Lilly and Company (Indianapolis, IN) for this purpose. Alternatively, one might empirically switch insulin preparations in an attempt to find a preparation that is less antigenic, remembering that in general purer preparations are less antigenic than cruder preparations, human insulin is less antigenic than insulins from other species, and short-acting preparations are less antigenic than sustained-action preparations. When a less antigenic insulin preparation cannot be identified, subcutaneous coinjection of 1 to 5 mg of diphenhydramine (Benadryl) or 2 to 10 mg of hydrocortisone with insulin may prevent or attenuate the appearance of a local allergic response. In cases in which local allergic reactions are of the delayed type, subcutaneous coinjection of a longer-acting glucocorticoid such as dexamethasone (0.1 to 0.5 mg) is often more efficacious. Since local insulin allergy is almost always a self-limited process, most patients will not require long-term treatment for cutaneous allergy; attempts should be made periodically to discontinue glucocorticoids or antihistamines.

Systemic Insulin Allergy: Diagnosis and Treatment

Symptoms of systemic insulin allergy, like those of local allergy, usually develop within the first weeks or months of therapy. The clinical manifestations of systemic insulin allergy may vary widely in severity and may be clinically indistinguishable from those observed with penicillin allergy.

Systemic allergy usually begins with an immediate localized reaction at the site of injection that spreads into a generalized urticarial pattern with pruritus and angioedema. Skin manifestations may be accompanied by rhinorrhea, nausea, and abdominal or uterine cramps. In more severe cases, laryngeal edema, bronchospasm, hypotension, and death may ensue.

The diagnosis of systemic insulin allergy is usually unambiguous. A thorough drug history should be elicited to exclude other possible offending antigens. Conditions such as idiopathic urticaria and idiopathic anaphylaxis can usually be excluded based on the temporal association of symptoms with insulin injection. Cutaneous skin testing may help to point away from the diagnosis of systemic insulin allergy when a negative test is elicited. However, because as many as 40 to 50 percent of patients receiving insulin may have a positive skin test in the absence of clinically significant systemic insulin allergy, a positive skin test is of limited diagnostic significance.

In patients manifesting mild to moderate symptoms of systemic insulin allergy such as pruritus or urticaria, skin testing may be helpful in identifying a less antigenic insulin preparation, which may then be substituted. Alternatively, a less antigenic preparation may be chosen empirically (e.g., monocomponent regular human insulin). Substitution of a less antigenic insulin preparation can result in improvement in symptoms in up to 70 percent of patients. Systemic treatment with an antihistamine (e.g., diphenhydramine, 25 to 50 mg orally every 6 hours) is useful in many patients.

Severe systemic insulin allergy or anaphylaxis may require immediate lifesaving therapy in an acute care setting. Urticaria and respiratory or hemodynamic compromise characteristic of anaphylaxis should be managed accordingly. Beta-adrenergic agents and glucocorticoids should be used as necessary, temporarily ignoring their insulin counter-regulatory actions.

As soon as the severe allergic reaction is under control, a key medical decision needs to be confronted: How essential is insulin for this particular patient? In a large series studied at the National Institutes of Health, about half of the patients with type II diabetes referred for management of insulin allergy did well after complete withdrawal of insulin.

When insulin therapy is required, it should be continued without interruption; the patient should be hospitalized promptly and closely observed while desensitization is carried out. Cutaneous skin testing may be helpful in identifying the least antigenic insulin preparation that may then be used for the desensitization.

When the patient has received insulin within the previous 24 hours, the first desensitization dose should be 20 percent of the patient's usual dose. Most patients tolerate this reduced dose without significant adverse effects. Should adverse effects occur, the dose may be decreased further. The insulin dose may be increased by 3 to 5 U each day until the desired therapeutic effect is achieved.

Patients who have not received insulin in the previous 24 hours need to be started at a much lower desensitization dose, since unbound IgE titers are much higher, increasing the likelihood of an allergic reaction. A typical desensitization schedule is outlined in Table 4. With this schedule, successful desensitization can be accomplished in most patients.

Localized Lipoatrophy and Lipohypertrophy

Insulin-induced lipoatrophy, the loss of subcutaneous fat at the site of insulin injection, is a localized adverse effect of insulin therapy. Insulin-induced lipoatrophy occurs more commonly in young females than males and is seen more frequently when less pure insulin preparations are used. With the advent of monocomponent insulins and the use of human and pork insulins rather than beef insulin, the prevalence of lipoatrophy has decreased substantially. Lipoatrophy may occur alone or may be accompanied by localized insulin allergy. It is thought that lipoatrophy is immunologically mediated.

Lipoatrophy is a benign process but may be cosmetically unacceptable for some patients. Preventive measures include the use of monocomponent insulin, preferably pork or human. In addition, localized lipoatrophy may be minimized by teaching patients to rotate their injection sites properly. In patients in whom lipoatrophy is already present, a purer insulin preparation should be substituted. Repeated injection of the purer preparation into the affected site can paradoxically result in dramatic resolution of lipoatrophy.

In some patients, repeated injection of the purer insulin preparations may result in localized lipohy-

TABLE 4 Typical Rapid Desensitization Schedule

Time (hr)	*Dose (units)*	*Route*
0	0.001	Intradermal
0.5	0.002	Intradermal
1	0.004	Subcutaneous
1.5	0.01	Subcutaneous
2	0.02	Subcutaneous
2.5	0.04	Subcutaneous
3	0.1	Subcutaneous
3.5	0.2	Subcutaneous
4	0.5	Subcutaneous
4.5	1	Subcutaneous
5	2	Subcutaneous
5.5	4	Subcutaneous
6	8	Subcutaneous

Follow by increase of dosage every 4 to 6 hr until desired therapeutic effect is achieved.

Adapted from Grammer L. Insulin allergy. Clin Rev Allergy 1986; 4:189–200.

pertrophy. When injection sites are rotated properly, this complication can usually be prevented as well.

INSULIN RESISTANCE

Insulin resistance may be defined as the lack of an adequate hypoglycemic response to a defined dose of exogenously administered insulin. Insulin resistance may coexist with normoglycemia when endogenous insulin overproduction is sufficient to compensate for the degree of insulin resistance. Alternatively, glucose intolerance or diabetes may ensue when the pancreatic response fails to match the insulin resistance.

Clinically, the diagnosis of insulin resistance is made when a patient with glucose intolerance or diabetes mellitus requires larger than expected quantities of exogenous insulin to achieve euglycemia. Based on the study of insulin requirements in pancreatectomized adults, and more recently using euglycemic clamp techniques, it has been determined that the average rate of endogenous insulin secretion in normal adults is 20 to 60 U per day. Thus, patients who require between 60 and 200 U of insulin per day may be considered to have mild to moderate insulin resistance. Patients with severe insulin resistance typically require more than 200 U of insulin per day. Fortunately, severe insulin resistance is quite rare and probably accounts for only about 0.01 percent of patients treated with insulin.

Insulin resistance has many causes (Fig. 1). Injected insulin may be hindered from entering the circulation because of a delay in subcutaneous absorption or an abnormally high rate of subcutaneous insulin degradation. Alternatively, once reaching the circulation, insulin may become bound to high-capacity anti-insulin immunoglobulins, impeding access to insulin-sensitive target tissues.

Once insulin reaches insulin-sensitive target tissues, resistance can occur when the target tissues cannot bind insulin properly because of a decrease in receptor number, decrease in receptor affinity, or both. Once insulin binds to its receptor, insulin action may be separated into a cascade with several distinct biochemical events that include (1) phosphorylation of the receptor (autophosphorylation), (2) phosphorylation of other cell proteins, and (3) increases in potential chemical mediators of insulin action (second messengers), such as inositol triphosphate and diacylglycerol. Clinically significant insulin resistance may result if there is a defect in any of these steps (see Fig. 1).

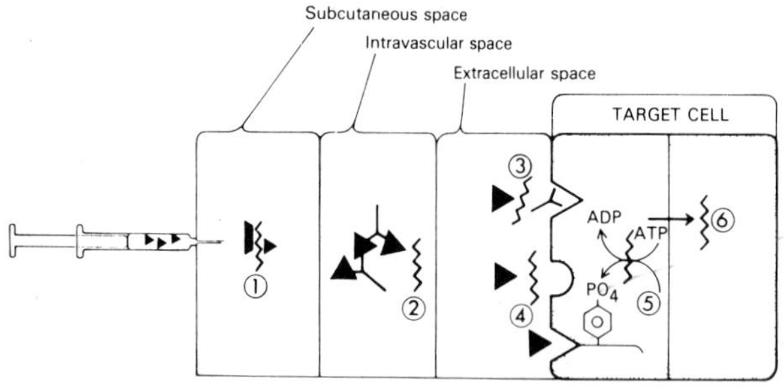

Figure 1 Mechanisms of insulin resistance. Resistance to exogenously administered insulin (▶) may occur if (1) there is increased insulin-degrading activity in subcutaneous tissue; (2) circulating high-capacity immunoglobulins bind insulin, preventing its delivery to target cells; (3) anti-insulin receptor antibodies bind to the insulin receptor, disrupting insulin action; (4) a genetically defective insulin receptor does not bind insulin properly; (5) insulin binding does not activate the insulin receptor tyrosine kinase; or (6) activation of the tyrosine kinase does not properly couple insulin binding to insulin action.

Mild to Moderate Insulin Resistance

Conditions associated with mild or moderate degrees of insulin resistance include obesity, non-insulin-dependent diabetes mellitus (type II), uremia, sepsis, acromegaly, glucocorticoid excess, and other metabolic diseases. The causes of insulin resistance in these conditions are either unknown or multifactorial. Patients with insulin resistance caused by these disorders usually have endogenous hyperinsulinemia, which is compensatory. Hyperinsulinemia may in turn lead to receptor down-regulation and further insulin resistance. Receptor abnormalities associated with some of the causes of mild to moderate insulin resistance are listed in Table 5.

Treatment for patients with mild to moderate insulin resistance who are glucose-intolerant should focus on insulin therapy to normalize the blood glucose level and, when possible, on identification and correction of the underlying cause of insulin resistance.

TABLE 5 Insulin Receptor Abnormalities in Mild to Moderate Insulin Resistance

Condition	*Insulin Binding*	*Receptor Number*	*Affinity*	*Cell Type*
Type II diabetes	→, ↓	→, ↓	→	Monocyte
Obesity	↓	↓	→	Monocyte, red blood cell
Pregnancy	↓	↓	→	Monocyte
Glucocorticoid excess	↓	→	↓	Liver
Acromegaly	→, ↑	↓	↑	Monocyte
Acidosis	↓	→	↓	Monocyte
Cirrhosis	↓	↓	→	Monocyte

(↑) increased; (↓) decreased; (→) normal or no change.
Adapted from Grunberger G, et al. Insulin receptors in normal and disease states. Clin Endocrinol Metab 1983; 12:191–219.

Severe Insulin Resistance

Subcutaneous Insulin Resistance Syndrome

In 1979, Paulsen and coworkers reported a patient with poorly controlled diabetes whose disease was resistant to subcutaneously administered insulin but had normal sensitivity to intravenously administered insulin which they ascribed to an elevated level of insulin-degrading activity in subcutaneous tissue. Subsequently several other similar patients have been described.

Although several of these case reports appear well documented, the true prevalence of subcutaneous insulin resistance is unknown. In one study, Shade and Duckworth were unable to identify a single case of subcutaneous insulin resistance after studying 16 patients referred to them with this presumptive diagnosis.

Once the diagnosis is secured, treatment of such patients may include alternative routes of insulin therapy (i.e., intravenous or intraperitoneal) or treatment with inhibitors of proteolysis such as aprotinin. Aprotinin has also been shown to cause vasodilation of the skin and may enhance subcutaneous insulin absorption by this mechanism as well. Alternatively, lysosomal membrane-stabilizing agents such as chloroquine have been used efficaciously. Since subcutaneous insulin resistance is quite rare and the assays required to make the diagnosis are not readily available, patients with presumptive subcutaneous insulin resistance should be referred to an appropriate research center to establish the diagnosis and for treatment.

Insulin Resistance Caused by Circulating Anti-insulin Antibodies

Within months to years of commencing insulin therapy, virtually all patients develop circulating anti-insulin antibodies. The clinical consequences of such antibodies are usually insignificant. Most have low affinity and are present at low concentration, designated low-capacity variety (i.e., less than 10 U of insulin bound per liter of plasma). Rarely, high-capacity circulating anti-insulin antibodies (i.e., 100 to 1,000 U of insulin bound per liter of plasma) may bind large quantities of the exogenously administered insulin, thus impairing its egress from the plasma and delivery to target tissues, thereby causing clinically significant insulin resistance. These antibodies, which are usually of the IgG subclass, are readily measured in vitro. The absolute binding capacity of circulating anti-insulin antibodies is well correlated with the degree of insulin resistance.

Treatment of insulin resistance caused by circulating anti-insulin antibodies may be difficult, since antibody titers may vary in unpredictable ways. Generally, the development of high-capacity anti-insulin antibodies is a transient phenomenon that can be treated by switching to a less antigenic preparation of insulin, such as pork or human insulin, and increasing the insulin dose as needed. When very high doses of insulin are required (i.e., more than 500 U per day), switching to U-500 insulin preparations may be useful. In some instances a switch to sulfated insulin or fish insulins may be efficacious. These insulins retain adequate bioactivity, but because they bind to the patient's antibodies much less well than unmodified mammalian insulins, they are more efficacious in vivo. These insulins are not available for clinical use outside of a research setting.

In circumstances in which glucose intolerance is severe despite these measures, administration of a systemic glucocorticoid (e.g., prednisone, 40 to 60 mg orally per day) may paradoxically result in a rapid decrease in insulin requirements. Since insulin resistance caused by anti-insulin antibodies is typically transient and resolves after several months, glucocorticoid therapy should only be used when necessary, and when instituted, attempts to taper the dose should be made early and repeatedly until successful.

Syndromes of Extreme Insulin Resistance

Syndromes of extreme insulin resistance are rare disorders in which patients manifest endogenous hyperinsulinemia that is compensatory and extreme resistance to exogenously administered insulin (e.g., more than 0.3 U per kilogram). Some patients have normal fasting glycemia and normal glucose tolerance, whereas others display varying degrees of glucose intolerance, including overt diabetes mellitus. Ketosis is rare but does occur. In association with extreme insulin resistance, these patients have acanthosis nigricans, a hyperpigmented hyperkeratotic rash commonly seen in the intertriginous areas of the body as well as over the elbows, base of the neck, and waist. In addition, premenopausal women with this syndrome often have high serum testosterone levels, thought to be due to a direct effect of hyperinsulinemia in impeding the normal conversion of testosterone to estradiol in the ovaries. Hypertestosteronemia is probably a major contributor to the amenorrhea, hirsutism, polycystic ovaries, and android habitus that is commonly seen in these disorders. Insulin resistance in these patients is caused by at least two distinct mechanisms, genetic (i.e., type A syndrome) and autoimmune (i.e., type B syndrome).

Genetic Syndromes of Extreme Insulin Resistance. Genetic syndromes of extreme insulin resistance are rare disorders with multiple modes of inheritance, although sporadic cases also occur. Although several phenotypic patterns are apparent, these syndromes have several biochemical similarities (Table 6).

Recently, using molecular biologic approaches, the DNA sequences of insulin receptor genes have been determined from a number of patients with ge-

TABLE 6 Syndromes of Extreme Insulin Resistance

Syndrome	*Phenotypic Distinction*
Genetic	
Type A syndrome	Nonobese, absence of phenotypic distinctions of other genetic syndromes
Leprechaunism	Congenital, small for gestational age, slow extrauterine growth, dysmorphic features, fasting hypoglycemia, death within first year of life
Lipoatrophic diabetes	Localized or generalized lipoatrophy, type V hypertriglyceridemia
Rabson-Mendenhall syndrome	Dystrophic nails and teeth, pineal hyperplasia
Autoimmune	
Type B syndrome	Evidence of autoimmunity such as lupus erythematosus, Sjögren's syndrome, elevated erythrocyte sedimentation rate, positive antinuclear antibody, decreased complement, pancytopenia, proteinuria

*Common features of all syndromes of extreme insulin resistance may include hyperinsulinemia, with or without glucose intolerance, and acanthosis nigricans. Premenopausal women may display amenorrhea, hirsutism, hypertestosteronemia, and polycystic ovaries.

netic forms of extreme insulin resistance. Several different mutations have been described that result in alteration of the amino acid sequence if the insulin receptor. Structural abnormalities in the insulin receptor may cause (1) inefficient receptor biosynthesis, resulting in a decreased number of receptors at the cell surface, (2) abnormal insulin binding, resulting in abnormal affinity, or (3) inability of insulin binding to stimulate receptor autophosphorylation and a marked defect in the coupling of insulin binding to insulin action. Most patients described are compound heterozygotes, since each allele contains a distinct mutation. Interestingly, family members who are heterozygous for one or the other mutant allele also contain a normal allele and may be normal or have only mild to moderate degrees of insulin resistance phenotypically similar to that of patients with type II diabetes mellitus.

Since there is no one diagnostic test that distinguishes genetic forms of extreme insulin resistance from other forms, the patient should be referred to an appropriate research center to secure the diagnosis. Treatment should focus on controlling the hyperglycemia. Doses of insulin higher than 10,000 U per day may be required. U-500 insulin is usually preferred when such high doses are needed. These patients are at risk for the end-organ complications of chronic diabetes, such as retinopathy, neuropathy, and nephropathy. Therefore, appropriate screening for end-organ complications should be instituted. Hirsutism may respond to estrogen therapy (e.g., Premarin 0.625 to 1.25 mg per day). Acanthosis nigricans may respond to topical retinoic acid (tretinoin).

Type B Syndrome of Extreme Insulin Resistance. Type B syndrome of extreme insulin resistance occurs predominantly in women who have a well-defined autoimmune disease such as lupus erythematosus or Sjögren's syndrome or a less well-defined constellation of features that suggest autoimmunity, e.g., elevated erythrocyte sedimentation rate, positive antinuclear antibody, decreased complement, pancytopenia, and proteinuria.

Insulin resistance in patients with type B syndrome is caused by polyclonal autoantibodies that bind to insulin receptors at or near the insulin binding site, thereby impairing their function. Removal of anti-insulin receptor antibodies in vitro restores normal insulin binding, implying that the underlying receptors are normal. These antibodies may be readily detected in vitro at some diabetes research centers, and the diagnosis may be secured.

Patients with severe glucose intolerance should be treated with insulin. The goal should be to decrease or prevent the symptoms of hyperglycemia. High doses of insulin (i.e., up to 100,000 U per day) may be required. Since the titer of anti-insulin receptor antibodies tends to change during the course of the disease and spontaneous remission is common, insulin requirements can vary dramatically and glycemic control may be problematic. Since patients with type B syndrome of extreme insulin resistance usually have evidence of systemic autoimmunity, problems such as nephritis, cerebritis, and thrombocytopenia must be closely monitored and if found treated aggressively.

In some patients the circulating titers of anti-insulin receptor antibodies may be insulinomimetic and lead to hypoglycemia. It appears that the same population of polyclonal antibodies may cause hyperglycemia at high titers but hypoglycemia at lower titers. Clinically, the patient my present initially with hyperglycemia, and in the face of fluctuating titers of anti-insulin receptor antibodies, he or she may later become hypoglycemic. Rarely, patients with anti-insulin receptor antibodies may initially manifest with hypoglycemia that is indistinguishable from other types of hypoglycemia, such as that caused by insulinoma and surreptitious insulin or sulfonylurea abuse. When the anti-insulin receptor antibodies are insulinomimetic, hypoglycemia may be life-threatening and should be treated with high doses of systemic glucocorticoids (prednisone, 60 to 100 mg orally per day).

In summary, insulin resistance may be considered to be present when high doses of exogenously administered insulin result in a less than expected response. The magnitude of insulin resistance and the extent to which the pancreas can secrete insulin in a compensatory fashion determine the clinical state of glycemia.

Acknowledgment. We wish to thank Drs. Simeon Taylor, Phillip Gorden, and Richard Eastman for their helpful discussions and comments.

SUGGESTED READING

Grammer L. Insulin allergy. Clin Rev Allergy 1986; 4:189–200.

Grunberger G, Roth J. Insulin interaction with its specific receptor on target cells. In: Davidson JK, ed. Clinical diabetes mellitus. New York: Thieme, 1986:64.

Grunberger G, Taylor SI, Dons RF, Gorden P. Insulin receptors in normal and disease states. Clin Endocrinol Metab 1983; 12:191–219.

Kahn CR. Insulin allergy and insulin resistance. In: Krieger DT, Bardin CW, eds. Current therapy in endocrinology and metabolism (1985–1986). Philadelphia: BC Decker, 1985:281.

Kahn CR, Rosenthal AS. Immunologic reactions to insulin: Insulin allergy, insulin resistance, and autoimmune insulin syndrome. Diabetes Care 1979; 2:283–295.

Paulsen EP, Courtney JW III, Duckworth WC. Insulin resistance caused by massive degradation of subcutaneous insulin. Diabetes 1979; 28:640–645.

Phillips T, Ratner RE, Steiner M. Persistent cutaneous insulin allergy resulting from insulin dimers (abstr). Indianapolis: American Diabetes Association, 1987:60A.

Shade DS, Duckworth WC. In search of the subcutaneous-insulin resistance syndrome. N Engl J Med 1986; 315:147–152.

Small P, Lerman S. Human insulin allergy. Ann Allergy 1984; 53:39–41.

Taylor SI, Dons RF, Hernandez E, et al. Insulin resistance associated with androgen excess in women with autoantibodies to the insulin receptor. Ann Intern Med 1982; 97:851–855.

Taylor SI, Grunberger G, Marcus-Samuels B, et al. Hypoglycemia associated with antibodies to the insulin receptor. N Engl J Med 1982; 307:1422–1426.

Taylor SI, Kadowaki T, Kadowaki H, et al. Mutations in insulin-receptor gene in insulin-resistant patients. Diabetes Care 1990; 13:257–279.

DIABETES AND PREGNANCY

LOIS JOVANOVIC-PETERSON, M.D.
CHARLES M. PETERSON, M.D.

Prior to 1922, infants of diabetic mothers rarely survived. With the advent of insulin and its use in a more physiologic fashion, infant mortality and morbidity has dropped to the rate that is seen in the general population. It is clear from this improvement that maternal glycemic levels play the major role in the outcome of pregnancies complicated by diabetes. When maternal glycemia is normal, the outcome of pregnancy is normal. The mainstay of management, therefore, is to achieve and maintain normoglycemia throughout the entirety of the pregnancy.

Glucose is transported to the fetus by facilitated diffusion, whereas amino acids are actively transported across the placenta. In addition, alanine is siphoned selectively to the fetus. The effect of maternal loss of glucose and gluconeogenic substrate to the fetus is a drop in maternal glucose levels below nonpregnant glycemia to 55 to 65 mg per deciliter in the fasting state. Simultaneously, plasma ketone concentrations are several fold higher and free fatty acid levels are elevated after an overnight fast. Thus, pregnancy stimulates a state of "accelerated starvation," leading to the use of alternate fuels for maternal metabolism while glucose is spared for fetal consumption. The second half of pregnancy is characterized by further lowering of glucose levels.

Although maternal fasting glucose levels remain below nonpregnant levels, insulin levels increase markedly, in part because of increasing anti-insulin hormonal activity. The major diabetogenic hormones of the placenta are human placental lactogen, estrogen, and progesterone. In addition, serum maternal cortisol levels (both bound and free) are increased and finally the pituitary hormone prolactin has a diabetogenic effect at the elevated levels seen during gestation. The normal pancreas can adapt to these factors by potentitation of insulin secretion. If the pancreas fails to respond adequately to these alterations, then gestational diabetes results. The net effect of these changes is a rise in the postprandial glucose levels which tend to be highest 1 hour after breakfast. Based on the glucose profiles of normal pregnant women, the glucose targets for diabetic pregnant women should be a fasting level of 55 to 65 mg per deciliter level, a mean of the pre- and post-meal glucose levels of 84 mg per deciliter, and no blood glucose level higher than 140 mg per deciliter (Table 1).

When maternal hyperglycemia is present, the fetus will be exposed to either sustained or intermittent pulses of hyperglycemia, both of which are mutagenic and teratogenic in the first trimester. Both situations also permaturely stimulate fetal insulin secretion. The Pederson hypothesis links maternal hyperglycemia-induced fetal hyperinsulinemia to morbidity of the infant. Thus, fetal hyperinsulinemia may

TABLE 1 Definition of Normoglycemia During Pregnancy

	*Whole Blood (mg/dl)**	*Plasma (mg/dl)+*
Fasting and Pre-meal values	55–65	64–74
Mean of pre- and Post-meal values	84	96
One-hour post-meal limit	140	160

* As measured by self-monitoring of blood glucose (capillary blood)
+ As measured by autoanalyzer (hexokinase) on venous blood

result in (1) increased fetal body fat (macrosomia) and, therefore, a difficult delivery; (2) inhibition of pulmonary maturation of surfactant and, therefore, respiratory distress of the newborn; (3) changing serum potassium concentration secondary to the elevated insulin and glucose levels, and thus a predisposition toward cardiac arrhythmias; and (4) neonatal hypoglycemia, which might result in permanent neurologic damage. Hyperglycemia in the mother may lead to maternal complications such as polyhydramnios, hypertension, urinary tract infections, candidal vaginitis, and recurrent spontaneous abortions. Thus, a vigorous effort should be made to diagnose diabetes early and to achieve and maintain normoglycemia throughout pregnancy (Fig. 1).

PREGESTATIONAL DIABETES: TYPE I AND TYPE II

Definition and Classification

Now that diabetic women live to childbearing years, classifications of pregestational diabetes have emerged in an attempt to help the physician predict the outcome of pregnancy for both the mother and the child (Table 2). White created a classification that labeled diabetic women based on the mode of therapy, duration, and age at onset of diabetes and on the degree of vascular compromise of each patient at the beginning of the pregnancy. This classification led to confusion because the "B" determination was given to both the patient with pregnancy-related diabetes (gestational diabetes) who necessitated insulin therapy and the pregestational woman with less than 5 years of insulin therapy. Many investigators have attempted to improve this classification only to create more confusion. Some have tried creating their own classification schemes. However, as the evidence mounts that maternal normoglycemia is necessary at the time of conception, organogenesis, and throughout gestation, a new classification emerges that places more emphasis on maternal glycemia (see Table 2).

Glycemic levels have been shown to be the major predictors of outcome in pregnancies complicated by diabetes. The outcome for mother or fetus need not be

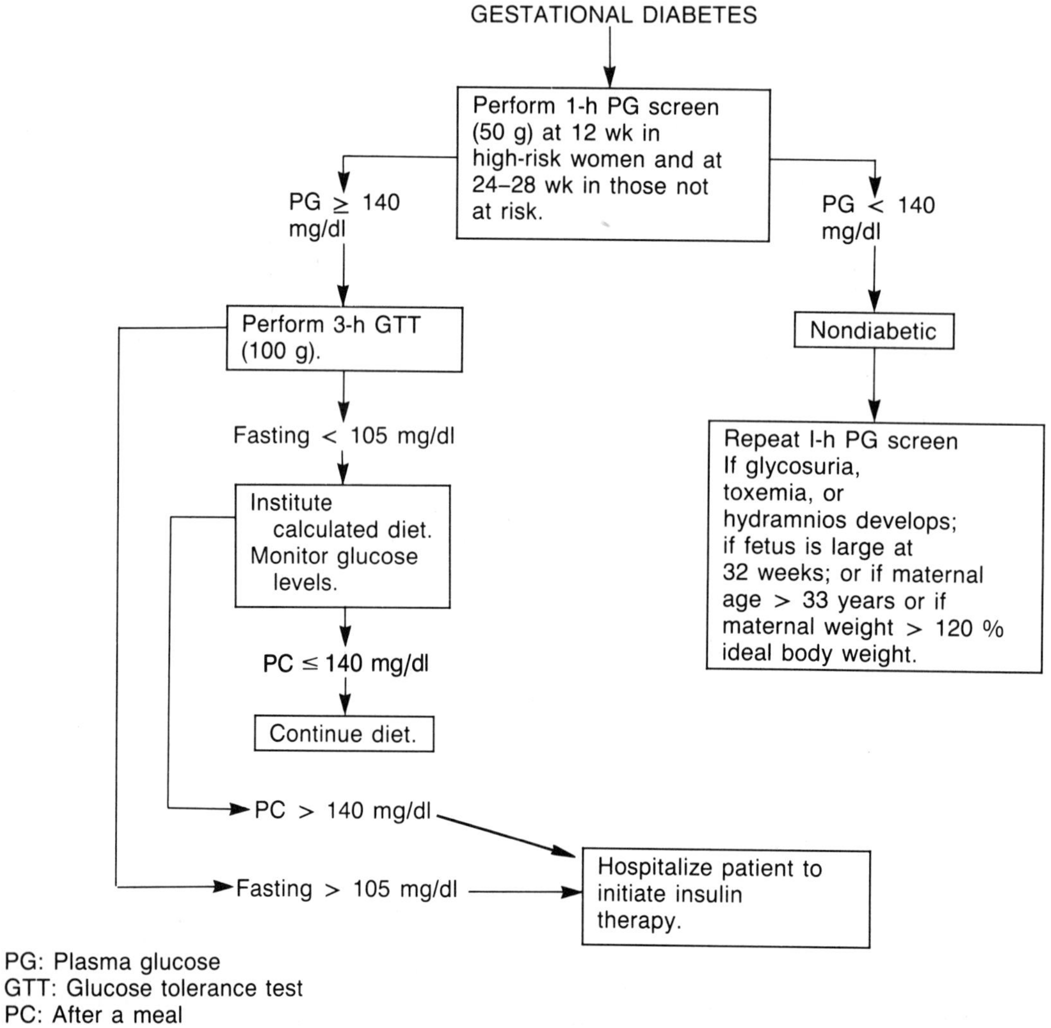

Figure 1 Triage procedure for gestational diabetes.

TABLE 2 Classifications of Diabetic Pregnancies

White Classification	
A.	Glucose tolerance test abnormal; no symptoms; euglycemia maintained with treament by appropriate diet but without insulin
B.	Adult onset (age 20 or older) and short duration (less than 10 years)
C.	Relatively young onset (age 10 to 19) or relatively long duration (10 to 19 years)
D.	Very young onset (age under 10) or very long duration (20 years or more) or evidence of background retinopathy
E.	Pelvic vascular disease (determined by radiography)
F.	Renal disease
RF.	Both renal disease and proliferative retinopathy
G.	Multiple failures in pregnancy
H.	Arteriosclerotic heart disease
T.	Pregnancy after renal transplantation
Pyke Classification	
	Gestational diabetes: starts during pregnancy and goes away after the pregnancy
	Pregestational diabetes: began before conception and continues after the pregnancy
	Pregestational diabetes complicated by vascular disease, retinopathy, nephropathy, pelvic vessel calcification, or peripheral vascular disease
Prognostically Bad Signs During Pregnancy	
	Clinical pyelonephritis: urinary tract infection (culture positive) with acute temperature elevation ($> 39^{\circ}$ C)
	Precoma (diabetic ketoacidosis with venous bicarbonate below 10 mEq/liter) or severe acidosis
	Pregnancy-induced hypertension
	Neglectors: pregnant women who are in labor when first admitted, who are psychopathic or of low intelligence, or who present less than 60 days before term
New Classification	
	Good diabetic control (whole blood, fingerstick self-determination of blood glucose criteria)
	Fasting 55–65 mg/dl; average blood glucose 84 mg/dl; 1 hr postprandial $<$ 140 mg/dl
	Less than optimal diabetic control
	a. Control not documented during pregnancy
	b. Blood glucose documented out of the ranges for good diabetic control

influenced by the presence of retinopathy, peripheral vascular disease, or nephropathy. In addition, kidney function seems to improve despite decreased function before pregnancy if normal glucose levels are maintained. However, the presence of hypertension confers an independent and worrisome risk. Type I diabetes presenting during gestation (generally presenting with maternal ketoacidosis) also implies a poor prognosis (see Table 2). The medical conditions of concern that frequently coexist in the patient with diabetes mellitus include hypertension, infection, thyroid dysfunction, retinopathy, and nephropathy. The paramount concern in the treatment of coexisting medical problems is that the treatment does not harm the fetus as it helps the mother.

Medical Related Problems

Hypertension

In the case of preexisting hypertension, all medication ideally should be discontinued during the time of organogenesis. If, however, the risk of accelerated hypertension is of concern, then the treatment of choice would be (1) salt and water restriction: 2 to 3 g of sodium per day, less than 2 L of oral fluid intake per 24 hours; (2) a thiazide diuretic with adequate natural potassium replacement; and (3) if more potent hypertensive medicine is needed, use of methyldopa and/or hydralazine. Both of these medicines seem not to interfere with organogenesis.

Urinary Tract Infection

In the case of a first-trimester urinary tract infection (reported to be 20 percent in some series), the infection-induced hyperglycemia must be vigorously treated, since the greatest harm to the fetus is the hyperglycemia not the infection. Antibiotic therapy should be used sparingly because the serum fetal levels could be significant. Antibiotics usually considered safe in pregnancy include the penicillins, cephalosporins, and erythromycin. Tetracycline and sulfa drugs should be avoided.

Thyroid Dysfunction

Forty percent of type I diabetic patients may have coexisting thyroid dysfunction. Because the stress of pregnancy may unmask a predisposition to thyroid disease, a radioimmunoassay for thyroid hormone paired with a thyroid-stimulating hormone (TSH), preferably the "extra-sensitive" TSH as assayed by monoclonal antibody, should be performed at pregnancy diagnosis and at each trimester. Hypothyroidism should be treated with L-thyroxine (T_4) in a dose titrated to the TSH level.

Hyperthyroidism diagnosed during pregnancy should be treated medically (preferably with propylthiouracil), after delivery definitive treatment can be given.

Retinopathy

Retinopathy is not a contraindication to pregnancy, but a retina specialist should clear the patient for a planned pregnancy and follow the patient closely (perhaps monthly) throughout pregnancy. Treatment with laser therapy may be necessary if neovascularization occurs or progresses.

Nephropathy

Nephropathy and proteinuria are also not contraindications to pregnancy. Kidney disease per se does not necessarily compromise or complicate the pregnancy unless superimposed hypertension intervenes.

Treatment

Diet Prescription for the Pregnant Diabetic Woman

The goal of management with diet is to maintain adequate nutrition and normoglycemia. In order to sustain normoglycemia, the food and the insulin must match. The "euglycemic diet," which is designed to prescribe enough calories to meet the nutritional needs of the pregnant woman but not cause postprandial hyperglycemia, is shown in Table 3.

A closer look at Table 3 reveals that less than 40 percent of the calories are prescribed in the form of carbohydrate since the carbohydrate content of foods accounts for the peak postprandial glucose level. The breakfast meal must be small and the carbohydrate portion of this meal minimal. Pregnancy produces severe morning carbohydrate intolerance. Later in the day, more carbohydrate can be tolerated. This diet of frequent small feedings is designed to avoid postprandial hyperglycemia and starvation ketosis. It promotes an average weight gain of 12.5 kg. In the first 8 to 10 weeks a pregnant woman needs 25 kcal per kilogram per 24 hours; thereafter, she needs 30 kcal per kilogram per 24 hours (present pregnant weight). For women who are greater than 120 percent ideal body weight, the diet should be calculated as 24 kcal per kilogram per 24 hours or less (present pregnant weight).

Monitoring for Hyperglycemia and Ketosis

Each woman should have her diet prescribed and the monitoring protocol explained at the same visit. She should check her urine for ketones on awakening and whenever a meal or snack is delayed. If ketonuria occurs, the intake of carbohydrate should be increased or an additional snack added. Until definitive studies show that ketosis or ketonuria is not harmful to the fetus, every attempt should be made to prevent ketonuria. For example, fasting ketonuria may be eliminated by a 3 AM glass of milk when the bedtime snack does not suffice to eliminate morning ketonuria of starvation.

TABLE 3 Diet Calculation

Time	*Meal*	*Fraction (kcal/24 h)*	*% of Daily Carbohydrate Allowed*
8:00 AM	Breakfast	2/18 D	10
10:30 AM	Snack	1/18 D	5
Noon	Lunch	5/18 D	30
3:00 PM	Snack	2/18 D	10
5:00 PM	Dinner	5/18 D	30
8:00 PM	Snack	2/18 D	10
11:00 PM	Snack	1/18 D	5

D = diet calculated to be 25 kcal/kg for the first 8 weeks of pregnancy and then raised to 30 kcal/kg for the duration of the pregnancy. In the case of women greater than 120% ideal body weight, then entire pregnancy is calculated as 24 kcal/kg.

Therapy Implementation

No matter how "educated" the pregestational woman is regarding diabetes management, metabolism is changed so greatly during pregnancy that reinforcement is always necessary. Ideally, this education to achieve and maintain normoglycemia should begin prior to conception. The education program usually requires 5 to 7 days to teach the patient the requisite goals and skills to normalize her blood glucose level throughout gestation through the use of insulin and food adjustments. The training process is best achieved in specialized centers for diabetes self-care or in the hospital.

Steps in a Normalization Program. The first step in the self-care program is to teach self-monitoring of blood glucose levels and to ensure (through a quality control program) that the values are accurate to within 10 percent of a laboratory standard. Most women prefer systems using reflectance meters because of the perceived accuracy over visually readable reagent strips.

The diet is maintained as described previously while insulin is administered to mimic normal pancreatic function. The normal pancreas secretes 50 percent of the insulin as mealtime "boluses." This delivery may be mimicked by four injections a day of combinations of NPH and regular insulin; however, it is possible to decrease the number of injections to three a day if the patient is willing to time lunch to coincide perfectly with the preinjected NPH insulin midday peak. The total daily dose of insulin is based on gestational week and the woman's current pregnant body weight (Table 4). The division of the insulin into three injections a day is also shown in Table 4. Following the initial insulin calculation, the dose is "tailored to fit" each woman by adjusting the dose until all the blood glucose levels before and 1 hour after each meal are normal (Table 5).

The division of the total daily insulin does take into account the basal needs of the pregnant woman and the mealtime insulin-to-food ratio. The most flexible plan prescribes four injections a day. If the total daily insulin requirement is represented by the letter "I" in the formulae below, then I = morning injection + lunch injection + dinner injection + bedtime injection:

Morning injection = NPH + regular (such that the NPH dose is 5/18 I and the regular is 4/18 I)
Lunch injection = regular (such that the regular insulin dose is 1/6 I)
Dinner injection = regular (such that the regular insulin dose is 1/6 I)
Bedtime injection = NPH (such that the NPH dose is 1/6 I)

If the patient prefers only three injections a day because she can eat exactly on time and not change her meal plan, then the I is divided such that the morning injection comprises a larger dose of NPH now equal to 8/18 I and the lunch injection is omitted. The doses of insulin are adjusted according to the blood glucose levels. Each blood glucose level determines a change in insulin (see Table 5).

In addition, the monitoring of blood glucose levels daily at this frequency (six per day: before and 1 hour after each meal), plus the use of titration procedures, ensures a smooth increase of insulin as the pregnancy progresses to a higher insulin requirement (up to 1 unit per kilogram per 24 hours at term (see Table 4). Twin gestations will result in a doubling of the insulin requirement throughout pregnancy. Each patient must also be taught her personal lag time between the injection and initiation of the meal. Simultaneous injection of insulin and ingestion of glucose will result in creating "brittle diabetes." The simple sugars in food will raise the blood glucose level before the subcutaneous insulin peaks. The quickly metabolized glucose will be gone when the insulin levels are at their maximum. To correct this problem, the insulin should be injected at least 30 to 45 minutes before the meal to allow the insulin and the food to "peak" together.

Follow-Up Visits. The visits on an outpatient basis should be frequent enough to provide the needed consultation, guidance, and emotional support to facilitate compliance. In addition, tests and therapy should be appropriate for gestational age (Table 6). The health care delivery team should give the impression that they, too, put forth an extra effort for this precious pregnancy. Therefore, each patient should have phone access to the team on a 24-hour basis for questions of insulin delivery, and visits should be spaced not longer than 2 weeks apart. A glycosylated hemoglobin level should be drawn at monthly intervals to confirm that the home blood glucose diary reflects maternal glycemia (see Table 6).

TABLE 4 Initial Calculation of Insulin and Sliding Scale for Regular Insulin Dosage

	7:30 AM	*4:30 PM*	*10:00 PM*
Type			
NPH	8/18 I		3/18 I
Regular	4/18 I	3/18 I	
Totals	2/3 I	1/6 I	1/6 I

Sliding Scale for Regular Insulin Dosage

7:30 AM *Blood Glucose*	*4:30 PM* *Blood Glucose*
< 60 = 3/18 I	< 60 = 2/18 I
60–100 = 4/18 I	60–100 = 3/18 I
100–140 = 5/18 I	100–140 = 4/18 I
> 140 = 6/18 I	> 140 = 5/18 I

I = 0.7 U/kg = total 24-h requirement for weeks 6–14
I = 0.8 U/kg = total 24-h requirement for weeks 14–26
I = 0.9 U/kg = total 24-h requirement for weeks 26–36
I = 1.0 U/kg = total 24-h requirement for weeks 36–40

Prevention of Hypoglycemia

Each patient should be taught to respond to symptoms of hypoglycemia (tingling sensations, diaphoresis, palpi-

TABLE 5 Insulin Titration

Time Insulin is Administered	*Insulin Type*	*Time of Blood Glucose Monitoring to Monitor Peak Action*	*Titration Procedure*
10:00 PM	NPH	7:30 AM	If fasting glucose is > 100 mg/dl, add 2 U to 10 PM NPH If fasting glucose is < 60 mg/dl, decrease 10 PM NPH by 2 U
7:30 AM	Regular	10:00 AM	If 1-hr postprandial glucose level is > 140 mg/dl, add 2 U of regular insulin to 7:30 AM dose of regular the following day. If 10 AM glucose level is < 60 mg/dl, increase pre-meal "lag time" or decrease dose
7:30 AM	NPH	4:00 PM	If 4 PM glucose level is > 100 mg/dl, add 2 U to 7:30 AM NPH dose If 4 PM glucose level is < 60 mg/dl, decrease 7:30 AM NPH by 2 U
4:30 PM	Regular	6:00 PM	If 6 PM blood glucose level is > 140 mg/dl, add 2 U to 4:30 PM regular insulin dose the following day

TABLE 6 Management of Diabetes and Pregnancy: Type I and Type II

Week of Gestation	*Test*	*Treatment*
-6	HbA_{1c} Self-monitoring of blood glucose Blood pressure Thyroid function testing	If HbA_{1c} is > 2 SD above the mean of nondiabetic control patients, normalize blood glucose levels
-2	HbA_{1c} Blood pressure Creatinine clearance + protein excretion	Recheck HbA_{1c} to ensure that it is normal prior to conception
	Clearance by Ophthalmologist Gynecologist Document normal blood pressure	Stop all medications if possible
+2	HbA_{1c} hCG by RIA T_4 RIA TSH Creatinine clearance plus total protein excretion CBC VDRL, toxoplasmosis Blood type Blood pressure Eye examination	

Table continues

TABLE 6 Continued

Week of Gestation	*Test*	*Treatment*
+2	Self-monitoring of blood glucose	Consider readmission if outpatient testing is too onerous and/or self-monitoring indicates a need for diet or insulin change. Diet: 25 kcal/kg/24 h Insulin: 0.7 U/kg/24 h
8–14	Every 2 weeks: HbA_{1c} Check blood glucose levels six times per day (before and 1 h after each meal Sonogram at 8 and 12 weeks	Increase Diet: 30 kcal/24 h Insulin: 0.7 U/kg/24h
14–18	HbA_{1c} every month Check blood glucose six times per day, Blood pressure	Diet: 30 kcal/kg/24 h Insulin: 0.7/kg/24 h
18–24	HbA_{1c} every month Check blood glucose levels six times per day. Repeat creatinine clearance, T_4 RIA, TSH, CBC, blood pressure Sonogram Begin kick count by mother	Diet: 30 kcal/kg/24 h Increase insulin: 0.8 U/kg/24 h
24–30	HbA_{1c} every month Check blood glucose levels six times per day Blood pressure	Diet: 30 kcal/kg/24 h Insulin: 0.8 U/kg/24 h
32	Creatinine clearance, T_4 RIA, CBC, HbA_{1c} every month. Check blood glucose levels six times per day Blood pressure	Admit for bed rest if blood pressure is rising Diet: 30 kcal/kg/24 h Insulin: 0.8 U/kg/24 h
34–36	Weekly visits for obstetric Assessment tests Uterine growth Fetal movement Kick count by mother daily	Diet: 30 kcal/kg/24 h Increase insulin: 0.9 U/kg/24 h
36–41	Visits two to three times per week for glucose control and obstetric check. Fetal movement kick count by mother daily.	Diet: 30 kcal/kg/24 h Increase insulin: 1 U/kg/24 h

HbA_{1c}, glycosylated hemoglobin; hCG, human chorionic gonadotropin; RIA, radioimmunoassay; T_4, thyroxine; TSH, thyroid-stimulating hormone; CBC, complete blood cell count; VDRL, Veneral Disease Research Laboratory test.

tations) by first checking her blood glucose level. If the blood glucose level is less than 70 mg per deciliter, she should drink 240 ml (8 ounces) of milk and recheck her blood glucose value 15 minutes later. This protocol is designed to return the blood glucose level to normal without rebound hyperglycemia.

In addition, patients and their families should be taught to inject glucagon subcutaneously to treat insulin reactions that cannot be corrected with food. During times of morning sickness and/or vomiting, judicious use of glucagon can be used to prevent hypoglycemia. In general, 0.15 mg (15 insulin units in a U-100 insulin syringe) of glucagon will raise blood glucose values 30 mg per deciliter within 15 minutes and maintain the levels for about 3 hours.

Timing of Delivery

When pregnancy is complicated by hyperglycemia, the risk of stillbirth increases as term approaches. In an attempt to decrease these losses, obstetricians have electively terminated such pregnancies between 35 and 38 weeks' gestation. However, this approach may have resulted in significant neonatal morbidity because of prematurity and hyaline membrane disease.

Recently it has been shown that even in poorly controlled pregnancies, neonatal morbidity can be markedly reduced if delivery is delayed until pulmonary maturity is documented in that 80 percent of preterm infants have some form of morbidity as compared with 40 percent of term infants. Therefore, watchful waiting is warranted and should be continued as long as maternal normoglycemia is maintained and the fetus is stable. Because programs of normoglycemia are relatively new and tools for fetal surveillance are improving rapidly, a protocol for optimal fetal surveillance is yet to be verified.

In pregnancies in which glucose control has been less than optimal, the lecithin-sphingomyelin ratio of the amniotic fluid should be assessed at 36 to 37 weeks' gestation. The presence of phosphatidylglycerol in the fluid is also indicative of pulmonary maturity. The fetus with documented pulmonary maturity and poor results on fetal surveillance protocols should be delivered. In the pregnancy in which glucose control is documented to be normal by six blood glucose determinations a day and normal glycosylated hemoglobin tests monthly, then the woman has the go-ahead for term delivery.

Labor and Delivery

With improvement in antenatal care, intrapartum events play an increasingly crucial role in the outcome of pregnancy. Before active labor, insulin requirements are present as noted previously, and glucose infusion is not necessary to maintain a blood glucose level of 70 to 90 mg per deciliter. With the onset of active labor, insulin requirements decrease to zero and glucose requirements are relatively consistent at 2.55 mg per kilogram per minute. From these data, a protocol for supplying the glucose needs of labor has been developed. The goal is to maintain the maternal blood glucose level between 70 and 90 mg per deciliter. The protocol for a planned induction is outlined in Table 7. In cases of the onset of active spontaneous labor, insulin is withheld and an intravenous dextrose infusion is begun at a rate of 2.55 mg per kilogram per minute (100 ml per hour in a 60 kg woman). If labor is latent, normal saline is usually sufficient to maintain normoglycemia until active labor begins, at which time dextrose is infused at 2.55 mg per kilogram per minute. The blood glucose level is then monitored hourly and if it is below 60 mg per deciliter, the infusion rate is doubled for the subsequent hour. If the blood glucose value rises to greater than 140 mg per deciliter, 2 to 4 units of regular insulin is given intravenously or subcutaneously each hour until the blood glucose level is 70 to 90 mg per deciliter. In the case of an elective cesarean secion, the bedtime dose of NPH insulin is repeated at 8 AM on the day of surgery and every 8 hours if the surgery is delayed. A dextrose infusion as described may be started if the blood glucose level falls below 60 mg per deciliter.

Postpartum Requirements

Maternal insulin requirements usually drop precipitously post partum; therefore, gestational diabetic women

TABLE 7 Insulin Titration

Protocol for Maintenance of Normoglycemia During Induction of Labor in Well-Controlled Insulin-Dependent Diabetic Pregnant Women
The evening before induction, give the usual bedtime dose of intermediate-acting insulin (NPH).
On morning of induction withhold the usual subcutaneous injection of insulin.
Start the intravenous line with normal saline.
Once active labor is achieved or the blood glucose level falls below 70 mg/dl, switch intravenous solutions to dextrose at a rate of 2.55 mg/kg/min.
Check blood glucose level by fingerstick and adjust dextrose infusion rate accordingly.

generally do not require further insulin. Pregestational diabetic women require resumption of insulin therapy; but insulin requirements may be decreased for up to 48 to 96 hours post partum. Insulin requirements should be recalculated at 0.6 units per kilogram per 24 hours based on the postpartum weight and should be started when the postprandial glucose level is above 150 mg per deciliter or the fasting glucose level is greater than 100 mg per deciliter. The postpartum caloric requirements are 25 kcal per kilogram per day based on postpartum weight. For the woman who wishes to breast feed her infant, the calculation is 27 kcal per kilogram per day and insulin requirements are still generally 0.6 unit per kilogram per day. Normoglycemia remains the goal for nursing diabetic women, since hyperglycemia results in elevated milk glucose levels.

Neonatal Care

If the blood glucose level is normalized throughout pregnancy in a woman with diabetes, there is no evidence that excess attention needs to be paid to her child. However, if a normal blood glucose level has not been documented throughout pregnancy, it is wise to monitor the infant in an intensive care situation for at least 24 hours post partum. The blood glucose level should be monitored hourly for 6 hours. If there are no signs of respiratory distress, hypocalcemia, or hyperbilirubinemia at 24 hours following delivery, the infant is discharged to the nursery.

GESTATIONAL DIABETES MELLITUS

Gestational diabetes is defined as carbohydrate intolerance of varying degree with onset or first recognition during pregnancy. Because methods for diagnosing gestational diabetes have varied greatly over the years, reports of the prevalence of this condition have varied from 0.15 to 12.3 percent. There are now internationally accepted guidelines for the method and treatment of gestational diabetes.

Universal Screening for Gestational Diabetes

The recommendation is that all pregnant women should be screened for gestational diabetes at 24 to 28 weeks of gestation. Selective screening based on clinical observations or past obstetric history have been shown to be inadequate. Screening should be by plasma glucose determination 1 hour after the ingestion of 50 g of oral glucose without regard for time of day or previous meal consumed. If the test result is greater than 140 mg per deciliter, a complete glucose tolerance test is recommended. Although up to 20 percent of all pregnant women may show a positive screening result, it is unlikely that a glucose-intolerant woman would be missed.

Diagnostic criteria for gestational diabetes are based on the 100-g glucose tolerance test. The results are taken from samples of venous plasma while fasting, and at 1-, 2-, and 3-hours after administration of glucose. The clinician should note that there is no half-hour value. In addition, 4- and 5-hour values are not part of the standard glucose tolerance test. The 3-hour test is strenuous, and the additional venipunctures are not necessary. The criteria for the diagnosis of gestational diabetes are presented in Table 8.

The majority of gestational diabetes is diagnosed between 24 and 28 weeks of gestation. However, up to 20 percent of gestational diabetic women do not show significant glucose intolerance until the 32nd week, when maximum counter-insulin hormonal levels have been reached. A negative glucose tolerance test at 24 to 28 weeks of gestation, therefore, does not guarantee a pregnancy free of metabolic problems. Rescreening the entire population to find these women would be difficult. The following criteria have been developed to help identify those women who are at risk for the development of diabetes during the third trimester:

1. A positive screen (greater than 140 mg per deciliter) at 24 to 28 weeks' gestation, with a negative glucose tolerance test
2. Maternal age greater than or equal to 33 years
3. Maternal obesity greater than or equal to 120 percent of ideal body weight

Therapy

The flow diagram (see Fig. 1) outlines the steps in establishing a treatment program toward optimal management.

Diet

The goal of management is to maintain normoglycemia. A nutritious meal for a mother and her unborn child usually results in at least a 40 mg per deciliter rise in blood glucose levels. Therefore, if a woman's fasting blood glucose is much above 100 mg per deciliter, she will not be able to maintain her postprandial glucose levels below 140 mg per deciliter. Fifteen percent of gestational diabetic women require insulin.

The "euglycemic diet" in pregnancy for the diabetic woman who is 80 to 120 percent of ideal body weight is the same as for the nondiabetic pregnant woman (see Table 3).

TABLE 8 Glucose Tolerance Test Criteria For Diagnosis And Classification

Two or more values above:	
A fasting plasma glucose > 105 mg/dl	
1 h > 190 mg/dl	
2 h > 165 mg/dl	
3 h > 145 mg/dl	
Treatment:	Diet therapy. Initiate insulin therapy if normoglycemia is not maintained on diet alone.

Monitoring for Hyperglycemia and Ketosis

The diet only "fits" if there is no postprandial hyperglycemia or preprandial ketosis. The diet and monitoring protocol should be explained to each woman during the same visit. Visually read reagent strips are an excellent means of self-monitoring both urine ketone and blood glucose levels. The patient should check her urine for ketones on awakening or whenever a meal or snack is delayed. If ketones are present, the caloric intake of carbohydrates should be cautiously increased. An additional snack of 12 g of carbohydrate (8 ounces of skim milk) is generally sufficient to prevent lipolysis. Fasting ketonuria may be cleared by a 3 AM glass of milk when the bedtime snack does not suffice until awakening.

Blood glucose levels can be monitored by self-testing of blood glucose levels. Only meals need to be monitored. However, the patient should monitor her snack if she fears it has been excessive. Since the goal is to remain below 140 mg per deciliter 1 hour after meals, if the patient's 1-hour blood glucose level is less than 140 mg per deciliter, she is "winning" on the diet.

Exercise Prescriptions

Recently it has been shown that an aerobic workout for 20 to 30 minutes three times a week for at least 6 weeks can improve glucose intolerance and reduce the need for insulin. The safest form of exercise is upper-body exercise, since lower-body and leg exercises precipitate uterine contractions.

Initiation of Insulin Therapy

Absolute indications for the initiation of insulin in a gestational diabetic woman are (1) elevated fasting plasma glucose levels greater than 105 mg per deciliter; (2) persistent ketonuria, which can only be cleared by increasing carbohydrates to the level causing postprandial hyperglycemia greater than 140 mg per deciliter; and (3) postprandial hyperglycemia greater than 140 mg per deciliter despite carbohydrate restriction.

Once it has been determined that insulin is required, hospitalization should be planned as soon as possible. Five to 7 days is usually required to teach the patient the necessary skills to understand and manage insulin administration.

The diet should be maintained while administering insulin injections designed to mimic normal pancreatic function. The insulin should be given in at least three injections a day as per Table 4. Since gestational diabetes occurs at the 24 to 28 weeks of gestation, the 24-hour insulin dose should be calculated as 0.8 unit times the present pregnant weight in kilograms. Insulin adjustment is based on six self-determinations of blood glucose level a day (Table 5).

Timing of Delivery

As in the case of a pregestational diabetic woman, when the maternal glucose levels are normal, the woman may proceed to term delivery. If the glucose levels are less than optimal, the same protocol as for the type I woman should be followed (see Table 4).

Postpartum

Ninety seven and one-half percent of all gestational diabetic women revert to normoglycemia post partum. The postpartum test should be a 75 g oral test according to the criteria of the National Diabetes Data Group. The recommended levels for the diagnosis of diabetes are fasting blood glucose greater than 140 mg per deciliter and/or any value after the 2-hour time point greater than or equal to 200 mg per deciliter. This test is generally performed at about 6 weeks post partum and provides an opportunity to discuss future pregnancies.

Most women should be warned that the probability that diabetes will recur with subsequent pregnancies is 90 percent. In addition, obese women who remain overweight have a 60 percent chance of manifesting overt diabetes within 20 years. This outcome may be improved if they reduce their weight to a normal range. Normal weight women have been found to have less than 25 percent prevalence of diabetes. Perhaps a positive outcome of pregnancy complicated by gestational diabetes is to prevent obesity-induced diabetes in the future.

SUGGESTED READING

Jovanovic L, Peterson CM, Saxena BB, Dawood MY, Saudek CD. Feasibility of maintaining euglycemia in insulin-dependent diabetic woman. Am J Med 1980; 68:105–112.

Jovanovic L, Druzin M, Peterson CM. The effect of euglycemia on the outcome of pregnancy in insulin-dependent diabetics as compared to normal controls. Am J Med 1981; 71:921–927.

Jovanovic L, Peterson CM. Insulin and glucose requirements during the first stage of labor in insulin-dependent diabetic women. Am J Med 1983; 75:607–612.

Jovanovic L, Peterson CM, eds. Contemporary issues in nutrition: diabetes mellitus. New York: Alan R Liss, 1985.

Jovanovic L, Peterson CM, eds. Diabetes in pregnancy: teratology, toxicology, and treatment. Philadelphia: Praeger, 1986.

Jovanovic L, Subak-Sharpe GL. The woman's answer book. New York: Atheneum, 1987.

Jovanovic L, Toohey B, Bieman J. The diabetic woman. Los Angeles: Jeremy P Tarcher, 1987.

Jovanovic L, ed. Controversies in the field of pregnancy and diabetes. New York: Springer-Verlag, 1987.

Jovanovic-Peterson L, Durak EP, Peterson CM. Randomized trial of diet versus diet plus cardiovascular conditioning on glucose levels in gestational diabetes. Am J Obstet Gynecol 1989; 161:415–419.

Jovanovic-Peterson L, Peterson CM. De novo hypothyroidism in pregnancies complicated by type I diabetes and proteinuria: A new syndrome. Am J Obstet Gynecol 1988; 159:441–446.

ADRENAL INSUFFICIENCY

DAVID N. ORTH, M.D., F.A.C.P.

Treatment of adrenal insufficiency is based on replacing the missing adrenal hormones and/or producing their effects under basal conditions as well as in situations of increased demand. The adrenal gland produces three major hormones: epinephrine in the medulla, cortisol in the middle zona fasciculata of the cortex, and aldosterone in the outer cortical zona glomerulosa. In addition, it produces adrenocortical androgens that are of some minor importance in women but are of little consequence in men, in whom the major androgen, testosterone, is produced by the testis. No attempt is made to replace adrenal androgens. Epinephrine, a catecholamine, has relatively unimportant cardiovascular effects, but it is the major acute counterregulatory hormone to insulin. The only clinical consequence of epinephrine deficiency may be postprandial reactive hypoglycemia. However, there are other glucogenic hormones (glucagon, cortisol, and growth hormone), so that symptoms of isolated epinephrine deficiency are usually mild, and no attempt is made to replace it.

Aldosterone and cortisol are the adrenal hormones that, when deficient, must be replaced. Cortisol (hydrocortisone) is the major glucocorticoid in humans. It is important to the proper function of virtually every cell in the body; it affects carbohydrate, protein, and fat metabolism; and it is one of the major mediators of the stress response. Nevertheless, one can function quite adequately for many years with a relatively low rate of cortisol production, as is the case in patients with chronic hypopituitarism. Cortisol is also a weak salt-retaining steroid, or mineralocorticoid, but the major mineralocorticoid in humans is aldosterone. Retention of sodium and reciprocal loss of potassium and hydrogen ions in the renal tubules, salivary glands, sweat glands, and gut under the influence of aldosterone maintains normal plasma volume, systemic arterial blood pressure, and electrolyte balance. Although one can survive without aldosterone under basal conditions by massive oral salt intake, one generally cannot survive major fluid loss, severe trauma, or surgery.

Primary adrenal insufficiency (Addison's disease) means that the adrenal glands are the target of the destructive disease process, whether it be an autoimmune disorder, metastatic neoplasm, granulomatous disease, or intraadrenal hemorrhage. Aldosterone, cortisol, adrenal androgens, and epinephrine are all partly or entirely deficient in primary adrenal insufficiency. Secondary adrenal insufficiency is due to lack of adrenocorticotropin (ACTH) stimulation. This disorder is most commonly the consequence of chronic suppression of hypothalamic-pituitary-adrenal axis function with pharmacologic doses of exogenous glucocorticoids (iatrogenous Cushing's syndrome); less commonly, primary tumors of the pituitary gland; relatively uncommonly, excessive production of endogenous glucocorticoids (endogenous or spontaneous Cushing's syndrome); and rarely, infections or metastatic disease of the pituitary or lack of hypothalamic corticotropin-releasing hormone (CRH) production or delivery to the pituitary gland. In terms of adrenal function, it is usually manifested by isolated cortisol deficiency, although aldosterone production may be diminished in chronic secondary adrenal insufficiency. The pattern of adrenal hormone deficiency affects both the manifestations of the disease and the rationale for its treatment.

Recommendations for withdrawing glucocorticoids from patients who have been taking pharmacologic doses of these drugs are discussed elsewhere in this volume (see chapter on *Corticosteroid Withdrawal*). Therefore, the discussion in this chapter is restricted to treatment of primary and other forms of secondary adrenal insufficiency.

ADRENAL CRISIS: ACUTE PRIMARY ADRENAL INSUFFICIENCY

Adrenal crisis is a life-threatening emergency. It occurs, virtually without exception, only in patients with primary adrenal insufficiency. Its major clinical manifestation is shock, and its major physiologic derangements are fluid and sodium depletion. It may be caused by trauma, blood loss, major infection, or failure to take prescribed steroid replacement therapy, especially when this is caused and complicated by vomiting and diarrhea, which accelerate loss of fluid and electrolytes. The underlying cause of the crisis must be addressed as quickly as possible, but the most urgent immediate need is to replace fluid volume and salt. I have outlined below a protocol for accomplishing this and, in the patient who is not known to have Addison's disease, a variation for simultaneously establishing the diagnosis. This treatment is summarized in Table 1.

1. Immediately insert a #19-gauge needle or an equivalent-sized catheter into a major vein. Obtain blood for immediate analysis of electrolytes. In patients

TABLE 1 Treatment of Adrenal Crisis

Establish 19-gauge intravenous line, obtain stat serum electrolytes, glucose, and cortisol values.
Infuse 3 L of normal saline solution or 5 percent dextrose in normal saline solution as quickly as possible. Observe central or peripheral venous pressure or monitor for development of pulmonary rales, reducing infusion rate if indicated.
Inject 4 mg dexamethasone at beginning of intravenous drip or give 100 mg cortisol (hydrocortisone) intravenously and 100 mg every 8 hours thereafter.
Use supportive measures as indicated.
Mineralocorticoids are unnecessary; ACTH is useless.
After initial fluid infusion, continue intravenous infusion at slower rate; identify and treat cause of crisis.

not known to have Addison's disease, other causes of shock must be considered.

2. Infuse 3 L of normal saline or 5 percent glucose in normal saline as fast as it will run in. Never infuse hypotonic saline or glucose alone, since the patient is already sodium depleted, and life-threatening hyponatremia can be induced in this manner. Many physicians balk at infusing this volume of fluid so rapidly, but it can be life-saving. One can easily monitor central or peripheral venous pressure or listen for development of pulmonary rales, slowing the infusion rate if needed, but this is rarely necessary, even in older patients.
3. Give 4 mg of dexamethasone phosphate intravenously at the beginning of the infusion. Although the immediate clinical problem is not glucocorticoid deficiency, glucocorticoids are important for responding adequately to a major stress and appear to be important in maintaining peripheral vascular tone, for example. This dose of dexamethasone will satisfy the patient's glucocorticoid requirements for the next 12 to 24 hours.
4. Keep the patient warm and use other supportive measures if indicated.
5. Do not worry about mineralocorticoid replacement until the patient is no longer in shock and is capable of taking oral medications. Intravenous saline administration is sufficient acutely. Mineralocorticoids can only retain sodium that is present in serum; they are of little value in the severely sodium-depleted patient.
6. After the first 3 L of fluid is infused and if the patient has responded to therapy, continue saline-plus-glucose infusion at a slower rate, monitor vital signs, and address the process that precipitated the crisis. When the patient is stable, begin maintenance oral glucocorticoid and mineralocorticoid therapy, discontinuing intravenous fluids when oral intake is adequate.
7. To diagnose previously undocumented Addison's disease, obtain the plasma cortisol concentration in the first blood sample, inject an ampule (250 μg) of cosyntropin (Cortrosyn) or 25 to 50 USP units of injectable ACTH (e.g., ACTHAR) and obtain plasma cortisol levels 30 and 60 minutes later. The first plasma cortisol value should be low, usually less than 5 μg per deciliter. It must be less than 20 μg per deciliter in all three specimens to confirm the diagnosis. Plasma ACTH should be high, usually greater than 200 pg per milliliter, if it is measured in the initial specimen. There is no point in measuring it after administering exogenous ACTH. It should be noted that dexamethasone does not interfere significantly in the measurement of immunoreactive plasma cortisol, nor does it interfere in the action of ACTH on the adrenal cortex. Therefore, one can simultaneously diagnose Addison's disease and treat adrenal crisis with fluid, salt, and dexamethasone. Hydrocortisone (cortisol) or cortisone (which is converted into cortisol) cannot be substituted for dexamethasone before performing this diagnostic test, because these agents will be measured as cortisol in plasma.

Once the patient's condition is stable, steroids can be decreased rapidly to a maintenance dosage. The rate depends on the nature and severity of the illness causing the crisis. If it is viral gastroenteritis, for example, it may be possible to discharge the patient on maintenance therapy within 24 hours. If it is a more serious illness, the dose of glucocorticoid may be halved each day, depending on symptoms, usually returning to maintenance dosage within 5 days.

CHRONIC PRIMARY ADRENAL INSUFFICIENCY

Perhaps the single most important aspect of chronic treatment is adequate education and reassurance of the patient as soon as the diagnosis is confirmed. My approach is to inform the patient that the condition is permanent but not progressive and that it will have absolutely no effect on the quality or duration of his life as long as he takes the medications as prescribed and follows a few commonsense precautions. I assure the patient that no activity, no matter how vigorous, is proscribed. I usually mention the names of some well-known persons who had Addison's disease, such as Dr. Roger Bannister, the English physician-athlete who first ran the mile in less than 4 minutes. I further note that my Addisonian patients are all so well that I have difficulty getting them to schedule occasional checkups and that in over 20 years I have had only two of my patients enter an emergency department with problems related to their adrenal insufficiency, both of whom were quickly treated and released. After answering all questions to the best of my ability, I describe the treatment of adrenal insufficiency, stressing that strict adherence to the prescribed regimen is the key to living a normal and healthy life. I have them repeat back to me, after I have finished, all aspects of the treatment that I have described to them.

There are four phases of treatment of chronic primary adrenocortical insufficiency: maintenance therapy, treatment during minor stress, measures to be taken in emergencies, and treatment during hospitalization for surgery or severe illness (Table 2).

Maintenance Therapy

Emergency Identification and Medication

Each patient should wear a Medic-Alert bracelet or necklace at all times. It should be inscribed with the disease ("adrenal insufficiency") and daily medications (e.g., "takes prednisone and fludrocortisone"). It also displays a "call collect" telephone number where medical records and the names of physicians and relatives to be contacted can be obtained 24 hours a day.

Each patient should also carry on his person at all times an Emergency Medical Information card (one is supplied with the Medic-Alert bracelet or necklace). It should list the patient's name, address, telephone number and date

TABLE 2 Treatment of Chronic Primary Adrenal Insufficiency*

Maintenance Therapy

Educate the patient.

Obtain Medic-Alert bracelet/necklace, Emergency Medical Information card, and preloaded syringes containing 4 mg dexamethasone in 1 ml saline.

Mineralocorticoid: fludrocortisone, 0.1 (0.05 to 0.2) mg orally daily. Double the dosage during hot summer months unless contraindicated. Increase normal liberal salt intake with excessive salt loss by sweating or mild diarrhea. Monitor serum electrolytes, supine and standing blood pressure, edema.

Glucocorticoid: dexamethasone, 0.5 (0.25 to 0.75) mg, or prednisone, 5 (2.5 to 7.5) mg orally daily, taken at bedtime. Supplement with cortisol 5 to 10 mg orally in midafternoon if indicated. monitor clinical response, morning plasma ACTH.

Minor Stress at Home (minor febrile or viral-type illness)

Can increase glucocorticoid twofold to threefold for no ore than 3 days without consulting a physician. Do not change mineralocorticoid.

If illness worsens during increased glucocorticoid treatment or persists more than 3 days, consult a physician.

Emergency (major trauma, myocardial infarction, inability to take oral medications because of vomiting, severe fluid loss)

Inject 4 mg dexamethasone from preloaded syringe subcutaneously. If in doubt, inject it.

Get to a physician as quickly as possible.

Surgery or Major Stress in Hospital (surgery, myocardial infarction, sepsis or other severe febrile illness, labor and delivery)

Increase glucocorticoid to ten times maintenance dose, beginning prior to anesthesia for scheduled surgery.

Taper rapidly, decreasing by half per day, to maintenance level: can adjust rate slightly according to signs and symptoms.

*Treatment of chronic secondary adrenal insufficiency is identical, except that mineralocorticoid replacement is only rarely required and replacement may be required for other pituitary hormones.

of birth, the name and telephone number of a physician and a relative to contact, the disease, daily medications and their dosages, and instructions for injecting dexamethasone ("Inject under the skin anywhere on the body in case of emergency and call a physician").

Each patient should have at least three preloaded dexamethasone syringes (4 mg dexamethasone sodium phosphate in 1 ml sterile saline solution). There should be one at home, one in each automobile, and one on his person at all times. Children need to leave one at school with the nurse or principal. These syringes are often difficult to obtain from the local pharmacist, who may require the patient to purchase an entire case of 24. They should be ordered well in advance or can be made up by the pharmacist with sterile 1-ml syringes and a multidose vial containing 4 mg per milliliter dexamethasone phosphate solution. The latter arrangement has the disadvantage of not having a ready-made package to prevent inadvertent depression of the plunger, but a suitable one can be constructed. Men and boys often like to have a holster made that fits on their belts; women usually carry theirs in their purses. The syringes should be replaced if used, if they leak, turn cloudy, or become discolored, or after about 1 year.

Mineralocorticoid and Salt Replacement

Aldosterone is not commercially available. Fludrocortisone acetate (Florinef) is a potent mineralocorticoid with significant glucocorticoid activity (about one-third that of dexamethasone, two and one-half times that of prednisone, and ten times that of cortisol, on a weight basis) (Table 3). The usual maintenance dose is 0.1 mg per day. Occasional patients require slightly more, others slightly less. Fludrocortisone can be taken at any time of day, but patients typically take it first thing in the morning. Dietary intake of salt should be normal. The best indices of adequate replacement are normal serum electrolyte values, especially that of potassium, normal supine blood pressure without orthostatic hypotension, and absence of dependent edema. Normal plasma renin activity, both supine and in response to 3 hours of upright posture, is a more quantitative measure of proper replacement. In general, the dosage should be modified only gradually, in 0.05-mg increments, and, once the correct dose is established, rarely requires changing. Addisonian patients can develop essential hypertension or congestive heart failure, however. Before treating them with a sodium-wasting diuretic, their dietary salt intake should be restricted and their fludrocortisone should be tapered or even discontinued, recognizing that, as in the non-Addison's patient taking a large dosage of diuretic, hyponatremic hyperkalemic acidosis may develop.

In situations in which accelerated loss of sodium may occur, the question arises as to whether the fludrocortisone dosage should be modified. These situations include increased sweating due to excessive summer heat or increased physical activity and fluid loss due to episodes of diarrhea. I am concerned that the patient may cause more harm than good by attempting to mimic the normal aldosterone response to acute fluid loss. I recommend doubling the usual daily maintenance dosage of fludrocortisone and liberaliz-

TABLE 3 Characteristics of Common Orally Administered Adrenal Steroids

Steroid	*Approximate Duration of Activity (hours)*	*Relative Glucocorticoid Activity*	*Relative Mineralocorticoid Activity*
Cortisol (hydrocortisone)	4–8	100	0.7
Cortisone	4–8	80	0.7
Prednisone	6–12	400	1.0
Prednisolone	6–12	400	1.0
Triamcinolone	6–12	500	0
Methylprednisolone	6–12	600	0.5
Dexamethasone	12–20	3,000–4,000	0
Fludrocortisone	12–20	1,000	100

ing dietary salt intake during the hot summer months, and anticipating losses due to exercise by taking increased salt in the diet or as salt tablets, 500 mg, with plenty of fluid immediately before and as often as every 2 hours during strenuous physical activity. I recommend increased salt intake only for mild diarrhea. A physician should be consulted if severe or prolonged diarrhea occurs.

Glucocorticoid Replacement

The first synthetic glucocorticoid to become commercially available was cortisone acetate (Cortone Acetate), and there are many physicians who still use it. Cortisone is biologically inactive and must be converted to cortisol by the liver. About 80 percent of orally administered cortisone is effectively converted to cortisol. Cortisol (Cortef) can also be administered. It seems attractive to replace missing endogenous cortisol with exogenous cortisol. At one time, I prescribed it with the notion that one could measure plasma and urinary cortisol and cortisol metabolites (17-hydroxycorticosteroids or 17-ketogenic steroids) as indices of adequacy of replacement. In practice, however, this provides very misleading information. These steroids are given occasionally as a single morning dose, more commonly as two divided doses with half or more given in the morning, and frequently as three divided doses. In each case, plasma cortisol rapidly exceeds the binding capacity of serum cortisol-binding globulin (CBG, or transcortin), which is about 25 μg per deciliter of total plasma cortisol. Cortisol concentrations in excess of about 25 μg per deciliter represent unbound, metabolically active, "free" cortisol. The free cortisol is rapidly cleared by glomerular filtration until the total plasma cortisol level falls to about 25 μg per deciliter, after which normal metabolism ("normal" because endogenous plasma cortisol concentration almost never exceeds 25 μg per deciliter) supervenes, and plasma cortisol falls more slowly to less than 5 μg per deciliter about 2.5 hours later. This "rollercoaster effect" on plasma cortisol concentrations is not infrequently reflected in the patient's symptoms several hours after the last dose, in the fact that plasma cortisol is only an index of when the last dose was given, and in the fact that the urinary-free cortisol level is much higher and urinary 17-hydroxycorticosteroid and 17-ketogenic steroid levels are lower than they would be for endogenous secretion of the same amount of cortisol. The usual daily adult maintenance dose is 37.5 mg of cortisone acetate or 25 mg of cortisol. Since they have significant mineralocorticoid activity (these doses are equivalent to about 0.2 mg of fludrocortisol) (see Table 3), mineralocorticoid replacement is not necessary. However, I find it preferable to manage glucocorticoid and mineralocorticoid therapy independently. Cortisol and cortisone are very useful when one wishes to administer a short-acting glucocorticoid, such as during recovery from chronic hypothalamic-pituitary-adrenal suppression by glucocorticoids in Cushing's syndrome. They have little if any role in the treatment of permanent primary or secondary adrenal insufficiency.

The appropriate replacement steroids are prednisone or dexamethasone (Decadron). The usual daily replacement doses are 5 and 0.5 mg, respectively (see Table 2). Occasional large adults require up to half-again this dosage, smaller adults may require somewhat smaller doses, and children's doses should be adjusted on the basis of estimated body surface area, which can be accomplished with smaller tablets or with elixirs of the drugs. Some patients may metabolize steroids more rapidly or more slowly than others. This may be a constitutional characteristic or may be caused by induction of hepatic enzyme systems by certain drugs, among them barbiturates, phenytoin, rifampin, mitotane, and aminoglutethimide. The last two agents may be used in certain patients with Cushing's syndrome and may complicate the process of estimating adequate replacement steroid dosage. In all patients, these considerations must be kept in mind when designing a glucocorticoid replacement regimen.

Unfortunately, there are neither established "normal" plasma levels of these synthetic glucocorticoids nor reliable indices for determining adequate replacement therapy. One possible index would be plasma ACTH levels: if plasma ACTH levels were in the normal range, the glucocorticoid replacement regimen might be judged adequate. In my experience, however, the majority of treated

Addison's patients have markedly elevated early morning plasma ACTH concentrations and variable but lower levels the remainder of the day. This is because the major daily stimulus for ACTH secretion occurs during the last 4 or 5 hours of sleep and the first 1 or 2 hours after awakening. Most patients take their first daily steroid dose after the major ACTH secretory period has ended and their last daily dose too long before the next morning's secretory period begins to affect its magnitude. Consequently, many Addison's patients never completely lose their hyperpigmentation, some of them develop extremely high, relatively nonsuppressible ACTH levels, and a few develop large ACTH-secreting pituitary tumors analogous to those observed in patients with Nelson's syndrome after treatment of pituitary Cushing's disease with bilateral adrenalectomy. Furthermore, a number of Addison's patients have symptoms of fatigue, lassitude, mild nausea, or headache on awakening that appear to be alleviated by glucocorticoid. What is needed is a timed-release glucocorticoid to be taken at bedtime. Since there is none, I treat Addison's patients with a single bedtime dose of dexamethasone or prednisone. This lowers their morning plasma ACTH into the normal range and alleviates the symptoms on awakening. In those very rare patients in whom it causes insomnia, I give the steroid in the morning. For those occasional patients who seem to require a little more steroid late the next afternoon, I prescribe a 5- to 10-mg dose of cortisol about an hour before they habitually develop symptoms, usually between 2 and 3 PM. Since none of us secretes significant amounts of cortisol between about 6 PM and 2 AM, there is no need for a dose of steroid later in the day. I adjust the dosage regimen to relieve symptoms of glucocorticoid deficiency, avoid signs and symptoms of Cushing's syndrome, and maintain early morning plasma ACTH levels in the normal range.

Treatment of Minor Stress

The patient should double or triple the maintenance dosage of glucocorticoid without consulting a physician for minor, febrile, virus-like syndromes. These episodes should typically occur no more than three or four times a year. The patient can continue the increased dosage for up to 3 days. Mineralocorticoid dosage should not be altered, but salt and fluid intake must be maintained and even augmented, if there is significant fever or diarrhea. If the illness gets worse during those 3 days or if it persists so that the patient cannot return to maintenance dosage by the fourth day, he should consult a physician for evaluation and possible treatment of the infectious disease. The patient should be assured that it is not necessary to augment the maintenance dosage of glucocorticoids for the minor psychological stresses of everyday life. This approach provides the patient with enough latitude to deal with most minor illnesses at home but prevents the anxious patient from developing the serious consequences of overuse of steroids.

Emergency Treatment

"Emergency" is defined as severe trauma, such as an automobile accident or injury involving fractures, lacerations, blood loss, or unconsciousness, myocardial infarction, or the inability to retain oral medications, as in vomiting due to an acute viral or bacterial gastroenteritis. In these situations, the conventional wisdom is that the patient requires increased glucocorticoid. In fact, there is little direct evidence for this, although it is clear that patients with Addison's disease have increased morbidity and mortality if they do not have maintenance doses of steroids administered during severe stress. Nevertheless, because there is almost no risk associated with brief administration of high doses of steroids, it is better to give them in order to eliminate glucocorticoid deficiency as a possible complicating factor.

The contents of one preloaded dexamethasone syringe (i.e., 4 mg dexamethasone sodium phosphate) should be injected under the skin on any part of the body, although the anterior thigh and forearm are the most convenient sites for self-administration. If the patient is unconscious or unable to self-administer the medication, paramedics or passersby must be relied on to find the Medic-Alert tag and follow the instructions on the card. If the patient is conscious, the responsibility is his. It is very important that the patient be instructed to inject it if in doubt about whether to do so, since the dexamethasone can do no harm. He should be told that it makes no difference whether the dexamethasone is injected subcutaneously, intramuscularly, intravenously, intra-arterially, into a viscus, or elsewhere, as long as it is under the skin. It can be injected through clothing. Skin preparation is unnecessary. Once it is injected, the patient needs to seek medical attention as quickly as possible to treat the emergency. The patient should be instructed on how to inject the drug to be certain he can do it.

I have never had a patient abuse injectable dexamethasone. Most patients use it only a few times in their lives. None should use it more than a few times each year. I know of only two of my patients who failed to inject it when they should have; one arrived in an emergency department in shock, and the other weathered a brief but severe bout of gastroenteritis.

Treatment for Surgery or Major Illness in Hospital

In my experience, most Addison's patients are overtreated in hospital. Indications for increased glucocorticoid dosage include surgery, myocardial infarction, sepsis, other severe febrile illnesses, and labor and delivery. On the day of surgery, the patient should receive three times his usual glucocorticoid maintenance dosage before leaving the floor for the operating room, because there may be a considerable delay before intravenous lines are established and there is a delay before steroids exert their effect. Glucocorticoid is most readily administered intravenously during and immediately after surgery as cortisol hemisuccinate (Solu-Cortef), prednisolone (Hydeltrasol Injection), the biologically active form of prednisone, or dexamethasone sodium phosphate. If one gives ten times the maintenance dosage during the 24 hours after the anesthesiologist establishes the intravenous lines (i.e., about 300 mg of cortisol hemisuccinate, 50 mg of prednisolone, or 5 mg of dexamethasone), any complication such as hypotension will not be due to glucocorticoid deficiency and causes such as hemorrhage, sepsis, pulmonary embolus, and myocardial infarction must be investigated and treated. The dosage can be halved the next day, halved again the day after that, and restored to maintenance on the third postoperative day, assuming that there are no major postoperative complications. This is a very conservative regimen. Most patients would do well most of the time with much less glucocorticoid given over a shorter time period. Conversely, occasional patients will require increased glucocorticoid for slightly longer periods of time to avoid anorexia, nausea, and occasional vomiting and postural hypotension. Within rather narrow limits, therefore, the rate of withdrawal must be individualized. The major risk is giving too much steroid for too long a time, masking fever, pain, or hypotension caused by nonendocrine complications that should be identified and treated.

Other severe illnesses should be treated in much the same manner. Uncomplicated infections with temperatures of less than 101° F do not require glucocorticoid adjustment in hospital. High doses of glucocorticoids will suppress fever and reduce pain but also inhibit cellular immunity, polymorphonuclear leukocyte response, and wound healing. They are not a substitute for surgical drainage of abscesses and other therapy directed at the infectious process itself, and they can mask the signs and symptoms of serious infection. Steroids can generally be reduced to the maintenance dosage within 1 or 2 days of uncomplicated labor and delivery.

In general, mineralocorticoid dosage need not be changed in hospital. If high doses of cortisol are being given, its mineralocorticoid activity is sufficient and the sodium in intravenous solutions is usually more than adequate to maintain normal serum electrolyte levels even without mineralocorticoid. However, Addison's disease patients can develop adrenal crisis while taking pure glucocorticoids, such as dexamethasone, when severely stressed. In such circumstances, they require increased salt and fluid, in addition to maintaining high glucocorticoid therapy. In rare patients, those on chronic parenteral nutrition, for example, desoxycorticosterone acetate (Doca, Percorten) may be given, 25 to 50 mg intramuscularly each month, as mineralocorticoid replacement therapy.

SECONDARY ADRENAL INSUFFICIENCY

Patients with secondary adrenal insufficiency should receive glucocorticoid replacement in the same way as patients with primary adrenal insufficiency. With only rare exceptions, however, they do not require mineralocorticoid. Because their renin–angiotensin–aldosterone system is functionally intact, they are not subject to developing adrenal crisis. However, they should wear a Medic-Alert bracelet or necklace, carry an Emergency Medical Information card, have dexamethasone syringes available, and be instructed in the use of glucocorticoid during minor stresses, emergencies, and hospitalizations just like the patient with primary adrenal insufficiency. Most of them will require maintenance therapy with other hormones, as indicated by clinical signs and symptoms and appropriate endocrine tests.

SUGGESTED READING

Baxter JD, Tyrrell JB. The adrenal cortex. In: Felig P, Baxter JD, Broadus AE, Frohman LA, eds. Endocrinology and metabolism. 2nd ed. New York: McGraw-Hill, 1987:581.

Bondy PK. Disorders of the adrenal cortex. In: Wilson JD, Foster DW, eds. Williams textbook of endocrinology. 7th ed. Philadelphia: WB Saunders, 1985:851.

Khalid BAK, Burke CW, Hurley DM, Funder JW, Stockigt JR. Steroid replacement in Addison's disease and in subjects adrenalectomized for Cushing's disease: comparison of various glucocorticoids. J Clin Endocrinol Metab 1982; 55:551–559.

CORTICOSTEROID WITHDRAWAL

NICHOLAS P. CHRISTY, M.D.

Successful withdrawal of a patient from corticosteroid therapy requires the physician to have a firm grasp of essential background information and to formulate clear answers to several questions. One must define "successful withdrawal." One needs to be fully acquainted with the disease the steroids have been used to suppress. One must be certain why corticosteroids were chosen in the first place and why they are now being stopped. The physician has to know in detail the duration of steroid treatment, the exact dosage schedule, and the pharmacologic characteristics of the specific corticosteroid the patient has been receiving. One must be prepared to identify and then deal with any of the various forms of the "corticosteroid withdrawal syndrome." Finally, it need hardly be said that the physician ought to possess intimate knowledge of all pertinent aspects of the patient's personality and the features of the underlying disease that are peculiar to that patient.

PRINCIPLES

Definition of Successful Steroid Withdrawal

An ideal course of steroid withdrawal would be a smooth and rapid transition from the induced state of "tissue" hyperadrenocorticism to total deprivation of exogenous corticosteroid without recrudescence of the basic disorder and without the emergence of either adrenocortical insufficiency due to adrenal suppression or of corticosteroid dependence (to be discussed). This untroubled state of affairs can often be achieved. For example, self-limited, short-lived disorders, such as severe penicillin reactions for which steroid treatment is highly effective, do not recur when corticosteroids are withdrawn. Neither adrenal suppression nor steroid dependence is likely to develop in patients given minute doses—the equivalent of prednisone, 5 mg or less per day even over periods as long as several years, a dosage schedule often used by gynecologists in treating mild forms of adrenal virilism. Nor does clinically significant suppression or dependence occur with large doses—the equivalent of 60 mg or more of prednisone daily—administered over periods as short as 7 to 10 days, a scheme frequently employed in treating, for example, severe acute *Rhus* dermatitides (poison ivy, poison oak, poison sumac).

These rules are generally applicable, but one must recognize that, as with other drugs, patients show wide individual variations in their responses to a given quantity of a given corticosteroid.

When the ideal smooth withdrawal from steroids cannot be achieved, successful management is then defined as gradual stepwise reduction of the corticosteroid dose, with intermittent increases when and if necessary to control flare-ups of the basic disorder or to palliate the symptoms and signs of adrenal insufficiency or corticosteroid dependence. This kind of interrupted downward titration demands vigilance on the part of the physician; in practical terms, frequent follow-up visits by the patient are required.

The Underlying Disease

As suggested before, knowledge of the disease being suppressed or controlled by the corticosteroids enables the physician to predict the likely course of steroid withdrawal and to gauge the probability that signs and symptoms of the disorder being treated will ensue. Such knowledge tells the physician how viligant he or she must be and provides the basic information necessary to design appropriate history taking, physical examination, and laboratory tests in order to detect evidence of recrudescence early, before symptomatically unpleasant or clinically threatening events occur or get out of control. In acute inflammatory or noninflammatory disorders that are immediately life-threatening, steroid withdrawal and the rate of steroid dosage reduction are dictated by the subsidence of the clinical condition. These disorders include, among other medical emergencies, acute adrenocortical insufficiency, allergic crises, shock associated with infection, hypoglycemic coma, water intoxication, central hyperthermia, thyroid storm, and myxedema coma. These conditions, with the exception of adrenal insufficiency, for which steroid therapy is crucial, *may* be improved by high-dose, short-term corticosteroid therapy, but *steroids are not the central element of therapy.* One must, of course, *treat the underlying disease with the appropriate primary modalities as well.* Steroid withdrawal can usually be abrupt without tapering, for the presence or absence of pharmacologic hypercortisolism is not the essential determinant of the patient's recovery.

Most of the patients the physician encounters who present major difficulties in steroid withdrawal suffer from serious hematologic, inflammatory, and immunologic diseases because the diseases themselves are systemic and more or less catastrophic and because high doses of corticosteroid are administered over long periods of time, usually as the principal means of palliating or suppressing the disease. These diseases include acute lymphoblastic leukemia, idiopathic thrombocytopenic purpura, and Hodgkin's disease; ulcerative colitis, chronic active and acute alcoholic hepatitis, and subacute hepatic necrosis; temporal (giant cell) arteritis, polymyositis, classic dermatomyositis, and disseminated lupus erythematosus; autoimmune hemolytic anemia; and severe asthma.

A detailed discussion of all the possible signs, symptoms, and abnormalities of laboratory tests that might mark the resurgence of these disorders during corticosteroid withdrawal would constitute a virtual textbook of internal medicine. The few essential points to be made follows. In many of these conditions, early signs of recurrence may be straightforward if rather general. For example, fever may characterize and be the first evidence of flare-up of leukemia, Hodgkin's disease, lupus, ulcerative colitis, the hepatitides, and the mesenchymal disorders. The physician, knowing this, regulates the rate of steroid withdrawal in part by the presence or absence of fever. Petechiae of skin and mucous membranes and dermal ecchymoses may mark a recurrence of idiopathic thrombocytopenic purpura; abdominal pain, diarrhea, and blood in the stool herald the return of colitis. Appearance of such signs dictates slowing the rate of steroid withdrawal and, in most instances, a temporary increase in steroid dosage. For other diseases, one resorts to a combination of clinical and laboratory findings. An example is the nephrotic syndrome of lupus. If ascites appears, the clinical need is obvious, but recurrent peripheral edema may be subtle. If it is, one is forced to measure the daily loss of urinary protein, which is a more sensitive and earlier marker for escape of the renal lesion from the suppressive effects of the diminishing quantity of circulating corticosteroid. In the hepatitides that can be treated with steroids, the most prudent course is to monitor hepatic function tests frequently. These are more likely to give early warning of recurrence than are clinical signs, such as fever or jaundice. Resorting to such subtleties is clearly not necessary in asthma; the obvious clinical sign, bronchial wheezing, informs patient and physician that the disorder is no longer controlled, and the steroid dosage is regulated accordingly.

Some patients with rheumatoid arthritis, many with regional enteritis (Crohn's disease), some with asthma, and the subset with disseminated lupus who have arthritis as the principal manifestation constitute another special group of steroid-responsive entities. These are treated with chronic low-dose palliative amounts of corticosteroids. They are troublesome to treat during withdrawal of corticosteroids, not because of adrenal suppression but because of apparent flare-ups of the disease upon the slightest reduction in dosage. I have had one patient with regional enteritis whose gastrointestinal symptoms were well controlled with a prednisone dose of 7.5 mg daily; reducing the amount to 5 mg was followed by recurrence of bloody diarrhea. Almost all rheumatologists have treated patients with rheumatoid arthritis who are satisfactorily free of articular pain and stiffness on daily prednisone doses as low as 2.0 and 2.5 mg of prednisone equivalent but whose arthritic symptoms become insupportable when the dosage of steroid is cut, not necessarily abruptly, to 1.0 mg or to zero.

Faced with the problem of withdrawing patients with these four conditions from corticosteroids, the physician is well advised to prepare the patient for a long and tedious period, usually which the dose of corticosteroid is diminished slowly and by minuscule degrees. One must also keep in mind the peculiar tendency of some rheumatoid patients to develop a panmesenchymal reaction, the so-called steroid pseudorheumatism, during steroid withdrawal. Such an occurrence may require the reinstitution of corticosteroids at far higher dosages than the palliative levels that had been used to suppress the basic rheumatoid disease.

Another category of patients, those receiving relatively low-dose chronic corticosteroid treatment to suppress the secretion of adrenocorticotropic hormone (ACTH) by the adenophypophysis, includes persons with idiopathic hirsutism, presumably due to acquired adrenal hyperplasia (acquired adrenal virilism) and those with the several forms of congenital adrenocortical hyperplasia with virilism. The first type, found in adolescent or adult women, requires only modest dosages of prednisone equivalent, on the order of 7.5 mg per day or less. These women generally need treatment only during reproductive life, except for those few who have associated hypertension. Further, the lower doses do not produce untoward effects, and their withdrawal can be accomplished abruptly without eliciting any of the manifestations of corticosteroid withdrawal syndrome, adrenal suppression, or corticosteroid dependence.

As for congenital adrenal hyperplasia, most patients can be treated with relatively low daily doses, so that difficulties with steroid withdrawal are generally not severe. However, this statement must be qualified. One must know precisely what type of adrenal enzymatic lesion is present. For the majority of subjects, the disorder is 21-hydroxylase deficiency with "relative," that is, usually incomplete, lack of cortisol biosynthesis and secretion. Once pituitary-adrenal suppressive therapy with corticoids has brought them successfully through the periods of growth, sexual development, and reproductive function, these individuals do not require further corticosteroid treatment into late adult life and old age. Withdrawal can be carried out abruptly and with impunity. One may wish to add extra steroid cover for intercurrent, severe, acute illness in patients still on suppressive therapy. For the other forms of congenital adrenal hyperplasia, characterized by more nearly complete cortisol deficiency and by blocked aldosterone biosynthesis or hypertension, corticosteroid therapy is both ACTH-suppressive and a form of adrenal steroid replacement. These patients—those with deficits of 3 beta-hydroxysteroid dehydrogenase, 17 alpha-hydroxylase, 11 beta-hydroxylase, and 18-hydroxysteroid dehydrogenase—are committed to a lifelong regimen of steroid medication. Like persons with Addison's disease, these people should never be subjected to steroid withdrawal.

A word should be said about patients, other than those just discussed, who are receiving lifelong adrenal replacement therapy. These are people with Addison's disease (primary adrenocortical insufficiency), those who have had total bilateral adrenalectomy (as for neoplastic disease), patients with secondary adrenocortical insufficiency due to hypopituitarism, and those few who are permanently adrenal-deficient because of hypothalamic-pituitary-adrenocortical (HPA) suppression caused by prolonged high-dose corticosteroid administration (see section on The Various Forms of Corticosteroid Withdrawal Syndrome). The main point to be made about these chronically adrenal-deficient patients is that the *replacement* doses of steroid, which are small and not associated with untoward effects, should *never* be withdrawn. The absolute contraindications to *pharmacologic* doses of corticosteroids—steroid-induced psychosis, herpes simplex, tuberculosis, and other infectious diseases—are not applicable to the small amounts needed for replacement, namely, the equivalent of cortisol, 25 mg per day (the normal daily secretion rate of cortisol normally not exceeding 20 mg). On the contrary, it is worth reemphasizing *the need for higher doses of steroid during most acute intercurrent infectious illnesses in these patients, not lower ones.* One other point concerning the secondary adrenal insufficiency states should be made: unlike in Addison's disease and the salt-losing forms of congenital adrenal hyperplasia, significant aldosterone deficiency does not occur. Measurements of plasma electrolytes are therefore normal in acute emergencies, but these findings do not signify that there is no cortisol deficiency.

Reasons for Starting and Stopping Corticosteroid Therapy

These reasons are plain enough when the managing physician has made all the decisions personally, less so when he or she has inherited a patient from another doctor or another locale. It is essential to familiarize oneself thoroughly with the rationale for the patient's receiving corticosteroids in the first place. We have seen that the basic indications for corticosteroid therapy may be summarized in this way: supportive-"curative," keeping a serious disease at bay, palliative, ACTH-suppressive, and a replacement. Knowing which of the categories a given patient occupies provides clear signals as to what has been expected of the steroid therapeutically, how long it has been given, and what dosage has been used, high or low. This information in turn permits accurate and detailed predictions concerning the likelihood and specific nature of possible recurrences and the probability of HPA suppression. Whether or not corticosteroid dependence supervenes appears to be an individual and unpredictable matter.

The rationale for withdrawal of pharmacologic —i.e., supraphysiologic—doses of corticosteroids should be clear and definite. If the corticosteroid is no longer deemed to be therapeutically effective, it should be discontinued. In cases of herpes simplex, corticosteroids are thought by most clinicians to be *absolutely* contraindicated and should be stopped as rapidly as possible. The appearance of most other viral, bacterial, fungal, protozoan, and metazoan infections during steroid therapy, which increases host susceptibility to all those infectious diseases, is regarded by most authorities as a *relative* contraindication. The procedure is to weigh the seriousness of the disease for which the steroid is being given against the threat posed by the intercurrent infectious insult. One cannot make a general rule.

As for the untoward effects of steroids themselves, for example, iatrogenic Cushing's syndrome (see the chapter *Cushing's Syndrome*), only a few dictate discontinuance of the drugs. The most definite of these is steroid-induced psychosis. Less commonly, the induction of uncontrollable diabetes in a patient with genetic diabetes forces one to stop corticosteroid treatment. The same is rarely true of steroid-related severe hypertension, which can usually be controlled by antihypertensive agents even if the steroid is continued at an undiminished dosage. Incapacitating osteopenia with pathologic fractures is an uncommon indication for withdrawing corticosteroids, as is pseudotumor cerebri (benign intracranial hypertension). Other untoward effects that may indicate withdrawal are peptic ulceration of the stomach or duodenum with hemorrhage or perforation, severe inhibition of growth in children, and crippling impairment of wound healing. The decision to withdraw steroids in each instance is again made by balancing the risks of the untoward effect against the benefit with respect to the underlying disease. As before, there is no simple rule applicable to all cases.

Duration of Therapy, Dosage Schedule, Specific Steroid Used

This information enables the physician to assess the likelihood of clinically significant steroid-induced HPA suppression with concomitant inability of the patient's HPA system to respond to clinical stress. It should be apparent that the longer the course of steroid therapy and the higher the dosage, the more likely is HPA suppression to occur. The relation between duration of dosage and magnitude of dose is complex, and information is incomplete. A few definite statements can be made. Patients' susceptibility to HPA suppression by steroids is extraordinarily variable. Some patients may receive corticosteroids for years without impairment in their response to provocative tests of HPA functions. Others, treated with prednisone, 15 mg daily for a week, show flattening of the adrenocortical response to ACTH. In general, patients treated with chronic low-dose palliation (as for rheumatoid arthritis), that is, with prednisone equivalent of 10 mg daily or less, show little or no impairment of HPA activity. Most patients with serious diseases treated with prolonged high-dose therapy (leukemia, lupus) have biochemical evidence of HPA suppression. Most people undergoing intensive short-term therapy (as for infectious shock) are not suppressed. People treated with high doses over long periods with the alternate-day schedule of corticosteroid administration have relative or partial preservation of HPA function, but given the present state of knowledge, they must still be considered at risk.

In numerical terms, any patient who has received the corticosteroid equivalent of 20 to 30 mg of prednisone per day for more than 3 to 4 weeks should be suspected of having biochemical (if not clinically significant) HPA suppression. Since so few data are available relating duration and amount of corticosteroid therapy to rate of recovery of a putatively suppressed HPA axis, a corticosteroid-treated patient should be considered to have possible HPA suppression, at least biochemically, for a year after cessation of the corticosteroid. This view is probably too conservative from the scientific point of view, but clinically it is prudent and thoroughly safe.

Further numerical data from stress tests (bacterial pyrogen) indicate that patients given 12.5 mg or more of prednisone equivalent daily for 1 month to 8 years uniformly show HPA suppression, whereas those receiving 4 mg or less for the same period do not. Suppressed patients are still suppressed 1 month after withdrawal from steroid therapy but have recovered by 5 months; alternate-day corticosteroid treatment usually does not suppress the HPA axis. One should note that the range of dosage between 4.0 and 12.5 mg of prednisone equivalent constitutes an area of ambiguity. The prudent therapist should probably consider such patients as having received the 12.5 mg or higher dose.

In the light of such information, one sees that detailed knowledge of duration and dosage schedule permits a fairly accurate calculation of probability that the HPA system will be suppressed.

The only point to be made about the specific corticosteroid used relates to the duration of drug action. Cortisone and cortisol (the "native" hormone), rarely used in pharmacotherapy because of their salt-retaining property in susceptible individuals, have short half-lives in plasma. The semisynthetic corticosteroid analogues are all less firmly bound to specific plasma corticosteroid-binding globulin (transcortin) and albumin than is cortisol, but all have longer plasma half-lives than cortisol; in the cases of prednisone, prednisolone, and methylprednisolone, slightly longer; triamcinolone, somewhat longer; and dexamethasone and betamethasone, much longer. Although the relationship between duration of action and plasma half-life is irregular, in general these properties mean that the longer-lasting steroids tend to induce a more constant state of "tissue" hyperadrenocorticism, a constancy conducive to a greater likelihood of HPA suppression for an equivalent dose.

The Various Forms of Corticosteroid Withdrawal Syndrome

The specific biologic type of steroid withdrawal syndrome determines its management. This section defines the types and sets out the methods for identifying them.

No Withdrawal Syndrome

Most patients of the millions receiving steroids undergo withdrawal without clinical difficulty. An unknown number may have subtle recrudescences of underlying disease or minor degrees of HPA suppression, but these are not clinically visible to patient or physician. No treatment is indicated.

Hypothalamic-Pituitary-Adrenocortical Suppression

The incidence and prevalence of true adrenocortical insufficiency due to HPA suppression are not known because the symptoms are often vague and difficult to distinguish from those of corticosteroid dependence, because systemic tests of HPA function are not routinely made, and because not enough data are available to allow a firm correlation between tests of HPA function and effective response of the HPA system to clinical stress. Normal biochemical behavior in a provocative test of the HPA system does not necessarily mean a normal adrenocortical capacity to withstand an acute episode of illness, and biochemical evidence of HPA suppression does not always predict an inability to make an adequate and appropriate hormonal response to acute illness, or trauma, or surgery. Nevertheless, tests of HPA response are the only objective guides available, and so such tests should be done where possible, and the results cautiously interpreted as if they were predictive (to be discussed).

The symptoms and signs of corticosteroid-induced adrenal insufficiency are much like those of Addison's disease. The most common manifestations are weakness, lassitude, easy fatigability, mental depression, hypotension, postural hypotension, and undue prostration in the face of minor illnesses, such as coryza and mild viral gastroenteritis. Addisonian pigmentation is not seen because pituitary ACTH secretion is suppressed, and hyponatremia and hyperkalemia do not occur because corticosteroid suppression of ACTH has no lasting or quantitatively major effect upon aldosterone production. The nonobjective elements of this clinical picture cannot easily be separated from those of psychological or physiologic dependence on corticosteroids except by provocative tests of HPA function.

The clinician has a choice of many procedures that test the whole HPA system: insulin hypoglycemia, vasopressin, bacterial pyrogen, and corticotropin-releasing hormone, for example. These are cumbersome, stressful, and require hospitalization. The adrenocortical response to ACTH is simpler, less traumatic, correlates well with the other tests of HPA function, and parallels most closely the response of the adrenal cortex to clinical stress. The preferred method is to withhold the corticosteroid for 12 to 24 hours, determine baseline plasma cortisol level at 8 AM, administer 250 μg of synthetic (proportional to amino acids 1 to 24) ACTH extra- or intramuscularly, and repeat the plasma cortisol measurement 60 and 120 minutes later. This procedure is safe and virtually devoid of side effects; the unexplained hypotension and prostration during administration of conventional ACTH to some patients with Addison's disease do not occur. Normal baseline values for plasma cortisol are 7 to 23 μg per deciliter, poststimulation values are 19 to 43 μg per deciliter, and the normal increment is greater than 6 to about 30. A deficient rise in plasma cortisol level after synthetic ACTH should be interpreted as evidence of HPA suppression; a subnormal cortisol response renders untenable the exclusive diagnosis of psychological dependence on corticosteroids.

Establishing the presence of HPA suppression rests on four elements: a plausible clinical syndrome, absence of recurrent disease whose symptoms mimic those of HPA suppression, rigorous laboratory demonstration of HPA insufficiency, and relief of the clinical syndrome by *replacement* doses of corticosteroid, not pharmacologic doses.

Psychological or Physical Dependence on Corticosteroids

The diagnosis of such dependence is made by elimination: recrudescent disease is absent, and HPA suppression is biochemically excluded. In those circumstances, a patient who cannot tolerate steroid withdrawal, or who demands increased doses, and who evinces weakness, lethargy, mood changes, or delirium when the amount of hormone is being reduced can be considered as corticosteroid-dependent or, in a sense, habituated. In the presence of anorexia; nausea; weight loss; fine desquamation of the skin of the face, hands, and feet; musculoskeletal aches; arthralgias; and fever, the clinician can reasonably suspect physical dependence on corticosteroids. The symptoms and signs are alleviated by *pharmacologic* doses of steroid, not by replacement or physiologic doses.

The psychological and subjective features of this type of withdrawal syndrome were originally ascribed to underlying and preexisting (that is presteroid) psychic disturbances. Longer experience has shown that the presteroid personality has no detectable bearing on the likelihood of corticosteroid habituation, with the single exception that persons known to be or to have been addicted to narcotics tend to become dependent upon steroids as well.

Symptomatic Flare-Up of the Underlying Disease

Detection of this kind of withdrawal syndrome depends on the reappearance of the subjective and objective manifestations of the disease being treated with steroids. The principles and methods have been outlined. If HPA function tests are normal, a given clinical picture cannot be attributed to adrenal insufficiency. Corticosteroid dependence is not always so easy to differentiate. For example, many of the symptoms and signs listed in the previous section on corticosteroid dependence would be indistinguishable from those of a recurrence of rheumatoid arthritis. But the distinction between disease flare-up and steroid dependence is usually clear and straightforward in patients with asthma and the severe illnesses for which long-term high-dose corticosteroid treatment is given.

Combination

Finally, perhaps the most common form of steroid withdrawal syndrome is a combination of the three syndromes just discussed. The best way to deal with this set of problems is to inject as much objectivity as possible into the clinical setting. One does this by routinely performing the simple ACTH-plasma cortisol test of HPA function and by undertaking careful physical and laboratory investigations for objective criteria of recrudescent disease.

Peculiarities of Patient and Disease

For optimal management of the patient undergoing steroid withdrawal, the physician must be aware of relevant aspects of that patient's personality; his or her tolerance for pain and willingness or unwillingness to undergo a long and tedious process of dosage reduction; the interplay of the patient's illness with his or her family, occupation, and social life; and whether or not there is a history of prior addiction to other pharmacologic agents. The physician must know about absolute and relative contraindications, for example, the status of tuberculin reactivity, which should be monitored every 6 months, and about the details of possible drug interactions between the corticosteroid and other medications the patient is receiving. With respect to the disease being treated with steroids, the therapist must know precisely what symptoms and signs predominate in the particular patient and which manifestations tend to appear earliest during recurrences. For most asthmatics, cough, dyspnea, or wheezing or combinations of these are the straightforward harbingers of recurrence. As suggested before, there is more variety in other diseases. One patient with leukemia may evince easy bruising, and another, fever, as the first sign that steroid treatment is failing. Some patients with rheumatoid arthritis may complain of myalgias and stiffness during corticosteroid withdrawal, others of objective arthritis in two or three joints. Knowledge of the natural history of the disease in the specific patient and of his or her specific reactions in the specific patient and of his or her specific reactions to treatment is thus essential to permit early detection of the need for slowing the rate of steroid reduction or for temporarily increasing the dose of corticosteroid.

THERAPEUTIC ALTERNATIVES

These alternatives consist of using other nonhormonal drugs in place of corticosteroids, small or homeopathic doses of steroids, the alternate-day schedule of glucocorticoid therapy, or ACTH.

In the severe diseases often treated with long-term, high-dose steroids, other immunosuppressive agents may enable the physician to avoid corticosteroids if there is good reason to do so, that is, if absolute or relative contraindications exist. Immunosuppressives may sometimes suffice in lupus, leukemia, and the hepatitides. In asthma, inhaled steroids may induce less HPA suppression than steroids given systemically; other nonsteroidal inhalants, cromolyn, or other bronchodilators, singly or in combination, may palliate the disease without steroids. As for rheumatoid arthritis, corticosteroids are being used less and less, and other anti-inflammatory agents, for example, indomethacin, are given instead.

Minute doses of corticosteroids may control the manifestations of inflammatory and immunologic disease, but such low doses are therapeutically ineffective. The physician may then resort to higher doses, but on the alternate-day schedule. It should be noted here that patients may be converted from the daily to the alternate-day schedule in mid-course of their treatment or of steroid withdrawal; this change permits HPA recovery to occur but does not accelerate that process.

Corticotropin (ACTH) has been used in intermittent dosage schedules *during steroid therapy* to prevent adrenocortical insufficiency due to HPA suppression. Although biochemical HPA response to both insulin and ACTH response tests is usually preserved, the subjective and objective signs of steroid withdrawal syndrome are as severe as with steroid therapy alone. The method has no value.

ACTH given *after* a course of steroids accelerates the return of adrenocortical function, but this return is transitory; the poststeroid hyporesponsiveness can be detected again within a week after the ACTH treatment. One would not expect to improve hypothalamic or pituitary function in these circumstances. In fact, ACTH may sometimes exert a negative feedback inhibitory influence on endogenous ACTH secretion, and anti-ACTH antibodies against the native hormone may be formed. This method is also without value.

ACTH given *instead of steroids* has some advantages. Allegedly there are fewer serious undesirable effects. Growth curves in children are more nearly normal. Some clinicians believe it is easier to withdraw patients from ACTH than from steroids. The HPA system is more likely to remain biochemically intact. *But these benefits are outweighed by the disadvantages.* ACTH has to be given by injection. No disease responds better clinically to ACTH than to steroid therapy. A moderate number of patients have sustained severe hypersensitivity reactions to ACTH, and a few have suffered intra-adrenal hemorrhage. Rarely, acute and catastrophic collapse, presumably due to adrenal failure, has occurred after a prolonged course of ACTH, especially in the face of simultaneous anticoagulant therapy. The maximum amount of endogenous cortisol secretion that can be stimulated by exogenous ACTH is not more than 250 mg per day (or the equivalent of 60 mg of prednisone); many diseases (acute leukemia, lupus nephritis) require more than that. Finally, there is some evidence that exogenous ACTH may interfere with the biosynthesis and release of pituitary ACTH. These seem sufficient reasons to discard this method.

PREFERRED APPROACH

Textbooks and treatises on therapeutics provide recommendations and recipes for corticosteroid withdrawal as if the only hazard were HPA suppression, but there are others as well (for example, recurrence of the disease for which the corticosteroid was being administered, psychosis, gastrointestinal bleeding, pathologic fracture, or other serious manifestations of iatrogenic Cushing's syndrome—see Reasons for Starting and Stopping Corticosteroid Therapy above). The foregoing analysis indicates that the disease that has been treated, its recurrence or failure to recur, the therapeutic indications for steroid therapy, the details of the corticosteroid regimen and its duration, the exact type of corticosteroid withdrawal syndrome, and the idiosyncrasies of the particular patient and the particular disease all influence the choice of method for withdrawing a patient from corticosteroids. No single, simple approach will do for all.

General Considerations

The category of disease dictates the intensity and duration of steroid treatment, and that regimen indicates in general the method of withdrawal.

For acute, catastrophic conditions (such as septic shock) treated for no more than 2 to 6 days with high-dose steroids (hundreds of milligrams to grams of prednisone equivalent daily), the physician can stop the steroid therapy as abruptly as it was started. The activity of the precipitating condition, not HPA suppression, dictates the rate of tapering the steroid dose.

For the serious inflammatory, immunologic, and hematologic disorders (such as disseminated lupus) treated with prolonged high-dose steroid therapy (more than 15 mg of prednisone daily), withdrawal must be gradual because of the dangers of acutely recurrent disease. HPA suppression is not an important consideration until the corticosteroid dose reaches or approaches zero. In those patients, acute secondary adrenal insufficiency may be precipitated or exacerbated if the disease flares up explosively during steroid withdrawal. If the patient has not been maintained throughout the course of steroid treatment on the alternate-day schedule, it does no good to switch to it as a prelude to steroid withdrawal, since the process of HPA recovery is not accelerated thereby. The integrity of the HPA system is more or less maintained by the alternate-day schedule only when alternation is continued throughout most of the course.

In the inflammatory disorders (e.g., rheumatoid arthritis) managed with prolonged low-dose palliative steroid therapy (2 to 10 mg of prednisone per day), corticosteroid withdrawal must be gradual, both because of recurrence of the disease and because of corticosteroid *dependence*. HPA suppression is probably not much of a factor. The doses have to be decreased by small steps and slowly, usually with intermittent plateaus or slight increases in dosage. Withdrawal may take a year or more, and a small portion of patients do not tolerate the total elimination of steroid therapy.

As suggested before, the low doses used in deliberate long-term inhibition of pituitary ACTH secretion (0.75 mg dexamethasone or equivalent daily as in congenital adrenal hyperplasia) do not seriously impair the cortisol-secreting facet of HPA function. Gradual lowering of steroid doses is therefore unnecessary.

Specific Methods of Corticosteroid Withdrawal

For Hypothalamic-Pituitary-Adrenal Suppression

Patients in this category are chiefly those with a serious disease that has been treated with prolonged high-dose daily steroid therapy. A good rule of thumb is that any patient who looks cushingoid probably has significant HPA suppression. The critical dose of corticosteroid above which cushingoid appearance almost universally occurs is 15 mg of prednisone daily or the equivalent. Since the dosage range for this category of patients is approximately 15 to 120 mg of prednisone per day and the duration of treatment is more than 3 to 4 weeks, one assumes that all patients in this group are biochemically HPA suppressed, whether the clinical degree of HPA suppression (generally difficult to detect) is significant or not.

A second rule depends on the reasons for stopping steroid treatment. The rate of withdrawal should be as rapid as possible in the face of major untoward effects of steroids or absolute contraindications to them, such as herpes simplex, varicella infections, or the abrupt appearance of psychosis. If the aim of withdrawal is to take advantage of a strong likelihood that the disease is in remission (for example, when it has been possible to lower the steroid dosage considerably without recurrence), then the rate of dosage reduction should be gradual. This is the procedure in many instances of disseminated lupus, ulcerative colitis, and acute lymphoblastic leukemia.

A third precept is that the physician should subdue his or her own excessive anxiety about corticosteroid withdrawal. With minimal vigilance, no patient dies from this process. Adrenal insufficiency does not happen suddenly, and HPA suppression as a cause of death has been proved only rarely. Disease recurrences, with the rare exception of such entities as grand mal seizures due to cerebral microvascular disease in lupus, are not fatal. The aim is to spare the patient avoidable sudden, intense flare-ups of disease. Since corticosteroids seldom eradicate the chronic disorders for which they are used, steroid removal merely allows a condition, hitherto apparently held in check, to show itself. During withdrawal, one wishes to blunt these manifestations as much as possible.

The fourth rule concerning this group of patients is that steroid dependence in a few, HPA suppression in a very few, and flare-up of disease in most govern the rate of withdrawal from steroids. This gradual lowering of dosage is directed toward reducing the probability of both clinically significant adrencortical insufficiency and recrudescent illness.

In this category of persons given long-term, high-dose steroid therapy, the clinical problem is that the disease (to the extent that one can separate disease from host) tolerates steroid withdrawal poorly; the host (with the same reservation) tolerates withdrawal relatively well.

Method. No prescription can be given that suits all patients and all diseases. What follows is a practical outline that is generally applicable but must be modified to fit individual needs.

For the patients whose steroid therapy is interrupted because of an acute emergency that contraindicates corticosteroid administration (generalized viral infection, psychotic break), the principle is to *cut the dose rapidly to an amount just enough above the physiologic level* (prednisone, 5 mg, or cortisone, 20 to 25 mg) to sustain a presumably HPA-suppressed, that is, adrenal-deficient patient through the stress of the intercurrent illness. Specifically, for the infectious complications, the daily steroid dosage is reduced from the maintenance level of 30 to 120 mg prednisone (for example) to 10 to 15 mg within 1 to 2 days, carefully observing vital signs and the activity of the basic disease. Since disseminated herpetic infection, for example, can be *immediately* fatal, whereas most of the steroid-treated systemic diseases are not, one errs on the low side of corticosteroid administration to minimize the immunosuppressive effect, that is, one lowers the dose still more to 5 to 10 mg of prednisone daily or 5 mg and 10 mg on alternate days, or less if possible. In managing steroid psychosis, the dosage can be at that level or lower—that is, physiologic—depending on the hyperactivity of the disturbed patient. In the event of severe trauma or a surgical emergency, patients receiving high-dose steroid therapy should be treated with parenterally administered corticosteroids.

For the majority of patients in this high-dose category whose steroids are being eliminated in anticipation of a partial or complete remission, withdrawal can usually be accomplished smoothly within 4 weeks. Before starting withdrawal, the physician carefully notes and records all objective physical signs of the basic disease and obtains the essential laboratory data that will be used as indices of its activity. If one starts from a dosage range of 15 to 40 mg of prednisone or equivalent daily, the amount of steroid can be reduced by decrements of 2.5 to 5 mg every second or third day until a physiologic level, 5 mg daily, is reached within 1 to 2 weeks. This reduction can usually be done with impunity. Beginning at the higher dosage ranges, above 40 to 120 mg of prednisone per day, the dosage is lowered by decrements of 10 to 40 mg every 3 to 7 days. The reduction can be discontinued through minor recurrences of the basic disease, but if the flare-up is serious or incapacitating, the dose is raised again to an amount just sufficient to suppress the clinical or laboratory manifestations, and a more gradual reduction is attempted. It may be necessary to add other therapeutic agents, for example, immunosuppressants or cytotoxic drugs, if these are not already being given. Switching the patient to the alternate-day steroid schedule during attempted steroid withdrawal is probably not useful and may only interpose another time-consuming step in an already lengthy procedure. By the third to fourth week, after a steady decrement of steroid dosage or after a series of decrements, brief increments, further decrements, or periods of plateau, the amount of steroid ought to have arrived at a physiologic level, 5 mg of prednisone daily or 0.75 mg of dexamethasone. At this point, after the patient has been shown to tolerate this dosage for 3 to 7 days, the steroid is changed to 20 to 25 mg of hydrocortisone or cortisone (a physiologic dose of the physiologic hormone, the steroid with the shortest biologic action), given as a single morning dose to allow the maximal opportunity for resurgence of the HPA system.

During the fourth week, a plasma cortisol determination is made at 8 AM, and that day's cortisone dose is withheld. Most patients then have a cortisol level of less than 10 μg per deciliter, a value likely to persist for 6 to 9 months after the initiation of corticosteroid withdrawal. At about the fourth to sixth week, the cortisone dosage is again reduced to 10 mg of cortisone, given as a single morning dose; this is not enough steroid to foster the continuance of iatrogenic Cushing's syndrome or to suppress the HPA system, but it is sufficient to provide a cushion against adrenocortical insufficiency under basal conditions. In medical emergencies, such as acute infections, trauma, or surgery, and in minor illnesses or small-scale interventive procedures (endoscopy, dental work), steroid cover is necessary. By the sixth to ninth month, the 8 AM plasma cortisol level, which may be measured about every 2 months, should have returned to a value greater than 10 μg per deciliter. Then the physician can assume that the basal HPA function has recovered and the morning dose of cortisone can be stopped, but steroid cover for emergencies is still required.

Nine or more months after the start of withdrawal, the integrity of the entire HPA system should have been restored. There is not much point in performing an ACTH stimulation test until this time because full HPA capacity to respond to provocative tests may take 9 to 12 months or more. During this period, a synthetic ACTH (Synacthen, cosyntropin) test is done; when the increment of plasma cortisol is in range of more than 6 to 30 μg per deciliter, HPA recovery is judged to be complete, and steroid cover for medical emergencies should theoretically not be required. Nevertheless, the correlation between biochemical tests of HPA function and HPA capacity to react to clinical stress is uncertain, so that for the first 12 to 16 months after the beginning of corticosteroid withdrawal, steroid cover should be instituted for acute stresses or in the event that manifestations suggesting adrenocortical insufficiency appear.

As stated previously, ACTH has no place in the treatment of the corticosteroid withdrawal syndrome or in the management of steroid withdrawal. Since the HPA-suppressed patient has an inadequate adrenocortical capacity to respond to endogenous or exogenous corticotropin, ACTH administration does not stimulate enough cortisol secretion to protect the patient from adrenal insufficiency during stress. Therefore, ACTH as a therapy has no value.

For Corticosteroid Dependence

This category includes patients with rheumatoid arthritis and some asthmatics maintained on long-term low-dose palliative therapy. Despite the low doses (less than 15 mg of prednisone daily), these people are more difficult to bring through withdrawal than are most of those receiving prolonged high-dose corticosteroid regimens. For unknown reasons, this group evinces a greater tendency to become dependent on corticosteroids. It is not known whether the dependence is psychological, physiologic, or both. The dangers of corticosteroid withdrawal are less than in patients on high does, but the likelihood of failure to achieve withdrawal is greater. The clinical problem is that the disease tolerates withdrawal relatively well, whereas the host tolerates it poorly or not at all.

For practical purposes, HPA suppression does not present difficulties during withdrawal, except that the cautious physician provides steroid cover if medical emergencies supervene during the process. Plasma cortisol measurement and ACTH tests are unnecessary. Particularly in rheumatoid arthritis, reduction of the steroid dose must be regular and deliberate. The physician has to make every effort to enlist the full cooperation and tolerance of the patient. Decrements in dosage should not exceed 1 mg of prednisone equivalent every 1 to 2 months; at that rate, withdrawal may require a year or more. The physician should not try to hasten the withdrawal process or attempt alternate-day schedules; such maneuvers may precipitate "steroid pseudo-rheumatism"—more likely a manifestation of corticosteroid withdrawal than of recurrent arthritis—which requires raising the steroid dose again, sometimes to levels above the starting dose. For mild to moderate exacerbations, increased amounts of salicylate may be given and indomethacin added. The physician must be careful about salicylates; corticosteroids enhance renal clearance of aspirin, and, when the steroid dosage is reduced, blood values of salicylate may rise to the toxic range in some patients. Monitoring of plasma salicylate levels permits appropriate titration of aspirin dosage.

Patients with asthma are almost as difficult to withdraw from steroids as those with rheumatoid arthritis. Reduction of the steroid dose must be gradual, but the decrements need not be as exquisitely small as for rheumatoid patients, and the variety of other effective medications (for example, systemic or inhaled bronchodilators) offers a broader choice in mitigating flare-ups during steroid withdrawal. As in the arthritis subjects, these patients must be persuaded to cooperate fully with the withdrawal procedure.

In this category of patients, the physician must be prepared to fail. An unknown proportion of people with these two diseases cannot or will not tolerate life without corticosteroids. In my opinion, this is because of corticosteroid dependence or habituation, not uncontrollable disease; but a clinical impression of steroid dependence does not give the physician license to adopt a high moral tone toward his dependent—some might say "addicted"—patient. The corticosteroid dependency syndrome, comprising objective and subjective signs, might as well be viewed as an organic illness. The only effective treatment is the lowest possible dosage of steroid, as little as 1 to 2.5 mg of prednisone daily. Such small amounts lie below the physiologic secretion rate of cortisol in equivalence. That these few milligrams effectively relieve symptoms is probably explained by the fact that the low dose of corticoid does not suppress the HPA system; therefore, the administered dose, given in the morning, is simply additive to the normal daily secretion rate of cortisol. Since there is no danger of HPA suppression or of iatrogenic Cushing's syndrome with such minute amounts of steroid, the physician has no good reason to withhold what the patient demands in any case.

For Flare-Ups of the Steroid-Treated Disease

Consideration of *recurrent* disease during steroid withdrawal is necessarily woven into the foregoing discussions concerning HPA suppression and corticosteroid dependence. This interweaving emphasizes the difficulty in separating, on clinical grounds, the manifestations of the three elements. This is not difficult in flagrant systemic diseases like ulcerative colitis and disseminated lupus or disorders like asthma, which are marked by some clear and unmistakable sign. But in rheumatoid arthritis, for example, a syndrome—occurring during steroid withdrawal—of weakness, lassitude, muscle aches, joint stiffness with only minimal swelling or redness, and low-grade fever can reasonably be interpreted as HPA insufficiency, corticosteroid dependence, or a mild recrudescence of the rheumatoid process. Serologic tests for mesenchymal disease may be somewhat informative but only rarely provide a definite diagnosis of recurrence. Provocative tests of HPA function may show normal or subnormal biochemical response, but the relation between test and clinical adequacy or deficiency of the HPA system is irregular and obscure. The physician must therefore be prepared to deal with some patients in whom the three threads—status of the HPA system, corticosteroid dependence, and mild flare-up of disease—are almost impossible to disentangle. In such people, the clinical syndrome is relieved by administration of low-dose corticosteroids. This maneuver is not intellectually rewarding for the physician but leads to a satisfactory clinical result for the patient.

SUGGESTED READING

Amatruda TT, Hurst MM, D'Esopo ND. Certain endocrine and metabolic facets of the steroid withdrawal syndrome. J Clin Endocrinol Metab 1965; 25:1207–1217.

Baxter, JD, Tyrell JB. Actions of glucocorticoids. In: Felig P, Baxter JD, Broadus AE, et al. Endocrinology and metabolism. 2nd ed. New York: McGraw-Hill, 1987:544.

Dixon RB, Christy NP. On the various forms of corticosteroid withdrawal syndrome. Am J Med 1980; 68:224–230.

Todd JK, Ressman M, Caston SA. Corticosteroid therapy for patients with toxic shock syndrome. JAMA 1984; 252:3399–3402.

HYPOALDOSTERONISM

JAMES C. MELBY, M.D.
GEORGE T. GRIFFING, M.D.

Isolated hypoaldosteronism, a selective deficiency of aldosterone secretion without alteration in cortisol production, results in a persistent hyperkalemia and modest renal salt wasting. The hyperkalemia may be associated with profound muscle weakness and cardiac arrhythmias, but these and other clinical manifestations are reversed by administration of exogenous mineralocorticoids such as fludrocortisone acetate. Isolated hypoaldosteronism may result from inborn errors in the biosynthesis or action of aldosterone, or it may be acquired. The following are the various causes of the isolated form of the disorder:

1. Mineralocorticoid resistance (pseudohypoaldosteronism).
2. Inborn errors in aldosterone biosynthesis (deficiencies in corticosterone methyloxidase [CMO] types I and II).
3. Failure of zona glomerulosa function of the adrenal gland: (a) pharmacologic (heparin and polysulfated glycosaminoglycan induced); (b) autoimmune, associated with idiopathic hypoparathyroidism.
4. Altered function of the renin-angiotensin system: (a) postunilateral adrenalectomy for an aldosterone-producing adenoma; (b) syndrome of hyporeninemic hypoaldosteronism.

Aldosterone resistance has been described in which the target cells (renal tubular epithelium) appear to be unable to respond to mineralocorticoids. This disorder has been called pseudohypoaldosteronism. Inborn errors in the CMO enzyme have been described for both CMO-I and CMO-II (Fig. 1), the most common of which is a CMO type II deficiency. This condition is inherited as an autosomal recessive; its onset, observed between 1 week and 3 months of age, is characterized by dehydration, vomiting, and failure to grow and thrive. Hyponatremia, hyperkalemia, and metabolic alkalosis are uniformly present; plasma renin activity (PRA) is elevated; and plasma aldosterone levels are low. On the other hand, plasma 18-hydroxycorticosterone levels are markedly elevated, and the ratio of 18-hydroxycorticosterone to alderosterone in plasma exceeds 5. The ratio of the urinary metabolite of 18-hydroxycorticosterone, 18-OH-THA, to the metabolite of aldosterone, TH-aldo, is also greater than 5.

Pharmacologic agents such as cyclosporine, heparin sodium, and calcium channel blockers specifically inhibit aldosterone biogenesis by the zona glomerulosa of the adrenal gland. Cyclosporin A produces hypoaldosteronism by dual effects on the adrenal cortex: first, an acute blockade of the angiotensin II-induced aldosterone production, and second, an inhibition of growth and steroidogenic capacity of adrenocortical cells. The latter effect may be caused by an impairment of protein synthesis.

Zona glomerulosa function can also be destroyed by an adrenalitis associated with idiopathic hypoparathyroidism, somewhat akin to idiopathic Addison's disease. Most commonly, isolated hypoaldosteronism results from or is part of altered function of the renin-angiotensin system.

The syndrome of hyporeninemic hypoaldosteronism is not uncommon and, in all probability, is caused either by prolonged impairment of renin secretion after juxtaglomerular cell destruction or by reduced conversion of inactive to active renin. Such hypoaldosteronism is also possibly due to impaired synthesis of the prostaglandins (PGE_2 and PGI_2) by the renal cortex; these prostaglandins are responsible for the stimulation of renin secretion. The syndrome of hyporeninemic hypoaldosteronism occurs in middle-aged and elderly individuals (median age 68 years) and in more males than females. Chronic insufficiency occurs in 80 percent of cases, and diabetes mellitus in less than 50 percent. Hyperkalemia has been observed in all, hyperchloremic metabolic acidosis in less than 70 percent, and mild to moderate hyponatremia in 50 percent. Both plasma aldosterone and PRA are low and (in nearly all cases) cannot be stimulated by appropriate maneuvers. Once recognized, the syndrome of hyporeninemic hypoaldosteronism should be treated with fludrocortisone acetate in a dose of between 0.1 mg and 1.0 mg per day. This dose is equivalent to between 200 and 2,000 μg of aldosterone. Ninety percent of patients then become normokalemic, but it is occasionally necessary to use potassium-wasting diuretics in addition.

Patients with the acquired immunodeficiency syndrome and persistent hyperkalemia may have ei-

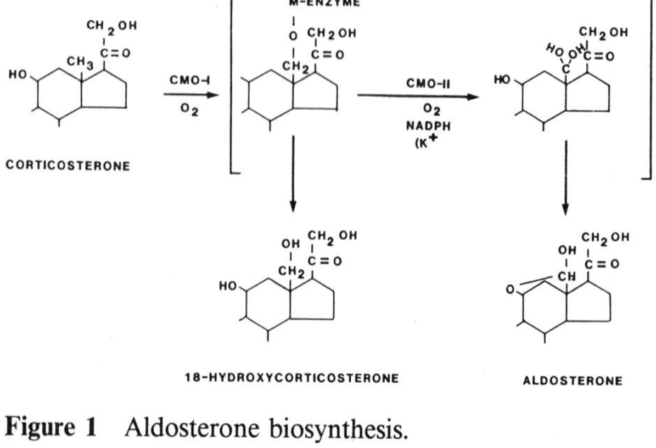

Figure 1 Aldosterone biosynthesis.

ther adrenal insufficiency or, less frequently, hyporeninemic hypoaldosteronism. The hypoaldosterone patients usually have adequate aldosterone stimulation, suggesting that inadequate renin was the cause of the hypoaldosteronism. Treatment with fludrocortisone (0.1 to 0.2 mg per day) produces normalization of serum potassium levels.

IgM monoclonal gammopathy has been associated with nodular glomerulosclerosis, a concentrating defect, and hyporeninemic hypoaldosteronism. The hyperaldosteronism is associated with decreasing renal function, suggesting that kappa light-chain nephropathy is a cause of this syndrome. Chemotherapy appears to have some beneficial effect in maintaining renal function.

PREVENTION AND ANCILLARY TREATMENT

Once the diagnosis of the syndrome of hyporeninemic hypoaldosteronism has been made, factors that precipitate or perpetuate suppression of renin biogenesis, aldosterone biogenesis, or both should be avoided. Diabetes mellitus is the most common cause of hyporeninemic hypoaldosteronism in the United States, and the successful treatment of diabetes mellitus improves nearly every level of the renin-aldosterone axis. It is also the most treatable cause.

Avoidance of Factors That Tend to Suppress Renin Secretion, Aldosterone Secretion, or Both

Volume Expansion

Chronic volume expansion is a well-known cause of renin suppression. It results in hypoaldosteronism and, in some clinical situations, hyperkalemia. Hypoaldosteronism from volume expansion occurs in postadrenalectomy patients following surgical excision of an aldosterone-producing adenoma. These patients can develop severe hyperkalemia and hypotension lasting several days to several weeks after surgery. Hypoaldosteronism also occurs in patients chronically ingesting sodium bicarbonate (baking soda), usually to treat gastrointestinal ulcer disease. Another rare cause of hypoaldosteronism is Gordon's syndrome. This syndrome is associated with renin suppression, hypoaldosteronism, and hyperkalemia and is believed to be caused by excessive sodium reabsorption at the distal tubule.

Medication

Many medications can interfere at multiple points in the renin-aldosterone axis. Avoidance of these drugs can be of major importance in the clinical management of hypoaldosteronism.

Beta-Blocking Adrenergic Drugs. These drugs interfere with renin secretion and are associated with hyporeninemic hypoaldosteronism. Juxtaglomerular cells that synthesize and secrete renin contain beta-adrenergic receptors. Either intrinsic neuronal or extrinsic adrenergic stimuli trigger these receptors, resulting in an immediate release of renin. Propranolol and similar agents are beta-adrenergic receptor blockers that prevent renin release and produce hyporeninemic hypoaldosteronism. These drugs should be avoided in patients with known hypoaldosteronism or in diabetic patients with latent hypoaldosteronism.

Prostaglandin Synthetase Inhibitors. These drugs, which specifically inhibit cyclo-oxygenase, block renin release and have been associated with severe hyperkalemia caused by hyporeninemic hypoaldosterone. PGE_2 directly stimulates renin release, probably by a direct action on the juxtaglomerular apparatus. Furosemide-induced renin release is blunted by indomethacin and other prostaglandin synthetase inhibitors. Use of indomethacin and similar prostaglandin inhibitors is widespread in clinical therapeutics. Use of these drugs should be avoided in patients with hypoaldosteronism and in diabetic patients with subclinical aldosterone insufficiency.

Angiotensin-Converting Enzyme Inhibitors. Captopril, enalapril, and other angiotensin-converting enzyme inhibitors act by inactivating angiotensin-converting enzyme. This action interrupts the renin-aldosterone axis, resulting in iatrogenic hypoaldosteronism. The clinical significance of hypoaldosteronism is unknown. Because of these unknown risks, the clinician must closely monitor high-risk patients on angiotensin-converting enzyme inhibitors for hyperkalemia. Recent studies have shown that the converting enzyme inhibitors may actually retard and even reverse the progress of diabetic nephropathy, so the renal insufficiency itself cannot now be considered an absolute contraindication for use.

Heparin Sodium. Polysulfated glycosaminoglycans, such as heparin sodium, impair aldosterone biosynthesis from the zona glomerulosa. With prolonged administration, heparin sodium can produce significant hypoaldosteronism with severe hyperkalemia because of a direct toxic effect on the zona glomerulosa, evidenced by a hyper-reninemic hypoaldosteronism and zona glomerulosa atrophy. The least toxic dose of heparin sodium is unknown, but a dose as small as 20,000 U per day for 5 days has been observed to reduce aldosterone secretion. This is an uncommon cause of hypoaldosteronism, but it is important because it is reversible and has been associated with lethal hyperkalemia. Heparin-induced aldosterone deficiency has been used therapeutically in some patients with chronic glomerulonephritis and initial hyperaldosteronism.

Potassium-Sparing Diuretics. Diuretics that conserve potassium include spironolactone, triamterene, and amiloride. Use of these drugs should be avoided in patients with hypoaldosteronism and are relatively contraindicated in patients with diabetes mellitus and chronic renal failure. Each of these drugs has a different mode of potassium conservation. Spironolactone has two effects: it is a mineralocorticoid receptor antagonist, and it inhibits aldosterone biosynthesis, presumably by competing with intermediates in corticosteroid biogenesis. Triamterene produces potassium retention by a direct action on nonaldosterone-mediated distal tubular exchange sites. Amiloride acts on the luminal surfaces of epithelial membranes to block sodium channels, resulting in less sodium resorption and potassium secretion.

Adrenolytic Therapy. Drugs that impair adrenal function are increasingly used for the hormonal treatment of breast cancer and medical management of Cushing's syndrome. These drugs include aminoglutethimide (Cytadren), mitotane, metyrapone (Metopirone), and trilostane. They block various enzymatic steps in impaired secretion of all classes of the corticosteroids: mineralocorticoids, glucocorticoids, and adrenal sex steroids. Lower doses of these drugs may not be associated with hyperkalemia, since secretion of aldosterone precursors may confer significant mineralocorticoid activity (deoxycorticosterone).

Other Drugs. As understanding of the pathophysiology of the renin-aldosterone system enlarges, some of the currently available and investigational drugs may be found to have adverse effects on the renin-aldosterone system. For example, drugs affecting the dopaminergic system have been shown to produce significant alterations in aldosterone secretion. Physicians believe at the present time that aldosterone is under tonic dopamine inhibition, and it is possible that administration of dopaminergic agonists, such as bromocriptine, could impair aldosterone secretion in certain physiologic situations. Also, calcium channel blockers like verapamil or nifedipine inhibit aldosterone biosynthesis and under certain clinical conditions may cause hypoaldosteronism.

Reduced Potassium Load

Reduction of extracellular potassium load can be the single most effective preventive measure in controlling hyperkalemia. Reducing dietary intake of potassium can be extremely helpful in avoiding hyperkalemia. Patients—and many physicians—have little awareness of the potassium content of many foods. Low salt foods and salt substitutes often contain potassium as the alternative cation. For example, low salt milk contains 60 mEq per liter of potassium. Other foods high in potassium include dried fruits (30 mEq per cup), meat (60 mEq per pound), decaffeinated coffee (4 mEq per cup), and a variety of other foods. Other sources of potassium include transfusions of bank blood (30 mEq per liter) and high-dose penicillin (1.7 mEq per 10^6 units).

Control of Diabetes Mellitus

As mentioned previously, this disorder is commonly associated with hyperkalemia and hypoaldosteronism due to multiple defects in the renin-aldosterone system. In addition to these factors, diabetic patients are predisposed to hyperkalemia because of insulin deficiency and hyperglycemia. Both insulin deficiency and hyperglycemia can independently produce a maldistribution of total body potassium. Hyperglycemia results in extracellular hyperosmolality, thereby producing an extracellular flux of potassium. Furthermore, insulin deficiency prevents cellular uptake of potassium, presumably related to the metabolic actions of this hormone. Both of these adverse effects, insulin deficiency and hyperglycemia, can be prevented by judicious control of the diabetes. Type II adult-onset, non-insulin-dependent diabetics should be encouraged to lose weight if they are obese, abstain from alcohol, and use oral hypoglycemic agents if necessary. Type I juvenile-onset, insulin-dependent diabetics may benefit from home glucose monitoring and split-dose insulin regimens.

Whatever the method of diabetic control, the level of blood glucose and normality of carbohydrate metabolism correlate directly with potassium homeostasis. Patients who are chronically hyperglycemic experience more hyperkalemia and, conversely, better controlled diabetics have a more normal potassium balance. Furthermore, the long-term control of glucose homeostasis in diabetes mellitus can reduce the risk of hypoaldosteronism. Autonomic insufficiency results in hyporeninemic hypoaldosteronism, and this risk is potentially avoidable in well-controlled diabetes mellitus. The degree of autonomic neuropathy correlates with the duration of hyperglycemia. If hyperglycemia can be prevented, it would remove an additional potential cause of hyporeninemic hypoaldosteronism in the diabetic patient.

Interstitial Nephritis

In interstitial nephritis, hyperkalemia occurs early, before chronic renal failure. This disease is associated with a high frequency of hyporeninemic hypoaldosteronism, presumably because of juxtaglomerular damage and impairment of renal synthesis and secretion. Early recognition of this disease is important because it is preventable and, in some cases, reversible. The leading causes of interstitial nephritis in many series are anatomic genitourinary abnormalities that, following early identification, are surgically correctable. Analgesic abuse with aspirin or phenacetin (greater than 2 kg) is a potentially reversible cause of interstitial nephritis. Other treatable causes of this disease include hyperuricemia, nephrocalcinosis, nephrolithiasis, and sickle cell disease.

TREATMENT

There is no ideal medical therapy for hypoaldosteronism. Many of the therapeutic modalities have limited benefits and are a calculated risk for selected patients. The majority of patients with mild selective hypoaldosteronism may require no therapy at all. When preventive measures are employed and patients are educated about their disease, specific therapy can be avoided. The decision to treat hypoaldosteronism and selection of a specific therapeutic agent depend on a number of factors, including the presence of diabetes mellitus, the degree of hyperkalemia, the age of the patient and his or her blood pressure, sodium balance, and renal function.

Mineralocorticoid Therapy

Mineralocorticoids are the mainstay of therapy for mineralocorticoid deficiency states. Fludrocortisone acetate (Florinef) is the most potent synthetic mineralocorticoid. It also has glucocorticoid activity, but it is not used as a systemic anti-inflammatory agent because of its salt-retaining qualities. It is absorbable from the gastrointestinal tract and can be administered as oral tablets (0.1 mg). Fludrocortisone acetate is used in dosages of 0.1 to 1.0 mg per day, which is equivalent to between 200 and 2,000 μg of aldosterone. Ninety percent of patients become normokalemic in this dosage range of fludrocortisone acetate.

Many patients with hypoaldosteronism have hypertension, mild renal failure, or incipient congestive heart failure. These patients cannot excrete a sodium load and are prone to excessive blood volume expansion. The use of fludrocortisone acetate in these patients would correct the hypokalemia but could lead to hazardous fluid accumulation. It is thus often wise either to avoid fludrocortisone acetate therapy or to combine it with a diuretic.

Diuretics

Diuretics may be the cardinal therapy for patients with hypoaldosteronism and coexisting diseases associated with sodium retention. Older patients with hypertension, mild renal impairment, and congestive heart failure in general respond better to diuretic therapy than to mineralocorticoid replacements. Since kaliuresis is the goal of diuretic therapy, the choice of a potent kaliuretic drug is of the utmost importance.

Chlorthalidone meets this requirement and may be administered in once-daily doses (25 mg per day). A cheaper but slightly less kaliuretic agent is hydrochlorothiazide. This drug has a shorter duration of action and should usually be administered in twice-daily doses (50 to 100 mg per day). The "loop" diuretics, such as furosemide or ethacrynic acid, are less potent kaliuretic agents but induce a greater degree of naturiuresis. These are short-acting drugs and should be administered in twice-daily doses (e.g., furosemide, 80 mg per day).

Although these drugs can correct the hyperkalemia associated with hypoaldosteronism, they are associated with side effects that may obviate their use. Both diabetes mellitus and hyperuricemia are frequently associated with hypoaldosteronism, and diuretics exacerbate both of these conditions. Thiazide drugs in particular impair insulin secretion and can necessitate initiation or increase of insulin therapy in some patients. Furthermore, thiazides are sometimes associated with precipitation of gout in hyperuricemic patients, which is a common coexisting problem in hypoaldosteronism. A potential benefit of diuretic therapy is stimulation of residual renin release in otherwise hyporeninemic patients. Patients with hyporeninism caused by autonomic insufficiency could be cured or at least experience an improvement of their hyporeninism following the use of diuretics.

Sodium Bicarbonate Therapy

Sodium bicarbonate cannot be recommended as routine therapy in the treatment of hyporeninemic hypoaldosteronism. This treatment is especially hazardous in elderly patients with coexisting renal impairment, congestive heart failure, and hypertension because of the increased sodium load. Children with defects in aldosterone biosynthesis may require sodium bicarbonate during the acute onset of the illness.

Kayexalate (Sodium Polystyrene Sulfonate)

Kayexalate is a cation exchange resin that can be given orally or via the rectum to correct hyperkalemia. Kayexalate removes approximately 1 mEq per gram resin by exchanging sodium for potassium in a 1:1 ratio. Administration of Kayexalate therefore increases sodium load and may be contraindicated in patients unable to tolerate an increase in sodium intake. Calcium-exchange resins have been under investigation for this problem, but they are currently unavailable for clinical use. The most efficient way of administering Kayexalate is by rectal enema. Approximately 50 g Kayexalate (2 teaspoons equal 10 g) is combined in solution with 25 percent sorbitol or 20 percent dextrose. The enema is retained for 60 minutes, and several enemas can be instituted if necessary. One enema can reduce the plasma potassium concentration by approximately 0.5 mEq per liter.

Patients often prefer oral Kayexalate, but it frequently produces nausea and constipation. Therefore diarrhea should be induced by cathartics prior to administration of Kayexalate. Fifty grams of Kayexalate are combined in a 20 percent sorbitol solution and given two to four times a day. The major problems with this therapy are the poor patient acceptance and the excessive sodium load administered. Thus clinicians treating hypoaldosteronism rarely use this agent.

SUGGESTED READING

Kalin MF, Poretsky L, Seres DS, Zumoff B. Hyporeninemic hypoaldosteronism associated with acquired immune deficiency syndrome. Am J Med 1987; 82.

Kutyrina IM, Nikishova TA, Tareyeva IE. Effects of heparin-induced aldosterone deficiency on renal function in patients with chronic glomerulonephritis. Nephrol Dial Transplant 1987; 2:219–223.

Nakamoto Y, Imai H, Hamanaka S, et al. IgM monoclonal gammopathy accompanied by nodular glomerulosclerosis, urine-concentrating defect, and hyporeninemic hypoaldosteronism. Am J Nephrol 1985; 5:53–58.

Rebuffat P, Kasprzak A, Andreis PG, et al. Effects of prolonged cyclosporine-A treatment on the morphology and function of rat adrenal cortex. Endocrinology 1989; 125:1407–1413.

CUSHING'S SYNDROME

RICHARD F. SPARK, M.D.

Cushing's syndrome is a generic diagnosis and is applicable to all patients with endogenous hypercorticolism. The designation Cushing's disease is reserved for those patients who have excessive cortisol levels as the result of inappropriate or disordered pituitary adrenocorticotropic hormone (ACTH) secretion. Other forms of Cushing's syndrome occur when unilateral adrenal adenomas or carcinomas function automously to synthesize and release unregulated and exorbitant amounts of cortisol into the peripheral circulation. The ACTH secreted by lung tumors (oat cells) and other malignancies is often bioactive and stimulates adrenal hypertrophy and cortisol hypersecretion. Recently, corticotropin-releasing hormone (CRH) secreting malignancies have been described. The CRH produced by these tumors stimulates otherwise normal pituitary corticotropes to hypertrophy and releases inappropriate amounts of ACTH, thereby causing adrenal hypertrophy and corticosteroid hypersecretion.

By consensus, there is now a "treatment of choice" for Cushing's disease and for each of the individual subsets of Cushing's syndrome. Unfortunately, the "treatment of choice" does not always provide maximum therapeutic benefit. When this occurs, physicians are obliged to resort to "fall-back" options and to restructure their therapeutic expectations.

The ideal treatment for Cushing's syndrome would obliterate chronic hypercorticolism permanently, allow for a return of normal circadian rhythm of cortisol secretion, and require no long-term hormone replacement therapy. Today one can anticipate that such therapeutic goals may be achieved in about 75 percent of the patients with Cushing's disease and almost all patients with benign adrenal adenomas. The outlook is considerably less optimistic for patients with adrenal carcinoma or the ectopic ACTH syndrome. Still, even for these patients, effective therapeutic intervention is available and can be implemented to maintain a eumetabolic state for a period of time.

TREATMENT OF CUSHING'S DISEASE

Cushing's disease is the result of a disorder in the central regulation of pituitary ACTH secretion and commonly associated with the development of a discrete pituitary adenoma. The term "pituitary basophilism" has lingered since Dr. Cushing's days. Today more specific immunocytologic studies with anti-ACTH antibodies are used to demonstrate the immunofluorescence of the pituitary corticotrope. Transsphenoidal hypophysectomy is the treatment of choice for patients with Cushing's disease. The transsphenoidal surgical approach is preferred, for it affords the neurosurgeon direct access to the pituitary. A small hole is drilled in the floor of the sella turcica, and the pituitary is examined under the operating microscope. In contrast to the prolactin-secreting pituitary microadenomas, which are readily visualized on the lateral portion of the pituitary, ACTH-secreting adenomas tend to hover near the midline of the pituitary and are only rarely immediately apparent. Often the neurosurgeon must bivalve the pituitary, taking care not to damage the normal gland or any vital structures. Then during further exploration, the ACTH-secreting adenoma may present as a small discrete mass or, alternatively, as a clump of grayish tissue distinct from the normal anterior pituitary.

Once identified, the neurosurgeon may selectively remove the corticotropin-secreting pituitary adenoma, leaving the normal pituitary behind. When pituitary surgery is fully successful and the ACTH-secreting pituitary adenoma is removed in toto, a condition of acute pituitary-adrenal insufficiency supervenes; chronic ACTH hypersecretion from the pituitary adenoma causes suppression of the other nontumorous corticotropes. These cells recover in time and, in response to pulses of hypothalamic CRH, eventually secrete ACTH to allow for a return of normal circadian ACTH and cortisol secretion.

However, the cells do not recover immediately and to ward off any untoward consequences of this abrupt change in cortisol dynamics, parenteral intravenous hydrocortisone (cortisol) should be given before, during, and for a brief time after pituitary surgery. The cortisol helps the soon to be pituitary-adrenal insufficient patient cope with the stress of surgery. I prefer to first administer hydrocortisone phosphate (or hemisuccinate) as a 50-mg bolus when the patient is "on call" to the operating room and then give 250 mg of hydrocortisone phosphate in 1,000 ml of saline during the day of surgery. Intravenous hydrocortisone is continued on the first postoperative day, but the dose is decreased to 150 mg every 24 hours, again in 1,000 ml of saline. The next day the total daily cortisol dose is reduced to 60 mg. By the second postoperative day, if the patient is taking fluids adequately, medication can be administered by mouth as 20 mg hydrocortisone three times a day, with the last dose given at 8:00 PM. The following day the dose of hydrocortisone is reduced to 40 mg given as 20 mg twice a day at 8:00 AM and 4:00 PM.

On the fourth postoperative day, fasting 8:00 AM plasma and serum samples are obtained to measure ACTH and cortisol levels. If surgery was fully successful, baseline ACTH and cortisol values should be suppressed fully. ACTH values of less than 25 pg per milliliter and cortisol values less than 5 μg per deciliter indicate that the ACTH-secreting adenoma is no longer present.

Recruitment of the remaining population of normal corticotropes will occur, but not immediately. The time course of recovery is variable and may not be fully normal until 1 year after surgery. More commonly, normal pituitary-adrenal function is evident between 4 and 7 months postoperatively. During the interval, supplemental physiologic doses of glucocorticoid are necessary. I prefer to give hydrocortisone 20 mg orally at 8:00 AM and 10 mg at 2:00 PM for at least 1 month. Thereafter I change to prednisone and administer that glucocorticoid in a dose of 5 mg every morning. Five milligrams of prednisone is equivalent to 20 mg of hydrocortisone. I maintain this schedule for another month, and then, in anticipation of discontinuing all medication, I alter the prednisone schedule to 10 mg every other day for approximately 2 months. A Cortrosyn stimulation test is performed on an alternate day, i.e., when the patient is not taking prednisone. The Cortrosyn test provides two critical pieces of information. A baseline serum cortisol level above 8 μg per deciliter indicates some return of endogenous pituitary-adrenal function. A postCortrosyn increment in serum cortisol of 8 to 10 μg per deciliter above baseline is considered normal.

The switch from hydrocortisone to prednisone is accomplished for two reasons. First, prednisone is both less expensive and more readily available than hydrocortisone in most pharmacies. Second, the somewhat longer half-life of prednisone allows the patient to remain comfortable and without any symptoms of adrenal insufficiency. The alternate-day regimen is usually well tolerated, and prednisone, when administered as a single morning dose, does not interfere with the following morning's serum cortisol level or Cortrosyn response. When results of these latter tests indicate return of normal pituitary-adrenal function, prednisone is tapered and discontinued.

In their initial series, Tyrell and Wilson reported that pituitary microadenectomy cured 90 percent of patients with Cushing's disease, and this report established transsphenoidal hypophysectomy as the "treatment of choice." Enthusiasm for transsphenoidal hypophysectomy persists although no single group has been able to match this extraordinary success rate. With an experienced neurosurgeon, successful resolution of Cushing's disease can be anticipated in about 75 percent of carefully selected patients. The operant phrase is "careful patient selection." Among patients with Cushing's disease, some are more and others less likely to benefit from pituitary microadenectomy. Unsatisfactory responses can be expected in patients with large pituitary adenomas. Surgical cure of Cushing's disease may be achieved in these individuals, but only by sacrificing other trophic hormones in the anterior pituitary. Unfortunately, such draconian surgery destroys not only the corticotrope-secreting pituitary adenoma, but also the thyrotropes, gonadotropes, and the normal nontumorous corticotropes, leaving the patient with chronic panhypopituitarism. Other factors may predispose to surgical failure.

Causes of Pituitary Surgery Failure

Within the realm of patients who fulfill the criteria required to establish a diagnosis of Cushing's disease, i.e., no suppression of 17 hydroxy corticosteroids, urinary free cortisol or plasma cortisol on low-dose dexamethasone but at least 50 percent suppression of these corticosteroids on high-dose dexamethasone testing, there are two subgroups who do not benefit from pituitary adenectomy.

One group does not have pituitary Cushing's at all, although their response to dexamethasone and other conventional studies would suggest that they do. These patients have benign bronchial adenomas or carcinoids and a form of the ectopic ACTH syndrome. The absolute level of ACTH is lower than usually observed in patients with malignant ectopic ACTH syndromes and more in line with values found in patients with Cushing's disease. The bronchial adenomas are small and may be detected only with extensive radiologic studies usually involving multiple computed tomography (CT) scans of the chest or selective venous catheterization.

A second group of surgery resistant patients have pituitary Cushing's disease, but the excessive ACTH secretion comes from hyperplastic corticotropes located in the intermediate lobe, not the anterior lobe of the pituitary. Discrete adenomas are uncommon. This subgroup of patients with intermediate lobe pituitary Cushing's disease are more likely to respond to bromocriptine with a prompt decrement in ACTH levels than those with anterior pituitary Cushing's disease.

Intraoperative bleeding is common during pituitary surgery for Cushing's disease. Bleeding or oozing may be extensive, and blood may well up in the operative field, thus completely obscuring the surgeon's view and rendering further exploration for the ACTH-secreting microadenoma impossible. The factors predisposing to such extensive bleeding in one patient and not in another are unclear. In some cases, bleeding is so extensive that surgery must be discontinued.

Finally, the highest percentage of surgical successes can be expected from those surgeons with the greatest experience. Neurosurgeons, like endocrinologists, are not all created equal. Some are simply more skilled at identifying and removing pituitary adenomas. As additional young neurosurgeons are trained by these more experienced hands, the variability in operative results may be less apparent. For the moment, however, it appears that neurosurgeon preselection is as important as patient preselection in obtaining optimum therapeutic results from pituitary surgery.

Long-Term Follow-Up After Successful "Microadenectomy"

For many patients the immediate postoperative response to pituitary surgery is dramatic. The physical manifestations of Cushing's disease resolve. Blood pressure and blood glucose return to normal, and menstruation and fertility return. In a distressing number of patients, this beneficial response is short-lived. Recurrent signs and symptoms of Cushing's disease indicate that the process thought to be cured was, in reality, only rendered transiently dormant. The time course of recurrence varies from series to series, but, in the aggregate, when recurrences occur, they apparently do so as early as 2 to 3 years after initially successful surgery. This phenomenon is similar to that observed in patients in whom recurrent hyperprolactinemia appears 4 to 5 years after initially successful surgery for prolactin-secreting pituitary microadenomas.

Several hypotheses have been advanced to explain the recurrence of Cushing's disease in patients originally thought to be "cured" after pituitary microadenectomy. Orth has speculated that more than one ACTH-secreting pituitary adenoma may have been present at the time of the original surgery, and only the dominant, i.e., the most prominent lesion was removed. Smaller microadenomas lurking nearby, but too small to identify, would remain after the dominant lesion was removed. With time, the smaller lesions, still capable of autonomous ACTH secretion, would grow and release ACTH at a slow but inexorable pace, resulting in a full recrudescence of Cushing's disease.

An alternate hypothesis implicates the hypothalamus as the culprit responsible for the recurrent Cushing's disease. In this scenario, CRH hypersecretion is the primary pathophysiologic abnormality in Cushing's disease. Persistent postmicroadenectomy CRH secretion results in recruitment of additional corticotropes, which, over time, coalesce into a new ACTH-secreting pituitary adenoma: a lesion that is fully capable of orchestrating the entire sequence of events that lead to a recurrence of Cushing's disease.

Complications of Transsphenoidal Microadenectomy

Surgical complications include those that occur intraoperatively, in the immediate postoperative period, and some that persist to remain as chronic problems, requiring lifelong treatment.

Bleeding into the surgical field is the most common intra-operative complication and prevents satisfactory completion of the surgical procedure (discussed before). The most common immediate postoperative problems are periorbital and circumoral ecchymoses and diabetes insipidus. Bruising is sufficiently common to be expected, and I usually alert my patients to this in advance lest they become alarmed when they look at their face in the mirror in the first few postoperative days. Also to be expected is a sensation of nasal stuffiness and a moderately severe "sinus type" headache. Liberal use of analgesic medications provides palliative relief for these distressing symptoms.

Diabetes insipidus is a common but fortunately evanescent problem. Even the most experienced neurosurgeons traumatize the posterior pituitary during surgery. Inadequate release of antidiuretic hormone (ADH) ensues, and polyuria of variable degree, sometimes as high as 6 to 12 liters per day, may occur. Dehydration can be avoided by careful attention to fluid balance and by maintenance of fluid intake to match output as closely as possible. On occasion, treatment with the ADH surrogate desmopressin is necessary. Ordinarily, this medication is administered intranasally, but intranasal administration of desmopressin should be avoided in the immediate postoperative period.

The technique of transsphenoidal hypophysectomy obliges the surgeon to drill a small hole in the sella turcica to visualize the pituitary. This hole is plugged with the patient's own fat of fascia at the conclusion of surgery to prevent cerebrospinal fluid (CSF) rhinorrhea. High-pressure nasal insufflation of desmopressin may dislodge this plug, leading to CSF rhinorrhea and so setting the stage for possible meningitis. If intravenous and oral fluid administration cannot keep pace with urine output, then desmopressin may be administered either by the intravenous or subcutaneous route. The usual dose is 2 to 4 μg (0.5 to 1.0 ml) daily.

Postoperative pituitary-adrenal insufficiency is to be expected and is not a complication but an indication of successful surgery. Support with glucocorticoid only is required. Mineralocorticoid replacement is unnecessary, for an intact renin-angiotensin system maintains aldosterone secretion and electrolyte homeostasis.

Long-Term Complications

The most troublesome long-term complications are panhypopituitarism and chronic diabetes insipidus. Both are more common after aggressive surgery for large pituitary adenomas. When extensive surgery results in panhypopituitarism, hormone replacement therapy is readily available. The diabetes insipidus that follows pituitary surgery is most often transient. When diabetes insipidus persists, long-term treatment with desmopressin or Pitressin is required.

Persistence of recurrence of Cushing's disease is more troublesome. When Cushing's disease persists or recurs, the physician is obliged to consider a series of "fall-back therapeutic options" including repeat pituitary surgery; pituitary radiotherapy; bilateral adrenalectomy; and medical therapy.

Repeat Pituitary Surgery

Repeat pituitary surgery is not recommended for patients in whom the first attempt at pituitary microadenectomy failed. However, for "cured" patients whose Cushing's disease recurs after 2 to 3 years, repeat surgery has been attempted with some success. Prior scarring in the surgical field makes a second exploration somewhat more difficult. Careful preoperative collaboration between patient, physician, and neurosurgeon is necessary so that appropriate expectations vis-à-vis the probability of success and the possibility of complications are reviewed in detail. Repeat surgery carries hazards similar to those outlined previously. No single series has reported extensive experience with reoperation, and, for the moment, decisions to proceed with a second surgical procedure must be made case by case.

Pituitary Radiotherapy

Pituitary radiotherapy can be accomplished with conventional megavoltage or heavy particle (proton beam) radiation. Conventional radiotherapy is more accessible. Total radiation dose is in the range of 4,500 to 4,800 rads and is administered in low fractional doses not exceeding 180 rads daily over a 4- to 5-week period. Heavy particle radiation is given as a single dose designed to deliver 8,000 to 12,000 rads to the pituitary. Conventional radiotherapy is considered the treatment of choice for youngsters and adolescents with Cushing's disease, but has not been used as the initial treatment for adults. Heavy particle radiation has been employed as a primary treatment for adults with mild Cushing's disease with singular effectiveness in some cases. However, even in areas of the country where this therapy is available, transsphenoidal hypophysectomy remains the treatment of choice. Conventional radiotherapy has been relegated to an adjunctive role and is used primarily for the following reasons:

1. Patients whose Cushing's disease persists after pituitary microadenectomy.
2. Patients whose Cushing's disease recurs after pituitary microadenectomy.
3. As a prophylactic maneuver to prevent the occurrence of Nelson's syndrome in patients who have had bilateral adrenalectomy for Cushing's disease.

Radiotherapy is not without its hazards. The radiotherapeutic field encompasses not only the pituitary but also the optic chiasm, the cavernous sinus, and the temporal lobe. Radiation-induced damage to the optic chiasm may cause blindness. The cavernous sinus contains the third, fourth, and sixth cranial nerves. Oculomotor palsies may occur, especially after heavy particle irradiation. The complication of temporal lobe malacia has been minimized to some degree by the current practice of delivering fractional doses of conventional radiotherapy through multiple arced ports. The normal pituitary is ordinarily relatively radioresistant, whereas the pituitary tumor tissue is sensitive to radiotherapy. However, the extraordinary high energy released by heavy particle irradiation may damage normal pituitary tissue, and hypopituitarism is common after treatment. Attempts to streamline the schedule of conventional radiotherapy by increasing the total daily fractional dose to complete the treatment schedule in 3 to 4 rather than 4 to 5 weeks has dire consequences, for it is in these patients that damage to the optic chiasm and blindness is most common.

Bilateral Adrenalectomy

Hypersecretion of cortisol and other adrenal steroids are responsible for all of the symptoms of Cushing's disease. Bilateral adrenalectomy removes the source of excessive glucocorticoid, mineralocorticoid, and androgen and provides a prompt resolution to symptoms caused by hypersecretion of these steroid hormones. Bilateral adrenalectomy is a formidable surgical procedure. I have found that the best results are achieved when the surgeons use a posterior rather than an anterior approach. The posterior approach affords better visualization of the adrenals and allows for the entire procedure to be done retroperitoneally. Postoperatively, the patient has complete adrenal insufficiency and requires support with both glucocorticoid and mineralocorticoid hormones for life. The steroid preparation before and during surgery is similar to that used for pituitary microadenectomy until the fourth or fifth postoperative day (see Treatment of Cushing's Disease). In the supraphysiologic doses administered, hydrocortisone provides some mineralocorticoid activity. However, when doses of hydrocortisone are tapered to 40 mg per day or lower, additional mineralocorticoid is needed. It is at this time that I add fludrocortisone acetate (Florinef) usually in a dose of 0.05 to 0.10 mg daily. Doses of Florinef are titrated in response to fluctuations in serum sodium and potassium levels, with increasing doses being administered when serum sodium falls and potassium increases and with decreasing doses for the converse.

Patients with Cushing's disease have poor wound healing as a result of their chronic hypercortisolism. Careful attention to suture lines is critical to avoid wound dehiscence. The approach to the adrenals through a posterior incision often requires the removal of all, or a portion of, a rib and not uncommonly invades, or comes dangerously close to, the pleura. I usually alert my patients to these problems preoperatively. The discomfort sustained from bilateral flank incisions and chest tubes is substantial. Postoperative respiratory therapy is often necessary to prevent the development of atelectasis or pneumonia. The immediate postoperative problems occur within a short period of time and can be handled most expeditiously with a coalition of physicians including an endocrinologist to manage steroid doses, a surgeon to cope with problems of wound healing, and a respiratory therapist to ensure that no postoperative pulmonary complications supervene. Following a tumultuous 3- to 4-day period, acute problems abate and plans for long-term management and treatment begin.

Chronic adrenal insufficiency is the result of bilateral adrenalectomy and therefore substitutes one chronic illness for another. Chronic adrenal insufficiency must be discussed in detail preoperatively. In the postoperative period, a program of patient education is initiated. Life-long glucocorticoid (hydrocortisone 20 to 30 mg per day or prednisone 5.0 to 7.5 mg per day and mineralocorticoid (Florinef 0.1 mg per day) is essential. The need to increase corticosteroid replacement above baseline during periods of physical and emotional stress is discussed. Patients are advised to obtain a Medic-Alert bracelet stating "Adrenal Insufficiency—In Emergency Give Hydrocortisone 100 mg IM." Prefilled syringes with that amount of hydrocortisone are available and prescribed for my patients. Acute illnesses, especially those associated with fever, trauma, and physical or emotional stress, can be managed with augmentation of a daily oral steroid dose. The steroid dose is titrated back to baseline once the stressful episode abates. When informed about the need to care for themselves properly, my patients become unusually facile in managing this aspect of their illness. Rarely, when an illness causes nausea or vomiting and an inability to retain steroid medication or fluids, hospitalization and parenteral fluid and steroid therapy is necessary.

A more pernicious problem following bilateral adrenalectomy is the development of an ACTH-secreting pituitary tumor (Nelson's syndrome). This disorder is characterized by inappropriate elevations in ACTH secretion from a progressively enlarging pituitary adenoma. The excessive ACTH secretion results in pigmentation, and Caucasian patients appear to be chronically suntanned. The enlarging pituitary adenoma may, like other pituitary lesions, cause compression of the optic chiasm and bitemporal hemianopsia or extend laterally and invade the cavernous sinus. Nelson's syndrome tumors are particularly prone to infarction, and pituitary apoplexy is common. That condition presents with acute onset of headache and, if the cavernous sinus is compromised, may cause damage to the oculomotor nerves, thus leading to ptosis, miosis, and diplopia. CT scan usually reveals an enlarged pituitary mass with a central hypolucent area reflecting the infarction and tissue necrosis. During neurosurgical evacuation, hemorrhagic tissue is removed and symptoms of headache and diplopia are alleviated with decompression.

Nelson's syndrome is said to occur in 15 to 30 percent of the patients who have had bilateral adrenalectomy. Stringent criteria for the diagnosis once demanded demonstration of both pigmentation and enlargement of the sella turcica on skull film. Today with availability of ACTH radioimmunoassay and CT scans, postadrenalectomy patients can be tracked more precisely. Following bilateral adrenalectomy for Cushing's disease, plasma ACTH levels are routinely elevated in most patients who are treated with "physiologic doses" of hydrocortisone. Mild to moderate elevations in plasma ACTH are not worrisome. However, progressive increases in plasma ACTH level are indicative of an enlarging pituitary tumor. Serial CT scans reveal the morphologic change in the pituitary. When a pattern of rising plasma ACTH levels and enlarging pituitary tumor is evident, one must consider neurosurgical intervention. Some have recommended that Nelson's syndrome can be avoided entirely by initiating pituitary radiotherapy immediately after bilateral adrenalectomy. I have not been enthusiastic about this approach, for radiotherapy carries its own baggage of adverse effects (see Pituitary Radiotherapy). Other than inappropriate tanning, the majority of patients with Nelson's syndrome do not experience any significant medical problems.

Medical Therapy

Among the pharmacologic agents used for treatment of Cushing's syndrome are compounds that act centrally and directly on the adrenal and at glucocorticoid receptors. Cyproheptadine hydrochloride and bromocriptine dampen or diminish pituitary ACTH release from the microadenoma by virtue of their respective anti-serotoninergic and dopaminergic actions. Cyproheptadine hydrochloride is more consistently effective, but even so produces sustained decreases in ACTH and cortisol secretion in no more than 15 percent of cases. Cyproheptadine hydrochloride in doses of 16 to 32 mg per day may be necessary. Drowsiness is the major side effect. Bromocriptine is partially effective and only in patients with intermediate lobe Cushing's syndrome.

Compounds acting directly on the adrenal glands include the adrenocytolytic agent mitotane (previously known as o,p'DDD) and adrenal enzyme inhibitors such as metyrapone, aminoglutethimide, trilostane, and ketoconazole. Mifepristone (RU-486) blocks the action of cortisol at the glucocorticoid receptor. I have restricted the use of mitotane to patients with adrenal cancer. In my experience, mitotane even when used in low doses (up to 4 g per day) causes substantial neurotoxicity, and I have not been comfortable in recommending its use for other forms of Cushing's syndrome. Adrenal enzyme inhibitors have been employed and found to be useful as palliative agents to control some of the symptoms and metabolic abnormalities associated with corticosteroid excess in Cushing's disease and the ectopic ACTH syndrome (see next section).

CUSHING'S SYNDROME CAUSED BY AN ADRENAL ADENOMA

Unilateral adrenalectomy is the treatment of choice when hypercorticolism is due to autonomous cortisol secretion from a unilateral adrenal adenoma. Again, a retroperitoneal flank incision is recommended. The schedule of steroid administration during surgery and in the immediate postoperative period is similar to that noted for pituitary microadenectomy. Once the cortisol-secreting adrenal adenoma is removed, the patient is thrust into a temporary state of acute pituitary-adrenal insufficiency. The contralateral adrenal gland, atrophic at this time, will recover normal function, but only after several months. Recovery involves not only reactivation of pituitary ACTH secretion, but also stimulation of the cells of the adrenal cortex. The trophic influences of ACTH facilitate the return of both morphologic and functional integrity to the zona fasciculata. Cortisol secretion resumes only when the complement of fasciculata cells approaches normal. A schedule of prednisone 5.0 to 7.5 mg orally daily is required for the first 2 postoperative months. Then the dose of prednisone is reduced to 5 mg daily; 1 month later, a schedule of 7.5 to 10.0 mg every other day is initiated. Two months later, the first Cortrosyn test is scheduled for an "alternate day" and may have to be repeated at periodic intervals over the next few months. When the Cortrosyn test is normal, prednisone is tapered and discontinued.

CUSHING'S SYNDROME CAUSED BY ADRENAL CARCINOMA

Adrenal carcinomas are often large, bulky masses with an unfortunate predilection for rapid growth, contiguous spread, and local and distant metastasis. Complete surgical removal of the primary carcinoma should be accomplished as early as possible. Tumor tissue may extend beyond the adrenal bed and into venous channels, thus invading the adjacent kidney. Simultaneous adrenalectomy and ipsilateral nephrectomy may be necessary. The anterior abdominal approach is preferred, for it affords the surgeon an adequate view of the primary tumor, contralateral adrenal gland and kidney, and the liver, which, with the lungs, are common sites of metastasis.

Adrenal cancers are notoriously inefficient steroid producers, and carcinoma may present without any evidence of adrenal hormone excess or only selective increases in the secretion of adrenal androgens. When increased glucocorticoid secretion is present, the classic clinical manifestations of Cushing's syndrome appear. Then physical and functional atrophy of the contralateral adrenal gland can be anticipated. The mechanism is similar to that described for adrenal adenoma. Glucocorticoid support during surgery and in the postoperative period is necessary. Remissions after surgery occur, but should not lull the physician into a sense of complacency. Adrenal carcinomas exhibit a capricious but ultimately an inexorable downhill course.

Local and distant metastases are common and are treated with the adrenocytolytic agent mitotane. Gastrointestinal distress is a common (80 percent) side effect, but is manageable with the liberal use of antacids. Mitotane is lipid-soluble and also causes significant central nervous system dysfunction including somnolence, confusion, dizziness, and anorexia (50 to 60 percent). One can minimize side effects to some degree by starting with low doses of mitotane and gradually advancing to therapeutic levels. I initially prescribe 250 mg four times a day and, as this dose is tolerated, increase by 1-g increments every 1 to 2 weeks. A tumoricidal dose is between 8 to 12 g daily. (Mitotane is available in 500-mg tablets, so that patients must take between 16 and 24 tablets each day.) Mitotane has a slow onset of action, and more rapid-acting adrenal enzyme inhibitors may be required to control symptoms of glucocorticoid and mineralocorticoid excess. These medications can be used in conjunction with mitotane. Eventually, mitotane's adrenocytolytic action may destroy all functioning adrenal tissue and so cause chronic adrenal insufficiency. This effect is to be anticipated and is an index of the therapeutic effectiveness of this agent.

CUSHING'S SYNDROME CAUSED BY ECTOPIC ADRENOCORTICOTROPIC HORMONE SYNDROME

The malignancies responsible for ACTH secretion in the ectopic ACTH syndrome are usually aggressive and not amenable to primary resection. On occasion, more benign lesions like bronchial adenomas and pheochromocytomas are responsible for excessive ACTH secretion and are removed readily. Many symptoms of the ectopic ACTH syndrome are caused by the primary malignancy, whereas others are the consequences of excessive secretion of adrenocortical hormones. Hyperglycemia and myopathy result from glucocorticoid excess; whereas electrolyte abnormalities, most commonly hypokalemic alkalosis, are a manifestation of adrenal mineralocorticoid excess. Medications that function to inhibit adrenal steroidogenesis are useful as palliative agents. Metyrapone, an 11 beta-hydroxylase inhibitor, blocks the final step in the synthesis of cortisol by preventing the conversion of 11-deoxycortisol to cortisol. Aminoglutethimide acts earlier in the steroid biosynthetic pathway by interfering with the conversion of cholesterol to pregnenolone succinate, the first step in steroid synthesis. Trilostane diminishes the conversion of pregnenolone to progesterone, another critical early step in cortisol biosynthesis. The antifungal agent ketoconazole inhibits mitochondrial cytochrome P-450 enzymes active in both 11 beta-hydroxylation and cholesterol side chain cleavage. A new compound, RU-486 blocks glucocorticoid action at the receptor level. Data on trilostane, ketoconazole, and RU-486 are limited. I have had more experience with aminoglutethimide and metyrapone in the management of patients with Cushing's syndrome to (1) lower cortisol production prior to bilateral adrenalectomy and (2) reduce total adrenal corticosteroid output in the ectopic ACTH syndrome or adrenal carcinoma.

Medical therapy is less effective in patients with Cushing's disease because any reduction in cortisol levels provokes a reflex increase in pituitary ACTH release that stimulates additional adrenal steroidogenesis, thereby vitiating the effectiveness of the pharmacologically induced enzymatic blockade. Increasing doses of medication maintain a higher level of enzyme inhibition and decrease cortisol levels further, but, in time, this effect is countered by compensatory increases in ACTH secretion. For this reason, pharmacologic treatment of patients with Cushing's disease is restricted to no more than 3 to 4 weeks prior to surgery and used primarily to establish or approach a euadrenal state to minimize postoperative complications.

In the ectopic ACTH syndrome, ACTH secretion is fixed and independent of circulating cortisol levels. Adrenal enzyme inhibitors are effective in controlling both glucocorticoid and mineralocorticoid secretion in this disorder. Treatment with metyrapone is initiated at a dose of 250 mg three times a day and gradually increased as needed to a maximum dose of 750 mg four times a day. Toxicity includes lightheadedness, dizziness, orthostatic hypotension, and hypoglycemia. Although metyrapone is commonly used for the pharmacologic treatment of Cushing's syndrome, it is not yet sanctioned for that indication and is approved only as a diagnostic test. Aminoglutethimide and trilostane are approved for the treatment of the hypercortisolism associated with Cushing's syndrome. Both are transiently effective in Cushing's disease, but more effective in controlling symptoms stemming from the corticosteroid excess of the ectopic ACTH syndrome. Either metyrapone or aminoglutethimide can be used as single therapeutic agents, but I prefer to use them together to achieve early and late pharmacologic inhibition of steroid synthesis. Further although the 11 beta-hydroxylation block induced by metyrapone lowers cortisol and aldosterone production, it increases production of another potent adrenal mineralocorticoid, desoxycorticosterone acetate (DCA). Aminoglutethimide by virtue of its earlier site of action limits the amount of steroid precursor available for conversion to DCA. Aminoglutethimide is introduced at a dose of 250 mg twice a day and then increased to 250 mg four times a day in order to maintain cortisol levels in an acceptable range. Somnolence is the major side effect, occurring in 70 percent of cases. Tolerance to the soporific effects of aminoglutethimide is evident after 3 to 4 weeks of therapy. An evanescent morbiliform rash apparent after 10 days usually disappears spontaneously.

Combined use of metyrapone and aminoglutethimide diminishes total steroid output. One can best assess the effectiveness of therapy by measuring specific plasma and urinary cortisol levels. Nonspecific measurements of urinary-17 hydroxy corticosteroids or other metabolites are to be avoided.

Hypokalemic alkalosis is a common cause of debilitating symptoms in the ectopic ACTH syndrome. Correction of the hypokalemia with potassium salts and potassium-retaining diuretics such as spironolactone or amiloride is helpful.

I have had good experience with the metyrapone-aminoglutethimide combination in treating the hypercortisolism associated with adrenal cancer and the ectopic ACTH syndrome. However, "success" is narrowly defined, with normalization of blood pressure, blood glucose, serum electrolyes, and patient comfort being the primary therapeutic goals.

SUGGESTED READING

Bertagna C, Orth DN. Clinical and laboratory findings and results of therapy in 58 patients with adrenocortical tumors admitted to a single medical center (1951 to 1978). Am J Med 1981; 71:855–875.

Howlett TA, Rees LH, Besser GM. Cushing's syndrome. Clin Endocrinol Metab 1985; 14:911–945.

Lamberts SW, Bons EG, Bruining HA, de Jong FH. Differential effects of the imidazole derivatives etomidate, ketoconazole and miconazole and of metyrapone on the secretion of cortisol and its precursors by human adrenocortical cells. J Pharmacol Exp Ther 1987; 240:259–264.

Luton JP, Mahoudeau JA, Bouchard P, et al. Treatment of Cushing's disease by o,p'DDD. Survey of 62 cases. N Engl J Med 1979; 300:459–464.

Orth DN, Liddis GW. Results of treatment in 108 patients with Cushing's syndrome. N Engl J Med 1971; 285:243–247.

Schteingart DE, Tsao HS, Taylor CI, et al. Sustained remission of Cushing's disease with mitotane and pituitary irradiation. Ann Intern Med 1980; 92:613–619.

Tyrrell JB, Brooks RM, Fitzgerald PA, et al. Cushing's disease. Selective trans-sphenoidal resection of pituitary microadenomas. N Engl J Med 1978; 298:753–758.

PRIMARY ALDOSTERONISM

GAIL K. ADLER, M.D., Ph.D.
GORDON H. WILLIAMS, M.D.

Primary aldosteronism, hypersecretion of aldosterone in the absence of definable stimulus, is most commonly associated with a unilateral adrenal adenoma. However, a significant minority of patients have bilateral adrenal hyperplasia. In rare cases, an adrenal carcinoma, an ectopic source of aldosterone, or glucocorticoid-suppressible cortical nodular hyperplasia can cause primary aldosteronism. Primary aldosteronism usually is detected in persons between the ages of 30 and 50 and has an incidence of approximately 1 percent in populations of unselected hypertensive patients. Since aldosterone causes sodium reabsorption and hydrogen and potassium ion excretion, signs and symptoms of primary aldosteronism are attributable to the hypertension (headache and infrequently visual disturbances) or, more commonly, to potassium depletion (fatigue, polyuria, muscle weakness, and cramps). Unfortunately, on the basis of the symptoms alone, patients with primary aldosteronism cannot be readily distinguished from patients with other forms of hypertension.

SCREENING

Even though primary aldosteronism occurs relatively infrequently, because it is a potentially curable disease it is important to have a simple, inexpensive screening test. In our opinion, no clinical characteristics distinguish the patient with primary aldosteronism. Studies conducted a number of years ago suggested that a low plasma renin activity may be an effective screen for primary aldosteronism. This was based on the observation that patients with primary aldosteronism are volume expanded and therefore would have suppressed renin levels. Unfortunately, we as well as others have not been particularly enchanted with plasma renin activity as a screening test since it is relatively expensive ($30 to $50) and not very specific (roughly 20 percent of patients with essential hypertension also have low renin levels). We believe that if certain precautions are taken, a more reliable, and certainly cheaper, screening test is a serum potassium level. In our experience, *spontaneous* hypokalemia in a hypertensive patient is almost invariably a sign of aldosterone excess. Whether it is primary or secondary, aldosteronism can readily be distinguished by measuring plasma renin activity (Fig. 1).

Unfortunately, spontaneous hypokalemia is unusual in hypertensive patients. In most instances a low serum potassium concentration is a result of treatment with potassium-wasting diuretics. Thus, if a patient is hypokalemic and taking potassium-wasting diuretics, the diuretics need to be discontinued for 10 to 14 days and the serum potassium concentration remeasured. If it is still low, this would suggest that the patient has mineralocorticoid excess.

What is the sensitivity of this procedure? Theoretically, all patients with primary aldosteronism should have hypokalemia unless they are on a low sodium diet (thereby preventing the reabsorption of sodium, a necessary prerequisite for the potassium wastage with aldosterone), are ingesting potassium-sparing diuretics, or have renal failure. Thus, in interpreting a serum potassium level, we take the following precautions to prevent a false-negative result. If patients are on potassium-sparing diuretics, these drugs are discontinued for 10 to 14 days and the serum potassium concentration is remeasured. During this period the patient should be maintained on a normal sodium (100 to 200 mEq) and potassium (60 to 100 mEq) intake. If the serum potassium level is normal while the patient is on a liberal sodium intake, off potassium-sparing diuretics, and free of evidence of renal failure (by blood

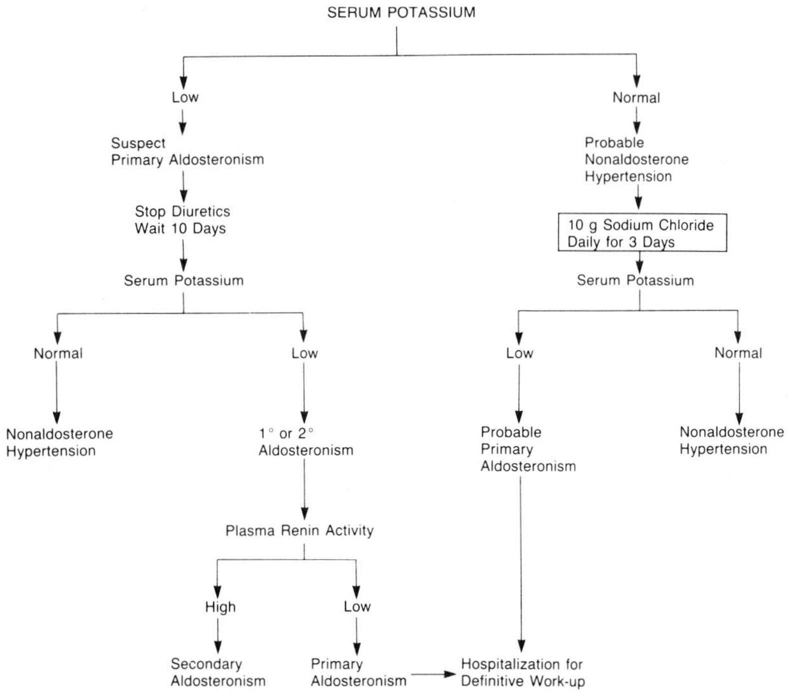

Figure 1 Flow sheet for office screening of hypertensive patients for hyperaldosteronism. (Reprinted with permission from Williams GH, Dluhy RG. How to evaluate and manage hypokalemic high blood pressure. In: Wolf GL, Eliot RS, eds. Contemporary problems in cardiology. Vol 2. Practical management of hypertension. Mt. Kisco, NY: Futura, 1975.)

urea nitrogen and/or creatinine), we believe that primary aldosteronism is effectively excluded.

Several concerns need to be addressed in performing what appears to be a relatively simple procedure. First, discontinuing diuretic therapy for 14 days may produce a rise in blood pressure that could be intolerable for the patient. Under these circumstances, if other antihypertensive agents are not effective and one is concerned about whether a low serum potassium level is secondary to potassium-losing diuretics or excess aldosterone, one could simply obtain a 24-hour urine potassium value after discontinuing the drug. Under most circumstances, if the hypokalemia is drug-induced, urinary potassium excretion declines markedly (less than 30 to 40 mEq per 24 hours). On the other hand, if the hypokalemia is secondary to aldosterone excess, the urinary potassium excretion rate remains elevated (greater than 50 to 60 mEq per 24 hours). Second, care should be taken when increasing a patient's dietary sodium intake, particularly in those who may have severe hypertension or incipient congestive heart failure. Finally, sodium should never be administered to a hypokalemic patient in whom you suspect primary aldosteronism. If the suspicion is correct, salt losing will promote further potassium loss, more hypokalemia, and potentially severe adverse cardiac manifestations of the hypokalemia.

A screening test for primary aldosteronism has been proposed in which patients are given 26 mg of captopril by mouth and their plasma aldosterone and renin levels measured 2 hours later. It is suggested that in patients with primary aldosteronism no change in renin or aldosterone levels will occur, whereas other patients show a rise in renin and a fall in aldosterone. A postcaptopril plasma aldosterone level greater than 15 ng per deciliter and a ratio of plasma aldosterone (ng per deciliter) to plasma renin activity (ng per milliliter per hour) greater than 50 indicate primary aldosteronism. We have had limited experience with this test but are concerned about two potential shortcomings: (1) the cost is probably greater than $100, and (2) the results are highly dependent on the reliability of blood sample collection and the processing of the laboratory samples. Both reasons in all probability exclude this test as a standard screening procedure.

DEFINITIVE DIAGNOSIS

If the techniques outlined previously reveal a hypertensive patient with spontaneous hypokalemia and a suppressed plasma renin activity, admission to a metabolic unit for a definitive work-up of primary aldosteronism should be arranged. In our experience, the definitive diagnosis of primary aldosteronism should be made on the basis of the following four criteria: (1) plasma or urinary aldosterone levels that do not suppress when salt loaded, (2) plasma renin activity that cannot be stimulated with salt restriction and upright posture, (3) potassium wasting and/or hypokalemia when salt loaded, and (4) normalization of serum potassium with sodium restriction. The easiest way to evaluate a patient suspected of having primary aldosteronism is as follows. The patient is admitted to a metabolic unit and placed on low (10 mEq) sodium and relatively high (100 to 150 mEq) potassium intake. After approximately 5 days when balance is achieved on this diet, supine and upright plasma renin activities are obtained. The patient is then given a saline load—3 L of normal saline intravenously over a 6-hour period. Plasma aldosterone and cortisol levels are obtained before starting the saline infusion and at 6 hours. In our laboratory the normal 6-hour aldosterone value should be less than 5 ng per deciliter. The cortisol level is obtained to rule out a false-positive elevation of aldosterone secondary to stress and adrenocorticotropic hormone (ACTH) stimulation.

The advantages of this approach are as follows:

1. The low sodium diet prepares the patient for the appropriate renin stimulation test. In our laboratory the upright plasma renin activity has been less than 2 ng angiotensin I per milliliter per hour in every patient with primary aldosteronism whom we have studied on a sodium-restricted diet.
2. Often, by first restricting the patient's salt, both blood pressure and potassium are normalized. The saline load now can be given with less potential danger to the patient (hypokalemia and/or hypertension).
3. Since approximately 40 percent of patients with essential hypertension have difficulty handling the sodium load and may take longer than 4 hours to suppress their plasma aldosterone levels, we prefer a 6-hour saline infusion and do not recommend a shorter 4-hour infusion. Because the renin levels also fail to suppress normally in these patients, the false-positive elevation of aldosterone usually becomes apparent if one obtains a simultaneous plasma renin activity.

Two other parameters are assessed during the course of the saline infusion: (1) urine potassium excretion (in primary aldosteronism the increment in 24-hour potassium excretion is at least 30 percent over basal) and (2) serum potassium levels. Although serum potassium levels can fall precipitously, we often do not observe a significant change in serum potassium at the conclusion of the 6-hour saline infusion but do observe it the following morning—24 hours after initiating the saline infusion. The reason we fail to see the rapid development of hypokalemia may be in part our preparation of the patients—high potassium, low sodium intake.

We have had an occasional patient in whom we were unable to carry out the foregoing procedures. These patients had concomitant mild-to-moderate renal failure; thus, the sodium-restricted intake produced a deterioration in renal function and the development of hyperkalemia. In these patients, we elected to perform a 4-hour saline infusion under closely monitored conditions both for blood pressure and potassium shifts. In each case, we observed no change in the plasma aldosterone levels over the 4-hour infusion. Each had an aldosterone-secreting adenoma removed at surgery, with lowering of blood pressure and normalization of the hypokalemia. However, each has required continued medication to normalize the blood pressure. The saline infusion should not be performed in patients with severe hypertension or in patients who have a stroke, myocardial infarction, or congestive heart failure within the past 6 months (Fig. 2).

BILATERAL ADRENAL HYPERPLASIA VERSUS AN ALDOSTERONE-PRODUCING ADENOMA

Once the diagnosis of primary aldosteronism is established, its etiology should be determined since the treatments for an adenoma and for bilateral adrenal hyperplasia differ. Initially, a high-resolution computed tomography (CT) scan should be obtained. The CT scan will detect approximately 90 percent of all adenomas with a less than 1 percent false-positive rate. In our experience, if both adrenal glands are visualized and a unilateral adrenal mass is found, further work-up is unnecessary, and the patient can be assumed to have an aldosterone-producing adenoma. Adenomas that are less than 1 cm in diameter are most difficult to detect by CT scan, especially if they are isodense with surrounding tissues and have not changed the contour of the gland. These small adenomas account for most of the 10 percent false-negative rate associated with CT scans.

If by CT scan both adrenals are of equal size, or if one adrenal is not seen, we believe that the patient should undergo adrenal vein sampling. This study should be performed by an experienced radiologist because technical

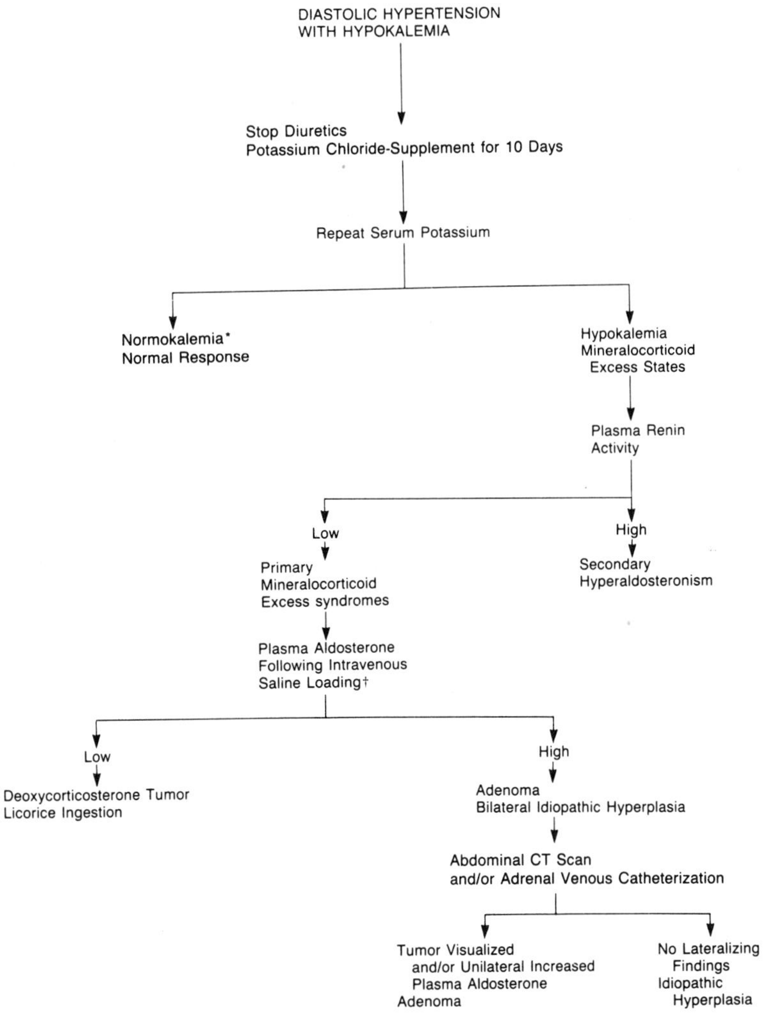

* Serum K^+ may be normal in some patients with hyperaldosteronism who are taking potassium-sparing diuretics (spironolactone, triamterene) or ingesting low sodium-high potassium intakes.

† This step should not be taken if hypertension is severe (diastolic greater than 115 mm Hg) or if cardiac failure is present. Also, serum potassium levels should be corrected before the infusion of saline.

Figure 2 Diagnostic flowchart for evaluating patients with suspected primary aldosteronism. (Reprinted with modifications from Williams GH, Dluhy RG. Diseases of the adrenal cortex. In: Petersdorf RG, Adams RD, eds. Harrison's principles of internal medicine. 10th ed. New York: McGraw-Hill, 1983.)

problems can lead to inadequate adrenal vein sampling and significant complications including adrenal vein thrombosis, adrenal infarction, rupture of the adrenal vein, and extravasation of contrast. The sensitivity of adrenal venous sampling is greater than 90 to 95 percent. Bilateral adrenal vein sampling for determination of aldosterone and cortisol concentrations should be obtained to look for lateralization of aldosterone secretion. Lateralization indicates an adenoma, and equal aldosterone levels indicate bilateral hyperplasia. The cortisol levels indicate whether the samples are adequate and should show no lateralization, although differences in levels between the two sides if samples are not obtained concomitantly may result from the normal episodic secretion of this steroid. Adrenal venography has a lower sensitivity of 75 to 90 percent with up to 30 percent false-positives and a slightly higher complication rate than just adrenal venous sampling. Because of the complication rate, the high cost of the procedure, and the relatively little added information obtained with adrenal venography, we no longer obtain this study.

The adrenal iodocholesterol scan is less sensitive (70 to 90 percent sensitivity) and more expensive, and it results in five to ten times more adrenal radiation than a CT scan. In addition, the radioisotopes used are not yet approved by the Food and Drug Administration except for research purposes. For these reasons, we do not perform adrenal iodocholesterol scintigraphy routinely. We have found that other procedures that have been advocated to distinguish an adenoma from hyperplasia are less reliable. They include plasma aldosterone response to upright posture. About 80 percent of patients with an aldosterone-producing adenoma have a decrease in their aldosterone level after 2 hours of upright posture. However, up to 25 percent of patients with bilateral hyperplasia also show this decrease in aldosterone. A second discriminant is an elevated 18-OH corticosterone level in a supine patient on an ad lib sodium intake. In our experience, there are both false-negatives and false-positives with this test.

Consideration should also be given to the rare causes of primary aldosteronism. An adrenal carcinoma probably would be detected by CT scan since these tumors tend to be inefficient producers of aldosterone and would be large by the time the patient developed symptoms of primary aldosteronism. Overproduction of additional adrenal hormones would also suggest carcinoma. Since our initial treatment for both adrenal adenomas and carcinomas is surgical removal of the affected adrenal, further preoperative testing to distinguish between these possibilities is seldom warranted. Finally, patients with a family history of primary aldosteronism should be evaluated for glucocorticoid-suppressible hyperaldosteronism. Prednisone, 5 mg twice a day for 4 to 6 weeks, will normalize blood pressure, potassium, plasma renin activity, and plasma aldosterone in patients with glucocorticoid-suppressible hyperaldosteronism. A *transient* decrease in aldosterone production during the first few days of prednisone suppression occurs in some patients with primary aldosteronism.

APPROACH TO TREATMENT

While waiting for study results, patients with suspected primary aldosteronism should be given a trial of medical therapy. Patients should be placed on less than an 80-mEq sodium diet. With less sodium available for exchange with potassium in the distal renal tubule, patients tend to conserve potassium. In addition, the mild volume depletion that accompanies a low sodium diet may lead to a decrease in the patient's blood pressure. Compliance with a low sodium diet can be monitored by obtaining a 12-hour urine for sodium and creatinine. At the same time, treatment with a potassium-sparing diuretic should be initiated (Table 1).

We usually use spironolactone, a competitive antagonist for the mineralocorticoid receptor. We start at 50 mg twice a day. The dose can be increased in increments of 100 mg at 1- or 2-week intervals up to 300 to 400 mg a day. The patient's blood pressure and serum potassium level should be followed weekly. With spironolactone there is an average increase in serum potassium levels of 1.5 mEq per liter. In addition, the majority of patients with primary aldosteronism become normotensive with spironolactone therapy. Unfortunately, up to 20 percent of patients develop side effects with spironolactone. In males these include decreased libido, impotence, gynecomastia, lassitude, and gastrointestinal disturbances. The gastrointestinal complaints can be minimized, however, if spironolactone is taken with meals.

TABLE 1 Drug Therapy for Patients with Primary Aldosteronism

Medication	*Initial Dose*	*Maximum Dose*	*Cost/Tablet**	*Side Efects*
Spironolactone	50 mg b.i.d.	200 mg b.i.d.	9¢–17¢ for 25 mg (generic) 29¢–40¢ for 25 mg (Aldactone) 95¢–$1.18 for 100 mg (Aldactone)	Impotence, decreased libido, gynecomastia, lassitude, gastrointestinal complaints
Amiloride	10 mg q.d.	40 mg q.d.	24¢–54¢ for 5 mg	Headaches, lassitude, muscle cramps, impotence, gastrointestinal complaints, increased blood urea nitrogen and uric acid levels

*Cost/tablet was obtained from a sampling of pharmacies in the Boston area.

An alternate potassium-sparing diuretic, amiloride, acts on the distal renal tubules to block sodium channels. Thus, sodium and chloride excretion is increased and potassium excretion decreased. Amiloride does not directly inhibit aldosterone's action. The initial oral dose is 10 mg a day, which may be increased at 10 mg intervals up to 40 mg a day. As with spironolactone therapy, average serum potassium levels rise by roughly 1.5 mEq per liter. Again the majority of patients with an aldosterone-producing adenoma become normotensive. A somewhat smaller decrease in blood pressure is seen in patients with bilateral adrenal hyperplasia. The side effects of amiloride are mild. They include headaches, lassitude, muscle cramps, gastrointestinal complaints, and occasionally impotence. A mild increase in blood urea nitrogen and uric acid levels can occur.

A combination of triamterene and thiazide has been tried, but in our opinion it is less effective than spironolactone or amiloride in reversing potassium depletion. The dose of triamterene-thiazide (50-mg-25 mg) tablets is up to two tablets twice a day. Side effects include blood dyscrasias, liver damage, gastrointestinal disturbances, weakness, headaches, and anaphylaxis.

Rarely, a low sodium diet and maximum therapy with either spironolactone or amiloride does not control a patient's hypokalemia. In these cases, we have begun potassium supplementation. Potassium supplementation and a potassium-sparing diuretic should not be started simultaneously because of the danger of hyperkalemia. Rather than initiating potassium supplementation, there is theoretical support for considering a combination of amiloride and spironolactone to control resistant hypokalemia. Spironolactone and amiloride exert their effects by different mechanisms and could have a synergistic effect on serum potassium. However, we have no practical experience with this approach.

If the patient's blood pressure is not controlled with a low-salt diet and a potassium-sparing diuretic, an aldosteronoma alone is unlikely. The patient has bilateral hyperplasia and/or renal damage secondary to the elevated blood pressure. In these patients, we have found a beta-blocker or a converting enzyme inhibitor (captopril) good first choices. Calcium-channel blockers decrease aldosterone levels in isolated glomerulosa cells and have been used with varying success in treating primary aldosteronism. Cyproheptadine, an antiserotoninergic agent, and bromocriptine, a dopamine agonist, have both proved to be ineffective in treating primary aldosteronism. Potential new drugs that exploit the ability of atrial natriuretic factor to inhibit aldosterone secretion may prove useful in the future. These medications were tested because of the hypotheses that aldosterone production is under tonic dopaminergic inhibition and that there exists a pituitary aldosterone-stimulating hormone under serotoninergic stimulation.

If test results indicate bilateral adrenal hyperplasia, patients should be continued on medical therapy. For unknown reasons, bilateral adrenalectomy, despite correcting the biochemical abnormalities in patients with bilateral adrenal hyperplasia, is generally ineffective in reversing hypertension, with only 15 percent of patients becoming normotensive after surgery. In addition, these patients face the problem of adrenal insufficiency. Because of the complications associated with long-term steroid administration, patients with glucocorticoid-suppressible hyperaldosteronism may need to be treated in the same way as patients with bilateral adrenal hyperplasia if a large glucocorticoid dose is required.

The treatment for a patient with an aldosterone-producing adenoma is surgical removal of the adenoma and the affected adrenal gland. Patients who refuse therapy or who are poor surgical candidates because of other medical problems may be treated medically. A posterior rather than a transabdominal surgical approach is preferred. With the posterior approach, patients tend to recover more rapidly and have fewer complications. In our experience, roughly 95 percent of patients who undergo adrenalectomy for an aldosterone-producing adenoma become normotensive and normokalemic in the first 3 to 6 months after surgery. Over the next 2 to 3 years, however, 20 to 25 percent again develop hypertension. When hypertension recurs, it is usually easier to control and is not associated with hypokalemia.

Preoperatively, patients should be treated with a low sodium diet, potassium-sparing diuretics, and antihypertensive agents as needed to control serum potassium and blood pressure. Intraoperatively, a patient's potassium level should be monitored, and because the remaining adrenal may not produce cortisol adequately, a patient should receive high-dose steroids. The intraoperative steroid dose is 10 mg hydrocortisone per hour by constant intravenous infusion. This dose also prevents rebound mineralocorticoid deficiency. Postoperatively, the patient can be switched to oral steroid supplementation and the dose gradually tapered to zero over a 2- to 6-week period. In the postoperative period, a patient may develop hypoaldosteronism with elevated serum potassium levels owing to inadequate functioning of the remaining adrenal cortex. It may take 3 to 6 months before the adrenal cortex fully recovers from the long-term suppressive effects of high aldosterone levels produced by the tumor. During this time a patient should follow a liberal sodium diet, follow daily weights, and be alert for signs of hypovolemia. Fluorohydrocortisone should be avoided since this can further suppress the adrenal cortex.

Finally, how does one treat a patient with an aldosteronoma who refuses surgery? We have had several such patients. All have been treated with spironolactone with normalization of blood pressure. The longest treatment has been 14 years. We have been successful with this approach only in women; no complications have occurred in them. We have not had any men who have tolerated the side effects, i.e., impotence, associated with long-term spironolactone therapy.

SUGGESTED READING

Drury PL. Disorders of mineralocorticoid activity. Clin Endocrinol Metab 1985; 14:175–202.

Hsueh WA. New insights into the medical management of primary aldosteronism. Hypertension 1986; 8:76–81.

Lyons DF, Kem DC, Brown RD, Hanson CS, Carollo ML. Single-dose captopril as a diagnostic test for primary aldosteronism. J Clin Endocrinol Metab 1983; 57:892–896.
Melby JC. Diagnosis and treatment of primary aldosteronism and isolated hypoaldosteronism. Clin Endocrinol Metab 1985; 14:977–995.
Williams GH, Dluhy RG. Diseases of the adrenal cortex. In: Braunwald E, Isselbacher KJ, Petersdorf RG, et al, eds. Harrison's principles of internal medicine. 11th ed. New York: McGraw Hill, 1987:1753.
Young WF, Klee GG. Primary aldosteronism—diagnostic evaluation. Endocrinol Metab Clin North Am 1988; 17:367–395.

PHEOCHROMOCYTOMA

STANLEY E. GITLOW, M.D.
DEMETRIUS PERTSEMLIDIS, M.D.
STANLEY W. DZIEDZIC, Ph.D, M.D.

Although it is considered to represent a medical curiosity, pheochromocytoma receives disproportionate attention because of the difficulty in differentiating it from one of the most common maladies, primary hypertension. We have had the opportunity to study 202 patients with proven pheochromocytomas who were originally referred for diagnostic evaluation, and one of us (D.P.) performed the required surgical procedures for patients in this group on 111 occasions.

The treatment of pheochromocytoma can be divided conveniently into four categories: (1) the therapeutic approach to a patient suspected of harboring this tumor of the neural crest, but for whom a biochemical diagnosis has not been obtained; (2) the preoperative management of a patient for whom a diagnosis has been ascertained; (3) management during and after surgery; and (4) care of patients whose tumors cannot be fully resected.

THERAPEUTIC APPROACH DURING DIAGNOSIS

Since a clinical presentation of hypertension in its accelerated phase increases the likelihood of the diagnosis of pheochromocytoma, one should always evaluate such a patient for an alpha-adrenergic crisis. The appropriate treatment of a patient who presents with *severe* hypertension, with or without substantive compromise of cerebral, cardiac, or renal function, consists of the intravenous administration by microdrip of two to four vials (10 to 20 mg) of phentolamine diluted in 250 ml of fluid. Within 3 or 4 minutes, the patient's response to alpha blockade is known: a marked lowering and optimal control of the arterial pressure (during which appropriate biochemical diagnostic studies may proceed while the patient remains at minimal risk), or a negligible hypotensive response that would lead at once to a therapeutic change to alternate antihypertensive agents. It should be emphasized that not every alpha-adrenergic crisis stems from a neural crest lesion. Central nervous system (CNS) lesions, neoplastic or vascular, as well as essential (primary) hypertension complicated by myocardial damage and beta-blockade administration may also lead to an alpha-adrenergic state that responds to treatment with alpha-adrenergic blockade. Such conditions may even be associated with elevated levels of circulating and urinary catecholamines and their metabolites. The use of phentolamine in this manner is not for diagnostic purposes other than to help the clinician realize that the patient is or is not hyperadrenergic. The technique results in minimal delay and enables the physician to avoid treating an alpha-hyperadrenergic subject with ineffectual or hazardous antihypertensive agents (i.e., beta blockers) while awaiting the results of diagnostic studies.

Although the majority of such patients ultimately prove to have essential hypertension, a sudden and violent onset of hypertension increases the statistical likelihood that a pheochromocytoma will be the etiology.

At no time should any patient be given phentolamine according to the manufacturer's prescription in the package insert. Intravenous administration of a few milligrams of phentolamine by direct "push" may result in irreversible shock in occasional patients with neural crest lesions; therefore, it should be avoided even in those patients with proven lesions and paroxysmal symptoms. It is not unusual for such a patient to require relatively high doses (10 to 100 mg per hour) or phentolamine for adequate control of the hyperadrenergic state, but this dose should always be administered by titration rather than as a bolus.

The relatively brittle clinical state of these patients must be emphasized. We know of subjects with these tumors who were treated with every antihypertensive agent currently available (even to the point of tumor resection during administration of the short-acting ganglioplegic trimethaphan). In some instances, modest control of the hypertension and symptoms was achieved; in others, the same drugs appeared to elicit no response, produced an exacerbation of symptoms, or even precipitated a demise. Unfortunately, sudden death of cardiac or cerebrovascular origin is still common in the presence of this tumor. *One should never induce a paroxysm, whether for diagnostic purposes or otherwise.* It is unfortunate that one can still read in journals recommendations for the use of diagnostic pharmacologic agents (currently glucagon) capable of inducing morbidity or even mortality in an unfortunate few with this tumor, despite the diagnostic inaccuracy of these methods and the current availability of accurate and reliable diagnostic biochemical assays. Only the failure of the majority of diagnostic clinical laboratories to use specific assay procedures frustrates the clinician in choosing between the pharmacologic and the biochemical diagnostic procedures. If the patient indicates that a hypertensive crisis may be induced by drinking beer or by assuming a certain body posture, he or she should be advised to avoid such actions until a reliable biochemical study has ruled out the presence of a pheochromocytoma. Similar caution extends to the physician's physical examination of a patient suspected of suffering from this tumor; avoid deep abdominal palpation.

Occasionally, patients with severe alpha adrenergia oscillate between extreme hypertension (diastolic pressures of 140 to 200 mm Hg) and shock. These swings in pressure may follow one another within minutes and represent either fluctuations in the peripheral release of alpha agonist or, more commonly, variations in cardiac competency in the face of continued severe peripheral vasoconstriction. Again, not all of these patients have neural crest lesions, but the treatment of choice is the intravenous administration of a dilute, rapidly acting alpha blocker (phentolamine). Other agents, such as nitroprusside, labetalol, or a calcium channel blocker may be used on occasion, but each suffers from some drawback, whether it is a limited duration for safe use, complicating effects on the heart, or restricted effectiveness.

Most patients suspected of having a pheochromocytoma do not present initially in the emergency room but rather in the company of and resembling subjects with essential hypertension, thyrotoxicosis, diabetes, and cardiomyopathy and those with recurrent paroxysmal symptoms often attributed to "nerves." Although their problems may seem to be of modest proportions, consider the advisability of administering an oral alpha-blocking drug while performing the required biochemical assays. Neither phentolamine nor phenoxybenzamine modifies catecholamine metabolism sufficiently to elicit diagnostic difficulties with assays of total metanephrines or vanillylmandelic acid excretion. There is no danger from the administration of oral phenoxybenzamine on an interim basis, and whatever slight orthostasis or stuffy nose that might occur is a small price to pay for the added safety.

If a choice is made to avoid alpha blockade, a beta-blocking drug (with the possible exception of labetalol) should not be administered under any circumstances until a pheochromocytoma has been ruled out. Bear in mind that about 15 percent of subjects with this tumor have no elevation of blood pressure at all. Some have no more than a paroxysmal arrhythmia but will be thrown violently into an episode of acute congestive heart failure upon administration of a beta blocker.

The commonly used diuretics as well as the antihypertensive drugs other than the beta blockers may not effectively control an alpha-hyperadrenergic state, but more important, they rarely result in direct injury to the patient. This is not the case with the beta-blocking drugs. The introduction of propranolol resulted in a number of deaths in patients with neural crest lesions before it became evident that the induced beta blockade resulted in substantively increased alpha sensitivity. Even in the presence of the less common epinephrine-secreting tumor, the toxicity of increased alpha sensitivity markedly outweighs any benefit to be derived from beta blockade. Those very patients with catecholamine myocardiopathy who might logically be expected to benefit the most from beta blockade may suffer calamitous results from the administration of these drugs. Even the most sanguine among us warn against their use before adequate alpha blockade has been achieved. It is our belief that there is rarely a need for using such a drug for a patient with or suspected of having a pheochromocytoma. Such patients who, during surgery or otherwise, suddenly develop premature contractions or other dysrhythmias are most commonly experiencing acute alpha adrenergia, the cardiac manifestations apparently resulting from an acute rise in systemic blood pressure. Increasing the rate of phentolamine infusion commonly controls such phenomena. Less frequently, these patients require lidocaine 50 to 100 mg intravenously, a deepening of the level of anesthesia, or, rarely, intravenous esmolol (50 mg) in the alpha-blocked patient.

Phentolamine is available not only as a parenteral preparation but as 50-mg oral tablets as well. This drug is less effective when given orally than the alternate alpha blocker, phenoxybenzamine. The latter, supplied as 10-mg capsules, demonstrates a relatively slower turnover but should be administered no less frequently than every 8 hours. The dosage should be titrated against the hypertension or other symptoms, starting with 30 to 40 mg per day in divided doses. Do not hesitate to prescribe this drug for a patient with normal blood pressure who is suspected of having a pheochromocytoma.

It is not uncommon for a patient to require as much as 160 to 200 mg of phenoxybenzamine daily to block adequately the catecholamine release of some pheochromocytomas. The unpleasant side effects of this drug may become difficult to bear with such high doses. Occasionally, the addition of prazosin assists such a patient, but in no case should the alpha blockade achievable with this drug be relied on as the sole protection against this tumor.

Alpha-methyl-para-tyrosine (metyrosine) was introduced as an inhibitor of catecholamine synthesis shortly after the role of tyrosine hydroxylase became appreciated. Unfortunately, the dosage required to modify substantively the biochemical behavior of these tumors commonly results in symptoms of extrapyramidal neural dysfunction (cogwheel rigidity, masked facies, weakness). We have rarely found this drug to be clinically useful, although putative improvement in hyperadrenergic ventricular dysfunction has been reported.

Disulfiram was considered a likely prospect to modify catecholamine synthesis by inhibition of dopamine-beta-hydroxylase. Our clinical studies failed to substantiate its usefulness, since significant enzyme inhibition required a dose far in excess of that tolerated by human subjects.

Although labetalol may be used for the treatment of hypertension before and during surgery for some of these patients (25 to 50 mg per hour intravenously), we have not used this drug as the sole long-term treatment of ambulatory subjects whose tumors could not be completely resected. Labetalol may result in falsely elevated values of both catecholamines and their metabolites when measured in urine.

Sensitive and specific assays of total metanephrines and vanillylmandelic acid excretion eventually lead to a biochemical diagnosis. Once reliable laboratory assays have established the presence of a neural crest lesion (and this can be accomplished in a noncomatose patient with 99 percent certainty), no unnecessary manipulation of that patient should be tolerated. We have witnessed paroxysms precipitated by as little as a carelessly performed sonography procedure from abdominal pressure with the probe.

Whereas the major advances in diagnosis of pheochromocytomas during the 1950s and 1960s stemmed from the biochemical laboratories, those of the past decade have obviously belonged to the newer techniques for demonstration of mass lesions. Sonography, computed tomography (CT) scan, magnetic resonance imaging (MRI), and ^{131}I-metaiodobenzylguanidine (MIBG) scintigraphy are the most reliable noninvasive techniques for the demonstration of a mass lesion. True, the use of such studies does not prove the presence of a biochemically active neural crest lesion, and they certainly do not relieve the surgeon of the necessity for using an anterior abdominal incision and performing a careful exploration to exclude the presence of unexpected lesions.

Small, nonfunctioning adrenocortical adenomas occur in about 5 percent of routine autopsies (a figure that would likely be higher among hypertensive individuals). Granulomatous and metastatic disease as well as a nonfunctioning adrenocortical carcinoma may result in mass lesions that may be mistaken for a pheochromocytoma. The importance of carefully performed biochemical studies is emphasized by the occasional false-negative mass study. The MIBG scans show false negative results in at least 15 percent of the benign and up to 50 percent of the malignant pheochromocytomas. Even 1 to 2 percent false positive studies with MIBG have been reported. Most important, about 15 to 20 percent of adults, 50 percent of children, and more than 75 percent of familial cases and those with multiple endocrine neoplasia (MEN II) or neurocutaneous syndromes have more than one pheochromocytoma. Some of these may be little more than 1 cm in diameter.

Efforts aimed at tumor localization became essential in those occasional patients who present with clinical and biochemical evidence of recurrent pheochromocytoma. Such cases often demand uncommon perseverance to delineate a lesion suitable for resection. Angiography and other invasive studies may be helpful, but none should be performed without the patients receiving intravenous phentolamine or in the absence of a clinician who is experienced in the management of this illness.

A few studies are essential, even for the patient presenting with a pheochromocytoma for the first time. A chest CT scan at the time of abdominal imaging rarely if ever misses the 1 to 2 percent of such lesions found above the diaphragm. With such a negative study, the surgeon may more securely prepare to enter and explore the abdomen as the source of excessive catecholamine synthesis. Finally, an intravenous pyelogram, an abdominal CT scan with contrast material, or a renogram in a dye-sensitive patient should be done to confirm the presence of two functioning kidneys prior to attempting the resection of a tumor that is often desmoplastic and occasionally so intimately related to the vasculature of one kidney that an unplanned nephrectomy is required during surgery for a neural crest lesion.

Only routine preoperative testing should be permitted beyond those studies just noted. It is unnecessary to evaluate blood volumes or perform special studies to rule out a concomitant medullary carcinoma of the thyroid prior to surgery, since this information does not change the management of the case until the removal of the pheochromocytoma. Only then should other endocrinologic studies (such as pentagastrin-stimulated calcitonin assays) begin. The not uncommon observation of cholelithiasis in a mass study of the abdomen might lead to resection of the gallbladder in a patient whose primary surgery proceeds without flaw, but in general one should not unnecessarily complicate these surgical procedures. There should also be no unnecessary delay in proceeding from diagnosis to resection. Our early hesitancy to perform these surgical resections in subjects whose status was complicated by serious cardiac disease (e.g., previous myocardial infarction, congestive heart failure, dysrhythmia with pacemaker) resulted in attempts to carry them through their illness with alpha blockade rather than tumor removal. Unfortunately, the illness tends to progress and leads to escape from effective alpha blockade and excessive side effects from high doses of phenoxybenzamine. A careful and experienced surgeon can rectify this problem.

At present, delay in tumor removal is tolerated only if the lesion is unresectable (malignant or anatomically obscure). We believe that this principle should be applied to the patient whose disease is complicated by pregnancy as well—prompt resection of the tumor with as little unnecessary manipulation of the patient as possible.

PREOPERATIVE MANAGEMENT

Parenteral phentolamine has been our drug of choice for alpha blockade immediately prior to and during the surgery of these patients. This is based on the likelihood that better moment-to-moment control of blood pressure was likely when using a short-acting alpha blocker. Removal of the tumor from the circulation, almost invariably resulting in an acute fall in blood pressure, was the moment when the short half-life of this agent was most appreciated. Rarely is it possible to attain such perfection of alpha blockade that a biochemically active tumor does not elicit some vasomotor response while it is being manipulated. Some physicians have expressed a preference for avoiding alpha blockade in order to ease the difficulty experienced by the surgeon in anatomically locating all of the neural crest tumors. In our opinion, nothing could be more hazardous to the patient. Permitting the patient to experience uncontrolled paroxysms, whether preoperatively or during surgery, can too easily lead to cardiac or cerebrovascular complications. Moreover, reasonable preoperative management demands that the patient's cardiovascular adjustment be returned to as close to normal status as possible. Circulating blood volumes, afterload levels, and cardiac function all improve during the few days in which alpha blockers are administered. The balance between the desire to achieve a reasonably normal physiologic state and the need to reduce the hazard of living with an unresected pheochromocytoma leads in practice to the use of oral alpha blockade with phenoxybenzamine during the 3 or 4 days required for adequate work-up, followed by administration of 24 to 48 hours of parenteral phentolamine immediately prior to surgery. The drawback of the latter step stems from the need for close monitoring. Thus, the patient is usually transferred to a critical care unit for titration of the drug versus hypertension, sweating, dysrhythmias, tremulousness, abdominal pain, or other paroxysmal symptoms. The infusion rate (by Harvard pump) is rarely changed by more than 5 mg per hour every 10 to 15 minutes until resection. Large variations in dosage should be avoided. The initial dosage is 10 mg per hour, and this commonly reaches about 35 mg per hour prior to induction. Excessive blockade is unlikely to result in any injury. Modest hypotension (systolic pressure of 90 mm Hg) is usually well tolerated in patients with reasonable cardiac and renal functions (evidence being that of maintenance of urinary output).

In some patients preparation for surgery can be accomplished with parenteral labetalol. Nitroprusside would be an unwise primary agent in view of the likely duration of its use, but its application as a potent hypotensive agent for short periods of time should not be ignored.

DURING AND AFTER SURGERY

Although the presence of an internist and an anesthesiologist informed in clinical pharmacology might be desirable at the operation, nothing takes the place of a surgeon experienced with neural crest lesions, their clinical behavior, pathophysiology, and anatomic distribution.

On the day of surgery, phentolamine solutions should be prepared in two dilutions in dextrose and water: 1 mg per milliliter (50 ampules in 250 ml) and 5 mg per milliliter (100 ampules in 100 ml). The weaker solution usually suffices for anesthetic induction, whereas the stronger one may be required during tumor manipulation. One hundred extra ampules of phentolamine should be readily available for procedures on large multiple tumors.

Preoperative use of atropine-like drugs should be avoided. Although there has been considerable comment about the potential untoward effect of anesthetics capable of sensitizing the myocardium to catecholamines, surgery can probably be accomplished with any of the anesthetic agents currently in use. It is more critical that portals be available for the immediate parenteral administration of antiarrhythmic, pressor, and alpha-blocking drugs. Volume replacement requires its own portal, since a disproportion between the vascular capacity and circulating volume can be expected to occur upon tumor removal (at the moment of loss of significant vasoconstriction). About 4 to 5 liters of crystalloid or colloid are usually needed to correct for this circumstance, with the bulk of volume repletion implemented after removal of the tumor. Fluid administration, however, should be initiated at the onset of surgery. A central venous line, or better, a Swan-Ganz catheter may be a better guide in the precise level of fluid replacement. Cardiac monitoring (electrocardiogram) and a direct arterial line complete the preoperative arrangements. It must be emphasized that the intravenous portal for drugs should be arranged with minimal dead space tubing so that one may switch from one substance or concentration to another without undue delay. A dilute solution of norepinephrine should be prepared but should rarely be required. Its required use usually signifies inadequate intraoperative volume replacement.

A sudden appearance of dysrhythmia, usually premature ventricular contractions, commonly results during surgery from an acute elevation of blood pressure. This may be treated most readily by increasing the rate of phentolamine infusion, deepening the anesthesia, or administering an intravenous bolus of 50 to 100 mg of lidocaine. Only in those rare instances in which these manipulations fail to yield a response is 50 mg of esmolol warranted.

For abdominal tumors, a transperitoneal approach is mandatory. An upper midline incision from the xiphoid process to below the umbilicus permits good access to both suprarenal areas, where 90 percent of pheochromocytomas are found (twice as often on the right as on the left). With large or extra-adrenal tumors, the type of incision is dictated primarily by the size and anatomic location; larger adrenal tumors are usually single and best approached by a subcostal incision. Thoracic lesions are resected via a posterolateral thoracotomy and neck tumors by an incision along the sternocleidomastoid muscle.

Thorough visual and manual exploration from the diaphragm to the pelvis is mandatory, with special focus on the adrenal glands and para-aortic regions. Complete exploration must be accomplished, regardless of the preoperative imaging results; there is no substitute for the surgeon's exploratory skills, particularly in view of the limited resolution of current imaging techniques.

Upon discovery of one adrenal tumor, resection is delayed until the other adrenal gland can be evaluated. This assists the surgeon in making a decision about the preservation of adrenocortical tissue. If the patient has a neurocutaneous (von Recklinghausen or von Hippel-Lindau) or a multiple endocrine neoplasia (MEN) type II syndrome, or is one of a kindred with pheochromocytomas, the incidence of bilateral lesions reaches almost 100 percent (synchronous or metachronous), and a preoperative decision might have been made to perform an elective bilateral adrenalectomy with autotransplantation of normal cortical tissue into a peripheral muscle compartment. Pertsemlidis has evidence of the effectiveness of such transplantation with twice-weekly adrenocorticotropic hormone stimulation (Fig. 1).

The main difficulties are posed by the retropancreatic location of the left adrenal gland and the retrocaval position of the right adrenal gland. Such proximities to large vessels and the pancreas may create problems during dissection. Adrenal or extra-adrenal tumors may grow near or around the renal vessels and may be difficult to remove without disrupting the renal blood supply. The right adrenal vein is short (about 5 mm), retrocaval, and enters the cava high, that is, about 6 to 7 cm from the level of the renal veins. Pheochromocytomas, like carcinoid tumors, occasionally display pericapsular desmoplasia; this fibrotic reaction may be severe enough to mimic malignancy and render dissection more difficult.

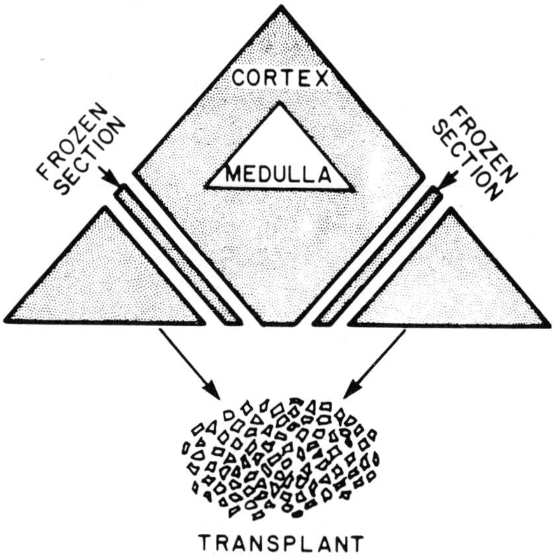

Figure 1 Technique of adrenocortical autotransplantation. Peripheral sections are preserved in iced saline and transplanted into rectus muscles after confirming absence of medulla in more central segments by frozen section.

Removal of each tumor from the vascular circuit usually results in a temporary fall in blood pressure. It is rarely great enough to compromise renal function, which can be monitored by measuring urine flow. Continued hypertension at this point usually signifies incomplete removal of the neural crest lesions. Somewhat fewer than 25 percent of patients have minimal residual hypertension, which rarely becomes evident until after discharge from the hospital. Its control should not pose any significant difficulty with ordinary antihypertensive drugs.

A continued requirement for postoperative pressor drugs, although possibly attributable to a myocardial infarction, sepsis, or adrenocortical insufficiency, is most likely related to retroperitoneal bleeding and represents an urgent indication for re-exploration. The swings in blood pressure during surgery make such bleeding more common. Deep retroperitoneal fluid collections, occasionally septic (often staphylococcal) after surgery, should be suspected when the patient moves one diaphragmatic leaflet poorly and becomes febrile. Bilateral adrenal resection obviously requires adrenocortical replacement.

On the one hand, total metanephrine excretion falls rapidly postoperatively but may remain above normal if the clinical course is stressful. On the other hand, excretion of vanillylmandelic acid almost always approaches normal about 2 to 4 days after a complete tumor resection.

Operative mortality should probably not exceed 1 percent. Even in the absence of persistent hypertension, all patients whose tumors have been resected require ongoing follow-up. Recurrent or additional pheochromocytomas, alternate neoplasms, evidence of MEN type II syndrome, neurocutaneous syndromes, or Carney's triad all demand periodic examinations, catecholamine catabolite assays, and calcitonin determinations. Family members should all be screened by means of total metanephrine excretion assays.

NONRESECTABLE TUMORS

Since pheochromocytomas are characterized by pleomorphism, the determination of anaplasia usually requires more than just a microscopic finding of mitotic figures. Rather, malignancy is suggested by (1) microscopic evidence of invasion of capsule, blood vessels, or lymphatics in the original specimen; (2) gross evidence of tumor spread at surgery; (3) evidence of metastases (liver, lungs, bone, local nodes) on imaging studies done prior to surgery; (4) elevated urinary excretion of homovanillic acid by an adult with a neural crest lesion; (5) local or distant recurrence of the pheochromocytoma (other than another primary lesion) after resection of the initial lesion. Pheochromocytomas fulfill these criteria for malignancy in approximately 10 percent of the cases. Although slow growth is common, it is not universal, and most of the tumors respond rather poorly or at least temporarily to cytotoxic agents. Radiotherapy occasionally succeeds in ameliorating such lesions, most commonly those involving bone. One of us (SEG) has had success in treating three such patients with streptozotocin, but the literature does not reflect similar experiences. A combination of cyclophosphamide, vincristine, and dacarbazine (CVD) has been observed to offer frequent although temporary response. As with any other sudden change in the status of these patients, one must be certain to administer alpha blockade prior to chemotherapy.

The slow growth pattern often yields to debulking procedures concomitantly with long-term treatment with alpha blockade (usually phenoxybenzamine). On occasion, metyrosine may be used for more complete reduction of alpha adrenergia; the authors have failed to observe much advantage in the use of this agent for patients with malignant lesions, since low doses are unavailing and at 3 g per day or more unacceptable basal ganglia dysfunction appears. Since only one-half of the malignant lesions concentrate MIBG and even these tend to be of low level, the therapeutic use of ^{131}I-labeled MIBG is only rarely beneficial. It may be that early detection and complete resection of these lesions offer the best prognosis, but there are no adequate data to prove such a supposition.

In the final analysis, pheochromocytoma represents the needle in the hypertensive haystack. It is worthy of our attention because its near 100 percent mortality rate may be reversed by biochemically precise evaluation, gentle and efficient preoperative preparation, and experienced surgical care.

SUGGESTED READING

Averbuch SD, Steakley CS, Young RC, et al. Malignant pheochromocytoma: Effective treatment with a combination of cyclophosphamide, vincristine, and dacarbazine. Ann Intern Med 1988; 109:267–273.

Elliott WJ, Murphy MB, Straus FH II, Jarabak J. Improved safety of glucagon testing for pheochromocytoma by prior alpha-receptor blockade. Arch Intern Med 1989; 149:214–216.

Gitlow SE, Mendlowitz M, Bertani LM. The biochemical techniques for detecting and establishing the presence of pheochromocytoma. Am J Cardiol 1970; 26:270–279.

Manager W, Gifford RW Jr. Pheochromocytoma. New York: Springer-Verlag, 1977.

Moulton JS. CT of the adrenal glands. Semin Roentgenol 1988; 23:288–303.

Samaan NA, Hickey RC, Shutts PE. Diagnosis, localization, and management of pheochromocytoma. Cancer 1988; 62:2451–2460.

Sheps SG, Jiang N, Klee GG, van Heerden JA. Recent developments in the diagnosis and treatment of pheochromocytoma. Mayo Clin Proc 1990; 65:88–95.

Turner MC, DeQuattro V, Falk R, et al. Childhood familial pheochromocytoma; conflicting results of localization techniques. Hypertension 1986; 8:851–858.

Villani A, Primieri P, DeCosmo G. Cardiomyopathy in pheochromocytoma. Eur J Anaesth 1989; 6:233–236.

Wells SA Jr, Dilley WG, Fandon JA, et al. Early diagnosis and treatment of medullary thyroid carcinoma. Arch Intern Med 1985; 145:1248–1252.

POLYCYSTIC OVARIAN DISEASE

JEFFREY R. CRAGUN, M.D.
R. JEFFREY CHANG, M.D.

Polycystic ovarian disease is a disorder of young women characterized by chronic anovulation and hirsutism. In 50 percent of cases, there is associated obesity and, to a lesser extent, acne. The diagnosis is generally implied by history of infrequent or absent menstruation and the gradual development of excessive hair growth. The distribution of increased hair usually involves the face, but may also include the lower abdomen (male pattern escutcheon) and chest. Classically, the ovaries are bilaterally enlarged and cystic, but may appear normal by pelvic examination. Endocrinologically, there are elevated levels of circulating androgens, of which the most biologically active arise from the ovaries. Adrenal androgens are increased in one-half of patients. These elevated androgens are peripherally converted to estrogens that are unopposed by progesterone since ovulation is suppressed. This hormonal environment can lead to chronic endometrial stimulation and even endometrial carcinoma.

The clinical and biochemical presentation of this syndrome points to three major areas of therapeutic concern: (1) abnormal stimulation of the pilosebaceous unit resulting in hirsutism and acne; (2) chronic anovulation leading to infertility; and (3) persistent exposure to uninterrupted estrogen secretion, posing an increased risk of endometrial hyperplasia and cancer.

HIRSUTISM

Pathophysiology

The development of hirsutism and acne in polycystic ovarian disease reflect three interrelated processes. First, there is excess production of androgen by either the ovary and/or the adrenal gland. The source of this increased androgen production has been studied for many years, and it now appears that the most biologically active compounds, androstenedione and testosterone, are derived from the ovary; whereas the relatively weaker androgens, dehydroepiandrosterone (DHA) and its sulfate (DHA-S), arise from the adrenal gland. This differentiation is important since it impacts upon therapy. Fortunately, the evaluation of hirsutism allows for this distinction to be made. When total serum testosterone is increased as measured by radioimmunoassay (RIA) with chromatographic separation, an ovarian source of increased androgen production is implied; whereas an increase in DHA-S suggests an adrenal source. If both hormones are elevated, treatment is directed toward the ovary. Adrenal suppression should be considered only if DHA-S alone is increased. Imaging of the ovary and adrenal is essential if high levels of androgens are measured since these high levels suggest the presence of a potentially life-threatening tumor.

The second aspect of excessive hair growth is the transport of androgens in the circulation. Transportation is particularly important for testosterone since sex-hormone binding globulin (SHBG) is reduced in hyperandrogenic states, which results in increased circulating free testosterone. The role of SHBG is clinically relevant since the magnitude of excess free testosterone correlates best with the severity of hirsutism.

The third consideration is target organ responsiveness to androgens. This responsiveness is dictated in part by ethnic background. In addition, some patients with hirsutism appear to have increased conversion of testosterone to dihydrotestosterone (DHT), which is the intracellular hormone primarily responsible for stimulation of hair growth. Thus hair growth is ultimately controlled not only by the intracellular conversion of testosterone to DHT, but also by the amount of free androgen present and the relative biologic activity of differing types of androgens.

It should be understood that the length of the hair life cycle on the beard area of the face is approximately 6 months. Thus any treatment should be continued for at least this interval and likely for 1 year before a therapeutic benefit derived from arresting new hair growth may become apparent. The severity of hirsutism at the initiation of treatment is also a consideration since mild hair growth is far more easily treated than severe hirsutism.

Treatment

The current mainstay of therapy for hirsutism in women with polycystic ovarian disease is ovarian suppression usually by administration of combination oral contraceptives (Table 1). Estrogen and progestin act in concert to suppress gonadotropin secretion. In addition, estrogen increases SHBG, which results in a reduction of serum free testosterone. Since the synthetic progestins contained in these formulations are 19-nortestosterone derivatives, it seems prudent to select a formulation that has the least androgenic effects based on a relative estrogenic and androgenic potential. This formulation is accomplished by the administration of ethynodiol diacetate, 1 mg, and ethinyl estradiol, 35 μg (Demulen 1 + 35).

Recently, it has been demonstrated that marked suppression of ovarian androgen steroidogenesis in polycystic ovarian disease may be achieved by administration of a long-acting gonadotropin-releasing hormone (Gn-RH) agonist. Whether this mode of therapy is practical or not is unclear since circulating estrogens were also decreased to castration levels, and there is concern of bone loss during this induced hypoestrogenic state. Further investigation is necessary before any recommendation can be made regarding therapy with Gn-RH agonists.

Adrenal suppression by dexamethasone administration has been shown to benefit some patients with polycystic ovarian disease and with mild hirsutism. However, its effectiveness for severe hair growth is limited since

TABLE 1 Treatment of Androgen Excess

	Mechanism of Action	Dose	Cost/Month ($)
Ovarian suppression			
Oral contraceptive pills	Suppresss LH and FSH Increases SHBG	Ethynodiol diacetate, 1 mg and ethinyl estradiol, 35 μg for 21 days of every 28 days	16–20
Gn-RH agonists	Suppresses LH and FSH	Experimental use only	—
Adrenal suppression			
Dexamethasone	Suppresses ACTH	0.5 mg qhs	6–9
Antiandrogens			
Cimetidine	Blocks androgen receptor Histamine (H2) antagonist	300 mg q4–6h	72–75
Spironolactone	Blocks androgen receptor Inhibits cytochrome P-450 (decreases androgen synthesis) Aldosterone antagonist	200 mg qd	8–44
Cyproterone acetate	Blocks androgen receptor Potent progestin action	25–100 mg × 10 days every month	N/A in USA
Local measures			
Dipilatories	Dissolves hair shafts	—	4–15
Electrolysis	Ablation of hair follicles	—	25–75

Abbreviations: ACTH = adrenocorticotropic hormone; LH = luteinizing hormone.

dexamethasone eliminates only the weak adrenal androgens, DHA and DHA-S, and not the major ovarian androgens, androstenedione and testosterone. In the past, combined ovarian and adrenal suppression was attempted in some cases of severe hirsutism, but this form of therapy has recently given way to the use of antiandrogenic agents either alone or in combination with oral contraceptive steroids.

Antiandrogens effectively reduce hair growth primarily by blocking the action of testosterone on the target organ through competitive binding of its receptor. Of this class of drugs, only cimetidine and spironolactone are used in the United States. Cyproterone acetate is approved in Europe. Spironolactone not only blocks the androgen receptor, but also interferes with cytochrome P-450, which results in defective steroidogenesis and a decrease in testosterone production. As an aldosterone antagonist, this compound may also be associated with a mild reduction in blood pressure and a mild elevation in serum potassium. Cimetidine has also been reported to reduce hair growth in hirsute individuals. However, the clinical benefit from this drug has been disappointing, and it is not used frequently.

Many patients bothered by excessive hair growth turn to local control measures. Depilatories are available without prescription and are used successfully by some, but they can be associated with adverse skin reactions, particularly when applied to delicate facial skin. Electrolysis by experienced technicians is an effective means of ablating abnormal hair follicles, but does not alter the hormonal stimulation of new hair follicle recruitment and may result in some scarring and discomfort.

Follow-up

The basic premise of therapy is directed toward improvement of hirsutism and patient satisfaction. Again, one is reminded of the life cycle of facial hair growth and the need to persist with treatment for a minimum of 6 months. With a successful response and near complete eradication of hirsutism, hormonal reassessment is probably unnecessary; however, if improvement is slow or absent and particularly if the patient worsens on therapy, reevaluation should be performed.

ANOVULATION

Pathophysiology

The precise mechanism for anovulation in polycystic ovarian disease is unknown. Studies to date have demonstrated diminished pituitary follicle-stimulating hormone (FSH) secretion, which presumably results from the negative feed-back effect of chronic estrogen stimulation. Whether or not the ovarian production of inhibin is sufficient to contribute to this suppression of FSH has not been established. The presence of increased serum androgens in polycystic ovarian disease may also cause a direct inhibitory effect on folliculogenesis. This effect may be mediated by either excessive adrenal androgen production or abnormal intraovarian androgen concentrations derived from ovarian stromal cells. Finally, 25 to 30 percent of patients with polycystic ovarian disease exhibit hyperprolactinemia, which may contribute to anovulation by mechanisms similar to those in amenorrheic women with prolactinomas.

Treatment

The standard method of ovulation induction in polycystic ovarian disease is by administration of clomiphene citrate (Table 2). Clomiphene citrate is similar in molecular structure to diethylstilbestrol and exhibits both estrogenic and antiestrogenic properties. In polycystic ovarian disease, clomiphene citrate presumably interferes with the negative feed-back of estrogen by binding to estrogen receptors in the hypothalmus and pituitary. This release from inhibition allows for increased FSH secretion with subsequent stimulation of follicular development and eventual ovulation. The initial dose is 50 mg per day for 5 days commencing on day 2 or 3 of a spontaneous or progesterone-induced menses. In amenorrheic patients, vaginal bleeding induced by progesterone in oil provides a convenient reference point, assures adequate estrogen levels, and safely confirms the lack of pregnancy. Indicative of a normal ovulatory response is a rise in the basal body temperature (BBT) of approximately 12 to 14 days followed by spontaneous vaginal bleeding or a serum progesterone level above 10 ng per milliliter in the midluteal phase. The same dose of clomiphene citrate is repeated in subsequent cycles. In the absence of spontaneous menses, the dose of clomiphene citrate may be increased by increments of 50 mg to 150 mg per day for 5 days until an ovulatory response is achieved as indicated by a biphasic BBT or elevated luteal progesterone. Higher doses of clomiphene citrate (up to 250 mg) have been recommended for resistant patients, but the success rate is minimal. Instead, it may be more appropriate to modify the regimen by lowering the dose of clomiphene citrate to 100 mg and adding human chorionic gonadotropin 10,000 IU on day 13 of administration of clomiphene citrate or extending the length of treatment with clomiphene citrate or imposing an incremental dose regimen.

An important adjunct to clomiphene citrate therapy is concomitant dexamethasone administration. It has previously been demonstrated that in patients with slightly increased DHA-S, both the ovulatory and pregnancy rate following administration of clomiphene citrate plus dexamethasone is significantly greater than that resulting from treatment with clomiphene citrate alone. The elevation of DHA-S need not necessarily exceed the upper normal range, but rather be higher than the mean concentration established by a given laboratory.

If there is coexistent hyperprolactinemia, it is unclear whether bromocriptine administration is beneficial or not. To date, no study has been able to demonstrate an advantage of bromocriptine alone or combined with clomiphene citrate compared to that of clomiphene citrate alone for induction of ovulation. Until more convincing data are available, it is not recommended to use bromocriptine for ovulation induction in polycystic ovarian disease.

Failure to ovulate or conceive in response to clomiphene citrate alone or in combination with other drugs warrants consideration of gonadotropin therapy. This therapy may be instituted by means of either human menopausal gonadotropins (Pergonal) or purified urinary

TABLE 2 Ovulation Induction

Agent	*Mechanism of Action*	*Dose*	*Cost/Month ($)*
Clomiphene citrate	Blocks estrogen binding Increases FSH	50–250 mg qd × 5d	20–90
Clomiphene citrate + hCG	Simulates LH surge	5,000–10,000 IU × 1 day	78–157
Clomiphene citrate + dexamethasone	Suppresses ACTH	0.5 mg qhs	26–99
Human menopausal gonadotropins (Pergonal)	Directly stimulates folliculogenesis	1–5 ampules qd prn	575–1,760
Purified FSH (Metrodin)	Same as human menopausal gonadotropin	1–5 ampules qd prn	590–2,870
Ovarian wedge resection	Temporary reduction in ovarian androgens	—	4,000–7,000

Abbreviations: ACTH = adrenocorticotropic hormone; LH = luteinizing hormone.

TABLE 3 Endometrial Protection

Agent	*Mechanism of Action*	*Dose*	*Cost ($)*
Oral contraceptive pills	See Table 1	See Table 1	See Table 1
Medroxyprogesterone acetate	Decreases estrogen receptors Increases estrogen metabolism Induces menstrual bleeding	10 mg qd × 10–14 days	12–15

FSH (Metrodin). Both regimens require careful clinical monitoring by means of ultrasonography for follicle development and hormonal assessment for ovarian steroid production. The dose of gonadotropins is adjusted according to each individual's follicular response.

For the few patients in whom all medical therapy fails, it is not unreasonable to consider an ovarian wedge resection. Traditionally, this has required an exploratory laparotomy with its inherent operative and anesthetic risks. As a result of this operative procedure, pelvic adhesions may form and further impede fertility. Recently, the effect of an ovarian wedge resection has been duplicated using laser laparoscopic techniques in which areas on the ovarian capsule are periodically vaporized. Although this procedure obviates some of the morbidity of a traditional wedge resection which requires a laparotomy, recent reports have shown a high incidence of ovarian adhesion formation following laser ovarian capsule puncture procedures. In addition, neither procedure assures ovulation, and if ovulation does occur, it may continue postoperatively for only a few months.

ENDOMETRIAL HYPERPLASIA

Pathophysiology

Amidst the immediate concerns about hair growth and infertility in polycystic ovarian disease, there exists an insidious process that poses the most serious threat to life to these women. With persistent unopposed estrogen, endometrial proliferation can occur, which may advance to endometrial hyperplasia or even frank carcinoma in some women. Therefore, not surprisingly, young women with endometrial cancer nearly always have a clinical history consistent with the diagnosis of polycystic ovarian disease, and the problem seems to be compounded in the presence of obesity. It is for this reason that endometrial sampling is mandatory in patients with a long history of chronic anovulation, and therapy must be directed toward prevention of endometrial proliferation.

Treatment

The needed protection may be provided by progesterone either endogenously through successful ovulation induction or exogenously by means of combination contraceptive steroids (Table 3). If endometrial hyperplasia is the sole therapeutic concern, medroxyprogesterone acetate (Provera) is administered at a dose of 10 mg a day for at least 12 days each month to induce menstrual bleeding. Other progestins, including 19-nortestosterone derivatives, may be considered, but their use is limited by their known adverse effects on high-density lipoproteins. Progestin therapy significantly reduces but does not exclude the risk of endometrial abnormalities. Therefore in the presence of abnormal bleeding, office endometrial biopsy or formal dilatation and curettage should be performed to rule out significant endometrial pathology.

SUGGESTED READING

Adashi ET, Rock JA, Guzick D, Wentz AC, Jones GS, Jones HW. Fertility following bilateral ovarian wedge resection: a critical analysis of 90 consecutive cases of the polycystic ovary syndrome. Fertil Steril 1981; 36:320–325.

Chang RJ, Lauffer LR, Meldrum DR, DeFazio J, Lu JKH, Vale WW, Rivier JE, Judd HL. Steroid secretion in polycystic ovarian disease after ovarian suppression by a long-acting gonadotropin-releasing hormone agonist. J Clin Endocrinol Metab 1983; 56:897–903.

Cumming DC, Yang JC, Rebar RW, Yen SSC. Treatment of hirsutism with spironolactone. JAMA 1982; 247:1295–1298.

Lobo RA, Goebelsmann V, Horton R. Evidence for the importance of peripheral tissue events in the development of hirsutism in polycystic ovary syndrome. J Clin Endocrinol Metab 1983; 57:393–397.

Pittaway DE, Maxson WS, Wentz AC. Spironolactone in combination drug therapy for unresponsive hirsutism. Fertil Steril 1985; 43:878–882.

Wang CF, Gemzell C. The use of human gonadotropins for the induction of ovulation in women with polycystic ovarian disease. Fertil Steril 1980; 33:479–486.

ORAL COMBINATION CONTRACEPTIVES

PAUL F. BRENNER, M.D.

More than 30 years have elapsed since oral steroid contraceptives were first tested clinically in Puerto Rico. More than 25 years have passed since the birth control pill was introduced clinically in the United States as a method of reversible family planning. The use of oral combination contraceptive formulations increased yearly through 1975. Since that time concerns pertaining to the risks of cancer, metabolic disease, and cardiovascular disease in oral contraceptive users and future fertility when the pill is discontinued have resulted in a decrease in the selection of the birth control pill as a method of family planning among American women. Many of these concerns are based on myth rather than scientific fact. The great expense needed to successfully defend the intrauterine device (IUD) against legal assaults led to the withdrawal of the first-generation IUDs (Lippes Loop and Saf-T-Coil) and second-generation copper IUDs (Copper T-200 and Copper 7) from the American market. Similar legal attacks attempting to link barrier contraceptive methods to an increased risk of teratogenicity threatens to force the removal from the American market of any barrier method of family planning that uses the spermicidal agent nonoxynol-9. As a result of these legal challenges to contraception as many as 5.5 million women in the United States are facing the potential loss of their family planning method of first choice. Another consequence of these legal actions is that the combination birth control pill will assume a more prominent role among contraceptive modalities. A decision to use oral steroid contraceptives should be made only after the myths associated with birth control pills are dispelled, the true risks and noncontraceptive benefits associated with this method are clearly defined, and women with absolute and relative contraindications to the use of the pill are identified.

CANCER MYTHS AND ORAL CONTRACEPTIVES

An increased risk of breast cancer, endometrial cancer, cervical cancer, liver cancer, malignant melanoma, and prolactin-secreting pituitary adenomas has been erroneously linked to the use of oral contraceptives. Careful scrutiny of the scientific data indicates that an increased risk of breast cancer, liver cancer, and prolactin-secreting pituitary adenomas are not associated with the ingestion of oral contraceptives. Because of problems in designing a study that would allow for the presence and influence of confounding factors, definite conclusions concerning cervical cancer and malignant melanoma and the use of birth control pills cannot be determined at this time. Most important of all there is a significant reduction in endometrial cancer and ovarian cancer in women who use oral contraceptives. The progestogen in the oral combination contraceptives decreases the synthesis of both estrogen and progesterone receptors by the endometrial cells. Clinically, the result of the reduced synthesis of estrogen receptors in the target organ leads to less endometrial cancer. The greatest mitotic activity in the ovary occurs at the time of ovulation. Contraceptive modalities that consistently inhibit ovulation decrease the risk of ovarian cancer. Overall, women receiving birth control pills have a decreased risk of cancer because they have a significant reduction in the risk of endometrial cancer and ovarian cancer.

METABOLIC DISORDER MYTHS AND ORAL CONTRACEPTIVES

Investigations of the metabolic changes produced by oral contraceptives demonstrated an increase in the serum glucose level, an increase in the serum insulin level, and a relative insulin insensitivity that led to impaired glucose tolerance. These alterations in carbohydrate metabolism are specifically associated with the synthetic progestogen component of the pill. From these studies concerns arose that oral contraceptive users would be more likely to develop diabetes mellitus. As the dose of progestogen used in oral contraceptives decreased and the phasic products were introduced clinically, there are now birth control pill formulations that do not produce any adverse changes in carbohydrate metabolism or may even result in a slight improvement in glucose tolerance. The use of birth control pills does not cause diabetes. The choice of a contraceptive method for insulin-dependent diabetics has always been a formidable decision. In general, these patients are best advised to have their desired number of children as soon as possible and then to use a permanent method of family planning. The dilemma has been the choice of a contraceptive method until they are ready to consider sterilization. Because diabetes is an intrinsic vascular disease known to signify a high-risk population for heart attacks there is great reluctance to use birth control pills in this group of women. Persons with diabetes have impaired defense mechanisms against infection. On this basis, the IUD was considered a poor choice. Other methods of family planning with lower use-effectiveness rates were less than optimal for insulin-dependent diabetic women. Since the IUD no longer remains an option for this group of women, one of the newer oral combination contraceptive formulations that does not adversely effect carbohydrate metabolism is the best choice for a temporary family planning method for the diabetic woman of childbearing age.

Post-pill amenorrhea is the failure of women to resume spontaneous menstrual cycles after discontinuing oral contraceptives. This condition is due to an abnormality of hypothalamic-pituitary function and is not related to the failure to have withdrawal bleeding while currently using birth control pills. The latter condition is related to insufficient exogenous hormonal stimulation of the endometrium. Post-pill amenorrhea of 6 months duration or longer should be evaluated. Post-pill amenorrhea associated with galactorrhea demands immediate investigation. Some women with post-pill amenorrhea-galactorrhea have a pituitary adenoma. Women with menstrual cycle irregularities prior to initiating oral contraceptive therapy are more likely to have post-pill amenorrhea than women with a history of regular menses prior to pill use. Some women are destined to develop secondary amenorrhea. If these women are given oral contraceptives they will have exogenous hormone withdrawal bleeding as long as they use the pill. When they stop using the pill the secondary amenorrhea may become clinically apparent. The incidence of secondary amenorrhea in former pill users is the same as in a population who never used pills. The use of oral steroid contraceptives does not increase the incidence of secondary amenorrhea.

There are more than 1 million teenage pregnancies each year in the United States, and most of these are unplanned and largely the result of the failure to use any method of contraception. The use of birth control pills by teenagers is accompanied by the myths that the pill causes premature epiphyseal closure and an ultimate reduction in height and that it leads to permanent dysfunction of the hypothalamic-pituitary axis. Both of these concerns are without scientific support. At menarche a woman's ultimate height is already predetermined and the administration of exogenous sex steroid even in large doses cannot shorten her stature. Once ovulatory menstrual cycles are established, use of birth control pills does not result in permanent impairment of the reproductive axis. Ideally a teenager should have at least three consecutive spontaneous menstrual cycles with intervals of less than 35 days before starting to use oral contraceptives. In practice, once menarche has occurred and the person is sexually active I am willing to prescribe birth control pills. I am far more concerned about the psychosocial and medical sequelae of teenage pregnancy than the effects of the birth control pills.

CARDIOVASCULAR DISEASE MYTHS AND ORAL CONTRACEPTIVES

Oral contraceptive users have an increased risk of death from both venous and arterial disease. Pill users have a threefold to fourfold increased risk of venous thromboembolic disease (deep vein thrombosis, pulmonary embolus, and thrombotic cerebrovascular accident) compared with non-pill users. The increased risk of venous vascular disease is related to the estrogen component of the pill in a dose-dependent manner. One of every 30,000 pill users are hospitalized annually because of a stroke, and one of every 200,000 pill users die each year from this disease. In the mid 1970s it was reported that all women currently using oral contraceptives had a significantly greater risk of myocardial infarction than non-pill users. Closer scrutiny of this study indicated that all pill users were not at an increased risk of a heart attack. This risk was limited to a specific population that included women with hypertension, diabetes, and hyperlipidemia, and the greatest risk was found in women over 35 years of age who were smokers. Nonsmokers may continue to use the pill until 45 years of age before there is a statistically significant increased risk of a myocardial infarction. The pathogenesis of the arterial vascular changes that lead to a heart attack may theoretically be thrombotic or atherogenic. An atherogenic phenomenon should be related to duration of use and should be present in former pill users. The risk of heart attacks is not related to the duration of use of oral contraceptives and is not increased in former pill users. The underlying pathology in the arterial vascular system must therefore be thrombotic and not atherogenic.

FERTILITY MYTHS AND ORAL CONTRACEPTIVES

The incidence of spontaneous abortion, birth defects, and chromosomal aberrations are not increased in former pill users even if they conceive in the first cycle after discontinuing birth control pills. There is no increase in sterility in women who have stopped using the pills. As a group it takes former pill users 2 to 3 months longer to conceive than women who have never used pills. Although there is a delay in the return of fertility in former pill users, 2 years after stopping the pill the same percentage of women are pregnant as in a group of women who discontinued barrier methods of family planning 2 years earlier. In the first cycle after stopping the pills, the follicular phase tends to be prolonged and there may be a corresponding delay in the return of ovulation. Women who conceive in this first cycle are not able to estimate their expected date of confinement with any precision. For this reason alone women who discontinue oral contraceptives are advised to delay at least one cycle before attempting to conceive, so that the gestational age may be more precisely calculated.

RISKS OF ORAL CONTRACEPTIVES

Family planning modalities are not imposed on acceptors but are dispensed after carefully weighing the risks and benefits of all options. The serious side effects associated with birth control pills include a twofold increased risk of cholelithiasis with an annual incidence of 1 in every 1,250 pill users; a threefold increased risk of myocardial infarction in smokers over the age of 35 years with an annual incidence of 1 in every 5,000 pill users; a threefold increased risk of deep vein thrombosis with an annual incidence of 1 in every 10,000 pill users; a fourfold increased risk of pulmonary embolism with an annual incidence of 1 in every 30,000 pill users; a threefold increased risk of stroke with an annual incidence of 1 in every 30,000 pill users; and liver adenoma with an estimated annual incidence of 1 in every 50,000 pill users.

The common side effects attributed to birth control pills occur most often in the first three treatment cycles and tend to diminish with continued use of the pill. Some of the common side effects are attributed to the synthetic estrogen component of the pill, some are related specifically to the synthetic progestogen, and a few are associated with both components. Those events related to the estrogen are nausea, breast tenderness, fluid retention, mood changes, and depression. The untoward events related to the progestogen are weight gain, acne, amenorrhea, and nervousness. Breakthrough bleeding, chloasma, and hypertension are related to both components. The common less-serious side effects disappear rapidly when the birth control pills are discontinued with the exception of the chloasma, which takes a relatively long period of time to fade.

NONCONTRACEPTIVE BENEFITS OF ORAL CONTRACEPTIVES

Much less attention has been directed to the benefits of oral contraceptives compared with the sensationalism and distorted reporting of the side effects associated with the pill. Indeed there are many very important, noncontraceptive benefits derived from the use of birth control pills, some of which are potentially lifesaving. Oral combination contraceptive users have regular menstrual cycles, fewer ovarian cysts, less benign breast disease, less iron deficiency anemia, less primary dysmenorrhea, and less acute salpingitis. Additional benefits afforded to birth control pill users include less endometrial and ovarian cancer and less rheumatoid arthritis. Oral contraceptive users are protected not only from unwanted intrauterine pregnancy but also from ectopic gestation.

CONTRAINDICATIONS TO THE USE OF ORAL CONTRACEPTIVES

For some women the risks of using oral contraceptives far outweigh any potential benefit and they should not receive the pill. These women are defined as having an absolute contraindication for the use of the combination oral contraceptives. One of the most important absolute contraindications for the use of the pill is a past history of thromboembolic disease. This includes a past history of deep vein thrombosis or thrombophlebitis, pulmonary embolus, cerebral thrombosis, systemic lupus erythematosus, and sickle cell disease. It does not include such events as varicose veins or sickle cell trait. Risk factors for myocardial infarction, including hypertension, diabetes, hyperlipidemia, women over 35 years of age who smoke, and organic heart disease, are absolute contraindications to the use of oral steroid contraceptives.

Women who had toxemia of pregnancy and following childbirth are normotensive can be considered candidates for birth control pills with the stipulation that their blood pressure is frequently monitored.

Gestational diabetics may be given birth control pills, but they must have periodic tests of glucose tolerance while taking the pill. Forty-five percent of patients with a past history of gestational diabetes develop impaired glucose tolerance while ingesting the birth control pills. Subjects who are at increased risk for diabetes mellitus (age more than 35 years, obesity, delivery of an infant weighing 4,000 g or more, unexplained stillbirth, previous abnormal blood glucose levels, family history of diabetes) should be screened for abnormal glucose tolerance before starting a steroid contraceptive.

Breast cancer and uterine cancer have long been considered absolute contraindications to the use of birth control pills. The presence of benign breast disease does not preclude the use of oral contraceptives. Women with vaginal adenosis, as the result of diethylestilbestrol (DES) exposure of their mothers during pregnancy, can take the pill.

Pregnancy is another absolute contraindication to the use of oral contraceptives. Undiagnosed abnormal uterine bleeding that might suggest either a complication of pregnancy or a possible genital malignancy negates the use of this medication.

Oral contraceptives should not be given to patients with active liver disease or to those with a history of jaundice or pruritus of pregnancy. Women with active liver disease may not be able to conjugate the estrogen, and as a result there is an increase in the free, biologically active form of estrogen. Patients with a past history of liver disease that is presently inactive as shown by normal results of liver function tests may take birth control pills.

The final absolute contraindications to oral contraceptive use include the rare conditions of intestinal malabsorption syndrome in which the sex steroids are not absorbed in the intestinal tract and the current use of the antituberculous drug rifampin. The concomitant use of rifampin and birth control pills significantly interferes with the metabolism of the steroids to the point that they are no longer effective.

Migraine headaches, severe depression, and oligomenorrhea-amenorrhea are not considered absolute contraindications to the selection of birth control pills but are certainly relative contraindications. Most women with migraine headaches experience an increased frequency and even severity of their headaches while taking oral contraceptives. An occasional patient reports no change in their headaches or even improvement while on the pill. If their migraine headaches become worse while using oral contraceptives, these women should discontinue this method of family planning. A patient seldom gets migraine headaches for the first time while taking the pill. Depression may be related to changes in tryptophan metabolism. The levels of several vitamins are known to decrease during the use of oral contraceptives. One of these vitamins is pyridoxine (vitamin B_6). Pyridoxine is a cofactor in the metabolism of tryptophan. As the levels of pyridoxine fall there is an increase in xanthurenic acid that is related to depression. Patients with oligomenorrhea or amenorrhea need to have the etiology of the absence of their menses determined before they select a contraceptive method. If a diagnosis of premature ovarian failure is established, these women do not require contraception. Women with polycystic ovarian disease and hirsutism may notice a decrease in the rate of hair growth from the use of an estrogen-dominant birth control pill in addition to the prevention of pregnancy. Furthermore, the synthetic progestogen in the combination pill inhibits the mitogenic effects of unopposed estrogen on the endometrium.

Leiomyomata uteri, seizure disorders, obesity, and candidal infections are not contraindications to the use of birth control pills. Uterine fibroids enlarge as circulating levels of estrogen increase in pregnancy or in response to large doses of exogenous estrogen. Oral contraceptives containing 30 to 35 μg of ethinylestradiol per tablet do not stimulate leiomyomata uteri to grow. Patients who have epilepsy and use oral contraceptives do not have an increase in the difficulty controlling their seizures. Phenytoin (Dilantin) may alter the metabolism of the estrogen component of the pill and adversely affect the efficacy of the oral contraceptives. Women taking phenytoin and choosing to use birth control pills should receive a formulation with 50 μg of estrogen per tablet. Women who are overweight but otherwise normotensive and healthy may use birth control pills. The dose of the pill is not adjusted for the weight of the patient. There is controversy concerning the use of birth control pills by women with vaginal candidiasis, but most women can use the oral contraceptives without an increase in candidal infections. There are a few pill users who develop vaginal or systemic candidiasis that cannot be cured until the birth control pills are discontinued.

ORAL CONTRACEPTIVE SELECTION

There are two types of oral steroid contraceptives. The first is the combination oral contraceptive in which one tablet containing both synthetic estrogen and progestogen is taken daily for 21 days. The second is the mini-pill, progestogen-only pill, in which a tablet containing only progestogen is taken continuously every day. This latter method has the advantage that there are no adverse effects attributed to estrogen. The mini-pill regimen has the disadvantages of frequent disruption of the menstrual cycle with episodes of both irregular bleeding and amenorrhea and diminished effectiveness when compared with the oral combination contraceptives. The mini-pill has a pregnancy rate of 2 to 8 percent because of the failure of this modality to inhibit ovulation consistently. Forty percent of women using the progestogen-only pill ovulate regularly, and another 20 percent ovulate irregularly. Only 40 percent of women using the mini-pill have a consistent inhibition of ovulation. About the only clinical situation suited for the mini-pill is postpartum women who are breastfeeding their child and desire a hormonal form of contraception that does not adversely affect the quantity or quality of the breast milk.

Therefore, the oral combination contraceptive is the first choice for nearly all women who want to use birth control pills. Until the 1980s all of the combination oral contraceptive formulations were monophasic. All of the 21 active steroid tablets in each cycle contained the same dose of estrogen and progestogen. The biphasic and triphasic oral contraceptives are now available for clinical use. The biphasic pills contain the same dose of estrogen in all 21 active tablets, but the dose of progestogen in each of the last 11 tablets is twice that found in each of the first 10 tablets. The triphasic formulations use three different doses of progestogen in the 21 tablets and may or may not alter the dose of estrogen. The particular oral combination contraceptive formulation to be prescribed is the one containing the lowest biologic activity, and the highest efficacy, safety, and cycle control. Oral contraceptive formulations in which the dose of estrogen in each tablet exceeds 50 μg should no longer be used in clinical contraception. For new oral contraceptive users the triphasic formulations are preferred since they offer the best opportunity for high efficacy, safety, and cycle control.

What has not changed in the past 30 years is that there is no family planning method available that is completely effective, free of any systemic or local untoward events, does not require patient supervision, and does not interrupt coitus. Therefore, each woman's and each couple's decision regarding the selection of a contraceptive method is a compromise.

SUGGESTED READING

Centers for Disease Control Cancer and Steroid Hormone Study: Long-term oral contraceptive use and the risk of breast cancer. JAMA 1983;249:1591–1595.

Centers for Disease Control Cancer and Steroid Hormone Study: Oral contraceptive use and the risk of endometrial cancer. JAMA 1983;249:1600–1604.

Centers for Disease Control Cancer and Steroid Hormone Study: Oral contraceptive use and the risk of ovarian cancer. JAMA 1983;249:1596–1599.

Diamond MP, Greene JW, Thompson JM, et al. Interaction of anticonvulsants and oral contraceptives in epileptic adolescents. Contraception 1985;31:623–632.

Klein TA, Mishell DR Jr. Gonadotropin, prolactin, and steroid hormone levels after discontinuation of oral contraceptives. Am J Obstet Gynecol 1977;172:585–589.

Meade TW, Greenberg G, Thompson SG. Progestogens and cardiovascular reactions associated with oral contraceptives and a comparison of the safety of 50- and 30-μg estrogen preparations. Br Med J 1980;280:1157–1161.

Ramcharan S, Pellegrin FA, Ray RM, et al. The Walnut Creek Contraceptive Drug Study: a prospective study of side effects of oral contraceptives, vol 3. National Institutes of Health publication #81-564. Washington, D.C.: U.S. Government Printing Office, 1981.

Royal College of General Practitioners' Oral Contraceptive Study: further analysis of mortality in oral contraceptive users. Lancet 1981;1:541–546.

Vessey MP, Wright NH, McPherson K, et al. Fertility after stopping different methods of contraception. Br Med J 1978;1:265–267.

MENOPAUSE

LUIGI MASTROIANNI Jr., M.D.

Management of the menopause is an increasingly important issue in practice today. Data from the 1980 census indicate that at that time there were 32 million women over the age of 50 in the United States. Symptoms vary substantially from woman to woman; in fact, some women have no symptoms at all. Decisions as to when and how to treat are based largely on good clinical judgment. Laboratory evaluation has limited usefulness.

Technically, menopause occurs with cessation of menstrual flow. The symptom complex associated with the menopause often begins much earlier, however, as the ovaries begin to show signs of ovulatory failure and transition from estrogen-producing to androgen-producing organs. In general, there are fewer ovulations as the time of the menopause approaches. In the United States, the mean age at menopause is 49.5 years, with tremendous variation around that number.

The menopause may or may not be predicted by changes in menstrual pattern. When a change does occur, it is related to variations in ovulation. Cycles may be irregular, with periods that are very heavy or very light. When flow is not preceded by ovulation, it is often heavy from an endometrium that has been stimulated with unopposed estrogen without benefit of progesterone effect.

In the early perimenopausal years, levels of circulating estradiol in the proliferative phase are actually somewhat increased. This may be related to the increase in gonadotropins, both follicle-stimulating hormone (FSH) and luteinizing hormone (LH), which occurs at about that time. The rise in FSH levels in the perimenopause is the most sensitive indicator of imminent ovarian failure. In practice, however, gonadotropin determinations are rarely useful to corroborate a clinical impression that menopause is impending. Gonadotropin determinations are somewhat helpful in the management of the amenorrheic patient in her 40s who wishes to know whether it is safe to stop contraception. If FSH and LH levels are consistently elevated, it is reasonable to assure the patient that she is postmenopausal. Sporadic ovulations occasionally occur after several months of amenorrhea associated with menopausal symptoms, and gonadotropins are most useful in the evaluation of amenorrhea to corroborate a diagnosis of premature ovarian failure.

Symptoms of the menopause do not present any really typical pattern. Hot flashes are an early symptom and among the most annoying. Another important symptom, one that may not surface except through direct questioning, is dyspareunia. This is the result of the atrophic vaginitis that is caused by estrogen deficiency. A common symptom is fatigue. This is a rather nondescript symptom, and there are many factors that could contribute to it. The usual explanation for menopause-related fatigue is the occurrence of nocturnal hot flashes and diaphoresis that interfere with sleep. Studies have shown a direct relationship between estrogen levels and sleep. As estrogen levels decline, there is an associated decrease in rapid eye movement (REM) sleep. Estrogen treatment promotes REM sleep.

Increasing awareness of the relationship between estrogen deficiency and osteoporosis has influenced attitudes toward estrogen treatment. Unfortunately, the patient is unaware that there is a problem until she experiences a fracture. Osteoporosis can begin during the perimenopausal interval and continue unabated as estrogen levels decline. Bone changes occur gradually, principally affecting the long bones and vertebrae. In some cases, spontaneous compression fractures of the vertebrae occur, producing the so-called dowager hump. Women who have bilateral oophorectomies are at greater risk and, with rare exceptions, should receive hormone replacement therapy. Some women, in fact, never experience hot flashes. They may be efficient converters of androgen to estrogen and may more effectively use the steroids produced by the adrenals. Thin women have less peripheral conversion of androstenedione to estrogen and generally experience earlier, more pronounced symptoms. There is now good evidence that smokers are at higher risk for osteoporosis.

Another organ system that may be affected adversely by the hormonal changes that occur at the menopause is the cardiovascular system. Data from several epidemiologic studies indicate that estrogen may exert a protective effect against cardiovascular disease. This effect may be mediated through the effect of estrogen on lipid profile, but a direct effect of estrogen on the cardiovascular system has not been ruled out.

TREATMENT

Treatment of the menopause requires considerable clinical skill. The most logical approach is to substitute for the estrogen that had previously been produced by the ovary. A strong case can be made for the use of replacement therapy unless there are contraindications. Since the troublesome symptoms are related directly to lack of estrogen, response is rapid. However, I have not made it a practice to treat patients who are completely asymptomatic. It is not unreasonable to assume that if a patient has no symptoms, i.e., no hot flashes or no atrophic vaginitis, she is probably producing sufficient circulating estrogen to protect her bones, although there are no data to support this position. When using estrogen, I like to start with a low dose. The dose is increased if the symptoms do not respond. The aim is to provide sufficient estrogen to eliminate the symptoms without causing bleeding. In practical terms, this means an initial dose of 0.3 mg of conjugated estrogens or its equivalent, 5 μg of ethinyl estradiol. It is usually necessary to increase the dose of conjugated estrogens to 0.625 mg or more.

A good case can be made for adding a progestational agent to the regimen. The most common estrogen-associated long-term complication is carcinoma of the endometrium. Progesterone down-regulates the estrogen receptors in the endometrial cells and therefore controls the growth-producing effect of estrogen on endometrial tissue. Evidence suggests that progesterone may be effective in a low dose, i.e., as little as 5.0 mg of medroxyprogesterone acetate daily. The estrogen is given cyclically, 25 days on and 5 days off, and the medroxyprogesterone acetate is added to the regimen in the last 12 days of each cycle. When the medication is given cyclically, continuous stimulation of the breast is avoided.

One of the difficulties associated with the use of the combination of estrogen and progesterone is the occurrence of withdrawal bleeding. Some women respond with cyclic menstrual periods and find these undesirable. One should try to regulate the dosage, making it high enough to prevent symptoms but low enough so that the endometrium is not stimulated sufficiently to bleed.

A continuous combined hormonal replacement regimen consisting of conjugated estrogen, 0.625 mg, and medroxyprogesterone acetate, 2.5 mg daily, has recently become popular. The suggested advantage is that in 90 percent or more of patients on this regimen, the monthly withdrawal menses are eliminated within the first 3 months of therapy. Long-term studies of this regimen have yet to be completed.

In addition to estrogen, diet is important in the prevention of osteoporosis. A daily intake of 1,500 mg of calcium is recommended. It is useful to provide the patient with a rundown on the calcium content of various foods and their caloric value. She can then review this in relation to her standard daily diet. If she is ingesting less than 1,500 mg of calcium daily, the diet should be modified or supplementary calcium prescribed. Yogurt is an excellent source of calcium and is low in calories. Calcium without estrogen is not very effective in preventing osteoporosis. Vitamin D and fluorides have been suggested, but there are few places in the United States where both vitamin D and fluoride intake is not adequate. High doses of fluoride would have to be taken to have any impact at all, and these could be associated with unacceptable side effects, including peptic ulcer and arthralgias. Furthermore, bone that is formed under the influence of fluoride alone tends to fracture easily. There is no evidence that the addition of fluoride to the diet offers any advantage.

Since endometrial carcinoma is a critical issue, endometrial sampling should be seriously considered in selected cases. A sample should certainly be taken from any postmenopausal patient who bleeds, unless bleeding is consistently associated temporarily with withdrawal flow. Certainly, any perimenopausal woman who is having irregular menses with variable menstrual flow should have her endometrium sampled before estrogen therapy is instituted. There is generally no need for a dilation and curettage, and some type of office aspiration procedure generally suffices. However, if it is not possible to obtain an endometrial sample in the office, a dilation and curettage should be carried out.

Unfortunately, there is no practical way to evaluate patients for osteoporosis and its progression. The most precise method is to measure bone mass periodically by photon absorption densitometry over a period of several months. The forearm, from the wrist to the elbow, is usually measured. The metacarpals also provide an excellent reference point. Dual-photon absorption densitometry or tomography of the spine is probably more reliable than the single-photon techniques, since these methods detect changes in trabecular bone. These changes usually precede those observed in the cortical bone (i.e., forearm or wrist). The equipment for these studies is expensive, and at this point the cost is unacceptably high to justify its routine use.

Increasing awareness of the potential adverse impact of progestin therapy on the estrogen-induced changes in lipid levels suggests that there is an advantage to the use of the lowest effective dose of progestin that will protect the endometrium. Using mathematical modeling, some investigators have shown that the beneficial impact of hormone replacement therapy on cardiovascular morbidity and mortality far outweighs any adverse effects of estrogen therapy.

The risks of prolonged estrogen treatment are a matter of some concern and should be thoroughly reviewed with the patient prior to treatment. She should be made aware of the possibility of future osteoporosis. She should know that a relationship between carcinoma of the endometrium and estrogen therapy has been established but that its incidence appears to be decreased when progesterone is added to the regimen. She should be advised that in the event of bleeding, endometrial sampling should be performed. The relationship between estrogen treatment and breast carcinoma should also be discussed. The combination of estrogen with a progestational agent has not been shown to be associated with an increased incidence of carcinoma of the breast, except in a small subset of patients, but periodic breast evaluation is important. The use of substitution therapy has relieved many women of the debilitating and discouraging symptoms of the menopause. It is hoped that this therapy, in combination with appropriate calcium intake, will also decrease the incidence of osteoporosis, with its debilitating sequelae.

SUGGESTED READING

Cutler WB, Garcia C-R. The medical management of menopause and postmenopause. Philadelphia: JB Lippincott, 1984.

Ettinger B, Genant HK, Cann CE. Post-menopausal bone loss is prevented by treatment with low dosage estrogen with calcium. Ann Intern Med 1987; 106:40.

Gambrell RD Jr, ed. The menopause. Obstet Gynecol Clin North Am 1987; 14:1–327.

Genant et al. Quantitative computed tomography of vertebral spongiosa: A sensitive method for detecting early bone loss after oophorectomy. Ann Intern Med 1982; 97:699–705.

Henderson BE, Ross RK, Lobo RA, et al. Re-evaluating the role of progestogen therapy after the menopause. Fertil Steril 1988; 49:95–155.

Hillner BE, Hollenberg JP, Pauker SG. Post menopausal estrogens in prevention of osteoporosis: Benefit virtually without risk if cardiovascular effects are considered. JAMA 1986; 80:1115–1127.

Lindsay et al. The minimum effective dose of estrogen for prevention of post-menopausal bone loss. Obstet Gynecol 1984; 63:759–763.

Nachtigall LE, Nachtigall RH, Nachtigall RB, et al. A 10-year prospective study in the relationship to osteoporosis. Obstet Gynecol 1979; 53–277.

Peck WA, Barrett-Conner E, Buckwalter JA, et al. Consensus conference: Osteoporosis. JAMA 1984; 252–799.

MEDICAL MANAGEMENT OF ENDOMETRIOSIS

RICHARD J. FALK, M.D.
SAFA M. RIFKA, M.D.

Endometriosis is one of the most frequently encountered gynecologic conditions. It is found at laparotomy in 10 to 25 percent of women of reproductive age. In our own practice, it is present in 35 percent of patients who undergo diagnostic laparoscopy for the evaluation of infertility.

The lesions consist of heterotopic, hormonally responsive, endometrium-like tissue, located most frequently in the pelvic peritoneum, ovaries, uterosacral ligaments, and cul de sac. When the lesion is found as a large cyst, usually in the ovary, it is called an endometrioma. Other pelvic structures such as the bowel and urinary tract may be involved, giving rise to cyclic symptoms that may include dysmenorrhea (usually premenstrual), dyspareunia, dysuria, tenesmus, and melena. Although endometriosis has been associated historically with infertility, a causal relationship has not been clearly demonstrated, except when extensive lesions or adhesions impede ovum pick-up or transport.

The condition may be suspected by history and/or physical examination, but the diagnosis is definitively made by direct observation or biopsy, usually via laparoscopy.

The following observations suggest that endometriosis is associated with the reproductive cycle. This condition (1) is rarely found in the premenarchal female; (2) is rarely found in anovulatory women; (3) improves after pregnancy both subjectively and objectively (the endometriotic tissue at first undergoes decidual changes, thought to be due to the high pregnancy progesterone levels, and then becomes necrotic); and (4) usually regresses after menopause. In view of these findings, early surgical therapy frequently included castration, which had therapeutic benefit in severe endometriosis. Today, surgery still plays a significant role in endometriosis therapy. It is reasonable to ablate lesions surgically with electrocautery or laser at the time of initial diagnostic laparoscopy, and if the condition is severe or if concomitant adhesions cause infertility or symptoms such as intestinal obstruction, surgery is also necessary. Surgical castration, however, is only performed at the time of hysterectomy, when more conservative methods have failed, or when fertility is no longer desired.

The aim of all available hormonal therapy for endometriosis is to inhibit the normal cyclic estrogen, with resultant atrophy of implants. Although currently the only medication specifically approved for the treatment of endometriosis is danazol, other agents utilized are estrogen-progestin combinations, progestins alone, and gonadotropin-releasing hormone agonists (GnRHa). Estrogens and androgens alone have also been used, but generally they are only of historical note. Although they are unavailable for clinical use in the United States, antiprogesterone agents represent a different and promising approach to therapy.

ESTROGENS

Administration of estrogens in high doses can suppress ovulation, and, in the 1940s and 1950s, they were utilized in treatment of endometriosis with some reported clinical success. The stimulatory effect on the endometrium frequently resulted in hyperplasia and breakthrough bleeding, however, and therefore estrogens alone have no place in managing endometriosis.

ANDROGENS

Androgens have also been employed in the treatment of endometriosis. Ten milligrams of sublingual methyltestosterone daily, for 30 days, followed by 5 mg daily for 2 to 3 months, can result in symptomatic relief. Interestingly, ovulation is frequently not inhibited at these doses, suggesting that the effect of the androgen is directly on the lesion. Side effects of androgenization (e.g., hirsutism, increased muscle mass, voice deepening) make this treatment undesirable for many patients, all of whom are young women in the reproductive age group.

Although methyltestosterone is infrequently used today because of its side effects, we have seen occasional patients who responded poorly to other medical therapy and for whom surgery was not feasible but who responded well to methyltestosterone.

ESTROGEN-PROGESTIN COMBINATIONS

In the late 1950s, the widespread use of oral contraceptives and the appreciation of their potent gonadotropin-suppressing activity spurred the use of these estrogen-progestin combinations for the treatment of endometriosis. Administered continuously for 6 to 9 months instead of cyclically as for contraception, they produce a pharmacologic "pseudopregnancy," and therefore they have become the principal hormonal treatment for endometriosis. The variety of preparations allows for individualization of treatment to minimize breakthrough bleeding, which is more common with the low dose estrogen pills. There is no convincing evidence that any single preparation is therapeutically superior. It is our policy to start treatment with a pill of moderate strength, containing the equivalent of 50 μg of mestranol (the 3-methyl ether of ethinyl estradiol) and 1 mg of norethindrone. Although breakthrough bleeding occurs almost invariably in the first few months of treatment, continued administration usually produces the desired amenorrhea. If amenorrhea does not occur or if the patient is upset by the inconvenience of the spotting, a preparation with 80 μg of mestranol may be substituted. If the vaginal bleeding continues, the patient is advised to double the dose for a few days. If this procedure is unsuccessful, the possibility of an anatomic uterine abnormality, such as a submucous leiomyoma, an endometrial polyp, or even a malignancy, should be ruled out by hysteroscopy and/or curettage before continuing the hormone therapy.

The efficacy of combination therapy is difficult to assess, since published studies often contain small numbers of patients with variable treatment regimens, but pain relief is attained in 80 to 90 percent of patients. The pregnancy rate following therapy in infertile patients is approximately 40 percent, not significantly different from expectant management in some studies.

The contraindications to this therapy, including hepatic disease, thromboembolic phenomena, hypertension, and the presence of estrogen-sensitive neoplasms, have been exhaustively reviewed over the past 20 years. If the patient has or is at risk for such conditions, progestins may be employed without estrogen.

Prophylaxis against progression of the disease by cyclic oral contraceptives has been widely used, and although there is no statistically significant proof of efficacy, this approach seems reasonable in the young patient who does not wish to become pregnant.

PROGESTINS

Medroxyprogesterone acetate in doses to inhibit ovulation (10 mg three times a day for 3 months) has been utilized with good relief from endometriosis-associated dysmenorrhea and dyspareunia. The principal problem with this therapy is irregular breakthrough bleeding. Breakthrough bleeding may be minimized by using the depot form, which can be administered at 400 mg intramuscularly every 2 weeks for four doses, then every 4 weeks for 5 months. Serious complications such as thromboembolic phenomena with "progestin-only" therapy have been reported only rarely. The most significant problem, and one that greatly limits the drug's usefulness, is the prolonged amenorrhea following cessation of treatment. The drug may be demonstrated in the blood more than 18 months after the last injection. Obviously, this prolonged presence makes depo-medroxyprogesterone acetate a poor choice for women whose therapeutic goal is fertility. Furthermore, studies have failed to show improved pregnancy rates. We have, however, utilized this treatment in the older woman with severe symptomatic disease who is not desirous of pregnancy, patients in whom the use of combined estrogen-progestin preparations is ill-advised, patients who could or would not undergo surgery, and patients for whom the financial burden of danazol (see below) was too great.

DANAZOL

Derived from the orally active synthetic androgen ethisterone, danazol was originally thought to decrease gonadotropin levels with concomitant reduction in estrogen and little or no demonstrable estrogenic or progestational activity. For these reasons, the hormone was believed to induce a pseudomenopause.

In actuality, however, studies on the hormonal effects of the drug have been conflicting. We now feel that danazol blocks the midcycle surge but does not significantly lower the baseline levels of gonadotropins. It exhibits significant androgenic activity, as suggested by its structure, and binds not only to androgen receptors but also to progesterone and glucocorticoid receptors. A progestin-like effect on the endometrium has also been demonstrated. Therefore the complex action of danazol on endometriosis is no longer held to be that of a pseudomenopause.

There are relatively few contraindications to the use of danazol. Pregnancy should be ruled out, since masculinization of a female fetus is possible with this agent. Nursing women should not be given the drug but are unlikely candidates in any event. The drug is metabolized in the liver and therefore should not be given to patients with hepatic dysfunction.

Doses of 200 to 800 mg per day have been advocated, but doses of 600 to 800 mg per day have been the most studied regimens. The usual duration of therapy is 6 months, but for patients whose continued symptoms demand more prolonged treatment, the drug may be maintained for longer periods of time.

Many studies have shown that approximately 90 percent of patients have symptomatic improvement after treatment with danazol, and in infertile patients, a pregnancy rate of 40 to 50 percent occurs, depending on the extent of the disease at the onset of treatment.

Side effects are common but usually not dangerous. In our experience, breakthrough bleeding and a weight gain of 2 to 5 kg occur in most patients. A transient decrease in breast size and hot flushes from hypoestrogenism are also common among our patients. Significant androgenization is rare but may be a problem in patients who are already plagued by oily skin, acne, or hirsutism. Deepening of the voice is rare but may be irreversible when it occurs. It would be ill-advised to prescribe this medication for a professional singer.

Depressed high-density lipoprotein levels, which are due in part to the lowered estrogen levels, have been demonstrated with chronic danazol administration. In addition, there may be a direct action of the drug on the liver, which decreases high-density lipoprotein. Thus there exists the theoretical but as yet unobserved possibility of cardiovascular disease in long-term users, especially in those with other high-risk factors such as diabetes, hypertension, or cigarette smoking.

Several studies suggest that danazol is more effective than pseudopregnancy for treatment of endometriosis, but there are few well-designed studies that definitively support this view.

GONADOTROPIN-RELEASING HORMONE AGONISTS

The GnRH analogues that have found the greatest clinical utility are the potent agonists that stimulate release of gonadotropins. After several weeks of administration, gonadotropin-releasing hormone agonist (GnRHa) induces receptor down-regulation, with resultant hypogonadotropinism and depression of serum estradiol to the castration range: a "medical oophorectomy." Currently available analogues are approved only for the diagnostic evaluation of derangements of the hypothalamic-pituitary-ovarian axis and for treatment of steroid-sensitive malignancies but are now widely used for treatment of endometriosis. Leuprolide, [D-Leu^6-Pro^9-NEt]-GnRH, originally administered in subcutaneous doses of 1 mg per day, is now available in depot form (3.75 to 7.5 mg intramuscularly monthly), which effectively produces pituitary-ovarian suppression. Nafarelin, [D-(2-Naph) Ala^6]-GnRH, is administered as an intranasal spray, 200 to 400 μg twice daily, and has actions similar to those of leuprolide.

Initial evidence suggests that GnRHa is as effective as danazol for relief of symptoms of endometriosis. Long-term benefits have yet to be assessed, and as with the other hormonal agents, GnRHa does not seem to improve pregnancy rates.

The hypoestrogenism associated with GnRHa suppression results in dyspareunia from vaginal atrophy and hot flushes that in the final analysis may be a significant limiting factor in patient acceptance of long-term clinical administration. We have found, however, that these side effects are generally better tolerated than those produced by danazol. Serum lipoprotein levels are not affected by GnRHa. Hypoestrogenic bone loss is a concern because there is an increase in urinary calcium and hydroxyproline excretion, but clinically significant bone loss does not appear to be a problem for the 6-month treatment period.

A not insignificant factor in the choice of drug may be price. Depot-leuprolide currently costs approximately \$390 per month, versus \$176 for generic danazol and approximately \$24 for estrogen-progestin combination pills.

ANTIPROGESTINS

The following two drugs are not available in the United States for clinical use. Gestrinone (R 2323), a derivative of 19-nortestosterone, has been widely used in Europe for the treatment of endometriosis. It inhibits pituitary function, with resultant endometrial atrophy. Perhaps more important, it has antiprogesterone activity, the mechanism of which is thought to be caused by a failure of the steroid-receptor complex to activate the chromatin. Good pain relief has been obtained at doses of 2.5 mg twice weekly for 6 months.

RU-486, the controversial French "abortion pill," has potent antiprogesterone activity, presumably as a result of receptor blockade. It has therefore been suggested as another possible treatment for endometriosis, but as yet no clinical data have been published.

SUGGESTED READING

Barbieri RL, Ryan KJ. Danazol: Endocrine pharmacology and therapeutic applications. Am J Obstet Gynecol 1981; 141:453.

Henzl MR, Corson SL, Moghissi KS, et al. Administration of nasal nafarelin as compared with oral danazol for endometriosis. N Engl J Med 1988; 318:485.

Katamaya KP, Manuel M, Jones HW Jr, et al. Methyltestosterone treatment of infertility associated with pelvic endometriosis. Fertil Steril 1976; 27:83.

Kokko E, Janne O, Kauppila A, et al. Danazol has progestin-like actions on the human endometrium. Acta Endocrinol (Copenh) 1982; 99:588.

Moghissi KS, Boyce BR. Management of endometriosis with oral medroxyprogesterone acetate. Obstet Gynecol 1976; 47:265.

Schenken RS (ed). Endometriosis: Contemporary concepts in clinical management. Philadelphia: JB Lippincott, 1989.

Tamaya T, Furuta N, Motoyama T, et al. Mechanism of antiprogestational action of synthetic steroids. Acta Endocrinol (Copenh) 1978; 88:190.

Tamaya T, Motoyama T, Ohono Y, et al. Steroid receptor levels and histology of endometriosis and adenomyosis. Fertil Steril 1979; 31:396.

HYPOGONADISM: ANDROGEN THERAPY

JURAJ OSTERMAN, M.D., Ph.D.

Testosterone deficiency is a common clinical problem encountered in the practice of general medicine, pediatrics, internal medicine, endocrinology, and urology. Testicular failure can result from abnormalities in hypothalamic synthesis and/or release of luteinizing hormone-releasing hormone (LHRH), dysfunction of pituitary gonadotropin-producing cells, or disease processes primarily affecting the testis. Before appropriate hormonal treatment is instituted, one should have a clear understanding of the pathophysiology of hypogonadism in every patient considered for androgen replacement therapy. This therapy is effective, safe, readily available, and generally affordable. Although various androgen preparations have been used for treatment of conditions other than documented testosterone deficiency, focus in this chapter is on issues of proper androgen replacement therapy for hypogonadism, which still remains the primary reason for their use.

BASIC CONSIDERATIONS

Pituitary luteinizing hormone (LH), released in pulsatile fashion, stimulates testicular Leydig cells to synthesize and release several steroids, the main one being testosterone. Adult human testes secrete 5 to 7 mg of testosterone per day and maintain a plasma level between 3 and 10 ng per milliliter. In normal men, plasma testosterone levels are 15 to 40 percent higher in the morning than in the late afternoon, an important consideration when assessing possible hormone deficiency. The majority of plasma testosterone is protein-bound: about 44 percent to testosterone-binding globulin, 50 percent to albumin, and about 4 percent to other proteins, mainly cortisol-binding globulin. About 2 percent of circulating testosterone is free and, until recently, was regarded as the only biologically active fraction. Evidence from several studies suggests that albumin-bound testosterone is also probably a biologically active form, based on kinetics of its dissociation and capillary transit time in several tissues. Testosterone can be viewed as both hormone and prohormone. In some tissue its binding to androgen receptors will initiate a cascade of biochemical events leading to specific physiologic effects. In other tissues (e.g., skin, prostate, seminal vesicles), initial conversion to dihydrotestosterone is required for initiation of biologic effects. In addition, testosterone serves as a precursor for peripheral (extragonadal) aromatization to estradiol. Changes in relative levels of these two hormones may lead to development of gynecomastia, a common problem seen in hypogonadal males and during initiation of androgen therapy in some patients.

GOALS IN ANDROGEN REPLACEMENT THERAPY

After appropriate clinical evaluation has established etiology and documented the existence of testosterone deficiency, androgen replacement therapy aims to restore or induce male sexual behavior (libido, potency), somatic development and sense of well-being (muscle mass, nitrogen balance), and development of male secondary sexual characteristics (genitalia, beard, body hair). Specific goals of this therapy and their results depend on the age of the patient when hypogonadism developed, the nature and the site of the pathologic process (testicular, pituitary, hypothalamic), and whether fertility is a desired goal. For instance, in a boy of pubertal age with hypogonadotropic hypogonadism, treatment with LHRH or gonadotropins (human chorionic gonadotropin [hCG] and follicle-stimulating hormone [FSH]) will aim to induce testicular growth and maturation and initiate development of secondary sexual characteristics. In an adult with primary testicular failure (e.g., secondary to mumps orchitis, trauma, or Klinefelter's syndrome), androgen replacement therapy to improve male sexual behavior and sense of well-being is an appropriate goal, since fertility may not be possible to achieve. When fertility is also a goal of treatment in a patient with acquired hypogonadotropic hypogonadism, administration of hCG and FSH (human menopausal gonadotropin) will be necessary to achieve adequate sperm concentration. Still, in an adult with prolactin-producing pituitary tumor and consequent hypogonadotropic hypogonadism, treatment with bromocriptine commonly will improve libido and potency and restore depressed plasma testosterone levels. In this situation, androgen therapy may not be necessary.

THERAPEUTIC ALTERNATIVES

LHRH and Gonadotropins

Long-term pulsatile administration of low doses of LHRH by portable infusion pumps is probably the most physiologic way to treat many patients with idiopathic hypogonadotropic hypogonadism. Unfortunately, this form of treatment is only available at several research centers conducting clinical trials with this hormone. Treatment with gonadotropins (hCG and FSH) represents an alternative approach to achieve pubertal development and spermatogenesis in a young boy with hypogonadotropic hypogonadism or to achieve fertility in an adult patient when this is a desired goal. These forms of therapy are discussed in more detail elsewhere in this book.

Testosterone

Although it is readily absorbed from the gastrointestinal tract or following injection, native testosterone is rapidly metabolized and degraded in the liver. For this reason, effective concentrations are difficult to achieve in the systemic circulation and acceptable androgenic effects are lacking. Two alternate means of testosterone delivery have been tried: subcutaneous implantation of testosterone-filled Silastic capsules and oral administration of high doses (200 to 400 mg per day) of a microparticulate form of testosterone. Although physiologic plasma levels of testosterone could be achieved by these two methods, neither form has received wide clinical acceptance.

A transdermal testosterone delivery system has been developed and clinically tested. Flexible polymeric membranes containing various doses (5, 10, or 15 mg) of testosterone have been applied to the scrotal skin, where hormone absorption is severalfold higher than at other skin sites. In one study conducted for 12 weeks, daily application of scrotal membranes was well tolerated without side effects. Following application of these membranes, the serum testosterone level reached a peak in 2 to 3 hours and then decreased slowly to 60 to 80 percent of the peak value by 22 hours. The mean 22-hour serum testosterone concentration was within the normal adult male range when membranes containing either 10 or 15 mg of testosterone were used. This form of testosterone delivery may have an advantage over currently preferred intramuscular injections of testosterone esters in that supraphysiologic peaks, observed during the first few days after injection, are avoided.

Several recent studies of chronic use (up to 14 months) of transdermal testosterone delivery in hypogonadal men demonstrated its effectiveness and the achievement of physiologic serum testosterone levels in the majority of patients. However, serum dihydrotestosterone concentration increased to a supraphysiologic level in all men during such treatment.

TABLE 1 Commonly Used Androgen Preparations

				Cost/Month†	
Medication	*Dose**	*Route*	*Schedule**	*Brand*	*Generic*
Testosterone					
Cypionate‡	200 mg	IM	Every 14 days	$13.00	$ 2.50
Enanthate‡	200 mg	IM	Every 14 days	$24.00	$ 3.00
Methyltestosterone	25–50 mg	Orally	Daily	$60.00	$ 5.40
	10–20 mg	Bucally	Daily	$30.00	$ 4.00
Fluoxymesterone	10–20 mg	Orally	Daily	$76.00	$25.00

*Dose schedule for adult hypogonadal men.
†Based on retail pharmacy costs in Columbia, South Carolina. Where applicable, cost was given for the highest dose listed.
‡Preferred preparations for chronic androgen replacement therapy of hypogonadal men.

The potential long-term effects of chronically elevated serum dihydrotestosterone concentration on prostate and other tissues are not known, and more investigation will be needed before this form of testosterone delivery can be generally recommended.

Synthetic Androgens

The goal of chemical modification of the testosterone molecule was to produce analogues of proven androgenic activity that will have slow and sustained absorption from the injection site and/or markedly reduced hepatic metabolism, so that effective and sustained circulating androgen levels can be maintained during chronic replacement therapy. Three types of chemical manipulation produced many currently available synthetic androgens. Esterification of the 17-beta-hydroxyl group with several carboxylic acids resulted in synthesis of four testosterone esters: testosterone propionate, cypionate, and enanthate for intramuscular use and testosterone undecanoate for oral use. Alkylation of the 17-alpha position and/or additional modification of the A, B, or C rings of testosterone made available several derivatives for oral or intramuscular administration.

Testosterone esters are less polar, are more lipid-soluble, and are released slowly from oily vehicles. Since they are hydrolyzed to testosterone before becoming biologically active, measurement of serum testosterone by radioimmunoassay allows monitoring and, if necessary, dose adjustment for effective therapy. Testosterone esters cross-react minimally in testosterone radioimmunoassay. Testosterone enanthate and cypionate have similar durations of action and can be conveniently injected every 2 to 3 weeks. Testosterone propionate has a relatively short duration of action and should be injected daily or every other day to maintain effective circulating levels. Testosterone undecanoate is not available in the United States. Several European studies showed it to be an effective and safe oral androgen. Measurement of plasma or salivary testosterone during treatment enables monitoring of systemic circulating levels. The reasons why this orally active testosterone ester has not been widely used for chronic replacement include the high doses required (120 to 160 mg per day), the considerable cost, and the need for twice-daily administration.

The 17-alpha-alkylated testosterone derivatives (i.e., ethylestrenol, methyltestosterone, fluoxymesterone, methandriol, oxandrolone, oxymetholone, and stanozolol) undergo slow catabolism in the liver following oral administration so that effective androgen levels can be achieved in the systemic circulation. However, these testosterone analogues are less potent than testosterone esters given parenterally, and full androgenic effects are usually not achieved. Since they variably cross-react in testosterone radioimmunoassay, monitoring of their circulating levels is difficult, and specific assays are not routinely available. Still, the major concern in their use is the potential of all 17-alpha-alkylated derivatives to produce severe hepatotoxicity. Although some of these testosterone analogues are claimed to be mainly anabolic and less androgenic, clear separation of androgenic and anabolic properties so far has not been achieved with any of the currently available derivatives. These preparations are also generally more expensive than injectable testosterone esters for chronic androgen replacement of hypogonadism (see Table 1).

PREFERRED APPROACH

Adult Therapy

The two long-acting testosterone esters for intramuscular use, testosterone cypionate and testosterone enanthate, are preparations of choice for chronic treatment of male hypogonadism. Over the years their use has been safe and free of significant side effects, they are more effective than oral preparations, and they have been the least costly. Although there is more information on the clinical pharmacokinetics of testosterone enanthate than cypionate, the general duration of action and effectiveness of these two preparations have been considered to be similar. Following intramuscular injections of testosterone enanthate in doses of 200 mg every 2 weeks or 300 mg every 3 weeks to hypogonadal men, circulating testosterone is frequently at supraphysiologic levels during the first 2 to 3 days. These levels then steadily decline but are usually maintained within the normal range. The dose of testosterone enanthate of 400 mg every 4 weeks did not maintain serum testosterone concentration within the normal range by the end of the fourth week. Studies using testosterone cypionate (200 mg every 2 weeks) in hypogonadal men showed that serum testosterone commonly declined to the basal level by the 10th to 14th day, suggesting that the duration of action of testosterone cypionate might be slightly shorter than that of testosterone enanthate.

Before initiating chronic androgen replacement therapy in the adult patient, careful examination of the prostate is performed to exclude the possibility of carcinoma that would contraindicate such treatment. Similar examinations are periodically performed (every 3 to 6 months) during replacement therapy. The patient and his wife are informed about expected somatic and behavioral changes of treatment. Psychological counseling is rarely required to deal with changing sexual behavior. I have used either testosterone enanthate or cypionate in the dosage of 200 mg every 2 weeks as standard treatment. Most of our patients learn to self-inject testosterone, or, alternatively, their wives are instructed in the techniques of deep intramuscular injection.

It is gratifying to learn from the patient about improvement of his general well-being, stamina, libido, and potency. These effects of androgen therapy develop within the first 1 to 2 months. If a patient's secondary sex features have regressed during prolonged undiagnosed and untreated hypogonadism, these will improve more slowly during the first 6 months of therapy. An occasional patient will report "recurrence" of his symptoms of hypogonadism during the last 2 to 4 days before the next testosterone dose. In such cases, the serum testosterone level is determined just before the next dose, and if it is found to be at a subnormal concentration, the frequency of injections is changed to every 10 days.

Testosterone propionate is used infrequently for routine replacement. Candidates for this short-acting preparation are older hypogonadal men complaining of symptoms of possible bladder neck obstruction and/or enlarged prostate. In such a clinical situation the advantage of a short-acting testosterone preparation is obvious and possible initial worsening of clinical symptoms after the injection is likely to improve within several days following discontinuation of therapy. An appropriate dosage of testosterone propionate is 25 to 50 mg intramuscularly three times a week.

As mentioned earlier, many patients with hypogonadotropic hypogonadism in the setting of prolactin-producing pituitary tumors regain normal circulating testosterone levels during treatment with dopaminergic-agonist bromocriptine. Those patients who remain hypogonadal on that therapy are usually treated with testosterone. In one report, a patient with an invasive prolactin-producing pituitary tumor treated with bromocriptine was described who developed exacerbation (increase in tumor size, neurologic symptoms, increase in prolactin level) temporarily related to injections of testosterone enanthate. Although this may or may not represent a rare complication of testosterone therapy, such a possibility should be kept in mind and anticipated in this clinical setting.

Transdermal testosterone delivery certainly appears a promising modality for the future and may be the way to achieve less variable levels of circulating testosterone during chronic therapy.

Pubertal Therapy

Treatment of a boy with delayed puberty is a more complicated issue. In general, lower doses of testosterone enanthate or cypionate (50 to 75 mg every 3 to 4 weeks) are adequate for initial androgen therapy lasting 4 to 6 months. Later on, these doses can be gradually increased to 100 to 150 mg every 3 to 4 weeks. The main concern is to interfere minimally with the natural height potential of the pubertal boy, in whom early and/or overzealous androgen replacement will cause premature closure of the epiphyses.

For those rare patients who refuse parenteral forms of testosterone replacement, oral forms (e.g., methyltestosterone, fluoxymesterone) can be instituted, but only with the patient's full appreciation for potential serious side effects. For pubertal boys, doses one-fourth to one-half of those listed in Table 1 should be adequate.

Corrective Surgical Therapy

Gynecomastia is a very common concern and reason for embarrassment of many, especially young, hypogonadal men; it may be a cause for their initial evaluation. Unfortunately, androgen therapy infrequently results in considerable reduction of markedly enlarged breasts. Therefore, it is appropriate to refer such patients for reduction mammoplasty when it is obvious that they continue to suffer psychologically. Small testes are another, although less frequent, cause of psychological embarrassment for some hypogonadal men, and surgical implantation of testicular prostheses can produce gratifying results.

SIDE EFFECTS

Androgenic Side Effects

As a result of their "anabolic" effects, therapy with androgens causes nitrogen, sodium, and fluid retention, which will manifest in mild weight gain. Significant edema can develop in patients with congestive cardiomyopathy, hepatic cirrhosis, or renal insufficiency. Development of acne is common in pubertal boys during the initial phase of testosterone treatment regardless of age; it tends to regress with progression of therapy. Excessive stimulation of libido and/or erections are uncommon complaints and are successfully managed by temporary reduction of testosterone dose. When considering treating elderly men, one should be concerned about the possible presence or development of prostate carcinoma when such therapy would be contraindicated. Androgens are also contraindicated in men with breast cancer.

Feminizing Side Effects

During testosterone replacement therapy there is an increase in plasma estradiol as a result of peripheral aromatization of testosterone. An elevation in the estradiol-testosterone ratio can cause development of gynecomastia. Pubertal children or elderly men with underlying hepatic cirrhosis are more likely to develop this complication.

Hepatotoxicity

In contrast to native testosterone and testosterone esters, all 17-alpha-alkylated testosterone derivatives have the potential for producing several abnormalities in liver function, including cholestasis, elevation in transaminases and alkaline phosphatase, and, less commonly, overt jaundice. Even more serious although rare complications are the development of peliosis hepatis, hepatocellular carcinoma, and possibly intrahepatic cholangiocarcinoma. A causative relationship between 17-alpha-alkylated testosterone derivatives and hepatocellular carcinoma is difficult to accept with certainty in view of the fact that many patients had Fanconi's anemia, a disease associated with an increased incidence of malignant tumors. Discontinuation of androgen therapy has caused regression of peliosis hepatis in some patients. An interesting side effect of 17-alpha-alklyated testosterone analogues is an elevation of several plasma proteins such as haptoglobin, plasminogen, and the inhibitor of the first component of complement. This last effect is conveniently used in treatment of hereditary angioneurotic edema in which the inhibitor of the first component of complement is markedly decreased.

Erythrocytosis

Androgens stimulate erythropoiesis by enhancing the production of erythropoietin. An occasional patient may develop marked elevation in hematocrit during testosterone replacement sufficient to warrant therapeutic phlebotomy. In such patients, replacement doses should be reduced on resuming therapy after the hematocrit has normalized. Development or worsening of obstructive sleep apnea has been described in some hypogonadal men receiving therapeutic doses of testosterone enanthate. Hypoxic ventilatory drive decreased significantly during testosterone replacement therapy in all patients studied; however, only some exhibited sleep apnea, oxygen desaturation, cardiac dysrhythmias, and marked elevation of hematocrit.

Allergic and Local Side Effects

Allergic reactions to oil vehicles (sesame oil, cottonseed oil) of testosterone esters are rare. Tetrazine, present in some 17-alpha-alkylated testosterones, can cause bronchospasm in susceptible persons. With proper techniques of intramuscular administration, skin reactions at the injection site are infrequent.

SUGGESTED READING

Ahmed SR, Boucher AE, Manni A, et al. Transdermal testosterone therapy of male hypogonadism. J Clin Endocrinol Metab 1988; 66:546–551.

Bals-Pratsch M, Langer K, Place VA, Nieschlag E. Substitution therapy of hypogonadal men with transdermal testosterone over one year. Acta Endocrinol 1988; 118:7–13.

Bals-Pratsch M, Yoon Y-D, Knuth VA, Nieschlag E. Transdermal testosterone substitution therapy for male hypogonadism. Lancet 1986; 2:943–945.

Findlay JC, Place VA, Snyder PJ. Transdermal delivery of testosterone. J Clin Endocrinol Metab 1987; 64:266–268.

Findlay JC, Place V, Snyder PJ. Treatment of primary hypogonadism in men by the transdermal administration of testosterone. J Clin Endocrinol Metab 1989; 68:369–373.

Korenman SG, Viosca S, Garza D, et al. Androgen therapy of hypogonadal men with transscrotal testosterone systems. Am J Med 1987; 83:471–478.

Mooradian AD, Morley JE, Korenman SG. Biological actions of androgens. Endocr Rev 1987; 8:1–28.

Nankin HR, Lin T, Osterman J. Chronic testosterone cypionate therapy in men with secondary impotence. Fertil Steril 1986; 46:300–307.

Snyder PJ. Clinical use of androgens. Annu Rev Med 1984; 35:207–217.

Wilson JD, Griffin JE. The use and misuse of androgens. Metabolism 1980; 29:1278–1295.

HYPOGONADOTROPIC HYPOGONADISM: GONADOTROPIN THERAPY

WYLIE C. HEMBREE, M.D.

The clinical manifestations of hypogonadism can each be attributed to a deficiency, absolute or relative, in the testicular production and secretion of testosterone. This syndrome occurs most commonly as a result of genetic, developmental, inflammatory, and, rarely, biosynthetic abnormalities of the testes. When androgen deficiency occurs in the absence of compensatory hypersecretion of gonadotropins, hypogonadotropism is presumed to be the cause and, after clinical evaluation of other indices of hypothalamic-pituitary function, treatment to correct the androgen deficiency is instituted. Treatment options for hypogonadotropism are far more complex than those available for treatment of hypergonadotropic hypogonadism. Thus, the type of treatment selected must first take into consideration the desired outcome of each patient and, second, a careful cost-benefit analysis of the several possible approaches. Principles that should be considered in this analysis are listed below:

1. Etiology/pathogenesis
2. Hypothalamic-pituitary-gonadal function
3. Desired outcome
4. Choice of medication
5. Acceptability

6. Duration
7. Cost management
8. Monitoring strategies
9. Maintenance

The diagnosis of hypogonadotropism may be made in association with a variety of clinical settings (Table 1). Discussion of the specific diagnostic categories that occasion consideration of hypogonadotropism is beyond the scope of this chapter. However, it must be emphasized that the disease processes that manifest themselves in hypogonadism should be carefully defined prior to the institution of treatment. Failure to do so can result in inappropriate treatment. Use of gonadotropins to treat hypogonadism associated with enzyme deficiencies such as 17-hydroxylase deficiency or 5-alpha-reductase deficiency would be inappropriate, although for different reasons. If hypogonadotropism is associated with other pituitary hormone deficiencies that go unrecognized, the response to gonadotropic stimulation may be limited. Some illnesses, such as autoimmune diseases, cirrhosis, and hemochromatosis, may be associated both with testicular dysfunction as well as with gonadotropin deficiencies. Thus, the status of the secretion of cortisone, as well as adrenal androgens, thyroid hormone, insulin, and prolactin, must be considered along with evaluation of the production of gonadotropin-releasing hormone (GnRH), luteinizing hormone (LH), follicle-stimulating hormone (FSH), testosterone, and estradiol. In addition, hypothalamic response to antiestrogens such as clomiphene citrate, gonadotrophic response to GnRH, and Leydig cell response to gonadotropin (LH) stimulation may need to be evaluated before the type of treatment can be appropriately selected. Finally, if the desired outcome includes stimulation of spermatogenesis for the purpose of impregnating the patient's sexual partner, the status of the germinal epithelium should be assessed, although qualitative and quantitative determination is difficult, even by testicular biopsy.

Hypogonadotropism that occurs after puberty is the type of problem most easily treated with gonadotropins, either with human chorionic gonadotropin (hCG) to maintain secondary sex characteristics and sexual function (androgen production) or with FSH to obtain fertility (spermatogenesis). This is true for two reasons. First, complete hypogonadotropism rarely occurs. Most cases of hypogonadotropism occurring in the adult are characterized by the disappearance of pulsatile LH secretion, as well as by decreases in the net production of LH. The consequent decrease in Leydig cell secretion of testosterone usually results in sexual dysfunction, in the diminution or disappearance of seminal emission, and in a reduction in sperm production and germ cell volume. Nonetheless, residual secretion of low levels of LH and FSH usually persists, thus maintaining an amount of intratesticular testosterone production sufficient to maintain spermatogonial turnover and limited degrees of meiosis and spermiogenesis. Second, this persistence of spermatogenesis despite low hormone levels is attributed to enhanced Leydig sensitivity induced by FSH as well as to the low levels of LH that serve to maintain testosterone biosynthesis. It is believed that the amount of residual gonadotropin found in adult hypogonadotropism would be insufficient to initiate spermatogenesis in the prepubertal boy. These patients behave in a manner similar to those with the unfortunate and inappropriate appellation of "fertile eunuch," i.e. men with low LH and testosterone levels, minimal secondary sexual characteristics, and normal testicular volume. Initiation or restoration of only androgen production and virilization, without using FSH, often results in sperm production sufficient for conception, even at testosterone levels generally considered to be below normal.

TABLE 1 Clinical Settings of Hypogonadotropism

Neonatal or childhood abnormalities, such as microphallus and/or cryptorchidism
Late onset of puberty
Arrested sexual development
Regression of sexual development in the adult
Sexual dysfunction
Infertility or disorders of sperm production
Acute and chronic systemic illness
Hypopituitarism

Knowledge of the etiology of the patient's hypogonadotropism and careful analysis of its pathophysiologic consequences on the endocrine system is essential to the appropriate choice of treatment and maintenance strategy. Although many cases of hypogonadotropism in the male result from pituitary or hypothalamic tumors, their incidence is lower than in women and occasions a higher proportion of congenital, idiopathic, and systemic causes in men. Even male patients with Kallman's syndrome exhibit varying degrees of basal LH and FSH secretion and of gonadotropin responsiveness. Thus, it often helps in the design of treatment to determine the extent to which GnRH, LH, FSH, and testosterone secretion can be increased by several diagnostic maneuvers. Standard testing regimens have been published for use of clomiphene citrate, GnRH, and hCG to assess hypothalamic (GnRH), gonadotropin and Leydig cell responsiveness, respectively (Table 2). Hormone assay methods vary so widely that it is wise for most clinicians to interpret the response with broad latitude. Published normal values may be useful diagnostically, but the purpose of using stimulation tests to aid in the design of therapy is to determine the ability of a medication and/or regimen to achieve normal hormone levels. Several standard tests serve this purpose well (see Table 2).

Stimulation of the hypothalamic-pituitary axis can be achieved by administration of clomiphene citrate, 50 mg three times a day for 7 days. Cases of hypogonadotropism in which clomiphene citrate treatment normalizes testosterone and gonadotropin levels are rare. Unusual instances of excess estrogen production in the male (e.g., massive

TABLE 2 Tests to Design Treatment

	Medication (Dose)	*Response (Times)*
Hypothalamus	Clomiphene citrate (50 mg t.i.d. for 7 days)	LH, FSH, testosterone (day 1 and day 7)
Pituitary	Gonadotropin releasing hormone (100 μg IV bolus)	LH and FSH (30-minute intervals for 30 to 120 minutes)
Leydig cells	Human chorionic gonadotropin (5,000 IU IM for 4 days)	Testosterone/estradiol (day 1 and day 5)

obesity, cirrhosis, excess peripheral aromatization) respond to clomiphene citrate. Occasionally, the resultant enhancement of Leydig cell secretion may also increase estradiol secretion disproportionately and thus inhibit sexual function (if peripheral levels increase) and/or spermatogenesis (if testicular tubule levels increase). Demonstration that clomiphene citrate can increase FSH levels may be useful as an adjunct to hCG treatment if fertility is desired. Use of this clomiphene test often clarifies the diagnosis of hypogonadism.

GnRH is available for testing in a dose of 100 μg. If chronic GnRH treatment is being considered, the ability of a test dose to normalize or, if assayed at the lower limit of normal, to double both LH and FSH provides sufficient data to make highly probable the potential efficiency of chronic pulsatile GnRH treatment. Patients with congenital hypogonadotropism, previously untreated with GnRH, often do not respond or respond poorly to a standard GnRH test. However, all patients with GnRH deficiency, when treated with pulsatile GnRH for 1 week, exhibit normal responses to a 100 μg bolus of GnRH. Lack of response after short-term GnRH priming suggests a deficiency of gonadotrophin or of GnRH receptors.

Ultimately, the efficacy of treatment designed to replace deficient gonadotropins depends on the ability of the LH or hCG to maintain Leydig cell testosterone production within the normal adult range found. To this end, daily administration of hCG for 4 days at 5,000 IU per day has served as a useful test for several reasons. First, it establishes the responsiveness of the Leydig cell; second, albeit a pharmacologic stimulus, this high dose enables normal Leydig cells to elevate testosterone levels into normal adult male range in both prepubertal and postpubertal gonadotropin deficiency. Finally, the estradiol response, if excessive, often alerts the physician to the possibility of estradiol excess during chronic treatment, thus potentially complicating treatment with gynecomastia, sexual dysfunction, and inhibition of spermatogenesis. This effect of hCG is usually dose dependent, and if anticipated, estradiol levels can be normalized.

Use of one or more of these tests will help to establish the functional status of the hormonal components of the reproductive endocrine system. Although treatment with GnRH will not be discussed here, the principles of management of gonadotropin treatment are the same whether gonadotropin stimulation of Leydig cell and/or the germinal epithelium is brought about by a one-step (hCG and/or menopausal gonadotropins), two-step (GnRH), or three-step (clomiphene citrate) mechanism. If treatment strategy is based on these principles, it may be possible to avoid unnecessary costs and time while minimizing the amount of medication required to achieve the desired outcome.

Choice of gonadotropin regimen is also largely determined by the desired outcome of the patient (or couple). If conception is sought, treatment requires not only management of hormone levels but also assessment of the man's sexual partner, of sperm production and function, of coital timing and frequency, and of other factors that may enhance or inhibit fertility. Although some have claimed that androgen therapy enhances fertility, the usual experience dictates that this approach does not effectively increase sperm production. However, if initiation or reestablishment of androgen production only is sought, the pros and cons of gonadotropin stimulation must be weighed against the potential benefits of lower costs, oral formulations, and/or less frequent administration. The age of the patient and the reason(s) enhanced androgen production is sought should be considered. The younger the patient, the more critical may be evaluation and monitoring of the psychological manifestations of treatment. In general, less invasive forms of administration and less rapid achievement of adult male levels are desirable in children and teenagers. For example, local application of androgen-containing cream would appear more appropriate in children with microphallus than hCG stimulation of endogenous androgen. Although increases in testicular volume and scrotal size by gonadotropins may facilitate stabilization of gonadal position in some cases of cryptorchidism, the dose, frequency, and duration of hCG treatment must be adjusted to minimize the systemic manifestations and the attendant complications of premature puberty.

In cases of delayed puberty, including forms of hypogonadotropism that present after age 20, a careful assessment must be made of the patient's prime concern, i.e., his chief complaint. From a physiologic point of view, the only harmful effects of remaining hypogonadal are the systemic consequences of chronic androgen deficiency, i.e., the low-grade chronic anemia, the orthopaedic consequences of the failure of epiphysial closure, and possibly osteoporosis. The treating physician must avoid imposing his own standards of "normalcy" of reproductive parameters on the patient and/or his family. In addition, the expectations of all concerned parties must be considered, although those of the patient should receive prime consideration. Gonadotropin deficiency is clinically manifested by a lack of the following: hirsutism, voice change, muscle development and strength, athletic prowess, sexual function, penile and/or testicular growth, and height. One or more of these findings may be perceived as of prime importance to the patient; failure to recognize and respond to this perception will jeopardize the effectiveness of the treatment.

The attainment of adult secondary sexual characteristics in the male is normally a process dependent on the gradual increase of testosterone levels into the adult range over 3 to 5 years and the subsequent achievement of adult height, virilization, psychosexual maturity, and fertility. This process begins with perceptible testicular growth as early as 8 years of age and continues until age 18 to 20 in some persons. Exact temporal recapitulation of pubertal development with gonadotropin treatment is difficult and, in most cases, inappropriate for a patient well beyond the usual age of puberty whose major concern is the absence of one or more manifestations of androgen production. Yet, rapid physical growth and development can be psychologically undesirable. Thus, initial efforts must be made to temper the patient's desire for a rapid change. At the other extreme, the patient with adult onset of gonadotropin deficiency responds best to a rapid return of androgen levels to normal. Once the specific nature of the treatment outcome is defined, it is essential that a timetable to achieve this goal be agreed on at the initiation of therapy.

In hypogonadotropic patients, oral and intramuscular androgen may be equally as effective as gonadotropin treatment for some patients. Thus, the acceptability of intramuscular administration should next be addressed. Intramuscular medications have the advantage that they permit measurement of the testosterone levels achieved so that they can be correlated, in turn, with the clinical responses. If the clinical response to oral medication is not satisfactory, it is not possible to verify the amount of active androgen present by blood tests. It is desirable that most teenagers be given the opportunity to assume responsibility for their treatment as fully as possible through self-administration. This usually facilitates their psychosexual development. Gonadotropin (hCG) injections can be given by the patient in a small volume of aqueous diluent, whereas the oil-based diluent of testosterone esters is more difficult to inject. Most adults find self-administration the most acceptable form of treatment while many teenagers are reluctant. It has been suggested that the relatively constant levels of testosterone that occur during hCG treatment may achieve more rapid and more complete virilization than that associated with the broad excursions of hormone levels derived from testosterone ester administration. Gonadotropin treatment also becomes more acceptable to adults who experience changes in their sense of general well-being, libido, and sexual function as testosterone levels decline. This potential advantage of gonadotropin treatment may be perceived by the patient given intramuscular androgen until he has the opportunity to compare his own response to the two medicines. In addition, patients who have been treated with both modalities often prefer the increased volume, weight, and lower scrotal position of the testes associated with gonadotropin therapy. Thus, the route of administration, the cost, the relative constancy of hormone levels, and the opportunity to monitor the effect of therapy on hormone levels weigh heavily in favor of using gonadotropin to achieve pubertal development or restoration of androgen levels in postpubertal hypogonadotropism.

The extent to which testicular growth is achieved by hCG treatment may be used as a "bioassay" for the presence of low levels of FSH. This response may also be a prognostic indicator for subsequent response of the germinal epithelium to FSH. Fertility is a potential complication of using hCG in the prepubertal hypogonadotropic patient. This possibility may reduce its acceptability. However, in conjunction with appropriate patient education, addressing this risk may serve as an opportunity to establish a more effective physician–patient relationship and to aid in the patient's psychosexual development. The potential for increasing sperm production makes hCG the treatment of choice for hypogonadotropic adult men desiring children. When fertility is the desired outcome, the consideration of both cost and route of administration often become secondary to the duration of treatment required to achieve a pregnancy.

As previously mentioned, when the gonadal (Leydig cell) response to gonadotropin is normal, adult levels of testosterone can be achieved by the appropriate regimen within 2 to 4 weeks. It is difficult to predict whether hCG alone will bring about a response of the germinal epithelium sufficient for conception. In general, the extent to which pretreatment testicular volume approaches that of normal adults correlates with the ability of hCG alone to stimuate sperm production. Because the cost increment associated with adding menopausal gonadotropin (LH/FSH or purified FSH alone) to the treatment program is so great, it is important to take sufficient time to allow hCG to "prime" the germ cell response to FSH. This usually takes 6 months. Although there are no data that satisfactorily define the optimal time needed to "prime" the testis for FSH treatment, the strong patient desire for his partner to become pregnant as soon as possible usually leads to earlier institution of FSH than required. It is critical not only that the time course of treatment of couples be agreed on at the onset but also that the importance of the monitoring strategy and the evaluation of the partner's reproductive potential be clearly understood.

Once the decision has been made to use gonadotropins to correct the manifestations of hypogonadotropism, the choice of medications is quite limited. Human chorionic gonadotropin (hCG) is used for its luteinizing hormone activity, i.e., direct stimulation of testosterone biosynthesis by the Leydig cells with consequent increases in peripheral testosterone concentration and massive increases in intratesticular testosterone. Research studies have shown that estradiol is also secreted by the Leydig cell in response to LH and hCG. In addition, animal data and feminizing germ cell/Sertoli cell tumors in the human suggest the potential for production of estradiol by the Sertoli cells, especially in the immature animals. High intratesticular concentrations of testosterone are essential for normal spermatogenesis, but, unlike data in other mammals, human spermatogenesis cannot be initiated and probably cannot be sustained by testosterone alone. Thus, patients desiring paternity as an outcome of gonadotropin treatment require not only hCG but also an FSH-containing preparation.

Extracted and purified urine from menopausal women has served as the source of LH and FSH for ovulation induction in women and, more lately, for induction of spermatogenesis. Until recently, the only commercially available menopausal gonadotropin preparation has contained equal amounts of LH and FSH, although the amount of LH is insufficient to maintain normal testosterone levels. Recently, a "purified" preparation with no LH activity has become available, designated "purified FSH." Either preparation can be used to induce spermatogenesis. Additional Leydig cell stimulation is provided by combining hCG with FSH. The dose of hCG required must be individualized and should be kept at a minimum. The standard schedule adopted for administration of gonadotropin has been three times a week. Variations have been used with success, although it is highly advisable to use a regimen clearly demonstrated to be successful in most gonadotropin-deficient patients, considering the expense of menopausal gonadotropins and the psychological cost of ineffective treatment. Whatever schedule is found to be acceptable, the schedule should be ridgidly maintained. Once sperm production is established, intermittent decline in androgen levels and/or FSH stimulation may result in prolonged decreases in sperm production. FSH should be given only if paternity is the desired outcome. The rare development of antibodies to FSH preclude its use for pubertal induction or to attempt to ascertain the potential for fertility.

Dose and frequency of gonadotropins are the most critical considerations for a successful outcome while minimizing costs. Human chorionic gonadotropin has a long half-life, and levels of hCG can be detected for 8 to 10 days after doses in excess of 2,000 units. The Leydig cell response to a large single dose of hCG (6,000 IU IM) is biphasic, peaking first within 12 hours, falling to a nadir at 24 to 36 hours, and rising again to a lower peak at 72 to 96 hours. This biphasic response is probably due to the rapid down-regulation of the Leydig cells within 12 to 24 hours by high levels of hCG and the subsequent recovery of sensitivity in the presence of declining hCG levels. Thus, it would appear that hCG administered once weekly would be sufficient to maintain testosterone secretion. On occasion, such strategy works. However, the large doses of hCG required for this prolonged response frequently cause a disproportionate increase in estradiol levels, which, in some patients, causes gynecomastia. These large doses of hCG, when given to normal men, chronically elevate estradiol production, suppress FSH, and lower sperm counts. In patients whose androgen deficiency is associated with short stature, high estradiol levels may limit the maximum height by premature closure of long-bone epiphyses. These adverse effects are dose dependent and can be prevented by careful monitoring. Most teenage and adult men with hypogonadotropism achieved testosterone levels within the normal range when given 500 IU of hCG three times per week. The time required to attain these levels may take longer in prepubertal teenagers first receiving treatment than in postpubertal adults. When testosterone levels of 200 ng per deciliter or greater are achieved within 2 to 3 months, maintenance of the hCG at this dose usually results in a progressive increase over 6 months are testicular volume increases. When doses greater than 500 IU three times per week are required, excess estradiol production is a frequent complication.

Ideally, FSH should be added to the hCG regimen when it is clear that testicular growth has reached a plateau or that sperm production, if present, has been stable for 3 months. Since the duration of one complete cycle of spermatogenesis is 75 days, and sperm transport takes approximately 15 days, one would not expect a stimulus to spermatogenesis to be manifested in seminal fluid for at least 90 days. One approach is to ask patients to submit monthly semen specimens after testosterone and estradiol levels have reached a satisfactory plateau. If six consecutive monthly specimens remain azoospermic and there is not evidence of continued testicular growth, FSH may be added. The dose of FSH required for sperm production sufficient for a pregnancy is between 37.5 and 75 units three times per week. I usually begin with the higher dose. The hCG and FSH are administered together. Despite a stable response to hCG prior to FSH, increases in both testosterone and estradiol are often observed after addition of FSH.

Management of the costs of gonadotropin therapy is quite difficult. Human chorionic gonadotropin at a dose of 500 IU three times per week should cost approximately $200 for 1 year of treatment; syringes and needles cost less than $100 annually; and menopausal gonadotropins 75 units three times per week cost $4,000 annually. Self-administration is mandatory to reduce costs. When stimulation of sperm production is required, the cost can be constrained by minimizing the amount of time required for FSH. This is accomplished by prolonging the pretreatment with hCG and careful monitoring of estradiol levels, with dose adjustment as required. Prior evaluation of the patient's partner prior to instituting FSH will avoid delays subsequently when sperm production has increased. Rigid adherence to the timing of the treatment protocol will avoid regression of germ cell response. FSH dose may be reduced once sperm production has reached a plateau. Regular monitoring incurs additional expense but consistently reduces costs by optimizing the therapy.

Monitoring the response to gonadotropin injections

TABLE 3 Monitoring Treatment

Hormone levels: routine	If pregnancy is desired:
Testosterone	Monthly semen analyses
Estradiol	Postcoital test
Special considerations	Hysterosalpingogram
17-OH Progesterone	Endometrial biopsy
hCG levels	Basal body temperature charts
Testicular volume	
Side effects	
Blood pressure	
Routine laboratory studies	
Complete blood cell count	
Liver function tests	
Cholesterol, triglycerides	

is the most critical of all the previously addressed considerations (Table 3). The monitoring protocol should be clearly reviewed, and preferably a written schedule should be given to the patient. Prepubertal patients should be told that significant physical changes will become apparent within the first 6 months and will continue to evolve for at least 24 months. Hormone levels should be assessed at 2 weeks, at 4 weeks, monthly for 6 months, and every 2 months thereafter, if stable. Blood samples should be drawn at the same time after injection for more precise assessment of the response (24 hours after an injection is the most useful time). In prepubertal patients, elevated testosterone levels greater than 300 ng per deciliter have been found to accelerate virilization to an unacceptable extent and require a reduction in dose. The amount of hCG given can most reasonably be reduced by diluting the hCG to obtain the desired dose (250 or 375 IU in 0.5 ml). The hCG should be increased if testosterone levels are less than 100 ng per deciliter by 4 weeks. It may also be helpful to assay hCG levels to make certain the injection technique is effective.

Estradiol levels should be measured regularly after 8 weeks of treatment. Levels in excess of 50 pg per milliliter, especially if increasing, may indicate an excess dose of hCG. Gradual reduction of the dose usually returns estradiol levels to an acceptably low range, thus preventing complications. If gynecomastia develops and persists despite "normal" estradiol levels, modest dose reduction should be attempted. On occasion, if the gynecomastia is physically or psychologically troublesome, antiestrogens or aromatase inhibitors may be used. Sexual dysfunction may occur during periods of high estradiol levels. It is wise to respond to such a complaint both with psychological support as well as with pharmacologic adjustments.

Adults treated with hCG usually achieve testosterone levels greater than 300 ng per deciliter by 4 to 8 weeks. If symptoms of decreased strength, depression, and low libido are increasing between 4 and 8 weeks, it may be wise to increase the dose at 8 weeks. In contrast to prepubertal hypogonadotropism, normal adult male testosterone levels should be attained as rapidly as possible in postpubertal gonadotropin-deficient patients. Some patients who require gonadotropin treatment for fertility will have been treated for long periods with testosterone esters. Because libido, sexual function, and other androgen-dependent symptoms will have been well established, many patients are reluctant to undergo a 1 to 2-month period of low androgen levels while the Leydig cell response to hCG is gradually returning testosterone levels to the normal range. This transient period of low testosterone levels can be avoided by monitoring the Leydig cell response to the hCG while continuing the testosterone injections.

Testosterone levels cannot be used reliably for this purpose. However, if adrenal secretion of 17-hydroxyprogesterone is obliterated by dexamethasone suppression, increases in the hormone can be used to verify an adequate Leydig cell response to the hCG. Dexamethasone, 0.5 mg taken orally at 12-hour intervals for three doses prior to the blood test has been effective in reducing adrenal secretion by more than 90 percent. Under this protocol, hCG-treated men with normal testosterone levels have 17-hydroxyprogesterone levels of 50 to 100 ng per deciliter. Once levels of greater than 50 ng per deciliter have been reached, exogenous testosterone administration can be stopped.

Testicular volume can be measured in a variety of ways. Ultrasound techniques are increasingly available for research protocols and may be useful clinically. Ellipsoids of increasing volume, called an orchidometer, are available to compare to actual volume of each testes. Rough estimates of volume can be made by measuring the length (*L*) and width (*W*) (not involving the epididymis) of the testes and calculating the volume according to the following formula:

$$L \times W^2 \times 0.52 = \text{Volume}$$

These values correlate well with other methods, and the measurements are sufficiently reproducible to document testicular growth. It is extemely important to have objective parameters of androgen effect. In prepubertal boys, height, weight, span, and pubis-to-floor measurements should be charted at each visit, whereas blood pressure, complete blood cell count, blood chemistries including liver function tests, and lipids should be checked quarterly in all patients in the first year and semiannually thereafter.

At each office visit, the clinical response to increased androgen and significant side effects should be assessed by a series of questions. Frequency of morning erections, spontaneous erections, masturbation, nocturnal emissions, sexual activity, and changes in libido are the earliest signs of increasing testosterone levels. Growth, voice change, facial hair growth, genital growth, body hair, temporal hair recession, and muscle development are late changes, and their significance will be dependent on the patient's stature at the intiation of therapy. Increased appetite and weight gain are frequent outcomes and may constitute undesirable side effects. Headaches, visual symptoms, acne, oily skin, gynecomastia, nausea, and increased blood pressure may be associated with high testosterone levels. Patients with adult-onset hypogonadotropism experience an increased sense of well-being, energy, and occasionally euphoria, as well as symptoms related to the reproductive system. Similarly, teenagers often develop mood swings, depression, and behavior problems, occasionally severe enough to require psychiatric intervention. I recommend that all parents and teenage patients have at least one interview with a psychiatrist skilled in psychosexual development prior to the initiation of treatment. It is not unusual for parents to request a reduction in dose as the patient's expression of his sexuality becomes a more dominant part of his relationship with parents and peers.

The high degree of variability in semen characteristics observed in men with apparently stable sperm production makes it imperative that semen specimens be analyzed at regular intervals beginning 2 to 3 months after the initiation of therapy. In addition, when couples seek conception as the desired outcome of treatment, the woman's ovulatory status and pelvic anatomy must be assessed. A hysterosalpingogram and an in-phase endometrial biopsy are usually sufficient. Normal receptivity of cervical mucus to sperm should also be confirmed if possible. When sperm are present in the ejaculate on several occasions, a postcoital test should be carried out. The sexual partner of a man being treated for hypogonadotropism regularly conceives when the patient's total sperm counts are 5 to 10 million per milliliter. Postcoital sperm survival assessed at mid cycle frequently exhibits larger number of sperm than would have been predicted from semen characteristics alone. If the woman's cervical mucus is poor and shows low degree of receptivity to sperm, it is essential that the reasons for the abnormality be defined and corrected. Early efforts to optimize postcoital sperm survival may save critical months of treatment time.

Options for maintenance of gonadotropin treatment should be discussed as part of the initial management strategy. Medication, frequency, and dose may be changed or left unaltered when the desired outcome has been achieved. However, when FSH therapy has been required, the cost and lack of its necessity after the partner is pregnant dictates a change. Since first-trimester miscarriage normally occur 15 percent of the time (the frequency is no higher in couples in whom sperm production requires gonatotropin treatment), couples often wait 2 to 3 months before decreasing or stopping FSH. Spermatogenesis may be maintained in some patients by continuing hCG alone at regular doses sufficient to maintain testosterone levels. Even if sperm counts decrease on maintenance, they can be restored more rapidly with FSH if hCG is maintained. However, patients may prefer to reduce the frequency of hCG to once weekly or to attempt testosterone ester injections every 3 to 4 weeks. Changing to exogenous testosterone should not reduce a patient's subsequent fertility with exogenous gonadotropins, although he should be advised to reinstitute hCG 6 to 12 months before the anticipated time of conception. The time to achieve the desired outcome in prepubertal hypogonadotropism may be 1 to 2 years or more. Most patients are willing to maintain hCG injections three times per week for this period. Many adults have found it possible to maintain androgen-dependent symptoms satisfactorily using 1,500 to 5,000 IU hCG once weekly, with the dose being dependent on Leydig cell number and sensitivity, height, and weight of the patient. It is important to monitor testosterone and estradiol levels in patients maintained on altered protocols of gonadotropin treatment. However, most patients after prolonged treatment will be very sensitive to significant decreases in testosterone and will request changes in dose or frequency. It is wise to document and to maintain control over the patient's access to hCG and/or testosterone since hypertension, lipid disorders, sleep apnea, and even stroke have been reported in association with apparent overdoses of androgens.

In conclusion, gonadotropin treatment of hypogonadotropism, although somewhat complicated by the individualization of medication, dose, and frequency required, is generally straightforward, highly successful, and rewarding. It requires complete knowledge of the patient's medical and psychosocial history, a good physician–patient relationship, and precise monitoring of the outcome. When cost is a major consideration, the accuracy of the diagnosis, understanding of the reproductive physiology involved, and thorough patient education are critical. If the reasons for the choice of medications and protocol, the monitoring strategy, and the projections for long-term maintenance are agreed on and understood initially, this type of endocrine treatment can be one of the most effective and satisfying, both for physician and patient.

SUGGESTED READING

Collins JA, Wrixon W, Janes LB, et al. Treatment-independent pregnancy among infertile couples. N Engl J Med 1983; 309(20):1201–1206.

Sherins RJ. Clinical aspects of treatment of male infertility with gonadotropins: testicular response of some men given hCG with and without Pergonal. In: Mancini RE, Martini L, eds. Male fertility and sterility. New York: Academic Press, 1974.

Vance JL, Thorner MO. Medical treatment of male infertility. Semin Urol 1984; 2:115.

MALE INFERTILITY OF UNDETERMINED ETIOLOGY

EMIL STEINBERGER, M.D.

The treatment of male infertility is difficult since frequently the physician is not only unable to make a specific diagnosis but also empiric treatment, in most instances, is either marginally effective or ineffective. Even at best, when infertility is not of "undetermined origin" and a specific diagnosis can be made, either there is no treatment available (e.g., Klinefelter's syndrome) or the treatment is unpredictable (e.g., hypogonadotropic hypogonadism, varicocele, excretory duct blockage).

The diagnosable disorders leading to male infertility include a broad spectrum of diseases, including, for example, systemic infections, specific organ or tissue disorders, genetic disorders, hypothalamic-pituitary disorders, thyroid disorders, prolactin disorders, and specific lesions in the steroidogenic pathways in Leydig cells. Although most of the diagnosable conditions are untreatable, some are amenable to therapy. For example, hypogonadotropic hypogonadism may respond to gonadotropin therapy. Varicocelectomy in patients with diagnosed varicocele leads to improvement in semen quality only in some cases; there are no effective diagnostic techniques to permit selection of patients with this condition who may benefit from surgery. Blocks in the excretory duct system (ductuli efferentia, epididymis, vas), although amenable to surgical correction, require highly skilled intervention, and results are unpredictable.

In the instance of male infertility of "undetermined origin," the frustration is magnified by the fact that current diagnostic tools are inadequate to carry out an evaluation, and even when an attempt is made to carry out a diagnostic evaluation, by definition, it lacks specific goals. Classically, men with infertility of "undetermined origin" present either with diminished sperm count or with diminished quality of the spermatozoa reflected by decreased or abnormal motility and/or an increase in the abnormal forms. The interpretation of these semen analysis parameters is fraught with uncertainties because of deficiencies in routine semen analysis technology (e.g., arbitrary and subjective evaluation of motility) and in the quality of its interpretation. Even if technologic aspects of semen analysis would be acceptable, the interpretation is controversial. For example, it is difficult to determine at what point diminution of sperm output can be equated with diagnosis of "male infertility." Similarly, it is poorly understood what degree of disturbance in the quality of motility interferes with the man's fertility potential. A similar statement can be made for morphology. In most instances, the male partner is referred for therapy for infertility when the semen analysis reveals deviation from "normal" or the evaluation of female fertility potential is interpreted to be normal but the female partner fails to become pregnant. Thus, for all practical purposes the diagnosis of "male infertility" is frequently an exclusion diagnosis rather than a positive diagnosis, unless the patient is azoospermic or severely oligospermic or asthenospermic. Extensive and sophisticated evaluation of the patient may reveal factors that could possibly be responsible for the interference with adequate sperm production, albeit there is usually no specific and effective treatment for it. Numerous investigators, including myself, have conducted studies in patients whose semen analysis results (sperm count and/or motility or morphology) were below standards. In some of these patients, one could detect an enzymatic defect in the steroidogenic pathways of Leydig cells resulting in testosterone levels in low normal range, "subclinical" hypogonadotropism, or suggestions of Sertoli cell damage as revealed by changes in the production by the Sertoli cell of specific macromolecular markers. However, in most instances, even in these patients the therapy is unsuccessful and, when the patient's partner does become pregnant, it is difficult to correlate with the diagnostic pattern or to establish a cause-and-effect relationship.

The problems in evaluating therapeutic success in "idiopathic infertility" relate to the fact that the sperm output and quality vary considerably in the same person. Therapy has been successful when post-therapy semen analysis appears to be somewhat "better" than before therapy. This frequently is simply an expression of physiologic variation rather than cause and effect of the treatment.

Second, the difficulties in evaluating the success of therapy are related to the fact that pregnancies do occur in couples in which the man's semen is "oligospermic" (less than 10 or 20 million per milliliter). A significant proportion (up to 35 percent) of men with sperm counts of less than 5 million are capable of fertility. Consequently, a pregnancy occurring after a course of empiric therapy may be the result of the treatment but also may be the result of chance. In addition, a totally different complicating factor enters into the picture when the man is treated by one physician and the woman by another. For instance, the woman may suffer with oligo-ovulation and therefore be receiving treatment from her gynecologist while the man is under the treatment of a urologist. It is impossible to determine whether the pregnancy that results is because of treatment of the man or treatment of the woman.

The various modalities of therapy used in treatment of idiopathic semen deficiency or "infertility of undetermined origin" can be placed in the following general categories:

1. Stimulation of spermatogenesis by administration of low doses of testosterone
2. Testosterone rebound therapy
3. Stimulation of endogenous testosterone production by administration of human chorionic gonadotropin (hCG)
4. Administration of both follicle-stimulating hormone

and luteinizing hormone in the form of Pergonal or other human gonadotropin preparations
5. Administration of clomiphene citrate
6. Administration of various vitamins
7. Administration of various amino acids and peptides
8. Administration of various gonadotropin-releasing factors
9. Administration of various ions (e.g., zinc)
10. Administration of antiestrogens
11. Administration of antibiotics
12. Administration of anti-inflammatory agents
13. Administration of immunosuppressants
14. Tying of the testicular veins

Reports in the literature by authors using any one or a combination of the previously listed forms of therapy reveal that a segment of couples in which the male partner has been treated with any of these modalities results in the female partner's pregnancy. The incidence of pregnancy in these couples is very low, usually less than 30 percent and frequently in the 7 to 15 percent range. On the other hand, incidence of pregnancy by the female partner in a large population of infertile couples in which the male partners had semen analyses of less than "normal" quality and were left untreated was reported to be better than 50 percent. Thus, reports in the literature suggesting therapeutic efficacy of any one of the previously listed modalities remain difficult to interpret, and no therapeutic cause and effect can be established. Unquestionably, a diagnostic evaluation of the man is a necessary exercise. However, in most instances, evaluation beyond semen analysis, fundamental hormonal studies, and thorough history and physical examination—unless some positive finding is uncovered—ends up to be primarily of academic interest. At times the patient insists on knowing the specific reasons why he is not producing adequate sperm and/or why he is not fertile. Under these circumstances, an extensive, sophisticated evaluation may be in order. I doubt, however, that such an investigation provides the physician with information useful in determining effective therapy.

Since I have been in the practice of treating infertile couples for 29 years, I have been able to observe the fads and fashions of therapeutic management of male infertility, which include low doses of testosterone, testosterone rebound, hCG therapy, pituitary or urinary gonadotropin therapy, clomiphene citrate therapy, antiestrogen therapy, ligation of the testicular veins, and cooling of the testes. By rather extensive and carefully conducted studies, I have been unable to prove that any of these forms of therapy are specifically effective, although some of the so-treated patients may show improvement in semen quality and some female partners may become pregnant. I was able to demonstrate clearly that the degree of success in the attainment of a pregnancy by an infertile couple, even when the couple is referred primarily for "male infertility," is dependent upon careful management of the couple as a unit in which one pays particular attention to improving the female partner's fertility potential. Thus, until diagnostic tools improve and specific forms of therapy are devised for cases of idiopathic male infertility (over 90 percent of all cases), the most effective form of management of deficient semen or male infertility of "undetermined origin," in our hands, has been careful diagnostic evaluation of the female partner and an effective treatment for her, resulting in an overall improvement of the fertility potential of the couple.

SUGGESTED READING

Aiman J, Griffin JE. The frequency of androgen receptor deficiency in infertile men. J Clin Endocrinol Metab 1982; 54:725–732.

Baker HWG, Burger HG, deKretser DM, Hudson B. Relative incidence of etiological disorders in male infertility. In: Santen R, Swerdloff R, eds. Male reproductive dysfunction. New York: Marcel Dekker, 1986:341.

Steinberger E, Rodriguez-Rigau LJ. The infertile couple. J Androl 1983; 4:111–118.

Steinberger E, Smith KD, Rodriguez-Rigau LJ. Relationship between the results of semen analysis and the fertility potential of the couple. In: Frajese G, Hafez ESE, Conti C, Fabbrini A, eds. Oligozoospermia: recent progress in andrology. New York: Raven Press, 1981:407.

ORGANIC IMPOTENCE

FREDERICK T. MURRAY, M.D.
IRA W. KLIMBERG, M.D.
MARC S. COHEN, M.D.

Impotence is defined as the inability to obtain or maintain a penile erection that is sufficient for vaginal penetration during intercourse. There is no age after puberty at which intercourse is not physiologic, and as such the development of impotence represents a pathologic process. Impotence may be an isolated form of sexual dysfunction or can also be accompanied by diminished libido and problems with ejaculation. Although a decade ago impotence was considered primarily psychogenic in over 90 percent of cases, our current state of knowledge as reported by most centers now estimates that the incidence of organic impotence is approximately 50 percent and rising. In general, organic impotence implies an endocrine, vascular, or neurologic basis or a combination of these factors that interferes with the normal physiology of the penis. Although great strides in our understanding of penile function have been made, the detailed interaction of hormones and other pharmacologic substances with blood flow and neurologic innervation remains a mystery. In addition, the interaction of these physiologic processes with a number of psychological factors in many cases makes the differentiation of organic and psychogenic impotence difficult if not impossible. For these reasons, many clinicians see impotence as a continuum that varies between primarily psychogenic and primarily organic processes. With this approach, psychological variables are considered to be important moderators of the patient's organic state. Understanding this model also allows us to consider additional forms of psychotherapy in treating primary organic impotence if unsatisfactory sexual function remains apparent even after treatment of the organic dysfunction.

CAUSES OF IMPOTENCE

Drugs

A large number of drugs have been associated with primary organic impotence and as an adverse reaction or a major cause of poor drug compliance. Although in a healthy patient the onset of impotence shortly following the introduction of a new medication may seem obvious, the insidious development of impotence may mask the association to both physician and patient. In addition, if the drug depresses libido initially before the development of impotence, this is even less recognizable. Even more confusing is the addition of more than one drug in a patient who also has a chronic disease process that contributes to the etiology of impotence.

A detailed list of all drugs that cause primary organic impotence is beyond the scope of this chapter. However, a discussion of the main groups of drugs causing primary organic impotence and alternative drugs unlikely to cause impotence is appropriate. It should be noted, however, that all drug associations may be causal or casual, since most reports are not placebo-controlled studies. Diuretics, antihypertensives, anticonvulsants, alcohol, narcotics, and psychotropic drugs are the major drug groups associated with primary organic impotence.

Many psychotropic drugs have been associated with impotence and other forms of sexual dysfunction (Table 1). Antipsychotic drugs commonly cause delayed or absent ejaculation at even low doses. Medium doses are associated with problems of impotence, and usually higher doses are required before the adverse reactions of painful orgasm or ejaculation are noted. There is no physiologic explanation for these two latter adverse reactions. Erectile dysfunction usually occurs shortly after the initiation of therapy, not uncommonly within 24 hours. Thioridazine and chlorpromazine appear to be the worst offenders, ac-

TABLE 1 Antipsychotic Drugs and Sexual Dysfunction

Drug	*Adverse Effect*	*Incidence (%)*	*Dose* (mg/day)*
Thioridazine (Mellaril)	Priapism	Uncommon	100
	Impaired ejaculation	30	150
	Obtaining erections	44	100
	Maintaining erections	35	150
Perphenazine (Triavil)	Painful orgasm	Rare	24
	Diminished or absent ejaculation	60	24
	Priapism	Rare	
Haloperidol	Impotence		10
	Absent ejaculation		
	Painful orgasm	Rare	5
Chlorpromazine	Erectile dysfunction	Rare	600
	Priapism	Uncommon	100
Thiothixene	Impotence		20
Fluphenazine	Erectile dysfunction	Rare	25
	Diminished ejaculation		
Trifluoperazine	Diminished ejaculation	100	20
	Painful orgasm		10
Butaperazine	Diminished ejaculation	100	40
Chlorprothixene	Diminished ejaculation	Rare	300
Piperacetazine	Diminished ejaculation	Rare	100
Mesoridazine	Diminished ejaculation	Rare	60
Pimozide	Priapism	Rare	400
	Delayed ejaculation		16
	Impotence		
Benperidol	Impotence		1–25
	Diminished ejaculation	60	3–17

*Minimum dose reported to produce adverse effect.

counting for an incidence as high as 40 to 60 percent in some studies. Other phenothiazines are reported to cause an incidence of impotence in 11 to 25 percent of cases. In some circumstances decreasing the dosage will eliminate symptoms, but more often it is necessary to substitute another phenothiazine. The mechanisms by which antipsychotic drugs interfere with sexual function are not well understood. The sedative effects and anticholinergic and antiadrenergic properties of these compounds appear to be important factors. Hyperprolactinemia is also common in these patients, although other alterations of the endocrine system may also occur. The antipsychotic agent most commonly associated with testosterone suppression secondary to hyperprolactinemia is thioridazine.

Tricyclic, tetracyclic, and monoamine oxidase inhibitors are all antidepressants associated with impotence and other problems of sexual dysfunction in men (Table 2). Although impotence is reported in 2 to 20 percent of patients on antidepressants, diminished or absent ejaculation is a much more common event, occurring in as many as 4 to 100 percent with certain drugs. Although reducing the dosage may improve or alleviate symptoms in some cases, discontinuation of the drug entirely may be required. Some studies have reported that bethanechol chloride, 20 mg, taken orally 1 to 2 hours prior to sexual activity permitted satisfactory erection and ejaculation during sexual intercourse.

Antihypertensive medications are the most common cause of drug-related impotence (Table 3). Impotence is frequently seen with thiazides, guanethidine, methyldopa, reserpine, clonidine, and most beta-adrenergic blockers. Prazosin, hydralazine, minoxidil, captopril, enalapril, nifedipine, and verapamil are all uncommonly associated with sexual dysfunction and impotence.

Several miscellaneous drugs have also been reported to be associated with impotence and sexual dysfunction (Table 4). Digoxin and glucocorticoids have been shown to decrease serum testosterone levels as much as 50 percent, with associated decrease in libido and impotence. Other drugs, including anticonvulsants, alcohol, narcotics, and cimetidine, radiation, and cytoxic and chemotherapeutic agents, all are associated with a significant incidence of impotence.

Endocrine Disease

A variety of primary endocrine diseases are associated with impotence and decreased libido. The majority of these disorders produce either a deficiency of serum testosterone or elevation of serum prolactin levels. Although serum testosterone levels below 250 ng per deciliter are often associated with decreased libido, several investigators have shown that even higher values are associated with problems of obtaining and maintaining erections. Serum prolactin levels above 50 ng per milliliter are usually associated with decreased serum testosterone values. However, serum prolactin levels above 25 ng per milliliter may be associated with problems of erection independent of any decrease in serum testosterone. Patients with hypothyroidism and primary adrenal insufficiency also usually have diminished serum testosterone levels.

TABLE 2 Antidepressant Drugs and Sexual Dysfunction

Drug	*Adverse Effect*	*Incidence (%)*	*Dose* (mg/day)*
Amitriptyline (Elavil)	Diminished ejaculation	4.5	75
	Impotence	7	50
	Reduced libido		50
	Reduced NPT†		75
Mianserin	Reduced NPT		30
Imipramine (Tofranil)	Libido diminished	30	290
	Decreased orgasm	30	290
	Decreased ejaculation	12	75
	Impotence	<7	20
Phenelzine	Diminished libido	40	60
	Diminished orgasm	40	60
	Diminished ejaculation	40	60
Protriptyline (Vivactil)	Impotence	<2	20
	Pain on ejaculation	Rare	20
Desmethylimipramine (Norpramin)	Impotence	<2	150
Mebanazine	Impotence	4	20–40
	Diminished ejaculation	100	40
Lithium	Impotence	20	0.6–0.8
Clomipramine	Impotence	20	75–125
	Diminished ejaculation	4	75

*Minimum dose reported to produce adverse effect.
NPT = nocturnal penile tumescence.

TABLE 3 Antihypertensive Drugs Associated with Sexual Dysfunction

Drug	*Adverse Effect*	*Incidence (%)*	*Dose* (mg/day)*
Thiazide diuretics	Impotence	4–32	50
Spironolactone	Gynecomastia	5.6	100
	Gynecomastia	11.8	200
	Impotence	2	150
Methyldopa	Impotence	20–80	1,000
	Impaired libido	15	500
	Impaired ejaculation	7	500
Clonidine	Impotence	17–30	0.075–4.8
Reserpine	Impotence	50	0.1
Guanethidine	Delayed or absent ejaculation	71	25
	Impotence and decreased libido	28–34	20
Prazosin	Impotence	0.6	0.5
Propranolol	Impotence	5–43	40
Labetalol	Decreased libido		
	Impotence	56	100

*Minimum dose reported to produce adverse effect.

Vascular Disease

Vascular disease is estimated to cause primary organic impotence with an incidence of 10 to 20 percent. Acute vascular lesions of the spinal cord from infarction as a result of occlusion of either the anterior spinal or the paired posterior spinal arteries can occur, and a similar etiology is responsible in prolonged ischemia because of systemic hypotension or dissecting aortic aneurysm. The myelopathy that sometimes occurs with systemic lupus erythematosus or polyarteritis nodosa is probably due to cord ischemia resulting from occlusion of small and medium-sized arteries reflecting the underlying vasculitis. Impotence may also be a prominent finding in the Leriche syndrome, appearing as a result of thrombotic or embolic occlusions of the aorta or of the iliac arteries. The hallmark symptom of the disease is intermittent claudication present in either the thigh, buttock, or calf muscles. Isolated atheromatous occlusion of the internal pudendal arteries and/or their penile branches is a cause of impotence, although its incidence is unknown. Recent evidence also suggests that essential hypertension independent of drugs may be associated with impotence.

TABLE 4 Miscellaneous Drugs Associated with Sexual Dysfunction

Drug	*Adverse Effect*	*Incidence (%)*	*Dose* (mg/day)*
Clofibrate	Impotence	3	1,500
	Erectile failure	<5	1,800
Glucocorticoids (prednisone and prednisolone)	Impotence	50	15
	Loss of libido		
Cimetidine	Impotence	50	1,200
	Gynecomastia or breast tenderness	50	
Methadone	Impotence	10–51	80
Digoxin	Impotence	30	0.25
Phenytoin	Impotence	30	300
Phenobarbital	Impotence	25	45
Carbamazepine	Impotence	15	200

*Minimum dose reported to produce adverse effect.

Primary Neurologic Disorders

Primary neurologic disorders probably are the cause of impotence in about 10 percent of cases (Table 5). The majority of these disorders involve primary injury to the spinal cord. Partial or total impotence has been observed in nearly 50 percent of men with an established diagnosis of multiple sclerosis. Although cerebrovascular disease, Parkinson's disease, and Alzheimer's disease involve centers of the brain associated with sexual function, the exact mechanisms relating to decreased libido and impotence are unknown. Reduced sexual activity has been observed

TABLE 5 Primary Neurologic Disease and Sexual Dysfunction

Multiple sclerosis
Spinal cord trauma
Pelvic trauma
Temporal lobe epilepsy
Alzheimer's disease
Primary and metastatic tumors
Parkinson's disease
Cervical spondylosis
Spinal arachnoiditis
Syphilis (tabes dorsalis)
Amyloidosis
Primary autonomic insufficiency
Cerebrovascular accidents

frequently in patients with Parkinson's disease, and an increase in sexual performance may follow therapy with levodopa.

Chronic Disease

A number of chronic medical diseases have been associated with impotence. Diabetes mellitus is by far the most common of such diseases and occurs in over 50 percent of all type II and type I diabetic males over the age of 50. In our experience this group of patients may constitute 20 to 30 percent of all men with sexual impotence. In our current series (Table 6), we have been able to separate this group into primary psychogenic (35 percent) and primary organic impotence (65 percent) using nocturnal penile tumescence (NPT; see evaluation of organic impotence). Diabetic patients with primary organic impotence appear to have low free and total testosterone values, high levels of urinary luteinizing hormone (LH), and blunted testosterone responses to human chorionic gonadotropin (hCG) stimulation. These endocrine changes are not seen in diabetic patients with primary psychogenic impotence. We have not seen any significant differences in endocrine function or NPT parameters in type I and type II diabetes. Duration of diabetes and impotence are also similar.

Patients with chronic liver disease, heart disease, chronic renal disease, chronic obstructive pulmonary disease, obesity, burn trauma, and essential hypertension also frequently complain of impotence. Patients with chronic liver disease and chronic alcoholics without liver disease frequently have low serum testosterone levels, increased estradiol concentrations, and, not infrequently, testicular atrophy. The serum LH level is generally normal or high, but some cases with hypogonadotropic hypogonadism have also been reported. In chronic renal disease testosterone levels may be low and serum prolactin levels elevated. Burn patients have low testosterone values that do not always return to normal even after long-term follow-up. In patients with essential hypertension, chronic obstructive pulmonary disease, and chronic heart diseases, the underlying causes of impotence are not clearly understood. Some of these patients do have low serum testosterone levels, but what proportion of this is due to medications or to the chronic disease process remains unclear.

Surgical Causes

Surgical trauma, particularly radical exenterative procedures performed for urologic malignancy, are associated with erectile dysfunction (Table 7). However, there may be adverse effects on erectile function following various general and vascular surgical procedures. Postoperative erectile failure is related to damage to the neural innervation of the penis, interruption of the penile vascular supply, or psychogenic factors.

Damage to the pelvic parasympathetic nerves is the most common cause of organic postoperative erectile failure. Arising from the spinal cord, the sacral roots S2 to S4 contribute nerve fibers to the pelvic parasympathetic plexus. These fibers then continue to sweep caudally along the pelvic side wall, passing lateral to the rectum. The principal parasympathetic fibers subserving erectile activity, the cavernous nerves, run dorsolateral and in close proximity to the prostate gland, to perforate the urogenital diaphragm and innervate the lacunar smooth muscle of the corpora cavernosa. The intimate association of these nerves with the prostatic capsule makes them particularly vulnerable to injury during radical prostatectomy or radical cystectomy performed for urologic malignancy.

The accurate mapping of the course of the cavernous nerves and modifications in surgical techniques allow for the intraoperative identification and preservation of these structures. Employing this nerve-sparing technique, researchers have indicated that erectile function can be preserved in 33 to 84 percent of patients undergoing radical prostatectomy. This same nerve-sparing technique may also be employed to maintain sexual function following radical cystectomy.

Postoperative erectile failure following surgery for lower bowel disease appears to be related to the extent of resection and the age of the patient. Impotence following these procedures is due primarily to damage to the pelvic parasympathetic nerves as they course from the pelvic wall along the rectum. The

TABLE 6 Nocturnal Penile Tumescence (NPT) in Normal Men and in Patients with Diabetes Mellitus and Impotence

	Total Tumescence Time (min)	*Total Sleep Time (min)*	*Maximum Penile Circumference Change (mm)*	*Number of Episodes*
Normal men (n = 17)	92 ± 8.8*	413.0 ± 11.1	17.9 ± 1.8	3.82 ± 0.36
Primary psychogenic impotence (n = 14)	87 ± 11.0	386 ± 8.0	13 ± 1.0†	3.9 ± 0.4
Primary organic impotence (n = 24)	21 ± 9.0†	382 ± 9.0	2.0 ± 0.6†	0.7 ± 0.2†

*Mean ± SEM.
†p < .01 (analysis of variance, one-way) when compared with controls.

TABLE 7 Surgical and Traumatic Causes of Impotence

Prostatectomy: radical or simple
Cystectomy
Penectomy
Prostate biopsy
Internal urethrotomy: sphincterotomy
Bilateral orchiectomy
Renal transplantation
Retroperitoneal lymphadenectomy
Sympathectomy
Aortoiliac surgery
Abdominoperineal resection
Proctocolectomy
Pelvic radiation therapy
Inguinoscrotal surgery
Spinal cord injury
Pelvic fractures
Genital trauma

incidence of impotence is much higher following abdominoperineal resection for carcinoma than for prostacolectomy for benign disease. This reflects the necessity for more extensive dissection in the presence of malignancy.

Aortoiliac surgery for vascular disease results in extensive dissection in the retroperitoneum and pelvis with possible neural and vascular disruption. Postoperative impotence has been reported in 21 to 80 percent of patients. Persistent impotence after renal transplantation or the onset of erectile failure following transplantation is probably related to abnormalities of the penile arterial supply. The frequency of this problem increases dramatically after a second renal transplant, particularly if both internal iliac arteries have been used for an end-to-end vascular anastomosis. Prostatectomy for benign disease, either transabdominal or transurethral, is uncommonly (0 to 13 percent) associated with erectile failure. The etiology of the postoperative impotence in these patients is unclear. Some suggest that the level of patient anxiety, comprehension of the surgical procedure and expected outcome, and overall psychological well-being may make the difference between postoperative potency and impotence. Reports of impotence following inguinal and scrotal operative procedures confirm that psychogenic factors may play a significant role in postoperative sexual dysfunction.

Resection of lumbar sympathetic ganglia during sympathectomy, aortic aneurysm repair, or retroperitoneal lymphadenectomy may lead to nonerectile sexual dysfunction. This is usually an isolated failure of ejaculation in the presence of normal libido, erection, or orgasm. Sympathectomy generally leads to failure of emission rather than retrograde ejaculation, and this may have adverse effects psychologically, resulting in secondary erectile dysfunction. Isolated sympathetic denervation of the penis does not appear to be a direct cause of erectile dysfunction.

EVALUATION OF PRIMARY ORGANIC IMPOTENCE

The most difficult problem in selecting the proper treatment for impotence is deciding whether the patient has primary organic impotence, primary psychogenic impotence, or primary organic and psychogenic impotence. This latter group may be as high as 30 percent in some clinic populations. Although sexual questionnaires, the Minnesota Multiphasic Personality Inventory (MMPI) test, and psychological and psychiatric interviews are clearly helpful in determining the presence of psychogenic factors, they rarely determine the presence or absence of organic impotence.

In our experience and that of others, the single most effective test to determine organic impotence is the use of NPT. Although initially this was described by using continuous sleep monitoring and measurements over 3 or more consecutive nights, such extensive monitoring is not required for most clinical purposes. In our sexual dysfunction clinic we routinely monitor patients in an outpatient overnight laboratory facility without continuous electroencephalographic monitoring. Approximately 25 percent of these patients return for a second evening of evaluation, usually because diminished sleep time was evident on the first evaluation. Total sleep time, number of tumescence episodes, total tumescence time, and maximal penile circumference change (MPCC) are measured on each patient, and results are reported as the best of both nights if two nights are recorded. Figure 1 summarizes MPCC in 26 men with normal sexual function ranging from 17 to 64 years of age. All of these normal volunteers had normal sexual function by history, normal semen analysis on three occasions, normal serum and urinary gonadotropin levels, and normal diurnal variation of serum prolactin, total testosterone, free testosterone, albumin-bound testosterone, beta-endorphins, and adrenocorticotropic hormone. Similar values are seen in the literature by a number of investigators. A value of 8 mm is two standard deviations from the mean and our most reliable parameter for the determination of primary organic impotence. The lowest MPCC change for any normal male evaluation was 11 mm (see Fig. 1). Other investigators have shown that MPCC from 7.5 to 10 mm using heparinized saline infusion in the corpus cavernosum is able to produce an erection that is sufficient for vaginal penetration. Ranges in the literature vary for MPCC from 7.5 to 12 mm using different NPT equipment and different controls. Figure 2 also indicates the significant relationship between serum testosterone (a pool of nine samples in 24 hours) and MPCC in normal men and those with pituitary-testicular dysfunction. Two men with Reifenstein's syndrome not included in this correlation having impotence, high testosterone levels, and decreased MPCC suggest that this correlation with testosterone is likely

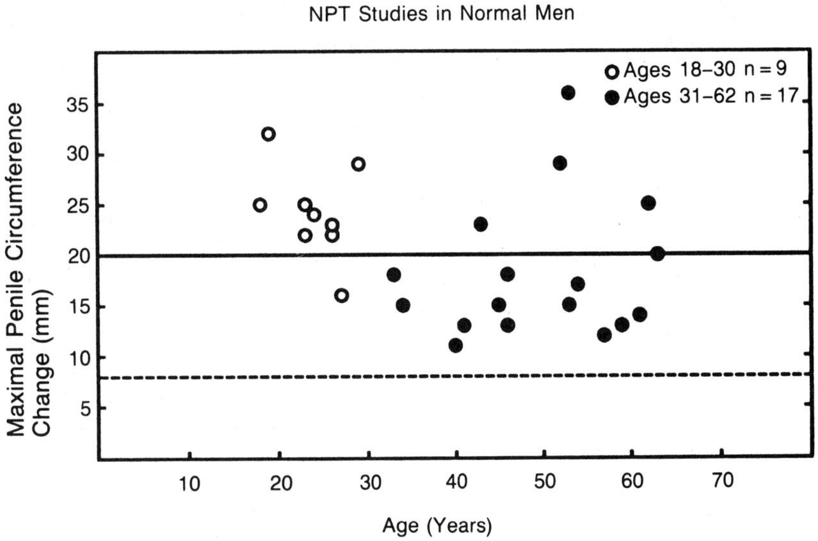

Figure 1 Maximal penile circumference change in normal men. The solid line indicates the mean of 26 normal men, and the dotted line is two standard deviations from the mean.

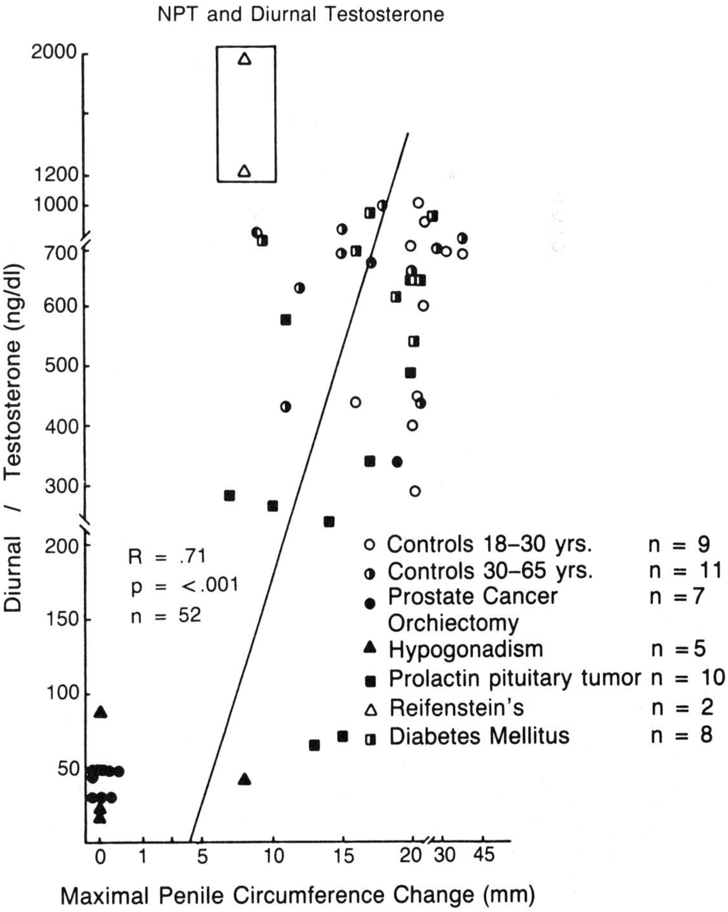

Figure 2 The mean of nine testosterone values over 24 hours is correlated (Pearson's coefficient) with MPCC in normal men, in diabetic men with normal sexual function, and in men with endocrine disorders of testosterone dysregulation. The two patients with Reifenstein's syndrome are not included in the correlation coefficient calculation.

TABLE 8 Disorders of Impotence Associated with Diminished Nocturnal Penile Tumescence

Chronic obstructive pulmonary disease
Drugs (cimetidine, amitriptyline, mianserin)
Diabetes mellitus
Chronic renal failure
Prolactin pituitary tumors
Reifenstein's syndrome
Hypogonadism
Peyronie's disease
Chronic alcoholism
Severe depression

to be androgen receptor–dependent. A number of disorders now reported in the literature associated with diminished NPT and impotence are listed in Table 8. In our experience NPT is clearly the single most important test to identify organic impotence. The cost of this procedure generally is $300 to $400 per night, although as much as $1,000 is generally charged in sleep laboratories that use electroencephalographic monitoring.

Once organic impotence is identified, a number of other tests are important to decide on the best mode of treatment (Fig. 3). Hormone studies generally include evaluating serum for testosterone, prolactin, and LH levels. Ideally these three samples should be drawn in the early morning at 10-minute intervals and pooled for a single radioimmunoassay. This is especially important in determining a low serum LH level. Because of the diurnal pattern of testosterone secretion, a late afternoon sample may be 50 percent lower than samples drawn before 10 AM. In our laboratory, a mean testosterone value of less than 400 ng per deciliter, collected over 24 hours, in a man under 65 years of age is considered abnormal. Although both free testosterone levels and albumin-bound testosterone (bioavailable testosterone) levels have been suggested in some clinical studies, it is not clear, particularly in patients with chronic disease, whether these additional blood measurements are more helpful for therapeutic decisions. From Figure 2 it would appear that a patient with normal NPT should not require additional androgen evaluation.

In patients with primary organic impotence demonstrated by NPT and normal endocrine studies, some assessment of the vascular supply to the penis is generally helpful for further therapeutic decisions (see Fig. 3). Penile brachial index (PBI) has been used to screen for macrovascular arteriogenic impotence. This is determined by measuring penile blood pressure by Doppler evaluation and expressing this over mean brachial pressure recorded in a similar manner. This is done on both sides, and the highest ratio is recorded. Normal values are above one. Minimal (0.80 to 0.90), mild (0.65 to 0.80), and severe (less than 0.65) arterial insufficiency can be determined by this methodology. Plethysmography of the penile arteries is less useful to screen for microvascular disease. In patients with a PBI index of 0.70 or less, selective internal pudendal arteriography should be assessed if vascular reconstruction surgery is to be considered. In the event of a normal PBI index and normal endocrine studies, further studies are warranted only if neurologic assessment is necessary before consideration of further therapy. These studies would include conduction velocity of the dorsal nerve of the penis, latency of the bulbocavernosus reflex, pudendal evoked potentials, cystometry, or sural electromyography.

Most recently, the intracavernosal injection of vasoactive, pharmacologic agents (papaverine with and without phentolamine, prostaglandin E_1)

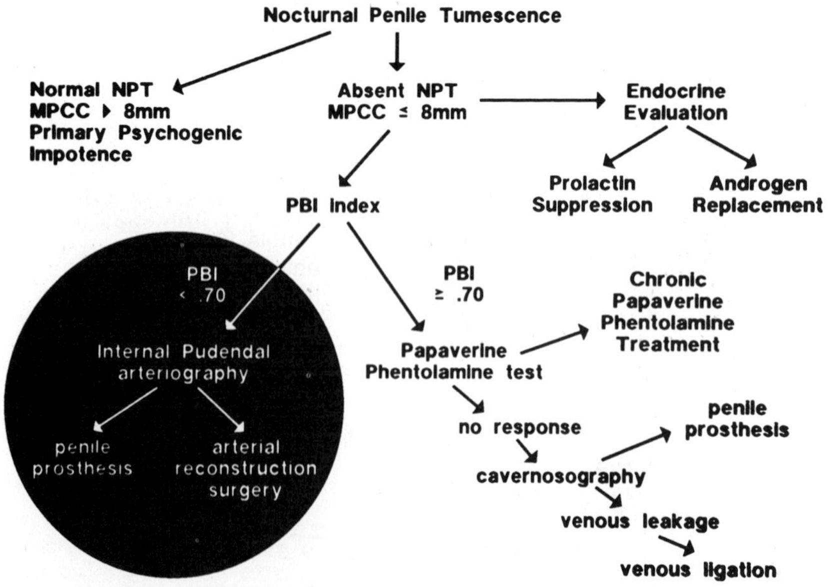

Figure 3 Evaluation and treatment of primary organic impotence. The area within the circle indicates an optional evaluation for those doing arterial reconstruction surgery. NPT, nocturnal penile tumescence; MPCC, maximal penile circumference change; PBI, penile brachial index.

has been employed in the evaluation of erectile dysfunction. Failure to achieve an erection within 10 minutes and to maintain an erection for 15 to 20 minutes after the administration of 10 μg of prostaglandin E_1 or 30 mg of papaverine may be taken as presumptive evidence of a vasculogenic etiology for dysfunction (although patient anxiety may induce enough sympathetic tone to override vasoactive effects).

The use of duplex sonography in association with intracavernosal injection represents a relatively noninvasive way of further evaluating presumed vasculogenic impotence. The penis is scanned in a flaccid state and then again after intracavernosal administration of papaverine with or without phentolamine. The diameter of the cavernosal arteries in response to injection and more important the velocity of blood flow (peak systolic velocity, mean peak velocity) may be determined, with decreased flow being indicative of arterial insufficiency.

Dynamic infusion cavernosometry and cavernosography are employed in an ever growing number of patients. This examination is combined with an initial injection of vasoactive agents (papaverine, phentolamine, prostaglandin E_1) into the cavernosa to induce a pharmacologic erection. Useful parameters obtained include changes in tumescence and intracorporal pressure in response to pharmacologic agents. In addition, the elapsed time until the equilibration of intracorporal pressure may be a useful indicator of underlying arterial pathophysiology. Inability to sustain tumescence may be seen with venous incompetence. The source and degree of venous leak may be confirmed by infusion of x-ray contrast material and fluoroscopy.

Cavernosometry allows accurate measurement of the cavernosal artery occlusion pressure and permits direct quantitation of the "blood trapping" (veno-occlusive) mechanisms that are important in normal erectile physiology. These studies permit a clearer understanding of the effects of systemic disorders on the vascular mechanisms of the penis. It is clear that local disorders of the hemodynamic process, either alone (arterial insufficiency or "venous leak"), or as is more commonly encountered, combined, are responsible for erectile problems in a substantial number of men formerly thought to have psychogenic erectile failure.

Cavernosometry is indicated in those individuals who fail to obtain good quality erections in response to intracorporal injections of vasoactive agents. The incidence of venous incompetence among this subgroup of patients is substantial.

MEDICAL TREATMENT

Our general approach to the evaluation and treatment of primary organic impotence is outlined in Figure 3. In the patient taking one or more medications that are known to cause or suspected of causing impotence in whom NPT has clearly demonstrated organic impotence, a consideration to decrease the dosage or substitute a different medication is warranted. NPT may be used to confirm efficacy of this treatment if the outcome is uncertain or if combined primary organic and psychogenic impotence is suspected.

Low testosterone levels or mild hyperprolactinemia may be related to drug medication as well as due to primary endocrine disease. Digoxin has been reported to reduce testosterone levels as much as 50 percent, and in those patients in whom this drug is truly warranted, testosterone replacement therapy should be considered. Many psychotropic drugs produce hyperprolactinemia, and in certain cases treatment with bromocriptine, 2.5 mg orally twice a day, may be necessary to restore normal sexual function. However, it should be cautioned that sellar computed tomography is necessary to determine whether the hyperprolactinemia is due to medication or sellar and suprasellar pathology.

The treatment of prolactin pituitary tumors is discussed in detail in the chapter entitled *Prolactinoma.* However, certain aspects relating to treatment in males will be discussed briefly. Although transsphenoidal surgery and medical therapy with bromocriptine appear equally effective in patients with microadenomas, data suggest that prolactin macroadenomas present a particular problem in men undergoing testosterone replacement therapy. It now appears that testosterone therapy, either directly or via conversion to estradiol, may increase the size of prolactin macroadenomas in which no previous radiation therapy or transsphenoidal surgery was performed. It should also be remembered that testosterone therapy will not restore normal sexual function unless hyperprolactinemia is reduced to levels below 50 ng per milliliter. We begin bromocriptine therapy in patients with prolactin microadenomas or macroadenomas with hyperprolactinemia above 50 ng per milliliter 4 to 6 weeks following transsphenoidal surgery. We start with 1.25 mg in the evening and increase by ½ tablets weekly to a dosage of 2.5 mg three times daily. In rare cases the dosage is increased further if the serum prolactin value remains above 25 ng per milliliter after 3 months. If testosterone values on repeat measurements are below 300 ng per deciliter in the presence of a normal serum prolactin value and complaints of impotence, we initiate testosterone parenteral therapy. If psychogenic impotence is strongly suspected, NPT evaluation is performed to document primary organic impotence. The treatment of hypogonadism with parenteral testosterone replacement is discussed in detail in the chapter entitled *Hypogonadism: Androgen Therapy.*

The most significant development in the medical treatment of impotence is pharmacologic erections.

The concept of intracavernous injection of vasoactive substances to reproduce pharmacologically the changes associated with physiologic erections was initially suggested by Brindley and Virag. Although various substances have been tried, the pharmacologic agents most often employed are papaverine, in combination with phentolamine with or without prostaglandin E_1. The mechanism by which these drugs cause erections is dilatation of the lacunar smooth muscle of the corpora cavernosa. Phentolamine is a beta-adrenergic antagonist.

Following complete evaluation for erectile dysfunction, eligible patients may undergo a test injection. Papaverine alone (10 to 30 mg) or in combination with phentolamine (1 mg) is administered directly into the corpus cavernosum at the base of the penis using a fine-gauge needle. Following the injection, the patient and his partner are instructed to attempt intercourse. In the event that plethysmography shows diminished blood flow on one side, the opposite side is used for injection.

Although some patients experience a rigid erection following injection, many have tumescence only. In these cases erection usually ensues with arousal and stimulation. Although the tumescence produced by the injection generally lasts 2 to 4 hours, the best results are seen if intercourse is attempted within the first hour.

Overall between 60 and 80 percent of patients are able to perform intercourse following injection. Some of these patients may be instructed in the technique of self-injection and use this technique to restore erectile function. In general, these patients require an injection prior to each sexual encounter in order to obtain a satisfactory erection. Anecdotal accounts of normal erections days or weeks following an injection have been reported. The significance of these reports is unclear at the present time.

Patients on this self-injection program require close urologic monitoring. There is no long-term knowledge concerning this treatment and possible untoward effects arising from repeated injection of the penis. Complications include dizziness, superficial hematoma, metallic taste, burning of the shaft, and sustained erection. Maximal follow-up time has been 24 months. Of the immediate problems encountered following intracavernous injections, the most significant have been prolonged erections. This condition is a surgical emergency and requires prompt treatment to prevent hypoxic damage and destruction of the penile substance.

Initial treatment of prolonged pharmacologically induced erections involves irrigation and aspiration of the corporeal bodies. Intracorporeal irrigation of a dilute solution of an adrenergic agonist (epinephrine, 1 mg per 1,000 ml; metaraminol, 2 mg; or dopamine) may produce rapid detumescence, since these agents appear to be able to reverse the effects of papaverine and phentolamine. Should these attempts at penile decompression fail, standard urologic surgical procedures for the treatment of priapism must be employed immediately. These procedures involve the construction of a cavernosal spongiosum or cavernosal venous fistula.

Intracorporeal injection appears to be most effective in patients in whom the PBI index is greater than 0.70. However, it should probably be tried even in situations in which the PBI is less than 0.70. Intracorporeal injections are also effective in a number of neurologic disorders, including diabetes mellitus, spinal cord injuries, multiple sclerosis, and Parkinson's disease.

Medical Treatment of Primary Organic Impotence in Chronic Disease

Diabetes mellitus is the most common chronic disease to present with primary organic impotence (see Table 6). Whether the primary etiology is vascular, neurologic, or endocrine still remains unknown. However, the majority of these patients respond favorably to papaverine-phentolamine intracorporeal injections. Our own preliminary studies would also indicate that testosterone cypionate or enanthate (200 mg given intramuscularly every 2 weeks) improves sexual function and NPT in selected patients without penile vascular disease and low serum testosterone levels. Other investigators have also reported improvement in sexual function with testosterone therapy in selected patients in randomized placebo-controlled studies. Studies using zinc, bromocriptine, or luteinizing hormone-releasing hormone have not been shown to be effective.

Chronic alcoholism with or without liver disease is also commonly associated with impotence. Studies suggest that only 25 percent of chronic alcoholics spontaneously recover normal sexual function following 6 months of abstinence from alcohol. Those who fail to respond have a high incidence of irreversible testicular atrophy. However, the majority of these patients respond favorably to parenteral testosterone therapy. Zinc therapy in chronic cirrhosis has not been shown to be effective in controlled placebo trials.

Uremia in patients often leads to sexual dysfunction, such as erectile failure and loss of libido. Many causes have been postulated, but exact mechanisms are unknown. However, hypogonadism with depression of steroidogenesis is a consistent feature of chronic renal failure. Animal data suggest that blood urea nitrogen directly infused intravenously into rodents diminishes serum testosterone. Most studies indicate that impotence significantly precedes chronic renal failure and is demonstrated often when the serum creatinine level exceeds 4 mg per deciliter. The data appear controversial as to whether sexual dysfunction worsens on chronic hemodialysis, and chronic hemodialysis alone does not clearly improve sexual dysfunction. In patients with mild chronic renal failure (creatinine 4 to 10 mg per deciliter), hCG therapy appears to improve sexual function significantly. However, once the patient is on hemodialysis, therapy with testosterone or hCG does not appear to be beneficial. In selected patients with chronic renal failure, bromocriptine, 1.25 mg twice daily, may be effective in improving sexual function, although adverse reactions are common. However, a positive response cannot always be related to either a fall in prolactin level or a rise in serum testosterone level. A negative response was seen frequently in patients who failed either at the onset or conclusion of therapy to have normal serum testosterone values. Several studies have looked at the use of zinc therapy in patients on chronic hemodialysis with sexual dysfunction. Only selected patients showed modest improvement in some studies, whereas many patients did not appear to benefit at all. In general, renal transplantation is the best treatment for impotence in patients with chronic renal failure. In patients with low serum testosterone levels, particularly if the serum creatinine value is less than 10 mg per deciliter, a trial of parenteral testosterone therapy may be beneficial. Papaverine intracorporeal injections in these patients are also usually effective.

Patients with chronic obstructive pulmonary disease and coronary artery disease frequently complain of impotence of unknown etiology. A significant proportion of these patients do have low serum testosterone levels and respond favorably to parenteral testosterone therapy. Again, papaverine intracorporeal injections are also beneficial.

TREATMENT WITH NONSURGICAL EXTERNAL DEVICES

For those patients who fail to respond to or do not wish medical treatment, a discussion of external devices is warranted.

Vacuum/entrapment devices were first patented in 1917 by Otto Lederer, and at present there are over six devices in this category available in the United States, with costs ranging from $200 to $500. Most of these devices require a physician's prescription and should not be prescribed for men with a history of or predisposition to priapism, those on anticoagulants, or those with bleeding diatheses. These devices generally consist of a plastic cylinder, a vacuum pump, tubing, and a plastic, rubber, or metal entrapment ring. An erection-like state is attained by placing the flaccid or semierect lubricated penis into the penile sleeve and applying vacuum pressure. The slower and smoother establishment of vacuum pressures minimizes potential complications such as petechiae and ecchymosis. Once the penis is engorged with blood, the patient slides an entrapment ring onto the base of the penis. In general, the manufacturers of vacuum/entrapment devices recommend that the inside of the device and the penis be lubricated prior to applying the vacuum. An empirical time limit of 30 minutes is recommended for use of the entrapment rings with all vacuum/entrapment devices. Generally, the presence of any entrapment ring does not allow the ejaculate to pass through the proximal urethra. The semen will drain out in a nonexpulsive manner once the occlusive band is removed. Ejaculation, although blocked by the ring, is not painful. Obviously, some patients may find external management options esthetically unacceptable, but they should still be discussed and at least offered as alternative choices. These devices generally require good manual dexterity, and people with arthritis or poor eye-hand coordination may have problems manipulating them.

SURGICAL TREATMENT

Surgical treatment of erectile dysfunction can be divided into vascular reconstructive procedures and placement of a penile prosthesis. All of the currently available penile prostheses consist of a pair of cylinders that are placed within the tunica albuginea of the corpora cavernosa to produce sufficient penile rigidity for intromission. There are two broad categories of these devices: semirigid and inflatable.

The semirigid devices all rely on the rigidity of the cylinder material to produce erection. There are numerous variations on the exact structure of the cylinders, but nearly all use a silicone rubber exterior that surrounds a core structure. These various devices are described as semirigid, flexible, or malleable. These are simple devices, and their appeal is based on reliability, ease of insertion, and economy. They provide adequate rigidity but do not have any mechanism to allow for flaccidity. The cost of these devices is approximately $1,500.

The semirigid prostheses have enjoyed tremendous popularity over the past 14 years. These devices have proved to be reliable and nearly free of mechanical failure. Infection (0 to 10 percent), malposition, erosion, and, in diabetics, persistent pain have been the most prevalent complications seen with these devices. Patient satisfaction has been excellent, with more than 80 percent of patients pleased with their result.

The inflatable penile prostheses comprise two inflatable pontoons, a pump, and a separate fluid reservoir or more recently a combined pump reservoir. These devices rely on hydraulic distention of the intracorporeal pontoons to provide rigidity during intercourse. The fluid can then be transported back into the reservoir following sexual activity to deflate the pontoons and allow a flaccid penis. These devices produce a more natural-appearing erection, which increases both penile length and girth and allows the patient to have a flaccid phallus between sexual encounters. The principal drawbacks to these devices have been related to their complex nature. They are prone to mechanical failure, require a more extensive surgical procedure to implant, and are expensive. The cost of these devices ranges from $2,500 to $3,000.

The inflatable prostheses have undergone numerous modifications in their design in an attempt to minimize the rate of mechanical failure, which was as high as 40 percent in early reports. Aneurysmal dilatation, input tube erosion, tube kinking, and connection failure have been drastically reduced in the currently implanted models, so that their overall complication rate approaches that of the simpler semirigid devices.

In the past year there have been two new self-contained inflatable penile prostheses introduced that have incorporated the pump and reservoir into the cylinders. These devices are implanted like the semirigid devices, and they are purported to be as reliable as those simpler devices because of their "self-contained" design.

Vascular reconstructive procedures have also been employed to restore erectile function in carefully selected patients. Patients must undergo additional invasive radiologic assessment of their penile vasculature prior to these procedures. These studies include selective internal pudendal arteriography as well as dynamic infusions for cavernosometry and cavernosography. These diagnostic studies are necessary to identify arterial lesions or cavernosal-venous leaks.

Arterial reconstructive procedures augment blood flow to the corpora cavernosa via microsurgical anastomosis of a neoarterial source to the corpora cavernosa, the deep dorsal penile vein, or the cavernosal artery. There are a multitude of these procedures, most based on the Michael and Virag operations. At the present time, they are performed only at a few centers, in a highly selected group of patients, and must be considered investigative procedures. Return of erectile activity has been reported in 30 to 80 percent of patients.

Surgical procedures for cavernosal-venous leaks are technically simpler to perform and consist of ligation or resection of the major venous channels draining the corpora. Postoperative recovery of erectile function has been reported in 50 to 80 percent of patients.

SUGGESTED READING

Bansal S. Sexual dysfunction in hypertensive men. Hypertension 1988; 12:1–10.

Handelsman DJ. Hypothalamic-pituitary gonadal dysfunction in renal failure, dialysis and renal transplantation. Endocr Rev 1985; 6:151–182.

Merrill DC. Clinical experience with mentor inflatable penile prosthesis in 206 patients. Urology 1986; 28:185–189.

Michael V. Arterial disease as a cause of impotence. Clin Endocrinol Metab 1982; 11:725–748.

Murray FT, Cameron DF, Ketchum C. Return of gonadal function in men with prolactin secreting pituitary tumors. J Clin Endocrinol Metab 1984; 59:79–85.

Murray FT, Wyss HU, Thomas R, et al. Gonadal dysfunction in diabetic men with organic impotence. J Clin Endocrinol Metab 1987; 65:127–135.

Murray FT, Sciadini M, Wyss HU. Is nocturnal penile tumescence (NPT) a test of pituitary-testicular function? J Androl 1987; 8:36.

Nadig PW, Ware JL, Blumhoff R. Noninvasive devices to produce and maintain an erection-like state. Urology 1986; 27:126–131.

Sidi AA, Cameron JS, Duffy LM, Lange PH. Intracavernosus drug-induced erections in the management of male erectile dysfunction: Experience with 100 patients. J Urol 1986; 135:704–706.

Smith PJ, Talbert RL. Sexual dysfunction with antihypertensive and antipsychotic agents. Clin Pharmacol 1986; 5:373–384.

Van Thiel DH, Gavaler JS, Sanghvi A. Recovery of sexual function in abstinent alcoholic men. Gastroenterology 1982; 84:672–682.

HYPOCALCEMIA AND HYPOPARATHYROIDISM

ROBERT K. RUDE, M.D.

Hypocalcemia can be due to a reduction in either the albumin-bound and/or ionized fraction of the serum calcium level. A reduction in the ionized serum calcium concentration is usually due to impairment in physiologic processes by which this fraction of the serum calcium is maintained, either through decreased flux of calcium into or an increased transfer of calcium out of the extracellular fluid compartment. The commonly encountered causes of hypocalcemia are listed in Table 1. Treatment of rickets and osteomalacia (due to vitamin D deficiency or resistance), and pseudohypoparathyroidism are not dealt with in this book. Reviews of the treatment of hypocalcemia in the setting of chronic renal failure and a general summary of the etiology and evaluation of hypocalcemia are covered in the suggested reading at the end of this chapter.

HYPOCALCEMIA NOT NEEDING TREATMENT

Hypoalbuminemia is frequently seen in patients with chronic liver disease, nephrotic syndrome, congestive heart failure, and malnutrition. Since approximately 50 percent of calcium in the circulation is bound to albumin, hypoalbuminemia will result in a low total serum calcium con-

TABLE 1 Differential Diagnosis of Hypocalcemia

Hypoalbuminemia
Chronic renal failure
Magnesium deficiency
Hypoparathyroidism
Pseudohypoparathyroidism
Osteomalacia and rickets due to vitamin D deficiency or resistance
Acute hemorrhagic and edematous pancreatitis
Healing phase of bone disease of treated hyperparathyroidism, hyperthyroidism, and hematologic malignancies (hungry bone syndrome)

centration. The ionized fraction is normal, and no therapy for the hypocalcemia is indicated. The serum calcium concentration should, therefore, be "corrected" for any decrease in the normal serum albumin concentration (4.0 g per deciliter). One gram of albumin per 100 ml of serum will bind 0.8 mg per deciliter of calcium.

$$\text{Corrected Ca} = \text{serum Ca} + 0.8\,(4.0 - \text{serum albumin}).$$

Example: A patient with hepatic cirrhosis was found to have a serum calcium level of 8.2 mg per deciliter. The serum albumin level was 2.5 g per deciliter. The corrected serum calcium value was 9.4 mg per deciliter. The serum calcium concentration corrects to normal, and no further evaluation or treatment of the hypocalcemia is necessary.

ACUTE SYMPTOMATIC HYPOCALCEMIA

A fall in the ionized fraction of the serum calcium will result in the characteristic symptoms of hypocalcemia. This is most commonly associated with neuromuscular hyperexcitability such as latent tetany (positive Chvostek's and Trousseau's signs), spontaneous tetany with carpopedal spasm and muscle cramps, paresthesias, and seizures. Regardless of the cause of the hypocalcemia, the acute management is the same (with the exception of hypocalcemia due to magnesium deficiency as discussed later).

Rapid relief of the symptoms of hypocalcemia is best achieved by intravenous injection of 10 to 20 ml of 10 percent calcium gluconate (90 to 180 mg elemental Ca^{2+}) over a 5- to 10-minute period. This usually produces improvement of symptoms for hours despite the observation that serum calcium concentration quickly (within 15 to 30 minutes) reverts to pretreatment levels after the injection is completed. The injection may be repeated as often as is needed to control the symptoms. Alternatively, following the initial calcium injection, an infusion of calcium, 2 to 3 mg elemental calcium per kilogram of ideal body weight, may be infused over a 4-hour period. This will result in a rise in the serum calcium concentration of 1 to 2 mg per deciliter and should relieve the symptoms of hypocalcemia. A low normal serum calcium concentration (8.0 to 8.5 mg per deciliter) is the ideal level so as to avoid the danger of hypercalcemia and hypercalciuria. The calcium infusion is especially useful in acute hypocalcemic states such as the hungry bone syndrome and hemorrhagic or edematous pancreatitis. The infusion may be repeated as needed to prevent symptomatic hypocalcemia.

MAGNESIUM DEFICIENCY

Many clinical problems may result in gastrointestinal or renal magnesium wasting, including diarrhea, malabsorption, alcoholism, diabetes mellitus and hypercalciuria. Additionally diuretic therapy, aminoglycoside therapy, cisplatin administration, and chronic parenteral fluid therapy may result in renal magnesium wasting and magnesium deficiency. The presence of hypocalcemia in any patient with these problems should alert the physician to the possibility of magnesium deficiency. A low serum magnesium concentration (less than 1.5 mEq per liter) indicates magnesium deficiency. Since less than 1 percent of body magnesium is in the extracellular fluid compartment, hypocalcemia due to magnesium deficiency may exist despite normal serum magnesium levels. A high index of suspicion must be present, therefore, in a patient with a known disorder that results in magnesium depletion in order to make the diagnosis.

Patients with magnesium deficiency must be treated with magnesium salts. It is important to recognize that the hypocalcemia of magnesium deficiency requires treatment with magnesium. Treatment with vitamin D or calcium alone is usually ineffective. Moderate to severe magnesium depletion is usually treated by the administration of parenteral magnesium, especially if there are continuing magnesium losses from the intestine or kidney. An effective treatment regimen is the administration of 2 g of $MgSO_4 \cdot 7H_2O$ (16.2 mEq Mg^{2+}) as a 50 percent solution every 8 hours intramuscularly. Since these injections may be painful, a continuous intravenous infusion of 48 mEq per 24 hours may be better tolerated. This treatment usually results in attainment of a serum magnesium concentration of 1.7 to 2.1 mEq per liter within a few hours of starting the magnesium infusion. Therapy should be continued to maintain the serum magnesium concentration within the normal range for at least 5 days or until the hypocalcemia is corrected. The serum calcium concentration usually normalizes in an average of 3 to 7 days of therapy. Continuing magnesium losses may require longer therapy to replace magnesium stores. If the patient is unable to eat, a maintenance dose of about 8 mEq should be continued daily in the intravenous fluids. If the patient has a reduced glomerular filtration rate (serum creatinine value greater than 1.5 mg per deciliter), the dose of magnesium given should be reduced (one-half) to avoid magnesium intoxication. Serum magnesium concentrations should be determined daily when a patient with azotemia is given magnesium replacement therapy.

Occasionally some patients may require long-term oral magnesium supplementation. Oral magnesium salts in the form of sulfate, lactate, oxide, hydroxide, chloride, or glycerophosphate can be used. An initial dose of about 300 mg of elemental magnesium is usually tolerated well. The dose may be increased to the desired amount until side effects such as diarrhea occur. If the magnesium is given in small doses three to four times a day, the cathartic effect of magnesium can be minimized.

HYPOPARATHYROIDISM

Hypoparathyroidism is usually due to prior neck surgery with removal or destruction of functioning parathyroid tissue, although idiopathic hypoparathyroidism is not uncommonly seen. Unusual causes include infiltrative disorders, postradioiodine therapy, and congenital aplasia. Regardless of the cause of hypoparathyroidism, the management is the same. The basic therapy involves the administration of vitamin D together with an oral calcium intake of 1 to 1.5 g (elemental calcium) per day. The calcium may be obtained through the dietary intake of dairy products or other calcium-rich foods. Calcium-rich foods and their respective calcium content are listed in Table 2. Alternatively, calcium supplements may be used if the patients cannot obtain the desired amount of calcium by dietary means because of caloric restriction or lactose intolerance. Some patients with hypoparathyroidism may have hyperphosphatemia. Since calcium-rich foods are also high in phosphate, calcium salts free of phosphate may be preferred.

TABLE 2 Calcium-Rich Foods

Food	*Amount*	*Elemental Calcium (mg)*
Dairy products		
Milk (whole or skim)	8 oz	298
Cheese	1 cu in	150
Cottage cheese (creamed)	12 oz	320
Ice cream	1 cup	204
Yogurt	1 cup	298
Seafood		
Oysters	1 cup	226
Salmon	3 oz	167
Sardines	3 oz	372
Vegetables		
Broccoli	1 stalk	158
Collards	1 cup	289
Mustard greens	1 cup	193
Spinach	1 cup	200
Turnip greens	1 cup	252
Fruits and nuts		
Dried apricots	1 cup	100
Dates, pitted	1 cup	105
Rhubarb, cooked	1 cup	212
Almonds	½ cup	160
Tofu (soybean curd)	3½ oz	128

TABLE 3 Oral Calcium Preparations

Salt	*Trade Name(s)*	*Calcium Content Per Gram*
Calcium carbonate	Titralac suspension, 1 g per 5 ml Titralac tablets, 420 mg OS-CAL, 650 mg and 1.25 g Tums tablets, 500 mg, 750 mg Biocal tablets, 625 mg, 1.25 g Cal-Sup, 750 mg Caltrate, 1.5 g	400 mg
Calcium glubionate	Neo-Calglucon syrup, 1.8 g per 5 ml	64 mg
Calcium gluconate	500-mg and 1-g tablets	90 mg
Calcium lactate	325-mg and 650-mg tablets	130 mg
Calcium (dibasic calcium phosphate)	500 mg	290 mg

Any calcium salt may be used. Some available calcium preparations are listed in Table 3. It is most important to recognize that the amount of elemental calcium will vary from compound to compound. For example, 40 percent of calcium carbonate is elemental calcium while only 6.4 percent of calcium glubionate is elemental calcium. Knowledge of the amounts of elemental calcium must be known to prescribe the correct amount of the salt to be given. Any compound may be given, but studies suggest that calcium carbonate is not well absorbed in patients with achlorhydria unless given with meals. Side effects are minimal and include constipation (calcium carbonate) and flatulence (calcium gluconate).

The major approach to the chronic treatment of hypoparathyroidism is the administration of vitamin D. Vitamin preparations available for use are listed in Table 4. Vitamin D_2 is the usual drug used. It is by far the least expensive agent. Initial therapy should be by daily administration of 50,000 units of vitamin D_2. This preparation has a prolonged onset of action so that full biologic activity may not be realized until 3 to 4 weeks of therapy. This may be due to the storage of vitamin in the body as well as to impaired metabolism of vitamin D to its active form in hypoparathyroidism. If after 4 weeks of therapy, the serum calcium concentration is not optimal (8 to 8.5 mg per deciliter) the dosage of vitamin D_2 should be increased to 75 to 100,000 units of vitamin D_2 per day and the serum calcium level reassessed again in 4 weeks. Such a stepwise approach to therapy will allow gradual titration of the vitamin D_2 dosage while lowering the risk of vitamin D_2 intoxication. The hydroxylated forms of vitamin D such as dihydrotachysterol, 25-hydroxyvitamin D_3 and 1,25-dihydroxyvitamin D_3 (Rocaltrol), have a shorter half-

TABLE 4 Vitamin D Preparations

	Trade Name	*Dosage in Hypoparathyroidism*	*Onset of Maximal Effect (approx)*
Vitamin D_2	Drisdol Calciferol	50,000–200,000 IU/day	30 days
Dihydrotachysterol	DHT	0.2–1 mg/day	15 days
25-Hydroxyvitamin D_3	Calderol	50 μg/day	15 days
1,25-Dihydroxyvitamin D_3	Rocaltrol	0.25–2 μg/day	2–3 days

life and faster onset of action (and metabolism in case of toxicity) but cost appreciably more. All these agents may be used, starting with the lower dosage given in Table 4, with stepwise increase depending on onset of maximal effect to achieve the desired serum calcium concentration. We have used 1,25-dihydroxyvitamin D_3 more as an adjunctive form of therapy at the onset of the treatment period. Rocaltrol may be given in a dose of 0.5 to 1.0 μg per day in patients who have symptomatic hypocalcemia in order to quickly resolve these disturbing symptoms. Vitamin D_2 may be started at the same time. After 3 to 4 weeks, when the vitamin D_2 level has reached its biologic potential, the Rocaltrol may be discontinued and the vitamin D_2 titrated as described above.

The therapeutic endpoint is to achieve a serum calcium concentration (corrected for the serum albumin concentration) of 8.0 to 8.5 mg per deciliter. Because of the absence of parathyroid hormone, fractional renal excretion of calcium is increased; at any given filtered calcium load, urinary calcium excretion will be greater in patients with hypoparathyroidism than in normal subjects. A "normal" serum calcium concentration of 9.5 mg per deciliter in a hypoparathyroid patient may therefore result in hypercalciuria and renal stone formation. It is recommended that once a stable serum calcium concentration of 8.0 to 8.5 mg per deciliter is achieved, the serum calcium level and 24-hour urinary calcium excretion should be determined every 3 to 4 months.

HYPOCALCEMIA FOLLOWING THYROID AND PARATHYROID SURGERY

Metabolites of vitamin D with faster onset of action may also be useful in the treatment of transient hypocalcemia following neck surgery. Although permanent hypoparathyroidism occurs in less than 5 percent of patients, transient hypocalcemia may develop in 30 percent. The hypocalcemia usually develops within 24 to 72 hours following surgery and resolves within 3 to 5 days. It may, however, persist for several weeks. Possible mechanisms for transient hypocalcemia include ischemia/damage to the parathyroid glands, hypercalcemia-induced atrophy of normal parathyroid glands, magnesium depletion, and the hungry bone syndrome. After appropriate diagnostic tests are done therapy may be instituted. An asymptomatic patient in whom the serum calcium value falls to less than 8 mg per deciliter but greater than 7.0 mg per deciliter may merely be started on 2 to 4 g of elemental calcium orally. If the serum calcium value is less than 7.0 mg per deciliter or the patient displays symptoms of neuromuscular hyperexcitability, Rocaltrol, 0.5 μg orally every 12 hours, may be given in addition to oral calcium. The aim of this therapy is to achieve a serum calcium concentration of approximately 8.0 mg per deciliter. This level will provide near maximal stimulation of parathyroid hormone secretion while relieving the symptoms of hypocalcemia. When the serum calcium value rises to greater than 8.5 mg per deciliter, the dose of Rocaltrol can be decreased or therapy discontinued and the serum calcium level monitored.

CONDITIONS THAT INFLUENCE VITAMIN D THERAPY

Change in Prescription

Vitamin D_2 may lose potency with prolonged shelf time. One of the most common causes of vitamin D intoxication or hypercalcemia in a patient with hypoparathyroidism is a refill of the prescription with a more recently manufactured vitamin D_2 preparation. Treatment of the hypercalcemia and retitration of the medication is then indicated. The serum and urinary calcium values should be checked 4 weeks after each new prescription is written.

Thiazide Diuretic

Thiazide diuretics will decrease urinary calcium excretion. Therefore, the serum calcium concentration may increase in a hypoparathyroid patient given a thiazide diuretic who is on vitamin D therapy. In such cases the dose of vitamin D may be decreased. Thiazide diuretics have been used as adjunctive therapy in hypoparathyroid patients whose disease is difficult to control with vitamin

D and calcium alone. This is not usually necessary, however.

Corticosteroid Therapy

Glucocorticoids antagonize the peripheral action of vitamin D. Administration of these agents to patients in vitamin D therapy results in a fall in the serum calcium concentration.

Estrogen Status

Because of the inhibitory effect of estrogens on bone resorption, the onset of the menopause in a previously stable hypoparathyroid patient may result in hypercalcemia. Correction of estrogen deficiency in a stable postmenopausal patient will produce the opposite response, a fall in serum calcium concentration.

Pregnancy and Lactation

Relief of tetany has been reported to occur during both pregnancy and lactation in hypoparathyroid women. Frank hypercalcemia may occur in patients treated with vitamin D during lactation. The mechanism of the reduced need for vitamin D therapy is not known.

Anticonvulsant Drugs

In patients who require anticonvulsant therapy the dose of vitamin D may have to be increased above the average. This may result from a combination of abnormal metabolism of vitamin D and a state of resistance to the peripheral actions of vitamin D.

Magnesium Deficiency

Occasionally patients with hypoparathyroidism develop resistance to vitamin D therapy. An increase of the dose severalfold may not raise the serum calcium concentration to the desired level. In such cases, hypomagnesemia and/or magnesium deficiency should be considered. Magnesium depletion may result in vitamin D resistance. Since patients treated with vitamin D are often hypercalciuric, and hypercalciuria results in renal magnesium wasting, this may explain magnesium depletion in such cases. I have found that the oral administration of magnesium (300 to 600 mg elemental magnesium per day) may decrease the dose of vitamin D required to control hypoparathyroidism.

TOXICITY OF VITAMIN D THERAPY

The major complications of vitamin D and calcium therapy of hypoparathyroidism are hypercalciuria and hypercalcemia. The patient may present with the usual symptoms of hypercalcemia, including nausea, vomiting, and mental confusion and obtundation. At this time, vitamin D therapy should be discontinued and therapy for the hypercalcemia instituted (rehydration with 0.9 percent saline followed by saline diuresis with furosemide therapy and glucocorticoid therapy). Chronic mild elevation of the serum calcium concentration and hypercalcemia may result in renal stones and/or nephrocalcinosis. These side effects are best prevented by careful titration of the vitamin D dose. The earliest indication of overdosage with vitamin D is hypercalciuria. During the initial phases of therapy with vitamin D_2 we obtain urinary calcium excretion and serum calcium estimates every 2 weeks until the desired serum calcium levels are achieved on two consecutive occasions. If 1,25-dihydroxyvitamin D_3 is used, urinary and serum calcium measurements should be made daily until the desired levels are reached. Subseuqently evaluations at least every 3 to 4 months are done if the patient is stable. The patients are asked to collect 24-hour urine specimens for calcium analysis rather than fasting specimens, since the former is a better reflection of intestinal calcium absorption. Creatinine is also measured to assess the adequacy of the collection. If the urinary calcium excretion is greater than 250 to 300 mg per day or the calcium/creatinine ratio is greater than 0.15 or fractional excretions of 0.15 mg per deciliter glomerular filtrate, the dose of vitamin D should be decreased. Therapy is successful when a serum calcium concentration of 8.0 to 8.5 mg per deciliter is achieved.

SUGGESTED READING

Slatopolsky E. Renal osteodystrophy. In: Wyngaarden JB, Smith LH, eds. Cecil textbook of medicine. 17th ed. Philadelphia: WB Saunders;1985: 1453.

Stewart AF, Broadus AE. Hypocalcemia. In: Broadus AE, ed. Endocrinology and metabolism. 2nd ed. New York: McGraw-Hill,1987: 1422.

PRIMARY HYPERPARATHYROIDISM

JOSEPH N. ATTIE, M.D., F.A.C.S.

Primary hyperparathyroidism (HPT) is a metabolic disorder in which there is hypersecretion of parathyroid hormone (PTH) from one or more adenomatous or hyperplastic parathyroid glands. There is usually an increase in the total mass of parathyroid tissue, representing an increase in both the size and the number of cells. The most consistent abnormal finding is hypercalcemia. The hypersecreting parathyroid glands are less sensitive to the suppressive effects of increased extracellular calcium and are relatively autonomous. Consequently, the findings of elevated or normal serum PTH levels (preferably C-terminal) by radioimmunoassay in the presence of elevated serum calcium levels (preferably ionized calcium) confirm the diagnosis.

In most patients, the cause of primary HPT is unknown. It has been suggested that an increase in the total mass of the parathyroid glands is a prerequisite for the development of the disease. Several reports have shown a relationship to prior irradiation. The radiation dose was generally between 300 and 1,200 rad; the latent period between irradiation and the development of primary HPT can be as long as 38 years. Primary HPT is more common in postmenopausal women; diminished estrogen levels may be responsible.

In a small percentage of cases the disease is hereditary. These patients display multiple endocrine neoplasia (MEN). The disease is autosomal dominant with a high penetrance and expressivity. In MEN type I, HPT accompanies lesions of the pancreatic islets and the pituitary gland. Patients with MEN type I have genetically directed glandular changes (hyperplasia, adenoma, or carcinoma), which result in clinical syndromes such as virulent peptic ulcer disease (Zollinger-Ellison syndrome) owing to hypergastrinemia produced by non-beta cells of the pancreatic islets and hyperinsulinemia derived from the beta islet cells. Most pituitary tumors found in MEN type I are chromophobe adenomas with no hormonal production or with prolactin secretion. Occasional cases of acromegaly have been reported.

Parathyroid lesions are found in 85 to 90 percent of patients with MEN type I. The most frequent finding is chief cell hyperplasia. Although surgical exploration may reveal single gland enlargement, it is generally agreed that subtotal parathyroidectomy (resection of three and one-half glands) is the proper treatment. Removal of less parathyroid tissue usually results in only temporary improvement; subsequent operations are required to alleviate recurrent hypercalcemia.

Multiple endocrine neoplasia type II is a genetically directed autosomal dominant disorder with variable expressivity characterized by medullary carcinoma of the thyroid, pheochromocytoma, and hyperparathyroidism. A rare subgroup, MEN type IIb, characterized by medullary carcinoma, pheochromocytoma, and multiple mucosal neuromas, is not associated with parathyroid disease.

The frequency and nature of the parathyroid pathology in MEN type II are variable. All patients with MEN type II have medullary carcinoma; about 50 percent have hyperparathyroidism and 50 percent have pheochromocytoma. In about 75 percent of those with hypercalcemia, there is more than one enlarged parathyroid gland. Some investigators have attempted to incriminate the amine precursor uptake decarboxylase (APUD) system as the etiologic factor in all cases of multiendocrine involvement. The fact that the parathyroids take origin from pharyngeal pouch endoderm and not from the neural crest would seem to contradict this view.

Occasionally, HPT with hypercalcemia can occur in the setting of advanced renal failure. Secondary HPT with normal or low serum calcium levels is often observed even in mild forms of renal disease. The increase in PTH secretion is part of the early response to nephron loss. In these cases there is four-gland hyperplasia. Rarely, one or more of the hyperplastic glands in secondary HPT may become autonomous and indistinguishable from a parathyroid adenoma. The HPT persists even after the renal failure is corrected (this is sometimes called tertiary HPT).

Until 20 years ago, primary HPT was considered to be a rare disease usually diagnosed in patients who presented with renal or osseous manifestations. Because of the widespread use of multichannel autoanalyzers, the diagnosis of primary HPT has become much more common. Routine screening of adults admitted to hospitals for unrelated conditions reveals an incidence of hypercalcemia of 1 in 2,000; approximately half of these prove to have primary HPT, or 1 in 4,000 subjects. Few cases have been reported in children and adolescents. In operated cases the sex ratio is 3:1, favoring females, with a peak incidence in the 51 to 60 age group.

PARAMETERS FOR MONITORING TREATMENT

Laboratory Findings

Hypercalcemia is the classic finding in nearly all cases of primary HPT. It may be intermittent in early or mild cases. The significant serum calcium measurement is the concentration of "ionized" serum calcium. Since most nonionized calcium is bound to albumin, abnormally high serum albumin binds more of the total calcium. Roughly, if serum albumin is 1 g per deciliter above the normal mean, 1 mg per deciliter should be subtracted from the figure for total calcium, with 2 mg per deciliter for 2 g per deciliter, and so on. When the serum albumin level is below the normal mean, one adds instead of subtracts.

Because of the variations among laboratories, the normal range for each laboratory used in evaluating patients should be known. Repeated readings of total serum calcium values (corrected if necessary for serum albumin) three standard deviations above the normal mean are an indication for more extensive diagnostic procedures to confirm HPT. For example, with a normal mean of 9.5 mg per deciliter and one standard deviation of 0.5, the upper limit would be 11.0.

Radioimmunoassay for PTH is of great help in the diagnosis of primary HPT. In normal subjects and in patients with hypercalcemia due to causes other than HPT, elevation of serum calcium levels above 10.5 mg per deciliter effectively shuts off PTH secretion. Consequently, the combination of hypercalcemia and elevated or normal serum PTH is diagnostic of primary HPT. PTH assays are even more variable and difficult to interpret than serum calcium levels. PTH is stored in the parathyroids generally as a peptide 84 amino acids long. The active portion contains the first 27 amino acids from the amino end, but serum contains either the intact hormone, the amino fragment, the inactive carboxyl fragment, or midregion fragments, which include neither terminal group. Most reliable laboratories supply correlations with clinically proved parathyroid disease. Carboxyl-terminal PTH assays (C-PTH) are most often used. It must be remembered that measurements of PTH can be distorted by renal insufficiency; the failure to excrete PTH fragments may lead to abnormally high serum PTH levels.

Rarely, one encounters normocalcemic hyperparathyroidism. I have operated on two such patients, who presented with recurrent renal calculi, hypercalciuria, and high serum PTH levels with normal serum calcium values. Both patients had single parathyroid adenomas, which were resected.

Although radioimmune PTH assay has proved useful in the preoperative evaluation of patients with primary HPT, postoperatively the PTH levels may remain elevated for prolonged periods of time, even though the calcium returns to normal and the patient remains clinically "cured."

The 24-hour urinary calcium excretion concentration is usually elevated in primary HPT. Low levels of calcium excretion may signify the presence of familial hypocalciuric hypercalcemia, in which one finds hypercalcemia in the presence of elevated or normal serum PTH levels and low urinary calcium levels. This may seem to be an indication for surgical exploration. The parathyroid glands are normal in appearance. Resection of one or more parathyroid glands does not influence the hypercalcemia. Treatment in this disease is rarely necessary, since the low urinary calcium excretion poses no threat of renal calculus formation.

Hyperchloremia (serum chloride level above 107 mEq per liter) in the presence of hypercalcemia is suggestive of primary HPT; the chloride-to-phosphate ratio above 33 is strongly indicative of the diagnosis.

Preoperative Localization of Abnormal Parathyroid Glands

Because 5 to 10 percent of parathyroid adenomas may be in abnormal positions in the neck or superior mediastinum, many techniques have been developed to attempt to localize the adenomas preoperatively or intraoperatively. Esophagograms may demonstrate large superior parathyroid adenomas located in the posterior mediastinum. Computed tomographic scanning has not been very useful in preoperative localization except in large or mediastinal adenomas.

In May 1987, I began to attempt to localize parathyroid adenomas preoperatively by one or more of three modalities: magnetic resonance imaging (MRI), technetium-thallium subtraction, and ultrasonography. In the first 64 patients subjected to preoperative localization, all three modalities were over 80 percent accurate; MRI proved to have the highest sensitivity and specificity. Up to December 1989, 155 patients were studied preoperatively by one or more of the three localization modalities. Ninety-six patients had all three studies performed. In 40 cases the parathyroid adenomas were accurately localized by all three modalities; in 36 cases, two of the three modalities were diagnostic; in 13 cases, one of the three tests were diagnostic; and in seven patients, all three tests were negative. Forty-nine patients had two of the three preoperative tests performed. In 25 cases both tests were positive; in 18 cases one of the two tests correctly localized the adenoma; and in six patients both tests were negative. Ten patients had only one preoperative test performed. Four had only MRI and all were positive; three had only technetium-thallium subtraction and all three were positive; three had only ultrasonography and one was positive and two were negative. In all 155 patients the abnormal parathyroid glands were found and removed, followed by a return of the serum calcium levels to normal.

Although the noninvasive localization techniques are not always diagnostic, they reduce operating time and demonstrate adenomas in ectopic locations, and in patients who have been explored surgically without success, they have greatly improved the success rate of reoperations.

The most accurate method of localization is the combination of venous sampling and arteriography. The high cost and rare accessibility of these procedures make their use valuable only in cases requiring reexploration after a failed initial operation when noninvasive localization techniques have been unsuccessful.

Some have advocated the intravenous use of phenothiazine dyes (e.g., toluidine blue) for intraoperative staining of parathyroid tissue. These dyes carry some risk and have therefore not been widely used.

TREATMENT

There is currently no medical treatment that can cure primary HPT. Surgery is the therapy of choice in most cases, since it offers the only opportunity for long-term cure. Once the diagnosis of primary HPT is made, prompt surgical exploration is generally indicated. The most constant findings confirming the diagnosis are hypercalcemia and elevated or normal serum PTH levels by radioimmunoassay. There is no controversy concerning surgery in patients who have signs or symptoms or in those with high levels of serum calcium. Many endocrinologists, however, choose to postpone or avoid surgery in patients who have mild or moderate hypercalcemia and are asymptomatic. I believe that all patients with hypercalcemia higher than 11 mg per deciliter or who have signs or symptoms, regardless of the degree of hypercalcemia, should be offered surgical therapy. It has been observed that long-term hypercalcemia is associated with increased morbidity, usually with worsening renal function.

Patients can develop renal colic or hypercalcemic coma while being observed and treated medically. At present there is no method available by which one can predict which patient with mild asymptomatic hypercalcemia will develop symptoms or suffer irreparable renal or osseous damage.

Medical Treatment

There are four situations in which temporary medical management may be undertaken. Some patients refuse surgery. Other patients may have serious medical conditions that make the risk of operative intervention too great. There is a small group of patients who have had several surgical procedures in an attempt to cure their HPT but who still have persistent or recurrent hypercalcemia. The fourth group are those who are usually normocalcemic except during periods when there is increased bone resorption (prolonged immobilization) or when calcium excretion is reduced (diuretic therapy).

There are several measures that may be instituted in patients with primary HPT in whom surgery is being postponed or not contemplated. Adequate hydration must be maintained. Diuretics should be used with great caution, since dehydration may raise the serum calcium level. Thiazides are to be avoided because they may increase the serum calcium level by reducing urinary calcium excretion. Nonthiazide diuretics, such as furosemide, increase urinary calcium excretion and thereby worsen the state of negative calcium balance. Dietary calcium in the form of dairy products is usually restricted or avoided. However, calcium restriction should only be advised if it results in reduction in serum or urinary calcium levels with no further increase in PTH levels.

Oral phosphate administration has long been used to lower elevated calcium values in HPT. The calcium-lowering effects of phosphates result from two modes of action. By increasing the calcium-phosphate product, there is increased deposition into bone with a reduction in serum calcium. More important, there is evidence to indicate that phosphate inhibits the production of 1,25-dihydroxyvitamin D, thereby decreasing absorption of calcium through the gastrointestinal tract. Thus, oral phosphates may be especially indicated in patients with a history of renal calculi.

Calcitonin has been tried in various hypercalcemic situations with only slight success. Its expense, the need for parenteral administration, and its transitory effects limit its usefulness. Preliminary experiments with dichlormethylene diphosphonate (Cl_2MDP) resulted in reduction of serum and urinary calcium levels and hydroxyproline excretion. The long-term effects are less encouraging. Other agents such as cimetidine have been tried with inconsistent results.

Occasionally hypercalcemia becomes acutely severe (hypercalcemic crisis), leading to coma, progressive uremia, and impending death. Aggressive treatment is imperative. If feasible, emergency surgery with removal of the causative parathyroid adenoma usually reverses the condition rapidly. Some prefer to improve the clinical state by lowering the serum calcium level prior to surgical intervention by means of intravenous fluids, furosemide, or judiciously administered plicamycin (formerly mithramycin). Plicamycin is effective in decreasing bone resorption. It is best administered intravenously (25 mg per kilogram in 100 ml of saline over a 1-hour period). It is contraindicated in the presence of thrombocytopenia or impaired hepatic or renal function. Furosemide is given in dosages ranging from 20 to 40 mg every 2 hours to a well-hydrated patient (to maintain a urine flow rate greater than 5 liters a day) until the desired calcium level is reached. Phosphates should not be given intravenously in the treatment of hypercalcemia.

Surgical Treatment

Surgery is the definitive treatment for primary HPT. The goal of therapy is to restore normal parathyroid function and avoid persistent hypercalcemia or permanent hypocalcemia. Once the diagnosis of primary HPT is made, the next most important decision is the choice of the surgeon. The patient's interest is best served by a surgeon with extensive experience in thyroid and parathyroid surgery. Thorough familiarity with the appearance and location (both usual and ectopic) of normal parathyroid glands is necessary for the removal of an appropriate amount of hyperfunctioning tissue without injuring residual normal glands.

The decision as to whether a parathyroid gland is abnormal or whether it is an adenoma or a hyperplastic gland must be made by the surgeon. There are no absolute histologic criteria that can be used by the pathologist to distinguish adenoma from hyperplasia or hyperplasia from normal parathyroid tissue. The routine use of minute biopsies of normal-looking parathyroids is not generally advocated; they are unreliable, except to identify parathyroid tissue.

At cervical exploration all four parathyroid glands should be sought and identified. If one large abnormal-looking gland and three normal-appearing glands are found, the enlarged parathyroid gland is resected and the other three are not disturbed, not even for biopsy. The excised gland is submitted for frozen section to confirm it as a parathyroid, and the procedure is terminated. Biopsy of normal-looking parathyroids in this situation is to be avoided because (1) there are no absolute histologic criteria to distinguish normal from hyperplastic parathyroids based on minute biopsy fragments; in the past the diagnosis of such glands as hyperplastic resulted in frequent performance of subtotal (three and one-half glands) parathyroidectomy with increased risk of permanent hypoparathyroidism; (2) routine normal gland biopsy may traumatize or devascularize the glands; and (3) no difference in results has been demonstrated after adenoma excision plus biopsy versus adenoma excision alone.

Some surgeons have advocated exploring one side of the neck and exposing two parathyroids; if one enlarged and one normal-appearing parathyroid are found, the large one is removed, the second one is subjected to biopsy, and the other side is not explored. I strongly oppose this approach. In my experience, a significant percentage of patients (5 percent) have two adenomas without having diffuse parathyroid hyperplasia, and in most patients with multiple adenomas the abnormal glands are bilateral in position. In one of my patients, resection of a large gland from one side of the neck resulted in only a partial decrease in the hypercalcemia; subsequent resection of a second enlarged parathyroid from the opposite side restored the serum calcium level to normal.

If three normal-looking parathyroids are identified and the missing parathyroid is one of the inferior glands, the thymus on that side is resected through the cervical wound. I have seen several intrathymic parathyroid adenomas. If four normal-appearing glands are found or if three normals are identified and the fourth is not intrathymic, tiny (2-mm fragments) biopsies are performed to confirm parathyroid tissue. The normal glands are then labeled with metal clips in order to aid subsequent reexplorations. Usually, the missing parathyroid (or in rare instances, an adenoma in a fifth parathyroid gland) is in the superior mediastinum. Prior to reexploration, localization studies should be performed. Selective venous sampling and PTH assay indicate the side of the lesion; thyroid arteriography demonstrates its precise location, thus facilitating the secondary operative procedure.

If all four glands are enlarged, a diagnosis of primary parathyroid hyperplasia is made and subtotal parathyroidectomy is performed, leaving behind about 50 mg of the smallest of the four glands. Some surgeons have advised total resection of all four parathyroids with autotransplantation of a small fragment into the forearm. There is risk of early or late failure of the graft as well as overgrowth of the transplanted tissue. Autotransplantation and/or cryopreservation of the tissue for possible subsequent transplantation is most useful in patients who have previously had three parathyroids removed.

At the first parathyroid operation, only the neck should be explored, with median sternotomy reserved for reexploration after localization studies have located the mediastinal adenoma. Most investigators agree that patients with MEN type I should undergo subtotal (three and one-half glands) parathyroidectomy even when single gland enlargement is found. Whether patients with familial hyperparathyroidism having one large parathyroid gland and three normal glands should have routine subtotal parathyroidectomy is debatable.

Cervical exploration is performed through a short, low, collar incision. The strap muscles are retracted and not divided. The entire anterior compartment of the neck is explored from larynx to sternum and from one carotid sheath to the other. The four parathyroids are sought. The superior parathyroid is found behind, or medial to, the upper portion of the thyroid lobe, in a plane behind the recurrent laryngeal nerve. When enlarged, the inferior parathyroid is more variable in position and may be found anterior, lateral, or posterior to the lower thyroid pole, always in front of the nerve, and often in association with the thymus gland either in the neck or in the anterior mediastinum. Whereas the normal parathyroids are pale tan, soft, and flattened, surrounded by varying amounts of fat, adenomas (or hyperplastic glands) are rounded or oval and are frequently dark brown or reddish.

Most parathyroid adenomas are larger, firmer, and more rounded than normal glands and weigh from 70 mg to several grams. In rare instances, "minute" adenomas (5 to 7 mm) are found and their removal results in normocalcemia.

Parathyroid adenomss may be found in the mediastinum, on the carotid sheath, along the larynx, or, rarely, intrathyroid. If three normal glands are found, some surgeons advise resection of the thyroid lobe on the side of the missing gland. Ligation and division of thyroid vessels should be avoided in patients with no apparent adenomas so that postoperative venous and arterial localization studies can be carried out.

AUTHOR'S EXPERIENCE

Between 1953 and December 1989, I operated successfully on 890 patients with HPT. In all these cases abnormal parathyroid tissue was removed, followed by return of serum calcium levels to normal. The clinical presentations of these patients are shown in Table 1. In recent years, the majority of patients have presented with asymptomatic hypercalcemia (Fig. 1). There were 612 females ranging in age from 16 to 83 years (mean age 54.3) and 278 males ranging in age from 18 to 88 years (mean age 50.9). The age-sex incidence is shown in Figure 2.

The pathologic findings in the 890 patients successfully operated on are seen in Table 2. In 786 cases, one enlarged gland (so-called adenoma) and three normal-looking glands were found; the single large gland was removed with resulting normocalcemia.

Two adenomas (i.e., two large and two normal-looking glands) were found in 35 patients and three adenomas (three large and one normal gland) were found in four patients. These 39 patients became and remained normocalcemic postoperatively after resection of the enlarged glands. Nineteen patients (2 percent) had primary hyperplasia, with all four glands enlarged; three and one-half glands were resected, and all the patients became normocalcemic. In one of the patients with two adenomas, one tumor was resected, resulting in only a slight drop in the serum calcium level. By the use of differential venous sampling for PTH radioimmunoassay and thyroid arteriography, a second adenoma was localized and resected, resulting in normocalcemia.

Four of the patients had a single adenoma resected with subsequent normocalcemia for 4 to 19 years. All became hypercalcemic again and on surgical reexploration were found to have a second adenoma. In each instance, the second tumor was removed followed by a return to normocalcemia. One of the patients required resection of a third adenoma because of recurrent hypercalcemia. In three additional patients, single adenomas had been removed elsewhere 7, 9, and 10 years previously, and following a period of normocalcemia, they again became hypercalcemic. I operated again on each of these patients and resected a second metachronous parathy-

TABLE 1 Primary Reasons for Initial Evaluation of Patients with Hyperparathyroidism (890 Operated Cases, 1953–1989)

Reason for Evaluation	*Number of Patients*
Asymptomatic hypercalcemia (intravenous pyelography revealed calculi in 4 patients)	564
Renal calculi	188
Secondary hyperparathyroidism	28
Incidental during thyroid operations	24
Gastrointestinal manifestations (ulcer, pancreatitis)	16
Minimal symptoms (e.g., fatigue, polyuria)	16
Skeletal manifestations	15
Coma	11
Tertiary hyperparathyroidism	8
Neurologic manifestations	5
Psychosis	5
Palpable mass only	5
Multiple endocrine neoplasia type I	4
Multiple endocrine neoplasia type II	1

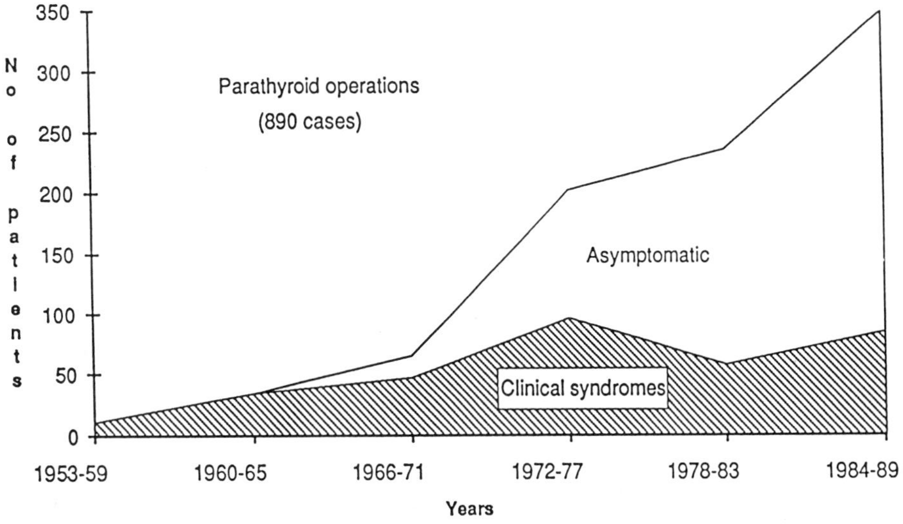

Figure 1 Changing proportion of asymptomatic patients versus patients with clinical manifestations of HPT at 5-year intervals.

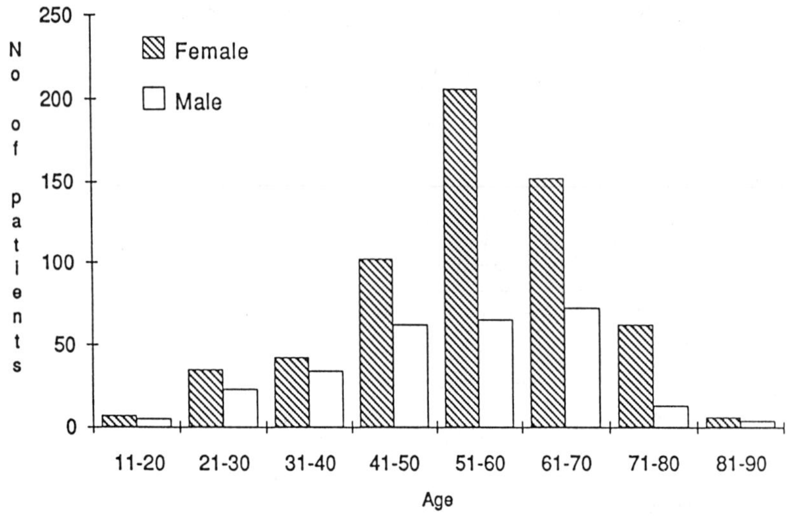

Figure 2 Age-sex incidence of 890 surgically treated patients with HPT.

roid adenoma; following the surgery the patients again became normocalcemic.

Thirty-six patients were operated on for secondary and tertiary hyperparathyroidism caused by renal failure. In 28 of these patients, there were varying degrees of bone resorption associated with hyperphosphatemia, hypocalcemia, and elevated PTH levels. Exploration revealed all four parathyroid glands to be enlarged. Subtotal parathyroidectomy (resection of three and one-half glands) was performed, and the patients improved. In two of these, severe symptoms of bone pain and elevated PTH levels recurred; the remaining half gland was resected and a portion of it was transplanted into the forearm. Eight of the 36 patients had hyperphosphatemia and hypercalcemia; a diagnosis of tertiary HPT was made. At operation three glands were diffusely enlarged, and the fourth was much larger and nodular, suggesting adenomatous change. Again subtotal parathyroidectomy effected a "cure," with return to a low serum calcium value.

Nine patients were found to have parathyroid carcinoma. One of these was operated on for recurrent parathyroid carcinoma; the neoplasm later recurred again and metastasized. One of the other carcinomas recurred during the follow-up period.

Four patients operated on had MEN type I. In one patient, only one large gland was found, and it was removed in each of two consecutive operations. Each time, the serum calcium level fell to normal, only to rise again to abnormal levels. A third operation completed the subtotal parathyroidectomy (resection of three and one-half glands). In a second patient, three large glands were removed elsewhere without causing the serum calcium level to drop. I operated on the patient again and removed the large hyperplastic fourth gland from the anterior mediastinum; this is the only patient in the series who developed permanent hypoparathyroidism. One patient, from whom two large glands were removed, died following total gastrectomy for Zollinger-Ellison syndrome; at autopsy, two more large parathyroids were found. In the fourth patient, three and one-half glands were resected with cure. One patient operated on had MEN type II. During thyroidectomy for medullary carcinoma, a large parathyroid adenoma was incidentally found and removed. The patient's mother also had medullary carcinoma and a parathyroid adenoma.

TABLE 2 Operative Findings in Hyperparathyroidism (890 Operated Cases, 1953–1989)

Single adenoma	786
Two adenomas	35
Three adenomas	4
Primary hyperplasia	19
Secondary hyperplasia	28
Tertiary hyperplasia	8
Carcinoma	9

In 16 patients, initial exploration failed to reveal abnormal parathyroid tissue. In two of these, four normal parathyroid glands were found; subsequent studies revealed lung cancer in one patient and liver cancer in the other. In three patients I found only three normal glands and no adenoma; following localization studies (computed tomography and sonography), I surgically reexplored these patients and successfully removed an adenoma in each instance. In two other patients, my initial operation failed to reveal an enlarged parathyroid; both patients went elsewhere, and after venous and arterial invasive localization procedures they underwent successful operations. In another patient, the adenoma was localized by arteriography, the tumor was destroyed by injection of excessive dye, and normocalcemia resulted. In the remaining eight patients three normal glands were found at operation and the patients remained hypercalcemic; two are awaiting reexploration, whereas the other six patients have refused reoperation.

In a significant number of patients, primary hyperparathyroidism was associated with benign or nonmedullary malignant lesions of the thyroid gland. Of the 890 operated patients, 170 had coincidental benign lesions and 20 had papillary or follicular carcinomas of the thyroid gland. Twenty-four patients underwent exploration for thyroid disease and were found to have incidental parathyroid adenomas.

SUGGESTED READING

Attie JN, Khafif RA. Surgical explorations in asymptomatic hypercalcemia. Am J Surg 1976; 132:449–452.

Attie JN, Khan A, Rumancik WM, et al. Preoperative localization of parathyroid adenomas. Am J Surg 1988; 156:323–326.

Attie JN, Wise L, Mir R, Ackerman LV. The rationale against routine subtotal parathyroidectomy for primary hyperparathyroidism. Am J Surg 1978; 136:437–444.

Clark OH. Endocrine surgery of the thyroid and parathyroid glands. St. Louis: CV Mosby, 1985.

Clark OH, Way LW, Hunt TK. Recurrent hyperparathyroidism. Ann Surg 1976; 184:391–402.

Goldman L, Gordon GS, Roof BS. The parathyroids: Progress, problems and practice. Curr Probl Surg 1971; August: 1–64.

Irvin GL, Newell DJ, Morgan SD. Parathyroid metabolism after operative treatment of hypercalcemic (primary) hyperparathyroidism. Surgery 1987; 102:898–902.

Purnell DC, Smith LH, Scholz. Primary hyperparathyroidism: A prospective clinical study. Am J Med 1971; 50:670–678.

Roses DF, Karp N, Sudarsky LA, et al. Primary hyperparathyroidism associated with two enlarged parathyroid glands. Arch Surg 1989; 124:1261–1265.

PAGET'S DISEASE OF BONE

ROBERT E. CANFIELD, M.D.
ETHEL S. SIRIS, M.D.

Paget's disease of bone is a localized disorder of skeletal remodeling that appears to be initiated by an increase in osteoclast-mediated bone resorption. It has been reported to occur in up to 3 percent of older persons in the United States. This disease is more common in patients of European ancestry, and many investigators have noted a familial association. Although the exact etiologic agent is unknown, the primary lesion appears to reside in pagetic osteoclasts that may have been transformed as a consequence of a viral infection earlier in life. This change in osteoclast activity leads to a marked increase in the resorption of bone, which is reflected by a rise in total urinary hydroxyproline excretion (UOHP) as an index of disease activity. There is a compensatory increase in the rate of new bone formation, and this is reflected by a rise in serum alkaline phosphatase (SAP) levels. There is a good correlation between these two indices in this disorder. The alteration in the skeletal remodeling rate eventually leads to architectural changes characterized by the development of nonlamellar, or "woven," bone that is frequently increased in size, more vascular, and less compact than normal bone.

Skeletal sites commonly affected by Paget's disease include the lumbar and thoracic spine, pelvis, skull, femur, and tibia; less commonly the humerus, clavicle, and scapula may also be involved. Frequently, only one or two sites are affected. Thus, depending on the location, extent, and metabolic activity in an individual patients, pagetic involvement of bone may typically cause no symptoms at all or may lead to deformity (e.g., skull enlargement or bowing of an extremity), cause a troublesome sensation of heat or frank pain, increase the susceptibility to traumatic or pathologic fracture, produce symptomatic joint dysfunction (especially at the hip or knee), or result in compression or impairment of adjacent neural structures (e.g., cranial and spinal nerve or cord compression syndromes). There is a very low incidence (less than 1 percent) of malignant degeneration in pagetic bone with the development of an osteogenic sarcoma.

PURPOSE AND GOALS OF TREATMENT

All of the accepted drug therapies for Paget's disease appear to act by decreasing the bone-resorbing activity of pagetic osteoclasts with subsequent restoration of more normal bone histology, and many patients who have specific symptoms resulting from their Paget's disease feel better with treatment. However, given the variability in presentation and symptomatic expression, it is essential that the goals of therapy be individualized for each patient. For example, pharmacologic treatment will not reverse the bowing deformity in a femur or tibia, but there is good evidence that it can prevent the progression and even reverse some of the neurologic symptoms that occur with apparent spinal cord compression.

The goals of treatment are to provide relief of current symptoms and to prevent the emergence of new problems or complications. Studies in many centers, including our own, have established that treatment has the potential to relieve certain symptoms, but there are no well-controlled, long-term studies to show that therapy will prevent the progression of the disease. Therefore, one is left to infer that the evidence for restoration of bone morphology toward normal, the improvement in the biochemical indices of the disease, and specific examples of reversal of neurologic compression syndromes offer promise that treatment for more than immediate symptomatic relief may be worthwhile. Thus, while we incorporate the goal of prevention in our rationale for instituting treatment of patients with Paget's disease, we recognize that there are a paucity of data providing guidelines for this indication.

The studies concerning the efficacy of treatment of Paget's disease of bone, which were conducted in a controlled double-blind design, not only provided support for symptomatic improvement but also revealed a high rate of placebo response. In exploring the basis for the subjective benefit in patients taking placebo, we gained the impression that patients with Paget's disease frequently have relatively little comprehension of the nature of their disorder. Thus, when they encounter a treatment program that not only provides a discussion of the character of the disease but also offers a specific treatment, they commonly achieve a marked relief of underlying anxiety that contributes to overall benefit. Therefore patient education and reassurance are important elements of treatment.

INDICATIONS FOR THERAPY

As noted earlier, the presence of symptoms referable to Paget's disease constitutes the primary indication for therapy. Ours is largely a referral practice made up of symptomatic patients; often in routine practice the disease is discovered incidentally and requires only observation.

In evaluating symptoms it is important to assess the likelihood that reduction in the activity of Paget's disease will provide relief. Bone pain, excessive warmth, arthritic symptoms, and neurologic compression syndromes have all been found to improve with therapy in many patients. Several studies have documented reduction in cardiac output as a consequence of treatment of Paget's disease, but a circumstance when this makes a difference in the treatment of a patient with congestive heart failure or angina is only encountered occasionally. Hearing loss is a relatively common symptom in patients with skull involvement, resulting from eighth nerve compression, otosclerosis, cochlear injury, or any combination of these. This problem is not reversible with treatment; only limited data are available concerning the effects of therapy on slowing the progression of loss. A final point regarding the evaluation of symptoms involves the situation in which new pain develops in a previously quiescent site or there is a recent increase in pain in a symptomatic area. Although this type of complaint most typically reflects changes in underlying pagetic involvement, it must be thoroughly evaluated, since these characteristics may herald an impending fracture or the development of an osteogenic sarcoma.

A second indication for treatment is to attempt to slow the pagetic process when it is active in an area of the skeleton where it may progress to produce symptoms in the future. This category includes patients with elevated biochemical indices more than two to three times normal who have involvement of a major weight-bearing bone, such as the femur or tibia, where there is a potential for bowing; those with disease of the vertebral column where there is a risk of spinal nerve or cord compression; those with extensive skull involvement where there is the possibility of basilar invagination; and those with involvement in the immediate vicinity of major joints—especially the knees or hips. In each of these categories there are no controlled studies to establish that therapy lessens the likelihood of these potential problems. However, the evidence for reversal of symptoms with treatment, coupled with the improvement that therapy produces in the histologic appearance of pagetic lesions and the decline of biochemical indices, leads us to recommend treatment for those patients in whom progression could potentially produce troublesome symptoms.

SPECIFIC PHARMACOLOGIC AGENTS AVAILABLE FOR THE TREATMENT OF PAGET'S DISEASE

Three classes of medications that inhibit osteoclast action in Paget's disease are in use. Each is capable of producing symptomatic improvement in many patients, and the use of each is associated with decreases in the UOHP and SAP and with restoration toward normal of bone architecture on biopsy specimens. Because of the high rates of bone turnover and perfusion in this disease, each of these therapies exhibits greater action at the sites of pagetic involvement than on other uninvolved areas of the skeleton.

Calcitonin

Calcitonin is a 32 amino acid polypeptide hormone that is secreted by the parafollicular cells of the thyroid gland in humans and other mammals and by the ultimobranchial body in birds and fish. Its action in decreasing bone resorption is thought to be mediated by recognition at specific receptors that are present in both normal and pagetic osteoclasts.

Early studies of this hormone in therapy for Paget's disease used porcine calcitonin, a preparation with a relatively high incidence of the development of neutralizing antibodies and one no longer used. The commercially available calcitonin that has been most widely used in this country is the synthetic form of the salmon hormone (Calcimar). After prolonged periods of treatment with salmon calcitonin, the SAP level may begin to rise toward pretreatment levels. This may reflect formation of neutralizing antibodies, in which case substitution of the human preparation will restore the effect. However, not all patients who demonstrate this "escape" phenomenon from calcitonin therapy have antibody formation, and it has been postulated that, with prolonged treatment, there is a loss of calcitonin receptors on the target cells and as a result a decrease in responsiveness to this agent.

A synthetic preparation of human calcitonin (Cibacalcin) has become commercially available in the United States over the past few years. This preparation has been widely used in Europe and in clinical trials in this country. It has the advantage over the salmon preparation that neutralizing antibodies should not occur over time, and a loss of efficacy of the agent on this basis would not be anticipated.

Both salmon and human calcitonin are expensive because their manufacture requires the synthesis of the entire polypeptide hormone. These agents require parenteral administration (by subcutaneous injection); a nasal spray formulation is still investigational. Side effects, consisting of nausea and occasionally diarrhea or unpleasant cutaneous flushing, may occur in a significant minority of patients following the injection of either of these medications.

Bisphosphonates

The bisphosphonates (also called diphosphonates) are structural analogues of pyrophosphate. They exhibit a strong affinity for sites of increased bone turnover, a property that has been used in bone scanning. When given in higher doses, they are bound at areas of high bone turnover, where they are apparently ingested by osteoclasts resorbing bone and then become toxic to these cells. These compounds impair osteoclast action and decrease the excessive rate of bone resorption in pagetic bone, but, to a variable extent, different diphosphonates also interfere with the mineralization of new bone, a fact that limits the dose and the duration of a given course of therapy. They are given orally, but only a small fraction (less than 10 percent) is absorbed from the gastrointestinal tract. Variability in absorption may account for some differences in patient response.

The bisphosphonate currently available for the treatment of Paget's disease is the sodium salt of ethane-1-hydroxy-1, 1-diphosphonic acid (commonly referred to as EHDP and sold as Didronel). In a dosage of 5 mg per kilogram per day (400 mg per day in an average patient) given for a 6-month period, EHDP produces a decrease in both symptoms and biochemical indices and an improvement in bone histology comparable to that noted with a similar time of treatment with salmon calcitonin, 100 IU per day, or human calcitonin, 0.5 mg per day. An intravenous formulation of EHDP has recently become available for use in hypercalcemia of malignancy, but this preparation has had limited use to date in Paget's disease.

Although EHDP has the advantage of oral administration and lower total cost to the patient, it has not been universally accepted as the therapy of choice in all patients with Paget's disease. Early clinical research studies with EHDP employed high dosages (20 mg per kilogram per day) for long periods of time (6 months or more), and some of the patients reported new pain in pagetic sites. In addition, although a tendency to develop pathologic fractures is part of the natural history of this disease, there appeared to be an increased incidence of this complication in these early studies in which patient therapy was prolonged. These side effects probably reflected an excessive suppression of bone remodeling that was dose related. As a consequence, we have been careful to limit our routine use of EHDP to low dosages (5 mg per kilogram per day) and to give the initial course of treatment for no more than 6 months. At these low dosages we have not encountered any serious side effects. It should be noted that higher doses of EHDP can cause diarrhea, but this is quite unusual at low doses. EHDP also decreases phosphate excretion in the urine; at low doses it usually leads to a rise in the serum phosphorus level of approximately 1 mg per deciliter. An increase of more than 2 mg per deciliter may be an indication that the patient is hyperabsorbing the drug from the gastrointestinal tract, and the dosage may have to be reduced.

Plicamycin

Plicamycin (previously termed mithramycin) is a compound that binds to DNA and inhibits RNA synthesis. Its potent cytotoxic effects on osteoclasts were first appreciated when it was noted that patients receiving this agent as chemotherapy for testicular neoplasms developed hypocalcemia. It is employed most often today in the treatment of hypercalcemia associated with a variety of cancers; presumably its main action in this setting is an inhibition of osteoclast-mediated bone destruction.

Plicamycin has significant toxic properties, and it must be administered intravenously, preferably over a 4- to 8-hour period. Its use is associated with nausea and transient elevations in the levels of liver enzymes and serum glutamic oxaloacetic and pyruvic transaminases in most patients. Less commonly, patients develop some degree of reversible nephrotoxicity, and at higher doses decreases in platelet counts can occur. For these reasons the calcitonins and bisphosphonates have become vastly preferred to plicamycin as therapeutic agents for Paget's disease. Nevertheless, despite the side effects, plicamycin may be a useful therapy for Paget's disease in certain specific situations because it is extremely potent and rapidly effective. For example, patients with rapidly progressive neurologic compression syndromes may experience quicker improvement in signs and symptoms following plicamycin therapy.

APPROACH TO THE INDIVIDUAL PATIENT

Establishing a Treatment Plan

The initial patient visit is usually devoted to the history and physical examination and to a careful assessment of the relationship of the patient's symptoms to the location and nature of pagetic lesions. A significant portion of that visit is used to assess the patient's comprehension of the disorder and to explain the nature of the disease. In this context the patient is introduced to our criteria for recommending therapy, the goals of treatment, and the drugs available. Since Paget's disease is a relatively benign disorder, it is important, when appropriate, to ease patient anxiety about the disease.

As part of the initial evaluation, a bone scan is performed to determine the distribution of the disease and roentgenograms of the affected sites are taken to characterize the lesions (e.g., lytic, sclerotic, cortical stress fractures, joint involvement). A multiphasic screening blood test that includes serum calcium and phosphorus measurements and indices of renal function is obtained. Duplicate baseline SAP values are determined, and it is important to be certain that the serum was adequately diluted for assay if the reported values are at the upper limits of measurement of the autoanalyzer. Since our practice has a research orientation, we also obtain duplicate UOHP values because this analysis provides a good reflection of bone resorption. Measurement of UOHP is not necessary in routine practice, but if available, it is recommended.

The second visit is scheduled at a time when all these data are available, and a decision is made concerning whether therapy is to be recommended. At that time the goals of treatment are reemphasized, especially with regard to the degree of symptomatic improvement that can reasonably be expected. We are more inclined to treat a younger person with relatively minor symptoms than a person in his or her 70s or 80s. Our rationale is that persons with Paget's disease have a normal life span and a younger person has a greater potential for progression.

Use of Specific Pharmacologic Agents

Therapy is usually begun with EHDP (Didronel) at a dosage of 5 mg per kilogram per day (either one 400-mg or two 200-mg tablets in the average patient, to be taken together with water at a time when the stomach has been and will remain empty for 2 hours), for a period of 6 months. It is the least expensive therapy and the only one that can be taken orally, so it enjoys the greatest patient acceptance. Ideally, the SAP (and an optional UOHP) is determined at the end of the 6 months of medication, and the initial course of treatment is discontinued at that time. The majority of patients will have had a decline in the biochemical indices (with a reduction by about 50 percent of the elevated portion of the SAP and UOHP) and will have experienced some improvement in their potentially reversible symptoms.

Although EHDP is considered to be the drug of choice in most situations, there are circumstances in which initial treatment with a calcitonin (Calcimar or Cibacalcin) is preferred. One example involves the patient with a fracture (or radiographic evidence of impending pathologic fracture) through pagetic bone, and another is that of the patient with Paget's disease who is immobilized and develops hypercalcemia, significant hypercalciuria, or both. A third situation is that of the patient with a large lytic lesion or an advancing lytic wedge in a weight-bearing region of the skeleton. There has been debate about the efficacy of EHDP in the treatment of patients in this last category. Some research groups experience no difficulty, whereas others find a significant incidence of increased osteolysis and new pain on treatment. Until this issue is resolved by more extensive clinical studies, it is best to use therapy with calcitonin for these types of patients. The calcitonins are injected subcutaneously, beginning with a dose of 100 IU of salmon calcitonin or 0.5 mg of human calcitonin daily. Some degree of symptomatic and biochemical improvement may be apparent as early as the first few weeks of therapy, if it is to occur, and improvement is usually evident after 2 to 3 months. As with EHDP, a 50 percent or greater reduction in the elevation of the biochemical values generally results, and symptoms are diminished to a variable extent; most of the improvement that is to be gained is achieved by the end of the first 6 months of treatment. Either calcitonin preparation can be continued indefinitely to sustain whatever benefit has been achieved, and usually, following the first 3 to 6 months of therapy, the dosage can be lowered without loss of effectiveness to 50 to 100 U of salmon calcitonin three times weekly, or a similar decrease in the human form. (Cibacalcin at present comes prepackaged in a prefilled syringe, so that a reduction in frequency of injection, rather than in the dosage per injection, will be most cost effective.)

Most patients will therefore be treated with either EHDP or a form of calcitonin. There are certain situations, however, in which alternative approaches may be useful. In cases of involvement of the thoracic spine that produces progressive neurologic dysfunction due to spinal cord compression, we prefer to hospitalize the patient, initiate a rapidly tapered course of dexamethasone, 4 mg four times daily, and give 15 to 20 μg per kilogram of plicamycin intravenously on alternate days for a maximum of five courses. If significant gastrointestinal or other toxicity intervenes, either the dose of plicamycin can be reduced or a longer interval between infusions may be substituted. At the same time that the plicamycin therapy is begun, treatment with calcitonin is started. The goal with plicamycin is to reverse the pagetic process rapidly, and the calcitonin treatment serves to sustain and add to the early benefit achieved with plicamycin. UOHP may decrease rapidly after the first plicamycin infusion. Additionally, since plicamycin tends to lower the serum calcium level, a dietary calcium intake of 1 g per day is advised and vitamin D supplements are given during the course of the plicamycin infusions. Patients with neurologic compression syndromes who are not showing a progressive deficit are in less urgent need of rapid reversal and are treated with a calcitonin, EHDP, or both, since there are numerous reports testifying to the efficacy of each of these agents in this situation.

It should also be noted that newer, investigational bisphosphonates inhibit bone resorption much more than bone formation, and these offer promise of even greater benefit in this disorder. Some can also be given intravenously to induce a rapid remission. Several of these agents are in active clinical trials in the United States and should become available in the next few years. Gallium nitrate, an agent recently studied for its use in hypercalcemia, is also in an early phase of investigation for efficacy and safety in Paget's disease.

Regardless of the choice of therapy in the more usual type of patient, after the first 6 months of treatment it is time to reassess the patient's status. As noted, data regarding objective and subjective benefit are obtained and the laboratory tests are repeated at this time. Except for the need to reexamine lytic disease or fractures, serial bone scans or roentgenograms are of little value in determining the benefit of therapy.

Following the evaluation of response to initial treatment, it is important to address the goals of long-term therapy. All of the drugs available only suppress the disease process; they do not cure it. If the first 6 months of treatment have produced significant relief of symptoms, that outcome testifies to the effectiveness of the treatment program, and a commitment to long-term therapy is usually indicated. Often, however, the physician is left to contemplate the meaning of a reduction during treatment of the biochemical indices, SAP and UOHP, in a patient with pagetic deformities whose symptomatic expression could not be expected to be reversed. If the abnormal elevation has been reduced by approximately 50 percent, it would indicate that the treatment has slowed the pagetic process significantly. The available data suggest that this correlates with a return of the microscopic elements of bone architecture toward a more normal, lamellar pattern. However, we do not believe that the goal of therapy is to reduce the SAP and UOHP to normal values. This is rarely achieved with calcitonin at the usual doses, and although high doses of bisphosphonates can reduce UOHP to normal levels, it is among this group of patients that we find persons who exhibit the largest number of disconcerting side effects. Normal bone remodeling requires maintenance of some degree of bone turnover. Thus in Paget's disease we are usually willing to accept a 50 percent reduction in the elevation of the SAP and UOHP values as an adequate therapeutic effect.

Unlike calcitonin, which may require continued administration indefinitely at the lowest effective dose, the essential point of long-term therapy with EHDP is that it must be given in a cyclic fashion. If the initial response to this drug was satisfactory, 5 mg per kilogram per day is given for 6 months of each year, allowing a 6-month drug-free period to adjust for its effects on normal bone remodeling and on mineralization in the pagetic lesion. The patients are evaluated at 6-month intervals and their biochemical indices determined. With this approach, the SAP level may tend to drift back toward the pretreatment value after several years, probably indicating either insufficient dose or the emergence of resistance. In some of these patients the drug was used in cycles of 1 month at 20 mg per kilogram per day followed by a 3-month drug-free interval to allow for the initiation and completion of one cycle of bone remodeling. Although this approach is within the guidelines that have been approved for the use of EHDP, there has been insufficient experience with it to evaluate the long-term effects and the potential for side effects. Patients on the higher dose of EHDP frequently report that it has a laxative effect and some experience frank diarrhea. When this occurs, treatment is usually discontinued for a few days until symptoms have cleared, and then medication is reintroduced for several days at one-half the dose, gradually returning to the full dose.

Some patients with only mild disease (e.g., a single site of involvement and only mild to moderate biochemical elevations) will have continued relief of symptoms and near-normal biochemical indices for a prolonged period after the initial 6-month course of low doses of EHDP. Such patients may be reevaluated at 6-month intervals with no further therapy until the SAP level again begins to rise or skeletal symptoms recur.

When a patient does not seem to achieve adequate suppression of the disease process with low-dose EHDP therapy, either initially or on a long-term program of cyclic therapy, treatment with one of the calcitonins, administered as described earlier, is recommended as an alternative. If this fails, then a calcitonin is given in addition to the EHDP cycles of treatment. Several clinical investigators have reported that, at low doses, a combination of EHDP and calcitonin appears to have an additive effect, and our experience is in agreement with this.

Many patients ask whether there is a role for calcium or vitamin D supplements in their treatment. Normally recommended dietary levels of these substances are probably adequate, taking into account the increased requirement for calcium that has been reported in postmenopausal women at risk for osteoporosis. During lytic phases of Paget's disease, patients may have periods of hypercalciuria with an increased propensity toward the development of renal calculi, and any prolonged use of very high doses of vitamin D might add to the likelihood of that complication.

Although Paget's disease is a localized disorder of the skeleton, the physician should be alert to two potential disturbances in mineral metabolism that may adversely affect the course of the disease. The first is the coincidence of another common problem, namely, a parathyroid adenoma. Hypercalcemia is not a feature of Paget's disease, except in occasional immobilized patients, and its presence should be evaluated because primary hyperparathyroidism can greatly increase the activity of pagetic osteoclasts and the expression of the disease. A second problem that has been noted is a tendency for patients with very active Paget's disease to develop secondary hyperparathyroidism, that is, with normal serum calcium values. This presumably arises as a result of prolonged parathyroid stimulation during blastic phases of the disease when there may be a relative calcium deficiency. It is manifested by slight to moderate elevations of serum parathyroid hormone levels (found in 18 percent of pagetic subjects in our own series) and biopsy evidence of a form of hyper-remodeling in uninvolved skeletal sites that is consistent with secondary hyperparathyroidism. The situation in these patients might provide a rationale for supplemental calcium therapy, but this is a subject for more extensive clinical investigation before any general recommendations are made.

Other Treatment Modalities

Anti-inflammatory Agents

Particularly when Paget's disease occurs in the spine or in the region of large joints, either by directly involving the areas of bone that comprise the joint or by causing a malalignment at the hip or knee (as might occur with bowing of the femur), significant symptomatic arthritis may ensue. The use of specific antipagetic therapy may readily decrease the metabolic indices in such a patient, but mechanical problems, such as bowing or protrusio acetabuli, are often not improved. If supplemental aspirin therapy is insufficient, considerable symptomatic relief may be afforded by treatment with the nonsteroidal anti-inflammatory agents. These agents have been quite helpful in some patients in relieving pain due to mild to moderate hip, knee, or ankle joint dysfunction and variably beneficial for symptoms resulting from spinal stenosis or for low back pain due to lumbar and sacral involvement by Paget's disease. A trial of these agents is definitely worth undertaking whenever there is a symptomatic arthritic component to Paget's disease, especially if the symptoms are refractory to calcitonin or EHDP therapy. It is also important to note that some patients who fail to respond to one anti-inflammatory drug may do very well with another, so some experimentation among the agents within this class can be tried.

Surgical Intervention

Several of the mechanical complications of Paget's disease can best be approached surgically. Severe joint dysfunction at the hip or the knee may respond only to joint replacement. If performed by orthopaedic surgeons with experience in the management of pagetic lesions, these operations can provide relatively good results with respect to pain relief and enhanced mobility. Internal stabilization of a weight-bearing bone that shows signs of an impending fracture is another procedure that is sometimes necessary, particularly when large cortical stress fractures persist or increase over time. Osteotomies of severely bowed limbs may be performed on those patients who have major gait disturbances or have severe pain due to stresses from the malalignment of the bone. This procedure may give symptomatic relief and additionally may lessen arthritis at the joints adjacent to the affected bone or in the opposite leg.

It is important to emphasize that many operations on pagetic bone may be quite difficult because the bone is very soft and vascular, and surgery should be considered only when there is a major mechanical problem causing symptoms that are refractory to medical treatment or that pose a serious risk of future complications, such as fracture. Prior to elective surgery on pagetic bone a course of salmon calcitonin therapy, at a dosage of 100 IU daily for up to 3 months preoperatively, may be of value in reducing the increased vascularity around the pagetic tissue, making the surgical procedure somewhat safer with respect to intraoperative blood loss.

Neurosurgical intervention may be required to relieve progressive spinal cord or root compression by pagetic bone if this complication fails to respond to drug therapy. Severe basilar invagination occasionally causes compression of posterior fossa structures or obstruction to cerebrospinal fluid flow and hydrocephalus, with the development of central nervous system symptoms. Computed tomography or magnetic resonance imaging of the skull is an excellent way to evaluate such patients periodically to detect these problems. In cases with hydrocephalus, rapid application of ventricular shunting may be imperative to decrease cerebrospinal fluid pressures.

SUGGESTED READING

Hosking DJ. Paget's disease of bone: An update on management. Drugs 1985; 30:156–173.

Paget's disease of bone. Proceedings of the Kroc Foundation Conference, March 24–March 28, 1980, Santa Ynez Valley, California. Arthritis Rheum 1980; 23:1073–1234.

Singer FR. Paget's disease of bone. New York: Plenum Press, 1977.

Siris ES. Indications for medical treatment of Paget's disease. In: Singer FR, Wallach S, eds. Paget's disease of bone: Clinical assessment, present and future therapies. New York: Elsevier, 1990: in press.

Siris ES, Jacobs TP, Canfield RE. Paget's disease of bone. Bull NY Acad Med 1980; 56:285–304.

Wallach S. Treatment of Paget's disease. Adv Intern Med 1982; 278:1–43.

OSTEOPOROSIS

LAWRENCE G. RAISZ, M.D.

Osteoporosis is defined as a decrease in bone mass and strength associated with an increased tendency of bones to fracture. It is a disease, or more likely a group of diseases, of unknown pathogenesis. However, a large number of risk factors have been identified that increase the likelihood of developing osteoporotic fractures. Although some of these risk factors are constitutional or genetic and cannot be altered, others, such as decreased physical activity, low calcium intake, estrogen deficiency, increased intake of alcohol, and smoking, can be reversed. Thus, a major therapeutic approach in osteoporosis is to develop an appropriate prevention program. This can be instituted after the first fracture, but it is clearly preferable to begin earlier. On this basis, osteoporosis prevention programs have been developed in a number of medical centers. When bone loss is severe and progressive and multiple fractures are likely to occur, the usual preventive programs may be insufficient and additional therapy is required.

The most common osteoporotic fractures are of the vertebrae and the proximal femur. These can occur in the same patient, but there are important differences in both the clinical characteristics and the therapeutic approach. The *vertebral crush fracture syndrome* has also been termed *type I* or *postmenopausal osteoporosis*. At least 90 percent of the patients are postmenopausal women, but crush fractures also can occur in men and in premenopausal women. The disease usually begins 10 to 15 years after the menopause, trauma is minimal or absent, and fractures are often multiple and recurrent. In contrast, *fracture of the proximal femur,* sometimes termed *type II* or *senile osteoporosis,* usually occurs later, with women affected more than men in a 2 to 1 ratio. This fracture is usually associated with a fall, although the trauma may be minimal. The major risk factors appear to increase the likelihood of both type of fractures, and prevention programs are thus aimed at decreasing both type I and type II osteoporosis. There are additional medical therapies for the progressive vertebral crush fracture syndrome, but these may not be appropriate for patients with a hip fracture. In this chapter a therapeutic approach is outlined in terms of (1) general preventive measures early in life, (2) risk factor analysis and prevention programs in premenopausal and postmenopausal women, (3) treatment of progressive vertebral crush fracture syndrome, (4) treatment of patients with hip fracture, and (5) treatment of atypical forms of osteoporosis and aggravating disorders.

GENERAL PREVENTIVE MEASURES

The increasing incidence of osteoporotic fractures is probably caused not only by the increase in the age of our population but also by changes in diet and lifestyle. Decreasing physical activity in an industrialized society may be associated with decreased caloric and calcium intake. This is aggravated in American women by an intense desire to be thin. The recommended daily allowance for calcium is 1,200 mg in teenagers and pregnant women and 800 mg for all other adults. The recommendation of the National Institutes of Health Osteoporosis Consensus Conference is a minimum intake of calcium of 1,000 mg per day in premenopausal women, which should be increased to 1,500 mg per day in postmenopausal women. The actual intake of calcium is much less, averaging about 600 mg per day in women and 800 mg per day in men. There is evidence that 30 minutes a day or more of moderate physical exercise will help to maintain or even increase bone mass. The majority of the population exercise less than 2 hours a week. Exercise and adequate calcium intake may be most important from early puberty until the mid 20s to early 30s when peak bone mass is established. In young women rigorous caloric restriction and exercise that lead to low body fat and decreased estrogen levels inhibit the development of optimal peak bone mass. This can occur in persons with anorexia nervosa, athletic amenorrhea, and prolactinoma.

RISK FACTOR ANALYSIS AND PREVENTION PROGRAM

Although there is some controversy concerning precise rates, age-related bone loss, particularly of trabecular bone in the spine, begins in women before the menopause. Thus, it is appropriate to begin to look for risk factors that predispose a person to osteoporosis and to develop a rational prevention program tailored to the person's risks before the menopause. Women with a thin, light frame, a family history of osteoporosis, a history of low calcium intake, decreased physical activity, increased alcohol intake, smoking, or prior menstrual dysfunction or who have been treated with glucocorticoid or anti-epileptic medications appear to be at higher risk. In women with one or more of these factors, measurement of bone density may provide further information as to risk. There is considerable controversy concerning the use of bone density measurements for osteoporosis prevention. The most established procedures are dual-energy photon absorptiometry (DPA) and computed tomography (CT) scanning of the lumbar spine. The newer dual-energy x-ray absorptiometry (DEXA) has replaced DPA and CT scanning in many centers because DEXA is more accurate and reproducible than DPA and is less expensive and involves less radiation exposure than CT. With DEXA, it should be possible to use serial measurements to assess changes in bone mass in individual patients. Moreover, the rapidity of DEXA scans makes it feasible to measure hip as well as spine bone density routinely. High-risk patients with low bone mass should be provided with a preventive regimen consisting of calcium supplementation and exercise before the menopause and hormone replacement added at the menopause. To the extent that these programs are carried out in centers where large numbers of patients are followed for prolonged periods of time, we will be able to gather the information needed to improve the precision of prediction and the efficacy of prevention; neither is well known at present.

Calcium Supplementation

Although the role of calcium in the prevention of osteoporosis is much debated, there is certainly enough evidence for some degree of protective effect to support a recommendation of adequate calcium intake throughout life. Probably, as indicated above, the most important time may be during puberty and the years thereafter, when maximal bone mass is achieved. High intakes during this period probably increase peak bone mass and appear to decrease the incidence of fractures much later in life. Calcium supplementation before and after menopause has not been shown to prevent loss of bone in the lumbar spine. Calcium supplementation does appear to slow cortical bone loss, although it is less effective than estrogen. An optimal postmenopausal calcium intake of 1,500 mg per day may allow the effective prevention of bone loss with lower doses of estrogen.

It is difficult to maintain a calcium intake of 1,000 mg per day in premenopausal women and even more difficult to maintain an intake of 1,500 mg per day in postmenopausal women by diet alone. Nevertheless, we urge patients to maximize their intake of milk products on the basis that these provide good general nutrition and good absorption of calcium. Dietary calcium is difficult to obtain from foods other than dairy products. Some vegetables, such as spinach, which are fairly rich in calcium, are also rich in oxalate so that the calcium is poorly absorbed. In patients who cannot get enough calcium from diet, a variety of calcium supplements are available in tablet form. If these are given with meals, there appears to be little difference in absorption of the different salts. However, patients with achlorhydria will not absorb calcium carbonate on an empty stomach. Many inexpensive generic calcium supplements are available. Chewable calcium carbonate antacids are inexpensive and widely used. Some supplements have enteric coatings that are slowly dissolved and hence are poorly absorbed, and others, such as bone meal and dolomite, should be avoided because they may contain heavy metals and other contaminants. It has been claimed that a large single dose of calcium at bedtime is particularly effective in inhibiting parathyroid hormone secretion and reducing nocturnal bone resorption, but this has not been proved. Although high doses of vitamin D were recommended in the past, intakes of 400 to 800 U per day or a sun exposure of 30 minutes per week appears to be quite adequate to maintain vitamin D levels.

There is relatively little risk from a high calcium intake. Patients with a family or personal history of renal stones should be checked for absorptive hypercalciuria. In these persons, calcium intake can be increased if a diuretic regimen with thiazide or amiloride plus thiazide is instituted to reduce urinary calcium excretion.

Side effects from increased calcium intake are rare, although some patients, particularly those with lactase deficiency, complain of intestinal upsets from milk products. Patients taking calcium carbonate often complain of constipation.

Exercise

The most appropriate exercise program for the prevention of osteoporosis involves a minimum of 3 hours per week of mild aerobic exercise with weight-bearing and specific exercises designed to improve the strength of the paraspinal muscles. Compliance with an exercise program appears to be greatest when there is supervision and group activity. However, it may be possible to obtain full compliance with only one period of supervised exercise per week. Among the unsupervised exercises that appear to be most effective, brisk walking, stair climbing, and use of a rowing machine or treadmill are appropriate and well accepted.

Hormone Replacement Therapy

The most difficult aspect of osteoporosis prevention is the selection of patients for hormone replacement therapy at the menopause. Certainly, patients who have an early menopause, either surgical or natural, should be placed on hormone therapy unless there are specific contraindications. For patients who enter menopause in the late 40s and early 50s, it is our practice to recommend prolonged replacement therapy with estrogen and progestin if there are multiple risk factors, particularly if bone mass is low by DPA, CT, or DEXA measurement. Once the decision to recommend hormone replacement therapy is made, the patient must be provided with complete information on risks and benefits and a program designed to maintain compliance with hormone therapy for at least 5 and probably up to 15 years. These patients should be followed with repeated measurements of bone density as well as gynecologic examinations. The major contraindications to hormone replacement therapy include a prior history of breast cancer, prior thromboembolic disease, and active liver disease. Hypertension is not a contraindication except in patients whose condition becomes much more difficult to treat on hormone replacement. The increased incidence of endometrial carcinoma with unopposed estrogen is probably not a consideration for those patients receiving combined estrogen and progestin therapy. In patients with an intact uterus, we recommend conjugated equine estrogens, 0.625 mg for 25 days of the month, with medroxyprogesterone, 5 or 10 mg, for the last 10 or 12 days of these cycles. Although the dose of 0.625 mg of conjugated estrogen or 25 μg of ethinyl estradiol has been required to prevent bone loss in prior studies, there is a study indicating that a dose of 0.3 mg of conjugated estrogen may be effective in patients on calcium intakes of 1,500 to 2,000 mg per day. Alternatively, 0.625 mg of conjugated estrogens can be given continuously and progestin given during the first 2 weeks of each month. In patients who wish to avoid regular menses, continuous estrogen with continuous progestin (2.5 or 5 mg of medroxyprogesterone daily) can be used. Irregular bleeding often occurs during the first few months of therapy but then stops.

The major drawback of hormone replacement is that this results in the return of menses in most patients. Continuous estrogen and progestin may resolve this problem, but the benefits and side effects of this regimen have not yet been fully evaluated. One major uncertainty concerning hormone replacement therapy is the effect on cardiovascular disease. Most studies suggest that the risk of cardiovascular disease is decreased by estrogen. If this is correct, it may be an even more important indication for hormone replacement than osteoporosis prevention. Progestins may increase the risk of heart disease, but this may be limited to synthetic progestins that have greater androgenic effects. In patients who have had a hysterectomy, progestin is not necessary for the prevention of endometrial carcinoma and estrogen can be given alone. Side effects of hormone replacement therapy are relatively uncommon even in those persons who previously had considerable symptoms with their normal menstrual cycle. When they occur, they can generally be controlled by reduction of dose.

TREATMENT OF PROGRESSIVE VERTEBRAL CRUSH FRACTURE SYNDROME

When a patient presents with one or more vertebral crush fractures, the first step is to rule out diseases that aggravate or mimic osteoporosis. These include hyperparathyroidism, hyperthyroidism, multiple myeloma, Cushing's disease, and osteomalacia. Once this is done, all patients should be put on as intense a preventive regimen as they can tolerate. Exercise programs should be developed carefully and cautiously. Analgesics and short periods of bed rest may be required to relieve pain. Back braces should be avoided or used only for short periods.

Conservative therapy alone may be adequate to prevent further fractures in a substantial proportion of patients. However, in patients with severe disease of continued bone loss and recurrent fractures, additional therapy is required. There is no established effective therapy for osteoporosis at this point. Calcitonin may also be useful, particularly in those patients who have high turnover and a rapid rate of bone loss. It is the only agent other than estrogen approved for use in osteoporosis. Fluoride therapy has been used extensively and can increase bone mass; however, there are frequent side effects and fluoride may not reduce the overall incidence of fractures. Most recently, intermittent bisphosphonate treatment has been shown to increase vertebral bone mass and decrease vertebral fractures. Other therapeutic approaches are under study. These include use of parathyroid hormone, 1,25-dihydroxyvitamin D (calcitriol), phosphate, and anabolic steroids.

Fluoride Therapy

Although sodium fluoride has been used in the treatment of osteoporosis for almost 20 years, we still do not have adequate evidence of its efficacy. The mechanism of action is not fully understood, but fluoride probably increases bone mass by stimulating the proliferation of osteoblasts, particularly on trabecular bone surfaces. This leads to an increase in the amount of trabecular bone. A recent prospective trial of long-term continuous high-dose fluoride therapy in the United States showed no significant decrease in vertebral fractures despite a marked increase in bone mass. Moreover, side effects were frequent and the incidence of fractures at other sites increased.

Fluoride must be given for long periods. It is most effective after a year of therapy. We usually employ continuous therapy for 1 to 2 years, but some clinics use 3 or 6 months of fluoride, alternating with free periods. Fluoride is given as 40 to 80 mg per day of sodium fluoride in divided doses. Gastrointestinal side effects can be decreased by giving fluoride as sodium monofluorophosphate or together with calcium carbonate. A slow-release form of fluoride has been tested and found to produce minimal gastrointestinal side effects, but it is not yet available for clinical use. Among the currently available forms, Florical tablets, containing 8.3 mg of sodium fluoride and 145 mg of calcium as carbonate, are available as an over-the-counter preparation. Alternatively, sodium fluoride can be made up by the hospital pharmacy in capsule or liquid form. Fluoride is also available as tablets containing 2.2 mg of sodium fluoride, which require that the patient take 20 to 36 tablets per day. Gastrointestinal side effects are also less frequent if fluoride is given with or 30 minutes after meals. Side effects can be markedly reduced by using preparations such as mono-fluoro phosphate or slow-release fluoride.

In addition to gastrointestinal side effects, fluoride therapy can produce musculoskeletal symptoms, particularly in the lower extremities. These side effects are often associated with areas of increased uptake or hot spots on bone scans and may represent stress fractures. Both musculoskeletal and gastrointestinal side effects may disappear despite continued therapy, especially with reduction of dose. Occasional patients do not tolerate therapy, and fluoride must be discontinued. A more important problem is that up to one-third of patients on fluoride therapy do not show a good therapeutic response. At present, there is no sure way of predicting these nonresponders. Measurement of bone-specific alkaline phosphatase, which should increase, as well as of serum fluoride levels, which should exceed 0.1 μM, may be helpful. Since fluoride stimulates bone formation, it would seem most appropriate for patients who have low turnover osteoporosis. In some clinics, bone biopsies are performed to help decide on fluoride therapy. However, this is probably not necessary since increased bone formation is desirable in any patient with severe bone loss.

In view of the recent negative results in controlled trials, fluoride therapy should probably be limited to patients with the most severe progressive vertebral fracture syndrome who do not respond to other forms of therapy. Patients with hip fractures or very low bone density in the proximal femur should probably not receive fluoride in view of the evidence that appendicular fractures may be increased.

Calcitonin Therapy

When calcitonin was identified as a potent inhibitor of bone resorption in the 1960s, it was expected that this hormone would provide a safe and effective therapy for preventing further bone loss in patients with osteoporosis. As with fluoride, there has been extensive clinical use of calcitonin without adequately controlled prospective trials. Calcitonin has been shown to increase bone mass in postmenopausal women with osteoporosis, although there is some evidence that the effect begins to reverse after 2 years of therapy. Since bone formation is normally coupled with bone resorption, it is possible that this reversal is due to a secondary decrease in bone formation. Alternatively, there may be a loss of sensitivity to calcitonin analogous to the escape or tolerance that is seen in patients with hypercalcemia of malignancy and Paget's disease.

At present, two forms of calcitonin are available for use in the United States. Salmon calcitonin has been available for some time, whereas human calcitonin has become available only recently. Both agents are effective inhibitors of bone resorption, although salmon calcitonin appears to be more potent and more long lasting. The major side effects are anorexia, nausea, and vomiting and are similar for both salmon and human calcitonin. We use calcitonin for patients who have evidence of increased bone turnover. In the past, bone biopsies have been used to assess bone turnover and to help decide whether or not to use calcitonin therapy. Although biopsy may still be indicated in some cases, noninvasive biochemical assessment of bone turnover is probably adequate for most patients. Measurement of fasting calcium and hydroxyproline excretion provides a rough index of bone resorption, whereas measurement of osteocalcin (bone gamma-carboxyglutamic acid containing protein) and bone-specific alkaline phosphatase provides an index of bone formation. Other methods are under development, including serum tartrate-resistant acid phosphatase and urine collagen cross-links to assess resorption and technetium diphosphonate bone scans to assess formation. Combining these, it is possible to separate osteoporotic patients into high turnover groups that are likely to show a substantial increase in bone mass in response to calcitonin and low turnover groups that may not. Calcitonin is probably worth trying in premenopausal women and younger men with rapidly progressive idiopathic osteoporosis, since they usually show accelerated bone resorption. Calcitonin may also be useful to prevent bone loss in patients who cannot take estrogen because of breast cancer or other contraindications and who are at high risk for developing osteoporosis.

Therapy should probably be continued for at least 6 months. Because of the possibility that intermittent therapy might delay escape and because it helps the patient to deal with the problem of anorexia, we have generally administered salmon calcitonin at bedtime for 3 or 5 days of the week in doses of 50 to 100 U. Cost and the requirement for subcutaneous injection are major drawbacks of calcitonin therapy. The latter may be circumvented in the future by the use of a nasal calcitonin spray, which is currently under clinical trial. Calcitonin administered by nasal spray clearly has a biologic effect and has fewer side effects than the injected form. We need more data on long-term efficacy before deciding whether this is a satisfactory alternative to subcutaneous injection.

Diphosphonate Therapy

Diphosphonates (bisphosphonates) have been used for many years in the therapy of Paget's disease and hypercalcemia of malignancy. These agents are potent inhibitors of bone resorption, which probably act by binding to the bone surface and then producing selective toxicity in the osteoclasts, which take up the mineral-diphosphonate complex. Sodium etidronate has been available in the United States for many years. Its major disadvantage is that at high doses it can inhibit mineralization and even produce osteomalacia. However, when used at lower doses (10 mg per kilogram per day or less) and intermittently, osteomalacia is not produced, but bone resorption is still inhibited. Recently, cyclic intermittent etidronate therapy has been tested in patients with vertebral crush fractures. Low doses (400 mg per day) are given for 2 weeks every 2 or 3 months. With this regimen, bone mass has been found to increase over a 3-year period, and there is evidence for a decrease in the number of new vertebral fractures. The greatest effects were seen in patients with low bone mass and multiple fractures.

Newer diphosphonates are being tested that are substantially more potent than etidronate and are clearly more effective in managing Paget's disease and hypercalcemia of malignancy. These compounds can also increase bone mass in osteoporosis, but it is not clear whether they have additional advantages over etidronate in long-term therapy. Although additional data are clearly needed, the diphosphonates could provide a safe and inexpensive substitute for calcitonin therapy. Based on our long experience with their use in Paget's disease, unexpected late side effects are not likely to appear. However, we need studies on the relative efficacy of calcitonin and diphosphonates in fracture prevention before we can select the best therapeutic approach.

Other Therapeutic Approaches

Among the therapeutic approaches under study for the treatment of osteoporosis, a combination of low-dose intermittent parathyroid hormone therapy with calcitriol seems promising, although it has not yet been evaluated in a controlled randomized prospective trial. The original rationale for parathyroid hormone therapy was that intermittent administration of relatively low doses had an anabolic effect in experimental animals. This effect has been demonstrated in patients with osteoporosis. The synthetic human parathyroid hormone fragment (amino acids 1 – 34) used is not yet approved for clinical use. However, it appears to be nontoxic and usually does not produce hypercalcemia in doses of 400 to 500 U per day. In the osteoporotic patient, low doses of 1,25-dihydroxyvitamin D (calcitriol, 0.25 μg) have been administered with parathyroid hormone to overcome the impaired intestinal calcium absorption characteristic of these patients.

The use of calcitriol alone has also been advocated. There is some evidence that this may increase bone mass, but further studies are needed to determine whether fractures are prevented. A major problem with calcitriol therapy is that the toxic-therapeutic ratio is quite low. With doses above 1.0 μg per day, hypercalciuria and hypercalcemia often occur. In most cases, this is transient and has no prolonged adverse effects, but vitamin D intoxication can lead to irreversible impairment of renal function.

Phosphate has been used by itself, but it is more often employed in combination with an inhibitor of bone resorption. The use of phosphate seems paradoxical because excess phosphate intake and resulting secondary hyperparathyroidism have been implicated as pathogenetic mechanisms in osteoporosis. However, intermittent phosphate administration may produce a transient increase in parathyroid hormone secretion that would increase bone turnover and might have the same anabolic effect as exogenous parathyroid hormone. However, the parathyroid hormone response to phosphate loading may be blunted in osteoporotic patients, and this could limit its therapeutic effectiveness. Phosphate may also have a direct effect to enhance bone formation. Although one small controlled trial did show increased bone mass with phosphate combined with calcitonin, a more recent study found that this combination was less effective than estrogen replacement.

Bone mass can also be increased by the administration of anabolic steroids. These agents are also androgenic. They produce some degree of masculinization, usually limited to a deepening of the voice and mild hirsutism. More important, they lower high density lipoprotein cholesterol, which could increase the risk of heart disease.

In assessing the newer forms of therapy for osteoporosis, it will be important to compare them with the standard conservative program of calcium, exercise, and estrogen. We need studies that combine new treatments with conservative therapy, particularly in patients who show continued loss of bone mass or recurrent fractures despite adequate conservative treatment. Thus far, none of the newer treatments has been adequately evaluated in this manner.

TREATMENT OF HIP FRACTURE

The surgical treatment of fractures of the femoral neck and greater trochanter has shortened the hospital stay and decreased morbidity and mortality. Although figures of as high as 10 or 20 percent excess mortality during the first year after hip fracture are frequently quoted, recent series have shown much lower figures. Since the majority of patients are over 65 and many are in the 80s and 90s, the life span after hip fracture is often short. The limitation of activity following hip fracture is a more persistent problem. Many patients who have had a hip fracture cannot return to their former level of activity. Functional outcomes can be improved by prolonged physical therapy and a carefully developed program of home care. Additional falls and recurrent fractures can be minimized by attention to risk factors such as neurologic disease, visual difficulty, and various hazards in the home and environment. Since a second hip fracture as well as vertebral crush fracture syndrome is more common in patients who have had one hip fracture, a preventive regimen should be begun. At the least, this should include calcium supplementation and an adequate intake of vitamin D. The question of whether to begin estrogen therapy in patients who have had a hip fracture has not been examined. Theoretically, further bone loss could be prevented and hormone replacement begun as late as the age of 70 or 75 years.

Since there is a subset of hip fracture patients who have vitamin D deficiency, it is important to identify and treat this group. Although they may show low 25-hydroxyvitamin D levels in the serum at the time of surgery, this can be due in part to blood loss and a decrease in vitamin D–binding protein. It seems reasonable to provide all hip fracture patients with a safe amount of vitamin D on the order of 400 to 1,000 U per day. One complication of hip fracture, which may be amenable to medical therapy, is heterotopic calcification. This occurs most often after larger surgical procedures such as hip replacement. Nonsteroidal anti-inflammatory agents have been shown to decrease the incidence of this disorder, presumably because prostaglandin production by the local tissues is important in stimulating cell replication and bone formation. Diphosphonates have also been used to inhibit heterotopic mineral deposition, but these agents can produce osteomalacia elsewhere and are, therefore, not recommended.

TREATMENT OF ATYPICAL FORMS OF OSTEOPOROSIS AND OF AGGRAVATING DISORDERS

One of the most difficult forms of osteoporosis to treat is that which develops in patients who require prolonged glucocorticoid therapy. Glucocorticoid osteoporosis is the combined result of inhibition of intestinal calcium absorption leading to secondary hyperparathyroidism with increased bone resorption and a direct inhibitory effect on osteoblast precursors that results in decreased bone formation. The calcium deficiency can be reversed by oral calcium and high doses of vitamin D. 25-Hydroxyvitamin D (calcidiol) in dosages of 20 to 50 μg per day has been used for this purpose. This results in a substantial increase in calcium absorption in the intestine. Although this may increase bone mass by reducing resorption, bone formation is still suppressed. Calcidiol therapy is often associated with hypercalciuria. The addition of a thiazide or an amiloride-thiazide combination can circumvent this problem and may result in a more positive calcium balance.

One rare but treatable cause of osteoporosis in younger men is hypogonadism. Here testosterone replacement therapy can produce a substantial increase in bone mass. Similarly, estrogen therapy can be used in women with anorexia nervosa, athletic amenorrhea, or prolactinoma.

Many postmenopausal women who present with osteoporosis give a history of treatment with thyroid hormone preparations, often those including triiodothyronine. Even ordinary replacement therapy for hypothyroidism with thyroxine and triiodothyronine has been shown to produce bone loss. Thus, hyperthyroidism should be treated promptly and excessive or unnecessary thyroid hormone therapy should be avoided in osteoporotic patients.

Osteomalacia is relatively uncommon in this country but should be considered in patients with gastrointestinal disease or a history of poor nutrition and inadequate sun exposure. Most patients show the typical biochemical changes, including low 25-hydroxyvitamin D as well as low calcium and phosphorus concentrations in the serum and low urinary calcium excretion. However, a definite diagnosis can only be made by bone biopsy with tetracycline labeling to assess mineralization.

SUGGESTED READING

Ettinger B, Genant HK, Cann CE. Postmenopausal bone loss as prevented by treatment with low dosage estrogen with calcium. Ann Intern Med 1987; 106:40–45.

Raisz LG. Osteoporosis. J Am Geriatr Soc 1982; 30:127–138.

Raisz LG. Local and systemic factors in the pathogenesis of osteoporosis. N Engl J Med 1988; 318:818–827.

Raisz LG, Smith JA. Pathogenesis, prevention, and treatment of osteoporosis. Annu Rev Med 1989; 40:251–267.

Riggs BL, Hodgson SF, O'Fallon WM, et al. Effect of fluoride treatment on the fracture rate in postmenopausal women with osteoporosis. N Engl J Med 1990; 322:802–809.

Riggs BL, Melton LG III. Involutional osteoporosis. N Engl J Med 1986; 314:1676–1685.

Riis B, Thomson K, Christiansen C. Does calcium supplementation prevent postmenopausal bone loss: Double-blind controlled study. N Engl J Med 1987; 316:173–177.

Silverberg SJ, Shane E, Dela Cruz L, et al. Abnormalities in parathyroid hormone secretion and 1,25-dihydroxyvitamin D_3 formation in women with osteoporosis. N Engl J Med 1989; 320:277–281.

Slovik DM, Rosenthal DI, Doppelt SH, et al. Restoration of spinal bone in osteoporotic men by treatment with human parathyroid hormone (1-34) and 1,25-dihydroxyvitamin D. J Bone Min Res 1986; 1:377–382.

HYPOGLYCEMIA: POSTPRANDIAL OR REACTIVE

PIERRE J. LEFEBVRE, M.D., Ph.D.

Postprandial or reactive hypoglycemia is often overdiagnosed and to a certain extent has become a fashionable disorder. Self-diagnosis of hypoglycemia, overdiagnosis by some physicians, and popularization in the lay literature have led to gross overestimation of the problem. Although useful in clinical investigation, the oral glucose tolerance test is not appropriate for the diagnosis of postprandial or reactive hypoglycemia. However, some patients indeed exhibit in everyday life postprandial symptoms suggesting hypoglycemia. If these symptoms are accompanied by blood glucose levels between 2.8 and 2.5 mmol per liter or below (determined by a specific method on capillary or arterialized venous blood), the diagnosis of postprandial or reactive hypoglycemia may be envisaged. In these patients, every effort should be made to document hypoglycemia under their everyday life conditions. In these cases, simultaneous relief of symptoms and correction of low blood glucose values are strong arguments in favor of the diagnosis. In some patients, postprandial or reactive hypoglycemia can occur as a consequence of gastric surgery, rapid gastric emptying, the simultaneous ingestion of sugar and ethanol, the presence of autoantibodies against insulin or against the insulin receptor (two extremely rare conditions) and other unidentified factors. The suggested therapeutic approach is summarized in Table 1.

DIETARY APPROACH

A regimen of multiple small, high-protein, low-carbohydrate feedings is classically recommended to patients with "alimentary" hypoglycemia. The most common form of alimentary hypoglycemia is that which occurs 2 to 3 hours after food ingestion in patients who have undergone gastrectomy or pyloroplasty whether or not associated with vagotomy. Rapid gastric emptying in patients who have not undergone such surgical procedures can also be identified by radiographic examination or isotopic investigations. When proven, alimentary hypoglycemia due to rapid gastric emptying is also a good indication of frequent small feedings low in rapidly absorbable carbohydrates. In the other forms of reactive hypoglycemia, the major dietary advice is avoidance of drinks rich in carbohydrates such as glucose or sucrose that have a high glycemic index and are potent stimulants of insulin secretion. The risk of reactive hypoglycemia is markedly enhanced by the simultaneous ingestion of ethanol and sucrose or glucose mainly in the fasting state. The risk of alcohol-induced reactive hypoglycemia is great when such drinks (beer, gin and tonic, rum and Coca-Cola, whisky and gingerale) are taken on an empty stomach. The incidence and severity of alcohol-provoked reactive hypoglycemia is decreased by decreasing the amount of sucrose (glucose) ingested and can be abolished by replacing it with either saccharin or the noninsulinotropic carbohydrate fructose.

PHARMACOLOGIC APPROACH

Besides dietary advice, the management of reactive hypoglycemia can make use of dietary fibers, anticholiner-

TABLE 1 Treatment of Postprandial or Reactive Hypoglycemia

1. Be critical before accepting the diagnosis.
2. Always try diet first: avoidance of rapidly adsorbable sugars, prescription of split meals, caution in associating sugar and alcohol.
3. Recommend fiber-rich food or add fiber to food.
4. Use glucosidase inhibitors or metformin if available.
5. Reconsider diagnosis periodically.

gic drugs, biguanides, alpha-glucosidase inhibitors, and, eventually, other drugs.

Dietary Fibers

Dietary soluble fibers as pectin and guar delay gastric emptying and prolong the intestinal transit time. The addition to the meal of 5 to 10 g hemicellulose, guar or pectin often improves postprandial hypoglycemia mainly when it is associated with decreased glucose tolerance or occurs after gastric surgery.

Anticholinergic Drugs

In view of the stimulatory control exerted by the vagus nerve on insulin secretion either directly or via the release of gut factors that potentiate glucose-stimulated insulin release, anticholinergic drugs may be useful in postprandial hypoglycemia. Atropine (0.25 mg) or Pro-Banthine (7.5 mg), taken before the meals, is indicated, keeping in mind the possible side effects of cholinergic blockade.

Biguanides

Alleviation of reactive hypoglycemia by phenformin, buformin, and metformin has been repeatedly reported. After the ban of phenformin and buformin in most countries, metformin remains in use in some others. Provided that the well-known contraindications of metformin are respected (kidney or liver insufficiency, peripheral vascular disease), I consider it as a useful adjunct to diet in the treatment of symptomatic reactive hypoglycemia. The dose is 500 to 850 mg orally taken with the meals. Nausea and diarrhea may occur as side effects; they are usually absent if low doses are taken initially and then progressively increased (start low—go slow).

Glucosidase Inhibitors

Acarbose, a complex oligosaccharide of microbial origin, delays starch digestion and possesses potent antisucrase and antimaltase activities. Acarbose is probably the most useful adjunct to diet in the treatment of reactive hypoglycemia. It should be ingested at the beginning of the meal at doses ranging 50 to 100 mg; the dose should be adapted to the amounts of carbohydrate present in the meal and adjusted according to individual tolerance. Side effects of this agent include meteorism and flatulence, which usually disappear after reduction of the dose. Additional drugs with glucosidase inhibitory properties are being developed.

Other Drugs

Other therapeutic approaches include the use of phenytoin, propranolol, calcium gluconate, diazoxide, and calcium antagonists such as nifedipine, diltiazem, and nicardipine. Controlled studies are lacking to assess their efficacy although anecdotal reports suggest that they might be useful in some patients.

SUGGESTED READING

American Diabetes Association. Statement on hypoglycemia. Diabetes 1973; 22:137.

Andreani D, Lefèbvre PJ, Marks V, eds. Current views on hypoglycemia and glucagon. London: Academic Press, 1980.

Andreani D, Marks V, Lefèbvre PJ, eds. Hypoglycemia. New York: Raven Press, 1987.

Gérard J, Luyckx AS, Lefèbvre PJ. Acarbose in reactive hypoglycemia: a double-blind study. Int J Clin Pharmacol Ther Toxicol 1984;22:25–31.

Lefèbvre PJ, Andreani D, Marks V, Creutzfeldt W. Statement on "postprandial" or "reactive" hypoglycemia. In: Andreani D, Marks V, Lefèbvre PJ, eds. Hypoglycemia. New York: Raven Press 1987:79. Also published in Acta Diabetol Lat 1987; 24:353; Diabetologia 1988; 31:68–69; Diab Med 1988; 5:200; and Diabetes Care 1988; 11:439.

Lefèbvre PJ, Luyckx AS. Hypoglycemia. In: Ellenberg M, Rifkin H, eds. Diabetes mellitus: theory and practice. New York: Medical Examination, 1983: 987.

Palardy J, Navrankova J, Lepage R, et al. Blood glucose measurements during symptomatic episodes in patients with suspected postprandial hypoglycemia. Engl J Med 1989; 321:1421–1425.

Marks V, Rose FC, eds. Hypoglycemia. Oxford: Blackwell, 1981.

Meador CK. The art and science of nondisease. N Engl J Med 1965; 272:92–95.

Service FJ, ed. Hypoglycemic disorders: pathogenesis, diagnosis and treatment. Boston: GK Hall, 1983.

Service FJ. Hypoglycemia and the postprandial syndrome. N Engl J Med 1989; 321:1472–1474.

Singer M, Arnold A, Fitzgerald M, Madden L, Voight von Legat C. Hypoglycemia: a controversial illness in U.S. society. Med Anthropol 1984; 8:1–35.

OBESITY

F. XAVIER PI-SUNYER, M.D.

The treatment of obesity is difficult and often discouraging, since the failure rate is extremely high. The primary emphasis must be on self-control rather than drugs, and what must be recognized by both patient and physician is that the primary agent for change is the patient rather than the physician. A self-motivated, committed patient is required, and a supportive, understanding physician is helpful.

Since physicians are accustomed to giving pharmacologic agents to treat most diseases, they are often not attuned to the tedious task of slow, difficult weight loss, with its slip-backs, plateaus, and disappointing statistics. Because of this, other health care professionals have become involved in treatment. Many dietitians, psychologists, social workers, and nurses advise and treat patients who want to lose weight. However, a physician still should monitor the patient's weight-loss program and treat any health problems that may develop.

Obesity is extremely common in the United States, and a physician usually requires nothing more than a quick look to determine the need for weight loss. However, since there is a great preoccupation with overweight and social, psychologic, and economic rewards are perceived to be derived from a trim look, patients who are not truly obese may wish to lose weight. A general table of weight standards for age and height is published by the Gerontology Research Center of the National Institute of Aging (Table 1). The percentage of body fat also can be calculated and followed during weight loss by using the sum of four skinfolds (Table 2).

Obesity aggravates or precipitates a number of other diseases, including diabetes mellitus, hypertension, coronary heart disease, congestive heart failure, thromboembolic disease, restrictive lung disease, pickwickian syndrome, gout, degenerative arthritis, gallbladder disease, infertility, and hyperlipoproteinemia. In cases in which one or more of these conditions is present, a more stringent standard seems appropriate, such as that used in the 1983 Metropolitan Life Insurance Company weight tables. In any case, the physician must recognize that although the loss of weight is likely to help any associated conditions, therapy targeted specifically for these disorders may be necessary.

TABLE 1 Age-Specific Weight-for-Height Tables

Height	*Weight Range for Men and Women by Age (Years)**				
	25	*35*	*45*	*55*	*65*
ft-in	lb				
4-10	84-111	92-119	99-127	107-135	115-142
4-11	87-115	95-123	103-131	111-139	119-147
5-0	90-119	98-127	106-135	114-143	123-152
5-1	93-123	101-131	110-140	118-148	127-157
5-2	96-127	105-136	113-144	122-153	131-163
5-3	99-131	108-140	117-149	126-158	135-168
5-4	102-135	112-145	121-154	130-163	140-173
5-5	106-140	115-149	125-159	134-168	144-179
5-6	109-144	119-154	129-164	138-174	148-184
5-7	112-148	122-159	133-169	143-179	153-190
5-8	116-153	126-163	137-174	147-184	158-196
5-9	119-157	130-168	141-179	151-190	162-201
5-10	122-162	134-173	145-184	156-195	167-207
5-11	126-167	137-178	149-190	160-201	172-213
6-0	129-171	141-183	153-195	165-207	177-219
6-1	133-176	145-188	157-200	169-213	182-225
6-2	137-181	149-194	162-206	174-219	187-232
6-3	141-186	153-199	166-212	179-225	192-238
6-4	144-191	157-205	171-218	184-231	197-244

* Values in this table are for height without shoes and weight without clothes. To convert inches to centimeters, multiply by 2.54; to convert pounds to kilograms, multiply by 0.455. Data from Andres R, Gerontology Research Center, National Institute for Aging, Baltimore, MD.

Obesity develops because energy intake exceeds energy expenditure. Once obesity has been attained, there may be a new weight plateau in which energy intake is equivalent to expenditure and weight is stable. To lose weight, one must decrease energy intake and increase energy expenditure to disequilibrate the energy balance equation.

The three approaches to weight reduction in order of importance are diet, exercise, and drugs.

DIET

The most important component of a weight-loss program is the diet. It is necessary for persons to lower caloric intake markedly and to sustain such a reduced intake for a prolonged period. It is usually preferable to encourage patients to document what they are eating and to try to develop a diet within the framework of what each person likes and is eating. This is sometimes impossible, because dietary habits are so poor that a radical restructuring must take place. However, better compliance occurs in those in whom it can be done. This is because the patient knows and is comfortable with the foods he is already eating. A diet should be adequate nutritionally, and this can occur without supplements only on diets of 1,000 to 1,200 kcal per day or more. To do this, patients must be taught to take certain micronutrient-rich foods that they are not used to eating, such as liver, once per week. In hypocaloric diets, the nutrients most likely to be deficient are iron, folacin, vitamin B_6, and zinc. If levels fall below 1,100 kcal per day, vitamin and mineral supplements become necessary.

In general, with weight reduction, protein intake should be maintained at a high level. The reason for this is that as weight falls, it is important to lose fat and retain lean body mass. There is some obligate loss of lean body mass, but it should be kept at a minimum. Thus, protein intake should be kept at a level of 1.0 to 1.5 kcal per kilogram of ideal body weight (calculated from Table 1). This would mean 60 to 90 g or 240 to 360 kcal per day of protein for a person of 60-kg ideal weight. The protein should be of high quality. The rest of the calories should come from fat and carbohydrate. Although no particular ratio is necessary, at least 20 percent of the dietary calories should come from carbohydrate and 20 percent from fat. This is important in order to get adequate amounts of fat-soluble vitamins and essential fatty acids from the fat and to obtain some of the fiber and the antiketogenic effect that comes with taking carbohydrate.

A patient must be taught that alcohol and sweets are not major sources of essential nutrients other than energy. They must be eliminated from weight reduction diets because they add calories without providing additional essential micronutrients. Fats in general also are high-energy, low-nutrient foods and should be restricted. It is important to teach patients that fat has a caloric concentration of 9 kcal per gram and carbohydrate 4 kcal per gram. Since carbohydrate often absorbs water when it is

TABLE 2 Equivalent Fat Content, as a Percentage of Body Weight, for a Range of Values for the Sum of Four Skinfolds (Biceps, Triceps, Subscapular, and Suprailiac) of Males and Females of Different Ages

Skinfolds (mm)	*MALES (age in years)*				*FEMALES (age in years)*			
	17–29	*30–39*	*40–49*	*50+*	*16–29*	*30–39*	*40–49*	*50+*
15	4.8				10.5			
20	8.1	12.2	12.2	12.6	14.1	17.0	19.8	21.4
25	10.5	14.2	15.0	15.6	16.8	19.4	22.2	24.0
30	12.9	16.2	17.7	18.6	19.5	21.8	24.5	26.6
35	14.7	17.7	19.6	20.8	21.5	23.7	26.4	28.5
40	16.4	19.2	21.4	22.9	23.4	25.5	28.2	30.3
45	17.7	20.4	23.0	24.7	25.0	26.9	29.6	31.9
50	19.0	21.5	24.6	26.5	26.5	28.2	31.0	33.4
55	20.1	22.5	25.9	27.9	27.8	29.4	32.1	34.6
60	21.2	23.5	27.1	29.2	29.1	30.6	33.2	35.7
65	22.2	24.3	28.2	30.4	30.2	31.6	34.1	36.7
70	23.1	25.1	29.3	31.6	31.2	32.5	35.0	37.7
75	24.0	25.9	30.3	32.7	32.2	33.4	35.9	38.7
80	24.8	26.6	31.2	33.8	33.1	34.3	36.7	39.6
85	25.5	27.2	32.1	34.8	34.0	35.1	37.5	40.4
90	26.2	27.8	33.0	35.8	34.8	35.8	38.3	41.2
95	26.9	28.4	33.7	36.6	35.6	36.5	39.0	41.9
100	27.6	29.0	34.4	37.4	36.4	37.2	39.7	42.6
105	28.2	29.6	35.1	38.2	37.1	37.9	40.4	43.3
110	28.8	30.1	35.8	39.0	37.8	38.6	41.0	43.9
115	29.4	30.6	36.4	39.7	38.4	39.1	41.5	44.5
120	30.0	31.1	37.0	40.4	39.0	39.6	42.0	45.1
125	31.0	31.5	37.6	41.1	39.6	40.1	42.5	45.7
130	31.5	31.9	38.2	41.8	40.2	40.6	43.0	46.2
135	32.0	32.3	38.7	42.4	40.8	41.1	43.5	46.7
140	32.5	32.7	39.2	43.0	41.3	41.6	44.0	47.2
145	32.9	33.1	39.7	43.6	41.8	42.1	44.5	47.7
150	33.3	33.5	40.2	44.1	42.3	42.6	45.0	48.2
155	33.7	33.9	40.7	44.6	42.8	43.1	45.4	48.7
160	34.1	34.3	41.2	45.1	43.3	43.6	45.8	49.2
165	34.5	34.6	41.6	45.6	43.7	44.0	46.2	49.6
170	34.9	34.8	42.0	46.1	44.1	44.4	46.6	50.0
175	35.3					44.8	47.0	50.4
180	35.6					45.2	47.4	50.8
185	35.9					45.6	47.8	51.2
190						45.9	48.2	51.6
195						46.2	48.5	52.0
200						46.5	48.8	52.4
205							49.1	52.7
210							49.4	53.0

Durnin JVGA, Womersley J. Body fat assessed from total body density and its estimation from skinfold thickness. Br J Nutr 1974;32:77.

cooked, in fact the caloric density of carbohydrate on the plate is often 1 to 2 kcal per gram. Thus, weight for weight, eliminating fat-containing food from the diet cuts many more calories than when carbohydrate-containing food is eliminated.

Many of the more popular media-touted diets are unbalanced diets. They focus on particular types of food and prohibit or deemphasize others; and they tend to group into diets emphasizing carbohydrate or fat. These diets are popular because their sponsors invest them with magical qualities. However, the marked imbalance of macronutrients generally also creates an imbalance of micronutrients. Such unbalanced diets are clearly a mistake. Since the diet has to be followed for a long period of time during weight loss and also during weight maintenance, micronutrient deficits must be prevented.

To help the patient eat a balanced diet in micronutrients and vitamins, it is wise to use the concept of the four food groups: (1) meat, fish, poultry, and meat substitutes; (2) milk and milk products; (3) cereals and cereal products; and (4) vegetables and fruits. By selecting from these groups, adequate nutrients are obtained as follows: (1) protein, fat, niacin, iron, thiamine; (2) protein, vitamins A and D, magnesium, calcium, and zinc; (3) carbohydrate, fat, protein, thiamine, niacin, vitamin E, calcium, iron, phosphorus, magnesium, zinc, and copper;

and (4) carbohydrate, vitamins A and C, iron, and magnesium.

Although short-term, severe hypocaloric diets are popular with some persons, they are not recommended. Quick weight loss occurs, but weight regain is the rule. These diets accomplish little except for a periodic loss of water and electrolytes. They also may cause loss of more lean body mass than the more conservative diets. Diets should be recognized as being long term, to be followed not only during weight loss but also for weight maintenance. Wishful thinking that a "quick fix" is possible is a mistake.

BEHAVIORAL THERAPY

The traditional technique of handing a patient a printed 1,200- or 1,500-kcal diet, complete with specific menus and specific portion sizes, was tried for many years but was generally unsuccessful. Since the patient had no investment in the diet, he quickly dispensed with it.

As an outgrowth of that failure, behavioral therapy has come into vogue. The goal in behavioral therapy is to accomplish two things: decrease food intake and increase activity. The behavior of a person is changed in ways that are possible, by reasonable steps, in concert with a physician or group therapy leader who helps one or, preferably, a group of patients.

The first step in such therapy is to describe the behavior to be controlled. This means making the patients aware of the amount, time, and circumstances of their eating and their activity (or inactivity) patterns. This increases awareness, which is required before corrective measures can be instituted. The second step is to practice control over stimuli that affect eating behavior. Typical stimuli would be persons or situations that increase stress, anxiety, or hostility. The particular stimuli need to be identified and an effort made to distance oneself from them. The third step is to develop techniques to control the act of eating. These include the places one eats, the speed of eating, the size of mouthfuls, the number of times eating occurs, and the attention paid to eating. Some therapists have suggested that prompt reinforcement of behaviors that delay or control eating are helpful. This would mean setting up some reward system (e.g., money, entertainment) as positive reinforcement for improved behavior.

The program is adapted to a patient's goals and skills rather than to a physician's idea of how a patient should behave. This individualization of treatment enhances the chances for success in a motivated person.

The advantage of a behavioral approach is that both patient and therapist (which may include the group) focus on the specific environmental variables that seem to govern a particular person's behavior. As Stunkard has suggested, "central to a behavioral analysis is the search by patient and therapist for solutions to problems which are at the same time both relatively modest and potentially soluble." This simplifies and focuses therapy. It has been the experience in the weight control program at St. Luke's-Roosevelt Hospital Center that conducting behavioral therapy in a group setting is highly efficacious. The group setting leads to a kind of inquiry and mutual support and encouragement that is conducive to success.

Another advantage of a behavioral approach is that by giving the patient the major responsibility for the weight loss strategy the patient can attribute increased power to himself. This tends to reinforce the treatment, since when subjects believe that the positive results are due to their own efforts, they gain increased confidence and desire to continue.

The final and most important advantage of a behavioral approach is that it allows patients to learn to eat under the natural social and environmental conditions with which they live day to day. Thus, the habits learned during weight loss can be continued during the difficult period of weight maintenance. This is not possible in programs of low calorie formula diets in which the patient is taken off natural foods for a period of time and then is suddenly confronted with returning to regular food and having to modify behavior at that point. The learning then comes too little and too late and most often leads to failure and weight gain.

It must be remembered that a behavioral program produces the slowest initial weight loss because calorie reduction is not radical and patients are encouraged to eat a hypocaloric but balanced and sensible diet. Patients must be advised to develop a long-term view. Goal weights should be set and perseverance encouraged. It is imperative that the patient remain in the treatment program until the goal weight is achieved and he or she is well into the weight maintenance period.

EXERCISE

Because exercise expends calories, it is a logical part of any weight-loss program. Overweight persons are generally very inactive, spending much of their day sitting or lying down. Many of them, particularly the heavier ones, have a real problem walking even short distances and climbing steps and tend to avoid occasions that require this. By staying as sedentary as they do, they are essentially almost at resting metabolic rate for most of the day. These persons must be taught to first walk, then walk faster, then run or cycle or do aerobic dance. An exercise program must start slowly. If an obese person is pushed too rapidly, discomfort and avoidance occurs. Careful observation for treatment of intertrigo, dependent edema, and foot or joint injuries is mandatory.

It is helpful to educate the patient about how many calories are spent in an individual exercise activity (Table 3). Most tables of calorie expenditure with given levels of activity have been compiled giving total caloric expenditure, not the amount over the basal metabolic rate. As a result, the caloric contribution of exercise must be calculated as the difference between the calories expended per minute while exercising and the calories the person would have expended just sitting. It is instructive and often disappointing to patients to discover just how much exercise they must do to expend a significant number of

TABLE 3 Approximate Energy Expenditure in Selected Activities for People of Different Weights (kcal per 30 minutes)

Activity	*Weight (pounds)*					
	110	*130*	*150*	*170*	*190*	*210*
Aerobic dancing						
Walking pace	99	114	132	150	168	186
Jogging pace	159	186	213	243	270	300
Running pace	204	240	276	315	351	387
Basketball	207	243	282	318	357	396
Canoeing—leisure	66	78	90	102	114	126
Canoeing—racing	156	183	210	237	267	294
Carpentry	78	93	105	120	135	147
Cycling—5.5 mph	96	114	132	147	165	183
Cycling—9.4 mph	150	177	204	231	258	285
Dancing—ballroom	78	90	105	117	132	144
Dancing—disco	156	183	210	237	267	294
Gardening	150	177	204	231	258	285
Golf	129	150	174	195	219	243
Judo	294	345	399	450	504	558
Lying or sitting down	33	39	45	51	57	63
Mopping floor	96	105	120	138	153	171
Running						
11.5 minutes per mile	204	240	276	315	351	387
9 minutes per mile	291	342	393	447	498	552
7 minutes per mile	366	417	468	522	573	624
5.5 minutes per mile	435	513	591	669	747	828
Skiing, cross-country	216	252	291	330	369	408
Standing quietly	39	45	51	57	66	72
Swimming						
Backstroke	255	300	345	390	435	486
Crawl	192	228	261	297	330	366
Table tennis	102	120	138	156	174	195
Tennis	165	192	222	252	282	312
Walking						
3 mph	102	114	126	138	153	165
4 mph	120	141	162	186	207	228

Adapted from Gutin B. The high energy factor. New York: Random House, 1983.

calories. For instance, if an overweight woman's basal metabolic rate is 1,400 kcal per day, lying down awake she expends 1.1 kcal per minute; sitting, about 1.2 kcal per minute; walking slowly, about 1.9 kcal per minute; and walking on a treadmill at 4.0 mph, 7.2 kcal per minute. Thus, the difference in caloric expenditure between sitting quietly and walking fast on a treadmill (at 4.0 mph) is 6.0 kcal per minute. In an hour, then, the calories expended by walking 4 miles is only 360 kcal higher than the subject would have expended just quietly sitting. It is important to emphasize that a significant and persistent commitment to exercise must be present for it to have any substantial effect on caloric balance and weight loss.

DRUGS

Although drugs have a definite role in weight-loss programs, they are often overused and abused. The important point about drug therapy is that it is never primary but always adjunctive. It should under no circumstances ever be the sole therapy but should always be used in conjunction with diet and exercise. Three principles must be kept in mind by the physician: First, tolerance occurs to many of the drugs used by many people, so that increasing doses may be necessary with time; second, only a modest effect on appetite occurs, so that using drugs as sole therapy will not work; third, all of the drugs have side effects and since it is unclear that any one drug is more effective than another, it seems reasonable to use those drugs that seem to have less potential for side effects, including the side effects of addiction or abuse.

The anorectic drugs have a central mode of action. Aside from mazindol, they share in common a phenethylamine group in their molecules. Amphetamine and its analogues (metamphetamine, phenmetrazine, phendimetrazine, benzphetamine, phenylpropanolamine, chlorphentermine, clortermine, diethylpropion, and phentermine) exert anorexia via brain catecholamines. Dopaminergic mechanisms also may be involved. Side effects of these drugs are insomnia, excitement, agitation, headache, tremor, dizziness, dry mouth, impotence, hallucinations, confusion, palpitations, tachycardia, assaultiveness, and panic. Fenfluramine is different in that its action is thought to be mediated via central serotoninergic satiety systems. It is not a stimulant but in fact is a sedative. Side effects are drowsiness and diarrhea.

At present, it is not possible to predict who will or will not have side effects of drug therapy and what they will be. Good therapeutic practice mandates that an appetite suppressant not be prescribed without a careful explanation of potential side effects. Also, it is not possible to predict who may become psychologically or physically dependent on these drugs. Careful monitoring of the patient is necessary.

While the above-mentioned drugs may be particularly helpful in getting a patient through certain difficult periods or times of weight "plateaus," they have generally not proven satisfactory in the long-term treatment of obesity.

Thyroid preparations, digitalis, and diuretics should not be used for weight loss. Inhibitors of carbohydrate absorption (α-amylase, α-glucosidase, and sucrase inhibitors) have not been successful as weight reduction agents. Interest in possible thermogenic agents is growing, but no satisfactory one is yet available.

GOALS OF THERAPY

It is common for patients beginning a weight-loss program to have faulty and unrealistic beliefs about how rapidly they can lose weight. It is important to instruct them in this regard in order to prevent disappointment and attrition.

One pound of fat is equivalent to 3,500 to 4,000 kcal. A caloric deficit of 350 kcal per day causes a 1-pound weight loss in 10 days; if the calorie deficit is 700 kcal it will take 5 days. (It may be a bit faster, because, particularly initially, a water diuresis also occurs). A diet and exercise regimen that creates a deficit of 700 to 1,000 kcal per day seems reasonable. Thus a man weighing 220 pounds whose calorie intake to maintain weight is 2,800 kcal needs to reduce intake to between 1,800 to 2,100 kcal. Such a diet should allow him to lose between 1 and 2 pounds per week assuming there is no increase in activity. It is clear that if this man's ideal body weight is 160 pounds, it will take him between 30 and 60 weeks to get to this weight. A clear realization at the start of the amount of time of sustained effort required to reach the goal is important to keep a patient motivated and positively reinforced.

WEIGHT MAINTENANCE

Maintaining weight once loss has been achieved is difficult. There is a persistent tendency to regain the weight, and there is experimental evidence, particularly in animal models, that the metabolic rate is abnormally depressed after weight loss and that lipogenic pathways enhancing the reaccretion of fat may be particularly efficient. Although diet may be liberalized after goal weight has been reached, it must be done gradually with daily weight monitoring. It is likely that a limitation of caloric intake will be required indefinitely. All the life-style changes learned during the weight-loss period should be continued, including a continuation of the exercise program.

SURGERY

Surgery may be indicated in patients who are massively obese and who have tried all other forms of therapy and have failed. Because of the significant morbidity and even mortality of the procedure, however, it is indicated only in those in whom the obesity itself or an associated condition is life threatening. The surgery should be done only in large centers with adequate support from anesthesia, pulmonary, cardiac, and metabolic divisions. Life-long follow-up is essential, and the surgeon must truly be interested in such follow-up. The surgery must be considered experimental, since no wholly adequate operation has been developed.

The initial procedure done was jejunoileal bypass, but it has been generally abandoned because its side effects were such as to make it unacceptable from a risk-benefit ratio. Problems included electrolyte and vitamin depletion, hepatic toxicity, renal stones, and polyarthritis. As a result, interest has moved to gastric procedures. In gastric bypass, a small 50-ml pouch is made in the proximal stomach with a small outlet into the small intestine, so that only a small amount of food can be eaten at any one time. In gastroplasty, a staple line partitions the stomach into two segments, which are connected by a narrow outlet. This staple line can be horizontal or vertical. Reports suggest that the side effects are less common and less serious than with the intestinal operations. However, this operation is technically more difficult to do. Also, success rates vary, and there have been quite a few failures. These can be related to poor operative technique or to a patient eating around the procedure by frequent ingestion of small meals that include high-calorie fluids.

In summary, an effective weight control program should include both a hypocaloric balanced diet and exercise presented in a behavior modification format. The program must make the patient the major agent of change. Education regarding the caloric content of foods and the caloric expenditure of various activities is important. Group therapy is often a distinct help, and drugs may be used with care as adjunctive therapy. Increasing the awareness and knowledge of the patient is key. The weight-maintenance part of the program is as important as the weight-loss part, and patients should be encouraged to stay in treatment even after goal weight has been reached.

SUGGESTED READING

Garrow JS. Treat obesity seriously. New York: Churchill Livingstone, 1981.

Sebrell WH. The nutritional adequacy of reducing diets. In: Howard A, ed. Recent advances in obesity research. London: Newman Publishing, 1975:286.

Stunkard AJ, Wadden TA. Behavior therapy and obesity. In: Conn HL Jr, DeFelice EA, Kuo P, eds. Health and obesity. New York: Raven Press, 1983:105.

Sullivan AC, Nauss-Karol C, Cheng L. Pharmacological treatment. In: Greenwood MRC, ed. Obesity. New York: Churchill Livingstone, 1983:123.

HYPERLIPOPROTEINEMIA

ELIOT A. BRINTON, M.D.

Hyperlipoproteinemia consists of an extremely heterogeneous group of abnormalities whose frequency ranges from very rare to very common and whose prognosis may range from death in infancy to pronounced longevity. The circulating lipoproteins are commonly divided by density and size into five classes. From the largest and least dense they are chylomicrons, very low density lipoprotein (VLDL), intermediate density lipoprotein (IDL), low density lipoprotein (LDL), and high density lipoprotein (HDL). These five lipoprotein classes fall into three groups according to increased, decreased, or neutral risk of atherosclerosis. Those lipoproteins positively associated with atherosclerosis are LDL, IDL, and VLDL. This association is approximately proportional to the quantity of cholesterol carried by the lipoproteins, and their link with atherosclerosis may be their tendency to transport cholesterol from the liver to peripheral tissues. In contrast, HDL is inversely associated with atherosclerosis, and this "protective" effect could relate to its ability to remove cholesterol from the periphery for transport to the liver. Elevated HDL levels, although by definition a hyperlipoproteinemia, are actually benign and are often associated with longevity. For HDL, diminished lipoprotein levels constitute the disease state. The third class of lipoproteins comprises chylomicrons, which are neutral with regard to atherosclerosis. This neutrality appears to result from a lack of effect on cholesterol stores in peripheral tissues. Chylomicrons carry dietary triglycerides from the intestines to the rest of the body and dietary cholesterol from the intestines to the liver. They are normally absent from fasting plasma. Despite the lack of atherosclerosis risk, excess chylomicrons frequently lead to abdominal pain from pancreatitis or bowel ischemia, hepatomegaly, and eruptive xanthomas, and occasionally they may cause emotional disturbances or peripheral neuropathy.

Three of the five lipoprotein fractions carry the vast majority of plasma cholesterol and are the most important in diagnosis and treatment. The total cholesterol level may be divided into these three cholesterol (C) subcategories designated by lipoprotein abbreviation: VLDL-C, LDL-C, and HDL-C. In this simplified but useful scheme, any chylomicron cholesterol is included with VLDL-C and the cholesterol of IDL is included with LDL-C. Thus, the sum of the three major fractions equals total cholesterol. For accurate assessment of these three fractions and for proper overall evaluation of lipid metabolism, three plasma measurements are required: triglycerides, HDL-C, and total cholesterol. Because plasma triglyceride values rise for a few hours after any fat-containing meal, blood should be sampled after an overnight fast. Even in the nonfasting state, however, a triglyceride level over 400 mg per deciliter is abnormal. The direct measurement of HDL-C is necessary for evaluation of the other lipoproteins and fortunately is widely available. In contrast, levels of the other two cholesterol subfractions, VLDL-C and LDL-C, are most practically obtained by calculations based on the three measured plasma lipid values. VLDL-C may be calculated by dividing the fasting triglyceride (TG) level by 5. This method is most accurate for a TG level below 400 mg per deciliter; however, VLDL-C may be estimated at high TG levels by dividing the TG level in excess of 700 mg per deciliter by 10 to reflect the lower cholesterol content of chylomicrons:

$$\text{VLDL-C} = \text{fasting TG} \div 5 \text{ (TG in excess of 700 is} \div 10)$$

LDL-C may then be estimated with some accuracy by subtracting VLDL-C and HDL-C from total cholesterol:

$$\text{LDL-C} = \text{total cholesterol} - \text{VLDL-C} - \text{HDL-C}$$

The usefulness of this method in assessing the contribution of the three cholesterol subfractions to total cholesterol is illustrated by the following examples:

$$\text{Total cholesterol} = 265 \text{ mg/dl, TG} = 125 \text{ mg/dl, HDL-C} = 40 \text{ mg/dl}$$
$$\text{VLDL-C} = 125 \div 5 = 25 \text{ mg/dl}$$
$$\text{LDL-C} = 265 - 25 - 40 = 200 \text{ mg/dl}$$

This patient has a high total cholesterol level secondary to an elevated LDL-C value, which is the most common and dangerous form of hypercholesterolemia. The patient requires vigorous LDL-lowering treatment, especially if he has other significant risk factors or is young.

A second example illustrates a different disorder:

$$\text{Total cholesterol} = 265 \text{ mg/dl, TG} = 900 \text{ mg/dl, HDL-C} = 20 \text{ mg/dl}$$
$$\text{VLDL-C} = (700 \div 5) + (200 \div 10) = 140 + 20 = 160 \text{ mg/dl}$$
$$\text{LDL-C} = 265 - 160 - 20 = 85 \text{ mg/dl}$$

For this patient, the high cholesterol level is due to elevated VLDL-C (including some chylomicrons) with low-normal LDL and very low HDL-C. If his triglyceride level increases, he will run a significant risk of pancreatitis and other hypertriglyceridemic complications. He also probably has an elevated risk of atherosclerosis and for both reasons should have therapy to lower his triglyceride levels.

The third example shows a contrasting case:

$$\text{Total cholesterol} = 265 \text{ mg/dl, TG} = 150 \text{ mg/dl, HDL-C} = 95 \text{ mg/dl}$$
$$\text{VLDL-C} = 150 \div 5 = 30 \text{ mg/dl}$$
$$\text{LDL-C} = 265 - 30 - 95 = 140 \text{ mg/dl}$$

This patient with an elevated total cholesterol value is found to have elevated HDL-C and normal LDL-C levels. His risk of atherosclerosis is low and he requires no treatment.

Each of these patients has an identical elevation of the total cholesterol value, but it is attributable to a different lipoprotein subfraction, carries a different prognosis, and requires a different management approach. Thus, it is essential to go beyond the measurement of total cholesterol and triglyceride alone. The range of normal by age and sex for cholesterol and triglyceride and the three cholesterol subfractions is given in Table 1; however, the optimal range for LDL-C is often lower as will be discussed.

In contrast to the sample cases, equivalent increases of both cholesterol and triglycerides may occasionally coexist. This suggests the presence of cholesterol-rich "beta" VLDL (type III hyperlipoproteinemia), elevated IDL, or simultaneous elevations of both VLDL and LDL.

TREATMENT OPTIONS

Dietary Intervention

Dietary modification is the cornerstone of all lipid-lowering treatment. In all cases of primary hypercholesterolemia and in most other cases in which the major goal is prevention or treatment of atherosclerosis, the most important single change is a reduction in saturated fat intake. Despite concerns about the palatability and efficacy of a low saturated fat diet, two important facts establish its primacy in cholesterol lowering. First, LDL decreases appreciably in nearly all patients, allowing reduction or elimination of a drug regimen. Second, in societies with

TABLE 1 Normal Lipoprotein Values (mg/dl): 10th to 90th Percentile for Age and Sex

Sex	*Age*	*Total Cholesterol*	*Triglyceride*	*VLDL-C*	*LDL-C*	*HDL-C*
Males	20–39	143–226	54–195	7–34	82–159	32–58
	40–59	168–258	70–231	8–43	102–184	32–61
	60+	168–263	66–207	3–35	103–190	33–71
Females	20–39	141–221	45–146	3–25	75–149	39–73
	40–59	168–261	57–190	5–33	91–181	41–83
	60+	182–277	66–207	3–32	104–195	40–85

Adapted from the Lipid Research Clinic's Prevalence Study, 1980.

low saturated fat intake atherosclerosis is uncommon and several populations have experienced increases or decreases in the incidence of atherosclerosis concordant with like changes in dietary saturated fat. Although the primary sources of saturated fat in the Western diet are red meats and dairy products, three common vegetable oils, coconut, palm, and palm kernel, are also high in saturated fat and should be avoided as much as possible. Unfortunately, their widespread use in restaurants and in prepared foods and snacks, in addition to ambiguous, misleading, or absent food labeling, makes restriction of intake difficult. Restriction of cholesterol in the diet is on average less potent in reducing plasma cholesterol levels than decreased saturated fat, and in some patients it may even appear to be without effect. Nevertheless, moderation of cholesterol intake is generally important, more so because cholesterol usually is found in foods with significant amounts of saturated fat. A few exceptions to this rule warrant specific mention. Egg yolks and organ meats are not particularly high in saturated fat but they are rich in cholesterol and should be avoided as much as possible. In contrast, most seafood, including shellfish, contains sufficient polyunsaturates that its cholesterol content may be ignored. Since LDL-C at any given time is a function of the average saturated fat and cholesterol intake over the preceding 1 or 2 weeks, occasional indulgence in "forbidden" foods has relatively little adverse effect and may greatly enhance long-term compliance to an otherwise strict dietary regimen.

In hypertriglyceridemia, isocaloric substitution of fat for carbohydrate or vice versa is effective only in certain specific situations. On the other hand, restriction of total calories is usually potent in lowering triglycerides. In addition, decreased intake of alcohol and sugar as well as liberal intake of fish and dietary fiber are often useful. In contrast, purified and concentrated supplements of fiber and fish oil, while perhaps more efficacious in some applications than their naturally occurring counterparts, may cause significant side effects. Their use should not be considered routine until further testing better establishes their long-term benefits and safety.

Medications

A variety of lipid-lowering drugs are now available. Because chronic preventive therapy in asymptomatic patients is commonly required, ease of administration, side effects, cost, long-term efficacy, and safety are of great importance in drug usefulness. A list of drugs by general categories with dosage and cost is given in Table 2. A more detailed discussion of their use follows.

LDL Lowering Drugs

The bile acid-binding resins cholestyramine (Questran) and colestipol (Colestid) are the agents most commonly prescribed for lowering of LDL. They lower LDL over a range of 10 to 50 percent, although they frequently increase triglyceride levels, at least temporarily. These drugs cause only a slight increase in HDL levels, but this increase is reported to contribute to their antiatherogenic effect. Their primary action is to bind bile acids and sterols in the proximal small intestine and prevent their reabsorption in the ileum. Because most of the bile is ordinarily reabsorbed for reuse by the liver, this intestinal loss greatly increases bile turnover and requires a large increase in bile synthesis. Since bile consists mostly of cholesterol or cholesterol products, there is a large increase in cholesterol use by the liver. This increased demand for cholesterol is met in part by increased hepatic clearance of plasma LDL via LDL receptor up-regulation, which lowers plasma LDL levels. The large prospective Lipid Research Clinic's trial found that LDL lowering by cholestyramine lowered cardiac and overall mortality in high-risk males. Because the resins are not absorbed, their side effects are usually limited to the gastrointestinal tract. Yellow dye, however, is present in Questran and may cause an allergic reaction in susceptible patients. Colestid has no added dye and can be substituted in these cases. Constipation occurs to some degree in most patients and may be severe; however, in almost every case it can be completely prevented or controlled by regular use of a bulk laxative such as wheat bran. It is rarely necessary for the physi-

TABLE 2 Lipid Lowering Drugs

	Generic (trade) Drug Name	*Average Dose (Usual Range)*	*Dosage Form*	*Monthly Cost of Average Dose**
Cholesterol lowering	Colestipol	10 g b.i.d.	5-g packet	$ 60
	(Colestid)	(5 g b.i.d. to 10 g t.i.d.)	5-g scoop	57
	Cholestyramine	8 g b.i.d.	4-g packet	90
	(Questran)	(4 g b.i.d. to 8 g t.i.d.)	4-g scoop	41
	Niacin	1,000 mg t.i.d.	500-mg tablet or capsule	
	(Nicobid)	(500 to 2,000 mg t.i.d.)	Timed release	72
	(Nicolar)		Regular release	50
	(generic)		Both forms	5
	Lovastatin	20 mg b.i.d.	20-mg tablet	75
	(Mevacor)	(20 mg h.s. to 40 mg b.i.d.)		
	Probucol	500 mg b.i.d.	250-mg tablet	47
	(Lorelco)	(250 to 500 mg b.i.d.)		
	Neomycin	1,000 mg b.i.d.	500-mg tablet	19
		(500 to 1,000 mg b.i.d.)		
	D-thyroxine	4 mg q.d.	4-mg tablet	23
	(Choloxin)	(4 to 8 mg q.d.)		
Triglyceride lowering	Gemfibrozil	600 mg b.i.d.	300-mg capsule	42
	(Lopid)	(300 to 600 mg b.i.d.)		
	Clofibrate	1,000 mg b.i.d.	500-mg capsule	32
	(Atromid S)	(500 to 1,000 mg b.i.d.)		
Cholesterol and triglyceride lowering	Niacin	see Cholesterol lowering		
	Lovastatin	see Cholesterol lowering		
	Gemfibrozil	see Triglyceride lowering		
	Clofibrate	see Triglyceride lowering		

*U.S. average wholesale price, 1987.

cian to withdraw these drugs, but patients may fail to comply in long-term use because of the expense and inconvenience and the disagreeable sandy texture of the resin powders.

Niacin (also called nicotinic acid, marketed as Nicobid, Nicolar, and others) constitutes another major type of LDL-lowering agent. Although it is a vitamin, it lowers lipid levels only in doses over a hundredfold higher than the usual vitamin requirements. Furthermore, niacinamide, while equally potent as a vitamin, has no effect on plasma lipids. Niacin is unique among well established lipid-lowering drugs in that it favorably affects all of the three major classes of lipoproteins: lowering VLDL and fasting plasma triglyceride levels in the range of 20 to 80 percent and lowering LDL levels to 10 to 20 percent while raising "protective" HDL levels from 10 to 50 percent. Its mechanisms of action appear to be primarily lowering of VLDL production by the liver and decreasing of HDL catabolism. LDL lowering results from decreased availability of its precursor VLDL. Presumably as a result of naicin's favorable effect on plasma lipoprotein levels, the Coronary Drug Project study showed that it reduces the incidence of both fatal and nonfatal coronary atherosclerosis and lowers overall mortality. Despite being the most widely applicable and also the least expensive lipid-lowering drug, its use is somewhat limited because of its frequent and bothersome side effects. When beginning niacin therapy, most patients notice transitory flushing of the face and trunk often accompanied by itching. This may be minimized by taking the drug with meals, by using the timed-release form (Nicobid and others) or by taking aspirin 30 minutes before the dose. Most importantly, one should start at a very low dose, such as 50 to 100 mg twice daily, and increase the amount gradually to allow development of tolerance to the flushing. A small number of patients may experience hyperuricemia, hyperglycemia, or peptic ulcer disease. Patients may develop elevated liver enzyme levels that are of concern only if greater than two to three times the upper limit of normal. Occasionally, this may present with the abrupt onset of severe nausea and weakness. When significant side effects occur, niacin must be discontinued, although a retrial might be attempted later at lower doses. The late-onset metabolic and gastrointestinal side effects appear to be less common with the regular-release form (Nicolar and others). Early- and late-onset side effects may be minimized by a regimen of timed-release niacin for the first month or so, then on nearing full dosage, a change to an equal dose of the regular-release form. With proper management and education, the majority of patients tolerate niacin well in chronic use. Furthermore, any significant side effects are readily reversible on discontinuation of the drug and there is no significant drug-related mortality.

Lovastatin (former generic name, mevinolin; trade name, Mevacor) is the first and only currently available cholesterol synthesis inhibitor, having been approved in 1987 by the Food and Drug Administration (FDA). By inhibiting hepatic cholesterol synthesis, lovastatin forces the liver to increase its uptake of lipoprotein cholesterol. This is achieved by up-regulated LDL receptor activity, which increases LDL fractional catabolic rate and lowers LDL levels. Except for a few resistant patients, lovastatin lowers LDL by 20 to 70 percent, exceeding the efficacy of the bile acid-binding resins or niacin. Furthermore, patient acceptance of lovastatin is far greater than for either of these standard cholesterol-lowering drugs. Lowering of triglyceride levels often occurs in contrast to the triglyceride elevation seen with the resins. The effect on HDL is small but tends to be positive. Despite these many promising aspects, early short-term studies in human subjects have also revealed some potentially significant side effects. Myositis with muscle pain and elevated serum creatine phosphokinase levels (CPK) may occur, often related to exertion or minor trauma. One case of rhabdomyolysis with acute renal failure has been reported. Elevated serum levels of liver enzymes may also occur, although these are rarely accompanied by symptoms of hepatitis. If any of these side effects becomes severe, therapy with lovastatin must be discontinued. Fortunately, the side effects appear reversible on termination of the drug. Cataract development has also been noted after lovastatin treatment, but the frequency and causality of this event are unclear. Despite these potential complications (and the resulting lack of "blanket approval" by the FDA), lovastatin has received extensive positive publicity and it will be prescribed frequently in the very near future. If after widespread use it is found to be safe and to prevent or reverse atherosclerosis, it will become the drug of choice for LDL excess and possibly other lipid disorders as well. Nevertheless, for the first few years of its availability, it is wise to reserve it for patients who cannot tolerate or fail to respond adequately to established diet and drug regimens. If the frequency or seriousness of side effects ultimately preclude its general use, it still will have narrow but important clinical application as an alternative or adjunct to other LDL-lowering therapy.

Probucol (Lorelco), a lipid-soluble drug, associates with LDL particles and accelerates their catabolism. As with niacin, the decrease in LDL is independent of the LDL receptor since efficacy is not diminished in receptor-absent states. LDL levels decrease only 5 to 20 percent, however, and the "protective" HDL fraction usually decreases to a greater degree, while triglyceride levels are usually unaffected. Because several epidemiologic studies have suggested that the LDL:HDL ratio is an important positive predictor of atherosclerosis risk, probucol's tendency to increase this ratio has greatly dampened enthusiasm for its use. Nevertheless, aside from its impact on lipid levels, probucol exerts a powerful influence against peroxidation of LDL lipids. There is considerable in vitro evidence that this antioxidant effect may protect against atherogenesis, and in two recent animal studies large decreases in atherosclerosis in vivo were shown as well. Interestingly, the protection occurred without a significant lipid effect in the animals, suggesting that the lackluster or even "adverse" lipid changes seen in humans may be irrelevant. Furthermore, a recent clinical study suggests probucol has a favorable effect on human atherosclerosis. Given its low side-effect profile, largely limited to occasional gastrointestinal discomfort, and evidence of its long-term safety, probucol may have great potential in prevention and treatment of atherosclerosis beyond its effect on plasma lipoprotein levels. Further clinical trials now in progress may confirm these important findings.

Neomycin is infrequently used as a cholesterol-lowering drug. It is an aminoglycoside antibiotic poorly absorbed from the intestine that, taken orally, binds bile acids in the gut. Its primary mode of action, therefore, is similar to that of the bile acid-binding resins, although its LDL lowering efficacy (decreases of 10 to 20 percent) is somewhat less. There are, in fact, several important differences between neomycin and the resins. Neomycin's potential advantages include a second mechanism for LDL lowering (decreased production), greater dosage convenience, an absence of constipation as a side effect, and considerable savings in price. Its drawbacks, in addition to lower efficacy, include a lack of synergistic or even additive effects with niacin or lovastatin, the potential for renal toxicity or ototoxicity, possible diarrhea, and a lack of data showing a reduction of atherosclerosis and overall mortality. Patients should have serum creatinine determinations and hearing tests before treatment and at least annually while on the drug, and it must be discontinued on significant deterioration of either parameter. Neomycin seems best considered an alternative for treatment of unusual cases rather than a first-line drug.

Dextrothyroxine is occasionally prescribed for lowering of cholesterol levels. Unfortunately, the change from the L to D stereoisomer seems of little help in separating lipid lowering from the other properties of thyroxine. Even when given cautiously to avoid symptoms of hyperthyroidism, there remains a significant risk of unmasking or exacerbating angina or other vascular insufficiency syndromes. In the one large trial studying its use, dextrothyroxine was quickly withdrawn because of the frequency and seriousness of adverse effects. Given the safer and more clearly effective alternatives available, use of this drug is rarely if ever indicated and its routine use is discouraged.

VLDL Lowering Drugs

One main class of drugs that lower VLDL levels is the fibric acid derivatives, which include clofibrate (Atromid S) and gemfibrozil (Lopid). They are almost always dramatically effective in lowering triglyceride and VLDL levels, often completely to the normal range. They also may raise HDL levels significantly (10 to 50 percent), although this effect is less with clofibrate. The mechanism of VLDL lowering appears to be decreased synthesis while HDL synthesis increases. LDL levels may be lowered but only in hypercholesterolemia. In treatment of hypertriglyceridemia, LDL levels usually increase substantially, although the total cholesterol level is often lowered because of the consistency and magnitude of VLDL cholesterol lowering. Symptomatic side effects are usually limited to an occasional episode of mild gastrointestinal distress. In the multicenter European World Health Organization study, clofibrate was given to a large number of patients with high cholesterol levels. Despite its poor efficacy as an LDL lowering agent, it reduced the incidence of nonfatal myocardial infarction proportional to cholesterol lowering. Unfortunately, cardiac sudden death and hepatobiliary mortality were higher with clofibrate, so overall survival did not improve. In the other major clinical trial of clofibrate, the Coronary Drug Project, only a nonsignificant trend toward decreased atherosclerotic complications was seen and there was no correlation with triglyceride reduction. Given the availability of safer and more effective lipid-lowering drugs, the general use of clofibrate is discouraged. However, in cases of type III hyperlipoproteinemia, in which clofibrate rapidly normalizes the lipid profile and may decrease morbidity and mortality, and in severe hypertriglyceridemia, in which it can prevent life-threatening pancreatitis, its use appears justified. In the recent prospective Helsinki Heart Study, gemfibrozil was associated with a 34 percent decline in the incidence of coronary heart disease. The drug showed no hepatobiliary or other serious side effects, in contrast to previous results with clofibrate. Unfortunately, 91 percent of the 4,081 men studied had hypercholesterolemia, for which two better-established treatments were already available. Not enough patients with elevated triglyceride and VLDL values were treated to show whether gemfibrozil may prevent atherosclerosis in this disorder; furthermore, since the drug raises LDL in these cases, such prevention cannot be assumed. Therefore, gemfibrozil should not yet be broadly recommended for atherosclerosis prevention in mild to moderate hypertriglyceridemia. It is, however, indicated for avoiding acute complications of severe hypertriglyceridemia and it may serve as an alternative to the resins and niacin in mild hypercholesterolemia.

The other major drug available for triglyceride lowering is niacin. Because of greater side effects and generally lower efficacy, this drug has been less often used for this purpose except when cholesterol levels are also elevated or when the patient fails to respond to a fibric acid derivative. However, another important indication may be the presence of mild to moderate hypertriglyceridemia as the sole lipid risk factor when the patient's personal or family history is positive for premature atherosclerosis.

With wider clinical experience, lovastatin may also prove to be a useful triglyceride-lowering drug. However, it cannot yet be recommended as a primary treatment for isolated hypertriglyceridemia.

HDL Raising Drugs

Two of the principal triglyceride-lowering drugs, gemfibrozil and niacin, also usually raise HDL levels. Their average efficacy is comparable, but HDL increases may vary between 10 and 50 percent, and the effect of the two drugs may be quite dissimilar in a given patient. Although niacin is somewhat better established both regarding efficacy against atherosclerosis and long-term safety, gemfibrozil is usually better tolerated. Unfortunately, in neither case has elevation of HDL been proven to play an important role in their prevention of vascular disease.

Extracorporeal Lipoprotein Removal

Plasma exchange has been used to lower LDL in cases of severe excess, but more specific means of direct removal of plasma LDL are now available. Plasmapheresis with exposure of plasma to an affinity column containing either heparin or anti-LDL antibodies rapidly removes almost all of the apo B containing lipoproteins (VLDL, IDL, and LDL) while leaving most of the HDL and other beneficial plasma components. These methods, often called LDL-pheresis, may lower even extreme LDL levels by 30 to 60 percent when used frequently over time, and they often provide the additional apparent benefit of increased HDL levels by an unknown mechanism. Nevertheless, their expense, inconvenience, and lack of widespread availability relegate them to use in a research context or in severe cases such as homozygous familial hypercholesterolemia.

Surgery

Three surgical procedures have been used in the treatment of elevated LDL levels. Ileal bypass is the surgical equivalent of the bile acid–binding resins in that it acts primarily by preventing reabsorption of bile from the gut. Although it is potentially useful in common polygenic hypercholesterolemia, operative complications and chronic side effects such as diarrhea and malabsorption have limited its application to a small number of severe cases. In the presence of ongoing advances in single- and multiple-drug treatment, this operation will likely continue to decline in usefulness.

Portacaval shunt acts somewhat like niacin in that it lowers VLDL and LDL levels by causing a decrease in hepatic VLDL synthesis and in that it also raises HDL levels, although the mechanism of the latter is not known. Probably as a result of these lipoprotein changes, body cholesterol pools have been shown to decrease postoperatively. Unfortunately, morbidity and mortality of the operation, as well as problems with long-term shunt patency, have limited this treatment to a few rare situations, such as homozygous familial hypercholesterolemia, in which extremely high LDL levels and a lack of LDL receptors render most other treatments ineffective or insufficient.

Liver transplantation from a normolipidemic cadaver donor has been successfully performed for homozygous familial hypercholesterolemia. Although, theoretically, it would be curative in a wide variety of disorders of hepatic lipid metabolism, the many acute and chronic dangers given current techniques, the expense, and the lack of donor organs clearly restrict this operation to experimental status for the near future.

PREFERRED APPROACH

A summary of the clinical presentation, etiology and treatment of the major lipid disorders is given in Table 3.

TABLE 3 Diagnosis and Treatment of Lipid Disorders

	Typical Plasma Lipid Levels (mg/dl)					*Treatment*		
							Medical and Surgical	
Disorder Name or Phenotype	*Cholesterol*	*Triglyceride*	*Lipoproteins in Excess*	*Clinical Risk**	*Causes*	*Dietary*	*First Choice*	*Alternative*
Hypercholesterolemias (all type IIa)								
Polygenic or secondary	250–400	50–250	LDL[†]	++CAD +AFD	Polygenic and/or secondary hypothyroidism (rarely nephrotic syndrome, biliary obstruction or dysglobulinemia)	Decreased saturated fat and cholesterol	Bile acid binding resin[‡]	Niacin, gemfibrozil, lovastatin,[§] probucol,[§] neomycin
Familial (heterozygote)	300–500	50–250	LDL	+++CAD +AFD	LDL receptor deficiency, monogenic codominant	Strict decrease in saturated fat and cholesterol	Bile acid-binding resin plus niacin	Lovastatin,[§] alone or with bile acid-binding resin; partial ileal bypass
Familial (homozygote)	450–900	50–250	LDL	++++CAD ++AFD	LDL receptor absence; monogenic codominant	Very strict decrease in saturated fat and cholesterol	LDL-pheresis	Niacin and/or probucol,[§] portocaval shunt
Hypertriglyceridemias								
Type I (lipoprotein lipase deficiency)	180–800	2,000–10,000	Chylomicrons (HDL strikingly decreased)	++++pancr	Deficiency of lipoprotein lipase activity, monogenic recessive	Very low fat (< 20% of calories), may supplement with medium-chain triglyceride oil	None	None
Type V[#]	250–1,200	700–7,000	Chylomicrons, VLDL (HDL strikingly decreased)	++pancr +to++CAD +AFD	Monogenic dominant or polygenic plus secondary factors: obesity, diabetes, alcohol, hypothyroidism (rarely estrogens)	Decreased calories (if obese), alcohol and sugar; increased fish and fiber	Gemfibrozil[‡]	Clofibrate, niacin
Type IV[#]	180–300	250–700	VLDL (HDL mildly decreased)	+to++CAD +AFD	As type V plus additional secondary factors: uremia, nephrotic syndrome, dysglobulinemias, glucocorticoids, or use of thiazide diuretics or beta-adrenergic blockers	As for type V	Niacin[‡]	Gemfibrozil[§]
Combined elevations of triglycerides and cholesterol								
Type III (familial dysbetalipoproteinemia)	250–600	250–600	Chylomicron remnants and IDL	+++CAD +++AFD	Abnormal apo E, monogenic recessive, plus unknown second factor	As for polygenic type IIa hypercholesterolemia, plus decreased calories (if obese)	Clofibrate	Niacin, gemfibrozil
Familial combined hyperlipidemia (hyperapobetalipoproteinemia	180–500	100–500	LDL and/or VLDL	++CAD	Possibly oversynthesis of apo B, monogenic dominant	As for polygenic type IIa hypercholesterolemia	Niacin	Bile acid binding resin, gemfibrozil,[§] lovastatin[§]

* Pancr, pancreatitis or other abdominal pain, neuropathy; CAD, coronary artery disease; AFD, aortofemoral disease; +mild risk; ++moderate risk; +++marked risk; ++++severe risk even in childhood.

† Rare cases due to excess HDL levels with normal LDL levels carry no risk and require no treatment.

‡ Drug treatment of this disorder should be reserved for cases in which available treatment of secondary causes is ineffective in normalizing the lipid levels.

§ Overall benefit from this drug in this case is unclear pending results of long-term studies.

\# Depending on the status of secondary factors and diet, a patient may interconvert between type IV and V; treatment should be based on the phenotype present after optimizing these factors.

A more detailed narrative explanation of treatment strategy follows.

When a high level of cholesterol or a mild-to-moderate elevation of triglyceride is first noted in a patient, the making of a firm diagnosis and the initiation of treatment can and should await testing of a second and possible third blood drawing at 2- to 4-week intervals. Given the indolent nature of atherogenesis, a delay in treatment of true chronic hyperlipidemia for even 2 to 4 months should have no adverse consequences. On the other hand, in the occasional case of laboratory error, acute physical or emotional stress, or temporary dietary indiscretion, the delay prevents erroneous diagnosis and unnecessary treatment. These same considerations also hold when evaluating response to dietary and pharmacologic therapy; repeated testing is always advisable to assess each treatment regimen employed. On initial presentation of the patient, the presence of hyperlipidemia should be confirmed and measurements or estimations of the various lipoprotein fractions made to reveal its extent and degree. The patient should be carefully educated in the appropriate diet and the prompt cessation of smoking. Also, hypertension and the secondary causes of hyperlipidemia (see Table 3) must either be excluded or treated. Considerable training, encouragement, and follow-up are usually required to attain a diet that is both optimally controlled and yet flexible and reasonable enough for lifetime use. Even in the ideal clinic setting, patients vary greatly in their willingness and ability to comply with dietary recommendations. This wide variety in dietary compliance coupled with the tremendous variability in physiologic response to a given dietary modification renders it impossible to predict the ultimate degree of dietary response. Depending on the number of remediable factors and the extent and speed of the changes made, one may need to follow the lipid levels for 3 to 6 months or longer before seeing the final response to altered life-style. If the levels thus obtained fail to reach the treatment goal, drug treatment, or rarely surgery, becomes necessary.

One very important exception to this approach is severe hypertriglyceridemia with levels greater than 1,000 mg per deciliter. Because of the risk of acute pancreatitis, which may be fatal, prompt assessment and treatment is necessary. A rapid provisional diagnosis is made by observing densely lipemic plasma. Immediate institution of appropriate diet and drug regimens ordinarily brings the triglycerides into a safe range within several days, at which time the usual follow-up schedule may be instituted.

Hypercholesterolemia

In the common case of moderate LDL excess and normal triglyceride levels (type IIa disease), which persists after optimal dietary intervention, the best agents have been the bile acid–binding resins cholestyramine and colestipol (4 or 5 g, respectively, per packet or scoop). The usual dosage is 1 to 2 packets three times daily, preferably taken at the start of each meal. In some cases niacin, 1 to 2 g three times daily, is as effective; however, because of its many side effects, it may be reserved for cases of resin failure or of concurrent hypertriglyceridemia and/or low HDL levels. Lovastatin is a good alternative in moderate to severe hypercholesterolemia when resistance or side effects preclude success with the first-line drugs. Experience with lovastatin over the next few years with widespread clinical use may prove it to be the drug of choice for high LDL levels; however, if significant side effects are found, it may continue to merit only secondary status. The usual regimen begins with 20 mg once daily in the evening, which may be increased to 20 or 40 mg twice daily as needed for further LDL lowering. Although gemfibrozil is not yet officially indicated for treatment of hypercholesterolemia, the Helsinki Heart Study has recently shown its efficacy in preventing coronary heart disease in patients with mild elevations of plasma cholesterol. Gemfibrozil, 600 mg twice daily, can be considered as an alternative agent for treatment or prevention of atherosclerosis in mild hypercholesterolemia. Since it usually does not normalize LDL-C levels, it may be best to add low doses of another LDL-lowering drug. If these drugs are contraindicated or ineffective, probucol, 250 to 500 mg twice daily, is an alternative medication with good patient tolerance and likely beneficial antioxidant properties counterbalanced by relatively weak LDL reduction and possibly harmful lowering of HDL levels. Neomycin is another treatment alternative but should not be used in patients with hearing deficits or renal insufficiency. Its indications are largely as for the resins, with the optimal dosage being 500 to 1,000 mg twice daily.

A combination of two or even three lipid-lowering drugs is often useful for resistance to single-drug regimens or to minimize side effects from a given drug. Nearly every conceivable combination has been tried, and most have been found beneficial under certain circumstances. For example, lower (and better tolerated) doses of niacin may be effective for elevated LDL levels if combined with a resin or probucol. The latter combination may be especially helpful in homozygous familial hypercholesterolemia. On the other hand, the addition of a fibric acid derivative or niacin to a resin may avoid the secondary increases in VLDL and triglyceride levels often noted during resin therapy. A resin may be added to probucol to enhance lowering of LDL levels and offset a decrease in HDL levels. Because of complementary modes of action, the combination of lovastatin and a resin is a potent LDL-C lowering regimen, which is particularly useful in cases of severe or resistant hypercholesterolemia, except the rare homozygous familial type. In contrast to the usual positive experience with multiple-drug regimens there are two apparently ineffective combinations: probucol plus clofibrate, and lovastatin or niacin plus neomycin. The latter drug in each pair is reported to add nothing to the LDL lowering while reducing potentially beneficial HDL levels. When lipid-lowering agents or other drugs are combined with bile acid–binding resins, the other medications should be taken at least 1 hour before or 2 hours after the resins. This is particularly important with thiazide diuretics, thyroxine, phenobarbital, warfarin, and digitalis since the resins are known to impede absorption of these drugs. If the regimen includes drugs such as niacin that should be taken with food, the patient may take those drugs immediately before a meal and the bile acid–binding resins at the end.

The assessment of cholesterol lowering first requires estimation of the LDL-C. The LDL treatment goal for a given patient depends on individual circumstances; thus, there is not just one universal target for LDL lowering but rather a range within which most cases fit. This range may be expressed as population percentiles by age and sex such as in Table 1. The LDL treatment-goal range extends from the 90th percentile (upper number of each pair in Table 1) to the 50th percentile (roughly the midpoint between each pair in Table 1). Alternatively, one may use a range of fixed LDL-C values from 180 to 120 mg per deciliter. The individual treatment goal varies within either range depending on many factors, including the patient's age, personal or family history, HDL-C and triglyceride levels, and extra risk factors such as diabetes mellitus, persistent hypertension, or smoking. In the older patient, side effects are likely to be greater and the benefit less. If the non-LDL lipid levels are normal and other risk factors for atherosclerosis are absent, the goal for the LDL level may be higher. Also, with a family history negative for atherosclerosis in relatives known to have elevated LDL levels, the atherosclerosis risk at a given LDL level would appear to be less than usual. In these cases, the treatment goal might be as high as 180 mg per deciliter or the 90th percentile for age and sex. On the other hand, in a young patient with a personal or family history of atherosclerosis and significant additional risk factors, LDL lowering as low as 120 mg per deciliter or the 50th percentile may be warranted. Although not proven, it is assumed that these guidelines for male patients apply equally to women, after allowing for the sex-related difference in atherosclerosis risk.

Excess HDL is the only other cause of normotriglyceridemic hypercholesterolemia. If HDL-C levels are high and LDL-C levels are normal, the risk of atherosclerosis is especially low and no treatment is indicated.

Hypertriglyceridemia

In the rare case of type I hyperlipidemia, the only effective treatment is strict reduction in the intake of long-chain fatty acids. Restriction of fat intake to 10 to 20 percent of total calories invariably decreases plasma triglycerides well below 1,000 mg per deciliter and, therefore, will essentially eliminate the risk of pancreatitis, bowel ischemia, hepatomegaly, eruptive xanthomas, and neuropathy. Addition of medium-chain triglyceride oil would not exacerbate the chylomicronemia and may enhance the palatability of the diet.

In the much more common case of type V disease, treatment best focuses initially on secondary causes such as obesity, diabetes, excess alcohol intake, hypothyroidism, or the use of certain medications such as thiazide diuretics or beta-adrenergic blockers lacking intrinsic sympathomimetic activity. Despite the effect of fat restriction in type I hypertriglyceridemia, this change is of limited use in type V disease. Rather, a decrease in total calories is a rapidly effective dietary maneuver in all patients at or above average body weight. A beneficial dietary adjunct is increased fish intake up to about one serving daily. Fish oil capsules might instead be tried, but owing to a lack of widespread experience their use is still somewhat experimental. Decreases of even moderate intake of alcohol and possibly of sucrose may be effective in certain cases. Increased physical activity is always helpful if the change can be maintained on a permanent basis. Long-term compliance is often best with a stationary bicycle at home in front of a television or next to a book or magazine holder. After the best achievable response from management of diet and exercise (or on initial presentation in severe cases), one may add twice-daily doses of gemfibrozil, 300 to 600 mg, or clofibrate, 500 to 1,000 mg, or, alternatively, niacin, 500 to 2,000 mg three times daily. Lovastatin may eventually prove to be another useful triglyceride-lowering drug. The minimum treatment goal should be to lower the plasma triglyceride levels well below 1,000 mg per deciliter, as for type I disease.

Below approximately 700 mg per deciliter, hypertriglyceridemia is termed type IV instead of type V (see Table 3). It is important to realize that these are not separate diseases but rather a continuum of one disease process, and many hypertriglyceridemic patients cross back and forth between the two types depending on various secondary factors. Although triglycerides approaching 1,000 mg per deciliter, must be treated to prevent abdominal and neuropathic complications, treatment of hypertriglyceridemia much into the type IV range, below about 500 mg per deciliter, must be justified on the basis of lowering the risk of atherosclerosis. Treatment of secondary factors, exercise, and dietary measures for type IV disease are basically as those for type V but may also include increased dietary fiber and should exclude the use of fish oil capsules. Decreased carbohydrate and increased fat intake usually lowers triglyceride values in patients with type IV disease, but the known hazards of high fat intake preclude its use for this purpose. Although there is no proof that pharmacologic lowering of moderate hypertriglyceridemia reduces the risk of atherosclerosis, in the presence of a personal or family history of premature atherosclerosis, medical treatment of the type IV pattern is probably indicated. Because it is known to decrease the risk of atherosclerosis and overall mortality, niacin is the first choice in this situation. Gemfibrozil is safe and well tolerated, but its effect on atherosclerosis in hypertriglyceridemia is unknown. Clofibrate and lovastatin show even less certainty of benefit. If the patient is taking thiazide diuretics or conventional beta-adrenergic blockers, triglyceride levels may decrease upon substitution with other agents, such as angiotensin-converting enzyme inhibitors, calcium-channel blockers, nitrates, or beta-adrenergic blockers with intrinsic sympathomimetic activity.

Combined Hyperlipidemia

Concurrent increases in cholesterol and triglyceride may be seen in at least two situations: type III and familial combined hyperlipidemia. The former may be suspected clinically by orange palmar creases, atherosclerosis frequently involving the peripheral vasculature, and sparing of premenopausal females and family members of both sexes under age 25. Confirmation may be obtained by lipoprotein electrophoresis showing the "broad beta" VLDL band and by apolipoprotein E phenotyping showing E_2 isoform homozygosity. Type III is traditionally and effectively treated with clofibrate; however, niacin and gemfibrozil are also effective. Drug treatment should be supplemented by weight loss in case of obesity or by low-dose estrogen supplementation in the postmenopausal female. In all cases a decrease in intake of saturated fat and cholesterol is indicated. In general, the cholesterol and triglyceride levels normalize with these treatments and significant improvement in symptoms and objective signs of atherosclerosis often occurs. Aside from type III hyperlipoproteinemia, elevated triglyceride and cholesterol levels may result from a poorly understood entity called familial combined hyperlipidemia. It can present with elevation of either cholesterol or triglyceride alone, or both together, and an excess of the major apolipoprotein of VLDL, IDL, and LDL, called apo B, may also be present. There may be still other cases of cholesterol and triglyceride elevation, including a coincidence of type V and IIa, apparenly unrelated to the other combined disorders. Nontype III disease generally responds to pharmacotherapy, but the best regimen usually cannot be determined without an empiric trial. Niacin probably should be tried first, but gemfibrozil was recently shown to be an attractive alternative. Other drugs, including clofibrate, a resin, lovastatin, or a combination of these, may also be considered.

Low HDL

Dietary intervention such as increased fish intake or substitution of monounsaturated for polyunsaturated fat and an aerobic exercise program are reported to raise HDL levels but are unlikely to have a significant effect in the ordinary clinical setting. Increases in intake of alcohol or saturated fat or use of fish oil capsules, while more potent in raising HDL levels, are potentially harmful and are therefore unwise. Given the extensive epidemiologic evidence for increased risk of atherosclerosis with low HDL levels and the limitations of nonpharmacologic means, the physician may be tempted to raise a low HDL level by drug therapy. Often the defect is associated with another lipid abnormality, and otherwise indicated treatment may normalize the HDL deficit. If a low HDL level is the sole lipoprotein problem, one must consider first that in contrast to studies of LDL lowering there is yet little proof that raising HDL levels by any method prevents atherosclerosis. Second, in a hyperlipidemic population, many patients are already on a diet low in saturated fat and cholesterol. Low HDL levels in these patients may often be entirely secondary to dietary alteration, and in such cases a low HDL level may not increase the risk of atherosclerosis.

Despite these negative considerations, the treatment of low HDL levels can be justified as potentially beneficial in high-risk patients with a personal or family history of premature atherosclerosis. Even then, however, the lack of strong evidence directly favoring this approach should be explained to the patient. Given its long-term safety and benefit, niacin is the drug of choice for this indication, although gemfibrozil is now a good alternative. Clofibrate, with its greater evidence for toxicity and its lesser efficacy in raising HDL levels, probably should not be considered. The resins and lovastatin may raise HDL levels slightly but are probably not indicated if the LDL level is competely normal.

SUGGESTED READING

American Heart Association. A joint statement of the Nutrition Committee and the Council on Arteriosclerosis of the American Heart Association: recommendations for the treatment of hyperlipidemia in adults. Circulation 1984; 69:443A–468A.

Blankenhorn DH, Nessim SA, Johnson RL, Sanmarco ME, Azen SP, Cashin-Hemphill L. Beneficial effects of combined colestipol–niacin therapy on coronary atherosclerosis and coronary venous bypass grafts. JAMA 1987; 257:3233–3240.

Brown MS, Goldstein JL. Drugs used in the treatment of hyperlipoproteinemias. In: Gilman AG, Goodman LS, Rall TW, Murad F, eds. The pharmacological basis of therapeutics, 7th ed. New York: Macmillan, 1985.

Frick MH, Elo O, Haapa K, et al. Helsinki heart study: primary-prevention trial with gemfibrozil in middle-aged men with dyslipidemia. N Engl J Med 1987; 317:1237–1245.

Kita T, Nagano Y, Yokode M, Ishii K, Kume N, Ooshima A, Yoshida H, Kawai C. Probucol prevents the progression of atherosclerosis in Watanabe heritable hyperlipidemic rabbit, an animal model for familial hypercholesterolemia. Proc Natl Acad Sci USA 1987; 84:5928–5931.

The Lovastatin Study Group II. Therapeutic response to lovastatin (mevinolin) in nonfamilial hypercholesterolemia. JAMA 1986; 256:2829–2834.

National Institutes of Health. Consensus development conference summary: treatment of hypertriglyceridemia. Arteriosclerosis 1984; 4:296–301.

Consensus Conference. Lowering blood cholesterol to prevent heart disease. JAMA 1985; 253:2080–2086.

GOUT

TS'AI-FAN YU, M.D.

Management of gout should be directed to prevention and treatment of acute gouty arthritis, tophaceous gout, uric acid nephropathy, and recurrent nephrolithiasis. With marked progress in the development of various therapeutic agents, it is important to know how to use these drugs intelligently.

TREATMENT OF ACUTE GOUTY ARTHRITIS

An attack of acute gouty arthritis must be treated with an appropriate anti-inflammatory drug without delay and in the correct dosage. An experienced sufferer of gout usually knows enough to begin taking medication even during the prodromal stage of an acute attack, and he also knows his exact degree of tolerance toward an anti-inflammatory drug. Nonetheless, the physician should guide him carefully so as to help ameliorate suffering as soon as possible and to prevent adverse reactions.

Various anti-inflammatory agents are of different chemical nature. All these agents nevertheless act as inhibitors of cyclo-oxygenase, the enzyme responsible for biosynthesis of prostaglandins, which lead to acute inflammations.

Colchicine

Colchicine used to be the sole agent for acute gouty arthritis. Owing to the introduction of new anti-inflammatory drugs and the toxic symptoms following a therapeutic course of colchicine, colchicine has lost its preeminent position.

Colchicine is an alkaloid derived from the corm and seeds of the autumn crocus (*Colchicum autumnale*). It is so named because it originally grew in Colchis, an ancient country is Asia Minor bordering the Black Sea. After oral administration, colchicine is absorbed from the gastrointestinal tract, metabolized in the liver, and excreted mostly by the bile, with approximately 20 percent excreted by the kidney. Colchicine is cleared from plasma rapidly, but it stays much longer in the leukocytes. The anti-inflammatory action of colchicine is through the inhibition of the crystal-induced chemotactic factor produced by polymorphonuclear leukocytes and a decrease in the release of lysozyme enzymes.

My experience in using colchicine to treat patients with acute gouty arthritis has been favorable. In order to avoid toxic effects of colchicine on the gastrointestinal tract, I prescribe 0.6 mg orally every 2 hours, after an initial dose of 1.2 mg. Most patients report improvement by taking colchicine, 0.6 mg every 2 hours, not to exceed five doses on day 1. The dosage may thereafter be reduced to three times a day for 1 or 2 days and finally to once or twice daily. The therapeutic program may be modified according to the progress in symptomatic relief. If the patients discontinue colchicine as soon as some suggestion of nausea or gastrointestinal discomfort appears, very few will develop alarming symptoms.

A colchicine preparation for intravenous use is available and may be employed in severe attacks, particularly if the patient is not able to tolerate the drug orally because of a coexisting gastrointestinal disorder. If given early in the course, a single injection of 0.6 or 1.2 mg is usually sufficient to terminate an attack. In some instances, a second injection of 0.6 mg or 1.2 mg may be necessary 4 to 5 hours after the first one. Although intravenously administered colchicine does not as a rule give rise to intestinal upset, nausea has been occasionally observed after repeated injections. Extravasation of colchicine could cause much pain and adjacent tissue necrosis.

Most physicians prescribe oral colchicine, 0.6 mg every hour, after an initial dose of 1.2 mg. If the drug is ordered to be given every hour until diarrhea, nausea, or vomiting develops, it may provoke a lot of unpleasant side effects. Many patients recall such experiences and develop abdominal cramps as soon as the word "colchicine" is mentioned.

Phenylbutazone

Phenylbutazone (Butazolidin), a pyrazolone derivative, is a potent anti-inflammatory agent. Following its ingestion, it is well absorbed from the gastrointestinal tract. The peak concentration in plasma is reached in 2 hours, and the biologic half-life is 72 hours in humans. Two metabolites are formed in the liver. One metabolite, oxyphenbutazone (Tandearil), formed with the introduction of a phenolic group to the *para*-position in one of the benzene rings has pharmacologic properties similar to those of phenylbutazone. With a dosage schedule of 200 mg three or four times a day for 1 or 2 days, the pain disappears promptly. Phenylbutazone is excreted after glucuronidation and hydroxylation of the phenyl rings of the butyl side chain. Phenylbutazone is extensively bound to plasma proteins. Drugs such as warfarin, oral hypoglycemics, or sulfonamides may be displaced from binding to plasma proteins by phenylbutazone, leading to increasing pharmacologic or toxic effects.

Phenylbutazone may sometimes cause bone marrow depression, but this is extremely rare after a brief period of use only. Since phenylbutazone tends to cause retention of sodium and water, its use is contraindicated in cases of cardiac insufficiency. It is also sometimes ulcerogenic. Because of such potential hazards, many physicians tend to use it in reduced dosages. As the efficacy is reduced with small dosages, an acute attack may become subacute. Accordingly, the drug may have to be used for a longer period of time, thus increasing the risk of undesirable side effects.

Indomethacin

Indomethacin (Indocin) is an indoleacetic acid derivative that inhibits prostaglandin synthetase, and it also interferes with the migration of leukocytes into sites of inflammation. Like phenylbutazone, it is rapidly and completely absorbed from the gastrointestinal tract, and it is strongly protein bound. However, the metabolites formed in the liver, unlike those from phenylbutazone, are inactive. Like phenylbutazone, it may cause peptic ulceration or gastrointestinal bleeding, but hematopoietic toxicity is rare. The most common side effects are dizziness and headache. In view of the undesirable side effects, I prefer to prescribe 25 mg instead of 50 mg, three or four times a day after meals for 2 to 4 days. An acute attack is usually terminated effectively without side effects.

Probenecid inhibits the renal tubular secretion of indomethacin. When both drugs are used together, the dosage of indomethacin should be reduced to avoid side effects. Combined use of salicylate and indomethacin, on the other hand, decreases the urinary excretion of indomethacin, which is diverted to bile, and thus increases excretion in the stool.

Naproxen

A propionic acid derivative, naproxen (Naprosyn) is another inhibitor of prostaglandin synthetase. Like the other anti-inflammatory drugs, naproxen is well absorbed from the gastrointestinal tract and is also strongly protein bound and metabolized in the liver. Its metabolite is a glucuronide, which is inactive. Its prolonged anti-inflammatory action is due to a long biologic half-life (exceeding 12 hours) and high drug concentration in synovial fluid. Naproxen, 250 mg twice daily for 2 to 3 days, is effective treatment for mild to moderate attacks of acute gouty arthritis. In patients with low-grade chronic pains, naproxen, 250 mg a day, may be continued for 1 or 2 weeks without apparent side effects. Some patients may develop gastrointestinal symptoms, but gastrointestinal bleeding has been rare.

Unlike phenylbutazone, naproxen has not been found to alter the effects of the oral hypoglycemic drugs or warfarin. Nevertheless, it is always better to adjust the dosage of warfarin since these drugs impair the platelet function and may cause gastrointestinal lesions.

Sulindac

Sulindac (Clinoril) is closely related to indomethacin. After oral administration there are two major biotransformations in addition to conjugation. It is first oxidized to the sulfone and then reversibly reduced to the sulfide, which is the active metabolite. Although the half-life of sulindac is about 7 hours, that of the sulfide metabolite is 18 hours. Like indomethacin, sulindac may cause drowsiness, dizziness, and headache.

Corticotropin

Hormonal therapy in acute gout has been in use for more than 3 decades. When there is failure to respond or when treatment is long delayed in patients who have very severe acute attacks involving several joints, corticotropin (ACTH) is the drug of choice. The initial dose should be 40 to 100 U intramuscularly on the first day, gradually lowering the dosage as the clinical picture dictates. Before discontinuing corticotropin, colchicine, 0.6 mg twice daily, should be added to the regimen.

PREVENTION OF ACUTE GOUTY ARTHRITIS

An attack of acute gouty arthritis may be incited by physical stress, emotional disturbance, excessive ingestion of rich food, or overindulgence in alcoholic drinks. Most of the time, however, no inciting cause may be recognized. In general, the daily use of colchicine to prevent recurrent attacks of acute gouty arthritis is well accepted by physicians and by sufferers of gout as well. However, the efficacy of prophylactic colchicine is not necessarily uniform. Factors contributing to failure of the prophylaxis are mostly related to associated uncontrolled medical complications, intemperate habits in eating and drinking, and irregular life-style, such as on-and-off starvation diet for weight reduction.

In most patients, colchicine, 0.6 mg once or twice a day, is sufficient to achieve satisfactory prophylaxis. Two tablets of colchicine taken at one time are usually more potent than one tablet taken twice a day. When one or two 0.6-mg tablets of colchicine are taken daily, the concentration of the drug in the body is extremely low. The possibility exists that such minute doses may affect the initiation of some immune responses, resulting in a gradual but steady suppression of chemotactic activity.

Long-term evaluation of the efficacy of colchicine prophylaxis in 540 patients revealed excellent results in 83 percent, satisfactory results in 12 percent, and unsatisfactory results in 5 percent. Very few patients were colchicine intolerant. No hematologic or renal toxic effects and no chromosomal aberration or infertility were observed.

Discontinuance of the colchicine prophylactic program may be attempted in patients who have been free from recurrent attacks for a reasonable period of time. The drug may be discontinued sooner in early uncomplicated gout with infrequent attacks, controlled uricemia, and adequate dietary programs. It is important to impress on those patients that acute attacks of gout may frequently be precipitated with sudden change in weight due to extreme dietary manipulations. Thus the prophylaxis should be continued longer in the obese patients who attempt weight reduction. As one gets older, the patient as a rule becomes less sensitive to provocative factors in precipitating acute gouty arthritis. However, if an elderly patient takes various drugs for controlling his associated medical conditions, he may be on the verge of getting an acute attack from time to time. Thus, continuation of the prophylactic program may also depend on the patient's general health other than gout.

TREATMENT OF TOPHACEOUS GOUT

Although acute gouty arthritis is usually brief and episodic, tophaceous gout is indeed a storage disease, in that the body is unable to excrete uric acid at a rate sufficient to balance the rate of formation. Human plasma is saturated with monosodium urate at a concentration of about 7 mg per deciliter. Precipitation of sodium urate sufficient to form tophi that are visible grossly or on a roentgenogram seems to require a plasma concentration well above 7 mg per deciliter; even then the process of precipitation is remarkably slow. The rate of overt tophaceous deposits in the joints is, in general, a function of both the degree and the duration of hyperuricemia. A retrospective study of a large number of gouty patients before appropriate drug therapy revealed 70 percent of patients remained free of tophi 1 to 5 years after the first attack of acute gouty arthritis. The proportion of nontophaceous cases slowly declined to 28 percent after 20 years. With a serum urate level or 7 or 8 mg per deciliter, more than 90 percent of the patients were free of tophi. When the serum urate level was maintained between 9 and 11 mg per deciliter, about 50 percent of them became tophaceous; with levels greater than 11 mg per deciliter, less than 30 percent remained free of tophi. Tophi are usually located at the periarticular areas of the peripheral joints where they appear as soft tissue swellings. Most frequently involved areas include first metatarsophalangeal joints, olecranon bursae, Achilles tendons, and finger joints. Minute juxta-articular punched-out erosions may be found on roentgenographic examination. Increasing destruction of articular ends of the bones may lead to narrowing of the joint space and eventually to chronic pains, joint deformity, and disability.

The principle of management for chronic tophaceous gout is to promote a negative balance between the production and the excretion of uric acid. With prolonged negative uric acid balance, joint mobility may be promoted. Tophi already present in the periarticular spaces may become smaller and eventually disappear. Further precipitation of sodium urate may be prevented.

Probenecid

Probenecid (Benemid) was originally developed to sustain high blood levels of penicillin by interfering with its renal tubular secretion at a time when penicillin was in short supply. Because of its similar capacity to inhibit the renal tubular reabsorption of uric acid, probenecid has been used as a uricosuric agent since 1949, thus ushering in the era of modern therapy for gout.

After its ingestion, probenecid is rapidly and completely absorbed from the gastrointestinal tract. It is about 90 percent protein bound. It has a pKa of 3.4 and a high lipid solubility; hence its excretion is pH dependent. In acid urine, it is mainly reabsorbed from tubular lumen by nonionic diffusion in relatively distal segments of the nephron. In alkaline urine, its excretion exceeds the amount filtered, and this is indicative of tubular secretion.

When probenecid is given to a person with gout, a profound uricosuric effect may be observed for a long time. Thus the expanded miscible uric acid pool is gradually reduced, and in turn, urate deposits in the tissues are mobilized. On the other hand, when probenecid is given to a normouricemic person, the uricosuric effect is short lived because of rapid exhaustion of the miscible uric acid pool. Probenecid is not an anti-inflammatory agent. Unfortunately this fact is often misunderstood. Probenecid is not indicated in patients who excrete an excessive amount of uric acid or who have a history of renal calculus. When probenecid is being used, maintenance of an adequate urine volume, at least 2 L daily, is important to prevent renal complications such as calculus formation.

Sulfinpyrazone

Sulfinpyrazone (Anturane) was discovered to be a potent uricosuric agent in a systematic evaluation of more than 80 phenylbutazone analogues. This sulfoxide derivative does not have anti-inflammatory or sodium- and water-retaining properties. After oral ingestion, gastrointestinal absorption is rapid and virtually complete. Sulfinpyrazone (pKa 2.8), is a more acidic compound than phenylbutazone, is almost totally bound to plasma proteins, and is largely confined to the extracellular compartment. Very little of the drug is filtered by the glomerulus; renal excretion is mainly by tubular secretion. Its rate of renal excretion is not affected by change in urine pH. The biologic half-life is short, averaging 3 hours. Its metabolite, *p*-hydroxy-sulfinpyrazone, is also uricosuric. Sulfinpyrazone is a much more potent uricosuric agent than probenecid, with a daily dosage of 200 to 400 mg of sulfinpyrazone being equivalent to 0.5 to 1.0 g of probenecid. Sulfinpyrazone may be used in patients who do not tolerate probenecid or do not respond satisfactorily to probenecid. Combined use of sulfinpyrazone and probenecid may exert additive uricosuric effects, in part because probenecid inhibits the tubular excretion of sulfinpyrazone, thus prolonging its uricosuric action.

Careful administration of appropriate dosages of probenecid or sulfinpyrazone in more recent years has not been associated with untoward side effects except for occasional complaints of gastrointestinal discomfort or drug allergy. Complete blood cell counts periodically are advisable.

Allopurinol

Allopurinol (Zyloprim) was originally selected as a prospective antitumor agent but proved to be ineffective. However, it was found to be effective in blocking the formation of uric acid from hypoxanthine and xanthine by inhibiting the enzyme xanthine oxidase. After its administration, a striking reduction in serum and urinary uric acid levels is found; yet hypoxanthine and xanthine do not accumulate in the blood because they are rapidly cleared by the kidneys. Allopurinol has a relatively short biologic half-life of 1 to 3 hours, being rapidly excreted by the kidneys and oxidized by xanthine oxidase to form oxipurinol. Oxipurinol noncompetitively inhibits xanthine oxidase, and it has a more prolonged half-life (17 to 40 hours). It is extensively reabsorbed in the kidney, and its renal clearance is about three times greater than the uric acid clearance. Because of the relatively longer half-life of oxipurinol, the effectiveness of allopurinol in reducing the rate of uric acid production is sustained for a long time. The reduction in uric acid excretion in most patients with gout does not correlate stoichiometrically with an increase in urinary excretion of hypoxanthine and xanthine. However, in Lesch-Nyhan syndrome and in gout with partial deficiency of hypoxanthine-guanine-phosphoribosyl transferase (HGPRT), the decreased excretion or uric acid is in balance with the increase in hypoxanthine and xanthine. This is apparently related to the loss of the feedback inhibition mechanism in purine biosynthesis.

Allopurinol offers an alternative to uricosuric drugs in preventing nephrolithiasis in patients with excessive urinary uric acid. It serves to prevent and mobilize tophaceous deposits, especially in patients who are intolerant or refractory to uricosuric agents. In order to facilitate the action on tophi, combined use of allopurinol and probenecid or sulfinpyrazone may be indicated in some patients.

The interaction between allopurinol and probenecid is rather complex. The biologic half-life of probenecid is usually prolonged with concurrent allopurinol administration. On the other hand, probenecid facilitates the renal excretion of oxipurinol as well as of uric acid, thus lowering the plasma oxipurinol level and hence diminishing the xanthine oxidase suppression. Because allopurinol is both a substrate and an inhibitor of xanthine oxidase, it can inhibit its own metabolism. Nevertheless, combined use of probenecid and allopurinol often facilitates the more rapid mobilization of urate deposits.

Concurrent use of allopurinol and dicumarol slows the metabolism of the latter by reducing the activity of hepatic microsomal drug-metabolizing enzyme systems. In a patient with gout and with associated coronary heart disease requiring both drugs, the dosage of allopurinol and dicumarol should be reduced and the prothrombin time determined regularly.

Although allopurinol is well tolerated, with a low order of toxicity, serious reactions such as drug rash, epidermal necrolysis, exfoliative dermatitis, hepatitis, vasculitis, and bone marrow suppression have been reported. It is therefore advisable to start allopurinol, 100 mg a day first for 1 to 2 weeks before dosage is increased to 200 mg daily. Most patients require only 200 mg daily, but secondary gout due to blood dyscrasia, HGPRT deficiency, or neoplastic disease with unusually excessive production of uric acid may require 300 mg of allopurinol daily. With 200 to 300 mg per day, untoward reactions are rare except for an occasional patient who manifests drug allergy. It is not advisable to place all patients with gout on 300 mg daily, regardless of the degree of hyperuricemia or the amount of urinary uric acid. With chronic use of allopurinol, periodic examination to check liver enzymes, blood cell counts, and blood and urine uric acid are indicated.

Indiscriminate use of probenecid, sulfinpyrazone, or allopurinol for just anyone with joint pains is to be discouraged. After prolonged use of either drug for a few years, normouricemia may last for weeks or months after its discontinuance. Drug dosage may have to be adjusted periodically. There is no justification for prescribing a particular drug indefinitely since the patient's biochemical state may change with time. Also, life-long commitment discourages patient compliance.

Aspirin

Acetylsalicylic acid was used widely for gout prior to the development of various antigout drugs. In more recent years, it has been used for prevention of coronary heart disease morbidity among elderly patients by virtue of its inhibition of platelet aggregation. Since many patients with gout belong to this age group, many are taking a small amount of aspirin daily.

Aspirin is rapidly hydrolyzed to salicylic acid after its administration, with a biologic half-life of 4 to 5 hours. Salicylic acid has a pKa of 3.0, and approximately 30 percent of plasma salicylate is not bound to plasma proteins in humans and is thus filtrable at the glomeruli. In acid urine, the filtered salicylate is reabsorbed by the proximal tubule. Of the salicylate appearing in acid urine, only a small part, about 20 percent or less, is excreted as free salicylate. The major portion is conjugated, 55 to 65 percent with glycine to form salicyluric acid and 20 to 30 percent with glucuronide; the remaining 20 percent or so is converted to gentisic acid and other degradation products. In alkaline urine, there is great enhancement of urinary excretion of free salicylate, which suppresses the tubular reabsorption of uric acid, resulting in a uricosuric effect. Hence, the competitive action between free salicylate and uric acid at the renal tubular level depends on the urinary free salicylate concentration, as determined by the salicylate dosage and on the pH of the urine.

Probenecid uricosuria, which is produced by inhibition of the tubular reabsorption of urate, is counteracted by small doses of salicylate, in part because of concurrent suppression of tubular secretion of urate. Probenecid likewise exerts a moderate inhibitory effect on the tubular secretion of free salicylate, which in turn affects the uric acid excretion. The interaction of salicylate with probenecid is complex.

In patients whose serum uric acid level has been satisfactorily maintained for a long time, it is not necessary to discourage the use of small doses of aspirin for a worthwhile purpose, such as inhibition of platelet aggregation.

Small doses of aspirin, 0.3 to 0.6 g per day, have only a minimal effect in elevating the serum uric acid value.

Aches and pains in chronic gouty arthritis associated with degenerative joint changes frequently require small doses of aspirin. When deformities are corrected with disappearance of tophi, the use of aspirin for analgesia can be discontinued. Physical therapy also helps.

Acetohexamide

Eight to 10 percent of patients with gout also have diabetes mellitus. Acetohexamide (Dymelor), a cyclohexyl derivative of sulfonylurea, is used in the treatment of diabetes. It has a uricosuric property in addition to its hypoglycemic action. Acetohexamide is readily metabolized with a short half-life of a little over an hour. The major metabolite is hydroxyhexamide, which is metabolically active, exerting a uricosuric action. Although the hypoglycemic action is due mainly to a metabolic effect on the cells of the islets of Langerhans, the uricosuric property depends on an inhibition of renal tubular reabsorption of uric acid. In patients with renal insufficiency, acetohexamide does not exert any uricosuric action. Thus, a dissociation of the hypoglycemic and uricosuric action may be observed in such patients. Acetohexamide is recommended for patients with gout and diabetes mellitus.

Surgical Intervention

With timely diagnosis and the availability of effective drugs to prevent and treat the tophaceous stage of the disorder, the deformities and disabilities of advanced chronic gouty arthritis have become much less common. However, surgical intervention may be indicated in a few patients. Débridement is useful in accelerating the disappearance of ulcerating and discharging superficial tophi. Impairment of joint mobility or joint deformity with structural erosion and destruction may require corrective surgery.

ASYMPTOMATIC HYPERURICEMIA

A common problem is how to treat the patient who is discovered to have hyperuricemia but who has never had symptoms referable to gout. Five to 10 percent of men past 30 years of age have some degree of asymptomatic hyperuricemia. Development of gout may be correlated with the degree of hyperuricemia, as observed in population and family studies.

A study of hyperuricemia among asymptomatic relatives of patients with primary gout reveals wide fluctuation of serum uric acid levels throughout the years of follow-up. Thus a single determination of serum uric acid can be misleading. Although the hyperuricemia trait may be inborn, it certainly can be modified by environmental changes. Appropriate dietary restriction and gradual weight reduction often lead to a decline in serum uric acid levels.

Alcohol consumption has traditionally been associated with hyperuricemia. Studies have indicated that it is related to elevation of blood lactate level, which leads to inhibition of urinary uric acid excretion. Other studies indicate that alcohol-induced hyperuricemia may be associated with hyperuricosuria due to enhancement of uric acid synthesis related to adenine nucleotide turnover. Normouricemia resumes when alcohol is entirely oxidized and eliminated from the body.

Hyperuricemia, sometimes of marked degree, may appear during starvation or after a high-fat diet. The induced ketosis apparently suppresses urinary uric acid excretion. A high-protein diet usually increases uric acid excretion, with a relatively modest increase in serum uric acid. The hyperuricemia may be greater when there is also some renal function impairment. With appropriate adjustment in diet, hyperuricemia should improve.

Hyperuricemia may be drug induced, such as after chlorothiazide or furosemide used for hypertension, or after pyrazinamide or ethambutol used in treating tuberculosis. Drug-induced hyperuricemia is apparently due to inhibition of renal uric acid excretion.

Hyperuricemia associated with blood dyscrasia, as in polycythemia and leukemia, is usually accompanied by excessive urinary uric acid excretion. Dietary regulation is frequently unable to control the hyperuricemia and hyperuricosuria. The use of allopurinol is rational, particularly when chemotherapy is contemplated.

In asymptomatic hyperuricemia and excessive hyperuricosuria among members of families with deficient HGPRT, and increased phosphoribosyl pyrophosphate synthetase or other purine metabolizing enzyme abnormalities, use of allopurinol again is indicated.

In general, in persistent hyperuricemia of more than 9 or 10 mg per deciliter, despite careful dietary restriction and modification of medications, or in hyperuricosuria on the order of 1.0 g or more per day, with the uric acid nitrogen to total nitrogen ratio of the 24-hour urine specimen being more than 2.0 percent, drug therapy using allopurinol is justified. If the ratio of urinary uric acid nitrogen to total nitrogen is within the normal range of 1.5 ± 0.3 percent, small doses of a uricosuric agent (either probenecid or sulfinpyrazone), may be used. When asymptomatic hyperuricemia is associated with reduced urinary uric acid levels and evidence of significant renal damage, it is more advisable to seek possible causes of intrinsic kidney disease first.

GOUT AND NEPHROPATHY

The number of patients with gout with severe renal damage is relatively small. Renal disease secondary to gout is not causally related to the severity of hyperuricemia and duration of gout, although a correlation does exist. Nephropathy in gout in most cases is due to associated independent conditions or to nephrolithiasis and infection.

In an analysis for a large number of patients with gout in the past 4 decades, underlying diseases causing nephropathy in gout are usually nongouty in nature. Forty to 50 percent of the patients had cardiovascular disease, particularly essential hypertension, and 30 to 40 percent had intrinsic renal disease including glomerulonephritis, pyelonephritis, or renal vascular abnormalities. Although hypertension is on the rise in more recent years, nephropathy in gout is on the decline, reflecting the benefits from more appropriate therapy for hypertension.

A substantial number of gout patients may have chronic renal disease antedating gout for many years. As renal damage progresses, hyperuricemia may become more extreme but not accompanied by increased uric acid excretion or higher incidence of renal calculi.

Nephropathy occurs in some variants of gout. In complete HGPRT deficiency (Lesch-Nyhan syndrome) and also those with partial deficiency of the enzyme, one may encounter extremely high serum uric acid and urine uric acid. Onset of gout may be early, and passage of uric acid calculi or gravel with obstructive uropathy is common. A few cases of familial gout with progressive renal failure but no enzyme deficiencies have been reported. In fulminating gout, no abnormal or deficient enzyme(s) can be detected. Gout and associated renal damage appear early in age. Hyperuricemia is marked, the uric acid level in urine is low, and tophi can be extensive but there are no renal calculi. Death from renal failure occurs in relatively young age.

Gout may occur in blood dyscrasia as polycythemia vera, particularly in its spent stage, and as leukemia in its blastic stage. The extreme hyperuricemia and hyperuricosuria lead to uric acid gravel and not uncommonly to obstruction of the urinary tract.

Saturnine gout is usually due to chronic lead poisoning from an industrial source or from lead intoxication from moonshine whiskey. Renal damage and hypertension are prominent features. Hyperuricemia is striking, but there is no high excretion of uric acid in urine. The damage to the interstitium and renal tubules frequently overshadows the hematopoietic changes. Allopurinol is the drug of choice since uricosuric therapy is not efficient in such cases with renal insufficiency. Deleading with edetate calcium disodium may help in some patients by enhancing lead mobilization and excretion.

SUGGESTED READING

Wyngaarden JB. Disorders of purine and pyrimidine metabolism—gout. In:Wyngaarden JB, Smith LH, eds. Cecil's textbook of medicine. 18th ed. Philadelphia: WB Saunders, 1985:1161.

Yu TF. Milestones in the treatment of gout. Am J Med 1974;56:676–685.

Yu TF, Berger L, Dorph DJ, Smith H. Renal function in gout: factors influencing the renal hemodynamics. Am J Med 1979;67:766–771.

Yu TF. The efficacy of colchicine prophylaxis in articular gout: a reappraisal after 20 years. Semin Arthritis Rheum 1982;12:256–264.

Yu TF. Nephrolithiasis. In: Yu TF, Berger L, eds. The kidney in gout and hyperuricemia. Mt. Kisco, NY: Futura, 1982:195.

Yu TF. Clinical aspects of nephropathy in gout and hyperuricemic states. In: Yu TF, Berger L, eds. The kidney in gout and hyperuricemia. Mt Kisco, NY: Futura, 1982:261.

ENDOCRINE SYNDROMES ASSOCIATED WITH NEOPLASMS

DAIVA R. BAJORUNAS, M.D.

Endocrine syndromes caused by an excessive production of peptide hormones by neoplastic tissue are recognized with increasing frequency to cause significant morbidity in the tumor-bearing patient. The more common clinical manifestations associated with "ectopic" hormone production by tumors are listed in Table 1. It should be recognized, however, that not in each instance is the syndrome the result of tumor hormonogenesis; moreover, the list of putative hormonal mediators of paraneoplastic syndromes is, at present, incompletely defined.

The only effective long-term means of reversing the malignancy-associated endocrine syndromes is tumor ablation or a reduction in the tumor burden; the success of a multimodality therapeutic regimen (surgical resection, chemotherapy, radiation therapy, or immunotherapy) is dependent on tumor histology and extent of disease and will not be further addressed here. In the absence of successful primary tumor therapy or while awaiting its outcome, specific measures that offset the hormonal systemic manifestations should be vigorously sought, since the endocrine aspects of palliative care in this population often form the mainstay of patient management.

CUSHING'S SYNDROME

Among patients presenting to an endocrine unit for evaluation of their clinical Cushing's syndrome, ectopic adrenocorticotropic hormone (ACTH) or corticotropin-releasing factor (CRF) production accounts for about 20 percent of ACTH-dependent disease. Although some of these patients have no obvious tumor ("occult ectopics") and pose a considerable diagnostic problem, when the full-blown syndrome

TABLE 1 Endocrine Syndromes Associated with Neoplasms

Clinical Presentation	*Pathogenesis*	*Tumor Type*
Cushing's syndrome	Ectopic ACTH, ectopic CRF	Lung (oat cell, bronchial adenoma), carcinoid, thymoma, pancreas, pheochromocytoma, thyroid (medullary), ovary, colon, prostate, cervix
Hyponatremia (syndrome of inappropriate antidiuresis)	Ectopic antidiuretic hormone or central arginine vasopressin secretion, vincristine or cyclophosphamide administration	Lung (oat cell, bronchogenic), pancreas, duodenum, bladder, sarcoma, lymphoma, thymoma
Hypercalcemia	Skeletal metastasis, systemic humoral bone-resorbing mediators (PTH, PTH-like peptide, or PTH-related protein; tumor-derived growth factors, such as TGF-alpha, interleukin-1, and TNF), local osteolytic factors (osteoclast-activating factors such as lymphotoxin, gamma-interferon, TGF-beta, interleukin-1, and TNF), 1, 25-dihydroxyvitamin D_3	Breast, multiple myeloma and other hematologic malignancies, squamous cell carcinoma (lung, head and neck, bladder), kidney, ovary, other (adrenal, pheochromocytoma, pancreas)
Hypoglycemia	Nonsuppressible insulin-like activity such as insulin-like growth factor II, glucose utilization by tumor, impaired hepatic glucose production, suppression of counterregulatory hormones	Mesenchymal (fibrosarcoma, mesothelioma) hepatoma, adrenocortical carcinoma, pheochromocytoma, other (breast, gastric, carcinoid, prostate, lymphoma, leukemia)
Acromegaly	Ectopic growth hormone, ectopic growth hormone releasing hormone	Pancreatic islet cell, carcinoid
Osteomalacia with hypophosphatemia	Unknown	Mesenchymal (osseous or soft tissue with giant cell vascular features), multiple myeloma, neurofibromatosis, carcinoma (prostate, oat cell, breast)
Hyperthyroidism	Human chorionic gonadotropin (very high levels)	Trophoblastic tumors (hydatidiform mole, choriocarcinoma)

ACTH = adrenocorticotropic hormone, CRF = corticotropin-releasing factor, PTH = parathyroid hormone, TGF = transforming growth factor, TNF = tumor necrosis factor

occurs it differs from that seen in patients with Cushing's disease in that the typical body habitus of Cushing's disease is masked in the context of a malignant wasting disease, and signs of excessive mineralocorticoid production predominate. Establishing the correct diagnosis may result in a complete cure if surgical resection of the tumor is feasible. In cases in which the tumor is deemed unresectable but can be expected to have a relatively indolent or prolonged course (e.g., in selected medullary carcinomas of the thyroid or islet cell carcinoid tumors) or in patients in whom the primary tumor has not been identified, bilateral adrenalectomy is not an unreasonable therapeutic option if the patient is an acceptable surgical candidate: it is associated with a low morbidity and mortality, and patient management is greatly simplified by definitive treatment of the Cushing's syndrome. In such patients, pretreatment with adrenal enzyme inhibitors should be tried to improve the metabolic derangements preoperatively and to hasten postoperative wound healing.

In patients with unresectable disease and a poor longterm prognosis, drugs that impair adrenal steroid biosynthesis can be tried to effect a medical adrenalectomy. Metyrapone acts by inhibition of 11-beta hydroxylase and thus lowers the production of cortisol and other 11-beta-hydroxylated corticosteroids; it has been reported to lower aldosterone secretion rates as well. In doses up to 4 g per day, given at frequent intervals, metyrapone should be titrated to achieve normal plasma cortisol/urinary free cortisol levels. I do not routinely administer dexamethasone at the start of metyrapone therapy in patients with fulminant hypercortisolemia; nevertheless, the possibility of drug-induced adrenal insufficiency should always be kept in mind. In a patient who develops significant gastrointestinal distress and/or dizziness, which are relatively common side effects of metyrapone, steroid replacement doses should be administered until laboratory indices of endogenous steroid production are available. Other less common side effects of therapy include a rash and hirsutism in women.

Aminoglutethimide is an inhibitor of steroid biosynthesis that acts by binding to cytochrome P-450 complexes to block several steroid hydroxylation steps, with the initial blockade occurring in the conversion of cholesterol to pregnenolone. In dosages up to 2 g per day (usual dosage: 750 to 1,000 mg per day), it suppresses estradiol synthesis (via aromatase inhibition) more than androgen production. Side effects are dose-dependent and consist of rash, sedation, headache, myalgia, and upper gastrointestinal symptoms. I have noted better patient tolerance and compliance when aminoglutethimide and metyrapone are administered in combination, in reduced dosage.

An adrenal enzyme inhibitor, *o,p′* -DDD (mitotane), is also uniquely adrenocorticolytic and thus presumably should be the most definitive pharmacologic agent in the treatment of tumor-induced Cushing's syndrome. Unfortunately, it has several major drawbacks. The effect of this drug on adrenal secretion is not immediate, with blood levels reaching a plateau at the eighth week. Variability in its clinical and biologic effects has been noted; only the drug-to-lipid ratio seems able to provide a reproducible index of drug entry into a tissue. Most important, its side effects of sedation, extreme depression, gastrointestinal symptoms, gynecomastia, and hypercholesterolemia make the drug poorly tolerated in a chronically ill and debilitated patient. I usually try to advance the drug fairly rapidly (increasing by 0.5 g every other day) to tolerance, then decrease the dose until the dose-limiting symptoms of nausea and gastrointestinal distress abate (usual maximal tolerated doses are 4 to 6 g per day, given with meals and at bedtime, although up to 12 g per day may be prescribed). Great care should be taken to avoid giving *o,p′* -DDD concomitantly with drugs that decrease the content of cytochrome P-450–dependent enzymes in the adrenal gland (such as spironolactone).

The substituted imidazole ketoconazole, an effective antimycotic agent, has been found to block gonadal and adrenal steroid synthesis by inhibition of cytochrome P-450–dependent enzymes; moreover, it can interfere with corticosteroid action at the receptor level. Although ketoconazole causes idiosyncratic liver toxicity rarely (with an incidence of 1 in 15,000 exposed subjects), it usually causes few nonhormone side effects when used in the antimycotic dose range (less than 600 mg per day). However, in the dose range used for inhibition of steroid synthesis (1,200 mg per day), nausea, vomiting, anorexia, and elevated liver enzymes are more common. Nevertheless, I believe that ketoconazole is a valuable palliative adjunct in malignancies associated with corticosteroid overproduction. In contrast to aminoglutethimide, ketoconazole appears to spare estrogen synthesis and primarily blocks androgen synthesis; thus, one rationale for choosing between the two agents would be the degree of tumor-induced androgenic-estrogenic manifestations.

Another imidazole, the intravenous sedative-hypnotic agent etomidate, used for the induction and/or maintenance of anesthesia, has been noted to be at least as potent as ketoconazole, on a mass basis, in inhibiting steroidogenesis. Its use in the management of patients with malignant hypercortisolemia currently would appear to be limited to patients requiring mechanical ventilation.

The potent competitive glucocorticoid antagonist RU 486 has been used successfully in two patients with ectopic ACTH syndrome, with the absence of side effects or toxicity. Currently the drug is costly to synthesize and thus is not available in quantities sufficient for extensive clinical evaluation; it may, however, offer therapeutic possibilities in the future.

The investigational drug suramin has been shown to be an active agent in the treatment of metastatic adrenocortical carcinoma. The drug has a unique mechanism of action. By inhibiting iduronate sulfatase, it causes accumulation of heparan sulfate, which appears to inhibit tumor growth. Preliminary reports on its response rates, however, have been somewhat disappointing, and the drug has considerable toxicity: reversible vortex keratopathy, severe demyelinating polyneuropathy, proteinuria, rash, reversible liver function abnormalities, and coagulopathy have been reported. Its role in the treatment of such patients therefore remains to be established.

When using steroidogenic blocking agents, in every case great care must be taken to detect adrenal insufficiency and treat it promptly. Unfortunately, more commonly, especially with progressive disease, tumor-produced ACTH or CRF levels are high enough to overcome the incomplete drug-induced blockade in steroid synthesis. In this setting, ancillary measures, such as potassium replacement, judicious diuretic administration, and reasonable glycemic control, become the mainstay of therapy in these highly catabolic and critically ill patients.

HYPONATREMIA

The syndrome of inappropriate antidiuretic hormone secretion (SIADH) has become recognized as the most prevalent cause of significant hyponatremia encountered in clinical practice. Tumors (see Table 1) remain the most common cause of non–drug-induced SIADH, and the cumulative evidence that tumors can synthesize and secrete antidiuretic hormone is now fairly conclusive, although immunologically recognizable antidiuretic hormone has been found in only about half the tumors studied to date. The clinical syndrome is characterized by hyponatremia and hypo-osmolality in the setting of normovolemia and an inappropriately concentrated urine. It should be remembered that not all tumor-associated hyponatremia represents SIADH, and a careful evaluation of the patient with cancer and a low serum sodium level may detect other potentially correctable causes of the electrolyte imbalance, such as solute depletion from vomiting or diarrhea, hypothyroidism, and hypoadrenalism.

Once the diagnosis of SIADH is firmly established, the choice of therapeutic interventions depends primarily on the clinical status of the patient. In the compliant patient with milder symptoms, such as anorexia, headache, irritability, personality changes, and muscle weakness, water restriction (total intake: 600 to 800 ml daily) remains the mainstay of therapy. However, the patient with cancer tolerates this poorly, since the chronic nature of the condition (unless tumor resectability and/or cure is possible), coupled with the patient's progressive debility, make this an increasingly difficult measure to enforce.

In the long-term treatment of chronic and mild tumor-induced SIADH, lithium, demeclocycline, loop diuretics, and urea have been advocated, although studies comparing the various long-term treatment regimens to one another are lacking, making the selection of a regimen of choice difficult. The tetracycline derivative demeclocycline has been shown to produce a predictable, reversible, and dose-dependent nephrogenic diabetes insipidus, resulting from impairment of both the generation and action of cyclic adenosine monophosphate (AMP) in the distal nephron. The use of 1,200 mg per day appears to be adequate in most cases of SIADH. The time of onset or response to the drug is variable, ranging from as little as 6 to 8 hours to as long as 4 weeks, and thus demeclocycline is not recommended for the acute emergency treatment of severe hyponatremia. Adverse effects of the therapy are uncommon, provided the patient has an intact thirst mechanism and adequate oral intake; skin photosensitivity has been noted and can be minimized by the use of sunscreen preparations. In patients with cirrhosis or congestive heart failure given demeclocycline, significant albeit reversible renal sodium wasting and renal insufficiency have been noted, and care should be used in this patient population. Superinfection has not been reported to occur with any regular frequency, but it remains a theoretical risk of this therapy, especially in the immunocompromised cancer patient.

Lithium, like demeclocycline, interferes with the normal effect of vasopressin to increase cyclic AMP in the renal tubules. Its clinical effect in producing diabetes insipidus is inconsistent, and it has been shown to be less effective than demeclocycline in the treatment of chronic SIADH. Moreover, the frequent and harmful incidence of gastrointestinal, cardiac, thyroid, and central nervous system toxicities as well as the hazard of lithium intoxication during drug-induced volume depletion has limited the clinical usefulness of this agent.

The use of oral urea (10 to 30 g per day) has been reported to relieve the symptoms of water intoxication via an osmotic diuresis. The advantages of this therapy are that urea acts immediately, is effective in patients with decreased creatinine clearance, and does not require mandatory salt ingestion because it actually decreases sodium urinary excretion; moreover, the development of hypokalemia is rare. However, gastrointestinal complaints are common, and patients are at risk of hypernatremic dehydration if they do not have an intact thirst mechanism; both these factors limit the usefulness of this agent in the patient with cancer.

The use of oral loop diuretics (furosemide or ethacrynic acid) along with sodium chloride tablets (adjusted to match urinary sodium output) has been shown to be effective in the chronic treatment of SIADH. The need to use a long loop diuretic has to be emphasized, since the inhibition of reabsorption of free water does not occur with thiazide diuretics. The patients are started on 40 mg of furosemide (or 50 mg ethacrynic acid) supplemented by 3 g of salt as tablets and 50 mg of triamterene; diuretic doses are doubled if the diuresis induced in the first 8 hours is less than 60 percent of the total daily urine output. From the reported literature, the time necessary to reverse the symptoms of water intoxication is not clear. Furthermore, there is also an inherent risk of developing a hypokalemic-hypochloremic alkalosis with this regimen. Thus there appears to be no demonstrated superiority over demeclocycline in the treatment of chronic SIADH.

More severe symptoms of hyponatremia, such as nausea, vomiting, confusion, and convulsions, in the presence of a serum sodium concentration less than 120 mEq per liter, particularly if the development of the hyponatremia was acute, require a more vigorous therapeutic approach. Hypertonic saline solutions provide the fastest means of correcting the serum sodium concentration and by rapidly raising the extracellular fluid osmolality create an osmotic gradient allowing for the movement of water out of brain cells. However, since patients with SIADH are already volume expanded, the possibility of further fluid overload in the elderly resulting in cardiopulmonary decompensation is real, a consideration that also limits the usefulness of the osmotic agents glycerol or mannitol. Also, the use of hypertonic sodium chloride solutions only transiently increases plasma sodium concentration, since these patients rapidly excrete nearly all the administered sodium. A safer alternative therapy appears to be the induction of a diuresis by a single dose of furosemide (1 mg per kilogram intravenously) with replacement of urinary electrolyte losses with a small volume of hypertonic (3 percent) saline; the net effect is to induce a negative water balance while avoiding expansion of the extracellular fluid volume. A dreaded result of acute and severe hyponatremia is the development of central pontine myelinolysis, a fatal neurologic sequel of the condition and/or its treatment. The dilemma the clinician faces is whether to initiate rapid versus slow repair of acute hyponatremia, currently an issue not resolved because of the paucity of carefully designed prospective protocols addressing this question. Until such information is forthcoming, it is reasonable to strive to limit the rate of the rise in the serum sodium level to 2 mEq per liter per hour until a level of 120 to 130 mEq per liter is reached in symptomatic patients with tumor-induced acute hyponatremia.

HYPERCALCEMIA

By far the most common endocrine paraneoplastic syndrome seen in a cancer hospital is hypercalcemia. It is estimated that this potentially lethal complication occurs in 10 to 20 percent of all patients with cancer at some time during the course of their disease. The most common malignancies associated with this complication and the probable pathogenic mechanisms are listed in Table 1. Urgent or emergent hypercalcemia is defined as a serum calcium level above 13 mg per deciliter when corrected for changes in the plasma proteins. Treatment for hypercalcemia, however, should also be urgent if the patient has symptoms of increasing severity that can be ascribed to the hypercalcemia. Although many of the symptoms, such as nausea, anorexia, weakness, fatigue, lethargy, and confusion, are nonspecific and may be seen in any patient with terminal illness, patients with cancer tolerate hypercalcemia less well than those with nonneoplastic causes of hypercalcemia, and vigorous treatment is usually mandated.

The only effective long-term means of reversing malignancy-associated hypercalcemia is tumor ablation or a reduction in the tumor burden. However, the more nonspecific measures in reducing malignant hypercalcemia are important and often lifesaving adjuvant measures, to be used on a short-term basis. Obviously, all agents capable of precipitating a hypercalcemic crisis should be looked for and stopped (pharmacologic ingestion of vitamin D or A, thiazide diuretics, hormonal therapy in patients with breast cancer, especially estrogens or antiestrogens). Vigorous rehydration remains a measure of primary importance, since dehydration is the rule in these patients. Restoring a normal effective plasma volume increases urinary calcium excretion by 100 to 300 mg per day. When intravenous saline is used as the replacement fluid, calciuresis can be enhanced by the provoked natriuresis. I prefer to alternate isotonic with hypotonic saline administration, since I have noted hypernatremia occurring in patients during vigorous rehydration with normal saline. The usual precautions regarding the patient's cardiopulmonary status must be observed. After partial rehydration has been accomplished, the addition of a potent loop diuretic (e.g., furosemide, 40 to 80 mg intravenously every 4 to 6 hours or 200 mg per 24 hours as a continuous infusion) may enhance calcium diuresis. This will only be effective if hypovolemia and consequent decreased glomerular filtration do not ensue; thus, attention to volume and electrolyte repletion is mandatory. A potential benefit of loop diuretics is to prevent inadvertent fluid overload during hydration; their hypocalcemic effectiveness is undoubtedly mild, and their use should not delay the start of more effective measures.

Rehydration with forced saline diuresis produces only transient effects because the proximal cause of the hypercalcemia, increased bone resorption, continues unabated. More specific measures therefore are usually necessary. Intravenous phosphate has been shown to be an effective inhibitor of bone resorption; it enhances calcium and phosphate deposition in soft tissues and probably also at the bone site. When given as a slow intravenous infusion of 50 mmol (1.5 mg) over 6 to 8 hours in hypercalcemic patients with neoplastic disease, it can acutely decrease the serum calcium concentration by more than 2 mg per deciliter. However, phosphate, when given by the parenteral route, is extremely toxic, being frequently associated with serious extraskeletal calcification in vital organs. Numerous deaths have now been ascribed to the use of intravenous phosphate, and I have seen fatalities in patients so treated. Therefore, there appears to be little role for the use of this agent in the management of hypercalcemia of malignancy.

Corticosteroids are capable of inhibiting bone resorption; their usefulness in hypercalcemic cancer patients has been variable, with the best results achieved in patients with multiple myeloma, non-Hodgkin's lymphoma, and breast carcinoma. In these patients the effectiveness of steroid therapy is probably attributable to direct inhibition of tumor growth, although an indirect effect may be that of prostaglandin or bone-resorbing lymphokine suppression. Another particular group of patients in whom glucocorticoids are often effective is patients with lymphoma and 1,25-dihydroxyvitamin D_3-mediated hypercalcemia, in whom the effect is dramatic and rapid. In most cases, however, the onset of corticosteroid action is not seen for at least 48 hours, and thus this regimen should not be used as sole therapy in an acute hypercalcemic emergency. Usually a trial of 7 to 10 days at doses of 40 to 60 mg of prednisone or 400 mg of hydrocortisone given intravenously should be attempted before it is concluded that the hypercalcemia is unresponsive.

Calcitonin is a 32-amino acid polypeptide that has been shown to inhibit bone resorption and so has been used in the treatment of patients with hypercalcemia and malignancy. In doses of 8 to 16 MRC units per kilogram given every 12 hours parenterally, it is relatively nontoxic, well tolerated, and particularly useful when fluid overload is a problem, since it enhances renal sodium excretion. Its effects are rapid but unfortunately transient, with a tachyphylaxis reportedly developing with continued use. Combination therapy with calcitonin plus glucocorticoids has been reported to prolong the calcium-lowering effect of calcitonin, although the morbidity of glucocorticoid administration may offset the minor advantage to be gained by this approach. Because of its safety and rapidity of action, I have found calcitonin to be an ideal agent as first-line therapy in the patient who is about to start a vigorous and definitive antineoplastic regimen.

Mithramycin, an antibiotic with cytotoxic activity, is uniformly effective in lowering serum calcium levels in hypercalcemia through an inhibitory effect on bone resorption. At doses of 25 μg per kilogram given intravenously, preferably as a slow infusion over 4 to 6 hours to minimize gastrointestinal symptoms, the calcium-lowering effect peaks at 48 to 96 hours and can persist for several days; a rapid rebound may provoke a hypercalcemic crisis, however, and patients should be closely monitored. Unfortunately, the agent is associated with significant toxicity, usually at higher doses or with repetitive administration, thus limiting its use in patients who are concomitantly receiving myelosuppressive doses of chemotherapy. Thrombocytopenia, hepatic dysfunction, a hemorrhagic diathesis, and nephrotoxicity have been reported with its use.

Several new agents offer promise in the management of the patient with malignancy-related hypercalcemia. Bisphosphonates, structural analogues of pyrophosphate, have been shown to be potent inhibitors of osteoclastic bone resorption. Intravenous etidronate disodium, having undergone clinical trials in the United States, was just made available for the management of this syndrome. It is given intravenously in a maximal dose of 7.5 mg per kilogram per day as a slow infusion over 4 hours, as acute renal failure has occurred with a more rapid infusion.

The more potent second-generation bisphosphonate pamidronate, which is not yet available in the United States, has been reported to achieve more consistent (87 percent) and more sustained (29 days) normocalcemia. Accumulated experience indicates that bisphosphonates are generally well tolerated and free of significant side effects. A major complication of the chronic use of etidronel is inhibition of normal skeletal mineralization, and long-term use has produced osteomalacia and nontraumatic bone fractures, a complication not reported with the newer agents. Gallium nitrate, still an investigational agent, is an antitumor drug that directly inhibits bone resorption; after administration, gallium accumulates in bone and reduces the solubility of bone crystal without affecting osteoclasts. At a dose of 200 mg per square meter per day given as a continuous infusion for 5 to 7 days, it effectively normalizes cancer-related hypercalcemia in 75 to 85 percent of patients and has been shown to be markedly superior to maximally approved doses of calcitonin. Nephrotoxicity is the major side effect, and a further disadvantage is the current requirement of several days of continuous intravenous infusions.

Therapy with oral phosphates or prostaglandin synthetase inhibitors has no place in the acute management of malignant hypercalcemia, since effectiveness is unpredictable and minor in this setting. In a patient in whom a reversible form of renal failure has developed, dialysis against a low-calcium bath may be indicated, since other therapies would surely be contraindicated or ineffective. It must be reiterated, however, that without promising therapy for the underlying cancer, management of the hypercalcemia will merely be a temporizing measure. Thus, the aggressiveness of the therapeutic approach depends on the potential for significant neoplastic palliation or cure.

HYPOGLYCEMIA

Hypoglycemia in the patient with a malignancy can develop as a consequence of the overall metabolic deterioration or be produced by the tumor itself (see Table 1). Superimposed malnutrition, with decreased glycogen stores and decreased substrate delivery, adrenal insufficiency, severe liver necrosis with hepatic failure, severe congestive heart failure, overwhelming sepsis, or terminal renal failure, especially in cancer patients with diabetes, can all cause profound fasting hypoglycemia.

In less critically ill patients, hypoglycemia can result as a consequence of the tumor itself, and, if profound and persistent, necessitates intensive care monitoring and vigorous therapy. Nonislet cell tumors are second only to islet cell tumors as a cause of chronic fasting hypoglycemia in the adult. It is clear that this paraneoplastic syndrome is rarely, if ever, caused by excessive insulin secretion by extrapancreatic tumors. Several mechanisms have been proposed: decreased hepatic glucose production, either by inhibitory substances produced by the tumor, such as a tryptophan-like substance, or by deficient glucagon secretion; increased glucose utilization, either by the tumor itself (especially when the tumor mass is large) or by other tissues; and increased production of an insulin-like substance that does not react in the insulin radioimmunoassay but does promote peripheral glucose uptake, such as NSILA-s. The latter's insulin-like activity can be largely accounted for by the two somatomedins, insulin-like growth factor I (IGF-I) and insulin-like growth factor II (IGF-II). The serum concentration of IGF-I of patients with nonislet cell tumor–associated hypoglycemia when measured by specific radioimmunoassay has almost invariably been low. IGF-II-like peptide was first noted in hypoglycemic nonislet tumor patients in 1974. Since that time, elevated levels in such patients have been noted by others, and extremely high levels of IGF-II mRNA have been detected in tumors of mesenchymal origin of patients with paraneoplastic hypoglycemia. In such patients a dual mechanism for hypoglycemia may be present: (1) increased glucose utilization mediated by the insulin-like actions of IGF-II, and (2) inhibition of growth hormone secretion, which may account in part for the decreased hepatic glucose production found in these patients.

Therapy for hypoglycemia is treatment of the tumor itself, even if widely metastatic disease precludes a complete cure, since a decreased tumor mass may greatly alleviate symptomatic, protracted hypoglycemia. For the acute management of the symptomatic patient, intravenous hyperalimentation with glucose concentrations of 20 to 30 percent is often required. For chronic management of these patients, enteral tube feeding formulations administered via a small-bore feeding tube in a continuous peristaltic pump delivery system have proved efficacious in optimizing outpatient care. The time of administration of such feedings can be varied to permit daytime mobility while ensuring nocturnal substrate delivery. The rate-limiting factor is usually gastrointestinal tolerance; diarrhea can be minimized by providing a formula less hyperosmotic, by a gradual titration of the rate and volume of delivery, and by the addition of 5 to 20 drops of tincture of opium to the formula preparation. Patients should be taught how to perform fingerstick glucose measurements so that nocturnal hypoglycemia can be prevented.

Hormones that have hyperglycemic effects, such as glucocorticoids or glucagon, are seldom of any prolonged benefit. Diazoxide, a drug that inhibits insulin secretion, decreases peripheral glucose utilization, and enhances hepatic glucogenesis, has been effective in patients with insulinomas; addition of thiazides potentiates the effect, and phenytoin may also be of some use. There is limited experience with the long-acting somatostatin analogue octreotide acetate (sandostatin) in islet cell tumor–induced hypoglycemia; patients need to be followed particularly closely because a disproportionate inhibition of glucagon or growth hormone secretion may in fact make the hypoglycemic episodes more severe. On average only about half the patients so treated have had symptomatic and hormonal responses. In nonpancreatic tumors, these agents are seldom effective.

ACROMEGALY

There has been great interest in the finding that neuroendocrine tumors, most often of foregut origin (islet cell tumors of the pancreas or carcinoids), produce acromegaly by elaborating either growth hormone or a peptide capable of stimulating growth hormone release, that is, growth hormone-releasing hormone (GHRH). Although it has been shown that extrahypothalamic GHRH secretion is a rare cause of acromegaly, it is important that an accurate diagnosis is made before the patient has unnecessary surgery and/or irradiation directed at the pituitary gland. The diagnostic problem is further compounded by the fact that patients with tumors secreting GHRH may have radiologic sellar abnormalities and a phenotype suggestive of multiple endocrine neoplasia type I. Since these tumors have been shown to exhibit immunoreactivity for a variety of other regulatory peptides and neurotransmitters, patients suspected of having this rare paraneoplastic disorder should be screened for the concomitant production of gastrin, insulin, glucagon, serotonin, substance P, somatostatin, pancreatic polypeptide, vasoactive intestinal peptide, or ACTH. Plasma and tumor arteriovenous gradients of growth hormone and immunoreactive GHRH may be of help in difficult cases.

Resection of the neuroendocrine neoplasm results in regression of acromegaly, and this is clearly the treatment of choice. In patients in whom residual tumor is unresponsive to a conventional chemotherapeutic regimen (including combinations of 5-fluorouracil, streptozocin, doxorubicin, dacarbazine, carmustine, or lomustine), bromocriptine therapy may be tried, although it is unlikely that, in the case of ectopic growth hormone production, ectopic tumors are subject to the same dopaminergic inhibition as adenomas within the pituitary gland itself. More recently, the somatostatin analogue octreotide acetate (sandostatin), with a shorter peptide sequence, high potency, and prolonged growth hormone inhibitory action, has been administered chronically in dosages of 100 to 300 μg per day given subcutaneously to patients with nonparaneoplastic acromegaly. A rapid amelioration of the clinical signs and symptoms and near-normalization of laboratory test results occurred in all patients. In order to achieve normalization of growth hormone secretion, higher dosages, up to 1,500 μg per day, may be required. Side effects, when reported, have been mild, although diarrhea and/or steatorrhea, altered carbohydrate tolerance, and potential development of gallstones with chronic use remain concerns.

ONCOGENIC HYPOPHOSPHATEMIC OSTEOMALACIA

Certain tumors (see Table 1) have been reported to cause a syndrome similar to that of vitamin D–resistant rickets. Patients present with bone pain, muscle weakness, and loss of height caused by vertebral collapse; hypophosphatemia is the rule, and in the oncogenic syndrome low plasma levels of 1,25-dihydroxyvitamin D_3 are usual and may therefore serve as a marker for the presence of a tumor. Since hypophosphatemia may occur in the cancer patient from a variety of causes (alkalosis, insulin administration, hyperalimentation, gastrointestinal losses, antacid administration), evidence of bone disease should be assiduously sought. Remission of the syndrome with removal of the tumor suggests a humoral origin, but direct demonstration of this pathogenetic mechanism is lacking.

A therapeutic regimen in patients whose neoplasm is unresectable should increase the serum phosphate concentration, prevent secondary hyperparathyroidism, suppress parathyroid hormone, and provide levels of 1,25-dihydroxyvitamin D_3 sufficient to promote bone healing. An adequate calcium intake should be provided, as well as at least 2 g per day of oral phosphorus (to normalize the serum phosphate level). High doses of Rocaltrol are usually necessary, initially in the range of 3 g per day. Once the bone lesions are healed, the dosage may need to be reduced so that hypercalcemia does not ensue. Urinary calcium excretion may rise on this regimen and needs to be monitored closely.

HYPERTHYROIDISM

In a cancer population, unusual causes of hyperthyroidism should be kept in mind. Iodine-induced thyrotoxicosis, although rare, should be considered in patients who have undergone radiologic studies with iodinated contrast media. Metastatic follicular thyroid carcinoma can rarely cause hyperthyroidism. Tumor metastases function suboptimally compared with normal thyroid tissue; however, hyperthyroidism can result if there is a large volume of tumor. Ovarian teratomas containing thyroid tissue (struma ovarii) are extremely uncommon; if they are present, hyperthyroidism caused by such ectopic thyroid tissues occurs with a frequency of 4 to 7 percent.

A humoral cause of hyperthyroidism in the cancer patient can be seen in patients with trophoblastic disease, either benign hydatidiform moles or malignant choriocarcinoma or one of its variants. The etiology is attributable to the thyroid-stimulating activity of human chorionic gonadotropin, which has 1 in 4,000 the bioactivity of thyroid-stimulating hormone. Although increased thyroid function is probably common in this population of patients, hyperthyroidism, which is severe and easily recognized, probably occurs in only a small minority of patients and depends primarily on the presence of a large tumor burden.

Surgical removal of the hydatidiform mole is the definitive treatment in this subgroup of patients and should be carried out as soon as possible, with intravenous sodium iodide and oral propranolol therapy serving as important preoperative adjunctive therapies. In patients with ovarian or testicular carcinomas containing trophoblastic elements, primary surgical resection, if possible, will result in complete cure of the hyperthyroidism. In those patients in whom complete resection is not feasible, existing chemotherapeutic regimens are usually effective in reducing levels of human chorionic gonadotropin and thus serve as the definitive treatment of the thyrotoxic state.

SUGGESTED READING

Agus ZS. Oncogenic hypophosphatemic osteomalacia. Kidney Int 1983; 24:113–123.

Baylin SB, Mendelsohn G. Ectopic (inappropriate) hormone production by tumors: Mechanisms involved and the biological and clinical implications. Endocr Rev 1980; 1:45–77.

Daughaday WH. Hypoglycemia in patients with non-islet cell tumors. Endocrinol Metab Clin North Am 1989; 18:91–101.

Imura H. Ectopic hormone syndromes. Clin Endocrinol Metab 1980; 9:235–260.

Jex RK, van Heerden JA, Carpenter PC, Grant CS. Ectopic ACTH syndrome: Diagnostic and therapeutic aspects. Am J Surg 1985; 149:276–283.

Miyagawa CI. The pharmacologic management of the syndrome of inappropriate secretion of antidiuretic hormone. Drug Intell Clin Pharm 1986; 20:527–531.

Mundy GR. Hypercalcemia of malignancy revisited. J Clin Invest 1988; 82:1–6.

IMMUNE, ALLERGIC, AND RHEUMATOLOGIC DISORDERS

ALLERGIC AND NONALLERGIC RHINITIS

HAROLD S. NELSON, M.D.

Rhinitis is a common affliction that varies in severity, producing nearly disabling symptoms in some patients, whereas in others producing such mild symptoms that they are not easily distinguished from heightened awareness of the normal mucus production of the nose. The types of rhinitis also present a broad spectrum. Seasonal allergic rhinitis is usually clearly distinguishable, but perennial rhinitis may be separated less precisely into (1) a group of disorders having an allergic basis, (2) a group that is nonallergic but clearly is associated with other allergic or potentially allergic conditions, and (3) the group formerly called vasomotor rhinitis. The last named could more accurately be called nonallergic, noneosinophilic rhinitis, since little is known of its cause or mechanisms. The importance of distinguishing among these types of rhinitis is that they affect the therapeutic approach. Clearly allergen avoidance and allergy immunotherapy are indicated only for rhinitis that truly has an allergic basis. Nonallergic rhinitis associated with asthma, eczema, or seasonal allergic rhinitis does not benefit from an allergen-directed therapy but often responds more satisfactorily to pharmacotherapy than does nonallergic rhinitis not sharing these associations.

CLASSIFICATION OF RHINITIS

Seasonal allergic rhinitis is characterized by symptoms of nasal and ocular pruritus, repetitive sneezing, watery rhinorrhea, and nasal obstruction occurring during a particular season corresponding to the appearance in the air of an allergen to which the subject can be demonstrated to be sensitive. Significant seasonal allergic rhinitis in the absence of skin test reactivity to the suspected allergen has not been convincingly demonstrated.

Perennial allergic rhinitis, in areas where the occurrence of frost ensures a season without significant outdoor aeroallergens, is primarily due to sensitivity to animal dander and insect allergens, particularly those from the house dust mite but perhaps more often than appreciated those from the cockroach. The importance of indoor molds in the etiology of perennial allergic rhinitis is suspected in some instances when damp areas exist in homes, but few studies have attempted to document their clinical importance. Ingestant allergens have been even less well studied, but the usual opinion is that they are of little importance as a cause of rhinitis beyond infancy and early childhood.

Perennial nonallergic eosinophilic (atopic) rhinitis is a condition that has only slowly been recognized, although the pace has been accelerated by several recent studies. It has been known for over 50 years that patients with nonallergic asthma have associated rhinitis and hypertrophic sinusitis with a tendency toward nasal polyps and that their nasal secretions, like their sputum and blood, are characterized by an excess of eosinophils. Nasal biopsies, or examination of tissue removed at the time of sinus surgery, has regularly shown an eosinophilic infiltration of the tissue. It is a reasonable assumption that the same nonallergic rhinitis, characterized by eosinophilic infiltration of the tissues and eosinophilia of the secretions, can occur alone as well as in conjunction with the other atopic diseases, such as seasonal allergic rhinitis, bronchial asthma, and atopic eczema. Also, just as patients with atopic eczema and bronchial asthma may have positive skin test results that are not clinically relevant to their disease, so, too, may patients with this atopic form of nonallergic rhinitis. Finally, since evidence has been presented that in patients with atopic diseases there may be enhanced mediator release in response to nonimmunologic stimuli, it should not be surprising that patients with nonallergic atopic rhinitis may experience symptoms suggesting the release of histamine, with itchy eyes and nose, sneezing, and rhinorrhea of a degree seen in seasonal allergic rhinitis.

Perennial nonallergic noneosinophilic (nonatopic) rhinitis formerly was termed vasomotor rhinitis, with the proposal that these patients experienced symptoms as a result of an excessive parasympathetic response to various noxious nonimmunologic stimuli. Although these patients do respond with symptoms to irritating odors and temperature changes, so, too, do virtually all patients with rhinitis. Since there is no convincing evidence that these patients' symptoms are caused by autonomic mechanisms or even that they constitute a single disease entity, a new term is needed that more accurately reflects the state of our knowledge. In general, the response of these patients to pharmacotherapy is not as favorable as it is in patients with the other types of rhinitis. However, there are a few well-categorized conditions that might be separated from this group, such as the rhinitis of pregnancy and hypothyroidism, and rhinitis medicamentosa due to either the topical use of decongestants or systemically administered medications. These conditions offer the prospect of a more successful resolution.

THERAPY OF ALLERGIC RHINITIS

The therapies of allergic and nonallergic rhinitis may be justifiably considered together. Measures directed toward allergens—avoidance and immunotherapy—are appropriate only in cases of rhinitis in which a significant allergic component has been demonstrated. Usually the treatment of rhinitis includes a major component of pharmacotherapy, and here the drugs employed are the same, although the response to the drug varies with the type of the rhinitis.

Avoidance

The first consideration in the treatment of allergic rhinitis should be an attempt to avoid completely or decrease the exposure to the offending allergen. Although with the exception of family pets complete elimination is seldom possible, substantial reduction in exposure often can be accomplished. In most pollen seasons the periods of peak counts are of limited duration, and these counts are generally highest during the midday or afternoon. Pollen concentrations are considerably reduced indoors, particularly if air conditioning is employed, allowing windows and doors to remain closed. For these reasons patients with pollen-induced seasonal allergic rhinitis often can avoid excessive symptoms by not undertaking outdoor recreational activities during the times of highest pollen counts. Although the season for the dry spore molds, such as *Alternaria* and *Cladosporium*, is more prolonged than it is for most pollens, peak counts are again encountered during dry, windy summer afternoons, allowing for some reduction in exposure by modification of activities at these times. The spores that particularly characterize periods of dampness and rain—basidiospores and ascospores—are especially numerous during the early morning hours. If they are suspected of causing allergic problems (a determination more dependent on history than testing because of the general lack of relevant extracts), closing windows at night, through the use of air conditioning if necessary, would be expected to effect a major reduction in exposure.

The most important allergens causing perennial allergy and the major components of "house dust" are animal danders and allergens derived from the house dust mite. The latter is ubiquitous except in the drier portions of the country, such as the Rocky Mountains and the southwest. An additional significant component—cockroach allergen—is encountered in areas where these insects are prevalent, such as the inner city areas of the north and the warmer portions of the country. Since house dust mites tend to accumulate in bedding, upholstered furniture, and adjacent carpeting, some control of allergen exposure is possible. When this has been undertaken in a thorough manner, a significant decrease in symptoms of asthma in both children and adults has been reported. The role of air cleaning devices in the avoidance of house dust mite allergen is not clear, since the allergen occurs predominantly in relatively large fecal pellets, which would be expected to fall rapidly from the air by gravity. Thus, local reservoirs, such as pillows, mattresses, and bed covers, appear more likely to be an important source than the allergen floating in the air.

Dander from pets, particularly cats and dogs, is a major perennial allergen. Clearly, complete avoidance should be possible, but emotional ties or the presence of pets in the homes of others often frustrates avoidance measures. It should be possible to "animal proof" the bedroom by excluding the pet from this room and keeping the door and heating ducts closed. There are no data that indicate whether under these circumstances the use of a room air-filtering device in the bedroom would be a worthwhile additional measure. However, dander remains airborne longer than mite antigen, and therefore some effect from air cleaner devices is likely. There is evidence that with the continued access of the pet to the bedroom, the concentration of allergen in the furnishings would negate any impact of the use of air filtration on the total allergen load. If only partial elimination of the family pet is possible, the more restricted the area in which the animal is allowed and the less furniture and carpeting to which it has access the better for the containment of allergens.

The role of indoor mold allergy in producing allergic rhinitis is unclear. Damp areas in the house that cause symptoms should be dehumidified if possible, and if humidifiers are employed, care should be taken that they are cleaned regularly and do not become a source of spore aerosols.

For all patients with rhinitis, nonimmunologic

irritants are a problem. Some can be avoided, and tobacco smoking within the home or workplace should be eliminated. It should also be possible, at least within the family, to avoid the use of strongly scented toiletries and cleaning products.

Pharmacotherapy

Antihistamines

Competitive antagonists of the histamine-1 (H_1) receptor have been the traditional basic treatment for allergic and nonallergic rhinitis. The older preparations have been grouped into six classes in part with the expectation that changing from one class to another might evade the tolerance that develops to this group of drugs. Recently it has been demonstrated that the tolerance is probably related to the histamine receptor and is not specific for the class of agent that induced it.

It has been suggested that subjects be provided with multiple samples of antihistamines to determine which they find most effective. However, several studies employing representatives from each of the antihistamine classes have confirmed a general pattern that the alkylamines, represented by chlorpheniramine and brompheniramine, are preferred by the largest number of subjects, and that hydroxyzine in the doses commonly employed appears to be slightly more effective than chlorpheniramine but also causes slightly more side effects, making it generally less satisfactory. A limited number of studies suggest that azatadine may also cause relatively few side effects.

The side effects of the traditional antihistamines are primarily of two types. There are direct central nervous system effects, which sometimes include stimulation, restlessness, and nervousness but much more often are characterized by drowsiness or incoordination. The second major group of side effects is related to anticholinergic actions of these drugs and includes dryness of the mouth, urinary retention, impotence, and blurring of vision. Tolerance to the central nervous system side effects develops rapidly, and by 4 to 10 days the incidence of drowsiness in many studies is similar to that with placebo. Tolerance to the desired antihistaminic properties also develops by 3 weeks, but this does not appear to be as profound in degree as the central tolerance, effectively improving the therapeutic ratio for these drugs. Recently, antihistamines have been developed that are nonsedating because they do not cross the blood-brain barrier. Furthermore, these drugs are free of anticholinergic action, thus avoiding some of the other side effects of the traditional antihistamines. This group includes terfenadine, astemizole, loratadine, and cetirizine.

Antihistamines block some but not all of the symptoms of allergic rhinitis. They effectively relieve pruritus, sneezing, and rhinorrhea, but they are largely ineffective for nasal congestion. Among the reasons offered for the latter is the demonstration that vasodilation in the nose is mediated largely by H_2 receptors. This has led to the suggestion that combined treatment with H_1 and H_2 antagonists might enhance symptomatic relief, and indeed the effectiveness of this combined treatment has been demonstrated both with nasal allergen challenge and in the course of seasonal allergic rhinitis. The use of H_1 and H_2 antagonists has not achieved widespread popularity, probably because of the availability of highly effective alternatives, such as topically applied corticosteroids. The availability of relatively pure H_1 antagonists, such as astemizole, has demonstrated that histamine is important in the production of symptoms in nonallergic as well as allergic rhinitis. The decision of whether to try antihistamine therapy is best made based on the types of symptoms the patient is experiencing rather than on the perception of whether the symptoms have an allergic basis.

Pharmacokinetic studies in adults have revealed unexpectedly long serum half-lives for a number of antihistamines. Hydroxyzine, chlorpheniramine, and brompheniramine all have serum half-lives of approximately 24 hours, suggesting that once daily dosing at bedtime with nonsustained release formulations should be adequate for the relief of symptoms. This dosing schedule has the advantage that maximal serum levels and therefore sedation occur while the patient is asleep. The use of single bedtime dosing, in addition to a gradual build-up of the dosage over 1 to 2 weeks, may allow the use of an inexpensive medication effectively with minimal side effects. In children the serum half-lives of these drugs are about 12 hours, perhaps accounting for the relatively higher doses of antihistamines employed in children but also making single daily dose therapy in children impractical. The new nonsedating antihistamine terfenadine has a half-life somewhat shorter than that of the preparations just listed, and twice daily dosing appears to be appropriate. Loratadine and cetirizine have longer half-lives consistent with once daily dosing. Astemizole, on the other hand, possesses pharmacokinetic properties of a different order, with a calculated half-life of 104 hours and with suppression of skin test reactions persisting for several months after the discontinuation of therapy.

In comparative trials, usually of only 1 or 2 weeks' duration, terfenadine, 60 mg twice daily, has produced control of symptoms equivalent to that with dosages of chlorpheniramine of 6 to 16 mg per day but with a lower incidence of side effects. Loratadine and cetirizine each at a dosage of 10 mg daily have been at least as effective as terfenadine, 60 mg twice a day. Astemizole, 10 mg once daily, on the other hand, has been consistently more effective than terfenadine, 60 mg twice daily, for both seasonal and perennial allergic rhinitis.

Astemizole has been compared in double-blind trials to both cromolyn and nasal beclomethasone dipropionate for the treatment of seasonal allergic rhinitis. It was found to be of equal effectiveness to a combination of nasal cromolyn six times daily and ocular cromolyn four times daily when administered as a once daily treatment. On the other hand, astemizole was found to be less effective than nasal beclomethasone for control of nasal symptoms although better for eye symptoms.

It is frequently stated that the antihistamines are more effective when administered on a regular basis rather than being taken as needed for the relief of already existing symptoms. Another argument for the regular use of the older preparations is that tolerance develops to the central nervous system side effects, improving their therapeutic ratio.

Decongestants

The drugs employed as decongestants are nonselective alpha-adrenergic agonists capable of constricting blood vessels elsewhere in the body. For that reason the preferred route of administration would be topical application to the nasal mucosa. Long-acting topical decongestant therapy is recommended for the treatment of nasal congestion associated with viral respiratory infections, to promote drainage during acute infections of the paranasal sinuses and middle ears, and to facilitate penetration during the first few days of topical corticosteroid therapy in patients with marked nasal obstruction. The limitation to their use is the well-recognized development of rebound obstruction, probably due to the induction of down regulation of the alpha-adrenergic receptors.

Orally administered alpha-adrenergic decongestants are also available, both as single drugs and in combination with antihistamines. They produce well-recognized side effects of tremor, restlessness, and agitation and can cause hypertension and urinary retention. Hypertension particularly has been reported with phenylpropanolamine, which appears to have a very narrow therapeutic range. Pseudoephedrine, the other commonly employed drug, has been implicated less frequently. Nevertheless a recent review concluded that there were inadequate studies to ensure the safety of oral decongestant therapy in patients with hypertension.

There also are few studies that have addressed the effectiveness of these drugs as decongestants during the course of long-term administration when some degree of alpha-adrenergic tolerance may be presumed to have developed. A reduction in nasal airway resistance was demonstrated following a dose of 60 mg of pseudoephedrine, but it persisted for only 2 hours. The sympathomimetics, however, have one advantage—their side effects tend to be directly opposed to those of the older antihistamines, making the combination attractive from the standpoint of reduced side effects.

Cromolyn Sodium

A nasal solution of 4 percent cromolyn sodium, administered four to six times daily, has been demonstrated to provide moderate relief of the symptoms of seasonal allergic rhinitis. As would be anticipated for a nasal spray, it does not alleviate eye symptoms. Cromolyn nasal solution also has been tested in patients with perennial rhinitis, in whom it produced a modest reduction in symptoms in those with positive skin test results but no better results than placebo in patients with negative skin test results, even in those who had profuse nasal eosinophilia. The topically applied steroid sprays have consistently demonstrated marked superiority over cromolyn in comparative trials and appear to be the preferred treatment except in patients with significant local side effects from the topical use of steroid preparations or those with marked "steroid phobia." Antihistamines have been demonstrated to be as effective as cromolyn and have the advantage of less frequent dosing, control of eye symptoms, and usually lower costs. Therefore, in patients tolerating antihistamines, they would appear to be the preferred initial treatment.

Cromolyn also is available as a 4 percent solution for use in the eyes. Again there is the inconvenience of six time daily use, but this preparation does provide good control of ocular symptoms as well as some effect on nasal symptoms and thus may complement topical nasal steroid therapy in the treatment of seasonal allergic rhinitis in patients whose ocular symptoms are prominent.

Corticosteroids

Two nasal steroids are available: beclomethasone dipropionate as a micronized powder in a freon-propelled vehicle or in an aqueous vehicle by pump spray and flunisolide as a propylene glycol solution delivered by a pump spray. The initial dosage of the former is usually four discharges into each nostril daily, and these can be delivered as one spray four times daily or two twice daily without affecting efficacy. Flunisolide therapy frequently has been initiated with two sprays into each nostril three times daily, but the dosage may be decreased to twice daily sprays without loss of control. In these dosages the two topically applied corticosteroids appear to be of similar efficacy. Both have some tendency to cause mucosal bleeding, but a particular problem with flunisolide for some patients is nasal burning, sufficient in a few patients to cause them to discontinue the medication.

Both drugs are very effective in seasonal allergic rhinitis, although symptom control is seldom complete. They do not relieve eye symptoms. Furthermore, there is a delay of several days for maximal effect. If marked nasal obstruction is present, they may be ineffective because of lack of access to the nasal mucosa, and initiation of therapy with 3 to 5 days of prednisone, 40 mg per day, or the topical use of a decongestant spray before each dose of corticosteroid for the same period may be necessary. Several studies suggest that antihistamines and topical corticosteroid therapy are complementary; there are no similar data for cromolyn and topical corticosteroid therapy.

It is clear that the topical corticosteroid therapy is more effective in "atopic (or nonallergic) eosinophilic rhinitis" than in rhinitis that is not related to the atopic diseases. Thus, a positive family history of atopic diseases, positive skin test results, pale swollen mucosa, or the presence of eosinophils in the nasal secretions all were predictors of a likely favorable response to topical corticosteroid therapy. The absence of these markers indicated perhaps at best a 24 percent chance of improvement. Despite this unpromising likelihood of a response, since these are generally patients who have failed to respond to other medications, a 2-week, carefully evaluated trial is indicated.

In patients with recurrent sinusitis or nasal polyps, the treatment of the associated nasal symptoms with topical corticosteroid therapy had been reported to diminish recurrences.

Miscellaneous Treatments

The vehicle of the flunisolide spray—propylene glycol—as well as saline nasal sprays and washes has been reported to diminish symptoms of perennial rhinitis, and in some cases this has been accompanied by an improvement in histopathologic findings.

The anticholinergic properties of the older antihistamines were thought to contribute to their efficacy by exerting a drying effect. Ipratropium bromide, a recently introduced anticholinergic, has been tried in selected cases of nonallergic perennial rhinitis characterized by marked rhinorrhea, with some decrease in symptoms.

Immunotherapy

Immunotherapy is reserved for last because that is its proper role in the treatment of allergic rhinitis. This is not a reflection of a lack of efficacy. Placebo controlled studies have clearly demonstrated that injection of extracts of pollens, animal danders, and house dust mite produces not only a decrease in clinical symptoms on natural exposure but also immunologic changes, which include a progressive decline in the levels of IgE specific for the substances being injected. Thus, unlike the other treatment modalities mentioned, allergy immunotherapy offers the promise of actually reversing the sensitized state.

Why then is the use of allergy immunotherapy deferred until other forms of therapy have first been tried and failed? The reason is the rigorous requirements placed upon the physician and the patient if allergy immunotherapy is to succeed: First the physician must determine that the symptoms are truly allergic—that the nature and timing of symptoms, the patient's exposure, and the patient's degree of sensitivity strongly suggest a causal relationship. Next the allergen must be specifically identified; this often is possible with pollens but rarely is possible with molds. Then potent extracts of these substances must be injected, ultimately at high concentrations, which carry the danger of serious or rarely even fatal reactions. The requirement on the patient's part is the investment in time and money over several years if lasting results are to be obtained. Anyone working in the field of allergy has to be concerned about the frequency with which immunotherapy is undertaken without these requisites being satisfied and the number of patients who report no decrease in symptoms after an investment of several years and many hundreds of dollars. Under present circumstances allergy immunotherapy should be reserved for clear-cut allergy to well-defined allergens in patients who have responded poorly to symptomatic therapy and have a prolonged season or perennial symptoms.

There are allergy extract preparations that have not yet been approved for release or that to some extent might restore the previous balance between symptomatic and allergy injection therapy. These are the modified extracts, allergenic extracts that have been treated to reduce their allergenicity, with preservation of their immunogenicity. These extracts hold the promise, should government approval be obtained for them, of allowing allergy immunotherapy to be offered with greater safety and with many fewer injections. These advantages, together with the fact that of the available modes of therapy of allergic rhinitis only allergy immunotherapy can promise to correct the underlying abnormality, would make injection therapy a much more attractive alternative than it is at present.

SUGGESTED READING

Hillas J, Booth RJ, et al. A comparative trial of intra-nasal beclomethasone dipropionate and sodium cromoglycate in patients with chronic perennial rhinitis. Clin Allergy 1980; 10:253–258.

Howarth PH, Holgate ST. Comparative trial or two non-sedating H_1 antihistamines, terfenadine and astemizole, for hay fever. Thorax 1984; 39:668–672.

Long WF, Taylor RJ, et al. Skin test suppression by antihistamines and the development of subsensitivity. J Allergy Clin Immunol 1985; 76:113–117.

Murray AB, Ferguson AC. Dust-free bedrooms in the treatment of asthmatic children with house dust or house dust mite allergy: A controlled trial. Pediatrics 1983; 71:418–422.

Sibbald B, Hilton S, et al. An open cross-over trial comparing two doses of astemizole and beclomethasone dipropionate in the treatment of perennial rhinitis. Clin Allergy 1986; 16:203–211.

Turkeltaub PC, Norman PS, et al. Treatment of seasonal and perennial rhinitis with intranasal flunisolide. Allergy 1982; 37:303–311.

Wohl J-A, Peterson BN, et al. Effect of the nonsedative H_1 receptor antagonist astemizole in perennial allergic and nonallergic rhinitis. J Allergy Clin Immunol 1985; 75:720–727.

ASTHMA

JOHN H. TOOGOOD, M.D., FRCPC, F.C.C.P.

To treat a patient with chronic asthma properly, the prerequisites cited in Table 1 must be met. All decisions about therapy are founded on these data.

TREATMENT

Three goals of treatment are common to all patients with asthma. These are to reduce exposure to identifiable "trigger" factors, both specific (i.e., allergic) and nonspecific (e.g., frosty air, tobacco smoke), to reverse or prevent bronchospasm using bronchodilator drugs, and to reduce the degree of nonspecific airway reactivity. The latter reflects, in part at least, the degree of airway inflammation. Regular treatment with a glucocorticoid, cromolyn, or immunotherapy (in appropriately selected cases) can each reduce nonspecific airway reactivity in addition to the more immediately perceptible bronchodilator action of beta-agonists or theophylline.

In patients with allergic asthma, it is also important to reduce the exposure to inhalant allergens. Rigorous environmental control of house dust, for example, can significantly improve nonspecific airway reactivity in asthmatics and reduce morbidity and the requirement for antiasthmatic drugs as well as the long-term costs of treatment.

It is convenient to consider the details of asthma therapy in terms of different levels of disease severity.

Chronic Asthma: Mild

Definition. No acute or chronic disability. Symptoms less frequent than daily. Prompt response to bronchodilator inhalant. No nocturnal asthma.

1. Eliminate any identifiable trigger factors, specific and nonspecific (e.g., a cat in the house).
2. Use albuterol, two puffs (200 μg), to relieve tightness of chest. Repeat every 2 hours as needed, up to a maximum of six doses per day.

TABLE 1 Diagnostic Prerequisites

Accuracy of asthma diagnosis?
Priority ranking in problem list?
Severity of pulmonary impairment?
Importance of allergic versus nonspecific "triggers"?
Clinical course: progressing, stable, labile?
Current therapy and drug intolerances?
Personality, lifestyle, social circumstances?
Expected results from therapy?

3. For predictable risk situations (e.g., exercise-induced asthma or occasional exposure to a known environmental allergen), premedicate with albuterol or cromolyn. The former is the more effective agent. Repeat four times daily for the duration of the exposure (e.g., a weekend stay in a household with cats).

Chronic Asthma: Moderate

Definition. Inhaled bronchodilator required almost daily. Nocturnal attacks. Restriction of lifestyle by exertional dyspnea or by periodic asthma exacerbations.

Plan

1. Eliminate identifiable trigger factors, specific and nonspecific.
2. Give sustained action theophylline preventively twice daily. Adjust the dosage to achieve a therapeutic serum concentration (55 to 110 μmol per liter). If the patient is symptom-free with levels less than 55 μmol per liter, do not increase the dosage.
3. As an alternative, the patient should inhale cromolyn, given as Intal, 20 mg (or Fivent, 2 mg) four times daily. This is the preferred regimen for children.
4. As an alternative to cromolyn, give beclomethasone dipropionate, 0.4 to 0.8 mg per day in four divided doses (or equivalent dose of budesonide, flunisolide, or triamcinolone). The patient should inhale the drug slowly. Aim for 5 to 10 seconds and breath-hold for 5 to 10 seconds after full inspiration.
5. To relieve "breakthrough" asthma symptoms, the patient inhales 200 μg of albuterol. Repeat every 2 hours as needed. If albuterol is required more than six times per day, this indicates the need for a change in the treatment plan. The physician should be contacted. If, on the other hand, the need for albuterol approximates zero, discontinue theophylline and continue the beclomethasone (except when compliance with the beclomethasone regimen is unsatisfactory).
6. To correct or avert disabling exacerbations, give prednisone, 40 to 60 mg per day for 5 to 7 days, in two to four divided doses. Reduce to zero over about 3 weeks. A 2- to 4-day burst may suffice if the asthmagenic challenge was short-lived. Abrupt withdrawal of prednisone after a short burst is safe.

Chronic Asthma: Severe

Definition. Lifestyle restricted by exertional dyspnea despite regular use of bronchodilators, cromolyn, or inhaled steroids in conventional doses. Bursts of prednisone are required more than three times per year to correct acute relapses.

Plan

1. Use aggressive prednisone therapy to correct disability and determine the maximal reversibility of

the obstructive impairment. Continue administration of 40 to 60 mg per day, if tolerated, until improvement plateaus. In older adults who have some chronic obstructive pulmonary disease associated with the asthma, this may require up to 3 weeks. Monitor the response objectively if possible by daily peak expiratory flow rate measurements at home or periodic spirometry in the office or hospital. After "plateauing," taper to a maintenance dosage level over 3 to 4 weeks.

2. Cotreat with sustained action theophylline twice daily. If low "trough" serum concentrations indicate a fast metabolizer, shift to three times daily dosing and increase the per diem dosage cautiously.

3. Increase the inhaled steroid dosage, e.g., to ≥1.0 mg per day of beclomethasone, and have the patient inhale the drug via a spacer. A large volume spacer such as the Inspir-Ease (about 700 ml) can double the intrapulmonary delivery of the drug. Titrate the oral and then the inhaled steroid dosage to determine the minimal dosages of each required to prevent disability and maintain symptom control. Provided minimal doses are used, there is no contraindication to the combined use of inhaled and oral steroid therapy (usually high-dose inhaled and low-dose, alternate-day oral). Some patients with labile severe asthma may require as much as 1 year of careful follow-up and dosage manipulation to achieve stable and optimal disease control.

4. Have the patient inhale albuterol immediately before each beclomethasone treatment. This improves the air flow and helps prevent the reflex cough that may be triggered if beclomethasone is inhaled too rapidly. Ipratropium may confer an additional advantage in the older asthmatic with associated chronic obstructive pulmonary disease. Use extra doses of albuterol to relieve breakthrough symptoms of bronchospasm. Ipratropium is also effective but takes about 20 minutes to act.

5. In a very few cases it may be necessary to administer nebulized albuterol at home, using an air compressor and mask (2.5 mg dissolved in about 2.0 ml of diluent, inhaled two to four times daily).

6. Cotreatment with cromolyn, administered via spincaps or a metered dose inhaler, does not add materially to the results that can be obtained with inhaled steroids alone. However, in labile asthmatics who are refractory to other treatment, especially those with atopic allergy, 1 percent cromolyn solution may be added, two to four times daily. The rationale for this treatment lies in its well-documented safety record, the reliable delivery system, and the drug's capacity to avoid seasonally recurrent increases in nonspecific airway reactivity consequent to periodic allergen exposure during long-term use.

Acute Asthma: Mild

Definition. Transient nondisabling bronchospasm.

TABLE 2 Beta-Agonist Bronchodilators

Albuterol	Isoproterenol
Epinephrine	Orciprenaline (metaproterenol)
Fenoterol	Terbutaline

Plan. Any of the inhaled beta-agonist drugs listed in Table 2 are effective. These are given by metered dose inhaler. Albuterol is the most efficient in terms of prompt action, sustained action, and minor adverse effects. Epinephrine is the least efficient.

If mild dyspneic attacks consistently fail to respond within 3 to 5 minutes to inhaled albuterol, they are probably not the result of asthma; functional dyspnea should be considered. If such attacks continue to recur despite explanation and reassurance, selected patients may benefit from relaxation breathing exercises, using autohypnosis techniques or a yoga type of regimen.

Acute Asthma: Moderate

Definition. The symptomatic response to bronchodilators is not sustained. Potentially disabling, recurrent exacerbations.

Plan

1. Abort exacerbations of infective asthma or asthmatic bronchitis by a burst of steroid administered systemically early in the illness: 20 mg of prednisone twice daily for about 5 days, reducing to zero after 10 days (longer, if necessary, depending on the severity of the attack). Use oral and inhaled bronchodilator administration concomitantly.

2. The infections that trigger these exacerbations are mostly viral. If an antibiotic is considered necessary, tetracycline, ampicillin, amoxicillin, cotrimoxazole, or erythromycin is a reasonable choice. However, erythromycin increases the risk of theophylline toxicity.

If a satisfactory response is not obtained after 1 week, repeated courses of antibiotic usually do not improve the situation. The persisting wheezy bronchitis commonly indicates the need for more aggressive steroid treatment, e.g., another week of prednisone, 20 to 40 mg per day.

Acute Asthma: Severe

Definition. Increasingly severe asthma, despite frequent (often excessive) bronchodilator use at home. Disabled.

Plan

1. Treat with oxygen and nebulized albuterol solution (2.5 mg inhaled at a flow rate of 6 to 8 L per minute over 5 to 10 minutes). If no response occurs in 30 minutes, repeat the albuterol treatment. In par-

TABLE 3 Characteristics of High-Risk Asthmatics Seen in Emergency Room

Previous life-threatening attack
Very labile asthma or gradually deteriorating air flows
Long delay before seeking medical attention
Pulsus paradoxus (systolic blood pressure drops > 12 mm Hg on inspiration)
PEFR* < 100 L per minute or FEV_1† < 0.7 L
Inadequate response 1 hour after nebulized albuterol administration (Δ PEFR < 60 L per minute or Δ FEV_1 < 0.4 L)
Respiratory alternans or paradoxic inspiratory diaphragmatic movement
Diminishing consciousness; increasing exhaustion
$PaCO_2$ normal, rising, or elevated
Presence of pneumothorax or mediastinum

*Peak expiratory flow rate.
†Forced expiratory volume in 1 second.

tially responsive cases, repeat as needed at 1 to 4 hour intervals. Check blood gas levels (off oxygen). Criteria for admission to hospital are shown in Table 3.

2. Cotreatment with theophylline intravenously may increase the toxicity of the treatment without a comparable increase in benefit. In patients with a history of recent theophylline ingestion, withhold intravenous therapy with theophylline until a failure to respond to combined albuterol-corticosteroid treatment clearly establishes the need for theophylline and the results of a theophylline serum concentration measurement are at hand.

3. Steroids should be used routinely for severe asthma. Because the steroid response is slow to appear (6 to 9 hours), bronchodilators must be used as well. Give 250 mg of hydrocortisone intravenously immediately and repeat every 8 hours (or 750 mg running continuously over 24 hours); 150 mg of methylprednisolone per 24 hours is equally effective and has less mineralocorticoid activity. Higher doses confer no additional benefit and on rare occasions may cause disastrous complications.

4. If narcotics and tranquilizers are avoided and aggressive bronchodilator-steroid-oxygen treatment is pursued, the need for assisted ventilation in uncomplicated asthma is rare.

COMPLICATIONS

Beta-Agonists

Muscle tremor can be minimized by using an inhaled rather than an oral formulation or substituting ipratropium inhalant.

The question of patients "abusing" their bronchodilator inhaler merits special attention. The increasingly frequent use of the metered dose inhaler usually signals a dangerous deterioration in ventilatory function due to beta-adrenergic tachyphylaxis or an increasing inflammatory component in the airway obstruction. Warnings about the danger of "inhaler abuse" are inappropriate in these circumstances. Steroids can reverse the problem and are urgently needed. Restoration of the airways responsiveness to adrenergics may begin within 1 hour. However, the widespread mucus plugging of small airways may take 1 week or more to resolve fully. Patients who have experienced such dangerous relapses should be committed to regular steroid treatment or given a home supply of prednisone with instructions outlining the indications for use and details of dosage.

Theophylline

Theophylline commonly leads to gastric reflux and occasionally to reflux esophagitis. When patients with active systems of reflux are given prednisone, ranitidine or cimetidine should also be prescribed preventively to inhibit gastric acid secretion. If the patient is symptomatic, add alginic acid compound (Gaviscon), three times daily after meals and at bedtime.

Insomnia, irritability, or nausea responds to lowering of the theophylline dosage. Major complications are avoidable if blood levels are kept below 110 μmol per liter. Erythromycin inhibits theophylline metabolism, and so do virus infections. Together or singly, these factors may trigger dangerous toxic effects. Avoid erythromycin in asthmatic patients taking theophylline.

Mood-Altering Drugs

Narcotics are contraindicated for asthma treatment. Tranquilizers are inappropriate for asthma and occasionally are dangerous. Typically, anxiety resolves spontaneously as severe asthma is brought under control with bronchodilators and steroids.

Steroid-Induced Bone Disease

To minimize the risk of steroid osteoporosis (and other systemic complications), follow the guidelines listed in Table 4. Postmenopausal women starting regular steroid therapy should maintain a high calcium intake (milk, cheese, supplemental calcium if necessary), ingest 800 IU of vitamin D daily, and exercise regularly outdoors. Estrogens, if started soon after the menopause, prevent excessive bone loss.

Treat patients with symptomatic vertebral fractures with calcium supplements, vitamin D, and

TABLE 4 Prevention of Systemic Complications of Steroid Therapy

Use prednisone in preference to slowly metabolized steroids, e.g., dexamethasone
Use the single-dose, alternate-morning regimen
Titrate dose to minimal effective level
Replace some or all of the prednisone with inhaled steroid
Give calcium supplement (to reduce osteoporosis)

enough codeine to facilitate walking (weight-bearing stress is essential for bone repair). After appropriate metabolic assessment, selected patients may benefit from estrogens (to decelerate bone loss), vitamin D (to increase calcium absorption), hydrochlorothiazide (to reduce urinary calcium loss), or fluoride (to stimulate bone formation). Monitor to avoid hypercalcemia. The safety of fluoride remains uncertain.

Steroid Withdrawal Syndrome

Abrupt or accelerated withdrawal of systemic doses of steroids after a long period of regular usage may precipitate disabling arthralgia, joint swelling, cellulitis, peripheral edema, lethargy, anorexia, and nausea—so-called "pseudorheumatism." The syndrome responds well to indomethacin and may be avoided altogether if the steroid dosage is tapered slowly, using an alternate-day regimen.

Use of Steroids in Asthmatics at Risk from Tuberculosis

When starting steroid treatment, routine isoniazid treatment is not indicated for asthmatic patients with a positive skin test to tuberculin unless they have clinically active tuberculosis or have recently converted to skin test positive status. Combined antituberculosis chemotherapy and beclomethasone have been used successfully in patients with active tuberculosis and asthma.

Treatment of the Pregnant Asthmatic

Treat the asthma of the pregnant patient to ensure optimal control. Topically active drugs such as beclomethasone, cromolyn, albuterol, or ipratropium are preferred. Systemic steroid treatment should be used as needed because the risk of steroid-induced adverse effects on the fetus or mother appears to be negligible, whereas uncontrolled asthma increases the incidence of maternal complications, premature delivery, and perinatal fetal morbidity and mortality.

Preoperative Preparation of the Steroid-Dependent Asthmatic

Anyone presenting for surgery with a history of use of oral or inhaled steroid therapy during the preceding year should receive 100 mg of cortisone acetate (2.0 ml) intramuscularly 24 hours preoperatively, as well as a repeat dose in 8 hours and 1 hour preoperatively. If the blood pressure drops, give hydrocortisone sodium succinate, 100 mg intravenously immediately. Repeat every 6 to 8 hours to prevent hypotensive crises. If emergency surgery is necessary, 4 mg of dexamethasone given intravenously at least 1 hour preoperatively may be preferable because it acts more quickly than cortisone and persists longer than hydrocortisone because of its slower metabolism.

Inhaled Steroids

High-dose inhaled steroid therapy in adults or conventional doses in children may suppress hypophysis-pituitary-adrenal axis function. Also, steroids inhaled in conventional doses may perpetuate adrenocortical hypofunction caused by earlier systemic steroid treatment. To minimize the problem, titrate the dosage to determine each patient's minimal needs.

A common complication of inhaled steroid treatment is reflex cough triggered by deposition of the drug in the central airways and carina region. To resolve the problem, peripheralize the dose by having the patient inhale the drug more slowly or via a spacer or by pretreatment with an inhaled beta-agonist. A 10-day burst of prednisone may be required in some cases to restore accessibility of the distal airways to the inhaled drug and thus eliminate the cough.

Dysphonia (huskiness) complicating inhaled steroid therapy is caused partly by irritation from the propellants and partly by dyskinesia of the muscles that control vocal cord tension. Therefore antifungal therapy is inappropriate. To alleviate or avoid huskiness, reduce deposition of the drug around the larynx by reducing the daily dosage, inhaling via a spacer, or reducing the speed of inspiration. Acute or chronic laryngeal stress, common in switchboard operators, sports coaches, and singers, aggravates the problem. Rigorous voice rest may be needed. Resumption of therapy with the drug is usually well tolerated if laryngeal stress is avoided.

To minimize the incidence of oropharyngeal thrush requiring nystatin, the patient should inhale the steroid via a spacer, avoid concomitant prednisone or antibiotic use as much as possible, and rinse the mouth after each treatment. Conversion from four times daily to twice daily dosing will largely eliminate thrush but may also reduce the drug's antiasthma efficacy. Esophageal candidiasis is an unusual complication that illustrates the interaction of multiple risk determinants (see below).

Systemic steroid treatment may be preferable to inhaling steroid for the long-term treatment of patients with advanced allergic bronchopulmonary aspergillosis. Asthmatics who have epithelialized cavities, cysts, or bronchiectatic segments may be at risk of mycotic superinfection if inhaled steroid therapy is used. In the immunocompromised patient, avoid any form of steroid therapy, oral or inhaled, or use it with great caution because of the risk of opportunistic infection.

Complicated Problems

Multiple factors may interact to produce complications in the particular patient. To deal effectively

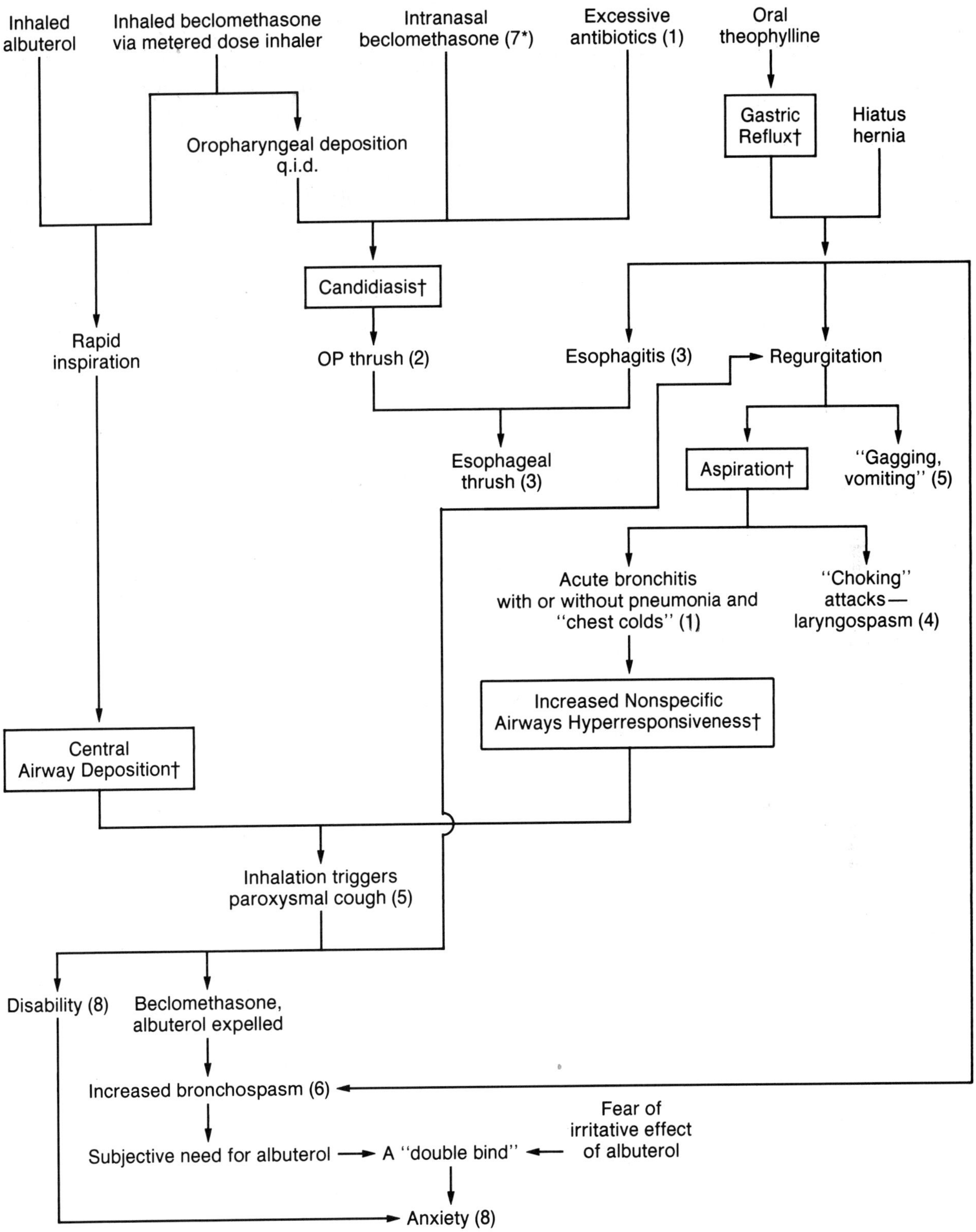

Figure 1 Pathogenesis of presenting complaints that led to a therapeutic impasse.
* Numbers can be referenced to the presenting complaint at initial visit (Table 5).
† See Table 6.
OP = oropharyngeal.

TABLE 5 Presenting Complaints*

1. Frequent "chest colds" (? pneumonia); constantly taking antibiotics for >6 months
2. Continuous nystatin for oral thrush for >6 months
3. Low substernal dysphagia, heartburn, bloating
   Endoscopic diagnosis: candidiasis of esophagus; no response to nystatin
4. Frightening "choking" attacks—about three per day
6. Cough, gagging, vomiting attacks, two or three each hour, triggered by any deep inhalation or by inhalation of an antiasthmatic drug (including albuterol)
6. Tight chest (but afraid to inhale albuterol)
7. Nose plugged, mouth breathing, anosmia
8. Unable to work for 4 months, depressed, anxious

*Complex drug interactions causing adverse symptoms: theophylline + BDP + antibiotics + albuterol (see Fig. 1).

TABLE 6 Treatment Plan*

1. Control reflux and aspiration:

   Quit theophylline. Substitute oral doses of albuterol. Elevate head of bed. Cimetidine b.i.d. + alginic acid compound q.i.d. (+ antacid prn)

2. Eliminate candidiasis:

   Avoid antibiotics (which stimulate *Candida* growth). Treat "chest colds" symptomatically only. Inhale beclomethasone via spacer (reduces oropharyngeal deposition 90%). Rinse mouth after each treatment.

   Quit intranasal beclomethasone. Use antihistamine orally instead. Switch beclomethasone dosage from q.i.d. to b.i.d. (conserves antifungal host defenses at mucosal surface).

3. Shift aerosol deposition away from upper airways, trachea, carina:

   Eliminate high-velocity impact on pharynx, larynx (by using spacer). Slow inhalation to 25 liters per minute—slower if necessary (to peripheralize inhaled drugs).
   Breath-hold 10 seconds after inhaling beclomethasone (to maximize antiasthmatic effect).

4. Reduce nonspecific airways hyperresponsiveness:

   Continue beclomethasone.
   Time.

Result:

At 2 months:	Improving. Nonspecific airways hyperresponsiveness still high.
At 5 months:	Much improved. Working.
At 14 months:	Unrestricted vigorous exercise. No longer taking antireflux drugs or antacids.
At 24 months:	Doing very well on beclomethasone and albuterol spray q.i.d. via spacer. Off oral albuterol. Antihistamine/decongestant prn for rhinitis. Prednisone weeks = 3/104. No antibiotics or nystatin in 2 years.

*Goals 1 to 4 can be referenced to the items enclosed by a rectangle in Figure 1.

with the problem, it is necessary to unravel these interactions. The data in Tables 5 and 6 and Figure 1 summarize the latter process in a young man with an array of complications that had led to a therapeutic impasse. Table 5 lists his presenting complaints. Figure 1 displays a flow chart of their pathogenesis. Constructing such a chart helps the physician to plan an effective strategic approach. The treatment plan and clinical results are shown in Table 6.

BEYOND DRUGS

Every patient with asthma brings three basic needs to the therapeutic encounter:

1. The need for an explanation of the mechanism of the symptoms and their prognostic significance. This explanation must be expressed in terms that are understandable to the patient, given his or her concepts of bodily function and disease. These concepts vary with social class and with cultural background and they may be radically different from those of the physician.

2. The need to be assured that there are things that he or she can do to control the illness.

3. The need to believe that the therapist is supportive and caring.

In meeting these needs, the good physician forges the "patient-physician" relationship—and the latter is at least as important as any drug for long-term therapeutic success.

A system of regular clinical follow-up strengthens the patient-physician bond. Furthermore, it shifts the emphasis of the therapeutic plan from intervention to prevention, from correcting illness to maintaining wellness. The process of follow-up also teaches the physician a great deal about the natural course of chronic asthma and how to deploy the various modalities of treatment to the greatest advantage of each patient.

SUGGESTED READING

Dolovich J, Hargreave FE, Wilson WM, et al. Control of asthma. Can Med Assoc J 1982; 126:613–618.
Littenberg B, Gluck EH. A controlled trial of methylprednisolone in the emergency treatment of acute asthma. N Engl J Med 1986; 314:150–152.
Mawhinney H, Spector SL. Optimum management of asthma in pregnancy. Drugs 1986; 32:178–187.
Rebuck AS, Chapman KR. Asthma. 1. Pathophysiologic features and evaluation of severity. Can Med Assoc J 1987; 136:351–354.
Rebuck AS, Chapman KR. Asthma. 2. Trends in pharmacologic therapy. Can Med Assoc J 1987; 136:483–488.
Siegel D, Sheppard D, Gelb A, Weinberg PF. Aminophylline increases the toxicity but not the efficacy of an inhaled beta-adrenergic agonist in the treatment of acute exacerbations of asthma. Am Rev Respir Dis 1985; 132:283–286.

STATUS ASTHMATICUS

HOMER A. BOUSHEY JR, M.D.

Status asthmaticus is defined as severe asthmatic bronchospasm that is unresponsive to acute bronchodilator therapy. It is not a distinct variant of asthma but rather a form in which the physiologic and pathologic changes of asthma are unusually severe. The treatment of status asthmaticus thus involves largely the vigorous, intensive application of therapies effective in relieving mild asthmatic bronchospasm, the use of measures to protect the patient against the consequences of severe obstruction to air flow, and the avoidance of injudicious therapies.

The clinical signs and symptoms of asthma are logical expressions of the underlying disease. In postmortem studies of patients dying of asthma the most impressive abnormality is the gross overinflation of the lungs due to widespread air trapping from diffuse obstruction of airways throughout the tracheobronchial tree. The airways themselves are filled with mucus, desquamated epithelial cells, and inflammatory cells, sometimes forming casts of small bronchi and their branches. The airway wall is thickened by an intense eosinophilic inflammatory infiltrate, and both airway smooth muscle and airway submucosal glands are hypertrophied and hyperplastic. These findings are not unique to patients dying of asthma, for similar but less pronounced changes are found in the lungs of people with asthma who die of other causes, as from accidents.

The physiologic consequences of diffuse airway narrowing include a reduction in maximal expiratory flow, an increase in the resistance to air flow, and an increase in lung volume. The increase in lung volume is due in part to the premature closure of narrowed peripheral airways (increasing residual volume) and is in part a compensatory mechanism, for the greater lung elastic recoil at high lung volumes tends to increase both the size of the airways and the driving force for expiration. Thus, the work that must be done to overcome both resistive and elastic forces is increased by diffuse airway narrowing, and hypoventilation occurs unless this increase in the work of breathing is matched by increases in respiratory drive and in the performance of the respiratory musculature.

The shift in functional residual capacity to a greater lung volume and the increased resistance to air flow result in a marked increase in the variation in pleural pressure from inspiration to expiration and thus to an exaggeration of the normal respiratory changes in arterial blood pressure (pulsus paradoxus). Alveolar pressure is markedly increased during the prolonged expiratory phase of breathing, and alveolar rupture with dissection of air within the pleural space or mediastinum sometimes occurs. Because small pulmonary vessels are exposed to this increased alveolar pressure, and because pulmonary arterial pressure must be greater than alveolar pressure to make possible pulmonary blood flow, pulmonary arterial pressure is increased and overload of the right ventricle may occur. Tests of the distribution of ventilation show that airway narrowing during an acute severe asthmatic attack is very uneven. This unevenness of ventilation inevitably leads to a mismatching of ventilation and perfusion, producing an increase in the alveolar-arterial oxygen difference, an increase in wasted ventilation, and compensatory vasoconstriction in poorly ventilated areas, further increasing pulmonary vascular resistance and pulmonary hypertension.

Despite the increases in the work of breathing and in wasted ventilation, alveolar and arterial P_{CO_2} values are characteristically below normal, indicating that the drive to maintain breathing is considerably increased. The increase in total ventilation helps to offset the fall in the P_{O_2} level caused by widening of the alveolar-arterial oxygen difference. The mechanisms responsible for alveolar hyperventilation are not precisely defined, but studies of animal models of asthma suggest that they depend on afferent innervation of the airways. Whatever the underlying mechanism, alveolar hyperventilation is typical in acute asthmatic attacks and means that carbon dioxide retention, or even a "normal" value for the P_{CO_2}, indicates extremely severe air flow obstruction, fatigue of respiratory muscles, or exhaustion of the patient and is thus an indication for urgent aggressive therapy. These physiologic disturbances have a characteristic clinical expression, and certain clinical manifestations are now recognized as hallmarks of severe life-threatening asthma.

Rebuck and Read, reasoning that death results from suffocation, suggested that the risk of death could be estimated from assessments of the degree of air flow limitation (the "load"), the arterial oxygen and carbon dioxide tensions (the "outcome"), and the physical costs of producing a given outcome in the face of a given load. In brief, they demonstrated that the clinical features of severe life-threatening asthmatic attacks are consequences of airway narrowing and include an FEV_1 of less than 0.5 liter, an FVC of less than 1.0 liter, alveolar hypoventilation, pulmonary hypertension and right heart strain, pulsus paradoxus greater than 18 mm Hg, hypoxemia (P_{O_2} less than 65 mm), exhaustion or any disturbance in consciousness, and pneumomediastinum or pneumothorax. Later studies have added tachycardia (pulse rate greater than 120 per minute), tachypnea (respiratory rate greater than 30 per minute), accessory muscle use, orthopnea, diaphoresis, and a history of severe attacks requiring intubation as other indices of severe, potentially lethal asthmatic attacks.

THERAPY

The intensity of initial therapy for asthmatic bronchospasm is adjusted according to the severity of the attack. For patients without the features of life-threatening asthma, the administration of a selective $beta_2$ adrenergic agonist by aerosol (e.g., 0.3 ml of 5 percent metaproterenol solution in 1.5 to 2.5 ml of normal saline) is effective as is the subcutaneous injection of 0.3 ml of a 1:1000 dilution of epinephrine, and both are more effective than the intravenous administration of aminophylline. The response should be assessed clinically and by repeat spirometry and the treatment repeated if no improvement is noted at 30 minutes. Those who respond to this initial treatment generally continue to improve and may be discharged if they have minimal symptoms at rest, an FEV_1 of more than 40 percent predicted, the ability to use outpatient medications (most often a selective $beta_2$ agonist given by metered dose inhaler and an orally administered theophylline compound), and a follow-up appointment.

For patients who present with two or more of the features of life-threatening asthma or who fail to respond to the initial bronchodilator therapy just described, a more aggressive approach must be taken. For these patients it is useful to record the key features of the severity of disease on a flow sheet. Serial recording of the general state of consciousness, heart rate, respiratory rate, pulsus paradoxus, FEV_1 and FVC (or peak expiratory flow) values, and arterial blood gas levels provides a useful, quickly comprehensible profile of the patient's condition and response to therapy. When the initial assessment has been completed, supplemental oxygen should be given by nasal prongs at a rate of 4 liters per minute. In acute severe asthma there is no need for concern about inducing hypercapnia by giving excessive oxygen as there is in patients with exacerbations of chronic obstructive lung disease. Aerosol treatment with an inhaled $beta_2$ selective adrenergic agonist should be given initially, 1 hour later, and at 1 to 2 hour intervals for the first 8 hours or until a response is seen. An intravenous line should be secured for the administration of aminophylline and a corticosteroid. The initial or loading dose of aminophylline is 5.6 mg per kg given over 20 to 30 minutes in 100 to 250 ml of 0.5 normal saline, followed by a maintenance dose of 0.6 mg per kg per hour given by continuous infusion.

Care must be taken with both the loading dose and the maintenance dose. Many different bronchodilator compounds (e.g., Tedral, Quibron, Uniphyllin, Theodur, and Marax) contain theophylline, and if a full loading dose is given to a patient who already has a nearly therapeutic blood level (10 to 20 μg per ml), toxic effects may occur (nausea, vomiting, diarrhea, tachycardia, cardiac arrhythmias, grand mal seizures) and complicate an already difficult clinical situation. When in doubt, it is wisest simply to start the maintenance dose by continuous infusion and await the result of a stat analysis of a baseline blood sample of theophylline. The maintenance dose must also be adjusted in some patients. Since an age over 50 years, congestive heart failure, and liver disease impair metabolism, the rate of infusion should be lowered to 0.4 mg per kg per hour in patients with those conditions. Children and current cigarette smokers metabolize theophylline more rapidly and may require 0.8 mg per kg per hour. Because the rates of metabolism vary widely even in healthy individuals, the blood level of theophylline should be checked in all patients 12 to 24 hours after therapy is started and the dose adjusted to achieve a therapeutic level.

Corticosteroids are effective in acute severe asthma and are credited by some experts for the fall in the mortality of hospitalized asthmatic patients since they were introduced in the 1950s. Their efficacy has been demonstrated in several prospective placebo controlled, double blind studies, but these studies also show that the greater improvement in the steroid treated group becomes apparent only 6 to 12 hours after steroids are given. The studies do not show clear dose dependency, but it is common practice to give 0.5 to 1.0 mg per kg (0.5 to 1.0 mg per kg) of methylprednisolone intravenously initially and every 6 hours thereafter for the first 24 to 48 hours or until clinical improvement is seen. Because one of the actions of corticosteroids is to potentiate beta-adrenergic responsiveness of airway smooth muscle, their effect may first be apparent as an increase in the change in FEV_1 provoked by aerosolized metaproterenol.

The pathologic abnormalities responsible for airway narrowing in asthma are not confined to smooth muscle contraction, of course, and corticosteroids have other important actions in relieving air flow obstruction. The inhibition of phospholipase A_2, for example, may prevent the metabolism of arachidonic acid in inflammatory cells and inhibit the production of the prostaglandins and leukotrienes that may be responsible for attracting and activating other inflammatory cells, for altering water transport across the epithelium, and for altering mucus secretion from submucosal glands and goblet cells. Only limited means are available for increasing the clearance of airway secretions more directly. Beta-adrenergic drugs may increase mucociliary clearance but are already being given to relax airway smooth muscle. Adequate hydration is probably important, and many patients may be dehydrated as a result of the increase in insensible water loss from the respiratory tract, but overhydration has not been shown to be helpful in mobilizing airway secretions.

Thus the standard initial therapy for acute severe asthma or for asthma unresponsive to two or three treatments with an injected or inhaled adrenergic drug is administration of supplemental oxygen, repeated administration of an adrenergic aerosol, intravenous administration of aminophylline and corticosteroids, and generous intravenous and oral replacement of fluids.

TOXIC REACTIONS

The regimen we have discussed is usually effective and well tolerated but carries some risk of toxicity. Most severe is the risk of cardiac arrhythmias. Myocardial irritability is directly increased by aminophylline and by adrenergic drugs and may be potentiated, especially in patients taking digitalis, by the hypokalemia sometimes produced by adrenergic drugs. Electrocardiographic monitoring therefore should be maintained in patients with premature beats on initial examination, in patients over 40, and in all patients with a history of heart disease or arrhythmias, and the serum potassium level should be measured at 4 and 24 hours to rule out hypokalemia.

A more common but less severe form of toxicity is skeletal muscle tremor, an additive effect of theophylline and adrenergic drugs. This may be minimized by substituting inhaled ipratropium bromide aerosol (Atrovent, 40 to 60 μg from a metered dose inhaler) for every other aerosol treatment with an adrenergic drug. Ipratropium is a derivative of atropine that is poorly absorbed and that also crosses the blood-brain barrier poorly. It does not appear to be a more effective bronchodilator than adrenergic drugs in asthmatic subjects, but it may have an additive effect on airway caliber and at the least offers a means of maintaining the bronchodilation achieved with adrenergic drugs without adding to their cardiac or muscular toxicity.

Another common side effect of the standard initial therapy for severe asthma, but one that is rarely of great clinical importance, is modest worsening of hypoxemia due to reversal of the compensatory vasoconstriction of pulmonary vessels supplying poorly ventilated lung regions. The resulting fall in the arterial Po_2 level is usually small and requires no intervention. It is simply important to recognize that a fall in the PaO_2 level in the absence of a rise in the $PaCO_2$ level does not indicate that bronchodilator therapy is ineffective or that the patient's condition is worsening.

Although viral respiratory infections are common precipitants of acute severe asthmatic attacks, bacterial infections are not, and antibiotics should be given only for specific indications. Sputum purulence is not itself sufficient, for it may simply reflect the airway mucosal inflammation associated with viral infections or possibly with late reactions to intense antigen exposure. Similarly a localized perihilar infiltrate revealed on the chest radiograph may reflect large mucus plugs in central airways. Moderate leukocytosis is common in uncomplicated asthmatic attacks, especially in patients treated with parenteral doses of epinephrine or high doses of corticosteroids. Fever is not typical of acute asthma, however, and requires explanation (fever may be overlooked if the rectal temperature is not obtained because oral breathing is invariable with severe bronchospasm). In patients with clinical or laboratory signs of infection, sputum and blood cultures should be done and treatment started with a broad spectrum antibiotic, such as erythromycin trimethoprim-sulfamethoxazole, or ampicillin. Care must be taken to ensure the absence of a history of allergy to the antibiotic chosen, for asthmatic patients are apt to develop immediate hypersensitivity reactions.

The use of oxygen, an adrenergic aerosol, and aminophylline and methylprednisolone intravenously is effective in the majority of patients, and serial measurements of the respiratory rate, pulsus paradoxus, spirometry, and blood gas levels show steady improvement. Controversies over treatment are most likely to arise in the care of patients who do not improve over the first few hours. In such patients it is useful to distinguish failure to improve from clinical deterioration. In general, the more abrupt the onset of bronchospasm, the more promptly it is reversed with therapy. The acute severe attack provoked by aspirin or sulfites in a sensitive asthmatic patient often starts to reverse within a few hours after the beginning of therapy, and pulmonary function test results may be nearly normal on the following day. In contrast, the attack provoked by a viral illness is typically more gradual in onset and less quickly reversible with therapy, perhaps because smooth muscle contraction is relatively less important, and inflammation and mucus plugging are relatively more important as causes of airway narrowing. This may be the reason that improvement is not seen in some patients until the third to fifth day of therapy.

It is sometimes the case, however, that the condition worsens despite therapy. The patient appears to be fatiguing, the $PaCO_2$ has increased to 40 mm or higher, and pulsus paradoxus has increased. In this event the patient must be under constant surveillance, and preparations must be made for intubation and mechanical ventilation, for deterioration can be abrupt and absolute when the patient is exhausted. It is at this point that other therapeutic measures are sometimes tried. Giving beta-adrenergic agonists intravenously (e.g., isoproterenol) is sometimes effective, perhaps because intravenous administration increases delivery of the drug to severely obstructed airways not reached by inhaled aerosols. Another measure that has been attempted but that is best avoided is intermittent positive pressure breathing, because it further increases intrathoracic pressure and thus further compromises cardiac output and increases the risk of pneumothorax. Chest physiotherapy is poorly tolerated by acutely dyspneic patients; delivery of an ultrasonic mist of distilled water aerosol achieves little hydration of airway mucus and increases bronchoconstriction (distilled water aerosol is used to provoke bronchoconstriction in research studies). Sedatives, which are sometimes given in the expectation that they will reduce motor activity and thus oxygen consumption and ventilatory demands, are contraindicated. Sedatives depress the respiratory center and increase fatigue; they frequently have been implicated as the cause of death in severe asthma.

Intubation and mechanical ventilation are indicated

for worsening hypercapnia, exhaustion, confusion, or impaired consciousness. Mechanical ventilation is hazardous in asthmatic patients, however, principally because of the high pressures needed to deliver an adequate tidal volume through narrowed airways into overdistended lungs. Pneumothorax, alveolar hypoventilation, and malfunction of the endotracheal tube or ventilator itself occur commonly. The risk of these complications can be reduced by using a volume cycled ventilator to ensure delivery of an adequate tidal volume and by taking measures to minimize inflation pressure: a large endotracheal tube, low inspiratory flow, and sedative and paralyzing drugs. Additional measures include using ketamine as a sedating, analgesic, and anesthetic drug with bronchodilating properties, and giving sodium bicarbonate to protect against respiratory acidosis if normal alveolar ventilation cannot be maintained except with dangerously high peak inspiratory pressures (60 cm H_2O and above). Cases have been reported in which bronchoscopy and lavage to remove mucus plugs from the airways were associated with clinical improvement, but they have yet to be shown to be effective in a prospective controlled study. The very low mortality in hospitalized asthmatic patients (estimated as 1 percent or less even for severe asthma) testifies to the effectiveness of current standard therapy. The reported recent increase in mortality from asthma seems not to be due to an increase in in-hospital deaths but to an increase in deaths in the hours before hospitalization.

The risk of sudden death appears to be increased in patients who have been hospitalized for asthma, especially if they have had attacks severe enough to require intubation, and especially in the first few weeks after discharge. Treatment therefore should be tapered slowly after discharge from the hospital and the severity of the disease should be monitored. It is our practice in hospitalized patients to switch from intravenous to oral therapy when objective signs show clear improvement, and not to discharge the patient until the response to oral and inhalation therapy has been observed for 24 hours. Oral doses of theophylline and the regular use of an inhaled beta-adrenergic drug are maintained, and the oral prednisone dosage is tapered over 7 to 10 days to 15 to 20 mg per day. The patient is then re-evaluated to determine the rate of further tapering. To permit this re-evaluation, tests of air flow obstruction must be carried out immediately prior to discharge and on return for outpatient evaluation. For patients with a history of abrupt attacks of severe bronchospasm without forewarning, twice daily measurements with a portable peak flow meter may show increased variability or progressive deterioration as the prednisone dosage is tapered, indicating the need for resumption of higher dosages or the institution of inhalation therapy with corticosteroids.

SUGGESTED READING

Fanta CH, Rossing TH, et al. Glucocorticoids in acute asthma—a critical controlled trial. Am J Med 1983; 74:845–851.

Haskell RJ, Wong BM, et al. A double-blind, randomized clinical trial of methylprednisolone in status asthmaticus. Arch Intern Med 1983; 143:1324–1327.

Huber HL, Koessler KK. The pathology of bronchial asthma. Arch Intern Med 1922; 30:689–760.

Minitove SM, Goldring RM. Combined ventilator and bicarbonate strategy in the management of status asthmaticus. Am J Med 1983; 74:898–901.

Rebuck AS, Read J. Assessment and management of severe asthma. Am J Med 1971; 51:788–798.

Rock MJ, De La Rocha S, et al. Use of ketamine in asthmatic children to treat respiratory failure refractory to conventional therapy. Crit Care Med 1986; 14:514–516.

Scoggin CH, Sahn SA, et al. Status asthmaticus: a nine-year experience. JAMA 1977; 238:1158–1162.

PENICILLIN ALLERGY

JOHN A. ANDERSON, M.D.

Benzylpenicillin G and semisynthetic penicillin (the penicillins) as well as the cephalosporin drugs are all classified as beta-lactam antibiotics because of a structural beta-lactam ring that all these drugs share. The penicillins, as a group, are among the most commonly prescribed drugs in the world today. The true incidence of allergic (immunologically mediated) reactions to the penicillin drugs in the world is not known. In continuing drug surveillance studies done in the United States among adult medical inpatients, however, the penicillin group of drugs is one of the most likely types of drugs to be involved in a significant adverse reaction. IgE-mediated systemic reactions complicate approximately 2 percent of the courses of penicillin therapy. In addition, since the prevalence of positive skin test reactions to penicillin drugs is estimated to be between 3 and 10 percent, a substantial proportion of the adult population is potentially at risk for anaphylactic reactions to these drugs. Anaphylaxis has been reported to occur with a frequency of 1 to 5 per 10,000 patient courses of penicillin treatment. Even if these incidence figures are inflated somewhat and even though the use of penicillins in the United States and other countries has declined in recent years because of the substitution of other less risky drugs in potentially susceptible patients, allergy to the penicillins and other beta-lactam antibiotics remains one of the most significant immunologically mediated adverse drug reactions.

Anaphylactic reactions to the penicillins occur most commonly in adults between the ages of 20 and 49, although anaphylaxis may occur at any age. Approximately 25 percent of these reactions occur within 48 hours after initial penicillin therapy. Seventy-five percent of the patients who have died of penicillin anaphylaxis had no history of allergy to these drugs. Sensitization to the penicillins can occur by any route, the topical route being most risky. Multiple short courses of administration of these drugs are most likely to result in sensitization. Once sensitization to the penicillins has occurred, the allergic reaction may occur following penicillin challenge by any route, but drug administration by the intramuscular route is most risky. The oral route is safest, since if reactions do occur, they tend to be mild, cutaneous in nature, and self-limited.

The patient's sex, race, and HLA phenotype do not appear to affect the incidence of penicillin allergy. A personal or family history of allergy to other substances does not correlate with penicillin reactivity. Skin test reactions to penicillin drug products in atopic and nonatopic individuals have been shown to occur with equal frequency. Most reported deaths due to penicillin drugs have occurred in nonatopic patients. Patients who are allergic to the penicillin group of molds are not at an increased risk of developing sensitization to the penicillin drugs.

PENICILLIN ALLERGENS: PENICILLIN SKIN TESTING AND IN VITRO METHODS

Penicillin is a simple structure with a low molecular weight of 300 daltons. As a hapten, it is itself not immunogenic, but it becomes so by combining with tissue proteins. The relative ease with which the parent drug, penicillin, and its drug metabolites combine with tissue proteins to become complete antigens (by forming stable covalent bonds) helps to explain the heightened "sensitivity" to this type of drug in humans compared with other drugs. The molecular nucleus of penicillin is 6-aminopenicillic acid, which contains a beta-lactam ring and a thiazolidine ring. Ninety-five percent of the parent penicillin drug is metabolized to the penicilloyl determinant (major penicillin determinant), and the rest of the drug is metabolized to minor haptenic determinants. The exact structures of all minor penicillin haptenic determinants are unknown, but they include sodium benzylpenicilloate and penilloate (when benzylpenicillin is processed to form a "minor determinant mixture").

In vivo the amino or the hydroxyl terminal group of tissue proteins combines with the beta-lactam ring of the penicillins. For allergy skin testing, the penicilloyl "major" determinant is combined with polylysine to produce penicilloyl-polylysine.* This antigenic material is usually used in a prick-scratch-puncture skin test followed by intradermal skin testing according to the manufacturer's instructions. This test is usually combined with penicillin G or individually produced minor determinant mixtures.

*Produced commercially by the Kremer-Urban Company.

Several protocols for allergy skin testing have been published. One common approach is to perform prick-scratch-puncture skin tests with penicilloyl-polylysine (6×10^{-5} molar), penicillin G (10,000 U per milliliter or 10^{-2} molar), or minor determinant mixture (10^{-2} molar) in addition to a histamine and saline control (Table 1). It is clearly desirable to do skin testing with the minor determinant mixture; however, since a validated standardized commercial minor determinant mixture is not available, many clinicians simply use a fresh solution of penicillin G as a partial substitute for the penicillin minor determinants at the present time. "Aging" penicillin has no advantage over freshly prepared penicillin allergens used for skin testing.

Prick-scratch-puncture skin tests are done with these reagents initially. If the results are negative, intradermal skin tests are performed. A prick-scratch-puncture or intradermal skin test is considered positive when a wheal develops that is at least 2 mm larger than the diluent control skin test reaction read 10 to 20 minutes after the penicillin or other beta-lactam antibiotic antigen presentation. In vitro solid phase immunoassays for antigen-specific IgE, such as the radioallergosorbent (RAST) or enzyme linked immunosorbent assay (ELISA), have been developed to detect antibodies to the penicilloyl determinant. No similar in vitro assay exists for routine testing for IgE antigen–specific antibodies to the minor penicillin haptenic determinants or to determinants to other beta-lactam antibiotics.

EVALUATION OF THE PATIENT WITH A HISTORY OF PENICILLIN ALLERGY

Penicillin skin testing is an extremely useful procedure in the evaluation of the patient with a history of an adverse reaction to penicillin and in whom an IgE-mediated immunologic mechanism for this reaction is suspected. If the penicillin skin test is positive, the presence of IgE antigen against penicillin products can be considered confirmed and the patient is at risk for a clinical reaction if challenged with penicillin. However, each patient who is history positive and penicillin skin test positive may not react clinically to a penicillin challenge on a given day (approximate risk, 60 to 70 percent). The chance of finding a positive penicillin skin test reaction varies with the length of time from the time the patient had a clinical reaction to penicillin. Patients in whom the clinical reaction occurred between 2 weeks and 3 months after drug exposure have been shown to develop a positive penicillin skin test 70 to 100 percent of the time. On

TABLE 1 Skin Testing for Beta-Lactam Antibiotic Allergy*

Skin Test Type	*Skin Test Reagent*	*Drug Test Concentration*	*Skin Test Volume*
Penicillin major determinant	Penicilloyl-polylysine†		
	1. Prick-scratch-puncture	Full skin test strength	One drop
	2. Intradermal	Full skin test strength	0.02 ml
Penicillin minor determinant	Fresh penicillin G‡		
	1. Prick-scratch-puncture	10,000 U/ml	One drop
	2. Intradermal	10,000 U/ml (serial skin testing optional, e.g., 10 U/ml followed by 100 U/ml and 1,000 U/ml)§	0.02 ml (each)
and/or			
	Penicillin minor determinant mixture		
	1. Prick-scratch-puncture	10^{-2} molar	One drop
	2. Intradermal	10^{-2} molar (individual schedules for serial testing optional)§	0.02 ml
Semisynthetic penicillin or cephalosporin	Specific drug		
	1. Prick-scratch-puncture	0.25, 2.5, 25 mg/ml serial skin tests§	One drop (each)
	2. Intradermal	2.5, 25 mg/ml serial skin tests §	0.02 ml (each)
Histamine (positive control)	Histamine phosphate		
	1. Prick-scratch-puncture	1:1,000 w/vol	One drop
	2. Intradermal	1:10,000 w/vol (1:100,000 w/vol optional)	0.02 ml
Saline (negative control)	Buffered saline on appropriate dilution		
	1. Prick-scratch-puncture	N/A	One drop
	2. Intradermal	N/A	0.02 ml

*All skin tests are considered as immediate reacting in nature and can be read in 10 to 20 minutes. Prick, scratch, or puncture skin tests always should be done first. If they are negative, intradermal skin testing can be done.

†Kremer Urban Co.—single skin test strength.

‡Freshly prepared (1 week) benzyl potassium penicillin (1 million U vial) mixed with 9.6 ml of sterile sodium chloride–penicillin stock solution (penn. stock on day of testing 0.5 ml of penn. stock + 4.5 ml of sodium chloride = 10,000 U/ml).

§Serial skin testing: Although the usual patient can be safely skin tested with single strength reagents, sensitive patients should be serially tested with weaker strengths first before proceeding with stronger reagents.

the other hand, positive penicillin skin test reactivity in patients shown to be allergic to penicillin decreases over time, approximately 50 percent being skin test negative 5 years following the allergic reaction and 70 to 80 percent being skin test negative 10 years or more after this allergic reaction.

In the majority of the studies involving patients who present to an allergist with a history of penicillin allergy at some time in the past, approximately 14 to 20 percent of the adults and no more than 10 percent of the children can be shown to be skin test positive to penicillin antigens. A single group of investigators reported, however, that 63 percent of 740 patients presenting with a positive history of penicillin sensitivity were shown to be skin test positive on penicillin skin testing (Sullivan et al, 1981).

If the penicillin skin test is negative, the patient generally can be considered to be not allergic to penicillin. The reliability of these tests has been reported to range between 96 and 99 percent in studies of patients who have had a history of penicillin reaction, who were skin test negative, and who were subsequently challenged. In one study, a 4 percent reaction rate was found after penicillin challenge in 370 history positive patients who tested negative with penicilloyl-polylysine and penicillin G (Green et al, 1977). In another, large National Institute of Allergy and Infectious Diseases collaborative study of adults, 1,173 patients with skin tests negative to penicilloyl-polylysine and a minor determinant mixture (615 of whom had positive histories of previous penicillin allergy), upon penicillin challenge only six patients (0.5 percent of the total and 1 percent of the penicillin history positive patients) had an adverse reaction compatible with an IgE-mediated immediate or "accelerated penicillin allergy" (Sogn et al, 1990). Patients who have had a significant reaction to penicillin cannot be reliably tested to penicillin within the immediate 2-week period following the clinical reaction. Although a positive penicillin skin test reaction during this period of time may provide useful information, negative skin test reactions are considered as unreliable indices of the lack of penicillin sensitivity. The exact reason for the existence of this refractory period in some penicillin-allergic patients is unknown.

In vitro penicilloyl RAST or ELISA assays may

be helpful in the diagnosis of penicillin allergy only if they are positive. If negative, these assays do not rule out sensitivity, since they detect only 60 to 95 percent of the patients who react in a positive fashion to penicilloyl-polylysine skin tests, and these in vitro assays do not detect circulating IgE antibodies directed against penicillin minor determinant haptens. A single investigator has reported a small number of patients who were shown to be clinically sensitive to penicillin and had circulating IgE antibodies directed against penicilloyl-polylysine by in vitro methods but who were also found to be skin test negative to penicilloyl-polylysine (Sullivan, personal communication).

These in vitro tests should be considered in situations in which reliable skin test reagents are not available, in which skin disease or conditions such as eczema or dermatographism preclude accurate determination of skin test reactivity, or in the presence of circulating drugs that affect the accuracy of skin test reactivity.

Some controversy surrounds the timing of the use of penicillin skin testing. Some allergists who deal primarily with adult patients recommend that skin testing with penicillin should be used only just before a therapeutic dose of penicillin is to be given. One of the reasons for this school of thought is that the penicillin skin test result is accurate only for that period of time or for that specific therapeutic endeavor. At any future time the patient may develop an initial penicillin sensitivity (or a renewed penicillin sensitivity). One investigator has recently shown that a select group of hospitalized patients who had a history of penicillin reactions but who were penicillin skin test negative following successful challenge with a full course of intravenous penicillin therapy had a high likelihood (60 percent) of developing subsequent positive penicillin skin test reactivity upon testing 2 to 3 months later (Earl et al, 1987).

Many allergists who deal primarily with children as patients advocate elective penicillin skin testing. The reasoning behind this school of thought centers on the fact that only one of 10 children (versus one of five or more adults) who have a history of penicillin allergy is likely to be shown to have positive penicillin skin test reactivity. Many of these children developed urticaria or other rashes at a young age during the treatment of an "infection" with a penicillin product. Often the reaction in the child, in retrospect, was due to factors other than an IgE immunologic reaction to penicillin (e.g., viral infection). One investigator has shown in a large number of patients (80 percent of whom were younger than 20 years of age) that elective skin testing can be done easily, is safe, and when followed by an oral challenge dose of penicillin is not likely to produce a clinical reaction in a skin test negative patient (Mendelson et al, 1984, 1987). Finally, when these patients were given a full therapeutic course of oral penicillin therapy, only a few developed a rash, and none experienced a systemic reaction to the antibiotic. Subsequently only 1 percent of the patients developed a positive skin test to penicillin when retested 4 weeks later. Thus elective skin testing, oral challenges in skin test negative patients, and oral penicillin therapy (in skin test negative, oral challenge negative patients) can help to "clear the air" for the physician who is in doubt about the patient who allegedly is sensitive to the drug. In the majority of the patients it is safe to give the penicillin again later without the necessity for retesting the patient for penicillin (before each treatment).

Some controversy also exists concerning the necessity for challenging a patient who has been found to be skin test negative. From the foregoing discussion it is evident that there is more risk of reaction in an adult who presents with a history of penicillin allergy than in a child. If the reaction is significant (e.g., life-threatening), it is probably wise to challenge the patient with a single oral dose of penicillin following a negative penicillin skin test reaction. Following a full course of antibiotics, it is probably also wise to retest the patient at a future date. These recommendations are particularly important when the minor determinant mixture has not been used in the skin test protocol. However, in children who have had a questionable history of a penicillin-allergic reaction at some time in the past, a negative penicillin skin test itself is a good index of the lack of penicillin sensitivity. In questionable cases, however, again an oral challenge under controlled conditions with a single dose of the penicillin product to be used is advised. It is wise also to advise the referring physician of the exact risk based on the percentage of the reliability of the testing procedure for each given patient.

EVALUATION OF THE PATIENT SUSPECTED OF BEING ALLERGIC TO SEMISYNTHETIC PENICILLIN

Patients who are proved to be sensitive to any one type of penicillin by the demonstration of IgE antibodies against the parent penicillin drug or the metabolic byproduct or by challenge with this drug should be considered allergic to all types of penicillins and semisynthetic penicillins. 6-Aminopenicilloic acid is the nucleus of the penicillin G molecule. This nucleus is present in all semisynthetic penicillins, and thus it should not be surprising that cross-allergenicity exists among these penicillins to some degree.

Routine skin testing procedures similar to those that have been recommended for the evaluation of the patient suspected of being allergic to penicillin G have not been perfected to the same degree for the evaluation of the patient suspected of being allergic to semisynthetic penicillins. Some investigators have shown that all reactors to the semisynthetic penicillins can be identified by skin testing with penicilloyl-polylysine, penicillin G, or minor determinant mixture. These methods are the most studied and most validated.

Other investigators contend that although defined cross-reactivity exists between penicillin G and the semisynthetic penicillins, there may be unique antigens associated with the latter penicillins and, for this reason, additional skin testing with the specific semisynthetic penicillin is recommended. No commercially available major or minor individual semisynthetic hapten determinant skin test material is available; therefore, usually the parent (semisynthetic penicillin) drug is used.

One suggested routine involves serial prick-scratch-puncture skin testing utilizing concentrations of the semisynthetic penicillin of 0.25, 2.5, and 25 mg per milliliter (see Table 1). These tests are done serially with the weakest concentration first and then are read at 10- to 20-minute intervals. A positive test includes any in which the wheal is 2 mm or more larger than the control. If the results of these prick-scratch-puncture tests are negative, serial intradermal skin testing is done with 2.5 mg per milliliter and then 25 mg per milliliter semisynthetic pencillin.

CEPHALOSPORIN AND OTHER BETA-LACTAM ANTIBIOTICS: SENSITIVITY AND CROSS-SENSITIVITY IN PATIENTS WHO ARE ALLERGIC TO PENICILLIN

The cephalosporins resemble the penicillins chemically; both drug nuclei contain a beta-lactam ring. However, in the case of the cephalosporins, the beta-lactam ring is attached to a six-membered dihydrothiazine ring instead of a five-membered thiazolidine ring, as is the situation with the penicillins. Cephalosporin breakdown during body metabolism results in a major cephaloyl determinant or grouping and probably is associated with other "minor" antigenic determinants.

The skin testing procedures used by various investigators in an attempt to demonstrate IgE antibodies against cephalosporin drugs involve utilizing various concentrations of the parent cephalosporin drug and almost exclusively utilizing the prick-scratch-puncture method. These methods are crude at best, and the experience of one investigator cannot be generalized (Anderson, 1986). If cephalosporin skin testing is done, care must be taken not to overinterpret a "positive" test, since nonspecific irritation is possible. Because so little clinical information exists about cephalosporins as skin test reagents, negative skin test reactions should be interpreted as "no information" rather than as a lack of cephalosporin allergy.

There are some clinical clues to the contention that each cephalosporin drug differs from the others in the degree of risk of an allergic reaction. Thus skin testing with these general types of drugs may depend on the use of several cephalosporin antigens when these methods are perfected in the future.

Anaphylaxis to cephalosporin does occur but much less often than with the penicillins. Reactions have been reported both to cephalothin and to cephaloridine—the latter in two patients who had no evidence of pencillin allergy. The continuing Boston Collaborative Drug Surveillance Program studying cutaneous drug reactions has demonstrated that among adult medical inpatients, cephalosporins account for only 1 percent of the cases of reactivity versus a 10 percent incidence with penicillin-semisynthetic penicillin (Bigby et al, 1986).

A recent study of children treated for otitis media with either amoxicillin or cefaclor demonstrated an allergy-like and nonallergy-like cutaneous reaction incidence with cefaclor of 5.4 percent versus 3.7 percent with amoxicillin (Anderson, 1986). The mechanism of reaction in this study was not investigated; however, it is possible that some cephalosporins will be shown to produce a toxic or idiopathic rash in a similar fashion to that shown for ampicillin. Although it is speculative, the incidence of such cutaneous allergy-like drug reactions may be increased by certain viral infections, as in the case of ampicillin rash with Epstein-Barr virus infection. If these speculations are true, many of the cutaneous reactions that are observed with the cephalosporins may be caused by mechanisms other than IgE and therefore do not constitute a risk when penicillin is a substitute.

The true incidence of cross-reactivity between penicillin–semisynthetic penicillin and the cephalosporin drugs is unknown. One investigator found in penicillin skin test positive patients that approximately half were allergic to ampicillin and half to cephalosporin utilizing prick-scratch-puncture and intradermal skin testing. None of the skin test positive (or negative) patients was challenged with these drugs, however. Another investigator challenged 27 patients known to be allergic to penicillin by history and skin testing (no cephalosporin skin testing), and none reacted. Furthermore, in the institution where the latter study was performed, it has become common practice to use cephalosporins in patients suspected of having penicillin allergy (without confirmation by either penicillin skin tests or challenges). Finally, in a recent study involving 19 patients shown to be penicillin allergic either by pencillin skin test, in vitro tests, or challenge, two (10.5 percent) were found to react on parenteral cephalosporin challenge.

With all the published information as a base, it would seem that the risk of reaction using cephalosporins in patients suspected of being allergic to penicillin is approximately 2 percent. Patients with a history of penicillin allergy should be skin tested with penicillin to define sensitivity. Most will be found to be nonallergic. In this group, cephalosporin administration is probably no more hazardous than it is in the general population. In confirmed penicillin-allergic patients (history positive, penicillin skin test positive), up to half may have a positive cephalosporin skin test reaction. The latter group should be presumed to be allergic to both drugs unless challenged, and alternative drugs should be considered.

Two new beta-lactam antibiotics have been developed: the monobactams (e.g., aztreonam) and the carbapenems (e.g., imipenem). Aztreonam has a monocyclic beta-lactam nucleus and a side chain identical to that of a third-generation cephalosporin, ceftazidime. Studies have shown no skin test reactivity to these drugs in patients who are allergic to penicillin and have a positive-reacting penicillin skin test. Recently, one patient, who failed oral penicillin desensitization, was successfully given Azactam utilizing a "rapid provocative dose challenge" (Loria et al, 1989).

Imipenem, a carbapenem that contains a bicyclic nuclear structure like that of the penicillins and the cephalosporins, has been studied in both normals and penicillin-allergic patients. Utilizing skin test strengths that do not produce an irritative response in normal patients, 50 percent of the penicillin-allergic patients reacted to one or more of the imipenem determinants on skin testing (approximately 80 percent of these penicillin-allergic patients were skin test positive to the penicillin minor determinant) (Saxon et al, 1988). Although the reported incidence of clinical reactions to imipenem is low, penicillin-allergic patients should be presumed to be allergic to this drug —unless challenged—since cross-sensitivity may be 50 percent.

DESENSITIZATION OF PATIENTS WHO ARE ALLERGIC (IgE SENSITIVITY) TO BETA-LACTAM ANTIBIOTICS (PENICILLIN G, SEMISYNTHETIC PENICILLIN, CEPHALOSPORINS, OR CARBAPENEMS)

The principal preventive therapy of allergy to the beta-lactam drugs is to avoid use of these drugs if possible. When infection requires treatment in the face of allergy to these medications, a safe alternative drug is recommended. This may include consideration of the use of the monobactam class of antibiotic. When this is not possible, and other beta-lactam antibiotic therapy is required, desensitization should be attempted. This procedure is not recommended for non-IgE-mediated reactions to the beta-lactam antibiotics, such as ampicillin rash, erythema multiforme, the Stevens-Johnson syndrome, toxic epidermal necrolysis or other exfoliative dermatitides, delayed (non-IgE-mediated) eczema, drug fever, hemolytic anemia, or intestinal nephritis.

The basic process of the acute desensitization procedure involves the serial, fairly rapid administration of doses of a beta-lactam antibiotic in small increments of increasing strength over a short time course. In the usual situation the penicillin drug-allergic patient is able to take a fixed amount of the medication to which he or she is allergic in this fashion without reaction or with minor controllable anaphylactic reactions.

The precise mechanism involved in the successful desensitization process to a drug like penicillin is not known. For many years it was assumed that mast cell-basophil preformed mediators (such as histamine) were being depleted. We now know that this does not completely explain the success of the desensitization procedure. Other hypotheses include antigen-specific desensitization of tissue mast cells, hapten inhibition by the induction of circulating monovalent drug conjugates, the binding of circulating antipenicillin IgE antibodies by small amounts of drug haptens, and, finally, some induction of IgG antipenicillin "blocking antibodies."

It is recognized that a refractory period exists immediately following a penicillin anaphylactic reaction. Such a refractory period also occurs in the case of reactions to drugs not involving an IgE mechanism (e.g., aspirin). In some way the refractory period is induced by the desensitization procedure, allowing a "window of opportunity" to administer a necessary drug. Once the cumulative drug dose necessary to fight the infection process has been reached in the patient, this top dose can be maintained in the allergic patient (chronic desensitization) as long as the interval between drug doses is not longer than 8 to 12 hours. If the interval of drug administration at this top dose is prolonged beyond this narrow time frame, life-threatening anaphylaxis may occur upon further drug administration as the refractory period or desensitized state dissolves.

DESENSITIZATION PROCEDURES: GENERAL PRINCIPLES

The desensitization procedure should be carried out with the appropriate informed consent of the patient, parent, or guardian. The procedure should be done under controlled conditions, such as in a hospital intensive care unit, so that not only can the patient be closely monitored but any adverse reaction to the drug administered during the procedure can be promptly recognized and appropriately treated. Whenever possible, the desensitization procedure should be performed on an elective basis instead of as an emergency—during the week and during regular hours so as to have the best chance of having available the optimal levels of support services and personnel for patient care. Any potential complicating factors should be corrected—if possible—before drug desensitization is started. This may include the control of urticaria, asthma, or shock and the discontinuation of beta-blocking drugs (and the control of disease by safer medications).

Premedication of the patient with antiallergic medications, such as those routinely used in patients with a history of adverse reactions to conventional radiocontrast media—antihistamines, cortisone, cimetidine, or ephedrine sulfate—is not recommended. It is important not to mask any early signs of anaphylaxis to the drug used in the desensitization process so that these reactions can be properly treated. The clinical status and vital signs should be monitored frequently throughout the procedure and throughout the first 12 hours of full dosage drug treatment. Finally, and most important, a knowledgeable physician should be present with the patient throughout the process.

DESENSITIZATION PROTOCOL: GUIDELINES

Individual protocols have been published by several authors over the years to help guide the less knowledgeable or less experienced physician through the desensitization procedure. The most widely published experience utilizing the desensitization procedure in patients who are allergic to penicillin involves the collective work of a single group of investigators (Sullivan et al, 1982; Stark et al, 1987). Table 2 represents an oral penicillin desensitization protocol devised by this group.

Although the initial dose in the protocol (step 1) indicates 100 U, the author indicated that desensitization in patients who are very sensitive (e.g., penicillin prick rather than intradermal skin test positive) may be started at even more dilute antigen concentrations of 10 U, 1 U, or 0.1 U. The recommended interval between dosing is 15 minutes. This can be lengthened, however, in the patient who demonstrates reactions. Following stabilization of the patient who does react during the procedure, the next dose of desensitizing drug should be at a strength no greater than that two steps below the dose that precipitated the reaction.

As far as penicillin allergy is concerned, desensitization utilizing the oral route has been shown to be safer than any parenteral route (fewer reactions during the procedure). In the case of allergy to the semisynthetic penicillins or cephalosporins, desensitization with oral penicillin therapy will not suffice. If oral drug forms of these other beta-lactam antibiotics are available, individual protocols should be made up, adapting to the general principles outlined in Table 2 for penicillin. On the other hand, when no oral beta-lactam antibiotic drug form exists, a parenteral desensitization protocol should be followed (Table 3). The experience of Stark and coworkers, utilizing the oral route of desensitization followed by beta-lactam antibiotic treatment in both adults and children for 1 to 40 days, shows a reaction incidence with the procedure of 38 percent. This incidence can be broken down further. Reactions during the acute desensitization process are as follows: pruritus, 4 percent; urticaria or angioedema, 5 percent; wheezing, 1 percent; total, 10 percent. Reactions during beta-lactam antibiotic therapy following attainment of the top dose during the desensitization process are as follows: pruritus, 3 percent; urticaria, 18 percent; large local reaction, 1 percent; serum sickness, 3 percent; hemolytic anemia, 1 percent; and glomerulonephritis, 1

TABLE 2 Oral Desensitization Protocol*

Step†	*Phenoxymethyl Penicillin (U/ml)*	*Amount (ml)*	*Dose (U)*	*Cumulative Dose (U)*
1	1,000	0.1	100	100
2	1,000	0.2	200	300
3	1,000	0.4	400	700
4	1,000	0.8	800	1,500
5	1,000	1.6	1,600	3,100
6	1,000	3.2	3,200	6,300
7	1,000	6.4	6,400	12,700
8	10,000	1.2	12,000	24,700
9	10,000	2.4	24,000	48,700
10	10,000	4.8	48,000	96,700
11	80,000	1.0	80,000	176,700
12	80,000	2.0	160,000	336,700
13	80,000	4.0	320,000	656,700
14	80,000	8.0	640,000	1,296,700
		Observe patient for 30 minutes		
	Change to benzylpenicillin G		IV	
15	500,000 U/ml	0.25	125,000	
16	500,000	0.50	250,000	
17	500,000	1.0	500,000	
18	500,000	2.25	1,125,000	

*From Sullivan TJ. Penicillin allergy. In: Lichtenstein LM, Fauci AS, eds. Current therapy in allergy, immunology and rheumatology. Toronto: BC Decker, 1985:60.
†Interval between steps: 15 minutes.

TABLE 3 Parenteral Desensitization Protocol*

Step†	*Concentration of Beta-Lactam Drug (mg/ml)*	*Amount (ml subcutaneously)*	*Dose (mg)*	*Cumulative Dose (mg)*
1	0.1	0.10	0.01	.01
2	0.1	0.20	0.02	.03
3	0.1	0.40	0.04	.07
4	0.1	0.80	0.08	.15
5	1	0.15	0.15	.30
6	1	0.30	0.3	.60
7	1	0.60	0.6	1.2
8	10	0.10	1	2.2
9	10	0.20	2	4.2
10	10	0.40	4	8.2
11	10	0.80	8	16.2
12	100	0.15	15	31.2
13	100	0.30	30	61.2
14	100	0.60	60	121.2
15	1,000	0.10	100	221.2
16	1,000	0.20	200	421.2
17	1,000	0.40	400	821.2
18	1,000	0.50	500	1,321.2
		Observe patient for 30 minutes		
19	1,000	IV	0.5 g	1,821.2
20	1,000	IV	1.5 g	3,321.2

*From Sullivan TJ. Penicillin allergy. In: Lichtenstein LM, Fauci AS, eds. Current therapy in allergy, immunology and rheumatology. Toronto: BC Decker, 1985:61.

percent. The total incidence of immunologic complications of the subsequent drug therapy was reported to be 27 percent. Stark and colleagues also have shown that following the acute desensitization procedure, patients needing antibiotics for long periods may be maintained in the refractory or desensitized state for 3 weeks to more than 2 years (median duration, 10 weeks' therapy). In all cases the full dosage of therapy was given orally in divided doses daily, no longer than 12 hours apart.

Once therapy with the beta-lactam antibiotics has been completed, and antibiotics used in the desensitization procedure or treatment have been stopped, the penicillin-allergic patient is again at risk for reaction to a beta-lactam antibiotic. At a future date, if beta-lactam antibiotics are again needed, retesting and, if appropriate, desensitization are indicated.

Newer antibiotics, such as the newer penicillins, cephalosporins, or structurally unique monobactams, may be less reactive than the commercially available beta-lactam antibiotics. In the future these safer substitute antibiotics may become available for beta-lactam sensitive individuals.

NON-IgE-MEDIATED IMMUNOLOGIC AND OTHER ADVERSE REACTIONS TO BETA-LACTAM ANTIBIOTICS

Other nonanaphylactic (but immunologic) reactions to the penicillins include hemolytic anemia, neutropenia and thrombocytopenia, serum sickness, glomerulonephritis, drug fever, and various cutaneous reactions. The antibody usually involved in the production of penicillin-induced hemolytic anemia is IgG, although IgM and IgA types of penicillin antibodies also have been implicated. Positive direct antiglobulin (Coombs') tests can develop in 3 percent of the patients who receive high intravenous doses of penicillins. Only a small percentage of these patients, however, actively develop hemolytic anemia. Inhibition of factor VII (blood coagulation factor) activity has been attributed to the presence of antipenicillin antibodies.

Penicillin is the most common cause of drug-induced serum sickness-like reactions today. This syndrome of fever, rash, arthralgia, and arthritis results from circulating IgG and IgM drug-antibody complexes. The local deposition of drug-antibody complexes is facilitated by IgE release of vasoactive amines. Antipenicillin IgE is involved in the urticarial rash associated with this condition. The reactions typically occur 7 to 14 days into therapy but may occur weeks following termination of the penicillin therapy. The majority of serum sickness-like reactions are mild and resolve spontaneously within a few days to weeks, although some may be treatable with cortisone.

Penicillin may induce drug fever. The penicillins, especially methicillin, have been associated with the induction of nephritis. One of the most common manifestations of an adverse reaction to a beta-lactam antibiotic is a maculopapular rash, which occurs with ampicillin therapy (approximately 5 percent risk). The risk of this rash has been reported to be higher in patients afflicted with Epstein-Barr virus (infectious mononucleosis) or cytomegalovirus infection than in those with chronic lymphocytic leukemia and hyperuricemia and patients receiving an allopurinol drug concomitantly. This rash is not associated with an IgE antibody; it has been shown to be safe to continue ampicillin in spite of this rash without adverse effects. However, since IgE drug antibody may involve a maculopapular rash, it may be impossible to determine definitively that the patient taking ampicillin who has a rash is not sensitive to penicillin. Therefore, in most cases ampicillin therapy should be discontinued in such situations. Two or more weeks following the episode involving the rash, and when the patient is stable, elective penicillin skin testing is recommended to determine the patient's allergic status. If penicillin skin testing is negative, reinstitution of any penicillin product should be considered safe for the immediate future.

Most serious cutaneous and mucocutaneous reactions to the beta-lactam antibiotics involve a rash such as erythema multiforme and either the Stevens-Johnson syndrome or toxic epidermal necrolysis or Lyell's syndrome. The latter types of febrile mucocutaneous syndromes are of particular importance in that they cannot be predicted, the prodrome is similar to that of an infectious disease, and in its severest form toxic epidermal necrolysis has been reported to be associated with up to a 30 percent mortality (Strom, 1977). Although these reactions are allergy-like, IgE immune reactions have not been shown to be involved. Skin testing to penicillins is not helpful. In the few instances in which penicillin has been given on another occasion in patients who had such reactions, a repeated episode of the reaction has been documented. Penicillin desensitization has not been shown to be successful in such reactions and is not recommended.

It is well to point out that the desensitization process is applicable only in instances in which IgE immune reactions to pencillin are involved. Furthermore, the IgE desensitization procedure does not prevent the onset of serum sickness-like reactions, hemolytic anemia, or glomerulonephritis, as has been shown by the work of Stark and associates. In all the cases of non-IgE adverse reactions to the beta-lactam antibiotics, data are insufficient to indicate that it is safe to readminister the beta-lactam antibiotics or to desensitize the patients, regardless of the specific mechanism of these reactions.

SUGGESTED READING

Anderson J. Cross-sensitivity to cephalosporins in patients allergic to penicillin. Pediatr Infect Dis 1986; 5:557–561.

Bigby M, Jick S, Jick H, Arndt K. Drug-induced cutaneous reactions—report from the Boston Collaborative Drug Surveillance Program on 15,438 consecutive inpatients, 1975–1982. JAMA 1986; 256:3358–3363.

Blanca M, Fernandez J, Miranda A, et al. Cross-reactivity between penicillins and cephalosporins: Clinical and immunologic studies. J Allergy Clin Immunol 1989; 83:381–385.

DeSwarte RD. Special consideration of allergic drug problems: The beta-lactam antibiotics—penicillins and cephalosporins. In: Paterson R, ed. Allergic diseases: Diagnosis and management. Philadelphia: JB Lippincott, 1985:595.

Earl H, Stark B, Sullivan T. Penicillin induced IgE re-sensitization. J Allergy Clin Immunol 1987; 79:200 (abstract).

Green G, Rosenblum A, Sweet L. Evaluation of penicillin hypersensitivity: Value of clinical history and skin testing with penicilloyl-polylysine and penicillin G. J Allergy Clin Immunol 1977; 60:339–345.

Loria R, Finnertz N, Wedner H. Successful use of aztreonam in a patient who failed oral penicillin desensitization J Allergy Clin Immunol 1989; 83:735–737.

Mendelson L, Ressler C, Page J, et al. Elective testing of penicillin allergic patients. J Allergy Clin Immunol 1987; 79:200 (abstract).

Mendelson L, Ressler C, Rosen J, Selcon J. Routine elective penicillin allergy skin testing in children and adolescents. J Allergy Clin Immunol 1984; 73:76–81.

Saxon A, Adelman D, Patel A, et al. Imipenem cross-reactivity with penicillin in humans. J Allergy Clin Immunol 1988; 82:213–217.

Sogn DD. Penicillin allergy. J Allergy Clin Immunol 1984; 74:589–593.

Sogn D, Evans R, Shepherd G, et al. Results of the NIAID collaborative clinical trial to test the predictive value of skin testing with major and minor penicillin derivatives in hospitalized adults. J Allergy Clin Immunol 1990; 191 (abstract).

Stark B, Earl H, Gross G, et al. Acute and chronic desensitization of penicillin-allergic patients using oral penicillin. J Allergy Clin Immunol 1987; 79:523–532.

Strom J. Aetiology of febrile mucocutaneous syndromes with special reference to the provocative role of infections and drugs. Acta Med Scand 1977; 201:131–136.

Sullivan T, Wedner H, Shatz G, et al. Skin testing to detect penicillin allergy. J Allergy Clin Immunol 1981; 68:171–180.

Sullivan T, Yecies L, Shatz G, et al. Desensitization of patients allergic to penicillin using orally administered beta-lactam antibiotics. J Allergy Clin Immunol 1982; 69:275–282.

INSECT STING ALLERGY

LAWRENCE M. LICHTENSTEIN, M.D., Ph.D.

Sensitivity to the venoms of Hymenoptera species (honeybee, yellow hornet, white hornet, yellow jacket, and Polistes wasp) is far more common than generally supposed. An epidemiologic study carried out by Golden at Johns Hopkins demonstrated that fully 20 to 25 percent of the population is sensitive as judged by a positive skin test result or a serum IgE antibody determination. Usually these two indices of sensitivity coexist. However, of this large group of sensitive individuals, only 3.3 percent have a history of systemic reactions, a larger number experiencing large local reactions. In a prospective study we found that approximately 20 percent of these skin test positive, history negative individuals have a systemic reaction when stung by the appropriate insect.

It is, of course, necessary to become sensitized by a sting before one can have a reaction on being stung again. However, individuals may become sensitized by one sting or may be stung repeatedly for many years before suddenly becoming sensitive. As with other types of atopy, we have no information regarding what causes a sting to sensitize an individual.

The clinical manifestations of insect sting allergy are quite variable. A large local reaction is defined as a reaction at the site of the sting that is 8 cm or larger; these evolve over 24 to 48 hours, resolving in the next 2 to 7 days. The majority of these large local reactions are IgE mediated and are accompanied by demonstrable IgE antibodies or positive skin test results to the appropriate venom. Individuals with large local reactions rarely (less than 5 percent) have a subsequent systemic reaction. Systemic reactions range from mild erythema to fatal shock. Although skin reactions are most common, the majority of adults also have respiratory symptoms, which may involve laryngeal edema or more diffuse bronchospasm, and approximately 30 percent have vascular symptoms, which may lead to hypotension and death. Individual patients may have many other manifestations, gastrointestinal symptoms of nausea, crampiness, or diarrhea probably being the next most common. In general, the pattern of the last reaction is repeated. That is, urticaria remains urticaria and bronchospasm remains bronchospasm. Although increases in severity can occur with successive stings, this is far rarer than is generally thought.

Study supported by grant A108270 from the National Institutes of Health, Bethesda, Maryland.

We have found in general that the patient's history in regard to the type of insect that caused the reaction is unreliable. It is also true that the common names for insects vary from country to country and perhaps from region to region. Many individuals have a characteristic prodrome, which is unique to the individual but repeats before each systemic reaction; the presence of this prodrome is a reliable diagnostic indicator.

DIAGNOSIS

The diagnosis of insect sting allergy is made by an appropriate history together with a positive skin test result. Skin test reagents in insect allergy are useful in a more narrow range than those in inhalant allergy, since the venoms are intrinsically irritating. With ragweed allergy, for example, 90 percent of clinically sensitive individuals have a positive skin test reaction with a concentration many orders of magnitude below that which causes irritation. With venoms this is not the case. Most individuals have a positive response only to 0.1 or 1 μg per ml, and the latter concentration is irritating in rare individuals. We have experimented with using 3 and 10 μg per ml concentrations in difficult patients, but this is not an established procedure. When a skin test result is equivocal or when for some reason this is not desirable, IgE antibody levels can be measured. These are found in about 85 percent of skin test positive individuals and often can be of real help when the skin test result is equivocal. We have seen virtually no individuals who have an appropriate and recent history in the absence of a positive skin test reaction or an increased IgE antibody level. Although others have reported this, it must be extremely rare.

In unusual circumstances individuals react to insect venoms that are not commercially available. Thus, for example, we have treated one individual who appears to be sensitive to sweat bee venom in addition to those of the other Hymenoptera species. A number of individuals are allergic to venom of the Polistes species, which have a very limited environmental niche.

One diagnostic test is of particular utility. In our area about 80 percent of the individuals who have a positive skin test reaction to yellow jacket venom are also sensitive to Polistes venom by skin testing. In most instances this is a cross reactivity and true Polistes sensitivity does not exist. This can be determined by doing a RAST inhibition test, a test that indicates whether a person has any antibodies to Polistes venom antigens, which do not cross react with yellow jacket antigens. Most patients tested are not truly sensitive to Polistes venom. Although this test is expensive, it can save the patient many thousands of dollars over the course of immunotherapy and eliminates immunization with an unneeded venom.

THERAPY

The treatment of an acute reaction to an insect sting is exactly the same as for anaphylaxis induced by any other cause; the treatment of this syndrome is covered in detail in another article in this volume. Epinephrine remains the treatment of choice. Although generalized cutaneous reactions do not necessarily require epinephrine, in the absence of a contraindication it may well stop a developing reaction. With mild reactions the patient must be observed for progression to more serious symptoms. Since most individuals, as noted, have a stereotypic response, epinephrine is used immediately in any individual who previously has had circulatory or respiratory distress. Individuals who are to be given immunotherapy (see following discussion) are supplied with an epinephrine injection kit, which they carry until their IgG antibody level has reached an adequate level. They are instructed to use this immediately and to report promptly to an emergency room. The dose of epinephrine initially is 0.3 to 0.5 cc subcutaneously. This is the only route of administration if the patient is conscious and has an obtainable blood pressure. This dose may be repeated every 10 to 15 minutes if it is not fully effective. Even with a good response to therapy, the patient with a severe reaction must be observed for at least 12 hours. In my opinion an individual who has had severe respiratory or circulatory distress should be hospitalized overnight, since a recurrence of symptoms 16 to 18 hours later may be life threatening.

As with any other sort of anaphylaxis, in addition to the use of epinephrine, the major therapeutic effort is designed to support airway function, applying artificial respiration or intubation if necessary. At times epinephrine does not restore the blood pressure, and in these instances it appears useful to provide large amounts of fluids using preparations that will maintain fluid in the vascular spaces, such as plasminate or albumin.

Most medical texts and emergency room manuals suggest that individuals suffering from anaphylaxis be treated with corticosteroids. There is no indication for corticosteroids during the acute reaction, since they are completely without efficacy. Some like to give these with the thought that they will abort a late phase relapse. Although this may be the case (and it has not been proven), I prefer observation, with prompt retreatment if a recurrence occurs.

Specific measures to prevent the occurrence of insect stings depend primarily on common sense. Patients should not walk barefoot and should avoid flowers, where honeybees may be active, or garbage cans, where yellow jackets are attracted. It is said that the wearing of bright clothes or perfumes can be dangerous.

Venom Immunotherapy

Patient Selection

Death from an insect sting is extremely rare. Literally millions of patients are sensitive, but the number of deaths that occur yearly probably does not exceed 100. However, to those of us who have seen a death or the far more common morbidity associated with the fear of insect stings, it is clear that venom immunotherapy plays a vital role in patient management. Since the therapy is not overly expensive (and should become much less expensive than it is), since it appears to be without serious toxicity, and particularly since it appears that it can be stopped after a number of years, I have no hesitation in recommending therapy to anyone with a serious systemic reaction. This recommendation is more or less forceful depending on the criteria to be discussed and summarized in Table 1. We recommend that all adults who have respiratory or vascular manifestations receive immunotherapy. However, in each case the possibilities and the risks are explored with each patient. Thus, for example, a 25 year old individual with minimal respiratory distress may wish not to undergo therapy, and we may respect this decision if we are sure that the pros and cons are understood.

We also recommend immunotherapy for most adults with merely cutaneous reactions. Age here is a major factor, since studies by our group have demonstrated that children with only cutaneous reactions do not require immunotherapy. We have been unable to study enough patients in the age range between 16 and 25 to determine whether they need therapy. However, in a young adult with only cutaneous reactions, we tend, after discussing the pros and cons, to be on the conservative side; whereas with an individual over 50, we tend to be more aggressive in suggesting immunotherapy.

In general, we do not recommend immunotherapy for large local reactions. However, I have offered such therapy to two kinds of individuals: those who are excessively fearful and the rare individual whose large local reaction is debilitating and in whom corticosteroid therapy may be contraindicated. We have not studied large local reactions specifically, but it seems likely from the data we have that immunotherapy is as effective in decreasing these reactions as it is in the systemic reaction.

TABLE 1 Patient Selection for Venom Immunotherapy*

Sting Reaction History	*Skin Test, RAST*	*Venom Immunotherapy*
Systemic (adult)	+	Yes
Systemic, life threatening (child)	+	Yes
Systemic, cutaneous (child)	+ or −	No
Systemic	−	No
Large local	+ or −	No
None	+ or −	No

* From Golden DBK. Insect sting allergy in adults. In: Lichtenstein LM, Fauci AS, eds. Current therapy in allergy and immunology 1983–1984. Toronto: BC Decker, 1983: 70–75.

We do not treat children who have only cutaneous reactions, although in cases in which there is excessive fear on the part of the parents or the child, this may be done. It might be argued that many children with mild respiratory or vascular effects from stings need not be treated. Although this is probably true, we have been unable to accumulate a large enough group of these individuals to study the problem and we continue to advise immunotherapy in these patients.

Mechanism of Immunotherapy

Our group has been studying the mechanisms by which immunotherapy is effective in a variety of clinical conditions for the last two decades. Only in venom immunotherapy is there a clear-cut relationship between the IgG blocking antibody and clinical projection. A number of studies have demonstrated that patients who have more than 3 to 5 μg of IgG against a venom have a reaction incidence well under 2 percent, whereas individuals with half this much antibody have a significantly higher incidence of reactions. Therefore, as is to be elucidated, we decide on the eventual therapeutic dose of venom and the interval between venom injections by following the IgG antibody level. The significance and utility of IgG antibody measurements begin to disappear in the fourth and fifth years of venom immunotherapy. It can be demonstrated that immunotherapy can be stopped after 5 years (to be discussed) and that clinical protection then bears no relationship to the IgG level. The mechanism of clinical protection after 5 years of immunotherapy is not known.

Method of Immunotherapy

The regimen developed at Johns Hopkins for venom immunotherapy is outlined in Table 2 and contrasted with other recommended regimens. Although achieving maintenance levels of venom is critical to the success of this treatment, it is to be emphasized that the actual schedule by which this dose of venom is achieved may be quite variable. We have chosen a more rapid regimen than that used in most other centers because we have demonstrated that this regimen causes the least number of adverse side reactions. However, in our initial studies of this subject we treated many patients from abroad and in order to limit the duration of their stay in Baltimore often completed venom immunotherapy to maintenance levels in 2 or 3 weeks. Alternatively, in Europe some 1 to 2 day "rush" regimens are used. We see no purpose in these regimens because they require hospitalization and cause many systemic reactions, but in theory there is nothing wrong with this type of approach. From an immunologic point of view it is probably most effective to repeat injections every 10 to 14 days when the IgG response to the previous injection has maximized; however, this extends the time required to reach maintenance levels.

The venoms to be used depend entirely on the skin test response. A rare patient is found who responds only to yellow jacket venom and not to hornet venoms. For practical reasons we rarely treat such individuals with only yellow jacket venom. The dose then would have to be 200 μg rather than 100 μg in many patients, and this would be more expensive than using the mixed vespid therapy. As noted, in most areas outside of Texas, Louisiana, and neighboring areas, true sensitivity

TABLE 2 Regimens for Hymenoptera Venom Immunotherapy: Dose (μg)*

Week No.	*Johns Hopkins Center for Allergic Diseases*	*Pharmalgen Package Insert*	*Albay Package Insert*
1	0.1+1+3=4.1	0.001+0.01+0.1=0.111	0.05
2	10	0.1+0.5+1.0=1.6	0.10
3	20	1+5+10=16	0.20
4	40	10+20=30	0.40
5	60	20+30=50	0.50
6	80	30+30=60	1.0
7	100	40+40=80	2
8	100	50+50=100	4
9	—	100	5
10	100	100	10
11	—	—	20
12	—	100	40
13	100	—	60
14	(Repeat monthly)	—	80
15		100	100

* From Golden DBK. Insect sting allergy in adults. In: Lichtenstein LM, Fauci AS, eds. Current therapy in allergy and immunology 1983–1984. Toronto: BC Decker, 1983: 70–75.

to Polistes venom is rare, and patients with positive skin test reactions to this insect venom should undergo RAST inhibition analysis, which in the majority of cases indicates that Polistes therapy is not needed.

As noted, the maintenance level of 100 μg of each venom was arrived at by trial and error. It is, however, extremely important to reach this level, since, after the fact, we found that half the dose of venom (50 μg) is only 80 percent as effective as the full dose, which gives 98 percent protection. The reader will note that the patient who is sensitive to yellow jacket venom receives 300 μg of mixed vespid venoms as the maintenance dose, which in terms of cross reactivity is about the same as 200 μg of yellow jacket venom. The honeybee sensitive individual, however, receives only 100 μg. In 15 to 20 percent of the cases this 100 μg is not sufficient to avoid mild systemic reactions and has to be increased to 200 μg.

Once a maintenance level is achieved, the interval between injections is gradually increased from 1 week to 1 month. After several months an IgG level is obtained. Most individuals have a level well above 5 μg per ml at this point, and the interval between injections can be increased to every 6 weeks with, again, an IgG level being measured after several months. In at least 10 percent of the cases the immune response on a once monthly regimen is not adequate and the interval must be reduced to 2 weeks or in even rarer circumstances weekly injections to maintain the IgG level at about 3 to 5 μg. As noted, Dr. Golden at our institution has carried out sting challenge studies of individuals with less than 3 μg of antibody and has established clearly that they are at a greater risk of sustaining a systemic reaction than those with higher antibody levels. Although the systemic reactions are rarely serious, it should be the goal of therapy to completely obviate adverse reactions to a sting.

Adverse Reactions

In our experience adverse reactions to venom immunotherapy occur no more frequently than reactions to injections of inhalant allergens. In that regard our experience apparently differs from that of other centers where the latter reactions are far less frequent. However, it is our opinion that the role of immunotherapy is to develop an adequate IgG antibody response, and if this is done with inhalant allergens, the dose of antigen required will lead to the same frequency of systemic and local reactions. The incidence of systemic reactions to venom immunotherapy is approximately 15 percent. These reactions usually occur at the initiation of venom immunotherapy when the dose is in the low microgram range. It is rare to see such a reaction once a dose above 25 to 50 μg of venom has been achieved. Most of these reactions are minor and, in experienced hands, do not require epinephrine therapy. There has been only one instance in the treatment of several thousand patients in which an injection induced a systemic response that appeared to be life threatening.

When an adverse reaction occurs, the dose is reduced to that (usually half) which caused no reaction and is then gradually increased. One important technique in getting past this point in the immunization regimen at which a systemic reaction occurs is to split the dose. That is, if a patient reacts to an injection of 5 μg of a venom, he will almost always not have an adverse reaction to 2.5 μg given twice at an interval of a half hour. In certain circumstances we have given individuals multiple injections at half hour intervals to expedite the immunization. We have never failed to get a patient to maintenance levels, and as mentioned elsewhere, it is critical to reach this level even in the patient who has severe and recurrent systemic reactions during therapy. In our worst case, reaching maintenance levels required 1 year's therapy with 30 or 40 significant systemic reactions. However, the dose was achieved and the patient has been taking this dose for many years without adverse reactions.

Large local reactions occur in approximately 50 percent of the individuals but rarely interfere with the progress of therapy. These reactions are much less common at doses under 15 μg or greater than 50 μg. In general, the presence of a large local reaction is not a contraindication to continuing the usual schedule of therapy, since it does not indicate that a more severe systemic reaction will occur at higher doses. We ask the patient to try to tolerate this reaction, and if it is overly bothersome, we may pretreat the patient with an antihistamine before the injection and continue this for 24 to 48 hours. In rare situations it has been necessary to pretreat a patient with prednisone to avoid a serious large local reaction. In this instance we would use 30 mg of prednisone 12 hours before the injection with a repeat dose 24 hours later.

Other adverse reactions to venom immunotherapy have not been observed. There are individuals who complain of malaise for a day after the injection, but it is not clear whether this incidence would be different following placebo injections. In a decade of administering venom immunotherapy to thousands of individuals, no long term toxic effect has been seen. Some years ago Yunginger studied beekeepers, who receive 100 to many thousands of times more venom over protracted periods of time, and found that the incidence of disease in this group was not different from that in control subjects. Thus, venom immunotherapy is quite safe.

Monitoring Immunotherapy

Table 3 indicates the way that we follow patients at Johns Hopkins. This is probably more intensive than is necessary in an office practice and is changing as we

TABLE 3 Monitoring Venom Immunotherapy*

Test	*Indication*	*Frequency*
Skin test (venom)	Diagnosis	Pretreatment
	Loss of sensitivity	Every 2 to 3 years
IgE (venom)	Diagnosis	Pretreatment
	Loss of sensitivity	Every 2 to 3 years
IgG (venom)	Response to induction	Pretreatment, achievement of maintenance
	Maintenance efficacy	Maintenance
	Prolonged interval	Every 12 months for 5 years
	Problems during therapy	
Sting challenge	Efficacy of therapy	Maintenance
Leukocyte histamine release	Diagnosis	Pretreatment
RAST inhibition	Vespid venom cross-reactivity	Pretreatment

* From Golden DBK. Insect sting allergy in adults. In: Lichtenstein LM, Fauci AS, eds. Current therapy in allergy and immunology 1983–1984. Toronto: BC Decker, 1983: 70–75.

gain more experience. At the outset of our studies we carried out RAST IgE antivenom analyses in every patient. As noted, this is now necessary only if the skin test result is equivocal or if there is another reason to use a serologic test. We also followed IgE antibody levels over the years of venom immunotherapy with the thought that a decrease in this antibody level or its disappearance would give us an indication of when to stop therapy. The IgE level has not proved useful in this regard and this practice has been largely abandoned.

As already mentioned, however, we believe that IgG antibody levels must be monitored closely. We generally draw blood for a baseline value and measure the IgG antibody level in this serum and in the serum obtained about 6 weeks after the maintenance dose of venom immunotherapy has been achieved. Earlier we emphasized the importance of a doubling or tripling of the baseline value. We now think that this is less important and focus on seeing that the patient has at least 5 μg of IgG venom antibody against each insect to which he is sensitive. This level is used to make the decision to increase the interval of venom immunotherapy injections to monthly and, later, every 6 weeks. It probably would be possible to spread injections to intervals of 8 to 10 weeks in a subset of patients who have a particularly good immune response. Since the duration of venom immunotherapy is limited, however, we have not pursued such studies. Once a maintenance regimen is established, IgG antibody levels should be obtained yearly for the first 4 or 5 years. As noted, they have little value after this period.

Cessation of Immunotherapy

To this point the diagnosis and treatment of venom hypersensitivity have been logical and based on firm immunologic principles. Information regarding the cessation of venom immunotherapy is based on clinical observations alone. To our surprise we found that after 5 years of immunotherapy, even in the face of continuing positive skin test results and elevated IgE antibody levels against venom, patients could tolerate a sting with no difficulty. The incidence of reactions is about 3 percent, which is not significantly different from what would be observed if the patient had continued with immunotherapy. These studies have just been completed. Dr. Golden has stung individuals after 1 year or 2 years without venom immunotherapy. He has also stung the first group at yearly intervals for 4 years and most recently repeated a sting 4 weeks after the first, trying to ascertain whether the first sting sensitized people. In all these studies the cited low incidence of reactions has been observed and no serious reactions have been encountered.

Our current position is to explain these data to the patients and advise them that in our opinion it is safe to stop immunotherapy after 5 years. It should be emphasized that this is new clinical information and that employing this strategy requires that both the patient and the physician feel comfortable. Certainly there are some individuals who do not wish to stop therapy (although well over 90 percent follow this course). Further, there are some individuals whose previous reactions have been of such a nature or whose physical condition is such that we would not feel comfortable taking the risk of even a mild systemic reaction. These patients, however, are rare.

The mechanism by which patients are protected after 5 years is not clear. I believe, however, that this protection is the result of the immunotherapy and not simply attributable to the passage of time. The only reliable data one can use to support this belief are derived from our study with children who had cutaneous manifestations. In those studies it was observed that patients taking venom immunotherapy had an incidence of systemic reactions of about 1 percent, whereas those given a placebo had a 10 percent reaction rate. This was highly significant, but since none of the placebo treated children had a reaction that was more serious than the initial reaction, we stopped this therapy after 5 to 7 years.

What is of great interest, however, is that in following these two groups of children with field stings, we discovered that the treated group had maintained its 1 percent reaction rate, whereas the untreated group had maintained its 10 percent reaction rate. This strongly suggests that venom immunotherapy had an effect over and above that due to the passage of time.

SUGGESTED READING

Golden DBK, Johnson K, Addison BI, Valentine MD, Kagey-Sobotka A, Lichtenstein LM. Clinical and immunologic observations in patients who discontinue venom immunotherapy. J Allergy Clin Immunol 1986; 77:435–442.

Golden DBK, Kagey-Sobotka A, Valentine MD, Lichtenstein LM. Dose dependence of Hymenoptera venom immunotherapy. J Allergy Clin Immunol 1981; 67:370–374.

Golden DBK, Marsh DG, Kagey-Sobotka A, Addison BI, Friedhoff L, Szklo M, Valentine MD, Lichtenstein LM. Epidemiology of insect sting allergy. JAMA (in press).

Golden DBK, Meyers DA, Kagey-Sobotka A, Valentine MD, Lichtenstein LM. Clinical relevance of the venom-specific immunoglobulin G antibody level during immunotherapy. J Allergy Clin Immunol 1982; 69:489–493.

Golden DBK, Valentine MD, Kagey-Sobotka A, Lichtenstein LM. Regimens of Hymenoptera venom immunotherapy. Ann Intern Med 1980; 92:620.

SYSTEMIC ANAPHYLAXIS

TIMOTHY J. SULLIVAN III, M.D.

Anaphylaxis is an acute, life endangering syndrome resulting from the sudden release of large amounts of diverse mediators from mast cells. The clinical manifestations include rapidly evolving respiratory tract obstruction or cardiovascular collapse. Anaphylaxis occurs in approximately one of every 2700 hospitalized patients, and the overall lifetime risk in the United States is approximately 1 percent.

The causes of anaphylaxis can be divided into four groups—antigens, direct mast cell activating agents, anaphylatoxin generating agents, and factors acting by mechanisms not currently understood (Table 1). IgE antibodies can initiate anaphylaxis by binding to complete antigens, such as insulin, or to determinants formed by covalent attachment of highly reactive drugs (e.g., penicillin) to large molecules, such as albumin or immunoglobulin. Some drugs can directly activate mast cell mediator release in the absence of specific IgE. Massive complement activation can generate formation of large amounts of the anaphylatoxins C3a and C5a. Anaphylatoxins bind to specific mast cell receptors and, as the name implies, can initiate marked mast cell mediator release. Several other causes of anaphylaxis are known, ranging from exercise to aspirin, that induce mast cell mediator release by unknown mechanisms.

These diverse stimuli induce similar pathophysiologic events. Activated mast cells secrete mediator containing granules and can form potent mediators from membrane lipids. Granule mediators include histamine, proteolytic enzymes such as mast cell tryptase, glycosidases, and granulocyte chemotactic factors. Newly formed lipid mediators include prostaglandin D_2, sulfidopeptide leukotrienes, and platelet activating factor. These mediators induce marked changes in the microenvironment and activate complex local reflex mechanisms. Histamine (acting through H_1 and H_2 receptors), PGD_2, the leukotrienes, and possibly platelet activating factor appear to be the principal mediators of anaphylaxis. These mediators can cause diminished arteriolar tone, increased permeability of postcapillary venules, increased venous capacitance, diminished force of ventricular contraction, cardiac rhythm disturbances, and ventricular conduction abnormalities, all of which can contribute to the hypotension occurring during anaphylaxis. Interstitial respiratory tract vessel engorgement, edema, contraction of respiratory tract smooth muscle, and increased bronchial gland secretion lead to the respiratory tract disorders noted during anaphylaxis.

CLINICAL MANIFESTATIONS OF ANAPHYLAXIS

As summarized in Table 2, characteristic clinical manifestations of anaphylaxis can appear in many organ systems. Anaphylaxis usually begins within minutes after exposure to the causative factor, although the onset may be delayed for several hours. Once under way, the reaction usually progresses in an explosive manner, reaching a peak intensity within 1 hour. Nonfatal reactions resolve over a period of up to 48 hours. Pruritic cutaneous reactions often are the first manifestations of anaphylaxis. Acute asthma, rhinitis, and conjunctivitis may occur. Acute perineal pruritus and a metallic taste in the mouth may be present.

Respiratory or cardiovascular dysfunction during anaphylaxis can be fatal. As noted in Table 3, respiratory failure may be the result of upper airway obstruction or

TABLE 1 Classification of Causes of Systemic Anaphylaxis*

- IgE mediated anaphylaxis
  - Haptens
    - Antimicrobial drugs
      - Penicillins and cephalosporins
      - Tetracyclines
      - Aminoglycosides
      - Nitrofurantoin
      - Amphotericin B
      - Sulfonamides
    - Other drugs
      - Ethylene oxide
      - Local anesthetics (some reactions)
  - Complete antigens
    - Proteins
      - Hymenoptera venoms
      - Chymopapain
      - Insulin
      - Streptokinase
      - Heterologous immunoglobulins (some reactions)
      - Allergen extracts
      - Protamine
      - Seminal fluid
      - Foods
        - Milk
        - Egg
        - Shellfish
        - Fish
        - Peanut
        - Nuts
        - Chocolate
      - Other agents
        - Quaternary ammonium muscle relaxants (some reactions)
- Direct activation of mast cell mediator release
  - Opiates
  - Radiocontrast media
  - Vancomycin
  - Polymyxin B
  - Dextran
  - Quaternary ammonium muscle relaxants (some reactions)
- Anaphylatoxin mediated anaphylaxis
  - Human plasma and blood products
  - Homologous and heterologous immunoglobulins (some reactions)
  - Dialysis membranes (some reactions)
- Anaphylaxis initiated by unknown mechanisms
  - Exercise
  - Mastocytosis
  - Nonsteroidal anti-inflammatory drugs, including aspirin
  - Synthetic steroid hormones
  - Recombinant immunoregulatory molecules
  - Cold exposure
  - Idiopathic anaphylaxis

*The substances, disease states, and activities noted are examples of common provocative factors. Numerous other agents are known or strongly suspected in each category.

TABLE 2 Clinical Manifestations of Anaphylaxis

System	*Manifestation*
Skin	Generalized, perineal, or vaginal pruritus; angioedema; urticaria and other pruritic rashes
Eye	Pruritus, conjunctival suffusion, lacrimation
Nose	Pruritus, congestion, sneezing, rhinorrhea
Mouth	Metallic taste
Upper airway	Sensation of narrowing airway, hoarseness, stridor, oropharyngeal or laryngeal edema, complete obstruction
Lower airway	Dyspnea, tachypnea, wheezing, use of accessory muscles of respiration, cyanosis, respiratory arrest
Cardiovascular	Tachycardia, hypotension, ventricular and supraventricular rhythm disturbances, cardiac arrest
Gastrointestinal	Nausea, vomiting, cramping abdominal pain, diarrhea, bloody diarrhea
Neurologic	Fear of impending death, weakness, dizziness, syncope, seizure

TABLE 3 Causes of Death from Anaphylaxis*

- Cardiovascular dysfunction
  - Peripheral vessel dysfunction
    - Loss of arteriolar tone
    - Increased vascular permeability
    - Increased capacitance of veins
  - Cardiac dysfunction
    - Diminished force of contraction
    - Diminished coronary blood flow
    - Rhythm disturbances
    - Conduction abnormalities
- Respiratory dysfunction
  - Upper respiratory tract obstruction
    - Angioedema
  - Pulmonary dysfunction
    - Airway narrowing from interstitial edema and smooth muscle contraction
    - Increased bronchial secretions

* Ischemia and hypoxia during anaphylaxis can cause extensive injury to the heart, brain, kidneys, and liver.

TABLE 4 Nonimmunologic Risk Factors for Severe or Fatal Anaphylaxis

Beta-adrenergic blockade
Bronchial asthma
Cardiac disease
Adrenal insufficiency

severe acute asthma. Cardiovascular collapse may be the result of peripheral vascular dysfunction or cardiac dysfunction. The relative frequencies of these disorders on presentation to a medical facility have been estimated to be as follows: hypotension, 68 percent; bronchial obstruction, 52 percent; laryngeal obstruction, 36 percent; respiratory arrest, 12 percent; and cardiac arrest, 12 percent.

Several nonimmunologic factors appear to increase the risk that anaphylaxis will progress to a severe or fatal outcome (Table 4). The presence of beta-adrenergic blocking drugs appears to increase the likelihood and severity of anaphylaxis and interferes with the use of beta-adrenergic agonists to treat anaphylaxis. Asthmatic patients appear to be twice as likely to die if anaphylaxis occurs. Anaphylaxis is more likely to be severe or fatal in patients with congestive heart failure or arteriosclerotic coronary artery disease.

DIAGNOSIS OF ANAPHYLAXIS

A diagnosis of anaphylaxis is based upon clinical and biochemical evidence of acute, life endangering secretion of mast cell mediators (Table 5). Essential to the diagnosis is the presence of acute upper airway obstruction, bronchial obstruction, or hypotension. The presence of other distinctive allergic symptoms and signs,

TABLE 5 Diagnosis of Anaphylaxis*

At least one of the following must be present: acute hypotension, bronchial obstruction, or upper airway obstruction (cardiac or respiratory arrest)
Presence of distinctive allergic symptoms and signs in other systems
Recent exposure to agents or activities known to be capable of inducing anaphylaxis
Evidence of IgE to an agent encountered just before onset of anaphylaxis
Absence of conditions that can mimic anaphylaxis
Elevated serum levels of mast cell tryptase
Elevated levels of other molecules associated with mast cell secretion: plasma and urinary histamine and metabolites, serum high molecular weight neutrophil chemotactic factor, and urinary PGD_2 metabolites

* Effective therapy of acute anaphylaxis requires accurate diagnosis based upon clinical criteria.

evidence of allergy to the agent in question, and elevated serum mast cell tryptase levels should suggest or support the diagnosis of anaphylaxis. Exposure to stimuli known to cause anaphylaxis immediately before the onset of the syndrome supports the diagnosis of anaphylaxis as does evidence of the presence of IgE to this agent.

Serum levels of mast cell tryptase are unequivocally elevated during most forms of anaphylaxis, providing a useful biochemical dimension for the diagnosis of anaphylaxis. Tryptase blood levels peak approximately 1 hour after the onset of the reaction and have an approximately 3 hour half-clearance time. Other possible biochemical markers of mast cell secretion include histamine and metabolites of histamine, and PGD_2 and metabolites of PGD_2, but measurements of these molecules have not yet been proven useful for routine clinical assessment.

Several illnesses that can be mistaken for anaphylaxis must be excluded. The differential diagnosis of anaphylaxis includes myocardial infarction, primary cardiac dysrhythmias, vasovagal syncope, pulmonary embolism, hypovolemic shock, stroke, aspiration pneumonia, adverse pharmacologic reactions to drugs, hereditary angioedema, foreign body in the airway, epiglottitis, other causes of upper airway obstruction, hyperventilation, anxiety attack, and Munchausen syndrome.

MANAGEMENT OF ANAPHYLAXIS

Assessment

The initial evaluation of a patient experiencing anaphylaxis should establish the nature and intensity of the clinical manifestations (see Table 2), the rate of progression of the reaction, medications the patient has received recently and for prolonged periods, and concurrent illnesses (particularly asthma and cardiac disease). Knowledge of the presence or absence of therapy with beta-adrenergic blocking drugs is especially important. Administration of any drug suspected of having caused the reaction should be discontinued. High priority must be given to assessment of the respiratory and cardiovascular systems: upper airway patency, pulmonary function, cardiac rhythm, and blood pressure (see Table 3). These four factors should be monitored (when feasible) by direct visualization, spirometry, electrocardiography, and serial blood pressure measurements.

The initial assessment permits formulation of a plan of management that takes into consideration the severity and nature of the anaphylaxis and individual patient factors. If the patient is receiving beta-adrenergic receptor blocking drugs, immediate institution of management approaches not dependent on beta-receptor activation by epinephrine or isoproterenol is mandatory (Table 6). Severe pulmonary problems should be anticipated and pharmacologically pre-empted in asthmatic patients (see Table 6). Steps should be taken to prepare for intubation, cricothyrotomy, assisted ventilation, cardiac monitoring, or intra-aortic balloon pumping as indicated by the initial examination. Delay in preparation for the use of potentially essential sophisticated measures, while assessing the effects of epinephrine or other initial medical therapy, can contribute to a fatal outcome.

Epinephrine

This adrenergic receptor agonist is the drug of choice for the initial management of anaphylaxis. The capacity of epinephrine to suppress mediator release from mast cells and basophils and to reverse many of the end organ effects of the mediators of anaphylaxis, while producing peripheral vasoconstriction, makes this a nearly ideal drug for initial therapy in most patients. Complete remission of the signs of anaphylaxis often occurs within minutes after the injection of epinephrine (Table 7).

TABLE 6 Management of Anaphylaxis

General therapeutic measaures
- Clinical assessment
- Epinephrine (subcutaneously or by infusion)

Specific interventions
- Hypotension
  - Peripheral vascular defects
    - Trendelenburg position
    - Intravenous administration of isotonic sodium chloride
    - Norepinephrine or other vasopressor infusion
    - H_1 and H_2 blocking drugs
  - Cardiac dysfunction
    - Conventional therapy of dysrhythmias
    - Isoproterenol infusion
    - H_1 and H_2 blocking drugs
    - Intra-aortic balloon pump or other cardiovascular assist devices
- Airway obstruction
  - Upper airway obstruction
    - Supplemental inspired oxygen
    - Extension of neck
    - Oropharyngeal airway
    - Endotracheal intubation
    - Cricothyrotomy
  - Lower airway obstruction
    - Supplemental inspired oxygen
    - Intravenous administration of theophylline
    - Aerosol bronchodilator therapy
    - Endotracheal intubation
    - Conventional treatment for status asthmaticus
    - Assisted ventilation

Biphasic anaphylaxis
- Monitor by direct observation for at least 12 hours after onset of anaphylaxis
- Systemic corticosteroid therapy after acute reaction has been treated and again 6 hours later
- H_1 and H_2 blocking drugs initially and again 6 hours later
- Recurrent anaphylaxis treated according to guidelines for acute anaphylaxis

TABLE 7 Epinephrine in Anaphylaxis

- Drug of choice in most cases
- Arrests mediator release and reverses many mediator actions
- Intravenous bolus therapy dangerous because of cardiac rhythm disturbances
- Subcutaneous therapy usually effective
- Intravenous infusions of 2 μg/ml usually safe in adults
- Failure to use epinephrine more dangerous than proper use of epinephrine

Subcutaneous doses of 300 to 500 μg (0.3 to 0.5 ml of a 1:1000 solution) for an adult usually are effective. Asthmatic adults should receive 500 μg, since they often are relatively insensitive to beta-adrenergic receptor stimulation. This dose can be repeated after 10 minutes if the first dose has not induced improvement or untoward effects. If serious manifestations of the reaction persist, an intravenous infusion of epinephrine at an initial infusion rate of 2 μg per minute (for an adult) can be instituted. One milligram of epinephrine (e.g., 1 ml of a 1:1000 solution or 10 ml of a 1:10,000 solution) can be diluted in 500 ml of fluid for intravenous infusion at a rate of 1 ml per minute. Intravenous bolus injections of epinephrine, in the context of anaphylaxis, often induce serious cardiac rhythm disturbances that can cause or contribute to a fatal outcome. Intravenous bolus therapy should be avoided. Excessive subcutaneous doses of epinephrine can induce similar cardiac complications. Inappropriately high doses of epinephrine also can induce hypertension, acute catecholamine cardiac toxicity, or other serious side effects.

Failure to use epinephrine early in the management of anaphylaxis increases the probability of a fatal outcome. The likelihood of prompt marked benefit is high, and the risk of serious untoward effects from properly administered epinephrine is low. The proper use of epinephrine remains the initial treatment of choice in most patients.

Hypotension

Peripheral Vascular Defects

Diminished arteriolar tone, increased postcapillary venule permeability with loss of intravascular volume, and vasodilation can contribute to hypotension during anaphylaxis. Epinephrine is the initial treatment of choice and usually is sufficient to restore vascular tone and normal permeability properties.

If epinephrine is not effective, or if the patient is being treated with beta-adrenergic blocking drugs, expansion of intravascular volume, vasopressor infusion, and combined H_1 and H_2 antihistamine therapy should be considered. A supine position with elevation of the legs (Trendelenburg position) may be helpful. Normal saline, or another salt containing fluid, can be administered rapidly to an adult at a rate of up to 100 ml per minute to a limit of 3 liters. Administration of fluid, especially amounts of more than 3 liters in an adult or the equivalent in a child, should be guided by the patient's response, cardiovascular status, age, and urine output.

If fluid administration and the Trendelenburg position are ineffective, or if hypotension is profound, a vasopressor may be needed. Norepinephrine appears to be the most consistently effective pressor in anaphylaxis, although success with other drugs has been reported. Norepinephrine should be diluted to a 4 μg per ml (4 ml of a 1 mg per ml solution in 1000 ml of 5 percent dextrose in water). The initial infusion rate for adults is 8 to 12 μg per minute (2 to 3 ml per minute). The rate of infusion should be adjusted to sustain a systolic blood pressure of 80 to 100 mm Hg. Previously hypertensive patients may require higher pressures, but the systolic pressure should be 40 mm Hg or more below the patient's usual systolic pressure. Conventional measures should be taken to avoid or treat extravasation of the drug.

Histamine, acting through both H_1 and H_2 receptors, appears to play a significant role in the peripheral vascular and cardiac disorders that contribute to hypotension. Concurrent blockage of H_1 and H_2 receptors appears to be necessary to block the hypotensive effects of histamine. Effective blockade can be achieved by using an H_1 antihistamine such as diphenhydramine (1 mg per kg of body weight in an adult, intravenously) and an H_2 antihistamine such as cimetidine (4 mg per kg infused intravenously over at least 5 minutes).

Cardiac Dysfunction

Dysrhythmias and diminished force of cardiac contraction can contribute to hypotension during anaphylaxis. Markedly decreased force of ventricular contraction may be the sole origin of hypotension in anaphylaxis. Complex and life endangering rhythm disturbances may arise from the combined impact of intercardiac mast cell mediator release, intravascular mediators, hypoxia, hypotension, or excessive doses of epinephrine. Electrocardiographic monitoring is desirable during anaphylaxis, when possible.

Epinephrine is the initial treatment of choice and usually is sufficient to restore normal cardiac function. Hypoxia and hypotension should be corrected immediately. Conventional therapy for ventricular rhythm disturbances usually is successful.

Cardiac contractility disorders may respond to the infusion of a beta$_1$-adrenergic agonist. Epinephrine is the usual drug of choice, but if a concurrent alpha-adrenergic effect is not desired, isoproterenol can be infused. For an adult, 1 mg of isoproterenol is dissolved in 500 ml of 5 percent dextrose in water (2 μg per ml) and administered at a rate of 0.25 to 2.50 ml per minute (0.5 to 5 μg per minute). The speed of infusion is adjusted according to the clinical response and the effect on heart rate. Dopamine has complex effects that could have both beneficial and undesirable effects on anaphylaxis. This drug appears to be less effective than other drugs for pressor or inotropic effects. Potent nonadrenergic inotropic drugs are available, but they often induce peripheral vasodilation that can be severe and difficult to reverse. This property renders available nonadrenergic inotropic drugs dangerous to use in anaphylaxis.

Cardiac dysfunction during anaphylaxis in a patient receiving beta-adrenergic blocking drugs presents an especially challenging problem. Attempts to overcome the block with high doses of epinephrine can cause excessive alpha-adrenergic effects. High doses of either epinephrine or isoproterenol can induce acute cardiac catecholamine toxicity despite beta-receptor blockade. General measures addressing hypoxia, ventricular rhythm disturbances, and hypotension should be applied. Combined blockade of H_1 and H_2 receptors may be beneficial.

Refractory hypotension may reflect acute myocardial infarction caused by acute hypoxia or hypotension during anaphylaxis.

Upper Airway Obstruction

The effective management of laryngeal or oropharyngeal angioedema depends upon aggressive use of the steps outlined in Tables 6 and 8. Epinephrine can induce remission rapidly, but direct intervention should be undertaken if significant obstruction is present. An H_1 antihistamine (e.g., diphenhydramine, 1 mg per kg intravenously in an adult) can be given. Aerosolized epinephrine may be used topically to complement parenteral doses of epinephrine. Supplemental inspired oxygen, extension of the neck, and insertion of an oropharyngeal airway may be helpful.

TABLE 8 Cricothyrotomy Procedure

1. Extend neck to place cricothyroid membrane and overlying skin under tension and to make membrane immediately accessible.
2. Locate cricothyroid membrane below thyroid cartilage and above cricoid cartilage.
3. Make small transverse incision in skin in anterior third of cricothyroid space just above upper border of cricoid cartilage (use vertical incision if patient is combative).
4. Puncture cricothyroid membrane in midline.
5. Enlarge opening with scalpel handle or another form of blunt dissection.
6. Insert endotracheal tube with internal diameter of 4 to 5 mm (smaller in children).

When initial measures are not sufficient or when severe obstruction is present at the beginning of therapy, endotracheal intubation is indicated. An endotracheal tube with a 4 or 5 mm internal diameter is sufficient to ventilate an adult and is more likely to be placed successfully than a conventional larger endotracheal tube. Airway needles and similar small aperture devices are not sufficient for the management of severe obstruction. If intubation is not possible, a cricothyrotomy should be performed. This procedure is much faster, safer, and more feasible in an emergency than a tracheotomy. Details of this intervention are presented in Table 8.

Lower Airway Obstruction

Pulmonary dysfunction in anaphylaxis can be managed with a stepwise approach similar to that used for severe acute asthma (see Table 6). Measurements of FEV_1, peak expiratory flow rate, pulsus paradoxus, and blood gas levels are useful in assessing the severity of the disease and the impact of therapy. Systemic epinephrine therapy may be sufficient to suppress pulmonary reactions. If epinephrine fails to halt the pulmonary reaction, if the reaction is severe at initial evaluations ($FEV_1 \leq 1.0$ liter, peak flow ≤ 299 liters per minute, pulsus paradoxus ≥ 18 mm Hg, $Pco_2 \geq 42$ mm Hg), or if the patient is being treated with beta-adrenergic blocking drugs, other measures are used to control the pulmonary dysfunction. Supplemental inspired oxygen should be administered by nasal cannula (5 liters per minute) or face mask (40 to 60 percent oxygen) as needed to sustain a Po_2 above 60 mm Hg (preferably 80 to 100 mm Hg).

Theophylline can exert powerful beneficial effects on pulmonary disorders in anaphylaxis, but a loading dose must be administered over 20 minutes and the therapeutic range of the drug is quite narrow. Decisions about dosages must be made with attention to prior theophylline therapy, concurrent illnesses, concurrent drug therapy, and other factors. In patients who are not taking theophylline therapy, an intravenous loading dose of 6 mg of aminophylline (the ethylene diamine salt of theophylline) per kg of body weight can be given over 20 minutes. If the patient has been receiving theophylline therapy, the dosage is selected according to the maintenance dosage being given, the time since the last dose, and the serum theophylline level; usually no more than half the usual loading dose is given. Theophylline blood levels of 10 to 20 μg per ml are maintained by infusions of aminophylline, usually 0.3 to 0.9 mg per kg per hour intravenously.

Theophylline clearance rates can vary markedly from patient to patient and are influenced by several intercurrent factors. Theophylline metabolism can be slow in cases of hepatic dysfunction, congestive heart failure, or concurrent therapy with drugs such as cimetidine or erythromycin. Cigarette smokers tend to metabolize theophylline more rapidly. The appearance of nausea, vomiting, or cardiac rhythm disturbances during theophylline infusion indicates possible theophylline toxicity; infusion should be halted until the blood level is determined. Clearly serial serum theophylline levels can be useful in achieving therapeutic but nontoxic blood levels.

Biphasic Anaphylaxis

The initial therapy of severe anaphylaxis induces prompt, complete, sustained clinical remissions in approximately half the cases. Protracted anaphylaxis (respiratory or cardiovascular manifestations at least partially resistant to therapy for hours to more than 1 day) occurs in approximately one fourth of the severe cases. A particularly dangerous pattern, biphasic anaphylaxis, occurs in approximately one fourth of the severe cases. Biphasic anaphylaxis is characterized by complete remission of symptoms and signs of anaphylaxis in response to initial therapy, followed by recurrence of potentially life endangering disorders after an asymptomatic interval of up to 8 hours.

Since no methods are available to predict whether the remission will be temporary or sustained, the patient should be observed for at least 12 hours after the onset of anaphylaxis. Laryngeal obstruction, bronchial obstruction, or hypotension may recur, but these disorders have not been observed to occur for the first time during the second episode. Thus, clinical monitoring is focused on possible recurrence of the life endangering features present during the initial phase.

Once the initial manifestations of anaphylaxis are controlled, systemic corticosteroid therapy can be given. Biphasic anaphylaxis can occur despite this intervention, but the use of corticosteroids is based upon studies of biphasic immediate hypersensitivity reactions in the lung, skin, and nose that demonstrate corticosteroid suppression of late reactions. The initial dose, equivalent to 60 mg of prednisone, should be given intravenously to permit a rapid onset of action. This dose should be repeated with oral medication 6 hours later.

Combined H_1 and H_2 blockade also should be considered. Although pruritus, wheal and flare reactions, and angioedema reactions are primarily H_1 receptor mediated, histamine induced hypotension is mediated by both H_1 and H_2 receptors. An H_1 antihistamine (e.g., diphenhydramine, 1 mg per kg intravenously in an adult) and an H_2 antihistamine (e.g., cimetidine, 4 mg per kg intravenously in an adult) should be given initially and again 6 hours later (a longer interval for long acting H_2 antihistamines).

Most of the reported instances of biphasic anaphylaxis have occurred in patients who received corticosteroids and H_1 antihistamine therapy, indicating that current prophylactic measures are not ideal. These reactions often are mild to moderate in severity, but immediately life endangering reactions do occur. Recurrent anaphylaxis is treated according to the same principles used to treat acute anaphylaxis.

Urticaria and Angioedema

Acute urticaria and angioedema associated with anaphylaxis usually remit with epinephrine therapy. Conventional therapy with an H_1 antihistamine or combined therapy with H_1 and H_2 antihistamines also exerts powerful suppressive effects. Corticosteroids suppress most continuing urticaria and angioedema reactions associated with anaphylaxis, but the onset of action is 4 to 6 hours after the first dose.

AVOIDANCE OF ANAPHYLAXIS

The incidence and severity of anaphylaxis can be reduced to a very low level by utilizing the approaches summarized in Table 9. Expanded precautions are indicated for patients who are at increased risk for severe anaphylaxis—those with a history of anaphylaxis, asthmatic patients, patients receiving beta-adrenergic blocking drugs, and those with cardiac disease. Patients with a history of multiple drug allergies may be at increased risk of anaphylaxis from other drugs. Immunologic tests are available to assist in the detection of IgE sensitivity to beta-lactam antibiotics, chymopapain, and a variety of other agents.

Immunization with specific Hymenoptera venoms can induce effective protection for approximately 98 percent of the patients who have had anaphylactic reactions to stings by bees, wasps, yellow jackets, or hornets. The efficacy and safety of similar therapy with fire ant materials are under investigation.

Premedication with corticosteroids and H_1 antihistamines has been proven effective in reducing the frequency and severity of anaphylactic reactions to radiocontrast media. This approach is ineffective against penicillin and other antigen induced anaphylaxis and should not be considered effective outside the context of radiocontrast reactions.

When strong indications for use of a drug are present in patients with anaphylactic sensitivity to that drug, acute desensitization can be considered. Acceptably safe oral desensitization protocols have been reported for beta-lactam drugs and sulfonamides. Similar approaches could be considered for other drugs available in an oral form. Parenteral desensitization, although associated with more frequent and more severe complications, has been successful for drugs such as insulin, aminoglycosides, and heteroantisera. Similar protocols could be considered for other drugs. In nearly all instances anaphylactic sensitivity can be bypassed by these procedures.

TABLE 9 Approaches to Avoidance of Anaphylaxis

General precautions
- Control exposure to factors known to have caused immediate hypersensitivity reactions in past (e.g., drugs, stinging insects, foods, exercise)
- Administer drugs by oral route when possible
- Observe for at least 30 minutes after first dose of drugs that are common causes of anaphylaxis
- Special precautions for patients at increased risk of severe anaphylaxis:
  - Discontinuation of beta-adrenergic blocking drugs during periods of risk (e.g., hospitalization, radiocontrast studies, stinging insect season)
  - Optimization of therapy of asthma before surgery; radiocontrast studies; new, high risk drug therapy
  - Immunologic screening for allergy before drug therapy when tests are available
  - Introduction of beta-lactam drug therapy with an oral dose when possible
  - Premedication before radiocontrast studies, general anesthesia, mediator releasing drugs

Immunologic screening for specific IgE before drug therapy

Immunization
- Hymenoptera venom sensitive patients

Premedication
- Before radiocontrast medium injections
  - Prednisone: 50 mg oral doses 13, 7, and 1 hour before procedure in adults
  - Diphenhydramine: 1 mg/kg 1 hour before procedure in adults

Acute desensitization of allergic patients
- Oral desensitization (e.g., penicillin, sulfonamides)
- Parenteral desensitization (e.g., insulin, aminoglycosides, heteroantisera)

Self-administered epinephrine

Self-administered epinephrine should be provided for patients who are likely to experience anaphylaxis outside a medical facility. The patient should be taught the indications and details of self-administration. These procedures should be reviewed with the patient and the patient's family on a regular basis. Speed and simplicity of administration favor the use of Epi-Pens for this purpose.

The patient and physicians involved in the patient's care should be thoroughly integrated into plans for avoidance and future therapy. These diverse strategies, carefully applied, can reduce the morbidity and mortality from episodes of recurrent anaphylaxis to a very low level.

SUGGESTED READING

Goldenberg IF, Cohn JN. New inotropic drugs for heart failure. JAMA 1987; 258:493–496.
Kravis TC, Warner CG, eds. Emergency medicine. Rockville: Aspen Publishers, 1987: 69, 1061–1063.
Patterson R, DeSwarte RD, Greenberger PA, Grammer LC. Drug allergy and protocols for management of drug allergies. N Engl Reg Allergy Proc 1986; 7:325–342.
Porter J, Jick H. Drug-induced anaphylaxis, convulsions, deafness, and extrapyramidal symptoms. Lancet 1977; 1:587–588.
Schwartz LB, Metcalfe DD, Sullivan TJ. Tryptase levels as an indicator of mast-cell activation in systemic anaphylaxis and mastocytosis. N Engl J Med 1987; 316:1622–1626.
Sheffer AL. Anaphylaxis. J Allergy Clin Immunol 1985; 75:227–233.
Stark BJ, Earl HS, Gross GN, Lumry WR, Goodman EL, Sullivan TJ. Acute and chronic desensitization of penicillin-allergic patients using oral penicillin. J Allergy Clin Immunol 1987; 79:523–532.
Stark BJ, Sullivan TJ. Biphasic and protracted anaphylaxis. J Allergy Clin Immunol 1986; 78:76–83.

HEREDITARY ANGIOEDEMA

ALLEN P. KAPLAN, M.D.

Hereditary angioedema is an autosomal dominant disorder associated with severe episodes of swelling of submucosal and subcutaneous tissues. Attacks may affect virtually any part of the body but most commonly involve the extremities or the face. Occasionally there may be edema of the submucosa of the small bowel that causes episodes of abdominal pain; the most severe of these may resemble an "acute abdomen." Episodes of swelling may also affect the upper respiratory tract to include the tongue, pharynx, and larynx. Laryngeal edema, in particular, can cause acute obstruction, stridor, and asphyxiation and therefore can present as a medical emergency. Attacks are sporadic and often occur in the absence of any precipitating event. However, in some patients there appears to be a preponderance of episodes in association with local trauma, concomitant illness, or emotional stress. The age of onset of episodes of angioedema can vary greatly; it most often occurs during childhood. However, episodes are seldom severe prior to puberty. The duration of attacks is typically 1 to 4 days; they are self-limited and most often require no therapy. However, attacks involving the upper airway or gastrointestinal tract require particular precautions, to be outlined.

Hereditary angioedema is caused by depressed function of the inhibitor of the activated first component of complement (C1 INH). Approximately 85 percent of the cases are attributable to diminished levels of the protein (typically less than 25 percent of normal), and 15 percent of the cases are attributable to synthesis of a dysfunctional protein and plasma levels may be normal or elevated. This protein is the only known physiologic inhibitor of the C1r and C1s components of the first component of complement. It is also the main plasma inhibitor of activated Hageman factor and kallikrein and is therefore the critical protein regulating the formation of the vasoactive peptide bradykinin. The swelling seen in hereditary angioedema is thought to be due to either a kinin-like molecule, which may be derived from one of the complement components, or to bradykinin (or both). Since the disease is transmitted as a dominant gene and patients are heterozygotes, one normal gene is present. The cause of C1 INH levels lower than 25 percent of normal (rather than the expected 50 percent) appears to be excessive catabolism. Similarly when an abnormal C1 INH is synthesized, small amounts of normal C1 INH are also present owing to transcription of the one normal gene.

In a patient presenting with angioedema, the diagnosis of hereditary angioedema is suspected if there is a positive family history. A low C4 level is suggestive regardless of the history, since sporadic cases or a new mutation occasionally may be found. A low C1 INH level is confirmatory. However, if the C1 INH level is normal or elevated in the presence of a low C4 level, a functional determination should be performed. During episodes of swelling the C4 level may approach zero and the C2 level also declines. Acquired angioedema with C1 INH deficiency is to be distinguished from the familial disorder. This is most often associated with B cell lymphomas or connective tissue diseases in which C1 INH levels are low as a result of unusual consumption. In these cases the C1q level is also often depressed; C1q levels are typically normal in hereditary angioedema. Therapy in acquired cases of C1 INH deficiency is directed to the underlying disease, but the modalities used to treat hereditary angioedema also can be utilized to prevent episodes of swelling.

Not all patients with hereditary angioedema require therapy. Some may have only mild attacks that do not have a major effect on life style. Others may have an attack frequency of less than one or two episodes per month. These do not require therapy unless severe episodes or life threatening situations are encountered. However, occasional patients such as these may be treated if the death of family members has created such anxiety that they prefer the risk of possible side effects associated with drug therapy. The clinical course of the patient should be the primary guide for therapy rather than the level of C4 or C1 INH.

TREATMENT OF ACUTE ATTACKS

Angioedema affecting the extremities requires no specific therapy, and the episode usually abates within a few days. Swelling affecting the face is more troublesome, and severe attacks can be aborted with repeated subcutaneous doses of epinephrine 1:1000. For example, 0.3 cc every 45 minutes for one to three doses would suffice for an otherwise healthy adult with prominent facial, lip, or tongue swelling. Abdominal attacks, although painful, require only supportive therapy. The main symptom is cramping abdominal pain, sometimes associated with nausea, vomiting, or diarrhea. These episodes are similarly self-limited, lasting for 1 to 4 days, but require careful observation if an episode is severe.

We admit patients with severe abdominal attacks, administer fluids intravenously (particularly if dehydration might result from fluid loss), and use mild analgesics. We generally avoid the use of narcotic analgesics; however, a single dose of Demerol administered early in an attack can be helpful. Repeated doses of epinephrine 1:1000 given every 1 to 2 hours sometimes can abort episodes after a few doses. An abdominal examination should be performed periodically with particular attention to the status of bowel sounds and evidence of rigidity. Typically a patient has areas of tenderness to palpation, or rebound may be elicited; bowel sounds are more often hyperactive than hypoactive. The areas of tenderness may vary over time as can rebound (likely the result of stretching of visceral but not parietal peritoneum). However, the abdominal wall remains soft. Fever, leukocytosis, an elevated sedimentation rate, and progressive rigidity of the abdominal wall are signs of an "acute abdomen" and alert one to the uncommon occurrence of another disease for which surgery might really be indicated.

Involvement of the airway is a true medical emergency, which is generally unresponsive to antihistamines or corticosteroids and may or may not respond to epinephrine. Early signs of laryngeal involvement include a change in voice, tone, or pitch or frank hoarseness. Pharyngeal involvement may cause a choking sensation and difficulty in swallowing food. This may not be an emergency, but careful observation is indicated because it can progress to difficulty in swallowing secretions, the risk of aspiration, or laryngeal symptoms. More severe laryngeal involvement can lead to inspiratory stridor and asphyxia. When angioedema of the airway appears likely, an otolaryngologic evaluation to examine the vocal cords and the laryngeal-pharyngeal area should be performed. Epinephrine should be administered (assuming that there are no contraindications)—about 0.3 ml of a 1:1000 dilution given repeatedly. Vital signs should be monitored to be sure that the cardiovascular effects of one dose have passed before another is given. Spacing can vary from every 45 to 120 minutes as indicated. Antihistamines or short acting corticosteroids may be given, but there is little rationale for their use and they are not likely to help.

The condition in a patient with airway involvement who is seen within hours after onset or during the first day may worsen during the ensuing 1 to 2 days before resolving by day 3 or 4. Such a patient should be observed, and if the attack appears to be progressive, admission to the hospital, the intravenous administration of fluids, and epinephrine are indicated. A patient seen at day 2 or 3 of an episode need not be admitted if the swelling is clearly nonprogressive after observation for many hours. Epsilon-aminocaproic acid can be used in an attempt to ameliorate the severity of edema of the airway. A dose of 8 g is given within the first 4 hours and then 16 g per day for the next 24 to 48 hours until the episode has ended. Thus a combination of subcutaneous doses of epinephrine administered periodically on day 1 with epsilon-aminocaproic acid for a few days is recommended. However, there is no truly reliable modality that one can count on and attacks may nevertheless progress in some patients.

In such a circumstance tracheostomy is indicated. An alternative is nasotracheal intubation in an operating room setting. The staff should be prepared to perform a tracheostomy if intubation is not successful. The tube remains in place until the episode abates.

The use of fresh frozen plasma in such circumstances is controversial. On the one hand C1 INH is being replenished and on the other hand substrate for circulating active enzyme is being given and generation of more permeability factor is possible. Fresh frozen plasma is best utilized as prophylactic therapy (to be discussed) and not administered during acute episodes.

SHORT TERM PROPHYLACTIC THERAPY

Patients with hereditary angioedema may require minor surgical or other invasive procedures, which could precipitate angioedema. Those involving the respiratory tract are of particular concern and include such circumstances as dental procedures (gingivectomy, extraction, root canal work, or even routine local anesthesia) and endoscopy. In such cases the use of fresh frozen plasma in a patient who is receiving no other therapy can prevent attacks. We recommend the infusion of 2 units of fresh frozen plasma the day prior to surgery and 2 units just before the procedure. One must be cautious because there is a finite risk of transmission of hepatitis or even AIDS, and all recommended precautions must be followed. Single doner volunteers who have been screened serologically may be used to allay patient anxiety. If such surgery is elective, the administration of androgens for 5 days prior to the procedure (e.g., 4 mg of stanozolol four times daily) should obviate the need for fresh frozen plasma and is a reasonable alternative. For major surgical procedures the approach is similar. In patients who are already taking maintenance dosages of androgens the dosage should be increased for the aforementioned 5 day period so that C4 and C1 INH levels rise.

MAINTENANCE THERAPY

The object of maintenance therapy is to prevent episodes of swelling by utilizing the least quantity of medication that is efficacious to minimize side effects and costs. The most effective drugs are androgens or androgen derivatives, such as methyltestosterone, danazol, and stanozolol. Methyltestosterone was the first androgenic compound shown to be effective in hereditary angioedema; its use is restricted to men but it is otherwise a satisfactory drug. It is efficacious, the cost is low, and the toxicity is minimal. One can start with 10 mg three times daily and, once the disease is quiescent, gradually decrease the dosage. The major danger in its use is cholestatic jaundice, and liver function should be assessed periodically—perhaps monthly at the start and then every few months.

For both women and men one can use attenuated androgens such as danazol or stanozolol. Both these drugs are capable of increasing synthesis of normal C1 INH and thereby correct the underlying biochemical defect. C4 levels also rise with therapy. In women taking birth control pills (estrogenic) there may be an increase in attacks, which can be reversed by discontinuing birth control tablets without further therapy. It has become clear that either drug can be effective for long term maintenance at dosages that produce little or no change in the plasma C4 or C1 INH level. It is not known whether the drug works by some other mechanism or whether small changes, perhaps within tissues, suffice in terms of protection. The main side effects of danazol use are weight gain (due in part to fluid retention and increased appetite), menometrorrhagia, headaches, muscle cramps, mild androgenic effects (voice deepening, hirsutism, alopecia, acne, altered libido), and a mild increase in the SGOT and SGPT levels.

The starting dosage is 600 mg per day and the dosage is then gradually decreased. As little as 50 mg every other day suffices for some patients, but this is highly variable. My experience with stanozolol is greater than that with danazol, and we utilize this as our first choice for long term therapy. Its efficacy is essentially the same as for danazol, the cost is less (about 10 to 20 percent), and the side effects, although similar in type, seem less prominent. An increase in SGOT, SGPT, or LDH levels can be seen but not frank jaundice or irreversible changes suggestive of chronic hepatitis or cirrhosis. Lowering the dosage or stopping therapy for a while leads to rapid reversal of the enzyme elevations. Stanozolol is marketed as a 2-mg tablet and most patients are controlled with 2 mg per day. For some, as little as 2 mg every other day is sufficient. One can proceed from 2 mg per day to 4 mg every other day and then to 2 mg every other day.

Epsilon-aminocaproic acid (7 to 8 g per day) also has been shown to control attacks of hereditary angioedema, although it has no effect on C4 or C1 INH levels, its mechanism of action is unclear. It is known to inhibit plasmin, plasminogen activation, and C1 activation even by immune complexes. Its effect is to decrease the severity of attacks of swelling rather than decreasing the frequency. It could be considered in severely ill patients who are unable to take any of the aforementioned androgens. It is clearly a "second line" drug and particular caution is needed when there is a predisposition to thrombosis because it is antifibrinolytic. Thus it could be dangerous if a patient were to have a myocardial infarction or cerebrovascular accident. Epsilon-aminocaproic acid can also cause severe muscle toxicity, with pain and elevation of the aldolase and creatine phosphokinase levels. Therapy should be discontinued immediately if this occurs.

It is uncommon for therapy to be required in children prior to puberty, although episodes of swelling may occur. However, severe or life threatening episodes are rare in this age group and avoiding treatment is best. If therapy is needed, the minimal androgenic dosage should be used. This is perhaps less of a problem for males. Therapy of prepubescent girls should be carried out in conjunction with an endocrinologist. Epsilon-aminocaproic acid can be considered in this circumstance, since it does not affect gonadal development. We have successfully treated young females (age 10 to 14) with 2 mg of stanozolol every other day, with a normal onset of puberty, normal menses, and no evident side effects. We assess liver function every 3 months during the first year of therapy and every 6 months thereafter.

SUGGESTED READING

Frank MM, Sergeant JS, Kane MA, Alling DW. Epsilon aminocaproic acid therapy of hereditary angioneurotic edema: a double blind study. N Engl J Med 1972; 286:808–812.

Gelfand JA, Boss GR, Conley CL, Reinhart R, Frank MM. Acquired C1 esterase deficiency and angioedema: a review. Medicine 1979; 58:321–328.

Gelfand JA, Sherms RJ, Alling DW, Frank MM. Treatment of hereditary angioedema with danazol: reversal of clinical and biochemical abnormalities. N Engl J Med 1976; 295:1444–1448.

Kaplan AP. Urticaria and angioedema. In: Kaplan AP, ed. Allergy. New York: Churchill Livingstone, 1985:439–471.

Sheffer AL, Fearon DT, Austen KF. Clinical and biochemical effects of stanazolol therapy for hereditary angioedema. J Allergy Clin Immunol 1981; 68:181–187.

Sheffer AL, Fearon DT, Austen KF. Hereditary angioedema: a decade of management with stanozolol. J Allergy Clin Immunol; (In press).

FOOD ALLERGY

BRETT V. KETTELHUT, M.D.
DEAN D. METCALFE, M.D.

Food allergy is an immunologically mediated reaction to an ingested food antigen. In adults food allergy is uncommon and may present with a wide variety of symptoms. Although gastrointestinal symptoms (nausea, vomiting, and diarrhea) and cutaneous symptoms (urticaria, hives, and angioedema) predominate, respiratory symptoms (bronchospasm and rhinitis) and anaphylaxis may be observed in allergic individuals. When entertaining the diagnosis of food allergy, non-immunologically mediated adverse reactions to food must be excluded (Table 1). Corroboration of the patient's history may be obtained by positive prick skin test reactions to food extracts demonstrating mast cell bound IgE to a food antigen, the elimination of symptoms on exclusion of the suspected food(s) from the diet, and in selected patients, the reproduction of the symptoms on double blinded oral food challenge. Because skin testing and diagnostic oral food challenges pose a potential risk to the patient, only physicians skilled in these procedures, with support facilities to manage severe allergic reactions, should perform these diagnostic tests.

TABLE 1 Examples of Adverse Food Reactions Due to Nonimmunologic Mechanisms

Enzyme deficiencies
Lactase deficiency
Sucrase deficiency
Phenylketonuria
Gastrointestinal disease
Hiatal hernia
Peptic ulcer
Gallbladder disease
Postsurgical dumping syndrome
Neoplasia
Inflammatory bowel disease
Pancreatic insufficiency
Additives and contaminants
Dyes
Tartrazine
Exogenous chemicals
Nitrates and nitrites
Monosodium glutamate
Sulfiting agents
Antibiotics
Endogenous chemicals
Caffeine
Tyramine
Phenylethylamine
Alcohol
Theobromine
Tryptamine
Histamine
Toxins
Bacterial toxins
Botulism
Staphylococcal toxin
Endogenous toxins
Certain mushrooms—α-amanitine
"Shellfish"—saxitoxin
Ichthyotoxin
Fungi
Aflatoxin
Ergot
Other disorders
Collagen vascular disease
Endocrine disorders
Psychologic reactions
Bulimia
Anorexia nervosa

THERAPY

Once a food allergy has been identified and confirmed, the management consists of dietary avoidance to prevent the allergic reaction and pharmacologic therapy of symptoms resulting from inadvertent ingestion. A treatment plan must be individualized to account for the number and types of food involved, the degree of sensitivity, and the nature and severity of the symptoms.

Diet

The treatment of choice in food allergy is elimination of the offending food(s) from the patient's diet. Care must be taken to provide optimal nutrition while completely eliminating the food(s) provoking adverse reactionis. Palatability is an important consideration, because the success of the diet depends upon patient compliance. Diets that eliminate one or two foods are generally easy to design, but may become difficult to employ when common foodstuffs are to be avoided. For example, the dietary sources of milk and egg are numerous because of their widespread use in common foodstuffs. Elimination of these two foods alone results in a major loss of common commercially prepared foods from the diet. Hidden sources of these foods and others must be identified by the patient to reduce unexpected exposure to an offending food. The patient should be instructed to be wary of meals prepared by others who may include foods to which the patient may be sensitive. Cases have been reported in which patients with extreme sensitivities have experienced anaphylaxis, with subsequent death after such inadvertent exposures. Knowledge of the botanical families, as well as the classification of foods from animal sources, is necessary, for cross reacting antigens sometimes may be found among foods in the same group. For example, patients sensitive to shrimp often exhibit symptoms after ingestion of other crustaceans, such as crab, lobster, and crayfish. Cross reactivity in other food groups is not uniform, and diets should be planned in accordance with the patient's history of tolerance to these foods. Examples of these classifications of food groups are listed in Tables 2 and 3.

The preparation of a diet for a food sensitive patient should involve the skill of a dietician who is experienced in the treatment of these patients. One approach to the design of a diet for a patient with multiple food sensitivities is the institution of a well defined, limited diet as presented in Table 4. Foods that are not suspected of causing a reaction are then added one at a time every 2 days. Foods that provoke symptoms should be withheld from the diet, whereas foods not leading to a recurrence

TABLE 2 Classification of Foods from Plant Sources

Family	Foods
Grain family	Wheat (Graham flour, Gluten flour, Bran, Wheat germ), Rye, Barley (Malt), Corn, Oats, Rice, Wild rice, Sorghum, Cane
Mustard family	Mustard, Cabbage, Cauliflower, Broccoli, Brussel sprouts, Turnip, Rutabaga, Kale, Collard, Celery cabbage, Kohlrabi, Radish, Horseradish, Watercress
Gourd family	Pumpkin, Squash, Cucumber, Cantaloupe, Muskmelon, Honeydew melon, Persian melon, Casaba, Watermelon
Apple family	Apple, Pear, Quince
Poppy family	Poppy seed
Plum family	Plum (Prune), Cherry, Peach, Apricot, Nectarine, Almond
Laurel family	Avocado, Cinnamon, Bay leaf
Olive family	Green olive, Ripe olive
Ginger family	Ginger, Turmeric, Cardamon
Pine family	Juniper
Orchid family	Vanilla
Madder family	Coffee
Tea family	Tea
Pedalium family	Sesame seed
Mallow family	Okra, Cottonseed
Spurge family	Tapioca
Arrowroot family	Arrowroot
Arum family	Taro
Buckwheat family	Buckwheat, Rhubarb
Potato family	Potato, Tomato, Eggplant, Red pepper, Green pepper, Bell pepper, Chili, Tabasco, Pimento
Lily family	Asparagus, Onion, Garlic, Leek, Chive, Aloes
Goosefoot family	Beet, Spinach, Swiss chard
Parsley family	Parsley, Parsnip, Carrot, Celery, Celeriac, Caraway, Anise, Dill, Coriander, Fennel
Heath family	Cranberry, Blueberry
Gooseberry family	Gooseberry, Currant
Honeysuckle family	Elderberry
Citrus family	Orange, Grapefruit, Lemon, Lime, Tangerine, Kumquat
Pineapple family	Pineapple
Papaw family	Papaya
Birch family	Filbert, Hazelnut
Mulberry family	Mulberry, Fig, Hop, Breadfruit
Maple family	Maple syrup
Palm family	Coconut, Date, Sago
Legythis family	Brazil nut
Composite family	Leaf lettuce, Head lettuce, Endive, Escarole, Artichoke, Dandelion, Oyster plant, Chicory
Legume family	Navy bean, Kidney bean, Lima bean, String bean, Soybean, Lentil, Black-eyed pea, Pea, Peanut, Licorice, Acacia, Senna
Morning glory family	Sweet potato, Yam
Sunflower family	Jerusalem artichoke, Sunflower seed
Pomegranate family	Pomegranate
Ebony family	Persimmon
Rose family	Raspberry, Blackberry, Loganberry, Boysenberry, Dewberry, Strawberry
Banana family	Banana, Plantain
Grape family	Grape (Raisin)
Myrtle family	Allspice, Cloves, Pimento, Paprika, Guava
Mint family	Mint, Peppermint, Spearmint, Thyme, Sage, Marjoram, Savory
Pepper family	Black pepper
Nutmeg family	Nutmeg
Walnut family	English walnut, Black walnut, Butternut, Hickory nut, Pecan
Cashew family	Cashew, Pistachio, Mango
Beech family	Beechnut, Chestnut
Fungi family	Mushroom, Yeast
Sterculia family	Cocoa (Chocolate)

TABLE 3 Classification of Foods from Animal Sources

Mollusks	*Crustaceans*	*Fish*
Abalone	Crab	Sturgeon
Mussel	Crayfish	Hake
Oyster	Lobster	Anchovy
Scallop	Shrimp	Sardine
Clam		Herring
Squid	*Reptiles*	Haddock
	Turtle	Bass
Amphibians	*Birds*	Trout
Frog	Chicken	Salmon
Mammals	Duck	Whitefish
Beef	Goose	Scrod
Pork	Turkey	Shad
Goat	Guinea hen	Eel
Mutton	Squab	Carp
Venison	Pheasant	Codfish
Horsemeat	Partridge	Halibut
Rabbit	Grouse	Catfish
Squirrel		Sole
		Pike
		Flounder
		Drum
		Mullet
		Weakfish
		Mackerel
		Tuna
		Pompano
		Bluefish
		Snapper
		Sunfish
		Swordfish

of symptoms may remain in the diet. This process is continued until enough foods have been reintroduced to provide a nutritious diet. Rarely a patient may be sensitive to numerous common foods. In these cases supplemental nutrition can be delivered by prescribing an elemental diet (e.g., Vivonex, Vital).

When treatment is first instituted, strict avoidance of all sources of the offending food should be observed. If the initial diagnosis is correct and compliance is maintained, improvement in the patient's condition should result. Eventually, in the absence of anaphylactic sensitivity, small amounts of the offending food may be tolerated upon cautious reintroduction into the diet. For example, small amounts of egg may be tolerated when used as an ingredient in the preparation of other foods. In addition, certain foods not tolerated raw or partially cooked may be ingested without difficulty when completely cooked. Usually by practical experience most patients learn the method of preparation and the volume of a particular food that may be ingested without inducing symptoms, thereby making the diet more manageable.

TABLE 4 Lamb and Rice Diet

Foods Allowed

Brown rice—natural long grain, short grain; parboiled
White rice—enriched, converted; cook without added fat
Brown or white rice, rice flour
Brown rice cakes—containing only brown rice and salt (if desired)
Puffed rice cereal—containing only brown rice
Lamb
Water
Salt

All food must be prepared without added fat. Rice, lamb, salt, and water are the only allowable foods. No food containing any other ingredients is to be eaten. Check labels. Salt or baking soda should be used to brush the teeth.

Eliminate

All foods not listed above, especially coffee, tea, soft drinks, and juices. Vitamins, aspirin, and any medication not ordered by a doctor must be eliminated.

Possible Menu

Breakfast	*Lunch*	*Dinner*	*Snack*
Rice mush	Rice patties Pan-fried lamb chops	Rice and lamb sauté	Rice cakes

Instructions

Stay on basic diet for ____ days.

Then, on ____ add ____________ all by itself, first thing in AM
Then, on ____ add ____________ all by itself, first thing in AM
Then, on ____ add ____________ all by itself, first thing in AM
Next, on ____ add ____________ all by itself, first thing in AM
Next, on ____ add ____________ all by itself, first thing in AM

Continue food additions one at a time at ____ day intervals until most or all other foods in the diet have been tested. Keep a diet diary as indicated. Add foods in large amounts, and eat them several times a day during addition period.

Drugs

Even the most careful patient may inadvertently ingest the food to which he is sensitive. When the resulting symptoms of this exposure involve sites distant from the gastrointestinal tract, the treatment for each specific symptom is the same as that for similar allergic reactions. For example, the treatment of food induced urticaria is the same as the treatment of idiopathic urticaria, and asthma resulting from food ingestion is managed in the same way as asthma provoked by other allergens. The treatment for anaphylaxis due to a food ingestion differs only slightly from the treatment of other anaphylactic reactions. In addition to the standard therapy of anaphylaxis, gastric lavage may be necessary to reduce further antigen absorption and exposure. The patient with anaphylactic sensitivity should be taught how to self-administer epinephrine and should have an epinephrine-containing syringe and antihistamine available at all times. An identification tag stating the patient's sensitivity is also mandatory.

Gastrointestinal symptoms following inadvertent food ingestion are usually treated with antihistamines. An H_1 antihistamine, such as diphenhydramine hydrochloride in 25 to 50 mg doses three to four times daily, may be administered. As with other members of the ethanolamine series, diphenhydramine has marked sedative properties that may be undesirable in certain patients. Chlorpheniramine, an alkylamine, has a distinctly less sedative effect in most patients and may be given initially in doses of 4 mg three to four times daily.

Antihistamines, in addition to sedative effects, occasionally cause other central nervous system side effects, such as ataxia, dizziness, and difficulty in concentration. The anticholinergic properties of these drugs may lead to manifestations of atropine poisoning in susceptible patients or when given in large doses. Recently the nonsedating antihistamine terfenadine has been licensed for use in the treatment of allergic disease in the United States. This antihistamine may be useful in patients who are unable to tolerate other H_1 antihistamines because of sedation. The role of H_2 antihistamines such as cimetidine in the treatment of gastrointestinal food reactions has not been determined.

Corticosteroids are rarely used in the treatment of food allergy. Eosinophilic gastroenteritis and protein-losing gastroenteropathy associated with food allergy are two conditions in which steroid use may be instituted and the dosage tapered as symptoms resolve. Prednisone in oral dosages up to 60 mg a day may be required initially to ameliorate symptoms. When prolonged steroid therapy is required, alternate day therapy with the minimal dosage required to control symptoms should be used. In these instances 5 to 10 mg of prednisone every other day is usually sufficient. Prolonged steroid therapy should be reserved for severe cases owing to the numerous side effects of this drug.

CONTROVERSIES IN FOOD ALLERGY

Controversy has arisen over the possible association of food allergy with poorly defined neurologic and behavioral complaints. It has been hypothesized for many years that symptoms such as depression, tension, and fatigue are associated with immunologically mediated reactions to foods. In spite of the long-standing nature of such claims, as yet no firm evidence has been presented to establish such an association. Thus, these problems should not be considered to be secondary to immunologically mediated food reactions.

Other areas of controversy center around two additional modes of treatment of food allergy. The first is either the parenteral or oral administration of dilute concentrations of food extract. No reasonable evidence exists to support this form of therapy. The second area of controversy concerns the prophylactic oral administration of cromolyn sodium or ketotifen. Insufficient clinical evidence exists to support use of cromolyn sodium use in food allergy, and it is not currently approved by the FDA for use in the disorder. Ketotifen, an antihistamine with mast cell stabilizing properties, has been suggested as being useful in the treatment of food allergy, although verification of this claim remains to be shown by careful clinical trials.

SUGGESTED READING

Atkins FM, Steinberg SS, et al. Evaluation of immediate adverse reactions to foods in adults. I. Correlation of demographic, laboratory, and prick skin test data with response to controlled oral challenge. J Allergy Clin Immunol 1985; 75:348–355.

Crawford LV. Allergy diets. In: Bierman CW, Pearlman DC, eds. Allergic diseases of infants, childhood and adolescence. Philadelphia: WB Saunders, 1980: 394.

Pearson DJ, Rix KJB. Allergy mimetic reactions to food and pseudofood allergy. In: Dokor P, et al., eds. Pseudoallergic reactions. Vol. 4. Basel: Kargev, 1985: 59.

Reisman RE. American Academy of Allergy position statement—controversial techniques. J Allergy Clin Immunol 1981; 67:333–338

Sogn D. Medications and their use in the treatment of adverse reaction to foods. J Allergy Clin Immunol 1986; 78:238–243.

Terrill EE, Hill SR, et al. A checklist of names for 3,000 vascular plants of economic importance. Agriculture handbook 505. Washington, D.C.: United States Department of Agriculture, Agricultural Research Service, October 1986.

ATOPIC DERMATITIS

KEVIN D. COOPER, M.D.
ALAIN TAÏEB, M.D.

Treating a patient with atopic dermatitis is largely a matter of teaching skills. Educating the patient—or the parents if the patient is a child—is a time consuming task, especially at the beginning, but generally turns out to be the most rewarding approach when a satisfactory degree of self-management can be achieved.

Atopic dermatitis is the most common chronic skin disorder in infancy and childhood. Later-onset cases may occur in early adulthood, are generally more recalcitrant, and bear an overall worse prognosis. Diagnostic criteria have been established for the diagnosis of atopic dermatitis. The major criteria include a positive family history of atopy, a chronic or chronically relapsing course, eczematous lesions of symmetrical distribution (involving mostly extensor surfaces in infants and flexural lichenification later), and low thresholds for pruritogenic stimuli, such as external irritants, sweating, and emotions. Before 3 months of age, pruritus is not noticeable and the rash may present as a recalcitrant bipolar seborrheic dermatitis.

Clinical and in vitro studies in atopic dermatitis point to a polygenic inherited defect involving abnormalities of the immune system, transduction of biochemical and hormonal signals into cells, and vascular reactivity. In combination with environmental influences these abnormalities result in a vicious cycle of self-perpetuating pathologic changes in the skin and immune system.

Certain of these abnormalities, listed in Table 1, offer potential sites of action for systemic drug therapy. However, there remains a large gap in the understanding of the relationship between the data gathered from in vitro studies and the clinical manifestations. Therefore, treatment remains largely supportive and palliative. The management of atopic dermatitis includes assessment of severity and factors of prognosis (summarized in Table 2), skin care and therapy adapted to age, type, site, and stage of lesions (acute versus chronic) and prevention of complications, with special emphasis on herpetic and staphylococcal superinfections, as well as prevention of exposure to irritants and allergens.

Two general principles ought to guide the physician. First, simplicity of therapeutic measures allows better adherence to prescriptions. The patient given too many topical medications may become confused as to their appropriate time and site of application, and accumulation of prescriptions may lead to long

TABLE 1 Pathophysiologic Data and Possible Targets for Therapy

Abnormal humoral immunity
Hyper IgE, frequent if atopic dermatitis is associated with asthma: Avoid exposure to airborne, contact, and food allergens? Specific desensitization beneficial only in rare cases.
Increased intestinal permeability and transient IgA deficiency in infancy: Elimination of potent food allergens in the first year of life? Treat any diarrhea vigorously.
Abnormal cell mediated immunity
Unrestrained eczematous dermatitis: Steroids, immunosuppressives, immunomodulators.
Decreased T suppressor-cytotoxic cells and cutaneous delayed type hypersensitivity: Immunomodulators? Antibiotics and antiviral therapy as needed for complications.
Impaired neutrophil and monocyte chemotaxis: Antibiotic therapy for infectious complications.
Pharmacologic and metabolic anomalies
Altered cyclic nucleotide (cAMP) metabolism in leukocytes: Development of specific phosphodiesterase inhibitors.
"Easy releasability" of mast cells: Avoidance of triggering agents and events, mast cell stabilization: Cromolyn? Steroids, antihistamines.

TABLE 2 Initial Assessment: Factors Influencing Prognosis and Management

Genetic background
Bilateral atopic heredity
Atopic dermatitis symptomatic of primary immunodeficiency (Wiskott-Aldrich syndrome, hyper IgE syndrome)
Associated ichthyosis vulgaris
Clinical features
Age at onset >2 yr
Inverted pattern of lesions
Hand eczema
Severity of rash (surface involved, acuteness of lesions, duration of attacks)
Delay and degree of response to correctly administered treatment
Severe herpetic infection
Environmental factors
Poor psychological environment
Exposure to irritants and allergens (inhalant or cutaneous)
Biologic features
Generally clinical evaluation and history suffice; high and very high (>10,000) IgE levels generally associated with severe disease

term storage, which in turn may compromise the efficacy of the drugs.

Second, clear and complete explanations about bathing, skin care, prescription use, and topical medicament use are needed. Prescriptions should be explained thoroughly, and a handout may be useful to reinforce the most important points (available from the American Academy of Dermatology, Evanston, IL, and from the Eczema Association for Science and Education [EASE], 1221 S.W. Yamhill, Suite 303, Portland, OR 97205). For example, even techniques for bathing infants require instructions in order to avoid adverse consequences. In severe cases demonstration of appropriate handling of topical treatment by specialized personnel on an outpatient basis is the best choice for children, but hospitalization is sometimes required for a more complete assessment of the disease and the therapeutic response.

DERMATOLOGIC MANAGEMENT

Since atopic dermatitis has a spontaneous course of relapsing acute exacerbations followed by more or less durable periods of improvement, a two step approach is detailed here (acute disease and maintenance management). Whatever the case, treatment is aimed at relieving pruritus, cutaneous inflammation, and superinfection. The rational use of topical corticosteroid therapy dominates all stages of therapy, but antibiotic therapy, skin hydration, the use of antihistamines, recognition of complicating conditions, and counseling are all important in the management of atopic dermatitis. Some of the myriad of corticosteroid preparations available are presented in Table 3, and an outline regarding their use can be found in Table 4. Familiarity with a single formulation from each category is generally sufficient. In the authors' experience combinations of corticosteroids with antimicrobial drugs for topical application are not particularly useful. Bases containing sensitizing compounds are also best avoided.

Acute Dermatitis

Acute flares of atopic dermatitis can occur as weeping crusted eruptions or in other cases may occur as erythema with or without scales, which can be so extensive as to constitute a generalized exfoliative erythroderma. The initial assessment should always survey previous treatments with special attention directed toward the possible deleterious effects of topical therapy. Application of nonprescription drugs can aggravate a case of moderate severity because of idiosyncratic intolerance, use of irritants or inappropriate drugs, or in rare instances allergic contact dermatitis. Examples of contact allergens include balsam of Peru, lanolin, neomycin, and preservatives contained in creams. In patients with rapid aggravation associated with wet vesiculopustular or crusted lesions, herpes simplex superinfection must be suspected (eczema herpeticum). Especially in cases of dramatic skin changes associated with fever and malaise in an infant, the most severe form of eczema herpeticum, Kaposi's varicelliform eruption, should be considered. Bacterial and viral culture results may take several days, but Giemsa or Wright's stained smears of scrapings of the base of vesiculopustular lesions (Tzanck smear) may provide rapid confirmation of the diagnosis by revealing the presence of multinucleated keratinocytes.

The rapid institution of combined antiherpetic-antistaphylococcal therapy is indicated. Parenteral administration of acyclovir (15 mg per kilogram per day) and methicillin (25 mg per kilogram every 6 hours) can be changed to oral therapy after 5 days. Milder forms of eczema herpeticum are not unusual in older patients; they are recognizable as punctate erosions that may be associated with more typical vesicles distributed over involved cutaneous areas. Simple acute bullous staphylococcal impetigo sometimes masquerades as eczema herpeticum.

Once these complications have been ruled out, treatment of acute flares of disease can proceed as follows:

Acute Weeping Crusted Eczematous Dermatitis

This manifestation is most frequent in children and is almost always associated with heavy colonization and superinfection with *Staphylococcus aureus*. Initial management should be directed toward reduction of cutaneous *Staphylococcus aureus*, since this is an inciting source of inflammation as well as a source of further recontamination through scratching.

1. An antibacterial liquid soap (chlorhexidine) can be applied by gently rubbing crusted areas with soap gauze.
2. Rinse completely in the tub, since retention of this type of soap results in dry itchy skin, gently removing remaining crusts after a few minutes of soaking.
3. The skin is partially dried by patting with a smooth towel. Then an antibiotic cream such as silver sulfadiazine or gentamicin is immediately applied to affected sites and covered with gauze (tubular gauze dressings are very convenient in infants).
4. This treatment is justified twice daily in severe cases for the first day or couple of days. After sufficient disinfection (24 to 36 hours), topical corticosteroid therapy can be introduced, using a cream at the beginning, twice a day, from the moderately potent category (Table 3).
5. Quantities should be monitored precisely. A recent survey of severe cases in infants admitted as inpatients showed that 30 to 50 g of a moderately

TABLE 3 Classification of Corticosteroids for Topical Use

Potency	*Concentration**	*Base†*	*Quantity Supplied‡*
Very potent			
Clobetasol propionate (Temovate)	0.05	C, O	15, 30
Betamethasone dipropionate (Diprolene)	0.05	O	15, 45
Potent			
Triamcinolone acetonide (Kenalog, Aristocort)	0.5	C O	15, 20, 240 15, 20
Halcinonide (Halog)	0.1 0.1	C, O L	15, 30, 60, 240 20, 60 ml
Fluocinonide (Lidex)	0.05 0.05 0.05	C, CE, O L Gel	15, 45, 110, 430 20, 60 ml 15, 30, 60, 120
Betamethasone 17-valerate (Valisone)	0.1 0.1 0.1	C O L	15, 45, 110, 430 15, 45 20, 60 ml
Desoximetasone (Topicort)	0.25 0.25	CE O	15, 60, 4 oz 15, 60
Diflorasone diacetate (Florone, Maxiflor)	0.05	C, O	15, 30, 60
Amcinonide (Cyclocort)	0.1	C, O	15, 30, 60
Moderately potent			
Triamcinolone acetonide (Aristocort, Kenalog)	0.1 0.1 0.1	C O L	15, 60, 80, 240; 1, 5 lb 15, 60, 80, 240; 1, 5 lb 15, 60
Fluocinolone acetonide (Fluonid, Synalar)	0.025 0.025	C, O L	15, 30, 60, 120, 425 20, 60 ml
Flurandrenolide (Cordan)	0.05	C, O L	15, 30, 60, 225 15, 60 ml
Clocortolone (Cloderm)	0.1	C	15, 45
Hydrocortisone butyrate (Locoid)§	0.1	C, O	15, 45
Mildy potent			
Triamcinolone acetonide (Aristocort, Kenalog)	0.025	C	15, 60, 80, 240; 1, 5 lb
Desonide (Tridesilon)§	0.05	C O	15, 60; 5 lb 15, 60
Mometasone (Elocon)	0.1	C, O	15, 45
Hydrocortisone valerate (Westcort)§	0.2	C O	15, 45, 60, 120 15, 45, 60
Alclometasone dipropionate (Aclovate)§	0.05	C, O	15, 45
Weak			
Hydrocortisone (Hytone, Texacort)§	1.0	C O	1, 4 oz 1 oz

*Concentration in % w/w. For clarity, only triamcinolone acetonide has been indicated in three different concentrations. The other molecules appear only in their highest available concentration.

†C, Cream. O, ointment. CE, cream-emollient. L, lotion.

‡Quantity supplied expressed in grams if no other mention.

§Non-fluorinated molecules.

TABLE 4 Topical Use of Corticosteroid in Atopic Dermatitis

Contraindications	
	Current cutaneous infection
	Potent fluorinated corticosteroid on face
	Diaper area: risk of systemic toxicity by plastic diaper occlusion: local side effects potentiated by maceration (infection, granuloma gluteale infantum)
General rules of use	
	Acute oozing lesions: creams, nonalcoholic lotions of moderate potency
	Chronic lichenified lesions and skin of extremities: cream or ointment of potent or very potent occlusion helpful in some instances
	Scalp: gels and lotions
	Consider comfort of patient: ointments indicated in cases of dry skin or associated ichthyosis but difficult to treat on an outpatient basis
	Prefer use of commercially available preparations rather than custom compounding
	Adapt quantity to involved surface
	Two applications per day are sufficient (tachyphylaxis); with potent and very potent derivatives, one application per day may suffice
Monitoring of prescription	
	Note quantity used at each follow-up visit
	Do not allow numerous automatic renewals
	Check for local side effects (atrophy, infection, depigmentation) and systemic side effects (hypercorticism), especially in infants or if large quantities and occlusion are required

potent corticosteroid cream can clear the rash within a 4 to 6 day period in most instances. The quantities used can be reduced by application to moist, lightly pat-dried skin, allowing better spreading.

6. Accessory measures include oral doses of antistaphylococcal antibiotics, mainly erythromycin, dicloxacillin, or an oral cephalosporin. In addition, antihistamines are useful to minimize pruritus and excoriation.

Maintenance Therapy

Once clearing of an acute flare occurs, proper skin care is essential for long term maintenance in chronic dermatitis. During the transition period topical steroid therapy is gradually tapered over several weeks. In moderate disease generally two to three applications per week of a moderately potent steroid suffices. In children a 30-g tube is often enough for 6 to 8 weeks, whereas adults may require up to two 60-g tubes for a similar period. To reduce costs, adult patients with extensive disease can be given prescriptions for generic triamcinolone, 0.025 or 0.1 percent cream in 1 pound sizes.

The patient's bathing habits should be strictly regulated: Bathing should be restricted to an every other day or every third day frequency. The patient should be instructed that the baths are not to be scalding, that the shower is preferable to the bath, and that the duration of the shower or bath should not be excessive. The patient should be instructed that soaps are to be used only in the axilla and groin, using a mild soap such as Dove or Basis, and that the soap is to be rinsed off completely. Foam or bubble baths should be avoided.

Immediately upon exiting from the bath or shower the patient should apply emollients, such as a heavy cream-based emollient (Eucerin cream). Some patients with heavily lichenified, thickened skin can tolerate heavier preparations, such as Aquaphor, but the occlusive properties of ointment-like preparations are uncomfortable for most patients with atopic dermatitis. Some cannot tolerate even a cream-based emollient such as Eucerin and can only tolerate lotions such as Shepherd's lotion, Lubriderm, or Keri lotion. Bath oils also can be directly applied to the skin. Emollients applied to inflamed skin can be irritating.

Patients should be instructed to repeat application of the emollient as many times during the day as is necessary to keep the skin moist. For extreme xerosis, as in atopic dermatitis associated with ichthyosis vulgaris, a lactic acid containing emollient is helpful (Lacticare, Lac-Hydrin). Recommendations for emollients may have to be altered in response to changing climatic conditions. The extreme dryness and low humidity of winter often require heavy creams and more frequent applications than in summer months. Steroid preparations for topical use should not be substituted for emollients. Children who are unable to be tapered off topical steroid therapy with proper skin care should be reevaluated.

As regards clothing, wool or acrylic sweaters should not be in direct contact with skin. Most patients do not tolerate handling raw foods or wet work with the hands, and patients who must be involved in such situations are advised to use cotton liners under protective rubber or plastic gloves. Atopic dermatitis is a common cause of occupational hand eczema. In some patients sweating associated with excessive physical exercise is poorly tolerated, but counseling in this respect should emphasize that the goal is to allow the patient a life as normal as possible.

SYSTEMIC THERAPY

Systemic Antihistamine Therapy

The systemic administration of sedating antihistamines can benefit the patient by reducing pruritus and excoriations, particularly at night. For adults, hydroxyzine 25 to 200 mg at bedtime, or diphenhydramine in similar doses is often a useful starting point. Pediatric doses of 5 mg per kilogram per day in syrup or elixir are used. However, the use of antihistamines in children should be limited to flares. Poor responses to these can be followed by the use of antihistamines from each of the major antihistamine categories. Another useful class of drugs is the tricyclic antidepressants, which exert potent anti-H_1 and H_2 activity. These can be used in adults in 25 to 75 mg oral doses at bedtime (e.g., doxepin hydrochloride or amitriptyline hydrochloride).

Nonsedating antihistamines can also bring relief to patients during the day. Terfenadine (Seldane), 120 mg orally two times per day, can be used for intermittent use, since it has a rapid onset of action. Astemizole (Hismanal) can also be used, but must be used on a regular basis because it takes several days to achieve its effects.

Antibiotics

As already stated, the use of antibiotics is helpful in acute exacerbations. In some cases with associated nummular lesions, the long-term administration of erythromycin, dicloxacillin, or a cephalosporin may reduce the frequency of flares. Culture of intact pustules may reveal a methicillin-resistant strain of *Staphylococcus aureus*. In this case, ciprofloxacillin or a combination of Septra (trimethoprim-sulfamethoxazole) and rifampin may be used.

Phototherapy

Patients with involvement of a large surface area and recalcitrant disease (adolescents and adults mostly, but also occasionally children) may benefit from a course of twice- or thrice-weekly exposure to banks of ultraviolet light–emitting bulbs. UVB, UVB with UVA, and UVA in combination with oral doses of methoxypsoralen (PUVA) have been used successfully. Results are not long-lasting.

Ketoconazole

Ketoconazole has been advocated for use in patients with prominent face and neck involvement and an immediate hypersensitivity to *Pityrosporum ovale*. Note, however, that ketoconazole inhibits corticosteroid metabolism, so that concurrent administration may increase the apparent dose of steroid (increased efficacy and complications).

Corticosteroids

In extremely severe, disabling cases that are unresponsive to topical management and in which compliance with all aspects of the regimen has been verified, systemic prednisone therapy can be used. A 2-week course of prednisone, 40 to 60 mg a day, will result in improvement. However, tapering of the prednisone dosage often results in a rebound flare, and repeated use of 2-week bursts of prednisone to manage acute flares of the disease often results in the inability to taper the patient off prednisone and the patient's commitment to long-term oral steroid therapy. For this reason it is best to avoid the systemic use of steroids for atopic dermatitis except in the most severe cases, when infection is under control.

Other Immunosuppressives and Immunomodulators

In truly recalcitrant, severe cases, experimental therapy with methotrexate, cyclosporine A, or azathioprine (Imuran) as an immunosuppressive, or with evening primrose oil or interferon, can be considered. However, these are currently unproved modalities with unknown risks in this patient group.

ALLERGY MANAGEMENT

The role of allergen avoidance in atopic dermatitis is at best controversial. Food allergy resulting in histamine release and skin lesions has been documented in a small percentage of patients with atopic dermatitis.

The food allergens most commonly implicated are cow's milk, eggs, fish, and nuts. Although conventional breast feeding does not seem to be superior to formula in clinical trials, in cases of a clear atopic hereditary predisposition a preventive diet avoiding those items may be recommended for both the feeding mother and her child. An artificial formula devoid of cow's milk proteins (soybean hydrolysate or a similar product) is an alternative. The introduction of potential allergens should be delayed for up to 6 months for cow's milk and 12 months for eggs and fish. In severe cases with a suspicion of food allergy, a more complete work-up may be indicated, including exclusion diets and food challenges. However, since the likelihood of successful therapy using dietary manipulation is low, this approach should be used rarely in order to avoid malnutrition in the child.

Maintaining a low level of airborne allergens in the environment is not easy, but preventing asthma or allergic rhinitis is perhaps worthwhile in the "at risk" baby. This can be achieved by frequent vacuum cleaning with water vacuum or wall vacuum vented to the outside to avoid aerosolization of small dust mite allergens, removing dust with a wet sponge, and avoiding carpets and other known shelters for house dust mites. Pet animals are not recommended. When present, they should be kept outside the home. An allergic cough or asthma may begin before the end of the second year and deserves a search for causative allergens. Allergen desensitization is generally not effective in clearing the skin of patients with active atopic dermatitis. Therefore, specific desensitization is rarely worth attempting, since only rare patients show some improvement.

PSYCHOLOGICAL SUPPORT

Psychological support is crucial for the patient and family. Flares are often associated with life stresses, and patients are often grateful to be asked about such recent stressful events. Presentation of an overly optimistic prognosis to patients and families of atopic patients may result in frustration. Patients and the families of patients with severe disease must make adjustments for dealing with a chronic disease. Patients or their parents should be given continued positive reinforcement and encouragement to maintain their efforts toward skin care, since this may affect the overall course of the disease, and since their efforts may provide an acceptable life for themselves or their child. However, it should be made clear to patients that despite their best efforts, flares will occur, and that it is not their "fault" or a failure on their part that the flare occurred. This will reduce anxiety and guilt that accelerate flares. Psychological counseling is indicated for families contending with frustration, depression, guilt, and manipulative behavior. An extremely useful resource for patients is to contact or join the patient advocacy group, EASE.

SUGGESTED READING

Hanifin JM, Cooper KD, Roth HL. Atopy and atopic dermatitis. J Am Acad Dermatol 1986; 15:703–706.

Rajka G, Braathen LR, eds. Proceedings of first international symposium on atopic dermatitis. Acta Dermatol Venereol (Suppl) (Stockh) 1980; 92:1–136.

Sampson HA, Jolie PL. Increased plasma histamine concentration after food challenges in children with atopic dermatitis. N Engl J Med 1984; 311:372–376.

Taieb A, Body S, Astar I, et al. Clinical epidemiology of symptomatic primary herpetic infection in children: A study of 50 cases. Acta Paediatr Scand 1987; 76:128–132.

SYSTEMIC LUPUS ERYTHEMATOSUS

JOHN H. KLIPPEL, M.D.

Systemic lupus erythematosus is a chronic, relapsing, and remitting inflammatory disease with multiple potential target organs. Although the cause, or perhaps more likely the causes, of the disease are unknown, sufficient knowledge of the clinical course and pathology exists to allow for the development of effective strategies for patient management. Medical therapies are directed primarily at suppression of inflammation or dysfunction of the immune system thought to be of basic importance in pathogenesis. The success of the management of patients has been a major factor in the progressive improvements in prognosis of the disease over the past several decades.

EDUCATION

Patient education is an essential part of lupus management that is far too often neglected. The need for education is perhaps most evident during the early months of disease. The newly diagnosed patient is typically overwhelmed to learn that the disease is incurable, chronic, potentially fatal, or requires drugs that have serious side effects. These, in fact, may be major issues in the seriously ill patient that need to be addressed promptly. However, in the majority of patients, emphasis on the general benign nature of the disease and reassurance that most patients respond well to management serve to minimize anxiety. Patient support groups and the distribution of appropriate patient literature concerning lupus are often very effective. Two of the better sources of patient information that can be highly recommended are *Living with S.L.E.: A Handbook for Patients with Systemic Lupus Erythematosus* (W. V. Epstein and G. Clewley, Millberry Union Bookstore, 500 Parnassus Avenue, San Francisco, CA 94143) and *Lupus Erythematosus: A Handbook for Physicians, Patients and Their Families* (Lupus Foundation of America, Inc., Suite 203, 1717 Massachusetts Avenue, N.W., Washington, D.C. 20036).

GENERAL MEDICAL MANAGEMENT

The physician caring for a patient with systemic lupus erythematosus must be prepared to deal with many problems that fall within the category of general internal medicine. The care and well-being of the patient are as much if not even more dependent on attention to these aspects of management as those few therapies directed at the disease per se. Among the more common medical needs of the patient with lupus is the treatment of infections, hypertension, seizures, and minor psychiatric illness. In addition, several general principles of preventive medical care that apply to essentially all lupus patients can be identified (Table 1).

DISEASE ACTIVITY

Therapy is guided by the concept of lupus disease activity. Although somewhat difficult to define precisely, disease activity is a composite of clinical and laboratory features reflective of active, ongoing inflammation (Table 2). On the basis of the potential for these features to cause serious morbidity or mortality, clinical manifestations or laboratory abnormalities can be divided into minor or major categories of disease activity. These may reflect direct evidence of continuing lupus organ disease (e.g., nephritis, cardiopulmonary disease, dermatitis, serositis), indirect nonspecific manifestations of systemic inflammation (e.g., fever, fatigue, elevated erythrocyte sedimentation rate), or simply evidence of a deranged immune system (antinuclear antibody, anti-DNA antibodies, or hypocomplementemia).

The assessment of lupus disease activity is used to plan appropriate therapy. In general, major disease activity warrants more intensive, aggressive approaches to management, whereas minor disease activity typically can be controlled with more conservative, less toxic forms of treatment. Changes in disease activity over time are useful in determining the effectiveness of therapy and whether more, less, or even another form of therapy is indicated. In most instances, objective measures of disease activity, such as urine sediment examination or renal function tests, or the detection of proteinuria in nephritis, or the hemoglobin level, white blood cell count, or platelet count for hematologic involvement, make the task of assessing disease activity for any given organ system affected by lupus relatively straightforward and easy.

TABLE 1 Important Preventive Measures in the Medical Management of Systemic Lupus Erythematosus

Regular monitoring	Patient should be evaluated every 6 months at a minimum to assess disease activity and review therapy; minimal standard laboratory studies should include blood urea nitrogen and creatinine, complete blood count, platelet count, urinalysis
Immunizations	Influenza vaccine should be given yearly Pneumococcal vaccine should be given to splenectomized patients
Antibiotic prophylaxis	Antibiotic prophylaxis should be used for all dental or genitourinary procedures
Photoprotection	Patients with photosensitivity should be reminded to avoid intense sun exposure and to use sunscreens
Birth control	Pregnancy should be avoided at times when the disease is active and uncontrolled or the patient is under treatment with major therapies

TABLE 2 Disease Activity in Systemic Lupus Erythematosus

	Clinical Features	*Laboratory Features*
Minor disease activity	Fatigue Fever Rash Oral and nasal ulcers Arthritis Alopecia	Elevated erythrocyte sedimentation rate Leukopenia Proteinuria Hematuria Red cell casts Antinuclear antibodies Anti-DNA antibodies Hypocomplementemia
Major disease activity	Serositis Myocarditis Pneumonitis Nephrotic syndrome Vasculitis Myositis Psychosis Status epilepticus Cranial neuropathy Transverse myelopathy	Thrombocytopenia Hemolytic anemia Rising blood urea nitrogen and creatinine levels

Far more complicated is the patient with multisystem disease. A patient may have multiple minor abnormalities that when combined clearly constitute a major serious illness. Moreover, in the course of therapy, certain features of the disease often decrease and others worsen.

To address this clinical problem, a number of different methods to quantify overall lupus disease activity have been proposed. These range from relatively simple, four-tier disease activity schemes (none, mild, moderate, severe) to more complex systems, which assign scores to individual measures, which are then summed to give a global disease activity index score.

Finally, it is important to note that measures of abnormal immunity should not by themselves be equated with disease activity. They may, however, provide supportive evidence of disease activity in conjunction with other chemical findings. The patient with high-titer antinuclear antibody, anti-DNA antibody, or depressed serum complement levels who is otherwise completely well should not be judged to have active lupus or have treatment initiated to correct the abnormalities.

DRUG THERAPY

The drug management of systemic lupus erythematosus is simplified by the limited number of drugs used in treatment. The pathologic changes seen in lupus as well as findings of abnormal immune function imply that drugs that suppress inflammation or immunity are likely to be of benefit. However, for the most part, detailed understanding of the exact mechanisms of action of drugs possessing either of these properties is lacking. Moreover, clinical use of these drugs is mostly empirical. With perhaps the single exception of lupus nephritis, there are no controlled trials upon which decisions can be based. Drug treatment thus comes to be based more on clinical experience and opinion than on scientific facts.

Nonsteroidal Anti-inflammatory Drugs

Minor clinical manifestations of lupus are commonly treated by means of nonsteroidal anti-inflammatory drugs (NSAIDs). In addition to various salicylate compounds, there are now a number of prescription drugs of this type available. There is no reason to believe that one such drug is preferable to another. In fact, the only comparative study that has been done to evaluate this class of drugs in lupus found aspirin and ibuprofen to be equally effective. The selection among these drugs thus is based on such factors as physician or patient preference, cost, patient tolerance, or, in individual patients, the apparent ability of one particular drug to best control the disease. The latter finding accounts for a good deal of changing from one drug to another until a nearly optimal drug is found. For unexplained reasons, certain patients appear to respond better to one drug, whereas others seem to experience no beneficial effect whatsoever from that drug. The combining of NSAIDs is strongly discouraged.

Several complications caused by NSAIDs may be mistaken for lupus activity. Since appropriate therapy under such circumstances is to discontinue the drug as opposed to intensifying drug therapy, these become important clinical considerations. Although fever, anaphylaxis, and pulmonary and cutaneous vasculitis have been rarely described with NSAIDs, the effects on the kidneys and the central nervous system are of particular importance in patients with lupus.

The inhibitory effect of these drugs on prostaglandins may produce a reduction in renal function with an elevation of the serum creatinine concentration or depression of creatinine clearance. The kidney with active or chronic lupus nephritis in which prostaglandins become an important adjunct to maintain renal function is particularly susceptible to NSAID-induced changes in renal function. In this setting, these drugs serve almost as a stress test to evaluate kidney involvement. In order to assess renal function accurately, it is therefore necessary that all nonsteroidal drug therapy be discontinued for several days prior to the study. This is of particular importance if the recent loss of renal function prompts considerations of further evaluation by renal biopsy or the need for major changes in therapy. If these drugs are contributing to the impairment of renal function, their discontinuation will result in a rapid improvement in function.

Several NSAIDs have been associated with the development of aseptic meningitis. Although these drugs appear to be capable of producing this reaction in patients without autoimmune disease, the majority of cases reported have involved patients with lupus or a lupus-like illness. The typical clinical presentation involves headaches, meningismus, and fever and rarely pruritus, facial edema, and conjunctivitis. Study of the cerebrospinal fluid reveals lymphocytosis, an elevated protein level, and a sterile culture.

Corticosteroids

Corticosteroids are the single most important class of drugs used in lupus treatment. They are used topically or intradermally for skin manifestations, in low doses for minor disease activity, and in high doses for major disease activity (Table 3). Ideally oral corticosteroid therapy should be given as a single daily morning dose. In the event that this is inadequate, the same total daily dosage should be divided into a two or three times a day schedule.

The reduction in the corticosteroid dosage (tapering) once the disease process is under control is of particular importance for high-dose corticosteroid programs. There are few agreed-upon rules as to how best to go about dosage reduction. An attempt to change to an alternate-day schedule after 4 to 6 weeks

TABLE 3 The Multiple Uses of Corticosteroids in Systemic Lupus Erythematosus

Indication	*Corticosteroid*
Rashes	Topical corticosteroid ointments and creams
	Short-acting Hydrocortisone (0.125–1.0%)
	Intermediate-acting Methylprednisolone (0.025–1.0%) Triamcinolone
	Long-acting Betamethasone (0.025–0.2%) Dexamethasone
Minor disease activity	Prednisone (equivalent) at a dose of <0.5 mg/kg in single or divided daily dose
Major disease activity	Prednisone (equivalent) at a dose of 1 mg/kg in single or divided daily dose
	Intravenous bolus megadose (1 g or 15 mg/kg) of methylprednisolone given over 30 minutes; often repeated for 3 consecutive days

of therapy is common practice. The rate of dose reduction should approximate 5 mg of prednisone (or equivalent) on alternate days weekly until the patient is on a pure alternate-day schedule. Some patients do not tolerate alternate-day corticosteroids and begin to show evidence of disease activity starting in the afternoon or evening of the off-corticosteroid day. NSAIDs are frequently used as a substitute; if these fail, efforts should be made to maintain the patient on the lowest possible daily corticosteroid dosage that controls the disease.

Many or perhaps even most rheumatologists reason that the risks of disease relapse when corticosteroids are discontinued far outweigh the potential long-term toxic effects of chronic low-dose corticosteroid therapy. Thus, the institution of corticosteroid therapy represents a lifelong treatment for many patients. There is, however, no evidence that low-dose corticosteroid therapy prevents lupus flares or is associated with a high incidence of relapse once discontinued in certain clinical settings. Thus, in patients with prolonged periods of disease remission, slow reduction of the corticosteroid dosage with an aim toward eventual discontinuation of corticosteroid therapy should be a goal of patient management.

Megadose bolus intravenous methylprednisolone therapy should be regarded as an alternative to traditional high-dose oral drug use in the treatment of major lupus activity. Several small randomized trials evaluating the efficacy of bolus methylprednisolone therapy appear to confirm at least the short-term benefits of this approach. A number of side effects of bolus megadose methylprednisolone not evident with high-dose oral corticosteroid therapy have been reported. Common minor events noted have included facial flushing, a metallic taste, hypertension, hyperglycemia, and noninflammatory arthritis.

Antimalarial Drugs

Antimalarial drugs are effective in the management of mild systemic, cutaneous, and musculoskeletal features of lupus. The mechanism of action of these drugs relevant to lupus is unknown; anti-inflammatory, immunosuppressive, photoprotective, and nucleoprotein stabilizing properties of antimalarial drugs have been described.

The antimalarial drugs commonly used in lupus include hydroxychloroquine or chloroquine (4-amino-quinolines) and less frequently mepacrine (a 9-aminoacridine compound; Table 4). Many advocate starting antimalarial therapy with a loading dose regimen (400 mg of hydroxychloroquine or 500 mg of chloroquine) for 4 weeks and then switching to a lower dosage maintenance schedule once the disease process is under control. The response to antimalarial drugs, particularly in terms of cutaneous manifestations, can be remarkably rapid, with improvement often evident in a matter of days after starting the drug. Patients taking long-term antimalarial therapy whose disease is in complete clinical remission pose a minor dilemma. As with corticosteroids, many believe that discontinuation of therapy often results in disease relapse. Thus there is, in general, a reluctance to ever discontinue therapy completely. Reduction of the dosage of antimalarial drugs to one or two tablets a week in these patients is worthwhile.

TABLE 4 Doses and Toxic Effects of Antimalarial Drugs in Systemic Lupus Erythematosus

	Tablet Size	*Daily Dosage*
Drugs and dose		
Hydroxychloroquine (Plaquenil)	200 mg	200–400 mg
Chloroquine phosphate (Aralen)	500 mg	250–500 mg
Mepacrine (Atabrine)	100 mg	100 mg
Toxic effects		
Gastrointestinal	Anorexia, cramps, nausea, diarrhea	
Cutaneous	Erythematous rashes, bleaching of hair, yellow staining (mepacrine)	
Neurologic	Headaches, dizziness, irritability, peripheral myopathy and neuropathy	
Ophthalmologic	Corneal deposits, retinopathy	
Hematologic	Leukopenia, toxic granulations, thrombocytopenia, aplastic anemia	
Cardiac	Cardiomyopathy	

There are a number of potential toxic effects of antimalarial therapy (see Table 4). However, with the low drug doses used in the treatment of lupus, the risks of most of these adverse effects are exceedingly small. The major concern is ocular toxicity, of which there are two types. Deposition of antimalarial drugs in the cornea is relatively common. This may be responsible for visual disturbances such as complaints of a halo effect around lights, often within several weeks after starting the drug. Corneal deposits can be detected by slit lamp examination and are not a contraindication to continued antimalarial therapy. In addition, corneal deposits are not in any way related to retinopathy, the other form of antimalarial eye toxicity. Clearly, antimalarial retinopathy has been the major concern regarding the long-term use of these drugs in lupus. The frequency with which antimalarial retinopathy occurs in the disease and whether daily drug doses or cumulative drug doses are the major important factors are not known. An ophthalmologic examination should be performed prior to therapy and then annually to detect any evidence of retinal toxicity early. Since antimalarial retinopathy has been reported to be exacerbated by light, patients treated with antimalarial drugs should be advised to wear sunglasses in bright sunlight.

Immunosuppressive Drugs

Various cytotoxic and antimetabolite drugs are used in the treatment of serious manifestations of systemic lupus, including nephritis, central nervous system disease, and hematologic involvement. The rationale for this approach stems from the concept that products of the immune system mediate the pathologic changes seen in lupus nephritis and that these agents suppress the heightened or exaggerated immune functions responsible for the observed disease. These drugs are not selective for the immune system, and the effects on other cells are responsible for a host of toxic effects associated with this approach. Immunosuppressive drugs are regarded as experimental and generally are reserved for patients who have failed to benefit from conservative therapies, including high-dose corticosteroid therapy.

Drugs of two different classes—alkylating drugs and purine analogues—are used most commonly (Table 5). These drugs should not be considered alternatives or substitutes for corticosteroids but rather are typically given in combination with corticosteroids. This approach to therapy has been studied best in patients with lupus nephritis. Recent data from an extensive long-term trial at the National Institutes of Health have suggested that immunosuppressive drugs, compared with prednisone alone, prevent the progression of irreversible sclerosing and atrophic renal disease and reduce the probability of end-stage renal failure. There has been no evidence that immunosuppressive drugs significantly alter patient survival. Intermittent intravenous doses of cyclophosphamide given over prolonged periods (every 3 months for an average of 4 years) appeared to be the most effective drug regimen in these studies.

The potential complications of immunosuppressive drug therapy arise from the direct consequences of suppression of immune function as well as adverse effects unique to individual drugs. There seems to be little doubt that in choosing between azathioprine and cyclophosphamide, the two drugs most commonly used in treatment of systemic lupus, cyclophosphamide is associated with many more complications. In particular, the risks of herpes zoster, gonadal failure, hemorrhagic cystitis, and carcinoma of the bladder are all significantly increased with the use of this drug. Of perhaps greatest concern with each of these drugs, however, is the risk of late developing neoplasia. Although it seems clear that there is a definite risk, its actual magnitude remains undefined and extensive cooperative efforts will be required over extended periods to establish a proper perspective on this issue.

SPECIAL THERAPEUTIC CONSIDERATIONS

Lupus Pregnancy

Potential complications in the mother and developing fetus require special considerations in managing the pregnant lupus patient. The increased risk of spontaneous abortion as well as rare manifestations of lupus in the newborn, such as skin, cardiac, and he-

TABLE 5 Immunosuppressive Drug Regimens Used in Treatment of Lupus Nephritis

	Schedule	*Toxic Effects*
Alkylating drugs		
Cyclophosphamide	PO: 1.0–4.0 mg/kg/day IV: 0.5–1.0 g/m²; give IV over 60 minutes, followed by hydration for 24 hours to induce diuresis; repeat every 1 to 3 months	Gastrointestinal distress, myelosuppression, amenorrhea-azoospermia, increased risk of infection and neoplasia Unique to cyclophosphamide—hemorrhagic cystitis, bladder fibrosis and carcinoma, cardiac and pulmonary toxicity, and inappropriate antidiuretic hormone secretion
Chlorambucil	PO: 0.1–0.2 mg/kg/day	
Mechlorethamine	IV: 0.2–0.4 mg/kg	
Purine analogues		
Azathioprine	PO: 1.0–4.0 mg/kg/day	Gastrointestinal distress, myelosuppression, hepatitis, pancreatitis, aseptic meningitis, increased risk of infection and neoplasia
Combination chemotherapy		
Cyclophosphamide + azathioprine	PO: 50 mg/day, each drug	Same as for individual drugs; ? additive toxicities

matologic involvement, requires that obstetric care be provided by a specialist in the management of high-risk pregnancies. Recurrent abortion in a patient with systemic lupus appears to be associated with antibody to cardiolipin. The treatment of these patients with high doses of prednisone combined with low-dose aspirin or anticoagulation therapy has been reported to be effective in preventing abortion.

For the expectant mother, there is a definite increased risk of worsening lupus throughout the pregnancy as well as in the postpartum period. Patients need to be followed more closely than usual during this period to monitor disease activity. The major treatment approach for increased lupus activity involves the use of prednisone. Although prednisone crosses the placenta, there is little evidence that the fetus is harmed even by high doses of prednisone. Stress doses of corticosteroids are often given to the mother for several days at the time of delivery to prevent a postpartum relapse of lupus. In general, other drugs used in the treatment of lupus are discontinued during pregnancy. Although it is common practice to discontinue antimalarial and immunosuppressive drugs for fear of damage to the fetus, the evidence that these drugs are teratogenic is meager.

Lupus Thrombocytopenia

Thrombocytopenia in systemic lupus represents a unique manifestation in which there are several alternatives to the general approaches to drug treatments already described. Chemotherapy with vinca alkaloids such as vinblastine and vincristine is an effective means of drug therapy. These drugs bind avidly to tubulin contained in platelets, and upon phagocytosis of the platelet the drug is selectively delivered to cells of the reticuloendothelial system (chemical splenectomy). Danazol, a synthetic analogue of androgenic steroids and progesterone, appears to play a potentially important role in the treatment of refractory lupus thrombocytopenia. Finally, high-dose intravenous therapy with monomeric gamma globulin has been used effectively to treat lupus thrombocytopenia. Although the effects on the platelet count are typically of short duration, prolonged responses have been observed.

The role of splenectomy in lupus thrombocytopenia has long been the subject of controversy, including at one time an allegation that splenectomy might actually promote dissemination of the disease. The recent literature regarding the effects of splenectomy in lupus thrombocytopenia is divided between studies advocating and those emphasizing the failure of the procedure to affect the short- or long-term outcome significantly. In selected patients, splenectomy has proved to be the only modality capable of managing lupus thrombocytopenia. However, it clearly should be reserved for patients who have failed to benefit from conventional medical approaches.

SUGGESTED READING

Austin HA, Klippel JH, Balow JE, et al. Therapy of lupus nephritis: Controlled trial of prednisone and cytotoxic drugs. N Engl J Med 1986; 314:614.

Kimberly RP. Treatment: Corticosteroids and anti-inflammatory drugs. Rheum Dis Clin North Am 1988:203.

McCune WJ, Golbus J, Zeldes W, et al. Clinical and immunologic effects of monthly administration of intravenous cyclophosphamide in severe systemic lupus erythematosus. N Engl J Med 1988; 318:1423.

Ramsey-Goldman R. Pregnancy in systemic lupus erythematosus. Rheum Dis Clin North Am 1988:169.

West SG, Johnson SC. Danazol for the treatment of refractory autoimmune thrombocytopenia in systemic lupus erythematosus. Ann Intern Med 1988; 108:703.

HASHIMOTO'S THYROIDITIS*

KENNETH D. BURMAN, M.D., Col. M.C.

Hashimoto's disease is a complex autoimmune disease in which perturbations of T and B lymphocytes result in the production of antithyroglobulin and antimicrosomal antibodies. It is presently speculated that hypothyroidism in this condition results from the interaction of antimicrosomal antibodies with thyroid peroxidase enzymes, thus inhibiting the generation of thyroxine (T_4) and triiodothyronine (T_3) and resulting in a compensatory increase in thyroid stimulating hormone (TSH) production and thyroidal enlargement. Despite this proposed scheme, most authorities believe that the precise temporal and pathophysiologic relationship between antithyroid antibodies and thyroidal enlargement or destruction is not yet completely understood.

Clinically, the diagnosis of Hashimoto's disease is documented by the presence in serum of high titers of antithyroglobulin or antimicrosomal antibodies or by cytologic or histologic study of a thyroid tissue sample that is characterized by lymphocytic infiltration, and

*The opinions or assertions contained herein are the private views of the author and are not to be construed as official or as reflecting the views of the Department of the Army or the Department of Defense.

perhaps germinal centers, with occasional macrophages or plasma cells. Thyroid follicles may be decreased in number and colloid accumulation may be scant; numerous large oxyphilic thyrocytes and inflammatory giant cells are usually present. Patients with Hashimoto's disease may be clinically euthyroid, hypothyroid, or even rarely hyperthyroid, and the thyroid gland may be normal in size, enlarged, or even not palpable. The specific goals of therapy usually are restoration of euthyroidism, when appropriate, and suppression of growth of an enlarged thyroid gland.

INTERPRETATION OF THYROID FUNCTION TESTS

The thyroid hormones, T_3 and T_4, circulate in serum bound to either albumin, thyroxine binding globulin, or prealbumin; only about 0.3 percent of the T_3 and 0.03 percent of the T_4 are unbound and thus available for binding to tissues. The serum TSH level, in a sensitive assay, is elevated in primary hypothyroidism and undetectable in thyrotoxicosis. The serum T_3 level by radioimmunoassay may be normal in many patients with hypothyroidism, but the serum T_4 level is usually decreased. Systemic illness of any nature may alter thyroid function test results, usually causing decreased serum T_4 and T_3 levels by radioimmunoassay and elevated resin T_3 uptake; these characteristic findings reflect the diminished binding of iodothyronines to serum proteins and also decreased serum T_4 to T_3 conversion. In this circumstance, as well as in healthy patients, the resin T_3 uptake does not reflect function but indicates the number of T_3 or T_4 binding sites available. In most laboratories a decrease in the number of binding sites is associated with low serum T_4 and T_3 radioimmunoassay levels and increased resin T_3 uptake; an increase in available binding sites is usually reflected by elevated serum T_4 and T_3 radioimmunoassay levels and by a decreased resin T_3 uptake.

Conditions that may elevate the number of thyroid hormone binding sites include estrogen administration, pregnancy, and birth control pills, and conditions that may decrease the number of binding sites include systemic illnesses, testosterone or glucocorticoid administration, and the nephrotic syndrome. A patient may also be born with decreased or increased thyroid hormone binding proteins. The typical alterations in T_4, T_3 radioimmunoassay, and resin T_3 uptake levels must be borne in mind in the interpretation of thyroid function test results in hypothyroid patients who also have other systemic illnesses. In general, a concordant change in T_4 and resin T_3 uptake levels suggests a bona fide alteration in thyroid function, and a discordant change suggests a binding abnormality. Of course, primary hypothyroidism also can occur in a patient who has decreased binding, in which case the T_4 level would be low, the resin T_3 uptake normal or elevated, and the TSH level increased; the serum TSH level is expected to be normal if there is a binding abnormality alone. Recent advances in technology have allowed the increasing clinical use of free T_4 (and free T_3) measurement, thus obviating in most cases the need for a total T_4 and resin T_3 uptake.

The proper interpretation of thyroid function tests relies on an understanding of the concept that the "normal range" is relative; not only can persons with normal thyroid function have abnormal serum T_4 levels, but an individual with abnormal thyroid function may have a normal serum T_4 level. Our interpretation of these tests is simplified by virtue of the fact that homeostatic mechanisms elevate the TSH level when insufficient T_4 or T_3 reaches the tissues. Thus, great importance is placed on T_4, T_3 radioimmunoassay, resin T_3 uptake, and especially TSH levels in the evaluation of a hypothyroid patient.

PRIMARY HYPOTHYROIDISM

Normally, in a 70 kg person, the thyroid gland secretes about 130 nmoles (100 μg) of T_4 daily. The total T_3 production is about 50 nmoles (32 μg); about 85 percent of this T_3 production is from peripheral T_4 conversion, and only about 15 percent is derived directly from thyroidal secretion. Serum T_4 and T_3 circulate bound to three proteins (thyroxine binding prealbumin, thyroxine binding globulin, and albumin), and, as noted earlier, only about 0.03 percent of T_4 and 0.3 percent of T_3 are bound and thus available to enter tissues to mediate biologic action. Serum TSH levels, as measured by a highly sensitive assay, are normally about 0.5 to 3.5 μU per ml and are elevated in patients with primary hypothyroidism. Therefore, a typical patient with primary hypothyroidism would have clinical symptoms that are consistent, decreased serum T_4 and T_3 radioimmunoassay and resin T_3 uptake levels, and an elevated TSH value. Consistent symptoms include cold intolerance, fatigue, constipation, slow speech, bradycardia, and decreased body temperature. Dry skin, loss of body hair, and hoarse voice may be present, and rarely patients may have pericardial or pleural effusions.

In such a patient synthetic levothyroxine (LT_4) usually should be used for treatment. The replacement dosage is about 1.7 μg per kg per day, which usually means 0.1 to 0.2 mg daily. The goal of therapy in this circumstance is a serum T_4 level between 6 and 12 μg per dl and a T_3 level between 120 and 180 ng per dl in a clinically euthyroid asymptomatic patient. The TSH value should be between 0.5 and 3.5 μU per ml when LT_4 is administered for the treatment of hypothyroidism.

In the treatment of hypothyroid subjects it is most prudent to institute levothyroxine therapy in a gradual manner. Gradual restoration of euthyroidism is indicated if the patient has accompanying atherosclerosis, known coronary artery disease, or angina. It may be useful to obtain an electrocardiogram in these patients prior to and during therapy.

A typical gradual regimen might be to administer 25 μg of LT_4 daily for 2 weeks and 50 μg daily for the next 2 weeks and then to increase the maintenance dosage to 75 μg daily. The patient continues with this daily dosage for 4 to 6 weeks and returns at that time for a repeat examination and thyroid function tests. If further increases are needed, they then can be instituted gradually. A patient must be receiving a given daily dosage of LT_4 for 4 to 6 weeks before blood tests represent an accurate assessment of the presumed biologic effect. After this close observation, patients receiving levothyroxine therapy for the treatment of primary hypothyroidism should be monitored with clinical examination and serum T_4, resin T_3 uptake, and TSH values about every 6 to 12 months. Patients who have autoimmune hypothyroidism are at higher risk for other autoimmune disorders and should be questioned about symptoms relevant to adrenal insufficiency, panhypopituitarism, systemic lupus erythematosus, rheumatoid arthritis, and scleroderma. Every patient with the diagnosis of hypothyroidism should have the serum TSH level measured, and in the case of primary hypothyroidism it should be elevated. If the patient has clinical hypothyroidism with decreased serum T_4 and resin T_3 uptake levels and a normal or low TSH level, secondary hypothyroidism should be suspected and a pituitary computed tomographic scan should be obtained.

SUBCLINICAL PRIMARY HYPOTHYROIDISM

Subclinical, latent, or biochemical hypothyroidism occurs when a patient does not have specific or notable signs or symptoms of hypothyroidism, and the serum T_4 and T_3 levels are within the normal range but the TSH concentration is mildly elevated, perhaps 5 to 15 μU per ml. Subclinical hypothyroidism is most frequent in elderly patients. This circumstance illustrates the clinical conundrum of whether to institute treatment with levothyroxine or simply to follow the patient at regular intervals. There is no simple answer to this problem.

I recommend a thorough history and physical examination, trying to elicit signs or symptoms related to hypothyroidism; I also measure the serum antithyroglobulin and antimicrosomal thyroid antibody levels. It is generally believed that the higher the antibody titer, the more likely it is that such cases will evolve into overt hypothyroidism. If there are specific symptoms or findings on physical examination that might be related to hypothyroidism, I consider instituting levothyroxine therapy. The presence of high titers of antithyroid antibodies makes me follow the patient more closely and consider levothyroxine therapy more strongly. Therapy is instituted with the full understanding and cooperation of the patient; the same precautions already noted with regard to gradual institution of therapy apply in these circumstances. Consideration also should be given to whether the patient has permanent primary hypothyroidism or whether the event may be transient, such as subacute thyroiditis or postpartum thyroiditis. Care should be taken to insure that the diagnosis of permanent primary hypothyroidism is correct prior to prescribing lifelong levothyroxine therapy.

HASHIMOTO'S DISEASE WITH AN ENLARGED THYROID GLAND

Some patients with Hashimoto's disease have an enlarged thyroid gland, which usually coexists with either euthyroidism or hypothyroidism. When a patient is hypothyroid, the guidelines already noted apply, except that careful attention must be given to whether the thyroid gland has areas of decreased function on radioisotopic scanning. If such areas exist and correspond to palpable nodules, an aspiration biopsy may be indicated. If the biopsy findings are indicative of malignancy, surgery may be advised, taking into consideration the general state of the patient. If the biopsy findings are benign and the nodular area is "cold" or hypofunctioning by scan, evaluation of the nodule's response to levothyroxine therapy is indicated. If the nodule does not decrease in size over several months, surgery should be considered. It must be kept in mind, however, that we are discussing only patients with known Hashimoto's disease, supported by either a high titer of antithyroid antibodies or a diagnostic aspiration. In this setting a nodular thyroid gland would be expected as an integral part of the disease process. Nevertheless it is still possible for a "cold" nodule to appear in a patient with Hashimoto's disease, and although it would be unusual, the possible co-occurrence of carcinoma should not be overlooked. The more usual circumstance is for the nodular enlargement to represent lymphocytic infiltration and fibrosis as a result of Hashimoto's disease; unnecessary surgery in this situation should be avoided. Growth of a nodule, lymphadenopathy in or around the thyroid gland, and symptoms of hoarseness, dysphagia, or pain may suggest a malignant process, since these findings usually do not occur in an uncomplicated routine case of Hashimoto's disease.

In a patient with Hashimoto's disease, generalized thyroid enlargement may occur in conjunction with a euthyroid state. If the patient does not have symptoms suggestive of rapid growth of the thyroid gland, such as dysphagia, hoarseness, or pain (in which case biopsy and surgery may be indicated), and if the patient is euthyroid clinically and chemically, levothyroxine therapy for suppression is usually indicated, with application of the precautions already noted. After stabilization, the patient is followed every 6 to 12 months with periodic examinations and thyroid function tests. The rationale for treating a patient with an enlarged thyroid gland with levothyroxine is based on the belief that levothyroxine suppression inhibits further growth or, perhaps, even shrinks the gland by inhibiting TSH secretion. Although this general course is followed by most clinicians, there are few definitive studies assessing this approach in patients with Hashimoto's disease.

"HASHITOXICOSIS"

"Hashitoxicosis" is an uncommon entity in which a patient has the usual manifestations of Hashimoto's disease, such as elevated antimicrosomal or antithyroglobulin antibody titers and an enlarged firm thyroid gland, yet displays clinical and biochemical evidence of hyperthyroidism, with elevated serum T_4 and T_3 and increased 24 hour radioactive iodine uptake. When it is documented that such a patient does not have other forms of thyrotoxicosis such as postpartum or subacute thyroiditis, appropriate treatment is indicated.

The pathophysiology of this hybrid entity between Hashimoto's disease and Graves' disease is unknown, but strikes at the basic causes of these two diseases. Some clinicians believe that Graves' disease and Hashimoto's disease represent different manifestations of the same or similar defects, presumably B cell escape from regulation, which then allows production of antithyroid antibodies. In some cases the antithyroglobulin and antimicrosomal antibodies predominate, resulting in clinical manifestations known as Hashimoto's disease, whereas in other circumstances the predominant antibodies are directed against the TSH receptor, and the clinical entity is Graves' disease. "Hashitoxicosis," or more accurately, the coexistence of Graves' disease and Hashimoto's disease, has not been adequately studied in order to document its natural history, the frequency of serum anti-TSH receptor antibodies, or the response to therapy.

With these reservations noted, when I encounter such a patient, I attempt to discern whether other factors (e.g., iodide ingestion, a recent history of childbirth) may be precipitating the thyrotoxicosis. If, for example, the thyrotoxicosis has occurred several weeks after a study in which radiographic contrast agents were used, I might believe that the patient has iodide induced thyrotoxicosis, and definitive therapy such as ^{131}I ablation or thyroidectomy should be avoided. I would treat such a patient with beta blocking drugs (e.g., Atenolol, 50 to 100 mg daily) and antithyroid drugs (propylthiouracil, 100 mg three times daily, or methimazole, 10 mg three times daily) for several months to induce euthyroidism. At the end of that time I would discontinue these drugs to determine whether thyrotoxicosis recurs. In the case of recurrent thyrotoxicosis, I still render the patient euthyroid with beta blocking drugs and antithyroid drugs, but when euthyroidism is restored, I discuss definitive management (i.e., surgery or ^{131}I) with the patient. For Graves' disease I prefer ^{131}I as therapy if the patient is over 25 to 30 years old, and I usually prefer surgical therapy if the patient is younger. "Hashitoxicosis" is a much rarer entity, but the same guidelines probably apply. Some clinicians also consider long term antithyroid drug treatment in an effort to induce a remission.

I would emphasize that individual patient preference should be given major consideration in this cooperative decision; the desirable goal of both these treatments is permanent hypothyroidism, and the patient then can be treated with levothyroxine replacement. Obviously ^{131}I therapy should not be given to a female patient who is or may shortly become pregnant. Further details regarding indications, methods, and objectives of the approaches can be obtained from recent references.

PREGNANCY

Hashimoto's disease with hypothyroidism can be treated during pregnancy with levothyroxine therapy. Because estrogens increase thyroxine binding globulin concentrations and binding capacity, the total serum T_4 and T_3 radioimmunoassay values may rise, but the resin T_3 uptake value decreases. A serum T_4 level between 8 and 18 μg per dl in most assays and a serum T_3 level between 120 and 240 ng per dl may be considered normal during pregnancy. These elevated total T_4 and T_3 radioimmunoassay values, as compared to the case in nonpregnant patients, are simply due to increases in binding proteins, and free hormone levels are expected to be normal and the patients clinically euthyroid. The dose of levothyroxine required is not believed to change significantly during pregnancy, and the rise in the serum T_4 level is expected and does not signify per se that the dose must be changed. Careful examination of the patient and evaluation of the laboratory tests will indicate whether modifications in therapy are needed. Occasionally it may be necessary to measure the free T_4 level directly.

POSTPARTUM THYROIDITIS

Postpartum thyroiditis is a recently recognized clinical syndrome in which alterations in thyroid function occur within the first year after delivery. This entity is very common, occurring in perhaps 5 to 8 percent of all women who have delivered babies. This syndrome may be characterized by transient hypothyroidism or hyperthyroidism, but a principal hallmark of the disease is that thyroid function evolves from one clinical state to another. Presentation at about 4 months post partum with hyperthyroidism, with evolution to hypothyroidism at 8 months and euthyroidism at 12 months, would be a common course. The clinician must be careful not to treat one clinical manifestation with definitive therapy (i.e., ^{131}I or surgery), since the natural history is so varied and the disease is usually transient. It is preferable to treat the clinical manifestations (e.g., with a beta blocker) when the patient is thyrotoxic, but then to consider withdrawing the drugs later to determine whether normal endogenous thyroid gland function has returned.

Because of its varied course and presentation, definitive treatment guidelines cannot be given. Rather the general advice to treat symptoms with short term therapy is prudent. To make matters even more complex, however, a small percentage of patients with postpartum thyroiditis have permanent hypothyroidism or permanent thyrotoxicosis. There is no method or test available to predict or detect such patients, and continued follow-up is mandatory. The cause of postpartum thyrotoxicosis is not known, but it does seem that such patients frequently have elevated serum titers of antithyroglobulin or antimicrosomal antibodies. The presence of anti-TSH receptor antibodies would be unusual and might signify the occurrence of permanent thyrotoxicosis, although further studies assessing these factors in postpartum thyroiditis are required.

LYMPHOMA

Primary thyroid lymphoma is a serious life threatening disorder that should be diagnosed as early as possible. This disease can arise in an otherwise normal gland, but it is now known that Hashimoto's disease predisposes to the development of thyroid lymphoma. There are no laboratory parameters that can help assess the likelihood that this disease will occur in a patient with Hashimoto's disease, although recent growth of the thyroid gland, pain in the neck, hoarseness, dyspnea, dysphagia, and the presence of lymphadenopathy proximal to the thyroid gland may all suggest that a thyroid lymphoma has arisen. The likelihood that a patient with Hashimoto's disease will develop thyroid lymphoma is not known to be related to the thyroid antibody titer or the size of the gland. Although thyroid lymphomas occur much more frequently in patients with Hashimoto's disease, the chance that an individual patient with Hashimoto's disease will develop thyroid lymphoma is still slight.

Aspiration biopsies of a suspected lymphomatous gland may be helpful if the infiltrating lymphocytes are found to be especially immature and if there are few plasma cells and Hürthle cells. However, in many cases the customary infiltrating lymphocytes and plasma cells that occur with Hashimoto's disease alone make it difficult to distinguish Hashimoto's disease from lymphoma. Surgical thyroidectomy or removal and examination of involved lymph nodes may be required for the correct diagnosis. Laboratory and radiographic studies to assess lymphoma elsewhere in the body are indicated either before surgery if the suspicion of thyroid lymphoma is high or after surgery for staging purposes. External radiation and chemotherapy are further customary treatment modalities used after the diagnosis is established.

THYROID MEDICATION

For either hypothyroidism or goiter suppression, levothyroxine is the drug of choice. The rationale for its use is that the half-life of T_4 is about 7 days, and this medication can be ingested only once daily. If the drug is taken in this manner, serum T_4 and T_3 levels are stable and thus give an accurate estimate of the dose ingested and absorbed. Further, when exogenous levothyroxine is given, the T_4 is converted to T_3, the more biologically active hormone, at a rate determined by the body's own homeostatic mechanism. The maintenance levothyroxine dose is about 1.7 μg per kg per day.

Cytomel (L-triiodothyronine, LT_3) should not be given for the long term treatment of hypothyroidism or for goiter suppression, because the half-life is only about 24 to 30 hours and therefore the pills must be ingested several times daily. Further, the serum levels after Cytomel administration fluctuate widely, for example, starting at an undetectable level prior to the morning T_3 dose (since the effects of the previous evening's dose are dissipated owing to its short half-life) and rising to several hundred ng per dl several hours after T_3 ingestion. These fluctuations result in a variable T_3 effect throughout the day and also may aggravate angina pectoris or arrhythmias in susceptible patients. Serum T_4 and T_3 levels cannot be used to help assess the adequacy of therapy when a patient is receiving T_3 but are helpful when T_4 is given. Other preparations such as LT_4-LT_3 mixtures and crude powdered thyroid gland should not be used for many of the same reasons.

CHILDREN

Hashimoto's disease with hypothyroidism can occur in children, and the plan already noted regarding diagnosis and treatment applies. In children a further consideration is the long term potentially adverse effects of hypothyroidism on growth. The recommended maintenance T_4 dosage in children is either 3 μg per kg of body weight per day or 100 μg per square meter. Therapy in a severely hypothyroid child should be initiated with a half-maintenance dosage for 1 to 2 weeks to help minimize adverse effects, such as tachycardia. Careful monitoring for the adequacy of therapy is critical, attention being given to growth curves, clinical examination, and thyroid function tests. Excessive T_4 dosage and resultant hyperthyroidism also should be avoided. The goal is serum T_4 and T_3 radioimmunoassay levels in the upper half of the normal range and a serum

TSH level that is normal. Although in neonates with hypothyroidism the capacity of T_4 to suppress the pituitary secretion of TSH may be defective, thus diminishing the usefulness of the serum TSH level as an effective monitor, children with Hashimoto's disease and hypothyroidism are expected to have normal feedback regulation while taking T_4.

THERAPEUTIC GOALS

The main objectives of therapy are to render a hypothyroid patient clinically and chemically euthyroid with normal or slightly elevated serum T_4, T_3 radioimmunoassay, and TSH levels or, when treating a patient with a goiter, to suppress the serum TSH to undetectable levels while maintaining a normal or only slightly elevated T_4 level, a normal serum T_3 level, and clinical euthyroidism.

A guideline for daily LT_4 dosage in adults is 1.7 μg per kg of body weight for replacement and 2.1 μg per kg of body weight for suppression. The serum T_4 level may be slightly elevated (perhaps as high as 14 μg per dl) when a person is ingesting exogenous thyroid hormone, and yet if the serum T_3 level is normal and the patient is clinically euthyroid, the dosage may be considered appropriate. A detectable serum TSH level in a supersensitive assay may indicate that pituitary suppression has not been achieved.

Occasionally thyrotropin-releasing hormone may be indicated. Following 200 to 500 μg of thyrotropin-releasing hormone given intravenously, normally there is a rise (usually at least a doubling) of the TSH level at 15 and 30 minutes; adequate suppression is indicated by undetectable basal values that do not rise after injection. Of course, this test cannot be used to distinguish a T_4 dosage that is excessive and causing clinical overt thyrotoxicosis from an appropriately suppressive dosage. The clinical examination and history give important information regarding the appropriateness of the dosage and, of course, serum T_4 and T_3 radioimmunoassay levels are also helpful. Symptoms suggestive of mild thyrotoxicosis (e.g., tachycardia, fine hand tremor, nervousness, and rapid return of reflexes) may suggest an excessive T_4 dosage; there are no diagnostic laboratory tests that can accurately reflect the excessive thyroid hormone levels presented to the tissues. When treating a patient for goiter suppression, finding the exogenous LT_4 dosage just sufficient to suppress TSH yet maintain relatively normal laboratory test results and clinical parameters is the goal. Thyroid function tests can be effectively interpreted only at about 4 to 6 weeks after alteration of the dosage.

TOXICITY

Each patient's response to excess thyroid hormone ingestion varies with dose and duration of therapy as well as individual patient characteristics. Most commonly palpitations, nervousness, anxiety, insomnia, heat intolerance, tremors, diarrhea, or menstrual irregularities are noted. Cardiac manifestations such as the presence or aggravation of angina pectoris, arrhythmia, or congestive heart failure may predominate when a patient has underlying atherosclerosis or coronary artery disease.

DRUG INTERACTIONS

Thyroid hormones should be administered with caution to patients who also are taking tricyclic antidepressants, adrenergic agonists, or oral anticoagulant therapy, since they may potentiate the action of these drugs. Cholestyramine can bind T_4 in the gastrointestinal tract and thus decrease its absorption; ingestion of these two drugs must be separated by at least 2 hours. Exogenous thyroid hormone administration to hypothyroid subjects may alter the biologic half-life of other drugs, and their doses must be carefully considered after a hypothyroid patient has become euthyroid.

SURGERY

Thyroidectomy is only rarely indicated or required in Hashimoto's disease and would be considered when there are palpable hypofunctioning nodules in the thyroid gland that are not suppressed with 1 to 3 months of thyroxine therapy or nodules that are found to be enlarged at a follow-up examination; when there are palpably enlarged lymph nodes surrounding the thyroid gland that are considered clinically significant; or when aspiration biopsy of the thyroid or surrounding lymph nodes is diagnostic or suggestive of cancer or lymphoma. Many coincident factors are also considered, including the presence of clinical symptoms (dysphagia, pain, and dyspnea) suggesting progressive thyroid enlargement. Aspiration biopsy findings consistent with uncomplicated Hashimoto's disease may be difficult to discriminate from the subtle features suggesting lymphomatous involvement.

DISEASES THAT MAY BE ASSOCIATED WITH HYPOTHYROIDISM

Hashimoto's disease may occur in association with other autoimmune diseases, including adrenocortical insufficiency, myasthenia gravis, systemic lupus erythematosus, scleroderma, and pernicious anemia. The pathophysiologic mechanism by which these autoimmune disorders occur together is unknown. The clinical courses of these diseases, as compared to that of Hashimoto's disease, may vary, with either disease occurring initially and either disease being more severe. A clinical history to detect the development of another autoimmune disease is taken during each visit of a patient with Hashimoto's disease. Examination of the patient also includes a search for orthostatic hypotension and increased skin and buccal mucosa pigmentation, each a manifestation of adrenal insufficiency. If there is sufficient clinical suspicion, a 24 hour urinary free cortisol level should be obtained; if it is decreased, an adrenocorticotropic hormone (ACTH) stimulation test should be performed. Some clinicians prefer to use the ACTH stimulation test as the initial screening test, rather than a 24 hour urinary free cortisol test.

In this test 25 units of synthetic ACTH is administered intravenously, a serum cortisol level being obtained immediately prior to ACTH injection and again 30 and 60 minutes later. A normal adrenal response is a basal serum cortisol level between 5 and 20 μg per dl (between 7:00 and 10:00 AM), which at least doubles after ACTH injection. Some authorities consider a post-ACTH serum cortisol level greater than 20 μg per dl also to be indicative of a normal response. Depending on the clinical circumstances and the degree of suspicion of adrenal insufficiency, either hydrocortisone therapy can be started when the ACTH response is clearly low or a longer ACTH infusion can be given to confirm the diagnosis. Clinical suspicion of the coexistence of one of the other autoimmune diseases should be confirmed by appropriate laboratory data.

SUGGESTED READING

Ahmann AJ, Burman KD. The role of T lymphocytes in autoimmune thyroid disease. Endocrinol Metab Clin North Am 1987; 16:287.

Borst GC, Eil C, Burman KD. Euthyroid hyperthyroxinemia. Ann Intern Med 1983; 98:366.

Burman KD, Baker JR Jr. Immune mechanisms in Graves' disease. Endocr Rev 1985; 6:183–232.

Graham GD, Burman KD. Radioiodine treatment of Graves' disease: an assessment of its potential risks. Ann Intern Med 1986; 105:901.

Hamburger JI, Miller JM, Kini SR. Lymphoma of the thyroid. Ann Intern Med 1983; 99:685–693.

Hennessey JV, Evaul JE, Tseng Y-C, Burman KD, Wartofsky L. L-thyroxine dosage: a re-evaluation of therapy with contemporary preparations. Ann Intern Med 1986; 105:11.

Wartofsky L, Burman KD. Alterations in thyroid patients with systemic illness: the "euthyroid sick syndrome." Endocr Rev 1982; 3:164–217.

Weetman AP, McGregor AM. Autoimmune thyroid disease: developments in our understanding. Endocr Rev 1984; 5:309–355.

RHEUMATOID ARTHRITIS

SHAUN RUDDY, M.D.
W. NEAL ROBERTS, M.D.

PROBLEMS IN PLANNING RHEUMATOID ARTHRITIS THERAPY

Rheumatoid arthritis is a chronic systemic inflammatory disease of unclear etiology, the sine qua non of which is joint inflammation. Other prominent characteristics are symmetry of joint involvement over time (although not necessarily at presentation), variability of presentation, and volatility of clinical course. Spontaneous partial remissions and exacerbations during the disease course characterize the course in three-quarters of the patients with rheumatoid arthritis; in another 10 percent the disease progresses relentlessly to debilitating deformity, and 15 percent have monocyclic disease with no recurrence after the first episode (Fig. 1). The joints involved during the first year or two tend to be the most troublesome joints throughout the course. Admixtures of inflammatory joint symptoms, secondary mechanical joint symptoms, nonarticular pain (fibrositis, bursitis, tendonitis), the psychological impact of chronic disease, an increased incidence of septic joints, and extra-articular features (including Sjögren's syndrome, scleritis, vasculitic skin ulcers, and Felty's syndrome) can all contribute to the variability of the clinical course, precluding a linear approach to the therapeutic choices.

The mainstays of long-term treatment are appropriate control of exercise and rest, including splinting, and the use of a relatively safe salicylate or nonsteroidal anti-inflammatory drug. Most patients have mild rheumatoid disease with only moderate threat of permanent structural damage to articular cartilage surfaces and respond satisfactorily to these two categories of treatment. Excessive pain and especially continued rapid loss of function or progression of deformity justify the use of more toxic, slow-acting antirheumatic drugs. The latter include primarily gold salts, penicillamine, and hydroxychloroquine. Hydroxychloroquine has special value in the control of moderately severe synovitis as an intermediate step between nonsteroidal anti-inflammatory drugs and other slow-acting antirheumatic drugs. Following the latter are the cytotoxic drugs methotrexate, azathioprine, and cyclophosphamide. Methotrexate now has become coequal with the slow-acting antirheumatic drugs owing to its relatively low toxicity; cyclophosphamide is generally withheld because of its recognized long-term risk of inducing cancer.

Of the patients who require a slow-acting anti-

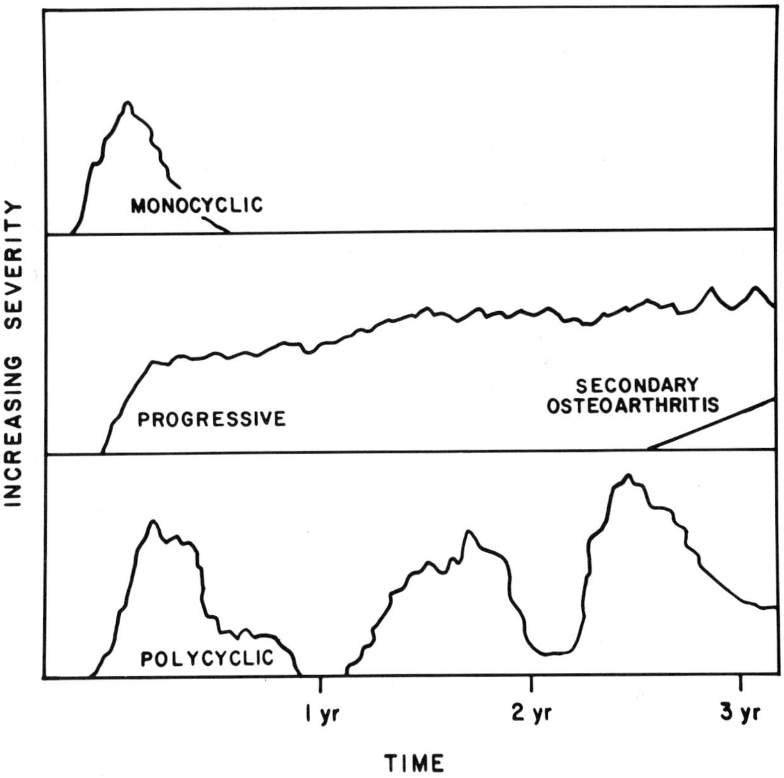

Figure 1 Clinical courses common in rheumatoid arthritis. Note secondary osteoarthritis beginning in the second panel.

rheumatic drug for rheumatoid arthritis, most will have ceased taking the medication within several years. The extensive dropout from this second line antirheumatic therapy is attributable partially to side effects and partially to a lack of efficacy, but in any case the overall impact of these drugs on the course of the disease probably is not as great as initial responses to therapy would lead one to suspect.

Treatments for which the efficacy in the usual clinical situation, the benefit-toxicity ratio, or the role relative to other established therapies is as yet poorly defined include low-dose daily oral therapy with prednisone, supplemental eicosopentanoic acid, sulfasalazine, thalidomide, therafectin, cyclosporine, total nodal irradiation, and low-dose combinations of cytotoxic drugs such as cyclophosphamide and methotrexate. Untraditional remedies, many with little or no apparent efficacy, add complexity.

Finally, surgical replacement of worn-out joints with extensive cartilage loss remarkably improves the function of hips and knees. The threshold for invoking this therapy continues to decrease every few years as technical improvements in joint replacement, particularly at the prosthesis-cement-bone interfaces, lengthen the half-lives of these implants. Therefore, in the face of slow-acting antirheumatic drug toxicity or lack of efficacy, a strategy of last resort for severe rheumatoid arthritis is to abandon the latter therapy, using only salicylates (or nonsteroidal anti-inflammatory drugs) and replacing joints as they fail.

SPECIFIC THERAPIES AND MANAGEMENT APPROACHES IN RHEUMATOID ARTHRITIS

Physical Measures

The goal of physical management—including formal physiotherapy as well as specific prescriptions for rest, exercise, and splinting of involved joints—is to steer a course between overuse of a joint leading to an increase in inflammatory symptoms and underuse permitting contractures of the surrounding joint capsule with loss of range of motion. The more actively involved a joint, the more immobilization it requires, sometimes requiring splinting accompanied by local steroid injection. With lessening inflammation, range of motion exercise should be intensified in order to recover range lost during the exacerbation.

The most frequent error in general physical management is failure to withdraw a prescription for rest after an exacerbation subsides. After several exacerbations and admonitions to rest, the patient forms the impression that activity should be restricted even when inflammation is minimal. The resulting generalized deconditioning and excessive fatigue may be difficult to distinguish from that of systemic disease activity.

The most frequent error in physical treatment of specific joints is failure to splint involved wrists in order to prevent excessive flexion while the patient is sleeping. Also important is the liberal use of metatarsal bars, orthotics, or metatarsal pads to decrease the load on the most involved metatarsophalangeal joints.

In two randomized trials comparing inpatient multidisciplinary treatment of flares of rheumatoid arthritis with vigorous outpatient team treatment with home visits, hospitalization proved to be more expensive and more effective, with benefits lasting for up to 1 year. The low priority accorded patients with rheumatoid arthritis by health planners and cost control schemes obviates this approach in most settings. In contrast to acute care hospitals, rehabilitation units are exempt from diagnosis related group regulations and may provide a setting for more prolonged care of patients with rheumatoid arthritis.

Family and Social Considerations

Support groups of patients with rheumatoid arthritis as well as other social services serve at least two important functions. First, they may define functional thresholds such as the appropriate degree of social activity in adolescents, the ability to remain on a job, and the ability to move around the house and carry out the activities of daily living sufficiently well to remain independent of the family. These thresholds should be vigorously defended with a multidisciplinary approach involving social services at the same time that toxic drugs are introduced for disease control. Even when the patient's course of deterioration has slowed and is not approaching one of these functional thresholds, a social support group can combat the unfavorable psychological aspects of chronic illness.

Second, social services, hospital admissions, and interviews with the family regarding drug toxicity serve to certify the patient in the sick role. Without this certification, the family may see no obvious deformity in the early stages and may conclude that the patient's fatigue and complaints are out of proportion to physical changes.

Salicylates and Nonsteroidal Anti-inflammatory Drugs

Of all the medications effective for rheumatoid arthritis, aspirin and nonsteroidal anti-inflammatory drugs are the safest and the ones with which physicians generally have the most experience. The traditional argument in favor of aspirin as an initial drug has been its lower cost. However, if costs of work-ups and treatment for peptic ulceration and gastrointestinal hemorrhage are counted, the cost advantage of aspirin over the nonsteroidal anti-inflammatory drugs may disappear. The availability of salicylate levels to monitor compliance constitutes another advantage of aspirin over nonsteroidal anti-inflammatory drugs. The toxic consequences of continuous, full anti-inflammatory dosages of aspirin include one death from gastrointestinal hemorrhage in every 100 patients every 5 years. The major advantage of the nonsteroidal anti-inflammatory drugs is their longer pharmacologic half-lives, which lengthen the dosing interval, thereby increasing compliance. For example, piroxicam can be given once a day, although the incidence of significant gastrointestinal bleeding may be high in older patients. In addition, once or twice a day dosing limits dosage flexibility. For example, stiffness may be much worse in the morning, suggesting weighting the major portion of the day's dosage toward the previous night. Indomethacin seems to cause a higher incidence of central nervous system side effects such as headache and dysphoria in older patients. Consequently, the first choice of many rheumatologists is a nonsteroidal anti-inflammatory drug, avoiding indomethacin in older patients. Sulindac may be particularly valuable in patients with mild renal insufficiency when a minimal effect on renal prostaglandins is desired, and when the patient is taking other medications that are renally excreted and whose toxicity may be augmented by any decrease in glomerular filtration rate. In patients over the age of 60 years in whom clearance is likely to be diminished despite an apparently normal serum creatinine concentration, intrarenal hemodynamic effects secondary to prostaglandin inhibition within the kidney may be more important. Many practitioners check serum creatinine concentration within a few weeks of starting nonsteroidal anti-inflammatory drugs in patients over 60 years old.

How long should therapy with an ineffective nonsteroidal anti-inflammatory drug be continued before one switches to another medication? The only prospective trial that specifically sought an answer to this question suggested that new responses still occurred 4 weeks into the therapy. The usual recommendation is for 2 weeks of full doses of nonsteroidal anti-inflammatory drug before concluding that there is a lack of efficacy. When patient noncompliance is factored in, the probable average trial is 7 to 10 days, however. This discrepancy between data and practice probably arises from differences between the patient's and the physician's concerns, the former being more interested in the analgesia and the latter in the anti-inflammatory effect. Combinations of nonsteroidal drugs with salicylates or other nonsteroidal drugs appear to increase the risk of toxic effects with no increase in efficacy. Most patients decide for themselves to use some additional medication for analgesia. In the majority of cases this is acetaminophen, but sometimes it is an aspirin-containing medication or over-the-counter ibuprofen.

When the first nonsteroidal anti-inflammatory drug employed proves ineffective after at least 2 weeks, what drug should replace it? Most rheumatologists would pick second and third choice nonsteroidal anti-inflammatory drugs on the basis of the principle of switching from one chemical class to another. There are six chemically distinct groups of nonsteroidal anti-inflammatory drugs, all of which inhibit cyclo-oxygenase activity. The major classes other than salicylates are propionic acids (ibuprofen, naproxen), indole related compounds (indomethacin, sulindac, tolmetin), which are structurally closest to phenylbutazone, arylacetic acids (diclofenac), anthranilic acids (meclofenamate), and oxicams (piroxicam). Data supporting the switching of classes over random choice of subsequent nonsteroidal anti-inflammatory drugs or their complete omission are lacking.

The main toxic effects of salicylates and nonsteroidal anti-inflammatory drugs are peptic gastritis, erosions, and ulcers. These lesions correlate imperfectly both with symptoms of upper gastrointestinal upset and with detectable gastrointestinal blood loss. For example, ulcers can occur, bleed, and heal while the patient continues to take nonsteroidal anti-inflammatory drugs without symptoms. By default most clinicians merely monitor symptoms to detect erosions and ulcers, although a case could be made for periodic monitoring of the hematocrit. Periodic testing of the stool for occult blood is of no value because positive test results occur in most patients taking these drugs for long periods. A strategy for handling gastrointestinal upset is to discontinue all nonsteroidal and salicylate medications until 5 days after all symptoms have subsided. Therapy with the same or a different drug then can be restarted. Extra meals, over-the-counter antacids, H_2 blockers, sucralfate, and, when available, prostaglandin congeners may permit continued nonsteroidal anti-inflammatory drug therapy. Nonacetylated salicylates (magnesium choline salicylate or salicyl salicylate) have the least effect on the gastric mucosa but may be less effective in moderate to severe inflammation.

Additional nonsteroidal anti-inflammatory drug effects for which there is no agreed upon detection strategy include drug-induced hepatitis and agranulocytosis. A complete blood count including a differential count and a chemistry battery should be carried out within the first 2 weeks after initiating nonsteroidal anti-inflammatory drug treatment.

A difficult to control feature of nonsteroidal anti-inflammatory drug prescribing is the patient's expectation for relief, which often exceeds what the medication can accomplish. The total effect of these drugs on the pain and inflammation of moderate rheumatoid arthritis may be in the range of 15 percent on a visual analogue scale, so that the medication may be of benefit but be seen by the patient as "only taking the edge off." The effect of the nonsteroidal drug may be evident only when it is discontinued. If pain is due to cartilage loss and secondary osteoarthritis, the patient almost certainly will be disappointed with the effect of the drug.

General Considerations in Therapy with Slow-Acting Anti-inflammatory Drugs

The therapy of rheumatoid arthritis with slow-acting anti-inflammatory drugs is one of the most unusual areas in modern medicine: the doctor gives the drug and then waits for 1 to 6 months for a clinical response. This delay in response makes the clinical effect of the drug difficult to differentiate from the natural history of a variable disease. Careful follow-up of certain clinical parameters is therefore imperative. Probably the easiest measurements to follow are the patient's global assessment, measured grip strength, length of the period of early morning stiffness, and the erythrocyte sedimentation rate. In general, slow-acting antirheumatic drugs have minimal immediate anti-inflammatory effects but in the long run are several-fold more effective against moderate rheumatoid inflammation than are nonsteroidal anti-inflammatory drugs. True remissions are rare, but approximately two-thirds of the patients who are able to take a full course of a given slow-acting antirheumatic drug improve and about half of these do so to a great degree. Adverse drug reactions requiring discontinuation of therapy occur in about one-third of the patients. Long-term benefit from these drugs is reduced because of the continuing occurrence of side effects throughout the period of drug use and the tendency of the disease to relapse when the drugs are withdrawn. It is possible but not certain that a patient who initially responds to a slow-acting antirheumatic drug can be "recaptured" with the same medication later. Failure to respond to one such drug does not predict a failure to respond to another; neither does toxicity with one accurately predict a recurrence of similar toxicity with another.

Some side effects of slow-acting antirheumatic drugs, particularly oral ulcers and mild skin rashes from gold, can be circumvented by discontinuing the medication long enough for the side effect to resolve and then reinstituting the same drug, perhaps by a different route of administration (e.g., oral instead of injectable doses of gold), at a low dosage, and slowly advancing the dosage over a period of weeks to months. Methotrexate hepatotoxicity can be "treated through" if it is manifested only by hepatocellular enzyme increases of two and a half-fold or less. Toxic effects for which this strategy definitely should not be tried include agranulocytosis, hydroxychloroquine retinopathy, proteinuria with a change in renal function (in contrast to mild proteinuria with a normal creatinine level), and gold colitis.

The choice of timing for beginning slow-acting antirheumatic drug therapy is complex (Table 1). The choice of such a drug is influenced by additional factors shown in Table 2. Hydroxychloroquine is clearly the least toxic, but it is also less effective than gold, penicillamine, and cytotoxic drugs. Of all the medications other than nonsteroidal anti-inflammatory

TABLE 1 The Decision to Begin Therapy with Slow-Acting Antirheumatic Drugs

In favor	
	Progressive deformity or loss of function
	Persistent active inflammation despite nonsteroidal anti-inflammatory drug therapy
	Radiographic evidence of erosions
	Steroid dependency
Against	
	No evidence of active synovitis on physical examination
	Questionable diagnosis
	Less than 6 months of disease
	Childbearing potential, off birth control therapy
	Lack of compliance or laboratory follow-up

drugs and aspirin, methotrexate and steroids in low oral doses act most rapidly. Penicillamine is the slowest. Despite the multiple in vitro mechanisms of action ascribed to each of the slow-acting antirheumatic drugs, it appears likely that gold and hydroxychloroquine operate by affecting monocyte function and that penicillamine interferes with T-lymphocyte function.

Hydroxychloroquine

Although the beneficial effects of hydroxychloroquine are not marked, this drug is the easiest of the slow-acting antirheumatic drugs to administer. It only rarely leads to gastrointestinal upset and otherwise causes a vanishingly small incidence of nuisance side effects. Skeletal muscle and myocardial toxic effects have been reported rarely. The abrupt onset of new heart failure in a patient taking hydroxychloroquine is reason to discontinue the drug. Unfortunately, rare instances of pigmentary macular degeneration in the retina occur with hydroxychloroquine. Most reported cases have occurred at high doses; it is recommended that the dosage not exceed 6.5 mg per kilogram per day. Dosage schedules that vary every other day may have to be used because the tablets come in only a 200-mg size. With this low dosage of one or two tablets per day, the incidence of pigmentary macular degeneration appears to be less than 1 percent and is related to the daily dosage rather than the total cumulative dose. Unfortunately, the prospect of visual loss, no matter how small statistically, often frightens patients. Nevertheless informed consent about visual loss is mandatory.

Appropriate monitoring of hydroxychloroquine includes a full retinal examination initially to exclude senile macular degeneration, which may be difficult to differentiate from pigmentary macular degeneration, along with an ophthalmologic follow-up examination every 6 months. It may take 3 months for the drug to have a beneficial effect. Patients who are in need of a rapid decrease in inflammatory symptoms are often given a more rapidly acting drug such as methotrexate. For those who need therapy in addition to nonsteroidal drugs but who can be expected to maintain function for a number of months, hydroxychloroquine is the slow-acting antirheumatic drug of choice.

Gold

Adverse drug reactions to gold include extensive skin eruptions, oral ulcers, and a membranous glomerulopathy, the latter manifested by proteinuria. There may be about a 0.5 percent incidence of mortality from agranulocytosis, aplastic anemia, or uncontrollable secretory diarrhea due to gold-induced colitis. Patients with HLA-DR3 disease may be more susceptible to gold-induced thrombocytopenia. Rarely, intramuscular doses of gold result in a "nitrotoid" reaction of acute vasodilation and hypotension when the rapidly absorbed aqueous solution (thiomalate salt) is used.

Most toxic reactions to gold occur during the first 4 months of treatment, but they may occur at any time during treatment, making complete blood counts with differential counts and urine tests for protein every 2 to 4 weeks the standard of monitoring for gold therapy, whether given by injection or orally. Hematuria without proteinuria probably is not gold membranous nephropathy and should be studied diagnostically as would any other hematuria.

Laboratory monitoring is the major expense in gold therapy. On the other hand, all the slow-acting antirheumatic drugs (with the exception of hydroxychloroquine) require similar monitoring. Monthly laboratory monitoring can be decreased in frequency to every 2 months in patients who are stable with gold therapy for years. Gold is the slow-acting antirheumatic drug for which the best case for protection of the patient from bone erosions can be made. High-dose prednisone, cyclophosphamide, or methotrexate may also prevent erosions, but the first two of these drugs are much more toxic than gold. Oral gold therapy may not be the equivalent of injectable therapy; the disease in patients who are stable with injectable gold therapy often flares when they are switched to the oral preparation.

D-Penicillamine

D-Penicillamine is a difficult drug to manage. In addition to the membranous nephropathy and bone marrow toxicity characteristic of gold, penicillamine produces the nuisance side effect of loss of taste in 20 percent of patients and rarely the more serious autoimmune side effects of a myasthenia gravis–like syndrome and pemphigus. If the dosage is accelerated rapidly (e.g., over 2 months rather than 6 months), the incidence of thrombocytopenia, gastrointestinal intolerance, and other adverse reactions increases significantly. On the "go low, go slow" regimen (125 mg

TABLE 2 Slow Acting Antirheumatic and Cytotoxic Drugs for the Treatment of Rheumatoid Arthritis

	Hydroxychloroquine	*Auranofin*	*Injectable Gold Salts*	*Methotrexate*	*Penicillamine*	*Azathioprine*
Indications	Mild to moderate synovitis Symptoms unresponsive to nonsteroidal anti-inflammatory drugs, splinting, physiotherapy, local steroid injections	Persistent or progressive disease despite hydroxychloroquine therapy	Persistent or progressive disease with hydroxychloroquine, diarrhea with auranofin	Failure of gold; need (often social or psychological) for rapid reliable response	Failure of gold and methotrexate	Failure of gold, methotrexate, and penicillamine
Relative contraindications	Pre-existing macular disease	Proteinuria, renal disease Expected poor compliance with monitoring	Proteinuria, renal disease; history of gold rash, oral lesions	Liver disease; alcohol consumption 4 oz/wk Renal disease Trimethoprim sulfa	Proteinuria, renal disease History of drug rash, oral lesions	Renal disease, liver disease
Usual dosage	200 mg q.d. or b.i.d.	3 mg b.i.d.	10 mg test dose, week 1 50 mg/wk × 20 wk Taper to 50 mg/mo	2.5 or 5.0 mg q 12 h ×3 doses weekly	125 mg daily, raising dose by 125 mg/mo	50 mg daily, raising dose by 25 mg/2 wk, guided by CBC
Maximal dosage	200 mg b.i.d.	3 mg t.i.d.	50 mg/wk	15 mg/wk	750 mg daily	200 mg daily
Major toxic effects	Pigmented macular degeneration (1%) Gastrointestinal upset (11%)	Mucocutaneous lesions (23%), rare exfoliation, diarrhea (25%), membranous nephropathy (2%), hematologic complication (7%)	Mucocutaneous lesions (48%), rare exfoliation, membranous nephropathy (6%), hematologic complication (7%)	Hepatic fibrosis, rarely cirrhosis (irreversible)	Mucocutaneous lesions (30%), membranous nephropathy (15–20%), hematologic complications (5%), autoimmune syndromes (1%)	Bone marrow suppression, hepatitis (1%)
Recommended monitoring	Baseline and q 6 mo retinal examinations with photographs and Ishikawa dot and Amsler grid tests	CBC, differential and platelet counts, urine dipstick for protein q 2 wk; may lengthen interval to q 3 wk at 2 mo	Same as oral gold, but check laboratory test results prior to each injection	CBC, differential and platelet counts, liver chemistries, creatinine q 2 wk May lengthen interval to q 3 wk at 2 mo	CBC, differential and platelet counts, urine dipstick for protein q 2 wk; may lengthen interval to monthly at 6 mo	CBC, differential and platelet counts prior to adjusting dose; liver chemistries monthly
Length of usual trial	3 mo	6–8 mo	4–6 mo	3 mo (many respond in first month)	7–9 mo	3 mo

as a starting dose with 125 mg monthly increments to a daily dose of 750 mg), it takes 6 months to reach the full dosage and another month to decide that the full dosage has been of no value. Patients who seem likely to tolerate the 6 to 9 months with no response are the best candidates for penicillamine. Penicillamine may be ineffective in seronegative rheumatoid arthritis.

Cytotoxic Drugs

Methotrexate

Cytotoxic drugs are probably as effective as or more effective, and also faster acting (see Table 2), than the slow-acting antirheumatic drugs against moderate to severe rheumatoid inflammation. However, the uncertain frequency and the known severity of adverse effects, including liver and lung toxicity in the case of methotrexate, make their exact role relative to the slow-acting antirheumatic drugs debatable. Methotrexate is a reasonable drug to try if hydroxychloroquine and gold have been of no value. For many therapists methotrexate is preferable to penicillamine. In two large trials methotrexate is being compared directly to oral therapy with gold and seems to be more effective and better tolerated than gold in the medium term (2 to 5 years). Responses to methotrexate tend to occur at 2 to 12 weeks of treatment in contrast to a longer period that may be needed for gold "loading" and the up to 9 months necessary for the evaluation of penicillamine treatment.

Experience with methotrexate in the treatment of psoriasis shows that it is not associated with any increase in malignant disease, but in animal models methotrexate breaks chromosomes at their fragile sites. The main clinical complications of methotrexate treatment are hepatic fibrosis and an interstitial-alveolar pulmonary infiltrate. These complications may occur in 1 to 2 percent of the patients, and there is no reliable way to predict when they will occur or to treat them when they do. Detection of hepatic toxicity is only marginally facilitated by carrying out the recommended liver chemistry panel every 2 to 4 weeks. The enzyme measurements should be made several days after the methotrexate dose. A decrease in the serum albumin level may also signify liver fibrosis due to methotrexate.

The role of liver biopsy in detecting hepatic toxicity is still unclear. Baseline liver biopsies are unnecessary, but rheumatologists still use needle biopsies of the liver as part of the routine monitoring when the total dose reaches 1 to 2 g. Bone marrow suppression is usually not a problem with the low dose of methotrexate used in the treatment of rheumatoid arthritis. However, renal insufficiency, seriously impaired pulmonary function, folate deficiency, severe infections, alcohol consumption greater than 4 ounces per week, and obesity great enough to preclude liver biopsy are contraindications to the use of methotrexate. Shortness of breath, a nonproductive cough, and fever are characteristics of methotrexate pulmonary toxicity. The clinical picture is one of a cold without rhinorrhea. A chest cold without a runny nose should be a red flag prompting physician evaluation for a patient taking methotrexate.

Other Cytotoxic Drugs

Anecdotal evidence indicates that azathioprine may be somewhat less effective than methotrexate and more apt to produce bone marrow suppression in the dosages commonly used. The one controlled comparison between methotrexate and azathioprine showed only a trend toward greater efficacy of methotrexate. Rarely, idiosyncratic hepatotoxicity from azathioprine occurs in the first few weeks of the course. An excess of lymphoreticular malignant disease has been observed among allograft recipients treated with azathioprine but not among patients with rheumatic diseases treated with this drug. Severe effects of rheumatoid vasculitis such as nonhealing lower extremity ulcers may require brief pulse treatment with cyclophosphamide for which there is an established protocol. Despite its efficacy, continuous use of cyclophosphamide for rheumatoid arthritis without vasculitis is precluded by an increased incidence of the development of neoplasia.

Oral Steroid Therapy

There is general agreement that the risks of osteoporosis and other adverse effects from pharmacologic doses of prednisone are great enough to counterbalance their beneficial effect in rheumatoid arthritis. Using steroids for rheumatoid arthritis is like buying an automobile on time: all the benefits occur in the first 2 years, and payment continues almost indefinitely. Nevertheless, as many as 15 or 20 percent of patients with moderately severe rheumatoid arthritis take steroids. There may be some role for low dosages of 5.0 to 7.5 mg a day. Every other day regimens usually fail owing to an exacerbation of symptoms on the "off" day ("every other day arthritis"). The role of steroid therapy hinges on the critical unanswered question of how much treatment with low dosages adds to the risk of osteoporosis. The risk-benefit ratio for low-dose prednisone treatment of rheumatoid arthritis therefore may be affected profoundly by increases in the use of estrogen for the prevention of postmenopausal osteoporosis or coronary artery disease. Prednisone given at a dosage of 7.5 mg daily is probably a reasonable addition to slow-acting antirheumatic drug treatment for patients with a lower baseline risk of osteoporosis, including those with high bone density determined by densitometry, large-framed individuals, men, and blacks.

Injectable Steroids

Steroid injections are most useful when one or a few joints dominate the clinical picture. Almost any joint or surrounding periarticular structure can be injected successfully by an experienced operator. Intra-articular injections should be limited to three or four per joint per year because animal evidence indicates that repeated intra-articular injections accelerate cartilage degeneration. Serious complications from steroid injections are rare, although "postinjection flares" from steroid crystal deposition can occur 2 to 8 hours following the injection and the vitiligo that occurs when some of the injectable steroid infiltrates the dermis in black patients is cosmetically undesirable. Local steroid injection is one of the most effective treatments for geographically limited rheumatoid arthritis.

Surgery in Rheumatoid Arthritis

Secondary osteoarthritis and "bone on bone" pain are indications for joint replacement. Open surgical synovectomy is no longer performed, but arthroscopic synovectomy of the knee may provide relief of symptoms if the knee dominates the clinical picture or is the remaining troublesome joint after successful slow-acting antirheumatic or cytotoxic drug therapy. Total joint replacement of the hips and the knees has a 95 percent certainty of affording pain relief, a 1 percent per year chance of resulting in loosening, and a 1 percent chance of resulting in postoperative infection.

Prosthetic replacements of other joints are less satisfactory. There is still no widely available prosthesis that withstands the stress put on an ankle. If the ankle joints or joints of the midfoot are destroyed by rheumatoid arthritis but remain painful, arthrodesis is the best option; the same is generally true of the wrist and elbow. Shoulder replacement eliminates pain as effectively as lower extremity joint replacements but adds little to function because the rotator cuff is usually destroyed and cannot be reconstructed. Silastic joint replacements in the small joints of the hands improve the hands cosmetically but often fracture and fail to increase strength even though they restore mechanical relationships. It is wise not to use hand surgery as a patient's first joint replacement surgery in order to avoid leaving the patient with an unrealistically pessimistic view of the functional value of joint replacement. Dorsal synovectomy to prevent rupture of the extensor tendons of the hands with consequent loss of function is an effective prophylactic surgical measure.

Experimental Treatments

There are a number of apparently effective treatments with major limitations imposed by side effects or inconvenience. Among these are radiation synovectomy with injected yttrium or dysprosium, which can be performed only in centers adjacent to a cyclotron or linear accelerator capable of creating these short-lived isotopes. Radiation synovectomy is 90 percent effective and may be superior to surgical synovectomy. Cyclosporine produces a partially reversible loss of renal function and is ineffective at doses that minimize this effect. Total nodal irradiation (2,000 to 3,000 rad) has produced remissions lasting 2 years but also deaths due to infection. Lower doses of total nodal irradiation (200 to 750 rad) are currently being investigated. Plasmapheresis is ineffective. Pulse methylprednisone offers no advantage over low-dose steroid therapy. Needed advances include more dosing information in regard to radiation, risk-to-benefit information delineating the role of low-dose prednisone therapy, and a clearer definition of the risk-to-benefit ratio inherent in the strategy of using cytotoxic and slow-acting antirheumatic drugs earlier in the course of the disease.

SPECIAL PROBLEMATIC SITUATIONS

Early Aggressive Disease

The patient who has severe synovitis during the first year of disease with considerable functional loss poses a major question. Does early aggressive treatment have a better chance of succeeding than late aggressive treatment? One point of view holds that as soon as one is certain of the diagnosis, one should use the drug most likely to suppress synovitis before the disease gets a foothold. The contrasting point of view suggests that slow-acting antirheumatic or cytotoxic drugs are rarely continued for many years consecutively and ultimately have little impact on the final outcome. One therefore should withhold them as long as possible in order to avoid unnecessary exposure to toxic drugs in patients in whom spontaneous remission might occur. Most rheumatologists have become increasingly aggressive in the early use of slow-acting antirheumatic drugs. Previous recommendations centered on the caution that one should avoid such drugs during the first year when the likelihood of spontaneous remission was the greatest. Most rheumatologists now place this limit at 6 months. Many use oral gold therapy even earlier. Hydroxychloroquine has always been available for early use.

The Discouraged Patient

The patient who adopts a therapeutically nihilistic attitude and gives up trying to maintain joint mobility is in a precarious situation. Flexion contractures may become permanent, and often function lost in this way cannot be regained even surgically. Two approaches greatly encourage the patient at almost zero cost. The first is to allow the patient as much control over the therapy as possible. Creating options of more or less equal value and presenting them to the patient as choices generate a sense of control on the part of the patient. Second, steroids can be injected into the two or three most actively inflamed joints. A long-lasting (e.g., 3 month) benefit from injection may occur, and the systemic spillover during the initial week after injection may also help the patient psychologically. The contrast between the response to intra-articular steroid therapy, even if it is short-lived, and the baseline to which the patient returns demonstrates that effective treatment is at least possible and that the situation is not hopeless.

Night Pain

Pain that awakens the patient at night usually leads to a specific treatment. The three most likely causes of night pain in patients with rheumatoid arthritis are: (1) bursitis-tendonitis in the shoulder, hip, or anserine bursa, which responds to local steroid injections (patients use the medial surface of the knees to push off against the mattress when turning over and may experience patellar and anserine bursa pain from this seemingly innocuous action); (2) compression neuropathy, which can be treated with steroid injection or decompression of the nerve (e.g., median nerve release); and (3) structurally diseased joints with bone on bone pain from cartilage loss (these patients may benefit from surgery).

The Patient Who Has Failed to Improve

The diagnosis of the patient who has failed to improve should be reviewed (Table 3). In the patient who has experienced failure with multiple slow-acting antirheumatic drugs as a result of toxicity, a detailed re-examination of the history should be made in order to determine whether the "toxicities" that led to discontinuing such a drug, particularly gold, are toxicities that definitely warrant abandoning the drug. These include nephrotoxicity with rising creatinine levels, cytopenias, and gold colitis. Mild (trace to 1+) proteinuria, stomatitis, or a mild skin rash sometimes can be "treated through" by restarting at a lower dosage and advancing the dosage more slowly. The probability of success using this strategy may be augmented by switching the route or form of administration of gold. Thus, if the toxic effect was minor and occurred with aurothioglucose, the patient is switched to gold sodium thiomalate, or auranofin. As an alternative to restarting slow-acting antirheumatic drug therapy, local steroid injections and nonsteroidal anti-inflammatory drugs may be used for the control of symptoms, using surgical replacements for joints as they fail. A patient with advanced widespread disease is sometimes paradoxically a very good candidate for multiple joint replacements, since the level of physical activity is so low that it puts little stress on the bone-cement interface. This conservative strategy of aspirin combined with replacement of joints as they fail from cumulative cartilage loss is often superior to repeated excursions into obscure areas of therapeutics such as plasmapheresis and long-term cyclophosphamide therapy.

TABLE 3 Rheumatic Diseases That May Resemble Rheumatoid Arthritis

Consider the following in seronegative rheumatoid arthritis that fails to respond to treatment:

Erosive interphalangeal osteoarthritis	Reiter's syndrome (especially if metacarpophalangeal involvement is asymmetric)
Calcium pyrophosphate deposition disease	Psoriatic arthritis
Chronic tophaceous gout (especially steroid treated)	Systemic lupus erythematosus
Ankylosing spondylitis (especially if metacarpophalangeal involvement is asymmetric)	

The "Burned Out" Patient

There is some debate about whether rheumatoid arthritis "burns" itself out. Fibrotic pannus may both insulate the examining hand from signs of inflammation in the joint and physically limit the volume of effusion. Some patients appear to have very limited inflammation on examination and yet have malaise and easy fatigability accompanied by laboratory evidence of disease activity, such as decreased albumin and hematocrit levels with increased erythrocyte sedimentation rate. These patients sometimes benefit from aggressive treatment even though they have long-standing rheumatoid arthritis with little apparent evidence of active synovitis on examination.

Generalized Fatigue and Aching Without Physical Signs

A patient who has had rheumatoid arthritis for a short period of time may not have the deformity and scarred pannus of the "burned out" patient but still may not be doing well. Such a person may have a mild synovitis or synovitis in a few joints but may complain of generalized aching, which may turn out to be secondary fibrositis or depression (treatable with amitriptyline). Comorbidity such as hypothyroidism is common. When symptoms of aching are disproportionate to physical findings or laboratory test results, special attention to the patient's home, family, or other social situation is indicated.

A Single Inflamed Joint or a Dominant Joint

This is the most important special situation in the treatment of patients with rheumatoid arthritis. A single dominant joint in a patient with rheumatoid arthritis should be aspirated the first time it is seen to effect symptomatic relief, diagnosis by culture, and drainage of a potentially infected joint space. Shoulders in particular require prompt aspiration. Unlike joints in the lower extremities, shoulders usually can be spared physical stress and are voluntarily and involuntarily splinted by the patient when a small effusion stretches the joint capsule. Therefore, a large palpable effusion makes the shoulder more likely to be infected even if it is not warm. In patients with rheumatoid arthritis, there may be several reasons why there is not so much warmth over a septic joint as in other patients. Nonsteroidal anti-inflammatory drugs, steroids, and generalized debility may contribute to decreasing the signs of inflammation.

In a particularly stubborn, culture-negative joint, especially one that is as anatomically complex as the shoulder, the failure of one local steroid injection to produce relief should prompt more careful examination of all the tendon and bursal structures around the joint. Injections directed at the structure that seems by physical examination to be most involved are more successful than steroid injections given intra-articularly by the anterior approach regardless of physical findings.

SUGGESTED READING

Furst DE, et al. A controlled study of concurrent therapy with nonacetylated salicylate and naproxen in rheumatoid arthritis. Arthritis Rheum 1987; 30:146–154.

Hamdy H, McKendry RJ, Mierins E, Liver JA. Low-dose methotrexate compared with azathioprine in the treatment of rheumatoid arthritis. Arthritis Rheum 1987; 30:361–368.

Healey LA. The current status of methotrexate use in rheumatic diseases. Bull Rheum Dis 1986; 36:4.

Helewa A, et al. Cost-effectiveness of in-patient and intensive out-patient treatment of rheumatoid arthritis: A randomized control trial. Arthritis Rheum 1989; 32:1505–1514.

Panush RS. Controversial arthritis remedies. Bull Rheum Dis 1985; 34:5.

Scott DGI, Bacon PA. Intravenous cyclophosphamide plus methylprednisolone in the treatment of systemic rheumatoid vasculitis. Am J Med 1984; 76:377–384.

JUVENILE RHEUMATOID ARTHRITIS

SUZANNE L. BOWYER, M.D.

Juvenile rheumatoid arthritis is an inflammatory disease of unknown etiology. In some patients systemic features may be present in addition to the arthritis. Pain at rest is extremely rare; moving a joint through its full range of motion seems to cause the most discomfort. Stiffness affecting the joints and adjacent soft tissues is usually a prominent symptom, and without constant attention to range of motion, contractures can and will result. The disease remains active for several years, but in the majority of children remission eventually occurs. Because of the chronic yet self-limited nature of this disease, which affects young children, safe, well-tested medications having no long-term side effects should be used. The patient and parents should have a good understanding of the disease process and work with the medical team in therapeutic planning.

The goals of treatment are to control the inflammation and stiffness, to prevent and correct any musculoskeletal deformities, and to ensure that the child reaches adulthood as functional as possible despite the illness. Throughout the treatment period the child's normal social, emotional, and intellectual development must continue. The problems encountered during the course of the illness are multidisciplinary in nature, and ideally these children should be cared for by a team of individuals familiar with the medical and psychological issues created by the disease. Such a team usually includes a pediatric rheumatologist, a nurse-clinician, a social worker, and physical and occupational therapists. A general approach to the treatment of juvenile rheumatoid arthritis is outlined in Table 1.

Juvenile rheumatoid arthritis has three distinct types of onset. The patients in each group differ in presentation, disease course, and prognosis (Table 2).

TABLE 1 Approach to Treatment in Juvenile Rheumatoid Arthritis

1. The patient and family should be educated regarding the nature of the disease, the expected disease course, and its prognosis
2. Adequate nutrition, rest, and exercise should be encouraged
3. Medications are prescribed to decrease inflammation and associated pain and stiffness
4. Exercises are prescribed to
   a. Preserve range of motion in involved joints
   b. Increase the strength of muscles crossing involved joints
   c. Prevent deformity
5. Splints may be prescribed to decrease stiffness and prevent contractures
6. The patient's ability to perform activities of daily living must be maximized
7. Potential complications should be screened for, dealt with, and prevented if possible
8. Emotional support must be provided to the patient and family

TABLE 2 Classification of Juvenile Rheumatoid Arthritis

Type of Onset	*Age at Onset*	*Males/Females*	*Clinical Characteristics*	*Laboratory Findings*	*Prognosis*
Systemic	Any	Equal	Rash, fever, lymphadenopathy, hepatosplenomegaly, pericarditis; may have a few or many joints involved	↑ ↑ESR ↑WBC ↓Hb Negative ANA, RF	All mortality (1–2%) in this group. 50% develop persistent arthritis and more than half of these have severe arthritis
Polyarticular					
Rheumatoid factor negative	Usually under 5 years old	Majority are female	More than five joints, symmetric, few systemic features	↑ESR ↑WBC ↓Hb May have positive ANA	10–15% develop severe arthritis
Rheumatoid factor positive	Usually older (teenage)	Majority are female	Symmetric polyarthritis, small joint involvement similar to adult rheumatoid arthritis, nodules	↑ESR ↑WBC ↓Hb RF positive, ANA negative	Prolonged course, rare remission, more than 50% with severe joint disease
Pauciarticular					
Type I	Usually under 5 years old	Majority are female	Fewer than five joints involved, usually lower extremity; uveitis in 20%	ESR slightly ↑ ANA frequently positive RF negative	Arthritis frequently goes into full remission. 10–20% have residual eye damage, some become polyarticular
Type II	Usually older (teenage)	Majority are male	Lower extremity involvement; hip commonly involved; enthesopathy; symptomatic acute iritis	HLA-B27 positive	Some may develop ankylosing spondylitis as adults

The general approach to treating arthritis is the same regardless of the subgroup into which the patient best fits. The severity and extent of joint involvement, which may vary between subtypes, determine the exact nature of the treatment regimen needed for any individual patient. Aggressive arthritis accompanied by early bone erosions implies the need for equally aggressive treatment. Drugs with the potential for causing side effects can be justified when the alternative is irreversible joint damage in a young patient. On the other hand, a more conservative regimen would be appropriate for a child with mild monoarticular arthritis, little functional disability, and no evidence of erosions on x-ray examination of the involved joints.

GENERAL MEASURES

Like children with any chronic inflammatory disease, patients with juvenile rheumatoid arthritis tend to be more tired than other children their own age. An after-school rest period can make a major difference in their disposition and ability to function in the evening.

Good nutrition is important for these children. No form of dietary manipulation has consistently been shown by rigorous scientific testing to alter the course of arthritis significantly. We recommend a regular balanced diet appropriate for the child's age. Because many children tend to have a poor appetite when the disease is active, administration of a multivitamin preparation is probably a good idea as well.

Children with juvenile rheumatoid arthritis stiffen up when they remain in one position for a long time. This process is called "gelling." It is most common in the morning, and a warm bath can be helpful in getting the child moving. When at school, the child should be allowed to get up, walk around, and stretch from time to time.

PHYSIOTHERAPY AND OCCUPATIONAL THERAPY

Pain and stiffness in joints and surrounding soft tissues keep children with juvenile rheumatoid arthritis from moving normally during the day, putting them at risk for contractures. Thus, physiotherapy becomes important as a means for maintaining joint range of motion. The type of therapy prescribed differs according to the level of disease activity present. Acutely inflamed joints should not be subjected to vigorous or weight-bearing exercise, for example. Therefore, during a flare only range of motion and isometric exercises are prescribed. Later, stretching and strengthening are added in order to preserve or increase the strength of the muscles surrounding the affected joints. Heat, provided as a warm bath, hot packs, paraffin, or ultrasound, can be helpful for increasing range of motion. Exercises such as swimming and pedaling a bicycle are excellent for preserving range of motion in a non-weight-bearing fashion.

Occupational therapists can assess a child's ability to carry out the activities of daily living. In order to maintain and improve their self-image, children with juvenile rheumatoid arthritis should be encouraged to do as much as possible for themselves. If functional deficits exist, an occupational therapist can provide assistive devices to help the child perform particularly difficult tasks.

Splints are used when a child is steadily losing range of motion in a particular joint. These devices are pieces of plastic molded to the areas of interest, padded, and held in place with Velcro straps. A resting splint temporarily immobilizes a joint in a comfortable but functional position. Splints often are worn at night during periods of active disease so that even though joint stiffening occurs, the joint will still be in a usable position. Functional splints can be worn during regular daily activities to support weakened joints and muscles.

COMPLICATIONS

Part of the physician's role in treating a child with juvenile rheumatoid arthritis is to anticipate and treat complications. The most common are joint contractures, leg length discrepancies, and chronic uveitis.

Prevention of contractures has been discussed in the previous section. If a contracture does occur, a vigorous program of stretching is indicated. Serial splinting and casting procedures have been successful in patients with contractures that have been unresponsive to more conservative measures. Rarely, a patient requires soft tissue release or balanced traction to relieve the contracture.

Children with pauciarticular arthritis affecting only one knee may develop overgrowth of the affected leg. If the leg becomes more than 1 inch longer than the other leg, a compensatory hip tilt and associated back problems may result. If this problem is identified, it can be easily treated by placing a small lift on the shoe on the unaffected side. In most patients the magnitude of the difference in leg lengths tends to diminish with time. Rarely, however, differences of as much as 3 to 4 cm may result. In these cases epiphyseal stapling procedures may be necessary.

Chronic uveitis occurs primarily in patients with antinuclear antibody positive pauciarticular juvenile rheumatoid arthritis. It can be seen, however, in antinuclear antibody negative patients as well. Because the condition is asymptomatic, screening must be performed at regular intervals in order to start treatment before permanent damage is done to the eye. A slit lamp examination done by an ophthalmologist will identify the earliest signs of inflammation. Treatment consisting of topical steroid therapy, mydriatics, and occasionally low-dose systemic steroid therapy should be supervised by an ophthalmologist.

DRUG THERAPY

Nonsteroidal Anti-inflammatory Drugs

Many nonsteroidal anti-inflammatory drugs are available for the treatment of arthritis (Table 3). In many areas aspirin still remains the drug of first choice in the treatment of juvenile rheumatoid arthritis. It has a long history of use, and its good and bad points are well characterized. This drug is given four times a day with a meal or snack. It is not necessary to awaken the child for a night-time dose, however, because a steady level is reached within the first week of therapy. Levels of 20 to 30 mg per deciliter are therapeutic.

In 50 percent of the children taking aspirin, the liver enzyme levels temporarily are increased to two to three times normal values. If the levels rise to five to ten times normal or if the child has abdominal pain, aspirin should be stopped and a nonsteroidal anti-inflammatory drug substituted. True hepatotoxicity occurs primarily in patients with systemic disease and in those with aspirin levels higher than 30 mg per deciliter. In some patients with systemic disease it is difficult to obtain a therapeutic aspirin level despite dosages in excess of 100 mg per kilogram per day. This phenomenon may be secondary to gastrointestinal absorption problems during the acute phase of the illness or may simply reflect an inability to measure accurate levels in the face of the hypoalbuminemia common to these patients. Raising the salicylate dose above 120 mg in an attempt to obtain therapeutic serum levels can result in *severe* toxicity.

Because of recent concern about the relationship between the use of salicylates and the development of Reye's syndrome, it is suggested that aspirin be stopped temporarily if the child develops chickenpox or influenza. It is not necessary to stop the drug for a mild upper respiratory infection. The Public Health Service recommends influenza vaccine for children taking long-term aspirin therapy.

Nonsteroidal anti-inflammatory drugs decrease the symptoms of inflammation via several mechanisms, among them suppression of prostaglandin synthesis. These drugs do not change the values of the laboratory tests measuring disease activity (erythrocyte sedimentation rate, rheumatoid factor titer, platelet count), nor do they alter the eventual course of the disease. They do provide relief of pain, swelling, warmth, and morning stiffness, however, and their effects are seen within days to weeks after starting the medications. The decrease in pain and stiffness allows the patient to do more effective range of motion exercises, thus preserving the ultimate functional state of the affected joints. The side effects of nonsteroidal anti-inflammatory drugs are listed in Table 3 as well.

In some cases it may be helpful to give two nonsteroidal anti-inflammatory drugs—each from a different drug class—for a short period. Although children do not seem to be as susceptible as adults to the adverse renal effects of nonsteroidal anti-inflammatory drugs, it is wise to monitor the blood urea nitrogen and creatinine levels and serial urinalyses frequently if two drugs are to be used for longer than 1 week.

Slow-Acting Antirheumatic Drugs

If arthritis remains active after 6 months of treatment with nonsteroidal anti-inflammatory drugs or if periarticular bone erosions are evident on x-ray examination, more aggressive treatment is indicated. This course is most common in patients with polyarticular juvenile rheumatoid arthritis. Slow-acting antirheumatic drugs are rarely indicated in patients with pauciarticular disease. They actually modify the course of the arthritis, decreasing the incidence of erosions and causing changes in laboratory values such as the erythrocyte sedimentation rate and the rheumatoid factor titer. These medications are given along with, not in place of, nonsteroidal anti-inflammatory drugs. No obvious improvement should be expected for about 2 to 4 months after starting therapy with one of these drugs; hence the name. If the patient is significantly disabled by the degree of disease activity, low-dose corticosteroid therapy can be used to allow the child to function while waiting for the slow-acting antirheumatic drugs to take effect.

Gold

Gold is the oldest and best-studied drug in this group. Intramuscular gold therapy has been used for years to treat adult and pediatric rheumatoid arthritis. It probably modifies disease activity by interfering with monocyte and macrophage function. Fifty to sixty percent of treated patients improve significantly, but some 25 percent are unable to tolerate the drug because of side effects. Guidelines for the administration of gold are given in Table 4.

Two gold salts are available for injection—gold sodium aurothiomalate (Myochrysine) and aurothioglucose (Solganal). Myochrysine tends to cause more pain on injection and causes a higher incidence of nitritoid reactions (flushing and dizziness) after injection than does Solganal.

The most common sites of gold toxicity are the skin and mucous membranes, bone marrow, and kidneys. If the patient develops a rash, mouth sores, eosinophilia, neutropenia, thrombocytopenia, hematuria, or proteinuria, the drug should be stopped. When the abnormality has completely resolved, the medication can be cautiously started again at a lower

TABLE 3 Nonsteroidal Anti-inflammatory Drugs Useful in Children Under 12 Years Old

Drug	*How Supplied*	*Dose*	*Dosing Interval*	*Side Effects*
Salicylates				
Aspirin	325 mg tablet	75–100 mg/kg/day	q.i.d.	Tinnitus, bruising, gastrointestinal irritation, hepatotoxicity, allergic reactions, papillary necrosis, decreased renal blood flow
Enteric-coated				
Ecotrin	325 and 500 mg tablets 325 and 500 mg capsules			Statistical association between aspirin administration and Reye's syndrome
Encaprin	325 and 500 mg capsules			
Baby aspirin	80 mg tablets (chewable)			
Choline salicylate (Arthropan)	600 mg/tsp liquid			
Choline-magnesium salicylate (Trilisate)	Scored 500, 750, 1000 mg tablets 500 mg/tsp liquid		t.i.d.	
Indomethacin Group				
Indomethacin (Indocin)	25 and 50 mg capsules, 25 mg/tsp liquid 75 mg sustained-release capsules	1.5–3.0 mg/kg/day	t.i.d.	Side effects common to all nonsteroidal anti-inflammatory drugs: gastrointestinal irritation, allergic reactions, papillary necrosis, fluid retention, headache, dizziness
Tolmetin sodium (Tolectin)	Scored 200 mg tablets (can be chewed or dissolved in 1 tsp milk) 400 mg capsules	15–30 mg/kg/day	t.i.d.	
Propionic Acid Derivatives				
Ibuprofen				
Motrin	400, 600, 800 mg tablets	30–50 mg/kg/day	q.i.d.	As above
Rufen	400,600 mg tablets			
Nuprin, Advil, Medipren	200 mg tablets available over the counter			
Pediaprofen	Liquid suspension 100 mg/tsp			
Naproxen (Naprosyn)	250, 375, 500 mg tablets 125 mg/tsp liquid	10–16 mg/kg/day	b.i.d.	

TABLE 4 Guidelines for Gold Administration

1. Check complete blood count, urinalysis, and liver function tests
2. Obtain baseline x-ray views of involved joints
3. Give test dose of 5 mg intramuscularly
4. If test dose is tolerated, increase weekly dose gradually to a maximum of 0.75–1.0 mg/kg/dose (maximal dose, 50 mg) per week
5. Prior to each injection, complete blood count and urinalysis should be checked and results obtained
6. Injection should not be given if
   a. WBC count is less than 4,500/mm^3
   b. Platelet count is less than 150,000
   c. Urine is positive for blood or protein
   d. Patient develops mouth sores, rash, or eosinophilia
7. If response is favorable after 20 weeks, intervals between injections may be lengthened to 2 weeks for next 3 months, 3 weeks for following 3 months, and eventually 4 weeks

TABLE 5 Guidelines for Treatment with Penicillamine

1. Obtain baseline complete blood count and urinalysis
2. Dosage: Begin at 125 mg/day; increase in increments of 125 mg every 2–3 months to a maximal dose of 10 mg/kg/day or 750 mg/day total (whichever value is less)
3. Monitor complete blood count and urinalysis weekly for 2 months, every other week for 6 months, then monthly
4. Dosage should be lowered if patient develops a decrease in white blood cells, mild proteinuria, or rash
5. Drug should be discontinued if patient develops a marked decrease in white blood cells or platelets, nephrotic range proteinuria, or autoimmune disease, or if the mild changes listed above do not clear on a lower dosage
6. Drug ideally should be taken on an empty stomach

dosage. The reappearance of gold toxicity should prompt the change to another drug. Extreme cytopenia and the development of exfoliative dermatitis are contraindications to restarting the drug.

An oral form of gold is now available (auranofin). Although it has not yet been approved by the FDA for use in children under 12 years of age, it has been studied in juvenile rheumatoid arthritis. The dosage is 0.1 to 0.2 mg per kilogram per day. Auranofin appears to be less effective than injectable gold in controlling the disease. The blood count and urinalysis should be monitored monthly in patients taking the drug.

Hydroxychloroquine (Plaquenil)

Although the exact mechanism of action of hydroxychloroquine is currently unknown, in vitro the drug has a stabilizing effect on the lysosomal membranes of inflammatory cells. The dosage is 7 mg per kilogram per day for 8 weeks and then 5 mg per kilogram per day. A recent multicenter collaborative study suggested that hydroxychloroquine was not effective for the treatment of childhood arthritis. Although the drug is not as effective as gold, it still plays a role in the treatment of selected patients. It is given in pill form and thus spares the child the pain of an intramuscular injection. Side effects are completely different from those associated with gold, and the drug thus can be used in patients who are intolerant of gold. The main toxic effect of this drug is retinopathy. A baseline eye examination should be obtained, and ophthalmologic screening should be done every 4 to 6 months. Although complications are rare in this dosage range, the drug should be stopped if signs of toxicity occur, because the damage is cumulative. The total duration of therapy probably should not exceed 2 years.

Penicillamine

Although penicillamine has many demonstrable effects on the immune system, the mechanism of its beneficial effect in the treatment of arthritis remains a mystery. Guidelines for the use of this drug are given in Table 5. The most common side effects of penicillamine are similar to those caused by gold. With both drugs, side effects are most often seen in patients who carry the HLA marker DR3. The penicillamine dose should be lowered at the first sign of bone marrow or renal toxicity. Autoimmune phenomena such as lupus erythematosus, polymyositis, myasthenia gravis, Goodpasture's syndrome, and pemphigoid are seen occasionally in patients treated with this drug. The spectrum of rare but serious side effects as well as a recent multicenter study that questions the usefulness of the drug in juvenile rheumatoid arthritis has resulted in fewer patients being given penicillamine.

Corticosteroids

The indications for steroid use in juvenile rheumatoid arthritis are given in Table 6. These drugs should be used in the lowest dosage possible for the shortest reasonable period of time. Steroids are not disease-modifying drugs. They do not prevent erosions or alter the disease course. However, they do mask the symptoms of the disease and give the patient a sense of well-being. Consequently they are useful in mobilizing a patient who would otherwise be confined to bed because of pain and stiffness.

When treating the pericarditis of systemic disease, dosages in the range of 1 to 2 mg per kilogram per day of prednisone are needed. Fever, arthritis, and uveitis, on the other hand, frequently respond to very

TABLE 6 Indications for Corticosteroid Use in Juvenile Rheumatoid Arthritis

Severe systemic symptoms unresponsive to nonsteroidal anti-inflammatory drugs
Symptomatic pericarditis unresponsive to nonsteroidal anti-inflammatory drugs
Symptomatic relief while starting slow-acting antirheumatic drug therapy
Intra-articular injection into a single troublesome joint
Topically for uveitis
Orally in low doses for patients with uveitis unresponsive to topical therapy

low dosages, on the order of 5 to 10 mg per day. For intra-articular injection, 10 to 30 mg of prednisone tebutate or 20 to 40 mg of triamcinolone hexacetonide is appropriate. A joint should not be injected more than three times in a year. In patients troubled by severe debilitating morning stiffness, giving all or most of the steroid dosage at night rather than in the morning can be helpful. With the low dosages used, giving the drug at night does not seem to increase the side effects. However, the arthritis associated with HLA-B27 positivity does not respond as well to steroids.

Once corticosteroids have been started, they are extremely difficult to taper. The decrease in dosage must be very slow—1 mg per day each week, for example, in order to avoid a flare of the underlying disease. The side effects of prolonged corticosteroid treatment are well known and are listed in Table 7.

Methotrexate

Methotrexate has been used by dermatologists since the 1950s for the treatment of psoriasis. The same dosing regimen was adopted for the treatment of adult rheumatoid arthritis during the 1970s. Methotrexate is now being tried in selected pediatric patients who have progressive erosive disease that is unresponsive to nonsteroidal anti-inflammatory and slow-acting antirheumatic drugs. It is also useful in patients with HLA-B27 positive arthritis. The drug is a folate antagonist and probably interferes with the immune phenomena associated with juvenile rheumatoid arthritis through its effect on DNA synthesis. It seems to have a direct anti-inflammatory effect as well.

The drug is given in a low-dosage oral regimen, beginning with 0.1 mg per kilogram per week given as one dose. The dosage may be increased to a maximum of 0.6 mg per kilogram per week. In most studies symptomatic relief has been noted within 2 to 4 weeks after starting the drug. Methotrexate's effect on the disease course will be clarified by continuing long-term studies; a multicenter pediatric study is currently in progress as well.

Although occasionally methotrexate causes a gastrointestinal irritation, liver toxicity has not been a major problem with this dosing regimen in the pediatric age group. Pulmonary toxicity also has not been a problem in children, but again experience is limited. In patients taking this drug, the complete blood count should be checked every other week and liver function tests monthly. If persistent elevation of liver enzyme levels is noted, the drug should be temporarily stopped. It is probably a good rule of thumb not to use the drug in patients with pre-existing lung disease.

TABLE 7 Side Effects of Corticosteroid Treatment

Growth suppression	Cataracts
Cushingoid body habitus	Osteoporosis
Weight gain and fluid retention	Gastric irritation
Striae	Myopathy
Hirsutism	

OTHER FORMS OF TREATMENT

Several forms of treatment that initially showed promise for patients with juvenile rheumatoid arthritis have fallen into disuse in recent years. Examples include pulse steroid therapy, plasmapheresis, leukapheresis, and cytotoxic drug therapy. The small additional therapeutic effects these modes of therapy offered did not seem to justify their increased toxicity except in very rare patients. Total lymphoid irradiation, which has been used in some adults with rheumatoid arthritis, is considered too toxic for use in juvenile rheumatoid arthritis.

Surgery

Soft tissue release can be helpful in severe contractures. Synovectomy is performed occasionally in cases of chronically active disease confined to a single joint (usually the knee). We have used the procedure in patients with severe pauciarticular disease unresponsive over a period of at least 1 year to therapeutic doses of nonsteroidal anti-inflammatory drugs and intra-articular corticosteroid injection. The ability to perform synovectomy via arthroscopy has shortened the recovery time significantly.

The availability of hip replacement for children with severe juvenile rheumatoid arthritis has made a vast difference in their ability to function as adults. Joint replacement should be delayed as long as possible in order to allow the child to reach maximal growth. Until the replacement is done, vigorous physiotherapy must be continued. Strengthening and range of motion exercises are necessary to maintain muscle tone and strength and to prevent contractures around the joint. If supporting structures are maintained, a return to good function is possible after joint replacement. If the muscles are allowed to become weak and contracted, however, even a new joint will not restore lost function to the limb.

The treatment of juvenile rheumatoid arthritis is vigorous, intense, and multidisciplinary in scope. It must include education of the patient and parent regarding the nature of the illness and the purpose of treatment. Medications are used to decrease pain and inflammation and to prevent long-term joint damage. Physiotherapy and occupational therapy are essential to keep the patient moving and functional. Screening for and treatment of complications are also important. Last but not least, normal social, emotional, and intellectual development should be encouraged.

SUGGESTED READING

Baum J. Aspirin in the treatment of juvenile arthritis. Am J Med 1983; 10–16.
Baum J. Treatment of juvenile arthritis. Hosp Pract 1983; 121–136.
Brewer EJ, Giannini EH, et al. Gold therapy in the management of juvenile rheumatoid arthritis. Arthritis Rheum 1983; 23: 404–410.
Brewer EJ, Nickeson RW. Diagnosis and management of juvenile rheumatoid arthritis. Part II. Drug treatment. Hosp Phys 1983; 30–35.
Howard-Lock HE, Lock CJL, et al. d-Penicillamine: Chemistry and clinical use in rheumatic disease. Semin Arthritis Rheum 1986; 15:261–281.
Wallace CA, Bleyer WA, et al. Toxicity and serum levels of methotrexate in chldren with juvenile rheumatoid arthritis. Arthritis Rheum 1989; 32:677–681.

ANKYLOSING SPONDYLITIS

JOSEPH H. KORN, M.D.

Ankylosing spondylitis, or Marie-Strümpell arthritis, is the prototype of the group of disorders known as the seronegative spondyloarthropathies. It is both a true arthritis or synovitis of diarthrodial joints and an enthesopathy, an inflammatory and destructive process involving tendinous and ligamentous attachments to bone. It differs from the other polyarthritides such as rheumatoid arthritis in the pattern of joint involvement. Although peripheral joint disease does occur in ankylosing spondylitis, the hallmark of the disease is axial involvement—the spine and the pelvic and shoulder girdles. It is this pattern of involvement that both distinguishes the disease from most inflammatory arthritides and leads to confusion with degenerative and muscular conditions of the lower back. Thus, diagnostic accuracy is important in selecting an appropriate approach to therapy.

In making the correct diagnosis, historical and physical findings are paramount. Clinical studies have shown that the patient's history is reliable in distinguishing inflammatory (e.g., spondylitic) back pain from mechanical back pain. An early age of onset, such as the late teens and early twenties, is found more commonly in ankylosing spondylitis. In addition, the back pain is more diffuse than in mechanical disorders, involving the entire spine and not just the lower back; thus, the symptoms are concordant with the radiographic and pathologic findings. Like other inflammatory arthritides, spondylitic back pain improves with activity, is made worse by prolonged recumbency, and is characterized by stiffness after sitting or lying in a single position (gelling). Night pain is a common associated feature. Finally, the presence of inflammatory peripheral arthritis, inflammatory enthesopathy, and extra-articular disease manifestations (see later discussion) distinguishes the spondyloarthropathies, including ankylosing spondylitis, from mechanical back pain.

The distinction between ankylosing spondylitis and other spondyloarthropathies is made largely on the basis of associated clinical findings. Extra-articular features of ankylosing spondylitis include uveitis, aortitis, apical pulmonary fibrosis, and enthesopathic findings (e.g., heel pain). Both uveitis and aortitis may be found in Reiter's syndrome, and the distinction between ankylosing spondylitis and Reiter's syndrome is often difficult. Such characteristic features of Reiter's syndrome as balanitis, keratodermia blennorrhagica, and urethritis, when present, differentiate the disorder from ankylosing spondylitis. Similarly, the presence of inflammatory bowel disease or psoriasis allows the distinction of spondyloarthropathy associated with these disorders from ankylosing spondylitis.

Early in the disease the symptom complex is a result of inflammatory processes in diarthrodial (synovial) joints, in synarthroses (nonsynovial joints), at cartilage-bone junctions, and at ligamentous and tendinous attachments to bone and cartilage. Thus, involvement of apophyseal and costovertebral joints leads to limited motion of the spine (at the intervertebral joints) and rib cage, respectively. Sacroiliac pain, often referred to the buttocks, is a result of involvement of both the true sacroiliac joints (approximately the lower two thirds of the sacroiliac articulation) and the synarthrosis of the upper articulation. Enthesopathy is common at ligamentous attachments to vertebrae, pelvic bones, ankles (Achilles tendon and plantar fascial attachment), and femurs. At the intervertebral discs, costochondral junctions, and symphysis pubis, inflammatory processes lead to pain, swelling, and erosive changes at the cartilage-bone interfaces. During the course of the disease there is both fusion of diarthrodial and synarthrodial joints and calcification of ligamentous structures leading to loss of mobility and function. These processes obviously are not amenable to medical therapy. The cauda equina syndrome with sphincter dysfunction secondary to root compression has been reported occasionally and may require surgery.

As noted earlier, the diagnosis of ankylosing spondylitis is best made on the basis of a characteristic symptom complex. In early disease both physical and radiographic findings may be normal. With progression, physical examination shows decreased chest expansion and decreased flexion of the lumbar spine. Physical maneuvers to elicit the pain of sacroiliitis, such as sacroiliac compression or hyperextension of the opposite hip, have not been of demonstrated value. With progressive disease there is often forward protrusion of the neck, kyphosis in the upper thoracic spine, and fixed flexion at the hips giving rise to a characteristic posture. Such features as iritis, aortic regurgitation, apical pulmonary fibrosis, and enthesopathic signs and symptoms (e.g., costochondral pain and tenderness) are unusual in mechanical back disease and in inflammatory arthritides other than the spondyloarthropathies, and their presence lends support to a diagnosis of ankylosing spondylitis. Laboratory tests show no consistent abnormalities that are diagnostically useful; the erythrocyte sedimentation rate, which is usually abnormal in other types of inflammatory arthritis, is often normal in ankylosing spondylitis.

Radiographic findings are helpful in the diagnosis. In the spine these include erosions at the vertebral corners and vertebral squaring, calcification in the outer border of the annulus fibrosus (syndesmophyte) followed by calcification of the anterior longitudinal ligament and other ligamentous structures giving the characteristic bamboo spine appearance, and erosion and fusion at apophyseal and costochondral joints. The sacroiliac joints may show definite erosions, which may be manifested as irregular widening of the joint, areas of narrowing and sclerosis, and, later, fusion. Calcification of ligamentous structures, heel spurs, and costochondral erosion are a few of the other radiographic changes that may be seen.

No discussion of ankylosing spondylitis would be complete without mention of the genetic associations of this disorder. In various studies, 90 to 95 percent of Caucasian patients with ankylosing spondylitis have the histocompatibility antigen HLA-B27; a similar association exists for B27 and Reiter's syndrome. In contrast, HLA-B27 is found in only 6 to 8 percent of the control population. Epidemiologic studies suggest that 1 to 2 percent of the population have symptoms attributable to ankylosing spondylitis; one may then calculate an attack incidence of approximately 20 percent for the B27 positive population. Interestingly, in epidemics of Reiter's syndrome associated with bacterial agents, susceptibility is largely limited to B27 positive individuals, and the attack incidence among these is approximately 20 percent.

Clinically overt ankylosing spondylitis is predominantly a male disease. Subclinical or undiagnosed disease occurs with considerable frequency in women; similarly, there is a reservoir of low grade disease—under the tip of the iceberg, so to speak—among B27 positive males. This is supported by the demonstration of radiographic evidence of sacroiliitis in B27 positive individuals who have not had symptoms of back pain requiring medical consultation. However, given the fact that approximately one of 14 individuals in the population is B27 positive, and given the high incidence of mechanical back pain in the population, a positive test for HLA-B27 does not sustain a diagnosis of ankylosing spondylitis. Indeed, in most instances testing for B27 is not diagnostically helpful.

Genetic linkage of a disorder raises questions in patients as to genetic transmission. Although half the children of B27 positive patients with ankylosing spondylitis are B27 positive, it is not clear that the risk of ankylosing spondylitis in these children is substantially greater than that in other B27 positive individuals. Although families with several cases of ankylosing spondylitis have been observed, it is clear that the disease is not transmitted in a typical mendelian dominant fashion.

THERAPY

In the treatment of the arthritis of ankylosing spondylitis the goals are to provide pain relief and to limit deformity, thus providing maximal function. It is not clear that any therapy, with the possible exception of axial irradiation (vide infra), halts the erosive, destructive, and ankylosing features of the disease. Nonetheless a program encompassing both anti-inflammatory therapy and physical therapy can prove of long term benefit to the patient. If ankylosis of the spine or other joints is to occur, these measures can help to insure that joint fusion will occur in the best functional position. The patient in whom the hips are fused in flexion and who has severe dorsal kyphosis and anterior protrusion at the neck represents a failure of medial management.

Physical Measures

Physical measures and physical therapy should be directed at mitigating the deformities just outlined and maintaining maximal mobility of the spine and hips. The physician's role in this regard is educating the patient as to possible long term consequences of the disease and the important role that the patient can play in treatment. Prolonged periods in any position are harmful, certainly in regard to immediate symptoms and probably long term outcome as well. Jobs requiring prolonged periods of sitting in one place, particularly while stooping forward, as over a desk or work bench, aggravate forward displacement of the head and dorsal kyphosis. The patient should make a point of arising from a sitting position at least hourly for a short walk. Standing jobs similarly require frequent changes of position and intermittent exercise. When possible, raising the work surface to obviate the need for leaning forward is helpful. Long drives, in the course of either work or leisure, should be interrupted hourly for brief periods of standing, stretching, or walking.

Furniture should be chosen for proper support of

the spine rather than for apparent immediate comfort. Chairs should be straight-backed and not deeply cushioned; furthermore, the patient should be instructed to sit with appropriate posture, not curled up or slouched. The patient should sleep on his back and not in a fetal position with hips flexed. Pillows should be thin and compressible, if used at all. Firm back support is essential; because one rarely encounters a patient who admits to anything other than a "firm" mattress, the most prudent course is to use a ¼ inch thickness of plywood even under "firm" mattresses.

"Physical therapy" should combine a generous measure of general physical activity along with specific exercises. Swimming provides excellent range of motion for most joints, including the spine, and at the same time protects joints from weight bearing stress. In this respect it is perhaps the best form of general exercise for arthritis. Depending on the individual patient, the severity and activity of the disease, and pre-existing deformity, activities ranging from walking to vigorous competitive sports may be appropriate.

Specific exercises should be directed at maximizing the range of motion of the spine and other joints and counteracting the direction in which deformities tend to develop. In the latter regard, instruction should be provided in exercises to counter forward propulsion of the head, to extend the dorsal spine, and to extend the hips. Other exercises should be directed at improving motion of the spine in all planes: rotation, flexion-extension, and lateral flexion. Breathing exercises to maintain the capacity for full chest expansion are often overlooked. A commitment of time for training with a physical therapist who understands the disease and the goals of physical therapy in ankylosing spondylitis is a worthwhile investment for the patient.

Drug Management

The ability of the patient to function normally in day to day activities and to follow an outlined program of physical activity is dependent upon the control of the inflammatory process. To the extent that physical therapy protects from or limits spinal and joint deformity and disability, control of acute symptoms of pain and stiffness permits the execution of a physical program that, we hope, leads to better spine and joint function in the long term. Conversely there is no evidence to indicate that anti-inflammatory therapy retards the destructive joint disease, and it is unlikely that ankylosis that would otherwise occur can be more than partially ameliorated.

The basis of therapy is the group of drugs called nonsteroidal anti-inflammatory drugs. The list of these drugs grows longer each year, and a comprehensive review of the benefits, side effects, and dollar cost of each is both beyond the scope of this article and unnecessary. Several general statements may be made. To varying degrees, all are effective in the management of ankylosing spondylitis. Indomethacin and phenylbutazone, in my experience and that of most others, are considerably more efficacious than other nonsteroidal anti-inflammatory drugs in most patients. Aspirin, for reasons that are unclear, is least effective in this disorder; this is in contrast with rheumatoid arthritis in which aspirin is effective on a par with all the newer nonsteroidal anti-inflammatory drugs. In general, the newer nonsteroidal anti-inflammatory drugs are equivalent to each other in effectiveness, although individual patients appear to respond better to one or another drug. In addition to effectiveness, both side effects and relative costs of the various drugs must be considered.

My preference is to initiate therapy with one of the new nonsteroidal anti-inflammatory drugs rather than with indomethacin and phenylbutazone, which, though generally more effective, are associated with greater toxicity. It is important to use these drugs at an adequate dosage (Table 1); too commonly they are prescribed at the lowest recommended dosage and the erroneous conclusion is drawn that they are ineffective. Within the group of available drugs the choice is based on drug half-life and cost. Drugs with short half-lifes are less effective in the management of morning stiffness, and the requirement for more frequent daily administration decreases compliance. It is important that patients take the drug around the clock and not only when they hurt. I would thus initiate treatment with a drug that requires no more than a three times daily dosage. It is worth advising the patient to check several pharmacies for relative cost as this may vary considerably in a given geographic area.

In my experience at least half the patients do not achieve sustained relief of symptoms with the newer group of nonsteroidal anti-inflammatory drugs, even when taken at maximal therapeutic dosages. Most of

TABLE 1 Nonsteroidal Anti-inflammatory Drugs for Ankylosing Spondylitis*

Drug	*Total Daily Dosage*	*Frequency of Administration*
Ibuprofen	2400–3200 mg†	t.i.d.-q.i.d.
Indomethacin	100–200 mg	b.i.d.-t.i.d.
Meclofenemate	300–400 mg	t.i.d.-q.i.d.
Naproxen	750–1500 mg	b.i.d.
Phenylbutazone	300–400 mg‡	t.i.d.-q.i.d.
Piroxicam	20 mg	q.d.
Sulindac	300–400 mg	b.i.d.
Tolectin	1200–1600 mg	t.i.d.-q.i.d.

*This is not an all encompassing list but rather those with which the author has had experience.
†Dosages of 3600 to 4200 mg daily have been used on rare occasion; 3200 mg represents upper limit of the officially recommended dosage.
‡400 mg only rarely required.

these respond well to indomethacin. Taken at a dosage of 150 to 200 mg daily initially, indomethacin provides good relief from pain and stiffness. The patient should be cautioned to take the drug with meals to ameliorate headache, light-headedness, and other neurologic symptoms. After an initial response the dosage of the drug may be tapered. It is not clear that "sustained release" formulations of the drug greatly enhance its effectiveness, but the incidence and severity of side effects may be lower. In patients who do not respond to indomethacin, phenylbutazone is usually effective. Despite the potential for serious side effects (to be outlined), ankylosing spondylitis is one disorder in which use of this drug is clearly indicated.

Side Effects of Therapy

Many of the adverse effects of therapy are shared, to greater or lesser extent, by all the nonsteroidal anti-inflammatory drugs and are a direct result of the pharmacology of drug action. All these drugs inhibit prostaglandin synthesis, and PGE_2 prevents back-diffusion of hydrogen ion in the gastric mucosa; this effect may be related to the high frequency of gastric irritation and, in some patients, gastrointestinal ulceration or bleeding. Bleeding is promoted by the inhibitory effects of these drugs on platelet function via inhibition of thromboxane and PGE synthesis. In patients with pre-existent gastric or duodenal ulcers, exacerbation of symptoms, new ulceration, and gastrointestinal bleeding should be carefully watched for. Some patients cannot tolerate any of the nonsteroidal anti-inflammatory drugs without the concomitant use of antacids, H_2 antagonists, or cytoprotective drugs. These, however, should not be used as a routine adjunct of nonsteroidal anti-inflammatory drug therapy in most patients.

Like the gastrointestinal side effects, renal toxicity may result from pharmacologic effects of the drug. Inhibition of renal prostaglandin synthesis results in decreased renal blood flow, an effect that is most often of clinical consequence in the elderly and those with pre-existent renal disease. The pharmacologic decrease in renal blood flow, however, is reversible, and a mild stable increase in the serum creatinine level should not require drug discontinuation. Sulindac, which is administered as a prodrug and not metabolized efficiently to an active metabolite in the kidney, appears to be associated with a lower incidence of decreased renal function.

More serious is the infrequent development of irreversible and, in rare instances, fatal renal disease. This has been reported with the majority, if not all, of the nonsteroidal anti-inflammatory drugs, is apparently due to an idiosyncratic reaction, and is usually manifested histologically as interstitial nephritis. Elderly patients and those with pre-existent renal disease may be at greater risk for the development of this side effect as well. In addition to the shared side effects already noted, individual drugs have unique but generally not serious side effects.

Indomethacin and phenylbutazone, because of their unique role in the treatment of ankylosing spondylitis and because of their generally greater toxicity, should be discussed separately. As noted, indomethacin causes neurologic side effects that are more pronounced in the elderly but are seen in all age groups, particularly when the drug is taken on an empty stomach. Thrombocytopenia has been reported as a consequence of indomethacin treatment, and platelet counts should be checked every few months, at least initially. Indomethacin is generally more gastric irritative than other nonsteroidal anti-inflammatory drugs, and gastric bleeding may be seen. Despite these side effects, indomethacin is a singularly useful drug in the management of ankylosing spondylitis.

Phenylbutazone is also associated with a greater frequency and severity of gastric intolerance than other nonsteroidal anti-inflammatory drugs and in the author's experience is associated with a greater frequency of gastrointestinal bleeding. Phenylbutazone may cause sodium retention to an extent sufficient to precipitate cardiac failure. Most worrying to many are the reported instances of agranulocytosis and general bone marrow depression due to this drug. Estimates suggest that this complication occurs in one of 10,000 treated patients each year and that half the reactions are fatal. For many patients, however, phenylbutazone is the only drug that provides relief from symptoms and allows physical mobility and function; the physician and patient therefore must weigh these benefits against the potential risk. If therapy with phenylbutazone is instituted, hematologic parameters should be followed regularly. Once an initial response is achieved, the patient may be able to be managed with another drug.

Corticosteroids and Immunosuppressive Drugs

There is no demonstrated benefit from corticosteroids in the management of spinal disease in ankylosing spondylitis. Occasional patients with peripheral arthritis may benefit from brief courses of steroids in low dosages (5 to 15 mg of prednisone daily) to suppress disease activity. When single peripheral joints are a persistent problem, intra-articular steroid instillation may be beneficial. Immunosuppressive drugs have not been shown to have a place in the treatment of ankylosing spondylitis. One exception may be in the rare patient who has predominant peripheral disease in whom weekly low dosage methotrexate (5 to 15 mg) may be tried. This approach is directed by analogy to Reiter's syndrome and psoriatic arthritis, as there is no published experience with methotrexate in ankylosing spondylitis. Whether axial disease might also respond to methotrexate is unknown, and the author has had no experience in this regard.

Recent evidence, from controlled studies, suggests that sulfasalazine is beneficial in the treatment of ankylosing spondylitis. It is clear that some patients show significant improvement with sulfasalazine therapy, while others are unresponsive. The mechanism of action of the drug is unknown. Gastrointestinal toxicity may be a limiting factor in therapy.

Irradiation

Irradiation of the axial skeleton can ameliorate spinal arthritis. This modality of treatment has been largely abandoned after reports of leukemia in patients with ankylosing spondylitis who had received irradiation. Nonetheless, in the patient who cannot tolerate any of the nonsteroidal anti-inflammatory drugs (e.g., because of activation of peptic ulcer disease), irradiation may be the only therapeutic intervention that will enable the patient to function. Administration of 400 to 600 rads to the axial skeleton over two sessions may provide good relief while leading to lower risks than previously encountered with higher dosages of radiation.

Surgery

The most common surgical procedure required in patients with ankylosing spondylitis is total hip replacement to correct or prevent hip ankylosis. These patients unfortunately have a tendency to develop periarticular calcium deposition and reankylosis following total hip replacement. The frequency of reankylosis has varied among different series, and the possibility of ankylosis should not preclude total hip replacement which is otherwise indicated. Surgery to correct spinal deformity is of limited utility and should not be attempted unless the deformity markedly limits function and the surgeon has had experience with these patients. There has been some experience with spinal osteotomy to correct severe kyphosis. Finally, it should be noted that many patients with ankylosing spondylitis, owing to a failure of diagnosis, have undergone surgical procedures for low back pain. The clinician should entertain the diagnosis of ankylosing spondylitis in young men with back disease and protect them from surgical procedures that will provide no therapeutic benefit.

Extra-articular Disease

Most extra-articular disease manifestations are not readily amenable to therapy. Thus the cardiac abnormalities of conduction disturbances and aortitis have not been treated medically except for control of arrhythmias; aortic valve replacement may be necessary, depending on the hemodynamic consequences of the lesion. There is little published experience about treatment of the pulmonary fibrotic lesion; although occasionally cavitary, it is more commonly a mild fibrosis. Acute iritis requires the use of topical corticosteroid therapy.

PATIENT EDUCATION

As with other disorders, taking the time to explain the disease to the patient—what we know about its course and its treatment, what the patient is free to do and what he should avoid, and how even if a disease is incurable, that does not mean that it is untreatable—is critically important. This is often best done over a period of several office visits rather than all at one time during the first encounter. Questions about the hereditary nature of the disease and the risk in offspring should be discussed frankly. Finally, in the course of a chronic disease it is a rare patient who does not seek second, third, or more opinions. This option should be discussed with the patient openly both so that care can be coherent and coordinated and so that the patient may be referred to knowledgeable specialists (lists are usually available from the local Arthritis Foundation). Otherwise many patients will find those who promise cures from diet, vitamins, enemas, or magic drugs, treatments that will have a great impact on the patient's wealth but no beneficial effect on his health.

SUGGESTED READING

Calin A, Fries JF. Striking prevalance of ankylosing spondylitis in healthy W27 positive males and females. N Engl J Med 1975; 293:835–839.

Calin A, Porta J, Fries JF. The clinical history as a screening test for ankylosing spondylitis. JAMA 1977; 237:2613–2617.

Carette S, Graham D, Little H, Rubenstein J, Rosen P. The natural disease course of ankylosing spondylitis. Arthritis Rheum 1983; 26:186–190.

Shanahan WR Jr, Kaprove RE, Major PA, Hunter T, Bargar FD. Assessment of longterm benefit of total hip replacement in patients with ankylosing spondylitis. J Rheumatol 1982; 9:101–114.

SYSTEMIC SCLEROSIS

ETHAN WEINER, M.D.
JOSEPH H. KORN, M.D.

Systemic sclerosis, or scleroderma, is a multisystem disease characterized by cutaneous and visceral fibrosis and obliteration of small vessels. Clinical expression of the disease is a reflection of these connective tissue and vascular processes. The skin is the most visible organ affected by this process, with thickening and induration usually beginning distally and extending proximally. Dermal fibrosis and atrophy of hair follicles and sweat glands are noted on histologic study of involved skin. A similar process in the gastrointestinal tract causes atrophy of the muscularis mucosae and of the longitudinal and circular layers of smooth muscle, resulting in loss of lower esophageal tone, motility disturbance, and malabsorption. In the lungs vascular obliteration or interstitial fibrosis can occur, leading to restrictive lung disease and cor pulmonale. Obliteration of the renal vascular bed can cause an abrupt hypertensive crisis, with the rapid onset of renal failure. The heart can be affected by pericarditis, restrictive cardiomyopathy, or conduction system disturbance. Obliteration of the vessels supplying peripheral nerves (vasa nervorum) can result in mononeuritis multiplex, often affecting the trigeminal nerve.

Almost all patients with scleroderma suffer from Raynaud's phenomenon, classically a triphasic vascular response to cold, emotion, or other stimuli manifested by pallor, cyanosis, and then reactive hyperemia of affected areas, most commonly the fingers. If no history of Raynaud's phenomenon is obtained, the diagnosis of scleroderma should be questioned. Likewise, if skin tightening proceeds from the trunk outward rather than from the extremities inward, other causes of skin tightening such as scleredema or eosinophilic fasciitis should be carefully ruled out before the diagnosis of scleroderma is made. Conversely, true scleroderma can present as a low grade myositis or arthritis, accompanied by edematous "puffy" skin that has not yet become hidebound. The diagnosis of scleroderma can be elusive until more characteristic cutaneous and visceral manifestations ultimately develop.

Scleroderma can present with a wide spectrum of organ involvement. In a subgroup of patients with what is often labeled the CREST syndrome (an acronym for calcinosis, Raynaud's phenomenon, esophageal dysmotility, sclerodactyly, and telangiectasia), skin changes are limited primarily to the fingers. In this subgroup pulmonary hypertension without fibrosis often develops late in the course of the disease, but other visceral involvement (except for esophageal) is uncommon. At the opposite end of the spectrum are patients who, within several months after the onset of Raynaud's phenomenon and sclerodactyly, develop thickened skin in more proximal areas such as the upper arms, thighs, and chest with or without associated involvement of the lungs, heart, kidneys, and gastrointestinal tract. Finally, many patients defy easy classification—they may have prominent CREST features but may have proximal skin disease or more aggressive organ system disease as well. Alternatively patients have associated features of other connective tissue diseases, such as systemic lupus erythematosus or rheumatoid arthritis, that only after some years develop into a single classic connective tissue disease. From a therapeutic viewpoint this means that the clinical manifestations that require treatment vary greatly from patient to patient, as does the pace of the disease, which can be indolent or rapidly life-threatening.

The pathogenesis of scleroderma is poorly understood. Fibroblasts isolated from patients with scleroderma produce more collagen than do normal cells. There is also both morphologic and functional evidence of endothelial cell dysfunction in scleroderma and associated evidence of platelet activation and aggregation in patients with active disease. However, there is no single underlying abnormality yet known to explain both the vascular and fibrotic phenomena that are the hallmarks of the disease.

There is no characteristic laboratory abnormality in scleroderma. Most patients have antinuclear antibodies, often with a speckled or nucleolar pattern, and some patients (particularly those with the CREST syndrome) have anticentromere antibodies. None of these antibodies is absolutely specific for scleroderma, however. Antibodies to topoisomerase I, formerly called Scl-70, are largely restricted to scleroderma. They are present in only about one third of the patients and therefore lack sufficient sensitivity to be diagnostically useful. Absence of all detectable autoantibodies does not rule out the diagnosis of scleroderma, but should invite closer scrutiny and further efforts to rule out other diseases with similar cutaneous manifestations. The erythrocyte sedimentation rate is often normal in scleroderma. Mild anemia or a low serum albumin level can occur if the patient has significant gastrointestinal involvement and is in a poor nutritional state. As a rule, complement levels are not depressed, and there is little evidence for immune complex disease.

Owing to the lack of understanding of the pathogenesis of scleroderma, treatment has been most successful when used to palliate specific organ system manifestations. Remittive therapies, designed to modulate the course of the disease in general, have yielded much less success, and their role in disease management remains to be clarified.

THERAPY FOR SPECIFIC ORGAN INVOLVEMENT (Table 1)

Skin Care

The skin should be kept warm and moisturizers should be used liberally, especially in the winter. Dry skin fissures easily and because of the poor vascular supply in scleroderma heals slowly. Wearing thin cotton gloves or glove liners under mittens provides optimal warmth and hand protection when mittens must be removed. Areas of calcinosis cutis should be kept clean, and local infections around calcium deposits should be treated early with systemic antibiotic therapy. Calcium deposits, which form niduses for recurrent or severe infections, may require surgical removal. Warfarin, probenecid, colchicine, and diphosphonates have been used to try to reduce the size of cutaneous calcium deposits or prevent the development of new ones. Unfortunately none of these drugs has been clearly successful. Pruritus in areas of involved skin is a common problem; although no treatment has proved uniformly successful, some patients benefit greatly from colchicine.

Raynaud's Phenomenon and Vascular Phenomenona

One of the most troublesome problems for scleroderma patients, both those with the CREST variant and those with diffuse systemic sclerosis, is Raynaud's phenomenon. Although typically episodic, it often can be severe and persistent, leading to painful digital ulcerations and resorption of the distal finger pads. Locally infected digital ulcerations should be treated with oral doses of antibiotics active against penicillinase producing staphylococci (dicloxacillin, erythromycin, or orally administered cephalosporins). Slowly healing ulcerations may conceal occult infection under scabs or crusts and may also benefit from antibiotics. In addition to scrupulous attention to keeping core and peripheral body temperature warm and keeping the skin lubricated, the use of vasodilators may be of significant benefit. We prefer to start with either nifedipine or topical nitrate therapy. Nifedipine therapy is initiated at low dosages (10 mg twice or three times daily) and gradually increased. Other calcium-channel blockers given in gradually increasing doses may be effective if nifedipine is not tolerated. Nitroglycerine ointment applied to the forearm or chest (½ to 1 inch every 4 to 6 hours) has been successful in many patients. Long acting nitrate patches, in our experience, have been much less successful perhaps because of tachyphylaxis in response to constant circulating drug levels. Pentoxifylline, a drug which lowers blood viscosity, is very useful in some patients. Alternative drugs such as alpha-adrenergic blocking drugs (prazosin, dibenzyline) or centrally acting drugs (methyldopa, reserpine) tend to be associated with more side effects. Prazosin, in particular, may be associated with syncope after the initial dose, and the patient should be warned and started on the lowest dosage (1 mg). Beta-blockers and other potentially vasoconstricting drugs should be avoided if substitute drugs are available. Some clinicians advocate the long term use of antiplatelet drugs such as aspirin and persantine to impede the platelet aggregation, release of vasoactive substances, and microthrombus formation that take place at sites of microvasculature injury in scleroderma. Such therapy has not been of demonstrated value but is appealing on theoretic grounds and, at least for low dose aspirin, is of little risk.

Occasionally patients need more aggressive intervention to save a digit from impending gangrene. Our initial approach was the intra-arterial infusion of reserpine (0.75 to 1.0 mg slowly) into the brachial artery of the affected side. Unfortunately reserpine for parenteral administration is no longer readily available. Local sympathetic blockage by repeated daily anesthetic injection has helped break the cycle of vasospasm, leading to ischemia and further vasospasm. Systemic intravenous infusion of PGE_1 (given by continuous central venous catheter infusion at doses of 6 to 10 ng per kilogram per minute for 3 days) also can be helpful in this situation. Surgical sympathectomies, however, are not recommended because their benefit is usually transient, lasting for weeks to months, and the patient is left with an uncomfortable, sometimes edematous, extremity. In our experience surgical amputation of digits is rarely necessary if the aggressive medical approaches just outlined are undertaken.

Gastrointestinal Dysmotility

Esophageal stricture formation can occur in scleroderma after prolonged acid reflux. In many but not all of these patients there is an antecedent history of reflux symptoms. It is reasonable therefore to apply antireflux measures in all patients with scleroderma to prevent potential stricture formation. These measures should include elevating the head of the bed 4 to 6 inches and the liberal use of antacids, particularly before sleep. Symptomatic patients may also benefit from the use of an H_2 blocker (cimetidine, famotidine, or ranitidine) at bedtime. Patients complaining of dysphagia or severe reflux symptoms may also benefit from metaclopramide, 5 to 10 mg, given before meals to increase lower esophageal sphincter pressure.

In the small bowel a malabsorption state may develop because of poor bowel motility, leading to stasis and bacterial overgrowth. This often is manifested as diarrhea and weight loss clinically and hypoalbuminemia on laboratory evaluation. Many patients benefit from the administration of tetracycline during exacerbations of this condition. Excessive use of tetracycline should be avoided, however, since alteration of the bacterial flora for extended periods may allow the development of

TABLE 1 Therapy for End Organ Involvement in Scleroderma

- Skin disease
  - Keep skin warm, lubricated, and protected from injury
  - Antibiotics (dicloxacillin, erythromycin, cephalexin) for infected or poorly healing digital ulcerations
  - Colchicine for pruritus due to calcinosis
- Raynaud's phenomenon
  - Vasodilators
    - Nifedipine, 10–20 mg b.i.d.-q.i.d.
    - Nitroglycerin ointment, 1/4 to 1 inch q 4–6 hr
    - Prazosin, 1 mg then 1 mg t.i.d. to start
    - Pentoxifylline, 400 mg t.i.d.
  - Persistent Raynaud's phenomenon or impending gangrene of a digit
    - Intravenous PGE_1 infusion via central catheter (6–10 ng/kg/minute continued for 3 days)
    - Sympathetic block repeated daily or every other day for several days
- Gastrointestinal disorders
  - Antireflux measures
    - Elevate head of bed
    - Antacids p.c. and h.s.
    - H_2 antagonists (ranitidine, 150 mg h.s.; famotidine, 40 mg h.s.; cimetidine 200 mg h.s.)
    - Metaclopramide, 5–10 mg before meals
  - Malabsorption, diarrhea
    - Trial of tetracycline, 500 mg q.i.d.
  - Constipation
    - Stool softeners
- Arthritis
  - Nonsteroidal anti-inflammatory drugs including aspirin and nonacetylated salicylates
  - Low doses of steroids for early puffy scleroderma (prednisone, 10–20 mg/day initially)
- Myositis (symptomatic)
  - Prednisone, 20–60 mg/day initially, tapering according to clinical and laboratory response
- Acute interstitial lung disease
  - Corticosteroids, 40–60 mg daily initially, tapering according to response
  - ? Cyclophosphamide for severe or steroid unresponsive disease
- Pericarditis
  - Prednisone, 20–60 mg/day for significant or symptomatic disease
- Hypertension and renal crisis
  - Enalapril, 5–20 mg b.i.d., or captopril, 25–150 mg t.i.d., increasing rapidly from starting dose until blood pressure control is achieved; after initial control, adjust dosage to maintain diastolic blood pressure ≤ 80 mm Hg
- Sjögren's syndrome
  - Artificial tears, t.i.d. to q.i.d.; lubricating ophthalmic ointment before bed
- Specialized dental care may be needed
- Psychologic and social support
  - Physician time, patient support groups

pseudomembranous colitis. Alternatively constipation can develop as a result of impaired bowel motility; it should be treated with stool softeners.

Musculoskeletal Disorders

Frank arthritis is an infrequent manifestation of scleroderma but may occur early in the disease. Management with aspirin or other nonsteroidal anti-inflammatory drugs often suffices, but small dosages of prednisone (5 to 10 mg per day) can be used on a short term basis if nonsteroidal drugs alone do not provide relief from pain and swelling. In patients with renal dysfunction nonsteroidal drugs generally should be avoided, except for the nonacetylated salycylates, which do not interfere with prostaglandin production. A common problem in patients with scleroderma is the development of flexion contractures at many joints due to the tightening of skin and ligaments around them. Regular physical therapy, with range of motion exercises at these joints, is vital both to prevent worsening of this condition and, it is hoped, to effect improvement.

Cardiac and Pulmonary Disease

Early aggressive therapy of the interstitial lung lesion of scleroderma with high dose steroid therapy (1 mg per kilogram per day of prednisone or the equivalent) or cytotoxic drugs may be beneficial in preventing or reducing the amount of pulmonary fibrosis. Such treatment should be undertaken only if there is ample evidence of active interstitial inflammation by gallium scan, bronchoalveolar lavage, and/or lung biopsy. Once established, however, pulmonary fibrosis is not reversible. In late disease supervening pulmonary hypertension may be treated by the use of pulmonary vasodilators, such as nifedipine or hydralazine, and by the use of supplemental oxygen if significant desaturation occurs with exercise.

Pleuritis or pericarditis frequently occurs during the course of the disease. These disorders respond well to moderate dosages of steroids (20 to 30 mg per day of prednisone), which are tapered when the patient is no longer symptomatic and pleural or pericardial fluid accumulation is resolving. All patients should be followed with periodic electrocardiograms, and if there is evidence of a conduction disturbance or the patient gives a history of palpitations or light-headedness, a 24 hour ambulatory electrocardiogram should be obtained. Some patients with scleroderma show evidence of a significant arrhythmia, which may be amenable to or require treatment by either drugs or pacemaker insertion.

Scleroderma Renal Crisis

Renal involvement in scleroderma is often abrupt in onset, manifesting as severe hypertension and progressing in days to weeks to renal failure. Rarely, progressive renal disease develops in the absence of associated hypertension. Associated proteinuria is common as is evidence of microangiopathy, including microangiopathic hemolysis resulting from fibrin thrombi occluding small vessels in the kidney and elsewhere. The pathophysiology involves marked narrowing or cortical renal vessels with associated areas of cortical infarction in severe cases.

Such renal involvement in scleroderma formerly (until 10 to 12 years ago) was almost uniformly and rapidly fatal. The advent of angiotensin converting enzyme inhibitors for the treatment of hypertension has dramatically reversed the previously poor prognosis in scleroderma renal disease. Thus, the currently available inhibitors enalapril and captopril are the initial drugs of choice in treating scleroderma associated hypertension. We also favor treating scleroderma renal failure without hypertension with angiotensin converting enzyme inhibitors on the assumption that there is disordered microvascular flow, which may respond to such therapy. In such instances other causes of renal insufficiency must first be considered and the diagnosis of scleroderma renal disease substantiated by the finding of microangiopathic changes on the peripheral blood smear or compatible renal angiographic or biopsy findings.

Aggressive treatment with angiotensin converting enzyme inhibitors has usually resulted in normalization of renal function when therapy has been initiated before there has been a two- to three-fold increase in the serum creatinine level (i.e., a 50 to 75 percent loss of renal function). Even in some patients whose renal disease has progressed to the point of requiring dialysis for acute scleroderma renal crisis, continued aggressive treatment with such inhibitors has resulted in the return of renal function to reasonable levels. It is our practice to "push" therapy to diastolic blood pressures of 80 mm Hg or lower, particularly in patients already showing impairment of renal function. Our experience has been that at such blood pressures improvement of renal function is more likely to occur. In most cases no additional therapy besides angiotensin converting enzyme inhibitors is required. We would particularly avoid diuretics because they tend to further decrease renal perfusion pressure and may aggravate what is often already a hyperreninemic state. Glucocorticoids have not been shown to be of any value in treatment and indeed may aggravate the hypertension and renal disease.

Ideally one would like to institute treatment of scleroderma hypertension before it becomes symptomatic. For this reason it is wise to teach patients to take their own blood pressure weekly. A trend toward rising blood pressures (e.g., from 110/70 to 150/90) would warrant treatment even if the diastolic blood pressure remained technically within the normal range. Here also we would be inclined to treat with angiotensin converting enzyme inhibitors rather than with milder antihypertensive drugs.

Sjögren's Syndrome

About 25 percent of the patients with scleroderma also suffer from Sjögren's syndrome, a polyglandular exocrinopathy resulting in decreased tear and saliva production. Increased dental caries often result from decreased saliva flow, and patients complaining of dry mouth should undergo frequent dental check-ups and should observe scrupulous dental hygeine. The decreased oral aperture in patients with scleroderma makes dental work and dental hygiene more difficult. Patients complaining of dry gritty eyes should be given artifical tears during the day and lubricating ophthalmic ointments for use at night. There is no systemic pharmacologic agent to increase tear and saliva production.

THE ROLE OF DISEASE MODIFYING DRUGS

Many drugs have been tried to alter the course of scleroderma in a global way. These have included antiinflammatory drugs, such as colchicine, immunosuppressive drugs, including corticosteroids and cytotoxic drugs, and p-aminobenzoate, which has been advocated as an antifibrosis drug. Unfortunately reports of success with these drugs have been largely anecdotal, and efficacy has not been reproducibly demonstrated. Preliminary studies suggest that recombinant gamma-interferon may ameliorate the disease, but await confirmation. Recent reports of the successful use of plasmapheresis, lymphoplasmapheresis, and photopheresis, are encouraging but require further documentation.

Attention has focused recently on D-penicillamine, a chelating drug that can prevent extracellular collagen fibril cross linking by reversibly blocking aldehyde groups on the fibril surface. D-penicillamine also may decrease the rate of collagen synthesis and increase the rate of collagen degradation. In addition, it has suppressive effects on T lymphocytes in vitro and could mediate an effect based on suppression of synthesis of lymphokines, which stimulate collagen synthesis.

All the studies with penicillamine have been uncontrolled and have largely been retrospective. There is, however, a suggestion that progression of skin disease can be slowed by the drug. Data suggesting that the development of renal crisis or pulmonary fibrosis may be prevented in some patients by the early use of penicillamine are inconclusive at best. The patients who have the most to gain from D-penicillamine are those with rapidly progressive, diffuse skin disease, since these are the patients for whom slowing of the skin progression would be most beneficial. This subgroup may also be the patients at greatest risk of developing pulmonary or renal involvement. The natural history of scleroderma is often one of gradual spontaneous skin softening after several years, and therefore patients with long-standing stable skin disease would be less likely to benefit from penicillamine. Likewise patients with the CREST syndrome, who have little skin involvement and who rarely develop renal crises or pulmonary fibrosis, would be less likely to benefit from penicillamine treatment. Penicillamine therefore should be reserved for patients with a recent onset of the disease (within 2 years) in whom noticeable progression of skin disease occurs over a period of months.

Treatment with penicillamine should not be undertaken lightly because its toxicity is great. The range of toxicity observed in patients with scleroderma who are taking penicillamine is similar to that observed in those with rheumatoid arthritis treated with this drug and includes rash, dysgeusia, stomatitis, blood dyscrasias, and proteinuria due to membranous nephritis. Patients with scleroderma seem to have a higher incidence than do patients with rheumatoid arthritis of developing pemphigus and myasthenia gravis secondary to penicillamine treatment. In about one patient in five the drug must be permanently discontinued within several months because of a serious side effect.

If treatment with penicillamine is begun, the initial dosage should be 250 mg per day for the average sized adult. The leukocyte count, hemoglobin level, platelet count, and urinalysis should be monitored weekly. If the drug is tolerated, the dosage should be increased gradually, no faster than 250 mg per day per month, until maximal dosages of 750 to 1500 mg per day are reached. Even with a maximal dosage it may take 6 months or more before any clinical effects are seen. There are no established guidelines for deciding when the drug dosage should be gradually tapered and then discontinued, but in patients who respond to the drug, therapy probably should be continued at the maximal dosage for at least 1 year before attempts are made to slowly reduce the daily dosage.

In general, corticosteroids and cytotoxic drugs do not have a role in the treatment of scleroderma. There are, however, several noteworthy exceptions. Corticosteroids in modest dosages (10 to 30 mg per day of prednisone) may provide symptomatic relief in the early edematous phase of skin involvement with scleroderma, before induration sets in; the dosage should be tapered rapidly to 10 mg daily or less. Likewise corticosteroids in high dosages or cytotoxic drugs may be of use in patients with early, rapidly progressive pulmonary interstitial fibrosis, as described earlier. Symptomatic myositis, with elevated muscle enzyme levels, requires corticosteroid therapy. However, many patients with scleroderma have persistent mild elevations (twice normal) of muscle enzyme levels, and corticosteroid therapy in these patients generally is not helpful. Pleuritis or pericarditis, which can accompany scleroderma, may respond to treatment with corticosteroids in modest doses.

In conclusion, systemic sclerosis presents a broad spectrum of disease activity. The underlying abnormalities causing the disease are poorly understood, and therefore therapies to treat the disease globally have so far been disappointing. With judicious use of medications to address abnormalities of specific organ systems, survival as well as the quality of life can be significantly improved. Finally the physician must spend the time to explain to the patient that although the disease cannot be cured, its worst manifestations can be controlled. Reassurance by the physician and emotional support remain an important part of the therapeutic armamentarium in this trying disease.

SUGGESTED READING

Clements PJ, et al. The relationship of arrhythmias and conduction disturbances to other manifestations of cardiopulmonary disease in progressive systemic sclerosis (PSS). Am J Med 1981; 71:38–46.

Korn JH, Leroy EC. Scleroderma. In: Cohen AS, ed. The principles and practice of medicine. Vol. 4. Rheumatology and immunology. New York: Grune & Stratton, 1979: 249–261.

Medsger TA Jr, et al. Survival with systemic sclerosis (scleroderma). A life table analysis of clinical and demographic factors in 309 patients. Ann Intern Med 1971; 75:369–376.

Smith CD, McKendry RJR. Controlled trial of nifedipende in the treatment of Raynaud's phenomenon. Lancet 1982; 2:1299–1301.

Steen VD, Medsger TA, Rodnan GP. D-penicillimine therapy in progressive systemic sclerosis (scleroderma), a retrospective analysis. Ann Intern Med 1982; 97:652–659.

Whitman HH, et al. Variable response to oral angiotensin-converting-enzyme blockade in hypertensive scleroderma patients. Arthritis Rheum 1982; 25:241–248.

DERMATOMYOSITIS AND POLYMYOSITIS

THOMAS R. CUPPS, M.D.

Polymyositis and dermatomyositis compose a heterogeneous group of clinical syndromes that have in common the diffuse nonsuppurative inflammatory damage of skeletal muscle. The term polymyositis is used when only skeletal muscle is involved; dermatomyositis is used when skin in addition to skeletal muscle is affected. Both may occur as isolated disease processes, or they may be associated with a number of collagen vascular diseases, including rheumatoid arthritis, systemic lupus erythematosus, scleroderma, systemic necrotizing vasculitis, and overlap syndromes. Inflammatory muscle disease in the pediatric age group is most commonly associated with a vasculitic component, with frequent involvement of the gastrointestinal tract. Involvement of organ systems other than skeletal muscles in the polymyositis-dermatomyositis complex is also recognized. Pulmonary involvement with a pattern of interstitial fibrosis or cardiac involvement with conduction or rhythm disturbances is present in a subset of these patients. The polymyositis-dermatomyositis complex in patients over the age of 40 years is associated with an increased incidence of malignant disease, the highest incidence being seen in patients who develop the disease after the age of 60 years.

The diagnosis of polymyositis-dermatomyositis is based on the finding of bilateral proximal muscle weakness with supportive laboratory findings, including elevated muscle enzyme levels (such as creatine kinase or aldolase); normal endocrine function; an electromyogram showing increased insertional activity, numerous fibrillation potentials and sharp waves at rest, and bizarre high frequency repetitive discharges; and characteristic muscle biopsy findings of a mononuclear cell infiltrate between the muscle fibers and around small vessels, necrosis, phagocytosis, and regeneration. The presence of cutaneous involvement of the eyelids, cheeks, the bridge of the nose, the front and back of the chest, and the extensor surfaces of the extremities with the characteristic erythematous to violaceous eruption completes the clinical spectrum of dermatomyositis.

The etiology of the polymyositis-dermatomyositis complex is unknown. Although viral agents have been suggested, there is little firmly established evidence of a causal role for any infectious agent. In the absence of an established infectious cause an immunologically mediated disease process has been postulated. Evidence to support a primary immunologically mediated mechanism is indirect. The presence of a predominantly mononuclear cell infiltrate in involved muscle supports the notion of immunologically mediated muscle damage. Cell mediated immune responses to myocytes have been reported in patients with inflammatory muscle disease. The association of the polymyositis-dermatomyositis complex with other apparently immunologically mediated disease processes also supports an immunologically mediated etiology.

THERAPY

General Considerations

Immunosuppressive drugs, including glucocorticosteroids and cytotoxic drugs, are the principle drugs used in the treatment of the polymyositis-dermatomyositis complex. These drugs are administered with the therapeutic goal of suppressing the inflammatory response in the skeletal muscles, restoring muscle strength and function, and preventing irreversible fibrotic changes. The use of immunosuppressive drugs in this disease is based on the assumption that the inflammatory muscle disease is immunologically mediated and on the improvement of certain patients during treatment with these drugs. There have been no long term double blinded prospective trials of these drugs to document therapeutic efficacy in the polymyositis-dermatomyositis complex. Despite this limitation, the use of immunosuppressive drugs remains the standard therapy for inflammatory muscle disease.

After the diagnosis of inflammatory muscle disease has been established, the possibility of an associated disease process should be considered as therapeutic decisions are being made. In the pediatric population the possibility of an associated vasculitic process, particularly of the bowel, should be considered. It is important to recognize that glucocorticosteroids may mask signs and symptoms of vasculitis induced bowel ischemia if present. In patients above the age of 40 years the possibility of associated malignant disease should be pursued as clinically indicated. The potential association with pulmonary and cardiac involvement should also be evaluated. The presence of an associated disease process may alter therapeutic decisions in individual patients.

Corticosteroid Therapy

Induction

Glucocorticosteroids in pharmacologic doses are the initial form of therapy in the majority of patients with the polymyositis-dermatomyositis complex. After the diagnosis has been established and an appropriate evaluation for associated disease processes considered, treatment should be expeditiously started. Prednisone therapy, started at 1 to 1.5 mg per kg as a single morning dose, is usually effective in patients with mild to moderately severe inflammatory muscle disease. Some subsets of patients may require more aggressive corticosteroid therapy.

Patients with cardiac or pulmonary involvement, severe muscle weakness, or functional impairment of the muscles of deglutition or respiration should be given split dose prednisone therapy. Prednisone, 20 mg orally four times a day, is one example of an aggressive therapeutic approach for the subset of patients with more severe involvement. In many patients started on therapy with split doses of prednisone, the dosage level can be rapidly tapered to a single daily dose during the initial weeks of therapy. It should be emphasized that the clinical response to corticosteroid therapy in this disease tends to be gradual and may not be apparent during the initial induction phase.

Management

The majority of patients with the polymyositis-dermatomyositis complex require prolonged treatment with pharmacologic doses of corticosteroids. To minimize the potential morbidity associated with long term corticosteroid therapy, the minimal effective dosage should be established for each patient. The monitoring of disease activity becomes crucial in decisions to modulate the corticosteroid dosage. Both clinical and laboratory parameters should be determined on a regular basis to define disease activity. Serial determinations of muscle strength should be recorded using the Medical Research Council scale (0, no movement of muscle groups; 1, flicker of movement; 2, movement with gravity eliminated; 3, movement against gravity but not against resistance; 4, movement against resistance; and 5, normal). In patients with impaired respiratory muscle function, serial determinations of the forced vital capacity also may be a useful parameter to follow.

The clinical response to corticosteroid therapy is characteristically slow and gradual. The majority of patients begin to show evidence of improved muscle strength 2 to 12 weeks after starting therapy. Delayed responses 4 to 6 months after starting therapy have been reported. In patients with dermatomyositis, the heliotrope pattern of the skin rash and the eruptions on the extensor surfaces may vary regardless of the muscle weakness; consequently the cutaneous involvement should not be used as a guide in therapeutic decisions.

Serial laboratory determinations provide useful information in evaluating disease activity. Although the creatine kinase determination is the single most sensitive and most specific muscle enzyme test in the diagnosis of the polymyositis-dermatomyositis complex, the test should be used advisedly in patients treated with corticosteroids. The use of pharmacologic doses of corticosteroids "nonspecifically" decreases the creatine kinase level. This corticosteroid associated reduction of the creatine kinase level has been noted in individuals with noninflammatory muscle disease as well as in those without muscle disease. A decrease in the level after starting corticosteroid therapy may reflect this nonspecific response rather than a true decrease in the skeletal muscle inflammation. Of note, another muscle associated enzyme, aldolase, does not appear to be affected "nonspecifically" by corticosteroid therapy. Serial aldolase levels, if initially elevated, may be a more reliable guide to underlying disease activity. Although elevated in some patients presenting with the polymyositis-dermatomyositis complex, the erythrocyte sedimentation rate is not a reliable indicator of disease activity in the majority of patients.

In cases of generally slow clinical responses to the corticosteroids, every effort should be made to establish the minimal effective dosage of this drug. Following the initial clinical improvement one should consider a gradual tapering of the corticosteroid dosage. The tapering should be carried out gradually because of the striking tendency to exacerbate the underlying inflammatory muscle disease during rapid tapering of corticosteroid dosages. An alternate day corticosteroid regimen produces less drug associated morbidity than the daily regimens and is preferable if this therapeutic approach is effective in treating the underlying disease.

Although the precise tapering schedule should be established on a patient by patient basis, the following approach is one example of a gradual tapering to an alternate day program. Starting from a single daily morning dose of 60 mg of prednisone, decrease the alternate day dosage of prednisone by 10 mg, resulting in a schedule of 60 mg as the single morning dose alternating with 50 mg as the single morning dose. After 2 weeks again drop the alternate day dose, resulting in a schedule of 60 mg alternating with 40 mg. Clinical and laboratory assessment of the disease activity should be carried out on a regular basis and the pace of the tapering adjusted accordingly. If the patient remains clinically stable, continue the tapering. A 10 mg dose of prednisone is dropped from the low day dosage regimen every 2 weeks until a dosage regimen of 60 mg alternating with 20 mg is established. At this point the tapering schedule is slowed to a reduction of 5 mg of prednisone from the low dose day every 2 weeks until a dosage of 60 mg alternating with 10 mg is obtained. Finally the alternate day low dosage is reduced by 2.5 mg every 3 to 4 weeks until a schedule of 60 mg alternating with an "off" day is established. The alternate day high dose may then be gradually tapered as tolerated. Not all patients tolerate tapering to an alternate day regimen. If the inflammatory muscle disease cannot be adequately controlled on an alternate day regimen, the prednisone dosage should be increased back to a level that was effective in controlling the disease and tapering to a low dosage daily regimen initiated once the disease process is adequately controlled.

The taper to a low dosage daily regimen should be done gradually also. The following is one example of such a prednisone taper. Starting from a single dose of 60 mg of prednisone, taper the dosage 10 mg every 2 weeks until the patient is taking 40 mg a day. At this point the tapering is slowed to lowering the dosage of prednisone by 5 mg every 2 weeks until a dosage of 20 mg a day is established. From 20 mg a day the prednisone dosage is tapered by 2.5 mg every 2 weeks until a maintenance dosage of 10 mg is reached. It is important to emphasize that these suggested corticosteroid tapering schedules are examples and will undoubtedly require some modification when used in individual patients.

Although the optimal duration of treatment varies with each patient, extended treatment periods are characteristically required. The majority of patients require treatment for 2 to 3 years. A subset of patients may respond to shorter periods of therapy. In patients who obtain complete clinical remission rapidly, an attempt to taper and discontinue the corticosteroids after 1 year of therapy should be considered. Although some patients require more prolonged therapy, approximately 75 percent can stop therapy within 5 years after starting treatment. A subset of patients require more prolonged corticosteroid therapy to suppress disease activity and may remain corticosteroid dependent for an extended period.

The management of patients with polymyositis-dermatomyositis who develop recurrent or progressive proximal muscle weakness after an established response to corticosteroid therapy requires special consideration. The use of daily pharmacologic doses of corticosteroids is associated with type 2 muscle fiber atrophy. In some patients progressive atrophy results in a clinically significant corticosteroid myopathy characterized by proximal weakness similar in pattern to the weakness seen in active myositis. The presence of prominent atrophy, proportionately greater weakness in the lower extremities, prolonged use of daily or split dose regimens, and normal serum muscle enzyme levels suggest the possibility of corticosteroid induced myopathy. Reduction of the corticosteroid dosage results in a gradual increase in muscle strength if the weakness is due to drug induced myopathy. By contrast, if the weakness is secondary to the underlying myositis, reduction of the corticosteroid dosage will result in increasing muscle weakness and rising enzyme levels.

In some patients the drug and inflammatory myopathies may contribute to clinical weakness; consequently a follow-up muscle biopsy may provide useful information by identifying the dominant pathologic process. In addition to drug induced myopathy, patients with the polymyositis-dermatomyositis complex associated with malignant disease may respond initially to corticosteroids and then develop progressive muscle weakness despite continued treatment with previously effective dosages of corticosteroids. In older patients with refractory myositis or progressive disease after an initial therapeutic response, the possibility of an underlying neoplastic process should be reconsidered.

Morbidity

Prolonged daily corticosteroid therapy can produce significant associated morbidity. The potential side effects of prolonged corticosteroid therapy are summarized in the chapter *Temporal Arteritis*. Although the nature and extent of adverse side effects vary from individual to individual, higher dosages, increased frequency of administration, and prolonged therapy increase the likelihood of corticosteroid induced morbidity. To minimize the morbidity associated with this drug, the minimal effective dosage should be established for each individual. Limiting the patient's exposure to corticosteroids decreases the likelihood of development of dose related side effects. Clinical concerns for the management of patients treated with corticosteroids are summarized in Table 1.

Cytotoxic Therapy

Cytotoxic drugs have been widely used in conjunction with corticosteroid therapy in polymyositis-dermatomyositis. There appears to be little difference in the therapeutic effects of the two most commonly used drugs, methotrexate and azathioprine. A cytotoxic drug is generally added to the prednisone regimen when the latter produces an inadequate response after 2 to 4 months. Anecdotal experience suggests that patients with disease that is more severe or of longer duration obtain greater benefit if combined therapy with prednisone and a cytotoxic drug such as azathioprine is started simultaneously. The cytotoxic immunosuppressive drugs may

TABLE 1 Management Considerations in Patients Treated with Corticosteroids

Problem	*Clinical Considerations*
Increased risk of infection	Intermediate PPD skin test with anergy panel prior to therapy; clinical follow-up of opportunistic infection
Glucose intolerance	Urinalysis for glucose; serum glucose level
Cushingoid features, truncal obesity	Dietary counseling to avoid weight gain; follow weights closely
Osteopenia	Prophylactic therapy: calcium 500 mg p.o., t.i.d., or q.i.d.; vitamin D 25,000 to 50,000 units twice weekly
Gastric distress	Antacids, H_2 blockers, sulcralfate
Hypothalamic-pituitary-adrenal axis suppression	Educate patient about the potential for Addisonian crisis and need for parenteral corticosteroid therapy if he is unable to take oral medication >24 h

produce an "additive" as well as a "corticosteroid sparing" therapeutic effect.

Methotrexate

Methotrexate is a folic acid analogue that inhibits thymidine and hence DNA synthesis by suppressing dihydrofolate reductase function. Therapy has been reported to result in clinical improvement in more than half the corticosteroid unresponsive patients. The drug can be administered with prednisone or by itself. Intravenous administration may cause fewer side effects. Drug administration is started on a once a week schedule with an initial dosage of 10 to 12 mg (approximately 0.2 mg per kg). The dosage is increased by the same weekly increment to a maximum of 40 to 50 mg (0.7 to 0.8 mg per kg). A clinical response may be seen as early as 6 weeks, but the maximal response may not be realized for 3 to 5 months. As the patient responds clinically, the frequency of administration can be decreased to every 2 weeks and then every 3 weeks until a maintenance schedule of once a month administration is realized. As the patient responds to the methotrexate, the prednisone dosage also can be tapered in the majority of cases. The total duration of therapy may extend from months to 2 years. Intramuscular administration should be avoided because of the potential for local muscle injury and noninflammatory elevations of muscle enzyme levels.

A program of intermittent oral administration of methotrexate has also been tried in patients with inflammatory muscle disease. Drug administration is started at 2.5 mg orally every 12 hours for a total of three doses over 1½ days once a week. If this level is tolerated, the individual dose can be increased to 5 mg. The total weekly dosage should not exceed 20 mg of methotrexate.

Information about the relative safety and efficacy of intravenous versus oral administration of methotrexate in patients with polymyositis-dermatomyositis is currently not available. Side effects such as stomatitis, diarrhea, and intestinal ulceration may necessitate dosage reduction, particularly in the setting of decreased renal function. More severe side effects of methotrexate therapy include necrotizing alveolitis and hepatic fibrosis leading to cirrhosis. Liver cirrhosis is a significant long term complication of methotrexate therapy and the risk is related to the cumulative dosage of the drug. Liver function studies are not particularly sensitive indicators of hepatic fibrosis, and some authors recommend liver biopsies after a total dosage of 1.5 to 2.0 g of the drug has been administered. Patients without risk factors for methotrexate-associated fibrosis may not require a liver biopsy until an even larger total dose of the drug has been administered. Optimal management of this potential drug related problem has not been clearly defined. Because ethanol consumption, diabetes mellitus, and obesity appear to be risk factors for the development of methotrexate associated fibrosis, the presence of these parameters is a relative contraindication to use of this drug. Patients with one of these risk factors who are treated with methotrexate should be followed with liver biopsies. Liver function studies should be carried out and a hemogram should be obtained every 2 to 4 weeks.

Azathioprine

Azathioprine is a purine analogue that inhibits purine biosynthesis. Therapy may be effective in one third of the patients with polymyositis-dermatomyositis that are refractory to corticosteroid therapy. Azathioprine generally is used in conjunction with prednisone to produce the so-called "corticosteroid sparing effect." The drug is administered orally at a dosage of 1.5 to 2.5 mg per kg. The clinical response to azathioprine does not appear to be as rapid as that with methotrexate, the maximal effect requiring 6 to 12 months. Attempts to taper the prednisone dosage can be initiated after about 3 months of azathioprine therapy. Prolonged use of low dose azathioprine therapy is feasible for several years if clinically indicated. The most common potential side effects include myelosuppression and drug induced hepatitis. Rare drug associated complications include pulmonary fibrosis, acute febrile reactions, and a slightly increased risk of malignant disease. Serial hemograms should be obtained and liver function studies done every 2 weeks during the initiation of therapy and every 4 weeks after the first 6 months of therapy.

Cyclophosphamide

Cyclophosphamide (a DNA alkylating drug) may be useful in treating refractory cases of inflammatory disease. Because of the potential for greater drug associated toxicity, the use of cyclophosphamide is reserved for patients who prove to be refractory to methotrexate, azathioprine, and prednisone. Cyclophosphamide therapy is started as a single morning dose of 2 mg per kg. Subsequently the dose is modified to maintain the total white cell count above 3,500 cells per cubic mm. The clinical response to cyclophosphamide is more rapid than that to azathioprine. Tapering to an alternate day prednisone regimen should be initiated 2 to 3 weeks after starting cyclophosphamide therapy. It should be emphasized that the combination of daily prednisone and cyclophosphamide is a very immunosuppressive regimen with a substantially increased risk of opportunistic infections. By contrast, a properly managed regimen of alternate day prednisone and cyclophosphamide therapy is generally well tolerated by the majority of patients. The side effects of cyclophosphamide include bone marrow suppression, hemorrhagic cystitis, bladder fibrosis, neoplastic transformation (acute myelocytic leukemia, bladder carcinoma), risk of infection, ovarian failure, sterility, and alopecia. The clinical management of patients treated with cyclophosphamide is discussed in more detail in the chapter on *Temporal Arteritis* in this book. Chlorambucil has been used in severe refractory cases and in patients who have developed unacceptable side effects with cyclophosphamide.

Alternative Therapies

A number of therapeutic approaches have been tried in patients with polymyositis-dermatomyositis who are refractory to the more standard forms of treatment. Anecdotal experience suggests that these approaches may work in selected individual cases, although none is uniformly successful in all refractory patients. High dose "pulse methylprednisolone" can be tried in unresponsive patients. Methylprednisolone (30 mg per kg) should be infused over 30 to 45 minutes. Different infusion protocols have been suggested. One approach is to carry out three infusions on 3 consecutive days. A second approach is infuse on alternating days for a total of six infusions. The infusion protocols generally are used in addition to other immunosuppressive therapy. The clinical management of patients treated with pulse methylprednisolone protocols is discussed in more detail in the chapter on *Temporal Arteritis* in this book.

Plasmapheresis has been used in refractory cases with limited success at some centers. Levamisole (a single 100 mg dose once a week) has been added to standard immunosuppressive regimens (prednisone with a cytotoxic drug) in refractory cases. The combination of corticosteroids, chlorambucil, and methotrexate has been used successfully in patients with refractory inflammatory muscle disease.

The successful use of cyclosporin A in the treatment of refractory polymyositis-dermatomyositis has also been reported. Drug therapy was started initially at a dosage of 7.5 to 10 mg per kg per day but was reduced to a level of 5 mg per kg per day because of associated renal toxicity. Rapid clinical and laboratory improvements after 1 to 2 weeks of therapy have been noted. Of particular importance is the high frequency of renal toxicity in patients treated with this particular protocol. Because marked individual variability in the metabolism of cyclosporin A has been reported, drug blood level determinations are required for safe administration. Close monitoring of the blood pressure and renal function parameters (blood urea nitrogen and creatinine levels) is advised.

Physical Medicine

Physiotherapy is an important aspect of the treatment of patients with the polymyositis-dermatomyositis complex. During the period of acute inflammation, excessive muscle strain should be avoided. It is, however, important to maintain flexibility with passive range of motion exercises. As the inflammatory process is controlled, the patient can progress to an active range of motion program. The increase in physical activity should be gradual as the disease is put into remission. Extreme muscle exertion should be avoided.

SUGGESTED READING

Ansell BM. Management of polymyositis and dermatomyositis. Clin Rheum Dis 1984; 10:205–213.

Bendtzen K, Tvede N, Andersen V, Bendixen G. Cyclosporin for polymyositis. Lancet 1984; 1:792–793.

Bradley GW. Inflammatory diseases of muscle. In: Kelley WN, Harris ED Jr, Ruddy S, Sledge CB, eds. Textbook of rheumatology. 2nd ed. Philadelphia: WB Saunders 1985.

Henriksson KG, Sandstedt P. Polymyositis—treatment and prognosis. A study of 107 patients. Acta Neurol Scand 1982; 65:280–300.

REITER'S SYNDROME

PAUL KATZ, M.D.

Historically the diagnosis of Reiter's syndrome was applied to patients with the clinical tetrad of arthritis, nongonococcal urethritis, conjunctivitis, and typical mucocutaneous lesions. However, it is now apparent that it may not only affect young males. It is recognized that "incomplete" forms of the disease exist in which not all these manifestations are present. Some females with oligoarthritis primarily involving the lower extremities who originally were misdiagnosed as having seronegative rheumatoid arthritis are afflicted with Reiter's syndrome. Furthermore, the disease may have manifestations other than those in the classic tetrad (Table 1).

Reiter's syndrome most frequently occurs in genetically susceptible individuals exposed to specific microorganisms. Thus, 60 to 80 percent of the patients have the HLA-B27 antigen. Infectious agents known to "trigger" Reiter's syndrome generally fall into two classes: postvenereal (or endemic) secondary to Chlamydia or Ureaplasma, and postdysenteric (or epidemic) related to Salmonella, *Shigella flexneri*, Yersinia, and Campylobacter. Nonetheless patients frequently have no history that suggests infection with either group of organisms. Perhaps 25 percent of HLA-B27 positive individuals

TABLE 1 Clinical Manifestations of Reiter's Syndrome During the Initial Attack

Signs or Symptoms	*Frequency (%)*
Musculoskeletal	100
Tendinitis	25
Back pain	50
Heel pain	40
Polyarthritis	80
Monarthritis	15
Sausage digits	20
Genitourinary	90
Urethritis	85
Cervicitis	70
Conjunctivitis	60
Skin lesions	50
Keratodermia blennorrhagica	15
Balanitis	40
Nail changes	10
Fever	35
Weight loss	40

exposed to these agents develop Reiter's syndrome. The manifestations of Reiter's syndrome are not secondary to persistence of the offending bacterium, but rather constitute an aberrant "reactive" host response to the infection, which can develop and recur despite absence of the organism.

Although many patients have an initial acute illness that does not reappear, most patients have chronic or recurrent symptoms. Five years after the onset approximately 80 percent of the patients with Reiter's syndrome are still symptomatic. Apart from an increased incidence of chronic uveitis and sacroiliitis in HLA-B27 positive individuals after 5 years, there is no difference in outcome between HLA-B27 positive and HLA-B27 negative patients or between males and females.

APPROACH TO THE PATIENT

Diagnosis

A primary problem in the approach to the patient with Reiter's syndrome is establishing the correct diagnosis. Unfortunately there may be significant delays in patients with atypical presentations or those lacking the clinical tetrad. As already noted and shown in Table 1, there may be confusion in the diagnosis or even a misdiagnosis because of the rarity of the disease and its protean manifestations. Additionally some patients with Reiter's syndrome have an acute and self-limited course; these patients are disserved by long term treatment with potentially toxic drugs.

Patient Education

The importance of patient education cannot be overemphasized. Because of the perceived stigma of a disease that may be sexually acquired, the inability to predict the natural history and outcome, the periods of remission and exacerbation, and the lack of a "cure," it is incumbent upon the physician treating patients with Reiter's syndrome to inform them of these potential problems. The concept of a disease initiated by an infection but not responsive to antibiotics is often difficult for patients to grasp. Affected individuals may benefit from a comparison of Reiter's syndrome to an "allergy" in which environmental agents "cause" the symptoms. It is probably imprudent to speak of the potential long term problems of the disease with patients who have been ill for less than 2 to 3 months, since some of these subjects will never have a recurrence.

Given the genetic predisposition to Reiter's syndrome, patients may express concern about the possibility of the disease in offspring. It should be emphasized that even if the affected individual is HLA-B27 positive, there is only a 50 percent chance that any child will carry this haplotype. Should the child have this antigen, there is only a 20 to 25 percent chance that he will develop Reiter's syndrome, and the likelihood of this is dependent upon contact with the offending agent. Therefore, patients should be told that the chance of "passing" the disease to a son or daughter is relatively low and that there is no reason to avoid childbearing.

Physical and Local Therapy

Articular and Periarticular Disorders

The importance of physical and local treatment in the management of Reiter's syndrome cannot be overemphasized. As is the case with any acute arthritis, inflamed joints initially should be rested and even splinted if necessary. Once the inflammation has begun to subside, range of motion exercises and maintenance of muscle strength should be instituted under the supervision of a physical therapist. Individuals afflicted with chronic arthritis and joint dysfunction should receive maintenance therapy and instruction in ways to carry out the activities of daily living.

Since Reiter's syndrome often involves the lower extremities, patients with foot symptoms may benefit from orthotics, shoe inserts, or custom shoes; this treatment often can be facilitated through consultation with an experienced podiatrist.

Patients with localized enthesopathies, tendinitis, or monarticular arthritis despite systemic therapy often can be aided by local corticosteroid injections. Tendon injection with corticosteroids should be performed carefully because of the danger of tendon rupture induced by overzealous infiltration. The use of a mixture of a local anesthetic and a depot corticosteroid preparation often can produce prompt and long lasting relief from tendinitis. Intra-articular corticosteroid injections in patients with one or two disproportionately "active" joints may be useful and may avoid changes in treatment in a patient who is otherwise doing well. My experience with corticosteroid injections in Reiter's syndrome is similar to that of others: although many patients respond, the results are usually not as dramatic or as lasting as those in rheumatoid arthritis or gout.

Ocular Disorders

The mild conjunctivitis that may accompany Reiter's syndrome usually does not require therapy; however, this determination should be made by an opthalmologist, who should also look for anterior uveitis. Symptomatic conjunctivitis or uveitis usually remits with topical or intralesional corticosteroid therapy. Some patients may report a response to systemic treatment with anti-inflammatory drugs; nonetheless topical treatment of the eye symptoms of Reiter's syndrome is preferable.

Mucocutaneous Lesions

The circinate balanitis, keratodermia blennorrhagica, and nail lesions of Reiter's syndrome are usually asymptomatic or mildly symptomatic and require no therapy. Because of the risk of corticosteroid induced skin atrophy, these compounds generally should be avoided except when lesions on the soles or palms are so severe as to limit function.

Pulmonary Disease

A late complication of Reiter's syndrome may be the development of apical fibrosis and cavitary disease similar to that in ankylosing spondylitis. This unusual condition needs to be recognized in order to avoid needless diagnostic intervention. The complication of a secondary mycetoma, or fungus ball, and the possible need for surgical resection should be appreciated.

Cardiac Disease

Pericarditis, conduction abnormalities, and aortic regurgitation are recognized complications of Reiter's syndrome. Pericarditis and conduction abnormalities are most common early in the disease and require systemic anti-inflammatory therapy such as the nonsteroidal drugs (see next section) or corticosteroids. Fewer patients develop chronic conduction disturbances or aortic regurgitation, and these problems and the need for invasive therapy should be guided by a cardiologist.

Systemic Therapy

Anti-inflammatory Therapy

The nonsteroidal anti-inflammatory drugs are the primary therapeutic modalities in Reiter's syndrome, and most patients require these drugs at some time during the course of the illness. Numerous drugs are available (Table 2), and a logical scheme is dependent upon the physician's familiarity with the drugs, side effects, efficacy, and cost. These drugs are not approved for use in Reiter's syndrome, yet their proven effectiveness is established. Unlike therapy in rheumatoid arthritis or osteoarthritis, salicylates are generally not useful in Reiter's syndrome. Historically indomethacin has been the drug used initially by most rheumatologists, since phenylbutazone has fallen into disfavor (to be discussed). It may be that indomethacin is considered the first drug of choice because it has been available longer than any of the "modern" nonsteroidal anti-inflammatory drugs. Nonetheless there are many rheumatologists, including myself, who generally begin treatment with indomethacin with the doses listed in Table 2. Therapy, if tolerated, is continued for at least 2 to 3 weeks, the time that may be required for a maximal response to be observed. If the patient has not responded to maximal doses of indomethacin, or if unacceptable side effects have occurred, I switch to another nonsteroidal anti-inflammatory drug, usually in a different chemical class (Table 2). Again a 2 to 3 week trial is mandatory with

TABLE 2 Commonly Used Nonsteroidal Anti-inflammatory Drugs for Reiter's Syndrome

Chemical Group	*Dosage Interval*	*Maximal Daily Dosage (mg)*
Propionic acid		
Ibuprofen	tid–qid	3,200
Naproxen	bid	1,500
Fenoprofen	tid–qid	2,400
Ketoprofen	tid–qid	300
Indole derivatives		
Indomethacin	tid–qid	200
Sulindac	bid	400
Tolectin	tid–qid	1,600
Pyrazolones		
Phenylbutazone	tid–qid	400
Fenamates		
Meclofenamate	tid–qid	400
Oxicams		
Piroxicam	qd	20

any of these drugs before considering the trial a "failure." It may be necessary to try multiple nonsteroidal anti-inflammatory drugs until one is found that is efficacious and well tolerated. Patients should be told that all these drugs are effective but that there is great variability in the response from patient to patient.

Although originally it was a first line drug for the treatment of Reiter's syndrome, the toxicity of phenylbutazone (to be discussed) as well as the availability of other nonsteroidal anti-inflammatory drugs has made it a second line choice. Nevertheless, I occasionally utilize this drug for a 1 to 2 week period in patients with severe Reiter's syndrome that has been unresponsive to other drugs. In this group, phenylbutazone may reduce the activity of a "flare" and permit the institution of therapy with another nonsteroidal anti-inflammatory drug.

Nonsteroidal anti-inflammatory drug therapy should be continued as long as the patient is symptomatic. It is desirable to utilize as low a dosage as possible to reduce the likelihood of complications. Some patients may be capable of achieving many "drug free" periods when the disease is quiescent.

Unfortunately the beneficial effects of the nonsteroidal anti-inflammatory drugs are often limited by their side effects, which in some instances may be life threatening. A partial list of the toxic effects of these drugs is contained in Table 3. Nonsteroidal anti-inflammatory drugs exert their effects on the inflammatory and immune responses through inhibition of the enzyme cyclooxygenase, which catalyzes an early step in the synthesis of prostaglandins. Thus, many (but not all) of the adverse effects of these drugs are secondary to local decreases in prostaglandin production.

Gastrointestinal symptoms are the most common side effects of this class of drugs and can include dyspepsia, nausea, vomiting, abdominal pain, constipation, diarrhea, erosions, ulcers, and hemorrhage. There is often poor correlation between abdominal symptoms and the severity of nonsteroidal anti-inflammatory drug induced lesions; thus patients with significant mucosal ulceration and massive hemorrhage may have no preceding symptoms, whereas patients with significant abdominal pain may have normal endoscopically visualized mucosa. Elderly patients or those with renal, liver, or cardiac disease may have significant reductions in glomerular filtration due to inhibition of prostaglandin dependent renal blood flow; in this group particular caution should be exercised when using a nonsteroidal anti-inflammatory drug. I generally avoid using longer acting drugs (e.g., piroxicam) in these individuals. There are data that suggest that sulindac may have less effect on renal blood flow, and this drug may be tried cautiously in patients at risk. The reduction in the glomerular filtration rate is generally reversible upon discontinuation of the nonsteroidal anti-inflammatory drug. Other renal side effects such as the nephrotic syndrome, allergic interstitial nephritis, and renal tubular acidosis can occur with any of these drugs.

TABLE 3 Side Effects of Nonsteroidal Anti-inflammatory Drugs

Gastrointestinal	Dyspepsia, nausea, vomiting, abdominal pain, constipation, diarrhea, ulcers, gastric erosions, hemorrhage
Renal	Edema, azotemia, proteinuria, nephrotic syndrome, allergic interstitial nephritis, renal tubular acidosis
Hematologic	Platelet dysfunction, agranulocytosis, aplasia, potentiation of anticoagulant action
Hepatic	Liver function abnormalities, jaundice
Cardiac	Congestive failure, hypertension
Central nervous system	Headache, cognitive dysfunction, depression, lethargy
Pulmonary	Asthma in aspirin sensitive individuals, hypersensitivity pneumonitis
Allergic	Hypersensitivity reactions, asthma in aspirin sensitive individuals

Platelet dysfunction related to prostaglandin inhibition is observed in the presence of active drug; this is reversible upon discontinuation of therapy with the offending drug. Hepatic toxicity with increased serum transaminase levels is not uncommon, but two- to threefold increases do not necessitate discontinuation of the drug. These elevations are reversible, however. Hyperbilirubinemia is more serious and calls for cessation of drug use.

Central nervous system symptoms are also observed, headache being the most common complaint. This is a particular problem with indomethacin. Cognitive dysfunction, depression, and lethargy are also reported, especially in older age groups. As is the case with most drugs, true allergic reactions can occur with nonsteroidal anti-inflammatory drugs; in such cases it may be relatively safe to switch to a drug in another chemical class.

As noted, the idiosyncratic and dose dependent toxic effects of phenylbutazone have limited its present day utility. The aplastic anemia originally reported was most commonly observed with long term use in the elderly. However, the unpredictable agranulocytosis that occurs within weeks after beginning therapy with the drug is of grave concern, and patients should be monitored with frequent white cell counts while receiving this drug.

Antibiotics

Despite the infectious "trigger" in most cases of Reiter's syndrome, there are no data indicating that persistent infection is responsible for symptoms. However, some patients with urethritis may respond to treatment with doxycycline or tetracycline.

Corticosteroids

Apart from topical, intra-articular, and periarticular treatment, corticosteroids are rarely indicated in patients with Reiter's syndrome. However, selected individuals with severe systemic symptoms may respond to short courses of low dose prednisone therapy (5 to 10 mg per day). This drug may be useful while awaiting the hoped-for beneficial effects of conventional drugs.

Cytotoxic Drugs

Although most patients with Reiter's syndrome respond to the foregoing therapies, there are a few whose arthritis and mucocutaneous disease mandate more aggressive treatment. In general, the remittive drugs used in rheumatoid arthritis are of no proven efficacy in Reiter's syndrome. Although there are few data regarding the controlled use of cytotoxic drugs, it appears that methotrexate and azathioprine may be useful in selected patients.

Because of similarities between the cutaneous lesions of psoriasis and those of Reiter's syndrome, there are reports of the successful use of methotrexate in Reiter's syndrome. I have used this drug in long term, low dose therapy (similar to the protocols for psoriasis and rheumatoid arthritis) and have found it to be efficacious in many patients. The drug can be given parenterally or orally as a single weekly dose. Treatment is usually begun with 5 mg per week, and the dosage is gradually increased in 2.5 to 5.0 mg increments; the usual maintenance dosage is approximately 15 to 20 mg per week. Joint symptoms usually decrease after the skin disease is controlled.

A number of side effects of methotrexate may curtail therapy. Included among these are mucositis, leukopenia, and pneumonitis. Liver fibrosis with prolonged methotrexate treatment has been reported in psoriasis, and this may not be detectable with liver function tests. Patients with pre-existing liver disease, hepatitis B antigenemia, or alcohol abuse should undergo a premethotrexate liver biopsy with a subsequent biopsy after a cumulative dosage of 1.5 g has been given. Liver biopsy in patients who are not at risk for liver disease is controversial; in general, I have not obtained tissue in these subjects.

Another cytotoxic drug that has been employed less frequently in Reiter's syndrome is azathioprine. Limited experience suggests that 1 to 2 mg per kg per day of this drug as a single oral dose may be effective in some patients with Reiter's syndrome. The major side effect of this drug, namely, leukopenia, may limit its use in this disease.

SUGGESTED READING

Fox R, Calin A, Gerber RC, Gibson D. The chronicity of symptoms and disability in Reiter's syndrome. An analysis of 131 consecutive cases. Ann Intern Med 1979; 91:190–193.

Keat A. Reiter's syndrome and reactive arthritis in perspective. N Engl J Med 1983; 309:1606–1615.

Lally EV, Ho G Jr. A review of methotrexate therapy in Reiter's syndrome. Sem Arthritis Rheum 1985; 15:139–145.

Willkens RF, Arnett FC, Bitter T, Calin A, Fisher L, Ford DK, Good AE, Masi AT. Reiter's syndrome. Evaluation of preliminary criteria for definite diagnosis. Bull Rheum Dis 1982; 32:31–34.

Wright V. Seronegative polyarthritis, a unified concept. Arthritis Rheum 1978; 21:619–633.

SJÖGREN'S SYNDROME

ELAINE L. ALEXANDER, M.D., Ph.D.

Sjögren's syndrome is a common autoimmune connective tissue disorder, which conservatively affects 2 percent of the adult population (more than 4 million Americans), the majority of whom are women (9:1). The disorder is often unrecognized or misdiagnosed by unsuspecting patients and physicians because of the characteristic insidious, slowly progressive, and subtle symptoms. The term autoimmune exocrinopathy has been used to describe the sicca (dryness) manifestations caused by progressive infiltration and destruction of salivary, lacrimal, and other glands by mononuclear inflammatory cells (predominantly lymphocytes and plasma cells). The syndrome has not only glandular (nonsystemic) but also extraglandular (systemic) manifestations. The disorder can occur alone (primary Sjögren's syndrome) or may be associated with another connective tissue disorder (secondary Sjögren's syndrome). Secondary Sjögren's syndrome most commonly is associated with rheumatoid arthritis and less commonly with systemic lupus erythematosus, progressive systemic sclerosis, or overlap syndromes or a lymphoproliferative disorder (benign [pseudolymphoma or angioblastic lymphadenopathy with dysproteinemia] or malignant [lymphoma or lymphosarcoma]). The management of the glandular and extraglandular manifestations is the same in primary and secondary Sjögren's syndrome.

The major clinical manifestations of the sicca complex are xerophthalmia (keratoconjunctivitis sicca [dry eyes]), xerostomia (dry mouth), and recurrent or chronic episodes of major salivary gland enlargement. Other glands may be affected, giving rise to dryness of mucous membranes in the nasopharynx and upper respiratory tract, dry skin (xerosis or cutaneous sicca), and vaginal dryness (vaginitis sicca). Extraglandular complications essentially can involve any organ in the body with associated mononuclear cell infiltrates, focal tissue damage, and organ dysfunction. Musculoskeletal symptoms including polyarthralgias-polyarthritis (nondeforming, nonerosive, often transient and migratory, and usually asymmetric) and myalgias are common. Their presence is not necessarily associated with more serious manifestations of systemic disease. Inflammation of blood vessels by either neutrophils or mononuclear cells also can cause cutaneous or systemic vasculitis. Basically the approach to the therapy of Sjögren's syndrome can be divided into the treatment of glandular and extraglandular manifestations.

GENERAL CONCEPTS

The management of the patient with Sjögren's syndrome requires a multidisciplinary approach. Successful treatment requires a working partnership between the patient and the physician. Patient education is of utmost importance. In patients with glandular manifestations alone, the rheumatologist, ophthalmologist, otolaryngologist, and dentist provide the basic support system. The rheumatologist is perhaps best qualified to monitor the patient for the potential emergence of extraglandular (systemic) disease and to coordinate diagnostic workups and therapeutic intervention. Because Sjögren's syndrome potentially may affect every organ in the body, additional consultation with appropriate specialists may be required for appropriate diagnosis and therapy. Ideally in complicated cases an internist should coordinate the multidimensional care recommended by specialists. Because of the diversity of symptoms, the patient with Sjögren's syndrome is often subject to the phenomena of "polydoctors" and "polypharmacy," which actually may impair optimal management.

There are several important general principles in the management of Sjögren's syndrome. First, most patients with Sjögren's syndrome can be treated successfully for sicca symptoms and other manifestations, such as musculoskeletal symptoms. Second, only a minority of patients require potent anti-inflammatory or immunosuppressive therapy. In fact, immunosuppressive therapy should be reserved for very specific indications (to be discussed). In particular, we do not recommend the use of these drugs for the treatment of sicca or musculoskeletal symptoms alone.

Sjögren's syndrome is a chronic disease. Because of the insidious and fluctuating pattern of sicca and musculoskeletal symptoms, the efficacy of a given therapeutic modality may be difficult to assess. Therefore, controlled blinded trials with serial assessment of objective parameters are required to verify the therapeutic efficacy of any given modality before it is incorporated into the therapeutic regimen. In some instances the patient's complaints may seem out of proportion to objective or pathologically defined documented abnormalities. In such cases physicians under pressure by patients for treatment should not resort to the use of immunosuppressive drugs but rather provide patient education and the appropriate utilization of conservative measures.

As with all chronic diseases, the symptoms of Sjögren's syndrome clearly are affected by stress. There may be important immunologic control mechanisms operative in the exacerbation of connective tissue disease by stress. The removal of stressful life situations is an important adjunct in the care of the patient with Sjögren's syndrome. Conversely, all the patient's symptoms and problems cannot be attributed to Sjögren's syndrome. Patient support groups appear to be an effective means for patient education and dissemination of information as well as serving as an important psychologic and emotional support system. Some patients, however, are uncomfortable with these groups and actually may react adversely with an increase in symptomatology and a decrease in subjective well-being and functional status. The physician may be helpful in assisting a patient in deciding whether a support group may be beneficial.

Most important in terms of therapy, there are numerous "common sense" alterations in the patient's behavior and life style that may result in a significant decrease in the symptom complex. Furthermore, there are a number of relatively minor therapeutic modalities that also may result in significant improvement. The patient may resist such a basic approach, searching instead for a "magic pill or remedy" to cure all symptoms.

TREATMENT OF GLANDULAR DISEASE

The management of glandular disease in Sjögren's syndrome is directed primarily at the treatment of ophthalmologic, oral, nasopharyngeal–upper respiratory tract, cutaneous, and vaginal sicca symptoms (Table 1).

Ophthalmologic Disease

The treatment of "dry eyes" is aimed primarily at alleviating symptoms, avoiding the development of superficial erosions of the corneal epithelium, preventing conjunctivitis and blepharitis, and appropriately treating complications as they develop.

The correction of environmental or extrinsic factors

TABLE 1 Glandular Manifestations (Symptomatic or Conservative Treatment): Sicca Manifestations

Ocular
Oral
Nasopharynx and upper respiratory tract
Skin
Vagina
Musculoskeletal syndrome

that may aggregate ocular sicca symptoms is important. The patient should be maintained in a high humidity environment year round. Air conditioning, forced heat, windy and dry environments, and high altitudes (including airplanes) worsen symptoms. Environmental toxins (tobacco smoke, fixatives, solvents) and other chemical agents also aggravate ocular dryness. Drugs, particularly those with anticholinergic side effects (phenothiazines, tricyclic antidepressants, antispasmodics, antiparkinsonian drugs, decongestants, and antihistamines), should be avoided.

The primary treatment for dry eyes is lubrication with artificial tears, which can be used as often as necessary. These preparations vary in viscosity and preservative content. The selection of an artificial tear product is usually an empiric choice by the patient. Eye irritation from these preparations may reflect the preservatives they contain, such as benzalkonium chloride, thimerosal, or chlorobutanol. Lubricating ointments can be used at night to provide protection over a longer period of time but may cause significant blurring of vision. Slow release capsules (Lacrisent, Merk, Sharp and Dohme) containing a polymer of hydroxypropyl cellulose can be inserted every 6 to 12 hours beneath the inferior tarsal margin. The capsule absorbs tears, dissolves slowly, and releases polymer. These capsules are particularly useful for patients who use artificial tears frequently. In some patients with extremely dry eyes, however, the capsule adheres to the conjunctiva and sclera and may not dissolve. Some investigators have suggested using the patient's own serum as an artificial tear. Data at present are insufficient to determine whether this approach is effective.

Drugs have had limited and inconsistent effects in the treatment of ocular sicca symptoms. Parasympathomimetics, especially the muscarines, serve to stimulate tear flow. The efficacy of pilocarpine in the treatment of ocular sicca is still under experimental investigation (see discussion of oral disease). Bromhexine (see discussion of oral disease) and acetylcysteine, a mucolytic drug, have not been documented to be effective consistently in controlled trials. The topical application of vitamin A has not proven effective in controlled trials. The topical use of corticosteroids in the treatment of corneal ulcers may actually worsen the condition and is not recommended. Uveitis can occur in Sjögren's syndrome and is treated with topical, or if necessary systemic, corticosteroid therapy.

The use of contact lenses in the treatment of ocular sicca symptoms is controversial. Some patients with emerging Sjögren's syndrome actually develop an intolerance to the use of contact lenses, which may be a subtle clue to the presence of the disorder. In others soft contact lenses actually may protect the cornea and prevent or treat corneal erosion or ulcers. Patients using contact lenses must observe meticulous hygienic standards and be followed very carefully, particularly since there is an increased risk of infection.

Surgical intervention is reserved for severe cases of keratoconjunctivitis sicca with progressive disease. Punctal occlusion of lacrimal canaliculi can be performed by electrolysis or diathermy but is irreversible. Less effective, but reversible, methods include strangling sutures of the canaliculi, laser photocoagulation of the lacrimal points, or the use of gelatine or silicone plugs. Recently diversion of the lacrimal canaliculus by surgical displacement of the punctum lacrimale onto the anterior edge of the lid, where it cannot collect tears, has been used and is reversible; the small quantity of residual tears is maintained in the lacrimal basin. Autografting of salivary glands to the lacrimal basin is an experimental procedure.

Oral Disease

The treatment of xerostomia in documented Sjögren's syndrome can be a difficult management problem. At the present time most treatment modalities are palliative. Identification of contributing factors that may aggravate xerostomia by further reducing salivary flow is important (sleep disorders, mouth breathing, cigarette and alcohol consumption, and drugs with anticholinergic side effects). Patients may consume increased quantities of liquids and may keep water at the bedside. The consumption of large quantities of fluid during the day may produce nocturia and disrupt normal sleep patterns. Unless fluid consumption is pushed to pathologic extremes, resulting in iatrogenic diabetes insipidus, however, there is no contraindication to liberal fluid intake. The majority of patients have residual salivary function and can stimulate salivary flow by using sugarless, highly flavored lozenges, chewing gum, candy, or beverages. The use of these agents prior to meals may enhance lubrication and the digestion of food. Dietary counseling to avoid dry food and the use of foods known to stimulate saliva production may be helpful. The slow ingestion of small pieces or portions of food, with complete chewing and wetting prior to swallowing, is an important practical aid.

Artificial saliva preparations are useful in some patients. The effects are transient, however, and the preparations are relatively expensive. Several preparations are available from different manufacturers, but essentially they are the same, containing sorbitol, sodium carboxymethylcellulose, and methylparaben in either liquid or spray form. Saliva substitutes should be used sparingly (approximately 2 ml) before and after meals, at bedtime, and following oral hygiene.

Dental care is an important cornerstone of the management of Sjögren's syndrome because of associated dental caries and periodontal disease with gum recession. Oral hygiene should be performed after meals and at bedtime with daily flossing. Dental check-ups and removal of dental plaque should be scheduled at least every 6 months and in some cases more frequently. When gingivitis is present, aggressive and persistent treatment is required to prevent the loss of teeth. Every attempt to maintain impeccable oral hygiene should be made because patients with Sjögren's syndrome have difficulty with the adequate fitting of dentures because of continuing problems with gum resorption. Single crystal aluminum oxide dental implants may be effective in preserving existing teeth. Topical or liquid treatment with stannous fluoride promotes mineralization and retards damage to tooth surfaces. The fluoride can be applied at night directly to the teeth from plastic trays, providing better coverage at the gingival margins.

Several preparations designed to stimulate the production of saliva have been used with variable success. Expectorants containing potassium iodide or iodinated glycerol may be useful. Parasympathomimetic drugs, such as pilocarpine (5 mg three to four times a day), recently have been shown in controlled trials to decrease xerostomia and increase salivary function. Pilocarpine may cause sweating approximately 30 minutes after ingestion and is contraindicated in patients taking beta-blockers or those with pulmonary or cardiac disease. Bromhexine, originally used as a mucolytic agent in cough syrups, and Efamol, derived from the evening primrose and containing gamma-linoleic acid, have been used in Scandinavia with reported success in decreasing xerostomia in some but not all patients. These drugs have not been studied in controlled trials in the United States. Efamol is available in the United States, but bromhexine is not. An electronic device for stimulating salivary flow has not undergone clinical research trials.

It is important to keep the mucous membranes of the mouth, nose, and upper tracheobronchial system moist. Normal saline nasal sprays used four to six times a day maintain moisture. Nasal irrigation with normal saline may prevent desiccation and crusting. Humidifiers should be attached to heating systems and a portable unit used within the bedroom at night. Adequate humidification decreases respiratory symptoms and decreases mouth breathing, which worsens xerostomia. Particular attention to increased fluid consumption and adequate humidification is needed in dry climates, with increased elevation, and during airplane flights.

Persistent or chronic salivary gland enlargement may occur. Infection, tumor, and obstruction are treatable causes. If these disorders are excluded and parotid gland enlargement is severe, a short course of moderate dose corticosteroid therapy may be effective.

Other Glandular Manifestations

Cutaneous sicca is a common and aggravating symptom in Sjögren's syndrome. Hot baths and showers should be avoided and the duration of exposure limited. Soaps containing a moisturizing cream are preferred. Moisturizing creams, particularly those that trap the body's natural moisture, should be applied while the skin is still wet. Avoidance of excessive sun exposure is important, and sun blocks should be used routinely to prevent premature aging of the skin. Hypoallergenic and nonscented cosmetics are preferred by some patients.

Vaginitis sicca is a serious symptom that may result in dyspareunia and impaired sexual performance and enjoyment. Standard lubricants are often effective in alleviating symptoms. Patients in whom symptoms are not controlled by this method should be evaluated by a gynecologist to assess the need for topical or systemic hormonal supplementation and to insure that there are no attendant infections (e.g., candidiasis).

TREATMENT OF EXTRAGLANDULAR DISEASE

There are two basic approaches to the treatment of the extraglandular manifestations of Sjögren's syndrome (Table 2). For extraglandular manifestations that result in end-organ damage and dysfunction, there is replacement therapy. For extraglandular manifestations second-

TABLE 2 Extraglandular Manifestations (Immunosuppressive or Replacement Therapy)

Organ Specific	
Thyroid	Graves' disease Hashimoto's thyroiditis
Pancreas	Pancreatitis, malabsorption
Stomach	Pernicious anemia
Liver	Chronic active hepatitis Primary biliary cirrhosis
Lung	Interstitial pulmonary fibrosis Bronchioalveolitis
Kidney	Interstitial nephritis Glomerulonephritis
Cytopenias	Neutropenia Thrombocytopenia Hemolytic anemia
Systemic	
Vasculitis, vasculopathy	Spectrum of small to medium sized, rarely large vessels
Neuromuscular disease	
Central nervous system	"Central nervous system Sjögren's syndrome"
Peripheral nervous system	Neuropathy
Muscle disease	Myositis
Lymph node disease	Pseudolymphoma Lymphoma Lymphosarcoma

ary to an active destructive inflammatory process, immunosuppressive therapy is used. Both approaches may be required in certain instances.

Organ Specific Disease

Sjögren's syndrome can affect any organ in the body. Organ specific involvement may result in an autoimmune process indistinguishable from a disorder occurring as an isolated manifestation (e.g., Graves' disease, Hashimoto's thyroiditis, pancreatitis, pernicious anemia, chronic active hepatitis, primary biliary cirrhosis, pulmonary fibrosis, interstitial nephritis). Cytopenias such as autoimmune thrombocytopenia or neutropenia and Coomb's positive autoimmune hemolytic anemia may be severe and require therapy. These disorders in Sjögren's syndrome are treated as if they occurred outside the setting of Sjögren's syndrome and with appropriate replacement therapy when indicated.

Two specific organ systems commonly involved in primary Sjögren's syndrome warrant special comment with respect to therapy. Interstitial pneumonitis resulting in pulmonary infiltrates, mild to moderate restrictive pulmonary disease, and decreased diffusing capacity usually does not require treatment. In some cases, however, the inflammatory process may be very aggressive and result in marked deterioration in pulmonary function. Obstructive lung disease secondary to inflammatory bronchioalveolitis may be severe and rapidly progressive. Lung biopsy should be performed in such cases to establish the presence of potentially treatable active inflammation or fibrosis, which is not treated.

Renal disease in Sjögren's syndrome is also common and usually does not require immunosuppressive therapy. The most common form of renal disease is interstitial nephritis, which results in overt or latent renal tubular acidosis and chronic sterile pyuria and hematuria. In rare instances this form of renal disease may be severe and associated with deteriorating renal function. Furthermore, patients with Sjögren's syndrome rarely can develop glomerulonephritis, particularly those with cryoglobulins. The latter two forms of aggressive renal disease need to be treated with immunosuppressive therapy.

TREATMENT OF SYSTEMIC DISEASE

Two other recently recognized systemic complications of Sjögren's syndrome may need to be treated with immunosuppressive therapy—inflammatory vascular disease (i.e., vasculitis) and neuromuscular disease (central and peripheral nervous system disease and inflammatory myopathies).

Cutaneous vasculitis, manifested most commonly by palpable purpura, petechiae, or chronic urticaria, is a common manifestation of Sjögren's syndrome. All patients with Sjögren's syndrome and cutaneous vasculitis should be carefully evaluated for systemic complications because of the potential for systemic or nervous system disease in such patients. Cutaneous vasculitis alone can be treated successfully with one or more drugs: hydroxychloroquine, dapsone, or low doses of corticosteroids. Patients should be monitored serially for the re-emergence of cutaneous lesions or the development of systemic complications.

Systemic vasculitis can occur in Sjögren's syndrome, often with nervous system involvement. Both histopathologic types of vasculitis (neutrophilic [leukocytoclastic] and mononuclear [lymphocytic]) can cause serious end-organ damage. Small to medium sized vessels are predominantly involved, but in some instances large vessels may be affected. Although vasculitis in the lungs, kidneys, gastrointestinal tract, heart, or nervous system (to be discussed) is most apt to result in clinically significant disease manifestations, vessels in any organ in the body can be affected. Patients with Sjögren's syndrome with systemic vasculitis require immunosuppressive therapy.

Recent investigations have indicated that central nervous system disease can occur in Sjögren's syndrome and may result in a multifocal neurologic disease affecting both the brain and the spinal cord, in addition to causing psychiatric or cognitive dysfunction. A spectrum of inflammatory insults are associated with neurologic disease in Sjögren's syndrome, ranging from frank vasculitis (predominantly small to medium sized vessels and rarely large vessels), to small vessel cerebral vasculopathy, to destructive lymphocytic infiltrates.

Currently we are recommending aggressive therapy only for patients with focal neurologic syndromes who have progressive disease documented by objective abnormalities by at least one of the following: magnetic resonance imaging study, multimodality evoked response testing, electroencephalography, cerebrospinal fluid analysis, or angiography. The abnormal parameter(s) can be followed serially to objectively assess the response to therapy. At present we do not recommend immunosuppressive therapy for patients with cognitive or psychiatric dysfunction alone. Inflammatory muscle disease (myositis) documented by biopsy associated with enzyme level elevation or electromyographic changes is another indication for immunosuppressive therapy.

The Musculoskeletal Syndrome

Many patients with Sjögren's syndrome have a recurrent transient symptom complex characterized by low grade fever, parotid gland enlargement, lymphadenopathy, malaise, fatigue, and musculoskeletal symptoms including arthralgias and myalgias. The syndrome may resemble a flu-like illness and can be very debilitating. The musculoskeletal symptoms and fatigue also may occur alone. Some patients have a soft tissue syndrome that resembles fibromyalgia or fibrositis. Nonsteroidal anti-inflammatory drugs, physical therapy, weight reduction (if indicated), an exercise program, and patient education are recommended for the management of these symptoms. Corticosteroids are not recommended for the management of these chronic recurrent musculoskeletal problems.

Frank arthritis is uncommon but does occur. Synovitis is usually transient, asymmetrical, migratory, and nondeforming. A transient symmetrical polyarthritis can occur. Nonsteroidal anti-inflammatory drugs usually are effective, but some patients may require a short course of low to moderate dose corticosteroid therapy. If rheumatoid arthritis coexists, the management of arthritis is the same as for rheumatoid arthritis alone.

Immunosuppressive Therapy

The approach to the treatment of systemic complications of Sjögren's syndrome is general and similar to that used in other autoimmune disorders, such as lupus erythematosus and multiple sclerosis. In general, Sjögren's syndrome appears to be a subtle, subacute, or insidious disease, but disease manifestations can be acute, devastating, and rapidly fatal.

There have been no controlled trials comparing the therapeutic efficacy of different approaches in treating the systemic complications of Sjögren's syndrome. Treatment is usually initiated with daily oral dosages of corticosteroids in the range of 0.5 to 1.0 mg per kg. More seriously ill patients initially may need intravenous therapy in divided doses. Treatment is continued for 3 to 6 months, and the dosage is tapered over several months to approximately half the starting dosage. Corticosteroids with little or no mineralocorticoid effects should be used at the lowest possible dosage and for the shortest possible duration; when possible, alternate day therapy should be used. Conversely, in patients with serious life threatening illness, adequate dosages of steroids should be given for appropriate periods of time without tapering too rapidly. Often such patients initially are not treated aggressively enough to control disease manifestations and dosages are tapered too quickly. There is no reported experience in the use and efficacy of pulse intravenous corticosteroid therapy in Sjögren's syndrome. Supplemental drugs that may permit lower corticosteroid dosages include salicylates, nonsteroidal anti-inflammatory drugs, hydroxychloroquine, and dapsone. Careful monitoring for potential steroid complications should be routine.

If corticosteroids are ineffective or toxic effects are unacceptable, there are several options. Antimetabolites, azathioprine, or an alkylating drug, cyclophosphamide, may be used in patients with potentially life threatening complications. Oral therapy with azathioprine or cyclophosphamide may be administered in the daily dosage of 1.0 to 3.0 mg per kg. To avoid corticosteroid side effects and the complications of daily immunosuppression, intravenous pulse cyclophosphamide therapy may be used for 6 to 12 months and every 3 to 4 months thereafter, depending on the severity of the disease and the therapeutic response. The starting dosage is 0.75 g per sq m, adjusting the dosage to maintain the white blood cell count nadir 10 days after administration at approximately 3000 cells per cubic mm. It appears to be important to induce leukopenia-lymphopenia for the successful treatment of the systemic complications of Sjögren's syndrome. This regimen should be accompanied by adequate hydration, intravenous corticosteroid therapy, and usually pretreatment with antiemetics. In very seriously ill patients therapy may be initiated with corticosteroids and cyclophosphamide concomitantly. Cyclosporine has been used in a small number of cases at low doses and is not recommended because of renal toxicity and the potential for the development of lymphoma.

Plasmapheresis is reserved for patients with systemic complications associated with hyperglobulinemia or cryoglobulinemia and is used in conjunction with corticosteroids and alkylating drugs, such as cyclophosphamide or chlorambucil, to prevent immunologic rebound. Newer experimental research approaches used in other autoimmune diseases, such as total body lymphoid radiation, monoclonal antibodies, and interferons, have not been studied in clinical trials in Sjögren's syndrome.

Lymphoma

Lymphoma is another systemic complication of Sjögren's syndrome requiring treatment. Patients with Sjögren's syndrome develop a spectrum of lymphoproliferative disease, from benign polyclonal gammopathy, to pseudolymphoma, to lymphoma (usually of the non-Hodgkin B cell type), to angioimmunoblastic lymphadenopathy with dysproteinemia. These disorders may be treated effectively with corticosteroids or cyclophosphamide. Patients with Sjögren's syndrome should be under constant surveillance for the development of lymphoma, for they have a 43-fold increased risk of developing lymphoma compared to normal individuals. Patients with rheumatoid arthritis with Sjögren's syndrome have a similar risk. The treatment of lymphoma or lymphosarcoma with chemotherapy or radiation therapy should be directed by experienced oncologists.

SUGGESTED READING

Alexander EL. Inflammatory vascular disease in Sjögren's syndrome. In: Talal N, Moutsopoulos HM, Kassan SS, eds. Sjögren's syndrome: clinical and immunological aspects. Heidelberg: Springer-Verlag, 1987:102.

Alexander EL. Neuromuscular complications of primary Sjögren's syndrome. In: Talal N, Moutsopoulos HM, Kassan SS, eds. Sjögren's syndrome: clinical and immunological aspects. Heidelberg: Springer-Verlag, 1987:61.
Alexander EL, Lijewski JE, Jerdan MS, Alexander GE. Evidence of an immunopathogenic basis for central nervous system disease in primary Sjögren's syndrome. Arthritis Rheum 1986; 29:1223–1231.
Alexander EL, Malinow K, Lijewski JE, Jerdan MS, Provost TT, Alexander GE. Primary Sjögren's syndrome with central nervous system dysfunction mimicking multiple sclerosis. Ann Intern Med 1986; 104:323–330.
Proceedings of 1st International Seminar on Sjögren's Syndrome. Chapter 8. Treatment. Scand J Rheum Suppl 1986; 61:237–270.
Talal N, Moutsopoulos HM. Treatment of Sjögren's syndrome. In: Talal N, Moutsopoulos HM, Kassan SS, eds. Sjögren's syndrome: clinical and immunological aspects. Heidelberg: Springer-Verlag, 1987:291.

SYSTEMIC VASCULITIS

ANTHONY S. FAUCI, M.D.
RANDI Y. LEAVITT, M.D., Ph.D.

Vasculitis is a clincopathologic process characterized by an inflammatory response within the blood vessel. Associated with this inflammatory process is a compromise of the vessel lumen with resulting ischemic changes in the tissues that are supplied by the blood vessels in question. It is predominantly this ischemia that constitutes the vasculitic syndrome. Since any size, location, and type of blood vessel may be involved in the vasculitic process, and since virtually any organ system can be involved, the vasculitic syndromes comprise a heterogeneous category of diseases, some of which have unique and distinguishing characteristics and others of which manifest overlapping clinical and pathologic features. Before one can apply a therapeutic protocol to a patient with a vasculitic syndrome, it is essential to appreciate the need to categorize as well as possible the syndrome with which one is dealing, particularly with regard to the real and potential extent of organ system involvement.

CATEGORIZATION OF THE VASCULITIC SYNDROMES

On one hand, the remarkable heterogeneity as well as the obvious overlap among the vasculitic syndromes must be appreciated by the treating physician, but on the other hand, it should not deter one from implementing the most appropriate therapeutic regimen for the particular syndrome the patient displays, as well as for the particular features within a given syndrome that the patient is manifesting. In approaching the classification of the vasculitic syndromes from the standpoint of therapy, it is helpful to realize that the vasculitis may be the primary disease process without an existing underlying disease to which it might be secondary; may be a secondary component of another underlying disease; may not be life threatening and, for example, may be limited to the skin without major organ system involvement; or may involve vital organ systems, leading to either irreversible organ system dysfunction or death. The latter type is referred to as severe systemic vasculitis, the treatment of which is the subject of this article.

An updated classification scheme for the vasculitic syndromes is shown in Table 1. Apart from the category referred to as "hypersensitivity vasculitis," which is generally associated either with a recognized antigenic stimulus, such as an infection, or with ingestion of a drug (particularly antibiotics such as penicillin and sulfa drugs), virtually all the other vasculitic syndromes are primary, i.e., unassociated with other underlying disease. In the latter groups, the major distinction to be

TABLE 1 Classification of the Vasculitic Syndromes

Systemic necrotizing vasculitis: involves multiple organ systems with potential for irreversible organ system dysfunction
- Systemic vasculitis of the polyarteritis nodosa group
  - Classic polyarteritis nodosa
  - Allergic angiitis and granulomatosis (Churg-Strauss disease)
  - Polyangiitis overlap syndrome
- Wegener's granulomatosis
- Giant cell arteritides
  - Cranial or temporal arteritis
  - Takayasu's arteritis
- Hypersensitivity vasculitis with predominantly extracutaneous involvement
  - Related to known antigenic stimulus, such as drug or infection
  - Secondary to another underlying disease
    - Associated with connective tissue disease, such as systemic lupus erythematosus, rheumatoid arthritis, or Sjögren's syndrome
    - Associated with neoplasm or infection
    - Associated with other underlying diseases
  - Unknown origin
- Miscellaneous systemic vasculitic syndromes
  - Behçet's disease
  - Mucocutaneous lymph node syndrome (Kawasaki's disease)

Predominantly cutaneous vasculitis
- Hypersensitivity vasculitis with predominantly cutaneous involvement
  - Related to known antigenic stimulus, such as drug or infection
  - Secondary to another underlying disease (see above)
  - Unknown origin

made regarding therapy is whether the disease is potentially life threatening and deserves an aggressive therapeutic approach or whether it will be confined to the skin and will not extensively and seriously involve other organ systems. This brings one to the most fundamental aspect of the treatment of the vasculitic syndromes. The physician must use information based on experience reported in the literature (to be summarized), together with clinical judgment related to the individual patient, in implementing a therapeutic regimen commensurate with the real and potential seriousness of the syndrome.

THERAPEUTIC APPROACH TO THE VASCULITIC SYNDROMES

The following discussion is directed toward the vasculitic syndromes that are truly systemic, i.e., those that involve multiple organ systems with the potential for serious organ system dysfunction. The approach to vasculitic syndromes that are confined to the skin or that manifest only minimal or insignificant renal involvement will not be discussed.

When possible, the treating physician should proceed in an orderly fashion from the most conservative therapeutic approach to a more aggressive approach, which, by definition, is generally associated with more serious toxic side effects. However, under certain circumstances when dealing with vasculitic syndromes, such as Wegener's granulomatosis and severe polyarteritis nodosa, whose usually fulminant courses are well recognized, the physician should immediately institute the aggressive therapeutic approaches (as will be discussed) that are of proved efficacy in these syndromes, as opposed to first attempting more conservative approaches. The obvious reason for this is that irreversible organ system dysfunction may occur during the period, however short, that conservative therapy is attempted. In addition, it is important to manage aggressively the hypertension that is frequently associated with the systemic vasculitides; this is often facilitated by the successful treatment of the underlying vasculitis. In Takayasu's arteritis, surgical bypass of a stenosed renal artery is sometimes required to treat the renovascular hypertension.

The following is a stepwise approach to the vasculitic syndromes.

Vasculitis Potentially Associated with a Recognized Antigen Stimulus

A substantial proportion of vasculitic syndromes associated with recognized antigenic stimuli, such as an infection or drug ingestion, manifest predominantly cutaneous features. Under certain circumstances, however, systemic and multiple organ system involvement is seen. The initial approach to this type of systemic vasculitis is the same as that for the cutaneous manifestations: withdrawal of the drug or specific treatment for the underlying infection. Unlike the cutaneous syndromes, however, which generally require only symptomatic treatment, in these cases it might be necessary to administer a brief course of corticosteroids, particularly if organ system dysfunction, such as renal function impairment, is seen. The corticosteroid administered should be prednisone, 1 mg per kilogram of body weight per day in three divided doses for 3 to 5 days, followed by consolidation to a single morning dose for an additional 2 to 3 days, followed by daily tapering by 10 mg decrements down to a total daily dosage of 30 mg per day, at which point the daily tapering should be by 5 mg decrements over a 3 week period until the dose is completely discontinued at approximately 1 month. If the patient cannot tolerate this relatively rapid tapering schedule, one can convert to an alternate day regimen, to be described, with tapering of the dosage according to the individual response. If the vasculitic process proves not to be self-limiting and organ system dysfunction persists without improvement over this period, the corticosteroid should be administered in the regimen described in Table 2 under Prednisone Component. A small percentage of patients with vasculitis associated with a recognized stimulus develop a vasculitic syndrome indistinguishable from the severe systemic necrotizing vasculitis group within which polyarteritis nodosa falls (see Table 1). Under these circumstances, the patient should be treated with the aggressive regimen described for that category (see Table 2).

Vasculitis Associated with Another Underlying Disease

Vasculitic syndromes may be a secondary manifestation of a recognized underlying disease, such as a connective tissue disease (rheumatoid arthritis, systemic lupus erythematosus, Sjögren's syndrome), an underlying neoplasm (particularly a lymphoproliferative disease), or an infection as already mentioned. Under these circumstances, the underlying disease should be specifically treated if possible, and if this is successful, the vasculitic syndrome usually resolves. If the vasculitis is confined predominantly to the skin, potential inciting antigens such as drugs are removed and therapy is primarily symptomatic. Since there is no consistently effective therapy for isolated cutaneous vasculitis, toxic regimens should be avoided. Occasionally short courses of corticosteroids are of benefit in this disorder. If the vasculitis involves multiple organ systems and does not resolve as the underlying disease is being treated, the approach should be similar to that already described, in which mild disease is treated with a brief course of corticosteroids and persistent or fulminant disease is treated more aggressively.

TABLE 2 Combined Cyclophosphamide-Prednisone Therapy for Severe Systemic Vasculitis*

Cyclophosphamide component: cyclophosphamide, 2 mg/kg per day orally; adjust dosage such that the leukocyte count remains above 3000–3500 per cubic mm (neutrophil count of 1000–1500 per cubic mm). Continue therapy with frequent downward adjustments of dosage so that severe neutropenia does not occur. Continue therapy for 1 year following induction of complete remission, at which point dose is tapered by 25 mg decrements every 2 months until discontinued.
Prednisone component: prednisone, 1 mg/kg per day in three to four divided doses for 7 to 10 days; consolidate to single morning dose by 2 to 3 weeks; continue single morning daily dose until 1 month of total corticosteroid treatment is reached. Convert to alternate day prednisone over the second month; maintain alternate day regimen over third month, followed by gradual tapering of alternate day dose over the next 3 to 6 months.

* Precise details of this regimen are given in the text. The cyclophosphamide and prednisone are begun simultaneously. For regimens that call for corticosteroids alone, the "prednisone component" of this protocol should be employed alone in the regimen indicated.

Primary Systemic or Multisystem Vasculitic Syndromes

An effective chemotherapeutic protocol for the severe systemic necrotizing vasculitides is a long term low dose therapy with a cytotoxic drug administered in combination with corticosteroids. The latter drug is given initially on a daily basis, with conversion to an alternate day regimen such that the patient is maintained on daily doses of the cytotoxic drug and alternate day corticosteroids. Clearly the cytotoxic drug of choice in these syndromes is cyclophosphamide, which is an alkylating agent, and the corticosteroid used most frequently is prednisone. The precise details for the initiation and modification of the cyclophosphamide-prednisone therapeutic protocol are outlined in Table 2. Certain systemic vasculitic syndromes can be successfully treated with just the prednisone component of the protocol. However, if rapid remission is not induced with prednisone alone and if organ system dysfunction progresses with this regimen, cyclophosphamide should be added. Furthermore, and most importantly, certain syndromes, such as Wegener's granulomatosis and fulminant systemic necrotizing vasculitis of the polyarteritis nodosa group (see Table 1), should be treated with the cyclophosphamide-prednisone combination from the beginning, since long term studies have now unequivocally demonstrated the superiority of the combination regimen over prednisone alone, particularly in the treatment of Wegener's granulomatosis.

Cyclophosphamide-Prednisone Combination

Cyclophosphamide should be administered in a dosage of 2 mg per kg of body weight per day orally. If the disease is rapidly fulminant, one can give 4 mg per kg per day for the first 2 to 3 days and then convert to the 2 mg per kg per day dosage. In individuals who cannot tolerate oral medications and in patients in whom there is a question of intestinal involvement with the vasculitic process, the drug should be administered intravenously; the intravenous dose is equivalent to the oral dose. The underlying strategy of cyclophosphamide therapy in patients with non-neoplastic diseases, such as systemic vasculitis, is to suppress the disease activity without lowering the peripheral leukocyte count below a level that would cause a significant host defense defect with regard to neutropenia. It is common experience that if the leukocyte count is maintained about 3000 to 3500 cells per cubic mm, which usually results in a neutrophil count of 1000 to 1500 cells per cubic mm, patients rarely, if ever, develop opportunistic infections provided they do not have a host defense defect for another reason, such as the administration of daily corticosteroid therapy. As is to be discussed, this is one of the major reasons for the use of alternate day prednisone in combination with cyclophosphamide. For reasons that are still unclear, the disease activity of the vasculitic syndromes is almost invariably suppressed prior to the point when the leukocyte count drops below the level of 3000 to 3500 per cubic mm. Given this observation, together with the fact that cytotoxic drug induced neutropenia is associated with a significant incidence of infectious disease complications, particularly with gram negative opportunistic infections, it is extremely important that the physician carefully monitor the leukocyte count and adjust the dosage frequently, if necessary, to maintain the count in the "safe" level. In this regard, it should be remembered that there is generally a lag of several days from a given dose to the time when the full effect on the leukocyte count is seen. In adjusting the dosage, the physician should be aware of the slope of the decline in leukocyte count as well as the absolute count so as to better guide the precise timing of the adjustment in dosage.

Daily cyclophosphamide should be continued with the frequent adjustments of dosage as already indicated for 6 months to 1 year from the time that it is believed that the patient has achieved a complete remission. When this point has been reached, the cyclophosphamide should be tapered by 25 mg decrements every 1 to 2 months until the drug has been discontinued. If flares of disease activity occur, the drug should be increased to 25 mg per day above the dosage that had been maintaining the remission. This dosage should be maintained for an additional 3 to 6 months, depending on the extent and severity of the relapse, and attempts at tapering should again be instituted as already indicated. Although there is a good deal of variability among patients with various systemic vasculitic diseases as well as among patients with a given vasculitic syndrome, it has been our experience that patients with Wegener's granulomatosis clearly require the full year of therapy following the induction of complete remission to avoid relapse. Despite the fact that the cyclophosphamide-prednisone therapeutic protocol has induced remissions in more than 90 percent of the patients with Wegener's granulomatosis, there is a substantial incidence of mild relapse if the drug is withdrawn too soon following induction of remission.

Prednisone therapy should be instituted together with the cyclophosphamide protocol, which is described herein, in the treatment of severe systemic vasculitis. The combination has proved to be quite effective, and mechanistically it is essential for prednisone to be included in the induction-of-remission protocol, since its anti-inflammatory and immunosuppressive effects are realized almost immediately, whereas cyclophosphamide in the dosage given takes 10 days to 3 weeks before producing significant immunosuppression. Therefore, the corticosteroid serves as an essential component of the early induction and can be withdrawn as the cyclophosphamide maintains the remission (as will be discussed).

Prednisone is given in a dosage of 1 mg per kg per day in divided doses for 7 to 10 days, with consolidation to a single morning dose by 2 to 3 weeks. This daily dosage is continued for an additional week, for the total daily corticosteroid regimen of 3 to 4 weeks. Over the second month of therapy, the prednisone is gradually converted to an alternate day regimen by decreasing the dose on the ultimate "off" day by 10 mg every one to two alternate day cycles. For example, on alternate days the patient is given 60 mg, 50 mg, 60 mg, 40 mg, 60 mg, and 30 mg. When 30 mg is reached on the "low" day, the tapering is changed to 5 mg decrements, that is, 60 mg, 30 mg, 60 mg, 25 mg, 60 mg, 20 mg, and so on. This is continued until the low dose is 10 mg, at which point the low day dose is tapered by 2.5 mg until the patient is receiving 60 mg alternatively with 0 mg, i.e., an alternate day regimen. The entire conversion to an alternate day regimen usually takes approximately 1 month, for a total corticosteroid treatment time of 2 months. Over the next (third) month the patient is maintained on 60 mg of prednisone on alternate days.

Hence, during the first 2 months of induction with cyclophosphamide, the patient receives 1 month of daily corticosteroid therapy to provide induction and 1 month of "modified daily" corticosteroid therapy over the period of time that the cyclophosphamide has achieved substantial immunosuppression. At the end of 2 months, the patient is receiving a true alternate day prednisone regimen with its significantly decreased incidence of opportunistic infections as well as other corticosteroid side effects (as will be discussed), which makes the synergistic host defense defect of corticosteroid and cyclophosphamide much less of a problem. Following this initial 3 month period of daily corticosteroid administration converted to alternate day therapy, the prednisone dosage is gradually tapered over 3 to 6 months until the drug is discontinued and the patient is receiving cyclophosphamide alone.

It is important to emphasize that during periods of corticosteroid tapering, the leukocyte count may decrease, necessitating appropriate reductions in cyclophosphamide dosage. As already mentioned, the cyclophosphamide should be continued for 6 months to preferably 1 year following the induction of complete remission. Since complete remission induction often takes several months, the total duration of therapy is usually about 2 years for patients with diseases such as Wegener's granulomatosis and somewhat less for others with the severe systemic necrotizing vasculitides.

The plan just delineated should be followed fairly strictly with regard to the induction phase. Once induction has been achieved, however, the precise timing of the tapering schedule should remain flexible and adjustments made according to the individual patient's response. For example, certain patients, although in complete remission, require much slower tapering of the alternate day prednisone, to the extent that it is difficult to get them off the final 10 to 20 mg every other day. Under these circumstances, one should merely be patient and continually attempt to taper the dose to the lowest possible level. Ultimately, virtually all patients who have achieved remission will be able to have their immunosuppressive regimen discontinued, or at least tapered to an extremely low dose regimen that maintains remission without causing serious side effects.

The capacity of the myeloid elements of the bone marrow to tolerate cyclophosphamide during induction and maintenance of remissions varies greatly from patient to patient and appears to be less in older patients. We have noticed in a few patients that neutropenia occurs sooner than expected; the patients may not yet have achieved remission, but the cyclophosphamide dose must be lowered owing to neutropenia. In these patients we increase the dose of alternate day prednisone or reinstitute alternate day prednisone if it had already been discontinued. This usually results in a significant marrow sparing effect such that a higher dose of cyclophosphamide then can be given without serious neutropenia.

Other Cytotoxic Drugs

Other cytotoxic drugs, such as azathioprine (purine analogue) and chlorambucil (alkylating agent), have been used in the vasculitic syndromes. Most studies, however, indicate that they are inferior to cyclophosphamide in the treatment of the vasculitic syndromes, particularly Wegener's granulomatosis. Nonetheless, one must remember that the real and potential toxic side effects and complications of cyclophosphamide therapy are substantial (as will be discussed), and this must be taken into account when one embarks upon such a therapeutic protocol. We have used alternative cytotoxic drugs, particularly azathioprine, in situations in which cyclophosphamide could not be used, as in patients who developed severe cystitis and who still needed longer treatment with a cytotoxic drug or patients who could not accept the almost invariable gonadal dysfunction associated with chronic cyclophosphamide therapy. The dosage of azathioprine is 2 mg per kg per day, with the same adjustments being made for leukopenia as indicated for cyclophosphamide. We have found that although azathioprine is clearly not as effective as cyclophosphamide in the induction of remission in the vasculitic syndromes, it can be quite useful in the maintenance of remission in someone whose disease has been put into remission by cyclophosphamide but who cannot tolerate the drug for an additional period of required therapy.

Chlorambucil has been used in the therapy of Wegener's granulomatosis but is somewhat less effective than cyclophosphamide, especially in patients with renal disease.

A few reports have indicated that methotrexate can be effective in the vasculitic syndromes, but the experience is not extensive.

Bolus Corticosteroid and Bolus Cyclophosphamide

Bolus corticosteroid administration in the form of 1 g of methylprednisolone intravenously for 1 to 3 consecutive days has been attempted in certain inflammatory and immune mediated diseases, including the vasculitic syndromes. Since controlled studies have not been performed, it is difficult to establish the efficacy of this regimen. Initial reports indicate that such an approach may be beneficial in patients with systemic lupus erythematosus with acutely deteriorating renal function and in patients with rapidly progressive glomerulonephritis. We have occasionally used a 1 g intravenous bolus of methylprednisolone during the first few days of the induction phase of therapy in patients with fulminant vasculitis while implementing the cyclophosphamide-prednisone protocol already described; the efficacy of this approach is not established. Nonetheless, since the side effects of 1 to 3 days of bolus corticosteroid administration are minimal, it is not unreasonable to employ this regimen during the first few days of treatment of life-threatening fulminant vasculitis.

Bolus cyclophosphamide in a dosage of 0.5 to 0.75 g per square meter of body surface has been employed with and without plasmapheresis in certain inflammatory diseases. It is currently being subjected to clinical trials in cases of systemic lupus erythematosus. It has not been used in controlled trials for the vasculitic syndromes, and our experience has been that bolus intravenous cyclophosphamide therapy is ineffective in inducing remissions in the vasculitic syndromes, which seem to require significant periods of prolonged low dose therapy. It is not known, however, whether the intravenous bolus approach would be effective on an intermittent basis to maintain a remission that has been induced by the standard regimens.

Plasmapheresis and Lymphoplasmapheresis

At the present time it is unclear whether plasmapheresis or lymphoplasmapheresis will have a useful role in the treatment of the systemic vasculitic syndromes. In general, this approach has not been effective in inducing and maintaining remissions in the severe vasculitic syndromes in the few uncontrolled reports that are available. However, we have noted several patients with severe systemic vasculitis associated with Sjögren's syndrome who have responded dramatically to plasmapheresis with or without concomitant bolus cyclophosphamide. We have employed daily 3 liter plasma exchanges for 1 to 2 weeks followed by alternate day exchanges for variable periods of time (up to a few weeks). This approach is currently being further evaluated in the vasculitis of Sjögren's syndrome and the severe vasculitis that can be seen with rheumatoid arthritis. However, plasmapheresis can be used in addition to corticosteroids and cyclophosphamide in patients with fulminant vasculitis.

Cyclosporin A

Cyclosporin A, a cyclic endecapeptide, is an effective immunosuppressive drug used in patients undergoing renal transplantation. It primarily affects T lymphocyte function and has been documented to inhibit the production of interleukin 2 in T cells. Cyclosporin A has been reported to be effective in certain patients with vasculitis, but the data are preliminary and no follow-up data are available.

Miscellaneous Therapy

A number of miscellaneous therapeutic approaches have been tried in patients with vasculitic syndromes, including dapsone, antihistamines, and indomethacin, and these are usually applicable to patients with isolated or predominant cutaneous disease.

In patients who have experienced end stage renal failure and in whom the disease activity has been subsequently suppressed, renal transplantation has proved to be an eminently feasible and successful modality of treatment for vasculitic syndromes, particularly Wegener's granulomatosis. Recurrence of disease in the graft, although it may occasionally occur, does not represent a contraindication to transplantation.

It should be mentioned that nonspecific symptoms of inflammation, such as joint manifestations, generally respond to nonsteroidal anti-inflammatory drugs, such as aspirin, 600 mg every 6 hours, or ibuprofen, 300 mg every 6 hours. However, these drugs should never be substituted for the immunosuppressive regimens described, since nonsteroidal anti-inflammatory drugs are not effective in treating the vasculitic components of the severe systemic vasculitic syndromes. The only clear exception to this appears to be the treatment of the mucocutaneous lymph node syndrome (Kawasaki's disease), in which corticosteroid therapy has been reported to result in an increased incidence of coronary artery aneurysm; aspirin therapy alone remains the treatment of choice at present.

It has been reported that several patients with Wegener's granulomatosis have responded to therapy with trimethoprim-sulfa. These reports are intriguing but anecdotal, and more data certainly need to be accumulated regarding the efficacy of trimethoprim-sulfa in the treatment of this disease before any conclusions can be drawn.

TOXIC SIDE EFFECTS AND COMPLICATIONS OF THERAPY

As discussed, the two mainstays of therapy for the severe systemic necrotizing vasculitides are corticosteroids and cytotoxic drugs, particularly cyclophosphamide. Although these drugs are effective in inducing and maintaining remissions in most of the systemic vasculitides, both are associated with significant toxic side effects (Table 3). It is essential for the physician to be aware of these side effects and to follow a regimen that will, when possible, minimize their occurrence. There is no question that most, if not all, of the side effects of daily corticosteroid therapy can be significantly minimized and in some cases avoided (as with infectious disease complications) if an alternate day regimen is employed as soon as feasible following induction of remission with daily corticosteroid therapy as already indicated. Certain of the toxic side effects of cyclophosphamide can also be avoided to some extent, although some are completely unavoidable. The toxic side effect that can best be controlled by physician awareness is severe leukopenia, which is avoided by careful monitoring of the leukocyte count and consequent adjustment of dosage as already detailed.

Avoidance of significant leukopenia together with the use of alternate day as opposed to daily corticosteroid therapy has resulted in virtually no increase in the incidence of opportunistic bacterial or fungal infections in patients with vasculitis treated with this regimen. However, we have noted an increased incidence of cutaneous herpes zoster infections in patients treated with cyclophosphamide, which was not related to leukopenia. The zoster never viscerally disseminated and did not require significant modification of the cyclophosphamide regimen. Careful attention to adequate hydration has been thought to lessen the incidence of hemorrhagic cystitis due to cyclophosphamide; however,

TABLE 3 Complications of Corticosteroid and Long Term Cyclophosphamide Therapy

Corticosteroid Therapy:
Central nervous system
Pseudotumor cerebri
Psychiatric disorders
Musculoskeletal
Osteoporosis with spontaneous fractures
Aseptic necrosis of bone
Myopathy
Ocular
Glaucoma
Cataracts
Gastrointestinal
Peptic ulceration
Intestinal perforation
Pancreatitis
Cardiovascular and fluid balance
Hypertension
Sodium and fluid retention
Hypokalemic alkalosis
Hypersensitivity reactions
Urticaria
Anaphylaxis
Endocrinologic
Suppression of hypothalamic-pituitary-adrenal axis
Growth failure
Secondary amenorrhea
Metabolic
Hyperglycemia and unmasking of genetic predisposition to diabetes mellitus
Nonketotic hyperosmolar states
Hyperlipidemia
Alterations of fat distribution (typical cushingoid appearance)
Fatty infiltration of liver
Drug interactions (decreased anticoagulant effect of ethyl biscoumacetate)
Fibroblast inhibition
Inhibition of wound healing
Subcutaneous tissue atrophy (striae, purpura, ecchymosis)
Suppression of host defenses
Immunosuppression, anergy
Effects on phagocyte kinetics and function
Increased incidence of infections
Chronic Cyclophosphamide Therapy:
Marrow suppression—particularly neutropenia with resulting secondary infection
Hemorrhagic cystitis
Gonadal dysfunction
Alopecia
Oncogenesis

the incidence of this complication is still disturbingly high. Both pulmonary and bladder fibrosis have been reported. Oncogenesis does not seem to occur as frequently as in patients who develop a second tumor following treatment of the original tumor with high dose cyclophosphamide, and this complication in patients who are treated with the long term low dose cyclophosphamide regimen outlined is surely rare. However, cases of leukemia, lymphoma, and bladder carcinoma following cyclophosphamide therapy for vasculitis have been reported, and this possibility should be recognized.

Gonadal dysfunction and sterility are serious and frequent problems in younger individuals treated with cyclophosphamide. Over the past few years, semen has been stored in sperm banks for male patients prior to the institution of cyclophosphamide therapy, and we have been administering birth control pills to women of childbearing age who wish to procreate after discontinuation of therapy. The latter approach is based on recent reports that suppression of cyclic ovarian function during therapy may protect the ovaries from the sterilizing effects of the drug. However, there are not sufficient data at present to determine the efficacy of this approach.

SUGGESTED READING

Cohen DJ, Loertscher R, Rubin MF, Tilney NL, Carpenter CB, Strom TB. Cyclosporin: a new immunosuppressive agent for organ transplantation. Ann Intern Med 1984; 101:667–682.

Fauci AS. Cytotoxic and other immunoregulatory agents. In: Kelly WN, Harris ED Jr, Ruddy S, Sledge CB, eds. Textbook of rheumatology. Philadelphia: WB Saunders, 1985: 833–857.

Fauci AS, Dale DC, Balow JE. Glucocorticosteroid therapy: mechanisms of action and clinical considerations. Ann Intern Med 1976; 84:304–315.

Fauci AS, Haynes BF, Katz P. The spectrum of vasculitis: clinical, pathologic, immunologic, and therapeutic considerations. Ann Intern Med 1978; 89:660–676.

Fauci AS, Haynes BF, Katz P, Wolff SM. Wegener's granulomatosis: prospective clinical and therapeutic experience with 85 patients for 21 years. Ann Intern Med 1983; 98:76–85.

TEMPORAL ARTERITIS

THOMAS R. CUPPS, M.D.

Temporal arteritis is a systemic panarteritis predominantly affecting elderly individuals. Although any medium or large sized muscular artery may be involved, the majority of clinical signs and symptoms result from vasculitis in the distribution of the cranial arteries. The terms cranial arteritis and giant cell arteritis are also used to describe this syndrome. Because this disease may present with a relatively nonspecific pattern, a high index of suspicion for the diagnosis of temporal arteritis should be maintained in evaluating elderly individuals with poorly characterized complaints.

The more common initial manifestations of temporal arteritis include, in descending order of frequency, headache, polymyalgia rheumatica (aching and morning stiffness of the proximal extremities, neck, and torso), fever, visual symptoms, and malaise. Less common presentations include myalgia, tenderness over the cranial arteries, jaw or tongue claudication, weight loss, and sore throat. The common laboratory findings include an abnormal erythrocyte sedimentation rate, marked elevations being characteristic. Elevations of other acute phase reactants (a_2 globulin, C reactive protein, and fibrinogen) have been reported. Other findings seen in some patients include a mild normochromic normocytic anemia with a chronic disease pattern and a mildly elevated alkaline phosphatase level.

The diagnosis is generally established by finding the characteristic pattern of panarteritis in a temporal artery biopsy specimen. The inflammatory infiltrate consists of mononuclear cells, polymorphonuclear leukocytes, and eosinophils. The major site of involvement is the media, with smooth muscle necrosis and interruption of the internal elastic membrane. Giant cells are present to varying degrees and may be relatively rare. Because of the segmental nature of the arterial inflammation, systematic evaluation of the biopsy specimen with multiple step sections increases the diagnostic yield.

THERAPY

General Considerations

Corticosteroids are the mainstay of therapy in patients with temporal arteritis. Although this group of drugs is not curative, appropriate use of corticosteroids generally suppresses the signs and symptoms of inflammation and prevents associated vascular complications. In most patients temporal arteritis is a self-limited disease with an average duration of 1 to 2 years. Although fluctuations of disease activity are commonly seen during the course of temporal arteritis, eventually the inflammatory process subsides. A subset of patients, however, may develop a more chronic process with well documented exacerbations years after the initial presentation of the disease. The therapeutic goal in the treatment of temporal arteritis is to suppress the signs and symptoms of inflammation and prevent vascular complications, particularly ischemia of the eye.

Because of the potential for adverse side effects of long term corticosteroid therapy in the elderly population affected by temporal arteritis, a systematic effort to minimize the morbidity associated with the use of this therapeutic agent is required. The potential for corticosteroid associated morbidity is related to the frequency, total dosage, and duration of therapy with this drug. Although general guidelines for the use of corticosteroids in temporal arteritis are reviewed in this article, the minimal effective corticosteroid dosage varies from patient to patient and must be established on an individual basis. The minimal effective dosage also may vary throughout the course of the disease. As disease activity decreases, the corticosteroid dosage should be adjusted accordingly, and when the condition resolves, the drug should be discontinued.

Corticosteroid Therapy Efficacy

Most patients with temporal arteritis respond dramatically to corticosteroid therapy. Within days, systemic symptoms of fever, malaise, and musculoskeletal pain begin to resolve. Focal complications of vascular disease, such as claudication, headache, or scalp tenderness, also respond. The efficacy of corticosteroid therapy in preventing blindness is well established. It should be emphasized that ischemic loss of vision, once it occurs, is frequently irreversible. Ischemia of one eye in temporal arteritis increases the risk of similar involvement in the other eye. In most cases clinical signs or symptoms of impending ocular involvement precede ischemic loss of vision by a variable period of time. In a clinical setting consistent with the diagnosis of temporal arteritis, the presence of ocular symptoms is an indication that appropriate therapy should be initiated immediately. With the exception of the ischemic loss of vision, the prognosis in temporal arteritis treated with corticosteroids is excellent. Most patients achieve complete remission and eventually can be tapered off the drug.

Induction

Once the diagnosis of temporal arteritis is made, corticosteroid therapy should be expeditiously initiated. Generally treatment is started with a dosage of 40 to 60 mg (1 mg per kg) of prednisone per day. In the absence of eye symptoms, ischemia, or severe constitutional symptoms, the prednisone therapy can be started as a single morning dose. In the presence of severe constitutional symptoms or continuing ischemia, more aggressive corticosteroid therapy is warranted. Splitting the prednisone regimen to 20 mg doses given three or four times per day increases the overall corticosteroid effect. In the setting of new onset (within 24 to 36 hours) or progressive loss of visual acuity despite use of the standard therapeutic regimen, ultrahigh dosages of corticosteroids (500 to 1,000 mg of methylprednisolone) have been used by some investigators. An aggressive induction regimen of 1,000 mg of intravenous pulse methylprednisolone therapy every 12 hours for 5 days (followed by standard high dose oral prednisone therapy) has been used to successfully treat ocular ischemia and impaired vision that developed during treatment with the more standard pharmacologic doses of corticosteroids. Although experience with ultrahigh doses of corticosteroids in temporal arteritis remains limited, a trial of high dose pulse intravenous methylprednisolone therapy should be considered in patients with new onset or progressive ocular ischemia.

In patients started on split doses of corticosteroids, the consolidation to a single daily dose should be initiated 10 to 14 days after the start of therapy. In most of these patients the consolidation to a single daily morning dose is complete in 2 additional weeks. An example of such a consolidation would be as follows: taper from 20 mg of prednisone four times a day to 40 mg of prednisone twice a day for 3 days, 60 mg in the morning and 20 mg in the evening for 3 days, 70 mg in the morning and 10 mg in the evening for 3 days, 80 mg in the morning for 3 days followed by tapering to 60 mg as a single dose in the morning. It should be emphasized that alternate day corticosteroid therapy is not effective in inducing remissions in patients with temporal arteritis. The initial induction therapy for temporal arteritis (in the absence of ocular ischemia or altered vision) consists of 40 to 60 mg of prednisone a day for approximately 1 month.

Management

The majority of patients with temporal arteritis are in remission after the completion of the 1 month induction phase and a gradual tapering of the corticosteroids can be initiated. The corticosteroid dosage should be tapered gradually over months. The goal is to taper to the minimal dosage of the drug that maintains the remission. One of several approaches may be considered. Although alternate day prednisone is not effective during the induction phase of treatment, alternate day corticosteroid therapy effectively maintains the disease in remission following the initial induction phase. If the patient rapidly enters remission and does not have significant eye involvement, an attempt to taper the corticosteroid dosage to an alternate day regimen should be considered. The alternate day corticosteroid regimen incurs less drug associated morbidity than the daily regimens and is preferable if this therapeutic approach is effective in treating the disease.

The following approach is one example of a gradual tapering to an alternate day regimen. Starting at a dosage of 60 mg per day, drop 10 mg from the daily dosage given on alternate days, resulting in a schedule of 60 mg as a single morning dose alternating with 50 mg as a single morning dose. After 2 weeks, again drop the alternate day dose, resulting in a schedule of 60 mg alternating with 40 mg. Then 10 mg of prednisone is dropped from the low day dose every 2 weeks until a dosage of 60 mg alternating with 20 mg is established. At this point the tapering schedule is slowed to a reduction of 5 mg of prednisone from the low dose day every 2 weeks until a dosage of 60 mg alternating with 10 mg is obtained. Finally the alternate day low dose is reduced by 2.5 mg every 2 weeks until a schedule of 60 mg alternating with an "off" day is established. The alternate day high dose then may be gradually tapered. Not all patients tolerate tapering to an alternate day regimen. If the patient develops evidence of reactivation of the disease during this tapering, the dosage of prednisone should be increased back to a level that was effective in controlling the disease and tapering to a low dose daily regimen is initiated once the patient is back in remission.

Tapering to a low dose daily regimen should be done gradually also. The following is one example of such a prednisone taper. Starting from a single morning dose of 60 mg of prednisone, taper the dosage by 10 mg every 2 weeks until the patient is taking 40 mg a day. At this point the tapering schedule is slowed to lowering the dosage of prednisone by 5 mg every 2 weeks until a dosage of 20 mg a day is established. From 20 mg a day the prednisone dosage is tapered by 2.5 mg every 2 weeks until a maintenance dosage of 10 mg (or less) is obtained. It is important to emphasize that these suggested corticosteroid tapering schedules are examples and will undoubtedly require some modification when used in individual patients.

As the corticosteroid dosage is tapered, the clinician will need to follow the disease activity. Serial laboratory studies reflecting inflammation, such as the erythrocyte sedimentation rate or the C reactive protein determination, are very useful adjuncts in assessing disease activity. A follow-up sedimentation rate determination should be carried out after successful induction of remission to provide a baseline determination for comparison. One should remember that the sedimentation rate, although very sensitive, is also a nonspecific indicator of inflammation. Some variation in the follow-up determinations is to be expected, and processes other than temporal arteritis may affect the test results. It is important to emphasize the patient's clinical status in making the final assessment of the disease activity when regulating the corticosteroid dosage.

The optimal duration of therapy varies from case to case. As mentioned earlier, corticosteroids suppress the signs and symptoms of inflammation as the disease runs a self-limited course. Although selected patients may require only 6 months of corticosteroid therapy to put the temporal arteritis into sustained remission, in many patients the disease is reactivated with such a short course of therapy. The majority of patients are successfully treated with a 12 month course of corticosteroids. After completing a 1 year course of prednisone therapy, an attempt to taper the patient off corticosteroids should be initiated. The patient should be monitored closely as the maintenance dosage is gradually tapered and discontinued over several months. If evidence of recurrent disease activity develops, prednisone therapy should be restarted at a level known to control the signs and symptoms. Treatment for an additional year followed by a second attempt to taper and discontinue the prednisone should be considered. A small subset of patients may require even more prolonged therapy.

Morbidity

Prolonged daily corticosteroid therapy can have significant associated morbidity. The potential side effects of prolonged corticosteroid therapy are summarized in Table 1. Although the nature and extent of adverse side effects vary from individual to individual, higher dosages, increased frequency of administration, and prolonged therapy increase the likelihood of developing corticosteroid induced morbidity. To minimize the morbidity of this drug, the minimal effective dosage should be established for each individual. Limiting the patient's exposure to the corticosteroids decreases the likelihood of developing dose related side effects.

Prior to initiating corticosteroid therapy, the patient should have a baseline intermediate purified protein derivative (PPD) skin test together with a control anergy panel to evaluate for evidence of exposure to tuberculosis. The skin test can be carried out coincidentally with the initiation of corticosteroid therapy without markedly decreasing the diagnostic yield. A delay in the application of the skin test decreases the potential diagnostic return of this study because corticosteroid induced anergy develops. Because most patients with temporal arteritis are over the age of 60 years at the onset of the disease, most have some degree of osteo-

TABLE 1 Complications of Glucocorticosteroid Therapy

Altered mood	Hypokalemic alkalosis
Pseudotumor cerebri	Suppression of the hypothalamic-pituitary-adrenal axis
Osteoporosis	Growth retardation
Aseptic necrosis	Hyperglycemia
Proximal myopathy	Weight gain
Cataracts	Cushingoid habitus
Glaucoma	Striae
Peptic ulceration	Purpura and ecchymosis
Hypertension	Immunosuppression
Fluid retention	Opportunistic infection

porosis when corticosteroid therapy is started. For this reason prophylactic therapy with calcium carbonate, 500 mg, on a three or four times daily schedule with vitamin D, 25,000 to 50,000 units twice weekly, is suggested. Because hypercalcemia or hypercalciuria may develop with this regimen, monitoring of the serum and urine calcium levels is advisable.

If high dose methylprednisolone infusion protocols are used, additional parameters should be evaluated. A number of sudden deaths have been reported in systemically ill patients in the postinfusion period. These deaths appear to be related to cardiac arrhythmias. A higher incidence of sudden death has been reported with rapid infusion of corticosteroids, particularly in patients with electrolyte abnormalities. During the infusion the patient may be at higher risk for developing bacteremia if an established localized infection is present. I have seen patients become bacteremic during the peri-infusion period as a result of low grade bladder infections. Finally patients with borderline or frank hypertension may develop hypertensive crises during the high dose methylprednisolone infusion protocol.

To avoid these potential complications, several precautions are suggested. Although there is some urgency in initiating corticosteroid therapy when visual symptoms are present in patients with temporal arteritis, the following parameters can be measured. While preparations are being made for the infusion, the blood pressure should be measured, baseline electrocardiography done, an electrolyte panel including a calcium and magnesium determination sent for analysis, and the urine examined for evidence of infection. If hypertension is present, appropriate therapy should be initiated. Any electrolyte abnormalities should be corrected. If there is evidence of infection, appropriate parenteral antibiotic coverage should be started. The corticosteroid should be infused slowly over a 30 to 60 minute period. The use of peripheral rather than deep central lines has also been suggested. If there is going to be any appreciable delay in safely starting the infusion, oral corticosteroid therapy should be started. When any existing problems have been addressed, the patient can then be switched to high dose infusion protocol if needed.

In the setting of continuing eye related symptoms, corticosteroid therapy may be started on the basis of a presumptive clinical diagnosis of temporal arteritis prior to carrying out a biopsy. However, the diagnostic yield in temporal artery biopsy may decrease following treatment with corticosteroids. In one series of 132 patients with a clinical diagnosis of temporal arteritis, the following biopsy results were obtained. Prior to corticosteroid therapy, patients with "clinically genuine temporal arteritis" had positive biopsy findings 82 percent of the time. During the first week of corticosteroid therapy the positive temporal artery incidence dropped to 60 percent. After 1 week of corticosteroid therapy the yield of positive results decreased dramatically to 10 percent. Thus, when corticosteroids are started on clinical grounds, a temporal artery biopsy should be performed as soon as possible after the medication has been started.

Alternative Therapies

In a very small subset of patients the dosage of corticosteroids with an acceptable morbidity does not totally suppress the signs and symptoms of temporal arteritis. This small percentage of patients represents a significant management problem, because no other group of drugs has manifested documented efficacy in the treatment of temporal arteritis. Although experience is limited, several drugs have been added to the corticosteroids to produce the so-called "steroid sparing effect." Anecdotal experience suggests that cytotoxic drugs, such as azathioprine or cyclophosphamide, when added to continuing corticosteroid therapy are effective in putting the refractory cases of temporal arteritis into clinical remission. Moreover, lower dosages of corticosteroids are generally effective when combined with cytotoxic drugs.

Azathioprine can be used at 1 to 2 mg per kg given as a single daily dose. Although this drug is generally well tolerated, hepatitis, bone marrow suppression, and an increased risk of neoplastic transformation have been reported. The patient should be appropriately monitored for these potential toxic effects. Alternatively, cyclophosphamide can be added at 1 to 2 mg per kg given as a single morning dose. Toxic effects associated with the use of cyclophosphamide include bone marrow suppression, hemorrhagic cystitis, bladder fibrosis, neoplastic transformation (acute myelocytic leukemia, bladder carcinoma), risk of infection, ovarian failure, sterility, and alopecia. Patients with temporal arteritis treated with cyclophosphamide should be monitored closely for drug related toxic effects.

During the induction phase with cyclophosphamide, the complete blood count should be monitored regularly for evidence of marrow suppression. Normally a reduction of the total leukocyte count to the 4,000 cells per cubic mm range is associated with a clinical response to cyclophosphamide. One should avoid letting the total granulocyte count drop below the 1,000 to 1,500 cells per cubic mm level because of the increased risk of infection.

The elderly population with temporal arteritis may be particularly sensitive to the marrow suppressive effects of this drug and may require a reduced dosage. The patient should be encouraged to drink enough fluid to maintain a urine output of approximately 3 liters per day. Drinking several glasses of water prior to retiring prevents the concentration of toxic metabolites in the overnight urine. Because incomplete emptying of the bladder may predispose a patient to cyclophosphamide induced bladder toxicity, a clinical history of obstructive urinary tract symptoms should be evaluated. If the patient is taking prednisone on a daily schedule when the cyclophosphamide is started, 2 weeks into the cyclophosphamide induction tapering to an alternate corticosteroid regimen should be initiated.

It should be emphasized that the prolonged daily use of prednisone and cyclophosphamide is associated with a substantial increase in the risk of opportunistic infections. By contrast, the use of cyclophosphamide and alternate day prednisone has been associated only with an increased risk of developing herpes zoster. The tapering to alternate day prednisone should be complete within 3 months after starting the cyclophosphamide therapy. During the tapering to an alternate day regimen there is a tendency for the leukocyte count to drop; consequently the dosage of cyclophosphamide must be decreased appropriately. Appropriate use and close monitoring for drug associated toxicity decrease the morbidity associated with the use of cyclophosphamide. The relative efficacy of azathioprine or cyclophosphamide when used as a corticosteroid sparing drug in temporal arteritis has not been systematically evaluated and should be considered only when it is absolutely clear that the corticosteroid regimen has failed.

Anecdotal experience with several other drugs used as "steroid sparing" therapy in temporal arteritis has also been reported. Dapsone at a dosage of 100 mg per day has been used with some success in reducing the corticosteroid dosage required to control the signs and symptoms of temporal arteritis. Cyclosporin A at a dosage of 3 mg per kg per day was used successfully in the treatment of a patient who was unresponsive to prednisone, cyclophosphamide, and dapsone. Patients treated with cyclosporin A require close monitoring, including drug level determinations and serial renal function studies. Treatment for the relatively rare case of corticosteroid resistant temporal arteritis should be evaluated on a case by case basis.

SUGGESTED READING

Allen NB, Studenski SA. Polymyalgia rheumatica and temporal arteritis. Med Clin North Am 1986; 70:369–384.

Allison MC, Gallagher PJ. Temporal artery biopsy and corticosteroid treatment. Ann Rheum Dis 1984; 43:416–417.

Cupps TR, Fauci AS. Giant cell arteritides. Major Probl Int Med 1981; 21:99–107.

Hunder GG, Hazelman BL. Giant cell arteritis and polymyalgia rheumatica. In: Kelley WN, Harris ED Jr, Ruddy LS, Sledge CB, eds. Textbook of rheumatology. 2nd ed. Philadelphia: WB Saunders, 1985.

Rosenfeld SI, Kosmorsky GS, Klingele TE, Burde RM. Treatment of temporal arteritis with ocular involvement. Am J Med 1986; 80:143–145.

HYPERSENSITIVITY PNEUMONITIS

RAYMOND G. SLAVIN, M.D.

Synonyms for hypersensitivity pneumonitis include pulmonary hypersensitivity syndrome and extrinsic allergic alveolitis. The latter term is perhaps the most appropriate because it is so descriptive. "Extrinsic" refers to an exogenous allergen as the cause of the problem. "Allergic" refers to the hypersensitivity basis for the disease. "Alveolitis" refers to the part of the lung that is most affected. Despite the different terms, they all refer to the same underlying pathogenetic entity, namely, a disease process that is caused by sensitivity to an organic dust that is inhaled. The clinical presentation of the disease depends on the circumstances and degree of exposure. In the more common acute form associated with intermittent intense exposure to the organic dust, the individual responds 4 to 6 hours after exposure with low grade fever, chills, chest pain, cough, and dyspnea. In the chronic form associated with prolonged low grade exposure, the clinical presentation is much more insidious, with progressively increasing cough, dyspnea, weakness, malaise, and weight loss.

The causative antigens responsible for hypersensitivity pneumonitis can be divided into several categories, including thermophilic actinomycetes, fungi, amebae, animal products, and small molecular weight chemicals. The majority of cases are associated with occupational exposure, such as farming, mushroom packing, or grain loading. However, offending antigens may contaminate home heating or humidification units or be associated with hobbies such as pigeon breeding.

The diagnosis of hypersensitivity pneumonitis should be suspected in any patient presenting with interstitial pneumonitis or pulmonary fibrosis. Pulmonary function testing reveals a largely restrictive dysfunction, including decreases in pulmonary compliance and in carbon monoxide diffusion capacity. A careful history eliciting the onset of symptoms following exposure with remission on avoidance together with positive serum precipitins to the appropriate antigen is presumptive evidence of hypersensitivity pneumonitis. In rare instances further confirmation may have to be made by inhalation challenge with the suspected antigen. A recently described diagnostic aid is bronchoalveolar lavage. In hypersensitivity pneumonitis the lavage fluid contains many T lymphocytes, with the predominant T-cell subset being the T8 positive or T-suppressor cell.

THERAPEUTIC APPROACH

Avoidance

Clearly the most important aspect in the management of hypersensitivity pneumonitis is recognition and avoidance of the causative antigen. The physician's diagnostic index of suspicion must be high, and in every case of interstitial pneumonitis or pulmonary fibrosis a careful environmental survey of the patient's occupational, home, and avocational life must be carried out, searching for the presence of offending antigens. Once the disease is diagnosed and the antigen recognized, early avoidance is the definitive therapy. Hypersensitivity pneumonitis ultimately may be a fatal disease due to progressive respiratory insufficiency. It is estimated that five acute episodes will be followed by pulmonary damage and progressive disease. Therefore, it is vital to make the diagnosis early and institute proper environmental precautions to prevent the inexorable consequences of pulmonary fibrosis and irreparable tissue damage.

A general approach to the prevention of hypersensitivity pneumonitis is seen in Table 1. A number of interventions will decrease the formation of antigens in conducive environments. For example, the growth of thermophilic actinomycetes spores in compost can be suppressed by treatment with a 1 percent solution of propionic acid. Water that remains for long periods of time in older air conditioning or humidification units may become a fertile source for the growth of thermophilic organisms. Therefore, the water needs to be changed and the unit cleaned on a regular basis. Contaminated ventilation systems have to be thoroughly cleaned or replaced. Blowing cool air through stored hay helps to prevent the growth of mold. Harvesting crops when the moisture content is low also results in less exposure to organic dusts.

In occupational situations in which organic dust generation is inevitable, every effort should be made to reduce the workers' exposure. In enclosed spaces extremely dusty material should be handled mechanically. The use of particular types of silos may allow for automated feeding of cattle. Materials such as sugar cane should be stored outside and cattle fed outside as much as possible so that the associated organic dusts can be diluted by the ambient air.

In terms of removal of dusts from the air, improved ventilation may aid considerably. Electrostatic air purifiers may be of help when the concentration of dust is not too great. They would be overwhelmed in an area where moldy hay is being handled in which it is estimated that there are 1600 million spores per cubic meter of air. A person doing light work with moldy hay inhales 10 liters of air per minute, which would deposit 750,000 spores per minute in the lung.

The use of personal dust respirators or masks is limited because of inconvenience. A type 2B filter is effective in filtering small particles but causes so much resistance to the flow of air that people hard at work are unable to wear them. An air stream helmet in which an electrical pump blows air through a filter and into the breathing zone is heavy and uncomfortable to wear. Even the best device has a maximal filtering capacity of 99 percent for fine particles. The remaining 1 percent can produce new attacks in a highly sensitive individual. If the disease is not yet manifest, even a filter with 95 percent filtering capacity is adequate. Good results have been reported with a 3M disposable mask model 8710.

When the foregoing environmental control measures cannot be carried out or are inadequate, the patient should be removed from that work area. This may entail a change in the work place or type of work or in extreme cases a change in occupation.

Drug Therapy (Table 2)

In many cases no treatment is necessary other than avoidance of the causative antigen. Corticosteroid therapy, however, can greatly accelerate clinical improve-

TABLE 1 Prevention of Hypersensitivity Pneumonitis*

Decrease formation of antigens
Add chemicals to prevent growth
Change water frequently in humidification or air conditioning units
Use storage dryers on hay and straw
Harvest crops when moisture content is low
Decrease exposure to organic dust
Mechanically handle dusty materials within closed spaces
Remove dusts from ambient air
Use personal respirators or masks
Remove worker from disease producing environment

* Modified from Terho EO. Extrinsic allergic alveolitis—management of established cases. Eur J Respir Dis 1982; 123:101.

TABLE 2 Treatment of Hypersensitivity Pneumonitis

Acute form
Remove patient from exposure; may entail hospitalization
Oxygen
Prednisone 40–60 mg/day with slow tapering
Supportive measures—rest, antitussives, antipyretics
Repeated acute or subacute form
Decrease exposure as much as possible
Long term corticosteroid therapy emphasizing alternate day therapy
Chronic form
Trial with corticosteroids but continue only if radiographic findings and physiologic testing indicate a response

ment and should be considered in very ill patients with gross radiographic or physiologic abnormalities, such as hypoxemia. Oral therapy with prednisone in an initial daily dosage of 40 to 60 mg is usually adequate and should be continued until there is significant clinical, radiographic, and pulmonary function test evidence of improvement. The prednisone dosage then may be tapered slowly until resolution of clinical and radiologic signs is complete. The total duration of therapy is generally no more than 4 to 6 weeks provided exposure to the antigen is prevented. Inhaled corticosteroids are of no value in the treatment of hypersensitivity pneumonitis nor are bronchodilators or cromolyn unless bronchospasm is also present.

The dramatic response of hypersensitivity pneumonitis to corticosteroids may be a two edged sword. The rapid relief afforded by steriods may result in a false sense of security, so much so that the patient may return to the same work environment. Re-exposure will result in progression of the lung disease. It therefore must be emphasized and re-emphasized to the patient that corticosteroids are not a substitute for antigen identification and avoidance.

In cases of severe hypoxemia in the acute stage, oxygen should be administered in amounts sufficient to keep the Po_2 level between 60 and 100 mm Hg. Other supportive measures include rest, antitussives, and antipyretics.

On occasion, despite the physician's best efforts, the patient may elect to return to the same work place or occupation. This seems to be especially true of farmers, who find it particularly difficult to leave farming because of age, a large financial investment, and a lack of training and skills in other occupations. In these instances long term continuous corticosteroid therapy may have to be administered. One should strive for an alternate day program utilizing the lowest dosage that still controls the patient's symptoms.

The chronic form of hypersensitivity pneumonitis develops insidiously and occurs either following repeated acute episodes or as a result of long term low grade exposure. A therapeutic trial of steroids can be given but should be continued only if radiographic findings and physiologic testing indicate a beneficial response.

Appropriate treatment of the acute episode of hypersensitivity pneumonitis with avoidance of further antigen exposure results in an uneventful recovery with no progression to chronic untreatable disease.

SUGGESTED READING

Fink JN. Hypersensitivity pneumonitis. J Allergy Clin Immunol 1984; 74:1–9.

Terho EO. Extrinsic allergic alveolitis—management of stable cases. Eur J Respir Dis 1982; 123:101 (Suppl.).

Schatz M, Patterson R. Hypersensitivity pneumonitis—general considerations. Clin Rev Allergy 1983; 1:451–467.

AMYLOIDOSIS*

MARTHA SKINNER, M.D.
ALAN S. COHEN, M.D.

The treatment of amyloidosis has been limited because of an incomplete knowledge of its biochemical nature and pathogenesis. In the past few years it has become clear that amyloid is the broad term for a protein that takes on a unique configuration when it is deposited in tissue and that multiple biochemical forms as well as clinical syndromes exist. With these more precise definitions, the current treatment program has evolved.

The common denominator of the various forms of amyloid are the appearance of green birefringence on polarization microscopy after Congo red staining, the electron microscopic display of nonbranching fibrils, and the cross beta pattern visible on x-ray diffraction. The physicochemical phenomena that lead the different proteins to this final common amyloid fibril pathway are far less understood than the nature of the individual amyloid proteins, and probably represent the major unknown problem whose elucidation would lead to the resolution of already established amyloid disease.

Although there may be generally applicable principles in amyloid therapy, it is likely that from the view of prevention of the accumulation of these different proteins, multiple approaches may be needed.

*Study supported by grants from the U.S. Public Health Service, NIAMDD (AM 04599 and AM07014), the General Clinical Research Centers Branch of the Division of Research Resources, National Institutes of Health (RR 533), the Multipurpose Arthritis Center, the National Institutes of Health (AM 20613), and the Arthritis Foundation.

TABLE 1 Differentiation of Amyloid Type

	Primary (AL)	*Secondary (AA)*	*Hereditary (AF)*	*Hemodialysis (AH)*
History	No underlying disease	Chronic inflammation	Family history	On dialysis many years
Physical examination	Macroglossia Cardiomyopathy Hepatomegaly Orthostatic hypotension	Associated with underlying disease Hepatomegaly Splenomegaly	Scalloped pupil, neuropathy, carpal tunnel syndrome, vitreous opacities	Carpal tunnel syndrome
Laboratory studies	Increased plasma cells in bone marrow; M component in serum	Elevated SAA protein in serum Proteinuria	Decreased transthyretin in serum	Elevated beta-2 microglobulin
Potassium permanganate-Congo red staining of biopsy specimen	Resistant	Sensitive	Resistant	
Immunohistochemical reaction of biopsy specmen	Not diagnostic	Positive reaction with anti-AA antiserum	Positive reaction with anti-transthyretin antiserum	Positive reaction with antibeta-2 microglobulin antiserum
Tissue isolation of fibrils	Light chains (N-terminal fragment or whole)	AA protein	Transthyretin	Beta-2 microblobulin

DIAGNOSIS

To treat any disorder properly, the diagnosis must be firmly established. A wide variety of clinical symptoms may lead the physician to suspect a diagnosis of systemic amyloidosis; however, its actual prevalence is low. The diagnosis must be made by tissue biopsy in which a specimen is stained with Congo red and examined in polarized light. Abdominal fat aspiration has become the screening biopsy method of choice because of its ease in performance and lack of risk to the patient. If the abdominal fat analysis is negative, a more invasive biopsy may need to be undertaken. Once the diagnosis is established, the amyloid disease is classified according to type by a number of parameters, including the history, physical examination, laboratory studies, and special staining of biopsy material (Table 1). The systemic types include AL (primary or immunoglobulin related), AA (secondary or reactive), AF (hereditary or transthyretin [TTR], formerly called prealbumin-related), and AH (associated with hemodialysis) amyloidosis. Localized types associated with endocrine organs, aging, or particular areas of the body also exist.

The patient's history can lead one to suspect primary amyloidosis if there is no history of preceding illness, or one may suspect secondary amyloidosis if chronic inflammation has been present, or the hereditary form if there is a family history of amyloidosis. The history, however, in our experience is often complicated and not always clear enough to define the biochemical type of disease present. The physical examination is important but likewise not diagnostic as to the type. It may show an enlarged liver and spleen in both primary and secondary amyloidosis, neuropathy in both primary and hereditary amyloidosis, and severe cardiac involvement in primary and hereditary types as well. However, two physical findings are more suggestive in the determination of type; they are macroglossia in primary amyloidosis and a scalloped pupil in hereditary amyloidosis (familial amyloid polyneuropathy).

No single laboratory test is in itself diagnostic of amyloid disease, including those that measure the amyloid fibril precursor protein. A serum monoclonal gammopathy is found in about 75 percent of the patients with primary (AL) amyloidosis, but its presence is not diagnostic, for a number of other conditions may be characterized by serum M components. Likewise an elevated serum amyloid A (SAA) protein level does not predict, or may not even always be found in, secondary (AA) amyloidosis. SAA concentrations in normal individuals are less than 1 μg per ml and in patients with AA amyloidosis have been normal to very high (0.6 to 100 μg per ml). SAA is an acute phase protein, and an elevated concentration is simply an indication of inflammation or cell necrosis. Similarly, although a lowered TTR level has been shown to be present in individuals with hereditary (AF) amyloidosis, it is not sufficiently depressed below normal values to be diagnostic in any one individual.

The biochemical classification of amyloid type can be determined to some extent on the basis of biopsy material. Paraffin embedded tissue sections can be treated with potassium permanganate prior to Congo red staining. If the amyloid fibrils are of the secondary (AA) type, they are "sensitive" by this test; i.e., they lose their capacity to stain with Congo red after treatment with potassium permanganate. Both primary (AL) and hereditary (AF) fibril types are "resistant," or retain their capacity to stain with Congo red after potassium permanganate treatment.

To differentiate the AL and AF fibril types one must perform immunohistochemical staining with specific antisera to TTR. This procedure identifies the hereditary (AF) amyloid fibril type. The immunohistochemical staining procedure can also confirm the identity of (AA) amyloid fibrils with an antibody specific for AA protein, but this procedure is available only in research laboratories. There is no specific antibody for AL amyloid fibrils, and biochemical classification is inferred by the lack of reaction to antibodies specific for the other types. In the hemodialysis associated (AH) type, the fibrils are "sensitive" in the potassium permanganate–Congo red staining procedure and by reactive immunohistochemical staining with antiserum to beta-2 microglobulin. When enough biopsy material is available, definitive identification of the amyloid type can be made by fibril isolation from the tissue followed by sequence analysis of the isolated protein. This requires a relatively large piece of unfixed biopsy material or, more frequently, autopsy tissue.

TREATMENT

There is as yet no adequate specific therapy for any form of established amyloid disease. A number of therapeutic interventions have been tried, and two were found to be helpful after being used in large series of patients. In addition, supportive measures directed at the specific problems associated with amyloidosis have increased the length of life and made life more comfortable for many individuals. For all patients it is important that the amyloid type be clearly defined biochemically at the outset. This information aids in determining the prognosis and in addressing family concerns regarding heredity and planning for eventual supportive therapies.

In primary (AL) amyloidosis the two therapeutic interventions most frequently used have been colchicine and melphalan combined with prednisone (Table 2). In clinical trials both colchicine and melphalan have been shown to prolong survival two to three times that in control patients given no treatment. Because primary amyloidosis is a plasma cell dyscrasia, the use of chemotherapeutic drugs has a logical basis. However, since it is not a true malignant disease, there has been some reluctance to subject patients with AL amyloidosis to the bone marrow suppression risks of chemotherapy. In addition, the long term risk of developing leukemia now approaches 11 percent for patients who have received large amounts of melphalan and who survive long enough (3 or more years). Nevertheless the large series of Kyle and coworkers and several single case reports have shown that in some patients treated with melphalan, there is improvement in measurable clinical parameters, i.e., urine protein excretion, hepatomegaly, bone marrow plasmacytosis, and monoclonal gammopathy.

The recommended dosage for melphalan has been 0.15 to 0.25 mg per kg per day with prednisone, 1.5 to 2.0 mg per kg per day. Both drugs are given for 4 days and the treatment repeated every 6 weeks. We recommend that treatment be discontinued after 1 year to maintain the total dosage of melphalan at less than 600 mg, at which level the risk of leukemia is minimal. This seems to be a reasonable approach, because many of the long term survivors with the AL form who have shown measurable improvement received only 1 year or less of therapy. A blood count must be obtained at midcycle and prior to the next course of therapy; the dosage of melphalan is altered accordingly.

The other therapeutic option for AL amyloidosis is treatment with colchicine. The rationale for this treatment is no more precisely defined, but in a large clinical trial it proved to be effective in improving survival. Colchicine is known to affect mitosis, to disrupt microtubule organization, and to potentially interfere with microtubule cell function. Owing to the presumed participation of the macrophage in the pathogenesis of AA amyloidosis, and the concept that in AL amyloid the immunoglobulin is processed by the macrophage prior to its tissue deposition, it seems reasonable to suspect that it might alter or delay fibril formation or deposition in AL amyloid. The recommended dosage of colchicine is 0.6 mg twice daily, with a reduction to 0.6 mg daily if gastrointestinal side effects occur.

Other major therapies that have been used for the treatment of amyloidosis include ascorbic acid, dimethyl sulfoxide, penicillamine, and cytoxan. Most of these therapies have been reported in single case studies and definitive benefit from therapy has been unconvincing.

Supportive measures relating to the treatment of involved organ systems are of the utmost importance, particularly since there is not yet a definitive major therapy. AL amyloidosis affects all organ systems to some degree, but is often marked in the cardiac, renal, autonomic nervous, and gastrointestinal systems. Each patient presents a unique set of symptoms and degree of organ involvement, and a supportive program for treatment must be individualized. Some guidelines for this treatment that have been helpful are presented in Table 2.

The degree of organ involvement should be measured by appropriate noninvasive tests prior to instituting therapy. In fact, even if a patient has no symptoms in a particular organ system, a number of tests are warranted to note whether asymptomatic involvement is present. Assessment of the heart by an electrocardiogram, an echocardiogram, and 24 hour Holter monitoring and the kidneys by function tests and a 24 hour urine protein analysis are important parts of the management for all patients. In some patients the gastrointestinal system should be examined by x-ray studies, a gastric emptying scan, and tests for malabsorption.

After the organ system involvement has been identified, the treatment program is symptomatic according to the physiologic problem presented. For example, the congestive heart failure of AL amyloidosis usually is due to a constrictive cardiomyopathy and is best treated with moderate salt restriction and vigorous diuretic therapy. The use of digitalis is not indicated. In fact, both digitalis and calcium channel blocking drugs have been

TABLE 2 Treatment for Primary (AL) Amyloidosis

Major therapy options:

Pharmacologic Therapy

1. Melphalan 0.15–0.25 mg/kg/day × 4 days
   Prednisone 1.5–2.0 mg/kg/day × 4 days
   Repeat administration every 6 weeks for 1 year with dosage changes according to CBC results
2. Colchicine 0.6 mg bid
   May be given as the major therapy alone or in combination with the above, omitting it on the days melphalan and prednisone are given

Supportive therapy (generally applicable to systemic amyloid of AL, AA, or AF types):

Organ System	*Symptom*	*Treatment*
Cardiac	Congestive failure	Salt restriction of 1–2 g/day (unless patient also has orthostatic hypotension)
		Diuretics
	Heart block	Pacemaker
Renal	Nephrotic syndrome	Salt restriction of 1–2 g/day
		Elastic stockings for edema
		Dietary increase of protein to 1.5 g/kg body weight
	Renal failure	Dialysis (chronic ambulatory peritoneal dialysis or hemodialysis)
Autonomic nervous	Orthostatic hypotension	Increase salt to at least 6 g/day (need to evaluate cardiac and renal systems first)
		Elastic stockings
		9-alpha-fluorohydrocortisone (Florinef)
	Gastric atony	Small frequent feedings (6/day) low in fat
		Metoclopramide hydrochloride (Reglan; use with caution if patient also has orthostatic hypotension)
		Jejunostomy tube for commercially prepared formula feeding
Gastrointestinal	Diarrhea	Dietary changes
		Medium chain triglyceride oil supplements of 60 ml/day
		Low fat diet of 40 g or less
		Medications
		Tetracycline
		Diphenoxylate hydrochloride with atropine (Lomotil)
		Psyllium hydrophilic muciloid (Metamucil)
		Total parenteral nutrition
	Macroglossia	Maintain airway
		Hemiglossectomy
Peripheral nervous	Neuropathy	Physical therapy
		Medications
		Amitriptyline
		Carbamazepine (Tegretol)
Hematologic	Intracutaneous bleeding	Avoid trauma
	Factor X deficiency	Splenectomy

shown to bind to amyloid fibrils, and their use has been associated with sudden death. Thus, unless a nonamyloid cardiac problem occurs coincidentally, their routine use is not recommended.

Major amyloid involvement of the kidneys poses another set of problems, with the nephrotic syndrome often associated with massive proteinuria, edema, and a low serum albumin concentration. Patients should be encouraged to increase the dietary protein to 1.5 g per kg body weight in an attempt to replace urinary protein loss and raise the serum albumin concentration. It is recommended that 80 percent of this protein be of high biologic value (meat, milk) and that, if necessary, the salt restriction be liberalized to make this diet palatable. The total caloric intake should be 30 to 50 cal per kg per day. Albumin infusions have been helpful, but because they are of very temporary benefit, they are not recommended. Rest periods during the day with the legs elevated and the use of elastic stockings decrease peripheral edema. If renal failure occurs, long term ambulatory peritoneal dialysis and hemodialysis are options for therapy, and both have been successful. Since amyloid involvement of many organ systems is often present, kidney transplantation is usually not considered, although it is not contraindicated.

Symptoms relating to the autonomic nervous system are the most difficult to treat. Orthostatic hypotension is treated initially by increasing the salt in the diet to 6 g per day or more and use of elastic stockings of the fitted antigravity type. Patients are also encouraged to stand up slowly and may be given 9-alpha-fluorohydrocortisone with some benefit. Symptoms of always feeling full and occasionally vomiting may represent gastric atony. If this is confirmed by a gastric emptying scan, treatment should start with small frequent feedings that are low in fat. Metoclopramide hydrochloride can be tried, but this drug may make orthostasis worse and should be used with caution. A surgically placed jejunostomy tube for enteral formula feeding may be lifesaving in providing adequate nutritional support in patients with gastric atony and can be used in place of or to supplement the oral intake.

Other supportive therapies in AL amyloidosis include changes in the dietary fat content or a trial of medications that slow the bowel or add bulk to combat diarrhea. Total parenteral nutrition is used as a last resort. Macroglossia has been a difficult problem to manage. Surgical intervention may be needed to maintain an airway or for cosmetic reasons if the tongue becomes so massive that the mouth cannot be closed.

Peripheral sensory neuropathy is mild in AL amyloidosis, and symptoms of pain disappear as the neuropathy worsens. Tranquilizing or antiseizure medications are helpful. Physical therapy is important in maintaining muscle mass and preventing contractures if motor neuropathy occurs.

Symptoms associated with bleeding can be mild or can constitute a serious hematologic emergency. Those of a mild nature include intracutaneous bleeding, for which there is no specific therapy other than avoiding trauma; intracutaneous bleeding is presumed to be due to the increased friability of small blood vessels with amyloid fibril deposits within their walls and is not a hematologic abnormality. Serious bleeding can occur with factor deficiencies, most commonly factor X, but all calcium dependent clotting factors can be deficient. This is believed to be the result of the affinity of anionic amyloid fibril deposits for clotting factors (as well as other proteins) and their removal from plasma by absorption onto the fibril deposit. It is important to assess the clotting status prior to all surgical procedures. In emergency bleeding situations patients can be given commercial clotting factor preparations. In a few patients with splenomegaly, removal of the spleen has corrected the factor deficiency, perhaps by removing a large deposit of amyloid fibrils.

In AA amyloidosis the major therapy depends on the underlying inflammatory or infectious disease (Table 3). The suppression or elimination of infection is of the utmost importance. Colchicine is the major therapy for patients with familial Mediterranean fever and is also used in AA amyloidosis due to other causes along with the major therapy appropriate for the underlying inflammation. If the disease is a form of arthritis, treatment with nonsteroidal anti-inflammatory drugs along with rest and exercises is appropriate. In addition a remittive drug should be given to completely suppress the underlying inflammation. If the patient has proteinuria (very common in AA amyloidosis), gold salts and D-penicillamine are not recommended, but methotrexate could be considered. It is not clear whether prednisone accelerates amyloid fibril deposition within tissues. Along with therapy it is wise to monitor the serum SAA level; it is a more accurate measure of inflammation than the sedi-

TABLE 3 Treatment for Secondary (AA) Amyloidosis

Major therapy:
1 Aggressive treatment of underlying inflammatory disease with monitoring of SAA level on a regular basis
2 Surgical excision of infectious process when feasible, i.e., lung lobectomy for bronchiectasis, bone resection for osteomyelitis, colectomy for chronic ulcerative colitis
3 Colchicine 0.6 mg bid

Supportive therapy (in addition to that outlined for AL amyloid):

Organ System	*Symptom*	*Treatment*
Renal	Renal failure	Avoid nonsteroidal anti-inflammatory drugs; if necessary use Aspirin or Clinoril
		Dialysis
		Kidney transplant should be considered

mentation rate, especially when the patient has the nephrotic syndrome.

If the underlying disease is an infection, surgical excision may be feasible, particularly if medical therapy has been ineffective. Usually after AA amyloidosis develops (it generally takes years), there is some urgency to resolve the infection. Surgical excision has been used with success in patients requiring partial pulmonary lobectomy for bronchiectasis, resection of bone affected with osteomyelitis, colectomy for chronic ulcerative colitis, and tooth extractions for dental abscesses. When surgery can be applied to remove a source of infection, it stops the progression of amyloid disease. In some patients who have already developed the nephrotic syndrome, progression of renal disease may continue.

Supportive therapy follows the recommendations given for AL amyloidosis when it is necessary. Because organ involvement with amyloidosis is usually considerably less, the need for supportive therapy is minimal. Renal involvement, however, is frequently present, and progression to renal failure occurs even when optimal therapy is given for the underlying disease. In these patients kidney transplantation should be strongly considered, for reports have shown that patients do well and in AA amyloidosis the survival is fairly long.

In hereditary (AF) amyloidosis the deposition of amyloid fibrils occurs because of a genetic variant structure of the protein TTR. No treatment has been defined that specifically interferes with or slows this process, and because patients with this condition survive 10 to 20 years, therapeutic benefit is difficult to measure. Colchicine has been given at a dosage of 0.6 mg twice daily because of its potential capacity to delay fibril processing noted earlier and its lack of toxicity. Supportive measures for the treatment of peripheral neuropathy, autonomic neuropathy, and diarrhea are frequently needed. They are used as outlined in Table 2 for AL amyloidosis. In addition, genetic counseling regarding the autosomal dominant nature of the genetic defect and the identification of "at risk" family members who are carriers of the trait can be offered. It is likely that technologic advances in genetic engineering will have more to offer for this form of amyloidosis in the future.

Amyloid associated with hemodialysis (AH) is a result of an excessively high serum level of beta-2 microglobulin, which is not filtered out by the cuprophan dialysis membrane. Normal levels of beta-2 microglobulin are less than 4 mg per liter, whereas in patients treated with hemodialysis, levels are from 45 to 189 mg per liter. It takes years of dialysis (usually 10 or more) for this type of amyloid to develop, and it forms in synovial membranes surrounding large joints (hips, shoulders, wrists) with erosive lesions within adjacent bones. Only rarely have amyloid deposits of the same biochemical composition been found in other tissues. Effective treatment will likely require a change in dialysis membrane that allows filtration of the 11,000 dalton protein, beta-2 microglobulin. It is reported that patients given hemodialysis with an AN 69 membrane, which currently has limited use in Europe, have beta-2 microglobulin levels consistently lower by 50 to 60 percent. It is known that in chronic ambulatory peritoneal dialysis the beta-2 levels are elevated to a lesser extent (range, 17 to 79 mg per liter) than in hemodialysis. It may be that patients given chronic ambulatory peritoneal dialysis will not get AH amyloidosis or that a longer time with dialysis treatment will be necessary for it to develop.

Localized amyloid deposits occasionally pose the need for surgical excision. These are most commonly located in the tracheobronchial tree, the urinary bladder, or the conjunctiva. The biochemical composition of this form of amyloid is not yet known. Biopsy staining patterns have always shown it to be potassium permanganate resistant, and immunohistochemical tests indicate that it is negative with antisera to AA protein and TTR. In patients suspected of having localized amyloidosis it is important to rule out a systemic form. If the amyloid deposit is localized, the treatment is usually observation. Enlargement of the amyloid deposit may take place; however, spreading to another site has never occurred. Local excision may be necessary to correct respiratory obstruction or for cosmetic purposes. Laser resecton is usually used for respiratory tract lesions because it minimizes the danger of excessive bleeding.

SUGGESTED READING

Cohen AS, Rubinow A, Anderson JJ, Skinner M, Mason JH, Libbey C, Kayne H. Survival of patients with primary (AL) amyloidosis: cases treated with colchicine from 1976–1983 compared with cases seen in previous years 1961–1973. Am J Med 1987; 82:1182–1190.

Cohen AS, Skinner M. The diagnosis of amyloid. In: Cohen AS, ed. Laboratory diagnostic procedures in the rheumatic diseases. 3rd ed. New York: Grune & Stratton, 1985; 377.

Kyle RA, Greipp PR. Primary systemic amyloidosis: comparison of melphalan and prednisone versus placebo. Blood 1978; 52:818–827.

Kyle RA, Greipp PR, Garton JP, Gertz MA. Primary systemic amyloidosis: comparison of melphalan/prednisone versus colchicine. Am J Med 1985; 79:708–716.

Zemer D, Pras M, Sohar E, Modan M, Cabili S, Gafni J. Colchicine in the prevention and treatment of the amyloidosis of familial Mediterranean fever. N Engl J Med 1986; 314:1001–1005.

SKIN DISEASES

ACNE

PETER E. POCHI, M.D.

Acne is a prevalent skin disorder, with a peak occurrence in the mid to late teens. However, adults are by no means immune from it, and some dermatologists' practices may actually comprise more adults than teenagers with the disease.

Although research on acne in the past two to three decades has elucidated a good deal of information about the pathogenic factors involved, two crucial matters about the disease remain elusive, namely, why it comes and why it goes. With time most cases of acne undergo complete or near complete involution, but the reason for it is a mystery. In terms of early development, susceptible pilosebaceous follicles of the face and trunk are affected, with abnormal keratinization occurring in the follicular epithelium. Again the reason for this follicle disturbance has not been adequately explained. Proliferation of anaerobic diphtheroids (*Propionibacterium acnes*) that require sebaceous lipids for subsistence is a central event in the induction of the inflammatory lesions of acne. These bacteria possess chemoattractant properties for neutrophils that initiate a series of events culminating in the expression of inflammation, both immune and nonimmune mediated. Characteristically an inflammatory lesion lasts 2 to 3 weeks, usually healing without a trace but occasionally leaving behind scars, mostly atrophic but occasionally hypertrophic.

GENERAL THERAPEUTIC APPROACH AND BASIS OF MANAGEMENT

From the foregoing brief summary of the etiologic events in acne, it is evident that such a multifactorial disorder would require a multifaceted therapeutic regimen. This is often desirable and necessary, although a unitarian approach may prove sufficient to control the disease, particularly mild cases or those early in their onset, or as maintenance therapy. Combination treatment may embrace the topical use of two or even three medications or the use of oral as well as topical therapy.

The decision about specific drugs or measures to use in acne depends on two broad considerations, namely, the severity of the acne and the type of acne present, i.e., whether it is predominantly inflammatory or noninflammatory. Before undertaking or recommending treatment it is important that time be taken to obtain an accurate history from the patient concerning the acne. Too often this aspect is overlooked or glossed over quickly. Important in this regard is the natural evolution of the acne and the response to prior treatments, including over the counter preparations. Women should be questioned about menstrual cycles and the presence of other possible manifestations of androgen excess, such as hirsutism or scalp hair recession or thinning. A history of drug ingestion can be important too, since certain medications such as lithium, excessive iodides, and anticonvulsants may aggravate existing acne. Even if little of the history obtained proves helpful for the overall management, the initial visit provides an important basis for a positive interaction between physician and patient. At times the patient, particularly a teenager, may seem indifferent to the physician's inquiry, but the opposite is more often the case.

After examination the disease should be explained to the patient, although the amount of time spent at this point depends on the simplicity or complexity of the problem and the physician's perception of how much of a "didactic" exercise the patient wishes to engage in. However, it is important to mention the general inutility of extrascrupulous cleansing, special diets, and the probable lack of association of the acne with the patient's sexual practices. Once a treatment plan is decided upon, the dermatologist should be sure that the following are explained to the patient: (1) Treatments by and large are suppressive rather than curative, so that therapy must be maintained, or changed if later necessary, until the condition undergoes natural involution, which it does in most cases. (2) Most treatments work by preventing the formation of new lesions rather than by healing more rapidly those lesions already present. Moreover, this preventive effect is not ordinarily observed until 3 to 6 weeks have elapsed. (3) Apropos to this, medications must be applied topically to all the affected areas rather than to individual lesions per se. (4) Trunk acne seems to be less well controlled by topical therapy than facial acne.

ANTIKERATINIZING (COMEDOLYTIC) EFFECT

Tretinoin (retinoic acid) is the most effective drug topically because of its capacity to reverse, at least in part, the abnormal follicular hyperkeratosis, the earliest known event in the formation of the acne lesion. By the same token it can help to prevent the transformation of early noninflammatory microcomedones (lesions not clinically visible) into inflammatory sequelae. Salicylic acid also has a keratolytic action, although its benefit in acne via this mechanism appears to be much less than that of tretinoin. Comedolytic assays have shown benzoyl peroxide to have a similar action, but its effect also seems to be comparatively weak.

The commonest objection patients have to the use of tretinoin is the primary irritant reaction it frequently causes. This can be lessened or even prevented by a number of measures that include waiting 20 to 30 minutes after washing before applying it; when using it at bedtime, not retiring until a half-hour has passed; using it every other day at first, rather than the recommended daily application, to allow for accommodation of the skin to its irritant effect; and at first, especially in the winter or dry climates, using the milder cream preparations. Tretinoin is available in creams (0.025, 0.05, and 0.1 percent) and gels (0.01 and 0.025 percent) and in a liquid formulation (0.05 percent) (Table 1).

Another complaint patients may have about tretinoin, which is less frequent but more annoying to the patient, is that there is a flare-up of the acne in the early weeks of treatment. In my experience this occurs to some extent in about 20 percent of the patients and at times can be quite marked. Fortunately the flare-up subsides within a few weeks or sooner, but very uncommonly the worsening may continue unabated and requires discontinuation of medication.

Oral therapy with isotretinoin, the 13-cis isomer of tretinoin, also, as one might expect, has antikeratinizing properties, but it has other antiacne actions as well. Treatment of acne with this drug is described later in this article.

ANTIMICROBIAL THERAPY

The therapy most commonly utilized for acne is antimicrobial therapy, owing in great measure to the availability of a wide variety of preparations for both topical and oral use. Implicit in the widespread use of antibacterial drugs is the recognition, mentioned earlier, that the inflammatory lesions of acne for which most patients seek a physician's attention result from the presence of *P. acnes* within acne susceptible pilosebaceous follicles. One could postulate, with reasonable certainty, that if these follicles could be depleted of these anaerobic diphtheroids, inflammatory acne could be reduced to zero, regardless of whether abnormal keratinization was affected. In actuality suppression of *P. acnes* by antimicrobial therapy, whether topical or oral, is only partially achievable, although sometimes just enough to effect marked or complete amelioration of the inflammatory lesions.

TABLE 1 Tretinoin Preparations

Form	*Concentration (%)*
Cream	0.025
	0.05
	0.1
Gel	0.01
	0.025
Liquid	0.05

For mild to moderate cases of inflammatory acne, benzoyl peroxide and topical antibiotic therapy have attained prominence in management. Benzoyl peroxide, longest in use for acne, is available in concentrations ranging from 2.5 to 10 percent and in a variety of vehicles—lotions, creams, gels, washes, and soaps. There are at least 30 different marketed preparations that are available with or without a prescription. The majority of nonprescription products are lotions and creams. There is no evidence that prescription products are more efficacious than over the counter preparations, although it is possible that gel formulations do possess some superiority.

Benzoyl peroxide may be applied one to two times daily, again being certain that the patient applies it to the entire affected area, although it has been reported (but not confirmed) that individual lesions may heal more quickly following its use. Benzoyl peroxide possesses two advantages over topical antibiotic therapy. First, it is, in general, more effective. Second, *P. acnes* resistance does not develop, so that if a patient's acne worsens during benzoyl peroxide therapy, it is because the acne has become more active rather than because the benzoyl peroxide somehow has been rendered less effective.

There are, however, disadvantages to the use of benzoyl peroxide compared with antibiotics. First, it is almost invariably more irritating than topically applied antibiotics, even if the lowest concentration, 2.5 percent, is used. Second, sensitization may occur (rare with topical antibiotic therapy), although the precise incidence has not been clearly established. In my experience fewer than one in 100 patients develop allergic contact dermatitis to benzoyl peroxide. Third, the irritant effect of benzoyl peroxide may accentuate the postinflammatory hyperpigmentation seen in dark skinned persons. Last, it may bleach hair and colored fabrics.

Topical antibiotic therapy has come to occupy a prominent niche in the treatment of minimal to moderately inflamed acne. Such preparations include, in order of their introduction into the clinical practice, tetracycline, clindamycin, erythromycin, and meclocycline sulfosalicylate (Table 2). All have been shown in controlled studies to be more effective in reducing the number of inflammatory lesions than control vehicles, although as a general rule, the percentage difference in inhibition between active drug and control vehicle is less than that between the vehicle and the baseline valves. Tetracycline is the least effective of this

TABLE 2 Antibiotics for Acne

Topical therapy
Clindamycin
Erythromycin
Meclocycline sulfosalicylate
Tetracycline
Oral therapy
Tetracycline
Erythromycin
Minocycline
Doxycycline
Trimethoprim-sulfamethoxazole
Clindamycin

group. Most of these antibiotics are in liquid vehicles, although some are available as pledgets, creams, and ointments. The latter two are better tolerated and more useful in patients with sensitive skin. Although, as noted, their effectiveness over a wide range of patients is less than that of benzoyl peroxide, one advantage is that the antibiotics are virtually devoid of allergenicity. A concern in regard to their use has been the potential for the development of resistant bacterial organisms, but to date this fear does not appear to have been realized, at least not at a clinical level.

The effect of benzoyl peroxide and of topical antibiotic therapy can be enhanced by the concomitant use of tretinoin. Often this combination, i.e., the use of each one daily or more frequently, is not well tolerated. However, if tolerated, a regimen of tretinoin with topical antibacterial therapy remains the most effective way, to date, of suppressing less than severe cases of acne. Benzoyl peroxide has also been combined with erythromycin in a single gel base preparation.

Systemic antibiotic therapy has been used for decades in the treatment of acne. The four that are clearly effective in the majority of cases of inflammatory acne are tetracycline, erythromycin, minocycline, and doxycycline (see Table 2). Also effective is clindamycin, although it is infrequently used nowadays because of the risk, albeit very small, of the development of pseudomembranous colitis. The indications for the oral use of antibiotics in acne are as follows: moderately severe to severe inflammatory acne; less severe cases of acne not adequately responsive to topical therapy; still milder cases of acne, in which the individual because of sensitive skin (atopics often) is unable to tolerate topical therapy or in which there is evidence of active scarring; and patients with predominantly truncal acne, which ordinarily does not respond satisfactorily to externally applied medications.

The oral doses of antibiotics used vary with the severity of the disease, although I tend to start with "full" dosages, viz., 1.0 g of tetracycline daily or its equivalent for other antibiotics, even if the acne is only of moderate severity. A more rapid response is achieved and is decidedly preferable if there is any evidence of the development of scarring. An exception to this starting dosage of antibiotic is minocycline, which in dosages of 200 mg per day can cause symptoms of ototoxicity. Only if the disease is severe would I start with this dosage. Tetracycline must be taken on an empty stomach and for logistic reasons can be taken in twice daily doses of 500 mg, although occasionally this amount is not tolerated by the upper gastrointestinal tract. Erythromycin is less affected by the ingestion of food and minocycline, the least.

The advantages and disadvantages of the different antibiotics vary. Gastrointestinal effects occur most frequently with erythromycin. Phototoxicity is moderately severe with doxycycline, moderate with tetracycline, minimal with minocycline, and absent with erythromycin. *Candida* vaginitis is most frequent with tetracycline, occurring in about 15 percent of the patients taking long term therapy. A special problem with minocycline is the occasional development of pigmentary changes, consisting either of small bluish tattoo-like macules on the face, often in scars, or less commonly a brownish hyperpigmentation elsewhere. These pigmentary changes are reversible on drug discontinuation.

The advantage shared by these three antibiotics is the very low incidence of allergic sensitization with their use. This is in contrast to trimethoprim-sulfamethoxazole, which is also effective for acne but with which allergic reactions are far more common.

Other antibiotics used in acne include ampicillin, amoxicillin, and the cephalosporin group of antibiotics. Controlled studies to assess their effectiveness are lacking. Ampicillin suppresses *P. acnes* weakly.

ANTI-INFLAMMATORY DRUGS

The most rapid and most predictable way of reducing the severity of inflammatory acne is the systemic use of corticosteroids in anti-inflammatory dosages, e.g., 30 to 50 mg of prednisone daily. Once the dosage is reduced to 10 to 15 mg per day, the acne begins to flare up. Obviously such treatment is replete with drawbacks, and its use is limited to patients who have periodic severe but infrequent and brief flare-ups.

The principal use of anti-inflammatory steroids is their injection into inflamed lesions to shorten their duration. I use triamcinolone acetonide suspension in a concentration of 2.5 to 10 mg per milliliter. The lower concentration is usually effective. In fact the results of one report have revealed that a concentration of 0.6 mg per milliliter is virtually as effective as higher ones. The risk of a 10 mg per milliliter concentration is the induction of atrophy, even though it almost always reverts with time.

Topical corticosteroid therapy seems to have little effect on acne, although the reason is not certain. The generally held view is that there is inadequate penetration of the steroid into the involved site. Moreover its use is thought to be contraindicated because of the weakening effect of the steroid on the follicular wall, with the possible consequent development of folliculitis ("steroid acne").

Studies with nonsteroidal anti-inflammatory drugs (e.g., naproxen, ibuprofen) have not shown an overwhelming benefit, even when administered in high dosages.

However, one study showed unequivocally that the administration of high dosages of ibuprofen (2.4 g per day) enhances the antiacne effect of concomitantly administered tetracycline in a dosage of 1.0 g daily.

SEBACEOUS GLAND INHIBITION

Sebum, the secretory product of the sebaceous glands, is an integral factor in the pathogenesis of acne. A substantive reduction in the activity of these androgen sensitive glands results in a decrease in the intensity of the disease. To date no topical therapy has been discovered that will effectively suppress sebaceous activity. Systemic therapy is required, involving the use of hormonal therapy for androgen suppression.

The drug longest in use for this purpose is estrogen, whose action is to inhibit the pituitary-ovarian axis, with consequent reduction of ovarian androgen production. Some effect on the adrenal gland may occur as well. The drugs are those marketed for oral contraception. Although no controlled studies have clearly delineated the effectiveness of oral estrogen treatment, clinical experience has disclosed that this form of therapy can be beneficial. However, uncomfortably high dosages of estrogen are usually needed, i.e., more than 50 μg of ethinyl estradiol or mestranol daily, to yield a reasonable chance of success. Preparations containing more than 50 μg of estrogen have been withdrawn from the market. The response is slow, requiring 2 to 4 months for clear-cut improvement to become evident. Moreover, as with virtually all other acne treatments, the effect is suppressive rather than curative, so that even if there is a good result, recurrence of the acne is the consequence of treatment discontinuance.

Another disadvantage of estrogen therapy is the problem of the concomitant use or need for oral antibiotic therapy for the acne or other medical conditions. There have been reports that antibiotics may decrease the level of the administered estrogen in the blood. As a consequence, if the estrogen is being taken for the dual purpose of acne treatment and contraception, protection against pregnancy might be reduced. The chance that such an interaction will lead to pregnancy is not known but is likely to be very low.

Another method for androgen suppression is low dose glucocorticoid administration to decrease adrenal elaboration of androgens, particularly dehydroepiandrosterone. In many studies this androgen, either free or sulfated, has been found to be increased in women with persistent acne, even without collateral signs of androgen excess. Treatment of such patients with dexamethasone, 0.25 to 0.5 mg daily, or with prednisone, 5 to 10 mg daily, has been reported to decrease the acne. However, as with estrogen, controlled studies are still lacking so that the true benefit from low dose steroid treatment remains unestablished. What has been demonstrated, however, is that combined estrogen-glucocorticoid treatment effects a marked reduction in sebum levels and very significant acne improvement.

Spironolactone in high dosages, i.e., 100 to 200 mg daily, has a peripheral antiandrogen effect. It has been reported to be helpful in women with acne. I have found it to be effective in approximately 50 percent of the patients, the remainder showing only modest to no improvement. Common side effects from spironolactone are menstrual irregularity and fatigue, symptoms that can decrease despite continued administration of the drug.

With any form of hormone therapy I generally try not to exceed 9 months of treatment but occasionally continue the therapy for up to 12 months. The occurrence of side effects in any given patient might curtail the use of whatever regimen has been selected.

ISOTRETINOIN

Introduced into clinical practice in 1982, the synthetic retinoid, isotretinoin, has proved to be superior in the treatment of acne and the drug to use in patients with severe nodulo-cystic acne in whom traditional regimens, including systemic antibiotic therapy, have failed. In fact, it is only in this class of patient that the drug has been approved for use. However, my inclination is to extend its use to the occasional patient who has less severe cystic acne or even noncystic acne but who is developing active scarring and has resisted the standard treatments. The oral dosage of isotretinoin is 0.5 to 2.0 mg per kilogram per day. The dosage that should suffice for most patients is 80 mg per day, although heavy individuals or those with predominantly truncal acne may require the higher dosages. The drug generally induces a high incidence of remission despite the severity of the disease and its previous recalcitrance to treatment.

Numerous side effects preclude the use of the drug in all forms of acne, although most of the reactions are more of a nuisance than a danger. These changes are chiefly in the skin and mucous membranes and most commonly consist of cheilitis, various types of dry skin rashes, dry eyes, minor degrees of scalp hair loss, and occasional musculoskeletal discomfort. Perhaps the most annoying side effect, insofar as the patient is concerned, is a temporary worsening of the acne, not dissimilar to that seen with tretinoin given topically, but more severe, and observed in about one-third of the patients treated with isotretinoin.

Minimal hyperostoses have been seen in spinal x-ray views in acne patients treated with conventional doses of isotretinoin. They have occurred in 10 percent of the patients, have been asymptomatic, and have not progressed on discontinuation of treatment. Decrease in dark adaptation has been experienced, which reverts to normal when the drug is stopped. The most serious side effect of isotretinoin is its teratogenic potential. One study demonstrates a 25-fold increase in the development of major fetal abnormalities in women who were pregnant or became pregnant while receiving the drug. Prevention of pregnancy while the patient is taking this treatment and for 1 month afterward is an absolute necessity, with the responsibility shared by the physician and the patient.

MISCELLANEOUS FORMS OF THERAPY

Cryotherapy

In addition to intralesional injections of steroid to combat inflammation in individual lesions, the use of cryotherapy is a useful alternative, although in my experience not as effective. Liquid nitrogen or dry ice is applied to individual lesions. Even less effective is the application of ice, but this has the advantage that the patient can do it at home. No standard regimen has been developed for lesional "ice cube" treatment, but I suggest to the patient that at the first evidence of a new inflammatory lesion forming, an ice cube be applied for 5 to 10 minutes to the lesion three to four times daily for 1 to 2 days. Some patients claim benefit from this treatment.

Surgical Measures

In active disease both noninflammatory and inflammatory lesions can be decreased by minor surgical procedures. Comedones can be removed with ease and little discomfort. Open comedones can be extracted directly, but closed comedones first need to have the small poral opening enlarged by inserting and rotating the opening with a 20 gauge needle.

Inflammatory lesions may be drained if pus is evident, but care must be taken not to incise widely. If the pustular contents cannot be drained easily following simple needle puncture, the lesion is best left alone or instead injected intralesionally with steroid.

A variety of procedures are used to improve the appearance of scars that may form during the healing of inflammatory lesions. If the scars are hypertrophic (usually on shoulders, upper back, and anterior chest), they can be injected with triamcinolone acetonide suspension in concentrations ranging from 10 to 40 mg per milliliter. Hypertrophic scars, however, have the tendency to decrease slowly in size spontaneously.

Atrophic scars are permanent. A variety of techniques are available for their removal, including dermabrasion, simple excision, excision with punch grafts, and bovine collagen implants.

ALLERGIC CONTACT DERMATITIS

WILLIAM P. JORDAN Jr., M.D.

Contact dermatitis is either an immunologic or nonimmunologic exogenous disorder that produces inflammatory changes ranging from acute eruptions (eczematous) to chronic secondary skin lesions. Since many strong haptenes are also irritating on contact, some cases of contact dermatitis can represent nearly simultaneous immunologic and nonimmunologic injuries. The dermatitis that is delayed, specific, acquired through exposure(s), and transferable (by cells) is universally referred to as allergic contact dermatitis. Irritant contact dermatitis cannot be transferred to a recipient by cells or serum. Contacts with potential irritants can suggest immunologic contact dermatitis, because exposure concentrations and schedules for irritants can create the appearance of specificity in some patients. Distinguishing between the two forms of contact dermatitis, and appreciating that the two may coexist in the same patient, can be critical to the patient, employer, or a third party responsible for medical payment or compensations. The United States Department of Labor reported that 45 percent of all cases of occupational illness in 1977 were caused by skin disorders, most of which are called contact dermatitis.

Under certain circumstances all substances, including water, can produce an inflammatory nonimmunologic dermatitis, but not every substance can produce allergic contact dermatitis. Some haptenes require only one exposure under some test conditions. The dermatitis appears approximately 14 days later (range, 7 to 21 days) and without a deliberate second exposure. A residuum of the first dose, applied 14 days earlier, is sufficient to elicit the dermatitis after the critical induction period is over. This induction dose flare is rarely seen in the clinical setting from poison ivy or hair dying, but could occur with prodigious amounts of a haptene.

Haptenes causing weak to moderate reactions require a catalogue to name. They typically induce allergic contact dermatitis when repeatedly applied to skin that has pre-existing inflammation or loss of corneal barrier integrity.

Nearly all cases of allergic contact dermatitis stem from exposures that have just taken place 1 to 5 days prior to the dermatitis in previously sensitized subjects. The exposures are covert or overt eliciting exposures. The median time until well developed dermatitis develops is about 2 days. Dermatitis can be observed as early as 8 hours. The time until the onset of a grossly observable reaction is between 8 hours and about 5 days; the patient's sensitivity and haptene flux are critical in determining this range.

ACUTE IRRITANT CONTACT DERMATITIS

Cutaneous injury from contact with strong irritating chemicals is almost always a self-evident diagnosis. Workplace exposures to strong irritants are common, but homes and offices contain many utility substances that rival those used in heavy industry in the irritation they cause. These injuries require copious aqueous washings and supportive therapy. Oral or topical steroid therapy has no beneficial effects in cases of significant chemically induced cytotoxic injury. Vigilon provides a nontraumatic changeable protective dressing that helps to alleviate pain associated with skin injuries that expose the dermis to air. The physician must feel confident that no residual chemical from the injury will be trapped under this type of dressing. The hydrofluoric acid skin burn is an example of a severe chemical burn that could conceivably be trapped under this type of dressing. Some burns require hours of aqueous irrigation. Reports in literature tend to favor intradermal and subcutaneous injections of 10 percent calcium gluconate in and around the burned areas as a preferred treatment for this type of burn. The injection dose is 0.5 ml per square centimeter of burned area, the injection is extended about 0.5 cm into the normal surrounding tissue margins of the burn.

Topical steroid therapy can decrease the clinical signs and symptoms of mild intact epidermal injuries from chemicals.

Locally Severe or Generalized Acute Allergic Contact Dermatitis

Acute allergic contact dermatitis can be a dermatologic emergency, requiring timely and aggressive therapy. Definitive therapy requires the use of large systemic doses of corticosteroids. Initial oral dosages of prednisone should be in the range of 1 to 1.2 mg per kilogram daily. The daily dosage is tapered after the initial doses have brought about significant clinical improvement. The initial dosage is reduced over a 7 to 14 day period. Occasionally severe rhus dermatitis rebounds 10 to 14 days after a good initial clearing and an apparently adequate reduction phase. This scenario is common with oral steroid therapy in a dose pack. Abrupt steroid withdrawal is not contraindicated when clearing can be accomplished within 3 weeks. In acute self-limited cases, as in accurately diagnosed rhus dermatitis, dividing the total day's dosage (AM and PM) gives a more even 24 hour coverage for the short half-life of prednisone.

Intermittent cool wet soaks or dressing applied for 5 to 10 minutes and followed by enhanced tepid air drying with a hair blower dramatically curtails weeping. These wet to dry periods are 20 to 40 minutes in duration and ideally are frequent (three or four times a day). Tap water, isotonic saline, and Burow's solution are the wetting agents commonly used.

Oral antihistamine therapy is time honored but only a secondary treatment consideration in acute significant allergic contact dermatitis. Hydroxyzine or diphenhydramine may alleviate pruritus and can function as a sedative at bedtime. In adults I prefer the short acting drug triazolam (0.25 to 0.5 mg) to ensure sleep and offset any steroid insomnia. Daytime sedation from antihistamines (terfinidine is not sedating) can be a significant problem, and none are dramatically antipruritic in acute allergic contact dermatitis. More is accomplished with an appropriate dosage of prednisone and a good short acting hypnotic at bedtime.

Mild and Moderate Acute Contact Dermatitis with Limited Involvement

Class 1 topical steroids suppress the signs and symptoms of allergic contact dermatitis in patients judged to be in this category. Those seen in the very early phases of dermatitis can worsen in days, and the topical therapy suddenly appears to be "too little, too late." Because topical therapy with class 1 steroids is costly, next day communication with the patient can correct undertreated contact dermatitis. Wet to dry compresses, as already described, are employed if weeping is present. Clobetasol and betamethasone diproprionate (in an optimized release vehicle) are applied in the intervening periods between the soaks. The goal of topical therapy in acute self-limited dermatitis is to mimic the power of occlusive therapy without risking the increase in heat, maceration, and higher bacterial counts from a synthetic membrane. Frequently applied (topically every 3 to 4 hours), unoccluded, potent steroid therapy is a step in this direction, particularly in areas that are not easy to occlude. Some anatomic sites are suitable for occlusive dressings for 24 to 48 hours. Topical therapy can be reduced to twice daily applications after significant improvement occurs.

CHRONIC CONTACT DERMATITIS

Chronic contact dermatitis presents a different problem: the cause must be identified. Haptene removal or substitution stops the dermatitis. If allergic contact dermatitis is a complicating feature of intrinsic eczema, treatment will be more gratifying when a secondary disorder is eliminated. If this is not done, treatment is nearly impossible. A thorough history of exposures to irritants or allergens is paramount. Every part of the patient's day is suspect and all treatments must be questioned. Patients do not volunteer information about some of their temporizing self-treatments. A correct diagnosis may require patch testing, which should be performed by experienced persons knowledgeable in this technique. Many items suspected of causing allergic contact dermatitis by the patient, or physician, cannot be tested in the form or concentration that is suspected of causing the dermatitis. Poorly performed patch testing is worse than no patch testing, for it may give the physician a false sense of security and undeserved confidence in the diagnosis. Severe false positive reactions create more than just physician embarrassment.

Topical corticosteroid therapy is standard treatment and, like the treatment of chronic intrinsic eczema, is used judiciously. Hydrocortisone (1 to 2.5 percent) and tridesilon (creams or ointments) are preferred for the face and intertriginous areas. Fluorinated steroids must be carefully monitored when used in these areas. "How long?" has not been defined. Some patients are more susceptible than others to the well publicized adverse effects. Steroid atrophy, when recognized reasonably early, improves significantly when fluorinated steroid administration is discontinued.

Antihistamines should be offered to relieve pruritus in patients who believe that they are beneficial. Hydroxyzine and doxepin are good choices as a first offering. The patient will soon let it be known if one or the other is cost effective. Ice pack compresses relieve itching, but are not always available when needed.

DERMATOPHYTE INFECTIONS

EVAN R. FARMER, M.D.

ESTABLISHING THE DIAGNOSIS

Dermatophytes are superficial fungi that infect the stratum corneum of the skin, hair shaft, or nail. They normally do not invade the viable tissue of the epidermis but still can elicit an inflammatory response, depending upon the immune competence of the host and prior exposure to the organism. The presence of a dermatophyte infection should always be suspected when scaling is a component of the lesion or when there is hair loss or nail dystrophy. The diagnosis of a dermatophyte infection should always be established prior to initiation of therapy by either direct visualization of the fungus on a potassium hydroxide wet mount or culture.

Since the fungus lives in keratin, scales, hair, or nail clippings can be placed on a glass slide with a drop of 20 percent potassium hydroxide in water, a coverslip applied, and the slide gently warmed with a flame and then examined for hyphae or spores. The addition of dimethyl sulfoxide or dyes to the potassium hydroxide solution may facilitate identification of the organism, but I do not find these additives a significant help. Similarly scale, hair, or nail may be placed on Sabouraud's medium or Dermatophyte Test Medium and incubated at room temperature. The culture should be examined weekly for growth of the fungus; identification is made on the basis of the morphology of the colony. If no growth has occurred by 6 weeks, the culture can be considered negative. Currently the most common dermatophyte cultured is *Trichophyton rubrum*, accounting for approximately 75 percent of the isolates.

The presence of a dermatophyte infection should always be considered in patients who present with erysipelas or lymphangitis of the lower extremities, especially those who have recurrent episodes. Since the bacterial infection can mask the dermatophyte infection, the patient should be reevaluated once the bacterial infection has resolved if the dermatophyte infection could not be documented on the initial presentation.

SITES OF INVOLVEMENT

Dermatophyte infections are named according to the anatomic site involved, generally irrespective of the specific fungus with only a few exceptions. For example, tinea capitis is an infection of scalp hair that may be due to either *Trichophyton tonsurans* or *Microsporum canis*. Tinea pedis, an infection of the feet, may be due to *Trichophyton rubrum*, *Trichophyton mentagrophytes* or *Epidermophyton floccosum*. Conversely, tinea imbricata is an unusual dermatophyte infection in the United States caused by *Trichophyton concentricum* and generally is seen in patients who have traveled for a prolonged period in the Far East or South America or who are immigrants to this country. This disorder is named for the imbricate or concentric pattern on the skin. (See Table 1 for designation of the sites and common dermatophytes.)

Tinea versicolor is a common disorder, of worldwide distribution, usually affecting large areas of the trunk and extremities and occasionally the hair follicles. The disease is caused by *Malassezia furfur* and is characterized by distinctive hypopigmented (rarely hyperpigmented) scaling macules that become confluent over large areas. The organism is somewhat difficult to culture but is easily demonstrated by a potassium hydroxide wet mount.

EVALUATING THE PATIENT

Once the diagnosis is established, the patient should be evaluated for predisposing factors such as atopy (asthma, hay fever, atopic dermatitis), diabetes mellitus, or immune deficiency. Patients with atopy tend to have chronic dermatophyte infections and tend to be infected with *Trichophyton rubrum.* The infection is difficult to eradicate, and it is difficult to prevent recurrences. Presumably these patients have an immune defect that permits dermatophyte infections to persist, although they are able to handle most other infections. Patients with diabetes mellitus, particularly when the blood sugar level is not under control, tend to have dermatophyte infections, especially in the groin region. Infection in this area may coexist with *Candida* and *Corynebacterium* infections of the skin. Immune deficiency may be primary, or as a result of an underlying disease, such as cancer, connective tissue disease, or genetic disease, or it may result from the

TABLE 1 Dermatophyte Infections

Site	*Designation*	*Dermatophyte*
Scalp	Tinea capitis	*Trichophyton tonsurans* *Microsporum canis**
Body	Tinea corporis	*Trichophyton rubrum* *Trichophyton verrucosum**
Body	Tinea versicolor	*Malassezia furfur*
Groin	Tinea cruris	*Trichophyton mentagrophytes* *Trichophyton rubrum* *Epidermophyton floccosum*
Feet	Tinea pedis	*Trichophyton mentagrophytes* *Trichophyton rubrum* *Epidermophyton floccosum*
Face	Tinea facei	*Trichophyton rubrum*
Beard	Tinea barbae	*Trichophyton rubrum* *Trichophyton mentagrophytes* *Trichophyton verrucosum** *Microsporum canis**
Nails	Tinea unguium	*Trichophyton rubrum* *Trichophyton mentagrophytes*
Follicles	Majocchi's granuloma	*Trichophyton rubrum*
Follicles	*Malassezia* folliculitis	*Malassezia furfur*

* Transmitted from animals.

administration of immunosuppressive drugs. Detection and treatment of an underlying immune deficiency disease and minimizing iatrogenic immunosuppression help in the management of the dermatophyte infection.

COINFECTION

As mentioned, dermatophyte infections may coexist with other fungal infections, especially in the diabetic or immunocompromised patient. Bacterial infections also may compound dermatophyte infections, particularly in the toe webs or skin folds. These infections may be due to either gram-positive or gram-negative micro-organisms and should be suspected whenever there is maceration or lesions are malodorous. Gram staining of the debris and culturing may be helpful in identifying these bacteria.

Corynebacterium infection may coexist in the groin and occasionally on the feet and can be detected by the presence of a coral-red fluoresence on examination with Wood's light. The patients tend to respond much more quickly to therapy for dermatophyte infection if these secondary infections are also treated.

THERAPY

The goals of therapy are to eradicate the fungus with a specific antifungal drug, to minimize the inflammatory response to the fungus when appropriate, to prevent recurrent disease, and to prevent transmission of the fungus.

Topical Therapy

Antifungal drugs in current use can be divided into those that are applied topically for localized disease and those that are given systemically for widespread, resistant, or adnexal (hair, nail) disease. The drugs that are most effective topically belong to the imidazole group and include 1 percent clotrimazole (Lotrimin, Mycelex), 2 percent miconazole (Monistat), and 1 percent econazole (Spectazole). These drugs are available in cream, solution, and lotion forms. One percent ciclopirox (Loprox) and 1 percent haloprogin (Halotex) are other effective drugs. Tolnaftate (Tinactin) and Desenex are over the counter drugs that are useful for mild disease but are much less effective than the prescription drugs in my experience. I generally use the cream preparation for most patients with localized disease and the solution preparation on hair-bearing skin, especially on the pubic region or genitalia. I have not found the powder formulations to be particularly helpful.

I recommend that the patient apply the cream twice daily to the affected area, rubbing it in well because these are vanishing creams. The skin does not have to be hydrated as when using a corticosteroid topically because the depth of penetration of the drug is not so critical. If there is maceration, I recommend comfortable temperature, tap water soaks using a small basin, linen, or terry cloth for 5 to 15 minutes before application of the cream. If there is maceration, I evaluate for *Candida* or bacterial infection and treat it at the same time. *Candida* infection of the skin usually responds to one of the imidazole drugs, but if the infection is in the groin or perineal region, I also prescribe a 7 to 10 day course of nystatin, 500,000 units orally four times daily. Nystatin vaginal suppositories (one twice daily) are also useful in women with dual *Candida* infections. For bacterial infection I usually take a culture and initiate therapy with enteric coated erythromycin, 500 mg twice daily for 10 days, and alter the drug, depending on the response, using cultures as a guide.

Dermatophyte infections usually respond quickly to this therapy, with clinical cures in 2 to 3 weeks and negative cultures in 4 to 6 weeks. Therefore, I usually expect to treat the patient for about 6 weeks with reevaluation at 3 weeks and again about 6 weeks if there is clinical activity at 3 weeks. If there is little or no response to this topical approach, I reevaluate for the presence of the fungus by potassium hydroxide examination and culture, evaluate for the presence of an associated bacterial infection, reevaluate for immune deficiency, consider alternative diagnoses, and review the patient's understanding and actual application of the drug.

For very inflammatory infections with significant pruritus, I add triamcinolone cream, 0.1 percent twice daily, for the first 7 days to be used concomitantly with topical application of the antifungal drug. Alternatively I may begin with Lotrisone cream (betamethasone dipropionate plus clotrimazole) for the first week and then switch to clotrimazole alone.

Systemic Therapy

Currently there are two systemically administered drugs—griseofulvin and ketoconazole—for use in the United States for dermatophyte infections, but other drugs are under investigation and show promise. Systemic therapy is indicated for the following situations: failure of topical therapy, widespread disease when topical therapy is impractical, infection of hair and hair follicles on either the scalp or the body as a folliculitis, and infection of the nails.

Griseofulvin is available in several different preparations, but I usually use the microsize tablets, 500 mg twice daily, for an average sized adult and adjust the dose downward for a smaller individual or child. Griseofulvin suspension is also available for children. In my experience the most common side effects of griseofulvin are headaches and gastrointestinal upset. These usually resolve in spite of continued therapy if the patient can tolerate the discomfort. Less frequent but potentially serious side effects include allergic reactions, photosensitivity, exacerbation of lupus erythematosus, and alteration of warfarin metabolism. The safety of griseofulvin in pregnancy has not been demonstrated.

Griseofulvin resistant dermatophytes are a problem and should be suspected if there is no clinical response within 1 month. An alternative explanation for the lack of response may be poor absorption of the drug or noncompliance. If resistance is most likely, I consider using ketoconazole at this point. Griseofulvin should be taken with food, and I usually recommend it with milk. Complete eradication of dermatophyte infections may take much longer than 1 month, especially if there is adnexal involvement; treatment should continue until there is a clinical cure, usually for several months. Confirmation of eradication of the infection can be made by a negative potassium hydroxide examination or culture.

Ketoconazole is the other currently available drug and in contradistinction to griseofulvin is effective against a wide variety of fungi in addition to dermatophytes. It is usually given in a single daily dose of 200 to 400 mg and generally is well tolerated. It is useful in mixed fungal infections with dermatophytes and *Candida*. It is also effective in tinea versicolor.

At present, when systemic therapy is indicated, I begin with griseofulvin, except for widespread tinea versicolor, and reserve ketoconazole for griseofulvin treatment failures. Ketoconazole, although generally well tolerated, may induce nondose-related hepatitis in 1 in 10,000 to 15,000 patients; transient elevation of liver function test results occurs more frequently, requiring careful laboratory monitoring. If these abnormalities are more than minor or are persistent, the drug should be discontinued immediately and the patient carefully monitored until the test results return to normal. If the test results do not normalize quickly or levels continue to rise after discontinuing the drug, consultation with a liver specialist may be indicated. Females and patients over 50 years of age seem to be most at risk for the complication of hepatitis. Liver function tests should be carried out prior to therapy and frequently for the duration of therapy. I usually carry out liver function tests every 2 weeks for the first 3 months and then monthly. The median time for the development of hepatitis is day 28 after the initiation of therapy. Ketoconazole also alters testosterone metabolism and may cause gynecomastia. The absorption of ketoconazole may be decreased when it is given in conjunction with cimetidine. Allergic reactions to ketoconazole have been reported, including a lichenoid eruption of the oral mucosa. Its safety in pregnancy has not been established. On the positive side, there seems to be minimal dermatophyte resistance to ketoconazole to date, and it may be more effective than griseofulvin in the treatment of tinea unguium and peristent *Trichophyton rubrum* infections.

TINEA VERSICOLOR

Tinea versicolor differs from tinea corporis in that in spite of widespread involvement, it usually responds well to topical therapy. My first choice is selenium sulfide lotion, 2.5 percent (Selsun), applied daily for 10 minutes and thoroughly washed off. Selenium sulfide can cause an irritant dermatitis if not completely removed. Applications should continue for 1 week with a second course in 1 month. Alternative regimens include clotrimazole cream, 1 percent twice daily for 7 days or 50 percent propylene glycol in water twice daily for 14 days. For patients who have extensive or recurrent tinea versicolor I now use a short course of ketoconazole, 200 mg daily for 7 to 14 days. Ketoconazole is also more effective than the topical approach for *Malassezia furfur* folliculitis.

IMMUNE REACTIONS

Two types of immune reactions are associated with dermatophyte infections—kerion and id reactions. A kerion is an acute pustular reaction forming an abscess-like lesion on the scalp in tinea capitis or in the beard in tinea barbae. The lesion is believed to be an immune reaction to dermatophyte antigen and not simply a rupture of the fungus into the dermis with a subsequent foreign-body response. A kerion responds best to a three-fold approach.

First, the fungus should be treated with either griseofulvin or ketoconazole because it usually does not respond to topical therapy. Second, these lesions tend to become secondarily infected with bacteria, and systemic antibiotic therapy, as with enteric coated erythromycin, 500 mg twice daily, or dicloxacillin, 500 mg twice daily, for 7 to 10 days is helpful. Third, I use a short course of prednisone, 0.5 to 1.0 mg per kg per day tapering to zero over 2 to 3 weeks. I continue the griseofulvin or ketoconazole for 2 to 3 months or until resolution of the dermatophyte infection occurs.

Most id reactions are manifested by a pruritic papulovesicular eruption, predominantly on the hands and feet, but it may become widespread. Id reactions occur most frequently in patients with inflammatory tinea pedis. Many patients have only toe web infections, and the id reaction involves the palms and soles. It is the id reaction that brings most of these patients to the physician. The id reaction by definition is an immune response and is potassium hydroxide and culture negative for dermatophytes. Once the dermatophyte infection has cleared, the id reaction spontaneously resolves. However, since eradication of the dermatophyte may take several weeks, I treat the id reaction with topical corticosteroid therapy, such as triamcinolone cream, 0.1 percent, or fluocinonide cream, 0.05 percent (Lidex), four times a day. The corticosteroid is applied following hydration of the affected area by soaking or compressing with cool tap water. An antihistamine at bedtime, such as hydroxyzine, 25 to 50 mg, or diphenhydramine, 25 to 50 mg, is helpful for the first 2 to 3 days. For severe id reactions a short course of prednisone, 0.5 to 1.0 mg per kg per day tapering to zero over 2 to 3 weeks, is indicated.

PREVENTION

Once a dermatophyte infection has been cleared, especially in patients with chronic widespread infection, prevention of a relapse or reinfection is desirable. In my experience the topical use of an antifungal drug, although probably effective, is not practical, and patients discontinue its use after a short time.

Recently I have been using 400 mg of ketoconazole in a single dose every 2 weeks, and it has been effective without side effects so far. I monitor liver function test results every 6 months. I have had no experience with griseofulvin used in a similar manner.

Since most dermatophyte infections occur in the groin region or feet, I recommend cotton underclothing and socks as well as a drying powder, such as Johnson's Baby Powder or Zeosorb, to decrease the moisture needed to promote fungal growth. Bathing and thorough drying after swimming or other sports activities are also helpful.

Spread of a dermatophyte infection to another family member normally is not a problem except in the case of tinea capitis. An individual's susceptibility to the organism seems to be the predominant factor. However, with tinea capitis the spores may be spread to other children, and thorough daily shampooing of the hair minimizes the number of loose spores. I also recommend restricting the use of combs, brushes, and towels to the patient alone. Notification of the local public health agency and the school nurse is also helpful in controlling spread.

Because some fungi are acquired from animals, especially dogs and cats (e.g., *Microsporum canis*), pets should be inspected and treated by a veterinarian.

CUTANEOUS DRUG REACTIONS

ANTOINETTE F. HOOD, M.D.

MAGNITUDE OF THE PROBLEM

Drugs are ubiquitous in our society. In the United States millions of people regularly ingest aspirin and other anti-inflammatory drugs, antibiotics, contraceptives, antihypertensives, diuretics, and tranquilizers. The exact incidence of adverse reactions to these and other medications is unknown. According to the Boston Collaborative Drug Surveillance Program, 30 percent of medical service inpatients had one or more complications as a result of drugs administered during hospitalization; 2 to 3 percent of the patients developed a "skin rash." Among hospitalized patients the incidence of cutaneous reactions per course of therapy has been reported to be 3 per 1,000. It has been estimated that 60,000 to 90,000 inpatients develop cutaneous drug reactions each year. Fortunately these reactions are rarely life-threatening; nonetheless they may produce significant morbidity and expense, especially in the form of prolonged hospitalization.

The Boston collaborative study reflects the incidence of drug reactions on an inpatient medical service. These figures may not accurately reflect the problem in other units of the hospital, such as surgery, pediatrics, and oncology. We casually surveyed one oncology ward in our hospital for a 2-month period and discovered that 50 percent of the patients developed one or more cutaneous eruptions that clinically were consistent with drug eruptions. These reactions often resulted in great discomfort to the patient and necessitated complex therapy manipulations on the part of the attending physicians.

Even less is known about the frequency of cutaneous reactions occurring in an outpatient setting. Attempts to monitor drug reactions are obviously fraught with difficulties. However, the American Academy of Dermatology has made an important effort to do this by sponsoring the Adverse Drug Reaction Reporting System. This system permits dermatologists to share their experience with adverse cutaneous reactions to drugs and to obtain information about such reactions as contained in the registry and in the medical literature.

PATHOGENESIS

Adverse drug reactions can be divided simplistically into two major categories: type A reactions, which are normal but augmented responses; and type B reactions, which are totally abnormal or bizarre responses. Type A reactions are pharmacologically predictable and dose-dependent. They generally are of high incidence and morbidity but low mortality. Examples of type A reactions in the skin include aspirin-induced purpura, mucositis, and alopecia caused by antimitotic chemotherapeutic drugs, striae associated with corticosteroid administration, and perhaps demeclocycline-induced phototoxicity. Type B (bizarre or idiosyncratic) reactions are less common, are pharmacologically unpredictable, and are not dose-dependent. They may be produced by a variety of chemicals, including the active constituent in the medication, decomposition or byproducts of the active ingredient, or the various additives, solubilizers, stabilizers, and colorizers in a preparation.

The pathobiology of most cutaneous drug reactions is not well understood; the overused terms "hypersensitivity" and "allergic" should be limited to describing reactions that are immunologically mediated or that can reasonably be presumed to be immunologically mediated. True allergic reactions usually affect a small percentage of the population receiving the drug, require a prior exposure or latent period for the development of an immune response, can occur at subtherapeutic or very low doses, and usually simulate other known hypersensitivity reactions. Examples of cutaneous allergic drug reactions are listed in Table 1.

Rashes of unknown etiology but that are presumed to be allergic include morbilliform-exanthematous eruptions, fixed drug eruptions, erythema multiforme, toxic epidermal necrolysis, exfoliative erythroderma, and erythema nodosum.

Few controlled or stringent studies have been done on drug reactions, and for practical purposes it is not convenient to categorize them by etiology. Traditionally drug reactions are classified morphologically. In terms of the frequency of types of drug rashes, the morbilliform pattern is seen most commonly, followed by urticarial eruptions, fixed drug eruptions, erythema multiforme, and others. There is a clinical dictum that states that any drug may produce any reaction, and although this may be true, it is also accepted that certain drugs are more likely to produce particular morphologic cutaneous reactions than others. Table 2 lists the various types of drug reactions and some of the more common drugs responsible for the eruptions.

PRACTICAL APPROACH TO THE DIAGNOSIS OF A SUSPECTED DRUG ERUPTION

As physicians we are aware that there are undoubtedly many more adverse reactions to drugs than are suspected and that, conversely, many reactions suspected of being drug-induced actually may be caused by other agents. In evaluating a suspected drug reaction, every effort should be directed toward diagnosis, discovery, and discontinuation.

Diagnosis requires a high index of suspicion, a detailed and directed history, careful examination, classification of the eruption by morphologic characteristics, evaluation of accompanying signs and symptoms, collection of adjuvant laboratory test results, and elimination of other causes of similar eruptions. Important historical information includes the onset and evolution of the eruption, any history of drug reactions, and detailed descriptions of all medications being taken, including proprietary drugs and vitamins. If a true allergic reaction is suspected, a history of similar medications taken systemically or applied topically may be important. Note any accompanying symptoms, such as pruritus (favors a drug reaction), sore throat (against a drug eruption), fever, and malaise (neither pro nor con). Categorizing the eruption by the morphologic appearance of the lesions is helpful in determining the type of reaction (allergic versus nonallergic) and in limiting the possible etiologic agents responsible for the eruption (see Table 2). Other physical findings such as mucosal involvement, lymphadenopathy, and temperature elevation are important.

Adjuvant tests may be helpful by pointing either toward or away from the diagnosis of drug-induced eruption (Table 3). Routine studies should include a complete blood cell count with a differential count urinalysis and a multiphasic screening panel; other tests such as skin biopsy and patch and light testing are important in categorizing the type and sometimes the cause of the reaction. Macrophage migration inhibition factor test and in vitro lymphocyte toxicity assays should be performed when available. Realistically,

TABLE 1 Allergic (Immunologically Mediated) Drug Eruptions*

Type	*Immunologic Mechanisms*	*Clinical Expression in Skin*	*Laboratory Testing*
Type I anaphylactic	IgE-mediated reactions to allergic haptens; involve mast cell activation and subsequent release of histamine, leukotrienes, and eosinophil-chemotactic factors of anaphylaxis; neutrophil chemotactic factors, platelet-activating factor, serotonin, and kinins may be involved	Urticaria Angioedema Transient cold urticaria Generalized pruritus	Radioallergosorbent test (RAST) Enzyme-linked immunosorbent assay (ELISA) Skin testing
Type II antibody-mediated (cytotoxic) injury	IgG or IgM antibodies activate complement through the classic pathway; under certain conditions, antigens and antibodies localized on circulating erythrocytes, leukocytes, or platelets cause drug-induced, antibody-dependent lysis of these cells	Thrombocytopenic reactions	
Type III antigen-antibody immune complex	IgG or IgM antibodies form circulating immune complexes with antigen and complement, activating complement-derived chemotactic factors and producing localized tissue inflammation	Serum sickness Leukocytoclastic vasculitis ?Drug-induced lupus erythematosus	Direct immunofluorescence performed on skin biopsy specimen
Type IV cell-mediated injury	Sensitized T lymphocytes react with allergen and thereby generate lymphokines	Allergic contact dermatitis Photoallergic reactions Granuloma formation following topical use of zirconium	Lymphocyte transformation Patch test

*Based on the Coombs and Gell classification.

although not necessarily practically, challenge by reintroduction of the suspected drug is still the most useful means of definitively diagnosing a drug eruption.

Current technology permits physicians ready access to current medical literature. In assessing a possible drug-induced reaction, a literature search may provide invaluable information and insight.

TREATMENT

The treatment of a drug reaction depends on the type of reaction, the severity and the presumed etiologic mechanism. With few exceptions, use of the suspected offender should be discontinued and the eruption treated symptomatically with antihistamines or antipruritics, compresses, and soothing lotions as needed. If the patient is taking multiple medications that are important to his or her health and well-being, I generally select the most likely causative drug and stop its administration. If the eruption persists or progresses over the next 48 hours, the next most likely medication is discontinued, and so on. Another approach is to discontinue all medications until the rash fades or clears completely and then reinstitute the medications one at a time at 48- to 72-hour intervals. This approach is not recommended in the treatment of IgE-mediated urticarial or angioedema episodes (since the challenging might induce a life-threatening anaphylactic reaction) or drug reactions, which concomitantly may involve the liver or kidneys.

Sever widespread or extremely symptomatic drug eruptions may require a short course of prednisone therapy to reduce inflammation and shorten the natural course of the reaction. Assuming that there are no medical contraindications, prednisone can be administered orally, 40 to 60 mg per day, in divided doses. As soon as it is apparent that the eruption is receding, the dosage may be tapered to 10 mg per day and discontinued.

At times it may be necessary to treat the patient through a drug-induced eruption. This may occur when the suspected medication is absolutely neces-

TABLE 2 Drugs Associated with Various Morphologic Cutaneous Patterns

Morbilliform-Exanthematous Eruptions
*Allopurinol
*Antibiotics (especially penicillin, penicillin derivatives, and sulfonamides)
Anticonvulsants
*Barbiturates
Benzodiazepines
*Gold salts
*Isoniazid
Meclofenamate sodium
Para-aminosalicylic acid
Phenylbutazone
Phenothiazines
Piroxicam
Quinidine
Thiazide diuretics
Urticaria
Enzymes (L-asparaginase)
Indomethacin
Insulin
Opiates
Penicillin and related antibiotics
Salicylates
Sulfonamides
X-ray contrast media
Fixed Drug Eruptions
*Barbiturates
Chlordiazepoxide
Phenacetin
*Phenolphthalein
*Phenylbutazone
Salicylates
*Sulfonamides
*Tetracycline
Erythema Multiforme
*Barbiturates
Chlorpropamide
Griseofulvin
Hydantoins
*Penicillin
Phenothiazines
*Sulfonamides
Thiazide diuretics
Leukocytoclastic Vasculitis
*Allopurinol
Gold salts
Hydantoins
Iodides
*Penicillin and related antibiotics
Phenothiazines
*Sulfonamides
Thiazide diuretics
Thiouracils
Photosensitivity Eruptions
Griseofulvin
Indomethacin
*Nalidixic acid
*Phenothiazines
Piroxicam
Sulindac
*Sulfonamides
*Tetracycline (demeclocycline)
*Thiazide diuretics
Toxic Epidermal Necrolysis
Allopurinol
*Barbiturates
*Hydantoins
Penicillin
Phenylbutazone
*Sulfonamides
Tetracycline
Lichenoid and Lichen Planus-like Eruptions
Antimalarials (chloroquine, hydroxychloroquine, quinacrine)
Chlordiazepoxide
Gold salts
Hydroxyurea
Para-aminosalicylic acid
Penicillamine
Quinidine
Thiazide diuretics
Exfoliative Dermatitis
Allopurinol
Carbamazepine
*Gold salts
Hydantoins
Isoniazid
Para-aminosalicylic acid
Phenylbutazone
*Sulfonamides
Streptomycin
Eczematous Eruptions (topical sensitizer/systemic medication)†
Ampicillin
(Chlorobutanol/chloral hydrate)
Diphenhydramine (Caladryl/Benadryl)
(Aminophylline/ethylenediamine)
Iodine/iodides
Neomycin sulfate/streptomycin, kanamycin
(Para-amino aromatic benzenes/para-aminobenzoic acid, sulfonamides, tolbutamide)
Penicillin
(Thiram/disulfiram)
Erythema Nodosum
Bromides
Codeine
Iodides
*Orally administered contraceptives
Penicillin
Salicylates
Sulfonamides

*Drugs that are frequent offenders.

†Drugs in parentheses may sensitize a patient by external application; subsequent systemic administration of immunochemically related chemicals may produce eczematous eruption.

sary and there are no unrelated drug substitutes of similar efficacy. We have had occasion to do this on the oncology unit or when treating other immunocompromised patients for life-threatening infections. In these situations the severity of the reaction may be diminished by switching modes of administration from intermittent to continuous intravenous administration of drugs (ticarcillin) or from daily administration to treatment three times a week (trimethoprim-sulfamethoxazole).

TABLE 3 Diagnostic Procedures

History
Physical examination
Laboratory tests
  Complete blood cell count with differential count
  Multiphasic screening panel
  Serum IgE RAST
Skin biopsy
Patch tests
Ultraviolet light testing

Once a drug has been implicated in a drug reaction, especially an allergic or presumed allergic reaction, the patient should be given the name of the drug and a list of similar chemical compounds to avoid in the future. The front of the chart should be clearly labeled, other physicians caring for the patient should be informed, and the manufacturers of the medication should be notified.

PHOTOALLERGIC CONTACT DERMATITIS

RICHARD D. GRANSTEIN, M.D.
ERNESTO GONZALEZ, M.D.

Photoallergic contact dermatitis (PCD) is an immune response to an offending exogenous chemical, in which participation of the immune system is necessary for the response to occur and in which photons are required with the chemical for immunologic activation. An epidemic of PCD occurred in the 1960s as a result of the use of the potent photoallergen tetrachlorsalicylanilide as an antimicrobial agent in soaps. Other halogenated salicylanilides and related compounds are still used in some toiletries, although their photosensitizing potential seems to be low. More recently musk ambrette and 6-methylcoumarin, contained in perfumes and other fragrance containing toiletries, have been implicated as a cause of PCD; this has required the U.S. Food and Drug Administration to remove 6-methylcoumarin from the market.

PCD is to be distinguished from phototoxic chemical photosensitivity states in which photosensitized damage occurs directly and does not involve the immune system. There is considerable controversy over this distinction in the clinical literature. Numerous drugs and chemicals have been reported in the past to be photoallergens, despite little or no evidence for immunologic involvement in the induced photosensitivity. Phototoxic reactions are characterized by occurrence on the first exposure to the offending agent, with a high incidence among those exposed (theoretically 100 percent if the dose of the chemical and radiation is sufficient) and with subsequent exposures at untreated sites mimicking the time course and intensity of the first exposure. By contrast, photoallergic reactions require previous exposure for sensitization to occur, with subsequent exposures resulting in more severe reactions than the initial exposure. The incidence of photoallergic reactions among those exposed is low, and the dose of chemical required to elicit the reaction in sensitive individuals is usually quite low. Table 1 summarizes these differences. In addition, many, if not most photoallergic agents are also phototoxic, yielding some confusion. Table 2 lists the major agents commonly implicated in PCD.

In recent years several animal models have been developed to study mechanisms involved in PCD. These models, utilizing guinea pigs or mice, have shown that PCD is a cell mediated immune response that can be induced in a naive animal by the adoptive transfer to T-lymphocytes from sensitive animals. Indeed PCD appears to be immunologically identical to ordinary allergic contact dermatitis except for the requirement for photons for initiation or elicitation of the response. In animal models it has been demonstrated that irradiation of chlorpromazine or sulfanilamide in vitro results in the production of a photoproduct that is capable of inducing or eliciting ordinary allergic contact dermatitis and that is cross reactive with induced PCD to these agents. Thus, in PCD the mechanism of antigen formation to these agents appears to be the generation of a hapten photoproduct.

Two other mechanisms have been proposed to account for the generation of the antigen in PCD. A photon could be necessary for the binding of a hapten to a carrier protein, or the photon with the chemical may alter a host protein, which becomes antigenic. There are no current experimental data to support these mechanisms.

TABLE 1 Characteristics of Photocontact Dermatitis

Characteristic	*Photoallergic*	*Phototoxic*
Occurs on first exposure	No	Yes
Requires previous sensitization	Yes	No
Incidence	Low	High
Dose of agent needed to elicit	Low	High
Flare at nonexposed, previously involved site	Possible	No
Skin changes	Eczematous	Similar to sunburn

TABLE 2 Agents Reported to Induce Photoallergic Contact Dermatitis *

Halogenated phenols	Sunscreens
Tetrachlorsalicylanilide	Para-aminobenzoic acid (PABA)
Tribromosalicylanilide	Glyceryl PABA
Dibromosalicylanilide	Digalloyl trioleate
Multifungin	Mexenone
Trichlorocarbanilide	Cinnamate
Bithionol	Various chemicals
Fenticlor	Moquizone
Hexachlorophene	Quindoxine
Buclosamide (Jadit)	Thiourea
Chloro-2-phenylphenol	Musk ambrette
Drugs	6-Methylcoumarin
Promethazine hydrochloride	Stilbenes
Chlorpromazine hydrochloride	Sandalwood oil
Sulphonamides	
Diphenhydramine	
Quinine	
Benzocaine	

* Inclusion of some of these agents is based on a single or very few reports.

CLINICAL DESCRIPTION

The majority of photoallergic reactions are eczematous. Early changes are acute eczema with vesiculation, which may progress to bullae, with scaling, crusting, and excoriations as variable features. In the chronic stage thick lichenified plaques are present. Urticarial papular and lichenoid eruptions have also been reported as photoallergic reactions, but these are unusual responses described in isolated case reports. The histology of the eruption is that of a spongiotic dermatitis with intercellular edema in the epidermis with or without vesicle formation, depending on the clinical pattern. A dense perivascular dermal lymphohistiocytic infiltrate is present, identical to that found in allergic contact dermatitis. Some authors believe that a biopsy in some cases may make it possible to distinguish a photoallergic reaction from a phototoxic one. The differences observed are those that distinguish allergic contact dermatitis from a primary irritant contact dermatitis.

PCD can occur at any age and in either sex. Males are more commonly affected than females, although it has been postulated that this may reflect differences in exposure to photoallergens. As in other diseases, the history and physical examination should begin the evaluation of the patient. The patient usually presents with a rash, restricted to exposed sites, which he attributes to sunlight exposure. The initial eruption frequently occurs a few days after long exposure to sunlight, but subsequent eruptions may occur within hours after exposure. The face, V of the neck, and dorsum of the hands and arms are usually involved. The areas behind the ears (Wilkinson's triangle), under the chin, between the fingers, and in the skin folds are usually spared. Facial involvement is sometimes surprisingly patchy. The actual distribution of the eruption and the time course are determined, of course, by the dose and site of exposure to the chemical and radiation. When a localized area is exposed to the offending agent as well as the relevant wavelengths of radiation and PCD ensues, a distant, previously involved area may demonstrate a flare of activity.

The differential diagnosis includes phototoxic reactions, contact dermatitis (especially airborne contact dermatitis), photosensitive eczema, and the eczematous form of polymorphous light eruption. Photoallergic reactions also may be a consequence of drugs administered systemically.

In addition to the physical findings and history, photopatch testing can be useful in making a diagnosis. There is no standard procedure, but the approach to testing is uniform. A battery of known photosensitizers is applied in duplicate to small areas of the back, and all sites are covered by an opaque material. Table 3 lists standard pho-

TABLE 3 Photopatch Testing Agents

Benzocaine	5% in petrolatum
Chlorpromazine	0.1% in petrolatum
Diphenhydramine	2% in petrolatum
Hydrochlorothiazide	1% in petrolatum
Musk ambrette	5% in petrolatum and 5% in alcohol
6-Methylcoumarin	10% in alcohol
Sandalwood oil	1% in petrolatum
Sulfanilamide	5% in petrolatum
Tribromosalicylanilide	1% in petrolatum
Bithionol	1% in petrolatum
Buclosamide (Jadit)	10% in water
Fenticlor	1% in petrolatum
Hexachlorophene	1% in petrolatum
Tetrachlorsalicylanilide	1% in petrolatum
Trichlorocarbanilide	1% in petrolatum
Quinine	1% in petrolatum
Para-aminobenzoic acid	1% in petrolatum
Cinnamate	1% in petrolatum
Benzophenone (Piz Buin sunscreen)	Commercial preparation as is

toallergy testing materials. Substances to be tested are prepared in petrolatum at the concentrations listed in Table 3.

After 24 hours one set of the applied substances is exposed to UVA (320 to 400 nm) radiation, because the action spectrum for most photoallergens is thought to be in this range. We use a bank of PUVA fluorescent bulbs filtered through mylar (to remove wavelengths below 320 nm) as the source of radiation in our clinic. The exposure dose is usually 10 J per square centimeter, a dose empirically selected because it is below the minimal erythema dose for most individuals and is presumed to be sufficient to elicit a photoallergic response. However, if the patient's minimal erythema dose for UVA is at or below this level, a lower exposure dose is used. We believe that it is mandatory to do phototesting prior to photopatch testing to ensure that a proper dose of UVA radiation is selected (see later discussion). The sites are then re-covered. Twenty-four and 48 hours later the sites are examined for a reaction. Erythema, edema, and vesiculation are considered positive responses that are graded on a 1+ to 4+ scale of severity. Positive responses of equal intensity at both the nonirradiated and the irradiated sites are interpreted as ordinary allergic contact dermatitis. A positive response at an irradiated site, or in the presence of allergic contact dermatitis, an enhanced response at the irradiated site are interpreted as being consistent with photocontact allergy.

Phototesting in which the minimal erythema dose to UVA and UVB radiation is determined may be helpful in differentiating idiopathic photosensitivity states from PCD (Table 4) and is necessary for determining the dose of radiation to use in photopatch testing, as already mentioned. All patients referred for photopatch testing undergo phototesting prior to photopatch testing. This is performed by exposing small areas of nonsun-exposed (buttock) skin to graded doses of radiation, shielding these sites from light exposure, and examining these areas 24 hours later. In our experience the skin type of the patient is not a reliable indicator of the "normal" minimal erythema dose. Generally a minimal erythema dose below 20 mJ per square centimeter for UVB or 20 J per square centimeter for UVA radiation is considered abnormal, depending on the circumstances and characteristics of the patient. We also examine sensitivity to visible radiation by exposing nonsun-exposed skin to graded doses of radiation from a tungsten lamp, shielding these areas from light exposure, and examining them 24 hours later. Any reaction is considered abnormal.

TABLE 4 Interpretation of Phototesting

Condition	*MED to UVA*	*MED to UVB*	*Photopatch Test*
PCD	Normal	Normal	Positive
Photosensitive eczema	Normal or decreased	Usually decreased	Negative
Persistent light reaction	Normal or decreased	Decreased	Positive
Actinic reticuloid	Usually decreased	Normal or decreased	Positive or negative

There are limitations to the use and interpretation of the photopatch test. Radiation sources used vary, but most investigators use a source with a main emission spectrum in the UVA range because, as already mentioned, the action spectra of photoallergic reactions to most chemicals are included in this waveband. However, the action spectra of some reactions probably involve UVB (280 to 320 nm) radiation. Therefore, a solar simulator that emits both UVA and UVB radiation is sometimes used. However, because UVB radiation is much more erythemogenic than UVA radiation, problems of dosimetry occur when using a solar simulator source for photopatch testing.

A suberythemal dose of radiation, chosen by testing the patient, is administered when the solar simulator is employed. To increase the probability of detecting a response, a dose of radiation just below the minimal erythema dose could be employed at each of several suspected wavelengths. This could clearly result in very large and impractical amounts of testing.

Other problems of phototesting include determining the amount of photosensitizer to apply and differentiating allergic contact dermatitis from photoallergic contact dermatitis when both occur. In addition, allergic contact dermatitis to some agents could be increased by exposure to ultraviolet radiation. Another problem relates to the possibility that photoallergic contact dermatitis to some chemicals might result from exposure to visible radiation. Finally, the differentiation of phototoxic responses from photoallergic responses can be difficult, although biopsy of test sites can sometimes distinguish these reactions, as already mentioned. Risks and complications of photopatch testing include inadvertant photosensitization to test agents, discomfort at positive test sites, occasional flares of disease activity at sites of previous involvement, and false-positive or false negative results due to incorrect amounts of chemical or radiation. Despite these caveats, in many circumstances photopatch testing can be very helpful in identifying the offending agent in a patient with PCD.

THERAPY

Avoidance of the offending agent is, of course, the single most important therapeutic maneuver. Thus, it is important to identify the offending agent if at all possible. This often can be done by means of the history, but when the history is ambiguous, photopatch testing can be useful. If more than one chemical is implicated by the history, photopatch testing can determine which among them is responsible for the eruption. It also can be used as a confirmatory test when the history suggests only one offending chemical, and occasionally it is useful in diagnosing photosensitivity states when the history does not clearly implicate any substance. Once an offending agent is identified, it is crucial to tell the patient what substances in his environment may contain that chemical or a cross reactive substance. In our clinic we provide the patient with a written list of common materials containing the agent to which he is sensitive.

The avoidance of sunlight can be important in the treatment of acute photoallergic contact dermatitis. This often must be extended beyond the period of acute dermatitis because the offending chemical may persist in the skin for some time. In severe cases confinement to a darkened room for several days may speed recovery. Since most offending agents are activated by exposure to wavelengths above 320 nm, sunlight penetrating window glass can aggravate the dermatitis. When the offending chemical cannot be identified, avoidance of sunlight may become a mainstay of treatment.

The utility of sunscreens is limited by the fact that most transparent sunscreens do not protect against photons of wavelengths in the UVA range. Although some of these agents, especially those that contain benzophenones, afford some protection above 320 nm, the most useful sunscreens are those that form an opaque barrier to all photons of solar radiation. These agents contain opaque powders, such as titanium oxide, kaolin, zinc oxide, or talc. Unfortunately these are usually not as cosmetically acceptable as sunscreens that are invisible. It should also be pointed out that some sunscreens, notably those that contain paraminobenzoic acid and its esters, can produce allergic contact dermatitis and sometimes, although rarely, photoallergic contact dermatitis. In addition, various inactive components of these preparations, such as preservatives and fragrances, may produce ACD or PCD.

Symptomatic Therapy

The acute treatment of photoallergic contact dermatitis is similar to that of ordinary allergic contact dermatitis. For vesicular and weeping areas, astringent soaks are appropriate as is topical steroid therapy. It is crucial to keep open areas clean to prevent superinfection. We often prescribe astringent soaks, such as Domeboro's solution, three or four times a day. If large areas are weeping, we also may advise the patient to clean these areas with an antimicrobial cleansing agent, such as Hibiclens antimicrobial cleanser, twice a day. Antihistamines may be helpful for pruritus. In severe cases a short course of systemic steroid therapy can be given. As already implied, removal of the offending photosensitizer and related compounds eliminates the problem once the acute eruption has resolved.

Persistent Light Reaction

A small number of patients with PCD display photosensitivity without apparent continuing exposure to a chemical or a cross-reacting agent to which they are demonstrably sensitive. This condition, termed persistent light reaction, was first recognized as a consequence of tetrachlorsalicylanilide exposure. Since that time it has been observed as a consequence of other photosensitizers. The eruption is a chronic eczematous dermatitis initially restricted to light exposed sites. Patients display marked photosensitivity with a lowered minimal erythema dose to UVB radiation, often to UVA radiation, and sometimes to visible light. Photopatch testing reveals a strongly positive response to a photoallergen. This disorder can be disabling, and severe depression and suicide have been reported among patients with photosensitivity states.

Various hypotheses have been presented to account for this condition. One is that patients continue to encounter the photoallergen or a cross-reacting substance. Another is that an induced photoantigen persists in the skin, and a third is that a normal skin constituent has undergone an alteration and has become antigenic, with subsequent exposure to ultraviolet radiation producing the same or a similar photoproduct without further exposure to an offending chemical. This last possible mechanism is perhaps, supported by the observation that tetrachlorsalicylanilide can photo-oxidize proteins. None of these hypotheses completely explains the broad spectrum of photosensitivity observed in some patients or the abnormal sensitivity of uninvolved skin on phototesting.

The treatment consists of using sunscreens, avoiding sun exposure and, when necessary, fluorescent light exposure. Topical and systemic steroid therapy is useful, especially for acute eruptions. Suppression of persistent light reaction (PLR) by 8-methoxypsoralen and sunlight has been reported. We find this interesting, because a patient with actinic reticuloid was treated in our clinic with PUVA and did very well for a prolonged period.

Patients with actinic reticuloid, photosensitive eczema, and PLR generally share a number of characteristics. They are usually male, middle-aged or older, and the eruption is usually eczematous. The relationship among these three disorders is not clear. For this reason it has been proposed by some authors that the present nomenclature be abandoned and that the term "chronic actinic dermatitis" with appropriate subdivisions be used to classify these diseases.

PSORIASIS

WARWICK L. MORISON, M.B., B.S., M.D.

We are all familiar with the concept of the "heartbreak" of psoriasis, although it is not clear whether the grief is felt by the physician, the patient, or both. The concept embodies the negative attitude toward treatment of the disease in so many patients and physicians. This negative attitude is unfounded because psoriasis can be successfully treated. However, to achieve this the physician must have a planned approach to the management of the disease. The plan must contain several key elements.

First, the physician must recognize, and explain to the patient, that psoriasis is a chronic disease that usually persists for years, that there is no quick fix or cure, but that there are some very successful treatments that can control the disease in most patients. Second, the initial visit must include a full evaluation of the patient and the disease. Sex, age, occupation, social environment, geographic location, and medical history are important factors in deciding upon the best treatment for the type and extent of disease present. This evaluation takes time, but is essential because the physician must know the patient, the disease, and how the patient feels about the disease. Third, the patient must be educated about the disease and all possible treatments; a handout is an invaluable addition but not a substitute for this explanation. Finally, the treatment program that is agreed upon with the patient must be tailored to the patient and to the disease. The patient must be "sold" on the treatment or it will not be used. The treatment must have a reasonable risk–benefit ratio and be effective for the type of disease being treated.

THERAPEUTIC AGENTS

Treatment modalities with antipsoriatic activity can be broadly divided into three groups: topical, ultraviolet radiation, and systemic. This sequence also roughly defines their risk–benefit ratios: topical agents are usually safest and of benefit only in limited disease, while systemic agents carry greatest risk and should be used only in extensive disease.

Topical Agents

Topically applied corticosteroids are the most frequently prescribed treatment for psoriasis, and this is probably more a tribute to advertising by drug companies rather than their true value as treatment. Only rarely do these agents convert psoriasis to normal skin, and as soon as the treatment is stopped, the psoriasis usually rapidly returns. Tachyphylaxis, permanent atrophy of the skin, and conversion of stable psoriasis to a more aggressive disease, are the chief problems associated with use of these agents. The introduction of clobetisol propionate and betamethasone dipropionate will undoubtedly add new adverse effects. Adrenal suppression and precipitation of generalized pustular psoriasis have been observed frequently in Europe with such potent agents. For all these reasons, corticosteroids should be used in psoriasis only as adjunctive treatment with other more effective agents, in special situations such as the treatment of nails, and in patients who will accept improvement rather than clearance of disease. Systemically administered corticosteroids have no place in the treatment of psoriasis, since rebound, spreading disease and serious adverse effects are almost inevitable.

There has been a resurgence of interest in using anthralin in the treatment of psoriasis, mainly because of the introduction of improved formulations and the discovery that its application for 30 minutes yields results as good as those from overnight application. Problems remain: Anthralin stains the skin a grayish color and this persists for several weeks. It also stains porcelain, and because this can be permanent, patients must be warned to wash it off in a fast flowing shower or to use a rubber basin for washing their hair. Anthralin is also a potent irritant and some patients cannot tolerate the treatment. Reducing the frequency of application and starting with a low strength are the main ways of minimizing the problems. However, despite these disadvantages, it has major advantages over topical corticosteroids: it can clear psoriasis, and remissions often last for months without treatment.

Tar is an effective antipsoriatic agent, but there are several reasons its use should be abandoned. First, it is only weakly effective. Second, it is messy and abhorrent to use. Third, it is carcinogenic in humans, and psoriatic patients are already exposed to enough other carcinogens and immunosuppressive agents. The so-called refined tar preparations appear to have little, if any, therapeutic effect.

Ultraviolet Radiation

The sun has probably been used in the treatment of psoriasis for as long as the disease has existed, since most patients know that they improve during the summer or a winter vacation in the tropics. The latter can be used as an effective and popular treatment in selected patients.

Phototherapy using ultraviolet B (UVB) radiation with prior application of a lubricant is an effective treatment for psoriasis. When erythemogenic doses of UVB radiation are used, about 95 percent of selected patients can be cleared in 20 to 30 treatments. This regimen requires, first, determining the minimal erythema dose, giving 70 percent of that dose as the first exposure dose, and then increasing the exposure dose by 17 percent each treatment. If there is significant disease on the limbs, the same dose is given as an extra exposure while the face and trunk are kept covered. Treatments are given three to five times each week. A lubricant must be applied to each psoriasis plaque that has a surface scale immediately before treatment, since this increases penetration of the radiation. Symptomatic erythema is the main short term problem. Over the long term this treatment is probably carcinogenic but the risk appears to be low. Photoaging of the skin is another long term problem. The main disadvantage of the treatment is the lack of a reasonable maintenance regimen. Twice-weekly treatment is usually necessary to maintain a clear state, and most patients find this frequency of treatment economically and socially unacceptable.

Low dose, nonerythemogenic UVB phototherapy has been used by some people with success. A starting dose well below an erythemal response is selected, and small increments are given with each treatment. A problem with this approach is that patients frequently finish a course of treatment tanned with psoriasis and, not surprisingly, unhappy.

Photochemotherapy, with ingestion of methoxsalen and subsequent exposure to ultraviolet A (UVA) radiation (PUVA therapy), is more effective than UVB phototherapy for both clearance and maintenance treatment. More than 95 percent of the patients with psoriasis can be cleared in 20 to 30 treatments. The treatment is given two to four times each week to clear disease, and the maintenance requirements vary from weekly to monthly treatments; most patients require two treatments each month.

The short term problems with this therapy are nausea and erythema. Nausea is due to methoxsalen and is dose related; reduction of the dose by 10 mg cures most people. Cataracts, skin cancer, and photoaging are the main long term concerns. Cataracts should not occur if patients wear ultraviolet-opaque glasses after ingesting methoxsalen. Skin cancer is a risk, especially if a patient has had superficial x-ray or grenz ray treatment, has had skin cancer, or is fair skinned. These risk factors must be evaluated in each patient. In addition, skin cancer is readily amenable to treatment provided the patient is carefully followed and regularly examined. The guidelines for PUVA therapy were published in the *Journal of the American Academy of Dermatology* (1979; 1:106).

Home phototherapy is useful in a few patients. A sunlamp from any drugstore can be used to augment topical treatment for localized psoriasis. Whole body treatment at home is not advisable for several reasons. First, it is not very effective, since patients frequently underdose or overdose themselves. Second, if the treatment is directed by a physician, he or she is taking some responsibility for its safety. Home built light boxes are unlikely to be electrically safe. Obviously if the physician supplies plans for the unit, he or she is even more involved. Finally, patients have a tendency to forget to come for follow-up examination until the first skin cancer appears.

The combination of the topical application of tar preparations and exposure to UVB radiation, the Goeckerman regimen, is still used in some centers. This treatment relies on the mild antipsoriatic effect of tar and the much more potent antipsoriatic effect of UVB radiation. On the positive side, the treatment is effective and safe. However, there is a negative side. The treatment is expensive, since it must be done in a hospital or a day care center. Second, because there is no provision for maintenance, the psoriasis gradually returns once the patient has been discharged. Finally, several studies have shown that tar given with UVB radiation is no more effective than a lubricant with UVB radiation; few patients have difficulty in choosing between a lubricant and a messy tar preparation.

Climatotherapy at the Dead Sea, a successful short term therapy for psoriasis, appears to involve a mixture of UVB phototherapy, psychotherapy, and topical treatment. The main component is phototherapy. Since the Dead Sea is below sea level, sunlight there passes through a greater thickness of atmosphere, which filters out the erythemogenic wavelengths shorter than 300 nm. Consequently, patients can expose themselves to sunlight for long periods each day and receive very high doses of radiation of wavelengths longer than 300 nm, which is more therapeutic for psoriasis. The psychotherapeutic effects of a vacation and association with other people with psoriasis, are also important factors. On the negative side, in many patients the disease does not clear completely, and the duration of a remission appears to be no longer than it is with the Goeckerman treatment. A winter vacation in the Caribbean is probably cheaper, more enjoyable, and equally effective.

Systemic Therapy

Methotrexate is the best systemically administered drug for the treatment of psoriasis. It is an excellent treatment, but it does have serious long term adverse effects. Therefore, this drug should be held in reserve until other less toxic therapeutic options have been exhausted and the patient has psoriasis of a sufficient severity to warrant taking the risks associated with the treatment. An exception is the short term use of methotrexate in combination with PUVA therapy or phototherapy.

Depression of the bone marrow is the main short term problem with methotrexate. The main long term problem is impairment of liver function, and this occurs in 25 to 40 percent of the patients. Methotrexate is teratogenic, and therefore it should not be used in women of child bearing age without adequate contraception during treatment and for 1 month after cessation of the drug. Another problem is that methotrexate appears to alter the nature of psoriasis, making it a more aggressive disease. Thus, a person may have had the ordinary plaque type of psoriasis but after receiving methotrexate for several years may develop unstable inflammatory psoriasis when an attempt is made to shift to another treatment. The guidelines for methotrexate therapy have been published in the *Journal of the American Academy of Dermatology* (1982; 6:145). Several different regimens are used, but the approach of dividing the weekly dose into 3 doses given at consecutive 12 hourly intervals appears to be the most effective and safest.

Retinoids have antipsoriatic activity. Etretinate is the preferred drug for the treatment of psoriasis because isotretinoin is much less effective. The main indications for etretinate are the erythrodermic and generalized pustular types of psoriasis, and in a daily dosage of 0.6 to 1 mg per kilogram of body weight this drug is equally as effective as methotrexate in the treatment of these two rare forms of the disease. Etretinate is not very useful in the treatment of the ordinary plaque type of psoriasis; in some patients the disease is partially controlled, but to achieve complete clearance, months of therapy are required. The major disadvantage of etretinate therapy is that it produces side effects in 100 percent of the patients. The most common adverse effects involve the skin and mucous membranes, and these are inconvenient rather than hazardous. However, hyperlipidemia, liver abnormalities, and calcification of tendons occur in 50 to 85 percent of the patients. The long term significance of some of these side effects is still unknown, and thus use of the drug should be restricted to the rare patient who is unresponsive to other less hazardous therapy. Etretinate is only slowly excreted over 12 to 18 months, and since it is markedly teratogenic, it should not be used in any women of child bearing age as it is impossible to guarantee contraception over such a long period.

Other Treatments

Trauma to the skin is a significant factor in inducing psoriasis, as evidenced by the Koebner phenomenon and localization of the disease to certain areas such as the elbows and knees. Telling patients to reduce the amount of trauma to the skin is good advice, but, except in specific instances, it is not a practical approach to treatment. Use of a condom in a person with psoriasis of the penis and protection of the hands, if they are affected, are two specific instances.

Emotional stress is also a trigger for psoriasis, but, again, telling patients to reduce the amount of stress in their lives is easy rather than practical advice. Perhaps the importance of emotional stress in exacerbating psoriasis is overemphasized. Certainly there are some patients who suffer a flare-up of disease whenever the social milieu becomes stormy. However, there are many other patients who go through deaths, divorces, operations, and other stressful experiences without fluctuation of the disease or requirement for increased treatment to control the disease. Alcohol abuse is an issue that has been raised in psoriatic patients. Anecodotal comments have claimed that alcohol exacerbates psoriasis, but there is no evidence to support this comment. It is possible that patients drink because they have severe psoriasis rather than vice versa, if indeed they do consume more alcohol than other people.

Several medications can induce or exacerbate psoriasis and should be avoided by patients if possible. Lithium and the antimalarial drugs are the main offenders. Beta-blockers can induce a psoriasiform eruption as a rare side effect, and there are a few reports of the exacerbation of existing psoriasis.

Finally, providing information about the National Psoriasis Foundation can be a worthwhile therapeutic measure in some patients. These patients have a desire to "do something" about finding a cause and cure for their disease, and contact with this organization provides an outlet for these feelings. Furthermore, patients feel that they are being kept up to date about psoriasis through information in the foundation's newsletter.

THERAPEUTIC REGIMENS

Psoriasis Vulgaris

From a therapeutic stand point, plaque-form and papular psoriasis of the trunk and limbs can be divided into three categories: minimal psoriasis involving an area less than the surface area of two palms, moderate psoriasis involving an area less than the surface area of one upper limb, and extensive psoriasis involving a surface area greater than one upper limb. Although the extent of disease is usually the main factor dictating a choice of treatment, other characteristics of the disease or the patient may dominate the decision; this applies particularly to patients with moderate disease.

Mild disease localized to a few plaques or papules is best managed by topical therapy. Drithocreme is the linchpin of treatment because it can clear disease and provide a remission for weeks or months. In fair skinned patients treatment should be started with the 0.25 percent strength, whereas in dark skinned patients 0.5 percent is a safe preparation as initial therapy. The patient is instructed to apply the preparation daily for 30 minutes and then to wash it off in a shower. Treatment should be reviewed every two weeks, and if the cream is not causing any irritation, a higher strength preparation is prescribed. If the Drithocreme is causing marked irritation, the frequency of application should be reduced until this ceases to be a problem.

A second treatment to be used overnight should always be given in addition to the short term application of Drithocreme. Keralyt gel under occlusion with Saran Wrap is useful if plaques are thick and hyperkeratotic. Cordran tape, or a medium potency corticosteroid cream under occlusion can be used in other patients and is helpful for the control of irritation from anthralin. Vioform-hydrocortisone cream should be substituted for intertriginous areas. A moisturizing preparation, selected by the preference of the patient for a cream, lotion, or ointment, should be used during the day. Intralesional steroid treatment is sometimes useful in patients with a few small thick lesions, but its use should always be combined with anthralin because otherwise the psoriasis will rapidly return once the effect of the corticosteroid has dissipated.

This regimen for the treatment of minimal psoriasis will be successful only if the physician exhibits enthusiasm and involvement and goals are defined at the initiation of treatment. The patient should be seen at least every 2 weeks, and the aim is to clear the psoriasis in 6 to 8 weeks. Short duration, focused treatment breeds enthusiasm and succeeds, whereas treatment with absence of deadlines and infrequent follow-up is bound to fail.

Psoriasis of moderate extent is a difficult therapeutic problem for two reasons. First, it is an economic and physical logistic problem for the patient to use topical therapy over a moderately extensive area and succeed in clearing the disease. Second, if a more potent therapy is used, such as UVB phototherapy in the office, the patient is frequently unhappy with the end result. The reason for this is simple. Phototherapy usually achieves 95 percent clearance of disease but rarely achieves 100 percent clearance. The patient with moderate disease usually wants 100 percent clearance, whereas a patient with much more extensive disease is usually delighted with 95 percent clearance. Despite these problems, the treatment of choice is topical therapy, as for minimal psoriasis, supplemented in most instances with the use of a small sunlamp at home or a course of UVB phototherapy in the office. The selection of treatment depends on assessment of the disease and the patient. Psoriasis confined mainly to exposed areas and concern about appearance because of employment and social factors are characteristics that weigh in favor of UVB phototherapy. Short term maintenance UVB treatment for a couple of months is useful in this type of patient to ensure a reasonable remission.

There are a number of therapeutic regimens available for treating psoriasis covering an extensive area. UVB phototherapy in the office is the treatment of choice in the following cases: children, nursing and pregnant women, patients unwilling to use eye protection or take psoralen, patients who have sustained extensive solar damage or who have had significant exposure to grenz rays or superficial x-rays, and patients with psoriasis of recent onset. Whether long term maintenance treatment is given after clearance of disease is a decision reached after a full discussion with the patient, since usually weekly or more frequent treatment is necessary.

In all other patients the treatment of choice is PUVA therapy alone or in combination with methotrexate. PUVA therapy is effective in clearing disease in almost all patients and provides convenient maintenance treatment to prevent a recurrence. In the maintenance phase the frequency of treatment is gradually reduced, and if there is no significant flare-up of disease on monthly treatment, the therapy can be suspended. A methotrexate-PUVA combination treatment is useful in patients with very thick plaques, in patients with very active disease, and in those in whom the disease cannot be cleared with PUVA therapy alone. Methotrexate is given for 3 weeks before commencing PUVA therapy and is gradually withdrawn as clearing is achieved.

An alternative combination treatment is UVB phototherapy with PUVA therapy, and this combination is particularly useful in patients in whom methotrexate is contraindicated. Full doses of both treatments are given, exposure to the two wave bands being administered consecutively on the same day. These two combination treatments are very effective, and virtually all patients with psoriasis vulgaris can be cleared of disease using single or multiple treatments.

The main problem with the combination treatments is a high incidence of phototoxicity, but this is a short term effect that is easily corrected by modifying the exposure dose. Although most patients can be cleared of disease using ultraviolet radiation, a small number cannot be maintained in a clear state using PUVA therapy alone. A combination of low dose methotrexate and PUVA therapy is often a better treatment for these patients. In addition, there are patients in whom PUVA therapy is contraindicated, and long term methotrexate treatment must be considered in these cases.

Psoriasis of the Scalp

The scalp requires specific attention when it is involved, except in patients being treated with methotrexate or etretinate. PUVA and UVB therapy are not effective for the treatment of psoriasis on the scalp, but if it is first cleared with topical therapy, UV therapy is often effective in keeping the scalp free of disease without continuation of topical therapy.

The best topical treatment is anthralin as Drithoscalp cream, which is formulated for application to the scalp. The application time is 30 minutes daily or as often as tolerated. A tar shampoo is used, because although the therapeutic effect from this brief exposure to tar is probably minimal, such preparations are labeled for the treatment of psoriasis and thus are favored by patients.

A corticosteroid lotion, such as Lidex solution, is applied overnight for its effect in reducing irritation from the Drithoscalp cream and its antipsoriatic action. If a patient has the thick asbestos type of psoriasis of the scalp, Keralyt gel under occlusion should be used initially to remove all the scale.

Psoriasis of the Palms and Soles

The treatment of choice is oral PUVA therapy. There is the temptation to use topical application of psoralen for this localized disease, but there is a high frequency of blistering burns with that treatment. Between 20 and 30 treatments with oral PUVA therapy are usually required to achieve clearance of disease. The only adjunctive treatment required is application of a keratolytic agent in patients with hyperkeratotic lesions so as to reduce the barrier to radiation. Specialized hand and foot UVA radiators are available and are very efficient, but the door panel of a stand-up unit is almost as effective. Ordinary topical therapy is ineffective in the treatment of psoriasis of the palms and soles. Topical corticosteroid therapy usually produces some improvement, but because it is seldom sustained, the patient is left a virtual cripple in these socially and physically important areas of the body. UVB phototherapy is also without effect because this wavelength cannot penetrate the thick stratum corneum of the palms and soles.

Psoriatic Nail Disease

Involvement of the nail bed or nail matrix by psoriasis is a difficult therapeutic problem. Pitting or a more severe dystrophy can be treated by application of Cordran tape to the skin over the matrix, but the treatment must be continued for months and the incidence of success is low. Onycholysis does not appear to respond to intralesional steroids applied into the nail bed. Nail disease clears in about 50 percent of the patients treated with PUVA therapy, but it usually requires 4 to 6 months of treatment. Local PUVA treatment, with exposure of the dorsa of the hands and feet, is a useful treatment in patients with severe nail disease.

Erythrodermic and Generalized Pustular Psoriasis

These rare forms of psoriasis are usually an indication for hospitalization, since, particularly in the case of the von Zumbusch form of pustular psoriasis, they can be life-threatening. If an infection or metabolic disturbance is present, this must be treated. Patients with pustular psoriasis that has been triggered by the abrupt withdrawal of large doses of high potency corticosteroid preparations must be tested for adrenocortical suppression and given appropriate supplementation. Local care of the skin should be confined to wet dressings and moisturizers. Methotrexate and etretinate are the specific drugs of choice, methotrexate being preferred provided there are no contraindications to its use. When the patient is stabilized, PUVA therapy should be commenced using low doses of UVA radiation and treatment on consecutive days followed by a rest day. Once the lesions have cleared, PUVA therapy usually can be continued as the sole treatment.

Acute Guttate Psoriasis

This variant of psoriasis typically follows an upper respiratory tract infection with a delay of 10 to 14 days. Streptococcal infection used to be the most common cause, but viral infections now seem to be almost as common. A 2 week course of penicillin is indicated if a streptococcal organism grows from a throat swab culture. Many cases of acute guttate psoriasis are said to clear spontaneously, but certainly some do not and the condition can become chronic. Thus, the treatment of choice is a course of UVB phototherapy to ensure that all lesions do clear. Maintenance therapy is usually unnecessary.

Psoriatic Arthritis

There is a form of arthritis that is peculiar to patients with psoriasis and afflicts about 5 percent of the patients. Psoriatic arthritis is rheumatoid factor negative, is usually asymmetric, and affects the distal interphalangeal and sacroiliac joints. A severe form, arthritis mutilans, is fortunately rare. In most instances dermatologists or their patients elect to have an internist or rheumatologist manage the arthritis, but for several reasons the dermatologist should keep in close contact with the progress of therapy for the arthritis. The activities of the skin disease and the arthritis are usually independent of each other, and treatment of the skin seldom affects the arthritis; however, the reverse is not true. Nonsteroidal anti-inflammatory drugs occasionally may exacerbate the skin disease, although this is probably a rare event. Oral doses of corticosteroids should be avoided if at all possible, as has been mentioned. Finally, some internists are not aware that methotrexate is a very effective drug for treating arthritis. Thus, in a patient with significant skin disease and arthritis, methotrexate is often the treatment of choice for both problems. Preliminary reports suggest that etretinate is also effective for psoriatic arthritis, but the toxicity of the treatment may limit its usefulness.

CONCLUSIONS

It is obvious from meeting many patients and from published surveys that many patients with psoriasis are displeased with the management of their disease. There are several common reasons for their displeasure. First, they perceive a lack of interest or a feeling of resignation on the part of many physicians. The "try this; it is new and it might work" attitude is hardly likely to boost morale and engender enthusiasm in a patient with a chronic disease. Second, patients do not like many of the treatments that are frequently used. Tying oneself into a layer of Saran Wrap over a film of grease is not really the nicest way to retire for the evening. Anointing oneself with foul smelling black goop is not a pleasant experience. Third, patients do not like to have psoriasis, any psoriasis, and yet many treatments leave them with a significant level of disease for long periods of time. Topical corticosteroid treatment improves but seldom clears psoriasis. Hospital treatment often flattens psoriasis without clearing it, and then the patient has to endure months of disease until its severity warrants another admission to a hospital or day care center. Finally, many physicians regard psoriasis as being only a cosmetic disturbance. Offering a red, scaly hand for a handshake and leaving a confetti trail of scale behind are more than cosmetic problems; not to mention the soreness and pruritus that can be present.

All these sources of displeasure on the part of the patient must be kept in mind when treating psoriasis. A positive, interested attitude on the part of the physician can work miracles. Selection of a treatment that works, and yet does not totally disrupt the patient's life, is possible with the therapeutic modalities available today. The end result is a happy patient who stays with that physician.

ERYTHEMA MULTIFORME

JOHN A. KAZMIEROWSKI, M.D.
KIRK D. WUEPPER, M.D.

Erythema multiforme (EM) is an acute self-limited inflammatory disorder of the skin and mucous membranes, with characteristic histopathologic changes, a tendency to recur, and sometimes a distinctive clinical appearance. A sizable body of evidence indicates that EM is a hypersensitivity disorder occurring in response to any one of a variety of precipitating factors, including drugs, neoplasms, and infections (especially herpes simplex and *Mycoplasma*). Both circulating immune complexes and sensitized lymphocytes have been implicated in the pathogenesis of EM.

A wide spectrum of manifestations are included in the clinical presentation of EM, and these may involve the skin alone, mucous membranes alone, or both skin and mucous membranes. Some patients present with a relatively mild disorder (EM minor) consisting of a few focally located erythematous skin lesions and mucosal inflammation. Others have severe mucocutaneous disease (EM major or Stevens-Johnson syndrome), with systemic symptoms as well as numerous inflammatory bullous and erythematous lesions on both mucosal and cutaneous surfaces. In some cases the nasal mucosa, urethra, vagina, trachea, and esophagus are involved in addition to the lips, oropharynx, and conjuctiva. The most common skin lesion is the iris or target lesion, which consists of a central violaceous or erythematous region surrounded by an erythematous and edematous ring. The necrotic areas sometimes evolve into hemorrhagic bullae. The clinical course of EM is variable, ranging from a mild acute syndrome lasting about 10 to 14 days to a severe disorder which lasts several weeks and in rare cases can be fatal.

THERAPY

The therapy of EM must take into account the clinical presentation of the patient and the severity of the disease. Although a precipitating cause cannot always be identified in cases of EM, when it can be treated or stopped, this should be done as soon as possible. Often, in mild disease with a known cause, no more therapy than removal of the initiating factor is necessary. Therefore, obvious mycoplasmal infections should be treated with erythromycin, offending drugs withdrawn, or neoplasms aggressively treated with appropriate chemotherapy or radiotherapy when these specific etiologies can be identified. In cases of EM associated with herpes simplex, prompt topical treatment of the initiating infection with antiviral drugs (e.g., acyclovir, 5 percent ointment applied 5 to 7 times per day) is recommended, but there are no specific data to suggest that this substantially alters the final course of the associated EM. Recurrent erythema multiforme associated with herpes simplex infection has been successfully treated by employing oral doses of acyclovir (200 mg five times per day for 7 to 10 days).

Oral acyclovir treatment also has been recommended prophylactically (200 mg three to five times per day) to treat frequent herpes simplex infections. This dosage should be given for no more than 4 to 6 months.

Some controversy exists about the treatment of patients with severe disease, but the literature seems to favor the use of systemic corticosteroid treatment. We use high dose corticosteroid therapy for severe disease, beginning with a single oral daily dose of 60 to 80 mg of prednisone or its equivalent, slowly tapering this dose over 2 to 4 weeks. Patients who are unable to take medications orally because of mucosal involvement can be treated with daily intravenous doses of corticosteroid preparations of similar potency and switched to an oral regimen once resolution of oral erosion begins. Intramuscular repository corticosteroid preparations are not recommended; they give the physician little control over situations in which dosage changes may be indicated, and they often do not provide a high enough steroid dose. Such side effects as fluid retention, gastrointestinal discomfort, psychiatric disturbances, muscle weakness and wasting, osteoporosis, glaucoma, and glucose intolerance must be kept in mind when treating patients with high dose corticosteroid regimens. Usually an initial favorable response can be seen after 3 to 5 days of corticosteroid therapy, but severe necrotic lesions may take weeks to resolve.

Although most patients do not require hospitalization, those with severe mucocutaneous involvement may need careful monitoring of the fluid and electrolyte balance and aggressive local care of lesions that can be provided only in a hospital setting. Occasionally secondary bacterial infection or septicemia may complicate EM, and this should be promptly and vigorously treated.

Antihistamine and antipruritic drugs may be used to treat itching in mild cases but have no effect on the long term course of the disease. Hydroxyzine hydrochloride, 25 to 50 mg orally every 6 to 8 hours, or Periactin, 4 mg orally every 6 to 8 hours may be helpful. Well established necrotic cutaneous lesions often are painful rather than itchy and are not helped by this therapy. Care must be taken to avoid the marked sedation caused by these drugs in some patients.

Local measures for cutaneous lesions are often not very effective, but bullous lesions should be treated with cleansing solutions and soaks (Burow's solution every 3 to 4 hours until drying occurs) to avoid secondary bacterial infection. If this is suspected, cultures should be taken and appropriate antibiotics started.

Oral lesions are frequently quite painful and require an aggressive treatment regimen, since secondary bacterial infection of severely damaged oral mucosa can readily occur. Hydrogen peroxide diluted 1:1 with water can be used regularly to remove necrotic material. Anesthetic drugs such as diphenhydramine elixir diluted 1:1 with water or viscous lidocaine, can help to control pain, especially when taken before meals. Bacterial superinfection should be treated with penicillin or erythromycin for 7 to 10 days, and candidal infection should be treated with nystatin, clotrimazole troches, or oral doses of ketoconazole, 200 mg per day, for 10 to 14 days.

Ophthalmic lesions require careful observation, and an ophthalmology consultation is indicated, since cicatrix formation can occur. Eye irrigation and wet compresses are sometimes indicated in severe cases, but usually topical instillation of corticosteroids is sufficient. Antibiotics are indicated when secondary infection occurs.

As already noted, there is some controversy concerning the use of corticosteroids in EM, but we believe that they are indicated early in the disease in most patients. Rarely, in patients with uncontrollable recurrent EM that is unresponsive to high dose corticosteroid therapy, we have added azathioprine, 100 mg per day, to the oral corticosteroid regimen, and results have been favorable. Caution is recommended in the long term use of corticosteroid therapy in patients with recurrent disease, especially disease associated with herpes infections. We have seen a marked increase in the frequency of herpes infection and associated EM in some patients taking corticosteroids regularly; only after the steroids were discontinued could both disorders be adequately controlled. In most patients with EM, however, short courses of corticosteroids are an important part of the therapeutic regimen.

ERYTHEMA NODOSUM

MARK E. UNIS, M.D.

Erythema nodosum is a distinctive clinical entity believed to represent a hypersensitivity reaction to a variety of stimuli and associated diseases. A typical patient presents with the sudden onset of crops of tender, painful, erythematous to purplish subcutaneous, usually pretibial, nodules, biopsy specimens of which show a predominantly septal panniculitis.

Although many cases are idiopathic, several associated diseases listed in Table 1 have been reported frequently. A history, physical examination, and appropriate laboratory evaluation are performed to exclude these associated diseases. If the history and physical findings are unremarkable except for cutaneous findings, a minimal initial evaluation would include a complete blood count, erythrocyte sedimentation rate, and chest x-ray examination. If there is an associated underlying disease, treatment or control of the underlying disease usually improves the erythema nodosum.

TABLE 1 Erythema Nodosum Associated Diseases

- Sarcoidosis
- Inflammatory bowel disease
  - Crohn's disease
  - Ulcerative colitis
- Collagen vascular diseases
- Drugs
  - Birth control pills
  - Sulfonamides
  - Antibiotics
  - Bromides
- Behçet's syndrome
- Infections
  - Streptococcal infection
  - Atypical mycobacterial infection
  - Fungal infections
  - Viral infections
  - Chlamydial infections
- Pregnancy
- Lymphoma and leukemia

PREFERRED APPROACH

Evaluation of any particular pharmacologic therapy in patients with erythema nodosum is difficult because of the tendency for spontaneous remission to occur in this disease. Nonetheless there are several modes of therapy that I have found effective. Nearly all patients with erythema nodosum find relief of symptoms with rest and leg elevation. The preferred approach includes attempts at treatment or control of an underlying disease, if present, bed rest, leg elevation, and pharmacologic therapy, usually potassium iodide or nonsteroidal anti-inflammatory drugs (NSAID).

Potassium Iodide

Although there are no established guidelines for the use of potassium iodide in treating erythema nodosum, the medication seems to inhibit mononuclear phagocytes, and this may be the reason for the response of erythema nodosum to therapy with iodides. The reason for their effectiveness is unclear, especially in light of the fact that iodides and bromides have been reported to induce erythema nodosum. I usually prescribe potassium iodide as the 300 mg enteric coated tablet taken three times daily with meals. Symptomatic improvement usually begins within a few days after starting therapy. If tablets are unavailable, a saturated solution of potassium iodide, 5 to 8 drops orally three times daily in juice or water, may be substituted.

Potassium iodide has a bitter taste. Dyspepsia and heartburn may result from its administration, and small bowel ulcerations have been associated with administration of the enteric coated potassium iodide preparations.

Potassium iodide is contraindicated during pregnancy because it can induce fetal goiter. Occasional patients display hypersensitivity reactions to iodides, including angioedema, fever, arthralgia, lymphadenopathy and eosinophilia.

Other effects of iodides are chronic and may include thyroid adenoma, goiter, and myxedema because the drug suppresses thyroid function. Chronic iodism may occur after prolonged treatment, and symptoms may include salivary gland enlargement, increased salivation, coryza, pain in the teeth and gingiva, swelling of the eyelids, headache, and pulmonary edema. Acne may develop or iododerma may occur.

In general, I do not use potassium iodide in chronic or refractory cases of erythema nodosum.

Nonsteroidal Anti-inflammatory Drugs

I have found several nonsteroidal anti-inflammatory drugs useful in the therapy of erythema nodosum. Their mode of action is not known, but it is believed that inhibition of prostaglandin synthesis by metabolites of NSAIDs may be involved in the anti-inflammatory action of these drugs.

The NSAID I most frequently prescribe is indomethacin in doses ranging from 25 to 75 mg orally three times daily with meals, depending on the age and size of the patient and the severity of the disease. Indomethacin is the most likely of the NSAIDs to cause gastrointestinal disturbance, including dyspepsia, ulceration, perforation, and hemorrhage. Patients should be monitored carefully for development of these problems. Indomethacin can precipitate renal insufficiency, particularly in those with pre-existing renal or hepatic dysfunction. Using the drug for only 2 or 3 weeks of continuous therapy in erythema nodosum usually helps avoid these problems.

Ibuprofen, 400 to 800 mg orally three or four times daily, also may be effective, but I have found it less useful than indomethacin. In general, gastrointestinal side effects are much less frequent with ibuprofen than with other nonsteroidal anti-inflammatory drugs. Its relative safety and efficacy in inflammatory diseases have been well established, as it has been a commonly prescribed medication.

Clinoril 200 mg orally daily or twice daily, might be considered for chronic or recurrent erythema nodosum. Many rheumatologists consider Clinoril to be the most efficacious NSAID with a good safety profile.

All nonsteroidal anti-inflammatory drugs are capable of causing adverse gastrointestinal reactions and platelet dysfunction and are contraindicated in aspirin sensitive patients.

MISCELLANEOUS THERAPIES

Aspirin can be effective in treating erythema nodosum, usually in doses of 10 to 15 grains taken orally every 4 hours. Use of enteric coated preparations again decreases the frequency of side effects, but the efficacy of nonsteroidal anti-inflammatory drugs seems to be greater.

I have had success in one patient with chronic and refractory erythema nodosum by treating with intermittent courses of phenylbutazone. It is usually prescribed in doses of 100 mg three or four times daily with meals. If there is no improvement in the condition within 1 week, the drug should be discontinued. When improvement is obtained, the dosage should be promptly decreased to the minimal effective level necessary to maintain relief, not exceeding 400 mg daily because of the possibility of cumulative toxicity, particularly in terms of bone marrow depression. Aplastic anemia and agranulocytosis have occurred in patients taking phenylbutazone. Like the nonsteroidal anti-inflammatory drugs, phenylbutazone causes gastrointestinal distress and may cause fluid retention. The patient should fail to respond to nonsteroidal anti-inflammatory drugs before one tries phenylbutazone.

I have treated four patients with colchicine, 0.6 mg orally twice daily, and I have had clinical responses in two patients. The most common side effects are nausea, diarrhea, and headache. Long-term use and high doses may be associated with bone marrow depression, among other complications.

I have not found systemic steroid therapy necessary in the treatment of patients with erythema nodosum, but I would not have any reservations about using steroids in patients who are unresponsive to any of the modalities listed, provided the erythema nodosum was not associated with infection. A burst of prednisone, 40 to 60 mg daily tapered over 2 to 3 weeks to avoid chronic side effects would be appropriate.

CHRONIC URTICARIA

MARTIN D. VALENTINE, M.D.

When a thoughtful medical evaluation of a patient in whom hives have been recurring for more than 6 weeks fails to reveal a specific cause, the condition is designated "chronic idiopathic urticaria." After systemic illness has been ruled out, the physician's role in such cases is to provide the therapeutic support that enables the patient to reduce symptoms to a manageable minimum while awaiting a spontaneous remission. Because chronic urticaria may adopt a cyclic pattern and usually regresses spontaneously, often to recur at a later date, what sometimes appears to be a therapeutic triumph may actually turn out to be the natural course of the disease. Although chronic urticaria is usually confined to the skin, mucosal and visceral symptoms occasionally occur, requiring separate therapeutic consideration, as noted later in this article.

Histamine is generally considered to be the primary mediator in most cases of chronic urticaria; thus, antihistamines taken systemically are the mainstay of therapy. Topical therapy with antihistamines or other drugs is rarely helpful, although certain general measures relating to skin care may help the patient feel more comfortable. These include avoidance of conditions that heat the skin, such as hot baths or showers and heavy bed clothing. Other items, such as chili peppers, spicy foods, and systemic ethyl alcohol also result in cutaneous vasodilation and increased susceptibility to urticaria. Clothing should be loose, comfortable, and no heavier than necessary. Skin dryness exacerbates pruritus and should be prevented with moisturizing lotions or creams.

Most H1 histamine antagonists also cause drowsiness. Some physicians believe that this is a desirable effect of a drug used for treating urticaria, but I disagree. The antihistamine that produces maximal effect in the skin with minimal sedation would be the drug of choice; several H1 antagonists are currently available, including ethanolamine derivatives, ethylenediamine derivatives, and alkylamines. Terfenadine (Seldane), an antihistamine with less sedative and anticholinergic effect than other H1 antagonists, is worth trying because of its reduced side effects. Astemizole (Hismanal), another new H1 antagonist with few side effects and a very long half-life, has shown some promise in clinical use. Although some patients do well with these drugs, I find hydroxyzine and cyproheptadine, and occasionally the cyproheptadine relative azatidine, generally superior to the other drugs. The phenothiazine drugs are generally avoided because of the side effects associated with this family of compounds, although one might consider their use in a patient in whom other H1 antihistamines had failed. Because of inherent differences in the pharmacology of hydroxyzine and cyproheptadine, their use is to be considered separately. Antihistamines work better when taken regularly in a prophylactic regimen; when taken after hives appear, they may relieve itching but do not reverse already visible lesions.

HYDROXYZINE

This drug is available as the pamoate (Vistaril and generic equivalents) and the hydrochloride (Atarax, Durrax, and generic equivalents). Either form may be used, both having inherently long durations of action when administered orally. The hydrochloride is available in smaller oral dosage forms, 10 mg being the smallest tablet dose available for the hydrochloride and 25 mg being the smallest capsule dose available of the pamoate. Both are available as liquids. Either form is relatively contraindicated in early pregnancy, because hydroxyzine has caused fetal abnormalities in rats when given in doses substantially above the human therapeutic range. Drowsiness may occur with hydroxyzine, although the duration of sedation with this drug seems to be far shorter than its duration of effect in the skin. Although most people tolerate 10 mg orally three to four times per day without drowsiness, some patients find this dosage to have sedative properties; for such patients an attempt may be made to give the entire day's dosage at bedtime. Some particularly sensitive patients may do well with as small a dosage as 10 mg at bedtime, although this is the exception. As a rule most patients improve with 20 to 40 mg daily, and some patients tolerate—and require—25 to 50 mg every 6 hours. Sedation is common but not universal with the higher dosages. In patients in whom hydroxyzine does not seem to be therapeutically successful, I try cyproheptadine.

CYPROHEPTADINE

In addition to being an antihistamine, this drug is also a serotonin antagonist whose nonapproved uses include prophylaxis against vascular headaches and maintenance therapy in certain patients with Cushing's syndrome. Although drowsiness is the major side effect associated with cyproheptadine, increased appetite or weight gain has also been associated with its use, and at one time it was approved for use as an appetite stimulating drug in children. In addition, I have found an occasional patient to experience otherwise unexplainable emotional depression while using this drug. It is not as inherently long acting as hydroxyzine and thus does not lend itself to single bedtime dosing. However, drowsiness does appear to be minimized if the drug is begun at a low dosage that is gradually increased. In practice, I suggest beginning with 2 mg twice a day, making incremental increases at 2- to 3-day intervals or as tolerated by the patient. After 2 mg twice daily the next dosages are 2 mg three times daily, 4 mg twice daily, and 4 mg three times daily to a maximum of 4 mg four times daily.

COMBINATION THERAPY AND H2 ANTAGONISTS

A single H1 antagonist may be insufficient in the management of patients with chronic urticaria. Although some advocate combinations of two or more H1 antagonists, I believe that other measures are more suitable. I would first consider maintaining the chosen dosage of the Hl antagonist, for example, hydroxyzine or cyproheptadine, and then adding an H2 antagonist, such a cimetidine or ranitidine. Some patients apparently respond to the combination of Hl and H2 antagonists with resolution of the urticaria. It is usually the case, however, that the patient who responds favorably to the addition of the H2 antagonist is the patient who has already responded partially to administration of the Hl antagonist. Certain patients may respond partially to the combination of Hl and H2 antagonists and still need additional therapy. Although steroid therapy may be considered for such patients, I would first consider adding ephedrine sulfate, 25 mg three to four times daily. The combination of alpha-adrenergic and B_1 and B_2 activities may be a useful adjunct in the patient with urticaria. Some authorities have favored B_2 agonists because of the inhibitory effects such drugs have on mediator release, but I believe that such selective drugs are less likely to be useful than the combination of alpha and mixed-beta effects of ephedrine.

TRICYCLIC ANTIDEPRESSANTS

It is known that drugs belonging to the tricyclic antidepressant family have great affinity for Hl receptors in certain binding assays in vitro. This has led to therapeutic trials in patients with chronic urticaria; some successes have been reported. In addition to Hl antagonism, some of the tricyclics, such as doxepin, have significant anti-H2 activity. A trial of doxepin may be warranted if a single conventional Hl antagonist is ineffectual in a patient with chronic urticaria.

CORTICOSTEROIDS

A minority of patients cannot be managed adequately even with a combination of Hl and H2 antagonists with ephedrine. In such patients it may be necessary to resort to systemic corticosteroid therapy. In cases of chronic urticaria one must keep in mind that since the condition may persist for months or even years, if steroids are employed, they may be necessary—with their attendant potential for side effects—for that period of time as well. In general, the rules for the use of steroids in urticaria are the same as they would be for asthma: one should use a drug that is short acting to avoid suppression of the pituitary-hypothalamic-adrenal axis, and should use the drug initially in a dosage sufficient to suppress symptoms completely and taper the dosage fairly rapidly until one can determine the dosage necessary to achieve satisfactory suppression of symptoms. A subgroup of the physical urticarias known as delayed pressure urticaria often responds poorly, if at all, to antihistamines and often requires steroid therapy.

The nonsteroidal anti-inflammatory drugs may have a beneficial therapeutic effect on physical urticaria and should be tried before steroids. Some clinicians believe that the nonsteroidal anti-inflammatory drugs are relatively contraindicated in chronic urticaria of the usual variety, however, and routinely advise against their use even if specific sensitivity to the drug in question is not suspected.

CUTANEOUS VASCULITIS

Cutaneous vasculitis may present as urticaria. This may be seen in the acute or chronic phase of viral hepatitis or other viral illnesses, and in other immunologically mediated syndromes, such as systemic lupus erythematosus, for which patients with urticaria should be screened. In both these examples the skin lesions appear to result from the local deposition of circulating immune complexes with an accompanying local inflammatory reaction, which may include the diapedesis of red blood cells into the skin, producing lesions that persist longer than 24 hours at individual sites and ecchymoses at the sites of individual lesions. This lesion is easily identified in a small punch skin biopsy specimen and also may be present in patients without any underlying systemic illness. In patients with cutaneous vasculitis an elevated erythrocyte sedimentation rate and abnormal serum complement levels are usually seen. Such patients are often unresponsive to conventional therapy for idiopathic urticaria until oral corticosteroid therapy is employed. If the cutaneous lesions are a manifestation of systemic vasculitis, consideration must be given to immunosuppressive therapy.

DRUGS NOT INDICATED

Patients with inherited or acquired deficiency of the inhibitor of C1 do not have urticaria but are susceptible to attacks of cutaneous and mucosal angioedema, which do not respond to epinephrine, antihistamines, or corticosteroids. In these syndromes, confirmed by appropriate immunochemical studies, various anabolic steroids ("impeded androgens") help prevent attacks by promoting biosynthesis of the normal C1 inhibitor protein. Such therapy is rarely indicated in chronic idiopathic urticaria because the risk of liver toxicity and tumors usually outweighs the possible benefit of this class of drug in this non-life-threatening condition.

ACUTE EXACERBATIONS

Occasionally the patient with chronic urticaria may experience an acute exacerbation requiring urgent treatment because a previously effective drug regimen has failed. Acute intervention may also be requested by a patient when urticaria involves an area that results in transient disfigurement, such as the lip or eyelid, causing embarrassment or social inability to continue normal activities. In such situations 0.3 mg (0.3 cc of a 1:1,000 solution) of aqueous epinephrine given by subcutaneous injection is often rapidly effective in reversing cutaneous lesions. Mucosal urticaria or angioedema may also require and benefit from such intervention to prevent airway compromise. Visceral urticaria can produce pain in the gut; esophageal lesions may produce pain that mimics angina but that is rapidly relieved with epinephrine.

PEMPHIGUS

GRANT J. ANHALT, M.D.

There are several different clinical syndromes, all of which are called pemphigus, and all of which share common features. These syndromes are pemphigus vulgaris, pemphigus foliaceus, pemphigus vegetans, pemphigus erythematosus, and endemic Brazilian pemphigus foliaceus (fogo selvagem). Specifically these syndromes present with blisters and erosions of the skin or mucous membranes, loss of normal cell–cell adhesion in the epidermis with the development of intraepidermal acantholytic blisters, and the presence of autoantibodies of the IgG class that bind to a cell surface protein of the epidermis. It is certain that these autoantibodies cause the cellular injury in the epidermis. Both in vitro and in vivo systems have been developed to study the mechanisms by which the autoantibodies induce acantholysis. There is still debate about these mechanisms, and it has not been possible so far to develop any specific way of significantly altering acantholysis in vivo when the autoantibodies are present. This means that all current therapies ultimately succeed by reducing autoantibody production rather than by affecting the events that occur after antibody binding in the skin. For this reason the efficacious therapy of pemphigus requires treatment of the bone marrow primarily, and the skin itself only secondarily.

Prior to the development of corticosteroids the disease was considered uniformly fatal, and if a patient survived the illness, the diagnosis was in doubt. Mortality is now uncommon, but morbidity from drug therapy of the disease remains a major problem and it can be severe. In general, pemphigus vulgaris is a serious disorder and requires aggressive therapy. Pemphigus vegetans is likely a variant of pemphigus vulgaris. Pemphigus foliaceus (including fogo selvagem and pemphigus erythematosus) is a more benign and more indolent disease and can be treated much less aggressively.

PEMPHIGUS VULGARIS

The diagnosis of pemphigus vulgaris is established by obtaining a histologic specimen showing suprabasilar intraepidermal acantholysis, direct immunofluorescence showing IgG (and often C3) bound to the cell surfaces of perilesional skin or mucosa, and demonstration of pemphigus antibodies in the serum by indirect immunofluorescence. If one excludes sampling and laboratory error, in my experience all patients with pemphigus have these three diagnostic features. Therefore, if any of these features is absent, the diagnosis or the laboratory results should be questioned.

Virtually all patients with pemphigus vulgaris develop painful oral erosions prior to developing cutaneous lesions. These patients are frequently misdiagnosed as having oral aphthae or other more common diseases and are treated with topical therapy or oral corticosteroid therapy. The possibility of oral pemphigus usually is entertained when the lesions persist or recur when the oral steroid dosage is decreased or when the patient develops cutaneous lesions. It has been my impression that patients with limited oral disease respond to therapy more quickly than those who have developed extensive lesions, but this may be due to variations in the aggressiveness of the disease itself.

Acute pemphigus requires early systemic drug treatment. A favorable response to treatment is demonstrated initially by halting formation of new lesions, the disappearance of the Nikolsky sign, and finally by re-epithelialization of existing lesions. I use serum pemphigus antibody titers initially as a diagnostic tool and occasionally to help evaluate the patient's status. It is generally not helpful to carry out numerous antibody determinations when treating acute disease, for one should never treat a titer. The response of the acute disease to treatment is determined by the clinical status of the patient, and in the majority of patients, as the disease improves clinically, the antibody titers gradually fall. I do find the titers helpful in management under certain circumstances. Specifically, if a patient is under good control on a stable dose of medication and develops a minor flare of the disease, if the antibody titer remains low, I feel more confident about not altering treatment. If the antibody titer is rising, however, it may be an indication that medication changes are required.

Systemic Therapy

Corticosteroids are the drugs of first choice in all patients with pemphigus vulgaris. It previously was popular to use a regimen with an initial dosage of prednisone of 80 mg per day. If satisfactory control of the disease was not observed in about 1 week, the dosage was doubled to 160 mg per day. If necessary, after 1 week the dosage was doubled again. With this regimen patients often were exposed to dosages of prednisone in the range of 200 to 400 mg per day. In my experience the potential for life threatening complications such as sepsis increases dramatically whenever the dose exceeds 2 mg per kilogram per day; consequently I never use this regimen.

Most patients can be controlled with prednisone, 1.0 to 2.0 mg per kilogram per day in divided doses. Subsequently this may be consolidated into a single daily dose and then tapered. The tapering may be relatively rapid at first (5 to 10 mg per week) but should proceed more slowly as the dosage reaches 40 mg per day. Once this dosage is achieved, an alternate day regimen should be started. This can be done by tapering the dosage administered on every other day until the values are 40 mg and 0 mg on alternate days. The alternate day high dosage then can be tapered. The disease is apt to develop flares of activity during this period, and treatment of such relapses must be individualized. Some patients can be maintained for decades on low doses of prednisone, and alternate day therapy reduces the well known side effects of steroids dramatically.

One must be careful about possible variability of generic preparations of prednisone. If a patient is not demonstrating a uniform response to oral prednisone therapy, it may be advisable to prescribe Deltasone rather than generic prednisone to eliminate variations in bioavailability of the drug. Prednisone is the corticosteroid used most frequently in the United States for pemphigus, but in other countries oral triamcinolone therapy is used because it is believed that there are fewer long term complications with this particular formulation. I have had no experience with this drug and cannot comment on this point.

Corticosteroid "pulse therapy" has also been used in certain patients. In this regimen 1 g of methylprednisolone is given daily in an intravenous infusion lasting 3 hours on 5 consecutive days. This is reported to provide rapid healing of lesions. I have not used this treatment because of the risk of sepsis, sudden death due to arrhythmias in elderly or debilitated patients, and possible aseptic necrosis of the femoral heads. I find that almost all patients can be controlled with lower doses of corticosteroids used in combination with immunosuppressive drugs.

I have found it necessary to use immunosuppressive drugs in addition to prednisone in about half the cases of pemphigus vulgaris that I have treated. Immunosuppressive drugs used in the treatment of pemphigus include cyclophosphamide (Cytoxan), azathioprine (Imuran), and methotrexate. They are listed here in order of their effectiveness (in my own experience). Immunosuppressive drugs are usually started when the prednisone tapering has begun. During initial therapy with large doses of prednisone, the addition of these drugs may produce profound immunosuppression with hazardous consequences.

I have found Cytoxan to be the most efficacious immunosuppressive drug. It has a greater effect in reducing immunoglobulin synthesis than does azathioprine or methotrexate, and I have found the side effects to be reasonably predictable. Cytoxan is given in a single dose of 1 to 2 mg per kilogram daily. The major side effects are bone marrow suppression, hemorrhagic cystitis, bladder fibrosis, sterility, and an increased risk of malignant disease. Marrow suppression is expected with the use of Cytoxan, and frequently one does not observe a clinical effect until the leukocyte count has decreased. It is important to remember, however, that the effect on the white cell count is masked by high doses of prednisone, that elderly patients are more sensitive to the drug than younger patients, and that the drug appears to kill hematopoietic stem cells, so that the longer a patient is treated with the drug, the lower the dose that is required. The risk of hemorrhagic cystitis and bladder fibrosis can be reduced by insisting on an oral fluid intake of 2 liters per day. The most serious potential side effects involve malignant change. The risk that such treatment will result in the emergence of a bladder carcinoma or other malignant tumor is not known exactly, but the possibility of this effect makes one reluctant to use this drug in a young patient.

Azathioprine, an alternative immunosuppressive drug, is preferred by some physicians. It is also administered in a dosage of 1 to 2 mg per kilogram daily and can be used if cyclophosphamide does not produce satisfactory results or if urinary tract complications develop. The side effects encountered with azathioprine are compared with those of Cytoxan in the chapter on *Bullous Pemphigoid* and are not reiterated here (Table 1). Like Cytoxan, the use of azathioprine has the potential for allowing the emergence of malignant disease, and it should be used judiciously.

Methotrexate initially was used more extensively because most dermatologists were more familiar with this drug than with either Cytoxan or Imuran, but it is not as effective as these other drugs.

The intramuscular administration of gold sodium thiomalate has also been used for both pemphigus vulgaris and pemphigus foliaceus. The mechanisms by which it works are unknown. The treatment regimen is similar to that for rheumatoid arthritis. A test dose of 5 or 10 mg is given, followed by 25 mg 1 week later. After that, 50 mg is given at 1 to 4 week intervals; a therapeutic effect usually is expected after a total dosage of 500 mg has been achieved. A complete blood count, urinalysis, and examination of the urine sediment must be done prior to each injection.

The possible side effects include a persistent and troublesome lichenoid dermatitis, acute nephritis, thrombocytopenia, and neutropenia. Nephritis usually is detected early only by an abnormal urinary sediment, often by the appearance of microscopic hematuria. Proteinuria and the nephrotic syndrome may progress even if the drug is discontinued, and rarely glomerulonephritis may occur. The probability of side effects requiring discontinuation of the drug is about one in four.

Reports in the literature indicate that chrysotherapy is of benefit in some patients, but the exact value of this

TABLE 1 Summary of Relative Effects and Side Effects of Immunosuppressive Drugs Employed in the Treatment of Bullous Pemphigoid

	Cyclophosphamide	*Azathioprine*
Effects		
Lymphopenia	++	+
Mitostatic effect	+	++
Depression of primary immune response	++	++
Depression of secondary immune response	++	+
Anti-inflammatory effects	+	++
Depression of cell mediated immunity	++	+
Side effects		
Bone marrow suppression	+	+
Hepatic damage	−	+
Teratogenesis	+	+
Gastrointestinal intolerance	+	−
Infection	+	+
Hair loss	++	−
Azoospermia	++	−
Anovulation	++	−
Oral ulcers	−	−
Cystitis	++	−

treatment is unclear. I have not been convinced that it is efficacious in pemphigus vulgaris, and two of my patients have developed sudden and significant complications. One patient developed allergic pneumonitis requiring admission to intensive care for a prolonged period; a second patient developed acute nephritis and proteinuria in excess of 4 g per day that persisted for 6 months. I have not had any experience as yet with oral gold therapy, but considering the unimpressive therapeutic effects of intramuscular gold therapy, I doubt that it will be more helpful.

Plasmapheresis also has been reported to be of benefit in the disease, and there is a rational basis for its use. It is proven that the IgG autoantibodies produce the cutaneous lesions; therefore removing large amounts of IgG from the circulation should decrease the autoantibody titer and control the disease. In brief, the treatment does just that, but there are substantive problems with this treatment modality. First, removal of the circulating antibody is expensive and requires multiple high volume exchanges to adequately affect the titers. Often six to 10 exchanges (about 3 liters per exchange) are required to produce healing of lesions. In our institution the first exchange costs $1000 and subsequent exchanges cost $600 each. Second, the effect of the plasmapheresis is very temporary. Because this only removes the end product (IgG), autoantibody production continues and actually can be stimulated by the procedure. Unless there is concomitant immunosuppression, there can be a rebound flare when the exchanges are discontinued. For these reasons plasmapheresis should be used only occasionally, when it is necessary to reduce antibody levels quickly while waiting for systemic drug therapy to become effective.

Additional Therapeutic Measures

During the acute phase frequent cultures and appropriate antibiotic therapy should be employed to reduce bacterial colonization. When extensive cutaneous erosions are present, topical treatment with Domeboro compresses three times daily followed by the application of silver sulfadiazine cream (Silvadene) also helps reduce colonization of the wounds and provides some pain relief. Recently I have used semipermeable dressings (Vigilon) on weeping erosions of acute pemphigus vulgaris with surprisingly good results. The dressing provided excellent pain relief, reduced serum exudation from the lesions, and allowed temporary re-epithelialization of the wound to occur. The benefits of these dressings are temporary, for as long as the disease is active, the regenerated epithelium will peel away with every dressing change. Therefore the use of these dressings is limited to the very acute phase of the disease and provides some relief for the patient while waiting for systemic drug therapy to become effective.

It has been stated that intralesional injections of Kenalog (10 mg per milliliter) promote healing of localized lesions, especially oral lesions that may persist despite overall improvement. I have found them not to be of much benefit. Topical steroid treatment can provide limited benefit in pemphigus vulgaris. Twice daily applications of Lidex gel can help reduce the crusting of scalp lesions and benefit oral lesions to a limited extent.

PEMPHIGUS FOLIACEUS

By light microscopy pemphigus foliaceus differs from pemphigus vulgaris in that the intraepidermal blister formation is very superficial, occurring just below the stratum corneum. Clinically it can also be differentiated. Oral lesions are rarely observed, and hyperkeratotic and crusted lesions are prominent. Fogo selvagem is an epidemic form of pemphigus foliaceus that occurs mainly in central Brazil.

In general the options available for the treatment of pemphigus foliaceus are similar to those used in pemphigus vulgaris, but one is much less aggressive with drug therapy because the disease has a better prognosis than pemphigus vulgaris. Most patients can be controlled with a combination of very low oral doses of corticosteroids and potent topical steroid therapy. The use of immunosuppressive drugs is rarely required, but in the rare severe case that requires a second drug, the choice of drugs and their usefulness are similar to that outlined for pemphigus vulgaris.

DRUG INDUCED PEMPHIGUS

Cases of pemphigus have been reported to occur during treatment with several different drugs. Most commonly a clinical disease resembling pemphigus foliaceus occurs during treatment with d-penicillamine and captopril. It is important to recognize that not all patients with drug induced pemphigus have demonstrable evidence of autoantibody production. The skin biopsy shows acantholysis, but direct immunofluorescence shows only complement components in the epidermal intercellular spaces, and indirect immunofluorescence examination for circulating antibodies will be negative. In these cases it is likely that the acantholysis is due to a direct action of the drug on the epidermis. In support of this theory it has been shown that penicillamine and captopril can produce acantholysis in organ cultures of skin without the addition of human antibodies. In these cases in which autoantibody production is not demonstrable, the disease resolves over a period of 6 to 8 weeks after withdrawal of the drug. It is not necessary to treat these patients with systemic steroid therapy or other drugs, although topical application of a potent steroid such as Topicort (desoximetasone, 0.25 percent) helps reduce crusting and discomfort in the lesions.

There are cases in which patients treated with these drugs do develop autoantibodies, both present in the perilesional epidermis and circulating in the serum. The relationship of drug treatment to the development of true autoimmunity in these patients is a challenging question for investigators. These patients appear to have true pemphigus and must be treated as if they have idiopathic pemphigus foliaceus.

BULLOUS PEMPHIGOID

HARISH P. PATEL, M.D.

Bullous pemphigoid is an autoimmune, inflammatory, subepidermal, blistering disease of the elderly. The blister formation in bullous pemphigoid occurs at the dermal-epidermal junction of the skin, and the individual blisters are characterized as being tense. In contradistinction to pemphigus vulgaris, the application of pressure to the blister or shearing force to the normal appearing skin does not produce extension of the existing blister or denuding of the skin.

These blisters arise in the axillary and inguinal regions and are characterized generally by the presence of significant surrounding erythema. This is a relatively benign, transient disease with low mortality, even in patients with untreated bullous pemphigoid. These patients, however, can develop widespread denuding of the skin accompanied by exudation and secondary infection.

Direct immunofluorescence examination of the skin of patients with bullous pemphigoid invariably demonstrates a linear deposition of IgG or the third component of complement along the dermal-epidermal junction of perilesional skin. In addition, other immunoglobulins are found together with both early and late components of the complement sequence—properdin, properdin factor B, and beta-1H globulin. The immunoreactants are localized to the lamina lucida of the dermal-epidermal junction of the skin. Approximately 75 to 80 percent of the patients with bullous pemphigoid demonstrate serum antibodies reactive against an antigen in the lamina lucida of the skin.

Recent in vitro studies reported by Gammon et al have shown that cryostat sections of human skin incubated in the presence of bullous pemphigoid serum, neutrophils, and a fresh source of complement bind pemphigoid antibodies and fix complement along the dermal-epidermal junction. Neutrophils are attracted to the dermal-epidermal junction and release their lysosomal enzymes, producing subepidermal separation of the epidermis from the dermis. This blister formation is similar, if not identical, to the blister formation of bullous pemphigoid.

Additional in vivo studies carried out in the rabbit cornea have also demonstrated the pathogenic role of bullous pemphigoid antibodies. The intraocular injection of the bullous pemphigoid sera results in deposition of human IgG and complement along the basement membrane zone separating the rabbit cornea from the stroma. Polymorphonuclear leukocytes attach to the epithelial-stromal junction, and a subepithelial blister identical to that seen in bullous pemphigoid occurs.

Clinical studies have also demonstrated that the bullous pemphigoid disease process almost always occurs in the presence of IgG or C3 deposition along the skin basement membrane zone. Furthermore, with successful treatment of the clinical disease, the pemphigoid antibody disappears from both the serum and the skin of the affected patient. With relapse of clinical disease activity there is a reappearance of the bullous pemphigoid antibody in the serum and the appearance of linear C3 basement membrane zone deposits.

These findings strongly suggest a cause and effect relationship between the bullous pemphigoid antibody and the bullous pemphigoid disease process. These studies also strongly support the hypothesis that the bullous pemphigoid antibody mediates the development of the characteristic blistering skin disease, at least in part, by the activation of the complement sequence. The aforementioned clinical and laboratory studies form the rationale for our therapeutic regimen, which is designed not only to eradicate the clinical disease but also to eliminate the bullous pemphigoid antibody.

The majority of the patients with bullous pemphigoid go into complete clinical remission following successful therapy. In addition, the bullous pemphigoid antibody disappears from the serum and, finally, from the skin of these patients. Once the pemphigoid antibody disappears from both the skin and the serum, all therapy can be gradually tapered completely. The majority of the patients with bullous pemphigoid need treatment for 4 to 6 months. Most remain in complete serologic and clinical remission, off all therapy. Recurrences are seen in approximately 15 to 20 percent of the patients.

TOPICAL THERAPY

Isolated bullous pemphigoid, generally localized to the lower extremities, may respond to saline or aluminum subacetate wet dressings and the frequent topical application of a potent fluorinated steroid (e.g., triamcinolone, 0.1 percent four to six times per day).

SYSTEMIC THERAPY

The mainstay of therapy for bullous pemphigoid is the parenteral administration of steroids. Forty to 60 mg of prednisone daily is generally an adequate oral dosage for the treatment of the majority of the patients with bullous pemphigoid. With this dosage of corticosteroids, the individual pemphigoid blisters generally heal within a 2 to 3 week period, and new blister formation ceases within approximately 3 weeks.

Immunosuppressants (azathioprine, 100 mg per day, and cyclophosphamide, 100 mg per day) alone or in combination with steroids may be used to suppress the blistering disease.

Prior to the institution of immunosuppressive or steroid therapy, a careful review of the patient's history is conducted to evaluate for a history of duodenal ulcer, diabetes, or exposure to tuberculosis. In addition to a routine CBC and differential counts and urinalysis, a chest roentgenogram is obtained. If evidence of tuberculosis is found, an infectious disease consultation is obtained. Generally, if there is a history of tuberculosis, the patient is treated with isoniazid, 300 mg per day, as long as he is receiving steroid or immunosuppressive therapy.

The immunosuppressive drugs are generally detoxified in the liver and the kidney; the function of these organs is evaluated by appropriate blood chemistry tests prior to the initiation of immunosuppressive therapy. In addition, potential bone marrow toxicity is monitored weekly with a complete blood count, including a platelet estimate during the first month of therapy and every 2 weeks thereafter (Table 1).

Clinically the combination of these drugs is thought to result in an additive therapeutic effect minimizing side effects of both the steroids and the immunosuppressive drug.

Azathioprine, 100 to 150 mg per day, appears to be an especially effective drug to be employed together with corticosteroids in the treatment of bullous pemphigoid. The combination of these drugs, i.e., prednisone, 20 to 30 mg per day, and azathioprine, 100 to 150 mg per day, is given until the patient ceases to demonstrate new blister formation and previous blisters heal. Following the disappearance of the bullous pemphigoid antibody from the serum, the presence of bullous pemphigoid antibody in the skin is determined by direct immunofluorescence examination of a skin biopsy specimen. If the bullous pemphigoid antibody is not detected, all therapy is gradually tapered completely. (Prednisone is completely tapered at a rate of 2.5 mg per week. Then azathioprine is tapered over a 1 to 2 month period after the steroids have been discontinued.) The patients are then examined for disease recurrence, clinically and serologically, every 3 to 4 months.

Dapsone (diaminodiphenylsulfone) alone, 100 mg per day, or in combination with steroids has been noted by some investigators to be of benefit in the treatment of bullous pemphigoid and its variant, benign mucous membrane pemphigoid. This, however, must be confirmed; its value in these two conditions appears to be marginal.

Before employing diaminodiphenylsulfone, a glucose-6-phosphate determination should be done with the patient's red blood cells. Older red blood cells, normally deficient in glucose-6-phosphate, hemolyze in the presence of diaminodiphenylsulfone. The presence of a deficiency in all red blood cells during sulfone therapy results in pronounced hemolytic anemia. Methemoglobinemia and sulfhemoglobinemia are also infrequent complications of sulfone therapy.

TABLE 1 Summary of Relative Effects and Side Effects of Immunosuppressive Drugs Employed in the Treatment of Bullous Pemphigoid

	Cyclophosphamide	*Azathioprine*
Effects		
Lymphopenia	++	+
Mitostatic effect	+	++
Depression of primary immune response	++	++
Depression of secondary immune response	++	+
Anti-inflammatory effects	+	++
Depression of cell mediated immunity	++	+
Side effects		
Bone marrow suppression	+	+
Hepatic damage	−	+
Teratogenesis	+	+
Gastrointestinal intolerance	+	−
Infection	+	+
Hair loss	++	−
Azoospermia	++	−
Anovulation	++	−
Oral ulcers	−	−
Cystitis	++	−

The mechanism of action of dapsone is unknown. Some evidence indicates that the sulfones interfere with the leukocyte myeloperoxidase system. Whether this mechanism is responsible for the mild anti-inflammatory effect of diaminodiphenylsulfones is unknown.

The major aim of present day therapy of bullous pemphigoid is to design therapeutic regimens that not only control the disease but also minimize the substantial morbidity and mortality potential related to the drug therapy. The combination of low doses of steroids with an immunosuppressive drug has been a successful form of treatment for this bullous disease. In addition, determination of the autoantibody disappearance in this disease has prevented needless maintenance therapy and minimized the morbidity of steroid and immunosuppressive therapy.

DERMATITIS HERPETIFORMIS

RUSSELL P. HALL III, M.D.

Dermatitis herpetiformis (DH) is a chronic, extremely pruritic papulovesicular disease, which generally begins in the second to fourth decade. Although periods of clinical remission occur, the disease should be considered to be lifelong and requires long-term therapy. DH is characterized clinically by very pruritic papules and vesicles, which occur in groups on extensor surfaces (elbows, knees, buttocks) and the scalp. Biopsy of an early lesion reveals a subepidermal blister with collections of neutrophils at the dermal papillary tips (papillary microabscesses). Although this histologic picture is characteristic of DH, a similar pattern can be seen in some patients with bullous pemphigoid and in those with the bullous eruption of systemic lupus erythematosus. In addition, biopsy of older vesicles or bullae in DH most often does not show the characteristic papillary microabscesses. Direct immunofluorescence of normal appearing perilesional skin reveals either granular deposits of IgA (85 percent of the patients) or a linear band of IgA at the dermal-epidermal junction (15 percent of the patients). Although the clinical and histologic presentation is, in general, identical in patients with either granular or linear deposits of IgA, the pattern of the cutaneous IgA deposits is important in planning therapy for patients with DH.

In patients with DH and granular IgA deposits there is a high prevalence of the histocompatibility antigens HLA B8, DR3, and DQw2 and an associated asymptomatic gluten sensitive enteropathy. In addition, the skin disease in these patients often responds to a gluten free diet (to be discussed). By contrast, DH patients with linear IgA deposits have a normal prevalence of HLA antigens B8, DR3, and DQw2 and do not appear to have associated gluten sensitive enteropathy, and there is no evidence suggesting that a gluten free diet is effective in treating the skin disease. It has been proposed that the name dermatitis herpetiformis be reserved for the disease in patients with granular IgA deposits and that those with linear IgA deposits be designated as having "linear IgA dermatosis."

THERAPY

The cornerstone of effective therapy for both DH and linear IgA dermatosis is establishment of the correct diagnosis. There should be appropriate clinical and histologic presentations and granular or linear IgA deposits should be evident on direct immunoflorescence. Most false negative results in immunofluorescence tests are a result of obtaining lesional skin for direct immunofluorescence examination. If the normal appearing perilesional skin does not reveal IgA deposits in a patient thought to have DH, direct immunofluorescence should be repeated using fresh tissue (without "transport media"), multiple sections being evaluated for IgA deposits. The clinical response to therapy with dapsone is not a useful criterion for the diagnosis of DH owing to the numerous other conditions that also respond to dapsone.

Dapsone (diaminodiphenylsulfone) is the drug of choice for both DH patients with granular IgA deposits and those with linear IgA dermatosis. Most patients respond quickly to dapsone, noting a marked decrease in the pruritus and a lack of new lesion formation within 12 to 48 hours after starting dapsone therapy. Although some patients with linear IgA dermatosis require systemic corticosteroid therapy and dapsone to control the disease, in my experience most of these patients have responded to dapsone therapy alone.

Dapsone, however, does have serious adverse hematologic effects that necessitate careful pretreatment evaluation and close follow-up. Dapsone causes dose related hemolysis, which can be severe in patients with glucose-6-phosphate dehydrogenase (G6PD) deficiency. G6PD deficiency occurs most frequently in blacks, Asians, and those of Southern Mediterranean descent, and in these individuals the G6PD level should be determined before therapy is begun. All individuals who take dapsone have a degree of hemolysis that results in a decreased hemoglobin level. This hemolysis is minimal at 25 to 50 mg of dapsone per day but can result in up to a 2 g reduction in hemoglobin at dosages of 150 to 200 mg per day. In patients who are not iron, folate, or vitamin B_{12} deficient, a compensatory reticulocytosis occurs and the hemoglobin rises nearly to pretreatment levels. Patients with cardiac or pulmonary disease should be evaluated carefully to determine that they will not be compromised by the expected drop in hemoglobin that occurs with dapsone therapy.

Methemoglobinemia also occurs during dapsone therapy in a dose related fashion. This can result in a slate blue discoloration in some patients but is generally well tolerated at the levels seen during dapsone therapy (12 percent methemoglobin or less). The patient needs to be made aware of this side effect and carry a card detailing his medications in order to avoid confusion during any possible medical emergency. Other symptoms of methemoglobinemia can include weakness, tachycardia, nausea, headache, and abdominal pain, but usually do not develop at methemoglobin levels lower than 20 percent. In patients with severe cardiopulmonary disease the effect of relatively low levels of methemoglobinemia may be more severe.

The other side effects of dapsone are either idiosyncratic or allergic and are listed in Table 1. For the most part these side effects disappear on discontinuation of the drug. Agranulocytosis has been reported in patients taking dapsone. This is a rare complication and has always occurred within the first 3 to 4 months of therapy. When agranulocytosis is recognized promptly, it appears to be reversible on withdrawal of the dapsone. Finally, although dapsone has been classified as a "weak carcinogen" in rats, evidence of carcinogenicity does not exist in humans.

TABLE 1 Adverse Reactions to Dapsone

Hemolysis
Methemoglobinemia
Headache
Gastric irritation
Anorexia
Hepatitis, infectious mononucleosis-like
Cholestatic jaundice
Morbilliform eruption
Erythema nodosum
Erythema multiforme
Toxic epidermal necrolysis
Psychosis
Leukopenia
Agranulocytosis
Hypoalbuminemia
Peripheral neuropathy (most commonly motor)

The pretreatment evaluation prior to dapsone therapy should include a history and physical examination, a complete blood count with a differential, liver and renal function tests, urinalysis, and, when indicated, a G6PD level. After this complete pretreatment evaluation, patients with DH or linear IgA dermatosis should be begun on 50 to 100 mg of dapsone per day. The long half-life of dapsone allows most patients to take a single daily dose. A complete blood count with a differential should be done weekly for the first 4 to 6 weeks, then biweekly for an additional 2 to 3 months, and finally at 8 to 12 week intervals while dapsone therapy is continued. This frequent follow-up allows for the potential early detection of agranulocytosis before serious morbidity occurs and for close monitoring of the hemolysis and resultant anemia that occur with dapsone. Liver and renal function should be assessed every 4 to 6 months. Patients also should be tested for distal motor weakness and sensory deficits on follow-up visits. Most patients respond within 24 to 48 hours after the institution of dapsone therapy with a marked decrease in itching and the cessation of new lesion formation. After 1 to 2 weeks the dosage of dapsone should be adjusted to the minimal dosage required to control the patient's symptoms by changing the daily dosage by 25 to 50 mg every 1 to 2 weeks.

Most patients' symptoms can be controlled with 100 to 150 mg of dapsone per day. Patients and physicians, however, should be aware that some lesions may still occur (two to three lesions every 1 to 2 weeks) at this dosage and that this normal variation in disease activity should not lead to an increase in the dapsone dosage. When a patient experiences long periods without any active skin disease, I recommend that the dosage of dapsone be decreased slowly in order to re-establish the minimal amount needed to control symptoms. It should be emphasized to the patient that dapsone is an effective drug that is well tolerated by most patients but that it has potentially severe side effects. It is important to discuss these side effects carefully with the patient and to explain that many are directly dose related. In this way the hazards of self-medication are emphasized as is the need for close and frequent follow-up care.

Patients who are unable to tolerate dapsone can be given sulfapyridine at initial oral doses of 500 mg twice daily. Although the side effects of sulfapyridine are less severe, the drug is also less effective. Sulfapyridine cannot be taken by patients who are allergic to sulfa drugs and must be taken with adequate fluid intake and close monitoring of renal function because renal calculi can occur. The dosage of sulfapyridine can be increased to 3 to 4 g per day, if needed, to control blistering; however, frequently even this dosage level is insufficient to control the disease.

In general, patients who are thought to be allergic to sulfapyridine can safely take dapsone and vice versa. Rare cases of cross reactivity have been reported, however, and such patients should be followed carefully when initiating therapy. Likewise the history of an allergic reaction to sulfa drugs is not thought to be an absolute contraindication to dapsone therapy, but these patients also should be observed closely for potential adverse effects.

A number of other drugs have been reported to be useful in DH. These include pyridoxine, cholestyramine, colchicine, nicotinic acid, and oral doses of antihistamines. In my experience these drugs have proven to be only minimally effective in most cases of DH. Topical steroid therapy, although not effective in controlling the eruption, occasionally is helpful in decreasing the symptoms associated with the sporadic lesions of DH that occur during therapy and perhaps may help in healing these lesions.

Since DH often affects women of child-bearing age, the question of the use of dapsone during pregnancy frequently is raised. There is little information documenting the safety of dapsone during pregnancy. It is my policy to discuss the issue with the patient at the time of the initial diagnosis and to suggest that she adhere to a gluten free diet during pregnancy (see next paragraph), which ideally should be started 6 to 12 months prior to the pregnancy. If this is not possible, the patient should be advised regarding the lack of data regarding the possible teratogenicity of dapsone. If the patient desires treatment, I favor low dose sulfapyridine (500 to 1,000 mg per day) or low dose dapsone (25 to 75 mg per day) therapy. The patient should be advised to take the minimal dose required to allow her to tolerate her symptoms. The patient's other physicians, including the pediatrician, should also be advised of the use of dapsone or sulfapyridine during the pregnancy. Finally the patient should be advised that dapsone is secreted in breast milk and can cause hemolytic anemia in the newborn and that she therefore should avoid breast feeding.

As mentioned previously, patients with DH and granular IgA deposits have an associated gluten sensitive enteropathy. This association has led to trials of a gluten free diet for control of the skin disease. It has been found by a number of investigators that patients with DH and granular IgA deposits who strictly adhere to a gluten free diet can decrease the dapsone requirement by 50 to 75 percent or more after 9 to 16 months with the diet. However, there is no evidence suggesting that a gluten free diet is of any value in the patient with linear IgA deposits (linear IgA dermatosis). The gluten free diet requires the total avoidance of all wheat containing foods for as long as 9 to 16 months before any substantial benefit to the patient can be noted. The patient should also be aware that as many as 25 to 30 percent of the cases of DH do not appear to respond to the gluten free diet and that it is currently not possible to predict who will respond to gluten restriction. It also appears that total gluten restriction is necessary for maximal benefit, even to the extent of avoiding the small amount of wheat additives found in some ice cream, sauces, and other foods. I advise my patients not to begin diets that eliminate only 50 to 75 percent of wheat protein, for in all probability this will offer little benefit. The complexity of this diet necessitates consultation with a dietitian who has been educated by dermatologists regarding DH as well as a well motivated patient. Patients should be made aware of resources available from the National Celiac-Sprue Society (5 Jeffrey Road, Wayland, MA 01778), which can help in planning and executing the gluten free diet.

EXFOLIATIVE DERMATITIS

HERMAN S. MOGAVERO Jr., M.D.

This entity, also known as erythroderma, is a cutaneous inflammation characterized by an initial erythema with the subsequent development of pronounced scaling or exfoliation. Although it is often initially localized, the process typically has spread to the majority of the cutaneous surfaces at the time of presentation.

There are multiple etiologies for this disorder, recognizing both a primary de novo clinical presentation and secondary underlying causes. These can be conveniently compartmentalized into the following classification:

1. Idiopathic.
2. Generalized or widespread cutaneous disease states such as atopic, contact, or seborrheic dermatitis, psoriasis, lichen planus, pemphigus foliaceus, or pityriasis rubra pilaris.
3. Systemic diseases with cutaneous manifestations such as leukemias, lymphomas (of both the T- and B-cell types), and some solid tumors (e.g., of the lung or rectum).
4. Adverse cutaneous reactions to drugs. This reaction can involve many classes of drugs, including but not limited to antibiotics, anti-inflammatory drugs, anticonvulsants, and metallic compounds.

The diagnosis of a pre-existing dermatologic condition in the erythrodermic patient relies on a detailed examination of the whole integument. Dermatologic consultation should be requested to assist in looking for distinct areas of "typical" morphology isolated from the surrounding "sea of erythema." It is in these areas that there is the highest yield of diagnostic skin biopsy findings in specific dermatologic entities. In addition, skin biopsy can be helpful in the diagnosis of underlying leukemia or lymphomas and is indicated in the evaluation of all cases of erythroderma.

The objective cutaneous manifestations of exfoliative dermatitis can extend beyond the obvious erythema and scaling. There can be complete or partial alopecia, onychodystrophy, deep painful fissuring of the skin, and desquamation of the palms and soles in broad thick sheets. Mucous membrane involvement is distinctly unusual in erythroderma.

There are major systemic components of exfoliative dermatitis, and in most cases these features warrant hospitalization for appropriate diagnostic evaluation and therapeutic intervention. Typically there are complaints referable to the inability to maintain thermostability. In spite of multiple layers of clothing, the patient is unable to keep warm at ambient temperatures that are uncomfortably hot for others. The patient reports chills and shaking sensations. On examination there may be either fever or hypothermia. In the latter instance it is important to be sure that the device measuring the temperature can register below 96°F (36°C). The remainder of the physical examination must be complete, with special attention paid to assessing lymphadenopathy, hepatomegaly, and splenomegaly. The distinction of lymphoma from dermatopathic lymphadenopathy often requires lymph node biopsy as well. Other signs of secondary infection, hypervolemia, tachycardia, edema, and high output cardiac failure must be sought. The laboratory evaluation can parallel that used in a severe burn with prominent fluid and electrolyte abnormalities, including hypoalbuminemia and hypernatremia if increased transepidermal water loss is not corrected. Accurate weight measurements and daily monitoring of fluid intake and output are also required.

TREATMENT

The treatment of exfoliative dermatitis is focused on the diagnostic entity responsible. Elimination of an offending drug usually initiates resolution of the dermatitis. Treatment of the underlying systemic disease is necessary to control erythroderma secondary to neoplastic processes. In this setting a consultation with a hematologist or oncologist is appropriate for therapeutic intervention.

The approach in cases of erythroderma related to widespread cutaneous disease or idiopathic exfoliative erythroderma is initially conservative. The patient is often best served by hospitalization in order to allow for the aforementioned diagnostic studies and systemic monitoring and also to remove him or her from any negative environmental factors (e.g., in cases of atopic dermatitis).

The mainstay of therapy is frequent lubrication of the skin with colloidal baths and bland ointments such as Aquaphor or petrolatum. If pruritus is a component of the eruption, antihistamines are given. I routinely employ hydroxyzine as an H_1 blocker and increase the dosage to maximal tolerance (up to 100 mg orally every 6 hours) before adding additional H_1 blockers (cyproheptadine, 4 mg orally every 8 hours, or terfenadine, 60 mg orally every 12 hours) or H_2 blockers (cimetidine, 300 mg orally three or four times daily).

The topical use of corticosteroid ointments is tempered by the realization that the widespread cutaneous inflammation and defective vasoconstriction allow for enhanced absorption percutaneously. I typically begin with 1 percent hydrocortisone ointment applied three times daily. If no response is noted after a brief period of time (while diagnostic studies are pending), one can advance to 0.1 percent triamcinolone ointment or its equivalents (class III or IV) three times daily. The topical use of more potent steroids (class I or II) is modulated by the extent of the cutaneous eruption because widespread disease allows for pituitary-adrenal axis suppression. If the diagnosis of psoriasis has been excluded and the risk versus benefit of systemic treatment of severe seborrheic or atopic dermatitis is considered, a course of systemic corticosteroid therapy is warranted, with initial doses of prednisone in the range of 1 to 1.5 mg per kilogram per day. Once control has been achieved the objective of therapy is to consolidate to a single daily dose and then taper to alternate day, low-dose steroid therapy to minimize the well-known complications of daily systemic steroid therapy.

The introduction of retinoids has added greatly to the therapeutic tools available to the dermatologist. In cases of erythrodermic psoriasis, etretinate has proved very effective. In contrast to pustular psoriasis, the approach in erythrodermic psoriasis is to use a low dose of etretinate (25 mg orally each day) and to increase gradually the amount if necessary. In a similar fashion, generalized or refractory cases of pityriasis rubra pilaris have been responsive to etretinate at doses of 0.5 to 1 mg per kilogram or to isotretinoin in the 1 to 2 mg per kilogram daily dosage range. The use of these retinoids requires a detailed knowledge of their biologic half-life and the associated risks of teratogenicity, skeletal abnormalities, and the signs and symptoms of hypervitaminosis A.

To some extent the use of cytotoxic drugs has been displaced by the retinoids. Methotrexate in the usual dosage of 2.5 to 5.0 mg every 12 hours for three consecutive doses per week remains an alternative for cases of idiopathic exfoliative dermatitis that are refractory to the foregoing approach.

Mortality from exfoliative dermatitis has been a prominent feature in a number of retrospective studies. The metabolic complications of exfoliative dermatitis have been discussed. There must also be constant vigilance for complications of systemic infections (sepsis, pneumonia, cellulitis), venous thrombosis or embolism, and complications caused by the underlying disease process or its treatment.

LEG ULCERS

DONALD P. LOOKINGBILL, M.D.

Leg ulcers can be due to a wide variety of etiologies, but the most common is stasis. This section deals primarily with the therapy of venous (stasis) ulcers, although some of the therapeutic measures can be applied to other types of leg ulcers as well.

PATIENT EVALUATION

Stasis ulcers result from sustained elevations in venous pressure in the lower extremities. Frequently there is a history of thrombophlebitis. The ulcers typically occur above the malleolus, usually on the medial side of the leg. Venous ulcers are often accompanied by petechiae and a brownish discoloration ("stasis changes") of the surrounding skin. Dermatitis may be present as well and is due either to the stasis itself or to secondary contact dermatitis. Dermatitis, if present, is sometimes confused with cellulitis in that both are manifested by erythematous skin;

but dermatitis is often vesicular and almost always pruritic, whereas cellulitis is warm and tender and sometimes is accompanied by fever.

In patients with venous ulcers, leg and pedal edema is usually present and is a critical factor that must be addressed if treatment is to succeed. In the general evaluation of the patient, consideration should be given to other possible causes of edema, including congestive heart failure and kidney disease. The blood pressure should also be obtained and pedal pulses examined to screen for other vascular causes or factors contributing to the leg ulcer. If pedal pulses are absent, a vascular surgery consultation is recommended. In chronic nonhealing ulcers, a biopsy specimen should be taken from the edge of the ulcer to rule out other etiologies, particularly malignant disease.

MEDICAL THERAPY

The preferred therapy for venous ulcers is medical. Surgical treatment may be needed if medical management fails or becomes unduly prolonged. The foremost consideration in medical management is to control edema. If this is not achieved, other measures will be of little value. The other measures include treatment of infection (if present), debridement, and wound dressings.

Edema Reduction

Edema control is more easily said than achieved, especially in an outpatient. For patients with severe disease, hospitalization may be necessary. In the hospital setting the patient is put at strict bed rest with the foot of the bed slightly elevated. Pneumatic compression devices such as the Jobst extremity pump can also be used to reduce edema and lymphedema more quickly. In our hospital this is done once or twice daily in the physical therapy department.

For most outpatients, strict bed rest is impossible to achieve, but patients are encouraged to maximize the amount of time they spend lying flat with their legs slightly elevated and minimize time spent sitting in a chair. We have found that in patients who comply with bed rest instructions the ulcers are much more likely to heal than those in patients who are noncompliant.

The judicious use of diuretics may help reduce edema in some patients, but this is not a mainstay of therapy. Unna boots and elastic stockings are also helpful for edema control (to be discussed).

Treatment of Infection

Most ulcers contain potentially pathogenic bacteria, which can be recovered on routine culture. However, cultures are not usually performed, and antibiotic treatment is not instituted, unless there is evidence of cellulitis around the ulcer. If cellulitis is present, a culture is taken empiric antibiotic therapy is begun to cover gram positive organisms. Erythromycin is most frequently employed. If there is no clinical response, the culture results may be of help in selecting alternative antibiotic therapy. When the cellulitis subsides, antibiotics are discontinued. Sterilization of the ulcer is an unrealistic goal; long-term antibiotic therapy only selects out resistant organisms.

Debridement

Necrotic debris enhances bacterial growth and impairs ulcer healing. Physical debridement can be done with a curette or scissors and forceps. Viscous lidocaine is often helpful for local anesthesia. We have not found the topical application of enzymatic preparations to be very useful and they can cause irritiation.

Medical measures for debridement include wet-to-dry dressings and Debrisan dressings. Occlusive dressings also provide for debridement and are discussed separately.

Wet Dressings

Wet dressings are most useful in the initial stages of treating ulcers that have abundant debris. Wet dressings are most conveniently used in patients who are at bed rest. For the "wetness" we use saline or quarter strength Burow's solution (aluminum acetate). Full strength Burow's solution is not used because evaporation can result in an ultimate concentration that will cause irritation. Since patients with venous ulcers have a predilection for developing contact dermatitis in the area of involvement, the use of potentially sensitizing chemicals should be avoided. This includes antiseptics such as povidone-iodine (Betadine) and topically applied antibiotics such as neomycin.

Wet dressings are applied as follows: Several layers of wet gauze are placed over the ulcer and held in place with tubular gauze. Since evaporation is desired, the dressing should not be occluded. Depending upon the amount of wetness to begin with, it takes 30 minutes to several hours for the dressings to dry. The dressings should be changed every 4 hours. At the time of removal, some of the debris will have stuck to the dressing and hence will have been removed. The ulcer base is then gently cleaned and another dressing applied. Wet-to-dry dressings are used mainly in the initial stages of ulcer therapy or in preparation for grafting.

Dextranomer (Debrisan)

Dextranomer is a hydrophilic dextran polymer that has been formulated into small spherical beads (Debrisan). It is of use in debriding moist ulcers, wherein fluid is absorbed into the beads and particulate matter is trapped between the swollen beads. Edema in the ulcer area may also be reduced by the hydrophilic action. Debrisan is available in loose beads or in a paste, either of which is applied to the moist ulcer in a ¼ inch layer and covered with a gauze dressing, closed on all four sides. Dressings are changed twice daily at which time the ulcer is thoroughly irrigated. Since Debrisan often tends to adhere to the ulcer base, vigorous irrigation is frequently needed, sometimes accompanied by gentle swabbing. Debrisan should be used only on moist ulcers; if they become dry, the medication should be discontinued. This method is relatively effective in treating ulcers, but it is expensive.

Occlusive Dressings

Occlusive dressings exploit the theory of "moist wound healing." A number of these dressings are now on the market, including Bioclusive, Duoderm, Op-Site, Synthaderm, Tegaderm, and Vigilon. Most are made of polyurethane, and all but Tegaderm and Vigilon are self-adhesive. All have in common the property of occlusion, which causes an accumulation of exudate (which aids debridement) and accelerates wound healing. We have mainly used either Duoderm or Op-site. Duoderm is easier to handle than Op-site, but Op-site is more adhesive. The dressing is applied to the ulcer and surrounding skin. With Duoderm, tape is used to further secure the edges. The dressing should not be removed until it loosens naturally or drainage leaks out from under the edges. Most dressings stay in place for at least several days (up to 1 week), but in ulcers with copious exudate, more frequent dressing changes may be necessary. Patients need to be advised that fluid will accumulate under the dressing and that the drainage may have a foul odor. Patient instruction booklets are available for some occlusive dressings (for example, Duoderm). The dressings are moderately expensive, and some patients need help in applying them. Development of cellulitic infection under the occlusive dressing is a theoretical concern, but surprisingly rarely occurs. A major advantage of occlusive dressings is that they usually provide excellent pain relief. Elastic stockings can be used over Op-site or Duoderm dressings. The use of occlusive dressings can be continued until complete healing occurs.

Unna Boot

The time tested Unna boot still has a place in the treatment of leg ulcers. It is best used after debridement and edema reduction. It protects the ulcers, provides partial occlusion, and helps to prevent edema. We use a Dome-Paste dressing, which is applied in accordance with the directions on the package. With the foot in a flexed position, the leg is wrapped from the forefoot to just below the knee, including the heel. Wrinkles and reverse turns should be avoided. The dressing should be applied in a "pressure gradient" fashion with more pressure at the ankle than at the knee, but care must be taken not to make the dressing too tight. The entire dressing is used and covers the leg in about three layers. It is then wrapped with a Kling bandage, which is held in place with tape applied to the top, bottom, and sides. Removal is accomplished by carefully cutting the dressing with bandage scissors on the side of the leg opposite the ulcer. At dressing changes, the ulcer and leg are gently cleaned, but no medications are applied except for the fresh dressing.

The Unna boot dressing is changed weekly until healing occurs (often months) or until no further progress is made. The Unna boot method has the advantage of requiring infrequent dressing changes with relatively inexpensive materials, but it is somewhat bulky and requires weekly office (or home) visits and a nurse skilled in its application.

SURGICAL THERAPY

With medical therapy many ulcers heal, albeit slowly. At each office visit the ulcer should be measured or traced so that progress can be monitored. The surrounding skin should be checked for edema, and if it is present, that aforementioned measures should be readdressed. If, in the absence of edema, the ulcer is enlarging or not improving over time, surgery should be considered. This is a time to also re-evaluate the original diagnosis. For example, if a biopsy had not been done initially, it might now be considered to rule out malignant disease.

In our hospital ulcer surgery is done by either plastic surgeons or vascular surgeons. An accurate assessment of the patient's vascular status is important prior to leg surgery. Some venous ulcerations occur over incompetent perforating veins in the lower legs, and sclerosing one or several of these vessels may be helpful. The arterial blood supply of course must also be adequate for successful grafting.

If the ulcer bed is clean, the ulcer may be covered directly with a split thickness skin graft. For necrotic ulcers with poor granulation tissue, excision is needed before grafting.

Properly performed and cared for, skin grafting can result in excellent coverage of long standing venous ulcers.

POSTULCER TREATMENT: ELASTIC SUPPORT STOCKINGS

The successful management of venous ulcers does not end with ulcer healing. Prevention is important. For this, the use of elastic stockings is strongly recommended. Several types are manufactured, and kits are now available for measuring patients in the office. We use knee length stockings and fit patients for either Jobst Fast-Fit or T.E.D. stockings. The Jobst Fast-Fit stockings are more expensive, but are flesh colored and provide venous pressure gradient support. Measurements are made at the calf and ankle, and the patient is fitted with one of six sizes. The T.E.D. stockings are white and are available in two lengths, each in small, medium, large, and extra large sizes. They are fitted on the basis of calf circumference and leg length measurements. Fitting measurements are preferably made when the patient has no or minimal edema; once fitted, patients are instructed to put the stockings on each morning before getting out of bed.

NEUROLOGIC DISEASES

DISORDERS OF CONSCIOUSNESS

MARTIN A. SAMUELS, M.D.

"Consciousness is a being such that in its being, its being is in question in so far as this being implies a being other than itself." (Sartre)

This impersonal concept of consciousness is the cornerstone of Jean-Paul Sartre's thought and represents one of the major principles underlying modern existentialism. Yet despite its profound importance, it has proved useless in the emergency department. Medical personnel require a more mundane definition—one capable of relating clinical phenomenology with anatomic and physiologic pathology. The concept of differential diagnosis fails when one is faced with a patient suffering from an altered level of responsiveness to external (and often internal) stimuli. The neurologist approaches the patient with a decreased level of responsiveness armed with a notion of consciousness which, although probably less profound than Sartre's, is practical and will allow one to localize the disorder, thereby reducing the plethora of possibilities to a realistic manageable number. To save time, some commonly encountered disorders may be treated simultaneously. The aim is to reach a diagnosis and or a definitive treatment within 1 hour of the patient's presentation.

AROUSAL AND AWARENESS

For our purposes, we shall assume that consciousness has two attributes, each of which has an anatomic substrate. These two attributes are arousal (or wakefulness) and awareness. Arousal (wakefulness) is that group of behavioral changes that occur when a person awakens from sleep. Of the array of changes that occur, the most conspicuous is that of opening of the eyes. Although one can be asleep with the eyes open or awake with the eyes closed, an organism with its eyes open is probably awake. Pathologic states associated with decreased responsiveness and closing of the eyes are therefore analogous to sleep in some respects. The neural system underlying this change in states is the fictitious ascending reticular activating system (ARAS), a conceptual array of nuclei and tracts, ascending in the core of the brainstem heading toward the nonspecific thalamic nuclei. These in turn relay information to the cerebral cortex. The inherent pacemaker rates of this centrocephalic system are the basis for the electroencephalogram. The ARAS is presumably part of the reticular formation in close proximity to other vegetative systems, such as those controlling respiration, cardiovascularity, eye movements, pupillary reaction, and cranial reflexes. Structural or metabolic processes that derange the function of the ARAS will probably have some effect on the neighboring systems that are dependent on reticular formation function. Thus, one cause of decreased consciousness would be failure of the ARAS. This category of decreased consciousness, also known as unarousal, is in a sense a state of pathologic sleep, and as such would share many of the behavioral manifestations of natural sleep, except that ordinary stimuli cannot arouse the patient.

Traditionally, the depth of unarousal is graded, largely to allow medical personnel to communicate with one another accurately in a shorthand fashion. Unfortunately, because the definitions of these grades have not been fully standardized, this has led to more rather than less confusion. It is best simply to describe the patient's appearance in plain English. For example: "Jones looks as if he were asleep. When I call his name he does not respond. When I pinch him he transiently awakens, curses, and falls back to sleep. I think he moves the left side less well than his right." This accurately describes the patient's state so that anyone can understand it. For those who must use shorthand, the following definitions of the various depths of unarousal may be used. *Confusion* (or inattention) refers to the inability to maintain a coherent stream of thought. This is the slightest abnormality in consciousness, and confused patients may appear to be awake or even hypervigilant with sympathetic hyperactivity (i.e., sweating with dilated pupils, tremor, and hypertension). This latter state, known as *delirium*, is generally seen in patients undergoing withdrawal from alcohol or sedatives or in states associated with excessive circulating sympathomimetic amines. *Drowsiness* is defined as a state of apparent sleep which can be overcome with a painful stimulus. For patients in a state of *stupor*, a simple pinch on the upper and lower extremities should elicit a response. If only reflex responses are elicited (e.g., decerebrate or decorticate posturing or triple flexion), one should not grade the state as stupor. *Coma* is defined as a state of apparent sleep in which there is only a reflex response (or no response at all) to a painful stimulus. Vague, undefined terms such as "obtundation" and "lethargy" should be avoided since generally no one, including the examining physician, knows what exactly they mean.

If a person is awake, does that mean that he or she is conscious? In humans, some aspects of consciousness are well beyond the brain stem's ken. It is these aspects of consciousness (which, for our purposes, we shall call "awareness") that are possibly unique to human beings. For the sake of our discussion, we will assume that the whole integrated function of the cerebral cortex is the anatomic substrate for awareness. We have learned from experience that in order to produce unawareness, there must be a diffuse bilateral lesion involving both sides of the cerebral cortex. Small lesions can produce profound deficits, such as aphasia, alexia, hemianopsia, and hemiparesis, but only a diffuse bilateral process, sparing the ARAS and diencephalic structures, can lead to unawareness or a vegetative state.

In summary, there are two kinds of unconsciousness: (1) unarousal caused by disease of the ARAS and (2) unawareness, caused by diffuse bilateral cerebral hemisphere disease. As far as we know, there are no other types of unconsciousness. Therefore, the problem of unconsciousness becomes a simple one for the physician. Is the trouble in the brain stem or is it diffusely present in the hemispheres? It should be obvious that failure of the arousal system renders it impossible to test the awareness system. Therefore, the question of whether there is consciousness when there is unarousal is a moot point.

MANAGEMENT OF THE UNCONSCIOUS PATIENT

Given this background, the evaluation of the unconscious person becomes simple. A few general practical rules should be kept in mind. The head or neck of the unconscious patient *must not be moved* until the cause of the loss of consciousness is determined. Head injuries are commonly associated with neck injuries. The latter may be the cause of the greatest permanent disability in an otherwise reversible concussion. At the scene of an accident, a collar should be placed on the neck in order to warn medical personnel not to move the head with respect to the torso until proper films can be taken. Naloxone, 0.01 mg per kilogram, administered by rapid intravenous (IV) infusion should be given immediately on the chance that an opiate overdose may be involved. Most adults should receive thiamine, 1 mg per kilogram, by rapid IV infusion in order to prevent exacerbation of possible Wernicke's encephalopathy. Dextrose, 1 g per kilogram, should be infused rapidly in order to reverse hypoglycemia. During the initial few minutes with the patient, a patent airway should be insured and the blood pressure measured. Most or all of the above maneuvers can be carried out in the field by emergency medical technicians.

When the patient reaches the emergency department, one should attempt to locate some person able to give a medical history. This is not always as easy as it sounds because often the unconscious patient has arrived in the emergency department unaccompanied. Family, police, ambulance personnel, or friends should be contacted and asked specifically about trauma, drugs (including alcohol, over-the-counter medications, and prescription drugs), headache, or other symptoms preceding the ictus, and whether such an attack has ever happened before. One good question to ask is: "Do you have any theories as to what may have caused the trouble?"

Examination of the unconscious patient is aimed at determining whether the process is a brain stem disease or is diffuse in both hemispheres. One does this by examining brain stem structures that are in close proximity to the ARAS. These include those controlling cranial reflexes, respiratory control centers, pupillary reaction, and eye movements.

Certain cranial reflexes or automatisms are signs of relatively good brain stem function. These include sneezing and yawning, both of which are probably respiratory reflexes requiring a relatively intact reticular formation. Swallowing and hiccoughing, on the other hand, are probably mainly gastrointestinal reflexes that require only medullary function and do not carry the same good prognosis.

Both normal and Cheyne-Stokes respiratory patterns are relatively good signs in the unconscious patient, reflecting intact respiratory control centers in the pons and medulla. Hyperventilation in an unconscious person should always alert one to a search for a cause of metabolic acidosis. Such causes include diabetic ketoacidosis, lactic acidosis, methanol intoxication, ethylene glycol intoxication, and aspirin poisoning, and are usually also the cause of the unconsciousness. Hyperventilation without a metabolic cause (i.e., central neurogenic hyperventilation) is not a precisely localizing sign and as such is not particularly useful. Apneustic breathing (i.e., deep breaths with inspiratory cramps at the end of each deep breath) is a reliable sign of pontine dam-

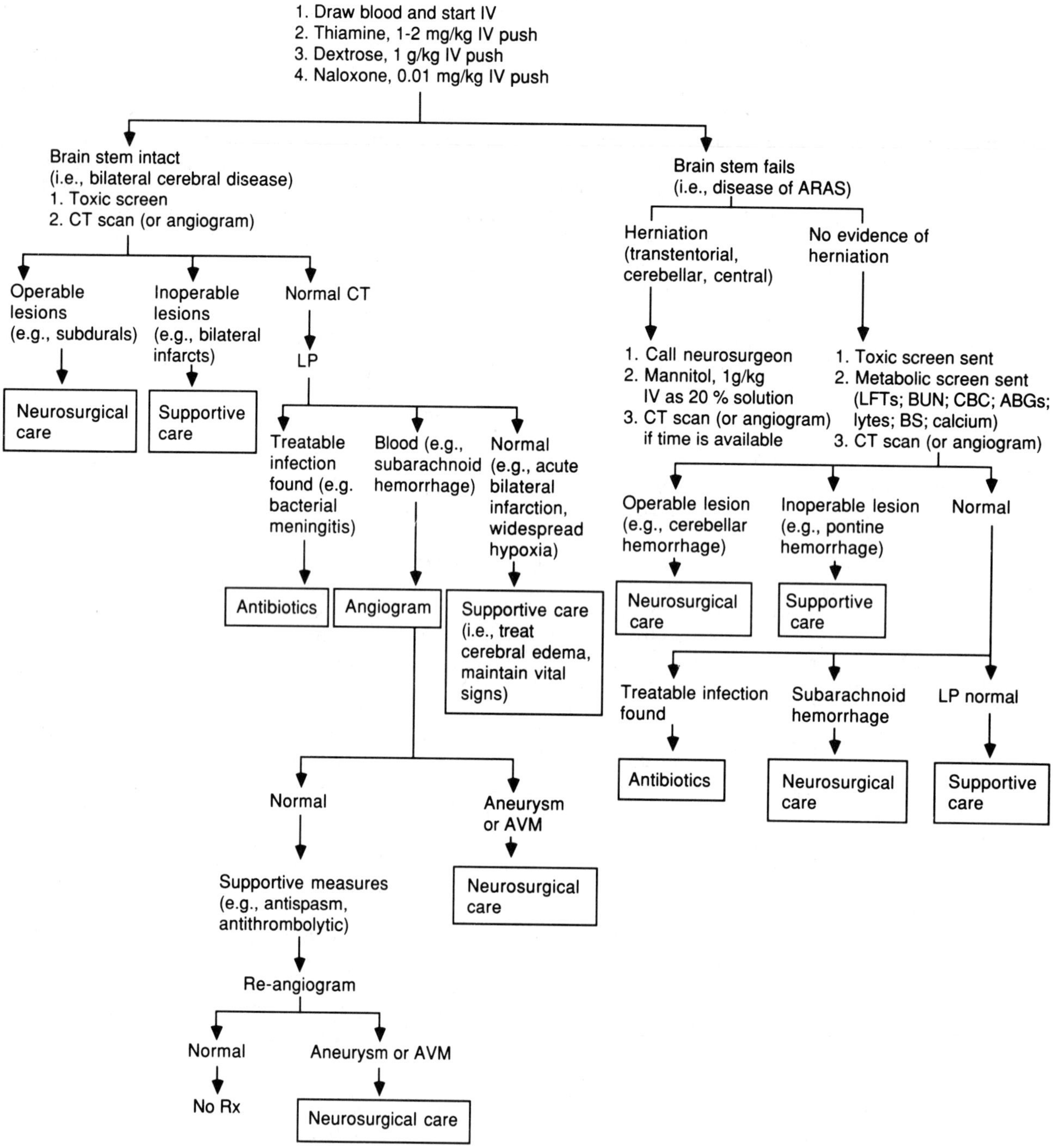

Figure 1 Diagnosis and treatment protocol in the comatose patient. LP = lumbar punctures; LFTs = liver function tests; ABGs = arterial blood gases; BS = blood sugar; AVM = arteriovenous malformation.

Republished with permission from Samuels MA, Aquino TM. Coma and other alterations of consciousness. In: Samuels MA, ed. Manual of neurologic therapeutics. 3rd ed. Boston: Little, Brown, & Co., 1986: 13.

age. Ataxic (or Biot) respiration is the poorly coordinated, mechanically ineffective breathing seen in patients with disease of the primary respiratory control centers in the medulla. In general, patients with apneustic and ataxic breathing should be intubated before the inevitable apnea occurs.

The pupils should be measured and the sizes recorded on the patient's chart. In general, sparing of the pupillary light reflex with simultaneous failure of other brainstem functions (e.g., breathing, eye movements) indicates a drug intoxication unless the drug in question has a direct effect on pupillary function (e.g., atropine). A dilating pupil in an unconscious patient with brain stem failure should be assumed to be caused by transtentorial herniation on the side of the large pupil. Such a patient should be hyperventilated (to a Pco_2 of about 25 mm Hg), and an imaging study (computed tomography or magnetic resonance imaging) should be performed while a neurosurgeon is called. Mannitol, 1 g per kilogram, may be given intravenously as a 20 percent solution if necessary. Unequal pupils in a conscious person is *never* caused by herniation of the brain. Most such patients are found to have a mydriatic drop in the eye, a migraine, or essential anisocoria. In no case should such a patient be treated for increased intracranial pressure.

The eye movements are examined to test the function of the brain stem from the level of the vestibular nuclei in the medulla to the oculomotor nuclei in the midbrain. There is no cause of brain stem unconsciousness—whether metabolic or structural—that does not also affect either the pupils, the eye movements, or both. First the patient is observed for spontaneous eye movement. If full conjugate eye movements occur without stimulus (so-called windshield-wiper eyes), this is strong evidence of a bihemisphere form of unconsciousness; the full-roving eye movements are prime fascia evidence of good brain stem function that has been disinhibited by the loss of input from the hemispheres above. If spontaneous eye movements are inadequate, the eyes should be stimulated to move using the vestibulo-ocular reflexes. The oculocephalic reflex cannot be used since, as I mentioned earlier, unconscious patients should not have their heads moved. The vestibulo-ocular reflex may be conveniently stimulated by infusing 20 to 50 ml of ice water into the ear. After a pause of a few seconds, the eyes should move conjugately and fully *toward* the side of the ice water infusion. If this occurs, the brain stem is partially functioning from the vestibular nuclei to the midbrain. If the hemispheres are functioning normally, they will issue a command to correct the vestibular-induced movement. This command probably comes from the frontal eye fields opposite the direction of the corrective fast eye movement. In physiologically explicable states of unconsciousness, there is always an abnormality in either the slow (vestibular) or fast (cortical) phase of the ice water–induced eye movement. If both phases are normal, the state of unconsciousness is caused by neither brain stem disease nor bilateral hemispheral disease. Because the traditional definition of unconsciousness attributes unconsciousness to only these two causes, this latter state is referred to as "functional" or "hysterical" unconsciousness. Unconsciousness is a relatively common conversion symptom, and is manifested by totally normal brain stem and hemispheral function as outlined above. It can usually be reversed through some type of strong suggestion that the patient will recover, thus allowing the patient a graceful way out of the emergency department.

Lastly, one should consider the presentation of a patient who is unresponsive but awake. In this case, the brain stem function is assumed to be intact, so the difficulty must be bihemispheral. If the ice water test shows intact slow (vestibular) phases but no fast (cortical) phases, one must conclude that the process is bilateral and diffuse in the hemispheres. This so-called vegetative state is distinct from brain death, since the latter includes brain stem death. The common processes leading to a chronic vegetative state are global hypoxic-ischemic damage such as cardiac arrest and chronic degenerative processes such as Alzheimer's disease. Other states in which patients appear to be awake but are unresponsive (akinetic mutism) include (1) the abulic state caused by bilateral prefrontal lobe disease (e.g., tumor, hemorrhage, hydrocephalus, degenerative disease, stroke), (2) the locked-in states (e.g., pontine hemorrhage), and (3) nonconvulsive status epilepticus, (4) catatonia, and (5) hysterical mutism.

Figure 1 shows a decision tree of the evaluation and treatment of unconscious patients based on the principles outlined in the text. It is designed so that the final diagnosis and/or definitive therapy is reached within 60 minutes.

SUGGESTED READING

Fisher CM. The neurological examination of the comatose patient. Acta Neurol Scand 1969; 45(suppl):5–56.

Levy DE, Caronna JJ, Singer BH, et al. Predicting outcome from hypoxic-ischemic coma. JAMA 1985; 253:1420–1426.

Plum F, Posner JB. The diagnosis of stupor and coma. 3rd ed. Philadelphia: Davis, 1980.

Ropper AH. Lateral displacement of the brain and level of consciousness in patients with an acute hemispheral mass. N Engl J Med 1986; 953–958.

SYNCOPE

GEORGE DAVID PERKIN, B.A., F.R.C.P.

Patients seldom use the term syncope to describe an episode of loss of consciousness. They are more likely to complain of experiencing blackouts or "passing out." A discussion of the management of syncope, restricting the term to episodes of altered consciousness triggered by a reduction of cerebral perfusion, is a relatively simple undertaking. In practice, however, many attacks of altered awareness cannot be so readily attributed to this cause, and their management becomes a more complex issue (Fig. 1). The problem is a common one. Between 1983 and 1987 I encountered 239 patients who had had one or more attacks of loss of consciousness that were not clearly epileptic in origin. The breakdown of their diagnoses is given in Table 1.

HISTORY

Patients usually appreciate that when they have had attacks of loss of consciousness, additional information about the episodes is required from a third party. If that information is not forthcoming at the first interview, the patient should be encouraged to bring a witness at their next visit. Close relatives are not necessarily best suited for this purpose. Often, concern over the attack limits their ability to give an accurate history. Estimates of the duration of the individual phases of the episode tend to be inaccu-

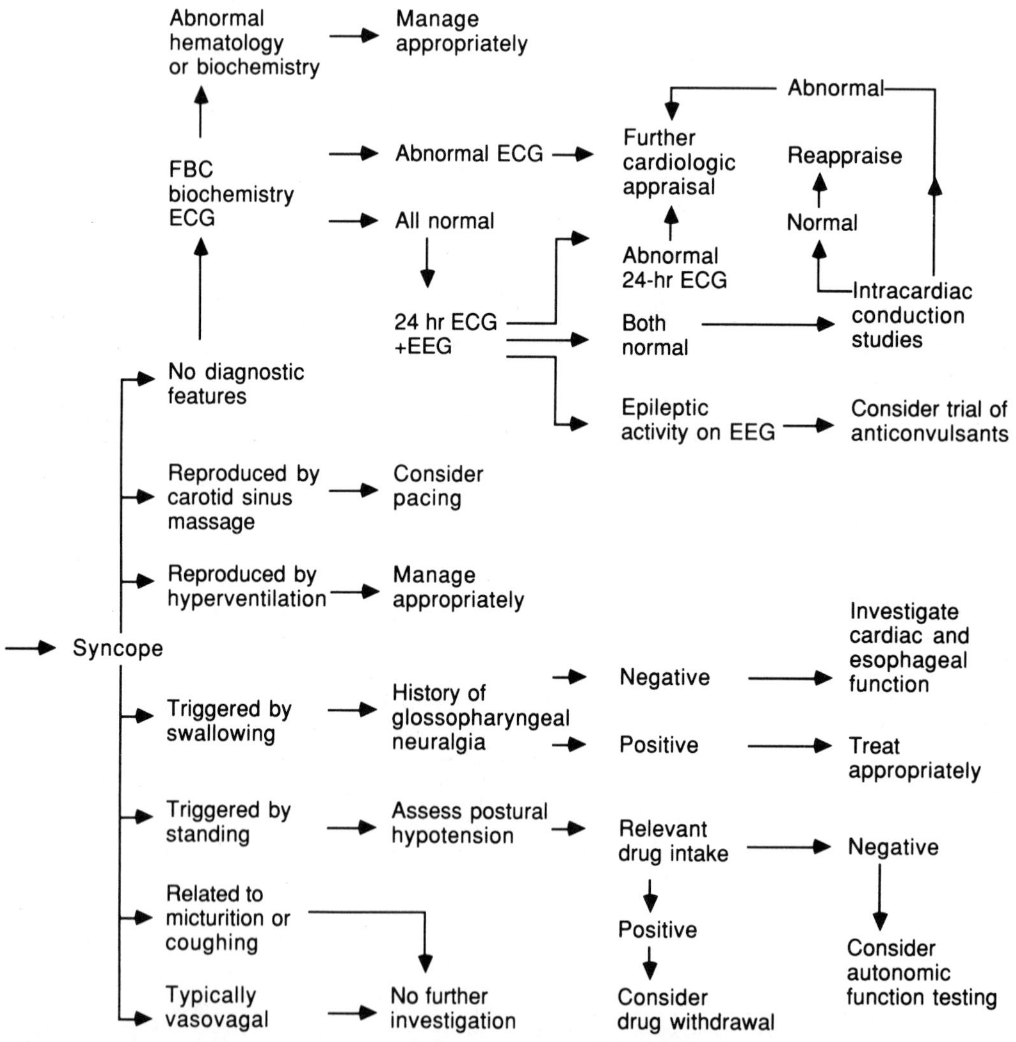

Figure 1 Evaluation and treatment of syncope. (Republished with permission from Perkin GD. Diagnostic tests in neurology. London: Chapman and Hall Medical, 1988:34.)

TABLE 1 Causes of Syncopal Attacks in a Series of 239 Patients

Causes	*No. of Patients*
Vasovagal attacks	76
Micturition syncope	6
Cough syncope	2
Vomiting syncope	1
Syncope secondary to anemia	1
Cardiac syncope	4
Orthostatic hypotension	1
Hyperventilation syndrome	21
Hysteria	7
Unknown	120
Total	239

rate, and elaborate descriptions sometimes owe more to the imagination of the witness than the reality of the event. Critical details aiding diagnosis include those describing the nature of any prodromal symptoms and the circumstances in which the attacks have occurred. Often these two pieces of information alone serve to establish the diagnosis. More problematic in terms of management is the group of patients in whom the initial history and examination fail to suggest a possible cause for the event.

VASOVAGAL ATTACKS

This is the most common form of diagnosable syncope encountered in clinical practice. The majority of attacks, which are more common in women than in men, occur during the 2nd and 3rd decades of life. There is a well-defined aura, with malaise, nausea, faintness, pallor, and sweating featuring prominently. The attacks are often triggered by specific events—for example, venesection or a stressful emotional experience. The loss of posture tends to be less abrupt than in epilepsy, and the patient lies quietly after such an attack. Patients giving a typical history do not require investigation. They should be advised to sit or (preferably) lie down as soon as symptoms appear. Loss of consciousness seldom occurs if the patient is already sitting, and never if they are lying, so that the effectiveness of posture change in influencing symptoms can serve as a diagnostic test. Individuals particularly liable to faint should lie down before having potentially painful procedures performed.

Under what circumstances may further investigation be necessary? Apparently typical attacks can occur in older patients; in my series, 5 percent were older than 40 years of age. The possibility of a cardiac dysrhythmia is higher in this group. If the cardiovascular system and electrocardiogram (ECG) are normal, I do not investigate further unless the episodes are recurrent. A brief tonic posture can occur during an attack of a vasovagal syncope but not clonic movements or a tonic-clonic progression, both of which suggest the diagnosis of a vasovagal syncope complicated by epilepsy. In this case, management depends on how closely related the attacks are to a specific stimulus; in some patients, avoidance of the relevant trigger may be a more rational approach than the use of anticonvulsants. Electroencephalography (EEG) is an appropriate means of investigation, but seldom computed tomography or magnetic resonance imaging scanning, since the occurrence of a vasovagal syncope complicated by epilepsy is rarely if ever the reflection of structural pathology within the central nervous system.

MICTURITION SYNCOPE

Attacks of micturition syncope are usually nocturnal, occur predominantly in men, and are more likely to occur after alcohol ingestion. Eyewitness accounts are seldom forthcoming and, when available, usually provide information only about the aftermath of the event. If the history is typical, no action is required other than that of suggesting to the patient (if male) that he be in a sitting position when micturating, particularly at night. Prostatic obstruction is seldom of importance in the genesis of this condition and should be investigated only if there are suggestive symptoms.

COUGH SYNCOPE

Cough syncope is rare. Typically, a bout of intractable coughing terminates in a syncope. I have encountered one patient in whom persistent retching had a similar effect. If the history is characteristic of patients with this condition, no further investigation is required. Management should be aimed at the underlying chest disorder. If the paroxysm of coughing that triggered the syncope was not particularly violent and if the attacks are recurrrent, it is advisable to perform ECG monitoring while the patient coughs. Sometimes this reveals that the syncope is caused by an atrioventricular block precipitated by coughing. If so, insertion of a pacemaker is required.

SWALLOW SYNCOPE

I have never seen a case of swallow syncope. Most patients with this complaint have structural disease of the esophagus readily revealed by barium swallow or endoscopy. Sometimes, however, the esophageal abnormality is subtle or even absent.

ECG monitoring should be performed while the patient swallows to identify the type of cardiac conduction defect responsible for the syncope. If there is overt esophageal disease, it is managed appropriately. If not, alternative treatments include either the use of anticholinergic drugs or cardiac pacing adjusted to the nature of the atrioventricular block. The latter approach is preferable.

CAROTID SINUS SYNCOPE

It has been suggested that this condition is underdiagnosed, although I have seldom encountered it in clinical practice. Cardioinhibitory and depressor forms are described in the literature, with the former producing a syncope by triggering asystole or atrioventricular block, and the latter by inducing hypotension. Reproduction of an attack by carotid sinus massage remains the cornerstone of diagnosis. ECG control is mandatory during this procedure. Symptomatic forms of the condition result from tumor invasion of the sinus, but the vast majority of cases are idiopathic. Therapeutic approaches include carotid sinus denervation and pacing. Theoretically, the former can deal with both the cardioinhibitory and depressor forms. Pacing, however, is probably the preferable option.

CARDIAC SYNCOPE

In some patients who experience syncope, a cardiac basis for the problem is suggested by a history of concurrent palpitations or by the presence of an abnormally slow heart rate on clinical examination. Additional support is provided if an observer is able to record an abnormal heart rate during subsequent attacks. A routine ECG may serve to establish a diagnosis, but if it does not, a period of Holter monitoring is justified. For patients with complete heart block or the sick sinus syndrome, the treatment of choice is cardiac pacing. Tachyarrhythmias are less likely to produce a syncope. If, on the basis of 24-hour monitoring or of clinical examination, I suspect a cardiologic abnormality, I refer the patient for an expert opinion. Other cardiac disorders sometimes presenting with syncope include aortic stenosis and atrial myxoma.

ORTHOSTATIC HYPOTENSION

Syncope caused by postural hypotension figures infrequently in a neurologist's case-load, but is a relatively common problem in the elderly. The history of attacks triggered by postural change is readily elicited, and the extent of the problem easily determined by measurement of blood pressure with the patient in the lying and standing positions. Drug therapy is often partly responsible; during the enquiry, one should look for ingestion of diuretics, hypotensive agents, phenothiazines and tricyclic antidepressants. Management should consist of either discontinuing the use of the offending agent or, if this is not possible, advice regarding changing posture. Full-length elastic stockings will help reduce venous pooling.

In some patients, orthostatic hypotension is the first manifestation of either pure autonomic failure or multisystem atrophy (Shy-Drager syndrome). The management of both conditions is unsatisfactory. The patient is advised to rise slowly from the sitting or recumbent posture. Micturition should be performed in the sitting position. The lavatory door must never be locked, as it may prevent access to the patient during a syncopal episode. Care-givers or relatives should be advised about what action to take if the patient complains of faintness. Therapeutic measures are of limited value. I advise patients to wear full-length elastic stockings, putting them on before rising in the morning, and prescribe fludrocortisone, 0.1 mg administered three times daily. The patients are encouraged to sleep at a slight "head up" tilt, slowly increasing to about 10 to 15 degrees. Beyond this, I have not been convinced that other forms of treatment influence the problem. Regimens advocated in the past have included administration of ephedrine, dihydroergotamine, a combination of tyramine and a monoamine oxidase inhibiter, and cardiac pacing at an artificially high rate. An antigravity suit successfully controls symptoms but is too cumbersome to be recommended.

HYPERVENTILATION SYNDROME

In most series, loss of consciousness has been an infrequent component of the hyperventilation syndrome. In my cases, encountered between 1983 and 1987, loss of consciousness occurred in one-fourth of patients, although for many of these, loss of consciousness was an isolated event despite multiple episodes of hyperventilation. The combination of a normal neurologic examination and the reproduction of an attack by overbreathing serves to establish the diagnosis, although some physicians also require the identification of hypocapnoea during the attack. Although rebreathing into a bag can rapidly terminate symptoms, I find many patients reluctant to use this measure. Where the symptoms are of recent onset and episodes are infrequent, discussion of the mechanism often helps alleviate the problem. In more chronic cases, formal breathing exercises are necessary. If there is evidence of an associated anxiety state, I favor psychiatric referral rather than simply prescribing anxiolytics.

CONVERSION HYSTERIA

Conversion hysteria is occasionally a cause of syncopal attacks. Pseudo-seizures are seen more commonly. The diagnosis can be difficult to establish and necessitates identification of other conversion reactions. Injuries sustained as a result of syncopal events do not exclude the diagnosis. The episodes are seldom brief, with the patient more often entering a fugue-like state lasting for hours. If the onset of conversion reactions has been relatively recent, and particularly if there are depressive features, I favor psychiatric referral. In my experience with patients who have longer-standing symptoms, attempts to modify their reactions have failed.

SYNCOPAL ATTACKS OF UNCERTAIN CAUSE

The protocol for the investigation and management of the conditions already described is straightforward (Fig. 1). There remains a substantial proportion of patients (almost exactly half in my series) in whom the cause of the syncopal event is not readily discernible. In other words, the attacks do not suggest epilepsy, nor are there the clinical characteristics that would identify one of the conditions discussed earlier in this chapter. Clinical examination is normal. In this case, the next step is to perform routine hematologic and biochemical investigations along with an ECG. In all likelihood, the results of these tests will be normal, but occasionally they suggest the probable basis for the events (as in the case of one of my patients with an unsuspected, but severe anemia). Further management should be influenced by whether the attack was isolated or recurrent. My policy is not to investigate further in patients who have had an isolated syncopal event with normal findings on the initial screening. If the attacks have recurred, I obtain an EEG and proceed to a 24-hour period of Holter monitoring. Unless they are very frequent, attacks rarely occur during the monitoring period, but certain abnormalities indicate the need for cardiologic appraisal. These include frequent or repetitive ventricular ectopy and periods of sinus arrest. In addition, high-resolution ECG monitoring, if available, should be performed in order to identify any low-amplitude signals in the terminal portion of the QRS complex or in the ST segment. Such potentials correlate with a susceptibility to spontaneous or inducible ventricular tachycardia and require cardiologic appraisal.

Remaining are a substantial number of patients with syncope whose investigations have yielded normal results. For these, the question of performing more invasive cardiologic procedures, including ventricular stimulation, arises. These techniques are not universally available and are more stressful for the patient. Furthermore uncertainty sometimes remains as to whether electrophysiologic abnormalities detected by such techniques necessarily explain the patient's attacks. I believe there is no justification for such investigation in patients who have had an isolated syncopal event or infrequently recurring events and in whom there are no cardiologic abnormalities. In patients who experience frequent syncope, the investigation is probably warranted, although further prospective studies in this field are required.

SUGGESTED READING

Morady F. The evaluation of syncope with electrophysiologic studies. Clin Cardiol 1986; 4:515–526.

Riley TZ, Roy A, eds. Pseudo-seizures. Baltimore: Williams and Wilkins, 1982.

Schellack J, Fulenwider JT, Olson RA, et al. The carotid sinus syndrome: a frequently overlooked cause of syncope in the elderly. J Vasc Surg 1986; 4:376–383.

VERTIGO

TIMOTHY C. HAIN, M.D.

Vertigo, the illusion of rotation, is nearly always caused by vestibular system dysfunction. Management of vertigo is easiest when an accurate localization and etiologic diagnosis are available. Unfortunately, however, an etiologic diagnosis cannot be established in the majority of patients with vertigo. In cases where a specific treatment is not available, symptomatic relief may be provided by antiemetics and drugs that depress peripheral vestibular function. Unfortunately, all vestibular suppressant medications have side effects that limit their use. Furthermore, reduction of vertigo is accomplished by reducing vestibular function on *both* the normal and abnormal side. Thus, vestibular suppressants can induce ataxia.

The inability of available medications to suppress vertigo effectively without unacceptable side effects has led clinicians to attempt other modes of treatment. Recently, greater emphasis has been placed on vestibular rehabilitation therapy in which recovery is promoted by exercises aimed at facilitating central adaptive mechanisms.

This chapter concentrates on common conditions that account for most of the referrals to a vertigo clinic and defines the role of medication or vestibular exercises in treating these disorders.

PATHOPHYSIOLOGY

The peripheral vestibular apparatus, which consists of the semicircular canals and otolith organs, senses angular and linear acceleration. Angular acceleration is related to rotation of the head and is registered by the canals. Linear acceleration is related to translation of the head as well as changes in the orientation of the head to gravity and is registered by the otoliths. Accordingly, illusions of rotation, translation, or tilt and symptoms initiated or aggravated by head movement are the hallmarks of vestibular system disease.

Symptoms of semicircular canal disturbance include a sensation of rotation as if the body were spinning, cartwheeling, or tumbling. Symptoms of otolith disturbance include sensations of tilt, levitation, or impulsion. If an otolithic disturbance is severe enough, the patient may be precipitated to the ground (e.g., the "otolithic crisis of Tumarkin" experienced by patients with Meniere's syndrome). Symptoms of autonomic overactivity such as sweating, pallor, nausea, and vomiting nearly always accompany vertigo of labyrinthine origin.

Central vestibular lesions, which may also cause vertigo, usually involve structures in which afferent activity from both labyrinths have been combined. The resulting pattern of imbalance in vestibular activity may more closely resemble naturally induced sensations of rotation and is usually associated with milder symptoms than peripheral vestibular imbalance.

ACUTE PERIPHERAL VESTIBULAR IMBALANCE

Most peripheral causes of vertigo result in distress caused by sensation of movement, nausea, and malaise for only 2 to 3 days. Even patients with vestibular nerve section are usually up and about within 1 week. Accordingly, even untreated, most patients with symptoms caused by a transient and incomplete paresis of vestibular function on one side will be ready to go back to their regular activities after 1 week.

In treating this condition, the dilemma of the physician is that, although patients want to be treated with a medication that will completely suppress their vertigo and somatic responses to vestibular imbalance, such treatment can harm the patient, by denying his nervous system the ability to compensate for a vestibular lesion. If the vestibular imbalance is covered up by a vestibular suppressant medication, little repair activity may be initiated. Even bedrest may be contraindicated. Animal studies have clearly shown that when experimental vestibular lesions are made, immobilization delays recovery.

The strategy is therefore to use as few medications as possible and to encourage head movement and early ambulation. When there appears to be no alternative to medication, I prefer to use antiemetics such as prochlorperazine (Compazine) or promethazine (Phenergan). These may be prescribed as suppositories. Brief usage of Antivert (meclizine) may also be helpful. If the patient appears to be dehydrated, he should be admitted. Tables 1 and 2 list commonly available drugs and dosages.

In the acute phase, generally on the 1st day, patients should be warned that sudden head movements and changing the position of the head relative to the gravitational axis may cause increased vertigo. However, once the patient is able to sit up and navigate about the room, he should be encouraged to attempt as much normal activity as is possible without triggering emesis. Medications, particularly sedatives, should be discontinued as soon as possible, as they may retard eventual compensation. Most patients recover spontaneously without the need for a formal vestibular rehabilitation program,

TABLE 1 Drugs Used for Nausea

Drug	*Dose*	*Comments*
Droperidol (Inapsine)	2.5 or 5 mg IM *or* sublingual q12h	May produce extra-pyramidal reaction
Prochlorperizine (Compazine)	10 mg IM or p.o. q4–6h *or* 25 mg rectal q12 h	May produce extra-pyramidal reaction
Promethazine (Phenergan)	25 mg p.o. q4–6h *or* 25 mg rectal q6h	Sedating

TABLE 2 Drugs Used to Decrease Vertigo

Drug	*Dose*	*Comments*
Diazepam (Valium)	5–10 mg p.o., IM, or IV (1 dose) given acutely	Sedating respiratory depressant
Dimenhydrinate (Dramamine)	50 mg p.o. q4–6h	Sedating
Meclizine (Antivert)	25 mg p.o. q4–6h	Sedating
Scopolamine Transdermscop	patch q3d	Anticholinergic side effects

because their vestibular impairment is transient rather than permanent.

What about the patients who don't recover spontaneously? Usually they have a fixed vestibular paresis or loss. Such patients can benefit from an organized physical therapy program incorporating the gait training and visual-vestibular exercises outlined in Table 3. This ensures that they receive adequate sensory input for their impaired vestibular system and develop appropriate strategies to deal with sensitivity to head motion and disequilibrium.

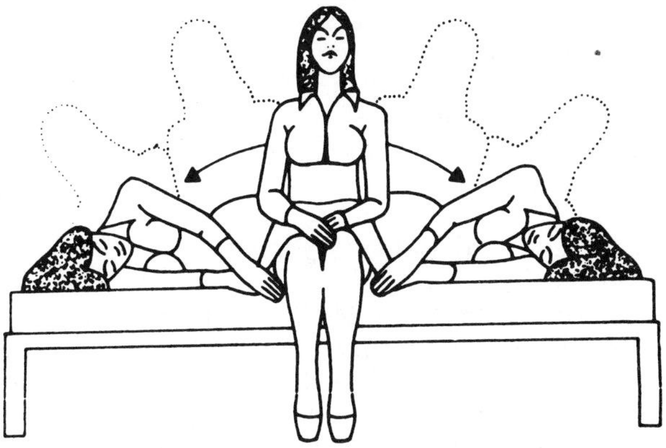

Figure 1 Positioning exercises for the treatment of benign paroxysmal positional vertigo (see Table 3 for details). (Republished with permission from Brandt T, Daroff RB. Physical therapy for benign paroxysmal positional vertigo. Arch Otolaryngol 1980; 106:484.

BENIGN PAROXYSMAL POSITIONAL VERTIGO

Benign paroxysmal positional vertigo (BPPV) is the most common cause of vertigo in the elderly. The diagnosis is easily made if the patient has had a history of vertigo elicited by turning over in bed and if there is a typical nystagmus pattern that appears on positional testing. The cause is currently believed to be small bits of free debris that are loose in the labyrinthine system and which settle to the bottom of the ear, causing nystagmus for certain head positions. These patients are sometimes troubled by mild gait ataxia, but they are always most concerned by their inability to control vertigo that arises when they roll over in bed at night, or when they get up in the morning.

Drugs are not useful in treating BPPV because, although the vertigo is severe, it lasts only for a few seconds. There are two available approaches to treatment.

Most patients benefit from exercises for BPPV (see Table 3), which consist essentially of repeatedly inducing the symptoms of the vertigo for 2 weeks or until the symptoms can no longer be induced. This approach is often successful, presumably because either (1) the debris is moved to an insensitive portion of the labyrinth, (2) the patient learns to tolerate his symptoms, or (3) the disease process remits spontaneously. Because BPPV is fatigable, some patients induce their symptoms purposefully at the beginning of the day so that they can go about their activities without trouble. If the exercises provoke nausea, patients can be premedicated with antiemetics. If patients do not benefit from the exercises, the diagnosis should be reconsidered as central positional nystagmus can be mistaken for BPPV.

A second treatment option is to cut the nerve to the posterior semicircular canal—that is, to perform a singular neurectomy. This procedure should be considered only in patients who have been sympto-

TABLE 3 Vestibular Exercises

Gait-training exercises
- Begin walking with feet at a comfortable distance apart, progress to tandem position, eyes closed tandem, and head up tandem.
- Perform the above exercise while standing on a slab of foam rubber about 4 inches off the floor.
- Walk across the room with the eyes open and then with the eyes closed.
- Walk from heel to toe across the room with the eyes open and then with the eyes closed.

Visual-Vestibular exercises
- View a small target (about 2 in. × 2 in.) containing written material (e.g., a match cover). Fix the target to the wall or other solid object—do *not* use a hand held object. While trying to keep the words on the target in clear focus, move your head, first from side to side (approximately ± 45 degrees) and then up and down (approximately ± 30 degrees) at progressively higher speeds. The speed of the head movement should be increased until the words on the target can no longer be read.
- Perform the above exercise with a large-patterned target.
- Hold a small target or a patterned piece of cardboard at arm's length. While trying to keep the pattern or target in focus, move the head and target horizontally in opposite directions approximately 20 degrees to either side.
- Play any game involving simultaneous movement of the head and use of vision.

Exercises for BPPV
- Assume an upright sitting position in bed, with your legs on the floor (see Fig. 1). Close your eyes and suddenly tilt yourself to one side so that one side of your body is against the bed. Turn the head slightly upward and wait for the vertigo to subside. Sit back up and wait for 30 seconds before tilting to the opposite side. If vertigo occurs in this position as well, wait until it subsides and then sit up again. Perform this exercise five times in the morning and five times at night until 2 days have passed during which you do not experience vertigo.

matic for more than 2 years, in whom the side of lesion is certain, and who have not benefitted from the exercises. Most patients decide against neurectomy because of the risk of hearing impairment associated with this surgery.

MENIERE'S SYNDROME

The diagnosis of Meniere's disease should be considered in any patient who has both intermittent vertigo combined with a static or intermittent hearing deficit, or vertigo combined with an abnormal sensation in one ear. Meniere's syndrome is probable when a brisk spontaneous nystagmus is observed on at least one occasion, fluctuations in hearing can be documented on audiometry, and studies necessary to exclude structural lesions of the labyrinth have been performed.

Two levels of therapy may be considered. For patients who have infrequent episodes of vertigo, vestibular suppressants, possibly combined with an antiemetic, are used for the acute attack, and no medications are used in the interim. Oral meclizine and promethazine are the most useful agents for mild attacks. For patients with severe attacks who present in the emergency room, prochlorperazine (which can be given intramuscularly) and diazepam are the most useful agents. If patients appear dehydrated, they should be admitted to the hospital. Vestibular exercises are not used, as adaptations made during the period of transient vestibular imbalance are inappropriate when the patient has recovered. Over the long-term, salt restriction and use of a mild sodium-wasting diuretic such as hydrochlorothiazide may reduce the frequency of attacks.

For patients who are troubled by frequent attacks of vertigo and who have hearing loss confined to one ear, vestibular neurectomy or labyrinthectomy may be considered. These operations must be considered with caution, since many patients with Meniere's syndrome have bilateral disease; in such patients, surgery will be ineffective. Furthermore, even if patients have disease confined to one side at the time of treatment, they may develop Meniere's syndrome in the opposite ear in the future. Nevertheless, given the ineffectiveness of drug therapy, vestibular neurectomy or labyrinthectomy may be the only practical form of relief to offer.

OTOTOXICITY

Ototoxic antibiotics can cause oscillopsia, ataxia, and vertigo. Usually the diagnosis of ototoxicity can be made on the basis of the history alone; patients with this condition include those receiving peritoneal dialysis or those whose bone marrow transplant has recently become infected and who have begun receiving ototoxic antibiotics. After they recover from their infection and try to get out of bed, they discover their ataxia. On examination, these patients can read the vision chart with their head still, but drop two or more lines of acuity when their heads are gently oscillated.

These patients usually respond well to physical therapy. Several avenues of adaptation to their deficit are available. First, there is considerable plasticity of the vestibulo-ocular reflex, and by having the patient perform maneuvers that exaggerate the mismatch between their head movements and compensatory eye responses (i.e., activities that elicit oscillopsia), their symptoms may be diminished (see Table 3).

Cognitive strategies provide a second avenue of help. Patients can "spot" or fixate a reference traget before making a head movement, and use their intact visual pursuit mechanism to provide visual stability. Before walking across a room in the dark, patients should form a mental map of the room before turning out the lights.

It is also important to optimize nonvestibular methods of obtaining orientation information and to develop better motor programs for dealing with instability. Improving vision through wearing proper eyeglasses or through cataract removal if indicated, and the use of appropriate (low-heeled) shoes can be very useful. The gait-training exercises such as those outlined in Table 3 may be used. Of course, medications that are ototoxic or which suppress the vestibular system (such as those listed in Table 2) and their pharmacologic relatives should be avoided.

CENTRAL VERTIGO

Vertigo and disequilibrium occur in patients with lesions of the cerebellum or brainstem and particularly of the area of the vestibular nucleus and the floor of the 4th ventricle. The vestibular nucleus is a large structure that extends from pons to medulla. While patients with peripheral vestibular asymmetry typically recover within months, patients with central vertigo may continue to be distressed by ataxia, nausea, and illusions of motion for years. Presumably the persistence of their symptoms reflects a lesion in the central mechanisms that usually compensate for vestibular lesions.

Although vestibular suppressants such as meclizine or scopolamine are usually unsuccessful in the treatment of central vertigo, they are worth a try. Ativan (lorazepam) in a dose of 1 to 2 mg twice daily helps in some cases. Gait training and visual-vestibular exercises such as those outlined in Table

3 should be attempted. In patients with craniocervical junction abnormalities such as the Chiari malformation, a two-post cervical collar may be tried.

VERTIGO OF UNKNOWN ORIGIN

The last, most difficult to treat, and unfortunately, most common group of patients are those who experience vertigo for which we have no clue as to the origin. Some of these patients have psychogenic causes of vertigo, and others simply have disorders for which our diagnostic technology is not adequate. There are probably a large number of patients in the latter group; although there are three semicircular canals and two otolith organs on each side of the head, we have specific tests for the lateral semicircular canals only—we have no good way of assessing function of the vertical canals or of the otolith organs.

My approach to these patients is to manage them symptomatically and follow them at 3- or 6-month intervals. I refer patients disabled by their vertigo for vestibular physical therapy. Patients with intermittent symptoms are prescribed vestibular suppressants which they are to use only when symptomatic. All vestibular suppressants are discontinued in patients with chronic disequilibrium or vertigo.

I see these patients emergently when they are acutely dizzy, hoping to be able to establish the side of lesion through observation of a nystagmus or hearing loss. Often, a trial of salt restriction and diuretics is useful because it is generally impossible to exclude the possibility of Meniere's syndrome. In patients with frequent headaches, an attempt at migraine prophylaxis is worthwhile.

SUGGESTED READING

Baloh RW. Dizziness, hearing loss, and tinnitus: the essentials of neurotology. Philadelphia: F.A. Davis, 1984.

Brandt T, Daroff RB. Physical therapy for benign paroxysmal positional vertigo. Arch Otolaryngol 1980; 106:484.

Wood CD, Graybiel A. Evaluation of sixteen anti-motion-sickness drugs under controlled laboratory conditions. Aerospace Med 1968; 39:1342.

IDIOPATHIC AUTONOMIC INSUFFICIENCY

KENNETH MAREK, M.D.

Autonomic failure causes a wide spectrum of symptoms, including prominent abnormalitites in regulation of blood pressure, heart rate, sweating and temperature control, gastrointestinal, bladder, sexual, and pupillary function, lacrimation, and salivary glands. Orthostatic hypotension is the most disabling feature of autonomic insufficiency. In this chapter, a multimodal approach to the management of blood pressure control in patients with autonomic failure is outlined. The goals of therapy are practical: to improve the patient's ability to stand for longer periods and to prevent syncope. Appropriate therapy frequently requires a combination of nonpharmacologic and pharmacologic treatment.

Disorders of the autonomic nervous system may be classified as either neurologic or non-neurologic. Non-neurologic etiologies remain the most common cause of autonomic dysfunction and are often treatable. An initial approach to any patient with orthostatic hypotension should include a thorough evaluation to determine whether there is volume depletion, cardiac dysrhythmia, or endocrine disorder (pheochromacytoma, adrenal insufficiency), and whether the patient is using hypotensive drugs (tricyclic antidepressants, antihypertensives, antiparkinsonians, alcohol). The neurologic causes of autonomic insufficiency may be characterized as either primary (generally involving the central nervous system) or secondary (generally part of a peripheral neuropathy). Common causes of secondary autonomic insufficiency include diabetes, amyloid, Guillain-Barré syndrome, porphyria, and paraneoplastic syndromes. In patients with these conditions, autonomic dysfunction may be improved by treating the underlying disease process. Primary autonomic insufficiency is most commonly caused by multisystem atrophy (MSA) or idiopathic orthostatic hypotension (IOH). In this chapter, I concentrate on the treatment of primary autonomic failure, but much of the treatment approach may be used to manage autonomic dysfunction of any cause.

APPROACH TO THERAPY

The first step in the treatment of autonomic insufficiency is to identify those patients with autonomic failure. While this may seem obvious, during the early stage of the disease, patients often report vague and intermittent symptoms. Orthostatic signs must be measured and autonomic insufficiency may be further confirmed at the bedside by measuring variability in heart rate caused by respiration or that follows a Valsalva maneuver. The degree of orthostatic hypotension that may evoke symptoms depends on both the absolute blood pressure and the rate of change of blood pressure. Therefore the goal of blood pressure management must be individualized. Early in the management of this problem, the patient's family or a friend should be instructed to take blood pressure measurements at home. Again, blood pressure values should serve only as a guide to disease, while the most important measure of disease progression and therapeutic response remains severity of symptoms.

Patients with autonomic failure develop hypotension in response to several stimuli in addition to that of standing. They may be sensitive to heat, exercise, large meals, or otherwise innocuous pharmacologic agents. In addition, they may develop supine hypertension. The therapeutic approach to these patients is multifaceted. Therapy begins with practical recommendations and continues with pharmacologic intervention, if necessary.

Nonpharmacologic Therapy

The initial management of mild orthostatic hypotension is based on several simple practical measures designed to optimize patients' functional capacity. The primary goal is to maximize circulating blood volume. Patient education is an essential component of therapy. Clear, specific instructions should be given regarding diet, activity, pressure garments, and nonprescription medications.

Patients should be encouraged to maintain adequate hydration with increased fluid and liberal salt intake. Salt tablets may be used to provide the patient with 3 to 4 g of sodium each day. The patient should be cautioned concerning fluid overload and the possibility of supine hypertension. The patient should eat several small meals since large meals may rapidly worsen orthostatic hypotension since blood flow shifts to the splanchnic bed and vasodilator substances may be secreted. Activity should be restricted after large meals to lessen symptoms. Patients rapidly learn to avoid sudden changes in posture and to avoid prolonged standing. Hypotension also may be worsened by prolonged bedrest. Tilting the head of the bed with 4-inch blocks may lessen orthostatic symptoms on rising in the morning. Supine hypertension may also be managed by tilting the head of the bed, thereby using the patient's orthostasis to reduce blood pressure. An alternative commonly used by patients is to sleep in a recliner, either during the day or night. A moderate-graded exercise program may be beneficial. Swimming is the best tolerated exercise, but patients should never be left alone and may experience hypotension on leaving the water. These patients should also avoid excessive heat, which they tolerate very poorly since increased temperature causes vasodilation that may be complicated by anhidrosis.

Pressure garments are a useful but poorly tolerated adjunct to therapy in patients with autonomic insufficiency. Generally, custom-fitted elastic stockings, either thigh-high or to the umbilicus (like panty hose) must be used. The stockings increase central blood volume by preventing pooling of blood in the legs. These stockings should be removed at night and put on before the patient arises from bed in the morning. However, these garments are difficult to put on (generally requiring the help of a family member or caretaker), are very uncomfortable in hot weather, and are quite expensive.

Patients should be advised to avoid all medications except those prescribed by a physician familiar with their autonomic disorder. These patients frequently have very poor regulation of blood pressure so that otherwise innocuous drugs may cause marked hypotension. Over-the-counter preparations such as cold remedies, allergy pills, diet pills, or nasal sprays are often problematic. Alcohol, a potent vasodilator, generally worsens symptoms substantially. Caffeine may lessen orthostatic symptoms, perhaps by reducing adenosine-induced vasodilation.

Pharmacologic Therapy

In patients with more severe autonomic insufficiency unresponsive to the practical measures detailed above, a variety of medications have been used to treat hypotension. These drugs are listed in Table 1. Most of the agents increase blood pressure through an increase in intravascular volume or a relative stimulation of vasoconstriction. Often these drugs are used in combination to manage severe symptoms. Patients may respond to therapy with marked fluctuations in blood pressure so that all changes in medications must be monitored carefully.

Treatment is generally initiated with fludrocortisone (Florinef) at a dose of 0.1 mg daily slowly titrated to approximately 1 mg daily. Fludrocortisone increases vascular volume and enhances the response of blood vessels to vasoconstrictors. Supine hypertension is often a limiting side effect. Hypokalemia frequently occurs but is easily managed with potassium supplementation. If symptoms persist in patients receiving adequate fludrocortisone, the next step is to add either indomethacin (Indocin) (25 mg three times per day) or ibuprofen (up to 800 mg four times per day). These drugs may increase blood pressure by inhibiting the vasodilator effects of prostaglandins. If the combination of Florinef and Indocin/ibuprofen is ineffective, the Indocin or ibuprofen should be discontinued.

TABLE 1 Drugs Used to Treat Orthostatic Hypotension

Drug	*Dose*	*Comments*
Volume expanders		
Fludrocortisone	0.1–0.5 mg t.i.d.	Supine hypertension, hypokalemia
Adrenergic agents		
Receptor agonists		
Phenylpropanolamine	25–75 mg t.i.d.	Supine hypertension
Ephedrine	25–50 mg t.i.d.	Supine hypertension
Phenylephrine	2–4 sprays q4h	Use only in nasal spray form
Midodrine		Experimental agent
Clonidine	0.2–0.6 mg b.i.d.	May worsen hypotension
Receptor antagonists		
Propranolol	10–40 mg q.i.d.	Higher doses may worsen hypotension, useful for orthostatic tachycardia
Pindolol	2.5 mg t.i.d.	Mixed agonist-antagonist
Yohimbine	5–10 mg b.i.d.	Central presynaptic receptor action
Increase synthesis		
L-threo-DOPS	100–600 mg/day	Use in dopamine beta-hydroxylase deficiency
Increase release		
Tyramine		Only bulk powder available
Decrease catabolism		
Monoamine oxidase (tranylcypromine)	10 mg t.i.d.	Potential severe hypertension
Vasodilator inhibitors		
Prostaglandin inhibitors		
Indomethacin	25–50 mg q.i.d.	GI distress, ulcers
Ibuprofen	400–800 mg q.i.d.	GI distress
Caffeine	250 mg before meals	Use for postprandial hypotension
Metaclopramide	10–20 mg t.i.d.	Dopamine receptor antagonist
Miscellaneous		
Vasopressin (DDAVP)	2–4 μg IM qhs	Prevents nocturnal diuresis

The next strategy is to combine Florinef with a vasoconstrictor agent. The mechanisms of action of the vasoconstrictor drugs generally involve adrenergic stimulation of blood vessels either by direct release of norepinephrine, adrenergic receptor–mediated interactions, or inhibition of norepinephrine catabolism. The first approach is to combine Florinef with an alpha-adrenergic receptor agonist, either phenylpropanolamine (25 mg daily increased to 75 mg three times per day) or ephedrine (12.5 mg twice per day increased to 50 mg four times per day). Unfortunately these agents act for only a short period and may be poorly absorbed. Furthermore, small doses of alpha-agonists may precipitate marked hypertension possibly because of denervation supersensitivity in patients with postganglionic neuronal lesions. If treatment with alpha-agonists is ineffective, these drugs should be discontinued and an alternative receptor-active drug should be tried. However, treatment of hypotension with other adrenergic receptor-active drugs is complex and must be individualized. In some patients, either clonidine or yohimbine (an alpha-2-adrenergic receptor agonist and antagonist, respectively) may lessen hypotension. The paradox of two drugs with opposing actions that both improve hypotensive symptoms may be explained by a potential peripheral action of clonidine and a central action of yohimbine. Beta-adrenergic blockade may also be effective in some patients. Propranolol at low doses (10 to 40 mg twice per day) may improve hypotensive symptoms through predominant beta-2-adrenergic antagonism, but treatment is limited because at higher doses, the net effect of both beta-1- and beta-2-adrenergic antagonism may worsen hypotension. Specific beta-2-adrenergic antagonists currently being developed may prove more useful.

If vasoactive agents are ineffective, a number of other medications (listed in Table 1) that have been reported to improve hypotension may be used. Two additional agents should be mentioned. Caffeine (250 mg) may alleviate symptoms related to postprandial hypotension, but patients frequently develop tolerance to its effects. Vasopressin by nasal spray may be effective in reducing the nocturnal diuresis in these patients and thereby alleviate symptoms.

Special Therapeutic Considerations

Orthostatic hypotension may be caused by several syndromes. Ideally, as the mechanisms of these syndromes are elucidated, specific effective treatments may be developed. Current biochemical and physiologic evaluations of patients have already identified several subsets of patients who should be treated in a manner differing from the general guidelines outlined above.

A group of patients with primary orthostatic hypotension may be distinguished by their marked tachycardia associated with standing. This condition has been postulated to represent a relative preservation of beta-adrenergic versus alpha-adrenergic receptors. These patients should be treated with a combination of Florinef and propranolol.

Two additional unusual hypotensive syndromes should be mentioned. Hyperbradykininism is a familial disorder associated with elevated levels of the vasodilator bradykinin. This disorder has been responsive to treatment with propranolol. Recently a specific dopamine beta-hydroxylase (an enzyme necessary for the synthesis of norepinephrine) deficiency has been identified in some patients with severe orthostatic hypotension. These patients have responded to treatment with L-threo-DOPS, which increases norepinephrine.

GUIDELINES FOR MANAGEMENT

The treatment of autonomic insufficiency in general and of orthostatic hypotension in particular remains a difficult problem. However, a combination of practical measures and pharmacologic interventions may alleviate symptoms and enable patients to continue some normal activities. The goals of treatment are simply to increase the length of time a patient can remain standing, without the development of unacceptable side effects. An approach to management is outlined in Figure 1. The general guideline is that blood pressure should be approximately 80 to 100/60 to 70 when the patient is standing and 160 to 180/90 to 100 when the patient is supine.

Several principles of therapy should be emphasized. Therapy should be a multifaceted "stepped" approach beginning with nonpharmacologic recommendations and, if necessary, proceeding to the use of a medication or a combination of medications. Florinef remains the most useful drug in most cases. Other drugs should be used in conjunction with Florinef and discontinued if ineffective. Treatment must be individualized and the side effects of drugs carefully monitored. Patients with autonomic insufficiency are particularly susceptible to the potential side effects of these drugs on bowel and bladder control in addition to the common problem of supine hypertension. Treatment is designed to reduce symptoms, but current therapy is not likely to reverse progression of disease or to enable patients to return to their normal lifestyle. Many of these patients require extensive psychosocial support in dealing with this enigmatic but disabling disease process. Finally, the value of the physician's role in educating patients by explaining their bewildering array of symptoms cannot be overestimated.

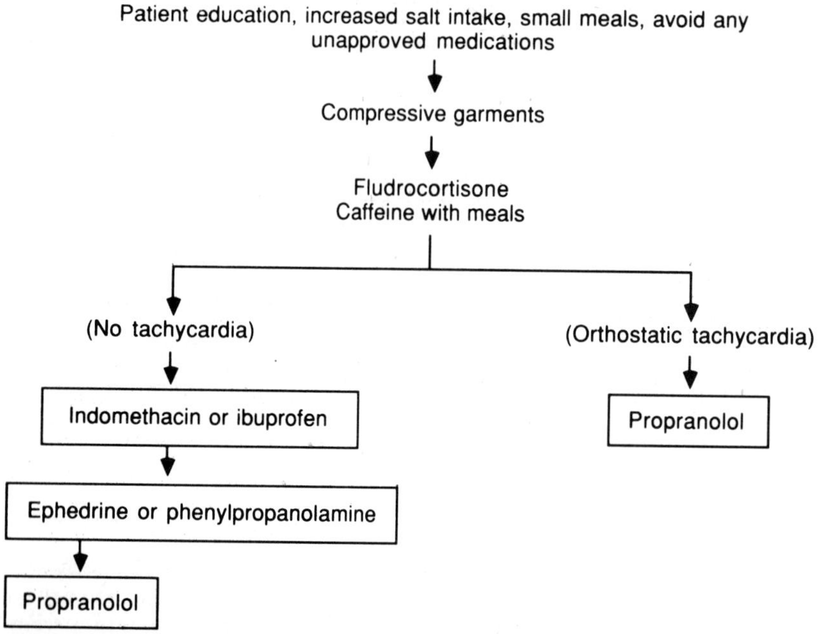

Figure 1 An ordered general strategy for the management of orthostatic hypotension. Management should be individualized to treat specific patient needs. Other drugs to treat orthostatic hypotension are listed in Table 1.

SUGGESTED READING

McLeod JG, Tuck RR. Disorders of the autonomic nervous system. Ann Neurol 1987; 21:519–529.

Onrot J, Goldberg MR, Holloster AS, et al. Management of chronic orthostatic hypotension. Am J Medicine 1986; 80:454–464.

Polinsky RJ, Kopin IJ, Ebert MH, Weise V. Pharmacologic distinction of different orthostatic hypotension syndromes. Neurology 1981; 31:1–7.

Schatz IJ. Orthostatic hypotension. Philadelphia: F.A. Davis Co., 1986.

PATIENT RESOURCE

Dysautonomia Foundation
270 Lexington Avenue
New York, New York 10017

FOCAL SEIZURE DISORDERS

THOMAS H. BURNSTINE, M.D.
RONALD P. LESSER, M.D.

Focal epileptic seizures originate in one or more discrete areas of the cerebral hemispheres. They are classified under the following headings: simple partial seizures, complex partial seizures, partial seizures with secondary generalization, and secondarily generalized seizures, which are generalized seizures of focal origin. Simple partial seizures do not impair consciousness; they consist of motor, sensory, autonomic, or psychic symptoms. Complex partial seizures do impair consciousness, although they may begin as simple partial seizures (e.g., an aura) consisting of any of the previously mentioned symptoms. Complex partial seizures may be accompanied by automatisms, which are complex motor activities occurring after consciousness is altered during the ictal or postictal phases of which the patient is amnestic. Whatever their manifestations, seizures that impair cognition or sensorimotor coordination often curtail educational, employment, and social opportunities. Therefore the goals of treatment should include eliminating as much seizure activity as possible and minimizing the disruption of the patient's personal life that epilepsy causes.

DIAGNOSIS

It is often difficult retrospectively to differentiate epileptic seizures from other paroxysmal events. For example, in the differential diagnosis of complex partial seizures, one takes into consideration almost any cause of alteration of consciousness, some of which may be nonepileptic disorders (Table 1), or other types of epilepsy such as petit mal seizures (i.e., absence seizures) (Table 2). Coexistence of more than one disorder is considered if more than one type of episode occurs. For instance, 10 to 20 percent of patients with psychogenic seizures also have epilepsy. However, when two diagnoses are suspected, each needs objective confirmation.

The clinical history is the most important initial diagnostic tool, since the physical examination usually is normal. The examiner should ask about the course of events during the seizure: the aura, the effect of the episode on consciousness, the duration of the episodes (including whether this duration was estimated or measured), and the number of different

TABLE 1 Nonepileptic Disorders That May Be Mistaken for Complex Partial Seizures

Syncope
Hyperventilation syndrome
Psychogenic seizures
Intoxications
Metabolic derangements/delirium
Migraine
Transient ischemic attacks
Sleep disorders

TABLE 2 A Comparison of Complex Partial Seizures and Absence Seizures

	Complex Partial Seizures	*Absence Seizures*
Aura	Usually	None
Duration	1–3 min	<30 sec
Automatisms	Often	Sometimes
Postictal phase	Usually	None
EEG findings	Focal epileptiform activity	Generalized 3/sec spike-and-slow wave complexes
Treatments	Carbamazepine Phenytoin Phenobarbital Primidone Valproic acid Clorazepate Resective surgery	Ethosuximide Valproic acid Clonazepam

types of episodes that occurred. Such subgroupings may indicate the site or sites of onset or the etiology of the seizures. One should then ask more specifically about motor activity, including focal clonic or tonic movements, or forced versive deviations; autonomic activity, such as diaphoresis, dyspnea, and palpitations; simple sensations of smell, taste, pain, abdominal discomfort or rising, and vertigo, tinnitus, or photopsias; more complex sensory perceptions, including well formed hallucinations; and psychic symptoms, such as emotional, language, and memory disturbances. Reserve questions about these phenomena until the end of the history to make the patient more comfortable with the history taking process and to obtain a spontaneous account unaffected by physician concerns. Also, some patients are reluctant to admit to having psychic and hallucinatory symptoms unless they are reassured that these experiences may be part of an epileptic seizure. One can then ask the patient or witnesses about occurrences that take place while the patient's awareness is decreased—e.g., facial expressions, repetitive or semipurposeful movements, altered speech, and the patient's reaction to being spoken to or touched. One should also assess the frequency of each seizure type, any cycling or clustering of seizures (e.g., during the perimenstrual period, ovulation, or pregnancy), and precipitating events, including stress and fatigue. Other clues to the etiology of the seizures may be in the history. One should ask about gestation and delivery, febrile seizures, head trauma, other central nervous system disorders, systemic illnesses, any medications that the patient is currently taking (including nonprescription preparations, alcohol, caffeine, and recreational drugs), sleeping habits, and a family history of seizures.

Ancillary tests may provide additional information. Since focal seizures arise from focal disease, computed axial tomography (CAT) studies or magnetic resonance imaging may show evidence of an underlying structural abnormality. Magnetic resonance imaging (MRI) may show small focal lesions or mesial temporal sclerosis not revealed by routine computed axial tomography. Occasionally, cardiac monitoring or echocardiography may be indicated if there is evidence for cardiogenic syncope.

The electroencephalogram (EEG) provides support for the diagnosis of epilepsy and aids in determining the appropriate anticonvulsant treatment, depending on the type of epileptiform discharges (focal onset versus primary generalized). Recordings should be obtained both while the patient is awake and asleep. The test may reveal epileptiform activity in either state, but sleep is often an activator of epileptiform discharges. An EEG obtained after a night of sleep deprivation also can increase the yield of epileptiform activity. Further abnormalities may occur with activation procedures such as hyperventilation and photic stimulation. These two techniques, useful for detecting generalized epileptiform activity, occasionally reveal focal epileptiform abnormalities as well. The yield also can be increased by adding extra electrodes: either over skin, especially over the temporal and orbito-frontal regions, or semiinvasively, using electrodes (sphenoidal, ethmoidal, and nasopharyngeal) which, again, record mainly from the anterior temporal or orbitofrontal regions. Only unequivocal spikes, polyspikes, sharp waves, and spike-and-slow-wave-complexes are indicative of epilepsy. Nonspecific abnormalities, such as focal or generalized slowing, may occur in patients with epilepsy, but also are seen in those with other conditions. Furthermore, several normal variants may be confused with epileptiform patterns: wicket spikes or rhythms; benign epileptiform transients of sleep or small sharp spikes; 14- and 6-Hz positive spikes; hyperventilation effects; hypnagogic and hypnopompic hypersynchrony; and slow wave transients of the elderly. Conversely, the EEG may be normal on repeated occasions in patients with epilepsy. In such cases, the diagnosis of epilepsy is not excluded by the normal EEG; additional recording, including prolonged monitoring, may be required.

TREATMENT

Once the diagnosis of a focal seizure disorder has been made, appropriate treatment is required. When prescribing antiepileptic medications, several principles should be considered:

1. Monotherapy is usually preferable to polypharmacy. Most patients with epilepsy can achieve seizure control through the use of a single anticonvulsant agent. Not only is monotherapy easier for the patient to use, there is a decreased risk of toxicity caused by drug-drug interactions: antiepileptic medications can potentiate each other's side effects and alter each other's serum concentration (Table 3).

2. In most cases, a single brand name antiepileptic drug should be used, since generic anticonvulsants are not necessarily bioequivalent, primarily because of differences in gastrointestinal absorption of the drugs. Therefore anticonvulsant levels may vary if the patient switches from one formulation to another. Also, differing preparations of the same brand may not have the same bioequivalency. For example, Dilantin capsules have a bioequivalency of approximately 90 percent, while Dilantin *tablets* have a bioequivalency of almost 100 percent. Therefore changing only the preparation, and not the dosage, of Dilantin could alter the amount of absorbed drug by 10 percent. Given the zero-order kinetics of phenytoin at higher blood levels, such an alteration

TABLE 3 Effect of Adding a Second Antiepileptic Drug on Serum Concentration of First Antiepileptic Drug

Initial Drug	*Second Drug*	*Effect of Second Drug on Serum Concentration of Initial Drug*
Carbamazepine	Phenobarbital	Decrease*
	Phenytoin	Decrease*
	Primidone	Decrease*
Phenobarbital	Carbamazepine	No change
	Phenytoin	Increase
	Valproic acid	Increase*
Phenytoin	Carbamazepine	Increase*
	Phenobarbital	Decrease, increase, or no change
	Primidone	No change
	Valproic acid	Decrease*
Primidone	Carbamazepine	Increased concentration of derived phenobarbital
	Phenytoin	Increased concentration of derived phenobarbital
	Valproic Acid	Increase
Valproic acid	Carbamazepine	Decrease*
	Phenobarbital	Decrease*
	Phenytoin	Decrease*
	Primidone	Decrease*

* Interactions particularly likely to be encountered in clinical practice. (Modified with permission from Brown TR, Feldman RG. Epilepsy: diagnosis and management. Boston: Little, Brown, and Co., 1983: 155.)

could lead to a significant change in the serum concentration of the drug.

3. The dosage of an anticonvulsant should be gradually increased to the point at which seizure control or toxicity is reached. If a patient does not achieve seizure control with the maximal tolerated dose of the initial medication, treatment with another anticonvulsant should be initiated. When the patient is taking an appropriate dose of the second drug, the initial drug may be gradually tapered and often may then be discontinued. Anticonvulsant medications should be tapered gradually because of the possibility of rebound seizures occurring during an abrupt withdrawal period.

4. If monotherapy with several first-line antiepileptic medications for partial seizures has been unsuccessful, polypharmacy becomes appropriate.

5. Serum concentrations of the antiepileptic medications should be obtained when a steady state has been achieved, which occurs after approximately five and a half serum half-lives. The so-called therapeutic ranges do not apply to all patients. Many patients need serum concentrations that are either below or above these ranges, depending on the clinical circumstances (i.e., the degree of clinical toxicity or seizure control).

6. When interpreting serum drug concentrations, one should consider the various factors that could affect the values obtained, such as (1) compliance, body weight, and age, (2) drug interactions, (3) systemic illnesses, (4) medication absorption, excretion, metabolism, protein binding, and serum half-life.

7. The total serum concentration represents the sum of the protein-bound and nonprotein-bound fractions. Excluding ethosuximide, all major anticonvulsants are partially protein bound, but only the nonprotein-bound (free) fraction penetrates the blood-brain barrier and exerts an anticonvulsant effect.

8. The free serum concentration may be altered by conditions affecting protein binding of the medication such as systemic illnesses (e.g., renal failure) and drug interactions. An example of the latter occurs when valproic acid is added to a phenytoin regimen. The free serum concentration of the phenytoin may rise since valproic acid is more tightly bound to serum proteins than phenytoin. Therefore the patients may have anticonvulsant toxicity because of an elevated free fraction while the total serum drug concentration is within or below the range usually employed.

Most antiepileptic medications cause similar signs and symptoms of neurologic dose-related toxicity. Higher cortical function and the vestibulocerebellar system are most commonly affected. If dose-related toxicity occurs, we try decreasing the dosage until the toxicity is no longer evident. We then gradually increase the dosage in small increments, using divided doses.

Certain anticonvulsants have nondosage-related hepatic and bone marrow toxicity. In patients using these agents, laboratory parameters such as the hepatic transaminases and complete blood counts should be monitored initially. Minor declines in values such as that of the white blood cell count should be expected. However, this decline should be maximal within the first few weeks of treatment, and partial recovery should occur by the end of the first few months. If there is a continuing trend of abnormalities in parameters such as the white blood cell count the responsible anticonvulsant drug should be discontinued and another one begun. Similarly, hepatic dysfunction usually occurs within the first few months of therapy. Again, the drug involved should be discontinued and another one begun. Of the first-line antiepileptic medications, carbamazepine is the one most often associated with bone marrow toxicity and valproic acid is the one most often associated with hepatic toxicity. However, fatalities from pancytopenia due to anticonvulsants, including carbamazepine, are extremely uncommon and do not constitute a contraindication to the use of carbamazepine in clinical practice. Rare cases of fatal hepatic necrosis have occurred, but almost all of these were in young children receiving polypharmaceutic therapy that included valproic acid. Therefore, valproic acid should be used with caution in young patients, especially those younger than 3 years of age.

Although antiepileptic medications have been associated with birth defects, much of the evidence is inconclusive. Valproic acid, however, has been associated with neural tube defects in as many as 1 percent of infants born to women who took this medication during the first trimester of pregnancy. Although the majority of infants born to such patients are normal, valproate is best avoided during pregnancy. Unfortunately, most women do not know that they are pregnant until after neural tube closure, which takes place at the end of the first month. Therefore, although most women taking valproate have offspring with no birth defects, whenever possible, substitution of another anticonvulsant for valproate should be considered if conception is likely.

The current consensus is that phenytoin and carbamazepine are the two best initial alternatives for the treatment of focal seizures, and some clinicians also report favorable results with valproic acid. Primidone and phenobarbital, although more sedating, may also be used. When monotherapy with these first-line antiepileptic drugs is unsuccessful, a second medication may be added. We usually prescribe either phenytoin or carbamazepine, depending on patient response, plus a second drug, usually valproic acid or clorazepate. It is generally better to administer two drugs with differing proposed mechanisms of action. However, there are occasional patients who respond best to combinations of medications with similar proposed mechanisms of action, such as the combination of phenytoin and carbamazepine. Other second-line anticonvulsants may be tried, but few patients respond well to them when the primary medications have been unsuccessful. These patients may be considered for enrollment in experimental drug protocols or for surgical therapy.

When treatment with antiepileptic drugs fails to control seizures or when the diagnosis is in doubt, the patient should undergo intensive monitoring that includes a video and EEG record of the patient over a period of hours or days. This may establish the diagnosis of epilepsy with certainty, determines the seizure type, and localizes the site or sites of epileptogenicity. Medication withdrawal initiated before admission or preferably on an inpatient basis is often necessary to increase the frequency of seizures. In addition, both sleep and sleep-deprivation studies are easily obtained during inpatient recordings. Also, using other electrodes in addition to the standard electrodes of the 10-20 system may increase the yield and improve the localization of epileptiform activity. Scalp electrodes may be placed between and below the standard electrode positions. Additional skin surface electrodes may be placed over the face and cheeks. Finally, nasopharyngeal, sphenoidal, and ethmoidal electrodes may be added.

Alternatively, 24-hour ambulatory outpatient EEG monitoring may be considered. However, while less expensive than inpatient monitoring, it has several disadvantages. No video record or precise second-by-second correlation of EEG and clinical events is obtained. The clinician must rely on the patient to keep a detailed diary of potentially ictal events for clinical-neurophysiologic correlations. There are typically only three to seven EEG channels, plus one often used for electrocardiography (ECG), limiting the amount of data that can be obtained and the precision with which epileptiform activity can be localized. However, one useful application of ambulatory EEG monitoring is as an event detector for the patient experiencing frequent episodes in a particular setting—for example, the patient's home or workplace.

Patients being considered for epilepsy surgery require an extensive preoperative evaluation, which begins with consistent localization of epileptic foci using prolonged video/surface EEG monitoring. If there is evidence of a potentially resectable epileptic focus and if the patient is willing to undergo a surgical procedure and understands the risks involved, further analysis is undertaken; this should include MRI of the head, neuropsychological testing, intracarotid sodium amobarbital (Wada) testing, and cerebral angiography in the context of the Wada testing. The neuropsychological and Wada tests are necessary to assess the integrity and lateralization of higher cortical functions such as memory and language. If the patient is a candidate for excisional epilepsy surgery, additional data obtained through the use of invasive (depth or subdural/epidural) electrodes may be required to delineate the epileptogenic region precisely.

Different types of invasive electrodes have somewhat different indications. If the issue is archicortical laterality, depth electrodes are usually employed since they can penetrate into the hippocampus or amygdala. These usually are excellent indicators of the side of seizure onset, but they provide limited sampling of the neocortex, and assessment of interictal epileptiform activity is difficult, in part because of the presence of normal variants that closely resemble seizure discharges. Alternatively, subdural strips or grids placed on the floor of the middle fossa can record similar information. When the laterality of a neocortical epileptogenic lesion is to be determined, either subdural/epidural or depth electrodes can be placed bilaterally to assess homologous areas of cortex. However, depth electrodes can record only from a few neocortical sites, and if more information beyond that of the laterality of a neocortical focus is required, subdural electrodes are preferable. Subdural grid, or strip, electrodes may aid in the planning of resective surgery by delineating the extent of epileptogenic cortex and by facilitating functional localization of primary speech, motor, and sensory regions.

The diagnosis and treatment of epilepsy often affects the lifestyle of the patient, many aspects of which must be discussed with the patient during the first visit. Patients should be cautioned to avoid situations that would be particularly dangerous to themselves or others if their consciousness or sensory-motor coordination should become impaired (e.g., operating a motor vehicle or machinery in certain working conditions). The laws pertaining to driving vary with each state and with the Interstate Commerce Commission. Physicians treating patients with epilepsy should be familiar with the regulations of the states in which they practice. Swimming and bathing should be discussed with the patient; because of the risk of drowning during an episode, others should be available to remove the patient from water if necessary, and showering may be preferable to taking a bath. One should inform the patient that his or her rights to employment and educational opportunities are not, in most cases, curtailed as a result of his disorder, and the patient should be counselled on how to minimize the disruption of their professional and personal lives that epilepsy causes.

The patient's family and/or friends need to be taught what to do when a seizure occurs. Patients often suffer oral injuries if a hard object, such as a spoon, is placed in their mouths during seizures in order to prevent the victims from "swallowing their tongues." Most non-health professionals need to be instructed to (1) remove the patient's eyeglasses, (2) remove furniture and potentially sharp objects from the immediate surrounding area, (3) loosen the patient's collar, (4) gently lay the patient on the side, if possible, and (5) place a pillow or rolled up jacket under the patient's head. The patient does not have to be taken to the emergency room unless the seizures are prolonged, repetitive, atypical, or of new onset.

Concerns about heredity should be dealt with. Many non-health professionals believe that all forms of epilepsy are primarily genetic in origin. It must be emphasized to the patients and their families that while there is strong evidence of a genetic component in certain types of primary generalized epilepsy, the vast majority of the children of epileptics do not have seizure disorders.

Aspects of reproduction that are affected by epilepsy and anticonvulsants also should be discussed. Patients using anticonvulsants need to be warned that the efficacy of birth control pills may be diminished, primarily because of the increased hepatic metabolism of hormones caused by many antiepileptic drugs. In practical terms, this means that low-dose formulations of birth control pills may become subtherapeutic. One should also stress the need for planning pregnancies, especially if the woman is taking valproate sodium, for the reasons stated earlier in this chapter. We warn patients that they may experience an increased frequency of seizures during pregnancy and caution them to monitor their serum medication concentrations closely. Although many women are worried about the possible deleterious effects of the anticonvulsant drugs on the fetus, they should be informed that most of the teratogenic effects have not been conclusively proven and occur in only a small minority of infants; seizure activity itself, because of either the hypoxia and acidosis of generalized tonic clonic seizures or the impaired motor coordination and consciousness of focal seizures, also poses a significant threat to the fetus. Finally, these risks appear to occur only when the mother (not the father) takes antiepileptic drugs.

SUGGESTED READING

Browne TR, Feldman RG. Epilepsy: diagnosis and management. Boston: Little, Brown and Co., 1983.

Dreifuss FE, Langer DH, Moline KA, Maxwell JE. Valproic acid hepatic fatalities. II. US experience since 1984. Neurology 1989; 39:201–207.

Engel J Jr. Surgical treatment of the epilepsies. New York: Raven Press, 1987.

Lesser RP. Psychogenic seizures. In: Pedley TA, Meldrum BS, eds. Recent advances in epilepsy–2. New York: Churchill Livingstone, 1985: 273.

Levy RH, Dreifuss FE, Mattson RH, et al. Antiepileptic drugs. 3rd ed. New York: Raven Press, 1989.

Lüders H, Lesser RP. Epilepsy: electroclinical syndromes. New York: Springer-Verlag, 1987.

PATIENT RESOURCE

Epilepsy Foundation of America
4351 Garden City Drive
Landover, Maryland 20785
Telephone: 1-800-332-1000

GENERALIZED SEIZURE DISORDERS

PETER W. KAPLAN, B.Sc. (Hons), M.D., M.B., B.S., M.R.C.P.

A generalized seizure is the clinical expression of a bihemispheric paroxysmal electrical disturbance that usually affects consciousness. Generalized seizures may present with different clinical signs, varying from a motionless stare to unresponsiveness accompanied by convulsions. Many brain functions including those subserving sensation, movement, speech, and awareness may be affected during the course of a seizure, although the patient is usually normal interictally. The term *epilepsy* is used to describe recurrent seizures resulting from persisting disease of the brain.

The seizure type and its frequency determine treatment and decisions regarding when and for how long medications should be given.

SEIZURE TYPES

Primary generalized nonconvulsive (absence), convulsive (tonic-clonic), and myoclonic epilepsies are probably largely genetically determined. Tonic, clonic, and atonic (astatic) seizures are frequently seen with diffuse cortical damage acquired during the perinatal and neonatal period (Table 1).

Clinical Manifestations of Epilepsy

In primary generalized epilepsy, the seizure discharges appear virtually synchronously over both hemispheres, in contrast to secondary generalized seizures, which begin in a localized area of the cortex. Although both types may present with tonic-clonic movements, primary generalized seizures are more frequently genetically determined or stem from a diffuse cortical insult. When a focal onset, whether sensory, autonomic, or motor, is determined or focal epileptiform activity is noted on the electroencephalogram (EEG), secondary generalized seizures should be suspected. A family history of seizures with no clinical focal onset or aura would suggest a primary generalized seizure disorder.

Even when a diagnosis of generalized seizures has been made (Table 2) and the patient has begun taking anticonvulsant medication, the seizures may continue. One may question then whether the correct diagnosis has been made. Psychogenic seizures may resemble tonic-clonic seizures and inpatient evaluation with video and EEG monitoring may be helpful in determining the nature, site, and frequency of the events so that appropriate management may be instituted.

Primary Generalized Tonic-Clonic (Grand Mal) Epilepsy

Primary generalized tonic-clonic seizures may appear at any age, although usually before the patient is 35 years old. No focal onset is noted. With

TABLE 1 Classification of Generalized Seizures (Bilaterally Symmetrical and Without Local Onset)

International Classification	*Previous Terminology*
Absence seizures	Petit mal seizures
Myoclonic seizures	Minor motor seizures
Clonic seizures	Grand mal seizures
Tonic seizures	Grand mal seizures
Tonic-clonic seizures	Grand mal seizures
Atonic seizures (astatic)	Akinetic, drop attacks

Adapted with permission from Commission on Classification and Terminology of the International League Against Epilepsy. Proposal for revised clinical and electroencephalographic classification of epileptic seizures. Epilepsia 1981; 22:489–501.

TABLE 2 Classification of the Generalized Epilepsy Syndromes

Idiopathic (age-related)
- Benign neonatal familial convulsions
- Benign neonatal convulsions
- West syndrome (idiopathic cases)
- Epilepsy with myoclonic-astatic seizures (Lennox-Gastaut syndrome)
- Childhood absence epilepsy (pyknolepsy)
- Epilepsy with (Myo)clonic absences
- Juvenile absence epilepsy
- Benign juvenile myoclonic epilepsy (impulsive petit mal)
- Epilepsy with generalized tonic-clonic seizures on awakening

Symptomatic
- Nonspecific etiology (age-related)
- Neonatal seizures
- Early myoclonic encephalopathy
- West syndrome (infantile spasms, Blitz-Nick-Salaam-Krampfe)

Special syndromes
- Occasional seizures
  - Febrile convulsions
  - Nonfebrile convulsions (in infancy or adolescence)
- Epilepsies characterized by specific modes of seizure precipitation
- Syndromes of chronic neuropsychologic suffering with status-like EEG activity
  - Syndromes of limited course
    - Epilepsy with continuous spike-waves during slow sleep

Adapted with permission from the Commission on Classification and Terminology of the International League Against Epilepsy. Proposal for classification of epilepsies and epileptic syndromes. Epilepsia 1985; 26:268–278.

the immediate generalization of the electrical discharge, the patient may cry out, roll the eyes upwards, and stiffen. There is an immediate loss of consciousness and frequently a fall to the ground with possible injury. An initial, predominantly symmetric, tonic contraction of musculature with cessation of breathing or forced expulsion of air with a "cry" is followed approximately one-half minute later by short, rapid, interrupted jerking movements of the limbs. This may be accompanied by foaming at the mouth and biting of the tongue. Urinary, and less frequently, fecal incontinence may follow the tonic or clonic phase. At the end of the clonic phase, limb contractions are less frequent, then cease and are followed by slow, labored breathing, lethargy, and amnesia. The patient may have a headache and sleep. The EEG, which is rarely obtained during the seizure, may show high-voltage, rapid, bilaterally synchronous spikes that decrease in frequency, stop, and are replaced by diffuse suppression of background activity.

Myoclonic Epilepsy

Seizures consist of brief, usually symmetric single or multiple jerks of the limbs or head. In the etiologically diverse progressive myoclonic epilepsies, the jerks are frequently stimulus-sensitive and may be induced by voluntary movements. They are associated with cognitive, cerebellar, and pyramidal tract abnormalities. More benign disorders, including essential myoclonus, tonic-clonic epilepsy with myoclonus (myoclonic epilepsy), and benign juvenile myoclonic epilepsy are not progressive. Myoclonic epilepsy may be photosensitive, with paroxysmal EEG abnormalities induced by photic stimulation. Essential myoclonus is usually not stimulus-sensitive and is not associated with convulsions or EEG abnormalities. The myoclonus may occur more frequently in the early morning and usually during wakefulness. Some patients have a family history of the disorder.

Clonic and Tonic Seizures

These seizures are rare and may represent a variation of generalized convulsive seizures, with one clinical characteristic predominating. Consciousness is usually lost during these seizures. In children, symmetric, bilateral tonic seizures frequently exhibit a slow hyperextension of the neck, torso, and legs with flexion of the arms. The EEG shows fast spikes at 9 to 10 Hz for both types. Clonic seizures may show spike-wave patterns.

Atonic Seizures

Atonic seizures are accompanied by a sudden loss of muscle tone with head or limb drop, frequently with falls to the ground and injury (drop attacks), and often a brief loss of consciousness. The EEG may show low-voltage fast activity, polyspikes, or voltage attenuation.

TREATMENT

General Management

Because of the frequent misperceptions regarding epilepsy, its causes, and its significance, it is essential to explain the nature of the disorder and lay to rest unwarranted feelings of guilt, inadequacy, and stigma (Table 3). The patient should be encouraged in every way to adapt to the disability and assume, as much as is possible, a normal life. General advice is aimed at regularizing the time and duration of sleep, as sleep deprivation may increase seizure tendency. Moderation in the use of alcohol and drugs with a central stimulant effect (amphetamines) or with possible epileptogenicity (antihistamines, tricyclic antidepressants, phenothiazines, theophylline) is also important (although when dosages are within the therapeutic range, these drugs may not significantly alter seizure threshold).

Adults, unless otherwise handicapped, should be able to maintain employment, although certain occupations involving heights, dangerous machinery, working near or in water, or driving must be carefully evaluated with respect to patient and public safety. Although there are risks to many facets of daily living, it is difficult to foresee them all. Moderate exercise does not increase seizure frequency.

Patients with severe disability, inadequately controlled convulsive seizures, or mental retardation may require supervised home care or institutionalization. Most communities have care centers or a local chapter of a group that provides help for people with epilepsy (see *Patient Resources* at the end of this chapter).

TABLE 3 Treatment of Epilepsy

1. Ascertain the diagnosis and type of seizure.
2. Discuss the diagnosis, implications, and therapeutic options with the patient or the patient's parent(s).
3. Based on the seizure type, select the most appropriate drug.
4. Increase the anticonvulsant dosage until seizures are controlled or until clinical toxicity appears.
5. If the anticonvulsant is ineffective at "toxic" levels, introduce a second anticonvulsant. When this drug produces a satisfactory blood level, gradually discontinue the first drug.
6. Monitor drug use frequently, as needed.
7. Provide information on local support groups, counseling, and educational materials.
8. After the patient has been without seizures for 2 to 5 years, consider tapering anticonvulsants.

In women with epilepsy, there is no formal contraindication to pregnancy, and although seizure control may vary during pregnancy, it usually can be adequately managed. All antiepileptic medications are thought to be potentially teratogenic during the first trimester of pregnancy, but valproate sodium and to a lesser extent phenytoin are most implicated. Neurotubular defects may be diagnosed antenatally with amniocentesis and measurement of alphafetoprotein levels. If at all possible, pregnancies should be planned and the physician alerted. Options for management without anticonvulsant medication or possibly with carbamazepine (which has a lower teratogenic potential) should be explored depending on seizure type and frequency. Although some epilepsies can carry a genetic component, it is not clear which pattern of inheritance predominates in a particular family. If inheritance can be assessed, this information may help prospective parents, but generally, a positive family history increases the risk two- to fourfold.

Management at Home

It is important that the family visit the physician to discuss the management of the patient at home. The family should be advised not to panic when a seizure occurs, but to turn the patient to the side or prone so as to avoid aspiration, and not to place any hard object or finger in the patient's mouth (the tongue cannot be "swallowed"). The family should also be asked to observe the seizure, as this may provide important information for determining the seizure type. They should seek acute medical attention if seizure activity continues for more than 10 minutes. In patients with known seizures and in the absence of fever and respiratory or cardiovascular problems, single or self-limited seizures probably do not warrant an emergency room evaluation.

Driving and Other Activities

The patient should be given specific advice regarding the driving laws in the state and a note should be placed in the patient's records to this effect. Most states prohibit individuals with generalized seizures from driving for periods of 3 to 24 months, depending on the locality, and some states require that all seizures be reported to the bureau of motor vehicles. All activities in which a momentary lapse of consciousness might endanger the patient or others, such as climbing, swimming, or working near moving machinery should be avoided if seizure control has not yet been achieved. Patients with nocturnal seizures only may be exempted from these restrictions.

Anticonvulsant Therapy

The Single Seizure

A single, idiopathic primary generalized tonic-clonic seizure does not necessarily imply a diagnosis of epilepsy or mandate chronic anticonvulsant therapy. Seizures associated with a precipitant cause (e.g., a toxic or metabolic disturbance) may be treated conservatively since the treatment of the underlying disturbance may suffice. When the patient has an "idiopathic" generalized convulsion, the decision to treat becomes more complex. About half of the patients in this group will have at least a second seizure. Those patients in whom further seizures pose significant social, employment, and driving problems might prefer the possible unpleasant side effects and bother of chronic medication. Conversely, some patients will wait until they have another seizure before deciding to take anticonvulsants. These concerns and treatment plans may vary from case to case and should be thoroughly discussed with the patient or the patient's family before planning therapy. Alcohol withdrawal seizures are difficult to manage, as frequently the patient discontinues both alcohol and anticonvulsants at the same time, thus precipitating seizures. In this group, resuming anticonvulsant therapy is often a futile experience.

Treatment of continued acute seizure activity is covered in the chapter *Focal Seizure Disorders.*

Recurrent Motor Seizures

The goal of therapy is to obtain optimal seizure control with the fewest medications and side effects. First-line therapy consists of the use of a single anticonvulsant (Table 4). Medication should be started at low doses and built up in gradual increments every 3 to 7 days. In order to reflect a steady state of the anticonvulsant, unless the patient is clinically toxic, serum anticonvulsant levels should be obtained no earlier than five drug half-lives after the full daily dose is reached or after changes in dosage have been made in order to reflect a steady state of the anticonvulsant. When either seizure control is reached or therapeutic levels are attained, I follow the patient monthly initially, and then at longer intervals while I monitor relevant hematologic or hepatic functions. Before considering changing to another single anticonvulsant or adding a second anticonvulsant, I gradually increase the dosage until "toxicity" appears (i.e., clinical side effects such as ataxia, somnolence, diplopia, marked malaise) or until seizure control is reached. The dosage, often above the therapeutic range, is then adjusted to be below the "toxic" dosage. Potential side effects should be fully explained, and the patient should

TABLE 4 Anticonvulsant Therapy for Seizures

Seizure Type	Drugs	Adult	Child	Usual Blood Levels*
Primary generalized tonic-clonic	Valproate sodium	1,000–3,000 mg	30–60 mg/kg	50–100 μg/ml
First-line therapy	Carbamazepine	600–2,000 mg	20–30 mg/kg	4–12 μg/ml
	Phenytoin	200–600 mg	4–7 mg/kg	10–25 μg/ml
Second-line therapy	Primidone	750–1,500 mg	10–25 mg/kg	6–12 μg/ml†
	Phenobarbital	90–250 mg	3–5 mg/kg	15–40 μg/ml
Myoclonic, atonic, tonic	Valproate sodium	1,000–3,000 mg	30–60 mg/kg	50–100 μg/ml
	Clonazepam	1.5–20 mg	0.01–0.2 mg/kg	0.013–0.072 μg/ml

* Higher levels are needed in some patients.
† With primidone monotherapy, primidone levels of approximately 20 μg/ml are frequently encountered.

understand that if skin rashes appear, the physician should be promptly notified.

If the initial anticonvulsant is unsatisfactory, the patient is prescribed a second anticonvulsant to be administered in a similar fashion, and the first agent is then discontinued. This may be repeated with three or four of the first-line agents before one progresses to multiple anticonvulsant therapy. During the overlap period, anticonvulsant drug interaction with resultant toxicity may develop and should be watched for.

First-Line Anticonvulsant Therapy

Valproic Acid (Depakene), Divalproex Sodium (Depakote)

Valproic acid is the drug of choice in patients with primary generalized tonic-clonic seizures, in patients with myoclonic seizures or seizures with a prominent myoclonic component. Depakote, somewhat more expensive, is believed to be better tolerated than Depakene, with less stomach upset. Depakote is available in 125-, 250-, and 500-mg tablets, and a common regimen is 250 to 500 mg taken orally two to four times per day. I start with 10 to 15 mg per kilogram per day and increase the dosage by 5 to 10 mg per kilogram per day at weekly intervals to a maximum dosage of 60 mg per kilogram per day, or 4,000 mg per day. The half-life is 8 to 12 hours, with peak blood levels reached within 1 to 4 hours after ingestion. A common goal is a level of 50 to 100 mg per liter, but higher levels are necessary in many patients. Common side effects include gastrointestinal upset, skin rashes, weight gain, ataxia, hyperactivity, drowsiness, tremor, headache, and hair loss. Serious side effects include liver failure, pancreatitis, and thrombocytopenia. Monitoring for marked changes in liver enzymes is important. When used as monotherapy in adults, fatal hepatic failure is virtually unknown.

Carbamazepine (Tegretol)

For cosmetic reasons, treatment with carbamazepine is preferable to that with phenytoin since gum hyperplasia (occurring in 10 to 30 percent of patients) is absent. Although more expensive than the nongeneric preparation, Tegretol avoids the wide spectrum of bioavailability and thus the problems of variable seizure control. An initial dosage of 100 to 200 mg administered once per day for 3 to 5 days, increased every 3 to 5 days to an initial plateau of 600 mg, may avoid some medication intolerance. The adult dosage may vary betwen 400 and 2,000 mg per day. The half-life is 10 to 25 hours, with the daily dosage divided into three to four doses. The therapeutic serum levels are approximately 4 to 12 mg per liter. Frequent side effects include fatigue, skin rashes, upset stomach, blurred and double vision, and ataxia as toxic levels are achieved. More serious side effects include the Stevens-Johnson syndrome, leukopenia, and thrombocytopenia, but a causal relationship to aplastic anemia is very rare.

Phenytoin (Dilantin)

Less expensive, but equally effective is Dilantin. Adult doses start at 100 mg administered once daily for 3 to 5 days, increasing gradually to an initial plateau of 300 mg per day. In urgent circumstances, an oral load of 1,000 mg may be given. The drug is absorbed within 4 to 8 hours and has a variable half-life of 7 to 42 hours (usually about 24 hours). Because it is protein-bound, low albumin levels may cause increased "free" levels and toxicity at lower dosages. The usual goal is to administer 10 to 20 mg per liter, but some patients may tolerate levels of 25 mg per liter or more without untoward effect. Although Dilantin is frequently administered three times daily, adequate control may sometimes be obtained with a once-daily regimen. Frequent side effects include coarsening of the facies caused by thickening of the subcutaneous tissue around the eyes and nose, facial and body hirsuties (occurring in 30 percent of young women), and gum hyperplasia (occurring in 30 percent of patients). Skin rashes (occurring in 2 to 10 percent of patients), stomach upset, mild drowsiness, and cognitive dysfunction are not unusual. Pseudolymphoma with arthralgia, fever, hepatosplenomegaly, and lymphadenopathy, as well as true lymphoma, have been described. Hepatitis, drug-induced lupus, peripheral neuropathy, folate deficiency, and osteoporosis are also seen. With 'toxic' levels, ataxia and behavioral disturbances may occur.

Second-Line Therapy

Primidone (Mysoline)

Primidone is less preferred as a first-line drug because of compliance problems caused by drowsiness and malaise, and less optimal seizure control. Advantages include a long half-life of the phenobarbital metabolite and low cost. After giving an initial test dose of 50 mg for hypersomnolence reaction, one should prescribe a dosage of 125 to 250 mg administered once daily, increasing this by 250 mg at 5- to 7-day intervals until a maximum of 1,500 mg, a therapeutic effect, or marked sedation is reached. The daily dosage is divided in two or three doses. These gradual increments are often necessary to avoid a marked sedative effect. Side effects include respiratory depression, confusion, behavioral and cognitive changes, and ataxia. Gastrointestinal upset and skin rashes may also be seen.

Phenobarbital

Phenobarbital is the least expensive of all anticonvulsants. Although it does not cause cosmetic side effects, it may cause behavioral problems, especially in children (it produces hyperactivity in 40 percent). With its prominent initial sedative effect and long half-life of 72 hours, it is best given once daily, at night. Peak blood levels are reached 10 to 12 hours after an oral dose with a therapeutic range of 15 to 40 mg per liter. I start with doses of 30 mg and increase these by 30 mg every 3 to 5 days until a total of 90 to 250 mg or 1 to 3 mg per kilogram per day is reached. Although excreted by the kidney, it is detoxified by the liver so that the dosage need only be slightly reduced in patients with renal insufficiency. These factors, as well as the interactions of phenobarbital with other medications and anticonvulsants, require that it be carefully monitored when changes in medication therapy are made. The side effects are much the same as those of primidone, although phenobarbital may be less sedating. Withdrawal of this anticonvulsant may be slow and problematic, as discussed later in this chapter.

Clonazepam (Klonopin)

This benzodiazepine is frequently used for myoclonic seizures. The serum half-life is 20 to 40 hours, with serum levels (5 to 70 ng per milliliter) correlating only approximately with clinical effectiveness. Side effects include drowsiness, dizziness, ataxia, personality changes, and drug tolerance. The drug is administered once daily, starting with a dosage of 0.01 to 0.03 mg per kilogram per day, which is then increased by 0.5 mg every 3 to 7 days to a maximum dosage of 0.1 to 0.2 mg per kilogram per day or 20 mg per day. Occasional exacerbation of other seizure types has been noted.

Interactions

All of the anticonvulsants may have interactions with each other and other intercurrent medications. (For interactions between anticonvulsants and other drugs, see 1989 edition of *The Medical Letter Handbook on Drugs and Therapeutics.*)

Polypharmacy and Patients Who Are Difficult to Control

The most common cause of poor control is noncompliance. For patients with poor compliance, written schedules, diaries, and plastic, compartmentalized daily pill boxes (available at most pharmacies) are helpful. Compliance may be assessed from the history, the testimony of witnesses of the seizures, blood levels, and by counting the number of tablets that the patient has not taken. Fine tuning of the daily dosage, readjustment of the frequency, the timing of intake, and attempts at producing drug levels above the laboratory "therapeutic" level but below clinical toxicity may be necessary. After most medication readjustments, repeated blood therapeutic monitoring is needed at five to eight half-lives after the time of medication change. Careful follow-up of patients receiving high doses is required.

When seizures are frequent while the patient is receiving the highest tolerated dose of a single anticonvulsant (and after each first-line anticonvulsant has been tried), a second agent may be added. Adding one of the first-line drugs is preferred, although primidone or phenobarbital may be satisfactory. However, problems with concurrent use of two first-line drugs may lead to more severe side effects. For example, when taken together, phenytoin and carbamazepine may lead to marked ataxia. Combining phenobarbital and primidone contribute little actual or theoretical improvement in seizure control and sedation may be further increased. The best combinations may prove to be medications with different mechanisms of action, such as valproate sodium and either phenytoin or carbamazepine. Interactions between the two anticonvulsants and other drugs may greatly alter blood levels, and frequent monitoring may be necessary since anticonvulsant levels may rise or fall. For example, if valproic acid is added to the regimen of a patient receiving phenobarbital, central nervous system depression caused by a rise in phenobarbital levels may result. Some combinations, such as that of valproic acid and clonazepam, may produce absence status epilepticus and therefore should be avoided. Patients should continue to take two anticonvulsants only if attempts to gradually wean the patient from one of the drugs leads to breakthrough seizures. In "brittle" (poorly controlled) patients, drug change-overs may necessitate hospitalization or intravenous loading of anticonvulsants. Most patients with primary generalized seizures are responsive to treatment with anticonvulsants, and epilepsy surgery is rarely helpful. If patients do not respond to anticonvulsants, the diagnosis should be re-examined for the possibility of secondary generalization, as poorly controlled seizures in patients with secondary generalization may make them eventual candidates for epilepsy surgery.

For clinic evaluation, a "seizure diary" is of great help in determining the frequency and type of seizures. If doubt persists, prolonged inpatient video and EEG monitoring or ambulatory monitoring helps determine the frequency, timing, and types of seizures, and helps distinguish these from other paroxysmal events such as syncope, panic attacks, or even pseudoseizures.

Anticonvulsant Withdrawal

After the patient has been without seizures for 2 to 5 years, I consider withdrawal of the single anticonvulsant. In patients who are seizure-free while receiving two anticonvulsants, one may attempt withdrawal of one of the anticonvulsants after 6 to 12 months. Even if the patient is seizure-free, however, caution should be exercised. Should seizures recur, medication should be resumed. The patient should be discouraged from driving an automobile during the months of anticonvulsant withdrawal. It is believed that epileptic discharges on a EEG obtained before withdrawal might herald an unfavorable outcome, but this is disputed. Although the seizure-free period is a good predictor of possible successful anticonvulsant withdrawal, previous unsuccessful attempts at withdrawal forebode a poor result. Rapid withdrawal of benzodiazepines or barbiturates may precipitate seizures even in a normal population and therefore should be withdrawn gradually. In the withdrawal of anticonvulsant medications such as phenytoin or carbamazepine, a common practice is to taper medications gradually, one at a time; however, there is little evidence to suggest that this forestalls withdrawal seizures. After initially reducing the dosage by one-third, one may decrease the phenobarbital dosage by 15 mg every 2 weeks in the most "brittle" patient. Sleep disturbances such as insomnia and anxiety are frequently encountered, especially in long-time users of anticonvulsants, and these problems should be anticipated and explained so that the patient can see the long-term benefit of an unpleasant withdrawal phase.

SUGGESTED READING

Drugs for epilepsy. Med Lett 1989; 31:1.

Fromm GH, Fisher RS, Dasheiff R, Hachinski V (discussants). Controversies in neurology: first seizure management reconsidered. Arch Neurol 1987; 44:1189–1191.

Laidlaw J, Richens A. A textbook of epilepsy. New York: Churchill Livingstone, 1982.

Ojemann LM, Baugh-Bookman C, Dudley DL. Effect of psychotropic medications on seizure control in patients with epilepsy. Neurology 1987; 37:1525–1527.

Solomon GE, Plum F. Clinical management of seizures: a guide for the physician. Philadelphia: WB Saunders, 1976.

PATIENT RESOURCES

Epilepsy Foundation of America
4351 Garden City Drive
Suite 406
Landover, Maryland 20785

Epilepsy International
Las Palmas C-160
2855 Apalachee Parkway
Tallahassee, Florida 32301

STATUS EPILEPTICUS

ROBERT J. DeLORENZO, M.D., Ph.D., M.P.H.

The International Classification of Epileptic Seizures defines status epilepticus as a seizure lasting for more than 30 minutes or intermittent seizures lasting for more than 30 minutes from which the patient does not regain consciousness. Thus, any seizure that lasts for more than 30 minutes must be diagnosed as status epilepticus. The first step in treating status epilepticus is making the diagnosis.

Many physicians are not sensitive to the importance of diagnosing this condition and making appropriate treatment initiations to avoid complications. Great care should be taken in determining the duration of any prolonged seizure; this as well as the time of seizure onset should be ascertained from ambulance drivers or emergency room staff. The importance of this in determining the diagnosis cannot be overemphasized.

Persistent generalized tonic-clonic seizures are the most common form of status epilepticus and are associated with the major risks of morbidity and mortality caused by this condition, and therefore this chapter focuses on the treatment of generalized tonic-clonic status epilepticus.

MORTALITY ASSOCIATED WITH STATUS EPILEPTICUS

One major reason for promptly diagnosing status epilepticus is that this condition is associated with high morbidity and mortality rates. Studies over the last 20 years involving more than 100 patients indicate that the mortality rate of status epilepticus ranges from 8 to 50 percent. Even a mortality rate as low as 8 to 10 percent is a significant risk.

Status epilepticus must be considered a major medical and neurologic emergency. In our experience at the Medical College of Virginia Epilepsy Research Center, where a large community and university–based study of status epilepticus is being conducted, we find that the mortality rate associated with status epilepticus in the community study parallels that of the university study. Thus, the high mortality rate associated with status epilepticus noted in previous university studies has recently been confirmed by our findings in a community-university environment.

Although our recent investigations indicate statistically valid correlations among seizure duration, etiology, and mortality, it is still too soon to base clinical decisions of treatment on these indicators. We are currently developing and testing a mortality relative risk scale and hope that this scale may lead to the identification of high-risk patients.

Once I have determined that the patient has prolonged seizures lasting more than 30 minutes and make the diagnosis of status epilepticus, I become concerned. Since these are patients at risk for death or developing serious complications, there is no room for missing this diagnosis or for not treating these patients aggressively.

CAUSES OF STATUS EPILEPTICUS

Once a diagnosis of status epilepticus has been made, the clinician must immediately consider the possible cause of the prolonged seizures. Treatment of status epilepticus, although directed at the control of seizures, must also take into account the underlying cause since these conditions often require aggressive treatment. Figure 1 presents the breakdown of etiologies of 280 cases of the Medical College of Virginia (MCV) series. These etiologies are typical of several other large studies.

The causes of status epilepticus shown in Figure 1 have been broken down into ten major etiologic subgroups: (1) withdrawal from anticonvulsants, (2) anoxia, (3) hypotension, (4) alcohol-related status, (5) metabolic, (6) infectious, (7) cerebrovascular disease, (8) tumor, (9) hemorrhage, (10) other causes. As can be seen from Figure 1, the three major etiologies associated with status epilepticus are cerebrovascular disease, alcohol-related causes, and withdrawal from anticonvulsants. Each of these

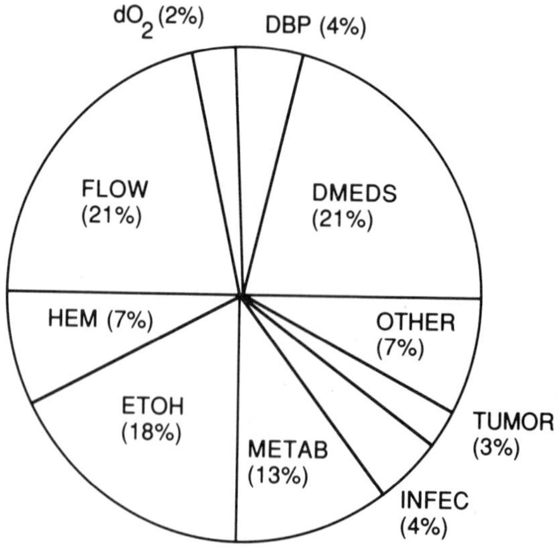

Figure 1 Etiologies of status epilepticus (percentage of patients). DMEDS = withdrawal from anticonvulsants; dO_2 = anoxia; DBP = hypotension; ETOH = alcohol-related causes; METAB = metabolic; INFEC = infectious; FLOW = cerebrovascular disease; HEM = hemorrhage.

categories represents one-fifth to one-fourth of the patients seen in most large series. Another major cause, representing anywhere from 10 to 15 percent of the cases, is metabolic disease.

Not all patients with status epilepticus have had previous seizures. Only about one-fifth of the patients who develop status epilepticus have a history of epilepsy. Many of the other causes of status epilepticus are of rather serious consequence, including central nervous system infection, vascular injury, tumor, and severe metabolic disease. Thus anytime a patient presents with status epilepticus, one should be greatly concerned because of the seriousness of the seizures and many of the underlying etiologies.

TREATMENT

Although it would be ideal to have a rigid protocol for the treatment of status epilepticus, this is not always possible because of the clinical variability in the presentation of status epilepticus, the patient's condition, and the possible idiosyncratic reactions to certain anticonvulsant drugs. Despite this inherent variability, we have developed a standard treatment plan for patients treated in the Greater Richmond Metropolitan area which includes care at the MCV Hospital Complex and surrounding community hospitals.

The protocol for treating adults with generalized tonic-clonic status epilepticus is based on years of clinical experience in treating this condition by physicians of the MCV Hospital and the surrounding community and on the protocols from other successful treatment plans. Thus by synthesizing the experience from our own patient population and that of the literature, we have developed a unified treatment plan that has been tested and utilized in both the MCV and community hospital. This standard recommended treatment protocol is summarized in Table 1.

The Diagnosis

As discussed earlier, the first major step in treating status epilepticus is to make the diagnosis. The most common error in missing the diagnosis is not obtaining a clear and detailed history of the duration of the seizures. Often the physician arrives in the emergency room or to the floor after the patient has been stabilized by the emergency room staff; the patient may have been undergoing a seizure for 20 to 30 minutes en route to the hospital and for another 20 to 30 minutes in the emergency room, but by the time the physician arrives, the seizures have been controlled with intravenous (IV) diazepam or phenytoin and the diagnosis of status epilepticus may not be made. Great care should be taken to avoid making this error.

Stabilizing the Patient

The second major treatment step is to stabilize the patient medically and to establish an IV line. Since a significant percentage of the causes of status epilepticus also produce severe cardiovascular and autonomic changes, it is essential that the patient's vital signs and medical condition be stabilized and the diagnosis or cause of status epilepticus be determined (see Table 1).

The IV line is ordinarily supported with normal saline containing vitamin B complex supplement. The only contraindication for the use of normal saline is a hypertensive patient or a patient requiring salt or fluid restriction. However, even in these situations, it is important to have a normal saline line piggybacked into the IV system so that phenytoin can be given with the normal saline in small volumes as needed. The MCV protocol recommends administration of a bolus of 50 ml of 50 percent glucose at this time. This is a routine emergency procedure. Once the line is obtained, the medical treatment of status epilepticus begins.

Figure 2, a decision tree for the initial treatment and stabilization of the patient, shows the basis for our diagnostic studies and hospitalized care. Most patients with status epilepticus arrive in the emergency room or present in the inpatient setting. After the stabilization of the patient, it is essential to obtain neurologic consultation whenever possible. The electroencephalogram (EEG) and computed tomography (CT) scan are invaluable in helping determine the etiology. Lumbar puncture (LP) is recommended for all status epilepticus patients if the CT scan and physical examination show no evidence of a mass lesion or other contraindications to performing the LP. If the patient stabilizes rapidly and regains consciousness during the diagnostic evaluation, admission to the neurology inpatient unit is recommended with good nursing care. If the patient does not regain consciousness or is medically unstable, admission to a neurological service intensive care unit (NSICU) is advisable. Careful observation and records of vital signs and the EEG are valuable in providing responsive care to these patients.

Anticonvulsants

The first anticonvulsant usually employed in the ambulance or emergency room setting is the IV injection of diazepam, administered at a rate not to exceed 2 mg/per minute until the seizures stop or a total of 20 mg has been given. The majority of our patients have received diazepam as the initial drug in this fashion. However, an alternative initial anticonvulsant that appears to be equally effective is lorazepam. Lorazepam is administered at a rate of 2 mg per minute (0.1 mg per kilogram) and repeated at 10- to 15- minute intervals if seizures persist. Experi-

TABLE 1 Status Epilepticus Treatment Protocol for Adults

Step	*Time Frame of Intervention*	*Procedure*
1	0–5 min	Determination of status epilepticus. As soon as the diagnosis is made, institute monitoring of blood pressure, temperature, pulse, respiratory ECG and EEG. Insert oral airway and administer 0_2 if necessary. Insert an IV catheter and draw venous blood for levels of anticonvulsant, glucose, electrolytes, Ca, Mg, BUN, CBC. Draw arterial blood for ABG. Obtain urine for urinalysis and toxic screen if indicated. If necessary, nasotracheal suction is performed.
2	6–9 min	Place an IV line with normal saline containing vitamin B complex. Administer a bolus of 50 ml of 50% glucose.
3	10–30 min	Infuse IV lorazepam given at a rate of 2 mg/min (0.1 mg/kg) to a maximum dose of 5 mg or alternatively administer IV diazepam given at a rate not to exceed 2 mg/min until seizures stop or to a total of 20 mg. This is followed by IV phenytoin, 20 mg/kg at a rate no faster than 50 mg/min. If seizures are not controlled, a repeat bolus of phenytoin of 10 mg/kg can be given before one proceeds to Step 4. Monitor ECG and blood pressure.
4	31–59 min	If seizures persist, perform elective endotracheal intubation before starting a bolus infusion of phenobarbital at a rate not to exceed 100 mg/min until seizures stop or to a loading dose of 20 mg/ng.
5	60 min	If control is still not achieved, other options include: 1) Pentobarbital with an initial IV loading dose of 5–10 mg/kg with additional amounts given to produce a "burst suppression" pattern on EEG. Maintenance of pentobarbital anesthesia is continued for approximately 4 hours by an infusion of 1–3 mg/kg/hr. The patients are then checked for the reappearance of seizure activity by decreasing the infusion rate. If clinical seizures and/or generalized EEG discharges persist, the procedure is repeated; if not, the pentobarbital is tapered over 12–24 hrs. 2) Paraldehyde is given either intravenously or rectally at a dose of 0.1–0.15 ml/kg after being diluted in normal saline every 2 to 4 hours if necessary. 3) Diazepam (50–100 mg) is diluted in a solution of 500 ml 0.9% NaCl or D_5W and run as a continuous infusion to achieve blood levels of 0.2–0.8 mg/ml. The IV solution is changed every 6 hours as advised by certain authors and short-length IV tubing is used.
6	61–80 min	If seizures are still not controlled, call the anesthesia department to begin general anesthesia with halothane and neuromuscular blockade.

Continuous EEG monitoring is recommended in the obtunded patient to assure that status elipticus has not recurred. In the management of intractable status, a neurologist who has expertise in status elipticus should be consulted and advice from a regional epilepsy center should be sought.

ence with lorazepam is not as extensive as with diazepam. A potential advantage of lorazepam is that it may have a more long-lasting effect. However, there must be more widespread experience with this drug before its relative benefits compared with those of diazepam can be established.

Immediately after the completion of benzodiazepine treatment, the next step is to provide a major anticonvulsant therapy. Diazepam, although having a long half-life in the body, is only effective in treating status epilepticus for approximately 30 minutes, during which time it reaches its peak blood level after the IV injection. Immediately after this peak blood level has been reached, diazepam is distributed in the fat of the body and its level comes down to a baseline level. As the diazepam level rapidly decreases, it is no longer effective as an anticonvulsant in controlling status epilepticus. A small percentage of patients taking diazepam or lorazepam will stop having seizures. However, the majority of patients require further anticonvulsant treatment before seizures are arrested. In those patients with seizures that stop rapidly with benzodiazepine treatment, an alternative anticonvulsant is still initiated to maintain the anticonvulsant effect. Thus the alternative anticonvulsant must be initiated before the anticonvulsant effects of diazepam subside, usually 20 to 30 minutes after injection.

The anticonvulsant of first choice is phenytoin. In a dose of 18 mg per kilogram, it is administered at a rate not to exceed 50 mg per minute. A significant percentage of patients will stop having seizures after benzodiazapine and phenytoin treatment. Phenytoin has been shown to be as effective as any other anticonvulsant in controlling status epilepticus. In addition, phenytoin is relatively nonsedative in the doses used to treat status epilepticus. Thus the patient who

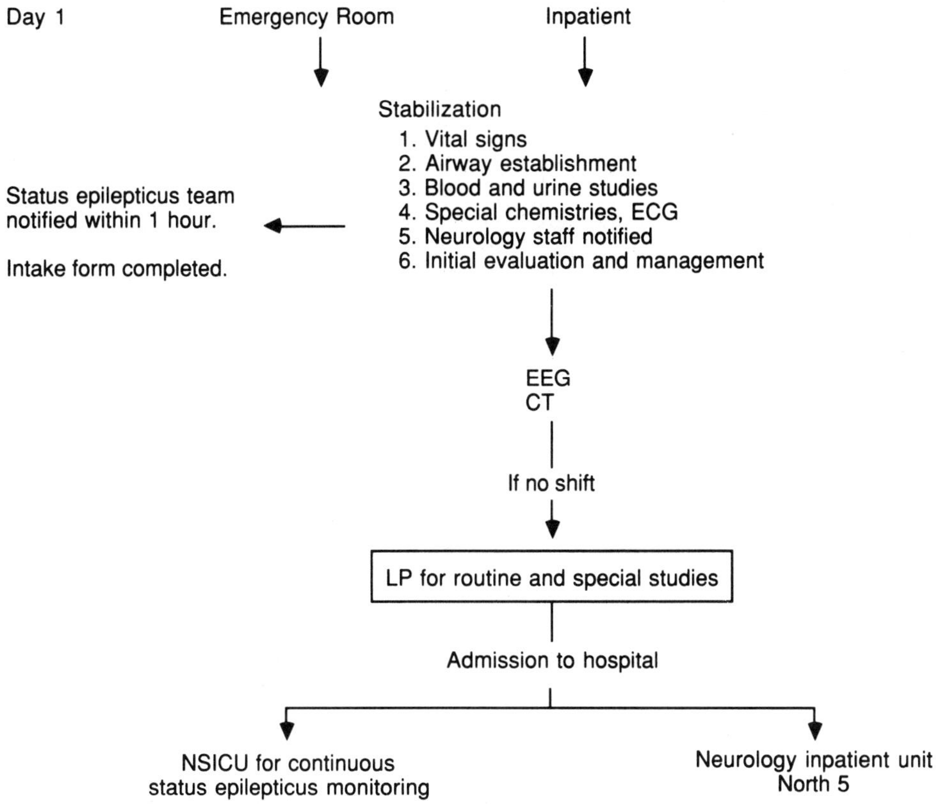

Figure 2 Flow chart for status epilepticus patients admitted to the Medical College of Virginia Hospital Complex.

is postictal will usually wake up after seizures depending upon the duration of the postictal coma. The lack of sedation caused by the phenytoin is a major advantage in patient care. Some patients successfully treated with diazepam and phenytoin will awaken within an hour or so after status epilepticus. Some patients may even wake up in the emergency room after status epilepticus.

Some disadvantages of employing phenytoin must also be addressed. Phenytoin is not soluble in 5 percent dextrose in water (D_5W) or other types of IV solutions that do not have a significant amount of normal saline. Normal saline is the preferred vehicle for IV infusion of phenytoin. If D_5W is used as the vehicle to infuse phenytoin, phenytoin crystals will immediately develop in the IV line as the phenytoin is injected. If one uses the recommended rate of injection, these crystals will form as the drug is administered and the clinician may not be able to see this in the IV line. In addition, mixing phenytoin with D_5W in a dripping reservoir will result in the patient receiving no drug at all since all of the phenytoin will precipitate out of the solution. When phenytoin comes out of solution during the injection, it has no significant anticonvulsant action.

It is essential that the clinician use the appropriate vehicle for IV phenytoin usage. If the patient cannot be administered saline because he requires salt restriction, D_5W can be run as the main IV line and normal saline solution can then be piggybacked into the system and opened into the system only when phenytoin is injected. After a limited injection of saline has been administered, the patient can be switched back to the appropriate IV treatment.

Care must be exercised in giving phenytoin to a patient who has epilepsy and may already have a therapeutic phenytoin blood level. Although this is an uncommon situation, it should be considered, since it can result in a high phenytoin blood level that in rare situations can cause cerebellar toxicity.

Another potential risk of phenytoin usage is hypotension and decreased cardiac output. In most normal healthy individuals, these side effects are not significant and are rarely of any consequence when the recommended dosage and rate of administration of phenytoin are used. However, more rapid rates of phenytoin administration can result in significant hypotension. In elderly patients with compromised cardiovascular status, phenytoin may produce hypotension and cerebrovascular collapse. Thus during phenytoin administration, electrocardiogram (ECG) or blood pressure monitoring is recommended, especially in the elderly patient.

Our protocol recommends that if a seizure persists after phenytoin infusion, elective endotracheal intubation be initiated before one starts a bolus infusion of phenobarbital. Phenobarbital is administered as a second anticonvulsant at a rate not to exceed 100 mg per minute until the seizures stop or until a loading dose of 20 mg per kilogram is reached.

Phenobarbital is an effective anticonvulsant in the treatment of status epilepticus. Before it was realized that phenytoin could be given rapidly through IV infusion, phenobarbital was widely used as the initial drug. Phenobarbital is effective and relatively safe in treating patients with status epilepticus. However, phenobarbital has a major side effect in that it is sedative and causes respiratory suppression. Most patients given a loading dose of 20 mg per kilogram of phenobarbital will be sedated for at least 24 hours. Thus this raises the difficulty of having to wait until the patient fully recovers from sedation before evaluation can begin. For this reason, phenobarbital is usually not given as the first major anticonvulsant and is a second-line agent after treatment with phenytoin.

Seizures Resistant to Treatment

In the more unlikely situation that seizure control is not achieved after benzodiazepine, phenytoin, and phenobarbital treatment, further anticonvulsant administration must be considered. At this time, either paraldehyde or a diazepam drip is used. Paraldehyde is preferably given rectally at a dose of 0.1 to 0.15 mg per kilogram after being mixed one-to-one with mineral oil. Paraldehyde can be conveniently mixed one-to-one part with mineral oil in a suspension and administered per rectum through a Foley catheter. The catheter is lubricated and carefully inserted into the rectum, and the catheter balloon is inflated. The paraldehyde and mineral oil mixture can be easily injected through the catheter. The catheter is then clamped. The paraldehyde is rapidly absorbed through the rectal route. Plastic containers should not be used for paraldehyde. Many forms of plastic are dissolved by this drug. Most IV tubing and Foley catheters are not soluble in paraldehyde.

The use of per rectal paraldehyde is also useful if an IV line cannot be placed. In the rare situation that an IV line cannot be started and benzodiazepine or phenytoin cannot be initially administered, per rectal paraldehyde is often the route of choice for obtaining initial control of status epilepticus. Paraldehyde can also be administered intravenously, but this is less desirable because of the potential complications. Unfortunately, it is becoming more difficult to obtain paraldehyde for patient use. This is a major obstacle for this useful treatment option.

If paraldehyde is not successful or if one prefers to use a diazepam drip initially, diazepam can be used again. Diazepam, 50 to 100 mg, is diluted in a solution of 500 ml of 0.9 percent sodium chloride or D_5W and run as a continuous infusion to achieve blood levels of 0.2 to 0.8 mg per milliliter. The use of diazepam has significant problems. For example, diazepam can come out of solution over time because it is not highly water soluble. Therefore the IV solution should be changed every 6 hours and short runs of IV tubing should be used. One must also be careful to control the continuous IV solution to avoid overdoses and rapid infusion rates. This procedure must be monitored in the intensive care unit setting so that overtreatment and resultant respiratory arrest do not occur.

In the rare patients in whom seizures are not controlled with this treatment protocol, a pentobarbital anesthetic is used with an initial IV loading dose of 5 mg per kilogram with additional amounts administered to produce a "burst suppression" pattern on the EEG. Maintenance of pentobarbital anesthesia is continued for approximately 4 hours by infusion of 1 to 3 mg per kilogram per hour. After this interval, the patient is checked for reappearance of seizure activity by decreasing the infusion rate. If clinical seizures and/or generalized EEG discharges persist, the procedure is repeated. If there are no repeat seizures, pentobarbital is tapered over the next 12 to 24 hours.

In remote cases in which this protocol is still not successful in controlling seizures, the anesthesia department is consulted and general anesthesia with halothane and neuromuscular blockade is initiated. This situation is extremely rare.

Treatment of Status Epilepticus in Children

Special considerations are often given to the treatment of children and infants with status epilepticus. Table 2 provides the status epilepticus treatment protocol for pediatric patients at the MCV Hospital Complex. This protocol is used in the same fashion as the adult protocol and has the same initial procedures. Table 2 gives the appropriate tests to be performed. After stabilization has been achieved, an IV line is placed with normal saline. A bolus of 2 ml per kilogram of 50 percent glucose is then given.

After the patient has been stabilized, initial anticonvulsant treatment is begun. The pediatric protocol recommends the use of IV lorazepam as the first-line treatment administered at a rate of 1 to 2 mg per minute to a maximum dose of 5 mg. The appropriate loading dose is 0.1 mg per kilogram.

After IV lorazepam has been administered, the patient is treated with IV phenytoin, 18 to 20 mg per

TABLE 2 Status Epilepticus Treatment Protocol for Children

Step	*Time Frame of Intervention*	*Procedure*
1	0–5 min	Determination of status elipticus. As soon as the diagnosis is made, institute monitoring of temperature, blood pressure, pulse, respiratory ECG and EEG. Insert oral airway and administer O_2 if necessary. Insert an IV catheter and draw venous blood for levels of anticonvulsants, glucose (check Dextrostik) electrolytes, calcium, BUN, CBC. Draw arterial antipyretics (acetaminophen). Perform frequent suction.
2	6–9 min	An IV line is placed with normal saline. Administer a bolus of 2 ml/kg 50% gluclose.
3	10–30 min	Initial treatment consists of an infusion of IV lorazepam given at a rate of 1–2 mg/min (0.1 mg/kg) to a maximum dose of 5 mg. This is followed by IV phenytoin, 18–20 mg/kg, infused at a rate not to exceed 1 mg/kg/min or 50 mg/min. Monitor ECG and blood pressure.
4	31–59 min	If seizures persist, administer a bolus infusion of phenobarbital at a rate not to exceed 50 mg/min until seizures stop or to a loading dose of 20 mg/kg.
5	60 min	If control is still not achieved, other options include: 1) Diazepam (50 mg) is diluted in a solution of 250 ml 0.9% NaCl or D_5W and run as a continuous infusion at 1 ml/kg/hr (2 mg/kg/hr) to achieve blood levels of 0.2–.8 mg/ml. The IV solution is changed every 6 hours as advised by certain authors, and short-length IV tubing is used. 2) Pentobarbital with an initial IV loading dose of 5 mg/kg with additional amounts given to produce a "burst suppression" pattern on EEG. Maintenance of pentobarbial anesthesia is continued for approximately 4 hours by an infusion of 1–3 mg/kg/hr. The patients are then checked for the reappearance of seizure activity by decreasing the infusion rate. If clinical seizures and/or generalized EEG discharges persist, the procedure is repeated; if not, the pentobarbital is tapered over 12–24 hours.
6	61–80 min	If seizures are still not controlled, call the anesthesia department to begin general anesthesia with halothane and neuromuscular blockage.

Continous EEG monitoring is recommended in the obtunded patient to assure that status elipticus has not recurred. In the management of intractable status, a neurologist who has expertise in status elipticus should be consulted and advice from a regional epilepsy center should be sought.

Lumbar puncture should be performed as soon as possible, especially in a febrile child or infant below 1 year.

For infants with a history of neonatal seizures, infantile spasms, or early onset seizures, pyridoxine, 100 mg IV, should be administered while EEG monitoring is being performed to diagnose and treat the rare patient with seizures with a vitamin B_6 deficiency.

kilogram, which is infused at a rate not to exceed 1 mg per kilogram per minute or a total of 50 mg per minute. ECG and blood pressure monitoring are recommended during phenytoin infusion.

If seizures persist, phenytoin therapy is followed by phenobarbital administration. Phenobarbital is administered at a rate not to exceed 50 mg per minute until the seizures stop or a loading dose of 20 mg per kilogram is given. This protocol is effective in stopping most cases of status epilepticus in children. In children seizures that are difficult to control and which do not respond to lorazepam, phenytoin, and phenobarbital require the same control as in adults. A diazepam drip followed by pentobarbital anesthesia is recommended. If seizures are still not controlled, general anesthesia is recommended.

Pyridoxine, 100 mg IV, is recommended for children or infants with a history of neonatal seizures, infantile spasms, or early onset seizures. The pyridoxine should be given while EEG monitoring is being performed. This allows the treatment and diagnosis of rare patients with seizures and a vitamin B_6 deficiency.

In our initial studies at the Medical College of Virginia, status epilepticus in children is a common problem, although it usually does not have as high a mortality rate as that of the adult population. Our findings also indicate that recurrent status epilepticus is more common in children. Further research needs to be developed to more definitively evaluate these observations.

As future research develops to define the risk management scale for mortality in status epilepticus in children and adults, the clinician will have a more definitive guideline for determining which patients need acute monitoring or follow-up. We recommend hospitalizing all patients who do not recover consciousness within 30 or 40 minutes after the cessation of status epilepticus in the neurologic intensive care unit. In this unit, the patients can have continuous EEG and vital sign monitoring. The patients who regain consciousness are hospitalized on the general neurology floor. Careful monitoring and follow-up of patients who do not recover rapidly from status epilepticus may often avoid complications that could be prevented by acute monitoring. This type of close observation may not be possible in all hospital settings, but it is recommended for patients who have prolonged seizures or significant associated medical complications.

SUGGESTED READING

Aminoff MJ, Simon RP. Status epilepticus: causes, clinical features and consequences in 98 patients. Am J Med 1980;69(5):657–666.

Delgado-Escueta AV, Waisterlain GC, Trieman DM, Porter RJ. Status epilepticus. New York: Raven Press, 1983.

Leppik IE, Derivan AT, Homan RW, et al. Double-blind study of lorazepam and diazepam in status epilepticus. JAMA 1983;249:1452–1454.

Rashkin MC, Youngs C, Penovich P. Pentobarbital treatment of refractory status epilepticus. Neurology 1987;37:500–502.

Wilder BJ, Ramsay E, Wilmore LJ, et al. Efficacy of intravenous phenytoin in the treatment of status epilepticus. Ann Neurol 1977;1:511–518.

PATIENT RESOURCES

Medical College of Virginia Epilepsy Center
Status Epilepticus Program Project
Robert J. DeLorenzo, M.D., Ph.D., M.P.H.
Department of Neurology
P.O. Box 599, MCV Station
Richmond, Virginia 23298

Epilepsy Foundation of American
4351 Garden City Drive
Landover, Maryland 20785

MIGRAINE AND CLUSTER HEADACHE

DEWEY K. ZIEGLER, M.D.

A problem in reaching a consensus on the optimum treatment of migraine is the difficulty in establishing criteria for diagnosis. There is no verifying biologic test; each clinician must rely on his or her clinical judgment. A universally agreed on criterion, however, is recurrence of attacks, and there are therefore two treatment considerations: treatment of an acute attack and prophylactic treatment for prevention of recurrent symptoms.

The first treatment necessity is to rule out any underlying disease of which headache is a symptom. Headache is a common symptom of increased intracranial pressure, meningeal irritation, and vasculitis and can occur in association with any kind of encephalopathy (e.g., that caused by electrolyte derangement or anemia). For this reason, all patients with severe, constant, or recurrent headache must undergo a careful neurologic examination and some laboratory tests—a complete blood count, a measurement of the sedimentation rate, and a profile of blood chemistry values. Minor degress of abnormality on neurologic examination must be suitably evaluated. Although usually if there are abnormalities on neurological examination, patients have referable symptoms, occasionally such symptoms are absent. Minor degrees of impairment of fine finger movement, rapid gait, or ability to hop may be found. Reflex asymmetry, abnormality of visual fields on confrontation, or any degree of impairment of higher functions (e.g., memory, flow of speech) may also be important.

Once a presumptive diagnosis of migraine is made on the basis of the history and a negative examination, I present to the patient a brief summary of migraine as it relates to his or her case. This "mini-lecture" usually covers the following points:

1. Based on a review of the history and the negative neurologic examination, there is minimal possibility of brain disease (often a patient has the unspoken apprehension that he or she is harboring a brain tumor; not infrequently the physician discovers that a family member or close friend has had this illness).
2. Migraine is defined as an illness characterized by recurrence of severe headache and, often but not always, one-sided location and occurrence of nausea and vomiting.
3. There is no single cause for this condition; many kinds of biochemical abnormalities and physiologic abnormalities have been found in some patients.
4. In many patients, migraine is associated with a hereditary tendency—probably a susceptibility to headache brought on by various stimuli through mechanisms still unknown.
5. Because migraine is characteristically recurrent, prophylactic treatment is often effective for varying periods of time; it can be discon-

tinued, but often later needs to be reinstituted.

6. Treatment of the acute attack and treatment to prevent recurrent attacks require different procedures.
7. Migraines are occasionally brought on by situations that can be avoided. Migraineurs should try not to skip meals since in some patients slight drops in blood sugar may precipitate attacks. Keeping regular sleeping hours is also important; some patients suffer attacks after missing sleep, others after particularly prolonged sleep (e.g., on weekends). Also to be avoided are excessive caffeine intake (contained in coffee and many soft drinks), chocolate, sharp cheeses, and red wine. In some individuals, a variety of other food substances have been reported to precipitate attacks.

TREATMENT OF ACUTE ATTACK

An urgent problem is the differentiation of an acute migraine attack from acute meningeal irritation caused by subarachnoid hemorrhage or bacterial meningitis. Distinguishing an acute attack from the latter is rarely a problem since infection is almost invariably characterized by fever and systemic signs of infection. Subarachnoid hemorrhage, however, presents more difficulties. Presence of any degree of nuchal rigidity, impairment of consciousness, or other abnormalities on neurologic examination mandates computed tomography (CT) scan of the head and a spinal fluid examination. The reason for the spinal fluid examination is that occasionally cases are seen before the blood is apparent on CT scan. Even without these clues, in a patient presenting with severe headache and no previous history of the same, these tests may be warranted—although clearly they cannot be made routine for each headache episode. I rely greatly on the previous history; if onset occurs at an early age, if attacks are fairly uniform, and particularly if the visual symptoms of classic migraine have occurred, I feel more confident that the attack is migraine. Positive family history also favors migraine to some degree.

I consider the treatment of the acute migraine attack to consist of five aspects: (1) avoidance of environmental stimuli, (2) antiemetics, (3) analgesics, (4) ergotamine, and (5) sedatives.

My first instruction to the patient with an acute attack is to initiate rest in a dark, quiet room. Most patients have discovered this treatment modality themselves, but some attempt to "tough it out"—go to work, often to a job that involves close visual work and causes "stress." Such an attempt invariably prolongs the headache.

The patient must decide when early symptoms herald a severe migraine attack and when they do not. Once migraine is diagnosed, administration of ergotamine is indicated (Fig. 1). Use of ergotamine early in the episode is far more effective than later. It can be given even during the aura of classical migraine. The caveat presented to the patient is that there is a danger of overuse of ergotamine; patients taking the drug when they are overly apprehensive may become psychologically dependent on larger amounts. The more psychologically unstable the patient, the greater the danger of such a dependence.

Often the severe migraine attack is accompanied by nausea and/or vomiting. These symptoms are intensified, if not initiated by, ergotamine. If the patient has a history of nausea with attacks, I recommend initiation of treatment with an antiemetic before administering ergotamine. If nausea has begun, a trimethobenzamide hydrochloride suppository (200 mg) is useful, or if considerable agitation is present, a phenothiazine such as prochlorperazine may be preferable, likewise in the form of a suppository. If the patient can anticipate the nausea and therefore receive medication orally, I prescribe metaclopramide, 10 to 20 mg by mouth, as the first therapeutic agent.

I prescribe ergotamine to be taken 20 to 30 minutes after the acute antiemetic. If nausea is not present, ergotamine can be taken orally in the tablet form combined with caffeine or with caffeine plus a small amount of phenobarbital and belladonna. Since it is desirable for migraine patients to sleep, one must remember that these preparations do contain the stimulant caffeine. I recommend 2 mg of ergotamine taken orally, followed by three additional 1-mg doses at hourly intervals if needed. I do not recommend more than 5 mg ergotamine for any single attack. I have no real opinion as to the additional benefit conferred to the ergotamine-caffeine by the addition of phenobarbital-belladonna. I rarely use sublingual ergotamine since the degree of its absorption is questionable. Ergotamine may also be taken via nasal inhalation; absorption is excellent, but the preparation is costly and I have not used it.

For some patients, ergotamine must be taken in suppository form. Often patients awaken with a severe headache accompanied by nausea and therefore cannot take medication by mouth. Some find the onset of nausea so rapid that there is no time for oral medication to take effect. Absorption of the drug from rectal mucosa is more complete than from gastric mucosa; rarely does a patient require more than one suppository.

Because ergotamine is a vasoconstrictor, it should probably never be used in patients who have a history of any arterial disease and should be used only with great caution in the elderly. It is particularly important to warn patients of these vasoconstrictive actions and of the symptoms of dangerous

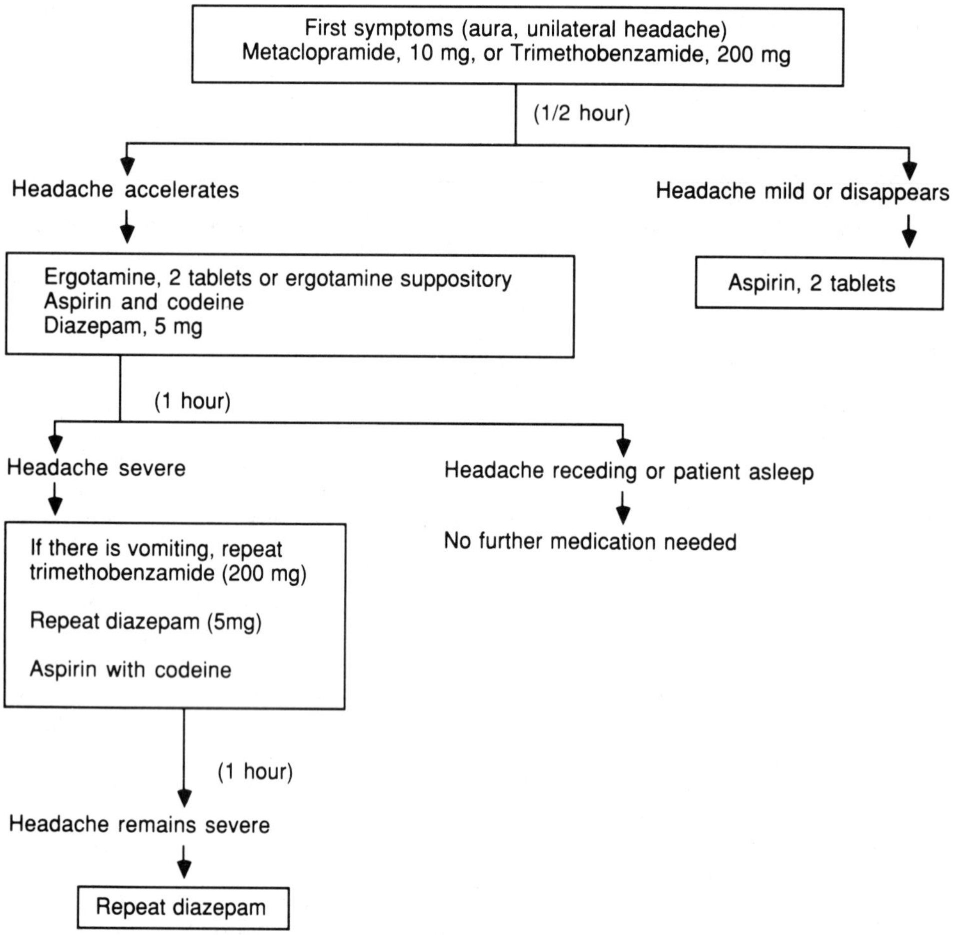

Figure 1 Treatment of acute migraine attack.

vasoconstriction (e.g., chest pain, extremity pain). As a general rule, after discussing with the patient the side effects of any medication prescribed, I provide him or her with one of the excellent American Medical Association (AMA) printed sheets (if available) discussing that particular class of drug.

Patients can develop a psychological habituation to ergotamine. This is probably not a true addiction, but it is nevertheless an effect that occasionally requires hospitalization to undo. I warn patients that the weekly limit of ergotamine is 8 to 10 mg. Occasional patients benefit from the compound Midrin, which also contains a vasoconstrictor of much weaker potency.

Analgesics are of course needed for the acute attack; some patients may achieve adequate relief with aspirin, acetaminophen, or ibuprofen. Although these agents should be tried alone first, in my experience there is usually adequate evidence of some attacks of pain severe enough to justify the occasional use of more potent agents such as codeine (e.g., 30 mg), or codeine derivatives combined with aspirin or acetaminophen. Of also greater analgesic potency is propoxyphene. Occasional patients achieve superior relief when a sedative is compounded with analgesics (e.g., butalbital [Fiorinal]). Such agents should be used for limited periods of time only, and the patient should be informed that they contain a sedative which can well be habit forming if taken continually.

I try to evaluate more or less intuitively the degree of probability of drug abuse in each individual patient. In those in whom there are clues of emotional instability, prescriptions for more potent analgesics should be given in only small amounts. All patients, of course, should receive a limited number of such tablets, both per single attack and per week.

One of the major decisions is whether to recommend or permit potent opiates (e.g., meperidine hydrochloride) parenterally for patients with severe attacks. I strongly discourage such treatment because of the frequency of dependence on these drugs. If patients become used to the euphoria and analgesia produced by opiates, they are progressively more unwilling to tolerate any headache pain, and demands for injections usually accelerate. I tell patients that they can almost always avoid the necessity of parenteral opiates by instituting prompt oral therapy that includes enough sedation to put them to sleep. I therefore instruct them to take a strong sedative with analgesics and ergotamine. (For the average adult, I have been prescribing diazepam 10 mg.) The dose is to be repeated in 1 hour if the patient is not asleep by that time. (Patients in pain frequently require large amounts of this medication to induce sleep.) It must be made clear to the patient that the diazepam is to be used only in the event of acute attacks and to induce sleep and that it must not be used with great frequency.

PROPHYLACTIC TREATMENT

The decision of whether to administer medication on a daily basis for prophylaxis of headache is often a difficult one. Certainly in the patients with one or two episodes per year such treatment is not justified. Conversely, in patients with one or more attacks weekly, such treatment regimens should be tried. The patient should share in the decision in questionable cases, the possible benefits of treatment being weighed against possible drug side effects.

Although the prophylactic agents to be discussed are reported to be effective in treating migraine and not "muscle tension headache," I have been liberal in their trial. In many patients, episodic headache has some (although far from all) of the characteristics of migraine, and in many of these patients, one of the drugs will be effective. We do not yet know which, if any, specific combinations of variables predict response to one or the other drug.

Frequently patients have several questions before beginning a daily drug regimen. Such questions may include the following:

1. "Will I have to stay on this for the rest of my life?" The answer I give is that migraine is an intermittent problem and that, although we cannot surgically "remove" migraine, many persons go without attacks for months and even years. After a long interval during which headaches are few or rare, I instruct patients to taper medication.
2. "Are the drugs addicting?" The answer to this is "no" in the sense that withdrawal is usually not difficult.
3. "Will these drugs interfere with any other medication I am taking—for example for cardiac disease?" The answer to this question is also usually "no," although drug interactions should be investigated for each combination in question.

If the decision is made to use prophylactic treatment, I tell patients that there is currently medical literature supporting the trial of several different agents for this purpose, the most generally used being propranolol, amitriptyline, methysergide, naproxen, and verapamil. There is little medical literature providing guidance as to which patient characteristics might indicate the preferential trial of one of these drugs or whether combinations of two or more drugs might be superior to one drug alone.

I instruct patients that, as a general principle, dosage should be increased gradually until one of three end-points is reached: (1) good reduction in headache (as determined by the patient), (2) the occurrence of unacceptable side effects, or (3) a dose is reached at the upper range of that reported in the medical literature. Only after failure with trials with each of the single prophylactic agents do I move to polypharmacy (two drugs).

I frequently select propranolol for a first trial unless there is a specific contraindication, such as hypotension, asthma, or diabetes. It is wise to start with a low dose—for example, 20 mg twice daily with an increase in dosage at biweekly intervals. I have seldom achieved better results with any daily dosage of more than 160 mg, although much larger doses are used in patients with hypertension and have been used in some patients with migraine. Once the effective daily dose is established, I offer the patient the option of using the once-daily long-acting preparation, which can be supplemented, if necessary, by one or more short-acting doses. I point out to the patient the possibility of such side effects as orthostatic hypotension (which usually occurs only with large doses), the usual bradycardia, and the occasional fatiguelike state often described as a "loss of drive" rather than as sedation. However, this latter side effect may be a consideration in the choice of a drug; if a modest tranquilizing effect occurs with the use of propranolol, it is natural to select this drug for those individuals with manifest anxiety. Propranolol has been used as an agent in prophylaxis of anxiety attacks and is commonly used by entertainers just before a performance.

Several other beta-adrenergic-blocking agents have been used effectively for migraine prophylaxis; these are the compounds of the series which lack sympathomimetic effects. However there is no published evidence that any of these are superior to propranolol either in efficacy or diminution of side effects, and to date, only propranolol is FDA-approved for migraine. Nevertheless, if propranolol is ineffective and the patient seems a particularly good candidate for beta-adrenergic blocking therapy, I occasionally give a brief trial with metoprolol, 50 to 150 mg per day.

Patients taking beta-adrenergic blocking agents, particularly the elderly, should be warned not to discontinue use of the drug abruptly. Such abrupt action can produce hypertensive reactions, although this is rare with the comparatively small doses used to treat migraine.

Amitriptyline can be used as an one-dose nighttime medication, and I have found it particularly effective when insomnia complicates migraine. I always begin this drug with a small dose (10 to 25 mg nightly) since side effects disturb many patients and are lessened if dose is increased gradually. The therapeutic range is usually 50 to 100 mg nightly, although occasional patients benefit from a higher dose. Common side effects are sedation and dryness of the mouth caused by anticholinergic action. Since headache patients are frequently depressed, it is wise to bear in mind the caveat that this drug has been used effectively as a suicidal agent. There is little published experience with other antidepressants in the treatment of migraine, and there is no indication of the superiority of any of them to amitriptyline.

Methysergide (Sansert) was first discovered to be effective as a migraine prophylactic several decades ago. It seems that the more typical the migraine, the more likely this drug is to be effective as a prophylactic agent. Again, I begin with a dose of 2 mg twice daily—a dose that is usually below the therapeutic range. The dose is increased to 2 mg three times daily after a few weeks, and if results are still unsatisfactory, it is increased to 2 mg four times daily. Its limitations are its side effects. Even with small doses, some patients have unpleasant subjective sensations that they find difficult to describe but which have hallucinatory elements. Methysergide can also cause nausea and insomnia. The drug also has vasoconstrictor properties, and patients should be told to report any symptoms suggestive of cardiac or limb ischemia. The most dangerous side effect is growth of fibrous tissue into various sites (retroperitoneal space, lungs, cardiac valves), which occurs with prolonged use of methysergide. Patients must be warned to take a "vacation" from the drug for 1 month after 6 months' use.

The calcium entry channel blocker, verapamil, is another effective drug in the prophylaxis of migraine and has the advantage of carrying less potentially serious side effects than many of the others. As my experience with this drug increases, I tend to consider it among the best of the agents to be used for this condition. The usual drug dose is 320 mg daily. The common side effect is constipation, and flushing of the skin is not uncommon. In my experience, neither of these have been severe enough to necessitate withdrawal of the drug. Patients should probably take bulk stool softeners while receiving this drug.

The nonsteroidal anti-inflammatory drug naproxen is another choice for trial in prophylaxis of migraine. The usual dose is 375 to 500 mg 3 times daily. It has the advantage of some analgesic properties and is particularly valuable if patients have additional pain problems (e.g., arthritis). Several side effects must be remembered, the most troublesome being irritation of gastric mucosa and activation of peptic ulcer. It is wise to tell patients to take it with food or an antacid. In patients with some degree of pre-existing disease, the drug may also cause serious renal or hepatic dysfunction.

In many patients, headache frequency and severity diminish with nonpharmacological treatment. The most commonly used such treatments are instruction in general psychic relaxation, muscle relaxation, and biofeedback of neck or forehead muscle contraction (to demonstrate to the patient that such relaxation *has* occurred) or of hand skin temperature (to demonstrate that he or she has succeeded in raising skin temperature). There are reports of improvement in both migraine and nonmigrainous headache with this treatment, particularly with nonmigrainous headache. Currently it is not known whether any biofeedback demonstration to the patient with a recording device of some change in a physiologic variable is superior to instruction in muscle relaxation. My practice is to judge from the patient's history and "body language" during examination the degree to which the patient is "tense." If the degree appears to be high or if the patient himself links the attacks to stress, I give some simple instructions on relaxation. I recommend that the patient allot three or four 15-minute periods per day to retiring to a quiet, dark place (often an extremely difficult undertaking). The patient should then concentrate on relaxing each limb in turn and should repeat a series of semi-self-hypnotic phrases (Table 1). I have not used formal biofeedback with metering devices.

When migraine attacks recur with great frequency despite high doses of medication, I recommend hospitalization. During the hospital stay, the high doses of medication to which the patient has become habituated are withdrawn (gradually in the case of beta-adrenergic blocking drugs) and the patient is kept heavily sedated for a few days. This maneuver is particularly important if patients are taking large amounts of analgesics or ergotamine. These measures should be accompanied by a program of psychological counseling to enable the patient to avoid recurrence of migraine.

CLUSTER HEADACHE

In most patients, the syndrome of cluster headache is clearly distinguishable from migraine and responds to different therapeutic agents. The acute attacks are characterized by retro-orbital pain and are always unilateral, severe, and usually brief in duration (lasting 0.5 to 1 hour). Attacks are of great

TABLE 1 Self-Administered Relaxation Phrases

I feel quite quiet . . . . I am beginning to feel quite relaxed . . . . My feet feel heavy and relaxed . . . . My solar plexus and the whole central portion of my body feel relaxed and quiet . . . . My hands, my arms, and my shoulders feel heavy, relaxed, and comfortable . . . . I feel all the tension in my neck letting go and relaxing . . . . My lower neck feels relaxed . . . . The upper neck at the base of my head is letting go . . . letting go . . . . My head feels free . . . . My jaws and my tongue are letting go . . . . The area around my eyes is letting go . . . . They feel relaxed . . . . I feel the areas around my mouth, my nose, and my forehead letting go and relaxing . . . . They feel comfortable and smooth . . . . My whole body feels quiet, heavy, comfortable, and relaxed.

I feel quite relaxed . . . . My arms and head are heavy and warm . . . . I feel quite quiet . . . . My whole body is relaxed and my hands are heavy and warm, relaxed and warm . . . . My hands are warm . . . . Warmth is flowing into my hands, they are warm . . . . I can feel the warmth flowing down my arms into my hands . . . . My hands are warm, relaxed and warm . . . . My forehead is relaxed . . . . I am relaxing every fiber . . . . The area around my eyes is soft, relaxed and letting go . . . . All the muscles in my face feel comfortable and smooth . . . .

My whole body feels quiet, heavy, comfortable, and relaxed . . . . My arms and hands are heavy and warm . . . . My forehead muscles are relaxed and smooth . . . . My mind is quiet . . . . I withdraw my thoughts from the surroundings and I feel serene and still . . . . My thoughts are turned inward and I am at ease . . . . Deep within my mind I am relaxed, comfortable, and still . . . . I am alert, but in an easy, quiet, inward-turned way . . . . My mind is calm and quiet . . . . I feel an inward quietness.

severity and characteristically repetitive during a short period of time. I have found few attacks to be responsive to treatment with ergotamine. Because the attacks are brief, oral analgesics do not have time to take effect. A further problem with the use of analgesics in patients with this condition is that the patients often take them in apprehension of the recurrent attacks. Occasional patients, however, do obtain relief from one of these agents, which must almost always be supplemented with codeine. I have found that inhalation of oxygen at 4 L/minute is effective in terminating attacks in most patients.

Patients with cluster headache should be warned to avoid alcohol; most of them have already discovered that even small amounts can precipitate attacks. Continuous prophylactic treatment is usually not needed since the "clusters" are separated by unpredictable intervals of time. Once the "bout" of headache attacks starts, I rely on adrenal steroid drugs to terminate the "cluster." I usually begin with 50 mg of prednisone administered daily and decrease the daily dose by 10 mg every week. When clusters are resistant to steroids or recur after only brief periods of relief, I have the patient begin taking lithium carbonate, beginning with one 300-mg tablet per day and rapidly increasing (over a period of 2 weeks) the dosage to 300 mg administered three times daily.

SUGGESTED READING

Jonsdottir BA, Meyer JS, Roger RL. Efficacy, side effects, and tolerance compared during headache treatment with three different calcium blockers. Headache 1987; 27:364–369.

Martin PR, Marie GV, Nathan PR. Behavioral research on headaches: a coded bibliography. Headache 1987; 27:555–570.

Tfelt-Hansen P. Efficacy of beta-blockers in migraine: a critical review. Cephalalgia 1986; 6 (suppl):15–24.

Ziegler DK, Ellis DJ. Naproxen in prophylaxis of migraine. Arch Neurol 1985; 42:582.

PATIENT RESOURCES

National Headache Foundation
5252 N. Western Avenue
Chicago, Illinois 60625

(There is a small membership fee. The organization provides up-to-date material concerning headache.)

Other sources of information:

Seymour Solomon, M.D.
Headache Clinic
Montefiore Hospital and Medical Center
111 East 210th St.
Bronx, New York 10467

Dewey K. Ziegler, M.D.
Headache Clinic
Department of Neurology
University of Kansas Medical Center
39th and Rainbow Blvd.
Kansas City, Kansas 66103

Neil Raskin, M.D.
Headache Clinic
Department of Neurology
University of California at San Francisco
505 Parnassus Avenue
San Francisco, California 94143

Joseph Sargent, M.D.
Menninger Headache Clinic
5800 West 6th Avenue
Topeka, Kansas 66604

Ninan Mathew, M.D.
Houston Headache Clinic
1213 Hermann Drive
Houston, Texas 77044

E.L. Speirings, M.D.
John R. Graham Headache Center
Faulkner Hospital
Allendale at Centre Street
Boston, Massachusetts 02130

Kenneth Welch, M.D.
Headache Clinic
Henry Ford Hospital
2799 West Grand Boulevard
Detroit, Michigan 48202

Seymour Diamond, M.D.
Diamond Headache Clinic
5252 N. Western Avenue
Chicago, Illinois, 66604

Joel Saper, M.D.
Michigan Headache and Neurological Institute
3120 Professional Drive
Ann Arbor, Michigan 48104

CERVICAL SPONDYLOSIS

ELLIOTT L. MANCALL, M.D.
MARK STACY, M.D.

Cervical spondylosis, an acquired disorder involving the intervertebral discs, the cervical vertebrae and processes themselves, and indirectly, the spinal roots and spinal cord, is a common degenerative disorder of midlife and old age. In this disorder, radiologic changes predominate in the fourth through seventh vertebral bodies; however, purely radiographic alterations, even when computed tomography (CT) scanning, magnetic resonance imaging (MRI), or myelography is used, often fail to explain fully the spectrum of clinical complaints. Pathologic examination may provide evidence of a complex assortment of changes, any or all of which may account for the symptomatology in a given patient. These include, *inter alia,* osteophyte formation, joint degeneration (spondyloarthropathy), central herniation of the intervertebral disc(s), and hypertrophy of the ligamentum flavum, all of which may narrow the spinal canal (and may potentially cause either direct cord compression or compromise of the spinal vascular network).

More laterally placed bony spurs involve the intervertebral foramina and compress the spinal roots; lateral extrusion of disc fragments may produce similar radicular affection. Osteophytic compromise of the vertebral foramina may also lead to compression of the vertebral artery, which is symptomatically manifest particularly with changes in position of the head and neck. Finally, entrapment of the greater occipital nerve may occur as a result of spasm of the cervical musculature. In such a complex setting, the patient's clinical symptoms and signs remain the most useful guide to the location, nature, and extent of the pathologic process.

From the therapeutic point of view, it is useful to divide the patients' complaints into several distinct groups, each reflecting a predominant, although not necessarily exclusive, constellation of clinical and pathologic alterations: headache, syncopal episodes, cervical radiculopathy, and cervical myelopathy. These may develop spontaneously in an insidious manner, or more acutely after trauma to the neck (e.g., a whiplash injury, the medicolegal implications of which should not be ignored in one's therapeutic approach).

HEADACHE

Spondolytic changes occurring superiorly at the cranio-cervical junction and within the upper cervical column may result in headache. In some patients, pain is lancinating in quality and radiates unilaterally or bilaterally from the neck or base of the skull to the vertex or forehead, sometimes into the orbit. Spontaneous pain may be reproduced by compression or percussion of the greater occipital nerve as it crosses the basiocciput. Spasm of the cervical musculature is almost invariably encountered; the pain in these instances of occipital neuralgia is likely caused by entrapment and compression of the occipital nerve as it traverses muscles of the posterior triangle of the neck.

More common is the aching or squeezing pain experienced at the occiput and radiating around the head in a band or viselike manner, and again reflecting spasm of the cervical musculature as so-called insertional or muscle-contraction pain. It may be extremely difficult to distinguish this pain from that of the classical tension headache syndrome; in fact, the mechanism of headache in both conditions is probably similar if not identical.

Treatment of headache in patients with cervical spondylosis is basically symptomatic, and includes the use of massage, ultrasonography, regular applications of moist heat, suitable muscle relaxants—e.g., chlorzoxazone (Parafon Forte DSC), 500 mg three times daily; cyclobenzaprine (Flexeril), 10 mg three times daily; or diazepam (Valium), 2 to 5 mg three times daily—and nonsteroidal anti-inflammatory agents. The use of narcotics should be avoided. Intermittent cervical traction may be helpful, particularly in patients with severe cervical spasm. In the face of neuralgic pain, agents such as amitriptyline hydrochloride (Elavil), 10 to 25 mg administered at bedtime, and/or carbamazepine (Tegretol), 800 mg per day or more as required, are helpful. In resistant cases of occipital neuralgia block of the greater occipital nerve, or as an extreme measure, avulsion of the nerve may be useful.

SYNCOPAL EPISODES

Syncope associated with head movements, particularly turning of the head with retroflexion, is associated with osteophyte formation with narrowing of the vertebral foramina, often with subluxation of the vertebral bodies. These changes result in compression—and sometimes frank occlusion—of the vertebral arteries. Symptoms are not confined to syncope alone; at times, a full-blown picture of vertebro-basilar insufficiency appears. Careful attention to the details of the patient's history should permit one to distinguish this osteophytic compromise of the vertebral arteries from the far more common transient ischemic attacks caused by atherosclerosis and stenosis of the posterior circulatory tree. If changes are demonstrated in the vertebral artery angiographically with changes in head posture, decompression of the vertebral canal may be beneficial.

CERVICAL RADICULOPATHY

Compression of the cervical roots, either by osteophyte formation within the intervertebral foramina or by traumatic lateral herniation of a disc fragment, results in cervical radiculopathy, characteristically presenting with severe lancinating pain that is generally referred in a dermatomal pattern to the shoulder, arm, or hand. Patients often complain of tingling paresthesias in the hand or arm. There may also be pain, particularly with a change in position of the neck or with coughing, sneezing, or other Valsalva maneuvers. Spasm of the cervical musculature with restriction of movement of the cervical spine is typically encountered, especially in acute cases of traumatic origin. Asymmetry or loss of the muscle stretch reflexes is common, and segmental weakness may be apparent. Sensory changes are more difficult to document, but in many cases, a dermatomal sensory loss is evident. Atrophy of muscle appropriate to the segmental level of the lesion may be noted.

The management of cervical radiculopathy is directed at relieving both pain and, ultimately, the nerve root compression itself. Cervical traction is useful, particularly in the face of cervical spasm and when supplemented by a cervical collar. Warm and/ or cold compresses, massage, and ultrasonography are often beneficial. Muscle relaxants (see preceding section) may be helpful, and relief of pain with appropriate analgesics is especially important; one must bear in mind that the pain itself will induce cervical spasm, and one must break this unfortunate cycle of pain-spasm-pain if at all possible. Ibuprofen (Motrin), 600 mg every 6 hours, or other nonsteroidal anti-inflammatory agents may be helpful; narcotics should be used only with caution.

Other treatment modalities such as acupuncture or transcutaneous nerve stimulation (TNS) may be used in some patients but are not uniformly helpful. TNS is probably more useful in acute cases than chronic cases. If painful radiculopathy has been present for a long period of time, amitriptyline is of benefit, beginning with 25 mg administered at bedtime, increasing to 100 mg, as required.

If conservative measures fail to relieve symptoms, surgical correction (foraminotomy) with decompression of the compromised spinal root(s) is necessary. It should be emphasized that the vast majority of patients respond to conservative management, with surgery being required only as a last resort.

CERVICAL MYELOPATHY

Myelopathy is the most serious of the complications of cervical spondylosis. Compression of the cervical cord is generally insidious in onset and slowly progressive; a more rapid course may follow trauma. Among the more common symptoms are tingling paresthesia and sensory impairment of the hands, often radicular in distribution; weakness, clumsiness, or atrophy of the hands, at times with segmental fasciculations; and spasticity and weakness of the lower extremities. Urinary urgency and frequency and impotence are not uncommon. Radicular pain and spasm of the cervical musculature may appear. Cervical myelopathy results from either or both of two mechanisms: (1) direct compression of the spinal cord by osteophytic processes or disc degeneration with central protrusion of soft disc material often with cartilaginous overgrowth, in many cases associated with thickening of the ligamentum flavum or (2) compromise of the vasculature of the cord with a seondary ischemic myelopathy.

The management of cervical myelopathy caused by spondylosis is often unsatisfactory. First, one must be careful in making the diagnosis since in the absence of significant pain or sensory changes, it may be difficult to distinguish this myelopathy from amyotrophic lateral sclerosis. Tumor of the cervical cord, multiple sclerosis, primary lateral sclerosis, and subacute combined degeneration of the cord caused by B_{12} deficiency are among the disorders which must be excluded. Even when the diagnosis is clear, management is difficult. Cervical traction, a cervical collar, warm or cold compresses, massage, ultrasonography and muscle relaxants all play a role in the treatment of this condition. If such measures fail, however, patients may require laminectomy with posterior decompression of the cord. In appropriately selected cases, anterior discectomy with removal of centrally protruded disc material and fusion may be the surgical approach of choice.

SUGGESTED READING

Brain L, Wilkinson M. Cervical spondylosis and other disorders of the cervical spine. Philadelphia: WB Saunders, 1967.

Herkowitz HN. The surgical management of cervical spondylotic radiculopathy and myelopathy. Clin Orthop 1989; 239:94–108.

Larsson E-M, Holtås S, Cronqvist S, Brandt L. Comparison of myelography, CT myelography and magnetic resonance imaging in cervical spondylosis and disc herniation. Acta Radiol 1989; 30:233–239.

Lestini WF, Wiesel SW. The pathogenesis of cervical spondylosis. Clin Orthop 1989; 239, 69–93.

Teresi LM, Lufkin RB, et al. Asymptomatic degenerative disc disease and spondylosis of the cervical spine: MRI imaging. Radiology 1987; 164:83–88.

ACUTE BACK PAIN AND DISC HERNIATION

RICHARD B. NORTH, M.D.

Low back pain is pandemic; a majority of adults experience a temporarily disabling episode. It is the most common cause of hospitalization, and its impact on the workplace is second only to that of upper respiratory infections, accounting for approximately one-quarter of lost work time. Associated health care and compensation costs, exclusive of lost productivity, are estimated to exceed $20 billion annually in the United States.

Degenerative lumbar disc disease is likewise ubiquitous, but it is only occasionally the cause of low back pain, and the need for surgical intervention is the exception rather than the rule. Even in patients with clear-cut disc herniation established clinically and by imaging studies, spontaneous recovery without surgery is common.

More than one-quarter million lumbar laminectomies and discectomies are performed annually in the United States, a rate which greatly exceeds that of other developed, industrialized countries. An estimated 30 to 40 percent of patients experience persistent pain after surgery; 25 percent are unable to return to their original occupations, and 10 to 15 percent undergo reoperation.

When the records and studies of patients with "failed back syndrome" (persistent, disabling pain occurring after one or more operations) are reviewed in detail, the original indications for surgery are commonly obscure. Secondary procedures are often necessary simply to correct the sequelae of primary procedures; in patients whose initial problem may have been a maladaptive or exaggerated response to minor pathology, the yield remains low.

Increasingly sophisticated imaging and other diagnostic tests are available for the evaluation of lumbosacral spine disease; however, clinical history and physical examination are of primary importance in the diagnosis and treatment of acute back pain, particularly during selection of patients for surgery. The sensitivity of modern diagnostic imaging (e.g., magnetic resonance imaging demonstration of disc degeneration) must be complemented by the specificity of a thorough clinical evaluation.

CLINICAL EVALUATION

Evaluation of the patient presenting with low back and/or lower extremity pain begins with a careful history. The patient's occupation, the circumstances under which symptoms developed (e.g., a lifting-related injury at work), and the effects of the condition on the patient's work and lifestyle should be recorded and considered. The relative magnitudes of low back and leg pain, the precise pattern of radiation, the quality of the pain, its aggravating and relieving factors, and associated neurologic symptoms should be noted. The latter include weakness, loss of sensation, abnormal sensations (e.g., paresthesias), changes in bladder or bowel habits or control, and changes in sexual function.

Pseudoradicular pain is a common manifestation of lumbosacral spine injury and degenerative disease. Experience with minor procedures involving paravertebral injections and radiofrequency denervations, with localization by electrical stimulation, shows that sciatica and other apparently radicular symptoms may occur in the absence of any nerve root compromise. On examination, referred pain syndromes of this sort are accompanied by mechanical signs, as opposed to neurologic or tension signs. Reproduction of pain by extension, for example, is a mechanical sign suggesting posterior element (facet joint) disease.

Although a detailed discussion of physical examination and differential diagnosis is beyond the scope of this chapter, some aspects of these deserve mention. The straight leg raising test, employed routinely in the physical examination, is often misinterpreted. If the patient complains only of low back pain with supine straight leg raising, this indicates a mechanical low back syndrome. A symptomatic disc herniation, on the other hand, should elicit complaints of ipsilateral (and sometimes contralateral) sciatica and should cause the patient to assume a protective position. When this occurs, the effects of simultaneous neck flexion and of dorsiflexion of the foot are noteworthy, as are the effects of popliteal and sciatic compression. Because of the variability between examiners in performing and interpreting these tests, recording the results as simply "positive" or "negative," as is done routinely, is of limited value. Explicit descriptions of these maneuvers and patient responses are much more informative.

Certain physical findings common in the "failed back" population predict a poor response to surgical treatment. As enumerated by Waddell, the most useful functional signs include the following:

1. Tenderness superficially (e.g., to gentle pinching of the skin of the low back) or in a nonanatomic pattern.
2. Simulated lumbosacral spine motion causing pain (e.g., axial loading at the vertex, trunk rotation).
3. Distraction (e.g., straight leg raising performed in the sitting position is well tolerated, but straight leg raising performed in the supine position is tolerated poorly).

4. Regional disturbances on neurologic examination (e.g., weakness or sensory loss that does not conform to a neuroanatomic pattern).
5. Overreaction to the examination, unexplained by cultural variability (e.g., pain behavior).

While it should be assumed that all patients complaining of low back pain have an organic basis for their complaint, individuals may vary greatly in their potential to respond to treatment for a given lesion. Patients with active workmen's compensation claims, personal injury litigation, or other issues of secondary gain are generally considered inferior candidates for surgery. Psychological tests have been developed or adapted for screening low back patients: the Minnesota Multiphasic Personality Inventory scales for depression, hypochondriasis, and hysteria, for example, are usually elevated in those who fail treatment. Personality disorders, somatization disorders, and other psychiatric diagnoses are common among patients with chronic low back pain or "failed back syndrome."

DIAGNOSTIC TESTS

Plain radiographs of the lumbosacral spine are the standard initial diagnostic study for patients with low back pain, although their yield and specificity are low. Findings of facet joint sclerosis, disc space narrowing or spurring, and other degenerative changes are of course ubiquitous even in asymptomatic patients, and should be interpreted accordingly. Not only the degenerative changes of spondylosis, but also those of spondylolysis and spondylolisthesis, are routinely assessed by plain films. Plain films also may disclose less common spinal conditions (e.g., infection or neoplasm) or extraspinal pathology (e.g., abdominal aortic aneurysm).

In patients presenting for initial evaluation, specialized diagnostic imaging such as magnetic resonance imaging (MRI), computed tomography (CT), and CT myelography should be reserved for those in whom there are specific indications that intervention may be required. As with plain radiographs, MRI, CT, and CT myelography commonly demonstrate signs of degenerative disease even in asymptomatic patients, but this does not contribute to the management of the acute low back syndrome. If, on the other hand, there are clinical indications of disc herniation or of another potential surgical problem, it is useful to obtain a definitive study early in the patient's management. If symptoms persist and are intractable, these studies are usually necessary to rule out significant pathology, even in the absence of a compelling clinical presentation.

As a noninvasive test that involves no exposure to ionizing radiation, MRI has obvious advantages over CT and CT myelography. Its ability to distinguish between soft tissues such as the thecal sac and the annulus and nucleus of the disc is a major advantage. It images cortical bone and calcifications poorly, however; CT provides a better demonstration of degenerative spurs, bony defects, and bony lateral recess and central stenosis of the spinal canal. While MRI is useful as a screening examination and may suffice as the sole imaging study (after plain films) for a clinically straightforward disc herniation, it has not replaced CT. With the addition of a small amount of water-soluble intrathecal contrast, CT remains the study of choice in demonstrating postsurgical arachnoid fibrosis.

Improvements in diagnostic imaging have reduced the need for ancillary electrophysiologic tests. Electromyography of lower extremity and paravertebral muscles remains useful, however, in confirming the diagnosis of radiculopathy (as opposed to pseudoradicular pain) in patients with equivocal clinical and imaging findings. Along with nerve conduction studies, it is useful in ruling out peripheral entrapment syndromes.

TREATMENT

Mechanical Low Back Syndrome

The patient presenting with acute onset of low back pain, with or without sciatica, with mechanical signs but without tension signs or neurologic symptoms or signs, may be diagnosed clinically as having an acute lumbosacral strain. Diagnostic evaluation may be limited to plain radiographs, and therapy to the traditional regimen of bedrest and analgesics. The duration of necessary bedrest is a matter of controversy; recent controlled studies suggest that restriction of activity is appropriate, but that the week or more of bedrest that has been prescribed routinely in the past is inferior to shorter periods.

If symptoms persist after the patient has undergone mobilization and low back education and exercise programs, further diagnostic study (CT or MRI) is indicated. In some patients with intractable mechanical low back pain, the lumbar facet joints are at fault. Facet joint syndrome may be defined empirically as mechanical low back pain that responds to medial branch posterior primary ramus blocks. Radiofrequency denervations are useful in this small subpopulation of patients.

Lumbar Disc Herniation

The patient presenting with radiculopathy—not only radiating pain, but tension signs and neurologic deficit—is a potential surgical candidate. However, even in patients with this condition, spontaneous recovery is common. Early diagnostic imaging is appropriate, to establish the diagnosis; but in the absence of a major neurologic deficit, conservative management is appropriate initially. As with acute lumbosacral strain injuries, even documented lumbar disc herniation will usually improve with conservative therapy and require no further intervention. Unlike the patient with acute lumbosacral strain, for whom prolonged bedrest and inactivity are not of proven benefit and may in fact be detrimental, the patient with acute lumbar disc herniation requires a more open-ended, individualized period of rest before mobilization.

The standard indication for surgical treatment of disc herniation is persistent, disabling pain despite an adequate trial of conservative care, with abnormal imaging studies sufficient to explain the patient's symptoms. The duration of an "adequate" trial is in general a matter of controversy and in each case a matter of clinical judgment. As spontaneous recovery is common, one might argue for extended conservative therapy. Another viewpoint, however, is that the results of surgery are less favorable after 6 to 9 weeks. Studies of these issues are difficult to interpret, particularly because of selection effects: Reported series of patients undergoing early surgery, for example, include some who might have improved spontaneously. On the other hand, those whose surgery has been delayed or postponed, whether by the physician or patient, would seem to be biased towards *a priori* inferior candidates for treatment. Prospective, randomized study data are scant; they suggest that there is short-term benefit for patients treated surgically, but little difference 1 year after presentation between those who have undergone operation and those who have not.

Lumbar disc herniation occasionally presents with a major neurologic deficit; this constitutes a neurosurgical emergency. Neurogenic bladder may occur with particularly large, central disc herniations, especially with pre-existing lumbar stenosis. Disabling weakness (e.g., foot drop) occurs more commonly. Although spontaneous recovery without surgery is possible, it is unpredictable; to maximize the chances of recovery, prompt surgical intervention is indicated.

Surgical Procedures

Although a detailed discussion of surgical techniques is beyond the scope of this chapter, some popular notions and procedures deserve discussion.

"Microsurgical" lumbar discectomy is common current terminology; it raises several technical issues: (1) the use of the operating microscope per se is considered less important than principles of microsurgical technique (i.e., gentle, meticulous dissection and hemostasis); (2) a small skin incision may permit adequate surgical exposure, but paravertebral muscle dissection should be of sufficient length to avoid traumatic focal retraction; and (3) if disc removal is limited to the herniated free fragment, the possibility of recurrent herniation may be greater, but if the surgeon must create a defect in the annulus to remove nuclear material, this may predispose to recurrence. Each side of these issues has its advocates and supporting case series; however, rigorous prospective study data are lacking.

In prospective studies, chymopapain chemonucleolysis has been found to compare favorably with placebo injections, although it compares unfavorably with traditional surgery in several respects. Its overall failure rate is higher, and the results of salvage surgery appear to be inferior to those of primary surgery—whether because of the effects of chemonucleolysis or because of the delay it introduces. It is occasionally complicated by catastrophic allergic reactions or toxic reactions to errant intrathecal injections. It may not be used for free fragment disc herniations that are sequestered and inaccessible to intradiscal injection. Percutaneous automated discectomy has been introduced recently as an alternative that may be used in the same subset of patients, but without the unique hazards of chymopapain.

Rehabilitation and Physical Therapy

Active participation in a daily exercise program is the most important aspect of rehabilitation after acute lumbosacral strain or postoperatively. The Williams flexion exercise program, which includes knee-chest stretching, pelvic tilts, and partial situps, is the best established and most widely applicable. The objective of any such program is strengthening deconditioned, strained paravertebral and abdominal muscles so as to provide necessary support and prevent further strain injury. After external bracing and prolonged disability and inactivity, exercises are a difficult undertaking for many patients, and a structured program is necessary to ensure compliance in many cases.

Education as to proper techniques for lifting and other activities of daily living is an important aspect of rehabilitation. Some patients with physically demanding jobs, despite compliance with these recommendations and with daily exercises, will continue to experience disabling lumbosacral strain injuries; for them, vocational rehabilitation may be appropriate.

SUGGESTED READING

King JS, Lagger R. Sciatica viewed as a referred pain symdrome. Surg Neurol 1976; 5:46–50.

Long DM, Filtzer DL, BenDebba M, Hendler NH. Clinical

features of the failed-back syndrome, J Neurosurg 1988; 69: 61–71.

Spitzer WO, LeBlanc FE, Dupuis M, et al. Scientific approach to the assessment and management of activity-related spinal disorders: a monograph for clinicians. Report of the Quebec Task Force on spinal disorders. Spine 1987; (suppl): S1–S60.

Waddell G, McCulloch JA, Kummel E, et al. Nonorganic physical signs in low-back pain. Spine 1980; 5:117–125.

Weber H. Lumbar disc herniation: a controlled, prospective trial with ten years of observation. Spine 1983; 8:131–140.

PATIENT RESOURCES

Back Basics: Managing Spine and Disc Problems with Self Care. Krames Communications, 312 90th Street, Daly City, California 94015-1898.

Back Care. Medic Publishing Co., Drawer O, Issaquah, Washington 98027.

CHRONIC LOW BACK PAIN AND FAILED BACK SYNDROME

LARRY EMPTING-KOSCHORKE, M.D.

Low back pain should be assessed and treated as a pain syndrome. There are multiple possible pathophysiologies for this condition, and these may be compounded further in a patient who has already undergone one or more low back operations. Pain in one anatomic area can be from any local tissue or may be radiated or referred. The pathologic source of the pain may be malignant or benign and may or may not be amenable to surgical intervention. As physicians, we are concerned that dangerous pathology may be missed and, conversely, that surgery performed to treat this pathology may worsen the patient's condition. There is also a stunning difference in the degree of pathologic impairment and the extent of disability in different patients that is based primarily on their psychiatric profile. Pain has an incredibly potent effect on psychological defenses, mood, and ultimately, the degree of disability. We have all seen patients who have either minor pathology but major disability or rather impressive pathology with minimized complaints and minor disability. The problem is deciding for which patients and to what extent our increasingly expensive diagnostic technology is required. In this chapter, I delineate the anatomic, pathophysiologic, and psychiatric syndromal features of the various sources of low back pain and "failed back" as determined by the traditional assessments and newer technologies, and finally, clarify treatment interventions.

BASIC PRINCIPLES OF PAIN SYNDROMES

One should assume that there is some physiologic source for the pain that the patient complains of; purely psychogenic pain is rare. The pathology may be minor, however, and the patient's response may be one of inappropriate disability. The converse may be true in a stoic person.

A general medical history and examination are essential for determining systemic factors causing local pathology. The neurologic and orthopedic examination will best define the syndromal signs. The neurologic examination must be complete in its screening for clues of a more widespread process presenting focally (e.g., mononeuritis multiplex presenting as sciatic and low back pain).

The psychological effects that pain has on personality, mood, and interpersonal relationships should be noted early on; this allows ease of intervention if the pain proves primarily psychogenic.

Physiologic and psychiatric components should be assessed concurrently rather than sequentially since both are inevitably operative and management of both will be necessary for whatever somatic pathology is found.

A familiarity with the local anatomy, referral patterns, and syndromal features of the pathophysiologic diagnoses is also important. One should start with simple and less invasive diagnostic testing, although one should use whatever testing is necessary to be as definitive as possible, whether making a diagnosis of inclusion or exclusion. One should define the source of pain and determine whether the lesion is surgically approachable. If it is not, physical therapy and/or pharmacologic and psychiatric interventions are indicated.

ANATOMIC CONSIDERATIONS

In treating chronic low back pain, each specialist focuses on his or her own "anatomy of interest"; for example, neurologists focus on the neural elements of the condition, orthopedic surgeons on correctable spinal and/or bony abnormalities. However, nearly all tissues in the low back are capable of producing pain locally. With the exception of the nucleus pulposus, the spinal, ligamentous, and neural elements are innervated by multilevel somatic and sympathetic nociceptive afferents. Hence there is little value in attempting to localize pain to one or another vertebral level. Historic and reproducible radicular paresthesias to a specific dermatome and facet pain syndrome induced by extension with radiation to posterior thigh or hip, anterolateral thigh, or groin (but rarely below the knee) are actually the only two pain patterns that are routinely helpful.

Bony Anatomy

The vertebral column anteriorly and facet joints posterolaterally are the stabilizing and most stressed bony components of the spine and hence the most susceptible to degenerative arthritic changes. As a disc degenerates and shrinks in height, the anatomic relationship of the articular surfaces is further altered and painful spondylosis and mechanically induced low back pain are hastened. Activity worsens the pain, whereas rest alleviates it. The posterior location of the facets tends to cause pain when the patient extends. Connecting anterior and posterior elements, the most vulnerable component is the pars interarticularis, which when fractured (spondylolysis) can allow shift of one vertebra (forward or back) on another (spondylolisthesis). Spondylosis posteriorly and laterally on the vertebral body causes central bony canal stenosis and lateral recess stenosis, respectively. Stenosis centrally creates "spinal claudication" syndromes with walking-induced back pain, leg pain, weakness, and/or change in reflexes.

Lateral recess stenosis of course narrows the foramen that the nerve root must take out of the bony canal. Facet spondylitic changes further narrow or even obliterate that foraminal opening, often causing classical radicular/dermatomal symptoms.

Disc Anatomy

Flexion places dorsally directed force on the disc, causing herniation either centrally or laterally, and thereby causing canal stenosis or lateral stenosis, respectively, with symptoms similar to those associated with bony changes. Of course they are not mutually exclusive, and often herniation is also seen with spondylolisthesis. Forcing a fragment through richly innervated ligaments causes low back pain in itself, regardless of whether or not the herniated portion of the disc impinges on nerve roots per se. When dorsal column stimulators are implanted, stimulation over the coverings of the cord can cause paresthesias many levels up, which partially explains why ligamentous pain can radiate quite high in the spinal column. With pressure on roots at any level, nociceptive afferents within its coverings and vessels as well as the somatic and sympathetic axons themselves can elicit painful radiating paresthesias without segmental findings on examination or electromyography (EMG). With sympathetic nociceptive afferents, the pain also is localized poorly or even "mirrored" contralaterally. Injury along the course of the lumbosacral plexus or even in the sciatic nerve as low as the pyriformis has been shown to cause referred pain to the low back. Hence one must consider pathology anywhere along the dermatomal course, from cord to peripheral nerve, especially if the patient has radicular symptoms.

Musculoligamentous Anatomy

Muscle and ligamentous injury or strain (e.g., myofascial syndrome) cannot be imaged and must be measured on clinical examination only.

Because underlying and correctable pathologies can be primary and spasm and muscular trigger points can be secondary, one is obligated to work up chronic "myofascial" or "musculoskeletal" syndromes that do not respond well to conservative therapy.

Referred Pain

Pelvic retroperitoneal lesions and, to a lesser extent, abdominal lesions can cause referred pain to the low back. However, history and review of systems usually helps determine the source of this pain.

Anatomy of the Failed Back

Surgery has many effects on normal anatomy, sometimes even at sites distant from the site of surgery. A herniated disc fragment can certainly recur at the same level. Scarring caused by the primary pathology or occurring postsurgically is common in the lateral recesses along the course of the roots' egress. More extensive scarring of the multiple roots may occur with even a single level disc resection (i.e., arachnoiditis). These scarred elements are restricted in mobility, pull on one another, and often progress with compressive scar. Laminectomies can resect much of the lateral lamina or facets, leading to later fracturing of facets or spondylitic nonanatomic joints. "Fusions" may fail to fuse originally, reabsorb, form pseudoarthroses, and fail to incorporate the facet joints. The low back with a solid fusion must make up for that lack of motion either above or below the fusion causing "transitional" changes such as laxity of ligaments behond physiologic norms and accelerated spondylitic changes. Again, some of these are suited to surgical correction, while others are not.

DIAGNOSTIC ASSESSMENT

Always let your neurologic examination guide your diagnostic testing and imaging. The clinician has a tremendous advantage over the radiologist in that the history and examination can focus on specific anatomic details that may not otherwise standout.

Plain Films

Lateral flexion and extension films may be the only way to show a dynamic spondylolisthesis. Oblique views are necessary for facet and foraminal anatomy and pars interarticularis fractures (especially in trauma cases). Plain films also indicate the amount and location of spondylitic changes as well as decreased disc height suggesting degenerative changes.

Electromyography/Nerve Conduction Velocity (EMG/NCV)

In a patient who has not undergone prior surgeries, radicular findings can be useful in bolstering a clinical opinion, but lesions on imaging will determine if a surgeon should operate. The main limitation of EMG/NCV is that it can be negative for slowing or denervation even while a painful irritative process that could be relieved by surgery (e.g., a foramenal decompression) remains active. Also, once the resection of the first laminectomy has been performed, the paraspinous EMG is not helpful. EMG/NCV will, however, help rule out more distal or widespread processes confusing the clinical picture (e.g., mononeuritis multiplex with radicular involvement). Similar arguments hold for somatosensory evoked potentials, which for the most part are less useful.

Thermography

On the whole, thermography has not provided more information on low back pain than a good neurologic examination.

Magnetic Resonance Imaging

Magnetic resonance imaging (MRI) has proven exceptionally useful in illustrating soft tissue intrathecal processes and disc herniations. The quality varies tremendously, however, and MRI is poor at illustrating the bony anatomy so important in spine pathology. MRI is most useful in patients who have not undergone prior surgeries. New contrast agents are evolving (e.g., gadolinium) that are useful in delineating recurrent disc (avascular) with scar tissue (vascularized, enhancing, and with a much poorer outcome for reoperation). MRI has been the most useful tool in illustrating pelvic and retroperitoneal processes that can refer to the low back.

Myelography with Computed Tomography

The most definitive study, plain myelography with postmyelogram computed tomography (CT) illustrates the bony features best as well as their relation to the neural elements. This is particularly true in patients who have undergone back operations or who have had fusions. Three-dimensional reconstruction has proven especially useful in patients with fusions, pseudoarthroses, foraminal stenosis, and occult facet and pars fractures. The software varies significantly for three-dimensional studies, and the actual films represent a surface view only, so that quality and utility may vary significantly. Myelogram CT and MRI can be quite complementary in defining of complex cases.

Nerve Blocks

Diagnostic facet and selected root blocks may help confirm clinical and imaging suspicions in a functional manner and support an argument for radiofrequency facet denervation or foramenotomy. Although recent literature has illustrated generic epidural steroid "therapeutic" blocks that are not effective for low back pain, selected root or arachnoiditis cases have still shown some response to steroid root or intrathecal injections.

PSYCHIATRIC VARIABLES

Personality types and disorders as well as cognitive ability determine not only the repertoire and adaptability of patients in dealing with pain, but also the degree of disability. Personality disorders that are most problematic (and which are preexistent to the low back pain syndrome) include histrionism, dependence, passive-aggressiveness, and borderline and antisocial personalities. Limited cognitive resources also decrease coping strategies.

Mood abnormalities and disorders include lifelong dysthymia, adjustment disorder with depressed mood, and major affective (depressive) disorder. Almost all patients with pain syndromes have depressive features, many of them evolved to the point that the patients are responsive to antidepressant medications, which often have serendipitous peripheral benefit on pain mechanisms. Some psychiatric or psychological input is essential to treating these complex, distressed and distressing patients. They often require psychological and psychopharmacologic management while the structural/pathophysiologic aspects are addressed.

ASSESSMENT STRATEGIES

Assessment should be definitive, whether or not the source of the low back pain is surgically approachable or even if the pathology is relatively minor and incongruous with the degree of disability. This enables one to define realistically the surgical, pharmacologic, and psychiatric strategies.

Although each work-up is guided by clinical judgment, the following generalizations can be made:

1. In clinically suspicious cases, the combination of plain films and regular MRI gives excellent data about both bony and soft tissues, and thus may guide further work-up or answer any questions regarding a surgical lesion.
2. In patients with failed backs, plain films followed directly by three-dimensional CT myelogram are the best diagnostic tools. If there is a question of scar versus recurrent disc herniation, a gadolinium MRI may be helpful with blocks useful in facet/root pathologies.
3. The more complex the diagnostic process and the more psychologically disabled the patient, the more desirable it is to assess and treat the patient in a chronic pain diagnostic unit or "Pain Treatment Center."
4. Many patients with chronic low back pain or a failed back syndrome are already taking narcotics or other addicting medications (e.g., benzodiazepines) at the time of presentation. Maintaining them on these medications during the diagnostic work-up is reasonable. Then once the pathology has been defined, decisions can be made regarding surgery, permanent blocks, and pharmacologic intervention. For detoxification of high-dose narcotics and benzodiazepines and/or addicting medications used over a long period of time, it is often necessary to hospitalize patients in an Inpatient Pain Treatment Center with psychiatric expertise.
5. Tricyclics, especially the lesser anticholinergics (e.g., nortriptyline hydrochloride and desipramine hydrochloride), are useful for peripheral pain. These should be started at low doses and increased slowly. Although pain may be alleviated with low doses, the dosage may need to be increased to typical antidepressant serum levels. The nontricyclic antidepressants are less useful except for an affective component. Carbamazepine, clonazepam, and phenytoin are useful for neuritic and radicular symptoms.
6. Posterior column stimulators may be quite useful in the treatment of arachnoiditis and focal multilevel scarring. In some cases, morphine pumps are useful in moderating pain. Thalamic stimulators may be most useful in patients with "central pain" states. All of these should be used in the setting of a controlled protocol and multidisciplinary workup.

ATHEROTHROMBOTIC CEREBROVASCULAR DISEASE

ALASTAIR BUCHAN, M.D., FRCPC
VLADIMIR HACHINSKI, M.D., D.Sc., FRCPC

DEFINITIONS

Cerebral ischemia can be either focal (i.e., in an arterial territory) or global, implying hypoperfusion of the entire brain. Ischemia is a reduction of cerebral blood flow either locally or globally. The outcome of ischemia depends on the severity of the reduced blood flow and its duration. Histologically, selective neuronal necrosis may occur after even brief periods of global ischemia, and after focal ischemia there may be regions of pan-necrosis in the territory of the affected artery.

The symptoms of ischemia define its location, severity, and duration. Patients may present with transient ischemic attacks, a progressing stroke, or a completed stroke. Although a *transient ischemic attack (TIA)* has by tradition been defined as symptoms of ischemia that last for 24 hours or less, most true TIAs that do not cause cerebral infarction last a few minutes and probably less than 1 hour. Deficits lasting longer than 1 hour are increasingly likely to be associated with cerebral infarction, although the patient may make a complete symptomatic recovery. *Minor stroke* and TIA are similar in terms of etiology and outcome, and for the purposes of treatment and investigation can be considered to be the same. *Progressing stroke* is an observed deterioration after the initial insult that can occur for as long as 48 hours if the stroke affects the anterior circulation and sometimes for as long as 96 hours in those of the posterior circulation. Progression is seen in about half of those patients whose stroke is partial at the outset. In a *partial stroke,* only a portion of the arterial territory has been afflicted, while in a progressing stroke, further thrombosis is occurring. A *completed stroke* occurs if the entire cerebral tissue perfused by an artery (e.g., the middle cerebral artery) is damaged at the onset of the stroke or if a partial stroke progresses to completion. Deterioration, however, may have several causes (Table 1) and should not be assumed to be the result of progressive thrombosis.

CAUSES

The causes of TIAs and stroke are best thought of in an anatomic context. They are embolic, resulting from either cardiac lesions, major arterial lesions (most commonly atherosclerotic disease at the carotid bifurcation), and (rarely) intracranial lesions such as aneurysm or arteriovenous malformation (AVM), which can give rise to distal embolization. Focal ischemia may also arise from small vessel disease or from diseases that promote a hypercoagulable state (e.g., the paradoxical lupus anticoagulant).

Episodes of hemodynamic ischemia may occur in watershed territories in the cortex between anterior, middle, and posterior cerebral artery territories and are being recognized increasingly in the white matter.

MANAGEMENT DIAGNOSIS

When the patient is admitted, a clear-cut diagnosis is necessary as to location, both in terms of central nervous system structure and the location of the vascular lesion. The clinical syndrome is then classified as a transient ischemic attack, a minor stroke which may become a progressive stroke or even a completed stroke. Investigations are based on the clinical evaluation, and include both essential routine investigations and "special" investigations that are needed to answer specific questions (Table 2).

A computed tomographic (CT) scan should be performed as soon as possible to rule out hemorrhage or an unsuspected space-occupying lesion that may mimic the sudden deficit resulting from vascular disease. Subsequent serial CT scans and magnetic resonance images (MRIs) are obtained if the location, existence, or nature of a lesion is in doubt. Frequent sensory symptoms result from seizures, hence the occasional need for an electroencephalogram (EEG), or from thalamic dysfunction, which is best demonstrated by MRI. In most instances, CT ensures that there is no hemorrhage or hemorrhagic conversion of an infarct and can demonstrate the evolution of the new lesion, or in the case of a TIA, the absence of cerebral infarction.

As can be seen in Table 2, most of the investigations revolve around the cause of the cerebral ischemia; although a careful clinical examination, normal chest x-ray examination, and electrocardiography might exclude the vast majority of potential cardiac emboli, we routinely perform echocardiography since it is cheap and noninvasive and since a large proportion of patients with cerebral ischemia have a source of cardiac emboli. Still more patients have coexistent coronary artery disease, even if their stroke is not related to abnormal structure and function of the heart. Only if there are paradoxical

TABLE 1 Causes of Deterioration in Stroke

Cerebral factors
- Infarction
  - Cerebral edema
  - Hemorrhagic infarction
  - Recurrent embolism
  - Progressive thrombosis
- (Postictal states)

Hemorrhage
- Cerebral edema
- Rebleeding
- Acute hydrocephalus
- (Postictal states)

Systemic factors
- Cardiac
  - Heart failure
  - Cardiac arrhythmias
- Pulmonary
  - Pneumonia
  - Pulmonary embolism
- Metabolic
  - Renal/hepatic failure
  - Syndrome of inappropriate antidiuretic hormone
  - Septicemia
  - Psychological
  - Drug use

TABLE 2 Investigations for Stroke

Affected Area	*Routine*	*Special*
Central nervous system	CT	MRI Lumbar puncture EEG
Vessels	Doppler	Angiography
Heart	ECG CXR Echocardiography	LV Wall Catheter Holter monitor
Systemic	CBC ESR VDRL Glucose Lipids Urea Liver function tests Urinanalysis	As needed

CBC = complete blood count; CXR = chest x-ray examination; ECG = electrocardiography; ESR = erythrocyte sedimentation rate; LV = left ventricle; VDRL = syphilis serology.

emboli through a patent atrial septal defect or the suggestion of dyskinesis on the echocardiogram do we go on to perform radionuclear angiography or angio-catheterization. In patients who have severe carotid artery disease as a cause of their cerebral symptoms (rather than heart disease), it may well be prudent to perform coronary stress tests, especially if the patient complains of angina.

Cerebral vessels are imaged in a variety of ways. Contrast-enhanced CT scans and MRI are indirect ways of looking for intracranial emboli and thrombosis. Although ultrasonography has proved to be a useful screening test for carotid artery disease, the use of transcranial doppler cannot yet be fully recommended. Cerebral angiography is the surest way of defining vascular lesions in both the extracranial and intracranial circulation. It allows us to see not only potential arterial sources of emboli, but if performed acutely, may show the distal occlusions. Patients with branch occlusions or hung-up vessels who have no arterial disease can then be investigated intensively from a cardiologic and hematologic standpoint. Hematologic tests are ordered on clinical suspicions, but a complete blood count, erythrocyte sedimentation rate, prothrombin time, partial thromboblastin time, VDRL, fasting glucose, and lipids are all deemed essential.

TREATMENT

Asymptomatic patients who are seen because of potential embolic sources such as atrial fibrillation or carotid stenosis are evaluated and treated for their risk factors. If appropriate, they are entered into prospective studies.

Transient Ischemic Attack

Patients who have been evaluated for a TIA or a minor stroke are treated with platelet anti-aggregants once cardiac and hematologic causes have been excluded. The arteries are then visualized with cerebral angiography, and if there is occlusive extracranial carotid disease appropriate to the symptom, and if there is no intracranial disease, these patients are then seen in consultation with either a vascular surgeon or a neurosurgeon. Carotid endarterectomy is an unproven prophylaxis against stroke in the ipsilateral territory, and we currently enter all of our appropriate patients into the North American Symptomatic Carotid Endarterectomy Trial (NASCET). We do not believe that there is any indication to operate on patients outside the study, (i.e., if they do not meet study criteria); we think it best that they be treated medically. There is no indication for prophylactic extracranial-intracranial bypass.

Aspirin, through its ability to acetylate platelet cyclooxygenase, thereby blocking thromboxane A_2 synthesis, inhibits platelet aggregation. Although the trials performed in patients with TIA and minor stroke have yielded mixed results, the overview as published by the antiplatelet trialists suggests through meta-analysis that there is a marked reduction in the risk of stroke or death for those patients treated with platelet anti-aggregants. New trials using Ticlopodine hydrochloride suggest that this agent is superior to aspirin, but the drug has not yet been approved by the Food and Drug Administration. Only in those patients whose carotid TIAs are uncontrolled by aspirin or whose angiography reveals intraluminal thrombus do we proceed to anticoagulation, initially with heparin and subsequent maintenance with warfarin sodium crystalline (Coumadin).

Completed Stroke

The treatment of completed stroke is essentially the prevention of further episodes, the detection and treatment of any complications, and ensuring that a complete cardiologic assessment has been made. Neurologically the only treatment that can be offered is supportive and rehabilitative. The prevention of recurrent stroke is essentially that of prevention after minor stroke or a TIA with the proviso that if the stroke is devastating, angiography, surgery, or anticoagulation should probably not be performed.

Progressive Stroke

Progressive stroke afflicts perhaps 30 to 40 percent of all patients being admitted urgently. It is essential to define the location and nature of the process. Although there are no good prospective trials assessing treatment for the progressing stroke, in the absence of contraindications such as hemorrhagic conversion on the CT, uncontrolled hypertension, or a potential source of hemorrhage, one may consider careful anticoagulation. However, the data supporting this are weak, and although a recent double-blind trial purported to show that there was no significant difference between those treated with heparin and those treated with placebo, the therapy was delayed until the stroke had been stabilized for at least 24 hours, negating the suggestion that heparin was not indicated in progressing stroke. Patients who have a partial stroke, particularly if they are progressing, can be treated with anticoagulation with minimal risk. The treatment of progressing stroke is limited to considering anticoagulation. Interestingly there are no studies to show the effects of aspirin on progressing stroke.

If angiography demonstrates intraluminal thrombus, then although the decision is empirical, we usually anticoagulate for at least the short-term before restudying the patient.

Complete Stroke

If there is a complete stroke, anticoagulation is of no benefit unless the stroke is of cardiogenic origin, in which case anticoagulation is performed after a 72-hour interval to ensure that spontaneous hemorrhagic conversion does not occur.

Hyperacute Stroke

Perhaps of most interest is the management of the patient with a hyperacute stroke. CT scanning and MRI or rapidly obtained angiography allow visualization not only of the brain but also of the vessels and the disease process underlying the deficit. Two strategies are currently being investigated: on the one hand, the return of cerebral perfusion through the use of a new generation of thrombolytic drugs such as *tissue plasminogen activator,* and on the other, the return of cerebral function through the treatment of ischemic tissue itself with both *calcium channel blockers* and *glutamate antagonists.* There may also be some scope during reperfusion for *lipid peroxidation inhibitors,* and during the recovery phase, for gangliosides.

Although hyperacute treatment of atherothrombotic cerebrovascular disease is still in the experimental stages, an understanding of the natural history of the acute stroke during the first 24 hours is evolving. A determined attempt is being made to learn how to manage patients with stroke more swiftly. Only through the development of such programs will it be possible to evaluate patients promptly so that active intervention can be attempted before the stroke is completed.

From clinical studies we now know that most patients with TIAs recover in less than an hour—an important fact given that treating TIAs with thrombolytic agents would be wholly undesirable. Angiography during the first 3 hours demonstrates that as many as 80 percent of patients will have evidence of embolic phenomena in the cerebral circulation. Two safety studies with tissue plasminogen activator are underway, one employing intravenous administration after CT but without angiography, and the other involving an arterial infusion of TPA after selective angiography. Both studies suggest that improvements can be achieved, but neither study has as yet involved a controlled group. The development of cytoprotective agents that block voltage-sensitive calcium channels (such as nimodipine) and glutamate-gated calcium channels (such as MK-801) mean that a combination of thrombolytic and cytoprotective agents may be used to resuscitate cerebral tissue. At present, however, these experimental strategies are not employed except under the auspices of experimental protocols.

It is not known whether aspirin on its own may be useful acutely, but we do have information suggesting that hemodilution, steroids, and barbituates are unnecessary. It makes sense to ensure that the blood pressure is judiciously stabilized and that the patient is normoglycemic. There is no evidence to suggest a deliberate reduction of blood sugar with insulin, unless hyperglycemia is producing hyperosmolar or ketotic states. At present, we have no reason to suggest that drugs such as mannitol should be given to prevent the formation of cytotoxic edema. If the stroke goes on to be large with consequent swelling of the hemisphere, the control of raised intracranial pressure with hyperventilation and mannitol may prove life-saving but we cannot recommend hemicraniectomies.

Cerebral venous stroke is now increasingly diagnosed with MRI showing sagittal and other sinus thromboses. Provided that significant cerebral hemorrhage is excluded, early anticoagulation is warranted and is effective in reducing the risk of both morbidity and mortality.

SUGGESTED READING

Anti-platelet Trialists Collaboration. Secondary prevention of vascular disease by prolonged anti-platelet treatment. Br Med J 1988; 296:320–331.

Buchan AM, Gates P, Pelz D, Barnett HJM. Intraluminal thrombus in the cerebral circulation. Stroke 1988; 19:681–687.

Cerebral Embolism Study Group. Brain hemorrhage and embolic stroke. Stroke 1984; 15:779–789.

Chambers BR, Norris JW, Shurvell B, Hachinski V. Prognosis of acute stroke. Neurology 1987; 37:221–225.

Delzopo G, Zeumer H, Harker L. Thrombolytic therapy in stroke: possibility and hazards. Stroke 1986; 17:595–607.

Duke RJ, Bloch RF, Turpie AGG, et al. Intravenous heparin for the prevention of stroke progression in acute partial stable stroke: a randomized controlled trial. Ann Int Med 1986; 105:825–828.

The EC/IC Bypass Study Group. Failure of extracranial-intracranial bypass to reduce the risk of ischemic stroke: results of an international randomized trial. New Engl J Med 1985; 313:1191–1200.

Levy DE. How transient are transient ischemic attacks. Neurology 1988; 38:674–677.

World Health Organization. Recommendations on stroke prevention: diagnosis and therapy. Stroke 1989; 20:1407–1431.

PATIENT RESOURCES

American Heart Association
7320 Greenville Avenue
Dallas, Texas 75231

Canadian Heart and Stroke Foundation
160 George Street, Suite 200
Ottawa, Ontario
Canada K1N 9M2

The Chest, Heart, and Stroke Association
Tavistock House North
Tavistock Square, London
United Kingdom WC1H 9JE

CAROTID ARTERY OCCLUSIVE DISEASE

THOMAS F. DODSON, M.D.
ROBERT B. SMITH III, M.D.

The majority of transient ischemic attacks (TIAs) and cerebrovascular accidents are thought to result from the embolization of material from ulcerated plaques in the carotid bifurcation, or from reduced regional blood flow related to a severely stenotic or occluded internal carotid artery. Over the past 30 years, carotid endarterectomy has become a widely accepted, generally effective, and relatively safe operation for prophylactic intervention in the stroke-prone patient. It is the most common vascular surgical procedure with more than 100,000 such operations performed yearly in the United States.

The surgical approach to atherosclerosis of the carotid artery is among the most controversial topics in medicine and surgery. Although the incidence of cardiovascular disease and cerebrovascular accidents is declining, there are still approximately 500,000 new stroke victims in the United States each year, and death occurs within the first 30 days after stroke in 40 percent of the patients. Although we have gained a great deal of information about carotid artery occlusive disease since the first carotid operations in the mid-1950s, the natural history of carotid disease is still not well-known. To better elucidate important clinical features in these patients, prospective randomized trials of carotid endarterectomy are now in progress but will not be completed for several years. In the meantime, physicians must respond to their patients' needs in a rational, consistent manner. The clinical problems of the asymptomatic patient with a carotid bruit, the symptomatic patient with TIAs or amaurosis fugax, and the symptomatic patient with a completed stroke comprise the majority of carotid-related problems that physicians must evaluate. Management perspectives of each of these conditions are presented in the following sections.

THERAPEUTIC ALTERNATIVES

In the case of atherosclerotic occlusive disease of the carotid bifurcation, the therapeutic alternatives are limited. Essentially, the choice is between carotid endarterectomy and medical therapy, as there are no other practical or safe treatment modalities. Extracranial-intracranial arterial bypasses are seldom performed today and direct disobliteration of the chronically occluded internal carotid is not a feasible approach. Remote interventional techniques such as transluminal balloon dilation, laser angioplasty, or intra-arterial atherectomy, all approaches that are used currently in other segments of the arterial system, are not suitable for use in the carotid artery because of the high risk of procedure-related embolization. Medical therapy requires a choice between antiplatelet medications such as aspirin and dipyridamole versus short-term heparin and long-term sodium warfarin (Coumadin) anticoagulation. Cessation of tobacco use, control of hypertension, and reduction of elevated serum cholesterol levels are forms of "medical therapy," but they are important steps that also should be taken in surgically treated patients.

PREFERRED APPROACH

Asymptomatic Patient with a Carotid Bruit

It is well-known that the mere presence of a carotid bruit does not signify hemodynamically significant carotid disease in one-half of patients. The converse is also true: patients with a hemodynamically significant lesion in their internal carotid artery have bruits only about one-half of the time. Although physician trainees are taught that auscultation of the carotids, the abdomen, and the area of the femoral arteries is an important part of the vascular exam, a bruit is an imprecise measure of the degree of stenosis of the underlying vessel. If a carotid bruit is detected, however, the next step should be an evaluation of the patient by duplex scanning of the carotid bifurcation. Whereas oculopneumoplethysmography (OPG) was formerly the noninvasive procedure of choice to evaluate carotid flow, it has now been largely supplanted by ultrasound technology. At the present time, ultrasonography results are categorized as follows: 1 to 39 percent stenosis is considered minimal; 40 to 59 percent stenosis is considered mild; 60 to 79 percent stenosis is considered moderate; and 80 to 99 percent stenosis is considered severe. These categories allow the physician to make an informed decision concerning proceeding with additional diagnostic studies. Experience from the University of Washington in Seattle suggests that the great majority of strokes, TIAs, and carotid thromboses are preceded by disease progression to an 80 percent stenosis, or greater. Additional information pertaining to plaque morphology, also obtainable at the time of ultrasonography, may be helpful in the decision process since a greater risk of symptoms correlates with plaques of lower density or heterogeneous composition.

In those asymptomatic patients shown to have severe stenosis (80 to 99 percent) by duplex scan, the next step is to recommend arch aortography with four-vessel arteriography. Even a lesser degree of stenosis of one internal carotid warrants angiography if the opposite internal carotid is totally occluded. The carotid system is studied to its terminal intracranial branches to gain complete information concerning both extracranial and intracranial lesions. Ordinarily this portion of the work-up is performed on an inpatient basis, although some centers are equipped to perform outpatient cerebral arteriography on selected patients. As a routine part of the complete evaluation, computed tomography (CT) of the brain is also done to detect the presence of unsuspected areas of infarction and to rule out other intracranial pathology. When CT of the head shows evidence of cerebral infarction, the patient is considered "symptomatic" and is transferred into the TIA management group.

In the majority of cases, angiography confirms the noninvasive duplex scan findings. If the carotid lumen is encroached by 80 percent or more, or if the lesion is severely ulcerated or irregular, operation should be considered (Hertzer, et al, 1984). As a regular part of preoperative preparation, cardiologic consultation is obtained to help assess the patient's perioperative risks. Approximately 50 percent of patients with asymptomatic carotid disease have significant coronary atherosclerosis, and myocardial infarction continues to be the most common cause of death in the early postoperative period. If there is any concern about the possibility of myocardial ischemia, a dipyridamole-thallium scintigraphy examination is performed to evaluate myocardial perfusion. A recent report from the Brigham and Women's Hospital in Boston suggests that preoperative electrocardiographic monitoring may be equally as effective as the dipyridamole-thallium test at greatly reduced cost.

Once an assessment of the cardiac risks of the procedure has been made and other factors such as underlying pulmonary disease, renal dysfunction, and uncontrolled hypertension have been addressed, a decision can be made regarding the patient's suitability for prophylactic carotid endarterectomy. The patient is then fully informed concerning the risks and uncertainties of operative intervention versus those associated with medical therapy. Based on the work of Roederer et al (1984) from Seattle, the risk of nonoperative therapy in patients with 80 percent or greater carotid stenosis is quite high: 35 percent of such patients had a stroke, TIA, or carotid occlusion within 6 months of the discovery of the lesion, and 45 percent had similar events within 1 year. In the otherwise good-risk patient, that course can be contrasted with our own figures of less than 1 percent operative mortality and approximately 1 percent perioperative stroke rate in asymptomatic patients. This is obviously the most important key to the puzzle: being able to offer patients who are asymptomatic an operation that has an extremely low morbidity and mortality rate, yet one that will favorably alter their risk of serious symptomatology or premature death over the ensuing years. With respect to the long-term outcome, our own statistics and those of others suggest that following operation the patient has an annual 1 percent risk of stroke in the ipsilateral cerebral hemisphere. In fact, in patients with bilateral carotid disease, the risk of stroke is five times greater in the unoperated side over time.

If the patient accepts carotid endarterectomy, operation is performed during the same admission, usually 1 day following the angiogram. Individuals with heart disease or evidence of myocardial ischemia have a Swan-Ganz catheter inserted to assess filling pressures and left ventricular function, and all patients have placement of a radial artery cannula for constant monitoring of blood pressure. The choice of anesthesia for carotid endarterectomy is variable in our institution. Patients who are at high risk for cardiac or pulmonary complications are usually done under monitored local anesthesia with minimal sedation. This form of anesthesia has the advantage of reducing the wide blood pressure fluctuations commonly associated with general anesthesia, and it also allows an exquisitely sensitive method of monitoring the patient neurologically during the operation. General anesthesia, on the other hand, reduces the metabolic demands of the brain while increasing cerebral perfusion, and it allows for a quiet surgical field. If general anesthesia is used, cerebral function is monitored by computed electroencephalography. Contraindications to local anesthesia are: (1) previous carotid surgery, (2) high carotid lesions requiring extended exposure, and (3) poor patient compliance.

Although only 15 to 20 percent of patients require placement of a shunt during carotid endarterectomy based upon observed responses during local anesthesia, the authors prefer to insert a shunt in all cases. The only exception to this preference would be anatomic constraints encountered at the time of operation. Since we routinely shunt, the EEG's chief value is to assess the adequacy of flow through the shunt. An EEG that shows loss of amplitude or slowing of rhythm may indicate shunt dysfunction or occlusion.

All patients are admitted to the Intensive Care Unit (ICU) after operation for overnight observation and monitoring. During the stay in the ICU, systemic blood pressure and neurologic status are carefully followed. The neck incision is also observed for development of an enlarging hematoma. Once the patient is released to the floor, the hospital stay is usually for another 3 to 4 days. All who can tolerate aspirin are instructed to take 80 mg per day on a permanent basis. Follow-up plans include office visits at 6 weeks, 6 months, and 1 year, with annual assessments thereafter. A carotid duplex scan is performed annually if the patient remains asymptomatic and is not shown to have a rapidly progressive recurrent stenosis. Patients with hemodynamically significant bilateral disease have staged operations, typically undergoing the second procedure 1 to 2 months after the first. At follow-up visits subjects are reminded to report new central nervous system symptoms or the reappearance of old deficits very promptly. They are also instructed to reduce known risk factors (smoking, hypertension, elevated cholesterol) as much as possible.

Symptomatic Patient with Transient Ischemic Attacks or Amaurosis Fugax

The presence of symptomatology adds a degree of urgency to the evaluation of carotid disease patients. Prospective studies in the literature indicate that patients experiencing TIAs have a risk of stroke of about 35 percent at 5 years, and that 50 percent of these strokes occur within the first year after the onset of symptoms (Wiebers and Whisnant, 1982). In light of these statistics, a TIA is a strong indicator of stroke risk. Accordingly, this clinical presentation has become the most widely accepted indication for operative intervention in patients with carotid artery occlusive disease.

The definition of a TIA is not uniform among disciplines treating patients with carotid disease; it is generally described as a focal neurologic deficit that usually lasts only minutes, but in all cases it resolves within 24 hours without residual neurologic deficit. The 24-hour limit for resolution of symptomatology must be acknowledged as arbitrary, bearing no known relationship to the underlying pathophysiology. Also important to remember is that the risk of myocardial infarction is quite high among patients who suffer from TIAs. Thus, an episode of cerebral ischemia should be interpreted as a warning signal of diffuse atherosclerosis.

With these factors in mind, when confronted with a patient who states that within the recent past he or she has experienced a brief loss of sensation or motor function of the face, arm, or leg, or is reported by an observer to have suffered a brief episode of inability to speak (aphasia) or even a short period of impairment of speech (dysphasia), the physician should infer that the clinical symptoms indicate a transient loss of blood supply to an area of the cortex. Another common presentation is the patient who reports a "shade" descending over the eye for a few seconds or minutes, suggesting a diagnosis of transient monocular blindness or amaurosis fugax. In symptomatic patients, we strongly suggest prompt admission to the hospital for carotid assessment and complete neurologic evaluation.

Although the most common etiology for TIAs is atherothrombotic disease in the cervical portion of the carotid artery, a host of other disease processes can be responsible for similar symptomatology. Other less common etiologies include spontaneous dissection of the carotid artery, temporal arteritis, fibromuscular dysplasia, vasculitis, coagulopathy, and cardiac pathology such as arrhythmias and valvular or ventricular emboli. A helpful clinical indicator is that embolic events from carotid atherothrombotic disease tend to be similar in repetitive episodes, whereas emboli from a cardiac source tend to be more variable in presentation. Other disease processes can masquerade as a TIA, including migraine, focal seizures, hypoglycemia, orthostatic hypotension, and simple fainting. During the patient's stay in the hospital these other potential diagnoses are considered while the primary focus of attention is directed toward the extracranial carotid circulation. As a routine part of the vascular examination, consultation is sought from the cardiology department to assess myocardial function. Since cardiac pathology may be an important part of the differential diagnosis, the cardiologist plays a significant role in the assessment of patients with TIAs. Neurologic consultation is also requested to assist in the interpretation of neurologic symptoms and help to exclude other nonvascular neurologic disorders.

Just as in the patient who is asymptomatic, initial examinations are noninvasive and designed to provide baseline information without discomfort or risk to the patient. Thus, among the early studies are duplex ultrasound scanning of both carotids and CT of the brain, the latter preferably with contrast. If the carotid ultrasound is entirely normal and another etiology is discovered for the TIA, we may conclude our workup after CT. On the other hand, if the carotid ultrasound is read as minimal or mild stenosis and no other etiology has been discovered for the patient's neurologic symptoms, four vessel cerebral angiography should be performed in the search for an ulcerated atheroma that may not be identified by duplex scanning. This aggressive diagnostic approach is justified in our institution by an experienced group of neuroradiologists with a low complication rate from cerebral angiography.

If the arteriogram confirms a smooth carotid stenosis of 50 percent or greater, or a lesser degree of stenosis with an ulcerated lesion, carotid endarterectomy is recommended to the patient. Once again, it is recognized that all such decisions are open to controversy, but this approach seems rational to us in light of the data now available. Patients who have experienced TIAs are at slightly greater risk of operative complications than symptomatic patients, but our experience suggests that the risk of death with operation is approximately 1 percent, and the perioperative stroke risk no more than 2 percent. The surgical approach to the symptomatic patient is essentially the same as in the asymptomatic individual. Because of the greater potential for cerebral embolization during dissection of the carotid artery in such circumstances, however, it is important to "dissect the patient from the carotid, rather than the carotid from the patient." Again it should be emphasized that risk factors such as smoking, hypertension, and hypercholesterolemia should be controlled postoperatively, and that the main thrust of care after operation should be educating both patient and family in risk reduction of vascular disease overall. In the case of an asymptomatic, but hemodynamically significant stenosis of the carotid opposite the one requiring endarterectomy for symptoms, surgical care should be consistent with that described in the foregoing section on asymptomatic lesions. Endarterectomy on the second side, if needed, is staged a number of weeks following the initial procedure.

Symptomatic Patient with a Completed Stroke

In 1969 a Joint Study of Extracranial Arterial Occlusion was performed in an attempt to answer some of the questions surrounding early operative intervention in patients with acute neurologic deficits. Of the 50 patients who were operated upon within the first 2 weeks after their acute stroke, 42 percent died; these figures contrasted with a mortality of 20 percent among those treated medically. This study strongly suggested that operation in the acute stroke patient was dangerous and contraindicated. Since that time, additional studies have been published that question the poor results of surgical management of patients with a complete stroke, but just as in other issues related to carotid artery occlusive disease, a consensus would be hard to obtain.

The acute stroke patient is typically a referral from within the hospital or from another hospital. Usually they have already been evaluated by a neurologist and initial diagnostic studies performed. The great majority of strokes are secondary to embolic or thrombotic events, whereas intracranial hemorrhage accounts for about 20 percent of such cases. Thus, the CT of the head is an important first step in the assessment of these patients to rule out intracranial hemorrhage. The next step should be duplex scanning of the carotid bifurcation. If severe occlusive disease is identified, and if the neurologic deficit is small or fluctuating, emergency carotid arteriography is performed. This step is obviously a prelude to possible early operation and would be undertaken only if the patient was felt to be an acceptable surgical candidate. If, on the other hand, the patient is stable and the carotid duplex scan does not indicate severe carotid stenosis, arteriography is delayed for 6 to 8 weeks during which time the patient undergoes supportive treatment and rehabilitation. At that point, he or she is readmitted to assess completeness of recovery and suitability for operative intervention. If a good neurologic recovery has occurred, the patient should be considered for endarterectomy to prevent recurrent ipsilateral strokes. The cardiologist and neurologist are invited to reevaluate their respective systems, and cerebral angiography is performed. If a significant lesion is confirmed by arteriography, carotid endarterectomy is planned during this second admission, 6 to 8 weeks from the initial cerebral event.

There are obvious permutations in the presentation of patients with a completed stroke, but our overall viewpoint is to be relatively aggressive in the patient with a small or fluctuating neurologic deficit and a "dangerous lesion," namely an ultra-tight stenosis or trailing intraluminal thrombus, and to be relatively conservative in patients with severe, fixed neurologic deficits. One major exception to this approach is the patient who undergoes carotid endarterectomy and who has the onset of a neurologic deficit during operation or in the early postoperative period. In this situation, reoperation is undertaken immediately in the effort to restore full internal carotid flow. Such occlusions are likely to be related to a technical error at the time of the initial operation, which may be identified and corrected at the second procedure. Another uncommon exception is the patient who develops an acute stroke in the hospital after having severe carotid disease identified angiographically a short time before. If carotid flow can be restored within 1 to 2 hours from the onset of symptoms, operative intervention should be considered. Some patients have dramatic neurologic clearing after an emergency thromboendarterectomy in this setting, but others fail to respond.

As emphasized at each step in this discussion, surgery for carotid artery occlusive disease is currently a highly controversial topic. Many physicians, particularly those who deal with cardiovascular disorders are confronted daily by patients with evidence of disease in the extracranial carotid circulation. It is not enough to say simply that we do not yet know the correct answers to all their problems. Each patient must be managed as an individual with compassion and candor, weighing the expected natural history of the disease against the risks inherent in surgical therapy. We have confidence in the system of care described but realize that all modes of therapy are subject to change as new data become available.

SUGGESTED READING

Blaisdell WF, Clauss RH, Galbraith JG, et al. Joint Study of Extracranial Arterial Occlusion. JAMA 1969; 209:1889.

Chambers BR, Norris JW. Outcome in patients with asymptomatic neck bruits. N Engl J Med 1986; 315:860.

Healy DA, Clowes AW, Zierler RE, et al. Immediate and long-term results of carotid endarterectomy. Stroke 1989; 20:49.

Hertzer NR, Beven EG, Young JR, et al. Coronary artery disease in peripheral vascular patients: A classification of 1000 coronary angiograms and results of surgical management. Ann Surg 1984; 199:223.

Johnson JM, Kennelly MM, Decesare D. Natural history of asymptomatic carotid plaque. Arch Surg 1985; 120:1010.

Meissner I, Wiebers DO, Whisnant JP, et al. The natural history of asymptomatic carotid artery occlusive lesions. JAMA 1987; 258:2704.

Mohr JP, Caplan LR, Melski JW, et al. The Harvard Cooperative Stoke Registry: A prospective registry. Neurology 1978; 28:754.

Moore WS. Indications for carotid endarterectomy. In: Moore WS, ed. Surgery for cerebrovascular disease. New York: Churchill-Livingstone, 1987:439.

Roederer GO, Langlois YE, Jager KA, et al. The natural history of carotid arterial disease in asymptomatic patients with cervical bruits. Stroke 1984; 15:605.

Rutherford RB, Patt A. Carotid endarterectomy following acute stroke: Must we always wait? Sem Vasc Surg 1989; 2:49.

Towne JB, Weiss DG, Hobson RW. First phase report of Cooperative Veterans Administration Asymptomatic Carotid Stenosis

Study—operative morbidity and mortality. J Vasc Surg 1990; 11:252.
Wallace DC. A study of the natural history of cerebral vascular disease. Med J Aust 1967; 1:90.
Wiebers DO, Whisnant JP. In: Warlow C, Morris PJ, eds. Transient ischemic attacks. New York: Marcel Dekker, 1982:8.
Winslow CM, Solomon DH, Chassin MR, et al. The appropriateness of carotid endarterectomy. N Engl J Med 1988; 318:721.

TRANSIENT ISCHEMIC ATTACK

JOSÉ BILLER, M.D.
HAROLD P. ADAMS Jr., M.D.

A transient ischemic attack (TIA) is an important predictor of the subsequent development of a stroke. If no therapy is instituted, cerebral infarction develops in one-third of patients with TIAs. The interval since the most recent TIA appears to be the single most important factor in forecasting the risk of cerebral infarction. Of those patients who will have a cerebral infarction, half do so within 1 year after a transient ischemic attack and approximately one-fifth during the first few months of follow-up. The rate of recurrence of TIAs or the risk of stroke during the first few days after a TIA is not clearly established, but appears to be greatest during this time. Because the risk of stroke cannot be predicted by the number of TIAs, the duration of symptoms, or the type of TIA, all patients are considered at risk, and those with recent onset (within the last 10 days) should be evaluated on an urgent basis. Likewise, although it is clear that TIAs are strong predictors of stroke, several studies have shown that myocardial infarction is the most common cause of death in these patients, accounting for a mortality rate of 5 percent per year.

DIAGNOSIS

The diagnosis of TIA is made on the basis of the history obtained from the patient or any observer. A TIA is characterized by a short-lived episode of focal, nonconvulsive loss of function caused by the reversible interference of the blood supply to an area of the retina or brain. Onset is abrupt and usually unprovoked, reaching maximal intensity almost immediately. A TIA usually persists for 2 to 20 minutes and only rarely for as long as 24 hours. An episode that lasts a few seconds is probably not a TIA. The 24-hour time frame that differentiates a TIA from an infarction is imprecise and does not reflect the mechanisms responsible for the development of transient focal brain ischemia. A TIA is part of the spectrum of ischemic stroke that includes events that produce neurologic signs that persist for more than 24 hours but resolve within 3 weeks: "reversible ischemic neurologic deficit" (RIND) and partial, nondisabling infarction. These conditions should be viewed as different expressions of the same dynamic process with probably similar underlying pathophysiology, and therefore investigations and treatment for each condition are essentially alike.

The symptoms of a TIA are outlined in Table 1.

TABLE 1 Symptoms of TIAs

Transient Focal Neurologic Deficits	*Symptoms: Carotid Artery Territory*	*Symptoms: Vertebrobasilar Artery Territory**
Motor deficit	Contralateral weakness, clumsiness or paralysis (primarily hands and face)	Bilateral or shifting weakness, clumsiness or paralysis Ataxia, imbalance or dysequilibrium not associated with vertigo
Sensory deficit	Contralateral numbness, paresthesias (including loss of sensation—primarily of hands and face)	Bilateral or shifting numbness, paresthesias (including loss of sensation)
Speech/language deficit	Dysphasia, dysarthria	Dysarthria
Visual deficit	Ipsilateral monocular blindness (amaurosis fugax), contralateral homonymous hemianopia	Diplopia, partial or complete blindness in both homonymous visual fields
Other	Combination of the above	Combination of the above

* Transient vertigo, diplopia, dysarthria, or dysphagia by themselves are insufficient to establish a diagnosis of vertebrobasilar artery territory TIA.

Because there is a differential diagnosis for TIAs, we refer to these symptoms as transient focal neurologic deficits and bear in mind that there are a variety of other conditions (i.e., seizures, neoplasms, arteriovenous malformations, subdural hematomas, metabolic derangements, demyelinating conditions, migraines, and vestibulopathies) that share these symptoms, mimicking TIAs. If the initiation or resolution of symptoms of a transient neurologic event is indistinct, the diagnosis of TIA should be questioned. A migration or "march" of symptoms from one body part to another is rare during a TIA and suggests a focal seizure or a migraine. Positive phenomena such as visual scintillations, fortification spectra, involuntary movements, or "seizurelike" activity are unusual during a TIA, as are loss of consciousness, confusion, sphincter incontinence, isolated episodic vertigo or wooziness, or drop-attacks. Although TIAs are often referred as "painless" episodes, headache occurs in approximately one-fifth of patients and is occipital in location with vertebrobasilar events, and hemicranial with carotid circulation TIAs.

Identification of the involved arterial territory influences investigation and management. Because of the several mechanisms responsible for the development of TIAs, we strive to determine the primary pathophysiologic mechanism of each case. Most patients with TIAs have atherosclerotic lesions of the carotid or vertebrobasilar arteries, and the mechanisms of ischemia are the result of either artery-to-artery embolization of atherosclerotic debris or fibrin-platelet emboli, or are hemodynamic disturbances causing focal hypoperfusion in areas of compromised circulation. Cardiac-to-artery embolism, small vessel (lacunar) disease, nonatherosclerotic vasculopathies, and a variety of hypercoagulable states account for the remainder of TIAs. Evaluation of a patient is aimed at excluding other conditions that may be causing the neurologic symptoms, establishing the mechanisms of the ischemic symptoms, and determining the presence of codeveloping vascular diseases. The neurologic, neurovascular, and cardiovascular examinations are emphasized. Between TIAs, the neurologic examination will be normal. Ophthalmoscopic examination may detect embolic retinal particles. An audible cervical bruit may be the first indication of extracranial atherosclerotic vascular disease. A cervical bruit ipsilateral to a carotid TIA is suggestive of an underlying arterial disease. Auscultation of the orbit, temple, or mastoid may disclose a bruit in a patient with stenosis of an intracranial artery. However, there is poor correlation between a bruit and underlying carotid stenosis. A bruit and atypical symptoms are not sufficient for diagnosing a carotid TIA. The absence of a bruit does not mean that the carotid artery is normal. The cardiac examination concentrates on the detection of structural cardiac lesions or rhythm abnormalities that may potentially account for the patient's symptoms. The blood pressure is measured in both arms. Orthostatic blood pressure changes are sought.

Figure 1 summarizes our approach to the diagnosis and management of patients with TIAs. Computed tomographic (CT) evaluation should be done in all patients because it detects hemorrhagic or mass lesions that can present as a TIA. The majority of TIA patients have a normal CT, although hypodense lesions are often found, particularly among those with protracted (>1 hour) events. Patients with TIAs should have a complete blood cell count with differential and platelet count, which may identify an underlying polycythemia or thrombocytosis. Coagulation studies including prothrombin time and activated partial thromboplastin time should also be performed. An abnormally prolonged, activated partial thromboplastin time that does not correct with the addition of normal plasma (1:1 mixing) suggests a circulating anticoagulant. The association between a circulating anticoagulant and clinical thrombosis should lead to the determination of antiphospholipid antibodies. Other investigations include serologic tests for syphilis, erythrocyte sedimendation rate, blood glucose, and lipid profile. Selected patients are evaluated for tests of platelet hyperfunction (platelet aggregation, circulating platelet aggregates, platelet factor IV activity, and platelet survival studies), antithrombin-III levels, protein-C levels, protein-S levels, fibrinogen, and hemoglobin electrophoresis.

Patients with TIAs should undergo chest roentgenography and baseline electrocardiography. Echocardiography and Holter monitoring are low-yield screening procedures that should be reserved for patients with clinical clues of cardiac disease. Noninvasive neurovascular testing in patients with TIAs is controversial. We use duplex scanning in combination with pressure oculoplethysmography as a complement to, although not as a replacement for, arteriography. These studies can be valuable during the follow-up evaluation.

Cerebral arteriography remains the most accurate means of determining the extent and site of atherosclerotic lesions. Selective cerebral arteriography is necessary to evaluate reliably the intracranial vasculature or to detect tandem large arterial lesions. Arteriography is not without complications. The risk of developing any complication (half of which are minor groin hematomas) is approximately 1 to 5 percent. The risk of developing permanent neurologic disability is 0.2 percent, whereas the risk of death is approximately 0.05 percent. Intra-arterial digital subtraction angiography (IA-DSA) provides adequate resolution for detection of extracranial disease and is generally useful for evaluating the intracranial circulation. IA-DSA is more economic than conventional film screen angiography and requires

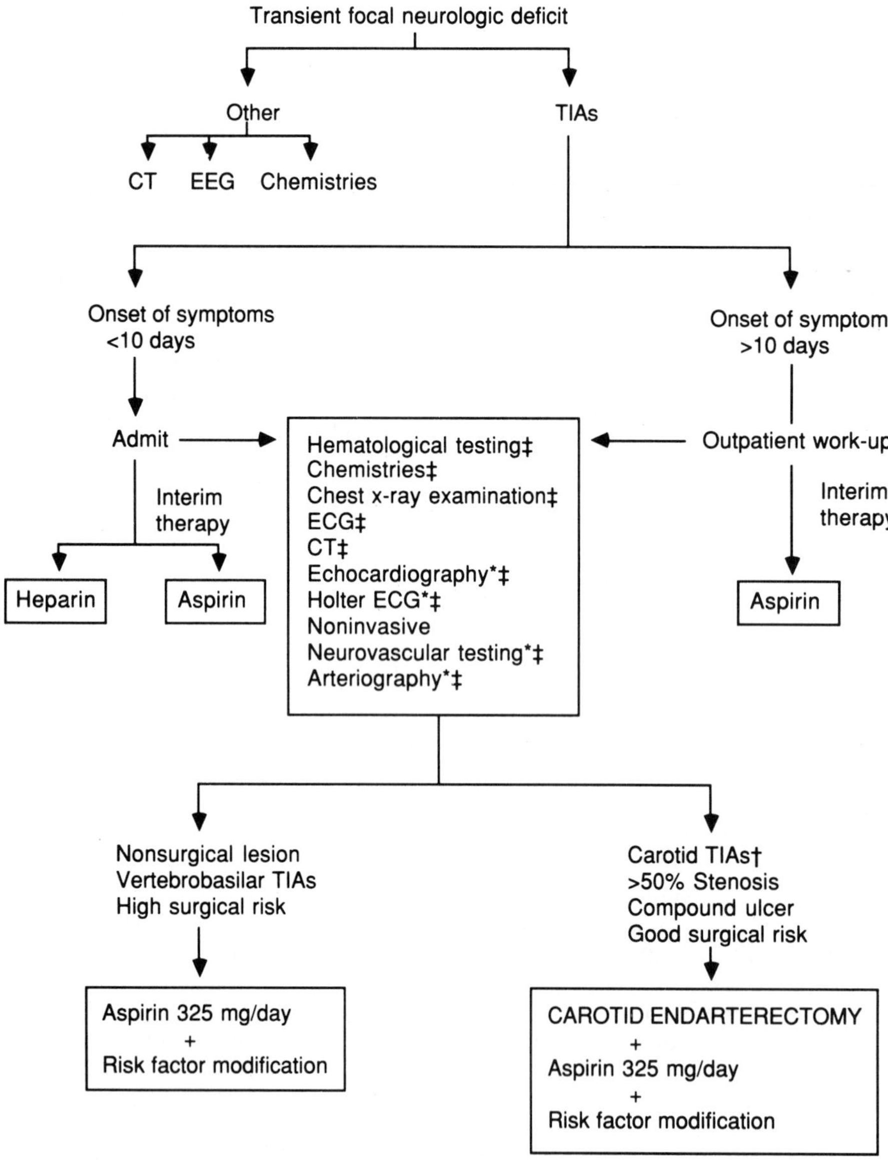

Figure 1 Diagnosis and management of patients with TIAs.
* Optional tests.
† For patients unwilling to participate in ongoing endarterectomy trial.
‡ See text for selected indications of anticoagulant therapy.

smaller volumes of contrast, although two injections are required for biplane views because most units are single plane. We favor conventional film screen angiography except for selected instances when we use IA-DSA. We undertake arteriography in good surgical-risk patients with bona fide carotid TIAs, selected cases in which we find it difficult to determine if the site of ischemia is the carotid or vertebrobasilar circulation, and in selected patients with vertebrobasilar TIAs in whom medical treatment with platelet antiaggregating agents has failed.

MANAGEMENT

Strategies for the treatment of TIAs include the use of platelet-antiaggregating agents, anticoagulants, and surgical revascularization and modification of atherosclerotic risk factors.

Modification of Atherosclerotic Risk Factors

Although the predisposing risk factors for ischemic stroke are not necessarily the same as the risk factors for coronary atherosclerosis, we avoid making a distinction because the main cause of death in patients with TIAs is cardiac disease. Advancing age, gender (male), and positive family history are fixed risk factors. A number of predisposing atherosclerotic risk factors such as arterial hypertension, diabetes mellitus, hypercholesterolemia, a low level of high-density lipoproteins, cigarette smoking, and obesity should be treated with a combination of drugs, dietary modification, and changes in lifestyle.

Platelet Antiaggregating Therapy

At present, aspirin is the best medical therapy in the management of TIAs. We currently use aspirin in a daily dose of 325 mg for both male and female patients. Aspirin inhibits platelet function by blocking cyclooxygenase, which converts arachidonic acid to prostaglandin endoperoxides and ultimately to thromboxane A_2. Several studies have evaluated the effectiveness of aspirin and other platelet antiaggregants in treating patients with threatened stroke. In most of these studies, doses of aspirin ranging from 900 to 1,300 mg daily were used.

The Canadian Cooperative Study Group evaluated 585 patients with TIAs or minor strokes and showed a 19 percent overall reduced incidence of TIAs, stroke, and death in all male patients. The use of aspirin yielded better results when overall stroke and death rates alone were analyzed, demonstrating a decrease in these rates of 31 percent, and even more favorable results in men without history of myocardial infarction (a 62 percent decrease in the incidence of stroke and death). This study did not show a benefit for women who received aspirin therapy.

A French study evaluated the effects of aspirin alone, aspirin in combination with dipyridamole, or placebo on 604 patients with either TIAs or stroke. At the end of the study, the cumulative rate of fatal and nonfatal stroke was 18 percent in the placebo group and 10.5 percent in each of the active-treatment groups. Dipyridamole did not provide additional benefit. Gender was not shown to influence the efficacy of aspirin in this study.

The American-Canadian Cooperative Study evaluated 890 patients with carotid TIAs to determine the potential benefit of a combination of aspirin plus dipyridamole versus aspirin alone. Dipyridamole did not supplement the effect of aspirin in reducing the risk of stroke, retinal infarction, or death.

The United Kingdom Trial evaluated the effects of two different dosages of aspirin (1,200 mg per day vs. 300 mg per day) and placebo among 2,435 patients with TIAs or minor strokes. The results of this study demonstrated that aspirin decreased the risk of myocardial infarction, major stroke, or death by 18 percent, and the risk of disabling stroke or vascular death by 7 percent. Aspirin benefited men only. No clear differences were noted between the two dosages of aspirin, except that fewer gastrointestinal side effects were associated with the lower dosage.

Ticlopidine hydrochloride, a new platelet antiaggregant, has been recently compared with aspirin in a study of more than 3,000 patients with TIAs or minor strokes. Ticlopidine hydrochloride appears to be approximately 15 percent better than aspirin in reducing strokes. The future role of this agent in the management of high-risk patients is yet to be defined.

Anticoagulant Therapy

The effectiveness of oral anticoagulant therapy is unknown. Anticoagulant therapy is risky and, in our opinion, should not be the first line of treatment, except in selected circumstances.

Although several nonrandomized and randomized trials have demonstrated a reduced incidence of cerebral infarction and TIA in treated patients, they have also shown a greater number of hemorrhages among them. Studies have failed to show a difference in the survival rates of the treated and control groups. The number of patients in these studies have been quite small, and all of the studies have had several flaws in their design.

We currently recommend warfarin therapy only for patients with a well-established cardiac source for TIA and for selected patients who continue to have TIAs despite treatment with platelet antiaggregants. If the TIAs are related to embolization from a left ventricular thrombus associated with a myocardial infarction, we use a 3- to 6-month course of warfarin to maintain the prothrombin time at 1.5 to 2 times control. In patients with rheumatic valvular heart disease, chronic atrial fibrillation, or dilated cardiomyopathy, we use a similar intensity of anticoagulation for the remainder of the patient's lifetime. In patients with mechanical prosthetic heart valves, we again use long-term anticoagulation of a similar intensity and add 300 to 400 mg of dipyridamole if the TIAs continue despite an adequate level of warfarin anticoagulation. When TIAs are attributed to mitral valve prolapse, we administer aspirin at a dosage of 325 mg daily.

Surgical Revascularization

There has been only one large controlled study evaluating the effectiveness of carotid endarterectomy, and it was inconclusive. At present, a large multicenter controlled trial underway in North America is comparing the efficacy of carotid endarterectomy supplementing best medical management with that of best medical management alone in the treatment of patients with TIAs or minor strokes in the carotid distribution and who have greater than 30 percent (but less than 100 percent) diameter stenosis with or without ulceration of the internal carotid artery. Until the results of this study and related trials are known, carotid endarterectomy is recommended only after careful consideration based on clinical judgment.

At present, we advise carotid endarterectomy on an "instinctual" basis for a suitable surgical-risk patient who has bona fide carotid distribution TIA and an ipsilateral carotid stenosis of greater than 50 percent diameter or a compound ulcerated lesion.

A recently completed trial of a superficial temporal-middle cerebral artery (extracranial-intracranial) bypass procedure demonstrated that the addition of surgery to medical therapy did not improve outcome for symptomatic patients with stenosis of the distal internal carotid artery, internal carotid artery occlusion, or middle cerebral artery stenosis or occlusion. We do not recommend this operation for patients with atherosclerotic cerebrovascular disease.

Interim Management for Patients Who Have Had Recent TIAs

We admit patients who have had recent TIAs (within the last 10 days) to the hospital for expeditious evaluation and treatment. We have been testing the usefulness of early medical therapy by randomly assigning these patients to receive either intravenous heparin or aspirin while evaluation is underway and until final recommendations can be made. For patients who are to receive heparin, we administer an intravenous bolus dose of 5,000 U followed by a constant maintenance infusion. The hourly dose of heparin is started at 1,000 U and is adjusted to maintain the activated partial thromboplastin time in the range of 1.5 to 2 times the preheparin controlled values. In patients undergoing cerebral arteriography, we discontinue the administration of heparin for 6 to 8 hours before the procedure.

SUGGESTED READING

The American-Canadian Co-operative Study Group. Persantine aspirin trial in cerebral ischemia. Part II: endpoint results. Stroke 1985; 16:406–415.

Bauer RB, Meyer JS, Fields WS, et al. Joint study of extracranial arterial occlusion. 3. Progress report of controlled study of long-term survival in patients with and without operation. JAMA 1969; 208:509–518.

Biller J, Bruno A, Adams HP Jr, et al. A randomized trial of aspirin or heparin in hospitalized patients with recent transient ischemic attacks: a pilot study. Stroke 1989; 20:441–447.

Bousser MG, Eschwege E, Haguenau M, et al. "AICLA" controlled trial of aspirin and dipyridamole in the secondary prevention of athero-thrombotic cerebral ischemia. Stroke 1983; 14:5–14.

Brust JC. Transient ischemic attacks: natural history and anticoagulation. Neurology 1977; 27:701–707.

The Bypass Study Group. Failure of extracranial-intracranial arterial bypass to reduce the risk of ischemic stroke: results of an international randomized trial. N Engl J Med 1985; 313:1191–1200.

The Canadian Cooperative Study Group. A randomized trial of aspirin and sulfinpyrazone in threatened stroke. N Engl J Med 1978; 299:53–59.

Hass WK, Easton JD, Adams HP Jr, et al. Randomized trial comparing ticlopidine hydrochloride with aspirin for the prevention of stroke in high-risk patients. N Engl J Med 1989; 521:501–507.

UK-TIA Study Group: United Kingdom Transient Ischemic Attack (UK-TIA) aspirin trial: interim results. Br Med J 1988; 296:316–320.

EMBOLIC STROKE OF CARDIAC ORIGIN

MERRILL C. KANTER, M.D.
DAVID G. SHERMAN, M.D.

Approximately 15 percent of all ischemic strokes are attributed to an embolus arising from the heart. The importance of cardiogenic embolus may in fact be much greater when one considers that several strokes are considered to be of "undetermined" etiology. The Stroke Data Bank found that one-third of their 1,805 patients had to be classified as "infarct, unknown cause." Approximately 30 percent of patients with an ischemic stroke have evidence of heart disease, and one-third of these have atherosclerotic cerebrovascular disease sufficient to have produced the stroke.

DIAGNOSIS

The diagnosis of a cardiogenic embolus to the brain is based on the best accumulated clinical and laboratory evidence. At times the nature of the heart disease and the patient's age and clinical presentation leave little doubt that the heart produced the stroke. Quite often, however, cardiac and noncardiac conditions coexist, making diagnosis difficult. The features of value in determining which strokes are caused by cardiogenic emboli and which strokes have other causes are outlined in Table 1. As demonstrated in the table, few features are both sensitive and specific for making this determination. Certain vascular-territory strokes are particularly suggestive of a cardiogenic embolism. In the middle cerebral artery territory, an isolated Wernicke's aphasia or global aphasia without hemiparesis appears to be a common sequela of embolic occlusion of the middle cerebral artery. The top of the basilar and posterior cerebral artery are sites of embolic occlusion in the vertebrobasilar territory.

CARDIAC EVALUATION

One of the first management questions confronting the physician caring for a stroke patient is how extensive a cardiac evaluation does this patient need? The cardiac studies most readily available are echocardiography and Holter monitoring. Most patients with a stroke do not need an extensive cardiac investigation unless the history, physical examination, chest roentgenogram, or electrocardiogram suggest a cardiac disorder. Patients older than 60 years of age with no clinical heart disease and a stroke onset and pattern suggestive of an atherothrombotic stroke are rarely (only 1 to 6 percent of such patients) found by echocardiography to have a possible cardiac abnormality. On the other hand, 11 to 25 percent of stroke patients who are younger than 50 years of age or have clinical evidence of heart disease or cardioembolic features suggestive of a cardiogenic embolus are found by echocardiography to have a possible source of embolus. Other promising technologies, as yet not widely available, for identifying intracardiac abnormalities include ultrafast cardiac computed tomography (CT), transesophageal echocardiography, cardiac magnetic resonance imaging (MRI), and labeled platelet scintigraphy.

CAUSES OF CARDIOGENIC EMBOLI

There are several cardiac abnormalities that can lead to intracardiac thrombus and embolization (Fig. 1). Atrial fibrillation with or without associated valvular disease accounts for approximately 45 percent of all cardioembolic strokes. Ischemic heart disease is the next most common cause, with 15 percent of cardioembolic strokes associated with an acute myocardial infarct and 10 percent related to intraventricular thrombi remote from a myocardial infarct. Rheumatic heart disease and prosthetic valves each cause 10 percent of cardiogenic emboli. The remaining 10 percent arise from any of several less common cardiac abnormalities whose propensity to embolize varies widely.

EVALUATION AND TREATMENT

Management decisions concerning antithrombotic therapy for patients with a potential or already demonstrated cardiac source of brain embolus are based on estimates of how great the risk of embolism is and how long this risk is apt to persist, as well as on the estimated degree of the risk involved in anticoagulant or antiplatelet therapy. We have attempted to estimate the risk of embolism associated with each of the most common cardiac abnormalities, and basing our guidelines on this estimate, determine whether the patient needs high-range or low-range anticoagulation or antiplatelet therapy, and how long such therapy should be continued (Ta-

TABLE 1 Clinical Features of Cardiogenic Embolism

	Frequency (%)		*Likelihood of CE* (%)*	
Clinical or Investigative Feature	*CE*	*Non-CE*	*Present*	*Absent*
Abrupt onset of maximal neurologic deficit	70	43	26	06
Loss of consciousness at onset	19	3	53	13
Concomitant systemic embolus	2.8	0	99	15
Prior transient ischemic attack	11	42	4	19
Past history of atrial fibrillation	37	6	52	10
History of myocardial infarction	33	15	28	12
History of congestive heart failure	36	7	48	10
CT scan showing hemorrhagic infarct	22	10	28	13
Cerebral angiography or noninvasive studies showing absent or insignificant disease	87	47	25	04

CE = Cardiogenic embolism.
* The likelihood of a cardiogenic embolism if the particular feature is "present" or "absent" is calculated using Bayes' theorem and assuming a pretest probability of cardiogenic embolism of 15% and of noncardiogenic embolism of 85%.

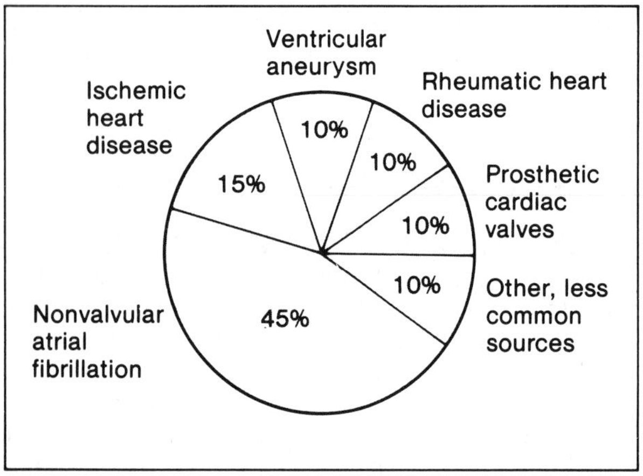

Figure 1 Sources of cardioembolism.

ble 2). Low-intensity warfarin therapy is that dose that prolongs the prothrombin time to 1.3 to 1.5 times the control value (International Normalized Ratio [INR] of 2 to 3). High-intensity warfarin therapy is that dose that prolongs the prothrombin time to 1.5 to 2 times the control value (INR of 3 to 4.5).

Each feature listed in Table 2 adds to the risk of embolism. Certain factors, such as intracardiac thrombi and atrial fibrillation, carry a higher risk of embolism. Patients with atrial fibrillation often have significant atherosclerotic cerebrovascular disease. The evaluation of the stroke mechanism is of paramount importance in selecting prevention strategies, as it determines whether treatment should be aimed at a cardioembolic event with anticoagulation or a stroke secondary to coexistent atherosclerotic vascular disease. In the latter case,

TABLE 2 Features and Treatment of Cardioembolic Stroke

Cardiac Disorder Features	*Primary Prevention*	*Secondary Prevention*	*Risk of Stroke/TIA (Untreated)**
Nonvalvular atrial fibrillation			
High risk	APA or AC (L)	AC (L)	6% per yr
SSS	LR	HR	
CHF			
LA thrombus			
LA >5.5 cm			
LV segmental wall dysfunction			
Cardiomyopathy (dilated/hypertrophic)			
Recent onset of sustained AF			
Thyrotoxicosis†	AC (S)	AC (L)	
	LR	HR	
Low risk	None	AC (L)	0.5% per yr
<60 yrs old		HR	
"Lone AF"			
Acute myocardial infarction			
High risk	AC (S)	AC (L)	2–6% per yr
Anterior MI	LR	HR	
LV thrombus			
AF			
CHF			
Apical akinesis/dyskinesis			
Low risk	None	AC (S)	1–3% per yr
Inferior MI		LR	
>6 weeks post-MI			
Ventricular aneurysm			
High risk	AC (S)	AC (L)	5% per yr
LV thrombus (protruding/freely mobile)	LR	HR	
<6 weeks post-MI		(+/− aneurysmectomy)	
Low risk	None	AC (S)	1–2% per yr
LV thrombus (flat/nonmobile)		LR	
No thrombus			
>6 weeks post-MI			
Rheumatic heart disease			
High risk	AC (L)	AC (L)	>5% per yr
Mitral stenosis	LR	HR	
AF		(+/− dipyridamole	
Left atrial diameter >5.5 cm		(225–400 mg/day)	
>45 yrs old			

Table continues

Cardiac Disorder Features	*Primary Prevention*	*Secondary Prevention*	*Risk of Stroke/TIA (Untreated)**
Low risk	None	AC (L)	<2% per yr
Mitral regurgitation		HR	
NSR			
<45 yrs old			
Infective endocarditis			
High risk			
Staphylococcus aureus	Treat infection	Reassess antibiotic R_x	20%
<48 hrs (i.e., uncontrolled infection)	(+/− valve surgery)	Valve surgery	
Mechanical valve	AC (L)	AC (L)	
Low risk	HR	HR	
Streptococcus	Treat infection	Reassess antibiotic R_x	6%
>48 hrs after antibiotics	(+/− valve surgery)	Valve surgery	
Native valve			
Prosthetic Valves			
High risk	AC (L)	AC (L)	15% (?)
Mechanical	HR	HR	(−AC)
Mitral valve		dipyridamole	3–4%
Bioprosthetic valve and AF, CHF, or LA >5.5 cm		(400 mg/day)	(+ AC)
Low risk	AC (S) LR, then	AC (S)	2–4%
Bioprosthetic valve	APA (L)	LR	
Mitral			
Nonmitral	APA (L)	AC (S)	
		LR	
Mitral valve prolapse			
High risk	None‡	APA (L)	?
>45 yrs old			
Male			
Redundant/thick or myxomatous valve			
Low risk	None‡	APA (L)	<0.01%
<45 yrs old			
Female			
Valvular Calcification			
High risk	Treatment of underlying disease	Treatment of underlying disease§	10%
Mitral annulus			
Atherosclerosis			
HTN			
AF			
IE			
Low risk	APA (?)	APA (?)	?
Aortic stenosis			
Nonbacterial thromboembolic endocarditis			
High risk	APA or AC (?)	APA or AC (?)	0.5–1%
Coagulation abnormality			
Valve vegetation			
Atrial myxoma			
High risk	Surgical removal	Surgical removal	27–55%
All atrial myxoma (intracavitary location/friability)			
Cardiomyopathy			
High risk	AC (L)	AC (L)	5–10%
CHF	HR	HR	
AF			
Thrombus			

High- and low-risk subgroups are based on the best available information (Cerebral Embolism Task Force).

* The percentages are based on a review of the literature. In several cases they may be modified by treatment and/or selection; however,we believe these are representative figures and have indicated where there is significant question.

† AC 2–4 weeks after conversion to NSR.

‡ General precautions against endocarditis.

§ Re-evaluate underlying disease as the cause of the infarct.

AC = Anticoagulation (Coumadin); AF = atrial fibrillation; APA = antiplatelet agent (ASA 1,300 mg/day divided dose); CHF = congestive heart failure; HR = High-range anticoagulation—PT ratio of 1.5–2 using a typical North American thromboplastin (INR of 3–4.5); HTN = hypertension; IE = infective endocarditis; (L) = long-term (indefinitely); LA = left atrium; LR = low-range anticoagulation—PT ratio of 1.3–1.5 using a typical North American thromboplastin (INR of 2–3); LV = left ventricle; MI = myocardial infarction; NSR = normal sinus rhythm; (S) = short-term (3 months); SSS = sick sinus syndrome.

platelet anti-aggregating agents are often advocated. The severity of embolic strokes and the recurrence rate, particularly during the first 2 weeks, determine the need for immediate intervention.

Nonvalvular Atrial Fibrillation

In patients with nonvalvular atrial fibrillation (NVAF), the underlying heart disease is treated and conversion to normal sinus rhythm is performed, thus eliminating the atrial fibrillation. Conversion to normal sinus rhythm should be approached cautiously, as the procedure itself may induce a cardioembolic event. We recommend low-range anticoagulation for 2 to 3 weeks before the electrical cardioversion of patients who have had atrial fibrillation for more than 3 days. This should be continued until the patient has had normal sinus rhythm for 2 to 4 weeks. Anticoagulation is not indicated for cardioversion of atrial flutter or supraventricular tachycardia. When it coexists with any of the cardiac problems listed, atrial fibrillation increases the risk of embolism. It is postulated that this increased risk correlates with the presence of left atrial thrombi, although this relationship has not been proved. The sensitivity of current noninvasive methods of thrombus detection (i.e., traditional echocardiography) is limited. Transesophageal echocardiography may enable us to detect atrial thrombi with a greater sensitivity, especially in the atrial appendage. Left atrial enlargement usually exists when thrombi are present, although it is sometimes seen when there is no evidence of thrombus or embolism. Left atrial enlargement of greater than 5.5 cm is associated with atrial fibrillation and is considered a high-risk factor for embolism because of this correlation with the atrial arrhythmia.

Cardiomyopathy

All patients with cardiomyopathy are at high risk for thromboembolism as the dilated hypokinetic ventricle predisposes them to form thrombi. Those patients at highest risk are those with secondary atrial fibrillation and/or identifiable thrombi in addition to the global wall abnormalities.

Mitral Valve Prolapse

Mitral valve prolapse (MVP) is the most common cardiac valvular abnormality in adults. Despite its frequency, the overall risk of thromboembolism is low and ischemic events are often transient. In the future, primary prevention for the high-risk group may include platelet antiaggregating agents. These patients appear to be at higher risk for developing platelet-fibrin emboli. Other potential causes of stroke should be sought, particularly in patients who are at low risk for thromboembolism. Specifically active endocarditis, the use of oral contraceptives, protein C and protein S deficiencies, and coexistent paroxysmal atrial fibrillation should not be overlooked.

Endocarditis

In patients with infective endocarditis, control of the infection dramatically decreases the risk of embolism. There is no correlation between emboli and the site of the valve affected in native valve endocarditis. Recurrent emboli are not common after adequate treatment of the underlying infection. Anticoagulation in patients with infective endocarditis is limited to those patients with mechanical prosthetic valves.

Embolism secondary to nonbacterial thromboembolic endocarditis (NBTE) is probably related to an underlying hypercoaguable hematologic state. The use of anticoagulation, at least on a short-term basis, is reasonable in patients with a prothrombotic state.

Atrial Myxomas

Atrial myxomas are friable intracardiac tumors and are the most common primary cardiac tumors to cause embolism. Approximately 1 percent of strokes that occur in young adults are caused by atrial myxomas. This tumor carries a high risk of embolism, although the overall incidence of atrial myxomas makes them an uncommon cause of cardiogenic brain embolism. Surgical therapy is usually curative. There is no clear indication for medical therapy in these patients.

Anticoagulation of Acute Cardioembolic Stroke

Approximately 20 percent of cardioembolic strokes undergo secondary hemorrhagic transformation. In the majority of cases, this occurs during the first 48 hours. In an untreated patient with a known source of embolus, the risk of reembolization during a 2-week period immediately after an embolic stroke is about 1 percent per day. Reviewing the risks versus the benefits of anticoagulation of an acute embolic stroke, we have developed the management plan outlined in Figure 2.

If cerebral hemorrhage is identified on the initial CT scan, the patient is re-evaluated after the hemorrhage has resolved. This difficult situation necessitates an individualized decision. Therapies that carry less risk, such as dipyridamole for the treatment of valvular disease, are often considered.

If no hemorrhage is identified on the initial CT

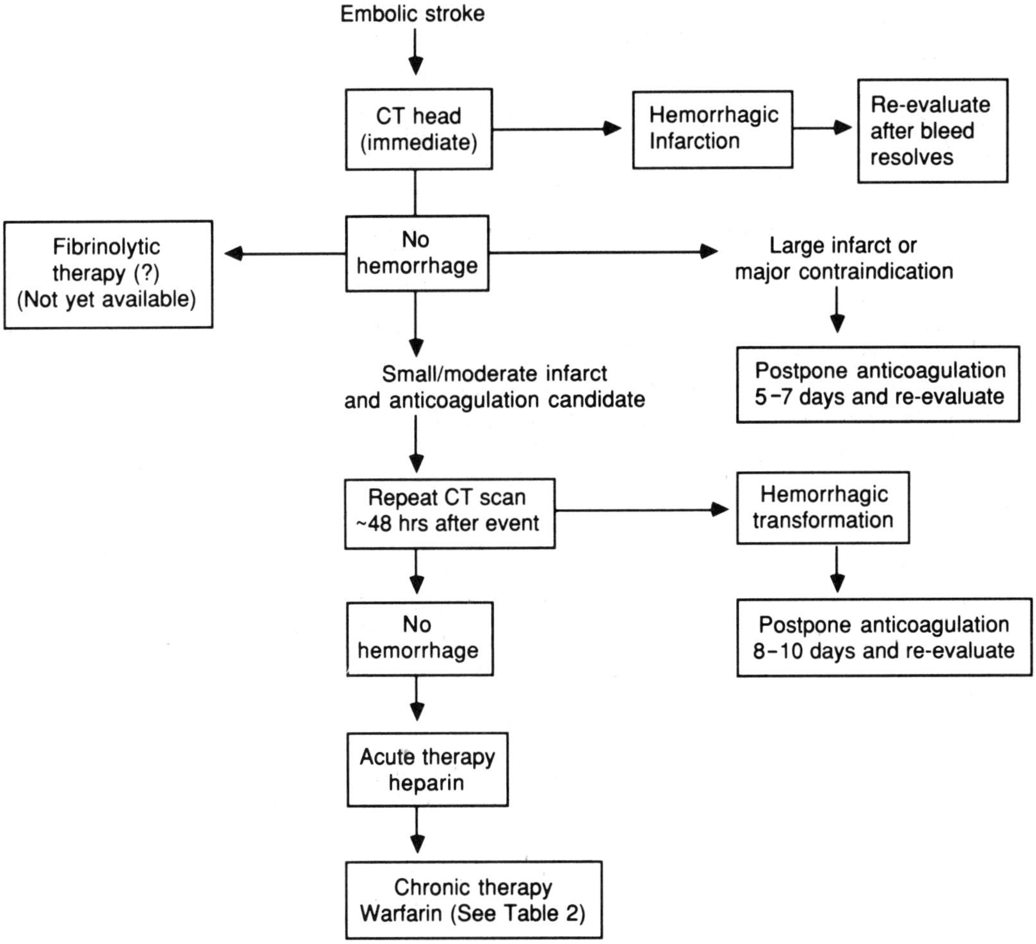

Figure 2 Anticoagulation of acute embolic stroke.

scan, there are currently two possible approaches to treatment. The first is used for patients with a large infarction or serious contraindication to anticoagulation. These patients are re-evaluated after 5 to 7 days. If they are candidates for anticoagulation therapy, their treatment is guided by their underlying cardiac disease (see Table 2). The second approach is used for patients with a small to moderate infarction and no serious contraindications to anticoagulation. We repeat the CT scan at approximately 48 hours after the event. If there is no hemorrhagic transformation, we begin acute anticoagulation followed by warfarin therapy. We begin with continuous infusion–heparin because of the higher risk of hemorrhagic complications and the lack of evidence for additional benefit with bolus therapy. Heparin should be administered via a continuous infusion pump to ensure accurate delivery. The partial thromboplastin time (PTT) should be maintained at 2 to 2.5 times the control value. Patients should continue to receive this level of anticoagulation while warfarin therapy is begun. Daily levels should be checked and used to adjust the infusion of heparin to maintain the therapeutic anticoagulated state. There are several options for changing from heparin to warfarin anticoagulation. We begin warfarin approximately 48 hours after heparin therapy. Warfarin started at a dosage of 10 to 15 mg per day usually brings the prothrombin time (PT) to near-therapeutic levels within 2 to 3 days. Heparin can then be tapered over 2 to 3 days. To ensure adequate anticoagulation, most physicians overlap the heparin and warfarin therapy for 2 to 6 days after the PT has reached therapeutic levels. We use low-intensity anticoagulation (PT = 1.3 to 1.5 times the control value) with warfarin after approximately 1 year of higher intensity therapy (PT = 1.5 to 2 times the control value) in patients who need anticoagulation indefinitely. This decreases the risk of serious side effects.

If hemorrhagic transformation has occurred, anticoagulation is postponed for 8 to 10 days. The source of embolization is sought and the patient is re-evaluated after the hemorrhage has resolved. The re-evaluation includes a repeat CT scan of the head and reassessment of the patient's medical, neurologic, and social risk factors for anticoagulation.

In the future we will have a third alternative that may include therapy with thrombolytic agents. It appears that this will carry the caveat of early detection and intervention. This approach is similar to the early use of fibrinolytic agents in acute coronary artery thrombosis. If therapy can be started within a therapeutic window (probably within 6 hours after the stroke), there is great promise for such intervention. Problems associated with early thrombolytic treatment include the potential for increased hemorrhagic transformation occurring most often during the first few days after embolic stroke. Controlled investigations are needed before there is widespread use of this therapy.

SUGGESTED READING

Dalen J, Hirsh J, eds. Second ACCP Conference on antithrombotic therapy. Chest 1989; 95(suppl).

PATIENT RESOURCES

Patient Information Guide for Neurology
American Academy of Neurology
(E. Wayne Massey, M.D.,
Coordinator AAN Practice Committee)
2221 University Avenue S.E., Suite 335
Minneapolis, Minnesota 55414

American Heart Association
7320 Greenville Avenue
Dallas, Texas 75231
Telephone: (214) 750-5300

National Stroke Association
1420 Ogden Street
Denver, Colorado 80218
Telephone: (303) 839-1992

INTRACRANIAL ANEURYSM

DAVID O. WIEBERS, M.D.

The most common mode of presentation of intracranial aneurysms is rupture resulting in subarachnoid hemorrhage (SAH) with or without intracerebral hemorrhage. Intracranial aneurysms are not congenital but rather develop with increasing age. The average annual incidence of aneurysmal rupture is approximately ten per 100,000 people in the same general population in which the autopsy prevalence of aneurysm is approximately 5 percent. These figures suggest that the vast majority of intracranial aneurysms never rupture or cause any other symptoms. Nevertheless, physicians are discovering more and more unruptured aneurysms from computed tomographic (CT) scans, magnetic resonance imaging (MRI) scans, and cerebral angiograms obtained for reasons other than aneurysmal rupture.

The management of intracranial aneurysm is quite different, depending on whether the aneurysm is discovered before or after the rupture. These two courses of action will therefore be addressed separately.

RUPTURED ANEURYSM

It is very important to be aware of the clinical picture of aneurysmal rupture, because as many as half of patients with fatal aneurysmal ruptures may have had previous warning leaks consisting of a partial or milder version of a typical SAH. The typical clinical picture of SAH includes the sudden onset of severe headache with or without stiff neck. Key diagnostic points are the suddenness of onset, the unusual quality of the headache for that particular patient, and the stiff neck, which is not merely a tightness or tenderness to direct palpation but usually includes meningismus and an inability to move the neck anteroposteriorly. In addition, the level of consciousness may be diminished, and focal neurologic signs, particularly cranial nerve palsies, such as a palsy of the third cranial nerve, may be present. Other recognized clinical features of SAH are nausea and vomiting, diffuse intellectual impairment, photophobia, seizures, and hemispheric symptoms, often related to hemorrhage extending into the brain parenchyma. Occasionally, SAH from an intracranial source may produce neck or low back pain with radicular features, particularly if the patient is sitting or standing and blood has pooled in the spinal subarachnoid space. A similar presentation may occur with spinal SAH.

Physical examination may reveal neck meningismus (especially if the examination is performed within hours of onset of even a minor leak), preretinal and subhyaloid hemorrhages, papilledema, fever, and other neurologic deficits, such as those mentioned above, depending on the location and severity of the hemorrhage. Patients with symptoms that raise the possibility of SAH should be examined with caution; specifically, the neurologic examination should not include strenuous muscle testing or Valsalva maneuvers that could precipitate another rupture.

Patients with symptoms consistent with SAH should undergo a CT scan of the head in an attempt to detect subarachnoid blood, which can be seen without the use of contrast medium in approximately 80 percent of patients. If the CT scan is negative for subarachnoid or intraparenchymal blood, a lumbar puncture should be performed. If the CT scan shows evidence of subarachnoid or intraparenchymal hemorrhage, a lumbar puncture need not be done, since it will not contribute significant additional diagnostic information and can sometimes be dangerous, particularly when intraparenchymal blood is present.

Traumatic lumbar puncture must be differentiated from true SAH. Three or four successive tubes of cerebrospinal fluid are collected, and if the specimens show progressively less blood, a traumatic puncture is suggested. Clotting of the specimen virtually never occurs with true SAH. Xanthochromia is present in the supernatant within hours of SAH and remains in the spinal fluid for an average of 3 to 4 weeks. Red blood cells often disappear within several days after SAH. The cerebrospinal fluid may not show xanthochromia if small numbers of red blood cells are present from SAH (approximately 400 or fewer), and xanthochromia has been reported in rare instances with traumatic lumbar puncture if the red blood cell count is more than 200,000.

After the diagnosis of SAH is established, patients are prescribed bedrest in a quiet, darkened room, and if the patient is to undergo operation, bedrest is continued for at least 2 to 3 weeks. The patient should be kept under close observation for at least the first few days, either in an intensive care unit or at least in a hospital room close to a nursing station. Vital signs and neurologic checks are recorded at least every 4 hours, and careful attention is placed on fluid and electrolyte balance.

If the patient is agitated, I often administer a sedative in the form of phenobarbital, 30 to 60 mg twice daily, or chloral hydrate, 500 mg three times daily. It is important not to oversedate since the effect of the medication may be indistinguishable from depressed level of consciousness caused by rehemorrhage or other complications of SAH.

It is important to provide analgesia for pain relief because extra pain often leads to agitation and an increased likelihood of additional hemorrhage. I usually use codeine, 60 mg IM or orally every 3 to 4 hours, as needed. The use of morphine should be avoided because it may depress respiration and level of consciousness.

Overhydration may produce cerebral edema and increased intracranial pressure, while underhydration can lead to cerebral vasospasm. Consequently, I recommend fluid replacement with approximately 2 L of 5 percent dextrose in ¼ isotonic saline per day. Patients are given laxatives to avoid straining when passing stool. For patients clearly suffering from increased intracranial pressure, mannitol (1 to 1.5 g per kilogram IV in 20 percent solution over 30 minutes) and glycerol (1 g per kilogram via a nasogastric tube) are sometimes used as temporary antiedema agents. Smaller doses of mannitol may be used at 4- to 6-hour intervals, and the glycerol dose may be given at these intervals if longer-term control of intracranial pressure is desired.

One must be very cautious about the use of antihypertensive agents in this situation, because at least part of the hypertension observed is often the result of Cushing's reflex, in which intracranial hypertension leads to peripheral hypertension to maintain cerebral perfusion. Most of the time, increased systemic blood pressure gradually decreases as the patient rests in the hospital with or without mild sedation and analgesia. Patients with previously treated hypertension should maintain their previous therapy. For patients who continue to have considerable hypertension (greater than 180/110 mm Hg) despite the general measures already mentioned, blood pressure can be controlled rather precisely by a continuous intravenous infusion of sodium nitroprusside titrated to pressures slightly below this level.

The use of antifibrinolytic agents, such as epsilon-aminocaproic acid (Amicar), may decrease mortality from rebleeding of aneurysms, but it also increases thrombotic side effects, including cerebral infarction, deep vein thrombosis, and pulmonary embolism. A delayed myopathy occurring with the use of epsilon-aminocaproic acid has also been reported. I generally do not administer antifibrinolytic agents after a single SAH, but I do recommend such treatment if there is any evidence of continued or recurrent hemorrhage after initial hemorrhage. Epsilon-aminocaproic acid is usually administered in a dosage of 24 to 36 g in 1,000 ml of 5 percent dextrose solution every 24 hours.

Another important complication of SAH is cerebral vasospasm, which involves spasm of one or more cerebral arteries, particularly in the area of extravasated blood. This may lead to focal cerebral infarction and sometimes to a more generalized or multifocal decreased cerebral perfusion. The peak time for the occurrence of vasospasm is between 4 and 14 days after SAH. When vasospasm occurs, I recommend blood volume expansion with plasma and whole blood transfusions. Human albumin (Albuminar) may also be used for this purpose. When central venous pressure is monitored, it is usually maintained between 8 and 12 cm H_2O. Dopamine infusion titration starting at doses of 5 to 10 μg per kilogram per minute to increase systolic blood pressure by 40 to 50 mm Hg may also be helpful in this circumstance, particularly if the patient is hypotensive. Recent studies have suggested that calcium-channel-blocking agents such as nimodipine and nicardipine hydrochloride may also be useful in this condition, but convincing confirmation of their efficacy awaits the completion of randomized clinical trials currently underway.

Surgical clipping of the ruptured aneurysm remains the definitive treatment for these lesions, and this is generally the ultimate goal in management. The overall mortality from aneurysmal SAH is approximately 59 percent at 30 days for each rupture, and the prognosis is clearly related to the patient's level of consciousness at the time of the first visit with the physician. Operative morbidity and mortality rates are much higher in patients who have depressed levels of consciousness or other severe neurologic deficits besides cranial nerve palsies. The peak time for rebleeding from intracranial aneurysm is 7 to 10 days after initial rupture, and as already mentioned, the peak time for vasospasm is 4 to 14 days after the initial rupture. Consequently, if at the time of the first examination patients with SAH have a normal or near-normal level of consciousness and no severe neurologic deficit other than cranial nerve palsy, I suggest that they undergo cerebral arteriography as soon as feasible so that the source for SAH may be clearly identified. When an intracranial aneurysm is identified, surgical clipping should be undertaken as soon as possible, preferably within the first 2 to 3 days after aneurysmal rupture to avoid the peak times for vasospasm and rebleeding. It is important to involve a neurosurgeon who is experienced and skilled in aneurysmal surgery, since these procedures are exceedingly difficult.

For patients with depressed levels of consciousness and severe neurologic deficits at the time of admission, medical management is generally undertaken until there is stabilization and improvement, at which time definitive surgical treatment has a lower probability of complications.

UNRUPTURED ANEURYSMS

Intracranial aneurysms may cause symptoms other than intracranial hemorrhage, particularly if they are 10 mm or greater in diameter. These symptoms may result from cranial nerve compression (most commonly compression of cranial nerves II, III, IV, V, and VI) or compression of other central nervous system structures, such as the pituitary on the brain stem. Seizure foci may result from impingement on supratentorial brain structures. In addition, aneurysms may rarely cause cerebral ischemia from embolization of a clot within the aneurysm to distal sites in the same arterial tree. When headache is caused by unruptured aneurysm, it may be produced by a sudden dilatation of the aneurysm or by chronic compression of pain-sensitive structures, such as the ophthalmic and maxillary divisions of the trigeminal nerve. Such headaches are often focal and unilateral, frontal, or orbital in location and may be associated with cranial nerve palsies.

Because the vast majority of intracranial aneurysms never rupture or cause any other symptoms, ideally the selection of patients for surgical treatment should depend on predicting which unruptured aneurysms will subsequently rupture. It is important to emphasize that this part of the discussion does not apply to patients with any suggestion of SAH (including warning leaks) before the discovery of the intracranial aneurysm.

Patients with unruptured aneurysms discovered by CT scan or MRI scan who are suitable surgical candidates should be considered for cerebral arteriography as soon as possible. Unruptured aneurysms 10 mm in angiographic diameter or larger have a fairly high probability of subsequent rupture, and many of these ruptures occur within a few months of identification of the aneurysm. Consequently, for patients with unruptured aneurysms of this size, an intracranial operation should be considered by a neurosurgeon experienced in aneurysmal surgery to isolate the aneurysm from the circulation as soon as possible.

For unruptured aneurysms less than 10 mm in diameter, there appears to be little likelihood of subsequent rupture. Only one such rupture has ever been reported (a 6-mm aneurysm), and it occurred after an ipsilateral carotid endarterectomy, which may have predisposed the aneurysm to rupture. Because there are no documented cases of clearly spontaneous subarachnoid hemorrhage in natural history studies for this patient group, it is difficult to recommend surgical intervention, particularly for patients with lesions 5 mm or less in diameter. Even in experienced hands, significant morbidity is associated with such aneurysmal surgery. Although data are limited, it also appears that carotid endarterectomy should be approached with increased caution in patients with unruptured intracranial aneurysms, particularly those that are >5 mm in diameter in the ipsilateral carotid system.

If compressive or embolic symptoms from an aneurysm develop after the original diagnosis, the aneurysm probably has enlarged and thus has a higher probability of rupture. In this circumstance, the patient should be restudied with cerebral arteriography and considered for neurologic surgery if enlargement has occurred. In recent years, high-resolution, dynamic, multiplane CT scanning techniques have made it possible to identify most intracranial aneurysms relatively noninvasively. Consequently, detection of aneurysmal enlargement has become easier and safer in many patients not treated surgically, even if they remain asymptomatic. In patients with normal renal function and no history of dye allergy who have not undergone operation, it seems reasonable to restudy at yearly intervals for 3 years, particularly if unruptured aneurysms are 6 to 9 mm in diameter. If no enlargement has occurred and no symptoms have developed after 3 years, it may be adequate to restudy at 5-year intervals.

SUGGESTED READING

Sengupta RP, McAllister VL. Subarachnoid haemorrhage. Berlin: Springer-Verlag, 1986.

Wiebers DO, Whisnant JP, Sundt TM Jr, O'Fallon WM. The significance of unruptured intracranial saccular aneurysms. J Neurosurg 1987; 66:23–29.

BRAIN ARTERIOVENOUS MALFORMATION

GERARD M. DEBRUN, M.D.

This chapter considers true arteriovenous malformations (AVMs), with a nidus of abnormal vessels interposed between the arterial feeders and the draining veins, and the fistulas with one direct communication between one artery and one vein, whether associated with a varix or not. It is interesting to note that there are also true fistulas inside the nidus of brain AVMs. The treatment of venous angiomas, cavernomas, and telangiectasias is not discussed in this chapter.

The therapeutic alternatives are conservative treatment, surgical excision alone, embolization alone, radiosurgery alone, embolization followed by surgical excision or radiosurgery, surgery followed by radiosurgery, and failure of radiosurgery followed by one of the previous therapeutic approaches. The decision of which approach to employ depends on many factors, most of which are objective, but some of which are subjective and have a psychological basis. We obviously need guidelines. In brief they are derived from: (1) the clinical presentation, (2) the location, size, anatomy and physiology of the AVM, and (3) the age and risk factors.

CLINICAL PRESENTATION

Patients who have already bled have a 2 percent chance of rebleeding per year. The cumulative risk increases if the patient's first occurrence of bleeding has taken place early in his life. It is therefore acceptable to be more aggressive in the treatment of young patients who have already bled.

If patients present with seizures that are well controlled with medical therapy without major side effects, conservative treatment should be considered whenever the risks of treatment seem to be greater than those associated with the natural history of the disease. Patients who have poorly controlled or uncontrollable seizures despite serious medical treatment are candidates for further treatment, if possible. Therapy is also indicated in patients with progressive neurologic deficit. Headaches and migraines are highly subjective factors; when they are isolated, the AVM should be treated only if the risks are low.

LOCATION, SIZE, ANATOMY, AND PHYSIOLOGY OF THE AVM

I have found it useful to use Spetzler's classification. This grading system is easy to apply and emphasizes the importance of whether or not the location of the AVM is in an eloquent area of the brain. The polar AVMs may be treated with less risk than a rolandic, internal capsule, basal ganglia, or brain stem AVM. The size of the AVM is also important, especially when radiosurgery is considered. The percentage of anatomic cure of an AVM at 2 years after radiotherapy is between 80 and 85 percent if the nidus is not larger than 2 cm. The dose to be delivered to the nidus and to its edge is controversial, but the number of cures percent at 2 years is probably dose dependent. The next decades will bring the answer when the results will be compared in function of the size of the nidus, the dose of radiation delivered, and the type of radiation used: cobalt ring, heavy particles, proton beam, or linear accelerator.

The geometry of the feeders and draining veins is an important factor when we consider embolization or surgical resection. The caliber and number of feeders are important to consider before attempting an embolization. When we consider embolization as a presurgical step, it is especially useful to embolize the feeders to which the neurosurgeon has difficulty obtaining access, while the feeders on the surface of the brain can be easily clipped and do not always need to be embolized, or sometimes cannot be embolized safely because they are too tortuous and distal.

The exact determination of the size of the nidus is probably the most difficult part of the radiologic evaluation. There is often a collateral circulation in the watershed areas with a highly tortuous abnormal network that should not be confused with the nidus and should be respected during embolization or surgery. Puck films with good subtractions, computed tomography (CT), and magnetic resonance imaging

(MRI) need to be juxtaposed in order to determine the nidus with accuracy.

The rapidity of blood shunting through the AVM is an important physiologic factor but also difficult to quantify. The vein is almost invariably reached within 2 seconds of the beginning of the filling of the carotid artery, and often within 1 second. The merit of recent superselective angiography with microcatheters advanced into the feeder of an AVM immediately before entering the nidus is to show direct fistulae inside the nidus of a brain AVM. This important discovery explains why particulate embolization might be contraindicated in this situation or should be performed only after closure of this fistula. It is difficult to determine whether there is relative ischemia of the surrounding normal tissue, even in the presence of an intense steal. The concept of normal pressure breakthrough phenomenon is controversial, as is the concept of loss of autoregulation of the normal adjacent tissue. Acute clipping or occlusion of the feeder of an AVM immediately increases the blood pressure into this feeder and may be putting the normal tissue fed by this artery at risk.

AGE AND RISK FACTORS

It seems that the older the patient, the less is the risk of bleeding if he has never bled before. This is why the patient's age at the onset of the first bleed is important to consider. A patient who first bled in early life should be treated whenever there is a reasonable degree of risk.

Other risks should be considered as in any surgical candidate (e.g., high blood pressure, diabetes, myocardial infarction, atheromatous disease). When all of the possible risks have been determined, a team made up of a neurologist, vascular and stereotaxic neurosurgeon, neuroradiologist, and a radiotherapist should discuss the indications for treatment in each particular case.

Conservative treatment is sometimes the only alternative for patients with hemispheric, basal ganglia, internal capsule, or brain stem AVMs. One difficult therapeutic decision is in advising a young patient, who is neurologically intact and has never bled and in whom an AVM has been discovered incidentally, after the first seizure or for unexplained headaches. We usually follow the patient unless his AVM is suitable for radiosurgery (the nidus is no larger than 2 cm) or operable with very low risk (a small polar AVM). The natural risk of bleeding is difficult to determine in this category of patients. However, some patients refuse the idea of living with the threat of rupture of their AVM and say that they want to take the risk of treatment. This is certainly one of the subjective factors that I was mentioning which may lead to a more aggressive therapeutic plan than what was initially considered.

SURGICAL RESECTION ALONE

Small AVMs in a noneloquent area of the brain are surgically resected with 0 percent mortality rate and a morbidity rate of almost 0 percent. The mortality and morbidity rates increase with the grading of the AVM. Very large AVMs (larger than 6 cm in diameter) in eloquent areas of the brain cannot be resected at one sitting and are usually not operated on without obliteration of the nidus with embolization as complete as possible.

RADIOSURGERY ALONE

We have already mentioned the ideal indications of radiosurgery. The size of the nidus should not be larger than 2 cm. For AVMs larger than 2 cm, radiosurgery is probably not the procedure of first choice but may be offered if no better choice for treatment is available. The dose delivered to the AVM is the second most important factor and is in fact closely related to the size of the nidus: the smaller the nidus, the larger the dose.

When one is considering radiosurgery as the only treatment, it is very important to know whether the patient has experienced any previous bleeding. Since in 80 percent of the patients with good indications it takes 2 years for an AVM to be cured after radiosurgery, this treatment is least attractive for a patient who has recently bled or has bled several times. A more expeditious way to cure the AVM should be considered in this particular situation.

EMBOLIZATION ALONE

Embolization alone may cure a brain AVM. The smaller the nidus, the better the chance of complete obliteration. Also, an AVM with one or a few feeders is easier to cure with this method than a larger one with multiple feeders coming from the three major trunks (middle, anterior, and posterior cerebral arteries). The materials used for embolization are also an important factor. There are actually three different techniques; the first technique uses cyanoacrylic glue (N Butyl Cyanoacrylate or Bucrylate), the second technique uses particles of IVALON (Polyvinyl alcohol foam) mixed with or without 30 percent ethanol, and the third technique uses coils. Only embolization with Bucrylate can offer a chance of complete occlusion of the nidus. I am not aware of a single case of brain AVM treated with any of the other materials that did not recanalize the previously occluded vessels or did not recruit "new" feeders from enlargement of tiny vessels that were present before embolization.

The highest complete cure rate of embolization alone of brain AVMs using Bucrylate that has been reported is 18 percent with an overall morbidity rate of 10 percent and a mortality rate of 1 or 2 percent (all AVM types are included). The main reason for this relatively low cure rate is that small AVMs with one or two feeders are rarely addressed to the neuroradiologist for embolization, but rather are surgically resected or treated with radiosurgery. Whatever materials are to be used for embolization, there are several strict rules to follow. The embolic material must be delivered into the nidus of the AVM from a microcatheter positioned into the feeder 1 or 2 cm proximal to the nidus. The presence or absence of a balloon at the tip of the catheter makes a great difference in the embolization. The presence of a balloon with a distal hole makes it possible to stop the flow into the feeder, to perform selective angiography under flow control, and to inject the glue in the same condition. More glue stays and solidifies into the nidus. There is less risk of gluing the vein or having part of the glue embolize to the lungs. The injection of glue is also sometimes done under moderate hypotension with a mean arterial pressure of approximately 60 mm of Hg. It is difficult to lower the blood pressure more in the sedated patient without risking nausea and an impossibility of injecting the glue. The inconvenience of using a balloon is the risk of rupturing the feeder with catastrophic subarachnoid or intracerebral hemorrhage. There is a 3 percent risk of mortality associated with this technique. Without a balloon at the tip of the catheter, injection of glue can be done without control of the flow. Therefore the injection is done when there is a true nidus interposed between feeder and vein. When there is a true fistula with fast shunting, the fistula can be closed with a small injection of 0.1 ml of pure nonradiopaque glue. Then embolization can be pursued with radiopaque glue as usual.

EMBOLIZATION FOLLOWED BY SURGICAL RESECTION OR RADIOSURGERY

The goal of the treatment of a brain AVM is to achieve a complete obliteration of the nidus with complete disappearance of any arteriovenous shunting. When we fail to achieve this goal, the risk of devastating hemorrhage is unchanged, even if only 1 percent of the nidus is left. The embolization is performed in patients with large AVMs, with multiple feeders from two or three major arterial trunks used as presurgical step. Several sittings of embolization separated by 3 or 4 weeks are often necessary. After embolization with glue, the feeder is closed. After embolization with particles, the feeder remains open. It is wise to occlude the feeder at the end of the embolization with a detachable balloon or with coils. The embolic material is delivered through a microcatheter with its tip positioned immediately proximal to the nidus. The same principles apply whatever the material used. The goal is to fill the nidus as much as we can with solid particles, glue, or coils. Obviously it is more difficult to fill the nidus with coils than with particles or glue. The use of coils is more likely to occlude the feeders and at a distance of the nidus than the nidus itself.

After embolization, surgical resection becomes easier and safer. When radiopaque glue has been used, the feeders of the AVM close to the nidus are filled with black material that helps the surgeon find the nidus. It has been said that an AVM embolized with glue is like a piece of rock, making surgical dissection more difficult and risky. This has not been my experience. The N Butyl Cyanoacrylate that we use today is less solid than isobutyl cyanoacrylate was. I wonder if the negative attitude held by a few neurosurgeons concerning this treatment is because they have operated on AVMs that were completely obliterated with a large amount of glue. It is questionable whether these AVMs should be operated on. I believe that it is dangerous and unnecessary to resect an AVM that has been totally cured with glue.

There is no doubt in my mind that performing embolization before surgery is extremely beneficial, allowing complete surgical resection of large AVMs and decreasing the mortality and morbidity rates of surgery. I have not seen any normal pressure breakthrough syndrome in any of the large AVMs resected after reduction of the shunt and the nidus size by embolization. This syndrome is controversial and may be rare. However, it is seen by neurosurgeons who have the experience of resection of very large AVMs of high grade in Spetzler's classification. It is unlikely to occur in patients with AVMs of smaller size and lower grade.

This category of AVMs treated with embolization and surgical resection corresponds to large AVMs. Neuroradiologists and neurosurgeons have a common commitment: first, to reduce the size of the nidus and the speed of arteriovenous shunting as much as possible, and second, to accept the risks of complete surgical resection after completion of the embolization.

The risks of embolization and surgical resection are higher in patients with large AVMs, carrying a mortality rate of 5 percent and a morbidity rate of 15 to 20 percent. We must always consider the quality of life that the patient will have at the completion of the treatment. Most patients are able to resume their professional activity, with few being greatly disabled. Most large AVMs of the occipital lobe involving the calcarine cortex will be left with a permanent hemianopic defect. We explain to the patient that he will almost certainly be left with a cortical field defect. I consider that it is an excellent result when the patient is totally cured despite his hemianopsia.

EMBOLIZATION, SURGICAL RESECTION, AND RADIOSURGERY

After embolization and surgical resection, a small remnant of the AVM may be left because it is located in an eloquent and highly risky area of the brain, as the internal capsule, the thalamus, or the deep cerebellar nuclei. Radiosurgery of this remnant of AVM may cure an AVM which cannot be cured by any other approach.

FAILURE OF RADIOSURGERY

More and more patients with large AVMs (i.e., with a nidus larger than 3 cm in every dimension) are not cured at 2 years postradiosurgery. This is because small doses of radiation were given in order to avoid brain radiation necrosis. Radiosurgery is not the first choice in large AVMs. Embolization and surgical resection should be considered first and radiosurgery second or as an adjunct to embolization and resection.

SUGGESTED READING

Batjer HH, Devous MD, Seibert GB, et al. Intracranial arteriovenous malformation: relationships between clinical and radiographic factors and ipsilateral steal severity. Neurosurgery 1988; 23:322–328.

Batjer HH, Devous MD, Seibert GB, et al. Intracranial arteriovenous malformation: relationship between clinical factors and surgical complications. Neurosurgery 1989; 24:75–79.

Brown RD, Wiebers DO, Forbes G, et al. The natural history of unruptured intracranial arteriovenous malformations. J Neurosurg 1988; 68:352–357.

Fisher WS. Decision analysis: a tool of the future—an application to unruptured arteriovenous malformations. Neurosurgery 1989; 24:129–135.

Fults D, Kelly DL. Natural history of arteriovenous malformations of the brain: a clinical study. Neurosurgery 1984; 15:658–662.

Graf CJ, Perret GE, Torner JC. Bleeding from cerebral arteriovenous malformations as part of their natural history. J Neurosurg 1983; 58:331–337.

Luessenhop AJ, Rosa L. Cerebral arteriovenous malformations: indications for and results of surgery, and the role of intravascular techniques. J Neurosurg 1984; 60:14–22.

Picard L, Moret J, Lepoire J. Endovascular treatment of cerebral AVM's. J Neuroradiology 1984; 11:9–28.

Spetzler RF, Martin NA. A proposed grading system for arteriovenous malformations. J Neurosurg 1986; 65:476–483.

Spetzler RF, Martin NA, Carter LP, et al. Surgical management of large AVM's by staged embolization and operative excision. J Neurosurg 1987; 67:17–28.

Troupp H, Marttila I, Halonen V. AVM's of the brain: prognosis without operation. Acta Neurochir 1970; 22:125–128.

Vinuela FV, Debrun GM, Fox AJ, et al. Dominant-hemisphere arteriovenous malformations: therapeutic embolization with isobutyl 2-Cyanoacrylate. AJNR 1983; 4:959–966.

INTRACEREBRAL HEMORRHAGE

MONROE COLE, M.D.

Decisions regarding the treatment of intracerebral hemorrhage must be based on acute appraisal of the clinical state; the site of the hemorrhage; the etiology of the hemorrhage; and the wishes of the patient (if able to act on his own behalf) or the patient's family.

ACUTE CARE

Cerebellar Hemorrhage

Typically the patient with cerebellar hemorrhage is first seen in the emergency room with coma and evidence of brain stem compression. The patient is hypertensive, and an adequate history of hypertension is obtained. No other causes of intracerebral hemorrhage (e.g., anticoagulation, antiplatelet agents, trauma) appear to play a role. If the hemorrhage is in the cerebellum, preparation should be made for immediate surgical evacuation of the cerebellar hematoma despite evidence of brain stem compromise (Fig. 1). While such preparation is being made, the following steps should be taken:

1. The patient should be intubated and supported by ventilator (i.e., hyperventilated) to reduce intracranial pressure.

2. A large-bore intravenous line should be inserted and kept open with 5 percent dextrose in water administered at a rate of 25 ml per minute, unless the patient is hypovolemic.

3. Blood pressure should be stabilized. I prefer a level of 140–160/80–100. If the pressure is much greater than these levels, a sodium nitroprusside drip is titrated under constant supervision (50 ml per 250 ml of 5 percent dextrose in water administered via an infusion pump at a rate of 3 μg per kilogram per minute ranging from 0.5 to 10 μg per kilogram per minute) (Table 1). The solution should be pro-

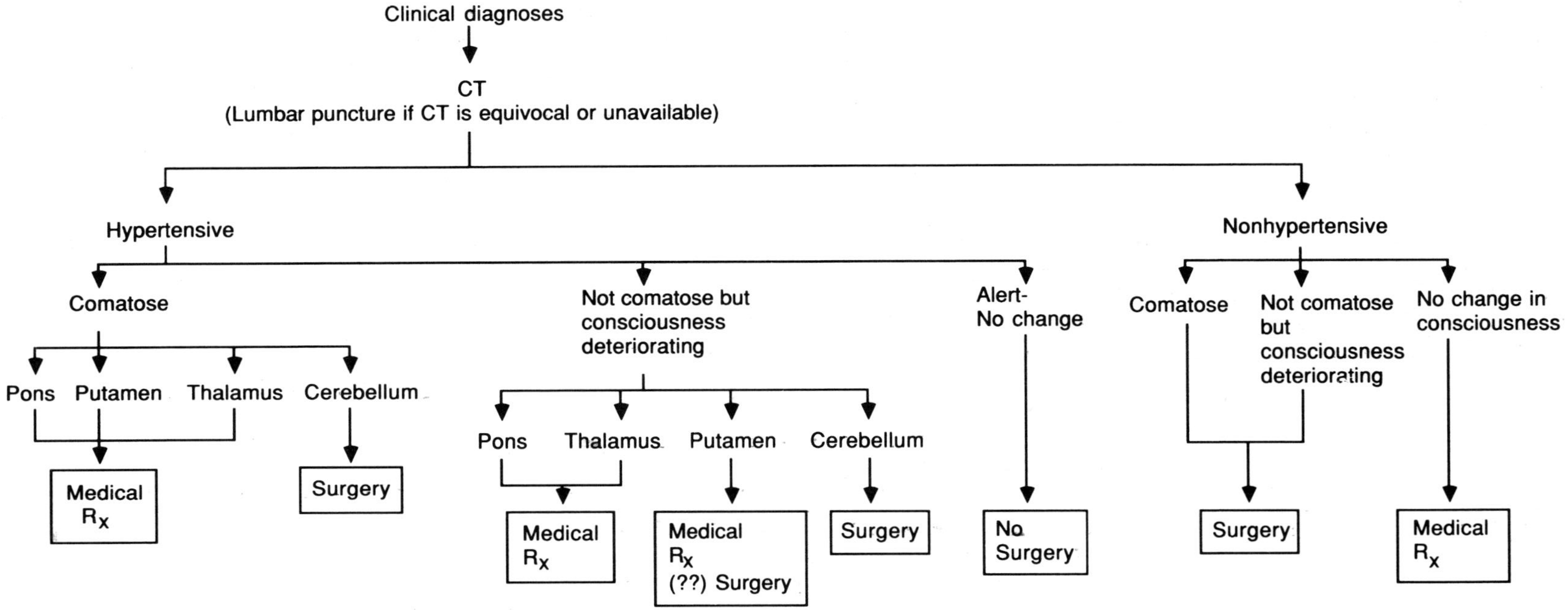

Figure 1 Treatment algorithm for intracerebral hemorrhage.

TABLE 1 Drugs Used in the Treatment of Intracerebral Hemorrhage

Drug	*Usual Dose*	*Range*	*Purpose*
Sodium Nitroprusside	3μ/kg/min (50 ml/250 ml 5% D/W)	0.5–10 μg/kg/min	Lower BP
Dopamine		2–20 μg/kg/min	Raise BP
Norepinephrine bitartrate (Levophed)	(4 ml/1,000 ml 5% D/W)	0.5–3 ml/min	Raise BP
Mannitol	20 g/hr (100 g/500 ml 5% D/W) or a 25–50-g bolus		Lower IICP
Dexamethasone	10 mg IV stat, then 4–6 mg IV or IM q6h		Lower IICP
Lidocaine	50--100-mg IV bolus, then 2 mg per min IV		Ventricle arrhythmia
Atropine	0.5–1 mg IV		Treat bradycardia
Dilantin	500–1,000 mg IV stat, then 100 mg IV q6h		Seizure Px
Carbamazepine (Tegretol)	200 mg via NG tube q6h		Treat seizure Px
Cimetidine	300 mg IV q6h		Treat ulcer Px
Alupent	0.3 ml in 2 ml saline q4h		Aerosol
Methyldopa	250–500 mg IV q6–8h		Lower BP
Ensure	Half-strength or full-strength at 75–100 ml/hr		Nutritional
Ensure Plus	75–100 ml/hr		Nutritional
Osmolite	Half-strength or full-strength at 75–100 ml/hr		Nutritional
Prochlorperazine	10 mg IM q4–6 h p.r.n.		Treat nausea
Vitamin K_1	25 mg IM		Reverse Coumadin
Nifedipine	10 mg SL q6h		Lower BP

BP = blood pressure; D/W = dextrose in water; IICP = increased intracranial pressure; NG = nasogastric; Px = prevention; SL = sublingual.

tected from light and freshly prepared. Hypotension is controlled by an infusion of dopamine (2 to 20 μg per kilogram per minute) or norepinephrine bitartrate (Levophed bitartrate) (4 ml per 1,000 ml in 5 percent dextrose in water at a rate of 0.5 to 1 ml per minute, average dose) (see Table 1).

4. Evidence of increasing intracranial pressure is treated with an infusion of a 20 percent mannitol solution (100 g of mannitol in 500 ml 5 percent dextrose in water) at a rate of 100 ml per hour or, more urgently, a bolus of 25 to 50 g of mannitol. I also immediately administer dexamethasone, 10 mg IV, although this treatment is controversial.

5. An indwelling urinary catheter should be placed and a baseline urinalysis and urine culture obtained.

6. Finally, the patient should be observed (by telemetry) for an arrhythmia while awaiting transfer to the operating room. Lidocaine (as a 50- to 100-mg bolus) should be administered for runs of premature ventricular contractions of three or more, or more than six per minute, followed by a drip of 2 mg per minute. Atropine, 0.5 to 1 mg IV, should be administered for a bradycardia of less than 50 beats per minute (see Table 1).

By the time these steps have been taken, preparations will have been made for the evacuation of the hematoma. If they have not, the patient should be transferred to an appropriate facility.

I have discussed the emergency treatment of a significant hypertensive intracerebellar hematoma first because it is a *treatable* lesion, often with a good prognosis for survival and acceptable function. The above scenario illustrates, with some exceptions (see below), the emergency neuromedical treatment necessary to support a patient in whom surgical treatment is indicated. However, the indications for surgical treatment may be uncertain or even contraindicated if the hypertensive hemorrhage is located at any of the other common sites.

Putaminal Hemorrhage

The comatose patient requires an intravenous line, stabilization, regulation of blood pressure, and an indwelling urinary catheter, and should be watched for cardiac arrhythmias, all as noted above. In addition I begin administering diphenylhydantoin (Dilantin) with a loading dose of 500 mg IV (if no seizures have occurred, otherwise 1,000 mg IV), specifying a rate of 50 mg per minute or less by direct push. A maintenance dose of 100 mg every 6 hours IV, by direct push, is continued with the same caveat, and serum Dilantin levels are obtained within 4 to 5 days. Finally, cimetidine, 300 mg every 6 hours IV, is administered to prevent a Cushing's ulcer.

Should the comatose patient with a putaminal hemorrhage be intubated and receive ventilatory support? In my experience, patients with a hypertensive putaminal hemorrhage severe enough to require artificial ventilation have such a poor prognosis that ventilatory support is not indicated. An airway (preferably) or intubation may be indicated for tracheal toilet only. This is, of course, an ethical as well as a medical (and medicolegal) decision and must be made after a frank discussion with the family, guardian, or attorney, if a "living will" is available indicating the wishes of the patient. I personally advise against the institution of ventilatory support. Frequently, however, this decision is moot, since the patient has already been intubated and is receiving ventilatory assistance by the time evaluation is made by a neurologist.

Similar considerations exist for surgical evacuation of a putaminal hematoma, which often involves more than the putamen, especially the internal capsule. If the patient is comatose and the brain stem embarrassed, evacuation of the hematoma is *not* indicated. If the patient is comatose, or consciousness is declining but the brain stem is intact, evacuation of the hematoma *may save life but functional recovery is usually poor*. I advise against surgery, but discuss the option frankly with the patient's family. I advise against evacuation of the hematoma as a means of improving a hemiparesis, aphasia, or other focal neurologic deficit.

Thalamic Hemorrhage

I do not consider evacuation of the hematoma indicated for preservation of life or for improving neurologic function. Considerations for respiratory support are the same as for putaminal hemorrhage. Blood pressure should be controlled as described above. Mannitol should be infused in an attempt to reduce intracranial pressure. I also continue to administer dexamethasone (a 10-mg IV bolus followed by 4 to 6 mg every 6 hours, IV or IM for the first 24 to 72 hours) in an attempt to reduce cerebral edema.

Pontine Hemorrhage

Usually a hypertensive pontine hemorrhage is a devastating event. The patient enters the hospital comatose, quadriplegic, with severe gaze palsies and bilateral Horner's syndrome. Because the prognosis is so poor, I do not advise surgery or respiratory support. If, however, the patient is already receiving ventilatory support, this should be continued. Once rapport is established with the family and the grave prognosis is outlined, the question of continuing ventilatory support may be addressed. Control and stabilization of blood pressure should be continued. Increased intracranial pressure is not a problem. The question of control of life-threatening cardiac arrhythmias should be agreed upon with the family as soon as possible.

SUBACUTE CARE

Hypertensive Intracerebral Hemorrhage

Cerebellar Hemorrhage

Of the common sites of hypertensive intracerebral hemorrhage, in my opinion only a cerebellar hemorrhage should be considered a surgically treatable disease. However, if the patient with a cerebellar hematoma remains alert with flexor plantar responses, neuromedical treatment with close observation is indicated. A diminution in level of consciousness and/or a reversion to extensor plantar responses (indicating brain stem compression) should lead to hematoma evacuation.

Putaminal Hemorrhage

If the level of consciousness of a previously alert patient with a putaminal hemorrhage deteriorates, evacuation of the hematoma may be offered to the family. I stress, however, that in my experience, functional results of surgery have been poor.

Thalamic Hemorrhage

If alertness diminishes because of thalamic hemorrhage, obstruction of the third ventricle of the cerebrum should be searched for by computed tomographic (CT) scan, and if it is documented, lateral ventricular shunting should be considered. Patients with hematomas large enough to obstruct the third ventricle usually have a poor prognosis, even if life is sustained.

Nonhypertensive Hemorrhage

Except for the intracerebral hemorrhage (or hemorrhages) of amyloid angiopathy, the other causes of nonhypertensive intracerebral hematoma warrant a more aggressive approach to treatment. Considerations including the patient's neurologic condition, the site of the lesion, the age of the patient, and the etiology of the hemorrhage should enter into the decision-making process.

Patient's Neurologic Condition. Deterioration of the level of consciousness warrants hematoma evacuation. Coma or other levels of seriously impaired consciousness, with intact pupillary responses, intact extraocular movements (demonstrable, if necessary, by caloric stimulation), and spontaneous respirations, also warrant hematoma evacuation. If the patient is reasonably alert, however, and remains so, surgical treatment is not indicated.

Site of Lesion. Cortical-subcortical or cerebellar hematomas are eminently suitable for evacuation. The hematoma of pituitary apoplexy may need transsphenoidal evacuation to relieve upward compression on optic chiasm or nerves, hypothalamus, or mesencephalon. Thalamic or pontine hematomas should be evacuated, particularly in the younger patient, if there is neurologic deterioration.

Age of Patient. The child or young adult is especially likely to benefit from hematoma evacuation.

Etiology of Hemorrhage. Intracerebral hematoma caused by aneurysm, arteriovenous malformation, idiopathic thrombocytopenic purpura, leukemia, trauma, vasculitis, anticoagulation, antiplatelet agents, clot-dissolving enzymes, or unknown cause all indicate hematoma evacuation, depending on the neurologic status and course. Decisions regarding hemorrhage into a known primary or secondary cerebral malignancy depends, at least to some degree, on the prognosis of the underlying tumor.

NEUROMEDICAL CARE

Respiratory

Nasopharyngeal or oropharyngeal suctioning should be performed every 1 to 2 hours, or more often if necessary. An aerosol of metaproterenol sulfate (Alupent), 0.3 ml in 2 ml saline every 4 hours (except during sleep), is ordered to prevent atelectasis. If the patient is alert, the aerosol is administered via a mouthpiece; if the patient is stuperous, it should be administered via a mask.

Blood Pressure

After 24 hours, an attempt is made to discontinue sodium nitroprusside, and methyldopa (250 to 500 mg every 6 to 8 hours IV) is started, unless oral medication (e.g., diuretics, captopril, nifedipine) can be taken and proves effective. Sublingual nifedipine, 10 mg every 6 hours, may be sufficient to control hypertension.

Activity

The patient is prescribed bedrest until vital signs and neurologic conditions are stable, and the patient is alert for at least 24 hours. Bedside range of motion is also ordered when the patient is neuromedically stable. If the patient is alert, a trapeze is put over the bed to enable him to change his own position. Unless the duration of bedrest is minimal, sitting in a chair is not permitted until vascular reflexes have proven adequate on a tilt table.

Increased Intracranial Pressure

Mannitol is used only on an urgent basis. If clinical evidence of increased intracranial pressure persists for more than 12 to 24 hours, the continuation of mannitol therapy is of little use. Rebound may occur when it is discontinued. Dexamethasone is continued at 4 to 6 mg every 6 hours for 3 to 5 days, and is then gradually discontinued by halving the dose every 2 days.

Anticonvulsants

Dilantin is continued intravenously until the patient can take medication by mouth, nasogastric tube, or percutaneous esophagogastrostomy (PEG). If an allergic rash develops, carbamazepine (Tegretol), 200 mg every 8 hours is administered via a nasogastric tube. In all patients with lesions involving cerebral cortex or subcortex, I continue to administer anticonvulsants for at least 1 year.

Nutrition

Intravenous fluids provide the sole source of nutrition for the first 96 hours. Thereafter, one must consider more adequate nutrition via oral, nasogastric, or PEG feeding. If the patient is alert and able to swallow, oral feeding is started as a liquid diet, advancing to mechanical soft, bland, and regular diets (in that order). I try to provide nourishment of at least 1,500 to 2,000 cal per day. If the patient is unable to swallow safely, feeding is accomplished by nasogastric tube or PEG. If the patient appears able to survive but the prognosis for oral feeding in the near future seems poor, a PEG is advised. If the prognosis for recovery is hopeful, nasogastric feeding is started.

There are several liquid feeding systems available. I usually start with Ensure or Osmolite (1.06 cal per milliliter) in equal parts with water by constant drip at a rate of 75 to 100 ml per hour. This is advanced to full strength, then to Ensure Plus (1.5 cal per milliliter) at a rate of 75 to 100 ml per hour.

Headache and Nausea

Headache is usually controllable with codeine, 32 mg IM every 4 to 6 hours; nausea with prochlorperazine 10 mg IM every 4 to 6 hours, as necessary.

Skin Care

It is the physician's responsibility to prevent the occurrence of a decubitus ulcer (bedsore). This must *never* occur. I order the following: (1) sheep's wool under torso and heels (inflatable pads or mattresses, in my opinion, are worse than useless, as most only make the patient perspire and thus contribute to the problem); (2) that the patient be turned *every hour;* and (3) that the patient's back be dry and powdered, with the skin inspected daily for erythema or other color change.

Specific Therapy

If hemorrhage is caused by warfarin sodium (Coumadin) therapy, vitamin K_1, 25 mg IM (not IV), should be administered. If it is caused by thrombocytopenia, platelet transfusion is indicated. If the cause is unknown, angiography should be performed, especially in younger patients, to search for an arteriovenous malformation, which, if demonstrated, requires surgical treatment. An aneurysm, demonstrated by angiography, requires definitive surgical treatment.

Rehabilitation

In my opinion, rehabilitation is more than a means of psychological support for the patient and family. A frank discussion of what neurorehabilitation is likely to accomplish in the individual patient is warranted. The family should not, for example, expect a hemiplegic arm to be restored to complete usefulness by the rehabilitation process. However, increased general strength and endurance, adaptation, substitution, bracing, the use of aids and appliances, and the alteration of the home environment may be expected to improve function. Intensive speech therapy is indicated in motivated individuals. I send my patients for physical, occupational, and if they are dysphasic, for speech therapy, starting at the bedside as soon as the patient is stable. Regular rounds in the rehabilitation department prove instructive to the physician and helpful to the patient.

SUGGESTED READING

Fisher CM, Picard EH, Polak A, et al. Acute hypertensive cerebellar hemorrhage: diagnosis and surgical treatment. J Nerv Ment Dis 1965;140:38.

McKissock W, Richardson A, Taylor J. Primary intracerebral hemorrhage: a controlled trial of surgical and conservative treatment in 180 unselected cases. Lancet 1961;2:221.

Humphreys RP, Hockley AD, Freedman MH, Saunders EF. Management of intracerebral hemorrhage in idiopathic thrombocytopenic purpura. J Neurosurg 1976;45:700.

Zervas NT, Mendelson G. Treatment of acute haemorrhage of pituitary tumours. Lancet 1975;1:604.

PATIENT RESOURCES

Stroke support groups:

National Stroke Association
1420 Ogden Street
Denver, Colorado 80218
Telephone: (303) 839-1992

Stroke Club International
805 12th Street
Galveston, Texas 77550
(Will give location of state or local chapter.)

ESSENTIAL TREMOR

WILLIAM C. KOLLER, M.D., Ph.D.

Essential tremor is a common disorder of the nervous system characterized by tremor of the hands, head, voice, and less often, the legs and trunk. Half of the cases occur sporadically and half are familial, transmitted as an autosomal dominant. Hand tremor is characteristically present during maintenance of a position (postural tremor) and during active movements (kinetic tremor). Patients complain of difficulty with handwriting, drinking liquids, and manipulative tasks. Hand tremor, and especially head tremor, result in embarrassment and potential social isolation. Essential voice tremor has a characteristic quavering intonation which results in a fluctuating and rhythmic dysphonia. Essential tremor is sometimes described as being benign. While the tremor may be a nuisance to some patients, the livelihood of others is threatened by it, and many experience functional disabilities. Effective treatment is available for many patients with essential tremor (Table 1).

ALCOHOL

Many patients relate that the ingestion of a small amount of alcohol will temporarily cause a substantial reduction of their tremor. Often patients find that a single glass of wine or even one beer will

TABLE 1 Treatment of Essential Tremor

Drugs with proven efficacy
Alcohol
Beta-adrenergic blockers
Primidone
Drugs with possible efficacy
Phenobarbital
Alprazolam
Drugs with limited efficacy
Diazepam
Clonazepam
Clonidine
Amantadine
Alpha-adrenergic blockers

check their tremor for 45 minutes to 1 hour. In 1949, McDonald Critchley stated that patients with essential tremor note that "a heavy dose of spirits will temporarily check the tremor." The effect of alcohol on essential tremor appears to be unique to this disorder. Patients with parkinsonian or cerebellar tremor do not find a dramatic reduction in their symptoms with alcohol intake. In several controlled studies, alcohol administered both orally and intravenously has been found to cause a dramatic reduction in essential tremor. All patients tested responded, and almost 75 percent of the patients experienced a reduction in their tremor. Alcohol would appear to be one of the most effective drugs in the treatment of essential tremor. Alcohol probably works through a central mechanism, as the local intra-arterial infusion of alcohol does not decrease tremor. However, exactly how alcohol works is unclear. Alcohol has a variety of actions on the central nervous system and affects many neurotransmitter systems. Yet an understanding of alcohol's action in the reduction of essential tremor could lead to the development of better pharmacologic agents for the treatment of this disorder.

A major concern with the use of alcohol to treat essential tremor is the fear that some patients might become chronic alcoholics. Critchley warned that alcohol was used to treat essential tremor "apparently all too often to serve as an excuse for habits of intemperance." Some considered the risk of addiction as a contraindication for the use of alcohol. The rate of chronic alcoholism in patients with essential tremor has been recently defined. A retrospective chart survey of former patients yielded a relatively high alcoholic rate. According to three subsequent prospective studies done in the United States, Sweden, and Finland, however, the prevalence of pathological drinking among patients with essential tremor did not differ from that among patients with other tremor disorders or chronic neurologic disease without tremor. As essential tremor often gets worse when the effect of alcohol wears off or the morning after heavy alcohol ingestion, it seems reasonable to assume that heavy alcohol consumption would not be a major problem for patients with essential tremor. Since chronic alcoholism and essential tremor are very common disorders, one would think that by chance alone these disorders may frequently coexist. Also, chronic alcoholism itself may result in a persistent tremor disorder lasting for as long as 1 year after complete abstinence. It can be concluded that the occasional use of alcohol in the treatment of essential tremor is not contraindicated and that the risk of alcoholism is low. The judicious use of small amounts of alcoholic beverages before meals or other events to reduce tremor appears reasonable. Many patients find that taking a glass of wine or some other alcoholic drink before meals helps them perform that task much more easily. Perhaps the recommendation of a glass of wine before dinner is a reasonable one for patients with tremor and those individuals without tremor alike.

BETA-ADRENERGIC BLOCKERS

Propranolol

In 1971, two groups independently reported that propranolol decreased essential tremor. Initially 24 patients were investigated in a double-blind crossover study using objective measurements. The average effective dose was 120 mg per day, with a range of 60 to 240 mg per day in divided doses. No side effects were encountered. Subsequent studies have also shown the efficacy of propranolol in the treatment of essential tremor. Some studies, however, have reported a lack of effect, but these results were probably due to inadequate dosage, small sample size, or lack of objective measures. Investigations that confirmed the efficacy of propranolol in reducing hand tremor used both subjective and objective (accelerometer recording) evaluations. According to these studies, tremor amplitude was decreased but tremor frequency was left unchanged.

Propranolol has become the drug of choice for the treatment of essential tremor. It is useful both for reducing essential tremor and for blocking stress-induced enhancement of the tremor. A sustained release preparation (long-acting propranolol) designed to be used in a once-daily dose is available and is preferred by many patients for ease of administration. Similar therapeutic results were obtained when this preparation was compared with multiple doses of propranolol. The drug is, however, somewhat more costly than generic propranolol. The clinical response of patients to propranolol is variable and often incomplete. A wide range of individual responses is to be expected. It is generally estimated that 50 to 70 percent of patients will have some symptomatic control. Dramatic improvement occurs in a much smaller percentage, and only in a rare individual is tremor totally suppressed. Unfortunately, some patients will have no response to this agent. In those patients who do respond, average tremor reduction is usually 50 to 60 percent, often allowing a patient to perform writing, eating, drinking, and other activities of daily living. The effective dose varies widely among individuals. In a dose response study, 120 to 320 mg per day in divided doses was found to be optimal. Doses greater than 320 mg per day provided no additional benefits and were associated with a higher incidence of side effects. There is no correlation between plasma drug levels and therapeutic response. No clinical characteristics have been identified that allow one to predict who will respond to the drug. A reasonable starting dose is 80 to 120 mg per day. This can be given in divided doses or, if the long-acting preparation is used, as a single dose. One question that is not totally resolved is the long-term efficacy of propranolol treatment. Some have suggested that tolerance to the drug occurs over time. In one recent study, however, loss of drug effect occurred in less than 15 percent of patients who were followed for 1 year. Propranolol therefore appears to have both short-term and long-term benefit.

Propranolol therapy is usually fairly well tolerated. Relative contraindications for propranolol use are (1) heart failure, especially if poorly controlled, (2) second-degree and third-degree atrioventricular block, (3) asthma or other bronchospastic disease, and (4) insulin-dependent diabetes, where propranolol may block the adrenergic manifestations of hypoglycemia. Many side effects of propranolol are related to beta-blockade. The pulse will be lowered in most patients. A pulse of 60 beats per minute is usually well tolerated. However, if the pulse is less than 50 beats per minute, it is probably wise to reduce the dose or discontinue the drug, even if the patient is asymptomatic. Other less common adverse reactions include fatigue, lassitude, nausea, diarrhea, skin rash, and impotence. A variety of mental status changes (e.g., depression) may also occur. It is important for the clinician to ascertain if these side effects are present, since often the patient may not volunteer this information when simply asked whether they are suffering any adverse reaction. If a patient does have adverse reactions with one beta-blocking drug, it may be possible to switch to another beta-blocking drug and retain the therapeutic efficacy without incurring the same type of side effect. The mechanism of action of propranolol in the treatment of essential tremor is unknown. Initially it was proposed that a central site of action was necessary because of a delay in the effect of chronic oral therapy. However, recent studies have shown that the effect of an oral dose of propranolol is almost immediate in reducing tremor. Beta-adrenergic–blocking drugs that have poor penetration of the central nervous system also decrease essential tremor, as do drugs that have pure beta-2–blocking properties. Therefore, it appears that propranolol acts at a peripheral site of action, probably through blockade of beta-2 adrenergic receptors, which are located on muscle spindles.

Other Beta-Adrenergic Blockers

Other beta-adrenergic blockers are currently available (Table 2). These drugs are also useful in the treatment of essential tremor. If essential tremor does not respond to propranolol, however, it will not respond to other beta-adrenergic–blocking drugs.

Metoprolol has been shown to reduce essential tremor. This drug differs from propranolol in preferentially antagonizing beta-1 adrenergic receptors. This selectivity for beta-1 receptors is, however, only relative. With higher doses, beta-2 adrenergic receptors are also blocked. Some degree of beta-2 blockade appears in patients receiving daily doses of more than 100 mg. Metoprolol is effective in the treatment of essential tremor in divided doses of 100 to 200 mg per day. It has been suggested that metoprolol is the preferred drug for patients with bronchospastic disease. Because of its relative lack of beta-2–blocking properties, metoprolol is theoretically better tolerated than propranolol or other nonspecific blockers. Several asthmatic patients with essential tremor have been reported to tolerate metoprolol but not propranolol. Metoprolol is also capable of causing respiratory distress, however, and should be used with caution in bronchospastic disease.

Because of its renal excretion, nadolol can be given in a single daily dosage and has been shown to significantly decrease essential tremor. Atenolol and timolol have been reported in several studies to have only a limited effect on essential tremor. Pindolol possesses partial agonist activity and may cause tremors.

PRIMIDONE

O'Brien and colleagues noted that when primidone was given to a patient with epilepsy and essential tremor, he reported marked reduction in

TABLE 2 Pharmacologic Properties of Beta-Adrenergic Blockers

Drug	*Beta-Blockage Potency*	*Cardioselectivity Relative Beta$_1$ Blockage*	*Partial Agonist Activity*	*Membrane Stabilization*	*Plasma Half-Life*	*Penetration Into Central Nervous System*	*Metabolism*
Propranolol	1	–	0	+	5–12 hrs	Good	Hepatic
Metoprolol	1	+	0	–	3–4 hrs	Good	Hepatic
Nadolol	0.5	–	0	–	20–24 hrs	Good	Renal
Atenolol	1	+	0	–	6–8 hrs	Poor	Hepatic
Timolol	6	–	+	–	4–5 hrs	Good	Hepatic
Pindolol	6	–	+	+	3–4 hrs	Good	Hepatic

tremor. They therefore gave the drug to 20 other patients, starting with a dose of 125 mg and increasing to 750 mg per day. In 1981, they reported that 12 patients had a good clinical response to the drug. Six patients, including four receiving the 125-mg dose, could not tolerate the drug because of side effects (vertigo, unsteadiness, and nausea). The addition of propranolol resulted in further clinical improvement in these patients. They concluded that primidone was more effective than propranolol, but that patients with essential tremor could not tolerate primidone as well as seizure patients. Several other studies have confirmed the efficacy of primidone in the treatment of essential tremor. It was found in one study that doses as low as 50 mg would reduce tremor and that doses of more than 250 mg were not associated with any greater reduction in tremor. The drug was given in a single night-time dosage. No correlation has been found between therapeutic response and serum drug levels. Several studies have found that primidone decreases essential tremor more than propranolol, and it is not uncommon to see very dramatic responses to primidone. However, some patients will not respond to the drug. There are no predictive factors that indicate which patients will respond to the drug. It has been suggested that the starting dose be 50 mg given at night-time, and that it then be increased, if necessary, to 125 mg and then to 250 mg taken as a single dose at night-time. The 50-mg dose is available as a pediatric dose form. The 250-mg tablet is scored and can be broken to provide the 125-mg dose. If the drug is taken before going to bed, there is less difficulty with daytime sedation and the therapeutic benefit tends to occur throughout the day.

A major problem with the use of primidone in the treatment of essential tremor is initial acute reactions. It has been estimated that 25 to 30 percent of the patients have a reaction the following day. This consists of an ''ill'' feeling involving nausea, malaise, and sometimes ataxia. This is a transient reaction that will last 1 to 3 days regardless of whether the drug is discontinued. This idiosyncratic reaction occurs even if a dose smaller than 50 mg is given. Many patients will attempt to discontinue the drug after the acute initial reaction. The patient should therefore be warned that such a reaction may occur; I often advise our patients to take the drug for the first time on a Friday when they have nothing planned for the weekend. If patients know that this reaction might occur and that it is transient and will not interfere with long-term drug treatment, they will probably not discontinue the drug. I ask that my patients call me if a reaction does occur, and encourage them to continue the drug and remind them that the reaction will soon go way. In a rare patient, adverse reactions may last for 1 week or longer, but the side effects often diminish quickly with time. Long-term side effects of primidone tend to be minimal when 250 mg at night-time is employed. There is also some controversy as to whether patients develop tolerance to primidone's effects. Some patients relate that their best tremor reduction occurs during the morning after the first night-time dose and that the tremor may still remain reduced below baseline levels thereafter. Some patients have been reported in whom the drug loses efficacy after several months of therapy. In one study, however, 85 percent of the patients still retained therapeutic benefit after 1 year of treatment. Tolerance does not appear to be a common problem with primidone therapy.

The mechanism of action of primidone's antitremor effect is unknown. Primidone is converted to two active metabolites: phenyethylmelomide (PEMA) with a half-life of 24 to 40 hours, and phenobarbital with a half-life of 50 to 120 hours. Primidone has a half-life of approximately 10 hours. PEMA has been administered to patients with essential tremor and has been found to have no effect. As discussed below, there is some controversy as to whether phenobarbital has an antitremor action. If primidone is given acutely, reduction of tremor is seen during the first several hours after administration. At this time, no phenobarbital is detected in the bloodstream, indicating that primidone's acute effect, at least, is not mediated through phenobarbital.

DRUG OF CHOICE

Both propranolol and primidone are effective drugs in the treatment of essential tremor. There is no concensus on the first drug that should be employed. For most patients, I prefer to start with primidone because it is effective in more patients and a greater degree of tremor reduction is often observed. The initial adverse reactions are problematic but, as I have discussed, if the patient is warned about this and encouraged to continue using the drug, the patient tends not to be deterred. The long-term side effects with primidone are generally minimal. Propranolol, on the other hand, is contraindicated in some patients, and the drug is not well tolerated by the many elderly patients. Mental changes that occur in some patients with propranolol and side effects with chronic therapy are additional negative aspects of this drug. I therefore prefer to give patients primidone in an initial dose of 50 mg at night, which I then increase to 125 or 250 mg after several weeks. If the patient has no response to 250 mg of primidone, I discontinue the drug. However, if the patient has some tremor reduction but still has functional disability, I will add propranolol to the dosage regimen. I prefer long-acting propranolol because of its ease of administration and good patient compliance. I usually give patients the long-acting preparation in an initial dose of 80 or 120 mg taken immediately on arising in the morning.

This dose can be increased to a total dose of 320 mg per day. Two drugs in combination will often cause tremor reduction and an increase in functional capabilities, with improvement in handwriting, drinking, and eating. Unfortunately, embarrassment and fine manual dexterity remain a problem for many patients even when tremor reduction can be demonstrated by objective measures.

PHENOBARBITAL

Phenobarbital has been used in the treatment of essential tremor for a long time and antedates the use of many other drugs. It is generally considered to have low efficacy. Although several studies have demonstrated that the drug does cause some tremor reduction, other studies have shown no effect. Sedation is often a major problem with the use of the drug. I therefore almost never employ this drug in the treatment of essential tremor.

ALPRAZOLAM

Recently a double-blind placebo-controlled parallel study of 24 patients was done showing that alprazolam (Xanax) causes reduction of essential tremor. However, mild fatigue and sedation occurred in 50 percent of these patients, and it is possible that tremor reduction could have been caused in part by the sedation. It was suggested that alprazolam may be effective in those needing only intermittent therapy. Further investigation is needed before this drug can be considered to have efficacy in the treatment of essential tremor. However, if propranolol and primidone have been found not to be effective, a trial of alprazolam may be indicated. The drug can be started at 0.25 mg twice per day and then slowly increased. Sedation often limits the ability to increase the dose to more than 1 to 2 mg per day.

OTHER DRUGS

Other benzodiazepines such as diazepam have often been employed in the treatment of essential tremor. Benzodiazepines may be more effective when used in combination with propranolol therapy and may block the enhancement of tremor by stress. However, these drugs have never been scientifically evaluated. It is my general impression that diazepam has very limited usefulness in the treatment of essential tremor and I never prescribe the drug. There are several anecdotal reports that clonidine and amantadine may be effective in reducing essential tremor. Similarly, there are reports of alpha-adrenergic blockers decreasing essential tremor. However, when studied in controlled trials, these drugs have been found to have no efficacy.

SURGERY

Surgical therapy (stereotaxic thalomotomy) is an option for those patients with severe tremor that causes marked functional disability that is unresponsive to all medications. Ablation of the ventral intermediate nucleus of the thalamus appears to alleviate parkinsonian, essential, and cerebellar type tremors equally well. Paresis, speech disturbances, hypertonus, and cerebellar dysfunction represent possible adverse reactions. Bilateral operations are rarely indicated because of the high incidence of speech abnormalities associated with this treatment. Tremor may recur in a certain percentage of patients. There has been no published long-term follow-up of stereotaxic thalomotomy in the treatment of essential tremor. My personal experience indicates that stereotaxic thalomotomy is efficacious in the treatment of essential tremor; however, not all patients will have good results. It is unclear how long the benefit will last. I have followed some patients for several years who have had continual benefit from the surgery. Therefore this option should be considered in patients with severe disabling tremor that has not responded to pharmacologic agents. With current technology, the procedure does appear to be associated with minimal risk only. Nevertheless, many patients are not inclined to undergo the procedure and refuse it when offered.

BEHAVIORAL THERAPY

A variety of behavior techniques including psychotherapy, biofeedback, and hypnosis have been employed in the treatment of movement disorders. Any benefit from these procedures has been minimal and short-lived. There is one anecdotal report of psychotherapy being helpful in the treatment of essential tremor. The reported improvement was believed to be caused by mental stabilization and relaxation of muscle tension. It is my opinion that behavioral therapy currently plays no role in the treatment of essential tremor.

ESSENTIAL TREMOR VARIANTS

A variety of atypical tremor disorders exist that appear to be related to essential tremor (Table 3). The association of these conditions with essential tremor is suggested by the high occurrence of a fam-

TABLE 3 Variants of Essential Tremor

Kinetic predominant hand tremor
Primary writing tremor
Orthostatic truncal tremor

ily history of essential tremor, the frequent presence of a mild postural tremor, and reduction in tremor noted to occur with alcohol ingestion. These tremor disorders have a different pharmacologic responsiveness than the more typical essential tremor. Most patients with essential tremor have varying degrees of postural and kinetic tremors. Marked dissociation occurs in what has been referred to as kinetic predominant tremor, where the postural component is minimal or absent. Cerebellar signs are also absent. Functional disability may be severe in patients with a marked kinetic tremor. These patients have been reported to have significant tremor reduction when taking clonazepam in doses of 1 to 2 mg per day. Drowsiness limits further dosage increase in many patients. Although propranolol is helpful in some of these patients, clonazepam appears to be the first drug of choice in the treatment of kinetic predominant essential tremor.

Primary writing tremor refers to a test-specific or selective action tremor in which pronation of the forearm elicits a pronation/supination tremor. Often it is not seen during other movements of the arm. The patient's chief complaint is "my hand shakes while writing." This disorder needs to be distinguished from writer's cramp or focal dystonia of the hand. Primidone or propranolol may be effective in some patients with this disorder. Anticholinergics have also been reported to reduce this tremor, and these drugs should be tried if the patient does not respond to primidone or propranolol.

Truncal tremors are sometimes observed in essential tremor as a late manifestation. An uncommon variant of essential tremor is orthostatic truncal tremor. In this condition, the sole symptom is a tremor of the trunk and proximal legs that occurs while standing. The tremor worsens the longer the patient stands, and may lead to falling. The tremor is absent when the patient is sitting, walking, or leaning against a firm support. Propranolol has been reported to be ineffective in the treatment of this disorder. However, clonazepam has been found to cause a marked reduction in a truncal tremor, and this has been confirmed by several reports. Clonazepam should be the first drug of choice in orthostatic truncal tremor.

GENERAL APPROACH

Treatment of essential tremor of the hand or head should start with primidone in a dose of 50 mg at bedtime, with the dose increased gradually to 250 mg per day. Propranolol at 80 to 120 mg should be added and increased to a maximum of 320 mg per day if the response remains inadequate. Long-acting propranolol can be used if once-daily administration is desired. Hand tremor tends to respond the best, and although head tremor may be reduced, it may still cause embarrassment for the patient. Tremor of the voice appears to respond poorly to both propranolol and primidone therapy. Rare variants of essential tremor may respond to clonazepam therapy. The use of these drugs frequently results in tremor reduction and increased functional abilities. However, some patients do not respond to any therapy and remain disabled.

SUGGESTED READING

Critchley M. Observations on an essential tremor. Brain 1949; 72:113–139.

Larsen TA, Calne DB. Essential tremor. Clin Neuropharmacol 1983; 6:285–306.

Koller WC. Diagnosis and treatment of tremors. In: Neurology Clinics. Jankovic J, ed. Philadelphia: WB Saunders Co. 1984:499.

Koller WC. Dose response relationship of propranolol in essential tremor. Arch Neurol 1986; 35:42–43.

Koller WC, Royse VL. Efficacy of primidone in the treatment of essential tremor. Neurology 1986; 26:121–124.

PATIENT RESOURCE

The International Tremor Foundation provides information on essential tremor and other tremor disorders and publishes a quarterly newsletter for patients with tremor disorders.

The International Tremor Foundation
360 West Superior
Chicago, Illinois 60610

PARKINSON'S DISEASE

STEPHEN G. REICH, M.D.
MAHLON R. DELONG, M.D.

Parkinson's disease (PD) is one of the most common movement disorders seen by primary care physicians and neurologists. The usual ease of diagnosis and the relatively few treatment options currently available suggest that management should be easy. However, the controversy about the optimal time to begin administering levodopa (Sinemet), the eventual emergence of motor fluctuations and drug-induced side effects in most patients, and the emotional and cognitive problems as well as the problems for the caregiver frequently encountered during long-term care of patients with PD present the physician with an intricate array of management options and dilemmas.

DIAGNOSIS

The classic signs of PD include tremor at rest, bradykinesia, stooped posture, masked face with diminished blink rate, cogwheel rigidity, shuffling gait, and postural instability. When all or most of these signs are present, the diagnosis is straightforward and is often made while the patient is observed in the waiting room; in his original essay *The Shaking Palsy* (1817) James Parkinson himself tells us that he encountered professionally only three of the six patients he reported, whereas the others were casually observed on the streets of London. We have observed three presentations of PD that occasionally lead to a delay in the diagnosis:

1. When the patient presents with a severe, dominant tremor without any other parkinsonian features or with other parkinsonian features that are subtle. In such patients, the essential tremor may be mistakenly diagnosed.
2. When tremor is absent in a patient presenting with unilateral rigidity and bradykinesia ("pseudo-hemiplegic" PD). In such cases, diagnoses of upper or lower motor neuron syndromes are entertained.
3. When patients with PD are younger than 50 years of age. PD may not be considered in the differential diagnosis, despite the fact that, while uncommon, PD may present as early as the fourth or fifth decade of life.

Although Parkinson's *disease* is the most common diagnosis among patients presenting with parkinsonian signs, there are a number of other diseases which must be considered in the differential diagnosis (Table 1). The appearance of cerebellar, corticospinal, lower motor neuron, autonomic, or ocular motor signs, particularly in patients with little or no response to antiparkinsonian medications, is a clue that another parkinsonian syndrome may be at hand.

GENERAL TREATMENT PRINCIPLES

The first step in effective treatment is education. Many patients are under the mistaken impression that the diagnosis of PD promises a future of complete dependency. We point out that although progressive, the rate is generally very slow, that effective treatment is available, and that most patients with PD live a normal life span and remain productive. Patient-oriented books and support groups should be prescribed with caution just after a patient is diagnosed, as they often serve only to emphasize the "worst case scenario." But as the disease progresses, both are useful, sometimes as much to the caregiver as to the patient.

From the beginning, emphasis is placed on the *activities of daily living* (ADLs) as the "barometer" for deciding when to initiate treatment and when

TABLE 1 Differential Diagnosis of Parkinsonism

Toxins
Manganese
Carbon monoxide
Carbon disulfide
Cyanide
Methanol
MPTP
Drugs
Neuroleptic
Metoclopramide
Multisystem degenerations
Progressive supranuclear palsy
Shy-Drager syndrome
Olivopontocerebellar atrophy
Striatonigral degeneration
Amyotrophic lateral sclerosis-PD-Dementia complex of Guam
Primary dementing illnesses
Alzheimer's disease
Creutzfeldt-Jakob disease
Heredofamilial diseases
Wilson's disease
Juvenile Huntington's disease
Hallervorden-Spatz syndrome
Multi-infarct state
Calcification of the basal ganglia
Idiopathic
Hypoparathyroidism

medication adjustments are needed in patients already receiving treatment. During routine follow-up visits, unless worsening symptoms translate into a *functional* decline, we do not make any changes in medication. The one exception to this rule is that when patients find the signs of PD embarrassing but not necessarily functionally limiting, we adjust antiparkinsonian medications accordingly. Before starting treatment we emphasize to patients that the goal is not to eliminate all of the symptoms and signs of PD, but rather to maintain an effective degree of functioning.

ANTIPARKINSONIAN THERAPY

Drugs used for the treatment of PD fall into one of two classes: anticholinergics and dopaminergics (Table 2). The latter group includes levodopa, which is usually combined with a decarboxylase inhibitor, carbidopa, and the direct dopamine receptor agonists bromocriptine and pergolide mesylate. Amantadine has both anticholinergic and dopaminergic activity.

Our treatment strategy is to begin administering an anticholinergic or amantadine when there is minimal impairment of the ADLs. As the disease progresses, we add Sinemet and increase toward a total daily levodopa dose of 400 mg, at which point bromocriptine or pergolide is added as adjunctive therapy. The goal is to use the least amount of medication necessary to maintain a reasonable degree of functioning.

Anticholinergics

Anticholinergics are helpful in the treatment of early PD, particularly when tremor is a predominant sign. No single preparation has been shown convincingly to be superior to the others, and as a group, anticholinergics are the least expensive of the antiparkinsonian medications. Although in modest doses they are generally well tolerated by younger patients, side effects include dry mouth, blurred vision, constipation, urinary retention, memory loss, and confusion. We try to avoid the use of anticholinergics in elderly or demented patients.

Amantadine Hydrochloride

Originally marketed as an anti-influenzal drug, amantadine (Symmetrel) was discovered by chance to improve PD. Although useful in the treatment of early PD, its beneficial effect is generally short-lived, and most patients will require additional treatment within 6 to 12 months. Once the patient begins taking Sinemet, amantadine can often be discontinued with no deterioration of the patient's condition. Common side effects include pedal edema, confusion, hallucinations, and livedo reticularis. Like the anticholinergics, amantadine is best avoided in elderly or demented patients. In later stages of PD, the addition of amantadine is occasionally useful, but again, the beneficial effect wanes after several months.

Dopaminergics

Levodopa (Sinemet)

Dopamine depletion is the biochemical hallmark of PD and its replacement is the mainstay of treatment. The inability of dopamine to cross the blood-brain barrier led to the use of its precursor, levodopa. In order to avoid the peripheral conversion of levodopa to dopamine, Sinemet combines levodopa with the decarboxylase inhibitor carbidopa. The optimal time to begin administering Sinemet remains controversial—proponents for early treatment with this agent have shown that this approach leads to a longer life span, slower progression of disease, and better preservation of function; others insist that the usefulness of Sinemet is limited and therefore that its use is best delayed as long as possible rather than "wasted" when symptoms and signs are minimal. Our approach is to delay the use of Sinemet until there is significant impairment of the ADLs, but at that point we do not hesitate to initiate treatment, particularly if the symptoms and signs cannot be controlled adequately with anticholinergics and amantadine.

We start with the 25/100 tablet twice per day and, depending on the patient's response, gradually increase the dose by half or full tablets to a maintenance dose of one tablet, administered 3 or 4 times per day. Most patients tolerate Sinemet well, with nausea being the most common early side effect. Although the nausea is generally self-limited, it can be prevented by having the patient take Sinemet with food and by making sure that at least 75 mg of carbidopa per day is used. Other side effects include orthostatic hypotension, confusion, hallucinations, and hypersexuality, but most resolve when the dose is reduced.

Dopamine Agonists

Bromocriptine and pergolide mesylate are ergot derivatives that have been shown to be useful adjuncts to Sinemet. To date, neither formulation has been shown to have a clear therapeutic advantage over the other. Although some advocate their use as initial monotherapy—and there is growing evidence that this may prevent or at least forestall motor fluctuations—our current approach is to add bromocriptine or pergolide mesylate when symptoms and signs cannot be controlled adequately by the use of 400 mg of levodopa per day. The starting dose of bromocriptine is 1.25 mg at bedtime; the dose is then increased

TABLE 2 Drugs Used for Parkinson's Disease

Drug	*Available Preparation*	*Dose (mg)*	*Schedule*	*Starting Dose (mg)*	*Maintenance Dose (mg)*
Anticholinergic agents (representative examples)					
Trihexyphenidyl hydrochloride Artane)	Scored tablets	2 mg, 5 mg	3 to 4 times daily	2 mg	2–10 mg
	Elixir	2 mg/5 ml			
	Timed-release capsule	5 mg	Once daily	(Timed-release capsule may be substituted for regular Artane after maintenance dose is determined)	
Benztropine mesylate (Cogentin)	Tablets	0.5 mg, 1 mg, 2 mg	Once or twice daily	1 mg	0.5–6 mg
Dopaminergic agents					
Carbidopa/levodopa (Sinemet)	Scored tablets 10/100, 25/100, 25/250		2 to 4 times daily	50/200 in two divided doses	400–500 mg levodopa
Bromocriptine (Parlodel)	Scored tablets	2.5 mg	2 to 3 times daily	1.25 mg daily	7.5–30 mg
	Capsules	5.0 mg			
Pergolide mesylate (Permax)	Scored tablets	0.05 mg, 0.25 mg, 1.0 mg	3 times daily	0.05 mg daily	1–3 mg
Deprenyl (Eldepryl, selegiline hydrochloride)	Tablets	5.0 mg	2 times daily	5 mg daily	10 mg
Amantadine (Symmetrel)	Capsules	100 mg	2 times daily	100 mg daily	200 mg

by increments of 1.25 mg, with the goal being an initial maintenance dose of 7.5 mg per day. Depending on the response and tolerance, the dose can be increased gradually every 2 to 4 weeks to as much as 30 mg per day. Pergolide mesylate is started at 0.05 mg at bedtime and gradually increased until a maintenance dose of 1 to 3 mg per day in 3 divided doses is achieved.

Patients should be warned that the optimal effect of bromocriptine or pergolide mesylate may not be seen until several weeks after a stable dose is reached and that the benefit is typically subtle, unlike the dramatic effect many patients experience when they initially receive Sinemet.

The side effects of bromocriptine and pergolide are similar to those of Sinemet; however, these agents are less well tolerated in elderly and demented patients because of their greater propensity to cause confusion, hallucinations, and psychosis. Dopamine agonists are the most expensive of the antiparkinsonian agents.

MOTOR FLUCTUATIONS

Most patients maintain an obvious beneficial response to Sinemet for the first 3 to 5 years of treatment. After that time, not only does the beneficial effect wane, but motor fluctuations also appear, and from this point onward, the management of PD becomes more difficult as the therapeutic window of Sinemet narrows. Variables contributing to dose fluctuations include erratic gastric emptying and intestinal absorption, competition between levodopa and dietary amino acids for transport across the blood-brain barrier, loss of the ability of the remaining nigral neurons to metabolize and store dopamine, and changes in the number and sensitivity of postsynaptic dopamine receptors.

The most common early fluctuation is end-of-dose deterioration ("wearing-off"). This is treated by decreasing the dosing interval while attempting to maintain the same total daily dose of levodopa, often accomplished by using half-tablets and adding an agonist.

The second category of dose-related fluctuations are dyskinesias, which take the form of choreoathetosis or dystonia and can effect the limbs as well as the face and trunk. Although many patients are unaware of their dyskinesia or find them preferable to akinetic periods, their appearance generally heralds the beginning of more problematic fluctuations. Peak dose dyskinesias occur 1.5 to 2 hours after each dose and is treated by decreasing the dose of Sinemet and using an agonist to maintain adequate antiparkinsonian control.

More problematic than the dose-related fluctuations are random fluctuations known as *"on–off"*, characterized by sudden, unpredictable, and occasionally dramatic motor oscillations, often accompanied by freezing episodes and falling. These fluctuations are difficult to treat but may diminish with the addition of an agonist, frequent Sinemet dosing, the use of long-acting Sinemet (controlled release), or a brief drug "holiday" during which the dose of Sinemet is temporarily decreased and then reintroduced at a slightly lower maintenance dose. Despite their one-time popularity, we do not advocate complete drug holidays, as they are potentially dangerous and the beneficial effect is short-lived. Several investigators have shown that continuous duodenal infusion of Sinemet or subcutaneous apomorphine is helpful in controlling motor fluctuations and these techniques may eventually become more widely available.

DEPRENYL

Deprenyl (Eldepryl, selegiline hydrochloride) is a monoamine oxidase B inhibitor that prevents the catabolism and re-uptake of dopamine and has been shown to be an effective adjunct to Sinemet for patients with response fluctuations. Because only the "B" form of the enzyme is inhibited, which exists exclusively in the central nervous system, it is not necessary to restrict dietary tyramine since systemic hypertension is not encountered. Although dyskinesias may be exacerbated, necessitating a reduction in the Sinemet dose, deprenyl is otherwise relatively free of side effects. Nevertheless, side effects have been reported, including nausea, insomnia, dry mouth, dizziness, psychosis, and confusion. The maintenance dose is 5 mg twice per day.

In addition to its effectiveness in diminishing motor fluctuations, Deprenyl has also recently been shown to slow the progression of early Parkinson's disease, specifically, delaying the length of time before treatment with Levodopa is required. The mechanism involved is believed to be due to the ability of Deprenyl to block the toxic transformation of unknown potential environmental substances such as 1-Methyl-4-Phenyl-1,2,3,6-Tetrahyropyridine (MPTP), thereby limiting the death of nigral neurons.

SURGERY

Renewed interest in the surgical treatment of PD was aroused by the initial report of dramatic clinical improvement occurring after implantation of autologous adrenal medullary tissue into the caudate nucleus. Subsequent series, including those using fetal nigral tissue, have been met with less enthusiasm. The current procedure is associated with an unacceptably high morbidity rate, a lack of extended follow-up, and failure to demonstrate viability of the graft. We consider implantation to be a strictly experimental procedure that should be performed only in carefully selected patients as part of a research protocol. By contrast, stereotaxtic thalamotomy, when performed at a center specializing in the procedure, is a safe, effective treatment for patients with disabling tremor unresponsive to medical therapy.

DEMENTIA

Based on the population studied, definition of dementia, and tools used to assess cognitive performance, the estimated frequency of dementia developing in patients with PD varies widely. A conservative estimate is that at least 15 to 20 percent of patients with PD develop dementia. Although the incidence of dementia in patients with PD is higher than in nonparkinsonian age-matched controls, it is crucial to appreciate that dementia is not an inevitable feature of PD and therefore must be approached with the same rigorous search for remediable causes as that used in patients without PD. All of the medications used to treat PD have cognitive and behavioral side effects, particularly the anticholinergics, and when dementia surfaces, an attempt should be made to reduce the dosages, and if possible, to discontinue the use of these drugs.

Dementia in patients with PD is occasionally complicated by bothersome hallucinations, agitation, and psychosis often coupled with insomnia or a reversal in the sleep-wake cycle. If these problems do not respond to a reduction in the dosage of antiparkinsonian medications or to the use of mild sedatives, a very low dose of a neuroleptic may be required. Although a worsening of parkinsonian signs may result, the suppression of intolerable behavior usually leads to an overall improvement in the patient's condition and eases the burden on the patient's caregiver.

DEPRESSION

Depression is common in PD, occurring in as many as 50 percent of patients. It is not clear to what extent depression is the result of an intrinsic neurochemical defect such as the mesolimbic loss of dopamine versus a reactive depression to the physical disability imposed by the disease. Patients (and physicians) commonly fail to recognize depression and often mistakenly ascribe a decline in function, particularly psychomotor retardation, to PD. Symptoms of depression, and specifically vegetative symptoms, should be rigorously sought during each outpatient visit. Psychiatric evaluation is helpful for most patients and essential for patients with severe depression.

Depression associated with PD can be effectively treated with tricyclic antidepressants. In severe cases, particularly when the depression is compounded by delusions or psychosis or when tricyclics are either ineffective or not tolerated, electroconvulsive therapy is the treatment of choice. As the depression resolves, there is often concurrent improvement of many parkinsonian symptoms and signs.

SUGGESTED READING

Brown RG, Marsden CD. How common is dementia in Parkinson's Disease? Lancet 1984; 1:1262–1265.

Jankovic J, Tolosa E, eds. Parkinson's disease and movement disorders. Baltimore: Urban & Schwarzenberg, Inc. 1988.

Koller WC, ed. Handbook of Parkinson's disease. New York: Marcel Dekker, 1987.

Lieberman AN. Update on Parkinson's disease. NY State J Med 1987; 87:147–153.

Marsden CD, Parkes JD. Success and problems of long-term levodopa therapy in Parkinson's disease. Lancet 1977; 1:345–349.

The Parkinson Study Group. Effect of Deprenyl on the progression of disability in early Parkinson's Disease. N Engl J Med 1989; 321:1364–1371.

PATIENT RESOURCES

Associations

United Parkinson Foundation (International)
360 West Superior Street
Chicago, Illinois 60610

The American Parkinson Disease Association, Inc.
116 John Street
New York, New York 10034

The Parkinson Disease Foundation
William Black Medical Research Building
640 West 168th Street
New York, New York 10032

National Parkinson Foundation, Inc.
1501 Ninth Avenue NW
Miami, Florida 33136

Literature

Duvoisin RC. Parkinson's disease: a guide for patient and family. New York: Raven Press, 1984.

HEPATIC ENCEPHALOPATHY

JEFFREY D. ROTHSTEIN, M.D., Ph.D.
GUY M. McKHANN, M.D.

Hepatic encephalopathy is a neuropsychiatric syndrome that complicates both acute and chronic liver disease. It is often seen in children with congenital urea cycle enzyme defects. Subtypes of this disorder are classified by the rate of progression and nature of the underlying hepatic disease. Fulminant hepatic failure results in hepatic encephalopathy within 8 weeks of the onset of liver injury and is associated with a high mortality rate. Subacute or chronic hepatic encephalopathy, which is associated with chronic hepatocellular disease, is episodic and milder.

Hepatic encephalopathy may be caused by potentially reversible metabolic abnormalities. Although the pathogenesis of hepatic encephalopathy remains obscure, it reflects direct or indirect central nervous system (CNS) exposure to substances not cleared by the liver.

TABLE 1 Signs and Symptoms of Hepatic Encephalopathy

Stage	*Mental status and behavior*	*Motor/Reflexes*
I	Diminished attention Mild confusion Anxiety Irritability Agitation Diminished attention Impaired serial 7's Altered sleep patterns Depression	Fine postural tremor Slowed coordination
II	Drowsiness Lethargy Gross personality changes Disorientation (time) Poor recall Inappropriate behavior	Asterixis Dysarthria Primitive reflexes (sucking, grasping) Paratonia Ataxia
III	Profound confusion Paranoia Disorientation of time and place Incomprehensible speech Somnolent but arousable	Hyperreflexia Seizures Babinski's sign Hyperventilation Incontinence Hypothermia Myoclonus
IV	Coma	Decerebrate posturing Brisk oculocephalic reflexes

CLINICAL AND LABORATORY FEATURES

The typical clinical course of hepatic encephalopathy is characterized by (1) alterations in behavior including inattention to personal hygiene and appearance and impairment of consciousness (delirium, coma); (2) alterations in motor tone and posture (tremor, paratonia, asterixis, hyperactive muscle stretch reflexes); (3) slowing of the electroencephalogram (EEG) ("triphasic" slow waves); and (4) characteristic elevations in fasting plasma ammonia and cerebrospinal fluid (CSF) glutamine concentrations. These signs and symptoms may vary, depending on the subtype of the hepatic encephalopathy.

Staging

Although manifestations of hepatic encephalopathy are protean, they are generally grouped into four clinical stages based on the severity of encephalopathy (Table 1). Signs and symptoms may vary within each stage. This staging may help in following patients and assessing the efficacy of therapy. Early hepatic encephalopathy, stage I or "incipient" encephalopathy, may be overlooked because of stable symptoms, such as reversal of sleep patterns or personality changes.

Asterixis and a worsening of mental status are seen in patients with stage II hepatic encephalopathy. Asterixis is a transient loss of postural tone of the extensors or the wrist when the hands are outstretched. It is not specific for hepatic encephalopathy and may be seen in patients with uremia, pulmonary disease, malnutrition, and polycythemia rubra vera.

Stage III of the disease heralds more profound and serious neurologic abnormalities. Focal or generalized seizures may develop. The patient may become somnolent or incontinent. Rapid, deep respirations may accompany hyperreflexia with extensor plantar reflexes. With stage IV coma, a diminished response to pain with decerebrate and decorticate posturing is seen. Unlike other diseases, with hepatic encephalopathy this posturing is reversible.

Establishing the Diagnosis

It is relatively easy to recognize encephalopathy in a patient with fulminant hepatic failure. When hepatic disease is not clinically obvious, however, the nonspecific characteristics of early hepatic encephalopathy make diagnosis more difficult. Abnormal laboratory tests of hepatic function may establish the presence of liver disease. An elevated plasma ammonia level may be useful in confirming the diagnosis of hepatic encephalopathy, but a normal plasma ammonia concentration does not exclude this diagnosis. Furthermore, the degree of elevation of plasma or cerebrospinal fluid (CSF) ammonia levels does not correlate with the severity of encephalopathy. An elevation in CSF glutamine concentration is the most specific and sensitive laboratory test for this disease and correlates well with the degree of hepatic encephalopathy. Unfortunately, glutamine assays are not performed in some clinical laboratories.

The coagulopathy and thrombocytopenia that can accompany hepatic disease may make lumbar puncture unsafe. If prothrombin time ratios are greater than 1.3 and/or platelet counts are less than 40,000, the physician should be prepared to administer fresh frozen plasma or platelets.

The EEG is abnormal in patients with hepatic encephalopathy, but the abnormalities are nonspecific. Symmetrical frontal slow waves that spread posteriorly are seen. Triphasic slow waves, commonly attributed to hepatic encephalopathy, may occur in patients with head injury, subdural hematomas, uremia, cerebral anoxia, and electrolyte abnormalities. Psychometric testing, although not particularly helpful in diagnosing hepatic encephalopathy, provides a semiquantitative means of following response to therapy. Easy bedside evaluations include trail-making (Reitan number connection) and tests using block designs or star constructions.

Differential Diagnosis

Since the neuropsychiatric manifestations of hepatic encephalopathy are nonspecific, it is important to rule out other causes of encephalopathy in patients with hepatic disease. Toxins, metabolic abnormalities, and structural lesions can cause similar clinical features. In patients with impaired liver function, cerebral depression caused by the use of sedatives, narcotics, or tranquilizers should be considered. The use of benzodiazepines should be avoided in patients with hepatic encephalopathy because of the increased sensitivities to these agents. The delirium of alcohol withdrawal may be confused with an agitated delirium of hepatic encephalopathy, and a recent history of alcohol abuse may help one make the necessary differentiation. Hypokalemia or hyponatremia are commonly seen in patients with cirrhosis and may produce a coma that can be rapidly reversed with electrolyte correction. Encephalopathy secondary to hypoxia, hypoglycemia, and uremia should also be considered.

Focal neurologic signs may occur, but these are unusual in patients with hepatic encephalopathy and should prompt a search for structural abnormalities. An EEG is essential to rule out subclinical status epilepticus. There are no characteristic computed tomographic (CT) changes of the brain. Patients with a subclinical stable lesion (head trauma, chronic subdural hematoma, stroke) may develop focal neurologic signs or symptoms when hepatic encephalopathy develops. Whenever a patient with hepatic encephalopathy develops focal neurologic signs, it is essential that CT scanning of the head be performed to exclude underlying structural disease (e.g., tumor or abscess). Meningitis should also be considered, especially in patients with alcoholic cirrhosis. Subarachnoid and intracerebral hemorrhage are not uncommon in patients with hepatic encephalopathy and are seen in 11 percent of autopsied patients after orthotopic liver transplantation.

PATHOGENESIS

Multiple hypotheses have been proposed to explain the pathogenesis of hepatic encephalopathy, but a specific cause is not known. Over the last several decades, several agents, including ammonia, short-chain fatty acids, mercaptans, phenols, false neurotransmitters (octopamine), and recently gamma-aminobutyric acid (GABA) have been proposed as candidate "toxins." No single agent is likely to be completely responsible for the disease.

Ammonia is the most commonly incriminated toxin. Its role as an important agent of hepatic encephalopathy is supported by the observation that encephalopathy develops in patients who have elevated ammonia concentrations from urea cycle enzyme defects but who have otherwise normal livers. Often patients with hepatic encephalopathy have elevated arterial ammonia levels. However, hepatic encephalopathy can clearly occur in the presence of normal blood and CSF ammonia levels. In addition, therapies that reduce plasma levels of ammonia ameliorate hepatic encephalopathy. Hyperammonemia is associated with seizures and may contribute to the encephalopathy of primary hyperammonemic disorders. The glutamine concentration is markedly increased in the CNS, probably reflecting brain ammonia detoxification. Although glutamine is inactive, it is an important precursor of amino acid neurotransmitters, including glutamate, aspartate, and GABA.

Hepatic encephalopathy can be rapidly reserved in animals and humans by benzodiazepine antagonists. Benzodiazepines produce their effects in the CNS by modulation of the inhibitory neurotransmitter GABA. New theories on the neurochemical etiology of hepatic encephalopathy suggest that increased inhibitory GABA tone, perhaps secondary to the use of endogenous benzodiazepines or benzodiazepine-like material, is responsible for the encephalopathy of hepatic failure.

TREATMENT

Recognition of Precipitating Causes

Treatment requires that the precipitating causes be addressed (Table 2). Agitated patients are often misdiagnosed as having insomnia rather than early encephalopathy and are treated with sedatives. Excessive diuretic therapy may cause a hypokalemic alkalosis. Hypokalemia causes increased renal am-

TABLE 2 Precipitants of Hepatic Encephalopathy

Drugs
Sedatives
Tranquilizers
Narcotics
Diuretics
Electrolyte imbalance
Hyponatremia
Hypokalemic alkalosis
Hypoxia
Hypovolemia
Excessive nitrogen load
Gastrointestinal hemorrhage
Excess dietary protein
Azotemia
Constipation
Infection

monia production, and alkalosis favors the diffusion of ammonia into the CNS. Intravascular volume depletion from diuretic therapy reduces renal blood flow and increases the blood urea nitrogen concentration. This excess urea diffuses into the gut, leading to increased ammonia production by bacterial ureases. Bacterial infections can precipitate encephalopathy and are often not suspected because patients with chronic liver disease are frequently hypothermic. Cultures of blood, urine, CSF, and ascites, if present, should be obtained for all cases of unexplained encephalopathy.

Specific Therapies

The therapy for hepatic encephalopathy is based on the premise that substances in the gastrointestinal tract are acted upon by intestinal bacteria and converted to "toxins" that are absorbed into the blood (Table 3). These toxins bypass the liver via collateral circulation, enter the brain, and presumably induce encephalopathy. Based on these principles, therapy is directed at (1) decreasing the colonic substrate for these putative comagenic toxins, (2) reducing the bacteria capable of producing these toxins, (3) diminishing the influx of these compounds into the CNS, and (4) decreasing the effect these compounds have on neurotransmitter activity and metabolism.

Reduction of Gastrointestinal Protein and Toxins

Reduction of dietary protein is a simple method for reducing gastrointestinal protein and should be the first step in therapy. Protein intake can be withheld for the first 1 to 2 days, and is gradually increased in increments of 10 g per day. Dietary intake should not be less than 40 g per day chronically, as negative nitrogen balance ensues with increased risk of infection and with diminished hepatic regeneration. Patients with hepatic encephalopathy secondary to gastrointestinal hemorrhage, constipation, or large protein loads should be treated with tap water

TABLE 3 Management of Hepatic Encephalopathy

Therapy
1. Eliminate predisposing factors:
   a. Sedatives, tranquilizers, analgesics
   b. Fluid/electrolyte dysfunction. (Correct hypokalemia/alkalosis, hyponatremia.)
   c. Gastrointestinal bleeding, commonly seen secondary to varices. (Determine if bleeding is occurring by nasogastric aspiration of stomach and stool heme monitoring. If there is gastrointestinal bleeding, frequent bowel movements need to be produced to help cleanse gut of proteinaceous blood—e.g., by repeated enemas.)
   Normalize intravascular volume (to prevent prerenal azotemia).
2. Dietary protein restriction
   a. Begin with protein-free diet (must provide enough calories to inhibit proteolysis—e.g., 10% D/W or nasogastric glucose + lipids; one should try to provide 1,500–2,000 cal/day; avoid hyperalimentation, as this will provide excess amino acids).
   b. With improvement, increase diet protein to 20 g/day and increase protein by 10 g/day increments every 2–3 days until maximum protein total is reached; for outpatients, maximum is usually 50 g/day.
   c. Administer cathartics to eliminate gut protein (e.g., oral magnesium citrate [200 ml] or sorbitol [50 g in 200 ml water).
   d. Administer vitamin supplementation: folate (1 mg/day), vitamin K (10 mg/day), thiamine, and multivitamins.
3. Diminish gastrointestinal ammonia absorption by using either:
   Neomycin (1 g p.o. q.i.d.; complicated by candidal gut overgrowth and malabsorption).
   or
   Lactulose (synthetic disaccharide that is not digested in the upper gastrointestinal tract) 10–30 ml p.o. or by retention enema t.i.d.

Monitoring
1. Stage patient.
2. Check arterial ammonia.
3. EEG.
4. CSF glutamine.

Chronic management/prevention
1. Prescribe low-protein diet (usually 50 g/day).
2. Administer vitamin supplementation: folate, vitamin K, multivitamins.
3. Administer lactulose (10–30 ml p.o. t.i.d. (at least one soft bowel movement/day).

enemas and lactulose to evacuate nitrogenous substrates.

Lactulose is the mainstay of therapy to prevent or diminish hepatic encephalopathy. Its cathartic action increases ammonia elimination. Bacterial metabolism of lactulose acidifies the colonic contents and converts ammonia to its ionized and less absorbable form. Lactulose may be administered orally or as retention enemas in obtunded patients. For patients with recurrent hepatic encephalopathy, lactulose can be used chronically (30 ml taken orally 3 times per day). In patients refractory to dietary protein restriction and lactulose therapy, the oral antibiotics neomycin and metronidazole have been used to promote colonic bacteriostasis.

Reduction of Gastrointestinal Bacteria

In patients who cannot be managed with dietary protein restriction and lactulose therapy, the elimination of gastrointestinal bacteria may prove useful. The premise of this therapy is that diminution of gastrointestinal flora diminishes the production of ammonia and other possible toxins. Neomycin can be taken orally in a dose of 1 to 2 g every 6 hours. Only small amounts of this drug can be absorbed, however, and since it is excreted primarily in urine, its use should be avoided in patients with renal insufficiency. Even in patients with normal renal function, prolonged therapy can produce ototoxicity and nephrotoxicity.

Alternatives to neomycin include metronidazole (250 mg taken orally three times per day), which has side effects that include leukopenia, peripheral neuropathy, metallic taste, and disulfiramlike reaction. Other bacteriostatic therapies include those using oral tetracycline or ampicillin.

Other Therapies

Because there have been so many theories concerning hepatic encephalopathy, several unproven therapies have been tried. These include levodopa and the dopamine agonist bromocriptine, both of which have arousal properties. In controlled clinical trials, these agents failed to produce reliable clinical benefits.

Because patients with hepatic encephalopathy have abnormal plasma and CSF amino acid concentrations, it has been suggested that the increased plasma aromatic amino acids producd in these patients may interfere with normal neurotransmitter synthesis. To that end, trials with solutions enriched with branched-chain amino acids, which compete with aromatic amino acids for transport into the CNS, have been tried. The results of these studies are mixed and controversial. For a variety of reasons, including the excessive cost of these solutions, the high osmolarity and fluid load, and the marginal benefit, this therapy is not routinely recommended.

An important, rare subset of patients with hepatic encephalopathy includes those suffering from inherited urea cycle defects (e.g., ornithine transcarbamoylase deficiency). In these patients, primarily children, accumulation of ammonia is believed to be responsible for the encephalopathy, and attempts to lower serum ammonia have proven useful. Infusions of sodium benzoate and sodium phenylacetate (as much as 0.25 g per kilogram per day of each) may be employed to control potentially fatal hyperammonemia successfully. Alternative therapies include the use of arginine or citrulline, depending on the specific enzyme deficiency.

Flumazenil (RO 15-1788) is a benzodiazepine receptor antagonist widely used in Europe. It is reported to reverse hepatic encephalopathy, eliminate relapsing encephalopathy, and allow the resumption of normal protein intake in patients with chronic hepatic failure. This agent is now being further evaluated in the United States, although it is not yet available.

PREVENTION

Preventative measures help minimize recurrent encephalopathy. Stool softeners reduce constipation and the use of outpatient lactulose serves both as a laxative and a means of eliminating gastrointestinal ammonia absorption. To anticipate the possibility for gastrointestinal hemorrhage, frequent stool Hemoccult can be employed, with the patient mailing test cards to their physician. Obviously, the use of sedatives (especially benzodiazepines) and narcotics should be avoided in patients with hepatic disease. The regular use of multivitamins, especially thiamine, should be encouraged.

FULMINANT HEPATIC FAILURE

Unlike chronic hepatic disease, fulminant hepatic failure (FHF) is associated with a high mortality rate (>50 percent). FHF is associated with a variety of hepatic insults including viral hepatitis, poison, chemical or drug exposure (e.g., acetaminophen), and ischemic hepatitis. Hyperammonemia as well as hypoglycemia, hypoxia secondary to cardiac failure, pulmonary infections, and uremia associated with hepatorenal syndrome all contribute to the encephalopathy. Intensive medical and neurologic management has, however, made inroads to decreasing overall mortality. In these patients, particular attention should be paid to electrolytes, acid-base balance, glucose, coagulation defects, and pulmonary, cardiac, and renal status. These patients may also develop coagulopathy, hypotension, hypoxia, pulmonary edema, hypoglycemia, and pancreatitis, and need to be monitored in an intensive care setting with central venous pressure monitoring as well as standard intensive care unit cardiac monitoring. Constant vigilance for infections must be maintained.

Cerebral Edema in Fulminant Hepatic Failure

Although this encephalopathy appears similar to that associated with chronic hepatic disease, the underlying mechanisms and the treatment may be quite different. Most importantly, FHF is associated with lethal cerebral edema, and that is the major extrahepatic lesion found at autopsy. Because papilledema may not be seen, there are no good clinical indices for cerebral edema. Sudden deterioration of consciousness, hyperactive reflexes along with plantar reflexes, and decerebrate/decorticate posturing may suggest increased intracranial pressure (ICP), but these can also be seen in patients with metabolic encephalopathy. Abnormal pupillary light responses and oculocephalic (''doll's eye'' maneuver) reflexes may be reversible; however, abnormal oculovestibular reflexes (cold caloric test) carry a poor prognosis. CT may reveal slitlike ventricles or other signs of an increased ICP. ICP transducers have been used by some to help monitor ICP, but their use may cause significant intracranial bleeding. Standard therapies aimed at controlling ICP, such as hyperventilation and furosemide therapy, can be employed. Mannitol has been used to reduce elevated pressure, but in patients with an ICP greater than 60 mm Hg, it may be deleterious. Mannitol should be used only when ICP transducers are in place. There is no proven value for the use of steroids.

Treatment

In addition to controlling ICP, one must still pay attention to the underlying hepatic abnormalities. Given the large number of metabolic problems, the approach to FHF is not as effective as that used for chronic hepatic disease. Most patients are obtunded or comatose, and therefore little dietary protein is ingested. Lactulose can be used to remove nitrogen waste from the gut initially, but can produce complicating electrolyte disturbances secondary to excessive diarrhea. Other therapies such as total body washout, charcoal hemoperfusion, and hemodialysis have not proved reliable. When available, orthotopic liver transplantation may be the most important therapeutic option.

SUGGESTED READING

Jones EA, Gammal SH. Hepatic encephalopathy. In: Arias IM, Jakoby WB, Popper H, et al, eds. The liver: biology and pathobiology. 2nd ed. New York: Raven Press, 1988:985.

Lockwood AH. Hepatic encephalopathy: experimental approaches to human metabolic encephalopathy. CRC Crit Rev Neurobiol 1987; 3:105–133.

Rothstein JD, Herlong FH. Neurological manifestations of hepatic disease. Neurol Clin 1989; 7:563–578.

Zieve L. Hepatic encephalopathy. In: Schiss O, Schiff ER, eds. Diseases of the liver. Philadelphia: JB Lippincott, 1987:925.

DRUG OVERDOSE AND WITHDRAWAL

WALTER ROYAL III, M.D.

The use of addictive substances for recreational or therapeutic purposes frequently results in the development of drug tolerance, the requirement of higher doses to achieve a desired effect, or drug dependence, the occurrence of undesirable physical or psychological symptoms after withdrawal from the substance. Drug abuse has been defined as the use of a chemical substance for more than 1 month resulting in impairment of social or occupational functioning or both. This chapter discusses the various classes of sedative, stimulant, and hallucinogenic agents and the recognition and treatment of the associated toxic and withdrawal syndromes.

OPIATES

The opiod (or narcotic analgesic) drugs include morphine, its semisynthetic derivatives, and structurally distinct classes of synthetic drugs with morphinelike pharmacologic properties. The opiods possess tremendous addictive potential. Their extensive use in medical therapy often leads to variable degrees of physical and psychological dependence. In the general population overt abuse may occur with any of these medications. Heroin is the mainstay of illegal street drug trafficking predominantly in urban areas. It is generally mixed with quinine or sugars such as lactose and mannose, and this results in variability of the final concentration of active drug. Individual use may vary from occasional small doses resulting in mild intoxication to large amounts used several times daily. It is therefore difficult to estimate an individual's tolerance and the amount of heroin used by an addict.

The signs of opiod intoxication include hypotension, bradycardia, slurred speech, miosis, and respiratory depression. Seizures may occur secondary to the use of meperidine hydrochloride, despite significant tolerance, and they may be caused by the severe anoxia induced by overdose of this drug. The signs of overdose include pinpoint pupils that are nevertheless reactive, respiratory depression, and coma; pulmonary edema may also occur. Treatment consists of prompt administration of naloxone and appropriate support of respiration and circulatory function. Naloxone is most effective when administered intravenously at a dose of 0.4 mg every 3 to 10 minutes until there is a clinical response. It may also be administered intramuscularly or subcutaneously, thus increasing the duration of its action. Repeated doses are often necessary and continuous infusions occasionally required to prevent recurrence of symptoms of overdose since the half-life of naloxone is less than that of both heroin and methadone. Ventricular arrhythmias associated with naloxone administration have been reported, and caution should therefore be exercised in treating patients with cardiac disease. The most frequent side effect, however, is the precipitation of withdrawal symptoms in addicts and reversal of analgesia in individuals with a history of a pain syndrome.

With the possible exception of meperidine-related seizures, the opiod withdrawal syndrome, although dramatic, is not life-threatening. The approximate time of onset of abstinence symptoms after the last dose of an opiate drug has been taken is as follows: 2 to 4 hours for meperidine, 4 to 8 hours for heroin, and 12 to 48 hours for methadone. Early symptoms include drug craving, anxiety, anorexia, and insomnia with muscular irritability, diaphoresis, rhinorrhea, lacrimation, dilated pupils, and piloerection. Abdominal cramping, diarrhea, nausea, vomiting, fever, hypertension, tachycardia, and tachypnea may develop later.

The symptoms of the abstinence syndrome may be attenuated with methadone in an initial dose of 10 to 20 mg and thereafter in doses of 5 to 10 mg administered as often as four times per day, as needed. After stabilization has been achieved, the dose may be reduced by 10 to 25 percent daily, with the clinician continuing to follow signs of withdrawal. Although it is difficult to achieve this in practice, the duration of methadone treatment should be equal to the time usually taken for abstinence symptoms to abate (7 to 10 days for heroin and as long as 3 weeks for morphine).

Clonidine (0.1 to 0.2 mg twice per day) has also been used for treatment of acute symptoms of opiate withdrawal, although it may not be as effective as methadone in relieving insomnia and lacrimation. Bradycardia and hallucinations may develop with clonidine treatment, and abrupt discontinuation may precipitate hypomania. Clonidine should be used cautiously in patients who have been receiving tricyclic antidepressants chronically. The methadone congener L-alpha acetyl methadol (methadyl acetate, LAAM) may also be effective in the treatment of opiate withdrawal. Buprenorphine is a mixed agonist antagonist that may be as effective as methadone for treating abstinence, but with lower toxicity and abuse potential.

SEDATIVES AND HYPNOTICS

This group of drugs includes the barbiturates, the nonbarbiturate sedative-hypnotics, and the benzodiazepines. These drugs are cross-tolerant within the group and with ethanol. The signs of sedative-hypnotic overdose and withdrawal are also similar to those seen with ethanol, with the shorter-acting drugs causing more severe withdrawal symptoms. Except in the case of withdrawal from the benzodiazepines, fatalities due to respiratory depression caused by the withdrawal from sedatives and hypnotics are common. Mild intoxication may be associated with drowsiness, nystagmus, slurred speech, and ataxia. Hyporeflexia, respiratory depression, hypotension, confusion, stupor, and coma may be seen in patients with moderate to severe intoxication. In patients with acute intoxication, electroencephalography initially shows diffuse fast activity. With progression to coma, the fast activity may be followed by generalized slowing and intermittent or sustained isoelectric periods.

Several unique signs and symptoms may be caused by the nonbarbiturate sedative-hypnotics, including seizures (caused by methaqualone and glutethimide), pupillary abnormalities (dilated, unreactive pupils with glutethimide, pinpoint pupils with chloral hydrate), psychosis and myoclonus (caused by methaqualone), cardiovascular collapse (caused by methaqualone, methyprylon, ethchlorvynol), metabolic acidosis, gastric bleeding, and pulmonary damage (caused by paraldehyde), and muscle spasm, ileus, and bladder atony (caused by glutethimide).

Treatment consists of respiratory and circulatory support and removal of unabsorbed drug. Emesis may be induced if the patient is conscious, while one observes closely for progressive drowsiness and aspiration. Unabsorbed gastrointestinal contents should be removed by performing gastric lavage and administering a cathartic and activated charcoal. Excretion or removal of the drug may be accomplished with urinary alkalinization and forced diuresis or dialysis. Because of its effect on urinary output, dopamine is the preferred pressor when poisoning is the result of ingestion of medium or long-acting barbiturates. Central stimulants may precipitate seizures and should therefore be avoided.

The abstinence syndrome associated with the use of barbiturates may occur after either total drug withdrawal or reduction of the usual dose. It is the most lethal of all withdrawal syndromes, with the most severe abstinence syndromes occurring with the shorter-acting drugs. Tremulousness, weakness, nausea, vomiting, agitation, insomnia, anorexia, pupillary dilatation, tachycardia, tachypnea, and orthostatic hypotension may develop within hours after the last dose of a short-acting barbiturate is taken. Seizures may occur after 24 to 72 hours and are generally brief single or multiple episodes, and less frequently, may be status epilepticus. A syndrome similar to delirium tremens may appear after 2 to 5 days, with agitation, confusion, delusions, hallucinations and formication, hyperthermia, and circulatory collapse.

Mild withdrawal symptoms caused by discontinuation of any of the barbiturate and nonbarbiturate sedative-hypnotics may be treated with pentobarbital. If the administration of 200 mg of pentobarbital does not lead to signs of intoxication, then significant tolerance to the drug is likely. The occurrence of mild ataxia and nystagmus 1 hour after the 200-mg dose suggests a daily tolerance to 600 mg of pentobarbital. In general, for patients who are physically dependent on sedative-hypnotics, withdrawal symptoms may be controlled with a dose of 200 to 400 mg of pentobarbital administered every 4 to 6 hours, with the drug withheld to watch for signs of intoxication. After 2 or 3 days, the drug may be tapered by 100 mg per day or in decrements of 10 percent of the initial dose or as tolerated.

Pentobarbital may also be used to treat hallucinations and delirium tremens. The latter is a medical emergency, and patients should be treated aggressively to control fever (exclude infection), fluid and electrolyte balance, and cardiac and renal status. Withdrawal seizures may be treated acutely with benzodiazepines such as diazepam (5 to 10 mg) or lorazepam (2 to 4 mg) while the clinician carefully monitors for hypotension and respiratory depression. It may be necessary to treat severe seizures with more than 1 g of phenobarbital.

Withdrawal of antianxiety doses of benzodiazepines has been associated with increased anxiety, depersonalization, visual disturbances, tinnitus, paresthesias, and muscle twitching. Disorientation and psychotic reactions as well as seizures have occurred after discontinuation of high doses of these drugs.

STIMULANTS

In cases of acute overdose of stimulants, there is a marked clinical presentation of prominent stimulatory effects on both the central and peripheral nervous systems, which these drugs produce. Included in this category of drugs are several sympathomimetics, such as amphetamine (Benzedrine), dextroamphetamine (Dexedrine), methamphetamine (Desoxyn or "speed"), and phenmetrazine (Preludin), as well as cocaine and its alkaloid derivative, "crack." All of these drugs produce an intense "rush" when used intravenously. The amphetamines are also taken orally. Cocaine is ineffective when taken orally but is effective when used intranasally, intravenously, or smoked ("free-based"). Crack is also smoked and has a profound effect that occurs within seconds, lasts for a few minutes, and is followed by a rapid and extremely unpleasant "crash." This results in an intense craving and is the reason for remarkably high addictive potential that is associated with crack.

The symptoms of amphetamine intoxication include a sense of well-being, elation, agitation, and occasionally aggressive, violent behavior. These symptoms may occur in association with hypertension, tachycardia, mydriasis, anorexia, insomnia, nausea, and vomiting. Stereotyped and repetitive movements may be seen as well. Severe overdose may be associated with cardiac arrythmia, high fever, delirium, hallucinations, seizures, coma, and death. Similar symptoms may also occur with cocaine intoxication, as may cardiac arrhythmias, myocardial infarction, and potentially fatal seizures.

Agitation caused by mild to moderate intoxication may be managed by the administration of benzodiazepines. Haloperidol may be administered in doses of 5 to 10 mg for patients with more severe overdose; however, it may also lower the seizure threshold. Because of the violent behavior sometimes induced by overdose of these drugs, patients may need to be restrained. To enhance excretion of the drug, the urine should be acidified to maintain a pH of 4 to 5.

Prolonged parenteral administration of large doses of stimulant or "runs" may be followed by sleep that may last for several days and severe depression, which may respond to treatment with antidepressants.

HALLUCINOGENS

Hallucinogens cause a wide range of effects, ranging from a mild euphoric state to marked modification of perception. Included in this category of drugs are lysergic acid diethylamide (LSD), dimethyltryptamine (DMT), 2,5-dimethoxy-4-methlyamphetamine (DOM or STP), trimethoxytryptamine (TMA), psilocybin, mescaline, phencyclidine (PCP), thiocyclodine (TCP) delta-9-tetrahydrocannabinol (THC), and marijuana (cannabis). The effects of these drugs begin several minutes to 1 hour after these substances have been taken, with individuals experiencing a euphoric or an altered perceptual state. Variable degrees of tolerance occur with the use of these drugs. With the exception of cannabis, which contains the active ingredient delta-

9-tetrahydrocannabinol, the drugs of this class have been associated with marked alteration of states of consciousness and behavior.

LSD, DOM, DMT, TMA, mescaline, and psilocybin may cause marked perceptual distortion, tachycardia, dilated and reactive pupils, tremor, hyperreflexia, piloerection, and incoordination. Acute intoxication may be managed by "talking down" (i.e., calming) the patient or with benzodiazepines or haloperidol. Overdoses are not known to be directly fatal. Slight tolerance may develop, and after abstaining from taking the drug, persistent anxiety, depression, or delusions may occur and persist for variable lengths of time. "Flashbacks," or brief hallucinations, may occur for weeks to years after a period of drug use.

PCP in low doses causes a sensation of numbness, emotional lability, and euphoria or dysphoria. High doses cause symptoms ranging from anxiety, confusion, and distorted perception and sensations, to rigidity, paranoid psychosis, a catatonic-like state, seizures, coma, and death. Toxicity may also result in hepatic necrosis, myoglobinuria, and severe hypertension that develops several days after the use of the drug. Treatment consists of continuous gastric suctioning, blood pressure control, and in the absence of myoglobinuria, urine acidification. If necessary, agitation may be acutely controlled with haloperidol, using caution since this may precipitate the neuroleptic malignant syndrome. Benzodiazepines may be subsequently administered intravenously. Patients should be placed in an environment with minimal external stimulation. The symptoms of acute toxicity usually clear within 3 to 6 hours, although the psychosis may last for weeks. In some cases, long-term abnormalities of speech and memory may occur.

THC may be smoked or ingested and commonly causes dry mouth, increased appetite, conjunctival injection, and tachycardia. Individuals using this drug may complain of significant anxiety or depression, a psychosis may occur at high doses. A significant degree of tolerance may develop. No specific abstinence syndrome has been identified for this drug.

INHALANTS

A common practice among older children and adolescents is the inhalation of vapors of various substances. Among the substances abused in this manner are glues, plastic and rubber cements, fingernail polish remover, furniture polish, lacquers, enamels, cleaning fluid, and gasoline. The symptoms commonly include mild euphoria, confusion, disorientation, and ataxia but may progress to develop into delirious or psychotic behavior, seizures, and coma. In general, the effects of acute intoxication resolve after several hours to days. However, damage may occur to the kidney, liver, and bone marrow which, in addition to cardiac arrhythmias, aspiration, and asphyxia, may result in death. There has been no abstinence syndrome associated with inhalant abuse.

Treatment consists of appropriate supportive measures to control impulsive behavior or neurologic or cardiac complications. A hematologic profile, determinations of electrolytes, blood urea nitrogen (BUN), creatinine, and urinary sediment, chest x-ray examination, and electrocardiography should be performed to search for specific organ damage.

SUGGESTED READING

Gossop M. Clonidine and the treatment of opiate withdrawal syndrome. Drug Alcohol Depend 1988; 21:253–259.

Millman RB. Evaluation and clinical management of cocaine abusers. Clin Psychiatry 1989; 49:27–33.

PATIENT RESOURCES

For information about drugs, drug use, and abuse:

National Clearing-House for Alcohol and Drug Information
P.O. Box 2345
Rockville, Maryland 20852
Telephone: (301) 468-2600

For information concerning treatment centers located throughout the United States:

National Institute on Drug Abuse
Treatment and Referral Hotline
1-800-662-HELP

WERNICKE'S ENCEPHALOPATHY AND ALCOHOL-RELATED NUTRITIONAL DISEASE

PETER L. CARLEN, M.D., FRCPC
JACK NEIMAN, M.D., Ph.D.

Chronic alcoholism predisposes to nutritional deficiencies for several reasons. When alcoholics go on a binge, frequently their only source of caloric intake is alcoholic beverages. The calories of alcoholic beverages are considered "empty" because alcoholics can ingest large quantities of calories in the form of alcohol and usually not show the expected weight gain, and because liquor, wine, and beer contain only insignificant amounts of vitamins and minerals and no other nutrients. Alcoholism per se is often associated with poor economic conditions, which also contributes to inadequate dietary intake. Impaired appetite secondary to alcohol-related gastrointestinal and liver disorders can also be a factor. Alcoholism can cause secondary malnutrition or deficient nutrient utilization through gastrointestinal damage causing maldigestion or malabsorption of nutrients, by energy wastage, and by decreased utilization of nutrients at the cellular level.

There are several diseases found in alcoholics that are attributed to nutritional deficiencies (Table 1). These are classified into probable and possible nutritional diseases. In this chapter, each disease entity is discussed in turn, and then a more general approach to the management of these alcoholic patients is presented. In addition to treating any specific nutritional deficiency, the physician is needed to assist alcoholics in altering their lifestyle and maintaining abstinence. To treat these alcoholism-related diseases, it is important to recognize the syndromes and the underlying alcoholism problem, sometimes difficult to spot in non-skid–row types, who, in fact, comprise the majority of alcohol abusers in the western world.

TABLE 1 Alcoholism-Related Nutritional Diseases of the Nervous System

Probable
Wernicke's encephalopathy
Korsakoff's syndrome
Alcoholic cerebellar degeneration
Alcoholic pellagra encephalopathy
Vitamin B_6 deficiency
Tobacco-alcohol amblyopia
Alcoholic neuropathy
Possible
Alcoholic cerebral atrophy (dementia)
Marchiafava-Bignami disease
Central pontine myelinolysis
Alcoholic myopathy

PROBABLE ALCOHOLISM-RELATED NUTRITIONAL DISEASES

Wernicke's Encephalopathy

Wernicke's encephalopathy (WE) is an underdiagnosed entity occurring mainly in chronic alcoholics, but also in other disease states including renal failure, renal dialysis, chronic bowel disease, persistent vomiting, or with intravenous hyperalimentation. It has a characteristic presentation of ophthalmoplegia, mental disturbance, and ataxia. The only signs that clearly differentiate WE from the acute alcoholic withdrawal state are the ophthalmoplegia found in WE and the tremulous-hyperexcitable state found in acute alcohol withdrawal. These two syndromes can coexist, however, and not all patients with WE have ophthalmoplegia. Nystagmus is common but is also part of alcohol withdrawal, as is ataxia. The ataxia associated with alcohol withdrawal is probably related to vestibular and cerebellar dysfunction. These patients can be hypothermic, presumably from hypothalamic involvement. The mental disturbance is usually a global confusional state with apathy and drowsiness, which can blend into an amnestic state characteristic of Korsakoff's amnesia. Confabulation is sometimes present. Often there is an associated peripheral neuropathy. It is thought that WE, as it becomes chronic, can persist as a Korsakoff's syndrome (KS). The topography of the pathologic changes are the same. The mammillary bodies are always involved. The other most consistently involved areas are the thalamus (especially the medial dorsal nuclei), hypothalamus, midbrain, pons, medulla, and midline cerebellar vermis. There is a symmetric, paraventricular distribution of lesions ranging from tissue necrosis to moderate neuronal and myelinated fiber loss with gliosis. In acute WE, there may be microhemorrhages.

Some classify WE as a medical emergency, since the danger of not treating this disease as soon as possible is the development of a chronic and possibly nonreversible KS. WE is due to thiamine (vitamin B_1) deficiency. With thiamine administration, there is a gratifyingly quick recovery from ophthalmoplegia within hours, followed by a clearing of the confusional state. Patients are slower to recover from nystagmus and ataxia. Although normally only a few milligrams of thiamine are required per day, much higher doses are used to treat WE, in part because cellular utilization of the vitamin may be impaired. Thiamine hydrochloride is initially given in a dose of 100 mg IV or IM followed by long-term administration of a multivitamin compound that includes all B vitamins and vitamin A, and a balanced diet. One must avoid giving patients susceptible to WE a sugar load before administering thiamine, since the increased glucose metabolism increases the central nervous system requirement for thiamine and can precipitate WE per se.

Korsakoff's Syndrome

KS is characterized by a memory deficit that is out of proportion to other cognitive functions. It can follow WE, but often there is no apparent history of WE. Superficially, these patients sometimes appear to converse and reason normally. However, they have limited insight into their condition and cannot remember events or comments that occurred even seconds or minutes previously. They have marked retrograde and anterograde amnesia. Their spontaneity and initiative are diminished.

Treatment consists of a nutritional diet and placing these patients in a properly supervised living situation. It is most important to follow up KS cases because some patients (10 to 25 percent) recover quite remarkably over several weeks to months and therefore may not require institutionalization.

Alcoholic Cerebellar Degeneration

Some alcoholics present primarily with a syndrome of ataxia of gait. Characteristically there is little impairment of finger-nose testing. Heel-shin testing is sometimes affected.

Alcoholic cerebellar degeneration is clinically considered a nutritionally related problem of chronic alcoholism, and it is frequently associated with a peripheral neuropathy. It can be seen both pathologically and clinically to coexist with WE and usually resolves with thiamine treatment. It can be chronic, however, and may not respond to thiamine administration. We have noted evidence of cerebellar atrophy on computed tomographic (CT) scans of alcoholics with no correlation to the degree of measured ataxia using the Heath Rails Test. In fact, the measured ataxia correlated better with the degree of supratentorial atrophy on CT scanning. Hence there may be more than one site of neuroanatomic damage to account for alcoholism-related ataxia. Finally, in acute alcohol withdrawal, there may be a profound ataxia syndrome that slowly resolves over weeks to months with maintained abstinence and an adequate diet.

Alcoholic Pellagra Encephalopathy

Pellagra is a nutritional disease associated with niacin deficiency. The hallmarks are dermatitis, diarrhea, and dementia. Pellagra can occur with malnutrition or secondarily with gastrointestinal tract disease, malignant carcinoid, isoniazid, G-mercaptopurine, S-fluorouracil, or puromycin treatment. Pellagra encephalopathy has also been reported in chronic alcoholics, often coexisting with other alcohol-related encephalopathies in the same patient. Pathologically one finds swollen neurons with eccentric nuclei and loss of Nissl particles in the cerebral cortex, reticular formation, pontine nuclei, and dentate nuclei. The major neurologic findings are a fluctuating confusional state that can progress to coma, hypertonus, and startle myoclonus. Severe deterioration and even death can be precipitated by thiamine and pyridoxine administration without niacin. Alcoholics often do not have the associated pellagra dermatitis or diarrhea. However, it is prudent to ensure that all encephalopathic alcoholics receive niacin in addition to other vitamins. The routine multivitamin therapy used in the western world to treat alcoholics is probably the reason that this disease is relatively uncommon today. There is some question as to whether all the symptoms and signs of alcoholic pellagra encephalopathy can be ascribed to niacin deficiency alone. Hence the treatment should be multivitamins that include niacin and an adequate nutritional diet.

Vitamin B_6 Deficiency

Pyridoxine (vitamin B_6) is converted to pyridoxal 5-phosphate (PLP) primarily in the liver. The level of PLP is often low in chronic alcoholics, especially those with liver disease. Its deficiency can be associated with a peripheral neuropathy and neuromuscular irritability, in addition to dermatitis, stomatitis, immune suppression, and a sideroblastic anemia. It is rare to find only pyridoxine deficiency in alcoholics, since this disease is usually associated with other nutritional deficiencies. Its treatment is multiple B vitamins and a nutritious diet.

Tobacco-Alcohol Amblyopia

This syndrome is characterized by bilateral decreased visual acuity, symmetric scotomata, impaired color vision, and usually normal fundi. There is uncertainty in the literature as to whether alcohol or tobacco alone can cause amblyopia. Patients are usually both alcohol abusers and heavy smokers.

Concomitant vitamin deficiencies and liver disease are probably the most important causative factors, although the specific pathogenesis has not yet been elucidated. The formerly cyanide-vitamin B_{12} hypothesis has been debunked. Vitamin A deficiency, which is associated with night blindness, is not uncommon in alcoholics, especially in those with liver disease. It could play a role in the tobacco-alcohol amblyopia. The recommended treatment is an adequate diet, multivitamin administration, and most important, maintained abstinence from alcohol.

Alcoholic Neuropathy

Almost all chronic alcoholics have a peripheral neuropathy to some degree, as evidenced by depressed ankle jerks and decreased vibration and cold sensation in the lower limbs. Usually these signs are not associated with sensory complaints. However, some alcoholics, particularly those with apparent dietary deficiency, do complain of weakness, paresthesia, and pain. These symptoms usually present insidiously. The weakness is often associated with distal wasting, which is usually more apparent in the lower limbs. The pain usually consists of a dull constant ache in the feet or legs, but brief lancinating pains can also occur. Patients may also complain of "burning feet" characterized by painful paresthesia, which is worsened by pressure on the soles and thus makes walking difficult. The cranial nerves are almost never involved, but an autonomic neuropathy and orthostatic hypotension can occur. Pathologically one sees a noninflammatory degeneration of the peripheral nerves with destruction of both myelin and axons. The evidence points to nutritional deficiency and alcohol toxicity as the major causative factors. The specific pathogenesis, however, has not yet been pinpointed. Treatment consists of alcohol abstinence, a nutritional diet, and administration of B vitamins. Symptomatic recovery can take several weeks to months because of the prolonged nature of nerve regeneration. As an aside, it should be noted that alcoholics are subject to pressure nerve palsies (ulnar, radial, peroneal) because of a probable subclinical neuropathy and the tendency of the patient to fall asleep in awkward positions when intoxicated, putting undue and prolonged pressure on the peripheral nerve.

POSSIBLE ALCOHOLISM-RELATED NUTRITIONAL DISEASES

Cerebral Atrophy (Dementia)

On CT or magnetic resonance imaging (MRI) scan, diffuse cerebral atrophy with cortical sulcal widening and enlarged ventricles is a common finding in most chronic alcoholics. There is a weak correlation between the degree of cerebral atrophy and cognitive impairment. Chronic alcohol intake in experimental animals is associated with some cerebral degenerative changes and decreased brain protein synthesis. Malnutrition in humans is associated with cerebral atrophy and cognitive changes. The exact relationship of chronic alcohol intake with alcoholism-related nutritional deficiencies, cerebral atrophy, and cognitive deficits is unclear. Alcoholics can develop a severe global dementia which some have distinguished from KS since more than memory is significantly impaired. However, recent pathologic evidence suggests that all autopsied alcoholics with a global dementia in fact have the pathology of KS. These alcoholics do not appear to have more cerebral cortical atrophy than patients with KS.

Practically speaking, it is important to follow these patients for several months after alcohol withdrawal since some show a marked improvement in their dementia syndrome. This can be associated with some reversibility in their cerebral atrophy and a concomitant increase in their mean cerebral tissue density on CT scan. We have seen several patients who were slated for nursing homes because of their dementia and who, over a few weeks, had improved to the point where chronic institutionalization was no longer necessary. It is presumed that a nutritious diet and lack of alcohol intake was helpful in these cases. However, many chronic alcoholics with a global dementia do not improve, and a small percentage continue to decline even with alcohol abstinence. Clearly other causes of encephalopathy and dementia must be considered. In alcoholics, the greatest danger is subdural hematoma, since its incidence among patients who have atrophied brains and a tendency to fall and suffer head injuries is inordinately high.

Marchiafava-Bignami Disease

This is a rare disease characterized by demyelination and destruction of the corpus callosum and is found in severe chronic alcoholics. Clinically, the presentation is quite variable, but often this pathology is associated with a frontal-lobe or dementia syndrome or with seizures, stupor, and coma.

Central Pontine Myelinolysis

This is another relatively rare entity pathologically defined by a noninflammatory demyelination of the basis pontis. Evidence of this disease can be seen on CT or MRI scans without significant accompanying clinical signs. It is often associated with other alcoholism-related encephalopathies such as Wernicke's encephalopathy, pellagra encephalopathy, or withdrawal seizures. When severe, it presents as a flaccid quadriparesis, dysarthia, and dysphagia. Recently, central pontine myelinolysis has been demonstrated to develop in patients with rapid correction of a significant hyponatremia. Hence in alcoholics with a low serum sodium, which can be associated with seizures and encephalopathy, judicious and slow correction of this metabolic defect is required. We would also advise a nutritious diet and multivitamin administration.

Alcoholic Myopathy

Many chronic alcoholics, especially those who appear malnourished or who have liver disease, present with diffuse proximal muscle weakness, wasting, and increased serum muscle enzymes. Both type I and type II muscle fibers are involved in light microscopic examination. Weakness usually resolves with adequate diet and abstinence. However, some patients may have a subacute or chronic, severe proximal myopathy that resolves only slowly. A few alcoholics develop an acute myopathy with rhabdomyolysis and myoglobinuria, sometimes followed by acute renal failure.

TREATMENT OF ALCOHOL ADDICTION

It is all well and good to diagnose and treat the nervous system disease caused by alcohol abuse. However, if the patient recovers, it is essential to address the underlying problem of the disease—namely, alcohol addiction. This is an extremely complex and difficult subject often ignored by the physician. Addiction management is now a legitimate, important, and difficult area of research. There are a wide variety of treatments available to choose from, depending on one's location and the socioeconomic stratum of the patient. With an alcoholic patient, it is first necessary to identify the problem. Today, many patients abuse other psychoactive drugs in addition to alcohol. Once the alcohol (and other drug abuse) problem is identified, it is important to discuss its consequences for the patient, and when relevant, for the patient's family.

The next step is to match available therapeutic options with the patient in an attempt to achieve behavioral modification such that the patient avoids alcohol abuse. This might sound obvious, but it is frequently overlooked. The recidivism rate is high among alcohol and drug abusers. In most North American communities, Alcoholics Anonymous is available. This organization, like many other programs, believes in total abstinence and uses a form of group therapy. There are also many different types of private and public treatment facilities, but detailed descriptions of these are beyond the scope of this chapter.

SUGGESTED READING

Carlen PL, Wilkinson DA. Reversibility of alcohol-related brain damage: clinical and experimental observations. Acta Med Scand 1987; 717 (suppl):19–26.

Krumsiek J, Kruger C, Patzold U. Tobacco-alcohol amblyopia neuro-ophthalmological findings and clinical course. Acta Neurol Scand 1985; 72:180–187.

Serdaru M, Hausser-Hauw C, LaPlante D, et al. The clinical spectrum of alcoholic pellagra encephalopathy. Brain 1988; 111:829–842.

Victor M. Neurologic disorders due to alcoholism and malnutrition. In: Baker AB, Baker LH. Clinical Neurology Vol. 2 (revised edition). Philadelphia: JB Lippincott, 1982:1.

MULTIPLE SCLEROSIS

ROBERT M. HERNDON, M.D.

DIAGNOSIS

Treatment of multiple sclerosis (MS) begins with diagnosis and classification. Approximately 10 percent of referrals to MS clinics are misdiagnosed. Although the spectrum of misdiagnosis has changed with the advent of magnetic resonance imaging (MRI), the rate of misdiagnosis has changed little. Misread and overinterpreted MRIs have become a common cause of misdiagnosis. *The diagnosis of MS remains a clinical diagnosis.* It is based on evidence of dissemination in time and clinical or paraclinical, *objective,* evidence of dissemination in location. It is important to realize that other disease processes can produce syndromes that meet formal diagnostic criteria for multiple sclerosis. Thus, atypical features such as absence of visual or oculomotor signs, normal cerebrospinal fluid, absence of bladder involvement, strictly posterior fossa signs, or a normal MRI should alert the physician to the possibility of misdiagnosis. Accurate diagnosis is especially important when more aggressive therapies are being considered, but it is also important in general, since many of the disorders that may be mistaken for MS can be effectively treated.

Classification

Once the diagnosis is clearly established, treatment depends on the type of disease and the severity of the process. Treatment can be divided into two categories; (1) treatment directed at the basic disease process and (2) symptomatic therapy. Treatment of the disease process is either immunosuppressive or immunomodulatory, and treatment selection is based on severity and classification (Fig. 1). In general, younger people with the disease are more likely to have an exacerbating remitting or exacerbating progressive course with relatively acute episodes of demyelination followed by periods of improvement or relative stability. In many of these cases, significant progression of the disease between attacks may be largely masked by the superimposed exacerbations and remissions. Improvement in one area after an acute attack will mask other symptoms that are continuing to progress, so that the patient may be improving in some areas and progressing in others simultaneously. In older patients, generally those older than 40 years of age, acute attacks are increasingly uncommon and the disease manifests itself primarily as a progressive loss of function without acute exacerbations or periods of remission.

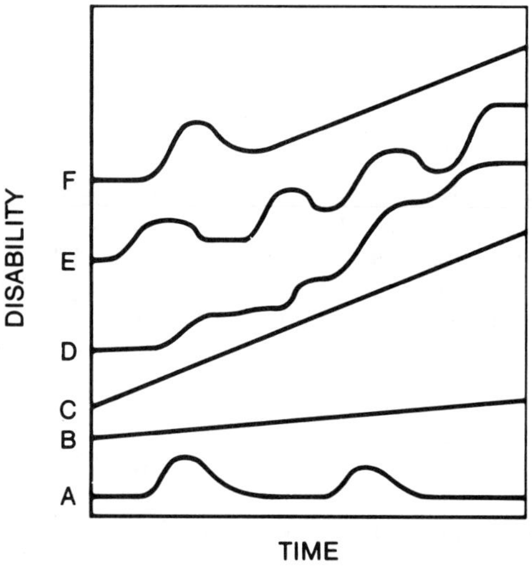

Figure 1 The varied course of multiple sclerosis. A = benign course; B = slowly progressive course; C = more rapid, steadily progressive course; D = intermittently progressive course; E = combined course with acute attacks, incomplete recovery, and a progressive component largely obscured by attacks and incomplete remissions; F = single acute attack followed by steady progression.

THERAPY DIRECTED AT THE DISEASE PROCESS

Diet

Numerous claims have been made regarding the therapeutic efficacy of a host of different diets, vitamin supplements, and mineral supplements. To date, the only credible evidence of the efficacy of diet in treating MS is that a dietary supplement of linoleic acid achieved with two tablespoons of sunflower seed oil daily produces a slight reduction in the frequency and/or severity of acute attacks. The effect is not great, but it has been seen in more than one properly controlled study. Aside from this, however, there are no convincing studies demonstrating that special diets have any beneficial effect on the course of the disease.

Caution should be taken in the use of mineral supplements since there is evidence suggesting that zinc can enhance immune responses, and also epidemiologic evidence suggesting that zinc might have an adverse effect on MS.

Rest

Bedrest, a time-honored treatment for MS, is frequently recommended. In the case of acute attacks in a person who is not severely handicapped, bedrest may provide some modest benefit in terms of reduced stress and anxiety. There is no evidence that it improves the rate of recovery. Bedrest is not recommended for individuals with progressive disease and especially for those with spastic paraparesis that has become chronic. Even 2 or 3 days in bed may be enough to convert an ambulatory patient with spastic paraparesis into a wheelchair-bound patient. Loss of muscle strength and tone occurs rapidly in paretic patients, and it is extremely difficult to make up lost ground.

Prevention of Acute Attacks

No treatment thus far reported is known to prevent acute attacks. Although there is preliminary evidence that beta-interferon and copolymer-1 (COP-1) reduce the number of acute attacks, these agents are still in the experimental stages. Therapeutic trials currently in progress may establish the place of these agents in the therapeutic armamentarium, but to date, they do not appear to be of much value in the treatment of progressive disease.

Azathioprine (Imuran) has been used to reduce the number of acute attacks of patients with MS, but controlled clinical trials have failed to demonstrate that it has a clear effect on exacerbation.

The Acute Attack

The acute attack of MS may be very mild with little impairment of important functions. In this case, and if the symptoms of the acute attack do not interfere with the patient's normal activities and are not uncomfortable for the patient, no treatment is necessary. There is no evidence that treatment of the acute attack improves the ultimate level of functional recovery. Although steroids will hasten the recovery process at the cost of side effects of varying severity, the ultimate level of recovery is probably not affected. The use of steroids in patients with optic neuritis may be an exception, however, because the optic nerve may become swollen and, since it passes through the restrictive optic canal, can be damaged by pressure and ischemia. Thus I believe that significant optic neuritis should be treated with steroids routinely, pending the outcome of the current multicenter optic neuritis treatment trial.

Severe acute attacks that interfere with the patient's livelihood or daily activities or that produce significant discomfort may be treated with adrenocorticotropic hormone (ACTH) or prednisone. Although many neurologists express a strong preference for one or the other, there is little evidence to support that one is significantly superior to the other. There is good evidence that ACTH shortens the duration of acute attacks, and the experience of most clinicians is that prednisone is equally efficacious. The two are by no means identical, and if one does not work, the other may. Individuals who have not been treated previously will often respond rapidly to prednisone in a dose of 60 mg daily, but with repeated courses, higher doses of as much as 100 mg daily or more may be required. Prednisone is best given as a single morning dose. I usually give the initial dose for 5 days, then taper. Recrudescence of symptoms is a common problem when the drug is tapered rapidly. When this happens, I find that resumption of full doses is usually required to regain the lost ground, and even then, the initial level of improvement may not be regained. Recrudescence during the taper can be minimized by using a slow taper (Table 1).

Acute attacks may also be treated with ACTH gel in a dosage of 40 to 80 U per day. In this case, the full dose is maintained for approximately 5 days, then decreased by 20 U every 3 days until the patient has discontinued the medication, or in some patients, may be completed with the patient receiving 20 U per day for 3 days followed by three alternate-day doses of 20 U each.

TABLE 1 Treatment with Prednisone

Day	*Dose (mg)*
1–4	100
5–7	80
8–10	60
11–13	40
14–16	30
17–20	20
21–23	15
24–26	10
27–29	5
30	0

Steroid Dependence

Steroid dependence occurs when the steroid dose cannot be decreased without a significant recrudescence of symptoms. This is unusual and occurs in no more than 1 to 3 percent of patients. If three successive attempts to taper the steroids result in recurrence of significant, disabling symptoms, the patient should be considered steroid dependent. When this is the case, I have found that a slow taper to 30 mg of prednisone daily and a slow taper to 30 mg every other day can usually be achieved without a flair in the symptoms. Levels of 20 to 30 mg of prednisone administered on an alternate-day schedule can be maintained for long periods of time with minimal side effects. My experience has been that these patients remain remarkably free of acute attacks on the alternate-day schedule. I do not advocate continuous therapy for patients who can be withdrawn from steroids without recurrence of symptoms. In addition, I usually try to reduce the alternate-day dose to the minimum that will keep the patient free of recurrence of the symptoms. After 1 year of the alternate-day schedule, I usually reattempt to decrease the dose, although my success rate in withdrawing these individuals from steroids without a recurrence of symptoms has been low.

Progressive Disease

Steroids and ACTH

The use of steroids and ACTH in the treatment of progressive MS has been disappointing. Transient improvement often occurs but usually disappears within a few days or weeks after treatment is discontinued. One can delay the onset of wheelchair dependence for several months by administering steroids continuously, but because of the high rate of complications and particularly of osteoporosis, I do not recommend this approach.

In patients with severe spastic paraparesis, high-dose methylprednisolone will significantly reduce spasticity for a substantial period. The drug is given in a dose of 1 g daily for 3 days by intravenous infusion. I prefer to administer this dose as 0.5 g twice daily for 3 days. Although the dose is usually well tolerated, complications have been seen. In particular, immobile patients with deep vein thrombosis are liable to develop pulmonary emboli if they begin to move their legs more freely. Such emboli are dangerous and can be fatal. If one is in doubt regarding the possibility of deep vein thrombosis, appropriate studies and/or anticoagulation should precede treatment. Aseptic necrosis of the head of the femur is also seen as an uncommon complication.

Immunosuppressive Therapy

Cyclophosphamide in combination with ACTH or a synthetic steroid has been reported to be useful in treating progressive MS. My experience suggests that, in a carefully selected group of patients, the treatment does have substantial benefit. It also carries significant risks, however, and deaths have occurred, particularly with the shorter, more intensive, 8-day course that some have advocated. I have not included a treatment protocol in this discussion because I do not recommend that this treatment be undertaken by clinicians not familiar with chemotherapy or by those who are treating only a small number of patients. It should be undertaken only after a thorough study of the literature on the subject, and preferably only after discussion with someone who has used this form of therapy. For patients in whom this approach is indicated, we recommend referral to a center that has an active treatment program.

Selection of appropriate patients to be referred for chemotherapy involves consideration of the following factors.

Age. Younger patients respond much better than older patients. We rarely use chemotherapy in patients older than 55 years of age. Younger patients are much more likely to show significant improvement than older patients. The few exceptions to this have been older patients with an unusually rapid course, which is rare in this age group.

Rate of Progression. The more rapidly the disease is progressing, the more effective immunosuppressive therapy is likely to be and the greater the probability of significant clinical improvement. In patients with an indolent or slowly progressive course, improvement is significantly less likely and, because of the slow rate at which the patient is changing, arrest of progression is difficult to observe.

Disability. The response to therapy is less and the complication rate much higher in severely disabled patients. I do not treat patients who are wheelchair-bound unless they have been using a wheelchair for only a short time and can still stand (bear weight) and self transfer. Patients who are effectively paraplegic usually have significant impairment of respiratory function and are at risk for pulmonary infection as well as for bladder infection.

Reproductive Status. Because cyclophosphamide therapy may cause sterility and may also damage DNA, it should not be used in individuals who plan to have children and should never be used in someone who is pregnant.

Complicating Medical Disorders. Patients with significant medical illness in addition to MS must be evaluated individually. Diabetes in particular presents a problem since steroids add to the difficulties in controlling the diabetes and because these patients are much more susceptible to infection, particularly if the diabetes is severe. In general, I prefer not to treat insulin-dependent diabetics. Other disorders such as malignancies and heart disease should be evaluated on a case-by-case basis.

Side Effects. To be selected for chemotherapy, patients should be able to accept side effects including hair loss, nausea, and vomiting, and other risks inherent in the treatment.

Azathioprine

Azathioprine (Imuran) has been widely used over the past two decades despite a paucity of studies demonstrating its effectiveness. Studies to date suggest that, in doses of approximately 100 mg per day, it is fairly well tolerated for long periods. The drug appears to have little effect on the exacerbation rate, but it appears to have some effect on the overall rate of progression. Although the effects of this drug on progression are not great, they may be sufficient to warrant its use in some patients. Further clinical trials are needed to better define its place in the therapeutic armamentarium.

Cyclosporin

Cyclosporin has been used in a recently completed clinical trial and appears to have some beneficial effect on the disease process; however, renal toxicity and hypertension appear to be a substantial problem when the doses that are used are high enough to be effective. Because of this, I do not recommend its use at this time.

Plasmapheresis

The role of plasmapheresis in the treatment of MS remains uncertain. Good results have been reported in at least one controlled study; however, other studies have shown much less clear-cut results. A large controlled trial is currently in progress and should help define the proper role of plasmapheresis in the treatment of MS. Until further research results become available, I do not recommend this expensive and unproven approach.

Several other therapies including hyperbaric oxygen and transfer factor have been recommended by some, but these have not proven useful when properly tested.

SYMPTOMATIC TREATMENT

Spasticity

Spasticity is very common and troublesome in patients with MS, but in patients with pyramidal weakness, it also plays a role in maintaining the ability to stand and walk. In patients with spastic paraparesis, the spasticity may provide the extensor strength for bearing weight. Thus effective drug therapy for spasticity often increases weakness and a balance must be found between the two.

Effective treatment of spasticity begins with physical therapy. Stretching is essential to prevent contractures and also reduces spasticity. Active exercise will help maintain strength and mobility. I regard physical therapy as the mainstay of therapy for spasticity.

Baclofen (Lioresal) has proven to be the most effective and useful drug for the treatment of spasticity. The proper dose is "enough but not too much." Some patients receive considerable relief from as little as 5 mg taken once or twice daily and become weak when taking 10 mg per dose, while others require much higher doses and do well with doses of as much as 200 mg (although the maximum recommended dose according to the manufacturer is 80 mg per day). Baclofen should be started in a dose of about 10 mg administered twice daily and increased by 10 mg per day until the spasticity is adequately relieved or weakness occurs. When weakness develops, the dose should be decreased to a point below that at which weakness occurs. If this does not produce significant reduction in spasticity, there is little point in continuing therapy unless the patient is willing to tolerate some weakness in return for reduced spasticity.

Diazepam (Valium) is another effective muscle relaxant and may be used when results with baclofen are unsatisfactory. It is usually started at a dosage of 5 mg twice daily and increased gradually. It is considerably more sedative than baclofen, is habituating, and may interfere with cognitive function. I reserve it for patients who cannot tolerate baclofen or, in some instances, as an adjunct to baclofen therapy, particularly in patients who have a high level of anxiety in addition to their spasticity.

Dantrolene has not proven useful in the therapy of spasticity in MS patients in my experience. It appears to be much less effective than baclofen or diazepam and carries a greater risk of toxicity, particularly liver toxicity.

More drastic measures may be needed for patients with spasticity that is refractory to drug treatment. I reserve such measures for patients with essentially complete paraplegia. These include chemical neurolysis by injection of phenol either into motor nerves (using electromyographic guidance) or into the motor point. Alternatively, ethanol can be injected intrathecally to block the lumbar nerve roots. Although this usually produces relief that lasts for at least 6 months and can be repeated if necessary, it should be reserved for patients who have lost bladder and bowel control. More permanent relief can be achieved with neurosurgical intervention either via dorsal rhizotomy or by Bischoff's myelotomy. These drastic procedures result in a flaccid paralysis that is permanent. Such procedures are rarely needed but may be used in patients with long-standing sensory loss, urinary retention, and flexor spasms or spasticity that is refractory and seriously interferes with patient care. Considerable attention to the prevention of decubitus ulcers is needed in patients with impaired sensation that is either a direct result of MS or a result of destructive treatment aimed at relieving spasticity.

Bladder Dysfunction

Frequently, both small spastic bladders with urgency and incontinence and large flaccid bladders with overflow incontinence are a problem in patients with MS.

Bowel Dysfunction

Constipation is a regular occurrence in patients with MS. Bowel motility is decreased, presumably because of altered autonomic function. This is aggravated in many patients by a low fluid intake, which is a common response in patients with urinary urgency, frequency, and incontinence. It is normally best to manage the bowel with stool softeners such as docusate sodium (Colace) in a dose of 50 to 200 mg per day and bulk laxatives such as bran. Increased fluid intake is also helpful. If these measures prove inadequate, bisacodyl (Dulcolax) may be useful. Bisacodyl tablets will usually work overnight and the suppositories within 1 to 2 hours. Severe constipation should not be ignored since obstipation with rupture of the bowel has been known to occur in patients with MS.

Cognitive and Emotional Aspects

While many MS patients have little clinically evident emotional or cognitive disturbance, most patients with well-established disease do have measurable changes in their cognitive abilities and many have disturbances in the emotional sphere. There are several relatively simple measures that can help in the management of these problems, although little can be done to help those few patients with serious cognitive impairment.

Depression, Euphoria, and Pathologic Laughing and Weeping

Depression. This is a common problem in patients with MS, and mania is also fairly common, particularly in patients receiving steroids. These affective disorders must be distinguished from the problems of exaggerated or perverted affective display described below. There is evidence of an increased incidence of true *bipolar disease* in MS patients and in relatives of MS patients, although the reason for this is unknown. These disorders usually respond to traditional treatment with lithium carbonate or with carbamazepine (Tegretol). Hypomanic episodes occurring during steroid treatment may usually be managed with Tegretol in a dose of 300 to 400 mg daily. This works more rapidly than lithium and can be easily introduced if sleeplessness and other signs of mania occur. If Tegretol does not work satisfactorily or cannot be used because of toxic side effects, lithium carbonate will usually prove effective.

Most depression associated with MS is probably situational, but endogenous depressions are also common. Tricyclic antidepressants are usually effective in the management of this disorder. The required dose is often much less than that traditionally used in the treatment of depression. I have found doses of amitriptyline hydrochloride of as little as 10 mg per day to be effective in some instances, and a dose of 25 to 50 mg at bedtime is typically adequate. The much higher doses traditionally used to treat depression are rarely required.

Pathologic Laughing and Weeping. Pathologic laughing and weeping are extreme examples of lability of affective display. In these extreme examples, the affective display (i.e., the laughter or crying) may bear little relationship to the feelings of the patient. The patient is unable to modulate affective expression, so that even relatively mild emotional stimuli bring on an affective display that is exaggerated in intensity and that may be inappropriate in relation to the patient's feelings or internal affective state. In milder cases, an exaggeration of the appropriate affective display is all that is seen.

These disorders of affective display, often described somewhat inaccurately as "emotional lability," are socially disabling and particularly prone to disrupt personal relationships since the patient's emotional displays are invariably interpreted as reflecting his or her feelings rather than recognized as an exaggerated and perhaps perverted expression of those feelings. It is extremely hard for the spouse, or indeed the physician, to recognize depression in someone who is laughing. We are taught from infancy to believe facial expression, and if the facial expression does not accurately reflect what the person is saying, we believe the expression. Thus emotional communication is disrupted for these patients, sometimes with devastating effects on interpersonal relations.

Both pathologic laughing and weeping and lability of affective display are responsive to treatment in the majority of cases. Amitriptyline hydrochloride in a dose of 10 to 50 mg daily, usually administered as a single bedtime dose, is effective in reducing lability of affective display in 80 to 90 percent of patients. The effect of this agent in treating these disorders is more rapid than in the treatment of depression. The result is a reduction in the extreme emotional expression so that the affective display is more consonant with the internal affective state. The use of L-dihydroxyphenylalanine(L-DOPA) has been recommended for pathologic laughing and weeping in patients with cerebrovascular disease, but its use in treating MS has not been reported.

Inability to Focus Attention

Many MS patients can do only one thing at a time. For example, many cannot walk and have a conversation at the same time because they need to concentrate on their walking. Such patients have a great deal of difficulty with concentration in a distracting environment. They are able to function reasonably well in a quiet, nondistracting environment but are unable to filter out distracting stimuli. This problem frequently leads to irritability and can significantly interfere with work performance. Such patients are extremely intolerant of typical family life in which children are running in and out, the television is often on, and multiple simultaneous conversations are taking place. The simple expedient of removing as much of the distraction as possible or of providing a quiet room where the patient can do one thing at a time without distraction will often greatly improve temper and allow him or her to cope with the frustrations of the disease much better. Similarly, removing distractions from the workplace may result in improved job performance.

SUGGESTED READING

McDonald WI, Silberberg DH. The diagnosis of multiple sclerosis. In: McDonald WI, Silberberg DH, eds. Multiple sclerosis. Boston: Butterworth Publishers, 1986:1.

Rudick RA, Schiffer RB, Schwetz K, Herndon RM. Multiple sclerosis: the problem of misdiagnosis. Arch Neurol 1986; 43:578–593.

Ellison GW, Myers LW, eds. Rationale for immunomodulating therapies of multiple sclerosis. Neurology 1988; 38 (suppl): 89.

Ellison GW. Treatment aimed at modifying the course of multiple sclerosis. In: McDonald WI, Silberberg DH, eds. Multiple sclerosis. Boston: Butterworth Publishers, 1986:153.

Sibley WA. Therapeutic claims in multiple sclerosis. New York: Demos Publications, 1988.

Schiffer RB, Rudick RA, Herndon RM. Pathological laughing and weeping: treatment with amitriptyline. N Engl J Med 1985; 312:1480–1482.

PATIENT RESOURCES

Literature

Scheinberg LS. Multiple sclerosis: a guide for patients and their families. New York: Raven Press, 1983.

Therapeutic claims in multiple sclerosis. Published by the International Federation of Multiple Sclerosis Societies (IFMSS).

Available from the National Multiple Sclerosis Society (see address below, under "Associations").
Wolf JK, ed. Mastering multiple sclerosis: a handbook for MSers and families. Chicago: Academy Books, 1984.

Associations
National Multiple Sclerosis Society
205 East 42nd Street
New York, New York 10017
Telephone: (212) 986-3240

(Local chapters throughout the United States are listed in telephone directories.

AMYOTROPHIC LATERAL SCLEROSIS

RALPH W. KUNCL, M.D., Ph.D.
LORA L. CLAWSON, R.N., B.S.N.

The work of the neurologist who *cares* for the ALS patient is to dissuade both the patient and himself from the idea that the patient is untreatable. In a recent article in the New England Journal of Medicine, Drs. Bulkin and Lukashok make the following observation on physicians' approach to the incurably ill.

> Physicians are trained to investigate, diagnose, prolong life, and cure. When these goals are no longer relevant, physicians often feel they have no skills to offer and distance themselves from the patient. Some turn the patient over to other care givers. Many, like the physician in Tolstoi's *Death of Ivan Ilyich,* continue to prescribe cures in an effort to hide the reality that the patient is dying. The family is then placed in the position of Ilyich's wife, insisting that the patient adhere to the doctor's protocol and refusing to acknowledge the truth. Thus, the patient's final act of living is denied validity, and the patient and family are deprived of the opportunity to come to terms with it and with each other. All are left with the perception that there is some sort of shame attached to being incurably ill, and the patient is left with a sense of having been abandoned at the time of greatest crisis. Yet in truth, there remains much that the physician can offer the patient when curing skills are no longer required.

Few patients are as needy as those with amyotrophic lateral sclerosis (ALS). Paradoxically, there are few patients for whom neurologists provide worse continuing care. Many patients with ALS—perhaps most—leave their doctor's office with the idea that they ("the average patient") will die in 3 years, and that ALS is "untreatable." Thus this chapter might be subtitled, "What to do when there is nothing to do," or "Treating the untreatable."

WHAT ALS PATIENTS SAY THEIR DOCTORS NEED TO KNOW

It is because of the sense of having been abandoned that ALS patients experience and the psychosocial problems that arise that we began an ALS support group in the early 1980s in Baltimore, with the collaboration of the Muscular Dystrophy Association. What the pressing needs of ALS patients are, which solutions work best, what unspoken questions patients harbor—these things we have learned best by simply listening to members of the support group, in a setting away from the formality of the office. When asked, "What is the worst part about having ALS," patients' answers have included the following: "I was in the dark for 6 months without a diagnosis." "Not being told about the MDA." "Nothing ever truly helps; things only become temporarily more tolerable." "The fear of the respirator—not being *on* it, but the machine itself, sort of like the fear some people have of using a computer. But it was much easier than I'd ever anticipated."

When asked "What are the most important things you learned and who did you learn them from?" patients answered as follows: "No physician can help." "We improvise—it's a matter of living with it . . . self-discovery." "I found out I was too afraid of the gastrostomy; it was no big deal." "I handled each symptom as it came up, through the support group and my doctor and my therapist." "Doctors need to learn how to talk to patients with ALS."

Talking to Patients With ALS

There seem to be two extremes in how doctors talk to patients with ALS. The first extreme is avoidance, whether active or unconscious. It naturally evolves from the doctor's feeling of helplessness about the disease. It leads to withdrawal from the patient, curtness, obfuscation concerning the diagnosis, a concentration on documenting the inevitable neuromuscular decline without discussing solutions to the problems of everyday living, and even to the formal discharge of the patient to the care of other previously unengaged specialists such as pulmonary physicians or internists. Of course, it often works in reverse. The patient may withdraw from the doctor in a sense of embarrassment or anger about the diagnosis or the way in which it was given or received. This combination of avoidance behaviors no doubt explains the common switching of doctors that occurs with this disease early in its course.

The opposite extreme is the physician who actively engages the patient, transmitting his or her great experience with the natural history of the disease or its multiple symptoms and treatments by launching into a nonstop treatise on every conceivable outcome. Such speeches are seldom heard during the clinician's first encounter with the patient, and if they are, they are probably very frightening. The advice of experienced ALS clinicians is always to schedule a second visit after a short time for reflection, in order to discuss the prognosis and its meaning regarding activities of daily living. It is then important to take the occupational therapists' approach and attempt to "fix" only what the patient perceives as "broken." To do otherwise leads to overload and a feeling of hopelessness. Thus, for example, extensive conversations or demonstrations about communication problems and the many devices available to aid communication are rarely of value to patients who have no trouble speaking. Despite our best intentions to prepare people well in advance for any contingency, human nature is such that most of us will not prepare for future risks. Inundating patients with information about their illness is to be avoided in favor of focusing on a single or a few distinct current problems.

A final point on talking to patients with ALS is that it pays to kneel or sit whenever talking to a patient in a wheelchair. This brings the doctor and patient eye to eye, removing the patient's need to strain his weak cervical paraspinal muscles while craning the neck during conversation, and removes the position-of-authority body language.

DIAGNOSIS

The diagnosis of ALS is usually straightforward. *Progressive* weakness accompanied by other lower motor neuron signs such as atrophy or fasciculation must be present. It is important to note that fasciculation is a lower motor neuron sign that accompanies many disorders and is *not* in and of itself pathognomonic of ALS. Further, although the tongue is always examined, it is only denervated in one-fourth of patients at the time of diagnosis. The definite diagnosis of ALS requires the presence of *widespread* denervation (Lambert's criteria) that is not explainable by neuropathy or radiculopathy and which occurs in the presence of upper motor neuron signs but in the absence of significant sensory, bowel, or bladder abnormalities. Although easy to recognize in approximately 80 percent of cases, ALS remains a diagnosis of exclusion. This requires the exclusion of disorders that may mimic it, such as cervical and lumbar spondylotic myeloradiculopathy, multifocal motor neuropathy with conduction block and antiganglioside antibodies, plasma cell dyscrasias, lead intoxication, adult hexosaminidase deficiency, hyperthyroidism, hyperparathyroidism, polymyositis, chronic inflammatory demyelinating polyneuropathy, and other primarily motor neuromuscular diseases. A few patients with ALS present with breathing difficulty from diaphragmatic paralysis as their first symptom. This is an important differential diagnostic point because few neuromuscular diseases present with predominant respiratory weakness. These include myasthenia gravis, polymyositis, adult acid maltase deficiency, amyloid myopathy, and ALS. Rarely are unusual presentations of multiple sclerosis or Parkinson's disease misdiagnosed as ALS.

THERAPEUTIC APPROACHES TO FOUR COMMON PROBLEM AREAS IN ALS

Weakness

The rule in treating weakness associated with ALS is that autonomy equals therapy. Weakness is only functionally important insofar as it prevents a particular activity. This is the premise of the occupational therapist who inquires about activities of daily living. One will never know that the patient needs a prescription for a raised toilet seat until the patient is asked whether he or she can rise from it and about his or her feelings of helplessness. One will never know that the patient needs a card-holding device until he or she is asked about hobbies and it is discovered that the patient's whole social life circles around the game of bridge. One will never know that the patient needs a wrist splint until it is learned that he can no longer shave by himself and that this depresses him. These basic but essential problems are not likely to be addressed in the course of a half-hour return visit to the hurried but compulsive neurologist who is busy documenting semeiologically how the patient's muscles have worsened since the last visit. The number of devices that can aid patients suffering from symptomatic weakness are as legion as the number of activities that can be impaired in this disease. The breadth of the problem and what we and our patients have found to be the most helpful solutions are shown in Tables 1 and 2. However, a picture is worth a thousand words. It is a good idea to lend your patient a catalogue of self help

TABLE 1 Most Useful Adaptive Aids for Weakness in ALS

Personal Hygiene
- Long-handled sponge
- Wash mitt
- Soap on a rope
- Lightweight built-up handles for toothbrush, comb, razor, nail file
- Electric toothbrush with suction brush device
- Electric razor
- Hand-held shower head
- Raised toilet seat

Dressing
- Button hook
- Zipper ring, hook, loop
- Dressing stick
- Long-handled shoehorn
- Velcro clothing closures
- Suspenders

Positioning
- Ankle-foot orthosis (AFO)
- Cock-up wrist splint
- Transfer board
- Foam wedge cushion (bed)
- Cervical collars: open Kydex frame collar with Plastozote padding; Philadelphia collar; soft collar
- Head strap
- Cervical pillow

Feeding
- Mobile arm support, ball-bearing feeder
- Non-skid foam (DYCEM)
- Plate guard
- Rocker knife
- Lightweight built-up silverware (tubular foam)
- Lightweight mugs with easy grip handles

Meal Preparation
- Long-lever jar opener with adaptive turning knob
- Lap tray (bean bag; bed tray/table)
- Lightweight built-up handles for cooking utensils, pots
- Adapted paring board
- Twist off bottle opener
- Milk carton holder

Other
- Lamp extension switch
- Triangular pencil grip
- Book holder
- Card holder
- Page turner (hand-held, mouth-held)
- Rubber thimble
- Speaker phone with automatic dialing
- Operator headset
- Lightweight reachers
- Adapted built-up key holder
- Doorknob extension lever
- Self-opening scissors
- Antiembolism stockings (Ted)

TABLE 2 Durable Medical Equipment

- Four-prong cane
- Forearm crutches
- Upright rolling walker (adapt with forearm supports, vertical grip handles, and basket)
- Manual wheelchair—measured and fitted by physical therapist (best choice is lightweight, portable, with removable armrests and swing-away removable leg supports; add high-density foam cushion and sheepskin)
- High-back recliner electric wheelchair—measured and fitted by physical therapist (should be adapted with changeable control switch—i.e., joystick, suck/blow controls—and with space under seat for respirator or computer as weakness progresses; should have removable armrests, swing-away removable leg supports, and cushion and sheepskin as above)
- Portable suction machine, with Yankar oral/tonsil adaptor
- Fracture bedpan/urinal
- Hand rails/safety bars for tub or shower and toilet
- Hospital bed (electric preferred; with high-density eggcrate mattress and sheepskin)
- Overbed table with tilting top
- Mechanical patient lift (portable preferred) with full body sling (e.g., Hoyer)
- Drop-arm bedside commode
- Accessible shower stall with rolling shower/commode chair (or tub chair)
- Electric reclining seat-lift chair
- Outdoor ramps
- Stairway glide
- Van adapted with electric hydrolic lift for wheelchair passenger

aids (such as that by Sammons) to thumb through at home, and to keep a copy as an office reference. The issue of excercise is discussed separately later in this chapter.

Swallowing

Conservative measures and helpful eating strategies (Table 3) go a long way towards improving swallowing and preventing aspiration. When swallowing is first jeopardized and aspiration is a risk, patients and their families should be trained in the Heimlich maneuver and cardiopulmonary resuscitation. They should obtain a portable suction machine to help clear secretions and retrieve from the posterior larynx boluses that cannot be expectorated and which jeopardize the airway. With the conservative measures outlined, many patients are surprisingly able to eat (though with great caution) despite severe corticobulbar dysfunction and severe impairment as measured by cine-esophagogram.

When the patient's intake of food provides inadequate nutrition, some form of tube feeding must be considered in consultation with a trained nutritionist. Patients may mistakenly think about feeding tubes in the same category as all tubes, including an endotracheal tube, as if it were a "heroic" measure.

TABLE 3 Swallowing: Helpful Strategies

Position	Sit upright at a 45- to 90-degree angle (high-Fowlers), with head bent slightly forward.
Attention	Concentrate on swallowing; avoid communication and other distractions at mealtime and eat in a comfortable, unhurried setting.
Adjustment of taste, texture, and temperature	Avoid excessively sweet or sour foods as they increase saliva production; avoid bitter and salty foods as they increase thirst.
	Use soft, cooked, moist foods and gelled, pureed, strained foods; add sauces.
	Avoid extremes of temperature.
Common sense	Have frequent, small feedings—six per day.
	Cut foods into small bite-size pieces.
	If adjustment of food texture limits nutrition, use high-calorie, high-protein supplements.
	Patient and family should be instructed in Heimlich maneuver.

This can be demystified by demonstrating the devices or referring the patient to another patient using the device. There are many options. Simple nasogastric tubes are often the easiest solution. Keough tubes have the advantage of smaller size and greater flexibility and comfort, but with chronic use they frequently become occluded. The most easily tolerated surgical procedure seems to be feeding gastrostomy, rather than cervical esophagostomy or feeding pharyngotomy with cricopharyngeal myotomy. One should emphasize the current best option, which is endoscopically guided gastrostomy performed with the patient under local anesthesia.

Sialorrhea is a difficult and humiliating problem. The problem with all treatments for drooling is that an excessively dry mouth may in fact make swallowing *more* difficult. We have only occasionally found permanent procedures such as parotid gland irradiation or tympanic neurectomy helpful. Unfortunately, such procedures may make residual saliva tenacious and difficult to expectorate or even inspissated—a cure worse than the original symptom. Most patients end up using a suction apparatus or a cloth in the mouth as the most practical solution. Over-the-counter antihistamines may be tried. Amitriptyline has the advantage of being a very potent anticholinergic agent for sialorrhea, as well as an antidepressant and hypnotic agent (although the drug is not indicated for sole use as a hypnotic over the long-term). There are, of course, many atropinic agents, but the most convenient is the scopolamine patch. Its convenience is its relatively constant therapeutic effect without the patient's needing to swallow anything, but its chief disadvantage, as with all atropinic agents, is potentiation of glaucoma, urinary retention, or adverse central nervous system (CNS) effects. The chief advantage of glycopyrrolate, a quaternary anticholinergic agent, is that it does not cross the blood-brain barrier.

Communication

Rarely is the low volume of the voice the only problem, so that amplification devices are rarely or briefly usable. For some patients with limited use of certain fingers, portable hand-held print-out devices such as the Canon Communicator are quick ways to produce a written output. For those with few recognizable spoken words and weakness of the hands there are still numerous strategies for communication (Table 4). Speed is the most frustrating aspect. ETRAN display boards are an old standard. Letters, phrases, or words can be indicated using eye movements or pointing. The pointer can be as simple as a soda straw held in the mouth if lip muscles or neck muscles are strong enough. A clear Lucite communication board is an ideal way to improve eye contact between the "speaker" and interpreter. Simple eye-blink (yes/no) strategies cost nothing and rely on the inventiveness of the patient and family in developing the quickest strategies for scanning the alphabet or developing codes. The disadvantages of such systems are that they become idiosyncratic and do not transfer to friends or multiple therapists. Personal computers have the potential for speed and permanent printout. Input can be linked to any residual movement (eyebrow, finger flicker, eye movement) via microswitch. Many kinds of software exist, and a popular one in our clinic is Words Plus. The more complex the algorithm of the software, such as the ability to predict the next letter or word from known common spelling patterns or rules of grammar and rhetoric, the more

TABLE 4 Communication Aids

Note pad
Magic slate
Call device (dinner bell, clicker, intercom system, Speak and Spell)
Letterboards (ETRAN, letter cuff [alphabet list worn on forearm])
Electric typewriter
Hand-held computers with print-out device (Canon Communicator)
Personal computer (desk top)
Computer augmentation devices
Specific software capabilities adapted to patient needs such as Words Plus
Voice synthesizer
Switches adaptable to head movement, eye blink, or suck/blow

speedy the output. Inefficiency and slowness of certain scanning programs make patients put their computers back in boxes and revert to simpler eye-blink and alphabet board strategies. An advantage of computers is the fact that the output can be linked to a speech synthesizer to add a human speech quality to communication, to printers to allow for correspondence, and to modems to allow telephone interaction. An important new national volunteer agency, Volunteers for Medical Engineering, is able to help provide and train handicapped patients with such devices. One should not forget that the old-fashioned pencil and note pad or the 29-cent magic slate are communication tools far superior to all the other "high tech" devices if the patient can use his or her hands.

Some speaking habits that caregivers develop are particularly irritating to ALS patients. These include speaking to family members rather than directly to the patient, speaking without eye-to-eye contact with the patient, standing far above the patient when addressing him or her, speaking loudly as if the patient were deaf, pretending to understand speech that is not understandable, completing patient's sentences and thoughts, or speaking in a manner or tone of voice as if one were speaking to a child.

Breathing

Respiratory impairment is the most serious sign in ALS. To the physician, the patient, and the family members it may appear to represent the beginning of the end. Pneumonia or aspiration, as secondary complications of severely weakened respiratory and bulbar muscles, are the usual causes of death.

Assessment

The two most important measurements for assessing neuromuscular respiratory impairment are vital capacity (VC) and negative inspiratory force (NIF). VC is the single-most important measurement, since it can be easily measured by spirometry (a hand-held Wright's spirometer is convenient). As a global indicator of lung function, VC should direct the physician's care in dealing with impending respiratory insufficiency. NIF begins to decline into a useful measurable range when the VC falls below 1.5 L or half of the patient's predicted baseline. It is a useful indicator of respiratory *muscle* status (with contributions from intercostals, diaphragm, and accessory muscles of respiration), exclusive of parenchymal lung disease. Arterial blood gas evaluations are rarely useful, since serious changes are only late indicators of respiratory muscle failure in ALS. PaO_2 levels remain well preserved until late in the course of the disease. CO_2 retention to levels greater than 45 mm Hg is a poor prognostic sign, common in patients presenting with severe respiratory failure (Fig. 1).

Symptomatic Care

Treatment should be directed toward maintaining and improving the patient's ventilation by instruction of family members in chest physiotherapy, nasopharyngeal suctioning, assistive cough techniques (Heimlich maneuver used synchronously with the patient's cough attempt), and use of intermittent positive pressure breathing (IPPB). Episodes of acute respiratory difficulty should not be automatically attributed to the progression of ALS but be properly diagnosed by examination of sputum, temperature, respiratory rate and effort, and by chest x-ray examination. Acute upper respiratory infection, aspiration, or dehydration should be treated early with intravenous fluids and/or antibiotics, as they further compromise an already poor respiratory status. Bronchodilators, such as metaproterenol sulfate or albuterol (preferably administered by a nebulizer), may be given if indicated by bronchospasm associated with mucus plugging. Long-acting theophylline compounds are used as well because of their putative direct effects on muscle to relieve respiratory muscle fatigue. Adequate hydration and nutrition to liquify secretions and maintain strength should be emphasized.

Mechanical Ventilation

The issue of mechanical ventilation should be openly and supportively discussed with the patient and the patient's family as soon as the involvement of respiratory muscle is observed. While symptomatic treatments may alleviate the initial symptoms, the underlying problem of respiratory muscle fatigue and eventual paralysis will not be solved until the decision regarding the use or refusal of mechanical ventilation is made. Although this decision is difficult, most patients and family members have difficulty grasping the consequences of their choices and are grateful to the physician for the opportunity to discuss them. There is no simple way to direct such a discussion other than to adopt an unhurried, honest approach. Discussion of a living will may be a catalyst in this conversation. The living will outlines in writing one's decision whether or not to use mechanical ventilation to sustain life. Many states have adopted the living will as a legal right; however, the patient should investigate if it is legal in his or her state. These documents can be obtained easily through a lawyer or directly from the Society for the Right to Die. The patient should understand that the decision does not have to be made immediately and is revocable.

The optimal family situation for home ventilator

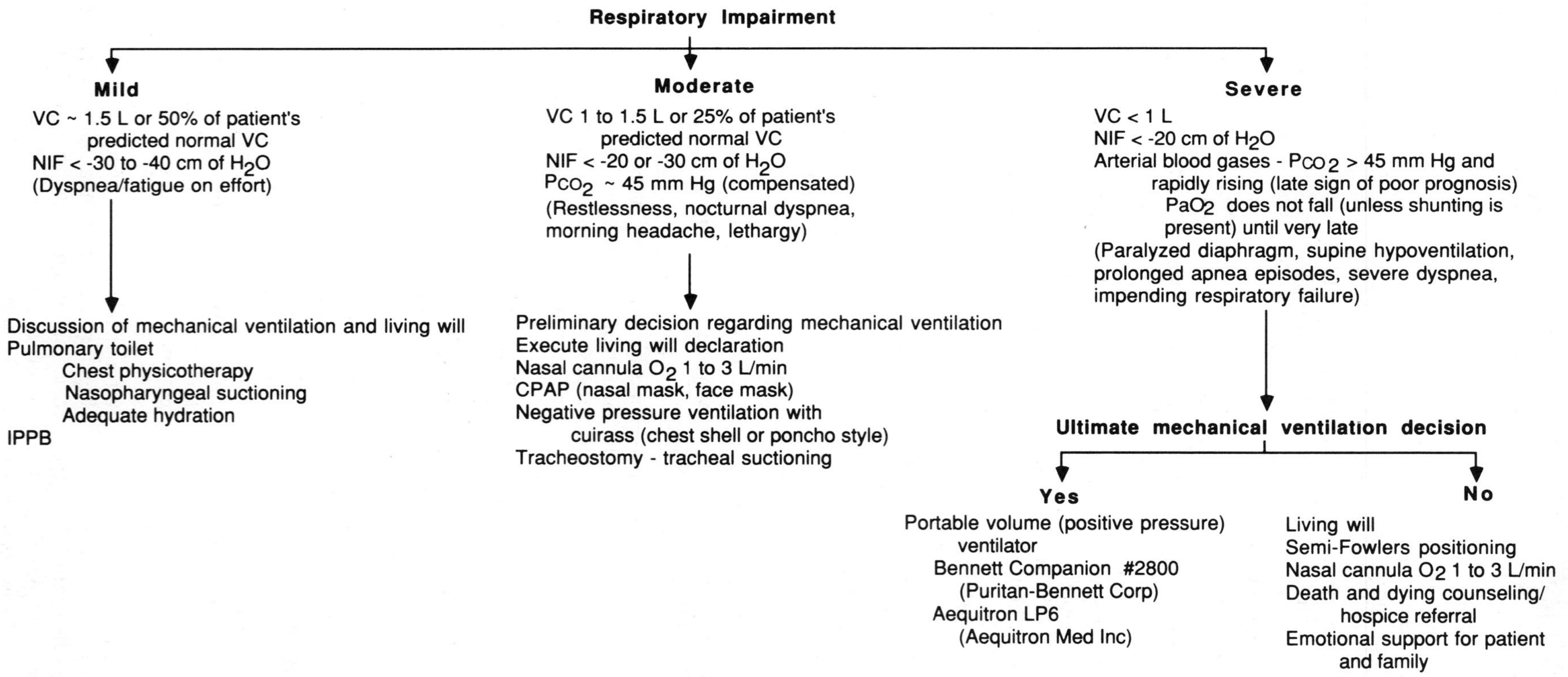

Figure 1 Treatment of respiratory impairment. The severity of respiratory impairment is determined by symptoms, signs, and the key measurements of vital capacity and negative inspiratory force, as listed across the top of the figure. Suggested treatment options follow below for each phase of severity.

VC = vital capacity; NIF = negative inspiratory force; IPPB = intermittent positive pressure breathing; ABG = arterial blood gas; CPAP = continuous positive airway pressure.

use requires many resources. Close proximity to an acute care hospital, supportive care by a dedicated nurse and physician, a home health agency, insurance coverage, financial support for that family member who will become the primary caretaker, respite care, emotional support for the patient and family members, and equipment and necessary electrical adaptations of the home are a few of the tangible and intangible resources necessary to improve the transition to total ventilator support. Most insurance companies assist financially with the cost of nursing care and respiratory therapy to allow the patient to remain in the home. Some agencies such as Muscular Dystrophy Association assist in the purchase of electric wheelchairs that, when modified, can include space for a portable ventilator to allow the patient mobility. After some initial adjustment, many patients can be weaned from the ventilator for several hours during the day. Travel to areas of interest is made possible by a wheelchair-accessible van equipped with a hydraulic lift. While the picture is not entirely rosy, it is not the same picture that one may envision of the patient attached to a large, noisy respirator in a socially isolated hospital ward. The patient can live a life of quality, albeit increasingly vicarious, if the appropriate support is available.

Tracheostomy by itself is an option for the patient whose problem with aspiration of food or secretions predominates over respiratory impairment. This procedure can be performed relatively easily and can increase comfort when the airway is jeopardized by aspiration. After a period of time, the patient can have a talking tracheostomy tube inserted, or in some cases, may be able to speak simply by deflating the tracheostomy cuff.

For the patient with moderate to severe respiratory difficulty who decides against using mechanical ventilation, other supportive measures can still be used (see Fig. 1). Negative pressure ventilation, although only a short-term solution, is possible with cuirass devices (chest shell or poncho style) that use a cage through which a vacuum motor provides negative pressure to the chest wall, thus enabling the patient's chest to rise and fall. Continuous positive airway pressure (CPAP) administered by a nasal mask or face mask, as recently used in the treatment of sleep apnea, can be successfully used in the ALS patient as well. In patients with otherwise marginal respiration, ventilation can be maintained for long periods, using CPAP at night and a continuous IPPB apparatus during the day to force otherwise atelectatic airways open. Low-flow oxygen (1 to 3 L per minute via nasal cannula) can be used, particularly at night to combat the typical supine hypoventilation that causes eventual hypoxia. Patients should sleep in a semi-Fowler's position (30 to 45 degrees) to aid in ventilation.

Sleeplessness and Breathing

In the context of respiratory insufficiency, sleeplessness may become a more significant problem. It can easily be treated with low-dose triazolam or flurazepam hydrochloride, but these should be used for a short time intermittently. Anxiety symptoms may be helped by these or other benzodiazepine derivatives when administered in low doses. If cough is the problem, short-term codeine also promotes rest. Alcohol or over-the-counter antihistamines should not be used routinely as hypnotics, since they are less effective, are prone to suppress rapid eye movement (REM) sleep, and cause adverse side effects when taken in overdose. In the moribund patient, administration of morphine—with the full knowledge of the potential for further respiratory suppression that exists with the use of all anxiolytics and hypnotics—allows patients partial mental detachment from their situation. However, at this stage of the disease, the majority of patients may be already naturally sedated or lethargic from CO_2 narcosis, and usually die quietly in their sleep. Referral to a local hospice agency long before this may provide much needed support for the patient and family members. The professional counseling and physical and emotional support that this multidisciplinary team can provide are invaluable resources for patients at this stage of ALS.

Any ALS patient has the right to change the decision regarding mechanical ventilation at any time. Whatever decision the patient makes, the physician should seek to understand it from the patient's perspective. In fact, the physician needs to become the student of the patient. Openness, flexibility, and most of all *caring* are essential in treating all aspects of this disease, but especially when treating the respiratory insufficiency that eventually progresses to respiratory failure.

QUESTIONS ALS PATIENTS ASK

"What Do I Have?"

The answer to this question should be simply "ALS." It is now the name that the lay public knows and uses in North America. A more generic and unfamiliar (e.g., British) term like "motor neuron disease" is often used as a form of medical obfuscation. Such a term should be reserved for truly atypical cases that fail to meet the criteria for the diagnosis of ALS. If a more specific form of motor neuron disease can be diagnosed, the specific correct term (e.g., progressive bulbar palsy, spinal muscular atrophy, primary lateral sclerosis, multifocal motor neuropathy) should be used and explained to the patient. To prevent common confusion, explicitly distinguish ALS from Alzheimer's disease (the other "A" disease), multiple sclerosis (the other "sclerosis"), and muscular dystrophy.

One should be honest when discussing the diagnosis and then let the patient limit the discussion during the first visit. One should allow an unhurried hour for this discussion. In explaining the meaning of ALS, avoid the impulse to say, "That's what Lou Gehrig had." Everyone is familiar with the picture of a stooped, tearful Lou Gehrig in his uniform. It evokes a sense of hopelessness, early retirement, and early death. Nowadays it is much more helpful to say something like "it's what Senator Jacob Javits had," since this evokes a sense of hopefulness, visibility, acceptance, and continued productivity.

"How Long Do I Have to Live?"

The wrong answer is "God only knows when *any* of us will die. We could be hit on the highway tomorrow by a truck. The average patient dies in 3 years." To someone who is assured of his death, it is not comforting to be told that they may be hit by a truck as well, and such a comment immediately conveys to the patient that the doctor does not really understand the dilemma. Further, quoting a specific time of survival is always wrong, since the patient can only assume that he is like the "average patient" spoken of. A much better answer evokes hope: "Half of the patients who come to us are alive 3 years after the onset of the disease, and many live for a much longer time—even for as long as 10 years or more." One may convincingly add at that point, "And all along the way there will be many treatments we can offer you for every problem that might arise." Such hopefulness is quite a different message to receive than the more typical 3-year "death sentence" that many patients end up hearing.

"Should I Exercise?"

One should resist the urge to answer in a scholarly way, "There is really no research on it, but if you do exercise, don't do too much—don't exert yourself to the point of fatigue." We see a surprising number of patients with ALS who have been forbidden by their physicians to exercise, even warned to quit active exercise programs to which they were previously accustomed, out ot some unspoken fear of the harmfulness of fatigue or an unfounded idea about motor units wearing out. Telling a patient to exercise but not to exert himself to the point of fatigue is like telling a child to have fun swimming but not to go near the water. ALS is in fact marked by reinnervation of muscle, as evidenced by electromyography and muscle biopsy. One should capitalize on this. Motor units *need* usage in order to prevent atrophy of innervated muscle fibers. Movement of joints is essential to prevent both disuse and contracture. The simplest of all reasons to prescribe exercise is that exercise *feels* good. It can produce a sense of euphoria and encourages hopefulness. Of course, there are no new converts to exercise; a sedentary person unaccustomed to exercising is unlikely to take up the challenge of a new way of coping with the diagnosis of ALS. Passive stretching exercises should certainly be encouraged. This is particularly important for families to learn in order to prevent contracture of shoulder joints, which, aside from being painful, can make such simple activities as dressing difficult.

When active exercise programs are undertaken, they should be designed and supervised by a physiotherapist or physiatrist who specializes in exercise evaluation and prescription. One common formula for a resistance exercise program begins by determining for the target muscle what the maximum resistance is for ten repetitions of an exercise. Prescribed exercise then consists of a series of graded efforts as follows: five to ten repetitions each at 50 percent maximum resistance, at 75 percent, and then 100 percent, with each cycle interspersed with 2 minutes of rest. Such programs, targeted at particular muscles that are functionally important for the individual patient, can be combined with cardiac fitness exercise programs using swimming, stationary bicycling, or other sustained activity, depending on the abilities of the patient at that stage of his illness. Overexertion can be prevented by using some fairly liberal rules of thumb, so that the level of exercise is reduced if any of the following occur: (1) tachycardia greater than two times the baseline heart rate, (2) persistent tachycardia of greater than 10 beats per minute over baseline heart rate at 10 minutes after exercise has ceased, (3) dyspnea for more than "a few" minutes, (4) angina, or (5) excessive pain and fatigue on the day *after* exercise.

"What Do I Do Now?"

Resources

In response to this question, the first advice one should give is to contact the Muscular Dystrophy Association, which is the single largest provider of money for research and patient services for this disease in the world. It is surprising how few patients are referred early to the Muscular Dystrophy Association or to the ALS Association (a fund-raising and educationally oriented association). Given the gravity of the diagnosis, the second piece of advice should be to obtain a responsible second opinion. One should then suggest that the entire family join a support group for ALS patients and families. Such support groups are now offered by every major clinic supported by the Muscular Dystrophy Association or the ALS Association. Support groups offer a place to vent anger and frustration, share common solutions to vexing problems (such as coping with insurance companies or determining which of the many available orthopedic and occupational aids are truly useful), deal with the sense of abandonment by physicians or friends or family, discuss the problem of respite care, and provide a forum where psychological needs can be heeded to carry patients and their families through phases of depression. In addition, probably the most important function such groups serve is that of creating a network that provides the most practical education about the disease and which provides friends with an understanding of what it feels like to have ALS.

Clinical Trials

The final prescription may be to encourage patients to participate in valid clinical research. One should strongly resist the urge to provide placebo therapy in the hope that it "might help keep the disease from progressing." The extensive menu of such placebos (from bee pollen to pancreatic enzymes) changes with time, but they are always used with the misguided rationale that "at least they won't do any harm." Expensive quack treatments like snake venom and transfer factor injections have been truly harmful by virtue of their expense alone. Placebo responses last from weeks to months. Their eventual failure leads to withdrawal of patients from health professionals and to hopelessness; they do not encourage attendance at clinic, nor do they provide the psychological support often intended. Rather, regular visits to a specialized multidisciplinary clinic that offers the services of social worker, patient service coordinator, nurse clinician, physician, occupational therapist, orthopedist, physiotherapist, speech therapist, and dietician offer infinitely better therapy and psychological support than all the prescribed cures of Ivan Ilyich's doctor.

A valid, controlled clinical trial is a real expression of hope. More than half of patients with ALS will want to participate in a clinical trial at least once. The physician's work is to be an advocate and to help the patient evaluate the validity of a particular trial. Quackery abounds with this disease as much as it does with cancer. Besides advocating participation in valid research, the physician needs to be a resource to help patients screen out quackery. The following can be offered to ALS families as obvious "red-flags" that should evoke their strong caution: (1) treatments that are good for many seemingly unrelated diseases, (2) treatments for which no formal protocol can be produced, (3) a rationale or an experimental trial that is neither written nor explainable to the referring physician, (4) the absence of controls, (5) supporting literature that relies on testimonials, (6) nonsponsored research that has not undergone some form of peer review, (7) high costs that are *all* borne by the patient. Any of these should evoke caution, but the presence of several should be indicative of quackery.

Current clinical research available to participants with ALS in the United States include trials of immunomodulators such as cyclophosphamide and neurotransmitter or neuropeptide modulators such as thyrotropin-releasing hormone, branched-chain amino acids, and N-methyl-d-aspartate receptor antagonists.

FINAL SUGGESTIONS

1. When you make the diagnosis of ALS, plan two sessions: first to give conclusions, and secondly to lay out your plans.
2. Know and connect the patient with essential public resources such as the Muscular Dystrophy Association.
3. Do not discuss all possible outcomes and available devices at an early stage. This only leads to information overload and feelings of helplessness.
4. Prescribe exercise. It is invigorating and encourages hopefulness. It prevents the development of frozen joints and subsequent pain, capitalizes on the potential for reinnervation of muscle, and is not harmful if certain rules of thumb regarding limits are followed.
5. Be knowledgeable about aids for activities of daily living; buy a Sammons catalogue or its equivalent. Read it and discuss it with a knowledgeable occupational therapist. Question patients on their needs and abilities, and when particular needs arise, have them try occupational aids. Use occupational therapists, nurse clinicians, or other professionals *experienced* and *interested* in ALS.
6. Start a support group for ALS patients and their families. Use other patients with ALS as a resource. You will learn everything that will be useful to you in treating these patients from the patients and families themselves.
7. Encourage the patient to participate in valid research. This fulfills altruistic motives and is morally rewarding for the patient to do at least once. It is an activity that inspires hopefulness. Become an active advocate to help patients screen various research opportunities.

ACKNOWLEDGMENTS

Acknowledgments. We gratefully acknowledge the dedicated assistance of Blair Ertel. Our ALS research and patient care have been generously supported by the Jay Slotkin Fund for Neuromuscular Research, the Baltimore Relief Foundation, and the Muscular Dystrophy Association. We are indebted to our colleagues in the Neuromuscular Division, and most of all to the many members of the Baltimore ALS Support Group and our ALS patients whose courage, patience, and guidance contributed greatly to the contents of this chapter.

SUGGESTED READING

Caroscio JT, ed. ALS: a guide to patient care. New York: Thieme, 1986.
Brooks BR, ed. Amyotrophic lateral sclerosis. Neurol Clin 1987; 5(1):1–195, 5(2):197–290.

PATIENT RESOURCES

Associations

The Muscular Dystrophy Association is a nonprofit national organization (information and referral agency) whose main focus is to provide funds for medical care, equipment, education, support groups, research, coordination, and financing of clinics for many neuromuscular diseases including ALS.

Muscular Dystrophy Association
810 Seventh Avenue
New York, New York 10019
Telephone: (212) 586–0808

The Amyotrophic Lateral Sclerosis Association is a nonprofit national organization (information and referral agency) whose main focus is to provide funds for education and research, and to sponsor chapter groups for patients with ALS.

Amyotrophic Lateral Sclerosis Association
21021 Ventura Boulevard Suite 321
Woodland Hills, California 91364
Telephone: (800) 782–4747

The Volunteers for Medical Engineering is a nonprofit national organization of engineers who donate equipment, time, and ingenuity to solving specific problems of the disabled.

Volunteers for Medical Engineering
The Good Samaritan Hospital
5601 Loch Raven Boulevard, 3 East 329
Baltimore, Maryland 21239
Telephone: (301) 532–4360

The Society for the Right to Die provides literature and documents related to living wills.

Society for the Right to Die
250 West 57th Street
New York, New York 10107
Telephone: (212) 246–6973

Literature

Appel V, Callender M, Sunter S. ALS: maintaining mobility—a guide to physical therapy and occupational therapy. MDA, Houston, Texas, 1988.
ALS Association: Five Manual Series. Manual I: Finding Help; Manual II: Muscular Weakness; Manual III: Swallowing Difficulty; Manual IV: Breathing Difficulty; Manual V: Communication Difficulty. Woodland Hills, California: ALS Association, 1986.
Fred Sammons Catalogue. 145 Tower Drive, Dept. #423, Burr Ridge, Illinois 60521-9842. Telephone: (312) 325-1700.
Sears & Roebuck Co. Catalogue.

MYASTHENIA GRAVIS

KLAUS V. TOYKA, M.D.

Myasthenia gravis (MG) is an autoimmune disease of the neuromuscular junction that is caused by an antibody-mediated immune attack against nicotinic acetylcholine receptors (AChR). The formation of autoantibodies may be caused indirectly by hyperactive T-helper lymphocytes or by reduced activity of suppressor cells. The exact mechanism of the disordered immunoregulation is incompletely understood. It has been speculated that the thymus may be a site at which the pivotal break in self-tolerance occurs.

The immunologic diagnostic tests and immunosuppressive treatment of MG are based on these immunopathologic concepts.

EVALUATION OF PATIENTS WITH MG

The diagnosis of MG is based on the typical clinical presentation, which includes muscle weakness of ocular, bulbar, truncal, and limb muscles. Muscle fatigue on exertion is usually present. If MG is suspected, pharmacologic testing with a cholinesterase (ChE) inhibitor such as edrophonium chloride (Tensilon) will show marked improvement of muscle strength in a typical patient. Equivocal test results may be seen in some patients with otherwise typical MG. In these patients, the diagnosis must be supported by antibody measurements.

The most sensitive and specific test for MG is the demonstration of circulating autoantibodies to AChR in the serum. Elevated titers can now be shown in several laboratories in more than 95 percent of patients with generalized MG. This applies to the modified double immunoprecipitation assay originally described by Lindstrom, which uses crude human muscle AChR. Other tests using nonhuman

AChR or enzyme-linked immunosorbent assay (ELISA) methods are less sensitive, and the titers may differ substantially. The test should be ordered in every patient with unexplained weakness or fatigue. A minority of patients with otherwise typical myasthenia may have titers in the normal range. In some laboratories, additional test methods are available for these patients. Absolute antibody titers do not correlate with severity of MG. In most patients, serial titers correlate with weakness in the individual.

Traditionally neurologists confirm the diagnosis by electrophysiologic testing. On repetitive stimulation of motor nerves, a typical fatigue reaction (decrement) can be recorded from proximal muscles in 70 percent of patients with generalized weakness. Single-fiber electromyography is more sensitive but is not specific for MG; it can be performed only by experienced examiners. In my opinion, it should be reserved for the "difficult patient," such as those with ocular myasthenia and antibody-negative cases.

Every patient is checked for thymic abnormalities by chest computed tomography (CT) or magnetic resonance imaging (MRI). In my patients with thymic hyperplasia, I have seen the enlargement on either scan in roughly 50 percent of patients preoperatively. With thymomas, the rate of discovery is usually higher but depends on the tumor size and type of malignancy.

MG may be associated with other autoimmune disorders that may have passed undiagnosed. A laboratory screen for other circulating autoantibodies, thyroid hormones, and diabetes mellitus should be done. Tuberculosis should be formally excluded if immunosuppressive treatment is planned.

MONITORING DISEASE ACTIVITY

Patients with MG should be seen at regular intervals, ranging from every 2 weeks in the more severely affected patient after the initiation of immunosuppressive treatment to every year in stable patients. I follow Drachman's suggestion of asking the patient to keep a diary in which one or two prominent clinical symptoms are recorded. Whenever possible, this self-testing should include a quantitative measurement such as a record of the length of time that the head can be lifted in the supine position and the length of time that the arms can be outstretched while standing.

Repeated tests for autoantibodies to AChR are needed only in patients with unexplained deterioration—in particular, when immunosuppressive drugs have been discontinued or the dose has been reduced. In my experience, rising antibody titers in immunosuppressed patients mean that the patient's condition may deteriorate after a lag phase of as long as 3 months.

TREATMENT MODALITIES

Most experts agree that patients with severe generalized myasthenia gravis should be treated vigorously with immunosuppressive drugs in combination with ChE inhibitors, and with plasmapheresis during critical deteriorations. Neither of these treatments has been studied by a prospective, double-blind, placebo-controlled trial, with the exception of cyclosporin A. The treatment of ocular MG and of the mildly or moderately affected patient is controversial. An important consideration is how much the physician and the patient expect from the treatment. In my experience, it has been possible in virtually every newly diagnosed patient to induce remission or near-remission. The only common exception is the elderly myasthenic patient with other severe disorders such as coronary artery disease, kidney failure, obstructive lung disease, strokes, and other life-threatening conditions; in these patients, treatment may improve myasthenic signs but may not result in general improvement.

I always discuss the possible outcome and the risks of treatment in great detail with the patient. Some patients prefer to have mild residual symptoms rather than to risk developing adverse reactions from immunosuppressive drugs. Most patients wish to be free of disease and to live a normal life, even if this requires having to take drugs for long periods.

Cholinesterase Inhibitors

Pharmacologic ChE inhibitors are the first-line treatment for almost all patients with symptomatic MG (Fig. 1). They enhance neuromuscular transmission by increasing effective transmitter concentrations and thus prolong the ligand (ACh)-receptor interaction. The compound most often used is pyridostigmine bromide (Mestinon), which is taken orally in 60-mg tablets. The average dose is 60 mg every 4 hours during the daytime. Action starts approximately 30 minutes after ingestion and lasts for about 4 to 6 hours, although the half-life is much longer. This regimen can be adjusted to the patient's needs. The intervals at which the drug is taken can be shortened to every 3 hours. Timing can be adjusted such that one single dose of 60 mg is given 30 to 60 minutes before major meals. A sustained-release tablet containing 180 mg of the drug is available (Mestinon Timespan). One such tablet taken at bedtime may be given to patients with marked weakness in the early morning. The maximum dosage of ChE

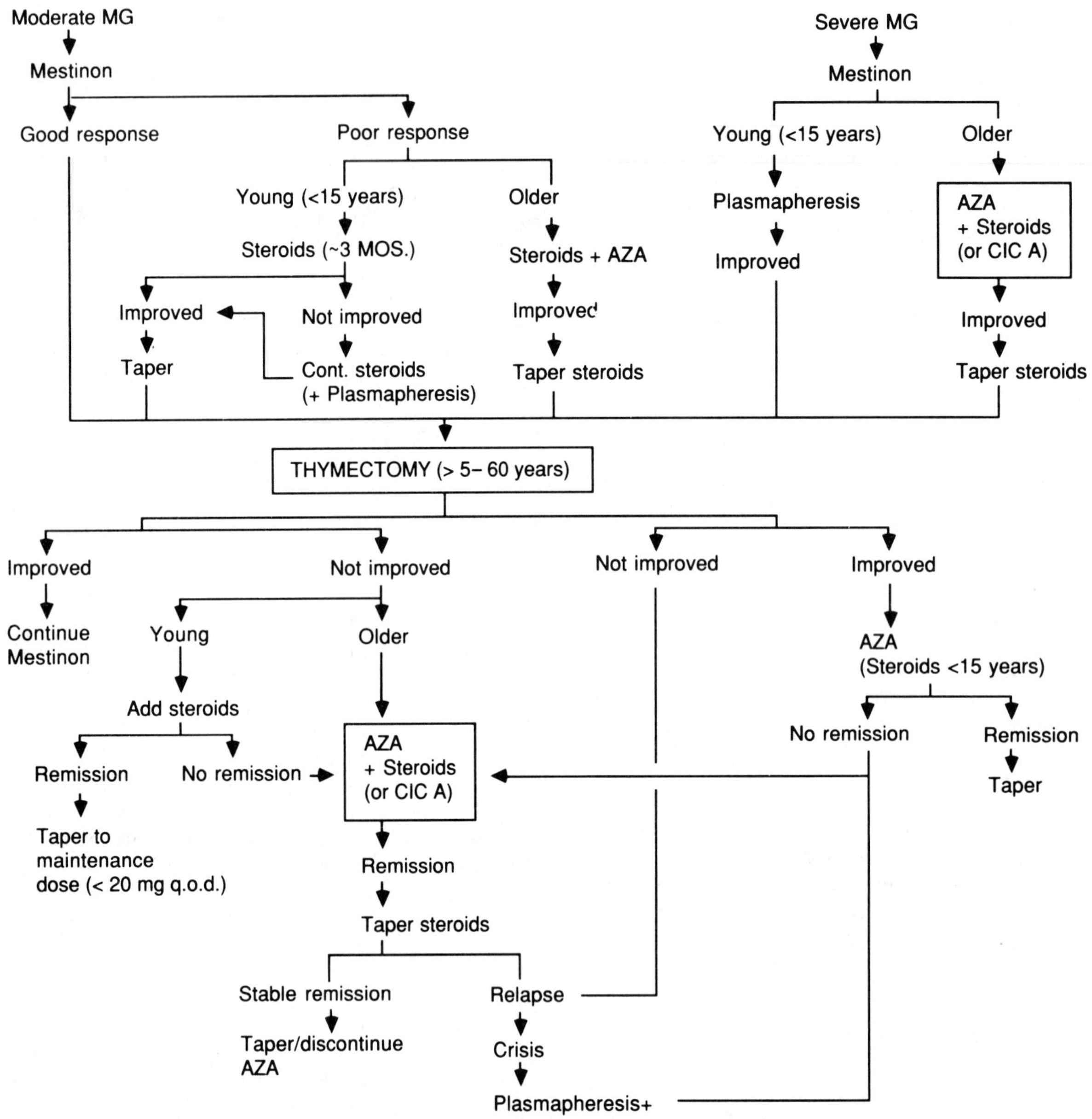

Figure 1 Steps in management of moderate and severe generalized MG. "Remission" includes near-remission; "moderate" includes at least two test items of the clinical MG score grade 2; "severe" incldues at least two test items or one vital sign (e.g., vital capacity) grade 3.

AZA=azathioprine; steroids=glucocorticosteroids; CIC A=cyclosporine.

inhibitors usually should not exceed 90 mg every 3 hours except over the short-term. The need for a steady increase of the dose of ChE inhibitors should alert the physician to the possibility of progressive deterioration.

ChE inhibitors can precipitate asthma. Other side effects are usually limited and reversible. I have rarely seen persistent diarrhea, but when I do, I treat it with atropine (0.2 to 0.5 mg) or by diphenoxylate hydrochloride with atropine (Lomotil) once or twice daily.

When stable remission has been achieved, I recommend that ChE inhibitors be withheld for a day or two. If no symptoms of MG recur, the patient may not need the drug anymore. Patients with double vision or severe ptosis may not respond satisfactorily to any dose of ChE inhibitors.

Thymectomy

Thymectomy is always indicated in patients with thymoma and is sometimes followed by x-irradiation, depending on the tumor type.

Performing thymectomy in patients with thymic

hyperplasia without thymoma is still controversial. In some centers, every patient is treated with thymectomy, and in others, only those with more severe disease who are also treated with immunosuppressive medication undergo this procedure. Even patients with pure ocular myasthenia are treated in this way at one institution. In a large clinical series, thymectomy has been shown to lead to marked improvement in roughly one-third of patients and to moderate improvement in another one-third. There is no controlled trial comparing thymectomy with immunosuppressive medication in terms of efficacy and adverse reactions.

I recommend thymectomy in conjunction with ChE inhibitors for all patients with mild MG who are between the ages of 6 and 60 years. If symptoms of MG persist for more than 3 months after thymectomy or if the patient's condition deteriorates, I discuss the possibility of immunosuppressive medication with the patient. For patients with moderate or marked MG, I recommend thymectomy only after pretreatment. For those younger than 15 years of age, this may be a short series of plasmapheresis. In older patients, I try to induce remission by immunosuppressive drugs first and have them thymectomized after reducing or stopping immunosuppression within the following 6 to 9 months. Plasmapheresis has also been used in older patients. Most experts recommend that thymectomy be performed early in the course of the disease.

The operation should be performed in a center that has experienced thoracic surgeons and a consulting neuromuscular physician available. If patients have been pretreated successfully, postoperative complications are virtually zero, as is mortality. Our patients are observed in an intensive care unit for 24 to 48 hours even though they all breathe spontaneously. Before the operation, patients are switched from oral pyridostigmine to intravenous neostigmine (Prostigmin) given via an infusion pump at 0.15 to 0.3 mg per hour. Sixty mg of pyridostigmine is roughly equivalent to 0.5 to 0.75 mg Prostigmin IV. Oral treatment can be given as soon as the patient is allowed to drink.

Immunosuppression

Before or after thymectomy, immunosuppressive drugs are now generally administered to patients not satisfactorily controlled by ChE inhibitors. In my opinion, the antimetabolite cytotoxic drug azathioprine is the first choice long-term drug for proper control of moderate, marked, and severe MG. To speed up recovery I generally give it in conjunction with corticosteroids for a few months until near-remission is achieved. Steroids are then gradually reduced and administered on alternate-day schedules until a dose of 20 mg or less every other day has been reached. In patients with stable remission or near-remission for more than 6 months, discontinuing the drug or decreasing the dose can be tried (see below). Long-term treatment with immunosuppressive drugs requires continual medical attention by physicians with experience in such treatment. Patients not followed in this way are at risk for developing potentially dangerous adverse reactions unnoted.

Corticosteroids

In patients with generalized moderate to marked MG, corticosteroids are used in conjunction with azathioprine, 60 to 100 mg per day, in a single morning dose. In young patients with mild generalized myasthenia, I occasionally use a short course of steroids alone if thymectomy has not improved myasthenic weakness satisfactorily within 3 months. Corticosteroids in high doses may transiently exacerbate myasthenic signs. Therefore Drachman has suggested slowly increasing doses of prednisone. In my experience, this is now rarely needed in the modern setting of available treatment modalities.

Steroids produce many unpleasant and serious side effects. It has been my experience that patients are reluctant to accept steroids if they know of another treatment. The most important side effects are cataracts, gastrointestinal ulcers, severe hypertension, and unusual bacterial or parasitic infections. Osteoporosis may be a problem in elderly patients even if the duration of high-dose treatment is restricted to a few months. Gastrointestinal discomfort is best dealt with by drinking skim milk during the day. I do not recommend antacids such as Maalox because they may interfere with intestinal absorption of drugs and mineral salts. A prescription of calcium gluconate, vitamin D supplements, and sodium fluoride may help prevent osteoporosis. If a patient has a history of recurrent ulcers or develops an ulcer during this treatment I now use ranitidine (Zantac). In patients with diabetes mellitus, I try to avoid administering corticosteroids and tend to administer cyclosporin A on a short-term basis instead.

Azathioprine

Azathioprine (Imuran, Imurek) is now the drug of first choice for patients with moderate and severe MG, and is used in conjunction with steroids and plasmapheresis for those in myasthenic crisis. In patients with moderate MG, I start with 3 mg per kilogram of body weight per day for several weeks and reduce this to 2.5 mg per kilogram thereafter. In patients with severe MG, one can start with 3.5 to 4 mg per kilogram and taper the dose gradually. A simple way of monitoring is to check total white blood cell (WBC) count, which should decrease to 3,500 to 4,000 per microliter. The lymphocyte count should be between 900 and 1,200 per microliter. If the WBC count is reduced to less than 3,200, the medication should be discontinued for a few days and treatment continued after it returns to more than 3,500. The long-term dose can be adjusted by checking these numbers. In patients receiving azathioprine plus steroids, the WBC count is two to three times as high and the above-mentioned counts can be used only after steroids have been discontinued. Another measure of drug effects is mean corpuscular volume of red cells (MCV), which is usually mildly elevated during long term treatment.

Adverse Reactions

In rare patients (less than 1 percent of my series), an acute idiosyncratic reaction including vomiting, fever, skin reactions, and general malaise has occurred. In this situation, the drug should be discontinued immediately. More commonly, milder gastrointestinal discomfort is reported. Splitting the dose into three divided doses, taking the drug after meals, and reducing the dose temporarily usually resolves these problems. Elevation of liver enzymes up to three times the baseline is also common and is reversible after the dose has been reduced. There is some evidence that long-term medication carries an increased risk of developing malignancies. In contrast to that of organ transplant patients, the risk seems to be very low in patients with MG. One estimated risk figure is four times the incidence compared with that of the general population. Theoretically, patients receiving azathioprine should be prone to serious infection. In my experience, however, this has rarely been a problem. Azathioprine is potentially teratogenic and mutagenic. I advise patients to use contraceptive measures during treatment and at least 6 months after its completion.

Cyclosporin A (Cyclosporine)

Cyclosporin A is the only immunosuppressive drug that has proved useful in a prospective, double-blind, placebo-controlled trial. This compound is more selective than azathioprine. It suppresses the activation and proliferation of T-helper lymphocytes. Cyclosporin A requires less time to act than azathioprine. This compound resembles corticosteroids in this regard. Because of its multiple and in part serious adverse reactions it is a third-choice drug. I use it in patients with marked or severe MG in conjunction with azathioprine when patients cannot take steroids (e.g., those with diabetes mellitus) or if azathioprine has induced idiosyncratic reactions. Whenever possible, cyclosporin A should be discontinued within the first 6 months of treatment. I do not use it in patients with a creatinine level of more than 1.5 mg per 100 ml. The starting dose is 5 mg per kilogram of bodyweight per day. This dose is corrected by measuring the trough level in whole blood or in plasma. Pharmacologic levels depend on the assay used (presently 40 to 60 ng per milliliter in plasma using a monoclonal antibody radioimmunoassay kit; one should check with a local laboratory.).

The major side effect of this drug is nephrotoxicity. This correlates with duration of treatment and with dose. If the creatinine level increases by 50 percent over baseline values or to more than 1.5 mg per 100 ml during treatment, the dose should be reduced or the drug discontinued. A more sensitive indicator is the measurement of creatinine clearance. There are many other adverse reactions, including arterial hypertension, tremor, hirsutism, and hepatic function abnormalities, which are usually reversible after cessation of treatment. The drug must be discontinued when idiosyncratic or allergic reactions develop. The risk of late malignancies is not firmly established. In patients with autoimmune disease, the risk may be similar to that carried by azathioprine.

Plasmapheresis

In therapeutic plasmapheresis, the plasma is separated from blood cells by centrifugation or, more commonly, by plasma filtration. All antibodies and other soluble factors are removed. Plasma is replaced by albumin-electrolyte solutions. Sometimes high-dose immunoglobulin G is added. Its main indication is myasthenic crisis. Less commonly it has been used for severe refractory MG and before an elective operation such as thymectomy is performed. Plasmapheresis should be carried out only in specialized centers because the number of serious adverse reactions is inversely correlated with experience. Most commonly one plasma volume is exchanged four to five times over a period of 6 to 8 days. Alternatively, one and a half plasma volumes can be exchanged three times every other day. There is practically no age limit for this treatment if the patient is in good general health. In my experience, it is only the elderly patient with multiple organ disease who carries a high risk for developing severe complications. Virtually all patients also receive combined immunosuppression with azathioprine and corticosteroids (or cyclosporin A) beginning at the time of plasma exchange. This is done to reduce antibody rebound and to prevent relapses.

A new alternative to plasmapheresis is selective immunoadsorption by tryptophan-linked polyvinylalcohol gels. This procedure is now licensed in Europe. We have treated 15 patients with this new procedure and found its efficacy virtually identical to that of plasmapheresis. No substitution with heterologous protein solutions is required.

Myasthenic Crisis

Myasthenic crisis is a neurologic emergency, with the patient unable to swallow and breathe. Progressive deterioration of muscle strength that cannot be improved with ChE inhibitors can result in rather sudden decompensation. Therefore any patient who is having difficulty breathing or swallowing should be tested for vital capacity and swallowing immediately. If the previous dosage of medication with ChE inhibitors has not exceeded 120 mg every 3 hours, the patient may receive 0.5 mg Prostigmin IV as a bolus injection and be admitted to the hospital immediately. Ventilatory support should be available during transfer. If the vital capacity drops to less than 1.5 L in males and 1.2 L in females, intubation and assisted ventilation should be provided. If the vital capacity cannot be measured accurately, artificial respiration is needed when arterial oxygen decreases to less than 85 mm Hg and arterial carbon dioxide increases to more than 45 mm Hg. In my experience, it is now rare that patients have been treated with excessive overdoses of ChE inhibitors, which is done to cope with myasthenic weakness but which instead accelerates the critical deterioration (this was formerly called cholinergic crisis).

Often viral infections are precipitating factors of rapid deterioration. Secondary bacterial infection is common if swallowing problems lead to aspiration. Early treatment with appropriate broad-spectrum antibiotics is indicated. After the infectious organism has been identified, the antibiotic regimen can be tailored more specifically. I see no restriction for aminoglycoside antibiotics under these circumstances.

Patients with myasthenic crisis receive the same respiratory support as patients with other breathing disorders. At my institution, patients with atelectases are treated invasively by bronchoscopy. Once patients are no longer receiving ventilation, they should not be treated with breathing devices that force them to breathe against a pressure gradient, as this will lead to early fatigue of respiratory muscles.

Specific Treatment of MG

I continue to administer ChE inhibitors (Prostigmin) to patients at pharmacologic doses of 0.2 to 0.4 mg per hour because some muscle groups may still respond satisfactorily. Others have recommended a "drug holiday" during artificial respiration.

Virtually every patient in myasthenic crisis is now treated with plasmapheresis and high-dose corticosteroids (150 to 1,000 mg prednisone or methylprednisolone) for the 1st week. The use of corticosteroids is controversial in patients with bacterial infection or septicemia. I add high-dose immunoglobulin G preparations (7 S globulin, 10 to 15 g per day) and immunoglobulin M (19 S globulin, 5 to 10 g per day) to substitute for losses during plasmapheresis. Immunoglobulin G has been shown to unspecifically downregulate formation of AChR antibodies, presumably by a Fc-mediated negative feedback mechanism. With immunoadsorption, this may not be necessary. A few days later, azathioprine is added to the regimen.

CHILDHOOD MYASTHENIA

Neonatal transitory myasthenia develops in 15 percent of newborns within a few days after birth. All newborn babies have circulating AChR antibodies if the mother has them. They may develop signs of MG regardless of whether the mother is symptomatic. I advise patients to schedule delivery in a specialized center where pediatricians and neurologists have experience with this condition. When a neonate develops sucking difficulties and muscle hypotonicity, Prostigmin is given intravenously (0.02 to 0.06 mg or more). The pharmacologic response supports the diagnosis. Later, oral pyridostigmine (Mestinon) can be given at a dosage of 2 to 10 mg every 4 hours. Weakness gradually wears off over the next weeks.

Childhood Autoimmune MG

In prepubescent patients, ChE inhibitors are the first-line drug and immunosuppressive agents are given with great care. Most physicians recommend thymectomy after the patient is 5 years of age. In myasthenic crisis, plasmapheresis may be performed with preloading albumin and immunoglobulin solutions. After puberty, treatment is essentially that given to adult patients. I recommend azathioprine for older children only in exceptional cases of severe and otherwise refractory MG.

OCULAR MG

This is often a difficult diagnosis to make. Only 50 to 60 percent of patients with clinically definite ocular MG have AChR antibodies. Several clinical signs need to be present to support the diagnosis, including lid twitch, ocular quiver movements, fatigue on sustained tonic deviation, pseudointernuclear ophthalmoplegia, and unequivocal response to ChE inhibitors. In the antibody-negative patients, other orbital or retro-orbital disorders that can masquerade as myasthenia need to be ruled out. In some centers, a low-dose curare test is performed. Single-fiber electromyography may detect subclinical disease in limb muscles. The majority of patients do not respond satisfactorily to treatment with ChE inhibitors. I recommend a short course of corticosteroids, starting with 30 to 50 mg per day until remission has been achieved, and then taper this to the lowest possible maintenance dose. The indication for azathioprine and thymectomy is still controversial.

ADDITIONAL REMARKS

If elective surgery is required, the patient is treated as before thymectomy. In view of the effective treatments now available, myasthenia rarely poses a problem for the anesthesiologist and surgeon. If an emergency operation has to be performed in a patient with still marked or severe signs of MG, succinylcholine or very low doses of curare—like muscle relaxants (less than 10 percent of the regular dose)—can be used if any relaxation is required at all.

I recommend that my patients become members of the National Muscular Dystrophy Association and obtain a medical ID indicating their diagnosis and medication. Several therapeutic agents have a potential for depressing neuromuscular transmission including beta-blockers, aminoglycoside antibiotics, chinidine, procainamide, and other antiarrhythmic compounds, as well as tranquilizers. In properly treated patients with at most mild signs of MG, I have not seen any problems with these drugs. Myasthenic patients are advised to contact our institution or any other specialized center immediately if uncommon problems arise. I do not recommend that patients receiving immunosuppressive drugs take trips to Third World countries because precautions such as live vaccines are contraindicated and a neuromuscular specialist may not be available. For other trips abroad, the patient is provided with name and address of the closest specialized center.

A small subgroup of patients remains that can be called "difficult" for various medical and psychological reasons. These patients often seek advice at many specialized centers. I strongly advise these patients to authorize the physicians to exchange their medical documents and opinions before profound changes in treatment are made, particularly if signs of MG are mild or absent. A similar recommendation applies to patients who have been misdiagnosed as having MG and are receiving treatment for MG.

SUGGESTED READING

Drachman DB, ed. Myasthenia gravis: biology and treatment. Ann NY Acad Sci 1987; 505:1–909.

Heininger K. Toyka KV, Gaczkowski A, et al. Selective removal of pathogenic factors in neurologic disease. Plasma Ther Transfus Technol 1986; 7: 351–357.

Hohlfeld R, Michels M, Heininger K, et al. Azathioprine toxicity during long-term immunosuppression of generalized myasthenia gravis. Neurology 1988; 38:258–261.

Hohlfeld R, Toyka KV, Besinger U, et al. Myasthenia gravis: reactivation of clinical disease and of autoimmune factors after discontinuation of long-term azathioprine. Ann Neurol 1987; 17:238–242.

Kissel JT, Levy RJ, Mendell JR, Griggs RC. Azathioprine toxicity in neuromuscular disease. Neurology 1986; 36:35–39.

Mertens HG, Hertel C, Reuther P, Ricker K. Effect of immunosuppressive drugs (azathioprine). Ann NY Acad Sci 1981; 377:691–699.

Michels M, Hohlfeld R, Hartung H-P, et al. Myasthenia gravis: discontinuation of long-term azathioprine. Ann Neurol 1988; 24:798.

National Institute of Health. The utility of therapeutic plasmapheresis for neurologic disorders. JAMA 1986; 256: 1333–1337.

Tindall RSA Rollins JA, Phillips JT, et al. Preliminary results of a double-blind, randomized, placebo-controlled trial of cyclosporine in myasthenia gravis. N Engl J Med 1987; 316:719–724.

PATIENT RESOURCES

Myasthenia Gravis Foundation
Suite 909
53 W. Jackson Blvd.
Chicago, Illinois 60604
(Provides information.)

Muscular Dystrophy Association
710 Seventh Avenue
New York, New York 10019
Telephone: (212) 586-0808
(Provides patient services).

European Alliance of Muscular Dystrophy Associations
Association de Myopathes de France (AMS)
13, Place Rungis
F-75650 Paris Cedex 13
Telephone: (33) 145651300
(Provides names and addresses of national European associations.

PERIODIC PARALYSIS

THERA P. LINKS, M.D.
HANS J.G.H. OOSTERHUIS, M.D., Ph.D.

Patients suffering from periodic paralysis have attacks of transient flaccid weakness of the extremities and trunk muscles. These attacks vary in intensity and duration. In severe attacks, the tongue and throat muscles may be involved and rarely the respiratory muscles; the eye muscles are never affected. During the attacks, muscle fibers become inexcitable to either direct or indirect stimulation. Serum potassium levels usually change in relation to the attacks; the classification in Table 1 is based on this phenomenon.

The molecular base of the membrane inexcitability in the different types of periodic paralysis is unknown, as is the exact mechanism of any of the treatment modalities used (except for the correction of serum potassium levels).

If a positive family history is known to the patient or to the physician, the diagnosis of a familial hypokalemic (less frequently hyperkalemic) periodic paralysis is easily confirmed by measuring serum potassium levels. In the absence of a family history, other diagnoses may be considered if a first episode of flaccid limb muscle weakness has occurred (Table 2). In general, these conditions have a more insidious onset than the periodic paralysis and they are accompanied by other signs and symptoms. The secondary forms of hypokalemic paralysis can be surmised if the patient's history reveals the use of laxatives or diuretics or gastrointestinal disturbances.

TABLE 1 Classification of the Periodic Paralyses*

Hypokalemic Periodic Paralysis
Primary:
familial
sporadic
Secondary:
to urinary and/or gastronintestinal potassium loss (laxatives, diuretics)
to intoxication by barium salts
Hyperkalemic Periodic Paralysis
Primary:
familial
sporadic
Secondary:
to renal or adrenal insufficiency to diuretics
Paramyotonia Congenita
Serum potassium level during attacks is variable
Thyrotoxic Periodic Paralysis
Serum potassium level during attacks is normal or low

*In normokalemic periodic paralysis, the appearance is based on description of some kinships. The clinical value of this entity is not yet clear.

HYPOKALEMIC PERIODIC PARALYSIS

In this disorder, paralytic attacks begin in the first or second decade of life, increase in frequency during early adult life, and become less frequent or cease after the fifth decade. Men are affected more seriously and more frequently than women. If untreated, these attacks may last from half a day to 7 days; very rarely, respiratory paralysis or cardiac arrhythmias lead to death. Hypokalemic periodic paralysis typically occurs as a dominant autosomal disease, although sporadic cases may occur. A permanent myopathy is not unusual in older patients, even in those who do not experience attacks. In an affected family, the present and *future* patients can be identified by a reduced muscle fiber conduction velocity.

Preventive Therapy

In patients with hypokalemic periodic paralysis, some changes in lifestyle can prevent paralytic attacks. These individuals have to restrict their daily carbohydrate and sugar intake and avoid heavy carbohydrate meals, especially in the evening. They also have to avoid exposure to cold and overexertion. Some patients can prevent an attack that would be precipitated by excercise or a heavy carbohydrate meal by taking a late evening dose of 20 to 40 mEq potassium chloride. Sometimes an incipient attack can be prevented by mild exercise; the patient can "walk off" the attack. In our personal experience, some patients can diminish their problem by eating fruit (an orange contains about 4 mEq potassium per 100 g). Therapuetic agents and/or medications include (1) *carbonic anhydrase inhibitors,* (2) *potassium-sparing diuretics,* (3) *beta blockers,* and (4) *potassium salts* (Table 3).

Carbonic Anhydrase Inhibitors

Acetazolamide. Acetazolamide, a carbonic anhydrase inhibitor, is the most useful and common drug in preventing attacks of hypolcalemic periodic paralysis. It may also increase the muscle strength and decrease the muscle stiffness in patients with weakness unrelated to attacks and not caused by permanent myopathy. Whether long-term treatment with acetazolamide reduces or prevents permanent late-onset myopathy is unknown. The way in which this agent is effective is still unclear. Acetazolamide inhibits the reabsorption of sodium, potassium, and bicarbonate ions in the renal tubules, which results in a significant potassium loss in the urine. A mild metabolic acidosis occurs in most patients, which may be the mechanism of action. Its possible influence on the glucose-insulin metabolism and conse-

TABLE 2 Differential Diagnosis of Acute Limb Muscle Weakness (Without Sensory Signs) Not Including the Periodic Paralyses

	History	*Clinical Picture*
Paralysis from tick bite	Tick bite	First weakness of the legs, later of the arms and the bulbar (respiratory) muscles
Paralysis from snake bite	Snake bite	First weakness of the ocular and bulbar muscles and weakness in the region of the bite, later of respiratory muscles
Paroxysmal myoglobinuria (Meyer-Betz)	Occasionally familial	Malaise, fever, vomiting, muscle pain, limb paralysis, elevated creatine kinase level, myoglobinuria
Rhabdomyolysis	Various conditions, e.g., trauma, drug abuse, excessive exertion	Dependent on various conditions; myoglobinuria, creatine kinase level elevated
Myasthenia gravis	Fever, provocation by medication, e.g., intravenous benzodiazepines	Limb muscles, eye muscles, and bulbar muscles are affected
Poliomyelitis (seldom coxsackie or echoviruses)	Fever, meningeal irritation	Weakness usually asymmetric
Botulism	Consumption of suspicious food	Ocular, bulbar weakness, autonomous signs
Conversion	History of acute emotion?	Reflexes preserved

quently on stabilizing the muscle membrane is another unclarified hypothesis.

A starting dose of 125 mg acetazolamide two to three times a day is preferred (in children half this dose is needed). The first effects on the frequency of attacks can be shown after 1 or 2 days, but an increase in the interictal strength takes place over a longer period (7 to 14 days). If the expected beneficial effect does not appear, the dosage can be increased 125 mg per dose up to a maximal daily dose of 1,000 to 1,200 mg. If a single dose is increased, the late evening dose is preferred, followed by the morning dose.

TABLE 3 Preventive Treatment in the Periodic Paralyses

Hypokalemic periodic paralysis
Acetazolamide 3 × 125 mg (max 1,200 mg)
Dichlorophenamide 2 × 50 mg (max 150 mg)
Potassium salts 15–50 mEq
Amiloride 2 × 5 mg (max 20 mg)
Triamterene 3 × 50 mg (max 200 mg)
Spironolactone 2 × 25 mg (max 100 mg)
Propranolol 2 × 40 mg (max 240 mg)
Hyperkalemic periodic paralysis
Acetazolamide 3 × 125 mg (max 1,200 mg)
Chlorothiazide 250 mg (max 500 mg)
Hydrochlorothiazide 25 mg (max 100 mg)
Hyperkalemic periodic paralysis with Myotonia
Tocainide 3 × 400 mg
Paramyotonia congenita
Tocainide 3 × 400 mg
Thyrotoxic periodic paralysis
Propranolol 3 × 20–40 mg

The most common side effects are paresthesias, dysgeusia, fatigue, and the formation of renal calculi. The paresthesias appear in the fingers, toes, and around the mouth, especially during transition from cold to warm temperatures, with a duration of some minutes. Most of the side effects decrease in severity after weeks of use. The risk of formation of renal calculi (family history of stones) makes it necessary to advise an adequate daily fluid intake.

Dichlorophenamide. This agent is another carbonic anhydrase inhibitor, with an inhibitory action of the enzyme 30 times greater than that of acetazolamide. Because of the induction of chloride excretion in the urine, this agent does not change the plasma pH; therefore the mechanism of action is even more puzzling.

The starting dose is 50 mg twice a day, with an increase to 50 mg 3 times a day if there is only a partial effect. If there is no response at this dosage, the medication should be discontinued. Side effects are the same as those for acetazolamide. Although the carbonic anhydrase inhibitors are the drugs of choice, in some cases it can be useful to have some alternatives, although in the treatment of hypokalemic periodic paralysis efficacy varies from patient to patient.

Potassium-Sparing Diuretics

The effect of potassium-sparing diuretics is possibly caused by a contribution to a permanent rise in plasma potassium level, which may be protective against a paralytic attack. Hyperkalemia can occur with or without using potassium salts, especially in older patients with impaired renal function; therefore regular control of electrolytes, blood urea nitrogen, and serum creatinine concentrations is necessary.

Amiloride. Amiloride directly interferes with tubular electrolyte transport, especially in the distal tubules. It should be given twice daily, 5 mg, increasing until a maximal daily dose of 20 mg is reached. Side effects include gastrointestinal disturbances, rashes, and disturbances of renal function (the last especially when it is administered in combination with nonsteroid, anti-inflammatory drugs).

Triamterene. Triamterene directly interferes with tubular electrolyte transport, especially in the distal renal tubules. The dosage is 50 mg, three times daily. If necessary, it is possible to increase to a maximal dose of 200 mg daily. Side effects are the same as those for amiloride.

Spironolactone. Spironolactone, an antagonist of aldosterone, acts in the distal renal tubules, decreasing the sodium reabsorption and sparing potassium. The specific drug regimen is 25 mg twice a day; if necessary it can be increased to 25 mg three times daily. The total dose should not exceed 100 mg. Side effects are gynecomastia, impotence, menstrual irregularities, gastrointestinal symptoms, and rashes.

Beta Blockers

Some case reports show a beneficial effect of beta blockers in reducing paralytic attacks. This effect could be ascribed to the inhibition of the activation of the sodium-potassium pump by catecholamines, which prevent a net shift of potassium to the intracellular space.

With propranolol, a nonselective beta blocker, 40 mg is given two or three times a day. If necessary, the dose can be doubled. Side effects include bronchospasm, bradycardia, hypotension, and cold and cyanotic extremities.

Potassium Salts

Potassium salts are widely used by patients with paralytic attacks. Although the intracellular shift of the potassium ions during an attack is not prevented, most likely the supply of extra potassium keeps the muscle membrane excitable. Based on our personal experience, potassium salts are only a supplemental therapy. Acetazolamide is still the drug of choice. However, some patients practically stay free of attacks while taking only potassium salts, in doses varying from 40 to 50 mEq divided over one day or only 15 mEq when symptoms are present.

Therapy of Acute Attacks

If total paralysis of the extremities is present without difficulties in deglutition or respiration, oral sips of potassium chloride solution can be given, 15 to 30 mEq (in children 10 to 14 mEq) over 30- to 60-minute intervals (the release from potassium chloride tablets is too slow). Often a patient will have taken several of these doses at home. (In patients using potassium-sparing diuretics or with renal function disturbances, serum potassium levels may rise rapidly after oral administration of potassium chloride.) If no improvement appears after four or five oral doses or if nausea or diarrhea accompanies the oral potassium chloride intake, intravenous administration is necessary. This also is preferable in patients with acute attacks of paralysis, difficulties in swallowing, and impaired respiration. In this situation, serial measurement of potassium and continued electrocardiographic monitoring are necessary. When using a peripheral vein, the concentration of the potassium chloride should not exceed 40 mEq per liter. Five percent mannitol is the preferred diluent; saline (0.9 percent) may be used, but not glucose. Infusion must be continued until the serum potassium level is normal and the patient's strength returns. Several hours of observation are necessary, during which potassium and muscle strength should be measured because sometimes the paralysis will return.

Patients with periodic paralysis who undergo surgery in which general anesthesia is required can develop paralytic attacks after the operation. Perioperative complications have not been reported. The anesthesiologist should use saline instead of 5 percent glucose, should prevent a decrease in the patient's temperature, and should monitor the patient for a longer period than usual.

HYPERKALEMIC PERIODIC PARALYSIS

This disease is transmitted as an autosomal dominant agent with high penetrance in both sexes. Attacks begin in the first or second decade and are often brief (10 to 20 minutes) but sometimes can last up to several days. Myotonic and nonmyotonic forms of hyperkalemic periodic paralysis can be distinguished. Myotonia can occur in the face, tongue and finger extensor and thenar muscles between attacks.

Preventive Therapy

The frequency of paralytic attacks can be lowered by many small meals of high carbohydrate content and avoidance of fasting. Exposure to cold and overexertion should also be avoided.

Drug treatment includes (1) acetazolamide, (2) thiazide diuretics, and (3) tocainide (see Table 3).

Acetazolamide. As in the hypokalemic form, of periodic paralysis, this drug has been found to be the most effective treatment. Its mechanism of action in hyperkalemic periodic paralysis can possibly be ascribed to the kaliuresis. However, because it is not the most effective kaliuretic diuretic, some other mechanism may play a role. Often patients with hyperkalemic periodic paralysis require a lower dose than those with hypokalemic periodic paralysis, but paresthesias occur more frequently in the former group.

Thiazide Diuretics. These drugs are also effective in hyperkalemic periodic paralysis probably because of the effect of kaliuresis. Specific drug regimens include chlorothiazide, 250 mg daily, or hydrochlorothiazide, 25 mg daily (children 6 months and older should receive chlorothiazide 20 mg per kilogram and hydrochlorothiazide 2 mg per kilogram daily, in two equal doses, but should not exceed the adult dosage). The lowest dose of diuretic required should be used. The serum potassium concentration should not fall below 3.7 mEq per liter.

Side effects include increased fasting blood glucose and uric acid levels, hypokalemia, hyponatremia, hypercalcemia, and occasionally blood dyscrasias.

Tocainide. Tocainide is an antiarrhythmic drug that blocks sodium channels and is useful in treating myotonic hyperkalemic periodic paralysis and in preventing the weakness and myotonia in paramyotonia congenita. It does not prevent hyperkalemic weakness. A dose of 400 mg 3 times daily is used. Side effects include gastrointestinal effects, blood dyscrasias, rash, and fever.

Acute Attacks

Acute attacks of weakness are often so brief that no treatment is necessary. Prompt ingestion of carbohydrates containing beverages at the first onset of weakness usually aborts the attack. Intravenous glucose is necessary only for prolonged and serious weakness. Sometimes a combination of oral glucose 1 to 2 g per kilogram with 10 to 20 U insulin subcutaneously is helpful. Paralytic attacks also respond favorably to beta-adrenergic agents. The mechanism of action may involve a beta-adrenergic –mediated increase of potassium transport via the sodium potassium pump. Case reports have appeared about the effective use of salbutamol (inhalation of 200 to 400 μg every 15 minutes) and metaproterenol (inhalations of 1.3 mg every 15 minutes for three doses. Calcium gluconate 0.5 to 2.0 g given intravenously has terminated attacks in some cases but has not been effective in others.

PARAMYOTONIA CONGENITA

This rare condition has an autosomal dominant inheritance and is characterized by myotonia and periods of weakness, both of which are provoked by exposure to cold and to a lesser degree by prior exercise. The onset is in childhood. Serum potassium levels may be elevated but also may be normal or even decreased.

Tocainide may reduce the myotonia and weakness (see Hyperkalemic Periodic Paralysis). Potassium-sparing diuretics can be useful in preventing paralytic attacks (see Hypokalemic Periodic Paralysis and Table 3).

THYROTOXIC PERIODIC PARALYSIS

This disease resembles hypokalemic periodic paralysis in clinical appearance and often in changes in serum potassium concentration. However, 95 percent of the cases are sporadic and occur among Orientals. The male:female ratio is 6:1, and the onset is usually in adult life. The most important part of therapy is the treatment of the hyperthyroidism and maintenance of the euthyroid state.

Preventive Treatment

Patients should avoid high carbohydrate intake, muscle cooling, or extreme exercise. Effective medications include (1) propranolol, at a dosage of 20 to 40 mg three times daily, which probably inhibits beta receptor–mediated actions of the thyroid hormones, (side effects are listed under Hypokalemic Periodic Paralysis), and (2) spironolactone (for details see Hypokalemic Periodic Paralysis and Table 3). In most of the reported cases, acetazolamide had a negative effect, and oral use of potassium does not prevent attacks of weakness.

Acute Attacks

The treatment of an acute attack of thyrotoxic periodic paralysis is the same for the hypokalemic form.

PERIODIC PARALYSIS WITH CARDIAC ARRHYTHMIA

In this disorder, treatment of the potentially fatal arrhythmia is of more importance than treatment of the paralytic attack. In these cases, tests to provoke the weakness (e.g., intravenous glucose and insulin) should not be used. Imipramine is the drug of choice in controlling cardiac arrhythmia, and low doses of acetazolamide are sometimes useful.

NORMOKALEMIC PERIODIC PARALYSIS

Although this is considered a distinct nosologic entity, no convincing therapeutic approach has been described. It is currently held that the therapy of choice is the same as for hyperkalemic periodic paralysis, but sometimes treatment with acetazolamide is not successful.

SUGGESTED READING

Gould RJ, Steeg CN, Eastwood AB, et al. Potentially fatal cardiac dysrhythmia and hyperkalemic periodic paralysis. Neurology 1985; 35:1208–1212.

Links TP, Zwarts MJ, Oosterhuis HJGH. Improvement of muscle strength in familial hypokalemic periodic paralysis with acetazolamide. Neurol Neurosurg Psychiatry 1988; 51:1142–1145.

Meyer-Lehnert H, Kramer HJ, Heck I, et al. Schwere periodische hypokaliämische Lähmung. Dtsch Med Wochenschr 1987; 112:1173–1177.

Streib EW. Paramyotonia congenita: Successful treatment with tocainide. Clinical and electrophysiologic findings in seven patients. Muscle Nerve 1987; 10:155–162.

Zwarts MJ, Van Weerden TW, Links TP, et al. The muscle fiber conduction velocity and power spectra in familial hypokalemic periodic paralysis. Muscle Nerve 1988; 11:166–173.

ENTRAPMENT NEUROPATHY

ASA J. WILBOURN, M.D.
PATRICK J. SWEENEY, M.D., FACP

Although the terms "entrapment neuropathy" and "compressive neuropathy" are often used interchangeably, they are not synonymous. A compressive neuropathy results when sustained pressure is applied to a localized region of the nerve. Most often this pressure derives from an external source and is transmitted through the tissues (including skin) overlying the nerve. However, occasionally pressure arises internally, such as from an expanding hematoma or neoplasm. An entrapment neuropathy, on the other hand, is one caused by constriction or mechanical distortion of the nerve within a fibrous or fibro-osseous tunnel, or by a fibrous band. In these situations, the source of injury is internal, and focal nerve compression may be less important in symptom production than nerve angulation and stretching.

MEDIAN NEUROPATHY AT OR DISTAL TO THE WRIST (CARPAL TUNNEL SYNDROME)

Although the characteristic clinical presentation of chronic entrapment of the median nerve beneath the transverse carpal ligament was first recognized only about 40 years ago, carpal tunnel syndrome (CTS) is the most common entrapment neuropathy by far and the most frequently encountered nontraumatic focal peripheral nerve lesion.

The initial step in the treatment of CTS is to confirm, by electrodiagnostic studies, that it is actually present. While its symptoms are often described as "characteristic" and frequently seem so, we have seen experienced clinicians confuse CTS with other entities (particularly C-6 or C-7 radiculopathies) often enough that such confirmation is warranted. When electrodiagnostic evaluation consists not only of the routine median motor and sensory nerve conduction studies (NCS), but also of median and ulnar (for comparison) palmar NCS, the procedure is highly sensitive for CTS. Electromyographic (EMG) studies are particularly important in patients with "atypical" CTS presentations. Frequently in these patients, either another focal neurogenic lesion is detected (e.g., a radiculopathy or a more proximal median nerve lesion) or, much more often, the studies are normal. Since CTS operations performed in patients of the latter group are likely to be failures, in our experience, the electrical data are helpful in management. Another useful benefit of electrodiagnostic studies in suspected CTS is that they identify those patients in whom CTS, while present, is not occurring in isolation but instead is superimposed on a generalized peripheral polyneuropathy, which can result in a very different diagnostic and therapeutic approach.

A variety of treatments are available for CTS. Wrist immobilization in the neutral position by an Ace bandage or a volar splint may offer considerable relief, by limiting flexion and extention movements at the wrist. Unfortunately, this compromises the functional use of the hand (which is often the dominant hand), thus limiting its use to periods of sleep. Also, symptom relief may be incomplete, symptoms often recur when splinting is discontinued, and few patients follow this regimen indefinitely. A short course of either nonsteroidal anti-inflammatory agents or diuretics helps some patients, but the symptoms frequently reappear after variable periods of time, and these medications cannot be given to some patients with CTS (e.g., pregnant women). A cortisone injection into the carpal tunnel is often beneficial, presumably because it decreases inflammation in the tendon sheaths. This treatment usually proves to be temporary, however, with relapses occurring after 2 to 3 months, and it is not without some risk. No attempt should be made to perform this procedure without first doing so under the direct supervision of an experienced clinician. We have seen patients whose median nerves were destroyed by the injudicious use of cortisone injections by clinicians unfamiliar with the technique.

Also, only a limited number of injections (probably 3 or less) should be attempted, and the patient should be reassessed at intervals. If the condition is worsening, clinically or electrically, this therapeutic approach should be abandoned. The most consistently helpful treatment by far (and the only one that usually provides permanent symptom relief) is sectioning of the transverse carpal ligament. This alleviates symptoms in more than 90 percent of patients, and most of the surgical failures are associated with inappropriate patient selection or improper surgical techniques. Patients in the former group are commonly those with atypical clinical findings and/or normal electrodiagnostic studies. Unsatisfactory surgical techniques generally result in incomplete sectioning of the ligament, and are usually associated with transverse or "micro" surgical wrist scars. A repeat operation by another surgeon is usually successful.

The clinical findings in these patients are generally more helpful in selecting surgical candidates than are the electrical findings. The symptoms, at least during the initial stages of the disorder, are caused primarily by small fiber involvement, while the electrical changes reflect only large myelinated nerve fiber compromise. Clinical signs of progression include pain increasing in frequency and occupying greater portions of the 24-hour day, (e.g., occurring more and more often during the wake cycle as well as during the sleep cycle), persistent sensory loss in a median nerve distribution (with subsequent finger clumsiness), and lateral thenar wasting. Lateral thenar wasting should be taken as an indication for prompt surgical intervention because it is a sign of a far-advanced problem. Many physicians consider certain electrical abnormalities to be indications for surgical treatment, since they, too, generally reflect advanced disease. These include (1) unelicitable median sensory nerve action potentials, (2) markedly prolonged median motor distal latency, (3) low-amplitude or unelicitable median motor compound muscle action potential, and (4) fibrillation potentials in the median-innervated thenar muscles.

Although CTS is sometimes self-limited (particularly in pregnant women and patients who have used their hands excessively for a restricted period of time), more often it is static or progressive. Hence if CTS does not appear serious enough to mandate therapy when it is first recognized, provision should be made for periodic reassessment. We have seen several patients over the years whose initially mild CTS ultimately culminated in total axon loss lesions, with permanent residuals, because they were not re-evaluated appropriately.

ULNAR NEUROPATHY AT THE ELBOW

Although these lesions have been recognized for much longer than CTS, in the majority of patients, their exact location along the ulnar nerve is unclear. For years, ulnar neuropathies at the elbow were attributed to nerve compromise at the ulnar groove. More recently, however, the cubital tunnel area, which lies immediately distal to the ulnar groove, has been implicated. To add to the confusion, some physicians are now referring to all ulnar neuropathies that occur at the elbow as "cubital tunnel syndrome," although there is no proof that even the majority of lesions actually occur at this site. Those within the groove are typically compressive or stretch lesions. By contrast, lesions within the cubital tunnel may be caused by either entrapment or external compression; both mechanisms may even be operative in the same patient. Electrodiagnostic studies are less sensitive for ulnar neuropathy at the elbow than for CTS. Although they are usually abnormal (a major exception being chronic lesions manifested solely as intermittent paresthesias), a focal demyelinating component (e.g., focal slowing, differential slowing, conduction block), detectable along the ulnar nerve and allowing localization to the elbow segment, is found in only about half of the patients. In the remaining patients, the lesions are "pure" axon loss in character and the EMG localization becomes much less precise. Hence the more severe ulnar neuropathies are more likely to be poorly localized by EMG examination.

With many ulnar neuropathies, the source of symptom production is as unclear as the lesion site. Some physicians attribute the symptoms to excessive elbow flexion/extension alone (somewhat comparable to carpal tunnel syndrome). Splinting the elbow region, particularly while the patient is asleep, with a removable rigid cast has been tried but is ineffective in many patients. In some patients a definite history of excessive elbow leaning can be elicited; they should be encouraged to cease this practice and be given elbow protection (elbow protectors worn by hockey or football players can be very helpful and can be obtained at any sporting goods store). A brief trial of a nonsteroidal anti-inflammatory drug occasionally relieves symptoms. If the symptoms are progressive, and particularly if a bony deformity is present at the elbow, surgical intervention should be considered. However, several aspects of the treatment of ulnar neuropathies stand in contrast to that of CTS: (1) several different surgical procedures are used to treat ulnar neuropathy at the elbow (depending largely on exactly where the particular surgeon believes the lesion is located), including medial epicondylectomy, cubital tunnel decompression, and nerve transposition; (2) the surgical success rate for ulnar neuropathies is much less predictable than that for CTS, although usually the milder the lesion, the better the result; and (3) the operations for ulnar neuropathies are not without risk. We have seen a few patients who had only sensory symptoms preoperatively, with little to no evidence of axon loss. However, after undergoing the operation, they had very severe axon loss ulnar neuropathies, presumably reflecting nerve infarction caused by stripping of nutrient arteries from the nerve while it was being prepared for transposition.

RADIAL NEUROPATHY AT THE SPIRAL GROOVE

These upper extremity nerve lesions are not commonly encountered. Those lesions not caused by obvious trauma rarely are due to nerve entrapment. Instead, they are usually caused by external compression. Because the type of pathophysiology at the lesion site is a major consideration in therapy, the electrodiagnostic evaluation is an important component of the initial assessment of these lesions. Since almost all patients present with extensor forearm muscle weakness (i.e., wrist and finger drop), the responsible process must be axon loss or demyelinating conduction block or a combination of both (demyelinating focal slowing and differential slowing are not associated with clinical weakness). These can be readily differentiated from one another if the appropriate studies are performed, thereby permitting early accurate prognostication and appropriate therapy. The most informative study is the radial motor NCS, with nerve stimulation at the elbow area and immediately distal and proximal to the spiral groove, while one records with a surface electrode over the proximal extensor forearm muscles. Radial neuropathies caused by external pressure (the so-called "Saturday night palsies") are usually demyelinating conduction block lesions and tend to resolve completely within approximately 6 to 8 weeks. Occasionally, however, they are axon loss in type, similar to those seen with midshaft humeral fractures and radial nerve injection injuries. Nonetheless, even these usually recover satisfactorily, although they are much slower in tempo because the nerve fibers must regenerate distally from the lesion site. Regeneration can be ascertained by electrodiagnostic studies several weeks before it is clinically evident, through needle electrode examination of the closest "target" muscle(s) distal to the injury site (i.e., the brachioradialis and extensor carpi radialis). A few motor unit potentials (MUPs) of low amplitude, with markedly increased duration and highly polyphasic in configuration ("reinnervation" MUPs) are seen in those muscles on attempted voluntary activation several weeks before enough reinnervation has occurred to produce a visible muscle twitch. If reinnervation is not progressing, (i.e., if "reinnervation" MUPs are not seen in the target muscles during 2 or 3 examinations, performed at 4-week intervals, with the first being performed at the time reinnervation was expected), surgical exploration is mandatory.

With all types of radial neuropathy at the spiral groove, sensory symptoms tend to be minimal and are overshadowed by the motor deficit, which results in wrist and finger drop. The latter should be treated with splinting, although the functional use of the hand is significantly impaired. For those relatively few patients with permanent axon loss radial neuropathies (i.e., those in whom no clinical or EMG evidence of reinnervation is present after approximately 1 year), reconstructive tendon transfers should be considered.

THORACIC OUTLET SYNDROME

At least 2 types of "neurogenic" thoracic outlet syndromes (TOS) have been described, but only one is noncontroversial. It is a rare entrapment lesion, limited to young and middle-aged females. It presents with weakness and wasting of the hand (particularly the lateral thenar eminence) and sometimes of the medial forearm, along with long standing aching pain along the medial forearm. Neck radiographs show a rudimentary cervical rib or at least an elongated C-7 transverse process (the lower trunk of the brachial plexus is stretched and angulated over a translucent band extending from the tip of this anomaly to the first rib). EMG examination is almost pathognomonic, showing a highly chronic, axon loss, lower-trunk brachial plexopathy. Appropriate treatment is sectioning of the band via a supraclavicular surigcal approach.

"Neurogenic" TOS is also diagnosed in a great number of patients (particularly women) who do not have the characteristic radiographic or EMG features described above. Frequently workman's compensation claims or personal injury lawsuits for minor automobile accidents are pending. For these patients, conservative therapy is indicated. Unfortunately, many of them undergo first rib removal or some other type of TOS surgery. This not only produces fleeting symptom relief in many (probably the majority), but also causes severe axon loss, lower-trunk brachial plexopathies in some.

PERONEAL NEUROPATHY AT THE FIBULAR HEAD

This is the most common mononeuropathy of the lower extremity. Most of these lesions are caused by compression or stretching of the common peroneal nerve fibers at the fibular head; entrapment is rarely the cause. Because these neuropathies characteristically present with foot drop (i.e., weakness of the tibialis anterior muscle), the pathophysiological process is either axon loss, demyelinating conduction block, or a combination of both. Clinically, it is difficult to distinguish between them, since each can produce any gradation of weakness, from mild to complete. Yet their prognosis with regard to time and degree of recovery is quite different. Hence, just as with radial neuropathies, electrodiagnostic studies (particularly peroneal motor NCS while recording from tibialis anterior) are of major importance in assessing these lesions. They not only reveal the pathophysiology at the lesion site, but also document that the cause of the patient's foot drop is a peroneal mononeuropathy, rather than a more proximal lesion, such as a sciatic neuropathy, sacral plexopathy, or particularly an L-5 radiculopathy. Any one of these would result in a different diagnostic and therapeutic regimen. Compressive peroneal neuropathies tend to be associated with recent, significant weight loss (>10 kg), chronic leg crossing, and/or major illness that causes prolonged hospitalization.

The most appropriate therapy is preventing additional nerve compression. In the hospital setting, this requires that adequate protection for the nerve at the fibular head be assured by proper padding and positioning. If the patient is a chronic leg-crosser, this habit must be discouraged. Because it is typically an unconscious act, merely advising the patient to stop crossing his legs is not sufficient. Instead, he should be instructed to tell his friends and close acquaintances to inform him each time they observe him doing this. Avoiding leg crossing can result in rapid resolution of symptoms in those patients with demyelinating conduction block. Hence during a subsequent visit, the patient often reports that his foot drop is improving while he simultaneously expresses displeasure concerning the number of times he has been told to uncross his legs by his associates and family members. Even when the nerve lesion is caused by traction, surgical nerve repair is rarely indicated. If the traction is mild and produces primarily demyelinating conduction block, recovery is relatively rapid and complete. Conversely, if the traction is severe enough to produce axon degeneration, the nerve segment affected is often so extensive as to preclude successful surgical repair. Nonetheless, if only for medicolegal reasons, a neurosurgical opinion should be obtained for any patient with an axon loss lesion that is not showing clinical or EMG improvement after 6 months.

Because most of these lesions are painless and produce few sensory complaints, the major disability is foot drop. This is corrected relatively easily by means of a dorsiflexor foot splint; of particular value are the light-weight, plastic foot splints that fit in the shoe. (However, these cannot be used with high-heeled shoes.) Orthopedic tendon transfers should be offered to those patients with permanent lesions, although many patients consider such surgery unnecessary.

MEDIAL/LATERAL PLANTAR ENTRAPMENT NEUROPATHY (TARSAL TUNNEL SYNDROME)

Although chronic entrapment of the terminal portions of the posterior tibial nerve—tarsal tunnel syndrome (TTS)—is well described in the literature, its incidence is uncertain. This entity is not the "CTS of the foot"; its electrical characteristics and response to surgical treatment are markedly different from those seen with CTS. As with all other compressive/entrapment neuropathies, other causes for the patient's symptoms (which in this case is predominantly or solely foot pain and paresthesia) must be excluded. Unilateral TTS can be confused with primary arthritic bone spurs in the foot, ischemic monomelic neuropathy, tibial neuropathies, sciatic neuropathies primarily affecting the tibial fibers, and sacral plexopathies affecting primarily the S-1, S-2 tibial fibers and, most often, S-1, S-2 radiculopathies. Bilateral TTS is most often confused with peripheral polyneuropathies and bilateral S-1, S-2 radiculopathies (cauda equina lesions).

Electrodiagnostic studies can be of help in the differential diagnosis. Although this syndrome has been reported to produce a characteristic electrodiagnostic pattern (slowing along the medial and/or lateral plantar nerves in a manner analogous to that of CTS), these findings can be demonstrated only rarely in patients referred to the EMG laboratory with a diagnosis of TTS. Much more often, when the lesion cannot be localized to a more proximal location, the EMG examination either is normal or demonstrates only axon loss in the distribution of one or both of these nerves. Because often the studies are performed in patients who have already undergone multiple unsuccessful TTS surgical procedures, there is no way to determine whether these electrical abnormalities antedated the operations or were caused by one or more of them. Since, in our experience, TTS surgery so often proves to be unsuccessful (i.e., the patient reports not only that the symptoms were unrelieved, but actually increased with each operation) possibly the best therapy a neurologist can provide for suspected TTS, once other diagnostic possibilities have been excluded, is avoidance of surgery. Those patients who have undergone multiple unsuccessful operations can present difficult management problems. Analgesics usually provide only temporary (if any) benefit, and carbamazepine (Tegretol), while helpful, seldom produces complete relief.

SUGGESTED READING

Dawson DM, Hallett M, Millender LH. Entrapment neuropathies. Boston: Little, Brown, and Co., 1983.

Gilliatt RW, Harrison MJG. Nerve compression and entrapment. In: Absury AK, Gilliatt RW, eds. Peripheral nerve disorders: a practical approach. Stoneham MA: Butterworths, 1984: 243.
Katirji MB, Wilbourn AJ. Common peroneal mononeuropathy: a clinical and electrophysiological study of 116 lesions. Neurology 1988; 38:1723–1728.
Stewart JD. Focal peripheral neuropathies. New York: Elsevier, 1987.

ACUTE INFLAMMATORY POLYNEUROPATHY

DAVID R. CORNBLATH, M.D.
DANIEL F. HANLEY, M.D.

Acute inflammatory polyneuropathy (AIP), commonly known as the Guillain-Barré syndrome, is an acute demyelinating disorder of the peripheral nervous system that affects individuals of all ages. Currently it is the most common acute neurologic disease leading to paralysis or respiratory failure within days. In two-thirds of patients, the disorder follows within 1 to 3 weeks a "viral" infection. AIP is also associated with several systemic disorders, including Hodgkin's disease, lymphoma, lupus erythematosus, and human immunodeficiency virus (HIV) infection. The disease typically begins with paresthesia in the hands or feet, but rapidly evolves to involve the motor system, with weakness usually progressing in an ascending fashion. Hyporeflexia or areflexia is always seen at some point in the course of the disease. Occasional patients have the rare Miller-Fisher variant of the disease (which includes ataxia, areflexia, and ophthalmoplegia), with preserved strength. The Miller-Fisher variant is considered part of the spectrum of AIP, and the treatment is the same as that for AIP.

DIAGNOSIS

Because of the reports of AIP occurring after the swine-influenza vaccine, standardized diagnostic criteria were developed by the National Institute of Neurologic Communication Disorders and Stroke. It is important to note that these criteria were developed primarily for epidemiologic and medicolegal purposes in response to the AIP-like syndrome associated with swine influenza vaccination, and thus may not include all cases that experienced neurologists would accept as AIP. Weakness and areflexia are required for diagnosis. Supportive features include progression after onset, relative symmetry, sensory and cranial nerve involvement, autonomic dysfunction, absence of fever at onset, and improvement after a nadir has been reached. Features that suggest an incorrect diagnosis include marked persistent asymmetry of weakness, persistent bowel or bladder dysfunction, significant bowel or bladder dysfunction at onset, cerebrospinal fluid (CSF) pleocytosis (>50 mononuclear cells per cubic millimeter), CSF polymorphonuclear cells, and a sharp sensory level. Disorders that may mimic AIP include conditions associated with hexacarbon abuse, porphyria, diphtheria, heavy metal intoxication, and botulism.

EVALUATION

In most patients, a relatively confident diagnosis can be made based on clinical criteria alone. Because of the clinical implications, however, diagnosis should be confirmed by a series of laboratory studies that can usually be completed within 1 to 2 days after admission to hospital. Evaluation serves 3 purposes: (1) to confirm the clinical diagnosis, (2) to eliminate other disorders, and (3) to look for associated diseases accompanying AIP. Blood studies should include a screening hematologic and biochemical battery, determinations of antinuclear antibodies (ANA) and antibodies to both hepatitis and HIV, and blood sent to a central laboratory for acute viral titers to be followed by a blood specimen obtained 2 weeks later for convalescent titers. Urine should be collected for evaluation of porphyria and heavy metal intoxication. CSF should be evaluated for glucose, protein, cell count, and VDRL. In classic AIP, there is little if any value in obtaining CSF for evidence of infection or for measuring of oligoclonal bands, myelin basic protein, or immunoglobulin synthesis. Early in the disorder, spinal fluid protein content may be normal, and for diagnostically difficult cases, it may be necessary to repeat the spinal fluid evaluation 7 to 14 days into the illness. Electrophysiologic studies are particularly important because, in addition to their use in diagnosis, they also have prognostic value (detailed later in this chapter). These studies should include sensory conduction studies, motor conduction studies including F-wave latencies, H-reflex latencies, and electromyography. Like the CSF protein level, routine electrophysiologic studies may rarely be normal early in the course of the disease.

THERAPY

All patients with AIP should be hospitalized. The disorder is highly variable, and in a seemingly well individual, the disease may rapidly progress over a period of hours to respiratory failure. Currently we admit most patients to a regular hospital bed near the nursing station. Those patients with respiratory embarrassment, bulbar weakness, or difficulty handling secretions are best managed in an intensive care unit. One cannot be cavalier about predicting the rate of progressive respiratory impairment for an individual patient.

Plasmapheresis

Three controlled studies comprising more than 450 patients now convincingly demonstrate that plasmapheresis is the treatment of choice for AIP. We use the plasmapheresis protocol developed in our initial studies of AIP: a set of 5 exchanges, each approximately 40 to 50 ml per kilogram, over a period of 7 to 14 days for a total volume exchange of 200 to 250 ml per kilogram. Our standard replacement fluid has been "plasma protein fraction." There is no advantage to fresh-frozen plasma. If possible, the use of a continuous-flow plasmapheresis machine is preferred. In approximately one-half of the patients undergoing pheresis, this can be readily accomplished through the use of peripheral venous access. In many patients, however, the large volumes and high flow rates required by continuous-flow plasmapheresis machines necessitate the placement of central venous catheters. These should be placed only by experienced clinicians and must be watched closely for signs of infection or thrombosis. We usually use a Shiley double-lumen catheter via the femoral venous route. One must pay careful attention to antiseptic technique. The catheter is discontinued after 3 days of use. The large lumenal diameter of these catheters has the additional advantage of allowing for the rapid infusion of fluid if hypotension occurs during pheresis.

One of the most frequently asked questions about plasmapheresis is who should undergo this procedure? We pherese those individuals who are unable to walk and who are able to tolerate plasmapheresis. Individuals whose disease appears to be rapidly progressing but who are still able to walk also undergo pheresis. It is unknown whether there is a lower limit to the age at which one should pherese a patient. Pregnancy is not a contraindication to pheresis if AIP supervenes during the course of the pregnancy. Individuals with antibodies to hepatitis or HIV can be pheresed safely. It is our practice to assume that all patients have antibodies to hepatitis and HIV until proven otherwise, so that appropriate precautions are taken in all patients. For patients with the Miller-Fisher variant, we follow the same guidelines for the use of plasmapheresis as in patients with more typical AIP.

Supportive Care

Prior to the advent of plasmapheresis therapy, the best therapy consisted of best medical and nursing supportive care. This includes attention to impending respiratory distress, frequent vital signs including measurement of respiratory parameters such as vital capacity and negative inspiratory force, maintenance of adequate nutrition, ongoing surveillance for the presence of infection, and particular attention to difficulties that arise in individuals who have had prolonged bedrest, such as orthostatic hypotension, atelectasis, and the development of decubitus ulcers.

Respiratory Therapy/Intubation

The majority of AIP patients do not require mechanical ventilation. However, because the illness is both unpredictable and reversible, mechanical ventilation should be used at the earliest sign of respiratory embarrassment. Both physicians and nurses perform frequent assessments of all aspects of ventilation (airway patency, mechanical effort, and gas exchange). Impairment of any of these 3 vital functions is an indication for artificial ventilation. We consider the inability to swallow secretions the major indicator of pharyngeal muscle dysfunction. Tidal volume and respiratory rate are the best indicators of mechanical effort. A tidal volume of less than 15 ml per kilogram of body weight or a respiratory rate 20 breaths per minute or greater are most often followed by complete respiratory failure. Systemic arterial hemoglobin desaturation ($\leq$90 percent saturation) via pulse oximetry or hypoxia/hypercapnia on arterial blood gas chemistry are equally important indicators of poor gas exchange. We attempt to identify all AIP patients with ventilatory failure before they achieve this degree of physiologic compromise.

Elective endotracheal intubation is best performed in anticipation of further decline rather than during rapidly progressive hypoxia and hypotension. We prefer to use ventilators that have "pressure support" capabilities, as this method of rate-supported and pressure-supported ventilation offers the ideal flexibility of ventilation settings for encouraging early diaphragmatic training and recovery. We extubate patients when their secretions can be well managed by swallowing, when cough and gag reflexes are present, when mechanical ventilatory effort is sustained at low respiratory rates and high tidal volumes, and when there is little or no parenchymal lung disease to impair gas exchange.

Autonomic Instability

Autonomic instability is frequently seen in patients with AIP. This may take the form of cardiac arrhythmias, hypertension or hypotension, pupillary dilatation, and sweat disturbances. The usual tendency is to rush to treat these manifestations of the disorder. Most are transitory, however, and are rarely life-threatening. Over-vigorous treatment of hypertension may be followed by potentially more threatening severe hypotension resulting from either overtreatment or increased sensitivity of blood pressure control mechanisms caused by the disease. Most patients tolerate their autonomic dysfunction.

Occupational and Physical Therapy

Some patients recover quickly from the disorder, requiring little bedrest or having a short recovery phase. However, the majority have a period of bedrest followed by a slower recovery phase. Early consultation with occupational and physical therapists regarding the maintenance of muscle tone and joint mobility is mandatory. The use of splints for both hands and feet may be useful in preventing contractures. Occupational therapists are particularly helpful for patients who have difficulty communicating and swallowing.

Pain

Pain may be particularly problematic at the onset of the disease. In most patients, it is centered in the lower back without radicular radiation. While the use of narcotic analgesics may depress respiration, one should not hesitate to use narcotics for controlling the pain. These patients generally receive narcotics for a short time and do not become addicted. During the recovery phase, occasional patients develop "neuritic pain," which responds best to tricyclic antidepressants or anticonvulsants. Tricyclic antidepressants have the added benefit of promoting sleep when nocturnal pain is prominent.

Psychological Support

Because the majority of individuals who develop AIP were previously healthy, they experience a great deal of psychic trauma in dealing with the fact that they have an acute devastating illness. Reassuring the patient that the disease is self-limited and that recovery usually occurs is helpful, but many patients are not convinced by this. It is more useful to have patients who have recovered visit currently ill patients in the hospital. Maintaining open lines of communication through the use of communication boards is extremely helpful and reasurring to the patient, who is frequently fearful of abandonment (by physicians and nurses). Rarely do patients need active psychiatric intervention or require major psychotropic drugs.

PROGNOSIS

Our prospective studies have elucidated important factors regarding the long-term prognosis (e.g., the ability to walk independently 6 months after the onset of the disease). Four of these are factors over which the physician has no control. These are the patient's age, the duration of the illness before treatment (≤7 days versus >7 days), respirator status (i.e., whether the patient is supported by a respirator), and mean distal motor amplitude (≤20 versus >20 percent of the lower limit of normal). A sample calculation of mean distal motor amplitude is shown in Table 1.

The only variable effecting prognosis over which the physician has influence is treatment. Our studies demonstrated that the prognosis was statistically improved by the use of plasmapheresis, even in the face of poor prognostic variables for the patient's age, the duration of the illness before treatment, respirator status, and mean distal motor amplitude.

In general, the prognosis for this illness is good. Most individuals make a complete or near-complete recovery. Residual signs and symptoms are frequent but rarely interefere with functional activities. In a subgroup, the disorder is more devastating and results in severe and permanent disability.

After the acute hospitalization, many patients are transferred to specialized rehabilitation centers for more intensive occupational and physical therapy than can be given in acute-care hospitals.

TABLE 1 Sample Calculations of Mean CMAP Amplitude From Distal Stimulation (Distal CMAP Amplitude)

Nerve	*Values*	*Laboratory Normal*	*Percentage of the Lower Limit of Normal*
Peroneal	500	2,000	25
Tibial	200	2,000	10
Median	5,000	4,000	125
Ulnar	4,000	4,000	100
Total			260
Mean distal CMAP amplitude			65

CMAP=compound muscle action potential.

Republished with permission from Cornblath, DR, Mellits ED, Griffin JW, et al (The GBS Study Group). Motor conduction studies in Guillan-Barré syndrome: description and prognostic value. Ann Neurol 1988; 23:354–359.

SUGGESTED READING

Ad Hoc NINCDS Committee. Criteria for the diagnosis of Guillain-Barré syndrome. Ann Neurol 1978; 3:565–566.
Cornblath DR, Mellits ED, Griffin JW, et al (The GBS Study Group). Motor conduction studies in Guillain-Barré syndrome: description and prognostic value. Ann Neurol 1988; 23:354–359.
French Cooperative Group on Plasma Exchange and Guillain-Barré Syndrome. efficiency of plasma exchange in Guillain-Barré syndrome: role of replacement fluids. Ann Neurol 1987; 22:753–761.
The Guillain-Barré Syndrome Study Group. Plasmapheresis and the acute Guillain-Barré syndrome. Neurology 1985; 35:1096–1104.
McKhann GM, Griffin JW, Cornblath DR, et al (GBS Study Group). Plasmapheresis and Guillain-Barré syndrome: prognostic factors and the effect of plasmapheresis. Ann Neurol 1988; 23:347–353.
Osterman PG, Ludemo G, Pirskanem R, et al. Beneficial effects of plasma exchange in acute inflammatory polyradiculoneuropathy. Lancet 1984; 2:1296–1299.

PATIENT RESOURCE

The Guillain-Barré Syndrome Support Group International is a patient-based organization providing information to individuals with AIP. The organization has chapters in the United States, Australia, Canada, Great Britain, and West Germany.

GBS Syndrome Support Group
P.O. Box 262
Wynnewood, PA 19096
Telephone: (215) 642–6855.

CHRONIC NEUROPATHY

DANNY F. WATSON, M.D., Ph.D.

DIAGNOSIS

Accurate etiologic diagnosis is vitally important for the primary treatment of a neuropathy; furthermore, many neuropathies are manifestations of systemic diseases that require treatment in their own right. Diagnostic efforts are appropriately directed to the identification of treatable disorders, despite the relatively frequent occurrence of neuropathies for which no specific treatment is available. Although a comprehensive review of the diagnosis of neuropathies is beyond the scope of this chapter, some principles that guide the diagnostic approach should be discussed.

The least specific pattern of neuropathy is distal degeneration of the longest axons of all fiber types (myelinated and unmyelinated, sensory, motor and autonomic) with subsequent dying-back to more proximal levels as the disease progresses. This pattern can be produced by a wide range of disorders, since any derangement in the complex processes of synthesis and transport of macromolecules from nerve cell bodies to their terminals produce distal axonal degeneration. By contrast, if a neuropathy differs from this common pattern (e.g., a primarily demyelinating neuropathy, a neuropathy with disproportionate involvement of the upper extremities, or a neuropathy with a single functional modality involved), there are fewer possible diagnoses and the chance of identifying a specific treatment is greatly enhanced. Recognition of special patterns of neuropathy requires that one obtain a careful history of the tempo and spatial distribution and perform a thorough examination of the function of different fiber classes: motor, large fiber sensory (vibration and joint position sense), small fiber sensory (pin and temperature), and autonomic (sympathetic and parasympathetic). Further characterization by nerve conduction testing and electromyography can be helpful in making these distinctions and may also prove valuable in identifying patients with discrete focal lesions of multiple nerves (a pattern with relatively few causes) as opposed to true polyneuropathy.

Systematic consideration of broad categories of etiologies helps the clinician avoid the pitfall of focusing on esoteric possibilities while forgetting more common ones. A list of common etiologies of neuropathy for which there exists some specific therapeutic intervention is shown in Table 1.

PRIMARY TREATMENT

The treatment of immune-mediated neuropathies is considered elsewhere in this text. The treatment of toxic and metabolic neuropathies is conceptually straightforward; the offending toxin is removed or the metabolic disorder is controlled. A few specific management problems are common enough to warrant comment.

Diabetes

In a patient with diabetes, identification of new onset neuropathy calls for careful re-evaluation of diabetic control. Mild reversible changes in nerve conduction velocities and slight associated paresthesias may resolve with adequate diabetic control. Diabetic lumbosacral plexopathy often undergoes significant improvement over some months, aided by good control of diabetes. More frequently, adequate diabetic control is useful for slowing the rate of progression of the weakness and numbness, but little improvement occurs. Very tight control, such as that which may be achieved with subcutaneous "insulin pump" therapy, has been disappointing

TABLE 1 Major Treatable Causes of Polyneuropathy

- Toxic
  - Medications
    - Amiodarone
    - Cisplatin
    - Colchicine
    - Dapsone
    - Gold salts
    - Hydralazine
    - Isoniazid
    - Metronidazole
    - Misonidazole
    - Nitrofurantoin
    - Pyridoxine
    - Vincristine
  - Environmental exposure
    - Lead
    - Mercury
    - Thallium
    - Acrylamide
    - Hexacarbons
    - Kepone
  - Intentional exposure
    - Alcohol
    - Nitrous oxide
    - Arsenic
- Metabolic
  - Diabetes
  - Nutritional deficiency
    - Thiamine
    - Pyridoxine
    - Niacin
    - Cobalamin (vitamin B_{12})
    - α-tocopherol (vitamin E)
  - Uremia
  - Porphyria
  - Endocrine
    - Hypothyroidism
    - Acromegaly
    - Hyperparathyroidism
  - Refsum's disease
- Paraneoplastic
- Immune-mediated

with regard to neuropathy; good control by conventional means should be pursued. Pancreatic transplantation may offer some advantages over insulin therapy, but there are still too few patients with adequate long-term follow-up. There are reports of modest improvement occurring in patients with diabetic neuropathy who have received aldose reductase inhibitors; however, the overall ratio of risk to benefit is not clearly favorable on the basis of studies to date.

Alcohol

Abstention from alcohol or even moderation of alcohol intake can produce considerable long-term improvement in patients with distal pain and weakness; however, this may take many months to several years. When obvious malnutrition is a conjoined cause, the response to vitamin repletion may occur more quickly, with improvement beginning within a few weeks. Because of the associated distal axonal degeneration, some residual weakness and sensory disturbance usually remain in alcohol-related neuropathies.

Paraproteinemia

Among patients with paraproteinemia leading to chronic axonal polyneuropathy, only a small proportion undergo a significant clinical improvement of their neuropathy with the use of plasma exchange and/or oral cytotoxic agents; however, it remains impossible to predict in advance which patients will improve. Usually the therapy must be intensive and achieve sustained reduction of circulating paraprotein levels. Decisions to initiate such treatment must be highly individualized with regard to the degree of potential benefit as compared with the potential risks of cytotoxic agents.

Paraneoplastic Syndromes

Stabilization of or improvement in paraneoplastic neuropathies may occur after effective surgical or chemotherapeutic treatment of the malignancy. Because of the demonstrated immunologic basis for certain other paraneoplastic neurologic syndromes, there is interest in treatment with corticosteroids or other immunosuppressive regimens. These treatments are experimental, however, and must not be viewed as established therapies.

SECONDARY COMPLICATIONS

Loss of Protective Sensation

Patients with altered sensation in the hands and especially in the feet should take precautions to avoid the trauma and sustained mechanical pressure that underlie "trophic" ulcers. If sensation is significantly impaired, the patient should change shoes (to redistribute pressure points) and inspect the feet several times per day. Persistent redness or breaks in the skin should be viewed with alarm and should lead to prompt measures to avoid all pressure until there is improvement. Procedures that break the skin should be avoided; well-intentioned orthopedic and podiatric procedures often lead to a wound that does not heal in the severly denervated foot. In order to avoid serious burns, the feet should not be immersed in bath water until the temperature is felt with a more normally innervated part of the body.

Altered Gait

Severe loss of proprioception is nearly as disabling as loss of motor power, and at its worst forces a patient to rely on a wheelchair. For lesser degrees of sensory difficulty, attempts at improving sensory feedback, such as use of a light cane and judicious placement of night-lights between the bed and bathroom, may be helpful. Foot drop may lead to an exaggerated steppage gait that predisposes to falls and degenerative joint disease of the hips and lower back. Appropriate ankle-foot orthoses may prove very helpful for foot drop, although they interfere with the patient's ability to point the foot downward and thereby may cause difficulty in walking down stairs and stepping down from curbs. Mechanical stabilization of weakened ankles, which is usually obtained with high-topped shoes, may improve steadiness of gait and may help prevent recurrent ankle sprains.

Pain

Unpleasant paresthesias are a common experience during the early stages of sensory neuropathy; fortunately, only a minority of patients experience significant chronic pain. In a few instances, a specific treatable cause of the pain can be remedied—for example, focal compression of the tibial nerve at the ankle. More frequently, chronic medical treatment for pain is required.

Narcotic analgesics are of limited usefulness, in part because neuropathic pains seem especially resistant to ordinary doses of narcotics, and in part because tolerance soon reduces the modest degree of relief obtained acutely. Anticonvulsants and tricyclic antidepressants are the mainstays of treatment. Carbamazepine may be helpful for a variety of neuropathic pain syndromes. Side effects of acute atoxia, drowsiness, and nausea are reduced when the dose is gradually increased from 100 mg twice daily to 200 mg three times daily over 10 days, thereby improving patient acceptance. Further adjustments can be made to achieve the same range of serum concentrations as those used in the treatment of epilepsy (8 to 12 mg per liter for most laboratories). Monitoring for hepatocellular injury or bone marrow dysfunction should be instituted early in the course of treatment. Maximum benefit at a single dose level is generally achieved in a few days. Phenytoin is a good second choice if carbamazepine is effective but is poorly tolerated.

If carbamazepine is not effective, or for selected patients who experience pain that is predominantly superficial and burning in quality or those patients with depression complicating the pain syndrome, desipramine hydrochloride administered at a dosage increased from 25 mg daily to 100 mg daily may prove helpful; usually 25 mg is added to the daily dose each week during initiation. Amitriptyline causes significant side effects in a greater proportion of patients than desipramine hydrochloride, but its sedative properties can prove useful for the not-unusual patient whose painful feet cause misery chiefly on retiring for the night. The effects of antidepressants tend to accrue gradually over several weeks and also wear off slowly, so that some patients appreciate the benefit only when neuropathic pains recur in full force a few weeks after the medication has been discontinued. In addition to the usual precautions and contraindications for tricyclic antidepressant use, the presence of a significant autonomic component to the neuropathy should be viewed as a relative contraindication. Constipation, urinary retention, and orthostatic hypotension are likely to become intolerable, and if the QT interval is already prolonged because of the autonomic neuropathy, tricyclic antidepressants might in principle predispose to serious cardiac arrhythmias.

Cardiac anti-arrhythmic drugs, especially mexiletine, have some ability to reduce neuropathic pains. Typical dosages are 150 to 200 mg three times daily.

Autonomic Dysfunction

Constipation, urinary retention, dry mouth, and other manifestations of cholinergic deficit seldom have a satisfactory long-range response to oral bethanecol or cholinomimetic drugs, although such drugs may prove helpful acutely. Diarrhea caused by abnormal gastrointestinal motility may be helped by metoclopramide; in addition, diarrhea sometimes results from bacterial overgrowth (initially because of stasis of enteric contents) and may be improved by occasional courses of antibiotics such as tetracycline. Erectile dysfunction can be managed by penile implants or, in selected cases, by injection of papaverine hydrochloride into the corpora cavernosa to produce erection.

Generally orthostatic hypotension is first managed by modest volume expansion through generous salt intake and mineralocorticoids such as fludocortisone. Tight elastic stockings must usually be extended to the proximal thighs or (ideally) to the abdomen to be effective. These are difficult for many patients to use, especially if the patient has weakness and hand incoordination. In young patients without significant coronary or peripheral vascular disease, ergotamines such as dihydroergotamine mesylate at a dosage of 0.5 to 1.0 mg intramuscularly daily or ergotamine tartrate at a dosage of approximately 1 mg taken orally twice daily may be helpful.

In the treatment of autonomic dysfunction, one must also avoid the therapeutic misadventures that ensue when slight supine hypertension is mistakenly treated in a patient with marked postural drop, or when sympathomimetic or anticholinergic medications act on partially denervated end-organs without effective reflex control of blood pressure and heart rate.

SUGGESTED READING

Bannister R, ed. Autonomic failure: a textbook of clinical disorders of the autonomic nervous system. New York: Oxford University, 1988.

Dyck PJ, Thomas PK, Lambert EH, Bunge RP, eds. Peripheral neuropathy. Philadelphia: WB Saunders, 1984.

Schaumburg HH, Spencer PS, Thomas PK, eds. Disorders of peripheral nerves. Philadelphia: FA Davis Company, 1983.

HERPES ZOSTER

RICHARD T. JOHNSON, M.D.

Herpes zoster is as easy to diagnose as it is difficult to treat. Indeed, the patient usually makes the correct diagnosis of "shingles," and simple inspection without laboratory studies confirms the diagnosis.

The varicella-zoster virus causes almost universal infection in childhood with the clinical disease of chickenpox. During the course of that generalized blood-borne infection, the virus moves from skin lesions up sensory nerves and establishes latency in the sensory ganglion neurons. It remains latent for life. With activation, the virus spreads down the nerve, causing infection with vesicular eruption over the appropriate cutaneous dermatome. The virus may spread to immediately adjacent dermatomes, but in the immunocompetent patient, activated infection remains localized. Activation can occur at any time, but it is more frequent with increasing age or when a patient is immunosuppressed. It is estimated that by 80 years of age, 50 percent of all people will have had at least one episode of shingles. Lesions are most common over the trigeminal distribution and thoracic dermatomes, where the chickenpox blisters were most prevalent. Zoster is usually a benign, self-limited disease, but it may lead to persistent segmental motor paralysis. In two circumstances the disease is more severe. With increasing age, the acute disease is more painful and there is a greater likelihood of the development of postherpetic neuralgia. This is defined as severe, segmental pain persisting for more than 4 weeks after the onset of blisters. Disease is also more severe in patients who are immunosuppressed, where dissemination within the central nervous system (CNS) and visceral involvement may lead to severe and fatal disease.

TREATMENT OF UNCOMPLICATED ZOSTER

The rash begins as red papules, which become clear vesicles, and after approximately 3 days the fluid becomes turbid with the entry of inflammatory cells; the vesicles usually crust between 5 and 10 days. During this period, treatment should be symptomatic and should include the use of drying or soothing lotion such as calamine, trimming the fingernails to avoid excoriation and secondary infections, and the use of aspirin or acetaminophen. (Aspirin should never be used in children with chickenpox or zoster, however, because of the association of varicella with Reye's syndrome.) Once lesions have dried, capsaicin lotion may be used. Although this lotion contains the active ingredient of hot peppers and burns on application, it does over time cause cutaneous anesthesia. Ethyl chloride spray can similarly be used for transient relief of cutaneous dysesthesia.

Secondary infections of the lesions frequently occur. If localized, they can usually be treated with neomycin ointment. If cellulitis occurs with fever, cephalexin (500 mg four times per day) or dicloxacillin sodium (500 mg four times per day) should be given for 5 to 7 days.

Although herpes zoster is associated with Hodgkin's disease, cancer, and other diseases causing immunosuppression, it is not a first disease manifestation frequently enough to justify a costly search for underlying neoplasms or immunodeficiency diseases.

OPHTHALMIC ZOSTER

Involvement of the first division of the trigeminal nerve is second in frequency only to that of the thoracic lesions. With this involvement, there is often nuchal rigidity, obtundation, and greater severity of illness. A major complication of ophthalmic zoster is keratoconjunctivitis or iridocyclitis. One is forewarned of this complication if vesicles appear along the distribution of the nasociliary nerve on the lateral side and to the tip of the nose. Patients with first division ophthalmic zoster are also those at highest risk for developing cerebral vasculitis (see below).

In patients older than 60 years of age who have prodromal symptoms of greater duration and severe pain at onset, as well as in patients who are acutely ill with ophthalmic zoster (particularly with nasociliary branch involvement), oral acyclovir (800 mg five times per day) should be used. Lower doses of acyclovir given orally have been shown to be ineffective. It has been established that this dose shortens the healing time of lesions and decreases the duration and severity of acute pain, but its effectiveness in decreasing the incidence of postherpetic neuralgia has not been proven. In the uncomplicated cases of shingles, particularly in those patients younger than 60 years of age, the benefits do not justify the expense of oral acyclovir. Prednisone given during the acute phase of shingles has been claimed to decrease the frequency of postherpetic neuralgia, but the data supporting this are inconsistent. I do not believe that this uncertain effect justifies the slight increased risk of dissemination or immunosuppression associated with the use of corticosteroids.

THE IMMUNOCOMPROMISED PATIENT

Exposure of the immunocompromised patient to patients with varicella or zoster should be prevented, since immunocompromised patients can develop disseminated zoster after external exposure as well as after internal reactivation. Hospitalized patients with varicella or zoster should be placed under strict isolation; this is done not to protect the staff and the patient's family, but to protect other patients in the hospital who may be immunocompromised by disease or medical therapy. Zoster immune globulin protects immunocompromised children from contracting chickenpox after exposure to chickenpox or zoster, but it does not protect against zoster in children and adults with a past history of chickenpox.

If the patient is immunocompromised (e.g., patients who have undergone organ transplants) or if the lesions spread or show dissemination over more than three contiguous dermatomes, intravenous acyclovir should be instituted. If given within the first 72 hours, the agent is clearly effective. Doses of 10 mg per kilogram every 8 hours infused over a 1-hour period should be continued for 7 days. Because intravenous acyclovir is potentially nephrotoxic, the creatine should be followed carefully and adequate hydration should be maintained, even during the night. CNS toxicity also occurs, accompanied by tremor and disorientation. Dosage must be modified in patients with renal disease (e.g., organ transplant patients). If the rate of creatinine clearance is 25 to 50 ml per minute, the drug should be given every 12 hours instead of every 8 hours; if the rate is less than 25 ml per minute, infusion should be given every 24 hours; and if the rate is less than 10 ml per minute, only half of the single dosage should be given. The drug is removed by hemodialysis, and therefore the doses must be administered after dialysis.

VASCULITIS

On rare occasions, acute hemiparesis develops 2 to 10 weeks after the onset of ophthalmic zoster. Lumbar puncture may show some mild signs of inflammation, and angiography may show a localized vasculitis in the carotid artery near the trigeminal ganglion, or diffuse, bilateral vasculitis. The time of onset and the histologic features suggest that this granulomatous angiitis may be immune-mediated; on the other hand, some morphologic evidence suggests that virus may be present in the vascular lesions. Because of this uncertainty of pathogenetic mechanisms and the potential catastrophic effects of a generalized granulomatous angiitis, simultaneous treatment with both anti-inflammatory and antiviral drugs is justified. Large doses of steroids and full doses of intravenous acyclovir may be given.

POSTHERPETIC NEURALGIA

A pain persisting for more than 4 weeks occurs in only 9 percent of patients who suffer from shingles. Fifty percent of these patients have spontaneous resolution of pain by 8 weeks; less than 2 percent of patients with herpes zoster have postherpetic neuralgia lasting for 1 year or more. Postherpetic neuralgia is extremely rare in patients younger than 50 years of age. The greater the duration of the preherpetic symptoms, the more severe the lesions; the older the patient, the more likely there is to be severe and protracted postherpetic neuralgia.

The first step is to explain to the patient that this is generally a self-limited disease, although no guarantee can be issued since some patients have been described who have had postherpetic neuralgia for 10 years or more. Nonetheless, the statistics justify reassurance. Second, the use of narcotics should be avoided. In addition to having addictive properties, they are relatively ineffective for this form of pain. Local analgesic ointments or sprays provide only transient and usually trivial relief.

The drug of choice is amitriptyline, started at doses of 10 mg four times per day. In patients who feel too sedated by these spaced doses, it may be given as 50 mg at bedtime. The dose is increased until relief is achieved or until toxicity limits dosage. Doses of approximately 100 mg per day provide effective reduction of pain in most patients. When administered in conjunction with amitriptyline, carbamazepine, 150 mg per day increasing to 1,200 mg per day, may give greater relief, but the use of carbamazepine alone has not been evaluated in controlled studies. A recent double-blind cross-over study indicated that pimozide (4 to 12 mg daily) was more effective than carbamazepine in refractory patients; because of its side effects of tardive dyskinesias, memory impairment, and parkinsonism, it should not be the first option in the treatment of postherpetic neuralgia.

Although transcutaneous nerve stimulation has been reported to benefit some patients, it has been shown to be inferior to the medical treatment in controlled studies. In patients who have had prolonged disabling postherpetic neuralgia for several months and who are refractive to medical treatment, surgical intervention may be considered. Local root section and injection of nerve roots are ineffective since the neuralgia originates from the ganglion or proximal to the ganglia. Surgical interventions include lesions in the sensory ganglia, dorsal root entry zone, or spinothalamic tracts. The most effective surgical approach appears to be placement of thermal lesions in the dorsal root entry zone at the appropriate dermatome as well as at the dermatomes above and below the site of pain, yet even this destructive surgical approach has limited success. Therefore, medical treatment should be aggressive and prolonged, in the hope that the patient will experience spontaneous abatement of pain.

SUGGESTED READING

Balfour H, et al. Acyclovir halts progression of herpes zoster in immunocompromised patients. N Engl J Med 1983; 308:1448–1453.

Friedman AH, Nashold BS, Ovelmen-Levitt J. Dorsal root entry zone lesions for the treatment of post-herpetic neuralgia. J Neurosurg 1984; 60:1258–1262.

Huff JC, et al. Therapy of herpes zoster with oral acyclovir. Am J Med 1988; 85 (suppl 2A):85–89.

Lechin F, et al. Pimozide therapy for trigeminal neuralgia. Arch Neurol 1989; 46:960–963.

Max MB, et al. Amitriptyline, but not torazepam, relieves post-herpetic neuralgia. Neurology 1988; 38:1427–1432.

Wood MJ, et al. Efficacy of oral acyclovir treatment of acute herpes zoster. Am J Med 1988; 85 (suppl 2A):79–83.

SUBACUTE COMBINED DEGENERATION AND OTHER VITAMIN B_{12} DEFICIENCY–INDUCED DISORDERS

BARBARA J. MARTIN, M.D.
MARK J. BROWN, M.D.

Vitamin B_{12} (cobalamin) deficiency can lead to myelopathy, encephalopathy, and optic and peripheral neuropathy. Therapy should begin only after one of the syndromes known to result from vitamin B_{12} deficiency has been demonstrated and it has been established that the deficit exists. Accurate laboratory diagnosis of viatmin B_{12} deficiency may be confounded by premature treatment. Therapy consists of lifelong parenteral vitamin B_{12} administration and, when possible, treatment of underlying or associated conditions.

SUBACUTE COMBINED DEGENERATION OF THE SPINAL CORD

The manifestations of vitamin B_{12} deficiency–induced subacute combined degeneration reflect the underlying dorsal and lateral spinal cord white matter abnormalities. Symptoms characteristically begin with paresthesia in the feet, with relative sparing of the hands and arms. Disproportionate vibratory and proprioceptive function loss in the legs and trunk is also characteristic, and small fiber modalities may be affected. Rarely, a thoracic sensory level suggests a segmental spinal cord disorder. Sensory symptoms may be followed by leg weakness and an ataxic or spastic gait. The plantar responses are typically extensor, and pathlolgic hyperreflexia may occur; however, when there is an associated neuropathy, ankle jerks and other reflexes may be depressed. Somatosensory-evoked potentials may indicate central nervous system disease, although signs of an associated axonal neuropathy may predominate in this test.

The characteristic early histologic finding in vitamin B_{12} deficiency–induced subacute combined degeneration is intra-myelin edema, followed by myelin sheath vacuolization. At this point, the process is likely to be reversible. Myelin breakdown follows, and lesions enlarge and coalesce to give a patchy spongiform appearance. The dorsal columns of the cervical and upper thoracic cord are most likely to be affected, with less severe involvement of the lateral and ventral white matter. Chronic lesions are characterized by axonal loss and fibrillary gliosis.

The differential diagnosis of subacute or chronic dorsal and lateral spinal cord dysfunction includes multiple sclerosis and tabes dorsalis. Lyme disease and human immunodeficiency virus (HIV) or human T-cell lymphotropic virus (HTLV)-1 may be considerations, especially if the peripheral nervous system is involved. Friedrich's ataxia patients may have hyporeflexia with extensor plantar responses. Prolonged nitrous oxide exposure may produce a clinical syndrome indistinguishable from subacute combined degeneration secondary to vitamin B_{12} deficiency.

SUBACUTE DEGENERATION OF THE BRAIN

Encephalopathy commonly accompanies subacute combined degeneration of the spinal cord, and appears to have the same neuropathologic basis. Brain myelin lesions and axonal loss are similar to those described for the spinal cord.

Neuropsychological manifestations of the encephalopathy range from mild personality and mood changes to severe dementia. Paranoia and hallucinations may occur, but psychosis is very rare. The severity of the encephalopathy and myelopathy may differ from patient to patient. Vitamin B_{12} encephalopathy can occur without other evidence of nervous system disease. However, because mild dementia and psychiatric disorders are common in the general population and vitamin B_{12} tests are requested frequently, the association between dementia and low levels of vitamin B_{12} may sometimes be coincidental.

PERIPHERAL NEUROPATHY

Peripheral neuropathy is frequently associated with subacute combined degeneration, although neuropathy makes a relatively small contribution to the symptomatology. Distal paresthesias, a symmetric stocking-glove sensory deficit, and orthostatic hypotension can be ascribed to either neuropathy or myelopathy; however, when looked for, hyporeflexia and depressed sensory potential amplitudes often confirm peripheral nervous system involvement. Although peripheral nerve demylination has been reported, more recently studies have demonstrated a predominance of axonal degeneration in biopsied sural nerves. This suggests that the mechanism of pathogenesis is different from that of the central nervous system lesions.

OPTIC NEUROPATHY

Ocular signs and symptoms can occur with subacute combined degeneration. The explanation for the reported severe disc edema, optic atrophy, and bilateral centrocecal scotomas is not clear. There are few neuropathologic reports of well-studied clinical cases, and the nature of the optic neuropathy remains uncertain. Nerve fiber layer hemorrhages are presumably related to the hematologic disorder. Ophthalmoplegia has been reported, but the association may be coincidental.

Tobacco-alcohol amblyopia presents with signs and symptoms similar to those of the optic neuropathy associated with subacute combined degeneration. Both are characterized by loss of visual acuity, dyschromatopsia, centrocecal scotomata, and optic disc pallor. Tobacco-alcohol amblyopia is believed to be secondary to vitamin B-complex deficiency, but is more likely linked to a deficiency of vitamin B_1 than a deficiency of viatmin B_{12}.

PATHOPHYSIOLOGY OF VITAMIN B_{12} DEFICIENCY IN THE NERVOUS SYSTEM

Vitamin B_{12} is a necessary coenzyme for the conversion of propionic acid to succinic acid through the intermediate metabolite methylmalonic acid. Vitamin B_{12} deficiency alters methylmalonic acid metabolism, resulting in abnormal fatty acid synthesis, presumably leading to abnormal myelin and other cell membranes. Serum levels and urinary excretion of methylmalonic acid are elevated with vitamin B_{12} deficiency, and this is used as a supportive diagnostic test. Vitamin B_{12} is also a necessary coenzyme for methionine synthetase which converts homocysteine to methionine by methylation. Serum homocysteine levels may be elevated in patients with neurologic manifestations of vitamin B_{12} deficiency. Notably, excess exposure to nitrous oxide, which inhibits methionine synthetase, can lead to a spinal cord syndrome indistinguishable from subacute combined degeneration.

LABORATORY DIAGNOSIS

The coexistence of anemia, macrocytosis, and neutrophil hypersegmentation strongly supports the diagnosis of vitamin B_{12} deficiency, but neurologic and hematologic manifestations may occur independently. The initial diagnostic step is measuring the serum vitamin B_{12} level through the use of a competitive binding radio-assay, which has supplanted the older bioassay. Serum is added to radio-labeled vitamin B_{12} bound to highly purified intrinsic factor; serum vitamin B_{12} displaces the labeled vitamin B_{12} from the intrinsic factor. The serum concentration is inversely proportional to the remaining bound vitamin B_{12} and can be calculated from the residual radioactivity of the complex. The sensitivity of this assay is approximately 98 percent with less than 0.1 percent false-positives.

Normal serum vitamin B_{12} levels are usually greater than 200 ng per liter although this varies among laboratories. Early vitamin B_{12} deficiency is indicated by levels of 160 to 200 ng per liter. Values for the elderly are consistently lower than those of younger patients, but are routinely greater than 150 ng per liter. Both serum methylmalonic acid and homocysteine levels may be elevated in subacute combined degeneration. These tests currently have limited availability, but may be used to confirm the diagnosis of vitamin B_{12} deficiency when results of standard tests are indeterminate. (Serum homocysteine levels may also be elevated with folate deficiency.) The laboratory diagnosis of vitamin B_{12} deficiency may be obscured by the widespread and nonspecific use of supplemental vitamin B_{12} in clinical practice. The administration of vitamin B_{12} within a week of the test may lead to misleading results and may warrant further studies.

CAUSES

Pernicious anemia (intrinsic factor deficiency) is by far the most important cause of vitamin B_{12} deficiency in the United States. The detection of antibodies to intrinsic factor is highly specific, and blocking antibodies are detected in approximately 50 to 60 percent of patients with pernicious anemia, with only rare false-positives. False-positives have resulted when another radioactive tracer, such as technetium, has been administered previously. False-negative results may be seen when supplemental vitamin B_{12} has been given within 1 week of testing. Causes of intrinsic factor deficiency other than pernicious anemia include atrophic gastritis, stomach neoplasia, and gastrectomy.

The Shilling test is the definitive method for diagnosing intrinsic factor deficiency. During the first stage of this test, radio-labeled oral vitamin B_{12} absorption is impaired, resulting in diminished urinary excretion of the isotope. If vitamin B_{12} excretion is demonstrably low, the second stage of the Shilling test should be performed. This consists of giving intrinsic factor orally along with labeled vitamin B_{12}, after which excretion is increased. Impaired urinary vitamin B_{12} excretion during both stages of the test is found in patients with malabsorption states, intrinsic factor–blocking antibody, severe renal insufficiency, and poor specimen collection. Twenty-five percent of patients with untreated true vitamin B_{12} deficiency show a "malabsorption" picture with the two-stage Shilling test. After prolonged vitamin B_{12} replacement therapy, the majority of these patients display improved vitamin B_{12} absorption and demonstrate repeat test results consistent with pernicious anemia. Pernicious anemia may be associated with other autoimmune diseases such as hypothyroidism. Approximately 20 percent of patients of Lambert-Eaton syndrome have intrinsic factor–blocking antibody without pernicious anemia, most likely reflecting altered autoimmunity in the pathogenesis of this illness.

The customary Western diet generally provides adequate amounts of vitamin B_{12} (approximately 2.5 μg per day). Poor diet and extreme vegetarianism, on the other hand, pose a risk for vitamin B_{12} deficiency. Malabsorption of vitamin B_{12} occurs with diseases such as sprue or inflammatory bowel diseases affecting the ileum, as well as with simple ileal resection. The fish tapeworm *Diphyllobothrium latum* creates a vitamin B_{12} deficient state by competing for vitamin B_{12} within the host's intestine. The blind loop syndrome is attributed to significant bacterial colonization in the small intestine with diversion of vitamin B_{12} from host absorption. Pregnancy may predispose toward vitamin B_{12} deficiency if increased vitamin B_{12} demands are not met with adequate intake. Coexisting folate deficiency should be considered in this context. Impaired B_{12} absorption from the gut may occur in conjunction with the usage of aminoglycosides, aspirin, colchicine, and chloramphenicol, as well as with excessive alcohol intake.

TREATMENT

The treatment of vitamin B_{12} deficiency should consist solely of intramuscular or subcutaneous vitamin B_{12} administration. Because of their limited absorption and high cost, oral vitamin B_{12} preparations with or without intrinsic factor are unacceptable alternatives, except for the rare vegetarian with dietary deficiency. Cyanocobalamin is currently the least expensive preparation available.

Initial treatment consists of 1,000 μg parenteral vitamin B_{12} daily or every other day for several weeks followed by weekly injections for 1 to 2 months. Thereafter, the same dose should be given monthly for life. Some have advised that initial dosages of greater than 30 μg daily afford little therapeutic advantage. However, we recommend continuing the higher dose because the extent to which vitamin B_{12} stores are repleted is directly related to the parenteral dose, and a higher dose poses no additional risk for the patient. Adverse effects of replacement are largely limited to the pain of intramuscular injection with allergic reactions reported very rarely. The hematologic response to vitamin B_{12} may be brisk, occurring at a tempo independent from that of the nervous system response.

Treatment with folate without vitamin B_{12} replacement is strictly contraindicated for patients with megaloblastic anemia with or without neurologic symptoms and signs. It is well known that the anemia of vitamin B_{12} deficiency responds to folate therapy, possibly via the mobilization of stores, while the neurologic symptoms of subacute combined degeneration may surface during this time or worsen if already present.

The success of treatment is related to the duration of neurologic dysfunction before therapy. Patients who have had symptoms for less than 3 months show the greatest improvement, and patients treated within weeks of onset may have a full recovery. Those treated after the first 3 to 6 months of symptoms have a less successful outcome. However, recent data indicate that all patients receive some benefit from replacement regardless of the duration of illness.

SUGGESTED READING

Agamanolis DP, Victor M, Harris JW, et al. An ultrastructural study of subacute combined degeneration of the spinal cord in vitamin B_{12}-deficient rhesus monkeys. J Neuropathol Exp Neurol 1978; 37:273–299.

Beck WS. Cobalamin and the nervous system, editorial. N Engl J Med 1988; 318; 1752–1754.

Lindenbaum J, Healton EB, Savage DG, et al. Neuropsychiatric disorders caused by cobalamin deficiency in the absence of anemia or macrocytosis. N Engl J Med 1988; 318:1720–1728.

Pant SS, Asbury AK, Richardson EP Jr. The myelopathy of pernicious anemia: a neuropathological reappraisal. Acta Neurol Scand 1968; 44 (suppl 35).

DEMENTIA

PETER V. RABINS, M.D., Ph.D.

EVALUATION

The treatment of dementia begins with the evaluation. Between 2 and 5 percent of individuals presenting for an assessment of memory complaints suffer from a potentially reversible disorder, and perhaps half of these experience a full recovery upon treatment. Thus at the initial assessment, the physician should explain to the family and patient that a full evaluation for treatable causes of dementia is appropriate but that there is little likelihood that a reversible condition will be found. Clinical experience suggests that the clinician can usually identify those patients with reversible dementias from the information gained during the history and physical examination; these patients have signs and symptoms of depression, thyroid disease, focal central nervous system lesions, or hydrocephalus or a history of head trauma, medication misuse, or alcoholism.

According to the recent National Institute of Health (NIH) Consensus Conference on Dementia, the evaluation for reversible dementia should include a complete blood count, electrolyte panel, screening metabolic panel, thyroid functions, vitamin B_{12}, folate, Venereal Disease Research Laboratory (VDRL), urinalysis, electrocardiogram, and chest x-ray examination. Most clinicians would include computed tomography (CT) of the head on this list. Many clinicians obtain electroencephalograms (EEGs) in all patients, although I do so only when symptoms have been present for less than 2 years, when the case is atypical, or if I have concerns about the possibility of seizures or a metabolic etiology. The EEG is useful in cases in which the etiology of the dementia is unclear and is most informative when the clinical picture and EEG are disparate. For example, marked diffuse slowing in mildly impaired individuals suggests a metabolic or toxic etiology. Conversely, a normal EEG in a person with definite cognitive impairment should prompt one to focus attention on searching for depression or other psychiatric etiologies. However, the EEG may be normal in patients with early Alzheimer's disease and other degenerative dementias.

A lumbar puncture should also be considered in the assessment of all patients with dementia. My practice is to recommend a lumbar puncture when the dementia has been present for less than 2 to 3 years. In more chronic cases, infectious etiology is unlikely.

Human immunodeficiency virus (HIV) testing should be considered in all patients with dementia; permission for testing should be sought in individuals with high-risk behaviors or exposures, in patients with signs and symptoms compatable with the acquired immunodeficiency syndrome (AIDS) spectrum, and in any patient in whom the cognitive and behavioral changes have been present for less than 6 months. Screening for other unusual causes of dementia depends on the patient's history and the clinical findings. The presence of movement disorders should raise the possibility of Wilson's disease or Huntington's disease. The presence of a neuropathy suggests a toxic or metabolic cause, and specific tests such as heavy metal screens and tests for deficiency diseases should be considered.

The role of magnetic resonance imaging (MRI) in the treatment of dementia is still under debate. In the elderly, MRI often presents information that is more confusing than helpful. I limit the use of MRI to patients for whom there is a high suspicion of focal lesion (including vascular disease) and those younger than 65 years of age, or if a condition is suspected for which the MRI is more specific than a CT scan (e.g., AIDS or multiple sclerosis).

The evaluation of dementia may well disclose other untreated or insufficiently treated medical conditions, and their proper management may improve cognition or prevent progression of the dementia, although it will not cure it. Patients with a vascular dementia caused by emboli should be assessed for a cardiac or extracranial carotid source and treated appropriately. Recent research suggests that patients with vascular dementia may benefit from the use of aspirin or other antiplatelet aggregation therapies.

Identification of Treatable Symptoms in Irreversible Dementia

After the diagnosis of an irreversible dementing disorder has been made, the next step is to identify comorbid medical, behavioral, or mood symptoms that might respond to treatment. The evaluation for reversible causes of dementia may disclose coexisting conditions such as heart failure, the treatment for which can improve the function of the patient. If a referring or family physician is involved, drawing his or her attention to these issues might be the most appropriate intervention.

Behavior disorder is common in dementias of various etiologies. Sleep disorder, hallucinations, delusions, and agitation are common. Some of these symptoms are clearly induced by the environment or by unrealistic expectations of the patient's family, friends, or treating institutions. For example, the behaviors resulting from apraxias, agnosias, perseveration, and apathy are often perceived of as willful refusal. Identifying these symptoms and the accompanying behaviors as arising from the brain disease can redirect caregivers to find ways to minimize their impact. Sometimes the most appropriate "treatment" is for the patient's family members or the staff of the treating institution to modify their expectations.

Some behavioral symptoms that arise from the brain disorder are upsetting, but because of the risk of drug side effects, pharmacotherapy is not justified. For example, if the demented patient accuses people of stealing money, the first intervention should be to help the family or nursing home to accept the fact that this symptom arises from the brain disease. However, if symptoms such as accusations cause significant distress to the patient or lead to dangerous behaviors such as striking others, then a cautious trial of a neuroleptic drug is indicated. No one neuroleptic drug is indicated over another, and the extrapyramidal side effects and orthostatic hypotension they commonly induce are often more troublesome than the behavior for which they are prescribed. However, some patients do respond to low doses of the neuroleptics and a time-limited trial (3 to 6 weeks) aimed at relieving a specific target symptom is sometimes appropriate.

A neuroleptic is chosen by determining which agent is least contraindicated based on its side effect profile. In patients for whom orthostasis is a serious risk or who are already receiving antihypertensive treatment, a high-potency, low-milligram neuroleptic such as haloperidol (starting dose of 0.5 to 1 mg twice daily), thiothixene (starting dose of 1 to 2 mg twice daily), or fluphenazine (starting dose of 1 mg twice daily) should be considered. For patients with frequent agitation in whom sedation would be desirable, thioridazine (starting dose of 10 to 20 mg three times daily or at bedtime) might first be tried. All neuroleptics may induce extrapyramidal symptoms that are often debilitating. However, when used judiciously (and in patients for whom nondrug treatments have failed or are unavailable), these medications can diminish severe behavior disorders.

Sleep disorder is common in many dementing illnesses. Behavioral interventions rarely seem to work in patients with this condition, and if the sleep disorder is not troublesome, it may be best not to treat it pharmacologically. However, sleep disorder can place the patient in danger of falling in a darkened home or cause extreme distress to an elderly family caregiver who cannot sleep at night because of it. In such cases, a judicious trial of chloral hydrate (500 to 1,500 mg at bedtime) or, in patients with sleep disorder who also have behavioral problems for which neuroleptics are indicated, a prescription of neuroleptics taken at night only might help.

Fifteen to 20 percent of patients with dementia of the Alzheimer type and vascular dementia suffer from depression. Patients who have been experiencing weight loss, frequent crying, behavioral disorder, and sleep disturbance should be considered for treatment with an antidepressant. Drugs with low anticholinergic side effect profiles such as nortriptyline (starting dose of 10 to 20 mg at bedtime) or desipramine hydrochloride (starting dose of 25 mg) are useful. If the patient is experiencing sleep disruption, this may be the only necessary treatment.

ASSESSMENT OF SUDDEN BEHAVIORAL CHANGE IN PATIENTS WITH DEMENTIA

Suddenly changing cognition and behavior in an individual with dementia suggests that the patient has suffered a new central nervous system insult, developed a new medical or psychiatric comorbidity (e.g., a new urinary tract infection, upper respiratory infection, or depression), or become delirious from a medication that has been added during the past month. Patients who undergo a change in behavior should therefore be assessed for each of these conditions. In the elderly, it may take as long as 30 days for a drug to accomplish the five half-lives necessary for it to reach steady state; thus medication changes during the previous 30 days should be reviewed when subacute or acute changes in conditions occur.

INVOLVEMENT OF THE FAMILY

Family members are usually involved at all stages of the patient's management. Often it is the family rather than the patient who initiates the assessment, and indeed, early on, patients often deny that there are problems. A clear, accurate diagnosis should be relayed to the family in such instances. When there are several diagnostic possibilities, the family should be informed of these and of their prognostic significance. Some families find that they are greatly benefited by referral to such organizations as the Alzheimer's Disease Association or the Huntington's Disease Association. They provide emotional support for the family and specific information about legal, social, and long-term health care resources.

LEGAL, SOCIAL, AND FINANCIAL ISSUES

Patients with early dementia may be able to drive an automobile safely, but no accurate means exists for identifying when driving becomes dangerous for these patients. In cases where motor impairment is prominent, visuospatial or perceptual abnormalities are significant, or judgment is impaired, the patient and family should be instructed that he or she must discontinue driving. The decision to notify the motor vehicle bureau rests on the clinician's judgment that the situation is indeed dangerous. One alternative is to suggest that the patient take a driving test at a local driving education agency. Because state requirements for notification vary, the clinician should be aware of the law in his or her locality.

Families also need to seek financial, legal, and social advice from individuals skilled in the practice of these disciplines, and physicians can make an important contribution by encouraging them to seek such counsel. Because of changing laws, it is important that families do so early. This is particularly important if the family and patient desire a durable power of attorney. This allows a competent person to appoint a person who can make major decisions for him if he becomes demented, without needing a judicial process to declare him incompetent. Once a demented person becomes incompetent, however, it is no longer possible to obtain such a document. Some families benefit from talking to a knowledgeable financial counselor.

Because nursing home placement is a difficult subject for many patients and families, recommending that they seek social work advice before placement becomes a necessity may prevent the complications that arise from last-minute decisions. Thus occasional office visits over time that identify new symptoms, treat behavioral comorbidity, and direct the family to needed social interventions can contribute to the well-being of the patient and his or her family, even in the face of progressive dementing illnesses.

SUGGESTED READING

Cummings J, Bensen DF. Dementia: a clinical approach. Stoneham, MA: Butterworth, 1984.

Drachman DA. Who may drive? Who may not? Who shall decide? Ann Neurol 1988; 24:787–788.

PATIENT RESOURCES

Literature

Mace NL, Rabins PV. The 36-hour day: a family guide to caring for persons with Alzheimer's disease, related dementing illnesses, and memory loss in later life. Baltimore: Johns Hopkins University Press, 1981.

Associations

Alzheimer's Disease and Related Disorders Association (ADRDA)
70 East Lake Street
Chicago, Illinois 60601
Telephone: 1-800-621-0379

Huntington's Disease Society of America (HDSA)
140 West 22nd Street
New York, New York 10011
Telephone: (212)242-1968

INDEX

Page numbers followed by *f* indicate figures; page numbers followed by *t* indicate tables.

H

I

S

T